T0073606

The Scofield® Study Bible

THE HOLY BIBLE

Containing the Old and New Testaments

AUTHORIZED KING JAMES VERSION

With a new system of connected topical references to all the greater themes of Scripture, with annotations, revised marginal renderings, summaries, definitions, chronology, and index, to which are added, helps at hard places, explanations of seeming discrepancies, and a new system of paragraphs

EDITED BY

REV. C. I. SCOFIELD, D.D.

CONSULTING EDITORS

REV. HENRY G. WESTON, D.D., LL.D.,
President Crozer Theological Seminary.

REV. JAMES M. GRAY, D.D.,
President Moody Bible Institute.

REV. WILLIAM J. ERDMAN, D.D.,
Author "The Gospel of John," etc., etc.

REV. ARTHUR T. PIERSON, D.D.,
Author, Editor, Teacher.

REV. W. G. MOOREHEAD, D.D.,
President Xenia (U.P.) Theological Seminary.

REV. ELMORE HARRIS, D.D.,
President Toronto Bible Institute.

REV. ARNO C. GAEBELEIN, D.D.,
Author "Harmony of Prophetic Word," etc., etc.

REV. WILLIAM L. PETTINGILL, D.D.,
Author, Editor, Teacher.

New and Improved Edition

NEW YORK

OXFORD UNIVERSITY PRESS

The Scofield® Reference Bible

The Scofield® Study Bible was previously published as *The Scofield Reference Bible.* Except for this change of title, the book remains as it was when Dr. C. I. Scofield finished his task. Not one word in Dr. Scofield's notes has been altered, added, or deleted.

This readers edition setting conforms page by page to the standard editions of *The Scofield® Study Bible* with a few format changes to enhance its use: (1) chapter and verse citations in the notes and references are separated with a colon, as opposed to a period or period and space, according to the most common use (e.g., 1.2 and 1. 2 are now 1:2); (2) the cross reference system has been enhanced with additional references from *The New Scofield Reference Bible,* although none of the subject reference chains have been altered.

28 30 29 27

PRINTED IN KOREA

INTRODUCTION.
(TO BE READ.)

THIS edition of the Bible had its origin in the increasing conviction of the Editor through thirty years' study and use of the Scriptures as pastor, teacher, writer, and lecturer upon biblical themes, that all of the many excellent and useful editions of the Word of God left much to be desired. Gradually the elements which must combine to facilitate the study and intelligent use of the Bible became clear to his mind. These he has, with the invaluable collaboration of a wide circle of spiritual and experienced Bible students and teachers, in England and the United States, endeavoured, with what measure of success others must now judge, to embody in the present work. The distinctive features are as follows:

I. It was felt that the old system of references, based solely upon the accident of the English words, was unscientific and often misleading. In the present edition, by a new system of connected topical references, all the greater truths of the divine revelation are so traced through the entire Bible, from the place of first mention to the last, that the reader may for himself follow the gradual unfolding of these, by many inspired writers through many ages, to their culmination in Jesus Christ and the New Testament Scriptures. This method imparts to Bible study an interest and vital reality which are wholly lacking in fragmentary and disconnected study.

II. The last fifty years have witnessed an intensity and breadth of interest in Bible study unprecedented in the history of the Christian Church. Never before have so many reverent, learned, and spiritual men brought to the study of the Scriptures minds so free from merely controversial motive. A new and vast exegetical and expository literature has been created, inaccessible for bulk, cost, and time to the average reader. The winnowed and attested results of this half-century of Bible study are embodied in the notes, summaries, and definitions of this edition. Expository novelties, and merely personal views and interpretations, have been rejected.

III. Helps have been provided, available for instant reference, on the very page where help is needed. For example, at every mention of a Hebrew month, weight, coin, or measure, the English equivalent is given in the margin. Obscure and difficult passages, alleged discrepancies or contradictions, and every important type or symbol are elucidated by new references, or made the subject of an explanatory footnote on the same page.

IV. All of the connected topical lines of reference end in analytic summaries of the whole teaching of Scripture on that subject, thus guarding the reader against hasty generalizations from a few passages or proof texts. The saying that "anything may be proved by the Bible" is both true and false—true if isolated passages are used; utterly false if the whole divine revelation is in view.

V. The great words of Scripture, as adoption, advocacy, assurance, atonement, church, conversion, death, election, eternal life, eternal punishment, faith, flesh, forgiveness, grace, hell (whether *sheol, hades,* or *gehenna*), imputation, justification, kingdom, propitiation, reconciliation, redemption, repentance, righteousness, salvation, sanctification, sin, world (in its four meanings), etc., etc., are defined in simple, non-technical terms. These definitions have been submitted to, and approved by, a very large number of eminent students and teachers of all the evangelical bodies.

VI. Each of the sixty-six books of the Bible is provided with an introduction and analysis, the latter so carried out in the text by appropriate sub-heads as greatly to facilitate the study and comprehension of the book.

VII. The entire Bible has been divided into paragraphs by italicized sub-heads while preserving the chapter and verse division which gives the Authorized Version, among many other superiorities, its unrivalled pre-eminence.

VIII. The remarkable results of the modern study of the Prophets, in recovering to the church not only a clear and coherent harmony of the predictive portions, but also great treasures of ethical truth, are indicated in expository notes. This portion of the Bible, nearly one-fourth of the whole, has been closed to the average reader by fanciful and allegorical schemes of interpretation. The method followed gives ready access also to the amazing literary riches of the Prophetical Books.

IX. The greater covenants of God which absolutely condition human life and the divine redemption, and about which the whole Bible gathers, are analyzed, and their relation to each other and to Christ made clear.

X. The Dispensations are distinguished, exhibiting the majestic, progressive order of the divine dealings of God with humanity, "the increasing purpose" which runs through and links together the ages, from the beginning of the life of man to the end in eternity. Augustine said: "Distinguish the ages, and the Scriptures harmonize."

XI. After mature reflection it was determined to use the Authorized Version. None of the many Revisions have commended themselves to the people at large. The Revised Version, which has now been before the public for twenty-seven years gives no indication of becoming in any general sense the people's Bible of the English-speaking world. The discovery of the Sinaitic MS. and the labours in the field of textual criticism of such scholars as Griesbach, Lachmann, Tischendorf, Tregelles, Winer, Alford, and Westcott and Hort, have cleared the Greek *textus receptus* of minor inaccuracies, while confirming in a remarkable degree the general accuracy of the Authorized Version of that text. Such emendations of the text as scholarship demands have been placed in the margins of this edition, which therefore combines the dignity, the high religious value, the tender associations of the past, the literary beauty and remarkable general accuracy of the Authorized Version, with the results of the best textual scholarship.

The Editor disclaims originality. Other men have laboured, he has but entered into their labours. The results of the study of God's Word by learned and spiritual men, in every division of the church and in every land, during the last fifty years, under the advantage of a perfected text, already form a vast literature, inaccessible to most Christian workers. The Editor has proposed to himself the modest if laborious task of summarizing, arranging, and condensing this mass of material.

That he has been able to accomplish this task at all is due in very large measure to the valuable suggestions and co-operation of the Consulting Editors, who have freely given of their time and the treasures of their scholarship to this work. It is due to them to say that the Editor alone is responsible for the final form of notes and definitions. The Editor's acknowledgments are also due to a very wide circle of learned and spiritual brethren in Europe and America to whose labours he is indebted for suggestions of inestimable value. It may not be invidious to mention among these Professor James Barrellet, of the Theological Faculty of Lausanne, Professors Sayce and Margoliouth, of Oxford, Mr. Walter Scott, the eminent Bible teacher, and Professor C. R. Erdman, of Princeton.

Finally, grateful thanks are due to those whose generous material assistance has made possible the preparation of a work involving years of time, and repeated journeys to the centres of biblical learning abroad.

The completed work is now dedicated to the service amongst men of that Loving and Holy God, whose marvellous grace in Christ Jesus it seeks to exalt.

Jan. 1, 1909. C. I. SCOFIELD.

PREFACE TO THE PRESENT EDITION.

The very large demand for the Scofield Reference Bible in every part of the world, and the consequent large and repeated printings, have made it necessary to reset the entire Bible in new type that the high standard of the Oxford University Press may be maintained, and the public furnished with this Bible in the highest form of the printer's art. To the attainment of this high purpose no labour of Editor or publishers has been counted too great.

The Scofield Reference Bible has now been nearly eight years in the hands of the Christian public. The editor would be more, or less, than human if he were not profoundly grateful, not only, nor chiefly, for the large sale accorded to it, but rather for the assurances which have reached him from every part of the earth of blessing through its use.

That this testimony has come in part from great biblical scholars has been most gratifying, but it has been an especial cause of gratitude to know that the plain people of God in their homes, and far away missionaries in heathen lands have been helped to a clearer and more spiritual apprehension of the Word of God.

But the very warmth of this welcome given to his labours has made the Editor solicitous that in any new typing of it he might find his opportunity to add, here and there, such further help as experience has shown to be desirable. This he has endeavoured here to do. The Panoramic View of the whole Bible will, it is believed, show the unity of the Book—a fact in danger of failing to be perceived in face of the other and more evident fact that it is made up of many books.

Chronological data have also been supplied; and, on the mechanical side, more distinct type; larger type in the reference columns; and the substitution of Arabic for Roman numerals will be noted as distinct improvements.

The Editor is especially grateful to the many eminent and spiritually minded brethren who have aided him by suggestions and counsel, and to those whose most Christian liberality has made such a work possible. He is sure that they, not less emphatically than himself, in again putting forth this testimony to Him whom having not seen we love, will say: "Yet not I, but the grace of God which was with me." C. I. SCOFIELD.

"Greyshingles," Douglaston, L. I., Jan. 1, 1917.

A PANORAMIC VIEW OF THE BIBLE.

The Bible, incomparably the most widely circulated of books, at once provokes and baffles study. Even the non-believer in its authority rightly feels that it is unintelligent to remain in almost total ignorance of the most famous and ancient of books. And yet most, even of sincere believers, soon retire from any serious effort to master the content of the sacred writings. The reason is not far to seek. It is found in the fact that no particular portion of Scripture is to be intelligently comprehended apart from some conception of its place in the whole. For the Bible story and message is like a picture wrought out in mosaics: each book, chapter, verse, and even word forms a necessary part, and has its own appointed place. It is, therefore, indispensable to any interesting and fruitful study of the Bible that a general knowledge of it be gained.

First. The Bible is one book. Seven great marks attest this unity. (1) From Genesis the Bible bears witness to *one God.* Wherever he speaks or acts he is consistent with himself, and with the total revelation concerning him. (2) The Bible forms one *continuous story*—the story of humanity in relation to God. (3) The Bible hazards the most unlikely *predictions* concerning the future, and, when the centuries have brought round the appointed time, records their fulfilment. (4) The Bible is a *progressive* unfolding of truth. Nothing is told all at once, and once for all. The law is, "first the blade, then the ear, after that the full corn." Without the possibility of collusion, often with centuries between, one writer of Scripture takes up an earlier revelation, adds to it, lays down the pen, and in due time another man moved by the Holy Spirit, and another, and another, add new details till the whole is complete. (5) From beginning to end the Bible testifies to *one redemption.* (6) From beginning to end the Bible has *one great theme*—the person and work of the Christ. (7) And, finally, these writers, some forty-four in number, writing through twenty centuries, have produced a *perfect harmony* of doctrine in progressive unfolding. This is, to every candid mind, the unanswerable proof of the Divine inspiration of the Bible.

Second. The Bible is a book of books. Sixty-six books make up the one Book. Considered with reference to the unity of the one book the separate books may be regarded as chapters. But that is but one side of the truth, for each of the sixty-six books is complete in itself, and has its own theme and analysis. In the present edition of the Bible these are fully shown in the introductions and divisions. It is therefore of the utmost moment that the books be studied in the light of their distinctive themes. Genesis, for instance, is the book of beginnings—the seed-plot of the whole Bible. Matthew is the book of the King, &c.

Third. The books of the Bible fall into groups. Speaking broadly there are five great divisions in the Scriptures, and these may be conveniently fixed in the memory by five key-words, Christ being the one theme (Luke 24:25-27):

PREPARATION.	MANIFESTATION.	PROPAGATION.
The O. T.	The Gospels.	The Acts.

EXPLANATION.	CONSUMMATION.
The Epistles.	The Apocalypse.

In other words, the Old Testament is the *preparation* for Christ; in the Gospels he is *manifested* to the world; in the Acts he is preached and his Gospel is *propagated* in the world; in the Epistles his Gospel is *explained;* and in the Revelation all the purposes of God in and through Christ are *consummated.* And these groups of books in turn fall into groups. This is especially true of the Old Testament, which is in four well defined groups. Over these may be written, as memory aids:

REDEMPTION.	ORGANIZATION.	POETRY.	SERMONS.	
Genesis	Joshua	Job	Isaiah	Jonah
Exodus	Judges	Psalms	Jeremiah	Micah
Leviticus	Ruth	Proverbs	Ezekiel	Nahum
Numbers	1, 2 Sam.	Ecclesiastes	Daniel	Habakkuk
Deuteronomy	1, 2 Kings	Song of Solomon	Hosea	Zephaniah
	1, 2 Chronicles	Lamentations	Joel	Haggai
	Ezra		Amos	Zechariah
	Nehemiah		Obadiah	Malachi
	Esther			

Again care should be taken not to overlook, in these general groupings, the distinctive messages of the several books composing them. Thus, while *redemption* is the *general* theme of the Pentateuch, telling as it does the story of the redemption of Israel out of bondage and into "a good land and large," each of the five books has its own distinctive part in the whole. Genesis is the book of beginnings, and explains the *origin* of Israel. Exodus tells the story of the *deliverance* of Israel; Leviticus of the *worship* of Israel as a delivered people; Numbers the wanderings and failures of the delivered people, and Deuteronomy warns and instructs that people in view of their approaching entrance upon their inheritance.

The Poetical books record the spiritual experiences of the redeemed people in the varied scenes and events through which the providence of God led them. The prophets were inspired preachers, and the prophetical books consist of sermons with brief connecting and explanatory passages. Two prophetical books, Ezekiel and Daniel, have a different character and are apocalyptic, largely.

Fourth. The Bible tells the Human Story. Beginning, logically, with the creation of the earth and of man, the story of the race sprung from the first human pair continues through the first eleven chapters of Genesis. With the twelfth chapter begins the history of Abraham and of the nation of which Abraham was the ancestor. It is that nation, Israel, with which the Bible narrative is thereafter chiefly concerned from the eleventh chapter of Genesis to the second chapter of the Acts of the Apostles. The Gentiles are mentioned, but only in connection with Israel. But it is made increasingly clear that Israel so fills the scene only because entrusted with the accomplishment of great world-wide purposes (Deut. 7:7).

The appointed mission of Israel was, (1) to be a witness to the unity of God in the midst of universal idolatry (Deut. 6:4; Isa. 43:10); (2) to illustrate to the nations the greater blessedness of serving the one true God (Deut. 33:26-29; 1 Chron. 17:20, 21; Psa. 102:15); (3) to receive and preserve the Divine revelation (Rom. 3:1, 2); and (4) to produce the Messiah, earth's Saviour and Lord (Rom. 9:4). The prophets foretell a glorious future for Israel under the reign of Christ.

The biblical story of Israel, past, present, and future, falls into seven distinct periods: (1) From the call of Abram (Gen. 12) to the Exodus (Ex. 1–20); (2) From the Exodus to the death of Joshua (Ex. 21 to Josh. 24); (3) from the death of Joshua to the establishment of the Hebrew monarchy under Saul; (4) the period of the kings from Saul to the Captivities; (5) the period of the Captivities; (6) the restored commonwealth from the end of the Babylonian captivity of Judah, to the destruction of Jerusalem, A.D. 70; (7) the present dispersion.

The Gospels record the appearance in human history and within the Hebrew nation of the promised Messiah, Jesus Christ, and tell the wonderful story of his manifestation to Israel, his rejection by that people, his crucifixion, resurrection, and ascension.

The Acts of the Apostles record the descent of the Holy Spirit, and the beginning of a new thing in human history, the Church. The division of the race now becomes threefold—the Jew, the Gentile, and the Church of God. Just as Israel is in the foreground from the call of Abram to the resurrection of Christ, so now the Church fills the scene from the second chapter of the Acts to the fourth chapter of the Revelation. The remaining chapters of that book complete the story of humanity and the final triumph of Christ.

Fifth. The Central Theme of the Bible is Christ. It is this manifestation of Jesus Christ, his Person as "God manifest in the flesh" (1 Tim. 3:16), his sacrificial death, and his resurrection, which constitute the Gospel. Unto this all preceding Scripture leads, from this all following Scripture proceeds. The Gospel is preached in the Acts and explained in the Epistles. Christ, Son of God, Son of man, Son of Abraham, Son of David, thus binds the many books into one Book. Seed of the woman (Gen. 3:15) he is the ultimate destroyer of Satan and his works; Seed of Abraham he is the world blesser; Seed of David he is Israel's King, "Desire of all Nations." Exalted to the right hand of God he is "head over all to the Church, which is his body," while to Israel and the nations the promise of his return forms the one and only rational expectation that humanity will yet fulfil itself. Meanwhile the Church looks momentarily for the fulfilment of his special promise: "I will come again and receive you unto myself" (John 14:1-3). To him the Holy Spirit throughout this Gospel age bears testimony. The last book of all, the Consummation book, is "The Revelation of Jesus Christ" (Rev. 1:1).

THE NAMES AND ORDER

OF ALL THE

BOOKS OF THE OLD AND NEW TESTAMENTS

WITH THE NUMBER OF THEIR CHAPTERS.

THE BOOKS OF THE OLD TESTAMENT

THE BOOKS OF THE NEW TESTAMENT.

HOW TO USE THE SUBJECT REFERENCES.

THE subject references lead the reader from the first clear mention of a great truth to the last. The first and last references (in parenthesis) are repeated each time, so that wherever a reader comes upon a subject he may recur to the first reference and follow the subject, or turn at once to the Summary at the last reference.

ILLUSTRATION
(at Mark 1:1)

b Gospel. vs. 1, 14, 15; Mk. 8:35. (Gen. 12:1-3; Rev. 14:6.)

Here *Gospel* is the subject; vs. 1, 14, 15 show where it is at that particular place; Mk. 8:35 is the next reference in the chain, and the references in parenthesis are the first and the last.

THE PENTATEUCH.

THE five books ascribed to Moses have a peculiar place in the structure of the Bible, and an order which is undeniably the order of the experience of the people of God in all ages. Genesis is the book of origins—of the beginning of life, and of ruin through sin. Its first word, "In the beginning God," is in striking contrast with the end, "In a coffin in Egypt." Exodus is the book of redemption, the first need of a ruined race. Leviticus is the book of worship and communion, the proper exercise of the redeemed. Numbers speaks of the experiences of a pilgrim people, the redeemed passing through a hostile scene to a promised inheritance. Deuteronomy, retrospective and prospective, is a book of instruction for the redeemed about to enter that inheritance.

That Babylonian and Assyrian monuments contain records bearing a grotesque resemblance to the majestic account of the creation and of the Flood is true, as also that these antedate Moses. But this confirms rather than invalidates the inspiration of the Mosaic account. *Some* tradition of creation and the Flood would inevitably be handed down in the ancient cradle of the race. Such a tradition, following the order of all tradition, would take on grotesque and mythological features, and these abound in the Babylonian records. Of necessity, therefore, the first task of inspiration would be to supplant the often absurd and childish tradition with a revelation of the true history, and such a history we find in words of matchless grandeur, and in an order which, rightly understood, is absolutely scientific.

In the Pentateuch,[a] therefore, we have a true and logical introduction to the entire Bible; and, in type, an epitome of the divine revelation.

[a] Cf. Mt. 8:4; 19:8; Mk. 12:26; Lk. 5:14; 16:29-31; John 3:14; 5:45, 46; 7:19.

The abbreviation cf. used throughout the Bible signifies compare.

THE FIRST BOOK OF MOSES
CALLED
GENESIS

GENESIS is the book of beginnings. It records not only the beginning of the heavens and the earth, and of plant, animal, and human life, but also of all human institutions and relationships. Typically, it speaks of the new birth, the new creation, where all was chaos and ruin.

With Genesis begins also that progressive self-revelation of God which culminates in Christ. The three primary names of Deity, Elohim, Jehovah, and Adonai, and the five most important of the compound names, occur in Genesis; and that in an ordered progression which could not be changed without confusion.

The problem of sin as affecting man's condition in the earth, and his relation to God, and the divine solution of that problem are here in essence. Of the eight great covenants which condition human life and the divine redemption, four, the Edenic, Adamic, Noahic, and Abrahamic Covenants, are in this book; and these are the fundamental covenants to which the other four, the Mosaic, Palestinian, Davidic, and New Covenants, are related chiefly as adding detail or development.

Genesis enters into the very structure of the New Testament, in which it is quoted above sixty times in seventeen books. In a profound sense, therefore, the roots of all subsequent revelation are planted deep in Genesis, and whoever would truly comprehend that revelation must begin here.

The inspiration of Genesis and its character as a divine revelation are authenticated by the testimony of history, and by the testimony of Christ (Mt. 19:4-6; 24:37-39; Mk. 10:4-9; Lk. 11:49-51; 17:26-29, 32; John 1:5; 7:21-23; 8:44, 56).

Genesis is in five chief divisions: I. Creation (1:1–2:25). II. The Fall and Redemption (3:1–4:7). III. The Diverse Seeds, Cain and Seth, to the Flood (4:8–7:24). IV. The Flood to Babel (8:1–11:9). V. From the call of Abram to the death of Joseph (11:10–50:26).

The events recorded in Genesis cover a period of 2,315 years (Ussher).

CHAPTER 1.

The original creation.

In the [a]beginning [1b]God [2]created the heaven and the earth.

Earth made waste and empty by judgment (Jer. 4:23–26).

2 And the earth was [3]without form, and void; and darkness *was* upon the face of the deep. And [c]the [d]Spirit of God moved upon the face of the waters.

The new beginning—the first day: light diffused.

3 And God said, Let there be [4]light: and there was light.

4 And God saw the light, that *it*

B.C. 4004.

a John 1:1.
b *Deity (names of).* Gen. 2:4, 7. (Gen. 1:1; Mal. 3:18.)
c *Holy Spirit,* Gen. 6:3. (Gen. 1:2; Mal. 2:15.)
d Job 26:13. Psa. 104:30.

---

[1](1:1) *Elohim* (sometimes *El* or *Elah*), English form "God," the first of the three primary names of Deity, is a uni-plural noun formed from *El* = strength, or the strong one, and *Alah,* to swear, to bind oneself by an oath, so implying faithfulness. This uni-plurality implied in the name is directly asserted in Gen. 1:26 (plurality), 27 (unity); see also Gen. 3:22. Thus the Trinity is latent in *Elohim.* As meaning primarily the Strong One it is fitly used in the first chapter of Genesis. Used in the O. T. about 2500 times. See also Gen. 2:4, *note;* 2:7; 14:18, *note;* 15:2, *note;* 17:1, *note;* 21:33, *note;* 1 Sam. 1:3, *note.*

[2](1:1) But three *creative* acts of God are recorded in this chapter: (1) the heavens and the earth, v. 1; (2) animal life, v. 21; and (3) human life, vs. 26, 27. The first creative act refers to the dateless past, and gives scope for all the geologic ages.

[3](1:2) Jer. 4:23-26, Isa. 24:1 and 45:18, clearly indicate that the earth had undergone a cataclysmic change as the result of a divine judgment. The face of the earth bears everywhere the marks of such a catastrophe. There are not wanting intimations which connect it with a previous testing and fall of angels. See Ezk. 28:12-15 and Isa. 14:9-14, which certainly go beyond the kings of Tyre and Babylon.

[4](1:3) Neither here nor in verses 14-18 is an original *creative* act implied. A different word is used. The sense is, made to *appear;* made *visible.* The sun and moon were *created* "in the beginning." The "light" of course came from the sun, but the vapour diffused the light. Later the sun appeared in an unclouded sky.

was good: and God divided the light
from the darkness.
5 And God called the light [1]Day, and
the darkness he called Night. And the
[2]evening and the morning were the first
day.

The second day: vapour above, water below.

6 And God said, Let there be a [a]firma-
ment in the midst of the waters, and let
it divide the waters from the waters.
7 And God made the firmament, and
divided the waters which *were* under the
firmament from the waters which *were*
above the firmament: and it was so.
8 And God called the [b]firmament
Heaven. And the evening and the morning were the second day.

The third day: land and sea;
plant life appears.

9 And God said, Let the waters under
the heaven be gathered together unto
one place, and let the dry *land* appear:
and it was so.
10 And God called the dry *land* Earth;
and the gathering together of the waters
called he Seas: and God saw that *it was*
good.
11 And God said, Let the earth [3]bring
forth grass, the herb yielding seed, *and*
the fruit tree yielding fruit after his kind,
whose seed *is* in itself, upon the earth:
and it was so.
12 And the earth brought forth grass,

B.C. 4004.

a Lit. *expanse* (i.e. of waters beneath, of vapour above).

b i.e. *the expanse above, the "heaven" of the clouds.* Gen. 7:11; 8:2.

c Psa. 136:5-9.

d The word does not imply a creative act; vs. 14-18 are declarative of function merely.

e i.e. the *"heaven" of the stars;* e.g. Gen. 15:5. See Lk. 23:43.

and herb yielding seed after his kind,
and the tree yielding fruit, whose seed
was in itself, after his kind: and God saw
that *it was* good.
13 And the evening and the morning
were the third day.

The fourth day: the sun, moon,
and stars became visible.

14 And God said, [c]Let there be lights
in the firmament of the heaven to divide
the day from the night; and let them be
for signs, and for seasons, and for days,
and years:
15 And let them be for lights in the firmament of the heaven to give light upon
the earth: and it was so.
16 And God [d]made two great lights;
the [4]greater light to rule the day, and the
lesser light to rule the night: *he made* the
stars also.
17 And God set them in the firmament
of the [e]heaven to give light upon the
earth,
18 And to rule over the day and over
the night, and to divide the light from the
darkness: and God saw that *it was* good.
19 And the evening and the morning
were the fourth day.

The fifth day: the second creative act—
animal life. (See Gen. 2:19.)

20 And God said, Let the waters
bring forth abundantly the moving
creature that hath life, and fowl

[1] **(1:5)** The word "day" is used in Scripture in three ways: (1) that part of the solar day of twenty-four hours which is light (Gen. 1:5, 14; John 9:4; 11:9); (2) such a day, set apart for some distinctive purpose, as, "day of atonement" (Lev. 23:27); "day of judgment" (Mt. 10:15); (3) a period of time, long or short, during which certain revealed purposes of God are to be accomplished, as "day of the LORD."

[2] **(1:5)** The use of "evening" and "morning" may be held to limit "day" to the solar day; but the frequent parabolic use of natural phenomena may warrant the conclusion that each creative "day" was a period of time marked off by a beginning and ending.

[3] **(1:11)** It is by no means necessary to suppose that the life-germ of seeds perished in the catastrophic judgment which overthrew the primitive order. With the restoration of dry land and light the earth would "bring forth" as described. It was *animal* life which perished, the traces of which remain as fossils. Relegate fossils to the primitive creation, and no conflict of science with the Genesis cosmogony remains.

[4] **(1:16)** The "greater light" is a type of Christ, the "Sun of righteousness" (Mal. 4:2). He will take this character at His second advent. Morally the world is now in the state between Gen. 1:3 and 1:16 (Eph. 6:12; Acts 26:18; 1 Pet. 2:9). The sun is not seen, but there is light. Christ is that light (John 1:4, 5, 9), but "shineth in darkness," comprehended only by faith. As "Sun of righteousness" He will dispel all darkness. Dispensationally the Church is in place as the "lesser light," the moon, reflecting the light of the unseen sun. The stars (Gen. 1:16) are individual believers who are "lights" (Phil. 2:15, 16). See John 1:5.

(A type is a divinely purposed illustration of some truth. It may be: (1) a person (Rom. 5:14); (2) an event (1 Cor. 10:11); (3) a thing (Heb. 10:20); (4) an institution (Heb. 9:11); (5) a ceremonial (1 Cor. 5:7). Types occur most frequently in the Pentateuch, but are found, more sparingly, elsewhere. The antitype, or fulfilment of the type, is found, usually, in the New Testament.)

that may fly above the earth in the open
firmament of heaven.
21 And God created great whales, and
every living [1]creature that moveth,
which the waters brought forth abundantly, after their kind, and every
winged fowl after his kind: and God saw
that *it was* good.
22 And God blessed them, saying, Be
fruitful, and multiply, and fill the waters
in the seas, and let fowl multiply in the
earth.
23 And the evening and the morning
were the fifth day.

The sixth day: (1) *the fecundity of the earth after the creative work of the fifth day.*

24 And God said, Let the earth bring
forth the living [2]creature after his kind,
cattle, and creeping thing, and beast of
the earth after his kind: and it was so.
25 And God made the beast of the
earth after his kind, and cattle after their
kind, and every thing that creepeth
upon the earth after his kind: and God
saw that *it was* good.

The sixth day: (2) *the creation of man* (described Gen. 2:7, 21–23).

26 And God said, Let [a]us make [3]man
in our image, after our likeness: and let
them have [b]dominion over the fish of
the sea, and over the fowl of the air, and
over the cattle, and over all the earth,
and over every creeping thing that
creepeth upon the earth.
27 So God created man in his *own*
image, in the image of God created he
him; [c]male and female created he them.

The First [4]*Dispensation: Innocency* (Gen. 1:38–3:13). *The First, or Edenic Covenant: conditioned the life of unfallen man.* (Add Gen. 2:8–17.)

28 [5]And God blessed them, and God
[d]said unto them, [6]Be fruitful, and

B.C. 4004.

a Gen. 11:7.

b Kingdom (O.T.). vs. 26-28; Gen. 9:6. (Gen. 1:26; Zech. 12:8.)

c Cf. Mt. 19:4; Mk. 10:6-8.

d *The Eight Covenants.* (1; Edenic). Gen. 2:15-17. (Gen. 1:28; Heb. 8:10.)

[1] **(1:21)** The second clause, "every living creature," as distinguished from fishes merely, is taken up again in verse 24, showing that in the second creative act all animal life is included.

[2] **(1:24)** "Creature," Heb. *nephesh,* trans. soul in 2:7 and usually. In itself *nephesh,* or soul, implies self-conscious life, as distinguished from plants, which have unconscious life. In the sense of self-conscious life animals also have "soul." See verses 26, 27, *note.*

[3] **(1:26)** Man. Gen. 1:26, 27, gives the *general,* Gen. 2:7, 21-23, the *particular,* account of the creation of man. The revealed facts are:

(1) Man was *created,* not *evolved.* This is *(a)* expressly declared, and the declaration is confirmed by Christ (Mt. 19:4; Mk. 10:6); *(b)* "an enormous gulf, a divergence practically infinite" (Huxley) between the lowest man and the highest beast, confirms it; *(c)* the highest beast has no trace of God-consciousness—the religious nature; *(d)* science and discovery have done nothing to bridge that "gulf."

(2) That man was made in the "image and likeness" of God. This "image" is found chiefly in man's tri-unity, and in his moral nature. Man is "spirit and soul and body" (1 Thes. 5:23). "Spirit" is that part of man which "knows" (1 Cor. 2:11), and which allies him to the spiritual creation and gives him God-consciousness. "Soul" in itself implies self-conscious life, as distinguished from plants, which have unconscious life. In that sense animals also have "soul" (Gen. 1:24). But the "soul" of man has a vaster content than "soul" as applied to beast life. It is the seat of his emotions, desires, affections (Psa. 42:1-6). The "heart" is, in Scripture usage, nearly synonymous with "soul." Because the natural man is, characteristically, the soulual or psychical man, "soul" is often used as synonymous with the individual, e. g. Gen. 12:5. The body, separable from spirit and soul, and susceptible to death, is nevertheless an integral part of man, as the resurrection shows (John 5:28, 29; 1 Cor. 15:47-50; Rev. 20:11-13). It is the seat of the senses (the means by which the spirit and soul have world-consciousness) and of the fallen Adamic nature (Rom. 7:23, 24).

[4] **(1:28, heading)** A dispensation is a period of time during which man is tested in respect of obedience to some *specific* revelation of the will of God. Seven such dispensations are distinguished in Scripture. See *note* 5.

[5] **(1:28)** The First Dispensation: Innocency. Man was created in innocency, placed in a perfect environment, subjected to an absolutely simple test, and warned of the consequence of disobedience. The woman fell through pride; the man, deliberately (1 Tim. 2:14). God restored His sinning creatures, but the dispensation of innocency ended in the judgment of the Expulsion (Gen. 3:24). See, for the other dispensations: *Conscience* (Gen. 3:23); *Human Government* (Gen. 8:20); *Promise* (Gen. 12:1); *Law* (Ex. 19:8); *Grace* (John 1:17); *Kingdom* (Eph. 1:10).

[6] **(1:28)** The Edenic Covenant, the first of the eight great covenants of Scripture which condition life

multiply, and replenish the earth, and
subdue it: and have dominion over the
fish of the sea, and over the fowl of the
air, and over every living thing that
moveth upon the earth.
29 And God said, Behold, I have given
you every herb bearing seed, which *is*
upon the face of all the earth, and every
tree, in the which *is* the fruit of a tree
yielding seed; to you it shall be for meat.
30 And to every beast of the earth, and
to every fowl of the air, and to every
thing that creepeth upon the earth,
wherein *there is* life, *I have given* every
green herb for meat: and it was so.
31 And God saw every thing that he
had made, and, behold, *it was* very good.
And the evening and the morning were
the sixth day.

B.C. 4004.

a Heb. 4:4; cf. Heb. 4:8-9

b *Sabbath.* Ex. 16:22-25. (Gen. 2:3; Mt. 12:1.)

c *Sanctify, holy* (O.T.). Ex. 19:23. (Gen. 2:3; Zech. 8:3.)

d *Deity (names of).* vs. 4, 7; Gen. 14:18. (Gen. 1:1; Mal. 3:18, *note.*)

CHAPTER 2.

The sabbath rest of God: type of the believer's rest in the finished work of redemption (Heb. 3–4).

Thus the heavens and the earth were
finished, and all the host of them.
2 And on the seventh day God ended
his work which he had made; and he
[a]rested on the seventh day from all his
work which he had made.
3 And God blessed the [b]seventh day,
and [1c]sanctified it: because that in it he
had rested from all his work which God
created and made.

Summary of the creation work of Chapter 1.

4 These *are* the generations of the
heavens and of the earth when they
were created, in the day that the [2d]LORD
God made the earth and the heavens,

and salvation, and about which all Scripture crystallizes, has seven elements. The man and woman in Eden were responsible:

(1) To replenish the earth with a new order—man; (2) to subdue the earth to human uses; (3) to have dominion over the animal creation; (4) to eat herbs and fruits; (5) to till and keep the garden; (6) to abstain from eating of the tree of knowledge of good and evil; (7) the penalty—death. See, for the other seven covenants: *Adamic* (Gen. 3:15); *Noahic* (Gen. 9:1); *Abrahamic* (Gen. 15:18) *Mosaic* (Ex. 19:25); *Palestinian* (Deut. 30:3); *Davidic* (2 Sam. 7:16); *New* (Heb. 8:8).

1 **(2:3)** In the O. T. the same Hebrew word *(qodesh)* is trans. sanctify, consecrate, dedicate, and holy. It means, set apart for the service of God. See *refs.* following "Sanctify," Gen. 2:3.

2 **(2:4)** LORD (Heb. *Jehovah*).

(1) The primary meaning of the name LORD (Jehovah) is "the self-existent One." Literally (as in Ex. 3:14), "He that is who He is, therefore the eternal I AM." But *Havah,* from which Jehovah, or *Yahwe,* is formed, signifies also "to become," that is, to become known, thus pointing to a continuous and increasing self-revelation. Combining these meanings of *Havah,* we arrive at the meaning of the name Jehovah. He is "the self-existent One who reveals Himself." The name is, in itself, an advance upon the name "God" *(El, Elah, Elohim),* which suggests certain *attributes* of Deity, as strength, etc., rather than His essential *being.*

(2) It is significant that the first appearance of the name Jehovah in Scripture follows the creation of man. It was God *(Elohim)* who said, "Let us make man in our image" (Gen. 1:26); but when man, as in the second chapter of Genesis, is to fill the scene and become dominant over creation, it is the LORD God *(Jehovah Elohim)* who acts. This clearly indicates a special relation of Deity, in His Jehovah character, to man, and all Scripture emphasizes this.

(3) Jehovah is distinctly the redemption name of Deity. When sin entered and redemption became necessary, it was Jehovah Elohim who sought the sinning ones (Gen. 3:9-13) and clothed them with "coats of skins" (Gen. 3:21), a beautiful type of a righteousness provided by the LORD God through sacrifice (Rom. 3:21, 22). The first distinct *revelation* of Himself by His name Jehovah was in connection with the redemption of the covenant people out of Egypt (Ex. 3:13-17).

As Redeemer, emphasis is laid upon those attributes of Jehovah which the sin and salvation of man bring into exercise. These are: *(a)* His holiness (Lev. 11:44, 45; 19:1, 2; 20:26; Hab. 1:12, 13); *(b)* His hatred and judgment of sin (Deut. 32:35-42; Gen. 6:5-7; Psa. 11:4-6; 66:18; Ex. 34:6, 7); *(c)* His love for and redemption of sinners, but always righteously (Gen. 3:21; 8:20, 21; Ex. 12:12, 13; Lev. 16:2, 3; Isa. 53:5, 6, 10). Salvation by Jehovah apart from sacrifice is unknown to Scripture.

5 And every plant of the field before it
was in the earth, and every herb of the
field before it grew: for the LORD God
had not caused it to rain upon the earth,
and *there was* not a man to till the
ground.
6 But there went up a mist from the
earth, and watered the whole face of the
ground.

The creative act of Gen. 1:27 *described.*

7 And the LORD God [a]formed man *of*
the dust of the ground, and breathed
into his nostrils the breath of life; and
man became a [a]living soul.

The habitation of unfallen man, and the Edenic Covenant. (Add Gen. 1:28–30.)

8 And the LORD God planted a garden
eastward in Eden; and there he put the
man whom he had formed.
9 And out of the ground made the
LORD God to grow every tree that is
pleasant to the sight, and good for food;
the tree of life also in the midst of the
garden, and the tree of knowledge of
good and evil.

B.C. 4004.

a Mt. 19:4; Mk. 10:6; 1 Cor. 15:45.

b *The Eight Covenants.* vs. 15-17; Gen. 3:14. (Gen. 1:28; Heb. 8:10.)

c Or, *Adam.*

d Cf. Rom. 5:12; 1 Cor. 15:21-22.

e *Death (spiritual)* Mt. 8:22. (Gen. 2:17; Eph. 2:5.)

f Hiddekel = ancient name of the Tigris.

10 And a river went out of Eden to
water the garden; and from thence it
was parted, and became into four heads.
11 The name of the first *is* Pison: that *is*
it which compasseth the whole land of
Havilah, where *there is* gold;
12 And the gold of that land *is* good:
there *is* bdellium and the onyx stone.
13 And the name of the second river *is*
Gihon: the same *is* it that compasseth the
whole land of Ethiopia.
14 And the name of the third river *is*
[f]Hiddekel: that *is* it which goeth toward
the east of Assyria. And the fourth river
is Euphrates.
15 [b]And the LORD God took the [c]man,
and put him into the garden of Eden to
dress it and to keep it.
16 And the LORD God commanded the
man, saying, Of every tree of the garden
thou mayest freely eat:
17 But of the tree of the knowledge of
good and evil, thou shalt not eat of it:
[d]for in the [e]day that thou eatest thereof
thou shalt surely die.

(4) In His redemptive relation to man, Jehovah has seven compound names which reveal Him as meeting every need of man from his lost state to the end. These compound names are: *(a) Jehovah-jireh,* "the LORD will provide" (Gen. 22:13, 14), i. e. will provide a sacrifice; *(b) Jehovah-rapha,* "the LORD that healeth" (Ex. 15:26). That this refers to physical healing the context shows, but the deeper healing of soul malady is implied. *(c) Jehovah-nissi,* "the LORD our banner" (Ex. 17:8-15). The name is interpreted by the context. The enemy was Amalek, a type of the flesh, and the conflict that day stands for the conflict of Gal. 5:17—the war of the Spirit against the flesh. Victory was wholly due to divine help. *(d) Jehovah-Shalom,* "the LORD our peace," or "the LORD send peace" (Jud. 6:24). Almost the whole ministry of Jehovah finds expression and illustration in that chapter. Jehovah hates and judges sin (vs. 1-5); Jehovah loves and saves sinners (vs. 7-18), but only through sacrifice (vs. 19-21) (see also Rom. 5:1; Eph. 2:14; Col. 1:20). *(e) Jehovah-rā-ah,* "the LORD my shepherd" (Psa. 23.). In Psa. 22 Jehovah makes peace by the blood of the cross; in Psa. 23. Jehovah is shepherding His own who are in the world (John. 10:7, *note*). *(f) Jehovah-tsidkenu,* "the LORD our righteousness" (Jer. 23:6). This name of Jehovah occurs in a prophecy concerning the future restoration and conversion of Israel. Then Israel will hail Him as Jehovah-tsidkenu—"the LORD our righteousness." *(g) Jehovah-shammah,* "the LORD is present" (Ezk. 48:35). This name signifies Jehovah's abiding presence with His people (see Ex. 33:14, 15; 1 Chr. 16:27, 33; Psa. 16:11; 97:5; Mt. 28:20; Heb. 13:5).

(5) LORD (Jehovah) is also the distinctive name of Deity as in covenant with Israel (Ex. 19:3; 20:1, 2; Jer. 31:31-34).

(6) LORD God (Heb. *Jehovah Elohim*) is the first of the *compound* names of Deity. LORD God is used distinctively: (1) of the relation of Deity to man *(a)* as Creator (Gen. 2:7-15); *(b)* as morally in authority over man (Gen. 2:16,17); *(c)* as creating and governing the earthly relationships of man (Gen. 2:18-24; 3:16-19, 22-24); and *(d)* as redeeming man (Gen. 3:8-15, 21); (2) of the relation of Deity to Israel (Gen. 24:7; 28:13; Ex. 3:15, 18; 4:5; 5:1; 7:6, etc.; Deut. 1:11, 21; 4:1; 6:3; 12:1, etc.; Josh. 7:13, 19, 20; 10:40, 42; Jud. 2:12; 1 Sam. 2:30; 1 Ki. 1:48; 2 Ki. 9:6; 10:31; 1 Chr. 22:19; 2 Chr. 1:9; Ezra 1:3; Isa. 21:17). See other names of Deity, Gen. 1:1, *note;* 2:4, *note;* 14:18, *note;* 15:2, *note;* 17:1, *note;* 21:33, *note;* 1 Sam. 1:3, *note.*

18 And the LORD God said, *It is* not good that the man should be alone; I will make him an help meet for him.

19 And out of the ground the LORD God formed every beast of the field, and every fowl of the air; and brought *them* unto Adam to see what he would call them: and whatsoever Adam called every living creature, that *was* the name thereof.

20 And Adam gave names to all cattle, and to the fowl of the air, and to every beast of the field; but for Adam there was not found an help meet for him.

The method of the creation of woman (Gen. 1: 27).

21 And the LORD God caused a deep sleep to fall upon Adam, and he slept: and he took one of his ribs, and closed up the flesh instead thereof;

22 And the rib, which the LORD God had taken from man, made he a woman, and brought her unto the man.

Eve, type of the church as bride of Christ (Eph. 5:28–32).

23 And Adam said, [1]This *is* now bone of my bones, and flesh of my flesh: she shall be called [a]Woman, because she was taken out of Man.

24 [b]Therefore shall a man leave his father and his mother, and shall cleave unto his wife: and they shall be one flesh.

25 And they were both naked, the man and his wife, and were not ashamed.

CHAPTER 3.

The temptation of Eve: (1) *the implied doubt of the benevolence of God.*

Now the [2c]serpent was more subtil than any beast of the field which the LORD God had made. And he said unto the woman, Yea, hath God [d]said, Ye shall not eat of every tree of the garden?

B.C. 4004.

a Isha, "because she was taken out of man" (Ish) (Hos. 2:16).

b Cf. Mt. 19:5; 1 Cor. 6:16; Eph. 5:31.

c Satan, vs. 1, 2, 4, 13, 14; 1 Chr. 21:1. (Gen. 3:1; Rev. 20:10.)

d Temptation. vs. 1-6, 12, 13; Gen. 22:1. (Gen. 3:1; Jas. 1:2.)

The temptation of Eve: (2) *adding to the Word of God.*

2 And the woman said unto the serpent, We may eat of the fruit of the trees of the garden:

3 But of the fruit of the tree which *is* in the midst of the garden, God hath said, Ye shall not eat of it, neither shall ye touch it, lest ye die.

The temptation of Eve: (3) *the first lie* (John 8:44).

4 And the serpent said unto the woman, Ye shall not surely die:

The temptation of Eve: (4) *the appeal to pride* (Isa. 14:12–14).

5 For God doth know that in the day ye eat thereof, then your eyes shall be opened, and ye shall be as gods, knowing good and evil.

The temptation of Eve: (5) *the fall* (1 Tim. 2:14).

6 And when the woman saw that the tree *was* good for food, and that it *was* pleasant to the eyes, and a tree to be desired to make *one* wise, she took of the fruit thereof, and did eat, and gave also unto her husband with her; and he did eat.

7 And the eyes of them both were opened, and they knew that they *were* naked; and they sewed fig leaves together, and made themselves aprons.

The seeking God. His sabbath rest broken; His new work begun (John 5:17; 9:4; 14:10).

8 And they heard the voice of the LORD God walking in the garden in the cool of the day: and Adam and his wife hid themselves from the presence of the LORD God amongst the trees of the garden.

9 And the LORD God called unto Adam, and said unto him, Where *art* thou?

10 And he said, I heard thy voice in the garden, and I was afraid, because I *was* naked; and I hid myself.

[1] **(2:23)** Eve, type of the Church as bride of Christ (John 3:28, 29; 2 Cor. 11:2; Eph. 5:25-32; Rev. 19:7, 8).

[2] **(3:1)** The serpent, in his Edenic form, is not to be thought of as a writhing reptile. That is the effect of the curse (Gen. 3:14). The creature which lent itself to Satan may well have been the most beautiful as it was the most "subtle" of creatures less than man. Traces of that beauty remain despite the curse. Every movement of a serpent is graceful, and many species are beautifully coloured. In the serpent, Satan first appeared "as an angel of light" (2 Cor. 11:14).

11 And he said, Who told thee that thou *wast* naked? Hast thou eaten of the tree, whereof I commanded thee that thou shouldest not eat?

12 And the man said, The woman whom thou gavest *to be* with me, she gave me of the tree, and I did eat.

13 And the LORD God said unto the woman, What *is* this *that* thou hast done? And the woman said, The serpent beguiled me, and I did eat.

The Second, or Adamic Covenant.

14 [1]And the LORD God [a]said unto the serpent, Because thou hast done this, thou *art* cursed above all cattle, and above every beast of the field; upon thy belly shalt thou go, and dust shalt thou eat all the days of thy life:

15 And I will put enmity between thee and the woman, and between thy seed and her seed; it shall bruise thy head, and [2]thou shalt [b]bruise [c]his heel.

16 Unto the woman he said, I will greatly multiply thy [d]sorrow and thy conception; in sorrow thou shalt bring forth children; and thy desire *shall be* to thy husband, and he shall [e]rule over thee.

17 And unto Adam he said, Because thou hast hearkened unto the voice of thy wife, and hast eaten of the tree, of which I commanded thee, saying, Thou shalt not eat of it: cursed *is* the ground for thy sake; in sorrow shalt thou eat *of* it all the days of thy life;

18 Thorns also and [f]thistles shall it bring forth to thee; and thou shalt eat the herb of the field;

19 In the sweat of thy face shalt thou eat bread, till thou return unto the ground; for out of it wast thou taken: for dust thou *art*, and unto dust shalt thou [g]return.

The faith of Adam.

20 And Adam [h]called his wife's name [i]Eve; because she was the mother of all living.

B.C. 4004.

a *The Eight Covenants.* Gen. 8:21. (Gen. 1:28; Heb. 8:10.)
b *Sacrifice (prophetic).* Psa. 2:1-3. (Gen. 3:15; Heb. 10:18.)
c *Christ (first advent).* Gen. 12:3. (Gen. 3:15; Acts. 1:9.)
d Or, *thy sorrow with thy conception.*
e Cf. 1 Cor. 11:3; 14:34; Eph. 5:22; Col. 3:18; 1 Tim. 2:11; Tit. 2:5; 1 Pet. 3:1, 5, 6.
f Cf. Rom. 8:22.
g *Death (physical).* Gen. 5:5. (Gen. 3:19; Heb. 9:27.)
h *Faith.* Gen. 4:4. (Gen. 3:20; Heb. 11:39.)
i i.e. *living,* or *life-giver.*

[1]**(3:14)** The Adamic Covenant conditions the life of fallen man—conditions which must remain till, in the kingdom age, "the creation also shall be delivered from the bondage of corruption into the glorious liberty of the sons of God" (Rom. 8:21). The elements of the Adamic Covenant are:

(1) The serpent, Satan's tool, is cursed (v. 14), and becomes God's illustration in nature of the effects of sin—from the most beautiful and subtle of creatures to a loathsome reptile! The deepest mystery of the atonement is intimated here. Christ, "made sin for us," in bearing our judgment, is typified by the brazen serpent (Num. 21:5-9; John 3:14, 15; 2 Cor. 5:21). Brass speaks of judgment—in the brazen altar, of God's judgment, and in the laver, of self-judgment.

(2) The first promise of a Redeemer (v. 15). Here begins the "highway of the Seed," Abel, Seth, Noah (Gen. 6:8-10), Shem (Gen. 9:26, 27), Abraham (Gen. 12:1-4), Isaac (Gen. 17:19-21), Jacob (Gen. 28:10-14), Judah (Gen. 49:10), David (2 Sam. 7:5-17), Immanuel-Christ (Isa. 7:9-14; Mt. 1:1, 20-23; 1 John 3:8; John 12:31).

(3) The changed state of the woman (v. 16). In three particulars: *(a)* Multiplied conception; *(b)* motherhood linked with sorrow; *(c)* the headship of the man (cf. Gen. 1:26, 27). The entrance of sin, which is disorder, makes necessary a headship, and it is vested in man (1 Tim. 2:11-14; Eph. 5:22-25; 1 Cor. 11:7-9).

(4) The earth cursed (v. 17) for man's sake. It is better for fallen man to battle with a reluctant earth than to live without toil.

(5) The inevitable sorrow of life (v. 17).

(6) The light occupation of Eden (Gen. 2:15) changed to burdensome labour (vs. 18, 19).

(7) Physical death (v. 19; Rom. 5:12-21). See Death (spiritual)" (Gen. 2:17; Eph. 2:5, *note*).

See for the other covenants: *Edenic* (Gen. 1:28); *Noahic* (Gen. 9:1); *Abrahamic* (Gen. 15:18); *Mosaic* (Ex. 19:25); *Palestinian* (Deut. 30:3); *Davidic* (2 Sam. 7:16); *New* (Heb. 8:8).

[2]**(3:15)** The chain of references which begins here includes the promises and prophecies concerning Christ which were fulfilled in His birth and works at His first advent. See, for line of unfulfilled promises and prophecies: "Christ (second advent)" (Deut. 30:3; Acts 1:9, *note*); "Kingdom" (Gen. 1:26-28: Zech. 12:8; "Kingdom (N. T.)" (Lk. 1:31; 1 Cor. 15:28); "Day of the Lord" (Isa. 2:10; Rev. 19:11).

The response of Jehovah Elohim to the faith of Adam.

21 Unto Adam also and to his wife did the LORD God make [1]coats of skins, and [a]clothed them.

The judgment of the Expulsion ends the First Dispensation.

22 And the LORD God said, Behold, the man is become as one of us, to know good and evil: and now, lest he put forth his hand, and take also of the tree of life, and eat, and live for ever:

The Second Dispensation: Conscience (Gen. 3:22–7:23).

23 [2]Therefore the LORD God sent him forth from the garden of Eden, to till the ground from whence he was taken.

24 So he drove out the man; and he placed at the east of the garden of Eden [b]Cherubims, and a flaming sword which turned every way, to keep the way of the tree of life.

B.C. 4003.

a *Righteousness (garment).* Job 29:14. (Gen. 3:21; Rev. 19:8.)

b Ezk. 1:5, *note.*

c Lit. *even Jehovah.*

d *Faith.* Gen. 5:22-24. (Gen. 3:20; Heb. 11:39)

e *Sacrifice (typical).* Gen. 8:20. (Gen. 4:4; Heb. 10:18.)

CHAPTER 4.

The first sons of Adam and Eve.

And Adam knew Eve his wife; and she conceived, and bare [3]Cain, and said, I have gotten a man [c]from the LORD.

2 And she again bare his brother [4]Abel. And Abel was a keeper of sheep, but Cain was a tiller of the ground.

3 And in process of time it came to pass, that Cain brought of the fruit of the ground an offering unto the LORD.

4 And Abel, he also [d]brought of the firstlings of his [5]flock and of the fat thereof. And the LORD had respect unto Abel and to his [e]offering:

5 But unto Cain and to his offering he had not respect. And Cain was very wroth, and his countenance fell.

Cain exhorted even yet to bring a sin-offering.

6 And the LORD said unto Cain, Why art thou wroth? and why is thy countenance fallen?

[1] **(3:21)** Coats of skins: Type of "Christ, made unto us righteousness"—a divinely provided garment that the first sinners might be made fit for God's presence. See *Righteousness, garment* (Gen. 3:21; Rev. 19:8).

[2] **(3:23)** The Second Dispensation: Conscience. By disobedience man came to a personal and experimental knowledge of good and evil—of good as obedience, of evil as disobedience to *the known will of God.* Through that knowledge conscience awoke. Expelled from Eden and placed under the second, or Adamic Covenant man was responsible to do all known good, to abstain from all known evil, and to approach God through sacrifice. The result of this second testing of man is stated in Gen. 6:5, and the dispensation ended in the judgment of the Flood. Apparently "the east of the garden" (v. 24), where were the cherubims and the flame, remained the place of worship through this second dispensation. See for the other six dispensations: *Innocence* (Gen. 1:28); *Human Government* (Gen. 8:20); *Promise* (Gen. 12:1); *Law* (Ex. 19:8); *Grace* (John 1:17); *Kingdom* (Eph. 1:10).

[3] **(4:1)** Cain ("acquisition") is a type of the mere man of the earth. His religion was destitute of any adequate sense of sin, or need of atonement. This religious type is described in 2 Pet. 2. Seven things are said of him: (1) he worships in self-will 2) is angry with God; (3) refuses to bring a sin-offering; (4) murders his brother; (5) lies to God; (6) becomes a vagabond; (7) is, nevertheless, the object of the divine solicitude.

[4] **(4:2)** Abel ("exhalation," or, "that which ascends") is a type of the spiritual man. His sacrifice, in which atoning blood was shed (Heb. 9:22), was therefore at once his confession of sin and the expression of his faith in the interposition of a substitute (Heb. 11:4).

[5] **(4:4)** Type of Christ, the Lamb of God, the most constant type of the *suffering* Messiah—"the Lamb of God that taketh away the sin of the world" (John 1:29). A lamb fitly symbolizes the unresisting innocency and harmlessness of the Lord Jesus (Isa. 53:7; Lk. 23:9; Mt. 26:53, 54). This type is brought into prominence by contrast with Cain's bloodless offering of the fruit of his own works, and proclaims, in the very infancy of the race, the primal truth that "without shedding of blood is no remission" (Heb. 9:22; 11:4).

7 If thou doest well, shalt thou not be accepted? and if thou doest not well, [1]sin lieth at the door. And unto thee *shall be* his desire, and thou shalt rule over him.

The first murder: history of Cain
(cf. Gen. 4:23).

8 And Cain talked with Abel his brother: and it came to pass, when they were in the field, that Cain rose up against Abel his brother, and [a]slew him.

9 And the LORD said unto Cain, Where *is* Abel thy brother? And he said, I know not: *Am* I my brother's keeper?

10 And he said, What hast thou done? the voice of thy brother's blood crieth unto me from the ground.

11 And now *art* thou cursed from the earth, which hath opened her mouth to receive thy brother's blood from thy hand;

12 When thou tillest the ground, it shall not henceforth yield unto thee her strength; a fugitive and a vagabond shalt thou be in the earth.

13 And Cain said unto the LORD, My punishment *is* greater than I can bear.

14 Behold, thou hast driven me out this day from the face of the earth; and from thy face shall I be hid; and I shall be a fugitive and a vagabond in the earth; and it shall come to pass, *that* every one that findeth me shall slay me.

15 And the LORD said unto him, Therefore whosoever slayeth Cain, vengeance shall be taken on him sevenfold. And the LORD set a [b]mark upon Cain, lest any finding him should kill him.

The first civilization.

16 And Cain went out from the presence of the LORD, and dwelt in the land of [c]Nod, on the east of Eden.

17 And Cain knew his wife; and she conceived, and bare Enoch: and he [2]builded a city, and called the name of the city, after the name of his son, Enoch.

18 And unto Enoch was born Irad: and Irad begat Mehujael: and Mehujael begat Methusael: and Methusael begat Lamech.

19 And Lamech took unto him two wives: the name of the one *was* Adah, and the name of the other Zillah.

20 And Adah bare Jabal: he was the father of such as dwell in tents, and *of such as have* cattle.

21 And his brother's name *was* Jubal: he was the father of all such as handle the harp and organ.

22 And Zillah, she also bare Tubal-cain, an instructer of every artificer in brass and iron: and the sister of Tubal-cain *was* Naamah.

23 And Lamech said unto his wives, Adah and Zillah, Hear my voice; ye wives of Lamech, hearken unto my speech: for I have slain a man [d]to my wounding, and a young man to my hurt.

24 If Cain shall be avenged sevenfold, truly Lamech seventy and sevenfold.

The birth of Seth:
the spiritual seed renewed.

25 And Adam knew his wife again; and she bare a son, and called his name

B.C. 3875.

a Mt. 23:35; Lk. 11:51; Heb. 11:4; 1 John 3:12.

b i.e. for Cain's protection. The law of Gen. 9:6 was not yet enacted.

c Lit. *wandering.*

d Or, *who wounded me.* Cain had slain an unoffending man and yet was protected by Jehovah; how much more Lamech, who had slain in self-defence.

[1]**(4:7)** Or, *sin-offering*. In Hebrew the same word is used for "sin," and "sin-offering," thus emphasizing in a remarkable way the complete identification of the believer's sin with his sin-offering (cf. John 3:14 with 2 Cor. 5:21). Here both meanings are brought together. "Sin lieth at the door," but so also "a sin-offering croucheth at the [tent] door." It is "*where* sin abounded" that "grace did much more abound" (Rom. 5:20). Abel's offering implies a previous instruction (cf. Gen. 3:21), for it was "by faith" (Heb. 11:4), and faith is taking God at His word; so that Cain's unbloody offering was a refusal of the divine way. But Jehovah made a last appeal to Cain (Gen. 4:7) even yet to bring the required offering.

[2]**(4:17)** The first civilization, that which perished in the judgment of the Flood, was Cainitic in origin, character, and destiny. Every element of material civilization is mentioned in verses 16-22, city and pastoral life, and the development of arts and manufactures. Enoch, after whom the first city was named, means "teacher." The *el* termination of the names of Enoch's son and grandson shows that for a time the knowledge of Elohim was preserved, but this soon disappears (Rom. 1:21-23). Adah means "pleasure," or "adornment"; Zillah, to "hide"; Lamech, "conqueror," or "wild man." (Cf. Rom. 1:21-25. See Gen. 6:4.) The Cainitic civilization may have been as splendid as that of Greece or Rome, but the divine judgment is according to the *moral* state, not the *material* (Gen. 6:5-7).

[a]Seth: For God, *said she*, hath appointed me another seed instead of Abel, whom Cain slew.

26 And to Seth, to him also there was born a son; and he called his name [b]Enos: then began men to [c]call upon the name of the LORD.

CHAPTER 5.

This *is* the book of the generations of [1]Adam. In the day that God created man, [d]in the likeness of God made he him;

2 [e]Male and female created he them; and blessed them, and called their name Adam, in the day when they were created.

3 And Adam lived an hundred and thirty years, and begat *a son* in his own likeness, after his image; and called his name Seth:

4 And the days of Adam after he had begotten Seth were eight hundred years: and he begat sons and daughters:

5 And all the days that Adam lived were nine hundred and thirty years: and he [f]died.

The family of Seth.

6 And Seth lived an hundred and five years, and begat Enos:

7 And Seth lived after he begat Enos eight hundred and seven years, and begat sons and daughters:

8 And all the days of Seth were nine hundred and twelve years: and he died.

9 And Enos lived ninety years, and begat Cainan:

10 And Enos lived after he begat Cainan eight hundred and fifteen years, and begat sons and daughters:

11 And all the days of Enos were nine hundred and five years: and he died.

12 And Cainan lived seventy years, and begat Mahalaleel:

13 And Cainan lived after he begat Mahalaleel eight hundred and forty years, and begat sons and daughters:

14 And all the days of Cainan were nine hundred and ten years: and he died.

15 And Mahalaleel lived sixty and five years, and begat Jared:

16 And Mahalaleel lived after he begat Jared eight hundred and thirty years, and begat sons and daughters:

17 And all the days of Mahalaleel were eight hundred ninety and five years: and he died.

18 And Jared lived an hundred sixty and two years, and he begat Enoch:

19 And Jared lived after he begat Enoch eight hundred years, and begat sons and daughters:

20 And all the days of Jared were nine hundred sixty and two years: and he died.

21 And Enoch lived sixty and five years, and begat Methuselah:

22 And [2]Enoch [g]walked with God after he begat Methuselah three hundred years, and begat sons and daughters:

23 And all the days of Enoch were three hundred sixty and five years:

24 And Enoch walked with God: and he *was* not; for God [h]took him.

25 And Methuselah lived an hundred eighty and seven years, and begat Lamech:

26 And Methuselah lived after he begat Lamech seven hundred eighty and two years, and begat sons and daughters:

27 And all the days of Methuselah were nine hundred sixty and nine years: and he died.

28 And Lamech lived an hundred eighty and two years, and begat a son:

29 And he called his name Noah, saying, This *same* shall comfort us concerning our work and toil of our hands, because of the ground which the LORD hath cursed.

30 And Lamech lived after he begat Noah five hundred ninety and five years, and begat sons and daughters:

B.C. 4004.

a i.e. *Sheth = appointed.*

b i.e. *mortal.*

c Or, *call themselves by the name of Jehovah.* Contra, Gen. 12:8; 26:25.

d Gen. 1:27.

e Mk. 10:6.

f *Death (physical).* Gen. 6:17. (Gen. 3:19; Heb. 9:27.)

g *Faith.* vs. 22-24; Gen. 6:22. (Gen. 3:20; Heb. 11:39.)

h *Miracles* (O.T.). Gen. 7:11. (Gen. 5:24; Jon. 2:1-10.)

[1] **(5:1)** Adam, as the natural head of the race (Lk. 3:38), is a *contrasting* type of Christ, the Head of the new creation. See Rom. 5:14; 1 Cor. 15:21, 22, 45-47.

[2] **(5:22)** Enoch, "translated that he should not see death" (Heb. 11:5) before the judgment of the Flood, is a type of those saints who are to be translated before the apocalyptic judgments (1 Thes. 4:14-17). Noah, left on the earth, but preserved through the judgment of the Flood, is a type of the Jewish people, who will be kept *through* the apocalyptic judgments (Jer. 30:5-9; Rev. 12:13-16) and brought as an earthly people to the new heaven and new earth (Isa. 65:17-19; 66:20-22; Rev. 21:1).

B.C. 2353.

31 And all the days of Lamech were seven hundred seventy and seven years: and he died.

32 And Noah was five hundred years old: and Noah begat Shem, Ham, and Japheth.

CHAPTER 6.

The Flood (Gen. 6:1–8:19);
(1) *The marriage of Cainites with Sethites.*

And it came to pass, when men began to multiply on the face of the earth, and daughters were born unto them,

2 That the sons of God saw the daughters of men that they *were* fair; and they took them wives of all which they chose.

(2) *The warning of Jehovah.*

3 And the LORD said, My [a]spirit shall not always strive with man, for that he also *is* flesh: yet his days shall be an hundred and twenty years.

(3) *The antediluvian civilization* (Lk. 17:27).

4 There were giants in the earth in those days; and also after that, when the [1]sons of God came in unto the daughters of men, and they bare *children* to them, the same *became* mighty men which *were* of old, men of renown.

(4) *The purpose of Jehovah in judgment.*

5 And God saw that the wickedness of man *was* great in the earth, and *that* every [b]imagination of the thoughts of his heart *was* only evil continually.

6 And it [c]repented the LORD that he had made man on the earth, and it grieved him at his heart.

7 And the LORD said, I will destroy man whom I have created from the face of the earth; both man, and beast, and the creeping thing, and the fowls of the air; for it [c]repenteth me that I have made them.

(5) *The purpose of Jehovah in grace.*

8 But Noah found grace in the eyes of the LORD.

9 These *are* the generations of Noah: Noah was a [d]just man *and* [e]perfect in his generations, *and* Noah [2]walked with God.

10 And Noah begat three sons, Shem, Ham, and Japheth.

11 The earth also was corrupt before God, and the earth was filled with violence.

12 And God looked upon the earth, and, behold, it was corrupt; for all flesh had corrupted his way upon the earth.

13 And God said unto Noah, The end of all flesh is come before me; for the earth is filled with violence through them; and, behold, I will destroy them with the earth.

14 Make thee an [3]ark of gopher wood; rooms shalt thou make in the ark, and shalt pitch it within and without with pitch.

a *Holy Spirit.* Ex. 28:3. (Gen. 1:2; Mal. 2:15.)

b Or, *the whole imagination.* The Hebrew word signifies not only *the imagination* but also *the purposes and desires.*

c Zech. 8:14, *note.*

d *Righteousness.* Gen. 7:1. (Gen. 6:9; Lk. 2:25.)

e i.e. *upright,* or *sincere.*

[1] **(6:4)** Some hold that these "sons of God" were the "angels which kept not their first estate" (Jude 6). It is asserted that the title is in the O. T. exclusively used of angels. But this is an error (Isa. 43:6). Angels are spoken of in a sexless way. No female angels are mentioned in Scripture, and we are expressly told that marriage is unknown among angels (Mt. 22:30). The uniform Hebrew and Christian interpretation has been that verse 2 marks the breaking down of the separation between the godly line of Seth and the godless line of Cain, and so the failure of the testimony to Jehovah committed to the line of Seth (Gen. 4:26). For *apostasy* there is no remedy but judgment (Isa. 1:2-7, 24, 25; Heb. 6:4-8; 10:26-31). Noah, "a preacher of righteousness," is given 120 years, but he won no convert, and the judgment predicted by his great-grandfather fell (Jude 14, 15; Gen. 7:11).

[2] **(6:9)** Noah and Enoch are the two antediluvians of whom it is said that they "walked with God" (Gen. 5:24; 6:9). Enoch, "translated that he should not see death" (Heb. 11:5), becomes a type of the saints who will be "caught up" before the great tribulation (1 Thes. 4:14-17; Rev. 3:10; Dan. 12:1; Mt. 24:21); Noah, preserved through the Flood, is a type of the Israelitish people who will be preserved through the tribulation (Jer. 30:5-9). See "Tribulation" (Psa. 2:5; Rev. 7:14).

[3] **(6:14)** "Ark": type of Christ as the refuge of His people from judgment (Heb. 11:7). In strictness of application this speaks of the preservation through the "great tribulation" (Mt. 24:21, 22) of the remnant of Israel who will turn to the Lord after the Church (typified by Enoch, who was translated to heaven before the judgment of the Flood) has been caught up to meet the Lord (Gen. 5:22-24; 1 Thes. 4:15-17; Heb. 11:5; Isa. 2:10,11; 26:20, 21). But the type has also a present reference to the position of the

15 And this *is the fashion* which thou
shalt make it *of*: The length of the ark
shall be three hundred [a]cubits, the
breadth of it fifty cubits, and the height
of it thirty cubits.
16 A window shalt thou make to the
ark, and in a cubit shalt thou finish it
above; and the door of the ark shalt thou
set in the side thereof; *with* lower, second, and third *stories* shalt thou make it.
17 And, behold, I, even I, do bring a
flood of waters upon the earth, to
destroy all flesh, wherein *is* the breath of
life, from under heaven; *and* every thing
that *is* in the earth shall [b]die.
18 But with thee will I establish my
covenant; and thou shalt come into the
ark, thou, and thy sons, and thy wife,
and thy sons' wives with thee.
19 And of every living thing of all
flesh, [1]two of every *sort* shalt thou bring
into the ark, to keep *them* alive with thee;
they shall be male and female.
20 Of fowls after their kind, and of cattle after their kind, of every creeping
thing of the earth after his kind, two of
every *sort* shall come unto thee, to keep
them alive.
21 And take thou unto thee of all food
that is eaten, and thou shalt gather *it* to
thee; and it shall be for food for thee,
and for them.
22 Thus [c]did Noah; according to all
that God commanded him, so did he.

CHAPTER 7.

(6) *The judgment of the Flood: end of testing under the Second Dispensation.*

And the LORD said unto Noah, Come
thou and all thy house into the ark;
for thee have I seen [d]righteous before me
in this generation.
2 Of every [e]clean beast thou shalt take
to thee by sevens, the male and his
female: and of beasts that *are* not clean
by two, the male and his female.
3 Of fowls also of the air by sevens,
the male and the female; to keep seed
alive upon the face of all the earth.
4 For yet seven days, and I will cause
it to rain upon the earth forty days and
forty nights; and every living substance
that I have made will I destroy from off
the face of the earth.
5 And Noah did according unto all
that the LORD commanded him.
6 And Noah *was* six hundred years old
when the flood of waters was upon the
earth.
7 And Noah [f]went in, and his sons,
and his wife, and his sons' wives with
him, into the ark, because of the waters
of the flood.
8 Of clean beasts, and of beasts that *are*
not clean, and of fowls, and of every
thing that creepeth upon the earth,
9 There went in two and two unto
Noah into the ark, the male and the
female, as God had commanded Noah.
10 And it came to pass after seven
days, that the waters of the flood were
upon the earth.
11 In the six hundredth year of Noah's
life, in the [g]second month, the seventeenth day of the month, the [h]same day
were all the fountains of the great deep
[i]broken up, and the windows of heaven
were opened.
12 And the rain was upon the earth
forty days and forty nights.
13 In the selfsame day entered Noah,
and Shem, and Ham, and Japheth, the
sons of Noah, and Noah's wife, and the
three wives of his sons with them, into
the ark;
14 They, and every beast after his kind,
and all the cattle after their kind, and
every creeping thing that creepeth upon
the earth after his kind, and every fowl
after his kind, every bird of every sort.
15 And they went in unto Noah

B.C. 2448.

a One cubit = 18 in.; also v. 16.

b *Death (physical).* Lk. 16:22, 23. (Gen. 3:19; Heb. 9:27.)

c *Faith.* Gen. 12:1-5. (Gen. 3:20; Heb. 11:39.)

d *Righteousness.* Gen. 15:6. (Gen. 6:9; Lk. 2:25.)

e Cf. Gen. 6:19, *note.*

f See Gen. 6:9, *note* 2.

g i.e. *May.*

h Mt. 24:27, 39; Lk. 17:26, 27; 1 Thes. 5:3; 2 Pet. 2:5; 2 Pet. 3:6.

i *Miracles* (O.T.). Gen. 8:2. (Gen. 5:24; Jon. 2:1-10.)

believer "in Christ" (Eph. 1), etc. It should be noted that the word translated "pitch" in Gen. 6:14 is the same word translated "atonement" in Lev. 17:11, etc. It is atonement that keeps out the waters of judgment and makes the believer's position "in Christ" safe and blessed.

1 **(6:19)** Cf. Gen. 7:2. In addition to two animals, etc., commanded (Gen. 6:19) to be preserved for future increase ("they shall be male and female"), the further command was given more than 100 years later to take of *clean beasts,* i. e. beasts acceptable for sacrifice, seven each. Exodus gives ten such beasts, or but seventy in all. Modern ships carry hundreds of live beasts, with their food, besides scores of human beings.

into the ark, two and two of all flesh, wherein *is* the breath of life.

16 And they that went in, went in male and female of all flesh, as God had commanded him: and the LORD shut him in.

17 And the flood was forty days upon the earth; and the waters increased, and bare up the ark, and it was lift up above the earth.

18 And the waters prevailed, and were increased greatly upon the earth; and the ark went upon the face of the waters.

19 And the waters prevailed exceedingly upon the earth; and all the high hills, that *were* under the whole heaven, were covered.

20 Fifteen [a]cubits upward did the waters prevail; and the mountains were covered.

21 And all flesh died that moved upon the earth, both of fowl, and of cattle, and of beast, and of every creeping thing that creepeth upon the earth, and every man:

22 All in whose nostrils *was* the breath of life, of all that *was* in the dry *land*, died.

23 And every living substance was destroyed which was upon the face of the ground, both man, and cattle, and the creeping things, and the fowl of the heaven; and they were destroyed from the earth: and Noah only remained *alive*, and they that *were* with him in the ark.

24 And the waters prevailed upon the earth an hundred and fifty days.

CHAPTER 8.

And God remembered Noah, and every living thing, and all the cattle that *was* with him in the ark: and God made a wind to pass over the earth, and the waters aswaged;

2 The fountains also of the deep and the windows of heaven were [b]stopped, and the rain from heaven was restrained;

3 And the waters returned from off the earth continually: and after the end of the hundred and fifty days the waters were abated.

4 And the ark rested in the [c]seventh month, on the seventeenth day of the month, upon the mountains of [d]Ararat.

5 And the waters decreased continually until the [e]tenth month: in the tenth *month*, on the first *day* of the month, were the tops of the mountains seen.

6 And it came to pass at the end of forty days, that Noah opened the window of the ark which he had made:

7 And he sent forth a [f]raven, which went forth to and fro, until the waters were dried up from off the earth.

8 Also he sent forth a [f]dove from him, to see if the waters were abated from off the face of the ground;

9 But the dove found no rest for the sole of her foot, and she returned unto him into the ark, for the waters *were* on the face of the whole earth: then he put forth his hand, and took her, and pulled her in unto him into the ark.

10 And he stayed yet other seven days; and again he sent forth the dove out of the ark;

11 And the dove came in to him in the evening; and, lo, in her mouth *was* an olive leaf pluckt off: so Noah knew that the waters were abated from off the earth.

12 And he stayed yet other seven days; and sent forth the dove; which returned not again unto him any more.

13 And it came to pass in the six hundredth and first year, in the [g]first *month*, the first *day* of the month, the waters were dried up from off the earth: and Noah removed the covering of the ark, and looked, and, behold, the face of the ground was dry.

14 And in the [h]second month, on the seven and twentieth day of the month, was the earth dried.

15 And God spake unto Noah, saying,

16 Go forth of the ark, thou, and thy wife, and thy sons, and thy sons' wives with thee.

17 Bring forth with thee every living thing that *is* with thee, of all flesh, *both* of fowl, and of cattle, and of every creeping thing that creepeth upon the earth; that they may breed abundantly in the earth, and be fruitful, and multiply upon the earth.

18 And Noah went forth, and his sons, and his wife, and his sons' wives with him:

19 Every beast, every creeping thing, and every fowl, *and* whatsoever creepeth upon the earth, after their kinds, went forth out of the ark.

B.C. 2349.

a One cubit = 18 in.

b *Miracles* (O.T.). Gen. 11:7-9. (Gen. 5:24; Jon. 2:1-10.)

c i.e. *October.*

d Lit. *holy ground,* answering to the "heavenly" of Eph. 2:4-6 for the Church, and to the "new heavens and new earth" for Israel. (Isa. 65:17-19; 66:22; Rev. 21:1).

e i.e. *January.*

f The raven and the dove have been thought to stand for the believer's two natures: the "old man" satisfied with a world under judgment; the "new man" finding satisfaction only in the things of the new creation.

g i.e. *April.*

h i.e. *May.*

The Third Dispensation: Human Government (Gen. 8:20–11:9). *The Third, or Noahic Covenant* (to Gen. 9:27).

20 And Noah builded an altar unto the
LORD; and took of every clean beast, and
of every clean fowl, and offered [a]burnt-
offerings on the altar.
21 And the LORD smelled a sweet
savour; and the LORD [1b]said in his heart,
I will not again curse the ground any
more for man's sake; for the imagination
of man's heart *is* evil from his youth; neither will I again smite any more every
thing living, as I have done.
22 While the earth remaineth, seed-
time and harvest, and cold and heat, and
summer and winter, and day and night
shall not cease.

CHAPTER 9.

And God blessed Noah and his sons,
and [2]said unto them, Be fruitful,
and multiply, and replenish the earth.
2 And the fear of you and the dread of
you shall be upon every beast of the
earth, and upon every fowl of the air,
upon all that moveth *upon* the earth, and
upon all the fishes of the sea; into your
hand are they delivered.
3 Every moving thing that liveth shall
be meat for you; even as the green herb
have I given you all things.
4 But flesh with the life thereof, *which*
is the blood thereof, shall ye not eat.
5 And surely your blood of your lives
will I require; at the hand of every beast
will I require it, and at the hand of man;
at the hand of every man's brother will I
require the life of man.
6 [c]Whoso sheddeth man's blood, by
man shall his blood be shed: for in the
image of God made he man.
7 And you, be ye fruitful, and

B.C. 2348.

a Sacrifice (typical). Gen. 12:7, 8. (Gen. 4:4; Heb. 10:18.)

b The Eight Covenants. Gen. 15:18. (Gen. 1:28; Heb. 8:10.)

c Kingdom (O.T.). Ex. 3:1-10. (Gen. 1:26; Zech. 12:8.)

[1] **(8:21)** The Third Dispensation: Human Government. Under Conscience, as in Innocency, man utterly failed, and the judgment of the Flood marks the end of the second dispensation and the beginning of the third. The declaration of the Noahic Covenant subjects humanity to a new test. Its distinctive feature is the institution, for the first time, of human government—the government of man by man. The highest function of government is the judicial taking of life. All other governmental powers are implied in that. It follows that the third dispensation is distinctively that of human government. Man is responsible to govern the world for God. That responsibility rested upon the whole race, Jew and Gentile, until the failure of Israel under the Palestinian Covenant (Deut. 28–30:1-10) brought the judgment of the Captivities, when "the times of the Gentiles" (See Lk. 21:24; Rev. 16:14) began, and the government of the world passed exclusively into Gentile hands (Dan. 2:36-45; Lk. 21:24; Acts 15:14-17). That both Israel and the Gentiles have governed for self, not God, is sadly apparent. The judgment of the confusion of tongues ended the *racial* testing; that of the captivities the *Jewish;* while the *Gentile* testing will end in the smiting of the Image (Dan. 2) and the judgment of the nations (Mt. 25:31-46). See, for the other six dispensations: *Innocence* (Gen. 1:28); *Conscience* (Gen. 3:23); *Promise* (Gen. 12:1); *Law* (Ex. 19:8); *Grace* (John 1:17); *Kingdom* (Eph. 1:10).

[2] **(9:1)** The Noahic Covenant. The elements are:

(1) The relation of man to the earth under the Adamic Covenant is confirmed (Gen. 8:21).

(2) The order of nature is confirmed (Gen. 8:22).

(3) Human government is established (Gen. 9:1-6).

(4) Earth is secured against another universal judgment by water (Gen. 8:21; 9:11)

(5) A prophetic declaration is made that from Ham will descend an inferior and servile posterity (Gen. 9:24, 25).

(6) A prophetic declaration is made that Shem will have a peculiar relation to Jehovah (Gen. 9:26, 27). All divine revelation is through Semitic men, and Christ, after the flesh, descends from Shem.

(7) A prophetic declaration is made that from Japheth will descend the "enlarged" races (Gen. 9:27). Government, science, and art, speaking broadly, are and have been Japhetic, so that history is the indisputable record of the exact fulfilment of these declarations. See, for the other seven covenants: *Edenic* (Gen. 1:28); *Adamic* (Gen. 3:15); *Abrahamic* (Gen. 15:18); *Mosaic* (Ex. 19:25); *Palestinian* (Deut. 30:3); *Davidic* (2 Sam. 7:16); *New* (Heb. 8:8).

B.C. 2348.

multiply; bring forth abundantly in the earth, and multiply therein.

8 And God spake unto Noah, and to his sons with him, [a]saying,

9 And I, behold, I establish my covenant with you, and with your seed after you;

10 And with every living creature that *is* with you, of the fowl, of the cattle, and of every beast of the earth with you; from all that go out of the ark, to every beast of the earth.

11 And I will establish my covenant with you; neither shall all flesh be cut off any more by the waters of a flood; neither shall there any more be a flood to destroy the earth.

12 And God said, This *is* the token of the covenant which I make between me and you and every living creature that *is* with you, for perpetual generations:

13 I do set my [b]bow in the cloud, and it shall be for a token of a covenant between me and the earth.

14 And it shall come to pass, when I bring a cloud over the earth, that the bow shall be seen in the cloud:

15 And I will remember my covenant, which *is* between me and you and every living creature of all flesh; and the waters shall no more become a flood to destroy all flesh.

16 And the bow shall be in the cloud; and I will look upon it, that I may remember the everlasting covenant between God and every living creature of all flesh that *is* upon the earth.

17 And God said unto Noah, This *is* the token of the covenant, which I have established between me and all flesh that *is* upon the earth.

18 And the sons of Noah, that went forth of the ark, were Shem, and Ham, and Japheth: and Ham *is* the father of Canaan.

19 These *are* the three sons of Noah: and of them was the whole earth overspread.

Parenthetical: the shame of Noah and the sin of Ham.

20 And Noah began *to be* an husbandman, and he planted a vineyard:

21 And he drank of the wine, and was drunken; and he was uncovered within his tent.

22 And Ham, the father of Canaan, saw the nakedness of his father, and told his two brethren without.

23 And Shem and Japheth took a garment, and laid *it* upon both their shoulders, and went backward, and covered the nakedness of their father; and their faces *were* backward, and they saw not their father's nakedness.

Conclusion of Noahic Covenant: the prophetic declaration.

24 And Noah awoke from his wine, and knew what his younger son had done unto him.

25 And he said, [c]Cursed *be* Canaan; a servant of servants shall he be unto his brethren.

26 And he said, Blessed *be* the LORD God of Shem; and Canaan shall be his servant.

27 God shall enlarge Japheth, and he shall dwell in the tents of Shem; and Canaan shall be his servant.

The family of Noah (Gen. 9:28–10:32).

28 And Noah lived after the flood three hundred and fifty years.

29 And all the days of Noah were nine hundred and fifty years: and he died.

CHAPTER 10.

Now these *are* the generations of the sons of Noah, Shem, Ham, and Japheth: and unto them were sons born after the flood.

2 The sons of Japheth; [1]Gomer, and [2]Magog, and [3]Madai, and [4]Javan, and [5]Tubal, and [6]Meshech, and [7]Tiras.

a See Gen. 8:21, *note;* 9:1, *note.*

b The bow is not said to have come into existence at this time, but only to have been here invested with the character of a *sign.* Cf. Ex. 31:13. Typically, the bow seen upon the storm clouds of judgment (Gen. 7:11), has been thought to speak of the cross where judgment, never to be repeated, has been visited upon the believer's sins (Gal. 3:10-14; Heb. 10:14-18).

c See Gen. 9:1. *note* 2, *subdiv.* 5-7.

[1] **(10:2)** Progenitor of the ancient Cimerians and Cimbri, from whom are descended the Celtic family.

[2] **(10:2)** From Magog are descended the ancient Scythians, or Tartars, whose descendants predominate in the modern Russia. See Ezk. 38:2; 39:6; Rev. 20:8.

[3] **(10:2)** Progenitor of the ancient Medes.

[4] **(10:2)** Progenitor of those who peopled Greece, Syria, etc.

[5] **(10:2)** Tubal's descendants peopled the region south of the Black Sea, from whence they spread north and south. It is probable that Tobolsk perpetuates the tribal name. A branch of this race peopled Spain.

[6] **(10:2)** Progenitor of a race mentioned in connection with Tubal, Magog, and other northern nations. Broadly speaking, Russia, excluding the conquests of Peter the Great and his successors, is the modern land of Magog, Tubal, and Meshech.

[7] **(10:2)** Progenitor of the Thracians.

3 And the sons of Gomer; Ashkenaz, and Riphath, and Togarmah.

4 And the sons of Javan; Elishah, and Tarshish, Kittim, and Dodanim.

5 By these were the [a]isles of the Gentiles divided in their lands; every one after his tongue, after their families, in their nations.

6 And the sons of Ham; Cush, and Mizraim, and Phut, and Canaan.

7 And the sons of Cush; Seba, and Havilah, and Sabtah, and Raamah, and Sabtecha: and the sons of Raamah; Sheba, and Dedan.

8 And Cush begat Nimrod: he began to be a mighty one in the earth.

9 He was a mighty hunter before the LORD: wherefore it is said, Even as Nimrod the mighty hunter before the LORD.

10 And the beginning of his kingdom was Babel, and Erech, and Accad, and Calneh, in the land of Shinar.

11 Out of that land [b]went forth Asshur, and builded [c]Nineveh, and the city Rehoboth, and Calah,

12 And Resen between [d]Nineveh and Calah: the same *is* a great city.

13 And Mizraim begat Ludim, and Anamim, and Lehabim, and Naphtuhim,

14 And Pathrusim, and Casluhim, (out of whom came Philistim,) and Caphtorim.

15 And Canaan begat Sidon his firstborn, and Heth,

16 And the Jebusite, and the Amorite, and the Girgasite,

17 And the Hivite, and the Arkite, and the Sinite,

18 And the Arvadite, and the Zemarite, and the Hamathite: and afterward were the families of the Canaanites spread abroad.

19 And the border of the Canaanites was from Sidon, as thou comest to Gerar, unto Gaza; as thou goest, unto Sodom, and Gomorrah, and Admah, and Zeboim, even unto Lasha.

B.C. 2347.

a Lit. *coasts.* Settlements would naturally follow the coasts first.

b Or, *he went out into Assyria.*

c Nah. 1:1, *note.*

d Isa. 13:1, *note.*

e *Arphaxad.* v. 24; Gen. 11:10; Lk. 3:36.

20 These *are* the sons of Ham, after their families, after their tongues, in their countries, *and* in their nations.

21 Unto Shem also, the father of all the children of Eber, the brother of Japheth the elder, even to him were *children* born.

22 The children of Shem; Elam, and Asshur, and [e]Arphaxad, and Lud, and Aram.

23 And the children of Aram; Uz, and Hul, and Gether, and Mash.

24 And Arphaxad begat Salah; and Salah begat Eber.

25 And unto Eber were born two sons: the name of one *was* Peleg; for in his days was the earth divided; and his brother's name *was* Joktan.

26 And Joktan begat Almodad, and Sheleph, and Hazarmaveth, and Jerah,

27 And Hadoram, and Uzal, and Diklah,

28 And Obal, and Abimael, and Sheba,

29 And Ophir, and Havilah, and Jobab: all these *were* the sons of Joktan.

30 And their dwelling was from Mesha, as thou goest unto Sephar a mount of the east.

31 These *are* the sons of Shem, after their families, after their tongues, in their lands, after their nations.

32 These *are* the families of the sons of Noah, after their generations, in their nations: and by these were the nations divided in the earth after the flood.

CHAPTER 11.

The failure of man under the Noahic Covenant.

And the whole earth was of [1]one language, and of one speech.

2 And it came to pass, as they journeyed from the east, that they found a plain in the land of Shinar; and they dwelt there.

3 And they said one to another, Go to,

From these seven sons of Japheth are descended the *goyim,* or Gentile, nations, trans. "heathen" 148 times in the A. V. The name implies nothing concerning religion, meaning simply, non-Israelite, or "foreigner."

[1]**(11:1)** The history of Babel ("confusion") strikingly parallels that of the professing Church. (1) Unity (Gen. 11:1)—the Apostolic Church (Acts 4:32, 33); (2) Ambition (Gen. 11:4), using worldly, not spiritual, means (Gen. 11:3), ending in a man-made unity—the papacy; (3) the confusion of tongues (Gen. 11:7)—Protestantism, with its innumerable sects. See Isa. 13:1, *note.*

let us make brick, and burn them throughly. And they had brick for stone, and slime had they for morter.

4 And they said, Go to, let us build us a city and a tower, whose top *may reach* unto heaven; and let us make us a name, lest we be scattered abroad upon the face of the whole earth.

The judgment of the confusion of tongues. Life continues under the Adamic and Noahic Covenants.

5 And the LORD came down to see the city and the tower, which the children of men builded.

6 And the LORD said, Behold, the people *is* one, and they have all one language; and this they begin to do: and now nothing will be restrained from them, which they have imagined to do.

7 Go to, let us go down, and there [a]confound their language, that they may not understand one another's speech.

8 So the LORD scattered them abroad from thence upon the face of all the earth: and they left off to build the city.

9 Therefore is the name of it called [b]Babel; because the LORD did there confound the language of all the earth: and from thence did the LORD scatter them abroad upon the face of all the earth.

The ancestry of Abram.

10 These *are* the [1]generations of Shem: Shem *was* an hundred years old, and begat [c]Arphaxad two years after the flood:

11 And Shem lived after he begat Arphaxad five hundred years, and begat sons and daughters.

12 And Arphaxad lived five and thirty years, and begat Salah:

13 And Arphaxad lived after he begat Salah four hundred and three years, and begat sons and daughters.

14 And Salah lived thirty years, and begat Eber:

15 And Salah lived after he begat Eber four hundred and three years, and begat sons and daughters.

16 And Eber lived four and thirty years, and begat Peleg:

17 And Eber lived after he begat Peleg four hundred and thirty years, and begat sons and daughters.

18 And Peleg lived thirty years, and begat Reu:

19 And Peleg lived after he begat Reu two hundred and nine years, and begat sons and daughters.

20 And Reu lived two and thirty years, and begat Serug:

21 And Reu lived after he begat Serug two hundred and seven years, and begat sons and daughters.

22 And Serug lived thirty years, and begat Nahor:

B.C. 2247.

a *Miracles* (O.T.). vs. 7-9; Gen. 12:17. (Gen. 5:24; Jon. 2:1-10.)

b i.e. *confusion.* See Gen. 11:1, note; Isa. 13:1, *note.*

c *Arphaxad.* vs. 10-13; 1 Chr. 1:17. (Gen. 10:22; Lk. 3:36.)

[1] **(11:10)** Genesis 11 and 12 mark an important turning point in the divine dealing. Heretofore the history has been that of the whole Adamic race. There has been neither Jew nor Gentile; all have been one in "the first man Adam." Henceforth, in the Scripture record, humanity must be thought of as a vast stream from which God, in the call of Abram and the creation of the nation of Israel, has but drawn off a slender rill, through which He may at last purify the great river itself. Israel was called to be a witness to the unity of God in the midst of universal idolatry (Deut. 6:4; Isa. 43:10-12); to illustrate the blessedness of serving the true God (Deut. 33:26-29); to receive and preserve the divine revelations (Rom. 3:1, 2; Deut. 4:5-8); and to produce the Messiah (Gen. 3:15; 21:12; 28:10, 14; 49:10; 2 Sam. 7:16, 17; Isa. 4:3, 4; Mt. 1:1.)

The reader of scripture should hold firmly in mind: (1) that from Gen. 12 to Mt. 12:45 the Scriptures have primarily in view Israel, the little rill, not the great Gentile river; though again and again the universality of the ultimate divine intent breaks into view (e. g. Gen. 12:3; Isa. 2:2, 4; 5:26; 9:1, 2; 11:10-12; 42:1-6; 49:6, 12; 52:15; 54:3; 55:5; 60:3, 5,11-16; 61:6, 9; 62:2; 66:12,18, 19; Jer. 16:19; Joel 3:9, 10; Mal. 1:11; Rom. 9, 10, 11; Gal. 3:8-14); (2) that the human race, henceforth called Gentile in distinction from Israel, goes on under the Adamic and Noahic covenants; and that for the race (outside Israel) the dispensations of Conscience and of Human Government continue. The moral history of the great Gentile world is told in Rom. 1:21-32, and its moral accountability in Rom. 2:1-16. Conscience never acquits: it either "accuses" or "excuses." Where the law is known to the Gentiles it is to them, as to Israel, "a ministration of death," a "curse" (Rom. 3:19, 20; 7:9, 10; 2 Cor. 3:7; Gal. 3:10). A wholly new responsibility arises when either Jew or Gentile knows the Gospel (John 3:18, 19, 36; 15:22-24; 16:9; 1 John 5:9-12).

23 And Serug lived after he begat Nahor two hundred years, and begat sons and daughters.

24 And Nahor lived nine and twenty years, and begat Terah:

25 And Nahor lived after he begat Terah an hundred and nineteen years, and begat sons and daughters.

26 And Terah lived seventy years, and begat Abram, Nahor, and Haran.

27 Now these *are* the generations of Terah: Terah begat Abram, Nahor, and Haran; and Haran begat Lot.

28 And Haran died before his father Terah in the land of his nativity, in Ur of the Chaldees.

29 And Abram and Nahor took them wives: the name of Abram's wife *was* Sarai; and the name of Nahor's wife, Milcah, the daughter of Haran, the father of Milcah, and the father of Iscah.

30 But Sarai was barren; she *had* no child.

Incomplete obedience: the wasted years at Haran.

31 And [a]Terah took Abram his son, and Lot the son of Haran his son's son, and Sarai his daughter in law, his son Abram's wife; and they went forth with them from Ur of the Chaldees, to go into the land of Canaan; and they came unto Haran, and dwelt there.

32 And the days of Terah were two hundred and five years: and Terah died in Haran.

CHAPTER 12.

The Fourth Dispensation: Promise: from the call of Abram to the giving of the law (Gen. 12:1–Ex. 19:8).
The Fourth, or Abrahamic Covenant.
(Add Gen. 13:14–18; 15:1–21; 17:4–8; 22:15–24; 26:1–5; 28:10–15.)

NOW [1]the LORD had said unto Abram, Get thee [b]out of thy country, and from thy kindred, and from thy father's house, unto a land that I will shew thee:

2 [2]And I will make of thee a great [c]nation, and I will bless thee, and make thy name great; and thou shalt be a blessing:

3 And I will bless them that bless thee, and curse him that curseth thee: and in [d]thee shall all families of the earth be [e]blessed.

Abram in the land: worship, communion, and promise.

4 So Abram departed, as the LORD had spoken unto him; and Lot went with him: and Abram *was* seventy and five years old when he departed out of Haran.

5 And Abram took Sarai his wife, and Lot his brother's son, and all their substance that they had gathered, and the souls that they had gotten in Haran; and they [f]went forth to go into the land of Canaan; and into the land of Canaan they came.

6 And Abram passed through the land unto the place of Sichem, unto the plain of Moreh. And the Canaanite *was* then in the land.

7 And the LORD [g]appeared unto Abram, and said, Unto thy seed will I

B.C. 2126.

a The name means *delay.*

b *Separation.* vs. 1-5; Gen. 13:7-11. (Gen. 12:1; 2 Cor. 6:14-17.)

c *Israel (origin)* vs. 2, 3; Gen. 13:15-17. (Gen. 12:2, 3; Rom. 11:26.)

d *Christ (first advent).* Gen. 17:19. (Gen. 3:15; Acts. 1:9.)

e *Gospel.* v. 3; Isa. 41:27. (Gen. 12:1-3; Rev. 14:6.)

f *Faith.* vs. 1-5; Gen. 13:14-18. (Gen. 3:20; Heb. 11:39.)

g *The theophanies.* Gen. 17:1. (Gen. 12:7; Rev. 1:10.)

[1]**(12:1)** The Fourth Dispensation: Promise. For Abraham and his descendants it is evident that the Abrahamic Covenant (Gen. 15:18, *note*) made a great change. They became distinctively the heirs of *promise.* That covenant is wholly gracious and unconditional. The descendants of Abraham had but to abide in their own land to inherit every blessing. In Egypt they lost their *blessings,* but not their *covenant.* The Dispensation of Promise ended when Israel rashly accepted the law (Ex. 19:8). Grace had prepared a deliverer (Moses), provided a sacrifice for the guilty, and by divine power brought them out of bondage (Ex. 19:4); but at Sinai they exchanged grace for law. The Dispensation of Promise extends from Gen. 12:1 to Ex. 19:8, and was exclusively Israelitish. The *dispensation* must be distinguished from the *covenant.* The former is a mode of testing; the latter is everlasting because unconditional. The law did not abrogate the Abrahamic Covenant (Gal. 3:15-18), but was an intermediate disciplinary dealing "till the Seed should come to whom the promise was made" (Gal. 3:19-29; 4:1-7). Only the *dispensation,* as a testing of Israel, ended at the giving of the law. See, for the other six dispensations: *Innocence* (Gen. 1:28); *Conscience* (Gen. 3:23); *Human Government* (Gen. 8:20); *Law* (Ex. 19:8); *Grace* (John 1:17); *Kingdom* (Eph. 1:10)

[2]**(12:2)** For analysis and summary of the Abrahamic Covenant, see Gen. 15:18.

give this land: and there builded he an [a]altar unto the LORD, who appeared unto him.

8 And he removed from thence unto a mountain on the east of Beth-el, and pitched his tent, *having* [1]Beth-el on the west, and Hai on the east: and there he builded an altar unto the LORD, and called upon the name of the LORD.

9 And Abram journeyed, going on still toward the south.

Under trial Abram forsakes the place of blessing.

10 And there was a [b]famine in the land: [2]and Abram went down into Egypt to sojourn there; for the famine *was* grievous in the land.

11 And it came to pass, when he was come near to enter into Egypt, that he [c]said unto Sarai his wife, Behold now, I know that thou *art* a fair woman to look upon:

12 Therefore it shall come to pass, when the Egyptians shall see thee, that they shall say, This *is* his wife: and they will kill me, but they will save thee alive.

13 Say, I pray thee, thou *art* my sister: that it may be well with me for thy sake; and my soul shall live because of thee.

14 And it came to pass, that, when Abram was come into Egypt, the Egyptians beheld the woman that she *was* very fair.

15 The princes also of Pharaoh saw her, and commended her before Pharaoh: and the woman was taken into Pharaoh's house.

16 And he entreated Abram well for her sake: and he had sheep, and oxen, and he asses, and menservants, and maidservants, and she asses, and camels.

17 And the LORD [d]plagued Pharaoh and his house with great plagues because of Sarai Abram's wife.

B.C. 1920.

a *Sacrifice, (typical).* vs. 7, 8; Gen. 13:18. (Gen. 4:4; Heb. 10:18.)

b Cf. Gen. 26:1-5; Ruth 1:1; *contra.* Psa. 33:18, 19.

c Cf. Gen. 20:1-18; 26:6-11.

d *Miracles* (O.T.). Gen. 15:17. (Gen. 5:24; Jon. 2:1-10.)

18 And Pharaoh called Abram, and said, What *is* this *that* thou hast done unto me? why didst thou not tell me that she *was* thy wife?

19 Why saidst thou, She *is* my sister? so I might have taken her to me to wife: now therefore behold thy wife, take *her*, and go thy way.

20 And Pharaoh commanded *his* men concerning him: and they sent him away, and his wife, and all that he had.

CHAPTER 13.

Abram returns to the land and the altar.

And Abram went up out of Egypt, he, and his wife, and all that he had, and Lot with him, into the south.

2 And Abram *was* very rich in cattle, in silver, and in gold.

3 And he went on his journeys from the south even to Beth-el, unto the place where his tent had been at the beginning, between Beth-el and Hai;

4 Unto the place of the altar, which he had made there at the first: and there Abram called on the name of the LORD.

Abram's separation from Lot.

5 And Lot also, which went with Abram, had flocks, and herds, and tents.

6 And the land was not able to bear them, that they might dwell together: for their substance was great, so that they could not dwell together.

7 And there was a strife between the herdmen of Abram's cattle and the herdmen of Lot's cattle: and the Canaanite and the Perizzite dwelled then in the land.

8 And Abram said unto Lot, Let there be no strife, I pray thee, between me and thee, and between my herdmen and thy herdmen; for we *be* brethren.

9 *Is* not the whole land before thee?

[1]**(12:8)** One of the sacred places of Canaan, meaning, *house of God* (Gen. 28:1-22; 35:1-7, *note.* It is characteristic of all apostasy that Jeroboam chose this sacred place in which to erect an idol (1 Ki. 12:28, 32. Cf. 1 Ki. 13:1-5); and of divine judgment upon apostasy that God should decree the destruction of Bethel, despite its sacred memories (1 Ki. 13:1-5; 2 Ki. 23:15-17; Amos 3:14, 15). God never hesitates to cast aside that which no longer serves His purpose (Rev. 2:5; 3:16).

[2]**(12:10)** A famine was often a disciplinary testing of God's people in the land. (Cf. Gen. 26:1; 42:5; Ruth 1:1; 2 Sam. 24:13; Psa. 105:16.) The resort to Egypt (the world) is typical of the tendency to substitute for lost spiritual power the fleshly resources of the world, instead of seeking, through confession and amendment, the restoration of God's presence and favour.

[a]separate thyself, I pray thee, from me: if *thou wilt take* the left hand, then I will go to the right; or if *thou depart* to the right hand, then I will go to the left.

Lot's first step in backsliding.
(Gen. 13:12; 19:1, 33.)

10 And Lot lifted up his eyes, and beheld all the plain of Jordan, that it *was* well watered every where, before the LORD destroyed Sodom and Gomorrah, *even* as the garden of the LORD, like the land of Egypt, as thou comest unto Zoar.

11 Then Lot chose him all the plain of Jordan; and Lot journeyed east: and they separated themselves the one from the other.

Lot's second step in backsliding.
(See Gen. 13:10; 19:1, 33.)

12 Abram dwelled in the land of Canaan, and Lot dwelled in the cities of the plain, and pitched *his* tent toward Sodom.

13 But the men of Sodom *were* wicked and sinners before the LORD exceedingly.

The Abrahamic Covenant: the land given; natural posterity promised (v. 16).

14 And the LORD said unto Abram, after that Lot was separated from him, Lift up now thine eyes, and look from the place where thou art northward, and southward, and eastward, and westward:

15 For all the land which thou seest, to thee will I give it, and to thy [b]seed for ever.

16 And I will make thy seed as the dust of the earth: so that if a man can number the dust of the earth, *then* shall thy seed also be numbered.

17 Arise, walk through the land in the length of it and in the breadth of it; for I will give it unto thee.

18 [c]Then Abram removed *his* tent, and came and dwelt in the plain of Mamre, which *is* in Hebron, and built there an [d]altar unto the LORD.

CHAPTER 14.

Abram delivers Lot.

And it came to pass in the days of Amraphel king of Shinar, Arioch king of Ellasar, Chedorlaomer king of Elam, and Tidal king of nations;

2 *That these* made war with Bera king of Sodom, and with Birsha king of Gomorrah, Shinab king of Admah, and

B.C. 1918.

a *Separation*, vs. 7, 11, 14-17; Ex. 6:6, 7. (Gen. 12:1, 2; 2 Cor. 6:14-17.)

b *Israel (covenant)*, vs. 15-17; Gen. 15:4, 5. (Gen. 12:2, 3; Rom. 11:26.)

c *Faith*, vs. 14-18; Gen. 14:22, 23. (Gen. 3:20; Heb. 11:39.)

d *Sacrifice, (typical)*. Gen. 22:8, 13. (Gen. 4:4; Heb. 10:18.)

e It is Abram the separated man who has power to help. See Gen. 19:29; 2 Tim. 2:20-21.

Shemeber king of Zeboiim, and the king of Bela, which is Zoar.

3 All these were joined together in the vale of Siddim, which is the salt sea.

4 Twelve years they served Chedorlaomer, and in the thirteenth year they rebelled.

5 And in the fourteenth year came Chedorlaomer, and the kings that *were* with him, and smote the Rephaims in Ashteroth Karnaim, and the Zuzims in Ham, and the Emims in Shaveh Kiriathaim,

6 And the Horites in their mount Seir, unto El-paran, which *is* by the wilderness.

7 And they returned, and came to En-mishpat, which *is* Kadesh, and smote all the country of the Amalekites, and also the Amorites, that dwelt in Hazezon-tamar.

8 And there went out the king of Sodom, and the king of Gomorrah, and the king of Admah, and the king of Zeboiim, and the king of Bela (the same *is* Zoar;) and they joined battle with them in the vale of Siddim;

9 With Chedorlaomer the king of Elam, and with Tidal king of nations, and Amraphel king of Shinar, and Arioch king of Ellasar; four kings with five.

10 And the vale of Siddim *was full of* slimepits; and the kings of Sodom and Gomorrah fled, and fell there; and they that remained fled to the mountain.

11 And they took all the goods of Sodom and Gomorrah, and all their victuals, and went their way.

12 And they took Lot, Abram's brother's son, who dwelt in Sodom, and his goods, and departed.

13 And there came one that had escaped, and told Abram the Hebrew; for he dwelt in the plain of Mamre the Amorite, brother of Eshcol, and brother of Aner: and these *were* confederate with Abram.

14 And [e]when Abram heard that his brother was taken captive, he armed his trained *servants*, born in his own house, three hundred and eighteen, and pursued *them* unto Dan.

15 And he divided himself against them, he and his servants, by night, and smote them, and pursued them unto Hobah, which *is* on the left hand of Damascus.

16 And he brought back all the

goods, and also brought again his brother Lot, and his goods, and the women
also, and the people.

The revelation of God as El Elyon,
"the most high God, possessor of
heaven and earth."

17 And the king of Sodom went out to
meet him after his return from the
slaughter of Chedorlaomer, and of the
kings that *were* with him, at the valley of
Shaveh, which *is* the king's dale.
18 And [1a]Melchizedek king of [b]Salem
brought forth bread and wine: and he
was the priest of the [c]most high [2]God.
19 And he blessed him, and said,
Blessed *be* Abram of the most high God,
possessor of heaven and earth:
20 And blessed be the most high God,
which hath delivered thine enemies into
thy hand. And he gave him tithes of all.
21 And the king of Sodom said unto
Abram, Give me the persons, and take
the goods to thyself.
22 And Abram [d]said to the king of
Sodom, I have lift up mine hand unto
the LORD, the most high God, the possessor of heaven and earth,
23 That I will not *take* from a thread
even to a shoelatchet, and that I will not
take any thing that *is* thine, lest thou
shouldest say, I have made Abram rich:
24 Save only that which the young
men have eaten, and the portion of the
men which went with me, Aner, Eshcol,
and Mamre; let them take their portion.

CHAPTER 15.

The Abrahamic Covenant confirmed:
a spiritual seed promised (v. 5).

After these things the word of the
LORD came unto Abram in a vision,
saying, Fear not, Abram: I *am* thy shield,
and thy exceeding great reward.

B.C. 1913.

a Meaning King of Righteousness. Cf. Heb. 7:2.

b Meaning Peace. Cf. Heb. 7:2

c *Deity (names of).* Gen. 15:2. (Gen. 1:1; Mal. 3:18.)

d *Faith,* vs. 22, 23; Gen. 15:6. (Gen. 3:20; Heb. 11:39.)

[1] **(14:18)** Melchizedek, type of Christ the King-Priest. The type strictly applies to the priestly work of Christ in *resurrection,* since Melchizedek presents only the *memorials* of sacrifice, bread and wine. "After the order of Melchizedek" (Heb. 6:20) refers to the royal *authority* and unending *duration* of Christ's high priesthood (Heb. 7:23, 24). The Aaronic priesthood was often interrupted by death. Christ is a priest after the *order* of Melchizedek, as King of righteousness King of peace (Isa. 11:4-9; Heb. 7:2), and in the *endlessness* of His priesthood, but the Aaronic priesthood typifies His priestly *work.*

[2] **(14:18)** "Most high," or "most high God" (Heb. *El Elyon*). "*Elyon*" means simply "highest."

(1) The first revelation of this name (v. 18) indicates its distinctive meanings. Abram, returning from his victory over the confederated kings (Gen. 14:1-17), is met by Melchizedek, King of Salem . . . the "priest of the most high God" (*El Elyon*), who blesses Abram in the name of *El Elyon,* "possessor of heaven and earth." This revelation produced a remarkable impression upon the patriarch. Not only did he at once give Melchizedek "tithes of all" the spoil of the battle, but when the King of Sodom offered other of that spoil to Abram, his answer was: "I have lift up mine hand unto the LORD [Jehovah], the most high God [*El Elyon*], the possessor of heaven and earth, that I will not take from a thread even to a shoelatchet," etc. (Gen. 14:18-23).

(a) The LORD (Jehovah) is known to a *Gentile* king (Melchizedek) by the name "most high God" (*El Elyon*); *(b)* a *Gentile* is the priest of *El Elyon* and *(c)* His distinctive character as most high God is "possessor of heaven and earth."

Appropriately to this Gentile knowledge of God by His name "Most High," we read that "the Most High divided to the nations [i.e. Gentiles] their inheritance, when he separated the sons of Adam," etc. (Deut. 32:8). As "*possessor* of heaven and earth," it was the prerogative of the Most High to distribute the earth among the nations according to whatever principle He chose. That principle is declared in Deut. 32:8. To the same purport is the use of the name in Daniel, the book of Gentile prophecy (Dan. 3:26; 4:17, 24, 25, 32, 34, 35; 5:18, 21).

(2) As "Possessor of heaven and earth," the most high God has and exercises authority in both spheres: *(a)* as the heavenly authority of *El Elyon* (e.g. Dan. 4:35, 37; Isa. 14:13, 14; Mt. 28:18); *(b)* the earthly authority of *El Elyon* (e.g. Deut. 32:8; Psa. 9:2-5; 21:7; 47:2-4; 56:2, 3; 82:6, 8; 83:16-18; 91:9-12; 2 Sam. 22:14, 15; Dan. 5:18). See, for other names of Deity: Gen. 1:1, *note;* 2:4, *note;* 2:7; 15:2, *note;* 17:1, *note;* 21:33, *note;* 1 Sam. 1:3, *note.*

2 [a]And Abram said, [1b]Lord [2]God, what wilt thou give me, seeing I go childless, and the steward of my house *is* this Eliezer of Damascus?

3 And Abram said, Behold, to me thou hast given no seed: and, lo, one born in my house is mine heir.

4 And, behold, the word of the LORD *came* unto him, saying, This shall not be thine heir; but he that shall come forth out of thine own bowels shall be thine heir.

5 And he brought him forth abroad, and said, Look now toward heaven, and tell the stars, if thou be able to number them: and he said unto him, [c]So shall thy [d]seed be.

6 And he [e]believed in the LORD; and he [f]counted it to him for [g]righteousness.

7 And he said unto him, I *am* the LORD that brought thee out of Ur of the Chaldees, to give thee this land to inherit it.

8 And he said, Lord God, whereby shall I know that I shall inherit it?

9 And he said unto him, Take me an heifer of three years old, and a she goat of three years old, and a ram of three years old, and a turtledove, and a young pigeon.

10 And he took unto him all these, and divided them in the midst, and laid each piece one against another: but the birds divided he not.

11 And when the fowls came down upon the carcases, Abram drove them away.

12 And when the sun was going down, a deep sleep fell upon Abram; and, lo, an horror of great darkness fell upon him.

13 And he said unto Abram, Know of a surety that thy seed shall be a stranger in a land *that is* not theirs, and shall serve them; and they shall afflict them four hundred years;

14 And also that nation, whom they shall serve, will I judge: and afterward shall they come out with great substance.

15 And thou shalt go to thy fathers in peace; thou shalt be buried in a good old age.

16 But in the fourth generation they shall come hither again: for the iniquity of the Amorites *is* not yet full.

17 And it came to pass, that, when the sun went down, and it was dark, behold a smoking furnace, and a burning lamp that [h]passed between those pieces.

18 In the same day the LORD made a [i]covenant with Abram, [3]saying, Unto

B.C. 1913.

a *Bible prayers* (O.T.). Gen. 17:17, 18. (Gen. 15:2; Hab. 3:1-16.)

b *Deity (names of).* Gen. 17:1. (Gen. 1:1; Mal. 3:18.)

c Rom. 4:18; cf. Heb. 11:12.

d *Israel (covenant).* vs. 4, 5; Gen. 17:15-19. (Gen. 12:2, 3; Rom. 11:26.)

e *Faith,* Gen. 21:1-6. (Gen. 3:20; Heb. 11:39.)

f Rom. 4:3; Gal. 3:6; Jas. 2:23.

g *Righteousness.* Prov. 21:15, 21. (Gen. 6:9; Lk. 2:25.)

h *Miracles* (O.T.). Gen. 19:24, 25, 26. (Gen. 5:24; Jon. 2:1-10.)

i *The Eight Covenants.* Ex. 19:25. (Gen. 1:28; Heb. 8:10.)

[1]**(15:2)** "Lord" (Heb. *Adon, Adonai*).

(1) The primary meaning of *Adon, Adonai,* is Master, and it is applied in the Old Testament Scriptures both to Deity and to man. The latter instances are distinguished in the English version by the omission of the capital. As applied to man, the word is used of two relationships: *master* and *husband* (Gen. 24:9, 10, 12, "master," may illustrate the former; Gen. 18:12, "lord," the latter). Both these relationships exist between Christ and the believer (John 13:13, "master"; 2 Cor. 11:2, 3, "husband").

(2) Two principles inhere in the relation of master and servant: *(a)* the Master's right to implicit obedience (John 13:13; Mt. 23:10; Lk. 6:46); *(b)* the servant's right to direction in service (Isa. 6:8-11). Clear distinction in the use of the divine names is illustrated in Ex. 4:10-12. Moses feels his weakness and incompetency, and "Moses said unto the LORD [Jehovah], O my Lord [*Adonai*], I am not eloquent," etc. Since *service* is in question, Moses (appropriately) addresses Jehovah as Lord. But now *power* is in question, and it is not the Lord *(Adonai)* but Jehovah (LORD) who answers (referring to creation power)—"and Jehovah said unto him, Who hath made man's mouth? . . . Now therefore go, and I will be with thy mouth." The same distinction appears in Josh. 7:8-11. See, for other names of Deity: Gen. 1:1, *note;* 2:4, *note;* 2:7; 14:18, *note;* 15:2, *note;* 17:1, *note;* 21:33, *note;* 1 Sam. 1:3, *note.*

[2]**(15:2)** "Lord GOD" (Heb. *Adonai Jehovah*). When used distinctively, this compound name, while gathering into one the special meanings of each (Gen. 2:4, *note;* 15:2, *note*) will be found to emphasize the *Adonai* rather than the *Jehovah* character of Deity. (The following passages may suffice to illustrate this: Gen. 15:2, 8; Deut. 3:24; 9:26; Josh. 7:7; Jud. 6:22; 16:28; 2 Sam. 7:18-20, 28, 29; 1 Ki. 2:26; Psa. 69:6; 71:5; Isa. 7:7). See, for other names of Deity: Gen. 1:1, *note;* 2:4, *note;* 2:7; 14:18, *note;* 15:2, *note;* 17:1, *note;* 21:33, *note;* 1 Sam. 1:3.

[3]**(15:18)** The Abrahamic Covenant as formed (Gen. 12:1-4) and confirmed (Gen. 13:14-17; 15:1-7; 17:1-8) is in seven distinct parts:

thy seed have I given this land, from the
river of Egypt unto the great river, the
river Euphrates:
19 The Kenites, and the Kenizzites,
and the Kadmonites,
20 And the Hittites, and the Perizzites,
and the Rephaims,
21 And the Amorites, and the
Canaanites, and the Girgashites, and the
Jebusites.

CHAPTER 16.

The birth of Ishmael.

Now Sarai Abram's wife bare him no
children: and she had an handmaid, an Egyptian, whose name *was*
Hagar.
2 And Sarai said unto Abram, Behold
now, the LORD hath restrained me from
bearing: I pray thee, go in unto my maid;
it may be that I may obtain children by
her. And Abram hearkened to the voice
of Sarai.
3 And Sarai Abram's wife took [1]Hagar
her maid the Egyptian, after Abram had
dwelt ten years in the land of Canaan,
and gave her to her husband Abram to
be his wife.
4 And he went in unto Hagar, and she
conceived: and when she saw that she
had conceived, her mistress was
despised in her eyes.
5 And Sarai said unto Abram, My
wrong *be* upon thee: I have given my
maid into thy bosom; and when she saw
that she had conceived, I was despised
in her eyes: the LORD judge between me
and thee.
6 But Abram said unto Sarai, Behold,
thy maid *is* in thy hand; do to her as it
pleaseth thee. And when Sarai dealt
hardly with her, she fled from her face.
7 And the [a]angel of the LORD found
her by a fountain of water in the wilderness, by the fountain in the way to Shur.
8 And he said, Hagar, Sarai's maid,
whence camest thou? and whither wilt
thou go? And she said, I flee from the
face of my mistress Sarai.
9 And the [a]angel of the LORD said unto
her, Return to thy mistress, and submit
thyself under her hands.
10 And the [a]angel of the LORD said
unto her, I will multiply thy seed
exceedingly, that it shall not be numbered for multitude.
11 And the [a]angel of the LORD said
unto her, Behold, thou *art* with child,
and shalt bear a son, and shalt call his
name [b]Ishmael; because the LORD hath
heard thy affliction.

B.C. 1913.

a Heb. 1:4, *note.*

b i.e. *God shall hear.*

(1) "I will make of thee a great nation." Fulfilled in a threefold way: *(a)* In a natural posterity—"as the dust of the *earth*" (Gen. 13:16; John 8:37), viz. the Hebrew people. *(b)* In a spiritual posterity—"look now toward *heaven* . . . so shall thy seed be" (John 8:39; Rom. 4:16,17; 9:7, 8; Gal. 3:6, 7, 29), viz. all men of faith, whether Jew or Gentile. *(c)* Fulfilled also through Ishmael (Gen. 17:18-20).

(2) "I will bless thee." Fulfilled in two ways: *(a)* temporally (Gen. 13:14, 15, 17; 15:18; 24:34, 35); *(b)* spiritually (Gen. 15:6; John 8:56).

(3) "And make thy name great." Abraham's is one of the universal names.

(4) "And thou shalt be a blessing" (Gal. 3:13, 14).

(5) "I will bless them that bless thee." In fulfilment closely related to the next clause.

(6) "And curse him that curseth thee." Wonderfully fulfilled in the history of the dispersion. It has invariably fared ill with the people who have persecuted the Jew—well with those who have protected him. The future will still more remarkably prove this principle (Deut. 30:7; Isa. 14:1, 2; Joel 3:1-8; Mic. 5:7-9; Hag. 2:22; Zech. 14:1-3; Mt. 25:40, 45).

(7) "In thee shall all the families of the earth be blessed." This is the great evangelic promise fulfilled in Abraham's Seed, Christ (Gal. 3:16; John 8:56-58). It brings into greater definiteness the promise of the Adamic Covenant concerning the Seed of the woman (Gen. 3:15).

NOTE.—The gift of the land is modified by prophecies of three dispossessions and restorations (Gen. 15:13,14, 16; Jer. 25:11, 12; Deut. 28:62-65; 30:1-3). Two dispossessions and restorations have been accomplished. Israel is now in the third dispersion, from which she will be restored at the return of the Lord as King under the Davidic Covenant (Deut. 30:3; Jer. 23:5-8; Ezk. 37:21-25; Lk. 1:30-33; Acts 15:14-17).

See, for the other seven covenants: *Edenic* (Gen. 1:28); *Adamic* (Gen. 3:15); *Noahic* (Gen. 9:1); *Mosaic* (Ex. 19:25); *Palestinian* (Deut. 30:3); *Davidic* (2 Sam. 7:16); *New* (Heb. 8:8).

[1] **(16:3)** Hagar is a type of the law "which gendereth to bondage" (Gal. 4:24, 25).

12 And he will be a wild man; his hand *will be* against every man, and every man's hand against him; and he shall dwell in the presence of all his brethren.

13 And she called the name of the LORD that spake unto her, Thou God seest me: for she said, Have I also here looked after him that seeth me?

14 Wherefore the well was called [a]Beer-lahai-roi; behold, *it is* between Kadesh and Bered.

15 And Hagar bare Abram a son: and Abram called his son's name, which Hagar bare, Ishmael.

16 And Abram *was* fourscore and six years old, when Hagar bare Ishmael to Abram.

CHAPTER 17.

The revelation of God as El Shaddai, Almighty God.

And when Abram was ninety years old and nine, the LORD [b]appeared to Abram, and said unto him, I *am* the [1]Almighty [c]God; walk before me, and be thou [d]perfect.

2 And I will make my covenant between me and thee, and will multiply thee exceedingly.

3 And Abram fell on his face: and God talked with him, saying,

Abram becomes Abraham.

4 As for me, behold, my covenant *is* with thee, and thou shalt be a father of many nations.

5 Neither shall thy name any more be called [e]Abram, but thy name shall be [f]Abraham; for a [g]father of many nations have I made thee.

The Abrahamic Covenant confirmed and made everlasting.

6 And I will make thee exceeding fruitful, and I will make nations of thee, and kings shall come out of thee.

7 And I will establish my covenant between me and thee and thy seed after thee in their generations for an everlasting covenant, to be a God unto thee, and to thy seed after thee.

8 And I will give unto thee, and to thy seed after thee, the land wherein thou art a stranger, all the land of Canaan, for an everlasting possession; and I will be their God.

Circumcision established as the sign of the Abrahamic Covenant.

9 And God said unto Abraham, Thou shalt keep my covenant therefore, thou, and thy seed after thee in their generations.

10 This *is* my covenant, which ye shall keep, between me and you and thy seed

B.C. 1911.

a i.e. *The well of him that liveth and seeth me.* Gen. 24:62; 25:11.

b *The theophanies.* Gen. 18:1. (Gen. 12:7; Rev. 1:9.)

c *Deity (names of).* Gen. 21:33. (Gen. 1:1; Mal. 3:18.)

d Or, *upright,* or *sincere.*

e Or, *high father.*

f Or, *father of many nations.*

g Rom. 4:17.

[1] **(17:1)** "Almighty God" (Heb. *El Shaddai.*)

(1) The etymological signification of Almighty God *(El Shaddai)* is both interesting and touching. God *(El)* signifies the "Strong One" (Gen. 1:1, *note*). The qualifying word *Shaddai* is formed from the Hebrew word "*shad,*" the breast, invariably used in Scripture for a *woman's* breast; e.g. Gen. 49:25; Job 3:12; Psa. 22:9; Song 1:13; 4:5; 7:3, 7, 8; 8:1, 8, 10; Isa. 28:9; Ezk. 16:7. *Shaddai* therefore means primarily "the breasted." God is "*Shaddai,*" because He is the Nourisher, the Strength-giver, and so, in a secondary sense, the Satisfier, who pours Himself into believing lives. As a fretful, unsatisfied babe is not only strengthened and nourished from the mother's breast, but also is quieted, rested, satisfied, so *El Shaddai* is that name of God which sets Him forth as the Strength-giver and Satisfier of His people. It is on every account to be regretted that "*Shaddai*" was translated "Almighty." The primary name *El* or *Elohim* sufficiently signifies almightiness. "All-sufficient" would far better express both the Hebrew meaning and the characteristic use of the name in Scripture.

(2) Almighty God *(El Shaddai)* not only enriches, but makes *fruitful.* This is nowhere better illustrated than in the first occurrence of the name (Gen. 17:1-8). To a man ninety-nine years of age, and "as good as dead" (Heb. 11:12), He said: "I am the Almighty God [*El Shaddai*] . . . I will . . . multiply thee exceedingly." To the same purport is the use of the name in Gen. 28:3, 4.

(3) As Giver of fruitfulness, Almighty God *(El Shaddai)* chastens His people. For the moral connection of chastening with fruit-bearing, see John 15:2; Heb. 12:10; Ruth 1:20. Hence, Almighty is the characteristic name of God in Job, occurring thirty-one times in that book. The hand of *El Shaddai* falls upon Job, the best man of his time, not in *judgment,* but in purifying unto greater fruitfulness (Job 5:17-25). See, for other names of Deity: Gen. 1:1, *note;* 2:4, *note;* 2:7; 14:18, *note;* 15:2, *note;* 21:33, *note;* 1 Sam. 1:3, *note.*

after thee; Every man child among you shall be circumcised.

11 And ye shall circumcise the flesh of your foreskin; and it shall be a [a]token of the covenant betwixt me and you.

12 And he that is eight days old shall be [b]circumcised among you, every man child in your generations, he that is born in the house, or bought with money of any stranger, which *is* not of thy seed.

13 He that is born in thy house, and he that is bought with thy money, must needs be circumcised: and my covenant shall be in your flesh for an everlasting covenant.

14 And the uncircumcised man child whose flesh of his foreskin is not circumcised, that soul shall be cut off from his people; he hath broken my covenant.

The promise of Isaac,
in whom the line of Christ runs.

15 And God said unto Abraham, As for Sarai thy wife, thou shalt not call her name Sarai, but [c]Sarah *shall* her name *be.*

16 And I will bless her, and give thee a son also of her: yea, I will bless her, and she shall be *a mother* of nations; kings of people shall be of her.

17 Then Abraham fell upon his face, and laughed, and said in his heart, Shall *a child* be born unto him that is an hundred years old? and shall Sarah, that is ninety years old, bear?

18 And Abraham [d]said unto God, O that Ishmael might live before thee!

19 And God said, Sarah thy wife shall bear thee a son indeed; and thou shalt call his name Isaac: and I will establish my [e]covenant with him for an everlasting covenant, *and* with his [f]seed after him.

Ishmael to be a nation.

20 And as for Ishmael, I have heard thee: Behold, I have blessed him, and will make him fruitful, and will multiply him exceedingly; [g]twelve princes shall he beget, and I will make him a great nation.

21 But my covenant will I establish with Isaac, which Sarah shall bear unto thee at this set time in the next year.

22 And he left off talking with him, and God went up from Abraham.

23 And Abraham took Ishmael his son, and all that were born in his house, and all that were bought with his money, every male among the men of Abraham's house; and circumcised the flesh of their foreskin in the selfsame day, as God had said unto him.

24 And Abraham *was* ninety years old and nine, when he was circumcised in the flesh of his foreskin.

25 And Ishmael his son *was* thirteen years old, when he was circumcised in the flesh of his foreskin.

26 In the selfsame day was Abraham circumcised, and Ishmael his son.

27 And all the men of his house, born in the house, and bought with money of the stranger, were circumcised with him.

CHAPTER 18.

Abraham, "the friend of God."
(Cf. John 3:29; 15:13–15.)

And the LORD [h]appeared unto him in the plains of Mamre: and he sat in the [i]tent door in the heat of the day;

2 And he lift up his eyes and looked, and, lo, three men stood by him: and when he saw *them*, he ran to meet them from the tent door, and bowed himself toward the ground,

3 And said, My Lord, if now I have found favour in thy sight, pass not away, I pray thee, from thy servant:

4 Let a little water, I pray you, be fetched, and wash your feet, and rest yourselves under the tree:

5 And I will fetch a morsel of bread, and comfort ye your hearts; after that ye shall pass on: for therefore are ye come to your servant. And they said, So do, as thou hast said.

6 And Abraham hastened into the tent unto Sarah, and said, Make ready quickly three measures of fine meal, knead *it*, and make cakes upon the hearth.

7 And Abraham ran unto the herd, and fetcht a calf tender and good, and gave *it* unto a young man; and he hasted to dress it.

8 And he took butter, and milk, and the calf which he had dressed, and set *it* before them; and he stood by them under the tree, and they did eat.

9 And they said unto him, Where

B.C. 1898.

a Rom. 4:9-12.

b Lk. 2:21; Rom. 2:25-29; 4:10-12; 1 Cor. 7:18-19; Gal. 5:2-3; cf. Col. 2:11.

c i.e. *princess.*

d *Bible prayers* (O.T.). Gen. 18:23. (Gen. 15:2; Hab. 3:1-16.)

e *Israel (covenant).* vs. 15-21; Gen. 22:16-18. (Gen. 12:2, 3; Rom. 11:26.)

f *Christ (first advent).* Gen. 24:60. (Gen. 3:15; Acts 1:9.)

g Gen. 16:10; 25:12-16.

h *The theophanies.* Gen. 26:2, 24. (Gen. 12:7; Rev. 1:9.)

i Cf. Gen. 19:1. For significance of Abraham's tent, Heb. 11:9, 10.

B.C. 1898.

is Sarah thy wife? And he said, Behold, in the tent.

10 And he said, I will certainly return unto thee according to the time of life; and, lo, [a]Sarah thy wife shall have a son. And Sarah heard *it* in the tent door, which *was* behind him.

11 Now Abraham and Sarah *were* old *and* well stricken in age; *and* it ceased to be with Sarah after the manner of women.

12 Therefore Sarah laughed within herself, saying, After I am waxed old shall I have pleasure, my lord being old also?

13 And the LORD said unto Abraham, Wherefore did Sarah laugh, saying, Shall I of a surety bear a child, which am old?

14 Is any thing too hard for the LORD? At the time appointed I will return unto thee, according to the time of life, and Sarah shall have a son.

15 Then Sarah denied, saying, I laughed not; for she was afraid. And he said, Nay; but thou didst laugh.

16 And the men rose up from thence, and looked toward Sodom: and Abraham went with them to bring them on the way.

17 And the LORD said, Shall I hide from Abraham that thing which I do;

18 Seeing that Abraham shall surely become a great and mighty nation, and all the nations of the earth shall be blessed in him?

19 For I know him, that he will command his children and his household after him, and they shall keep the way of the LORD, to do justice and judgment; that the LORD may bring upon Abraham that which he hath spoken of him.

20 And the LORD said, Because the cry of Sodom and Gomorrah is great, and because their sin is very grievous;

21 I will go down now, and see whether they have done altogether according to the cry of it, which is come unto me; and if not, I will know.

22 And the men turned their faces from thence, and went toward Sodom: but Abraham stood yet before the LORD.

Abraham the intercessor.

23 And Abraham drew [b]near, and said, [c]Wilt thou also destroy the righteous with the wicked?

24 Peradventure there be fifty righteous within the city: wilt thou also destroy and not spare the place for the fifty righteous that *are* therein?

25 That be far from thee to do after this manner, to slay the righteous with the wicked: and that the righteous should be as the wicked, that be far from thee: Shall not the Judge of all the earth do right?

26 And the LORD said, If I find in Sodom fifty righteous within the city, then I will spare all the place for their sakes.

27 And Abraham answered and said, Behold now, I have taken upon me to speak unto the Lord, which *am but* dust and ashes:

28 Peradventure there shall lack five of the fifty righteous: wilt thou destroy all the city for *lack of* five? And he said, If I find there forty and five, I will not destroy *it*.

29 And he spake unto him yet again, and said, Peradventure there shall be forty found there. And he said, I will not do *it* for forty's sake.

30 And he said *unto him*, Oh let not the Lord be angry, and I will speak: Peradventure there shall thirty be found there. And he said, I will not do *it*, if I find thirty there.

31 And he said, Behold now, I have taken upon me to speak unto the Lord: Peradventure there shall be twenty found there. And he said, I will not destroy *it* for twenty's sake.

32 And he said, Oh let not the Lord be angry, and I will speak yet but this once: Peradventure ten shall be found there. And he said, I will not destroy *it* for ten's sake.

33 And the LORD went his way, as soon as he had left communing with Abraham: and Abraham returned unto his place.

CHAPTER 19.

The destruction of Sodom. The third step in Lot's backsliding: a great man in Sodom (v. 1). (See Gen. 13:10, 12; 19:33.)

And there [d]came two [e]angels to Sodom at even; and Lot [f]sat in the gate of Sodom: and Lot seeing *them* rose up to meet them; and he bowed himself with his face toward the ground;

a Cf. Rom. 9:9.

b Communion (vs. 1-8) and intercession go together.

c *Bible prayers* (O.T.). Gen. 24:12. (Gen. 15:2; Hab. 3:1-16.)

d Cf. Gen. 18:2, 16, 22.

e Heb. 1:4, *note*.

f Lot was a great man (Deut. 21:19, 20) in a place devoted to judgment. Cf. Acts 17:31.

B.C. 1898.

2 And he said, Behold now, my lords, turn in, I pray you, into your servant's house, and tarry all night, and wash your feet, and ye shall rise up early, and go on your ways. And they said, Nay; but we will abide in the street all night.

3 And he pressed upon them greatly; and they turned in unto him, and entered into his house; and he made them a feast, and did bake [a]unleavened bread, and they did eat.

4 But before they lay down, the men of the city, *even* the men of Sodom, compassed the house round, both old and young, all the people from every quarter:

5 And they called unto Lot, and said unto him, Where *are* the men which came in to thee this night? bring them out unto us, that we may know them.

6 And Lot went out at the door unto them, and shut the door after him,

7 And said, I pray you, brethren, do not so wickedly.

8 Behold now, I have two daughters which have not known man; let me, I pray you, bring them out unto you, and do ye to them as *is* good in your eyes: only unto these men do nothing; for therefore came they under the shadow of my roof.

9 And they said, Stand back. [b]And they said *again*, This one *fellow* came in to sojourn, and he will needs be a judge: now will we deal worse with thee, than with them. And they pressed sore upon the man, *even* Lot, and came near to break the door.

10 But the men put forth their hand, and pulled Lot into the house to them, and shut to the door.

11 And they smote the men that *were* at the door of the house with blindness, both small and great: so that they wearied themselves to find the door.

12 And the men said unto Lot, Hast thou here any besides? son in law, and thy sons, and thy daughters, and whatsoever thou hast in the city, bring *them* out of this place:

13 For we will destroy this place, because the cry of them is waxen great before the face of the LORD; and the LORD hath sent us to destroy it.

14 And [c]Lot went out, and spake unto his sons in law, which married his daughters, and said, Up, get you out of this place; for the LORD will destroy this city. But he seemed as one that mocked unto his sons in law.

15 And when the morning arose, then the [d]angels hastened Lot, saying, Arise, take thy wife, and thy two daughters, which are here; lest thou be consumed in the iniquity of the city.

16 And while he lingered, the men laid hold upon his hand, and upon the hand of his wife, and upon the hand of his two daughters; the LORD being merciful unto him: and they brought him forth, and set him without the city.

17 And it came to pass, when they had brought them forth abroad, that he said, Escape for thy life; look not behind thee, neither stay thou in all the plain; escape to the mountain, lest thou be consumed.

18 And Lot said unto them, Oh, not so, my Lord:

19 Behold now, thy servant hath found grace in thy sight, and thou hast magnified thy mercy, which thou hast shewed unto me in saving my life; and I cannot escape to the mountain, lest some evil take me, and I die:

20 Behold now, this city *is* near to flee unto, and it *is* a little one: Oh, let me escape thither, (*is* it not a little one?) and my soul shall live.

21 And he said unto him, See, I have accepted thee concerning this thing also, that I will not overthrow this city, for the which thou hast spoken.

22 Haste thee, escape thither; for I cannot do any thing till thou be come thither. Therefore the name of the city was called Zoar.

23 The sun was risen upon the earth when Lot entered into Zoar.

24 Then the LORD [e]rained upon Sodom and upon Gomorrah brimstone and fire from the LORD out of heaven;

25 And he overthrew those cities, and all the plain, and all the inhabitants of the cities, and that which grew upon the ground.

26 But his [f]wife looked back from behind him, and she became a pillar of salt.

27 And Abraham gat up early in the morning to the place where he stood before the LORD:

a *Leaven.* Ex. 12:8, 15-20, 34, 39. (Gen. 19:3; Mt. 13:33.)

b The world's contempt for a worldly believer.

c Lot had utterly lost his testimony. In gaining *influence* (Gen. 19:1) he had lost *power*, even in his own family.

d Heb. 1:4, *note.*

e *Miracles* (O.T.), vs. 24-26; Gen. 20:17, 18. (Gen. 5:24; Jon. 2:1-10.)

f Lk. 17:32.

28 And he looked toward Sodom and Gomorrah, and toward all the land of the plain, and beheld, and, lo, the smoke of the country went up as the smoke of a furnace.

29 And it came to pass, [a]when God destroyed the cities of the plain, that God remembered Abraham, and sent Lot out of the midst of the overthrow, when he overthrew the cities in the which Lot dwelt.

30 And Lot went up out of Zoar, and dwelt in the mountain, and his two daughters with him; for he feared to dwell in Zoar: and he dwelt in a cave, he and his two daughters.

31 And the firstborn said unto the younger, Our father *is* old, and *there is* not a man in the earth to come in unto us after the manner of all the earth:

32 [b]Come, let us make our father drink wine, and we will lie with him, that we may preserve seed of our father.

The last step in Lot's backsliding. (See Gen. 13:10, 12; 19:1. Cf. Lk. 22:31–62.)

33 And they made their father drink wine that night: and the firstborn went in, and lay with her father; and he perceived not when she lay down, nor when she arose.

34 And it came to pass on the morrow, that the firstborn said unto the younger, Behold, I lay yesternight with my father: let us make him drink wine this night also; and go thou in, *and* lie with him, that we may preserve seed of our father.

35 And they made their father drink wine that night also: and the younger arose, and lay with him; and he perceived not when she lay down, nor when she arose.

36 [1]Thus were both the daughters of Lot with child by their father.

37 And the firstborn bare a son, and called his name Moab: the same *is* the father of the Moabites unto this day.

38 And the younger, she also bare a son, and called his name Benammi: the same *is* the father of the children of Ammon unto this day.

B.C. 1898.

a See v. 36, *note*.

b Lot "pitched toward Sodom" (Gen. 13:12) for worldly advantage; then became a great man in Sodom (Gen. 19:1), at the cost of his daughters' accepting the morals of Sodom.

CHAPTER 20.

Abraham's lapse at Gerar.
(Cf. Gen. 26:6–32.)

And Abraham journeyed from thence toward the south country, and dwelled between Kadesh and Shur, and sojourned in Gerar.

2 And Abraham said of Sarah his wife, She *is* my sister: and Abimelech king of Gerar sent, and took Sarah.

3 But God came to Abimelech in a dream by night, and said to him, Behold, thou *art but* a dead man, for the woman which thou hast taken; for she *is* a man's wife.

4 But Abimelech had not come near her: and he said, Lord, wilt thou slay also a righteous nation?

5 Said he not unto me, She *is* my sister? and she, even she herself said, He *is* my brother: in the integrity of my heart and innocency of my hands have I done this.

6 And God said unto him in a dream, Yea, I know that thou didst this in the integrity of thy heart; for I also withheld thee from sinning against me: therefore suffered I thee not to touch her.

7 Now therefore restore the man *his* wife; for he *is* a prophet, and he shall pray for thee, and thou shalt live: and if thou restore *her* not, know thou that thou shalt surely die, thou, and all that *are* thine.

8 Therefore Abimelech rose early in the morning, and called all his servants, and told all these things in their ears: and the men were sore afraid.

9 Then Abimelech called Abraham, and said unto him, What hast thou done unto us? and what have I offended thee, that thou hast brought on me and on my kingdom a great sin? thou hast done deeds unto me that ought not to be done.

[1]**(19:36)** Abraham and Lot are contrasted characters. Of the same stock (Gen. 11:31), subjected to the same environment, and both justified men (Gen. 15:6; 2 Pet. 2:7, 8), the contrast in character and career is shown to be the result of their respective *choices* at the crisis of their lives. Lot "chose him all the plain of Jordan" for present advantage; Abraham "looked for a city which hath foundations" (Heb. 11:10), and (Gen. 13:18) "came and dwelt in the plain of Mamre *(fatness)*, which is in Hebron" *(communion)*. The men remain types of the worldly and the spiritual believer.

B.C. 1898.

10 And Abimelech said unto Abraham, What sawest thou, that thou hast done this thing?

11 And Abraham said, Because I thought, Surely the [a]fear of God *is* not in this place; and they will slay me for my wife's sake.

12 And yet indeed *she is* my sister; she *is* the daughter of my father, but not the daughter of my mother; and she became my wife.

13 And it came to pass, when God caused me to wander from my father's house, that I said unto her, This *is* thy kindness which thou shalt shew unto me; at every place whither we shall come, say of me, He *is* my brother.

14 And Abimelech took sheep, and oxen, and menservants, and womenservants, and gave *them* unto Abraham, and restored him Sarah his wife.

15 And Abimelech said, Behold, my land *is* before thee: dwell where it pleaseth thee.

16 And unto Sarah he said, Behold, I have given thy brother a thousand *pieces* of silver: behold, he *is* to thee a covering of the eyes, unto all that *are* with thee, and with all *other*: thus she was reproved.

17 So Abraham prayed unto God: and God [b]healed Abimelech, and his wife, and his maidservants; and they bare *children*.

18 For the LORD had fast closed up all the wombs of the house of Abimelech, because of Sarah Abraham's wife.

CHAPTER 21.

The birth of Isaac.

And the LORD visited Sarah as he had [c]said, and the LORD did unto Sarah as he had spoken.

2 For Sarah [d]conceived, and bare Abraham a son in his old age, at the set time of which God had spoken to him.

3 And Abraham called the name of his son that was born unto him, whom [1]Sarah bare to him, [2]Isaac.

4 And Abraham circumcised his son Isaac being eight days old, as God had commanded him.

5 And Abraham was an hundred years old, when his son Isaac was born unto him.

6 And Sarah said, God hath made me to laugh, *so that* all that hear will laugh with me.

7 And she said, Who would have said unto Abraham, that Sarah should have given children suck? for I have born *him* a son in his old age.

8 And the child grew, and was weaned: and Abraham made a great feast the *same* day that Isaac was weaned.

The bondwoman and her son cast out
(Gal. 4:21–31).

9 And Sarah saw the son of Hagar the Egyptian, which she had born unto Abraham, mocking.

10 Wherefore she said unto Abraham, [e]Cast out this bondwoman and her son: for the son of this bondwoman shall not be heir with my son, *even* with Isaac.

11 And the thing was very grievous in Abraham's sight because of his son.

12 And God said unto Abraham, Let it not be grievous in thy sight because of the lad, and because of thy bondwoman; in all that Sarah hath said unto thee, hearken unto her voice; for in Isaac shall thy seed be called.

13 And also of the son of the bondwoman will I make a nation, because he *is* thy seed.

14 And Abraham rose up early in the morning, and took bread, and a bottle of water, and gave *it* unto Hagar, putting *it* on her shoulder, and the child, and sent her away: and she departed, and wandered in the wilderness of Beer-sheba.

15 And the water was spent in the bottle, and she cast the child under one of the shrubs.

16 And she went, and sat her down over against *him* a good way off, as it were a bowshot: for she said, Let me not see the death of the child. And she sat over against *him*, and lift up her voice, and wept.

a Psa. 19:9, *note*.

b *Miracles* (O.T.), vs. 17, 18; Gen. 21:2. (Gen. 5:24; Jon. 2:1-10.)

c *Faith*. vs. 1-6; Gen. 22:1-14. (Gen. 3:20; Heb. 11:39.)

d *Miracles* (O.T.). Ex. 4:3, 4, 6, 7. (Gen. 5:24; Jon. 2:1-10.)

e Gal. 3:18; 4:30; 1 Tim. 1:7-10.

[1] **(21:3)** Sarah. type of grace, "the freewoman," and of the "Jerusalem which is above." See Gen. 17:15-19; Gal. 4:22-31.

[2] **(21:3)** Isaac is typical in a fourfold way: (1) of the Church as composed of the spiritual children of Abraham (Gal. 4:28); (2) of Christ as the Son "obedient unto death" (Gen. 22:1-10; Phil. 2:5-8; (3) of Christ as the Bridegroom of a called-out bride (see Gen. 24; also, "Church," Mt. 16:18 and *refs.*); (4) of the new nature of the believer as "born after the Spirit" (Gal. 4:29).

B.C. 1892.

17 And God heard the voice of the lad; and the [a]angel of God called to Hagar out of heaven, and said unto her, What aileth thee, Hagar? fear not; for God hath heard the voice of the lad where he *is*.

18 Arise, lift up the lad, and hold him in thine hand; for I will make him a great nation.

19 And God opened her eyes, and she saw a well of water; and she went, and filled the bottle with water, and gave the lad drink.

20 And God was with the lad; and he grew, and dwelt in the wilderness, and became an archer.

21 And he dwelt in the wilderness of Paran: and his mother took him a wife out of the land of Egypt.

Abraham at Beer-sheba.

22 And it came to pass at that time, that Abimelech and Phichol the chief captain of his host spake unto Abraham, saying, God *is* with thee in all that thou doest:

23 Now therefore swear unto me here by God that thou wilt not deal falsely with me, nor with my son, nor with my son's son: *but* according to the kindness that I have done unto thee, thou shalt do unto me, and to the land wherein thou hast sojourned.

24 And Abraham said, I will swear.

25 And Abraham reproved Abimelech because of a well of water, which Abimelech's servants had violently taken away.

a Heb. 1:4, *note*.

b *Deity (names of).* Gen. 35:11. (Gen. 1:1; Mal. 3:18.)

c *Temptation.* Ex. 17:2, 7. (Gen. 3:1; Jas. 1:2.)

26 And Abimelech said, I wot not who hath done this thing: neither didst thou tell me, neither yet heard I *of it*, but to day.

27 And Abraham took sheep and oxen, and gave them unto Abimelech; and both of them made a covenant.

28 And Abraham set seven ewe lambs of the flock by themselves.

29 And Abimelech said unto Abraham, What *mean* these seven ewe lambs which thou hast set by themselves?

30 And he said, For *these* seven ewe lambs shalt thou take of my hand, that they may be a witness unto me, that I have digged this well.

31 Wherefore he called that place Beer-sheba; because there they sware both of them.

32 Thus they made a covenant at Beer-sheba: then Abimelech rose up, and Phichol the chief captain of his host, and they returned into the land of the Philistines.

33 And *Abraham* planted a grove in Beer-sheba, and called there on the name of the LORD, the [b]everlasting [1]God.

34 And Abraham sojourned in the Philistines' land many days.

CHAPTER 22.

The offering of Isaac.

[2]And it came to pass after these things, that God did [c]tempt Abraham, and said unto him, Abraham: and he said, Behold, *here* I *am*.

[1]**(21:33)** "Everlasting God" (Heb. *El Olam*).

(1) The Hebrew *Olam* is used in Scripture: *(a)* of secret or hidden things (e.g. Lev. 5:2, "hidden"; 2 Ki. 4:27, "hid"; Psa. 10:1, "hidest"); *(b)* an indefinite time or age (Lev. 25:32, "at any *time*"; Josh. 24:2, "in old *time*). *Hence* the word is used to express the eternal duration of the being of God (Psa. 90:2, "From everlasting to everlasting"), and is the Hebrew synonym of the Greek *aion*, age or dispensation. See Gen. 1:27, 28, *note* 4.

(2) The ideas therefore of things kept secret and of indefinite duration combine in this word. Both ideas inhere in the doctrine of the dispensations or ages. They are among the "mysteries" of God (Eph. 1:9, 10; 3:2-6; Mt. 13:11). The "everlasting" God *(El Olam)* is, therefore, that name of Deity in virtue of which He is the God whose wisdom has divided all time and eternity into the mystery of successive ages or dispensations. It is not merely that He is everlasting, but that He is God *over* everlasting things. See, for other names of Deity: Gen. 1:1, *note;* 2:4, *note;* 2:7; 14:18, *note;* 15:2, *note;* 17:1, *note;* 1 Sam. 1:3, *note*.

[2]**(22:1)** The spiritual experience of Abraham was marked by four great crises, each of which involved a surrender of something *naturally* most dear. These were: (1) Country and kindred (Gen. 12:1. Cf. Mt. 10:34-39; 2 Cor. 6:14-18). (2) His nephew, Lot; especially dear to Abraham by nature, as a possible heir and as a fellow believer (2 Pet. 2:7, 8; Gen. 13:1-18). The completeness of Abraham's separation from one who, though a believer, was a "vessel unto dishonour," is shown by Gen. 15:1-3. Cf. 2 Tim. 2:20, 21; Acts 15:36-40. (3) His own plan about Ishmael (Gen. 17:17, 18. Cf. 1 Chr. 13:1-14; 15:1, 2). (4) Isaac, "thy son, thine only son Isaac, whom thou lovest" (Gen. 22:1-19. Cf. Heb. 11:17, 18).

2 And he said, Take now thy son, thine
only *son* Isaac, whom thou lovest, and get
thee into the land of Moriah; and offer
him there for a burnt-offering upon one
of the mountains which I will tell thee of.
3 [a]And Abraham rose up early in the
morning, and saddled his ass, and took
two of his young men with him, and Isaac
his son, and clave the wood for the burnt-
offering, and rose up, and went unto the
place of which God had told him.
4 Then on the third day Abraham lifted
up his eyes, and saw the place afar off.
5 And Abraham said unto his young
men, Abide ye here with the ass; and I
and the lad will go yonder and worship,
and [b]come again to you.
6 And Abraham took the wood of the
burnt-offering, and laid *it* upon Isaac his
son; and he took the fire in his hand, and a
knife; and they went both of them together.
7 And Isaac spake unto Abraham his
father, and said, My father: and he said,
Here *am* I, my son. And he said, Behold
the fire and the wood: but where *is* the
lamb for a burnt-offering?
8 And Abraham said, My son, God
will provide himself a lamb for a [c]burnt-
offering: so they went both of them
together.
9 And they came to the place which
God had told him of; and Abraham built
an altar there, and laid the wood in
order, and bound Isaac his son, and [1]laid
him on the altar upon the wood.
10 And Abraham stretched forth his
hand, and took the knife to slay his son.
11 And the [d]angel of the LORD called
unto him out of heaven, and said,
Abraham, Abraham: and he said, Here
am I.
12 And he said, Lay not thine hand
upon the lad, neither do thou any thing
unto him: for now I know that thou
[e]fearest God, seeing thou hast not withheld thy son, thine only *son* from me.
13 And Abraham lifted up his eyes,
and looked, and behold behind *him* a
ram caught in a thicket by his horns: and

B.C. 1872.

a *Faith*. vs. 1-14; Gen. 50:24, 25. (Gen. 3:20; Heb. 11:39.)

b *Resurrection*. 2 Ki. 4:32-35. (Job 19:25; 1 Cor. 15:52.)

c *Sacrifice (typical)*, vs. 8, 13; Ex. 12:3-11, 27. (Gen. 4:4; Heb. 10:18.)

d Heb. 1:4, *note*.

e Psa. 19:9, *note*.

f *Israel (covenant)*, vs. 16-18; Gen. 26:2-5. (Gen. 12:2, 3; Rom. 11:26.)

Abraham went and took the ram, and
offered him up for a burnt-offering in
the stead of his son.
14 And Abraham called the name of that
place Jehovah-jireh: as it is said *to* this day,
In the mount of the LORD it shall be seen.

The Abrahamic Covenant confirmed.

15 And the [d]angel of the LORD called
unto Abraham out of heaven the second
time,
16 And [f]said, By myself have I sworn,
saith the LORD, for because thou hast
done this thing, and hast not withheld
thy son, thine only *son*:
17 That in blessing I will bless thee, and
in multiplying I will multiply thy seed as
the stars of the heaven, and as the sand
which *is* upon the sea shore; and thy seed
shall possess the gate of his enemies;
18 And in thy seed shall all the nations
of the earth be blessed; because thou
hast obeyed my voice.
19 So Abraham returned unto his
young men, and they rose up and went
together to Beer-sheba; and Abraham
dwelt at Beer-sheba.
20 And it came to pass after these
things, that it was told Abraham, saying,
Behold, Milcah, she hath also born children unto thy brother Nahor;
21 Huz his firstborn, and Buz his
brother, and Kemuel the father of Aram,
22 And Chesed, and Hazo, and
Pildash, and Jidlaph, and Bethuel.
23 And Bethuel begat Rebekah: these
eight Milcah did bear to Nahor,
Abraham's brother.
24 And his concubine, whose name
was Reumah, she bare also Tebah, and
Gaham, and Thahash, and Maachah.

CHAPTER 23.

The death and burial of Sarah.

And Sarah was an hundred and
seven and twenty years old: *these
were* the years of the life of Sarah.
2 And Sarah died in Kirjath-arba; the
same *is* Hebron in the land of Canaan:

[1] **(22:9)** The typical lessons here are: (1) Isaac, type of Christ "obedient unto death" (Phil. 2:5-8); (2) Abraham, type of the Father, who "spared not His own son, but delivered Him up for us all" (John 3:16: Rom. 8:32); (3) the ram, type of substitution—Christ offered as a burnt-offering in our stead (Heb. 10:5-10); (4) cf. resurrection (Heb. 11:17-19). See also Jas. 2:21-23.

and Abraham came to mourn for Sarah, and to weep for her.

3 And Abraham stood up from before his dead, and spake unto the sons of Heth, saying,

4 I *am* a stranger and a sojourner with you: give me a possession of a [1]buryingplace with you, that I may bury my dead out of my sight.

5 And the children of Heth answered Abraham, saying unto him,

6 Hear us, my lord: thou *art* a mighty prince among us: in the choice of our sepulchres bury thy dead; none of us shall withhold from thee his sepulchre, but that thou mayest bury thy dead.

7 And Abraham stood up, and bowed himself to the people of the land, *even* to the children of Heth.

8 And he communed with them, saying, If it be your mind that I should bury my dead out of my sight; hear me, and intreat for me to Ephron the son of Zohar,

9 That he may give me the cave of Machpelah, which he hath, which *is* in the end of his field; for as much money as it is worth he shall give it me for a possession of a buryingplace amongst you.

10 And Ephron dwelt among the children of Heth: and Ephron the Hittite answered Abraham in the audience of the children of Heth, *even* of all that went in at the gate of his city, saying,

11 Nay, my lord, hear me: the field give I thee, and the cave that *is* therein, I give it thee; in the presence of the sons of my people give I it thee: bury thy dead.

12 And Abraham bowed down himself before the people of the land.

B.C. 1860.

a One shekel = 2*s*. 9*d*. , or 65 cents; also v. 16.

b v. 4, *note.*

13 And he spake unto Ephron in the audience of the people of the land, saying, But if thou *wilt give it*, I pray thee, hear me: I will give thee money for the field; take *it* of me, and I will bury my dead there.

14 And Ephron answered Abraham, saying unto him,

15 My lord, hearken unto me: the land *is worth* four hundred [a]shekels of silver; what *is* that betwixt me and thee? bury therefore thy dead.

16 [b]And Abraham hearkened unto Ephron; and Abraham weighed to Ephron the silver, which he had named in the audience of the sons of Heth, four hundred shekels of silver, current *money* with the merchant.

17 And the field of Ephron, which *was* in Machpelah, which *was* before Mamre, the field, and the cave which *was* therein, and all the trees that *were* in the field, that *were* in all the borders round about, were made sure

18 Unto Abraham for a possession in the presence of the children of Heth, before all that went in at the gate of his city.

19 And after this, Abraham buried Sarah his wife in the cave of the field of Machpelah before Mamre: the same *is* Hebron in the land of Canaan.

20 And the field, and the cave that *is* therein, were made sure unto Abraham for a possession of a buryingplace by the sons of Heth.

CHAPTER 24.

A bride for Isaac.

[2] And Abraham was old, *and* well stricken in age: and the LORD had blessed Abraham in all things.

[1] **(23:4)** Cf. Gen. 33:19; 50:13; Josh. 24:32; Acts 7:15, 16. A discrepancy in these statements has been fancied. It disappears entirely before the natural supposition that in the interval of about eighty years between the purchase by Abraham of the family sepulchre (Gen. 23:4-20) and Jacob's purchase (Gen. 33:19), the descendants of Hamor (or "Emmor," Acts 7:15, 16) had resumed possession of the field in which the burial-cave was situated. Instead of asserting an ancient title by inheritance, Jacob repurchased the field. Heth was the common ancestor.

[2] **(24:1)** The entire chapter is highly typical: (1) Abraham, type of a certain king who would make a marriage for his son (Mt. 22:2; John 6:44); (2) the unnamed servant, type of the Holy Spirit, who does not "speak of himself," but takes of the things of the Bridegroom with which to win the bride (John 16:13, 14); (3) the servant, type of the Spirit as enriching the bride with the Bridegroom's gifts (Gal 5:22; 1 Cor. 12:7-11); (4) the servant, type of the Spirit as bringing the bride to the meeting with the Bridegroom (Acts 13:4; 16:6, 7; Rom. 8:11; 1 Thes. 4:14-16); (5) Rebekah, type of the Church, the *ecclesia,* the "called out" virgin bride of Christ (Gen. 24:16; 2 Cor. 11:2; Eph. 5:25-32); (6) Isaac, type of the Bridegroom, "whom not having seen," the bride loves through the testimony of the unnamed Servant (1 Pet. 1:8); (7) Isaac, type of the Bridegroom who goes out to meet and receive His bride (Gen. 24:63; 1 Thes. 4:14-16).

2 And Abraham said unto his eldest servant of his house, that ruled over all that he had, Put, I pray thee, thy hand under my thigh:

3 And I will make thee swear by the LORD, the God of heaven, and the God of the earth, that thou shalt not take a wife unto my son of the daughters of the Canaanites, among whom I dwell:

4 But thou shalt go unto my country, and to my kindred, and take a wife unto my son Isaac.

5 And the servant said unto him, Peradventure the woman will not be willing to follow me unto this land: must I needs bring thy son again unto the land from whence thou camest?

6 And Abraham said unto him, Beware thou that thou bring not my son thither again.

7 The LORD God of heaven, which took me from my father's house, and from the land of my kindred, and which spake unto me, and that sware unto me, saying, Unto thy seed will I give this land; he shall send his [a]angel before thee, and thou shalt take a wife unto my son from thence.

8 And if the woman will not be willing to follow thee, then thou shalt be clear from this my oath: only bring not my son thither again.

9 And the servant put his hand under the thigh of Abraham his master, and sware to him concerning that matter.

10 And the servant took ten camels of the camels of his master, and departed; for all the goods of his master *were* in his hand: and he arose, and went to Mesopotamia, unto the city of Nahor.

11 And he made his camels to kneel down without the city by a well of water at the time of the evening, *even* the time that women go out to draw *water*.

12 And he [b]said, O LORD God of my master Abraham, I pray thee, send me good speed this day, and shew kindness unto my master Abraham.

13 Behold, I stand *here* by the well of water; and the daughters of the men of the city come out to draw water:

14 And let it come to pass, that the damsel to whom I shall say, Let down thy pitcher, I pray thee, that I may drink; and she shall say, Drink, and I will give thy camels drink also: *let the same be* she *that* thou hast appointed for thy servant Isaac; and [c]thereby shall I know that thou hast shewed kindness unto my master.

15 And it came to pass, before he had done speaking, that, behold, Rebekah came out, who was born to Bethuel, son of Milcah, the wife of Nahor, Abraham's brother, with her pitcher upon her shoulder.

16 And the damsel *was* very fair to look upon, a virgin, neither had any man known her: and she went down to the well, and filled her pitcher, and came up.

17 And the servant ran to meet her, and said, Let me, I pray thee, drink a little water of thy pitcher.

18 And she said, Drink, my lord: and she hasted, and let down her pitcher upon her hand, and gave him drink.

19 And when she had done giving him drink, she said, I will draw *water* for thy camels also, until they have done drinking.

20 And she hasted, and emptied her pitcher into the trough, and ran again unto the well to draw *water*, and drew for all his camels.

21 And the man wondering at her held his peace, to wit whether the LORD had made his journey prosperous or not.

22 And it came to pass, as the camels had done drinking, that the man took a golden earring of half a [d]shekel weight, and two bracelets for her hands of ten *shekels* weight of gold;

23 And said, Whose daughter *art* thou? tell me, I pray thee: is there room *in* thy father's house for us to lodge in?

24 And she said unto him, I *am* the daughter of Bethuel the son of Milcah, which she bare unto Nahor.

25 She said moreover unto him, We have both straw and provender enough, and room to lodge in.

26 And the man bowed down his head, and worshipped the LORD.

27 And he said, Blessed *be* the LORD God of my master Abraham, who hath not left destitute my master of his mercy and his truth: I *being* in the way, the LORD led me to the house of my master's brethren.

28 And the damsel ran, and told *them* *of* her mother's house these things.

29 And Rebekah had a brother,

B.C.1857.

a Heb. 1:4, *note.*

b *Bible prayers* (O.T.). Gen. 32:9. (Gen. 15:2; Hab. 3:1-16.)

c Jud. 6:17, 37; 2 Ki. 20:9; Prov. 16:33; Acts 1:26. Cf. Mt. 12:39. Signs are given to faith, not to doubt.

d One shekel = 1/2 oz. troy.

and his name *was* Laban: and Laban ran
out unto the man, unto the well.
30 And it came to pass, when he saw
the earring and bracelets upon his sister's hands, and when he heard the
words of Rebekah his sister, saying,
Thus spake the man unto me; that he
came unto the man; and, behold, he
stood by the camels at the well.
31 And he said, Come in, thou blessed
of the LORD; wherefore standest thou
without? for I have prepared the house,
and room for the camels.
32 And the man came into the house:
and he ungirded his camels, and gave
straw and provender for the camels, and
water to wash his feet, and the men's
feet that *were* with him.
33 And there was set *meat* before him to
eat: but he said, I will not eat, until I have
told mine errand. And he said, Speak on.
34 And he said, I *am* Abraham's servant.
35 And the LORD hath blessed my master greatly; and he is become great: and
he hath given him flocks, and herds, and
silver, and gold, and menservants, and
maidservants, and camels, and asses.
36 And Sarah my master's wife bare a
son to my master when she was old: and
unto him hath he given all that he hath.
37 And my master [a]made me swear,
saying, Thou shalt not take a wife to my
son of the daughters of the Canaanites,
in whose land I dwell:
38 But thou shalt go unto my father's
house, and to my kindred, and take a
wife unto my son.
39 And I said unto my master, Peradventure the woman will not follow me.
40 And he said unto me, The LORD,
[b]before whom I walk, will send his [c]an-
gel with thee, and prosper thy way; and
thou shalt take a wife for my son of my
kindred, and of my father's house:
41 Then shalt thou be clear from *this*
my oath, when thou comest to my kindred; and if they give not thee *one*, thou
shalt be clear from my oath.
42 And I came this day unto the well,
and said, O [d]LORD God of my master
Abraham, if now thou do prosper my
way which I go:
43 Behold, I stand by the well of water;
and it shall come to pass, that when the
virgin cometh forth to draw *water*, and I
say to her, Give me, I pray thee, a little
water of thy pitcher to drink;

B.C. 1857.

a v. 3.
b 1 Ki. 8:23.
c Heb. 1:4, *note.*
d v. 12.
e 1 Sam. 1:13.

44 And she say to me, Both drink
thou, and I will also draw for thy
camels: *let* the same *be* the woman
whom the LORD hath appointed out for
my master's son.
45 And before I had done speaking in
mine [e]heart, behold, Rebekah came forth
with her pitcher on her shoulder; and
she went down unto the well, and drew
water: and I said unto her, Let me drink,
I pray thee.
46 And she made haste, and let down
her pitcher from her *shoulder*, and said,
Drink, and I will give thy camels drink
also: so I drank, and she made the
camels drink also.
47 And I asked her, and said, Whose
daughter *art* thou? And she said, The
daughter of Bethuel, Nahor's son, whom
Milcah bare unto him: and I put the earring upon her face, and the bracelets
upon her hands.
48 And I bowed down my head, and
worshipped the LORD, and blessed the
LORD God of my master Abraham, which
had led me in the right way to take my
master's brother's daughter unto his son.
49 And now if ye will deal kindly and
truly with my master, tell me: and if not,
tell me; that I may turn to the right hand,
or to the left.
50 Then Laban and Bethuel answered
and said, The thing proceedeth from the
LORD: we cannot speak unto thee bad or
good.
51 Behold, Rebekah *is* before thee, take
her, and go, and let her be thy master's
son's wife, as the LORD hath spoken.
52 And it came to pass, that, when
Abraham's servant heard their words,
he worshipped the LORD, *bowing himself*
to the earth.
53 And the servant brought forth jewels
of silver, and jewels of gold, and raiment,
and gave *them* to Rebekah: he gave also to
her brother and to her mother precious
things.
54 And they did eat and drink, he and
the men that *were* with him, and tarried
all night; and they rose up in the morning, and he said, Send me away unto my
master.
55 And her brother and her mother said,
Let the damsel abide with us *a few* days, at
the least ten; after that she shall go.

56 And he said unto them, Hinder me
not, seeing the LORD hath prospered my
way; send me away that I may go to my
master.
57 And they said, We will call the
damsel, and inquire at her mouth.
58 And they called Rebekah, and said
unto her, Wilt thou go with this man?
And she said, I will go.
59 And they sent away Rebekah their
sister, and her nurse, and Abraham's servant, and his men.
60 And they blessed Rebekah, and
said unto her, Thou *art* our sister, be
thou *the mother* of thousands of millions,
and let thy [a]seed possess the gate of
those which hate them.
61 And Rebekah arose, and her
damsels, and they rode upon the camels,
and followed the man: and the servant
took Rebekah, and went his way.
62 And Isaac came from the way of
the well [b]Lahai-roi; for he dwelt in the
south country.
63 And Isaac went out to meditate in
the field at the eventide: and he lifted up
his eyes, and saw, and, behold, the
camels *were* coming.
64 And Rebekah lifted up her eyes,
and when she saw Isaac, she lighted off
the camel.
65 For she *had* said unto the servant,
What man *is* this that walketh in the
field to meet us? And the servant *had*
said, It *is* my master: therefore she took a
vail, and covered herself.
66 And the [1]servant told Isaac all
things that he had done.
67 And Isaac brought her into his
mother Sarah's tent, and took Rebekah,
and she became his wife; and he loved
her: and Isaac was comforted after his
mother's *death*.

B.C. 1857.

a *Christ (first advent).* Gen. 28:14. (Gen. 3:15; Acts 1:9.)

b i.e. *"the well of him that liveth and seeth me."* Gen. 16:14; 25:11.

CHAPTER 25.

Abraham weds Keturah.

Then again Abraham took a wife, and
her name *was* [2]Keturah.
2 And she bare him Zimran, and
Jokshan, and Medan, and Midian, and
Ishbak, and Shuah.
3 And Jokshan begat Sheba, and
Dedan. And the sons of Dedan were
Asshurim, and Letushim, and Leummim.
4 And the sons of Midian; Ephah, and
Epher, and Hanoch, and Abida, and
Eldaah. All these *were* the children of
Keturah.

Isaac heir of all things (Heb. 1:2).

5 And Abraham gave all that he had
unto Isaac.
6 But unto the sons of the concubines,
which Abraham had, Abraham gave
gifts, and sent them away from Isaac his
son, while he yet lived, eastward, unto
the east country.

The death of Abraham.

7 And these *are* the days of the years
of Abraham's life which he lived, an
hundred threescore and fifteen years.
8 Then Abraham gave up the ghost,
and died in a good old age, an old man,
and full *of years*; and was gathered to his
people.
9 And his sons Isaac and Ishmael
buried him in the cave of Machpelah, in
the field of Ephron the son of Zohar the
Hittite, which *is* before Mamre;
10 The field which Abraham purchased of the sons of Heth: there was
Abraham buried, and Sarah his wife.
11 And it came to pass after the death of
Abraham, that God blessed his son Isaac;
and Isaac dwelt by the well Lahai-roi.

The generations of Ishmael.

12 Now these *are* the generations of
Ishmael, Abraham's son, whom Hagar
the Egyptian, Sarah's handmaid, bare
unto Abraham:

[1] **(24:66)** This is the model servant: (1) he does not run unsent, vs. 2-9; (2) goes where he is sent, vs. 4, 10; (3) does nothing else; (4) is prayerful and thankful, vs. 12-14, 26, 27; (5) is wise to win, vs. 17, 18, 21. Cf. John 4:7; (6) speaks not of himself, but of his master's riches and Isaac's heirship, vs. 22, 34-36; Acts 1:8; (7) presents the true issue, and requires clear decision, v. 49.

[2] **(25:1)** As Sarah stands for "the mother of *us* all," i.e. of those who, by grace, are one with the true Son of promise, of whom Isaac was the type (John 3:6-8; Gal. 4:26, 28, 29- Heb. 2:11-13); and joint heirs of His wealth (Heb. 1:2; Rom. 8:16, 17), so Keturah (wedded after the full blessing of Isaac) and her children by Abraham may well stand for the fertility of Israel the natural seed, Jehovah's wife (Hos. 2:1-23) after the future national restoration under the Palestinian covenant (Deut. 30:1-9, *note*).

B.C. 1800.

13 And these *are* the names of the sons of Ishmael, by their names, according to their generations: the firstborn of Ishmael, Nebajoth; and Kedar, and Adbeel, and Mibsam,

14 And Mishma, and Dumah, and Massa,

15 Hadar, and Tema, Jetur, Naphish, and Kedemah:

16 These *are* the sons of Ishmael, and these *are* their names, by their towns, and by their castles; twelve princes according to their nations.

17 And these *are* the years of the life of Ishmael, an hundred and thirty and seven years: and he gave up the ghost and died; and was gathered unto his people.

18 And they dwelt from Havilah unto Shur, that *is* before Egypt, as thou goest toward Assyria: *and* he died in the presence of all his brethren.

The generations of Isaac.

19 And these *are* the generations of Isaac, Abraham's son: Abraham begat Isaac:

20 And Isaac was forty years old when he took Rebekah to wife, the daughter of Bethuel the Syrian of Padan-aram, the sister to Laban the Syrian.

21 And Isaac intreated the LORD for his wife, because she *was* barren: and the LORD was intreated of him, and Rebekah his wife conceived.

22 And the children struggled together within her; and she said, If *it be* so, why *am* I thus? And she went to enquire of the LORD.

23 And the LORD said unto her, Two nations *are* in thy womb, and two manner of people shall be separated from thy bowels; and *the one* people shall be stronger than *the other* people; and the [a]elder shall serve the younger.

The birth of Esau and Jacob.

24 And when her days to be delivered were fulfilled, behold, *there were* twins in her womb.

25 And the first came out red, all over like an hairy garment; and they called his name [1]Esau.

26 And after that came his brother out, and his hand took hold on Esau's heel; and his name was called Jacob: and Isaac *was* threescore years old when she bare them.

The sale of the birthright.

27 And the boys grew: and Esau was a cunning hunter, a man of the field; and Jacob *was* a plain man, dwelling in tents.

28 And Isaac loved Esau, because he did eat of *his* venison: but Rebekah loved Jacob.

29 And Jacob sod pottage: and Esau came from the field, and he *was* faint:

30 And Esau said to Jacob, Feed me, I pray thee, with that same red *pottage*; for I *am* faint: therefore was his name called [b]Edom.

31 And Jacob said, Sell me this day thy [2]birthright.

32 And Esau said, Behold, I *am* at the point to die: and what profit shall this birthright do to me?

33 And Jacob said, Swear to me this day; and he sware unto him: and he sold his birthright unto Jacob.

34 Then Jacob gave Esau bread and pottage of lentiles; and he did eat and drink, and rose up, and went his way: thus Esau despised *his* birthright.

CHAPTER 26.

The Abrahamic Covenant confirmed to Isaac.

And there was a [c]famine in the land, beside the first famine that was in the days of Abraham. And Isaac went unto Abimelech king of the Philistines unto Gerar.

2 And the LORD [d]appeared unto him, and said, [e]Go not down into Egypt; dwell in the land which I shall tell thee of:

a Cf. Rom. 9:12.

b i.e. *red.*

c See Gen. 12:10, *note.*

d *The theophanies.* vs. 2, 24; Gen. 35:9 (Gen. 12:7; Rev. 1:10.)

e Cf. Gen. 46:3, *note.*

[1] **(25:25)** Esau stands for the mere man of the earth (Heb. 12:16, 17). In many respects a nobler man, naturally, than Jacob, he was destitute of faith, and despised the birthright because it was a spiritual thing, of value only as there was faith to apprehend it.

[2] **(25:31)** The "birthright" had three elements: (1) Until the establishment of the Aaronic priesthood the head of the family exercised priestly rights. (2) The Abrahamic family held the Edenic promise of the Satan-Bruiser (Gen. 3:15)—Abel, Seth, Shem, Abraham, Isaac, *Esau.* (3) Esau, as the firstborn, was in the direct line of the Abrahamic promise of the Earth-Blesser (Gen. 12:3). For all that was revealed, in Esau might have been fulfilled those two great Messianic promises. This birthright Esau sold for a momentary fleshly gratification. Jacob's conception of the birthright at that time was, doubtless, carnal and inadequate, but his desire for it evidenced true faith.

3 [a]Sojourn in this land, and I will be with thee, and will bless thee; for unto thee, and unto thy seed, I will give all these countries, and I will perform the oath which I sware unto Abraham thy father;

4 And I will make thy seed to multiply as the stars of heaven, and will give unto thy seed all these countries; and in thy seed shall all the nations of the earth be blessed;

5 Because that Abraham obeyed my voice, and kept my charge, my commandments, my statutes, and my laws.

The lapse of Isaac. (Cf. Gen. 20:1–18.)

6 And Isaac dwelt in Gerar:

7 And the men of the place asked *him* of his wife; and he said, She *is* my sister: for he feared to say, *She is* my wife; lest, *said he,* the men of the place should kill me for Rebekah; because she *was* fair to look upon.

8 And it came to pass, when he had been there a long time, that Abimelech king of the Philistines looked out at a window, and saw, and, behold, Isaac *was* sporting with Rebekah his wife.

9 And Abimelech called Isaac, and said, Behold, of a surety she *is* thy wife: and how saidst thou, She *is* my sister? And Isaac said unto him, Because I said, Lest I die for her.

10 And Abimelech said, What *is* this thou hast done unto us? one of the people might lightly have lien with thy wife, and thou shouldest have brought guiltiness upon us.

11 And Abimelech charged all *his* people, saying, He that toucheth this man or his wife shall surely be put to death.

12 Then Isaac sowed in that land, and received in the same year an hundredfold: and the LORD blessed him.

13 And the man waxed great, and went forward, and grew until he became very great:

14 For he had possession of flocks, and possession of herds, and great store of servants: and the Philistines envied him.

B.C. 1804.

a *Israel (covenant).* vs. 2-5; Gen. 28:13-15. (Gen. 12:2, 3; Rom. 11:26.)

15 For all the wells which his father's servants had digged in the days of Abraham his father, the Philistines had stopped them, and filled them with earth.

16 And Abimelech said unto Isaac, Go from us; for thou art much mightier than we.

Isaac the well-digger.

17 And Isaac departed thence, and pitched his tent in the valley of Gerar, and dwelt there.

18 And Isaac digged again the wells of water, which they had digged in the days of Abraham his father; for the Philistines had stopped them after the death of Abraham: and he called their names after the names by which his father had called them.

19 And Isaac's servants digged in the valley, and found there a well of springing water.

20 And the herdmen of Gerar did strive with Isaac's herdmen, saying, The water *is* ours: and he called the [1]name of the well Esek; because they strove with him.

21 And they digged another well, and strove for that also: and he called the name of it Sitnah.

22 And he removed from thence, and digged another well; and for that they strove not: and he called the name of it Rehoboth; and he said, For now the LORD hath made room for us, and we shall be fruitful in the land.

23 And he went up from thence to Beer-sheba.

24 And the LORD appeared unto him the same night, and said, I *am* the God of Abraham thy father: fear not, for I *am* with thee, and will bless thee, and multiply thy seed for my servant Abraham's sake.

25 And he builded an altar there, and called upon the name of the LORD, and pitched his tent there: and there Isaac's servants digged a well.

26 Then Abimelech went to him from Gerar, and Ahuzzath one of his friends, and Phichol the chief captain of his army.

[1]**(26:20)** The wells of Genesis have significant names, and are associated with significant events: (1) Beer-lahai-roi, *the well of him that liveth and seeth me* (Gen. 16:14; 24:62; 25:11). (2) Beer-sheba, *the well of the oath* or *covenant* Gen. 21:25-33; 22:19; 26:23-25; 46:1-5). (3) Esek, *contention* (Gen. 26:20). (4) Sitnah *hatred* (Gen. 26:21). Esek and Sitnah were Isaac's own attempts at well-digging. Afterward, he dwelt by the old wells of his father. (5) Rehoboth, *enlargement* (Gen. 26:22).

B.C. 1804.

27 And Isaac said unto them, Wherefore come ye to me, seeing ye hate me, and have sent me away from you?

28 And they said, We saw certainly that the LORD was with thee: and we said, Let there be now an oath betwixt us, *even* betwixt us and thee, and let us make a covenant with thee;

29 That thou wilt do us no hurt, as we have not touched thee, and as we have done unto thee nothing but good, and have sent thee away in peace: thou *art* now the blessed of the LORD.

30 And he made them a feast, and they did eat and drink.

31 And they rose up betimes in the morning, and sware one to another: and Isaac sent them away, and they departed from him in peace.

32 And it came to pass the same day, that Isaac's servants came, and told him concerning the well which they had digged, and said unto him, We have found water.

33 And he called it Shebah: therefore the name of the city *is* Beer-sheba unto this day.

34 And Esau was forty years old when he took to wife Judith the daughter of Beeri the Hittite, and Bashemath the daughter of Elon the Hittite:

35 Which were a grief of mind unto Isaac and to Rebekah.

CHAPTER 27.

The stolen blessing.

And it came to pass, that when Isaac was old, and his eyes were dim, so that he could not see, he called Esau his eldest son, and said unto him, My son: and he said unto him, Behold, *here am* I.

2 And he said, Behold now, I am old, I know not the day of my death:

3 Now therefore take, I pray thee, thy weapons, thy quiver and thy bow, and go out to the field, and take me *some* venison;

4 And make me savoury meat, such as I love, and bring *it* to me, that I may eat; that my soul may bless thee before I die.

5 And Rebekah heard when Isaac spake to Esau his son. And Esau went to the field to hunt *for* venison, *and* to bring *it*.

6 And Rebekah spake unto Jacob her son, saying, Behold, I heard thy father speak unto Esau thy brother, saying,

7 Bring me venison, and make me savoury meat, that I may eat, and bless thee before the LORD before my death.

8 Now therefore, my son, obey my voice according to that which I command thee.

9 Go now to the flock, and fetch me from thence two good kids of the goats; and I will make them savoury meat for thy father, such as he loveth:

10 And thou shalt bring *it* to thy father, that he may eat, and that he may bless thee before his death.

11 And Jacob said to Rebekah his mother, Behold, Esau my brother *is* a hairy man, and I *am* a smooth man:

12 My father peradventure will feel me, and I shall seem to him as a deceiver; and I shall bring a curse upon me, and not a blessing.

13 And his mother said unto him, Upon me *be* thy curse, my son: only obey my voice, and go fetch me *them*.

14 And he went, and fetched, and brought *them* to his mother: and his mother made savoury meat, such as his father loved.

15 And Rebekah took goodly raiment of her eldest son Esau, which *were* with her in the house, and put them upon Jacob her younger son:

16 And she put the skins of the kids of the goats upon his hands, and upon the smooth of his neck:

17 And she gave the savoury meat and the bread, which she had prepared, into the hand of her son Jacob.

18 And he came unto his father, and said, My father: and he said, Here *am* I; who *art* thou, my son?

19 And Jacob said unto his father, I *am* Esau thy firstborn; I have done according as thou badest me: arise, I pray thee, sit and eat of my venison, that thy soul may bless me.

20 And Isaac said unto his son, How *is it* that thou hast found *it* so quickly, my son? And he said, Because the LORD thy God brought *it* to me.

21 And Isaac said unto Jacob, Come near, I pray thee, that I may feel thee, my son, whether thou *be* my very son Esau or not.

22 And Jacob went near unto Isaac his father; and he felt him, and said, The

voice *is* Jacob's voice, but the hands *are* the hands of Esau.

23 And he discerned him not, because his hands were hairy, as his brother Esau's hands: so he blessed him.

24 And he said, *Art* thou my very son Esau? And he said, I *am*.

25 And he said, Bring *it* near to me, and I will eat of my son's venison, that my soul may bless thee. And he brought *it* near to him, and he did eat: and he brought him wine, and he drank.

The blessing of Jacob.

26 And his father Isaac said unto him, Come near now, and kiss me, my son.

27 And he came near, and kissed him: and he smelled the smell of his raiment, and blessed him, and said, See, the smell of my son *is* as the smell of a field which the LORD hath blessed:

28 Therefore God give thee of the dew of heaven, and the fatness of the earth, and plenty of corn and wine:

29 Let people serve thee, and nations bow down to thee: be lord over thy brethren, and let thy mother's sons bow down to thee: [a]cursed *be* every one that curseth thee, and blessed *be* he that blesseth thee.

30 And it came to pass, as soon as Isaac had made an end of blessing Jacob, and Jacob was yet scarce gone out from the presence of Isaac his father, that Esau his brother came in from his hunting.

31 And he also had made savoury meat, and brought it unto his father, and said unto his father, Let my father arise, and eat of his son's venison, that thy soul may bless me.

32 And Isaac his father said unto him, Who *art* thou? And he said, I *am* thy son, thy firstborn Esau.

33 And [b]Isaac trembled very exceedingly, and said, Who? where *is* he that hath taken venison, and brought *it* me, and I have eaten of all before thou camest, and have blessed him? yea, *and* he shall be blessed.

Esau's unavailing remorse.
(See Heb. 12:16, 17.)

34 And when Esau heard the words of his father, he cried with a great and exceeding bitter cry, and said unto his father, Bless me, *even* me also, O my father.

35 And he said, Thy brother came with subtilty, and hath taken away thy blessing.

36 And he said, Is not he rightly named [c]Jacob? for he hath supplanted me these two times: he took away my birthright; and, behold, now he hath taken away my blessing. And he said, Hast thou not reserved a blessing for me?

37 And Isaac answered and said unto Esau, Behold, I have made him thy lord, and all his brethren have I given to him for servants; and with corn and wine have I sustained him: and what shall I do now unto thee, my son?

38 And Esau said unto his father, Hast thou but one blessing, my father? bless me, *even* me also, O my father. [d]And Esau lifted up his voice, and wept.

39 And Isaac his father answered and said unto him, Behold, thy dwelling shall be the fatness of the earth, and of the dew of heaven from above;

40 And by thy sword shalt thou live, and shalt serve thy brother; and it shall come to pass when thou shalt have the dominion, that thou shalt break his yoke from off thy neck.

41 And Esau hated Jacob because of the blessing wherewith his father blessed him: and Esau said in his heart, The days of mourning for my father are at hand; then will I slay my brother Jacob.

42 And these words of Esau her elder son were told to Rebekah: and she sent and called Jacob her younger son, and said unto him, Behold, thy brother Esau, as touching thee, doth comfort himself, *purposing* to kill thee.

43 Now therefore, my son, obey my voice; and arise, flee thou to Laban my brother to Haran;

44 And tarry with him a few days, until thy brother's fury turn away;

45 Until thy brother's anger turn away from thee, and he forget *that* which thou hast done to him: then I will send, and fetch thee from thence: why should I be deprived also of you both in one day?

46 And Rebekah said to Isaac, I am weary of my [e]life because of the daughters of Heth: if Jacob take a wife of the daughters of Heth, such as these *which are* of the daughters of the land, what good shall my life do me?

B.C. 1760.

a Gen. 12:3; 15:18, note 3, (5). Cf. Num. 24:9.

b trembled with a great trembling; greatly.

c i.e. *supplanter.*

d Esau wept because of a lost advantage, but found no way to change his mind, though he sought it carefully with tears" (Heb. 12:17)—so far may regret or remorse be from true repentance.

e Gen. 26:34-35. Heth was ancestor of the Hittites.

CHAPTER 28.

Jacob at Bethel: the Abrahamic Covenant confirmed to him.

B.C. 1760.

AND Isaac called Jacob, and blessed him, and charged him, and said unto him, Thou shalt not take a wife of the daughters of Canaan.

2 Arise, go to Padan-aram, to the house of Bethuel thy mother's father; and take thee a wife from thence of the daughters of Laban thy mother's brother.

3 And God Almighty bless thee, and make thee fruitful, and multiply thee, that thou mayest be a multitude of people;

4 And give thee the blessing of Abraham, to thee, and to thy seed with thee; that thou mayest inherit the land wherein thou art a stranger, which God gave unto Abraham.

5 And Isaac sent away Jacob: and he went to Padan-aram unto Laban, son of Bethuel the Syrian, the brother of Rebekah, Jacob's and Esau's mother.

6 When Esau saw that Isaac had blessed Jacob, and sent him away to Padan-aram, to take him a wife from thence; and that as he blessed him he gave him a charge, saying, Thou shalt not take a wife of the daughters of Canaan;

7 And that Jacob obeyed his father and his mother, and was gone to Padan-aram;

8 And Esau seeing that the daughters of Canaan pleased not Isaac his father;

9 Then went Esau unto Ishmael, and took unto the wives which he had [a]Mahalath the daughter of Ishmael Abraham's son, the sister of Nebajoth, to be his wife.

10 [1]And Jacob went out from Beer-sheba, and went toward Haran.

11 And he lighted upon a certain place, and tarried there all night, because the sun was set; and he took of the stones of that place, and put *them for* his pillows, and lay down in that place to sleep.

12 And he dreamed, and behold a ladder set up on the earth, and the top of it reached to heaven: and behold the [b]angels of God ascending and descending on it.

13 And, behold, the LORD stood above it, and said, I *am* the LORD God of Abraham thy father, and the God of Isaac: the [c]land whereon thou liest, to thee will I give it, and to thy seed;

14 And thy seed shall be as the dust of the earth, and thou shalt spread abroad to the west, and to the east, and to the north, and to the south: and in thee and in thy [d]seed shall all the families of the earth be blessed.

15 And, behold, I *am* with [e]thee, and will keep thee in all *places* whither thou goest, and will bring thee again into this land; for I will not leave thee, until I have done *that* which I have spoken to thee of.

16 And Jacob awaked out of his sleep, and he said, Surely the LORD is in this place; and I knew *it* not.

17 And he was afraid, and said, How dreadful *is* this place! this *is* none other but the house of God, and this *is* the gate of heaven.

18 And Jacob rose up early in the morning, and took the stone that he had put *for* his pillows, and set it up *for* a pillar, and poured oil upon the top of it.

19 And he called the name of that place [f]Beth-el: but the name of that city *was called* Luz at the first.

20 And Jacob vowed a vow, saying, If God will be with me, and will keep me in this way that I go, and will give me bread to eat, and raiment to put on,

21 So that I come again to my father's house in peace; then shall the LORD be my God:

22 And this stone, which I have set *for* a pillar, shall be God's house: and of all that thou shalt give me I will surely give the [g]tenth unto thee.

a Gen. 36:3 is called *Bashemath.*

b Heb. 1:4, *note.*

c *Israel (covenant).* vs. 13-15; Gen. 35:9-12. (Gen. 12:2, 3; Rom. 11:26.)

d *Christ (first advent).* Gen. 49:10. (Gen. 3:15; Acts 1:9.)

e Heb. 13:5.

f *i.e. the house of God.* Cf. Gen. 35:7.

g Gen. 14:20; Lev. 27:30.

[1] **(28:10)** Bethel becomes, because of Jacob's vision there, one of the significant places of Scripture. To the Christian it stands for a realization, however imperfect, of the heavenly and spiritual contents of faith, answering to Paul's prayer in Eph. 1:17-23. Dispensationally, the scene speaks of Israel the nation, cast out of the Land of Promise because of evil-doing there, but holding the promise of restoration and blessing (Gen. 28:15; Deut. 30:1-10, *refs.*). To "an Israelite indeed" Christ speaks of Jacob's vision as to be fulfilled in the Son of man (cf. Gen. 28:12; John 1:47-51).

CHAPTER 29.

B.C. 1760.

Jacob's years at Haran (to Gen. 31:10).

THEN Jacob went on his journey, and [1]came into the land of the people of the east.

2 And he looked, and behold a well in the field, and, lo, there *were* three flocks of sheep lying by it; for out of that well they watered the flocks: and a great stone *was* upon the well's mouth.

3 And thither were all the flocks gathered: and they rolled the stone from the well's mouth, and watered the sheep, and put the stone again upon the well's mouth in his place.

4 And Jacob said unto them, My brethren, whence *be* ye? And they said, Of Haran *are* we.

5 And he said unto them, Know ye Laban the son of Nahor? And they said, We know *him*.

6 And he said unto them, *Is* he well? And they said, *He is* well: and, behold, Rachel his daughter cometh with the sheep.

7 And he said, Lo, *it is* yet high day, neither *is it* time that the cattle should be gathered together: water ye the sheep, and go *and* feed *them*.

8 And they said, We cannot, until all the flocks be gathered together, and *till* they roll the stone from the well's mouth; then we water the sheep.

9 And while he yet spake with them, Rachel came with her father's sheep: for she kept them.

10 And it came to pass, when Jacob saw Rachel the daughter of Laban his mother's brother, and the sheep of Laban his mother's brother, that Jacob went near, and rolled the stone from the well's mouth, and watered the flock of Laban his mother's brother.

11 And Jacob kissed Rachel, and lifted up his voice, and wept.

12 And Jacob told Rachel that he *was* her father's brother, and that he *was* Rebekah's son: and she ran and told her father.

13 And it came to pass, when Laban heard the tidings of Jacob his sister's son, that he ran to meet him, and embraced him, and kissed him, and brought him to his house. And he told Laban all these things.

14 And Laban said to him, Surely thou *art* my bone and my flesh. And he abode with him the space of a month.

15 And Laban said unto Jacob, Because thou *art* my brother, shouldest thou therefore serve me for nought? tell me, what *shall* thy wages *be*?

16 And Laban had two daughters: the name of the elder *was* Leah, and the name of the younger *was* Rachel.

17 Leah *was* tender eyed; but Rachel was beautiful and well favoured.

18 And Jacob loved Rachel; and said, I will serve thee seven years for Rachel thy younger daughter.

19 And Laban said, *It is* better that I give her to thee, than that I should give her to another man: abide with me.

20 And Jacob served seven years for Rachel; and they seemed unto him *but* a few days, for the love he had to her.

21 And Jacob said unto Laban, Give *me* my wife, for my days are fulfilled, that I may go in unto her.

22 And Laban gathered together all the men of the place, and made a feast.

23 And it came to pass in the evening, that he took Leah his daughter, and brought her to him; and he went in unto her.

24 And Laban gave unto his daughter Leah Zilpah his maid *for* an handmaid.

25 And it came to pass, that in the morning, behold, it *was* Leah: and he said to Laban, What *is* this thou hast done unto me? did not I serve with thee for Rachel? wherefore then hast thou beguiled me?

26 And Laban said, It must not be so done in our country, to give the younger before the firstborn.

27 Fulfil her week, and we will give thee this also for the service which thou

[1]**(29:1)** Jacob at Haran becomes a striking illustration, if not type, of the nation descended from him in its present long dispersion. Like Israel, he was: (1) Out of the *place* of blessing (Gen. 26:3); (2) without an altar (Hos. 3:4, 5); (3) gained an evil name (Gen. 31:1; Rom. 2:17-24); (4) but was under the covenant care of Jehovah (Gen. 28:13, 14; Rom. 11:1, 25-30); (5) and was ultimately brought back (Gen. 31:3; 35:1-4; Ezk. 37:21-23).

The *personal* lesson is obvious: while Jacob is not forsaken, he is permitted to reap the shame and sorrow of his self-chosen way.

B.C. 1753.

shalt serve with me yet seven other years.

28 And Jacob did so, and fulfilled her week: and he gave him Rachel his daughter to wife also.

29 And Laban gave to Rachel his daughter Bilhah his handmaid to be her maid.

30 And he went in also unto Rachel, and he [a]loved also Rachel more than Leah, and served with him yet seven other years.

31 And when the LORD saw that Leah *was* hated, he opened her womb: but Rachel *was* barren.

32 And Leah conceived, and bare a son, and she called his name [b]Reuben: for she said, Surely the LORD hath looked upon my affliction; now therefore my husband will love me.

33 And she conceived again, and bare a son; and said, Because the LORD hath heard that I *was* hated, he hath therefore given me this *son* also: and she called his name [c]Simeon.

34 And she conceived again, and bare a son; and said, Now this time will my husband be joined unto me, because I have born him three sons: therefore was his name called [d]Levi.

35 And she conceived again, and bare a son: and she said, Now will I praise the LORD: therefore she called his name [e]Judah; and left bearing.

CHAPTER 30.

And when Rachel saw that she bare Jacob no children, Rachel envied her sister; and said unto Jacob, Give me children, or else I die.

2 And Jacob's anger was kindled against Rachel: and he said, *Am* I in God's stead, who hath withheld from thee the fruit of the womb?

3 And she said, Behold my maid Bilhah, go in unto her; and she shall bear upon my knees, that I may also have children by her.

4 And she gave him Bilhah her handmaid to wife: and Jacob went in unto her.

5 And Bilhah conceived, and bare Jacob a son.

6 And Rachel said, God hath judged me, and hath also heard my voice, and hath given me a son: therefore called she his name [f]Dan.

7 And Bilhah Rachel's maid conceived again, and bare Jacob a second son.

8 And Rachel said, With great wrestlings have I wrestled with my sister, and I have prevailed: and she called his name [g]Naphtali.

9 When Leah saw that she had left bearing, she took Zilpah her maid, and gave her Jacob to wife.

10 And Zilpah Leah's maid bare Jacob a son.

11 And Leah said, A troop cometh: and she called his name [h]Gad.

12 And Zilpah Leah's maid bare Jacob a second son.

13 And Leah said, Happy am I, for the daughters will call me blessed: and she called his name [i]Asher.

14 And Reuben went in the days of wheat harvest, and found mandrakes in the field, and brought them unto his mother Leah. Then Rachel said to Leah, Give me, I pray thee, of thy son's mandrakes.

15 And she said unto her, *Is it* a small matter that thou hast taken my husband? and wouldest thou take away my son's mandrakes also? And Rachel said, Therefore he shall lie with thee to night for thy son's mandrakes.

16 And Jacob came out of the field in the evening, and Leah went out to meet him, and said, Thou must come in unto me; for surely I have hired thee with my son's mandrakes. And he lay with her that night.

17 And God hearkened unto Leah, and she conceived, and bare Jacob the fifth son.

18 And Leah said, God hath given me my hire, because I have given my maiden to my husband: and she called his name [j]Issachar.

19 And Leah conceived again, and bare Jacob the sixth son.

20 And Leah said, God hath endued me *with* a good dowry; now will my husband dwell with me, because I have born him six sons: and she called his name [k]Zebulun.

21 And afterwards she bare a daughter, and called her name [l]Dinah.

22 And God remembered Rachel, and God hearkened to her, and opened her womb.

23 And she conceived, and bare a son; and said, God hath taken away my reproach:

24 And she called his name [m]Joseph; and said, The LORD shall add to me another son.

25 And it came to pass, when Rachel had born Joseph, that Jacob said unto

a v. 20; cf. Deut. 21:15-17.
b i.e. *see, a son.*
c i.e. *hearing.*
d i.e. *joined.* Num. 18:2-4.
e i.e. *praise.*
f i.e. *judging.*
g i.e. *wrestling.*
h i.e. *a troop.*
i i.e. *happy.*
j i.e. *hire.*
k i.e. *dwelling.*
l i.e. *judgment.*
m i.e. *adding.*

Laban, Send me away, that I may go unto
mine own place, and to my country.
26 Give *me* my wives and my children,
for whom I have served thee, and let me
go: for thou knowest my service which I
have done thee.
27 And Laban said unto him, I pray
thee, if I have found favour in thine eyes,
tarry: for I have learned by experience that
the LORD hath blessed me for thy sake.
28 And he said, Appoint me thy
wages, and I will give *it*.
29 And he said unto him, Thou knowest how I have served thee, and how thy
cattle was with me.
30 For *it was* little which thou hadst
before I *came*, and it is *now* increased unto
a multitude; and the LORD hath blessed
thee since my coming: and now when
shall I provide for mine own house also?
31 And he said, What shall I give thee?
And Jacob said, Thou shalt not give me
any thing: if thou wilt do this thing for
me, I will again feed *and* keep thy flock:
32 I will pass through all thy flock to
day, removing from thence all the speckled and spotted cattle, and all the brown
cattle among the sheep, and the spotted
and speckled among the goats: and *of
such* shall be my [a]hire.
33 So shall my righteousness answer for
me in time to come, when it shall come
for my hire before thy face: every one that
is not speckled and spotted among the
goats, and brown among the sheep, that
shall be counted stolen with me.
34 And Laban said, Behold, I would it
might be according to thy word.
35 And he removed that day the he
goats that were ringstraked and spotted,
and all the she goats that were speckled
and spotted, *and* every one that had *some*
white in it, and all the brown among the
sheep, and gave *them* into the hand of
his sons.
36 And he set three days' journey
betwixt himself and Jacob: and Jacob fed
the rest of Laban's flocks.
37 And Jacob took him rods of green
poplar, and of the hazel and chesnut
tree; and pilled white strakes in them,
and made the white appear which *was* in
the rods.
38 And he set the rods which he had
pilled before the flocks in the gutters in
the watering troughs when the flocks

B.C. 1746.

a Gen. 31:8.

b Gen. 31:9-12.

c v. 30.

d Gen. 28:15; 46:4.

e vs. 2, 3.

f vs. 38-41; cf. Gen. 30:29.

came to drink, that they should conceive
when they came to drink.
39 And the flocks conceived before the
rods, and brought forth cattle [b]ring-
straked, speckled, and spotted.
40 And Jacob did separate the lambs,
and set the faces of the flocks toward the
ringstraked, and all the brown in the
flock of Laban; and he put his own
flocks by themselves, and put them not
unto Laban's cattle.
41 And it came to pass, whensoever
the stronger cattle did conceive, that
Jacob laid the rods before the eyes of the
cattle in the gutters, that they might conceive among the rods.
42 But when the cattle were feeble, he
put *them* not in: so the feebler were
Laban's, and the stronger Jacob's.
43 And the [c]man increased exceedingly,
and had much cattle, and maidservants,
and menservants, and camels, and asses.

CHAPTER 31.

And he heard the words of Laban's
sons, saying, Jacob hath taken
away all that *was* our father's; and of
that which *was* our father's hath he gotten all this glory.
2 And Jacob beheld the countenance
of Laban, and, behold, it *was* not toward
him as before.
3 And the LORD said unto Jacob,
Return unto the land of thy fathers, and
to thy kindred; and I will [d]be with thee.
4 And Jacob sent and called Rachel
and Leah to the field unto his flock,
5 And said unto them, I see your
father's countenance, that it *is* not
toward me as before; but the God of my
father [e]hath been with me.
6 And ye know that with all my
power I have [f]served your father.
7 And your father hath deceived me,
and changed my wages ten times; but
God suffered him not to hurt me.
8 If he said thus, The speckled shall be
thy wages; then all the cattle bare speckled: and if he said thus, The ringstraked
shall be thy hire; then bare all the cattle
ringstraked.
9 Thus God hath taken away the cattle
of your father, and given *them* to me.
10 And it came to pass at the time

that the cattle conceived, that I lifted up
mine eyes, and saw in a dream, and,
behold, the rams which leaped upon the
cattle *were* ringstraked, speckled, and
grisled.

Parenthesis: the call back to Bethel
(vs. 11–13).

11 And the [a]angel of God spake unto
me in a dream, *saying*, Jacob: And I said,
Here *am* I.
12 And he said, Lift up now thine
eyes, and see, all the rams which leap
upon the cattle *are* ringstraked, speckled,
and grisled: for I have seen all that
Laban doeth unto thee.
13 I *am* the [b]God of Beth-el, where
thou anointedst the pillar, *and* where
thou vowedst a vow unto me: now arise,
get thee out from this land, and [c]return
unto the land of thy kindred.

The flight of Jacob.

14 And Rachel and Leah answered and
said unto him, *Is there* yet any portion or
inheritance for us in our father's house?
15 Are we not counted of him
strangers? for he hath sold us, and hath
quite devoured also our money.
16 For all the riches which God hath
taken from our father, that *is* ours, and
our children's: now then, whatsoever
God hath said unto thee, do.
17 Then Jacob rose up, and set his sons
and his wives upon camels;
18 And he carried away all his cattle,
and all his goods which he had gotten,
the cattle of his getting, which he had
gotten in Padan-aram, for to go to Isaac
his father in the land of Canaan.
19 And Laban went to shear his sheep:
and Rachel had stolen the images that
were her father's.
20 And Jacob stole away unawares to
Laban the Syrian, in that he told him not
that he fled.
21 So he fled with all that he had; and
he rose up, and passed over the river,
and set his face *toward* the mount Gilead.
22 And it was told Laban on the third
day that Jacob was fled.
23 And he took his brethren with him,
and pursued after him seven days' journey; and they overtook him in the
mount Gilead.
24 And God came to Laban the Syrian
in a [d]dream by night, and said unto him,
Take heed that thou speak not to Jacob
either good or bad.
25 Then Laban overtook Jacob. Now
Jacob had pitched his tent in the mount:
and Laban with his brethren pitched in
the mount of Gilead.
26 And Laban said to Jacob, What hast
thou done, that thou hast stolen away
unawares to me, and carried away my
daughters, as captives *taken* with the
sword?
27 Wherefore didst thou flee away
secretly, and steal away from me; and
didst not tell me, that I might have sent
thee away with mirth, and with songs,
with tabret, and with harp?
28 And hast not suffered me to kiss
my sons and my daughters? thou hast
now done foolishly in *so* doing.
29 It is in the power of my hand to do
you hurt: but the God of your father
spake unto me yesternight, saying, Take
thou heed that thou speak not to Jacob
either good or bad.
30 And now, *though* thou wouldest
needs be gone, because thou sore
longedst after thy father's house, *yet*
wherefore hast thou [e]stolen my gods?
31 And Jacob answered and said to
Laban, Because I was afraid: for I said,
Peradventure thou wouldest take by
force thy daughters from me.
32 With whomsoever thou findest thy
gods, let him not live: before our
brethren discern thou what *is* thine with
me, and take *it* to thee. For Jacob knew
not that Rachel had stolen them.
33 And Laban went into Jacob's tent,
and into Leah's tent, and into the two
maidservants' tents; but he found *them*
not. Then went he out of Leah's tent,
and entered into Rachel's tent.
34 Now Rachel had taken the images,
and put them in the camel's furniture,
and sat upon them. And Laban searched
all the tent, but found *them* not.
35 And she said to her father, Let it not
displease my lord that I cannot rise up
before thee; for the custom of women *is*
upon me. And he searched, but found
not the images.
36 And Jacob was wroth, and chode
with Laban: and Jacob answered and
said to Laban, What *is* my trespass?

B.C. 1739.

a Heb. 1:4, *note*.
b Gen. 28:16-22.
c v. 3.
d Cf. v. 10; Gen. 20:3; 46:2-4.
e v. 19.

what *is* my sin, that thou hast so hotly
pursued after me?
37 Whereas thou hast searched all my
stuff, what hast thou found of all thy
household stuff? set *it* here before my
brethren and thy brethren, that they may
judge betwixt us both.
38 This twenty years *have* I *been* with
thee; thy ewes and thy she goats have
not cast their young, and the rams of thy
flock have I not eaten.
39 That which was torn *of beasts* I
brought not unto thee; I bare the [a]loss of
it; of my hand didst thou require it,
whether stolen by day, or stolen by night.
40 *Thus* I was; in the day the drought
consumed me, and the frost by night;
and my sleep departed from mine eyes.
41 Thus have I been twenty years in
thy house; I served thee fourteen years
for thy two daughters, and six years for
thy cattle: and thou hast changed my
wages ten times.
42 Except the God of my father, the
God of Abraham, and the fear of Isaac,
had been with me, surely thou hadst
sent me away now empty. God hath
seen mine affliction and the labour of
my hands, and rebuked *thee* yesternight.
43 And Laban answered and said unto
Jacob, *These* daughters *are* my daughters,
and *these* children *are* my children, and
these cattle *are* my cattle, and all that thou
seest *is* mine: and what can I do this day
unto these my daughters, or unto their
children which they have born?
44 Now therefore come thou, let us
make a covenant, I and thou; and let it
be for a witness between me and thee.
45 And Jacob took a stone, and set it
up *for* a pillar.
46 And Jacob said unto his brethren,
Gather stones; and they took stones, and
made an heap: and they did eat there
upon the heap.
47 And Laban called it [b]Jegar-
sahadutha: but Jacob called it [c]Galeed.
48 And Laban said, This heap *is* a witness between me and thee this day.
Therefore was the name of it called
Galeed;
49 And [d]Mizpah; for he said, The
LORD watch between me and thee, when
we are absent one from another.
50 If thou shalt afflict my daughters,

B.C. 1739.

a Ex. 22:10-13.

b Chald. *the heap of witness.*

c Heb. *the heap of witness.*

d i.e. *beacon, in the sense of watch-tower.*

e Heb. 1:4, *note.*

f i.e. *two hosts, or bands*—the visible band, Jacob and his servants; the invisible band, God's angels. Cf. 2 Ki. 6:13-17.

g i.e. *Esau's country.* Gen. 25:30. See Gen. 36:1, *note.*

or if thou shalt take *other* wives beside
my daughters, no man *is* with us; see,
God *is* witness betwixt me and thee.
51 And Laban said to Jacob, Behold
this heap, and behold *this* pillar, which I
have cast betwixt me and thee;
52 This heap *be* witness, and *this* pillar
be witness, that I will not pass over this
heap to thee, and that thou shalt not
pass over this heap and this pillar unto
me, for harm.
53 The God of Abraham, and the God
of Nahor, the God of their father, judge
betwixt us. And Jacob sware by the fear
of his father Isaac.
54 Then Jacob offered sacrifice upon
the mount, and called his brethren to eat
bread: and they did eat bread, and tarried all night in the mount.
55 And early in the morning Laban
rose up, and kissed his sons and his
daughters, and blessed them: and Laban
departed, and returned unto his place.

CHAPTER 32.

Jacob ("supplanter") becomes Israel ("a prince with God").

And Jacob went on his way, and the
[e]angels of God met him.
2 And when Jacob saw them, he said,
This *is* God's host: and he called the
name of that place [f]Mahanaim.
3 And Jacob sent messengers before
him to Esau his brother unto the land of
Seir, the country of [g]Edom.
4 And he commanded them, saying,
Thus shall ye speak unto my lord Esau;
Thy servant Jacob saith thus, I have
sojourned with Laban, and stayed there
until now:
5 And I have oxen, and asses, flocks,
and menservants, and womenservants:
and I have sent to tell my lord, that I
may find grace in thy sight.
6 And the messengers returned to
Jacob, saying, We came to thy brother
Esau, and also he cometh to meet thee,
and four hundred men with him.
7 Then Jacob was greatly afraid and
distressed: and he divided the people
that *was* with him, and the flocks, and
herds, and the camels, into two bands;
8 And said, If Esau come to the

one company, and smite it, then the other company which is left shall escape.

9 And [a]Jacob said, O God of my father Abraham, and God of my father Isaac, the LORD which saidst unto me, Return unto thy country, and to thy kindred, and I will deal well with thee:

10 I am not worthy of the least of all the mercies, and of all the truth, which thou hast shewed unto thy servant; for with my staff I passed over this Jordan; and now I am become two bands.

11 Deliver me, I pray thee, from the hand of my brother, from the hand of Esau: for I fear him, lest he will come and smite me, *and* the mother with the children.

12 And thou saidst, I will surely do thee good, and make thy seed as the sand of the sea, which cannot be numbered for multitude.

13 And he lodged there that same night; and took of that which came to his hand a present for Esau his brother;

14 Two hundred she goats, and twenty he goats, two hundred ewes, and twenty rams,

15 Thirty milch camels with their colts, forty kine, and ten bulls, twenty she asses, and ten foals.

16 And he delivered *them* into the hand of his servants, every drove by themselves; and said unto his servants, Pass over before me, and put a space betwixt drove and drove.

17 And he commanded the foremost, saying, When Esau my brother meeteth thee, and asketh thee, saying, Whose *art* thou? and whither goest thou? and whose *are* these before thee?

18 Then thou shalt say, *They be* thy servant Jacob's; it *is* a present sent unto my lord Esau: and, behold, also he *is* behind us.

19 And so commanded he the second, and the third, and all that followed the droves, saying, On this manner shall ye speak unto Esau, when ye find him.

20 And say ye moreover, Behold, thy servant Jacob *is* behind us. For he said, I will appease him with the present that goeth before me, and afterward I will see his face; peradventure he will accept of me.

21 So went the present over before him: and himself lodged that night in the company.

22 And he rose up that night, and took his two wives, and his two womenservants, and his eleven sons, and passed over the ford Jabbok.

23 And he took them, and sent them over the brook, and sent over that he had.

24 And Jacob was left alone; [b]and there wrestled a man with him until the breaking of the day.

25 And when he saw that he prevailed not against him, he touched the hollow of his thigh; and the hollow of Jacob's thigh was out of joint, as he wrestled with him.

26 And he said, Let me go, for the day breaketh. And he said, I will not let thee go, except thou bless me.

27 And he said unto him, What *is* thy name? And he said, Jacob.

28 And he said, Thy name shall be called no more [1]Jacob, but [c]Israel: for as a prince hast thou power with God and with men, and hast prevailed.

29 And Jacob asked *him*, and said, Tell *me*, I pray thee, thy name. And he said, Wherefore *is* it *that* thou dost ask after my name? And he blessed him there.

30 And Jacob called the name of the place [d]Peniel: for I have [e]seen God face to face, and my life is preserved.

31 And as he passed over Penuel the sun rose upon him, and he halted upon his thigh.

32 Therefore the children of Israel eat not *of* the sinew which shrank, which *is* upon the hollow of the thigh, unto this day: because he touched the hollow of Jacob's thigh in the sinew that shrank.

CHAPTER 33.

Jacob meets Esau.

And Jacob lifted up his eyes, and looked, and, behold, Esau came, and with him four hundred men.

B.C. 1739.

a *Bible prayers* (O.T.). vs. 9-11; Ex. 32:11. (Gen. 15:2; Hab. 3:1-16.)

b Jacob's crisis. Cf. Josh. 5:13-15; Job 42:5-6; Isa. 6:1-8; Jer. 1:4-9; Ezk. 1:28; 2:1-7; Dan. 10:1-12; Acts 9:1-6; Rev. 1:13-18.

c i.e. *a prince of (or with) God.*

d i.e. *the face of God.*

e Ex. 24:11; 33:20; Deut. 34:10; Jud. 13:22, 23; Isa. 6:5; John 1:18.

[1] **(32:28)** Both names are applied to the nation descended from Jacob. When used *characteristically* "Jacob" is the name for the natural posterity of Abraham, Isaac, and Jacob; "Israel" for the spiritual part of the nation. See, e.g. Isa. 9:8. The "word" was sent to all the people, "Jacob," but it "lighted upon *Israel*," i.e. was comprehended by the spiritual part of the people. See "Israel" (Gen. 12:2, 3; Rom. 11:26, *summary*).

And he divided the children unto Leah, and unto Rachel, and unto the two handmaids.

2 And he put the handmaids and their children foremost, and Leah and her children after, and Rachel and Joseph hindermost.

3 And he passed over before them, and bowed himself to the ground seven times, until he came near to his brother.

4 And Esau ran to meet him, and embraced him, and fell on his neck, and kissed him: and they wept.

5 And he lifted up his eyes, and saw the women and the children; and said, Who *are* those with thee? And he said, The children which God hath graciously given thy servant.

6 Then the handmaidens came near, they and their children, and they bowed themselves.

7 And Leah also with her children came near, and bowed themselves: and after came Joseph near and Rachel, and they bowed themselves.

8 And he said, What *meanest* thou by all this drove which I met? And he said, *These are* to find grace in the sight of my lord.

9 And Esau said, I have enough, my brother; keep that thou hast unto thyself.

10 And Jacob said, Nay, I pray thee, if now I have found grace in thy sight, then receive my present at my hand: for therefore I have seen thy face, as though I had seen the face of God, and thou wast pleased with me.

11 Take, I pray thee, my blessing that is brought to thee; because God hath dealt graciously with me, and because I have enough. And he urged him, and he took *it*.

12 And he said, Let us take our journey, and let us go, and I will go before thee.

13 And he said unto him, [a]My lord knoweth that the children *are* tender, and the flocks and herds with young *are* with me: and if men should overdrive them one day, all the flock will die.

14 Let my lord, I pray thee, pass over before his servant: and I will lead on softly, according as the cattle that goeth before me and the children be able to endure, until I come unto my lord unto Seir.

15 And Esau said, Let me now leave with thee *some* of the folk that *are* with me. And he said, What needeth it? let me find grace in the sight of my lord.

16 So Esau returned that day on his way unto Seir.

B.C. 1739.

17 And Jacob journeyed to Succoth, and built him an house, and made booths for his cattle: therefore the name of the place is called [b]Succoth.

Jacob's worship in self-will.

18 And Jacob came to Shalem, a city of Shechem, which *is* in the land of Canaan, when he came from Padan-aram; and pitched his tent before the city.

19 And he bought a parcel of a field, where he had spread his tent, at the hand of the children of Hamor, [c]Shechem's father, for an hundred pieces of money.

20 And he erected there an altar, and called it [d]El-elohe-Israel.

CHAPTER 34.

Jacob reaps the harvest of his evil years (Gal. 6:7, 8).

And Dinah the daughter of Leah, which she bare unto Jacob, went out to see the daughters of the land.

2 And when Shechem the son of Hamor the Hivite, prince of the country, saw her, he took her, and lay with her, and defiled her.

3 And his soul clave unto Dinah the daughter of Jacob, and he loved the damsel, and spake kindly unto the damsel.

4 And Shechem spake unto his father Hamor, saying, Get me this damsel to wife.

5 And Jacob heard that he had defiled Dinah his daughter: now his sons were with his cattle in the field: and Jacob held his peace until they were come.

6 And Hamor the father of Shechem went out unto Jacob to commune with him.

7 And the sons of Jacob came out of the field when they heard *it*: and the men were grieved, and they were very wroth, because he had wrought folly in Israel in lying with Jacob's daughter; which thing ought not to be done.

8 And Hamor communed with them, saying, The soul of my son Shechem longeth for your daughter: I pray you give her him to wife.

9 And make ye marriages with us, *and* give your daughters unto us, and take our daughters unto you.

10 And ye shall dwell with us: and the land shall be before you; dwell and

a Not all at once does "Jacob" cease to dominate the walk of "Israel." Cf. Gen. 35:1-10, where the walk becomes according to the new *name*.

b i.e. *booths (of branches).*

c Called "*Sychem,*" Acts 7:16.

d i.e. *God, the God of Israel.* Jacob's act of faith, appropriating his new name, but claiming Elohim in this new sense as the God through whom alone he could walk according to his new name. See Gen. 14:18-23, *note,* for a similar appropriation by Abraham.

trade ye therein, and get you possessions therein.

11 And Shechem said unto her father and unto her brethren, Let me find grace in your eyes, and what ye shall say unto me I will give.

12 Ask me never so much dowry and gift, and I will give according as ye shall say unto me: but give me the damsel to wife.

13 And the sons of Jacob answered Shechem and Hamor his father deceitfully, and said, because he had defiled Dinah their sister:

14 And they said unto them, We cannot do this thing, to give our sister to one that is uncircumcised; for that *were* a reproach unto us:

15 But in this will we consent unto you: If ye will be as we *be*, that every male of you be circumcised;

16 Then will we give our daughters unto you, and we will take your daughters to us, and we will dwell with you, and we will become one people.

17 But if ye will not hearken unto us, to be circumcised; then will we take our daughter, and we will be gone.

18 And their words pleased Hamor, and Shechem Hamor's son.

19 And the young man deferred not to do the thing, because he had delight in Jacob's daughter: and he *was* more honourable than all the house of his father.

20 And Hamor and Shechem his son came unto the gate of their city, and communed with the men of their city, saying,

21 These men *are* peaceable with us; therefore let them dwell in the land, and trade therein; for the land, behold, *it is* large enough for them; let us take their daughters to us for wives, and let us give them our daughters.

22 Only herein will the men consent unto us for to dwell with us, to be one people, if every male among us be circumcised, as they *are* circumcised.

23 *Shall* not their cattle and their substance and every beast of theirs *be* ours? only let us consent unto them, and they will dwell with us.

24 And unto Hamor and unto Shechem his son hearkened all that went out of the gate of his city; and every male was circumcised, all that went out of the gate of his city.

B.C. 1732.

25 And it came to pass on the third day, when they were sore, that two of the sons of Jacob, Simeon and Levi, Dinah's brethren, took each man his sword, and came upon the city boldly, and slew all the males.

26 And they slew Hamor and Shechem his son with the edge of the sword, and took Dinah out of Shechem's house, and went out.

27 The sons of Jacob came upon the slain, and spoiled the city, because they had defiled their sister.

28 They took their sheep, and their oxen, and their asses, and that which *was* in the city, and that which *was* in the field,

29 And all their wealth, and all their little ones, and their wives took they captive, and spoiled even all that *was* in the house.

30 And Jacob said to Simeon and Levi, Ye have troubled me to make me to stink among the inhabitants of the land, among the Canaanites and the Perizzites: and I *being* few in number, they shall gather themselves together against me, and slay me; and I shall be destroyed, I and my house.

31 And they said, Should he deal with our sister as with an harlot?

CHAPTER 35.

Jacob's return to Bethel: communion and promise restored.

And God said unto Jacob, Arise, go up to Beth-el, and dwell there: and make there an altar unto God, that appeared unto thee when thou fleddest from the face of Esau thy brother.

2 Then Jacob said unto his household, and to all that *were* with him, Put away the strange gods that *are* among you, and be clean, and change your garments:

3 And let us arise, and go up to Beth-el; and I will make there an altar unto God, who answered me in the day of my distress, and was with me in the way which I went.

4 And they gave unto Jacob all the strange gods which *were* in their hand, and *all their* earrings which *were* in their ears; and Jacob hid them under the oak which *was* by Shechem.

5 And they journeyed: and the terror of God was upon the cities that *were* round about them, and they did not pursue after the sons of Jacob.

6 So Jacob came to Luz, which *is*

in the land of Canaan, that *is,* Beth-el, he and all the people that *were* with him.

7 And he built there an altar, and called the place [1]El-beth-el: because there God appeared unto him, when he fled from the face of his brother.

8 But Deborah Rebekah's nurse died, and she was buried beneath Beth-el under an oak: and the name of it was called [a]Allon-bachuth.

9 And God [b]appeared unto Jacob again, when he came out of Padan-aram, and blessed him.

10 And God said unto him, Thy name *is* Jacob: thy name shall not be called any more Jacob, but Israel shall be thy name: and he called his name Israel.

11 And God said unto him, I *am* [c]God Almighty: be fruitful and multiply; a nation and a company of nations shall be of thee, and kings shall come out of thy loins;

12 And the land which I gave Abraham and Isaac, to thee I will give it, and to thy seed after thee will I give the land.

13 And God went up from him in the place where he talked with him.

14 And Jacob set up a pillar in the place where he talked with him, *even* a pillar of stone: and he poured a [2]drink-offering thereon, and he poured oil thereon.

15 And Jacob called the name of the place where God spake with him, Beth-el.

Death of Rachel and birth of Benjamin.

16 And they journeyed from Beth-el; and there was but a little way to come to Ephrath: and Rachel travailed, and she had hard labour.

17 And it came to pass, when she was in hard labour, that the midwife said unto her, Fear not; thou shalt have this son also.

18 And it came to pass, as her soul was in departing, (for she died) that she called his name [d]Ben-oni: but his father called him [3]Benjamin.

19 And Rachel died, and was buried in the way to Ephrath, which *is* Beth-lehem.

20 And Jacob set a pillar upon her grave: that *is* the pillar of Rachel's grave unto this day.

21 And Israel journeyed, and spread his tent beyond the tower of Edar.

22 And it came to pass, when Israel dwelt in that land, that Reuben went and lay with Bilhah his father's concubine: and Israel heard *it.* Now the sons of Jacob were twelve:

23 The sons of Leah; Reuben, Jacob's firstborn, and Simeon, and Levi, and Judah, and Issachar, and Zebulun:

24 The sons of Rachel; Joseph, and Benjamin:

25 And the sons of Bilhah, Rachel's handmaid; Dan, and Naphtali:

26 And the sons of Zilpah, Leah's handmaid; Gad, and Asher: these *are* the sons of Jacob, which were born to him in Padan-aram.

Death of Isaac.

27 And Jacob came unto Isaac his father unto Mamre, unto the city of Arbah, which *is* Hebron, where Abraham and Isaac sojourned.

28 And the days of Isaac were an hundred and fourscore years.

29 And Isaac gave up the ghost, and died, and was gathered unto his people,

B.C. 1732.

a i.e. *the oak of weeping.*

b *The theophanies.* Ezk. 40:3. (Gen. 12:7; Rev. 1:9.)

c *Deity (names of).* Ex. 3:13-15. (Gen. 1:1; Mal. 3:18.)

d i.e. *son of sorrow.*

[1] **(35:7)** i.e. *the God of Bethel.* Cf. Gen. 28:19. There it was the *place* as scene of the ladder-vision which impressed Jacob. He called the place "Bethel," i.e. *the house of God.* Now it is the *God* of the place, rather than the *place,* and he calls it El-Bethel, i.e. *"the God of the house of God."* Cf. Gen. 33:20, *ref.*

[2] **(35:14)** The first mention of the drink-offering. It is not mentioned among the Levitical offerings of Lev. 1–7, though included in the instructions for sacrifice *in the land* (Num. 15:5-7). It was always "poured out," never drunk, and may be considered a type of Christ in the sense of Psa. 22:14; Isa. 53:12.

[3] **(35:18)** i.e. *son of my right hand.* Benjamin, *"son of sorrow"* to his mother, but *"son of my right hand"* to his father, becomes thus a double type of Christ. As Ben-oni He was the suffering One because of whom a sword pierced His mother's heart (Lk. 2:35); as Benjamin, head of the warrior tribe (Gen. 49:27), firmly joined to Judah the kingly tribe (Gen. 49:8-12; 1 Ki. 12:21), he becomes a type of the victorious One. It is noteworthy that Benjamin was especially honoured among the Gentiles (Gen. 45:22).

So manifold are the distinctions of Christ that *many* personal types of Him are needed. Joseph is most complete, Benjamin standing only for Christ the sorrowful One (Isa. 53:3, 4) yet to have power on earth. Cf. Gen. 43:34, *note.*

being old and full of days: and his sons Esau and Jacob buried him.

CHAPTER 36.

The generations of Esau (Edom).

NOW these *are* the generations of Esau, who *is* [1]Edom.

2 Esau took his wives of the daughters of Canaan; Adah the daughter of Elon the Hittite, and Aholibamah the daughter of Anah the daughter of Zibeon the Hivite;

3 And Bashemath Ishmael's daughter, sister of Nebajoth.

4 And Adah bare to Esau Eliphaz; and Bashemath bare Reuel;

5 And Aholibamah bare Jeush, and Jaalam, and Korah: these *are* the sons of Esau, which were born unto him in the land of Canaan.

6 And Esau took his wives, and his sons, and his daughters, and all the persons of his house, and his cattle, and all his beasts, and all his substance, which he had got in the land of Canaan; and went into the country from the face of his brother Jacob.

7 For their riches were more than that they might dwell together; and the land wherein they were strangers could not bear them because of their cattle.

8 Thus dwelt Esau in mount Seir: Esau *is* Edom.

9 And these *are* the generations of Esau the father of the Edomites in mount Seir:

10 These *are* the names of Esau's sons; Eliphaz the son of Adah the wife of Esau, Reuel the son of Bashemath the wife of Esau.

11 And the sons of Eliphaz were Teman, Omar, Zepho, and Gatam, and Kenaz.

12 And Timna was concubine to Eliphaz Esau's son; and she bare to Eliphaz [a]Amalek: these *were* the sons of Adah Esau's wife.

13 And these *are* the sons of Reuel; Nahath, and Zerah, Shammah, and Mizzah: these were the sons of Bashemath Esau's wife.

B.C. 1796.

a 1 Sam. 15:1-33. See Ex. 17:8, *note.*

b Lit. *chiefs of thousands.*

c Lit. *Rock dweller.*

14 And these were the sons of Aholibamah, the daughter of Anah the daughter of Zibeon, Esau's wife: and she bare to Esau Jeush, and Jaalam, and Korah.

15 These *were* [b]dukes of the sons of Esau: the sons of Eliphaz the firstborn *son* of Esau; duke Teman, duke Omar, duke Zepho, duke Kenaz,

16 Duke Korah, duke Gatam, *and* duke Amalek: these *are* the dukes *that came* of Eliphaz in the land of Edom; these *were* the sons of Adah.

17 And these *are* the sons of Reuel Esau's son; duke Nahath, duke Zerah, duke Shammah, duke Mizzah: these *are* the dukes *that came* of Reuel in the land of Edom; these *are* the sons of Bashemath Esau's wife.

18 And these *are* the sons of Aholibamah Esau's wife; duke Jeush, duke Jaalam, duke Korah: these *were* the dukes *that came* of Aholibamah the daughter of Anah, Esau's wife.

19 These *are* the sons of Esau, who *is* Edom, and these *are* their dukes.

20 These *are* the sons of Seir the [c]Horite, who inhabited the land; Lotan, and Shobal, and Zibeon, and Anah,

21 And Dishon, and Ezer, and Dishan: these *are* the dukes of the Horites, the children of Seir in the land of Edom.

22 And the children of Lotan were Hori and Hemam; and Lotan's sister *was* Timna.

23 And the children of Shobal *were* these; Alvan, and Manahath, and Ebal, Shepho, and Onam.

24 And these *are* the children of Zibeon; both Ajah, and Anah: this *was that* Anah that found the mules in the wilderness, as he fed the asses of Zibeon his father.

25 And the children of Anah *were* these; Dishon, and Aholibamah the daughter of Anah.

26 And these *are* the children of Dishon; Hemdan, and Eshban, and Ithran, and Cheran.

27 The children of Ezer *are* these; Bilhan, and Zaavan, and Akan.

[1]**(36:1)** Edom (called also "Seir," Gen. 32:3; 36:8) is the name of the country lying south of the ancient kingdom of Judah, and extending from the Dead Sea to the Gulf of Akaba. It includes the ruins of Petra, and is bounded on the north by Moab. Peopled by descendants of Esau (Gen. 36:1-19), Edom has a remarkable prominence in the prophetic word as (together with Moab) the scene of the final destruction of Gentile world-power in the day of the Lord. See "Armageddon" (Rev. 16:14; Rev. 19:21) and "Times of the Gentiles" (Lk. 21:24; Rev. 16:14). Cf. Psa. 137:7; Oba. 8-16; Isa. 34:1-8; 63:1-6; Jer. 49:14-22; Ezk. 25:12-14.

28 The children of Dishan *are* these;
Uz, and Aran.
29 These *are* the dukes *that came* of the
Horites; duke Lotan, duke Shobal, duke
Zibeon, duke Anah,
30 Duke Dishon, duke Ezer, duke
Dishan: these *are* the dukes *that came* of
Hori, among their dukes in the land of
Seir.
31 [1]And these *are* the kings that
reigned in the land of Edom, before
there reigned any king over the children
of Israel.
32 And Bela the son of Beor reigned in
Edom: and the name of his city *was*
Dinhabah.
33 And Bela died, and Jobab the son of
Zerah of Bozrah reigned in his stead.
34 And Jobab died, and Husham of
the land of Temani reigned in his stead.
35 And Husham died, and Hadad the
son of Bedad, who smote Midian in the
field of Moab, reigned in his stead: and
the name of his city *was* Avith.
36 And Hadad died, and Samlah of
Masrekah reigned in his stead.
37 And Samlah died, and Saul of
Rehoboth *by* the river reigned in his
stead.
38 And Saul died, and Baal-hanan the
son of Achbor reigned in his stead.
39 And Baal-hanan the son of Achbor
died, and Hadar reigned in his stead:
and the name of his city *was* Pau; and his
wife's name *was* Mehetabel, the daughter of Matred, the daughter of Mezahab.
40 And these *are* the names of the
dukes *that came* of Esau, according to
their families, after their places, by their
names; duke Timnah, duke Alvah, duke
Jetheth,

B.C. 1780.

a Cf. vs. 9, 10, and Gen. 40:5-23.

b Cf. Gen. 27:41; John 15:18-20.

c Gen. 42:6; 44:14; Hos. 3:4, 5; cf. Phil. 2:10.

41 Duke Aholibamah, duke Elah, duke
Pinon,
42 Duke Kenaz, duke Teman, duke
Mibzar,
43 Duke Magdiel, duke Iram: these *be*
the dukes of Edom, according to their
habitations in the land of their possession:
he *is* Esau the father of the Edomites.

CHAPTER 37.

The history of Jacob resumed.

And Jacob dwelt in the land wherein
his father was a stranger, in the
land of Canaan.

Joseph, the beloved of his father.

2 These *are* the generations of Jacob.
[2]Joseph, *being* seventeen years old, was
feeding the flock with his brethren; and
the lad *was* with the sons of Bilhah, and
with the sons of Zilpah, his father's
wives: and Joseph brought unto his
father their evil report.
3 Now Israel loved Joseph more than
all his children, because he *was* the son
of his old age: and he made him a coat of
many colours.
4 And when his brethren saw that
their father loved him more than all his
brethren, they hated him, and could not
speak peaceably unto him.
5 And [a]Joseph dreamed a dream, and
he told *it* his brethren: and they [b]hated
him yet the more.
6 And he said unto them, Hear, I pray
you, this dream which I have dreamed:
7 For, behold, we *were* binding sheaves
in the field, and, lo, my sheaf arose, and
also stood upright; and, behold, your
sheaves stood round about, and made
[c]obeisance to my sheaf.

[1] **(36:31)** It is characteristic of Scripture that the kings of Edom should be enumerated before the kings of Israel. The *principle* is stated in 1 Cor. 15:46. First things are "natural," man's best, and always fail; second things are "spiritual," God's things, and succeed. Adam—Christ; Cain—Abel; Cain's posterity—Seth's posterity; Saul—David; Israel—the true Church, etc.

[2] **(37:2)** While it is nowhere asserted that Joseph was a type of Christ, the analogies are too numerous to be accidental. They are: (1) both were especial objects of a father's love (Gen. 37:3; Mt. 3:17; John 3:35; 5:20); (2) both were hated by their brethren (Gen. 37:4; John 15:25); (3) the superior claims of both were rejected by their brethren (Gen. 37:8; Mt. 21:37-39; John 15:24, 25); (4) the brethren of both conspired against them to slay them (Gen. 37:18; Mt. 26:3, 4); (5) Joseph was, in intent and figure, slain by his brethren, as was Christ (Gen. 37:24; Mt. 27:35-37); (6) each became a blessing among the Gentiles, and gained a Gentile bride (Gen. 41:1-45; Acts 15:14; Eph. 5:25-32); (7) as Joseph reconciled his brethren to himself, and afterward exalted them, so will it be with Christ and His Jewish brethren (Gen. 45:1-15; Deut. 30:1-10; Hos. 2:14-18; Rom. 11:1, 15, 25, 26).

Joseph hated and rejected by his brethren.

8 And his brethren said to him, Shalt thou indeed reign over us? or shalt thou indeed have [a]dominion over us? And they hated him yet the more for his dreams, and for his words.

9 And he dreamed yet another dream, and told it his brethren, and said, Behold, I have dreamed a dream more; and, behold, the sun and the moon and the eleven stars made obeisance to me.

10 And he told *it* to his father, and to his brethren: and his father rebuked him, and said unto him, What *is* this dream that thou hast dreamed? Shall I and thy mother and thy brethren indeed come to bow down ourselves to thee to the earth?

11 And his brethren [b]envied him; but his father observed the saying.

12 And his brethren went to feed their father's flock in Shechem.

13 [c]And Israel said unto Joseph, Do not thy brethren feed *the flock* in Shechem? come, and I will send thee unto them. And he said to him, Here *am I*.

14 And he said to him, Go, I pray thee, see whether it be well with thy brethren, and well with the flocks; and bring me word again. So he [d]sent him out of the vale of Hebron, and he came to Shechem.

15 And a certain man found him, and, behold, *he was* wandering in the field: and the man asked him, saying, What seekest thou?

16 And he said, I seek my brethren: tell me, I pray thee, where they feed *their flocks*.

17 And the man said, They are departed hence; for I heard them say, Let us go to Dothan. And Joseph went after his brethren, and found them in Dothan.

18 And when they saw him afar off, even before he came near unto them, they [e]conspired against him to slay him.

19 And they said one to another, Behold, this dreamer cometh.

Joseph cast into the place of death.

20 Come now therefore, and let us slay him, and cast him into some pit, and we will say, Some evil beast hath devoured him: and we shall see what will become of his dreams.

21 And Reuben heard *it*, and he delivered him out of their hands; and said, Let us not kill him.

22 And Reuben said unto them, Shed no blood, *but* cast him into this pit that *is* in the wilderness, and lay no hand upon him; that he might rid him out of their hands, to deliver him to his father again.

23 And it came to pass, when Joseph was come unto his brethren, that they [f]stript Joseph out of his coat, *his* coat of *many* colours that *was* on him;

24 And they took him, and cast him into a pit: and the pit *was* empty, *there was* no water in it.

25 And they sat down to eat bread: and they lifted up their eyes and looked, and, behold, a company of Ishmeelites came from Gilead with their camels bearing spicery and balm and myrrh, going to carry *it* down to Egypt.

26 And Judah said unto his brethren, What profit *is it* if we slay our brother, and conceal his blood?

27 Come, and let us sell him to the Ishmeelites, and let not our hand be upon him; for he *is* our brother *and* our flesh. And his brethren were content.

Joseph, drawn up from the pit, goes to the Gentiles.

28 Then there passed by Midianites merchantmen; and they drew and lifted up Joseph out of the pit, and [g]sold Joseph to the Ishmeelites for twenty *pieces* of silver: and they brought Joseph into Egypt.

29 And Reuben returned unto the pit; and, behold, Joseph *was* not in the pit; and he rent his clothes.

30 And he returned unto his brethren, and said, The child *is* not; and I, whither shall I go?

31 And they took Joseph's coat, and killed a kid of the goats, and dipped the coat in the blood;

32 And they sent the coat of *many* colours, and they brought *it* to their father; and said, This have we found: know now whether it *be* thy son's coat or no.

33 And he knew it, and said, *It is* my son's coat; an evil beast hath devoured him; Joseph is without doubt rent in pieces.

34 And Jacob rent his clothes, and put sackcloth upon his loins, and mourned for his son many days.

B.C. 1729.

a Cf. John 19:15.

b Mt. 27:17-18; Acts 7:9.

c *Israel (history).* vs. 13-28; Gen. 46:1-6. (Gen. 12:2, 3; Rom. 11:26.)

d Cf. 1 Sam. 17:17-18; Lk. 20:13-15; John 3:16.

e Cf. Mt. 21:38; 26:3-4.

f Mt. 27:28.

g Cf. Mt. 26:15; 27:9.

35 And all his sons and all his daughters rose up to comfort him; but he refused to be comforted; and he said, For I will go down into the [a]grave unto my son mourning. Thus his father wept for him.

36 And the Midianites sold him into Egypt unto Potiphar, an officer of Pharaoh's, *and* captain of the guard.

CHAPTER 38.

Parenthesis: the shame of Judah.

And it came to pass at that time, that Judah went down from his brethren, and turned in to a certain Adullamite, whose name *was* Hirah.

2 And Judah saw there a daughter of a certain Canaanite, whose name *was* Shuah; and he took her, and went in unto her.

3 And she conceived, and bare a son; and he called his name Er.

4 And she conceived again, and bare a son; and she called his name Onan.

5 And she yet again conceived, and bare a son; and called his name Shelah: and he was at Chezib, when she bare him.

6 And Judah took a wife for Er his firstborn, whose name *was* Tamar.

7 And Er, Judah's firstborn, was wicked in the sight of the [b]LORD; and the LORD slew him.

8 And Judah said unto Onan, Go in unto thy brother's wife, and marry her, and raise up seed to thy brother.

9 And Onan knew that the seed should not be his; and it came to pass, when he went in unto his brother's wife, that he spilled *it* on the ground, lest that he should give seed to his brother.

10 And the thing which he did [c]displeased the LORD: wherefore he slew him also.

11 Then said Judah to Tamar his daughter in law, Remain a widow at thy father's house, till Shelah my son be grown: for he said, Lest peradventure he die also, as his brethren *did*. And Tamar went and dwelt in her father's house.

12 And in process of time the daughter of Shuah Judah's wife died; and Judah was comforted, and went up unto his sheepshearers to Timnath, he and his friend Hirah the Adullamite.

13 And it was told Tamar, saying, Behold thy father in law goeth up to Timnath to shear his sheep.

14 And she put her widow's garments off from her, and covered her with a vail, and wrapped herself, and sat in an open place, which *is* by the way to Timnath; for she saw that Shelah was grown, and she was not given unto him to wife.

15 When Judah saw her, he thought her *to be* an harlot; because she had covered her face.

16 And he turned unto her by the way, and said, Go to, I pray thee, let me come in unto thee; (for he knew not that she *was* his daughter in law.) And she said, What wilt thou give me, that thou mayest come in unto me?

17 And he said, I will send *thee* a kid from the flock. And she said, Wilt thou give *me* a pledge, till thou send *it*?

18 And he said, What pledge shall I give thee? And she said, Thy signet, and thy bracelets, and thy staff that *is* in thine hand. And he gave *it* her, and came in unto her, and she conceived by him.

19 And she arose, and went away, and laid by her vail from her, and put on the garments of her widowhood.

20 And Judah sent the kid by the hand of his friend the Adullamite, to receive *his* pledge from the woman's hand: but he found her not.

21 Then he asked the men of that place, saying, Where *is* the harlot, that *was* openly by the way side? And they said, There was no harlot in this *place*.

22 And he returned to Judah, and said, I cannot find her; and also the men of the place said, *that* there was no harlot in this *place*.

23 And Judah said, Let her take *it* to her, lest we be [d]shamed: behold, I sent this kid, and thou hast not found her.

24 And it came to pass about three months after, that it was told Judah, saying, Tamar thy daughter in law hath played the harlot; and also, behold, she *is* with child by whoredom. And Judah said, Bring her forth, and let her be burnt.

25 When she *was* brought forth, she sent to her father in law, saying, By the man, whose these *are*, *am* I with child: and she said, Discern, I pray thee, whose *are* these, the signet, and bracelets, and staff.

B.C. 1729.

a Heb. *sheol.* See Hab. 2:5, *note.*

b 1 Chr. 2:3.

c Lit. *was evil in the eyes of the Lord.*

d Lit. *become a contempt.*

26 And Judah acknowledged *them,* and said, She hath been more righteous than I; because that I gave her not to Shelah my son. And he knew her again no more.

27 And it came to pass in the time of her travail, that, behold, twins *were* in her womb.

28 And it came to pass, when she travailed, that *the one* put out *his* hand: and the midwife took and bound upon his hand a scarlet thread, saying, This came out first.

29 And it came to pass, as he drew back his hand, that, behold, his brother came out: and she said, How hast thou broken forth? *this* breach *be* upon thee: therefore his name was called Pharez.

30 And afterward came out his brother, that had the scarlet thread upon his hand: and his name was called Zarah.

CHAPTER 39.

Joseph tested by adversity.

And Joseph was brought down to Egypt; and Potiphar, an officer of Pharaoh, captain of the guard, an Egyptian, [a]bought him of the hands of the Ishmeelites, which had brought him down thither.

2 And the LORD was with Joseph, and he was a prosperous man; and he was in the house of his master the Egyptian.

3 And his master saw that the LORD *was* with him, and that the LORD made all that he did to prosper in his hand.

4 And Joseph found grace in his sight, and he served him: and he made him overseer over his house, and all *that* he had he put into his hand.

5 And it came to pass from the time *that* he had made him overseer in his house, and over all that he had, that the LORD [b]blessed the Egyptian's house for Joseph's sake; and the blessing of the LORD was upon all that he had in the house, and in the field.

6 And he left all that he had in Joseph's hand; and he knew not ought he had, save the bread which he did eat. And Joseph was a goodly *person,* and well favoured.

7 And it came to pass after these things, that his master's wife cast her eyes upon Joseph; and she said, Lie with me.

8 But he refused, and said unto his master's wife, Behold, my master wotteth not what *is* with me in the house, and he hath committed all that he hath to my hand;

9 *There is* none greater in this house than I; neither hath he kept back any thing from me but thee, because thou *art* his wife: how then can I do this great [c]wickedness, and sin [d]against God?

10 And it came to pass, as she spake to Joseph day by day, that he hearkened not unto her, to lie by her, *or* to be with her.

11 And it came to pass about this time, that *Joseph* went into the house to do his business; and *there was* none of the men of the house there within.

12 And she caught him by his garment, saying, Lie with me: and he left his garment in her hand, and fled, and got him out.

13 And it came to pass, when she saw that he had left his garment in her hand, and was fled forth,

14 That she called unto the men of her house, and spake unto them, saying, See, he hath brought in an Hebrew unto us to mock us; he came in unto me to lie with me, and I cried with a loud voice:

15 And it came to pass, when he heard that I lifted up my voice and cried, that he left his garment with me, and fled, and got him out.

16 And she laid up his garment by her, until his lord came home.

17 And she spake unto him according to these words, saying, The Hebrew servant, which thou hast brought unto us, came in unto me to mock me:

18 And it came to pass, as I lifted up my voice and cried, that he left his garment with me, and fled out.

19 And it came to pass, when his master heard the words of his wife, which she spake unto him, saying, After this manner did thy servant to me; that his wrath was kindled.

20 And Joseph's master took him, and put him into the prison, a place where the king's prisoners *were* bound: and he was there in the prison.

21 But the LORD was with Joseph, and shewed him mercy, and gave him [e]favour in the sight of the keeper of the prison.

22 And the keeper of the prison committed to Joseph's hand all the prisoners that *were* in the prison; and

B.C. 1727.

a Gen. 37:28; 45:4; Psa. 105:17.

b Gen. 18:26; 30:27; 2 Sam. 6:11.

c Lev. 20:10.

d Psa. 51:4.

e Dan. 1:9; Acts 7:9-10.

whatsoever they did there, he was the doer *of it*.

23 The keeper of the prison looked not to any thing *that was* under his hand; because the LORD was with him, and *that* which he did, the LORD made *it* to prosper.

CHAPTER 40.

And it came to pass after these things, *that* the butler of the king of Egypt and *his* baker had offended their lord the king of Egypt.

2 And Pharaoh was wroth against two *of* his officers, against the chief of the butlers, and against the chief of the bakers.

3 And he put them in ward in the house of the captain of the guard, into the [a]prison, the place where Joseph *was* bound.

4 And the captain of the guard charged Joseph with them, and he served them: and they continued a season in ward.

5 And they dreamed a dream both of them, each man his dream in one night, each man according to the interpretation of his dream, the butler and the baker of the king of Egypt, which *were* bound in the prison.

6 And Joseph came in unto them in the morning, and looked upon them, and, behold, they *were* sad.

7 And he asked Pharaoh's officers that *were* with him in the ward of his lord's house, saying, Wherefore look ye *so* sadly to day?

8 And they said unto him, We have dreamed a dream, and *there is* no interpreter of it. And Joseph said unto them, *Do* not [b]interpretations *belong* to God? tell me *them*, I pray you.

9 And the chief butler told his dream to Joseph, and said to him, In my dream, behold, a vine *was* before me;

10 And in the vine *were* three branches: and it *was* as though it budded, *and* her blossoms shot forth; and the clusters thereof brought forth ripe grapes:

11 And Pharaoh's cup *was* in my hand: and I took the grapes, and pressed them into Pharaoh's cup, and I gave the cup into Pharaoh's hand.

12 And Joseph said unto him, This *is* the [c]interpretation of it: The three branches *are* three days:

13 Yet within three days shall Pharaoh lift up thine [d]head, and restore thee unto thy place: and thou shalt deliver Pharaoh's cup into his hand, after the former manner when thou wast his butler.

14 But think on me when it shall be well with thee, and shew kindness, I pray thee, unto me, and make mention of me unto Pharaoh, and bring me out of this house:

15 For indeed I was stolen away out of the land of the Hebrews: and here also have I done nothing that they should put me into the dungeon.

16 When the chief baker saw that the interpretation was good, he said unto Joseph, I also *was* in my dream, and, behold, *I had* three white baskets on my head:

17 And in the uppermost basket *there was* of all manner of bakemeats for Pharaoh; and the birds did eat them out of the basket upon my head.

18 And Joseph answered and said, This *is* the interpretation thereof: The three baskets *are* three days:

19 Yet within three days shall Pharaoh lift up thy head from off thee, and shall hang thee on a tree; and the birds shall eat thy flesh from off thee.

20 And it came to pass the third day, *which was* Pharaoh's birthday, that he made a feast unto all his servants: and he lifted up the head of the chief butler and of the chief baker among his servants.

21 And he restored the chief butler unto his butlership again; and he gave the [e]cup into Pharaoh's hand:

22 But he hanged the chief baker: as Joseph had interpreted to them.

23 Yet did not the chief butler remember Joseph, but forgat him.

CHAPTER 41.

The dream of Pharaoh.

And it came to pass at the end of two full years, that Pharaoh dreamed: and, behold, he stood by the river.

2 And, behold, there came up out of the river seven well favoured kine and fatfleshed; and they fed in a meadow.

3 And, behold, seven other kine came up after them out of the river, ill favoured and leanfleshed; and stood by the *other* kine upon the brink of the river.

B.C. 1729.

a Gen. 39:20, 23.
b Dan. 2:20-22.
c Dan. 2:36.
d 2 Ki. 25:27; Jer. 52:31.
e Cf. Neh. 2:1.

4 And the ill favoured and leanfleshed kine did eat up the seven well favoured and fat kine. So Pharaoh awoke.

5 And he slept and dreamed the second time: and, behold, seven ears of corn came up upon one stalk, rank and good.

6 And, behold, seven thin ears and blasted with the east wind sprung up after them.

7 And the seven thin ears devoured the seven rank and full ears. And Pharaoh awoke, and, behold, *it was* a dream.

8 And it came to pass in the morning that his [a]spirit was troubled; and he sent and called for all the magicians of Egypt, and all the wise men thereof: and Pharaoh told them his dream; but *there was* none that could interpret them unto Pharaoh.

9 Then spake the chief butler unto Pharaoh, saying, I do remember my faults this day:

10 Pharaoh was wroth with his servants, and put me in ward in the captain of the guard's house, *both* me and the chief baker:

11 And we dreamed a dream in one night, I and he; we dreamed each man according to the interpretation of his dream.

12 And *there was* there with us a young man, an Hebrew, servant to the captain of the guard; and we told him, and he interpreted to us our dreams; to each man according to his dream he did interpret.

13 And it came to pass, as he interpreted to us, so it was; me he restored unto mine office, and him he hanged.

Joseph's exaltation in Egypt.

14 Then Pharaoh sent and called Joseph, and they brought him hastily [b]out of the dungeon: and he shaved *himself*, and changed his raiment, and came in unto Pharaoh.

15 And Pharaoh said unto Joseph, I have dreamed a dream, and *there is* none that can interpret it: and I have heard say of thee, *that* thou canst understand a dream to interpret it.

16 And Joseph answered Pharaoh, saying, *It is* not in me: God shall give Pharaoh an answer of peace.

17 And Pharaoh said unto Joseph, In my dream, behold, I stood upon the bank of the river:

18 And, behold, there came up out of the river seven kine, fatfleshed and well favoured; and they fed in a meadow:

19 And, behold, seven other kine came up after them, poor and very ill favoured and leanfleshed, such as I never saw in all the land of Egypt for badness:

20 And the lean and the ill favoured kine did eat up the first seven fat kine:

21 And when they had eaten them up, it could not be known that they had eaten them; but they *were* still ill favoured, as at the beginning. So I awoke.

22 And I saw in my dream, and, behold, seven ears came up in one stalk, full and good:

23 And, behold, seven ears, withered, thin, *and* blasted with the east wind, sprung up after them:

24 And the thin ears devoured the seven good ears: and I told *this* unto the magicians; but *there was* none that could declare *it* to me.

25 And Joseph said unto Pharaoh, The dream of Pharaoh *is* one: God hath shewed Pharaoh what he *is* [c]about to do.

26 The seven good kine *are* seven years; and the seven good ears *are* seven years: the dream *is* one.

27 And the seven thin and ill favoured kine that came up after them *are* seven years; and the seven empty ears blasted with the east wind shall be seven years of famine.

28 This *is* the thing which I have spoken unto Pharaoh: What God *is* about to do he sheweth unto Pharaoh.

29 Behold, there come seven years of great plenty throughout all the land of Egypt:

30 And there shall arise after them seven years of famine; and all the plenty shall be forgotten in the land of Egypt; and the famine shall consume the land;

31 And the plenty shall not be known in the land by reason of that famine following; for it *shall be* very grievous.

32 And for that the dream was doubled unto Pharaoh twice; *it is* because the thing *is* established by God, and God will shortly bring it to pass.

33 Now therefore let Pharaoh look out a man discreet and wise, and set him over the land of Egypt.

B.C. 1715.

a Dan. 2:1, 3; 4:5, 19; 7:28; 8:27.

b Cf. 1 Sam. 2:8.

c Cf. Dan. 2:29, 45.

34 Let Pharaoh do *this*, and let him appoint officers over the land, and take up the fifth part of the land of Egypt in the seven plenteous years.

35 And let them gather all the food of those good years that come, and lay up corn under the hand of Pharaoh, and let them keep food in the cities.

36 And that food shall be for store to the land against the seven years of famine, which shall be in the land of Egypt; that the land perish not through the famine.

37 And the thing was good in the eyes of Pharaoh, and in the eyes of all his servants.

38 And Pharaoh said unto his servants, Can we find *such a one* as this *is*, a man in whom the Spirit of God *is*?

39 And Pharaoh said unto Joseph, Forasmuch as God hath shewed thee all this, *there is* none so discreet and wise as thou *art*:

40 Thou shalt be [a]over my house, and according unto thy word shall all my people be ruled: only in the throne will I be greater than thou.

41 And Pharaoh said unto Joseph, See, I have set thee over all the land of Egypt.

42 And Pharaoh took off his ring from his hand, and put it upon Joseph's hand, and arrayed him in vestures of fine linen, and put a gold chain about his neck;

43 And he made him to ride in the second chariot which he had; and they cried before him, Bow the knee: and he made him *ruler* over all the land of Egypt.

44 And Pharaoh said unto Joseph, I *am* Pharaoh, and without thee shall no man lift up his hand or foot in all the land of Egypt.

Joseph, rejected by his brethren, receives a Gentile bride.

45 And Pharaoh called Joseph's name [b]Zaphnath-paaneah; and he gave him to wife [1]Asenath the daughter of Poti-pherah priest of On. And Joseph went out over *all* the land of Egypt.

46 And Joseph *was* thirty years old when he stood before Pharaoh king of Egypt. And Joseph went out from the presence of Pharaoh, and went throughout all the land of Egypt.

47 And in the seven plenteous years the earth brought forth by handfuls.

48 And he gathered up all the food of the seven years, which were in the land of Egypt, and laid up the food in the cities: the food of the field, which *was* round about every city, laid he up in the same.

49 And Joseph gathered corn as the sand of the sea, very much, until he left numbering; for *it was* without number.

50 And unto Joseph were born two sons before the years of famine came, which Asenath the daughter of Poti-pherah priest of On bare unto him.

51 And Joseph called the name of the firstborn [c]Manasseh: For God, *said he*, hath made me forget all my toil, and all my father's house.

52 And the name of the second called he [d]Ephraim: For God hath caused me to be fruitful in the land of my affliction.

53 And the seven years of plenteousness, that was in the land of Egypt, were ended.

54 And the seven years of dearth began to come, according as Joseph had said: and the dearth was in all lands; but in all the land of Egypt there was bread.

55 And when all the land of Egypt was famished, the people cried to Pharaoh for bread: and Pharaoh said unto all the Egyptians, Go unto Joseph; what he saith to you, do.

56 And the famine was over all the face of the earth: And Joseph opened all the storehouses, and sold unto the Egyptians; and the famine waxed sore in the land of Egypt.

57 And all countries came into Egypt to Joseph for to buy *corn*; because that the famine was *so* sore in all lands.

CHAPTER 42.

Joseph, rejected by his brethren, preserves them (cf. Ezk. 11:16).

Now when Jacob saw that there was corn in Egypt, Jacob said unto his sons, Why do ye look one upon another?

B.C. 1715.

a Isa. 11:10; Rev. 11:15; 15:2-4.

b Coptic, *revealer of secret things.*

c i.e. *forgetting.* Gen. 46:20.

d i.e. *fruitful.* Gen. 48:5.

[1] **(41:45)** Asenath, the Gentile bride espoused by Joseph the rejected one (John 19:15), type of the Church, called out from the Gentiles to be the bride of Christ during the time of His rejection by His brethren, Israel (Acts 15:14; Eph. 5:31, 32). See Gen. 37:2, *note*.

2 And he said, Behold, I have heard that there is corn in Egypt: get you down thither, and buy for us from thence; that we may live, and not die.

3 And Joseph's ten brethren went down to buy corn in Egypt.

4 But Benjamin, Joseph's brother, Jacob sent not with his brethren; for he said, Lest peradventure mischief befall him.

5 And the sons of Israel came to buy *corn* among those that came: for the [a]famine was in the land of Canaan.

6 And Joseph *was* the governor over the land, *and* he *it was* that sold to all the people of the land: and Joseph's brethren came, and [b]bowed down themselves before him *with* their faces to the earth.

7 And Joseph saw his brethren, and he knew them, but made himself [c]strange unto them, and spake roughly unto them; and he said unto them, Whence come ye? And they said, From the land of Canaan to buy food.

8 And Joseph knew his brethren, but they knew not him.

9 And Joseph remembered the dreams which he dreamed of them, and said unto them, Ye *are* spies; to see the nakedness of the land ye are come.

10 And they said unto him, Nay, my lord, but to buy food are thy servants come.

11 We *are* all one man's sons; we *are* true *men*, thy servants are no spies.

12 And he said unto them, Nay, but to see the nakedness of the land ye are come.

13 And they said, Thy servants *are* twelve brethren, the sons of one man in the land of Canaan; and, behold, the youngest *is* this day with our father, and one *is* not.

14 And Joseph said unto them, That *is it* that I spake unto you, saying, Ye *are* spies:

15 Hereby ye shall be proved: By the life of Pharaoh ye shall not go forth hence, except your youngest brother come hither.

16 Send one of you, and let him fetch your brother, and ye shall be kept in prison, that your words may be proved, whether *there be any* truth in you: or else by the life of Pharaoh surely ye *are* spies.

17 And he put them all together into ward three days.

18 And Joseph said unto them the third day, This do, and live; *for* I [d]fear God:

B.C. 1707.

a Gen. 12:10, *note.*

b Cf. Gen. 37:8.

c Cf. Gen. 45:1-2; Mt. 23:37-39.

d Gen 22:12; Ex. 1:17; Prov. 1:7; 9:10; see Psa. 19:9, *note.*

19 If ye *be* true *men*, let one of your brethren be bound in the house of your prison: go ye, carry corn for the famine of your houses:

20 But bring your youngest brother unto me; so shall your words be verified, and ye shall not die. And they did so.

21 And they said one to another, We *are* verily guilty concerning our brother, in that we saw the anguish of his soul, when he besought us, and we would not hear; therefore is this distress come upon us.

22 And Reuben answered them, saying, Spake I not unto you, saying, Do not sin against the child; and ye would not hear? therefore, behold, also his blood is required.

23 And they knew not that Joseph understood *them*; for he spake unto them by an interpreter.

24 And he turned himself about from them, and wept; and returned to them again, and communed with them, and took from them Simeon, and bound him before their eyes.

25 Then Joseph commanded to fill their sacks with corn, and to restore every man's money into his sack, and to give them provision for the way: and thus did he unto them.

26 And they laded their asses with the corn, and departed thence.

27 And as one of them opened his sack to give his ass provender in the inn, he espied his money; for, behold, it *was* in his sack's mouth.

28 And he said unto his brethren, My money is restored; and, lo, *it is* even in my sack: and their heart failed *them*, and they were afraid, saying one to another, What *is* this *that* God hath done unto us?

29 And they came unto Jacob their father unto the land of Canaan, and told him all that befell unto them; saying,

30 The man, *who is* the lord of the land, spake roughly to us, and took us for spies of the country.

31 And we said unto him, We *are* true *men*; we are no spies:

32 We *be* twelve brethren, sons of our father; one *is* not, and the youngest *is* this day with our father in the land of Canaan.

33 And the man, the lord of the country, said unto us, Hereby shall I know that ye *are* true *men*; leave one of your

brethren *here* with me, and take *food for* the famine of your households, and be gone:
34 And bring your youngest brother unto me: then shall I know that ye *are* no spies, but *that* ye *are* true *men: so* will I deliver you your brother, and ye shall traffick in the land.
35 And it came to pass as they emptied their sacks, that, behold, every man's bundle of money *was* in his sack: and when *both* they and their father saw the bundles of money, they were afraid.
36 And Jacob their father said unto them, Me have ye bereaved *of my children*: Joseph *is* not, and Simeon *is* not, and ye will take Benjamin *away*: all these things are against me.
37 And Reuben spake unto his father, saying, Slay my two sons, if I bring him not to thee: deliver him into my hand, and I will bring him to thee again.
38 And he said, My son shall not go down with you; for his brother is dead, and he is left alone: if mischief befall him by the way in the which ye go, then shall ye bring down my gray hairs with sorrow to the [a]grave.

CHAPTER 43.

And the [b]famine *was* sore in the land.
2 And it came to pass, when they had eaten up the corn which they had brought out of Egypt, their father said unto them, Go again, buy us a little food.
3 And Judah spake unto him, saying, The man did solemnly protest unto us, saying, Ye shall not [c]see my face, except your brother *be* with you.
4 If thou wilt send our brother with us, we will go down and buy thee food:
5 But if thou wilt not send *him*, we will not go down: for the man said unto us, Ye shall not see my face, except your brother *be* with you.
6 And Israel said, Wherefore dealt ye *so* ill with me, *as* to tell the man whether ye had yet a brother?
7 And they said, The man asked us straitly of our state, and of our kindred, saying, *Is* your father yet alive? have ye *another* brother? and we told him according to the tenor of these words: could we

B.C. 1707.

a Heb. *sheol.* See Hab. 2:5, *note.* Cf. Gen. 37:35; 44:29, 31.

b See Gen. 12:10, *note;* 42:5; 45:6, 11.

c Gen. 44:23.

d Gen. 44:32.

e Gen. 37:25.

f Gen. 42:25.

g Cf. Gen. 42:28.

certainly know that he would say, Bring your brother down?
8 And Judah said unto Israel his father, Send the lad with me, and we will arise and go; that we may live, and not die, both we, and thou, *and* also our little ones.
9 I will be [d]surety for him; of my hand shalt thou require him: if I bring him not unto thee, and set him before thee, then let me bear the blame for ever:
10 For except we had lingered, surely now we had returned this second time.
11 And their father Israel said unto them, If *it must be* so now, do this; take of the best fruits in the land in your vessels, and carry down the man a present, a little [e]balm, and a little honey, spices, and myrrh, nuts, and almonds:
12 And take double money in your hand; and the money that was brought [f]again in the mouth of your sacks, carry *it* again in your hand; peradventure it *was* an oversight:
13 Take also your brother, and arise, go again unto the man:
14 And God Almighty give you mercy before the man, that he may send away your other brother, and Benjamin. If I be bereaved *of my children*, I am bereaved.
15 And the men took that present, and they took double money in their hand, and Benjamin; and rose up, and went down to Egypt, and stood before Joseph.
16 And when Joseph saw Benjamin with them, he said to the ruler of his house, Bring *these* men home, and slay, and make ready; for *these* men shall dine with me at noon.
17 And the man did as Joseph bade; and the man brought the men into Joseph's house.
18 And the men were [g]afraid, because they were brought into Joseph's house; and they said, Because of the money that was returned in our sacks at the first time are we brought in; that he may seek occasion against us, and fall upon us, and take us for bondmen, and our asses.
19 And they came near to the steward of Joseph's house, and they communed with him at the door of the house,
20 And said, O sir, we came indeed down at the first time to buy food:

B.C. 1707.

21 And it came to pass, when we came to the inn, that we opened our sacks, and, behold, *every* man's money *was* in the mouth of his sack, our money in full weight: and we have brought it again in our hand.

22 And other money have we brought down in our hands to buy food: we cannot tell who put our money in our sacks.

23 And he said, Peace *be* to you, fear not: your God, and the God of your father, hath given you treasure in your sacks: I had your money. And he brought Simeon out unto them.

24 And the man brought the men into Joseph's house, and gave *them* water, and they washed their feet; and he gave their asses provender.

25 And they made ready the present against Joseph came at noon: for they heard that they should eat bread there.

26 And when Joseph came home, they brought him the present which *was* in their hand into the house, and bowed themselves to him to the earth.

27 And he asked them of *their* welfare, and said, *Is* your father well, the old man of whom ye spake? *Is* he yet alive?

28 And they answered, Thy servant our father *is* in good health, he *is* yet alive. And they bowed down their heads, and made obeisance.

29 And he lifted up his eyes, and saw his brother Benjamin, his mother's son, and said, *Is* this your younger brother, of whom ye spake unto me? And he said, God be gracious unto thee, my son.

30 And Joseph made haste; for his bowels did yearn upon his brother: and he sought *where* to weep; and he entered into *his* chamber, and wept there.

31 And he washed his face, and went out, and refrained himself, and said, Set on bread.

32 And they set on for him by himself, and for them by themselves, and for the Egyptians, which did eat with him, by themselves: because the Egyptians might not eat bread with the Hebrews; for that *is* an abomination unto the Egyptians.

33 And they sat before him, the firstborn according to his birthright, and the youngest according to his youth: and the men marvelled one at another.

34 And he took *and sent* messes unto them from before him: [1]but Benjamin's mess was five times so much as any of theirs. And they drank, and were merry with him.

CHAPTER 44.

And he commanded the steward of his house, saying, Fill the men's sacks *with* food, as much as they can carry, and put every man's money in his sack's mouth.

2 And put my cup, the silver cup, in the sack's mouth of the youngest, and his corn money. And he did according to the word that Joseph had spoken.

3 As soon as the morning was light, the men were sent away, they and their asses.

4 *And* when they were gone out of the city, *and* not *yet* far off, Joseph said unto his steward, Up, follow after the men; and when thou dost overtake them, say unto them, Wherefore have ye rewarded evil for good?

5 *Is* not this *it* in which my lord drinketh, and whereby indeed he divineth? ye have done evil in so doing.

6 And he overtook them, and he spake unto them these same words.

7 And they said unto him, Wherefore saith my lord these words? God forbid that thy servants should do according to this thing:

8 Behold, the money, which we found in our sacks' mouths, we brought again unto thee out of the land of Canaan: how then should we steal out of thy lord's house silver or gold?

[1] **(43:34)** Cf. Gen. 35:18, *note.* It is important to observe that Benjamin now becomes prominent. Joseph is peculiarly the type of Christ in His first advent, rejection, death, resurrection, and present exaltation among the Gentiles, but unrecognized of Israel. As the greater Benjamin, "Son of sorrow," but also "Son of my right hand," He is to be revealed in power in the Kingdom (see Gen. 1:26-28; Zech. 12:8, *note.* It is then, and not till then, that Israel is to be restored and converted (see Deut. 30:1-9, *note*). *Typically* Gen. 45:1, 2 anticipates the revelation *prophetically* described, Ezk. 20:33-36; Hos. 2:14-23, at which time the Benjamin type of Christ will be fulfilled.

9 With whomsoever of thy servants it be found, both let him die, and we also will be my lord's bondmen.

10 And he said, Now also *let* it *be* according unto your words: he with whom it is found shall be my servant; and ye shall be blameless.

11 Then they speedily took down every man his sack to the ground, and opened every man his sack.

12 And he searched, *and* began at the eldest, and left at the youngest: and the cup was found in Benjamin's sack.

13 Then they rent their clothes, and laded every man his ass, and returned to the city.

14 And Judah and his brethren came to Joseph's house; for he *was* yet there: and they fell [a]before him on the ground.

15 And Joseph said unto them, What deed *is* this that ye have done? wot ye not that such a man as I can certainly divine?

16 And Judah said, What shall we say unto my lord? what shall we speak? or how shall we clear ourselves? God hath found out the iniquity of thy servants: behold, we *are* my lord's servants, both we, and *he* also with whom the cup is found.

17 And he said, God forbid that I should do so: *but* the man in whose hand the cup is found, he shall be my servant; and as for you, get you up in peace unto your father.

18 Then Judah came near unto him, and said, Oh my lord, let thy servant, I pray thee, speak a word in my lord's ears, and let not thine anger burn against thy servant: for thou *art* even as Pharaoh.

19 My lord asked his servants, saying, Have ye a father, or a brother?

20 And we said unto my lord, We have a father, an old man, and a child of his old age, a little one; and his brother is dead, and he [b]alone is left of his mother, and his [c]father loveth him.

21 And thou saidst unto thy servants, Bring him down unto me, that I may set mine eyes upon him.

22 And we said unto my lord, The lad cannot leave his father: for *if* he should leave his father, *his father* would die.

23 And thou saidst unto thy servants, Except your youngest brother come down with you, ye shall see my face no more.

B.C. 1707.

a Gen. 37:7.
b Gen. 46:19.
c Gen. 37:3; 42:4.
d Gen. 30:22-24; 35:16-18; 46:19.
e Gen. 37:33.
f Heb. *sheol.* See Hab. 2:5, *note.*
g 1 Sam. 18:1; 25:29.
h Hos. 2:14-23.
i i.e. *terrified.*
j Cf. Zech. 12:10-14.

24 And it came to pass when we came up unto thy servant my father, we told him the words of my lord.

25 And our father said, Go again, *and* buy us a little food.

26 And we said, We cannot go down: if our youngest brother be with us, then will we go down: for we may not see the man's face, except our youngest brother *be* with us.

27 And thy servant my father said unto us, Ye know that my wife bare me [d]two *sons*:

28 And the one went out from me, and I said, [e]Surely he is torn in pieces; and I saw him not since:

29 And if ye take this also from me, and mischief befall him, ye shall bring down my gray hairs with sorrow to the [f]grave.

30 Now therefore when I come to thy servant my father, and the lad *be* not with us; seeing that his life is [g]bound up in the lad's life;

31 It shall come to pass, when he seeth that the lad *is* not *with us*, that he will die: and thy servants shall bring down the gray hairs of thy servant our father with sorrow to the [f]grave.

32 For thy servant became surety for the lad unto my father, saying, If I bring him not unto thee, then I shall bear the blame to my father for ever.

33 Now therefore, I pray thee, let thy servant abide instead of the lad a bondman to my lord; and let the lad go up with his brethren.

34 For how shall I go up to my father, and the lad *be* not with me? lest peradventure I see the evil that shall come on my father.

CHAPTER 45.

Joseph reveals himself to his brethren.

Then Joseph could not refrain himself before all them that stood by him; and he cried, Cause every man to go out from me. And there stood no man with him, [h]while Joseph made himself known unto his brethren.

2 And he wept aloud: and the Egyptians and the house of Pharaoh heard.

3 And Joseph said unto his brethren, I *am* Joseph; doth my father yet live? And his brethren could not answer him; for they were [ij]troubled at his presence.

B.C. 1707.

4 And Joseph said unto his brethren, Come near to me, I pray you. And they came near. And he said, I *am* Joseph your brother, whom [a]ye sold into Egypt.

5 Now therefore be not grieved, nor angry with yourselves, that ye sold me hither: for God did send me before you to preserve life.

6 For these two years *hath* the famine *been* in the land: and yet *there are* five years, in the which *there shall* neither *be* earing nor harvest.

7 And God [b]sent me before you to [c]preserve you a posterity in the earth, and to save your lives by a great deliverance.

8 So now *it was* not you *that* sent me hither, but God: and he hath made me a father to Pharaoh, and lord of all his house, and a ruler throughout all the land of Egypt.

9 Haste ye, and go up to my father, and say unto him, Thus saith thy son Joseph, God hath made me lord of all Egypt: come down unto me, tarry not:

10 And thou shalt dwell in the land of [d]Goshen, and thou shalt be near unto me, thou, and thy children, and thy children's children, and thy flocks, and thy herds, and all that thou hast:

11 And there will I nourish thee; for yet *there are* five years of famine; lest thou, and thy household, and all that thou hast, come to poverty.

12 And, behold, your eyes see, and the eyes of my brother Benjamin, that *it is* my mouth that speaketh unto you.

13 And ye shall tell my father of all my glory in Egypt, and of all that ye have seen; and ye shall haste and [e]bring down my father hither.

14 And he fell upon his brother Benjamin's neck, and wept; and Benjamin wept upon his neck.

15 Moreover he kissed all his brethren, and wept upon them: and after that his brethren talked with him.

Joseph's brethren blessed and sent to Jacob.

16 And the fame thereof was heard in Pharaoh's house, saying, Joseph's brethren are come: and it pleased Pharaoh well, and his servants.

17 And Pharaoh said unto Joseph, Say unto thy brethren, This do ye; lade your beasts, and go, get you unto the land of Canaan;

18 And take your father and your households, and come unto me: and I will give you the good of the land of Egypt, and ye shall [f]eat the fat of the land.

19 Now thou art commanded, this do ye; take you wagons out of the land of Egypt for your little ones, and for your wives, and bring your father, and come.

20 Also regard not your stuff; for the good of all the land of Egypt *is* yours.

21 And the children of Israel did so: and Joseph gave them wagons, according to the commandment of Pharaoh, and gave them provision for the way.

22 To all of them he gave each man changes of raiment; but to Benjamin he gave three hundred *pieces* of silver, and five changes of raiment.

23 And to his father he sent after this *manner*; ten asses laden with the good things of Egypt, and ten she asses laden with corn and bread and meat for his father by the way.

24 So he sent his brethren away, and they departed: and he said unto them, See that ye fall not out by the way.

25 And they went up out of Egypt, and came into the land of Canaan unto Jacob their father,

26 And told him, saying, Joseph *is* yet alive, and he *is* governor over all the land of Egypt. And Jacob's heart fainted, for he believed them not.

27 And they told him all the words of Joseph, which he had said unto them: and when he saw the wagons which Joseph had sent to carry him, the spirit of Jacob their father revived:

28 And Israel said, *It is* enough; Joseph my son *is* yet alive: I will go and see him before I die.

CHAPTER 46.

Jacob journeys to Egypt.

And [g]Israel took his journey with all that he had, and came to [h]Beer-sheba, and offered sacrifices unto the God of his father Isaac.

2 And God spake unto Israel in the visions of the night, and said, Jacob, Jacob. And he said, Here *am* I.

---

a Gen. 37:28; 39:1; Psa. 105:17.

b Gen. 50:20; Acts 2:23.

c Heb. *to make you a remnant.* See Isa. 1:9; Rom. 11:5, *note.*

d Gen. 47:6; Ex. 9:26.

e Gen. 46:6-28; Acts 7:14.

f Gen. 47:6; Deut. 32:9-14.

g *Israel (history),* vs. 1-6; Ex. 3:15-17. (Gen. 12:2, 3; Rom. 11:26.)

h Gen. 21:33; 26:32-33; 28:10.

3 And he said, [1]I *am* God, the God of thy
father: fear not to go down into Egypt; for
I will [a]there make of thee a great nation:
4 I will go down with thee into Egypt;
and I will also surely [b]bring thee up
again: and Joseph shall put his hand
upon thine eyes.
5 And Jacob rose up from Beer-sheba:
and the sons of Israel carried Jacob their
father, and their little ones, and their
wives, in the wagons which Pharaoh
had sent to carry him.
6 And they took their cattle, and their
goods, which they had gotten in the land
of Canaan, and came into Egypt, Jacob,
and all his seed with him:
7 His sons, and his sons' sons with
him, his daughters, and his sons' daughters, and all his seed brought he with
him into Egypt.
8 And these *are* the names of the children
of Israel, which came into Egypt, Jacob and
his sons: Reuben, Jacob's firstborn.
9 And the sons of Reuben; Hanoch,
and Phallu, and Hezron, and Carmi.
10 And the sons of Simeon; Jemuel, and
Jamin, and Ohad, and Jachin, and Zohar,
and Shaul the son of a Canaanitish
woman.
11 And the sons of Levi; Gershon,
Kohath, and Merari.
12 And the sons of Judah; Er, and
Onan, and Shelah, and Pharez, and
Zerah: but Er and Onan died in the land
of Canaan. And the sons of Pharez were
Hezron and Hamul.
13 And the sons of Issachar; Tola, and
Phuvah, and Job, and Shimron.
14 And the sons of Zebulun; Sered,
and Elon, and Jahleel.
15 These *be* the sons of Leah, which she
bare unto Jacob in Padan-aram, with his
daughter Dinah: all the souls of his sons
and his daughters *were* thirty and three.
16 And the sons of Gad; Ziphion, and
Haggi, Shuni, and Ezbon, Eri, and Arodi,
and Areli.
17 And the sons of Asher; Jimnah, and
Ishuah, and Isui, and Beriah, and Serah
their sister: and the sons of Beriah;
Heber, and Malchiel.
18 These *are* the sons of Zilpah, whom
Laban gave to Leah his daughter, and
these she bare unto Jacob, *even* sixteen
souls.
19 The sons of Rachel Jacob's wife;
Joseph, and Benjamin.
20 And unto Joseph in the land of
Egypt were born Manasseh and
Ephraim, which Asenath the daughter of
Poti-pherah priest of On bare unto him.
21 And the sons of Benjamin *were*
Belah, and Becher, and Ashbel, Gera,
and Naaman, Ehi, and Rosh, Muppim,
and Huppim, and Ard.
22 These *are* the sons of Rachel, which
were born to Jacob: all the souls *were*
fourteen.
23 And the sons of Dan; Hushim.
24 And the sons of Naphtali; Jahzeel,
and Guni, and Jezer, and Shillem.
25 These *are* the sons of Bilhah, which
Laban gave unto Rachel his daughter,
and she bare these unto Jacob: all the
souls *were* seven.
26 All the [2]souls that came with Jacob
into Egypt, which came out of his loins,
besides Jacob's sons' wives, all the souls
were threescore and six;
27 And the sons of Joseph, which were
born him in Egypt, *were* two souls: all the
souls of the house of Jacob, which came
into Egypt, *were* threescore and ten.
28 And he sent Judah before him unto
Joseph, to direct his face unto Goshen;
and they came into the land of Goshen.

B.C. 1706.

a Ex. 12:37; Deut. 26:5; cf. Gen 35:11; 48:4.

b Gen. 15:16; 50:13, 25; Ex. 3:8.

[1] **(46:3)** It is important to distinguish between the *directive* and the *permissive* will of God. In the first sense the place for the covenant family was Canaan (Gen. 26:1-5). Gen. 46:3 is a touching instance of the permissive will of God. Jacob's family, broken, and in part already in Egypt, the tenderness of Jehovah would not forbid the aged patriarch to follow. God will take up His people and, so far as possible, bless them, even when they are out of His best. In Israel's choice of a king (1 Sam. 8:7-9); in the turning back from Kadesh (Deut. 1:19-22); in the sending of the spies; in the case of Balaam—illustrations of this principle are seen. It is needless to say that God's permissive will never extends to things morally wrong. The highest blessing is ever found in obedience to His directive will.

[2] **(46:26)** Cf. v. 27. A discrepancy has been imagined. The "souls that came with Jacob" were 66. The "souls of the *house* of Jacob" (v. 27, i.e. the entire Jacobean family) were 70, viz. the 66 which came with Jacob, Joseph and his two sons, already in Egypt=69; Jacob himself=70. See Acts 7:14, *note*.

B.C. 1706.

29 And Joseph made ready his chariot, and went up to meet Israel his father, to Goshen, and presented himself unto him; and he fell on his neck, and wept on his neck a good while.

30 And Israel said unto Joseph, Now [a]let me die, since I have seen thy face, because thou *art* yet alive.

31 And Joseph said unto his brethren, and unto his father's house, I will go up, and shew Pharaoh, and say unto him, My brethren, and my father's house, which *were* in the land of Canaan, are come unto me;

32 And the men *are* shepherds, for their trade hath been to feed cattle; and they have brought their flocks, and their herds, and all that they have.

33 And it shall come to pass, when Pharaoh shall call you, and shall say, What *is* your occupation?

34 That ye shall say, Thy servants' trade hath been about cattle from our youth even until now, both we, *and* also our fathers: that ye may dwell in the land of Goshen; for every shepherd *is* an abomination unto the Egyptians.

CHAPTER 47.

Jacob and his descendants exalted.

Then Joseph came and told Pharaoh, and said, My father and my brethren, and their flocks, and their herds, and all that they have, are come out of the land of Canaan; and, behold, they *are* in the land of Goshen.

2 And he took some of his brethren, *even* five men, and presented them unto Pharaoh.

3 And Pharaoh said unto his brethren, What *is* your occupation? And they said unto Pharaoh, Thy servants *are* shepherds, both we, *and* also our fathers.

4 They said moreover unto Pharaoh, For to sojourn in the land are we come; for thy servants have no pasture for their flocks; for the famine *is* sore in the land of Canaan: now therefore, we pray thee, let thy servants dwell in the land of Goshen.

5 And Pharaoh spake unto Joseph, saying, Thy father and thy brethren are come unto thee:

6 The land of Egypt *is* before thee; in the best of the land make thy father and brethren to dwell; in the land of Goshen let them dwell: and if thou knowest *any* men of [b]activity among them, then make them rulers over my cattle.

7 And Joseph brought in Jacob his father, and set him before Pharaoh: and Jacob [c]blessed Pharaoh.

8 And Pharaoh said unto Jacob, How old *art* thou?

9 And Jacob said unto Pharaoh, The days of the years of my pilgrimage *are* an hundred and thirty years: few and evil have the days of the years of my life been, and have not [d]attained unto the days of the years of the life of my fathers in the days of their pilgrimage.

10 And Jacob blessed Pharaoh, and went out from before Pharaoh.

11 And Joseph placed his father and his brethren, and gave them a possession in the land of Egypt, in the best of the land, in the land of Rameses, as Pharaoh had commanded.

12 And Joseph nourished his father, and his brethren, and all his father's household, with bread, according to *their* families.

13 And *there was* no bread in all the land; for the famine *was* very sore, so that the land of Egypt and *all* the land of Canaan fainted by reason of the famine.

14 And Joseph gathered up all the money that was found in the land of Egypt, and in the land of Canaan, for the corn which they bought: and Joseph brought the money into Pharaoh's house.

15 And when money failed in the land of Egypt, and in the land of Canaan, all the Egyptians came unto Joseph, and said, Give us bread: for why should we die in thy presence? for the money faileth.

16 And Joseph said, Give your cattle; and I will give you for your cattle, if money fail.

17 And they brought their cattle unto Joseph: and Joseph gave them bread *in exchange* for horses, and for the flocks, and for the cattle of the herds, and for the asses: and he fed them with bread for all their cattle for that year.

18 When that year was ended, they came unto him the second year, and said unto him, We will not hide *it* from my lord, how that our money is spent; my lord also hath our herds of cattle; there is not ought left in the sight of my lord, but our bodies, and our lands:

a Lk. 2:29, 30.

b Lk. 12:42-44.

c Gen. 48:15, 20; cf. Heb. 7:7.

d Gen. 5:5; 11:10-11; 25:7-8.

19 Wherefore shall we die before thine eyes, both we and our land? buy us and our land for bread, and we and our land will be servants unto Pharaoh: and give *us* seed, that we may live, and not die, that the land be not desolate.

20 And Joseph [a]bought all the land of Egypt for Pharaoh; for the Egyptians sold every man his field, because the famine prevailed over them: so the land became Pharaoh's.

21 And as for the people, he removed them to cities from *one* end of the borders of Egypt even to the *other* end thereof.

22 Only the land of the priests bought he not; for the priests had a portion *assigned them* of Pharaoh, and did eat their portion which Pharaoh gave them: wherefore they sold not their lands.

23 Then Joseph said unto the people, Behold, I have bought you this day and your land for Pharaoh: lo, *here is* seed for you, and ye shall sow the land.

24 And it shall come to pass in the increase, that ye shall give the fifth *part* unto Pharaoh, and four parts shall be your own, for seed of the field, and for your food, and for them of your households, and for food for your little ones.

25 And they said, Thou hast saved our lives: let us find grace in the sight of my lord, and we will be Pharaoh's servants.

26 And Joseph made it a law over the land of Egypt unto this day, *that* Pharaoh should have the fifth *part*; except the land of the priests only, *which* became not Pharaoh's.

The last days of Jacob.

27 And Israel dwelt in the land of Egypt, in the country of Goshen; and they had possessions therein, and grew, and [b]multiplied exceedingly.

28 And Jacob lived in the land of Egypt seventeen years: so the [c]whole age of Jacob was an hundred forty and seven years.

29 And the [d]time drew nigh that Israel must die: and he called his son Joseph, and said unto him, If now I have found grace in thy sight, [e]put, I pray thee, thy hand under my thigh, and deal kindly and truly with me; bury me not, I pray thee, in Egypt:

30 But I will [f]lie with my fathers, and thou shalt carry me out of Egypt, and bury me in their buryingplace. And he said, I will do as thou hast said.

31 And he said, Swear unto me. And he sware unto him. And Israel bowed himself upon the bed's head.

B.C. 1702.

a Rev. 5:5-10; 11:15.

b Gen. 15:13-16; Ex. 1:7-12; 12:37; Heb. 11:12.

c Or, *days of the years of his life.* Gen. 47:9.

d Job 14:14; John 7:8; 19:11.

e Gen. 24:2-4.

f Gen. 50:5-13; Heb. 11:21.

CHAPTER 48.

And it came to pass after these things, that *one* told Joseph, Behold, thy father *is* sick: and he took with him his two sons, Manasseh and Ephraim.

2 And *one* told Jacob, and said, Behold, thy son Joseph cometh unto thee: and Israel strengthened himself, and sat upon the bed.

3 And Jacob said unto Joseph, God Almighty appeared unto me at Luz in the land of Canaan, and blessed me,

4 And said unto me, Behold, I will make thee fruitful, and multiply thee, and I will make of thee a multitude of people; and will give this land to thy seed after thee *for* an everlasting possession.

5 And now thy two sons, Ephraim and Manasseh, which were born unto thee in the land of Egypt before I came unto thee into Egypt, *are* mine; as Reuben and Simeon, they shall be mine.

6 And thy issue, which thou begettest after them, shall be thine, *and* shall be called after the name of their brethren in their inheritance.

7 And as for me, when I came from Padan, Rachel died by me in the land of Canaan in the way, when yet *there was* but a little way to come unto Ephrath: and I buried her there in the way of Ephrath; the same *is* Beth-lehem.

8 And Israel beheld Joseph's sons, and said, Who *are* these?

9 And Joseph said unto his father, They *are* my sons, whom God hath given me in this *place*. And he said, Bring them, I pray thee, unto me, and I will bless them.

10 Now the eyes of Israel were dim for age, *so that* he could not see. And he brought them near unto him; and he kissed them, and embraced them.

11 And Israel said unto Joseph, I had not thought to see thy face: and, lo, God hath shewed me also thy seed.

12 And Joseph brought them out from between his knees, and he bowed himself with his face to the earth.

13 And Joseph took them both, Ephraim in his right hand toward Israel's left hand, and Manasseh in his left hand toward Israel's right hand, and brought *them* near unto him.

14 And Israel stretched out his right hand, and laid *it* upon Ephraim's head, who *was* the younger, and his left hand upon Manasseh's head, guiding his hands wittingly; for Manasseh *was* the firstborn.

15 And he blessed Joseph, and said, God, before whom my fathers Abraham and Isaac did walk, the God which fed me all my life long unto this day,

16 The [a]Angel which [b]redeemed me from all evil, bless the lads; and let my name be named on them, and the name of my fathers Abraham and Isaac; and let them grow into a multitude in the midst of the earth.

17 And when Joseph saw that his father laid his right hand upon the head of Ephraim, it displeased him: and he held up his father's hand, to remove it from Ephraim's head unto Manasseh's head.

18 And Joseph said unto his father, Not so, my father: for this *is* the firstborn; put thy right hand upon his head.

19 And his father refused, and said, I know *it*, my son, I know *it*: he also shall become a people, and he also shall be great: but truly his younger brother shall be greater than he, and his seed shall become a multitude of nations.

20 And he blessed them that day, saying, In thee shall Israel bless, saying, God make thee as Ephraim and as Manasseh: and he set Ephraim before Manasseh.

21 And Israel said unto Joseph, Behold, I die: but God shall be with you, and bring you again unto the land of your fathers.

22 Moreover I have given to thee one portion above thy brethren, which I took out of the hand of the Amorite with my sword and with my bow.

CHAPTER 49.

Jacob's dying blessing: prophetic of the tribes of Israel.

And Jacob called unto his sons, and said, Gather yourselves together, that I may tell you *that* which shall befall you in the last days.

2 Gather yourselves together, and hear, ye sons of Jacob; and hearken unto Israel your father.

3 Reuben, thou *art* my firstborn, my might, and the beginning of my strength, the excellency of dignity, and the excellency of power:

4 Unstable as water, thou shalt not excel; because thou wentest up to thy father's bed; then defiledst thou *it*: he went up to my couch.

5 Simeon and Levi *are* brethren; instruments of cruelty *are in* their habitations.

6 O my soul, come not thou into their secret; unto their assembly, mine honour, be not thou united: for in their anger they slew a man, and in their selfwill they digged down a wall.

7 Cursed *be* their anger, for *it was* fierce; and their wrath, for it was cruel: I will divide them in Jacob, and scatter them in Israel.

8 [c]Judah, thou *art he* whom thy brethren shall praise: thy hand *shall be* in the neck of thine enemies; thy father's children shall bow down before thee.

9 Judah *is* a lion's whelp: from the prey, my son, thou art gone up: he stooped down, he couched as a lion, and as an old lion; who shall rouse him up?

10 The sceptre shall not depart from Judah, nor a lawgiver from between his feet, until [d]Shiloh come; and unto him *shall* the gathering of the people *be*.

11 Binding his foal unto the vine, and his ass's colt unto the choice vine; he washed his garments in wine, and his clothes in the blood of grapes:

12 His eyes *shall be* red with wine, and his teeth white with milk.

13 Zebulun shall dwell at the haven of the sea; and he *shall be* for an haven of ships; and his border *shall be* unto Zidon.

14 [e]Issachar *is* a strong ass couching down between two burdens:

15 And he saw that rest *was* good, and the land that *it was* pleasant; and bowed his shoulder to bear, and became a servant unto tribute.

16 Dan shall judge his people, as one of the tribes of Israel.

17 Dan shall be a serpent by the way, an adder in the path, that biteth the horse heels, so that his rider shall fall backward.

B.C. 1689.

a Heb. 1:4, *note.*

b Heb. *goel, Redemp. (Kinsman type).* Isa. 59:20, *note.*

c vs. 8, 10; Rev. 5:5.

d *Christ (first advent).* 2 Sam. 7:16. (Gen. 3:15; Acts 1:9.)

e v. 15; 1 Chr. 12:32.

18 I have waited for thy salvation, O LORD.

19 [a]Gad, a troop shall overcome him: but he shall overcome at the last.

20 Out of [b]Asher his bread *shall be* fat, and he shall yield royal dainties.

21 Naphtali *is* a hind let loose: he giveth goodly words.

22 Joseph *is* a fruitful bough, *even* a fruitful bough by a well; *whose* branches run over the wall:

23 The archers have sorely grieved him, and shot *at him*, and hated him:

24 But his bow abode in strength, and the arms of his hands were made strong by the hands of the mighty *God* of Jacob; (from thence *is* the shepherd, the stone of Israel:)

25 *Even* by the God of thy father, who shall help thee; and by the Almighty, who shall bless thee with blessings of heaven above, blessings of the deep that lieth under, blessings of the breasts, and of the womb:

26 The blessings of thy father have prevailed above the blessings of my progenitors unto the utmost bound of the everlasting hills: they shall be on the head of Joseph, and on the crown of the head of him that was separate from his brethren.

27 Benjamin shall ravin *as* a wolf: in the morning he shall devour the prey, and at night he shall divide the spoil.

28 All these *are* the twelve tribes of Israel: and this *is it* that their father spake unto them, and [1]blessed them; every one according to his blessing he blessed them.

29 And he charged them, and said unto them, I am to be gathered unto my people: bury me with my fathers in the cave that *is* in the field of Ephron the Hittite,

30 In the cave that *is* in the field of [c]Machpelah, which *is* before Mamre, in the land of Canaan, which Abraham bought with the field of Ephron the Hittite for a possession of a buryingplace.

31 There they buried Abraham and Sarah his wife; there they buried [d]Isaac and Rebekah his wife; and there I buried Leah.

32 The purchase of the field and of the cave that *is* therein *was* from the children of Heth.

33 And when Jacob had made an end of commanding his sons, he gathered up his feet into the bed, and yielded up the ghost, and was gathered unto his people.

CHAPTER 50.

The burial of Jacob.

And [e]Joseph fell upon his father's face, and wept upon him, and kissed him.

2 And Joseph commanded his servants the physicians to [f]embalm his father: and the physicians embalmed Israel.

3 And forty days were fulfilled for him; for so are fulfilled the days of those which are embalmed: and the Egyptians [g]mourned for him threescore and ten days.

4 And when the days of his mourning were past, Joseph spake unto the house of Pharaoh, saying, If now I have found grace in your eyes, speak, I pray you, in the ears of Pharaoh, saying,

5 My father made me swear, saying, Lo, I die: in my grave which I have digged for me in the land of Canaan, there shalt thou bury me. Now therefore let me go up, I pray thee, and bury my father, and I will come again.

6 And Pharaoh said, Go up, and bury thy father, according as he made thee swear.

7 And Joseph went up to bury his father: and with him went up all the servants of Pharaoh, the elders of his house, and all the elders of the land of Egypt,

8 And all the house of Joseph, and his brethren, and his father's house: only their little ones, and their flocks, and their herds, they left in the land of Goshen.

B.C. 1689.

a Gen. 30:11.
b Josh. 19:24-31.
c Gen. 23:4, *note.*
d Gen. 35:29.
e Gen. 46:4.
f v. 26.
g Gen. 37:34; Num. 20:29; Deut. 34:8.

[1] **(49:28)** Jacob's life, ending in serenity and blessing, testifies to the power of God to transform character. His spiritual progress has six notable phases: (1) the first exercise of faith, as shown in the purchase of the birthright (Gen. 25:28-34; 27:10-22); (2) the vision at Bethel (Gen. 28:10-19); (3) walking in the flesh (Gen. 29:1–31:55); (4) the transforming experience (Gen. 32:24-31); (5) the return to Bethel: idols put away (Gen. 35:1-7); (6) the walk of faith (Gen. 37:1-49:33).

9 And there went up with him both
chariots and horsemen: and it was a
very great company.
10 And they came to the threshingfloor of Atad, which *is* beyond Jordan,
and there they mourned with a great
and very sore lamentation: and he made
a mourning for his father seven days.
11 And when the inhabitants of the
land, the Canaanites, saw the mourning
in the floor of Atad, they said, This *is* a
grievous mourning to the Egyptians:
wherefore the name of it was called
Abel-mizraim, which *is* beyond Jordan.
12 And his sons did unto him according as he commanded them:
13 For his sons carried him into the
land of Canaan, and [a]buried him in the
cave of the field of Machpelah, which
Abraham bought with the field for a
possession of a buryingplace of Ephron
the Hittite, before Mamre.
14 And Joseph returned into Egypt,
he, and his brethren, and all that went
up with him to bury his father, after he
had buried his father.

The fear of Joseph's brethren.

15 And when Joseph's brethren saw
that their father was dead, they said,
Joseph will peradventure hate us, and
will certainly requite us all the evil
which we did unto him.
16 And they sent a messenger unto
Joseph, saying, Thy father did command
before he died, saying,
17 So shall ye say unto Joseph,
Forgive, I pray thee now, the trespass of
thy brethren, and their sin; for they did
unto thee evil: and now, we pray thee,
forgive the trespass of the servants of the
God of thy father. And Joseph wept
when they spake unto him.
18 And his brethren also went and fell
down before his face; and they said,
Behold, we *be* thy servants.
19 And Joseph said unto them, Fear
not: for *am* I in the place of God?
20 But as for you, ye thought evil
against me; *but* God meant it unto good,
to bring to pass, as *it is* this day, to save
much people alive.
21 Now therefore fear ye not: I will
nourish you, and your little ones. And
he comforted them, and spake [b]kindly
unto them.

The last days and death of Joseph.

22 And Joseph dwelt in Egypt, he, and
his father's house: and Joseph lived an
hundred and ten years.
23 And Joseph saw Ephraim's children of the third *generation*: the children
also of Machir the son of Manasseh were
brought up upon Joseph's knees.
24 And Joseph [c]said unto his brethren,
I die: and God will surely visit you, and
bring you out of this land unto the land
which he sware to Abraham, to Isaac,
and to Jacob.
25 And Joseph took an [d]oath of the
children of Israel, saying, God will surely visit [e]you, and ye shall carry up my
bones from hence.
26 So Joseph died, *being* an hundred
and ten years old: and they embalmed
him, and he was put in a coffin in Egypt.

B.C. 1689.

a Gen. 23:4, *note*; 49:30-31.

b i.e. *to their hearts.*

c *Faith.* vs. 24, 25; Ex. 1:17. (Gen. 3:20; Heb. 11:39.)

d Ex. 13:19; Josh. 24:32; Acts 7:15-16; Heb. 11:22.

e Gen. 17:8; 26:3; 28:13; 35:12; Deut. 1:8; 30:1-9, *refs.*

THE SECOND BOOK OF MOSES CALLED EXODUS

EXODUS, "going out," records the redemption out of Egyptian bondage of the descendants of Abraham, and sets forth, in type, all redemption. It is therefore peculiarly the book of redemption. But as all redemption is unto a relationship with God of which worship, fellowship, and service are expressions, so Exodus, in the giving of the law and the provisions of sacrifice and priesthood, becomes not only the book of redemption, but also, in type, of the conditions upon which all relationships with God exist.

Broadly, the book teaches that redemption is essential to any relationship with a holy God; and that even a redeemed people cannot have fellowship with Him unless constantly cleansed from defilement.

In Exodus, God, hitherto connected with the Israelitish people only through His covenant with Abraham, brings them to Himself *nationally* through redemption, puts them under the Mosaic Covenant, and dwells among them in the cloud of glory. Galatians explains the relation of the law to the Abrahamic Covenant. In the Commandments God taught Israel His just demands. Experience under the Commandments convicted Israel of sin; and the provision of priesthood and sacrifice (filled with precious types of Christ) gave a guilty people a way of forgiveness, cleansing, restoration to fellowship, and worship.

Exodus falls into three chief divisions: I. Israel in Egypt (1–15). II. From the Red Sea to Sinai (16–18). III. Israel at Sinai (19–40).

The events recorded in Exodus cover a period of 216 years (Ussher).

CHAPTER 1.

B.C. 1706.

Israel in Egypt.

Now these *are* the names of the children of Israel, which came into Egypt; every man and his household came with Jacob.

2 Reuben, Simeon, Levi, and Judah,

3 Issachar, Zebulun, and Benjamin,

4 Dan, and Naphtali, Gad, and Asher.

5 And all the souls that came out of the loins of Jacob were seventy souls: for Joseph was in Egypt *already*.

6 And Joseph died, and all his brethren, and all that generation.

The Egyptian bondage.

7 And the children of Israel were fruitful, and increased abundantly, and multiplied, and waxed exceeding mighty; and the land was filled with them.

8 Now there arose up a new king over Egypt, which knew not Joseph.

9 And he said unto his people, Behold, the people of the children of Israel *are* more and mightier than we:

10 Come on, let us deal wisely with them; lest they multiply, and it come to pass, that, when there falleth out any war, they join also unto our enemies, and fight against us, and *so* get them up out of the land.

11 Therefore they did set over them taskmasters to afflict them with their burdens. And they built for Pharaoh treasure cities, Pithom and Raamses.

12 But the more they afflicted them, the more they multiplied and grew. And they were grieved because of the children of Israel.

13 And the Egyptians made the children of Israel to serve with rigour:

14 And they made their lives bitter with hard bondage, in morter, and in brick, and in all manner of service in the field: all their service, wherein they made them serve, *was* with rigour.

15 And the king of Egypt spake to the Hebrew midwives, of which the name of the one *was* Shiphrah, and the name of the other Puah:

16 And he said, When ye do the office of a midwife to the Hebrew women, and see *them* upon the stools; if it *be* a son, then ye shall kill him: but if it *be* a daughter, then she shall live.

17 But the midwives [a]feared God, and did not as the king of Egypt commanded them, [b]but saved the men children alive.

18 And the king of Egypt called for the midwives, and said unto

a Psa. 19:19, *note*.

b *Faith*. Ex. 2:1-3. (Gen. 3:20; Heb. 11:39.)

B.C. 1635.

them, Why have ye done this thing, and have saved the men children alive?

19 And the midwives said unto Pharaoh, Because the Hebrew women *are* not as the Egyptian women; for they *are* lively, and are delivered ere the midwives come in unto them.

20 Therefore God dealt well with the midwives: and the people multiplied, and waxed very mighty.

21 And it came to pass, because the midwives feared God, that he made them houses.

22 And Pharaoh charged all his people, saying, Every son that is born ye shall cast into the river, and every daughter ye shall save alive.

CHAPTER 2.

The preparation of the deliverer (Ex. 2:1–4:28). *The birth of Moses.*

And there went a man of the house of Levi, and took *to wife* a daughter of Levi.

2 And the woman conceived, and bare a [1]son: and when she saw him that he *was a* goodly *child,* [a]she [b]hid him three months.

3 And when she could not longer hide him, she took for him an ark of bulrushes, and daubed it with slime and with pitch, and put the child therein; and she laid *it* in the flags by the river's brink.

4 And his sister stood afar off, to wit what would be done to him.

5 And the daughter of Pharaoh came down to wash *herself* at the river; and her maidens walked along by the river's side; and when she saw the ark among the flags, she sent her maid to fetch it.

6 And when she had opened *it,* she saw the child: and, behold, the babe wept. And she had compassion on him, and said, This *is one* of the Hebrews' children.

7 Then said his sister to Pharaoh's daughter, Shall I go and call to thee a nurse of the Hebrew women, that she may nurse the child for thee?

8 And Pharaoh's daughter said to her, Go. And the maid went and called the child's mother.

9 And Pharaoh's daughter said unto her, Take this child away, and nurse it for me, and I will give *thee* thy wages. And the woman took the child, and nursed it.

10 And the child grew, and she brought him unto Pharaoh's daughter, and he became her son. And she called his name [c]Moses: and she said, [d]Because I drew him out of the water.

Moses identifies himself with Israel.

11 And it came to pass in those days, when Moses was grown, that he went out unto his brethren, and looked on their burdens: and he spied an Egyptian smiting an Hebrew, one of his brethren.

12 And he looked this way and that way, and when he saw that *there was* no man, he slew the Egyptian, and hid him in the sand.

13 And when he went out the second day, behold, two men of the Hebrews strove together: and he said to him that did the wrong, Wherefore smitest thou thy fellow?

14 And he said, Who made thee a prince and a judge over us? intendest thou to kill me, as thou killedst the Egyptian? And Moses feared, and said, Surely this thing is known.

15 Now when Pharaoh heard this thing, he sought to slay Moses. But Moses fled from the face of Pharaoh, and dwelt in the land of Midian: and he sat down by a well.

16 Now the priest of Midian had seven daughters: and they came and drew *water,* and filled the

a Faith. vs. 1-3; Ex. 12:21-28. (Gen. 3:20; Heb. 11:39.)

b Acts 7:20-28; Heb. 11:23.

c Heb. *Mosheh.*

d Heb. *mashah,* to draw out.

1 (2:2) Moses, type of Christ the Deliverer (Isa. 61:1; Lk. 4:18; 2 Cor. 1:10; 1 Thes. 1:10): (1) A divinely chosen deliverer (Ex. 3:7-10; Acts 7:25; John 3:16). (2) Rejected by Israel he turns to the Gentiles (Ex. 2:11-15; Acts 7:25; 18:5, 6; 28:17-28). (3) During his rejection he gains a Gentile bride (Ex. 2:16-21; Mt. 12:14-21; 2 Cor. 11:2; Eph. 5:30-32). (4) Afterward he again appears as Israel's deliverer, and is accepted (Ex. 4:29-31; Rom. 11:24-26; Acts 15:14-17). (5) Officially, Moses typifies Christ as Prophet (Acts 3:22, 23), Advocate (Ex. 32:31-35; 1 John 2:1, 2), Intercessor (Ex. 17:1-6; Heb. 7:25), and Leader, or King (Deut. 33:4, 5; Isa. 55:4; Heb. 2:10); while, in relation to the house of God, he is in contrast with Christ. Moses was faithful as a servant over another's house; Christ as a Son over His own house (Heb. 3:5, 6).

troughs to water their father's flock.
17 And the shepherds came and drove
them away: but Moses stood up and
helped them, and watered their flock.
18 And when they came to [a]Reuel
their father, he said, How *is it that* ye are
come so soon to day?
19 And they said, An Egyptian delivered us out of the hand of the shepherds,
and also drew *water* enough for us, and
watered the flock.
20 And he said unto his daughters, And
where *is* he? why *is* it *that* ye have left the
man? call him, that he may eat bread.

Moses, rejected by his brethren, takes a Gentile bride.
(Cf. Acts 18:5, 6; Eph. 5:30–32.)

21 And Moses was content to dwell
with the man: and he gave Moses
Zipporah his daughter.
22 And she bare *him* a son, and he
called his name Gershom: for he said, I
have been a stranger in a strange land.
23 And it came to pass in process of
time, that the king of Egypt died: and
the children of Israel sighed by reason of
the bondage, and they cried, and their
cry came up unto God by reason of the
bondage.
24 And God heard their groaning, and
God remembered his covenant with
Abraham, with Isaac, and with Jacob.
25 And God looked upon the children
of Israel, and God had respect unto *them*.

CHAPTER 3.

The call of Moses: the burning bush.

[b]Now Moses kept the flock of
Jethro his father in law, the priest
of Midian: and he led the flock to the
backside of the desert, and came to the
mountain of God, *even* to Horeb.
2 And the [c]angel of the LORD appeared
unto him in a flame of fire out of the
midst of a bush: and he looked, and,
behold, the bush burned with fire, and
the bush *was* not consumed.
3 And Moses said, I will now turn
aside, and see this great sight, why the
bush is not burnt.
4 And when the LORD saw that he
turned aside to see, God called unto him
out of the midst of the bush, and said,
Moses, Moses. And he said, Here *am* I.
5 And he said, Draw not nigh hither:
put off thy shoes from off thy feet, for
the place whereon thou standest *is* holy
ground.
6 Moreover he said, I *am* the God of
thy father, [d]the God of Abraham, the
God of Isaac, and the God of Jacob. And
Moses hid his face; for he was afraid to
look upon God.
7 And the LORD said, I have surely
seen the affliction of my people which
are in Egypt, and have heard their cry by
reason of their taskmasters; for I know
their sorrows;
8 And I am come down to deliver
them out of the hand of the Egyptians,
and to bring them up out of that land
unto a good land and a large, unto a land
flowing with milk and honey; unto the
place of the Canaanites, and the Hittites,
and the Amorites, and the Perizzites, and
the Hivites, and the Jebusites.
9 Now therefore, behold, the cry of the
children of Israel is come unto me: and I
have also seen the oppression wherewith the Egyptians oppress them.
10 Come now therefore, and I will
send thee unto Pharaoh, that thou
mayest bring forth my people the children of Israel out of Egypt.
11 And Moses said unto God, Who *am*
I, that I should go unto Pharaoh, and
that I should bring forth the children of
Israel out of Egypt?
12 And he said, Certainly I will be with
thee; and this *shall be* a token unto thee,
that I have sent thee: When thou hast
brought forth the people out of Egypt, ye
shall serve God upon this mountain.

The revelation of the name Jehovah.

13 And Moses said unto God, Behold,
when I come unto the children of Israel,
and shall say unto them, The God of
your fathers hath sent me unto you; and
they shall say to me, What *is* his name?
what shall I say unto them?
14 And God said unto Moses, [e]I AM
THAT I AM: and he said, Thus shalt
thou say unto the children of Israel, I
AM hath sent me unto you.

The commission of Moses.

15 And God said moreover unto
Moses, Thus shalt thou say unto the
children of [f]Israel, The LORD God

B.C. 1531.

a Called *Raguel*, Num. 10:29.

b *Kingdom* (O.T.). vs. 1-10; Ex. 19:9. (Gen. 1:26; Zech. 12:8.)

c Heb. 1:4, *note*.

d Mt. 22:32; Mk. 12:26; Acts 7:32.

e *Deity* (*names of*). Ex. 34:6, 7. (Gen. 1:1; Mal. 3:18.)

f *Israel* (*history*). vs. 15-17; Ex. 12:1-13. (Gen. 12:2, 3; Rom. 11:26.)

of your fathers, the God of Abraham, the God of Isaac, and the God of Jacob, hath sent me unto you: this *is* my name for ever, and this *is* my memorial unto all generations.

16 Go, and gather the elders of Israel together, and say unto them, The LORD God of your fathers, the God of Abraham, of Isaac, and of Jacob, appeared unto me, saying, I have surely visited you, and *seen* that which is done to you in Egypt:

17 And I have said, I will bring you up out of the affliction of Egypt unto the land of the Canaanites, and the Hittites, and the Amorites, and the Perizzites, and the Hivites, and the Jebusites, unto a land flowing with milk and honey.

18 And they shall hearken to thy voice: and thou shalt come, thou and the elders of Israel, unto the king of Egypt, and ye shall say unto him, The LORD God of the Hebrews hath met with us: and now let us go, we beseech thee, three days' journey into the wilderness, that we may sacrifice to the LORD our God.

19 And I am sure that the king of Egypt will not let you go, no, not by a mighty hand.

20 And I will stretch out my hand, and smite Egypt with all my wonders which I will do in the midst thereof: and after that he will let you go.

21 And I will give this people favour in the sight of the Egyptians: and it shall come to pass, that, when ye go, ye shall not go empty:

22 But every woman shall [a]borrow of her neighbour, and of her that sojourneth in her house, jewels of silver, and jewels of gold, and raiment: and ye shall put *them* upon your sons, and upon your daughters; and ye shall spoil the Egyptians.

CHAPTER 4.

Moses' two objections:
(1) *the unbelief of the people.*

AND Moses answered and said, But, behold, they will not believe me, nor hearken unto my voice: for they will say, The LORD hath not appeared unto thee.

B.C. 1491.

a Lit. *ask.*

b The use of little things. Cf. Jud. 3:31; 1 Ki. 17:12-16; John 6:9; 1 Cor. 1:25-31.

c Sign of the rod = power (Psa. 110:2; 2:9; Rev. 2:27). It was Moses' shepherd's crook, the tool of his calling. Cast down it became a serpent; taken up in faith, it became "the rod of God" (Ex. 4:20. Cf. Ex. 7:12, *note*).

d *Miracles* (O.T.). vs. 3, 4, 6, 7; Ex. 7:10-12. (Gen. 5:24; Jon. 2:1-10.)

2 And the LORD said unto him, What *is* that in thine [b]hand? And he said, A [c]rod.

3 And he said, Cast it on the ground. And he cast it on the ground, and it [d]became a serpent; and Moses fled from before it.

4 And the LORD said unto Moses, Put forth thine hand, and take it by the tail. And he put forth his hand, and caught it, and it became a rod in his hand:

5 That they may believe that the LORD God of their fathers, the God of Abraham, the God of Isaac, and the God of Jacob, hath appeared unto thee.

6 And the LORD said furthermore unto him, [1]Put now thine hand into thy bosom. And he put his hand into his bosom: and when he took it out, behold, his hand *was* leprous as snow.

7 And he said, Put thine hand into thy bosom again. And he put his hand into his bosom again; and plucked it out of his bosom, and, behold, it was turned again as his *other* flesh.

8 And it shall come to pass, if they will not believe thee, neither hearken to the voice of the first sign, that they will believe the voice of the latter sign.

9 And it shall come to pass, if they will not believe also these two signs, neither hearken unto thy voice, that thou shalt take of the water of the river, and pour *it* upon the dry *land*: and the water which thou takest out of the river shall become blood upon the dry *land.*

Moses' two objections:
(2) *his lack of eloquence.*

10 And Moses said unto the LORD, O my Lord, I *am* not eloquent, neither heretofore, nor since thou hast spoken unto thy servant: but I *am* slow of speech, and of a slow tongue.

11 And the LORD said unto him, Who hath made man's mouth? or who maketh the dumb, or deaf, or the seeing, or the blind? have not I the LORD?

12 Now therefore go, and I will be with thy mouth, and teach thee what thou shalt say.

[1] **(4:6)** The sign of leprosy. The heart ("bosom") stands for what we *are,* the hand for what we *do.* What we are, that ultimately we do. It is a sign of Lk. 6:43-45. The two signs, rod and hand, speak of preparation for service: (1) consecration—our capacity taken up for God; (2) the hand that holds the rod of God's power must be a cleansed hand swayed by a new heart (Isa. 52:11).

13 And he said, O my Lord, send, I pray thee, by the hand *of him whom* thou wilt send.

Aaron joined with Moses.

14 And the anger of the LORD was kindled against Moses, and he said, *Is* not [a]Aaron [1]the Levite thy brother? I know that he can speak well. And also, behold, he cometh forth to meet thee: and when he seeth thee, he will be glad in his heart.

15 And thou shalt speak unto him, and put words in his [b]mouth: and I will be with thy mouth, and with his mouth, and will teach you what ye shall do.

16 And he shall be thy spokesman unto the people: and he shall be, *even* he shall be to thee instead of a mouth, and thou shalt be to him instead of God.

17 And thou shalt take this rod in thine hand, wherewith thou shalt do signs.

18 And Moses went and returned to Jethro his father in law, and said unto him, Let me go, I pray thee, and return unto my brethren which *are* in Egypt, and see whether they be yet alive. And Jethro said to Moses, Go in peace.

The return of Moses to Egypt.

19 And the LORD said unto Moses in Midian, Go, return into Egypt: for all the men are dead which sought thy life.

20 And Moses took his wife and his sons, and set them upon an ass, and he returned to the land of Egypt: and Moses took the rod of God in his hand.

21 And the LORD said unto Moses, When thou goest to return into Egypt, see that thou do all those wonders before Pharaoh, which I have put in thine hand: but I will [2]harden his heart, that he shall not let the people go.

22 And thou shalt [c]say unto Pharaoh, Thus saith the LORD, Israel *is* my son, *even* my firstborn:

23 And I say unto thee, Let my son go, that he may serve me: and if thou refuse to let him go, behold, I will slay thy son, *even* thy firstborn.

24 And it came to pass by the way in the inn, that the LORD met him, and sought to [3]kill him.

25 Then Zipporah took a sharp stone, and cut off the foreskin of her son, and cast *it* at his feet, and said, Surely a bloody husband *art* thou to me.

26 So he let him go: then she said, A bloody husband *thou art*, because of the circumcision.

27 And the LORD said to Aaron, Go into the wilderness to meet Moses. And he went, and met him in the mount of God, and kissed him.

28 And Moses told Aaron all the words of the LORD who had sent him, and all the signs which he had commanded him.

Deliverance announced to the elders of Israel.

29 And Moses and Aaron went and gathered together all the elders of the children of Israel:

30 And Aaron spake all the words which the LORD had spoken unto Moses, and did the signs in the sight of the people.

31 And the people believed: and when they heard that the LORD had visited the children of Israel, and that he had looked upon their affliction, then they bowed their heads and worshipped.

CHAPTER 5.

The contest with Pharaoh: the first demand; the increased burdens.

And afterward Moses and Aaron went in, and told Pharaoh, Thus saith the LORD God of Israel, [d]Let my people go, that they may hold a feast unto me in the wilderness.

B.C. 1491.

a Cf. Ex. 32:21.

b *Inspiration.* vs. 15, 28, 30. Ex. 17:14. (Ex. 4:15; Rev. 22:29.)

c Cf. Ex. 5:1.

d Cf. Ex. 4:22, 23. Possibly Moses and Aaron shrank from delivering the message concerning the firstborn.

[1] **(4:14)** Cf. Ex. 28:1, *note.*

[2] **(4:21)** Cf. Ex. 8:15, 32; 9:34. In the face of the righteous demand of Jehovah and of the tremendous attestations by miracle that He was indeed God, and that Moses and Aaron were His representatives, Pharaoh "hardened his heart." *Instrumentally* God hardened Pharaoh's heart by forcing him to an issue against which he hardened his own heart in refusal. Light rejected, rightful obedience refused, inevitably hardens conscience and heart. See Rom. 9:17-24.

[3] **(4:24)** Cf. Gen. 17:14. The context (v. 25) interprets v. 24. Moses was forgetful of the very foundation sign of Israel's covenant relation to Jehovah. On the eve of delivering Israel he was thus reminded that without circumcision an Israelite was cut off from the covenant. See Josh. 5:3-9.

B.C. 1491.

2 And Pharaoh said, Who *is* the LORD,
that I should obey his voice to let Israel
go? I know not the LORD, neither will I
let Israel go.
3 And they said, The God of the
Hebrews hath met with us: let us go, we
pray thee, [a]three days' journey into the
desert, and sacrifice unto the LORD our
God; lest he fall upon us with pestilence,
or with the sword.
4 And the king of Egypt said unto
them, Wherefore do ye, Moses and
Aaron, let the people from their works?
get you unto your burdens.
5 And Pharaoh said, Behold, the people of the land now *are* many, and ye
make them rest from their burdens.
6 And Pharaoh commanded the same
day the taskmasters of the people, and
their officers, saying,
7 Ye shall no more give the people
straw to make brick, as heretofore: let
them go and gather straw for themselves.
8 And the tale of the bricks, which they
did make heretofore, ye shall lay upon
them; ye shall not diminish *ought* thereof:
for they *be* idle; therefore they cry, saying, Let us go *and* sacrifice to our God.
9 Let there more work be laid upon
the men, that they may labour therein;
and let them not regard vain words.
10 And the taskmasters of the people
went out, and their officers, and they
spake to the people, saying, Thus saith
Pharaoh, I will not give you straw.
11 Go ye, get you straw where ye can
find it: yet not ought of your work shall
be diminished.
12 So the people were scattered
abroad throughout all the land of Egypt
to gather stubble instead of straw.
13 And the taskmasters hasted *them*,
saying, Fulfil your works, *your* daily
tasks, as when there was straw.
14 And the officers of the children of
Israel, which Pharaoh's taskmasters had
set over them, were beaten, *and* demanded, Wherefore have ye not fulfilled your
task in making brick both yesterday and
to day, as heretofore?
15 Then the officers of the children of
Israel came and cried unto Pharaoh, saying, Wherefore dealest thou thus with
thy servants?
16 There is no straw given unto thy
servants, and they say to us, Make brick:
and, behold, thy servants *are* beaten; but
the fault *is* in thine own people.
17 But he said, Ye *are* idle, *ye are* idle:
therefore ye say, Let us go *and* do sacrifice to the LORD.
18 Go therefore now, *and* work; for
there shall no straw be given you, yet
shall ye deliver the tale of bricks.
19 And the officers of the children of
Israel did see *that* they *were* in evil *case*,
after it was said, Ye shall not minish
ought from your bricks of your daily task.
20 And they met Moses and Aaron,
who stood in the way, as they came forth
from Pharaoh:
21 And they said unto them, The
LORD look upon you, and judge;
because ye have made our savour to be
abhorred in the eyes of Pharaoh, and
in the eyes of his servants, to put a
sword in their hand to slay us.
22 And Moses returned unto the LORD,
and said, Lord, wherefore hast thou *so*
evil entreated this people? why *is* it *that*
thou hast sent me?
23 For since I came to Pharaoh to
speak in thy name, he hath done evil to
this people; neither hast thou delivered
thy people at all.

CHAPTER 6.

The answer of Jehovah
to Moses' first prayer.

Then the LORD said unto Moses, Now
shalt thou see what I will do to
Pharaoh: for with a strong hand shall he
let them go, and with a strong hand shall
he drive them out of his land.
2 And God spake unto Moses, and
said unto him, I *am* the LORD:
3 And I appeared unto Abraham, unto
Isaac, and unto Jacob, by *the name of* God
Almighty, but by my name JEHOVAH
was I not known to them.
4 And I have also established my
covenant with them, to give them the
land of Canaan, the land of their pilgrimage, wherein they were strangers.
5 And I have also heard the groaning
of the children of Israel, whom the
Egyptians keep in bondage; and I have
remembered my covenant.
6 Wherefore say unto the children of
Israel, I *am* the LORD, and I will bring

a Cf. Mt. 12:38-40. By death and resurrection will God have his people separated from Egypt—the world (Rom. 6:1-11; Gal. 6:14, 15; Heb. 13:12, 13).

you [a]out from under the burdens of the
Egyptians, and I will rid you out of their
bondage, and I will [b]redeem you with a
stretched out arm, and with great judgments:
7 And I will take you to me for a people, and I will be to you a God: and ye
shall know that I *am* the LORD your God,
which bringeth you out from under the
burdens of the Egyptians.
8 And I will bring you in unto the
land, concerning the which I did [c]swear
to give it to Abraham, to Isaac, and to
Jacob; and I will give it you for an heritage: I *am* the LORD.
9 And Moses spake so unto the children of Israel: but they hearkened not
unto Moses for anguish of spirit, and for
cruel bondage.
10 And the LORD spake unto Moses,
saying,
11 Go in, speak unto Pharaoh king of
Egypt, that he let the children of Israel
go out of his land.
12 And Moses spake before the LORD,
saying, Behold, the children of Israel
have not hearkened unto me; how then
shall Pharaoh hear me, who *am* of uncircumcised lips?
13 And the LORD spake unto Moses
and unto Aaron, and gave them a [d]charge
unto the children of Israel, and unto
Pharaoh king of Egypt, to bring the children of Israel out of the land of Egypt.

The families of Israel.

14 These *be* the heads of their fathers'
houses: The sons of Reuben the firstborn
of Israel; Hanoch, and Pallu, Hezron, and
Carmi: these *be* the families of Reuben.
15 And the sons of Simeon; Jemuel, and
Jamin, and Ohad, and Jachin, and Zohar,
and Shaul the son of a Canaanitish
woman: these *are* the families of Simeon.
16 And these *are* the names of the sons
of Levi according to their generations;
Gershon, and Kohath, and Merari: and
the years of the life of Levi *were* an hundred thirty and seven years.
17 The sons of Gershon; Libni, and
Shimi, according to their families.
18 And the sons of Kohath; Amram,
and Izhar, and Hebron, and Uzziel: and
the years of the life of Kohath *were* an
hundred thirty and three years.
19 And the sons of Merari; Mahali and

B.C. 1491.

a *Separation.* vs. 6, 7; Ex. 8:25-27. (Gen. 12:1; 2 Cor. 6:14-17.)

b Heb. *goel*, *Redemp.* (*Kinsman type*). Isa. 59:20, *note.*

c v. 4; Gen. 15:18; 26:3; 35:12.

d Num. 27:19, 23; Deut. 31:14.

e Ex. 5:1; 7:4.

Mushi: these *are* the families of Levi
according to their generations.
20 And Amram took him Jochebed his
father's sister to wife; and she bare him
Aaron and Moses: and the years of the
life of Amram *were* an hundred and thirty and seven years.
21 And the sons of Izhar; Korah, and
Nepheg, and Zichri.
22 And the sons of Uzziel; Mishael,
and Elzaphan, and Zithri.
23 And Aaron took him Elisheba,
daughter of Amminadab, sister of
Naashon, to wife; and she bare him
Nadab, and Abihu, Eleazar, and Ithamar.
24 And the sons of Korah; Assir, and
Elkanah, and Abiasaph: these *are* the
families of the Korhites.
25 And Eleazar Aaron's son took him
one of the daughters of Putiel to wife;
and she bare him Phinehas: these *are* the
heads of the fathers of the Levites
according to their families.
26 These *are* that Aaron and Moses, to
whom the LORD said, [e]Bring out the children of Israel from the land of Egypt
according to their armies.
27 These *are* they which spake to
Pharaoh king of Egypt, to bring out the
children of Israel from Egypt: these *are*
that Moses and Aaron.

The renewed commission.

28 And it came to pass on the day
when the LORD spake unto Moses in the
land of Egypt,
29 That the LORD spake unto Moses,
saying, I *am* the LORD: speak thou unto
Pharaoh king of Egypt all that I say unto
thee.
30 And Moses said before the LORD,
Behold, I *am* of uncircumcised lips, and
how shall Pharaoh hearken unto me?

CHAPTER 7.

And the LORD said unto Moses, See, I
have made thee a god to Pharaoh:
and Aaron thy brother shall be thy
prophet.
2 Thou shalt speak all that I command
thee: and Aaron thy brother shall speak
unto Pharaoh, that he send the children
of Israel out of his land.
3 And I will harden Pharaoh's heart,
and multiply my signs and my wonders
in the land of Egypt.

4 But Pharaoh shall not hearken unto you, that I may lay my hand upon Egypt, and bring forth mine armies, *and* my people the children of Israel, out of the land of Egypt by great judgments.

5 And the Egyptians shall know that I *am* the LORD, [a]when I stretch forth mine hand upon Egypt, and bring out the children of Israel from among them.

6 And Moses and Aaron did as the LORD commanded them, so did they.

7 And Moses *was* fourscore years old, and Aaron fourscore and three years old, when they spake unto Pharaoh.

8 And the LORD spake unto Moses and unto Aaron, saying,

9 When Pharaoh shall speak unto you, saying, Shew a miracle for you: then thou shalt say unto Aaron, Take thy rod, and cast *it* before Pharaoh, *and* it shall become a serpent.

The contest with Pharaoh: the second demand; the first miracle.

10 And Moses and Aaron went in unto Pharaoh, and they did so as the LORD had commanded: and Aaron cast down his rod before Pharaoh, and before his servants, and it [b]became a serpent.

11 Then Pharaoh also called the wise men and the sorcerers: now the magicians of Egypt, they also did in [c]like manner with their enchantments.

12 For they cast down every man his rod, and they became serpents: but Aaron's [1]rod swallowed up their rods.

13 And he hardened Pharaoh's heart, that he hearkened not unto them; as the LORD had said.

The contest with Pharaoh: the third demand.

14 And the LORD said unto Moses, Pharaoh's heart *is* hardened, he refuseth to let the people go.

15 Get thee unto Pharaoh in the morning; lo, he goeth out unto the water; and thou shalt stand by the river's brink against he come; and the rod which was turned to a serpent shalt thou take in thine hand.

16 And thou shalt say unto him, The LORD God of the Hebrews hath sent me unto thee, saying, Let my people go, that they may serve me in the wilderness: and, behold, hitherto thou wouldest not hear.

17 Thus saith the LORD, In this thou shalt know that I *am* the LORD: behold, I will smite with the rod that *is* in mine hand upon the waters which *are* in the river, and they shall be turned to blood.

18 And the fish that *is* in the river shall die, and the river shall stink; and the Egyptians shall lothe to drink of the water of the river.

19 And the LORD spake unto Moses, Say unto Aaron, Take thy rod, and stretch out thine hand upon the waters of Egypt, upon their streams, upon their rivers, and upon their ponds, and upon all their pools of water, that they may become blood; and *that* there may be blood throughout all the land of Egypt, both in *vessels of* wood, and in *vessels of* stone.

The contest with Pharaoh: the second miracle; the first judgment.

20 And Moses and Aaron did so, as the LORD commanded; and he lifted up the rod, and smote the waters that *were* in the river, in the sight of Pharaoh, and in the sight of his servants; and all the waters that *were* in the river were turned to blood.

21 And the fish that *was* in the river died; and the river stank, and the Egyptians could not drink of the water of the river; and there was blood throughout all the land of Egypt.

22 And the magicians of Egypt did [d]so with their enchantments: and Pharaoh's heart was hardened, neither did he hearken unto them; [e]as the LORD had said.

23 And Pharaoh turned and went into his house, neither did he set his heart to this also.

24 And all the Egyptians digged round about the river for water to drink; for they could not drink of the water of the river.

B.C. 1491.

a A prophetic sign also. The nations shall know Jehovah when He restores and blesses Israel in the kingdom (Isa. 2:1-3; 11:10-12; 14:1; 60:4, 5; Ezk. 37:28).

b *Miracles* (O.T.). vs. 10-12, 20-25; Ex. 8:5-14. (Gen. 5:24; Jon. 2:1-10.)

c Cf. 2 Tim. 3:8. See Ex. 8:18. Neither Satan nor his tools can create *life*. Rev. 13:15 will be a "lying wonder" (2 Thes. 2:9).

d vs. 11.

e Ex. 3:19.

[1] **(7:12)** Cf. Ex. 4:2. As Moses' rod was the rod of *power*, the rod of the King (Deut. 33:4, 5), so Aaron's was the rod of *life*, the rod of the Priest. As here the serpents, symbols of Satan, who had the power of death (Rev. 12:9, Heb. 2:14), are swallowed up, so in resurrection death will be "swallowed up in victory" (1 Cor. 15:54). See Num. 17:8.

25 And seven days were fulfilled, after that the LORD had smitten the river.

CHAPTER 8.

The contest with Pharaoh: the fourth demand.

And the LORD spake unto Moses, Go unto Pharaoh, and say unto him, Thus saith the LORD, Let my people go, that they may serve me.

2 And if thou refuse to let *them* go, behold, I will smite all thy borders with frogs:

3 And the river shall bring forth frogs abundantly, which shall go up and come into thine house, and into thy bedchamber, and upon thy bed, and into the house of thy servants, and upon thy people, and into thine ovens, and into thy kneadingtroughs:

4 And the frogs shall come up both on thee, and upon thy people, and upon all thy servants.

5 And the LORD spake unto Moses, Say unto Aaron, Stretch forth thine hand with thy rod over the streams, over the rivers, and over the ponds, and cause frogs to come up upon the land of Egypt.

The contest with Pharaoh: the third miracle; the second judgment.

6 And Aaron stretched out his hand over the waters of Egypt; [a]and the frogs came up, and covered the land of Egypt.

7 And the magicians did [b]so with their enchantments, and brought up frogs upon the land of Egypt.

8 Then Pharaoh called for Moses and Aaron, and said, Intreat the LORD, that he may take away the frogs from me, and from my people; and I will let the people go, that they may do sacrifice unto the LORD.

9 And Moses said unto Pharaoh, Glory over me: when shall I intreat for thee, and for thy servants, and for thy people, to destroy the frogs from thee and thy houses, *that* they may remain in the river only?

10 And he said, To morrow. And he said, *Be it* according to thy word: that thou mayest know that *there is* none like unto the LORD our God.

11 And the frogs shall depart from thee, and from thy houses, and from thy servants, and from thy people; they shall remain in the river only.

B.C. 1491.

a *Miracles* (O.T.). vs. 5-14, 16-18, 20-24; Ex. 9:3-6. (Gen. 5:24; Jon. 2:1-10.)

b Ex. 7:11.

c Ex. 7:13.

d Cf. Ex. 7:11.

e Ex. 2:5.

The fourth miracle.

12 And Moses and Aaron went out from Pharaoh: and Moses cried unto the LORD because of the frogs which he had brought against Pharaoh.

13 And the LORD did according to the word of Moses; and the frogs died out of the houses, out of the villages, and out of the fields.

14 And they gathered them together upon heaps: and the land stank.

15 But when Pharaoh saw that there was respite, he [c]hardened his heart, and hearkened not unto them; as the LORD had said.

The contest with Pharaoh: the fifth miracle; the third judgment.

16 And the LORD said unto Moses, Say unto Aaron, Stretch out thy rod, and smite the dust of the land, that it may become lice throughout all the land of Egypt.

17 And they did so; for Aaron stretched out his hand with his rod, and smote the dust of the earth, and it became lice in man, and in beast; all the dust of the land became lice throughout all the land of Egypt.

18 And the magicians did so with their enchantments to bring forth lice, but they [d]could not: so there were lice upon man, and upon beast.

19 Then the magicians said unto Pharaoh, This *is* the finger of God: and Pharaoh's heart was hardened, and he hearkened not unto them; as the LORD had said.

The contest with Pharaoh: the fifth demand.

20 And the LORD said unto Moses, Rise up early in the morning, and stand before Pharaoh; lo, he [e]cometh forth to the water; and say unto him, Thus saith the LORD, Let my people go, that they may serve me.

21 Else, if thou wilt not let my people go, behold, I will send swarms *of flies* upon thee, and upon thy servants, and upon thy people, and into thy houses: and the houses of the Egyptians shall be full of swarms *of flies*, and also the ground whereon they *are*.

22 And I will sever in that day the land of Goshen, in which my people dwell, that no swarms *of flies* shall be there; to the end thou mayest know

that I *am* the LORD in the midst of the earth.

23 And I will put a [a]division between my people and thy people: to morrow shall this sign be.

The contest with Pharaoh: the sixth miracle; the fourth judgment.

24 And the LORD did so; and there came a grievous swarm *of flies* into the house of Pharaoh, and *into* his servants' houses, and into all the land of Egypt: the land was corrupted by reason of the swarm *of flies*.

The contest with Pharaoh: the first compromise refused.

25 And Pharaoh called for Moses and for Aaron, and said, Go ye, sacrifice to your God [1]in the land.

26 And Moses [b]said, It is not meet so to do; for we shall sacrifice the abomination of the Egyptians to the LORD our God: lo, shall we sacrifice the abomination of the Egyptians before their eyes, and will they not stone us?

27 We will go three days' journey into the wilderness, and sacrifice to the LORD our God, as he shall command us.

The contest with Pharaoh: the second compromise refused.

28 And Pharaoh said, I will let you go, that ye may sacrifice to the LORD your God in the wilderness; only ye shall not go [c]very far away: intreat for me.

29 And Moses said, Behold, I go out from thee, and I will intreat the LORD that the swarms *of flies* may depart from Pharaoh, from his servants, and from his people, to morrow: but let not Pharaoh deal deceitfully any more in not letting the people go to sacrifice to the LORD.

The seventh miracle.

30 And Moses went out from Pharaoh, and intreated the LORD.

31 And the LORD did according to the word of Moses; and he removed the swarms *of flies* from Pharaoh, from his servants, and from his people; there remained not one.

32 And Pharaoh hardened his heart at this time also, neither would he let the people go.

B.C. 1491.

a Heb. *peduth*, trans. "redemtion," Psa. 111:9; 130:7. It is, in type, Gal. 6:14.

b *Separation*. vs. 25-27; Ex. 10:8-11; 24-26. (Gen. 12:1; 2 Cor. 6:14-17.)

c The second compromise is a modification merely of the first. "Do not be *too* unworldly:" Cf. 1 Sam. 15:3, 9, 13-15, 19-23.

d *Miracles* (O.T.). vs. 3-6, 8-11, 22-26, 33-35; Ex. 10:12-19. (Gen. 5:24; Jon. 2:1-10.)

e Deut. 28:27; Job 2:7; Rev. 16:1, 2.

CHAPTER 9.

The contest with Pharaoh: the sixth demand; the eighth miracle; the fifth judgment.

Then the LORD said unto Moses, Go in unto Pharaoh, and tell him, Thus saith the LORD God of the Hebrews, Let my people go, that they may serve me.

2 For if thou refuse to let *them* go, and wilt hold them still,

3 Behold, the hand of the LORD is upon thy cattle which *is* in the field, upon the horses, upon the asses, upon the camels, upon the oxen, and upon the sheep: *there shall be* a very grievous [d]murrain.

4 And the LORD shall sever between the cattle of Israel and the cattle of Egypt: and there shall nothing die of all *that is* the children's of Israel.

5 And the LORD appointed a set time, saying, To morrow the LORD shall do this thing in the land.

6 And the LORD did that thing on the morrow, and all the cattle of Egypt died: but of the cattle of the children of Israel died not one.

7 And Pharaoh sent, and, behold, there was not one of the cattle of the Israelites dead. And the heart of Pharaoh was hardened, and he did not let the people go.

The contest with Pharaoh: the ninth miracle; the sixth judgment.

8 And the LORD said unto Moses and unto Aaron, Take to you handfuls of ashes of the furnace, and let Moses sprinkle it toward the heaven in the sight of Pharaoh.

9 And it shall become small dust in all the land of Egypt, and shall be a boil breaking forth *with* blains upon man, and upon beast, throughout all the land of Egypt.

10 And they took ashes of the furnace, and stood before Pharaoh; and Moses sprinkled it up toward heaven; and it became a boil breaking forth *with* blains upon man, and upon beast.

11 And the magicians could not stand before Moses because of the [e]boils; for the boil was upon the magicians, and upon all the Egyptians.

[1] **(8:25)** The compromises proposed by Pharaoh are those urged upon Christians to day. The first says in effect: "Be a Christian if you will, but not a 'narrow' one—stay in Egypt." Invariably it ends in world-conformity, world-pleasing, and seeking the world's money for God (Psa. 50:9-17). Cf. 2 Cor. 6:14-18; Gal. 1:4.

B.C. 1491.

12 And the LORD hardened the heart of Pharaoh, and he hearkened not unto them; as the LORD had spoken unto Moses.

The contest with Pharaoh: the seventh demand.

13 And the LORD said unto Moses, Rise up early in the morning, and stand before Pharaoh, and say unto him, Thus saith the LORD God of the Hebrews, Let my people go, that they may serve me.

14 For I will at this time send all my plagues upon thine heart, and upon thy servants, and upon thy people; that thou mayest know that *there is* none like me in all the earth.

15 For now I will stretch out my hand, that I may smite thee and thy people with pestilence; and thou shalt be cut off from the earth.

16 And in very deed for [a]this *cause* have I raised thee up, for to shew *in* thee my power; and that my name may be declared throughout all the earth.

17 As yet exaltest thou thyself against my people, that thou wilt not let them go?

18 Behold, to morrow about this time I will cause it to rain a very grievous hail, such as hath not been in Egypt since the foundation thereof even until now.

19 Send therefore now, *and* gather thy cattle, and all that thou hast in the field; *for upon* every man and beast which shall be found in the field, and shall not be brought home, the hail shall come down upon them, and they shall die.

20 He that feared the word of the LORD among the servants of Pharaoh made his servants and his cattle flee into the houses:

21 And he that regarded not the word of the LORD left his servants and his cattle in the field.

The contest with Pharaoh: the tenth miracle; the seventh judgment.

22 And the LORD said unto Moses, Stretch forth thine hand toward heaven, that there may be hail in all the land of Egypt, upon man, and upon beast, and upon every herb of the field, throughout the land of Egypt.

23 And Moses stretched forth his rod toward heaven: and the LORD sent thunder and hail, and the fire ran along upon the ground; and the LORD rained hail upon the land of Egypt.

24 So there was hail, and fire mingled with the hail, very grievous, such as there was none like it in all the land of Egypt since it became a nation.

25 And the hail smote throughout all the land of Egypt all that *was* in the field, both man and beast; and the hail smote every herb of the field, and brake every tree of the field.

26 Only in the land of Goshen, [b]where the children of Israel *were*, was there no hail.

27 And Pharaoh sent, and called for Moses and Aaron, and said unto them, I have sinned this time: the LORD *is* righteous, and I and my people *are* wicked.

28 Intreat the LORD (for *it is* enough) that there be no *more* mighty thunderings and hail; and I will let you go, and ye shall stay no longer.

29 And Moses said unto him, As soon as I am gone out of the city, I will spread abroad my hands unto the LORD; *and* the thunder shall cease, neither shall there be any more hail; that thou mayest know how that the earth *is* the LORD'S.

30 But as for thee and thy servants, I know that ye will not yet fear the LORD God.

31 And the flax and the barley was smitten: for the barley *was* in the ear, and the flax *was* bolled.

32 But the wheat and the rie were not smitten: for they *were* not grown up.

33 And Moses went out of the city from Pharaoh, and spread abroad his hands unto the LORD: and the thunders and hail ceased, and the rain was not poured upon the earth.

34 And when Pharaoh saw that the rain and the hail and the thunders were ceased, he sinned yet more, and hardened his heart, he and his servants.

35 And the heart of Pharaoh was hardened, neither would he let the children of Israel go; as the LORD had spoken by Moses.

CHAPTER 10.

The contest with Pharaoh: the eighth demand.

And the LORD said unto Moses, Go in unto Pharaoh: for I have hardened his heart, and the heart of his servants,

a Rom. 9:16, 17; 2 Cor. 2:16; cf. 1 Pet. 2:8.

b Cf. Ex 8:23.

that I might shew these my signs before him:

2 And that thou mayest tell in the ears of thy son, and of thy son's son, what things I have wrought in Egypt, and my signs which I have done among them; that ye may know how that I *am* the LORD.

3 And Moses and Aaron came in unto Pharaoh, and said unto him, Thus saith the LORD God of the Hebrews, How long wilt thou refuse to humble thyself before me? let my people go, that they may serve me.

4 Else, if thou refuse to let my people go, behold, to morrow will I bring the [a]locusts into thy coast:

5 And they shall cover the face of the earth, that one cannot be able to see the earth: and they shall eat the residue of that which is escaped, which remaineth unto you from the hail, and shall eat every tree which groweth for you out of the field:

6 And they shall fill thy houses, and the houses of all thy servants, and the houses of all the Egyptians; which neither thy fathers, nor thy fathers' fathers have seen, since the day that they were upon the earth unto this day. And he turned himself, and went out from Pharaoh.

7 And Pharaoh's servants said unto him, How long shall this man be a snare unto us? let the men go, that they may serve the LORD their God: knowest thou not yet that Egypt is destroyed?

The contest with Pharaoh:
the third compromise refused.

8 And Moses and Aaron were brought again unto Pharaoh: and he said unto them, [b]Go, serve the LORD your God: *but* who *are* they that shall go?

9 And Moses said, We will go with our young and with our old, with our sons and with our daughters, with our flocks and with our herds will we go; for we *must hold* a feast unto the LORD.

10 And he said unto them, Let the LORD be so with you, as I will let you go, and your little ones: look *to it*; for evil *is* before you.

11 Not so: go now [c]ye *that are* men, and serve the LORD; for that ye did desire. And they were driven out from Pharaoh's presence.

The contest with Pharaoh:
the eleventh miracle; the eighth judgment.

12 And the LORD said unto Moses, Stretch out thine hand over the land of Egypt for the locusts, that they may come up upon the land of Egypt, and eat every herb of the land, *even* all that the hail hath left.

13 And Moses stretched forth his rod over the land of Egypt, and the LORD brought an east wind upon the land all that day, and all *that* night; *and* when it was morning, the east wind brought the [d]locusts.

14 And the locusts went up over all the land of Egypt, and rested in all the coasts of Egypt: very grievous *were they;* before them there were no such locusts as they, neither after them shall be such.

15 For they covered the face of the whole earth, so that the land was darkened; and they did eat every herb of the land, and all the fruit of the trees which the hail had left: and there remained not any green thing in the trees, or in the herbs of the field, through all the land of Egypt.

16 Then Pharaoh called for Moses and Aaron in haste; and he said, I have sinned against the LORD your God, and against you.

17 Now therefore forgive, I pray thee, my sin only this once, and intreat the LORD your God, that he may take away from me this death only.

18 And he went out from Pharaoh, and intreated the LORD.

19 And the LORD turned a mighty strong west wind, which took away the locusts, and cast them into the Red sea; there remained not one locust in all the coasts of Egypt.

20 But the LORD hardened Pharaoh's heart, so that he would not let the children of Israel go.

The contest with Pharaoh:
the twelfth miracle; the ninth judgment.

21 And the LORD said unto Moses, Stretch out thine hand toward heaven, that there may be darkness over the land of Egypt, even darkness *which* may be felt.

22 And Moses stretched forth his hand toward heaven; and there was a thick darkness in all the land of Egypt three days:

23 They saw not one another, neither rose any from his place for three days: [e]but all the children of Israel had light in their dwellings.

The contest with Pharaoh:
the fourth compromise refused.

24 And Pharaoh called unto Moses, and [f]said, Go ye, serve the LORD; only let

B.C. 1491.

a Prov. 30:27; Rev. 9:2, 3.

b *Separation.* vs. 8-11, 24-26; Ex. 11:7. (Gen. 12:1; 2 Cor. 6:14-17.)

c The third compromise proposed by Pharaoh is, perhaps, as applied to believers, the subtlest and most successful of them all. The most godly parents desire worldly prosperity and position for their children (Mt. 20:20, 21).

d *Miracles* (O.T.). vs. 12-19, 21-23; Ex. 12:29, 30. (Gen. 5:24; Jon. 2:1-10.)

e Cf. Ex. 8:23.

f i.e. "Leave your property in the world." Cf. Mt. 16:25-27; Lk. 18:18-25.

B.C. 1491.

your flocks and your herds be stayed: let your little ones also go with you.

25 And Moses said, Thou must give us also sacrifices and burnt-offerings, that we may sacrifice unto the LORD our God.

26 Our cattle also shall go with us; there shall not an hoof be left behind; for thereof must we take to serve the LORD our God; and we know not with what we must serve the LORD, until we come thither.

27 But the LORD hardened Pharaoh's heart, and he would not let them go.

The contest with Pharaoh: the king abandoned to judgment.

28 And Pharaoh said unto him, Get thee from me, take heed to thyself, see my face no more; for in *that* day thou seest my face thou shalt die.

29 And Moses said, Thou hast spoken well, I will see thy face again no more.

CHAPTER 11.

The contest with Pharaoh: the judgment upon the firstborn foretold.

And the LORD said unto Moses, Yet will I bring one plague *more* upon Pharaoh, and upon Egypt; afterwards he will let you go hence: when he shall let *you* go, he shall surely thrust you out hence altogether.

2 Speak now in the ears of the people, and let every man [a]borrow of his neighbour, and every woman of her neighbour, jewels of silver, and jewels of gold.

3 And the LORD gave the people favour in the sight of the Egyptians. Moreover the man Moses *was* very great in the land of Egypt, in the sight of Pharaoh's servants, and in the sight of the people.

4 And Moses said, Thus saith the LORD, About midnight will I go out into the midst of Egypt:

5 And all the firstborn in the land of Egypt shall die, from the firstborn of Pharaoh that sitteth upon his throne, even unto the firstborn of the maidservant that *is* behind the mill; and all the firstborn of beasts.

6 And there shall be a great cry throughout all the land of Egypt, such as there was none like it, nor shall be like it any more.

7 But against any of the children of Israel shall not a dog move his tongue, against man or beast: that ye may know how that the LORD doth put a [b]difference between the Egyptians and Israel.

8 And all these thy servants shall come down unto me, and bow down themselves unto me, saying, Get thee out, and all the people that follow thee: and after that I will go out. And he went out from Pharaoh in a great anger.

9 And the LORD said unto Moses, Pharaoh shall not hearken unto you; that my wonders may be multiplied in the land of Egypt.

10 And Moses and Aaron did all these wonders before Pharaoh: and the LORD hardened Pharaoh's heart, so that he would not let the children of Israel go out of his land.

CHAPTER 12.

The contest with Pharaoh: Parenthesis—the Passover.

And the LORD spake unto Moses and Aaron in the land of Egypt, [c]saying,

2 This month *shall be* unto you the beginning of months: it *shall be* the [d]first month of the year to you.

3 Speak ye unto all the congregation of Israel, saying, In the tenth *day* of this month they shall take to them every man a [e]lamb, according to the house of *their* fathers, a lamb for an house:

4 And if the household be too little for the lamb, let him and his neighbour next unto his house take *it* according to the number of the souls; every man according to his eating shall make your count for the lamb.

5 Your lamb shall be without blemish, a male of the first year: ye shall take *it* out from the sheep, or from the goats:

6 And ye shall keep it up until the fourteenth day of the same month: and the whole assembly of the congregation of Israel shall kill it in the evening.

7 And they shall take of the blood, and strike *it* on the two side posts and on the upper door post of the houses, wherein they shall eat it.

8 And they shall eat the flesh in that night, roast with fire, and [f]unleavened bread; *and* with bitter *herbs* they shall eat it.

a Lit. *ask.*

b *Separation.* Ex. 19:4. (Gen. 12:1; 2 Cor. 6:14-17.)

c *Israel* (*history*). vs. 1-13; Ex. 13:17-22. (Gen. 12:2, 3; Rom. 11:26.)

d i.e. *April.*

e *Sacrifice* (*typical*). vs. 3-11, 27; Ex. 17:15. (Gen. 4:4; Heb. 10:18.)

f *Leaven.* vs. 8, 15-20, 34, 39; Ex. 13:3, 6, 7. (Gen. 19:3; Mt. 13:33.)

9 Eat not of it raw, nor sodden at all with water, but roast *with* fire; his head with his legs, and with the purtenance thereof.

10 And ye shall let nothing of it remain until the morning; and that which remaineth of it until the morning ye shall burn with fire.

11 And thus shall ye eat it; *with* your loins girded, your shoes on your feet, and your staff in your hand; and ye shall eat it in haste: it *is* the LORD'S [1]passover.

Redemption (*typical*): (1) *by blood.*

12 For I will pass through the land of Egypt this night, and will smite all the firstborn in the land of Egypt, both man and beast; and against all the gods of Egypt I will execute judgment: I *am* the LORD.

13 And the blood shall be to you for a token upon the houses where ye *are*: and when I see the blood, I will pass over you, and the plague shall not be upon you to destroy *you*, when I smite the land of Egypt.

The memorial of redemption by blood.

14 And this day shall be unto you for a memorial; and ye shall keep it a feast to the LORD throughout your generations; ye shall keep it a feast by an ordinance for ever.

15 [a]Seven days shall ye eat unleavened bread; even the first day ye shall put away leaven out of your houses: for whosoever eateth leavened bread from the first day until the seventh day, that soul shall be cut off from Israel.

16 And in the first day *there shall be* an holy convocation, and in the seventh day there shall be an holy convocation to you; no manner of work shall be done in them, save *that* which every man must eat, that only may be done of you.

B.C. 1491.

a Ex. 13:6.

b Heb. 11:28.

c Heb. 12:24.

d 2 Sam. 24:16; Heb. 12:24.

17 And ye shall observe *the feast of* unleavened bread; for in this selfsame day have I brought your armies out of the land of Egypt: therefore shall ye observe this day in your generations by an ordinance for ever.

18 In the first *month*, on the fourteenth day of the month at even, ye shall eat unleavened bread, until the one and twentieth day of the month at even.

19 Seven days shall there be no leaven found in your houses: for whosoever eateth that which is leavened, even that soul shall be cut off from the congregation of Israel, whether he be a stranger, or born in the land.

20 Ye shall eat nothing leavened; in all your habitations shall ye eat unleavened bread.

21 Then Moses called for all the elders of Israel, and said unto them, Draw out and take you a lamb according to your families, and kill the passover.

22 And ye shall take a bunch of hyssop, and dip *it* in the blood that *is* in the bason, and [b]strike the lintel and the two side posts with the blood that *is* in the bason; and none of you shall go out at the door of his house until the morning.

23 For the LORD will pass through to smite the Egyptians; and when he seeth the [c]blood upon the lintel, and on the two side posts, the LORD will pass over the door, and will not [d]suffer the destroyer to come in unto your houses to smite *you*.

24 And ye shall observe this thing for an ordinance to thee and to thy sons for ever.

25 And it shall come to pass, when ye be come to the land which the LORD will give you, according as he hath promised, that ye shall keep this service.

26 And it shall come to pass, when

[1] **(12:11)** The Passover, type of Christ our Redeemer (Ex. 12:1-28; John 1:29; 1 Cor. 5:6, 7; 1 Pet. 1:18, 19): (1) The lamb must be without blemish, and to test this it was kept up four days (Ex. 12:5, 6). So our Lord's public life, under hostile scrutiny, was the testing which proved His holiness (Lk. 11:53, 54; John 8:46; 18:38). (2) The Lamb thus tested must be slain (Ex. 12:6: John 12:24; Heb. 9:22). (3) The blood must be applied (Ex. 12:7). This answers to appropriation by personal faith, and refutes universalism (John 3:36). (4) The blood thus applied of itself, without anything in addition, constituted a perfect protection from judgment (Ex. 12:13; 1 John 1:7; Heb. 10:10, 14). (5) The *feast* typified Christ the bread of life, answering to the memorial supper (Mt. 26:26-28; 1 Cor. 11:23-26). To observe the feast was a *duty* and *privilege*, but not a condition of safety. As a matter of fact, the bread was not eaten by the Israelites on the night in which, nevertheless, they were preserved from the judgment upon the firstborn (Ex. 12:34-39).

your children shall say unto you, What
mean ye by this service?
27 That ye shall say, It *is* the sacrifice
of the LORD'S passover, who passed over
the houses of the children of Israel in
Egypt, when he smote the Egyptians,
and delivered our houses. And the people bowed the head and worshipped.
28 And the children of Israel went
away, and [a]did as the LORD had commanded Moses and Aaron, so did they.

The contest with Pharaoh:
the tenth judgment; death of the firstborn.

29 And it came to pass, that at midnight the LORD [b]smote all the firstborn in
the land of Egypt, from the firstborn of
Pharaoh that sat on his throne unto the
firstborn of the captive that *was* in the
dungeon; and all the firstborn of cattle.
30 And Pharaoh rose up in the night,
he, and all his servants, and all the
Egyptians; and there was a great cry in
Egypt; for *there was* not a house where
there was not one dead.
31 And he called for Moses and Aaron
by night, and said, Rise up, *and* get you
forth from among my people, both ye
and the children of Israel; and go, serve
the LORD, as ye have said.
32 Also take your flocks and your
herds, as ye have said, and be gone; and
bless me also.
33 And the Egyptians were urgent
upon the people, that they might send
them out of the land in haste; for they
said, We *be* all dead *men*.
34 And the people took their dough
before it was leavened, their kneadingtroughs being bound up in their
clothes upon their shoulders.
35 And the children of Israel did
according to the word of Moses; and they
[c]borrowed of the Egyptians jewels of silver, and jewels of gold, and raiment:
36 And the LORD gave the people
favour in the sight of the Egyptians, so
that they [d]lent unto them *such things as
they required*. And they spoiled the
Egyptians.

Redemption: (2) by power;
the first stage of the journey.

37 And the children of Israel journeyed from Rameses to Succoth, about
six hundred thousand on foot *that were*
men, beside children.
38 And a [e]mixed multitude went up
also with them; and flocks, and herds,
even very much cattle.
39 And they baked unleavened cakes
of the dough which they brought forth
out of Egypt, for it was not leavened;
because they were thrust out of Egypt,
and could not tarry, neither had they
prepared for themselves any victual.
40 Now the sojourning of the children
of Israel, who dwelt in Egypt, *was* four
hundred and thirty years.
41 And it came to pass at the end of
the four hundred and thirty years, even
the selfsame day it came to pass, that all
the hosts of the LORD went out from the
land of Egypt.
42 It *is* a night to be much observed
unto the LORD for bringing them out
from the land of Egypt: this *is* that night
of the LORD to be observed of all the children of Israel in their generations.
43 And the LORD said unto Moses and
Aaron, This *is* the ordinance of the
passover: There shall no stranger eat
thereof:
44 But every man's servant that is
bought for money, when thou hast circumcised him, then shall he eat thereof.
45 A foreigner and an hired servant
shall not eat thereof.
46 In one house shall it be eaten; thou
shalt not carry forth ought of the flesh
abroad out of the house; neither shall ye
break a [f]bone thereof.
47 All the congregation of Israel shall
keep it.
48 And when a stranger shall sojourn
with thee, and will keep the passover to
the LORD, let all his males be circumcised, and then let him come near and
keep it; and he shall be as one that is
born in the land: for no uncircumcised
person shall eat thereof.
49 One law shall be to him that is
homeborn, and unto the stranger that
sojourneth among you.
50 Thus did all the children of Israel;
as the LORD commanded Moses and
Aaron, so did they.
51 And it came to pass the selfsame
day, *that* the LORD did bring the children
of Israel out of the land of Egypt by their
armies.

B.C. 1491.

a *Faith.* vs. 21-28; Ex. 14:21, 22. (Gen. 3:20; Heb. 11:39.)

b *Miracles* (O.T.). vs. 29, 30; Ex. 14:21-31. (Gen. 5:24; Jon. 2:1-10.)

c Lit. *asked.*

d Lit. *gave.*

e This mixed multitude, standing for unconverted church-members, was a source of weakness and division, then as now (see Num. 11:4-6). There had been a manifestation of divine power, and men were drawn to it without change of heart. Cf. Lk. 14:25-27.

f See John 19:36.

CHAPTER 13.

Parenthetical: The firstborn set apart for Jehovah.

And the LORD spake unto Moses,
saying,
2 Sanctify unto me all the firstborn,
whatsoever openeth the womb among
the children of Israel, *both* of man and of
beast: it *is* mine.
3 And Moses said unto the people,
Remember this day, in which ye came
out from Egypt, out of the house of
bondage; for by strength of hand the
LORD brought you out from this *place*:
[a]there shall no leavened bread be eaten.
4 This day came ye out in the month
[b]Abib.
5 And it shall be when the LORD shall
bring thee into the land of the
Canaanites, and the Hittites, and the
Amorites, and the Hivites, and the
Jebusites, which he sware unto thy
fathers to give thee, a land flowing with
milk and honey, that thou shalt keep this
service in this month.
6 Seven days thou shalt eat unleavened bread, and in the seventh day *shall
be* a feast to the LORD.
7 Unleavened bread shall be eaten
seven days; and there shall no leavened
bread be seen with thee, neither shall
there be leaven seen with thee in all thy
quarters.
8 And thou shalt shew thy son in that
day, saying, *This is done* because of that
which the LORD did unto me when I
came forth out of Egypt.
9 And it shall be for a sign unto thee
upon thine hand, and for a memorial
between thine eyes, that the LORD'S law
may be in thy mouth: for with a strong
hand hath the LORD brought thee out of
Egypt.
10 Thou shalt therefore keep this ordinance in his season from year to year.
11 And it shall be when the LORD shall
bring thee into the land of the
Canaanites, as he sware unto thee and to
thy fathers, and shall give it thee,
12 That thou shalt set [c]apart unto the
LORD all that openeth the matrix, and
every firstling that cometh of a beast
which thou hast; the males *shall be* the
LORD'S.
13 And every [d]firstling of an ass thou
shalt redeem with a lamb; and if thou
wilt not redeem it, then thou shalt break
his neck: and all the firstborn of man
among thy children shalt thou redeem.
14 And it shall be when thy son asketh
thee in time to come, saying, What *is*
this? that thou shalt say unto him, By
strength of hand the LORD brought us out
from Egypt, from the house of bondage:
15 And it came to pass, when Pharaoh
would hardly let us go, that the LORD
slew all the firstborn in the land of
Egypt, both the firstborn of man, and the
firstborn of beast: therefore I sacrifice to
the LORD all that openeth the matrix,
being males; but all the firstborn of my
children I redeem.
16 And it shall be for a token upon
thine hand, and for frontlets between
thine eyes: for by strength of hand the
LORD brought us forth out of Egypt.
17 And it came to pass, when Pharaoh
had let the people go, that God led them
not *through* the way of the land of the
Philistines, although that *was* near; for
God said, Lest peradventure the people
[e]repent when they see war, and they
return to Egypt:
18 But God led the people about,
through the way of the wilderness of the
Red sea: and the children of Israel went
up harnessed out of the land of Egypt.
19 And Moses took the bones of
Joseph with him: for he had straitly
sworn the children of Israel, saying, God
will surely visit you; and ye shall carry
up my bones away hence with you.

Redemption: (2) by power; the second stage of the journey.

20 And they took their journey from
Succoth, and encamped in Etham, in the
edge of the wilderness.

Redemption: (2) by power; the divine presence and guidance.

21 And the LORD went before them by
day in a pillar of a cloud, to lead them the
way; and by night in a pillar of fire, to
give them light; to go by day and night:
22 He took not away the pillar of the
cloud by day, nor the pillar of fire by
night, *from* before the [f]people.

CHAPTER 14.

Redemption: (2) by power; the third stage of the journey.

And the LORD spake unto Moses,
saying,
2 Speak unto the children of Israel,

B.C. 1491.

a *Leaven.* vs. 3, 6, 7; Ex. 23:15, 18. (Gen. 19:3; Mt. 13:33.)

b i.e. *April.*

c Cf. Lk. 2:23.

d The redemption of the firstlings made a memorial sign to Israel of their own redemption.

e Zech. 8:14, *note.*

f *Israel* (*history*). vs. 17-22; Ex. 14:19-31. (Gen. 12:2, 3; Rom. 11:26.)

that they turn and encamp before [a]Pi-hahiroth, between Migdol and the sea, over against Baal-zephon: before it shall ye encamp by the sea.

3 For Pharaoh will say of the children of Israel, They *are* entangled in the land, the wilderness hath shut them in.

4 And I will harden Pharaoh's heart, that he shall follow after them; and I will be honoured upon Pharaoh, and upon all his host; that the Egyptians may know that I *am* the LORD. And they did so.

5 And it was told the king of Egypt that the people fled: and the heart of Pharaoh and of his servants was turned against the people, and they said, Why have we done this, that we have let Israel go from serving us?

6 And he made ready his chariot, and took his people with him:

7 And he took six hundred chosen chariots, and all the chariots of Egypt, and captains over every one of them.

8 And the LORD hardened the heart of Pharaoh king of Egypt, and he pursued after the children of Israel: and the children of Israel went out with an high hand.

9 But the Egyptians pursued after them, all the horses *and* chariots of Pharaoh, and his horsemen, and his army, and overtook them encamping by the sea, beside Pi-hahiroth, before Baal-zephon.

10 And when Pharaoh drew nigh, the children of Israel lifted up their eyes, and, behold, the Egyptians marched after them; and they were sore afraid: and the children of Israel cried out unto the LORD.

11 And they said unto Moses, Because *there were* no graves in Egypt, hast thou taken us away to die in the wilderness? wherefore hast thou dealt thus with us, to carry us forth out of Egypt?

12 *Is* not this the word that we did tell thee in Egypt, saying, Let us alone, that we may serve the Egyptians? For *it had been* better for us to serve the Egyptians, than that we should die in the wilderness.

Redemption: (2) *by power;*
Jehovah's victory over pursuing Egypt.

13 And Moses said unto the people, Fear ye not, [b]stand still, and see the salvation of the LORD, which he will shew to you to day: for the Egyptians whom ye have seen to day, ye shall see them again no more for ever.

14 The LORD shall fight for you, and ye shall hold your peace.

15 And the LORD said unto Moses, Wherefore criest thou unto me? speak unto the children of Israel, that they go forward:

16 But lift thou up thy rod, and stretch out thine hand over the sea, and divide it: and the children of Israel shall go on dry *ground* through the midst of the sea.

17 And I, behold, I will harden the hearts of the Egyptians, and they shall follow them: and I will get me honour upon Pharaoh, and upon all his host, upon his chariots, and upon his horsemen.

18 And the Egyptians shall know that I *am* the LORD, when I have gotten me honour upon Pharaoh, upon his chariots, and upon his horsemen.

19 And the [c]angel of God, which went before the camp of [d]Israel, removed and went [e]behind them; and the pillar of the cloud went from before their face, and stood behind them:

20 And it came between the camp of the Egyptians and the camp of Israel; and it was a cloud and darkness *to them,* but it gave light by night *to these*: so that the one came not near the other all the night.

21 And Moses stretched out his hand over the sea; and the LORD [f]caused the sea to go *back* by a strong east wind all that night, and made the sea dry *land,* and the waters were divided.

22 And the children of Israel [g]went into the midst of the sea upon the dry *ground*: and the waters *were* a wall unto them on their right hand, and on their left.

23 And the Egyptians pursued, and went in after them to the midst of the sea, *even* all Pharaoh's horses, his chariots, and his horsemen.

24 And it came to pass, that in the morning watch the LORD looked unto the host of the Egyptians through the pillar of fire and of the cloud, and troubled the host of the Egyptians,

25 And took off their chariot wheels, that they drave them heavily: so that the Egyptians said, Let us flee from the face of Israel; for the LORD fighteth for them against the Egyptians.

B.C. 1491.

a Num. 33:7.

b 2 Chr. 20:17; Psa. 46:10, 11; Isa. 30:15; Rom. 4:5; 1 Pet. 2:24.

c Heb. 1:4, *note.*

d *Israel* (*history*). vs. 19-31; Ex. 19:1-8. (Gen. 12:2, 3; Rom. 11:26.)

e Isa. 52:12; 58:8.

f *Miracles* (O.T.). vs. 21-31; Ex. 15:23-25. (Gen. 5:24; Jon. 2:1-10.)

g *Faith.* vs. 21, 22; Josh. 6:20. (Gen. 3:20; Heb. 11:39.)

B.C. 1491.

26 And the LORD said unto Moses, Stretch out thine hand over the sea, that the waters may come again upon the Egyptians, upon their chariots, and upon their horsemen.

27 And Moses stretched forth his hand over the sea, and the sea returned to his strength when the morning appeared; and the Egyptians fled against it; and the LORD overthrew the Egyptians in the midst of the sea.

28 And the waters returned, and covered the chariots, and the horsemen, *and* all the host of Pharaoh that came into the sea after them; there remained not so much as one of them.

Redemption: (2) *by power; the fourth stage of the journey.*

29 But the children of Israel walked upon dry *land* in the midst of the sea; and the waters *were* a wall unto them on their right hand, and on their left.

30 [1]Thus the LORD saved Israel that day out of the hand of the Egyptians; and Israel saw the Egyptians dead upon the sea shore.

31 And Israel saw that great work which the LORD did upon the Egyptians: and the people [a]feared the LORD, and believed the LORD, and his servant Moses.

CHAPTER 15.

Redemption: complete (1)*by blood;* (2) *by power. The song of the redeemed.*

Then sang Moses and the children of Israel this song unto the LORD, and spake, saying, I will sing unto the LORD, for he hath triumphed gloriously: the horse and his rider hath he thrown into the sea.

2 The LORD *is* my strength and song, and he is become my salvation: he *is* my God, and I will prepare him an habitation; my father's God, and I will exalt him.

3 The LORD *is* a man of war: the LORD *is* his name.

4 Pharaoh's chariots and his host hath he cast into the sea: his chosen captains also are drowned in the Red sea.

5 The depths have covered them: they sank into the bottom as a stone.

6 Thy right hand, O LORD, is become glorious in power: thy right hand, O LORD, hath dashed in pieces the enemy.

7 And in the greatness of thine excellency thou hast overthrown them that rose up against thee: thou sentest forth thy wrath, *which* consumed them as stubble.

8 And with the blast of thy nostrils the waters were gathered together, the floods stood upright as an heap, *and* the depths were congealed in the heart of the sea.

9 The enemy said, I will pursue, I will overtake, I will divide the spoil; my lust shall be satisfied upon them; I will draw my sword, my hand shall destroy them.

10 Thou didst blow with thy wind, the sea covered them: they sank as lead in the mighty waters.

11 Who *is* like unto thee, O LORD, among the gods? who *is* like thee, glorious in holiness, fearful *in* praises, doing wonders?

12 Thou stretchedst out thy right hand, the earth swallowed them.

13 Thou in thy mercy hast led forth the people *which* thou hast [b]redeemed: thou hast guided *them* in thy strength unto thy holy habitation.

14 The people shall hear, *and* be afraid: sorrow shall take hold on the inhabitants of Palestina.

15 Then the dukes of Edom shall be amazed; the mighty men of Moab, trembling shall take hold upon them; all the inhabitants of Canaan shall melt away.

16 Fear and dread shall fall upon them; by the greatness of thine arm they shall be *as* still as a stone; till thy people pass over, O LORD, till the people pass over, *which* thou hast purchased.

17 Thou shalt bring them in, and plant them in the mountain of thine

a Psa. 19:9, *note.*

b Heb. *gaal, Redemp.* (*Kinsman type*). Isa. 59:20, *note.*

[1] **(14:30)** Redemption: (Exodus type) Summary. Exodus is the book of redemption, and teaches: (1) redemption is *wholly of God* (Ex. 3:7, 8; John 3:16); (2) redemption is *through a person* (Ex. 2:2, *note;* John 3:16, 17); (3) redemption is *by blood* (Ex. 12:13, 23, 27; 1 Pet. 1:18); (4) redemption is *by power* (Ex. 6:6; 13:14; Rom. 8:2. See Isa. 59:20, *note;* Rom. 3:24, *note*).

The blood of Christ redeems the believer from the *guilt* and *penalty* of sin (1 Pet. 1:18) as the power of the Spirit delivers from the *dominion* of sin (Rom. 8:2; Eph. 2:2).

inheritance, *in* the place, O LORD, *which*
thou hast made for thee to dwell in, *in*
the Sanctuary, O Lord, *which* thy hands
have established.
18 The LORD shall reign for ever and
ever.
19 For the horse of Pharaoh went in
with his chariots and with his horsemen
into the sea, and the LORD brought again
the waters of the sea upon them; but the
children of Israel went on dry *land* in the
midst of the sea.
20 [a]And Miriam the prophetess, the
sister of Aaron, took a timbrel in her
hand; and all the women went out after
her with timbrels and with dances.
21 And Miriam answered them, [b]Sing
ye to the LORD, for he hath triumphed
gloriously; the horse and his rider hath
he thrown into the sea.

Redemption: (3) *experience;*
fifth stage of the journey.

22 So Moses brought Israel from the
Red sea, and they went out into the
wilderness of [c]Shur; and they went three
days in the wilderness, and found no
water.

Redemption: (3) *experience; sixth stage of*
the journey—how bitter becomes sweet.

23 And when they came to Marah,
they could not drink of the waters of
Marah, for they *were* bitter: therefore the
name of it was called [d]Marah.
24 And the people murmured against
Moses, saying, What shall we drink?
25 And he cried unto the LORD; and
the LORD shewed him a tree, *which*
[1]when he had cast into the waters, the
waters were made [e]sweet: there he made
for them a statute and an ordinance, and
there he proved them,
26 And said, If thou wilt diligently
hearken to the voice of the LORD thy God,
and wilt do that which is right in his
sight, and wilt give ear to his commandments, and keep all his statutes, I will put
none of these diseases upon thee, which I
have brought upon the Egyptians: for I
am the LORD that healeth thee.

B.C. 1491.

a 2 Sam. 6:5.

b v. 1.

c Gen. 16:7.

d i.e. *bitter.*

e *Miracles* (O.T.). vs. 23-25; Ex. 16:14-35. (Gen. 5:24; Jon. 2:1-10.)

f i.e. *trees.* Cf. Psa. 92:12; 1:3. After trial accepted as the Father's will, blessing and growth.

g i.e. *May.*

Redemption: (3) *experience; rest after trial.*

27 And they came to [f]Elim, where *were*
twelve wells of water, and threescore
and ten palm trees: and they encamped
there by the waters.

CHAPTER 16.

Redemption: (3) *experience;*
seventh stage of the journey; hunger.

And they took their journey from
Elim, and all the congregation of
the children of Israel came unto the
wilderness of Sin, which *is* between Elim
and Sinai, on the fifteenth day of the
[g]second month after their departing out
of the land of Egypt.
2 And the whole congregation of the
children of Israel murmured against
Moses and Aaron in the wilderness:
3 And the children of Israel said unto
them, Would to God we had died by the
hand of the LORD in the land of Egypt,
when we sat by the flesh pots, *and* when
we did eat bread to the full; for ye have
brought us forth into this wilderness, to
kill this whole assembly with hunger.
4 Then said the LORD unto Moses,
Behold, I will rain bread from heaven for
you; and the people shall go out and
gather a certain rate every day, that I
may prove them, whether they will walk
in my law, or no.
5 And it shall come to pass, that on the
sixth day they shall prepare *that* which
they bring in; and it shall be twice as
much as they gather daily.
6 And Moses and Aaron said unto all
the children of Israel, At even, then ye
shall know that the LORD hath brought
you out from the land of Egypt:
7 And in the morning, then ye shall see
the glory of the LORD; for that he heareth
your murmurings against the LORD: and
what *are* we, that ye murmur against us?
8 And Moses said, *This shall be,* when
the LORD shall give you in the evening
flesh to eat, and in the morning bread to

[1] **(15:25)** These bitter waters were in the very path of the Lord's leading, and stand for the trials of God's people, which are educatory and not punitive. The "tree" is the cross (Gal. 3:13), which became sweet to Christ as the expression of the Father's will (John 18:11). When our Marahs are so taken we cast the "tree" into the waters (Rom. 5:3, 4).

the full; for that the LORD heareth your
murmurings which ye murmur against
him: and what *are* we? your murmurings
are not against us, but against the LORD.
9 And Moses spake unto Aaron, Say
unto all the congregation of the children
of Israel, Come near before the LORD: for
he hath heard your murmurings.
10 And it came to pass, as Aaron
spake unto the whole congregation of
the children of Israel, that they looked
toward the wilderness, and, behold, the
glory of the LORD appeared in the cloud.
11 And the LORD spake unto Moses,
saying,
12 I have heard the murmurings of the
children of Israel: speak unto them, saying, At even ye shall eat flesh, and in the
morning ye shall be filled with bread;
and ye shall know that I *am* the LORD
your God.
13 And it came to pass, that at even
the quails came up, and covered the
camp: and in the morning the dew lay
round about the host.

The manna: type of Christ the giver and sustainer of life (John 6:30–63).

14 And when the dew that lay was
gone up, behold, upon the face of the
wilderness *there lay* a [a]small round thing,
as small as the hoar frost on the ground.
15 And when the children of Israel saw
it, they said one to another, It *is* [b]manna:
for they wist not what it *was*. And Moses
said unto them, This *is* the bread which
the LORD hath [c]given you to eat.
16 This *is* the thing which the LORD
hath commanded, Gather of it every
man [d]according to his eating, an [e]omer
for every man, *according to* the number
of your persons; take ye every man for
them which *are* in his tents.
17 And the children of Israel did so,
and gathered, some more, some less.
18 And when they did mete *it* with an
omer, he that gathered much had nothing over, and he that gathered little had
no lack; they gathered every man
according to his eating.
19 And Moses said, Let no man leave
of it till the morning.
20 Notwithstanding they hearkened
not unto Moses; but some of them [f]left
of it until the morning, and it bred
worms, and stank: and Moses was wroth
with them.
21 And they gathered it every morning, every man according to his eating:
and when the sun waxed hot, it melted.
22 And it came to pass, *that* on the
sixth day they gathered twice as much
bread, two omers for one *man*: and all
the rulers of the congregation came and
told Moses.

The Sabbath given to Israel; type of Israel's kingdom (Heb. 4:8, 9).

23 And he said unto them, This *is that*
which the LORD hath said, To morrow *is*
the rest of the holy sabbath unto the
LORD: bake *that* which ye will bake *to
day*, and seethe that ye will seethe; and
that which remaineth over lay up for
you to be kept until the morning.
24 And they laid it up till the morning,
as Moses bade: and it did not stink, neither was there any worm therein.
25 And Moses said, Eat that to day; for
to day *is* a [g]sabbath unto the LORD: to
day ye shall not find it in the field.
26 Six days ye shall gather it; but on
the seventh day, *which is* the sabbath, in
it there shall be none.
27 And it came to pass, *that* there went
out *some* of the people on the seventh
day for to gather, and they found none.
28 And the LORD said unto Moses,
How long refuse ye to keep my commandments and my laws?
29 See, for that the LORD hath given you
the sabbath, therefore he giveth you on
the sixth day the bread of two days; abide
ye every man in his place, let no man go
out of his place on the seventh day.
30 So the people rested on the seventh
day.
31 And the house of Israel called the
name thereof Manna: and it *was* like
coriander seed, white; and the taste of it
was like wafers *made* with honey.
32 And Moses said, This *is* the thing
which the LORD commandeth, Fill an
omer of it to be kept for your generations; that they may see the bread
wherewith I have fed you in the wilderness, when I brought you forth from the
land of Egypt.

B.C. 1491.

a Isa. 53:2; Mk. 6:3.

b Ex. 16:35, *note*.

c *Miracles* (O.T.). vs. 14-35; Ex. 17:5-7. (Gen. 5:24; Jon. 2:1-10.)

d Cf. John 6:33 with John 6:41, 42, 52. Christ gives himself unreservedly, but we have no more of Him than faith appropriates, v. 18. Cf. v. 2, Josh. 1, with v. 3. V. 2 is our title; v. 3, the law of possession.

e One omer = 6:70 pints; also vs. 18, 22, 32, 33, 36.

f As we are not nourished by the memory of food, so neither can spirituality be sustained on past appropriations of Christ.

g *Sabbath*. vs. 22-25; Ex. 20:8-11. (Gen. 2:3; Mt. 12:1.)

33 And Moses said unto Aaron, Take a pot, and put an omer full of manna therein, and lay it up before the LORD, to be kept for your generations.

34 As the LORD commanded Moses, so Aaron laid it up before the Testimony, to be kept.

35 And the children of Israel did eat [1]manna forty years, until they came to a land inhabited; they did eat manna, until they came unto the borders of the land of Canaan.

36 Now an omer *is* the tenth *part* of an [a]ephah.

CHAPTER 17.

Redemption: (3) *experience;*
eighth stage of the journey; thirst.

And all the congregation of the children of Israel journeyed from the wilderness of Sin, after their journeys, according to the commandment of the LORD, and pitched in Rephidim: and *there was* no water for the people to drink.

2 Wherefore the people did chide with Moses, and said, Give us water that we may drink. And Moses said unto them, Why chide ye with me? wherefore do ye [b]tempt the LORD?

3 And the people thirsted there for water; and the people murmured against Moses, and said, Wherefore *is* this *that* thou hast brought us up out of Egypt, to kill us and our children and our cattle with thirst?

4 And Moses cried unto the LORD, saying, What shall I do unto this people? they be almost ready to stone me.

Redemption: (3) *experience;*
water from the rock; type of Christ,
the giver of the Spirit (John 7:37–39).

5 And the LORD said unto Moses, Go on before the people, and take with thee of the elders of Israel; and thy rod, wherewith thou smotest the river, take in thine hand, and go.

6 Behold, I will stand before thee there upon the [2c]rock in Horeb; and thou shalt [d]smite the rock, and there shall come [e]water out of it, that the people may drink. And Moses did so in the sight of the elders of Israel.

7 And he called the name of the place [f]Massah, and Meribah, because of the chiding of the children of Israel, and because they tempted the LORD, saying, Is the LORD among us, or not?

Redemption: (3) *experience;*
the conflict with Amalek.

8 [g]Then came [3]Amalek, and fought with Israel in Rephidim.

9 And Moses said unto Joshua, Choose us out men, and go out, fight

B.C. 1491.

a 1 bu. 3 pts.

b *Temptation.* vs. 2, 7; Num. 14:22. (Gen3:1; Jas. 1:2.)

c *Christ* (*as Stone*). 1 Cor. 10:4. (Ex. 17:6; 1 Pet. 2:8.)

d Cf. Num. 20:8; Psa. 105:41; 114:8; Zech. 13:7, 8; 1 Cor. 10:4, 6.

e *Miracles* (O.T.). vs. 5-7; Lev. 10:1, 2. (Gen. 5:24; Jon. 2:1-10.)

f Deut. 6:16.

g Gen. 36:12; Num. 24:20; Deut. 25:17; 1 Sam. 15:2.

---

[1]**(16:35)** Manna, type of Christ as "the bread of life," come down from heaven to die "for the life of the world" (John 6:35, 48-51). A "small" thing (Ex. 16:14), having but the taste of "fresh oil" (Num. 11:8), or "wafers with honey" (Ex. 16:31), it typifies Christ in humiliation as presented in Matthew, Mark, and Luke; "having no form nor comeliness; . . . no beauty that we should desire him" (Isa. 53:2). But *as such* He must be received by faith if we would be saved (John 6:53-58). To meditate upon Christ as He went about among men, doing not His own will but the will of the Father (John 6:38-40), is to feed on the manna. This is, of necessity, the spiritual food of young believers, and answers to "milk" (1 Cor. 3:1, 2). But Christ in glory, and the believer's present and eternal association with Him there, answers to "the old corn of the land" (Josh. 5:11), the "meat" of Heb. 5:13,14, or Christ as presented in the Epistles of Paul. Cf. 2 Cor. 5:16.

[2]**(17:6)** The rock, type of life through the Spirit by grace: (1) Christ the Rock (1 Cor. 10:4). (2) The people utterly unworthy (Ex. 17:2; Eph. 2:1-6). (3) Characteristics of life through grace: *(a)* free (John 4:10; Rom. 6:23; Eph. 2:8); *(b)* abundant (Rom. 5:20; Psa. 105:41; John 3:16); *(c)* near (Rom. 10:8); *(d)* the people had only to take (Isa. 55:1) The smitten-rock aspect of the death of Christ looks toward the outpouring of the Holy Spirit as a result of accomplished redemption, rather than toward our *guilt.* It is the affirmative side of John 3:16. "Not perish" speaks of atoning blood; "but have" speaks of life bestowed.

[3]**(17:8)** Amalek, grandson of Esau (Gen. 36:12), who was "born after the flesh" (Gal. 4:22-29) and progenitor of the Amalekites, Israel's persistent enemy, is a type of the flesh in the believer (Gal. 4:29). But the conflict with Amalek in chapter 17 sets forth the resources of the man under law, rather than those of the believer under grace. The man under law could fight and pray (vs. 9-12). Under grace the Holy Spirit gains the victory over the flesh in the believer's behalf (Rom. 8:2-4; Gal. 5:16, 17); but this

with Amalek: to morrow I will stand on the top of the hill with the rod of God in mine hand.

10 So Joshua did as Moses had said to him, and fought with Amalek: and Moses, Aaron, and Hur went up to the top of the hill.

11 And it came to pass, [a]when Moses held up his hand, that Israel prevailed: and when he let down his hand, Amalek prevailed.

12 But Moses' hands *were* heavy; and they took a stone, and put *it* under him, and he sat thereon; and Aaron and Hur [b]stayed up his hands, the one on the one side, and the other on the other side; and his hands were steady until the going down of the sun.

13 And Joshua discomfited Amalek and his people with the edge of the sword.

14 And the LORD said unto Moses, Write this *for* a memorial in a [c]book, and rehearse *it* in the ears of Joshua: for I will utterly put out the remembrance of Amalek from under heaven.

15 And Moses built an [d]altar, and called the name of it Jehovah-nissi:

16 For he said, Because the LORD hath sworn *that* the LORD *will have* war with Amalek from generation to generation.

CHAPTER 18.

Redemption: (3) *experience; leaning on the arm of flesh.*

When Jethro, the priest of Midian, Moses' father in law, heard of all that God had done for Moses, and for Israel his people, *and* that the LORD had brought Israel out of Egypt;

2 Then Jethro, Moses' father in law, took Zipporah, Moses' wife, after he had sent her back,

3 And her two sons; of which the name of the one *was* [e]Gershom; for he said, I have been an alien in a strange land:

4 And the name of the other *was* [f]Eliezer; for the God of my father, *said he, was* mine help, and delivered me from the sword of Pharaoh:

5 And Jethro, Moses' father in law, came with his sons and his wife unto Moses into the wilderness, where he encamped at the mount of God:

6 And he said unto Moses, I thy father in law Jethro am come unto thee, and thy wife, and her two sons with her.

7 And Moses went out to meet his father in law, and did obeisance, and kissed him; and they asked each other of *their* welfare; and they came into the tent.

8 And Moses told his father in law all that the LORD had done unto Pharaoh and to the Egyptians for Israel's sake, *and* all the travail that had come upon them by the way, and *how* the LORD delivered them.

9 And Jethro rejoiced for all the goodness which the LORD had done to Israel, whom he had delivered out of the hand of the Egyptians.

10 And Jethro said, Blessed *be* the LORD, who hath delivered you out of the hand of the Egyptians, and out of the hand of Pharaoh, who hath delivered the people from under the hand of the Egyptians.

11 Now I know that the LORD *is* greater than all gods: for in the thing wherein they dealt proudly *he was* above them.

12 And Jethro, Moses' father in law, took a burnt-offering and sacrifices for God: and Aaron came, and all the elders of Israel, to eat bread with Moses' father in law before God.

13 And it came to pass on the morrow, that Moses sat to judge the people: and the people stood by Moses from the morning unto the evening.

14 And when Moses' father in law saw all that he did to the people, he said, What *is* this thing that thou doest to the people? why sittest thou thyself alone, and all the people stand by thee from morning unto even?

15 And Moses said unto his father in law, Because the people come unto me to enquire of God:

16 When they have a matter, they come unto me; and I judge between one and another, and I do make *them* know the statutes of God, and his laws.

17 And Moses' father in law said unto

B.C. 1491.

a Heb. 7:25.

b Deut. 33:27; Isa. 40:28-31

c *Inspiration.* Ex. 19:6, 7. (Ex. 4:15; Rev. 22:19.)

d *Sacrifice (typical).* Lev. 1:3-17. (Gen. 4:4; Heb. 10:18.)

e i.e. *a stranger.*

f i.e. *God is help.*

victory is only as the believer walks in the Spirit. Acting in independency or disobedience, Amalek gains an easy victory (Num. 14:42-45). Like Saul we are prone to spare the flesh (1 Sam. 15:8, 9), forgetting Rom. 7:18. See "Flesh," John 1:13; Jude 23.

him, The thing that thou doest *is* not
good.
18 Thou wilt surely wear away, both
thou, and this people that *is* with thee:
for this thing *is* too heavy for thee; thou
art not able to perform it thyself alone.
19 Hearken now unto my voice, [1]I will
give thee counsel, and God shall be with
thee: Be thou for the people to God-
ward, that thou mayest bring the causes
unto God:
20 And thou shalt teach them ordinances and laws, and shalt shew them
the way wherein they must walk, and
the work that they must do.
21 Moreover thou shalt provide out of
all the people able men, such as [a]fear
God, men of truth, hating covetousness;
and place *such* over them, *to be* rulers of
thousands, *and* rulers of hundreds,
rulers of fifties, and rulers of tens:
22 And let them judge the people at all
seasons: and it shall be, *that* every great
matter they shall bring unto thee, but
every small matter they shall judge: so
shall it be easier for thyself, and they
shall bear *the burden* with thee.
23 If thou shalt do this thing, and God
command thee *so*, then thou shalt be
able to endure, and all this people shall
also go to their place in peace.
24 So Moses hearkened to the voice of
his father in law, and did all that he had
said.
25 And Moses chose able men out of all
Israel, and made them heads over the
people, rulers of thousands, rulers of hundreds, rulers of fifties, and rulers of tens.
26 And they judged the people at all
seasons: the hard causes they brought
unto Moses, but every small matter they
judged themselves.
27 And Moses [b]let his father in law
depart; and he went his way into his
own land.

CHAPTER 19.

Redemption: (3) *experience;*
ninth stage of the journey; Israel at Sinai.

In the [c]third [2]month, when the children
of [d]Israel were gone forth out of the
land of Egypt, the same day came they
into the wilderness of [e]Sinai.
2 For they were departed from
Rephidim, and were come *to* the desert
of Sinai, and had pitched in the wilderness; and there Israel [f]camped before the
mount.

Redemption: (3) *experience;*
grace given up for law.

3 And Moses went up unto God, and
the LORD called unto him out of the
mountain, saying, [3]Thus shalt thou say
to the house of Jacob, and tell the children of Israel;
4 Ye have seen what I did unto the
Egyptians, and *how* I bare you on eagles'
wings, and brought you unto [g]myself.
5 Now therefore, [4]if ye will obey my
voice indeed, and keep my covenant,
then ye shall be a peculiar treasure unto

B.C. 1491.

a Psa. 19:9, *note.*
b Cf. Num. 10:31.
c i.e. *June.*
d *Israel* (*history*). vs. 1-8; Ex. 20:1-17. (Gen. 12:2, 3; Rom. 11:26.)
e *Law* (*of Moses*). Ex. 20:1-17. (Ex. 19:1; Gal. 3:1-29.)
f Cf. Ex. 3:12.
g *Separation.* Ex. 33:16. (Gen. 12:1; 2 Cor. 6:14-17.)

[1]**(18:19)** Cf. Num. 11:14-17. Jehovah entirely ignored this worldly-wise organization, substituting His own order.

[2]**(19:1)** At Sinai Israel learned the lessons: (1) of the holiness of Jehovah through the Commandments; (2) of their own sinfulness and weakness through failure; (3) and of the goodness of Jehovah through the provision of priesthood and sacrifice. The Christian learns through the experience of Rom. 7:7-24 what Israel learned at Sinai. This division of Exodus should be read in the light of Rom. 3:19-26; 7:7-24; Gal. 4:1-3. Gal. 3:6-25 explains the relation of the law to the Abrahamic Covenant: (1) the law cannot disannul that covenant; (2) it was "added" to convict of sin; (3) it was a child-leader unto Christ; (4) it was but a preparatory discipline "till the Seed should come."

[3]**(19:3)** It is exceedingly important to observe: (1) that Jehovah reminded the people that hitherto they had been the objects of His free grace; (2) that the law is not proposed as a means of life, but as a means by which Israel might become "a peculiar treasure" and a "kingdom of priests"; (3) that the law was not *imposed* until it had been *proposed* and voluntarily accepted. The *principle* is stated in Gal. 5:1-4.

[4]**(19:5)** Cf. 1 Pet. 2:9; Rev. 1:6; 5:10. What, under law, was *condition,* is under grace, freely *given* to every believer. The "if" of v. 5 is the essence of law as a method of divine dealing, and the fundamental reason why "the law made nothing perfect" (Rom. 8:3; Heb. 7:18, 19). The Abrahamic (Gen. 15:18, *note*) and New (Heb. 8:8-12, *note*) covenants minister salvation and assurance because they impose but one condition, faith.

me above all people: for all the earth *is* mine:

6 And ye shall be unto me a kingdom of priests, and an holy nation. These *are* the [a]words which thou shalt speak unto the children of Israel.

7 And Moses came and called for the elders of the people, and laid before their faces all these words which the LORD commanded him.

The Fifth Dispensation, Law (extends to the Cross). (From Ex. 19:8 to Mt. 27:35.)

8 And all the people answered together, and said, All that the LORD hath spoken we will [1]do. And Moses returned the words of the people unto the LORD.

Redemption: (3) *experience. To a people under law, God is "in a thick cloud," and unapproachable* (vs. 9–23).

9 And the LORD said unto Moses, Lo, I come unto thee in a thick cloud, that the people may hear when I speak with thee, [b]and believe thee for ever. And Moses told the words of the people unto the LORD.

10 And the LORD said unto Moses, Go unto the people, and sanctify them to day and to morrow, and let them wash their clothes,

11 And be ready against the third day: for the third day the LORD will come down in the sight of all the people upon mount Sinai.

12 And thou shalt set bounds unto the people round about, saying, Take heed to yourselves, *that ye* go *not* up into the mount, or touch the border of it: whosoever toucheth the mount shall be surely put to death:

13 There shall not an hand touch it, but he shall surely be stoned, or shot through; whether *it be* beast or man, it shall not live: when the trumpet soundeth long, they shall come up to the mount.

B.C. 1491.

a *Inspiration.* vs. 6, 7; Ex. 20:1. (Ex. 4:15; Rev. 22:19.)

b *Kingdom* (O.T.). Ex. 24:12. (Gen. 1:26; Zech. 12:8.)

c *Sanctify, holy* (O.T.). Ex. 28:1-3. (Gen. 2:3; Zech. 8:3.)

14 And Moses went down from the mount unto the people, and sanctified the people; and they washed their clothes.

15 And he said unto the people, Be ready against the third day: come not at *your* wives.

16 And it came to pass on the third day in the morning, that there were thunders and lightnings, and a thick cloud upon the mount, and the voice of the trumpet exceeding loud; so that all the people that *was* in the camp trembled.

17 And Moses brought forth the people out of the camp to meet with God; and they stood at the nether part of the mount.

18 And mount Sinai was altogether on a smoke, because the LORD descended upon it in fire: and the smoke thereof ascended as the smoke of a furnace, and the whole mount quaked greatly.

19 And when the voice of the trumpet sounded long, and waxed louder and louder, Moses spake, and God answered him by a voice.

20 And the LORD came down upon mount Sinai, on the top of the mount: and the LORD called Moses *up* to the top of the mount; and Moses went up.

21 And the LORD said unto Moses, Go down, charge the people, lest they break through unto the LORD to gaze, and many of them perish.

22 And let the priests also, which come near to the LORD, sanctify themselves, lest the LORD break forth upon them.

23 And Moses said unto the LORD, The people cannot come up to mount Sinai: for thou chargedst us, saying, Set bounds about the mount, and [c]sanctify it.

24 And the LORD said unto him, Away, get thee down, and thou shalt come up, thou, and Aaron with thee: but let not the priests and the people break through to come up unto the LORD, lest he break forth upon them.

[1](19:8) The Fifth Dispensation: Law. This dispensation extends from Sinai to Calvary—from the Exodus to the Cross. The history of Israel in the wilderness and in the land is one long record of the violation of the law. The testing of the *nation* by law ended in the judgment of the Captivities, but the dispensation itself ended at the Cross. (1) Man's state at the beginning (Ex. 19:1-4). (2) His responsibility (Ex. 19:5, 6; Rom. 10:5). (3) His failure (2 Ki. 17:7-17, 19; Acts 2:22, 23). (4) The judgment (2 Ki. 17:1-6, 20; 25:1-11; Lk. 21:20-24).

See, for the other six dispensations: *Innocence* (Gen. 1:28); *Conscience* (Gen. 3:23); *Human Government* (Gen. 8:20); *Promise* (Gen. 12:1); *Grace* (John 1:17); *Kingdom* (Eph. 1:10).

25 So [1]Moses went down unto the people, and [a]spake unto them.

CHAPTER 20.

Redemption: (3) *experience; self known through the revelation of God's holy law* (Rom. 7:7–24).

The Law: (1) *the Commandments; the Fifth, or Mosaic, Covenant.*

And God [b]spake all these [c]words, [d]saying,

2 I *am* the LORD thy God, which have brought thee out of the land of Egypt, out of the house of bondage.

3 Thou shalt have no other gods before me.

4 Thou [2]shalt not make unto thee any graven image, or any likeness *of any thing* that *is* in heaven above, or that *is* in the earth beneath, or that *is* in the water under the earth:

5 Thou shalt not bow down thyself to them, nor serve them: for I the LORD thy God *am* a jealous God, visiting the iniquity of the fathers upon the children unto the third and fourth *generation* of them that hate me;

6 And shewing mercy unto thousands of them that love me, and keep my commandments.

7 Thou shalt not take the name of the LORD thy God in vain; for the LORD will not hold him guiltless that taketh his name in vain.

8 Remember the [e]sabbath day, to keep it holy.

9 Six days shalt thou labour, and do all thy work:

10 But the seventh day *is* the sabbath of the LORD thy God: *in it* thou shalt not do any work, thou, nor thy son, nor thy daughter, thy manservant, nor thy maidservant, nor thy cattle, nor thy stranger that *is* within thy gates:

11 For *in* six days the LORD made heaven and earth, the sea, and all that in them *is*, and rested the seventh day: wherefore the LORD blessed the sabbath day, and hallowed it.

12 [f]Honour thy father and thy mother: that thy days may be long upon the land which the LORD thy God giveth thee.

13 [g]Thou shalt not kill.

14 [h]Thou shalt not commit adultery.

15 Thou shalt not steal.

B.C. 1491.

a *The Eight Covenants.* Deut. 30:1. (Gen. 1:28; Heb. 8:10.)

b *Law* (*of Moses*). vs. 1-17. Ex. 31:18. (Ex. 19:1; Gal. 3:1-29.)

c *Inspiration.* Ex. 24:3, 4, 7, 8, 12. (Ex. 4:15; Rev. 22:19.)

d *Israel* (*history*). vs. 1-17; Ex. 40:1-38. (Gen. 12:2, 3; Rom. 11:26.)

e *Sabbath.* vs. 8-11; Ex. 31:13-16. (Gen. 2:3; Mt. 12:1.)

f Mt. 15:4; 19:19; Mk. 7:10.

g Mt. 5:21; 19:18; Lk. 18:20; Mk. 10:19.

h Mt. 5:27; Mk. 10:19; Lk. 18:20; Rom. 13:9; Jas. 2:11.

[1] **(19:25)** The Mosaic Covenant, (1) given to Israel (2) in three divisions, each essential to the others, and together forming the Mosaic Covenant, viz.: the Commandments, expressing the righteous will of God (Ex. 20:1-26); the "judgments," governing the social life of Israel (Ex. 21:1-24:11); and the "ordinances," governing the religious life of Israel (Ex. 24:12-31:18). These three elements form "the law," as that phrase is generically used in the New Testament (e.g. Mt. 5:17, 18). The Commandments and the ordinances formed one religious system. The Commandments were a "ministry of condemnation" and of "death" (2 Cor. 3:7-9); the ordinances gave, in the high priest, a representative of the people with Jehovah; and in the sacrifices a "cover" (see "Atonement," Lev. 16:6, *note*) for their sins in anticipation of the Cross (Heb. 5:1-3; 9:6-9; Rom. 3:25, 26). The Christian is not under the conditional Mosaic Covenant of works, the law, but under the unconditional New Covenant of grace (Rom. 3:21-27; 6:14, 15; Gal. 2:16; 3:10-14, 16-18, 24-26; 4:21-31; Heb. 10:11-17). See *New Covenant* (Heb. 8:8, *note*).

See, for the other seven covenants: *Edenic* (Gen. 1:28); *Adamic* (Gen. 3:15); *Noahic* (Gen. 9:1); *Abrahamic* (Gen. 15:18); *Palestinian* (Deut. 30:3); *Davidic* (2 Sam. 7:16); *New* (Heb. 8:8).

[2] **(20:4)** There is a threefold giving of the law. First, orally, in Ex. 20:1-17. This was pure law, with no provision of priesthood and sacrifice for failure, and was accompanied by the "judgments" (Ex. 21:1-23:13) relating to the relations of Hebrew with Hebrew; to which were added (Ex. 23:14-19) directions for keeping three annual feasts, and (Ex. 23:20-33) instructions for the conquest of Canaan. These *words* Moses communicated to the people (Ex. 24:3-8). Immediately, in the persons of their elders, they were admitted to the fellowship of God (Ex. 24:9-11). Second, Moses was then called up to receive the *tables* of stone (Ex. 24:12-18). The story then divides. Moses, in the mount, receives the gracious instructions concerning the tabernacle, priesthood, and sacrifice (Ex. 25-31). Meantime (Ex. 32), the people, led by Aaron, break the first commandment. Moses, returning, breaks the tables "written with the finger of God" (Ex. 31:18; 32:16-19). Third, the *second* tables were made by Moses, and the law again written by the hand of Jehovah (Ex. 34:1, 28, 29; Deut. 10:4).

16 Thou shalt not bear false witness against thy neighbour.

17 Thou shalt not [a]covet thy neighbour's house, thou shalt not covet thy neighbour's wife, nor his manservant, nor his maidservant, nor his ox, nor his ass, nor any thing that *is* thy neighbour's.

18 And all the people saw the thunderings, and the lightnings, and the noise of the trumpet, and the mountain smoking: and when the people saw *it*, they removed, and stood [b]afar off.

19 And they said unto Moses, Speak thou with us, and we will hear: but let not God speak with us, lest we die.

20 And Moses said unto the people, Fear not: for God is come to prove you, and that his [c]fear may be before your faces, that ye sin not.

21 And the people stood afar off, and Moses drew near unto the thick darkness where God *was*.

22 And the LORD said unto Moses, Thus thou shalt say unto the children of Israel, Ye have seen that I have talked with you from heaven.

23 Ye shall not make with me gods of silver, neither shall ye make unto you gods of gold.

24 An altar of earth thou shalt make unto me, and shalt sacrifice thereon thy burnt-offerings, and thy peace-offerings, thy sheep, and thine oxen: in all places where I record my name I will come unto thee, and I will bless thee.

25 And if thou wilt make me an altar of stone, thou shalt not build it of hewn stone: for if [d]thou lift up thy tool upon it, thou hast polluted it.

26 Neither shalt thou go up by steps unto mine altar, that thy nakedness be not discovered thereon.

CHAPTER 21.

The Law: (2) *the "judgments"; master and servant.*

NOW these *are* the judgments which thou shalt set before them.

2 If thou buy an [e]Hebrew servant, six years he shall serve: and in the seventh he shall go out free for nothing.

3 If he came in by himself, he shall go out by himself: if he were married, then his wife shall go out with him.

B.C. 1491.

a Cf. Rom. 7:7.

b For contrast between law and grace cf. Eph. 2:13; Lk. 1:10, with Heb. 10:19-22.

c Psa. 19:9, *note*.

d Josh. 8:30, 31; Rom. 4:4-8; Eph. 2:8-10.

e Deut. 15:12-18; Jer. 34:8-11.

f Psa. 40:6; Heb. 10:5.

g Gen. 9:6.

h Num. 35:11.

i 1 Ki. 2:29.

j Deut. 24:7.

k Prov. 20:20; Mt. 15:4; Mk. 7:10.

4 If his master have given him a wife, and she have born him sons or daughters; the wife and her children shall be her master's, and he shall go out by himself.

5 And if the servant shall plainly say, I love my master, my wife, and my children; I will not go out free:

6 Then his master shall bring him unto the judges; he shall also bring him to the door, or unto the door post; and his master shall bore his [f]ear through with an aul; and he shall serve him for ever.

7 And if a man sell his daughter to be a maidservant, she shall not go out as the menservants do.

8 If she please not her master, who hath betrothed her to himself, then shall he let her be redeemed: to sell her unto a strange nation he shall have no power, seeing he hath dealt deceitfully with her.

9 And if he have betrothed her unto his son, he shall deal with her after the manner of daughters.

10 If he take him another *wife*; her food, her raiment, and her duty of marriage, shall he not diminish.

11 And if he do not these three unto her, then shall she go out free without money.

The Law: (2) *the "judgments"; injuries to the person.*

12 He that smiteth a man, so that he die, shall be surely put to [g]death.

13 And if a man lie not in wait, but God deliver *him* into his hand; then I will appoint thee [h]a place whither he shall flee.

14 But if a man come presumptuously upon his neighbour, to slay him with guile; thou shalt [i]take him from mine altar, that he may die.

15 And he that smiteth his father, or his mother, shall be surely put to death.

16 And he that [j]stealeth a man, and selleth him, or if he be found in his hand, he shall surely be put to death.

17 And he that [k]curseth his father, or his mother, shall surely be put to death.

18 And if men strive together, and one smite another with a stone, or with *his* fist, and he die not, but keepeth *his* bed:

19 If he rise again, and walk abroad upon his staff, then shall he that smote *him* be quit: only he shall pay *for* the loss

B.C. 1491.

of his time, and shall cause *him* to be thoroughly healed.

20 And if a man smite his servant, or his maid, with a rod, and he die under his hand; he shall be surely punished.

21 Notwithstanding, if he continue a day or two, he shall not be punished: for he *is* his money.

22 If men strive, and hurt a woman with child, so that her fruit depart *from her*, and yet no mischief follow: he shall be surely punished, according as the woman's husband will lay upon him; and he shall pay as the judges *determine*.

23 And if *any* mischief follow, then thou shalt give life for life,

24 [a]Eye for eye, tooth for tooth, hand for hand, foot for foot,

25 Burning for burning, wound for wound, stripe for stripe.

26 And if a man smite the eye of his servant, or the eye of his maid, that it perish; he shall let him go free for his eye's sake.

27 And if he smite out his manservant's tooth, or his maidservant's tooth; he shall let him go free for his tooth's sake.

28 If an ox gore a man or a woman, that they die: then the ox shall be surely stoned, and his flesh shall not be eaten; but the owner of the ox *shall be* quit.

29 But if the ox were wont to push with his horn in time past, and it hath been testified to his owner, and he hath not kept him in, but that he hath killed a man or a woman; the ox shall be stoned, and his owner also shall be put to death.

30 If there be laid on him a sum of money, then he shall give for the ransom of his life whatsoever is laid upon him.

31 Whether he have gored a son, or have gored a daughter, according to this judgment shall it be done unto him.

32 If the ox shall push a manservant or a maidservant; he shall give unto their master thirty [b]shekels of silver, and the ox shall be stoned.

33 And if a man shall open a pit, or if a man shall dig a pit, and not cover it, and an ox or an ass fall therein;

34 The owner of the pit shall make *it* good, *and* give money unto the owner of them; and the dead *beast* shall be his.

35 And if one man's ox hurt another's, that he die; then they shall sell the live ox, and divide the money of it; and the dead *ox* also they shall divide.

36 Or if it be known that the ox hath used to push in time past, and his owner hath not kept him in; he shall surely pay ox for ox; and the dead shall be his own.

CHAPTER 22.

The Law: (2) the "judgments"; rights of property.

If a man shall steal an ox, or a sheep, and kill it, or sell it; he shall restore five oxen for an ox, and four [c]sheep for a sheep.

2 If a thief be found breaking up, and be smitten that he die, *there shall* no blood *be shed* for him.

3 If the sun be risen upon him, *there shall be* blood *shed* for him; *for* he should make full restitution; if he have nothing, then he shall be sold for his theft.

4 If the theft be certainly found in his hand alive, whether it be ox, or ass, or sheep; he shall restore double.

5 If a man shall cause a field or vineyard to be eaten, and shall put in his beast, and shall feed in another man's field; of the best of his own field, and of the best of his own vineyard, shall he make restitution.

6 If fire break out, and catch in thorns, so that the stacks of corn, or the standing corn, or the field, be consumed *therewith*; he that kindled the fire shall surely make restitution.

7 If a man shall deliver unto his neighbour money or stuff to keep, and it be stolen out of the man's house; if the thief be found, let him pay double.

8 If the thief be not found, then the master of the house shall be brought unto the judges, *to see* whether he have put his hand unto his neighbour's goods.

9 For all manner of trespass, *whether it be* for ox, for ass, for sheep, for raiment, *or* for any manner of lost thing, which *another* challengeth to be his, the cause of both parties shall come before the judges; *and* whom the judges shall condemn, he shall pay double unto his neighbour.

10 If a man deliver unto his neighbour an ass, or an ox, or a sheep, or any beast,

a Lev. 24:20; Deut. 19:21; cf. Mt. 5:38-44; 1 Pet. 2:19-21. The provision in Exodus is *law*, and righteous; the N.T. passages, *grace*, and merciful.

b One shekel = 2*s*. 9*d*., or 65 cents.

c 2 Sam. 12:6.

to keep; and it die, or be hurt, or driven away, no man seeing *it*:

11 *Then* shall an oath of the LORD be between them both, that he hath not put his hand unto his neighbour's goods; and the owner of it shall accept *thereof*, and he shall not make *it* good.

12 And if it be stolen from him, he shall make restitution unto the owner thereof.

13 If it be torn in pieces, *then* let him bring it *for* witness, *and* he shall not make good that which was torn.

14 And if a man borrow *ought* of his neighbour, and it be hurt, or die, the owner thereof *being* not with it, he shall surely make *it* good.

15 *But* if the owner thereof *be* with it, he shall not make *it* good: if it *be* an hired *thing*, it came for his hire.

The Law: (2) the "judgments"; crimes against humanity.

16 And if a man entice a maid that is not betrothed, and lie with her, he shall surely endow her to be his wife.

17 If her father utterly refuse to give her unto him, he shall pay money according to the dowry of virgins.

18 Thou shalt not suffer a [a]witch to live.

19 Whosoever lieth with a beast shall surely be put to death.

20 He that sacrificeth unto *any* [b]god, save unto the LORD only, he shall be utterly destroyed.

21 Thou shalt neither [c]vex a stranger, nor oppress him: for ye were strangers in the land of Egypt.

22 Ye shall not [d]afflict any widow, or fatherless child.

23 If thou afflict them in any wise, and they cry at all unto me, I will surely hear their cry;

24 And my wrath shall wax hot, and I will kill you with the sword; and your wives shall be widows, and your children fatherless.

25 If thou lend money to *any of* my people *that is* poor by thee, thou shalt not be to him as an usurer, neither shalt thou lay upon him usury.

26 If thou at all take thy neighbour's raiment to pledge, thou shalt deliver it unto him by that the sun goeth down:

27 For that *is* his covering only, it *is* his raiment for his skin: wherein shall he sleep? and it shall come to pass, when he crieth unto me, that I will hear; for I *am* [e]gracious.

28 Thou shalt not revile the gods, nor curse the [f]ruler of thy people.

29 Thou shalt not delay *to offer* the first of thy ripe fruits, and of thy liquors: [g]the firstborn of thy sons shalt thou give unto me.

30 Likewise shalt thou do with thine oxen, *and* with thy sheep: seven days it shall be with his dam; on the eighth day thou shalt give it me.

31 And ye shall be holy men unto me: neither shall ye eat *any* flesh *that is* torn of beasts in the field; ye shall cast it to the dogs.

B.C. 1491.

a Deut. 18:10, 11. Cf. 1 Sam. 28:3-10.

b Deut. 13:6-16.

c Ex. 23:9; Mal. 3:5.

d Deut. 24:17, 18.

e Ex. 34:6, 7.

f Acts 23:5.

g Ex. 13:12, 15.

h v. 6; Lev. 19:15.

CHAPTER 23.

Thou shalt not raise a false report: put not thine hand with the wicked to be an unrighteous witness.

2 Thou shalt not follow a multitude to *do* evil; neither shalt thou speak in a cause to decline after many to wrest *judgment*:

3 Neither shalt thou countenance a [h]poor man in his cause.

4 If thou meet thine enemy's ox or his ass going astray, thou shalt surely bring it back to him again.

5 If thou see the ass of him that hateth thee lying under his burden, and wouldest forbear to help him, thou shalt surely help with him.

6 Thou shalt not wrest the judgment of thy poor in his cause.

7 Keep thee far from a false matter; and the innocent and righteous slay thou not: for I will not justify the wicked.

8 And thou shalt take no gift: for the gift blindeth the wise, and perverteth the words of the righteous.

9 Also thou shalt not oppress a stranger: for ye know the heart of a stranger, seeing ye were strangers in the land of Egypt.

The Law: (2) the "judgments"; the land and the Sabbath.

10 And six years thou shalt sow thy land, and shalt gather in the fruits thereof:

11 But the seventh *year* thou shalt let it rest and lie still; that the poor of thy people may eat: and what they leave the beasts of the field shall eat. In like

manner thou shalt deal with thy vineyard, *and* with thy oliveyard.
12 Six days thou shalt do thy work,
and on the seventh day thou shalt rest:
that thine ox and thine ass may rest, and
the son of thy handmaid, and the
stranger, may be refreshed.
13 And in all *things* that I have said
unto you be circumspect: and make no
mention of the name of other gods, neither let it be heard out of thy mouth.

The three national feasts: unleavened bread; firstfruits; ingathering.

14 [a]Three times thou shalt keep a feast
unto me in the year.
15 Thou shalt keep the feast of [b]unleav-
ened bread: (thou shalt eat unleavened
bread seven days, as I commanded thee,
in the time appointed of the month [c]Abib;
for in it thou camest out from Egypt: and
none shall appear before me empty:)
16 And the feast of harvest, the firstfruits of thy labours, which thou hast
sown in the field: and the feast of ingathering, *which is* in the end of the year,
when thou hast gathered in thy labours
out of the field.
17 Three times in the year all thy
males shall appear before the Lord GOD.
18 Thou shalt not offer the blood of
my sacrifice with leavened bread; neither shall the fat of my sacrifice remain
until the morning.
19 The first of the firstfruits of thy
land thou shalt bring into the house of
the LORD thy God. Thou shalt not seethe
a kid in his mother's milk.

Instructions and promises concerning the conquest of the land.

20 Behold, I send an [d]Angel before
thee, to keep thee in the way, and to
bring thee into the place which I have
prepared.
21 Beware of him, and obey his voice,
provoke him not; for he will not pardon
your transgressions: for my name *is* in
him.
22 But if thou shalt indeed obey his
voice, and do all that I speak; then I will
be an enemy unto thine enemies, and an
adversary unto thine adversaries.
23 For mine Angel shall go before thee,
and bring thee in unto the Amorites, and
the Hittites, and the Perizzites, and the
Canaanites, the Hivites, and the
Jebusites: and I will cut them off.
24 Thou shalt not bow down to their
gods, nor serve them, nor do after their
works: but thou shalt utterly overthrow
them, and quite break down their images.
25 And ye shall serve the LORD your
God, and he shall bless thy bread, and
thy water; and I will take sickness away
from the midst of thee.
26 There shall nothing cast their
young, nor be barren, in thy land: the
number of thy days I will fulfil.
27 I will send my fear before thee, and
will destroy all the people to whom thou
shalt come, and I will make all thine enemies turn their backs unto thee.
28 And I will send hornets before thee,
which shall drive out the Hivite, the
Canaanite, and the Hittite, from before
thee.
29 I will not drive them out from
before thee in one year; lest the land
become desolate, and the beast of the
field multiply against thee.
30 By little and little I will drive them
out from before thee, until thou be
increased, and inherit the land.
31 And I will set thy bounds from the
Red sea even unto the sea of the
Philistines, and from the desert unto the
river: for I will deliver the inhabitants of
the land into your hand; and thou shalt
drive them out before thee.
32 Thou shalt make no covenant with
them, nor with their gods.
33 They shall not dwell in thy land,
lest they make thee sin against me: for if
thou serve their gods, it will surely be a
snare unto thee.

CHAPTER 24.

The order of worship pending the building of the tabernacle.

And he said unto Moses, Come up
unto the LORD, thou, and Aaron,
Nadab, and Abihu, and seventy of the
elders of Israel; and worship ye afar off.
2 And Moses alone shall come near
the LORD: but they shall not come nigh;
neither shall the people go up with him.

The people accept the covenant: the worship of the people.

3 And Moses came and told the people
all the [e]words of the LORD, and all the

B.C. 1491.

a Cf. Lev. 23:4-44. Exodus for the wilderness; Leviticus for the land.

b *Leaven.* vs. 15, 18; Ex. 29:2, 23. (Gen. 19:3; Mt. 13:33.)

c i.e. *April.*

d Heb. 1:4, *note.*

e *Inspiration.* vs. 3, 4, 7, 8, 12; Ex. 32:16. (Ex. 4:15; Rev. 22:19.)

judgments: and all the people answered
with one voice, and said, All the words
which the LORD hath said will we do.
4 And Moses wrote all the words of
the LORD, and rose up early in the morning, and [a]builded an altar under the hill,
and twelve pillars, according to the
twelve tribes of Israel.
5 And he sent young men of the children of Israel, which offered burnt-offerings, and sacrificed peace-offerings of
oxen unto the LORD.
6 And Moses took half of the blood,
and put *it* in basons; and half of the
blood he sprinkled on the altar.
7 And he took the book of the
covenant, and read in the audience of the
people: and they said, All that the LORD
hath said will we do, and be obedient.
8 And Moses took the blood, and
sprinkled *it* on the people, and said,
Behold the [b]blood of the covenant,
which the LORD hath made with you
concerning all these words.

The worship of Moses, the priests, and the elders.

9 Then went up Moses, and Aaron,
Nadab, and Abihu, and seventy of the
elders of Israel:
10 And they saw the God of Israel: and
there was under his feet as it were a
paved work of a sapphire stone, and as it
were the body of heaven in *his* clearness.
11 And upon the nobles of the children of Israel he laid not his hand: also
they saw God, and did [c]eat and drink.
12 And the LORD said unto Moses,
Come up to me into the mount, and be
there: and I will give thee tables of stone,
and a law, and commandments which I
have written; that [d]thou mayest teach
them.
13 And Moses rose up, and his minister Joshua: and Moses went up into the
mount of God.

B.C. 1491.

a Cf. Ex. 33:7-11. This arrangement for worship was temporarily called the "tabernacle."

b Heb. 9:20.

c Symbol of communion. Cf. Lk. 22:15-18. A blood-sprinkled people (see Heb. 9:19-22) who had not yet broken the law could thus commune with God. Never again was this repeated. Cf. Ex. 24:9-11 with Lev. 16:2 and Heb. 9:6-8. But cf., under grace, Eph. 2:13; Heb. 10:19, 20.

d *Kingdom* (O.T.). Deut. 30:1-9. (Gen. 1:26; Zech. 12:8.)

e See 2 Cor. 8:1, *note.*

f i.e. *acacia.*

14 And he said unto the elders, Tarry
ye here for us, until we come again unto
you: and, behold, Aaron and Hur *are*
with you: if any man have any matters
to do, let him come unto them.
15 And Moses went up into the
mount, and a cloud covered the mount.
16 And the glory of the LORD abode
upon mount Sinai, and the cloud covered
it six days: and the seventh day he called
unto Moses out of the midst of the cloud.
17 And the sight of the glory of the
LORD *was* like devouring fire on the top
of the mount in the eyes of the children
of Israel.
18 And Moses went into the midst of
the cloud, and gat him up into the
mount: and Moses was in the mount
forty days and forty nights.

CHAPTER 25.

Moses in the mount. The tabernacle: (1) the materials.

And [1]the LORD spake unto Moses,
saying,
2 Speak unto the children of Israel,
that they bring me an offering: of every
man that giveth it [e]willingly with his
heart ye shall take my offering.
3 And this *is* the offering which ye
shall take of them; gold, and silver, and
brass,
4 And blue, and purple, and scarlet,
and fine linen, and goats' *hair,*
5 And rams' skins dyed red, and badgers' skins, and [f]shittim wood,
6 Oil for the light, spices for anointing
oil, and for sweet incense,
7 Onyx stones, and stones to be set in
the ephod, and in the breastplate.
8 And let them make me a sanctuary;
that I may dwell among them.
9 According to all that I shew thee,

[1]**(25:1)** The *general* authority for the types of Exodus is found: (1) as to the *persons* and *events,* in 1 Cor. 10:1-11; (2) as to the *tabernacle,* in Heb. 9:1-24. Having the assurance that in the tabernacle everything is typical, the details must of necessity be received as such. Two warnings are necessary: (1) Nothing may be dogmatically asserted to be a type without explicit New Testament authority; and (2) all types not so authenticated must be recognized as having the authority of *analogy,* or spiritual *congruity,* merely. The typical meanings of the *materials* and *colours* of the tabernacle are believed to be as follows: Gold, Deity in manifestation—divine glory; silver, redemption (Ex. 30:12-16; 38:27, *note*); brass, symbol of judgment, as in the brazen altar and in the serpent of brass (Num. 21:6-9); blue, heavenly in nature or origin; purple, royalty; scarlet, sacrifice.

after the pattern of the [1]tabernacle, and the pattern of all the instruments thereof, even so shall ye make *it*.

The tabernacle: (2) *the ark.*

10 And they shall [a]make an [2]ark *of* [b]shittim wood: two [c]cubits and a half *shall be* the length thereof, and a cubit and a half the breadth thereof, and a cubit and a half the height thereof.

11 And thou shalt overlay it with pure gold, within and without shalt thou overlay it, and shalt make upon it a crown of gold round about.

12 And thou shalt cast four rings of gold for it, and put *them* in the four corners thereof; and two rings *shall be* in the one side of it, and two rings in the other side of it.

13 And thou shalt make staves *of* [b]shittim wood, and overlay them with gold.

14 And thou shalt put the staves into the rings by the sides of the ark, that the ark may be borne with them.

15 The staves shall be in the rings of the ark: they shall not be taken from it.

16 And thou shalt put into the ark the testimony which I shall give thee.

17 And thou shalt make a [d]mercy seat *of* pure gold: two cubits and a half *shall be* the length thereof, and a cubit and a half the breadth thereof.

18 And thou shalt make two [e]cherubims *of* gold, *of* beaten work shalt thou make them, in the two ends of the mercy seat.

19 And make one cherub on the one end, and the other cherub on the other end: *even* of the mercy seat shall ye make the cherubims on the two ends thereof.

B.C. 1491.

a The most inclusive type of Christ. Gold = Deity; wood = humanity. History: Num. 3:31; 10:33; Josh. 3:3-15; 6:11; Jud. 20:27; 1 Sam. 3:3; 4:1-11; 5:1-10; 6:1-21; 7:1, 2; 2 Sam. 6:2-17; 7:2; 15:24-29; 1 Ki. 8:1-21; *not* carried to Babylon, 2 Ki. 24:13; 2 Chr. 35:3; *not* mentioned in Ezra or Neh. Where is it? Rev. 11:19.

b i.e. *acacia.*

c One cubit = 1 ft. 5.48 in.; see also vs. 17, 23.

d See "*Propitiation.*" Rom. 3:25, *note.*

e Ezk. 1:5, *note;* 1 Ki. 6:23; Psa. 99:1; Rev. 4:6.

20 And the cherubims shall stretch forth *their* wings on high, covering the mercy seat with their wings, and their faces *shall look* one to another; toward the mercy seat shall the faces of the cherubims be.

21 And thou shalt put the mercy seat above upon the ark; and in the ark thou shalt put the testimony that I shall give thee.

22 And there I will meet with thee, and I will commune with thee from above the mercy seat, from between the two cherubims which *are* upon the ark of the testimony, of all *things* which I will give thee in commandment unto the children of Israel.

The tabernacle:

(3) *the table of shewbread* (Lev. 24:5–9).

23 Thou shalt also make a table *of* [b]shittim wood: two cubits *shall be* the length thereof, and a cubit the breadth thereof, and a cubit and a half the height thereof.

24 And thou shalt overlay it with pure gold, and make thereto a crown of gold round about.

25 And thou shalt make unto it a border of an hand breadth round about, and thou shalt make a golden crown to the border thereof round about.

26 And thou shalt make for it four rings of gold, and put the rings in the four corners that *are* on the four feet thereof.

27 Over against the border shall the rings be for places of the staves to bear the table.

28 And thou shalt make the staves *of* [b]shittim wood, and overlay them with

[1]**(25:9)** The tabernacle, speaking comprehensively, is explained in the N. T. as typical in three ways: (1) of the Church as a habitation of God through the Spirit (Ex. 25:8; Eph. 2:19-22); (2) of the believer (2 Cor. 6:16); (3) as a figure of things in the heavens (Heb. 9:23, 24). In *detail,* all speaks of Christ: (1) The ark, in its *materials,* acacia-wood (see Ex. 26:15, *note*) and gold, is a type of the humanity and deity of Christ. (2) In its *contents,* a type of Christ, as: *(a)* having God's law in His heart (Ex. 25:16); *(b)* the wilderness food (or portion) of His people (Ex. 16:33); *(c)* Himself the resurrection, of which Aaron's rod is the symbol (Num. 17:10). (3) In its *use* the ark, especially the mercy-seat, was a type of God's throne. That it was, to the sinning Israelite, a throne of grace and not of judgment was due to the mercy-seat formed of gold and sprinkled with the blood of atonement, which vindicated the law, and the divine holiness guarded by the cherubim (Gen. 3:24; Ezk. 1:5, *note*). See *Propitiation,* Rom. 3:25, *note.*

[2]**(25:10)** All begins with the ark, which, in the completed tabernacle, was placed in the holy of holies, because, in *revelation,* God begins from Himself, working outward toward man; as, in *approach,* the worshipper begins from himself, moving toward God in the holy of holies. The same order is followed in the Levitical offerings (Lev. 1-5). In *approach* man begins at the brazen altar, type of the Cross, where, in the fire of judgment, atonement is made.

gold, that the table may be borne with them.
29 And thou shalt make the dishes thereof, and spoons thereof, and covers thereof, and bowls thereof, to cover withal: *of* pure gold shalt thou make them.
30 And thou shalt set upon the table [1]shewbread before me alway.

The tabernacle: (4) *the golden candlestick.*

31 And thou shalt [2]make a [a]candlestick *of* pure gold: *of* beaten work shall the candlestick be made: his shaft, and his branches, his bowls, his knops, and his flowers, shall be of the same.
32 And six branches shall come out of the sides of it; three branches of the candlestick out of the one side, and three branches of the candlestick out of the other side:
33 Three bowls made like unto almonds, *with* a knop and a flower in one branch; and three bowls made like almonds in the other branch, *with* a knop and a flower: so in the six branches that come out of the candlestick.
34 And in the candlestick *shall be* four bowls made like unto almonds, *with* their knops and their flowers.
35 And *there shall be* a knop under two branches of the same, and a knop under two branches of the same, and a knop under two branches of the same, according to the six branches that proceed out of the candlestick.
36 Their knops and their branches shall be of the same: all it *shall be* one beaten work *of* pure gold.
37 And thou shalt make the seven lamps thereof: and they shall light the lamps thereof, that they may give light over against it.
38 And the tongs thereof, and the snuffdishes thereof, *shall be of* pure gold.
39 *Of* a [b]talent of pure gold shall he make it, with all these vessels.
40 And look that thou make *them* after their [c]pattern, which was shewed thee in the mount.

CHAPTER 26.

The tabernacle: (5) *the curtains of linen.*

Moreover thou shalt make the tabernacle *with* ten curtains *of* [d]fine twined linen, and [e]blue, and purple, and scarlet: *with* [f]cherubims of cunning work shalt thou make them.
2 The length of one curtain *shall be* eight and twenty [g]cubits, and the breadth of one curtain four cubits: and every one of the curtains shall have one measure.
3 The five curtains shall be coupled together one to another; and *other* five curtains *shall be* coupled one to another.
4 And thou shalt make loops of blue upon the edge of the one curtain from the selvedge in the coupling; and likewise shalt thou make in the uttermost edge of *another* curtain, in the coupling of the second.
5 Fifty loops shalt thou make in the one curtain, and fifty loops shalt thou make in the edge of the curtain that *is* in the coupling of the second; that the loops may take hold one of another.
6 And thou shalt make fifty taches of gold, and couple the curtains together with the taches: and it shall be one tabernacle.

The tabernacle:
(6) *the curtains of goats' hair.*

7 And thou shalt make curtains *of* [h]goats' *hair* to be a covering upon the tabernacle: eleven curtains shalt thou make.
8 The length of one curtain *shall be* thirty cubits, and the breadth of one

B.C. 1491.

a Or, *lampstand.* Cf. Rev. 1:12, 13, 20.

b £6150, or $29, 085.

c Cf. Heb. 8:5.

d Fine linen typifies personal righteousness (Rev. 19:8). The fine linen here typifies the sinless life of Christ.

e *Blue,* Christ's heavenly origin; *purple,* His royalty as David's son; *scarlet,* His sacrifice.

f See Ezk. 1:5, *note.*

g One cubit = 1 ft. 5.48 in.; also vs. 8, 13, 16.

h Cf. Lev. 16:5, 7-10. The reference seems to be to the result of the ordinance of the two goats as "covering" (Lev. 16:5, *note*), thus speaking of Christ in atonement (cf. Gen. 3:21, *note*). This thought is intensified in the colour of the rams' skins, v. 14.

[1] **(25:30)** Showbread, type of Christ, the Bread of God, nourisher of the Christian's life as a believer-priest (1 Pet. 2:9; Rev. 1:6). In John 6:33-58 our Lord has more in mind the manna, that food which "came down"; but all typical meanings of "bread" are there gathered into His words. The manna is the life-giving Christ; the showbread, the life-sustaining Christ. The showbread typifies Christ as the "corn of wheat" (John 12:24) ground in the mill of suffering (John 12:27) and brought into the fire of judgment (John 12:31-33). We, as priests, by faith feed upon Him as having undergone that in our stead and for our sakes. It is meditation upon Christ, as in Heb. 12:2, 3.

[2] **(25:31)** Candlestick, type of Christ our Light, shining in the fullness of the power of the sevenfold Spirit (Isa. 11:2; Heb. 1:9; Rev. 1:4). Natural light was excluded from the tabernacle. Cf. 1 Cor. 2:14, 15. See Gen. 1:16, *note,* and John 1:4.

curtain four cubits: and the eleven curtains *shall be all* of one measure.

9 And thou shalt couple five curtains by themselves, and six curtains by themselves, and shalt double the sixth curtain in the forefront of the tabernacle.

10 And thou shalt make fifty loops on the edge of the one curtain *that is* outmost in the coupling, and fifty loops in the edge of the curtain which coupleth the second.

11 And thou shalt make fifty taches of brass, and put the taches into the loops, and couple the tent together, that it may be one.

12 And the remnant that remaineth of the curtains of the tent, the half curtain that remaineth, shall hang over the backside of the tabernacle.

13 And a cubit on the one side, and a cubit on the other side of that which remaineth in the length of the curtains of the tent, it shall hang over the sides of the tabernacle on this side and on that side, to cover it.

The tabernacle:
(7) *the covering of rams' skins.*

14 And thou shalt make a covering for the tent *of* [a]rams' skins dyed red, and a covering above *of* badgers' skins.

The tabernacle: (8) *the boards and sockets.*

15 And thou shalt make [1]boards for the tabernacle *of* [b]shittim wood standing up.

16 Ten cubits *shall be* the length of a board, and a cubit and a half *shall be* the breadth of one board.

17 Two tenons *shall there be* in one board, set in order one against another: thus shalt thou make for all the boards of the tabernacle.

B.C. 1491.

a See v. 7, *ref.*

b i.e. *acacia.*

c Rom. 8:9; 1 Cor. 6:19.

18 And thou shalt make the boards for the tabernacle, twenty boards on the south side southward.

19 And thou shalt make forty [2]sockets of silver under the twenty boards; two sockets under one board for his two tenons, and two sockets under another board for his two tenons.

20 And for the second side of the tabernacle on the north side *there shall be* twenty boards:

21 And their forty sockets *of* silver; two sockets under one board, and two sockets under another board.

22 And for the sides of the tabernacle westward thou shalt make six boards.

23 And two boards shalt thou make for the corners of the tabernacle in the two sides.

24 And they shall be coupled together beneath, and they shall be coupled together above the head of it unto one ring: thus shall it be for them both; they shall be for the two corners.

25 And they shall be eight boards, and their sockets *of* silver, sixteen sockets; two sockets under one board, and two sockets under another board.

The tabernacle: (9) *the outside bars.*

26 And thou shalt make bars *of* [b]shittim wood; five for the boards of the one side of the tabernacle,

27 And five bars for the boards of the other side of the tabernacle, and five bars for the boards of the side of the tabernacle, for the two sides westward.

The tabernacle: (10) *the bar in the midst.*

28 And the [c]middle bar in the midst of the boards shall reach from end to end.

[1]**(26:15)** The typical meaning of the boards is clear as to Christ. Acacia wood, a desert growth, is a fitting symbol of Christ in His humanity as "a root out of dry ground" (Isa. 53:2). The covering, gold, typifies Deity in manifestation, speaks of His divine glory. As applied to the individual believer the meaning of the boards is less clear. The connection may be found in John 17:21, 22, 23; Eph. 1:4, 6; 1 John 4:13. Only as seen "in Him" could the boards be taken as representing the believer. So viewed the type is beautiful. In the world, and yet separated from it by the silver of redemption (Gal. 1:4; Ex. 30:11;16; 38:25-27), as the boards of the tabernacle were separated from the earth by the sockets of silver, and united by the "middle bar" (v. 28), representing both the one life (Gal. 2:20) and one Spirit (Eph. 4:3), "all the building, fitly framed together, groweth unto an holy temple in the Lord" (Eph. 2:21).

[2]**(26:19)** Silver symbolizes redemption (Ex. 25:1, *note;* 38:27, *note*). All the tabernacle rests upon silver except the hangings of the *gate,* the way of access (Ex. 27:17, *note*).

The tabernacle: (11) *the overlay of gold.*

29 And thou shalt overlay the boards with gold, and make their rings *of* gold *for* places for the bars: and thou shalt overlay the bars with gold.

30 And thou shalt rear up the tabernacle according to the fashion thereof which was shewed thee in the mount.

The tabernacle: (12) *the inner vail.*

31 And thou shalt make a [1]vail *of* blue, and purple, and scarlet, and fine twined linen of cunning work: with cherubims shall it be made:

32 And thou shalt hang it upon four pillars of [a]shittim *wood* overlaid with gold: their hooks *shall be of* gold, upon the four sockets of silver.

33 And thou shalt hang up the vail under the taches, that thou mayest bring in thither within the vail the ark of the testimony: and the vail shall divide unto you between the holy *place* and the most holy.

34 And thou shalt put the mercy seat upon the ark of the testimony in the most holy *place*.

35 And thou shalt set the table without the vail, and the candlestick over against the table on the side of the tabernacle toward the south: and thou shalt put the table on the north side.

The tabernacle: (13) *the outer vail.*

36 And thou shalt make an hanging for the door of the tent, *of* blue, and purple, and scarlet, and fine twined linen, wrought with needlework.

37 And thou shalt make for the hanging five pillars *of* [a]shittim *wood*, and overlay them with gold, *and* their hooks *shall be of* gold: and thou shalt cast five sockets of [b]brass for them.

B.C. 1491.

a i.e. *acacia.*

b See Ex. 27:17, *note.*

c The wood (Christ's humanity), completely inclosed in brass, must have become completely charred by sacrificial fires. Cf. Heb. 10:5-7.

d One cubit = 1 ft. 5:48 in.; also vs. 9, 12-16, 18.

e Cf. Num. 21:9; John 3:14 with John 12:31-33; thus fixing the symbolic meaning of brass as *divine manifestation in judgment.*

CHAPTER 27.

The tabernacle: (14) *the brazen altar.*

And thou shalt make an [2]altar *of* [a]shittim [c]wood, five [d]cubits long, and five cubits broad; the altar shall be foursquare: and the [3]height thereof *shall be* three cubits.

2 And thou shalt make the horns of it upon the four corners thereof: his horns shall be of the same: and thou shalt overlay it with [e]brass.

3 And thou shalt make his pans to receive his ashes, and his shovels, and his basons, and his fleshhooks, and his firepans: all the vessels thereof thou shalt make *of* brass.

4 And thou shalt make for it a grate of network *of* brass; and upon the net shalt thou make four brasen rings in the four corners thereof.

5 And thou shalt put it under the compass of the altar beneath, that the net may be even to the midst of the altar.

6 And thou shalt make staves for the altar, staves *of* [a]shittim wood, and overlay them with brass.

7 And the staves shall be put into the rings, and the staves shall be upon the two sides of the altar, to bear it.

8 Hollow with boards shalt thou make it: as it was shewed thee in the mount, so shall they make *it*.

The tabernacle: (15) *the court.*

9 And thou shalt make the court of the tabernacle: for the south side southward *there shall be* hangings for the court *of* [4]fine

[1] **(26:31)** The inner veil, type of Christ's human body (Mt. 26:26; 27:50; Heb. 10:20). This veil, barring entrance into the holiest, was the most expressive symbol of the truth that "by the deeds of the law shall no flesh be justified" (Rom. 3:20; Heb. 9:8). Rent by an unseen hand when Christ died (Mt. 27:51), thus giving instant access to God to all who come by faith in Him, it was the end of all legality; the way to God was open. It is deeply significant that the priests must have patched together again the veil that God had rent, for the temple services went on yet for nearly forty years. That patched veil is Galatianism—the attempt to put saint or sinner back under law. (Cf. Gal. 1:6-9.) *Anything* but "the *grace* of Christ" is "another gospel," and under anathema.

[2] **(27:1)** Brazen altar type of the Cross upon which Christ, our whole burnt-offering, offered Himself without spot to God (Heb. 9:14).

[3] **(27:1)** Cf. Ex. 25:10. The altar of burnt-offering is double the height of the mercy-seat. The atonement more than saves *us*—it glorifies God (John 17: 4).

[4] **(27:9)** The fine linen commonly typifies personal righteousness (Ex. 26:1, *ref. d*), and in the hangings of the court stands for that measure of righteousness which God demands of any who would, in his own righteousness, approach. Christ, figuratively speaking, put up the hangings of the court in

twined linen of an hundred cubits long for one side:

10 And the twenty pillars thereof and their twenty sockets *shall be of* brass; the hooks of the pillars and their fillets *shall be of* silver.

11 And likewise for the north side in length *there shall be* hangings of an hundred *cubits* long, and his twenty pillars and their twenty sockets *of* brass; the hooks of the pillars and their fillets *of* silver.

12 And *for* the breadth of the court on the west side *shall be* hangings of fifty cubits: their pillars ten, and their sockets ten.

13 And the breadth of the court on the east side eastward *shall be* fifty cubits.

14 The hangings of one side *of the gate shall be* fifteen cubits: their pillars three, and their sockets three.

15 And on the other side *shall be* hangings fifteen *cubits*: their pillars three, and their sockets three.

The tabernacle:
(16) *the hanging for the gate of the court.*

16 And for the [1]gate of the court *shall be* an hanging of twenty cubits, *of* blue, and purple, and scarlet, and fine twined linen, wrought with needlework: *and* their pillars *shall be* four, and their sockets four.

17 All the [2]pillars round about the court *shall be* filleted with silver; their hooks *shall be of* silver, and their sockets *of* brass.

18 The length of the court *shall be* an hundred cubits, and the breadth fifty every where, and the height five cubits *of* fine twined linen, and their sockets *of* brass.

19 All the vessels of the tabernacle in all the service thereof, and all the pins thereof, and all the pins of the court, *shall be of* [a]brass.

The tabernacle: (17) *the oil for the light.*

20 And thou shalt command the children of Israel, that they bring thee pure [3]oil olive beaten for the light, to cause the lamp to burn always.

21 In the tabernacle of the congregation without the vail, which *is* before the testimony, Aaron and his sons shall order it from evening to morning before the LORD: *it shall be* a statute for ever unto their generations on the behalf of the children of Israel.

B.C. 1491.

a Num. 21:9, *note.*

Lk. 10:25-28. The only way of approach was the "gate" (v. 16, John 10:9). The hangings of the court bar out equally the self-righteous man and the open sinner, for the height was above seven feet (Ex. 27:18).

[1] **(27:16)** In the hangings of the court (v. 9, *ref.*) representing that practical righteousness which God demands in the law, and which, therefore, bars out all men (Rom. 3:19, 20; 10:3-5), no colours are inwrought. But the "gate" is Christ (John 10:9), and so the colours reappear as in the veil (Ex. 26:31).

[2] **(27:17)** The fillets and hooks upholding the linen hangings are of silver (Ex. 38:27, *note*), for it is in virtue of His redemptive work that Christ is our way of access, and not by virtue of His righteous *life* (symbolized by the fine linen); but the *pillars* of the court rest upon brass sockets, not silver as in the case of the boards (Ex. 26:19, *note*), and brass symbolizes divine righteousness in judgment (Num. 21:9, *note*). Redemption not only displays God's *mercy*, but vindicates His *righteousness* in showing that mercy (Rom. 3:21-26).

[3] **(27:20)** Oil is a symbol of the Holy Spirit (Cf. John 3:34, with Heb. 1:9). In Christ the oil-fed Light ever burns, the Light of the world (John 8:12). But here we have not the world, but the sanctuary. It is a question, not of testimony in and to the world, but of our communion and worship as believer-priests in the holiest (Heb. 10:19, 20). In the Tabernacle there were two compartments, two lights: the holy place with the candlestick (Ex. 25:31, *note*); the holy of holies with the shekinah, or manifested glory of God. These two places are now one (Mt. 27:50, 51; Heb. 9:6-8; 10:19-21), but it is important to see that there are still two lights: Christ, the Light of life (John 8:12), through the Spirit giving light upon the holy things of God, the showbread and altar of incense; and also the shekinah, now on the face of Jesus Christ (2 Cor. 4:6). Into this twofold light we, as believer priests, are brought (1 Pet. 2:9). We "walk in the light," not merely which He *gives*, but in which He lives (1 John 1:7). But what of the command to "*bring* pure oil" (Ex. 27:20)? Because our access, apprehension, communion, and transformation are by the Spirit (Eph. 2:18; 1 Cor. 2:14, 15; 2 Cor. 13:14; Phil. 2:1; 2 Cor. 3:18). Our *title* to His presence is the blood (Eph. 2:13), but only as filled with the Spirit (Eph. 5:18) do we really walk in the light.

CHAPTER 28.

The priesthood: (1) *the high priest and the priests; types of Christ and* [a]*believers of the Church age.*

And take thou unto thee [1]Aaron thy
brother, and his sons with him,
from [b]among the children of Israel, that
he may minister unto me in the priest's
office, *even* Aaron, Nadab and Abihu,
Eleazar and Ithamar, Aaron's sons.
2 And thou shalt make [2]holy garments
for Aaron thy brother for glory and for
beauty.
3 And thou shalt speak unto all *that*
are wise hearted, whom I have filled
with the [c]spirit of wisdom, that they
may make Aaron's garments to [2]conse-
crate him, that he may minister unto me
in the priest's office.

The priesthood:
(2) *the garments of the high priest.*

4 And these *are* the [d]garments which
they shall make; a breastplate, and an
ephod, and a robe, and a broidered coat,
a mitre, and a girdle: and they shall
make holy garments for Aaron thy
brother, and his sons, that he may minister unto me in the priest's office.

The materials.

5 And they shall [e]take gold, and blue,
and purple, and scarlet, and fine linen.

The ephod.

6 And they shall make the [e]ephod *of*
gold, *of* blue, and *of* purple, *of* scarlet, and
fine twined linen, with cunning work.
7 It shall have the two shoulderpieces
thereof joined at the two edges thereof;
and *so* it shall be joined together.
8 And the curious girdle of the ephod,
which *is* upon it, shall be of the same,
according to the work thereof; *even of*
gold, *of* blue, and purple, and scarlet,
and fine twined linen.
9 And thou shalt take two onyx
stones, and grave on them the names of
the children of Israel:

B.C. 1491.

a See 1 Pet. 2:9; Rev. 1:6.

b *Sanctify, holy* (O.T.). vs. 1-3; Ex. 29:37, 44. (Gen. 2:3; Zech. 8:3.)

c *Holy Spirit.* Ex. 31:3. (Gen. 1:2; Mal. 2:15.)

d See Ex. 29:5, *note.*

e *Gold,* Deity in manifestation; *blue,* heavenly; *purple,* royalty; *scarlet,* sacrifice; *fine linen,* personal righteousness (Ex. 26:1, *ref.*)

f The place of strength, Isa. 9:6; Lk. 15:4, 5.

g One span = 8:737 inches.

10 Six of their names on one stone,
and *the other* six names of the rest on the
other stone, according to their birth.
11 With the work of an engraver in
stone, *like* the engravings of a signet, shalt
thou engrave the two stones with the
names of the children of Israel: thou shalt
make them to be set in ouches of gold.
12 And thou shalt put the two stones
upon the shoulders of the ephod *for*
stones of memorial unto the children of
Israel: and Aaron shall bear their names
before the LORD upon his two [f]shoulders
for a memorial.
13 And thou shalt make ouches *of*
gold;
14 And two chains *of* pure gold at the
ends; *of* wreathen work shalt thou make
them, and fasten the wreathen chains to
the ouches.

The breastplate.

15 And thou shalt make the breastplate of judgment with cunning work;
after the work of the ephod thou shalt
make it; *of* [e]gold, *of* blue, and *of* purple,
and *of* scarlet, and *of* fine twined linen,
shalt thou make it.
16 Foursquare it shall be *being* doubled; a [g]span *shall be* the length thereof,
and a span *shall be* the breadth thereof.
17 And thou shalt set in it settings of
stones, *even* four rows of stones: *the first*
row *shall be* a sardius, a topaz, and a carbuncle: *this shall be* the first row.
18 And the second row *shall be* an
emerald, a sapphire, and a diamond.
19 And the third row a ligure, an
agate, and an amethyst.
20 And the fourth row a beryl, and an
onyx, and a jasper: they shall be set in
gold in their inclosings.
21 And the stones shall be with the
names of the children of Israel, twelve,
according to their names, *like* the engravings of a signet; every one with his name
shall they be according to the twelve
tribes.

[1]**(28:1)** Type of Christ, our High Priest. Christ is a priest after the order of Melchizedek, but He executes his priestly office after the *pattern* of Aaron. Heb. 7. gives the *order;* Heb. 9, the *pattern.* See Gen. 14:18-20, *note.*

[2]**(28:2)** Heb. *qodesh* = "set apart" for God. Trans. "holy," v. 2; "consecrate," v. 3. Often trans. "sanctify." See summary, Zech. 8:3, *note.* This is always the fundamental idea of a holy, consecrated, separated, or sanctified person or thing—something set apart for God. Infinite confusion would have been spared the reader if *qodesh* had been uniformly trans. "set apart."

22 And thou shalt make upon the breastplate chains at the ends *of* wreathen work *of* pure gold.

23 And thou shalt make upon the breastplate two rings of gold, and shalt put the two rings on the two ends of the breastplate.

24 And thou shalt put the two wreathen *chains* of gold in the two rings *which are* on the ends of the breastplate.

25 And *the other* two ends of the two wreathen *chains* thou shalt fasten in the two ouches, and put *them* on the shoulderpieces of the ephod before it.

26 And thou shalt make two rings of gold, and thou shalt put them upon the two ends of the breastplate in the border thereof, which *is* in the side of the ephod inward.

27 And two *other* rings of gold thou shalt make, and shalt put them on the two sides of the ephod underneath, toward the forepart thereof, over against the *other* coupling thereof, above the curious girdle of the ephod.

28 And they shall bind the breastplate by the rings thereof unto the rings of the ephod with a lace of blue, that *it* may be above the curious girdle of the ephod, and that the breastplate be not loosed from the ephod.

29 And Aaron shall bear the names of the children of Israel in the breastplate of judgment upon his [a]heart, when he goeth in unto the holy *place*, for a memorial before the LORD continually.

The Urim and Thummim.

30 And thou shalt put in the breastplate of judgment the [1]Urim and the Thummim; and they shall be upon Aaron's heart, when he goeth in before the LORD: and Aaron shall bear the judgment of the children of Israel upon his heart before the LORD continually.

The robe of the Ephod.

31 And thou shalt make the [b]robe of the ephod all *of* blue.

B.C. 1491.

a The place of affection Cf. v. 12, *ref.*

b See Ex. 29:5, *note.*

c i.e. be responsible for every neglect or offense respecting "the holy things," etc.

32 And there shall be an hole in the top of it, in the midst thereof: it shall have a binding of woven work round about the hole of it, as it were the hole of an habergeon, that it be not rent.

33 And *beneath* upon the hem of it thou shalt make pomegranates *of* blue, and *of* purple, and *of* scarlet, round about the hem thereof; and bells of gold between them round about:

34 A golden bell and a pomegranate, a golden bell and a pomegranate, upon the hem of the robe round about.

35 And it shall be upon Aaron to minister: and his sound shall be heard when he goeth in unto the holy *place* before the LORD, and when he cometh out, that he die not.

The "holy crown" (Ex. 29:6).

36 And thou shalt make a plate *of* pure gold, and grave upon it, *like* the engravings of a signet, HOLINESS TO THE LORD.

37 And thou shalt put it on a blue lace, that it may be upon the mitre; upon the forefront of the mitre it shall be.

38 And it shall be upon Aaron's forehead, that Aaron may [c]bear the iniquity of the holy things, which the children of Israel shall hallow in all their holy gifts; and it shall be always upon his forehead, that they may be accepted before the LORD.

The ordinary garments of high priest and priests, over which the garments for glory and beauty were put on.

39 And thou shalt embroider the coat of fine linen, and thou shalt make the mitre *of* fine linen, and thou shalt make the girdle *of* needlework.

40 And for Aaron's sons thou shalt make coats, and thou shalt make for them girdles, and bonnets shalt thou make for them, for glory and for beauty.

[1]**(28:30)** Urim and Thummim, meaning "lights and perfections." Some make these to be simply a collective name for the stones of the breastplate, so that the total effect of the twelve stones is to manifest the "lights and perfections" of Him who is the antitype of the Aaronic high priest. *Per contra,* Lev. 8:8. This would seem to be conclusive that "the Urim and Thummim" are additional to the stones of the breastplate. In *use* the U and T were connected, in some way not clearly expressed, with the ascertainment of the divine will in particular cases (Num. 27:21; Deut. 33:8; 1 Sam. 28:6; Ezra 2:63).

41 And thou shalt put them upon Aaron thy brother, and his sons with him; and shalt anoint them, and consecrate them, and sanctify them, that they may minister unto me in the priest's office.

42 And thou shalt make them linen breeches to cover their nakedness; from the loins even unto the thighs they shall reach:

43 And they shall be upon Aaron, and upon his sons, when they come in unto the tabernacle of the congregation, or when they come near unto the altar to minister in the holy *place*; that they bear not iniquity, and die: *it shall be* a statute for ever unto him and his seed after him.

CHAPTER 29.

The priesthood: (3) *the consecration of the priests; the offerings.*

And this *is* the thing that thou shalt [1]do unto them to hallow them, to minister unto me in the priest's office: [a]Take one young bullock, and two [b]rams without blemish,

2 And [c]unleavened bread, and [d]cakes unleavened tempered with oil, and wafers unleavened anointed with oil: *of* wheaten flour shalt thou make them.

3 And thou shalt put them into one basket, and bring them in the basket, with the bullock and the two rams.

4 And [2]Aaron and his sons thou shalt bring unto the door of the tabernacle of the congregation, and shalt [e]wash them with water.

The order for the high priest.

5 And thou shalt take the [3]garments, and put upon Aaron the coat, and the robe of the ephod, and the ephod, and the breastplate, and gird him with the curious girdle of the ephod:

6 And thou shalt put the mitre upon his head, and put the holy crown upon the mitre.

B.C. 1491.

a Cf. Heb. 7:26-28.

b See Lev. 1:2, *note.*

c *Leaven.* vs. 2, 23; Ex. 34:18, 25. (Gen. 19:3; Mt. 13:33.)

d See Ex. 25:30, *note;* Lev. 2:1, *note* 3.

e Distinguish the *washing* from the use of the *laver.* Ex. 30:18-21. This washing typifies regeneration (Tit. 3:5); the laver, daily cleansing (1 John 1:9.) See both, John 13:10.

[1] **(29:1)** The priest type of consecration. (Cf. the temple type, 1 Ki. 8:1-11; 2 Chr. 5:4-14). The order in Leviticus (8:1–9:24) differs from the order here. In Leviticus the filling the hands precedes the sprinkling.

[2] **(29:4)** Aaron shares in the washing (i.e. symbol of regeneration, Tit. 3:5; John 3:5-6): (1) as needing it, being in this in *contrast* with Christ (Heb. 7:26-28); (2) to typify Christ's action, who received the baptism of John, not as needing it, but as thus identifying Himself with sinners, and as fulfilling the Aaronic type. As in Aaron's case, His anointing followed the washing (Ex. 29:4, 7; Mt. 3:14-16).

[3] **(29:5)** The high priest's garments were put on in reverse order of the instructions for making them:

(1) The "coat" (Ex. 28:39), the oriental long garment worn next the person, made of fine linen (Ex. 27:9, *ref.*).

(2) The "robe of the ephod" (Ex. 28:31-35), a long seamless garment of blue linen with an opening for the head, worn over the "coat." Pomegranates, symbol of fruitfulness, were embroidered on the skirt of the robe in blue, purple and scarlet, alternated with golden bells, symbol of testimony, which gave a sound as the high priest went in and out of the sanctuary. The robe was secured by an embroidered girdle.

(3) The ephod (Ex. 28:5-12) was next put on. A short garment made of linen, embroidered with gold, blue, purple, and scarlet, it consisted of two pieces, front and back, united by two shoulder-pieces and by a band about the bottom. Two onyx stones, set in gold and fastened upon the shoulder-pieces of the ephod, were engraved with the names of the twelve tribes: "and Aaron shall bear their names before Jehovah upon his two shoulders (the place of strength) for a memorial." Cf. Isa. 9:6; Lk. 15: 4, 5.

(4) The breastplate was a square pouch (Ex. 28:16) of linen to contain the Urim and Thummim (Ex. 28:30, *note*). To the linen pouch was attached the oblong gold setting containing four rows of precious stones, three in each row, with the names of the twelve tribes engraved thereon, on each stone a tribal name. The breastplate with the jewel work was attached at the upper corners to the shoulder-pieces of the ephod by golden chains. Golden rings were sewn on ephod and breastplate, and the latter was further secured to the ephod by laces of blue through the rings. Altogether, it was called "the breastplate of judgment" because worn by the high priest when judging the causes of the people (Ex. 28:30, *note, refs.*).

(5) A mitre (or "turban") of fine linen was made (Ex. 28:37) to cover the head, bearing upon the front a gold plate engraved, "Holiness to the LORD" (v. 36).

B.C. 1491.

7 Then shalt thou take the anointing oil, and pour *it* upon his head, and anoint him.

The order for the priests.

8 And thou shalt bring his sons, and put coats upon them.

9 And thou shalt [a]gird them with girdles, Aaron and his sons, and put the bonnets on them: and the priest's office shall be theirs for a perpetual statute: and thou shalt consecrate Aaron and his sons.

The order for the sacrifices.

10 And thou shalt cause a bullock to be brought before the tabernacle of the congregation: and Aaron and his sons shall [b]put their hands upon the head of the bullock.

11 And thou shalt kill the bullock before the LORD, *by* the door of the tabernacle of the congregation.

12 And thou shalt take of the blood of the bullock, and put *it* upon the horns of the altar with thy finger, and pour all the blood beside the bottom of the altar.

13 And thou shalt take all the [c]fat that covereth the inwards, and the caul *that is* above the liver, and the two kidneys, and the fat that *is* upon them, and burn *them* upon the altar.

14 But the flesh of the bullock, and his skin, and his dung, shalt thou burn with fire [d]without the camp: it *is* a sin-offering.

15 Thou shalt also take one ram; and Aaron and his sons shall put their hands upon the head of the ram.

16 And thou shalt slay the ram, and thou shalt take his blood, and sprinkle *it* round about upon the altar.

17 And thou shalt cut the ram in pieces, and wash the inwards of him, and his legs, and put *them* unto his pieces, and unto his head.

18 And thou shalt burn the whole ram upon the altar: it *is* a burnt-offering unto the LORD: it *is* a sweet savour, an offering made by fire unto the LORD.

19 And thou shalt take the other ram; and Aaron and his sons shall put their hands upon the head of the ram.

20 Then shalt thou kill the ram, and take of his blood, and put *it* upon the tip of the right ear of Aaron, and upon the tip of the right ear of his sons, and upon the thumb of their right hand, and upon the great toe of their right foot, and sprinkle the blood upon the altar round about.

21 And thou shalt take of the blood that *is* upon the altar, and of the anointing oil, and sprinkle *it* upon Aaron, and upon his garments, and upon his sons, and upon the garments of his sons with him: and he shall be hallowed, and his garments, and his sons, and his sons' garments with him.

22 Also thou shalt take of the ram the fat and the rump, and the fat that covereth the inwards, and the caul *above* the liver, and the two kidneys, and the fat that *is* upon them, and the right shoulder; for it *is* a ram of consecration:

23 And one loaf of bread, and one cake of oiled bread, and one wafer out of the basket of the unleavened bread that *is* before the LORD:

24 And thou shalt put all in the [e]hands of Aaron, and in the hands of his sons; and shalt wave them *for* a wave-offering before the LORD.

25 And thou shalt receive them of their hands, and burn *them* upon the altar for a burnt-offering, for a sweet savour before the LORD: it *is* an offering made by fire unto the LORD.

The priesthood: (4) *the food of the priests.* (See also vs. 29–33; Lev. 2:6; 6:14–18, 24–29; 7:6–11, 34.)

26 And thou shalt take the breast of the ram of Aaron's consecration, and wave it *for* a wave-offering before the LORD: and it shall be thy part.

27 And thou shalt sanctify the breast of the wave-offering, and the shoulder of the heave-offering, which is waved, and which is heaved up, of the ram of the consecration, *even* of *that* which *is* for Aaron, and of *that* which is for his sons:

28 And it shall be Aaron's and his

a Symbol of service. Lk. 12:37; 17:8; John 13:4; Rev. 1:13.

b Lev. 1:4, *note.*

c Lev. 1:8, *ref.*

d Lev. 4:11, 12, *ref.*

e Lit. *fill the hands.*

(6) To these were added linen breeches, "from the loins even to the thighs" (Ex. 28:42).

The "coat" and linen breeches were made for the priests, also, and were the ordinary garments of high priest and priests as distinguished from the other garments, which were "for glory and beauty."

sons' by a statute for ever from the children of Israel: for it *is* an heave-offering: and it shall be an heave-offering from the children of Israel of the sacrifice of their peace-offerings, *even* their heave-offering unto the LORD.

29 And the holy garments of Aaron shall be his sons' after him, to be anointed therein, and to be consecrated in them.

30 *And* that son that is priest in his stead shall put them on seven days, when he cometh into the tabernacle of the congregation to minister in the holy *place*.

31 And thou shalt take the ram of the consecration, and seethe his flesh in the holy place.

32 And Aaron and his sons shall eat the flesh of the ram, and the bread that *is* in the basket, *by* the door of the tabernacle of the congregation.

33 And they shall eat those things wherewith the [1]atonement was made, to consecrate *and* to sanctify them: but a stranger shall not eat *thereof*, because they *are* holy.

34 And if ought of the flesh of the consecrations, or of the bread, remain unto the morning, then thou shalt burn the remainder with fire: it shall not be eaten, because it *is* holy.

35 And thus shalt thou do unto Aaron, and to his sons, according to all *things* which I have commanded thee: seven days shalt thou consecrate them.

36 And thou shalt offer every day a bullock *for* a sin-offering for [a]atonement: and thou shalt cleanse the altar, when thou hast made an atonement for it, and thou shalt anoint it, to sanctify it.

37 Seven days thou shalt make an [a]atonement for the altar, and [b]sanctify it; and it shall be an altar most holy: whatsoever toucheth the altar shall be holy.

B.C. 1491.

a v. 33, *note.*

b *Sanctify, holy* (O.T.). vs. 37, 44; Ex. 30:30, 37. (Gen. 2:3; Zech. 8:3.)

c One hin = about 6 quarts.

d Lit. *meal.*

e i.e. *acacia.*

The continued burnt-offering.

38 Now this *is that* which thou shalt offer upon the altar; two lambs of the first year day by day continually.

39 The one lamb thou shalt offer in the morning; and the other lamb thou shalt offer at even:

40 And with the one lamb a tenth deal of flour mingled with the fourth part of an [c]hin of beaten oil; and the fourth part of an hin of wine *for* a drink-offering.

41 And the other lamb thou shalt offer at even, and shalt do thereto according to the [d]meat-offering of the morning, and according to the drink-offering thereof, for a sweet savour, an offering made by fire unto the LORD.

42 *This shall be* a continual burnt-offering throughout your generations *at* the door of the tabernacle of the congregation before the LORD: where I will meet you, to speak there unto thee.

43 And there I will meet with the children of Israel, and *the tabernacle* shall be sanctified by my glory.

44 And I will sanctify the tabernacle of the congregation, and the altar: I will sanctify also both Aaron and his sons, to minister to me in the priest's office.

45 And I will dwell among the children of Israel, and will be their God.

46 And they shall know that I *am* the LORD their God, that brought them forth out of the land of Egypt, that I may dwell among them: I *am* the LORD their God.

CHAPTER 30.

The tabernacle: (18) *the altar of incense; the great worship chapter.*

And thou shalt make an altar to burn [2]incense upon: *of* [e]shittim wood shalt thou make it.

[1] **(29:33)** Heb. *kaphar,* "to cover." The English word "atonement" (at-one-ment) is not a *translation* of the Heb. *kaphar,* but a translator's *interpretation.* According to Scripture the legal sacrifice "covered" the offerer's *sin* and secured the divine *forgiveness;* according to the translators it made God' and the sinner at-one. But the O.T. sacrifices did *not* at-one the sinner and God. "It is not possible that the blood of bulls and goats should take away sins" (Heb. 10:4). The Israelite's offering implied confession of sin and of its due desert, death; and God "covered" ("passed over," Rom. 3:25) his sin, in anticipation of *Christ's* sacrifice, which did, finally, "put away" the sins "done aforetime in the forbearance of God" (Rom. 3:25; Heb. 9:15). See Rom. 3:25, *note.* The word "atonement" does not occur in the N.T.; Rom. 5:11, meaning reconciliation, and so rendered in the R.V. See "Sacrifice," Gen. 4:4, and *refs.* See *note* on atonement, Lev. 16.

[2] **(30:1)** Altar of incense, type of Christ our intercessor (John 17:1-26; Heb. 7:25), through whom our

2 A [a]cubit *shall be* the length thereof, and a cubit the breadth thereof; foursquare shall it be: and two cubits *shall be* the height thereof: the horns thereof *shall be* of the same.

3 And thou shalt overlay it with pure gold, the top thereof, and the sides thereof round about, and the horns thereof; and thou shalt make unto it a crown of gold round about.

4 And two golden rings shalt thou make to it under the crown of it, by the two corners thereof, upon the two sides of it shalt thou make *it*; and they shall be for places for the staves to bear it withal.

5 And thou shalt make the staves *of* [b]shittim wood, and overlay them with gold.

6 And thou shalt put it before the vail that *is* by the ark of the testimony, before the mercy seat that *is* over the testimony, where I will meet with thee.

7 And Aaron shall burn thereon sweet incense every morning: when he dresseth the lamps, he shall burn incense upon it.

8 And when Aaron lighteth the lamps at even, he shall burn incense upon it, a perpetual incense before the LORD throughout your generations.

9 Ye shall offer no [1]strange incense thereon, nor burnt sacrifice, nor [c]meat-offering; neither shall ye pour drink-offering thereon.

10 And Aaron shall make an [d]atonement upon the horns of it once in a year with the blood of the sin-offering of atonements: once in the year shall he make [d]atonement upon it throughout your generations: it *is* most holy unto the LORD.

Who may worship? (1) *the redeemed* (Psa. 107:1, 2; Ex. 15:1–21).

11 And the LORD spake unto Moses, saying,

12 When thou takest the sum of the children of Israel after their number, then shall they give every man a ransom for his soul unto the LORD, when thou numberest them; that there be no plague among them, when *thou* numberest them.

13 [e]This they shall give, every one that passeth among them that are numbered, half a [f]shekel after the shekel of the sanctuary: (a shekel *is* twenty [g]gerahs:) an half shekel *shall be* the offering of the LORD.

14 Every one that passeth among them that are numbered, from twenty years old and above, shall give an offering unto the LORD.

15 The rich shall not give more, and the poor shall not give less than half a [f]shekel, when *they* give an offering unto the LORD, to make an [d]atonement for your souls.

16 And thou shalt take the [d]atonement money of the children of Israel, and shalt appoint it for the service of the tabernacle of the congregation; that it may be a memorial unto the children of Israel before the LORD, to make an [d]atonement for your souls.

Who may worship? (2) *the cleansed* (Heb. 10:22; John 13:3–10; 1 John 1:9).

17 And the LORD spake unto Moses, saying,

18 Thou shalt also make a [2]laver *of* brass, and his foot *also of* brass, to wash *withal*: and thou shalt put it between the tabernacle of the congregation and the altar, and thou shalt put water therein.

19 For Aaron and his sons shall [h]wash their hands and their feet thereat:

20 When they go into the tabernacle of the congregation, they shall wash with water, that they die not; or when they come near to the altar to minister, to burn offering made by fire unto the LORD:

21 So they shall wash their hands and

B.C. 1491.

a One cubit = 1 ft. 5:48 in.

b i.e. *acacia.*

c Lit. *meal.*

d See Ex. 29:33, *note.*

e Cf. Ex. 38:25-27. Silver thus becomes a type of redemption (Ex. 26:19, *note*).

f One shekel = 2*s.* 9*d.*, or 65 cents.

g One gerah = 11.2 grains.

h John 13:8.

own prayers and praises ascend to God (Heb. 13:15; Rev. 8:3, 4), and of the believer-priest's sacrifice of praise and worship (Heb. 13:15).

[1] **(30:9)** Cf. Lev. 10:1-3. Two prohibitions are given concerning worship: (1) No "strange" incense is to be offered. This speaks of simulated or purely formal worship: (2) No "strange" fire was permitted. This refers to the excitation of "religious" feelings by merely sensuous means, and to the substitution for devotion to Christ of any other devotion, as to religious causes, or sects. Cf. 1 Cor. 1:11-13; Col. 2:8, 16-19. See Ex. 30:38, *note.*

[2] **(30:18)** Laver, type of Christ cleansing us from defilement, and from "every spot or wrinkle or any such thing" (John 13:2-10; Eph. 5:25-27). It is significant that the priests could not enter the holy place after serving at the brazen altar till hands and feet were cleansed.

their feet, that they die not: and it shall be a statute for ever to them, *even* to him and to his seed throughout their generations.

Who may worship? (3) *the anointed* (John 4:23; Eph. 2:18; 5:18, 19).

22 Moreover the LORD spake unto Moses, saying,

23 Take thou also unto thee principal spices, of pure myrrh five hundred [a]*shekels*, and of sweet cinnamon half so much, *even* two hundred and fifty *shekels*, and of sweet calamus two hundred and fifty *shekels*,

24 And of cassia five hundred *shekels*, after the shekel of the sanctuary, and of oil olive an [b]hin:

25 And thou shalt make it an oil of holy ointment, an ointment compound after the art of the apothecary: it shall be an holy anointing oil.

26 And thou shalt anoint the tabernacle of the congregation therewith, and the ark of the testimony,

27 And the table and all his vessels, and the candlestick and his vessels, and the altar of incense,

28 And the altar of burnt-offering with all his vessels, and the laver and his foot.

29 And thou shalt sanctify them, that they may be most holy: whatsoever toucheth them shall be holy.

30 And thou shalt anoint Aaron and his sons, and [c]consecrate them, that *they* may minister unto me in the priest's office.

31 And thou shalt speak unto the children of Israel, saying, This shall be an holy anointing [1]oil unto me throughout your generations.

32 Upon man's flesh shall it not be poured, neither shall ye make *any other* like it, after the composition of it: it *is* holy, *and* it shall be holy unto you.

33 Whosoever compoundeth *any* like it, or whosoever putteth *any* of it upon a stranger, shall even be cut off from his people.

Worship: the incense, type of prayer and praise. It is for the Lord, v. 37; *spiritual, not sensuous*, v. 38.

34 And the LORD said unto Moses, Take unto thee sweet spices, stacte, and onycha, and galbanum; *these* sweet spices with pure [2]frankincense: of each shall there be a like *weight*:

35 And thou shalt make it a perfume, a confection after the art of the apothecary, tempered together, pure *and* holy:

36 And thou shalt beat *some* of it very small, and put of it before the testimony in the tabernacle of the congregation, where I will meet with thee: it shall be unto you most holy.

37 And *as for* the perfume which thou shalt make, ye shall not make to yourselves according to the composition thereof: it shall be unto thee holy for the LORD.

38 Whosoever shall make like unto that, to [3]smell thereto, shall even be cut off from his people.

CHAPTER 31.

The tabernacle: (19) *the workmen.*

And the LORD spake unto Moses, saying,

2 See, I have called by name Bezaleel the son of Uri, the son of Hur, of the tribe of Judah:

3 And I have filled him with the [d]spirit of God, in wisdom, and in understanding, and in knowledge, and in all manner of workmanship,

4 To devise cunning works, to work in gold, and in silver, and in brass,

5 And in cutting of stones, to set *them*, and in carving of timber, to work in all manner of workmanship.

6 And I, behold, I have given with him Aholiab, the son of Ahisamach, of the tribe of Dan: and in the hearts of all that

B.C. 1491.

a One shekel = 2*s*. 9*d*., or 65 cents.

b One hin = about 6 quarts.

c *Sanctify, holy* (O.T.). vs. 30, 37; Lev. 8:15. (Gen. 2:3; Zech. 8:3.)

d *Holy Spirit*. Ex. 35:31. (Gen. 1:2; Mal. 2:15.)

[1] **(30:31)** Anointing oil, type of the Holy Spirit for service (Acts 1:8).

[2] **(30:34)** Frankincense is not to be confounded with incense (to which it was to be added), as it is often used apart from incense. We are told what composed the incense—never in Scripture what the frankincense was. All speaks of Christ—the sweet spices of those perfections which we may apprehend, the frankincense of that which God saw in Jesus ineffable.

[3] **(30:38)** What is condemned here is making worship a mere pleasure to the natural man, whether sensuous, as in beautiful music to please the ear, or eloquence, merely to give delight to the natural mind. Cf. John 4:23, 24.

are wise hearted I have put wisdom, that
they may make all that I have commanded thee;
7 The tabernacle of the congregation,
and the ark of the testimony, and the
mercy seat that *is* thereupon, and all the
furniture of the tabernacle,
8 And the table and his furniture, and
the pure candlestick with all his furniture, and the altar of incense,
9 And the altar of burnt-offering with
all his furniture, and the laver and his
foot,
10 And the cloths of service, and the
holy garments for Aaron the priest, and
the garments of his sons, to minister in
the priest's office,
11 And the anointing oil, and sweet
incense for the holy *place*: according to
all that I have commanded thee shall
they do.

The Sabbath a sign between Jehovah and Israel.

12 And the LORD spake unto Moses,
saying,
13 Speak thou also unto the children
of Israel, saying, Verily my [a]sabbaths ye
shall keep: for it *is* a sign between me
and you throughout your generations;
that *ye* may know that I *am* the LORD that
doth sanctify you.
14 Ye shall keep the sabbath therefore;
for it *is* holy unto you: every one that
defileth it shall surely be put to death:
for whosoever doeth *any* work therein,
that soul shall be cut off from among his
people.
15 Six days may work be done; but in
the seventh *is* the sabbath of rest, holy to
the LORD: whosoever doeth *any* work in
the sabbath day, he shall surely be put to
death.
16 Wherefore the children of Israel
shall keep the sabbath, to observe the
sabbath throughout their generations, *for*
a perpetual covenant.
17 It *is* a sign between me and the children of Israel for ever: for *in* six days the
LORD made heaven and earth, and on the
seventh day he rested, and was refreshed.
18 And he gave unto Moses, when he
had made an end of communing with
him upon mount Sinai, two tables of testimony, [b]tables of stone, [c]written with
the finger of God.

B.C. 1491.

a *Sabbath.* vs. 13-16; Ex. 35:2, 3. (Gen. 2:3; Mt. 12:1.)

b See Ex. 20:4, *note.*

c *Law (of Moses).* Ex. 34:18-28. (Ex. 19:1; Gal. 3:1-29.)

d Acts 7:40.

e Cf. 1 Cor. 10:7.

f Deut. 9:8-22.

g Cf. v. 11.

CHAPTER 32.

Parenthetical: the broken law.

And when the people saw that Moses
delayed to come down out of the
mount, the people gathered themselves
together unto Aaron, and said unto him,
Up, [d]make us gods, which shall go before
us; for *as for* this Moses, the man that
brought us up out of the land of Egypt,
we wot not what is become of him.
2 And Aaron said unto them, Break off
the golden earrings, which *are* in the ears
of your wives, of your sons, and of your
daughters, and bring *them* unto me.
3 And all the people brake off the
golden earrings which *were* in their ears,
and brought *them* unto Aaron.
4 And he received *them* at their hand,
and fashioned it with a graving tool, after
he had made it a molten calf: and they
said, These *be* thy gods, O Israel, which
brought thee up out of the land of Egypt.
5 And when Aaron saw *it*, he built an
altar before it; and Aaron made proclamation, and said, To morrow *is* a feast to
the LORD.
6 And they rose up early on the morrow,
and offered burnt-offerings, and brought
peace-offerings; [e]and the people sat down
to eat and to drink, and rose up to play.

The condemnation of Jehovah.

7 [f]And the LORD said unto Moses, Go,
get thee down; for [g]thy people, which
thou broughtest out of the land of Egypt,
have corrupted *themselves*:
8 They have turned aside quickly out
of the way which I commanded them:
they have made them a molten calf, and
have worshipped it, and have sacrificed
thereunto, and said, These *be* thy gods,
O Israel, which have brought thee up
out of the land of Egypt.
9 And the LORD said unto Moses, I
have seen this people, and, behold, it *is* a
stiffnecked people:
10 Now therefore [1]let me alone, that
my wrath may wax hot against them,

[1] **(32:10)** This whole scene affords a striking contrast between law and grace. Cf. Moses' intercession with Christ's (John 17). Israel was a *nation,* under *probation* (Ex. 19:5, 6); believers under grace are a *family,* awaiting *glory* (John 20:17; Rom. 5:1, 2). For them there is "an advocate with the *Father,*" whose propitiatory sacrifice never loses efficacy (1 John 2:1, 2). Moses pleads a *covenant* (Ex. 32:13); Christ points to a *sacrifice* (John 17:4).

and that I may consume them: and I will make of thee a great nation.

The advocacy of Moses (1 John 2:1).

11 And Moses besought the LORD his God, and [a]said, LORD, why doth thy wrath wax hot against thy people, which thou hast brought forth out of the land of Egypt with great power, and with a mighty hand?

12 Wherefore should the Egyptians speak, and say, For mischief did he bring them out, to slay them in the mountains, and to consume them from the face of the earth? Turn from thy fierce wrath, and [b]repent of this evil against thy people.

13 Remember Abraham, Isaac, and Israel, thy servants, to whom thou swarest by thine own self, and saidst unto them, I will multiply your seed as the stars of heaven, and all this land that I have spoken of will I give unto your seed, and they shall inherit *it* for ever.

14 And the LORD [b]repented of the evil which he thought to do unto his people.

Disciplinary judgment.

15 And Moses turned, and went down from the mount, and the two tables of the testimony *were* in his hand: the tables *were* written on both their sides; on the one side and on the other *were* they written.

16 And the [c]tables *were* the work of God, and the [d]writing *was* the writing of God, graven upon the tables.

17 And when Joshua heard the noise of the people as they shouted, he said unto Moses, *There is* a noise of war in the camp.

18 And he said, *It is* not the voice of *them that* shout for mastery, neither *is it* the voice of *them that* cry for being overcome: *but* the noise of *them that* sing do I hear.

19 And it came to pass, as soon as he came nigh unto the camp, that he saw the calf, and the dancing: and Moses' anger waxed hot, and he cast the tables out of his hands, and brake them beneath the mount.

20 And he took the calf which they had made, and burnt *it* in the fire, and ground *it* to powder, and strawed *it* upon the water, and made the children of Israel drink *of it*.

21 And Moses said unto Aaron, What did this people unto thee, that thou hast brought so great a sin upon them?

22 And Aaron said, Let not the anger of my lord wax hot: thou knowest the people, that they *are set* on mischief.

23 For they said unto me, Make us gods, which shall go before us: for *as for* this Moses, the man that brought us up out of the land of Egypt, we wot not what is become of him.

24 And I said unto them, Whosoever hath any gold, let them break *it* off. So they gave *it* me: then I cast it into the fire, and there came out this calf.

25 And when Moses saw that the people *were* naked; (for Aaron had made them naked unto *their* shame among their enemies:)

26 Then Moses stood in the gate of the camp, and said, Who *is* on the LORD'S side? *let him come* unto me. And all the sons of Levi gathered themselves together unto him.

27 And he said unto them, Thus saith the LORD God of Israel, Put every man his sword by his side, *and* go in and out from gate to gate throughout the camp, and slay every man his brother, and every man his companion, and every man his neighbour.

28 And the children of Levi did according to the word of Moses: and there fell of the people that day about three thousand men.

The missed blessing.

29 For Moses had said, Consecrate yourselves to day to the LORD, even every man upon his son, and upon his brother; that he may bestow upon you a blessing this day.

The confession and intercession of Moses.

30 And it came to pass on the morrow, that Moses said unto the people, Ye have sinned a great sin: and now I will go up unto the LORD; peradventure I shall make an [e]atonement for your sin.

31 And Moses returned unto the LORD, and said, Oh, this people have sinned a great sin, and have made them gods of gold.

32 Yet now, if thou wilt forgive their sin—; and if not, blot me, I pray thee, out of thy book which thou hast written.

33 And the LORD said unto Moses,

B.C. 1491.

a *Bible prayers* (O.T.). Ex. 33:12. (Gen. 15:2; Hab. 3:1-16.)

b Zech. 8:14, *note.*

c See Ex. 20:4, *note.*

d *Inspiration.* Ex. 34:1, 27, 28. (Ex. 4:15; Rev. 22:19.)

e See Ex. 29:33, *note.*

Whosoever hath sinned against me, him will I blot out of my book.

34 Therefore now go, lead the people unto *the place* of which I have spoken unto thee: behold, mine [a]Angel shall go before thee: nevertheless in the day when I visit I will visit their sin upon them.

35 And the LORD plagued the people, because they made the calf, which Aaron made.

CHAPTER 33.

The journey to be resumed.

And the LORD said unto Moses, Depart, *and* go up hence, thou and the people which thou hast brought up out of the land of Egypt, unto the land which I sware unto Abraham, to Isaac, and to Jacob, saying, Unto thy seed will I give it:

2 And I will send an [a]angel before thee; and I will drive out the Canaanite, the Amorite, and the Hittite, and the Perizzite, the Hivite, and the Jebusite:

3 Unto a land flowing with milk and honey: for I will not go up in the midst of thee; for thou *art* a stiffnecked people: lest I consume thee in the way.

4 And when the people heard these evil tidings, they mourned: and no man did put on him his ornaments.

5 For the LORD had said unto Moses, Say unto the children of Israel, Ye *are* a stiffnecked people: I will come up into the midst of thee in a moment, and consume thee: therefore now put off thy ornaments from thee, that I may know what to do unto thee.

6 And the children of Israel stripped themselves of their ornaments by the mount Horeb.

The "tent of meeting" outside the camp.

7 And Moses took the [b]tabernacle, and pitched it without the camp, afar off from the camp, and called it the Tabernacle of the congregation. And it came to pass, *that* every one which sought the LORD went out unto the tabernacle of the congregation, which *was* without the camp.

8 And it came to pass, when Moses went out unto the tabernacle, *that* all the people rose up, and stood every man *at* his tent door, and looked after Moses, until he was gone into the tabernacle.

9 And it came to pass, as Moses entered into the tabernacle, the cloudy pillar descended, and stood *at* the door of the tabernacle, and *the LORD* talked with Moses.

10 And all the people saw the cloudy pillar stand *at* the tabernacle door: and all the people rose up and worshipped, every man *in* his tent door.

11 And the LORD spake unto Moses face to face, as a man speaketh unto his friend. And he turned again into the camp: but his servant Joshua, the son of Nun, a young man, departed not out of the tabernacle.

Moses' prayer; Jehovah's answer.

12 And Moses [c]said unto the LORD, See, thou sayest unto me, Bring up this people: and thou hast not let me know whom thou wilt send with me. Yet thou hast said, I know thee by name, and thou hast also found grace in my sight.

13 Now therefore, I pray thee, if I have found grace in thy sight, shew me now thy way, that I may know thee, that I may find grace in thy sight: and consider that this nation *is* thy people.

14 And he said, My presence shall go *with thee*, and I will give thee rest.

15 And he said unto him, If thy presence go not *with me*, carry us not up hence.

16 For wherein shall it be known here that I and thy people have found grace in thy sight? *is it* not in that thou goest with us? so shall we be [d]separated, I and thy people, from all the people that *are* upon the face of the earth.

17 And the LORD said unto Moses, I will do this thing also that thou hast spoken: for thou hast found grace in my sight, and I know thee by name.

Moses seeks a new vision for the new task.

18 And he said, I beseech thee, shew me thy glory.

19 And he said, I will make all my [e]goodness pass before thee, and I will proclaim the name of the LORD before thee; and [f]will be gracious to whom I will be gracious, and will shew mercy on whom I will shew mercy.

20 And he said, Thou canst not see [g]my face: for there shall no man see me, and live.

B.C. 1491.

a Heb. 1:4, *note*.

b Cf. Ex. 24:4. This "tabernacle" is not to be confounded with that afterward made by commandment of God, but not yet made.

c *Bible prayers* (O.T.). Num. 6:22-26. (Gen. 15:2; Hab. 3:1-16.)

d *Separation*. Lev. 20:24-26. (Gen. 12:1; 2 Cor. 6:14-17.)

e i.e. Ex. 34:6, 7.

f Rom. 9:15.

g Cf. John 1:18, *note*.

B.C. 1491.

21 And the LORD said, Behold, *there is* a place by me, and thou shalt stand upon a rock:

22 And it shall come to pass, while my glory passeth by, that I will put thee in a [a]clift of the rock, and will cover thee with my [b]hand while I pass by:

23 And I will take away mine hand, and thou shalt see my back parts: but my face shall not be seen.

CHAPTER 34.

The second tables of the law.

And the LORD said unto Moses, [c]Hew thee two tables of stone like unto the first: and I will write upon *these* tables the [d]words that were in the first tables, which thou brakest.

2 And be ready in the morning, and come up in the morning unto mount Sinai, and present thyself there to me in the top of the mount.

3 And no man shall come up with thee, neither let any man be seen throughout all the mount; neither let the flocks nor herds feed before that mount.

4 And he hewed two tables of stone like unto the first; and Moses rose up early in the morning, and went up unto mount Sinai, as the LORD had commanded him, and took in his hand the two tables of stone.

The new vision. (Cf.Ex. 33:18–23.)

5 And the LORD descended in the cloud, and stood with him there, and proclaimed the name of the LORD.

6 And the LORD passed by before him, and proclaimed, [e]The LORD, The LORD God, merciful and gracious, longsuffering, and abundant in goodness and truth,

7 Keeping mercy for thousands, forgiving iniquity and transgression and sin, and that will by no means clear *the guilty;* visiting the iniquity of the fathers upon the children, and upon the children's children, unto the third and to the fourth *generation.*

8 And Moses made haste, and bowed his head toward the earth, and worshipped.

9 And he said, If now I have found grace in thy sight, O Lord, let my Lord, I pray thee, go among us; for it *is* a stiffnecked people; and pardon our iniquity and our sin, and take us for thine inheritance.

The renewed commission.

10 And he said, Behold, I make a covenant: before all thy people I will do marvels, such as have not been done in all the earth, nor in any nation: and all the people among which thou *art* shall see the work of the LORD: for it *is* a terrible thing that I will do with thee.

11 Observe thou that which I command thee this day: behold, I drive out before thee the Amorite, and the Canaanite, and the Hittite, and the Perizzite, and the Hivite, and the Jebusite.

12 Take heed to thyself, lest thou make a [f]covenant with the inhabitants of the land whither thou goest, lest it be for a snare in the midst of thee:

13 But ye shall destroy their altars, break their images, and cut down their [g]groves:

14 For thou shalt worship no other god: for the LORD, whose name *is* Jealous, *is* a jealous God:

15 Lest thou make a covenant with the inhabitants of the land, and they go a whoring after their gods, and do sacrifice unto their gods, and *one* call thee, and thou eat of his sacrifice;

16 And thou take of their daughters unto thy sons, and their daughters go a whoring after their gods, and make thy sons go a whoring after their gods.

17 Thou shalt make thee no molten gods.

The feasts and the sabbaths again enjoined. (Cf. Lev. 23:4–44.)

18 The feast of [h]unleavened bread shalt thou keep. Seven days thou shalt eat unleavened bread, as I commanded thee, in the time of the month [i]Abib: for in the month Abib thou camest out from [j]Egypt.

19 All that openeth the matrix *is* mine; and every firstling among thy cattle, *whether* ox or sheep, *that is male.*

20 But the firstling of an ass thou shalt redeem with a lamb: and if thou redeem *him* not, then shalt thou break his neck. All the firstborn of thy sons thou shalt redeem. And none shall appear before me empty.

21 Six days thou shalt work, but on the seventh day thou shalt rest:

a Song 2:14.

b Cf. John 10:28, 29.

c See Ex. 20:4, *note.*

d *Inspiration.* vs. 1, 27, 28; Ex. 35:1. (Ex. 4:15; Rev. 22:19.)

e *Deity* (*names of*). 1 Sam. 1:3. (Gen. 1:1; Mal. 3:18.)

f Josh. 23:12; Psa. 106:34-38; 2 Cor. 6:14; 2 Tim. 2:20, 21;Jas. 4:4.

g See Deut. 16:21.

h *Leaven.* vs. 18, 25; Lev. 2:4, 5, 11. (Gen. 19:3; Mt. 13:33.)

i i.e. *April.*

j *Law* (*of Moses*). vs. 18-28; Lev. 1:1-16, 34. (Ex. 19:1; Gal. 3:1-29.)

in earing time and in harvest thou shalt
rest.
22 And thou shalt observe the feast of
weeks, of the firstfruits of wheat harvest,
and the feast of ingathering at the year's
end.
23 Thrice in the year shall all your
men children appear before the Lord
GOD, the God of Israel.
24 For I will cast out the nations before
thee, and enlarge thy borders: neither
shall any man desire thy land, when
thou shalt go up to appear before the
LORD thy God thrice in the year.
25 Thou shalt not offer the blood of
my sacrifice with leaven; neither shall
the sacrifice of the feast of the passover
be left unto the morning.
26 The first of the firstfruits of thy
land thou shalt bring unto the house of
the LORD thy God. Thou shalt not seethe
a kid in his mother's milk.
27 And the LORD said unto Moses,
Write thou these words: for after the
tenor of these words I have made a
covenant with thee and with Israel.
28 And he was there with the LORD
forty days and forty nights; he did neither eat bread, nor drink water. And he
wrote upon the tables the words of the
covenant, the ten commandments.
29 And it came to pass, when Moses
came down from mount Sinai with the
two tables of testimony in Moses' hand,
when he came down from the mount,
that Moses [a]wist not that the skin of his
face shone while he talked with him.
30 And when Aaron and all the children of Israel saw Moses, behold, the
skin of his face shone; and they were
afraid to come nigh him.
31 And Moses called unto them; and
Aaron and all the rulers of the congregation returned unto him: and Moses
talked with them.
32 And afterward all the children of
Israel came nigh: and he gave them in
commandment all that the LORD had
spoken with him in mount Sinai.
33 And *till* Moses had done speaking
with them, he put a [b]vail on his face.
34 But when Moses went in before the
LORD to speak with him, he took the vail
off, until he came out. And he came out,
and spake unto the children of Israel *that*
which he was commanded.
35 And the children of Israel saw the
face of Moses, that the skin of Moses'
face shone: and Moses put the vail upon
his face again, until he went in to speak
with him.

CHAPTER 35.

The Sabbath in Israel.

And Moses gathered all the congregation of the children of Israel together, and said unto them, These *are* the
[c]words which the LORD hath commanded, that *ye* should do them.
2 Six days shall work be done, but on
the seventh day there shall be to you an
holy day, a [d]sabbath of rest to the LORD:
whosoever doeth work therein shall be
put to death.
3 Ye shall kindle no fire throughout
your habitations upon the sabbath day.

The tabernacle: Moses instructs the people.

4 And Moses spake unto all the congregation of the children of Israel, saying, This *is* the thing which the LORD
commanded, saying,
5 Take ye from among you an offering
unto the LORD: whosoever *is* of a [e]will-
ing heart, let him bring it, an offering of
the LORD; gold, and silver, and brass,

The gifts of the people. (Cf. Ex. 25:1–8.)

6 And blue, and purple, and scarlet,
and fine linen, and goats' *hair*,
7 And rams' skins dyed red, and badgers' skins, and [f]shittim wood,
8 And oil for the light, and spices for
anointing oil, and for the sweet incense,
9 And onyx stones, and stones to be set
for the ephod, and for the breastplate.
10 And every wise hearted among you
shall come, and make all that the LORD
hath commanded;
11 The tabernacle, his tent, and his
covering, his taches, and his boards, his
bars, his pillars, and his sockets,
12 The ark, and the staves thereof, *with*
the mercy seat, and the vail of the covering,
13 The table, and his staves, and all his
vessels, and the [g]shewbread,
14 The candlestick also for the light,
and his furniture, and his lamps, with
the oil for the light,
15 And the incense altar, and his
staves, and the anointing oil, and the

B.C. 1491.

a See Jud. 16:20.

b Cf. 2 Cor. 3:13-16.

c *Inspiration.* Num. 11:24. (Ex. 4:15; Rev. 22:19.)

d *Sabbath.* vs. 2, 3; Lev. 19:3:30. (Gen. 2:3; Mt. 12:1.)

e vs. 21, 22, 26, 29; Ex. 36:3-6; 1 Chr. 29:14; Mk. 12:41-44; 2 Cor. 8:10-12; 2 Cor. 9:15.

f i.e. *acacia*

g Ex. 25:30, *note.*

B.C. 1491.

sweet incense, and the hanging for the door at the entering in of the tabernacle,

16 The altar of burnt-offering, with his brasen grate, his staves, and all his vessels, the laver and his foot,

17 The hangings of the court, his pillars, and their sockets, and the hanging for the door of the court,

18 The pins of the tabernacle, and the pins of the court, and their cords,

19 The cloths of service, to do service in the holy *place*, the holy garments for Aaron the priest, and the garments of his sons, to minister in the priest's office.

20 And all the congregation of the children of Israel departed from the presence of Moses.

21 And they came, every one whose heart stirred him up, and every one whom his spirit made willing, *and* they brought the LORD'S offering to the work of the tabernacle of the congregation, and for all his service, and for the holy garments.

22 And they came, both men and women, as many as were willing hearted, *and* brought bracelets, and earrings, and rings, and tablets, all jewels of gold: and every man that offered *offered* an offering of gold unto the LORD.

23 And every man, with whom was found blue, and purple, and scarlet, and fine linen, and goats' *hair*, and red skins of rams, and badgers' skins, brought *them*.

24 Every one that did offer an offering of silver and brass brought the LORD'S offering: and every man, with whom was found [a]shittim wood for any work of the service, brought *it*.

25 And all the women that were wise hearted did spin with their hands, and brought that which they had spun, *both* of blue, and of purple, *and* of scarlet, and of fine linen.

26 And all the women whose heart stirred them up in wisdom spun goats' *hair*.

27 And the rulers brought onyx stones, and stones to be set, for the ephod, and for the breastplate;

28 And spice, and oil for the light, and for the anointing oil, and for the sweet incense.

29 The children of Israel brought a willing offering unto the LORD, every man and woman, whose heart made them willing to bring for all manner of work, which the LORD had commanded to be made by the hand of Moses.

Bezaleel and Aholiab to devise and teach.
(Cf. Ex. 31:1–11.)

30 And Moses said unto the children of Israel, See, the LORD hath called by name Bezaleel the son of Uri, the son of Hur, of the tribe of Judah;

31 And he hath filled him with the [b]spirit of God, in wisdom, in understanding, and in knowledge, and in all manner of workmanship;

32 And to devise curious works, to work in gold, and in silver, and in brass,

33 And in the cutting of stones, to set *them*, and in carving of wood, to make any manner of cunning work.

34 And he hath put in his heart that he may teach, *both* he, and Aholiab, the son of Ahisamach, of the tribe of Dan.

35 Them hath he filled with wisdom of heart, to work all manner of work, of the engraver, and of the cunning workman, and of the embroiderer, in blue, and in purple, in scarlet, and in fine linen, and of the weaver, *even* of them that do any work, and of those that devise cunning work.

CHAPTER 36.

More than enough: the work begun.

Then wrought Bezaleel and Aholiab, and every [c]wise hearted man, in whom the LORD put wisdom and understanding to know how to work all manner of work for the service of the sanctuary, according to all that the LORD had commanded.

2 And Moses called Bezaleel and Aholiab, and every wise hearted man, in whose heart the LORD had put wisdom, *even* every one whose [d]heart stirred him up to come unto the work to do it:

3 And they received of Moses all the offering, which the children of Israel had brought for the work of the service of the sanctuary, to make it *withal*. And they brought yet unto him [e]free offerings every morning.

4 And all the wise men, that wrought all the work of the sanctuary, came every man from his work which they made;

a i.e. *acacia*

b *Holy Spirit.* Num. 11:17, 25, 26, 29. (Gen. 1:2; Mal. 2:15.)

c Ex. 28:3; 31:6; 35:10, 35.

d Ex. 35:25, 26; 1 Chr. 29:5, 9, 17.

e i.e. *free will.* 2 Cor. 8:1. *note.*

B.C. 1491.

5 And they spake unto Moses, saying, The people bring much more than enough for the service of the work, which the LORD commanded to make.

6 And Moses gave commandment, and they caused it to be proclaimed throughout the camp, saying, Let neither man nor woman make any more work for the offering of the sanctuary. So the people were restrained from bringing.

7 For the stuff they had was sufficient for all the work to make it, and too much.

The linen curtains (Ex. 26:1–6).

8 And every wise hearted man among them that wrought the work of the tabernacle made ten curtains *of* fine twined linen, and blue, and purple, and scarlet: *with* cherubims of cunning work made he them.

9 The length of one curtain *was* twenty and eight [a]cubits, and the breadth of one curtain four cubits: the curtains *were* all of one size.

10 And he coupled the five curtains one unto another: and *the other* five curtains he coupled one unto another.

11 And he made loops of blue on the edge of one curtain from the selvedge in the coupling: likewise he made in the uttermost side of *another* curtain, in the coupling of the second.

12 [b]Fifty loops made he in one curtain, and fifty loops made he in the edge of the curtain which *was* in the coupling of the second: the loops held one *curtain* to another.

13 And he made fifty taches of gold, and coupled the curtains one unto another with the taches: so it became one tabernacle.

The curtains of goats' hair. (Cf. Ex. 26:7.)

14 And he made curtains *of* goats' *hair* for the tent over the tabernacle: eleven curtains he made them.

15 The length of one curtain *was* thirty cubits, and four cubits *was* the breadth of one curtain: the eleven curtains *were* of one size.

16 And he coupled five curtains by themselves, and six curtains by themselves.

17 And he made fifty loops upon the uttermost edge of the curtain in the coupling, and fifty loops made he upon the edge of the curtain which coupleth the second.

18 And he made fifty taches *of* brass to couple the tent together, that it might be one.

The covering of rams' skins.
(Cf. Ex. 26:14.)

19 And he made a [c]covering for the tent *of* rams' skins dyed red, and a covering *of* badgers' skins above *that*.

The boards and sockets. (Cf. Ex. 26:15.)

20 And he made boards for the tabernacle *of* [d]shittim wood, standing up.

21 The length of a board *was* ten cubits, and the breadth of a board one cubit and a half.

22 One board had two tenons, equally distant one from another: thus did he make for all the boards of the tabernacle.

23 And he made boards for the tabernacle; twenty boards for the south side southward:

The sockets of silver. (Cf. Ex. 26:19.)

24 And forty sockets of silver he made under the twenty boards; two sockets under one board for his two tenons, and two sockets under another board for his two tenons.

25 And for the other side of the tabernacle, *which is* toward the north corner, he made twenty boards,

26 And their forty sockets of silver; two sockets under one board, and two sockets under another board.

27 And for the sides of the tabernacle westward he made six boards.

28 And two boards made he for the corners of the tabernacle in the two sides.

29 And they were coupled beneath, and coupled together at the head thereof, to one ring: thus he did to both of them in both the corners.

30 And there were eight boards; and their sockets *were* sixteen sockets of silver, under every board two sockets.

The bars. (Cf. Ex. 26:26.)

31 And he made bars of [d]shittim wood; five for the boards of the one side of the tabernacle,

32 And five [e]bars for the boards of the other side of the tabernacle, and five bars for the boards of the tabernacle for the sides westward.

33 And he made the middle bar to shoot through the boards from the one end to the other.

a One cubit = 1 ft. 5.48 in.; also vs. 15, 21.

b Ex. 26:5.

c Ex. 26:14.

d i.e. *acacia*

e Ex. 26:26.

The gold overlay. (Cf. Ex. 26:29.)

34 And he overlaid the boards with gold, and made their rings *of* gold *to be* places for the bars, and overlaid the bars with gold.

The inner vail. (Cf. Ex. 26:31.)

35 And he made a [a]vail *of* blue, and purple, and scarlet, and fine twined linen: *with* cherubims made he it of cunning work.

36 And he made thereunto four pillars *of* [b]shittim *wood*, and overlaid them with gold: their hooks *were of* gold; and he cast for them four sockets of silver.

The outer vail. (Cf. Ex. 26:36.)

37 And he made an [c]hanging for the tabernacle door *of* blue, and purple, and scarlet, and fine twined linen, of needlework;

38 And the five pillars of it with their hooks: and he overlaid their chapiters and their fillets with gold: but their five sockets *were of* brass.

CHAPTER 37.

The ark. (Cf. Ex. 25:10.)

And [d]Bezaleel made the ark *of* [b]shittim wood: two [e]cubits and a half *was* the length of it, and a cubit and a half the breadth of it, and a cubit and a half the height of it:

2 And he overlaid it with pure gold within and without, and made a crown of gold to it round about.

3 And he cast for it four rings of gold, *to be set* by the four corners of it; even two rings upon the one side of it, and two rings upon the other side of it.

4 And he made staves *of* [b]shittim wood, and overlaid them with gold.

5 And he put the staves into the rings by the sides of the ark, to bear the ark.

The mercy seat. (Cf. Ex. 25:17.)

6 And he made the mercy seat *of* pure gold: two cubits and a half *was* the length thereof, and one cubit and a half the breadth thereof.

7 And he made two [f]cherubims *of* gold, beaten out of one piece made he them, on the two ends of the mercy seat;

8 One cherub on the end on this side, and another cherub on the *other* end on that side: out of the mercy seat made he the cherubims on the two ends thereof.

9 And the cherubims spread out *their* wings on high, *and* covered with their wings over the [g]mercy seat, with their faces one to another; *even* to the mercy seatward were the faces of the cherubims.

The table of shewbread. (Cf. Ex. 25:23.)

10 And he made the [h]table *of* [b]shittim wood: two cubits *was* the length thereof, and a cubit the breadth thereof, and a cubit and a half the height thereof:

11 And he overlaid it with pure gold, and made thereunto a crown of gold round about.

12 Also he made thereunto a border of an handbreadth round about; and made a crown of gold for the border thereof round about.

13 And he cast for it four rings of gold, and put the rings upon the four corners that *were* in the four feet thereof.

14 Over against the border were the rings, the places for the staves to bear the table.

15 And he made the staves *of* [b]shittim wood, and overlaid them with gold, to bear the table.

16 And he made the vessels which *were* upon the table, his dishes, and his spoons, and his bowls, and his covers to cover withal, *of* pure gold.

The golden candlestick. (Cf. Ex. 25:31.)

17 And he made the candlestick *of* pure gold: *of* beaten work made he the [i]candlestick; his shaft, and his branch, his bowls, his knops, and his flowers, were of the same:

18 And six branches going out of the sides thereof; three branches of the candlestick out of the one side thereof, and three branches of the candlestick out of the other side thereof:

19 Three bowls made after the fashion of almonds in one branch, a knop and a flower; and three bowls made like almonds in another branch, a knop and a flower: so throughout the six branches going out of the candlestick.

20 And in the candlestick *were* four bowls made like almonds, his knops, and his flowers:

21 And a knop under two branches of the same, and a knop under two branches of the same, and a knop under two branches of the same, according to the six branches going out of it.

B.C. 1491.

a Ex. 26:31; 30:6; Heb. 10:20.

b i.e. *acacia.*

c Ex. 26:36.

d Ex. 25:10; 40:3, 21; Num. 10:33, 35.

e One cubit = 1 ft. 5.48 in.; also vs. 6, 10, 25.

f 1 Ki. 6:23; Ezk. 1:5, *note.*

g Ex. 25:20.

h Ex. 25:23; 35:13; 40:4, 22.

i Ex. 25:31; 40:24, 25; Heb. 9:2.

22 Their knops and their branches were of the same: all of it *was* one beaten work *of* pure gold.

23 And he made his seven lamps, and his snuffers, and his snuffdishes, *of* pure gold.

24 *Of* a [a]talent of pure gold made he it, and all the vessels thereof.

The incense altar. (Cf. Ex. 30:1.)

25 And he made the incense altar *of* [b]shittim wood: the length of it *was* a cubit, and the breadth of it a cubit; *it was* foursquare; and two cubits *was* the height of it; the horns thereof were of the same.

26 And he overlaid it with pure gold, *both* the top of it, and the sides thereof round about, and the horns of it: also he made unto it a crown of gold round about.

27 And he made two rings of gold for it under the crown thereof, by the two corners of it, upon the two sides thereof, to be places for the staves to bear it withal.

28 And he made the staves *of* [b]shittim wood, and overlaid them with gold.

The holy anointing oil. (Cf. Ex. 30:23–38.)

29 And he made the [c]holy anointing oil, and the pure incense of sweet spices, according to the work of the apothecary.

CHAPTER 38.

The altar of burnt-offering. (Cf. Ex. 27:1.)

And he made the altar of burnt-offering *of* [b]shittim wood: five [d]cubits *was* the length thereof, and five cubits the breadth thereof; *it was* foursquare; and three cubits the height thereof.

2 And he made the horns thereof on the four corners of it; the horns thereof were of the same: and he overlaid it with brass.

3 And he made all the vessels of the altar, the pots, and the shovels, and the basons, *and* the fleshhooks, and the firepans: all the vessels thereof made he *of* brass.

4 And he made for the altar a brasen grate of network under the compass thereof beneath unto the midst of it.

5 And he cast four rings for the four ends of the grate of brass, *to be* places for the staves.

6 And he made the staves *of* [b]shittim wood, and overlaid them with brass.

7 And he put the staves into the rings on the sides of the altar, to bear it withal; he made the altar hollow with boards.

The laver of brass. (Cf. Ex. 30:18.)

8 And he made the laver *of* brass, and the foot of it *of* brass, of the lookingglasses of *the women* assembling, which assembled *at* the door of the tabernacle of the congregation.

The court. (Cf. Ex. 27:9.)

9 And he made the court: on the south side southward the hangings of the court *were of* fine twined linen, an hundred cubits:

10 Their pillars *were* twenty, and their brasen sockets twenty; the hooks of the pillars and their fillets *were of* silver.

11 And for the north side *the hangings were* an hundred cubits, their pillars *were* twenty, and their sockets of brass twenty; the hooks of the pillars and their fillets *of* silver.

12 And for the west side *were* hangings of fifty cubits, their pillars ten, and their sockets ten; the hooks of the pillars and their fillets *of* silver.

13 And for the east side eastward fifty cubits.

14 The hangings of the one side *of the gate were* fifteen cubits; their pillars three, and their sockets three.

15 And for the other side of the court gate, on this hand and that hand, *were* hangings of fifteen cubits; their pillars three, and their sockets three.

16 All the hangings of the court round about *were* of fine twined linen.

17 And the sockets for the pillars *were of* brass; the hooks of the pillars and their fillets *of* silver; and the overlaying of their chapiters *of* silver; and all the pillars of the court *were* filleted with silver.

The gate of the court. (Cf. Ex. 27:16.)

18 And the hanging for the gate of the court *was* needlework, *of* blue, and purple, and scarlet, and fine twined linen: and twenty cubits *was* the length, and the height in the breadth *was* five

B.C. 1491.

a £6150, or $29, 085.

b i.e. *acacia.*

c Ex. 30:23.

d One cubit = 1 ft. 5.48 in.; also vs. 9, 11-15, 18.

cubits, answerable to the hangings of the court.

19 And their pillars *were* four, and their sockets *of* brass four; their hooks *of* silver, and the overlaying of their chapiters and their fillets *of* silver.

20 And all the pins of the tabernacle, and of the court round about, *were of* brass.

21 This is the sum of the tabernacle, *even* of the tabernacle of testimony, as it was counted, according to the commandment of Moses, *for* the service of the Levites, by the hand of Ithamar, son to Aaron the priest.

22 And Bezaleel the son of Uri, the son of Hur, of the tribe of Judah, made all that the LORD commanded Moses.

23 And with him *was* Aholiab, son of Ahisamach, of the tribe of Dan, an engraver, and a cunning workman, and an embroiderer in blue, and in purple, and in scarlet, and fine linen.

24 All the gold that was occupied for the work in all the work of the holy *place*, even the gold of the offering, was twenty and nine [a]talents, and seven hundred and thirty [b]shekels, after the shekel of the sanctuary.

25 And the silver of them that were numbered of the congregation *was* an hundred [c]talents, and a thousand seven hundred and threescore and fifteen shekels, after the shekel of the sanctuary:

26 A [d]bekah for every man, *that is*, half a shekel, after the shekel of the sanctuary, for every one that went to be numbered, from twenty years old and upward, for six hundred thousand and three thousand and five hundred and fifty *men*.

27 And of the hundred talents of [1]silver were cast the [e]sockets of the sanctuary, and the sockets of the vail; an hundred sockets of the hundred talents, a talent for a socket.

28 And of the thousand seven hundred seventy and five *shekels* he made hooks for the pillars, and overlaid their chapiters, and filleted them.

29 And the brass of the offering *was* seventy talents, and two thousand and four hundred shekels.

30 And therewith he made the sockets to the door of the tabernacle of the congregation, and the brasen altar, and the brasen grate for it, and all the vessels of the altar,

31 And the sockets of the court round about, and the sockets of the court gate, and all the pins of the tabernacle, and all the pins of the court round about.

B.C. 1491.

a One talent = £6150, or $29,085.

b One shekel = 2s. 9d., or 65 cents; also v. 29.

c One silver talent = £410, or $1940; also v. 27.

d One bekah = 1s. 4 1/2d., or 33 cents.

e Ex. 26:19, *note.*

f Ex. 25:4; 35:23.

g Ex. 31:10; 35:19.

h Ex. 28:6; Lev. 8:7.

i Ex. 28:9, 12.

j Ex. 28:29; Josh. 4:7.

k One span = 8.737 inches

CHAPTER 39.

The holy garments for Aaron.
(Cf. Ex. 31:10.)

AND of the [f]blue, and purple, and scarlet, they made [g]cloths of service, to do service in the holy *place*, and made the holy garments for Aaron; as the LORD commanded Moses.

2 And he made the [h]ephod *of* gold, blue, and purple, and scarlet, and fine twined linen.

3 And they did beat the gold into thin plates, and cut *it into* wires, to work *it* in the blue, and in the purple, and in the scarlet, and in the fine linen, *with* cunning work.

4 They made shoulderpieces for it, to couple *it* together: by the two edges was it coupled together.

5 And the curious girdle of his ephod, that *was* upon it, *was* of the same, according to the work thereof; *of* gold, blue, and purple, and scarlet, and fine twined linen; as the LORD commanded Moses.

6 And they wrought onyx stones inclosed in ouches of gold, graven, as signets are [i]graven, with the names of the children of Israel.

7 And he put them on the shoulders of the ephod, *that they should be* stones for a [j]memorial to the children of Israel; as the LORD commanded Moses.

8 And he made the breastplate *of* cunning work, like the work of the ephod; *of* gold, blue, and purple, and scarlet, and fine twined linen.

9 It was foursquare; they made the breastplate double: a [k]span *was* the length thereof, and a span the breadth thereof, *being* doubled.

10 And they set in it four rows of stones: *the first* row *was* a sardius, a topaz, and a carbuncle: this *was* the first row.

11 And the second row, an emerald, a sapphire, and a diamond.

[1] **(38:27)** Silver thus receives its symbolic meaning—redemption. The sockets were made of the redemption money of the children of Israel. Cf. Ex. 26:19; 30:13-16; Num. 3:44-51.

B.C. 1491.

12 And the third row, a ligure, an agate, and an amethyst.

13 And the fourth row, a beryl, an onyx, and a jasper: *they were* inclosed in ouches of gold in their inclosings.

14 And the stones *were* according to the names of the children of Israel, [a]twelve, according to their names, *like* the engravings of a signet, every one with his name, according to the twelve tribes.

15 And they made upon the breastplate chains at the ends, *of* wreathen work *of* pure gold.

16 And they made two ouches *of* gold, and two gold rings; and put the two rings in the two ends of the breastplate.

17 And they put the two wreathen chains of gold in the two rings on the ends of the breastplate.

18 And the two ends of the two wreathen chains they fastened in the two ouches, and put them on the shoulderpieces of the ephod, before it.

19 And they made two rings of gold, and put *them* on the two ends of the breastplate, upon the border of it, which *was* on the side of the ephod inward.

20 And they made two *other* golden rings, and put them on the two sides of the ephod underneath, toward the forepart of it, over against the *other* coupling thereof, above the curious girdle of the ephod.

21 And they did bind the breastplate by his rings unto the rings of the ephod with a lace of blue, that it might be above the curious girdle of the ephod, and that the breastplate might not be loosed from the ephod; as the LORD commanded Moses.

22 And he made the robe of the ephod *of* woven work, all *of* blue.

23 And *there was* an hole in the midst of the robe, as the hole of an habergeon, *with* a band round about the hole, that it should not rend.

24 And they made upon the hems of the robe pomegranates *of* blue, and purple, and scarlet, *and* twined *linen*.

25 And they made [b]bells *of* pure gold, and put the bells between the pomegranates upon the hem of the robe, round about between the pomegranates;

26 A bell and a pomegranate, a bell and a pomegranate, round about the hem of the robe to minister *in*; as the LORD commanded Moses.

27 And they made [c]coats *of* fine linen *of* woven work for Aaron, and for his sons,

28 And a [d]mitre *of* fine linen, and goodly bonnets *of* fine linen, and [e]linen breeches *of* fine twined linen,

29 And a [f]girdle *of* fine twined linen, and blue, and purple, and scarlet, *of* needlework; as the LORD commanded Moses.

30 And they made the plate of the holy crown *of* pure gold, and wrote upon it a writing, *like to* the engravings of a signet, [g]HOLINESS TO THE LORD.

31 And they tied unto it a lace of blue, to fasten *it* on high upon the mitre; as the LORD commanded Moses.

32 Thus was all the work of the tabernacle of the tent of the congregation finished: and the children of Israel did according to all that the LORD commanded Moses, so did they.

33 And they brought the tabernacle unto Moses, the tent, and all his furniture, his taches, his boards, his bars, and his pillars, and his sockets,

34 And the covering of rams' skins dyed red, and the covering of badgers' skins, and the vail of the covering,

35 The ark of the testimony, and the staves thereof, and the mercy seat,

36 The table, *and* all the vessels thereof, and the [h]shewbread,

37 The pure candlestick, *with* the lamps thereof, *even with* the lamps to be set in order, and all the vessels thereof, and the oil for light,

38 And the golden altar, and the anointing oil, and the sweet incense, and the hanging for the tabernacle door,

39 The brasen altar, and his grate of brass, his staves, and all his vessels, the laver and his foot,

40 The hangings of the court, his pillars, and his sockets, and the hanging for the court gate, his cords, and his pins, and all the vessels of the service of the tabernacle, for the tent of the congregation,

41 The cloths of service to do service in the *holy place*, and the holy garments for Aaron the priest, and his sons' garments, to minister in the priest's office.

42 According to all that the LORD

a Rev. 21:12.
b Ex. 28:33.
c Ex. 28:39, 40.
d Ex. 28:4, 39.
e Ex. 28:42.
f Ex. 28:39.
g Zech. 14:20.
h Ex. 25:23-30.

B.C. 1491.

commanded Moses, so the children of Israel made all the work.

43 And Moses did look upon all the work, and, behold, they had done it as the LORD had commanded, even so had they done it: and Moses blessed them.

CHAPTER 40.

The tabernacle set up.

And the LORD [a]spake unto Moses, [b]saying,

2 On the first day of the [c]first month shalt thou set up the tabernacle of the tent of the congregation.

3 And thou shalt put therein the ark of the testimony, and cover the ark with the vail.

4 And thou shalt bring in the table, and set in order the things that are to be set in order upon it; and thou shalt bring in the candlestick, and light the lamps thereof.

5 And thou shalt set the altar of gold for the incense before the ark of the testimony, and put the hanging of the door to the tabernacle.

6 And thou shalt set the altar of the burnt-offering before the door of the tabernacle of the tent of the congregation.

7 And thou shalt set the laver between the tent of the congregation and the altar, and shalt put water therein.

8 And thou shalt set up the court round about, and hang up the hanging at the court gate.

9 And thou shalt take the anointing oil, and anoint the tabernacle, and all that *is* therein, and shalt hallow it, and all the vessels thereof: and it shall be holy.

10 And thou shalt anoint the altar of the burnt-offering, and all his vessels, and sanctify the altar: and it shall be an altar most holy.

11 And thou shalt anoint the laver and his foot, and sanctify it.

12 And thou shalt bring Aaron and his sons unto the door of the tabernacle of the congregation, and wash them with water.

13 And thou shalt put upon Aaron the holy garments, and anoint him, and sanctify him; that he may minister unto me in the priest's office.

14 And thou shalt bring his sons, and clothe them with coats:

15 And thou shalt anoint them, as thou didst anoint their father, that they may minister unto me in the priest's office: for their anointing shall surely be an everlasting priesthood throughout their generations.

16 Thus did Moses: according to all that the LORD commanded him, so did he.

17 And it came to pass in the [c]first month in the second year, on the first *day* of the month, *that* the tabernacle was reared up.

18 And Moses reared up the tabernacle, and fastened his sockets, and set up the boards thereof, and put in the bars thereof, and reared up his pillars.

19 And he spread abroad the tent over the tabernacle, and put the covering of the tent above upon it; as the LORD commanded Moses.

20 And he took and put the testimony into the ark, and set the staves on the ark, and put the mercy seat above upon the ark:

21 And he brought the ark into the tabernacle, and set up the vail of the covering, and covered the ark of the testimony; as the LORD commanded Moses.

22 And he put the table in the tent of the congregation, upon the side of the tabernacle northward, without the vail.

23 And he set the bread in order upon it before the LORD; as the LORD had commanded Moses.

24 And he put the candlestick in the tent of the congregation, over against the table, on the side of the tabernacle southward.

25 And he lighted the lamps before the LORD; as the LORD commanded Moses.

26 And he put the golden altar in the tent of the congregation before the vail:

27 And he burnt sweet incense thereon; as the LORD commanded Moses.

28 And he set up the hanging *at* the door of the tabernacle.

29 And he put the altar of burnt-offering *by* the door of the tabernacle of the tent of the congregation, and offered upon it the burnt-offering and the [d]meat-offering; as the LORD commanded Moses.

30 And he set the laver between the tent of the congregation and the altar, and put water there, to wash *withal*.

31 And Moses and Aaron and his sons washed their hands and their feet thereat:

32 When they went into the tent of the

a Cf. Ex. 25-29.

b *Israel (history).* vs. 1-38; Lev. 16:1-34. (Gen. 12:2, 3; Rom. 11:26.)

c i.e. *April.*

d Lit. *meal.*

congregation, and when they came near
unto the altar, they washed; as the LORD
commanded Moses.
33 And he reared up the court round
about the tabernacle and the altar, and
set up the hanging of the court gate. So
Moses [a]finished the work.
34 [b]Then a [c]cloud covered the tent of
the congregation, and the [1]glory of the
LORD filled the tabernacle.
35 And Moses was not able to enter
into the tent of the congregation, because
the cloud abode thereon, and the glory
of the LORD filled the tabernacle.
36 And when the cloud was taken up
from over the tabernacle, the children of
Israel went onward in all their journeys:
37 But if the cloud were not taken up,
then they journeyed not till the day that
it was taken up.
38 For the [d]cloud of the LORD *was* upon
the tabernacle by day, and fire was on it
by night, in the sight of all the house of
Israel, throughout all their journeys.

B.C. 1490.

a Heb. 3:2, 3.

b Cf. 1 Ki. 8:10, 11.

c Lev. 16:2; Num. 9:15; 1 Ki. 8:10; 2 Chr. 5:13.

d Neh. 9:12; Psa. 78:14; Isa. 4:5.

[1] **(40:34)** Cf. Eph. 2:22. What the shekinah glory was to tabernacle and temple, that the Spirit is to the "holy temple," the Church, and to the temple which is the believer's body (1 Cor. 6:19).

THE THIRD BOOK OF MOSES
CALLED
LEVITICUS

LEVITICUS stands in the same relation to Exodus, that the Epistles do to the Gospels. Exodus is the record of redemption, and lays the foundation of the cleansing, worship, and service of a redeemed people. Leviticus gives the detail of the walk, worship, and service of that people. In Exodus God speaks out of the mount to which approach was forbidden; in Leviticus He speaks out of the tabernacle in which He dwells in the midst of His people, to tell them that which befits His holiness in their approach to, and communion with, Himself.

The key-word of Leviticus is holiness, occurring 87 times. Key-verse, 19:2.

Leviticus is in nine chief divisions: I. The Offerings, 1:1–6:7. II. The Law of the Offerings, 6:8–7:38. III. Consecration, 8:1–9:24. IV. A Warning Example, 10:1-20. V. A Holy God must have a Cleansed People, 11–15. VI. Atonement, 16, 17. VII. The Relationships of God's People, 18–22. VIII. The Feasts of Jehovah, 23. IX. Instructions and Warnings, 24–27.

CHAPTER 1.

The sweet savour offerings:
(1) *the burnt-offering: Christ offering Himself without spot to God.*
See Law of this offering, Lev. 6:8–13.

B.C. 1490.

AND the LORD called unto [a]Moses, and spake unto him out of the tabernacle of the congregation, saying,
2 Speak unto the children of Israel, and say unto them, If any man of you bring an offering unto the LORD, ye shall bring your offering of the cattle, *even* of the herd, and of the flock.

a *Law (of Moses).* v. 1 to ch. 16:34. (Ex. 19:1; Gal. 3:1-29.)

b *Sacrifice (typical).* vs. 3-17; Lev. 2:1-16. (Gen. 4:4; Heb. 10:18.)

c See Ex. 29:33, *note.*

3 If his offering *be* a [1b]burnt-sacrifice of the herd, let him offer a male without blemish: he shall offer it of his own voluntary will at the door of the tabernacle of the congregation before the LORD.
4 And he shall put his [2]hand upon the head of the burnt-offering; and it shall be accepted for him to make [c]atonement for him.
5 And he shall kill the bullock before the LORD: and the priests, Aaron's sons, shall bring the blood,

[1] **(1:3)** The burnt-offering (1) typifies Christ offering Himself without spot to God in delight to do His Father's will even in death. (2) It is *atoning* because the believer has *not* had this delight in the will of God; and (3) *substitutionary* (v. 4) because Christ did it in the sinner's stead. But the thought of *penalty* is not prominent (Heb. 9:11-14; 10:5-7, Psa. 40:6-8; Phil. 2:8). The emphatic words (Lev. 1:3-5) are "burnt-sacrifice," "voluntary," "it shall be accepted for him," and "atonement."

The creatures acceptable for sacrifice are five:

(1) The bullock, or ox, typifies Christ as the patient and enduring Servant (1 Cor. 9:9, 10; Heb. 12:2, 3), "obedient unto death" (Isa. 52:13-15; Phil. 2:5-8). His offering in this character is substitutionary, for this we have not been.

(2) The sheep, or lamb, typifies Christ in unresisting self-surrender to the death of the cross (Isa. 53:7; Acts 8:32-35).

(3) The goat typifies the sinner (Mt. 25:33) and, when used sacrificially, Christ, as "numbered with the transgressors" (Isa. 53:12; Lk. 23:33), and "made sin," and "a curse" (Gal. 3:13; 2 Cor. 5:21), as the sinner's substitute.

(4, 5) The turtle-dove or pigeon. Naturally a symbol of mourning innocency (Isa. 38:14; 59:11; Mt. 23:37; Heb. 7:26), is associated with poverty in Lev. 5:7, and speaks of Him who for our sakes became poor (Lk. 9:58), and whose pathway of poverty which began with laying aside "the form of God," ended in the sacrifice through which we became rich (2 Cor. 8:9; Phil. 2:6-8). The sacrifice of the poor Man becomes the poor man's sacrifice (Lk. 2:24).

These grades of typical sacrifice test the measure of our apprehension of the varied aspects of Christ's one sacrifice on the cross. The mature believer should see Christ crucified in all these aspects.

[2] **(1:4)** The laying on of the offerer's hand signified *acceptance* and *identification*

and sprinkle the blood round about
upon the altar that *is by* the door of the
tabernacle of the congregation.
6 And he shall flay the burnt-offering,
and cut it into his pieces.
7 And the sons of Aaron the priest
shall put fire upon the altar, and lay the
wood in order upon the fire:
8 And the priests, Aaron's sons, shall
lay the parts, the head, and the [a]fat, in
order upon the wood that *is* on the [1]fire
which *is* upon the altar:
9 But his inwards and his legs shall he
wash in water: and the priest shall burn
all on the altar, *to be* a burnt-sacrifice, an
offering made by fire, of a [2]sweet
[b]savour unto the LORD.
10 And if his offering *be* of the flocks,
namely, of the sheep, or of the goats, for a
burnt-sacrifice; he shall bring it a male
without blemish.
11 And he shall kill it on the side of
the altar northward before the LORD: and
the priests, Aaron's sons, shall sprinkle
his blood round about upon the altar.
12 And he shall cut it into his pieces,
with his head and his fat: and the priest
shall lay them in order on the wood that
is on the fire which *is* upon the altar:
13 But he shall wash the inwards and
the legs with water: and the priest shall
bring *it* all, and burn *it* upon the altar: it
is a burnt-sacrifice, an offering made by
fire, of a sweet savour unto the LORD.
14 And if the burnt-sacrifice for his
offering to the LORD *be* of fowls, then he
shall bring his offering of turtledoves, or
of young pigeons.
15 And the priest shall bring it unto the
altar, and wring off his head, and burn *it*
on the altar; and the blood thereof shall be
wrung out at the side of the altar:
16 And he shall pluck away his crop
with his feathers, and cast it beside the
altar on the east part, by the place of the
ashes:
17 And he shall cleave it with the wings
thereof, *but* shall not divide *it* asunder:
and the priest shall burn it upon the altar,
upon the wood that *is* upon the fire: it *is* a
burnt-sacrifice, an offering made by fire,
of a sweet savour unto the LORD.

B.C. 1490.

a That which burns most quickly—devotedness, zeal. Lev. 3:3-4; 7:23-24.

b *Savour of satisfaction.*

c Lit. *meal.*

CHAPTER 2.

The sweet savour offerings:
(2) *the meat-offering; Christ in His human perfections tested by suffering.*
See Law of this offering, Lev. 6:14–23.

AND when any will offer a [c]meat-offering unto the LORD, his offering shall be *of* [3]fine flour; and he shall pour oil upon it, and put frankincense thereon:

of himself with his offering. In type it answered to the believer's faith accepting and identifying himself with Christ (Rom. 4:5; 6:3-11). The believer is justified by faith, and his faith is reckoned for righteousness, because his faith identifies him with Christ, who died as his sin-offering (2 Cor 5:21; 1 Pet. 2:24).

[1] **(1:8)** Fire. Essentially a symbol of God's holiness. As such it expresses God in three ways: (1) In judgment upon that which His holiness utterly condemns (e.g. Gen. 19:24; Mk. 9:43-48; Rev. 20:15); (2) in the manifestation of Himself, and of that which He approves (e.g. Ex. 3:2; 1 Pet. 1:7; Ex. 13:21); and (3) in purification (e.g. 1 Cor. 3:12-14; Mal. 3:2, 3). So, in Leviticus, the fire which only manifests the sweet savour of the burnt-, meal-, and peace-offerings, wholly consumes the sin-offering.

[2] **(1:9)** The sweet savour offerings are so called because they typify Christ in His own perfections, and in His affectionate devotion to the Father's will. The non-sweet savour offerings typify Christ as bearing the whole demerit of the sinner. Both are substitutional. In our place Christ, in the burnt-offering, makes good our lack of devotedness, and, in the sin- and trespass-offerings, suffers because of our disobedience.

[3] **(2:1)** The meal-offering. The *fine flour* speaks of the evenness and balance of the character of Christ; of that perfection in which no quality was in excess, none lacking; *the fire,* of His testing by suffering, even unto death; *frankincense,* the fragrance of His life Godward (see Ex. 30:34); *absence of leaven,* His character as "the Truth" (see Ex. 12:8, *refs.*) *absence of honey;*—His was not that mere natural sweetness which may exist quite apart from grace; *oil mingled,* Christ as born of the Spirit (Mt. 1:18-23); *oil upon,* Christ as baptized with the Spirit (John 1:32; 6:27); *the oven,* the unseen sufferings of Christ—His inner agonies (Heb. 2:18; Mt. 27:45,46); *the pan,* His more evident sufferings (e.g. Mt. 27:27-31); *salt,* the pungency of the truth of God—that which arrests the action of leaven.

2 And he shall bring it to Aaron's sons the priests: and he shall take thereout his handful of the flour thereof, and of the oil thereof, with all the frankincense thereof; and the priest shall burn the memorial of it upon the altar, *to be* an [a]offering made by fire, of a sweet savour unto the LORD:

3 And the remnant of the [b]meat-offering *shall be* Aaron's and his sons': *it is* a thing most holy of the offerings of the LORD made by fire.

4 And if thou bring an oblation of a [b]meat-offering baken in the oven, *it shall be* [c]unleavened cakes of fine flour mingled with oil, or unleavened wafers anointed with oil.

5 And if thy oblation *be* a [b]meat-offering *baken* in a pan, it shall be *of* fine flour unleavened, mingled with oil.

6 Thou shalt part it in pieces, and pour oil thereon: it *is* a [b]meat-offering.

7 And if thy oblation *be* a [b]meat-offering *baken* in the fryingpan, it shall be made *of* fine flour with oil.

8 And thou shalt bring the [b]meat-offering that is made of these things unto the LORD: and when it is presented unto the priest, he shall bring it unto the altar.

9 And the priest shall take from the [b]meat-offering a memorial thereof, and shall burn *it* upon the altar: *it is* an offering made by fire, of a sweet savour unto the LORD.

10 And that which is left of the [b]meat-offering *shall be* Aaron's and his sons': *it is* a thing most holy of the offerings of the LORD made by fire.

11 No [b]meat-offering, which ye shall bring unto the LORD, shall be made with [1]leaven: for ye shall burn no leaven, nor any [2]honey, in any offering of the LORD made by fire.

12 As for the oblation of the firstfruits, ye shall offer them unto the LORD: but they shall not be burnt on the altar for a sweet savour.

13 And every oblation of thy [b]meat-offering shalt thou season with [3]salt; neither shalt thou suffer the salt of the covenant of thy God to be lacking from thy [b]meat-offering: with all thine offerings thou shalt offer salt.

14 And if thou offer a [b]meat-offering of thy firstfruits unto the LORD, thou shalt offer for the [b]meat-offering of thy firstfruits green ears of corn dried by the fire, *even* corn beaten out of full ears.

15 And thou shalt put oil upon it, and lay frankincense thereon: it *is* a [b]meat-offering.

16 And the priest shall burn the memorial of it, *part* of the beaten corn thereof, and *part* of the oil thereof, with all the frankincense thereof: *it is* an offering made by fire unto the LORD.

CHAPTER 3.

The sweet savour offerings:
(3) the peace-offering: Christ our peace (Eph. 2:14–18).

See Law of this offering, Lev. 7:11–21.

AND if his oblation *be* a [d]sacrifice of [4]peace-offering, if he offer *it* of the herd; whether *it be* a male or female, he shall offer it without blemish before the LORD.

2 And he shall [e]lay his hand upon the head of his offering, and kill it *at* the door of the tabernacle of the congregation: and Aaron's sons the priests shall sprinkle the blood upon the altar round about.

3 And he shall offer of the sacrifice of the peace-offering an offering made by fire unto the LORD; the fat that covereth the inwards, and all the fat that *is* upon the inwards,

4 And the two kidneys, and the fat

B.C. 1490.

a *Sacrifice (typical).* vs. 1-16; Lev. 3:1-17. (Gen. 4:4; Heb. 10:18.)

b Lit. *meal.*

c *Leaven.* vs. 4, 5, 11; Lev. 6:16, 17. (Gen. 19:3; Mt. 13:33.)

d *Sacrifice (typical).* vs. 1-17; Lev. 4:3-35. (Gen. 4:4; Heb. 10:18.)

e Lev. 1:4; 16:21; cf. Isa. 53:6.

[1]**(2:11)** For meanings of leaven see Mt. 13:33. Also Lev. 7:13, *note.*

[2]**(2:11)** Honey is mere natural sweetness and could not symbolize the divine graciousness of the Lord Jesus.

[3]**(2:13)** Cf. Num. 18:19; Mk. 9:49, 50; Col. 4:6.

[4]**(3:1)** The peace-offering. The whole work of Christ in relation to the believer's *peace* is here in type. He *made* peace, Col. 1:20; *proclaimed* peace, Eph. 2:17; and *is* our peace, Eph. 2:14. In Christ God and the sinner meet in peace; God is propitiated, the sinner reconciled—both alike satisfied with what Christ has done. But all this at the cost of blood and fire. The details speak of fellowship. This brings in prominently the thought of *fellowship* with God through Christ. Hence the peace-offering is set forth as affording food for the priests (Lev. 7:31-34). Observe that it is the breast (affections) and shoulders (strength) upon which we as priests (1 Pet. 2:9) feed in fellowship with the Father. This it is which makes the peace-offering especially a *thank-offering* (Lev. 7:11, 12).

that *is* on them, which *is by* the flanks,
and the [a]caul above the liver, with the
kidneys, it shall he take away.
5 And Aaron's sons shall [b]burn it on
the altar upon the burnt-sacrifice, which
is upon the wood that *is* on the fire: *it is*
an offering made by fire, of a sweet
savour unto the LORD.
6 And if his offering for a sacrifice of
peace-offering unto the LORD *be* of the
flock; male or female, he shall offer it
without blemish.
7 If he offer a lamb for his offering,
then shall he [c]offer it before the LORD.
8 And he shall lay his hand upon the
head of his offering, and kill it before the
tabernacle of the congregation: and
Aaron's sons shall sprinkle the blood
thereof round about upon the altar.
9 And he shall offer of the sacrifice of
the peace-offering an offering made by
fire unto the LORD; the fat thereof, *and*
the whole rump, it shall he take off hard
by the backbone; and the fat that covereth the inwards, and all the fat that *is*
upon the inwards,
10 And the two kidneys, and the fat
that *is* upon them, which *is* by the flanks,
and the [d]caul above the liver, with the
kidneys, it shall he take away.
11 And the priest shall burn it upon
the altar: *it is* the [e]food of the offering
made by fire unto the LORD.
12 And if his offering *be* a goat, then
he shall offer it before the LORD.
13 And he shall lay his hand upon the
head of it, and kill it before the tabernacle of the congregation: and the sons of
Aaron shall sprinkle the blood thereof
upon the altar round about.
14 And he shall offer thereof his offering, *even* an offering made by fire unto the
LORD; the fat that covereth the inwards,
and all the fat that *is* upon the inwards,
15 And the two kidneys, and the fat
that *is* upon them, which *is* by the flanks,
and the caul above the liver, with the
kidneys, it shall he take away.
16 And the priest shall burn them
upon the altar: *it is* the food of the offering made by fire for a sweet savour: all
the fat *is* the LORD'S.
17 *It shall be* a perpetual statute for
your generations throughout all your
dwellings, that ye eat neither fat nor
blood.

CHAPTER 4.

The non-sweet savour offerings:
(1) *the sin-offering; Christ atoning for the guilt of sin* (Heb. 13:11, 12).
See Law of this offering, Lev. 6:25–30.

And the LORD spake unto Moses,
saying,
2 Speak unto the children of Israel, saying, If a soul shall sin through ignorance
against any of the commandments of the
LORD *concerning things* which ought not to
be done, and shall do against any of them:
3 If the priest that is anointed do sin
according to the sin of the people; then
let him [f]bring for his sin, which he hath
sinned, a young bullock without blemish
unto the LORD for a [1]sin-offering.
4 And he shall bring the bullock unto
the door of the tabernacle of the congregation before the LORD; and shall lay his
hand upon the bullock's head, and kill
the bullock before the LORD.
5 And the priest that is anointed shall
take of the bullock's blood, and bring it
to the tabernacle of the congregation:
6 And the priest shall dip his finger in
the blood, and sprinkle of the blood
seven times before the LORD, before the
vail of the sanctuary.
7 And the priest shall put *some* of the
blood upon the horns of the altar of
sweet incense before the LORD, which *is*
in the tabernacle of the congregation;
and shall pour all the blood of the bullock at the bottom of the altar of the
burnt-offering, which *is at* the door of
the tabernacle of the congregation.
8 And he shall take off from it all the

B.C. 1490.

a *Fat appendage.*
b 2 Chr. 35:14.
c 1 Ki. 8:62.
d v. 4.
e Lev. 21:6, 8, 17; Num. 28:2.
f *Sacrifice (typical).* vs. 3-35; Lev. 5:1-19. (Gen. 4:4; Heb. 10:18.)

1 **(4:3)** The sin-offering, though still Christ, is Christ seen laden with the believer's sin, absolutely in the sinner's place and stead, and not, as in the sweet savour offerings, in His own perfections. It is Christ's death as viewed in Isa. 53; Psa. 22; Mt. 26:28; 1 Pet. 2:24; 3:18. But note (Lev. 6:24-30) how the essential holiness of Him who was "made sin for us" (2 Cor. 5:21) is guarded. The sin-offerings are *expiatory, substitutional, efficacious* (Lev. 4:12, 29, 35); and have in view the vindication of the law through substitutional sacrifice.

fat of the bullock for the sin-offering; the
fat that covereth the inwards, and all the
fat that *is* upon the inwards,
9 And the two kidneys, and the fat
that *is* upon them, which *is* by the flanks,
and the caul above the liver, with the
kidneys, it shall he take away,
10 As it was taken off from the bullock
of the sacrifice of peace-offerings: and
the priest shall burn them upon the altar
of the burnt-offering.
11 And the skin of the bullock, and all
his flesh, with his head, and with his
legs, and his inwards, and his dung,
12 Even the whole bullock shall he
carry forth [1]without the camp unto a
clean place, where the ashes are poured
out, and burn him on the wood with
fire: where the ashes are poured out
shall he be burnt.
13 And if the whole congregation of
Israel sin through ignorance, and the
thing be hid from the eyes of the assembly, and they have done *somewhat against*
any of the commandments of the LORD
concerning things which should not be
done, and are guilty;
14 When the sin, which they have
sinned against it, is known, then the congregation shall offer a young bullock for
the sin, and bring him before the tabernacle of the congregation.
15 And the elders of the congregation
shall lay their hands upon the head of
the bullock before the LORD: and the
bullock shall be killed before the LORD.
16 And the priest that is anointed shall
bring of the bullock's blood to the tabernacle of the congregation:
17 And the priest shall dip his finger
in some of the blood, and sprinkle *it*
seven times before the LORD, *even* before
the vail.
18 And he shall put *some* of the blood
upon the horns of the altar which *is*
before the LORD, that *is* in the tabernacle
of the congregation, and shall pour out
all the blood at the bottom of the altar of
the burnt-offering, which *is at* the door
of the tabernacle of the congregation.
19 And he shall take all his fat from
him, and burn *it* upon the altar.
20 And he shall do with the bullock as
he did with the bullock for a sin-offering, so shall he do with this: and the
priest shall make an [a]atonement for
them, and it shall be [b]forgiven them.
21 And he shall carry forth the bullock
without the camp, and burn him as he
burned the first bullock: it *is* a sin-offering for the congregation.
22 When a ruler hath sinned, and
done *somewhat* through ignorance *against*
any of the commandments of the LORD
his God *concerning things* which should
not be done, and is guilty;
23 Or if his sin, wherein he hath
sinned, come to his knowledge; he shall
bring his offering, a kid of the goats, a
male without blemish:
24 And he shall lay his hand upon the
head of the goat, and kill it in the place
where they kill the burnt-offering before
the LORD: it *is* a sin-offering.
25 And the priest shall take of the
blood of the sin-offering with his finger,
and put *it* upon the horns of the altar of
burnt-offering, and shall pour out his
blood at the bottom of the altar of burnt-
offering.

B.C. 1490.

a Lev. 1:4. See Ex. 29:33, *note.*

b *Forgiveness.* vs. 20, 26, 31, 35; Lev. 5:10, 13, 16, 18. (Lev. 4:20; Mt. 26:28.)

[1]**(4:12)** Cf. Ex. 29:14; Lev. 16:27; Num. 19:3; Heb. 13:10-13. The last passage is the interpretative one. The "camp" was Judaism—a religion of forms and ceremonies. "Jesus, also, that He might sanctify [separate, or set apart for God] the people with [or 'through'] His own blood, suffered without the gate" [temple gate, city gate. i.e. Judaism civil and religious]; Heb. 13:12. But how does this sanctify, or set apart, a people? "Let us go forth therefore unto Him without the camp [Judaism then, Judaized Christianity now—anything *religious* which denies Him as our sin-offering] bearing His reproach" (Heb. 13:13). The sin-offering, "burned without the camp," typifies this aspect of the death of Christ. The cross becomes a new altar, in a new place, where, without the smallest merit in themselves, the redeemed gather to offer, as believer-priests, spiritual sacrifices (Heb. 13:15: 1 Pet. 2:5). The bodies of the sin-offering beasts were not burned without the camp, as some have fancied, because "saturated with sin," and unfit for a holy camp. Rather, an unholy camp was an unfit place for a holy sin-offering. The dead body of our Lord was not "saturated with sin," though in it our sins had been borne (1 Pet. 2:24).

26 And he shall burn all his fat upon
the altar, as the fat of the sacrifice of
peace-offerings: and the priest shall
make an [a]atonement for him as concerning his sin, and it shall be forgiven him.
27 And if any one of the common people sin through ignorance, while he doeth
somewhat against any of the commandments of the LORD *concerning things* which
ought not to be done, and be guilty;
28 Or if his sin, which he hath sinned,
come to his knowledge: then he shall
bring his offering, a kid of the goats, a
female without blemish, for his sin
which he hath sinned.
29 And he shall lay his hand upon the
head of the sin-offering, and slay the sin-
offering in the place of the burnt-offering.
30 And the priest shall take of the
blood thereof with his finger, and put *it*
upon the horns of the altar of burnt-
offering, and shall pour out all the blood
thereof at the bottom of the altar.
31 And he shall take away all the fat
thereof, as the fat is taken away from off
the sacrifice of peace-offerings; and the
priest shall burn *it* upon the altar for a
sweet savour unto the LORD; and the
priest shall make an [a]atonement for him,
and it shall be forgiven him.
32 And if he bring a lamb for a sin-
offering, he shall bring it a female without blemish.
33 And he shall lay his hand upon the
head of the sin-offering, and slay it for a
sin-offering in the place where they kill
the burnt-offering.
34 And the priest shall take of the
blood of the sin-offering with his finger,
and put *it* upon the horns of the altar of
burnt-offering, and shall pour out all the
blood thereof at the bottom of the altar:
35 And he shall take away all the fat
thereof, as the fat of the lamb is taken
away from the sacrifice of the peace-
offerings; and the priest shall burn them
upon the altar, according to the offerings
made by fire unto the LORD: and the
priest shall make an [a]atonement for his
sin that he hath committed, and it shall
be forgiven him.

B.C. 1490.

a See Ex. 29:33, *note*.

b *Sacrifice (typical)*. vs. 1-19; Lev. 6:1-7. (Gen. 4:4; Heb. 10:18.)

c Num. 5:7; Psa. 32:5; 1 John 1:9; cf. Lev. 16:21; Josh. 7:19.

d Lev. 12:8; 14:21.

CHAPTER 5.

The non-sweet savour offerings:
(2) *the trespass-offerings;*
Christ atoning for the injury of sin.
See Law of this offering, Lev. 7:1–7.

And if a soul [b]sin, and hear the voice
of swearing, and *is* a witness,
whether he hath seen or known *of it*; if
he do not utter *it*, then he shall bear his
iniquity.
2 Or if a soul touch any unclean thing,
whether *it be* a carcase of an unclean
beast, or a carcase of unclean cattle, or
the carcase of unclean creeping things,
and *if* it be hidden from him; he also
shall be unclean, and guilty.
3 Or if he touch the uncleanness of
man, whatsoever uncleanness *it be* that a
man shall be defiled withal, and it be hid
from him; when he knoweth *of it*, then
he shall be guilty.
4 Or if a soul swear, pronouncing with
his lips to do evil, or to do good, whatsoever *it be* that a man shall pronounce
with an oath, and it be hid from him;
when he knoweth *of it*, then he shall be
guilty in one of these.
5 And it shall be, when he shall be
guilty in one of these *things*, that he shall
[c]confess that he hath sinned in that *thing*:
6 And he shall bring his [1]trespass-
offering unto the LORD for his sin which
he hath sinned, a female from the flock,
a lamb or a kid of the goats, for a sin-
offering; and the priest shall make an
[a]atonement for him concerning his sin.
7 And if he be [d]not able to bring a
lamb, then he shall bring for his trespass,
which he hath committed, two turtledoves, or two young pigeons, unto the
LORD; one for a sin-offering, and the
other for a burnt-offering.
8 And he shall bring them unto the
priest, who shall offer *that* which *is* for
the sin-offering first, and wring off his
head from his neck, but shall not divide
it asunder:
9 And he shall sprinkle of the blood of
the sin-offering upon the side of the
altar; and the rest of the blood shall be
wrung out at the bottom of the altar: it *is*
a sin-offering.

[1] **(5:6)** The trespass-offerings have in view rather the *injury* which sin does than its *guilt*—which is the sin-offering aspect. What is due to God's rights in every human being is here meant. Psa. 51:4 is a perfect expression of this.

10 And he shall offer the second *for* a burnt-offering, according to the manner: and the priest shall make an [a]atonement for him for his sin which he hath sinned, and it shall be [b]forgiven him.

11 But if he be not able to bring two turtledoves, or two young pigeons, then he that sinned shall bring for his offering the tenth part of an [c]ephah of fine flour for a sin-offering; he shall put no oil upon it, neither shall he put *any* frankincense thereon: for it *is* a sin-offering.

12 Then shall he bring it to the priest, and the priest shall take his handful of it, *even* a memorial thereof, and burn *it* on the altar, according to the offerings made by fire unto the LORD: it *is* a sin-offering.

13 And the priest shall make an [a]atonement for him as touching his sin that he hath sinned in one of these, and it shall be forgiven him: and *the remnant* shall be the priest's, as a [d]meat-offering.

14 And the LORD spake unto Moses, saying,

15 If a soul commit a trespass, and sin through ignorance, in the holy things of the LORD; then he shall bring for his trespass unto the LORD a ram without blemish out of the flocks, with thy estimation by [e]shekels of silver, after the shekel of the sanctuary, for a trespass-offering:

16 And he shall make amends for the harm that he hath done in the holy thing, and shall add the fifth part thereto, and give it unto the priest: and the priest shall make an [a]atonement for him with the ram of the trespass-offering, and it shall be forgiven him.

17 And if a soul sin, and commit any of these things which are forbidden to be done by the commandments of the LORD; though he wist *it* not, yet is he guilty, and shall bear his iniquity.

18 And he shall bring a ram without blemish out of the flock, with thy estimation, for a trespass-offering, unto the priest: and the priest shall make an [a]atonement for him concerning his ignorance wherein he erred and wist *it* not, and it shall be forgiven him.

19 It *is* a trespass-offering: he hath certainly trespassed against the LORD.

B.C. 1490.

a See Ex. 29:33, *note.*

b *Forgiveness.* vs. 10, 13, 16, 18; Lev. 6:7. (Lev. 4:20; Mt. 26:28.)

c One ephah = 1 bu. 3 pts.

d Lit. *meal.*

e One shekel = 2*s.* 9*d.* or 65 cents.

f *Sacrifice (typical).* vs. 1-7; Lev. 16:1-24. (Gen. 4:4; Heb. 10:18.)

g *Forgiveness.* Lev. 19:22. (Lev. 4:20; Mt. 26:28.)

CHAPTER 6.

The trespass-offering and restitution. See Law of this offering, Lev. 7:1–7.

AND the LORD spake unto Moses, saying,

2 [f]If a soul sin, and commit a trespass against the LORD, and lie unto his neighbour in that which was delivered him to keep, or in fellowship, or in a thing taken away by violence, or hath deceived his neighbour;

3 Or have found that which was lost, and lieth concerning it, and sweareth falsely; in any of all these that a man doeth, sinning therein:

4 Then it shall be, because he hath sinned, and is guilty, that he shall restore that which he took violently away, or the thing which he hath deceitfully gotten, or that which was delivered him to keep, or the lost thing which he found,

5 Or all that about which he hath sworn falsely; he shall even restore it in the principal, and shall add the fifth part more thereto, *and* give it unto him to whom it appertaineth, in the day of his trespass-offering.

6 And he shall bring his trespass-offering unto the LORD, a ram without blemish out of the flock, with thy estimation, for a trespass-offering, unto the priest:

7 And the priest shall make an [a]atonement for him before the LORD: and it shall be [g]forgiven him for any thing of all that he hath done in trespassing therein.

The law of the offerings:
(1) *the burnt-offering* (Lev. 1:1–17).

8 And the LORD spake unto Moses, saying,

9 Command Aaron and his sons, saying, This *is* the law of the burnt-offering: It *is* the burnt-offering, because of the burning upon the altar all night unto the morning, and the fire of the altar shall be burning in it.

10 And the priest shall put on his linen garment, and his linen breeches shall he put upon his flesh, and take up the ashes which the fire hath consumed with the burnt-offering on the altar, and he shall put them beside the altar.

11 And he shall put off his garments, and put on other garments, and carry forth the ashes without the camp unto a clean place.

B.C. 1490.

12 And the fire upon the altar shall be burning in it; it shall not be put out: and the priest shall burn wood on it every morning, and lay the burnt-offering in order upon it; and he shall burn thereon the fat of the peace-offerings.

13 The [1]fire shall ever be burning upon the altar; it shall never go out.

The law of the offerings:
(2) *the meat-offering* (Lev. 2:1–16).

14 And this *is* the law of the [a]meat-offering: the sons of Aaron shall offer it before the LORD, before the altar.

15 And he shall take of it his handful, of the flour of the [a]meat-offering, and of the oil thereof, and all the frankincense which *is* upon the [a]meat-offering, and shall burn *it* upon the altar *for* a sweet savour, *even* the memorial of it, unto the LORD.

16 And the remainder thereof shall Aaron and his sons eat: with [b]unleavened bread shall it be eaten in the holy place; in the court of the tabernacle of the congregation they shall eat it.

17 It shall not be baken with leaven. I have given it *unto them for* their portion of my offerings made by fire; it *is* most holy, as *is* the sin-offering, and as the trespass-offering.

18 All the males among the children of Aaron shall eat of it. *It shall be* a statute for ever in your generations concerning the offerings of the LORD made by fire: every one that toucheth them shall be holy.

(*The priests' meat-offering.*)

19 And the LORD spake unto Moses, saying,

20 This *is* the offering of Aaron and of his sons, which they shall offer unto the LORD in the day when he is anointed; the tenth part of an [c]ephah of fine flour for a [a]meat-offering perpetual, half of it in the morning, and half thereof at night.

21 In a pan it shall be made with oil; *and when it is* baken, thou shalt bring it in: *and* the baken pieces of the [a]meat-offering shalt thou offer *for* a sweet savour unto the LORD.

22 And the priest of his sons that is anointed in his stead shall offer it: *it is* a statute for ever unto the LORD; it shall be wholly burnt.

23 For every [a]meat-offering for the priest shall be wholly burnt: it shall not be eaten.

The law of the offerings:
(3) *the sin-offering* (Lev. 4:1–35).

24 And the LORD spake unto Moses, saying,

25 Speak unto Aaron and to his sons, saying, This *is* the law of the sin-offering: In the place where the burnt-offering is killed shall the sin-offering be killed before the LORD: it *is* most holy.

26 The priest that offereth it for sin shall eat it: in the holy place shall it be eaten, in the court of the tabernacle of the congregation.

27 Whatsoever shall touch the flesh thereof shall be holy: and when there is sprinkled of the blood thereof upon any garment, thou shalt wash that whereon it was sprinkled in the holy place.

28 But the earthen vessel wherein it is sodden shall be broken: and if it be sodden in a brasen pot, it shall be both scoured, and rinsed in water.

29 All the males among the priests shall eat thereof: it *is* most holy.

30 And no sin-offering, whereof *any* of the blood is brought into the tabernacle of the congregation to [d]reconcile *withal* in the holy *place*, shall be eaten: it shall be burnt in the fire.

CHAPTER 7.

The law of the offerings:
(4) *the trespass-offering* (Lev. 5:1 to 6:7).

Likewise this *is* the law of the trespass-offering: it *is* most holy.

2 In the place where they kill the burnt-offering shall they kill the trespass-offering: and the blood thereof shall he sprinkle round about upon the altar.

3 And he shall offer of it all the fat thereof; the rump, and the fat that covereth the inwards,

4 And the two kidneys, and the fat that *is* on them, which *is* by the flanks, and the caul *that is* above the liver, with the kidneys, it shall he take away:

5 And the priest shall burn them upon the altar *for* an offering made by

a Lit. *meal.*

b *Leaven.* vs. 16, 17; Lev. 7:12, 13. (Gen. 19:3; Mt. 13:33.)

c One ephah = 1 bu. 3 pts.

d Heb. *kaphar, to cover.* See Dan. 9:24, note; Ex. 29:33; *note.*

[1] **(6:13)** See Lev. 1:8, *note.* Here the fire expresses also the undying devotedness of Christ.

fire unto the LORD: it *is* a trespass-offering.

6 Every male among the priests shall eat thereof: it shall be eaten in the holy place: it *is* most holy.

7 As the sin-offering *is*, so *is* the trespass-offering: *there is* one law for them: the priest that maketh [a]atonement therewith shall have *it*.

8 And the priest that offereth any man's burnt-offering, *even* the priest shall have to himself the skin of the burnt-offering which he hath offered.

9 And all the [b]meat-offering that is baken in the oven, and all that is dressed in the fryingpan, and in the pan, shall be the priest's that offereth it.

10 And every [b]meat-offering, mingled with oil, and dry, shall all the sons of Aaron have, one *as much* as another.

The law of the offerings:
(5) the peace-offering (Lev. 3:1–17).

11 And this *is* the law of the sacrifice of [1]peace-offerings, which he shall offer unto the LORD.

12 If he offer it for a thanksgiving, then he shall offer with the sacrifice of thanksgiving [c]unleavened cakes mingled with oil, and unleavened wafers anointed with oil, and cakes mingled with oil, of fine flour, fried.

13 Besides the cakes, he shall offer *for* his offering [2c]leavened bread with the sacrifice of thanksgiving of his peace-offerings.

14 And of it he shall offer one out of the whole oblation *for* an heave-offering unto the LORD, *and* it shall be the priest's that sprinkleth the blood of the peace-offerings.

15 And the flesh of the sacrifice of his peace-offerings for thanksgiving shall be eaten the same day that it is offered; he shall not leave any of it until the morning.

16 But if the sacrifice of his offering *be* a vow, or a voluntary offering, it shall be eaten the same day that he offereth his sacrifice: and on the morrow also the remainder of it shall be eaten:

17 But the remainder of the flesh of the sacrifice on the third day shall be burnt with fire.

18 And if *any* of the flesh of the sacrifice of his peace-offerings be eaten at all on the third day, it shall not be accepted, neither shall it be imputed unto him that offereth it: it shall be an [d]abomination, and the soul that eateth of it shall bear his iniquity.

19 And the flesh that toucheth any unclean *thing* shall not be eaten; it shall be burnt with fire: and as for the flesh, all that be clean shall eat thereof.

20 But the soul that eateth *of* the flesh of the sacrifice of peace-offerings, that *pertain* unto the [e]LORD, having his uncleanness upon him, even that soul shall be cut off from his people.

21 Moreover the [f]soul that shall touch any unclean *thing, as* the uncleanness of man, or *any* unclean beast, or any abominable unclean *thing*, and eat of the flesh of the sacrifice of peace-offerings, which *pertain* unto the LORD, even that soul shall be cut off from his people.

22 And the LORD spake unto Moses, saying,

23 Speak unto the children of Israel,

B.C. 1490.

a See Ex. 29:33, *note.*
b Lit. *meal.*
c *Leaven.* vs. 12, 13; Lev. 8:2, 26. (Gen. 19:3; Mt. 13:33.)
d Lev. 11:10, 41; 19:7.
e Lev. 15:3; cf. Heb. 2:17.
f Lev. 11:24, 28.

[1] **(7:11)** In the "law of the offerings," the peace-offering is taken out of its place as third of the sweet savour offerings, and placed alone, and after all the non-sweet savour offerings. The explanation is as simple as the fact is beautiful. In *revealing* the offerings Jehovah works from Himself *out* to the sinner (see Ex. 25:10, *note*). The whole burnt-offering comes first as meeting what is due to the divine affections, and the trespass-offering last as meeting the simplest aspect of sin—its *injuriousness.* But the sinner begins of necessity with that which lies nearest to a newly awakened conscience—a sense, namely, that because of sin he is at *enmity* with God. His first need, therefore, is peace with God. And that is precisely the Gospel order. Christ's first message is, "Peace" (John 20:19), *afterward* He shows them His hands and His side. It is the order of 2 Cor. 5:18-21: first "the word of reconciliation," verse 19, then the trespass- and sin-offering, verse 21. *Experience* thus reverses the order of *revelation.*

[2] **(7:13)** The use of leaven here is significant. Peace with God is something which the believer *shares* with God. Christ is our peace-offering (Eph. 2:13). Any thanksgiving for peace *must,* first of all, present *Him.* In verse 12 we have this, in type, and so leaven is excluded. In verse 13 it is the *offerer* who gives thanks for *his* participation in the peace, and so leaven fitly signifies, that though having peace with God through the work of another, there is still evil in him. This is illustrated in Amos 4:5, where the evil in Israel is before God.

saying, Ye shall eat no manner of fat, of ox, or of sheep, or of goat.

24 And the fat of the beast that dieth of itself, and the fat of that which is torn with beasts, may be used in any other use: but ye shall in no wise eat of it.

25 For whosoever eateth the fat of the beast, of which men offer an offering made by fire unto the LORD, even the soul that eateth *it* shall be cut off from his people.

26 Moreover ye shall eat no manner of blood, *whether it be* of fowl or of beast, in any of your dwellings.

27 Whatsoever soul *it be* that eateth any manner of blood, even that soul shall be [a]cut off from his people.

28 And the LORD spake unto Moses, saying,

29 Speak unto the children of Israel, saying, He that offereth the sacrifice of his peace-offerings unto the LORD shall bring his oblation unto the LORD of the sacrifice of his peace-offerings.

30 His own hands shall bring the offerings of the LORD made by fire, the fat with the breast, it shall he bring, that the breast may be waved *for* a [b]wave-offering before the LORD.

31 And the priest shall burn the fat upon the altar: but the breast shall be Aaron's and his sons'.

32 And the right shoulder shall ye give unto the [c]priest *for* an heave-offering of the sacrifices of your peace-offerings.

33 He among the sons of Aaron, that offereth the blood of the peace-offerings, and the fat, shall have the right shoulder for *his* part.

34 For the wave breast and the heave shoulder have I taken of the children of Israel from off the sacrifices of their peace-offerings, and have given them unto Aaron the priest and unto his sons by a statute for ever from among the children of Israel.

35 This *is the portion* of the anointing of Aaron, and of the anointing of his sons, out of the offerings of the LORD made by fire, in the day *when* he presented them to minister unto the LORD in the priest's office;

36 Which the LORD commanded to be given them of the children of Israel, in the day that [d]he anointed them, *by* a statute for ever throughout their generations.

37 This *is* the [e]law of the burnt-offering, of the [f]meat-offering, and of the sin-offering, and of the trespass-offering, and of the consecrations, and of the sacrifice of the peace-offerings;

38 Which the LORD commanded Moses in mount Sinai, in the day that he commanded the children of Israel to offer their oblations unto the LORD, in the wilderness of Sinai.

CHAPTER 8.

Consecration of the priests.

And the LORD spake unto Moses, saying,

2 Take [1]Aaron and his sons with him, and the garments, and the anointing oil, and a bullock for the sin-offering, and two rams, and a basket of [g]unleavened bread;

3 And gather thou all the congregation together unto the door of the tabernacle of the congregation.

4 And Moses did as the LORD commanded him; and the assembly was gathered together unto the door of the tabernacle of the congregation.

5 And Moses said unto the congregation, This *is* the thing which the LORD commanded to be done.

Consecration: (1) *cleansing* (Eph. 5:25–27; John 13:3–10).

6 And Moses brought Aaron and his sons, and washed them with water.

Consecration: (2) *the high priest clothed.*

7 And he put upon him the coat, and girded him with the girdle, and clothed him with the robe, and put the ephod upon him, and he girded him with the curious girdle of the ephod, and bound *it* unto him therewith.

8 And he put the breastplate upon him: also he put in the breastplate the [h]Urim and the Thummim.

9 And he put the mitre upon his head; also upon the mitre, *even* upon his fore-front, did he put the golden plate, the holy crown; as the LORD commanded Moses.

B.C. 1490.

a v. 20.

b Lev. 8:27; 9:21; Ex. 29:24-27.

c Num. 6:20.

d Ex. 40:13, 15; Lev. 8:12, 30.

e Lev. 6:9, 14, 25.

f Lit. *meal.*

g *Leaven.* vs. 2, 26; Lev. 10:12. (Gen. 19:3; Mt. 13:33.)

h See Ex. 28:30, *note.*

U-rim 'lights:' *Thum*-mim, 'perfection:'

[1] **(8:2)** The priests did not consecrate themselves, all was done by another, in this instance Moses, acting for Jehovah. The priests simply presented their bodies in the sense of Rom. 12:1.

Consecration:
(3) *the high priest's anointing.*

10 And Moses took the anointing oil, and anointed the tabernacle and all that *was* therein, and sanctified them.

11 And he sprinkled thereof upon the altar seven times, and anointed the altar and all his vessels, both the laver and his foot, to sanctify them.

12 And he [1]poured of the anointing oil upon Aaron's head, and anointed him, to sanctify him.

Consecration: (4) *the priests clothed.*

13 And Moses brought Aaron's sons, and put coats upon them, and girded them with girdles, and put bonnets upon them; as the LORD commanded Moses.

Consecration: (5) *the offerings.*

14 And he brought the bullock for the sin-offering: and Aaron and his sons laid their hands upon the head of the bullock for the sin-offering.

15 And he slew *it*; and Moses took the blood, and put *it* upon the horns of the altar round about with his finger, and purified the altar, and poured the blood at the bottom of the altar, and [a]sanctified it, to make [b]reconciliation upon it.

16 And he took all the fat that *was* upon the inwards, and the caul *above* the liver, and the two kidneys, and their fat, and Moses burned *it* upon the altar.

17 But the bullock, and his hide, his flesh, and his dung, he burnt with fire without the camp; as the LORD commanded Moses.

18 And he brought the ram for the burnt-offering: and Aaron and his sons laid their hands upon the head of the ram.

19 And he killed *it*; and Moses sprinkled the blood upon the altar round about.

20 And he cut the ram into pieces; and Moses burnt the head, and the pieces, and the fat.

21 And he washed the inwards and the legs in water; and Moses burnt the whole ram upon the altar: it *was* a burnt-sacrifice for a sweet savour, *and* an offering made by fire unto the LORD; as the LORD commanded Moses.

B.C. 1490.

a *Sanctify, holy* (O.T.). Lev. 27:14-22. (Gen. 2:3; Zech. 8:3.)

b Heb. *kaphar, to cover.* See Dan. 9:24, *note.*

c Ex. 29:19, 31.

d Lev. 14:14.

e Ex. 29:20; cf. Heb. 9:13-14, 22-23.

f Ex. 29:22.

g Ex. 29:26.

22 And he brought the [c]other ram, the ram of consecration: and Aaron and his sons laid their hands upon the head of the ram.

Consecration: (6) *the blood applied.*

23 And he slew *it*; and Moses took of the [d]blood of it, and put *it* upon the tip of Aaron's right ear, and upon the thumb of his right hand, and upon the great toe of his right foot.

24 And he brought Aaron's sons, and Moses put of the [e]blood upon the tip of their right ear, and upon the thumbs of their right hands, and upon the great toes of their right feet: and Moses sprinkled the blood upon the altar round about.

25 And he [f]took the fat, and the rump, and all the fat that *was* upon the inwards, and the caul *above* the liver, and the two kidneys, and their fat, and the right shoulder:

26 And out of the basket of unleavened bread, that *was* before the LORD, he took one unleavened cake, and a cake of oiled bread, and one wafer, and put *them* on the fat, and upon the right shoulder:

Consecration: (7) *the hands filled.*

27 And he put all upon Aaron's hands, and upon his sons' hands, and waved them *for* a wave-offering before the LORD.

28 And Moses took them from off their hands, and burnt *them* on the altar upon the burnt-offering: they *were* consecrations for a sweet savour: it *is* an offering made by fire unto the LORD.

29 And Moses took the [g]breast, and waved it *for* a wave-offering before the LORD: *for* of the ram of consecration it was Moses' part; as the LORD commanded Moses.

Consecration:
(8) *the anointing of the priests.*

30 And Moses took of the anointing

[1] **(8:12)** Two important distinctions are made in the case of the high priest, thus confirming his typical relation to Christ the anti-type: (1) Aaron is anointed before the sacrifices are slain, while in the case of the priests the application of blood precedes the anointing. Christ the sinless One required no preparation for receiving the anointing oil, symbol of the Holy Spirit; (2) upon the high priest only was the anointing oil poured. "God giveth not the Spirit by measure unto him" (John 3:34). "Thy God hath anointed Thee with the oil of gladness above Thy fellows" (Heb. 1:9).

oil, and of the blood which *was* upon the
altar, and sprinkled *it* upon Aaron, *and*
upon his garments, and upon his sons,
and upon his sons' garments with him;
and sanctified Aaron, *and* his garments,
and his sons, and his sons' garments
with him.

Consecration: (9) *the food of the priests.*
(Ex. 29:26, and *refs.*)

31 And Moses said unto Aaron and to
his sons, Boil the flesh *at* the door of the
tabernacle of the congregation: and there
eat it with the bread that *is* in the basket
of consecrations, as I commanded, saying, Aaron and his sons shall eat it.
32 And that which remaineth of the
flesh and of the bread shall ye burn with
fire.

Consecration:
(10) *the priests separated unto God.*

33 And ye shall not go out of the door
of the tabernacle of the congregation *in*
seven days, until the days of your consecration be at an end: for seven days shall
he consecrate you.
34 As he hath done this day, *so* the
LORD hath commanded to do, to make
an [a]atonement for you.
35 Therefore shall ye abide *at* the door
of the tabernacle of the congregation day
and night seven days, and keep the
charge of the LORD, that ye die not: for so
I am commanded.
36 So Aaron and his sons did all things
which the LORD commanded by the
hand of Moses.

CHAPTER 9.

The priests begin their ministry.

And it came to pass on the eighth day,
that Moses called Aaron and his
sons, and the elders of Israel;
2 And he said unto Aaron, Take thee a
young calf for a sin-offering, and a ram
for a burnt-offering, without blemish,
and offer *them* before the LORD.
3 And unto the children of Israel thou
shalt speak, saying, Take ye a kid of the
goats for a sin-offering; and a calf and a
lamb, *both* of the first year, without
blemish, for a burnt-offering;
4 Also a bullock and a ram for peace-
offerings, to sacrifice before the LORD;
and a [b]meat-offering mingled with oil:
for to day the LORD will appear unto you.
5 And they brought *that* which Moses
commanded before the tabernacle of the
congregation: and all the congregation
drew near and stood before the LORD.
6 And Moses said, This *is* the thing
which the LORD commanded that ye
should do: and the glory of the LORD
shall appear unto you.
7 And Moses said unto Aaron, Go
unto the altar, and offer thy sin-offering,
and thy burnt-offering, and make an
[a]atonement for thyself, and for the people: and offer the offering of the people,
and make an [a]atonement for them; as
the LORD commanded.
8 Aaron therefore went unto the altar,
and slew the calf of the sin-offering,
which *was* for himself.
9 And the sons of Aaron brought the
[c]blood unto him: and he dipped his finger in the blood, and put *it* upon the
horns of the altar, and poured out the
blood at the bottom of the altar:
10 But the fat, and the kidneys, and
the caul above the liver of the sin-offering, he burnt upon the altar; as the LORD
commanded Moses.
11 And the flesh and the hide he burnt
with fire without the camp.
12 And he slew the burnt-offering;
and Aaron's sons presented unto him
the blood, which he sprinkled round
about upon the altar.
13 And they presented the burnt-offering unto him, with the pieces thereof,
and the head: and he burnt *them* upon
the altar.
14 And he did wash the inwards and
the legs, and burnt *them* upon the burnt-
offering on the altar.
15 And he brought the people's offering, and took the goat, which *was* the
sin-offering for the people, and slew it,
and [d]offered it for sin, as the first.
16 And he brought the burnt-offering,
and offered it according to the manner.
17 And he brought the [e]meat-offering,
and took an handful thereof, and burnt
it upon the altar, beside the [f]burnt-sacri-
fice of the morning.
18 He slew also the bullock and the
ram *for* a sacrifice of peace-offerings,
which *was* for the people: and Aaron's
sons presented unto him the blood,
which he sprinkled upon the altar round
about,
19 And the fat of the bullock and of
the ram, the rump, and that which

B.C. 1490.

a See Ex. 29:33, *note.*

b Lit. *meal.*

c Heb. 9:22, 23.

d Isa. 53:10; Heb. 2:17; 5:3.

e Lit. *meal.*

f Ex. 29:38.

covereth *the inwards,* and the kidneys, and the caul *above* the liver:

20 And they put the fat upon the breasts, and he burnt the fat upon the altar:

21 And the breasts and the right shoulder Aaron waved *for* a wave-offering before the LORD; as Moses commanded.

22 And Aaron lifted up his hand toward the people, and blessed them, and came down from offering of the sin-offering, and the burnt-offering, and peace-offerings.

23 And Moses and Aaron went into the tabernacle of the congregation, and came out, and blessed the people: and the glory of the LORD appeared unto all the people.

24 And there came a fire out from before the LORD, and consumed upon the altar the burnt-offering and the fat: *which* when all the people saw, they shouted, and fell on their faces.

CHAPTER 10.

The strange fire of Nadab and Abihu.

And Nadab and Abihu, the sons of Aaron, took either of them his censer, and put fire therein, and put incense thereon, and offered strange [1]fire before the LORD, which he commanded them not.

2 And there went out fire from the LORD, and devoured them, and they [a]died before the LORD.

3 Then Moses said unto Aaron, This *is it* that the LORD spake, saying, I will be sanctified in them that come nigh me, and before all the people I will be glorified. And Aaron held his peace.

4 And Moses called Mishael and Elzaphan, the sons of Uzziel the uncle of Aaron, and said unto them, Come near, carry your brethren from before the sanctuary out of the camp.

5 So they went near, and carried them in their coats out of the camp; as Moses had said.

6 And Moses said unto Aaron, and unto Eleazar and unto Ithamar, his sons, Uncover not your heads, neither rend your clothes; lest ye die, and lest [b]wrath come upon all the people: but let your brethren, the whole house of Israel, bewail the burning which the LORD hath kindled.

7 And ye shall not go out from the door of the tabernacle of the congregation, lest ye die: for the anointing oil of the LORD *is* upon you. And they did according to the word of Moses.

8 And the LORD spake unto Aaron, saying,

9 Do not drink wine nor strong drink, thou, nor thy sons with thee, when ye go into the tabernacle of the congregation, lest ye die: *it shall be* a statute for ever throughout your generations:

10 And that ye may put difference between holy and unholy, and between unclean and clean;

11 And that ye may teach the children of Israel all the statutes which the LORD hath spoken unto them by the hand of Moses.

12 And Moses spake unto Aaron, and unto Eleazar and unto Ithamar, his sons that were left, Take the [c]meat-offering that remaineth of the offerings of the LORD made by fire, and eat it without [d]leaven beside the altar: for it *is* most holy:

13 And ye shall eat it in the [e]holy place, because it *is* thy due, and thy sons' due, of the sacrifices of the LORD made by fire: for so I am commanded.

14 And the wave breast and heave shoulder shall ye eat in a clean place; thou, and thy sons, and thy daughters with thee: for *they be* thy due, and thy sons' due, *which* are given out of the sacrifices of peace-offerings of the children of Israel.

15 The heave shoulder and the wave breast shall they bring with the offerings made by fire of the fat, to wave *it for* a wave-offering before the LORD; and it shall be thine, and thy sons' with thee, by a statute for ever; as the LORD hath commanded.

16 And Moses diligently sought the goat of the sin-offering, and, behold, it

B.C. 1490.

a *Miracles* (O.T.). vs. 1, 2; Num. 11:1-3. (Gen. 5:24; Jon. 2:1-10.)

b Num. 16:46; Josh. 7:1; 22:18, 20; 2 Sam. 24:1, 15.

c Lit. *meal.*

d *Leaven.* Lev. 23:6-17. (Gen. 19:3; Mt. 13:33.)

e Num. 18:10.

Na-dab, *'liberal.'*

A-*bi*-hu, 'God is father.'

Mish-a-el, one with God.

El-*za*-phan, '*God protects.*'

Uz-zi-el, '*power of God.*'

El-e-*a-zar*, '*God has helped.*'

Ith-a-mar, '*isle of palms.*'

[1] **(10:1)** Strange fire. Fire "from before the Lord" had kindled upon the altar of *burnt-offering* the fire which the care of the priests was to keep burning (Lev. 6:12). No commandment had yet been given (Lev. 16:12) how the *incense* should be kindled. The sin of Nadab and Abihu was in acting in the things of God without seeking the mind of God. It was "will worship" (Col. 2:23), which often has a "show of wisdom and humility." It typifies any use of carnal means to kindle the fire of devotion and praise.

was burnt: and he was angry with Eleazar and Ithamar, the sons of Aaron *which*
were left *alive*, saying,
17 Wherefore have ye not eaten the sin-
offering in the holy place, seeing it *is* most
holy, and *God* hath given it you to bear the
iniquity of the congregation, to make
[a]atonement for them before the LORD?
18 Behold, the blood of it was not
brought in within the [b]holy *place*: ye
should indeed have eaten it in the holy
place, as I commanded.
19 And Aaron said unto Moses,
Behold, this day have they offered their
sin-offering and their burnt-offering
before the LORD; and such things have
befallen me: and *if* I had eaten the sin-
offering to day, should it have been [c]ac-
cepted in the sight of the LORD?
20 And when Moses heard *that*, he
was content.

CHAPTER 11.

A holy God—a holy people: (1) *their food.*

And the LORD spake unto Moses and
to Aaron, saying unto them,
2 Speak unto the children of Israel,
saying, [1]These *are* the beasts which ye
shall eat among all the beasts that *are* on
the earth.
3 Whatsoever parteth the hoof, and is
clovenfooted, *and* cheweth the cud,
among the beasts, that shall ye eat.
4 Nevertheless these shall ye not eat of
them that chew the cud, or of them that
divide the hoof: *as* the camel, because he
cheweth the cud, but divideth not the
hoof; he *is* unclean unto you.
5 And the coney, because he cheweth
the cud, but divideth not the hoof; he *is*
unclean unto you.
6 And the [2]hare, because he cheweth
the cud, but divideth not the hoof; he *is*
unclean unto you.
7 And the swine, though he divide the
hoof, and be clovenfooted, yet he
cheweth not the cud; he *is* unclean to you.
8 Of their flesh shall ye not eat, and
their carcase shall ye not touch; they *are*
unclean to you.
9 These shall ye eat of all that *are* in
the waters: whatsoever hath fins and
scales in the waters, in the seas, and in
the rivers, them shall ye eat.
10 And all that have not fins and
scales in the seas, and in the rivers, of all
that move in the waters, and of any living thing which *is* in the waters, they
shall be an abomination unto you:
11 They shall be even an abomination
unto you; ye shall not eat of their flesh,
but ye shall have their carcases in abomination.
12 Whatsoever hath no fins nor scales
in the waters, that *shall be* an abomination unto you.
13 And these *are they which* ye shall
have in abomination among the fowls;
they shall not be eaten, they *are* an abomination: the eagle, and the ossifrage, and
the ospray,
14 And the vulture, and the kite after
his kind;
15 Every raven after his kind;
16 And the owl, and the night hawk,
and the cuckow, and the hawk after his
kind,
17 And the little owl, and the cormorant, and the great owl,
18 And the swan, and the pelican, and
the gier eagle,
19 And the stork, the heron after her
kind, and the lapwing, and the bat.
20 All fowls that creep, going upon *all*
four, *shall be* an abomination unto you.
21 Yet these may ye eat of every flying
creeping thing that goeth upon *all* four,
which have legs above their feet, to leap
withal upon the earth;
22 *Even* these of them ye may eat; the
locust after his kind, and the bald locust

B.C. 1490.

a See Ex. 29:33, *note*.

b Lev. 6:26, 30.

c Isa. 1:11, 15; Jer. 6:20; 14:12; Hos. 9:4; Mal. 1:10, 13.

[1] **(11:2)** The dietary regulations of the covenant people must be regarded *primarily* as sanitary. Israel it must be remembered, was a nation living on the earth under a theocratic government. Of necessity the divine legislation concerned itself with the social as well as with the religious life of that people. To force upon every word of that legislation a typical meaning is to strain 1 Cor. 10:1-11 and Heb. 9:23, 24 beyond all reasonable interpretation.

[2] **(11:6)** Heb. *arnebeth,* an unidentified animal, but certainly not a hare, possessing as it is said to, characteristics not possessed by the hare. The supposed error in the *text* is due entirely to the translators' assumption that the English hare and the ancient "arnebeth" were identical.

after his kind, and the beetle after his
kind, and the grasshopper after his kind.
23 But all *other* flying creeping things,
which have four feet, *shall be* an abomination unto you.
24 And for these ye shall be unclean:
whosoever [a]toucheth the carcase of them
shall be unclean until the even.
25 And whosoever beareth *ought* of
the carcase of them shall [b]wash his
clothes, and be unclean until the even.
26 *The carcases* of every beast which
divideth the hoof, and *is* not clovenfooted, nor cheweth the cud, *are* unclean
unto you: every one that toucheth them
shall be unclean.
27 And whatsoever goeth upon his
paws, among all manner of beasts that
go on *all* four, those *are* unclean unto
you: whoso toucheth their carcase shall
be unclean until the even.
28 And he that beareth the carcase of
them shall [c]wash his clothes, and be
unclean until the even: they *are* unclean
unto you.
29 These also *shall be* unclean unto you
among the creeping things that creep
upon the earth; the weasel, and the
mouse, and the tortoise after his kind,
30 And the ferret, and the chameleon,
and the lizard, and the snail, and the
mole.
31 These *are* unclean to you among all
that creep: whosoever doth [d]touch them,
when they be dead, shall be unclean
until the even.
32 And upon whatsoever *any* of them,
when they are dead, doth fall, it shall be
unclean; whether *it be* any vessel of
wood, or raiment, or skin, or sack, whatsoever vessel *it be*, wherein *any* work is
done, it must be put into water, and it
shall be unclean until the even; so it shall
be cleansed.
33 And every earthen vessel, whereinto *any* of them falleth, whatsoever *is* in it
shall be unclean; and ye shall [e]break it.
34 Of all meat which may be eaten,
that on which *such* water cometh shall be
unclean: and all drink that may be
drunk in every *such* vessel shall be
unclean.
35 And every *thing* whereupon *any part*
of their carcase falleth shall be unclean;
whether it be oven, or ranges for pots, they
shall be broken down: *for* they *are*
unclean, and shall be unclean unto you.

B.C. 1490.

a v. 8; Lev. 17:15, 16; 1 Cor. 15:33.

b Num. 19:10, 22; 31:24; cf. Zech. 13:1; Heb. 9:10; 10:22.

c vs. 24-25.

d v. 8; Hag. 2:13.

e Psa. 2:9; Jer. 48:38.

f 1 Pet. 1:16.

36 Nevertheless a fountain or pit,
wherein there is plenty of water, shall be
clean: but that which toucheth their carcase shall be unclean.
37 And if *any part* of their carcase fall
upon any sowing seed which is to be
sown, it *shall be* clean.
38 But if *any* water be put upon the
seed, and *any part* of their carcase fall
thereon, it *shall be* unclean unto you.
39 And if any beast, of which ye may
eat, die; he that toucheth the carcase
thereof shall be unclean until the even.
40 And he that eateth of the carcase of
it shall wash his clothes, and be unclean
until the even: he also that beareth the
carcase of it shall wash his clothes, and
be unclean until the even.
41 And every creeping thing that
creepeth upon the earth *shall be* an
abomination; it shall not be eaten.
42 Whatsoever goeth upon the belly,
and whatsoever goeth upon *all* four, or
whatsoever hath more feet among all
creeping things that creep upon the
earth, them ye shall not eat; for they *are*
an abomination.
43 Ye shall not make yourselves abominable with any creeping thing that
creepeth, neither shall ye make yourselves unclean with them, that ye should
be defiled thereby.
44 For I *am* the LORD your God: ye
shall therefore sanctify yourselves, and
ye shall be holy; for I *am* [f]holy: neither
shall ye defile yourselves with any manner of creeping thing that creepeth upon
the earth.
45 For I *am* the LORD that bringeth you
up out of the land of Egypt, to be your
God: ye shall therefore be holy, for I *am*
holy.
46 This *is* the law of the beasts, and of
the fowl, and of every living creature
that moveth in the waters, and of every
creature that creepeth upon the earth:
47 To make a difference between the
unclean and the clean, and between the
beast that may be eaten and the beast
that may not be eaten.

CHAPTER 12.

A holy God—a holy people:
(2) *the law of motherhood*
(Psa. 51:5; John 3:6).

And the LORD spake unto Moses,
saying,

2 Speak unto the children of Israel,
saying, If a woman have conceived seed,
and born a man child: then she shall be
unclean seven days; according to the
days of the separation for her infirmity
shall she be unclean.
3 And in the eighth day the flesh of his
foreskin shall be circumcised.
4 And she shall then continue in the
blood of her purifying three and thirty
days; she shall touch no hallowed thing,
nor come into the sanctuary, until the
days of her purifying be fulfilled.
5 But if she bear a maid child, then she
shall be unclean two weeks, as in her
separation: and she shall continue in the
blood of her purifying threescore and six
days.
6 And when the days of her purifying
are fulfilled, for a son, or for a daughter,
she shall bring a [a]lamb of the first year
for a burnt-offering, and a young
pigeon, or a turtledove, for a sin-offering,
unto the door of the tabernacle of
the congregation, unto the priest:
7 Who shall offer it before the LORD,
and make an [b]atonement for her; and
she shall be cleansed from the issue of
her blood. This *is* the law for her that
hath born a male or a female.
8 And if she be not [c]able to bring a
lamb, then she shall [d]bring two turtles, or
two young pigeons; the one for the burnt-offering,
and the other for a sin-offering:
and the priest shall make an [b]atonement
for her, and she shall be clean.

CHAPTER 13.

A holy God—a holy people:
(3) *leprosy—Type of sin as in*
Rom. 6:12–14; 1 John 1:8.

AND the LORD spake unto Moses and
Aaron, saying,
2 When a man shall have in the skin of
his flesh a rising, a scab, or bright spot,
and it be in the skin of his flesh *like* the
plague of [1]leprosy; then he shall be
brought unto Aaron the [e]priest, or unto
one of his sons the priests:
3 And the [2]priest shall look on the
plague in the skin of the flesh: and *when*
the hair in the plague is turned white,
and the plague in sight *be* deeper than
the skin of his flesh, it *is* a plague of leprosy:
and the priest shall look on him,
and pronounce him unclean.
4 If the bright spot *be* white in the skin
of his flesh, and in sight *be* not deeper
than the skin, and the hair thereof be not
turned white; then the priest shall shut
up *him that hath* the plague seven days:
5 And the priest shall look on him the
seventh day: and, behold, *if* the plague
in his sight be at a stay, *and* the plague
spread not in the skin; then the priest
shall shut him up seven days more:
6 And the priest shall look on him
again the seventh day: and, behold, *if* the
plague *be* somewhat dark, *and* the plague
spread not in the skin, the priest shall
pronounce him clean: it *is but* a scab: and
he shall [f]wash his clothes, and be clean.
7 But if the scab spread much abroad
in the skin, after that he hath been seen
of the priest for his cleansing, he shall be
seen of the priest again:
8 And *if* the priest see that, behold, the
scab spreadeth in the skin, then the
priest shall pronounce him unclean: it *is*
a leprosy.
9 When the plague of leprosy is in a
man, then he shall be brought unto the
priest;
10 And the [g]priest shall see *him*: and,
behold, *if* the rising *be* white in the skin,
and it have turned the hair white, and
there be quick raw flesh in the rising;
11 It *is* an old leprosy in the skin of his
flesh, and the priest shall pronounce him
unclean, and shall not shut him up: for
he *is* unclean.
12 And if a leprosy break out abroad
in the skin, and the leprosy cover all the
skin of *him that hath* the plague from his
head even to his foot, wheresoever the
priest looketh;

B.C. 1490.

a Cf. John 1:29; 1 Pet. 1:18-19.
b See Ex. 29:33, *note.*
c Lev. 5:7.
d Lk. 2:22-24.
e Deut. 17:8, 9; 24:8; Mal. 2:7; Lk. 17:14.
f Psa. 19:12; John 13:8, 10.
g Num. 12:10, 12; 2 Ki. 5:27; 2 Chr. 26:19-20; John 3:19, 20.

[1] **(13:2)** Leprosy speaks of sin as (1) in the blood; (2) becoming overt in loathsome ways; (3) incurable by human means. The anti-type as applied to the people of God is "sin," demanding self-judgment (1 Cor. 11:31); and "sins," demanding confession and cleansing (1 John 1:9).

[2] **(13:3)** Some have found in the regulations of this chapter concerning an inquest by the priests of a case of leprosy, elaborate provisions for the exercise of discipline in the local church. No little self-righteousness and cruelty have come in thereby. The *explicit* instructions of the N.T. are the alone and sufficient rule of discipline.

B.C. 1490.

13 Then the priest shall consider: and, behold, *if* the leprosy have covered all his flesh, he shall pronounce *him* clean *that hath* the plague: it is all turned white: he *is* clean.

14 But when raw flesh appeareth in him, he shall be unclean.

15 And the priest shall see the raw flesh, and pronounce him to be unclean: *for* the raw flesh *is* unclean: it *is* a leprosy.

16 Or if the raw flesh turn again, and be changed unto white, he shall come unto the priest;

17 And the priest shall see him: and, behold, *if* the plague be turned into white; then the priest shall pronounce *him* clean *that hath* the plague: he *is* clean.

18 The flesh also, in which, *even* in the skin thereof, was a boil, and is healed,

19 And in the place of the boil there be a white rising, or a bright spot, white, and somewhat reddish, and it be shewed to the priest;

20 And if, when the priest seeth it, behold, it *be* in sight lower than the skin, and the hair thereof be turned white; the priest shall pronounce him unclean: it *is* a plague of leprosy broken out of the boil.

21 But if the priest look on it, and, behold, *there be* no white hairs therein, and *if* it *be* not lower than the skin, but *be* somewhat dark; then the priest shall shut him up seven days:

22 And if it spread much abroad in the skin, then the priest shall pronounce him unclean: it *is* a plague.

23 But if the bright spot stay in his place, *and* spread not, it *is* a burning boil; and the priest shall pronounce him clean.

24 Or if there be *any* flesh, in the skin whereof *there is* a hot [a]burning, and the quick *flesh* that burneth have a white bright spot, somewhat reddish, or white;

25 Then the priest shall look upon it: and, behold, *if* the hair in the bright spot be turned white, and it *be in* sight deeper than the skin; it *is* a leprosy broken out of the burning: wherefore the priest shall pronounce him unclean: it *is* the plague of leprosy.

26 But if the priest look on it, and, behold, *there be* no white hair in the bright spot, and it *be* no lower than the *other* skin, but *be* somewhat dark; then the priest shall shut him up seven days:

27 And the priest shall look upon him the seventh day: *and* if it be spread much abroad in the skin, then the priest shall pronounce him unclean: it *is* the plague of leprosy.

28 And if the bright spot stay in his place, *and* spread not in the skin, but it *be* somewhat dark; it *is* a rising of the burning, and the priest shall pronounce him clean: for it *is* an inflammation of the burning.

29 If a man or woman have a [b]plague upon the head or the beard;

30 Then the priest shall see the plague: and, behold, if it *be* in sight deeper than the skin; *and there be* in it a yellow thin hair; then the priest shall pronounce him unclean: it *is* a dry scall, *even* a leprosy upon the head or beard.

31 And if the priest look on the plague of the scall, and, behold, it *be* not in sight deeper than the skin, and *that there is* no black hair in it; then the priest shall shut up *him that hath* the plague of the scall [c]seven days:

32 And in the seventh day the priest shall look on the plague: and, behold, *if* the scall spread not, and there be in it no yellow hair, and the scall *be* not in sight deeper than the skin;

33 He shall be shaven, but the scall shall he not shave; and the priest shall shut up *him that hath* the scall seven days more:

34 And in the seventh day the priest shall look on the scall: and, behold, *if* the scall be not spread in the skin, nor *be* in sight deeper than the skin; then the priest shall pronounce him clean: and he shall wash his clothes, and be clean.

35 But if the scall [d]spread much in the skin after his cleansing;

36 Then the priest shall look on him: and, behold, if the scall be spread in the skin, the priest shall not seek for yellow hair; he *is* unclean.

37 But if the scall be in his sight at a stay, and *that* there is black hair grown up therein; the scall is healed, he *is* clean: and the priest shall pronounce him clean.

38 If a man also or a woman have in the skin of their flesh bright spots, *even* white bright spots;

39 Then the priest shall look: and, behold, *if* the bright spots in the skin of

a Isa. 3:24.
b 1 Ki. 8:38; 2 Chr. 6:29; Isa. 1:5.
c vs. 4, 6.
d vs. 7, 27.

their flesh *be* darkish white; it *is* a freckled
spot *that* groweth in the skin; he *is* clean.
40 And the man whose hair is fallen
off his head, he *is* bald; *yet is* he clean.
41 And he that hath his hair fallen off
from the part of his head toward his
face, he *is* forehead bald: *yet is* he clean.
42 And if there be in the bald head, or
bald forehead, a white reddish sore; it *is*
a leprosy sprung up in his bald head, or
his bald forehead.
43 Then the priest shall look upon it:
and, behold, *if* the rising of the sore *be*
white reddish in his bald head, or in his
bald forehead, as the leprosy appeareth
in the skin of the flesh;
44 He is a leprous man, he *is* unclean:
the priest shall pronounce him utterly
unclean; his plague *is* in his [a]head.
45 And the leper in whom the plague
is, his clothes shall be [b]rent, and his head
[c]bare, and he shall put a covering upon
his upper lip, and shall cry, [d]Unclean,
unclean.
46 All the days wherein the plague
shall be in him he shall be defiled; he *is*
unclean: he shall dwell [e]alone; without
the camp *shall* his habitation *be*.
47 The garment also that the plague of
leprosy is in, *whether it be* a woollen garment, or a linen garment;
48 Whether *it be* in the warp, or woof;
of linen, or of woollen; whether in a
skin, or in any thing made of skin;
49 And if the plague be greenish or
reddish in the garment, or in the skin,
either in the warp, or in the woof, or in
any thing of skin; it *is* a plague of leprosy,
and shall be shewed unto the priest:
50 And the priest shall look upon the
plague, and shut up *it that hath* the
plague seven days:
51 And he shall look on the plague on
the seventh day: if the plague be spread
in the garment, either in the warp, or in
the woof, or in a skin, *or* in any work
that is made of skin; the plague *is* a fretting leprosy; it *is* unclean.
52 He shall therefore burn that garment, whether warp or woof, in woollen
or in linen, or any thing of skin, wherein

B.C. 1490.

a Isa. 1:5.

b 2 Sam. 13:19; Ezra 9:3; Job 1:20; Jer. 36:24; Joel 2:13.

c Lev. 10:6; 21:10.

d Cf. Job 40:4; 42:6; Psa. 51:3, 5; Isa. 6:5; 64:6; Lk. 5:8.

e 2 Chr. 26:21; Psa. 38:11.

the plague is: for it *is* a fretting leprosy; it
shall be burnt in the fire.
53 And if the priest shall look, and,
behold, the plague be not spread in the
garment, either in the warp, or in the
woof, or in any thing of skin;
54 Then the priest shall command that
they wash *the thing* wherein the plague *is*,
and he shall shut it up seven days more:
55 And the priest shall look on the
plague, after that it is washed: and,
behold, *if* the plague have not changed
his colour, and the plague be not spread;
it *is* unclean; thou shalt burn it in the
fire; it *is* fret inward, *whether* it *be* bare
within or without.
56 And if the priest look, and, behold,
the plague *be* somewhat dark after the
washing of it; then he shall rend it out of
the garment, or out of the skin, or out of
the warp, or out of the woof:
57 And if it appear still in the garment,
either in the warp, or in the woof, or in
any thing of skin; it *is* a spreading *plague*:
thou shalt burn that wherein the plague
is with fire.
58 And the garment, either warp, or
woof, or whatsoever thing of skin *it be*,
which thou shalt wash, if the plague be
departed from them, then it shall be
washed the second time, and shall be
clean.
59 This *is* the law of the plague of leprosy in a garment of woollen or linen,
either in the warp, or woof, or any thing
of skins, to pronounce it clean, or to pronounce it unclean.

CHAPTER 14.

A holy God—a holy people:
(4) the law of the leper's cleansing.

And the LORD spake unto Moses,
saying,
2 This shall be the law of the leper in
the day of his cleansing: He shall be
brought unto the priest:
3 And the priest shall go [1]forth out of
the camp; and the priest shall look, and,
behold, *if* the plague of leprosy be
healed in the leper;
4 Then shall the priest command to

[1] **(14:3)** As a type of Gospel salvation the points are: (1) The leper does nothing (Rom. 4:4, 5); (2) the priest seeks the leper, not the leper the priest (Lk. 19:10), (3) "without shedding of blood is no remission" (Heb. 9:22); (4) "and if Christ be not raised, your faith is vain (1 Cor. 15:17).

B.C. 1490.

take for him that is to be cleansed two
[1]birds alive *and* clean, [a]and cedar wood,
and scarlet, and hyssop:
5 And the priest shall command that
one of the birds be killed in an earthen
[2]vessel over running water:
6 As for the living bird, he shall take it,
and the cedar wood, and the scarlet, and
the hyssop, and shall dip them and the
living bird in the blood of the bird *that*
was killed over the running water:
7 And he shall sprinkle upon him that
is to be cleansed from the leprosy seven
times, and shall pronounce him clean,
and shall let the living bird loose into the
open field.
8 And he that is to be cleansed shall
wash his clothes, and shave off all his
hair, and wash himself in water, that he
may be clean: and after that he shall
come into the camp, and shall tarry
abroad out of his tent seven days.
9 But it shall be on the seventh day, that
he shall shave all his hair off his head and
his beard and his eyebrows, even all his
hair he shall shave off: and he shall wash
his clothes, also he shall wash his flesh in
water, and he shall be clean.
10 And on the eighth day he shall take
two he lambs without blemish, and one
ewe lamb of the first year without blemish, and three tenth deals of fine flour *for*
a [b]meat-offering, mingled with oil, and
one [c]log of oil.
11 And the priest that maketh *him*
clean shall present the man that is to be
made clean, and those things, before the
LORD, *at* the door of the tabernacle of the
congregation:
12 And the [d]priest shall take one he
lamb, and offer him for a [e]trespass-offer-
ing, and the log of oil, and wave them *for*
a wave-offering before the LORD:
13 And he shall slay the lamb in the
place where he shall kill the sin-offering
and the burnt-offering, in the holy place:
for as the sin-offering *is* the priest's, *so is*
the trespass-offering: it *is* most holy:
14 And the priest shall take *some* of the
blood of the trespass-offering, and the
priest shall put *it* upon the tip of the
right ear of him that is to be cleansed,
and upon the thumb of his right hand,
and upon the great toe of his right foot:
15 And the priest shall take *some* of the
log of oil, and pour *it* into the palm of
his own left hand:
16 And the priest shall dip his right
finger in the oil that *is* in his left hand,
and shall sprinkle of the oil with his finger seven times before the LORD:
17 And of the rest of the oil that *is* in his
hand shall the priest put upon the tip of
the right ear of him that is to be cleansed,
and upon the thumb of his right hand,
and upon the great toe of his right foot,
upon the blood of the trespass-offering:
18 And the remnant of the oil that *is* in
the priest's hand he shall pour upon the
head of him that is to be cleansed: and
the priest shall make an [f]atonement for
him before the LORD.
19 And the priest shall offer the [g]sin-
offering, and make an [f]atonement for
him that is to be cleansed from his
uncleanness; and afterward he shall kill
the burnt-offering:
20 And the priest shall offer the burnt-
offering and the [b]meat-offering upon the
altar: and the priest shall make an [f]atone-
ment for him, and he shall be clean.
21 And if he *be* poor, and cannot get so
much; then he shall take one lamb *for* a
trespass-offering to be waved, to make
an [f]atonement for him, and one tenth
deal of fine flour mingled with oil for a
[b]meat-offering, and a log of oil;
22 And two turtledoves, or two young
pigeons, such as he is able to get; and the
one shall be a sin-offering, and the other
a burnt-offering.
23 And he shall bring them on the
eighth day for his cleansing unto the
priest, unto the door of the tabernacle of
the congregation, before the LORD.
24 And the priest shall take the lamb
of the trespass-offering, and the log of

a Num. 19:6; Heb. 9:19.
b Lit. *meal.*
c One log = .96 pts.; also vs. 12, 15, 21, 24.
d Lev. 5:18; 6:6.
e Isa. 53:10.
f See Ex. 29:33, *note.*
g Cf. 2 Cor. 5:21.

[1]**(14:4)** The bird slain, and the live bird, dipped in blood and released, present the two aspects of salvation in Rom. 4:25; "delivered for our offences, and raised again for our justification."

[2]**(14:5)** The earthen vessel typifies the humanity of Christ, as the running water typifies the Holy Spirit as the "Spirit of life" (Rom. 8:2): "put to death in the flesh, but quickened by the Spirit" (1 Pet. 3:18).

B.C. 1490.

oil, and the priest shall wave them *for* a
wave-offering before the LORD:
25 And he shall kill the lamb of the
trespass-offering, and the priest shall
take *some* of the blood of the trespass-
offering, and put *it* upon the tip of the
right ear of him that is to be cleansed,
and upon the thumb of his right hand,
and upon the great toe of his right foot:
26 And the priest shall pour of the oil
into the palm of his own left hand:
27 And the priest shall sprinkle with
his right finger *some* of the oil that *is* in his
left hand seven times before the LORD:
28 And the priest shall put of the oil
that *is* in his hand upon the tip of the right
ear of him that is to be cleansed, and upon
the thumb of his right hand, and upon the
great toe of his right foot, upon the place
of the blood of the trespass-offering:
29 And the rest of the oil that *is* in the
priest's hand he shall put upon the head
of him that is to be cleansed, to make an
[a]atonement for him before the LORD.
30 And he shall offer the one of the
turtledoves, or of the young pigeons,
such as he can get;
31 *Even* such as he is able to get, the
one *for* a sin-offering, and the other *for* a
burnt-offering, with the [b]meat-offering:
and the priest shall make an [a]atonement
for him that is to be cleansed before the
LORD.
32 This *is* the law *of him* in whom *is* the
plague of leprosy, whose hand is not
[c]able to get *that which pertaineth* to his
cleansing.
33 And the LORD spake unto Moses
and unto Aaron, saying,
34 When ye be come into the land of
Canaan, which I give to [d]you for a possession, and I put the plague of leprosy
in a house of the land of your possession;
35 And he that owneth the house shall
come and tell the priest, saying, It
seemeth to me *there is* as it were a plague
in the house:
36 Then the priest shall command that
they [e]empty the house, before the priest
go *into it* to see the plague, that all that *is*
in the house be not made unclean: and
afterward the priest shall go in to see the
house:
37 And he shall look on the plague,
and, behold, *if* the plague *be* in the walls
of the house with hollow strakes, greenish or reddish, which in sight *are* lower
than the wall;
38 Then the priest shall go out of the
house to the door of the house, and shut
up the house seven days:
39 And the priest shall come again the
seventh day, and shall look: and, behold,
if the plague be spread in the walls of the
house;
40 Then the priest shall command that
they take away the stones in which the
plague *is*, and they shall cast them into
an unclean place without the city:
41 And he shall cause the house to be
scraped within round about, and they
shall pour out the dust that they scrape
off without the city into an unclean place:
42 And they shall take other stones,
and put *them* in the place of those stones;
and he shall take other morter, and shall
plaister the house.
43 And if the plague come again, and
break out in the house, after that he hath
taken away the stones, and after he hath
scraped the house, and after it is plaistered;
44 Then the priest shall come and
look, and, behold, *if* the plague be
spread in the house, [f]it *is* a fretting leprosy in the house: it *is* unclean.
45 And he shall [g]break down the
house, the stones of it, and the timber
thereof, and all the morter of the house;
and he shall carry *them* forth out of the
city into an unclean place.
46 Moreover he that goeth into the
house all the while that it is shut up
shall be unclean until the even.
47 And he that lieth in the house shall
wash his clothes; and he that eateth in
the house shall wash his clothes.
48 And if the priest shall come in, and
look *upon it*, and, behold, the plague
hath not spread in the house, after the
house was plaistered: then the priest
shall pronounce the house clean,
because the plague is healed.
49 And he shall take to cleanse the
house two birds, and cedar wood, and
scarlet, and hyssop:
50 And he shall kill the one of the
birds in an earthen vessel over running
water:
51 And he shall take the cedar wood,
and the hyssop, and the scarlet, and the
living bird, and dip them in the blood of
the slain bird, and in the running water,
and sprinkle the house seven times:
52 And he shall cleanse the house with
the blood of the bird, and with the

a See Ex. 29:33, *note.*
b Lit. *meal.*
c Psa. 72:12, 14.
d Gen. 12:7; 13:17; 17:8; Deut. 32:49.
e Or, *prepare.*
f Lev. 13:51; Zech. 5:4.
g 1 Ki. 9:6, 9; 2 Ki. 10:27; 18:4; Jer. 52:13.

running water, and with the living bird, and with the cedar wood, and with the hyssop, and with the scarlet:

53 But he shall let go the living bird out of the city into the open fields, and make an [a]atonement for the house: and it shall be clean.

54 This *is* the law for all manner of [b]plague of leprosy, and scall,

55 And for the leprosy of a garment, and of a house,

56 And for a rising, and for a scab, and for a bright spot:

57 To teach when *it is* unclean, and when *it is* clean: this *is* the law of leprosy.

CHAPTER 15.

A holy God—a holy people:
(5) *the imperative of cleansing*
(John 13:3–10; Eph. 5:25–27; 1 John 1:9).

And the LORD spake unto Moses and to Aaron, saying,

2 Speak unto the children of Israel, and say unto them, When any man hath a running [c]issue out of his flesh, *because of* his issue he *is* unclean.

3 And this shall be his uncleanness in his issue: whether his flesh run with his issue, or his flesh be stopped from his issue, it *is* his uncleanness.

4 Every bed, whereon he lieth that hath the issue, is unclean: and every thing, whereon he sitteth, shall be unclean.

5 And whosoever toucheth his bed shall wash his [d]clothes, and bathe *himself* in water, and be unclean until the even.

6 And he that sitteth on *any* thing whereon he sat that hath the issue shall wash his clothes, and bathe *himself* in water, and be unclean until the even.

7 And he that toucheth the flesh of him that hath the issue shall wash his clothes, and bathe *himself* in water, and be unclean until the even.

8 And if he that hath the issue spit upon him that is clean; then he shall wash his clothes, and bathe *himself* in water, and be unclean until the even.

9 And what saddle soever he rideth upon that hath the issue shall be unclean.

10 And whosoever toucheth any thing that was under him shall be unclean until the even: and he that beareth *any of* those things shall wash his clothes, and bathe *himself* in water, and be unclean until the even.

11 And whomsoever he toucheth that hath the issue, and hath not rinsed his hands in water, he shall wash his clothes, and bathe *himself* in water, and be unclean until the even.

12 And the [e]vessel of earth, that he toucheth which hath the issue, shall be broken: and every vessel of wood shall be rinsed in water.

13 And when he that hath an issue is cleansed of his issue; then he shall number to [f]himself seven days for his cleansing, and wash his clothes, and bathe his flesh in running water, and shall be clean.

14 And on the eighth day he shall take to him [g]two turtledoves, or two young pigeons, and come before the LORD unto the door of the tabernacle of the congregation, and give them unto the priest:

15 And the priest shall offer them, the one *for* a sin-offering, and the other *for* a burnt-offering; and the priest shall make an [a]atonement for him before the LORD for his issue.

16 And if any man's seed of copulation go out from him, then he shall wash all his flesh in water, and be unclean until the even.

17 And every garment, and every skin, whereon is the seed of copulation, shall be washed with water, and be unclean until the even.

18 The woman also with whom man shall lie *with* seed of copulation, they shall *both* bathe *themselves* in water, and be unclean until the even.

19 And if a woman have an issue, *and* her issue in her flesh be blood, she shall be put apart seven days: and whosoever toucheth her shall be unclean until the even.

20 And every thing that she lieth upon in her separation shall be unclean: every thing also that she sitteth upon shall be unclean.

21 And whosoever toucheth her bed shall wash his clothes, and bathe *himself* in water, and be unclean until the even.

22 And whosoever toucheth any thing that she sat upon shall wash his clothes, and bathe *himself* in water, and be unclean until the even.

23 And if it *be* on *her* bed, or on any thing whereon she sitteth, when he

B.C. 1490.

a See Ex. 29:33, *note.*

b Lev. 13:30.

c Lev. 22:4; Num. 5:2; 2 Sam. 3:29.

d Lev. 22:4; Deut. 23:10.

e Lev. 6:28; 11:33.

f v. 28; Lev. 14:8; Num. 19:11-12.

g Lev. 14:22, 30-31.

toucheth it, he shall be unclean until the even.

24 And if any man lie with her at all, and her flowers be upon him, he shall be unclean seven days; and all the bed whereon he lieth shall be unclean.

25 And if a woman have an issue of her blood many days out of the time of her separation, or if it run beyond the time of her separation; all the days of the issue of her uncleanness shall be as the days of her separation: she *shall be* unclean.

26 Every bed whereon she lieth all the days of her issue shall be unto her as the bed of her separation: and whatsoever she sitteth upon shall be unclean, as the uncleanness of her separation.

27 And whosoever toucheth those things shall be unclean, and shall wash his clothes, and bathe *himself* in water, and be unclean until the even.

28 But if she be cleansed of her issue, then she shall number to herself seven days, and after that she shall be clean.

29 And on the eighth day she shall take unto her two turtles, or two young pigeons, and bring them unto the priest, to the door of the tabernacle of the congregation.

30 And the priest shall offer the one *for* a sin-offering, and the other *for* a burnt-offering; and the priest shall make an [a]atonement for her before the LORD for the issue of her uncleanness.

31 Thus shall ye separate the children of Israel from their uncleanness; that they die not in their uncleanness, when they defile my tabernacle that *is* among them.

32 This *is* the law of him that hath an issue, and *of him* whose seed goeth from him, and is defiled therewith;

33 And of her that is sick of her flowers, and of him that hath an issue, of the man, and of the woman, and of him that lieth with her that is unclean.

CHAPTER 16.

The day of atonement:
Christ as High Priest and sacrifice
(Heb. 9:1–14).

AND the LORD spake unto [b]Moses after the death of the [c]two sons of Aaron, when they offered before the LORD, and died;

2 And the LORD said unto Moses, Speak unto Aaron thy brother, that he come not at all [d]times into the holy *place* within the vail before the mercy seat, which *is* upon the ark; that he die not: for I will appear in the cloud upon the mercy seat.

3 Thus shall Aaron come into the holy *place*: with a young bullock for a sin-offering, and a ram for a burnt-offering.

4 He shall put on the holy linen coat, and he shall have the linen breeches upon his flesh, and shall be girded with a linen girdle, and with the linen mitre shall he be attired: these *are* holy garments; therefore shall he wash his flesh in water, and *so* put them on.

5 And he shall take of the congregation of the children of Israel two kids of the [1]goats for a [e]sin-offering, and one ram for a burnt-offering.

B.C. 1490.

a See Ex. 29:33, *note.*

b *Israel (history).* vs. 1-34; Num. 3:1-10. (Gen. 12:2, 3; Rom. 11:26.)

c Lev. 10:1-2.

d Ex. 30:10; Lev. 16:34; Heb. 9:7-8; cf. Heb. 4:16; 10:19.

e *Sacrifice (typical).* vs. 2-34; Lev. 17:11. (Gen. 4:4; Heb. 10:18.)

1(16:5) The two goats. The offering of the high priest for himself has no anti-type in Christ (Heb. 7:26, 27). The *typical* interest centres upon the two goats and the high priest. Typically (1) all is done by the high priest (Heb. 1:3, "by Himself"), the people only bring the sacrifice (Mt. 26:47; 27:24, 25). (2) The goat slain (Jehovah's lot) is that aspect of Christ's death which vindicates the holiness and righteousness of God as expressed in the law (Rom. 3:24-26), and is *expiatory.* (3) The living goat typifies that aspect of Christ's work which puts *away* our sins from before God (Heb. 9:26; Rom. 8:33, 34). (4) The high priest entering the holiest, typifies Christ entering "heaven itself" with "His own blood" for us (Heb. 9:11, 12). His blood makes that to be a "throne of grace," and "mercy seat," which else must have been a throne of judgment. (5) For us, the priests of the New Covenant, there is what Israel never had, a rent veil (Mt. 27:51; Heb. 10:19, 20). So that, for worship and blessing, we enter, in virtue of His blood, where He is, into the holiest (Heb. 4:14-16; 10:19-22).

The atonement of Christ, as interpreted by the O.T. sacrificial types, has these necessary elements: (1) It is substitutionary—the offering takes the offerer's place in death. (2) The law is not evaded but honored—every sacrificial death was an execution of the sentence of the law. (3) The sinlessness of Him who bore our sins is expressed in every animal sacrifice—it must be without blemish. (4) The

B.C. 1490.

6 And Aaron shall offer his bullock of the sin-offering, which *is* for himself, and make an [1a]atonement for himself, and for his house.

7 And he shall take the two goats, and present them before the LORD *at* the door of the tabernacle of the congregation.

8 And Aaron shall cast lots upon the two goats; one lot for the LORD, and the other lot for the scapegoat.

9 And Aaron shall bring the goat upon which the LORD'S lot fell, and offer him *for* a sin-offering.

10 But the goat, on which the lot fell to be the scapegoat, shall be presented alive before the LORD, to make an [b]atonement with him, *and* to let him go for a scapegoat into the wilderness.

11 And Aaron shall bring the bullock of the sin-offering, which *is* for himself, and shall make an [a]atonement for himself, and for his house, and shall kill the bullock of the sin-offering which *is* for himself:

12 And he shall take a censer full of burning coals of fire from off the altar before the LORD, and his hands full of sweet incense beaten small, and bring *it* within the vail:

13 And he shall put the incense upon the fire before the LORD, that the cloud of the incense may cover the mercy seat that *is* upon the testimony, that he die not:

14 And he shall take of the blood of the bullock, and sprinkle *it* with his finger upon the mercy seat eastward; and before the mercy seat shall he sprinkle of the blood with his finger seven times.

15 Then shall he kill the goat of the sin-offering, that *is* for the people, and bring his blood within the vail, and do with that blood as he did with the blood of the bullock, and sprinkle it upon the mercy seat, and before the mercy seat:

16 And he shall make an [a]atonement for the holy *place*, because of the uncleanness of the children of Israel, and because of their transgressions in all their sins: and so shall he do for the tabernacle of the congregation, that remaineth among them in the midst of their uncleanness.

17 And there shall be no man in the tabernacle of the congregation when he goeth in to make an [a]atonement in the holy *place*, until he come out, and have made an atonement for himself, and for his household, and for all the congregation of Israel.

18 And he shall go [2]out unto the altar that *is* before the LORD, and make an [a]atonement for it; and shall take of the blood of the bullock, and of the blood of the goat, and put *it* upon the horns of the altar round about.

19 And he shall sprinkle of the blood upon it with his finger seven times, and cleanse it, and hallow it from the uncleanness of the children of Israel.

20 And when he hath made an end of [c]reconciling the holy *place*, and the tabernacle of the congregation, and the altar, he shall bring the live goat:

21 And Aaron shall lay both his hands

a See Ex. 29:33, *note.*
b Cf. Isa. 53:5-6; Heb. 7:27; 9:23-24.
c Heb. *kaphar* = covering. See Dan. 9:24, *note.*

effect of the atoning work of Christ is typified *(a)* in the promises, "it shall be forgiven him"; and *(b)* in the peace-offering, the expression of fellowship—the highest privilege of the saint. See Ex. 29:33, *note.*

[1]**(16:6)** Atonement. The biblical use and meaning of the word must be sharply distinguished from its use in theology. In theology it is a term which covers the whole sacrificial and redemptive work of Christ. In the O.T. atonement is the English word used to translate the Hebrew words which mean "cover," "coverings," or "to cover." Atonement (at-one-ment) is, therefore, not a translation of the Hebrew, but a purely theologic concept. The Levitical offerings "covered" the sins of Israel until, and in anticipation of the Cross, but did not "take away" (Heb. 10:4) those sins. These were the "sins done aforetime" ("covered" meantime by the Levitical sacrifices), which God "passed over" (Rom. 3:25)—for which "passing over" God's righteousness was never vindicated until, in the Cross, Jesus Christ was "set forth a propitiation." See "Propitiation," Rom. 3:25, *note.* It was the Cross, not the Levitical sacrifices which made "at-one-ment." The O.T. sacrifices enabled God to go on with a guilty people because they typified the Cross. To the *offerer* they were the confession of his desert of death, and the expression of his faith; to God they were the "shadows" (Heb. 10:1) of which Christ was the reality.

[2]**(16:18)** Dispensationally, for Israel, this is yet future; the High Priest is still in the holiest. When He comes out to His ancient people they will be converted and restored (Rom. 11:23-27; Zech. 12:10, 12; 13:1; Rev. 1:7). Meantime, believers of this dispensation as priests (1 Pet. 2:9) enter into the holiest where He is (Heb. 10:19-22).

B.C. 1490.

upon the head of the live goat, and confess over him all the iniquities of the
children of Israel, and all their transgressions in all their sins, putting them upon
the head of the goat, and shall send *him*
away by the hand of a fit man into the
wilderness:
22 And the goat shall bear upon him
all their iniquities unto a land not inhabited: and he shall let go the goat in the
wilderness.
23 And Aaron shall come into the
tabernacle of the congregation, and shall
put off the linen garments, which he put
on when he went into the holy *place*, and
shall leave them there:
24 And he shall wash his flesh with
water in the holy place, and put on his
garments, and come forth, and offer his
burnt-offering, and the burnt-offering of
the people, and make an [a]atonement for
himself, and for the people.
25 And the [b]fat of the sin-offering
shall he burn upon the altar.
26 And he that let go the goat for the
scapegoat shall wash his clothes, and
bathe his flesh in water, and afterward
come into the camp.
27 And the bullock *for* the sin-offering,
and the goat *for* the sin-offering, whose
blood was brought in to make [a]atone-
ment in the holy *place*, shall *one* carry
forth without the camp; and they shall
burn in the fire their skins, and their
flesh, and their dung.
28 And he that burneth them shall
wash his clothes, and bathe his flesh in
water, and afterward he shall come into
the camp.
29 And *this* shall be a statute for ever
unto you: *that* in the [c]seventh month, on
the tenth *day* of the month, ye shall
afflict your souls, and do no work at all,
whether it be one of your own country, or
a stranger that sojourneth among you:
30 For on that day shall *the priest* make
an [a]atonement for you, to cleanse you,
that ye may be clean from all your sins
before the LORD.
31 It *shall be* a sabbath of rest unto you,
and ye shall afflict your souls, by a
statute for ever.
32 And the priest, whom he shall
anoint, and whom he shall consecrate to
minister in the priest's office in his
father's stead, shall make the [a]atone-
ment, and shall put on the linen clothes,
even the holy garments:
33 And he shall make an [a]atonement
for the holy sanctuary, and he shall make
an [a]atonement for the tabernacle of the
congregation, and for the altar, and he
shall make an [a]atonement for the priests,
and for all the people of the congregation.
34 And this shall be an everlasting
statute unto you, to make an [a]atonement
for the children of Israel for all their sins
once a year. And he did as the LORD
commanded [d]Moses.

CHAPTER 17.

But one place of sacrifice.

And the LORD spake unto Moses,
saying,
2 Speak unto Aaron, and unto his sons,
and unto all the children of Israel, and
say unto them; This *is* the thing which
the LORD hath commanded, saying,
3 What man soever *there be* of the
house of Israel, that killeth an ox, or
lamb, or goat, in the camp, or that killeth
it out of the camp,
4 And bringeth it not unto the door of
the tabernacle of the congregation, to
offer an offering unto the LORD before
the tabernacle of the LORD; blood shall
be imputed unto that man; he hath shed
blood; and that man shall be cut off from
among his people:
5 To the [e]end that the children of Israel
may bring their sacrifices, which they
offer in the open field, even that they
may bring them unto the LORD, unto the
door of the tabernacle of the congregation, unto the priest, and offer them *for*
peace-offerings unto the LORD.
6 And the priest shall sprinkle the
blood upon the altar of the LORD *at* the
door of the tabernacle of the congregation, and [f]burn the fat for a sweet savour
unto the LORD.
7 And they shall no more offer their
sacrifices unto [g]devils, after whom they
have gone a whoring. This shall be a
statute for ever unto them throughout
their generations.
8 And thou shalt say unto them,
Whatsoever man *there be* of the house of
Israel, or of the strangers which sojourn
among you, that offereth a burnt-offering or sacrifice,
9 And [h]bringeth it not unto the door
of the tabernacle of the congregation, to
offer it unto the LORD; even that man
shall be cut off from among his people.

a See Ex. 29:33, *note.*

b Lev. 1:8, *ref.*

c i.e. *October.*

d *Law (of Moses).* Lev. 26:2. (Ex. 19:1; Gal. 3:1-29.)

e Psa. 87:2; Ezk. 20:28; Mal. 1:11; Heb. 13:10; cf. Deut. 12:1-27.

f Ex. 29:13.

g *Hairy one.* Deut. 32:17; 2 Chr. 11:15.

h v. 4.

The explanation and sanctity of "blood."

10 And whatsoever man *there be* of the house of Israel, or of the strangers that sojourn among you, that eateth any manner of blood; I will even set my face against that soul that eateth blood, and will cut him off from among his people.

11 For the life of the flesh *is* in the blood: and I have given it to you upon the [1]altar to make an [a]atonement for your [b]souls: for it *is* the [2]blood *that* maketh an [a]atonement for the soul.

12 Therefore I said unto the children of Israel, No soul of you shall eat blood, neither shall any stranger that sojourneth among you eat blood.

13 And whatsoever man *there be* of the children of Israel, or of the strangers that sojourn among you, which hunteth and catcheth any beast or fowl that may be eaten; he shall even pour out the blood thereof, and cover it with dust.

14 For *it is* the life of all flesh; the blood of it *is* for the life thereof: therefore I said unto the children of Israel, Ye shall eat the blood of no manner of flesh: for the life of all flesh *is* the blood thereof: whosoever eateth it shall be cut off.

15 And every soul that eateth that which died *of itself*, or that which was torn *with beasts, whether it be* one of your own country, or a stranger, he shall both wash his clothes, and bathe *himself* in water, and be unclean until the even: then shall he be clean.

16 But if he wash *them* not, nor bathe his flesh; then he shall bear his iniquity.

CHAPTER 18.

The relationships and walk of God's earthly people.

And the LORD spake unto Moses, saying,

2 Speak unto the children of Israel, and say unto them, I am the LORD your God.

3 After the doings of the land of Egypt, wherein ye dwelt, shall ye not do: and after the doings of the land of Canaan, whither I bring you, shall ye not do: neither shall ye walk in their ordinances.

4 Ye shall do my judgments, and keep mine ordinances, to walk therein: I *am* the LORD your God.

5 Ye shall therefore keep my statutes, and my judgments: which if a man do, he shall live in [c]them: I *am* the LORD.

6 None of you shall approach to any that is near of kin to him, to uncover *their* nakedness: I *am* the LORD.

7 The nakedness of thy father, or the nakedness of thy mother, shalt thou not uncover: she *is* thy mother; thou shalt not uncover her nakedness.

8 The nakedness of thy father's wife shalt thou not uncover: it *is* thy father's nakedness.

9 The nakedness of thy sister, the daughter of thy father, or daughter of thy mother, *whether she be* born at home, or born abroad, *even* their nakedness thou shalt not uncover.

10 The nakedness of thy son's daughter, or of thy daughter's daughter, *even* their nakedness thou shalt not uncover: for theirs *is* thine own nakedness.

11 The nakedness of thy father's wife's daughter, begotten of thy father, she *is* thy sister, thou shalt not uncover her nakedness.

12 Thou shalt not uncover the nakedness of thy father's sister: she *is* thy father's near kinswoman.

13 Thou shalt not uncover the nakedness of thy mother's sister: for she *is* thy mother's near kinswoman.

14 Thou shalt not uncover the nakedness of thy father's brother, thou shalt

B.C. 1490.

a See Ex. 29:33, *note.*

b *Sacrifice (typical).* See *prophetic,* Gen. 3:15. (Gen. 4:4; Heb. 10:18.)

c Rom. 10:5; Gal. 3:12.

[1]**(17:11)** (1) The value of the "life" is the measure of the value of the "blood." This gives the blood of Christ its inconceivable value. When it was shed the sinless God-man gave His life. "It is not possible that the blood of bulls and of goats could take away sins" (Heb. 10:4). (2) It is not the blood in the veins of the sacrifice, but the blood *upon the altar* which is efficacious. The Scripture knows nothing of salvation by the imitation or influence of Christ's life, but only by that life yielded up on the cross.

[2]**(17:11)** The meaning of all sacrifice is here explained. Every offering was an execution of the sentence of the law upon a substitute for the offender, and every such offering pointed forward to that substitutional death of Christ which alone vindicated the righteousness of God in passing over the sins of those who offered the typical sacrifices (Rom. 3:24, 25; Ex. 29:36, *refs.*).

not approach to his wife: she *is* thine
aunt.
15 Thou shalt not uncover the nakedness of thy daughter in law: she *is* thy
son's wife; thou shalt not uncover her
nakedness.
16 Thou shalt not uncover the nakedness of thy brother's wife: it *is* thy
brother's nakedness.
17 Thou shalt not uncover the nakedness of a woman and her daughter, neither shalt thou take her son's daughter,
or her daughter's daughter, to uncover
her nakedness; *for* they *are* her near
kinswomen: it *is* wickedness.
18 Neither shalt thou take a wife to her
sister, to vex *her*, to uncover her nakedness, beside the other in her life *time*.
19 Also thou shalt not approach unto a
woman to uncover her nakedness, as
[a]long as she is put apart for her uncleanness.
20 [b]Moreover thou shalt not lie carnally with thy neighbour's wife, to defile
thyself with her.
21 And thou shalt not let any of thy
seed pass through *the* [c]*fire* to [d]Molech,
neither shalt thou profane the name of
thy God: I *am* the LORD.
22 Thou shalt not lie with [e]mankind,
as with womankind: it *is* abomination.
23 Neither shalt thou lie with any
beast to defile thyself therewith: neither
shall any woman stand before a beast to
lie down thereto: it *is* confusion.
24 Defile not ye yourselves in any of
these things: for in all these the nations
are defiled which I cast out before you:
25 And the land is defiled: therefore I
do visit the iniquity thereof upon it, and
the land itself vomiteth out her inhabitants.
26 Ye shall therefore keep my statutes
and my judgments, and shall not commit *any* of these abominations; *neither*
any of your own nation, nor any
stranger that sojourneth among you:
27 (For all these abominations have
the men of the land done, which *were*
before you, and the land is defiled;)
28 That the land spue not you out also,
when ye defile it, as it spued out the
nations that *were* before you.
29 For whosoever shall commit any of
these abominations, even the souls that
commit *them* shall be cut off from among
their people.
30 Therefore shall ye keep mine ordinance, that *ye* commit not *any one* of
these abominable customs, which were
committed before you, and that ye defile
not yourselves therein: I *am* the LORD
your God.

CHAPTER 19.

The relationships and walk
of God's earthly people, continued.

AND the LORD spake unto Moses,
saying,
2 Speak unto all the congregation of
the children of Israel, and say unto them,
Ye shall be holy: for I the LORD your God
am holy.
3 Ye shall fear every man his [f]mother,
and his father, and [g]keep my [h]sabbaths:
I *am* the LORD your God.
4 Turn ye not unto [i]idols, nor make to
yourselves molten gods: I *am* the LORD
your God.
5 And if ye offer a sacrifice of peace-
offerings unto the LORD, ye shall offer it
at your own will.
6 It shall be eaten the same day ye
offer it, and on the morrow: and if ought
remain until the third day, it shall be
burnt in the fire.
7 And if it be eaten at all on the third
day, it *is* abominable; it shall not be
accepted.
8 Therefore *every one* that eateth it
shall bear his iniquity, because he hath
profaned the hallowed thing of the
LORD: and that soul shall be cut off from
among his people.
9 And when ye reap the harvest of
your land, thou shalt not wholly reap
the corners of thy field, neither shalt
thou gather the gleanings of thy harvest.
10 And thou shalt not glean thy vineyard, neither shalt thou gather *every*
grape of thy vineyard; thou shalt leave
them for the poor and stranger: I *am* the
LORD your God.
11 Ye shall not steal, neither deal falsely, neither lie one to another.
12 And ye shall not swear by my
name [j]falsely, neither shalt thou profane
the name of thy God: I *am* the LORD.
13 Thou shalt not defraud thy neighbour, neither rob *him*: the wages of him
that is hired shall not abide with thee all
night until the morning.
14 Thou shalt not curse the deaf, nor
put a stumblingblock before the blind,
but shalt [k]fear thy God: I *am* the LORD.

B.C. 1490.

a Ezk. 18:6.
b Prov. 6:25-33.
c 2 Ki. 16:3.
d Called *Moloch*, Acts 7:43.
e Rom. 1:27.
f Ex. 20:12; Mt. 15:4; Eph. 6:2.
g Ex. 16:23; 20:8.
h *Sabbath.* vs. 3, 30; Lev. 23:3. (Gen. 2:3; Mt. 12:1.)
i Ex. 20:4; Psa. 96:5; 115:4-7; 1 Cor. 10:14; Col. 3:15.
j Mt. 5:33.
k Psa. 19:9, *note*.

B.C. 1490.

15 Ye shall do no unrighteousness in judgment: thou shalt not respect the person of the poor, nor honour the person of the mighty: *but* in righteousness shalt thou judge thy neighbour.

16 Thou shalt not go up and down *as* a talebearer among thy people: neither shalt thou stand against the blood of thy neighbour: I *am* the LORD.

17 Thou shalt not hate thy brother in thine heart: thou shalt in any wise rebuke thy neighbour, and not suffer sin upon him.

18 Thou shalt not avenge, nor bear any grudge against the children of thy people, but thou shalt [a]love thy neighbour as thyself: I *am* the LORD.

19 Ye shall keep my statutes. Thou shalt not let thy cattle gender with a diverse kind: thou shalt not sow thy field with mingled seed: neither shall a garment mingled of linen and woollen come upon thee.

20 And whosoever lieth carnally with a woman, that *is* a bondmaid, betrothed to an husband, and not at all redeemed, nor freedom given her; she shall be scourged; they shall not be put to death, because she was not free.

21 And he shall bring his trespass-offering unto the LORD, unto the door of the tabernacle of the congregation, *even* a ram for a trespass-offering.

22 And the priest shall make an [b]atonement for him with the ram of the trespass-offering before the LORD for his sin which he hath done: and the sin which he hath done shall be [c]forgiven him.

23 And when ye shall come into the land, and shall have planted all manner of trees for food, then ye shall count the fruit thereof as uncircumcised: three years shall it be as uncircumcised unto you: it shall not be eaten of.

24 But in the fourth year all the fruit thereof shall be holy to praise the LORD *withal*.

25 And in the fifth year shall ye eat of the fruit thereof, that it may yield unto you the increase thereof: I *am* the LORD your God.

26 Ye shall not eat *any thing* with the blood: neither shall ye use enchantment, nor observe times.

27 Ye shall not round the corners of your heads, neither shalt thou mar the corners of thy beard.

28 Ye shall not make any cuttings in your flesh for the dead, nor print any marks upon you: I *am* the LORD.

29 Do not prostitute thy daughter, to cause her to be a whore; lest the land fall to whoredom, and the land become full of wickedness.

30 Ye shall keep my sabbaths, and reverence my sanctuary: I *am* the LORD.

31 Regard not them that have familiar spirits, neither seek after wizards, to be defiled by them: I *am* the LORD your God.

32 Thou shalt rise up before the hoary head, and honour the face of the old man, and [d]fear thy God: I *am* the LORD.

33 And if a stranger sojourn with thee in your land, ye shall not vex him.

34 *But* the stranger that dwelleth with you shall be unto you as one born among you, and thou shalt love him as thyself; for ye were strangers in the land of Egypt: I *am* the LORD your God.

35 Ye shall do no unrighteousness in judgment, in meteyard, in weight, or in measure.

36 Just balances, just weights, a just [e]ephah, and a just [f]hin, shall ye have: I *am* the LORD your God, which brought you out of the land of Egypt.

37 Therefore shall ye observe all my statutes, and all my judgments, and do them: I *am* the LORD.

CHAPTER 20.

The relationships and walk of God's earthly people, continued.

And the LORD spake unto Moses, saying,

2 Again, thou shalt say to the children of Israel, Whosoever *he be* of the children of Israel, or of the strangers that sojourn in Israel, that giveth *any* of his seed unto Molech; he shall surely be put to death: the people of the land shall stone him with stones.

3 And I will set my face against that man, and will cut him off from among his people; because he hath given of his seed unto Molech, to defile my sanctuary, and to profane my holy name.

4 And if the people of the land do any ways hide their eyes from the man, when he giveth of his seed unto Molech, and [g]kill him not:

5 Then I will set my face against that

a Mt. 5:43; 19:19; 22:39; Mk. 12:31; Lk. 10:27; Gal. 5:14; Jas. 2:8.

b See Ex. 29:33, *note.*

c *Forgiveness.* Num. 15:25, 26, 28. (Lev. 4:20; Mt. 26:28.)

d Psa. 19:9, *note.*

e One ephah = 1 bu. 3 pts.

f One hin = about 6 qts.

g Deut. 17:2-5.

man, and against his [a]family, and will
cut him off, and all that go a whoring
after him, to commit whoredom with
Molech, from among their people.
6 [b]And the soul that turneth after such
as have familiar spirits, and after wizards, to go a whoring after them, I will
even set my face against that soul, and
will cut him off from among his people.
7 [c]Sanctify yourselves therefore, and
be ye holy: for I *am* the LORD your God.
8 And ye shall keep my statutes, and do
them: [d]I *am* the LORD which sanctify you.
9 For [e]every one that curseth his father
or his mother shall be surely put to
death: he hath cursed his father or his
mother; his [f]blood *shall be* upon him.
10 And the man that committeth adultery with *another* man's wife, *even he* that
committeth adultery with his neighbour's wife, the adulterer and the adulteress shall surely be put to death.
11 And the man that lieth with his
father's wife hath uncovered his father's
nakedness: both of them shall surely be
put to death; their blood *shall be* upon
them.
12 And if a man lie with his daughter
in law, both of them shall surely be put
to death: they have wrought confusion;
their blood *shall be* upon them.
13 If a man also lie with mankind, as
he lieth with a woman, both of them
have committed an abomination: they
shall surely be put to death; their blood
shall be upon them.
14 And if a man take a wife and her
mother, it *is* wickedness: they shall be
burnt with fire, both he and they; that
there be no wickedness among you.
15 And if a man lie with a beast, he
shall surely be put to death: and ye shall
slay the beast.
16 And if a woman approach unto any
beast, and lie down thereto, thou shalt
kill the woman, and the beast: they shall
surely be put to death; their blood *shall
be* upon them.
17 And if a man shall take his sister, his
father's daughter, or his mother's daughter, and see her nakedness, and she see
his nakedness; it *is* a wicked thing; and
they shall be cut off in the sight of their
people: he hath uncovered his sister's
nakedness; he shall bear his iniquity.

B.C. 1490.

a Ex. 20:5.
b Lev. 19:31.
c Heb. 12:14.
d Ex. 31:13; Deut. 14:2; Ezk. 37:28.
e Ex. 21:17; Prov. 20:20.
f vs. 11, 13, 16, 17.
g *Separation.* vs. 24-26; Num. 6:1-8. (Gen. 12:1; 2 Cor. 6:14-17.)
h Lev. 19:31; 1 Sam. 28:9.

18 And if a man shall lie with a woman
having her sickness, and shall uncover
her nakedness; he hath discovered her
fountain, and she hath uncovered the
fountain of her blood: and both of them
shall be cut off from among their people.
19 And thou shalt not uncover the
nakedness of thy mother's sister, nor of
thy father's sister: for he uncovereth his
near kin: they shall bear their iniquity.
20 And if a man shall lie with his
uncle's wife, he hath uncovered his
uncle's nakedness: they shall bear their
sin; they shall die childless.
21 And if a man shall take his
brother's wife, it *is* an unclean thing: he
hath uncovered his brother's nakedness;
they shall be childless.
22 Ye shall therefore keep all my
statutes, and all my judgments, and do
them: that the land, whither I bring you
to dwell therein, spue you not out.
23 And ye shall not walk in the manners of the nation, which I cast out
before you: for they committed all these
things, and therefore I abhorred them.
24 But I have said unto you, Ye shall
inherit their land, and I will give it unto
you to possess it, a land that floweth
with milk and honey: I *am* the LORD your
God, which have [g]separated you from
other people.
25 Ye shall therefore put difference
between clean beasts and unclean, and
between unclean fowls and clean: and ye
shall not make your souls abominable
by beast, or by fowl, or by any manner
of living thing that creepeth on the
ground, which I have separated from
you as unclean.
26 And ye shall be holy unto me: for I
the LORD *am* holy, and have severed you
from *other* people, that ye should be mine.
27 A man also or woman that hath a
familiar [h]spirit, or that is a wizard, shall
surely be put to death: they shall stone
them with stones: their blood *shall be*
upon them.

CHAPTER 21.

The relationships and walk of the priests.

And the LORD said unto Moses, Speak
unto the priests the sons of Aaron,

and say unto them, [a]There shall none be defiled for the dead among his people:

2 But for his kin, that is near unto him, *that is*, for his mother, and for his father, and for his son, and for his daughter, and for his brother,

3 And for his sister a virgin, that is nigh unto him, which hath had no husband; for her may he be defiled.

4 *But* he shall not defile himself, *being* a chief man among his people, to profane himself.

5 They shall not make baldness upon their head, neither shall they shave off the corner of their beard, nor make any cuttings in their flesh.

6 They shall be [b]holy unto their God, and not profane the name of their God: for the offerings of the LORD made by fire, *and* the bread of their God, they do offer: [c]therefore they shall be holy.

7 They shall not take a wife *that is* a whore, or profane; neither shall they take a woman put away from her husband: for he *is* holy unto his God.

8 [1]Thou shalt [d]sanctify him therefore; for he offereth the bread of thy God: he shall be [d]holy unto thee: for I the LORD, which [d]sanctify you, *am* [d]holy.

9 And the daughter of any priest, if she profane herself by playing the whore, she profaneth her father: she shall be burnt with fire.

10 And *he that is* the high priest among his brethren, upon whose head the anointing oil was poured, and that is consecrated to put on the garments, shall not [e]uncover his head, nor rend his clothes;

11 Neither shall he go [f]in to any dead body, nor defile himself for his father, or for his mother;

12 Neither shall he go out of the sanctuary, nor profane the sanctuary of his God; for the [g]crown of the anointing oil of his God *is* upon him: I *am* the LORD.

13 And he shall take a [h]wife in her virginity.

14 A widow, or a divorced woman, or profane, *or* an harlot, these shall he not take: but he shall take a virgin of his own people to wife.

15 Neither shall he [i]profane his seed among his people: for I the LORD do sanctify him.

B.C. 1490.

a Ezk. 44:25.
b Ex. 22:31; 1 Pet. 2:9.
c Isa. 52:11.
d Heb. *qodesh.* Gen. 2:3, *note.*
e Lev. 10:6, 7.
f Num. 19:14.
g Lev. 8:9, 12; Ex. 29:6, 7.
h v. 7.
i Gen. 18:19.
j Lev. 22:23.
k Num. 6:3.
l Lev. 18:21.
m Lev. 16:19; 25:10.
n Lev. 7:20.
o Lev. 15:2.

The physical disqualifications of a priest.

16 And the LORD spake unto Moses, saying,

17 Speak unto Aaron, saying, Whosoever *he be* of thy seed in their generations that hath *any* blemish, let him not approach to offer the bread of his God.

18 For whatsoever man *he be* that hath a blemish, he shall not approach: a blind man, or a lame, or he that hath a flat nose, or any thing [j]superfluous,

19 Or a man that is brokenfooted, or brokenhanded,

20 Or crookbackt, or a dwarf, or that hath a blemish in his eye, or be scurvy, or scabbed, or hath his stones broken;

21 No man that hath a blemish of the seed of Aaron the priest shall come nigh to offer the offerings of the LORD made by fire: he hath a blemish; he shall not come nigh to offer the bread of his God.

22 He shall eat the bread of his God, *both* of the most holy, and of the holy.

23 Only he shall not go in unto the vail, nor come nigh unto the altar, because he hath a blemish; that he profane not my sanctuaries: for I the LORD do sanctify them.

24 And Moses told *it* unto Aaron, and to his sons, and unto all the children of Israel.

CHAPTER 22.

The separation of the priests (Heb. 7:26).

And the LORD spake unto Moses, saying,

2 Speak unto Aaron and to his sons, that they [k]separate themselves from the holy things of the children of Israel, and [l]that they profane not my holy name *in those things* which they [m]hallow unto me: I *am* the LORD.

3 Say unto them, Whosoever *he be* of all your seed among your generations, that goeth unto the holy things, which the children of Israel hallow unto the LORD, [n]having his uncleanness upon him, that soul shall be cut off from my presence: I *am* the LORD.

4 What man soever of the seed of Aaron *is* a leper, or [o]hath a running issue; he shall not eat of the holy things,

[1] **(21:8)** Verse 8 illustrates the O.T. holiness or sanctification—a person set apart for the service of God.

until he be [a]clean. And [b]whoso toucheth
any thing *that is* unclean *by* the dead, or
a man whose seed goeth from him;
5 Or whosoever toucheth any creeping
thing, whereby he may be made unclean,
or a man of whom he may take uncleanness, whatsoever uncleanness he hath;
6 The soul which hath touched any
such shall be unclean until even, and
shall not eat of the holy things, unless he
[c]wash his flesh with water.
7 And when the sun is down, he shall
be clean, and shall afterward eat of the
holy things; [d]because it *is* his food.
8 That which dieth of itself, or is torn
with beasts, he shall not eat to defile himself therewith: I *am* the LORD.
9 They shall therefore keep mine ordinance, [e]lest they bear sin for it, and die
therefore, if they profane it: I the LORD
do sanctify them.
10 There shall no stranger eat *of* the
holy thing: a sojourner of the priest, or
an hired servant, shall not eat *of* the holy
thing.
11 But if the priest buy *any* soul with
his money, he shall eat of it, and he that
is born in his house: they shall eat of his
meat.
12 If the priest's daughter also be *mar-*
ried unto a stranger, she may not eat of
an offering of the holy things.
13 But if the priest's daughter be a
widow, or divorced, and have no child,
and is [f]returned unto her father's house,
as in her youth, she shall eat of her
father's meat: but there shall no stranger
eat thereof.
14 And if a man eat *of* the holy thing
unwittingly, then he shall put the fifth
part thereof unto it, and shall give *it* unto
the priest with the holy thing.
15 And they shall not profane the
[g]holy things of the children of Israel,
which they offer unto the LORD;
16 Or suffer them to bear the iniquity
of trespass, when they eat their holy
things: for I the LORD do sanctify them.

Sacrifices must be physically perfect—
type of the moral perfections of Christ
(Heb. 9:14).

17 And the LORD spake unto Moses,
saying,
18 Speak unto Aaron, and to his sons,
and unto all the children of Israel, and
say unto them, Whatsoever *he be* of the

B.C. 1490.

a Lev. 15:13.

b Lev. 11:24-28, 39-40; Num. 19:11.

c Heb. 10:22.

d Lev. 21:22; Num. 18:11, 13.

e Ex. 28:43.

f Gen. 38:11.

g Num. 18:32.

h Num. 16:40.

i Lev. 19:37; Num. 15:40; Deut. 4:40.

house of Israel, or of the strangers in
Israel, that will offer his oblation for all
his vows, and for all his freewill offerings, which they will offer unto the LORD
for a burnt-offering;
19 *Ye shall offer* at your own will a male
without blemish, of the beeves, of the
sheep, or of the goats.
20 *But* whatsoever hath a blemish, *that*
shall ye not offer: for it shall not be
acceptable for you.
21 And whosoever offereth a sacrifice
of peace-offerings unto the LORD to
accomplish *his* vow, or a freewill offering
in beeves or sheep, it shall be perfect to
be accepted; there shall be no blemish
therein.
22 Blind, or broken, or maimed, or
having a wen, or scurvy, or scabbed, ye
shall not offer these unto the LORD, nor
make an offering by fire of them upon
the altar unto the LORD.
23 Either a bullock or a lamb that hath
any thing superfluous or lacking in his
parts, that mayest thou offer *for* a
freewill offering; but for a vow it shall
not be accepted.
24 Ye shall not offer unto the LORD that
which is bruised, or crushed, or broken,
or cut; neither shall ye make *any offering*
thereof in your land.
25 Neither from a [h]stranger's hand
shall ye offer the bread of your God of
any of these; because their corruption *is*
in them, *and* blemishes *be* in them: they
shall not be accepted for you.
26 And the LORD spake unto Moses,
saying,
27 When a bullock, or a sheep, or a
goat, is brought forth, then it shall be
seven days under the dam; and from the
eighth day and thenceforth it shall be
accepted for an offering made by fire
unto the LORD.
28 And *whether it be* cow or ewe, ye
shall not kill it and her young both in
one day.
29 And when ye will offer a sacrifice
of thanksgiving unto the LORD, offer *it* at
your own will.
30 On the same day it shall be eaten
up; ye shall leave none of it until the
morrow: I *am* the LORD.
31 [i]Therefore shall ye keep my commandments, and do them: I *am* the LORD.
32 Neither shall ye profane my holy
name; but I will be hallowed among the

children of Israel: I *am* the LORD which hallow you,

33 That brought you out of the land of Egypt, to be your God: I *am* the LORD.

CHAPTER 23.

The feasts of Jehovah: the sabbath and the feasts.

And the LORD spake unto Moses, saying,

2 Speak unto the children of Israel, and say unto them, *Concerning* the [1]feasts of the LORD, which ye shall proclaim *to be* holy convocations, *even* these *are* my feasts.

3 Six days shall work be done: but the seventh day *is* the [a]sabbath of rest, an holy convocation; ye shall do no work *therein*: it *is* the sabbath of the LORD in all your dwellings.

The feasts of Jehovah:
(1) *the Passover; Christ our Redeemer*
(1 Cor. 5:7; 1 Pet. 1:19).

4 These *are* the feasts of the LORD, *even* holy convocations, which ye shall proclaim in their seasons.

5 In the fourteenth *day* of the [b]first month at even *is* the LORD'S [2]passover.

The feasts of Jehovah: (2) *unleavened bread. Memorial feast* (1 Cor. 11:23–26; 5:6–8; 2 Cor. 7:1; Gal. 5:7–9).

6 And on the fifteenth day of the same month *is* the feast of [c]unleavened [3]bread unto the LORD: seven days ye must eat unleavened bread.

7 In the first day ye shall have an holy convocation: ye shall do no servile work therein.

8 But ye shall offer an offering made by fire unto the LORD seven days: in the seventh day *is* an holy convocation: ye shall do no servile work *therein*.

B.C. 1490.

a Sabbath. Num. 15:32-36. (Gen. 2:3; Mt. 12:1.)

b i.e. *April.*

c Leaven. vs. 6-17; Num. 6:15, 17, 19. (Gen. 19:3; Mt. 13:33.)

d Lit. *meal.*

e One hin = about 6 qts.

The feasts of Jehovah: (3) *Firstfruits; Christ risen* (1 Cor. 15:23).

9 And the LORD spake unto Moses, saying,

10 Speak unto the children of Israel, and say unto them, When ye be come into the land which I give unto you, and shall reap the harvest thereof, then ye shall bring a sheaf of the [4]firstfruits of your harvest unto the priest:

11 And he shall wave the sheaf before the LORD, to be accepted for you: on the morrow after the sabbath the priest shall wave it.

12 And ye shall offer that day when ye wave the sheaf an he lamb without blemish of the first year for a burnt-offering unto the LORD.

13 And the [d]meat-offering thereof *shall be* two tenth deals of fine flour mingled with oil, an offering made by fire unto the LORD *for* a sweet savour: and the drink-offering thereof *shall be* of wine, the fourth *part* of an [e]hin.

14 And ye shall eat neither bread, nor parched corn, nor green ears, until the selfsame day that ye have brought an offering unto your God: *it shall be* a statute for ever throughout your generations in all your dwellings.

The feasts of Jehovah: (4) *the wave-loaves; the church at Pentecost, fifty days after the resurrection of Christ*
(1 Cor. 10:16, 17; 12:12, 13, 20).

15 And ye shall count unto you from the morrow after the sabbath, from the day that ye brought the sheaf of the wave-offering; seven sabbaths shall be complete:

16 Even unto the morrow after the seventh sabbath shall ye number [5]fifty days; and ye shall offer a new [d]meat-offering unto the LORD.

17 Ye shall bring out of your habitations

[1] **(23:2)** The feasts of Jehovah. As given to Israel, these were simply seven great religious festivals which were to be observed every year. The first three verses of Lev. 23 do not relate to the *feasts*, but separate the sabbath from the feasts.

[2] **(23:5)** The Passover, vs. 4, 5. This feast is memorial and brings into view *redemption*, upon which all blessing rests. Typically, it stands for "Christ our passover, sacrificed for us" (1 Cor. 5:7).

[3] **(23:6)** The feast of Unleavened Bread, vs. 6-8. This feast speaks of communion with Christ, the unleavened wave-loaf, in the full blessing of His redemption, and of a holy walk. The divine order here is beautiful; first, redemption, then a holy walk. See 1 Cor. 5:6-8; 2 Cor. 7:1; Gal. 5:7-9.

[4] **(23:10)** The feast of Firstfruits, vs. 10-14. This feast is typical of resurrection—first, of Christ, then of "them that are Christ's at His coming" (1 Cor. 15:23; 1 Thes. 4:13-18).

[5] **(23:16)** The feast of Pentecost, vs. 15-22. The anti-type is the descent of the Holy Spirit to form the church. For this reason leaven is present, because there is evil in the church (Mt. 13:33; Acts 5:1, 10; 15:1).

two [1]wave loaves of two tenth deals: they shall be of fine flour; they shall be baken with leaven; *they are* the firstfruits unto the LORD.
18 And ye shall offer with the bread seven lambs without blemish of the first year, and one young bullock, and two rams: they shall be *for* a burnt-offering unto the LORD, with their [a]meat-offering, and their drink-offerings, *even* an offering made by fire, of sweet savour unto the LORD.
19 Then ye shall sacrifice one kid of the goats for a [b]sin-offering, and two lambs of the first year for a sacrifice of peace-offerings.
20 And the priest shall wave them with the bread of the firstfruits *for* a wave-offering before the LORD, with the two lambs: they shall be holy to the LORD for the priest.
21 And ye shall proclaim on the selfsame day, *that* it may be an holy convocation unto you: ye shall do no servile work *therein: it shall be* a statute for ever in all your dwellings throughout your generations.
22 And when ye reap the harvest of your land, thou shalt not make clean riddance of the corners of thy field when thou reapest, neither shalt thou gather any gleaning of thy harvest: thou shalt leave them unto the poor, and to the stranger: I *am* the LORD your God.

B.C. 1490.

a Lit. *meal.*

b Num. 28:30; cf. 2 Cor. 5:21.

c i.e. *October;* also vs. 27, 34, 39, 41.

d See Ex. 29:33, *note.*

e Cf. Isa. 22:12; Jer. 31:9; Ezk. 7:16.

The feasts of Jehovah: (5) *Trumpets; prophetic of the future regathering of Israel* (Isa. 18:3, 7; 27:12, 13; 58:1–14; Joel 2:15–32).

23 And the LORD spake unto Moses, saying,
24 Speak unto the children of Israel, saying, In the [c]seventh month, in the first *day* of the month, shall ye have a sabbath, a memorial of blowing of [2]trumpets, an holy convocation.
25 Ye shall do no servile work *therein*: but ye shall offer an offering made by fire unto the LORD.

The feasts of Jehovah: (6) *the day of Atonement* (Heb. 9:1–16).

26 And the LORD spake unto Moses, saying,
27 Also on the tenth *day* of this seventh month *there shall be* a day of [3d]atonement: it shall be an holy convocation unto you; and ye shall afflict your souls, and offer an offering made by fire unto the LORD.
28 And ye shall do no work in that same day: for it *is* a day of [d]atonement, to make an [d]atonement for you before the LORD your God.
29 For whatsoever soul *it be* that shall not be [e]afflicted in that same day, he shall be cut off from among his people.
30 And whatsoever soul *it be* that doeth any work in that same day, the

Observe, it is now *loaves;* not a sheaf of separate growths loosely bound together, but a real union of particles making one homogeneous *body.* The descent of the Holy Spirit at Pentecost united the separate disciples into one organism (1 Cor. 10:16, 17; 12:12, 13, 20).

[1]**(23:17)** The wave-loaves were offered fifty days after the wave-sheaf. This is precisely the period between the resurrection of Christ and the formation of the church at Pentecost by the baptism of the Holy Spirit (Acts 2:1-4; 1 Cor. 12:12, 13). See "Church" (Mt. 16:18; Heb. 12:22, 23). With the wave-sheaf no leaven was offered, for there was no evil in Christ; but the wave-loaves, typifying the church, are "baken with leaven," for in the church there is still evil.

[2]**(23:24)** The feast of Trumpets, vs. 23-25. This feast is a prophetical type and refers to the future regathering of long-dispersed Israel. A long interval elapses between Pentecost and Trumpets, answering to the long period occupied in the pentecostal work of the Holy Spirit in the present dispensation. Study carefully Isa. 18:3; 27:13 (with contexts); 58 (entire chapter), and Joel 2:1 to 3:21 in connection with the "trumpets," and it will be seen that these trumpets, always symbols of testimony, are connected with the regathering and repentance of Israel after the church, or pentecostal, period is ended. This feast is immediately followed by the day of atonement.

[3]**(23:27)** The day of Atonement, vs. 26-32. The *day* is the same described in Lev. 16, but here the stress is laid upon the sorrow and repentance of Israel. In other words, the *prophetical* feature is made prominent, and that looks forward to the repentance of Israel after her regathering under the Palestinian Covenant, Deut. 30:1-10, preparatory to the second advent of Messiah and the establishment of the kingdom. See the connection between the "trumpet" in Joel 2:1 and the mourning which follows in verses 11-15. Also Zech. 12:10-13 in connection with the atonement of Zech. 13:1.

same soul will I [a]destroy from among
his people.
31 Ye shall do no manner of work: *it*
shall be a statute for ever throughout
your generations in all your dwellings.
32 It *shall be* unto you a sabbath of rest,
and ye shall afflict your souls: in the ninth
day of the month at even, from even unto
even, shall ye celebrate your sabbath.

The feasts of Jehovah: (7) *Tabernacles*
(Ezra 3:4; Zech. 14:16–19; Rev. 21:3).

33 And the LORD spake unto Moses,
saying,
34 Speak unto the children of Israel,
saying, The fifteenth day of this seventh
month *shall be* the [b]feast of tabernacles
for seven days unto the LORD.
35 On the first day *shall be* an holy convocation: ye shall do no servile work
therein.
36 Seven days ye shall offer an offering made by fire unto the LORD: on the
eighth day shall be an holy convocation
unto you; and ye shall offer an offering
made by fire unto the LORD: it *is* a
solemn assembly; *and* ye [c]shall do no
servile work *therein*.
37 These *are* the feasts of the LORD,
which ye shall proclaim *to be* holy convocations, to offer an offering made by
fire unto the LORD, a burnt-offering, and
a [d]meat-offering, a sacrifice, and drink-
offerings, every thing upon his day:
38 Beside the sabbaths of the LORD,
and beside your gifts, and beside all
your vows, and beside all your freewill
offerings, which ye give unto the LORD.
39 Also in the fifteenth day of the seventh month, when ye have gathered in
the fruit of the land, ye shall keep a feast
unto the LORD seven days: on the first
day *shall be* a sabbath, and on the eighth
day *shall be* a sabbath.
40 And ye shall take you on the first
day the boughs of goodly trees, branches
of palm trees, and the boughs of thick
trees, and willows of the brook; and ye
shall rejoice before the LORD your God
seven days.
41 And ye shall keep it a feast unto the
LORD seven days in the year. *It shall be* a
statute for ever in your generations: ye
shall celebrate it in the seventh month.
42 Ye shall [e]dwell in [1]booths seven
days; [f]all that are Israelites born shall
dwell in booths:
43 That your [g]generations may know
that I made the children of Israel to dwell
in booths, when I brought them out of the
land of Egypt: I *am* the LORD your God.
44 And Moses declared unto the children of Israel the feasts of the LORD.

CHAPTER 24.

The oil for the light in the holy place
(Ex. 25:6.)

AND the LORD spake unto Moses,
saying,
2 [h]Command the children of Israel,
that they bring unto thee pure oil olive
beaten for the light, to cause the lamps
to burn continually.
3 Without the vail of the testimony, in
the tabernacle of the congregation, shall
Aaron order it from the evening unto the
morning before the LORD continually: *it*
shall be a statute for ever in your generations.
4 He shall order the lamps upon the
pure [i]candlestick before the LORD continually.

The shewbread (Ex. 25:23–30).

5 And thou shalt take fine flour, and
bake [j]twelve cakes thereof: two tenth
deals shall be in one cake.
6 And thou shalt set them in two rows,
six on a row, upon the pure table before
the LORD.
7 And thou shalt put pure frankincense upon *each* row, that it may be on
the bread for a memorial, *even* an offering made by fire unto the LORD.
8 Every sabbath he shall set it in order
before the LORD continually, *being taken*
from the children of Israel by an everlasting covenant.
9 And it shall be Aaron's and his sons';

B.C. 1490.

a Lev. 20:3-6.
b Ex. 23:16; 34:22; Zech. 14:16-19; Heb. 11:9.
c Continued at v. 39.
d Lit. *meal*.
e Heb. 11:13, 16.
f Neh. 8:14-18.
g Ex. 13:14.
h Ex. 27:20.
i Ex. 31:8; Zech. 4:2, 11.
j Ex. 25:30.

Historically the "fountain" of Zech. 13:1 was opened at the crucifixion, but rejected by the Jews of that and the succeeding centuries. After the regathering of Israel the fountain will be *efficaciously* "opened" to Israel.

[1]**(23:42)** The feast of Tabernacles, vs. 34-44, is (like the Lord's Supper for the church) both memorial and prophetic—memorial as to redemption out of Egypt (v. 43); prophetic as to the kingdom-rest of Israel after her regathering and restoration, when the feast again becomes memorial, not for Israel alone, but for all nations (Zech. 14:16-21).

and they shall eat it in the holy place: for
it *is* most holy unto him of the offerings
of the LORD made by fire by a perpetual
statute.

The penalty of blasphemy
(John 8:59; 10:31).

10 And the son of an Israelitish woman,
whose father *was* an Egyptian, went out
among the children of Israel: and this son
of the Israelitish *woman* and a man of
Israel strove together in the camp;
11 And the Israelitish woman's son
blasphemed the name *of the LORD*, and
cursed. And they [a]brought him unto
Moses: (and his mother's name *was*
Shelomith, the daughter of Dibri, of the
tribe of Dan:)
12 And they put him in ward, that the
[b]mind of the LORD might be shewed them.
13 And the LORD spake unto Moses,
saying,
14 Bring forth him that hath cursed
without the camp; and let all that heard
him lay their [c]hands upon his head, and
let all the congregation stone him.
15 And thou shalt speak unto the children of Israel, saying, Whosoever
curseth his God shall bear his sin.
16 And [d]he that blasphemeth the
name of the LORD, he shall surely be put
to death, *and* all the congregation shall
certainly stone him: as well the stranger,
as he that is born in the land, when he
blasphemeth the name *of the LORD*, shall
be put to death.
17 And he that [e]killeth any man shall
surely be put to death.
18 And he that killeth a beast shall
make it good; beast for beast.
19 And if a man cause a blemish in his
neighbour; as he hath done, so shall it be
done to him;
20 Breach for breach, eye for eye, tooth
for tooth: as he hath caused a blemish in
a man, so shall it be done to him *again*.
21 And he that killeth a beast, he shall
restore it: and he that killeth a man, he
shall be put to death.
22 Ye shall have one manner of law, as
well for the stranger, as for one of your
own country: for I *am* the LORD your
God.
23 And Moses spake to the children of
Israel, that they should bring forth him
that had cursed out of the camp, and
stone him with stones. And the children
of Israel did as the LORD commanded
Moses.

B.C. 1490.

a Ex. 18:26.
b Num. 27:5.
c Deut. 13:9.
d Ex. 20:7.
e Num. 35:31.
f Cf. Heb. 4:9.
g 2 Ki. 19:29.
h i.e. *October.*
i See Ex. 29:33, *note.*

CHAPTER 25.

The law of the land: (1) *the sabbatic year.*

And the LORD spake unto Moses in
mount Sinai, saying,
2 Speak unto the children of Israel,
and say unto them, When ye come into
the land which I give you, then shall the
land keep a sabbath unto the LORD.
3 Six years thou shalt sow thy field,
and six years thou shalt prune thy vineyard, and gather in the fruit thereof;
4 But in the seventh year shall be a
sabbath of [f]rest unto the land, a sabbath
for the LORD: thou shalt neither sow thy
field, nor prune thy vineyard.
5 [g]That which groweth of its own
accord of thy harvest thou shalt not
reap, neither gather the grapes of thy
vine undressed: *for* it is a year of rest
unto the land.
6 And the sabbath of the land shall be
meat for you; for thee, and for thy servant, and for thy maid, and for thy hired
servant, and for thy stranger that sojourneth with thee,
7 And for thy cattle, and for the beast
that *are* in thy land, shall all the increase
thereof be meat.

The law of the land: (2) *the year of jubile.*

8 And thou shalt number seven sabbaths of years unto thee, seven times
seven years; and the space of the seven
sabbaths of years shall be unto thee forty
and nine years.
9 Then shalt thou cause the trumpet of
the jubile to sound on the tenth *day* of
the [h]seventh month, in the day of [i]atone-
ment shall ye make the trumpet sound
throughout all your land.
10 And ye shall hallow the fiftieth
year, and proclaim liberty throughout *all*
the land unto all the inhabitants thereof:
it shall be a jubile unto you; and ye shall
return every man unto his possession,
and ye shall return every man unto his
family.
11 A jubile shall that fiftieth year be
unto you: ye shall not sow, neither reap
that which groweth of itself in it, nor
gather *the grapes* in it of thy vine
undressed.
12 For it *is* the jubile; it shall be holy
unto you: ye shall eat the increase thereof out of the field.
13 In the year of this jubile ye shall

return every man unto his possession.
14 And if thou sell ought unto thy
neighbour, or buyest *ought* of thy neighbour's hand, ye shall not oppress one
another:
15 According to the number of years
after the jubile thou shalt buy of thy
neighbour, *and* according unto the number of years of the fruits he shall sell
unto thee:
16 According to the multitude of years
thou shalt increase the price thereof, and
according to the fewness of years thou
shalt diminish the price of it: for *according* to the number *of the years* of the fruits
doth he sell unto thee.
17 Ye shall not therefore oppress one
another; but thou shalt [a]fear thy God: for
I *am* the LORD your God.
18 Wherefore ye shall do my statutes,
and keep my judgments, and do them;
and ye shall dwell in the land in safety.
19 And the land shall yield her fruit,
and ye shall eat your fill, and dwell
therein in safety.
20 And if ye shall say, What shall we
eat the seventh year? behold, we shall
not sow, nor gather in our increase:
21 Then I will [b]command my blessing
upon you in the sixth year, and it shall
bring forth fruit for three years.
22 And ye shall sow the eighth year,
and eat *yet* of old fruit until the ninth
year; until her fruits come in ye shall eat
of the old *store*.
23 The land shall not be sold for ever:
for the land *is* [c]mine; for ye *are*
[d]strangers and sojourners with me.
24 And in all the land of your possession ye shall grant a redemption for the
land.

The law of the land:
(3) *the redemption of the inheritance.*

25 If thy brother be waxen poor, and
hath sold away *some* of his possession,
[e]and if any of his kin come to [f]redeem it,
then shall he redeem that which his
brother sold.
26 And if the man have none to
redeem it, and himself be able to redeem
it;
27 Then let him count the years of the
sale thereof, and restore the overplus
unto the man to whom he sold it; that he
may return unto his possession.
28 But if he be not able to restore *it* to
him, then that which is sold shall remain
in the hand of him that hath bought it
until the year of jubile: and in the jubile
it shall go out, and he shall return unto
his possession.
29 And if a man sell a dwelling house
in a walled city, then he may redeem it
within a whole year after it is sold; *within* a full year may he redeem it.
30 And if it be not [f]redeemed within
the space of a full year, then the house
that *is* in the walled city shall be established for ever to him that bought it
throughout his generations: it shall not
go out in the jubile.
31 But the houses of the villages which
have no wall round about them shall be
counted as the fields of the country: they
may be redeemed, and they shall go out
in the jubile.
32 Notwithstanding the cities of the
Levites, *and* the houses of the cities of
their possession, may the Levites
redeem at any time.
33 And if a man purchase of the
Levites, then the house that was sold,
and the city of his possession, shall go
out in *the year of* jubile: for the houses of
the cities of the Levites *are* their possession among the children of Israel.
34 But the field of the suburbs of their
cities may not be sold; for it *is* their perpetual possession.

The law of the land: (4) *the poor brother.*

35 And if thy brother be waxen poor,
and fallen in decay with thee; then thou
shalt relieve him: *yea, though he be* a
stranger, or a sojourner; that he may live
with thee.
36 Take thou no usury of him, or
increase: but [g]fear thy God; that thy
brother may live with thee.
37 Thou shalt not give him thy money
upon usury, nor lend him thy victuals
for increase.
38 I *am* the LORD your God, which
brought you forth out of the land of
Egypt, to give you the land of Canaan,
and to be your God.
39 And if thy brother *that dwelleth* by
thee be waxen poor, and be sold unto
thee; thou shalt not compel him to serve
as a bondservant:
40 *But* as an hired servant, *and* as a
sojourner, he shall be with thee, *and* shall
serve thee unto the year of jubile:

B.C. 1491.

a Psa. 19:9, *note.*
b Deut. 28:8.
c Ex. 19:5; Dt. 11:12; 2 Chr. 7:20.
d Ex. 6:4; Psa. 39:12; Heb. 11:13, 16.
e Num. 5:8; Job 19:25; Jer. 32:7, 8.
f Heb. *goel, Redemp. (Kinsman type).* Isa. 59:20, *note.*
g Psa. 19:9, *note.*

41 And *then* shall he depart from thee,
both he and his children with him, and
shall return unto his own family, and
unto the possession of his fathers shall
he return.
42 For they *are* my servants, which I
brought forth out of the land of Egypt:
they shall not be sold as bondmen.
43 Thou shalt not rule over him with
rigour; but shalt [a]fear thy God.
44 Both thy bondmen, and thy bondmaids, which thou shalt have, *shall be* of
the [b]heathen that are round about you;
of them shall ye buy bondmen and
bondmaids.
45 Moreover of the children of the
strangers that do sojourn among you, of
them shall ye buy, and of their families
that *are* with you, which they begat in
your land: and they shall be your possession.
46 And ye shall take them as an inheritance for your children after you, to
inherit *them for* a possession; they shall
be your bondmen for ever: but over your
brethren the children of Israel, ye shall
not rule one over another with rigour.

The law of the land:
(5) *the redemption of the poor brother—*
Christ our Kinsman- Redeemer.

47 And if a sojourner or stranger wax
rich by thee, and thy brother *that dwelleth*
by him wax poor, and sell himself unto
the stranger *or* sojourner by thee, or to
the stock of the stranger's family:
48 After that he is sold he may be [c]re-
deemed again; one of his brethren may
[d]redeem him:
49 Either his uncle, or his uncle's son,
may [c]redeem him, or *any* that is nigh of
[1]kin unto him of his family may redeem
him; or if he be able, he may redeem
himself.
50 And he shall [e]reckon with him that
bought him from the year that he was
sold to him unto the year of jubile: and
the price of his sale shall be according
unto the number of years, according to
the time of an hired servant shall it be
with him.
51 If *there be* yet many years *behind*,

B.C. 1491.

a Psa. 19:9, *note.*

b Lit. *nations.*

c Heb. *goel, Redemp. (Kinsman type).* Isa. 59:20, *note.*

d Gal. 4:4, 5.

e *Imputation.* Lev. 27:18. (Lev. 25:50; Jas. 2:23.)

f *Law (of Moses).* Lev. 27:1-34. (Ex. 19:1; Gal. 3:1-29.)

g Psa. 4:8.

h 2 Ki. 17:25; cf. Hos. 2:18.

i Deut. 32:30; Jud. 7:7, 12; 1 Sam. 14:14.

according unto them he shall give again
the price of his redemption out of the
money that he was bought for.
52 And if there remain but few years
unto the year of jubile, then he shall
count with him, *and* according unto his
years shall he give him again the price of
his redemption.
53 *And* as a yearly hired servant shall
he be with him: *and the other* shall not
rule with rigour over him in thy sight.
54 And if he be not [c]redeemed in these
years, then he shall go out in the year of
jubile, *both* he, and his children with him.
55 For unto me the children of Israel
are servants; they *are* my servants whom
I brought forth out of the land of Egypt:
I *am* the LORD your God.

[2]CHAPTER 26.

The law of the land: (6) conditions of
blessing; warnings of chastisement.

Ye shall make you no idols nor graven
image, neither rear you up a standing image, neither shall ye set up *any*
image of stone in your land, to bow down
unto it: for I *am* the LORD your God.
2 Ye shall [f]keep my sabbaths, and reverence my sanctuary: I *am* the LORD.

Conditions of blessing.

3 If ye walk in my statutes, and keep
my commandments, and do them;
4 Then I will give you rain in due season, and the land shall yield her
increase, and the trees of the field shall
yield their fruit.
5 And your threshing shall reach unto
the vintage, and the vintage shall reach
unto the sowing time: and ye shall eat
your bread to the full, and dwell in your
land safely.
6 And I will give peace in the land,
and ye shall [g]lie down, and none shall
make *you* afraid: and I will rid evil
[h]beasts out of the land, neither shall the
sword go through your land.
7 And ye shall chase your enemies,
and they shall fall before you by the
sword.
8 And [i]five of you shall chase an

[1]**(25:49)** The Kinsman-Redeemer. The word *goel* is used to indicate both the *redemption*—"to free by paying," and the Redeemer—"the one who pays." The case of Ruth and Boaz (Ruth 2:1; 3:10-18; 4:1-10) perfectly illustrates this beautiful type of Christ. See "Redemption," Isa. 59:20, *note.*

[2]**(26, heading)** Chapter 26 should be read in connection with Deut. 28, 29, 30, the Palestinian Covenant.

hundred, and an hundred of you shall
put ten thousand to flight: and your enemies shall fall before you by the sword.
9 For I will have [a]respect unto you,
and make you fruitful, and multiply you,
and establish my covenant with you.
10 And ye shall eat old store, and
bring forth the old because of the new.
11 And I will set my tabernacle among
you: and my soul shall not abhor you.
12 And I will walk among you, and will
be your [b]God, and ye shall be my people.
13 I *am* the LORD your God, which
brought you forth out of the land of
Egypt, that ye should not be their bondmen; and I have broken the bands of
your yoke, and made you go upright.

Warnings of chastisement.

14 But if ye will not hearken unto me,
and will not do all these commandments;
15 And if ye shall despise my statutes,
or if your soul abhor my judgments, so
that ye will not do all my commandments, *but* that ye break my covenant:

The first chastisement.

16 I also will do this unto you; I will
even appoint over you terror, consumption, and the burning ague, that shall
consume the eyes, and cause sorrow of
heart: and ye shall sow your seed in
vain, for your enemies shall eat it.
17 And I will set my face against you,
and ye shall be [c]slain before your enemies: they that hate you shall reign over
you; and ye shall flee when none pursueth you.

The second chastisement.

18 And if ye will not yet for all this
hearken unto me, then I will punish you
seven times more for your sins.
19 And I will break the pride of your
power; and I will make your [d]heaven as
iron, and your earth as brass:
20 And your strength shall be spent in
vain: for your land shall not yield her
increase, neither shall the trees of the
land yield their fruits.

The third chastisement.

21 And if ye walk contrary unto me,
and will not hearken unto me; I will
bring seven times more plagues upon
you according to your sins.
22 I will also send [e]wild beasts among
you, which shall rob you of your children, and destroy your cattle, and make
you few in number; and your *high* ways
shall be desolate.

The fourth chastisement.

23 And if ye will not be reformed by
me by these things, but will walk contrary unto me;
24 Then will I also walk contrary unto
you, and will punish you yet seven
times for your sins.
25 And I will bring a sword upon you,
that shall avenge the quarrel of *my*
covenant: and when ye are gathered
together within your cities, I will send
the [f]pestilence among you; and ye shall
be delivered into the hand of the enemy.
26 *And* when I have broken the staff of
your bread, ten women shall bake your
bread in one oven, and they shall deliver
you your bread again by weight: and ye
shall eat, and not be [g]satisfied.

The fifth chastisement.

27 And if ye will not for all this hearken unto me, but walk contrary unto me;
28 Then I will walk contrary unto you
also in fury; and I, even I, will chastise
you seven times for your sins.
29 And ye shall [h]eat the flesh of your
sons, and the flesh of your daughters
shall ye eat.
30 And I will [i]destroy your high
places, and cut down your images, and
cast your carcases upon the carcases of
your idols, and my soul shall abhor you.
31 And I will make your [j]cities waste,
and bring your [k]sanctuaries unto desolation, and I will not smell the savour of
your sweet odours.

The dispersion predicted.

(Cf. Deut. 28:58–67.)

32 And I will bring the land into desolation: and your enemies which dwell
therein shall be astonished at it.
33 And I will [l]scatter you among the
[m]heathen, and will draw out a sword
after you: and your land shall be desolate, and your cities waste.
34 Then shall the land enjoy her sabbaths, as long as it lieth desolate, and ye

B.C. 1491.

a 2 Ki. 13:23.
b Jer. 7:23; 2 Cor. 6:16.
c 1 Sam. 4:10; 31:1.
d Deut. 28:23; cf. 1 Ki. 17:1.
e Deut. 32:24; 2 Ki. 17:25; Ezk. 14:21.
f Num. 16:49; 2 Sam. 24:15.
g Hag. 1:6.
h 2 Ki. 6:28-29.
i 2 Ki. 23:8, 20.
j 2 Ki. 25:4, 10.
k 2 Chr. 36:19.
l Psa. 44:11.
m Lit. *nations.*

be in your enemies' land; *even* then shall the land rest, and enjoy her sabbaths.

35 As long as it lieth desolate it shall rest; because it did not rest in your sabbaths, when ye dwelt upon it.

36 And upon them that are left *alive* of you I will send a faintness into their hearts in the lands of their enemies; and the sound of a shaken leaf shall chase them; and they shall flee, as fleeing from a sword; and they shall fall when none pursueth.

37 And they shall fall one upon another, as it were before a sword, when none pursueth: and ye shall have no power to stand before your enemies.

38 And ye shall perish among the [a]heathen, and the land of your enemies shall eat you up.

39 And they that are left of you shall pine away in their iniquity in your enemies' lands; and also in the iniquities of their fathers shall they pine away with them.

The Abrahamic Covenant remains, despite the disobedience and dispersion.

40 If they shall [b]confess their iniquity, and the iniquity of their fathers, with their trespass which they trespassed against me, and that also they have walked contrary unto me;

41 And *that* I also have walked contrary unto them, and have brought them into the land of their enemies; if then their uncircumcised hearts be [c]humbled, and they then [d]accept of the punishment of their iniquity:

42 Then will I [e]remember my covenant with Jacob, and also my covenant with Isaac, and also my covenant with Abraham will I remember; and I will remember the land.

43 The land also shall be left of them, and shall enjoy her sabbaths, while she lieth desolate without them: and they shall accept of the punishment of their iniquity: because, even because they despised my judgments, and because their soul abhorred my statutes.

44 And yet for all that, when they be in the land of their enemies, I will not cast them away, neither will I abhor them, to destroy them utterly, and to break my covenant with them: for I *am* the LORD their God.

45 But I will for their sakes remember the covenant of their ancestors, whom I brought forth out of the land of Egypt in the sight of the [a]heathen, that I might be their God: I *am* the LORD.

46 These *are* the statutes and judgments and laws, which the LORD made between him and the children of Israel in mount Sinai by the hand of Moses.

CHAPTER 27.

Concerning vowed (dedicated) persons and things.

And the LORD spake unto [f]Moses, saying,

2 Speak unto the children of Israel, and say unto them, When a man shall make a singular vow, the persons *shall be* for the LORD by thy estimation.

3 And thy estimation shall be of the male from twenty years old even unto sixty years old, even thy estimation shall be fifty [g]shekels of silver, after the shekel of the sanctuary.

4 And if it *be* a female, then thy estimation shall be thirty shekels.

5 And if *it be* from five years old even unto twenty years old, then thy estimation shall be of the male twenty shekels, and for the female ten shekels.

6 And if *it be* from a month old even unto five years old, then thy estimation shall be of the male five shekels of silver, and for the female thy estimation *shall be* three shekels of silver.

7 And if *it be* from sixty years old and above; if *it be* a male, then thy estimation shall be fifteen shekels, and for the female ten shekels.

8 But if he be poorer than thy estimation, then he shall present himself before the priest, and the priest shall value him; according to his ability that vowed shall the priest value him.

9 And if *it be* a beast, whereof men bring an offering unto the LORD, all that *any man* giveth of such unto the LORD shall be holy.

10 He shall not alter it, nor change it, a good for a bad, or a bad for a good: and if he shall at all change beast for beast, then it and the exchange thereof shall be holy.

11 And if *it be* any unclean beast, of which they do not offer a sacrifice unto the LORD, then he shall present the beast before the priest:

B.C. 1491.

a Lit. *nations.*

b 1 Ki. 8:33-34; Neh. 9:2; 1 John 1:9.

c 2 Chr. 12:6, 7, 12; 1 Pet. 5:5-6.

d Psa. 39:9; 51:3, 4; Dan. 9:7.

e Psa. 106:45.

f *Law (of Moses).* vs. 1-34; Deut. 5:1-22. (Ex. 19:1; Gal. 3:1-29.)

g One shekel = 2*s.* 9*d.*, or 65 cents; also vs. 4, 5, 6, 7, 16, 25.

12 And the priest shall value it, whether it be good or bad: as thou valuest it, *who art* the priest, so shall it be.

13 But if he will at all [a]redeem it, then he shall add a fifth *part* thereof unto thy estimation.

14 And when a man shall [b]sanctify his house *to be* holy unto the LORD, then the priest shall estimate it, whether it be good or bad: as the priest shall estimate it, so shall it stand.

15 And if he that sanctified it will [a]redeem his house, then he shall add the fifth *part* of the money of thy estimation unto it, and it shall be his.

16 And if a man shall sanctify unto the LORD *some part* of a field of his possession, then thy estimation shall be according to the seed thereof: an [c]homer of barley seed *shall be valued* at fifty shekels of silver.

17 If he sanctify his field from the year of jubile, according to thy estimation it shall stand.

18 But if he sanctify his field after the jubile, then the priest shall [d]reckon unto him the money according to the years that remain, even unto the year of the jubile, and it shall be abated from thy estimation.

19 And if he that sanctified the field will in any wise [a]redeem it, then he shall add the fifth *part* of the money of thy estimation unto it, and it shall be assured to him.

20 And if he will not [a]redeem the field, or if he have sold the field to another man, it shall not be redeemed any more.

21 But the field, when it goeth out in the jubile, shall be holy unto the LORD, as a field devoted; the possession thereof shall be the priest's.

22 And if *a man* sanctify unto the LORD a field which he hath bought, which *is* not of the fields of his possession;

23 Then the priest shall reckon unto him the worth of thy estimation, *even* unto the year of the jubile: and he shall give thine estimation in that day, *as* a holy thing unto the LORD.

24 In the year of the jubile the field shall return unto him of whom it was bought, *even* to him to whom the possession of the land *did belong*.

25 And all thy estimations shall be according to the shekel of the sanctuary: twenty [e]gerahs shall be the shekel.

The three things which are the Lord's absolutely: (1) *the firstling of the beasts.*

26 Only the firstling of the beasts, which should be the LORD'S firstling, no man shall sanctify it; whether *it be* ox, or sheep: it *is* the LORD'S.

27 And if *it be* of an unclean beast, then he shall [a]redeem *it* according to thine estimation, and shall add a fifth *part* of it thereto: or if it be not redeemed, then it shall be sold according to thy estimation.

(2) *Any dedicated thing.*

28 Notwithstanding no devoted thing, that a man shall devote unto the LORD of all that he hath, *both* of man and beast, and of the field of his possession, shall be sold or [a]redeemed: every devoted thing *is* most holy unto the LORD.

29 None devoted, which shall be devoted of men, shall be redeemed; *but* shall surely be put to death.

(3) *All the tithe of the land, tree, and beast.*

30 And [f]all the [g]tithe of the land, *whether* of the seed of the land, *or* of the fruit of the tree, *is* the LORD'S: *it is* holy unto the LORD.

31 And if a man will at all [a]redeem *ought* of his tithes, he shall add thereto the fifth *part* thereof.

32 And concerning the tithe of the herd, or of the flock, *even* of whatsoever [h]passeth under the rod, the tenth shall be holy unto the LORD.

33 He shall not search whether it be good or bad, neither shall he change it: and if he change it at all, then both it and the [i]change thereof shall be holy; it shall not be [a]redeemed.

34 [j]These *are* the commandments, which the LORD commanded Moses for the children of Israel in mount [k]Sinai.

B.C. 1491.

a Heb. *goel, Redemp. (Kinsman type).* Isa. 59:20, *note.*

b *Sanctify, holy* (O.T.). vs. 14-22; Josh. 5:15. (Gen. 2:3; Zech. 8:3.)

c About 86 gals.

d *Imputation.* vs. 18:23; 1 Sam. 22:15. (Lev. 25:50; Jas. 2:23.)

e One gerah = 11.2 grains, or 3 1-4 cts.

f Gen. 28:22; Num. 18:21, 24.

g 2 Cor. 8:1, *note.*

h Cf. Jer. 33:13; Ezk. 20:37; Mic. 7:14.

i v. 10.

j Mal. 4:4.

k Ex. 19:1-6, 25; Heb. 12:8, 18-29.

THE FOURTH BOOK OF MOSES CALLED

NUMBERS

THE book derives its name from the fact that it records the enumeration of Israel. Historically, Numbers takes up the story where Exodus left it, and is the book of the wilderness wanderings of the redeemed people consequent upon their failure to enter the land at Kadesh-barnea.

Typically, it is the book of service and walk, and thus completes, with the preceding books, a beautiful moral order: Genesis, the book of the creation and fall; Exodus, of redemption; Leviticus, of worship and fellowship; and Numbers, of that which should follow—service and walk.

It is important to see that nothing was left to self-will. Every servant was numbered, knew his place in the family, and had his own definitely assigned service. The N.T. parallel is 1 Cor. 12.

The second typical lesson is that, tested by wilderness circumstances, Israel utterly failed.

Numbers is in five chief divisions: I. The Order of the Host, 1:1–10:10. II. From Sinai to Kadesh-barnea, 10:11-12:16. III. Israel at Kadesh-barnea, 13:1–19:22. IV. The Wilderness Wanderings, 20:1-33:49. V. Closing Instructions, 33:50–36:13.

The events recorded in Numbers cover a period of 39 years (Ussher).

CHAPTER 1.

The order of the host: (1) *Moses commanded to number the people.*

AND the LORD spake unto Moses in the wilderness of [a]Sinai, in the tabernacle of the congregation, on the first *day* of the [b]second month, in the second year after they were come out of the land of Egypt, saying,

2 [c]Take ye the sum of all the congregation of the children of Israel, after their families, by the house of their fathers, with the number of *their* names, every male by their polls;

3 From twenty years old and upward, all that are able to go forth to war in Israel: thou and Aaron shall number them by their armies.

4 And with you there shall be a man of every tribe; every one head of the house of his fathers.

5 And these *are* the names of the men that shall stand with you: of *the tribe of* Reuben; Elizur the son of Shedeur.

6 Of Simeon; Shelumiel the son of Zurishaddai.

7 Of Judah; Nahshon the son of Amminadab.

8 Of Issachar; Nethaneel the son of Zuar.

9 Of Zebulun; Eliab the son of Helon.

10 Of the children of Joseph: of Ephraim; Elishama the son of Ammihud: of Manasseh; Gamaliel the son of Pedahzur.

11 Of Benjamin; Abidan the son of Gideoni.

12 Of Dan; Ahiezer the son of Ammishaddai.

13 Of Asher; Pagiel the son of Ocran.

14 Of Gad; Eliasaph the son of Deuel.

15 Of Naphtali; Ahira the son of Enan.

16 [d]These *were* the renowned of the congregation, princes of the tribes of their fathers, [e]heads of thousands in Israel.

17 And Moses and Aaron took these men which are expressed by *their* names:

18 And they assembled all the congregation together on the first *day* of the second month, and they declared their pedigrees after their families, by the house of their fathers, according to the number of the names, from twenty years old and upward, by their polls.

19 [f]As the LORD commanded Moses, so he numbered them in the wilderness of Sinai.

20 And the children of Reuben, Israel's eldest son, by their generations, after their families, by the house of their fathers, according to the number of the names, by their polls, every male from twenty years old and upward, all that were able to go forth to war;

B.C. 1490.

a Num. 10:12; Ex. 19:1. Cf. Heb. 12:18.

b i.e. *May;* also v. 18.

c Num. 26:1-63; Ex. 30:12; 2 Sam. 24:2; 1 Chr. 21:2.

d Num. 7:2; 1 Chr. 27:16, 22; Jer. 9:23, 24.

e Ex. 18:21, 25; Jer. 5:5; Mic. 3:1, 9; 5:2.

f v. 2.

B.C. 1490.

21 Those that were numbered of them, *even* of the tribe of Reuben, *were* forty and six thousand and five hundred.

22 Of the children of Simeon, by their generations, after their families, by the house of their fathers, those that were numbered of them, according to the number of the names, by their polls, every male from twenty years old and upward, all that were able to go forth to war;

23 Those that were numbered of them, *even* of the tribe of Simeon, *were* fifty and nine thousand and three hundred.

24 Of the children of Gad, by their generations, after their families, by the house of their fathers, according to the number of the names, from twenty years old and upward, all that were able to go forth to war;

25 Those that were numbered of them, *even* of the tribe of Gad, *were* forty and five thousand six hundred and fifty.

26 Of the children of Judah, by their generations, after their families, by the house of their fathers, according to the number of the names, from twenty years old and upward, all that were able to go forth to war;

27 Those that were numbered of them, *even* of the tribe of Judah, *were* threescore and fourteen thousand and six hundred.

28 Of the children of Issachar, by their generations, after their families, by the house of their fathers, according to the number of the names, from twenty years old and upward, all that were able to go forth to war;

29 Those that were numbered of them, *even* of the tribe of Issachar, *were* fifty and four thousand and four hundred.

30 Of the children of Zebulun, by their generations, after their families, by the house of their fathers, according to the number of the names, from twenty years old and upward, all that were able to go forth to war;

31 Those that were numbered of them, *even* of the tribe of Zebulun, *were* fifty and seven thousand and four hundred.

32 Of the children of Joseph, *namely*, of the children of Ephraim, by their generations, after their families, by the house of their fathers, according to the number of the names, from twenty years old and upward, all that were able to go forth to war;

33 Those that were numbered of them, *even* of the tribe of Ephraim, *were* forty thousand and five hundred.

34 Of the children of Manasseh, by their generations, after their families, by the house of their fathers, according to the number of the names, from twenty years old and upward, all that were able to go forth to war;

35 Those that were numbered of them, *even* of the tribe of Manasseh, *were* thirty and two thousand and two hundred.

36 Of the children of Benjamin, by their generations, after their families, by the house of their fathers, according to the number of the names, from twenty years old and upward, all that were able to go forth to war;

37 Those that were numbered of them, *even* of the tribe of Benjamin, *were* thirty and five thousand and four hundred.

38 Of the children of Dan, by their generations, after their families, by the house of their fathers, according to the number of the names, from twenty years old and upward, all that were able to go forth to war;

39 Those that were numbered of them, *even* of the tribe of Dan, *were* threescore and two thousand and seven hundred.

40 Of the children of Asher, by their generations, after their families, by the house of their fathers, according to the number of the names, from twenty years old and upward, all that were able to go forth to war;

41 Those that were numbered of them, *even* of the tribe of Asher, *were* forty and one thousand and five hundred.

42 Of the children of Naphtali, throughout their generations, after their families, by the house of their fathers, according to the number of the names, from twenty years old and upward, all that were able to go forth to war;

43 Those that were numbered of them, *even* of the tribe of Naphtali, *were* fifty and three thousand and four hundred.

44 These *are* those that were numbered, which Moses and Aaron numbered, and the princes of Israel, *being*

twelve men: each one was for the house
of his fathers.
45 So were all those that were numbered of the children of Israel, by the
house of their fathers, from twenty years
old and upward, all that were able to go
forth to war in Israel;
46 Even all [a]they that were numbered
were six hundred thousand and three
thousand and five hundred and fifty.
47 [b]But the Levites after the tribe of
their fathers were not numbered among
them.
48 For the LORD had spoken unto
Moses, saying,
49 Only thou shalt not number the
tribe of Levi, neither take the sum of
them among the children of Israel:
50 But thou shalt appoint the Levites
over the tabernacle of testimony, and
over all the vessels thereof, and over all
things that *belong* to it: they shall bear the
tabernacle, and all the vessels thereof;
and they shall minister unto it, and shall
encamp round about the tabernacle.
51 And when the tabernacle setteth forward, the [c]Levites shall take it down: and
when the tabernacle is to be pitched, the
Levites shall set it up: and the stranger
that cometh nigh shall be put to death.
52 And the children of Israel shall
pitch their tents, [d]every man by his own
camp, and every man by his own standard, throughout their hosts.
53 But the Levites shall pitch round
about the tabernacle of testimony, that
there be no wrath upon the congregation
of the children of Israel: and the Levites
shall keep the charge of the tabernacle of
testimony.
54 And the children of Israel did
according to all that the LORD commanded Moses, so did they.

CHAPTER 2.

The order of the host:
(2) *arrangement of the camp.*

AND the LORD spake unto Moses and
unto Aaron, saying,
2 [e]Every man of the children of Israel
shall pitch by his own standard, with the
ensign of their father's house: [f]far off
about the tabernacle of the congregation
shall they pitch.
3 And on the east side toward the rising of the sun shall they of the standard

B.C. 1490.

a Num. 2:32; 14:22-38; 26:63-65; Ex. 12:37; 38:26; Deut. 10:22; Heb. 11:12. Cf. Rev. 7:4-9.

b Num. 2:33; cf. 3:14-22; 26:57-62; Ex. 38:21; 1 Chr. 6:1-48; 21:6.

c Num. 10:17-21.

d Num. 2:2; 24:2.

e Num. 1:52; Psa. 16:6.

f Josh. 3:4.

g Num. 1:7; 10:14; 1 Chr. 2:10.

h Num. 10:14.

i Num. 10:18.

j Num. 10:17, 21.

of the camp of Judah pitch throughout
their armies: and [g]Nahshon the son of
Amminadab *shall be* captain of the children of Judah.
4 And his host, and those that were
numbered of them, *were* threescore and
fourteen thousand and six hundred.
5 And those that do pitch next unto
him *shall be* the tribe of Issachar: and
Nethaneel the son of Zuar *shall be* captain of the children of Issachar.
6 And his host, and those that were
numbered thereof, *were* fifty and four
thousand and four hundred.
7 *Then* the tribe of Zebulun: and Eliab
the son of Helon *shall be* captain of the
children of Zebulun.
8 And his host, and those that were
numbered thereof, *were* fifty and seven
thousand and four hundred.
9 All that were numbered in the camp
of Judah *were* an hundred thousand and
fourscore thousand and six thousand
and four hundred, throughout their
armies. These shall [h]first set forth.
10 On the south side *shall be* the standard of the camp of Reuben according to
their armies: and the captain of the children of Reuben *shall be* Elizur the son of
Shedeur.
11 And his host, and those that were
numbered thereof, *were* forty and six
thousand and five hundred.
12 And those which pitch by him *shall
be* the tribe of Simeon: and the captain of
the children of Simeon *shall be* Shelumiel
the son of Zurishaddai.
13 And his host, and those that were
numbered of them, *were* fifty and nine
thousand and three hundred.
14 Then the tribe of Gad: and the captain of the sons of Gad *shall be* Eliasaph
the son of Reuel.
15 And his host, and those that were
numbered of them, *were* forty and five
thousand and six hundred and fifty.
16 All that were numbered in the
camp of Reuben *were* an hundred thousand and fifty and one thousand and
four hundred and fifty, throughout their
armies. And they shall set forth in the
[i]second rank.
17 [j]Then the tabernacle of the congregation shall set forward with the camp
of the Levites in the midst of the camp:
as they encamp, so shall they set

forward, every man in his place by their standards.

18 On the west side *shall be* the standard of the camp of Ephraim according to their armies: and the captain of the sons of Ephraim *shall be* Elishama the son of Ammihud.

19 And his host, and those that were numbered of them, *were* forty thousand and five hundred.

20 And by him *shall be* the tribe of Manasseh: and the captain of the children of Manasseh *shall be* Gamaliel the son of Pedahzur.

21 And his host, and those that were numbered of them, *were* thirty and two thousand and two hundred.

22 Then the tribe of Benjamin: and the captain of the sons of Benjamin *shall be* Abidan the son of Gideoni.

23 And his host, and those that were numbered of them, *were* thirty and five thousand and four hundred.

24 All that were numbered of the camp of Ephraim *were* an hundred thousand and eight thousand and an hundred, throughout their armies. And they shall go forward in the [a]third rank.

25 The standard of the camp of Dan *shall be* on the north side by their armies: and the captain of the children of Dan *shall be* Ahiezer the son of Ammishaddai.

26 And his host, and those that were numbered of them, *were* threescore and two thousand and seven hundred.

27 And those that encamp by him *shall be* the tribe of Asher: and the captain of the children of Asher *shall be* Pagiel the son of Ocran.

28 And his host, and those that were numbered of them, *were* forty and one thousand and five hundred.

29 Then the tribe of Naphtali: and the captain of the children of Naphtali *shall be* Ahira the son of Enan.

30 And his host, and those that were numbered of them, *were* fifty and three thousand and four hundred.

31 All they that were numbered in the camp of Dan *were* an hundred thousand and fifty and seven thousand and six hundred. They shall go hindmost with their standards.

32 These *are* those which were numbered of the children of Israel by the house of their fathers: [b]all those that were numbered of the camps throughout their hosts *were* six hundred thousand and three thousand and five hundred and fifty.

33 But the Levites were not numbered among the children of Israel; as the LORD commanded Moses.

34 And the children of Israel did according to all that the LORD commanded Moses: [c]so they pitched by their standards, and so they set forward, every one after their families, according to the house of their fathers.

CHAPTER 3.

The order of the host: (3) *the priests.*

These also *are* the generations of Aaron and Moses in the day *that* the LORD spake with Moses in mount [d]Sinai.

2 And these *are* the names of the sons of Aaron; Nadab the firstborn, and Abihu, Eleazar, and Ithamar.

3 These *are* the names of the sons of Aaron, the priests which were anointed, whom he consecrated to minister in the priest's office.

4 And Nadab and [e]Abihu died before the LORD, when they offered strange fire before the LORD, in the wilderness of Sinai, and they had no children: and Eleazar and Ithamar ministered in the priest's office in the sight of Aaron their father.

The order of the host: (4) *the tribe of Levi.*

5 And the LORD spake unto Moses, saying,

6 [f]Bring the tribe of Levi near, and present them before Aaron the priest, that they may minister unto him.

7 And they shall keep his charge, and the charge of the whole congregation before the tabernacle of the congregation, to do the service of the tabernacle.

8 And they shall keep all the instruments of the tabernacle of the congregation, and the charge of the children of Israel, to do the service of the tabernacle.

9 And thou shalt [g]give the Levites unto Aaron and to his sons: they *are* wholly given unto him out of the children of Israel.

10 And thou shalt appoint Aaron and his sons, and they shall wait on their priest's office: and the stranger that cometh nigh shall be put to death.

B.C. 1490.

a Num. 10:22.

b Num. 1:46, 47; 11:21; Ex. 38:26.

c Num. 24:2, 5, 6.

d *Israel (history).* vs. 1-10; Deut. 1:6-8, 19-40. (Gen. 12:2, 3; Rom. 11:26.)

e Num. 26:61; Lev. 10:1, 2; 1 Chr. 24:2.

f Num. 8:6-19; 18:2-4; Ex. 32:26-28; Deut. 33:8-11.

g Num. 8:19; 18:6, 7.

11 And the LORD spake unto Moses,
saying,
12 And I, behold, I have taken the
Levites from among the children of Israel
instead of all the firstborn that openeth
the matrix among the children of Israel:
therefore the Levites shall be mine;
13 Because all the firstborn *are* mine; *for*
on the day that I smote all the firstborn in
the land of Egypt I hallowed unto me all
the firstborn in Israel, both man and
beast: mine shall they be: I *am* the LORD.

The order of host: (5) *the families of Levi.*

14 And the LORD spake unto Moses in
the wilderness of Sinai, saying,
15 Number the children of Levi after
the house of their fathers, by their families: every male from a month old and
upward shalt thou number them.
16 And Moses numbered them according to the word of the LORD, as he was
commanded.
17 And these were the sons of Levi by
their names; Gershon, and Kohath, and
Merari.
18 And these *are* the names of the sons
of Gershon by their families; Libni, and
Shimei.
19 And the sons of Kohath by their
families; Amram, and Izehar, Hebron,
and Uzziel.
20 And the sons of Merari by their
families; Mahli, and Mushi. These *are* the
families of the Levites according to the
house of their fathers.
21 Of Gershon *was* the family of the
Libnites, and the family of the Shimites:
these *are* the families of the Gershonites.
22 Those that were numbered of them,
according to the number of all the males,
from a month old and upward, *even*
those that were numbered of them *were*
seven thousand and five hundred.
23 The families of the Gershonites shall
pitch behind the tabernacle westward.
24 And the chief of the house of the
father of the Gershonites *shall be*
Eliasaph the son of Lael.

The order of the host:
(6) *the charges of the sons of Levi.*

25 And the charge of the sons of
[a]Gershon in the tabernacle of the congregation *shall be* the [b]tabernacle, and the
tent, the covering thereof, and the hanging for the door of the tabernacle of the
congregation,

B.C. 1490.

a Num. 4:24, 26.
b Ex. 25:9.
c Ex. 35:18.
d 1 Chr. 26:23.
e Num. 1:53.
f Num. 1:53.
g Num. 4:31, 32.

26 And the hangings of the court, and
the curtain for the door of the court,
which *is* by the tabernacle, and by the
altar round about, and the [c]cords of it
for all the service thereof.
27 And of [d]Kohath *was* the family of
the Amramites, and the family of the
Izeharites, and the family of the
Hebronites, and the family of the
Uzzielites: these *are* the families of the
Kohathites.
28 In the number of all the males, from
a month old and upward, *were* eight
thousand and six hundred, keeping the
charge of the sanctuary.
29 The families of the [e]sons of Kohath
shall pitch on the side of the tabernacle
southward.
30 And the chief of the house of the
father of the families of the Kohathites
shall be Elizaphan the son of Uzziel.
31 And their charge *shall be* the ark,
and the table, and the candlestick, and
the altars, and the vessels of the sanctuary wherewith they minister, and the
hanging, and all the service thereof.
32 And Eleazar the son of Aaron the
priest *shall be* chief over the chief of the
Levites, *and have* the oversight of them
that keep the charge of the sanctuary.
33 Of Merari *was* the family of the
Mahlites, and the family of the Mushites:
these *are* the families of Merari.
34 And those that were numbered of
them, according to the number of all the
males, from a month old and upward,
were six thousand and two hundred.
35 And the chief of the house of the
father of the families of Merari *was* Zuriel
the son of Abihail: [f]*these* shall pitch on
the side of the tabernacle northward.
36 And *under* the [g]custody and charge
of the sons of Merari *shall be* the boards
of the tabernacle, and the bars thereof,
and the pillars thereof, and the sockets
thereof, and all the vessels thereof, and
all that serveth thereto,
37 And the pillars of the court round
about, and their sockets, and their pins,
and their cords.
38 But those that encamp before the
tabernacle toward the east, *even* before
the tabernacle of the congregation eastward, *shall be* Moses, and Aaron and his

sons, [a]keeping the charge of the sanctuary for the charge of the children of Israel; and the stranger that cometh nigh shall be put to death.

39 [b]All that were numbered of the Levites, which Moses and Aaron numbered at the commandment of the LORD, throughout their families, all the males from a month old and upward, *were* twenty and two thousand.

The order of the host: (7) *the firstborn redeemed* (Ex. 38:27, *note*).

40 And the LORD said unto Moses, [c]Number all the firstborn of the males of the children of Israel from a month old and upward, and take the number of their names.

41 [d]And thou shalt take the Levites for me (I *am* the LORD) instead of all the firstborn among the children of Israel; and the cattle of the Levites instead of all the firstlings among the cattle of the children of Israel.

42 And Moses numbered, as the LORD commanded him, all the firstborn among the children of Israel.

43 And all the firstborn males by the number of names, from a month old and upward, of those that were numbered of them, were twenty and two thousand two hundred and threescore and thirteen.

44 And the LORD spake unto Moses, saying,

45 Take the Levites instead of all the firstborn among the children of Israel, and the cattle of the Levites instead of their cattle; and the Levites shall be mine: I *am* the LORD.

46 And for those that are to be redeemed of the two hundred and threescore and thirteen of the firstborn of the children of Israel, which are more than the Levites;

47 Thou shalt even take five [e]shekels apiece by the poll, after the shekel of the sanctuary shalt thou take *them*: (the shekel *is* twenty [f]gerahs:)

48 And thou shalt give the money, wherewith the odd number of them is to be redeemed, unto Aaron and to his sons.

49 And Moses took the redemption money of them that were over and above them that were redeemed by the Levites:

50 Of the firstborn of the children of Israel took he the money; a thousand three hundred and threescore and five *shekels*, after the shekel of the sanctuary:

51 And Moses gave the money of them that were [g]redeemed unto Aaron and to his sons, according to the word of the LORD, as the LORD commanded Moses.

CHAPTER 4.

The order of the host: (8) *service of the Kohathites.*

And the LORD spake unto Moses and unto Aaron, saying,

2 Take the sum of the sons of Kohath from among the sons of Levi, after their families, by the house of their fathers,

3 From thirty years old and upward even until fifty years old, all that enter into the host, to do the work in the tabernacle of the congregation.

4 This *shall be* the service of the sons of Kohath in the tabernacle of the congregation, *about* the most holy things:

5 And when the camp setteth forward, Aaron shall come, and his sons, and they shall take down the covering [h]vail, and cover the [i]ark of testimony with it:

6 And shall put thereon the covering of badgers' skins, and shall spread over *it* a cloth wholly of blue, and shall put in the [j]staves thereof.

7 And upon the table of [k]shewbread they shall spread a cloth of blue, and put thereon the dishes, and the spoons, and the bowls, and covers to cover withal: and the continual bread shall be thereon:

8 And they shall spread upon them a cloth of scarlet, and cover the same with a covering of badgers' skins, and shall put in the staves thereof.

9 And they shall take a cloth of blue, and cover the [l]candlestick of the light, and his lamps, and his tongs, and his snuffdishes, and all the oil vessels thereof, wherewith they minister unto it:

10 And they shall put it and all the vessels thereof within a covering of badgers' skins, and shall put *it* upon a bar.

11 And upon the [m]golden altar they shall spread a cloth of blue, and cover it with a covering of badgers' skins, and shall put to the staves thereof:

12 And they shall take all the [n]instruments of ministry, wherewith they minister in the sanctuary, and put *them* in a

B.C. 1490.

a vs. 7, 8.

b Num. 26:62.

c v. 15.

d vs. 12, 45.

e one shekel=2*s.* 9*d.*, or 65 cts.; also v. 50.

f One gerah=11:2 grains, or 3 1-4 cts.

g Ex. 38:27, *note.*

h Ex. 26:31; Isa. 25:7; Heb. 9:3; 10:20.

i Ex. 25:10, 16.

j 1 Ki. 8:7, 8.

k Ex. 25:30, *note.*

l Ex. 25:31-38.

m Ex. 30:1-5.

n Ex. 25:9; 1 Chr. 9:29.

cloth of blue, and cover them with a covering of badgers' skins, and shall put *them* on a bar:

13 And they shall take away the ashes from the altar, and spread a purple cloth thereon:

14 And they shall put upon it all the vessels thereof, wherewith they minister about it, *even* the censers, the fleshhooks, and the shovels, and the basons, all the vessels of the altar; and they shall spread upon it a covering of badgers' skins, and put to the staves of it.

15 And when Aaron and his sons have made an end of covering the sanctuary, and all the vessels of the sanctuary, as the camp is to set forward; after that, the sons of [a]Kohath shall come to bear *it*: but they shall not touch *any* holy thing, lest they die. These *things are* the burden of the sons of Kohath in the tabernacle of the congregation.

The order of the host:
(9) *the office of Eleazar.*

16 And to the office of Eleazar the son of Aaron the priest *pertaineth* the [b]oil for the light, and the [c]sweet incense, and the daily [d]meat-offering, and the [e]anointing oil, *and* the oversight of all the tabernacle, and of all that therein *is*, in the sanctuary, and in the vessels thereof.

17 And the LORD spake unto Moses and unto Aaron, saying,

18 Cut ye not off the tribe of the families of the Kohathites from among the Levites:

19 But thus do unto them, that they may live, and not die, when they approach unto the most [f]holy things: Aaron and his sons shall go in, and appoint them every one to his service and to his burden:

20 But they shall not go in to see when the holy things are covered, lest they die.

The order of the host:
(10) *the service of the Gershonites.*

21 And the LORD spake unto Moses, saying,

22 Take also the sum of the sons of Gershon, throughout the houses of their fathers, by their families;

23 From thirty years old and upward until fifty years old shalt thou number them; all that enter in to perform the service, to do the work in the tabernacle of the congregation.

24 This *is* the service of the families of the Gershonites, to serve, and for burdens:

25 [g]And they shall bear the curtains of the tabernacle, and the tabernacle of the congregation, his covering, and the covering of the [h]badgers' skins that *is* above upon it, and the hanging for the door of the tabernacle of the congregation,

26 And the hangings of the court, and the hanging for the door of the gate of the court, which *is* by the tabernacle and by the altar round about, and their cords, and all the instruments of their service, and all that is made for them: so shall they serve.

27 At the appointment of Aaron and his sons shall be all the service of the sons of the Gershonites, in all their burdens, and in all their service: and ye shall appoint unto them in charge all their burdens.

28 This *is* the service of the families of the sons of Gershon in the tabernacle of the congregation: and their charge *shall be* under the hand of [i]Ithamar the son of Aaron the priest.

The order of the host:
(11) *the service of the Merarites.*

29 As for the sons of Merari, thou shalt number them after their families, by the house of their fathers;

30 From [j]thirty years old and upward even unto fifty years old shalt thou number them, every one that entereth into the service, to do the work of the tabernacle of the congregation.

31 And [k]this *is* the charge of their burden, according to all their service in the tabernacle of the congregation; the [l]boards of the tabernacle, and the bars thereof, and the pillars thereof, and sockets thereof,

32 And the pillars of the court round about, and their sockets, and their pins, and their cords, with all their [m]instruments, and with all their service: and by name ye shall reckon the instruments of the charge of their burden.

33 This *is* the service of the families of the sons of Merari, according to all their service, in the tabernacle of the [n]congregation, under the hand of Ithamar the son of Aaron the priest.

34 And Moses and Aaron and the chief of the congregation numbered the

B.C. 1490.

a Num. 7:9; 10:21; Deut. 31:9; Josh. 4:10; 2 Sam. 6:13; 1 Chr. 15:2, 15.
b Ex. 25:6; Lev. 24:2.
c Ex. 30:34.
d Lit. *meal.*
e Ex. 30:23-25.
f v. 4.
g Num. 3:25, 26.
h Ex. 26:14.
i v. 33.
j v. 3.
k Num. 3:36, 37.
l Ex. 26:15.
m Ex. 25:9.
n v. 28.

sons of the Kohathites after their families, and after the house of their fathers,

35 From [a]thirty years old and upward even unto fifty years old, every one that entereth into the service, for the work in the tabernacle of the congregation:

36 And those that were numbered of them by their families were two thousand seven hundred and fifty.

37 These *were* they that were numbered of the families of the Kohathites, all that might do service in the tabernacle of the congregation, which Moses and Aaron did number according to the commandment of the LORD by the hand of Moses.

38 And those that were numbered of the sons of Gershon, throughout their families, and by the house of their fathers,

39 From thirty years old and upward even unto fifty years old, every one that entereth into the service, for the work in the tabernacle of the congregation,

40 Even those that were numbered of them, throughout their families, by the house of their fathers, were two thousand and six hundred and thirty.

41 [b]These *are* they that were numbered of the families of the sons of Gershon, of all that might do service in the tabernacle of the congregation, whom Moses and Aaron did number according to the commandment of the LORD.

42 And those that were numbered of the families of the sons of Merari, throughout their families, by the house of their fathers,

43 From thirty years old and upward even unto fifty years old, every one that entereth into the service, for the work in the tabernacle of the congregation,

44 Even those that were numbered of them after their families, were three thousand and two hundred.

45 These *be* those that were numbered of the families of the sons of Merari, whom Moses and Aaron numbered according to the word of the [c]LORD by the hand of Moses.

46 All those that were numbered of the Levites, whom Moses and Aaron and the chief of Israel numbered, after their families, and after the house of their fathers,

47 [d]From thirty years old and upward even unto fifty years old, every one that came to do the service of the ministry, and the service of the burden in the tabernacle of the congregation,

B.C. 1490.

a v. 47.

b v. 22.

c v. 29.

d vs. 3, 23, 30; 1 Chr. 23:3, 27.

e vs. 15, 24, 31.

f Lev. 15:2.

g 2 Ki. 7:3; 2 Chr. 26:21.

h Lev. 6:2.

i Lev. 5:5; Psa. 32:5; 1 John 1:9.

j Heb. *goel, Redemp. (Kinsman type).* Isa. 59:20, *note.*

k See Ex. 29:33, *note.*

48 Even those that were numbered of them, were eight thousand and five hundred and fourscore.

49 According to the commandment of the LORD they were numbered by the hand of Moses, every one according to his [e]service, and according to his burden: thus were they numbered of him, as the LORD commanded Moses.

CHAPTER 5.

The order of the host:
(12) *defilement of the camp.*

And the LORD spake unto Moses, saying,

2 Command the children of Israel, that they put out of the camp every leper, and every one that hath an [f]issue, and whosoever is defiled by the dead:

3 Both male and female shall ye put out, [g]without the camp shall ye put them; that they defile not their camps, in the midst whereof I dwell.

4 And the children of Israel did so, and put them out without the camp: as the LORD spake unto Moses, so did the children of Israel.

5 And the LORD spake unto Moses, saying,

6 Speak unto the children of Israel, [h]When a man or woman shall commit any sin that men commit, to do a trespass against the LORD, and that person be guilty;

7 Then they shall [i]confess their sin which they have done: and he shall recompense his trespass with the principal thereof, and add unto it the fifth *part* thereof, and give *it* unto *him* against whom he hath trespassed.

8 But if the man have no [j]kinsman to recompense the trespass unto, let the trespass be recompensed unto the LORD, *even* to the priest; beside the ram of the [k]atonement, whereby an atonement shall be made for him.

9 And every offering of all the holy things of the children of Israel, which they bring unto the priest, shall be his.

10 And every man's hallowed things shall be his: whatsoever any man giveth the priest, it shall be his.

11 And the LORD spake unto Moses, saying,

12 Speak unto the children of Israel, and say unto them, If any man's wife go

aside, and commit a trespass against him,
13 And a man lie with her carnally, and it be hid from the eyes of her husband, and be kept close, and she be defiled, and *there be* no witness against her, neither she be taken *with the manner*;
14 And the spirit of jealousy come upon him, and he be jealous of his wife, and she be defiled: or if the spirit of jealousy come upon him, and he be jealous of his wife, and she be not defiled:
15 Then shall the man bring his wife unto the priest, and he shall bring her [a]offering for her, the tenth *part* of an [b]ephah of barley meal; he shall pour no oil upon it, nor put frankincense thereon; for it *is* an offering of jealousy, an offering of memorial, [c]bringing iniquity to remembrance.
16 And the priest shall bring her near, and set her before the LORD:
17 And the priest shall take holy water in an earthen vessel; and of the dust that is in the floor of the tabernacle the priest shall take, and put *it* into the water:
18 And the priest shall set the woman before the [d]LORD, and uncover the woman's head, and put the offering of memorial in her hands, which *is* the jealousy offering: and the priest shall have in his hand the [e]bitter water that causeth the curse:
19 And the priest shall charge her by an oath, and say unto the woman, If no man have lain with thee, and if thou hast not gone aside to uncleanness *with another* instead of thy husband, be thou free from this bitter water that causeth the curse:
20 But if thou hast gone aside *to another* instead of thy husband, and if thou be defiled, and some man have lain with thee beside thine husband:
21 Then the priest shall [f]charge the woman with an oath of cursing, and the priest shall say unto the woman, The LORD make thee a curse and an oath among thy people, when the LORD doth make thy thigh to rot, and thy belly to swell;
22 And this water that causeth the curse shall go into thy bowels, to make *thy* belly to swell, and *thy* thigh to rot: And the woman shall say, Amen, amen.
23 And the priest shall write these curses in a book, and he shall blot *them* out with the bitter water:
24 And he shall cause the woman to drink the bitter water that causeth the curse: and the water that causeth the curse shall enter into her, *and become* bitter.
25 Then the priest shall take the jealousy offering out of the woman's hand, and shall [g]wave the offering before the LORD, and offer it upon the altar:
26 And the priest shall take an handful of the offering, [h]even the memorial thereof, and burn *it* upon the altar, and afterward shall cause the woman to drink the water.
27 And when he hath made her to drink the water, then it shall come to pass, *that*, if she be defiled, and have done trespass against her husband, that the water that causeth the curse shall enter into her, *and become* bitter, and her belly shall swell, and her thigh shall rot: and the woman shall be a [i]curse among her people.
28 And if the woman be not defiled, but be clean; then she shall be free, and shall conceive seed.
29 This *is* the law of jealousies, when a wife goeth aside *to another* instead of her husband, and is defiled;
30 Or when the spirit of jealousy cometh upon him, and he be jealous over his wife, and shall set the woman before the LORD, and the priest shall execute upon her all this law.
31 Then shall the man be guiltless from iniquity, and this woman shall bear her iniquity.

CHAPTER 6.

The order of the host: (13) *the Nazarites.*

AND the LORD spake unto Moses, [1]saying,
2 Speak unto the children of Israel, and say unto them, When either man or woman shall [j]separate *themselves* to vow a vow of a [2k]Nazarite, to separate *themselves* unto the LORD:

B.C. 1490.

a Lev. 5:11.
b One ephah=1 bu. 3 pts.
c 1 Ki. 17:18; Ezk. 29:16; Heb. 10:3.
d Heb. 13:4.
e vs. 17, 22, 24.
f Josh. 6:26; 1 Sam. 14:24; Neh. 10:29.
g Lev. 8:27.
h Lev. 2:2, 9.
i Deut. 28:37; Isa. 65:15; Jer. 24:9; 29:18, 22; 42:18.
j *Separation.* vs.1-8; Num. 16:20-26. (Gen. 12:1; 2 Cor. 6:14-17.)
k Jud. 13:5; Lam. 4:7; Amos 2:11-12; Heb. 7:26.

[1] **(6:1)** There is a beautiful moral order in chapters 6–7; *separation,* 6:1-12; *worship,* 6:13-21; *blessing,* 6:22-27; *service,* 7:1-89. See Heb. 13:12-16.

[2] **(6:2)** The Nazarite (more accurately Nazirite, *one separated*) was a person of either sex separated wholly unto the LORD. Abstention from wine, the symbol of mere natural joy (Psa. 104:15), was the expression of a devotedness which found all its joy in the LORD (cf. Psa. 87:7; 97:12; Hab. 3:18; Phil. 3:1, 3;

3 He shall separate *himself* from wine and strong drink, and shall drink no vinegar of wine, or vinegar of strong drink, neither shall he drink any liquor of grapes, nor eat moist grapes, or dried.

4 All the days of his separation shall he eat nothing that is made of the vine tree, from the kernels even to the husk.

5 All the days of the vow of his separation there shall no razor come upon his head: until the days be fulfilled, in the which he separateth *himself* unto the LORD, he shall be holy, *and* shall let the locks of the hair of his head grow.

6 All the days that he separateth *himself* unto the LORD he shall come at no dead body.

7 He shall not make himself unclean for his father, or for his mother, for his brother, or for his sister, when they die: because the consecration of his God *is* upon his head.

8 All the days of his separation he *is* holy unto the LORD.

9 And if any man die very suddenly by him, and he hath defiled the head of his consecration; then he shall shave his head in the day of his cleansing, on the seventh day shall he shave it.

10 And on the eighth day he shall bring [a]two turtles, or two young pigeons, to the priest, to the door of the tabernacle of the congregation:

11 And the priest shall offer the one for a sin-offering, and the other for a burnt-offering, and make an [b]atonement for him, for that he sinned by the dead, and shall hallow his head that same day.

12 And he shall consecrate unto the LORD the days of his separation, and shall bring a lamb of the first year for a trespass-offering: but the days that were before shall be lost, because his separation was defiled.

13 And this *is* the law of the Nazarite, when the days of his separation are fulfilled: he shall be brought unto the door of the tabernacle of the congregation:

B.C. 1490.

a Lev. 5:7.

b See Ex. 29:33, *note.*

c *Leaven.* vs. 15, 17, 19; Num. 9:11. (Gen. 19:3; Mt. 13:33.)

d Lit. *meal.* Num. 15:1-7.

e Lev. 4:30.

f 1 Sam. 2:15.

g Ex. 29:23, 28.

h Eccl. 9:7.

i *Bible prayers* (O.T.) vs. 22-26; Num. 10:35, 36 (Gen. 15:2; Hab. 3:1-16.)

14 And he shall offer his offering unto the LORD, one he lamb of the first year without blemish for a burnt-offering, and one ewe lamb of the first year without blemish for a sin-offering, and one ram without blemish for peace-offerings,

15 And a basket of [c]unleavened bread, cakes of fine flour mingled with oil, and wafers of unleavened bread anointed with oil, and their [d]meat-offering, and their drink-offerings.

16 And the priest shall bring *them* before the LORD, and shall [e]offer his sin-offering, and his burnt-offering:

17 And he shall offer the ram *for* a sacrifice of peace-offerings unto the LORD, with the basket of unleavened bread: the priest shall offer also his [d]meat-offering, and his drink-offering.

18 And the Nazarite shall shave the head of his separation *at* the door of the tabernacle of the congregation, and shall take the hair of the head of his separation, and put *it* in the fire which *is* under the sacrifice of the peace-offerings.

19 And the priest shall take the [f]sodden shoulder of the ram, and one unleavened cake out of the basket, and one [g]unleavened wafer, and shall put *them* upon the hands of the Nazarite, after *the hair of* his separation is shaven:

20 And the priest shall wave them *for* a wave-offering before the LORD: this *is* holy for the priest, with the wave breast and heave shoulder: and [h]after that the Nazarite may drink wine.

21 This *is* the law of the Nazarite who hath vowed, *and of* his offering unto the LORD for his separation, beside *that* that his hand shall get: according to the vow which he vowed, so he must do after the law of his separation.

22 And the LORD spake unto Moses, saying,

23 Speak unto Aaron and unto his sons, saying, [i]On this wise ye shall bless the children of Israel, saying unto them,

4:4, 10). The long hair, naturally a reproach to man (1 Cor. 11:14), was at once the visible sign of the Nazarite's separation, and of his willingness to bear reproach for Jehovah's sake. The type found its perfect fulfillment in Jesus, who was "holy, harmless, undefiled and separate from sinners" (Heb. 7:26); who was utterly separated unto the Father (John 1:18; 6:38); who allowed no mere natural claim to hinder or divert Him (Mt. 12:46-50).

24 The LORD bless thee, and keep thee:

25 The LORD make his [a]face shine upon thee, and be gracious unto thee:

26 The LORD [b]lift up his countenance upon thee, and give thee [c]peace.

27 And they shall put my name upon the children of Israel; and I will bless them.

CHAPTER 7.

The order of the host:
(14) *the gifts of the princes.*

And it came to pass on the day that Moses had fully set up the tabernacle, and had [d]anointed it, and sanctified it, and all the instruments thereof, both the altar and all the vessels thereof, and had anointed them, and sanctified them;

2 That the [e]princes of Israel, heads of the house of their fathers, who *were* the princes of the tribes, and were over them that were numbered, offered:

3 And [1]they brought their offering before the LORD, six covered wagons, and twelve oxen; a wagon for two of the princes, and for each one an ox: and they brought them before the tabernacle.

4 And the LORD spake unto Moses, saying,

5 Take *it* of them, that they may be to do the service of the tabernacle of the congregation; and thou shalt give them unto the Levites, to every man according to his service.

6 And Moses took the wagons and the oxen, and gave them unto the Levites.

7 Two wagons and four oxen he gave unto the sons of [f]Gershon, according to their service:

8 And four wagons and eight oxen he gave unto the sons of Merari, according unto their service, under the hand of Ithamar the son of Aaron the priest.

9 But unto the sons of Kohath he gave none: because the [g]service of the sanctuary belonging unto them *was that* they should bear upon their shoulders.

10 And the princes offered for dedicating of the altar in the day that it was anointed, even the princes offered their offering before the altar.

B.C. 1490.

a Psa. 31:16; 80:3, 7, 19; Dan. 9:17.
b Psa. 89:15.
c Lev. 26:6; Isa. 26:3, 12.
d Lev. 8:10, 11.
e Num. 1:4.
f Num. 4:24, 28.
g Num. 4:4, 15.
h One shekel=2*s.* 9*d.*, or 65 cts.; also vs. 19, 25, 31, 37, 43, 49, 55, 61, 67, 73, 79, 85, 86.
i Lit. *meal.*
j Ex. 30:34.
k Lev. 1:2, 3.
l Lev. 4:23.
m Lev. 3:1.
n v. 13.

11 And the LORD said unto Moses, They shall offer their offering, each prince on his day, for the dedicating of the altar.

12 And he that offered his offering the first day was Nahshon the son of Amminadab, of the tribe of Judah:

13 And his offering *was* one silver charger, the weight thereof *was* an hundred and thirty [h]*shekels*, one silver bowl of seventy shekels, after the shekel of the sanctuary; both of them *were* full of fine flour mingled with oil for a [i]meat-offering:

14 One spoon of ten *shekels* of gold, full of [j]incense:

15 One young bullock, one ram, one lamb of the first year, for a [k]burnt-offering:

16 One kid of the goats for a [l]sin-offering:

17 And for a sacrifice of [m]peace-offerings, two oxen, five rams, five he goats, five lambs of the first year: this *was* the offering of Nahshon the son of Amminadab.

18 On the second day Nethaneel the son of Zuar, prince of Issachar, did offer:

19 He [n]offered *for* his offering one silver charger, the weight whereof *was* an hundred and thirty *shekels*, one silver bowl of seventy shekels, after the shekel of the sanctuary; both of them full of fine flour mingled with oil for a [i]meat-offering:

20 One spoon of gold of ten *shekels*, full of incense:

21 One young bullock, one ram, one lamb of the first year, for a burnt-offering:

22 One kid of the goats for a sin-offering:

23 And for a sacrifice of peace-offerings, two oxen, five rams, five he goats, five lambs of the first year: this *was* the offering of Nethaneel the son of Zuar.

24 On the third day Eliab the son of Helon, prince of the children of Zebulun, *did offer*:

25 His offering *was* one silver charger, the weight whereof *was* an hundred and thirty *shekels*, one silver bowl of seventy shekels, after the shekel of the sanctuary; both of them full of fine flour mingled with oil for a [i]meat-offering:

[1]**(7:3)** It is beautiful to observe that, though the offerings of the princes were identical, each is separately recorded by the pen of inspiration. Cf. Mk. 12:41-44.

26 One golden spoon of ten *shekels*, full of incense:
27 One young bullock, one ram, one lamb of the first year, for a burnt-offering:
28 One kid of the goats for a sin-offering:
29 And for a sacrifice of peace-offerings, two oxen, five rams, five he goats, five lambs of the first year: this *was* the offering of Eliab the son of Helon.
30 On the fourth day [a]Elizur the son of Shedeur, prince of the children of Reuben, *did offer*:
31 His offering *was* one silver charger of the weight of an hundred and thirty *shekels*, one silver bowl of seventy shekels, after the shekel of the sanctuary; both of them full of fine flour mingled with oil for a [b]meat-offering:
32 One golden spoon of ten *shekels*, full of incense:
33 One young bullock, one ram, one lamb of the first year, for a burnt-offering:
34 One kid of the goats for a sin-offering:
35 And for a sacrifice of peace-offerings, two oxen, five rams, five he goats, five lambs of the first year: this *was* the offering of Elizur the son of Shedeur.
36 On the fifth day Shelumiel the son of Zurishaddai, prince of the children of Simeon, *did offer*:
37 His [c]offering *was* one silver charger, the weight whereof *was* an hundred and thirty *shekels*, one silver bowl of seventy shekels, after the shekel of the sanctuary; both of them full of fine flour mingled with oil for a [b]meat-offering:
38 One golden spoon of ten *shekels*, full of incense:
39 One young bullock, one ram, one lamb of the first year, for a burnt-offering:
40 One kid of the goats for a sin-offering:
41 And for a sacrifice of peace-offerings, two oxen, five rams, five he goats, five lambs of the first year: this *was* the offering of Shelumiel the son of Zurishaddai.
42 On the sixth day [d]Eliasaph the son of [e]Deuel, prince of the children of Gad, *offered*:
43 His [f]offering *was* one silver charger of the weight of an hundred and thirty *shekels*, a silver bowl of seventy shekels, after the shekel of the sanctuary; both of them full of fine flour mingled with oil for a [b]meat-offering:

B.C. 1490.

a Num. 1:5; 2:10.
b Lit. *meal.*
c v. 13.
d Num. 1:14; 2:14.
e Called *Reuel;* Num. 2:14.
f v. 13.
g v. 13.
h Num. 1:10; 2:20.
i v. 13.

44 One golden spoon of ten *shekels*, full of incense:
45 One young bullock, one ram, one lamb of the first year, for a burnt-offering:
46 One kid of the goats for a sin-offering:
47 And for a sacrifice of peace-offerings, two oxen, five rams, five he goats, five lambs of the first year: this *was* the offering of Eliasaph the son of Deuel.
48 On the seventh day Elishama the son of Ammihud, prince of the children of Ephraim, *offered*:
49 His [g]offering *was* one silver charger, the weight whereof *was* an hundred and thirty *shekels*, one silver bowl of seventy shekels, after the shekel of the sanctuary; both of them full of fine flour mingled with oil for a [b]meat-offering:
50 One golden spoon of ten *shekels*, full of incense:
51 One young bullock, one ram, one lamb of the first year, for a burnt-offering:
52 One kid of the goats for a sin-offering:
53 And for a sacrifice of peace-offerings, two oxen, five rams, five he goats, five lambs of the first year: this *was* the offering of Elishama the son of Ammihud.
54 On the eighth day [h]*offered* Gamaliel the son of Pedahzur, prince of the children of Manasseh:
55 His [i]offering *was* one silver charger of the weight of an hundred and thirty *shekels*, one silver bowl of seventy shekels, after the shekel of the sanctuary; both of them full of fine flour mingled with oil for a [b]meat-offering:
56 One golden spoon of ten *shekels*, full of incense:
57 One young bullock, one ram, one lamb of the first year, for a burnt-offering:
58 One kid of the goats for a sin-offering:
59 And for a sacrifice of peace-offerings, two oxen, five rams, five he goats, five lambs of the first year: this *was* the offering of Gamaliel the son of Pedahzur.
60 On the ninth day Abidan the son of Gideoni, prince of the children of Benjamin, *offered*:
61 His offering *was* one silver charger, the weight whereof *was* an hundred and thirty *shekels*, one silver bowl of seventy

shekels, after the shekel of the sanctuary;
both of them full of fine flour mingled
with oil for a [a]meat-offering:
62 One golden spoon of ten *shekels*,
full of incense:
63 One young bullock, one ram, one
lamb of the first year, for a burnt-offering:
64 One kid of the goats for a sin-offering:
65 And for a sacrifice of peace-offerings, two oxen, five rams, five he goats,
five lambs of the first year: this *was* the
offering of Abidan the son of Gideoni.
66 On the tenth day Ahiezer the son of
Ammishaddai, prince of the children of
Dan, *offered*:
67 His offering *was* one silver charger,
the weight whereof *was* an hundred and
thirty *shekels*, one silver bowl of seventy
shekels, after the shekel of the sanctuary;
both of them full of fine flour mingled
with oil for a [a]meat-offering:
68 One golden spoon of ten *shekels*,
full of incense:
69 One young bullock, one ram, one
lamb of the first year, for a burnt-offering:
70 One kid of the goats for a sin-offering:
71 And for a sacrifice of peace-offerings, two oxen, five rams, five he goats,
five lambs of the first year: this *was* the
offering of Ahiezer the son of
Ammishaddai.
72 On the eleventh day [b]Pagiel the son
of Ocran, prince of the children of Asher,
offered:
73 His [c]offering *was* one silver charger,
the weight whereof *was* an hundred and
thirty *shekels*, one silver bowl of seventy
shekels, after the shekel of the sanctuary;
both of them full of fine flour mingled
with oil for a [a]meat-offering:
74 One golden spoon of ten *shekels*,
full of incense:
75 One young bullock, one ram, one
lamb of the first year, for a burnt-offering:
76 One kid of the goats for a sin-offering:
77 And for a sacrifice of peace-offerings, two oxen, five rams, five he goats,
five lambs of the first year: this *was* the
offering of Pagiel the son of Ocran.
78 On the twelfth day Ahira the son of
Enan, prince of the children of Naphtali,
offered:
79 His offering *was* one silver charger,
the weight whereof *was* an hundred and
thirty *shekels*, one silver bowl of seventy
shekels, after the shekel of the sanctuary;
both of them full of fine flour mingled
with oil for a [a]meat-offering:
80 One golden spoon of ten *shekels*,
full of incense:
81 One young bullock, one ram, one
lamb of the first year, for a burnt-offering:
82 One kid of the goats for a sin-offering:
83 And for a sacrifice of peace-offerings, two oxen, five rams, five he goats,
five lambs of the first year: this *was* the
offering of Ahira the son of Enan.
84 This *was* the dedication of the altar,
in the day when it was anointed, by the
princes of Israel: twelve chargers of silver, twelve silver bowls, twelve spoons
of gold:
85 Each charger of silver *weighing* an
hundred and thirty *shekels*, each bowl
seventy: all the silver vessels *weighed*
two thousand and four hundred *shekels*,
after the shekel of the sanctuary:
86 The golden spoons *were* twelve, full
of incense, *weighing* ten *shekels* apiece,
after the shekel of the sanctuary: all the
gold of the spoons *was* an hundred and
twenty *shekels*.
87 All the oxen for the burnt-offering
were twelve bullocks, the rams twelve,
the lambs of the first year twelve, with
their [a]meat-offering: and the kids of the
goats for sin-offering twelve.
88 And all the oxen for the sacrifice of
the peace-offerings *were* twenty and four
bullocks, the rams sixty, the he goats
sixty, the lambs of the first year sixty.
This *was* the dedication of the altar, after
that it was [d]anointed.
89 And when Moses was gone into the
tabernacle of the congregation to [e]speak
with him, then he heard the voice of one
speaking unto him from off the [f]mercy
seat that *was* upon the ark of testimony,
from between the two cherubims: and he
spake unto him.

CHAPTER 8.

The order of the host:
(15) *the lamps and the candlestick.*

And the LORD spake unto Moses,
saying,
2 Speak unto Aaron, and say unto
him, When thou lightest the lamps, the
seven [g]lamps shall give light over
against the candlestick.

B.C. 1490.

a Lit. *meal.*
b Num. 1:13; 2:27.
c v. 13.
d v. 1.
e Num. 12:8; Ex. 33:9, 11.
f Ex. 25:22.
g Ex. 25:37; 40:25.

B.C. 1490.

3 And Aaron did so; he lighted the lamps thereof over against the candlestick, as the LORD commanded Moses.

4 And this work of the [a]candlestick *was of* beaten gold, unto the shaft thereof, unto the flowers thereof, *was* beaten work: according unto the [b]pattern which the LORD had shewed Moses, so he made the candlestick.

The order of the host:
(16) *cleansing the Levites.*

5 And the LORD spake unto Moses, saying,

6 Take the Levites from among the children of Israel, and [c]cleanse them.

7 And thus shalt thou do unto them, to cleanse them: Sprinkle [d]water of purifying upon them, and let them shave all their flesh, and let them wash their clothes, and *so* make themselves clean.

8 Then let them take a young bullock with his [e]meat-offering, *even* fine flour mingled with oil, and another young bullock shalt thou take for a sin-offering.

9 And thou shalt bring the Levites before the tabernacle of the congregation: and thou shalt gather the whole assembly of the children of Israel together:

10 And thou shalt bring the Levites before the LORD: and the children of Israel shall put their hands upon the Levites:

11 And Aaron shall [f]offer the Levites before the LORD *for* an offering of the children of Israel, that they may execute the service of the LORD.

12 And the Levites shall lay their hands upon the heads of the bullocks: and thou shalt offer the one *for* a sin-offering, and the other *for* a burnt-offering, unto the LORD, to make an [g]atonement for the Levites.

13 And thou shalt set the Levites before Aaron, and before his sons, and offer them *for* an offering unto the LORD.

14 Thus shalt thou separate the Levites from among the children of Israel: and the Levites shall be mine.

15 And after that shall the Levites go in to do the service of the tabernacle of the congregation: and thou shalt cleanse them, and offer them *for* an offering.

16 For they *are* wholly given unto me from among the children of Israel; instead of such as open every womb, *even instead of* the firstborn of all the children of Israel, have I taken them unto me.

17 For all the firstborn of the children of Israel *are* mine, *both* man and beast: on the day that I smote every firstborn in the land of Egypt I sanctified them for myself.

18 And I have taken the Levites for all the firstborn of the children of Israel.

19 And I have given the Levites *as* a gift to Aaron and to his sons from among the children of Israel, to do the service of the children of Israel in the tabernacle of the congregation, and to make an [g]atonement for the children of Israel: that there be no plague among the children of Israel, when the children of Israel come nigh unto the sanctuary.

20 And Moses, and Aaron, and all the congregation of the children of Israel, did to the Levites according unto all that the LORD commanded Moses concerning the Levites, so did the children of Israel unto them.

21 And the Levites were purified, and they washed their clothes; and Aaron offered them *as* an offering before the LORD; and Aaron made an [g]atonement for them to cleanse them.

22 And after that went the Levites in to do their service in the tabernacle of the congregation before Aaron, and before his sons: as the LORD had commanded Moses concerning the Levites, so did they unto them.

23 And the LORD spake unto Moses, saying,

24 This *is it* that *belongeth* unto the Levites: from twenty and five years old and upward they shall go in to wait upon the service of the tabernacle of the congregation:

25 And from the age of fifty years they shall cease waiting upon the service *thereof*, and shall serve no more:

26 But shall minister with their brethren in the tabernacle of the congregation, to keep the charge, and shall do no service. Thus shalt thou do unto the Levites touching their charge.

CHAPTER 9.

The order of the host: (17) *the Passover.*

And the LORD spake unto Moses in the wilderness of Sinai, in the

a Ex. 25:31.
b Ex. 25:40.
c 2 Cor. 7:1.
d Num. 19:9, 17; Psa. 51:2, 7; Heb. 9:13, 14.
e Lit. *meal.*
f vs. 11-22; cf. Rom. 15:16.
g See Ex. 29:33, *note.*

B.C. 1490.

[a]first month of the second year after they were come out of the land of Egypt, saying,

2 Let the children of Israel also keep the passover at his appointed [b]season.

3 In the fourteenth day of this month, at even, ye shall keep it in his appointed season: according to all the rites of it, and according to all the ceremonies thereof, shall ye keep it.

4 And Moses spake unto the children of Israel, that they should keep the passover.

5 And they kept the passover on the fourteenth day of the first month at even in the wilderness of Sinai: according to all that the LORD commanded Moses, so did the children of Israel.

6 And there were certain men, who were defiled by the dead body of a man, that they could not keep the passover on that day: and they came before Moses and before Aaron on that day:

7 And those men said unto him, We *are* defiled by the dead body of a man: wherefore are we kept back, that we may not offer an offering of the LORD in his appointed season among the children of Israel?

8 And Moses said unto them, Stand still, and I will hear what the LORD will command concerning you.

9 And the LORD spake unto Moses, saying,

10 Speak unto the children of Israel, saying, If any man of you or of your posterity shall be unclean by reason of a dead body, or *be* in a journey afar off, yet he shall keep the passover unto the LORD.

11 The fourteenth day of the [c]second month at even they shall keep it, *and* eat it with [d]unleavened bread and bitter *herbs*.

12 They shall leave none of it unto the morning, nor break any [e]bone of it: according to all the ordinances of the passover they shall keep it.

13 But the man that *is* clean, and is not in a journey, and forbeareth to keep the passover, even the same [f]soul shall be cut off from among his people: because he brought not the offering of the LORD in his appointed season, that man shall bear his sin.

14 And if a [g]stranger shall sojourn among you, and will keep the passover unto the LORD; according to the ordinance of the passover, and according to the manner thereof, so shall he do: ye shall have one ordinance, both for the stranger, and for him that was born in the land.

The order of the host:
(18) *the guiding cloud.*

15 And on the day that the tabernacle was reared up the cloud [h]covered the tabernacle, *namely*, the tent of the testimony: and at even there was upon the tabernacle as it were the appearance of fire, until the morning.

16 So it was alway: the cloud covered it *by day*, and the appearance of fire by night.

17 And when the [i]cloud was taken up from the tabernacle, then after that the children of Israel journeyed: and in the place where the cloud abode, there the children of Israel pitched their tents.

18 At the commandment of the LORD the children of Israel journeyed, and at the commandment of the LORD they pitched: as long as the cloud abode upon the tabernacle they rested in their tents.

19 And when the cloud tarried long upon the tabernacle many days, then the children of Israel kept the [j]charge of the LORD, and journeyed not.

20 And *so* it was, when the cloud was a few days upon the tabernacle; according to the commandment of the LORD they abode in their tents, and according to the commandment of the LORD they journeyed.

21 And *so* it was, when the cloud abode from even unto the morning, and *that* the cloud was taken up in the morning, then they journeyed: whether *it was* by day or by night that the cloud was taken up, they journeyed.

22 Or *whether it were* two days, or a month, or a year, that the cloud tarried upon the tabernacle, remaining thereon, the children of Israel [k]abode in their tents, and journeyed not: but when it was taken up, they journeyed.

23 At the commandment of the LORD they rested in the tents, and at the commandment of the LORD they journeyed: they kept the charge of the LORD, at the commandment of the LORD by the hand of Moses.

a i.e. *April;* also v. 5.
b Ex. 12:3; Deut. 16:1; 2 Chr. 30:1-15; Lk. 22:7; 1 Cor. 5:7-8.
c i.e. *May.*
d *Leaven.* Num. 28:17. (Gen. 19:3; Mt. 13:33.)
e Fulfilled. John 19:36.
f Heb. 10:29; 12:25.
g Isa. 56:6, 7.
h Isa. 4:5.
i Num. 10:11, 33, 34; Ex. 33:14, 15; Ex. 40:36, 38.
j Num. 1:53; 3:8; Zech. 3:7.
k Ex. 40:36, 37.

B.C. 1490.

CHAPTER 10.

The order of the host
(19) *the silver assembly-trumpets.*

And the LORD spake unto Moses, saying,

2 Make thee two trumpets of silver; of a whole piece shalt thou make them: that thou mayest use them for the calling of the assembly, and for the journeying of the camps.

3 And when they shall blow with them, all the assembly shall assemble themselves to thee at the door of the tabernacle of the congregation.

4 And if they blow *but* with one *trumpet*, then the princes, *which are* [a]heads of the thousands of Israel, shall gather themselves unto thee.

5 When ye blow an [b]alarm, then the camps that lie on the east parts shall go forward.

6 When ye blow an alarm the second time, then the camps that lie on the [c]south side shall take their journey: they shall blow an alarm for their journeys.

7 But when the congregation is to be gathered together, ye shall blow, but ye shall not sound an alarm.

8 And the sons of Aaron, the [d]priests, shall blow with the trumpets; and they shall be to you for an ordinance for ever throughout your generations.

9 And if ye go to war in your land against the enemy that oppresseth you, then ye shall blow an alarm with the trumpets; and ye shall be remembered before the LORD your God, and ye shall be saved from your enemies.

10 [e]Also in the day of your gladness, and in your solemn days, and in the beginnings of your months, ye shall blow with the trumpets over your burnt-offerings, and over the sacrifices of your peace-offerings; that they may be to you for a [f]memorial before your God: I *am* the LORD your God.

From Sinai to Kadesh-barnea:
(1) *the first march; the halt in Paran.*

11 And it came to pass on the twentieth *day* of the [g]second month, in the second year, that the cloud was taken up from off the tabernacle of the testimony.

12 And the children of Israel took their journeys out of the wilderness of Sinai; and the cloud rested in the wilderness of Paran.

13 And they first took their journey according to the commandment of the LORD by the hand of Moses.

14 In the first *place* went the standard of the camp of the children of Judah according to their armies: and over his host *was* Nahshon the son of Amminadab.

15 And over the host of the tribe of the children of Issachar *was* Nethaneel the son of Zuar.

16 And over the host of the tribe of the children of Zebulun *was* Eliab the son of Helon.

17 And the tabernacle was taken down; and the sons of Gershon and the sons of Merari set forward, bearing the tabernacle.

18 And the standard of the camp of Reuben set forward according to their armies: and over his host *was* Elizur the son of Shedeur.

19 And over the host of the tribe of the children of Simeon *was* Shelumiel the son of Zurishaddai.

20 And over the host of the tribe of the children of Gad *was* Eliasaph the son of Deuel.

21 And the Kohathites set forward, bearing the sanctuary: and *the other* did set up the tabernacle against they came.

22 And the standard of the camp of the children of Ephraim set forward according to their armies: and over his host *was* Elishama the son of Ammihud.

23 And over the host of the tribe of the children of Manasseh *was* Gamaliel the son of Pedahzur.

24 And over the host of the tribe of the children of Benjamin *was* Abidan the son of Gideoni.

25 And the standard of the camp of the children of Dan set forward, *which was* the rereward of all the camps throughout their hosts: and over his host *was* Ahiezer the son of Ammishaddai.

26 And over the host of the tribe of the children of Asher *was* Pagiel the son of Ocran.

27 And over the host of the tribe of the children of Naphtali *was* Ahira the son of Enan.

28 Thus *were* the journeyings of the children of Israel according to their armies, when they set forward.

29 And Moses said unto Hobab, the son of [h]Raguel the [i]Midianite, Moses' father in law, We are journeying unto the place of which the LORD said, I will give it you: come thou with us, and we will

a Num. 1:16; Ex. 18:21.
b Joel 2:1.
c Num. 2:10.
d Num. 31:6; 1 Chr. 15:24; 2 Chr. 13:12.
e Num. 29:1; Lev. 23:24; 2 Chr. 5:12; Psa. 81:3; 89:15; Isa. 18:3-7; 27:13.
f Ex. 28:29.
g i.e. *May.*
h Called *Reuel,* Ex. 2:18.
i Cf. Ex. 18:15-27.

do thee good: for the LORD hath spoken
good concerning Israel.
30 And he said unto him, I will not go;
but I will depart to mine own land, and
to my kindred.
31 And he said, Leave us not, I pray
thee; forasmuch as thou knowest how
we are to encamp in the wilderness, and
[a]thou mayest be to us instead of eyes.
32 And it shall be, if thou go with us,
yea, it shall be, that what goodness the
LORD shall do unto us, the same will we
do unto thee.
33 And they departed from the mount
of the LORD three days' journey: and the
ark of the covenant of the LORD went
before them in the three days' journey, to
search out a resting place for them.
34 And the cloud of the LORD *was*
upon them by day, when they went out
of the camp.
35 And it came to pass, when the ark set
forward, that Moses said, Rise up, LORD,
and let thine enemies be scattered; and let
them that hate thee flee before thee.
36 And when it rested, he [b]said,
Return, O LORD, unto the many thousands of Israel.

CHAPTER 11.

From Sinai to Kadesh-barnea:
(2) *the fire of the Lord at Taberah.*

And *when* the people complained, it
displeased the LORD: and the LORD
heard *it*; and his anger was kindled; and
the fire of the LORD burnt among them,
and [c]consumed *them that were* in the
uttermost parts of the camp.
2 And the people cried unto Moses;
and when Moses prayed unto the LORD,
the fire was quenched.
3 And he called the name of the place
[d]Taberah: because the fire of the LORD
burnt among them.

From Sinai to Kadesh-barnea:
(3) *the flesh-pots of Egypt.*

4 And [e]the mixt multitude that *was*
among them fell a lusting: and the children of Israel also wept again, and said,
Who shall give us flesh to eat?
5 We remember the fish, which we did
eat in Egypt freely; the cucumbers, and
the melons, and the leeks, and the
onions, and the garlick:
6 But now our soul *is* dried away: *there*
is nothing at all, beside this [f]manna,
before our eyes.
7 And the manna *was* as coriander
seed, and the colour thereof as the
colour of bdellium.
8 *And* the people went about, and
gathered *it*, and ground *it* in mills, or
beat *it* in a mortar, and baked *it* in pans,
and made cakes of it: and the taste of it
was as the taste of fresh oil.
9 And when the dew fell upon the
camp in the night, the manna fell upon it.

From Sinai to Kadesh-barnea:
(4) *the complaint of Moses.*

10 Then Moses heard the people weep
throughout their families, every man in
the door of his tent: and the anger of the
LORD was kindled greatly; Moses also
was displeased.
11 And Moses said unto the LORD,
Wherefore hast thou afflicted thy servant? and wherefore have I not found
favour in thy sight, that thou layest the
burden of all this people upon me?
12 Have I conceived all this people?
have I begotten them, that thou
shouldest say unto me, Carry them in
thy bosom, as a nursing father beareth
the sucking child, unto the land which
thou swarest unto their fathers?
13 Whence should I have flesh to give
unto all this people? for they weep unto
me, saying, Give us flesh, that we may
eat.
14 I am not able to bear all this people
alone, because *it is* too heavy for me.
15 And if thou deal thus with me, kill
me, I [g]pray thee, out of hand, if I have
found favour in thy sight; and let me not
see my wretchedness.

From Sinai to Kadesh-barnea:
(5) *the seventy elders.* (Cf. Ex. 18:19.)

16 And the LORD said unto Moses,
Gather unto me seventy men of the
elders of Israel, whom thou knowest to
be the elders of the people, and officers
over them; and bring them unto the
tabernacle of the congregation, that they
may stand there with thee.
17 And I will come down and talk
with thee there: and I will take of the
[h]spirit which *is* upon thee, and will put
it upon them; and they shall bear the
burden of the people with thee, that
thou bear *it* not thyself alone.
18 And say thou unto the people,
Sanctify yourselves against to morrow,
and ye shall eat flesh: for ye have wept

B.C. 1490.

a But see Ex. 13:21, 22. What need had Moses of Hobab's eyes? Cf. Jer. 17:5.

b *Bible prayers* (O.T.). Num. 11:11-15. (Gen. 15:2; Hab. 3:1-16.)

c *Miracles* (O.T.). vs. 1-3; Num. 16:31-35. (Gen. 5:24; Jon. 2:1-10.)

d *a burning.*

e Cf. Ex. 12:38, *note.* Unconverted church members, unable to desire or understand Christ as the Bread of God (Ex. 16:35, note), will clamour for things pleasing to the flesh in the work and way of the church: sumptuous buildings, ornate ritual, an easy doctrine. Alas! they led away the unspiritual believers also.

f Ex. 16:35, *note.*

g *Bible prayers* (O.T.). vs. 11-15; Num. 12:13. (Gen. 15:2; Hab. 3:1-16.)

h *Holy Spirit.* vs. 17, 25, 26, 29; Num. 24:2. (Gen. 1:2; Mal. 2:15.)

in the ears of the LORD, saying, Who shall give us flesh to eat? for *it was* well with us in Egypt: therefore the LORD will give you flesh, and ye shall eat.

19 Ye shall not eat one day, nor two days, nor five days, neither ten days, nor twenty days;

20 *But* even a whole month, until it come out at your nostrils, and it be loathsome unto you: because that ye have despised the LORD which *is* among you, and have wept before him, saying, Why came we forth out of Egypt?

21 And Moses said, The people, among whom I *am*, *are* six hundred thousand footmen; and thou hast said, I will give them flesh, that they may eat a whole month.

22 Shall the flocks and the herds be slain for them, to suffice them? or shall all the fish of the sea be gathered together for them, to suffice them?

23 And the LORD said unto Moses, Is the LORD'S hand waxed short? thou shalt see now whether my word shall come to pass unto thee or not.

24 And Moses went out, and told the people the [a]words of the LORD, and gathered the seventy men of the elders of the people, and set them round about the tabernacle.

25 And the LORD came down in a cloud, and spake unto him, and took of the [b]spirit that *was* upon [1]him, and gave *it* unto the seventy elders: and it came to pass, *that*, when the spirit rested upon them, they prophesied, and did not cease.

From Sinai to Kadesh-barnea:
(6) *Eldad and Medad prophesy.*

26 But there remained two *of the* men in the camp, the name of the one *was* Eldad, and the name of the other Medad: and the [b]spirit rested upon them; and they *were* of them that were written, but went not out unto the tabernacle: and they prophesied in the camp.

27 And there ran a young man, and told Moses, and said, Eldad and Medad do prophesy in the camp.

B.C. 1490.

a *Inspiration.* Num. 22:38. (Ex. 4:15; Rev. 22:19.)

b *Holy Spirit.* vs. 17, 25, 26, 29; Num. 24:2. (Gen. 1:2; Mal. 2:15.)

c One cubit=1 ft. 5.48 in.

d One homer=about 86 gals.

e Num. 33:17.

f i.e. *graves of lust.* Num. 33:17.

g Ex. 15:20, 21; Num. 20:1. Cf. Acts 22:21, 22.

h Cf. Song 1:5.

i Cf. Lk. 9:33-36.

28 And Joshua the son of Nun, the servant of Moses, *one* of his young men, answered and said, My lord Moses, forbid them.

29 And Moses said unto him, Enviest thou for my sake? would God that all the LORD'S people were prophets, *and* that the LORD would put his [b]spirit upon them!

30 And Moses gat him into the camp, he and the elders of Israel.

From Sinai to Kadesh-barnea:
(7) *the quails and the plague.*

31 And there went forth a wind from the LORD, and brought quails from the sea, and let *them* fall by the camp, as it were a day's journey on this side, and as it were a day's journey on the other side, round about the camp, and as it were two [c]cubits *high* [2]upon the face of the earth.

32 And the people stood up all that day, and all *that* night, and all the next day, and they gathered the quails: he that gathered least gathered ten [d]homers: and they spread *them* all abroad for themselves round about the camp.

33 And while the flesh *was* yet between their teeth, ere it was chewed, the wrath of the LORD was kindled against the people, and the LORD smote the people with a very great plague.

34 And he called the name of that place Kibroth-hattaavah: because there they buried the people that lusted.

35 *And* the people [e]journeyed from [f]Kibroth-hattaavah unto Hazeroth; and abode at Hazeroth.

CHAPTER 12.

From Sinai to Kadesh-barnea:
(8) *the murmuring of Miriam and Aaron.*

And [g]Miriam and Aaron spake against Moses because of the [h]Ethiopian woman whom he had married: for he had married an Ethiopian woman.

2 And they said, Hath the LORD indeed spoken [i]only by Moses? hath he

[1]**(11:25)** There was no more *power* than before—only more *machinery.* Moses had murmured (v. 11) because of the burden that God had laid upon him. God, in distributing the burden, shows that Moses' power had, all along, been in proportion to his burden.

[2]**(11:31)** The correct rendering is, "about two cubits above the face of the earth," that is, within reach of the people that they might slay them for food. The statement is not that the quails were piled up from the face of the earth two cubits *deep.* The *level of their flight* was two cubits above the earth.

not spoken also by us? And the LORD heard *it*.

3 (Now the man Moses *was* very [a]meek, above all the men which *were* upon the face of the earth.)

4 And the LORD spake suddenly unto Moses, and unto Aaron, and unto Miriam, Come out ye three unto the tabernacle of the congregation. And they three came out.

5 And the LORD came down in the pillar of the cloud, and stood *in* the door of the tabernacle, and called Aaron and Miriam: and they both came forth.

6 And he said, Hear now my words: If there be a [b]prophet among you, *I* the LORD will make myself known unto him in a vision, *and* will speak unto him in a dream.

7 My servant Moses *is* not so, [c]who *is* faithful in all mine house.

8 With him will I speak mouth to mouth, even apparently, and not in dark speeches; and the similitude of the LORD shall he behold: wherefore then were ye not [d]afraid to speak against my servant Moses?

9 And the anger of the LORD was kindled against them; and he departed.

10 And the cloud departed from off the tabernacle; and, behold, Miriam *became* [e]leprous, *white* as snow: and Aaron looked upon Miriam, and, behold, *she was* leprous.

11 And Aaron said unto Moses, Alas, my lord, I beseech thee, lay not the sin upon us, wherein we have done foolishly, and wherein we have sinned.

12 Let her not be as one dead, of whom the flesh is half consumed when he cometh out of his mother's womb.

13 And Moses cried unto the LORD, saying, Heal her now, O God, I [f]beseech thee.

14 And the LORD said unto Moses, If her father had but spit in her face, should she not be ashamed seven days? let her be [g]shut out from the camp seven days, and after that let her be received in *again*.

15 And Miriam was shut out from the camp seven days: and the people journeyed not till Miriam was brought in *again*.

16 And afterward the people removed from Hazeroth, and [h]pitched in the wilderness of Paran.

B.C. 1490.

a See Num. 20:10; 1 Pet. 2:23; 2 Cor. 10:1.

b Cf. Num. 11:25.

c Heb. 3:1-6.

d Psa. 105:15.

e Cf. 2 Ki. 5:27; 2 Chr. 26:19.

f *Bible prayers* (O.T.). Num. 14:13-19. (Gen. 15:2; Hab. 3:1-16.)

g Lev. 13:4-46; Heb. 12:9.

h Deut. 1:19.

i Cf. Deut. 1:19-28.

j i.e. *Saviour*, or *Deliverer*.

CHAPTER 13.

At Kadesh-barnea: (1) the spies sent in.

And the LORD spake unto Moses, saying,

2 [i]Send thou men, that they may search the land of Canaan, which I give unto the children of Israel: of every tribe of their fathers shall ye send a man, every one a ruler among them.

3 And Moses by the commandment of the LORD sent them from the wilderness of Paran: all those men *were* heads of the children of Israel.

4 And these *were* their names: of the tribe of Reuben, Shammua the son of Zaccur.

5 Of the tribe of Simeon, Shaphat the son of Hori.

6 Of the tribe of Judah, Caleb the son of Jephunneh.

7 Of the tribe of Issachar, Igal the son of Joseph.

8 Of the tribe of Ephraim, Oshea the son of Nun.

9 Of the tribe of Benjamin, Palti the son of Raphu.

10 Of the tribe of Zebulun, Gaddiel the son of Sodi.

11 Of the tribe of Joseph, *namely*, of the tribe of Manasseh, Gaddi the son of Susi.

12 Of the tribe of Dan, Ammiel the son of Gemalli.

13 Of the tribe of Asher, Sethur the son of Michael.

14 Of the tribe of Naphtali, Nahbi the son of Vophsi.

15 Of the tribe of Gad, Geuel the son of Machi.

16 These *are* the names of the men which Moses sent to spy out the land. And Moses called Oshea the son of Nun [j]Jehoshua.

17 And Moses sent them to spy out the land of Canaan, and said unto them, Get you up this *way* southward, and go up into the mountain:

18 And see the land, what it *is*; and the people that dwelleth therein, whether they *be* strong or weak, few or many;

19 And what the land *is* that they dwell in, whether it *be* good or bad; and what cities *they be* that they dwell in, whether in tents, or in strong holds;

20 And what the land *is*, whether it *be* fat or lean, whether there be wood therein, or not. And be ye of good courage, and bring of the fruit of the land. Now

B.C. 1490.

the time *was* the time of the firstripe grapes.

21 So they went up, and searched the land from the wilderness of Zin unto Rehob, as men come to Hamath.

22 And they ascended by the south, and came unto Hebron; where Ahiman, Sheshai, and Talmai, the children of [a]Anak, *were*. (Now Hebron was built seven years before Zoan in Egypt.)

23 And they came unto the brook of [b]Eshcol, and cut down from thence a branch with one cluster of grapes, and they bare it between two upon a staff; and *they brought* of the pomegranates, and of the figs.

24 The place was called the brook Eshcol, because of the cluster of grapes which the children of Israel cut down from thence.

25 And they returned from searching of the land after forty days.

At Kadesh-barnea:
(2) *the report of the spies.*

26 And they went and came to Moses, and to Aaron, and to all the congregation of the children of Israel, unto the [c]wilderness of Paran, to [d]Kadesh; and brought back word unto them, and unto all the congregation, and shewed them the fruit of the land.

27 And they told him, and said, We came unto the land whither thou sentest us, and surely it [e]floweth with milk and honey; and this *is* the fruit of it.

28 Nevertheless the [f]people *be* strong that dwell in the land, and the cities *are* walled, *and* very great: and moreover we saw the children of [g]Anak there.

29 The Amalekites dwell in the land of the south: and the Hittites, and the Jebusites, and the Amorites, dwell in the mountains: and the Canaanites dwell by the sea, and by the coast of Jordan.

30 And Caleb stilled the people before Moses, and said, Let us go up at once, and possess it; for we are well able to overcome it.

31 But the men that went up with him said, We be not able to go up against the people; for they *are* stronger than we.

32 And they brought up an evil report of the land which they had searched unto the children of Israel, saying, The land, through which we have gone to search it, *is* a land that eateth up the inhabitants thereof; and all the people that we saw in it *are* men of a great stature.

33 And there we saw the giants, the sons of [h]Anak, *which come* of the giants: and we were in our own sight as grasshoppers, and so we were in their sight.

CHAPTER 14.

At Kadesh-barnea: (3) *the unbelief of Israel*
(1 Cor. 10:1–5; Heb. 3:7–19).

And all the congregation lifted up their voice, and cried; and the people wept that night.

2 And all the children of Israel [i]murmured against Moses and against Aaron: and the whole congregation said unto them, Would God that we had died in the land of Egypt! or would God we had died in this wilderness!

3 And wherefore hath the LORD brought us unto this land, to fall by the sword, that our wives and our children should be a prey? were it not better for us to return into Egypt?

4 And they said one to another, Let us make a captain, and let us return into Egypt.

5 Then Moses and Aaron fell on their faces before all the assembly of the congregation of the children of Israel.

6 And Joshua the son of Nun, and Caleb the son of Jephunneh, *which were* of them that searched the land, rent their clothes:

7 And they spake unto all the company of the children of Israel, saying, The land, which we passed through to search it, *is* an exceeding good land.

8 If the LORD delight in us, then he will bring us into this land, and give it us; a land which floweth with milk and honey.

9 Only [j]rebel not ye against the LORD, neither fear ye the people of the land; for they *are* bread for us: their defence is departed from them, [k]and the LORD *is* with us: fear them not.

10 But all the congregation bade stone them with stones. And the glory of the LORD appeared in the tabernacle of the congregation before all the children of Israel.

11 And the LORD said unto Moses, How long will this people [l]provoke me?

a Josh. 11:21, 22;15:13, 14.
b i.e. *cluster.*
c v. 3.
d Num. 20:1, 16; 32:8; 33:36; Deut. 1:19; Josh. 14:6.
e Ex. 3:8; 33:3.
f Deut. 1:28; 9:1, 2.
g v. 33.
h Josh. 11:21, 22.
i Ex. 16:2; 17:3; Num. 16:41; Psa. 106:25.
j Deut. 9:7; 20:3; 1 Sam. 15:22, 23.
k Gen. 48:21; Ex. 33:16; Deut. 20:1, 3, 4; 31:6-8; Josh. 1:5; Jud. 1:22; 2 Chr. 13:12; Psa. 46:7-11; Zech. 8:23.
l v. 23; Deut. 9:7, 8, 22; Heb. 3:8, 16.

and how long will it be ere they believe me, for all the signs which I have shewed among them?

12 I will smite them with the pestilence, and disinherit them, and will [a]make of thee a greater nation and mightier than they.

13 [b]And Moses said unto the LORD, [c]Then the Egyptians shall hear *it*, (for thou broughtest up this people in thy might from among them;)

14 And they will tell *it* to the inhabitants of this land: *for* they have heard that thou LORD *art* among this people, that thou LORD art seen face to face, and *that* thy cloud standeth over them, and *that* thou goest before them, by day time in a pillar of a cloud, and in a pillar of fire by night.

15 Now *if* thou shalt kill *all* this people as one man, then the nations which have heard the fame of thee will speak, saying,

16 Because the LORD was not able to bring this people into the land which he sware unto them, therefore he hath slain them in the wilderness.

17 And now, I beseech thee, let the power of my Lord be great, according as thou hast spoken, saying,

18 The LORD *is* longsuffering, and of great mercy, forgiving iniquity and transgression, and by no means clearing *the guilty*, visiting the iniquity of the fathers upon the children unto the third and fourth *generation*.

19 Pardon, I beseech thee, the iniquity of this people according unto the greatness of thy mercy, and as thou hast forgiven this people, from Egypt even until now.

20 And the LORD said, I have pardoned according to thy word:

21 But *as* truly *as* I live, all the earth shall be [d]filled with the glory of the LORD.

22 Because all those men which have seen my glory, and my miracles, which I did in Egypt and in the wilderness, and have [e]tempted me now these ten times, and have not hearkened to my voice;

23 [1]Surely they shall not see the land which I sware unto their fathers, neither shall any of them that provoked me see it:

24 But my servant Caleb, because he had another spirit with him, and hath followed me fully, him will I bring into the land whereinto he went; and his seed shall possess it.

25 (Now the Amalekites and the Canaanites dwelt in the valley.) To morrow turn you, and get you into the wilderness by the way of the Red sea.

26 And the LORD spake unto Moses and unto Aaron, saying,

27 How long *shall I bear with* this evil congregation, which murmur against me? I have heard the murmurings of the children of Israel, which they murmur against me.

28 Say unto them, *As truly as* I live, saith the LORD, as ye have spoken in mine ears, so will I do to you:

29 Your carcases shall fall in this wilderness; and all that were numbered of you, according to your whole number, from twenty years old and upward, which have murmured against me,

30 Doubtless ye shall not come into the land, *concerning* which I sware to make you dwell therein, [f]save Caleb the son of Jephunneh, and Joshua the son of Nun.

31 But your little ones, which ye said should be a prey, them will I bring in, and they shall know the land which ye have despised.

32 But *as for* you, your carcases, they shall fall in this wilderness.

33 And your children shall wander in the wilderness forty years, and bear your whoredoms, until your carcases be wasted in the wilderness.

34 After the number of the days in which ye searched the land, *even* forty days, each day for a year, shall ye bear your iniquities, *even* forty years, and ye shall know my breach of promise.

35 I the LORD have said, I will surely do it unto all this evil congregation, that are gathered together against me: in this wilderness they shall be consumed, and there they shall die.

36 And the men, which Moses sent to search the land, who returned, and

B.C. 1490.

a Cf. Ex. 32:10.

b *Bible prayers* (O.T.). Num. 27:15. (Gen. 15:2; Hab. 3:1-16.)

c Ex. 32:12; Deut. 9:26-28; 32:27.

d Psa. 72:19; Isa. 66:18, 19; Hab. 2:14; Mt. 6:10.

e *Temptation*. Deut. 6:16. (Gen. 3:1; Jas. 1:2.)

f v. 38; Num. 26:65; 32:12; Deut. 1:36-38; Josh. 14:6-15.

[1]**(14:23)** Kadesh-barnea is, by the unbelief of Israel there, and the divine comment on that unbelief (Num. 14:22-38; Deut. 1:19-40; 1 Cor. 10:1-5; Heb. 3:12-19), invested with immense spiritual significance. The people had faith to sprinkle the blood of atonement (Ex. 12:28) and to come out of Egypt (the world), but had not faith to enter their Canaan rest. Therefore, though redeemed, they were a forty years' grief to Jehovah. The spiritual application is made in Heb. 6:3-11, *note*.

made all the congregation to murmur
against him, by bringing up a slander
upon the land,
37 Even those men that did bring up
the evil report upon the land, died by
the plague before the LORD.
38 But Joshua the son of Nun, and
Caleb the son of Jephunneh, *which were*
of the men that went to search the land,
lived *still*.
39 And Moses told these sayings unto
all the children of Israel: and the people
mourned greatly.
40 And they rose up early in the morning, and gat them up into the top of the
mountain, saying, Lo, we *be here*, and
will go up unto the place which the LORD
hath promised: for we have sinned.
41 And Moses said, Wherefore now do
ye transgress the commandment of the
LORD? but it shall not prosper.
42 Go not up, for the LORD *is* not
among you; that ye be not smitten before
your enemies.
43 For the Amalekites and the
Canaanites *are* there before you, and ye
shall fall by the sword: because ye are
turned away from the LORD, therefore
the LORD will not be with you.
44 But they [a]presumed to go up unto
the hill top: nevertheless the ark of the
covenant of the LORD, and Moses,
departed not out of the camp.
45 Then the Amalekites came down,
and the Canaanites which dwelt in that
hill, and smote them, and discomfited
them, *even* unto Hormah.

CHAPTER 15.

The years of [1]*wandering:*
(1) *the end anticipated.*

And the LORD spake unto Moses,
saying,
2 Speak unto the children of Israel,
and say unto them, [2]When ye be come
into the land of your habitations, which I
give unto you,
3 And will make an offering by fire
unto the LORD, a burnt-offering, or a sacrifice in performing a vow, or in a
freewill offering, or in your solemn
feasts, to make a sweet savour unto the
LORD, of the herd, or of the flock:
4 Then shall he that offereth his offering unto the LORD bring a [b]meat-offering
of a tenth deal of flour mingled with the
fourth *part* of an [c]hin of oil.
5 And the fourth *part* of an hin of wine
for a drink-offering shalt thou prepare
with the burnt-offering or sacrifice, for
one lamb.
6 Or for a ram, thou shalt prepare *for* a
[b]meat-offering two tenth deals of flour
mingled with the third *part* of an hin of
oil.
7 And for a drink-offering thou shalt
offer the third *part* of an hin of wine, *for*
a sweet savour unto the LORD.
8 And when thou preparest a bullock
for a burnt-offering, or *for* a sacrifice in
performing a vow, or peace-offerings
unto the LORD:
9 Then shall he bring with a bullock a
[b]meat-offering of three tenth deals of
flour mingled with half an hin of oil.
10 And thou shalt bring for a drink-
offering half an hin of wine, *for* an offering made by fire, of a sweet savour unto
the LORD.
11 Thus shall it be done for one bullock, or for one ram, or for a lamb, or a
kid.
12 According to the number that ye
shall prepare, so shall ye do to every one
according to their number.
13 All that are born of the country
shall do these things after this manner,

B.C. 1490.

a Cf. Josh. 7:1-8.

b Lit. *meal.*

c One hin=about 6 qts.; also vs. 5, 6, 7, 9, 10.

[1]**(15, heading)** The *wilderness* was part of the necessary discipline of the redeemed people, but not the years of *wandering*. The latter were due wholly to the unbelief of the people at Kadesh-barnea. The Red Sea, Marah, Elim, Sinai, were God's ways, in development and discipline, and have, of necessity, their counterpart in Christian experience. The Red Sea speaks of the cross as that which—death to Christ but life for us—separates us from Egypt, the world (Gal. 6:14); Marah of God's power to turn untoward things into blessing; Elim of God's power to give rest and refreshment by the way; Sinai of God's holiness and our deep inherent evil, the experience of Rom. 7:7-24. So far the path was and is of God. But from Kadesh-barnea to Jordan all save the grace of God toward an unbelieving people, is for warning, not imitation (1 Cor. 10:1-11; Heb. 3:17-19). There is a present rest of God, of which the Sabbath and Canaan were types, into which believers may, and therefore should, enter by faith (Heb. 3–4).

[2]**(15:2)** It is remarkable that just when the *people* are turning in unbelief from the land, *God*

in offering an offering made by fire, of a sweet savour unto the LORD.

14 And if a stranger sojourn with you, or whosoever *be* among you in your generations, and will offer an offering made by fire, of a sweet savour unto the LORD; as ye do, so he shall do.

15 One ordinance *shall be both* for you of the congregation, and also for the stranger that sojourneth *with you*, an ordinance for ever in your generations: as ye *are*, so shall the stranger be before the LORD.

16 One law and one manner shall be for you, and for the stranger that sojourneth with you.

17 And the LORD spake unto Moses, saying,

18 Speak unto the children of Israel, and say unto them, When ye come into the land whither I bring you,

19 Then it shall be, that, when ye eat of the bread of the land, ye shall offer up an heave-offering unto the LORD.

20 Ye shall offer up a cake of the first of your dough *for* an heave-offering: as *ye do* the heave-offering of the threshingfloor, so shall ye heave it.

21 Of the first of your dough ye shall give unto the LORD an heave-offering in your generations.

22 And if ye have erred, and not observed all these commandments, which the LORD hath spoken unto Moses,

23 *Even* all that the LORD hath commanded you by the hand of Moses, from the day that the LORD commanded *Moses*, and henceforward among your generations;

24 Then it shall be, if *ought* be committed by ignorance without the knowledge of the congregation, that all the congregation shall offer one young bullock for a burnt-offering, for a sweet savour unto the LORD, with his [a]meat-offering, and his drink-offering, according to the manner, and one kid of the goats for a sin-offering.

25 And the priest shall make an [b]atonement for all the congregation of the children of Israel, and it shall be [c]forgiven them; for it *is* ignorance: and they shall bring their offering, a sacrifice made by fire unto the LORD, and their sin-offering before the LORD, for their ignorance:

26 And it shall be forgiven all the congregation of the children of Israel, and the stranger that sojourneth among them; seeing all the people *were* in ignorance.

27 And if any soul sin through ignorance, then he shall bring a she goat of the first year for a sin-offering.

28 And the priest shall make an [b]atonement for the soul that sinneth ignorantly, when he sinneth by ignorance before the LORD, to make an [b]atonement for him; and it shall be forgiven him.

29 Ye shall have one law for him that sinneth through ignorance, *both for* him that is born among the children of Israel, and for the stranger that sojourneth among them.

30 But the soul that doeth *ought* presumptuously, *whether he be* born in the land, or a stranger, the same reproacheth the LORD; and that soul shall be cut off from among his people.

31 Because he hath despised the word of the LORD, and hath broken his commandment, that soul shall utterly be cut off; his iniquity *shall be* upon him.

What the law really is (Rom. 3:19; 7:7–11; 2 Cor. 3:7, 9; Gal. 3:10).

32 And while the children of Israel were in the wilderness, they found a man that gathered sticks upon the [d]sabbath day.

33 And they that found him gathering sticks brought him unto Moses and Aaron, and unto all the congregation.

34 And they put him in ward, because it was not declared what should be done to him.

35 And the LORD said unto Moses, The man shall be surely put to death: all the congregation shall stone him with stones without the camp.

36 And all the congregation brought him without the camp, and stoned him with stones, and he died; as the LORD commanded Moses.

The ribband of blue, the heavenly color—reminder of a separated walk.

37 And the LORD spake unto Moses, saying,

B.C. 1490.

a Lit. *meal.*

b See Ex. 29:33, *note.*

c *Forgiveness.* vs. 25, 26, 28; Psa. 32:5. (Lev. 4:20; Mt. 26:28.)

d *Sabbath.* vs. 32-36; Neh. 9:13, 14. (Gen. 2:3; Mt. 12:1.)

gives directions for conduct when they shall have entered it. See Rom. 11:29; Phil. 1:6.

38 Speak unto the children of Israel, and bid them that they make them fringes in the borders of their garments throughout their generations, and that they put upon the fringe of the borders a ribband of [1]blue:

39 And it shall be unto you for a fringe, that ye may look upon it, and remember all the commandments of the LORD, and do them; and that ye seek not after your own heart and your own eyes, after which ye use to go a whoring:

40 That ye may remember, and do all my commandments, and be holy unto your God.

41 I *am* the LORD your God, which brought you out of the land of Egypt, to be your God: I *am* the LORD your God.

CHAPTER 16.

The years of wandering: (2) *the "gainsaying of Korah"* (vs. 8–10; Jude 11).

Now [a]Korah, the son of Izhar, the son of Kohath, the son of Levi, and Dathan and Abiram, the sons of Eliab, and On, the son of Peleth, sons of Reuben, took *men*:

2 And they rose up before Moses, with certain of the children of Israel, two hundred and fifty princes of the assembly, famous in the congregation, men of renown:

3 And they gathered themselves together against Moses and against Aaron, and said unto them, *Ye take* too much upon you, seeing all the congregation *are* holy, every one of them, and the LORD *is* among them: wherefore then lift ye up yourselves above the congregation of the LORD?

4 And when Moses heard *it*, he fell upon his face:

5 And he spake unto Korah and unto all his company, saying, Even to morrow the LORD will shew who *are* his, [b]and *who is* holy; and will cause *him* to come near unto him: even *him* whom he hath chosen will he cause to come near unto him.

6 This do; Take you censers, Korah, and all his company;

7 And put fire therein, and put incense in them before the LORD to morrow: and it shall be *that* the man whom the LORD doth choose, he *shall be* holy: *ye take* too much upon you, ye sons of Levi.

8 And Moses said unto Korah, Hear, I pray you, ye sons of Levi:

9 *Seemeth it but* a small thing unto you, that the God of Israel hath separated you from the congregation of Israel, to bring you near to himself to [c]do the service of the tabernacle of the LORD, and to stand before the congregation to minister unto them?

10 And he hath brought thee near *to him*, and all thy brethren the sons of Levi with thee: and [2]seek ye the priesthood also?

11 For which cause *both* thou and all thy company *are* gathered together against the LORD: and what *is* Aaron, that ye murmur against him?

12 And Moses sent to call Dathan and Abiram, the sons of Eliab: which said, We will not come up:

13 *Is it* a small thing that thou hast brought us up out of a land that floweth with milk and honey, to kill us in the wilderness, except thou make thyself altogether a prince over us?

14 Moreover thou hast not brought us into a land that floweth with milk and honey, or given us inheritance of fields and vineyards: wilt thou put out the eyes of these men? we will not come up.

15 And Moses was very wroth, and said unto the LORD, Respect not thou their offering: I have not taken one ass from them, neither have I hurt one of them.

16 And Moses said unto Korah, Be thou and all thy company before the LORD, thou, and they, and Aaron, to morrow:

17 And take every man his censer, and put incense in them, and bring ye before

B.C. 1490.

a Ex. 6:21; Jude 11..

b 2 Tim. 2:19.

c Num. 3:41-45; 8:13-16; Deut. 10:8.

[1] **(15:38)** The ribband of blue. Blue, the heavenly colour, used upon the borders of the priests' garments signified that the servants of God were to be heavenly in obedience and character, and separate from earthly ambitions and desires.

[2] **(16:10)** The "gainsaying of Korah" was intrusion into the priest's office ("no man taketh this honour unto himself," Heb. 5:4). It was an attempt to create a priestly order without the divine authority (5:10). The modern analogue is Nicolaitanism (Rev. 2:6, 15), the division of an equal brotherhood (Mt. 23:8) into "clergy" and "laity"; a vastly different thing from the due recognition of ministry-gifts (1 Cor, 12:4-31; Eph. 4:8, 11, 12), or of elders and deacons (1 Tim. 3:1-13; Tit. 1:5-9).

B.C. 1471.

the LORD every man his censer, two hundred and fifty censers; thou also, and Aaron, each *of you* his censer.

18 And they took every man his censer, and put fire in them, and laid incense thereon, and stood in the door of the tabernacle of the congregation with Moses and Aaron.

19 And Korah gathered all the congregation against them unto the door of the tabernacle of the congregation: and the glory of the LORD appeared unto all the congregation.

20 And the LORD spake unto Moses and unto Aaron, saying,

21 [a]Separate yourselves from among this congregation, that I may consume them in a moment.

22 And they fell upon their faces, and said, O God, the God of the spirits of all flesh, shall one man sin, and wilt thou be wroth with all the congregation?

23 And the LORD spake unto Moses, saying,

24 Speak unto the congregation, saying, Get you up from about the tabernacle of Korah, Dathan, and Abiram.

25 And Moses rose up and went unto Dathan and Abiram; and the elders of Israel followed him.

26 And he spake unto the congregation, saying, Depart, I pray you, from the tents of these wicked men, and touch nothing of theirs, lest ye be consumed in all their sins.

27 So they gat up from the tabernacle of Korah, Dathan, and Abiram, on every side: and Dathan and Abiram came out, and stood in the door of their tents, and their wives, and their sons, and their little children.

28 And Moses said, Hereby ye shall know that the LORD hath sent me to do all these works; for *I have* not *done them* of mine own mind.

29 If these men die the common death of all men, or if they be visited after the visitation of all men; *then* the LORD hath not sent me.

30 But if the LORD make a new thing, and the earth open her mouth, and swallow them up, with all that *appertain* unto them, and they go down quick into the [b]pit; then ye shall understand that these men have provoked the LORD.

31 And it came to pass, as he had made an end of speaking all these words, that the ground [c]clave asunder that *was* under them:

32 And the earth opened her mouth, and swallowed them up, and their houses, and all the men that *appertained* unto Korah, and all *their* goods.

33 They, and all that *appertained* to them, went down alive into the [b]pit, and the earth closed upon them: and they perished from among the congregation.

34 And all Israel that *were* round about them fled at the cry of them: for they said, Lest the earth swallow us up *also*.

35 And there came out a fire from the LORD, and consumed the two hundred and fifty men that offered incense.

36 And the LORD spake unto Moses, saying,

37 Speak unto Eleazar the son of Aaron the priest, that he take up the censers out of the burning, and scatter thou the fire yonder; for they are [d]hallowed.

38 The censers of these sinners against their own souls, let them make them broad plates *for* a covering of the altar: for they offered them before the LORD, therefore they are hallowed: and they shall be a sign unto the children of Israel.

39 And Eleazar the priest took the brasen censers, wherewith they that were burnt had offered; and they were made broad *plates for* a covering of the altar:

40 *To be* a memorial unto the children of Israel, [e]that no stranger, which *is* not of the seed of Aaron, come near to offer incense before the LORD; that he be not as Korah, and as his company: as the LORD said to him by the hand of Moses.

41 But on the morrow all the congregation of the children of Israel murmured against Moses and against Aaron, saying, Ye have killed the people of the LORD.

42 And it came to pass, when the congregation was gathered against Moses and against Aaron, that they looked toward the tabernacle of the congregation: and, behold, the cloud covered it, and the glory of the LORD appeared.

43 And Moses and Aaron came before the tabernacle of the congregation.

a *Separation.* vs. 20-26; Deut. 22:10. (Gen. 12:1; 2 Cor. 6:14-17.)

b Heb. *sheol.*

c *Miracles* (O.T.). vs. 31-35; Num. 17:8. (Gen. 5:24; Jon. 2:1-10.)

d Lev. 27:28.

e Cf. 1 Sam. 13:9; Heb. 5:4; Jude 11.

44 And the LORD spake unto Moses, saying,

45 Get you up from among this congregation, that I may consume them as in a moment. And they fell upon their faces.

46 And Moses said unto Aaron, Take a censer, and put fire therein from off the altar, and put on incense, and go quickly unto the congregation, and make an [a]atonement for them: for there is wrath gone out from the LORD; the plague is begun.

47 And Aaron took as Moses commanded, and ran into the midst of the congregation; and, behold, the plague was begun among the people: and he put on incense, and made an [a]atonement for the people.

48 And he stood between the dead and the living; and the plague was stayed.

49 Now they that died in the plague were fourteen thousand and seven hundred, [b]beside them that died about the matter of Korah.

50 And Aaron returned unto Moses unto the door of the tabernacle of the congregation: and the plague was stayed.

CHAPTER 17.

The years of wandering:
(3) *Aaron's rod that budded.*

And the LORD spake unto Moses, saying,

2 Speak unto the children of Israel, and take of every one of them a rod according to the house of *their* fathers, of all their princes according to the house of their fathers twelve rods: write thou every man's name upon his rod.

3 And thou shalt write Aaron's name upon the rod of Levi: for one rod *shall be* for the head of the house of their fathers.

4 And thou shalt lay them up in the tabernacle of the congregation before the testimony, [c]where I will meet with you.

5 And it shall come to pass, *that* the man's rod, whom I shall [d]choose, shall blossom: and I will make to cease from me the murmurings of the children of Israel, whereby they murmur against you.

6 And Moses spake unto the children of Israel, and every one of their princes gave him a rod apiece, for each prince one, according to their fathers' houses, *even* twelve rods: and the rod of Aaron *was* among their rods.

7 And Moses laid up the rods before the LORD in the tabernacle of witness.

8 And it came to pass, that on the morrow Moses went into the tabernacle of witness; and, behold, the [1]rod of Aaron for the house of Levi was [e]budded, and brought forth buds, and bloomed blossoms, and yielded almonds.

9 And Moses brought out all the rods from before the LORD unto all the children of Israel: and they looked, and took every man his rod.

10 And the LORD said unto Moses, Bring Aaron's rod again before the testimony, to be [f]kept for a token against the rebels; and thou shalt quite take away their murmurings from me, that they die not.

11 And Moses did *so*: as the LORD commanded him, so did he.

12 And the children of Israel spake unto Moses, saying, Behold, we die, we perish, we all perish.

13 Whosoever cometh any thing near unto the tabernacle of the LORD shall die: shall we be consumed with dying?

CHAPTER 18.

The years of wandering:
(4) *Aaron and the Levites confirmed in their privileges and responsibilities.*

And the LORD said unto Aaron, Thou and thy sons and thy father's house with thee shall bear the iniquity of the sanctuary: and thou and thy sons with thee shall [g]bear the iniquity of your priesthood.

2 And thy brethren also of the [h]tribe of Levi, the tribe of thy father, bring thou with thee, that they may be joined unto thee, and minister unto thee: but thou and thy sons with thee *shall minister* before the tabernacle of witness.

B.C. 1471.

a See Ex. 29:33, *note.*

b v. 35.

c Ex. 25:22; 29:42, 43; 30:36.

d Num. 16:5.

e *Miracles* (O.T.). Num. 20:7-11. (Gen. 5:24; Jon. 2:1-10.)

f Num. 16:38; Heb. 9:4.

g i.e. be responsible for every neglect or offence relating to. Cf. Ex. 28:38.

h Num. 1:47, *ref.*

[1] **(17:8)** Aaron's rod that budded: Type of Christ in resurrection, owned of God as High Priest. Aaron's priesthood had been questioned in the rebellion of Korah, so God Himself will confirm it (v. 5). Each of the tribe-heads brought a perfectly dead rod; God put life into Aaron's only. So all the authors of religions have died, Christ among them, but only Christ was raised from the dead, and exalted to be a high priest (Heb. 4:14; 5:4-10).

3 And they shall keep thy charge, and the charge of all the tabernacle: only they shall not come nigh the vessels of the sanctuary and the altar, that neither they, nor ye also, die.

4 And they shall be joined unto thee, and keep the charge of the tabernacle of the congregation, for all the service of the tabernacle: and a stranger shall not come nigh unto you.

5 And ye shall keep the charge of the sanctuary, and the charge of the altar: that there be no wrath any more upon the children of Israel.

6 And I, behold, I have taken your brethren the Levites from among the children of Israel: to you *they are* given *as* a gift for the LORD, to do the service of the tabernacle of the congregation.

7 Therefore thou and thy sons with thee shall keep your priest's office for every thing of the altar, and within the vail; and ye shall serve: I have given your priest's office *unto you as* a service of gift: and the stranger that cometh nigh shall be put to death.

8 And the LORD spake unto Aaron, Behold, I also have given thee the charge of mine heave-offerings of all the hallowed things of the children of Israel; unto thee have I given them by reason of the anointing, and to thy sons, by an ordinance for ever.

9 This shall be thine of the most holy things, *reserved* from the fire: every oblation of theirs, every [a]meat-offering of theirs, and every sin-offering of theirs, and every trespass-offering of theirs, which they shall render unto me, *shall be* most holy for thee and for thy sons.

10 In the most holy *place* shalt thou eat it; every male shall eat it: it shall be holy unto thee.

11 And this *is* thine; the heave-offering of their gift, with all the wave-offerings of the children of Israel: I have given them unto thee, and to thy sons and to thy daughters with thee, by a statute for ever: every one that is clean in thy house shall eat of it.

12 All the best of the oil, and all the best of the wine, and of the wheat, the firstfruits of them which they shall offer unto the LORD, them have I given thee.

13 *And* whatsoever is first ripe in the land, which they shall bring unto the LORD, shall be thine; every one that is clean in thine house shall eat *of* it.

14 Every thing devoted in Israel shall be thine.

15 Every thing that openeth the matrix in all flesh, which they bring unto the LORD, *whether it be* of men or beasts, shall be thine: nevertheless the [b]firstborn of man shalt thou surely redeem, and the firstling of unclean beasts shalt thou redeem.

16 And those that are to be redeemed from a month old shalt thou redeem, according to thine estimation, for the money of five [c]shekels, after the shekel of the sanctuary, which *is* twenty [d]gerahs.

17 But the firstling of a cow, or the firstling of a sheep, or the firstling of a goat, thou shalt not redeem; they *are* holy: thou shalt sprinkle their blood upon the altar, and shalt burn their fat *for* an offering made by fire, for a sweet savour unto the LORD.

18 And the flesh of them shall be thine, [e]as the wave breast and as the right shoulder are thine.

19 All the heave-offerings of the holy things, which the children of Israel offer unto the LORD, have I given thee, and thy sons and thy daughters with thee, by a statute for ever: it *is* a covenant of [f]salt for ever before the LORD unto thee and to thy seed with thee.

20 And the LORD spake unto Aaron, Thou shalt have [g]no inheritance in their land, neither shalt thou have any part among them: [h]I *am* thy part and thine inheritance among the children of Israel.

21 And, behold, I have given the children of Levi all the [i]tenth in Israel for an inheritance, for their service which they serve, *even* the service of the tabernacle of the congregation.

22 Neither must the children of Israel henceforth come nigh the tabernacle of the congregation, lest they bear sin, and die.

23 But the Levites shall do the service of the tabernacle of the congregation, and they shall bear their iniquity: *it shall be* a statute for ever throughout your generations, that among the children of Israel they have no inheritance.

24 But the tithes of the children of Israel, which they offer *as* an heave-offering unto the LORD, I have given to the Levites to inherit: therefore I have

B.C. 1471.

a Lit. *meal.*

b Ex. 13:2-13; 34, 20; Lk. 2:22-24.

c One shekel=2*s.* 9*d.*, or 65 cts.

d One gerah=11.2 grains, or 3 1-4 cts.

e Ex. 29:26-28; Lev. 7:31-36.

f Lev. 2:13; 2 Chr. 13:5; Mk. 9:49, 50; Col. 4:6.

g Deut. 10:8, 9; 12:12; 14:27-29; 18:1, 2; Josh. 13:14, 33; 14:3; 18:7.

h Psa. 16:5; Ezk. 44:28.

i vs. 24, 26; Lev. 27:30, 32; Neh. 10:37; 12:44; Mal. 3:8-10; Heb. 7:5, 8, 9.

said unto them, Among the children of Israel they shall have no inheritance.

25 And the LORD spake unto Moses, saying,

26 Thus speak unto the Levites, and say unto them, When ye take of the children of Israel the tithes which I have given you from them for your inheritance, then ye shall offer up an heave-offering of it for the LORD, *even* a tenth *part* of the tithe.

27 And *this* your heave-offering shall be reckoned unto you, [a]as though *it were* the corn of the threshingfloor, and as the fulness of the winepress.

28 Thus ye also shall offer an heave-offering unto the LORD of all your tithes, which ye receive of the children of Israel; and ye shall give thereof the LORD'S heave-offering to Aaron the priest.

29 Out of all your gifts ye shall offer every heave-offering of the LORD, of all the best thereof, *even* the hallowed part thereof out of it.

30 Therefore thou shalt say unto them, When ye have heaved the best thereof from it, then it shall be counted unto the Levites as the increase of the threshingfloor, and as the increase of the winepress.

31 And ye shall eat it in every place, ye and your households: for it *is* your reward for your service in the tabernacle of the congregation.

32 And ye shall bear no sin by reason of it, when ye have heaved from it the best of it: neither shall ye pollute the holy things of the children of Israel, lest ye die.

CHAPTER 19,

The years of wandering:
(5) *the ordinance of the red heifer.*

And the LORD spake unto Moses and unto Aaron, saying,

2 This *is* the ordinance of the law which the LORD hath commanded, saying, Speak unto the children of Israel, that they bring thee a [1]red heifer without spot, wherein *is* no blemish, *and* [b]upon which never came yoke:

3 And ye shall give her unto Eleazar the priest, that he may bring her forth [c]without the camp, and *one* shall slay her before his face:

4 And Eleazar the priest shall take of her blood with his finger, and [d]sprinkle of her blood directly before the tabernacle of the congregation seven times:

5 And *one* shall burn the heifer in his sight; her skin, and her flesh, and her blood, with her dung, shall he burn:

6 And the priest shall take [e]cedar wood, and [f]hyssop, and scarlet, and cast *it* into the midst of the burning of the heifer.

7 Then the priest shall wash his clothes, and he shall bathe his flesh in water, and afterward he shall come into the camp, and the priest shall be unclean until the even.

8 And he that burneth her shall wash his clothes in water, and bathe his flesh in water, and shall be unclean until the even.

9 And a man *that is* clean shall gather up the [g]ashes of the heifer, and lay *them* up without the camp in a clean place, and it shall be kept for the congregation of the children of Israel for a [h]water of separation: it *is* a purification for sin.

10 And he that gathereth the ashes of the heifer shall wash his clothes, and be unclean until the even: and it shall be unto the children of Israel, and unto the stranger that sojourneth among them, for a statute for ever.

11 He that toucheth the dead body of

B.C. 1471.

a 2 Cor. 8:12.
b Deut. 21:3; 1 Sam. 6:7.
c Lev. 4:12, 21; 16:27; Heb. 13:11.
d Lev. 4:6; 16:14-19.
e Lev. 14:4, 6, 49.
f Ex. 12:22; 1 Ki. 4:33.
g Heb. 9:13.
h vs. 13, 20, 21; Num. 31:23.

[1]**(19:2)** The red heifer: Type of the sacrifice of Christ as the *ground* of the cleansing of the believer from the defilement contracted in his pilgrim walk through this world, and illustration of the *method* of his cleansing. The order is: (1) The *slaying* of the sacrifice; (2) the sevenfold sprinkling of the blood, typical public testimony before the eyes of all of the complete and never-to-be-repeated putting away of all the believer's sins as *before God* (Heb. 9:12-14; 10:10-12); (3) the reduction of the sacrifice to ashes which are preserved and become a *memorial* of the sacrifice; (4) the cleansing from defilement (sin has two aspects—*guilt* and *uncleanness*) by sprinkling with the ashes mingled with water. Water is a type of both the Spirit and the Word (John 7:37-39; Eph. 5:26). The operation typified is this: the Holy Spirit uses the Word to convict the believer of some evil allowed in his life to the hindering of his joy, growth, and service. Thus convicted, he remembers that the *guilt* of his sin has been met by the sacrifice of Christ (1 John 1:7). Instead, therefore, of despairing, the convicted believer judges and confesses the defiling thing as unworthy a saint, and is forgiven and cleansed (John 13:3-10; 1 John 1:7-10.

any man shall be unclean seven days.
12 He shall [a]purify himself with it on
the third day, and on the seventh day he
shall be clean: but if he purify not himself the third day, then the seventh day
he shall not be clean.
13 Whosoever toucheth the dead body
of any man that is dead, and purifieth
not himself, defileth the tabernacle of the
LORD; and that soul shall be cut off from
Israel: because the water of separation
was not sprinkled upon him, he shall be
unclean; his uncleanness *is* yet upon him.
14 This *is* the law, when a man dieth in
a tent: all that come into the tent, and all
that *is* in the tent, shall be unclean seven
days.
15 And every open vessel, which hath
no covering bound upon it, *is* unclean.
16 And whosoever toucheth one that
is slain with a sword in the open fields,
or a dead body, or a bone of a man, or a
grave, shall be unclean seven days.
17 And [b]for an unclean *person* they
shall take of the ashes of the burnt heifer
of purification for sin, and running
water shall be put thereto in a vessel:
18 And a clean person shall take hyssop, and dip *it* in the water, and sprinkle
it upon the tent, and upon all the vessels,
and upon the persons that were there,
and upon him that touched a bone, or
one slain, or one dead, or a grave:
19 And the clean *person* shall sprinkle
upon the unclean on the third day, and
on the seventh day: and on the seventh
day he shall purify himself, and wash
his clothes, and bathe himself in water,
and shall be clean at even.
20 But the man that shall be unclean,
and shall not purify himself, that soul
shall be cut off from among the congregation, because he hath defiled the sanctuary of the LORD: the water of separation hath not been sprinkled upon him;
he *is* unclean.
21 And it shall be a perpetual statute
unto them, that he that sprinkleth the
water of separation shall wash his
clothes; and he that toucheth the water
of separation shall be unclean until even.
22 And whatsoever the unclean *person*
toucheth shall be unclean; and the soul
that toucheth *it* shall be unclean until
even.

CHAPTER 20.

The years of wandering:
(6) *death of Miriam.*

Then came the children of Israel, *even*
the whole congregation, into the
desert of Zin in the [c]first month: and the
people abode in Kadesh; and [d]Miriam
died there, and was buried there.

The years of wandering:
(7) *thirst in Meribah – Kadesh.*
(Deut. 32:51. Cf. Ex. 17:1–7.)

2 And there was no water for the congregation: and they gathered themselves
together [e]against Moses and against
Aaron.
3 And the people [f]chode with Moses,
and spake, saying, Would God that we
had died when our brethren died before
the LORD!
4 And why have ye brought up the
congregation of the LORD into this
wilderness, that we and our cattle
should die there?
5 And wherefore have ye made us to
come up out of Egypt, to bring us in unto
this evil place? it *is* no place of seed, or of
figs, or of vines, or of pomegranates; neither *is* there any [g]water to drink.
6 And Moses and Aaron went from the
presence of the assembly unto the door
of the tabernacle of the congregation, and
they fell upon their faces: and the glory
of the LORD appeared unto them.

Water from the rock, and Moses' sin.

7 And the LORD spake unto Moses,
saying,
8 Take the [h]rod, and gather thou the
assembly together, thou, and Aaron thy
brother, and [1]speak ye unto the rock
before their eyes; and it shall give forth
his water, and thou shalt bring forth to

B.C. 1471.

a Lit. *purge himself from sin.*
b See v. 2, *note.* Cf. John 13:1-10, *note.*
c i.e. *April.*
d Ex. 15:20; Num. 26:59.
e Num. 16:19, 42.
f Ex. 17:2; Num. 14:2.
g v. 8, *note.*
h Num. 17:10; see v. 9.

[1] **(20:8)** See Ex. 17:5, and *refs.* The rock (Christ, 1 Cor. 10:4) once smitten, needs not to be smitten (crucified) again. Moses' act exalted himself (v. 10), and implied (in type) that the one sacrifice was ineffectual, thus denying the eternal efficacy of the blood (Heb. 9:25, 26; 10:3, 11, 12). The abundant water (grace reaching the need of the people, despite the error of their leader) tells of refreshing and power through the Spirit.

them water out of the [a]rock: so thou
shalt give the congregation and their
beasts drink.
9 And Moses took the rod from before
the LORD, as he commanded him.
10 And Moses and Aaron gathered the
congregation together before the rock,
and he said unto them, Hear now, ye
rebels; must we fetch you water out of
this rock?
11 And Moses lifted up his hand, and
with his rod he smote the rock twice: and
the [b]water came out abundantly, and the
congregation drank, and their beasts *also*.
12 And the LORD spake unto Moses
and Aaron, Because ye believed me not,
to sanctify me in the eyes of the children
of Israel, therefore ye shall not bring this
congregation into the land which I have
given them.
13 This *is* the water of [c]Meribah;
because the children of Israel strove with
the LORD, and he was sanctified in them.

The years of wandering: (8) *the never-forgiven sin of Edom* (Gen. 25:30).

14 And Moses sent messengers from
Kadesh [d]unto the king of Edom, Thus
saith thy brother Israel, Thou knowest
all the travail that hath befallen us:
15 How our fathers went down into
Egypt, and we have dwelt in Egypt a
long time; and the Egyptians vexed us,
and our fathers:
16 And when we cried unto the LORD,
he heard our voice, and sent an [e]angel,
and hath brought us forth out of Egypt:
and, behold, we *are* in Kadesh, a city in
the uttermost of thy border:
17 Let us pass, I pray thee, through thy
country: we will not pass through the
fields, or through the vineyards, neither
will we drink *of* the water of the wells:
we will go by the king's *high* way, we
will not turn to the right hand nor to the
left, until we have passed thy borders.
18 And Edom said unto him, Thou
shalt not pass by me, lest I come out
against thee with the sword.
19 And the children of Israel said unto
him, We will go by the high way: and if I
and my cattle drink of thy water, then I
will pay for it: I will only, without *doing*
any thing *else*, go through on my feet.

B.C. 1453.

a Neh. 9:15; Psa. 78:15, 16; 105:41; 1 Cor. 10:4.

b *Miracles* (O.T.). vs. 7-11; Num. 21:8, 9. (Gen. 5:24; Jon. 2:1-10.)

c i.e. *strife*. (Ex. 17:7.)

d Jud. 11:16, 17.

e Heb. 1:4, *note*.

f Psa. 137:7; Ezk. 25:12, 13; Oba. 10-15.

g Deut. 32:50.

h Cf. Deut. 32:48-52.

i Cf. Gen. 28:20; Jud. 11:30.

20 And he said, Thou shalt not go
through. And Edom came out against
him with much people, and with a
strong hand.
21 Thus [f]Edom refused to give Israel
passage through his border: wherefore
Israel turned away from him.
22 And the children of Israel, *even* the
whole congregation, journeyed from
Kadesh, and came unto mount Hor.

The death of Aaron.

23 And the LORD spake unto Moses
and Aaron in mount Hor, by the coast of
the land of Edom, saying,
24 [g]Aaron shall be gathered unto his
people: for he shall not enter into the land
which I have given unto the children of
Israel, [h]because ye rebelled against my
word at the water of Meribah.
25 Take Aaron and Eleazar his son,
and bring them up unto mount Hor:
26 And strip Aaron of his garments,
and put them upon Eleazar his son: and
Aaron shall be gathered *unto his people*,
and shall die there.
27 And Moses did as the LORD commanded: and they went up into mount
Hor in the sight of all the congregation.
28 And Moses stripped Aaron of his
garments, and put them upon Eleazar
his son; and Aaron [1]died there in the top
of the mount: and Moses and Eleazar
came down from the mount.
29 And when all the congregation saw
that Aaron was dead, they mourned for
Aaron thirty days, *even* all the house of
Israel.

CHAPTER 21.

The march of Israel: (1) *victory.*

And *when* king Arad the Canaanite,
which dwelt in the south, heard
tell that Israel came by the way of the
spies; then he fought against Israel, and
took *some* of them prisoners.
2 And Israel vowed a vow unto the
LORD, and said, [i]If thou wilt indeed

[1](20:28) The death of Aaron marks the end of the *wanderings*. Henceforth Israel marches or halts, but does not wander (see Num. 15, *note* 1).

deliver this people into my hand, then I will utterly destroy their cities.

3 And the LORD hearkened to the voice of Israel, and delivered up the Canaanites; and they utterly destroyed them and their cities: and he called the name of the place [a]Hormah.

4 And they journeyed from mount Hor by the way of the Red sea, to compass the land of Edom: and the soul of the people was much discouraged because of the way.

The march of Israel:
(2) *the serpent of brass* (Gen. 3:1, *note;* John 3:14, 15; 2 Cor. 5:20).

5 And the people [b]spake against God, and against Moses, [c]Wherefore have ye brought us up out of Egypt to die in the wilderness? for *there is* no bread, neither *is there any* water; [d]and our soul loatheth [e]this light bread.

6 And the LORD [f]sent fiery serpents among the people, and they bit the people; and much people of Israel died.

7 Therefore the people came to Moses, and said, We have sinned, for we have spoken against the LORD, and against thee; pray unto the LORD, that he take away the serpents from us. And Moses prayed for the people.

8 And the LORD said unto Moses, [g]Make thee a fiery serpent, and set it upon a pole: and it shall come to pass, that every one that is bitten, when he looketh upon it, shall live.

9 And Moses made a [1]serpent of [h]brass, and put it upon a pole, and it came to pass, that if a serpent had bitten any man, when he beheld the serpent of brass, he [i]lived.

10 And the children of Israel set forward, and pitched in Oboth.

11 And they journeyed from Oboth, and pitched at [j]Ije-abarim, in the wilderness which *is* before Moab, toward the sunrising.

12 From thence they removed, and pitched in the valley of Zared.

13 From thence they removed, and pitched on the other side of Arnon, which *is* in the wilderness that cometh out of the coasts of the Amorites: for Arnon *is* the border of Moab, between Moab and the Amorites.

14 Wherefore it is said in the book of the wars of the LORD, What he did in the Red sea, and in the brooks of Arnon,

15 And at the stream of the brooks that goeth down to the dwelling of Ar, and lieth upon the border of Moab.

16 And from thence *they went* to Beer: that *is* the well whereof the LORD spake unto Moses, Gather the people together, and I will give them water.

17 [2]Then Israel sang this song, Spring up, O well; sing ye unto it:

18 The princes digged the well, the nobles of the people digged it, by *the direction of* the lawgiver, with their staves. And from the wilderness *they went* to Mattanah:

19 And from Mattanah to Nahaliel: and from Nahaliel to Bamoth:

20 And from Bamoth *in* the valley, that *is* in the country of Moab, to the top of [k]Pisgah, which looketh toward [l]Jeshimon.

The march of Israel: (3) *two victories.*

21 And Israel sent messengers unto Sihon king of the Amorites, saying,

22 Let me pass through thy land: we will not turn into the fields, or into the vineyards; we will not drink *of* the waters of the well: *but* we will go along by the king's *high* way, until we be past thy borders.

23 And Sihon would not suffer Israel to pass through his border: but Sihon gathered all his people together, and went out against Israel into the wilderness: and he came to Jahaz, and fought against Israel.

24 And Israel smote him with the edge of the sword, and possessed his land from Arnon unto Jabbok, even unto the children of Ammon: for the border of the children of Ammon *was* strong.

B.C. 1452.

a i.e. *utter destruction.*
b Psa. 78:19.
c Cf. Ex. 16:3; 17:3.
d Cf. Num. 11:4-6
e Cf. John 6:48-52, 60-64.
f 1 Cor. 10:9; Deut. 8:15.
g John 3:14, 15.
h 2 Ki. 18:4.
i *Miracles* (O.T.). vs. 8, 9; Josh. 3:14-17. (Gen. 5:24; Jon. 2:1-10.)
j i.e. *ruins of Abarim.*
k i.e. *the hill.*
l i.e. *the wilderness.*

[1] **(21:9)** See Gen. 3:14, *note.* The serpent is a symbol of sin *judged;* brass speaks of the divine judgment, as in the brazen altar (Ex. 27:2, *refs.* and *note*), and self-judgment, as in the laver of brass. The brazen serpent is a type of Christ "made sin for us" (John 3:14, 15; 2 Cor. 5:21) in bearing our judgment. Historically, the moment is indicated in the cry: "My God, My God, why hast Thou forsaken Me?" (Mt. 27:46).

[2] **(21:17)** The spiritual order here is beautiful: (1) atonement (vs. 8, 9; John 3:14, 15); (2) water, symbol of the Spirit bestowed (v. 16; John 7:37-39); (3) joy (vs. 17, 18; Rom. 14:17); (4) power (vs. 21-24).

25 And Israel took all these cities: and Israel dwelt in all the cities of the Amorites, in Heshbon, and in all the villages thereof.

26 For Heshbon *was* the city of Sihon the king of the Amorites, who had fought against the former king of Moab, and taken all his land out of his hand, even unto Arnon.

27 Wherefore they that speak in proverbs say, Come into Heshbon, let the city of Sihon be built and prepared:

28 For there is a fire gone out of Heshbon, a flame from the city of Sihon: it hath consumed Ar of Moab, *and* the lords of the high places of Arnon.

29 Woe to thee, Moab! thou art undone, O people of Chemosh: he hath given his sons that escaped, and his daughters, into captivity unto Sihon king of the Amorites.

30 We have shot at them; Heshbon is perished even unto Dibon, and we have laid them waste even unto Nophah, which *reacheth* unto Medeba.

31 Thus Israel dwelt in the land of the Amorites.

32 And Moses sent to spy out Jaazer, and they took the villages thereof, and drove out the Amorites that *were* there.

33 [a]And they turned and went up by the way of Bashan: and Og the king of Bashan went out against them, he, and all his people, to the battle at Edrei.

34 And the LORD [b]said unto Moses, Fear him not: for I have delivered him into thy hand, and all his people, and his land; and thou shalt do to him as thou didst unto Sihon king of the Amorites, which dwelt at Heshbon.

35 So they smote him, and his sons, and all his people, until there was none left him alive: and they possessed his land.

B.C. 1452.

a Deut. 3:1; 29:7.

b Deut. 3:2.

c Josh. 24:9; Jud. 11:25; Mic. 6:5; Rev. 2:14.

d Num. 31:8, 16; Josh. 13:22; Neh. 13:2; 2 Pet. 2:15; Jude 11; Rev. 2:14.

CHAPTER 22.

The march of Israel: (4) *Balaam* (2 Pet. 2:15; Jude 11; Rev. 2:14).

And the children of Israel set forward, and pitched in the plains of Moab on this side Jordan *by* Jericho.

2 And [c]Balak the son of Zippor saw all that Israel had done to the Amorites.

3 And Moab was sore afraid of the people, because they *were* many: and Moab was distressed because of the children of Israel.

4 And Moab said unto the elders of Midian, Now shall this company lick up all *that are* round about us, as the ox licketh up the grass of the field. And Balak the son of Zippor *was* king of the Moabites at that time.

5 He sent messengers therefore unto [1d]Balaam the son of Beor to Pethor, which *is* by the river of the land of the children of his people, to call him, saying, Behold, there is a people come out from Egypt: behold, they cover the face of the earth, and they abide over against me:

6 Come now therefore, I pray thee, curse me this people; for they *are* too mighty for me: peradventure I shall prevail, *that* we may smite them, and *that* I may drive them out of the land: for I wot that he whom thou blessest *is* blessed, and he whom thou cursest is cursed.

7 And the elders of Moab and the elders of Midian departed with the rewards of divination in their hand; and they came unto Balaam, and spake unto him the words of Balak.

8 And he said unto them, Lodge here this night, and I will bring you word again, as the LORD shall speak unto me: and the princes of Moab abode with Balaam.

9 And God came unto Balaam, and said, What men *are* these with thee?

10 And Balaam said unto God, Balak

[1] **(22:5)** Balaam is the typical hireling prophet, seeking only to make a market of his gift. This is "the *way* of Balaam" (2 Pet. 2:15), and characterizes false teachers. The "*error* of Balaam" (Jude 11) was that he could see only the natural morality—a holy God, he reasoned, *must* curse such a people as Israel. Like all false teachers he was ignorant of the higher morality of vicarious atonement, by which God could be just and yet the justifier of *believing* sinners (Rom. 3:26). The "*doctrine* of Balaam" (Rev. 2:14) refers to his teaching Balak to corrupt the people whom he could not curse (Num. 31:16, with Num. 25:1-3 and Jas. 4:4). Spiritually, Balaamism in teaching never rises above natural reasonings; in practice, it is easy world-conformity. See Rev. 2:14, *note*.

the son of Zippor, king of Moab, hath sent unto me, *saying*,

11 Behold, *there is* a people come out of Egypt, which covereth the face of the earth: come now, curse me them; peradventure I shall be able to overcome them, and drive them out.

12 And God said unto Balaam, Thou shalt [a]not go with them; thou shalt not curse the people: for they *are* blessed.

13 And Balaam rose up in the morning, and said unto the princes of Balak, Get you into your land: for the LORD refuseth to give me leave to go with you.

14 And the princes of Moab rose up, and they went unto Balak, and said, Balaam refuseth to come with us.

15 And Balak sent yet again princes, more, and more honourable than they.

16 And they came to Balaam, and said to him, Thus saith Balak the son of Zippor, Let nothing, I pray thee, hinder thee from coming unto me:

17 For I will promote thee unto very great honour, and I will do whatsoever thou sayest unto me: come therefore, I pray thee, curse me this people.

18 And Balaam answered and said unto the servants of Balak, If Balak would give me his house full of silver and gold, I cannot go beyond the word of the LORD my God, to do less or more.

19 Now therefore, I pray you, tarry ye also here this night, that I may know what the LORD will say unto me more.

20 And God came unto Balaam at night, and said unto him, [b]If the men come to call thee, rise up, *and* go with them; but yet the word which I shall say unto thee, that shalt thou do.

21 And Balaam rose up in the morning, and saddled his ass, and went with the princes of Moab.

22 And God's [1]anger was kindled because he went: and the [c]angel of the LORD stood in the way for an adversary against him. Now he was riding upon his ass, and his two servants *were* with him.

B.C. 1452.

a Cf. v. 20. See Gen. 46:3, *note*.

b See v. 12, *ref*.

c Heb. 1:4, *note*.

d See Gen. 21:19; 2 Ki. 6:17; Lk. 24:16, 31.

e See 2 Pet. 2:14-16.

23 And the ass saw the [c]angel of the LORD standing in the way, and his sword drawn in his hand: and the ass turned aside out of the way, and went into the field: and Balaam smote the ass, to turn her into the way.

24 But the [c]angel of the LORD stood in a path of the vineyards, a wall *being* on this side, and a wall on that side.

25 And when the ass saw the [c]angel of the LORD, she thrust herself unto the wall, and crushed Balaam's foot against the wall: and he smote her again.

26 And the angel of the LORD went further, and stood in a narrow place, where *was* no way to turn either to the right hand or to the left.

27 And when the ass saw the angel of the LORD, she fell down under Balaam: and Balaam's anger was kindled, and he smote the ass with a staff.

28 And the LORD opened the mouth of the ass, and she said unto Balaam, What have I done unto thee, that thou hast smitten me these three times?

29 And Balaam said unto the ass, Because thou hast mocked me: I would there were a sword in mine hand, for now would I kill thee.

30 And the ass said unto Balaam, *Am* not I thine ass, upon which thou hast ridden ever since *I was* thine unto this day? was I ever wont to do so unto thee? And he said, Nay.

31 Then the LORD [d]opened the eyes of Balaam, and he saw the angel of the LORD standing in the way, and his sword drawn in his hand: and he bowed down his head, and fell flat on his face.

32 And the angel of the LORD said unto him, Wherefore hast thou smitten thine ass these three times? behold, I went out to withstand thee, because *thy* way is [e]perverse before me:

33 And the ass saw me, and turned from me these three times: unless she

[1] **(22:22)** Cf. Gen. 46:3, *note*. In v. 12 the directive will of Jehovah is made known to Balaam, in v. 20 Jehovah's *permissive* will. The prophet is now free to go, but knows the true mind of the Lord about it. The matter is wholly one between Jehovah and His servant. The permission of v. 20 really constitutes a testing of Balaam. He chose the path of self-will and self-advantage, and Jehovah could not but gravely disapprove. The whole scene, vs. 22-35, prepared Balaam for what was to follow.

had turned from me, surely now also I had slain thee, and saved her alive.

34 And Balaam said unto the [a]angel of the LORD, I have sinned; for I knew not that thou stoodest in the way against me: now therefore, if it [b]displease thee, I will get me back again.

35 And the [a]angel of the LORD said unto Balaam, Go with the men: [c]but only the word that I shall speak unto thee, that thou shalt speak. So Balaam went with the princes of Balak.

36 And when Balak heard that Balaam was come, he went out to meet him unto a city of Moab, [d]which *is* in the border of Arnon, which *is* in the utmost coast.

37 And Balak said unto Balaam, Did I not earnestly send unto thee to call thee? wherefore camest thou not unto me? am I not able indeed to promote thee to honour?

38 And Balaam said unto Balak, Lo, I am come unto thee: have I now any power at all to say any thing? the [e]word that God putteth in my mouth, that shall I [f]speak.

39 And Balaam went with Balak, and they came unto [g]Kirjath-huzoth.

40 And Balak offered oxen and sheep, and sent to Balaam, and to the princes that *were* with him.

41 And it came to pass on the morrow, that Balak took Balaam, and brought him up into the high places of Baal, that thence he might see the [1]utmost *part* of the people.

CHAPTER 23.

Balaam: the prophecy from the high places of Baal. The separation of Israel.

AND Balaam said unto Balak, Build me here seven altars, and prepare me here seven oxen and seven rams.

2 And Balak did as Balaam had spoken; and Balak and Balaam offered on *every* altar a bullock and a ram.

3 And Balaam said unto Balak, Stand by thy burnt-offering, and I will go: peradventure the LORD will come to meet me: and whatsoever he sheweth me I will tell thee. And he went to an high place.

4 And God met Balaam: and he said unto him, I have prepared seven altars, and I have offered upon *every* altar a bullock and a ram.

5 And the LORD put a [h]word in Balaam's mouth, and said, Return unto Balak, and thus thou shalt speak.

6 And he returned unto him, and, lo, he stood by his burnt sacrifice, he, and all the princes of Moab.

7 And he took up his parable, and [2]said, Balak the king of Moab hath brought me from Aram, out of the mountains of the east, *saying*, Come, curse me Jacob, and come, defy Israel.

8 How shall I curse, whom God hath not cursed? or how shall I defy, *whom* the LORD hath not defied?

9 For from the top of the rocks I see him, and from the hills I behold him: lo, the people shall dwell alone, and shall not be reckoned among the nations.

10 Who can count the dust of Jacob, and the number of the fourth *part* of Israel? Let me die the death of the righteous, and let my last end be like his!

11 And Balak said unto Balaam, What hast thou done unto me? I took thee to curse mine enemies, and, behold, thou hast blessed *them* altogether.

B.C. 1452.

a Heb. 1:4, *note.*

b i.e. *be evil in thine eyes.*

c See v. 20.

d Num. 21:13.

e *Inspiration.* Num. 23:5, 12-16. (Ex. 4:15; Rev. 22:19.)

f Num. 23:26; 24:13; 1 Ki. 22:14; 2 Chr. 18:13.

g Or, *a city of streets.*

h *Inspiration.* vs. 5:12-16; Deut. 4:2, 13. (Ex. 4:15; Rev. 22:19.)

[1] **(22:41)** "Utmost part " etc., means the end of the encampment, the "fourth part of Israel" (Num. 23:10). Balak's thought, as Grant (following Keil) points out, was not at all to permit Balaam to see the whole of the Hebrew host. In bringing Balaam to Pisgah (vs. 13, 14), Balak corrects what, evidently, he thought a blunder (Num. 23:13, 14). But when the hireling sees the whole camp he must utter a grander word than before, "He hath not beheld iniquity in Jacob," and that with the nation in full view! What an illustration of the truth of Rom. 4:5-8!

[2] **(23:7)** In the prophecies of Balaam God testifies on *behalf* of His people rather than (as usual) *to* them. It is the divine testimony to their standing as a redeemed people in view of the serpent "lifted up," and of the water from the smitten rock (Num. 21:5-9; 20:11). Their *state* was morally bad, but this was a matter concerning the *discipline* of God, not His *judgment.* The interpretation of the prophecies is literal as to Israel, typical as to Christians. Through Christ "lifted up" (John 3:14) our standing is eternally secure and perfect, though our state may require the Father's discipline (1 Cor. 11:30-32; 2 Cor. 1:4-9; cf. vs. 10-13); meantime, against all enemies, God is "for us" (Rom. 8:31).

12 And he answered and said, Must I
not take heed to speak that which the
LORD hath put in my mouth?

Balaam: the prophecy from Pisgah: the justification and power of Israel.

13 And Balak said unto him, Come, I
pray thee, with me unto another place,
from whence thou mayest see them:
[a]thou shalt see but the utmost part of
them, and shalt not see them all: and
curse me them from thence.
14 And he brought him into the field
of Zophim, to the top of Pisgah, and
built seven altars, and offered a bullock
and a ram on *every* altar.
15 And he said unto Balak, Stand here
by thy burnt-offering, while I meet *the
LORD* yonder.
16 And the LORD met Balaam, and put
a word in his mouth, and said, Go again
unto Balak, and say thus.
17 And when he came to him, behold,
he stood by his burnt-offering, and the
princes of Moab with him. And Balak said
unto him, What hath the LORD spoken?
18 And he took up his parable, and
said, Rise up, Balak, and hear; hearken
unto me, thou son of Zippor:
19 God *is* not a man, that he should
lie; neither the son of man, that he
should [b]repent: hath he said, and shall
he not do *it*? or hath he spoken, and
shall he not make it good?
20 Behold, I have received *commandment* to bless: and he hath blessed; and I
cannot reverse it.
21 He hath not beheld iniquity in
Jacob, neither hath he seen perverseness
in Israel: the LORD his God *is* with him,
and the shout of a king *is* among them.
22 God brought them out of Egypt; he
hath as it were the strength of an [c]uni-
corn.
23 Surely *there is* no enchantment
[d]against Jacob, neither *is there* any divination [d]against Israel: according to this
time it shall be said of Jacob and of
Israel, [e]What hath God wrought!
24 Behold, the people shall rise up as a
great lion, and lift up himself as a young
lion: he shall not lie down until he eat *of*
the prey, and drink the blood of the slain.
25 And Balak said unto Balaam,
Neither curse them at all, nor bless them
at all.
26 But Balaam answered and said
unto Balak, Told not I thee, saying, All
that the LORD speaketh, that I must do?

Balaam: the prophecy from Peor:
(1) *the beauty and order of Israel.*

27 And Balak said unto Balaam,
Come, I pray thee, I will bring thee unto
another place; peradventure it will
please God that thou mayest curse me
them from thence.
28 And Balak brought Balaam unto
the top of Peor, that looketh [f]toward
[g]Jeshimon.
29 And Balaam said unto Balak, Build
me here seven altars, and prepare me
here seven bullocks and seven rams.
30 And Balak did as Balaam had said,
and offered a bullock and a ram on *every*
altar.

CHAPTER 24.

And when Balaam saw that it pleased
the LORD to bless Israel, he went
not, as at other times, to seek for [h]en-
chantments, but he set his face toward
the wilderness.
2 And Balaam lifted up his eyes, and
he saw Israel [i]abiding *in his tents* according to their tribes; and [j]the [k]spirit of God
came upon him.
3 [l]And he took up his parable, and said,
Balaam the son of Beor hath said, and the
man whose eyes are open hath said:
4 He hath said, which heard the words
of God, which saw the vision of the
Almighty, [m]falling *into a trance*, but having his eyes open:
5 How goodly are thy tents, O Jacob,
and thy tabernacles, O Israel!
6 As the valleys are they spread forth,
as gardens by the river's side, as the trees
of lign aloes which the LORD hath planted, *and* as cedar trees beside the waters.
7 He shall pour the water out of his
buckets, and his seed *shall be* [n]in many
waters, and his king shall be higher than
[o]Agag, and his [p]kingdom shall be exalted.
8 God brought him forth out of Egypt;
he hath as it were the strength of an unicorn: he shall [q]eat up the nations his enemies, and shall break their bones, and
pierce *them* through with his arrows.
9 He couched, he lay down as a lion,
and as a great lion: who shall stir him

B.C. 1452.

a *Better, thou seest but the extremity of them, and dost not see them all.*
b Zech. 8:14, *note.*
c i.e. *the aurochs, or wild ox.*
d Or, *in.*
e Psa. 31:19; 44:1.
f Num. 21:20.
g Or, *the waste.*
h Or, *to the meeting of enchantments.*
i Num. 2:2, etc.
j Num. 11:25; 1 Sam. 19:20, 23; 10:10; 2 Chr. 15:1.
k *Holy Spirit.* Num. 27:18. (Gen. 1:2; Mal. 2:15.)
l Num. 23:7, 18.
m i.e. *prostrated by the prophetic impulse.* See 1 Sam. 19:24; Ezk. 1:28; Dan. 8:18; 10:15, 16; 2 Cor. 12:2-4; Rev. 1:10, 17.
n See Jer. 51:13; Rev. 17:1, 15.
o 1 Sam. 15:9.
p 2 Sam. 5:12; 1 Chr. 14:2.
q Num. 14:9; 23:24.

up? [a]Blessed *is* he that blesseth thee, and cursed *is* he that curseth thee.

10 And Balak's anger was kindled against Balaam, and he smote his hands together: and Balak said unto Balaam, I called thee to curse mine enemies, and, behold, thou hast altogether blessed *them* these three times.

11 Therefore now flee thou to thy place: [b]I thought to promote thee unto great honour; but, lo, the LORD hath kept thee back from honour.

12 And Balaam said unto Balak, Spake I not also to thy messengers which thou sentest unto me, saying,

13 If Balak would give me his house full of silver and gold, I cannot go beyond the commandment of the LORD, to do *either* good or bad of mine own mind; *but* what the LORD saith, that will I speak?

14 And now, behold, I go unto my people: come *therefore, and* I will advertise thee what this people shall do to thy people in the latter days.

Balaam: the prophecy from Peor:
(2) the Messianic kingdom.

15 And he took up his parable, and said, Balaam the son of Beor hath said, and the man whose eyes are open hath said:

16 He hath said, which heard the words of God, and knew the knowledge of the most High, *which* saw the vision of the Almighty, falling *into a trance*, but having his eyes open:

17 I shall see him, but not now: I shall behold him, but not nigh: there shall come a Star out of Jacob, and a [c]Sceptre shall rise out of Israel, and shall smite the corners of Moab, and destroy all the children of Sheth.

18 And Edom shall be a possession, Seir also shall be a possession for his enemies; and Israel shall do valiantly.

19 Out of Jacob shall come he that shall have dominion, and shall destroy him that remaineth of the city.

20 And when he looked on Amalek, he took up his parable, and said, Amalek *was* the first of the [d]nations; but his latter end *shall be* that he perish for ever.

21 And he looked on the Kenites, and took up his parable, and said, Strong is thy dwellingplace, and thou puttest thy nest in a rock.

22 Nevertheless the Kenite shall be wasted, until Asshur shall carry thee away captive.

23 And he took up his parable, and said, Alas, who shall live when God doeth this!

24 And ships *shall come* from the coast of [e]Chittim, and shall afflict Asshur, and shall afflict Eber, and he also shall perish for ever.

25 And Balaam rose up, and went and [f]returned to his place: and Balak also went his way.

CHAPTER 25.

"The doctrine of Balaam"
(Num. 31:16; Rev. 2:14; Jas. 4:4).

And Israel abode in Shittim, and [g]the people began to commit whoredom with the daughters of Moab.

2 And they called the people unto [h]the sacrifices of their gods: and the people did eat, and [i]bowed down to their gods.

3 And Israel joined himself unto [j]Baal-peor: and the anger of the LORD was kindled against Israel.

4 And the LORD said unto Moses, Take all the heads of the people, and hang them up before the LORD against the sun, that the fierce anger of the LORD may be turned away from Israel.

5 And Moses said unto the judges of Israel, Slay ye every one his men that were joined unto Baal-peor.

6 And, behold, one of the children of Israel came and brought unto his brethren a Midianitish woman in the sight of Moses, and in the sight of all the congregation of the children of Israel, who *were* weeping *before* the door of the tabernacle of the congregation.

7 And when Phinehas, the son of Eleazar, the son of Aaron the priest, saw *it*, he rose up from among the congregation, and took a javelin in his hand;

8 And he went after the man of Israel into the tent, and thrust both of them through, the man of Israel, and the woman through her belly. [k]So the plague was stayed from the children of Israel.

9 And those that [l]died in the plague were twenty and four thousand.

10 And the LORD spake unto Moses, saying,

11 Phinehas, the son of Eleazar, the

B.C. 1452.

a Gen. 12:3; 27:29.

b Num. 22:17, 37.

c See *"Kingdom:"* (Gen. 1:26-28; Zech. 12:8.)

d Or, *the first of the nations that warred against Israel.* Ex. 17:8.

e Pronounced *Kittim.* Gen. 10:4; Dan. 11:30.

f Num. 31:8.

g Num. 31:16; 1 Cor. 10:8.

h Ex. 34:15, 16; 1 Cor. 10:8.

i Ex. 20:5.

j Or, *Baal of Peor.* See Num. 23:28; Psa. 106:28-29; Hos. 9:10.

k Psa. 106:30.

l Deut. 4:3; cf. 1 Cor. 10:8, *note.*

son of Aaron the priest, hath turned my wrath away from the children of Israel, while he was zealous for my sake among them, that I consumed not the children of Israel in my [a]jealousy.

12 Wherefore say, [b]Behold, I give unto him my covenant of peace:

13 And he shall have it, and his seed after him, *even* the covenant of an everlasting priesthood; because he was zealous for his God, and made an [c]atonement for the children of Israel.

14 Now the name of the Israelite that was slain, *even* that was slain with the Midianitish woman, *was* Zimri, the son of Salu, a prince of a chief house among the Simeonites.

15 And the name of the Midianitish woman that was slain *was* Cozbi, the daughter of Zur; he *was* head over a people, *and* of a chief house in Midian.

16 And the LORD spake unto Moses, saying,

17 Vex the Midianites, and smite them:

18 For they vex you with their wiles, wherewith they have beguiled you in the matter of Peor, and in the matter of Cozbi, the daughter of a prince of Midian, their sister, which was slain in the day of the plague for Peor's sake.

CHAPTER 26.

The new generation of Israel numbered (vs. 64, 65).

And it came to pass after the plague, that the LORD spake unto Moses and unto Eleazar the son of Aaron the priest, saying,

2 Take the sum of all the congregation of the children of Israel, from twenty years old and upward, throughout their fathers' house, all that are able to go to war in Israel.

3 And Moses and Eleazar the priest spake with them in the plains of Moab by Jordan *near* Jericho, saying,

4 *Take the sum of the people,* from twenty years old and upward; as the LORD [d]commanded Moses and the children of Israel, which went forth out of the land of Egypt.

5 [e]Reuben, the eldest son of Israel: the children of Reuben; Hanoch, *of whom cometh* the family of the Hanochites: of Pallu, the family of the Palluites:

6 Of Hezron, the family of the Hezronites: of Carmi, the family of the Carmites.

7 These *are* the families of the Reubenites: and they that were numbered of them were forty and three thousand and seven hundred and thirty.

8 And the sons of Pallu; Eliab.

9 And the sons of Eliab; Nemuel, and Dathan, and Abiram. This *is that* Dathan and Abiram, *which were* famous in the congregation, who strove against Moses and against Aaron in the company of Korah, when they strove against the LORD:

10 [f]And the earth opened her mouth, and swallowed them up together with Korah, when that company died, what time the fire devoured two hundred and fifty men: [g]and they became a sign.

11 Notwithstanding the children of [h]Korah died not.

12 The sons of Simeon after their families: of Nemuel, the family of the Nemuelites: of Jamin, the family of the Jaminites: of Jachin, the family of the Jachinites:

13 Of Zerah, the family of the Zarhites: of Shaul, the family of the Shaulites.

14 These *are* the families of the Simeonites, twenty and two thousand and two hundred.

15 The children of Gad after their families: of Zephon, the family of the Zephonites: of Haggi, the family of the Haggites: of Shuni, the family of the Shunites:

16 Of Ozni, the family of the Oznites: of Eri, the family of the Erites:

17 Of Arod, the family of the Arodites: of Areli, the family of the Arelites.

18 These *are* the families of the children of Gad according to those that were numbered of them, forty thousand and five hundred.

19 The sons of [i]Judah *were* Er and Onan: and Er and Onan died in the land of Canaan.

20 And the sons of Judah after their families were; of Shelah, the family of the Shelanites: of Pharez, the family of the Pharzites: of Zerah, the family of the Zarhites.

21 And the sons of Pharez were; of Hezron, the family of the Hezronites: of Hamul, the family of the Hamulites.

22 These *are* the families of Judah according to those that were numbered

B.C. 1452.

a Cf. Ex. 20:5; Deut. 32:16, 21; 1 Ki. 14:22.
b Mal. 2:4, 5; 3:1
c See Ex. 29:33, *note.*
d See Num. 1:1, 2.
e Gen. 46:8; Ex. 6:14; 1 Chr. 5:1-3.
f Num. 16:32-35.
g 1 Cor. 10:6; 2 Pet. 2:6.
h Ex. 6:24; 1 Cor. 6:22.
i Gen. 38:2, etc.; 46:12.

of them, threescore and sixteen thousand and five hundred.

23 *Of* the sons of [a]Issachar after their families: *of* Tola, the family of the Tolaites: of Pua, the family of the Punites:

24 Of Jashub, the family of the Jashubites: of Shimron, the family of the Shimronites.

25 These *are* the families of Issachar according to those that were numbered of them, threescore and four thousand and three hundred.

26 *Of* the sons of [b]Zebulun after their families: of Sered, the family of the Sardites: of Elon, the family of the Elonites: of Jahleel, the family of the Jahleelites.

27 These *are* the families of the Zebulunites according to those that were numbered of them, threescore thousand and five hundred.

28 The sons of [c]Joseph after their families *were* Manasseh and Ephraim.

29 Of the sons of Manasseh: of Machir, the family of the Machirites: and Machir begat Gilead: of Gilead *come* the family of the Gileadites.

30 These *are* the sons of Gilead: *of* Jeezer, the family of the Jeezerites: of Helek, the family of the Helekites:

31 And *of* Asriel, the family of the Asrielites: and *of* Shechem, the family of the Shechemites:

32 And *of* Shemida, the family of the Shemidaites: and *of* Hepher, the family of the Hepherites.

33 And Zelophehad the son of Hepher had no sons, but daughters: and the names of the daughters of Zelophehad *were* Mahlah, and Noah, Hoglah, Milcah, and Tirzah.

34 These *are* the families of Manasseh, and those that were numbered of them, fifty and two thousand and seven hundred.

35 These *are* the sons of Ephraim after their families: of Shuthelah, the family of the Shuthalhites: of Becher, the family of the Bachrites: of Tahan, the family of the Tahanites.

36 And these *are* the sons of Shuthelah: of Eran, the family of the Eranites.

37 These *are* the families of the sons of Ephraim according to those that were numbered of them, thirty and two thousand and five hundred. These *are* the sons of Joseph after their families.

B.C. 1452.

a Gen. 46:13; 1 Chr. 7:1; 8:1-2.

b Gen. 46:14.

c Gen. 46:20.

d Gen. 46:21; 1 Chr. 7:6.

e Gen. 46:23.

f Gen. 46:17; 1 Chr. 7:30.

g Gen. 46:24; 1 Chr. 7:13.

h See Num. 1:46.

i Josh. 11:23; 14:1.

38 The sons of [d]Benjamin after their families: of Bela, the family of the Belaites: of Ashbel, the family of the Ashbelites: of Ahiram, the family of the Ahiramites:

39 Of Shupham, the family of the Shuphamites: of Hupham, the family of the Huphamites.

40 And the sons of Bela were Ard and Naaman: *of Ard*, the family of the Ardites: *and* of Naaman, the family of the Naamites.

41 These *are* the sons of Benjamin after their families: and they that were numbered of them *were* forty and five thousand and six hundred.

42 These *are* the sons of [e]Dan after their families: of Shuham, the family of the Shuhamites. These *are* the families of Dan after their families.

43 All the families of the Shuhamites, according to those that were numbered of them, *were* threescore and four thousand and four hundred.

44 *Of* the children of [f]Asher after their families: of Jimna, the family of the Jimnites: of Jesui, the family of the Jesuites: of Beriah, the family of the Beriites.

45 Of the sons of Beriah: of Heber, the family of the Heberites: of Malchiel, the family of the Malchielites.

46 And the name of the daughter of Asher *was* Sarah.

47 These *are* the families of the sons of Asher according to those that were numbered of them; *who were* fifty and three thousand and four hundred.

48 *Of* the sons of [g]Naphtali after their families: of Jahzeel, the family of the Jahzeelites: of Guni, the family of the Gunites:

49 Of Jezer, the family of the Jezerites: of Shillem, the family of the Shillemites.

50 These *are* the families of Naphtali according to their families: and they that were numbered of them *were* forty and five thousand and four hundred.

51 These *were* the numbered of the children of [h]Israel, six hundred thousand and a thousand seven hundred and thirty.

52 And the LORD spake unto Moses, saying,

53 [i]Unto these the land shall be divided for an inheritance according to the number of names.

B.C. 1452.

54 To [a]many thou shalt give the more inheritance, and to [b]few thou shalt give the less inheritance: to every one shall his inheritance be given according to those that were numbered of him.

55 Notwithstanding the land shall be divided by lot: according to the names of the tribes of their fathers they shall inherit.

56 According to the lot shall the possession thereof be divided between many and few.

57 And these *are* they that were numbered of the Levites after their families: of Gershon, the family of the Gershonites: of Kohath, the family of the Kohathites: of Merari, the family of the Merarites.

58 These *are* the families of the Levites: the family of the Libnites, the family of the Hebronites, the family of the Mahlites, the family of the Mushites, the family of the Korathites. And Kohath begat Amram.

59 And the name of Amram's wife *was* Jochebed, the daughter of Levi, whom *her mother* bare to Levi in Egypt: and she bare unto Amram Aaron and Moses, and Miriam their sister.

60 And unto Aaron was born Nadab, and Abihu, Eleazar, and Ithamar.

61 And [c]Nadab and Abihu died, when they offered strange fire before the LORD.

62 And those that were numbered of them were twenty and three thousand, all males from a month old and upward: for they were not numbered among the children of Israel, because there was no inheritance given them among the children of Israel.

63 These *are* they that were numbered by Moses and Eleazar the priest, who numbered the children of Israel in the plains of Moab by Jordan *near* Jericho.

64 But among these there was not a man of them whom Moses and Aaron the priest numbered, when they numbered the children of Israel in the wilderness of Sinai.

65 For the LORD had said of them, [d]They shall surely die in the wilderness. And there was not left a man of them, [e]save Caleb the son of Jephunneh, and Joshua the son of Nun.

CHAPTER 27.

The law of inheritance.

Then came the daughters of Zelophehad, the son of Hepher, the son of Gilead, the son of Machir, the son of Manasseh, of the families of Manasseh the son of Joseph: and these *are* the names of his daughters; Mahlah, Noah, and Hoglah, and Milcah, and Tirzah.

2 And they stood before Moses, and before Eleazar the priest, and before the [f]princes and all the congregation, *by* the door of the tabernacle of the congregation, saying,

3 Our father died in the wilderness, and he was not in the company of them that gathered themselves together against the LORD in the company of Korah; but died in his own sin, and had no sons.

4 Why should the name of our father be done away from among his family, because he hath no son? [g]Give unto us *therefore* a possession among the brethren of our father.

5 And Moses [h]brought their cause before the LORD.

6 And the LORD spake unto Moses, saying,

7 The daughters of Zelophehad speak right: thou shalt surely give them a possession of an inheritance among their father's brethren; and thou shalt cause the inheritance of their father to pass unto them.

8 And thou shalt speak unto the children of Israel, saying, If a man die, and have no son, then ye shall cause his inheritance to pass unto his daughter.

9 And if he have no daughter, then ye shall give his inheritance unto his brethren.

10 And if he have no brethren, then ye shall give his inheritance unto his father's brethren.

11 And if his father have no brethren, then ye shall give his inheritance unto his kinsman that is next to him of his family, and he shall possess it: and it shall be unto the children of Israel a statute of [i]judgment, as the LORD commanded Moses.

Moses to prepare for death.

12 And the LORD said unto Moses, Get thee up into this mount Abarim, and see the land which I have given unto the children of Israel.

13 And when thou hast seen it, thou

a i.e. *the greater.*
b i.e. *the smaller.*
c Lev. 10:1, 2; Num. 3:4; 1 Chr. 24:2.
d Num. 14:28, 29; 1 Cor. 10:5, 6.
e Num. 14:30.
f Or, *Chiefs.*
g Josh. 17:4.
h Ex. 18:15, 19.
i Or, *right.*

also [a]shalt be gathered unto thy people,
as Aaron thy brother was gathered.
14 For ye [b]rebelled against my commandment in the desert of Zin, in the
strife of the congregation, to sanctify me
at the water before their eyes: that *is* the
water of Meribah in Kadesh in the
wilderness of Zin.

Joshua appointed in Moses' place.

15 And Moses spake unto the LORD,
[c]saying,
16 Let the LORD, the God of the spirits
of all flesh, set a man over the congregation,
17 Which may go out before them, and
which may go in before them, and which
may lead them out, and which may bring
them in; that the congregation of the LORD
be not as [d]sheep which have no shepherd.
18 And the LORD said unto Moses,
Take thee Joshua the son of Nun, a man
in whom *is* the [e]spirit, and lay thine
hand upon him;
19 And set him before Eleazar the
priest, and before all the congregation;
and give him a charge in their sight.
20 And thou shalt put *some* of thine
honour upon him, that all the congregation of the children of Israel may be obedient.
21 And he shall stand before Eleazar
the priest, who shall ask *counsel* for him
[f]after the judgment of Urim before the
LORD: [g]at his word shall they go out, and
at his word they shall come in, *both* he,
and all the children of Israel with him,
even all the congregation.
22 And Moses did as the LORD commanded him: and he took Joshua, and
set him before Eleazar the priest, and
before all the congregation:
23 And he laid his hands upon him,
[h]and gave him a charge, as the LORD
commanded by the hand of Moses.

CHAPTER 28.

The order of offerings.

And the LORD spake unto Moses,
saying,
2 Command the children of Israel, and
say unto them, My offering, *and* my
bread for my sacrifices made by fire, *for* a
[i]sweet savour unto me, shall ye observe
to offer unto me in their due season.
3 And thou shalt say unto them, This
is the offering made by fire which ye
shall offer unto the LORD; two lambs of
the first year without spot day by day,
for a continual burnt-offering.
4 The one lamb shalt thou offer in the
morning, and the other lamb shalt thou
offer at even;
5 And a tenth *part* of an [j]ephah of
flour for a [k]meat-offering, mingled with
the fourth *part* of an [l]hin of beaten oil.
6 *It is* a [m]continual burnt-offering,
which was ordained in mount Sinai for a
sweet savour, a sacrifice made by fire
unto the LORD.
7 And the drink-offering thereof *shall
be* the fourth *part* of an [l]hin for the one
lamb: in the holy *place* shalt thou cause
the strong wine to be poured unto the
LORD *for* a drink-offering.
8 And the other lamb shalt thou offer
at even: as the [k]meat-offering of the
morning, and as the drink-offering thereof, thou shalt offer *it*, a sacrifice made by
fire, of a sweet savour unto the LORD.
9 And on the sabbath day two lambs
of the first year without spot, and two
tenth deals of flour *for* a [k]meat-offering,
mingled with oil, and the drink-offering
thereof:
10 *This is* the burnt-offering of every
sabbath, beside the continual burnt-
offering, and his drink-offering.
11 And in the beginnings of your
months ye shall offer a burnt-offering
unto the LORD; two young bullocks, and
one ram, seven lambs of the first year
without spot;
12 And three tenth deals of flour *for* a
[k]meat-offering, mingled with oil, for one
bullock; and two tenth deals of flour *for*
a [k]meat-offering, mingled with oil, for
one ram;
13 And a several tenth deal of flour
mingled with oil *for* a [k]meat-offering
unto one lamb; *for* a burnt-offering of a
sweet savour, a sacrifice made by fire
unto the LORD.
14 And their drink-offerings shall be
half an [l]hin of wine unto a bullock, and
the third *part* of an hin unto a ram, and a
fourth *part* of an hin unto a lamb: this *is*
the burnt-offering of every month
throughout the months of the year.
15 And one kid of the goats for a sin-
offering unto the LORD shall be offered,
beside the continual burnt-offering, and
his drink-offering.
16 And in the fourteenth day of the
[n]first month *is* the [o]passover of the LORD.

B.C. 1452.

a Num. 20:24, 28; 31:2; Deut. 10:6.

b Num. 20:12, 24; Deut. 1:37; 32:51; Psa. 106:33.

c *Bible prayers* (O.T.). Deut. 3:24. (Gen. 15:2; Hab. 3:1-16.

d 1 Ki. 22:17; Zech. 10:2; Mt. 9:36; Mk. 6:34.

e *Holy Spirit.* Deut. 34:9. (Gen. 1:2; Mal. 2:15.)

f Ex. 28:30, *note.*

g Josh. 9:14; 1 Sam. 22:10, 13, 15.

h Deut. 3:28; 31:7, 8.

i Or, *savour of satisfaction.* Lev. 1:9, *note.*

j One ephah = 1 bu. 3 pts.

k Lit. *meal.*

l One hin = about 6 qts.

m Ex. 29:42; see Amos 5:25.

n i.e. *April.*

o Ex. 12:3-18; Lev. 23:5; Num. 9:2-5; Deut. 16:1; Ezk. 45:21.

17 And in the fifteenth day of this month *is* the feast: seven days shall [a]unleavened bread be eaten.

18 In the first day *shall be* an holy convocation; ye shall do no manner of servile work *therein*:

19 But ye shall offer a sacrifice made by fire *for* a burnt-offering unto the LORD; two young bullocks, and one ram, and seven lambs of the first year: they shall be unto you without blemish:

20 And their [b]meat-offering *shall be of* flour mingled with oil: three tenth deals shall ye offer for a bullock, and two tenth deals for a ram;

21 A several tenth deal shalt thou offer for every lamb, throughout the seven lambs:

22 And one goat *for* a sin-offering, to make an [c]atonement for you.

23 Ye shall offer these beside the burnt-offering in the morning, which *is* for a continual burnt-offering.

24 After this manner ye shall offer daily, throughout the seven days, the meat of the sacrifice made by fire, of a sweet savour unto the LORD: it shall be offered beside the continual burnt-offering, and his drink-offering.

25 And [d]on the seventh day ye shall have an holy convocation; ye shall do no servile work.

26 Also [e]in the day of the firstfruits, when ye bring a new [b]meat-offering unto the LORD, after your weeks *be out*, ye shall have an holy convocation; ye shall do no servile work:

27 But ye shall offer the burnt-offering for a sweet savour unto the LORD; two young bullocks, one ram, seven lambs of the first year;

28 And their [b]meat-offering of flour mingled with oil, three tenth deals unto one bullock, two tenth deals unto one ram,

29 A several tenth deal unto one lamb, throughout the seven lambs;

30 *And* one kid of the goats, to make an [c]atonement for you.

31 Ye shall offer *them* beside the continual burnt-offering, and his [b]meat-offering, (they shall be unto you without blemish) and their drink-offerings.

CHAPTER 29.

And in the [f]seventh month, on the first *day* of the month, ye shall have an holy convocation; ye shall do no servile work: [g]it is a day of blowing the trumpets unto you.

2 And ye shall offer a burnt-offering for a sweet savour unto the LORD; one young bullock, one ram, *and* seven lambs of the first year without blemish:

3 And their [b]meat-offering *shall be of* flour mingled with oil, three tenth deals for a bullock, *and* two tenth deals for a ram,

4 And one tenth deal for one lamb, throughout the seven lambs:

5 And one kid of the goats *for* a sin-offering, to make an [c]atonement for you:

6 Beside the burnt-offering of the month, and his [b]meat-offering, and the daily burnt-offering, and his [b]meat-offering, and their drink-offerings, according unto their manner, for a sweet savour, a sacrifice made by fire unto the LORD.

7 And ye shall have on the tenth *day* of this [f]seventh month an holy convocation; and ye shall [h]afflict your souls: ye shall not do any work *therein*:

8 But ye shall offer a burnt-offering unto the LORD *for* a sweet savour; one young bullock, one ram, *and* seven lambs of the first year; they shall be unto you without blemish:

9 And their [b]meat-offering *shall be of* flour mingled with oil, three tenth deals to a bullock, *and* two tenth deals to one ram,

10 A several tenth deal for one lamb, throughout the seven lambs:

11 One kid of the goats *for* a sin-offering; beside the [i]sin-offering of [c]atonement, and the continual burnt-offering, and the [b]meat-offering of it, and their drink-offerings.

12 And [j]on the fifteenth day of the seventh month ye shall have an holy convocation; ye shall do no servile work, and ye shall keep a feast unto the LORD seven days:

13 And [k]ye shall offer a burnt-offering, a sacrifice made by fire, of a sweet savour unto the LORD; thirteen young bullocks, two rams, *and* fourteen lambs of the first year; they shall be without blemish:

14 And their [b]meat-offering *shall be of* flour mingled with oil, three tenth deals unto every bullock of the thirteen bullocks, two tenth deals to each ram of the two rams,

15 And a several tenth deal to each lamb of the fourteen lambs:

16 And one kid of the goats *for* a sin-offering; beside the continual burnt-offering, his [b]meat-offering, and his drink-offering.

B.C. 1452.

a *Leaven.* Deut. 16:3, 4, 8, 16. (Gen. 19:3; Mt. 13:33.)

b Lit. *meal.*

c See Ex. 29:33, *note.*

d Ex. 12:16; 13:6; Lev. 23:8.

e Ex. 23:16; 34:22; Lev. 23:10-15; Deut. 16:10; Acts 2:1.

f i.e. *October;* also vs. 7, 12.

g Lev. 23:24.

h Psa. 35:13; Isa. 58:5.

i Lev. 16:3, 5.

j Lev. 23:34; Deut. 16:13; Ezk. 45:25.

k Ezra 3:4.

17 And on the second day *ye shall offer* twelve young bullocks, two rams, fourteen lambs of the first year without spot:

18 And their [a]meat-offering and their drink-offerings for the bullocks, for the rams, and for the lambs, *shall be* according to their number, [b]after the manner:

19 And one kid of the goats *for* a sin-offering; beside the continual burnt-offering, and the [a]meat-offering thereof, and their drink-offerings.

20 And on the third day eleven bullocks, two rams, fourteen lambs of the first year without blemish;

21 And their [a]meat-offering and their drink-offerings for the bullocks, for the rams, and for the lambs, *shall be* according to their number, after the manner:

22 And one goat *for* a sin-offering; beside the continual burnt-offering, and his [a]meat-offering, and his drink-offering.

23 And on the fourth day ten bullocks, two rams, *and* fourteen lambs of the first year without blemish:

24 Their [a]meat-offering and their drink-offerings for the bullocks, for the rams, and for the lambs, *shall be* according to their number, after the manner:

25 And one kid of the goats *for* a sin-offering; beside the continual burnt-offering, his [a]meat-offering, and his drink-offering.

26 And on the fifth day nine bullocks, two rams, *and* fourteen lambs of the first year without spot:

27 And their [a]meat-offering and their drink-offerings for the bullocks, for the rams, and for the lambs, *shall be* according to their number, after the manner:

28 And one goat *for* a sin-offering; beside the continual burnt-offering, and his [a]meat-offering, and his drink-offering.

29 And on the sixth day eight bullocks, two rams, *and* fourteen lambs of the first year without blemish:

30 And their [a]meat-offering and their drink-offerings for the bullocks, for the rams, and for the lambs, *shall be* according to their number, after the manner:

31 And one goat *for* a sin-offering; beside the continual burnt-offering, his [a]meat-offering, and his drink-offering.

32 And on the seventh day seven bullocks, two rams, *and* fourteen lambs of the first year without blemish:

33 And their [a]meat-offering and their drink-offerings for the bullocks, for the rams, and for the lambs, *shall be* according to their number, after the manner:

34 And one goat *for* a sin-offering; beside the continual burnt-offering, his [a]meat-offering, and his drink-offering.

35 On the eighth day ye shall have a [c]solemn assembly: ye shall do no servile work *therein*:

36 But ye shall offer a burnt-offering, a sacrifice made by fire, of a sweet savour unto the LORD: one bullock, one ram, seven lambs of the first year without blemish:

37 Their [a]meat-offering and their drink-offerings for the bullock, for the ram, and for the lambs, *shall be* according to their number, after the manner:

38 And one goat *for* a sin-offering; beside the continual burnt-offering, and his [a]meat-offering, and his drink-offering.

39 These *things* ye shall do unto the LORD in your [d]set feasts, beside your [e]vows, and your freewill offerings, for your burnt-offerings, and for your [a]meat-offerings, and for your drink-offerings, and for your peace-offerings.

40 And Moses told the children of Israel according to all that the LORD commanded Moses.

CHAPTER 30.

The law of vows. (Cf. Mt. 5:33–37.)

And Moses spake [f]unto the heads of the tribes concerning the children of Israel, saying, This *is* the thing which the LORD hath commanded.

2 [g]If a man vow a vow unto the LORD, or [h]swear an oath to bind his soul with a bond; he shall not break his word, he shall do according to all that proceedeth out of his mouth.

3 If a woman also vow a vow unto the LORD, and bind *herself* by a bond, *being* in her father's house in her youth;

4 And her father hear her vow, and her bond wherewith she hath bound her soul, and her father shall hold his peace at her: then all her vows shall stand, and every bond wherewith she hath bound her soul shall stand.

B.C. 1452.

a Lit. *meal.*

b vs. 3, 4, 9, 10; Num. 15:12; 28:7, 14.

c Lev. 23:36.

d Lev. 23:1-44; 1 Chr. 23:31; 2 Chr. 31:3; Ezra 3:5; Neh. 10:33; Isa. 1:14.

e Lev. 7:11, 16; 21:22, 23.

f Num. 1:4, 16; 7:2.

g Lev. 27:2; Deut. 23:21; Jud. 11:30, 35; Eccl. 5:4.

h Lev. 5:4; Mt. 14:9; Acts 23:14.

B.C. 1452.

5 But if her father disallow her in the day that he heareth; not any of her vows, or of her bonds wherewith she hath bound her soul, shall stand: and the LORD shall forgive her, because her father disallowed her.

6 And if she had at all an husband, when she vowed, or uttered ought out of her lips, wherewith she bound her soul;

7 And her husband heard *it*, and held his peace at her in the day that he heard *it*: then her vows shall stand, and her bonds wherewith she bound her soul shall stand.

8 But if her husband [a]disallowed her on the day that he heard *it*; then he shall make her vow which she vowed, and that which she uttered with her lips, wherewith she bound her soul, of none effect: and the LORD shall forgive her.

9 But every vow of a widow, and of her that is divorced, wherewith they have bound their souls, shall stand against her.

10 And if she vowed in her husband's house, or bound her soul by a bond with an oath;

11 And her husband heard *it*, and held his peace at her, *and* disallowed her not: then all her vows shall stand, and every bond wherewith she bound her soul shall stand.

12 But if her husband hath utterly made them void on the day he heard *them; then* whatsoever proceeded out of her lips concerning her vows, or concerning the bond of her soul, shall not stand: her husband hath made them void; and the LORD shall forgive her.

13 Every vow, and every binding oath to afflict the soul, her husband may establish it, or her husband may make it void.

14 But if her husband altogether hold his peace at her from day to day; then he establisheth all her vows, or all her bonds, which *are* upon her: he confirmeth them, because he held his peace at her in the day that he heard *them*.

15 But if he shall any ways make them void after that he hath heard *them*; then he shall bear her iniquity.

16 These *are* the statutes, which the LORD commanded Moses, between a man and his wife, between the father and his daughter, *being yet* in her youth in her father's house.

CHAPTER 31.

The judgment on Midian (Num. 25:6–18).

And the LORD spake unto Moses, saying,

2 [b]Avenge the children of Israel of the Midianites: afterward shalt thou [c]be gathered unto thy people.

3 And Moses spake unto the people, saying, Arm some of yourselves unto the war, and let them go against the Midianites, and avenge the LORD of Midian.

4 Of every tribe a thousand, throughout all the tribes of Israel, shall ye send to the war.

5 So there were delivered out of the thousands of Israel, a thousand of *every* tribe, twelve thousand armed for war.

6 And Moses sent them to the war, a thousand of *every* tribe, them and Phinehas the son of Eleazar the priest, to the war, with the holy instruments, and [d]the [e]trumpets to blow in his hand.

7 And they warred against the Midianites, as the LORD commanded Moses; and they slew all the [f]males.

8 And they slew the kings of Midian, beside the rest of them that were slain; *namely*, Evi, and Rekem, and Zur, and Hur, and Reba, five kings of Midian: [g]Balaam also the son of Beor they slew with the sword.

9 And the children of Israel took *all* the women of Midian captives, and their little ones, and took the spoil of all their cattle, and all their flocks, and all their goods.

10 And they burnt all their cities wherein they dwelt, and all their goodly [h]castles, with fire.

11 And [i]they took all the spoil, and all the prey, *both* of men and of beasts.

12 And they brought the captives, and the prey, and the spoil, unto Moses, and Eleazar the priest, and unto the congregation of the children of Israel, unto the camp at the plains of Moab, which *are* by Jordan *near* Jericho.

13 And Moses, and Eleazar the priest, and all the princes of the congregation, went forth to meet them without the camp.

14 And Moses was wroth with the officers of the host, *with* the captains over

a Gen. 3:16.
b Num. 25:17.
c Num. 27:13.
d Num. 10:9.
e i.e. *alarm clarions.*
f See Jud. 6:1, 2, 33.
g Josh. 13:22.
h i.e. *encampments.*
i Deut. 20:14.

thousands, and captains over hundreds, which came from the battle.

15 And Moses said unto them, Have ye [a]saved all the women alive?

16 Behold, [b]these caused the children of Israel, through the [c]counsel of Balaam, to commit trespass against the LORD in the matter of Peor, and there was a plague among the congregation of the LORD.

17 Now therefore kill every male among the little ones, and kill every woman that hath known man by lying with him.

18 But all the women children, that have not known a man by lying with him, keep alive for yourselves.

19 And do ye abide without the camp seven days: whosoever hath killed any person, and whosoever hath touched any slain, purify *both* yourselves and your captives on the third day, and on the seventh day.

20 And purify all *your* raiment, and all that is made of skins, and all work of goats' *hair*, and all things made of wood.

21 And Eleazar the priest said unto the men of war which went to the battle, This *is* the ordinance of the law which the LORD commanded Moses;

22 Only the gold, and the silver, the brass, the iron, the tin, and the lead,

23 Every thing that may abide the fire, ye shall make *it* go through the fire, and it shall be clean: nevertheless it shall be purified with the water of separation: and all that abideth not the fire ye shall make go through the water.

24 And ye shall wash your clothes on the seventh day, and ye shall be clean, and afterward ye shall come into the camp.

25 And the LORD spake unto Moses, saying,

26 Take the sum of the prey that was taken, *both* of man and of beast, thou, and Eleazar the priest, and the chief fathers of the congregation:

27 And [d]divide the prey into two parts; between them that took the war upon them, who went out to battle, and between all the congregation:

28 And levy a tribute unto the LORD of the men of war which went out to battle: [e]one soul of five hundred, *both* of the persons, and of the beeves, and of the asses, and of the sheep:

29 Take *it* of their half, and give *it* unto Eleazar the priest, *for* an heave-offering of the LORD.

30 And of the children of Israel's half, thou shalt take [f]one portion of fifty, of the persons, of the beeves, of the asses, and of the flocks, of all manner of beasts, and give them unto the Levites, [g]which keep the charge of the tabernacle of the LORD.

31 And Moses and Eleazar the priest did as the LORD commanded Moses.

32 And the booty, *being* the rest of the prey which the men of war had caught, was six hundred thousand and seventy thousand and five thousand sheep,

33 And threescore and twelve thousand beeves,

34 And threescore and one thousand asses,

35 And thirty and two thousand persons in all, of women that had not known man by lying with him.

36 And the half, *which was* the portion of them that went out to war, was in number three hundred thousand and seven and thirty thousand and five hundred sheep:

37 And the LORD'S tribute of the sheep was six hundred and threescore and fifteen.

38 And the beeves *were* thirty and six thousand; of which the LORD'S tribute *was* threescore and twelve.

39 And the asses *were* thirty thousand and five hundred; of which the LORD'S tribute *was* threescore and one.

40 And the persons *were* sixteen thousand; of which the LORD'S tribute *was* thirty and two persons.

41 And Moses gave the tribute, *which was* the LORD'S heave-offering, unto Eleazar the priest, [h]as the LORD commanded Moses.

42 And of the children of Israel's half, which Moses divided from the men that warred,

43 (Now the half *that pertained unto* the congregation was three hundred thousand and thirty thousand *and* seven thousand and five hundred sheep,

44 And thirty and six thousand beeves,

45 And thirty thousand asses and five hundred,

46 And sixteen thousand persons;)

47 Even [i]of the children of Israel's

B.C. 1452.

a See Deut. 20:14; 1 Sam. 15:3:.
b Num. 25:2.
c 2 Pet. 2:15; Rev. 2:14.
d Josh. 22:8; 1 Sam. 30:26.
e See vs. 30, 47; and Num. 18:26.
f See vs. 42-47.
g Num. 3:7, 8, 25, 31, 36; 18:3, 4.
h See Num. 18:8-19.
i v. 30.

half, Moses took one portion of fifty, *both* of man and of beast, and gave them unto the Levites, which kept the charge of the tabernacle of the LORD; as the LORD commanded Moses.

48 And the officers which *were* over thousands of the host, the captains of thousands, and captains of hundreds, came near unto Moses:

49 And they said unto Moses, Thy servants have taken the sum of the men of war which *are* under our charge, and there lacketh not one man of us.

50 We have therefore brought an oblation for the LORD, what every man hath gotten, of jewels of gold, chains, and bracelets, rings, earrings, and [a]tablets, to make an [b]atonement for our [c]souls before the LORD.

51 And Moses and Eleazar the priest took the gold of them, *even* all wrought jewels.

52 And all the gold of the offering that they offered up to the LORD, of the captains of thousands, and of the captains of hundreds, was sixteen thousand seven hundred and fifty [d]shekels.

53 (For [e]the men of war had taken spoil, every man for himself.)

54 And Moses and Eleazar the priest took the gold of the captains of thousands and of hundreds, and brought it into the tabernacle of the congregation, [f]*for* a memorial for the children of Israel before the LORD.

CHAPTER 32.

The choice of the world-borderers (Gen. 11:31; Jud. 5:16; Josh. 7:7; 2 Tim. 4:10).

Now the children of [1]Reuben and the children of Gad had a very great multitude of cattle: and when they saw the land of [g]Jazer, and the land of Gilead, that, behold, the place *was* a place for cattle;

2 The children of Gad and the children of Reuben came and spake unto Moses, and to Eleazar the priest, and unto the princes of the congregation, saying,

3 Ataroth, and Dibon, and Jazer, and Nimrah, and Heshbon, and Elealeh, and Shebam, and Nebo, and Beon,

4 *Even* the country which the LORD smote before the congregation of Israel, *is* a land for cattle, and thy servants have cattle:

5 Wherefore, said they, if we have found grace in thy sight, let this land be given unto thy servants for a possession, *and* bring us not over Jordan.

6 And Moses said unto the children of Gad and to the children of Reuben, Shall your brethren go to war, and shall ye sit here?

7 And wherefore discourage ye the heart of the children of Israel from going over into the land which the LORD hath given them?

8 Thus did your fathers, [h]when I sent them from [i]Kadesh-barnea to see the land.

9 For [j]when they went up unto the valley of Eshcol, and saw the land, they discouraged the heart of the children of Israel, that they should not go into the land which the LORD had given them.

10 And the LORD'S anger was kindled the same time, and he sware, saying,

11 Surely none of the men that came up out of Egypt, from twenty years old and upward, shall see the land which I sware unto Abraham, unto Isaac, and unto Jacob; because they have not wholly followed me:

12 Save Caleb the son of Jephunneh the Kenezite, and Joshua the son of Nun: [k]for they have wholly followed the LORD.

13 And the LORD'S anger was kindled against Israel, and he made them wander in the wilderness forty years, until all the generation, that had done evil in the sight of the LORD, was consumed.

14 And, behold, ye are risen up in your fathers' stead, an increase of sinful men, to augment yet the [l]fierce anger of the LORD toward Israel.

15 For if ye [m]turn away from after him, he will yet again leave them in the wilderness; and ye shall destroy all this people.

16 And they came near unto him, and said, We will build sheepfolds here for our cattle, and cities for our little ones:

17 But [n]we ourselves will go ready armed before the children of Israel, until we have brought them unto their place:

B.C. 1452.

a Or, *necklaces.*
b See Ex. 29:33, *note.*
c Ex. 30:12-16.
d One shekel = 1/2 ounce Troy.
e Deut. 20:14.
f Ex. 30:16.
g Num. 21:32; Josh. 13:25; 2 Sam. 24:5.
h Num. 13:3-26.
i Deut. 1:22.
j Num. 13:24, 31; Deut. 1:24, 28.
k Num. 14:24; Deut. 1:36; Josh. 14:8, 9.
l Deut. 1:34.
m Deut. 30:17; Josh. 22:16, 18; 2 Chr. 7:19; 15:2.
n Josh. 4:12, 13.

[1] **(32:1)** *The Reubenites, Gadites, and half-tribe of Manasseh,* who chose their inheritance just outside the land, are types of world-borderers—carnal Christians. What their descendants were when Messiah came is seen in Mk. 5:1-17.

B.C. 1452.

and our little ones shall dwell in the fenced cities because of the inhabitants of the land.

18 [a]We will not return unto our houses, until the children of Israel have inherited every man his inheritance.

19 For we will not inherit with them on yonder side Jordan, or forward; [b]because our inheritance is fallen to us on this side Jordan eastward.

20 And [c]Moses said unto them, If ye will do this thing, if ye will go armed before the LORD to war,

21 And will go all of you armed over Jordan before the LORD, until he hath driven out his enemies from before him,

22 And the land be subdued before the LORD: then afterward ye shall return, and be guiltless before the LORD, and before Israel; and this land shall be your possession before the LORD.

23 But if ye will not do so, behold, ye have sinned against the LORD: and be sure [d]your sin will find you out.

24 Build you cities for your little ones, and folds for your sheep; and do that which hath proceeded out of your mouth.

25 And the children of Gad and the children of Reuben spake unto Moses, saying, Thy servants will do as my lord commandeth.

26 Our little ones, our wives, our flocks, and all our cattle, shall be there in the cities of Gilead:

27 But thy servants will pass over, every man armed for war, before the LORD to battle, as my lord saith.

28 So concerning them Moses commanded Eleazar the priest, and Joshua the son of Nun, and the chief fathers of the tribes of the children of Israel:

29 And Moses said unto them, If the children of Gad and the children of Reuben will pass with you over Jordan, every man armed to battle, before the LORD, and the land shall be subdued before you; then ye shall give them the land of Gilead for a possession:

30 But if they will not pass over with you armed, they shall have possessions among you in the land of Canaan.

31 And the children of Gad and the children of Reuben answered, saying, As the LORD hath said unto thy servants, so will we do.

32 We will pass over armed before the LORD into the land of Canaan, that the possession of our inheritance on this side Jordan *may be* ours.

33 And Moses gave unto them, *even* to the children of Gad, and to the children of Reuben, and unto half the tribe of Manasseh the son of Joseph, the kingdom of Sihon king of the Amorites, and the kingdom of Og king of Bashan, the land, with the cities thereof in the coasts, *even* the cities of the country round about.

34 And the children of Gad built Dibon, and Ataroth, and Aroer,

35 And Atroth, Shophan, and Jaazer, and Jogbehah,

36 And Beth-nimrah, and Beth-haran, fenced cities: and folds for sheep.

37 And the children of Reuben built Heshbon, and Elealeh, and Kirjathaim,

38 And Nebo, and Baal-meon, (their names being changed,) and Shibmah: and gave other names unto the cities which they builded.

39 And the children of Machir the son of Manasseh went to Gilead, and took it, and dispossessed the Amorite which *was* in it.

40 And Moses gave Gilead unto Machir the son of Manasseh; and he dwelt therein.

41 And Jair the son of Manasseh went and took the small [e]towns thereof, and called them [f]Havoth-jair.

42 And Nobah went and took Kenath, and the villages thereof, and called it Nobah, after his own name.

CHAPTER 33.

Summary of the journeys from Egypt to Jordan.

These *are* the journeys of the children of Israel, which went forth out of the land of Egypt with their armies under the hand of Moses and Aaron.

2 And Moses wrote their goings out according to their journeys by the commandment of the LORD: and these *are* their journeys according to their goings out.

3 And they [g]departed from Rameses in the [h]first month, on the fifteenth day of the first month; on the morrow after the passover the children of Israel went out [i]with an high hand in the sight of all the Egyptians.

4 For the Egyptians buried all *their*

a Josh. 22:3, 4.
b v. 33. Josh. 12:1; 13:8.
c Deut. 3:18; Josh. 1:14; 4:12, 13.
d Gen. 4:7; 44:16; Josh. 7:1-26; Isa. 59:12.
e Or, *tent-villages.*
f Or, *the tent-villages of Jair.*
g Ex. 12:37.
h i.e. *April.*
i Ex. 14:8.

firstborn, which the LORD had smitten
among them: [a]upon their gods also the
LORD executed judgments.
5 [b]And the children of Israel removed
from Rameses, and pitched in Succoth.
6 And they departed from [c]Succoth,
and pitched in Etham, which *is* in the
edge of the wilderness.
7 And they [d]removed from Etham,
and turned again unto Pi-hahiroth,
which *is* before Baal-zephon: and they
pitched before Migdol.
8 And they departed from before Pi-
hahiroth, and [e]passed through the midst
of the sea into the wilderness, and went
three days' journey in the wilderness of
Etham, and pitched in Marah.
9 And they removed from Marah, and
[f]came unto Elim: and in Elim *were*
twelve fountains of water, and threescore and ten palm trees; and they
pitched there.
10 And they removed from Elim, and
encamped by the Red sea.
11 And they removed from the Red sea,
and encamped in the [g]wilderness of Sin.
12 And they took their journey out of
the wilderness of Sin, and encamped in
Dophkah.
13 And they departed from Dophkah,
and encamped in Alush.
14 And they removed from Alush, and
encamped at [h]Rephidim, where was no
water for the people to drink.
15 And they departed from Rephidim,
and pitched in the wilderness of Sinai.
16 And they removed from the desert
of Sinai, and pitched [i]at [j]Kibroth-
hattaavah.
17 And they departed from Kibroth-
hattaavah, and encamped at Hazeroth.
18 And they departed from Hazeroth,
and pitched in Rithmah.
19 And they departed from Rithmah,
and pitched at Rimmon-parez.
20 And they departed from Rimmon-
parez, and pitched in Libnah.
21 And they removed from Libnah,
and pitched at Rissah.
22 And they journeyed from Rissah,
and pitched in Kehelathah.
23 And they went from Kehelathah,
and pitched in mount Shapher.
24 And they removed from mount
Shapher, and encamped in Haradah.
25 And they removed from Haradah,
and pitched in Makheloth.
26 And they removed from Makheloth, and encamped at Tahath.

B.C. 1452.

27 And they departed from Tahath,
and pitched at Tarah.
28 And they removed from Tarah, and
pitched in Mithcah.
29 And they went from Mithcah, and
pitched in Hashmonah.
30 And they departed from Hashmonah, and [k]encamped at Moseroth.
31 And they departed from Moseroth,
and pitched in Bene-jaakan.
32 And they removed from Bene-
jaakan, and [l]encamped at Hor-hagidgad.
33 And they went from Hor-hagidgad,
and pitched in Jotbathah.
34 And they removed from Jotbathah,
and encamped at Ebronah.
35 And they departed from Ebronah,
and encamped at Ezion-gaber.
36 And they removed from Ezion-
gaber, and pitched in the [m]wilderness of
Zin, which *is* Kadesh.
37 And they removed from Kadesh,
and pitched in mount Hor, in the edge of
the land of Edom.
38 And Aaron the priest went up into
mount Hor at the commandment of the
LORD, and died there, in the fortieth year
after the children of Israel were come
out of the land of Egypt, in the first *day*
of the [n]fifth month.
39 And Aaron *was* an hundred and
twenty and three years old when he
died in mount Hor.
40 And king Arad the Canaanite,
which dwelt in the south in the land of
Canaan, heard of the coming of the children of Israel.
41 And they departed from mount
Hor, and pitched in Zalmonah.
42 And they departed from Zalmonah,
and pitched in Punon.
43 And they departed from Punon,
and pitched in Oboth.
44 And they departed from Oboth,
and pitched in [o]Ije-abarim, in the border
of Moab.
45 And they departed from Iim, and
pitched in Dibon-gad.
46 And they removed from Dibon-gad,
and encamped in Almon-diblathaim.
47 And they removed from Almon-
diblathaim, and pitched in the mountains of Abarim, before Nebo.
48 And they departed from the mountains of Abarim, and pitched in the
plains of Moab by Jordan *near* Jericho.
49 And they pitched by Jordan, from

a Ex. 12:12; 18:11; Isa. 19:1.
b Ex. 12:37.
c Ex. 13:20.
d Ex. 14:2, 9.
e Ex. 14:22; 15:22, 23.
f Ex. 15:27.
g Ex. 16:1.
h Ex. 17:1; 19:2.
i Num. 11:34.
j i.e. *the graves of lust.*
k Deut. 10:6.
l Deut. 10:7.
m Num. 20:1; 27:14.
n i.e. *August.*
o i.e. *the ruins of Abarim.*

Beth-jesimoth *even* unto [a]Abel-shittim in the plains of Moab.

50 And the LORD spake unto Moses in the plains of Moab by Jordan *near* Jericho, saying,

The law of the possession of the land.

51 Speak unto the children of Israel, and say unto them, [b]When ye are passed over Jordan into the land of Canaan;

52 [c]Then ye shall drive out all the inhabitants of the land from before you, and destroy all their pictures, and destroy all their molten images, and quite pluck down all their high places:

53 And ye shall dispossess *the inhabitants* of the land, and dwell therein: for I have given you the land to possess it.

54 And ye shall divide the land by lot for an inheritance among your families: *and* to the [d]more ye shall give the more inheritance, and to the [e]fewer ye shall give the less inheritance: every man's *inheritance* shall be in the place where his lot falleth; according to the tribes of your fathers ye shall inherit.

55 But if ye will not drive out the inhabitants of the land from before you; then it shall come to pass, that those which ye let remain of them *shall be* [f]pricks in your eyes, and thorns in your sides, and shall vex you in the land wherein ye dwell.

56 Moreover it shall come to pass, *that* I shall do unto you, as I thought to do unto them.

CHAPTER 34.

Preparations to enter the land.

And the LORD spake unto Moses, saying,

2 Command the children of Israel, and say unto them, When ye come into the land of [g]Canaan; (this *is* the land that shall fall unto you for an inheritance, *even* the land of Canaan with the coasts thereof:)

3 Then [h]your south quarter shall be from the wilderness of Zin along by the coast of Edom, and your south border shall be the outmost coast of [i]the salt sea eastward:

4 And your border shall turn from the south to the ascent of Akrabbim, and pass on to Zin: and the going forth thereof shall be from the south to Kadesh-barnea, and shall go on to Hazar-addar, and pass on to Azmon:

B.C. 1452.

a i.e. *the plains of Shittim.*

b Deut. 7:1, 2; 9:1; Josh. 3:17.

c Ex. 23:24, 33; 34:13; Deut. 7:2, 5; 12:3; Josh. 11:12; Jud. 2:2.

d i.e. *greater.*

e i.e. *smaller.*

f Josh. 23:13; Jud. 2:3; Psa. 106:34-36; see Ex. 23:33; Ezk. 28:14.

g Gen. 17:8; Deut. 1:7, 8; Psa. 78:55; 105:11; Ezk. 47:14.

h Josh. 15:1; see Ezk. 47:13, etc.

i Gen. 14:3; Josh. 15:2.

j Gen. 15:18; Josh. 15:4, 47; 1 Ki. 8:65; Isa. 27:12.

k Ezk. 47:15.

l Ezk. 47:17.

m 2 Ki. 23:33; Jer. 39:5, 6.

n Deut. 3:17; Josh. 11:2; 12:3; 13:27; 19:35; Mt. 14:34; Lk. 5:1; John 6:1.

5 And the border shall fetch a compass from Azmon [j]unto the river of Egypt, and the goings out of it shall be at the sea.

6 And *as for* the western border, ye shall even have the great sea for a border: this shall be your west border.

7 And this shall be your north border: from the great sea ye shall point out for you mount Hor:

8 From mount Hor ye shall point out *your border* unto the entrance of Hamath; and the goings forth of the border shall be to [k]Zedad:

9 And the border shall go on to Ziphron, and the goings out of it shall be at [l]Hazar-enan: this shall be your north border.

10 And ye shall point out your east border from Hazar-enan to Shepham:

11 And the coast shall go down from [m]Shepham to Riblah, on the east side of Ain; and the border shall descend, and shall reach unto the side of the sea [n]of Chinnereth eastward:

12 And the border shall go down to Jordan, and the goings out of it shall be at the salt sea: this shall be your land with the coasts thereof round about.

13 And Moses commanded the children of Israel, saying, This *is* the land which ye shall inherit by lot, which the LORD commanded to give unto the nine tribes, and to the half tribe:

14 For the tribe of the children of Reuben according to the house of their fathers, and the tribe of the children of Gad according to the house of their fathers, have received *their inheritance*; and half the tribe of Manasseh have received their inheritance:

15 The two tribes and the half tribe have received their inheritance on this side Jordan *near* Jericho eastward, toward the sunrising.

16 And the LORD spake unto Moses, saying,

17 These *are* the names of the men which shall divide the land unto you: Eleazar the priest, and Joshua the son of Nun.

18 And ye shall take one prince of every tribe, to divide the land by inheritance.

19 And the names of the men *are* these: Of the tribe of Judah, Caleb the son of Jephunneh.

20 And of the tribe of the children of

Simeon, Shemuel the son of Ammihud.

21 Of the tribe of Benjamin, Elidad the son of Chislon.

22 And the prince of the tribe of the children of Dan, Bukki the son of Jogli.

23 The prince of the children of Joseph, for the tribe of the children of Manasseh, Hanniel the son of Ephod.

24 And the prince of the tribe of the children of Ephraim, Kemuel the son of Shiphtan.

25 And the prince of the tribe of the children of Zebulun, Elizaphan the son of Parnach.

26 And the prince of the tribe of the children of Issachar, Paltiel the son of Azzan.

27 And the prince of the tribe of the children of Asher, Ahihud the son of Shelomi.

28 And the prince of the tribe of the children of Naphtali, Pedahel the son of Ammihud.

29 These *are they* whom the LORD commanded to divide the inheritance unto the children of Israel in the land of Canaan.

CHAPTER 35.

The cities of refuge.

And the LORD spake unto Moses in the plains of Moab by Jordan *near* Jericho, saying,

2 [a]Command the children of Israel, that they give unto the Levites of the inheritance of their possession cities to dwell in; and ye shall give *also* unto the Levites suburbs for the cities round about them.

3 And the cities shall they have to dwell in; and the [b]suburbs of them shall be for their cattle, and for their goods, and for all their beasts.

4 And the suburbs of the cities, which ye shall give unto the Levites, *shall reach* from the wall of the city and outward a thousand [c]cubits round about.

5 And ye shall measure from without the city on the east side two thousand cubits, and on the south side two thousand cubits, and on the west side two thousand cubits, and on the north side two thousand cubits; and the city *shall be* in the midst: this shall be to them the suburbs of the cities.

6 And among the cities which ye shall give unto the Levites *there shall be* six cities for [1]refuge, which ye shall appoint for the manslayer, that he may flee thither: and to them ye shall add forty and two cities.

7 *So* all the cities which ye shall give to the Levites *shall be* forty and eight cities: them *shall ye give* with their suburbs.

8 And the cities which ye shall give *shall be* of the possession of the children of Israel: from *them that have* many ye shall give many; but from *them that have* few ye shall give few: every one shall give of his cities unto the Levites according to his inheritance which he inheriteth.

9 And the LORD spake unto Moses, saying,

10 Speak unto the children of Israel, and say unto them, When ye be come over Jordan into the land of Canaan;

11 Then ye shall appoint you cities to be cities of refuge for you; that the slayer may flee thither, which killeth any person at [d]unawares.

12 And they shall be unto you cities for refuge from the [e]avenger; [f]that the manslayer die not, until he stand before the congregation in judgment.

13 And of these cities which ye shall give six cities shall ye have for refuge.

14 [g]Ye shall give three cities on this side Jordan, and three cities shall ye give in the land of Canaan, *which* shall be cities of refuge.

15 These six cities shall be a refuge, *both* for the children of Israel, and for the stranger, and for the sojourner among them: that every one that killeth any person unawares may flee thither.

16 [h]And if he smite him with an instrument of iron, so that he die, he *is* a murderer: the murderer shall surely be put to death.

17 And if he smite him with throwing a stone, wherewith he may die, and he die, he *is* a murderer: the murderer shall surely be put to death.

18 Or *if* he smite him with an hand weapon of wood, wherewith he may

B.C. 1452.

a Josh. 14:3, 4; 21:2. See Ezk. 45:1; 48:8, etc.

b i.e. *pasture grounds.*

c One cubit = 1 ft. 5.48 in.; also v. 5.

d i.e. *by error; unwittingly.*

e Heb. *goel, Redemp. (Kinsman type).* Isa. 59:20, *note.*

f Deut. 19:6; Josh. 20:3, 5, 6.

g Deut. 4:41; Josh. 20:8.

h Ex. 21:12, 14; Lev. 24:17; Deut. 19:11, 12.

[1] **(35:6)** The cities of refuge are types of Christ sheltering the sinner from judgment (Psa. 46:1; 142:5; Isa. 4:6; Ex. 21:13; Deut. 19:2-9; Rom. 8:1, 33, 34; Phil. 3:9; Heb. 6:18, 19).

B.C. 1451.

die, and he die, he *is* a murderer: the murderer shall surely be put to death.

19 The [a]revenger of blood himself shall slay the murderer: when he meeteth him, he shall slay him.

20 But if he thrust him of hatred, or hurl at him [b]by laying of wait, that he die;

21 Or in enmity smite him with his hand, that he die: he that smote *him* shall surely be put to death; *for* he *is* a murderer: the [a]revenger of blood shall slay the murderer, when he meeteth him.

22 But if he thrust him suddenly [c]without enmity, or have cast upon him any thing without laying of wait,

23 Or with any stone, wherewith a man may die, seeing *him* not, and cast *it* upon him, that he die, and *was* not his enemy, neither sought his harm:

24 Then the congregation shall judge between the slayer and the revenger of blood according to these judgments:

25 And the congregation shall deliver the slayer out of the hand of the [a]revenger of blood, and the congregation shall restore him to the city of his refuge, whither he was fled: and he shall abide in it unto the death of the high priest, [d]which was anointed with the holy oil.

26 But if the slayer shall at any time come without the border of the city of his refuge, whither he was fled;

27 And the [a]revenger of blood find him without the borders of the city of his refuge, and the [a]revenger of blood kill the slayer; he shall not be guilty of blood:

28 Because he should have remained in the city of his refuge until the death of the high priest: but after the death of the high priest the slayer shall return into the land of his possession.

29 So these *things* shall be for a statute of judgment unto you throughout your generations in all your dwellings.

30 Whoso killeth any person, the murderer shall be put to death by the [e]mouth of witnesses: but one witness shall not testify against any person *to cause him* to die.

31 Moreover ye shall take no [f]satisfaction for the life of a murderer, which *is* guilty of death: but he shall be surely put to death.

32 And ye shall take no satisfaction for him that is fled to the city of his refuge, that he should come again to dwell in the land, until the death of the priest.

33 So ye shall not pollute the land wherein ye *are*: for blood [g]it defileth the land: and the land cannot be [h]cleansed of the [i]blood that is shed therein, but by the blood of him that shed it.

34 Defile not therefore the land which ye shall inhabit, wherein I dwell: for [j]I the LORD dwell among the children of Israel.

CHAPTER 36.

As to inheritances.

And the chief fathers of the families of the children of Gilead, the son of Machir, the son of Manasseh, of the families of the sons of Joseph, came near, and spake before Moses, and before the princes, the chief fathers of the children of Israel:

2 And they said, The LORD commanded my lord to give the land for an inheritance by lot to the children of Israel: and my lord was commanded by the LORD to give the inheritance of Zelophehad our brother unto his daughters.

3 And if they be married to any of the sons of the *other* tribes of the children of Israel, then shall their inheritance be taken from the inheritance of our fathers, and shall be put to the inheritance of the tribe whereunto they are received: so shall it be taken from the lot of our inheritance.

4 And when the [k]jubile of the children of Israel shall be, then shall their inheritance be put unto the inheritance of the tribe whereunto they are received: so shall their inheritance be taken away from the inheritance of the tribe of our fathers.

5 And Moses commanded the children of Israel according to the word of the LORD, saying, The tribe of the sons of Joseph [l]hath said well.

6 This *is* the thing which the LORD doth command concerning the daughters of Zelophehad, saying, Let them marry to whom they think best; only to the family of the tribe of their father shall they marry.

7 So shall not the inheritance of the children of Israel remove from tribe to tribe: for every one of the children of Israel shall [m]keep

a Heb. *goel, Redemp. (Kinsman type).* Isa. 59:20, *note.*

b Ex. 21:12, 14; Lev. 24:17; Deut. 19:11, 12.

c Ex. 21:13.

d Ex. 29:7; Lev. 4:3; 21:10.

e Deut. 17:6; 19:15; Mt. 18:16; 2 Cor. 13:1; Heb. 10:28.

f i.e. *ransom.*

g Psa. 106:38; Mic. 4:11; cf. Deut. 21:7-8.

h Or, *have atonement made for.*

i Gen. 9:6.

j Ex. 29:45, 46.

k Lev. 25:10.

l Num. 27:7.

m 1 Ki. 21:3.

himself to the inheritance of the tribe of his fathers.

8 And [a]every daughter, that possesseth an inheritance in any tribe of the children of Israel, shall be wife unto one of the family of the tribe of her father, that the children of Israel may enjoy every man the inheritance of his fathers.

9 Neither shall the inheritance remove from *one* tribe to another tribe; but every one of the tribes of the children of Israel shall keep himself to his own inheritance.

10 Even as the LORD commanded Moses, so did the daughters of Zelophehad:

11 For Mahlah, Tirzah, and Hoglah, and Milcah, and Noah, the daughters of Zelophehad, were married unto their father's brothers' sons:

12 *And* they were married into the families of the sons of Manasseh the son of Joseph, and their inheritance remained in the tribe of the family of their father.

13 These *are* the commandments and the judgments, which the LORD commanded by the hand of Moses unto the children of Israel [b]in the plains of Moab by Jordan *near* Jericho.

B.C. 1451.

a 1 Chr. 23:22.

b Num. 26:3; 33:48.

THE FIFTH BOOK OF MOSES
CALLED
DEUTERONOMY

DEUTERONOMY consists of the parting counsels of Moses delivered to Israel in view of their impending entrance upon their covenanted possession. It contains a summary of the wilderness wanderings of Israel, which is important as unfolding the moral judgment of God upon those events; repeats the Decalogue to a generation which had grown up in the wilderness; gives needed instruction as to the conduct of Israel in the land, and contains the Palestinian Covenant (30:1-9). The book breathes the sternness of the Law. Key-words, "Thou shalt"; key-verses, 11:26-28.

It is important to note that, while the land of promise was unconditionally given to Abraham and to his seed in the Abrahamic Covenant (Gen. 13:15; 15:7), it was under the conditional Palestinian Covenant (Deut. 28:1–30:9) that Israel entered the land under Joshua. Utterly violating the conditions of that covenant, the nation was first disrupted (1 Ki. 12) and then cast out of the land (2 Ki. 17:1-18; 24:1–25:11). But the same covenant unconditionally promises a national restoration of Israel which is yet to be fulfilled (Gen. 15:18, *note*).

Deuteronomy is in seven divisions: I. Summary of the history of Israel in the wilderness, 1:1–3:29. II. A restatement of the Law, with warnings and exhortations, 4:1–11:32. III. Instructions, warnings, and predictions, 12:1–27:26. IV. The great closing prophecies summarizing the history of Israel to the second coming of Christ, and containing the Palestinian Covenant, 28:1–30:20. V. Last counsels to Priests, Levites, and to Joshua, 31. VI. The Song of Moses and his parting blessings, 32, 33. VII. The death of Moses, 34.

The time covered by this retrospect is approximately forty years.

CHAPTER 1.

The failure at Kadesh-barnea.

These *be* the words which Moses
spake unto all [a]Israel on this [b]side
Jordan in the wilderness, in the plain
over against the Red *sea*, between Paran,
and Tophel, and Laban, and Hazeroth,
and Dizahab.
2 (*There are* [c]eleven days' *journey* from
Horeb by the way of mount Seir unto
Kadesh-barnea.)
3 And it came to pass in the fortieth
year, in the [d]eleventh month, on the first
day of the month, *that* Moses spake unto
the children of Israel, according unto all
that the LORD had given him in commandment unto them;
4 After he had slain [e]Sihon the king of
the Amorites, which dwelt in Heshbon,
and Og the king of Bashan, which dwelt
at Astaroth in Edrei:
5 On this side Jordan, in the land of
Moab, began Moses to declare this law,
saying,
6 The LORD our God [f]spake unto us in
Horeb, saying, Ye have [g]dwelt long
enough in this mount:
7 Turn you, and take your journey, and
go to the mount of the Amorites, and
unto all *the places* nigh thereunto, in the
plain, in the hills, and in the vale, and in
the south, and by the sea side, to the land
of the Canaanites, and unto Lebanon,
unto the great river, the river Euphrates.
8 Behold, I have set the land before
you: go in and possess the [h]land which
the LORD sware unto your fathers,
Abraham, Isaac, and Jacob, to give unto
them and to their seed after them.
9 And I [i]spake unto you at that time,
saying, I am not able to bear you myself
alone:
10 The LORD your God hath multiplied
you, and, behold, ye *are* this day [j]as the
stars of heaven for multitude.
11 (The LORD God of your fathers
make you a thousand times so many
more as ye *are*, and bless you, as he hath
promised you!)
12 How can I myself alone bear your
cumbrance, and your burden, and your
strife?
13 Take you wise men, and understanding, and known among your tribes,
and I will make them rulers over you.
14 And ye answered me, and said, The
thing which thou hast spoken *is* good *for*
us to do.
15 So I took the chief of your

B.C. 1451.

a *Israel (history).* vs. 6-8, 19-40; Deut. 7:6-8. (Gen. 12:2, 3; Rom. 11:26.)

b Josh. 9:1-10; 22:4-7.

c Prolonged by one act of unbelief to forty years. Num. 14:23, *note.*

d i.e. *February.*

e Num. 21:23-24, 33-35.

f Ex. 3:1.

g Cf. Gen. 31:3; Num. 10:11.

h Gen. 12:7; 15:18; 17:7, 8; 26:4; 28:13. Cf. Isa. 11:10, 11; Jer. 23:5-8; Ezk. 37:21-26.

i Ex. 18:18; Num. 11:14.

j Cf. Gen. 15:5; Deut. 28:62.

tribes, wise men, and known, and made
them heads over you, captains over thousands, and captains over hundreds, and
captains over fifties, and captains over
tens, and officers among your tribes.
16 And I charged your judges at that
time, saying, Hear *the causes* between
your brethren, and judge righteously
between *every* man and his brother, and
the stranger *that is* with him.
17 [a]Ye shall not respect persons in
judgment; *but* ye shall hear the small as
well as the great; ye shall not be afraid of
the face of man; for the judgment *is*
God's: and the cause that is too hard for
you, bring *it* unto me, and I will hear it.
18 And I commanded you at that time
all the things which ye should do.
19 And when we departed from
Horeb, we went through all that great
and terrible wilderness, which ye saw by
the way of the mountain of the Amorites,
as the LORD our God commanded us;
and we [b]came to Kadesh-barnea.
20 And I said unto you, Ye are come
unto the mountain of the Amorites, which
the LORD our God doth give unto us.
21 Behold, the LORD thy God hath set
the land before thee: go up *and* possess *it*,
as the LORD God of thy fathers hath said
unto thee; fear not, neither be discouraged.
22 And ye came near unto me every
one of you, and said, We will send men
before us, and they shall search us out
the land, and bring us word again by
what way we must go up, and into what
cities we shall come.
23 And the saying pleased me well:
and I [c]took twelve men of you, one of a
tribe:
24 [d]And they turned and went up into
the mountain, and came unto the valley
of Eshcol, and searched it out.
25 And they took of the fruit of the
land in their hands, and brought *it* down
unto us, and brought us word again, and
said, *It is* [e]a good land which the LORD
our God doth give us.
26 [f]Notwithstanding ye would not go
up, but rebelled against the commandment of the LORD your God:
27 And ye murmured in your tents,
and said, Because the LORD hated us, he
hath brought us forth out of the land of
Egypt, to deliver us into the hand of the
Amorites, to destroy us.
28 Whither shall we go up? our
brethren have discouraged our heart,
saying, [g]The people *is* greater and taller
than we; the cities *are* great and walled
up to heaven; and moreover we have
seen the sons of the Anakims there.
29 Then I said unto you, Dread not,
neither be afraid of them.
30 The LORD your God which goeth
before you, he shall fight for you,
according to all that he did for you in
Egypt before your eyes;
31 And in the wilderness, where thou
hast seen how that the LORD thy God
bare thee, as a man doth bear his son, in
all the way that ye went, until ye came
into this place.
32 Yet in this thing [h]ye did not believe
the LORD your God,
33 Who went in the way before you, to
search you out a place to pitch your tents
in, in fire by night, to shew you by what
way ye should go, and in a cloud by day.
34 And the LORD heard the voice of
your words, and was wroth, and sware,
saying,
35 [i]Surely there shall not one of these
men of this evil generation see that good
land, which I sware to give unto your
fathers,
36 [j]Save Caleb the son of Jephunneh;
he shall see it, and to him will I give the
land that he hath trodden upon, and to
his children, because he hath wholly followed the LORD.
37 [k]Also the LORD was angry with me
for your sakes, saying, Thou also shalt
not go in thither.
38 *But* [l]Joshua the son of Nun, which
standeth before thee, he shall go in thither: encourage him: for he shall cause
Israel to inherit it.
39 Moreover your little ones, which ye
said should be a prey, and your children,
which in that day had no knowledge
between good and evil, they shall go in
thither, and unto them will I give it, and
they shall possess it.
40 But *as for* you, turn you, and take
your journey into the wilderness by the
way of the Red sea.
41 Then ye answered and said unto
me, We have sinned against the LORD,
we will go up and fight, according to all
that the LORD our God commanded us.
And when ye had girded on every man
his weapons of war, ye were ready to go
up into the hill.
42 And the LORD said unto me,

B.C. 1451.

a Deut. 16:19; Lev. 19:15; 1 Sam. 16:7; Prov. 24:23; Jas. 2:1.

b Num. 13:26.

c Num. 13:2.

d Num. 13:22-24.

e Num. 13:2.

f Num. 14:1-4; Psa. 106:24, 25.

g Num. 13:28, 31-33; Deut. 9:1, 2.

h Psa. 106:24; Heb. 3:7-19; 4:1, 2.

i Num. 14:22, 23; Psa. 95:11.

j Num. 14:24, 30; Josh. 14:9, 10.

k Num. 20:12; 27:14; Deut. 3:26; 4:21; 34:4; Psa. 106:32.

l Num. 14:30.

Say unto them, Go not up, neither fight;
for I *am* not among you; lest ye be smitten before your enemies.
43 So I spake unto you; and ye would
not hear, but rebelled against the commandment of the LORD, and went presumptuously up into the hill.
44 And the Amorites, which dwelt in
that mountain, came out against you, and
chased you, as bees do, and destroyed
you in Seir, *even* unto Hormah.
45 And ye returned and wept before
the LORD; [a]but the LORD would not hearken to your voice, nor give ear unto you.
46 So ye abode in Kadesh many days,
according unto the days that ye abode
there.

CHAPTER 2.

The wanderings and conflicts of the wilderness.

Then we turned, [b]and took our
journey into the wilderness by the
way of the Red sea, as the LORD spake
unto me: and we compassed mount Seir
many days.
2 And the LORD spake unto me, saying,
3 Ye have compassed this mountain
[c]long enough: turn you northward.
4 And command thou the people, saying, Ye *are* to pass through the coast of
your brethren the children of Esau,
which dwell in Seir; and they shall be
afraid of you: take ye good heed unto
yourselves therefore:
5 Meddle not with them; for I will not
give you of their land, no, not so much
as a foot breadth; because I have [d]given
mount Seir unto Esau *for* a possession.
6 Ye shall buy meat of them for money,
that ye may eat; and ye shall also buy
water of them for money, that ye may
drink.
7 For the LORD thy God hath blessed
thee in all the works of thy hand: he
[e]knoweth thy walking through this great
wilderness: these forty years the LORD
thy God *hath been* with thee; thou hast
lacked nothing.
8 And when we passed by from our
brethren the children of Esau, which
dwelt in Seir, through the way of the
plain from [f]Elath, and from Ezion-gaber,
we turned and passed by the way of the
[g]wilderness of Moab.
9 And the LORD said unto me, Distress
not the Moabites, neither contend with
them in battle: for I will not give thee of
their land *for* a possession; because I
have [h]given Ar unto the children of Lot
for a possession.
10 The [i]Emims dwelt therein in times
past, a people great, and many, and tall,
as the [j]Anakims;
11 Which also were accounted giants,
as the Anakims; but the Moabites call
them Emims.
12 The [k]Horims also dwelt in Seir
beforetime; but the children of Esau succeeded them, when they had destroyed
them from before them, and dwelt in
their stead; as Israel did unto the land of
his possession, which the LORD gave unto
them.
13 Now rise up, *said I*, [l]and get you
over the brook Zered. And we went over
the brook Zered.
14 And the space in which we came
from [m]Kadesh-barnea, until we were
come over the brook Zered, *was* thirty and
eight years; [n]until all the generation of the
men of war were wasted out from among
the host, [o]as the LORD sware unto them.
15 For indeed the hand of the LORD was
against them, to destroy them from among
the host, until they were consumed.
16 So it came to pass, when all the
men of war were consumed and dead
from among the people,
17 That the LORD spake unto me, saying,
18 Thou art to pass over through Ar,
the coast of Moab, this day:
19 And *when* thou comest nigh over
against the children of Ammon, distress
them not, nor meddle with them: for I
will not give thee of the land of the children of Ammon *any* possession; because
I have given it unto the children of Lot
for a possession.
20 (That also was accounted a land
of giants: giants dwelt therein in old
time; and the Ammonites call them
[p]Zamzummims;
21 A people great, and many, and tall,
as the Anakims; but the LORD destroyed
them before them; and they succeeded
them, and dwelt in their stead:
22 As he did to the children of Esau,
which dwelt in Seir, when he destroyed
the Horims from before them; and they
succeeded them, and dwelt in their stead
even unto this day:

B.C. 1491.

a Cf. Zech. 7:11-13.
b Deut. 1:40; Num. 14:25.
c Cf. Deut. 1:6, 7.
d Gen. 36:8; Josh. 24:4.
e Psa. 1:6; 37:18; 44:21; 69:5; 94:11; 103:14; Mt. 6:8, 32; 2 Pet. 2:9.
f 1 Ki. 9:26.
g A region east of the Dead Sea.
h Gen. 19:36-38.
i Gen. 14:5.
j Deut. 9:2; Num. 13:22, 33.
k v. 22; Gen. 14:6; 36:20.
l Num. 21:12.
m Num. 13:26.
n Num. 14:33; 26:64; Deut. 1:34-35.
o Num. 14:35; Ezk. 20:15; Heb. 3:17, 18.
p Gen. 14:5.

23 And the Avims which dwelt in Hazerim, *even* unto Azzah, the Caphtorims, which came forth out of Caphtor, destroyed them, and dwelt in their stead.)

24 Rise ye up, take your journey, and pass over the river Arnon: behold, I have given into thine hand Sihon the Amorite, king of Heshbon, and his land: begin to possess *it*, and contend with him in battle.

25 This day will I begin to put the dread of thee and the fear of thee upon the nations *that are* under the whole heaven, who shall hear report of thee, and shall tremble, and be in anguish because of thee.

26 And I sent messengers out of the wilderness of Kedemoth unto Sihon king of Heshbon with words of peace, saying,

27 Let me pass through thy land: I will go along by the high way, I will neither turn unto the right hand nor to the left.

28 Thou shalt sell me meat for money, that I may eat; and give me water for money, that I may drink: only I will pass through on my feet;

29 (As the children of Esau which dwell in Seir, and the Moabites which dwell in Ar, did unto me;) until I shall pass over Jordan into the land which the LORD our God giveth us.

30 But Sihon king of Heshbon would not let us pass by him: for the LORD thy God hardened his spirit, and made his heart obstinate, that he might deliver him into thy hand, as *appeareth* this day.

31 And the LORD said unto me, Behold, I have begun to give Sihon and his land before thee: begin to [a]possess, that thou mayest inherit his land.

32 Then Sihon came out against us, he and all his people, to fight at Jahaz.

33 And the LORD our God delivered him before us; and we smote him, and his sons, and all his people.

34 And we took all his cities at that time, and utterly destroyed the men, and the women, and the little ones, of every city, we left none to remain:

35 Only the cattle we took for a prey unto ourselves, and the spoil of the cities which we took.

36 From [b]Aroer, which *is* by the brink of the river of Arnon, and *from* the city that *is* by the river, even unto Gilead, there was not one city too strong for us: the LORD our God delivered all unto us:

37 Only unto the land of the children of Ammon thou camest not, *nor* unto any place of the river Jabbok, nor unto the cities in the mountains, nor unto whatsoever the LORD our God forbad us.

CHAPTER 3.

Then we turned, and went up the way to Bashan: and [c]Og the king of Bashan came out against us, he and all his people, to battle at [d]Edrei.

2 And the LORD said unto me, Fear him not: for I will deliver him, and all his people, and his land, into thy hand; and thou shalt do unto him as thou didst unto [e]Sihon king of the Amorites, which dwelt at Heshbon.

3 So the LORD our God delivered into our hands Og also, the king of Bashan, and all his people: and we smote him until none was left to him remaining.

4 And we took all his cities at that time, there was not a city which we took not from them, threescore cities, all the region of Argob, the kingdom of Og in Bashan.

5 All these cities *were* fenced with high walls, gates, and bars; beside unwalled towns a great many.

6 And we utterly destroyed them, as we did unto Sihon king of Heshbon, utterly destroying the men, women, and children, of every city.

7 But all the cattle, and the spoil of the cities, we took for a prey to ourselves.

8 And we took at that time out of the hand of the two kings of the Amorites the land that *was* on this side Jordan, from the river of Arnon unto mount [f]Hermon;

9 (*Which* Hermon the Sidonians call Sirion; and the Amorites call it Shenir;)

10 All the cities of the plain, and all Gilead, and all Bashan, unto Salchah and Edrei, cities of the kingdom of Og in Bashan.

11 For only Og king of Bashan remained of the remnant of giants; behold, his bedstead *was* a bedstead of iron; *is* it not in Rabbath of the children of Ammon? nine [g]cubits *was* the length thereof, and four cubits the breadth of it, after the cubit of a man.

12 And this [h]land, *which* we possessed

B.C. 1451.

a Josh. 1:3.

b Deut. 3:12; 4:48; Josh. 13:9.

c Num. 21:33, etc.; Deut. 29:7.

d Deut. 1:4.

e Num. 21:34.

f Deut. 4:48; 1 Chr. 5:23; Psa. 29:6.

g One cubit = 1 ft. 5.48 in.

h Num. 32:33; Josh. 12:6; 13:8-12.

at that time, from Aroer, which *is* by the river Arnon, and half mount Gilead, and the cities thereof, gave I unto the Reubenites and to the Gadites.

13 [a]And the rest of Gilead, and all Bashan, *being* the kingdom of Og, gave I unto the half tribe of Manasseh; all the region of Argob, with all Bashan, which was called the land of giants.

14 Jair the son of Manasseh took all the country of Argob unto the coasts of Geshuri and Maachathi; and called them after his own name, Bashan-havoth-jair, unto this day.

15 And I gave [b]Gilead unto Machir.

16 And unto the Reubenites and unto the Gadites I gave from Gilead even unto the river Arnon half the valley, and the border even unto the river Jabbok, *which is* the border of the children of Ammon;

17 The plain also, and Jordan, and the coast *thereof*, from Chinnereth even unto the sea of the plain, *even* the salt sea, under [c]Ashdoth-pisgah eastward.

18 And I commanded you at that time, saying, The LORD your God hath given you this land to possess it: [d]ye shall pass over armed before your brethren the children of Israel, all *that are* meet for the war.

19 But your wives, and your little ones, and your cattle, (*for* I know that ye have much cattle,) shall abide in your cities which I have given you;

20 Until the LORD have given rest unto your brethren, as well as unto you, and *until* they also possess the land which the LORD your God hath given them beyond Jordan: and *then* shall ye [e]return every man unto his possession, which I have given you.

21 And [f]I commanded Joshua at that time, saying, Thine eyes have seen all that the LORD your God hath done unto these two kings: so shall the LORD do unto all the kingdoms whither thou passest.

22 Ye shall not fear them: for [g]the LORD your God he shall fight for you.

23 And I [h]besought the LORD at that time, saying,

24 O Lord GOD, thou hast begun to shew thy servant thy greatness, and thy mighty hand: for what God *is there* in heaven or in earth, that can do according to thy works, and according to thy might?

25 I pray thee, let me go over, and see the good land that *is* beyond Jordan, that goodly mountain, and Lebanon.

B.C. 1451.

a Josh. 13:29-31; 17:1.

b Num. 32:39.

c i.e. *the springs of Pisgah, or the hill.*

d Num. 32:20, etc.

e Josh. 22:4.

f Num. 27:18.

g Ex. 14:14; Deut. 1:30; 20:4.

h *Bible prayers* (O.T.). Deut. 9:26. (Gen. 15:2; Hab. 3:1-16.)

i Num. 20:12; 27:14; Deut. 1:37; 31:2; 32:51, 52; 34:4; Psa. 106:32, 33.

j Or, *ravine.*

k Lev. 19:37; 20:8; 22:31; Deut. 5:1; 8:1; Ezk. 20:11; Rom. 10:5.

l Deut. 12:32; Josh. 1:7; Prov. 30:6; Rev. 22:18, 19.

m *Inspiration.* vs. 2, 13; Deut. 5:22. (Ex. 4:15; Rev. 22:19.)

n Num. 25:4, etc.; Josh. 22:17; Psa. 106:28, 29.

o Lit. *gods.*

p Psa. 46:1; 145:18; 148:14; Isa. 55:6.

26 But the LORD [i]was wroth with me for your sakes, and would not hear me: and the LORD said unto me, Let it suffice thee; speak no more unto me of this matter.

27 Get thee up into the top of Pisgah, and lift up thine eyes westward, and northward, and southward, and eastward, and behold *it* with thine eyes: for thou shalt not go over this Jordan.

28 But charge Joshua, and encourage him, and strengthen him: for he shall go over before this people, and he shall cause them to inherit the land which thou shalt see.

29 So we abode in the [j]valley over against Beth-peor.

CHAPTER 4.

The new generation taught the lessons of Sinai.

NOW therefore hearken, O Israel, unto the [k]statutes and unto the judgments, which I teach you, for to do *them*, that ye may live, and go in and possess the land which the LORD God of your fathers giveth you.

2 [l]Ye shall not add unto the [m]word which I command you, neither shall ye diminish *ought* from it, that ye may keep the commandments of the LORD your God which I command you.

3 Your eyes have seen what the LORD did because of [n]Baal-peor: for all the men that followed Baal-peor, the LORD thy God hath destroyed them from among you.

4 But ye that did cleave unto the LORD your God *are* alive every one of you this day.

5 Behold, I have taught you statutes and judgments, even as the LORD my God commanded me, that ye should do so in the land whither ye go to possess it.

6 Keep therefore and do *them;* for this *is* your wisdom and your understanding in the sight of the nations, which shall hear all these statutes, and say, Surely this great nation *is* a wise and understanding people.

7 For what nation *is there so* great, who *hath* [o]God so [p]nigh unto them, as the LORD our God *is* in all *things that* we call upon him *for*?

8 And what nation *is there so* great, that hath statutes and judgments

B.C. 1451.

so righteous as all this law, which I set before you this day?

9 Only take heed to thyself, and keep thy soul diligently, lest thou forget the things which thine eyes have seen, and lest they depart from thy heart all the days of thy life: but teach them thy sons, and thy sons' sons;

10 *Specially* the day that thou stoodest before the LORD thy God in Horeb, when the LORD said unto me, Gather me the people together, and I will make them hear my words, that they may learn to [a]fear me all the days that they shall live upon the earth, and *that* they may teach their children.

11 And ye came near and stood under the mountain; and the mountain burned with fire unto the midst of heaven, with darkness, clouds, and thick darkness.

12 And the LORD spake unto you out of the midst of the fire: ye heard the voice of the words, but saw no similitude; [b]only *ye heard* a voice.

13 And he declared unto you his covenant, which he commanded you to perform, *even* ten commandments; and he wrote them upon two tables of stone.

14 And the LORD commanded me at that time to teach you statutes and judgments, that ye might do them in the land whither ye go over to possess it.

15 Take ye therefore good heed unto yourselves; for ye [c]saw no manner of similitude on the day *that* the LORD spake unto you in Horeb out of the midst of the fire:

16 Lest ye corrupt *yourselves*, and make you a graven image, the similitude of any figure, the [d]likeness of male or female,

17 The likeness of any beast that *is* on the earth, the likeness of any winged fowl that flieth in the air,

18 The likeness of any thing that creepeth on the ground, the likeness of any fish that *is* in the waters beneath the earth:

19 And lest thou lift up thine eyes unto heaven, and when thou seest the sun, and the moon, and the stars, *even* all the host of heaven, shouldest be [e]driven to worship them, and serve them, which the LORD thy God hath divided unto all nations under the whole heaven.

20 But the LORD hath taken you, and [f]brought you forth out of the iron furnace, *even* out of Egypt, to be unto him a people of inheritance, as *ye are* this day.

21 Furthermore the LORD was angry with me for your sakes, and sware that I should not go over Jordan, and that I should not go in unto that good land, which the LORD thy God giveth thee *for* an inheritance:

22 But I must die in this land, I must not go over Jordan: but ye shall go over, and possess that good land.

23 Take heed unto yourselves, lest ye forget the covenant of the LORD your God, which he made with you, and make you a graven image, *or* the likeness of any *thing*, which the LORD thy God hath forbidden thee.

24 For the LORD thy God *is* a consuming fire, *even* a jealous God.

25 When thou shalt beget children, and children's children, and ye shall have remained long in the land, and shall corrupt *yourselves*, and make a graven image, *or* the likeness of any *thing*, and shall do evil in the sight of the LORD thy God, to provoke him to anger:

26 [g]I call heaven and earth to witness against you this day, that ye shall soon utterly perish from off the land whereunto ye go over Jordan to possess it; ye shall not prolong *your* days upon it, but shall utterly be destroyed.

27 And the LORD shall [h]scatter you among the [i]nations, and ye shall be left few in number among the [j]heathen, whither the LORD shall lead you.

28 And there ye shall serve gods, the work of men's hands, wood and stone, [k]which neither see, nor hear, nor eat, nor smell.

29 But if from thence thou shalt seek the LORD thy God, thou shalt find *him*, if thou seek him with all thy heart and with all thy soul.

30 When thou art in tribulation, and all these things are come upon thee, [l]*even* in the latter days, if thou turn to the LORD thy God, and shalt be obedient unto his voice;

31 (For the LORD thy God *is* a merciful God;) he will not forsake thee, neither destroy thee, nor forget the covenant of thy fathers which he sware unto them.

32 For ask now of the days that are past, which were before thee, since the day that God created man upon the earth, and *ask* from the one side of heaven unto the other, whether there hath

a Psa. 19:9, *note.*
b Ex. 20:22; 1 Ki. 19:12.
c Cf. John 1:18, *note.*
d Rom. 1:23.
e Or, *drawn away.*
f 1 Ki. 8:51; Jer. 11:4.
g Deut. 30:18, 19; Isa. 1:2; Mic. 6:2.
h Lev. 26:33; Deut. 28:62, 64; Neh. 1:8.
i i.e. *Gentiles.*
j i.e. *nations.*
k Psa. 115:4, 5; 135:15-17; Isa. 44:9; 46:7.
l Gen. 49:1; Deut. 31:29; Jer. 23:20; Hos. 3:5.

been *any such thing* as this great thing *is*, or hath been heard like it?

33 Did *ever* people hear the voice of God speaking out of the midst of the fire, as thou hast heard, and live?

34 Or hath God assayed to go *and* take him a nation from the midst of *another* nation, by temptations, by signs, and by wonders, and by war, and by a mighty hand, and by a stretched out arm, and by great terrors, according to all that the LORD your God did for you in Egypt before your eyes?

35 Unto thee it was shewed, that thou mightest know that the LORD he *is* God; *there is* none else beside him.

36 [a]Out of heaven he made thee to hear his voice, that he might instruct thee: and upon earth he shewed thee his great fire; and thou heardest his words out of the midst of the fire.

37 And because he loved thy fathers, therefore he chose their seed after them, and brought thee out in his sight with his mighty power out of Egypt;

38 To drive out nations from before thee greater and mightier than thou *art*, to bring thee in, to give thee their land *for* an inheritance, as *it is* this day.

39 Know therefore this day, and consider *it* in thine heart, that the LORD he *is* God in heaven above, and upon the earth beneath: *there is* none else.

40 Thou shalt keep therefore his statutes, and his commandments, which I command thee this day, that it may go well with thee, and with thy children after thee, and that thou mayest prolong *thy* days upon the earth, which the LORD thy God giveth thee, for ever.

Three of the cities of refuge designated.

41 Then Moses [b]severed three cities on this side Jordan toward the sunrising;

42 [c]That the slayer might flee thither, which should kill his neighbour unawares, and hated him not in times past; and that fleeing unto one of these cities he might live:

43 *Namely,* [d]Bezer in the wilderness, in the plain country, of the Reubenites; and Ramoth in Gilead, of the Gadites; and Golan in Bashan, of the Manassites.

44 And this *is* the law which Moses set before the children of Israel:

45 These *are* the testimonies, and the statutes, and the judgments, which Moses spake unto the children of Israel, after they came forth out of Egypt,

46 On this side Jordan, in the valley over against Beth-peor, in the land of Sihon king of the Amorites, who dwelt at Heshbon, whom Moses and the children of Israel [e]smote, after they were come forth out of Egypt:

47 And they possessed his land, and the land of Og king of Bashan, two kings of the Amorites, which *were* on this side Jordan toward the sunrising;

48 From Aroer, which *is* by the bank of the river Arnon, even unto mount Sion, which *is* Hermon,

49 And all the plain on this side Jordan eastward, even unto the sea of the plain, under the springs of Pisgah.

CHAPTER 5.

The new generation taught the Mosaic covenant. (Cf. Ex. 20:4, *note.*)

AND Moses called all Israel, and said unto them, Hear, O Israel, the statutes and judgments which I speak in your ears this day, that ye may learn them, and keep, and [f]do them.

2 The LORD our God made a [g]covenant with us in Horeb.

3 The LORD [h]made not this covenant with our fathers, but with us, *even* us, who *are* all of us here alive this day.

4 The LORD talked with you face to face in the mount out of the midst of the fire,

5 ([i]I stood between the LORD and you at that time, to shew you the word of the LORD: for ye were afraid by reason of the fire, and went not up into the mount;) saying,

6 I *am* the LORD thy God, which brought thee out of the land of Egypt, from the house of bondage.

7 Thou shalt have none other gods before me.

8 Thou shalt not make thee *any* graven image, *or* any likeness *of any thing* that *is* in heaven above, or that *is* in the earth beneath, or that *is* in the waters beneath the earth:

9 Thou shalt not bow down thyself

B.C. 1451.

a Ex. 19:9, 19; 20:18-22; 24:16; Heb. 12:19.

b Num. 35:6, 14.

c Deut. 19:4.

d Josh. 20:8.

e Num. 21:24; Deut. 1:4.

f *Law (of Moses).* vs. 1-22; Deut. 6:1-5. (Ex. 19:1; Gal. 3:1-29.)

g Ex. 19:5; Deut. 4:23; Mal. 4:4.

h Heb. 8:9.

i Ex. 20:21; Gal. 3:19.

unto them, nor serve them: for I the LORD thy God *am* a jealous God, visiting the iniquity of the fathers upon the children unto the third and fourth *generation* of them that hate me,

10 And shewing [a]*mercy* unto thousands of them that love me and keep my commandments.

11 Thou shalt not take the name of the LORD thy God in vain: for the LORD will not hold *him* guiltless that taketh his name in vain.

12 Keep the sabbath day to sanctify it, as the LORD thy God hath commanded thee.

13 [b]Six days thou shalt labour, and do all thy work:

14 But the seventh day *is* the sabbath of the LORD thy God: *in it* thou shalt not do any work, thou, nor thy son, nor thy daughter, nor thy manservant, nor thy maidservant, nor thine ox, nor thine ass, nor any of thy cattle, nor thy stranger that *is* within thy gates; that thy manservant and thy maidservant may rest as well as thou.

15 And remember that thou wast a servant in the land of Egypt, and *that* the LORD thy God brought thee out thence through a mighty hand and by a stretched out arm: therefore the LORD thy God commanded thee to keep the sabbath day.

16 Honour thy father and thy [c]mother, as the LORD thy God hath commanded thee; that thy days may be prolonged, and that it may go well with thee, in the land which the LORD thy God giveth thee.

17 Thou shalt not kill.

18 Neither shalt thou commit adultery.

19 Neither shalt thou steal.

20 Neither shalt thou bear false witness against thy neighbour.

21 Neither shalt thou desire thy neighbour's wife, neither shalt thou covet thy neighbour's house, his field, or his manservant, or his maidservant, his ox, or his ass, or any *thing* that *is* thy neighbour's.

22 These [d]words the LORD spake unto all your assembly in the mount out of the midst of the fire, of the cloud, and of the thick darkness, with a great voice: and he added no more. And he wrote them in two tables of stone, and delivered them unto me.

23 And it came to pass, when ye heard the voice out of the midst of the darkness, (for the mountain did burn with fire,) that ye came near unto me, *even* all the heads of your tribes, and your elders;

24 And ye said, Behold, the LORD our God hath shewed us his glory and his greatness, and we have heard his voice out of the midst of the fire: we have seen this day that God doth talk with man, and he [e]liveth.

25 Now therefore why should we die? for this great fire will consume us: if we hear the voice of the LORD our God any more, then we shall die.

26 For who *is there of* all flesh, that hath heard the voice of the living God speaking out of the midst of the fire, as we *have*, and lived?

27 Go thou near, and hear all that the LORD our God shall say: and [f]speak thou unto us all that the LORD our God shall speak unto thee; and we will hear *it*, and do *it*.

28 And the LORD heard the voice of your words, when ye spake unto me; and the LORD said unto me, I have heard the voice of the words of this people, which they have spoken unto thee: they have well said all that they have spoken.

29 [g]O that there were such an heart in them, that they would [h]fear me, and keep all my commandments always, that it might be well with them, and with their children for ever!

30 Go say to them, Get you into your tents again.

31 But as for thee, stand thou here by me, and I will speak unto thee all the commandments, and the statutes, and the judgments, which thou shalt teach them, that they may do *them* in the land which I give them to possess it.

32 Ye shall observe to do therefore as the LORD your God hath commanded you: ye shall not turn aside to the right hand or to the left.

33 Ye shall walk in [i]all the ways which the LORD your God hath commanded you, that ye may live, and *that it may be* well with you, and *that* ye may prolong *your* days in the land which ye shall possess.

CHAPTER 6.

Now these *are* the commandments, the statutes, and the judgments, which the LORD your God commanded

B.C. 1451.

a Jer. 32:18; Dan. 9:4.

b Ex. 23:12; 35:2; Ezk. 20:12.

c Eph. 6:2, 3; Col. 3:20.

d *Inspiration.* Deut. 10:1-4. (Ex. 4:15; Rev. 22:19.)

e Deut. 4:33; Jud. 13:22.

f Ex. 20:19; Heb. 12:19.

g Deut. 32:29; Psa. 81:13; Isa. 48:18; Mt. 23:37; Lk. 19:42.

h Psa. 19:9, *note.*

i Deut. 10:12; Psa. 119:3; Jer. 7:23; Lk. 1:6.

to teach you, that ye might [a]do *them* in the land whither ye go to possess it:

2 That thou mightest [b]fear the LORD thy God, to keep all his statutes and his commandments, which I command thee, thou, and thy son, and thy son's son, all the days of thy life; and that thy days may be prolonged.

3 Hear therefore, O Israel, and observe to do *it*; that it may be well with thee, and that ye may increase mightily, as the LORD God of thy fathers hath promised thee, in the land that floweth with milk and honey.

The "great commandment."

4 Hear, O Israel: The LORD our God *is* one [c]LORD:

5 And thou shalt [d]love the LORD thy God with all thine heart, and with all thy soul, and with all thy might.

Instruction and warning.

6 And these words, which I command thee this day, shall be in thine heart:

7 And thou shalt teach them diligently unto thy children, and shalt talk of them when thou sittest in thine house, and when thou walkest by the way, and when thou liest down, and when thou risest up.

8 And thou shalt bind them for a sign upon thine hand, and they shall be as frontlets between thine eyes.

9 And thou shalt write them upon the posts of thy house, and on thy gates.

10 And it shall be, when the LORD thy God shall have brought thee into the land which he sware unto thy fathers, to Abraham, to Isaac, and to Jacob, to give thee great and goodly cities, which thou buildedst not,

11 And houses full of all good *things*, which thou filledst not, and wells digged, which thou diggedst not, vineyards and olive trees, which thou plantedst not; when thou shalt have eaten and be full;

12 *Then* beware lest thou forget the LORD, which brought thee forth out of the land of Egypt, from the house of bondage.

13 Thou shalt [b]fear the LORD thy God, and serve [e]him, and shalt swear by his name.

14 Ye shall not go after other gods, of the gods of the people which *are* round about you;

15 (For the LORD thy God *is* a jealous God among you) lest the anger of the LORD thy God be kindled against thee, and destroy thee from off the face of the earth.

16 Ye shall not [f]tempt the LORD your [g]God, as ye tempted *him* in Massah.

17 Ye shall diligently keep the commandments of the LORD your God, and his testimonies, and his statutes, which he hath commanded thee.

18 And thou shalt do *that which is* right and good in the sight of the LORD: that it may be well with thee, and that thou mayest go in and possess the good land which the LORD sware unto thy fathers,

19 [h]To cast out all thine enemies from before thee, as the LORD hath spoken.

20 *And* when thy son asketh thee in time to come, saying, What *mean* the testimonies, and the statutes, and the judgments, which the LORD our God hath commanded you?

21 Then thou shalt say unto thy son, We were Pharaoh's bondmen in Egypt; and the LORD brought us out of [i]Egypt with a mighty hand:

22 And the LORD shewed signs and wonders, great and sore, upon Egypt, upon Pharaoh, and upon all his household, before our eyes:

23 And he brought us out from thence, that he might bring us in, to give us the land which he sware unto our fathers.

24 And the LORD commanded us to do all these statutes, to [b]fear the LORD our God, [j]for our good always, that he might preserve us alive, as *it is* at this day.

25 And [k]it shall be our righteousness, if we observe to do all these commandments before the LORD our God, as he hath commanded us.

CHAPTER 7.

The command to be separate.

When the LORD thy God shall bring thee into the land whither thou goest to possess it, and hath cast out many nations before thee, [l]the Hittites, and the Girgashites, and the Amorites, and the Canaanites, and the Perizzites, and the Hivites, and the Jebusites, seven nations greater and mightier than thou;

B.C. 1451.

a *Law (of Moses).* vs. 1-5; Psa. 1:2. (Ex. 19:1; Gal. 3:1-29.)

b Psa. 19:9, *note.*

c Mk. 12:29.

d Mt. 22:37; Mk. 12:29, 30; Lk. 10:27.

e Mt. 4:10; Lk. 4:8.

f *Temptation.* Psa. 78:18, 41, 56. (Gen. 3:1; Jas. 1:2.)

g Mt. 4:7; Lk. 4:12.

h Num. 33:52, 53.

i Ex. 3:19; 13:3.

j Deut. 10:13; Job 35:7, 8; Jer. 32:39.

k Lev. 18:5; Deut. 24:13; Rom. 10:3, 5.

l Gen. 15:19, etc.; Ex. 33:2.

B.C. 1451.

2 And when the LORD thy God shall deliver them before thee; thou shalt smite them, *and* utterly destroy them; thou shalt make no covenant with them, nor shew mercy unto them:

3 [a]Neither shalt thou make marriages with them; thy daughter thou shalt not give unto his son, nor his daughter shalt thou take unto thy son.

4 For they will turn away thy son from following me, that they may serve other gods: so will the anger of the LORD be kindled against you, and destroy thee suddenly.

5 But thus shall ye deal with them; ye shall destroy their altars, and break down their images, and cut down their [b]groves, and burn their graven images with fire.

6 For thou *art* an holy [c]people unto the LORD thy God: the LORD thy God hath [d]chosen thee to be a special people unto himself, above all people that *are* upon the face of the earth.

7 The LORD did not set his love upon you, nor choose you, because ye were more in number than any people; for ye *were* the fewest of all people:

8 But because the LORD loved you, and because he would keep the oath which he had sworn unto your fathers, hath the LORD brought you out with a mighty hand, and [e]redeemed you out of the house of bondmen, from the hand of Pharaoh king of Egypt.

9 Know therefore that the LORD thy God, he *is* God, the faithful God, [f]which keepeth covenant and mercy with them that love him and keep his commandments to a thousand generations;

10 And repayeth them that hate him to their face, to destroy them: he will not be slack to him that hateth him, he will repay him to his face.

11 Thou shalt therefore keep the commandments, and the statutes, and the judgments, which I command thee this day, to do them.

The promise of victory.

12 Wherefore it shall come to pass, if ye hearken to these judgments, and keep, and do them, that the LORD thy God shall keep unto thee the covenant and the mercy which he sware unto thy fathers:

13 And he will [g]love thee, and bless thee, and multiply thee: he will also bless the fruit of thy womb, and the fruit of thy land, thy corn, and thy wine, and thine oil, the increase of thy kine, and the flocks of thy sheep, in the land which he sware unto thy fathers to give thee.

14 Thou shalt be blessed above all people: there shall not be male or female barren among you, or among your cattle.

15 And the LORD will take away from thee all sickness, and will put none of the [h]evil diseases of Egypt, which thou knowest, upon thee; but will lay them upon all *them* that hate thee.

16 And thou shalt consume all the people which the LORD thy God shall deliver thee; thine eye shall have no pity upon them: neither shalt thou serve their gods; for that *will be* a [i]snare unto thee.

17 If thou shalt say in thine heart, These nations *are* more than I; how can I dispossess them?

18 Thou shalt not be afraid of them: *but* shalt well remember what the LORD thy God did unto Pharaoh, and unto all Egypt;

19 The great temptations which thine eyes saw, and the signs, and the wonders, and the mighty hand, and the stretched out arm, whereby the LORD thy God brought thee out: so shall the LORD thy God do unto all the people of whom thou art afraid.

20 Moreover the LORD thy God will send the hornet among them, until they that are left, and hide themselves from thee, be destroyed.

21 Thou shalt not be affrighted at them: for the LORD thy God *is* among you, a mighty God and terrible.

22 And the LORD thy God will put out those nations before thee by little and little: thou mayest not consume them at once, lest the beasts of the field increase upon thee.

23 But the LORD thy God shall deliver them unto thee, and shall destroy them with a mighty destruction, until they be destroyed.

24 And he [j]shall deliver their kings into thine hand, and thou shalt destroy their name from under heaven: there shall no man be able to stand before thee, until thou have destroyed them.

25 The graven images of their gods shall ye burn with fire: thou shalt not desire the silver or gold *that is* on them,

a Josh. 23:12; 1 Ki. 11:2; Ezra 9:2.

b See Deut. 16:21.

c *Israel (history).* vs. 6-8; Deut. 28:58-68. (Gen. 12:2, 3; Rom. 11:26.)

d *Election (corporate).* vs. 6, 7; Psa. 33:12. (Deut. 7:6; 1 Pet. 1:2.)

e Ex. 14:30, *note.*

f Ex. 20:6; Deut. 5:10; Neh. 1:5; Dan. 9:4.

g John 14:21.

h Ex. 9:14; 15:26; Deut. 28:27, 60.

i Ex. 23:33; Deut. 7:4, 5; 12:30; Jud. 8:27; Psa. 106:36.

j Josh. 10:24, 25, 42; 12:1, etc.

B.C. 1451.

nor take *it* unto thee, lest thou be [a]snared therein: for it *is* an abomination to the LORD thy God.

26 Neither shalt thou bring an abomination into thine house, lest thou be a cursed thing like it: *but* thou shalt utterly detest it, and thou shalt utterly abhor it; for it *is* a cursed thing.

CHAPTER 8.

Warnings and exhortations.

All the commandments which I command thee this day shall ye observe to do, that ye may live, and multiply, and go in and possess the land which the LORD sware unto your fathers.

2 And thou shalt remember all the way which the LORD thy God [b]led thee these forty years in the wilderness, to humble thee, *and* to prove thee, to know what *was* in thine heart, whether thou wouldest keep his commandments, or no.

3 And he humbled thee, and suffered thee to hunger, and fed thee with manna, which thou knewest not, neither did thy fathers know; that he might make thee know that man doth not live by bread [c]only, but by every *word* that proceedeth out of the mouth of the LORD doth man live.

4 Thy [d]raiment waxed not old upon thee, neither did thy foot swell, these forty years.

5 [e]Thou shalt also consider in thine heart, that, as a man chasteneth his son, *so* the LORD thy God chasteneth thee.

6 Therefore thou shalt keep the commandments of the LORD thy God, to walk in his ways, and to [f]fear him.

7 For the LORD thy God bringeth thee into a good land, a land of brooks of water, of fountains and depths that spring out of valleys and hills;

8 A land of wheat, and barley, and vines, and fig trees, and pomegranates; a land of oil olive, and honey;

9 A land wherein thou shalt eat bread without scarceness, thou shalt not lack any *thing* in it; a land whose stones *are* iron, and out of whose hills thou mayest dig brass.

10 When thou hast eaten and art full, then thou shalt bless the LORD thy God for the good land which he hath given thee.

11 Beware that thou forget not the LORD thy God, in not keeping his commandments, and his judgments, and his statutes, which I command thee this day:

12 [g]Lest *when* thou hast eaten and art full, and hast built goodly houses, and dwelt *therein*;

13 And *when* thy herds and thy flocks multiply, and thy silver and thy gold is multiplied, and all that thou hast is multiplied;

14 [h]Then thine heart be lifted up, and thou [i]forget the LORD thy God, which brought thee forth out of the land of Egypt, from the house of bondage;

15 Who led thee through that great and terrible wilderness, *wherein were* fiery serpents, and scorpions, and drought, where *there was* no water; who brought thee forth water out of the rock of flint;

16 Who fed thee in the wilderness with manna, which thy fathers knew not, that he might humble thee, and that he might prove thee, [j]to do thee good at thy latter end;

17 And thou say in thine heart, My power and the might of *mine* hand hath gotten me this wealth.

18 But thou shalt remember the LORD thy God: for *it is* he that giveth thee power to get wealth, that he may establish his covenant which he sware unto thy fathers, as *it is* this day.

19 And it shall be, if thou do at all forget the LORD thy God, and walk after other gods, and serve them, and worship them, I testify against you this day that ye shall surely perish.

20 As the nations which the LORD destroyeth before your face, [k]so shall ye perish; because ye would not be obedient unto the voice of the LORD your God.

CHAPTER 9.

Warnings and exhortations.

Hear, O Israel: Thou *art* to pass over Jordan this day, to go in to possess nations greater and mightier than thyself, cities great and fenced up to heaven,

2 A people great and tall, [l]the children of the Anakims, whom thou knowest, and *of whom* thou hast heard *say*, Who can stand before the children of Anak!

3 Understand therefore this day, that the LORD thy God *is* he which [m]goeth over before thee; *as* a consuming fire he

a Jud. 8:27; Zeph. 1:3.
b Deut. 2:7; 29:5; Psa. 136:16; Amos 2:10.
c Psa. 104:29; Mt. 4:4; Lk. 4:4.
d Deut. 29:5; Neh. 9:21.
e 2 Sam. 7:14-15; Psa. 89:30-33; Prov. 3:11-12; Heb. 12:5-11; Rev. 3:19.
f Psa. 19:9, *note.*
g Deut. 28:47; 32:15; Prov. 30:9; Hos. 13:6.
h Ezk. 28:17; 1 Cor. 4:7.
i Psa. 106:21.
j Jer. 24:5, 6; Heb. 12:11.
k Dan. 9:11-14.
l Num. 13:22, 28, 32, 33.
m Deut. 31:3; Josh. 3:11; John 10:4.

shall destroy them, and he shall bring them down before thy face: so shalt thou drive them out, and destroy them quickly, as the LORD hath said unto thee.

4 [a]Speak not thou in thine heart, after that the LORD thy God hath cast them out from before thee, saying, For my righteousness the LORD hath brought me in to possess this land: but for the wickedness of these nations the LORD doth drive them out from before thee.

5 Not for thy righteousness, or for the uprightness of thine heart, dost thou go to possess their land: but for the wickedness of these nations the LORD thy God doth drive them out from before thee, and that he may perform the word which the LORD sware unto thy fathers, Abraham, Isaac, and Jacob.

6 Understand therefore, that the LORD thy God giveth thee not this good land to possess it for thy righteousness; for thou *art* a stiffnecked people.

7 Remember, *and* forget not, how thou provokedst the LORD thy God to wrath in the wilderness: from the day that thou didst depart out of the land of Egypt, until ye came unto this place, ye have been rebellious against the LORD.

8 Also in [b]Horeb ye provoked the LORD to wrath, so that the LORD was angry with you to have destroyed you.

9 When I was gone up into the mount to receive the tables of stone, *even* the tables of the covenant which the LORD made with you, then I abode in the mount forty days and forty nights, I neither did eat bread nor drink water:

10 [c]And the LORD delivered unto me two tables of stone written with the finger of God; and on them *was written* according to all the words, which the LORD spake with you in the mount out of the midst of the fire in the day of the assembly.

11 And it came to pass at the end of forty days and forty nights, *that* the LORD gave me the two tables of stone, *even* the tables of the covenant.

12 And the LORD said unto me, Arise, get thee down quickly from hence; for thy people which thou hast brought forth out of Egypt have corrupted *themselves*; they are quickly turned aside out of the way which I commanded them; they have made them a molten image.

B.C. 1451.

a Deut. 8:17; Rom. 11:6, 20; 1 Cor. 4:4, 7.

b Ex. 32:4; Psa. 106:19.

c Ex. 20:4, *note.*

d Num. 14:12.

e Ex. 34:28; Psa. 106:23.

13 Furthermore the LORD spake unto me, saying, I have seen this people, and, behold, it *is* a stiffnecked people:

14 Let me alone, that I may destroy them, and blot out their name from under heaven: [d]and I will make of thee a nation mightier and greater than they.

15 So I turned and came down from the mount, and the mount burned with fire: and the two tables of the covenant *were* in my two hands.

16 And I looked, and, behold, ye had sinned against the LORD your God, *and* had made you a molten calf: ye had turned aside quickly out of the way which the LORD had commanded you.

17 And I took the two tables, and cast them out of my two hands, and brake them before your eyes.

18 And I [e]fell down before the LORD, as at the first, forty days and forty nights: I did neither eat bread, nor drink water, because of all your sins which ye sinned, in doing wickedly in the sight of the LORD, to provoke him to anger.

19 For I was afraid of the anger and hot displeasure, wherewith the LORD was wroth against you to destroy you. But the LORD hearkened unto me at that time also.

20 And the LORD was very angry with Aaron to have destroyed him: and I prayed for Aaron also the same time.

21 And I took your sin, the calf which ye had made, and burnt it with fire, and stamped it, *and* ground *it* very small, *even* until it was as small as dust: and I cast the dust thereof into the brook that descended out of the mount.

22 And at Taberah, and at Massah, and at Kibroth-hattaavah, ye provoked the LORD to wrath.

23 Likewise when the LORD sent you from Kadesh-barnea, saying, Go up and possess the land which I have given you; then ye rebelled against the commandment of the LORD your God, and ye believed him not, nor hearkened to his voice.

24 Ye have been rebellious against the LORD from the day that I knew you.

25 Thus I fell down before the LORD forty days and forty nights, as I fell down *at the first*; because the LORD had said he would destroy you.

26 I [a]prayed therefore unto the LORD, and said, O Lord GOD, destroy not thy people and thine inheritance, which thou hast [b]redeemed through thy greatness, which thou hast brought forth out of Egypt with a mighty hand.

27 Remember thy servants, Abraham, Isaac, and Jacob; look not unto the stubbornness of this people, nor to their wickedness, nor to their sin:

28 Lest the land whence thou broughtest us out say, Because the LORD was not able to bring them into the land which he promised them, and because he hated them, he hath brought them out to slay them in the wilderness.

29 Yet they *are* thy people and thine inheritance, which thou broughtest out by thy mighty power and by thy stretched out arm.

CHAPTER 10.

Warnings and exhortations.

At that time the LORD [c]said unto me, Hew thee two tables of stone like unto the first, and come up unto me into the mount, and make thee an ark of wood.

2 And I will write on the tables the words that were in the first tables which thou brakest, and thou shalt put them in the ark.

3 And I made an ark *of* [d]shittim wood, and hewed two tables of stone like unto the first, and went up into the mount, having the two tables in mine hand.

4 And he wrote on the tables, according to the first writing, the ten commandments, which the LORD spake unto you in the mount out of the midst of the fire in the day of the assembly: and the LORD gave them unto me.

5 And I turned myself and came down from the mount, and put the tables in the ark which I had made; and there they be, as the LORD commanded me.

6 And the children of Israel took their journey from Beeroth of the children of Jaakan to Mosera: there Aaron died, and there he was buried; and Eleazar his son ministered in the priest's office in his stead.

7 From thence they journeyed unto Gudgodah; and from Gudgodah to Jotbath, a land of rivers of waters.

8 At that time the LORD separated the tribe of Levi, to bear the ark of the covenant of the LORD, to stand before the LORD to minister unto him, and to bless in his name, unto this day.

9 Wherefore Levi hath no part nor inheritance with his brethren; the LORD *is* his inheritance, according as the LORD thy God promised him.

10 And I stayed in the mount, according to the first time, forty days and forty nights; and the LORD hearkened unto me at that time also, *and* the LORD would not destroy thee.

11 And the LORD said unto me, Arise, take *thy* journey before the people, that they may go in and possess the land, which I sware unto their fathers to give unto them.

12 And now, Israel, [e]what doth the LORD thy God require of thee, but to [f]fear the LORD thy God, to walk in all his ways, and to love him, and to serve the LORD thy God with all thy heart and with all thy soul,

13 To keep the commandments of the LORD, and his statutes, which I command thee this day for thy good?

14 Behold, the heaven and the heaven of heavens *is* the LORD'S thy God, the earth *also*, with all that therein *is*.

15 Only the LORD had a delight in thy fathers to love them, and he chose their seed after them, *even* you above all people, as *it is* this day.

16 Circumcise therefore the foreskin of your heart, and be no more stiffnecked.

17 For the LORD your God *is* [g]God of gods, and Lord of lords, a great God, a mighty, and a terrible, which regardeth not persons, nor taketh reward:

18 He doth execute the judgment of the fatherless and widow, and loveth the stranger, in giving him food and raiment.

19 Love ye therefore the stranger: for ye were strangers in the land of Egypt.

20 Thou shalt [h]fear the LORD thy God; him shalt thou serve, and to him shalt thou cleave, and swear by his name.

21 He *is* thy praise, and he *is* thy God, that hath done for thee these great and terrible things, which thine eyes have seen.

22 Thy fathers went down into [i]Egypt with threescore and ten persons; and

B.C. 1451.

a *Bible prayers* (O.T.). Deut. 21:6-8. (Gen. 15:2; Hab. 3:1-16.)

b Ex. 14:30, *note.*

c *Inspiration.* vs. 1-4; Deut. 29:29. (Ex. 4:15; Rev. 22:19.)

d i.e. *acacia.*

e Mic. 6:8.

f Psa. 19:9, *note.*

g Josh. 22:22; Psa. 136:2; Isa. 44:8; Dan. 2:47; 11:36.

h Psa. 19:9, *note.*

i Gen. 46:27; Ex. 1:5; Acts 7:14.

now the LORD thy God hath made thee as the stars of heaven for multitude.

CHAPTER 11.

Warnings and exhorations.

Therefore thou shalt love the LORD thy God, and keep his charge, and his statutes, and his judgments, and his commandments, alway.

2 And know ye this day: for *I speak* not with your children which have not known, and which have not seen the chastisement of the LORD your God, his greatness, his mighty hand, and his stretched out arm,

3 [a]And his miracles, and his acts, which he did in the midst of Egypt unto Pharaoh the king of Egypt, and unto all his land;

4 And what he did unto the army of Egypt, unto their horses, and to their chariots; how he made the water of the Red sea to overflow them as they pursued after you, and *how* the LORD hath destroyed them unto this day;

5 And what he did unto you in the wilderness, until ye came into this place;

6 And [b]what he did unto Dathan and Abiram, the sons of Eliab, the son of Reuben: how the earth opened her mouth, and swallowed them up, and their households, and their tents, and all the substance that *was* in their possession, in the midst of all Israel:

7 But your eyes have seen all the great acts of the LORD which he did.

8 Therefore shall ye keep all the commandments which I command you this day, that ye may be strong, and go in and possess the land, whither ye go to possess it;

9 And that ye may prolong *your* days in the land, which the LORD sware unto your fathers to give unto them and to their seed, a land that floweth with milk and honey.

10 For the land, whither thou goest in to possess it, *is* not as the land of Egypt, from whence ye came out, where thou sowedst thy seed, and wateredst *it* with thy foot, as a garden of herbs:

11 But the land, whither ye go to possess it, *is* a land of hills and valleys, *and* drinketh water of the rain of heaven:

12 A land which the LORD thy God careth for: the eyes of the LORD thy God *are* always upon it, from the beginning of the year even unto the end of the year.

13 And it shall come to pass, if ye shall hearken diligently unto my commandments which I command you this day, to love the LORD your God, and to serve him with all your heart and with all your soul,

14 That I will give *you* the rain of your land in his due season, the first rain and the latter rain, that thou mayest gather in thy corn, and thy wine, and thine oil.

15 And I will send grass in thy fields for thy cattle, that thou mayest eat and be full.

16 Take heed to yourselves, that your heart be not deceived, and ye turn aside, and serve other gods, and worship them;

17 And *then* the LORD'S wrath be kindled against you, and he shut up the heaven, that there be no rain, and that the land yield not her fruit; and *lest* ye perish quickly from off the good land which the LORD giveth you.

18 Therefore shall ye lay up these my words in your heart and in your [c]soul, and bind them for a sign upon your hand, that they may be as frontlets between your eyes.

19 And ye shall teach them your children, speaking of them when thou sittest in thine house, and when thou walkest by the way, when thou liest down, and when thou risest up.

20 And thou shalt write them upon the door posts of thine house, and upon thy gates:

21 That your days may be multiplied, and the days of your children, in the land which the LORD sware unto your fathers to give them, [d]as the days of heaven upon the earth.

22 For if ye shall diligently keep all these commandments which I command you, to do them, to love the LORD your God, to walk in all his ways, and to cleave unto him;

23 Then will the LORD drive out all these nations from before you, and ye shall possess greater nations and mightier than yourselves.

24 [e]Every place whereon the soles of your feet shall tread shall be yours: from the wilderness and Lebanon, from the river, the river Euphrates, even unto the uttermost sea shall your coast be.

25 There shall no man be able to stand before you: *for* the LORD your God shall lay the fear of you and the dread of you

B.C. 1451.

a Psa. 78:12; 135:9.

b Num. 16:1, 31; 27:3; Psa. 106:17.

c Psa. 119:2, 34.

d Psa. 72:5; 89:29.

e Josh. 1:3; 14:9.

upon all the land that ye shall tread
upon, as he hath said unto you.
26 [a]Behold, I set before you this day a
blessing and a curse;
27 A blessing, if ye obey the commandments of the LORD your God,
which I command you this day:
28 And a curse, if ye will not obey the
commandments of the LORD your God,
but turn aside out of the way which I
command you this day, to go after other
gods, which ye have not known.
29 And it shall come to pass, when the
LORD thy God hath brought thee in unto
the land whither thou goest to possess it,
that thou shalt put [b]the blessing upon
mount Gerizim, and the curse upon
mount Ebal.
30 *Are* they not on the other side Jordan,
by the way where the sun goeth down, in
the land of the Canaanites, which dwell in
the champaign over against Gilgal, beside
the plains of Moreh?
31 For ye shall pass over Jordan to go
in to possess the land which the LORD
your God giveth you, and ye shall possess it, and dwell therein.
32 And ye shall observe to do all the
statutes and judgments which I set
before you this day.

CHAPTER 12.

Conditions of blessing in the land.

These *are* the statutes and judgments,
which ye shall observe to do in the
land, which the LORD God of thy fathers
giveth thee to possess it, all the days that
ye live upon the earth.
2 Ye shall utterly destroy all the places,
wherein the nations which ye shall possess served their gods, upon the high
mountains, and upon the hills, and
under every green tree:
3 And ye shall overthrow their altars,
and break their pillars, and burn their
[c]groves with fire; and ye shall hew
down the graven images of their gods,
and destroy the names of them out of
that place.
4 Ye shall not do so unto the LORD
your God.
5 But unto the place which the LORD
your God shall choose out of all your
tribes to put his name there, *even* unto
his habitation shall ye seek, and thither
thou shalt come:

B.C. 1451.

a Deut. 30:1, 15, 19.

b Deut. 27:12, 13; Josh. 8:33.

c See Deut. 16:21.

d Lev. 17:3, 4.

e Jud. 17:6; 21:25.

f v. 7.

g Gen. 9:4; Lev. 7:26; 17:10; Deut. 15:23; vs. 23, 24.

6 And [d]thither ye shall bring your
burnt-offerings, and your sacrifices, and
your tithes, and heave-offerings of your
hand, and your vows, and your freewill
offerings, and the firstlings of your herds
and of your flocks:
7 And there ye shall eat before the
LORD your God, and ye shall rejoice in
all that ye put your hand unto, ye and
your households, wherein the LORD thy
God hath blessed thee.
8 Ye shall not do after all *the things* that
we do here this day, [e]every man whatsoever *is* right in his own eyes.
9 For ye are not as yet come to the rest
and to the inheritance, which the LORD
your God giveth you.
10 But *when* ye go over Jordan, and
dwell in the land which the LORD your
God giveth you to inherit, and *when* he
giveth you rest from all your enemies
round about, so that ye dwell in safety;
11 Then there shall be a place which
the LORD your God shall choose to cause
his name to dwell there; thither shall ye
bring all that I command you; your
burnt-offerings, and your sacrifices,
your tithes, and the heave-offering of
your hand, and all your choice vows
which ye vow unto the LORD:
12 And [f]ye shall rejoice before the
LORD your God, ye, and your sons, and
your daughters, and your menservants,
and your maidservants, and the Levite
that *is* within your gates; forasmuch as
he hath no part nor inheritance with you.
13 Take heed to thyself that thou offer
not thy burnt-offerings in every place
that thou seest:
14 But in the place which the LORD shall
choose in one of thy tribes, there thou
shalt offer thy burnt-offerings, and there
thou shalt do all that I command thee.
15 Notwithstanding thou mayest kill
and eat flesh in all thy gates, whatsoever
thy soul lusteth after, according to the
blessing of the LORD thy God which he
hath given thee: the unclean and the
clean may eat thereof, as of the roebuck,
and as of the hart.
16 [g]Only ye shall not eat the blood; ye
shall pour it upon the earth as water.
17 Thou mayest not eat within thy
gates the tithe of thy corn, or of thy wine,
or of thy oil, or the firstlings of thy herds
or of thy flock, nor any of thy

vows which thou vowest, nor thy
freewill offerings, or heave-offering of
thine hand:
18 But thou must eat them before the
LORD thy God in the place which the
LORD thy God shall choose, thou, and thy
son, and thy daughter, and thy manservant, and thy maidservant, and the
Levite that *is* within thy gates: and thou
shalt rejoice before the LORD thy God in
all that thou puttest thine hands unto.
19 Take heed to thyself that thou forsake not the Levite as long as thou livest
upon the earth.
20 When the LORD thy God shall
enlarge thy border, as he hath promised
thee, and thou shalt say, I will eat flesh,
because thy soul longeth to eat flesh;
thou mayest eat flesh, whatsoever thy
soul lusteth after.
21 If the place which the LORD thy God
hath chosen to put his name there be too
far from thee, then thou shalt kill of thy
herd and of thy flock, which the LORD
hath given thee, as I have commanded
thee, and thou shalt eat in thy gates
whatsoever thy soul lusteth after.
22 Even as the roebuck and the hart is
eaten, so thou shalt eat them: the unclean
and the clean shall eat *of* them alike.
23 Only be sure that thou eat not the
[a]blood: for the blood *is* the life; and thou
mayest not eat the life with the flesh.
24 Thou shalt not eat it; thou shalt
pour it upon the earth as water.
25 Thou shalt not eat it; that it may go
well with thee, and with thy children
after thee, when thou shalt do *that which*
is right in the sight of the LORD.
26 Only thy holy things which thou
hast, and thy vows, thou shalt take, and
go unto the place which the LORD shall
choose:
27 And [b]thou shalt offer thy burnt-
offerings, the flesh and the blood, upon
the altar of the LORD thy God: and the
blood of thy sacrifices shall be poured
out upon the altar of the LORD thy God,
and thou shalt eat the flesh.
28 Observe and hear all these words
which I command thee, that it may go
well with thee, and with thy children
after thee for ever, when thou doest *that*
which is good and right in the sight of
the LORD thy God.
29 When the [c]LORD thy God shall cut
off the nations from before thee, whither
thou goest to possess them, and thou
succeedest them, and dwellest in their
land;
30 Take heed to thyself that thou be
not snared by following them, after that
they be destroyed from before thee; and
that thou enquire not after their gods,
saying, How did these nations serve
their gods? even so will I do likewise.
31 Thou shalt not do so unto the LORD
thy God: for every abomination to the
LORD, which he hateth, have they done
unto their gods; for even their sons and
their daughters they have burnt in the
fire to their gods.
32 What thing soever I command you,
observe to do it: [d]thou shalt not add
thereto, nor diminish from it.

CHAPTER 13.

The test of false prophets.

If there arise among you a prophet, or a
[e]dreamer of dreams, [f]and giveth thee
a sign or a wonder,
2 And the sign or the wonder come to
pass, whereof he spake unto thee, saying,
Let us go after other gods, which thou
hast not known, and let us serve them;
3 Thou shalt not hearken unto the
words of that prophet, or that dreamer
of dreams: for the LORD your God
proveth you, to know whether ye love
the LORD your God with all your heart
and with all your soul.
4 Ye shall walk after the LORD your
God, and [g]fear him, and keep his commandments, and obey his voice, and ye
shall serve him, and cleave unto him.
5 And that prophet, or that dreamer of
dreams, shall be put to death; because he
hath spoken to turn *you* away from the
LORD your God, which brought you out
of the land of Egypt, and [h]redeemed you
out of the house of bondage, to thrust
thee out of the way which the LORD thy
God commanded thee to walk in. So
shalt thou put the evil away from the
midst of thee.
6 If thy brother, the son of thy mother,
or thy son, or thy daughter, or the wife
of thy bosom, or thy friend, which *is* as
thine own soul, entice thee secretly, saying, Let us go and serve other gods,

B.C. 1451.

a Gen. 9:4; Lev. 17:11, 14.

b Lev. 1:5, 9, 13, 17; 17:11.

c Ex. 23:23; Deut. 19:1; Josh. 23:4.

d Deut. 4:2; 13:18; Josh. 1:7; Prov. 30:6; Rev. 22:18-19.

e Jer. 23:28; Zech. 10:2.

f Mt. 24:24; 2 Thes. 2:9; cf. Heb. 2:4.

g Psa. 19:9, *note.*

h Ex. 14:30, *note.*

which thou hast not known, thou, nor
thy fathers;
7 *Namely*, of the gods of the people
which *are* round about you, nigh unto
thee, or far off from thee, from the *one*
end of the earth even unto the *other* end
of the earth;
8 Thou shalt not consent unto him, nor
hearken unto him; neither shall thine
eye pity him, neither shalt thou spare,
neither shalt thou conceal him:
9 But thou shalt surely kill him; thine
hand shall be first upon him to put him
to death, and afterwards the hand of all
the people.
10 And thou shalt stone him with
stones, that he die; because he hath
sought to thrust thee away from the LORD
thy God, which brought thee out of the
land of Egypt, from the house of bondage.
11 And all Israel shall hear, and fear,
and shall do no more any such wickedness as this is among you.
12 If thou shalt hear *say* in one of thy
cities, which the LORD thy God hath
given thee to dwell there, saying,
13 *Certain* men, the children of Belial,
are gone out from among you, and have
withdrawn the inhabitants of their city,
saying, Let us go and serve other gods,
which ye have not known;
14 Then shalt thou enquire, and make
search, and ask diligently; and, behold, *if*
it be truth, *and* the thing certain, *that* such
abomination is wrought among you;
15 Thou shalt surely smite the inhabitants of that city with the edge of the
sword, destroying it utterly, and all that
is therein, and the cattle thereof, with the
edge of the sword.
16 And thou shalt gather all the spoil
of it into the midst of the street thereof,
and shalt [a]burn with fire the city, and all
the spoil thereof every whit, for the LORD
thy God: and it shall be an heap for ever;
it shall not be built again.
17 And there shall cleave nought of
the cursed thing to thine hand: that the
LORD may turn from the fierceness of his
anger, and shew thee mercy, and have
compassion upon thee, and multiply
thee, as he hath sworn unto thy fathers;
18 When thou shalt hearken to the
voice of the LORD thy God, to keep all
his commandments which I command
thee this day, to do *that which is* right in
the eyes of the LORD thy God.

B.C. 1451.

a Josh. 6:24.
b Gal. 3:26.
c 1 Pet. 2:9.
d Ezk. 4:14; Acts 10:13, 14.
e See Lev. 11:6, *note*.
f Lev. 11:13.

CHAPTER 14.

Ye *are* the [b]children of the LORD your
God: ye shall not cut yourselves,
nor make any baldness between your
eyes for the dead.
2 [c]For thou *art* an holy people unto the
LORD thy God, and the LORD hath chosen
thee to be a peculiar people unto himself, above all the nations that *are* upon
the earth.

The dietary laws.

3 [d]Thou shalt not eat any abominable
thing.
4 These *are* the beasts which ye shall
eat: the ox, the sheep, and the goat,
5 The hart, and the roebuck, and the fallow deer, and the wild goat, and the
pygarg, and the wild ox, and the chamois.
6 And every beast that parteth the
hoof, and cleaveth the cleft into two
claws, *and* cheweth the cud among the
beasts, that ye shall eat.
7 Nevertheless these ye shall not eat of
them that chew the cud, or of them that
divide the cloven hoof; *as* the camel, and
the [e]hare, and the coney: for they chew
the cud, but divide not the hoof; *therefore*
they *are* unclean unto you.
8 And the swine, because it divideth
the hoof, yet cheweth not the cud, it *is*
unclean unto you: ye shall not eat of
their flesh, nor touch their dead carcase.
9 These ye shall eat of all that *are* in
the waters: all that have fins and scales
shall ye eat:
10 And whatsoever hath not fins and
scales ye may not eat; it *is* unclean unto
you.
11 *Of* all clean birds ye shall eat.
12 [f]But these *are they* of which ye shall
not eat: the eagle, and the ossifrage, and
the ospray,
13 And the glede, and the kite, and the
vulture after his kind,
14 And every raven after his kind,
15 And the owl, and the night hawk,
and the cuckow, and the hawk after his
kind,
16 The little owl, and the great owl,
and the swan,
17 And the pelican, and the gier eagle,
and the cormorant,
18 And the stork, and the heron after
her kind, and the lapwing, and the bat.

19 And every creeping thing that flieth *is* unclean unto you: they shall not be eaten.
20 *But of* all clean fowls ye may eat.
21 [a]Ye shall not eat *of* any thing that dieth of itself: thou shalt give it unto the stranger that *is* in thy gates, that he may eat it; or thou mayest sell it unto an alien: for thou *art* an holy people unto the LORD thy God. Thou shalt not seethe a kid in his mother's milk.
22 [b]Thou shalt truly tithe all the increase of thy seed, that the field bringeth forth year by year.
23 And thou shalt eat before the LORD thy God, in the place which he shall choose to place his name there, the tithe of thy corn, of thy wine, and of thine oil, and the firstlings of thy herds and of thy flocks; that thou mayest learn to [c]fear the LORD thy God always.
24 And if the way be too long for thee, so that thou art not able to carry it; *or* if the place be too far from thee, which the LORD thy God shall choose to set his name there, when the LORD thy God hath blessed thee:
25 Then shalt thou turn *it* into money, and bind up the money in thine hand, and shalt go unto the place which the LORD thy God shall choose:
26 And thou shalt bestow that money for whatsoever thy soul lusteth after, for oxen, or for sheep, or for wine, or for strong drink, or for whatsoever thy soul desireth: and thou shalt eat there before the LORD thy God, and thou shalt rejoice, thou, and thine household,
27 And the Levite that *is* within thy gates; thou shalt not forsake him; for he hath no part nor inheritance with thee.
28 [d]At the end of three years thou shalt bring forth all the tithe of thine increase the same year, and shalt lay *it* up within thy gates:
29 And the Levite, (because he hath no part nor inheritance with thee,) and the stranger, and the fatherless, and the widow, which *are* within thy gates, shall come, and shall eat and be satisfied; that [e]the LORD thy God may bless thee in all the work of thine hand which thou doest.

CHAPTER 15.

The sabbatic year.

At the end of [f]*every* seven years thou shalt make a release.
2 And this *is* the manner of the release: Every creditor that lendeth *ought* unto his neighbour shall release *it*; he shall not exact *it* of his neighbour, or of his brother; because it is called the LORD'S release.
3 Of a foreigner thou mayest exact *it again*: but *that* which is thine with thy brother thine hand shall release;
4 Save when there shall be no poor among you; for the LORD shall greatly bless thee in the land which the LORD thy God giveth thee *for* an inheritance to possess it:
5 Only if thou carefully hearken unto the voice of the LORD thy God, to observe to do all these commandments which I command thee this day.
6 For the LORD thy God blesseth thee, as he promised thee: and thou shalt lend unto many nations, but thou shalt not borrow; and thou shalt reign over many nations, but they shall not reign over thee.
7 If there be among you a poor man of one of thy brethren within any of thy gates in thy land which the LORD thy God giveth thee, thou shalt not harden thine heart, nor shut thine hand from thy poor brother:
8 But [g]thou shalt open thine hand wide unto him, and shalt surely lend him sufficient for his need, *in that* which he wanteth.
9 Beware that there be not a thought in thy wicked heart, saying, The seventh year, the year of release, is at hand; and thine eye be evil against thy poor brother, and thou givest him nought; and he cry unto the LORD against thee, and it be sin unto thee.
10 Thou shalt surely give him, and thine heart shall not be grieved when thou givest unto him: because that for this thing the LORD thy God shall bless thee in all thy works, and in all that thou puttest thine hand unto.
11 For the [h]poor shall never cease out of the land: therefore I command thee, saying, Thou shalt open thine hand wide unto thy brother, to thy poor, and to thy needy, in thy land.
12 *And* [i]if thy brother, an Hebrew man, or an Hebrew woman, be sold unto thee, and serve thee six years; then in the seventh year thou shalt let him go free from thee.
13 And when thou sendest him out

B.C. 1451.

a Lev. 17:15; 22:8; Ezk. 4:14.
b Lev. 27:30; Deut. 12:6, 17; Neh. 10:37.
c Psa. 19:9, *note.*
d Deut. 26:12; Amos 4:4.
e See Mal. 3:10.
f Ex. 21:2; 23:10, 11; Jer. 34:14.
g 1 John 3:17.
h Mt. 26:11; Mk. 14:7; John 12:8.
i Ex. 21:2; Lev. 25:39; Jer. 34:14.

free from thee, thou shalt not let him go
away empty:
14 Thou shalt furnish him liberally out
of thy flock, and out of thy floor, and out
of thy winepress: *of that* wherewith the
LORD thy God hath blessed thee thou
shalt give unto him.
15 And thou shalt remember that thou
wast a bondman in the land of Egypt, and
the LORD thy God [a]redeemed thee: therefore I command thee this thing to day.

The perpetual servant.

16 And it shall be, if he say unto thee, I
will not go away from thee; because he
loveth thee and thine house, because he
is well with thee;
17 Then thou shalt take an aul, and
thrust *it* through his ear unto the door,
and he shall be thy servant for ever. And
also unto thy maidservant thou shalt do
likewise.
18 It shall not seem hard unto thee,
when thou sendest him away free from
thee; for he hath been worth a double
hired servant *to thee,* in serving thee six
years: and the LORD thy God shall bless
thee in all that thou doest.
19 All the firstling males that come of
thy herd and of thy flock thou shalt sanctify unto the LORD thy God: thou shalt do
no work with the firstling of thy bullock,
nor shear the firstling of thy sheep.
20 Thou shalt eat *it* before the LORD
thy God year by year in the place which
the LORD shall choose, thou and thy
household.
21 And if there be *any* blemish therein,
as if it be lame, or blind, *or have* any ill
blemish, thou shalt not sacrifice it unto
the LORD thy God.
22 Thou shalt eat it within thy gates:
the unclean and the clean *person shall eat
it* alike, as the roebuck, and as the hart.
23 Only thou shalt not eat the blood
thereof; thou shalt pour it upon the
ground as water.

CHAPTER 16.

The Passover.

Observe the month of [b]Abib, and
[1]keep the passover unto the LORD
thy God: for in the month of Abib the
LORD thy God brought thee forth out of
Egypt by night.
2 Thou shalt therefore sacrifice the
passover unto the LORD thy God, of the
flock and the herd, in the place which the
LORD shall choose to place his name there.
3 Thou shalt eat no [c]leavened bread
with it; seven days shalt thou eat unleavened bread therewith, *even* the bread of
affliction; for thou camest forth out of
the land of Egypt in haste: that thou
mayest remember the day when thou
camest forth out of the land of Egypt all
the days of thy life.
4 And there shall be no leavened
bread seen with thee in all thy coast
seven days; neither shall there *any thing*
of the flesh, which thou sacrificedst the
first day at even, remain all night until
the morning.
5 Thou mayest not sacrifice the
passover within any of thy gates, which
the LORD thy God giveth thee:
6 But at the place which the LORD thy
God shall choose to place his name in,
there thou shalt sacrifice the passover at
even, at the going down of the sun, at
the season that thou camest forth out of
Egypt.
7 And thou shalt roast and eat *it* in the
place which the LORD thy God shall
choose: and thou shalt turn in the morning, and go unto thy tents.
8 Six days thou shalt eat unleavened
bread: and on the seventh day *shall be* a
solemn assembly to the LORD thy God:
thou shalt do no work *therein.*

The feast of Weeks.

9 Seven weeks shalt thou number unto
thee: begin to number the seven weeks
from *such time as* thou beginnest *to put*
the sickle to the corn.
10 And thou shalt keep the feast of
weeks unto the LORD thy God with a
tribute of a freewill offering of thine
hand, which thou shalt give *unto the
LORD thy God,* [d]according as the LORD thy
God hath blessed thee:

B.C. 1451.

a Ex. 14:30, *note.*

b i.e. *April.*

c *Leaven.* vs. 3, 4, 8, 16; Amos 4:5. (Gen. 19:3; Mt. 13:33.)

d v. 17; 1 Cor. 16:2; 2 Cor. 8:12.

[1] **(16:1)** Cf. the order of the feasts in Lev. 23. Here the Passover and Tabernacles are given especial emphasis as marking the beginning and the consummation of God's ways with Israel; the former speaking of redemption, the foundation of all: the latter, of re-gathered Israel blessed in the kingdom. Between, in Deut. 16:9-12, comes the Feast of Weeks—the joy of a redeemed people, anticipating greater blessing yet to come. It is, morally, Rom. 5:1, 2.

B.C. 1451.

11 And thou shalt rejoice before the LORD thy God, thou, and thy son, and thy daughter, and thy manservant, and thy maidservant, and the Levite that *is* within thy gates, and the stranger, and the fatherless, and the widow, that *are* among you, in the place which the LORD thy God hath chosen to place his name there.

12 And thou shalt remember that thou wast a bondman in Egypt: and thou shalt observe and do these statutes.

The feast of Tabernacles.

13 [a]Thou shalt observe the feast of tabernacles seven days, after that thou hast gathered in thy corn and thy wine:

14 And thou shalt rejoice in thy feast, thou, and thy son, and thy daughter, and thy manservant, and thy maidservant, and the Levite, the stranger, and the fatherless, and the widow, that *are* within thy gates.

15 [b]Seven days shalt thou keep a solemn feast unto the LORD thy God in the place which the LORD shall choose: because the LORD thy God shall bless thee in all thine increase, and in all the works of thine hands, therefore thou shalt surely rejoice.

The gifts of the males.

16 Three times in a year shall all thy males appear before the LORD thy God in the place which he shall choose; in the feast of unleavened bread, and in the feast of weeks, and in the feast of tabernacles: and they shall not appear before the LORD empty:

17 Every man *shall give* as he is able, according to the blessing of the LORD thy God which he hath given thee.

Judges in the gates.

18 Judges and officers shalt thou make thee in all thy gates, which the LORD thy God giveth thee, throughout thy tribes: and they shall judge the people with just judgment.

19 Thou shalt not wrest judgment; thou shalt not respect persons, neither take a gift: for a gift doth blind the eyes of the wise, and pervert the words of the righteous.

20 That which is altogether just shalt thou follow, that thou mayest live, and inherit the land which the LORD thy God giveth thee.

21 Thou shalt not plant thee a [c]grove of any trees near unto the altar of the LORD thy God, which thou shalt make thee.

22 Neither shalt thou set thee up *any* image; which the LORD thy God hateth.

CHAPTER 17.

Offerings must be unblemished.

Thou shalt not sacrifice unto the LORD thy God *any* bullock, or sheep, wherein is blemish, *or* any evilfavouredness: for that *is* an abomination unto the LORD thy God.

Idolaters to be stoned.

2 If there be found among you, within any of thy gates which the LORD thy God giveth thee, man or woman, that hath wrought wickedness in the sight of the LORD thy God, in transgressing his covenant,

3 And hath gone and served other gods, and worshipped them, either the sun, or moon, or any of the host of heaven, which I have not commanded;

4 And it be told thee, and thou hast heard *of it*, and enquired diligently, and, behold, *it be* true, *and* the thing certain, *that* such abomination is wrought in Israel:

5 Then shalt thou bring forth that man or that woman, which have committed that wicked thing, unto thy gates, *even* that man or that woman, and shalt [d]stone them with stones, till they die.

6 At the mouth of two witnesses, or three witnesses, shall he that is worthy of death be put to death; *but* at the mouth of one witness he shall not be put to death.

7 The hands of the witnesses shall be first upon him to put him to death, and afterward the hands of all the people. So thou shalt put the evil away from among you.

Obedience to authority.

8 If there arise a matter too hard for thee in judgment, between blood and blood, between plea and plea, and between stroke and stroke, *being* matters of controversy within thy gates: then shalt thou arise, and get thee up into the place which the LORD thy God shall choose;

9 And [e]thou shalt come unto the priests the Levites, and unto the judge that shall be in those days, and enquire; and they shall shew thee the sentence of judgment:

a Ex. 23:16; Lev. 23:34; Num. 29:12.

b Lev. 23:39-41.

c The groves (Heb. *Asherim*) so often mentioned in the O.T. were devoted to the worship of Ashtereth, the Babylonian goddess Ishtar, the Aphrodite of the Greeks, the Roman Venus. Cf. Jud. 2:13, *note.*

d Lev. 24:14, 16; Josh. 7:25.

e See Jer. 18:18.

10 And thou shalt do according to the sentence, which they of that place which the LORD shall choose shall shew thee; and thou shalt observe to do according to all that they inform thee:

11 According to the sentence of the law which they shall teach thee, and according to the judgment which they shall tell thee, thou shalt do: thou shalt not decline from the sentence which they shall shew thee, *to* the right hand, nor *to* the left.

12 And [a]the man that will do presumptuously, and will not hearken unto the priest that standeth to minister there before the LORD thy God, or unto the judge, even that man shall die: and thou shalt put away the evil from Israel.

13 And all the people shall hear, and fear, and do no more presumptuously.

Concerning a king.

14 When thou art come unto the land which the LORD thy God giveth thee, and shalt possess it, and shalt dwell therein, and shalt say, [b]I will set a king over me, like as all the nations that *are* about me;

15 Thou shalt in any wise set *him* king over thee, [c]whom the LORD thy God shall choose: *one* from among thy brethren shalt thou set king over thee: thou mayest not set a stranger over thee, which *is* not thy brother.

16 But he shall not multiply horses to himself, nor cause the people to return to Egypt, to the end that he should multiply horses: forasmuch as the LORD hath said unto you, Ye shall henceforth return no more that way.

17 Neither shall he multiply wives to himself, that [d]his heart turn not away: neither shall he greatly multiply to himself silver and gold.

18 [e]And it shall be, when he sitteth upon the throne of his kingdom, that he shall write him a copy of this law in a book out of *that which is* before the priests the Levites:

19 And it shall be with him, and he shall read therein all the days of his life: that he may learn to [f]fear the LORD his God, to keep all the words of this law and these statutes, to do them:

20 That his heart be not lifted up above his brethren, and that he turn not aside from the commandment, *to* the right hand, or *to* the left: to the end that he may prolong *his* days in his kingdom, he, and his children, in the midst of Israel.

B.C. 1451.

a Num. 15:30; Deut. 1:43; Ezra 10:8; Hos. 4:4.

b 1 Sam. 8:5, 19, 20.

c See 1 Sam. 9:15; 10:24; 16:12; 1 Chr. 22:10.

d See 1 Ki. 11:3, 4.

e 2 Ki. 11:12.

f Psa. 19:9, *note.*

CHAPTER 18.

The tribe of Levi.

The priests the Levites, *and* all the tribe of Levi, shall have no part nor inheritance with Israel: they shall eat the offerings of the LORD made by fire, and his inheritance.

2 Therefore shall they have no inheritance among their brethren: the LORD *is* their inheritance, as he hath said unto them.

The priest's due.

3 And this shall be the priest's due from the people, from them that offer a sacrifice, whether *it be* ox or sheep; and they shall give unto the priest the shoulder, and the two cheeks, and the maw.

4 The firstfruit *also* of thy corn, of thy wine, and of thine oil, and the first of the fleece of thy sheep, shalt thou give him.

5 For the LORD thy God hath chosen him out of all thy tribes, to stand to minister in the name of the LORD, him and his sons for ever.

6 And if a Levite come from any of thy gates out of all Israel, where he sojourned, and come with all the desire of his mind unto the place which the LORD shall choose;

7 Then he shall minister in the name of the LORD his God, as all his brethren the Levites *do*, which stand there before the LORD.

8 They shall have like portions to eat, beside that which cometh of the sale of his patrimony.

Idolatrous practices forbidden.

9 When thou art come into the land which the LORD thy God giveth thee, thou shalt not learn to do after the abominations of those nations.

10 There shall not be found among you *any one* that maketh his son or his daughter to pass through the fire, *or* that useth divination, *or* an observer of times, or an enchanter, or a witch,

11 Or a charmer, or a consulter with familiar spirits, or a wizard, or a necromancer.

12 For all that do these things *are* an abomination unto the LORD: and because

B.C. 1451.

of these abominations the LORD thy God doth drive them out from before thee.

13 Thou shalt be [a]perfect with the LORD thy God.

14 For these nations, which thou shalt possess, hearkened unto observers of times, and unto diviners: but as for thee, the LORD thy God hath not suffered thee so *to do.*

The great prophecy of Messiah the Prophet (Acts 3:22, 23).

15 The LORD thy God will raise up unto thee a [b]Prophet from the midst of thee, of thy brethren, like unto me; unto him ye shall hearken;

16 According to all that thou desiredst of the LORD thy God in Horeb in the day of the assembly, saying, Let me not hear again the voice of the LORD my God, neither let me see this great fire any more, that I die not.

17 And the LORD said unto me, They have well *spoken that* which they have spoken.

18 I will raise them up a Prophet from among their brethren, like unto thee, and will put my words in his mouth; and he shall speak unto them all that I shall command him.

19 [c]And it shall come to pass, *that* whosoever will not hearken unto my words which he shall speak in my name, I will require *it* of him.

The test of the prophets.

20 But [d]the prophet, which shall presume to speak a word in my name, which I have not commanded him to speak, or [e]that shall speak in the name of other gods, even that prophet shall die.

21 And if thou say in thine heart, How shall we know the word which the LORD hath not spoken?

22 When a [f]prophet speaketh in the name of the LORD, if the thing follow not, nor come to pass, that *is* the thing which the LORD hath not spoken, *but* the prophet hath spoken it presumptuously: thou shalt not be afraid of him.

CHAPTER 19.

Cities of refuge
(Num. 35:1–34; Deut. 4:41–49).

When the LORD thy God hath cut off the nations, whose land the LORD thy God giveth thee, and thou succeedest them, and dwellest in their cities, and in their houses;

2 [g]Thou shalt separate three cities for thee in the midst of thy land, which the LORD thy God giveth thee to possess it.

3 Thou shalt prepare thee a way, and divide the coasts of thy land, which the LORD thy God giveth thee to inherit, into three parts, that every slayer may flee thither.

4 And [h]this *is* the case of the slayer, which shall flee thither, that he may live: Whoso killeth his neighbour ignorantly, whom he hated not in time past;

5 As when a man goeth into the wood with his neighbour to hew wood, and his hand fetcheth a stroke with the axe to cut down the tree, and the head slippeth from the helve, and lighteth upon his neighbour, that he die; he shall flee unto one of those cities, and live:

6 Lest the [i]avenger of the blood pursue the slayer, while his heart is hot, and overtake him, because the way is long, and slay him; whereas he *was* not worthy of death, inasmuch as he hated him not in time past.

7 Wherefore I command thee, saying, Thou shalt separate three cities for thee.

8 And if the LORD thy God enlarge thy coast, as he hath sworn unto thy fathers, and give thee all the land which he promised to give unto thy fathers;

9 If thou shalt keep all these commandments to do them, which I command thee this day, to love the LORD thy God, and to walk ever in his ways; then shalt thou add three cities more for thee, beside these three:

10 That innocent blood be not shed in thy land, which the LORD thy God giveth thee *for* an inheritance, and *so* blood be upon thee.

11 But if any man hate his neighbour, and lie in wait for him, and rise up against him, and smite him mortally that he die, and fleeth into one of these cities:

12 Then the elders of his city shall send and fetch him thence, and deliver him into the hand of the avenger of blood, that he may die.

13 Thine eye shall not pity him, but thou shalt put away *the guilt of* innocent blood from Israel, that it may go well with thee.

a i.e. *upright* or *sincere.*

b vs. 15, 18, 19; John 1:21-45; 7:16; 8:28; 12:49, 50; 14:10, 24; 17:8; Acts 3:22, 23; 7:37.

c Acts 3:23; Heb. 12:25.

d Deut. 13:5; Jer. 14:14, 15; Zech. 13:3.

e Deut. 13:1, 2; Jer. 2:8.

f Jer. 28:9.

g Ex. 21:13; Num. 35:10, 14; Josh. 20:2.

h Num. 35:15; Deut. 4:42.

i Heb. *goel, Redemp. (Kinsman type).* Isa. 59:20, *note.*

The sacred landmark.

14 Thou shalt not remove thy neighbour's landmark, which they of old time have set in thine inheritance, which thou shalt inherit in the land that the LORD thy God giveth thee to possess it.

The terror of the law.

15 One witness shall not rise up against a man for any iniquity, or for any sin, in any sin that he sinneth: at the mouth of two witnesses, or at the mouth of three [a]witnesses, shall the matter be established.

16 If a false witness rise up against any man to testify against him *that which is* wrong;

17 Then both the men, between whom the controversy *is,* shall stand before the LORD, before the priests and the judges, which shall be in those days;

18 And the judges shall make diligent inquisition: and, behold, *if* the witness *be* a false witness, *and* hath testified falsely against his brother;

19 Then shall ye do unto him, as he had thought to have done unto his brother: so shalt thou put the evil away from among you.

20 And those which remain shall hear, and fear, and shall henceforth commit no more any such evil among you.

21 And thine eye shall not pity; *but* [b]life *shall go* for life, eye for eye, tooth for tooth, hand for hand, foot for foot.

CHAPTER 20.

The law of warfare.

When thou goest out to battle against thine enemies, and seest horses, and chariots, *and* a people more than thou, be not afraid of them: for the LORD thy God *is* with thee, which brought thee up out of the land of Egypt.

2 And it shall be, when ye are come nigh unto the battle, that the priest shall approach and speak unto the people,

3 And shall say unto them, Hear, O Israel, ye approach this day unto battle against your enemies: let not your hearts faint, fear not, and do not tremble, neither be ye terrified because of them;

4 For the LORD your God *is* he that goeth with you, [c]to fight for you against your enemies, to save you.

5 And the officers shall speak unto the people, saying, What man *is there* that hath built a new house, and hath not dedicated it? let him go and return to his house, lest he die in the battle, and another man dedicate it.

6 And what man *is he* that hath planted a vineyard, and hath not *yet* eaten of it? let him *also* go and return unto his house, lest he die in the battle, and another man eat of it.

7 And what man *is there* that hath betrothed a wife, and hath not taken her? let him go and return unto his house, lest he die in the battle, and another man take her.

8 And the officers shall speak further unto the people, and they shall say, [d]What man *is there that is* fearful and fainthearted? let him go and return unto his house, lest his brethren's heart faint as well as his heart.

9 And it shall be, when the officers have made an end of speaking unto the people, that they shall make captains of the armies to lead the people.

10 When thou comest nigh unto a city to fight against it, [e]then proclaim peace unto it.

11 And it shall be, if it make thee answer of peace, and open unto thee, then it shall be, *that* all the people *that is* found therein shall be tributaries unto thee, and they shall serve thee.

12 And if it will make no peace with thee, but will make war against thee, then thou shalt besiege it:

13 And when the LORD thy God hath delivered it into thine hands, [f]thou shalt smite every male thereof with the edge of the sword:

14 But the women, and the little ones, and [g]the cattle, and all that is in the city, *even* all the spoil thereof, shalt thou take unto thyself; and thou shalt eat the spoil of thine enemies, which the LORD thy God hath given thee.

15 Thus shalt thou do unto all the cities *which are* very far off from thee, which *are* not of the cities of these nations.

16 But of the cities of these people, which the LORD thy God doth give thee *for* an inheritance, thou shalt save alive nothing that breatheth:

17 But thou shalt utterly destroy them; *namely,* the Hittites, and the Amorites, the Canaanites, and the Perizzites, the

B.C. 1451.

a 2 Cor. 13:1.
b Ex. 21:23-25; Lev. 24:20; Mt. 5:38, 39.
c Deut. 1:30; 3:22; Josh. 23:10.
d Jud. 7:3.
e 2 Sam. 20:18, 20.
f Num. 31:7.
g Josh. 8:2.

Hivites, and the Jebusites; as the LORD thy God hath commanded thee:

18 That they teach you not to do after all their abominations, which they have done unto their gods; so should ye [a]sin against the LORD your God.

19 When thou shalt besiege a city a long time, in making war against it to take it, thou shalt not destroy the trees thereof by forcing an axe against them: for thou mayest eat of them, and thou shalt not cut them down (for the tree of the field *is* man's *life*) to employ *them* in the siege:

20 Only the trees which thou knowest that they *be* not trees for meat, thou shalt destroy and cut them down; and thou shalt build bulwarks against the city that maketh war with thee, until it be subdued.

CHAPTER 21.

Inquest for the slain.

If *one* be found slain in the land which the LORD thy God giveth thee to possess it, lying in the field, *and* it be not known who hath slain him:

2 Then thy elders and thy judges shall come forth, and they shall measure unto the cities which *are* round about him that is slain:

3 And it shall be, *that* the city *which is* next unto the slain man, even the elders of that city shall take an heifer, which hath not been wrought with, *and* which hath not drawn in the yoke;

4 And the elders of that city shall bring down the heifer unto a rough valley, which is neither eared nor sown, and shall strike off the heifer's neck there in the valley:

5 And the priests the sons of Levi shall come near; for them the LORD thy God hath chosen to minister unto him, and to bless in the name of the LORD; and by their word shall every controversy and every stroke be *tried*:

6 And all the elders of that city, *that are* next unto the slain *man*, shall wash their hands over the heifer that is beheaded in the valley:

7 And they shall answer and say, Our hands have not shed this blood, neither have our eyes seen *it*.

8 Be [b]merciful, O LORD, unto thy people [c]Israel, whom thou hast redeemed, and lay not innocent blood unto thy people of Israel's charge. And the blood shall be forgiven them.

9 So shalt thou put away the *guilt of* innocent blood from among you, when thou shalt do *that which is* right in the sight of the LORD.

Domestic regulations.

10 When thou goest forth to war against thine enemies, and the LORD thy God hath delivered them into thine hands, and thou hast taken them captive,

11 And seest among the captives a beautiful woman, and hast a desire unto her, that thou wouldest have her to thy wife;

12 Then thou shalt bring her home to thine house; and she shall shave her head, and pare her nails;

13 And she shall put the raiment of her captivity from off her, and shall remain in thine house, and bewail her father and her mother a full month: and after that thou shalt go in unto her, and be her husband, and she shall be thy wife.

14 And it shall be, if thou have no delight in her, then thou shalt let her go whither she will; but thou shalt not sell her at all for money, thou shalt not make merchandise of her, because thou hast humbled her.

15 If a man have two wives, one beloved, [d]and another hated, and they have born him children, *both* the beloved and the hated; and *if* the firstborn son be hers that was hated:

16 Then it shall be, when he maketh his sons to inherit *that* which he hath, *that* he may not make the son of the beloved firstborn before the son of the hated, *which is indeed* the firstborn:

17 But he shall acknowledge the son of the hated *for* the firstborn, [e]by giving him a double portion of all that he hath: for he *is* the beginning of his strength; [f]the right of the firstborn *is* his.

A prodigal son under law.
(Cf. Lk. 15:11–23.)

18 If a man have a stubborn and rebellious son, which will not obey the voice of his father, or the voice of his mother, and *that*, when they have chastened him, will not hearken unto them:

19 Then shall his father and his mother lay hold on him, and bring him out unto the elders of his city, and unto the gate of his place;

B.C. 1451.

a Ex. 23:33.

b *Bible prayers* (O.T.). Deut. 26:5-10. (Gen. 15:2; Hab. 3:1-16.)

c Ex. 14:30, *note.*

d Gen. 29:33.

e See 1 Chr. 5:1.

f Gen. 25:31-33.

20 And they shall say unto the elders
of his city, This our son *is* stubborn and
rebellious, he will not obey our voice; *he*
is a glutton, and a drunkard.
21 And all the men of his city shall
stone him with stones, that he die: so
shalt thou put evil away from among
you; and all Israel shall hear, and fear.
22 And if a man have committed a sin
worthy of death, and he be to be put to
death, and thou hang him on a tree:
23 [a]His body shall not remain all night
upon the tree, but thou shalt in any wise
bury him that day; (for he that is hanged
is accursed of [b]God;) that thy land be not
defiled, which the LORD thy God giveth
thee *for* an inheritance.

CHAPTER 22.

The law of brotherhood.

Thou [c]shalt not see thy brother's ox or
his sheep go astray, and hide thyself
from them: thou shalt in any case bring
them again unto thy brother.
2 And if thy brother *be* not nigh unto
thee, or if thou know him not, then thou
shalt bring it unto thine own house, and
it shall be with thee until thy brother
seek after it, and thou shalt restore it to
him again.
3 In like manner shalt thou do with his
ass; and so shalt thou do with his raiment;
and with all lost thing of thy
brother's, which he hath lost, and thou
hast found, shalt thou do likewise: thou
mayest not hide thyself.
4 Thou [d]shalt not see thy brother's ass
or his ox fall down by the way, and hide
thyself from them: thou shalt surely help
him to lift *them* up again.
5 The woman shall not wear that
which pertaineth unto a man, neither
shall a man put on a woman's garment:
for all that do so *are* abomination unto
the LORD thy God.
6 If a bird's nest chance to be before
thee in the way in any tree, or on the
ground, *whether they be* young ones, or
eggs, and the dam sitting upon the
young, or upon the eggs, [e]thou shalt not
take the dam with the young:
7 *But* thou shalt in any wise let the
dam go, and take the young to thee; that
it may be well with thee, and *that* thou
mayest prolong *thy* days.
8 When thou buildest a new house,
then thou shalt make a battlement for
thy roof, that thou bring not blood upon
thine house, if any man fall from thence.

The law of separation.

9 [f]Thou shalt not sow thy vineyard
with divers seeds: lest the fruit of thy
seed which thou hast sown, and the fruit
of thy vineyard, be defiled.
10 [g]Thou shalt not plow with an ox
and an ass [h]together.
11 [i]Thou shalt not wear a garment of
divers sorts, *as* of woollen and linen
together.
12 Thou shalt make thee [j]fringes upon
the four quarters of thy vesture, wherewith
thou coverest *thyself*.

The innocent wife protected.

13 If any man take a wife, and go in
unto her, and hate her,
14 And give occasions of speech
against her, and bring up an evil name
upon her, and say, I took this woman,
and when I came to her, I found her not
a maid:
15 Then shall the father of the damsel,
and her mother, take and bring forth *the*
tokens of the damsel's virginity unto the
elders of the city in the gate:
16 And the damsel's father shall say
unto the elders, I gave my daughter unto
this man to wife, and he hateth her;
17 And, lo, he hath given occasions of
speech *against her*, saying, I found not
thy daughter a maid; and yet these *are*
the tokens of my daughter's virginity.
And they shall spread the cloth before
the elders of the city.
18 And the elders of that city shall
take that man and chastise him;
19 And they shall amerce him in an
hundred *shekels* of silver, and give *them*
unto the father of the damsel, because he
hath brought up an evil name upon a
virgin of Israel: and she shall be his wife;
he may not put her away all his days.

The guilty wife to be stoned.

20 But if this thing be true, *and the*
tokens of virginity be not found for the
damsel:
21 Then they shall bring out the
damsel to the door of her father's house,
and the men of her city shall stone her

B.C. 1451.

a Josh. 8:29; John 19:31.
b Gal. 3:13.
c Ex. 23:4.
d Ex. 23:5.
e Lev. 22:28.
f Lev. 19:19
g See 2 Cor. 6:14-16.
h *Separation.* 1 Ki. 8:53. (Gen. 12:1; 2 Cor. 6:14-17.)
i Lev. 19:19.
j Num. 15:38; Mt. 23:5.

B.C. 1451.

with stones that she die: because she hath [a]wrought folly in Israel, to play the whore in her father's house: so shalt thou put evil away from among you.

22 If a man be found lying with a woman married to an husband, then they shall both of them die, *both* the man that lay with the woman, and the woman: so shalt thou put away evil from Israel.

23 If a damsel *that is* a virgin be betrothed unto an husband, and a man find her in the city, and lie with her;

24 Then ye shall bring them both out unto the gate of that city, and ye shall stone them with stones that they die; the damsel, because she cried not, *being* in the city; and the man, because he hath humbled his neighbour's wife: so thou shalt put away evil from among you.

25 But if a man find a betrothed damsel in the field, and the man force her, and lie with her: then the man only that lay with her shall die:

26 But unto the damsel thou shalt do nothing; *there is* in the damsel no sin *worthy* of death: for as when a man riseth against his neighbour, and slayeth him, even so *is* this matter:

27 For he found her in the field, *and* the betrothed damsel cried, and *there was* none to save her.

28 If a man find a damsel *that is* a virgin, which is not betrothed, and lay hold on her, and lie with her, and they be found;

29 Then the man that lay with her shall give unto the damsel's father fifty *shekels* of silver, and she shall be his wife; because he hath humbled her, he may not put her away all his days.

30 A man shall not take his father's wife, nor discover his father's skirt.

CHAPTER 23.

Divers regulations.

He that is wounded in the stones, or hath his privy member cut off, shall not enter into the congregation of the LORD.

2 A bastard shall not enter into the congregation of the LORD; even to his tenth generation shall he not enter into the congregation of the LORD.

3 An [b]Ammonite or Moabite shall not enter into the congregation of the LORD; even to their tenth generation shall they not enter into the congregation of the LORD for ever:

4 [c]Because they met you not with bread and with water in the way, when ye came forth out of Egypt; and [d]because they hired against thee Balaam the son of Beor of Pethor of Mesopotamia, to curse thee.

5 Nevertheless the LORD thy God would not hearken unto Balaam; but the LORD thy God turned the curse into a blessing unto thee, because the LORD thy God loved thee.

6 [e]Thou shalt not seek their peace nor their prosperity all thy days for ever.

7 Thou shalt not abhor an Edomite; [f]for he *is* thy brother: thou shalt not abhor an Egyptian; because [g]thou wast a stranger in his land.

8 The children that are begotten of them shall enter into the congregation of the LORD in their third generation.

9 When the host goeth forth against thine enemies, then keep thee from every wicked thing.

10 If there be among you any man, that is not clean by reason of uncleanness that chanceth him by night, then shall he go abroad out of the camp, he shall not come within the camp:

11 But it shall be, when evening cometh on, he shall wash *himself* with water: and when the sun is down, he shall come into the camp *again*.

12 Thou shalt have a place also without the camp, whither thou shalt go forth abroad:

13 And thou shalt have a paddle upon thy weapon; and it shall be, when thou wilt ease thyself abroad, thou shalt dig therewith, and shalt turn back and cover that which cometh from thee:

14 For the LORD thy God [h]walketh in the midst of thy camp, to deliver thee, and to give up thine enemies before thee; therefore shall thy camp be holy: that he see no unclean thing in thee, and turn away from thee.

15 Thou shalt not [i]deliver unto his master the servant which is escaped from his master unto thee:

16 He shall dwell with thee, *even* among you, in that place which he shall choose in one of thy gates, where it liketh him best: thou shalt not oppress him.

a Gen. 34:7; Jud. 20:6, 10; 2 Sam. 13:12, 13.
b Neh. 13:1, 2.
c See Deut. 2:27-30.
d Num. 22:5, 6.
e Ezra 9:12.
f Gen. 25:24, 25, 26; Oba. 10, 12.
g Ex. 22:21; 23:9; Lev. 19:34.
h Lev. 26:12.
i 1 Sam. 30:15.

17 There shall be no whore of the daughters of Israel, nor a sodomite of the sons of Israel.

18 Thou shalt not bring the hire of a whore, or the price of a dog, into the house of the LORD thy God for any vow: for even both these *are* abomination unto the LORD thy God.

19 Thou shalt not lend upon usury to thy brother; usury of money, usury of victuals, usury of any thing that is lent upon usury:

20 Unto a stranger thou mayest lend upon usury; but unto thy brother thou shalt not lend upon usury: that the LORD thy God may bless thee in all that thou settest thine hand to in the land whither thou goest to possess it.

21 When thou shalt vow a vow unto the LORD thy God, thou shalt not slack to pay it: for the LORD thy God will surely require it of thee; and it would be sin in thee.

22 But if thou shalt forbear to vow, it shall be no sin in thee.

23 [a]That which is gone out of thy lips thou shalt keep and perform; *even* a freewill offering, according as thou hast vowed unto the LORD thy God, which thou hast promised with thy mouth.

24 When thou comest into thy neighbour's vineyard, then thou mayest eat grapes thy fill at thine own pleasure; but thou shalt not put *any* in thy vessel.

25 When thou comest into the standing corn of thy neighbour, [b]then thou mayest pluck the ears with thine hand; but thou shalt not move a sickle unto thy neighbour's standing corn.

CHAPTER 24.

The Mosaic law of divorce
(Mt. 19:8; cf. 1 Cor. 7:12–15).

When a man hath taken a wife, and married her, and it come to pass that she find no favour in his eyes, because he hath found some uncleanness in her: then let him write her a bill of divorcement, and give *it* in her hand, and send her out of his [c]house.

2 And when she is departed out of his house, she may go and be another man's *wife*.

3 And *if* the latter husband hate her, and write her a bill of divorcement, and giveth *it* in her hand, and sendeth her out of his house; or if the latter husband die, which took her *to be* his wife;

4 Her former husband, which sent her away, may not take her again to be his wife, after that she is defiled; for that *is* abomination before the LORD: and thou shalt not cause the land to sin, which the LORD thy God giveth thee *for* an inheritance.

5 When a man hath taken a new wife, he shall not go out to war, neither shall he be charged with any business: *but* he shall be free at home one year, and shall cheer up his wife which he hath taken.

6 No man shall take the nether or the upper millstone to pledge: for he taketh *a man's* life to pledge.

7 [d]If a man be found stealing any of his brethren of the children of Israel, and maketh merchandise of him, or selleth him; then that thief shall die; and thou shalt put evil away from among you.

8 Take heed in [e]the plague of leprosy, that thou observe diligently, and do according to all that the priests the Levites shall teach you: as I commanded them, *so* ye shall observe to do.

9 [f]Remember what the LORD thy God did unto Miriam by the way, after that ye were come forth out of Egypt.

10 When thou dost lend thy brother any thing, thou shalt not go into his house to fetch his pledge.

11 Thou shalt stand abroad, and the man to whom thou dost lend shall bring out the pledge abroad unto thee.

12 And if the man *be* poor, thou shalt not sleep with his pledge:

13 In any case thou shalt deliver him the pledge again when the sun goeth down, that he may sleep in his own raiment, and bless thee: and it shall be righteousness unto thee before the LORD thy God.

14 Thou shalt not oppress an hired servant *that is* poor and needy, *whether he be* of thy brethren, or of thy strangers that *are* in thy land within thy gates:

15 At his day thou shalt give *him* his hire, neither shall the sun go down upon it; for he *is* poor, and setteth his heart upon it: [g]lest he cry against thee unto the LORD, and it be sin unto thee.

16 The fathers shall not be put to death for the children, neither shall the children be put to death for the fathers:

B.C. 1451.

a Num. 30:2; Psa. 66:13, 14.
b Mt. 12:1; Mk. 2:23; Lk. 6:1.
c Mt. 5:31.
d Ex. 21:16.
e Lev. 13:2; 14:2.
f See Lk. 17:32; 1 Cor. 10:6.
g Jas. 5:4.

every man shall be put to death for his
own sin.
17 Thou shalt not pervert the judgment
of the stranger, *nor* of the fatherless; nor
take a widow's raiment to pledge:
18 But thou shalt remember that thou
wast a bondman in Egypt, and the LORD
thy God [a]redeemed thee thence: therefore I command thee to do this thing.
19 When thou cuttest down thine harvest in thy field, and hast forgot a sheaf
in the field, thou shalt not go again to
fetch it: it shall be for the stranger, for
the fatherless, and for the widow: that
the LORD thy God may [b]bless thee in all
the work of thine hands.
20 When thou beatest thine olive tree,
thou shalt not go over the boughs again:
it shall be for the stranger, for the fatherless, and for the widow.
21 When thou gatherest the grapes of
thy vineyard, thou shalt not glean *it*
afterward: it shall be for the stranger, for
the fatherless, and for the widow.
22 And thou shalt remember that thou
wast a bondman in the land of Egypt:
therefore I command thee to do this thing.

CHAPTER 25.

Divers regulations.

If there be a controversy between men,
and they come unto judgment, that
the judges may judge them; then they
shall justify the righteous, and condemn
the wicked.
2 And it shall be, if the wicked man *be*
worthy to be beaten, that the judge shall
cause him to lie down, and to be beaten
before his face, according to his fault, by
a certain number.
3 Forty stripes he may give him, *and* not
exceed: lest, *if* he should exceed, and beat
him above these with many stripes, then
thy brother should seem vile unto thee.
4 Thou shalt not muzzle the ox when
he treadeth out *the* [c]*corn.*
5 If brethren dwell together, and one
of them die, and have no [d]child, the wife
of the dead shall not marry without unto
a stranger: her husband's brother shall
go in unto her, and take her to him to
wife, and perform the duty of an husband's brother unto her.
6 And it shall be, *that* the firstborn
which she beareth [e]shall succeed in the
name of his brother *which is* dead, that
his name be not put out of Israel.
7 And if the man like not to take his
brother's wife, then let his brother's wife
go up to the [f]gate unto the elders, and
say, My husband's brother refuseth to
raise up unto his brother a name in
Israel, he will not perform the duty of
my husband's brother.
8 Then the elders of his city shall call
him, and speak unto him: and *if* he stand
to it, and say, [g]I like not to take her;
9 Then shall his brother's wife come
unto him in the presence of the elders,
and [h]loose his shoe from off his foot, and
spit in his face, and shall answer and say,
So shall it be done unto that man that
will not [i]build up his brother's house.
10 And his name shall be called in
Israel, The house of him that hath his
shoe loosed.
11 When men strive together one with
another, and the wife of the one draweth
near for to deliver her husband out of
the hand of him that smiteth him, and
putteth forth her hand, and taketh him
by the secrets:
12 Then thou shalt cut off her hand,
thine eye shall not pity *her*.
13 Thou shalt not have in thy bag
divers weights, a great and a small.
14 Thou shalt not have in thine house
divers measures, a great and a small.
15 *But* thou shalt have a perfect and
just weight, a perfect and just measure
shalt thou have: [j]that thy days may be
lengthened in the land which the LORD
thy God giveth thee.
16 For [k]all that do such things, *and* all
that do unrighteously, *are* an abomination unto the LORD thy God.
17 [l]Remember what Amalek did unto
thee by the way, when ye were come
forth out of Egypt;
18 How he met thee by the way, and
smote the hindmost of thee, *even* all *that*
were feeble behind thee, when thou *wast*
faint and weary; and he feared not God.
19 Therefore it shall be, when the LORD
thy God hath given thee rest from all
thine enemies round about, in the land
which the LORD thy God giveth thee *for*
an inheritance to possess it, *that* thou
shalt blot out the remembrance of
Amalek from under heaven; thou shalt
not forget *it*.

B.C. 1451.

a Ex. 14:30, *note.*
b Deut. 15:10; Psa. 41:1; Prov. 19:17.
c 1 Cor. 9:9; 1 Tim. 5:18.
d Mt. 22:24; Mk. 12:19; Lk. 20:28.
e Gen. 38:9.
f Ruth 4:1, 2.
g Ruth 4:6.
h Ruth 4:7.
i Ruth 4:11.
j Ex. 20:12.
k Prov. 11:1; 1 Thes. 4:6.
l Ex. 17:8; 1 Sam. 15:1-3.

CHAPTER 26.

The law of the offering of firstfruits.
(Cf. Ex. 23:16–19.)

AND it shall be, when thou *art* come in unto the land which the LORD thy God giveth thee *for* an inheritance, and possessest it, and dwellest therein;

2 That thou shalt take of the first of all the fruit of the earth, which thou shalt bring of thy land that the LORD thy God giveth thee, and shalt put *it* in a basket, and shalt go unto the place which the LORD thy God shall choose to place his name there.

3 And thou shalt go unto the priest that shall be in those days, and say unto him, I profess this day unto the LORD thy God, that I am come unto the country which the LORD sware unto our fathers for to give us.

4 And the priest shall take the basket out of thine hand, and set it down before the altar of the LORD thy God.

5 And thou shalt speak and [a]say before the LORD thy God, A [b]Syrian [c]ready to perish *was* my father, and he went down into Egypt, and sojourned there with a [d]few, and became there a nation, great, mighty, and populous:

6 And the [e]Egyptians evil entreated us, and afflicted us, and laid upon us hard bondage:

7 And [f]when we cried unto the LORD God of our fathers, the LORD heard our voice, and looked on our affliction, and our labour, and our oppression:

8 And the [g]LORD brought us forth out of Egypt with a mighty hand, and with an outstretched arm, and with great [h]terribleness, and with signs, and with wonders:

9 And he hath brought us into this place, and hath given us this land, *even* a [i]land that floweth with milk and honey.

10 And now, behold, I have brought the firstfruits of the land, which thou, O LORD, hast given me. And thou shalt set it before the LORD thy God, and worship before the LORD thy God:

11 And [j]thou shalt rejoice in every good *thing* which the LORD thy God hath given unto thee, and unto thine house, thou, and the Levite, and the stranger that *is* among you.

12 When thou hast made an end of tithing all the tithes of thine increase the third year, *which is* the year of tithing, and hast given *it* unto the Levite, the stranger, the fatherless, and the widow, that they may eat within thy gates, and be filled;

13 Then thou shalt [k]say before the LORD thy God, I have brought away the hallowed things out of *mine* house, and also have given them unto the Levite, and unto the stranger, to the fatherless, and to the widow, according to all thy commandments which thou hast commanded me: I have not transgressed thy commandments, neither have I forgotten *them*:

14 [l]I have not eaten thereof in my mourning, neither have I taken away *ought* thereof for *any* unclean *use*, nor given *ought* thereof for the dead: *but* I have hearkened to the voice of the LORD my God, *and* have done according to all that thou hast commanded me.

15 [m]Look down from thy holy habitation, from heaven, and bless thy people Israel, and the land which thou hast given us, as thou swarest unto our fathers, a land that floweth with milk and honey.

16 This day the LORD thy God hath commanded thee to do these statutes and judgments: thou shalt therefore keep and do them with all thine heart, and with all thy soul.

17 Thou hast avouched the LORD this day to be thy God, and to walk in his ways, and to keep his statutes, and his commandments, and his judgments, and to hearken unto his voice:

18 And the LORD hath avouched thee this day to be his peculiar people, as he hath promised thee, and that *thou* shouldest keep all his commandments;

19 And to make thee high above all nations which he hath made, in praise, and in name, and in honour; and that thou mayest be an holy people unto the LORD thy God, as he hath spoken.

CHAPTER 27.

The stones of the law in Mount Ebal.

AND Moses with the elders of Israel commanded the people, saying, Keep all the commandments which I command you this day.

B.C. 1451.

a *Bible prayers* (O.T.). Deut. 26:13-15. (Gen. 15:2; Hab. 3:1-16.)
b Hos. 12:12.
c Gen. 43:1, 2; 45:7, 11.
d Gen. 46:27; Deut. 10:22.
e Ex. 1:11, 14.
f Ex. 2:23-25; 3:9; 4:31.
g Ex. 12:42, 51; 13:3, 14, 16; Deut. 5:15.
h Deut. 4:34.
i Ex. 3:8.
j Deut. 12:7, 12, 18; 16:11.
k *Bible prayers* (O.T.). Josh. 7:7-9. (Gen. 15:2; Hab. 3:1-16.)
l Lev. 7:20; Hos. 9:4.
m Isa. 63:15; Zech. 2:13.

B.C. 1451.

2 And it shall be on the [a]day when ye shall pass over Jordan unto the land which the LORD thy God giveth thee, that thou shalt [b]set thee up great stones, and plaister them with plaister:

3 And thou shalt write upon them all the words of this law, when thou art passed over, that thou mayest go in unto the land which the LORD thy God giveth thee, a land that floweth with milk and honey; as the LORD God of thy fathers hath promised thee.

4 Therefore it shall be when ye be gone over Jordan, *that* ye shall set up these stones, which I command you this day, in mount [c]Ebal, and thou shalt plaister them with plaister.

5 And there shalt thou build an altar unto the LORD thy God, an altar of stones: [d]thou shalt not lift up *any* iron *tool* upon them.

6 Thou shalt build the altar of the LORD thy God of whole stones: and thou shalt offer burnt-offerings thereon unto the LORD thy God:

7 And thou shalt offer peace-offerings, and shalt eat there, and rejoice before the LORD thy God.

8 And thou shalt write upon the stones all the words of this law very plainly.

Blessings and curses from Ebal and Gerizim.

9 And Moses and the priests the Levites spake unto all Israel, saying, Take heed, and hearken, O Israel; this day [e]thou art become the people of the LORD thy God.

10 Thou shalt therefore obey the voice of the LORD thy God, and do his commandments and his statutes, which I command thee this day.

11 And Moses charged the people the same day, saying,

12 These shall stand [f]upon mount Gerizim to bless the people, when ye are come over Jordan; Simeon, and Levi, and Judah, and Issachar, and Joseph, and Benjamin:

13 And these shall stand [g]upon mount Ebal to curse; Reuben, Gad, and Asher, and Zebulun, Dan, and Naphtali.

14 And [h]the Levites shall speak, and say unto all the men of Israel with a loud voice,

15 [i]Cursed *be* the man that maketh *any* graven or molten image, an abomination unto the LORD, the work of the hands of the craftsman, and putteth *it* in *a* secret *place*. And all the people shall answer and say, Amen.

16 Cursed *be* he that setteth light by his father or his mother. And all the people shall say, Amen.

17 Cursed *be* he that removeth his neighbour's landmark. And all the people shall say, Amen.

18 Cursed *be* he that maketh the blind to wander out of the way. And all the people shall say, Amen.

19 Cursed *be* he that perverteth the judgment of the stranger, fatherless, and widow. And all the people shall say, Amen.

20 Cursed *be* he that lieth with his father's wife; because he uncovereth his father's skirt. And all the people shall say, Amen.

21 Cursed *be* he that lieth with any manner of beast. And all the people shall say, Amen.

22 Cursed *be* he that lieth with his sister, the daughter of his father, or the daughter of his mother. And all the people shall say, Amen.

23 Cursed *be* he that lieth with his mother in law. And all the people shall say, Amen.

24 Cursed *be* he that smiteth his neighbour secretly. And all the people shall say, Amen.

25 Cursed *be* he that taketh reward to slay an innocent person. And all the people shall say, Amen.

26 Cursed *be* he that confirmeth not *all* the words of this law to do [j]them. And all the people shall say, Amen.

CHAPTER 28.

Conditions of blessing in the land.

AND it shall come to [k]pass, [1]if thou shalt hearken diligently unto the voice of the LORD thy God, to observe *and* to do all his commandments which I command thee this day, that the LORD thy God will set thee on high above all nations of the earth:

2 And all these blessings shall come on thee, and [l]overtake thee, if thou shalt hearken unto the voice of the LORD thy God.

3 Blessed *shalt* thou *be* in the city, and blessed *shalt* thou *be* in the field.

a Josh. 4:1.
b Josh. 8:32.
c Deut. 11:29; Josh. 8:30.
d Ex. 20:25; Josh. 8:31.
e Deut. 26:18.
f Deut. 11:29; Josh. 8:33; Jud. 9:7; Dan. 9:11.
g Deut. 11:29; Josh. 8:33.
h Deut. 33:10; Josh. 8:33; Dan. 9:11.
i Ex. 20:4, 23; Ex. 34:17; Lev. 19:4; 26:1.
j Gal. 3:10.
k Ex. 15:26; Lev. 26:3; Isa. 55:2.
l v. 15; Zech. 1:6.

[1] **(28:1)** Chapters 28–29. are, properly, an integral part of the Palestinian Covenant (Deut. 30:1-9, *note*).

4 Blessed *shall be* the fruit of thy body,
and the fruit of thy ground, and the fruit
of thy cattle, the increase of thy kine, and
the flocks of thy sheep.
5 Blessed *shall be* thy basket and thy
store.
6 Blessed *shalt* thou *be* when thou
comest in, and blessed *shalt* thou *be*
when thou goest out.
7 The LORD shall cause thine enemies
that rise up against thee to be smitten
before thy face: they shall come out
against thee one way, and flee before
thee seven ways.
8 The LORD shall [a]command the blessing upon thee in thy storehouses, and in
all that thou settest thine hand unto; and
he shall bless thee in the land which the
LORD thy God giveth thee.
9 The LORD shall establish thee an holy
people unto himself, as he hath sworn
unto thee, if thou shalt keep the commandments of the LORD thy God, and
walk in his ways.
10 And all people of the earth shall see
that thou art [b]called by the name of the
LORD; and they shall be afraid of thee.
11 And the LORD shall make thee plenteous in goods, in the fruit of thy body,
and in the fruit of thy cattle, and in the
fruit of thy ground, in the land which the
LORD sware unto thy fathers to give thee.
12 The LORD shall open unto thee his
good treasure, the heaven to give the
rain unto thy land in his season, and to
bless all the work of thine hand: and
thou shalt lend unto many nations, and
thou shalt not borrow.
13 And the LORD shall make thee the
[c]head, and not the tail; and thou shalt be
above only, and thou shalt not be
beneath; if that thou hearken unto the
commandments of the LORD thy God,
which I command thee this day, to
observe and to do *them*:
14 And thou shalt not go aside from
any of the words which I command thee
this day, *to* the right hand, or *to* the left,
to go after other gods to serve them.

Conditions which will bring chastisement in the land.

15 But it shall come to pass, [d]if thou wilt
not hearken unto the voice of the LORD
thy God, to observe to do all his commandments and his statutes which I command thee this day; that all these curses
shall come upon thee, and overtake thee:
16 Cursed *shalt* thou *be* in the city, and
cursed *shalt* thou *be* in the field.
17 Cursed *shall be* thy basket and thy
store.
18 Cursed *shall be* the fruit of thy body,
and the fruit of thy land, the increase of
thy kine, and the flocks of thy sheep.
19 Cursed *shalt* thou *be* when thou
comest in, and cursed *shalt* thou *be* when
thou goest out.
20 The LORD shall send upon thee
[e]cursing, [f]vexation, and [g]rebuke, in all
that thou settest thine hand unto for to
do, until thou be destroyed, and until
thou perish quickly; because of the
wickedness of thy doings, whereby thou
hast forsaken me.
21 The LORD shall make the pestilence
cleave unto thee, until he have consumed thee from off the land, whither
thou goest to possess it.
22 The LORD shall smite thee with a
consumption, and with a fever, and with
an inflammation, and with an extreme
burning, and with the sword, and with
[h]blasting, and with mildew; and they
shall pursue thee until thou perish.
23 And thy heaven that *is* over thy
head shall be brass, and the earth that *is*
under thee *shall be* iron.
24 The LORD shall make the rain of thy
land powder and dust: from heaven
shall it come down upon thee, until thou
be destroyed.
25 The LORD shall cause thee to be smitten before thine enemies: thou shalt go
out one way against them, and flee seven
ways before them: and shalt be removed
into all the kingdoms of the earth.
26 And thy carcase shall be meat unto
all fowls of the air, and unto the beasts of
the earth, and no man shall fray *them*
away.
27 The LORD will smite thee with the
botch of Egypt, and with the emerods,
and with the scab, and with the itch,
whereof thou canst not be healed.
28 The LORD shall [i]smite thee with
madness, and blindness, and astonishment of heart:
29 And thou shalt grope at noonday,
as the blind gropeth in darkness, and
thou shalt not prosper in thy ways: and

B.C. 1451.

a Lev. 25:21.

b Num. 6:27; 2 Chr. 7:14; Isa. 63:19; Dan. 9:18, 19.

c Cf. v. 44; Isa. 9:14, 15.

d Lev. 26:14; Dan. 9:10-14; Mal. 2:2.

e Mal. 2:2.

f 1 Sam. 14:20; Zech. 14:13.

g Isa. 30:17; 51:20; 66:15.

h Amos 4:9.

i *Times of the Gentiles.* vs. 28, 49-52, 63-68; 2 Ki. 18:9-12. (Lk. 21:24; Rev. 16:19.)

thou shalt be only oppressed and spoiled evermore, and no man shall save *thee.*

30 Thou shalt betroth a wife, and another man shall lie with her: thou shalt build an house, and thou shalt not dwell therein: thou shalt plant a vineyard, and shalt not gather the grapes thereof.

31 Thine ox *shall be* slain before thine eyes, and thou shalt not eat thereof: thine ass *shall be* violently taken away from before thy face, and shall not be restored to thee: thy sheep *shall be* given unto thine enemies, and thou shalt have none to rescue *them.*

32 Thy sons and thy daughters *shall be* given unto another people, and thine eyes shall look, and fail *with longing* for them all the day long: and *there shall be* no might in thine hand.

33 The fruit of thy land, and all thy labours, shall a nation which thou knowest not eat up; and thou shalt be only oppressed and crushed alway:

34 So that thou shalt be mad for the sight of thine eyes which thou shalt see.

35 The LORD shall smite thee in the knees, and in the legs, with a sore botch that cannot be healed, from the sole of thy foot unto the top of thy head.

36 The LORD shall [a]bring thee, and thy king which thou shalt set over thee, unto a nation which neither thou nor thy fathers have known; and there shalt thou serve other gods, wood and stone.

37 And thou shalt become [b]an astonishment, a proverb, and a byword, among all nations whither the LORD shall lead thee.

38 Thou shalt carry much seed out into the field, and shalt gather *but* little in; for the locust shall consume it.

39 Thou shalt plant vineyards, and dress *them,* but shalt neither drink *of* the wine, nor gather *the grapes;* for the worms shall eat them.

40 Thou shalt have olive trees throughout all thy coasts, but thou shalt not anoint *thyself* with the oil; for thine olive shall cast *his fruit.*

41 Thou shalt beget sons and daughters, but thou shalt not enjoy them; for they shall go into captivity.

42 All thy trees and fruit of thy land shall the locust consume.

43 The stranger that *is* within thee shall get up above thee very high; and thou shalt come down very low.

44 He shall lend to thee, and thou shalt not lend to him: he shall be the [c]head, and thou shalt be the tail.

45 Moreover all these curses shall come upon thee, and shall pursue thee, and overtake thee, till thou be destroyed; because thou hearkenedst not unto the voice of the LORD thy God, to keep his commandments and his statutes which he commanded thee:

46 And they shall be upon [d]thee for a sign and for a wonder, and upon thy seed for ever.

47 Because thou servedst not the LORD thy God with joyfulness, and with gladness of heart, for the abundance of all *things;*

48 Therefore shalt thou serve thine enemies which the LORD shall send against thee, in hunger, and in thirst, and in nakedness, and in want of all *things:* and he [e]shall put a yoke of iron upon thy neck, until he have destroyed thee.

49 The LORD shall bring [f]a nation against thee from far, from the end of the [g]earth, *as swift* as the eagle flieth; a nation whose tongue thou shalt not understand;

50 A nation of fierce countenance, which shall not regard the person of the old, nor shew favour to the young:

51 And he shall eat the fruit of thy cattle, and the fruit of thy land, until thou be destroyed: which *also* shall not leave thee *either* corn, wine, or oil, *or* the increase of thy kine, or flocks of thy sheep, until he have destroyed thee.

52 And he shall besiege thee in all thy gates, until thy high and fenced walls come down, wherein thou [h]trustedst, throughout all thy land: and he shall besiege thee in all thy gates throughout all thy land, which the LORD thy God hath given thee.

53 And thou shalt eat [i]the fruit of thine own body, the flesh of thy sons and of thy daughters, which the LORD thy God hath given thee, in the siege, and in the straitness, wherewith thine enemies shall distress thee:

54 *So that* the man *that is* tender among you, and very delicate, his eye shall be evil toward his brother, and toward the wife of his bosom, and

B.C. 1451.

a 2 Ki. 17:4, 6; 24:12, 14; 25:7, 11; 2 Chr. 33:11; 36:6, 20.

b 1 Ki. 9:7, 8; Jer. 24:9; 25:9; Zech. 8:13.

c v. 13; Lam. 1:5.

d Isa. 8:18; Ezk. 14:8.

e Jer. 28:14.

f *Times of the Gentiles.* vs. 49-68; Dan. 2:29-45. (Lk. 21:24; Rev. 16:19.)

g Jer. 48:40; 49:22; Lam. 4:19; Ezk. 17:3, 12; Hos. 8:1.

h Psa. 2:12, *note.*

i 2 Ki. 6:28, 29.

toward the remnant of his children which he shall leave:

55 So that he will not give to any of them of the flesh of his children whom he shall eat: because he hath nothing left him in the siege, and in the straitness, wherewith thine enemies shall distress thee in all thy gates.

56 The tender and delicate woman among you, which would not adventure to set the sole of her foot upon the ground for delicateness and tenderness, her eye shall be evil toward the husband of her bosom, and toward her son, and toward her daughter,

57 And toward her young one that cometh out from between her feet, and toward her children which she shall bear: for she shall eat them for want of all *things* secretly in the siege and straitness, wherewith thine enemy shall distress thee in thy gates.

58 If thou wilt not observe to do all the words of this law that are written in this book, that [a]thou mayest [b]fear this [c]glorious and fearful name, THE LORD THY GOD;

59 Then the LORD will make thy plagues wonderful, and the plagues of thy seed, *even* great plagues, and of long continuance, and sore sicknesses, and of long continuance.

60 Moreover he will bring upon thee all the diseases of Egypt, which thou wast afraid of; and they shall cleave unto thee.

61 Also every sickness, and every plague, which *is* not written in the book of this law, them will the LORD bring upon thee, until thou be destroyed.

62 And ye shall be left few in number, whereas ye were [d]as the stars of heaven for multitude; because thou wouldest not obey the voice of the LORD thy God.

Continued disobedience to be punished by a world-wide dispersion.

63 And it shall come to pass, *that* as the LORD rejoiced over you to do you good, and to multiply you; so the LORD [e]will rejoice over you to destroy you, and to bring you to nought; and ye shall be plucked from off the land whither thou goest to possess it.

64 And the LORD shall [f]scatter thee among all people, from the one end of the earth even unto the other; and there thou shalt serve other gods, which neither thou nor thy fathers have known, *even* wood and stone.

65 And [g]among these nations shalt thou find no ease, neither shall the sole of thy foot have rest: but the LORD shall give thee there a trembling heart, and failing of eyes, and sorrow of mind:

66 And thy life shall hang in doubt before thee; and thou shalt fear day and night, and shalt have none assurance of thy life:

67 In the morning thou shalt say, Would God it were even! and at even thou shalt say, Would God it were morning! for the fear of thine heart wherewith thou shalt fear, and for the sight of thine eyes which thou shalt see.

68 And the LORD shall bring thee into Egypt again with ships, by the way whereof I spake unto thee, Thou shalt see it no more again: and there ye shall be sold unto your enemies for bondmen and bondwomen, and no man shall buy *you*.

CHAPTER 29.

The Palestinian Covenant:
(1) *introductory words.*

These *are* the words of the covenant, which the LORD commanded Moses to make with the children of Israel in the land of Moab, beside the covenant which he made with them in Horeb.

2 And Moses called unto all Israel, and said unto them, [h]Ye have seen all that the LORD did before your eyes in the land of Egypt unto Pharaoh, and unto all his servants, and unto all his land;

3 The great temptations which thine eyes have seen, the signs, and those great miracles:

4 Yet [i]the LORD hath not given you an heart to perceive, and eyes to see, and ears to hear, unto this day.

5 And I have led you forty years in the wilderness: your clothes are not waxen old upon you, and thy shoe is not waxen old upon thy foot.

6 Ye have not eaten bread, neither have ye drunk wine or strong drink: that ye might know that I *am* the LORD your God.

7 And when ye came unto this place, Sihon the king of Heshbon, and Og the king of Bashan, came out against us unto battle, and we smote them:

B.C. 1451.

a *Israel (history).* vs. 58-68; Deut. 30:1-7. (Gen. 12:2, 3; Rom. 11:26.)

b Psa. 19:9, *note.*

c Ex. 6:3.

d Deut. 10:22; Neh. 9:23.

e Isa. 1:24.

f Jer. 16:13; Amos 9:9.

g Amos 9:4.

h Ex. 19:4.

i 2 Cor. 3:14-16; Eph. 4:18.

B.C. 1451.

8 And we took their land, and gave it
for an inheritance unto the Reubenites,
and to the Gadites, and to the half tribe
of Manasseh.
9 Keep therefore the words of this
covenant, and do them, that ye may
prosper in all that ye do.
10 Ye stand this day all of you before
the LORD your God; your captains of
your tribes, your elders, and your officers, *with* all the men of Israel,
11 Your little ones, your wives, and
thy stranger that *is* in thy camp, from the
hewer of thy wood unto the drawer of
thy water:
12 That thou shouldest enter into
covenant with the LORD thy God, and
into his oath, which the LORD thy God
maketh with thee this day:
13 That he may establish thee to day
for a people unto himself, and *that* he
may be unto thee a God, as he hath said
unto thee, and as he hath sworn unto
thy fathers, to Abraham, to Isaac, and to
Jacob.
14 Neither with you [a]only do I make
this covenant and this oath;
15 But with *him* that standeth here
with us this day before the LORD our
God, and also with *him* that *is* not here
with us this day:
16 (For ye know how we have dwelt
in the land of Egypt; and how we came
through the nations which ye passed by;
17 And ye have seen their abominations, and their idols, wood and stone, silver and gold, which *were* among them:)
18 Lest there should be among you
man, or woman, or family, or tribe,
whose heart turneth away this day from
the LORD our God, to go *and* serve the
gods of these nations; [b]lest there should
be among you a root that beareth gall
and wormwood;
19 And it come to pass, when he
heareth the words of this curse, that he
bless himself in his heart, saying, I shall
have peace, though I walk in the imagination of mine heart, to add drunkenness to thirst:
20 The LORD will not spare him, but
then the anger of the LORD and his jealousy shall smoke against that man, and
all the curses that are written in this book
shall lie upon him, and the LORD shall
blot out his name from under heaven.
21 And the LORD shall separate him
unto evil out of all the tribes of Israel,
according to all the curses of the covenant
that are written in this book of the law:
22 So that the generation to come of
your children that shall rise up after you,
and the stranger that shall come from a
far land, shall say, when they see the
plagues of that land, and the sicknesses
which the LORD hath laid upon it;
23 *And that* the whole land thereof *is*
brimstone, and salt, *and* burning, *that* it
is not sown, nor beareth, nor any grass
groweth therein, like the overthrow of
Sodom, and Gomorrah, Admah, and
Zeboim, which the LORD overthrew in
his anger, and in his wrath:
24 Even all nations shall say,
Wherefore hath the LORD done thus unto
this land? what *meaneth* the heat of this
great anger?
25 Then men shall say, Because they
have forsaken the covenant of the LORD
God of their fathers, which he made
with them when he brought them forth
out of the land of Egypt:
26 For they went and served other
gods, and worshipped them, gods
whom they knew not, and *whom* he had
not given unto them:
27 And the anger of the LORD was kindled against this land, to bring upon it all
the curses that are written in this book:
28 And the LORD rooted them out of
their land in anger, and in wrath, and in
great indignation, and cast them into
another land, as *it is* this day.
29 The secret *things belong* unto the
LORD our God: but those *things which are*
[c]revealed *belong* unto us and to our children for ever, that *we* may do all the
words of this law.

CHAPTER 30.

The Sixth, or Palestinian Covenant:
(2) *the covenant declared.*

[d]AND it shall come to pass, when all
these things are come upon [e]thee,
the blessing and the curse, which I have
set before thee, and thou shalt call *them*
to mind among all the nations, whither
the [f]LORD thy God hath driven thee,
2 And shalt return unto the LORD thy
God, and shalt obey his voice according
to all that I command thee this day, thou
and thy children, with all thine heart,
and with all thy soul;

a Jer. 31:31-33; Heb. 8:7, 8.

b Acts 8:23; Heb. 12:15.

c *Inspiration.* Deut. 31:24. (Ex. 4:15; Rev. 22:19.)

d *The Eight Covenants.* 2 Sam. 7:8. (Gen. 1:28; Heb. 8:10.)

e *Israel (history).* vs. 1-7; Deut. 31:16-23. (Gen. 12:2, 3; Rom. 11:26.)

f *Kingdom* (O.T.). vs. 1-9; Deut. 33:4, 5. (Gen. 1:26; Zech. 12:8.)

3 That then the LORD thy God will
[1]turn thy captivity, and have compassion upon thee, and will [a]return and
gather thee from all the nations, whither
the LORD thy God hath scattered thee.
4 If *any* of thine be driven out unto the
outmost *parts* of heaven, from thence
will the LORD thy God gather thee, and
from thence will he fetch thee:
5 And the LORD thy God will bring
thee into the land which thy fathers possessed, and thou shalt possess it; and he
will do thee good, and multiply thee
above thy fathers.
6 And [b]the LORD thy God will circumcise thine heart, and the heart of thy
seed, to love the LORD thy God with all
thine heart, and with all thy soul, that
thou mayest live.
7 And the LORD thy God will put all
these [c]curses upon thine enemies, and
on them that hate thee, which persecuted thee.
8 And thou shalt [d]return and obey the
voice of the LORD, and do all his commandments which I command thee this
day.
9 And the LORD thy God will make
thee plenteous in every work of thine
hand, in the fruit of thy body, and in the
fruit of thy cattle, and in the fruit of thy
land, for good: for the LORD will again
[e]rejoice over thee for good, as he rejoiced
over thy fathers:
10 If thou shalt hearken unto the voice
of the LORD thy God, to keep his commandments and his statutes which are
written in this book of the law, *and* if
thou turn unto the LORD thy God with
all thine heart, and with all thy soul.

The final warning.

11 For this commandment which I
command thee this day, it *is* not hidden
from thee, neither *is* it far off.
12 It *is* not in heaven, that thou
shouldest say, Who shall go up for us to
[f]heaven, and bring it unto us, that we
may hear it, and do it?
13 Neither *is* it beyond the sea, that
thou shouldest say, Who shall go over
the sea for us, and bring it unto us, that
we may hear it, and do it?
14 But the word *is* very nigh unto thee,
in thy [g]mouth, and in thy heart, that
thou mayest do it.
15 See, I have set before thee this day
life and good, and death and evil;
16 In that I command thee this day to
love the LORD thy God, to walk in his
ways, and to keep his commandments
and his statutes and his judgments, that
thou mayest live and multiply: and the
LORD thy God shall bless thee in the land
whither thou goest to possess it.
17 But if thine heart turn away, so that
thou wilt not hear, but shalt be drawn
away, and worship other gods, and
serve them;
18 I denounce unto you this day, that
ye shall surely perish, *and that* ye shall
not prolong *your* days upon the land,
whither thou passest over Jordan to go
to possess it.
19 I call heaven and earth to record
this day against you, *that* I have set
before you life and death, blessing and
cursing: therefore choose life, that both
thou and thy seed may live:
20 That thou mayest love the LORD thy
God, *and* that thou mayest obey his
voice, and that thou mayest cleave unto
him: for he *is* thy [h]life, and the length of
thy days: that thou mayest dwell in the
land which the LORD sware unto thy

B.C. 1451.

a *Christ (second advent).* Psa. 2:1-9. (Deut. 30:3; Acts 1:9-11.)

b Jer. 32:39; Ezk. 11:19; 36:26.

c Zeph. 3:19. See *Abrahamic Covenant.* Gen. 15:18, *note.*

d Zeph. 3:20. See *Palestinian Covenant.* Deut. 30:1-9, *note.*

e Jer. 32:41.

f Rom. 10:6, 7.

g Rom. 10:8.

h John 11:25; 14:6; Col. 3:4.

[1] **(30:3)** The Palestinian Covenant gives the conditions under which Israel entered the land of promise. It is important to see that the nation has never as yet taken the land under the unconditional Abrahamic Covenant, nor has it ever possessed the whole land (cf. Gen. 15:18, with Num. 34:1-12). The Palestinian Covenant is in seven parts:

(1) Dispersion for disobedience, v. 1 (Deut. 28:63-68. See Gen. 15:18, *note*).
(2) The future repentance of Israel while in the dispersion, v. 2.
(3) The return of the Lord, v. 3 (Amos 9:9-14; Acts 15:14-17).
(4) Restoration to the land, v. 5 (Isa. 11:11, 12; Jer. 23:3-8; Ezk. 37:21-25).
(5) National conversion, v. 6 (Rom. 11:26, 27; Hos. 2:14-16).
(6) The judgment of Israel's oppressors, v. 7 (Isa. 14:1, 2; Joel 3:1-8; Mt. 25:31-46).
(7) National prosperity, v. 9 (Amos 9:11-14).

See, for the other seven covenants: *Edenic,* Gen. 1:28; *Adamic,* Gen. 3:15; *Noahic,* Gen. 9:1; *Abrahamic,* Gen. 15:18; *Mosaic,* Ex. 19:25; *Davidic,* 2 Sam. 7:16; *New,* Heb. 8:8.

fathers, to Abraham, to Isaac, and to
Jacob, to give them.

CHAPTER 31.

Moses' last counsels to the priests,
Levites, and Joshua.

And Moses went and spake these
words unto all Israel.
2 And he said unto them, I *am* an hundred and twenty years old this day; I can
no more go out and come in: also the
LORD hath said unto me, Thou shalt not
go over this Jordan.
3 The LORD thy God, he will go over
before thee, *and* he will destroy these
nations from before thee, and thou shalt
possess them: *and* Joshua, he shall go
over before thee, as the LORD hath said.
4 And the LORD shall do unto them as
he did to Sihon and to Og, kings of the
Amorites, and unto the land of them,
whom he destroyed.
5 And the LORD shall give them up
before your face, that ye may do unto
them according unto all the commandments which I have commanded you.
6 [a]Be strong and of a good courage, fear
not, nor be afraid of them: for the LORD
thy God, he *it is* that doth go with thee;
[b]he will not fail thee, nor forsake thee.
7 And Moses called unto Joshua, and
said unto him in the sight of all Israel, Be
strong and of a good courage: for thou
must go with this people unto the land
which the LORD hath sworn unto their
fathers to give them; and thou shalt
cause them to inherit it.
8 And the LORD, he *it is* that doth go
before thee; [c]he will be with thee, he will
not fail thee, neither forsake thee: fear
not, neither be dismayed.
9 And Moses wrote this law, and delivered it unto the priests the sons of Levi,
which bare the ark of the covenant of the
LORD, and unto all the elders of Israel.
10 And Moses commanded them, saying, At the end of *every* seven years, in
the solemnity of the year of release, in
the feast of tabernacles,
11 When all Israel is come to appear
before the LORD thy God in the place
which he shall choose, thou shalt read
this law before all Israel in their hearing.
12 Gather the people together, men,
and women, and children, and thy
stranger that *is* within thy gates, that
they may hear, and that they may learn,
and [d]fear the LORD your God, and
observe to do all the words of this law:
13 And *that* their children, which have
not known *any thing*, may hear, and
learn to [d]fear the LORD your God, as long
as ye live in the land whither ye go over
Jordan to possess it.

Jehovah warns Moses of the apostasy
of Israel. (Cf. 1 Tim. 4:1–3;
2 Tim. 3: 1–8; Jude 1–19.)

14 And the LORD said unto Moses,
Behold, thy days approach that thou
must die: call Joshua, and present yourselves in the tabernacle of the congregation, that I may give him a charge. And
Moses and Joshua went, and presented
themselves in the tabernacle of the congregation.
15 And the LORD appeared in the
tabernacle in a pillar of a cloud: and the
pillar of the cloud stood over the door of
the tabernacle.
16 And the LORD said unto Moses,
Behold, thou shalt sleep with thy fathers;
and this people will rise up, and go a
whoring after the gods of the strangers
of the land, whither they go *to be* among
them, and will forsake me, and break my
covenant which I have made with them.
17 Then my anger shall be kindled
against them in that day, and I will forsake them, and I will hide my face from
them, and they shall be devoured, and
many evils and troubles shall befall
them; so that they will say in that day,
Are not these evils come upon us,
because our God *is* not among us?
18 And I will surely hide my face in
that day for all the evils which they shall
have wrought, in that they are turned
unto other gods.
19 Now therefore write ye this song
for you, and teach it the children of
[e]Israel: put it in their mouths, that this
song may be a witness for me against
the children of Israel.
20 For when I shall have brought them
into the land which I sware unto their
fathers, that floweth with milk and
honey; and they shall have eaten and
filled themselves, and waxen fat; then
will they turn unto other gods, and serve
them, and provoke me, and break my
covenant.

B.C. 1451.

a Josh. 10:25; 1 Chr. 22:13.

b Heb. 13:5.

c Josh. 1:5, 9; 1 Chr. 28:20.

d Psa. 19:9, *note.*

e *Israel (history).* vs. 16-23; Deut. 32:8, 9. (Gen. 12:2, 3; Rom. 11:26.)

21 And it shall come to pass, when many evils and troubles are befallen them, that this song shall testify against them as a witness; for it shall not be forgotten out of the mouths of their seed: for I know their imagination [a]which they go about, even now, before I have brought them into the land which I sware.

22 Moses therefore wrote this song the same day, and taught it the children of Israel.

23 And he gave Joshua the son of Nun a charge, and said, Be strong and of a good courage: for thou shalt bring the children of Israel into the land which I sware unto them: and I will be with thee.

Moses instructs the Levites.

24 And it came to pass, when Moses had made an end of writing the [b]words of this law in a book, until they were finished,

25 That Moses commanded the Levites, which bare the ark of the covenant of the LORD, saying,

26 Take this book of the law, [c]and put it in the side of the ark of the covenant of the LORD your God, that it may be there for a witness against thee.

27 For I know thy rebellion, and thy stiff neck: behold, while I am yet alive with you this day, ye have been rebellious against the LORD; and how much more after my death?

28 Gather unto me all the elders of your tribes, and your officers, that I may speak these words in their ears, and call heaven and earth to record against them.

29 For I know that after my death ye will utterly corrupt *yourselves*, and turn aside from the way which I have commanded you; and evil will befall you in the latter days; because ye will do evil in the sight of the LORD, to provoke him to anger through the work of your hands.

30 And Moses spake in the ears of all the congregation of Israel the words of this song, until they were ended.

CHAPTER 32.

The song of Moses.

Give ear, O ye heavens, and I will speak; and hear, O earth, the words of my mouth.

2 [d]My doctrine shall drop as the rain, my speech shall distil as the dew, as the small rain upon the tender herb, and as the showers upon the grass:

3 Because I will publish the name of the LORD: ascribe ye greatness unto our God.

4 *He is* the Rock, his work *is* perfect: for [e]all his ways *are* judgment: a God of truth and without iniquity, just and right *is* he.

5 They have corrupted themselves, their spot *is* not *the spot* of his children: *they are* a perverse and crooked generation.

6 Do ye thus requite the LORD, O foolish people and unwise? *is* not he thy father *that* hath bought thee? hath he not made thee, and established thee?

7 Remember the days of old, consider the years of many generations: ask thy father, and he will shew thee; thy elders, and they will tell thee.

8 When the most High divided to the nations their [f]inheritance, when he separated the sons of Adam, he set the bounds of the people according to the number of the children of Israel.

9 For the LORD'S portion *is* his people; Jacob *is* the lot of his inheritance.

10 He found him [g]in a desert land, and in the waste howling wilderness; he led him about, he instructed him, he kept him as the apple of his eye.

11 As an eagle stirreth up her nest, fluttereth over her young, spreadeth abroad her wings, taketh them, beareth them on her wings:

12 *So* the LORD alone did lead him, and *there was* no strange god with him.

13 He made him ride on the high places of the earth, that he might eat the increase of the fields; and he made him to suck honey out of the rock, and oil out of the flinty rock;

14 Butter of kine, and milk of sheep, with fat of lambs, and rams of the breed of Bashan, and goats, with the fat of kidneys of wheat; and thou didst drink the pure blood of the grape.

15 But Jeshurun waxed fat, and kicked: thou art waxen fat, thou art grown thick, thou art covered *with fatness*; then he forsook God *which* made him, and lightly esteemed the Rock of his salvation.

16 They provoked him to jealousy with strange *gods*, with abominations provoked they him to anger.

B.C. 1451.

a Amos 5:25, 26.

b *Inspiration.* 2 Sam. 23:2. (Ex. 4:15; Rev. 22:19.)

c See 2 Ki. 22:8.

d Isa. 55:10, 11; 1 Cor. 3:6-8.

e Dan. 4:37; Rev. 15:3.

f *Israel (history).* vs. 8, 9; Deut. 34:1-5. (Gen. 12:2, 3; Rom. 11:26.)

g Jer. 2:6; Hos. 13:5.

B.C. 1451.

17 They sacrificed unto [a]devils, not to
God; to gods whom they knew not, to
new *gods that* came newly up, whom
your fathers feared not.
18 [b]Of the Rock *that* begat thee thou
art unmindful, and hast forgotten God
that formed thee.
19 [c]And when the LORD saw *it*, he
abhorred *them*, because of the provoking
of his sons, and of his daughters.
20 And he said, I will hide my face
from them, I will see what their end *shall*
be: for they *are* a very froward generation, children in whom *is* no faith.
21 They have moved me to [d]jealousy
with *that which is* not God; they have
provoked me to anger with their vanities: and I will move them to [d]jealousy
with *those which are* not a people; I will
provoke them to anger with a foolish
nation.
22 For a fire is kindled in mine anger,
and shall burn unto the lowest hell, and
shall consume the earth with her
increase, and set on fire the foundations
of the mountains.
23 I will heap mischiefs upon them; I
will spend mine arrows upon them.
24 *They shall be* burnt with hunger, and
devoured with burning heat, and with
bitter destruction: I will also send the
teeth of beasts upon them, with the poison of serpents of the dust.
25 The sword without, and terror
within, shall destroy both the young
man and the virgin, the suckling *also*
with the man of gray hairs.
26 [e]I said, I would scatter them into
corners, I would make the remembrance
of them to cease from among men:
27 Were it not that I feared the wrath
of the enemy, lest their adversaries
should behave themselves strangely, *and*
lest they should say, Our hand *is* high,
and the LORD hath not done all this.
28 For they *are* a nation void of counsel, neither *is there any* understanding in
them.
29 [f]O that they were wise, *that* they
understood this, *that* they would consider their latter end!
30 How should one chase a thousand,
and two put ten thousand to flight,
except their Rock had sold them, and the
LORD had shut them up?
31 For their rock *is* not as our Rock,
[g]even our enemies themselves *being*
judges.
32 For their vine *is* of the vine of
Sodom, and of the fields of Gomorrah:
their grapes *are* grapes of gall, their clusters *are* bitter:
33 Their wine *is* the poison of dragons,
and the cruel venom of asps.
34 *Is* not this [h]laid up in store with me,
and sealed up among my treasures?
35 To me *belongeth* vengeance, and
[i]recompence; their foot shall slide in *due*
time: for the day of their calamity *is* at
hand, and the things that shall come
upon them make haste.
36 For the LORD shall judge his people,
and [j]repent himself for his servants,
when he seeth that *their* power is gone,
and *there is* none shut up, or left.
37 And he shall say, Where *are* their
gods, *their* rock in whom they [k]trusted,
38 Which did eat the fat of their sacrifices, *and* drank the wine of their drink-
offerings? let them rise up and help you,
and be your protection.
39 See now that I, *even* I, *am* he, and
there is no god with me: I kill, and I make
alive; I wound, and I heal: neither *is there*
any that can deliver out of my hand.
40 For I lift up my hand to heaven,
and say, I live for ever.
41 If I whet my glittering sword, and
mine hand take hold on judgment; I will
render vengeance to mine enemies, and
will reward them that hate me.
42 I will make mine arrows drunk
with blood, and my sword shall devour
flesh; *and that* with the blood of the slain
and of the captives, from the beginning
of revenges upon the enemy.
43 Rejoice, O ye nations, *with* his [l]peo-
ple: for he will avenge the blood of his
servants, and will render vengeance to
his adversaries, and will be merciful
unto his land, *and* to his people.
44 And Moses came and spake all the
words of this song in the ears of the people, he, and Hoshea the son of Nun.

The exhortation.

45 And Moses made an end of speaking all these words to all Israel:

a *Spoiler, destroyer.*
b Isa. 17:10.
c Jud. 2:14.
d Rom. 10:19; 11:11.
e Ezk. 20:13, 14, 23.
f Psa. 81:13; Lk. 19:42.
g 1 Sam. 4:7-8; Jer. 40:2-3.
h Hos. 13:12; Rom. 2:5.
i Rom. 12:19; Heb. 10:30.
j Zech. 8:14, *note.*
k Psa. 2:12, *note.*
l Rom. 15:10.

46 And he said unto them, [a]Set your hearts unto all the words which I testify among you this day, which ye shall command your children to observe to do, all the words of this law.

47 For it *is* not a vain thing for you; because it *is* your life: and through this thing ye shall prolong *your* days in the land, whither ye go over Jordan to possess it.

48 And the LORD spake unto Moses that selfsame day, saying,

49 Get thee up into this mountain Abarim, *unto* mount Nebo, which *is* in the land of Moab, that *is* over against Jericho; and behold the land of Canaan, which I give unto the children of Israel for a possession:

50 And die in the mount whither thou goest up, and be gathered unto thy people; as Aaron thy brother died in mount Hor, and was gathered unto his people:

51 Because ye trespassed against me among the children of Israel at the waters of Meribah-Kadesh, in the wilderness of Zin; because ye sanctified me not in the midst of the children of Israel.

52 Yet thou shalt see the land before *thee*; but thou shalt not go thither unto the land which I give the children of Israel.

CHAPTER 33.

The blessing of the tribes.

And this *is* [b]the blessing, wherewith Moses the man of God blessed the children of Israel before his death.

2 And he said, The LORD came from Sinai, and rose up from Seir unto them; he shined forth from mount Paran, and he came with ten thousands of saints: from his right hand *went* a fiery law for them.

3 Yea, he loved the people; all his saints *are* in thy hand: and they [c]sat down at thy feet; *every one* shall receive of thy words.

4 [d]Moses commanded us a law, *even* the inheritance of the congregation of Jacob.

5 And he was [e]king in Jeshurun, when the heads of the people *and* the tribes of Israel were gathered together.

6 Let Reuben live, and not die; and let *not* his men be few.

7 And this *is the blessing* of Judah: and he said, Hear, LORD, the voice of Judah, and bring him unto his people: let his hands be sufficient for him; and be thou an help *to him* from his enemies.

8 And of Levi he said, *Let* thy [f]Thummim and thy Urim *be* with thy holy one, whom thou didst prove at Massah, *and with* whom thou didst strive at the waters of Meribah;

9 Who said unto his father and to his mother, I have not seen him; neither did he acknowledge his brethren, nor knew his own children: for they have observed thy word, and kept thy covenant.

10 They shall teach Jacob thy judgments, and Israel thy law: they shall put incense before thee, and whole burnt sacrifice upon thine altar.

11 Bless, LORD, his substance, and accept the work of his hands: smite through the loins of them that rise against him, and of them that hate him, that they rise not again.

12 *And* of Benjamin he said, The beloved of the LORD shall dwell in safety by him; *and the LORD* shall cover him all the day long, and he shall dwell between his shoulders.

13 And of Joseph he said, Blessed of the LORD *be* his land, for the precious things of heaven, for the dew, and for the deep that coucheth beneath,

14 And for the precious fruits *brought forth* by the sun, and for the precious things put forth by the moon,

15 And for the chief things of the ancient mountains, and for the precious things of the lasting hills,

16 And for the precious things of the earth and fulness thereof, and *for* the good will of him that dwelt in the bush: let *the blessing* come upon the head of Joseph, and upon the top of the head of him *that was* separated from his brethren.

17 His glory *is like* the firstling of his bullock, and his horns *are like* the horns of unicorns: with them he shall push the people together to the ends of the earth: and they *are* the ten thousands of Ephraim, and they *are* the thousands of Manasseh.

18 And of Zebulun he said, Rejoice, Zebulun, in thy going out; and, Issachar, in thy tents.

19 They shall [g]call the people unto the mountain; there they shall offer sacrifices of righteousness: for they shall suck *of* the abundance of the seas, and *of* treasures hid in the sand.

B.C. 1451.

a Ezk. 40:4.

b Gen. 49:28.

c Lk. 10:39; Acts 22:3.

d John 1:17; 7:19.

e *Kingdom* (O.T.). vs. 4, 5; Josh. 1:1-5. (Gen. 1:26; Zech. 12:8.)

f See Ex. 28:30, *note*.

g Isa. 2:3.

20 And of Gad he said, Blessed *be* he
that enlargeth Gad: he dwelleth as a lion,
and teareth the arm with the crown of
the head.
21 And he provided the first part for
himself, because there, *in* a portion of
the lawgiver, *was he* seated; and he came
with the heads of the people, he executed the justice of the LORD, and his judgments with Israel.
22 And of Dan he said, Dan *is* a lion's
whelp: he shall leap from Bashan.
23 And of Naphtali he said, O
Naphtali, satisfied with favour, and full
with the blessing of the LORD: possess
thou the west and the south.
24 And of Asher he said, *Let* Asher *be*
blessed with children; let him be acceptable to his brethren, and let him dip his
foot in oil.
25 Thy shoes *shall be* iron and brass;
and as thy days, *so shall* thy strength *be*.
26 *There is* none like unto the God of
Jeshurun, *who* rideth upon the heaven in
thy help, and in his excellency on the
sky.
27 The eternal God *is thy* [a]refuge, and
underneath *are* the everlasting arms: and
he shall thrust out the enemy from
before thee; and shall say, Destroy *them*.
28 [b]Israel then shall dwell in safety
alone: the fountain of Jacob *shall be* upon
a land of corn and wine; also his heavens shall drop down dew.
29 Happy *art* thou, O Israel: who *is* like
unto thee, O people saved by the LORD,
the shield of thy help, and who *is* the
sword of thy excellency! and thine enemies shall be found liars unto thee; and
thou shalt tread upon their high places.

CHAPTER 34.

The vision and death of Moses.

And Moses went up from the plains
of Moab unto the mountain of
Nebo, to the top of Pisgah, that *is* over
against Jericho. And the LORD [c]shewed
him all the land of Gilead, unto Dan,
2 And all Naphtali, and the land of
Ephraim, and Manasseh, and all the
land of Judah, unto the utmost sea,
3 And the south, and the plain of the
valley of Jericho, the city of palm trees,
unto Zoar.
4 And the LORD said unto him, This *is*
the land which I sware unto Abraham,
unto Isaac, and unto Jacob, saying, I will
give it unto thy seed: I have caused thee
to see *it* with thine eyes, but thou shalt
not go over thither.
5 So Moses the servant of the LORD
died there in the land of Moab, according to the word of the LORD.
6 And he buried him in a valley in the
land of Moab, over against Beth-peor:
but [d]no man knoweth of his sepulchre
unto this day.
7 And Moses *was* an hundred and
twenty years old when he died: his eye
was not dim, nor his natural force abated.
8 And the children of Israel wept for
Moses in the plains of Moab [e]thirty
days: so the days of weeping *and* mourning for Moses were ended.

After Moses, Joshua.

9 And Joshua the son of Nun was full
of the [f]spirit of wisdom; for Moses had
[g]laid his hands upon him: and the children of Israel hearkened unto him, and
did as the LORD commanded Moses.
10 And there arose not a prophet since
in Israel like unto Moses, [h]whom the
LORD knew face to face,
11 In all the signs and the wonders,
which the LORD sent him to do in the
land of Egypt to Pharaoh, and to all his
servants, and to all his land,
12 And in all that mighty hand, and in
all the great terror which Moses shewed
in the sight of all Israel.

B.C. 1451.

a Psa. 90:1; 91:2, 9.

b Jer. 23:6; 33:16.

c *Israel (history).* vs. 1-5; Josh. 3:9-17. (Gen. 12:2, 3; Rom. 11:26.)

d Jude 9.

e Gen. 50:3, 10.

f *Holy Spirit.* Jud. 3:10. (Gen. 1:2; Mal. 2:15.)

g Num. 27:3; Acts 8:17; 1 Tim. 4:14.

h Ex. 33:11; Num. 12:6, 8.

THE HISTORICAL BOOKS

THE Historical Books of the Old Testament, usually so called, are twelve in number, from Joshua to Esther inclusive. It should, however, be remembered that the entire Old Testament is filled with historical material. The accuracy of these writings, often questioned, has been in recent years completely confirmed by the testimony of the monuments of contemporaneous antiquity.

The story of the Historical Books is the story of the rise and fall of the Commonwealth of Israel, while the prophets foretell the future restoration and glory of that people under King Messiah.

The history of Israel falls into seven distinct periods:

I. From the call of Abraham to the Exodus, Gen. 12:1–Ex. 1:22 (with Acts 7). The book of Job belongs to this period and shows the maturity and depth of philosophic and religious thought, and the extent of revelation of the age of the Patriarchs.

II. From the Exodus to the death of Joshua. The history of this period is gathered from the books of Exodus, Numbers, Deuteronomy, Joshua, and such parts of Leviticus as relate to the story of Israel. The great figures of Moses, Aaron, and Joshua dominate this period.

III. The period of the Judges, from the death of Joshua to the call of Saul, Jud. 1:1–1 Sam. 10:24.

IV. The period of the Kings, from Saul to the Captivities, 1 Sam. 11:1–2 Ki. 17:6; 25:30–2 Chr. 36:23.

V. The period of the Captivities, Esther, and the historical parts of Daniel. With the captivity of Judah began "the times of the Gentiles," the mark of which is the political subjection of Israel to the Gentile world-powers (Lk. 21:24).

VI. The restored Commonwealth, always under Gentile over-lordship, from the end of the seventy years' captivity and the return of the Jewish remnant to the destruction of Jerusalem, A.D. 70. The inspired history of this period is found in Ezra, Nehemiah, Haggai, Zechariah, and Malachi in the Old Testament, and in the historical and biographical material found in the New Testament. During this period Christ, the promised King of the Davidic Covenant, and the Seed of the Adamic and Abrahamic Covenants, appeared, was rejected as king, was crucified, rose again from the dead, and ascended to heaven. Toward the end of this period, also, the church came into being, and the New Testament Scriptures, save the Gospel of John, John's Epistles, and the Revelation, were written.

VII. The present dispersion (Lk. 21:20-24), which according to all the Old Testament prophets is to be ended by the final national regathering promised in the Palestinian Covenant (Deut. 30:1-9). The partial restoration at the end of the 70 years was foretold only by Daniel and Jeremiah, and was to the end that Messiah might come and fulfil the prophecies of His sufferings. In the year A.D. 70 Jerusalem was again destroyed, and the descendants of the remnant of Judah sent to share the national dispersion which still continues.

HOW TO USE THE SUBJECT REFERENCES.

THE subject references lead the reader from the first clear mention of a great truth to the last. The first and last references (in parenthesis) are repeated each time, so that wherever a reader comes upon a subject he may recur to the first reference and follow the subject, or turn at once to the Summary at the last reference.

ILLUSTRATION

(at Mark 1:1.)

b Gospel. vs. 1, 14, 15; Mk. 8:35. (Gen. 12:1-3; Rev. 14:6.)

Here *Gospel* is the subject; vs. 1, 14, 15 show where it is at that particular place; Mk. 8:35 is the next reference in the chain, and the references in parenthesis are the first and last.

THE BOOK OF JOSHUA

JOSHUA records the consummation of the redemption of Israel out of Egypt; for redemption has two parts: "out," and "into" (Deut. 6:23). The key-phrase is "Moses My servant is dead" (Josh. 1:2). Law, of which Moses is the representative, could never give a sinful people victory (Heb. 7:19; Rom. 6:14; 8:2-4)

In a spiritual sense the book of Joshua is the Ephesians of the Old Testament. "The heavenly" of Ephesians is to the Christian what Canaan was to the Israelite—a place of conflict, and therefore not a type of heaven, but also a place of victory and blessing through divine power (Josh. 21:43-45; Eph. 1:3).

The government, as before, was theocratic; Joshua succeeding Moses as the ruler under God.

Joshua falls into four parts: I. The conquest, 1–12. II. The partition of the inheritance, 13–21. III. Incipient discord, 22. IV. Joshua's last counsels and death, 23, 24.

The events recorded in Joshua cover a period of 26 years (Ussher).

CHAPTER 1.

Now after the [a]death of Moses the servant of the LORD it came to pass, that the LORD spake unto [1b]Joshua the [c]son of Nun, Moses' minister, saying,

Joshua commissioned.

2 Moses my servant is dead; now therefore arise, go over this Jordan, thou, and all this people, unto the land which I do give to them, *even* to the children of Israel.

3 [d]Every place that the sole of your foot shall tread upon, that have I given unto you, as I said unto Moses.

4 From the wilderness and this Lebanon even unto the great river, the river Euphrates, all the land of the Hittites, and unto the great sea toward the going down of the sun, shall be your coast.

5 There shall not any man be able to stand before thee all the days of thy life: as I was with Moses, *so* [e]I will be with thee: I will not fail thee, nor forsake thee.

6 Be [f]strong and of a good courage: for unto this people shalt thou divide for an inheritance the land, which I sware unto their fathers to give them.

7 Only be thou strong and very courageous, that thou mayest observe to do according to all the law, which Moses my servant commanded thee: [g]turn not from it *to* the right hand or *to* the left, that thou mayest prosper whithersoever thou goest.

8 [h]This book of the law shall not depart out of thy mouth; but thou shalt [i]meditate therein day and night, that thou mayest observe to do according to all that is written therein: for then thou shalt make thy way prosperous, and then thou shalt have good success.

9 Have not I commanded thee? Be strong and of a good courage; be not afraid, neither be thou dismayed: for the LORD thy God *is* with thee whithersoever thou goest.

Joshua assumes command.

10 Then Joshua commanded the officers of the people, saying,

11 Pass through the host, and command the people, saying, Prepare you victuals; for within three days ye shall pass over this Jordan, to go in to possess the land, which the LORD your God giveth you to possess it.

12 And to the Reubenites, and to the Gadites, and to half the tribe of Manasseh, spake Joshua, saying,

13 Remember the word which Moses the servant of the LORD commanded you, saying, The LORD your God hath

B.C. 1451.

a Deut. 34:5; Cf. Rev. 1:18.

b *Kingdom* (O.T.). vs. 1-5; Jud. 2:16-18. (Gen. 1:26; Zech. 12:8.)

c Num. 13:16; 14:6, 29, 30, 37, 38; Acts 7:45.

d The law of appropriation. God gives, but we must take.

e Deut. 31:6-7; Heb. 13:5.

f Phil. 4:13.

g 1 Cor. 9:26, 27.

h Cf. Col. 3:16, 17.

i Psa. 1:2, 3; 143:5; Jer. 15:16, 17; Ezk. 3:1-4; *contra*, Hos. 10:13.

[1]**(1:1)** Joshua (Je-hoshua, meaning Jehovah-Saviour) is a type of Christ, the "Captain of our salvation" (Heb. 2:10, 11). The more important points are: (1) He comes after Moses (John 1:17; Rom. 8:3, 4; 10:4, 5; Heb. 7:18, 19; Gal. 3:23-25). (2) He leads to victory (Rom. 8:37; 2 Cor. 1:10; 2:14). (3) He is our Advocate when we have suffered defeat (Josh. 7:5-9; 1 John 2:1). (4) He allots our portions (Eph. 1:11, 14; 4:8-11).

given you rest, and hath given you this land.

14 Your wives, your little ones, and your cattle, shall remain in the land which Moses gave you on this side Jordan; but ye shall pass before your brethren armed, all the mighty men of valour, and help them;

15 Until the LORD have given your brethren rest, as *he hath given* you, and they also have possessed the land which the LORD your God giveth them: then ye shall return unto the land of your possession, and enjoy it, which Moses the LORD'S servant gave you on this side Jordan toward the sunrising.

16 And they answered Joshua, saying, All that thou commandest us we will do, and whithersoever thou sendest us, we will go.

17 According as we hearkened unto Moses in all things, so will we hearken unto thee: only the LORD thy God be with thee, as he was with Moses.

18 Whosoever *he be* that doth rebel against thy commandment, and will not hearken unto thy words in all that thou commandest him, he shall be put to death: only be strong and of a good courage.

CHAPTER 2.

Rahab and the spies.

And Joshua the son of Nun sent out of Shittim two men to spy secretly, saying, Go view the land, even Jericho. And they went, and came into an harlot's house, named [a]Rahab, and lodged there.

2 And it was told the king of Jericho, saying, Behold, there came men in hither to night of the children of Israel to search out the country.

3 And the king of Jericho sent unto Rahab, saying, Bring forth the men that are come to thee, which are entered into thine house: for they be come to search out all the country.

4 And the woman took the two men, and hid them, and said thus, There came men unto me, but I wist not whence they *were*:

5 And it came to pass *about the time* of shutting of the gate, when it was dark, that the men went out: whither the men went I wot not: pursue after them quickly; for ye shall overtake them.

6 But she had [b]brought them up to the roof of the house, and hid them with the stalks of flax, which she had laid in order upon the roof.

7 And the men pursued after them the way to Jordan unto the fords: and as soon as they which pursued after them were gone out, they shut the gate.

8 And before they were laid down, she came up unto them upon the roof;

9 And she said unto the men, [c]I know that the LORD hath given you the land, and that your [d]terror is fallen upon us, and that all the inhabitants of the land faint because of you.

10 For we have heard how the LORD [e]dried up the water of the Red sea for you, when ye came out of Egypt; and what ye [f]did unto the two kings of the Amorites, that *were* on the other side Jordan, Sihon and Og, whom ye utterly destroyed.

11 And as soon as we had heard *these things*, our hearts did melt, neither did there remain any more courage in any man, because of you: for the LORD your God, he *is* God in heaven above, and in earth beneath.

12 Now therefore, I pray you, swear unto me by the LORD, since I have shewed you kindness, that ye will also shew kindness unto my father's house, and give me a true [g]token:

13 And *that* ye will save [h]alive my father, and my mother, and my brethren, and my sisters, and all that they have, and deliver our lives from death.

14 And the men answered her, Our life for yours, if ye utter not this our business. And it shall be, when the LORD hath given us the land, that we will deal kindly and truly with thee.

15 Then she let them down by a cord through the window: for her house *was* upon the town wall, and she dwelt upon the wall.

16 And she said unto them, Get you to the mountain, lest the pursuers meet you; and hide yourselves there three days, until the pursuers be returned: and afterward may ye go your way.

17 And the men said unto her, We *will be* blameless of this thine oath which thou hast made us swear.

18 Behold, *when* we come into the land, thou shalt bind this [i]line of scarlet thread in the window which thou didst

B.C. 1451.

a Heb. 11:31; Jas. 2:25.
b Jas. 2:24, 25; Heb. 11:31.
c Deut. 1:8.
d Deut. 2:25.
e Ex. 14:21.
f Num. 21:21.
g v. 18.
h Josh. 6:23-25.
i v. 12.

let us down by: and thou shalt bring thy
father, and thy mother, and thy brethren,
and all thy father's household, home
unto thee.
19 And it shall be, *that* whosoever
shall go out of the doors of thy house
into the street, his blood *shall be* upon his
head, and we *will be* guiltless: and
whosoever shall be with thee in the
house, his blood *shall be* on our head, if
any hand be upon him.
20 And if thou utter this our business,
then we will be quit of thine oath which
thou hast made us to swear.
21 And she said, According unto your
words, so *be* it. And she sent them away,
and they departed: and she bound the
scarlet [1]line in the window.
22 And they went, and came unto the
mountain, and abode there three days,
until the pursuers were returned: and
the pursuers sought *them* throughout all
the way, but found *them* not.
23 So the two men returned, and
descended from the mountain, and
passed over, and came to Joshua the son
of Nun, and told him all *things* that
befell them:
24 And they said unto Joshua, Truly
the LORD hath delivered into our hands
all the land; for even all the inhabitants
of the country do faint because of us.

CHAPTER 3.

The Passage of Jordan.

And Joshua rose early in the morning;
and they removed from Shittim,
and came to [2]Jordan, he and all the children of Israel, and lodged there before
they passed over.
2 And it came to pass after three days,
that the officers went through the host;
3 And they commanded the people,
saying, When ye see the ark of the
covenant of the LORD your God, and the
priests the Levites bearing it, then ye shall
remove from your place, and go after it.
4 Yet there shall be a [a]space between
you and it, about two thousand [b]cubits
by measure: come not near unto it, that
ye may know the way by which ye must
go: for ye have not passed *this* way
heretofore.
5 And Joshua said unto the people,
[c]Sanctify yourselves: for to morrow the
LORD will do wonders among you.
6 And Joshua spake unto the priests,
saying, Take up the ark of the covenant,
and pass over before the people. And
they took up the ark of the covenant,
and went before the people.
7 And the LORD said unto Joshua, This
day will I begin to magnify thee in the
sight of all Israel, that they may know
that, as I was with Moses, *so* I will be
with thee.
8 And thou shalt command the priests
that bear the ark of the covenant, saying,
When ye are come to the brink of the
water of Jordan, ye shall stand still in
Jordan.
9 And Joshua said unto the children of
[d]Israel, Come hither, and hear the words
of the LORD your God.
10 And Joshua said, Hereby ye shall
know that the living God *is* among you,
and *that* he will without fail drive out
from before you the Canaanites, and the
Hittites, and the Hivites, and the
Perizzites, and the Girgashites, and the
Amorites, and the Jebusites.
11 Behold, the ark of the covenant of
the Lord of all the earth passeth over
[e]before you into Jordan.
12 Now therefore take you twelve
men out of the tribes of Israel, out of
every tribe a man.
13 And it shall come to pass, as soon as
the soles of the feet of the priests that bear
the ark of the LORD, the Lord of all the
earth, shall rest in the waters of Jordan,
that the waters of Jordan shall be cut off
from the waters that come down from
above; and they shall stand upon an heap.
14 And it came to pass, when the people removed from their tents, to pass
over Jordan, and the priests bearing the
ark of the covenant before the people;
15 And as they that bare the ark were
come unto Jordan, and the feet of the
priests that bare the ark were dipped in
the brim of the water, (for Jordan

B.C. 1451.

a Heb. 10:19-22.

b One cubit = about 18 in.

c Ex. 19:10-15; Josh. 7:13; Job 1:5; Joel 2:16.

d *Israel* (*history*). vs. 9-17; Josh. 24:29-33. (Gen. 12:2, 3; Rom. 11:26.)

e Ex. 13:21, 22; John 10:4; Heb. 2:14-18; 12:2-4.

[1]**(2:21)** The scarlet line of Rahab speaks, by its color, of safety through *sacrifice* (Heb. 9:19, 22).

[2]**(3:1)** The passage of Jordan, type of our death with Christ (Rom. 6:6-11; Eph. 2:5, 6; Col. 3:1-3).

overfloweth all his banks all the time of
harvest,)
16 That the [a]waters which came down
from above stood *and* rose up upon an
heap very far from the city Adam, that *is*
beside Zaretan: and those that came down
toward the sea of the plain, *even* the salt
sea, failed, *and* were cut off: and the people passed over right against Jericho.
17 And the priests that bare the ark of
the covenant of the LORD stood firm on
dry ground in the midst of Jordan, and
all the Israelites passed over on dry
ground, until all the people were passed
clean over Jordan.

CHAPTER 4.

The two memorials.

And it came to pass, when all the people were clean passed over Jordan,
that the LORD spake unto Joshua, saying,
2 Take you twelve men out of the people, out of every tribe a man,
3 And command ye them, saying,
Take you hence out of the midst of
Jordan, out of the place where the
priests' feet stood firm, twelve [1]stones,
and ye shall carry them over with you,
and leave them in the lodging place,
where ye shall lodge this night.
4 Then Joshua called the twelve men,
whom he had prepared of the children
of Israel, out of every tribe a man:
5 And Joshua said unto them, Pass
over before the ark of the LORD your
God into the midst of Jordan, and take
ye up every man of you a stone upon his
shoulder, according unto the number of
the tribes of the children of Israel:
6 That this may be a [b]sign among you,
that when your children ask *their fathers*
in time to come, saying, What *mean* ye
by these stones?
7 Then ye shall answer them, That the
waters of Jordan were cut off before the
ark of the covenant of the LORD; when it
passed over Jordan, the waters of Jordan
were cut off: and these stones shall be
for a memorial unto the children of
Israel for ever.
8 And the children of Israel did so as

B.C. 1451.

a *Miracles* (O.T.). vs. 14-17; Josh. 4:1-18. (Gen. 5:24; Jon. 2:1-10.)

b Deut. 27:2; Psa. 103:2.

c *Miracles* (O.T.). vs. 1-18; Josh. 6:6-25. (Gen. 5:24; Jon. 2:1-10.)

Joshua commanded, and took up twelve
stones out of the midst of Jordan, as the
LORD spake unto Joshua, according to
the number of the tribes of the children
of Israel, and carried them over with
them unto the place where they lodged,
and laid them down there.
9 And Joshua set up twelve stones in
the midst of Jordan, in the place where
the feet of the priests which bare the ark
of the covenant stood: and they are there
unto this day.
10 For the priests which bare the ark
stood in the midst of Jordan, until every
thing was finished that the LORD commanded Joshua to speak unto the people, according to all that Moses commanded Joshua: and the people hasted
and passed over.
11 And it came to pass, when all the
people were clean passed over, that the
ark of the LORD passed over, and the
priests, in the presence of the people.
12 And the children of Reuben, and
the children of Gad, and half the tribe of
Manasseh, passed over armed before the
children of Israel, as Moses spake unto
them:
13 About forty thousand prepared for
war passed over before the LORD unto
battle, to the plains of Jericho.
14 On that day the LORD magnified
Joshua in the sight of all Israel; and they
feared him, as they feared Moses, all the
days of his life.
15 And the LORD spake unto Joshua,
saying,
16 Command the priests that bear the
ark of the testimony, that they come up
out of Jordan.
17 Joshua therefore commanded the
priests, saying, Come ye up out of
Jordan.
18 And it came to pass, when the
priests that bare the ark of the covenant
of the LORD were come up out of the
midst of [c]Jordan, *and* the soles of the
priests' feet were lifted up unto the dry
land, that the waters of Jordan returned
unto their place, and flowed over all his
banks, as *they did* before.

[1]**(4:3)** The two memorials. The twelve stones taken out of Jordan and erected by Joshua in Gilgal, and the twelve stones left in Jordan to be overwhelmed by its waters, are memorials marking the distinction between Christ's death under judgment in the believer's place (Psa. 42:7; 88:7; John 12:31-33), and the believer's perfect deliverance from judgment. The stones in Jordan stand, typically, for Psa. 22:1-18.

The encampment at Gilgal.

19 And the people came up out of Jordan on the tenth *day* of the [a]first month, and encamped in Gilgal, in the east border of Jericho.

20 And those twelve stones, which they took out of Jordan, did Joshua pitch in Gilgal.

21 And he spake unto the children of Israel, saying, When your children shall ask their fathers in time to come, saying, What *mean* these stones?

22 Then [b]ye shall let your children know, saying, Israel came over this Jordan on dry land.

23 For the LORD your God dried up the waters of Jordan from before you, until ye were passed over, as the LORD your God did to the Red sea, which he dried up from before us, until we were gone over:

24 That all the people of the earth might know the hand of the LORD, that it *is* mighty: that ye might fear the LORD your God for ever.

CHAPTER 5.

And it came to pass, when all the kings of the Amorites, which *were* on the side of Jordan westward, and all the kings of the Canaanites, which *were* by the sea, heard that the LORD had dried up the waters of Jordan from before the children of Israel, until we were passed over, that their heart melted, neither was there spirit in them any more, because of the children of Israel.

The reproach of Egypt rolled away.

2 At that time the LORD said unto Joshua, Make thee sharp knives, and [1]circumcise again the children of Israel the second time.

3 And Joshua made him sharp knives, and [c]circumcised the children of Israel at the hill of the foreskins.

4 And this *is* the cause why Joshua did circumcise: All the people that came out of Egypt, *that were* males, *even* all the men of war, died in the wilderness by the way, after they came out of Egypt.

5 Now all the people that came out were circumcised: but all the people *that were* born in the wilderness by the way as they came forth out of Egypt, *them* they had not circumcised.

6 For the children of Israel walked forty years in the wilderness, till all the people *that were* men of war, which came out of Egypt, were consumed, because they obeyed not the voice of the LORD: unto whom the LORD sware that he would not shew them the land, which the LORD sware unto their fathers that he would give us, a land that floweth with milk and honey.

7 And their children, *whom* he raised up in their stead, them Joshua circumcised: for they were uncircumcised, because they had not circumcised them by the way.

8 And it came to pass, when they had done circumcising all the people, that they abode in their places in the camp, till they were whole.

9 And the LORD said unto Joshua, This day have I rolled away the reproach of Egypt from off you. Wherefore the name of the place is called [d]Gilgal unto this day.

10 And the children of Israel encamped in Gilgal, and kept the passover on the fourteenth day of the [e]month at even in the plains of Jericho.

The new food for the new place.

11 And they did eat of the old [2]corn of the land on the morrow after the

B.C. 1451.

a i.e. *April.*

b Ex. 12:26, 27; 13:8-14; Deut. 26:5-9; 1 Cor. 11:23-26.

c Gen. 17:10-14; Deut. 30:6; Jer. 9:25, 26; Rom. 2:28, 29; 1 Cor. 7:19; Gal. 5:6; 6:15; Phil. 3:3; Col. 2:11.

d *A rolling.*

e See Josh. 4:19.

[1](5:2) Circumcision is the "sign" of the Abrahamic Covenant (Gen. 17:7-14; Rom. 4:11). "The reproach of Egypt" was that, during the later years of the Egyptian bondage, this separating sign had been neglected (cf. Ex. 4:24-26), and this neglect had continued during the wilderness wanderings. The N.T. analogue is world conformity; the failure openly to take a believer's place with Christ in death and resurrection (Rom. 6:2-11; Gal. 6:14-16). Spiritually it is mortifying the deeds of the body through the Spirit (Rom. 8:13; Gal. 5:16, 17; Col. 2:11, 12; 3:5-10).

[2](5:11) The manna is a type of Christ in humiliation, known "after the flesh," giving his flesh that the believer might have life (John 6:49-51); while the "old corn of the land" is Christ apprehended as risen, glorified, and seated in the heavenlies. Occupation with Christ on earth, "crucified through weakness," tends to a wilderness experience. An experience befitting the believer's place in the heavenlies demands an apprehension of the power of His resurrection (2 Cor. 5:16; 13:4; Phil. 3:10; Eph. 1:15-23). It is the contrast between "milk" and "meat" in Paul's writings (1 Cor. 3:1, 2; Heb. 5:12-14; 6:1-3).

passover, unleavened cakes, and parched *corn* in the selfsame day.

12 And the manna ceased on the morrow after they had eaten of the old corn of the land; neither had the children of Israel manna any more; but they did eat of the fruit of the land of Canaan that year.

The unseen Captain.

13 And it came to pass, when Joshua was by Jericho, that he lifted up his eyes and looked, and, behold, there stood a [a]man over against him with his sword drawn in his hand: and Joshua went unto him, and said unto him, *Art* thou for us, or for our adversaries?

14 And he said, Nay; but *as* captain of the host of the LORD am I now come. And Joshua fell on his face to the earth, and did worship, and said unto him, What saith my lord unto his servant?

15 And the captain of the LORD'S host said unto Joshua, Loose thy shoe from off thy foot; for the place whereon thou standest [b]*is* [c]holy. And Joshua did so.

CHAPTER 6.

The conquest of Jericho.

Now Jericho was straitly shut up because of the children of Israel: none went out, and none came in.

2 And the LORD said unto Joshua, See, I have given into thine hand Jericho, and the king thereof, *and* the mighty men of valour.

3 And ye shall compass the city, all *ye* men of war, *and* go round about the city once. Thus shalt thou do six days.

4 And seven priests shall bear before the ark seven trumpets of rams' horns: and the seventh day ye shall compass the city seven times, and the priests shall blow with the trumpets.

5 [1]And it shall come to pass, that when they make a long *blast* with the ram's horn, *and* when ye hear the sound of the trumpet, all the people shall shout with a great shout; and the wall of the city shall fall down flat, and the people shall ascend up every man straight before him.

6 And Joshua the son of Nun called the priests, and said unto them, Take up the ark of the covenant, and let seven priests bear seven trumpets of rams' horns before the ark of the LORD.

7 And he said unto the people, Pass on, and compass the city, and let him that is armed pass on before the ark of the LORD.

8 And it came to pass, when Joshua had spoken unto the people, that the seven priests bearing the seven trumpets of rams' horns passed on before the LORD, and blew with the trumpets: and the ark of the covenant of the LORD followed them.

9 And the armed men went before the priests that blew with the trumpets, and the rereward came after the ark, *the priests* going on, and blowing with the trumpets.

10 And Joshua had commanded the people, saying, Ye shall not shout, nor make any noise with your voice, neither shall *any* word proceed out of your mouth, until the [d]day I bid you shout; then shall ye shout.

11 So the ark of the LORD compassed the city, going about *it* once: and they came into the camp, and lodged in the camp.

12 And Joshua rose early in the morning, and the priests took up the ark of the LORD.

13 And seven priests bearing seven trumpets of rams' horns before the ark of the LORD went on continually, and blew with the trumpets: and the armed men went before them; but the rereward came after the ark of the LORD, *the priests* going on, and blowing with the trumpets.

14 And the second day they compassed the city once, and returned into the camp: so they did six days.

15 And it came to pass on the seventh day, that they rose early about the dawning of the day, and compassed the city after the same manner seven times: only on that day they compassed the city seven times.

16 And it came to pass at the seventh time, when the priests blew with the trumpets, Joshua said unto the people, Shout; for the LORD hath given you the city.

17 And the city shall be accursed, *even* it, and all that *are* therein, to the LORD:

B.C. 1451.

a Cf. Job 42:5, 6; Isa. 6:5; Jer. 1:5, 6; Ezk. 1:28; Dan. 10:5-8; Acts 9:3-6; Rev. 1:17.

b Sanctify, holy (O.T.). Josh. 6:19. (Gen. 2:3; Zech. 8:3.)

c Trans. *"consecrated,"* Josh. 6:19; in R.V. *holy.*

d Cf. Jer. 14:14, 15; 27:14, 15; Jon. 3:2.

[1]**(6:5)** The central truth here is that spiritual victories are won by means and upon principles utterly foolish and inadequate in the view of human wisdom (1 Cor. 1:17-29; 2 Cor. 10:3-5).

only Rahab the harlot shall live, she and all that *are* with her in the house, because she hid the messengers that we sent.

18 And ye, in any wise keep *yourselves* from the accursed thing, lest ye make *yourselves* accursed, when ye take of the accursed thing, and make the camp of Israel a curse, and trouble it.

19 But all the silver, and gold, and vessels of brass and iron, *are* [a]consecrated unto the LORD: they shall come into the treasury of the LORD.

20 So the [b]people shouted when *the priests* blew with the trumpets: and it came to pass, when the people heard the sound of the trumpet, and the people shouted with a great shout, that the wall [c]fell down flat, so that the people went up into the city, every man straight before him, and they took the city.

21 And they utterly destroyed all that *was* in the city, both man and woman, young and old, and ox, and sheep, and ass, with the edge of the sword.

22 But Joshua had said unto the two men that had spied out the country, Go into the harlot's house, and bring out thence the woman, and all that she hath, as ye sware unto her.

23 And the young men that were spies went in, and brought out Rahab, and her father, and her mother, and her brethren, and all that she had; and they brought out all her kindred, and left them without the camp of Israel.

24 And they burnt the city with fire, and all that *was* therein: only the silver, and the gold, and the vessels of brass and of iron, they put into the treasury of the house of the LORD.

25 And Joshua saved Rahab the harlot alive, and her father's household, and all that she had; and she dwelleth in Israel *even* unto this day; because she hid the messengers, which Joshua sent to spy out Jericho.

26 And Joshua adjured *them* at that time, saying, [d]Cursed *be* the man before the LORD, that riseth up and buildeth this city Jericho: he shall lay the foundation thereof in his firstborn, and in his youngest *son* shall he set up the gates of it.

27 So the LORD was with Joshua; and his fame was *noised* throughout all the country.

CHAPTER 7.

The sin of Achan.

But the children of Israel committed a [e]trespass in the accursed thing: for [f]Achan, the son of Carmi, the son of Zabdi, the son of Zerah, of the tribe of Judah, took of the accursed thing: and the anger of the LORD was kindled against the children of Israel.

2 And Joshua sent men from Jericho to Ai, which *is* beside Beth-aven, on the east side of Beth-el, and spake unto them, saying, Go up and view the country. And the men went up and viewed Ai.

3 And they returned to Joshua, and said unto him, Let not all the people go up; but let about two or three thousand men go up and smite Ai; *and* make not all the people to labour thither; for they *are but* few.

4 So there went up thither of the people about three thousand men: and they fled before the men of Ai.

5 And the men of Ai smote of them about thirty and six men: for they chased them *from* before the gate *even* unto Shebarim, and smote them in the going down: wherefore the hearts of the people [g]melted, and became as water.

6 And Joshua rent his clothes, and fell to the earth upon his face before the ark of the LORD until the eventide, he and the elders of Israel, and put dust upon their heads.

7 And Joshua [h]said, Alas, O Lord GOD, [i]wherefore hast thou at all brought this people over Jordan, to deliver us into the hand of the Amorites, to destroy us? would to God we had been content, and dwelt on the other side Jordan!

8 O Lord, what shall I say, when Israel turneth their backs before their enemies!

9 For [j]the Canaanites and all the inhabitants of the land shall hear *of it*, and shall environ us round, and cut off our name from the earth: and what wilt thou do unto thy great name?

10 And the LORD said unto Joshua, Get thee up; wherefore liest thou thus upon thy face?

11 [1]Israel hath sinned, and they have

B.C. 1451.

a *Sanctify, holy* (O.T.). Josh. 7:13. (Gen. 2:3; Zech. 8:3.)

b *Faith.* vs. 20, 25; Psa. 2:12. (Gen. 3:20; Heb. 11:39.)

c *Miracles* (O.T.). vs. 6-25; Josh. 10:12-14. (Gen. 5:24; Jon. 2:1-10.)

d See 1 Ki. 16:34.

e vs. 20, 21.

f Called Achar, Josh. 22:20; 1 Chr. 2:7.

g Cf. Josh. 2:11.

h *Bible prayers* (O.T.). Jud. 13:8, 9. (Gen. 15:2; Hab. 3:1-16.)

i Cf. Ex. 5:22; 14:11; 16:3; 17:3; Num. 21:5.

j Ex. 32:12; Num. 14:13.

[1]**(7:11)** The sin of Achan and its results teach the great truth of the oneness of the people of God, 7:11. "Israel hath sinned." See in illustration 1 Cor. 5:1-7; 12:12-14, 26. The whole cause of Christ is injured by the sin, neglect, or unspirituality of one believer.

B.C. 1451.

also transgressed my covenant which I [a]commanded them: for they have even [b]taken of the accursed thing, and have also stolen, and [c]dissembled also, and they have put *it* even among their own stuff.

12 Therefore the children of Israel could not stand before their enemies, *but* turned *their* backs before their enemies, because they were accursed: neither will I be with you any more, except ye destroy the accursed from among you.

13 Up, sanctify the people, and say, [d]Sanctify yourselves against to morrow: for thus saith the LORD God of Israel, *There is* an accursed thing in the midst of thee, O Israel: thou canst not stand before thine enemies, until ye take away the accursed thing from among you.

14 In the morning therefore ye shall be brought according to your tribes: and it shall be, *that* the tribe which the LORD taketh shall come according to the families *thereof*; and the family which the LORD shall take shall come by households; and the household which the LORD shall take shall come man by man.

15 And it shall be, *that* he that is taken with the accursed thing shall be burnt with fire, he and all that he hath: because he hath transgressed the covenant of the LORD, and because he hath wrought folly in Israel.

16 So Joshua rose up early in the morning, and brought Israel by their tribes; and the tribe of Judah was taken:

17 And he brought the family of Judah; and he took the family of the Zarhites: and he brought the family of the Zarhites man by man; and Zabdi was taken:

18 And he brought his household man by man; and Achan, the son of Carmi, the son of Zabdi, the son of Zerah, of the tribe of Judah, was taken.

19 And Joshua said unto Achan, My son, give, I pray thee, glory to the LORD God of Israel, and make [e]confession unto him; and tell me now what thou hast done; hide *it* not from me.

20 And Achan answered Joshua, and said, Indeed I have sinned against the LORD God of Israel, and thus and thus have I done:

21 When I saw among the spoils a goodly Babylonish garment, and two hundred [f]shekels of silver, and a wedge of gold of fifty shekels weight, then I coveted them, and took them; and, behold, they *are* hid in the earth in the midst of my tent, and the silver under it.

22 So Joshua sent messengers, and they ran unto the tent; and, behold, *it was* hid in his tent, and the silver under it.

23 And they took them out of the midst of the tent, and brought them unto Joshua, and unto all the children of Israel, and laid them out before the LORD.

24 And Joshua, and all Israel with him, took Achan the son of Zerah, and the silver, and the garment, and the wedge of gold, and his sons, and his daughters, and his oxen, and his asses, and his sheep, and his tent, and all that he had: and they brought them unto the valley of Achor.

25 And Joshua said, Why hast thou troubled us? the LORD shall trouble thee this day. And all Israel stoned him with stones, and burned them with fire, after they had stoned them with stones.

26 And they raised over him a great heap of stones unto this day. So the LORD turned from the fierceness of his anger. Wherefore the name of that place was called, The [g]valley of Achor, unto this day.

CHAPTER 8.

The conquest of Ai.

And the LORD said unto Joshua, [h]Fear not, neither be thou dismayed: take all the people of war with thee, and arise, go up to Ai: see, I have [i]given into thy hand the king of Ai, and his people, and his city, and his land:

2 And thou shalt do to Ai and her king as thou didst unto Jericho and her king: only the [j]spoil thereof, and the cattle thereof, shall ye take for a prey unto yourselves: lay thee an ambush for the city behind it.

3 So Joshua arose, and all the people of war, to go up against Ai: and Joshua chose out thirty thousand mighty men of valour, and sent them away by night.

4 And he commanded them, saying, Behold, ye shall lie in wait against the

a Josh. 6:17, 18.

b v. 21.

c Acts 5:1, 2; Heb. 4:13.

d *Sanctify, holy* (O.T.). 1 Ki. 7:51. (Gen. 2:3; Zech. 8:3.)

e Num. 5:6, 7; 2 Chr. 30:22; Psa. 32:5; Prov. 28:13; Jer. 3:12, 13.

f One shekel = 2*s.* 9*d.*, or 65 cts.

g Isa. 65:10; Hos. 2:15.

h Josh. 1:9; 10:8.

i Josh. 6:2.

j Cf. Deut. 20:14.

city, *even* behind the city: go not very far from the city, but be ye all ready:

5 And I, and all the people that *are* with me, will approach unto the city: and it shall come to pass, when they come out against us, as at the first, that we will flee before them,

6 (For they will come out after us) till we have drawn them from the city; for they will say, They flee before us, as at the first: therefore we will flee before them.

7 Then ye shall rise up from the ambush, and seize upon the city: for the LORD your God will deliver it into your hand.

8 And it shall be, when ye have taken the city, *that* ye shall set the city on fire: [a]according to the commandment of the LORD shall ye do. See, I have commanded you.

9 Joshua therefore sent them forth: and they went to lie in ambush, and abode between Beth-el and Ai, on the west side of Ai: but Joshua lodged that night among the people.

10 And Joshua rose up early in the morning, and numbered the people, and went up, he and the elders of Israel, before the people to Ai.

11 And all the people, *even the people* of war that *were* with him, went up, and drew nigh, and came before the city, and pitched on the north side of Ai: now *there was* a valley between them and Ai.

12 And he took about five thousand men, and set them to lie in ambush between Beth-el and Ai, on the west side of the city.

13 And when they had set the people, *even* all the host that *was* on the north of the city, and their liers in wait on the west of the city, Joshua went that night into the midst of the valley.

14 And it came to pass, when the king of Ai saw *it*, that they hasted and rose up early, and the men of the city went out against Israel to battle, he and all his people, at a time appointed, before the plain; but he wist not that *there were* liers in ambush against him behind the city.

15 And Joshua and all Israel made as if they were beaten before them, and fled by the way of the wilderness.

16 And all the people that *were* in Ai were called together to pursue after them: and they pursued after Joshua,

B.C. 1451.

a Deut. 20:16-18; cf. Josh. 15:13; 1 Chr. 12:23.

b Ex. 14:16; Psa. 44:3.

c Deut. 7:2.

and were drawn away from the city.

17 And there was not a man left in Ai or Beth-el, that went not out after Israel: and they left the city open, and pursued after Israel.

18 And the LORD said unto Joshua, [b]Stretch out the spear that *is* in thy hand toward Ai; for I will give it into thine hand. And Joshua stretched out the spear that *he had* in his hand toward the city.

19 And the ambush arose quickly out of their place, and they ran as soon as he had stretched out his hand: and they entered into the city, and took it, and hasted and set the city on fire.

20 And when the men of Ai looked behind them, they saw, and, behold, the smoke of the city ascended up to heaven, and they had no power to flee this way or that way: and the people that fled to the wilderness turned back upon the pursuers.

21 And when Joshua and all Israel saw that the ambush had taken the city, and that the smoke of the city ascended, then they turned again, and slew the men of Ai.

22 And the other issued out of the city against them; so they were in the midst of Israel, some on this side, and some on that side: and they smote them, so that they let none [c]of them remain or escape.

23 And the king of Ai they took alive, and brought him to Joshua.

24 And it came to pass, when Israel had made an end of slaying all the inhabitants of Ai in the field, in the wilderness wherein they chased them, and when they were all fallen on the edge of the sword, until they were consumed, that all the Israelites returned unto Ai, and smote it with the edge of the sword.

25 And *so* it was, *that* all that fell that day, both of men and women, *were* twelve thousand, *even* all the men of Ai.

26 For Joshua drew not his hand back, wherewith he stretched out the spear, until he had utterly destroyed all the inhabitants of Ai.

27 Only the cattle and the spoil of that city Israel took for a prey unto themselves, according unto the word of the LORD which he commanded Joshua.

28 And Joshua burnt Ai, and made it an heap for ever, *even* a desolation unto this day.

29 And the king of Ai he hanged on a tree until eventide: and as soon as the sun was down, Joshua commanded that they should take his carcase down from the tree, and cast it at the entering of the gate of the city, and raise thereon a great heap of stones, *that remaineth* unto this day.

The blessings and cursings.

30 Then Joshua built an [a]altar unto the LORD God of Israel in mount Ebal,

31 As Moses the servant of the LORD commanded the children of Israel, as it is written in the book of the law of Moses, an [b]altar of whole stones, over which no man hath lift up *any* iron: and they offered thereon burnt-offerings unto the LORD, and sacrificed peace-offerings.

32 And he [c]wrote there upon the stones a copy of the law of Moses, which he wrote in the presence of the children of Israel.

33 And all Israel, and their elders, and officers, and their judges, stood on this side the ark and on that side before the priests the Levites, which bare the ark of the covenant of the LORD, as well the stranger, as he that was born among them; [d]half of them over against mount Gerizim, and half of them over against mount Ebal; as Moses the servant of the LORD had commanded before, that they should bless the people of Israel.

34 And afterward he [e]read all the words of the law, the blessings and cursings, according to all that is written in the book of the law.

35 There was not a word of all that Moses commanded, which Joshua read not before all the congregation of Israel, with the women, and the little ones, and the strangers that were conversant among them.

CHAPTER 9.

The league with the Gibeonites.

And it came to pass, when all the kings which *were* on this side Jordan, in the hills, and in the valleys, and in all the coasts of the great sea over against Lebanon, the Hittite, and the Amorite, the Canaanite, the Perizzite, the Hivite, and the Jebusite, heard *thereof;*

2 That they gathered themselves together, to fight with Joshua and with Israel, with one accord.

3 And when the inhabitants of [f]Gibeon heard what Joshua had done unto Jericho and to Ai,

4 They did work wilily, and went and made as if they had been ambassadors, and took old sacks upon their asses, and wine bottles, old, and rent, and bound up;

5 And old shoes and clouted upon their feet, and old garments upon them; and all the bread of their provision was dry *and* mouldy.

6 And they went to Joshua unto the [g]camp at Gilgal, and said unto him, and to the men of Israel, We be come from a far country: now therefore make ye a league with us.

7 And the men of Israel said unto the Hivites, Peradventure ye dwell among us; and how shall we make a league with you?

8 And they said unto Joshua, We *are* thy servants. And Joshua said unto them, Who *are* ye? and from whence come ye?

9 And they said unto him, From a very far country thy servants are come because of the name of the LORD thy God: for we have heard the fame of him, and all that he did in Egypt,

10 And all that he did to the two kings of the Amorites, that *were* beyond Jordan, to Sihon king of Heshbon, and to Og king of Bashan, which *was* at Ashtaroth.

11 Wherefore our elders and all the inhabitants of our country spake to us, saying, Take victuals with you for the journey, and go to meet them, and say unto them, We *are* your servants: therefore now make ye a league with us.

12 This our bread we took hot *for* our provision out of our houses on the day we came forth to go unto you; but now, behold, it is dry, and it is mouldy:

13 And these bottles of wine, which we filled, *were* new; and, behold, they be rent: and these our garments and our shoes are become old by reason of the very long journey.

14 And the men took of their victuals, and asked not *counsel* at [h]the mouth of the LORD.

15 And Joshua made peace with them, and made a league with them, to let them live: and the princes of the congregation sware unto them.

16 And it came to pass at the end of three days after they had made a league with them, that they heard that they *were* their neighbours, and *that* they dwelt among them.

B.C. 1451.

a Deut. 27:4-6.
b Ex. 20:25.
c Deut. 27:2, 3, 8.
d Deut. 11:29; 27:12, 13.
e Deut. 31:11; 28:1-30:20.
f Josh. 2:9, 11; 10:2.
g Josh. 5:10.
h 1 Sam. 23:11; 30:8; 2 Sam. 2:1; 5:19.

17 And the children of Israel journeyed, and came unto their cities on the
third day. Now their cities *were* Gibeon,
and Chephirah, and Beeroth, and
Kirjath-jearim.
18 And the children of Israel smote
them not, because the princes of the congregation had sworn [a]unto them by the
LORD God of Israel. And all the congregation murmured against the princes.
19 But all the princes said unto all the
congregation, We have sworn unto them
by the LORD God of Israel: now therefore
we may not touch them.
20 This we will do to them; we will
even let them live, lest wrath be upon
us, because of the oath which we sware
unto them.
21 And the princes said unto them, Let
them live; but let them be hewers of wood
and drawers of water unto all the congregation; as the princes had promised them.
22 And Joshua called for them, and he
spake unto them, saying, Wherefore
have ye beguiled us, saying, We *are* very
far from you; when ye dwell among us?
23 Now therefore ye *are* cursed, and
there shall none of you be freed from
being bondmen, and hewers of wood
and drawers of water for the house of
my God.
24 And they answered Joshua, and
said, Because it was certainly told thy
servants, how that the LORD thy God
commanded his servant Moses to give
you all the land, and to destroy all the
inhabitants of the land from before you,
therefore we were sore afraid of our lives
because of you, and have done this thing.
25 And now, behold, we *are* in thine
hand: as it seemeth good and right unto
thee to do unto us, do.
26 And so did he unto them, and delivered them out of the hand of the children
of Israel, that they slew them not.
27 And Joshua made them that day
hewers of wood and drawers of water
for the congregation, and for the altar of
the LORD, even unto this day, in the place
which he should choose.

CHAPTER 10.

The victory at Gibeon.

Now it came to pass, when Adoni-
zedek king of Jerusalem had heard
how Joshua had taken Ai, and had utterly destroyed it; as he had done to Jericho
and her king, so he had done to Ai and
her king; and how the inhabitants of
Gibeon had made peace with Israel, and
were among them;
2 That they feared [b]greatly, because
Gibeon *was* a great city, as one of the royal
cities, and because it *was* greater than Ai,
and all the men thereof *were* mighty.
3 Wherefore Adoni-zedek king of
Jerusalem sent unto Hoham king of
Hebron, and unto Piram king of Jarmuth,
and unto Japhia king of Lachish, and
unto Debir king of Eglon, saying,
4 Come up unto me, and help me, that
we may smite Gibeon: for it hath made
peace with Joshua and with the children
of Israel.
5 Therefore the five kings of the
Amorites, the king of Jerusalem, the
king of Hebron, the king of Jarmuth, the
king of Lachish, the king of Eglon, gathered themselves together, and went up,
they and all their hosts, and encamped
before Gibeon, and made war against it.
6 And the men of Gibeon sent unto
Joshua to the camp to Gilgal, saying,
Slack not thy hand from thy servants;
come up to us quickly, and save us, and
help us: for all the kings of the Amorites
that dwell in the mountains are gathered
together against us.
7 So Joshua ascended from Gilgal, he,
and all the people of war with him, and
all the mighty men of valour.
8 And the LORD said unto Joshua, Fear
them not: for I have delivered them into
thine hand; there shall not a man of
them stand before thee.
9 Joshua therefore came unto them suddenly, *and* went up from Gilgal all night.
10 And the LORD discomfited them
before Israel, and slew them with a great
slaughter at Gibeon, and chased them
along the way that goeth up to Beth-
horon, and smote them to Azekah, and
unto Makkedah.
11 And it came to pass, as they fled
from before Israel, *and* were in the going
down to Beth-horon, that the LORD cast
down great stones from heaven upon
them unto Azekah, and they died: *they*
were more which died with hailstones
than *they* whom the children of Israel
slew with the sword.

B.C. 1451.

a Psa. 15:4; Eccl. 5:6.

b Ex. 15:14; Deut. 11:25; 1 Chr. 14:17; Heb. 10:27.

12 Then spake Joshua to the LORD in the day when the LORD delivered up the Amorites before the children of Israel, and he said in the sight of Israel, Sun, stand thou still upon Gibeon; and thou, Moon, in the valley of Ajalon.

13 And the sun [a]stood still, and the moon stayed, until the people had avenged themselves upon their enemies. *Is* not this written in the book of Jasher? So the sun stood still in the midst of heaven, and hasted not to go down about a whole day.

14 And there was no day like that before it or after it, that the LORD hearkened unto the voice of a man: for the LORD fought for Israel.

15 And Joshua returned, and all Israel with him, unto the camp to Gilgal.

16 But these five kings fled, and hid themselves in a cave at Makkedah.

17 And it was told Joshua, saying, The five kings are found hid in a cave at Makkedah.

18 And Joshua said, Roll great stones upon the mouth of the cave, and set men by it for to keep them:

19 And stay ye not, *but* pursue after your enemies, and smite the hindmost of them; suffer them not to enter into their cities: for the LORD your God hath delivered them into your hand.

20 And it came to pass, when Joshua and the children of Israel had made an end of slaying them with a very great slaughter, till they were consumed, that the rest *which* remained of them entered into fenced cities.

21 And all the people returned to the camp to Joshua at Makkedah in peace: none moved his [b]tongue against any of the children of Israel.

22 Then said Joshua, Open the mouth of the cave, and bring out those five kings unto me out of the cave.

23 And they did so, and brought forth those five kings unto him out of the cave, the king of Jerusalem, the king of Hebron, the king of Jarmuth, the king of Lachish, *and* the king of Eglon.

24 And it came to pass, when they brought out those kings unto Joshua, that Joshua called for all the men of Israel, and said unto the captains of the men of war which went with him, Come near, put your [c]feet upon the necks of these kings. And they came near, and put their feet upon the necks of them.

25 And Joshua said unto them, [d]Fear not, nor be dismayed, be strong and of good courage: for thus shall the LORD do to all your enemies against whom ye fight.

26 And afterward Joshua smote them, and slew them, and hanged them on five trees: and they were hanging upon the trees until the evening.

27 And it came to pass at the time of the going down of the sun, *that* Joshua commanded, and they took them down off the trees, and cast them into the cave wherein they had been hid, and laid great stones in the cave's mouth, *which remain* until this very day.

Victories at Makkedah, etc.

28 And that day Joshua took Makkedah, and smote it with the edge of the sword, and the king thereof he utterly [e]destroyed, them, and all the souls that *were* therein; he let none remain: and he did to the king of Makkedah as he did unto the king of Jericho.

29 Then Joshua passed from Makkedah, and all Israel with him, unto Libnah, and fought against [f]Libnah:

30 And the LORD delivered it also, and the king thereof, into the hand of Israel; and he smote it with the edge of the sword, and all the souls that *were* therein; he let none remain in it; but did unto the king thereof as he did unto the king of Jericho.

31 And Joshua passed from Libnah, and all Israel with him, unto Lachish, and encamped against it, and fought against it:

32 And the LORD delivered Lachish into the hand of Israel, which took it on the second day, and smote it with the edge of the sword, and all the souls that *were* therein, according to all that he had done to Libnah.

33 Then Horam king of Gezer came up to help Lachish; and Joshua smote him and his people, until he had left him none remaining.

34 And from Lachish Joshua passed unto [g]Eglon, and all Israel with him; and they encamped against it, and fought against it:

35 And they took it on that day, and smote it with the edge of the sword, and all the souls that *were* therein he utterly

B.C. 1451.

a *Miracles* (O.T.). vs. 12-14; Jud. 14:5, 6, 19. (Gen. 5:24; Jon. 2:1-10.)

b Ex. 11:7.

c Psa. 110:1; Isa. 26:5, 6; Mal. 4:3; Heb. 2:8.

d Josh. 1:9; Deut. 31:6, 8; 2 Tim. 4:17, 18.

e Deut. 7:2, 16; 1 Cor. 15:25.

f Josh. 15:42; 21:13; 2 Ki. 8:22; 19:8.

g v. 3.

destroyed that day, according to all that he had done to Lachish.

36 And Joshua went up from Eglon, and all Israel with him, unto Hebron; and they fought against it:

37 And they took it, and smote it with the edge of the sword, and the king thereof, and all the cities thereof, and all the souls that *were* therein; he left none remaining, according to all that he had done to Eglon; but destroyed it utterly, and all the souls that *were* therein.

38 And Joshua returned, and all Israel with him, to [a]Debir; and fought against it:

39 And he took it, and the king thereof, and all the cities thereof; and they smote them with the edge of the sword, and utterly destroyed all the souls that *were* therein; he left none remaining: as he had done to Hebron, so he did to Debir, and to the king thereof; as he had done also to Libnah, and to her king.

40 So Joshua smote all the country of the hills, and of the south, and of the vale, and of the springs, and all their kings: he left none remaining, but utterly destroyed all that breathed, as the LORD God of Israel commanded.

41 And Joshua smote them from [b]Kadesh-barnea even unto Gaza, and all the country of Goshen, even unto Gibeon.

42 And all these kings and their land did Joshua take at one [1]time, because the LORD God of Israel fought for Israel.

43 And Joshua returned, and all Israel with him, unto the camp to Gilgal.

CHAPTER 11.

Final conquest of Canaan.

And it came to pass, when Jabin king of Hazor had heard *those things*, that he sent to Jobab king of Madon, and to the king of Shimron, and to the king of Achshaph,

2 And to the kings that *were* on the north of the mountains, and of the plains south of Chinneroth, and in the valley, and in the borders of Dor on the west,

3 *And to* the Canaanite on the east and on the west, and *to* the Amorite, and the Hittite, and the Perizzite, and the Jebusite in the mountains, and *to* the Hivite under Hermon in the land of Mizpeh.

4 And they went out, they and all their hosts with them, much people, even as the [c]sand that *is* upon the sea shore in multitude, with horses and chariots very many.

5 And when all these kings were met together, they came and pitched together at the waters of Merom, to fight against Israel.

6 And the LORD said unto Joshua, Be not afraid because of them: for to morrow about this time will I deliver them up all slain before Israel: thou shalt hough their horses, and burn their chariots with fire.

7 So Joshua came, and all the people of war with him, against them by the waters of Merom suddenly; and they fell upon them.

8 And the LORD delivered them into the hand of Israel, who smote them, and chased them unto great Zidon, and unto Misrephoth-maim, and unto the valley of Mizpeh eastward; and they smote them, until they left them none remaining.

9 And Joshua did unto them as the LORD bade him: he houghed their horses, and burnt their chariots with fire.

10 And Joshua at that time turned back, and took Hazor, and smote the king thereof with the sword: for Hazor beforetime was the head of all those kingdoms.

11 And they smote all the souls that *were* therein with the edge of the sword, utterly destroying *them*: there was not any left to breathe: and he burnt Hazor with fire.

12 And all the cities of those kings, and all the kings of them, did Joshua take, and smote them with the edge of the sword, *and* he utterly destroyed them, as Moses the servant of the LORD commanded.

13 But *as for* the cities that stood still in their strength, Israel burned none of them, save Hazor only; *that* did Joshua burn.

14 And all the spoil of these cities, and the cattle, the children of Israel took for a prey unto themselves; but every man they smote with the edge of the sword, until they had destroyed them, neither left they any to breathe.

15 As the LORD commanded Moses his servant, so did Moses command Joshua,

B.C. 1451.

a Josh. 11:21; 15:15; Jud. 1:11.

b Deut. 9:23.

c Jud. 7:12; 1 Sam. 13:5; Psa. 2:2.

[1]**(10:42)** Cf. Josh. 11:18. As the context shows, the verses refer to different parts of Palestine and different kings.

and so did Joshua; he left nothing undone of all that the LORD commanded Moses.

16 So Joshua took all that land, the hills, and all the south country, and all the land of Goshen, and the valley, and the plain, and the mountain of Israel, and the valley of the same;

17 *Even* from the mount Halak, that goeth up to Seir, even unto Baal-gad in the valley of Lebanon under mount Hermon: and all their kings he took, and smote them, and slew them.

18 Joshua made war a [a]long time with all those kings.

19 There was not a city that made peace with the children of Israel, save the Hivites the inhabitants of Gibeon: all *other* they took in battle.

20 For it was of the LORD to harden their hearts, that they should come against Israel in battle, that he might destroy them utterly, *and* that they might have no favour, but that he might destroy them, as the LORD commanded Moses.

21 And at that time came Joshua, and cut off the [b]Anakims from the mountains, from Hebron, from Debir, from Anab, and from all the mountains of Judah, and from all the mountains of Israel: Joshua destroyed them utterly with their cities.

22 There was none of the Anakims left in the land of the children of Israel: only in Gaza, in Gath, and in Ashdod, there remained.

23 So Joshua took the whole land, according to all that the LORD [c]said unto Moses; and Joshua gave it for an inheritance unto Israel according to their divisions by their tribes. And the land rested from war.

CHAPTER 12.

The roster of the kings of Canaan.

Now these *are* the kings of the land, which the children of Israel smote, and possessed their land on the other side Jordan toward the rising of the sun, from the river Arnon unto mount Hermon, and all the plain on the east:

2 [d]Sihon king of the Amorites, who dwelt in Heshbon, *and* ruled from Aroer, which *is* upon the bank of the river Arnon, and from the middle of the river, and from half Gilead, even unto the river Jabbok, *which is* the border of the children of Ammon;

3 And from the plain to the sea of Chinneroth on the east, and unto the sea of the plain, *even* the salt sea on the east, the way to Beth-jeshimoth; and from the south, under Ashdoth-pisgah:

4 And the coast of Og king of Bashan, *which was* of the remnant of the giants, that dwelt at Ashtaroth and at Edrei,

5 And reigned in mount [e]Hermon, and in Salcah, and in all Bashan, unto the border of the Geshurites and the Maachathites, and half Gilead, the border of Sihon king of Heshbon.

6 Them did Moses the servant of the LORD and the children of Israel smite: and Moses the servant of the LORD gave [f]it *for* a possession unto the Reubenites, and the Gadites, and the half tribe of Manasseh.

7 And these *are* the kings of the country which Joshua and the children of Israel smote on this side Jordan on the west, from Baal-gad in the valley of Lebanon even unto the mount Halak, that goeth up to Seir; which Joshua gave unto the tribes of Israel *for* a possession according to their divisions;

8 In the mountains, and in the valleys, and in the plains, and in the springs, and in the wilderness, and in the south country; the [g]Hittites, the Amorites, and the Canaanites, the Perizzites, the Hivites, and the Jebusites:

9 The king of [h]Jericho, one; the king of Ai, which *is* beside Beth-el, one;

10 The king of [i]Jerusalem, one; the king of Hebron, one;

11 The king of Jarmuth, one; the king of Lachish, one;

12 The king of Eglon, one; the king of Gezer, one;

13 The king of Debir, one; the king of Geder, one;

14 The king of Hormah, one; the king of Arad, one;

15 The king of Libnah, one; the king of Adullam, one;

16 The king of Makkedah, one; the king of [j]Beth-el, one;

17 The king of Tappuah, one; the king of [k]Hepher, one;

18 The king of Aphek, one; the king of Lasharon, one;

19 The king of Madon, one; the king of Hazor, one;

20 The king of Shimron-meron, one; the king of Achshaph, one;

21 The king of Taanach, one; the king of Megiddo, one;

B.C. 1450.

a Cf. Josh. 10:42, *note.*

b Num. 13:22; Deut. 9:2.

c Ex. 33:2; Num. 34:2; Deut. 9:3.

d Deut. 2:33, 36; 3:6, 16, 17.

e Deut. 3:8, 14.

f Num. 32:29, 33.

g Ex. 23:23.

h Josh. 6:2.

i Josh. 10:23.

j Jud. 1:22.

k 1 Ki. 4:10.

22 The king of Kedesh, one; the king of Jokneam of Carmel, one;

23 The king of Dor in the coast of Dor, one; the king of the nations of Gilgal, one;

24 The king of Tirzah, one: all the kings thirty and one.

CHAPTER 13.

The Lord instructs Joshua concerning the division of the land.

Now Joshua was old *and* stricken in years; and the LORD said unto him, Thou art old *and* stricken in years, and there remaineth yet very much land to be possessed.

2 This *is* the land that yet remaineth: all the borders of the Philistines, and all Geshuri,

3 From Sihor, which *is* before Egypt, even unto the borders of Ekron northward, *which* is counted to the Canaanite: five lords of the Philistines; the Gazathites, and the Ashdothites, the Eshkalonites, the Gittites, and the Ekronites; also the Avites:

4 From the south, all the land of the Canaanites, and Mearah that *is* beside the Sidonians, unto Aphek, to the borders of the Amorites:

5 And the land of the Giblites, and all Lebanon, toward the sunrising, from Baal-gad under mount Hermon unto the entering into Hamath.

6 All the inhabitants of the hill country from Lebanon unto Misrephoth-maim, *and* all the Sidonians, them will I drive out from before the children of Israel: only divide thou it by lot unto the Israelites for an inheritance, as I have commanded thee.

7 Now therefore divide this land for an inheritance unto the nine tribes, and the half tribe of Manasseh,

8 With whom the Reubenites and the Gadites have received their inheritance, which [a]Moses gave them, beyond Jordan eastward, *even* as Moses the servant of the LORD gave them;

9 From Aroer, that *is* upon the bank of the river Arnon, and the city that *is* in the midst of the river, and all the plain of Medeba unto Dibon;

10 And all the cities of Sihon king of the Amorites, which reigned in Heshbon, unto the border of the children of Ammon;

11 And [b]Gilead, and the border of the Geshurites and Maachathites, and all mount Hermon, and all Bashan unto Salcah;

12 All the kingdom of Og in Bashan, which reigned in Ashtaroth and in Edrei, who remained of the remnant of the giants: for [c]these did Moses smite, and cast them out.

13 Nevertheless the children of Israel expelled [d]not the Geshurites, nor the Maachathites: but the Geshurites and the Maachathites dwell among the Israelites until this day.

14 Only unto the tribe of Levi he gave [e]none inheritance; the sacrifices of the LORD God of Israel made by fire *are* their inheritance, as he said unto them.

15 And Moses gave unto the tribe of the children of Reuben *inheritance* according to their families.

16 And their coast was from [f]Aroer, that *is* on the bank of the river Arnon, and the city that *is* in the midst of the river, and all the plain by Medeba;

17 [g]Heshbon, and all her cities that *are* in the plain; Dibon, and Bamoth-baal, and Beth-baal-meon,

18 And [h]Jahazah, and Kedemoth, and Mephaath,

19 And Kirjathaim, and Sibmah, and Zareth-shahar in the mount of the valley,

20 And Beth-peor, and Ashdoth-pisgah, and Beth-jeshimoth,

21 And all the cities of the plain, and all the kingdom of Sihon king of the Amorites, which reigned in Heshbon, whom Moses smote with the princes of [i]Midian, Evi, and Rekem, and Zur, and Hur, and Reba, *which were* dukes of Sihon, dwelling in the country.

22 [j]Balaam also the son of Beor, the soothsayer, did the children of Israel slay with the sword among them that were slain by them.

23 And the border of the children of Reuben was Jordan, and the border *thereof*. This *was* the inheritance of the children of Reuben after their families, the cities and the villages thereof.

24 And Moses gave *inheritance* unto the tribe of Gad, *even* unto the children of Gad according to their families.

25 And their coast was Jazer, and all the cities of Gilead, and half the land of the children of Ammon, unto Aroer that *is* before Rabbah;

26 And from Heshbon unto Ramath-mizpeh, and Betonim; and from

B.C. 1451.

a Num. 32:33.
b Josh. 12:5.
c Num. 21:34.
d Josh. 23:12, 13; Num. 33:55; Jud. 2:2, 3.
e Deut. 18:1; Josh. 14:3, 4.
f Josh. 12:2.
g Num. 21:28, 30.
h Num. 21:23.
i Num. 31:8.
j Num. 22:5; 31:8.

Mahanaim unto the border of Debir;

27 And in the valley, Beth-aram, and Beth-nimrah, and Succoth, and Zaphon, the rest of the kingdom of Sihon king of Heshbon, Jordan and *his* border, *even* unto the edge of the sea of Chinnereth on the other side Jordan eastward.

28 This *is* the inheritance of the children of Gad after their families, the cities, and their villages.

29 And Moses gave *inheritance* unto the half tribe of Manasseh: and *this* was *the possession* of the half tribe of the children of Manasseh by their families.

30 And their coast was from Mahanaim, all Bashan, all the kingdom of Og king of Bashan, and all the towns of Jair, which *are* in Bashan, threescore cities:

31 And half Gilead, and Ashtaroth, and Edrei, cities of the kingdom of Og in Bashan, *were pertaining* unto the children of Machir the son of Manasseh, *even* to the one half of the children of Machir by their families.

32 These *are the countries* which Moses did distribute for inheritance in the plains of Moab, on the other side Jordan, by Jericho, eastward.

33 But unto the tribe of Levi Moses gave not *any* inheritance: the LORD God of Israel *was* their inheritance, as he said unto them.

CHAPTER 14.

The land divided: the portion of Caleb.

And these *are the countries* which the children of Israel inherited in the land of Canaan, which Eleazar the priest, and Joshua the son of Nun, and the heads of the fathers of the tribes of the children of Israel, distributed for inheritance to them.

2 By [a]lot *was* their inheritance, as the LORD commanded by the hand of Moses, for the nine tribes, and *for* the half tribe.

3 For Moses had given the inheritance of two tribes and an half tribe on the other side Jordan: but unto the Levites he gave none inheritance among them.

4 For the children of Joseph [b]were two tribes, Manasseh and Ephraim: therefore they gave no part unto the Levites in the land, save cities to dwell *in*, with their suburbs for their cattle and for their substance.

5 As the LORD commanded Moses, so the children of Israel did, and they divided the land.

6 Then the children of Judah came unto Joshua in Gilgal: and [c]Caleb the son of Jephunneh the Kenezite said unto him, Thou knowest the thing that the LORD said unto Moses the man of God concerning me and thee in Kadesh-barnea.

7 Forty years old *was* I when Moses the servant of the LORD [d]sent me from Kadesh-barnea to espy out the land; and I brought him word again as *it was* in mine heart.

8 Nevertheless my brethren that went up with me made the heart of the people melt: but I [e]wholly followed the LORD my God.

9 And Moses sware on that day, saying, Surely the land whereon thy feet have trodden shall be thine inheritance, and thy children's for ever, because thou hast wholly followed the LORD my God.

10 And now, behold, the LORD hath kept me alive, as he [f]said, these forty and five years, even since the LORD spake this word unto Moses, while *the children of* Israel wandered in the wilderness: and now, lo, I *am* this day fourscore and five years old.

11 As yet I *am as* strong this day as I *was* in the day that Moses sent me: as my strength *was* then, even so *is* my strength now, for war, both to go out, and to come in.

12 Now therefore give me this mountain, whereof the LORD spake in that day; for thou heardest in that day [g]how the Anakims *were* there, and *that* the cities *were* great *and* fenced: if so be the LORD *will be* with me, then I shall be able to drive them out, as the LORD said.

13 And Joshua blessed him, and gave unto Caleb the son of Jephunneh Hebron for an inheritance.

14 Hebron therefore became the inheritance of Caleb the son of Jephunneh the Kenezite unto this day, because that he wholly followed the LORD God of Israel.

15 And the name of Hebron before *was* Kirjath-arba; *which Arba was* a great man among the Anakims. And the land had rest from war.

B.C. 1455.

a Num. 26:55; 33:54; 34:13; Psa. 16:5, 6; 47:4.

b Gen. 48:5; 1 Chr. 5:1, 2.

c Num. 32:12.

d Num. 13:6, 26.

e Num. 14:24.

f Num. 14:30.

g Num. 13:28, 33.

CHAPTER 15.

B.C. 1444.

The land divided: the portion of Judah.

This then was the lot of the tribe of the children of Judah by their families; *even* to the border of Edom the wilderness of Zin southward *was* the uttermost part of the south coast.

2 And their south border was from the shore of the salt sea, from the bay that looketh southward:

3 And it went out to the south side to Maaleh-acrabbim, and passed along to Zin, and ascended up on the south side unto Kadesh-barnea, and passed along to Hezron, and went up to Adar, and fetched a compass to Karkaa:

4 *From thence* it passed toward Azmon, and went out unto the river of Egypt; and the goings out of that coast were at the sea: this shall be your south coast.

5 And the east border *was* the salt sea, *even* unto the end of Jordan. And *their* border in the north quarter *was* from the bay of the sea at the uttermost part of Jordan:

6 And the border went up to Beth-hogla, and passed along by the north of Beth-arabah; and the border went up to the stone of Bohan the son of Reuben:

7 And the border went up toward Debir from the valley of Achor, and so northward, looking toward Gilgal, that *is* before the going up to Adummim, which *is* on the south side of the river: and the border passed toward the waters of En-shemesh, and the goings out thereof were at En-rogel:

8 And the border went up by the valley of the son of Hinnom unto the south side of the Jebusite; the same *is* Jerusalem: and the border went up to the top of the mountain that *lieth* before the valley of Hinnom westward, which *is* at the end of the valley of the giants northward:

9 And the border was drawn from the top of the hill unto the [a]fountain of the water of Nephtoah, and went out to the cities of mount Ephron; and the border was drawn to [b]Baalah, which *is* Kirjath-jearim:

10 And the border compassed from Baalah westward unto mount Seir, and passed along unto the side of mount Jearim, which *is* Chesalon, on the north side, and went down to Beth-shemesh, and passed on to [c]Timnah:

11 And the border went out unto the side of Ekron northward: and the border was drawn to Shicron, and passed along to mount Baalah, and went out unto Jabneel; and the goings out of the border were at the sea.

12 And the west border *was* to the great sea, and the coast *thereof*. This *is* the coast of the children of Judah round about according to their families.

13 And unto Caleb the son of Jephunneh he gave a part among the children of Judah, according to the commandment of the LORD to Joshua, *even* the city of [d]Arba the father of Anak, which *city is* Hebron.

14 And Caleb drove thence the three [e]sons of Anak, Sheshai, and Ahiman, and Talmai, the children of Anak.

15 And he went up thence to the inhabitants of [f]Debir: and the name of Debir before *was* Kirjath-sepher.

16 And Caleb said, He that smiteth Kirjath-sepher, and taketh it, to him will I give Achsah my daughter to wife.

17 And Othniel the [g]son of Kenaz, the brother of Caleb, took it: and he gave him Achsah his daughter to wife.

18 And it came to pass, as she came *unto him*, that she moved him to ask of her father a field: and she lighted off *her* ass; and Caleb said unto her, What wouldest thou?

19 Who answered, Give me a blessing; for thou hast given me a south land; give me also springs of water. And he gave her the upper springs, and the nether springs.

20 This *is* the inheritance of the tribe of the children of Judah according to their families.

21 And the uttermost cities of the tribe of the children of Judah toward the coast of Edom southward were Kabzeel, and Eder, and Jagur,

22 And Kinah, and Dimonah, and Adadah,

23 And Kedesh, and Hazor, and Ithnan,

24 Ziph, and Telem, and Bealoth,

25 And Hazor, Hadattah, and Kerioth, *and* Hezron, which *is* Hazor,

26 Amam, and Shema, and Moladah,

27 And Hazar-gaddah, and Heshmon, and Beth-palet,

a Josh. 18:15.
b 2 Sam. 6:2; 1 Chr. 13:6.
c Gen. 38:13; Jud. 14:1.
d *Kirjath-arba.*
e Num. 13:22; Jud. 1:10, 20.
f Josh. 10:38.
g Num. 32:12; Jud. 1:13.

B.C. 1444.

28 And Hazar-shual, and Beer-sheba, and Bizjothjah,

29 [a]Baalah, and Iim, and Azem,

30 And Eltolad, and Chesil, and Hormah,

31 And [b]Ziklag, and Madmannah, and Sansannah,

32 And Lebaoth, and Shilhim, and Ain, and Rimmon: all the cities *are* twenty and nine, with their villages:

33 *And* in the valley, Eshtaol, and Zoreah, and Ashnah,

34 And Zanoah, and En-gannim, Tappuah, and Enam,

35 Jarmuth, and Adullam, Socoh, and Azekah,

36 And Sharaim, and Adithaim, and Gederah, and Gederothaim; fourteen cities with their villages:

37 Zenan, and Hadashah, and Migdal-gad,

38 And Dilean, and Mizpeh, and Joktheel,

39 Lachish, and Bozkath, and Eglon,

40 And Cabbon, and Lahmam, and Kithlish,

41 And Gederoth, Beth-dagon, and Naamah, and Makkedah; sixteen cities with their villages:

42 Libnah, and Ether, and Ashan,

43 And Jiphtah, and Ashnah, and Nezib,

44 And Keilah, and Achzib, and Mareshah; nine cities with their villages:

45 Ekron, with her towns and her villages:

46 From Ekron even unto the sea, all that *lay* near Ashdod, with their villages:

47 Ashdod with her towns and her villages, Gaza with her towns and her villages, unto the river of Egypt, and the great sea, and the border *thereof*:

48 And in the mountains, Shamir, and Jattir, and Socoh,

49 And Dannah, and Kirjath-sannah, which *is* Debir,

50 And Anab, and Eshtemoh, and Anim,

51 And Goshen, and Holon, and Giloh; eleven cities with their villages:

52 Arab, and Dumah, and Eshean,

53 And Janum, and Beth-tappuah, and Aphekah,

54 And Humtah, and Kirjath-arba, which *is* Hebron, and Zior; nine cities with their villages:

55 Maon, Carmel, and Ziph, and Juttah,

56 And Jezreel, and Jokdeam, and Zanoah,

57 Cain, Gibeah, and Timnah; ten cities with their villages:

58 Halhul, Beth-zur, and Gedor,

59 And Maarath, and Beth-anoth, and Eltekon; six cities with their villages:

60 [c]Kirjath-baal, which *is* Kirjath-jearim, and Rabbah; two cities with their villages:

61 In the wilderness, Beth-arabah, Middin, and Secacah,

62 And Nibshan, and the city of Salt, and [d]En-gedi; six cities with their villages.

63 As for the [e]Jebusites the inhabitants of Jerusalem, the children of Judah could not drive them out: but the Jebusites dwell with the children of Judah at Jerusalem unto this day.

CHAPTER 16.

The land divided: the portion of Manasseh and Ephraim.

And the lot of the children of Joseph fell from Jordan by Jericho, unto the water of Jericho on the east, to the wilderness that goeth up from Jericho throughout mount Beth-el,

2 And goeth out from Beth-el to Luz, and passeth along unto the borders of Archi to Ataroth,

3 And goeth down westward to the coast of Japhleti, unto the coast of [f]Beth-horon the nether, and to Gezer: and the goings out thereof are at the sea.

4 So the children of Joseph, Manasseh and Ephraim, took their inheritance.

5 And the border of the children of Ephraim according to their families was *thus*: even the border of their inheritance on the east side was Ataroth-addar, unto Beth-horon the upper;

6 And the border went out toward the sea to [g]Michmethah on the north side; and the border went about eastward unto Taanath-shiloh, and passed by it on the east to Janohah;

7 And it went down from Janohah to Ataroth, and to Naarath, and came to Jericho, and went out at Jordan.

8 The border went out from Tappuah westward unto the river [h]Kanah; and the goings out thereof were at the sea.

a v. 9.
b 1 Sam. 27:6.
c Josh. 18:14.
d 1 Sam. 23:29.
e Jud. 1:8, 21; 2 Sam. 5:6.
f 2 Chr. 8:5.
g Josh. 17:7.
h Josh. 17:9.

This *is* the inheritance of the tribe of the
children of Ephraim by their families.
9 And the separate cities for the children of Ephraim *were* among the inheritance of the children of Manasseh, all the
cities with their villages.
10 And they drave not out the
Canaanites that dwelt in Gezer: but the
Canaanites dwell among the Ephraimites
unto this day, and serve under tribute.

CHAPTER 17.

The land divided:
the separate portion of Manasseh.

There was also a lot for the tribe of
Manasseh; for he *was* the firstborn
of Joseph; *to wit*, for Machir the firstborn
of Manasseh, the father of Gilead:
because he was a man of war, therefore
he had Gilead and Bashan.
2 There was also *a lot* for the rest of the
children of Manasseh by their families;
for the children of Abiezer, and for the
children of Helek, and for the children of
Asriel, and for the children of Shechem,
and for the children of Hepher, and for
the children of Shemida: these *were* the
male children of Manasseh the son of
Joseph by their families.
3 But Zelophehad, the son of Hepher,
the son of Gilead, the son of Machir, the
son of Manasseh, had no sons, but
daughters: and these *are* the names of his
daughters, Mahlah, and Noah, Hoglah,
Milcah, and Tirzah.
4 And they came near before Eleazar
the priest, and before Joshua the son of
Nun, and before the princes, saying, The
LORD commanded Moses to give us an
inheritance among our brethren.
Therefore according to the commandment of the LORD he gave them an inheritance among the brethren of their father.
5 And there fell ten portions to
Manasseh, beside the land of Gilead and
Bashan, which *were* on the other side
Jordan;
6 Because the daughters of Manasseh
had an inheritance among his sons: and
the rest of Manasseh's sons had the land
of Gilead.
7 And the coast of Manasseh was from
Asher to Michmethah, that *lieth* before
Shechem; and the border went along on
the right hand unto the inhabitants of
En-tappuah.
8 *Now* Manasseh had the land of
Tappuah: but Tappuah on the border of
Manasseh *belonged* to the children of
Ephraim;
9 And the coast descended unto the
river Kanah, southward of the river:
[a]these cities of Ephraim *are* among the
cities of Manasseh: the coast of Manasseh
also *was* on the north side of the river,
and the outgoings of it were at the sea:
10 Southward *it was* Ephraim's, and
northward *it was* Manasseh's, and the
sea is his border; and they met together
in Asher on the north, and in Issachar on
the east.
11 And Manasseh had in Issachar and
in Asher [b]Beth-shean and her towns,
and Ibleam and her towns, and the
inhabitants of Dor and her towns, and
the inhabitants of Endor and her towns,
and the inhabitants of Taanach and her
towns, and the inhabitants of Megiddo
and her towns, *even* three countries.
12 Yet the children of Manasseh could
not drive out *the inhabitants of* those
cities; but the Canaanites would dwell in
that land.
13 Yet it came to pass, when the children of Israel were waxen strong, that
they put the Canaanites to tribute; but
did not utterly drive them out.
14 And the children of Joseph spake
unto Joshua, saying, Why hast thou given
me *but* one lot and one portion to inherit,
seeing I *am* a great people, forasmuch as
the LORD hath blessed me hitherto?
15 And Joshua answered them, If thou
be a great people, *then* get thee up to the
wood *country*, and cut down for thyself
there in the land of the Perizzites and of
the [c]giants, if mount Ephraim be too
narrow for thee.
16 And the children of Joseph said,
The hill is not enough for us: and all the
Canaanites that dwell in the land of the
valley have chariots of iron, *both they*
who *are* of Beth-shean and her towns,
and *they* who *are* of the valley of Jezreel.
17 And Joshua spake unto the house
of Joseph, *even* to Ephraim and to
Manasseh, saying, Thou *art* a great people, and hast great power: thou shalt not
have one lot *only*:
18 But the mountain shall be thine; for
it *is* a wood, and thou shalt cut it down:
and the outgoings of it shall be thine: for

B.C. 1444.

a Josh. 16:9.

b Jud. 1:27; 1 Sam. 31:10; 1 Ki. 4:12.

c Or, *Rephaims*.

B.C. 1444.

thou shalt drive out the Canaanites, though they have iron chariots, *and* though they *be* strong.

CHAPTER 18.

The tabernacle set up at Shiloh.

And the whole congregation of the children of Israel assembled together at [a]Shiloh, and set up the tabernacle of the congregation there. And the land was subdued before them.

The land divided: the portion of the seven tribes.

2 And there remained among the children of Israel seven tribes, which had not yet received their inheritance.

3 And Joshua said unto the children of Israel, How long *are* ye [b]slack to go to possess the land, which the LORD God of your fathers hath given you?

4 Give out from among you three men for *each* tribe: and I will send them, and they shall rise, and [c]go through the land, and describe it according to the inheritance of them; and they shall come *again* to me.

5 And they shall divide it into seven parts: [d]Judah shall abide in their coast on the south, and the house of Joseph shall abide in their coasts on the north.

6 Ye shall therefore describe the land *into* seven parts, and bring *the description* hither to me, that I may cast lots for you here before the LORD our God.

7 But the Levites have no part among you; for the priesthood of the LORD *is* their inheritance: and Gad, and Reuben, and half the tribe of Manasseh, have received their inheritance beyond Jordan on the east, which Moses the servant of the LORD gave them.

8 And the men arose, and went away: and Joshua charged them that went to describe the land, saying, Go and walk [e]through the land, and describe it, and come again to me, that I may here cast lots for you before the LORD in Shiloh.

9 And the men went and passed through the land, and described it by cities into seven parts in a book, and came *again* to Joshua to the host at Shiloh.

10 And Joshua cast [f]lots for them in Shiloh before the LORD: and there Joshua divided the land unto the children of Israel according to their divisions.

11 And the lot of the tribe of the children of Benjamin came up according to their families: and the coast of their lot came forth between the children of Judah and the children of Joseph.

12 And their border on the north side was from Jordan; and the border went up to the side of Jericho on the north side, and went up through the mountains westward; and the goings out thereof were at the wilderness of Beth-aven.

13 And the border went over from thence toward Luz, to the side of [g]Luz, which *is* Beth-el, southward; and the border descended to Ataroth-adar, near the hill that *lieth* on the south side of the nether [h]Beth-horon.

14 And the border was drawn *thence*, and compassed the corner of the sea southward, from the hill that *lieth* before Beth-horon southward; and the goings out thereof were at Kirjath-baal, which *is* Kirjath-jearim, a city of the children of Judah: this *was* the west quarter.

15 And the south quarter *was* from the end of [i]Kirjath-jearim, and the border went out on the west, and went out to the well of [j]waters of Nephtoah:

16 And the border came down to the end of the mountain that *lieth* before the valley of the son of Hinnom, *and* which *is* in the valley of the giants on the north, and descended to the valley of Hinnom, to the side of Jebusi on the south, and descended to En-rogel,

17 And was drawn from the north, and went forth to En-shemesh, and went forth toward Geliloth, which *is* over against the going up of Adummim, and descended to the stone of Bohan the son of Reuben,

18 And passed along toward the side over against Arabah northward, and went down unto Arabah:

19 And the border passed along to the side of Beth-hoglah northward: and the outgoings of the border were at the north bay of the salt sea at the south end of Jordan: this *was* the south coast.

20 And Jordan was the border of it on the east side. This *was* the inheritance of the children of Benjamin, by the coasts thereof round about, according to their families.

21 Now the cities of the tribe of the

a Josh. 19:51; Jer. 7:12.
b Jud. 18:9; Eccl. 9:10.
c v. 8.
d Josh. 15:1.
e Gen. 13:17.
f Acts 13:19.
g Gen. 28:19; Jud. 1:23.
h Josh. 16:3.
i 1 Chr. 13:5, 6.
j Josh. 15:9.

B.C. 1444.

children of Benjamin according to their
families were Jericho, and Beth-hoglah,
and the valley of Keziz,
22 And Beth-arabah, and Zemaraim,
and Beth-el,
23 And Avim, and Parah, and Ophrah,
24 And Chephar-haammonai, and
Ophni, and Gaba; twelve cities with
their villages:
25 [a]Gibeon, and [b]Ramah, and Beeroth,
26 And Mizpeh, and Chephirah, and
Mozah,
27 And Rekem, and Irpeel, and
Taralah,
28 And Zelah, Eleph, and Jebusi,
which *is* Jerusalem, Gibeath, *and* Kirjath;
fourteen cities with their villages. This *is*
the inheritance of the children of
Benjamin according to their families.

CHAPTER 19.

And the second lot came forth to
Simeon, *even* for the tribe of the
children of Simeon according to their
families: and their inheritance was within
the inheritance of the [c]children of Judah.
2 And they had in their inheritance
[d]Beer-sheba, or Sheba, and Moladah,
3 And Hazar-shual, and Balah, and
Azem,
4 And Eltolad, and Bethul, and
Hormah,
5 And Ziklag, and Beth-marcaboth,
and [e]Hazar-susah,
6 And Beth-lebaoth, and Sharuhen;
thirteen cities and their villages:
7 Ain, Remmon, and Ether, and
Ashan; four cities and their villages:
8 And all the villages that *were* round
about these cities to Baalath-beer,
[f]Ramath of the south. This *is* the inheritance of the tribe of the children of
Simeon according to their families.
9 Out of the portion of the children of
Judah *was* the inheritance of the children
of Simeon: for the part of the children of
Judah was too much for [g]them: therefore
the children of Simeon had their inheritance within the inheritance of them.
10 And the third lot came up for the
children of Zebulun according to their
families: and the border of their inheritance was unto Sarid:
11 And their border went up toward
the [h]sea, and Maralah, and reached to
Dabbasheth, and reached to the river
that *is* before Jokneam;
12 And turned from Sarid eastward
toward the sunrising unto the border of
[i]Chisloth-tabor, and then goeth out to
Daberath, and goeth up to Japhia,
13 And from thence passeth on along
on the east to [j]Gittah-hepher, to Ittah-
kazin, and goeth out to Remmon-
methoar to Neah;
14 And the border compasseth it on
the north side to Hannathon: and the
outgoings thereof are in the valley of
Jiphthah-el:
15 And Kattath, and Nahallal, and
Shimron, and Idalah, and Beth-lehem:
twelve cities with their villages.
16 This *is* the inheritance of the children of Zebulun according to their families, these cities with their villages.
17 *And* the fourth lot came out to
Issachar, for the children of Issachar
according to their families.
18 And their border was toward
[k]Jezreel, and Chesulloth, and Shunem,
19 And Hapharaim, and Shion, and
Anaharath,
20 And Rabbith, and Kishion, and
Abez,
21 And Remeth, and En-gannim, and
En-haddah, and Beth-pazzez;
22 And the coast reacheth to Tabor,
and Shahazimah, and Beth-shemesh; and
the outgoings of their border were at
Jordan: sixteen cities with their villages.
23 This *is* the inheritance of the tribe of
the children of Issachar according to their
families, the cities and their villages.
24 And the fifth lot came out for the
tribe of the children of Asher according
to their families.
25 And their border was Helkath, and
Hali, and Beten, and Achshaph,
26 And Alammelech, and Amad, and
Misheal; and reacheth to [l]Carmel westward, and to Shihor-libnath;
27 And turneth toward the sunrising
to Beth-dagon, and reacheth to Zebulun,
and to the valley of Jiphthah-el toward
the north side of Beth-emek, and Neiel,
and goeth out to Cabul on the left hand,
28 And Hebron, and Rehob, and
Hammon, and Kanah, *even* unto great
Zidon;
29 And *then* the coast turneth to

a Josh. 11:19; 21:17; 1 Ki. 3:4, 5.
b Jer. 31:15.
c v. 9.
d Gen. 21:31; 1 Chr. 4:28.
e Josh. 15:28.
f 1 Sam. 30:27.
g v. 1.
h Gen. 49:13.
i Jud. 4:6, 12; Psa. 89:12.
j 2 Ki. 14:25.
k 1 Ki. 21:1.
l 1 Sam. 15:12; 1 Ki. 18:20; Isa. 33:9; 35:2; Jer. 46:18.

Ramah, and to the strong city Tyre; and the coast turneth to Hosah; and the outgoings thereof are at the sea from the coast to Achzib:

30 Ummah also, and Aphek, and Rehob: twenty and two cities with their villages.

31 This *is* the inheritance of the tribe of the children of Asher according to their families, these cities with their villages.

32 The sixth lot came out to the children of Naphtali, *even* for the children of Naphtali according to their families.

33 And their coast was from Heleph, from Allon to Zaanannim, and Adami, Nekeb, and Jabneel, unto Lakum; and the outgoings thereof were at Jordan:

34 And *then* the coast turneth westward to Aznoth-tabor, and goeth out from thence to Hukkok, and reacheth to Zebulun on the south side, and reacheth to Asher on the west side, and to Judah upon Jordan toward the sunrising.

35 And the fenced cities *are* Ziddim, Zer, and Hammath, Rakkath, and Chinnereth,

36 And Adamah, and Ramah, and Hazor,

37 And Kedesh, and Edrei, and En-hazor,

38 And Iron, and Migdal-el, Horem, and Beth-anath, and Beth-shemesh; nineteen cities with their villages.

39 This *is* the inheritance of the tribe of the children of Naphtali according to their families, the cities and their villages.

40 *And* the seventh lot came out for the tribe of the children of Dan according to their families.

41 And the coast of their inheritance was Zorah, and Eshtaol, and Ir-shemesh,

42 And Shaalabbin, and Ajalon, and Jethlah,

43 And Elon, and Thimnathah, and Ekron,

44 And Eltekeh, and Gibbethon, and Baalath,

45 And Jehud, and Bene-berak, and Gath-rimmon,

46 And Me-jarkon, and Rakkon, with the border before Japho.

47 And the coast of the children of Dan went out *too little* for them: therefore the children of Dan went up to fight against Leshem, and took it, and smote it with the edge of the sword, and possessed it, and dwelt therein, and called Leshem, Dan, after the name of Dan their father.

48 This *is* the inheritance of the tribe of the children of Dan according to their families, these cities with their villages.

49 When they had made an end of dividing the land for inheritance by their coasts, the children of Israel gave an inheritance to Joshua the son of Nun among them:

50 According to the word of the LORD they gave him the city which he asked, *even* Timnath-serah in mount Ephraim: and he built the city, and dwelt therein.

51 These *are* the inheritances, which Eleazar the priest, and Joshua the son of Nun, and the heads of the fathers of the tribes of the children of Israel, divided for an inheritance by lot in Shiloh before the LORD, at the door of the tabernacle of the congregation. So they made an end of dividing the country.

CHAPTER 20.

The cities of refuge.

The LORD also spake unto Joshua, saying,

2 Speak to the children of Israel, saying, Appoint out for you cities of refuge, whereof I [a]spake unto you by the hand of Moses:

3 That the slayer that killeth *any* person unawares *and* unwittingly may flee thither: and they shall be your refuge from the [b]avenger of blood.

4 And when he that doth flee unto one of those cities shall stand at the [c]entering of the gate of the city, and shall declare his cause in the ears of the elders of that city, they shall take him into the city unto them, and give him a place, that he may [d]dwell among them.

5 And if the [e]avenger of blood pursue after him, then they shall not deliver the slayer up into his hand; because he smote his neighbour unwittingly, and hated him not beforetime.

6 And he shall dwell in that city, until he stand before the congregation for judgment, *and* until the death of the high priest that shall be in those days: then shall the slayer return, and come unto his own city, and unto his own house, unto the city from whence he fled.

7 And they appointed [f]Kedesh in Galilee in mount Naphtali, and Shechem

B.C. 1444.

a Num. 35:6, *refs.*

b Heb. *goel*, *Redemp.* (*Kinsman type*). Isa. 59:20, *note.*

c Ruth 4:1, 2.

d Heb. 6:18.

e Num. 35:12, 25.

f Josh. 21:32; 1 Chr. 6:76.

in mount Ephraim, and Kirjath-arba, which *is* Hebron, in the mountain of Judah.

8 And on the other side Jordan by Jericho eastward, they assigned [a]Bezer in the wilderness upon the plain out of the tribe of Reuben, and Ramoth in Gilead out of the tribe of Gad, and Golan in Bashan out of the tribe of Manasseh.

9 These were the cities appointed for all the children of Israel, and for the stranger that sojourneth among them, that whosoever killeth *any* person at unawares might flee thither, and not die by the hand of the avenger of blood, until he stood before the congregation.

CHAPTER 21.

Division of the land: the portion of the Levites.

Then came near the heads of the fathers of the Levites unto [b]Eleazar the priest, and unto Joshua the son of Nun, and unto the heads of the fathers of the tribes of the children of Israel;

2 And they spake unto them at Shiloh in the land of Canaan, saying, The [c]LORD commanded by the hand of Moses to give us cities to dwell in, with the suburbs thereof for our cattle.

3 And the children of Israel gave unto the Levites out of their inheritance, at the commandment of the LORD, these cities and their suburbs.

4 And the lot came out for the families of the Kohathites: and the children of [d]Aaron the priest, *which were* of the Levites, had by lot out of the tribe of Judah, and out of the tribe of Simeon, and out of the tribe of Benjamin, thirteen cities.

5 And the rest of the children of [e]Kohath *had* by lot out of the families of the tribe of Ephraim, and out of the tribe of Dan, and out of the half tribe of Manasseh, ten cities.

6 And the children of Gershon *had* by lot out of the families of the tribe of Issachar, and out of the tribe of Asher, and out of the tribe of Naphtali, and out of the half tribe of Manasseh in Bashan, thirteen cities.

7 The children of Merari by their families *had* out of the tribe of Reuben, and out of the tribe of Gad, and out of the tribe of Zebulun, twelve cities.

8 And the children of Israel gave by lot unto the Levites these cities with their suburbs, as the LORD commanded by the hand of Moses.

9 And they gave out of the tribe of the children of Judah, and out of the tribe of the children of Simeon, these cities which are *here* mentioned by name,

10 Which the children of Aaron, *being* of the families of the Kohathites, *who were* of the children of Levi, had: for theirs was the first lot.

11 And [f]they gave them the city of Arba the father of Anak, which *city is* Hebron, in the hill *country* of Judah, with the suburbs thereof round about it.

12 But the fields of the city, and the villages thereof, gave they to [g]Caleb the son of Jephunneh for his possession.

13 Thus they gave to the children of Aaron the priest Hebron with her suburbs, *to be* a city of refuge for the slayer; and Libnah with her suburbs,

14 And Jattir with her suburbs, and Eshtemoa with her suburbs,

15 And [h]Holon with her suburbs, and Debir with her suburbs,

16 And [i]Ain with her suburbs, and Juttah with her suburbs, *and* Beth-shemesh with her suburbs; nine cities out of those two tribes.

17 And out of the tribe of Benjamin, Gibeon with her suburbs, Geba with her suburbs,

18 Anathoth with her suburbs, and Almon with her suburbs; four cities.

19 All the cities of the children of Aaron, the priests, *were* thirteen cities with their suburbs.

20 And the families of the children of Kohath, the Levites which remained of the children of Kohath, even they had the cities of their lot out of the tribe of Ephraim.

21 For they gave them Shechem with her suburbs in mount Ephraim, *to be* a city of refuge for the slayer; and Gezer with her suburbs,

22 And Kibzaim with her suburbs, and Beth-horon with her suburbs; four cities.

23 And out of the tribe of Dan, Eltekeh with her suburbs, Gibbethon with her suburbs,

24 Aijalon with her suburbs, Gath-rimmon with her suburbs; four cities.

25 And out of the half tribe of Manasseh, Tanach with her suburbs, and Gath-rimmon with her suburbs; two cities.

26 All the cities *were* ten with their

B.C. 1444.

a Josh. 21:36; Deut. 4:43; 1 Chr. 6:78.

b Josh. 14:1; 17:4.

c Num. 35:2; 1 Cor. 9:14.

d vs. 8, 19; Josh. 24:33.

e v. 20.

f 1 Chr. 6:54-60.

g Josh. 14:14.

h Josh. 15:51; 1 Chr. 6:58, *Hilen.*

i Josh. 15:42; 1 Chr. 6:59, *Ashan.*

suburbs for the families of the children
of Kohath that remained.
27 And unto the children of Gershon,
of the families of the Levites, out of the
other half tribe of Manasseh *they gave*
Golan in Bashan with her suburbs, *to be*
a city of refuge for the slayer; and Beesh-
terah with her suburbs; two cities.
28 And out of the tribe of Issachar,
Kishon with her suburbs, Dabareh with
her suburbs,
29 Jarmuth with her suburbs, En-gannim with her suburbs; four cities.
30 And out of the tribe of Asher,
Mishal with her suburbs, Abdon with
her suburbs,
31 Helkath with her suburbs, and
Rehob with her suburbs; four cities.
32 And out of the tribe of Naphtali,
[a]Kedesh in Galilee with her suburbs, *to*
be a city of refuge for the slayer; and
Hammoth-dor with her suburbs, and
Kartan with her suburbs; three cities.
33 All the cities of the Gershonites
according to their families *were* thirteen
cities with their suburbs.
34 And unto the families of the children
of [b]Merari, the rest of the Levites, out of
the tribe of Zebulun, Jokneam with her
suburbs, and Kartah with her suburbs,
35 Dimnah with her suburbs, Nahalal
with her suburbs; four cities.
36 And out of the tribe of [c]Reuben,
Bezer with her suburbs, and Jahazah
with her suburbs,
37 Kedemoth with her suburbs, and
Mephaath with her suburbs; four cities.
38 And out of the tribe of Gad,
Ramoth in Gilead with her suburbs, *to be*
a city of refuge for the slayer; and
Mahanaim with her suburbs,
39 Heshbon with her suburbs, Jazer
with her suburbs; four cities in all.
40 So all the cities for the children of
Merari by their families, which were
remaining of the families of the Levites,
were *by* their lot twelve cities.
41 All the cities of the Levites within the
possession of the children of Israel *were*
[d]forty and eight cities with their suburbs.
42 These cities were every one with
their suburbs round about them: thus
were all these cities.
43 And the LORD gave unto Israel all
the land which he [e]sware to give unto
their fathers; and they possessed it, and
dwelt therein.
44 [f]And the LORD gave them rest
round about, according to all that he
sware unto their fathers: and there stood
not a man of all their enemies before
them; the LORD delivered all their enemies into their hand.
45 [g]There failed not ought of any good
thing which the LORD had spoken unto
the house of Israel; all came to pass.

CHAPTER 22.

The schismatic altar of Reuben and Gad.

Then Joshua called the Reubenites,
and the Gadites, and the half tribe
of Manasseh,
2 And said unto them, Ye have kept all
that Moses the servant of the LORD commanded you, and have obeyed my voice
in all that I commanded you:
3 Ye have not left your brethren these
many days unto this day, but have kept
the charge of the commandment of the
LORD your God.
4 And now the LORD your God hath
given rest unto your brethren, as he
promised them: therefore now return ye,
and get you unto your tents, *and* unto
the land of your possession, which
Moses the servant of the LORD gave you
on the other side Jordan.
5 But take diligent heed to do the commandment and the law, which Moses the
servant of the LORD charged you, to love
the LORD your God, and to walk in all his
ways, and to keep his commandments,
and to cleave unto him, and to serve him
with all your heart and with all your soul.
6 So Joshua blessed them, and sent
them away: and they went unto their
tents.
7 Now to the *one* half of the tribe of
Manasseh Moses had given *possession* in
Bashan: but unto the *other* half thereof
gave Joshua among their brethren on
this side Jordan westward. And when
Joshua sent them away also unto their
tents, then he blessed them,
8 And he spake unto them, saying,
Return with much riches unto your
tents, and with very much cattle, with
silver, and with gold, and with brass,
and with iron, and with very much raiment: divide the spoil of your enemies
with your brethren.
9 And the children of Reuben and the

B.C. 1444.

a Josh. 20:7.
b v. 7; 1 Chr. 6:77.
c Josh. 20:8.
d Num. 35:7.
e Gen. 12:7; 26:3, 4; 28:4, 13, 14.
f Deut. 7:23, 24.
g Josh. 23:14; Num. 23:19; 1 Ki. 8:56; 1 Cor. 1:9; 1 Thes. 5:24; Tit. 1:2.

children of Gad and the half tribe of
Manasseh returned, and departed from
the children of Israel out of Shiloh,
which *is* in the land of Canaan, to go
unto the country of Gilead, to the land of
their possession, whereof they were possessed, according to the word of the
LORD by the hand of Moses.
10 And when they came unto the borders of Jordan, that *are* in the land of
Canaan, the children of Reuben and the
children of Gad and the half tribe of
Manasseh built there an altar by Jordan,
a great altar to see to.
11 And the children of Israel [a]heard
say, Behold, the children of Reuben and
the children of Gad and the half tribe of
Manasseh have built an altar over
against the land of Canaan, in the borders of Jordan, at the passage of the children of Israel.
12 And when the children of Israel
heard *of it*, the whole congregation of the
children of Israel gathered themselves
together at Shiloh, to go up to war
against them.
13 And the children of Israel sent unto
the children of Reuben, and to the children of Gad, and to the half tribe of
Manasseh, into the land of [b]Gilead,
Phinehas the son of Eleazar the priest,
14 And with him ten princes, of each
chief house a prince throughout all the
tribes of Israel; and each one *was* an
head of the house of their fathers among
the thousands of Israel.
15 And they came unto the children of
Reuben, and to the children of Gad, and
to the half tribe of Manasseh, unto the
land of Gilead, and they spake with
them, saying,
16 Thus saith the whole congregation
of the LORD, What [c]trespass *is* this that
ye have committed against the God of
Israel, to turn away this day from following the LORD, in that ye have builded
you an altar, that ye might rebel this day
against the LORD?
17 *Is* the iniquity of Peor too little for
us, from which we are not cleansed until
this day, although there was a plague in
the congregation of the LORD,
18 But that ye must turn away this day
from following the LORD? and it will be,
seeing ye rebel to day against the LORD,
that to morrow he will be wroth with the
whole congregation of Israel.

19 Notwithstanding, if the land of
your possession *be* unclean, *then* pass ye
over unto the land of the possession of
the LORD, wherein the LORD'S tabernacle
dwelleth, and take possession among us:
but rebel not against the LORD, nor rebel
against us, in building you an altar
beside the altar of the LORD our God.
20 Did not Achan the son of Zerah
commit a trespass in the accursed thing,
and wrath fell on all the congregation of
Israel? and that man perished not alone
in his iniquity.
21 Then the children of Reuben and
the children of Gad and the half tribe of
Manasseh answered, and said unto the
heads of the thousands of Israel,
22 The LORD God of gods, the LORD
God of gods, he knoweth, and Israel he
shall know; if *it be* in rebellion, or if in
transgression against the LORD, (save us
not this day,)
23 That we have built us an altar to
turn from following the LORD, or if to
offer thereon burnt-offering or [d]meat-
offering, or if to offer peace-offerings
thereon, let the LORD himself require *it*;
24 And if we have not *rather* done it
for fear of *this* thing, saying, In time to
come your children might speak unto
our children, saying, What have ye to do
with the LORD God of Israel?
25 For the LORD hath made Jordan a
border between us and you, ye children
of Reuben and children of Gad; ye have
no part in the LORD: so shall your children make our children cease from [e]fear-
ing the LORD.
26 Therefore we said, Let us now prepare to build us an altar, not for burnt-
offering, nor for sacrifice:
27 But *that* it *may be* a [f]witness between
us, and you, and our generations after
us, that we might do the service of the
[g]LORD before him with our burnt-offerings, and with our sacrifices, and with
our peace-offerings; that your children
may not say to our children in time to
come, Ye have no part in the LORD.
28 Therefore said we, that it shall be,
when they should *so* say to us or to our
generations in time to come, that we
may say *again*, Behold the pattern of the
altar of the LORD, which our fathers
made, not for burnt-offerings, nor for

B.C. 1444.

a Deut. 13:12-18; Jud. 20:1, 12.

b Ex. 6:25; Num. 25:7.

c Deut. 12:5-14.

d Lit. *meal.*

e Psa. 19:9, *note.*

f v. 34.

g Deut. 12:5, 6.

B.C. 1444.

sacrifices; but it *is* a [a]witness between us
and you.
29 God forbid that we should rebel
against the LORD, and turn this day from
following the LORD, to build an altar for
burnt-offerings, for [b]meat-offerings, or
for sacrifices, beside the altar of the LORD
our God that *is* before his tabernacle.
30 And when Phinehas the priest, and
the princes of the congregation and
heads of the thousands of Israel which
were with him, heard the words that the
children of Reuben and the children of
Gad and the children of Manasseh
spake, it pleased them.
31 And Phinehas the son of Eleazar the
priest said unto the children of Reuben,
and to the children of Gad, and to the children of Manasseh, This day we perceive
that the [c]LORD *is* among us, because ye
have not committed this trespass against
the LORD: now ye have delivered the children of Israel out of the hand of the LORD.
32 And Phinehas the son of Eleazar the
priest, and the princes, returned from the
children of Reuben, and from the children of Gad, out of the land of Gilead,
unto the land of Canaan, to the children
of Israel, and brought them word again.
33 And the thing pleased the children
of Israel; and the children of Israel
blessed God, and did not intend to go
up against them in battle, to destroy the
land wherein the children of Reuben and
Gad dwelt.
34 And the children of Reuben and the
children of Gad called the altar [d]*Ed:* for
it *shall be* a witness between us that the
LORD *is* God.

CHAPTER 23.

The last counsels of Joshua.

And it came to pass a long time after
that the LORD had given [e]rest unto
Israel from all their enemies round about,
that Joshua waxed old *and* stricken in age.
2 And Joshua [f]called for all Israel, *and*
for their elders, and for their heads, and
for their judges, and for their officers,
and said unto them, I am old *and* strick-
en in age:
3 And ye have seen all that the [g]LORD
your God hath done unto all these
nations because of you; for the LORD
your God *is* he that hath fought for you.
4 Behold, I have divided unto you by
lot these nations that remain, to be an
inheritance for your tribes, from Jordan,
with all the nations that I have cut off,
even unto the great sea westward.
5 And the LORD your God, he shall
expel them from before you, and drive
them from out of your sight; and ye shall
possess their land, as the LORD your God
hath [h]promised unto you.
6 Be ye therefore very courageous to
keep and to do all that is written in the
book of the law of Moses, that ye turn
not aside therefrom *to* the right hand or
to the left;
7 That ye come not among these
nations, these that remain among you;
neither make [i]mention of the name of
their gods, nor cause to swear *by them,*
neither serve them, nor bow yourselves
unto them:
8 But cleave unto the LORD your God,
as ye have done unto this day.
9 For the LORD hath driven out from
before you great nations and strong: but
as for you, no man hath been able to
stand before you unto this day.
10 One man of you shall chase a thousand: for the LORD your God, he *it is* that
fighteth for you, as he hath promised you.
11 Take good heed therefore unto yourselves, that ye love the LORD your God.
12 Else if ye do in any wise go back, and
cleave unto the remnant of these nations,
even these that remain among you, and
shall make marriages with them, and go
in unto them, and they to you:
13 Know for a certainty that the LORD
your God will no more drive out *any of*
these nations from before you; but they
shall be snares and traps unto you, and
scourges in your sides, and thorns in
your eyes, until ye perish from off this
good land which the LORD your God
hath given you.
14 And, behold, this day I *am* going the
way of all the earth: and ye know in all
your hearts and in all your souls, that not
one thing hath failed of all the good
things which the LORD your God spake
concerning you; all are come to pass unto
you, *and* not one thing hath failed thereof.
15 Therefore it shall come to pass, *that*
as all good things are come upon you,
which the LORD your God promised you;

a Gen. 31:44, 48.
b Lit. *meal.*
c Lev. 26:11, 12; Zech. 8:23.
d i.e. *a witness;* so Josh. 24:27.
e Josh. 22:4.
f Deut. 31:28; 1 Chr. 28:1.
g Psa. 44:3.
h Num. 33:53.
i Psa. 16:4; Hos. 2:17.

so shall the LORD bring upon you all evil things, until he have destroyed you from off this good land which the LORD your God hath given you.

16 When ye have transgressed the covenant of the LORD your God, which he commanded you, and have gone and served other gods, and bowed yourselves to them; then shall the [a]anger of the LORD be kindled against you, and ye shall perish quickly from off the good land which he hath given unto you.

CHAPTER 24.

Joshua's last charge to Israel: his death.

And Joshua gathered all the tribes of Israel to Shechem, and [b]called for the elders of Israel, and for their heads, and for their judges, and for their officers; and they presented themselves before God.

2 And Joshua said unto all the people, Thus saith the LORD God of Israel, [c]Your fathers dwelt on the other side of the flood in old time, *even* Terah, the father of Abraham, and the father of Nachor: and they served other gods.

3 And I [d]took your father Abraham from the other side of the flood, and led him throughout all the land of Canaan, and multiplied his seed, and gave him Isaac.

4 And I gave unto Isaac Jacob and Esau: and I gave unto Esau mount Seir, to possess it; but Jacob and his children went down into Egypt.

5 I sent Moses also and Aaron, and I plagued Egypt, according to that which I did among them: and afterward I brought you out.

6 And I brought your fathers out of Egypt: and ye came unto the sea; and the Egyptians pursued after your fathers with chariots and horsemen unto the Red sea.

7 And when they cried unto the LORD, he put darkness between you and the Egyptians, and brought the sea upon them, and covered them; and your eyes have seen what I have done in Egypt: and ye dwelt in the wilderness a long season.

8 And I brought you into the land of the Amorites, which dwelt on the other side Jordan; and they fought with you: and I gave them into your hand, that ye might possess their land; and I destroyed them from before you.

9 Then Balak the son of Zippor, king of Moab, arose and warred against [e]Israel, and sent and called Balaam the son of Beor to curse you:

10 But I would not hearken unto Balaam; therefore he blessed you still: so I delivered you out of his hand.

11 And ye went over Jordan, and came unto Jericho: and the men of Jericho fought against you, the Amorites, and the Perizzites, and the Canaanites, and the Hittites, and the Girgashites, the Hivites, and the Jebusites; and I delivered them into your hand.

12 And I sent the hornet before you, which drave them out from before you, *even* the two kings of the Amorites; *but* not with thy sword, nor with thy bow.

13 And I have given you a land for which ye did not labour, and cities which ye built not, and ye dwell in them; of the vineyards and oliveyards which ye planted not do ye eat.

14 Now therefore [f]fear the LORD, and serve him in sincerity and in truth: and put away the gods which your fathers served on the other side of the flood, and in Egypt; and serve ye the LORD.

15 And if it seem evil unto you to serve the LORD, choose you this day whom ye will serve; [g]whether the gods which your fathers served that *were* on the other side of the flood, or the gods of the Amorites, in whose land ye dwell: [h]but as for me and my house, we will serve the LORD.

16 And the people answered and said, God forbid that we should forsake the LORD, to serve other gods;

17 For the LORD our God, he *it is* that brought us up and our fathers out of the land of Egypt, from the house of bondage, and which did those great signs in our sight, and preserved us in all the way wherein we went, and among all the people through whom we passed:

18 And the LORD drave out from before us all the people, even the Amorites which dwelt in the land: [i]*therefore* will we also serve the LORD; for he *is* our God.

19 And Joshua said unto the people, Ye cannot serve the LORD: for he *is* an holy God; he *is* a jealous God; he will not forgive your transgressions nor your sins.

B.C. 1427.

a Deut. 4:24-28; 2 Ki. 24:20.

b Josh. 23:2.

c Gen. 11:26.

d Gen. 12:1.

e *Israel* (*history*). vs. 1-33; Jud. 2:8-18. (Gen. 12:2, 3; Rom. 11:26.)

f Psa. 19:9, *note.*

g Ezk. 20:39.

h Gen. 18:19; Psa. 101:2; 1 Tim. 3:4, 5.

i Psa. 116:16.

20 [a]If ye forsake the LORD, and serve strange gods, then he will turn and do you hurt, and consume you, [b]after that he hath done you good.

21 And the people said unto Joshua, Nay; but we will serve the LORD.

22 And Joshua said unto the people, Ye *are* witnesses against yourselves that ye have [c]chosen you the LORD, to serve him. And they said, *We are* witnesses.

23 Now therefore [d]put away, *said he,* the strange gods which *are* among you, and incline your heart unto the LORD God of Israel.

24 And the people [e]said unto Joshua, The LORD our God will we serve, and his voice will we obey.

25 So Joshua made a covenant with the people that day, and set them a statute and an ordinance in Shechem.

26 And Joshua wrote these words in the book of the law of God, and took a great stone, and set it up [f]there under an oak, that *was* by the sanctuary of the LORD.

27 And Joshua said unto all the people, Behold, this stone shall be a witness unto us; for it hath heard all the words of the LORD which he spake unto us: it shall be therefore a witness unto you, lest ye deny your God.

28 So Joshua let the people depart, every man unto his inheritance.

The death of Joshua.

29 And it [g]came to pass after these things, that Joshua the son of Nun, the servant of the LORD, died, *being* an hundred and ten years old.

30 And they buried him in the border of his [h]inheritance in Timnath-serah, which *is* in mount Ephraim, on the north side of the hill of Gaash.

31 And Israel served the LORD all the days of Joshua, and all the days of the elders that [i]overlived Joshua, and which had known all the works of the LORD, that he had done for Israel.

32 And the [j]bones of Joseph, which the children of Israel brought up out of Egypt, buried they in Shechem, in a parcel of ground which Jacob bought of the sons of Hamor the father of Shechem for an hundred pieces of silver: and it became the inheritance of the children of Joseph.

33 And Eleazar the son of Aaron died; and they buried him in a hill *that pertained to* Phinehas his son, which was given him in mount Ephraim.

B.C. 1427.

a 1 Chr. 28:9; Ezra 8:22; Isa. 63:10; 65:11, 12.

b Ezk. 18:24.

c Psa. 119:173.

d Jud. 10:15, 16; 1 Sam. 7:3; 2 Cor. 6:16-18.

e Deut. 5:28, 29.

f Jud. 9:6.

g *Israel* (*history*). vs. 29-33; Jud. 2:8-18. (Gen. 12:2, 3; Rom. 11:26.)

h Josh. 19:50.

i *prolonged their days after.*

j Gen. 50:25; Heb. 11:22.

THE BOOK OF JUDGES

THIS book takes its name from the thirteen men raised up to deliver Israel in the declension and disunion which followed the death of Joshua. Through these men Jehovah continued His personal government of Israel. The key-verse to the condition of Israel is (17:6), "Every man did that which was right in his own eyes." Two facts stand out—the utter failure of Israel; the persistent grace of Jehovah. In the choice of the Judges is illustrated Zechariah's great word (4:6), "not by might, nor by power, but by My Spirit, saith the Lord"; and Paul's word (1 Cor. 1:25), "not many wise men after the flesh, not many mighty, not many noble, are called."

The book records seven apostasies, seven servitudes to seven heathen nations, seven deliverances. The spiritual parallel is found in the history of the professing church since the Apostles, in the rise of sects and the lost sense of the unity of the one body (1 Cor. 12:12, 13).

Judges is in two parts: I. 1–16 inclusive; key-verse, 2:18. II. 17–21; key verse, 21:25.

The events recorded in Judges cover a period of 305 years (Ussher).

CHAPTER 1.

B.C. 1425.

The incomplete victory of Judah.

NOW after the [a]death of Joshua it
came to pass, that the children of
Israel asked the LORD, saying, Who shall
go up for us against the Canaanites first,
to fight against them?
2 And the LORD said, [b]Judah shall go
up: behold, I have delivered the land
into his hand.
3 And Judah said unto Simeon his
brother, Come up with me into my lot,
that we may fight against the
Canaanites; and I likewise will go with
thee into thy lot. So Simeon went with
him.
4 And Judah went up; and the LORD
delivered the Canaanites and the
Perizzites into their hand: and they slew
of them in Bezek ten thousand men.
5 And they found Adoni-bezek in
Bezek: and they fought against him, and
they slew the Canaanites and the
Perizzites.
6 But Adoni-bezek fled; and they pursued after him, and caught him, and cut
off his thumbs and his great toes.
7 And Adoni-bezek said, Threescore
and ten kings, having their thumbs and
their great toes cut off, gathered *their
meat* under my table: as I have done, so
God hath requited me. And they
brought him to Jerusalem, and there he
died.
8 Now the children of Judah had
fought against Jerusalem, and had taken
it, and smitten it with the edge of the
sword, and set the city on fire.
9 And [c]afterward the children of
Judah went down to fight against the
Canaanites, that dwelt in the mountain,
and in the south, and in the valley.
10 And Judah went against the
Canaanites that dwelt in [d]Hebron: (now
the name of Hebron before *was* Kirjath-arba:) and they slew Sheshai, and
Ahiman, and Talmai.
11 And from thence he went against
the inhabitants of Debir: and the name of
Debir before *was* Kirjath-sepher:
12 And [e]Caleb said, He that smiteth
Kirjath-sepher, and taketh it, to him will
I give Achsah my daughter to wife.
13 And Othniel the son of Kenaz,
Caleb's younger brother, took it: and he
gave him Achsah his daughter to wife.
14 And it came to pass, when she
came *to him*, that she moved him to ask
of her father a field: and she lighted
from off *her* ass; and Caleb said unto her,
What wilt thou?
15 And she said unto him, Give me a
blessing: for thou hast given me a south
land; give me also springs of water. And
Caleb gave her the upper springs and
the nether springs.
16 And the children of the Kenite,
Moses' father in law, went up out
of the city of [f]palm trees with the children of Judah into the wilderness

a Josh. 24:29.
b Gen. 49:8, 9; Rev. 5:5.
c Josh. 11:21.
d Josh. 15:13.
e Josh. 15:16, 17.
f Deut. 34:3.

B.C. 1425.

of Judah, which *lieth* in the south of Arad; and they went and dwelt among the people.

17 And Judah went with Simeon his brother, and they slew the Canaanites that inhabited Zephath, and utterly destroyed it. And the name of the city was called Hormah.

18 Also Judah took Gaza with the coast thereof, and Askelon with the coast thereof, and Ekron with the coast thereof.

19 And the LORD was with Judah; and he drave out *the inhabitants of* the mountain; but could not drive out the inhabitants of the valley, because they had chariots of iron.

20 And they gave [a]Hebron unto Caleb, as Moses said: and he expelled thence the three sons of Anak.

The incomplete victory of Benjamin.

21 And the children of Benjamin did not drive out the Jebusites that inhabited Jerusalem; but the Jebusites dwell with the children of Benjamin in Jerusalem unto this day.

22 And the house of Joseph, they also went up against Beth-el: and the LORD *was* with them.

23 And the house of Joseph sent to descry Beth-el. (Now the name of the city before *was* Luz.)

24 And the spies saw a man come forth out of the city, and they said unto him, Shew us, we pray thee, the entrance into the city, and [b]we will shew thee mercy.

25 And when he shewed them the entrance into the city, they smote the city with the edge of the sword; but they let go the man and all his family.

26 And the man went into the land of the [c]Hittites, and built a city, and called the name thereof Luz: which *is* the name thereof unto this day.

The incomplete victory of Manasseh.

27 Neither did Manasseh drive out *the inhabitants of* Beth-shean and her towns, nor Taanach and her towns, nor the inhabitants of Dor and her towns, nor the inhabitants of Ibleam and her towns, nor the inhabitants of Megiddo and her towns: but the Canaanites would dwell in that land.

28 And it came to pass, when Israel was strong, that they put the Canaanites to tribute, and did not utterly drive them out.

29 Neither did Ephraim drive out the Canaanites that dwelt in Gezer; but the Canaanites dwelt in Gezer among them.

30 Neither did Zebulun drive out the inhabitants of Kitron, nor the inhabitants of Nahalol; but the Canaanites dwelt among them, and became tributaries.

31 Neither did Asher drive out the inhabitants of Accho, nor the inhabitants of Zidon, nor of Ahlab, nor of Achzib, nor of Helbah, nor of Aphik, nor of Rehob:

32 But the Asherites dwelt among the Canaanites, the inhabitants of the land: for they did not drive them out.

33 Neither did Naphtali drive out the inhabitants of Beth-shemeth, nor the inhabitants of Beth-anath; but he dwelt among the Canaanites, the inhabitants of the land: nevertheless the inhabitants of Beth-shemeth and of Beth-anath became tributaries unto them.

34 And the Amorites forced the children of Dan into the mountain: for they would not suffer them to come down to the valley:

35 But the Amorites would dwell in mount Heres in Aijalon, and in Shaalbim: yet the hand of the house of Joseph prevailed, so that they became tributaries.

36 And the coast of the Amorites *was* from the going up to Akrabbim, from the rock, and upward.

CHAPTER 2.

Review of the Israelitish invasion of Canaan to the death of Joshua.

And an [d]angel of the LORD came up from Gilgal to Bochim, and said, I made you to go up out of Egypt, and have brought you unto the land which I sware unto your fathers; and I [e]said, I will never break my covenant with you.

2 And ye shall make no league with the inhabitants of this land; ye shall throw down their altars: [f]but ye have not obeyed my voice: why have ye done this?

3 Wherefore I also said, I will not drive them out from before you; but they shall be *as thorns* in your sides, and their gods shall be a snare unto you.

4 And it came to pass, when the angel of the LORD spake these words unto all the children of Israel, that the people lifted up their voice, and wept.

a Josh. 14:9, 14.
b Josh. 2:12; 1 Sam. 30:15.
c 2 Ki. 7:6.
d Heb. 1:4, *note.*
e Gen. 17:7; Ex. 23:20; Psa. 89:34.
f Psa. 106:34.

B.C. 1425.

5 And they called the name of that place [a]Bochim: and they sacrificed there unto the LORD.

6 And when Joshua had let the people go, the children of Israel went every man unto his inheritance to possess the land.

7 And the people served the LORD all the days of Joshua, and all the days of the elders that outlived Joshua, who had seen all the great works of the LORD, that he did for Israel.

8 And [b]Joshua the son of Nun, the servant of the LORD, died, *being* an hundred and ten years old.

9 And they buried him in the border of his inheritance in [c]Timnath-heres, in the mount of Ephraim, on the north side of the hill Gaash.

10 And also all that generation were gathered unto their fathers: and there arose another generation after them, which knew not the LORD, nor yet the works which he had done for Israel.

11 And the children of Israel did evil in the sight of the LORD, and served Baalim:

12 And they forsook the LORD God of their fathers, which brought them out of the land of Egypt, and followed other gods, of the gods of the people that *were* round about them, and bowed themselves unto them, and provoked the LORD to anger.

13 And they forsook the LORD, and served Baal and [1]Ashtaroth.

14 And the anger of the LORD was hot against Israel, and he delivered them into the hands of spoilers that spoiled them, and he sold them into the hands of their enemies round about, so that they could not any longer stand before their enemies.

15 Whithersoever they went out, the hand of the LORD was against them for evil, as the LORD had said, and as the LORD had sworn unto them: and they were greatly distressed.

Institution of the Judges.

16 Nevertheless the LORD raised up [d]judges, which delivered them out of the hand of those that spoiled them.

17 And yet they would not hearken unto their judges, but they went a whoring after other gods, and bowed themselves unto them: they turned quickly out of the way which their fathers walked in, obeying the commandments of the LORD; *but* they did not so.

18 And when the LORD raised them up [2]judges, then the LORD was with the judge, and delivered them out of the hand of their enemies all the days of the judge: for it [e]repented the LORD because of their groanings by reason of them that oppressed them and vexed them.

19 And it came to pass, when the judge was dead, *that* they returned, and corrupted *themselves* more than their fathers, in following other gods to serve them, and to bow down unto them; they ceased not from their own doings, nor from their stubborn way.

Result of Israel's incomplete obedience.

20 And the anger of the LORD was hot against Israel; and he said, Because that this people hath transgressed my covenant which I commanded their fathers, and have not hearkened unto my voice;

21 I also will not henceforth drive out any from before them of the nations which Joshua left when he died:

22 That through them I may prove Israel, whether they will keep the way of the LORD to walk therein, as their fathers did keep *it*, or not.

a i.e. *weepers.*

b *Israel* (*history*). vs. 8-18; 1 Sam. 8:1-8. (Gen. 12:2, 3; Rom. 11:26.)

c Josh. 19:50, *Timnath-serah.*

d *Kingdom* (O.T.). vs. 16-18; 1 Sam. 8:1-7. (Gen. 1:26; Zech. 12:8.)

e Zech. 8:14, *note.*

[1] **(2:13)** Ashtaroth, plural of Ashtoreth (1 Ki. 11:5), were figures of Ashtoreth the Phoenician goddess (the Astarte of the Greeks), which were worshipped as idols during times of spiritual declension in Israel (Jud. 10:6; 1 Sam. 7:3, 4; 12:10; 31:10; 1 Ki. 11:5, 33; 2 Ki. 23:13). Jeremiah refers (44:18, 19) to Ashtoreth as the "queen of heaven."

[2] **(2:18)** The judges were tribesmen in Israel upon whom the Lord laid the burden of Israel's apostate and oppressed state. They were the spiritual ancestors of the prophets; that is to say, men raised up of God, the theocratic King, to represent Him in the nation. They were patriots and religious reformers because national security and prosperity were inseparably connected with loyalty and obedience to Jehovah. Not one of the chosen deliverers had anything whereof to glory in the flesh. Othniel was but the son of the younger brother of Caleb; Ehud was a left-handed man and an assassin; Shamgar, a rustic with an ox-goad; Deborah, a woman; Gideon, of an obscure family in the smallest tribe, etc. Each of the classes mentioned in 1 Cor. 1:27, 28 is illustrated among the judges.

23 Therefore the LORD left those nations,
without driving them out hastily; neither
delivered he them into the hand of
Joshua.

CHAPTER 3.

NOW these *are* the nations which the
LORD left, to prove Israel by them,
even as many *of Israel* as had not known
all the wars of Canaan;
2 Only that the generations of the children of Israel might know, to teach them
war, at the least such as before knew
nothing thereof;
3 *Namely*, five lords of the Philistines,
and all the Canaanites, and the Sidonians, and the Hivites that dwelt in mount
Lebanon, from mount Baal-hermon unto
the entering in of Hamath.
4 And they were to prove Israel by
them, to know whether they would
hearken unto the commandments of the
LORD, which he commanded their
fathers by the hand of Moses.

The first apostasy and servitude.

5 And the children of Israel dwelt
among the Canaanites, Hittites, and
Amorites, and Perizzites, and Hivites,
and Jebusites:
6 And they took their daughters to be
their wives, and gave their daughters to
their sons, and served their gods.
7 And the children of Israel did evil in
the sight of the LORD, and forgat the
LORD their God, and served Baalim and
the [1a]groves.
8 Therefore the anger of the LORD was
hot against Israel, and he sold them into
the hand of Chushan-rishathaim king of
Mesopotamia: and the children of Israel
served Chushan-rishathaim eight years.

Othniel, the first Judge.

9 And when the children of Israel
cried unto the LORD, the LORD raised up
a [b]deliverer to the children of Israel, who
delivered them, *even* Othniel the son of
Kenaz, Caleb's younger brother.
10 And the [c]Spirit of the LORD came
upon him, and he judged Israel, and
went out to war: and the LORD delivered
Chushan-rishathaim king of Mesopotamia into his hand; and his hand prevailed
against Chushan-rishathaim.
11 And the land had rest forty years.
And Othniel the son of Kenaz died.

The second apostasy and servitude.

12 And the children of Israel did evil
again in the sight of the LORD: and the
[d]LORD strengthened Eglon the king of
Moab against Israel, because they had
done evil in the sight of the LORD.
13 And he gathered unto him the children of Ammon and Amalek, and went
and smote Israel, and possessed the city
of palm trees.
14 So the children of Israel served
Eglon the king of Moab eighteen years.

Ehud, the second Judge.

15 But when the children of Israel
cried unto the LORD, the LORD raised
them up a deliverer, Ehud the son of
Gera, a Benjamite, a man lefthanded:
and by him the children of Israel sent a
present unto Eglon the king of Moab.
16 But Ehud made him a dagger
which had two edges, of a [e]cubit length;
and he did gird it under his raiment
upon his right thigh.
17 And he brought the present unto
Eglon king of Moab: and Eglon *was* a
very fat man.
18 And when he had made an end to
offer the present, he sent away the people that bare the present.
19 But he himself turned again from
the quarries that *were* by Gilgal, and
said, I have a secret errand unto thee, O
king: who said, Keep silence. And all
that stood by him went out from him.
20 And Ehud came unto him; and he
was sitting in a summer parlour, which
he had for himself alone. And Ehud
said, I have a message from God unto
thee. And he arose out of *his* seat.
21 And Ehud put forth his left hand,
and took the dagger from his right thigh,
and thrust it into his belly:
22 And the haft also went in after the

B.C. 1406.

a See Deut. 16:21.
b *saviour.*
c *Holy Spirit.* Jud. 6:34. (Gen. 1:2; Mal. 2:15.)
d 2 Ki. 5:1; Isa. 10:5, 6; 45:1-6.
e About 18 in.

[1](3:7) Groves, like high places, have been associated with idolatrous worship from time immemorial. The Heb. *asherah,* trans. "grove," means also the idol enshrined there (Deut. 16:21). This idol seems often to have been a sacred tree, the figure of which is constantly found on Assyrian monuments. In apostate Israel, however, such groves were associated with every form of idolatry (e.g. 2 Ki. 17:16, 17). See, also, "high places" (1 Ki. 3:2, *note*), and "Ashtaroth," Jud. 2:13, *note.*

blade; and the fat closed upon the blade, so that he could not draw the dagger out of his belly; and the dirt came out.

23 Then Ehud went forth through the porch, and shut the doors of the parlour upon him, and locked them.

24 When he was gone out, his servants came; and when they saw that, behold, the doors of the parlour *were* locked, they said, Surely he [a]covereth his feet in his summer chamber.

25 And they tarried till they were ashamed: and, behold, he opened not the doors of the parlour; therefore they took a key, and opened *them*: and, behold, their lord *was* fallen down dead on the earth.

26 And Ehud escaped while they tarried, and passed beyond the quarries, and escaped unto Seirath.

27 And it came to pass, when he was come, that he blew a trumpet in the mountain of Ephraim, and the children of Israel went down with him from the mount, and he before them.

28 And he said unto them, Follow after me: for the LORD hath delivered your enemies the Moabites into your hand. And they went down after him, and took the fords of Jordan toward Moab, and suffered not a man to pass over.

29 And they slew of Moab at that time about ten thousand men, all lusty, and all men of valour; and there escaped not a man.

30 So Moab was subdued that day under the hand of Israel. And the land had rest fourscore years.

Shamgar, the third Judge.

31 And after him was [b]Shamgar the son of Anath, which slew of the Philistines six hundred men with an ox goad: and he also delivered Israel.

CHAPTER 4.

The third apostasy and servitude.

And the children of Israel [c]again did evil in the sight of the LORD, when Ehud was dead.

2 And the LORD [d]sold them into the hand of Jabin king of Canaan, that reigned in Hazor; the captain of whose host *was* Sisera, which dwelt in [e]Harosheth of the Gentiles.

3 And the children of Israel cried unto the LORD: for he had nine hundred chariots of iron; and twenty years he mightily oppressed the children of Israel.

Deborah and Barak, the fourth and fifth Judges.

4 And Deborah, a prophetess, the wife of Lapidoth, she judged Israel at that time.

5 And she dwelt under the palm tree of [f]Deborah between Ramah and Beth-el in mount Ephraim: and the children of Israel came up to her for judgment.

6 And she sent and called Barak the son of Abinoam out of Kedesh-naphtali, and said unto him, Hath not the LORD God of Israel commanded, *saying*, Go and draw toward mount Tabor, and take with thee ten thousand men of the children of Naphtali and of the children of Zebulun?

7 And [g]I will draw unto thee to the river Kishon Sisera, the captain of Jabin's army, with his chariots and his multitude; and I will deliver him into thine hand.

8 And Barak said unto her, If thou wilt go with me, then I will go: but if thou wilt not go with me, *then* I will not go.

9 And she said, I will surely go with thee: notwithstanding the journey that thou takest shall not be for thine honour; for the LORD shall sell Sisera into the hand of a [h]woman. And Deborah arose, and went with Barak to Kedesh.

10 And Barak called Zebulun and Naphtali to Kedesh; [i]and he went up with ten thousand men at his feet: and Deborah went up with him.

11 Now Heber the Kenite, *which was* of the children of Hobab the father in law of Moses, had severed himself from the Kenites, and pitched his tent unto the plain of Zaanaim, which *is* by Kedesh.

12 And they shewed Sisera that Barak the son of Abinoam was gone up to mount Tabor.

13 And Sisera [j]gathered together all his chariots, *even* nine hundred chariots of iron, and all the people that *were* with him, from Harosheth of the Gentiles unto the river of Kishon.

14 And Deborah said unto Barak, Up; for this *is* the day in which the LORD hath delivered Sisera into thine hand: is not the LORD gone out before thee? So Barak went down from mount Tabor, and ten thousand men after him.

15 And the LORD discomfited Sisera,

B.C. 1336.

a 1 Sam. 24:3.

b Jud. 5:6.

c Jud. 2:19.

d Jud. 2:14; 1 Sam. 12:9; Psa. 83:9. It seems to concern only north Israel.

e vs. 13:16.

f Gen. 35:8.

g Ex. 14:4; Psa. 83:9.

h vs. 18, 21.

i Deut. 20:1.

j *gathered by cry, or, proclamation.*

and all *his* chariots, and all *his* host, with
the edge of the sword before Barak; so
that Sisera lighted down off *his* chariot,
and fled away on his feet.
16 But Barak pursued after the chariots, and after the host, unto Harosheth
of the Gentiles: and all the host of Sisera
fell upon the edge of the sword; *and*
there was not a man left.
17 Howbeit Sisera fled away on his
feet to the tent of Jael the wife of Heber
the Kenite: for *there was* peace between
Jabin the king of Hazor and the house of
Heber the Kenite.
18 And Jael went out to meet Sisera,
and said unto him, Turn in, my lord,
turn in to me; fear not. And when he had
turned in unto her into the tent, she covered him with a mantle.
19 And he said unto her, Give me, I
pray thee, a little water to drink; for I am
thirsty. And she opened a bottle of milk,
and gave him drink, and covered him.
20 Again he said unto her, Stand in the
door of the tent, and it shall be, when
any man doth come and enquire of thee,
and say, Is there any man here? that thou
shalt say, No.
21 Then Jael Heber's wife took a nail
of the tent, and took an hammer in her
hand, and went softly unto him, and
smote the nail into his temples, and fastened it into the ground: for he was fast
asleep and weary. So he died.
22 And, behold, as Barak pursued
Sisera, Jael came out to meet him, and
said unto him, Come, and I will shew thee
the man whom thou seekest. And when
he came into her *tent*, behold, Sisera lay
dead, and the nail *was* in his temples.
23 So God subdued on that day Jabin
the king of Canaan before the children of
Israel.
24 And the hand of the children of
Israel prospered, and prevailed against
Jabin the king of Canaan, until they had
destroyed Jabin king of Canaan.

CHAPTER 5.

The song of Deborah and Barak.

[a]Then sang Deborah and Barak the
son of Abinoam on that day, saying,
2 Praise ye the LORD for the avenging
of Israel, when the people willingly
offered themselves.

B.C. 1296.

3 Hear, O ye kings; give ear, O ye
princes; I, *even* I, will sing unto the LORD;
I will sing *praise* to the LORD God of Israel.
4 LORD, when thou wentest out of Seir,
when thou marchedst out of the field of
Edom, the earth trembled, and the heavens dropped, the clouds also dropped
water.
5 The mountains [b]melted from before
the LORD, *even* that Sinai from before the
LORD God of Israel.
6 In the days of [c]Shamgar the son of
Anath, in the days of Jael, the highways
were unoccupied, and the travellers
walked through byways.
7 *The inhabitants of* the villages ceased,
they ceased in Israel, until that I Deborah
arose, that I arose a mother in Israel.
8 They chose new gods; then *was* war
in the gates: was there a shield or spear
seen among forty thousand in Israel?
9 My heart *is* toward the governors of
Israel, that offered themselves willingly
among the people. Bless ye the LORD.
10 Speak, ye that ride on white asses, ye
that sit in judgment, and walk by the way.
11 *They that are delivered* from the noise
of archers in the places of drawing
water, there shall they rehearse the
[d]righteous acts of the LORD, *even* the
righteous acts *toward the inhabitants* of
his villages in Israel: then shall the people of the LORD go down to the gates.
12 [e]Awake, awake, Deborah: awake,
awake, utter a song: arise, Barak, and
lead thy captivity captive, thou son of
Abinoam.
13 Then he made him that remaineth
have dominion over the nobles among
the people: the LORD made me have
dominion over the mighty.
14 Out of Ephraim *was there* a root of
them against Amalek; after thee,
Benjamin, among thy people; out of
Machir came down governors, and out
of Zebulun they that handle the pen of
the writer.
15 And the princes of Issachar *were*
with Deborah; even Issachar, and also
Barak: he was sent on foot into the valley. For the divisions of Reuben *there
were* great thoughts of heart.
16 Why abodest thou among the
sheepfolds, to hear the bleatings of the

a Ex. 15:1-19; Psa. 18, *title;* Rev. 15:3, 4.

b *flowed.*

c Jud. 3:31.

d *righteousnesses.*

e Psa. 103:1, 2.

flocks? For the divisions of Reuben *there*
were great searchings of heart.
17 Gilead abode beyond Jordan: and
why did Dan remain in ships? Asher
continued on the sea shore, and abode in
his breaches.
18 Zebulun and Naphtali *were* a people *that* jeoparded their lives unto the
death in the high places of the field.
19 The kings came *and* fought, then
fought the kings of Canaan in Taanach
by the waters of Megiddo; they took no
gain of money.
20 They fought from heaven; the stars
in their courses fought against Sisera.
21 The river of Kishon swept them
away, that ancient river, the river
Kishon. O my soul, thou hast trodden
down strength.
22 Then were the horsehoofs broken
by the means of the pransings, the
pransings of their mighty ones.
23 Curse ye Meroz, said the [a]angel of
the LORD, curse ye bitterly the inhabitants thereof; because they came not to
the help of the LORD, to the help of the
LORD against the mighty.
24 Blessed above women shall Jael the
wife of Heber the Kenite be, blessed
shall she be above women in the tent.
25 He asked water, *and* she gave *him*
milk; she brought forth butter in a lordly
dish.
26 She put her hand to the nail, and her
right hand to the workmen's hammer;
and with the hammer she smote Sisera,
she smote off his head, when she had
pierced and stricken through his temples.
27 At her feet he bowed, he fell, he lay
down: at her feet he bowed, he fell: where
he bowed, there he fell down dead.
28 The mother of Sisera looked out at
a window, and cried through the lattice,
Why is his chariot *so* long in coming?
why tarry the wheels of his chariots?
29 Her wise ladies answered her, yea,
she returned [b]answer to herself,
30 Have they not sped? have they *not*
divided the prey; to every man a damsel
or two; to Sisera a prey of divers colours,
a prey of divers colours of needlework,
of divers colours of needlework on both
sides, *meet* for the necks of *them that take*
the spoil?
31 So let all thine enemies [c]perish, O
LORD: but *let* them that love him *be* as the
[d]sun when he goeth forth in his might.
And the land had rest forty years.

B.C. 1296.

a Heb. 1:4, *note*.

b *her words*.

c Psa. 92:9.

d Psa. 37:6; 89:36-37.

e Psa. 50:15; Hos. 5:15.

CHAPTER 6.

The fourth apostasy and servitude.

And the children of Israel did evil in
the sight of the LORD: and the LORD
delivered them into the hand of Midian
seven years.
2 And the hand of Midian prevailed
against Israel: *and* because of the Midianites the children of Israel made them
the dens which *are* in the mountains, and
caves, and strong holds.
3 And *so* it was, when Israel had sown,
that the Midianites came up, and the
Amalekites, and the children of the east,
even they came up against them;
4 And they encamped against them,
and destroyed the increase of the earth,
till thou come unto Gaza, and left no
sustenance for Israel, neither sheep, nor
ox, nor ass.
5 For they came up with their cattle and
their tents, and they came as grasshoppers for multitude; *for* both they and their
camels were without number: and they
entered into the land to destroy it.
6 And Israel was greatly impoverished
because of the Midianites; and the children of Israel [e]cried unto the LORD.
7 And it came to pass, when the children of Israel cried unto the LORD
because of the Midianites,
8 That the LORD sent a prophet unto the
children of Israel, which said unto them,
Thus saith the LORD God of Israel, I
brought you up from Egypt, and brought
you forth out of the house of bondage;
9 And I delivered you out of the hand
of the Egyptians, and out of the hand of
all that oppressed you, and drave them
out from before you, and gave you their
land;
10 And I said unto you, I *am* the LORD
your God; fear not the gods of the
Amorites, in whose land ye dwell: but
ye have not obeyed my voice.

Gideon, the sixth Judge.

11 And there came an [a]angel of the
LORD, and sat under an oak which *was* in
Ophrah, that *pertained* unto Joash the
Abi-ezrite: and his son Gideon threshed

wheat by the winepress, to hide *it* from
the Midianites.
12 And the angel of the LORD appeared
unto him, and said unto him, The LORD *is*
with thee, thou mighty man of valour.
13 And Gideon said unto him, Oh my
Lord, [a]if the LORD be with us, why then
is all this befallen us? and where *be* all
his miracles which our fathers told us of,
saying, Did not the LORD bring us up
from Egypt? but now the LORD hath forsaken us, and delivered us into the
hands of the Midianites.
14 And the LORD looked upon him,
and said, Go in this thy might, and thou
shalt save Israel from the hand of the
Midianites: have not I sent thee?
15 And he said unto him, Oh my Lord,
wherewith shall I save Israel? behold,
my family *is* poor in Manasseh, and I *am*
the least in my father's house.
16 And the LORD said unto him, Surely
I will be with thee, and thou shalt smite
the Midianites as one man.
17 And he said unto him, If now I
have found grace in thy sight, then shew
me a sign that thou talkest with me.
18 Depart not hence, I pray thee, until
I come unto thee, and bring forth my
present, and set *it* before thee. And he
said, I will tarry until thou come again.
19 And Gideon went in, and made
ready a kid, and unleavened cakes of an
[b]ephah of flour: the flesh he put in a basket, and he put the broth in a pot, and
brought *it* out unto him under the oak,
and presented *it*.
20 And the [c]angel of God said unto
him, Take the flesh and the unleavened
cakes, and lay *them* upon this rock, and
pour out the broth. And he did so.
21 Then the [c]angel of the LORD put
forth the end of the staff that *was* in his
hand, and touched the flesh and the
unleavened cakes; and there rose up fire
out of the rock, and consumed the flesh
and the unleavened cakes. Then the [c]an-
gel of the LORD departed out of his sight.
22 And when Gideon perceived that he
was an [c]angel of the LORD, Gideon said,
Alas, O Lord GOD! for because I have
seen an [c]angel of the LORD face to face.
23 And the LORD said unto him, Peace
be unto thee; fear not: thou shalt not die.
24 Then Gideon built an altar there
unto the LORD, and called it Jehovah-
shalom: unto this day it *is* yet in Ophrah
of the Abi-ezrites.
25 And it came to pass the same night,
that the LORD said unto him, Take thy
father's young bullock, even the second
bullock of seven years old, and throw
down the altar of Baal that thy father
hath, and cut down the [d]grove that *is* by
it:
26 And build an altar unto the LORD
thy God upon the top of this rock, in the
ordered place, and take the second bullock, and offer a burnt sacrifice with the
wood of the [d]grove which thou shalt cut
down.
27 Then Gideon took ten men of his
servants, and did as the LORD had said
unto him: and *so* it was, because he
feared his father's household, and the
men of the city, that he could not do *it* by
day, that he did *it* by night.
28 And when the men of the city arose
early in the morning, behold, the altar of
Baal was cast down, and the [d]grove was
cut down that *was* by it, and the second
bullock was offered upon the altar *that*
was built.
29 And they said one to another, Who
hath done this thing? And when they
enquired and asked, they said, Gideon
the son of Joash hath done this thing.
30 Then the men of the city said unto
Joash, Bring out thy son, that he may
die: because he hath cast down the altar
of Baal, and because he hath cut down
the [d]grove that *was* by it.
31 And Joash said unto all that stood
against him, Will ye plead for Baal? will
ye save him? he that will plead for him,
let him be put to death whilst *it is yet*
morning: if he *be* a god, let him plead for
himself, because *one* hath cast down his
altar.
32 Therefore on that day he called him
[e]Jerubbaal, saying, Let Baal plead
against him, because he hath thrown
down his altar.
33 Then all the Midianites and the
Amalekites and the children of the east
were gathered together, and went over,
and pitched in the valley of Jezreel.
34 But the [f]Spirit of the LORD came
upon Gideon, and he blew a trumpet;
and Abi-ezer was gathered after him.

B.C. 1249.

a Gen. 25:22; Psa. 44:9-25.

b One ephah = 1 bu. 3 pts.

c Heb. 1:4, *note.*

d See Deut. 16:21; Jud. 3:7, *note.*

e i.e. *let Baal plead.*

f *Holy Spirit.* Jud. 11:29. (Gen. 1:2; Mal. 2:15.)

35 And he sent messengers throughout
all Manasseh; who also was gathered after
him: and he sent messengers unto Asher,
and unto Zebulun, and unto Naphtali;
and they came up to meet them.
36 And Gideon said unto God, If thou
wilt save Israel by mine hand, as thou
hast said,
37 Behold, I will put a fleece of wool
in the floor; *and* if the dew be on the
fleece only, and *it be* dry upon all the
earth *beside*, then shall I know that thou
wilt save Israel by mine hand, as thou
hast said.
38 And it was so: for he rose up early
on the morrow, and thrust the fleece
together, and wringed the dew out of the
fleece, a bowl full of water.
39 And Gideon said unto God, Let not
thine anger be hot against me, and I will
speak but this once: let me prove, I pray
thee, but this once with the fleece; let it
now be dry only upon the fleece, and
upon all the ground let there be dew.
40 And God did so that night: for it
was dry upon the fleece only, and there
was dew on all the ground.

CHAPTER 7.

The preparation for battle.

Then Jerubbaal, who *is* Gideon, and all
the people that *were* with him, rose
up early, and pitched beside the well of
Harod: so that the host of the Midianites
were on the north side of them, by the
hill of Moreh, in the valley.
2 And the LORD said unto Gideon, The
people that *are* with thee *are* too many
for me to give the Midianites into their
hands, lest Israel [a]vaunt themselves
against me, saying, Mine own hand hath
saved me.
3 Now therefore go to, proclaim in the
ears of the people, saying, [b]Whosoever *is*
fearful and afraid, let him return and
depart early from mount Gilead. And
there returned of the people twenty and
two thousand; and there remained ten
thousand.
4 And the LORD said unto Gideon, The
people *are* yet *too* many; bring them
down unto the water, and I will try them
for thee there: and it shall be, *that* of
whom I say unto thee, This shall go with
thee, the same shall go with thee; and of
whomsoever I say unto thee, This shall
not go with thee, the same shall not go.

B.C. 1249.

a Deut. 8:17; 1 Sam. 14:6; Isa. 10:13; Rom. 11:18; 1 Cor. 1:29; 2 Cor. 4:7; Jas. 4:6.

b Deut. 20:8.

c 1 Sam. 14:6.

5 So he brought down the people unto
the water: and the LORD said unto
Gideon, Every one that lappeth of the
water with his tongue, as a dog lappeth,
him shalt thou set by himself; likewise
every one that boweth down upon his
knees to drink.
6 And the number of them that
lapped, *putting* their hand to their
mouth, were three hundred men: but all
the rest of the people bowed down upon
their knees to drink water.

Gideon's three hundred.

7 And the LORD said unto [c]Gideon, By
the three hundred men that lapped will I
save you, and deliver the Midianites into
thine hand: and let all the *other* people
go every man unto his place.
8 So the people took victuals in their
hand, and their trumpets: and he sent all
the rest of Israel every man unto his tent,
and retained those three hundred men:
and the host of Midian was beneath him
in the valley.
9 And it came to pass the same night,
that the LORD said unto him, Arise, get
thee down unto the host; for I have
delivered it into thine hand.
10 But if thou fear to go down, go thou
with Phurah thy servant down to the
host:
11 And thou shalt hear what they say;
and afterward shall thine hands be
strengthened to go down unto the host.
Then went he down with Phurah his servant unto the outside of the armed men
that *were* in the host.
12 And the Midianites and the
Amalekites and all the children of the
east lay along in the valley like
grasshoppers for multitude; and their
camels *were* without number, as the sand
by the sea side for multitude.
13 And when Gideon was come,
behold, *there was* a man that told a dream
unto his fellow, and said, Behold, I
dreamed a dream, and, lo, a cake of barley bread tumbled into the host of
Midian, and came unto a tent, and smote
it that it fell, and overturned it, that the
tent lay along.
14 And his fellow answered and said,
This *is* nothing else save the sword of
Gideon the son of Joash, a man of Israel:
for into his hand hath God delivered
Midian, and all the host.

15 And it was *so*, when Gideon heard
the telling of the dream, and the interpretation thereof, that he worshipped,
and returned into the host of Israel, and
said, Arise; for the LORD hath delivered
into your hand the host of Midian.

The victory over Midian.

16 And he divided the three hundred
men *into* three companies, and he put a
trumpet in every man's hand, with empty
pitchers, and [a]lamps within the pitchers.
17 And he said unto them, Look on
me, and do likewise: and, behold, when
I come to the outside of the camp, it
shall be *that*, as I do, so shall ye do.
18 When I blow with a trumpet, I and
all that *are* with me, then blow ye the
trumpets also on every side of all the
camp, and say, *The sword* of the LORD,
and of Gideon.
19 So Gideon, and the hundred men
that *were* with him, came unto the outside
of the camp in the beginning of the middle watch; and they had but newly set the
watch: and they blew the trumpets, and
brake the pitchers that *were* in their hands.
20 And the three companies blew the
trumpets, and brake the pitchers, and
held the lamps in their left hands, and
the trumpets in their right hands to blow
withal: and they cried, The sword of the
LORD, and of Gideon.
21 And they [b]stood every man in his
place round about the camp: and all the
host ran, and cried, and fled.
22 And the three hundred blew the
trumpets, and the LORD set every man's
sword against his fellow, even throughout all the host: and the host fled to
Beth-shittah in Zererath, *and* to the border of Abel-meholah, unto Tabbath.
23 And the men of Israel gathered
themselves together out of Naphtali, and
out of Asher, and out of all Manasseh,
and pursued after the Midianites.
24 And Gideon sent messengers
throughout all mount Ephraim, saying,
Come down against the Midianites, and
take before them the waters unto Beth-
barah and Jordan. Then all the men of
Ephraim gathered themselves together,
and took the waters unto [c]Beth-barah
and Jordan.
25 And they took two princes of the
[d]Midianites, Oreb and Zeeb; and they
slew Oreb upon the rock Oreb, and Zeeb
they slew at the winepress of Zeeb, and
pursued Midian, and brought the heads
of Oreb and Zeeb to Gideon on the other
side Jordan.

CHAPTER 8.

The jealousy of Ephraim.
Events to the death of Gideon.

And the men of [e]Ephraim said unto
him, Why hast thou served us thus,
that thou calledst us not, when thou
wentest to fight with the Midianites?
And they did chide with him sharply.
2 And he said unto them, What have I
done now in comparison of you? *Is* not
the gleaning of the grapes of Ephraim
better than the vintage of Abi-ezer?
3 God hath delivered into your hands
the princes of Midian, Oreb and Zeeb:
and what was I able to do in comparison
of you? Then their anger was abated
toward him, when he had said that.
4 And Gideon came to Jordan, *and*
passed over, he, and the three hundred
men that *were* with him, faint, yet pursuing *them*.
5 And he said unto the men of
Succoth, Give, I pray you, loaves of
bread unto the people that follow me;
for they *be* faint, and I am pursuing after
Zebah and Zalmunna, kings of Midian.
6 And the princes of [f]Succoth said, *Are*
the hands of Zebah and Zalmunna now
in thine hand, that we should give bread
unto thine army?
7 And Gideon said, Therefore when
the LORD hath delivered Zebah and
Zalmunna into mine hand, then I will
tear your flesh with the thorns of the
wilderness and with briers.
8 And he went up thence to Penuel,
and spake unto them likewise: and the
men of Penuel answered him as the men
of Succoth had answered *him*.
9 And he spake also unto the men of
Penuel, saying, When I come again in
peace, I will break down this tower.
10 Now Zebah and Zalmunna *were* in
Karkor, and their hosts with them, about
fifteen thousand *men*, all that were left of
all the hosts of the children of the east:
for there fell an hundred and twenty
thousand men that drew sword.

B.C. 1249.

a Or, *firebrands*, or, *torches*.

b Ex. 14:13, 14; 2 Chr. 20:17.

c John 1:28.

d Psa. 83:11, 12; Isa. 10:26.

e Cf. Jud. 12:1; 2 Sam. 2:8; 1 Ki. 12:16. Here begins that deep rooted division in Israel which culminated in the division of Solomon's kingdom under Jeroboam and Rehoboam.

f 1 Sam. 25:11; 1 Ki. 20:11.

B.C. 1249.

11 And Gideon went up by the way of
them that dwelt in tents on the east of
Nobah and Jogbehah, and smote the
host: for the host was secure.
12 And when Zebah and Zalmunna
fled, he pursued after them, and took the
two kings of Midian, Zebah and
Zalmunna, and discomfited all the host.
13 And Gideon the son of Joash
returned from battle before the sun *was*
up,
14 And caught a young man of the
men of Succoth, and enquired of him:
and he described unto him the princes of
Succoth, and the elders thereof, *even*
threescore and seventeen men.
15 And he came unto the men of
Succoth, and said, Behold Zebah and
Zalmunna, with whom ye did upbraid
me, saying, *Are* the hands of Zebah and
Zalmunna now in thine hand, that we
should give bread unto thy men *that are*
weary?
16 And he took the elders of the city,
and thorns of the wilderness and briers,
and with them he taught the men of
Succoth.
17 And he beat down the [a]tower of
Penuel, and slew the men of the city.
18 Then said he unto Zebah and
Zalmunna, What manner of men *were*
they whom ye slew at [b]Tabor? And they
answered, As thou *art*, so *were* they; each
one resembled the children of a king.
19 And he said, They *were* my
brethren, *even* the sons of my mother: *as*
the LORD liveth, if ye had saved them
alive, I would not slay you.
20 And he said unto Jether his firstborn, Up, *and* slay them. But the youth
drew not his sword: for he feared,
because he *was* yet a youth.
21 Then Zebah and Zalmunna said,
Rise thou, and fall upon us: for as the
man *is, so is* his strength. And Gideon
arose, and slew Zebah and Zalmunna,
and took away the ornaments that *were*
on their camels' necks.
22 Then the men of Israel said unto
Gideon, Rule thou over us, both thou,
and thy son, and thy son's son also: for
thou hast delivered us from the hand of
Midian.
23 And Gideon said unto them, I will
not rule over you, neither shall my son
rule over you: the [c]LORD shall rule over
you.
24 And Gideon said unto them, I
would desire a request of you, that ye
would give me every man the earrings
of his prey. (For they had golden earrings, because they *were* [d]Ishmaelites.)
25 And they answered, We will willingly give *them*. And they spread a garment, and did cast therein every man the
earrings of his prey.
26 And the weight of the golden earrings that he requested was a thousand
and seven hundred *shekels* of gold;
beside ornaments, and collars, and purple raiment that *was* on the kings of
Midian, and beside the chains that *were*
about their camels' necks.
27 And Gideon made an ephod there-
of, and put it in his city, *even* in [e]Ophrah:
and all Israel went thither a whoring
after it: which thing became a snare unto
Gideon, and to his house.
28 Thus was Midian subdued before
the children of Israel, so that they lifted
up their heads no more. And the country
was in quietness forty years in the days
of Gideon.
29 And Jerubbaal the son of Joash
went and dwelt in his own house.
30 And Gideon had threescore and ten
sons of his body begotten: for he had
many wives.
31 And his concubine that *was* in
Shechem, she also bare him a son, whose
name he called Abimelech.
32 And Gideon the son of Joash died
in a good old age, and was buried in the
sepulchre of Joash his father, in Ophrah
of the Abi-ezrites.

The fifth apostasy: the time of confusion.

33 And it came to pass, as soon as
Gideon was dead, that the children of
Israel turned again, and went a whoring
after Baalim, and made Baal-berith their
god.
34 And the children of Israel remembered not the LORD their God, who had
delivered them out of the hands of all
their enemies on every side:
35 Neither shewed they kindness to
the house of Jerubbaal, *namely*, Gideon,
according to all the goodness which he
had shewed unto Israel.

a v. 9.
b Psa. 89:12.
c 1 Sam. 8:7; 10:19; Isa. 33:22.
d Gen. 25:13.
e Jud. 6:24.

CHAPTER 9.

The conspiracy of Abimelech.

And Abimelech the son of Jerubbaal went to [a]Shechem unto his mother's brethren, and communed with them, and with all the family of the house of his mother's father, saying,

2 Speak, I pray you, in the ears of all the men of Shechem, Whether *is* better for you, either that all the sons of Jerubbaal, *which* [b]*are* threescore and ten persons, reign over you, or that one reign over you? remember also that I *am* your bone and your flesh.

3 And his mother's brethren spake of him in the ears of all the men of Shechem all these words: and their hearts inclined to follow Abimelech; for they said, He *is* our brother.

4 And they gave him threescore and ten *pieces* of silver out of the house of [c]Baal-berith, wherewith Abimelech hired vain and light persons, which followed him.

5 And he went unto his father's house at Ophrah, and [d]slew his brethren the sons of Jerubbaal, *being* threescore and ten persons, upon one stone: notwithstanding yet Jotham the youngest son of Jerubbaal was left; for he hid himself.

6 And all the men of Shechem gathered together, and all the house of Millo, and went, and made Abimelech king, by the plain of the pillar that *was* in Shechem.

7 And when they told *it* to Jotham, he went and stood in the top of mount [e]Gerizim, and lifted up his voice, and cried, and said unto them, Hearken unto me, ye men of Shechem, that God may hearken unto you.

8 The [f]trees went forth *on a time* to anoint a king over them; and they said unto the olive tree, Reign thou over us.

9 But the olive tree said unto them, Should I leave my fatness, wherewith by me they honour God and man, and go to be promoted over the trees?

10 And the trees said to the fig tree, Come thou, *and* reign over us.

11 But the fig tree said unto them, Should I forsake my sweetness, and my good fruit, and go to be promoted over the trees?

12 Then said the trees unto the vine, Come thou, *and* reign over us.

13 And the vine said unto them, Should I leave my wine, which cheereth God and man, and go to be promoted over the trees?

14 Then said all the trees unto the bramble, Come thou, *and* reign over us.

15 And the bramble said unto the trees, If in truth ye anoint me king over you, *then* come *and* put your [g]trust in my shadow: and if not, let fire come out of the bramble, and devour the cedars of Lebanon.

16 Now therefore, if ye have done truly and sincerely, in that ye have made Abimelech king, and if ye have dealt well with Jerubbaal and his house, and have done unto him according to the deserving of his hands;

17 (For my [h]father fought for you, and adventured his life far, and delivered you out of the hand of Midian:

18 And [i]ye are risen up against my father's house this day, and have slain his sons, threescore and ten persons, upon one stone, and have made Abimelech, the son of his maidservant, king over the men of Shechem, because he *is* your brother;)

19 If ye then have dealt truly and sincerely with Jerubbaal and with his house this day, *then* rejoice ye in Abimelech, and let him also rejoice in you:

20 But if not, let fire come out from Abimelech, and devour the men of Shechem, and the house of Millo; and let fire come out from the men of Shechem, and from the house of Millo, and devour Abimelech.

21 And Jotham ran away, and fled, and went to Beer, and dwelt there, for fear of Abimelech his brother.

22 When Abimelech had reigned three years over Israel,

23 Then God [j]sent an evil spirit between Abimelech and the men of Shechem; and the men of Shechem dealt treacherously with Abimelech:

24 That the cruelty *done* to the threescore and ten sons of Jerubbaal might come, and their blood be laid upon Abimelech their brother, which slew them; and upon the men of Shechem, which aided him in the killing of his brethren.

25 And the men of Shechem set liers in wait for him in the top of the mountains,

B.C. 1209.

a Jud. 8:31.
b Jud. 8:30.
c Jud. 8:33.
d 2 Ki. 10:7; 11:1, 2.
e Josh. 8:33.
f *Parables* (O.T.). vs. 7-15; 2 Sam. 12:1-4. (Jud. 9:7-15; Zech. 11:7-14.)
g Psa. 2:12, *note.*
h Jud. 7.
i Jud. 8:35.
j 1 Ki. 12:15; Isa. 19:14.

and they robbed all that came along that way by them: and it was told Abimelech.

26 And Gaal the son of Ebed came with his brethren, and went over to Shechem: and the men of Shechem put their confidence in him.

27 And they went out into the fields, and gathered their vineyards, and trode *the grapes*, and made merry, and went into the house of their god, and did eat and drink, and cursed Abimelech.

28 And Gaal the son of Ebed said, Who [a]*is* Abimelech, and who *is* Shechem, that we should serve him? *is* not *he* the son of Jerubbaal? and Zebul his officer? serve the men of Hamor the father of Shechem: for why should we serve him?

29 And [b]would to God this people were under my hand! then would I remove Abimelech. And he said to Abimelech, Increase thine army, and come out.

30 And when Zebul the ruler of the city heard the words of Gaal the son of Ebed, his anger was kindled.

31 And he sent messengers unto Abimelech [c]privily, saying, Behold, Gaal the son of Ebed and his brethren be come to Shechem; and, behold, they fortify the city against thee.

32 Now therefore up by night, thou and the people that *is* with thee, and lie in wait in the field:

33 And it shall be, *that* in the morning, as soon as the sun is up, thou shalt rise early, and set upon the city: and, behold, *when* he and the people that *is* with him come out against thee, then mayest thou do to them as thou shalt find occasion.

34 And Abimelech rose up, and all the people that *were* with him, by night, and they laid wait against Shechem in four companies.

35 And Gaal the son of Ebed went out, and stood in the entering of the gate of the city: and Abimelech rose up, and the people that *were* with him, from lying in wait.

36 And when Gaal saw the people, he said to Zebul, Behold, there come people down from the top of the mountains. And Zebul said unto him, Thou seest the shadow of the mountains as *if they were* men.

37 And Gaal spake again and said, See there come people down by the middle of the land, and another company come along by the plain of Meonenim.

B.C. 1206.

a 1 Sam. 25:10; 1 Ki. 12:16.

b 2 Sam. 15:4; Psa. 10:3.

c *craftily.*

d vs. 28, 29.

e v. 20.

f 2 Ki. 3:25.

38 Then said Zebul unto him, Where *is* now thy mouth, wherewith thou [d]saidst, Who *is* Abimelech, that we should serve him? *is* not this the people that thou hast despised? go out, I pray now, and fight with them.

39 And Gaal went out before the men of Shechem, and fought with Abimelech.

40 And Abimelech chased him, and he fled before him, and many were overthrown *and* wounded, *even* unto the entering of the gate.

41 And Abimelech dwelt at Arumah: and Zebul thrust out Gaal and his brethren, that they should not dwell in Shechem.

42 And it came to pass on the morrow, that the people went out into the field; and they told Abimelech.

43 And he took the people, and divided them into three companies, and laid wait in the field, and looked, and, behold, the people *were* come forth out of the city; and he rose up against them, and smote them.

44 And Abimelech, and the company that *was* with him, rushed forward, and stood in the entering of the gate of the city: and the two *other* companies ran upon all *the people* that *were* in the fields, and slew them.

45 And Abimelech fought against the city all that day; [e]and he took the city, and slew the people that *was* therein, and beat [f]down the city, and sowed it with salt.

46 And when all the men of the tower of Shechem heard *that*, they entered into an hold of the house of the god Berith.

47 And it was told Abimelech, that all the men of the tower of Shechem were gathered together.

48 And Abimelech gat him up to mount Zalmon, he and all the people that *were* with him; and Abimelech took an axe in his hand, and cut down a bough from the trees, and took it, and laid *it* on his shoulder, and said unto the people that *were* with him, What ye have seen me do, make haste, *and* do as I *have done*.

49 And all the people likewise cut down every man his bough, and followed Abimelech, and put *them* to the hold, and set the hold on fire upon them;

so that all the men of the tower of
Shechem died also, about a thousand
men and women.
50 Then went Abimelech to Thebez,
and encamped against Thebez, and took
it.
51 But there was a strong tower within
the city, and thither fled all the men and
women, and all they of the city, and shut
it to them, and gat them up to the top of
the tower.
52 And Abimelech came unto the
tower, and fought against it, and went
hard unto the door of the tower to burn
it with fire.
53 [a]And a certain woman cast a piece
of a millstone upon Abimelech's head,
and all to brake his skull.
54 [b]Then he called hastily unto the
young man his armourbearer, and said
unto him, Draw thy sword, and slay me,
that men say not of me, A woman slew
him. And his young man thrust him
through, and he died.
55 And when the men of Israel saw
that Abimelech was dead, they departed
every man unto his place.
56 Thus God [c]rendered the wickedness
of Abimelech, which he did unto his
father, in slaying his seventy brethren:
57 And all the evil of the men of
Shechem did God render upon their
heads: and upon them came the [d]curse
of Jotham the son of Jerubbaal.

CHAPTER 10.

Tola, the seventh Judge.

And after Abimelech there arose to
[e]defend Israel Tola the son of Puah,
the son of Dodo, a man of Issachar; and
he dwelt in Shamir in mount Ephraim.
2 And he judged Israel twenty and
three years, and died, and was buried in
Shamir.

Jair, the eighth Judge.

3 And after him arose Jair, a Gileadite,
and judged Israel twenty and two years.
4 And he had thirty sons that rode on
thirty ass colts, and they had thirty
cities, which are called [f]Havoth-jair unto
this day, which *are* in the land of Gilead.
5 And Jair died, and was buried in
Camon.

The sixth apostasy and servitude.

6 And the children of Israel did evil
again in the sight of the LORD, and
served Baalim, and Ashtaroth, and the
gods of Syria, and the gods of Zidon,
and the gods of Moab, and the gods of
the children of Ammon, and the gods of
the Philistines, and forsook the LORD,
and served not him.
7 And the anger of the LORD was hot
against Israel, and he sold them into the
hands of the Philistines, and into the
hands of the children of Ammon.
8 And that year they vexed and
oppressed the children of Israel: eighteen years, all the children of Israel that
were on the other side Jordan in the land
of the Amorites, which *is* in Gilead.
9 Moreover the children of Ammon
passed over Jordan to fight also against
Judah, and against Benjamin, and
against the house of Ephraim; so that
Israel was sore distressed.
10 And the children of Israel cried
unto the LORD, saying, We have sinned
against thee, both because we have forsaken our God, and also served Baalim.
11 And the LORD said unto the children of Israel, *Did* not *I deliver you* from
the Egyptians, and from the Amorites,
from the children of Ammon, and from
the Philistines?
12 The Zidonians also, and the Amalekites, and the Maonites, did oppress
you; and ye cried to me, and I delivered
you out of their hand.
13 Yet ye have forsaken me, and
served other gods: wherefore I will
deliver you no more.
14 Go and cry unto the gods which ye
have chosen; let them deliver you in the
time of your tribulation.
15 And the children of Israel said unto
the LORD, We have sinned: do thou unto
us whatsoever seemeth good unto thee;
deliver us only, we pray thee, this day.
16 And they put away the strange
gods from among them, and served the
LORD: and his soul was grieved for the
misery of Israel.
17 Then the children of Ammon were
gathered together, and encamped in
Gilead. And the children of Israel assembled themselves together, and encamped
in Mizpeh.
18 And the people *and* princes of
Gilead said one to another, What man *is*
he that will begin to fight against the
children of Ammon? he shall be head
over all the inhabitants of Gilead.

B.C. 1206.

a 2 Sam. 11:21.
b 1 Sam. 31:4.
c v. 24.
d vs. 20, 45. Cf. Gen. 27:12.
e *Save,* or, *deliverer.*
f Or, *The villages of Jair.* Num. 32:41.

CHAPTER 11.

Jephthah, the ninth Judge.

Now [a]Jephthah the Gileadite was a
mighty man of valour, and he *was*
the son of an harlot: and Gilead begat
Jephthah.
2 And Gilead's wife bare him sons; and
his wife's sons grew up, and they thrust
out Jephthah, and said unto him, Thou
shalt [b]not inherit in our father's house; for
thou *art* the son of a strange woman.
3 Then Jephthah fled from his
brethren, and dwelt in the land of Tob:
and there were gathered vain men to
Jephthah, and went out with him.
4 And it came to [c]pass in process of
time, that the children of Ammon made
war against Israel.
5 And it was so, that when the children of Ammon made war against
Israel, the elders of Gilead went to fetch
Jephthah out of the land of Tob:
6 And they said unto Jephthah, Come,
and be our captain, that we may fight
with the children of Ammon.
7 And Jephthah said unto the elders of
Gilead, Did not ye hate me, and expel
me out of my father's house? and why
are ye come unto me now when ye are in
distress?
8 And the elders of Gilead said unto
Jephthah, Therefore we turn again to
thee now, that thou mayest go with us,
and fight against the children of
Ammon, and be our head over all the
inhabitants of Gilead.
9 And Jephthah said unto the elders of
Gilead, If ye bring me home again to
fight against the children of Ammon,
and the LORD deliver them before me,
shall I be your head?
10 And the elders of Gilead said unto
Jephthah, The LORD be witness between
us, if we do not so according to thy
words.
11 Then Jephthah went with the elders
of Gilead, and the people made him
head and captain over them: and
Jephthah uttered all his words before the
LORD in Mizpeh.
12 And Jephthah sent messengers
unto the king of the children of Ammon,
saying, [d]What hast thou to do with me,
that thou art come against me to fight in
my land?
13 And the king of the children of
Ammon answered unto the messengers
of Jephthah, Because [e]Israel took away
my land, when they came up out of
Egypt, from Arnon even unto Jabbok,
and unto Jordan: now therefore restore
those *lands* again peaceably.
14 And Jephthah sent messengers
again unto the king of the children of
Ammon:
15 And said unto him, Thus saith
Jephthah, Israel [f]took not away the land
of Moab, nor the land of the children of
Ammon:
16 But when Israel came up from
Egypt, and walked through the wilderness unto the Red sea, and came to
Kadesh;
17 Then Israel sent messengers unto
the king of Edom, saying, Let me, I pray
thee, pass through thy land: but the king
of Edom would not hearken *thereto*. And
in like manner they sent unto the king of
Moab: but he would not *consent*: and
Israel abode in Kadesh.
18 Then they went along through the
wilderness, and [g]compassed the land of
Edom, and the land of Moab, and came
by the east side of the land of Moab, and
pitched on the other side of Arnon, but
came not within the border of Moab: for
Arnon *was* the border of Moab.
19 And Israel [h]sent messengers unto
Sihon king of the Amorites, the king of
Heshbon; and Israel said unto him, Let
us pass, we pray thee, through thy land
into my place.
20 But Sihon trusted not Israel to pass
through his coast: but Sihon gathered all
his people together, and pitched in
Jahaz, and fought against Israel.
21 And the LORD God of Israel delivered Sihon and all his people into the
hand of Israel, and they smote them: so
Israel possessed all the land of the
Amorites, the inhabitants of that country.
22 And they possessed all the coasts of
the Amorites, from Arnon even unto
Jabbok, and from the wilderness even
unto Jordan.
23 So now the LORD God of Israel hath
dispossessed the Amorites from before
his people Israel, and shouldest thou
possess it?
24 Wilt not thou possess that which
Chemosh thy god giveth thee to possess? So whomsoever the LORD our God
shall drive out from before us, them will
we possess.
25 And now *art* thou any thing better
than Balak the son of Zippor, king of

B.C. 1161.

a Heb. 11:32, called *Jephthae.*
b Gen. 21:10; Deut. 23:2.
c *after days.*
d Deut. 20:10, 12.
e Num. 21:24.
f Deut. 2:9, 19.
g Num. 21:4.
h Num. 21:21; Deut. 2:26-36.

B.C. 1143.

Moab? did he ever strive against Israel, or did he ever fight against them,

26 While Israel dwelt in Heshbon and her towns, and in Aroer and her towns, and in all the cities that *be* along by the coasts of Arnon, three hundred years? why therefore did ye not recover *them* within that time?

27 Wherefore I have not sinned against thee, but thou doest me wrong to war against me: the LORD the Judge be judge this day between the children of Israel and the children of Ammon.

28 Howbeit the king of the children of Ammon hearkened not unto the words of Jephthah which he sent him.

29 Then the [a]Spirit of the LORD came upon [b]Jephthah, and he passed over Gilead, and Manasseh, and passed over Mizpeh of Gilead, and from Mizpeh of Gilead he passed over *unto* the children of Ammon.

Jephthah's awful vow.

30 And Jephthah [c]vowed a vow unto the LORD, and said, If thou shalt without fail deliver the children of Ammon into mine hands,

31 Then it shall be, that whatsoever cometh forth of the doors of my house to meet me, when I return in peace from the children of Ammon, [d]shall surely be the LORD'S, and I will offer it up for a burnt-offering.

32 So Jephthah passed over unto the children of Ammon to fight against them; and the LORD delivered them into his hands.

33 And he smote them from Aroer, even till thou come to Minnith, *even* twenty cities, and unto the plain of the vineyards, with a very great slaughter. Thus the children of Ammon were subdued before the children of Israel.

34 And Jephthah came to [e]Mizpeh unto his house, and, behold, his daughter came out to meet him with timbrels and with dances: and she *was his* only child; beside her he had neither son nor daughter.

35 And it came to pass, when he saw her, that he rent his clothes, and said, Alas, my daughter! thou hast brought me very low, and thou art one of them that trouble me: for I have opened my mouth unto the LORD, and I [f]cannot go back.

36 And she said unto him, My father, *if* thou hast opened thy mouth unto the LORD, do to me according to that which hath proceeded out of thy mouth; forasmuch as the LORD hath taken vengeance for thee of thine enemies, *even* of the children of Ammon.

37 And she said unto her father, Let this thing be done for me: let me alone two months, that I may go up and down upon the mountains, and bewail my virginity, I and my fellows.

38 And he said, Go. And he sent her away *for* two months: and she went with her companions, and bewailed her virginity upon the mountains.

39 And it came to pass at the end of two months, that she returned unto her father, who did with her *according* to his vow which he had vowed: and she knew no man. And it was a custom in Israel,

40 *That* the daughters of Israel went yearly to [g]lament the daughter of Jephthah the Gileadite four days in a year.

CHAPTER 12.

The second jealousy of Ephraim.

And the men of [h]Ephraim gathered themselves together, and went northward, and said unto Jephthah, Wherefore passedst thou over to fight against the children of Ammon, and didst not call us to go with thee? we will burn thine house upon thee with fire.

2 And Jephthah said unto them, I and my people were at great strife with the children of Ammon; and when I called you, ye delivered me not out of their hands.

3 And when I saw that ye delivered *me* not, I put my life in my hands, and passed over against the children of Ammon, and the LORD delivered them into my hand: wherefore then are ye come up unto me this day, to fight against me?

4 Then Jephthah gathered together all the men of Gilead, and fought with Ephraim: and the men of Gilead smote Ephraim, because they said, Ye Gileadites *are* fugitives of Ephraim among the Ephraimites, *and* among the Manassites.

5 And the Gileadites took the passages of Jordan before the Ephraimites: and it was *so*, that when those Ephraimites which were escaped said, Let me go over; that the men of Gilead said unto him, *Art* thou an Ephraimite? If he said, Nay;

a *Holy Spirit.* Jud. 13:25. (Gen. 1:2; Mal. 2:15.)

b Jephthah seems to have been judge only of northeast Israel.

c Gen. 28:20; Num. 30:2; 1 Sam. 1:11.

d Lev. 27:2, 3, 28.

e v. 11.

f Num. 30:2.

g Or, *celebrate.*

h Jud. 8:1, *note.*

6 Then said they unto him, Say now
[a]Shibboleth: and he said Sibboleth: for
he could not frame to pronounce *it* right.
Then they took him, and slew him at the
passages of Jordan: and there fell at that
time of the Ephraimites forty and two
thousand.
7 And Jephthah judged Israel six years.
Then died Jephthah the Gileadite, and
was buried in *one of* the cities of Gilead.

Ibzan, the tenth Judge.

8 And after him [b]Ibzan of Beth-lehem
judged Israel.
9 And he had thirty sons, and thirty
daughters, *whom* he sent abroad, and took
in thirty daughters from abroad for his
sons. And he judged Israel seven years.
10 Then died Ibzan, and was buried at
Beth-lehem.

Elon, the eleventh Judge.

11 And after him Elon, a Zebulonite,
judged Israel; and he judged Israel ten
years.
12 And Elon the Zebulonite died, and
was buried in Aijalon in the country of
Zebulun.

Abdon, the twelfth Judge.

13 And after him Abdon the son of
Hillel, a Pirathonite, judged Israel.
14 And he had forty sons and thirty
nephews, that rode on threescore and ten
ass colts: and he judged Israel eight years.
15 And Abdon the son of Hillel the
Pirathonite died, and was buried in
Pirathon in the land of Ephraim, in the
mount of the Amalekites.

CHAPTER 13.

The seveth apostasy and servitude.

And the children of Israel did evil
again in the sight of the LORD; and
the LORD delivered them into the hand
of the Philistines forty years.

The parents of Samson.

2 And there was a certain man of
Zorah, of the family of the Danites,
whose name *was* Manoah; and his wife
was barren, and bare not.
3 And the [c]angel of the LORD appeared
unto the woman, and [d]said unto her,
Behold now, thou *art* barren, and bearest
not: but thou shalt conceive, and bear a
son.

B.C. 1143.

a Signifying a *stream* or *flood.* Psa. 69:2, 15; Isa. 27:12.

b He seems to have been only a civil judge in northeast Israel.

c Heb. 1:4, *note.*

d 1 Sam. 1:19, 20.

e Num. 6:2.

f *Bible prayers* (O.T.). Jud. 16:28. (Gen. 15:2; Hab. 3:1-16.)

4 Now therefore beware, I pray thee,
and drink not wine nor strong drink,
and eat not any unclean *thing*:
5 For, lo, thou shalt conceive, and bear
a son; and no razor shall come on his
head: for the child shall be a [e]Nazarite
unto God from the womb: and he shall
begin to deliver Israel out of the hand of
the Philistines.
6 Then the woman came and told her
husband, saying, A man of God came
unto me, and his countenance *was* like
the countenance of an [c]angel of God,
very terrible: but I asked him not whence
he *was*, neither told he me his name:
7 But he said unto me, Behold, thou
shalt conceive, and bear a son; and now
drink no wine nor strong drink, neither
eat any unclean *thing*: for the child shall
be a Nazarite to God from the womb to
the day of his death.
8 Then Manoah [f]intreated the LORD,
and said, O my Lord, let the man of God
which thou didst send come again unto
us, and teach us what we shall do unto
the child that shall be born.
9 And God hearkened to the voice of
Manoah; and the [c]angel of God came
again unto the woman as she sat in the
field: but Manoah her husband *was* not
with her.
10 And the woman made haste, and
ran, and shewed her husband, and said
unto him, Behold, the man hath appeared
unto me, that came unto me the *other* day.
11 And Manoah arose, and went after
his wife, and came to the man, and said
unto him, *Art* thou the man that spakest
unto the woman? And he said, I *am*.
12 And Manoah said, Now let thy
words come to pass. How shall we order
the child, and *how* shall we do unto him?
13 And the [c]angel of the LORD said
unto Manoah, Of all that I said unto the
woman let her beware.
14 She may not eat of any *thing* that
cometh of the vine, neither let her drink
wine or strong drink, nor eat any
unclean *thing*: all that I commanded her
let her observe.
15 And Manoah said unto the [c]angel
of the LORD, I pray thee, let us detain
thee, until we shall have made ready a
kid for thee.
16 And the [c]angel of the LORD said
unto Manoah, Though thou detain me, I
will not eat of thy bread: and if thou wilt

offer a burnt-offering, thou must offer it unto the LORD. For Manoah knew not that he *was* an angel of the LORD.

17 And Manoah said unto the [a]angel of the LORD, What *is* thy name, that when thy sayings come to pass we may do thee honour?

18 And the [a]angel of the LORD said unto him, Why askest thou thus after my name, seeing it *is* secret?

19 So Manoah took a kid with a [b]meat-offering, and offered *it* upon a rock unto the LORD: and *the angel* did wondrously; and Manoah and his wife looked on.

20 For it came to pass, when the flame went up toward heaven from off the altar, that the [a]angel of the LORD ascended in the flame of the altar. And Manoah and his wife looked on *it*, and fell on their faces to the ground.

21 But the [a]angel of the LORD did no more appear to Manoah and to his wife. Then Manoah knew that he *was* an [a]angel of the LORD.

22 And Manoah said unto his wife, We shall surely die, because we have seen [c]God.

23 But his wife said unto him, If the LORD were pleased to kill us, he would not have received a burnt-offering and a [b]meat-offering at our hands, neither would he have shewed us all these *things*, nor would as at this time have told us *such things* as these.

The birth of Samson.

24 And the woman bare a son, and called his name Samson: and the child grew, and the LORD blessed him.

25 And the [d]Spirit of the LORD began to move him at times in the camp of Dan between Zorah and Eshtaol.

CHAPTER 14.

Samson, the thirteenth Judge.

And Samson went down to Timnath, and saw a woman in Timnath of the daughters of the Philistines.

2 And he came up, and told his father and his mother, and said, I have seen a woman in Timnath of the daughters of the Philistines: now therefore get her for me to wife.

3 Then his father and his mother said unto him, *Is there* never a woman among the daughters of thy brethren, or among all my people, that thou goest to take a wife of the uncircumcised Philistines? And Samson said unto his father, Get her for me; for she pleaseth me well.

4 But his father and his mother knew not that it *was* of the LORD, that he sought an occasion against the Philistines: for at that time the Philistines had dominion over Israel.

Samson and the lion.

5 Then went Samson down, and his father and his mother, to Timnath, and came to the vineyards of Timnath: and, behold, a young lion roared against him.

6 And the [e]Spirit of the LORD came mightily upon him, and he [f]rent him as he would have rent a kid, and *he had* nothing in his hand: but he told not his father or his mother what he had done.

7 And he went down, and talked with the woman; and she pleased Samson well.

Samson's riddle.

8 And after a time he returned to take her, and he turned aside to see the carcase of the lion: and, behold, *there was* a swarm of bees and honey in the carcase of the lion.

9 [g]And he took thereof in his hands, and went on eating, and came to his father and mother, and he gave them, and they did eat: but he told not them that he had taken the honey out of the [h]carcase of the lion.

10 So his father went down unto the woman: and Samson made there a feast; for so used the young men to do.

11 And it came to pass, when they saw him, that they brought thirty companions to be with him.

12 And Samson said unto them, I will now put forth a riddle unto you: if ye can certainly declare it me within the seven days of the feast, and find *it* out, then I will give you thirty [i]sheets and thirty change of garments:

13 But if ye cannot declare *it* me, then shall ye give me thirty [i]sheets and thirty change of garments. And they said unto him, Put forth thy riddle, that we may hear it.

14 And he said unto them, Out of the eater came forth meat, and out of the strong came forth sweetness. And they could not in three days expound the riddle.

B.C. 1161.

a Heb. 1:4, *note.*

b Lit. *meal.*

c See John 1:18, *note.*

d *Holy Spirit.* Jud. 14:6, 19. (Gen. 1:2; Mal. 2:15.)

e *Holy Spirit.* vs. 6, 19; Jud. 15:14. (Gen. 1:2; Mal. 2:15.)

f *Miracles* (O.T.). vs. 5, 6, 19; Jud. 15:14-17. (Gen. 5:24; Jon. 2:1-10.)

g 1 Sam. 14:25, 26.

h Lev. 11:27.

i Or, *shirts.*

B.C. 1141.

15 And it came to pass on the seventh day, that they said unto Samson's wife, [a]Entice thy husband, that he may declare unto us the riddle, [b]lest we burn thee and thy father's house with fire: have ye called us to take that we have? *is it* not *so*?

16 And Samson's wife wept before him, and said, [c]Thou dost but hate me, and lovest me not: thou hast put forth a riddle unto the children of my people, and hast not told *it* me. And he said unto her, Behold, I have not told *it* my father nor my mother, and shall I tell *it* thee?

17 And she wept before him the seven days, while their feast lasted: and it came to pass on the seventh day, that he told her, because she lay sore upon him: and she told the riddle to the children of her people.

18 And the men of the city said unto him on the seventh day before the sun went down, What *is* sweeter than honey? and what *is* stronger than a lion? And he said unto them, If ye had not plowed with my heifer, ye had not found out my riddle.

Samson at Ashkelon.

19 And the [d]Spirit of the LORD came upon him, and he went down to Ashkelon, and slew thirty men of them, and took their spoil, and gave change of garments unto them which expounded the riddle. And his anger was kindled, and he went up to his father's house.

20 But Samson's wife was [e]*given* to his companion, whom he had used as his friend.

CHAPTER 15.

But it came to pass within a while after, in the time of wheat harvest, that Samson visited his wife with a kid; and he said, I will go in to my wife into the chamber. But her father would not suffer him to go in.

2 And her father said, I verily thought that thou hadst utterly hated her; [f]therefore I gave her to thy companion: *is* not her younger sister fairer than she? take her, I pray thee, instead of her.

The foxes and firebrands.

3 And Samson said concerning them, Now shall I be more blameless than the Philistines, though I do them a displeasure.

4 And Samson went and caught three hundred foxes, and took firebrands, and turned tail to tail, and put a firebrand in the midst between two tails.

5 And when he had set the brands on fire, he let *them* go into the standing corn of the Philistines, and burnt up both the shocks, and also the standing [g]corn, with the vineyards *and* olives.

6 Then the Philistines said, Who hath done this? And they answered, Samson, the son in law of the Timnite, because he had taken his wife, and given her to his companion. And the Philistines came up, and [h]burnt her and her father with fire.

7 And Samson said unto them, Though ye have done this, yet will I be avenged of you, and after that I will cease.

8 And he smote them hip and thigh with a great slaughter: and he went down and dwelt in the top of the rock Etam.

9 Then the Philistines went up, and pitched in Judah, and spread themselves in Lehi.

10 And the men of Judah said, Why are ye come up against us? And they answered, To bind Samson are we come up, to do to him as he hath done to us.

11 Then three thousand men of Judah went to the top of the rock Etam, and said to Samson, Knowest thou not that the Philistines *are* rulers over us? what *is* this *that* thou hast done unto us? And he said unto them, As they did unto me, so have I done unto them.

12 And they said unto him, We are come down to bind thee, that we may deliver thee into the hand of the Philistines. And Samson said unto them, Swear unto me, that ye will not fall upon me yourselves.

13 And they spake unto him, saying, No; but we will bind thee fast, and deliver thee into their hand: but surely we will not kill thee. And they bound him with two new cords, and brought him up from the rock.

Samson slays a thousand Philistines.

14 *And* when he came unto Lehi, the Philistines shouted against him: and the [i]Spirit of the LORD came mightily upon him, and the cords that *were* upon his arms became as flax that was burnt with

a Jud. 16:5.
b Jud. 15:6.
c Jud. 16:15.
d v. 6.
e Jud. 15:2.
f Jud. 14:20.
g 2 Sam. 14:30.
h Jud. 14:15.
i *Holy Spirit.* 1 Sam. 10:6, 10. (Gen. 1:2; Mal. 2:15.)

fire, and his bands [a]loosed from off his
hands.
15 And he found a new [b]jawbone of
an ass, and put forth his hand, and took
it, and slew a thousand men therewith.
16 And Samson said, With the jawbone
of an ass, heaps upon heaps, with the jaw
of an ass have I slain a thousand men.
17 And it came to pass, when he had
made an end of speaking, that he cast
away the jawbone out of his hand, and
called that place [c]Ramath-lehi.
18 And he was sore athirst, and called
on the LORD, and said, Thou hast given
this great deliverance into the hand of thy
servant: and now shall I die for thirst, and
fall into the hand of the uncircumcised?
19 But God clave an hollow place that
was in the jaw, and there came water
thereout; and when he had drunk, his
spirit came again, and he revived: wherefore he called the name thereof [d]En-
hakkore, which *is* in Lehi unto this day.
20 And he judged Israel in the days of
the Philistines twenty years.

CHAPTER 16.

Samson at Gaza.

Then went Samson to Gaza, and saw
there an harlot, and went in unto her.
2 *And it was told* the Gazites, saying,
Samson is come hither. And they compassed *him* in, and laid wait for him all
night in the gate of the city, and were
quiet all the night, saying, In the morning, when it is day, we shall kill him.
3 And Samson lay till midnight, and
arose at midnight, and took the doors of
the gate of the city, and the two posts,
and went away with them, bar and all,
and put *them* upon his shoulders, and
carried them up to the top of an hill that
is before Hebron.

Samson and Delilah.

4 And it came to pass afterward, that
he loved a [e]woman in the valley of
Sorek, whose name *was* Delilah.
5 And the lords of the Philistines came
up unto her, and said unto her, Entice
him, and see wherein his great strength
lieth, and by what *means* we may prevail
against him, that we may bind him to
afflict him: and we will give thee every
one of us eleven hundred *pieces* of silver.
6 And Delilah said to Samson, Tell me,
I pray thee, wherein thy great strength
lieth, and wherewith thou mightest be
bound to afflict thee.
7 And Samson said unto her, If they
bind me with seven green withs that
were never dried, then shall I be weak,
and be as another man.
8 Then the lords of the Philistines
brought up to her seven green withs
which had not been dried, and she
bound him with them.
9 Now *there were* men lying in wait,
abiding with her in the chamber. And
she said unto him, The Philistines *be*
upon thee, Samson. And he brake the
withs, as a thread of tow is broken when
it toucheth the fire. So his strength was
not known.
10 And Delilah said unto Samson,
Behold, thou hast mocked me, and told
me lies: now tell me, I pray thee, wherewith thou mightest be bound.
11 And he said unto her, If they bind
me fast with new ropes that never were
occupied, then shall I be weak, and be as
another man.
12 Delilah therefore took new ropes,
and bound him therewith, and said unto
him, The Philistines *be* upon thee,
Samson. And *there were* liers in wait
abiding in the chamber. And he brake
them from off his arms like a thread.
13 And Delilah said unto Samson,
Hitherto thou hast mocked me, and told
me lies: tell me wherewith thou mightest
be bound. And he said unto her, If thou
weavest the seven locks of my head with
the web.
14 And she fastened *it* with the pin,
and said unto him, The Philistines *be*
upon thee, Samson. And he awaked out
of his sleep, and went away with the pin
of the beam, and with the web.
15 And she said unto him, [f]How canst
thou say, I love thee, when thine heart *is*
not with me? thou hast mocked me these
three times, and hast not told me wherein thy great strength *lieth*.
16 [g]And it came to pass, when she
pressed him daily with her words, and
urged him, *so* that his soul was vexed
unto death;
17 That he told her all his heart, and
said unto her, There hath not come a
razor upon mine head; for I *have been* a

B.C. 1140.

a *Miracles* (O.T.). vs. 14-17, 18, 19; Jud. 16:28-30. (Gen. 5:24; Jon. 2:1-10.)

b 1 Cor. 1:27, 28.

c *The hill of the jawbone.*

d *The well of him that cried.*

e 1 Ki. 11:1.

f Jud. 14:16.

g Gen. 39:10.

Nazarite unto God from my mother's
womb: if I be shaven, then my strength
will go from me, and I shall become
weak, and be like any *other* man.
18 And when Delilah saw that he had
told her all his heart, she sent and called
for the lords of the Philistines, saying,
Come up this once, for he hath shewed
me all his heart. Then the lords of the
Philistines came up unto her, and
brought money in their hand.
19 And she made him sleep upon her
knees; and she called for a man, and she
caused him to shave off the seven locks
of his head; and she began to afflict him,
and his strength went from him.
20 And she said, The Philistines *be*
upon thee, Samson. And he awoke out
of his sleep, and said, I will go out as at
other times before, and shake myself.
And he [a]wist not that the LORD was
departed from him.
21 But the Philistines took him, and
[b]put out his eyes, and brought him
down to Gaza, and bound him with fetters of brass; and he did grind in the
prison house.
22 Howbeit the hair of his head began
to grow again after he was shaven.

The death of Samson.

23 Then the lords of the Philistines
gathered them together for to offer a great
sacrifice unto Dagon their god, and to
rejoice: for they said, Our god hath delivered Samson our enemy into our hand.
24 And when the people saw him,
they praised their god: for they said, Our
god hath delivered into our hands our
enemy, and the destroyer of our country,
which slew many of us.
25 And it came to pass, when their
hearts were merry, that they said, Call
for Samson, that he may make us sport.
And they called for Samson out of the
prison house; and he made them sport:
and they set him between the pillars.
26 And Samson said unto the lad that
held him by the hand, Suffer me that I
may feel the pillars whereupon the house
standeth, that I may lean upon them.
27 Now the house was full of men and
women; and all the lords of the
Philistines *were* there; and *there were*
upon the roof about three thousand men
and women, that beheld while Samson
made sport.
28 And Samson [c]called unto the LORD,
and said, O Lord GOD, remember me, I
pray thee, and strengthen me, I pray
thee, only this once, O God, that I may
be at once avenged of the Philistines for
my two eyes.
29 And Samson took hold of the two
middle pillars upon which the house
stood, and on which it was borne up, of
the one with his right hand, and of the
other with his left.
30 And Samson said, Let me die with
the Philistines. And he bowed himself
with *all his* might; and the house [d]fell
upon the lords, and upon all the people
that *were* therein. So the dead which he
slew at his death were more than *they*
which he slew in his life.
31 Then his brethren and all the house
of his father came down, and took him,
and brought *him* up, and buried him
between Zorah and Eshtaol in the buryingplace of Manoah his father. And he
[1]judged Israel twenty years.

CHAPTER 17.

Confusion, civil and religious.

And there was a man of mount
Ephraim, whose name *was* Micah.

(1) *Micah's worship in self-will.*

2 And he said unto his mother, The
eleven hundred *shekels* of silver that
were taken from thee, about which thou
cursedst, and spakest of also in mine
ears, behold, the silver *is* with me; I took
it. And his mother said, Blessed *be thou*
of the LORD, my son.
3 And when he had restored the
eleven hundred *shekels* of silver to his
mother, his mother said, I had wholly
dedicated the silver unto the LORD from
my hand for my son, to make a graven

B.C. 1120.

a *Contra,* Ex. 34:29.

b *Bored out.*

c *Bible prayers* (O.T.). 1 Sam. 1:11. (Gen. 15:2; Hab. 3:1-16.)

d *Miracles* (O.T.). vs. 28-30; 1 Sam. 5:3-12. (Gen. 5:24; Jon. 2:1-10.)

[1] **(16:31)** The character and work of Samson are alike enigmatical. Announced by an angel (13:1-21) he was a Nazarite (Num. 6; Jud. 13:5) who constantly defiled his Nazarite separation through fleshly appetites. Called of God to judge Israel, and endued wonderfully with the Spirit, he wrought no abiding work for Israel and perished in captivity to his enemies the Philistines. What was real in the man was his mighty faith in Jehovah in a time of doubt and apostasy, and this faith God honoured (Heb. 11:32).

image and a molten image: now therefore I will restore it unto thee.
4 Yet he restored the money unto his
mother; and his mother took two hundred *shekels* of silver, and gave them to
the founder, who made thereof a graven
image and a molten image: and they
were in the house of Micah.
5 And the man Micah had an house of
gods, and made an ephod, and teraphim,
and consecrated one of his sons, who
became his priest.
6 In those days *there was* no king in
Israel, *but* every man did *that which was*
right in his own eyes.
7 And there was a young man out of
Beth-lehem-judah of the family of Judah,
who *was* a Levite, and he sojourned there.
8 And the man departed out of the
city from Beth-lehem-judah to sojourn
where he could find *a place*: and he came
to mount Ephraim to the house of
Micah, as he journeyed.
9 And Micah said unto him, Whence
comest thou? And he said unto him, I *am*
a Levite of Beth-lehem-judah, and I go to
sojourn where I may find *a place*.
10 And Micah said unto him, Dwell
with me, and be unto me a father and a
priest, and I will give thee ten *shekels* of
silver by the year, and a suit of apparel,
and thy victuals. So the Levite went in.
11 And the Levite was content to
dwell with the man; and the young man
was unto him as one of his sons.
12 And Micah consecrated the Levite;
and the young man became his priest,
and was in the house of Micah.
13 Then said Micah, Now [1]know I that
the LORD will do me good, seeing I have
a Levite to *my* priest.

CHAPTER 18.

Confusion, civil and religious:
(2) *and Danite invasion.*

In those days *there was* no king in Israel:
and in those days the tribe of the
Danites sought them an inheritance to
dwell in; for unto that day *all their* inheritance had not fallen unto them among
the tribes of Israel.
2 And the children of Dan sent of their
family five men from their coasts, men
of valour, from Zorah, and from Eshtaol,
to spy out the land, and to search it; and
they said unto them, Go, search the land:
who when they came to mount Ephraim,
to the house of Micah, they lodged there.
3 When they *were* by the house of
Micah, they knew the voice of the young
man the Levite: and they turned in thither, and said unto him, Who brought thee
hither? and what makest thou in this
place? and what hast thou here?
4 And he said unto them, Thus and
thus dealeth Micah with me, and hath
hired me, and I am his priest.
5 And they said unto him, [a]Ask counsel, we pray thee, of God, that we may
know whether our way which we go
shall be prosperous.
6 And the priest said unto [b]them, Go
in peace: before the LORD *is* your way
wherein ye go.
7 Then the five men departed, and
came to [c]Laish, and saw the people that
were therein, how they dwelt careless,
after the manner of the Zidonians, quiet
and secure; and *there was* no magistrate
in the land, that might put *them* to
shame in *any* thing; and they *were* far
from the Zidonians, and had no business
with *any* man.
8 And they came unto their brethren
to [d]Zorah and Eshtaol: and their
brethren said unto them, What *say* ye?
9 And they said, Arise, that we may go
up against them: for we have seen the
land, and, behold, it *is* very good: and
are ye still? be not slothful to go, *and* to
enter to possess the land.
10 When ye go, ye shall come unto a
people secure, and to a large land: for
[e]God hath given it into your hands; a
place where *there is* no want of any thing
that *is* in the earth.
11 And there went from thence of the
family of the Danites, out of Zorah and
out of Eshtaol, six hundred men
appointed with weapons of war.
12 And they went up, and pitched in

B.C. 1406.

a Jud. 1:1; 20:18; Hos. 4:12.
b 1 Ki. 22:6.
c Jud. 18:29; Josh. 19:47, called *Leshem*.
d v. 2.
e Josh. 2:23, 24.

[1] **(17:13)** A striking illustration of all apostasy. With his entire departure from the revealed will of God concerning worship and priesthood, there is yet an exaltation of false priesthood. Saying, "Blessed be thou of Jehovah," Micah's mother makes an idol; and Micah expects the blessing of Jehovah because he has linked his idolatry to the ancient levitical order.

Kirjath-jearim, in Judah: wherefore they called that place [a]Mahaneh-dan unto this day: behold, *it is* behind Kirjath-jearim.

13 And they passed thence unto mount Ephraim, and came unto the house of Micah.

14 Then answered the five men that went to spy out the country of Laish, and said unto their brethren, Do ye know that there is in these houses an [b]ephod, and teraphim, and a graven image, and a molten image? now therefore consider what ye have to do.

15 And they turned thitherward, and came to the house of the young man the Levite, *even* unto the house of Micah, and saluted him.

16 And the six hundred men appointed with their weapons of war, which *were* of the children of Dan, stood by the entering of the gate.

17 And the five men that went to spy out the land went up, *and* came in thither, *and* took the graven image, and the ephod, and the teraphim, and the molten image: and the priest stood in the entering of the gate with the six hundred men *that were* appointed with weapons of war.

18 And these went into Micah's house, and fetched the carved image, the ephod, and the teraphim, and the molten image. Then said the priest unto them, What do ye?

19 And they said unto him, Hold thy peace, lay thine hand upon thy mouth, and go with us, and be to us a father and a priest: *is it* better for thee to be a priest unto the house of one man, or that thou be a priest unto a tribe and a family in Israel?

20 And the priest's heart was glad, and he took the ephod, and the teraphim, and the graven image, and went in the midst of the people.

21 So they turned and departed, and put the little ones and the cattle and the carriage before them.

22 *And* when they were a good way from the house of Micah, the men that *were* in the houses near to Micah's house were gathered together, and overtook the children of Dan.

23 And they cried unto the children of Dan. And they turned their faces, and said unto Micah, [c]What aileth thee, that thou comest with such a company?

24 And he said, Ye have taken away my gods which I made, and the priest, and ye are gone away: and what have I more? and what *is* this *that* ye say unto me, What aileth thee?

25 And the children of Dan said unto him, Let not thy voice be heard among us, lest angry fellows run upon thee, and thou lose thy life, with the lives of thy household.

26 And the children of Dan went their way: and when Micah saw that they *were* too strong for him, he turned and went back unto his house.

27 And they took *the things* which Micah had made, and the priest which he had, and came unto Laish, unto a people *that were* at quiet and secure: and they smote them with the edge of the sword, and burnt the city with fire.

28 And *there was* no deliverer, because it *was* far from Zidon, and they had no business with *any* man; and it was in the valley that *lieth* by Beth-rehob. And they built a city, and dwelt therein.

29 [d]And they called the name of the city Dan, after the name of Dan their father, who was born unto Israel: howbeit the name of the city *was* Laish at the first.

Confusion, civil and religious:
(3) *the Danite idolatry.*

30 And the children of Dan set up the graven image: and Jonathan, the son of Gershom, the son of Manasseh, he and his sons were priests to the tribe of Dan until the day of the captivity of the land.

31 And they set them up Micah's graven image, which he made, all the time that the house of God was in Shiloh.

CHAPTER 19.

Confusion, civil and religious:
(4) *the Levite and his concubine.*

And it came to pass in those days, when *there was* no king in Israel, that there was a certain Levite sojourning on the side of mount Ephraim, who took to him a concubine out of Beth-lehem-judah.

2 And his concubine played the whore against him, and went away from him unto her father's house to Beth-lehem-judah, and was there four whole months.

3 And her husband arose, and went after her, to speak friendly unto her, *and* to bring her again, having his servant with him, and a couple of asses: and she

B.C. 1406.

a 2 Chr. 1:4.
b Jud. 17:5.
c 2 Ki. 6:28.
d Gen. 14:14; Josh. 19:47; 1 Ki. 12:29, 30; 15:20.

brought him into her father's house: and
when the father of the damsel saw him,
he rejoiced to meet him.
4 And his father in law, the damsel's
father, retained him; and he abode with
him three days: so they did eat and
drink, and lodged there.
5 And it came to pass on the fourth
day, when they arose early in the morning, that he rose up to depart: and the
damsel's father said unto his son in law,
Comfort thine [a]heart with a morsel of
bread, and afterward go your way.
6 And they sat down, and did eat and
drink both of them together: for the
damsel's father had said unto the man,
Be content, I pray thee, and tarry all
night, and let thine heart be merry.
7 And when the man rose up to
depart, his father in law urged him:
therefore he lodged there again.
8 And he arose early in the morning on
the fifth day to depart: and the damsel's
father said, Comfort thine heart, I pray
thee. And they tarried until afternoon,
and they did eat both of them.
9 And when the man rose up to depart,
he, and his concubine, and his servant,
his father in law, the damsel's father, said
unto him, Behold, now the day draweth
toward evening, I pray you tarry all
night: behold, the day groweth to an end,
lodge here, that thine heart may be
merry; and to morrow get you early on
your way, that thou mayest go home.
10 But the man would not tarry that
night, but he rose up and departed, and
came over against Jebus, which *is*
Jerusalem; and *there were* with him two
asses saddled, his concubine also *was*
with him.
11 *And* when they *were* by Jebus, the
day was far spent; and the servant said
unto his master, Come, I pray thee, and
let us turn in into this city of the
Jebusites, and lodge in it.
12 And his master said unto him, We
will not turn aside hither into the city of
a stranger, that *is* not of the children of
Israel; we will pass over to Gibeah.
13 And he said unto his servant,
Come, and let us draw near to one of
these places to lodge all night, in Gibeah,
or in Ramah.
14 And they passed on and went their
way; and the sun went down upon them

B.C. 1406.

a Psa. 104:15.

b Josh. 18:1; 1 Sam. 1:3, 7.

c Jud. 6:23; 1 Sam. 25:6.

d vs. 6, 9; Jud. 16:25.

e *the matter of this folly.*

when they were by Gibeah, which
belongeth to Benjamin.
15 And they turned aside thither, to go
in *and* to lodge in Gibeah: and when he
went in, he sat him down in a street of
the city: for *there was* no man that took
them into his house to lodging.
16 And, behold, there came an old
man from his work out of the field at
even, which *was* also of mount Ephraim;
and he sojourned in Gibeah: but the men
of the place *were* Benjamites.
17 And when he had lifted up his eyes,
he saw a wayfaring man in the street of
the city: and the old man said, Whither
goest thou? and whence comest thou?
18 And he said unto him, We *are* passing from Beth-lehem-judah toward the
side of mount Ephraim; from thence *am* I:
and I went to Beth-lehem-judah, but I *am*
now going to the [b]house of the LORD; and
there *is* no man that receiveth me to
house.
19 Yet there is both straw and provender for our asses; and there is bread and
wine also for me, and for thy handmaid,
and for the young man *which is* with thy
servants: *there is* no want of any thing.
20 And the old man said, [c]Peace *be*
with thee; howsoever *let* all thy wants *lie*
upon me; only lodge not in the street.
21 So he brought him into his house,
and gave provender unto the asses: and
they washed their feet, and did eat and
drink.
22 *Now* as they were making their
[d]hearts merry, behold, the men of the
city, certain sons of Belial, beset the
house round about, *and* beat at the door,
and spake to the master of the house, the
old man, saying, Bring forth the man
that came into thine house, that we may
know him.
23 And the man, the master of the
house, went out unto them, and said unto
them, Nay, my brethren, *nay*, I pray you,
do not *so* wickedly; seeing that this man
is come into mine house, do not this folly.
24 Behold, *here is* my daughter a maid-
en, and his concubine; them I will bring
out now, and humble ye them, and do
with them what seemeth good unto you:
but unto this man do not so [e]vile a thing.
25 But the men would not hearken to
him: so the man took his concubine, and
brought her forth unto them; and they

knew her, and abused her all the night
until the morning: and when the day
began to spring, they let her go.
26 Then came the woman in the
dawning of the day, and fell down at the
door of the man's house where her lord
was, till it was light.
27 And her lord rose up in the morning, and opened the doors of the house,
and went out to go his way: and, behold,
the woman his concubine was fallen
down *at* the door of the house, and her
hands *were* upon the threshold.
28 And he said unto her, Up, and let us
be going. But none answered. Then the
man took her *up* upon an ass, and the
man rose up, and gat him unto his place.
29 And when he was come into his
house, he took a knife, and laid hold on
his concubine, and divided her, *together*
with her bones, into twelve pieces, and
sent her into all the coasts of Israel.
30 And it was so, that all that saw it
said, There was no such deed done nor
seen from the day that the children of
Israel came up out of the land of Egypt
unto this day: consider of it, take advice,
and speak *your minds*.

CHAPTER 20.

Confusion, civil and religious:
(5) *the civil*[a] *war.*

Then all the children of Israel went
out, and the congregation was gathered together as one man, from [b]Dan
even to Beer-sheba, with the land of
Gilead, unto the LORD in Mizpeh.
2 And the chief of all the people, *even*
of all the tribes of Israel, presented themselves in the assembly of the people of
God, four hundred thousand footmen
that drew sword.
3 (Now the children of Benjamin heard
that the children of Israel were gone up
to Mizpeh.) Then said the children of
Israel, Tell *us*, how was this wickedness?
4 And the Levite, the husband of the
woman that was slain, answered and
said, I [c]came into Gibeah that *belongeth* to
Benjamin, I and my concubine, to lodge.
5 And the men of Gibeah rose against
me, and beset the house round about
upon me by night, *and* thought to have
slain me: and my concubine have they
forced, that she is dead.
6 And I took my concubine, and cut
her in pieces, and sent her throughout
all the country of the inheritance of
Israel: for they have committed lewdness and [d]folly in Israel.
7 Behold, ye *are* all children of Israel;
give here your advice and counsel.
8 And all the people arose as one man,
saying, We will not any *of us* go to his
tent, neither will we any *of us* turn into
his house.
9 But now this *shall be* the thing which
we will do to Gibeah; *we will go up* by lot
against it;
10 And we will take ten men of an
hundred throughout all the tribes of
Israel, and an hundred of a thousand,
and a thousand out of ten thousand, to
fetch victual for the people, that they
may do, when they come to Gibeah of
Benjamin, according to all the folly that
they have wrought in Israel.
11 So all the men of Israel were gathered against the city, knit together as one
man.
12 And the tribes of Israel sent men
through all the tribe of Benjamin, saying,
What wickedness *is* this that is done
among you?
13 Now therefore deliver *us* the [e]men,
the children of Belial, which *are* in Gibeah,
that we may put them to death, and put
away evil from Israel. But the children of
Benjamin would not hearken to the voice
of their brethren the children of Israel:
14 But the children of Benjamin gathered themselves together out of the cities
unto Gibeah, to go out to battle against
the children of Israel.
15 And the children of Benjamin were
numbered at that time out of the cities
twenty and six thousand men that drew
sword, beside the inhabitants of Gibeah,
which were numbered seven hundred
chosen men.
16 Among all this people *there were*
seven hundred chosen men [f]lefthanded;
every one could sling stones at an hair
breadth, and not miss.
17 And the men of Israel, beside
Benjamin, were numbered four hundred
thousand men that drew sword: all these
were men of war.
18 And the children of Israel arose,
and went up to the house of God, and
asked counsel of God, and said, Which
of us shall go up first to the battle

B.C. 1406.

a Cf. 2 Sam. 2:12.
b 1 Sam. 3:20; 2 Sam. 3:10; 24:2.
c Jud. 19:15.
d Josh. 7:15.
e Jud. 19:22.
f Jud. 3:15; 1 Chr. 12:2.

against the children of Benjamin? And the LORD said, Judah *shall go up* first.

19 And the children of Israel rose up in the morning, and encamped against Gibeah.

20 And the men of Israel went out to battle against Benjamin; and the men of Israel put themselves in array to fight against them at Gibeah.

21 And the children of Benjamin came forth out of Gibeah, and destroyed down to the ground of the Israelites that day twenty and two thousand men.

22 And the people the men of Israel encouraged themselves, and set their battle again in array in the place where they put themselves in array the first day.

23 (And the children of Israel went up and wept before the LORD until even, and asked counsel of the LORD, saying, Shall I go up again to battle against the children of Benjamin my brother? And the LORD said, Go up against him.)

24 And the children of Israel came near against the children of Benjamin the second day.

25 And Benjamin went forth against them out of Gibeah the second day, and destroyed down to the ground of the children of Israel again eighteen thousand men; all these drew the sword.

26 [a]Then all the children of Israel, and all the people, went up, and came unto the house of God, and wept, and sat there before the LORD, and fasted that day until even, and offered burnt-offerings and peace-offerings before the LORD.

27 And the children of Israel enquired of the LORD, (for the ark of the covenant of God *was* there in those days,

28 And [b]Phinehas, the son of Eleazar, the son of Aaron, stood before it in those days,) saying, Shall I yet again go out to battle against the children of Benjamin my brother, or shall I cease? And the LORD said, Go up; for to morrow I will deliver them into thine hand.

29 And Israel set liers in wait round about Gibeah.

30 And the children of Israel went up against the children of Benjamin on the third day, and put themselves in array against Gibeah, as at other times.

31 And the children of Benjamin went out against the people, *and* were drawn away from the city; and they began to smite of the people, *and* kill, as at other times, in the highways, of which one goeth up to the house of God, and the other to Gibeah in the field, about thirty men of Israel.

32 And the children of Benjamin said, They *are* smitten down before us, as at the first. But the children of Israel said, Let us flee, and draw them from the city unto the highways.

33 And all the men of Israel rose up out of their place, and put themselves in array at Baal-tamar: and the liers in wait of Israel came forth out of their places, *even* out of the meadows of Gibeah.

34 And there came against Gibeah ten thousand chosen men out of all Israel, and the battle was sore: [c]but they knew not that evil *was* near them.

35 And the LORD smote Benjamin before Israel: and the children of Israel destroyed of the Benjamites that day twenty and five thousand and an hundred men: all these drew the sword.

36 So the children of Benjamin saw that they were smitten: for the men of [d]Israel gave place to the Benjamites, because they trusted unto the liers in wait which they had set beside Gibeah.

37 And the liers in wait hasted, and rushed upon Gibeah; and the liers in wait drew *themselves* along, and smote all the city with the edge of the sword.

38 Now there was an appointed sign between the men of Israel and the liers in wait, that they should make a great flame with smoke rise up out of the city.

39 And when the men of Israel retired in the battle, Benjamin began to smite *and* kill of the men of Israel about thirty persons: for they said, Surely they are smitten down before us, as *in* the first battle.

40 But when the flame began to arise up out of the city with a pillar of smoke, the Benjamites looked behind them, and, behold, the flame of the city ascended up to heaven.

41 And when the men of Israel turned again, the men of Benjamin were amazed: for they saw that evil was come upon them.

42 Therefore they turned *their backs* before the men of Israel unto the way of

B.C. 1406.

a vs. 18, 23.

b Num. 25:7, 13; Josh. 24:33.

c Josh. 8:14.

d Josh. 8:15.

B.C. 1406.

the wilderness; but the battle overtook them; and them which *came* out of the cities they destroyed in the midst of them.

43 *Thus* they inclosed the Benjamites round about, *and* chased them, *and* trode them down with ease over against Gibeah toward the sunrising.

44 And there fell of Benjamin eighteen thousand men; all these *were* men of valour.

45 And they turned and fled toward the wilderness unto the rock of [a]Rimmon: and they gleaned of them in the highways five thousand men; and pursued hard after them unto Gidom, and slew two thousand men of them.

46 So that all which fell that day of Benjamin were twenty and five thousand men that drew the sword; all these *were* men of valour.

47 [b]But six hundred men turned and fled to the wilderness unto the rock Rimmon, and abode in the rock Rimmon four months.

48 And the men of Israel turned again upon the children of Benjamin, and smote them with the edge of the sword, as well the men of *every* city, as the beast, and all that came to hand: also they set on fire all the cities that they came to.

CHAPTER 21.

Confusion, civil and religious:
(6) *mourning for a lost tribe.*

Now the men of Israel had sworn in Mizpeh, saying, There shall not any of us give his daughter unto Benjamin to wife.

2 And the people came to the house of God, and abode there till even before God, and lifted up their voices, and wept sore;

3 And said, O LORD God of Israel, why is this come to pass in Israel, that there should be to day one [c]tribe lacking in Israel?

4 And it came to pass on the morrow, that the people rose early, and built there an altar, and offered burnt-offerings and peace-offerings.

5 And the children of Israel said, Who *is there* among all the tribes of Israel that came not up with the congregation unto the LORD? For they had made a great oath concerning him that came not up to the LORD to Mizpeh, saying, He shall surely be put to death.

6 And the children of Israel [d]repented them for Benjamin their brother, and said, There is one tribe cut off from Israel this day.

7 How shall we do for wives for them that remain, seeing we have sworn by the LORD that we will not give them of our daughters to wives?

8 And they said, What one *is there* of the tribes of Israel that came not up to Mizpeh to the LORD? And, behold, there came none to the camp from Jabesh-gilead to the assembly.

9 For the people were numbered, and, behold, *there were* none of the inhabitants of Jabesh-gilead there.

10 And the congregation sent thither twelve thousand men of the valiantest, and commanded them, saying, [e]Go and smite the inhabitants of Jabesh-gilead with the edge of the sword, with the women and the children.

11 And this *is* the thing that ye shall do, [f]Ye shall utterly destroy every male, and every woman that hath lain by man.

12 And they found among the inhabitants of Jabesh-gilead four hundred young virgins, that had known no man by lying with any male: and they brought them unto the camp to Shiloh, which *is* in the land of Canaan.

13 And the whole congregation sent *some* to speak to the children of Benjamin that *were* in the rock Rimmon, and to call peaceably unto them.

14 And Benjamin came again at that time; and they gave them wives which they had saved alive of the women of Jabesh-gilead: and yet so they sufficed them not.

15 And the people [d]repented them for Benjamin, because that the LORD had made a breach in the tribes of Israel.

16 Then the elders of the congregation said, How shall we do for wives for them that remain, seeing the women are destroyed out of Benjamin?

17 And they said, *There must be* an inheritance for them that be escaped of Benjamin, that a tribe be not destroyed out of Israel.

18 Howbeit we may not give them wives of our daughters: for the children of Israel have sworn, saying, Cursed *be* he that giveth a wife to Benjamin.

a Josh. 15:32; 1 Chr. 6:77; Zech. 14:10.

b Jud. 21:13.

c There is here no mourning for sin, no humbling because of national transgression, no return to Jehovah. Accordingly, no word from Jehovah comes to them. They act wholly in self-will (v. 10). Cf. Dan. 9:3-13.

d Zech. 8:14, *note.*

e v. 5; Jud. 5:23; 1 Sam. 11:7.

f Num. 31:17; Deut. 20:13-14.

B.C. 1406.

19 Then they said, Behold, *there is* a
feast of the LORD in Shiloh yearly *in a*
place which *is* on the north side of Beth-
el, on the east side of the highway that
goeth up from Beth-el to Shechem, and
on the south of Lebonah.
20 Therefore they commanded the
children of Benjamin, saying, Go and lie
in wait in the vineyards;
21 And see, and, behold, if the daughters of Shiloh come out to [a]dance in
dances, then come ye out of the vineyards, and catch you every man his wife
of the daughters of Shiloh, and go to the
land of Benjamin.
22 And it shall be, when their fathers or
their brethren come unto us to complain,
that we will say unto them, Be favourable
unto them for our sakes: because we
reserved not to each man his wife in the
war: for ye did not give unto them at this
time, *that* ye should be guilty.
23 And the children of Benjamin did
so, and took *them* wives, according to
their number, of them that danced,
whom they caught: and they went and
returned unto their inheritance, and
repaired the [b]cities, and dwelt in them.
24 And the children of Israel departed
thence at that time, every man to his
tribe and to his family, and they went
out from thence every man to his inheritance.
25 In those days *there was* no king in
Israel: every man did *that which was* right
in his own eyes.

a Jud. 11:34.
b Jud. 20:48.

THE BOOK OF RUTH

THIS lovely story should be read in connection with the first half of Judges, as it presents a picture of life in Israel at that time.

Typically, the book may be taken as a foreview of the church (Ruth), as the Gentile bride of Christ, the Bethlehemite who is able to redeem. Ruth also gives a normal Christian experience: I. Ruth deciding, 1. II. Ruth serving, 2. III. Ruth resting, 3. IV. Ruth rewarded, 4.

The events recorded in Ruth cover a period of 10 years (Ussher).

CHAPTER 1.

B.C. 1322.

Ruth deciding.

NOW it came to [a]pass in the days when the judges ruled, that there was a [b]famine in the land. And a certain man of [c]Beth-lehem-judah went to sojourn in the country of [d]Moab, he, and his wife, and his two sons.

2 And the name of the man *was* [e]Elimelech, and the name of his wife [f]Naomi, and the name of his two sons [g]Mahlon and [h]Chilion, [i]Ephrathites of Beth-lehem-judah. And they came into the country of Moab, and continued there.

3 And Elimelech Naomi's husband died; and she was left, and her two sons.

4 And they took them wives of the women of Moab; the name of the one *was* [j]Orpah, and the name of the other [k]Ruth: and they dwelled there about ten years.

5 And Mahlon and Chilion died also both of them; and the woman was left of her two sons and her husband.

6 Then she arose with her daughters in law, that she might return from the country of Moab: for she had heard in the country of Moab how that the LORD had visited his people in giving them bread.

7 Wherefore she went forth out of the place where she was, and her two daughters in law with her; and they went on the way to return unto the land of Judah.

8 And Naomi said unto her two daughters in law, Go, return each to her mother's house: the LORD deal kindly with you, as ye have dealt with the dead, and with me.

9 The LORD grant you that ye may find rest, each *of you* in the house of her husband. Then she kissed them; and they lifted up their voice, and wept.

10 And they said unto her, Surely we will return with thee unto thy people.

11 And Naomi said, Turn again, my daughters: why will ye go with me? *are* there yet *any more* sons in my womb, that they may be your husbands?

12 Turn again, my daughters, go *your way*; for I am too old to have an husband. If I should say, I have hope, *if* I should have an husband also to night, and should also bear sons;

13 Would ye tarry for them till they were grown? would ye stay for them from having husbands? nay, my daughters; for it grieveth me much for your sakes that the [l]hand of the LORD is gone out against me.

14 And they lifted up their voice, and wept again: and Orpah kissed her mother in law; but Ruth clave unto her.

15 And she said, Behold, thy sister in law is gone back unto her people, and unto her [m]gods: return thou after thy sister in law.

16 And Ruth said, Intreat me not to leave thee, *or* to return from following after thee: for whither thou goest, I will go; and where thou lodgest, I will lodge: [n]thy people *shall be* my people, and thy God my God:

17 Where thou diest, will I die, and there will I be buried: [o]the LORD do so to me, and more also, *if ought* but death part thee and me.

18 When she saw that she was stedfastly minded to go with her, then she left speaking unto her.

19 So they two went until they came to Beth-lehem. And it came to pass, when they were come to Beth-lehem, that all the city

a Jud. 2:16, 18
b Gen. 12:10, *note.*
c *House of Bread and Praise.*
d Gen. 19:37.
e i.e. *My God is King.*
f *Pleasant*
g *Sick.*
h *Pining.*
i Gen. 35:19.
j *Hind* or *Fawn.*
k *Friendship* or *Beauty*
l Psa. 38:2.
m Jud. 11:24.
n Ruth 2:11, 12
o 1 Sam. 3:17.

was moved about them, and they said, *Is* this [a]Naomi?

20 And she said unto them, Call me not Naomi, call me [b]Mara: for the Almighty hath dealt very bitterly with me.

21 I went out full, and the LORD hath brought me home again empty: why *then* call ye me Naomi, seeing the LORD hath testified against me, and the Almighty hath afflicted me?

22 So Naomi returned, and Ruth the Moabitess, her daughter in law, with her, which returned out of the country of Moab: and they came to Beth-lehem in the beginning of barley harvest.

CHAPTER 2.

Ruth serving.

And Naomi had a [c]kinsman of her husband's, a mighty man of wealth, of the family of Elimelech; and his name *was* Boaz.

2 And Ruth the Moabitess said unto Naomi, Let me now go to the field, and glean ears of corn after *him* in whose sight I shall find grace. And she said unto her, Go, my daughter.

3 And she went, and came, and gleaned in the field after the reapers: and her hap was to light on a part of the field *belonging* unto Boaz, who *was* of the kindred of Elimelech.

4 And, behold, Boaz came from Beth-lehem, and said unto the reapers, The LORD *be* with you. And they answered him, The LORD bless thee.

5 Then said Boaz unto his servant that was set over the reapers, Whose damsel *is* this?

6 And the servant that was set over the reapers answered and said, It *is* the Moabitish damsel that came back with Naomi out of the country of Moab:

7 And she said, I pray you, let me glean and gather after the reapers among the sheaves: so she came, and hath continued even from the morning until now, that she tarried a little in the house.

8 Then said Boaz unto Ruth, Hearest thou not, my daughter? Go not to glean in another field, neither go from hence, but abide here fast by my maidens:

9 *Let* thine eyes *be* on the field that they do reap, and go thou after them: have I not charged the young men that they shall not touch thee? and when thou art athirst, go unto the vessels, and drink of *that* which the young men have drawn.

10 Then she fell on her face, and bowed herself to the ground, and said unto him, Why have I found grace in thine eyes, that thou shouldest take knowledge of me, seeing I *am* a stranger?

11 And [d]Boaz answered and said unto her, It hath fully been shewed me, all that thou hast done unto thy mother in law since the death of thine husband: and *how* thou hast left thy father and thy mother, and the land of thy nativity, and art come unto a people which thou knewest not heretofore.

12 The LORD recompense thy work, and a full reward be given thee of the LORD God of Israel, under whose wings thou art come to [e]trust.

13 Then she said, Let me find favour in thy sight, my lord; for that thou hast comforted me, and for that thou hast spoken friendly unto thine handmaid, though I be not like unto one of thine handmaidens.

14 And Boaz said unto her, At mealtime come thou hither, and eat of the bread, and dip thy morsel in the vinegar. And she sat beside the reapers: and he reached her parched *corn*, and she did eat, and was sufficed, and left.

15 And when she was risen up to glean, Boaz commanded his young men, saying, Let her glean even among the sheaves, and reproach her not:

16 And let fall also *some* of the handfuls of purpose for her, and leave *them*, that she may glean *them*, and rebuke her not.

17 So she gleaned in the field until even, and beat out that she had gleaned: and it was about an [f]ephah of barley.

18 And she took *it* up, and went into the city: and her mother in law saw what she had gleaned: and she brought forth, and gave to her that she had reserved after she was sufficed.

19 And her mother in law said unto her, Where hast thou gleaned to day? and where wroughtest thou? blessed be he that did take knowledge of thee. And she shewed her mother in law with whom she had wrought, and said, The man's name with whom I wrought to day *is* Boaz.

B.C. 1312.

a i.e. *Pleasant.*

b i.e. *Bitter.*

c Ruth 3:2, 12.

d Called *Booz*, Mt. 1:5.

e Psa. 2:12, *note.*

f One ephah = 1 bu. 3 pts.

B.C. 1312.

20 And Naomi said unto her daughter in law, Blessed *be* he of the LORD, who hath not left off his kindness to the living and to the dead. And Naomi said unto her, The man *is* near of kin unto us, one of our next [a]kinsmen.

21 And Ruth the Moabitess said, He said unto me also, Thou shalt keep fast by my young men, until they have ended all my harvest.

22 And Naomi said unto Ruth her daughter in law, *It is* good, my daughter, that thou go out with his maidens, that they meet thee not in any other field.

23 So she kept fast by the maidens of Boaz to glean unto the end of barley harvest and of wheat harvest; and dwelt with her mother in law.

CHAPTER 3.

Ruth resting.

Then Naomi her mother in law said unto her, My daughter, shall I not seek rest for thee, that it may be well with thee?

2 And now *is* not Boaz of our kindred, with whose maidens thou wast? Behold, he winnoweth barley to night in the threshingfloor.

3 Wash thyself therefore, and [b]anoint thee, and put thy raiment upon thee, and get thee down to the floor: *but* make not thyself known unto the man, until he shall have done eating and drinking.

4 And it shall be, when he lieth down, that thou shalt mark the place where he shall lie, and thou shalt go in, and uncover his feet, and lay thee down; and he will tell thee what thou shalt do.

5 And she said unto her, All that thou sayest unto me I will do.

6 And she went down unto the floor, and did according to all that her mother in law bade her.

7 And when Boaz had eaten and drunk, and his heart was merry, he went to lie down at the end of the heap of corn: and she came softly, and uncovered his feet, and laid her down.

8 And it came to pass at midnight, that the man was afraid, and turned himself: and, behold, a woman lay at his feet.

9 And he said, Who *art* thou? And she answered, I *am* Ruth thine handmaid: spread therefore thy skirt over thine handmaid; for thou *art* a near [a]kinsman.

10 And he said, Blessed *be* thou of the LORD, my daughter: *for* thou hast shewed more kindness in the latter end than at the beginning, inasmuch as thou followedst not young men, whether poor or rich.

11 And now, my daughter, fear not; I will do to thee all that thou requirest: for all the [c]city of my people doth know that thou *art* a virtuous woman.

12 And now it is true that I *am thy* near [a]kinsman: [d]howbeit there is a kinsman nearer than I.

13 Tarry this night, and it shall be in the morning, *that* if he will perform unto thee the part of a [a]kinsman, well; let him do the kinsman's part: but if he will not do the part of a kinsman to thee, then will I do the part of a kinsman to thee, *as* the LORD liveth: lie down until the morning.

14 And she lay at his feet until the morning: and she rose up before one could know another. And he said, Let it not be known that a woman came into the floor.

15 Also he said, Bring the [e]vail that *thou hast* upon thee, and hold it. And when she held it, he measured six *measures* of barley, and laid *it* on her: and she went into the city.

16 And when she came to her mother in law, she said, Who *art* thou, my daughter? And she told her all that the man had done to her.

17 And she said, These six *measures* of barley gave he me; for he said to me, Go not empty unto thy mother in law.

18 Then said she, Sit still, my daughter, until thou know how the matter will fall: for the man will not be in rest, until he have finished the thing this day.

CHAPTER 4.

Ruth rewarded.

Then went Boaz up to the gate, and sat him down there: and, behold, the kinsman of whom Boaz [f]spake came by; unto whom he said, Ho, such a one! turn aside, sit down here. And he turned aside, and sat down.

2 And he took ten men of the [g]elders of the city, and said, Sit ye down here. And they sat down.

3 And he said unto the kinsman, Naomi, that is come again out of the

a Heb. *goel, Redemp. (Kinsman type).* Isa. 59:20, *note.*
b Eccl. 9:8.
c *Gate.*
d Ruth 4:1.
e Or, *sheet,* or, *apron.*
f Ruth 3:12.
g 1 Ki. 21:8.

country of Moab, selleth a parcel of land, which *was* our brother Elimelech's:

4 And I thought to advertise thee, saying, Buy *it* before the inhabitants, and before the elders of my people. If thou wilt [a]redeem *it*, redeem *it*: but if thou wilt not redeem *it*, *then* tell me, that I may know: for *there is* none to redeem *it* beside thee; and I *am* after thee. And he said, I will redeem *it*.

5 Then said Boaz, What day thou buyest the field of the hand of Naomi, thou must buy *it* also of Ruth the Moabitess, the wife of the dead, to raise up the name of the dead upon his inheritance.

6 And the [a]kinsman said, I cannot [a]redeem *it* for myself, lest I mar mine own inheritance: redeem thou my right to thyself; for I cannot redeem *it*.

7 Now [b]this *was the manner* in former time in Israel concerning redeeming and concerning changing, for to confirm all things; a man plucked off his shoe, and gave *it* to his neighbour: and this *was* a testimony in Israel.

8 Therefore the [a]kinsman said unto Boaz, Buy *it* for thee. So he drew off his shoe.

9 And Boaz said unto the elders, and *unto* all the people, Ye *are* witnesses this day, that I have bought all that *was* Elimelech's, and all that *was* Chilion's and Mahlon's, of the hand of Naomi.

10 Moreover Ruth the Moabitess, the wife of Mahlon, have I purchased to be my wife, to raise up the name of the dead upon his inheritance, that the name of the dead be not cut off from among his brethren, and from the gate of his place: ye *are* witnesses this day.

11 And all the people that *were* in the gate, and the elders, said, *We are* witnesses. The LORD make the woman that is come into thine house like Rachel and like Leah, which [c]two did build the house of Israel: and do thou worthily in Ephratah, and be famous in Beth-lehem:

12 And let thy house be like the house of Pharez, whom [d]Tamar bare unto Judah, of the seed which the LORD shall give thee of this young woman.

13 So Boaz took Ruth, and she was his wife: and when he went in unto her, the LORD gave her conception, and she bare a son.

14 And the women said unto Naomi, Blessed *be* the LORD, which hath not left thee this day without a [a]kinsman, that his name may be famous in Israel.

15 And he shall be unto thee a restorer of *thy* life, and a nourisher of thine old age: for thy daughter in law, which loveth thee, which is [e]better to thee than seven sons, hath born him.

16 And Naomi took the child, and laid it in her bosom, and became nurse unto it.

17 And the [f]women her neighbours gave it a name, saying, There is a son born to Naomi; and they called his name [g]Obed: he *is* the father of Jesse, the father of [h]David.

18 Now these *are* the generations of Pharez: Pharez begat Hezron,

19 And Hezron begat Ram, and Ram begat Amminadab,

20 And Amminadab begat Nahshon, and Nahshon begat Salmon,

21 And [i]Salmon begat Boaz, and Boaz begat Obed,

22 And Obed begat Jesse, and Jesse begat David.

B.C. 1312.

a Heb. *goel, Redemp. (Kinsman type).* Isa. 59:20, *note.*

b Deut. 25:7-9.

c Gen. 29:30.

d Gen. 38:29.

e 1 Sam. 1:8.

f Lk. 1:58.

g i.e. *Worshipper.*

h i.e. *Beloved.*

i Or, *Salmah.*

THE FIRST BOOK OF SAMUEL

OTHERWISE CALLED
THE FIRST BOOK OF THE KINGS

THIS book presents the personal history of Samuel, last of the Judges. It records the moral failure of the priesthood under Eli and of the Judges in Samuel's attempt to make the office hereditary (1 Sam. 8:1). In his prophetic office Samuel was faithful, and in him begins the line of writing prophets. Henceforth the prophet, not the priest, is conspicuous in Israel. In this book the theocracy, as exercised through judges, ends (8:7), and the line of kings begins with Saul.

The book is in four parts: I. The story of Samuel to the death of Eli, 1:1–4:22. II. From the taking of the ark to the demand for a king, 5:1–8:22. III. The reign of Saul to the call of David, 9:1–15:35. IV. From the call of David to the death of Saul, 16:1–31:13.

The events recorded in First Samuel cover a period of 115 years (Ussher).

CHAPTER 1.

The mother of Samuel.

NOW there was a certain man of Ramathaim-zophim, of mount Ephraim, and his name *was* Elkanah, the son of Jeroham, the son of Elihu, the son of Tohu, the son of Zuph, an Ephrathite:
2 And he had two wives; the name of the one *was* Hannah, and the name of the other Peninnah: and Peninnah had children, but Hannah had no children.
3 And this man went up out of his city yearly to [a]worship and to sacrifice unto the [b]LORD of [1]hosts in Shiloh. And the two sons of Eli, Hophni and Phinehas, the priests of the LORD, *were* there.
4 And when the time was that Elkanah offered, he gave to Peninnah his wife, and to all her sons and her daughters, portions:
5 But unto Hannah he gave a worthy portion; for he loved Hannah: but the LORD had shut up her womb.
6 And her adversary also provoked her sore, for to make her fret, because the LORD had shut up her womb.
7 And *as* he did so year by year, when she went up to the house of the LORD, so she provoked her; therefore she wept, and did not eat.
8 Then said Elkanah her husband to her, Hannah, why weepest thou? and why eatest thou not? and why is thy heart grieved? *am* not I better to thee than ten sons?
9 So Hannah rose up after they had eaten in Shiloh, and after they had drunk. Now Eli the priest sat upon a seat by a post of the temple of the LORD.

B.C. 1171.

a Ex. 23:14; Deut. 12:5-7.

b Deity (names of). Mal. 2:16. (Gen. 1:1; Mal. 3:18.)

[1] **(1:3)** Jehovah (LORD) of Hosts, Heb. *Jehovah Sabaoth.* For the distinctive meanings of Jehovah, see Gen. 2:4, *note. Sabaoth* means simply host or hosts, but with especial reference to warfare or service. In use the two ideas are united, Jehovah is LORD of (warrior) hosts. It is the name, therefore, of Jehovah in manifestation of *power.* "The LORD of Hosts, He is the King of glory" (Psa. 24:10), and accordingly in Old Testament Scripture this name is revealed in the time of Israel's *need.* It is never found in the Pentateuch, nor directly in Joshua or Judges, and occurs but rarely in the Psalms; but Jeremiah, the prophet of approaching national judgment, uses the name about eighty times. Haggai in two chapters uses the name fourteen times; Zechariah in fourteen chapters calls upon the LORD of hosts about fifty times. In Malachi the name occurs about twenty-five times. In the utmost extremity, the Psalmist twice comforts his heart with the assurance "the LORD of hosts is with us" (Psa. 46:7, 11). The meanings and uses of this name may be thus summarized: (1) The "hosts" are heavenly. Primarily the angels are meant, but the name gathers into itself the idea of *all* divine or heavenly power as available for the need of God's people (Gen. 32:1, 2; Isa. 6:1-5; 1 Ki. 22:19; Lk. 2:13-15). (2) In use this is the distinctive name of Deity for Israel's help and comfort in the time of her division and failure (1 Ki. 18:15; 19:14; Isa. 1:9; 8:11-14; 9:13-19; 10:24-27; 31:4, 5; Hag. 2:4; Mal. 3:16, 17; Jas. 5:4). See other names of Deity, Gen. 1:1, *note;* 2:4, *note;* 2:7; 14:18, *note;* 15: 2, *note;* 17:1, *note;* 21:33, *note.*

The vow of Hannah.

10 And she *was* in bitterness of soul, and prayed unto the LORD, and wept sore.

11 And she vowed a vow, and [a]said, O LORD of hosts, if thou wilt indeed look on the affliction of thine handmaid, and remember me, and not forget thine handmaid, but wilt give unto thine handmaid a man child, then I will give him unto the LORD all the days of his life, and there shall no [b]razor come upon his head.

12 And it came to pass, as she continued praying before the LORD, that Eli marked her mouth.

13 Now Hannah, she spake in her heart; only her lips moved, but her voice was not heard: therefore Eli thought she had been drunken.

14 And Eli said unto her, How long wilt thou be drunken? put away thy wine from thee.

15 And Hannah answered and said, No, my lord, I *am* a woman of a sorrowful spirit: I have drunk neither wine nor strong drink, but have [c]poured out my soul before the LORD.

16 Count not thine handmaid for a daughter of Belial: for out of the abundance of my complaint and grief have I spoken hitherto.

17 Then Eli answered and said, Go in peace: and the God of Israel grant *thee* thy petition that thou hast asked of him.

18 And she said, Let thine handmaid find grace in thy sight. So the woman went her way, and did eat, and her countenance was no more *sad*.

19 And they rose up in the morning early, and worshipped before the LORD, and returned, and came to their house to Ramah: and Elkanah knew Hannah his wife; and the LORD remembered her.

The birth of Samuel.

20 Wherefore it came to pass, when the time was come about after Hannah had conceived, that she bare a son, and called his name [d]Samuel, *saying*, Because I have asked him of the LORD.

21 And the man Elkanah, and all his house, [e]went up to offer unto the LORD the yearly sacrifice, and his vow.

22 But Hannah went not up; for she said unto her husband, *I will not go up* until the child be weaned, and *then* I will bring him, that he may appear before the LORD, and there abide for ever.

23 And Elkanah her husband said unto her, Do what seemeth thee good; tarry until thou have weaned him; only the LORD establish his word. So the woman abode, and gave her son suck until she weaned him.

Hannah brings Samuel to Eli.

24 And when she had weaned him, she took him up with her, with three bullocks, and one [f]ephah of flour, and a bottle of wine, and brought him unto the house of the LORD in Shiloh: and the child *was* young.

25 And they slew a bullock, and brought the child to Eli.

26 And she said, Oh my lord, *as* thy soul liveth, my lord, I *am* the woman that stood by thee here, praying unto the LORD.

27 For this child I prayed; and the LORD hath given me my petition which I asked of him:

28 Therefore also I have lent him to the LORD; as long as he liveth he shall be lent to the LORD. And he worshipped the LORD there.

CHAPTER 2.

Hannah's prophetic prayer.

And Hannah [g]prayed, and said, My heart [h]rejoiceth in the LORD, mine horn is exalted in the LORD: my mouth is enlarged over mine enemies; because I rejoice in thy salvation.

2 [i]*There is* none holy as the LORD: for *there is* none beside thee: neither *is there* any [j]rock like our God.

3 Talk no more so exceeding proudly; let *not* arrogancy come out of your mouth: for the LORD *is* a God of knowledge, and by him actions are weighed.

4 The bows of the mighty men *are* broken, and they that stumbled are girded with strength.

5 *They that were* full have hired out themselves for bread; and *they that were* hungry ceased: so that the barren hath born seven; and she that hath many children is waxed feeble.

6 The LORD [k]killeth, and maketh alive: he bringeth down to the [l]grave, and bringeth up.

7 The LORD maketh poor, and maketh rich: he bringeth low, and lifteth up.

B.C. 1171.

a *Bible prayers* (O.T.). 1 Sam. 2:1. (Gen. 15:2; Hab. 3:1-16.)

b Num. 6:5.

c Psa. 62:8.

d i.e. *asked of God.*

e Gen. 18:19; Josh. 24:15; Psa. 101:2.

f One ephah = 1 bu. 3 pts.

g *Bible prayers* (O.T.). 2 Sam. 7:18. (Gen. 15:2; Hab. 3:1-16.)

h Psa. 97:11, 12.

i Rev. 15:4.

j Psa. 18:2.

k Psa. 116:3.

l Heb. *Sheol.* See Hab. 2:5, *note.*

8 He raiseth up the poor out of the dust, *and* lifteth up the beggar from the dunghill, to set *them* among princes, and to make them inherit the throne of glory: for the pillars of the earth *are* the LORD'S, and he hath set the world upon them.

9 He will [a]keep the feet of his saints, and the [b]wicked shall be silent in darkness; for by strength shall no man prevail.

10 The adversaries of the LORD shall be broken to pieces; out of heaven shall he thunder upon them: the LORD shall judge the ends of the earth; and [c]he shall give strength unto his king, and exalt the horn of his [d]anointed.

11 And Elkanah went to Ramah to his house. And the child did minister unto the LORD before Eli the priest.

The evil sons of Eli.

12 Now the sons of Eli *were* sons of Belial; they knew not the LORD.

13 And the priests' custom with the people *was, that,* when any man offered sacrifice, the priest's servant came, while the flesh was in seething, with a fleshhook of three teeth in his hand;

14 And he struck *it* into the pan, or kettle, or caldron, or pot; all that the fleshhook brought up the priest took for himself. So they did in Shiloh unto all the Israelites that came thither.

15 Also before they burnt the fat, the priest's servant came, and said to the man that sacrificed, Give flesh to roast for the priest; for he will not have sodden flesh of thee, but raw.

16 And *if* any man said unto him, Let them not fail to burn the fat presently, and *then* take *as much* as thy soul desireth; then he would answer him, *Nay;* but thou shalt give *it me* now: and if not, I will take *it* by force.

17 Wherefore the sin of the young men was very great before the LORD: for men abhorred the offering of the LORD.

The child Samuel in the tabernacle.

18 But Samuel ministered before the LORD, *being* a child, girded with a linen ephod.

19 Moreover his mother made him a little coat, and brought *it* to him from year to year, when she came up with her husband to offer the yearly sacrifice.

20 And Eli blessed Elkanah and his wife, and said, The LORD give thee seed of this woman for the loan which is lent to the LORD. And they went unto their own home.

21 And the LORD visited Hannah, so that she conceived, and bare three sons and two daughters. And the child Samuel grew before the LORD.

22 Now Eli was very old, and heard all that his sons did unto all Israel; and how they lay with the women that assembled *at* the door of the tabernacle of the congregation.

23 And he said unto them, Why do ye such things? for I hear of your evil dealings by all this people.

24 Nay, my sons; for *it is* no good report that I hear: ye make the LORD'S people to transgress.

25 If one man sin against another, the judge shall judge him: but if a man sin against the [e]LORD, who shall intreat for him? Notwithstanding they hearkened not unto the voice of their father, because the LORD would slay them.

26 And the child Samuel grew on, and was in favour both with the LORD, and also with men.

The warning to Eli.

27 And there came a [f]man of God unto Eli, and said unto him, Thus saith the LORD, Did I plainly appear unto the house of thy father, when they were in Egypt in Pharaoh's house?

28 And did I [g]choose him out of all the tribes of Israel *to be* my priest, to offer upon mine altar, to burn incense, to wear an ephod before me? and did I give unto the house of thy father all the offerings made by fire of the children of Israel?

29 Wherefore kick ye at my sacrifice and at mine offering, which I have commanded *in my* habitation; and honourest thy sons above me, to make yourselves fat with the chiefest of all the offerings of Israel my people?

30 Wherefore the LORD God of Israel saith, I [h]said indeed *that* thy house, and the house of thy father, should walk before me for ever: but now the LORD saith, Be it far from me; for them that honour me I will honour, and they that despise me shall be lightly esteemed.

31 Behold, the [i]days come, that I will

B.C. 1165.

a Psa. 37:23, 24; 91:11-12; 94:18; 121:3; 1 Pet. 1:5.

b Rom. 3:19.

c Mt. 28:18.

d A prophecy of Christ as King. Cf. Psa. 2:1-9.

e Num. 15:30; Psa. 51:4, 16.

f Deut. 33:1.

g Ex. 28:1, 4.

h Ex. 29:9.

i 1 Ki. 2:27, 35.

cut off thine arm, and the arm of thy father's house, that there shall not be an old man in thine house.

32 And thou shalt see an enemy *in my* habitation, in all *the wealth* which *God* shall give Israel: and there shall not be an old man in thine house for ever.

33 And the man of thine, *whom* I shall not cut off from mine altar, *shall be* to consume thine eyes, and to grieve thine heart: and all the increase of thine house shall die in the flower of their age.

34 And this *shall be* a sign unto thee, that shall come upon thy two sons, on Hophni and Phinehas; in one day they shall [a]die both of them.

35 And I will [b]raise me up a faithful priest, *that* shall do according to *that* which *is* in mine heart and in my mind: and I will build him a sure house; and he shall walk before mine anointed for ever.

36 And it shall come to pass, *that* every one that is left in thine house shall come *and* crouch to him for a piece of silver and a morsel of bread, and shall say, Put me, I pray thee, into one of the priests' offices, that I may eat a piece of bread.

CHAPTER 3.

Samuel becomes Jehovah's prophet-priest.

And the child Samuel ministered unto the LORD before Eli. And [c]the word of the LORD was precious in those days; *there was* no open vision.

2 And it came to pass at that time, when Eli *was* laid down in his place, and his eyes began to wax dim, *that* he could not see;

3 And ere the [d]lamp of God went out in the temple of the LORD, where the ark of God *was*, and Samuel was laid down *to sleep*;

4 That the LORD called Samuel: and he answered, Here *am* I.

5 And he ran unto Eli, and said, Here *am* I; for thou calledst me. And he said, I called not; lie down again. And he went and lay down.

6 And the LORD called yet again, Samuel. And Samuel arose and went to Eli, and said, Here *am* I; for thou didst call me. And he answered, I called not, my son; lie down again.

7 Now Samuel did not yet know the LORD, neither was the word of the LORD yet revealed unto him.

8 And the LORD called Samuel again the third time. And he arose and went to Eli, and said, Here *am* I; for thou didst call me. And Eli perceived that the LORD had called the child.

9 Therefore Eli said unto Samuel, Go, lie down: and it shall be, if he call thee, that thou shalt say, [e]Speak, LORD; for thy servant heareth. So Samuel went and lay down in his place.

10 And the LORD came, and stood, and called as at other times, Samuel, Samuel. Then Samuel answered, Speak; for thy servant heareth.

11 And the LORD said to Samuel, Behold, I will do a thing in Israel, at which both the ears of every one that heareth it shall tingle.

12 In that day I will perform against Eli all *things* which I have [f]spoken concerning his house: when I begin, I will also make an end.

13 For I have told him that I will judge his house for ever for the iniquity which he knoweth; because his [g]sons made themselves vile, and he restrained them not.

14 And therefore I have sworn unto the house of Eli, that the iniquity of Eli's house shall not be [h]purged with sacrifice nor offering for ever.

15 And Samuel lay until the morning, and opened the doors of the house of the LORD. And Samuel feared to shew Eli the vision.

16 Then Eli called Samuel, and said, Samuel, my son. And he answered, Here *am* I.

17 And he said, What *is* the thing that *the* LORD hath said unto thee? I pray thee hide *it* not from me: God do so to thee, and more also, if thou hide *any* thing from me of all the things that he said unto thee.

18 And Samuel told him every whit, and hid nothing from him. And he said, It *is* the LORD: let him do what seemeth him good.

19 And Samuel grew, and the LORD was with him, and did let none of his words fall to the ground.

20 And all Israel from Dan even to Beer-sheba knew that Samuel *was* established *to be* a prophet of the LORD.

21 And the LORD appeared again in

B.C. 1165.

a 1 Sam. 4:11.

b Heb. 2:17; 7:26-28.

c Or, *a word from the LORD was unusual in those days; there was no public vision.*

d Ex. 27:20, 21.

e Psa. 85:8.

f 1 Sam. 2:29-36.

g 1 Sam. 2:12, 23.

h Num. 15:30; Isa. 22:14; Heb. 10:4, 26, 31.

Shiloh: for the LORD revealed himself to
Samuel in Shiloh by the word of the LORD.

CHAPTER 4.

The ark taken by the Philistines.

And the word of Samuel came to all
Israel. Now Israel went out against
the Philistines to battle, and pitched
beside Eben-ezer: and the Philistines
pitched in Aphek.
2 And the Philistines put themselves in
array against Israel: and when they
joined battle, Israel was smitten before
the Philistines: and they slew of the army
in the field about four thousand men.
3 And when the people were come
into the camp, the elders of Israel said,
[a]Wherefore hath the LORD smitten us to
day before the Philistines? [b]Let us fetch
the ark of the covenant of the LORD out
of Shiloh unto us, that, when it cometh
among us, it may save us out of the
hand of our enemies.
4 So the people sent to Shiloh, that
they might bring from thence the ark of
the covenant of the LORD of hosts, which
[c]dwelleth *between* the cherubims: and
the two sons of Eli, Hophni and
Phinehas, *were* there with the ark of the
covenant of God.
5 And when the ark of the covenant of
the LORD came into the camp, all Israel
shouted with a great shout, so that the
earth rang again.
6 And when the Philistines heard the
noise of the shout, they said, What
meaneth the noise of this great shout in
the camp of the Hebrews? And they
understood that the ark of the LORD was
come into the camp.
7 And the Philistines were afraid, for
they said, God is come into the camp.
And they said, Woe unto us! for there
hath not been such a thing heretofore.
8 Woe unto us! who shall deliver us out
of the hand of these mighty Gods? these
are the Gods that smote the Egyptians
with all the plagues in the wilderness.
9 Be strong, and quit yourselves like
men, O ye Philistines, that ye be not servants unto the Hebrews, as they have
been to you: quit yourselves like men,
and fight.
10 And the Philistines fought, and
Israel was smitten, and they fled every
man into his tent: and there was a very
great slaughter; for there fell of Israel
thirty thousand footmen.
11 And the ark of God was taken; and
the two sons of Eli, Hophni and
Phinehas, were slain.
12 And there ran a man of Benjamin
out of the army, and came to Shiloh the
same day with his clothes rent, and with
earth upon his head.
13 And when he came, lo, Eli sat upon
a seat by the wayside watching: for his
heart trembled for the ark of God. And
when the man came into the city, and
told *it*, all the city cried out.
14 And when Eli heard the noise of
the crying, he said, What *meaneth* the
noise of this tumult? And the man came
in hastily, and told Eli.
15 Now Eli was ninety and eight years
old; and his eyes were dim, that he
could not see.
16 And the man said unto Eli, I *am* he
that came out of the army, and I fled to
day out of the army. And he said, What
is there done, my son?
17 And the messenger answered and
said, Israel is fled before the Philistines,
and there hath been also a great slaughter among the people, and thy two sons
also, Hophni and Phinehas, are dead,
and the ark of God is taken.
18 And it came to pass, when he made
mention of the ark of God, that he fell
from off the seat backward by the side of
the gate, and his neck brake, and he
died: for he was an old man, and heavy.
And he had judged Israel forty years.
19 And his daughter in law, Phinehas'
wife, was with child, *near* to be delivered: and when she heard the tidings
that the ark of God was taken, and that
her father in law and her husband were
dead, she bowed herself and travailed;
for her pains came upon her.
20 And about the time of her death the
women that stood by her said unto her,
Fear not; for thou hast born a son. But she
answered not, neither did she regard *it*.
21 And she named the child I-chabod,
saying, The glory is departed from
Israel: because the ark of God was taken,
and because of her father in law and her
husband.
22 And she said, The glory is departed
from Israel: for the ark of God is taken.

B.C. 1141.

a Josh. 7:7-8; Prov. 19:3.

b Deut. 12:11.

c Ex. 25:18, 22.

B.C. 1141.

CHAPTER 5.

The ark of God a curse to the Philistines.

And the Philistines took the ark of
God, and brought it from [a]Eben-
ezer unto [b]Ashdod.
2 When the Philistines took the ark of
God, they brought it into the house of
Dagon, and set it by [c]Dagon.
3 And when they of Ashdod arose
early on the morrow, behold, Dagon *was*
fallen upon his face to the earth before
the ark of the LORD. And they took
Dagon, and set him in his place again.
4 And when they arose early on the
morrow morning, behold, Dagon *was*
fallen upon his face to the ground before
the ark of the LORD; and the head of
Dagon and both the palms of his hands
were cut off upon the threshold; only *the*
stump of Dagon was left to him.
5 Therefore neither the priests of
Dagon, nor any that come into Dagon's
house, tread on the threshold of Dagon
in Ashdod unto this day.
6 But the [d]hand of the LORD was heavy
upon them of Ashdod, and he destroyed
them, and [e]smote them with emerods,
even Ashdod and the coasts thereof.
7 And when the men of Ashdod saw
that *it was* so, they said, The ark of the
God of Israel shall not abide with us: for
his hand is sore upon us, and upon
Dagon our god.
8 They sent therefore and gathered all
the lords of the Philistines unto them,
and said, What shall we do with the ark
of the God of Israel? And they answered,
Let the ark of the God of Israel be carried about unto Gath. And they carried
the ark of the God of Israel about *thither*.
9 And it was *so*, that, after they had
carried it about, the [f]hand of the LORD
was against the city with a very great
destruction: and he smote the men of the
city, both small and great, and they had
emerods in their secret parts.
10 Therefore they sent the ark of God
to Ekron. And it came to pass, as the ark
of God came to Ekron, that the Ekronites
cried out, saying, They have brought
about the ark of the God of Israel to us,
to slay us and our people.
11 So they sent and gathered together
all the lords of the Philistines, and said,
Send away the ark of the God of Israel,
and let it go again to his own place, that
it slay us not, and our people: for there
was a deadly destruction throughout all
the city; the [g]hand of God was very
heavy there.
12 And the men that died not were
smitten with the emerods: and the [h]cry
of the city went up to heaven.

CHAPTER 6.

The ark brought to
Joshua the Beth-shemite.

And the ark of the LORD was in the
country of the Philistines seven
months.
2 And the Philistines called for the
priests and the [i]diviners, saying, What
shall we do to the ark of the LORD? tell us
wherewith we shall send it to his place.
3 And they said, If ye send away the
ark of the God of Israel, send it not
[j]empty; but in any wise return him a
[k]trespass-offering: [l]then ye shall be
healed, and it shall be known to you
why his hand is not removed from you.
4 Then said they, What *shall be* the trespass-offering which we shall return to
him? They answered, Five golden
emerods, and five golden mice, *according*
to the number of the lords of the
Philistines: for one plague *was* on you
all, and on your lords.
5 Wherefore ye shall make images of
your emerods, and images of your mice
that mar the land; and ye shall give
glory unto the God of Israel: peradventure he will [m]lighten his hand from off
you, and from off your gods, and from
off your land.
6 Wherefore then do ye harden your
hearts, as the Egyptians and Pharaoh
hardened their hearts? when he had
wrought wonderfully among them, did
they not let the people go, and they
departed?
7 Now therefore make a new [n]cart,
and take two milch kine, on which there
hath come no yoke, and tie the kine to
the cart, and bring their calves home
from them:
8 And take the ark of the LORD, and
lay it upon the cart; and put the jewels of
gold, which ye return him *for* a trespass-
offering, in a coffer by the side thereof;
and send it away, that it may go.
9 And see, if it goeth up by the way of
his own coast to Beth-shemesh, *then* he
hath done us this great evil: but if not,

a 1 Sam. 7:12.
b Acts 8:40.
c 1 Chr. 10:10.
d vs. 7, 11; Ex. 9:3; Psa. 32:4.
e *Miracles* (O.T.). vs. 3-12; 2 Sam. 6:7. (Gen. 5:24; Jon. 2:1-10.)
f 1 Sam. 7:13; 12:15; Deut. 2:15.
g vs. 6, 9.
h 1 Sam. 9:16; Jer. 14:2.
i Gen. 41:8; Ex. 7:11; Isa. 47:13.
j Deut. 16:16.
k *Contra*, Lev.5:15, 16.
l *Contra*, Heb. 9:22.
m 1 Sam. 5:6, 11.
n Cf. 2 Sam. 6:3.

B.C. 1140.

then we shall know that *it is* not his
hand *that* smote us; it *was* a chance *that*
happened to us.
10 And the men did so; and took two
milch kine, and tied them to the cart,
and shut up their calves at home:
11 And they laid the ark of the LORD
upon the cart, and the coffer with the mice
of gold and the images of their emerods.
12 And the kine took the straight way
to the way of Beth-shemesh, *and* went
along the highway, lowing as they went,
and turned not aside *to* the right hand or
to the left; and the lords of the Philistines
went after them unto the border of Beth-
shemesh.
13 And *they of* Beth-shemesh *were*
reaping their wheat harvest in the valley: and they lifted up their eyes, and
saw the ark, and rejoiced to see *it*.
14 And the cart came into the field of
Joshua, a Beth-shemite, and stood there,
where *there was* a great stone: and they
clave the wood of the cart, and offered
the kine a burnt-offering unto the LORD.
15 And the Levites took down the ark
of the LORD, and the coffer that *was* with
it, wherein the jewels of gold *were*, and
put *them* on the great stone: and the men
of Beth-shemesh offered burnt-offerings
and sacrificed sacrifices the same day
unto the LORD.
16 And when the five lords of the
Philistines had seen *it*, they returned to
Ekron the same day.
17 And these *are* the golden emerods
which the Philistines returned *for* a trespass-offering unto the LORD; for Ashdod
one, for Gaza one, for Askelon one, for
Gath one, for Ekron one;
18 And the golden mice, *according to*
the number of all the cities of the
Philistines *belonging* to the five lords,
both of fenced cities, and of country villages, even unto the great *stone of* Abel,
whereon they set down the ark of the
LORD: *which stone remaineth* unto this day
in the field of Joshua, the Beth-shemite.
19 And he smote the men of Beth-
shemesh, [a]because they had looked into
the ark of the LORD, even he smote of the
people fifty thousand and threescore
and ten men: and the people lamented,
because the LORD had smitten *many* of
the people with a great slaughter.
20 And the men of Beth-shemesh said,
Who is able to stand before this holy
LORD God? and to whom shall he go up
from us?
21 And they sent messengers to the
inhabitants of Kirjath-jearim, saying, The
Philistines have brought again the ark of
the LORD; come ye down, *and* fetch it up
to you.

CHAPTER 7.

The ark brought to the house of Abinadab.
The revival at Mizpeh.

And the men of Kirjath-jearim came,
and fetched up the ark of the LORD,
and brought it into the house of Abinadab
in the hill, and sanctified Eleazar his son
to keep the ark of the LORD.
2 And it came to pass, while the ark
abode in Kirjath-jearim, that the time was
long; for it was twenty years: and all the
house of Israel [b]lamented after the LORD.
3 And Samuel spake unto all the
house of Israel, saying, If ye do [c]return
unto the LORD with all your hearts, *then*
put away the strange gods and
[d]Ashtaroth from among you, and prepare your hearts unto the LORD, and
serve him only: and he will deliver you
out of the hand of the Philistines.
4 Then the children of Israel did put
away Baalim and Ashtaroth, and served
the LORD only.
5 And Samuel said, Gather all Israel to
Mizpeh, and I will pray for you unto the
LORD.
6 And they gathered together to
Mizpeh, and drew water, and poured *it*
out before the LORD, and fasted on that
day, and said there, We have sinned
against the LORD. And Samuel judged
the children of Israel in Mizpeh.
7 And when the Philistines heard that
the children of Israel were gathered
together to Mizpeh, the lords of the
Philistines went up against Israel. And
when the children of Israel heard *it*, they
were afraid of the Philistines.
8 And the children of Israel said to
Samuel, Cease not to cry unto the LORD
our God for us, that he will save us out
of the hand of the Philistines.

The Israelites victorious at Eben-ezer.

9 And Samuel took a sucking lamb,
and offered *it for* a burnt-offering wholly

a Num. 4:15, 16; 1 Chr. 13:9, 10.
b Zech. 12:10, 11.
c Deut. 30:2, 10; 2 Chr. 30:6-9; Joel 2:13.
d See Jud. 2:13, *note*.

unto the LORD: and Samuel cried unto the
LORD for Israel; and the LORD heard him.
10 And as Samuel was offering up the
burnt-offering, the Philistines drew near
to battle against Israel: but the LORD thundered with a great thunder on that day
upon the Philistines, and [a]discomfited
them; and they were smitten before Israel.
11 And the men of Israel went out of
Mizpeh, and pursued the Philistines,
and smote them, until *they came* under
Beth-car.
12 Then Samuel took a stone, and set *it*
between Mizpeh and Shen, and called
the name of it [b]Eben-ezer, saying,
Hitherto hath the LORD helped us.
13 So the Philistines were subdued, and
they came no more into the coast of Israel:
and the hand of the LORD was against the
Philistines all the days of Samuel.
14 And the cities which the Philistines
had taken from Israel were restored to
Israel, from Ekron even unto Gath; and
the coasts thereof did Israel deliver out
of the hands of the Philistines. And there
was peace between Israel and the
Amorites.

Samuel, prophet, priest, and Judge.

15 And Samuel judged Israel all the
days of his life.
16 And he went from year to year in
circuit to Beth-el, and Gilgal, and Mizpeh,
and judged Israel in all those places.
17 And his return *was* to Ramah; for
there *was* his house; and there he judged
Israel; and there he built an altar unto
the LORD.

CHAPTER 8.

Israel demands a king.

And it [c]came to pass, when Samuel
was old, that he made his sons
[d]judges over Israel.
2 Now the name of his firstborn was
Joel; and the name of his second, Abiah:
they were judges in Beer-sheba.
3 And his sons walked not in his
ways, but turned aside after lucre, and
took [e]bribes, and perverted judgment.
4 Then all the elders of Israel gathered
themselves together, and came to
Samuel unto Ramah,
5 And said unto him, Behold, thou art
old, and thy sons walk not in thy ways:
now [f]make us a king to judge us like all
the nations.
6 But the thing displeased Samuel,
when they said, Give us a king to judge
us. And Samuel prayed unto the LORD.

The theocracy rejected.

7 And the LORD said unto Samuel,
Hearken unto the voice of the people in
all that they say unto thee: [g]for they have
not rejected thee, but they have rejected
me, that I should not reign over them.
8 According to all the works which
they have done since the day that I
brought them up out of Egypt even unto
this day, wherewith they have forsaken
me, and served other gods, so do they
also unto thee.
9 Now therefore hearken unto their
voice: howbeit yet protest solemnly unto
them, and shew them the manner of the
king that shall reign over them.
10 And Samuel told all the words of
the LORD unto the people that asked of
him a king.
11 And he said, This will be the manner of the king that shall reign over you:
He will take your sons, and appoint *them*
for himself, for his chariots, and *to be* his
horsemen; and *some* shall run before his
chariots.
12 And he will appoint him captains
over thousands, and captains over
fifties; and *will set them* to ear his
ground, and to reap his harvest, and to
make his instruments of war, and instruments of his chariots.
13 And he will take your daughters *to
be* confectionaries, and *to be* cooks, and *to
be* bakers.
14 And he will take your [h]fields, and
your vineyards, and your oliveyards,
even the best *of them*, and give *them* to his
servants.
15 And he will take the tenth of your
seed, and of your vineyards, and give to
his officers, and to his servants.
16 And he will take your menservants,
and your maidservants, and your goodliest young men, and your asses, and put
them to his work.
17 He will take the tenth of your
sheep: and ye shall be his servants.
18 And ye shall cry out in that day
because of your king which ye shall
have chosen you; and the LORD will not
[i]hear you in that day.

B.C. 1120.

a Psa. 18:14.

b i.e. *The stone of help.*

c *Israel (history).* vs. 1-8; 2 Sam. 7:8-17. (Gen. 12:2, 3; Rom. 11:26.)

d *Kingdom* (O.T.). vs. 1-7; 1 Sam. 9:15-17. (Gen. 1:26; Zech. 12:8.)

e 1 Sam. 12:3; Prov. 29:4.

f Deut. 17:14, 15; Hos. 13:10, 11.

g Ex. 16:8.

h 1 Ki. 21:7.

i Isa. 1:15; Mic. 3:4.

19 Nevertheless the people refused to
obey the voice of Samuel; and they said,
Nay; but we will have a king over us;
20 That we also may be like all the
nations; and that our king may judge us,
and go out before us, and fight our battles.
21 And Samuel heard all the words of
the people, and he rehearsed them in the
ears of the LORD.
22 And the LORD said to Samuel,
Hearken unto their voice, and make them
a king. And Samuel said unto the men of
Israel, Go ye every man unto his city.

CHAPTER 9.

Saul chosen to be king.

Now there was a man of Benjamin,
whose name *was* Kish, the son of
Abiel, the son of Zeror, the son of
Bechorath, the son of Aphiah, a
Benjamite, a mighty man of power.
2 And he had a son, whose name *was*
Saul, a choice young man, and a goodly:
and *there was* not among the children of
Israel a goodlier person than he: from
his shoulders and upward *he* [a]*was* higher
than any of the people.
3 And the asses of Kish Saul's father
were lost. And Kish said to Saul his son,
Take now one of the servants with thee,
and arise, go seek the asses.
4 And he passed through mount
Ephraim, and passed through the land
of [b]Shalisha, but they found *them* not:
then they passed through the land of
Shalim, and *there they were* not: and he
passed through the land of the
Benjamites, but they found *them* not.
5 *And* when they were come to the
land of Zuph, Saul said to his servant
that *was* with him, Come, and let us
return; lest my father leave *caring* for the
asses, and take thought for us.
6 And he said unto him, Behold now,
there is in this city a man of God, and *he
is* an honourable man; all that he saith
cometh surely to pass: now let us go
thither; peradventure he can shew us
our way that we should go.
7 Then said Saul to his servant, But,
behold, *if* we go, what shall we bring the
man? for the bread is spent in our vessels, and *there is* not a present to bring to
the man of God: what have we?
8 And the servant answered Saul
again, and said, Behold, I have here at
hand the fourth part of a [c]shekel of silver: *that* will I give to the man of God, to
tell us our way.
9 (Beforetime in Israel, when a man
went to enquire of God, thus he spake,
Come, and let us go to the seer: for *he
that is* now *called* a Prophet was beforetime called a Seer.)
10 Then said Saul to his servant, Well
said; come, let us go. So they went unto
the city where the man of God *was*.
11 *And* as they went up the hill to the
city, they found young [d]maidens going
out to draw water, and said unto them,
Is the seer here?
12 And they answered them, and said,
He is; behold, *he is* before you: make
haste now, for he came to day to the city;
for *there is* a sacrifice of the people to day
in the [e]high place:
13 As soon as ye be come into the city,
ye shall straightway find him, before he
go up to the high place to eat: for the
people will not eat until he come,
because he doth bless the sacrifice; *and*
afterwards they eat that be bidden. Now
therefore get you up; for about this time
ye shall find him.
14 And they went up into the city: *and*
when they were come into the city,
behold, Samuel came out against them,
for to go up to the high place.
15 Now the LORD had told Samuel in
his ear a day before Saul came, saying,
16 To morrow about this time I will
send thee a man out of the land of
Benjamin, and thou shalt [f]anoint him *to
be* captain over my people Israel, that he
may save my people out of the hand of
the Philistines: for I have [g]looked upon
my people, because their cry is come
unto me.
17 And when Samuel saw Saul, the
LORD said unto him, Behold the man
whom I spake to thee of! this same shall
[h]reign over my people.
18 Then Saul drew near to Samuel in
the gate, and said, Tell me, I pray thee,
where the seer's house *is*.
19 And Samuel answered Saul, and
said, I *am* the seer: go up before me unto
the high place; for ye shall eat with me
to day, and to morrow I will let thee go,
and will tell thee all that *is* in thine heart.
20 And as for thine asses that were
lost three days ago, set not thy mind on

B.C. 1095.

a 1 Sam. 10:23.

b 2 Ki. 4:42.

c One shekel = 2*s*. 9*d*., or 65 cts

d Gen. 24:11; Ex. 2:16.

e 1 Ki. 3:2.

f 1 Sam. 10:1.

g Ex. 2:23-25.

h *Kingdom* (O.T.). vs. 15-17; 1 Sam. 10:17-25. (Gen. 1:26; Zech. 12:8.)

them; for they are found. And on whom *is* all the desire of Israel? *Is it* not on thee, and on all thy father's house?

21 And Saul answered and said, *Am* not I a Benjamite, of the smallest of the tribes of Israel? and my family the least of all the families of the tribe of Benjamin? wherefore then speakest thou so to me?

22 And Samuel took Saul and his servant, and brought them into the parlour, and made them sit in the chiefest place among them that were bidden, which *were* about thirty persons.

23 And Samuel said unto the cook, Bring the portion which I gave thee, of which I said unto thee, Set it by thee.

24 And the cook took up the shoulder, and *that* which *was* upon it, and set *it* before Saul. And *Samuel* said, Behold that which is left! set *it* before thee, *and* eat: for unto this time hath it been kept for thee since I said, I have invited the people. So Saul did eat with Samuel that day.

25 And when they were come down from the high place into the city, *Samuel* communed with Saul upon the top of the house.

26 And they arose early: and it came to pass about the spring of the day, that Samuel called Saul to the top of the house, saying, Up, that I may send thee away. And Saul arose, and they went out both of them, he and Samuel, abroad.

27 *And* as they were going down to the end of the city, Samuel said to Saul, Bid the servant pass on before us, (and he passed on,) but stand thou still a while, that I may shew thee the word of God.

CHAPTER 10.

Saul anointed king.

Then [a]Samuel took a vial of oil, and poured *it* upon his head, and kissed him, and said, *Is it* not because the LORD hath anointed thee *to be* [b]captain over his inheritance?

2 When thou art departed from me to day, then shalt thou find two men by Rachel's [c]sepulchre in the border of Benjamin at Zelzah; and they will say unto thee, The asses which thou wentest to seek are found: and, lo, thy father hath left the care of the asses, and sorroweth for you, saying, What shall I do for my son?

3 Then shalt thou go on forward from thence, and thou shalt come to the plain of Tabor, and there shall meet thee three men going up to God to Beth-el, one carrying three kids, and another carrying three loaves of bread, and another carrying a bottle of wine:

4 And they will salute thee, and give thee two *loaves* of bread; which thou shalt receive of their hands.

5 After that thou shalt come to the hill of God, where *is* the garrison of the Philistines: and it shall come to pass, when thou art come thither to the city, that thou shalt meet a company of prophets coming down from the high place with a psaltery, and a tabret, and a pipe, and a harp, before them; and they shall prophesy:

6 And the [d]Spirit of the LORD will come upon thee, and thou shalt prophesy with them, and shalt be turned into another man.

7 And let it be, when these signs are come unto thee, *that* thou do as occasion serve thee; for God *is* with thee.

8 And thou shalt go down before me to Gilgal; and, behold, I will come down unto thee, to offer burnt-offerings, *and* to sacrifice sacrifices of peace-offerings: seven days shalt thou tarry, till I come to thee, and shew thee what thou shalt do.

9 And it was *so*, that when he had turned his back to go from Samuel, God gave him another heart: and all those signs came to pass that day.

10 And when they came thither to the hill, behold, a company of prophets met him; and the [e]Spirit of God came upon him, and he prophesied among them.

11 And it came to pass, when all that knew him beforetime saw that, behold, he prophesied among the prophets, then the people said one to another, What *is* this *that* is come unto the son of Kish? *Is* Saul also among the prophets?

12 And one of the same place answered and said, But who *is* their father? Therefore it became a proverb, *Is* Saul also among the prophets?

13 And when he had made an end of prophesying, he came to the high place.

14 And Saul's uncle said unto him and

B.C. 1095.

a 1 Sam. 9:16; 16:13; 2 Ki. 9:3, 6.

b 2 Sam. 5:2.

c Gen. 35:19, 20.

d *Holy Spirit*. vs. 6, 10; 1 Sam. 11:6. (Gen. 1:2; Mal. 2:15.)

e 1 Sam. 11:6.

to his servant, Whither went ye? And he
said, To seek the asses: and when we
saw that *they were* no where, we came to
Samuel.
15 And Saul's uncle said, Tell me, I
pray thee, what Samuel said unto you.
16 And Saul said unto his uncle, He
told us plainly that the asses were
found. But of the matter of the kingdom,
whereof Samuel spake, he told him not.
17 And Samuel called the people
together unto the LORD to Mizpeh;
18 And said unto the children of Israel,
Thus saith the LORD God of Israel, I
brought up Israel out of Egypt, and delivered
you out of the hand of the Egyptians,
and out of the hand of all kingdoms, *and*
of them that oppressed you:
19 And ye have this day rejected your
God, who himself saved you out of all
your adversities and your tribulations;
and ye have said unto him, *Nay*, but set
a king over us. Now therefore present
yourselves before the LORD by your
tribes, and by your thousands.
20 And when Samuel had caused all
the tribes of Israel to come near, the tribe
of Benjamin was taken.
21 When he had caused the tribe of
Benjamin to come near by their families,
the family of Matri was taken, and Saul
the son of Kish was taken: and when
they sought him, he could not be found.
22 Therefore they enquired of the
LORD further, if the man should yet come
thither. And the LORD answered, Behold,
he hath hid himself among the stuff.
23 And they ran and fetched him
thence: and when he stood among the
people, he was higher than any of the
people from his shoulders and upward.
24 And Samuel said to all the people,
See ye him whom the LORD hath chosen,
that *there is* none like him among all the
people? And all the people shouted, and
said, God save the king.
25 Then Samuel told the people the
manner of the [a]kingdom, and wrote *it* in
a book, and laid *it* up before the LORD.
And Samuel sent all the people away,
every man to his house.
26 And Saul also went home to
Gibeah; and there went with him a band
of men, whose hearts God had touched.
27 But the children of Belial said, How
shall this man save us? And they
despised him, and brought him no presents.
But he held his peace.

CHAPTER 11.

Saul's victory at Jabesh-gilead.

Then [b]Nahash the Ammonite came
up, and encamped against Jabesh-gilead:
and all the men of Jabesh said
unto Nahash, Make a [c]covenant with us,
and we will serve thee.
2 And Nahash the Ammonite
answered them, On this *condition* will I
make *a covenant* with you, that I may
thrust out all your right eyes, and lay it
for a reproach upon all Israel.
3 And the elders of Jabesh said unto
him, Give us seven days' respite, that we
may send messengers unto all the coasts
of Israel: and then, if *there be* no man to
save us, we will come out to thee.
4 Then came the messengers to Gibeah
of Saul, and told the tidings in the ears
of the people: and all the people lifted
up their voices, and wept.
5 And, behold, Saul came after the
herd out of the field; and Saul said,
What *aileth* the people that they weep?
And they told him the tidings of the
men of Jabesh.
6 And the [d]Spirit of God came upon
Saul when he heard those tidings, and
his anger was kindled greatly.
7 And he took a yoke of oxen, and
hewed them in pieces, and sent *them*
throughout all the coasts of Israel by the
hands of messengers, saying, Whosoever
cometh not forth after Saul and after
Samuel, so shall it be done unto his oxen.
And the fear of the LORD fell on the people,
and they came out with one consent.
8 And when he numbered them in
Bezek, the children of Israel were three
hundred thousand, and the men of
Judah thirty thousand.
9 And they said unto the messengers
that came, Thus shall ye say unto the
men of Jabesh-gilead, To morrow, by *that*
time the sun be hot, ye shall have help.
And the messengers came and shewed *it*
to the men of Jabesh; and they were glad.
10 Therefore the men of Jabesh said,
To morrow we will come out unto you,

B.C. 1095.

a *Kingdom* (O.T.). 1 Sam. 15:1-23. (Gen. 1:26; Zech. 12:8.)

b 1 Sam. 12:12.

c Isa. 36:16; cf. Ex. 23:31-33.

d *Holy Spirit.* 1 Sam. 16:13, 14. (Gen. 1:2; Mal. 2:15.)

and ye shall do with us all that seemeth good unto you.

11 And it was *so* on the morrow, that Saul put the people in three companies; and they came into the midst of the host in the morning watch, and slew the Ammonites until the heat of the day: and it came to pass, that they which remained were scattered, so that two of them were not left together.

12 And the people said unto Samuel, Who *is* he that said, Shall Saul reign over us? bring the men, that we may put them to death.

13 And Saul said, There shall not a man be put to death this day: for to day the LORD hath wrought salvation in Israel.

14 Then said Samuel to the people, Come, and let us go to Gilgal, and renew the kingdom there.

The kingdom renewed at Gilgal.

15 And all the people went to Gilgal; and there they made Saul king before the LORD in Gilgal; and there they sacrificed sacrifices of peace-offerings before the LORD; and there Saul and all the men of Israel rejoiced greatly.

CHAPTER 12.

Samuel's proclamation of the kingdom.

And Samuel said unto all Israel, Behold, I have hearkened unto your voice in all that ye said unto me, and have made a king over you.

2 And now, behold, the king walketh before you: and I am old and grayheaded; and, behold, my sons *are* with you: and I have walked before you from my childhood unto this day.

3 Behold, here I *am*: witness against me before the LORD, and before his anointed: whose ox have I taken? or whose ass have I taken? or whom have I defrauded? whom have I oppressed? or of whose hand have I received *any* bribe to [a]blind mine eyes therewith? and I will restore it you.

4 And they said, [b]Thou hast not defrauded us, nor oppressed us, neither hast thou taken ought of any man's hand.

5 And he said unto them, The LORD *is* witness against you, and his anointed *is* witness this day, that ye have not found ought in my hand. And they answered, *He is* witness.

Samuel rehearses the deliverances of Jehovah.

6 And Samuel said unto the people, *It is* the LORD that advanced Moses and Aaron, and that brought your fathers up out of the land of Egypt.

7 Now therefore stand still, that I may [c]reason with you before the LORD of all the righteous acts of the LORD, which he did to you and to your fathers.

8 When Jacob was come into Egypt, and your fathers cried unto the LORD, then the LORD [d]sent Moses and Aaron, which brought forth your fathers out of Egypt, and made them dwell in this place.

9 And when they forgat the LORD their God, he sold them into the hand of [e]Sisera, captain of the host of Hazor, and into the hand of the [f]Philistines, and into the hand of the king of [g]Moab, and they fought against them.

10 And they cried unto the LORD, and [h]said, We have sinned, because we have forsaken the LORD, and have served Baalim and [i]Ashtaroth: but now deliver us out of the hand of our enemies, and we will serve thee.

11 And the LORD sent [j]Jerubbaal, and Bedan, and [k]Jephthah, and [l]Samuel, and delivered you out of the hand of your enemies on every side, and ye dwelled safe.

12 And [m]when ye saw that Nahash the king of the children of Ammon came against you, ye said unto me, Nay; but a king shall reign over us: when the LORD your God *was* your king.

13 Now therefore behold the king whom ye have chosen, *and* whom ye have desired! and, behold, the LORD hath set a king over you.

14 If ye will [n]fear the LORD, and serve him, and obey his voice, and not rebel against the commandment of the LORD, then shall both ye and also the king that reigneth over you continue following the LORD your God:

15 But if ye will not obey the voice of the LORD, but rebel against the commandment of the LORD, then shall the hand of the LORD be against you, as *it was* against your fathers.

B.C. 1095.

a Deut. 16:19.
b Psa. 37:5, 6; cf. 2 Cor. 7:2.
c Isa. 1:18; Mic. 6:2, 3.
d Ex. 3:10.
e Jud. 4:2.
f Jud. 10:7.
g Jud. 3:12.
h Jud. 10:10.
i Jud. 2:13, *note.*
j Jud. 6:14, 23.
k Jud. 11:1.
l 1 Sam. 7:13.
m 1 Sam. 11:2.
n Psa. 19:9, *note.*

The sign of thunder and rain.

16 Now therefore stand and see this
great thing, which the LORD will do
before your eyes.
17 *Is it* not wheat harvest to day? I will
call unto the LORD, and he shall send
thunder and rain; that ye may perceive
and see that your wickedness *is* great,
which ye have done in the sight of the
LORD, in asking you a king.
18 So Samuel called unto the LORD;
and the LORD sent thunder and rain that
day: and all the people greatly feared the
LORD and Samuel.
19 And all the people said unto
Samuel, Pray for thy servants unto the
LORD thy God, that we die not: for we
have added unto all our sins *this* evil, to
ask us a king.
20 And Samuel said unto the people,
Fear not: ye have done all this wickedness: yet turn not aside from following
the LORD, but serve the LORD with all
your heart;
21 And turn ye not aside: for *then
should ye go* after vain *things*, which cannot profit nor deliver; for they *are* vain.
22 For the LORD will not forsake his
people for his great name's sake:
because it hath pleased the LORD to
make you his people.
23 Moreover as for me, God forbid
that I should sin against the LORD in
ceasing to pray for you: but I will teach
you the good and the right way:
24 Only [a]fear the LORD, and serve him
in truth with all your heart: for consider
how great *things* he hath done for you.
25 But if ye shall still do wickedly, ye
shall be consumed, both ye and your
king.

CHAPTER 13.

The self-will of Saul.

Saul reigned one year; and when he
had reigned two years over Israel,
2 Saul chose him three thousand *men*
of Israel; *whereof* two thousand were with
Saul in Michmash and in mount Beth-el,
and a thousand were with Jonathan in
[b]Gibeah of Benjamin: and the rest of the
people he sent every man to his tent.
3 And Jonathan smote the garrison of
the Philistines that *was* in Geba, and the
Philistines heard *of it*. And Saul blew the
trumpet throughout all the land, saying,
Let the Hebrews hear.
4 And all Israel heard say *that* Saul had
smitten a garrison of the Philistines, and
that Israel also was had in abomination
with the Philistines. And the people were
called together after Saul to [c]Gilgal.
5 And the Philistines gathered themselves together to fight with Israel, thirty
thousand chariots, and six thousand
horsemen, and people as the sand which
is on the sea shore in multitude: and
they came up, and pitched in Michmash,
eastward from [d]Beth-aven.
6 When the men of Israel saw that they
were in a strait, (for the people were distressed,) then the people did [e]hide themselves in caves, and in thickets, and in
rocks, and in high places, and in pits.
7 And *some of* the Hebrews went over
Jordan to the land of [f]Gad and Gilead.
As for Saul, he *was* yet in Gilgal, and all
the people followed him trembling.

Saul intrudes into the priest's office.

8 And he tarried seven days, according to the set time that Samuel *had
appointed*: but Samuel came not to Gilgal;
and the people were scattered from him.
9 And Saul said, Bring hither a burnt-
offering to me, and peace-offerings. And
[g]he offered the burnt-offering.
10 And it came to pass, that as soon as
he had made an end of offering the
burnt-offering, behold, Samuel came;
and Saul went out to meet him, that he
might salute him.

The divine rejection of Saul announced.

11 And Samuel said, What hast thou
done? And Saul said, Because I saw that
the people were scattered from me, and
that thou camest not within the days
appointed, and *that* the Philistines gathered themselves together at Michmash;
12 Therefore said I, The Philistines will
come down now upon me to Gilgal, and
I have not made supplication unto the
LORD: I forced myself therefore, and
offered a burnt-offering.
13 And Samuel said to [h]Saul, Thou
hast done foolishly: thou hast not kept
the commandment of the LORD thy God,
which he [i]commanded thee: for now

B.C. 1095.

a Psa. 19:9, *note*.
b 1 Sam. 10:26.
c Josh. 5:9.
d Josh. 7:2.
e 1 Sam. 14:11; Jud. 6:2.
f Num. 32:1-42.
g Num. 16:1-3, 32-40.
h 2 Chr. 16:9.
i 1 Sam. 15:11, 28.

would the LORD have established thy kingdom upon Israel for ever.

14 But now thy kingdom shall not continue: the LORD hath sought him a man [a]after his own heart, and the LORD hath commanded him *to be* captain over his people, because thou hast not kept *that* which the LORD commanded thee.

15 And Samuel arose, and gat him up from Gilgal unto Gibeah of Benjamin. And Saul numbered the people *that were* present with him, about six hundred men.

16 And Saul, and Jonathan his son, and the people *that were* present with them, abode in Gibeah of Benjamin: but the Philistines encamped in Michmash.

17 And the spoilers came out of the camp of the Philistines in three companies: one company turned unto the way *that leadeth to* [b]Ophrah, unto the land of Shual:

18 And another company turned the way *to* [c]Beth-horon: and another company turned *to* the way of the border that looketh to the valley of Zeboim toward the wilderness.

19 Now there was no smith found throughout all the land of Israel: for the Philistines said, Lest the Hebrews make *them* swords or spears:

20 But all the Israelites went down to the Philistines, to sharpen every man his share, and his coulter, and his axe, and his mattock.

21 Yet they had a file for the mattocks, and for the coulters, and for the forks, and for the axes, and to sharpen the goads.

22 So it came to pass in the day of battle, that there was neither sword nor spear found in the hand of any of the people that *were* with Saul and Jonathan: but with Saul and with Jonathan his son was there found.

23 And the garrison of the Philistines went out to the passage of Michmash.

CHAPTER 14.

Jonathan's great victory.

Now it came to pass upon a day, that Jonathan the son of Saul said unto the young man that bare his armour, Come, and let us go over to the Philistines' garrison, that *is* on the other side. But he told not his father.

2 And Saul tarried in the uttermost part of Gibeah under a pomegranate tree which *is* in Migron: and the people that *were* with him *were* about six hundred men;

3 And [d]Ahiah, the son of Ahitub, I-chabod's brother, the son of Phinehas, the son of Eli, the LORD'S priest in Shiloh, [e]wearing an ephod. And the people knew not that Jonathan was gone.

4 And between the passages, by which Jonathan sought to go over unto the Philistines' garrison, *there was* a sharp rock on the one side, and a sharp rock on the other side: and the name of the one *was* Bozez, and the name of the other Seneh.

5 The forefront of the one *was* situate northward over against Michmash, and the other southward over against Gibeah.

6 And Jonathan said to the young man that bare his armour, Come, and let us go over unto the garrison of these uncircumcised: it may be that the LORD will work for us: for *there is* no restraint to the LORD to [f]save by many or by few.

7 And his armourbearer said unto him, Do all that *is* in thine heart: turn thee; behold, I *am* with thee according to thy heart.

8 Then said Jonathan, Behold, we will pass over unto *these* men, and we will discover ourselves unto them.

9 If they say thus unto us, Tarry until we come to you; then we will stand still in our place, and will not go up unto them.

10 But if they say thus, Come up unto us; then we will go up: for the LORD hath delivered them into our hand: and this *shall be* a sign unto us.

11 And both of them discovered themselves unto the garrison of the Philistines: and the Philistines said, Behold, the Hebrews come forth out of the holes where they had [g]hid themselves.

12 And the men of the garrison answered Jonathan and his armourbearer, and said, Come up to us, and we will shew you a thing. And Jonathan said unto his armourbearer, Come up after me: for the LORD hath delivered them into the hand of Israel.

13 And Jonathan climbed up upon his hands and upon his feet, and his armourbearer after him: and they

B.C. 1093.

a Psa. 89:20; Acts 13:22.

b Josh. 18:23.

c Josh. 16:3.

d Called *Ahimelech,* 1 Sam. 22:9, 11, 20.

e Cf. 1 Sam. 2:27-33; Num. 16:1-3; 32-40; Jude 11.

f Deut. 32:36; Jud. 7:4, 7; 2 Chr. 14:11; Rom. 8:31.

g 1 Sam. 13:6.

B.C. 1087.

[a]fell before Jonathan; and his armourbearer slew after him.

14 And that first slaughter, which Jonathan and his armourbearer made, was about twenty men, within as it were an half acre of land, *which* a yoke *of oxen might plow*.

15 And there was [b]trembling in the host, in the field, and among all the people: the garrison, and the spoilers, they also trembled, and the earth quaked: so it was a very great trembling.

16 And the watchmen of Saul in Gibeah of Benjamin looked; and, behold, the multitude melted away, and they went on beating down *one another*.

17 Then said Saul unto the people that *were* with him, Number now, and see who is gone from us. And when they had numbered, behold, Jonathan and his armourbearer *were* not *there*.

18 And Saul said unto Ahiah, Bring hither the ark of God. For the ark of God was at that time with the children of Israel.

19 And it came to pass, while Saul talked unto the priest, that the noise that *was* in the host of the Philistines went on and increased: and Saul said unto the priest, Withdraw thine hand.

20 And Saul and all the people that *were* with him assembled themselves, and they came to the battle: and, behold, every man's sword was against his fellow, *and there was* a very great discomfiture.

21 Moreover the Hebrews *that* were with the Philistines before that time, which went up with them into the camp *from the country* round about, even they also *turned* to be with the Israelites that *were* with Saul and Jonathan.

22 Likewise all the men of Israel which had hid themselves in mount Ephraim, *when* they heard that the Philistines fled, even they also followed hard after them in the battle.

23 So the LORD saved Israel that day: and the battle passed over unto Beth-aven.

24 And the men of Israel were distressed that day: for Saul [c]had adjured the people, saying, Cursed *be* the man that eateth *any* food until evening, that I may be avenged on mine enemies. So none of the people tasted *any* food.

25 And all *they of* the land came to a wood; and there was [d]honey upon the ground.

26 And when the people were come into the wood, behold, the honey dropped; but no man put his hand to his mouth: for the people feared the oath.

27 But Jonathan heard not when his father charged the people with the oath: wherefore he put forth the end of the rod that *was* in his hand, and dipped it in an honeycomb, and put his hand to his mouth; and his eyes were [e]enlightened.

28 Then answered one of the people, and said, Thy father straitly charged the people with an oath, saying, Cursed *be* the man that eateth *any* food this day. And the people were faint.

29 Then said Jonathan, My father hath troubled the land: see, I pray you, how mine eyes have been enlightened, because I tasted a little of this honey.

30 How much more, if haply the people had eaten freely to day of the spoil of their enemies which they found? for had there not been now a much greater slaughter among the Philistines?

31 And they smote the Philistines that day from Michmash to Aijalon: and the people were very faint.

32 And the people flew upon the spoil, and took sheep, and oxen, and calves, and slew *them* on the ground: and the people did eat *them* with the [f]blood.

33 Then they told Saul, saying, Behold, the people sin against the LORD, in that they eat with the blood. And he said, Ye have transgressed: roll a great stone unto me this day.

34 And Saul said, Disperse yourselves among the people, and say unto them, Bring me hither every man his ox, and every man his sheep, and slay *them* here, and eat; and sin not against the LORD in eating with the blood. And all the people brought every man his ox with him that night, and slew *them* there.

35 And Saul built an altar unto the LORD: the same was the first altar that he built unto the LORD.

36 And Saul said, Let us go down after the Philistines by night, and spoil them until the morning light, and let us not leave a man of them. And they said, Do whatsoever seemeth good unto thee.

a Lev. 26:8.
b Deut. 28:7; 2 Ki. 7:6 Job 18:11.
c Cf. Josh. 6:26.
d Ex. 3:8; Num. 13:27; Mt. 3:4.
e 1 Sam. 30:12.
f Lev. 3:17; 17:10; Deut. 12:23, 24; Ezk. 33:25; Acts 15:19, 20.

Then said the priest, Let us draw near hither unto God.

37 And Saul asked counsel of God, Shall I go down after the Philistines? wilt thou deliver them into the hand of Israel? But he answered him not that day.

38 And Saul said, Draw ye near hither, all the chief of the people: and know and see wherein this sin hath been this day.

39 For, *as* the LORD liveth, which saveth Israel, [a]though it be in Jonathan my son, he shall surely die. But *there was* not a man among all the people *that* answered him.

40 Then said he unto all Israel, Be ye on one side, and I and Jonathan my son will be on the other side. And the people said unto Saul, Do what seemeth good unto thee.

41 Therefore Saul said unto the LORD God of Israel, [b]Give a perfect *lot*. And Saul and Jonathan were taken: but the people escaped.

42 And Saul said, Cast *lots* between me and Jonathan my son. And Jonathan was taken.

43 Then Saul said to Jonathan, Tell me what thou hast done. And Jonathan told him, and said, I did but taste a little honey with the end of the rod that *was* in mine hand, *and*, lo, I must die.

44 And Saul answered, God do so and more also: [c]for thou shalt surely die, Jonathan.

45 And the people said unto Saul, Shall Jonathan die, who hath wrought this great salvation in Israel? God forbid: *as* the LORD liveth, there shall not one hair of his head fall to the ground; for he hath wrought [d]with God this day. So the people rescued Jonathan, that he died not.

46 Then Saul went up from following the Philistines: and the Philistines went to their own place.

47 So Saul took the kingdom over Israel, and fought against all his enemies on every side, against Moab, and against the children of Ammon, and against Edom, and against the kings of Zobah, and against the Philistines: and whithersoever he turned himself, he vexed *them*.

48 And he gathered an host, and smote the [e]Amalekites, and delivered Israel out of the hands of them that spoiled them.

49 Now the sons of Saul were Jonathan, and Ishui, and Melchi-shua: and the names of his two daughters *were these*; the name of the firstborn Merab,

B.C. 1087.

a Cf. v. 44.

b Cf. Josh. 7:14-18.

c Cf. v. 39.

d 2 Chr. 19:11; Isa. 13:3; 2 Cor. 6:1; Phil. 2:12, 13.

e Ex. 17:16.

f 1 Sam. 9:16.

g *Kingdom* (O.T.). vs. 1-23; 1 Sam. 16:1-13. (Gen. 1:26; Zech. 12:8.)

h Ex. 17:8-14; Deut. 25:17-19.

i Num. 24:20.

j Jud. 1:16; 4:11-22; 1 Chr. 2:55.

k v. 18.

and the name of the younger Michal:

50 And the name of Saul's wife *was* Ahinoam, the daughter of Ahimaaz: and the name of the captain of his host *was* Abner, the son of Ner, Saul's uncle.

51 And Kish *was* the father of Saul; and Ner the father of Abner *was* the son of Abiel.

52 And there was sore war against the Philistines all the days of Saul: and when Saul saw any strong man, or any valiant man, he took him unto him.

CHAPTER 15.

Saul's incomplete obedience.
(Cf. Gen. 11:31.)

Samuel also said unto [f]Saul, The LORD sent me to anoint thee *to be* [g]king over his people, over Israel: now therefore hearken thou unto the voice of the words of the LORD.

2 Thus saith the LORD of hosts, I remember *that* which [h]Amalek did to Israel, how he laid *wait* for him in the way, when he came up from Egypt.

3 Now go and smite Amalek, and utterly [i]destroy all that they have, and spare them not; but slay both man and woman, infant and suckling, ox and sheep, camel and ass.

4 And Saul gathered the people together, and numbered them in Telaim, two hundred thousand footmen, and ten thousand men of Judah.

5 And Saul came to a city of Amalek, and laid wait in the valley.

6 And Saul said unto the [j]Kenites, Go, depart, get you down from among the Amalekites, lest I destroy you with them: for ye shewed kindness to all the children of Israel, when they came up out of Egypt. So the Kenites departed from among the Amalekites.

7 And Saul smote the Amalekites from Havilah *until* thou comest to Shur, that *is* over against Egypt.

8 And he took Agag the king of the Amalekites alive, and utterly destroyed all the people with the edge of the sword.

9 [k]But Saul and the people spared Agag, and the best of the sheep, and of the oxen, and of the fatlings, and the lambs, and all *that was* good, and would not utterly destroy them: but every thing *that was* vile and refuse, that they destroyed utterly.

10 Then came the word of the LORD
unto Samuel, saying,
11 It [a]repenteth me that I have set up
Saul *to be* king: for he is turned back from
following me, and hath not performed my
commandments. And it grieved Samuel;
and he cried unto the LORD all night.
12 And when Samuel rose early to
meet Saul in the morning, it was told
Samuel, saying, Saul came to Carmel,
and, behold, he set him up a place, and
is gone about, and passed on, and gone
down to Gilgal.
13 And Samuel came to Saul: and Saul
said unto him, Blessed *be* thou of the
LORD: I have performed the commandment of the LORD.
14 And Samuel said, What *meaneth* then
this bleating of the sheep in mine ears,
and the lowing of the oxen which I hear?
15 And Saul said, They have brought
them from the Amalekites: for the people
spared the best of the sheep and of the
oxen, to sacrifice unto the LORD thy God;
and the rest we have utterly destroyed.
16 Then Samuel said unto Saul, Stay,
and I will tell thee what the LORD hath
said to me this night. And he said unto
him, Say on.
17 And Samuel said, When thou *wast*
little in thine own sight, *wast* thou not
made the head of the tribes of Israel, and
the LORD anointed thee king over Israel?
18 And the LORD sent thee on a journey, and said, Go and utterly destroy the
sinners the Amalekites, and fight against
them until they be consumed.
19 Wherefore then didst thou not obey
the voice of the LORD, but didst fly upon
the spoil, and didst evil in the sight of
the LORD?
20 And Saul said unto Samuel, Yea, I
have [b]obeyed the voice of the LORD, and
have gone the way which the LORD sent
me, and have brought Agag the king of
Amalek, and have utterly destroyed the
Amalekites.
21 But the people took of the spoil,
sheep and oxen, the chief of the things
which should have been utterly
destroyed, to sacrifice unto the LORD thy
God in Gilgal.
22 And Samuel said, [c]Hath the LORD *as*
great delight in burnt-offerings and sacrifices, as in obeying the voice of the LORD?
Behold, to obey *is* better than sacrifice,
and to hearken than the fat of rams.
23 For rebellion *is as* the sin of
witchcraft, and stubbornness *is as* iniquity and idolatry. [d]Because thou hast
rejected the word of the LORD, he hath
also rejected thee from *being* king.
24 And Saul said unto Samuel, I have
sinned: for I have transgressed the commandment of the LORD, and thy words:
because I feared the people, and obeyed
their voice.
25 Now therefore, I pray thee, pardon
my sin, and turn again with me, that I
may worship the LORD.
26 And Samuel said unto Saul, I will
not return with thee: for thou hast rejected
the word of the LORD, and the LORD hath
rejected thee from being king over Israel.
27 And as Samuel turned about to go
away, he laid hold upon the skirt of his
mantle, and it rent.
28 And Samuel said unto him, The
LORD hath rent the kingdom of Israel from
thee this day, and hath given it to a neighbour of thine, *that is* better than thou.
29 And also the Strength of Israel will
not lie nor [a]repent: for he *is* not a man,
that he should repent.
30 Then he said, I have sinned: *yet*
honour me now, I pray thee, before the
elders of my people, and before Israel,
and turn again with me, that I may worship the LORD thy God.
31 So Samuel turned again after Saul;
and Saul worshipped the LORD.
32 Then said Samuel, Bring ye hither
to me Agag the king of the Amalekites.
And Agag came unto him delicately.
And Agag said, Surely the bitterness of
death is past.
33 And Samuel said, As thy sword
hath made women childless, so shall thy
mother be childless among women. And
Samuel hewed Agag in pieces before the
LORD in Gilgal.
34 Then Samuel went to Ramah; and
Saul went up to his house to Gibeah of
Saul.
35 And Samuel came no more to see
Saul until the day of his death: nevertheless Samuel mourned for Saul: and the
LORD [a]repented that he had made Saul
king over Israel.

CHAPTER 16.

The choice of David to be king.

AND the LORD said unto Samuel, How
long wilt thou mourn for Saul, seeing I have rejected him from reigning

B.C. 1079.

a Zech. 8:14, *note.*

b Prov. 28:13.

c Psa. 50:8, 9; 51:16, 17; Prov. 21:3; Isa. 1:11-17; Jer. 7:22, 23; Mic. 6:6-8; Heb. 10:4-10.

d John 6:38, 63, 64; 8:47; 10:26; 12:48; 15:22.

over Israel? fill thine horn with oil, and
go, I will send thee to Jesse the Beth-
lehemite: for I have provided me a [a]king
among his sons.
2 And Samuel said, How can I go? if
Saul hear *it*, he will kill me. And the
LORD said, Take an heifer with thee, and
say, I am come to sacrifice to the LORD.
3 And call Jesse to the sacrifice, and I
will shew thee what thou shalt do: and
thou shalt anoint unto me *him* whom I
name unto thee.
4 And Samuel did that which the LORD
spake, and came to Beth-lehem. And the
elders of the town trembled at his coming, and said, Comest thou peaceably?
5 And he said, Peaceably: I am come
to sacrifice unto the LORD: sanctify yourselves, and come with me to the sacrifice. And he sanctified Jesse and his
sons, and called them to the sacrifice.
6 And it came to pass, when they were
come, that he looked on Eliab, and said,
Surely the LORD'S anointed *is* before him.
7 But the LORD said unto Samuel, Look
not on his countenance, or on the height
of his stature; because I have refused
him: [b]for *the LORD seeth* not as man seeth;
for man looketh on the [c]outward appearance, but the LORD looketh on the heart.
8 Then Jesse called Abinadab, and
made him pass before Samuel. And he
said, Neither hath the LORD chosen this.
9 Then Jesse made Shammah to pass
by. And he said, Neither hath the LORD
chosen this.
10 Again, Jesse made seven of his sons
to pass before Samuel. And Samuel said
unto Jesse, The LORD hath not chosen
these.
11 And Samuel said unto Jesse, Are
here all *thy* children? And he said, There
remaineth yet the youngest, and, behold,
he keepeth the [d]sheep. And Samuel said
unto Jesse, Send and fetch him: for we
will not sit down till he come hither.

David anointed to be king.

12 And he sent, and brought him in.
Now he *was* ruddy, *and* withal of a beautiful countenance, and goodly to look to.
And the LORD said, Arise, anoint him:
for this *is* he.
13 Then Samuel took the horn of oil,
and anointed him in the midst of his
brethren: and the [e]Spirit of the LORD
came upon David from that day forward.
So Samuel rose up, and went to Ramah.

David is brought to Saul.

14 But the Spirit of the LORD departed
from Saul, and an evil spirit from the
LORD troubled him.
15 And Saul's servants said unto him,
Behold now, an evil spirit from God
troubleth thee.
16 Let our lord now command thy servants, *which are* before thee, to seek out a
man, *who is* a cunning player on an harp:
and it shall come to pass, when the evil
spirit from God is upon thee, that he
shall play with his hand, and thou shalt
be well.
17 And Saul said unto his servants,
Provide me now a man that can play
well, and bring *him* to me.
18 Then answered one of the servants,
and said, Behold, I have seen a son of
Jesse the Beth-lehemite, *that is* cunning in
playing, and a mighty valiant man, and a
man of war, and prudent in matters, and a
comely person, and the LORD *is* with him.
19 Wherefore Saul sent messengers
unto Jesse, and said, Send me David thy
son, which *is* with the sheep.
20 And Jesse took an ass *laden* with
bread, and a bottle of wine, and a kid,
and sent *them* by David his son unto Saul.
21 And David [1]came to Saul, and
stood before him: and he loved him
greatly; and he became his armourbearer.
22 And Saul sent to Jesse, saying, Let
David, I pray thee, stand before me; for
he hath found favour in my sight.
23 And it came to pass, when the *evil*
spirit from God was upon Saul, that
David took an harp, and played with his

B.C. 1063.

a *Kingdom* (O.T.). vs. 1-13; 2 Sam. 2:1-4. (Gen. 1:26; Zech. 12:8.)

b Isa. 55:8, 9.

c 2 Cor. 10:7; 1 Pet. 2:4.

d 2 Sam. 7:8; Psa. 78:70-72

e *Holy Spirit.* vs. 13, 14; 1 Sam. 19:20, 23. (Gen. 1:2; Mal. 2:15.)

[1] **(16:21)** Cf. 1 Sam. 17:55, 56. The order of events is: (1) David, whose skill on the harp, and valour in the combat with the lion and bear (1 Sam. 17:34, 36) were known to "one of the servants" of Saul, was brought to play before the king (1 Sam. 16:17, 18). (2) David returns to Bethlehem (1 Sam. 17:15). (3) David is sent to Saul's camp (1 Sam. 17:17, 18) and performs his great exploit. (4) Saul's question (1 Sam. 17:55, 56) implies only that he had forgotten the name of David s father—not remarkable certainly in an oriental king.

hand: so Saul was refreshed, and was
well, and the evil spirit departed from
him.

CHAPTER 17.

The defiance of Israel by Goliath.

Now the Philistines gathered together
their armies to battle, and were
gathered together at Shochoh, which
belongeth to Judah, and pitched between
Shochoh and Azekah, in Ephes-dammim.
2 And Saul and the men of Israel were
gathered together, and pitched by the
valley of Elah, and set the battle in array
against the Philistines.
3 And the Philistines stood on a
mountain on the one side, and Israel
stood on a mountain on the other side:
and *there was* a valley between them.
4 And there went out a champion out
of the camp of the Philistines, named
Goliath, of Gath, whose height *was* six
[a]cubits and a [b]span.
5 And *he had* an helmet of brass upon
his head, and he *was* armed with a coat
of mail; and the weight of the coat *was*
five thousand shekels of brass.
6 And *he had* greaves of brass upon his
legs, and a target of brass between his
shoulders.
7 And the staff of his spear *was* like a
weaver's beam; and his spear's head
weighed six hundred shekels of iron: and
one bearing a shield went before him.
8 And he stood and cried unto the
armies of Israel, and said unto them,
Why are ye come out to set *your* battle in
array? *am* not I a Philistine, and ye servants to Saul? choose you a man for you,
and let him come down to me.
9 If he be able to fight with me, and to
kill me, then will we be your servants: but
if I prevail against him, and kill him, then
shall ye be our servants, and serve us.
10 And the Philistine said, I defy the
armies of Israel this day; give me a man,
that we may fight together.
11 When Saul and all Israel heard
those words of the Philistine, they were
dismayed, and greatly afraid.
12 Now David *was* the [c]son of that
Ephrathite of Beth-lehem-judah, whose
name *was* Jesse; and he had [d]eight sons:
and the man went among men *for* an old
man in the days of Saul.
13 And the three eldest sons of Jesse
went *and* followed Saul to the battle: and
the names of his three sons that went to
the battle *were* Eliab the firstborn, and
next unto him Abinadab, and the third
Shammah.
14 And David *was* the youngest: and
the three eldest followed Saul.

David is sent to the army of Saul.

15 But David went and returned from
Saul to [e]feed his father's sheep at Beth-
lehem.
16 And the Philistine drew near morning and evening, and presented himself
forty days.
17 And Jesse said unto David his son,
Take now for thy brethren an [f]ephah of
this parched *corn*, and these ten loaves,
and run to the camp to thy brethren;
18 And carry these ten cheeses unto the
captain of *their* thousand, and [g]look how
thy brethren fare, and take their pledge.
19 Now Saul, and they, and all the
men of Israel, *were* in the valley of Elah,
fighting with the Philistines.
20 And David rose up early in the
morning, and left the sheep with a keeper, and took, and went, as Jesse had commanded him; and he came to the trench,
as the host was going forth to the fight,
and shouted for the battle.
21 For Israel and the Philistines had put
the battle in array, army against army.
22 And David left his carriage in the
hand of the keeper of the carriage, and
ran into the army, and came and saluted
his brethren.
23 And as he talked with them,
behold, there came up the champion, the
Philistine of Gath, Goliath by name, out
of the armies of the Philistines, and
spake according to the same words: and
David heard *them*.
24 And all the men of Israel, when
they saw the man, fled from him, and
were sore afraid.
25 And the men of Israel said, Have ye
seen this man that is come up? surely to
defy Israel is he come up: and it shall be,
that the man who killeth him, the king
will enrich him with great riches, and
will give him his daughter, and make his
father's house free in Israel.
26 And David spake to the men that

B.C. 1063.

a One cubit = 1 ft. 5 in.
b One span = about 9 in.
c Ruth 4:22.
d 1 Sam. 16:10, 11.
e 1 Sam. 16:11, 19.
f One ephah = 1 bu. 3 pts.
g Gen. 37:14.

stood by him, saying, What shall be
done to the man that killeth this
Philistine, and taketh away the reproach
from Israel? for who *is* this uncircumcised Philistine, that he should defy the
armies of the [a]living God?
27 And the people answered him after
this manner, saying, So shall it be done
to the man that killeth him.
28 And Eliab his eldest brother heard
when he spake unto the men; and
Eliab's [b]anger was kindled against
David, and he said, Why camest thou
down hither? and with whom hast thou
left those few sheep in the wilderness? I
know thy pride, and the naughtiness of
thine heart; for thou art come down that
thou mightest see the battle.
29 And David said, What have I now
done? *Is there* not a cause?
30 And he turned from him toward
another, and spake after the same manner: and the people answered him again
after the former manner.

David's victory over Goliath.

31 And when the words were heard
which David spake, they rehearsed *them*
before Saul: and he sent for him.
32 And David said to Saul, Let no
man's heart [c]fail because of him; thy servant will go and fight with this Philistine.
33 And Saul said to David, Thou art
not able to go against this Philistine to
fight with him: for thou *art but* a youth,
and he a man of war from his youth.
34 And David said unto Saul, Thy servant kept his father's sheep, and there
came a lion, and a bear, and took a lamb
out of the flock:
35 And I went out after him, and
smote him, and delivered *it* out of his
mouth: and when he arose against me, I
caught *him* by his beard, and smote him,
and slew him.
36 Thy servant slew both the lion and
the bear: and this uncircumcised
Philistine shall be as one of them, seeing
he hath defied the armies of the living
God.
37 David said moreover, The LORD
that delivered me out of the paw of the
lion, and out of the paw of the bear, he
will deliver me out of the hand of this
Philistine. And Saul said unto David,
Go, and the [d]LORD be with thee.
38 And Saul armed David with his
armour, and he put an helmet of brass

B.C. 1063.

a Deut. 5:26; Josh. 3:10.

b Gen. 37:4, 8.

c Deut. 20:2, 3.

d 1 Sam. 20:13; 1 Chr. 22:11.

e 2 Sam. 3:8; 2 Ki. 8:13.

f 1 Ki. 20:10-11.

g 2 Sam. 22:33; Psa. 124:8; Heb. 11:32-34.

h v. 10.

i v. 51.

j Josh. 4:24; 1 Ki. 8:43; 18:36; 2 Ki. 19:19; Psa. 46:10; Isa. 52.10.

k Psa. 44:6, 7; Hos. 1:7; Zech. 4:6.

upon his head; also he armed him with a
coat of mail.
39 And David girded his sword upon
his armour, and he assayed to go; for he
had not proved *it*. And David said unto
Saul, I cannot go with these; for I have
not proved *them*. And David put them
off him.
40 And he took his staff in his hand,
and chose him five smooth stones out of
the brook, and put them in a shepherd's
bag which he had, even in a scrip; and
his sling *was* in his hand: and he drew
near to the Philistine.
41 And the Philistine came on and
drew near unto David; and the man that
bare the shield *went* before him.
42 And when the Philistine looked
about, and saw David, he disdained
him: for he was *but* a youth, and ruddy,
and of a fair countenance.
43 And the Philistine said unto David,
Am I a [e]dog, that thou comest to me with
staves? And the Philistine cursed David
by his gods.
44 And the Philistine [f]said to David,
Come to me, and I will give thy flesh
unto the fowls of the air, and to the
beasts of the field.
45 Then said David to the Philistine,
Thou comest to me with a sword, and
with a spear, and with a shield: but [g]I
come to thee in the name of the LORD of
hosts, the God of the armies of Israel,
whom thou hast [h]defied.
46 This day will the LORD deliver thee
into mine hand; and I will smite thee,
and [i]take thine head from thee; and I
will give the carcases of the host of the
Philistines this day unto the fowls of the
air, and to the wild beasts of the earth;
that all the earth may [j]know that there is
a God in Israel.
47 And all this assembly shall [k]know
that the LORD saveth not with sword and
spear: for the battle *is* the LORD'S, and he
will give you into our hands.
48 And it came to pass, when the
Philistine arose, and came and drew
nigh to meet David, that David hasted,
and ran toward the army to meet the
Philistine.
49 And David put his hand in his bag,
and took thence a stone, and slang *it*,
and smote the Philistine in his forehead,
that the stone sunk into his forehead;
and he fell upon his face to the earth.

B.C. 1063.

50 So David prevailed over the
Philistine with a [a]sling and with a stone,
and smote the Philistine, and slew him;
but *there was* no sword in the hand of
David.
51 Therefore David ran, and stood
upon the Philistine, and took his sword,
and drew it out of the sheath thereof,
and slew him, and cut off his head therewith. And when the Philistines saw their
champion was dead, they [b]fled.
52 And the men of Israel and of Judah
arose, and shouted, and pursued the
Philistines, until thou come to the valley,
and to the gates of Ekron. And the
wounded of the Philistines fell down by
the way to Shaaraim, even unto Gath,
and unto Ekron.
53 And the children of Israel returned
from chasing after the Philistines, and
they spoiled their tents.
54 And David took the head of the
Philistine, and brought it to Jerusalem;
but he put his armour in his tent.
55 And when Saul saw David go forth
against the Philistine, he said unto
Abner, the captain of the host, Abner,
whose son *is* this youth? And Abner said,
As thy soul liveth, O king, I cannot tell.
56 And the king said, Enquire thou
whose [c]son the stripling *is*.
57 And as David returned from the
slaughter of the Philistine, Abner took
him, and brought him before Saul with
the head of the Philistine in his hand.
58 And Saul said to him, Whose son
art thou, *thou* young man? And David
answered, *I am* the son of thy servant
Jesse the Beth-lehemite.

CHAPTER 18.

The love-covenant of Jonathan and David.

And it came to pass, when he had
made an end of speaking unto
Saul, that the soul of Jonathan was knit
with the soul of David, and Jonathan
loved him as his own soul.
2 And Saul took him that day, and
would let him go no more home to his
father's house.
3 Then Jonathan and David made a
covenant, because he loved him as his
own soul.
4 And Jonathan stripped himself of
the robe that *was* upon him, and gave it
to David, and his garments, even to his
sword, and to his bow, and to his girdle.
5 And David went out whithersoever
Saul sent him, *and* behaved himself
wisely: and Saul set him over the men of
war, and he was accepted in the sight of
all the people, and also in the sight of
Saul's servants.
6 And it came to pass as they came,
when David was returned from the
slaughter of the Philistine, that the
women came out of all cities of Israel,
singing and dancing, to meet king Saul,
with tabrets, with joy, and with instruments of musick.
7 And the women answered *one another* as they played, and said, Saul hath
[d]slain his thousands, and David his ten
thousands.

Saul's jealousy of David,
whom he endeavours twice to kill.

8 And Saul was very wroth, and the
saying displeased him; and he said,
They have ascribed unto David ten
thousands, and to me they have ascribed
but thousands: and *what* can he have
more but the [e]kingdom?
9 And Saul eyed David from that day
and forward.
10 And it came to pass on the morrow,
that the [f]evil spirit from God came upon
Saul, and he [g]prophesied in the midst of
the house: and David played with his
hand, as at other times: and *there was* a
[h]javelin in Saul's hand.
11 And Saul cast the javelin; for he
said, I will smite David even to the wall
with it. And David avoided out of his
presence twice.
12 And Saul was afraid of David,
because the LORD was with him, and
was departed from Saul.
13 Therefore Saul removed him from
him, and made him his captain over a
thousand; and he went out and came in
before the people.
14 And David behaved himself wisely
in all his ways; and the LORD *was* with
him.
15 Wherefore when Saul saw that he
behaved himself very wisely, he was
afraid of him.
16 But all Israel and Judah loved
David, [i]because he went out and came
in before them.
17 And Saul said to David, Behold my
elder daughter [j]Merab, her will I give
thee to wife: only be thou valiant for me,
and [k]fight the LORD'S battles. For Saul

a Jud. 3:31; 15:15.
b Heb. 11:34.
c Cf. 1 Sam. 16:21, *note*.
d 1 Sam. 21:11.
e 1 Sam. 15:28.
f 1 Sam. 16:14.
g 1 Sam. 19:24.
h 1 Sam. 19:9, 10.
i Num. 27:16-17; 2 Sam. 5:2; 1 Ki. 3:7.
j 1 Sam. 17:25.
k 1 Sam. 25:28.

said, Let not mine hand be upon him, but let the [a]hand of the Philistines be upon him.

18 And David said unto [b]Saul, Who *am* I? and what *is* my life, *or* my father's family in Israel, that I should be son in law to the king?

19 But it came to pass at the time when Merab Saul's daughter should have been given to David, that she was given unto [c]Adriel the Meholathite to wife.

Michal, Saul's daughter, given to David.

20 And Michal Saul's daughter loved David: and they told Saul, and the thing pleased him.

21 And Saul said, I will give him her, that she may be a snare to him, and that the [d]hand of the Philistines may be against him. Wherefore Saul said to David, Thou shalt this day be my son in law in *the one of* the twain.

22 And Saul commanded his servants, *saying*, Commune with David secretly, and say, Behold, the king hath delight in thee, and all his servants love thee: now therefore be the king's son in law.

23 And Saul's servants spake those words in the ears of David. And David said, Seemeth it to you *a* light *thing* to be a king's son in law, seeing that I *am* a poor man, and lightly esteemed?

24 And the servants of Saul told him, saying, On this manner spake David.

25 And Saul said, Thus shall ye say to David, The king desireth not any dowry, but an hundred foreskins of the Philistines, to be [e]avenged of the king's enemies. But Saul thought to make David fall by the hand of the Philistines.

26 And when his servants told David these words, it pleased David well to be the king's son in law: and the days were not expired.

27 Wherefore David arose and went, he and his men, and slew of the Philistines two hundred men; and David brought their [f]foreskins, and they gave them in full tale to the king, that he might be the king's son in law. And Saul gave him Michal his daughter to wife.

28 And Saul saw and knew that the LORD *was* with David, and *that* Michal Saul's daughter loved him.

29 And Saul was yet the more afraid of David; and Saul became David's enemy continually.

B.C. 1063.

a vs. 21, 25; 2 Sam. 12:9.
b v. 23; 1 Sam. 9:21; 2 Sam. 7:18.
c 2 Sam. 21:8.
d v. 17.
e 1 Sam. 14:24.
f 2 Sam. 3:14.
g v. 5.
h 1 Sam. 18:1.
i Jud. 12:3.
j 1 Sam. 14:49; 17:49, 50.
k 1 Chr. 11:14.
l 1 Sam. 16:14.

30 Then the princes of the Philistines went forth: and it came to pass, after they went forth, *that* David behaved himself more [g]wisely than all the servants of Saul; so that his name was much set by.

CHAPTER 19.

Saul's third attempt to kill David: David's flight.

And Saul spake to Jonathan his son, and to all his servants, that they should kill David.

2 But Jonathan Saul's son delighted [h]much in David: and Jonathan told David, saying, Saul my father seeketh to kill thee: now therefore, I pray thee, take heed to thyself until the morning, and abide in a secret *place*, and hide thyself:

3 And I will go out and stand beside my father in the field where thou *art*, and I will commune with my father of thee; and what I see, that I will tell thee.

4 And Jonathan spake good of David unto Saul his father, and said unto him, Let not the king sin against his servant, against David; because he hath not sinned against thee, and because his works *have been* to thee-ward very good:

5 For he [i]did put his life in his hand, and [j]slew the Philistine, and the [k]LORD wrought a great salvation for all Israel: thou sawest *it*, and didst rejoice: wherefore then wilt thou sin against innocent blood, to slay David without a cause?

6 And Saul hearkened unto the voice of Jonathan: and Saul sware, *As* the LORD liveth, he shall not be slain.

7 And Jonathan called David, and Jonathan shewed him all those things. And Jonathan brought David to Saul, and he was in his presence, as in times past.

8 And there was war again: and David went out, and fought with the Philistines, and slew them with a great slaughter; and they fled from him.

9 And the [l]evil spirit from the LORD was upon Saul, as he sat in his house with his javelin in his hand: and David played with *his* hand.

10 And Saul sought to smite David even to the wall with the javelin; but he slipped away out of Saul's presence, and he smote the javelin into the wall: and David fled, and escaped that night.

B.C. 1063.

11 Saul also sent messengers unto David's house, to watch him, and to slay him in the morning: and Michal David's wife told him, saying, If thou save not thy life to night, to morrow thou shalt be slain.
12 So Michal [a]let David down through a window: and he went, and fled, and escaped.
13 And Michal took an image, and laid *it* in the bed, and put a pillow of goats' *hair* for his bolster, and covered *it* with a cloth.
14 And when Saul sent messengers to take David, she said, He *is* sick.
15 And Saul sent the messengers *again* to see David, saying, Bring him up to me in the bed, that I may slay him.
16 And when the messengers were come in, behold, *there was* an image in the bed, with a pillow of goats' *hair* for his bolster.
17 And Saul said unto Michal, Why hast thou deceived me so, and sent away mine enemy, that he is escaped? And Michal answered Saul, He said unto me, Let me go; why should I kill thee?

The Spirit of God protects David.

18 So David fled, and escaped, and came to Samuel to Ramah, and told him all that Saul had done to him. And he and Samuel went and dwelt in Naioth.
19 And it was told Saul, saying, Behold, David *is* at Naioth in Ramah.
20 And Saul sent messengers to take David: and when they [b]saw the company of the prophets prophesying, and Samuel standing *as* appointed over them, the [c]Spirit of God was upon the messengers of Saul, and they also prophesied.
21 And when it was told Saul, he sent other messengers, and they prophesied likewise. And Saul sent messengers again the third time, and they prophesied also.
22 Then went he also to Ramah, and came to a great well that *is* in Sechu: and he asked and said, Where *are* Samuel and David? And *one* said, Behold, *they be* at Naioth in Ramah.
23 And he went thither to Naioth in Ramah: and the Spirit of God was upon him also, and he went on, and prophesied, until he came to Naioth in Ramah.
24 And he stripped off his clothes also, and prophesied before Samuel in like manner, and lay down naked all that day and all that night. Wherefore they say, *Is* [d]Saul also among the prophets?

CHAPTER 20.

Jonathan protects David.

And David fled from Naioth in Ramah, and came and said before Jonathan, What have I done? what *is* mine iniquity? and what *is* my sin before thy father, that he seeketh my life?
2 And he said unto him, God forbid; thou shalt not die: behold, my father will do nothing either great or small, but that he will shew it me: and why should my father hide this thing from me? it *is* not *so*.
3 And David sware moreover, and said, Thy father certainly knoweth that I have found grace in thine eyes; and he saith, Let not Jonathan know this, lest he be grieved: but [e]truly *as* the LORD liveth, and *as* thy soul liveth, *there is* but a step between me and death.
4 Then said Jonathan unto David, Whatsoever thy soul desireth, I will even do *it* for thee.
5 And David said unto Jonathan, Behold, to morrow *is* the new moon, and I should not fail to sit with the king at meat: but let me go, that I may hide myself in the [f]field unto the third *day* at even.
6 If thy father at all miss me, then say, David earnestly asked *leave* of me that he might run to [g]Beth-lehem his city: for *there is* a yearly sacrifice there for all the family.
7 If he say thus, *It is* well; thy servant shall have peace: but if he be very wroth, *then* be sure that evil is [h]determined by him.
8 Therefore thou shalt deal kindly with thy servant; for thou hast brought thy servant into a [i]covenant of the LORD with thee: notwithstanding, if there be in me iniquity, slay me thyself; for why shouldest thou bring me to thy father?
9 And Jonathan said, Far be it from thee: for if I knew certainly that evil were determined by my father to come upon thee, then would not I tell it thee?
10 Then said David to Jonathan, Who shall tell me? or what *if* thy father answer thee roughly?
11 And Jonathan said unto David, Come, and let us go out into the field.

a Josh. 2:15; cf. 2 Cor. 11:33.
b 1 Sam. 10:5, 6.
c *Holy Spirit.* vs. 20, 23; 2 Sam. 23:2. (Gen. 1.2; Mal. 2.15.)
d 1 Sam. 10:1, 12.
e 1 Sam. 27:1.
f 1 Sam. 19:2.
g John 7:42.
h 1 Sam. 25:17.
i 1 Sam. 18:3; 23:18.

And they went out both of them into the
field.
12 And Jonathan said unto David, O
LORD God of Israel, when I have sounded my father about to morrow any time,
or the third *day*, and, behold, *if there be*
good toward David, and I then send not
unto thee, and shew it thee;
13 The LORD do so and much more to
Jonathan: but if it please my father *to do*
thee evil, then I will shew it thee, and
send thee away, that thou mayest go in
peace: and the LORD be with thee, as he
hath [a]been with my father.
14 And thou shalt not only while yet I
live shew me the kindness of the LORD,
that I die not:
15 But [b]*also* thou shalt not cut off thy
kindness from my house for ever: no,
not when the LORD hath cut off the enemies of David every one from the face of
the earth.
16 So Jonathan made *a covenant* with
the house of David, *saying*, Let the LORD
even [c]require *it* at the hand of David's
enemies.
17 And Jonathan caused David to
swear again, because he loved him: for
he loved him as he loved his own soul.
18 Then Jonathan said to David, To
morrow *is* the new moon: and thou shalt
be missed, because thy seat will be empty.
19 And *when* thou hast stayed three
days, *then* thou shalt go down quickly,
and come to the place where thou didst
hide thyself when the business was *in*
hand, and shalt remain by the stone Ezel.
20 And I will shoot three arrows on the
side *thereof*, as though I shot at a mark.
21 And, behold, I will send a lad, *say-*
ing, Go, find out the arrows. If I expressly say unto the lad, Behold, the arrows
are on this side of thee, take them; then
come thou: for *there is* peace to thee, and
no hurt; *as* the LORD liveth.
22 But if I say thus unto the young
man, Behold, the arrows *are* beyond
thee; go thy way: for the LORD hath sent
thee away.
23 And *as touching* the [d]matter which
thou and I have spoken of, behold, the
LORD *be* between thee and me for ever.
24 So David hid himself in the field:
and when the new moon was come, the
king sat him down to eat meat.
25 And the king sat upon his seat, as at
other times, *even* upon a seat by the wall:
and Jonathan arose, and Abner sat by
Saul's side, and David's place was empty.
26 Nevertheless Saul spake not any
thing that day: for he thought,
Something hath befallen him, he *is* not
[e]clean; surely he *is* not clean.
27 And it came to pass on the morrow,
which was the second *day* of the month,
that David's place was empty: and Saul
said unto Jonathan his son, Wherefore
cometh not the son of Jesse to meat, neither yesterday, nor to day?
28 And Jonathan answered [f]Saul,
David earnestly asked *leave* of me *to go*
to Beth-lehem:
29 And he said, Let me go, I pray thee;
for our family hath a sacrifice in the city;
and my brother, he hath commanded me
to be there: and now, if I have found
favour in thine eyes, let me get away, I
pray thee, and see my brethren. Therefore
he cometh not unto the king's table.
30 Then Saul's anger was kindled
against Jonathan, and he said unto him,
Thou son of the perverse rebellious
woman, do not I know that thou hast
chosen the son of Jesse to thine own confusion, and unto the confusion of thy
mother's nakedness?
31 For as long as the son of Jesse liveth
upon the ground, thou shalt not be
established, nor thy kingdom. Wherefore now send and fetch him unto [g]me,
for he shall surely die.
32 And Jonathan answered Saul his
father, and said unto him, Wherefore
shall he be slain? what hath he done?
33 And Saul cast a [h]javelin at him to
smite him: whereby Jonathan knew that
it was determined of his father to slay
David.
34 So Jonathan arose from the table in
fierce anger, and did eat no meat the second day of the month: for he was grieved for David, because his father had
done him shame.
35 And it came to pass in the morning,
that Jonathan went out into the field at
the time appointed with David, and a little lad with him.
36 And he said unto his lad, Run, find
out now the arrows which I shoot. *And* as
the lad ran, he shot an arrow beyond him.

B.C. 1062.

a 1 Sam. 10:7; 11:6; 2 Sam. 7:15.
b 1 Sam. 24:21; 2 Sam. 9:1, 7.
c 2 Sam. 4:7.
d vs. 14, 15.
e Lev. 15:5.
f v. 6.
g 1 Sam. 19:6, 11.
h 1 Sam. 18:11.

37 And when the lad was come to the
place of the arrow which Jonathan had
shot, Jonathan cried after the lad, and
said, *Is* not the arrow [a]beyond thee?
38 And Jonathan cried after the lad,
Make speed, haste, stay not. And
Jonathan's lad gathered up the arrows,
and came to his master.
39 But the lad knew not any thing: only
Jonathan and David knew the matter.
40 And Jonathan gave his artillery
unto his lad, and said unto him, Go,
carry *them* to the city.
41 *And* as soon as the lad was gone,
David arose out of *a place* toward the
south, and fell on his face to the ground,
and bowed himself three times: and they
kissed one another, and wept one with
another, until David exceeded.
42 And Jonathan said to David, Go in
peace, forasmuch as we have sworn both
of us in the name of the LORD, saying,
The LORD be between me and thee, and
between my seed and thy seed for ever.
And he arose and departed: and
Jonathan went into the city.

CHAPTER 21.

David flees to Ahimelech and to Achish.

Then came David to Nob to [b]Ahi-
melech the priest: and Ahimelech
was afraid at the meeting of David, and
said unto him, Why *art* thou alone, and
no man with thee?
2 And David said unto Ahimelech the
priest, The king hath commanded me a
business, and hath said unto me, Let no
man know any thing of the business
whereabout I send thee, and what I have
commanded thee: and I have appointed
my servants to such and such a place.
3 Now therefore what is under thine
hand? give *me* five *loaves of* bread in
mine hand, or what there is present.
4 And the priest answered David, and
said, *There is* no common bread under
mine hand, but there is [c]hallowed bread;
if the young men have kept themselves
at least from women.
5 And David answered the priest, and
said unto him, Of a truth women *have
been* kept from us about these three days,
since I came out, and the vessels of the
young men are holy, and *the bread is* in a
manner common, yea, though it were
sanctified this day in the vessel.

B.C. 1062.

6 So the priest gave him hallowed
bread: for there was no bread there but
the [d]shewbread, that was taken from
before the LORD, to put hot bread in the
day when it was taken away.
7 Now a certain man of the servants of
Saul *was* there that day, detained before
the LORD; and his name *was* [e]Doeg, an
Edomite, the chiefest of the herdmen
that *belonged* to Saul.
8 And David said unto Ahimelech, And
is there not here under thine hand spear
or sword? for I have neither brought my
sword nor my weapons with me, because
the king's business required haste.
9 And the priest said, The sword of
Goliath the Philistine, [f]whom thou
slewest in the valley of Elah, behold, it *is
here* wrapped in a cloth behind the ephod:
if thou wilt take that, take *it*: for *there is* no
other save that here. And David said,
There is none like that; give it me.
10 And David arose, and fled that day
for fear of Saul, and went to Achish the
king of Gath.
11 And the servants of Achish said
unto him, *Is* not this David the king of
the land? did they not sing one to another of him in dances, saying, Saul hath
slain his thousands, and David his ten
thousands?
12 And David laid up these words in
his heart, and was [g]sore afraid of Achish
the king of Gath.
13 And he changed his behaviour
before them, and feigned himself mad in
their hands, and scrabbled on the doors
of the gate, and let his spittle fall down
upon his beard.
14 Then said Achish unto his servants,
Lo, ye see the man is mad: wherefore
then have ye brought him to me?
15 Have I need of mad men, that ye
have brought this *fellow* to play the mad
man in my presence? shall this *fellow*
come into my house?

CHAPTER 22.

David in rejection gathers his mighty men.

David therefore departed thence, and
escaped to the cave [h]Adullam: and
when his brethren and all his father's

a vs. 21, 22.

b 1 Sam. 14:3, called *Ahiah*, also *Abithar*, Mk. 2:26.

c Ex 25:30; Lev. 24:5-9.

d Ex. 25:30, *note*.

e 1 Sam. 22:9; Psa. 52, *title*.

f 1 Sam. 17:2, 50.

g Psa. 34:4; 56:3.

h 2 Sam. 23:13; Mic. 1:15; Heb. 11:38.

house heard *it*, they went down thither to him.

2 [a]And every one *that was* in distress, and every one that *was* in debt, and every one *that was* discontented, gathered themselves unto him; and he became a [b]captain over them: and there were with him about four hundred men.

David's wanderings and dangers.

3 And David went thence to Mizpeh of Moab: and he said unto the king of Moab, Let my father and my mother, I pray thee, come forth, *and be* with you, till I know what God will do for me.

4 And he brought them before the king of Moab: and they dwelt with him all the while that David was in the hold.

5 And the prophet Gad said unto David, Abide not in the hold; depart, and get thee into the land of Judah. Then David departed, and came into the forest of Hareth.

6 When Saul heard that David was discovered, and the men that *were* with him, (now Saul abode in Gibeah under a tree in Ramah, having his spear in his hand, and all his servants *were* standing about him;)

7 Then Saul said unto his servants that stood about him, Hear now, ye Benjamites; will the [c]son of Jesse give every one of you fields and vineyards, *and* make you all captains of thousands, and captains of hundreds;

8 That all of you have conspired against me, and *there is* none that sheweth me that my son hath made a league with the son of Jesse, and *there is* none of you that is sorry for me, or sheweth unto me that my son hath stirred up my servant against me, to lie in wait, as at this day?

9 Then answered Doeg the Edomite, which was set over the servants of Saul, and said, I saw the son of Jesse coming to Nob, to Ahimelech the son of Ahitub.

10 And he [d]enquired of the LORD for him, and gave him victuals, and gave him the sword of Goliath the Philistine.

11 Then the king sent to call Ahimelech the priest, the son of Ahitub, and all his father's house, the priests that *were* in Nob: and they came all of them to the king.

12 And Saul said, Hear now, thou son of Ahitub. And he answered, Here I *am*, my lord.

13 And Saul said unto him, Why have ye conspired against me, thou and the son of Jesse, in that thou hast given him bread, and a sword, and hast enquired of God for him, that he should rise against me, to lie in wait, as at this day?

14 Then Ahimelech answered the king, and said, And who *is so* [e]faithful among all thy servants as David, which is the king's son in law, and goeth at thy bidding, and is honourable in thine house?

15 Did I then begin to enquire of God for him? be it far from me: let not the king [f]impute *any* thing unto his servant, *nor* to all the house of my father: for thy servant knew nothing of all this, less or more.

16 And the king said, Thou shalt surely die, Ahimelech, thou, and all [g]thy father's house.

17 And the king said unto the footmen that stood about him, Turn, and slay the priests of the LORD; because their hand also *is* with David, and because they knew when he fled, and did not shew it to me. But the servants of the king would not put [h]forth their hand to fall upon the priests of the LORD.

18 And the king said to Doeg, Turn thou, and fall upon the priests. And Doeg the Edomite turned, and he fell upon the priests, and slew on that day fourscore and five persons that did wear a linen ephod.

19 And [i]Nob, the city of the priests, smote he with the edge of the sword, both men and women, children and sucklings, and oxen, and asses, and sheep, with the edge of the sword.

20 And one of the sons of Ahimelech the son of Ahitub, named [j]Abiathar, escaped, and fled after David.

21 And Abiathar shewed David that Saul had slain the LORD'S priests.

22 And David said unto Abiathar, I knew *it* that day, when Doeg the Edomite *was* there, that he would surely tell Saul: I have occasioned *the death* of all the persons of thy father's house.

23 Abide thou with me, fear not: for he that seeketh my life seeketh thy life: but with me thou *shalt be* in safeguard.

CHAPTER 23.

David's wanderings and adventures.

Then they told David, saying, Behold, the Philistines fight against Keilah, and they rob the threshingfloors.

B.C. 1062.

a Jud. 11:3.
b Heb. 2:10.
c 1 Sam. 8:14.
d Num. 27:21.
e 1 Sam. 19:4, 5; 24:11.
f *Imputation.* 2 Sam. 19:18, 19. (Lev. 25:50; Jas. 2:23.)
g Deut. 24:16.
h Ex. 1:17.
i vs. 9, 11.
j 1 Sam. 23:6; 1 Ki. 2:26, 27.

2 Therefore David enquired of the
LORD, saying, Shall I go and smite these
Philistines? And the LORD said unto
David, Go, and smite the Philistines, and
save Keilah.
3 And David's men said unto him,
Behold, we be afraid here in Judah: how
much more then if we come to Keilah
against the armies of the Philistines?
4 Then David enquired of the LORD yet
again. And the LORD answered him and
said, Arise, go down to Keilah; for I will
deliver the Philistines into thine hand.
5 So David and his men went to
Keilah, and fought with the Philistines,
and brought away their cattle, and
smote them with a great slaughter. So
David saved the inhabitants of Keilah.
6 And it came to pass, when Abiathar
the son of Ahimelech fled to David to
Keilah, *that* he came down *with* an
ephod in his hand.
7 And it was told Saul that David was
come to Keilah. And Saul said, God hath
delivered him into mine hand; for he is
shut in, by entering into a town that hath
gates and bars.
8 And Saul called all the people
together to war, to go down to Keilah, to
besiege David and his men.
9 And David knew that Saul secretly
practised mischief against him; and he
[a]said to Abiathar the priest, Bring hither
the ephod.
10 Then said David, O LORD God of
Israel, thy servant hath certainly heard
that Saul seeketh to come to Keilah, to
destroy the city for my sake.
11 Will the men of Keilah deliver me
up into his hand? will Saul come down,
as thy servant hath heard? O LORD God
of Israel, I beseech thee, tell thy servant.
And the LORD said, He will come down.
12 Then said David, Will the men of
Keilah deliver me and my men into the
hand of Saul? And the LORD said, They
will deliver *thee* up.
13 Then David and his men, *which*
were about six hundred, arose and
departed out of Keilah, and went whithersoever they could go. And it was told
Saul that David was escaped from
Keilah; and he forbare to go forth.
14 And David abode in the wilderness
in strong holds, and remained in a
mountain in the wilderness of Ziph. And
Saul sought him every day, but God
delivered him not into his hand.
15 And David saw that Saul was come
out to seek his life: and David *was* in the
wilderness of Ziph in a wood.
16 And Jonathan Saul's son arose, and
went to David into the wood, and
[b]strengthened his hand in God.
17 And he said unto him, [c]Fear not:
for the hand of Saul my father shall not
find thee; and thou shalt be king over
Israel, and I shall be next unto thee; and
that also [d]Saul my father knoweth.
18 And they two made a [e]covenant
before the LORD: and David abode in the
wood, and Jonathan went to his house.
19 [f]Then came up the Ziphites to Saul
to Gibeah, saying, Doth not David hide
himself with us in strong holds in the
wood, in the hill of Hachilah, which *is*
on the south of Jeshimon?
20 Now therefore, O king, come down
according to all the desire of thy soul to
come down; and our part *shall be* to
deliver him into the king's hand.
21 And Saul said, [g]Blessed *be* ye of the
LORD; for ye have compassion on me.
22 Go, I pray you, prepare yet, and
know and see his place where his haunt
is, *and* who hath seen him there: for it is
told me *that* he dealeth very subtilly.
23 See therefore, and take knowledge
of all the lurking places where he hideth
himself, and come ye again to me with
the certainty, and I will go with you: and
it shall come to pass, if he be in the land,
that I will [h]search him out throughout
all the thousands of Judah.
24 And they arose, and went to Ziph
before Saul: but David and his men *were*
in the wilderness of [i]Maon, in the plain
on the south of Jeshimon.
25 Saul also and his men went to seek
him. And they told David: wherefore he
came down into a rock, and abode in the
wilderness of Maon. And when Saul
heard *that*, he pursued after David in the
wilderness of Maon.
26 And Saul went on this side of the
mountain, and David and his men on
that side of the mountain: and David
made haste to get away for fear of Saul;
for Saul and his men compassed David
and his men round about to take them.

B.C. 1062.

a Num. 27:21; 1 Sam. 18:3; 20:12-17.
b Heb. 12:12.
c Psa. 27:1, 3; Isa. 54:17; Heb. 13:6.
d 1 Sam. 24:20.
e 2 Sam. 21:7.
f 1 Sam. 26:1.
g Jud. 17:2; Mic. 3:11.
h 1 Ki. 18:10.
i 1 Sam. 25:2.

27 But there [a]came a messenger unto Saul, saying, Haste thee, and come; for the Philistines have invaded the land.

28 Wherefore Saul returned from pursuing after David, and went against the Philistines: therefore they called that place [b]Sela-hammahlekoth.

29 And David went up from thence, and dwelt in strong holds at En-gedi.

CHAPTER 24.

David's mercy to Saul in En-gedi.

And it came to pass, when Saul was returned from following the Philistines, that it was told him, saying, Behold, David *is* in the wilderness of En-gedi.

2 Then Saul took three thousand chosen men out of all Israel, and went to seek David and his men upon the rocks of the wild goats.

3 And he came to the sheepcotes by the way, where *was* a cave; and Saul went in to [c]cover his feet: and David and his men remained in the sides of the cave.

4 And the men of David said unto him, [d]Behold the day of which the LORD said unto thee, Behold, I will deliver thine enemy into thine hand, that thou mayest do to him as it shall seem good unto thee. Then David arose, and cut off the skirt of Saul's robe privily.

5 And it came to pass afterward, that David's heart [e]smote him, because he had cut off Saul's skirt.

6 And he said unto his men, The LORD forbid that I should do this thing unto my master, the LORD'S anointed, to stretch forth mine hand against him, seeing he *is* the anointed of the LORD.

7 So David stayed his servants with these words, and suffered them not to rise against Saul. But Saul rose up out of the cave, and went on *his* way.

8 David also arose afterward, and went out of the cave, and cried after Saul, saying, My lord the king. And when Saul looked behind him, David stooped with his face to the earth, and bowed himself.

9 And David said to Saul, Wherefore hearest thou men's words, saying, Behold, David seeketh thy hurt?

10 Behold, this day thine eyes have seen how that the LORD had delivered thee to day into mine hand in the cave: and *some* bade *me* kill thee: but *mine eye* spared thee; and I said, I will not put forth mine hand against my lord; for he *is* the LORD'S anointed.

11 Moreover, my father, see, yea, see the skirt of thy robe in my hand: for in that I cut off the skirt of thy robe, and killed thee not, know thou and see that *there is* neither evil nor transgression in mine hand, and I have not sinned against thee; yet thou huntest my soul to take it.

12 The LORD judge between me and thee, and the LORD avenge me of thee: but mine hand shall not be upon thee.

13 As saith the proverb of the ancients, Wickedness proceedeth from the wicked: but mine hand shall not be upon thee.

14 After whom is the king of Israel come out? after whom dost thou pursue? after a dead dog, after a flea.

15 The LORD therefore be judge, and judge between me and thee, and see, and plead my cause, and deliver me out of thine hand.

16 And it came to pass, when David had made an end of speaking these words unto Saul, that Saul said, *Is* this thy voice, my son David? And Saul lifted up his voice, and wept.

17 And he said to David, Thou *art* more righteous than I: for thou hast rewarded me good, whereas I have rewarded thee evil.

18 And thou hast shewed this day how that thou hast dealt well with me: forasmuch as when the LORD had delivered me into thine hand, thou killedst me not.

19 For if a man find his enemy, will he let him go well away? wherefore the LORD reward thee good for that thou hast done unto me this day.

20 And now, behold, I know well that thou shalt surely be king, and that the kingdom of Israel shall be established in thine hand.

21 Swear now therefore unto me by the LORD, [f]that thou wilt not cut off my seed after me, and that thou wilt not destroy my name out of my father's house.

22 And David sware unto Saul. And Saul went home; but David and his men gat them up unto the hold.

B.C. 1061.

a 2 Ki. 19:9.

b i.e. *The Crag (or Cliff) of Divisions.*

c Jud. 3:24.

d 1 Sam. 26:8, 11.

e 2 Sam. 24:10.

f 2 Sam. 21:6-8.

B.C. 1060.

CHAPTER 25.

The death of Samuel.

And Samuel died; [a]and all the Israelites were gathered together, and lamented him, and buried him in his house at Ramah. And David arose, and went down to the wilderness of [b]Paran.

David and Nabal.

2 And *there was* a man in Maon, whose possessions *were* in Carmel; and the man *was* very great, and he had three thousand sheep, and a thousand goats: and he was shearing his sheep in Carmel.

3 Now the name of the man *was* [c]Nabal; and the name of his wife Abigail: and *she was* a woman of good understanding, and of a beautiful countenance: but the man *was* [d]churlish and evil in his doings; and he *was* of the house of Caleb.

4 And David heard in the wilderness that Nabal did [e]shear his sheep.

5 And David sent out ten young men, and David said unto the young men, Get you up to Carmel, and go to Nabal, and greet him in my name:

6 And thus shall ye say to him that liveth *in prosperity*, Peace *be* both to thee, and peace *be* to thine house, and peace *be* unto all that thou hast.

7 And now I have heard that thou hast shearers: now thy shepherds which were with us, we hurt them not, neither was there ought missing unto them, all the while they were in Carmel.

8 Ask thy young men, and they will shew thee. Wherefore let the young men find favour in thine eyes: for we come in a good day: give, I pray thee, whatsoever cometh to thine hand unto thy servants, and to thy son David.

9 And when David's young men came, they spake to Nabal according to all those words in the name of David, and ceased.

10 And Nabal answered David's servants, and said, Who *is* David? and who *is* the son of Jesse? there be many servants now a days that break away every man from his master.

11 [f]Shall I then take my bread, and my water, and my flesh that I have killed for my shearers, and give *it* unto men, whom I know not whence they *be*?

12 So David's young men turned their way, and went again, and came and told him all those sayings.

13 And David said unto his men, Gird ye on every man his sword. And they girded on every man his sword; and David also girded on his sword: and there went up after David about four hundred men; and two hundred [g]abode by the stuff.

14 But one of the young men told Abigail, Nabal's wife, saying, Behold, David sent messengers out of the wilderness to salute our master; and he railed on them.

15 But the men *were* very good unto us, and [h]we were not hurt, neither missed we any thing, as long as we were conversant with them, when we were in the fields:

16 They were a wall unto us both by night and day, all the while we were with them keeping the sheep.

17 Now therefore know and consider what thou wilt do; for evil is determined against our master, and against all his household: for he *is such* a son of [i]Belial, that *a man* cannot speak to him.

18 Then Abigail made haste, and took two hundred loaves, and two bottles of wine, and five sheep ready dressed, and five [j]measures of parched *corn*, and an hundred clusters of raisins, and two hundred cakes of figs, and laid *them* on asses.

19 And she said unto her servants, Go on before me; behold, I come after you. But she told not her husband Nabal.

20 And it was *so, as* she rode on the ass, that she came down by the covert of the hill, and, behold, David and his men came down against her; and she met them.

21 Now David had said, Surely in vain have I kept all that this *fellow* hath in the wilderness, so that nothing was missed of all that *pertained* unto him: and he hath requited me evil for good.

22 So and more also do God unto the enemies of David, if I leave of all that *pertain* to him by the morning light any that pisseth against the wall.

23 And when Abigail saw David, she hasted, and [k]lighted off the ass, and fell before David on her face, and bowed herself to the ground,

24 And fell at his feet, and said, Upon me, my lord, *upon* me *let this* iniquity *be*: and let thine handmaid, I pray thee,

a Num. 20:29; Deut. 34:8.
b Gen. 21:21; Num. 10:12.
c i.e. *fool*.
d vs. 10, 11, 17.
e Gen. 38:13; 2 Sam. 13:23.
f Jud. 8:6.
g 1 Sam. 30:24.
h v. 7.
i 2 Sam. 23:6, 7.
j One measure = about 4 pecks.
k Josh. 15:18.

speak in thine audience, and hear the
words of thine handmaid.
25 Let not my lord, I pray thee, regard
this man of Belial, *even* Nabal: for as his
name *is*, so *is* he; Nabal *is* his name, and
folly *is* with him: but I thine handmaid
saw not the young men of my lord,
whom thou didst send.
26 Now therefore, my lord, *as* the
LORD liveth, and *as* thy soul liveth, seeing the LORD hath withholden thee from
coming to *shed* blood, and from avenging thyself with thine own hand, now let
thine enemies, and they that seek evil to
my lord, be as Nabal.
27 And now this blessing which thine
handmaid hath brought unto my lord,
let it even be given unto the young men
that follow my lord.
28 I pray thee, forgive the trespass of
thine handmaid: for the LORD will certainly make my lord a sure house;
because my lord [a]fighteth the battles of
the LORD, and evil hath not been found
in thee *all* thy days.
29 Yet a man is risen to pursue thee,
and to seek thy soul: but the soul of my
lord shall be [b]bound in the bundle of life
with the LORD thy God; and the souls of
thine enemies, them shall he sling out, *as*
out of the middle of a sling.
30 And it shall come to pass, when the
LORD shall have done to my lord according to all the good that he hath spoken
concerning thee, and shall have appointed thee ruler over Israel;
31 That this shall be no grief unto thee,
nor offence of heart unto my lord, either
that thou hast shed blood causeless, or
that my lord hath avenged himself: but
when the LORD shall have dealt well with
my lord, then remember thine handmaid.
32 And David said to Abigail, Blessed
be the LORD God of Israel, which sent
thee this day to meet me:
33 And blessed *be* thy advice, and
blessed *be* thou, which hast kept me this
day from coming to *shed* blood, and from
avenging myself with mine own hand.
34 For in very deed, *as* the LORD God
of Israel liveth, which hath kept me back
from hurting thee, except thou hadst
hasted and come to meet me, surely
there had not been left unto Nabal by
the morning light any that pisseth
against the wall.
35 So David received of her hand *that*
which she had brought him, and said
unto her, Go up in peace to thine house;
see, I have hearkened to thy voice, and
have accepted thy person.
36 And Abigail came to Nabal; and,
behold, he held a feast in his house, like
the feast of a king; and Nabal's heart *was*
merry within him, for he *was* very
drunken: wherefore she told him nothing, less or more, until the morning
light.
37 But it came to pass in the morning,
when the wine was gone out of Nabal,
and his wife had told him these things,
that his heart died within him, and he
became *as* a stone.
38 And it came to pass about ten days
after, that the LORD [c]smote Nabal, that he
died.

Abigail becomes David's wife.

39 And when David heard that Nabal
was dead, he said, [d]Blessed *be* the LORD,
that hath [e]pleaded the cause of my
reproach from the hand of Nabal, and
hath kept his servant from evil: for the
LORD hath returned the wickedness of
Nabal upon his own head. And David
sent and communed with Abigail, to
take her to him to wife.
40 And when the servants of David
were come to Abigail to Carmel, they
spake unto her, saying, David sent us
unto thee, to take thee to him to wife.
41 And she arose, and bowed herself
on *her* face to the earth, and said, Behold,
let thine handmaid *be* a servant to wash
the feet of the servants of my lord.
42 And Abigail hasted, and arose, and
rode upon an ass, with five damsels of
hers that went after her; and she went
after the messengers of David, and
became his wife.

Ahinoam becomes David's wife.

43 David also took [f]Ahinoam of
Jezreel; and they were also both of them
his wives.
44 But Saul had given Michal his
daughter, David's wife, to Phalti the son
of Laish, which *was* of Gallim.

B.C. 1060.

a 1 Sam. 18:17.
b Psa. 66:9; Mal. 3:17; Col. 3:3.
c 2 Ki, 15:5.
d v. 32.
e Prov. 22:23.
f 1 Sam. 27:3.

CHAPTER 26.

David spares Saul the second time.

And the Ziphites came unto Saul to
Gibeah, saying, Doth not David
hide himself in the hill of Hachilah,
which is before Jeshimon?
2 Then Saul arose, and went down to
the wilderness of Ziph, having three
thousand chosen men of Israel with him,
to seek David in the wilderness of Ziph.
3 And Saul pitched in the hill of
Hachilah, which *is* before Jeshimon, by
the way. But David abode in the wilderness, and he saw that Saul came after
him into the wilderness.
4 David therefore sent out spies, and
understood that Saul was come in very
deed.
5 And David arose, and came to the
place where Saul had pitched: and
David beheld the place where Saul lay,
and [a]Abner the son of Ner, the captain of
his host: and Saul lay in the trench, and
the people pitched round about him.
6 Then answered David and said to
Ahimelech the Hittite, and to Abishai
the son of Zeruiah, brother to Joab, saying, Who will go down with me to Saul
to the camp? And Abishai said, I will go
down with thee.
7 So David and Abishai came to the
people by night: and, behold, Saul lay
sleeping within the trench, and his spear
stuck in the ground at his bolster: but
Abner and the people lay round about
him.
8 Then said Abishai to David, God
hath delivered thine enemy into thine
hand this day: now therefore let me
smite him, I pray thee, with the spear
even to the earth at once, and I will not
smite him the second time.
9 And David said to Abishai, Destroy
him not: for [b]who can stretch forth his
hand against the LORD'S anointed, and
be guiltless?
10 David said furthermore, *As* the
LORD liveth, the LORD shall smite him; or
his day shall come to die; or he shall
descend into battle, and [c]perish.
11 The LORD [d]forbid that I should
stretch forth mine hand against the
LORD'S anointed: but, I pray thee, take
thou now the spear that *is* at his bolster,
and the cruse of water, and let us go.
12 So David took the spear and the
cruse of water from Saul's bolster; and
they gat them away, and no man saw *it*,
nor knew *it*, neither awaked: for they
were all asleep; because a deep sleep
from the LORD was fallen upon them.
13 Then David went over to the other
side, and stood on the top of an hill afar
off; a great space *being* between them:
14 And David cried to the people, and
to Abner the son of Ner, saying,
Answerest thou not, Abner? Then Abner
answered and said, *Who art* thou *that*
criest to the king?
15 And David said to Abner, *Art* not
thou a *valiant* man? and who *is* like to
thee in Israel? wherefore then hast thou
not kept thy lord the king? for there
came one of the people in to destroy the
king thy lord.
16 This thing *is* not good that thou
hast done. *As* the LORD liveth, ye *are*
worthy to die, because ye have not kept
your master, the LORD'S anointed. And
now see where the king's spear *is*, and
the cruse of water that *was* at his bolster.
17 And Saul knew David's voice, and
said, [e]*Is* this thy voice, my son David?
And David said, *It is* my voice, my lord,
O king.
18 And he said, Wherefore doth my
lord thus pursue after his servant? for
what have I done? or what evil *is* in
mine hand?
19 Now therefore, I pray thee, let my
lord the king hear the words of his servant. If the [f]LORD have stirred thee up
against me, let him accept an offering:
but if *they be* the children of men, cursed
be they before the LORD; for they have
driven me out this day from abiding in
the [g]inheritance of the LORD, saying, Go,
serve other gods.
20 Now therefore, let not my blood fall
to the earth before the face of the LORD:
for the king of Israel is come out to seek
a flea, as when one doth hunt a partridge in the mountains.
21 Then said Saul, I have sinned:
return, my son David: for I will no more
do thee harm, because my [h]soul was
precious in thine eyes this day: behold, I
have played the fool, and have erred
exceedingly.
22 And David answered and said,
Behold the king's spear! and let one of
the young men come over and fetch it.
23 The [i]LORD render to every man his

B.C. 1060.

a 1 Sam. 14:50.
b 1 Sam. 24:6; 2 Sam. 1:16.
c 1 Sam. 31:6.
d 1 Sam. 24:6-12.
e 1 Sam. 24:16.
f 2 Sam. 16:11.
g 2 Sam. 14:16.
h v. 24.
i Psa. 7:8.

righteousness and his faithfulness: for the LORD delivered thee into *my* hand to day, but I would not stretch forth mine hand against the LORD'S anointed.

24 And, behold, as thy life was much set by this day in mine eyes, so let my life be much set by in the eyes of the LORD, and let him deliver me out of all tribulation.

25 Then Saul said to David, Blessed *be* thou, my son David: thou shalt both do great *things*, and also shalt still prevail. So David went on his way, and Saul returned to his place.

CHAPTER 27.

David's lapse of faith. He goes to Philistia.

And David [a]said in his heart, I shall now perish one day by the hand of Saul: *there is* nothing better for me than that I should speedily escape into the land of the Philistines; and Saul shall despair of me, to seek me any more in any coast of Israel: so shall I escape out of his hand.

2 And David arose, and he passed over with the six hundred [b]men that *were* with him unto Achish, the son of Maoch, king of Gath.

3 And David dwelt with Achish at Gath, he and his men, every man with his household, *even* David with his two wives, Ahinoam the Jezreelitess, and Abigail the Carmelitess, Nabal's wife.

4 And it was told Saul that David was fled to Gath: and he sought no more again for him.

5 And David said unto Achish, If I have now found grace in thine eyes, let them give me a place in some town in the country, that I may dwell there: for why should thy servant dwell in the royal city with thee?

6 Then Achish gave him [c]Ziklag that day: wherefore Ziklag pertaineth unto the kings of Judah unto this day.

7 And the time that David dwelt in the country of the Philistines was a full year and four months.

8 And David and his men went up, and invaded the Geshurites, and the [d]Gezrites, and the Amalekites: for those *nations were* of old the inhabitants of the land, as thou goest to Shur, even unto the land of Egypt.

9 And David smote the land, and left neither man nor woman alive, and took away the sheep, and the oxen, and the asses, and the camels, and the apparel, and returned, and came to Achish.

10 And Achish said, Whither have ye made a road to day? And David said, Against the south of Judah, and against the south of the Jerahmeelites, and against the south of the Kenites.

11 And David saved neither man nor woman alive, to bring *tidings* to Gath, saying, Lest they should tell on us, saying, So did David, and so *will be* his manner all the while he dwelleth in the country of the Philistines.

12 And Achish believed David, saying, He hath made his people Israel utterly to abhor him; therefore he shall be my servant for ever.

CHAPTER 28.

David among Israel's enemies.

And it came to pass in those days, that the Philistines gathered their armies together for warfare, to fight with Israel. And Achish said unto David, Know thou assuredly, that thou shalt go out with me to battle, thou and thy men.

2 And David said to Achish, Surely thou shalt know what thy servant can do. And Achish said to David, Therefore will I make thee keeper of mine head for ever.

3 Now [e]Samuel was dead, and all Israel had lamented him, and buried him in Ramah, even in his own city. And Saul had put away those that had familiar spirits, and the wizards, out of the land.

4 And the Philistines gathered themselves together, and came and pitched in [f]Shunem: and Saul gathered all Israel together, and they pitched in Gilboa.

5 And when Saul saw the host of the Philistines, he was afraid, and his heart greatly trembled.

6 And when Saul enquired of the LORD, the LORD answered him not, neither by dreams, nor by [g]Urim, nor by prophets.

Saul and the witch of En-dor.

7 Then said Saul unto his servants, Seek me a woman that hath a familiar spirit, [h]that I may go to her, and enquire

B.C. 1060.

a Cf. 1 Chr. 29:28.
b 1 Sam. 25:13.
c Josh. 19:5; 1 Chr. 12:1.
d Jud. 1:29.
e 1 Sam. 25:1.
f Josh. 19:18; 2 Ki. 4:8.
g See Ex. 28:30, *note.*
h 1 Chr. 10:13; Isa. 8:19.

of her. And his servants said to him,
Behold, *there is* a woman that hath a
familiar spirit at Endor.
8 And Saul disguised himself, and put
on other raiment, and he went, and two
men with him, and they came to the
woman by night: and he said, I pray
thee, divine unto me by the familiar
spirit, and bring me *him* up, whom I
shall name unto thee.
9 And the woman said unto him,
Behold, thou knowest what Saul hath
done, how he hath [a]cut off those that
have familiar spirits, and the wizards, out
of the land: wherefore then layest thou a
snare for my life, to cause me to die?
10 And Saul sware to her by the LORD,
saying, *As* the LORD liveth, there shall no
punishment happen to thee for this thing.
11 Then said the woman, Whom shall
I bring up unto thee? And he said, Bring
me up Samuel.
12 And when the woman saw Samuel,
she cried with a loud voice: and the
woman spake to Saul, saying, Why hast
thou deceived me? for thou *art* Saul.
13 And the king said unto her, Be not
afraid: for what sawest thou? And the
woman said unto Saul, I saw gods
ascending out of the earth.
14 And he said unto her, What form *is*
he of? And she said, An old man cometh
up; and he *is* covered with a mantle.
And Saul perceived that it *was* Samuel,
and he stooped with *his* face to the
ground, and bowed himself.
15 And Samuel said to Saul, Why hast
thou disquieted me, to bring me up?
And Saul answered, I am sore distressed; for the Philistines make war
against me, and God is departed from
me, and [b]answereth me no more, neither
by prophets, nor by dreams: therefore I
have called thee, that thou mayest make
known unto me what I shall do.
16 Then said Samuel, Wherefore then
dost thou ask of me, seeing the LORD is
departed from thee, and is become thine
enemy?
17 And the LORD hath done to him, as
he [c]spake by me: for the LORD hath rent
the kingdom out of thine hand, and
given it to thy neighbour, *even* to David:
18 [d]Because thou obeyedst not the voice
of the LORD, nor executedst his fierce
wrath upon Amalek, therefore hath the

B.C. 1056.

a v. 3.

b v. 6.

c 1 Sam. 15:28

d 1 Sam. 13:9, 13; 15:1-26; 1 Chr. 10:13.

LORD done this thing unto thee this day.
19 Moreover the LORD will also deliver
Israel with thee into the hand of the
Philistines: and to morrow *shalt* thou
and thy sons *be* with me: the LORD also
shall deliver the host of Israel into the
hand of the Philistines.
20 Then Saul fell straightway all along
on the earth, and was sore afraid, because
of the words of Samuel: and there was no
strength in him; for he had eaten no
bread all the day, nor all the night.
21 And the woman came unto Saul, and
saw that he was sore troubled, and said
unto him, Behold, thine handmaid hath
obeyed thy voice, and I have put my life
in my hand, and have hearkened unto thy
words which thou spakest unto me.
22 Now therefore, I pray thee, hearken
thou also unto the voice of thine handmaid, and let me set a morsel of bread
before thee; and eat, that thou mayest
have strength, when thou goest on thy
way.
23 But he refused, and said, I will not
eat. But his servants, together with the
woman, compelled him; and he hearkened unto their voice. So he arose from
the earth, and sat upon the bed.
24 And the woman had a fat calf in the
house; and she hasted, and killed it, and
took flour, and kneaded *it*, and did bake
unleavened bread thereof:
25 And she brought *it* before Saul, and
before his servants; and they did eat. Then
they rose up, and went away that night.

CHAPTER 29.

David providentially saved from fighting against Israel.

Now the Philistines gathered together
all their armies to Aphek: and the
Israelites pitched by a fountain which *is*
in Jezreel.
2 And the lords of the Philistines
passed on by hundreds, and by thousands: but David and his men passed on
in the rereward with Achish.
3 Then said the princes of the
Philistines, What *do* these Hebrews *here*?
And Achish said unto the princes of the
Philistines, *Is* not this David, the servant
of Saul the king of Israel, which hath
been with me these days, or these years,
and I have found no fault in him since
he fell *unto me* unto this day?

4 And the princes of the Philistines were wroth with him; and the princes of the Philistines said unto him, Make this fellow return, that he may go again to his place which thou hast appointed him, and let him not go down with us to [a]battle, lest in the battle he be an adversary to us: for wherewith should he [b]reconcile himself unto his master? *should it* not *be* with the heads of these men?

5 *Is* not this David, of whom [c]they sang one to another in dances, saying, Saul slew his thousands, and David his ten thousands?

6 Then Achish called David, and said unto him, Surely, *as* the LORD liveth, thou hast been upright, and thy going out and thy coming in with me in the host *is* good in my sight: [d]for I have not found evil in thee since the day of thy coming unto me unto this day: nevertheless the lords favour thee not.

7 Wherefore now return, and go in peace, that thou displease not the lords of the Philistines.

8 And David said unto Achish, But what have I done? and what hast thou found in thy servant so long as I have been with thee unto this day, that I may not go fight against the enemies of my lord the king?

9 And Achish answered and said to David, I know that thou *art* good in my sight, as an [e]angel of God: notwithstanding the princes of the Philistines have said, He shall not go up with us to the battle.

10 Wherefore now rise up early in the morning with thy master's servants that are come with thee: and as soon as ye be up early in the morning, and have light, depart.

11 So David and his men rose up early to depart in the morning, to return into the land of the Philistines. And the Philistines went up to Jezreel.

CHAPTER 30.

David avenges the distruction of Ziklag.

And it came to pass, when David and his men were come to Ziklag on the third day, that the Amalekites had invaded the south, and Ziklag, and smitten Ziklag, and burned it with fire;

2 And had taken the women captives, that *were* therein: they slew not any, either great or small, but carried *them* away, and went on their way.

3 So David and his men came to the city, and, behold, *it was* burned with fire; and their wives, and their sons, and their daughters, were taken captives.

4 Then David and the people that *were* with him lifted up their voice and wept, until they had no more power to weep.

5 And David's two [f]wives were taken captives, Ahinoam the Jezreelitess, and Abigail the wife of Nabal the Carmelite.

6 And David was greatly distressed; for the people spake of stoning him, because the soul of all the people was grieved, every man for his sons and for his daughters: but David [g]encouraged himself in the LORD his God.

7 And David said to Abiathar the priest, Ahimelech's son, I pray thee, [h]bring me hither the ephod. And Abiathar brought thither the ephod to David.

8 And David enquired at the LORD, saying, Shall I pursue after this troop? shall I overtake them? And he answered him, Pursue: for thou shalt surely overtake *them*, and without fail recover *all*.

9 So David went, he and the six hundred men that *were* with him, and came to the brook Besor, where those that were left behind stayed.

10 But David pursued, he and four hundred men: for two hundred abode behind, which were so faint that they could not go over the brook Besor.

11 And they found an Egyptian in the field, and brought him to David, and gave him bread, and he did eat; and they made him drink water;

12 And they gave him a piece of a cake of figs, and two clusters of raisins: and when he had eaten, his [i]spirit came again to him: for he had eaten no bread, nor drunk *any* water, three days and three nights.

13 And David said unto him, To whom *belongest* thou? and whence *art* thou? And he said, I *am* a young man of Egypt, servant to an Amalekite; and my master left me, because three days agone I fell sick.

14 We made an invasion *upon* the south of the [j]Cherethites, and upon *the coast* which *belongeth* to Judah, and upon the south of Caleb; and we burned Ziklag with fire.

15 And David said to him, Canst thou bring me down to this company? And he

B.C. 1056.

a 1 Sam. 14:21.

b Or, *make himself pleasing.* See Dan. 9:24, *note.*

c 1 Sam. 18:7.

d v. 3.

e Heb. 1:4, *note.*

f 1 Sam. 25:42, 43.

g Psa. 18:6; 25:1, 2; 34:1-8; 40:1, 2; 42:5-11; 56:1-4; Isa. 25:4; Jer. 16:19; Hab. 3:17-19.

h 1 Sam. 23:2, 9.

i 1 Sam. 14:27; Jud. 15:19.

j 2 Sam. 8:18; 1 Ki. 1:38.

B.C. 1056.

said, Swear unto me by God, that thou
wilt neither kill me, nor deliver me into
the hands of my master, and I will bring
thee down to this company.
16 And when he had brought him
down, behold, *they were* spread abroad
upon all the earth, eating and drinking,
and dancing, because of all the great spoil
that they had taken out of the land of the
Philistines, and out of the land of Judah.
17 And David smote them from the
twilight even unto the evening of the
next day: and there escaped not a man of
them, save four hundred young men,
which rode upon camels, and fled.
18 And David recovered all that the
Amalekites had carried away: and
David rescued his two wives.
19 And there was nothing lacking to
them, neither small nor great, neither
sons nor daughters, neither spoil, nor
any *thing* that they had taken to them:
David [a]recovered all.
20 And David took all the flocks and
the herds, *which* they drave before those
other cattle, and said, This *is* David's spoil.
21 And David came to the two hun-
dred men, which were so faint that they
could not follow David, whom they had
made also to abide at the brook Besor:
and they went forth to meet David, and
to meet the people that *were* with him:
and when David came near to the people, he saluted them.
22 Then answered all the wicked men
and *men* of Belial, of those that went with
David, and said, Because they went not
with us, we will not give them *ought* of
the spoil that we have recovered, save to
every man his wife and his children, that
they may lead *them* away, and depart.
23 Then said David, Ye shall not do so,
my brethren, with that which the LORD
hath given us, who hath preserved us,
and delivered the company that came
against us into our hand.
24 For who will hearken unto you in
this matter? [b]but as his part *is* that goeth
down to the battle, so *shall* his part *be* that
tarrieth by the stuff: they shall part alike.
25 And it was *so* from that day forward, that he made it a statute and an
ordinance for Israel unto this day.
26 And when David came to Ziklag,
he sent of the spoil unto the elders of
Judah, *even* to his friends, saying, Behold
a present for you of the spoil of the enemies of the LORD;
27 To *them* which *were* in Beth-el, and
to *them* which *were* in south [c]Ramoth,
and to *them* which *were* in Jattir,
28 And to *them* which *were* in [d]Aroer,
and to *them* which *were* in Siphmoth, and
to *them* which *were* in [e]Eshtemoa,
29 And to *them* which *were* in Rachal,
and to *them* which *were* in the cities of
the [f]Jerahmeelites, and to *them* which
were in the cities of the [g]Kenites,
30 And to *them* which *were* in [h]Hormah,
and to *them* which *were* in Chor-ashan,
and to *them* which *were* in Athach,
31 And to *them* which *were* in [i]Hebron,
and to all the places where David himself and his men were wont to haunt.

CHAPTER 31.

The death of Saul.

[j]Now the Philistines fought against
Israel: and the men of Israel fled
from before the Philistines, and fell
down slain in mount [k]Gilboa.
2 And the Philistines followed hard
upon Saul and upon his sons; and the
Philistines slew Jonathan, and Abinadab,
and Melchi-shua, [l]Saul's sons.
3 And the battle went sore against
Saul, and the archers [1]hit him; and he
was sore wounded of the archers.
4 [m]Then said Saul unto his armourbearer, Draw thy sword, and thrust me
through therewith; lest these uncircumcised come and thrust me through, and
abuse me. But his armourbearer would
not; for he was sore afraid. Therefore
Saul took a sword, and fell upon it.
5 And when his armourbearer saw
that Saul was dead, he fell likewise upon
his sword, and died with him.

a v. 8.
b Num. 31:27; Josh. 22:8.
c Josh. 19:8.
d Josh. 13:16.
e Josh. 15:50.
f 1 Sam. 27:10.
g Jud. 1:16.
h Jud. 1:17.
i Josh. 14:13; 2 Sam. 2:1.
j 1 Chr. 10:1.
k 1 Sam. 28:4.
l 1 Sam. 14:49; 1 Chr. 8:33.
m Jud. 9:54.

[1] **(31:3)** Cf. 2 Sam. 1:10; 21:12. The order is: (1) Saul is "hit"—wounded mortally, potentially "slain," by the Philistines; (2) either to escape agony, or insult by the enemy, he falls upon his sword, and his armour-bearer, supposing him to be dead, slew himself; (3) but Saul was not dead; raising himself upon his spear, he besought the Amalekite to put him to death.

6 So Saul died, and his three sons, and his armourbearer, and all his men, that same day together.

7 And when the men of Israel that *were* on the other side of the valley, and *they* that *were* on the other side Jordan, saw that the men of Israel fled, and that Saul and his sons were dead, they forsook the cities, and fled; and the Philistines came and dwelt in them.

8 And it came to pass on the morrow, when the Philistines came to strip the slain, that they found Saul and his three sons fallen in mount Gilboa.

9 And they cut off his head, and stripped off his armour, and sent into the land of the Philistines round about, to publish *it in* the house of their idols, and among the people.

10 And they put his [a]armour in the house of [b]Ashtaroth: and they fastened his [c]body to the wall of Beth-shan.

11 And when the inhabitants of Jabesh-gilead heard of that which the Philistines had done to Saul;

12 All the valiant men arose, and went all night, and took the body of Saul and the bodies of his sons from the wall of Beth-shan, and came to Jabesh, and [d]burnt them there.

13 And they took their bones, and [e]buried *them* under a tree at Jabesh, and fasted seven days.

B.C. 1056.

a 1 Sam. 21:9.

b Jud. 2:13; 2 Sam. 21:12.

c Josh. 17:11; Jud. 1:27.

d *Contra*, 2 Chr. 16:14.

e 2 Sam. 2:4, 5; 2 Sam. 21:12-14.

THE SECOND BOOK OF SAMUEL

OTHERWISE CALLED
THE SECOND BOOK OF THE KINGS

AS First Samuel marks the failure of man in Eli, Saul, and even Samuel, so Second Samuel marks the restoration of order through the enthroning of God's king, David. This book also records the establishment of Israel's political centre in Jerusalem (2 Sam. 5:6-12), and her religious centre in Zion (2 Sam. 5:7; 6:1-17). When all was thus ordered, Jehovah established the great Davidic Covenant (7:8-17) out of which all kingdom truth is henceforth developed. David, in his "last words" (23:1-7), describes the millennial kingdom yet to be.

The book is in four parts: I. From the death of Saul to the anointing of David over Judah, in Hebron, 1:1-27. II. From the anointing in Hebron to the establishment of David over united Israel, 2:1–5:25. III. From the conquest of Jerusalem to the rebellion of Absalom, 6:1–14:33. IV. From the rebellion of Absalom to the purchase of the temple-site, 15:1–24:25.

The events recorded in II Samuel cover a period of 38 years (Ussher).

CHAPTER 1.

David hears of Saul's death.

NOW it came to pass after the death of
Saul, when David was returned
from the [a]slaughter of the Amalekites,
and David had abode two days in Ziklag;
2 It came even to pass on the third day,
that, behold, a man came out of the
camp from Saul with his clothes rent,
and earth upon his head: and *so* it was,
when he came to David, that he fell to
the earth, and did obeisance.
3 And David said unto him, From
whence comest thou? And he said unto
him, Out of the camp of Israel am I
escaped.
4 And David said unto him, [b]How
went the matter? I pray thee, tell me.
And he answered, That the people are
fled from the battle, and many of the
people also are fallen and dead; and Saul
and Jonathan his son are dead also.
5 And David said unto the young man
that told him, How knowest thou that
Saul and Jonathan his son be dead?
6 And the young man that told him
said, As I happened by chance upon
mount Gilboa, behold, Saul leaned upon
his spear; and, lo, the chariots and horsemen followed hard after him.
7 And when he looked behind him, he
saw me, and called unto me. And I
answered, Here *am* I.
8 And he said unto me, Who *art* thou?
And I answered him, I *am* an Amalekite.
9 He said unto me again, Stand, I pray
thee, upon me, and slay me: for anguish
is come upon me, because my life *is* yet
whole in me.
10 So I [c]stood upon him, and slew
him, because I was sure that he could
not live after that he was fallen: and I
took the crown that *was* upon his head,
and the bracelet that *was* on his arm, and
have brought them hither unto my lord.
11 Then David took hold on his
clothes, and rent them; and likewise all
the men that *were* with him:
12 And they mourned, and wept, and
fasted until even, for Saul, and for
Jonathan his son, and for the people of
the LORD, and for the house of Israel;
because they were fallen by the sword.
13 And David said unto the young
man that told him, Whence *art* thou?
And he answered, I *am* the son of a
stranger, an Amalekite.
14 And David [d]said unto him, How
wast thou not afraid to stretch forth thine
hand to destroy the LORD'S anointed?
15 And David called one of the young
men, and said, Go near, *and* fall upon
him. And he smote him that he died.
16 And David said unto him, Thy
[e]blood *be* upon thy head; for thy mouth
hath testified against thee, saying, I have
slain the LORD'S anointed.

David mourns the death of Saul and Jonathan.

17 And David lamented with this
lamentation over Saul and over Jonathan
his son:

B.C. 1056.

a 1 Sam. 30:17-26.

b 1 Sam. 4:16.

c Cf. 1 Sam. 31:4, 5, *note*.

d 1 Sam. 24:6; 26:9; Psa. 105:15.

e 1 Ki. 2:32, 33, 37.

18 (Also he bade them teach the children of Judah *the use of* the bow: behold,
it is written in the book of Jasher.)
19 The beauty of Israel is slain upon thy
high places: how are the mighty fallen!
20 Tell *it* not in Gath, publish *it* not in
the streets of Askelon; lest the daughters
of the Philistines [a]rejoice, lest the daughters of the uncircumcised triumph.
21 Ye mountains of Gilboa, *let there be*
no dew, neither *let there be* rain, upon
you, nor fields of offerings: for there the
shield of the mighty is vilely cast away,
the shield of Saul, *as though he had* not
been anointed with oil.
22 From the blood of the slain, from
the fat of the mighty, the bow of
Jonathan turned not back, and the sword
of Saul returned not empty.
23 Saul and Jonathan *were* lovely and
pleasant in their lives, and in their
[b]death they were not divided: they were
swifter than eagles, they were stronger
than lions.
24 Ye daughters of Israel, weep over
Saul, who clothed you in scarlet, with
other delights, who put on ornaments of
gold upon your apparel.
25 How are the mighty fallen in the
midst of the battle! O Jonathan, *thou wast*
slain in thine high places.
26 I am distressed for thee, my brother
Jonathan: very pleasant hast thou been
unto me: thy love to me was wonderful,
passing the love of women.
27 How are the mighty fallen, and the
weapons of war perished!

CHAPTER 2.

David received as king by Judah.

And it came to pass after this, that
[c]David enquired of the LORD, saying, Shall I go up into any of the cities of
Judah? And the LORD said unto him, Go
up. And David said, Whither shall I go
up? And he said, Unto [d]Hebron.
2 So David went up thither, and his
two wives also, Ahinoam the Jezreelitess,
and Abigail Nabal's wife the Carmelite.
3 And his [e]men that *were* with him did
David bring up, every man with his
household: and they dwelt in the cities
of Hebron.
4 And the men of Judah came, and
there they anointed David king over the
house of Judah. And they told David,
saying, *That* the men of [f]Jabesh-gilead
were they that buried Saul.

David's message to the men of Jabesh-gilead.

5 And David sent messengers unto the
men of Jabesh-gilead, and said unto them,
Blessed *be* ye of the LORD, that ye have
shewed this kindness unto your lord, *even*
unto Saul, and have buried him.
6 And now the LORD shew kindness
and truth unto you: and I also will
requite you this kindness, because ye
have done this thing.
7 Therefore now let your hands be
strengthened, and be ye valiant: for your
master Saul is dead, and also the house of
Judah have anointed me king over them.

Abner makes Ish-bosheth king over eleven tribes.

8 But [g]Abner the son of Ner, captain of
Saul's host, took Ish-bosheth the son of
Saul, and brought him over to Mahanaim;
9 And made him king over Gilead,
and over the Ashurites, and over Jezreel,
and over Ephraim, and over Benjamin,
and over all Israel.
10 Ish-bosheth Saul's son *was* forty
years old when he began to reign over
Israel, and reigned two years. But the
house of Judah followed David.
11 And the time that David was king
in Hebron over the house of Judah was
seven years and six months.

The second civil [h]war.

12 And Abner the son of Ner, and the
servants of Ish-bosheth the son of Saul,
went out from Mahanaim to [i]Gibeon.
13 And Joab the son of Zeruiah, and
the servants of David, went out, and met
together by the [j]pool of Gibeon: and
they sat down, the one on the one side of
the pool, and the other on the other side
of the pool.
14 And Abner said to Joab, Let the
young men now arise, and play before
us. And Joab said, Let them arise.
15 Then there arose and went over by
number twelve of Benjamin, which *pertained* to Ish-bosheth the son of Saul, and
twelve of the servants of David.
16 And they caught every one his

B.C. 1056.

a Jud. 16:23.

b 1 Sam. 31:2, 4.

c *Kingdom.* (O.T.). vs. 1-4; 2 Sam. 5:1-3. (Gen. 1:26; Zech. 12:8.)

d 2 Sam. 5:1, 3.

e 1 Sam. 27:2, 3; 1 Chr. 12:1.

f 1 Sam. 31:11, 13.

g Jud. 8:1, *note.*

h Cf. Jud. 20:1.

i Joshua 10:2, 4, 12.

j Jer. 41:12.

fellow by the head, and *thrust* his sword
in his fellow's side; so they fell down
together: wherefore that place was called
[a]Helkath-hazzurim, which *is* in Gibeon.
17 And there was a very sore battle that
day; and Abner was beaten, and the men
of Israel, before the servants of David.
18 And there were three sons of
Zeruiah there, Joab, and Abishai, and
Asahel: and Asahel *was as* light of foot as
a wild roe.
19 And Asahel pursued after Abner;
and in going he turned not to the right
hand nor to the left from following Abner.
20 Then Abner looked behind him,
and said, *Art* thou Asahel? And he
answered, I *am*.
21 And Abner said to him, Turn thee
aside to thy right hand or to thy left, and
lay thee hold on one of the young men,
and take thee his armour. But Asahel
would not turn aside from following of
him.
22 And Abner said again to Asahel,
Turn thee aside from following me:
wherefore should I smite thee to the
ground? how then should I hold up my
face to [b]Joab thy brother?
23 Howbeit he refused to turn aside:
wherefore Abner with the hinder end of
the spear [c]smote him under the fifth *rib*,
that the spear came out behind him; and
he fell down there, and died in the same
place: and it came to pass, *that* as many
as came to the place where Asahel fell
down and died stood still.
24 Joab also and Abishai pursued after
Abner: and the sun went down when
they were come to the hill of Ammah,
that *lieth* before Giah by the way of the
wilderness of Gibeon.
25 And the children of Benjamin gathered themselves together after Abner,
and became one troop, and stood on the
top of an hill.
26 Then Abner called to Joab, and
said, Shall the sword devour for ever?
knowest thou not that it will be bitterness in the latter end? how long shall it
be then, ere thou bid the people return
from following their brethren?
27 And Joab said, *As* God liveth,
unless thou hadst spoken, surely then in
the morning the people had gone up
every one from following his brother.
28 So Joab blew a trumpet, and all the
people stood still, and pursued after Israel
no more, neither fought they any more.
29 And Abner and his men walked all
that night through the plain, and passed
over Jordan, and went through all
Bithron, and they came to [d]Mahanaim.
30 And Joab returned from following
Abner: and when he had gathered all the
people together, there lacked of David's
servants nineteen men and Asahel.
31 But the servants of David had smitten of Benjamin, and of Abner's men, *so
that* three hundred and threescore men
died.
32 And they took up Asahel, and
buried him in the sepulchre of his father,
which *was in* Beth-lehem. And Joab and
his men went all night, and they came to
Hebron at break of day.

CHAPTER 3.

Now there was long war between the
house of Saul and the house of
David: but David waxed stronger and
stronger, and the house of Saul waxed
weaker and weaker.

David's family in [e]Hebron (1 Chr. 3:1-4).

2 And unto David were sons [f]born in
Hebron: and his firstborn was Amnon,
of [g]Ahinoam the Jezreelitess;
3 And his second, Chileab, of Abigail
the wife of Nabal the Carmelite; and the
third, [h]Absalom the son of Maacah the
daughter of Talmai king of [i]Geshur;
4 And the fourth, Adonijah the son of
Haggith; and the fifth, Shephatiah the
son of Abital;
5 And the sixth, Ithream, by Eglah
David's wife. These were born to David
in Hebron.
6 And it came to pass, while there was
war between the house of Saul and the
house of David, that Abner made himself strong for the house of Saul.

Abner deserts to David.

7 And Saul had a concubine, whose
name *was* [j]Rizpah, the daughter of Aiah:
and *Ish-bosheth* said to Abner, Wherefore
hast thou gone in unto my father's concubine?
8 Then was Abner very wroth for
the words of Ish-bosheth, and said,

B.C. 1053.

a i.e. *Field of Swords.*
b 2 Sam. 3:27.
c 2 Sam. 3:27; 4:6; 20:10.
d v. 12.
e Cf. 2 Sam. 5:13-16.
f 1 Chr. 3:1, 4.
g 1 Sam. 25:43.
h 2 Sam. 15:1-18.
i Josh. 13:13; 2 Sam. 13:37; 1 Sam 27:8.
j 2 Sam. 21:8.

[a]*Am* I a dog's head, which against Judah do shew kindness this day unto the house of Saul thy father, to his brethren, and to his friends, and have not delivered thee into the hand of David, that thou chargest me to day with a fault concerning this woman?

9 So do God to Abner, and more also, except, [b]as the LORD hath sworn to David, even so I do to him;

10 To translate the kingdom from the house of Saul, and to set up the throne of David over Israel and over Judah, from Dan even to Beer-sheba.

11 And he could not answer Abner a word again, because he feared him.

12 And Abner sent messengers to David on his behalf, saying, Whose *is* the land? saying *also*, Make thy league with me, and, behold, my hand *shall be* with thee, to bring about all Israel unto thee.

13 And he said, Well; I will make a league with thee: but one thing I require of thee, that is, Thou shalt not see my face, except thou first bring [c]Michal Saul's daughter, when thou comest to see my face.

14 And David sent messengers to [d]Ish-bosheth Saul's son, saying, Deliver *me* my wife Michal, which I espoused to me [e]for an hundred foreskins of the Philistines.

15 And Ish-bosheth sent, and took her from *her* husband, *even* from [f]Phaltiel the son of Laish.

16 And her husband went with her along weeping behind her to [g]Bahurim. Then said Abner unto him, Go, return. And he returned.

17 And Abner had communication with the elders of Israel, saying, Ye sought for David in times past *to be* king over you:

18 Now then do *it*: for the LORD hath spoken of David, saying, By the hand of my servant David I will save my people Israel out of the hand of the Philistines, and out of the hand of all their enemies.

19 And Abner also spake in the ears [h]of Benjamin: and Abner went also to speak in the ears of David in Hebron all that seemed good to Israel, and that seemed good to the whole house of Benjamin.

20 So Abner came to David to Hebron, and twenty men with him. And David made Abner and the men that *were* with him a feast.

B.C. 1053.

a 1 Sam. 24:14.
b 1 Sam. 15:28.
c 1 Sam. 18:20.
d 2 Sam. 2:10.
e 1 Sam. 18:25, 27.
f 1 Sam. 25:44, *Phalti.*
g 2 Sam. 19:16.
h 1 Chr. 12:29
i vs. 10, 12.
j 1 Sam. 29:6.
k 1 Ki. 2:5.
l 1 Ki. 2:32, 33.
m 2 Sam. 1:2, 11; Josh. 7:6.

21 And Abner said unto David, I will arise and go, [i]and will gather all Israel unto my lord the king, that they may make a league with thee, and that thou mayest reign over all that thine heart desireth. And David sent Abner away; and he went in peace.

22 And, behold, the servants of David and Joab came from *pursuing* a troop, and brought in a great spoil with them: but Abner *was* not with David in Hebron; for he had sent him away, and he was gone in peace.

23 When Joab and all the host that *was* with him were come, they told Joab, saying, Abner the son of Ner came to the king, and he hath sent him away, and he is gone in peace.

24 Then Joab came to the king, and said, What hast thou done? behold, Abner came unto thee; why *is* it *that* thou hast sent him away, and he is quite gone?

25 Thou knowest Abner the son of Ner, that he came to deceive thee, and to know thy [j]going out and thy coming in, and to know all that thou doest.

26 And when Joab was come out from David, he sent messengers after Abner, which brought him again from the well of Sirah: but David knew *it* not.

Joab's murder of Abner.

27 And when Abner was returned to Hebron, Joab took him [k]aside in the gate to speak with him quietly, and smote him there under the fifth *rib*, that he died, for the blood of Asahel his brother.

28 And afterward when David heard *it*, he said, I and my kingdom *are* guiltless before the LORD for ever from the blood of Abner the son of Ner:

29 Let it [l]rest on the head of Joab, and on all his father's house; and let there not fail from the house of Joab one that hath an issue, or that is a leper, or that leaneth on a staff, or that falleth on the sword, or that lacketh bread.

30 So Joab and Abishai his brother slew Abner, because he had slain their brother Asahel at Gibeon in the battle.

31 And David said to Joab, and to all the people that *were* with him, [m]Rend your clothes, and gird you with sackcloth, and mourn before Abner. And king David *himself* followed the bier.

32 And they buried Abner in Hebron: and the king lifted up his voice, and wept at the grave of Abner; and all the people wept.

33 And the king lamented over Abner, and said, Died Abner as a fool dieth?

34 Thy hands *were* not bound, nor thy feet put into fetters: as a man falleth before wicked men, *so* fellest thou. And all the people wept again over him.

35 And when all the people came to cause David to eat meat while it was yet day, David sware, saying, So do God to me, and more also, if I taste bread, or ought else, [a]till the sun be down.

36 And all the people took notice *of it*, and it pleased them: as whatsoever the king did [b]pleased all the people.

37 For all the people and all Israel understood that day that it was not of the king to slay Abner the son of Ner.

38 And the king said unto his servants, Know ye not that there is a prince and a great man fallen this day in Israel?

39 And I *am* this day weak, though anointed king; and these men the sons of Zeruiah *be* [c]too hard for me: the LORD shall reward the doer of evil according to his wickedness.

CHAPTER 4.

The murder of Ish-bosheth.

And when Saul's son heard that Abner was dead in Hebron, his hands were feeble, and all the Israelites were troubled.

2 And Saul's son had two men *that were* captains of bands: the name of the one *was* Baanah, and the name of the other Rechab, the sons of Rimmon a Beerothite, of the children of Benjamin: (for [d]Beeroth also was reckoned to Benjamin:

3 And the Beerothites fled to [e]Gittaim, and were sojourners there until this day.)

4 And Jonathan, Saul's son, had a son *that was* lame of *his* feet. He was five years old when the tidings came of Saul and Jonathan out of [f]Jezreel, and his nurse took him up, and fled: and it came to pass, as she made haste to flee, that he fell, and became lame. And his name *was* Mephibosheth.

5 And the sons of Rimmon the Beerothite, Rechab and Baanah, went, and came about the heat of the day to the house of Ish-bosheth, who lay on a bed at noon.

6 And they came thither into the midst of the house, *as though* they would have fetched wheat; and they smote him under the fifth *rib*: and Rechab and Baanah his brother escaped.

7 For when they came into the house, he lay on his bed in his bedchamber, and they smote him, and slew him, and beheaded him, and took his head, and gat them away through the plain all night.

8 And they brought the head of Ish-bosheth unto David to Hebron, and said to the king, Behold the head of Ish-bosheth the son of Saul thine enemy, [g]which sought thy life; and the LORD hath avenged my lord the king this day of Saul, and of his seed.

9 And David answered Rechab and Baanah his brother, the sons of Rimmon the Beerothite, and said unto them, *As* the LORD liveth, who hath [h]redeemed my soul out of all adversity,

10 [i]When one told me, saying, Behold, Saul is dead, thinking to have brought good tidings, I took hold of him, and slew him in Ziklag, who *thought* that I would have given him a reward for his tidings:

11 How much more, when wicked men have slain a righteous person in his own house upon his bed? shall I not therefore now [j]require his blood of your hand, and take you away from the earth?

12 And David commanded his young men, and they slew them, and cut off their hands and their feet, and hanged *them* up over the pool in Hebron. But they took the head of Ish-bosheth, and buried *it* in the sepulchre of Abner in Hebron.

CHAPTER 5.

David becomes king over Israel
(1 Chr. 11:1-3).

Then came all the tribes of Israel to [k]David unto Hebron, and spake, saying, Behold, we *are* thy bone and thy flesh.

2 Also in time past, when Saul was king over us, thou wast he that leddest out and broughtest in Israel: and the LORD said to thee, Thou shalt feed my people Israel, and thou shalt be a captain over Israel.

3 So all the [l]elders of Israel came to the king to Hebron; and king David made a

B.C. 1048.

a Jud. 20:26.
b *was good in their eyes.*
c 2 Sam. 19:5-7.
d Josh. 18:25.
e Neh. 11:33.
f 1 Sam. 29:1, 11.
g 1 Sam. 19:2; 23:15; 25:29.
h Ex. 14:30, *note;* Isa. 59:20, *note.*
i 2 Sam. 1:2, 16.
j Gen. 9:5, 6.
k *Kingdom* (O.T.). vs. 1-3; 2 Sam. 7:8-16. (Gen. 1:26; Zech. 12:8.)
l Cf. 1 Chr. 12:23-40.

league with them in Hebron before the LORD: and they anointed David king over Israel.

4 David *was* thirty years old when he began to reign, *and* he reigned forty years.

5 In Hebron he reigned over Judah seven years and six months: and in Jerusalem he reigned thirty and three years over all Israel and Judah.

Jerusalem made the capital of the united kingdom (1 Chr. 11:4-9).

6 And the king and his men went to [a]Jerusalem unto the Jebusites, the inhabitants of the land: which spake unto David, saying, Except thou take away the blind and the lame, thou shalt not come in hither: thinking, David cannot come in hither.

7 Nevertheless David took the strong hold of Zion: the same *is* the city of David.

8 And David said on that day, Whosoever getteth up to the gutter, and smiteth the Jebusites, and the lame and the blind, *that are* hated of David's soul, *he shall be chief and captain*. Wherefore they said, The blind and the lame shall not come into the house.

9 So David dwelt in the fort, and called it the city of David. And David built round about from Millo and inward.

10 And David went on, and grew great, and the LORD God of hosts *was* with him.

11 And Hiram [b]king of Tyre sent messengers to David, and cedar trees, and carpenters, and masons: and they built David an house.

12 And David perceived that the LORD had established him king over Israel, and that he had exalted his kingdom for his people Israel's sake.

Children of David born in Jerusalem. (Cf. 2 Sam. 3:2-5; 1 Chr. 3:1-4.)

13 And David took *him* more concubines and wives out of Jerusalem, after he was come from Hebron: and there were yet sons and daughters born to David.

14 And these *be* the names of those that were born unto him in Jerusalem; Shammua, and Shobab, and Nathan, and Solomon,

15 Ibhar also, and Elishua, and Nepheg, and Japhia,

16 And Elishama, and Eliada, and Eliphalet.

War with the Philistines (1 Chr. 14:8-17).

17 But when the Philistines heard that they had anointed David king over Israel, all the Philistines came up to seek David; and David heard *of it*, and went down to the [c]hold.

(Here, in the order of time, comes 2 Sam. 23:13-17; 1 Chr. 11:15-19; 12:8-15.)

18 The [d]Philistines also came and spread themselves in the valley of Rephaim.

19 And David [e]enquired of the LORD, saying, Shall I go up to the Philistines? wilt thou deliver them into mine hand? And the LORD said unto David, Go up: for I will doubtless deliver the Philistines into thine hand.

20 And David came to Baal-perazim, and David smote them there, and said, The LORD hath broken forth upon mine enemies before me, as the breach of waters. Therefore he called the name of that place [f]Baal-perazim.

21 And there they left their images, and David and his men burned them.

22 And the Philistines came up yet again, and spread themselves in the valley of Rephaim.

23 And when David enquired of the LORD, he said, Thou shalt not go up; *but* fetch a compass behind them, and come upon them over against the mulberry trees.

24 And let it be, when thou hearest the sound of a going in the tops of the mulberry trees, that then thou shalt bestir thyself: for then shall the LORD go out before thee, to smite the host of the Philistines.

25 And David did so, as the LORD had commanded him; and smote the Philistines from [g]Geba until thou come to Gazer.

CHAPTER 6.

David seeks to bring the ark to Jerusalem.

Again, David gathered together all *the* chosen *men* of Israel, thirty thousand.

2 And David arose, and went with all the people that *were* with him from [h]Baale of Judah, to bring up from thence the ark of God, whose name is called by the name of the LORD of hosts that dwelleth *between* the cherubims.

B.C. 1048.

a Josh. 15:63.
b 1 Chr. 14:1, 2.
c 2 Sam. 23:14.
d 1 Chr. 11:15.
e Jas. 4:15.
f i.e. *The plain of breaches.*
g 1 Chr. 14:16, *Gibeon.*
h Josh. 15:9, 60, *Kirjath-jearim*

3 And they set the ark of God upon a
new [1]cart, and brought it out of the
house of Abinadab that *was* in Gibeah:
and Uzzah and Ahio, the sons of
Abinadab, drave the new cart.
4 And they brought it out of the house
of Abinadab which *was* at Gibeah,
accompanying the ark of God: and Ahio
went before the ark.
5 And David and all the house of Israel
played before the LORD on all manner of
instruments made of fir wood, even on
harps, and on psalteries, and on timbrels,
and on cornets, and on cymbals.
6 And when they came to [a]Nachon's
threshingfloor, Uzzah put forth *his* [b]*hand*
to the ark of God, and took hold of it; for
the oxen shook *it*.
7 And the anger of the LORD was kindled against Uzzah; and God [c]smote
him there for *his* error; and there he died
by the ark of God.
8 And David was displeased, because
the LORD had made a breach upon
Uzzah: and he called the name of the
place Perez-uzzah to this day.
9 And David was afraid of the LORD
that day, and said, How shall the ark of
the LORD come to me?
10 So David would not remove the ark
of the LORD unto him into the city of
David: but David carried it aside into
the house of Obed-edom the Gittite.
11 And the ark of the LORD continued
in the house of Obed-edom the Gittite
three months: and the LORD blessed
Obed-edom, and all his household.

David brings up the ark
(1 Chr. 15:25-29; 16:1).

12 And it was told king David, saying,
The LORD hath blessed the house of
Obed-edom, and all that *pertaineth* unto
him, because of the ark of God. So David
went and brought up the ark of God
from the house of Obed-edom into the
city of David with gladness.
13 And it was *so*, that when they that
bare the ark of the LORD had gone six
[d]paces, he sacrificed oxen and fatlings.
14 And David danced before the LORD
with all *his* might; and David *was* girded
with a linen ephod.
15 So David and all the house of Israel
brought up the ark of the LORD with
shouting, and with the sound of the
trumpet.
16 And as the ark of the LORD came into
the city of David, Michal Saul's daughter
looked through a window, and saw king
David leaping and dancing before the
LORD; and she despised him in her heart.
17 [e]And they brought in the ark of the
LORD, and set it in his place, in the midst
of the tabernacle that David had pitched
for it: and David offered burnt-offerings
and peace-offerings before the LORD.
18 And as soon as David had made an
end of offering burnt-offerings and
peace-offerings, he blessed the people in
the name of the LORD of hosts.
19 And he dealt among all the people,
even among the whole multitude of Israel,
as well to the women as men, to every
one a cake of bread, and a good piece *of*
flesh, and a flagon *of wine*. So all the people departed every one to his house.
20 Then David returned to bless his
household. And Michal the daughter of
Saul came out to meet David, and said,
How glorious was the king of Israel to
day, who uncovered himself to day in
the eyes of the handmaids of his servants, as one of the vain fellows shame-
lessly uncovereth himself!
21 And David said unto Michal, *It was*
before the LORD, [f]which chose me before
thy father, and before all his house, to
appoint me ruler over the people of the
LORD, over Israel: therefore will I play
before the LORD.
22 And I will yet be more vile than thus,
and will be base in mine own sight: and of
the maidservants which thou hast spoken
of, of them shall I be had in honour.
23 Therefore Michal the daughter of
Saul had no [g]child unto the day of her
death.

B.C. 1042.

a 1 Chr. 13:9, *Chidon*.

b Num. 4:15.

c *Miracles* (O.T.). 1 Ki. 13:4-6. (Gen. 5:24; Jon. 2:1-10.)

d One pace = about 5 ft.

e 1 Chr. 16:1.

f 1 Sam. 13:14; 15:28.

g Cf. 2 Sam. 21:8.

[1] **(6:3)** The story of David's new cart and its results is a striking illustration of the spiritual truth that blessing does not follow even the best intentions in the service of God except as that service is rendered in God's *way*. It is a constant point of failure. God had given explicit directions how the ark should be borne (Num. 4:1-15), but David adopted a Philistine expedient (1 Sam. 6:7, 8). The church is full of Philistine ways of doing service to Christ. Cf. 1 Cor. 1:17-31; 2 Cor. 10:4, 5. See, also, 1 Chr. 15:2.

CHAPTER 7.

David's desire to build the LORD's house
(1 Chr. 17:1-3).

And it came to pass, when the king sat in his house, and the LORD had given him rest round about from all his enemies;

2 That the king said unto Nathan the prophet, See now, I dwell in an house of cedar, but the ark of God dwelleth within curtains.

3 And Nathan said to the king, Go, do all that *is* in thine heart; for the LORD *is* with thee.

The Seventh or Davidic Covenant
(1 Chr. 17:4-15).

4 And it came to pass that night, that the word of the LORD came unto Nathan, saying,

5 Go and tell my servant David, Thus saith the LORD, Shalt thou build me an house for me to dwell in?

6 Whereas I have not dwelt in *any* house since the time that I brought up the children of Israel out of Egypt, even to this day, but have walked in a tent and in a tabernacle.

7 In all *the places* wherein I have walked with all the children of Israel spake I a word with any of the tribes of Israel, whom I commanded to feed my people Israel, saying, Why build ye not me an house of cedar?

8 Now therefore [a]so shalt thou say unto my servant [b]David, Thus saith the LORD of hosts, I took thee from the sheepcote, from following the sheep, to be ruler over my people, over Israel:

9 And I was with thee whithersoever thou wentest, and have cut off all thine enemies out of thy sight, and have made thee a great name, like unto the name of the great *men* that *are* in the earth.

10 Moreover I will appoint a place for my people Israel, and will plant them, that they may dwell in a place of their own, and move no more; neither shall the children of wickedness afflict them any more, as beforetime,

11 And as since the time that I commanded judges *to be* over my people Israel, and have caused thee to rest from all thine enemies. Also the LORD telleth thee that he will make thee an house.

12 And when thy days be fulfilled, and thou shalt sleep with thy fathers, I will set up thy seed after thee, which shall proceed out of thy bowels, and I will establish his kingdom.

13 He shall build an house for my name, and I will stablish the throne of his kingdom for ever.

14 [c]I will be his father, and he shall be my son. If he commit iniquity, I will [d]chasten him with the rod of men, and with the stripes of the children of men:

15 But [1]my mercy shall not depart away from him, as I took *it* from Saul, whom I put away before thee.

16 And thine [e]house and thy kingdom [2]shall be established for ever before

B.C. 1042.

a *The Eight Covenants.* Hebrews 8:8 (Gen. 1:28; Heb 8:10.)

b *Israel (history).* vs. 8-17; 2 Ki. 17:6-23. (Gen. 12:2, 3; Rom. 11:26.)

c Heb. 1:5.

d *Judgments (the seven).* vs. 14, 15; 2 Sam. 12:13, 14. (2 Sam. 7:14; Rev. 22:12.)

e *Christ (first advent).* Psa. 2:2. (Gen. 3:15; Acts 1:9.)

[1] **(7:15)** Verses 14 and 15 state the principle of judgment within the *family* of God (see 1 Cor. 11:31, *note*). It is always remedial, not penal (Heb. 12:5-11). Judgment of the wicked is penal, not remedial.

[2] **(7:16)** The Davidic Covenant (vs. 8-17). This covenant, upon which the glorious kingdom of Christ "of the seed of David according to the flesh" is to be founded, secures:

(1) A Davidic "house"; i.e. posterity, family.
(2) A "throne"; i.e. royal authority.
(3) A kingdom; i.e. sphere of rule.
(4) In perpetuity; "for ever."
(5) And this fourfold covenant has but one condition: disobedience in the Davidic family is to be visited with chastisement, but *not* to the abrogation of the covenant (2 Sam. 7:15; Psa. 89:20-37; Isa. 24:5; 54:3). The chastisement fell; first in the division of the kingdom under Rehoboam, and, finally, in the captivities (2 Ki. 25:1-7). Since that time but one King of the Davidic family has been crowned at Jerusalem and He was crowned with thorns. But the Davidic Covenant confirmed to David by the oath of Jehovah, and renewed to Mary by the angel Gabriel, is immutable (Psa. 89:30-37), and the Lord God will yet give to that thorn-crowned One "the throne of his father David" (Lk. 1:31-33; Acts 2:29-32; 15:14-17).

See, for the other seven covenants: *Edenic,* Gen. 1:28; *Adamic,* Gen. 3:15; *Noahic,* Gen. 9:1; *Abrahamic,* Gen. 15:18; *Mosaic,* Ex. 19:25; *Palestinian,* Deut. 30:3; *New,* Heb. 8:8.

thee: thy [a]throne shall be established for
ever.
17 According to all these words, and
according to all this vision, so did
Nathan speak unto David.

David's worship and prayer
(1 Chr. 17:16-27).

18 Then went king David in, and sat
before the LORD, and he [b]said, Who *am* I,
O Lord GOD? and what *is* my house, that
thou hast brought me hitherto?
19 And this was yet a small thing in
thy sight, O Lord GOD; but thou hast
spoken also of thy servant's house for a
great while to come. And *is* this the manner of man, O Lord GOD?
20 And what can David say more unto
thee? for thou, Lord GOD, knowest thy
servant.
21 For thy word's sake, and according
to thine own heart, hast thou done all
these great things, to make thy servant
know *them*.
22 Wherefore thou art great, O LORD
God: for *there is* none like thee, neither *is*
there any God beside thee, according to
all that we have heard with our ears.
23 And what one nation in the earth *is*
like thy people, *even* like Israel, whom
God went to [c]redeem for a people to
himself, and to make him a name, and to
do for you great things and terrible, for
thy land, before thy people, which thou
redeemedst to thee from Egypt, *from* the
nations and their gods?
24 For thou hast confirmed to thyself
thy people Israel *to be* a people unto thee
for ever: and thou, LORD, art become
their God.
25 And now, O LORD God, the word
that thou hast spoken concerning thy servant, and concerning his house, establish
it for ever, and do as thou hast said.
26 And let thy name be magnified for
ever, saying, The LORD of hosts *is* the
God over Israel: and let the house of thy
servant David be established before thee.
27 For thou, O LORD of hosts, God of
Israel, hast revealed to thy servant, saying, I will build thee an house: therefore
hath thy servant found in his heart to
pray this prayer unto thee.
28 And now, O Lord GOD, thou *art*
that God, and thy words be true, and
thou hast promised this goodness unto
thy servant:
29 Therefore now let it please thee to
bless the house of thy servant, that it
may continue for ever before thee: for
thou, O Lord GOD, hast spoken *it*: and
with thy blessing let the house of thy
servant be blessed for ever.

CHAPTER 8.

The full establishment of David's kingdom
(1 Chr. 18:1-17).

And after this it came to pass, that
David smote the Philistines, and
subdued them: and David took Metheg-
ammah out of the hand of the Philistines.
2 And he smote [d]Moab, [e]and measured
them with a line, casting them down to
the ground; even with two lines measured
he to put to death, and with one full line
to keep alive. And *so* the Moabites became
David's servants, *and* brought gifts.
3 David smote also Hadadezer, the son
of Rehob, king of Zobah, as he went to
recover his border at the river Euphrates.
4 And David took from him a thousand [f]*chariots*, and seven hundred horsemen, and twenty thousand footmen: and
David houghed all the chariot *horses*, but
reserved of them *for* an hundred chariots.
5 And when the Syrians of Damascus
came to succour Hadadezer king of
Zobah, David slew of the Syrians two
and twenty thousand men.
6 Then David put garrisons in Syria of
Damascus: and the Syrians became servants to David, *and* brought gifts. And
the LORD preserved David whithersoever he went.
7 And David took the shields of gold
that were on the servants of Hadadezer,
and brought them to Jerusalem.
8 And from [g]Betah, and from Berothai,
cities of Hadadezer, king David took
exceeding much brass.
9 When Toi king of Hamath heard that
David had smitten all the host of
Hadadezer,
10 Then Toi sent Joram his son unto
king David, to salute him, and to bless
him, because he had fought against
Hadadezer, and smitten him: for
Hadadezer had wars with Toi. And
Joram brought with him vessels of silver,
and vessels of gold, and vessels of brass:
11 Which also king David did [h]dedi-
cate unto the LORD, with the silver and

B.C. 1042.

a *Kingdom (O.T.).* vs. 8-16; 2 Sam. 23:1-5. (Gen. 1:26; Zech. 12:8.)

b *Bible prayers* (O.T.). 2 Sam. 24:17. (Gen. 15:2; Hab. 3:1-16.)

c Ex. 14:30, *note.*

d Num. 24:17.

e 2 Sam. 12:31.

f 1 Chr. 18:4.

g or, *Tibhath.*

h 1 Ki. 7:51; 1 Chr. 18:11.

B.C. 1040.

gold that he had dedicated of all nations which he subdued;

12 Of Syria, and of Moab, and of the children of Ammon, and of the Philistines, and of Amalek, and of the spoil of Hadadezer, son of Rehob, king of Zobah.

13 And David gat *him* a name when he returned from smiting of the Syrians in the valley of salt, *being* eighteen thousand *men*.

14 And he put garrisons in Edom; throughout all Edom put he garrisons, and all they of [a]Edom became David's servants. And the LORD preserved David whithersoever he went.

15 And David reigned over all Israel; and David executed judgment and justice unto all his people.

16 And Joab the son of Zeruiah *was* over the host; and [b]Jehoshaphat the son of Ahilud *was* recorder;

17 And Zadok the son of Ahitub, and Ahimelech the son of Abiathar, *were* the priests; and Seraiah *was* the scribe;

18 And [c]Benaiah the son of Jehoiada *was over* both the Cherethites and the Pelethites; and David's sons were chief rulers.

CHAPTER 9.

David and Mephibosheth.

And David said, Is there yet any that is left of the house of Saul, that I may shew him [d]kindness for Jonathan's sake?

2 And *there was* of the house of Saul a servant whose name *was* Ziba. And when they had called him unto David, the king said unto him, *Art* thou Ziba? And he said, Thy servant *is he*.

3 And the king said, *Is* there not yet any of the house of Saul, that I may shew the kindness of God unto him? And Ziba said unto the king, Jonathan hath yet a son, *which is* lame on *his* feet.

4 And the king said unto him, Where *is* he? And Ziba said unto the king, Behold, he *is* in the house of Machir, the son of Ammiel, in Lo-debar.

5 Then king David sent, and fetched him out of the house of Machir, the son of Ammiel, from Lo-debar.

6 Now when Mephibosheth, the son of Jonathan, the son of Saul, was come unto David, he fell on his face, and did reverence. And David said, Mephibosheth. And he answered, Behold thy servant!

7 And David said unto him, Fear not: for I will surely shew thee kindness for Jonathan thy father's sake, and will restore thee all the land of Saul thy father; and thou shalt eat bread at my table continually.

8 And he bowed himself, and said, What *is* thy servant, that thou shouldest look upon such a dead [e]dog as I *am*?

9 Then the king called to Ziba, Saul's servant, and said unto him, I have [f]given unto thy master's son all that pertained to Saul and to all his house.

10 Thou therefore, and thy sons, and thy servants, shall till the land for him, and thou shalt bring in *the fruits*, that thy master's son may have food to eat: but Mephibosheth thy master's son shall eat bread [g]alway at my table. Now Ziba had fifteen sons and twenty servants.

11 Then said Ziba unto the king, According to all that my lord the king hath commanded his servant, so shall thy servant do. As for Mephibosheth, *said the king*, he shall eat at my table, as one of the king's sons.

12 And Mephibosheth had a young son, whose name *was* [h]Micha. And all that dwelt in the house of Ziba *were* servants unto Mephibosheth.

13 So Mephibosheth dwelt in Jerusalem: for he did eat continually at the king's [i]table; and was lame on both his feet.

CHAPTER 10.

The Ammonite-Syrian war
(1 Chr. 19:1-19).

And it came to pass after this, that the king of the children of Ammon died, and Hanun his son reigned in his stead.

2 Then said David, I will shew kindness unto Hanun the son of Nahash, as his father shewed kindness unto me. And David sent to comfort him by the hand of his servants for his father. And David's servants came into the land of the children of Ammon.

3 And the princes of the children of Ammon said unto Hanun their lord, Thinkest thou that David doth honour thy father, that he hath sent comforters unto thee? hath not David *rather* sent his

a Gen. 27:29; Num. 24:18; 1 Ki. 11:15.

b 1 Ki. 4:3.

c 1 Ki. 1:8; 1 Chr. 18:17.

d A lovely picture of salvation by grace. (1) What grace is—kindness to a helpless one for another's sake, vs. 1-3. (1 John 2:12.) (2) Grace gives the highest place, v. 11. (Eph. 1:1-6.) (3) Grace keeps the saved one, v. 13. (John 10:28, 29.)

e 2 Sam. 16:9.

f 2 Sam. 19:29.

g vs. 7, 13.

h 1 Chr. 8:34.

i 2 Ki. 25:29.

servants unto thee, to search the city, and to spy it out, and to overthrow it?

4 Wherefore Hanun took David's servants, and shaved off the one half of their beards, and cut off their garments in the middle, *even* to their buttocks, and sent them away.

5 When they told *it* unto David, he sent to meet them, because the men were greatly ashamed: and the king said, Tarry at Jericho until your beards be grown, and *then* return.

6 And when the children of Ammon saw that they stank before David, the children of Ammon sent and hired the [a]Syrians of Beth-rehob, and the Syrians of Zoba, twenty thousand footmen, and of king Maacah a thousand men, and of Ish-tob twelve thousand men.

7 And when David heard of *it*, he sent Joab, and all the host of the [b]mighty men.

8 And the children of Ammon came out, and put the battle in array at the entering in of the gate: and the Syrians of Zoba, and of Rehob, and Ish-tob, and Maacah, *were* by themselves in the field.

9 When Joab saw that the front of the battle was against him before and behind, he chose of all the choice *men* of Israel, and put *them* in array against the Syrians:

10 And the rest of the people he delivered into the hand of Abishai his brother, that he might put *them* in array against the children of Ammon.

11 And he said, If the Syrians be too strong for me, then thou shalt help me: but if the children of Ammon be too strong for thee, then I will come and help thee.

12 Be of good [c]courage, and let us play the men for our people, and for the cities of our God: and the LORD do that which seemeth him good.

13 And Joab drew nigh, and the people that *were* with him, unto the battle against the Syrians: and they fled before him.

14 And when the children of Ammon saw that the Syrians were fled, then fled they also before Abishai, and entered into the city. So Joab returned from the children of Ammon, and came to Jerusalem.

15 And when the Syrians saw that they were smitten before Israel, they gathered themselves together.

16 And Hadarezer sent, and brought out the Syrians that *were* beyond the river: and they came to Helam; and [d]Shobach the captain of the host of Hadarezer *went* before them.

17 And when it was told David, he gathered all Israel together, and passed over Jordan, and came to Helam. And the Syrians set themselves in array against David, and fought with him.

18 And the Syrians fled before Israel; and David slew *the men of* seven hundred chariots of the Syrians, and forty thousand [e]horsemen, and smote Shobach the captain of their host, who died there.

19 And when all the kings *that were* servants to Hadarezer saw that they were smitten before Israel, they made peace with Israel, and served them. So the Syrians feared to help the children of Ammon any more.

CHAPTER 11.

David's great sin.

And it came to pass, after the year was expired, at the time when kings go forth *to battle*, that David sent [f]Joab, and his servants with him, and all Israel; and they destroyed the children of Ammon, and besieged Rabbah. But David tarried still at Jerusalem.

2 And it came to pass in an eveningtide, that David arose from off his bed, and walked upon the roof of the king's house: and from the roof he saw a woman washing herself; and the woman *was* very beautiful to look upon.

3 And David sent and enquired after the woman. And *one* said, *Is* not this [g]Bath-sheba, the daughter of Eliam, the wife of Uriah the Hittite?

4 And David sent messengers, and took her; and she came in unto him, and he lay with her; for she was purified from her uncleanness: and she returned unto her house.

5 And the woman conceived, and sent and told David, and said, I *am* with child.

6 And David sent to Joab, *saying*, Send me Uriah the Hittite. And Joab sent Uriah to David.

7 And when Uriah was come unto him, David demanded *of him* how Joab did, and how the people did, and how the war prospered.

8 And David said to Uriah, Go down to thy house, and wash thy feet. And Uriah departed out of the king's house, and there followed him a mess *of meat* from the king.

B.C. 1037.

a 2 Sam. 8:3, 5.

b 2 Sam. 23:8.

c Deut. 31:6; Josh. 1:6, 7, 9; Neh. 4:14.

d 1 Chr. 19:16, 18, *Shophach.*

e 1 Chr. 19:18.

f 1 Chr. 20:1.

g 1 Chr. 3:5.

B.C. 1035.

9 But Uriah slept at the door of the king's house with all the servants of his lord, and went not down to his house.

10 And when they had told David, saying, Uriah went not down unto his house, David said unto Uriah, Camest thou not from *thy* journey? why *then* didst thou not go down unto thine house?

11 And Uriah [a]said unto David, The ark, and Israel, and Judah, abide in tents; and my lord Joab, and the servants of my lord, are encamped in the open fields; shall I then go into mine house, to eat and to drink, and to lie with my wife? *as* thou livest, and *as* thy soul liveth, I will not do this thing.

12 And David said to Uriah, Tarry here to day also, and to morrow I will let thee depart. So Uriah abode in Jerusalem that day, and the morrow.

13 And when David had called him, he did eat and drink before him; and he made him drunk: and at even he went out to lie on his bed with the servants of his lord, but went not down to his house.

14 And it came to pass in the morning, that David wrote a [b]letter to Joab, and sent *it* by the hand of Uriah.

15 And he wrote in the letter, saying, Set ye Uriah in the forefront of the hottest battle, and retire ye from him, that he may be [c]smitten, and die.

16 And it came to pass, when Joab observed the city, that he assigned Uriah unto a place where he knew that valiant men *were*.

17 And the men of the city went out, and fought with Joab: and there fell *some* of the people of the servants of David; and Uriah the Hittite died also.

18 Then Joab sent and told David all the things concerning the war;

19 And charged the messenger, saying, When thou hast made an end of telling the matters of the war unto the king,

20 And if so be that the king's wrath arise, and he say unto thee, Wherefore approached ye so nigh unto the city when ye did fight? knew ye not that they would shoot from the wall?

21 Who smote Abimelech the son of [d]Jerubbesheth? did not a woman cast a piece of a millstone upon him from the wall, that he died in Thebez? why went ye nigh the wall? then say thou, Thy servant Uriah the Hittite is dead also.

22 So the messenger went, and came and shewed David all that Joab had sent him for.

23 And the messenger said unto David, Surely the men prevailed against us, and came out unto us into the field, and we were upon them even unto the entering of the gate.

24 And the shooters shot from off the wall upon thy servants; and *some* of the king's servants be dead, and thy servant Uriah the Hittite is dead also.

25 Then David said unto the messenger, Thus shalt thou say unto Joab, Let not this thing displease thee, for the sword devoureth one as well as another: make thy battle more strong against the city, and [e]overthrow it: and encourage thou him.

26 And when the wife of Uriah heard that Uriah her husband was dead, she mourned for her husband.

27 And when the mourning was past, David sent and fetched her to his house, and she became his wife, and bare him a son. But the thing that David had done [f]displeased the LORD.

CHAPTER 12.

David's repentance.

And the LORD sent [g]Nathan unto David. And he came unto him, and said unto him, There were two men in one city; the one rich, and the other poor.

2 The rich *man* had exceeding many flocks and herds:

3 But the poor *man* had nothing, save one little ewe lamb, which he had bought and nourished up: and it grew up together with him, and with his children; it did eat of his own meat, and drank of his own cup, and lay in his bosom, and was unto him as a daughter.

4 And there came a traveller unto the rich man, and he spared to take of his own flock and of his own herd, to dress for the wayfaring man that was come unto him; but took the poor man's lamb, and dressed it for the man that was come to him.

5 And David's anger was greatly kindled against the man; and he said to Nathan, *As* the LORD liveth, the man that hath done this *thing* shall surely die:

a 2 Sam. 7:2, 6.

b 1 Ki. 21:8, 9.

c 2 Sam. 12:9.

d *Jerubbaal*, Jud. 6:32.

e 2 Sam. 12:26.

f 1 Chr. 21:7; Heb. 13:4.

g *Parables* (O.T.). vs. 1-4; 2 Sam. 14:1-4. (Jud. 9:7-15; Zech. 11:7-14.

B.C. 1034.

6 And he shall restore the lamb fourfold, because he did this thing, and
because he had no pity.
7 And Nathan said to David, Thou *art*
the man. Thus saith the LORD God of
Israel, I anointed thee king over Israel,
and I delivered thee out of the hand of
Saul;
8 And I gave thee thy master's house,
and thy master's wives into thy bosom,
and gave thee the house of Israel and of
Judah; and if *that had been* too little, I
would moreover have given unto thee
such and such things.
9 Wherefore hast thou despised the
commandment of the LORD, to do evil in
his sight? thou hast killed Uriah the
Hittite with the sword, and hast taken his
wife *to be* thy wife, and hast slain him
with the sword of the children of Ammon.
10 Now therefore the sword shall never
depart from thine house; because thou
hast despised me, and hast taken the wife
of Uriah the Hittite to be thy wife.
11 Thus saith the LORD, Behold, I will
raise up evil against thee out of thine
own house, and I will take thy wives
before thine eyes, and give *them* unto thy
neighbour, and he shall lie with thy
wives in the sight of this sun.
12 For thou didst *it* secretly: but I will
do this thing before all Israel, and before
the sun.
13 And David said unto Nathan, I
have [a]sinned against the LORD. And
Nathan said unto David, The LORD also
hath put away thy sin; thou shalt not die.
14 Howbeit, because by this deed thou
hast given great occasion to the enemies
of the LORD to blaspheme, the child also
that is born unto thee [b]shall surely die.
15 And Nathan departed unto his
house. And the LORD struck the child
that Uriah's wife bare unto David, and it
was very sick.
16 David therefore besought God for
the child; and David fasted, and went in,
and lay all night upon the earth.
17 And the elders of his house arose,
and went to him, to raise him up from the
earth: but he would not, neither did he
eat bread with them.
18 And it came to pass on the seventh
day, that the child died. And the servants
of David feared to tell him that the child
was dead: for they said, Behold, while
the child was yet alive, we spake unto
him, and he would not hearken unto our
voice: how will he then vex himself, if we
tell him that the child is dead?
19 But when David saw that his servants whispered, David perceived that
the child was dead: therefore David said
unto his servants, Is the child dead? And
they said, He is dead.
20 Then David arose from the earth,
and washed, and anointed *himself*, and
changed his apparel, and came into the
house of the LORD, and worshipped:
then he came to his own house; and
when he required, they set bread before
him, and he did eat.
21 Then said his servants unto him,
What thing *is* this that thou hast done?
thou didst fast and weep for the child,
while it was alive; but when the child was
dead, thou didst rise and eat bread.
22 And he said, While the child was
yet alive, I fasted and wept: for I said,
[c]Who can tell *whether* GOD will be gracious to me, that the child may live?
23 But now he is dead, wherefore
should I fast? can I bring him back
again? I shall go to him, but he shall not
return to me.

The birth of Solomon.

24 And David comforted Bath-sheba
his wife, and went in unto her, and lay
with her: and she bare a son, and he
called his name Solomon: and the LORD
loved him.
25 And he sent by the hand of Nathan
the prophet; and he called his name
[d]Jedidiah, because of the LORD.

David and Joab take Rabbah
(1 Chr. 20:1-3).

26 And Joab fought against Rabbah of
the children of Ammon, and took the
royal city.
27 And Joab sent messengers to
David, and said, I have fought against
Rabbah, and have taken the city of
waters.
28 Now therefore gather the rest of the
people together, and encamp against the
city, and take it: lest I take the city, and it
be called after my name.
29 And David gathered all the people
together, and went to Rabbah, and
fought against it, and took it.

a Here read Psa. 51.

b *Judgments (the seven).* vs. 13, 14; Psa. 50:1-22. (2 Sam. 7:14; Rev. 22:12.)

c Isa. 38:2, 3; Joel 2:14; Jon. 3:9.

d i.e. *Beloved of the LORD.* Neh. 13:26; Mt. 3:17.

30 And he took their king's crown
from off his head, the weight whereof
was a [a]talent of gold with the precious
stones: and it was *set* on David's head.
And he brought forth the spoil of the
city in great abundance.
31 And he brought forth the people
that *were* therein, and put *them* under
saws, and under harrows of iron, and
under axes of iron, and made them pass
through the brickkiln: and thus did he
unto all the cities of the children of
Ammon. So David and all the people
returned unto Jerusalem.

CHAPTER 13.

Amnon's crime.

And it came to pass after this, that
Absalom the son of David had a
fair sister, whose name *was* [b]Tamar; and
Amnon the son of David loved her.
2 And Amnon was so [c]vexed, that he
fell sick for his sister Tamar; for she *was*
a virgin; and Amnon thought it hard for
him to do any thing to her.
3 But Amnon had a friend, whose
name *was* Jonadab, the son of [d]Shimeah
David's brother: and Jonadab *was* a very
subtil man.
4 And he said unto him, Why *art* thou,
being the king's son, lean from day to
day? wilt thou not tell me? And Amnon
said unto him, I love Tamar, my brother
Absalom's sister.
5 And Jonadab said unto him, Lay
thee down on thy bed, and make thyself
sick: and when thy father cometh to see
thee, say unto him, I pray thee, let my
sister Tamar come, and give me meat,
and dress the meat in my sight, that I
may see *it*, and eat *it* at her hand.
6 So Amnon lay down, and made himself sick: and when the king was come to
see him, Amnon said unto the king, I
pray thee, let Tamar my sister come, and
make me a couple of [e]cakes in my sight,
that I may eat at her hand.
7 Then David sent home to Tamar,
saying, Go now to thy brother Amnon's
house, and dress him meat.
8 So Tamar went to her brother
Amnon's house; and he was laid down.
And she took flour, and kneaded *it*, and
made cakes in his sight, and did bake
the cakes.
9 And she took a pan, and poured *them*
out before him; but he refused to eat. And
Amnon said, Have out all men from me.
And they went out every man from him.
10 And Amnon said unto Tamar, Bring
the meat into the chamber, that I may eat
of thine hand. And Tamar took the cakes
which she had made, and brought *them*
into the chamber to Amnon her brother.
11 And when she had brought *them*
unto him to eat, he took hold of her, and
said unto her, Come lie with me, my sister.
12 And she answered him, Nay, my
brother, do not force me; for no such
thing ought to be done in [f]Israel: do not
thou this folly.
13 And I, whither shall I cause my
shame to go? and as for thee, thou shalt
be as one of the fools in Israel. Now therefore, I pray thee, speak unto the king; for
he will not withhold me from thee.
14 Howbeit he would not hearken
unto her voice: but, being stronger than
she, forced her, and lay with her.
15 Then Amnon hated her exceedingly; so that the hatred wherewith he
hated her *was* greater than the love
wherewith he had loved her. And
Amnon said unto her, Arise, be gone.
16 And she said unto him, *There is* no
cause: this evil in sending me away *is*
greater than the other that thou didst unto
me. But he would not hearken unto her.
17 Then he called his servant that ministered unto him, and said, Put now this
woman out from me, and bolt the door
after her.
18 And *she had* a garment of divers
colours upon her: [g]for with such robes
were the king's daughters *that were* virgins apparelled. Then his servant brought
her out, and bolted the door after her.
19 And Tamar put [h]ashes on her head,
and rent her garment of divers colours
that *was* on her, and laid her hand on her
head, and went on crying.
20 And Absalom her brother said unto
her, Hath Amnon thy brother been with
thee? but hold now thy peace, my sister:
he *is* thy brother; regard not this thing.
So Tamar remained desolate in her
brother Absalom's house.
21 But when king David heard of all
these things, he was very wroth.
22 And Absalom spake unto his
brother Amnon neither good nor bad:

B.C. 1033.

a One talent = £6150, or in dollars $29,085
b 1 Chr. 3:9.
c 1 Ki 21:4.
d 1 Sam. 16:9. *Shammah.*
e Gen. 18:6.
f Lev. 18:9-11; 20:17.
g Psa. 45:13, 14.
h 2 Sam. 1:2; Josh. 7:6; Job 2:12; 42:6.

for Absalom hated Amnon, because he
had forced his sister Tamar.

Absalom's vengeance for Tamar's wrong.

23 And it came to pass after two full
years, that Absalom had sheepshearers
in Baal-hazor, which *is* beside Ephraim:
and Absalom invited all the king's sons.
24 And Absalom came to the king, and
said, Behold now, thy servant hath
sheepshearers; let the king, I beseech thee,
and his servants go with thy servant.
25 And the king said to Absalom, Nay,
my son, let us not all now go, lest we be
chargeable unto thee. And he pressed
him: howbeit he would not go, but
blessed him.
26 Then said Absalom, If not, I pray
thee, let my brother Amnon go with us.
And the king said unto him, Why
should he go with thee?
27 But Absalom pressed him, that he
let Amnon and all the king's sons go
with him.
28 Now Absalom had commanded his
servants, saying, Mark ye now when
Amnon's heart is merry with wine, and
when I say unto you, Smite Amnon; then
kill him, fear not: have not I commanded
you? be courageous, and be valiant.
29 And the servants of Absalom did
unto Amnon as Absalom had commanded. Then all the king's sons arose, and
every man gat him up upon his mule,
and fled.
30 And it came to pass, while they
were in the way, that tidings came to
David, saying, Absalom hath slain all
the king's sons, and there is not one of
them left.
31 Then the king arose, and tare his garments, and lay on the earth; and all his
servants stood by with their clothes rent.
32 And Jonadab, the son of Shimeah
David's brother, answered and said, Let
not my lord suppose *that* they have slain
all the young men the king's sons; for
Amnon only is dead: for by the appointment of Absalom this hath been determined from the day that he forced his
sister Tamar.
33 Now therefore let not my lord the
king take the thing to his heart, to think
that all the king's sons are dead: for
Amnon only is dead.
34 But Absalom fled. And the young
man that kept the watch lifted up his
eyes, and looked, and, behold, there
came much people by the way of the hill
side behind him.
35 And Jonadab said unto the king,
Behold, the king's sons come: as thy servant said, so it is.
36 And it came to pass, as soon as he
had made an end of speaking, that,
behold, the king's sons came, and lifted
up their voice and wept: and the king
also and all his servants wept very sore.

Absalom's flight to Geshur.

37 But Absalom fled, and went to
Talmai, the son of Ammihud, king of
[1]Geshur. And *David* mourned for his son
every day.
38 So Absalom fled, and went to
Geshur, and was there three years.
39 And *the soul of* king David [a]longed
to go forth unto Absalom: for he was
comforted concerning Amnon, seeing he
was dead.

CHAPTER 14.

The recall of Absalom: (1) *Joab's craft.*

Now Joab the son of Zeruiah perceived that the king's heart *was*
toward Absalom.
2 And Joab sent to [b]Tekoah, and
fetched thence a wise woman, and said
unto her, I pray thee, feign thyself to be a
mourner, and put on now mourning
apparel, and anoint not thyself with oil,
but be as a woman that had a long time
mourned for the dead:
3 And come to the king, and [c]speak on
this manner unto him. So Joab put the
words in her mouth.
4 And when the woman of Tekoah
spake to the king, she fell on her face to
the ground, and did obeisance, and said,
Help, O king.
5 And the king said unto her, What
aileth thee? And she answered, I *am*
indeed a widow woman, and mine husband is dead.

B.C. 1032.

a Lit. *was consumed.*

b 2 Chr. 11:6.

c *Parables* (O.T.). vs. 1-14; 1 Ki. 20:35-40. (Jud. 9:7-15; Zech. 11:7-14.)

[1] **(13:37)** See 1 Sam. 27:8. David, in the years of his wanderings, made a savage raid upon Geshur, and evidently bore away Maacah, daughter of the king of Geshur. Of her was born Absalom, and in him was her wild Bedouin blood, and the blood of a father who had been the reckless chief of a handful of desperate men (2 Sam. 3:3; 23:8-39), and whom only the divine love could tame (2 Sam. 22:36). In Absalom David reaped from his own sowing.

B.C. 1027.

6 And thy handmaid had two sons,
and they two strove together in the field,
and *there was* none to part them, but the
one smote the other, and slew him.
7 And, behold, the whole family is
risen against thine handmaid, and they
said, Deliver him that smote his brother,
that we may kill him, for the life of his
brother whom he slew; and we will
destroy the heir also: and so they shall
quench my coal which is left, and shall
not leave to my husband *neither* name
nor remainder upon the earth.
8 And the king said unto the woman,
Go to thine house, and I will give charge
concerning thee.
9 And the woman of Tekoah said unto
the king, My lord, O king, the iniquity *be*
on me, and on my father's house: and
the king and his throne *be* guiltless.
10 And the king said, Whosoever saith
ought unto thee, bring him to me, and he
shall not touch thee any more.
11 Then said she, I pray thee, let the
king remember the LORD thy God, that
thou wouldest not suffer the [a]revengers
of [b]blood to destroy any more, lest they
destroy my son. And he said, *As* the
LORD liveth, there shall not one hair of
thy son fall to the earth.
12 Then the woman said, Let thine
handmaid, I pray thee, speak *one* word
unto my lord the king. And he said, Say
on.
13 And the woman said, Wherefore
then hast thou thought such a thing
against the people of God? for the king
doth speak this thing as one which is
faulty, in that the king doth not fetch
home again his banished.
14 For we must needs die, and *are* as
water spilt on the ground, which cannot
be gathered up again; neither doth God
[c]respect *any* person: yet doth he devise
means, that his banished be not expelled
from him.
15 Now therefore that I am come to
speak of this thing unto my lord the
king, *it is* because the people have made
me afraid: and thy handmaid said, I will
now speak unto the king; it may be that
the king will perform the request of his
handmaid.
16 For the king will hear, to deliver his
handmaid out of the hand of the man
that would destroy me and my son
together out of the inheritance of God.
17 Then thine handmaid said, The word
of my lord the king shall now be comfortable: for as an [d]angel of God, so *is* my lord
the king to discern good and bad: therefore the LORD thy God will be with thee.
18 Then the king answered and said
unto the woman, Hide not from me, I
pray thee, the thing that I shall ask thee.
And the woman said, Let my lord the
king now speak.
19 And the king said, *Is not* the hand
of Joab with thee in all this? And the
woman answered and said, *As* thy soul
liveth, my lord the king, none can turn
to the right hand or to the left from
ought that my lord the king hath spoken: for thy servant Joab, he bade me,
and he put all these words in the mouth
of thine handmaid:
20 To fetch about this form of speech
hath thy servant Joab done this thing:
and my lord *is* wise, according to the
wisdom of an [d]angel of God, to know all
things that *are* in the earth.

David's half-hearted forgiveness of Absalom.

21 And the king said unto Joab, Behold
now, I have done this thing: go therefore,
bring the young man Absalom again.
22 And Joab fell to the ground on his
face, and bowed himself, and thanked the
king: and Joab said, To day thy servant
knoweth that I have found grace in thy
sight, my lord, O king, in that the king
hath fulfilled the request of his servant.
23 So Joab arose and went to [e]Geshur,
and brought Absalom to Jerusalem.
24 And the king said, Let him turn to
his own house, and let him not see my
face. So Absalom returned to his own
house, and [1]saw not the king's face.

David forgives Absalom.

25 But in all Israel there was none to
be so much praised as Absalom for his

a Heb. *goel*, *Redemp. (Kinsman type).* Isa. 59:20, *note*.
b Num. 35:19.
c 2 Sam. 13:37; Job 34:19; Mt. 22:16; Acts 10:34; Rom. 2:11.
d Heb. 1:4, *note*.
e 2 Sam. 13:37.

[1] **(14:24)** Not so had God taught David to forgive. Legalists have thought Absalom's wilfulness to have been due to over-indulgence on the part of David. There is no such intimation in Scripture. Rather it would seem that had David at this time taken Absalom into intimacy, the rebellion might have been averted.

beauty: from the sole of his foot even to the crown of his head there was no blemish in him.

26 And when he polled his head, (for it was at every year's end that he polled *it*: because *the hair* was heavy on him, therefore he polled it:) he weighed the hair of his head at two hundred shekels after the king's weight.

27 And unto Absalom there were born three [a]sons, and one daughter, whose name *was* Tamar: she was a woman of a fair countenance.

28 So Absalom dwelt two full years in Jerusalem, and saw not the king's face.

29 Therefore Absalom sent for Joab, to have sent him to the king; but he would not come to him: and when he sent again the second time, he would not come.

30 Therefore he said unto his servants, See, Joab's field is near mine, and he hath barley there; go and set it on fire. And Absalom's servants set the field on fire.

31 Then Joab arose, and came to Absalom unto *his* house, and said unto him, Wherefore have thy servants set my field on fire?

32 And Absalom answered Joab, Behold, I sent unto thee, saying, Come hither, that I may send thee to the king, to say, Wherefore am I come from Geshur? *it had been* good for me *to have been* there still: now therefore let me see the king's face; and if there be *any* iniquity in me, let him kill me.

33 So Joab came to the king, and told him: and when he had called for Absalom, he came to the king, and bowed himself on his face to the ground before the king: and the king kissed Absalom.

CHAPTER 15.

Absalom steals the love of the ten tribes ("Israel").

And it came to pass after this, that Absalom [b]prepared him chariots and horses, and fifty men to run before him.

2 And Absalom rose up early, and stood beside the way of the gate: and it was *so*, that when any man that had a controversy came to the king for judgment, then Absalom called unto him, and said, Of what city *art* thou? And he said, Thy servant *is* of one of the tribes of Israel.

B.C. 1027.

a See 2 Sam. 18:18, *note*.

b 1 Ki. 1:5.

c Jud. 9:29.

d Some authorities read "four."

e 1 Sam. 16:2.

3 And Absalom said unto him, See, thy matters *are* good and right; but *there is* no man *deputed* of the king to hear thee.

4 Absalom [c]said moreover, Oh that I were made judge in the land, that every man which hath any suit or cause might come unto me, and I would do him justice!

5 And it was *so*, that when any man came nigh *to him* to do him obeisance, he put forth his hand, and took him, and kissed him.

6 And on this manner did Absalom to all Israel that came to the king for judgment: so Absalom stole the hearts of the men of Israel.

Outbreak of Absalom's rebellion.

7 And it came to pass after [d]forty years, that Absalom said unto the king, I pray thee, let me go and [e]pay my vow, which I have vowed unto the LORD, in Hebron.

8 For thy servant vowed a vow while I abode at Geshur in Syria, saying, If the LORD shall bring me again indeed to Jerusalem, then I will serve the LORD.

9 And the king said unto him, Go in peace. So he arose, and went to Hebron.

10 But Absalom sent spies throughout all the tribes of Israel, saying, As soon as ye hear the sound of the trumpet, then ye shall say, Absalom reigneth in Hebron.

11 And with Absalom went two hundred men out of Jerusalem, *that were* called; and they went in their simplicity, and they knew not any thing.

12 And Absalom sent for Ahithophel the Gilonite, David's counsellor, from his city, *even* from Giloh, while he offered sacrifices. And the conspiracy was strong; for the people increased continually with Absalom.

Flight of David from Jerusalem.

13 And there came a messenger to David, saying, The hearts of the men of Israel are after Absalom.

14 And David said unto all his servants that *were* with him at Jerusalem, Arise, and let us flee; for we shall not *else* escape from Absalom: make speed to depart, lest he overtake us suddenly, and bring evil upon us, and smite the city with the edge of the sword.

15 And the king's servants said unto the king, Behold, thy servants *are ready to*

B.C. 1023.

do whatsoever my lord the king shall appoint.

16 And the king went forth, and all his household after him. And the king left ten women, *which were* [a]concubines, to keep the house.

17 And the king went forth, and all the people after him, and tarried in a place that was far off.

18 And all his servants passed on beside him; and all the [b]Cherethites, and all the Pelethites, and all the Gittites, six hundred men which came after him from Gath, passed on before the king.

19 Then said the king to [c]Ittai the Gittite, Wherefore goest thou also with us? return to thy place, and abide with the king: for thou *art* a stranger, and also an exile.

20 Whereas thou camest *but* yesterday, should I this day make thee go up and down with us? seeing I [d]go whither I may, return thou, and take back thy brethren: mercy and truth *be* with thee.

21 And Ittai answered the king, and said, *As* the LORD liveth, and *as* my lord the king liveth, surely in what place my lord the king shall be, whether in death or life, even there also will thy servant be.

22 And David said to Ittai, Go and pass over. And Ittai the Gittite passed over, and all his men, and all the little ones that *were* with him.

23 And all the country wept with a loud voice, and all the people passed over: the king also himself passed over the brook Kidron, and all the people passed over, toward the way of the [e]wilderness.

24 And lo Zadok also, and all the Levites *were* with him, bearing the [f]ark of the covenant of God: and they set down the ark of God; and Abiathar went up, until all the people had done passing out of the city.

25 And the king said unto Zadok, Carry back the ark of God into the city: if I shall find favour in the eyes of the LORD, he will bring me again, and shew me *both* it, and his habitation:

26 But if he thus say, I have no [g]delight in thee; behold, *here am* I, [h]let him do to me as seemeth good unto him.

27 The king said also unto Zadok the priest, *Art not* thou a [i]seer? return into the city in peace, and your two sons with you, Ahimaaz thy son, and Jonathan the son of Abiathar.

28 See, I will tarry in the plain of the [j]wilderness, until there come word from you to certify me.

29 Zadok therefore and Abiathar carried the ark of God again to Jerusalem: and they tarried there.

30 And David went up by the ascent of *mount* Olivet, and wept as he went up, and had his [k]head covered, and he went barefoot: and all the people that *was* with him covered every man his head, and they went up, weeping as they went up.

31 And *one* told David, saying, [l]Ahithophel *is* among the conspirators with Absalom. And David said, O LORD, I pray thee, [m]turn the counsel of Ahithophel into foolishness.

32 And it came to pass, that *when* David was come to the top *of the mount,* where he worshipped God, behold, Hushai the [n]Archite came to meet him with his coat rent, and earth upon his head:

33 Unto whom David said, If thou passest on with me, then thou shalt be a burden unto me:

34 But if thou return to the city, and say unto Absalom, I will be thy servant, O king; *as* I *have been* thy father's servant hitherto, so *will* I now also *be* thy servant: then mayest thou for me defeat the counsel of Ahithophel.

35 And *hast thou* not there with thee [o]Zadok and Abiathar the priests? therefore it shall be, *that* what thing soever thou shalt hear out of the king's house, thou shalt tell *it* to Zadok and Abiathar the priests.

36 Behold, *they have* there with them their two sons, Ahimaaz Zadok's *son,* and Jonathan Abiathar's *son;* and by them ye shall send unto me every thing that ye can hear.

37 So Hushai David's friend came into the city, and Absalom came into Jerusalem.

CHAPTER 16.

The false servant of Mephibosheth.

And when David was a little [p]past the top *of the hill,* behold, Ziba the servant of Mephibosheth met him, with a couple of asses saddled, and upon them two hundred *loaves* of bread, and an hundred bunches of raisins, and an hundred of summer fruits, and a bottle of wine.

a 2 Sam. 12:11; 16:21, 22.
b 2 Sam. 8:18.
c 2 Sam. 18:2.
d 1 Sam. 23:13.
e 2 Sam. 16:2.
f Num. 4:15.
g Num. 14:8; 1 Ki. 10:9.
h 1 Sam. 3:18.
i 1 Sam. 9:9.
j 2 Sam. 17:16.
k 2 Sam. 19:4.
l v. 12.
m 2 Sam. 16:23; 17:14-23.
n Josh. 16:2.
o 2 Sam. 17:15, 16.
p 2 Sam. 15:30, 32.

B.C. 1023.

2 And the king said unto Ziba, What
meanest thou by these? And Ziba said,
The asses *be* for the king's household to
ride on; and the bread and summer fruit
for the young men to eat; and the wine,
that such as be faint in the wilderness
may drink.
3 And the king said, And where *is* thy
master's son? And Ziba said unto the
[a]king, Behold, he abideth at Jerusalem: for
he said, To day shall the house of Israel
restore me the kingdom of my father.
4 Then said the king to Ziba, Behold,
thine *are* all that *pertained* unto
Mephibosheth. And Ziba said, I humbly
beseech thee *that* I may find grace in thy
sight, my lord, O king.

Shimei curses David.

5 And when king David came to
Bahurim, behold, thence came out a man
of the family of the house of Saul, whose
name *was* Shimei, the son of Gera: he
came forth, and cursed still as he came.
6 And he cast stones at David, and at
all the servants of king David: and all
the people and all the mighty men *were*
on his right hand and on his left.
7 And thus said Shimei when he
cursed, Come out, come out, thou
bloody man, and thou man of Belial:
8 The LORD hath returned upon thee
all the [b]blood of the house of Saul, in
whose stead thou hast reigned; and the
LORD hath delivered the kingdom into
the hand of Absalom thy son: and,
behold, thou *art taken* in thy mischief,
because thou *art* a bloody man.
9 Then said Abishai the son of Zeruiah
unto the king, Why should this dead
[c]dog curse my lord the king? let me go
over, I pray thee, and take off his head.
10 And the king said, What have I to
do with you, ye sons of Zeruiah? so let
him curse, because the LORD hath said
unto him, Curse David. Who shall then
say, Wherefore hast thou done so?
11 And David said to Abishai, and to
all his servants, Behold, my son, which
came forth of my bowels, seeketh my
life: how much more now *may this*
Benjamite *do it*? let him alone, and let
him curse; for the LORD hath bidden him.
12 It may be that the LORD will look on
mine affliction, and that the LORD will
requite me [d]good for his cursing this day.
13 And as David and his men went by
the way, Shimei went along on the hill's
side over against him, and cursed as he
went, and threw stones at him, and cast
dust.
14 And the king, and all the people
that *were* with him, came weary, and
refreshed themselves there.

Absalom enters Jerusalem.

15 And Absalom, and all the people
the men of Israel, came to Jerusalem,
and Ahithophel with him.
16 And it came to pass, [e]when Hushai
the Archite, David's friend, was come
unto Absalom, that Hushai said unto
Absalom, God save the king, God save
the king.
17 And Absalom said to Hushai, *Is*
this thy kindness to thy friend? why
wentest thou not with thy [f]friend?
18 And Hushai said unto Absalom,
Nay; but whom the LORD, and this people, and all the men of Israel, choose, his
will I be, and with him will I abide.
19 And again, whom should I serve?
should I not *serve* in the presence of his
son? as I have served in thy father's
presence, so will I be in thy presence.
20 Then said Absalom to [g]Ahithophel,
Give counsel among you what we shall
do.
21 And Ahithophel said unto
Absalom, Go in unto thy father's concubines, which he hath left to keep the
house; and all Israel shall hear that thou
art abhorred of thy father: then shall the
[h]hands of all that *are* with thee be strong.
22 So they spread Absalom a tent
upon the top of the house; and Absalom
went [i]in unto his father's concubines in
the sight of all Israel.
23 And the counsel of Ahithophel,
which he counselled in those days, *was*
as if a man had enquired at the oracle of
God: so *was* all the counsel of Ahithophel
both with David and with Absalom.

CHAPTER 17.

The diverse counsel of
Ahithophel and Hushai.

Moreover Ahithophel said unto
Absalom, Let me now choose out
twelve thousand men, and I will arise
and pursue after David this night:
2 And I will come upon him while he
is [j]weary and weak handed, and will

a 2 Sam. 19:27.
b 2 Sam. 1:16; 3:28, 29; 4:8-12; cf. 21:1-9.
c 2 Sam. 9:8.
d Rom. 8:28; Heb. 12:10, 12.
e 2 Sam. 15:37.
f 2 Sam. 15:33, 34.
g 2 Sam. 15:12.
h 2 Sam. 2:7.
i 2 Sam. 12:11, 12.
j 2 Sam. 16:14; Deut. 25:18.

B.C. 1023.

make him afraid: and all the people that
are with him shall flee; and I will smite
the king only:
3 And I will bring back all the people
unto thee: the man whom thou seekest *is*
as if all returned: *so* all the people shall
be in peace.
4 And the saying pleased Absalom
well, and all the elders of Israel.
5 Then said Absalom, Call now
Hushai the Archite also, and let us hear
likewise what he saith.
6 And when Hushai was come to
Absalom, Absalom spake unto him, saying, Ahithophel hath spoken after this
manner: shall we do *after* his saying? if
not; speak thou.
7 And Hushai said unto Absalom, The
counsel that Ahithophel hath given *is*
not good at this time.
8 For, said Hushai, thou knowest thy
father and his men, that they *be* mighty
men, and they *be* chafed in their minds,
as a bear robbed of her whelps in the
field: and thy father *is* a man of war, and
will not lodge with the people.
9 Behold, he is hid now in some pit, or
in some *other* place: and it will come to
pass, when some of them be overthrown
at the first, that whosoever heareth it
will say, There is a slaughter among the
people that follow Absalom.
10 And he also *that is* valiant, whose
heart *is* as the heart of a lion, shall utterly [a]melt: for all Israel knoweth that thy
father *is* a mighty man, and *they* which
be with him *are* valiant men.
11 Therefore I counsel that all Israel be
generally gathered unto thee, from Dan
even to Beer-sheba, [b]as the sand that *is*
by the sea for multitude; and that thou
go to battle in thine own person.
12 So shall we come upon him in some
place where he shall be found, and we
will light upon him as the dew falleth on
the ground: and of him and of all the
men that *are* with him there shall not be
left so much as one.
13 Moreover, if he be gotten into a city,
then shall all Israel bring ropes to that city,
and we will draw it into the river, until
there be not one small stone found there.
14 And Absalom and all the men of
Israel said, The counsel of Hushai the
Archite *is* better than the counsel of
Ahithophel. For the [c]LORD had appointed to defeat the good counsel of
Ahithophel, to the intent that the LORD
might bring evil upon Absalom.
15 Then said Hushai unto Zadok and
to Abiathar the priests, Thus and thus
did Ahithophel counsel Absalom and
the elders of Israel; and thus and thus
have I counselled.
16 Now therefore send quickly, and tell
David, saying, Lodge not this night in
the plains of the wilderness, but speedily
pass over; lest the king be swallowed up,
and all the people that *are* with him.
17 Now [d]Jonathan and Ahimaaz
stayed by [e]En-rogel; for they might not
be seen to come into the city: and a
wench went and told them; and they
went and told king David.
18 Nevertheless a lad saw them, and
told Absalom: but they went both of
them away quickly, and came to a man's
house in [f]Bahurim, which had a well in
his court; whither they went down.
19 And the woman took and spread a
covering over the well's mouth, and
spread ground corn thereon; and the
thing was not known.
20 And when Absalom's servants
came to the woman to the house, they
said, Where *is* Ahimaaz and Jonathan?
And the woman said unto them, They be
gone over the brook of water. And when
they had sought and could not find
them, they returned to Jerusalem.
21 And it came to pass, after they were
departed, that they came up out of the
well, and went and told king David, and
said unto David, Arise, and pass quickly
over the water: for thus hath Ahithophel
counselled against you.
22 Then David arose, and all the people that *were* with him, and they passed
over Jordan: by the morning light there
lacked not one of them that was not
gone over Jordan.
23 And when Ahithophel saw that his
counsel was not followed, he saddled *his*
ass, and arose, and gat him home to his
house, to his city, and put his household
in order, and hanged himself, and died,
and was buried in the sepulchre of his
father.
24 Then David came to [g]Mahanaim.
And Absalom passed over Jordan, he
and all the men of Israel with him.
25 And Absalom made Amasa captain
of the host instead of Joab: which Amasa

a Josh. 2:11.
b Josh. 11:4; 1 Ki. 20:10.
c 2 Sam. 15:31.
d 2 Sam. 15:27, 36; 1 Ki. 1:42, 43.
e Josh. 15:7.
f 2 Sam. 16:5.
g 2 Sam. 2:8.

was a man's son, whose name *was* Ithra
an Israelite, that went in to Abigail the
daughter of Nahash, sister to Zeruiah
Joab's mother.
26 So Israel and Absalom pitched in
the land of Gilead.
27 And it came to pass, when David
was come to Mahanaim, that [a]Shobi the
son of Nahash of Rabbah of the children
of Ammon, and [b]Machir the son of
Ammiel of Lo-debar, and [c]Barzillai the
Gileadite of Rogelim,
28 Brought beds, and basons, and
earthen vessels, and wheat, and barley,
and flour, and parched *corn*, and beans,
and lentiles, and parched *pulse*,
29 And honey, and butter, and sheep,
and cheese of kine, for David, and for
the people that *were* with him, to eat: for
they said, The [d]people *is* hungry, and
weary, and thirsty, in the wilderness.

CHAPTER 18.

The battle of Mount Ephraim.

And David numbered the people that
were with him, and set captains of
thousands and captains of hundreds
over them.
2 And David sent forth a third part of
the people under the hand of Joab, and a
third part under the hand of Abishai the
son of Zeruiah, Joab's brother, and a third
part under the hand of [e]Ittai the Gittite.
And the king said unto the people, I will
surely go forth with you myself also.
3 But the [f]people answered, Thou
shalt not go forth: for if we flee away,
they will not care for us; neither if half of
us die, will they care for us: but now
thou art worth ten thousand of us: therefore now *it is* better that thou succour us
out of the city.
4 And the king said unto them, What
seemeth you best I will do. And the king
stood by the gate side, and all the people
came out by hundreds and by thousands.
5 And the king commanded Joab and
Abishai and Ittai, saying, *Deal* gently for
my sake with the young man, *even* with
Absalom. And all the people heard
when the king gave all the captains
charge concerning Absalom.
6 So the people went out into the field
against Israel: and the battle was in the
wood of Ephraim;

B.C. 1023.

a 2 Sam. 10:1.

b 2 Sam. 9:4.

c 2 Sam. 19:31, 32; 1 Ki. 2:7.

d 2 Sam. 16:2, 14.

e 2 Sam. 15:19.

f 2 Sam. 21:17.

g v. 5.

h 2 Sam. 14:19, 20.

7 Where the people of Israel were slain
before the servants of David, and there
was there a great slaughter that day of
twenty thousand *men*.
8 For the battle was there scattered
over the face of all the country: and the
wood devoured more people that day
than the sword devoured.

The slaying of Absalom.

9 And Absalom met the servants of
David. And Absalom rode upon a mule,
and the mule went under the thick
boughs of a great oak, and his head
caught hold of the oak, and he was taken
up between the heaven and the earth; and
the mule that *was* under him went away.
10 And a certain man saw *it*, and told
Joab, and said, Behold, I saw Absalom
hanged in an oak.
11 And Joab said unto the man that
told him, And, behold, thou sawest *him*,
and why didst thou not smite him there
to the ground? and I would have given
thee ten *shekels* of silver, and a girdle.
12 And the man said unto Joab, Though
I should receive a thousand *shekels* of silver in mine hand, *yet* would I not put
forth mine hand against the king's son:
for in [g]our hearing the king charged thee
and Abishai and Ittai, saying, Beware that
none *touch* the young man Absalom.
13 Otherwise I should have wrought
falsehood against mine own life: [h]for
there is no matter hid from the king, and
thou thyself wouldest have set thyself
against *me*.
14 Then said Joab, I may not tarry thus
with thee. And he took three darts in his
hand, and thrust them through the heart
of Absalom, while he *was* yet alive in the
midst of the oak.
15 And ten young men that bare
Joab's armour compassed about and
smote Absalom, and slew him.
16 And Joab blew the trumpet, and the
people returned from pursuing after
Israel: for Joab held back the people.
17 And they took Absalom, and cast
him into a great pit in the wood, and laid
a very great heap of stones upon him:
and all Israel fled every one to his tent.
18 Now Absalom in his lifetime had
taken and reared up for himself a pillar,
which *is* in the king's dale: for he said,

[1]I have no son to keep my name in remembrance: and he called the pillar after his own name: and it is called unto this day, Absalom's place.

David is told of Absalom's death.

19 Then said Ahimaaz the son of Zadok, Let me now run, and bear the king tidings, how that the LORD hath avenged him of his enemies.

20 And Joab said unto him, Thou shalt not bear tidings this day, but thou shalt bear tidings another day: but this day thou shalt bear no tidings, because the king's son is dead.

21 Then said Joab to Cushi, Go tell the king what thou hast seen. And Cushi bowed himself unto Joab, and ran.

22 Then said Ahimaaz the son of Zadok yet again to Joab, But howsoever, let me, I pray thee, also run after Cushi. And Joab said, Wherefore wilt thou run, my son, seeing that thou hast no tidings ready?

23 But howsoever, *said he*, let me run. And he said unto him, Run. Then Ahimaaz ran by the way of the plain, and overran Cushi.

24 And David [a]sat between the two gates: and the [b]watchman went up to the roof over the gate unto the wall, and lifted up his eyes, and looked, and behold a man running alone.

25 And the watchman cried, and told the king. And the king said, If he *be* alone, *there is* tidings in his mouth. And he came apace, and drew near.

26 And the watchman saw another man running: and the watchman called unto the porter, and said, Behold *another* man running alone. And the king said, He also bringeth tidings.

27 And the watchman said, Me thinketh the running of the foremost is like the running of Ahimaaz the son of Zadok. And the king said, He *is* a [c]good man, and cometh with good tidings.

28 And Ahimaaz called, and said unto the king, All is well. And he fell down to the earth upon his face before the king, and said, [d]Blessed *be* the LORD thy God, which hath delivered up the men that lifted up their hand against my lord the king.

29 And the king said, Is the young man Absalom safe? And Ahimaaz answered, When [e]Joab sent the king's servant, and *me* thy servant, I saw a great tumult, but I knew not what *it was*.

30 And the king said *unto him*, Turn aside, *and* stand here. And he turned aside, and stood still.

31 And, behold, Cushi came; and Cushi said, Tidings, my lord the king: for the LORD hath avenged thee this day of all them that rose up against thee.

32 And the king said unto Cushi, *Is* the young man Absalom safe? And Cushi answered, The enemies of my lord the king, and all that rise against thee to do *thee* hurt, be as *that* young man *is*.

The touching grief of King David.

33 And the king was much moved, and went up to the chamber over the gate, and wept: and as he went, thus he said, O my son [f]Absalom, my son, my son Absalom! would God I had died for thee, O Absalom, my son, my son!

CHAPTER 19.

Joab reproaches David.

And it was told Joab, Behold, the king weepeth and mourneth for Absalom.

2 And the victory that day was *turned* into [g]mourning unto all the people: for the people heard say that day how the king was grieved for his son.

3 And the people gat them by stealth that day into the city, as people being ashamed steal away when they flee in battle.

4 But the king covered his face, and the king cried with a loud voice, O my son Absalom, O Absalom, my son, my son!

5 And [h]Joab came into the house to the king, and said, Thou hast shamed this day the faces of all thy servants, which this day have saved thy life, and the lives of thy sons and of thy daughters, and the lives of thy wives, and the lives of thy concubines;

6 In that thou lovest thine enemies, and hatest thy friends. For thou hast declared this day, that thou regardest neither princes nor servants: for this day

B.C. 1023.

a 1 Sam 4:13.
b 2 Ki. 9:17.
c 1 Ki. 1:42.
d 2 Sam. 16:12.
e vs. 14-17.
f 2 Sam. 12:10.
g Jud. 21:2.
h 2 Sam. 18:14.

[1] **(18:18)** The pillar mentioned must have been reared before the birth of sons to Absalom. Cf. 2 Sam. 14:27. Another view is that his sons died in youth. They are not mentioned in the genealogies.

I perceive, that if Absalom had lived,
and all we had died this day, then it had
pleased thee well.
7 Now therefore arise, go forth, and
speak comfortably unto thy servants: for
I swear by the LORD, if thou go not forth,
there will not tarry one with thee this
night: and that will be worse unto thee
than all the evil that befell thee from thy
youth until now.
8 Then the king arose, and sat in the
gate. And they told unto all the people,
saying, Behold, the king doth sit in the
gate. And all the people came before the
king: for Israel had [a]fled every man to
his tent.

David's return to Jerusalem.

9 And all the people were at strife
throughout all the tribes of Israel, saying, The king saved us out of the hand of
our enemies, and he delivered us out of
the hand of the Philistines; and now [b]he
is fled out of the land for Absalom.
10 And Absalom, whom we anointed
over us, is dead in battle. Now therefore
why speak ye not a word of bringing the
king back?
11 And king David sent to Zadok and
to Abiathar the priests, saying, Speak
unto the elders of Judah, saying, Why
are ye the last to bring the king back to
his house? seeing the speech of all Israel
is come to the king, *even* to his house.
12 Ye *are* my brethren, ye *are* my
[c]bones and my flesh: wherefore then are
ye the last to bring back the king?
13 And say ye to [d]Amasa, *Art* thou not
of my bone, and of my flesh? God do so
to me, and more also, if thou be not captain of the host before me continually in
the room of Joab.
14 And he bowed the heart of all the
men of Judah, even as *the heart of* one
man; so that they sent *this word* unto the
king, Return thou, and all thy servants.
15 So the king returned, and came to
Jordan. And Judah came to [e]Gilgal, to go
to meet the king, to conduct the king
over Jordan.
16 And Shimei the son of Gera, a
Benjamite, which *was* of Bahurim, hasted
and came down with the men of Judah
to meet king David.
17 And *there were* a thousand men of
Benjamin with him, and [f]Ziba the servant
of the house of Saul, and his fifteen sons
and his twenty servants with him; and
they went over Jordan before the king.
18 And there went over a ferry boat to
carry over the king's household, and to
do what he thought good. And Shimei
the son of Gera fell down before the
king, as he was come over Jordan;
19 And said unto the king, Let not my
lord [g]impute iniquity unto me, neither
do thou remember that which thy servant did [h]perversely the day that my
lord the king went out of Jerusalem, that
the king should take it to his [i]heart.
20 For thy servant doth know that I
have sinned: therefore, behold, I am come
the first this day of all the house of Joseph
to go down to meet my lord the king.
21 But Abishai the son of Zeruiah
answered and said, Shall not Shimei be
put to death for this, because he [j]cursed
the LORD'S anointed?
22 And David said, What have I to do
with you, ye sons of Zeruiah, that ye
should this day be adversaries unto me?
shall there any man be put to death this
day in Israel? for do not I know that I *am*
this day king over Israel?
23 Therefore the king said unto
Shimei, Thou shalt not die. And the king
sware unto him.
24 And Mephibosheth the son of Saul
came down to meet the king, and had
neither dressed his feet, nor trimmed his
beard, nor washed his clothes, from the
day the king departed until the day he
came *again* in peace.
25 And it came to pass, when he was
come to Jerusalem to meet the king, that
the king said unto him, Wherefore wentest not thou with me, Mephibosheth?
26 And he answered, My lord, O king,
my servant deceived me: for thy servant
said, I will saddle me an ass, that I may
ride thereon, and go to the king; because
thy servant *is* lame.
27 And he hath slandered thy servant
unto my lord the king; but my lord the
king *is* as an [k]angel of God: do therefore
what is good in thine eyes.
28 For all *of* my father's house were
but dead men before my lord the king:
yet didst thou [l]set thy servant among
them that did eat at thine own table.
What right therefore have I yet to cry
any more unto the king?

B.C. 1023.

a 2 Sam. 18:6, 8, 17.
b 2 Sam. 15:14.
c 2 Sam. 5:1; 1 Chr. 11:1.
d 2 Sam. 17:25; 1 Chr. 2:17.
e Josh. 5:9.
f 2 Sam. 9:2, 10.
g *Imputation.* vs. 18, 19; Psa. 32:2. (Lev. 25:50; Jas. 2:23.)
h 2 Sam. 16:5.
i 2 Sam. 13:33.
j 1 Sam. 26:9.
k Heb. 1:4, *note.*
l 2 Sam. 9:7, 10, 13.

29 And the king said unto him, Why speakest thou any more of thy matters? I have said, Thou and Ziba divide the land.

30 And Mephibosheth said unto the king, Yea, let him take all, forasmuch as my lord the king is come again in peace unto his own house.

31 And Barzillai the Gileadite came down from Rogelim, and went over Jordan with the king, to conduct him over Jordan.

32 Now Barzillai was a very aged man, *even* fourscore years old: and he had provided the king of sustenance while he lay at Mahanaim; for he *was* a very great man.

33 And the king said unto Barzillai, Come thou over with me, and I will feed thee with me in Jerusalem.

34 And Barzillai said unto the king, How long have I to live, that I should go up with the king unto Jerusalem?

35 I *am* this day fourscore years old: *and* can I discern between good and evil? can thy servant taste what I eat or what I drink? can I hear any more the voice of singing men and singing women? wherefore then should thy servant be yet a burden unto my lord the king?

36 Thy servant will go a little way over Jordan with the king: and why should the king recompense it me with such a reward?

37 Let thy servant, I pray thee, turn back again, that I may die in mine own city, *and be buried* by the grave of my father and of my mother. But behold thy servant [a]Chimham; let him go over with my lord the king; and do to him what shall seem good unto thee.

38 And the king answered, Chimham shall go over with me, and I will do to him that which shall seem good unto thee: and whatsoever thou shalt require of me, *that* will I do for thee.

39 And all the people went over Jordan. And when the king was come over, the king kissed Barzillai, and blessed him; and he returned unto his own place.

40 Then the king went on to Gilgal, and Chimham went on with him: and all the people of Judah conducted the king, and also half the people of Israel.

The old strife begins anew.

41 And, behold, all the men of Israel came to the king, and said unto the king, Why have our brethren the men of Judah stolen thee away, and have [b]brought the king, and his household, and all David's men with him, over Jordan?

42 And all the men of Judah answered the men of Israel, Because the king *is* near of kin to us: wherefore then be ye angry for this matter? have we eaten at all of the king's *cost*? or hath he given us any gift?

43 And the men of Israel answered the men of Judah, and said, We have ten parts in the king, and we have also more *right* in David than ye: why then did ye despise us, that our advice should not be first had in bringing back our king? And the words of the men of Judah were fiercer than the words of the men of Israel.

CHAPTER 20.

And there happened to be there a man of Belial, whose name *was* Sheba, the son of Bichri, a Benjamite: and he blew a trumpet, and said, We have no [c]part in David, neither have we inheritance in the son of Jesse: every man to his tents, O Israel.

2 So every man of Israel went up from after David, *and* followed Sheba the son of Bichri: but the men of Judah clave unto their king, from Jordan even to Jerusalem.

3 And David came to his house at Jerusalem; and the king took the ten women *his* [d]concubines, whom he had left to keep the house, and put them in ward, and fed them, but went not in unto them. So they were shut up unto the day of their death, living in widowhood.

Joab murders Amasa.

4 Then said the king to Amasa, Assemble me the men of Judah within three days, and be thou here present.

5 So Amasa went to [e]assemble *the men of* Judah: but he tarried longer than the set time which he had appointed him.

6 And David said to Abishai, Now shall Sheba the son of Bichri do us more harm than *did* Absalom: take thou thy lord's servants, and pursue after him, lest he get him fenced cities, and escape us.

7 And there went out after him Joab's men, and the Cherethites, and the Pelethites, and all the mighty men: and

B.C. 1023.

a 1 Ki. 2:7; Jer. 41:17.
b vs. 11, 15.
c 1 Ki. 12:16.
d 2 Sam. 15:16.
e 2 Sam. 19:13.

they went out of Jerusalem, to pursue
after Sheba the son of Bichri.
8 When they *were* at the great stone
which *is* in Gibeon, Amasa went before
them. And Joab's garment that he had
put on was girded unto him, and upon it
a girdle *with* a sword fastened upon his
loins in the sheath thereof; and as he
went forth it fell out.
9 And Joab said to Amasa, *Art* thou in
health, my brother? And Joab took
Amasa by the beard with the right hand
to kiss him.
10 But Amasa took no heed to the
sword that *was* in Joab's hand: so he
[a]smote him therewith in the fifth *rib*, and
shed out his bowels to the ground, and
struck him not again; and he died. So
Joab and Abishai his brother pursued
after Sheba the son of Bichri.
11 And one of Joab's men stood by him,
and said, He that favoureth Joab, and he
that *is* for David, *let him go* after Joab.
12 And Amasa wallowed in blood in
the midst of the highway. And when the
man saw that all the people stood still,
he removed Amasa out of the highway
into the field, and cast a cloth upon him,
when he saw that every one that came
by him stood still.

Suppression of Sheba's revolt.

13 When he was removed out of the
highway, all the people went on after
Joab, to pursue after Sheba the son of
Bichri.
14 And he went through all the tribes
of Israel unto [b]Abel, and to Beth-
maachah, and all the Berites: and they
were gathered together, and went also
after him.
15 And they came and besieged him in
Abel of Beth-maachah, and they cast up a
[c]bank against the city, and it stood in the
trench: and all the people that *were* with
Joab battered the wall, to throw it down.
16 Then cried a wise woman out of the
city, Hear, hear; say, I pray you, unto
Joab, Come near hither, that I may speak
with thee.
17 And when he was come near unto
her, the woman said, *Art* thou Joab? And
he answered, I *am he*. Then she said unto
him, Hear the words of thine handmaid.
And he answered, I do hear.
18 Then she spake, saying, They were
wont to speak in old time, saying, They
shall surely ask *counsel* at Abel: and so
they ended *the matter*.
19 I *am one of them that are* peaceable
and faithful in Israel: thou seekest to
destroy a city and a mother in Israel:
why wilt thou swallow up the inheritance of the LORD?
20 And Joab answered and said, Far
be it, far be it from me, that I should
swallow up or destroy.
21 The matter *is* not so: but a man of
mount Ephraim, Sheba the son of Bichri
by name, hath lifted up his hand against
the king, *even* against David: deliver him
only, and I will depart from the city. And
the woman said unto Joab, Behold, his
head shall be thrown to thee over the
wall.
22 Then the woman went unto all the
people in her wisdom. And they cut off
the head of Sheba the son of Bichri, and
cast *it* out to Joab. And he blew a trumpet, and they retired from the city, every
man to his tent. And Joab returned to
Jerusalem unto the king.
23 Now [d]Joab *was* over all the host of
Israel: and Benaiah the son of Jehoiada
was over the Cherethites and over the
Pelethites:
24 And Adoram *was* over the [e]tribute:
and Jehoshaphat the son of Ahilud *was*
recorder:
25 And Sheva *was* scribe: and Zadok
and Abiathar *were* the priests:
26 And Ira also the Jairite was a chief
ruler about David.

CHAPTER 21.

The three years' famine.

Then there was a famine in the days of
David three years, year after year;
and David enquired of the LORD. And
the LORD answered, *It is* for Saul, and for
his bloody house, because he slew the
Gibeonites.
2 And the king called the Gibeonites,
and said unto them; (now the Gibeonites
were [f]not of the children of Israel, but of
the remnant of the Amorites; and the
children of Israel had sworn unto them:
and Saul sought to slay them in his zeal
to the children of Israel and Judah.)
3 Wherefore David said unto the
Gibeonites, What shall I do for you? and
wherewith shall I make the [g]atonement,
that ye may bless the inheritance of the
LORD?

B.C. 1022.

a 1 Ki. 2:5; 2 Sam. 3:27.
b 2 Ki. 15:29.
c 2 Ki. 19:32.
d 2 Sam. 8:16, 18.
e 1 Ki. 4:6.
f Josh. 9:3, 21.
g See Ex. 29:33, *note.*

4 And the Gibeonites said unto him, We will have no silver nor gold of Saul, nor of his house; neither for us shalt thou kill any man in Israel. And he said, What ye shall say, *that* will I do for you.

5 And they answered the king, The man that consumed us, and that devised against us *that* we should be destroyed from remaining in any of the coasts of Israel,

6 Let seven men of his sons be delivered unto us, and we will hang them up unto the LORD in [a]Gibeah of Saul, *whom* the LORD did choose. And the king said, I will give *them*.

7 But the king spared Mephibosheth, the son of Jonathan the son of Saul, because of the [b]LORD'S oath that *was* between them, between David and Jonathan the son of Saul.

8 But the king took the two sons of Rizpah the daughter of Aiah, whom she bare unto Saul, Armoni and Mephibosheth; and the five [c]sons of Michal the daughter of Saul, whom she brought up for Adriel the son of Barzillai the Meholathite:

9 And he delivered them into the hands of the Gibeonites, and they hanged them in the hill before the LORD: and they fell *all* seven together, and were put to death in the days of harvest, in the first *days*, in the beginning of barley harvest.

10 And Rizpah the daughter of Aiah took sackcloth, and spread it for her upon the rock, from the beginning of harvest until water dropped upon them out of heaven, and suffered neither the birds of the air to rest on them by day, nor the beasts of the field by night.

11 And it was told David what Rizpah the daughter of Aiah, the concubine of Saul, had done.

12 And David went and took the bones of Saul and the bones of Jonathan his son from the men of Jabesh-gilead, which had stolen them from the street of Beth-shan, where the [d]Philistines had hanged them, when the Philistines had slain Saul in Gilboa:

13 And he brought up from thence the bones of Saul and the bones of Jonathan his son; and they gathered the bones of them that were hanged.

14 And the bones of Saul and Jonathan his son buried they in the country of Benjamin in [e]Zelah, in the sepulchre of Kish his father: and they performed all that the king commanded. And after that God was [f]intreated for the land.

A war with the Philistines.

15 Moreover the Philistines had yet war again with Israel; and David went down, and his servants with him, and fought against the Philistines: and David waxed faint.

16 And Ishbi-benob, which *was* of the sons of the giant, the weight of whose spear *weighed* three hundred *shekels* of brass in weight, he being girded with a new *sword*, thought to have slain David.

17 But Abishai the son of Zeruiah succoured him, and smote the Philistine, and killed him. Then the men of David sware unto him, saying, [g]Thou shalt go no more out with us to battle, that thou quench not the [h]light of Israel.

18 And it came to pass after this, that there was again a battle with the Philistines at Gob: then [i]Sibbechai the Hushathite slew Saph, which *was* of the sons of the giant.

19 And there was again a battle in Gob with the Philistines, where Elhanan the son of Jaare-oregim, a Beth-lehemite, slew *the brother of* Goliath the Gittite, the staff of whose spear *was* like a weaver's beam.

20 And there was yet a battle in Gath, where was a man of *great* stature, that had on every hand six fingers, and on every foot six toes, four and twenty in number; and he also was born to the giant.

21 And when he defied Israel, Jonathan the son of [j]Shimea the brother of David slew him.

22 These four were born to the giant in Gath, and fell by the hand of David, and by the hand of his servants.

CHAPTER 22.

David's song of deliverance.

And David spake unto the LORD the words of this [k]song in the day *that* the LORD had delivered him out of the hand of all his enemies, and out of the hand of Saul:

2 And he said, The LORD *is* my rock, and my [l]fortress, and my deliverer;

3 The God of my rock; in him will I [m]trust: *he is* my [n]shield, and the horn of

B.C. 1021.

a 1 Sam. 10:26.
b 1 Sam. 20:15.
c Cf. 2 Sam. 6:23. The "five sons" were children of Michal's sister Merab, wife of Adriel, "whom she brought up for Adriel," (1 Sam. 18:19).
d Cf. 1 Sam. 31:4, 5, *note*.
e Josh, 18:28.
f 2 Sam. 24:25.
g 2 Sam. 18:3.
h 1 Ki. 11:36.
i 1 Chr. 20:4.
j 1 Sam. 16:9, *Shammah*.
k Psa. 18.
l Psa. 91:2.
m Psa. 2:12, *note*.
n Psa. 84:11.

my salvation, my high tower, and my
[a]refuge, my saviour; thou savest me
from violence.
4 I will call on the LORD, *who is* worthy
to be praised: so shall I be saved from
mine enemies.
5 When the waves of death compassed
me, the floods of ungodly men made me
afraid;
6 The sorrows of hell compassed me
about; the snares of death prevented me;
7 In my distress I called upon the
LORD, and cried to my God: and he did
[b]hear my voice out of his temple, and
my cry *did enter* into his ears.
8 Then the earth shook and trembled;
the foundations of heaven moved and
shook, because he was wroth.
9 There went up a smoke out of his
nostrils, and [c]fire out of his mouth
devoured: coals were kindled by it.
10 He bowed the heavens also, and
came down; and darkness *was* under his
feet.
11 And he rode upon a cherub, and
did fly: and he was seen upon the wings
of the wind.
12 And he made darkness pavilions
round about him, dark waters, *and* thick
clouds of the skies.
13 Through the brightness before him
were coals of fire kindled.
14 The LORD [d]thundered from heaven,
and the most High uttered his voice.
15 And he sent out [e]arrows, and scattered them; lightning, and discomfited
them.
16 And the channels of [f]the sea
appeared, the foundations of the world
were discovered, at the rebuking of the
LORD, at the blast of the breath of his
nostrils.
17 He sent from above, he took me; he
drew me out of many [g]waters;
18 He delivered me from my strong
enemy, *and* from them that hated me: for
they were too strong for me.
19 They prevented me in the day of
my calamity: but the LORD was my stay.
20 He brought me forth also into a
large place: he delivered me, because he
delighted in [h]me.
21 The LORD rewarded me [i]according
to my righteousness: according to the

B.C. 1018.

a Psa. 46:1, 7, 11.
b Psa. 34:6, 15.
c Psa. 97:3, 4.
d Psa. 29:3.
e Deut. 32:23.
f Nah. 1:4.
g Isa. 43:2.
h 2 Sam. 15:26.
i 1 Sam. 26:23.
j Job 17:9.
k Psa. 2:12, *note.*
l Hab. 3:19.

[j]cleanness of my hands hath he recompensed me.
22 For I have kept the ways of the
LORD, and have not wickedly departed
from my God.
23 For all his judgments *were* before
me: and *as for* his statutes, I did not
depart from them.
24 I was also upright before him, and
have kept myself from mine iniquity.
25 Therefore the LORD hath recompensed me according to my righteousness; according to my cleanness in his
eye sight.
26 With the merciful thou wilt shew
thyself merciful, *and* with the upright
man thou wilt shew thyself upright.
27 With the pure thou wilt shew thyself pure; and with the froward thou wilt
shew thyself unsavoury.
28 And the afflicted people thou wilt
save: but thine eyes *are* upon the haughty,
that thou mayest bring *them* down.
29 For thou *art* my lamp, O LORD: and
the LORD will lighten my darkness.
30 For by thee I have run through a
troop: by my God have I leaped over a
wall.
31 *As for* God, his way *is* perfect; the
word of the LORD *is* tried: he *is* a buckler
to all them that [k]trust in him.
32 For who *is* God, save the LORD? and
who *is* a rock, save our God?
33 God *is* my strength *and* power: and
he maketh my way perfect.
34 He maketh my [l]feet like hinds' *feet*:
and setteth me upon my high places.
35 He teacheth my hands to war; so that
a bow of steel is broken by mine arms.
36 Thou hast also given me the shield
of thy salvation: and thy gentleness hath
made me great.
37 Thou hast enlarged my steps under
me; so that my feet did not slip.
38 I have pursued mine enemies, and
destroyed them; and turned not again
until I had consumed them.
39 And I have consumed them, and
wounded them, that they could not
arise: yea, they are fallen under my feet.
40 For thou hast girded me with
strength to battle: them that rose up
against me hast thou subdued under me.
41 Thou hast also given me the necks
of mine enemies, that I might destroy
them that hate me.

B.C. 1018.

42 They looked, but *there was* none to save; *even* unto the LORD, but he answered them not.

43 Then did I beat them as small as the dust of the earth, I did stamp them as the mire of the street, *and* did spread them abroad.

44 Thou also hast delivered me from the [a]strivings of my people, thou hast kept me *to be* head of the [b]heathen: a people *which* I knew not shall serve me.

45 Strangers shall submit themselves unto me: as soon as they hear, they shall be obedient unto me.

46 Strangers shall fade away, and they shall be afraid out of their close places.

47 The LORD liveth; and blessed *be* my rock; and exalted be the God of the rock of my salvation.

48 It *is* God that avengeth me, and that bringeth down the people under me,

49 And that bringeth me forth from mine enemies: thou also hast lifted me up on high above them that rose up against me: thou hast delivered me from the violent man.

50 Therefore I will give thanks unto thee, O LORD, among the [b]heathen, and I will sing praises unto thy name.

51 *He is* the tower of salvation for his king: and sheweth mercy to his anointed, unto David, and to his seed for evermore.

CHAPTER 23.

The last words of David.

NOW these *be* the last words of David. [c]David the son of Jesse said, and the man *who was* raised up on high, the anointed of the God of Jacob, and the sweet psalmist of Israel, said,

2 The [d]Spirit of the LORD spake by me, and his [e]word *was* in my tongue.

3 The God of Israel said, the Rock of Israel spake to me, He that ruleth over men *must be* just, ruling in the [f]fear of God.

4 And *he shall be* as the light of the morning, *when* the sun riseth, *even* a morning without clouds; *as* the tender grass *springing* out of the earth by clear shining after rain.

5 Although my house *be* not so with God; yet he hath made with me an everlasting covenant, ordered in all *things*, and sure: for *this is* all my salvation, and all *my* desire, although he make *it* not to grow.

6 But *the sons* of Belial *shall be* all of them as thorns thrust away, because they cannot be taken with hands:

7 But the man *that* shall touch them must be fenced with iron and the staff of a spear; and they shall be utterly burned with fire in the *same* place.

David's mighty men. (Cf. 1 Chr. 11:10-47.)

8 These *be* the names of the mighty men whom David had: The Tachmonite that sat in the seat, chief among the captains; the same *was* Adino the [g]Eznite: *he lift up his spear* against eight hundred, whom he slew at one time.

9 And after him *was* Eleazar the son of Dodo the Ahohite, *one* of the three mighty men with David, when they defied the Philistines *that* were there gathered together to battle, and the men of Israel were gone away:

10 He arose, and smote the Philistines until his hand was [h]weary, and his hand clave unto the sword: and the LORD wrought a great victory that day; and the people returned after him only to [i]spoil.

11 And after him *was* Shammah the son of Agee the Hararite. And the Philistines were gathered together into a troop, where was a piece of ground full of lentiles: and the people [j]fled from the Philistines.

12 But he stood in the midst of the ground, and defended it, and slew the Philistines: and the LORD wrought a great victory.

13 And [k]three of the thirty chief went down, and came to David in the harvest time unto the cave of Adullam: and the troop of the Philistines pitched in the valley of Rephaim.

14 And David *was* then in an hold, and the garrison of the Philistines *was* then *in* Beth-lehem.

15 And David longed, and said, Oh that one would give me drink of the water of the well of Beth-lehem, which *is* by the gate!

16 And the three mighty men brake through the host of the Philistines, and drew water out of the well of Beth-lehem, that *was* by the gate, and took *it*, and brought *it* to David: nevertheless he would not drink thereof, but poured it out unto the LORD.

a 2 Sam. 3:1.

b i.e. *nations.*

c *Kingdom.* (O.T.) vs. 1-5; 1 Ki. 8:20. (Gen. 1:26; Zech. 12:8.)

d *Holy Spirit.* 2 Ki. 2:9. (Gen. 1:2; Mal. 2:15.)

e *Inspiration.* Job 6:10. (Ex. 4:15; Rev. 22:19.)

f Psa. 19:9, *note.*

g i.e. *one belonging to Etsen.*

h Jud. 8:4.

i 1 Sam. 30:24, 25.

j 1 Sam. 17:24.

k See 2 Sam. 5:18; 1 Chr. 11:15-19.

17 And he said, Be it far from me, O
LORD, that I should do this: *is not this* the
blood of the men that went in jeopardy
of their lives? therefore he would not
drink it. These things did these three
mighty men.
18 And Abishai, the brother of Joab,
the son of Zeruiah, was chief among
three. And he lifted up his spear against
three hundred, *and* slew *them*, and had
the name among three.
19 Was he not most honourable of
three? therefore he was their captain:
howbeit he attained not unto the *first*
three.
20 And Benaiah the son of Jehoiada,
the son of a valiant man, of Kabzeel,
who had done many acts, he slew two
lionlike men of Moab: [a]he went down
also and slew a lion in the midst of a pit
in time of snow:
21 And he slew an Egyptian, a [b]good-
ly man: and the Egyptian had a spear in
his hand; but he went down to him with
a staff, and plucked the spear out of the
Egyptian's hand, and slew him with his
own spear.
22 These *things* did Benaiah the son of
Jehoiada, and had the name among three
mighty men.
23 He was more honourable than the
thirty, but he attained not to the *first*
three. And David set him [c]over his guard.
24 [d]Asahel the brother of Joab *was* one
of the thirty; Elhanan the son of Dodo of
Beth-lehem,
25 Shammah the Harodite, Elika the
Harodite,
26 Helez the Paltite, Ira the son of
Ikkesh the Tekoite,
27 Abiezer the Anethothite, Mebunnai
the Hushathite,
28 Zalmon the Ahohite, Maharai the
Netophathite,
29 Heleb the son of Baanah, a
Netophathite, Ittai the son of Ribai out
of Gibeah of the children of Benjamin,
30 Benaiah the Pirathonite, Hiddai of
the brooks of [e]Gaash,
31 Abi-albon the Arbathite, Azmaveth
the Barhumite,
32 Eliahba the Shaalbonite, of the sons
of Jashen, Jonathan,
33 Shammah the Hararite, Ahiam the
son of Sharar the Hararite,
34 Eliphelet the son of Ahasbai, the
son of the Maachathite, Eliam the son of
Ahithophel the Gilonite,
35 Hezrai the Carmelite, Paarai the
Arbite,
36 Igal the son of Nathan of Zobah,
Bani the Gadite,
37 Zelek the Ammonite, Naharai the
Beerothite, armourbearer to Joab the son
of Zeruiah,
38 [f]Ira an Ithrite, Gareb an Ithrite,
39 [g]Uriah the Hittite: thirty and seven
in all.

CHAPTER 24.

David's sin in numbering the people
(1 Chr. 21:1-6).

AND [h]again the anger of the LORD was
kindled against Israel, and [i]he
moved David against them to say, Go,
number Israel and Judah.
2 For the king said to Joab the captain
of the host, which *was* with him, Go now
through all the tribes of Israel, [j]from Dan
even to Beer-sheba, and number ye the
people, that [k]I may know the number of
the people.
3 And Joab said unto the king, Now
the LORD thy God add unto the people,
how many soever they be, an hundredfold, and that the eyes of my lord the
king may see *it*: but why doth my lord
the king delight in this thing?
4 Notwithstanding the king's word
prevailed against Joab, and against the
captains of the host. And Joab and the
captains of the host went out from the
presence of the king, to number the people of Israel.
5 And they passed over Jordan, and
pitched in [l]Aroer, on the right side of the
city that *lieth* in the midst of the river of
Gad, and toward [m]Jazer:
6 Then they came to Gilead, and to the
land of Tahtim-hodshi; and they came to
Dan-jaan, and about to [n]Zidon,
7 And came to the strong hold of Tyre,
and to all the cities of the Hivites, and of
the Canaanites: and they went out to the
south of Judah, *even* to Beer-sheba.
8 So when they had gone through all
the land, they came to Jerusalem at the
end of nine months and twenty days.
9 And Joab gave up the sum of the
number of the people unto the king: and
there were [1]in Israel eight hundred

B.C. 1018.

a Ex. 15:15; 1 Chr. 11:22.
b 1 Chr. 11:23.
c 2 Sam. 8:18; 20:23.
d 2 Sam. 2:18.
e Jud. 2:9.
f 2 Sam. 20:26.
g 2 Sam. 11:3, 6.
h 2 Sam. 21:1.
i 1 Chr. 21:1.
j Jud. 20:1.
k Jer. 17:5.
l Deut. 2:36; Josh. 13:9.
m Num. 32:1, 3.
n Josh. 19:28; Jud. 18:28.

1(24:9) Cf. 1 Chr. 21:5. The total military strength of Israel (the northern kingdom) was 1,100,000, and of Judah 500,000. The numbers actually set in array were, of Israel, 800,000; of Judah, 470,000.

thousand valiant men that drew the
sword; and the men of Judah *were* five
hundred thousand men.

David's choice of punishment
(1 Chr. 21:7-17).

10 And David's heart smote him after
that he had numbered the people. And
[a]David said unto the LORD, I have
sinned greatly in that I have done: and
now, I beseech thee, O LORD, take away
the iniquity of thy servant; for I have
done very foolishly.
11 For when David was up in the
morning, the word of the LORD came
unto the prophet [b]Gad, David's seer,
saying,
12 Go and say unto David, Thus saith
the LORD, I offer thee three *things*; choose
thee one of them, that I may *do it* unto
thee.
13 So Gad came to David, and told
him, and said unto him, Shall seven
years of [c]famine come unto thee in thy
land? or wilt thou flee three months
before thine enemies, while they pursue
thee? or that there be three days' pestilence in thy land? now advise, and see
what answer I shall return to him that
sent me.
14 And David said unto Gad, I am in a
great strait: let us fall now into the hand
of the LORD; for his mercies *are* great:
and let me not fall into the hand of man.
15 So the LORD sent a pestilence upon
Israel from the morning even to the time
appointed: and there died of the people
from Dan even to Beer-sheba seventy
thousand men.
16 And when the [d]angel stretched out
his hand upon Jerusalem to destroy it,
the LORD [e]repented him of the evil, and
said to the angel that destroyed the people, It is enough: stay now thine hand.
And the angel of the LORD was by the
threshingplace of Araunah the Jebusite.
17 And David [f]spake unto the LORD
when he saw the angel that smote the
people, and said, Lo, I have sinned, and
I have done wickedly: but these sheep,
what have they done? let thine hand, I
pray thee, be against me, and against my
father's house.

David buys Araunah's threshingfloor;
erects and altar (1 Chr. 21:18-30).

18 And Gad came that day to David,
and said unto him, Go up, rear an altar
unto the LORD in the threshingfloor of
Araunah the Jebusite.
19 And David, according to the saying
of Gad, went up as the LORD commanded.
20 And Araunah looked, and [g]saw the
king and his servants coming on toward
him: and Araunah went out, and bowed
himself before the king on his face upon
the ground.
21 And Araunah said, Wherefore is
my lord the king come to his servant?
And David said, To buy the threshingfloor of thee, to build an altar unto
the LORD, that the plague may be stayed
from the people.
22 And Araunah said unto David, Let
my lord the king take and offer up what
seemeth good unto him: behold, *here be*
oxen for burnt sacrifice, and threshing
instruments and *other* instruments of the
oxen for wood.
23 All these *things* did Araunah, *as* a
king, give unto the king. And Araunah
said unto the king, The LORD thy God
accept thee.
24 And the king said unto Araunah,
Nay; but I will surely buy *it* of thee at a
price: neither will I [h]offer burnt-offerings
unto the LORD my God of that which
doth cost me nothing. So David bought
the [i]threshingfloor and the oxen for fifty
[j]shekels of silver.
25 And David built there an altar unto
the LORD, and offered burnt-offerings
and peace-offerings. So the LORD was
intreated for the land, and the plague
was stayed from Israel.

B.C. 1017.

a 1 Sam. 24:5.
b 1 Sam. 9:9; 1 Chr. 29:29.
c Gen. 12:10, *note.*
d Heb. 1:4, *note.*
e Zech. 8:14, *note.*
f *Bible prayers* (O.T.). 1 Ki. 3:5-9. (Gen. 15:2; Hab. 3:1-16.)
g Here read 1 Chr. 21:20.
h 2 Cor. 8:1, *note.*
i Cf. 1 Chr. 21:25, *note.*
j One shekel = 2*s.* 9*d.*, or 65 cts.

THE FIRST BOOK OF THE KINGS

COMMONLY CALLED
THE THIRD BOOK OF THE KINGS

FIRST KINGS records the death of David, the reign of Solomon, the building of the temple, death of Solomon, division of the kingdom under Rehoboam and Jeroboam, and the history of the two kingdoms to the reign of Jehoram over Judah, and Ahaziah over Samaria. Includes the mighty ministry of Elijah.

The book is in seven parts: I. From the rebellion of Adonijah to the death of David, 1:1–2:11. II. From the accession of Solomon to the dedication of the temple, 2:12–8:66. III. From the confirmation of the Davidic Covenant to the death of Solomon, 9:1–11:43. IV. From the division of the kingdom to the death of Jeroboam and Rehoboam, 12:1–14:31. V. The kingdoms to the accession of Ahab, 15:1–16:28. VI. Accession of Ahab to his death, 16:29–22:40. VII. From the reign of Jehoshaphat to the accession of Jehoram over Judah, and Ahaziah over Samaria, 22:41-53.

The events recorded in First Kings cover a period of 118 years (Ussher).

CHAPTER 1.

David's declining strength.

NOW king David was old *and* stricken
in years; and they covered him
with clothes, but he gat no heat.
2 Wherefore his servants said unto
him, Let there be sought for my lord the
king a young virgin: and let her stand
before the king, and let her cherish him,
and let her lie in thy bosom, that my lord
the king may get heat.
3 So they sought for a fair damsel
throughout all the coasts of Israel, and
found Abishag a [a]Shunammite, and
brought her to the king.
4 And the damsel *was* very fair, and
cherished the king, and ministered to
him: but the king knew her not.

Adonijah plots to seize the kingdom.

5 Then Adonijah [b]the son of Haggith
exalted himself, saying, I will be king:
and [c]he prepared him chariots and
horsemen, and fifty men to run before
him.
6 And his father had not displeased
him at any time in saying, Why hast
thou done so? and he also *was a* very
goodly *man*; [d]and *his mother* bare him
after Absalom.
7 And he conferred with Joab the son
of Zeruiah, and with [e]Abiathar the priest:
and [f]they following Adonijah helped *him*.
8 But Zadok the priest, and Benaiah
the son of Jehoiada, and Nathan the
prophet, and [g]Shimei, and Rei, and the
[h]mighty men which *belonged* to David,
were not with Adonijah.
9 And Adonijah slew sheep and oxen
and fat cattle by the stone of Zoheleth,
which *is* by En-rogel, and called all his
brethren the king's sons, and all the men
of Judah the king's servants:

The counter-plot of Nathan and Bath-sheba.

10 But Nathan the prophet, and Benaiah,
and the mighty men, and Solomon
his brother, he called not.
11 Wherefore Nathan spake unto Bath-
sheba the mother of Solomon, saying,
Hast thou not heard that Adonijah the
son of [i]Haggith doth reign, and David
our lord knoweth *it* not?
12 Now therefore come, let me, I pray
thee, give thee counsel, that thou mayest
save thine own life, and the life of thy
son Solomon.
13 Go and get thee in unto king David,
and say unto him, Didst not thou, my
lord, O king, swear unto thine handmaid,
saying, [j]Assuredly Solomon thy son shall
reign after me, and he shall sit upon my
throne? why then doth Adonijah reign?
14 Behold, while thou yet talkest there
with the king, I also will come in after
thee, and confirm thy words.
15 And Bath-sheba went in unto the
king into the chamber: and the king was
very old; and Abishag the Shunammite
ministered unto the king.
16 And Bath-sheba bowed, and did
obeisance unto the king. And the king
said, What wouldest thou?
17 And she said unto him, My

B.C. 1015.

a Josh. 19:18.
b 2 Sam. 3:4.
c 2 Sam. 15:1.
d 2 Sam. 3:3, 4.
e 1 Sam. 22:20-23; 2 Sam. 20:25.
f 1 Ki. 2:22, 28.
g 1 Ki. 4:18.
h 2 Sam. 23:8.
i 2 Sam. 3:4.
j 1 Chr. 22:9, 10.

lord, thou swarest by the LORD thy God
unto thine handmaid, *saying*, Assuredly
Solomon thy son shall reign after me,
and he shall sit upon my throne.
18 And now, behold, Adonijah
reigneth; and now, my lord the king,
thou knowest *it* not:
19 And he hath slain oxen and fat cattle and sheep in abundance, and hath
called all the sons of the king, and
Abiathar the priest, and Joab the captain
of the host: but Solomon thy servant
hath he not called.
20 And thou, my lord, O king, the eyes
of all Israel *are* upon thee, that thou
shouldest tell them who shall sit on the
throne of my lord the king after him.
21 Otherwise it shall come to pass,
when my lord the king shall [a]sleep with
his fathers, that I and my son Solomon
shall be counted offenders.
22 And, lo, while she yet talked with
the king, Nathan the prophet also came
in.
23 And they told the king, saying,
Behold Nathan the prophet. And when
he was come in before the king, he
bowed himself before the king with his
face to the ground.
24 And Nathan said, My lord, O king,
hast thou said, Adonijah shall reign after
me, and he shall sit upon my throne?
25 For he is gone down this day, and
hath slain oxen and fat cattle and sheep
in abundance, and hath called all the
king's sons, and the captains of the host,
and Abiathar the priest; and, behold,
they eat and drink before him, and say,
God save king Adonijah.
26 But me, *even* me thy servant, and
Zadok the priest, and Benaiah the son of
Jehoiada, and thy servant Solomon, hath
he not called.
27 Is this thing done by my lord the
king, and thou hast not shewed *it* unto
thy servant, who should sit on the
throne of my lord the king after him?
28 Then king David answered and
said, Call me Bath-sheba. And she came
into the king's presence, and stood
before the king.
29 And the king sware, and said, [b]*As*
the LORD liveth, that hath [c]redeemed my
soul out of all distress,
30 Even as I sware unto thee by the
LORD God of Israel, saying, Assuredly
Solomon thy son shall reign after me,
and he shall sit upon my throne in my
stead; even so will I certainly do this day.
31 Then Bath-sheba bowed with *her*
face to the earth, and did reverence to
the king, and said, [d]Let my lord king
David live for ever.
32 And king David said, Call me
Zadok the priest, and Nathan the
prophet, and Benaiah the son of
Jehoiada. And they came before the king.
33 The king also said unto them, [e]Take
with you the servants of your lord, and
cause Solomon my son to ride upon mine
own mule, and bring him down to Gihon:
34 And let Zadok the priest and Nathan
the prophet [f]anoint him there king over
Israel: and [g]blow ye with the trumpet,
and say, God save king Solomon.
35 Then ye shall come up after him,
that he may come and sit upon my
throne; for he shall be king in my stead:
and I have appointed him to be ruler
over Israel and over Judah.
36 And Benaiah the son of Jehoiada
answered the king, and said, Amen: the
LORD God of my lord the king say so *too*.
37 As the LORD hath been with my
lord the king, even so be he with
Solomon, and make his throne greater
than the throne of my lord king David.
38 So Zadok the priest, and Nathan
the prophet, and [h]Benaiah the son of
Jehoiada, and the Cherethites, and the
Pelethites, went down, and caused
Solomon to ride upon king David's
mule, and brought him to Gihon.

Solomon anointed king (1 Chr. 29:22).

39 And Zadok the priest took an horn
of oil out of the tabernacle, and [i]anoint-
ed Solomon. And they blew the trumpet;
and [j]all the people said, God save king
Solomon.
40 And all the people came up after
him, and the people piped with pipes,
and rejoiced with great joy, so that the
earth rent with the sound of them.

Adonijah's submission.

41 And Adonijah and all the guests
that *were* with him heard *it* as they had
made an end of eating. And when Joab
heard the sound of the trumpet, he said,
Wherefore *is this* noise of the city being
in an uproar?
42 And while he yet spake,
behold, Jonathan the son of Abiathar
the priest came: and Adonijah said
unto him, Come in; for [k]thou *art* a

B.C. 1015.

a Deut. 31:16; 1 Ki. 2:10.
b 2 Sam. 4:9.
c Ex. 14:30, *note*; Isa. 59:20, *note*.
d Neh. 2:3; Dan. 2:4.
e 2 Sam. 20:6.
f 1 Sam. 10:1; 1 Chr. 29:22.
g 2 Sam. 15:10; 2 Ki. 9:13; 11:14.
h 2 Sam. 8:18.
i 1 Chr. 29:22.
j 1 Sam. 10:24.
k 2 Sam. 18:27.

valiant man, and bringest good tidings.
43 And Jonathan answered and said to
Adonijah, Verily our lord king David
hath made Solomon king.
44 And the king hath sent with him
Zadok the priest, and Nathan the
prophet, and Benaiah the son of
Jehoiada, and the Cherethites, and the
Pelethites, and they have caused him to
ride upon the king's mule:
45 And Zadok the priest and Nathan
the prophet have anointed him king in
Gihon: and they are come up from thence
rejoicing, so that the city rang again. This
is the noise that ye have heard.
46 And also Solomon [a]sitteth on the
throne of the kingdom.
47 And moreover the king's servants
came to bless our lord king David, saying, God make the name of Solomon better than thy name, and make his throne
greater than thy throne. And the king
bowed himself upon the bed.
48 And also thus said the king,
Blessed *be* the LORD God of Israel, which
hath [b]given *one* to sit on my throne this
day, mine eyes even seeing *it*.
49 And all the guests that *were* with
Adonijah were afraid, and rose up, and
went every man his way.
50 And Adonijah feared because of
Solomon, and arose, and went, and
caught hold on the horns of the altar.
51 And it was told Solomon, saying,
Behold, Adonijah feareth king Solomon:
for, lo, he hath caught hold on the horns
of the altar, saying, Let king Solomon
swear unto me to day that he will not
slay his servant with the sword.
52 And Solomon said, If he will shew
himself a worthy man, [c]there shall not an
hair of him fall to the earth: but if wickedness shall be found in him, he shall die.
53 So king Solomon sent, and they
brought him down from the altar. And
he came and bowed himself to king
Solomon: and Solomon said unto him,
Go to thine house.

CHAPTER 2.

David's charge to Solomon.

Now the [d]days of David drew nigh
that he should die; and he charged
Solomon his son, saying,
2 [e]I go the way of all the earth: be thou
strong therefore, and shew thyself a man;
3 And keep the charge of the LORD thy
God, to walk in his ways, to keep his
statutes, and his commandments, and
his judgments, and his testimonies, as it
is written in the law of Moses, that thou
mayest [f]prosper in all that thou doest,
and whithersoever thou turnest thyself:
4 That the LORD may [g]continue his
word which he spake concerning me,
saying, If thy children take heed to their
way, to [h]walk before me in truth with all
their heart and with all their soul, [i]there
shall not fail thee (said he) a man on the
throne of Israel.
5 Moreover thou knowest also what
Joab the son of Zeruiah [j]did to me, *and*
what he did to the two captains of the
hosts of Israel, unto [k]Abner the son of
Ner, and unto Amasa the son of Jether,
whom he slew, and shed the blood of
war in peace, and put the blood of war
upon his girdle that *was* about his loins,
and in his shoes that *were* on his feet.
6 Do therefore according to thy wisdom, and let not his hoar head go down
to the [l]grave in peace.
7 But shew kindness unto the sons of
[m]Barzillai the Gileadite, and let them be
of those that eat at thy table: for so [n]they
came to me when I fled because of
Absalom thy brother.
8 And, behold, *thou hast* with thee
[o]Shimei the son of Gera, a Benjamite of
Bahurim, which cursed me with a grievous curse in the day when I went to
Mahanaim: but [p]he came down to meet
me at Jordan, and I sware to him by the
LORD, saying, I will not put thee to death
with the sword.
9 Now therefore [q]hold him not guiltless: for thou *art* a wise man, and knowest what thou oughtest to do unto him;
but his hoar head bring thou down to
the [l]grave with blood.

The death of David (1 Chr. 29:26-30).

10 So David slept with his fathers, and
was buried in the city of David.
11 And the days that David reigned
over Israel *were* forty years: seven years
reigned he in Hebron, and thirty and
three years reigned he in Jerusalem.

B.C. 1015.

a 1 Ki. 2:12; 1 Chr. 29:23.
b 1 Ki. 3:6; Psa. 132:11, 12.
c 1 Sam. 14:45; 2 Sam. 14:11; Acts 27:34.
d Gen. 47:29; Deut. 31:14.
e Josh. 23:14.
f Deut. 29:9; Josh. 1:7; 1 Chr. 22:12, 13.
g 2 Sam. 7:25.
h 2 Ki. 20:3.
i 2 Sam. 7:12, 13; 1 Ki. 8:25.
j 2 Sam. 3:39; 18:5, 12, 14.
k 2 Sam. 3:27.
l Heb. *Sheol.* See Hab. 2:5.
m 2 Sam. 19:31, 38.
n 2 Sam. 17:27.
o 2 Sam. 16:5.
p 2 Sam. 19:18.
q Ex. 20:7; Job 9:28.

Solomon's accession (1 Chr. 29:23-25).

12 Then sat Solomon upon the throne of David his father; and his kingdom was established greatly.

Execution of Adonijah.

13 And Adonijah the son of Haggith came to Bath-sheba the mother of Solomon. And she said, Comest thou peaceably? And he said, Peaceably.

14 He said moreover, I have somewhat to say unto thee. And she said, Say on.

15 And he said, Thou knowest that the kingdom was mine, and *that* all Israel set their faces on me, that I should reign: howbeit the kingdom is turned about, and is become my brother's: for [a]it was his from the LORD.

16 And now I ask one petition of thee, deny me not. And she said unto him, Say on.

17 And he said, Speak, I pray thee, unto Solomon the king, (for he will not say thee nay,) that he give me Abishag the Shunammite to wife.

18 And Bath-sheba said, Well; I will speak for thee unto the king.

19 Bath-sheba therefore went unto king Solomon, to speak unto him for Adonijah. And the king rose up to meet her, and bowed himself unto her, and sat down on his throne, and caused a seat to be set for the king's mother; and she sat on his right hand.

20 Then she said, I desire one small petition of thee; *I pray thee,* say me not nay. And the king said unto her, Ask on, my mother: for I will not say thee nay.

21 And she said, Let Abishag the Shunammite be given to Adonijah thy brother to wife.

22 And king Solomon answered and said unto his mother, And why dost thou ask Abishag the Shunammite for Adonijah? ask for him the kingdom also; for he *is* mine elder brother; even for him, and for [b]Abiathar the priest, and for Joab the son of Zeruiah.

23 Then king Solomon sware by the LORD, saying, God do so to me, and more also, if Adonijah have not spoken this word against his own life.

24 Now therefore, *as* the LORD liveth, which hath established me, and set me on the throne of David my father, and who hath made me an house, as he [c]promised, Adonijah shall be put to death this day.

25 And king Solomon sent by the hand of Benaiah the son of Jehoiada; and he fell upon him that he died.

Abiathar removed from the priesthood.

26 And unto Abiathar the priest said the king, Get thee to [d]Anathoth, unto thine own fields; for thou *art* worthy of death: but I will not at this time put thee to death, because thou barest the ark of the Lord GOD before David my father, and [e]because thou hast been afflicted in all wherein my father was afflicted.

27 So Solomon thrust out Abiathar from being priest unto the LORD; that he might [f]fulfil the word of the LORD, which he spake concerning the house of Eli in Shiloh.

The flight and death of Joab.

28 Then tidings came to Joab: for Joab had turned after Adonijah, though he turned not after Absalom. And Joab fled unto the tabernacle of the LORD, and [g]caught hold on the horns of the altar.

29 And it was told king Solomon that Joab was fled unto the tabernacle of the LORD; and, behold, *he is* by the altar. Then Solomon sent Benaiah the son of Jehoiada, saying, Go, fall upon him.

30 And Benaiah came to the tabernacle of the LORD, and said unto him, Thus saith the king, Come forth. And he said, Nay; but I will die here. And Benaiah brought the king word again, saying, Thus said Joab, and thus he answered me.

31 And the king said unto him, Do as he hath said, and fall upon him, and bury him; [h]that thou mayest take away the innocent blood, which Joab shed, from me, and from the house of my father.

32 And the LORD shall [i]return his blood upon his own head, who fell upon two men more righteous and better than he, and slew them with the sword, my father David not knowing *thereof, to wit,* Abner the son of Ner, captain of the host of Israel, and Amasa the son of Jether, captain of the host of Judah.

33 Their blood shall therefore return upon the head of Joab, and [j]upon the head of his seed for ever: but upon David, and upon his seed, and upon his

B.C. 1015.

a 1 Chr. 22:9, 10; 28:5-7; Dan. 2:21.
b 1 Ki. 1:7.
c 2 Sam. 7:11, 13; 1 Chr. 22:10.
d Josh. 21:18.
e 1 Sam. 23:6; 2 Sam. 15:24, 29.
f 1 Sam. 2:31-35.
g 1 Ki. 1:50.
h Num. 35:33; Deut. 19:13; 21:8, 9.
i Jud. 9:24, 57.
j 2 Sam. 3:29.

house, and upon his throne, shall there
be peace for ever from the LORD.
34 So Benaiah the son of Jehoiada
went up, and fell upon him, and slew
him: and he was buried in his own
house in the wilderness.

Benaiah made chief captain,
and Zadok priest.

35 And the king put Benaiah the son
of Jehoiada in his room over the host:
and Zadok the priest did the king put in
the room of Abiathar.

Execution of Shimei.

36 And the king sent and called for
[a]Shimei, and said unto him, Build thee
an house in Jerusalem, and dwell there,
and go not forth thence any whither.
37 For it shall be, *that* on the day thou
goest out, and passest over the brook
Kidron, thou shalt know for certain that
thou shalt surely die: thy blood shall be
upon thine own head.
38 And Shimei said unto the king, The
saying *is* good: as my lord the king hath
said, so will thy servant do. And Shimei
dwelt in Jerusalem many days.
39 And it came to pass at the end of
three years, that two of the servants of
Shimei ran away unto Achish son of
Maachah king of Gath. And they told
Shimei, saying, Behold, thy servants *be*
in Gath.
40 And Shimei arose, and saddled his
ass, and went to Gath to Achish to seek
his servants: and Shimei went, and
brought his servants from Gath.
41 And it was told Solomon that
Shimei had gone from Jerusalem to
Gath, and was come again.
42 And the king sent and called for
Shimei, and said unto him, Did I not
make thee to swear by the LORD, and
protested unto thee, saying, Know for a
certain, on the day thou goest out, and
walkest abroad any whither, that thou
shalt surely die? and thou saidst unto
me, The word *that* I have heard *is* good.
43 Why then hast thou not kept the
oath of the LORD, and the commandment
that I have charged thee with?
44 The king said moreover to Shimei,
Thou knowest all the wickedness which
thine heart is privy to, that thou didst to
David my father: therefore the LORD
shall return thy wickedness upon thine
own head;
45 And king Solomon *shall be* blessed,
and the throne of David shall be established before the LORD for ever.
46 So the king commanded Benaiah the
son of Jehoiada; which went out, and fell
upon him, that he died. And the kingdom
was established in the hand of Solomon.

CHAPTER 3.

Solomon makes alliance with Pharaoh,
and marries his daughter.

And [b]Solomon made affinity with
Pharaoh king of Egypt, and took
Pharaoh's daughter, and brought her
into the [c]city of David, until he had
made an end of building his own house,
and [d]the house of the LORD, and the
[e]wall of Jerusalem round about.
2 Only the people sacrificed [1]in high
places, because there was no house built
unto the name of the LORD, until those
days.
3 And Solomon loved the LORD, walking in the statutes of David his father:
only he sacrificed and burnt incense in
high places.

Solomon sacrifices at Gibeon
(2 Chr. 1:2-6).

4 And the king went to Gibeon to sacrifice there; for that *was* the great high
place: a thousand burnt-offerings did
Solomon offer upon that altar.

B.C. 1014.

a v. 8; 2 Sam. 16:5-13.
b 1 Ki. 7:8; 9:24.
c 2 Sam. 5:7.
d 1 Ki. 6.
e 1 Ki. 9:15, 19.

[1](3:2) Cf. Lev. 26:30; Deut. 12:11-14. The use of commanding elevations for altars seems to have been immemorial and universal. In itself the practice was not evil (Gen. 12:7, 8; 22:2-4; 31:54; Jud. 6:25, 26; 13:16-23). After the establishment of Mount Moriah and the temple as the centre of divine worship (Deut. 12:5, with 2 Chr. 7:12) the pentateuchal prohibition of the use of high places (Deut. 12:11-14), which had looked forward to the setting up of such a centre, came into effect, and high places became identified with idolatrous practices. The constant recurrence to the use of high places, even for Jehovistic worship (1 Ki. 15:14, *note*), and after the building of the temple, proves how deeply rooted the custom was. See 2 Ki. 18:4-22; 23; 2 Chr. 33:3, 17, 19. See, also, note on "groves," Jud. 3:7.

Solomon's prayer for wisdom
(2 Chr. 1:7-13).

B.C. 1014.

5 In Gibeon the LORD appeared to Solomon in a dream by night: and God said, [a]Ask what I shall give thee.

6 [b]And Solomon said, Thou hast shewed unto thy servant David my father great mercy, according as he [c]walked before thee in truth, and in righteousness, and in uprightness of heart with thee; and thou hast kept for him this great kindness, that thou hast given him a son to sit on his throne, as *it is* this day.

7 And now, O LORD my God, thou hast made thy servant king instead of David my father: and I *am but* a little child: I know not *how* to go out or come in.

8 And thy servant *is* in the midst of thy people which thou [d]hast chosen, a great people, [e]that cannot be numbered nor counted for multitude.

9 Give therefore thy servant an [f]understanding heart to judge thy people, that I may [g]discern between good and bad: for who is able to judge this thy so great a people?

10 And the speech pleased the Lord, that Solomon had asked this thing.

11 And God said unto him, Because thou hast asked this thing, and hast not asked for thyself long life; neither hast asked riches for thyself, nor hast asked the life of thine enemies; but hast asked for thyself understanding to discern judgment;

12 Behold, I have done according to thy words: [h]lo, I have given thee a wise and an understanding heart; so that there was none like thee before thee, neither after thee shall any arise like unto thee.

13 And I have also given thee that which thou hast not asked, both riches, and honour: so that there [i]shall not be any among the kings like unto thee all thy days.

14 And if thou wilt walk in my ways, to keep my statutes and my commandments, [j]as thy father David did walk, then I will lengthen thy days.

15 And Solomon awoke; and, behold, *it was* a dream. And he came to Jerusalem, and stood before the ark of the covenant of the LORD, and offered up burnt-offerings, and offered peace-offerings, and made a feast to all his servants.

The wisdom of Solomon.

16 Then came there two women, *that were* harlots, unto the king, and [k]stood before him.

17 And the one woman said, O my lord, I and this woman dwell in one house; and I was delivered of a child with her in the house.

18 And it came to pass the third day after that I was delivered, that this woman was delivered also: and we *were* together; *there was* no stranger with us in the house, save we two in the house.

19 And this woman's child died in the night; because she overlaid it.

20 And she arose at midnight, and took my son from beside me, while thine handmaid slept, and laid it in her bosom, and laid her dead child in my bosom.

21 And when I rose in the morning to give my child suck, behold, it was dead: but when I had considered it in the morning, behold, it was not my son, which I did bear.

22 And the other woman said, Nay; but the living *is* my son, and the dead *is* thy son. And this said, No; but the dead *is* thy son, and the living *is* my son. Thus they spake before the king.

23 Then said the king, The one saith, This *is* my son that liveth, and thy son *is* the dead: and the other saith, Nay; but thy son *is* the dead, and my son *is* the living.

24 And the king said, Bring me a sword. And they brought a sword before the king.

25 And the king said, Divide the living child in two, and give half to the one, and half to the other.

26 Then spake the woman whose the living child *was* unto the king, for her bowels [l]yearned upon her son, and she said, O my lord, give her the living child, and in no wise slay it. But the other said, Let it be neither mine nor thine, *but* divide *it*.

27 Then the king answered and said, Give her the living child, and in no wise slay it: she *is* the mother thereof.

28 And all Israel heard of the judgment which the king had judged; and they feared the king: for they saw that the wisdom of God *was* [m]in him, to do judgment

a *Bible prayers* (O.T.). 1 Ki. 8:23. (Gen. 15:2; Hab. 3:1-16.)
b 2 Chr. 1:8.
c 1 Ki. 2:4; 9:4.
d Deut. 7:6.
e Gen. 13:16; 15:5.
f Heb. *hearing.*
g Heb. 5:14.
h 1 Ki. 4:29, 30, 31; 5:12; 10:24; Eccl. 1:16.
i Or, *hath not been.*
j 1 Ki. 15:5.
k Num. 27:2.
l Heb. *were hot.*
m Heb. *in the midst of him.*

CHAPTER 4.

The princes of Israel in Solomon's reign.

So king Solomon was king over all
Israel.
2 And these *were* the princes which he
had; Azariah the son of Zadok the priest,
3 Elihoreph and Ahiah, the sons of
Shisha, scribes; [a]Jehoshaphat the son of
Ahilud, the recorder.
4 And [b]Benaiah the son of Jehoiada
was over the host: and Zadok and
[c]Abiathar *were* the priests:
5 And Azariah the son of Nathan *was*
over the officers: and Zabud the son of
Nathan *was* [d]principal officer, *and* the
[e]king's friend:
6 And Ahishar *was* over the household: and [f]Adoniram the son of Abda
was over the tribute.

The twelve commissaries.

7 And Solomon had twelve officers
over all Israel, which provided victuals
for the king and his household: each man
his month in a year made provision.
8 And these *are* their names: The [g]son
of Hur, in mount Ephraim:
9 The son of Dekar, in Makaz, and in
Shaalbim, and Beth-shemesh, and Elon-
beth-hanan:
10 The [h]son of Hesed, in Aruboth; to
him *pertained* Sochoh, and all the land of
Hepher:
11 The [i]son of Abinadab, in all the
region of Dor; which had Taphath the
daughter of Solomon to wife:
12 Baana the son of Ahilud; *to him pertained* Taanach and Megiddo, and all Beth-
shean, which *is* by Zartanah beneath
Jezreel, from Beth-shean to Abel-meholah,
even unto *the place that is* beyond Jokneam:
13 The son of Geber, in Ramoth-gilead;
to him *pertained* the towns of Jair the son
of Manasseh, which *are* in Gilead; to him
also pertained [j]the region of Argob, which
is in Bashan, threescore great cities with
walls and brasen bars:
14 Ahinadab the son of Iddo *had*
Mahanaim:
15 Ahimaaz *was* in Naphtali; he also
took Basmath the daughter of Solomon
to wife:
16 Baanah the son of Hushai *was* in
Asher and in Aloth:
17 Jehoshaphat the son of Paruah, in
Issachar:
18 Shimei the son of Elah, in Benjamin:
19 Geber the son of Uri *was* in the
country of Gilead, *in* [k]the country of
Sihon king of the Amorites, and of Og
king of Bashan; and *he was* the only officer which *was* in the land.
20 Judah and Israel *were* many, [l]as the
sand which *is* by the sea in multitude,
eating and drinking, and making merry.
21 And [m]Solomon reigned over all
kingdoms from the river unto the land
of the Philistines, and unto the border of
Egypt: they brought presents, and
served Solomon all the days of his life.
22 And Solomon's [n]provision for one
day was thirty [o]measures of fine flour,
and threescore measures of meal,
23 Ten fat oxen, and twenty oxen out
of the pastures, and an hundred sheep,
beside harts, and roebucks, and fal-
lowdeer, and fatted fowl.
24 For he had dominion over all *the
region* on this side the river, from
Tiphsah even to Azzah, over all the
kings on this side the river: and [p]he had
peace on all sides round about him.
25 And Judah and Israel [q]dwelt [r]safe-
ly, [s]every man under his vine and under
his fig tree, from Dan even to Beer-
sheba, all the days of Solomon.
26 And [t]Solomon had forty thousand
stalls of [u]horses for his chariots, and
twelve thousand horsemen.
27 And those officers provided victual
for king Solomon, and for all that came
unto king Solomon's table, every man in
his month: they lacked nothing.
28 Barley also and straw for the horses
and dromedaries brought they unto the
place where *the officers* were, every man
according to his charge.

The wisdom of Solomon.

29 And God gave Solomon wisdom
and understanding exceeding much,
and largeness of heart, even as the sand
that *is* on the sea shore.
30 And Solomon's wisdom excelled
the wisdom of all the children of the east
country, and [v]all the wisdom of Egypt.
31 For he was [w]wiser than all men;
than Ethan the Ezrahite, and Heman,
and Chalcol, and Darda, the sons of
Mahol: and his fame was in all nations
round about.

B.C. 1014.

a 2 Sam. 8:16; 20:24.
b 1 Ki. 2:35.
c 1 Ki. 2:27.
d 2 Sam. 8:18; 20:26.
e 2 Sam. 15:37; 16:16; 1 Chr. 27:33.
f 1 Ki. 5:14.
g Or, *Ben-hur.*
h Or, *Ben-hesed.*
i Or, *Ben-abinadab.*
j Deut. 3:4.
k Deut. 3:8.
l Gen. 22:17; 1 Ki. 3:8.
m 2 Chr. 9:26; Psa. 72:8.
n Heb. *bread.*
o One measure = about 10 bu.
p 1 Ki. 5:4; 1 Chr. 22:9.
q Jer. 23:6.
r Heb. *confidently.*
s Mic. 4:4; Zech. 3:10.
t 1 Ki. 10:26; 2 Chr. 1:14; 9:25.
u Deut. 17:16.
v Acts 7:22.
w I Ki. 3:12.

32 And he spake three thousand proverbs: and his [a]songs were a thousand and five.

33 And he spake of trees, from the cedar tree that *is* in Lebanon even unto the hyssop that springeth out of the wall: he spake also of beasts, and of fowl, and of creeping things, and of fishes.

34 And there came of all people to hear the wisdom of Solomon, from all kings of the earth, which had heard of his wisdom.

CHAPTER 5.

Solomon prepares to build the temple (2 Chr. 2:1-16).

And [b]Hiram king of Tyre sent his servants unto Solomon; for he had heard that they had anointed him king in the room of his father: for Hiram was ever a lover of David.

2 And [c]Solomon sent to Hiram, saying,

3 Thou knowest how that David my father could not build an house unto the name of the LORD his God [d]for the wars which were about him on every side, until the LORD put them under the soles of his feet.

4 But now the LORD my God hath given me rest on every side, *so that there is* neither adversary nor evil occurrent.

5 And, behold, I purpose to build an house unto the name of the LORD my God, as the LORD spake unto David my father, saying, Thy son, whom I will set upon thy throne in thy room, he shall build an house unto my name.

6 Now therefore command thou that they hew me cedar trees out of Lebanon; and my servants shall be with thy servants: and unto thee will I give hire for thy servants according to all that thou shalt appoint: for thou knowest that *there is* not among us any that can skill to hew timber like unto the Sidonians.

7 And it came to pass, when Hiram heard the words of Solomon, that he rejoiced greatly, and said, Blessed *be* the LORD this day, which hath given unto David a wise son over this great people.

8 And Hiram sent to Solomon, saying, I have considered the things which thou sentest to me for: *and* I will do all thy desire concerning timber of cedar, and concerning timber of fir.

B.C. 1014.

a Song 1:1.

b vs. 10, 18; 2 Chr. 2:3, *Huram.*

c 2 Chr. 2:3.

d 1 Chr. 22:8; 28:3.

e One measure = about 10 bu.

f One measure (liquid) = about 86 gals.

9 My servants shall bring *them* down from Lebanon unto the sea: and I will convey them by sea in floats unto the place that thou shalt appoint me, and will cause them to be discharged there, and thou shalt receive *them*: and thou shalt accomplish my desire, in giving food for my household.

10 So Hiram gave Solomon cedar trees and fir trees *according to* all his desire.

11 And Solomon gave Hiram twenty thousand [e]measures of wheat *for* food to his household, and twenty [f]measures of pure oil: thus gave Solomon to Hiram year by year.

12 And the LORD gave Solomon wisdom, as he promised him: and there was peace between Hiram and Solomon; and they two made a league together.

Preparations for building the temple: the labourers and their work (2 Chr. 2:2).

13 And king Solomon raised a levy out of all Israel; and the levy was thirty thousand men.

14 And he sent them to Lebanon, ten thousand a month by courses: a month they were in Lebanon, *and* two months at home: and Adoniram *was* over the levy.

15 And Solomon had threescore and ten thousand that bare burdens, and fourscore thousand hewers in the mountains;

16 Beside the chief of Solomon's officers which *were* over the work, three thousand and three hundred, which ruled over the people that wrought in the work.

17 And the king commanded, and they brought great stones, costly stones, *and* hewed stones, to lay the foundation of the house.

18 And Solomon's builders and Hiram's builders did hew *them*, and the stonesquarers: so they prepared timber and stones to build the house.

CHAPTER 6.

Solomon begins to build the temple (2 Chr. 3:1, 2).

And it came to pass in the four hundred and eightieth year after the children of Israel were come out of the land of Egypt, in the fourth year of Solomon's reign over Israel, in the

month [a]Zif, which *is* the second month,
that he began to build the [1]house of the
LORD.

Dimensions and materials of the temple
(2 Chr. 3:3 to 4:22).

2 And the house which king Solomon
built for the LORD, the length thereof *was*
threescore [b]cubits, and the breadth
thereof twenty *cubits*, and the height
thereof thirty cubits.
3 And the porch before the temple of
the house, twenty cubits *was* the length
thereof, according to the breadth of the
house; *and* ten cubits *was* the breadth
thereof before the house.
4 And for the house he made [2]win-
dows of narrow lights.
5 And against the wall of the house he
built chambers round about, *against* the
walls of the house round about, *both* of
the temple and of the oracle: and he
made chambers round about:
6 The nethermost chamber *was* five
cubits broad, and the middle *was* six
cubits broad, and the third *was* seven
cubits broad: for without *in the wall* of
the house he made narrowed rests
round about, that *the beams* should not
be fastened in the walls of the house.
7 And the [c]house, when it was in
building, was built of stone made ready
before it was brought thither: so that
there was neither hammer nor axe *nor*
any tool of iron heard in the house,
while it was in building.
8 The door for the middle chamber
was in the right [d]side of the house: and
they went up with winding stairs into
the middle *chamber*, and out of the middle into the third.
9 [e]So he built the house, and finished
it; and covered the house with beams
and boards of cedar.
10 And *then* he built chambers against
all the house, five cubits high: and they
rested on the house with timber of cedar.
11 And the word of the LORD came to
Solomon, saying,
12 *Concerning* this house which thou
art in building, [f]if thou wilt walk in my
statutes, and execute my judgments, and
keep all my commandments to walk in
them; then will I perform my word with
thee, [g]which I spake unto David thy
father:
13 And [h]I will dwell among the children of Israel, and will not [i]forsake my
people Israel.
14 So Solomon built the house, and
finished it.
15 And he built the walls of the house
within with boards of cedar, both the
floor of the house, and the walls of the
cieling: *and* he covered *them* on the
inside with wood, and covered the floor
of the house with planks of fir.
16 And he built twenty cubits on the
sides of the house, both the floor and the
walls with boards of cedar: he even built
them for it within, *even* for the oracle,
even for the most holy *place*.
17 And the house, that *is*, the temple
before it, was forty cubits *long*.
18 And the cedar of the house within
was carved with knops and open flowers:
all *was* cedar; there was no stone seen.
19 And the oracle he prepared in the
house within, to set there the ark of the
covenant of the LORD.
20 And the oracle in the forepart *was*
twenty cubits in length, and twenty
cubits in breadth, and twenty cubits in
the height thereof: and he overlaid it
with pure gold; and *so* covered the altar
which was of cedar.
21 So Solomon overlaid the house
within with pure gold: and he made a
partition by the chains of gold before the
oracle; and he overlaid it with gold.
22 And the whole house he overlaid with gold, until he had finished all
the house: also the [j]whole altar

B.C. 1012.

a i.e. *May.*

b One cubit = about 18 in.; also vs. 3, 6, 10, 17, 20, 23, 24, 25, 26.

c Deut. 27:5, 6; 1 Ki. 5:18.

d Heb. *shoulder.*

e vs. 14, 38.

f 1 Ki. 2:4; 9:4.

g 2 Sam. 7:13; 1 Chr. 22:10.

h Ex. 25:8; Lev. 26:11; 2 Cor. 6:16; Rev. 21:3.

i Deut. 31:6.

j Ex. 30:1-6.

[1]**(6:1)** The typology of the temple, if indeed it has any typical significance, is most obscure and difficult. The N.T. invariably expounds the typology of the tabernacle, not of the temple. The symbolism of the latter may be revealed in the kingdom-age (see "Kingdom" [O.T.], Gen. 1:26; Zech. 12:8; [N.T.], Lk. 1:32; 1 Cor. 15:28). In the N.T. the usual Gk. word for *sanctuary* (*naos*) is used (1) of the temple in Jerusalem (Mt. 23:16); (2) of the believer's body (1 Cor. 3:16, 17; 6:19); (3) of the local church (2 Cor. 6:16); and (4) of the true church (Eph. 2:21). But in all these instances the thought is simply of *a habitation of God.* No reference to the structure of the temple, as in the case of the tabernacle (Heb. 9–10), is traceable.

[2]**(6:4)** Cf. 2 Chr. 4:20. In the holy of holies in the tabernacle no light but the shekinah glory was provided. In many ways Solomon's temple manifests the spiritual deterioration of the people, and Jehovah's condescension to it in grace.

that *was* by the oracle he overlaid with
gold.
23 And within the oracle he made two
cherubims *of* olive tree, *each* ten cubits
high.
24 And five cubits *was* the one wing of
the cherub, and five cubits the other
wing of the cherub: from the uttermost
part of the one wing unto the uttermost
part of the other *were* ten cubits.
25 And the other cherub *was* ten
cubits: both the cherubims *were* of one
measure and one size.
26 The height of the one cherub *was* ten
cubits, and so *was it* of the other cherub.
27 And he set the cherubims within the
inner house: and [a]they stretched forth the
wings of the cherubims, so that the wing
of the one touched the *one* wall, and the
wing of the other cherub touched the
other wall; and their wings touched one
another in the midst of the house.
28 And he overlaid the cherubims
with gold.
29 And he carved all the walls of the
house round about with carved figures
of cherubims and palm trees and open
flowers, within and without.
30 And the floor of the house he overlaid with gold, within and without.
31 And for the entering of the oracle
he made doors *of* olive tree: the lintel *and*
side posts *were* [b]a fifth part *of the wall*.
32 The two doors also *were of* olive
tree; and he carved upon them carvings
of cherubims and palm trees and open
flowers, and overlaid *them* with gold,
and spread gold upon the cherubims,
and upon the palm trees.
33 So also made he for the door of the
temple posts *of* olive tree, [c]a fourth part
of the wall.
34 And the two doors *were of* fir tree:
the two leaves of the one door *were* folding, and the two leaves of the other door
were folding.
35 And he carved *thereon* cherubims
and palm trees and open flowers: and
covered *them* with gold fitted upon the
carved work.
36 And he built the inner court with
three rows of hewed stone, and a row of
cedar beams.
37 In the fourth year was the foundation of the house of the LORD laid, in the
month [d]Zif:
38 And in the eleventh year, in the
month [e]Bul, which *is* the eighth month,
was the house finished throughout all
the parts thereof, and according to all
the fashion of it. So was he [f]seven years
in building it.

CHAPTER 7.

But Solomon was building his own
house thirteen years, and he finished all his house.
2 He built also the house of the forest
of Lebanon; the length thereof *was* an
hundred [g]cubits, and the breadth thereof
fifty cubits, and the height thereof thirty
cubits, upon four rows of cedar pillars,
with cedar beams upon the pillars.
3 And *it was* covered with cedar above
upon the [h]beams, that *lay* on forty five
pillars, fifteen *in* a row.
4 And *there were* windows *in* three rows,
and light *was* against light *in* three ranks.
5 And all the [i]doors and posts *were*
square, with the windows: and light *was*
against light *in* three ranks.
6 And he made a porch of pillars; the
length thereof *was* fifty cubits, and the
breadth thereof thirty cubits: and the
porch *was* before them: and the *other* pillars and the thick beam *were* before them.
7 Then he made a porch for the throne
where he might judge, *even* the porch of
judgment: and *it was* covered with cedar
[j]from one side of the floor to the other.
8 And his house where he dwelt *had*
another court within the porch, *which* was
of the like work. Solomon made also an
house for Pharaoh's daughter, [k]whom he
had taken *to wife*, like unto this porch.
9 All these *were of* costly stones,
according to the measures of hewed
stones, sawed with saws, within and
without, even from the foundation unto
the coping, and *so* on the outside toward
the great court.
10 And the foundation *was of* costly
stones, even great stones, stones of ten
cubits, and stones of eight cubits.
11 And above *were* costly stones, after
the measures of hewed stones, and
cedars.
12 And the great court round about
was with three rows of hewed stones,
and a row of cedar beams, both for the
inner court of the house of the LORD, and
[l]for the porch of the house.

B.C. 1005.

a Or, *the cherubim stretched forth their wings.*

b Or, *fivesquare.*

c Or, *foursquare.*

d i.e. *May.*

e i.e. *November.*

f Cf. v. 1.

g One cubit = about 18 in.; also vs. 6, 10, 15, 16, 19, 23, 24, 27, 31, 32, 35, 38.

h Heb. *ribs.*

i Or, *spaces and pillars were square in prospect.*

j Heb. *from floor to floor.*

k 1 Ki. 3:1; 2 Chr. 8:11.

l John 10:23; Acts 3:11.

B.C. 1005.

13 And king Solomon sent and fetched
Hiram out of Tyre.
14 He *was* a widow's son of the tribe
of Naphtali, and [a]his father *was* a man of
Tyre, a worker in brass: and [b]he was
filled with wisdom, and understanding,
and cunning to work all works in brass.
And he came to king Solomon, and
wrought all his work.
15 For he cast two pillars of brass, of
eighteen cubits high apiece: and a line of
twelve cubits did compass either of
them about.
16 And he made two chapiters *of*
molten brass, to set upon the tops of the
pillars: the height of the one chapiter *was*
five cubits, and the height of the other
chapiter *was* five cubits:
17 *And* nets of checker work, and
wreaths of chain work, for the chapiters
which *were* upon the top of the pillars;
seven for the one chapiter, and seven for
the other chapiter.
18 And he made the pillars, and two
rows round about upon the one network, to cover the chapiters that *were*
upon the top, with pomegranates: and
so did he for the other chapiter.
19 And the chapiters that *were* upon
the top of the pillars *were* of lily work in
the porch, four cubits.
20 And the chapiters upon the two pillars *had pomegranates* also above, over
against the belly which *was* by the network: and the pomegranates *were* two
hundred in rows round about upon the
other chapiter.
21 And he set up the pillars in the
porch of the temple: and he set up the
right pillar, and called the name thereof
[c]Jachin: and he set up the left pillar, and
called the name thereof [d]Boaz.
22 And upon the top of the pillars *was*
lily work: so was the work of the pillars
finished.
23 And he made a [e]molten sea, ten
cubits [f]from the one brim to the other: *it*
was round all about, and his height *was*
five cubits: and a line of thirty cubits did
compass it round about.
24 And under the brim of it round
about *there were* knops compassing it, ten
in a cubit, compassing the sea round
about: the knops *were* cast in two rows,
when it was cast.
25 It stood upon twelve oxen, three
looking toward the north, and three
looking toward the west, and three looking toward the south, and three looking
toward the east: and the sea *was set*
above upon them, and all their hinder
parts *were* inward.
26 And it *was* an hand breadth thick,
and the brim thereof was wrought like
the brim of a cup, with flowers of lilies:
it contained two thousand [g]baths.
27 And he made ten bases of brass;
four cubits *was* the length of one base,
and four cubits the breadth thereof, and
three cubits the height of it.
28 And the work of the bases *was* on
this *manner*: they had borders, and the
borders *were* between the ledges:
29 And on the borders that *were*
between the ledges *were* lions, oxen, and
cherubims: and upon the ledges *there*
was a base above: and beneath the lions
and oxen *were* certain additions made of
thin work.
30 And every base had four brasen
wheels, and plates of brass: and the four
corners thereof had undersetters: under
the laver *were* undersetters molten, at the
side of every addition.
31 And the mouth of it within the
chapiter and above *was* a cubit: but the
mouth thereof *was* round *after* the work
of the base, a cubit and an half: and also
upon the mouth of it *were* gravings with
their borders, foursquare, not round.
32 And under the borders *were* four
wheels; and the axletrees of the wheels
were [h]*joined* to the base: and the height of
a wheel *was* a cubit and half a cubit.
33 And the work of the wheels *was*
like the work of a chariot wheel: their
axletrees, and their naves, and their fel-
loes, and their spokes, *were* all molten.
34 And *there were* four undersetters to
the four corners of one base: *and* the
undersetters *were* of the very base itself.
35 And in the top of the base *was there*
a round compass of half a cubit high: and
on the top of the base the ledges thereof
and the borders thereof *were* of the same.
36 For on the plates of the ledges
thereof, and on the borders thereof, he
graved cherubims, lions, and palm trees,
according to the proportion of every
one, and additions round about.
37 After this *manner* he made the ten

a 2 Chr. 4:16.
b Ex. 31:3; 36:1.
c i.e. *He shall establish.*
d i.e. *in it is strength.*
e 2 Ki. 25:13; 2 Chr. 4:2; Jer. 52:17; cf. Ex. 30:19.
f Heb. *from his brim to his brim.*
g One bath = about 8 gals.; also v.38.
h Heb. *in the base.*

bases: all of them had one casting, one measure, *and* one size.

38 Then [a]made he ten lavers of brass: one laver contained forty baths: *and* every laver was four cubits: *and* upon every one of the ten bases one laver.

39 And he put five bases on the right side of the house, and five on the left side of the house: and he set the sea on the right side of the house eastward over against the south.

40 And [b]Hiram made the lavers, and the shovels, and the basons. So Hiram made an end of doing all the work that he made king Solomon for the house of the LORD:

41 The two pillars, and the *two* bowls of the chapiters that *were* on the top of the two pillars; and the two networks, to cover the two bowls of the chapiters which *were* upon the top of the pillars;

42 And four hundred pomegranates for the two networks, *even* two rows of pomegranates for one network, to cover the two bowls of the chapiters that *were* upon the pillars;

43 And the ten bases, and ten lavers on the bases;

44 And one sea, and twelve oxen under the sea;

45 And the pots, and the shovels, and the basons: and all these vessels, which Hiram made to king Solomon for the house of the LORD, *were of* bright brass.

46 In the plain of Jordan did the king cast them, in the clay ground between Succoth and Zarthan.

47 And Solomon left all the vessels *unweighed*, [c]because they were exceeding many: neither was the weight of the brass found out.

48 And Solomon made all the vessels that *pertained* unto the house of the LORD: the [d]altar of gold, and the [e]table of gold, whereupon the [f]shewbread *was*,

49 And the candlesticks of pure gold, five on the right *side*, and five on the left, before the oracle, with the flowers, and the lamps, and the tongs *of* gold,

50 And the bowls, and the snuffers, and the basons, and the spoons, and the censers *of* pure gold; and the hinges *of* gold, *both* for the doors of the inner house, the most holy *place, and* for the doors of the house, *to wit*, of the temple.

51 So was ended all the work that king Solomon made for the house of the LORD. And Solomon brought in the things which David his father had [g]dedicated; *even* the silver, and the gold, and the vessels, did he put among the treasures of the house of the LORD.

B.C. 1005.

a 2 Chr. 4:6.

b v. 13.

c Heb. *for the exceeding multitude.*

d Ex. 37:25, 26.

e Ex. 37:10, 11.

f Ex. 25:30, *note.*

g *Sanctify, holy* (O.T.). 2 Chr. 2:4. (Gen. 2:3; Zech. 8:3.)

h i.e. *October.*

CHAPTER 8.

The ark brought in: the shekinah-glory fills the house (2 Chr. 5:2-14).

[1]Then Solomon assembled the elders of Israel, and all the heads of the tribes, the chief of the fathers of the children of Israel, unto king Solomon in Jerusalem, that they might bring up the ark of the covenant of the LORD out of the city of David, which *is* Zion.

2 And all the men of Israel assembled themselves unto king Solomon at the feast in the month [h]Ethanim, which *is* the seventh month.

3 And all the elders of Israel came, and the priests took up the ark.

4 And they brought up the ark of the LORD, and the tabernacle of the congregation, and all the holy vessels that *were* in the tabernacle, even those did the priests and the Levites bring up.

5 And king Solomon, and all the congregation of Israel, that were assembled unto him, *were* with him before the ark, sacrificing sheep and oxen, that could not be told nor numbered for multitude.

6 And the priests brought in the ark of the covenant of the LORD unto his place,

[1]**(8:1)** The consecration of the temple illustrates all consecration. The temple, like the believer (1 Thes. 5:23), was threefold: the court, that which was outward, visible, answered to the body; the holy place, where everything appealed to the sacred emotions, answered to the soul; the holy of holies, the place of communion with God (Ex. 25:22), answered to the spirit of man. The ark was the most all-inclusive type of Christ of any one of the vessels of the tabernacle (Ex. 25:9, *note*). When, therefore, the priests brought the ark into the court, the holy place, and the holy of holies, they were, in type, enthroning Christ over the body, with its powers and appetites; the soul, seat of the emotions and desires; and the mind, seat of the capacity to know and commune with God. See Gen. 1:26, *note* 3. In Christian experience this answers to Rom. 12:1-3; Eph. 5:18.

into the oracle of the house, to the most holy *place, even* under the wings of the cherubims.

7 For the cherubims spread forth *their* two wings over the place of the ark, and the cherubims covered the ark and the staves thereof above.

8 And they drew out the staves, that the ends of the staves were seen out in the holy *place* before the oracle, and they were not seen without: and there they are unto this day.

9 *There was* nothing in the ark save the two tables of stone, which Moses put there at Horeb, when the LORD made *a covenant* with the children of Israel, when they came out of the land of Egypt.

10 And it came to pass, when the priests were come out of the holy *place,* that the [a]cloud filled the house of the LORD,

11 So that the priests could not stand to minister because of the cloud: for the glory of the LORD had filled the house of the LORD.

The sermon of Solomon (2 Chr. 6:1-11).

12 Then spake Solomon, The LORD said that he would dwell in the thick darkness.

13 I have surely built thee an house to dwell in, a settled place for thee to abide in for ever.

14 And the king turned his face about, and blessed all the congregation of Israel: (and all the congregation of Israel stood;)

15 And he said, Blessed *be* the LORD God of Israel, which spake with his mouth unto David my father, and hath with his hand fulfilled *it,* saying,

16 Since the day that I brought forth my people Israel out of Egypt, I chose no city out of all the tribes of Israel to build an house, that my name might be therein; but I chose David to be over my people Israel.

17 And it was in the heart of David my father to build an house for the name of the LORD God of Israel.

18 And the LORD said unto David my father, Whereas it was in thine heart to build an house unto my name, thou didst well that it was in thine heart.

19 Nevertheless thou shalt not build the house; but thy son that shall come forth out of thy loins, he shall build the house unto my name.

B.C. 1004.

a vs. 10, 11; Ex. 40:34, *note.*

b Kingdom (O.T.). 1 Ki. 11:9-13, 32, 36. (Gen. 1:26-28; Zech. 12:8.)

c Bible prayers (O.T.). 1 Ki. 17:20. (Gen. 15:2; Hab. 3:1-16.)

d 2 Chr. 2:6; Isa. 66:1; Jer. 23:24; Acts 7:49; 17:24.

e Deut. 12:11.

20 And the LORD hath performed his word that he spake, and I am risen up in the room of [b]David my father, and sit on the throne of Israel, as the LORD promised, and have built an house for the name of the LORD God of Israel.

21 And I have set there a place for the ark, wherein *is* the covenant of the LORD, which he made with our fathers, when he brought them out of the land of Egypt.

Solomon's prayer of dedication
(2 Chr. 6:12-42).

22 And Solomon stood before the altar of the LORD in the presence of all the congregation of Israel, and spread forth his hands toward heaven:

23 And he [c]said, LORD God of Israel, *there is* no God like thee, in heaven above, or on earth beneath, who keepest covenant and mercy with thy servants that walk before thee with all their heart:

24 Who hast kept with thy servant David my father that thou promisedst him: thou spakest also with thy mouth, and hast fulfilled *it* with thine hand, as *it is* this day.

25 Therefore now, LORD God of Israel, keep with thy servant David my father that thou promisedst him, saying, There shall not fail thee a man in my sight to sit on the throne of Israel; so that thy children take heed to their way, that they walk before me as thou hast walked before me.

26 And now, O God of Israel, let thy word, I pray thee, be verified, which thou spakest unto thy servant David my father.

27 But [d]will God indeed dwell on the earth? behold, the heaven and heaven of heavens cannot contain thee; how much less this house that I have builded?

28 Yet have thou respect unto the prayer of thy servant, and to his supplication, O LORD my God, to hearken unto the cry and to the prayer, which thy servant prayeth before thee to day:

29 That thine eyes may be open toward this house night and day, *even* toward the place of which thou hast said, [e]My name shall be there: that thou mayest hearken unto the prayer which thy servant shall make toward this place.

30 And hearken thou to the supplication of thy servant, and of thy people

Israel, when they shall pray toward this
place: and hear thou in heaven thy
dwelling place: and when thou hearest,
forgive.
31 If any man trespass against his
neighbour, and [a]an oath be laid upon
him to cause him to swear, and the oath
come before thine altar in this house:
32 Then hear thou in heaven, and do,
and judge thy servants, condemning the
wicked, to bring his way upon his head;
and justifying the righteous, to give him
according to his righteousness.
33 When thy people Israel be smitten
down before the enemy, because they
have sinned against thee, and shall turn
again to thee, and confess thy name, and
pray, and make supplication unto thee in
this house:
34 Then hear thou in heaven, and forgive the sin of thy people Israel, and
bring them again unto the land which
thou gavest unto their fathers.
35 When heaven is shut up, and there
is no rain, because they have sinned
against thee; if they pray toward this
place, and confess thy name, and turn
from their sin, when thou afflictest them:
36 Then hear thou in heaven, and forgive the sin of thy servants, and of thy
people Israel, that thou teach them [b]the
good way wherein they should walk, and
give rain upon thy land, which thou hast
given to thy people for an inheritance.
37 [c]If there be in the land famine, if
there be pestilence, blasting, mildew,
locust, *or* if there be caterpiller; if their
enemy besiege them in the land of their
cities; whatsoever plague, whatsoever
sickness *there be*;
38 What prayer and supplication soever be *made* by any man, *or* by all thy people Israel, which shall know every man
the plague of his own heart, and spread
forth his hands toward this house:
39 Then hear thou in heaven thy
dwelling place, and forgive, and do, and
give to every man according to his ways,
whose heart thou knowest; (for thou,
even thou only, knowest the hearts of all
the children of men;)
40 That they may [d]fear thee all the
days that they live in the land which
thou gavest unto our fathers.
41 Moreover concerning a stranger, that

B.C. 1004.

a Heb. *and he requires an oath of him.*

b 1 Sam. 12:23.

c Lev. 26:16, 25, 26; Deut. 28:21, 22, 27, 38, 42, 52; 2 Chr. 20:9.

d Psa. 19:9, *note.*

e Deut. 3:24.

f 1 Sam. 17:46; 2 Ki. 19:19; Psa. 67:2.

g Or, *right.*

h Lev. 26:34, 44; Deut. 28:36, 64; 2 Ki. 17:6, 18; 25:21.

i Neh. 1:6; Psa. 106:6; Dan. 9:5.

j Dan. 6:10.

is not of thy people Israel, but cometh out
of a far country for thy name's sake;
42 (For they shall hear of thy great
name, and of [e]thy strong hand, and of
thy stretched out arm;) when he shall
come and pray toward this house;
43 Hear thou in heaven thy dwelling
place, and do according to all that the
stranger calleth to thee for: [f]that all people
of the earth may know thy name, to [d]fear
thee, as *do* thy people Israel; and that they
may know that this house, which I have
builded, is called by thy name.
44 If thy people go out to battle
against their enemy, whithersoever thou
shalt send them, and shall pray unto the
LORD toward the city which thou hast
chosen, and *toward* the house that I have
built for thy name:
45 Then hear thou in heaven their
prayer and their supplication, and maintain their [g]cause.
46 If they sin against thee, (for *there is*
no man that sinneth not,) and thou be
angry with them, and deliver them to
the enemy, so that they carry them away
captives [h]unto the land of the enemy, far
or near;
47 *Yet* if they shall bethink themselves
in the land whither they were carried
captives, and repent, and make supplication unto thee in the land of them that
carried them captives, [i]saying, We have
sinned, and have done perversely, we
have committed wickedness;
48 And *so* return unto thee with all
their heart, and with all their soul, in the
land of their enemies, which led them
away captive, and pray unto thee [j]to-
ward their land, which thou gavest unto
their fathers, the city which thou hast
chosen, and the house which I have built
for thy name:
49 Then hear thou their prayer and
their supplication in heaven thy dwelling
place, and maintain their cause,
50 And forgive thy people that have
sinned against thee, and all their transgressions wherein they have transgressed against thee, and give them
compassion before them who carried
them captive, that they may have compassion on them:
51 For they *be* thy people, and thine
inheritance, which thou broughtest forth

B.C. 1004.

out of Egypt, [a]from the midst of the furnace of iron:
52 That thine eyes may be open unto
the supplication of thy servant, and unto
the supplication of thy people Israel, to
hearken unto them in all that they call
for unto thee.
53 For thou didst [b]separate them from
among all the people of the earth, *to be*
thine inheritance, as thou spakest by the
hand of Moses thy servant, when thou
broughtest our fathers out of Egypt, O
Lord GOD.

Solomon's blessing after the prayer.

54 And it was *so*, that when Solomon
had made an end of praying all this
prayer and supplication unto the LORD,
he arose from before the altar of the
LORD, from kneeling on his knees with
his hands spread up to heaven.
55 And he stood, and blessed all the
congregation of Israel with a loud voice,
saying,
56 Blessed *be* the LORD, that hath given
rest unto his people Israel, according to
all that he promised: there hath not
failed one word of all his good promise,
which he promised by the hand of
Moses his servant.
57 The LORD our God be with us, as he
was with our fathers: let him not leave
us, nor forsake us:
58 That he may incline our hearts unto
him, to walk in all his ways, and to keep
his commandments, and his statutes,
and his judgments, which he commanded our fathers.
59 And let these my words, wherewith I
have made supplication before the LORD,
be nigh unto the LORD our God day and
night, that he maintain the cause of his
servant, and the cause of his people Israel
at all times, as the matter shall require:
60 That all the people of the earth may
know that the LORD *is* God, *and that there
is* none else.
61 Let your heart therefore be [c]perfect
with the LORD our God, to walk in his
statutes, and to keep his commandments, as at this day.

Sacrifice and rejoicing (2 Chr. 7:4-10).

62 And the king, and all Israel with
him, offered sacrifice before the LORD.
63 And Solomon offered a sacrifice of
peace-offerings, which he offered unto
the LORD, two and twenty thousand oxen,
and an hundred and twenty thousand
sheep. So the king and all the children of
Israel dedicated the house of the LORD.
64 The same day did the king hallow
the middle of the court that *was* before
the house of the LORD: for there he
offered burnt-offerings, and [d]meat-offer-
ings, and the fat of the peace-offerings:
because the brasen altar that *was* before
the LORD *was* too little to receive the
burnt-offerings, and meat-offerings, and
the fat of the peace-offerings.
65 And at that time Solomon held a
feast, and all Israel with him, a great
congregation, from the entering in of
Hamath unto the river of Egypt, before
the LORD our God, seven days and seven
days, *even* fourteen days.
66 On the eighth day he sent the people away: and they blessed the king, and
went unto their tents joyful and glad of
heart for all the goodness that the LORD
had done for David his servant, and for
Israel his people.

CHAPTER 9.

Jehovah appears the second time to Solomon (2 Chr. 7:12-22).

And [e]it came to pass, when Solomon
had finished the building of the
house of the LORD, [f]and the king's
house, and [g]all Solomon's desire which
he was pleased to do,
2 That the LORD appeared to Solomon
the second time, [h]as he had appeared
unto him at Gibeon.
3 And the LORD said unto him, [i]I have
heard thy prayer and thy supplication,
that thou hast made before me: I have
hallowed this house, which thou hast
built, [j]to put my name there for ever;
and [k]mine eyes and mine heart shall be
there perpetually.
4 And if thou wilt [l]walk before me, as
David thy father walked, in integrity of
heart, and in uprightness, to do according
to all that I have commanded thee, *and*
wilt keep my statutes and my judgments:
5 Then I will establish the throne of
thy kingdom upon Israel for ever, as I
promised to David thy father, saying,
There shall not fail thee a man upon the
throne of Israel.

a Deut. 4:20; Jer. 11:4.
b *Separation.* Ezra 6:21. (Gen. 12:1; 2 Cor. 6:14-17.)
c The word implies whole-heartedness for God, single-mindedness, sincerity—not sinless perfection.
d Lit. *meal.*
e 2 Chr. 7:11.
f 1 Ki. 7:1.
g 2 Chr. 8:6.
h 1 Ki. 3:5.
i 2 Ki. 20:5; Psa. 10:17.
j 1 Ki. 8:29.
k Deut. 11:12.
l Gen. 17:1.

B.C. 992.

6 *But* if ye shall at all turn from following me, ye or your children, and will not keep my commandments *and* my statutes which I have set before you, but go and serve other gods, and worship them:

7 [a]Then will I cut off Israel out of the land which I have given them; and this house, which I have hallowed [b]for my name, will I cast out of my sight; and [c]Israel shall be a proverb and a byword among all people:

8 And at this house, *which* is high, every one that passeth by it shall be astonished, and shall hiss; and they shall say, [d]Why hath the LORD done thus unto this land, and to this house?

9 And they shall answer, Because they forsook the LORD their God, who brought forth their fathers out of the land of Egypt, and have taken hold upon other gods, and have worshipped them, and served them: therefore hath the LORD brought upon them all this evil.

The energy and fame of Solomon
(2 Chr. 8:1-18).

10 And it came to pass at the end of twenty years, when Solomon had built the two houses, the house of the LORD, and the king's house,

11 (*Now* Hiram the king of Tyre had furnished Solomon with cedar trees and fir trees, and with gold, according to all his desire,) that then king Solomon gave Hiram twenty cities in the land of Galilee.

12 And Hiram came out from Tyre to see the cities which Solomon had given him; and they pleased him not.

13 And he said, What cities *are* these which thou hast given me, my brother? And he called them the land of Cabul unto this day.

14 And Hiram sent to the king sixscore [e]talents of gold.

15 And this *is* the reason of the [f]levy which king Solomon raised; for to build the house of the LORD, and his own house, and [g]Millo, and the wall of Jerusalem, and [h]Hazor, and [i]Megiddo, and [j]Gezer.

16 *For* Pharaoh king of Egypt had gone up, and taken Gezer, and burnt it with fire, and slain the Canaanites that dwelt in the city, and given it *for* a present unto his daughter, Solomon's wife.

17 And Solomon built Gezer, and Beth-horon the nether,

18 And Baalath, and Tadmor in the wilderness, in the land,

a Deut. 4:26; 2 Ki. 17:23; 25:21.

b Jer. 7:14.

c Deut. 28:37; Psa. 44:14.

d Deut. 29:24-26; Jer. 22:8, 9.

e One talent = £6150, or $29,085; also v. 28.

f 1 Ki. 5:13.

g v. 24; 2 Sam. 5:9.

h Josh. 19:36.

i Josh. 17:11.

j Josh. 16:10; Jud. 1:29.

k 1 Ki. 3:1; 2 Chr. 8:11.

l 2 Sam. 5:9; 1 Ki. 11:27; 2 Chr. 32:5.

m 2 Chr. 9:1; Mt. 12:42; Lk. 11:31.

19 And all the cities of store that Solomon had, and cities for his chariots, and cities for his horsemen, and that which Solomon desired to build in Jerusalem, and in Lebanon, and in all the land of his dominion.

20 *And* all the people *that were* left of the Amorites, Hittites, Perizzites, Hivites, and Jebusites, which *were* not of the children of Israel,

21 Their children that were left after them in the land, whom the children of Israel also were not able utterly to destroy, upon those did Solomon levy a tribute of bondservice unto this day.

22 But of the children of Israel did Solomon make no bondmen: but they *were* men of war, and his servants, and his princes, and his captains, and rulers of his chariots, and his horsemen.

23 These *were* the chief of the officers that *were* over Solomon's work, five hundred and fifty, which bare rule over the people that wrought in the work.

24 But [k]Pharaoh's daughter came up out of the city of David unto her house which *Solomon* had built for her: [l]then did he build Millo.

25 And three times in a year did Solomon offer burnt-offerings and peace-offerings upon the altar which he built unto the LORD, and he burnt incense upon the altar that *was* before the LORD. So he finished the house.

26 And king Solomon made a navy of ships in Ezion-geber, which *is* beside Eloth, on the shore of the Red sea, in the land of Edom.

27 And Hiram sent in the navy his servants, shipmen that had knowledge of the sea, with the servants of Solomon.

28 And they came to Ophir, and fetched from thence gold, four hundred and twenty talents, and brought *it* to king Solomon.

CHAPTER 10.

Solomon and the queen of Sheba
(2 Chr. 9:1-12).

And when the [m]queen of Sheba heard of the fame of Solomon concerning the name of the LORD, she came to prove him with hard questions.

2 And she came to Jerusalem with a very great train, with camels that bare

spices, and very much gold, and precious stones: and when she was come to
Solomon, she communed with him of all
that was in her heart.
3 And Solomon told her all her questions: there was not *any* thing hid from
the king, which he told her not.
4 And when the queen of Sheba had
seen all Solomon's wisdom, and the
house that he had built,
5 And the meat of his table, and the
sitting of his servants, and the attendance of his ministers, and their apparel,
and his cupbearers, [a]and his ascent by
which he went up unto the house of the
LORD; there was no more spirit in her.
6 And she said to the king, It was a
true report that I heard in mine own
land of thy acts and of thy wisdom.
7 Howbeit I believed not the words,
until I came, and mine eyes had seen *it*:
and, behold, the half was not told me:
thy wisdom and prosperity exceedeth
the fame which I heard.
8 Happy *are* thy men, happy *are* these
thy servants, which stand continually
before thee, *and* that hear thy wisdom.
9 [b]Blessed be the LORD thy God, which
delighted in thee, to set thee on the
throne of Israel: because the LORD loved
Israel for ever, therefore made he thee
king, to do judgment and justice.
10 And she [c]gave the king an hundred
and twenty [d]talents of gold, and of
spices very great store, and precious
stones: there came no more such abundance of spices as these which the queen
of Sheba gave to king Solomon.
11 And the navy also of Hiram, that
brought gold from Ophir, brought in
from Ophir great plenty of almug trees,
and precious stones.
12 And the king made of the almug
trees pillars for the house of the LORD,
and for the king's house, harps also and
psalteries for singers: there came no such
[e]almug trees, nor were seen unto this day.
13 And king Solomon gave unto the
queen of Sheba all her desire, whatsoever she asked, beside *that* which Solomon
gave her of his royal bounty. So she
turned and went to her own country, she
and her servants.

B.C. 992.

a 2 Chr. 9:4.

b 1 Ki. 5:7.

c Psa. 72:10, 15.

d One talent = £6150, or $29,085; also v. 14.

e 2 Chr. 9:10.

f 2 Chr. 9:24; Psa. 72:10.

g 2 Chr. 9:20.

h Gen. 10:4; 2 Chr. 20:36.

i 1 Ki. 3:12, 13; 4:30.

j 1 Ki. 4:26; 2 Chr. 1:14; 9:25.

k 2 Chr. 1:15-17.

l Heb. *gave*.

Solomon's revenue and splendour (2 Chr. 9:13-28).

14 Now the weight of gold that came
to Solomon in one year was six hundred
threescore and six talents of gold,
15 Beside *that he had* of the merchantmen, and of the traffick of the spice merchants, and [f]of all the kings of Arabia,
and of the governors of the country.
16 And king Solomon made two hundred targets *of* beaten gold: six hundred
shekels of gold went to one target.
17 And *he made* three hundred shields
of beaten gold; three pound of gold went
to one shield: and the king put them in
the house of the forest of Lebanon.
18 Moreover the king made a great
throne of ivory, and overlaid it with the
best gold.
19 The throne had six steps, and the
top of the throne *was* round behind: and
there were stays on either side on the
place of the seat, and two lions stood
beside the stays.
20 And twelve lions stood there on the
one side and on the other upon the six
steps: there was not the like made in any
kingdom.
21 [g]And all king Solomon's drinking
vessels *were of* gold, and all the vessels of
the house of the forest of Lebanon *were of*
pure gold; none *were of* silver: it was nothing accounted of in the days of Solomon.
22 For the king had at sea a navy of
Tharshish with the navy of Hiram: once
in three years came the navy of
[h]Tharshish, bringing gold, and silver,
ivory, and apes, and peacocks.
23 [i]So king Solomon exceeded all the
kings of the earth for riches and for wisdom.
24 And all the earth sought to
Solomon, to hear his wisdom, which
God had put in his heart.
25 And they brought every man his
present, vessels of silver, and vessels of
gold, and garments, and armour, and
spices, horses, and mules, a rate year by
year.
26 [j]And Solomon gathered together
chariots and horsemen: and he had a
thousand and four hundred chariots,
and twelve thousand horsemen, whom
he bestowed in the cities for chariots,
and with the king at Jerusalem.
27 [k]And the king [l]made silver *to be* in

Jerusalem as stones, and cedars made he *to be* as the sycomore trees that *are* in the vale, for abundance.

28 And Solomon had horses brought out of Egypt, and linen yarn: the king's merchants received the linen yarn at a price.

29 And a chariot came up and went out of Egypt for six hundred *shekels* of silver, and an horse for an hundred and fifty: and so for all the kings of the Hittites, [a]and for the kings of Syria, did they bring *them* out by their means.

CHAPTER 11.

Solomon's heart turned away from Jehovah.

But king Solomon loved many strange women, together with the daughter of Pharaoh, women of the Moabites, Ammonites, Edomites, Zidonians, *and* Hittites;

2 Of the nations *concerning* which the LORD said unto the children of Israel, Ye shall not go in to them, neither shall they come in unto you: *for* surely they will turn away your heart after their gods: Solomon clave unto these in love.

3 And he had seven hundred wives, princesses, and three hundred concubines: and his wives turned away his heart.

4 For it came to pass, when Solomon was old, *that* his wives turned away his heart after other gods: and his heart was not [b]perfect with the LORD his God, as *was* the heart of David his father.

5 For Solomon went after [c]Ashtoreth the goddess of the Zidonians, and after [d]Milcom the abomination of the Ammonites.

6 And Solomon did evil in the sight of the LORD, and went not fully after the LORD, as *did* David his father.

7 Then did Solomon build an high place for Chemosh, the abomination of Moab, in the hill that *is* before Jerusalem, and for Molech, the abomination of the children of Ammon.

8 And likewise did he for all his strange wives, which burnt incense and sacrificed unto their gods.

The anger and chastening of Jehovah.

9 And the LORD was angry with Solomon, because his heart was turned from the LORD God of [e]Israel, which had appeared unto him twice,

10 And [f]had commanded him concerning this thing, that he should not go after other gods: but he kept not that which the LORD commanded.

11 Wherefore the LORD said unto Solomon, Forasmuch as this is done of thee, and thou hast not kept my covenant and my statutes, which I have commanded thee, [g]I will surely rend the kingdom from thee, and will give it to thy servant.

12 Notwithstanding in thy days I will not do it for David thy father's sake: *but* I will rend it out of the hand of thy son.

13 Howbeit I will not rend away all the kingdom; *but* will give one tribe to thy son for David my servant's sake, and for Jerusalem's sake which I have chosen.

14 And the LORD stirred up an adversary unto Solomon, Hadad the Edomite: he *was* of the king's seed in Edom.

15 For it came to pass, when David was in Edom, and Joab the captain of the host was gone up to bury the slain, [h]after he had smitten every male in Edom;

16 (For six months did Joab remain there with all Israel, until he had cut off every male in Edom:)

17 That Hadad fled, he and certain Edomites of his father's servants with him, to go into Egypt; Hadad *being* yet a little child.

18 And they arose out of Midian, and came to Paran: and they took men with them out of Paran, and they came to Egypt, unto Pharaoh king of Egypt; which gave him an house, and appointed him victuals, and gave him land.

19 And Hadad found great favour in the sight of Pharaoh, so that he gave him to wife the sister of his own wife, the sister of Tahpenes the queen.

20 And the sister of Tahpenes bare him Genubath his son, whom Tahpenes weaned in Pharaoh's house: and Genubath was in Pharaoh's household among the sons of Pharaoh.

21 [i]And when Hadad heard in Egypt that David slept with his fathers, and that Joab the captain of the host was dead, Hadad said to Pharaoh, Let me depart, that I may go to mine own country.

22 Then Pharaoh said unto him, But what hast thou lacked with me, that,

B.C. 992.

a Josh. 1:4; 2 Ki. 7:6.
b See 1 Ki. 8:61.
c v. 33; Jud. 2:13, *note.*
d Called *Molech*, v. 7.
e 1 Ki. 3:5; 9:2.
f 1 Ki. 6:12; 9:6, 7.
g v. 31; 1 Ki. 12:15, 16.
h Num. 24:19; Deut. 20:13.
i 1 Ki. 2:10, 34.

behold, thou seekest to go to thine own country? And he answered, Nothing: howbeit let me go in any wise.

23 And God stirred him up *another* adversary, Rezon the son of Eliadah, which fled from his lord [a]Hadadezer king of Zobah:

24 And he gathered men unto him, and became captain over a band, [b]when David slew them *of Zobah*: and they went to Damascus, and dwelt therein, and reigned in Damascus.

25 And he was an adversary to Israel all the days of Solomon, beside the mischief that Hadad *did*: and he abhorred Israel, and reigned over Syria.

The rise of Jeroboam.

26 And [c]Jeroboam the son of Nebat, an Ephrathite of Zereda, Solomon's servant, whose mother's name *was* Zeruah, a widow woman, even he [d]lifted up *his* hand against the king.

27 And this *was* the cause that he lifted up *his* hand against the king: [e]Solomon built Millo, *and* [f]repaired the breaches of the city of David his father.

28 And the man Jeroboam *was* a mighty man of valour: and Solomon seeing the young man that he was industrious, he made him ruler over all the charge of the house of Joseph.

29 And it came to pass at that time when Jeroboam went out of Jerusalem, that the prophet [g]Ahijah the Shilonite found him in the way; and he had clad himself with a new garment; and they two *were* alone in the field:

30 And Ahijah caught the new garment that *was* on him, and [h]rent it *in* twelve pieces:

31 And he said to Jeroboam, Take thee ten pieces: for [i]thus saith the LORD, the God of Israel, Behold, I will rend the kingdom out of the hand of Solomon, and will give ten tribes to thee:

32 (But he shall have one tribe for my servant David's sake, and for Jerusalem's sake, the city which I have chosen out of all the tribes of Israel:)

33 [j]Because that they have forsaken me, and have worshipped Ashtoreth the goddess of the Zidonians, Chemosh the god of the Moabites, and Milcom the god of the children of Ammon, and have not walked in my ways, to do *that which is* right in mine eyes, and *to keep* my statutes and my judgments, as *did* David his father.

34 Howbeit I will not take the whole kingdom out of his hand: but I will make him prince all the days of his life for David my servant's sake, whom I chose, because he kept my commandments and my statutes:

35 But I will take the kingdom out of his son's hand, and will give it unto thee, *even* ten tribes.

36 And unto his son will I give one tribe, that [k]David my servant may have a light alway before me in Jerusalem, the city which I have chosen me to put my name there.

37 And I will take thee, and thou shalt reign according to all that thy soul desireth, and shalt be king over Israel.

38 And it shall be, if thou wilt hearken unto all that I command thee, and wilt walk in my ways, and do *that is* right in my sight, to keep my statutes and my commandments, as David my servant did; that I will be with thee, and [l]build thee a sure house, as I built for David, and will give Israel unto thee.

39 And I will for this afflict the seed of David, but not for ever.

40 Solomon sought therefore to kill Jeroboam. And Jeroboam arose, and fled into Egypt, unto Shishak king of Egypt, and was in Egypt until the death of Solomon.

The death of Solomon (2 Chr. 9:29-31).

41 And the [m]rest of the acts of Solomon, and all that he did, and his wisdom, *are* they not written in the book of the acts of Solomon?

42 And the time that Solomon reigned in Jerusalem over all Israel *was* forty years.

43 And [n]Solomon slept with his fathers, and was buried in the city of David his father: and [o]Rehoboam his son reigned in his stead.

CHAPTER 12.

Accession and folly of Rehoboam
(2 Chr. 10:1-11).

And [p]Rehoboam went to Shechem: for all Israel were come to Shechem to make him king.

2 And it came to pass, when [q]Jeroboam the son of Nebat, who was yet in Egypt, heard *of it*, (for he was fled

B.C. 984.

a 2 Sam. 8:3; 10:16.
b 2 Sam. 8:3; 10:8-18.
c 1 Ki. 12:2; 2 Chr. 13:6.
d 2 Sam. 20:21.
e I Ki. 9:24.
f Heb. *closed.*
g 1 Ki. 14:2; 2 Chr. 9:29.
h 1 Sam. 15:27; 24:5.
i vs. 11, 13.
j vs. 5-7.
k *Kingdom* (O.T.). 2 Ki. 25:1-7. (Gen. 1:26-28; Zech. 12:8.)
l 2 Sam. 7:11, 27.
m 2 Chr. 9:29.
n 2 Chr. 9:31.
o Mt. 1:7, called *Roboam.*
p 2 Chr. 10:1.
q 1 Ki. 11:26.

from the presence of king Solomon, and
Jeroboam dwelt in [a]Egypt;)
3 That they sent and called him. And
Jeroboam and all the congregation of
Israel came, and spake unto Rehoboam,
saying,
4 Thy father made our [b]yoke grievous:
now therefore make thou the grievous
service of thy father, and his heavy yoke
which he put upon us, lighter, and we
will serve thee.
5 And he said unto them, Depart yet
for three days, then come again to me.
And the people departed.
6 And king Rehoboam consulted with
the old men, that stood before Solomon
his father while he yet lived, and said,
How do ye advise that I may answer
this people?
7 And they spake unto him, saying, [c]If
thou wilt be a servant unto this people
this day, and wilt serve them, and answer
them, and speak good words to them,
then they will be thy servants for ever.
8 But he forsook the counsel of the old
men, which they had given him, and
consulted with the young men that were
grown up with him, *and* which stood
before him:
9 And he said unto them, What counsel give ye that we may answer this people, who have spoken to me, saying,
Make the yoke which thy father did put
upon us lighter?
10 And the young men that were
grown up with him spake unto him, saying, Thus shalt thou speak unto this people that spake unto thee, saying, Thy
father made our yoke heavy, but make
thou *it* lighter unto us; thus shalt thou
say unto them, My little *finger* shall be
thicker than my father's loins.
11 And now whereas my father did
lade you with a heavy yoke, I will add to
your yoke: my father hath chastised you
with whips, but I will chastise you with
scorpions.
12 So Jeroboam and all the people
came to Rehoboam the third day, as the
king had appointed, saying, Come to me
again the third day.
13 And the king answered the people
[d]roughly, and forsook the old men's
counsel that they gave him;
14 And spake to them after the counsel of the young men, saying, My father
made your yoke heavy, and I will add to
your yoke: my father *also* chastised you
with whips, but I will chastise you with
scorpions.
15 Wherefore the king hearkened not
unto the people; for the [e]cause was from
the LORD, that he might perform his saying, which the LORD spake by Ahijah the
Shilonite unto Jeroboam the son of Nebat.

Division of the kingdom: accession of Jeroboam over Israel
(2 Chr. 10:12-19; 11:1-4).

16 So when all Israel saw that the king
hearkened not unto them, the people
answered the king, [f]saying, [g]What portion have we in David? neither *have we*
inheritance in the son of Jesse: to your
tents, O Israel: now see to thine own
house, David. So Israel departed unto
their tents.
17 But [h]*as for* the children of Israel
which dwelt in the cities of Judah,
Rehoboam reigned over them.
18 Then king Rehoboam [i]sent
Adoram, who *was* over the tribute; and
all Israel stoned him with stones, that he
died. Therefore king Rehoboam made
speed to get him up to his chariot, to flee
to Jerusalem.
19 So Israel rebelled against the house
of David unto this day.
20 And it came to pass, when all Israel
heard that Jeroboam was come again, that
they sent and called him unto the congregation, and made him king over all Israel:
there was none that followed the house of
David, but the tribe of Judah only.
21 And when Rehoboam was come to
Jerusalem, he assembled all the house of
Judah, with the tribe of Benjamin, an hundred and fourscore thousand chosen men,
which were warriors, to fight against the
house of Israel, to bring the kingdom
again to Rehoboam the son of Solomon.
22 But the word of God came unto
Shemaiah the man of God, saying,
23 Speak unto Rehoboam, the son of
Solomon, king of Judah, and unto all the
house of Judah and Benjamin, and to the
remnant of the people, saying,
24 Thus saith the LORD, Ye shall not go
up, nor fight against your brethren the
children of Israel: return every man to
his house; for this thing is from me. They
hearkened therefore to the word of the
LORD, and returned to depart, according
to the word of the LORD.

B.C. 975.

a 1 Ki. 11:40.
b 1 Sam. 8:11-18; 1 Ki. 4:7; 5:13-15.
c 2 Chr. 10:7; Prov. 15:1.
d Heb. *hardly.*
e v. 24; Jud. 14:4; 2 Chr. 10:15; 22:7; 25:20.
f Jud. 8:1, *note.*
g 2 Sam. 20:1.
h 1 Ki. 11:13, 36.
i 1 Ki. 4:6; 5:14.

Jeroboam destroys the religious unity of the nation.

25 Then Jeroboam [a]built Shechem in
mount Ephraim, and dwelt therein; and
went out from thence, and built [b]Penuel.
26 And Jeroboam said in his heart,
Now shall the kingdom return to the
house of David:
27 If this people go up to do sacrifice in
the house of the LORD at Jerusalem, then
shall the heart of this people turn again
unto their lord, *even* unto Rehoboam
king of Judah, and they shall kill me, and
go again to Rehoboam king of Judah.
28 Whereupon the king took counsel,
and made two calves *of* gold, and said
unto them, It is too much for you to go
up to Jerusalem: behold thy gods, O
Israel, which brought thee up out of the
land of Egypt.
29 And he set the one in Beth-el, and
the other put he in Dan.
30 And this thing became a sin: for the
people went *to worship* before the one,
even unto Dan.
31 And he made an house of high
[c]places, and made priests of the lowest
of the people, which were not of the sons
of Levi.
32 And Jeroboam ordained a feast in
the [d]eighth month, on the fifteenth day
of the month, like unto the feast that *is* in
Judah, and he offered upon the [e]altar. So
did he in Beth-el, sacrificing unto the
calves that he had made: and he placed
in Beth-el the priests of the high places
which he had made.
33 So he offered upon the altar which
he had made in Beth-el the fifteenth day
of the eighth month, *even* in the month
which he had devised of his own heart;
and ordained a feast unto the children of
Israel: and he offered upon the altar, and
burnt incense.

CHAPTER 13.

Prophecy against Jeroboam's false altar.

And, behold, [f]there came a man of
God out of Judah by the word of
the LORD unto Beth-el: [g]and Jeroboam
stood by the altar to burn incense.
2 And he cried against the altar in the
word of the LORD, and said, O altar, altar,
thus saith the LORD; Behold, a child shall
be born unto the house of David, [h]Josiah
by name; and upon thee shall he offer
the priests of the high places that burn
incense upon thee, and men's bones
shall be burnt upon thee.
3 And he gave a [i]sign the same day,
saying, This *is* the sign which the LORD
hath spoken; Behold, the altar shall be
rent, and the ashes that *are* upon it shall
be poured out.

The sign from God upon Jeroboam.

4 And it came to pass, when king
Jeroboam heard the saying of the man of
God, which had cried against the altar in
Beth-el, that he put forth his hand from
the altar, saying, Lay hold on him. And
his hand, which he put forth against
him, [j]dried up, so that he could not pull
it in again to him.
5 The altar also was rent, and the
ashes poured out from the altar, according to the sign which the man of God
had given by the word of the LORD.
6 And the king answered and said
unto the man of God, Intreat now the
face of the LORD thy God, and pray for
me, that my hand may be restored me
again. And the man of God besought the
LORD, and the king's hand was restored
him again, and became as *it was* before.
7 And the king said unto the man of
God, Come home with me, and refresh
thyself, and I will give thee a [k]reward.
8 And the man of God said unto the
king, [l]If thou wilt give me half thine
house, I will not go in with thee, neither
will I eat bread nor drink water in this
place:
9 For so was it charged me by the
word of the LORD, saying, Eat no bread,
nor drink water, nor turn again by the
same way that thou camest.
10 So he went another way, and
returned not by the way that he came to
Beth-el.

Disobedience and death of the man of God.

11 Now there dwelt an old prophet in
Beth-el; and his sons came and told him
all the works that the man of God had
done that day in Beth-el: the words
which he had spoken unto the king,
them they told also to their father.
12 And their father said unto them,
What way went he? For his sons had

B.C. 975.

a Jud. 9:45.
b Jud. 8:17.
c Cf. 2 Chr. 11:15.
d i.e. *November;* also v. 33.
e vs. 25-33; see Amos 4:4, *note;* Deut. 12:4-14.
f 2 Ki. 23.17.
g 1 Ki. 12:32, 33.
h 2 Ki. 23:15, 16.
i Isa. 7:14; John 2:18; 1 Cor. 1:22.
j *Miracles* (O.T.). vs. 4-6; 1 Ki. 17:14-16. (Gen. 5:24; Jon. 2:1-10.)
k 1 Sam. 9:7; 2 Ki. 5:15.
l Num. 22:18; 24:13.

B.C. 975.

seen what way the man of God went, which came from Judah.

13 And he said unto his sons, Saddle me the ass. So they saddled him the ass: and he rode thereon,

14 And went after the man of God, and found him sitting under an oak: and he said unto him, *Art* thou the man of God that camest from Judah? And he said, I *am*.

15 Then he said unto him, Come home with me, and eat bread.

16 And he said, [a]I may not return with thee, nor go in with thee: neither will I eat bread nor drink water with thee in this place:

17 For it was said to me by the word of the LORD, Thou shalt eat no bread nor drink water there, nor turn again to go by the way that thou camest.

18 He said unto him, I *am* a prophet also as thou *art*; [b]and an [c]angel spake unto me by the word of the LORD, saying, Bring him back with thee into thine house, that he may eat bread and drink water. *But* he lied unto him.

19 So he went back with him, and did eat bread in his house, and drank water.

20 And it came to pass, as they sat at the table, that the word of the LORD came unto the prophet that brought him back:

21 And he cried unto the man of God that came from Judah, saying, Thus saith the LORD, Forasmuch as thou hast disobeyed the mouth of the LORD, and hast not kept the commandment which the LORD thy God commanded thee,

22 But camest back, and hast eaten bread and drunk water in the [d]place, of the which *the LORD* did say to thee, Eat no bread, and drink no water; thy carcase shall not come unto the sepulchre of thy fathers.

23 And it came to pass, after he had eaten bread, and after he had drunk, that he saddled for him the ass, *to wit*, for the prophet whom he had brought back.

24 And when he was gone, [e]a lion met him by the way, and slew him: and his carcase was cast in the way, and the ass stood by it, the lion also stood by the carcase.

25 And, behold, men passed by, and saw the carcase cast in the way, and the lion standing by the carcase: and they came and told *it* in the city where the old prophet dwelt.

26 And when the prophet that brought him back from the way heard *thereof*, he said, It *is* the man of God, who was disobedient unto the word of the LORD: therefore the LORD hath delivered him unto the lion, which hath torn him, and slain him, according to the word of the LORD, which he spake unto him.

27 And he spake to his sons, saying, Saddle me the ass. And they saddled *him*.

28 And he went and found his carcase cast in the way, and the ass and the lion standing by the carcase: the lion had not eaten the carcase, nor torn the ass.

29 And the prophet took up the carcase of the man of God, and laid it upon the ass, and brought it back: and the old prophet came to the city, to mourn and to bury him.

30 And he laid his carcase in his own grave; and they mourned over him, *saying*, [f]Alas, my brother!

31 And it came to pass, after he had buried him, that he spake to his sons, saying, When I am dead, then bury me in the sepulchre wherein the man of God *is* buried; [g]lay my bones beside his bones:

32 [h]For the saying which he cried by the word of the LORD against the altar in Beth-el, and against all the houses of the high places which *are* in the cities of [i]Samaria, shall surely come to pass.

Jeroboam persists in evil.

33 After this thing Jeroboam returned not from his evil way, but made again of the lowest of the people priests of the high places: whosoever would, he consecrated him, and he became *one* of the priests of the high places.

34 And this thing became sin unto the house of Jeroboam, even [j]to cut *it* off, and to destroy *it* from off the face of the earth.

CHAPTER 14.

Prophecy against Jeroboam: partial fulfilment.

At that time Abijah the son of Jeroboam fell sick.

2 And Jeroboam said to his wife, Arise, I pray thee, and disguise thyself, that thou be not known to be the wife of Jeroboam; and get thee to Shiloh:

a vs. 8, 9.
b An impressive illustration of Gal. 1:.8, 9.
c Heb. 1:4, *note.*
d v. 9.
e 1 Ki. 20:36.
f Jer. 22:18.
g 2 Ki. 23:17, 18.
h v. 2; 2 Ki. 23:16, 17.
i 1 Ki. 16:24.
j 1 Ki. 14:10; cf. 14:16.

behold, there *is* Ahijah the prophet, which told me that [a]*I should be* king over this people.

3 [b]And take with thee ten loaves, and cracknels, and a cruse of honey, and go to him: he shall tell thee what shall become of the child.

4 And Jeroboam's wife did so, and arose, and went to Shiloh, and came to the house of Ahijah. But Ahijah could not see; for his eyes were set by reason of his age.

5 And the LORD said unto Ahijah, Behold, the wife of Jeroboam cometh to ask a thing of thee for her son; for he *is* sick: thus and thus shalt thou say unto her: for it shall be, when she cometh in, that she shall feign herself *to be* another *woman*.

6 And it was *so*, when Ahijah heard the sound of her feet, as she came in at the door, that he said, Come in, thou wife of Jeroboam; why feignest thou thyself *to be* another? for I *am* sent to thee *with* [c]heavy *tidings*.

7 Go, tell Jeroboam, Thus saith the LORD God of Israel, [d]Forasmuch as I exalted thee from among the people, and made thee prince over my people Israel,

8 And [e]rent the kingdom away from the house of David, and gave it thee: and *yet* thou hast not been as my servant David, [f]who kept my commandments, and who followed me with all his heart, to do *that* only *which was* right in mine eyes;

9 But hast done evil above all that were before thee: [g]for thou hast gone and made thee other gods, and molten images, to provoke me to anger, and hast cast me behind thy back:

10 Therefore, behold, I will bring evil upon the house of Jeroboam, and will cut off from Jeroboam him that pisseth against the wall, *and* him that is shut up and left in Israel, and will take away the remnant of the house of Jeroboam, as a man taketh away dung, till it be all gone.

11 Him that dieth of Jeroboam in the city shall the dogs eat; and him that dieth in the field shall the fowls of the air eat: for the LORD hath spoken *it*.

12 Arise thou therefore, get thee to thine own house: *and* when thy feet enter into the city, the child shall die.

13 And all Israel shall mourn for him, and bury him: for he only of Jeroboam shall come to the grave, because in him there is found *some* good thing toward

B.C. 956.

a 1 Ki. 11:31.
b 1 Sam. 9:7, 8..
c Heb. *hard*.
d 2 Sam. 12:7, 8; 1 Ki. 16:2.
e 1 Ki. 11:31.
f 1 Ki. 11:33, 38; 15:5.
g 1 Ki. 12:28; 2 Chr. 11:15.
h See Deut. 16:21.

the LORD God of Israel in the house of Jeroboam.

14 Moreover the LORD shall raise him up a king over Israel, who shall cut off the house of Jeroboam that day: but what? even now.

15 For the LORD shall smite Israel, as a reed is shaken in the water, and he shall root up Israel out of this good land, which he gave to their fathers, and shall scatter them beyond the river, because they have made their [h]groves, provoking the LORD to anger.

16 And he shall give Israel up because of the sins of Jeroboam, who did sin, and who made Israel to sin.

17 And Jeroboam's wife arose, and departed, and came to Tirzah: *and* when she came to the threshold of the door, the child died;

18 And they buried him; and all Israel mourned for him, according to the word of the LORD, which he spake by the hand of his servant Ahijah the prophet.

Death of Jeroboam (2 Chr. 13:20).

19 And the rest of the acts of Jeroboam, how he warred, and how he reigned, behold, they *are* written in the book of the chronicles of the kings of Israel.

20 And the days which Jeroboam reigned *were* two and twenty years: and he slept with his fathers, and Nadab his son reigned in his stead.

Judah's apostasy under Rehoboam (2 Chr. 12:1).

21 And Rehoboam the son of Solomon reigned in Judah. Rehoboam *was* forty and one years old when he began to reign, and he reigned seventeen years in Jerusalem, the city which the LORD did choose out of all the tribes of Israel, to put his name there. And his mother's name *was* Naamah an Ammonitess.

22 And Judah did evil in the sight of the LORD, and they provoked him to jealousy with their sins which they had committed, above all that their fathers had done.

23 For they also built them high places, and images, and [h]groves, on every high hill, and under every green tree.

24 And there were also sodomites in the land: *and* they did according to all the abominations of the nations which the LORD cast out before the children of Israel.

Invasion of Sishak (2 Chr. 12:2-12).

25 And it came to pass in the fifth year
of king Rehoboam, *that* Shishak king of
Egypt came up against Jerusalem:
26 And he took away the treasures of
the house of the LORD, and the treasures
of the king's house; he even took away
all: and he took away all the shields of
gold which Solomon had made.
27 And king Rehoboam made in their
stead brasen shields, and committed *them*
unto the hands of the chief of the guard,
which kept the door of the king's house.
28 And it was *so*, when the king went
into the house of the LORD, that the
guard bare them, and brought them
back into the guard chamber.
29 Now the rest of the acts of
Rehoboam, and all that he did, *are* they
not written in the book of the chronicles
of the kings of Judah?
30 And there was war between
Rehoboam and Jeroboam all *their* days.

Death of Rehoboam (2 Chr. 12:13-16).

31 And Rehoboam slept with his
fathers, and was buried with his fathers
in the city of David. And his mother's
name *was* Naamah an Ammonitess. And
Abijam his son reigned in his stead.

CHAPTER 15.

Accession of Abijam (2 Chr. 13:1, 2).

Now in the eighteenth year of king
Jeroboam the son of Nebat reigned
[a]Abijam over Judah.
2 Three years reigned he in Jerusalem.
And his mother's name *was* Maachah,
the daughter of Abishalom.
3 And he walked in all the sins of his
father, which he had done before him: and
his heart was not [b]perfect with the LORD
his God, as the heart of David his father.
4 Nevertheless for David's sake did
the LORD his God give him a lamp in
Jerusalem, to set up his son after him,
and to establish Jerusalem:
5 Because David did *that which was*
right in the eyes of the LORD, and turned
not aside from any *thing* that he commanded him all the days of his life, save
only in the matter of Uriah the Hittite.
6 And there was [c]war between
Rehoboam and Jeroboam all the days of
his life.
7 [d]Now the rest of the acts of Abijam,
and all that he did, *are* they not written
in the book of the chronicles of the kings
of Judah? And there was war between
Abijam and Jeroboam.

Death of Abijam (2 Chr. 14:1).

8 And [e]Abijam slept with his fathers;
and they buried him in the city of David:
and Asa his son reigned in his stead.

Accession of Asa (2 Chr. 14:1).

9 And in the twentieth year of Jeroboam
king of Israel reigned Asa over Judah.
10 And forty and one years reigned he
in Jerusalem. And his mother's name *was*
Maachah, the daughter of Abishalom.
11 [f]And Asa did *that which was* right in
the eyes of the LORD, as *did* David his
father.
12 [g]And he took away the sodomites
out of the land, and removed all the
idols that his fathers had made.
13 And also Maachah his mother, even
her he removed from *being* queen,
because she had made an idol in a
[h]grove; and Asa destroyed her idol, and
burnt *it* by the brook Kidron.
14 But [1]the high places were not
removed: nevertheless Asa's heart was
[b]perfect with the LORD all his days.
15 And he brought in the things which
his father had dedicated, and the things
which himself had dedicated, into the
house of the LORD, silver, and gold, and
vessels.

The war with Baasha: Asa's league with Syria (2 Chr. 16:1-6).

16 And there was war between Asa
and Baasha king of Israel all their days.
17 And [i]Baasha king of Israel
went up against Judah, and built

B.C. 951.

a Called *Abijah*, 2 Chr. 13:1, etc.

b See 1 Ki. 8:61.

c See 2 Chr. 13:2-22.

d 2 Chr. 13:2, 3, 22.

e 2 Chr. 14:1.

f 2 Chr. 14:2.

g 1 Ki. 14:24; 22:46.

h See Deut. 16:21.

i 2 Chr. 16:1.

[1]**(15:14)** Cf. 2 Chr. 14:3. It appears that local sacrifices to Jehovah (though not according to the divine order) were offered in the times of the kings upon "high places" (cf. 1 Sam. 9:12). Apparently Asa's mother had defiled one of these with an idol (1 Ki. 15:13). Asa destroyed the idol and the idolatrous (but not the Jehovistic) "high places." But see "high places," 1 Ki. 3:2, *note*.

B.C. 951.

[a]Ramah, [b]that he might not suffer any to go out or come in to Asa king of Judah.

18 Then Asa took all the silver and the gold *that were* left in the treasures of the house of the LORD, and the treasures of the king's house, and delivered them into the hand of his servants: and king Asa sent them to Ben-hadad, the son of Tabrimon, the son of Hezion, king of Syria, that dwelt at [c]Damascus, saying,

19 *There is* a league between me and thee, *and* between my father and thy father: behold, I have sent unto thee a present of silver and gold; come and break thy league with Baasha king of Israel, that he may depart from me.

20 So Ben-hadad hearkened unto king Asa, and sent the captains of the hosts which he had against the cities of Israel, and smote [d]Ijon, and [e]Dan, and [f]Abel-beth-maachah, and all Cinneroth, with all the land of Naphtali.

21 And it came to pass, when Baasha heard *thereof*, that he left off building of Ramah, and dwelt in Tirzah.

22 Then king Asa made a proclamation throughout all Judah; none *was* exempted: and they took away the stones of Ramah, and the timber thereof, wherewith Baasha had builded; and king Asa built with them Geba of Benjamin, and Mizpah.

Illness and death of Asa (2 Chr. 16:12-14). *Accession of Jehoshaphat* (2 Chr. 17:1).

23 The rest of all the acts of Asa, and all his might, and all that he did, and the cities which he built, *are* they not written in the book of the chronicles of the kings of Judah? Nevertheless in the time of his old age he was diseased in his feet.

24 And Asa slept with his fathers, and was buried with his fathers in the city of David his father: [g]and [h]Jehoshaphat his son reigned in his stead.

Accession of Nadab over Israel.

25 And Nadab the son of Jeroboam began to reign over Israel in the second year of Asa king of Judah, and reigned over Israel two years.

26 And he did evil in the sight of the LORD, and walked in the way of his father, and in his sin wherewith he made Israel to sin.

Rebellion and accession of Baasha over Israel.

27 And Baasha the son of Ahijah, of the house of Issachar, conspired against him; and Baasha smote him at [i]Gibbethon, which *belonged* to the Philistines; for Nadab and all Israel laid siege to Gibbethon.

28 Even in the third year of Asa king of Judah did Baasha slay him, and reigned in his stead.

29 And it came to pass, when he reigned, *that* he smote all the house of Jeroboam; he left not to Jeroboam any that breathed, until he had destroyed him, according unto the [j]saying of the LORD, which he spake by his servant Ahijah the Shilonite:

30 Because of the sins of Jeroboam which he sinned, and which he made Israel sin, by his provocation wherewith he provoked the LORD God of Israel to anger.

31 Now the rest of the acts of Nadab, and all that he did, *are* they not written in the book of the chronicles of the kings of Israel?

War between Asa, king of Judah, and Baasha, king of Israel.

32 And there was war between Asa and Baasha king of Israel all their days.

33 In the third year of Asa king of Judah began Baasha the son of Ahijah to reign over all Israel in Tirzah, twenty and four years.

34 And he did evil in the sight of the LORD, and walked in the way of Jeroboam, and in his sin wherewith he made Israel to sin.

CHAPTER 16.

Prophecy against Baasha: his death.

Then the word of the LORD came to [k]Jehu the son of Hanani against Baasha, saying,

2 [l]Forasmuch as I exalted thee out of the dust, and made thee prince over my people Israel; and thou hast walked in the way of Jeroboam, and hast made my people Israel to sin, to provoke me to anger with their sins;

3 Behold, I will [m]take away the posterity of Baasha, and the posterity of his house; and will make thy house like the [n]house of Jeroboam the son of Nebat.

a Josh. 18:25.
b 1 Ki. 12:27.
c 1 Ki. 11:23, 24.
d 2 Ki. 15:29.
e Jud. 18:29.
f 2 Sam. 20:14.
g 2 Chr. 17:1.
h Called *Josaphat*, Mt. 1:8.
i Josh. 19:44; 21:23; 1 Ki. 16:15.
j 1 Ki. 14:10, 14.
k v. 7; 2 Chr 19:2; 20:34.
l 1 Ki. 14:7.
m v. 11.
n 1 Ki. 14:10; 15:29.

4 [a]Him that dieth of Baasha in the city shall the dogs eat; and him that dieth of his in the fields shall the fowls of the air eat.

5 Now the rest of the acts of Baasha, and what he did, and his might, [b]*are* they not written in the book of the chronicles of the kings of Israel?

6 So Baasha slept with his fathers, and was buried in [c]Tirzah: and Elah his son reigned in his stead.

7 And also by the hand of the prophet Jehu the son of Hanani came the word of the LORD against Baasha, and against his house, even for all the evil that he did in the sight of the LORD, in provoking him to anger with the work of his hands, in being like the house of Jeroboam; and because [d]he killed him.

Accession of Elah over Israel.

8 In the twenty and sixth year of Asa king of Judah began Elah the son of Baasha to reign over Israel in Tirzah, two years.

9 [e]And his servant Zimri, captain of half *his* chariots, conspired against him, as he was in Tirzah, drinking himself drunk in the house of Arza steward of *his* house in Tirzah.

10 And Zimri went in and smote him, and killed him, in the twenty and seventh year of Asa king of Judah, and reigned in his stead.

The reign of Zimri over Israel.

11 And it came to pass, when he began to reign, as soon as he sat on his throne, *that* he slew all the house of Baasha: he left him [f]not one that pisseth against a wall, neither of his [g]kinsfolks, nor of his friends.

12 Thus did Zimri destroy all the house of Baasha, according to the word of the LORD, which he spake against Baasha by Jehu the prophet,

13 For all the sins of Baasha, and the sins of Elah his son, by which they sinned, and by which they made Israel to sin, in provoking the LORD God of Israel to anger with their vanities.

14 Now the rest of the acts of Elah, and all that he did, *are* they not written in the book of the chronicles of the kings of Israel?

15 In the twenty and seventh year of Asa king of Judah did Zimri reign seven days in Tirzah. And the people *were* encamped against Gibbethon, which *belonged* to the Philistines.

16 And the people *that were* encamped heard say, Zimri hath conspired, and hath also slain the king: wherefore all Israel made Omri, the captain of the host, king over Israel that day in the camp.

17 And Omri went up from Gibbethon, and all Israel with him, and they besieged Tirzah.

18 And it came to pass, when Zimri saw that the city was taken, that he went into the palace of the king's house, and burnt the king's house over him with fire, and died,

19 For his sins which he sinned in doing evil in the sight of the LORD, [h]in walking in the way of Jeroboam, and in his sin which he did, to make Israel to sin.

20 Now the rest of the acts of Zimri, and his treason that he wrought, *are* they not written in the book of the chronicles of the kings of Israel?

Tibni and Omri rival kings of Israel: death of Tibni.

21 Then were the people of Israel divided into two parts: half of the people followed Tibni the son of Ginath, to make him king; and half followed Omri.

22 But the people that followed Omri prevailed against the people that followed Tibni the son of Ginath: so Tibni died, and Omri reigned.

Reign of Omri over Israel: he makes Samaria the capital.

23 In the thirty and first year of Asa king of Judah began Omri to reign over Israel, twelve years: six years reigned he in Tirzah.

24 And he bought the hill Samaria of Shemer for two [i]talents of silver, and built on the hill, and called the name of the city which he built, after the name of Shemer, owner of the hill, Samaria.

25 But Omri wrought evil in the eyes of the LORD, and did worse than all that *were* before him.

26 For he walked in all the way of Jeroboam the son of Nebat, and in his sin wherewith he made Israel to sin, to provoke the LORD God of Israel to anger with their vanities.

27 Now the rest of the acts of Omri which he did, and his might that he shewed, *are* they not written in the book of the chronicles of the kings of Israel?

B.C. 930.

a 1 Ki. 14:11.
b 2 Chr. 16:1.
c 1 Ki. 14:17; 15:21.
d 1 Ki. 15:27-29; Hos. 1:4.
e 2 Ki. 9:31.
f 1 Sam. 25:22.
g Heb. *goel*, *Redemp. (Kinsman type).* Isa. 59:20, *note.*
h 1 Ki. 12:28; 15:26, 34.
i One talent = £410, or $1940.

Accession of Ahab over Israel: he marries Jezebel.

28 So Omri slept with his fathers, and was buried in Samaria: and Ahab his son reigned in his stead.

29 And in the thirty and eighth year of Asa king of Judah began Ahab the son of Omri to reign over Israel: and Ahab the son of Omri reigned over Israel in Samaria twenty and two years.

30 And Ahab the son of Omri did evil in the sight of the LORD above all that *were* before him.

31 And it came to pass, as if it had been a light thing for him to walk in the sins of Jeroboam the son of Nebat, that he took to wife Jezebel the daughter of Ethbaal king of the Zidonians, and went and served Baal, and worshipped him.

32 And he reared up an altar for Baal in the house of Baal, which he had built in Samaria.

33 And Ahab made a [a]grove; and Ahab did more to provoke the LORD God of Israel to anger than all the kings of Israel that were before him.

34 In his days did Hiel the Beth-elite build Jericho: he laid the foundation thereof in Abiram his firstborn, and set up the gates thereof in his youngest *son* Segub, according to the [b]word of the LORD, which he spake by Joshua the son of Nun.

CHAPTER 17.

Ministry of Elijah: his prediction of three years' drought.

And [c]Elijah the Tishbite, *who was* of the inhabitants of Gilead, said unto [d]Ahab, *As* the LORD God of Israel liveth, before whom I stand, there shall not be dew nor rain these years, but according to my word.

Elijah fed at Cherith.

2 And the word of the LORD came unto him, saying,

3 Get thee hence, and turn thee eastward, and hide thyself by the brook Cherith, that *is* before Jordan.

4 And it shall be, *that* thou shalt drink of the brook; and I have commanded the ravens to feed thee there.

5 So he went and did according unto the word of the LORD: for he went and dwelt by the brook Cherith, that *is* before Jordan.

6 And the ravens brought him bread and flesh in the morning, and bread and flesh in the evening; and he drank of the brook.

7 And it came to pass after a while, that the brook dried up, because there had been no rain in the land.

Elijah fed at Zarephath.

8 And the word of the LORD came unto him, saying,

9 Arise, get thee to [e]Zarephath, which *belongeth* to Zidon, and dwell there: behold, I have commanded a widow woman there to sustain thee.

10 So he arose and went to Zarephath. And when he came to the gate of the city, behold, the widow woman *was* there gathering of sticks: and he called to her, and said, Fetch me, I pray thee, a little water in a vessel, that I may drink.

11 And as she was going to fetch *it*, he called to her, and said, Bring me, I pray thee, a morsel of bread in thine hand.

12 And she said, *As* the LORD thy God liveth, I have not a cake, but an handful of meal in a barrel, and a little oil in a cruse: and, behold, I *am* gathering two sticks, that I may go in and dress it for me and my son, that we may eat it, and die.

13 And Elijah said unto her, Fear not; go *and* do as thou hast said: but make me thereof a little cake first, and bring *it* unto me, and after make for thee and for thy son.

14 For thus saith the LORD God of Israel, The barrel of meal shall not waste, neither shall the cruse of oil fail, until the day *that* the LORD sendeth rain upon the earth.

15 And she went and did according to the saying of Elijah: and she, and he, and her house, did eat *many* days.

16 *And* the barrel of meal wasted not, neither did the cruse of oil fail, [f]according to the word of the LORD, which he spake by Elijah.

Elijah raises the widow's son.

17 And it came to pass after these things, *that* the son of the woman, the mistress of the house, fell sick; and his sickness was so sore, that there was no breath left in him.

18 And she said unto Elijah, What have I to do with thee, O thou man of God? art thou come unto me to call my sin to remembrance, and to slay my son?

B.C. 925.

a See Deut. 16:21.

b See Josh. 6:26.

c Heb. *Elijahu*, Lk. 1:17; Lk. 4:25, called *Elias*.

d It was a small thing for a man whose life was passed in Jehovah's presence to stand before Ahab.

e Oba. 20; Lk. 4:26, called *Sarepta*.

f *Miracles* (O.T.). vs. 14-16, 17-24; 1 Ki. 18:30-38. (Gen. 5:24; Jon. 2:1-10.)

19 And he said unto her, Give me thy son. And he took him out of her bosom, and carried him up into a loft, where he abode, and laid him upon his own bed.

20 And he [a]cried unto the LORD, and said, O LORD my God, hast thou also brought evil upon the widow with whom I sojourn, by slaying her son?

21 And he stretched himself upon the child three times, and cried unto the LORD, and said, O LORD my God, I pray thee, let this child's soul come into him again.

22 And the LORD heard the voice of Elijah; and the soul of the child came into him again, and he revived.

23 And Elijah took the child, and brought him down out of the chamber into the house, and delivered him unto his mother: and Elijah said, See, thy son liveth.

24 And the woman said to Elijah, Now by this I know that thou *art* a man of God, *and* that the word of the LORD in thy mouth *is* truth.

CHAPTER 18.

Elijah goes to meet Ahab.

And it came to pass *after* many days, that the word of the LORD came to Elijah in the third year, saying, Go, shew thyself unto Ahab; and I will send rain upon the earth.

2 And Elijah went to shew himself unto Ahab. And *there was* a sore famine in Samaria.

A believer out of touch with God.

3 And Ahab called [b]Obadiah, which *was* the governor of *his* house. (Now Obadiah [c]feared the LORD greatly:

4 For it was *so*, when Jezebel cut off the prophets of the LORD, that Obadiah took an hundred prophets, and hid them by fifty in a cave, and fed them with bread and water.)

5 And Ahab said unto Obadiah, Go into the land, unto all fountains of water, and unto all brooks: peradventure we may find grass to save the horses and mules alive, that we lose not all the beasts.

6 So they divided the land between them to pass throughout it: Ahab went one way by himself, and Obadiah went another way by himself.

7 And as Obadiah was in the way, behold, Elijah met him: and he knew him, and fell on his face, and said, *Art* thou that my lord Elijah?

8 And he answered him, I *am*: go, tell thy lord, Behold, Elijah *is here*.

9 And he said, What have I sinned, that thou wouldest deliver thy servant into the hand of Ahab, to slay me?

10 *As* the LORD thy God liveth, there is no nation or kingdom, whither my lord hath not sent to seek thee: and when they said, *He is* not *there*; he took an oath of the kingdom and nation, that they found thee not.

11 And now thou sayest, Go, tell thy lord, Behold, Elijah *is here*.

12 And it shall come to pass, *as soon as* I am gone from thee, that the [d]Spirit of the LORD shall carry thee whither I know not; and *so* when I come and tell Ahab, and he cannot find thee, he shall slay me: but I thy servant [c]fear the LORD from my youth.

13 Was it not told my lord what I did when Jezebel slew the prophets of the LORD, how I hid an hundred men of the LORD'S prophets by fifty in a cave, and fed them with bread and water?

14 And now thou sayest, Go, tell thy lord, Behold, Elijah *is here*: and he shall slay me.

15 And Elijah said, *As* the LORD of hosts liveth, before whom I stand, I will surely shew myself unto him to day.

16 So Obadiah went to meet Ahab, and told him: and Ahab went to meet Elijah.

Elijah meets Ahab: the prophet's challenge.

17 And it came to pass, when Ahab saw Elijah, that Ahab said unto him, [e]*Art* thou he that [f]troubleth Israel?

18 And he answered, I have not troubled Israel; but thou, and thy father's house, [g]in that ye have forsaken the commandments of the LORD, and thou hast followed Baalim.

19 Now therefore send, *and* gather to me all Israel unto mount [h]Carmel, and the prophets of Baal four hundred and fifty, and the prophets of the [i]groves four hundred, which eat at Jezebel's table.

20 So Ahab sent unto all the children of Israel, and gathered the prophets together unto mount Carmel.

21 And Elijah came unto all the people, and said, [j]How long halt ye between two opinions? if the LORD *be* God, follow

B.C. 910.

a *Bible prayers* (O.T.). 1 Ki. 18:36. (Gen. 15:2; Hab. 3:1-16.)

b In such a time as the reign of Ahab and Jezebel a believer's true place was by Elijah's side. Obadiah is a warning type of the men of God who adhere to the world while still seeking to serve God. The secret of the Lord, and the power of the Lord were with Elijah, the separated servant. Cf. 2 Tim. 2:20, 21.

c Psa. 19:9, *note*.

d 2 Ki. 2:16; Ezk. 3:12, 14.

e 1 Ki. 21:20.

f Josh. 7:25.

g 2 Chr. 15:2.

h Josh. 19:26.

i Deut. 16:21.

j 2 Ki. 17:41; Mt. 6:24.

him: but if Baal, *then* follow him. And
the people answered him not a word.
22 Then said Elijah unto the people, [a]I,
even I only, remain a prophet of the
LORD; but Baal's prophets *are* four hundred and fifty men.
23 Let them therefore give us two bullocks; and let them choose one bullock
for themselves, and cut it in pieces, and
lay *it* on wood, and put no fire *under*:
and I will dress the other bullock, and
lay *it* on wood, and put no fire *under*:
24 And call ye on the name of your
gods, and I will call on the name of the
LORD: and the God that [b]answereth by
fire, let him be God. And all the people
answered and said, It is well spoken.

Jehovah versus Baal.

25 And Elijah said unto the prophets
of Baal, Choose you one bullock for
yourselves, and dress *it* first; for ye *are*
many; and call on the name of your
gods, but put no fire *under*.
26 And they took the bullock which
was given them, and they dressed *it*, and
called on the name of Baal from morning
even until noon, saying, O Baal, hear us.
But *there was* no voice, nor any that
answered. And they leaped upon the
altar which was made.
27 And it came to pass at noon, that
Elijah mocked them, and said, Cry
aloud: for he *is* a god; either he is talking, or he is pursuing, or he is in a journey, *or* peradventure he sleepeth, and
must be awaked.
28 And they cried aloud, and cut
themselves after their manner with
knives and lancets, till the blood gushed
out upon them.
29 And it came to pass, when midday
was past, and they prophesied until the
time of the offering of the *evening* sacrifice, that *there was* neither voice, nor any
to answer, nor any that regarded.
30 And Elijah said unto all the people,
Come near unto me. And all the people
came near unto him. And he repaired the
altar of the LORD *that was* broken down.
31 And Elijah took twelve stones,
according to the number of the tribes of
the sons of Jacob, unto whom the word
of the LORD came, saying, Israel shall be
thy name:
32 And with the stones he built an
altar in the name of the LORD: and he
made a trench about the altar, as great as
would contain two [c]measures of seed.
33 And he put the wood in order, and
cut the bullock in pieces, and laid *him* on
the wood, and said, Fill four barrels with
water, and pour *it* on the burnt sacrifice,
and on the wood.
34 And he said, Do *it* the second time.
And they did *it* the second time. And he
said, Do *it* the third time. And they did *it*
the third time.
35 And the water ran round about the
altar; and he filled the trench also with
water.
36 And it came to pass at *the time of* the
offering of the *evening* sacrifice, that
Elijah the prophet came near, and [d]said,
LORD God of Abraham, Isaac, and of
Israel, let it be known this day that thou
art God in Israel, and *that* I *am* thy servant, and *that* I have done all these
things at thy word.
37 Hear me, O LORD, hear me, that this
people may know that thou *art* the LORD
God, and *that* thou hast turned their
heart back again.
38 Then the fire of the LORD [e]fell, and
consumed the burnt sacrifice, and the
wood, and the stones, and the dust, and
licked up the water that *was* in the trench.
39 And when all the people saw *it*,
they fell on their faces: and they said,
The LORD, he *is* the God; the LORD, he *is*
the God.
40 And Elijah said unto them, Take the
prophets of Baal; let not one of them
escape. And they took them: and Elijah
brought them down to the brook
Kishon, and slew them there.
41 And Elijah said unto Ahab, Get
thee up, eat and drink; for *there is* a
sound of abundance of rain.

Elijah on Carmel.

42 So Ahab went up to eat and to drink.
And Elijah went up to the top of Carmel;
and he cast himself down upon the earth,
and put his face between his knees,
43 And said to his servant, Go up now,
look toward the sea. And he went up,
and looked, and said, *There is* nothing.
And he said, Go again seven times.
44 And it came to pass at the seventh
time, that he said, Behold, there ariseth a
little cloud out of the sea, like a man's

B.C. 906.

a 1 Ki. 19:10, 14.

b v. 38; 1 Chr. 21:26.

c One measure = about 4 pecks.

d *Bible prayers* (O.T.). 1 Ki. 19:4. (Gen. 15:2; Hab. 3:1-16.)

e *Miracles* (O.T.). vs. 30-38; 2 Ki. 1:10-12. (Gen. 5:24; Jon. 2:1-10.)

B.C. 906.

hand. And he said, Go up, say unto Ahab, Prepare *thy chariot*, and get thee down, that the rain stop thee not.

45 And it came to pass in the mean while, that the heaven was black with clouds and wind, and there was a great rain. And Ahab rode, and went to Jezreel.

46 And the hand of the LORD was on Elijah; and he girded up his loins, and ran before Ahab to the entrance of Jezreel.

CHAPTER 19.

Jehovah's tender care of His overwrought prophet.

And Ahab told Jezebel all that Elijah had done, and withal how he had slain all the prophets with the sword.

2 Then Jezebel sent a messenger unto Elijah, saying, So let the gods do *to me*, and more also, if I make not thy life as the life of one of them by to morrow about this time.

3 And when he saw *that*, he arose, and went for his life, and came to Beer-sheba, which *belongeth* to Judah, and left his servant there.

4 But he himself went a day's journey into the wilderness, and came and sat down under a juniper tree: and he [a]requested for himself that he might die; and said, It is enough; now, O LORD, take away my life; for I *am* not better than my fathers.

5 And as he lay and slept under a juniper tree, behold, then an [b]angel touched him, and said unto him, Arise *and* eat.

6 And he looked, and, behold, *there was* a cake baken on the coals, and a cruse of water at his head. And he did eat and drink, and laid him down again.

7 And the angel of the LORD came again the second time, and touched him, and said, Arise *and* eat; because the journey *is* too great for thee.

Elijah on Horeb.

8 And he arose, and did eat and drink, and went in the strength of that meat forty days and forty nights unto Horeb the mount of God.

9 And he came thither unto a cave, and lodged there; and, behold, the word of the LORD *came* to him, and he said unto him, What doest thou here, Elijah?

10 And he said, I have been very jealous for the LORD God of hosts: for the children of Israel have forsaken thy covenant, thrown down thine altars, and slain thy [c]prophets with the sword; and I, *even* I only, am left; and they seek my life, to take it away.

11 And he said, Go forth, and stand upon the mount before the LORD. And, behold, the LORD passed by, and a [d]great and strong wind rent the mountains, and brake in pieces the rocks before the LORD; *but* the LORD *was* not in the wind: and after the wind an earthquake; *but* the LORD *was* not in the earthquake:

12 And after the earthquake a fire; *but* the LORD *was* not in the fire: and after the fire a still small voice.

13 And it was *so*, when Elijah heard *it*, that he [e]wrapped his face in his mantle, and went out, and stood in the entering in of the cave. [f]And, behold, *there came* a voice unto him, and said, What doest thou here, Elijah?

14 [g]And he said, I have been very jealous for the LORD God of hosts: because the children of Israel have forsaken thy covenant, thrown down thine altars, and slain thy prophets with the sword; and I, *even* I only, am left; and they seek my life, to take it away.

15 And the LORD said unto him, Go, return on thy way to the wilderness of Damascus: [h]and when thou comest, anoint Hazael *to be* king over Syria:

16 And [i]Jehu the son of Nimshi shalt thou anoint *to be* king over Israel: and [j]Elisha the son of Shaphat of Abel-meholah shalt thou anoint *to be* prophet in thy room.

17 And it shall come to pass, *that* him that escapeth the sword of Hazael shall Jehu slay: and him that escapeth from the sword of Jehu shall Elisha slay.

18 Yet [k]I have [l]left *me* seven thousand in Israel, all the knees which have not bowed unto Baal, and every mouth which hath not kissed him.

The call of Elisha.

19 So he departed thence, and found Elisha the son of Shaphat, who *was* plowing *with* twelve yoke *of oxen* before him, and he with the twelfth: and Elijah

a *Bible prayers* (O.T.). 2 Ki. 6:17. (Gen. 15:2; Hab. 3:1-16.)

b Heb. 1.4, *note.*

c v. 14; Rom. 11:3.

d Ezk. 1:4; 37:9.

e Ex. 3:6; Isa. 6:2.

f v. 9.

g v. 10.

h 2 Ki. 8:12, 13.

i 2 Ki. 9:1-3.

j 2 Ki. 2:9-15. Called *Eliseus*, Lk. 4:27.

k Rom. 11:4.

l See *Remnant* (Isa. 1:9; Rom. 11:5).

passed by him, and cast his mantle upon him.

20 And he left the oxen, and ran after Elijah, and said, Let me, I pray thee, kiss my father and my mother, and *then* I will follow thee. And he said unto him, Go back again: for what have I done to thee?

21 And he returned back from him, and took a yoke of oxen, and slew them, and boiled their flesh with the instruments of the oxen, and gave unto the people, and they did eat. Then he arose, and went after Elijah, and ministered unto him.

CHAPTER 20.

Ahab's first Syrian campaign.

And Ben-hadad the king of Syria gathered all his host together: and *there were* thirty and two kings with him, and horses, and chariots: and he went up and besieged Samaria, and warred against it.

2 And he sent messengers to Ahab king of Israel into the city, and said unto him, Thus saith Ben-hadad,

3 Thy silver and thy gold *is* mine; thy wives also and thy children, *even* the goodliest, *are* mine.

4 And the king of Israel answered and said, My lord, O king, according to thy saying, I *am* thine, and all that I have.

5 And the messengers came again, and said, Thus speaketh Ben-hadad, saying, Although I have sent unto thee, saying, Thou shalt deliver me thy silver, and thy gold, and thy wives, and thy children;

6 Yet I will send my servants unto thee to morrow about this time, and they shall search thine house, and the houses of thy servants; and it shall be, *that* whatsoever is pleasant in thine eyes, they shall put *it* in their hand, and take *it* away.

7 Then the king of Israel called all the elders of the land, and said, Mark, I pray you, and see how this *man* seeketh mischief: for he sent unto me for my wives, and for my children, and for my silver, and for my gold; and I denied him not.

8 And all the elders and all the people said unto him, Hearken not *unto him,* nor consent.

9 Wherefore he said unto the messengers of Ben-hadad, Tell my lord the king, All that thou didst send for to thy servant at the first I will do: but this thing I may not do. And the messengers departed, and brought him word again.

10 And Ben-hadad sent unto him, and said, The [a]gods do so unto me, and more also, if the dust of Samaria shall suffice for handfuls for all the people that [b]follow me.

11 And the king of Israel answered and said, Tell *him,* Let not him that girdeth on *his harness* boast himself as he that putteth it off.

12 And it came to pass, when *Ben-hadad* heard this message, as he *was* drinking, he and the kings in the pavilions, that he said unto his servants, Set *yourselves in array*. And they set *themselves in array* against the city.

God's promise of victory.

13 And, behold, there came a prophet unto Ahab king of Israel, saying, Thus saith the LORD, Hast thou seen all this great multitude? behold, [c]I will deliver it into thine hand this day; and thou shalt know that I *am* the LORD.

14 And Ahab said, By whom? And he said, Thus saith the LORD, *Even* by the young men of the princes of the provinces. Then he said, Who shall order the battle? And he answered, Thou.

Ahab's victory over the Syrians.

15 Then he numbered the young men of the princes of the provinces, and they were two hundred and thirty two: and after them he numbered all the people, *even* all the children of Israel, *being* seven thousand.

16 And they went out at noon. But Ben-hadad *was* [d]drinking himself drunk in the pavilions, he and the kings, the thirty and two kings that helped him.

17 And the young men of the princes of the provinces went out first; and Ben-hadad sent out, and they told him, saying, There are men come out of Samaria.

18 And he said, Whether they be come out for peace, take them alive; or whether they be come out for war, take them alive.

19 So these young men of the princes of the provinces came out of the city, and the army which followed them.

20 And they slew every one his man: and the Syrians fled; and Israel pursued them: and Ben-hadad the king of Syria escaped on an horse with the horsemen.

B.C. 906.

a 1 Ki. 19:2.

b Heb. *are at my feet.*

c v. 28.

d v. 12; 1 Ki. 16:9.

21 And the king of Israel went out, and smote the horses and chariots, and slew the Syrians with a great slaughter.

The prophet warns Ahab.

22 And the prophet came to the king of Israel, and said unto him, Go, strengthen thyself, and mark, and see what thou doest: [a]for at the return of the year the king of Syria will come up against thee.

Ahab's second Syrian campaign.

23 And the servants of the king of Syria said unto him, Their gods *are* gods of the hills; therefore they were stronger than we; but let us fight against them in the plain, and surely we shall be stronger than they.

24 And do this thing, Take the kings away, every man out of his place, and put captains in their rooms:

25 And number thee an army, like the army that thou hast lost, horse for horse, and chariot for chariot: and we will fight against them in the plain, *and* surely we shall be stronger than they. And he hearkened unto their voice, and did so.

26 And it came to pass at the return of the year, that Ben-hadad numbered the Syrians, and went up to [b]Aphek, to fight against Israel.

27 And the children of Israel were numbered, and were all present, and went against them: and the children of Israel pitched before them like two little flocks of kids; but the Syrians filled the country.

28 And there came a man of God, and spake unto the king of Israel, and said, Thus saith the LORD, Because the Syrians have said, The LORD *is* God of the hills, but he *is* not God of the valleys, therefore [c]will I deliver all this great multitude into thine hand, and ye shall know that I *am* the LORD.

29 And they pitched one over against the other seven days. And *so* it was, that in the seventh day the battle was joined: and the children of Israel slew of the Syrians an hundred thousand footmen in one day.

30 But the rest fled to Aphek, into the city; and *there* a wall fell upon twenty and seven thousand of the men *that were* left. And Ben-hadad fled, and came into the city, into an inner chamber.

31 And his servants said unto him, Behold now, we have heard that the kings of the house of Israel *are* merciful kings: let us, I pray thee, [d]put sackcloth on our loins, and ropes upon our heads, and go out to the king of Israel: peradventure he will save thy life.

32 So they girded sackcloth on their loins, and *put* ropes on their heads, and came to the king of Israel, and said, Thy servant Ben-hadad saith, I pray thee, let me live. And he said, *Is* he yet alive? he *is* my brother.

33 Now the men did diligently observe whether *any thing would come* from him, and did hastily catch *it*: and they said, Thy brother Ben-hadad. Then he said, Go ye, bring him. Then Ben-hadad came forth to him; and he caused him to come up into the chariot.

34 And *Ben-hadad* said unto him, The [e]cities, which my father took from thy father, I will restore; and thou shalt make streets for thee in Damascus, as my father made in Samaria. Then *said Ahab*, I will send thee away with this covenant. So he made a covenant with him, and sent him away.

Ahab's sin in sparing Ben-hadad.

35 [f]And a certain man of the sons of the prophets said unto his neighbour in the word of the LORD, Smite me, I pray thee. And the man refused to smite him.

36 Then said he unto him, Because thou hast not obeyed the voice of the LORD, behold, as soon as thou art departed from me, a lion shall slay thee. And as soon as he was departed from him, a lion found him, and slew him.

37 Then he found another man, and said, Smite me, I pray thee. And the man smote him, so that in smiting he wounded *him*.

38 So the prophet departed, and waited for the king by the way, and disguised himself with ashes upon his face.

39 And as the king passed by, he cried unto the king: and he said, Thy servant went out into the midst of the battle; and, behold, a man turned aside, and brought a man unto me, and said, Keep this man: if by any means he be missing, then shall thy life be for his life, or else thou shalt pay a [g]talent of silver.

40 And as thy servant was busy here and there, [h]he was gone. And the king of

B.C. 901.

a 2 Sam. 11:1.

b 2 Ki. 13:17; Josh. 13:4.

c v. 13.

d Gen. 37:34.

e 1 Ki. 15:20.

f *Parables* (O.T.). vs. 35-40; 1 Ki. 22:19-23. (Jud. 9:7-15; Zech. 11:7-14.)

g One talent = £410, or $1940.

h Heb. *he was not.*

Israel said unto him, So *shall* thy judgment *be;* thyself hast decided *it*.
41 And he hasted, and took the ashes
away from his face; and the king of Israel
discerned him that he *was* of the prophets.
42 And he said unto him, Thus saith
the LORD, [a]Because thou hast let go out
of *thy* hand a man whom I appointed to
utter destruction, therefore thy life shall
go for his life, and thy people for his
people.
43 And the king of Israel [b]went to his
house heavy and displeased, and came
to Samaria.

CHAPTER 21.

Ahab covets Naboth's vineyard.

And it came to pass after these things,
that Naboth the Jezreelite had a
vineyard, which *was* in Jezreel, hard by
the palace of Ahab king of Samaria.
2 And Ahab spake unto Naboth, saying, Give me thy [c]vineyard, that I may
have it for a garden of herbs, because it
is near unto my house: and I will give
thee for it a better vineyard than it; *or*, if
it seem good to thee, I will give thee the
worth of it in money.
3 And Naboth said to Ahab, The LORD
forbid it me, [d]that I should give the
inheritance of my fathers unto thee.
4 And Ahab came into his house heavy
and displeased because of the word
which Naboth the Jezreelite had spoken
to him: for he had said, I will not give thee
the inheritance of my fathers. And he laid
him down upon his bed, and turned
away his face, and would eat no bread.
5 But Jezebel his wife came to him,
and said unto him, Why is thy spirit so
sad, that thou eatest no bread?
6 And he said unto her, Because I spake
unto Naboth the Jezreelite, and said unto
him, Give me thy vineyard for money; or
else, if it please thee, I will give thee
another vineyard for it: and he answered, I
will not give thee my vineyard.
7 And Jezebel his wife said unto him,
Dost thou now govern the kingdom of
Israel? arise, *and* eat bread, and let thine
heart be merry: I will give thee the vineyard of Naboth the Jezreelite.
8 So she wrote letters in Ahab's name,
and sealed *them* with his seal, and sent
the letters unto the elders and to the
nobles that *were* in his city, dwelling
with Naboth.
9 And she wrote in the letters, saying,
Proclaim a fast, and set Naboth on high
among the people:
10 And set two men, sons of Belial,
before him, to bear witness against him,
saying, Thou didst [e]blaspheme God and
the king. And *then* carry him out, and
[f]stone him, that he may die.
11 And the men of his city, *even* the
elders and the nobles who were the
inhabitants in his city, did as Jezebel had
sent unto them, *and* as it *was* written in
the letters which she had sent unto them.
12 [g]They proclaimed a fast, and set
Naboth on high among the people.
13 And there came in two men, children of Belial, and sat before him: and
the men of Belial witnessed against him,
even against Naboth, in the presence of
the people, saying, Naboth did blaspheme God and the king. Then they carried him forth out of the city, and stoned
him with stones, that he died.
14 Then they sent to Jezebel, saying,
Naboth is stoned, and is dead.
15 And it came to pass, when Jezebel
heard that Naboth was stoned, and was
dead, that Jezebel said to Ahab, Arise,
take possession of the vineyard of
Naboth the Jezreelite, which he refused
to give thee for money: for Naboth is not
alive, but dead.
16 And it came to pass, when Ahab
heard that Naboth was dead, that Ahab
rose up to go down to the vineyard of
Naboth the Jezreelite, to take possession
of it.

Elijah announces Ahab's doom.

17 [h]And the word of the LORD came to
Elijah the Tishbite, saying,
18 Arise, go down to meet Ahab king
of Israel, [i]which *is* in Samaria: behold, *he*
is in the vineyard of Naboth, whither he
is gone down to possess it.
19 And thou shalt speak unto him,
saying, Thus saith the LORD, Hast thou
killed, and also taken possession? And
thou shalt speak unto him, saying, Thus
saith the LORD, [j]In the place where dogs
licked the blood of Naboth shall dogs
lick thy blood, even thine.
20 And Ahab said to Elijah, [k]Hast thou

B.C. 900.

a 1 Ki. 22:31-37.
b 1 Ki. 21:4.
c 1 Sam. 8:14
d Lev. 25:23; Num. 36:7; Ezk. 46:18.
e Ex. 22:28; Lev. 24:15, 16; Acts 6:11.
f Lev. 24:14.
g Isa. 58:4.
h Psa. 9:12.
i 1 Ki. 13:32; 2 Chr. 22:9.
j 1 Ki. 22:38.
k 1 Ki. 18:17.

found me, O mine enemy? And he answered, I have found *thee*: because [a]thou hast sold thyself to work evil in the sight of the LORD.

21 Behold, [b]I will bring evil upon thee, and will take away thy [c]posterity, and will cut off from Ahab him that pisseth against the wall, and him that is shut up and left in Israel,

22 And will make thine house like the house of Jeroboam the son of Nebat, and like the house of Baasha the son of Ahijah, for the provocation wherewith thou hast provoked *me* to anger, and made Israel to sin.

23 And [d]of Jezebel also spake the LORD, saying, The dogs shall eat Jezebel by the wall of Jezreel.

24 [e]Him that dieth of Ahab in the city the dogs shall eat; and him that dieth in the field shall the fowls of the air eat.

25 But there was none like unto Ahab, which did sell himself to work wickedness in the sight of the LORD, whom Jezebel his wife stirred up.

26 And he did very abominably in following idols, according to all *things* as did the Amorites, whom the LORD cast out before the children of Israel.

Ahab's repentance gains him a respite.

27 And it came to pass, when Ahab heard those words, that he rent his clothes, and put [f]sackcloth upon his flesh, and fasted, and lay in sackcloth, and went softly.

28 And the word of the LORD came to Elijah the Tishbite, saying,

29 Seest thou how Ahab humbleth himself before me? because he humbleth himself before me, I will not bring the evil in his days: *but* [g]in his son's days will I bring the evil upon his house.

CHAPTER 22.

The three years' peace between Syria and Israel.

And they continued three years without war between Syria and Israel.

Ahab, aided by Jehoshaphat, makes his third Syrian campaign.

2 And it came to pass in the third year, that [h]Jehoshaphat the king of Judah came down to the king of Israel.

3 And the king of Israel said unto his servants, Know ye that [i]Ramoth in Gilead *is* ours, and we *be* [j]still, *and* take it not out of the hand of the king of Syria?

4 And he said unto Jehoshaphat, Wilt thou go with me to battle to Ramoth-gilead? And Jehoshaphat said to the king of Israel, I *am* as thou *art*, my people as thy people, my horses as thy horses.

5 And Jehoshaphat said unto the king of Israel, Enquire, I pray thee, at the word of the LORD to day.

The lying prophets of Ahab (2 Chr. 18:4-11).

6 Then the king of Israel gathered the prophets together, about four hundred men, and said unto them, Shall I go against Ramoth-gilead to battle, or shall I forbear? And they said, Go up; for the Lord shall deliver *it* into the hand of the king.

7 And Jehoshaphat said, *Is there* not here a prophet of the LORD besides, that we might enquire of him?

8 And the king of Israel said unto Jehoshaphat, *There is* yet one man, Micaiah the son of Imlah, by whom we may enquire of the LORD: but I hate him; for he doth not prophesy good concerning me, but evil. And Jehoshaphat said, Let not the king say so.

9 Then the king of Israel called an officer, and said, Hasten *hither* Micaiah the son of Imlah.

10 And the king of Israel and Jehoshaphat the king of Judah sat each on his throne, having put on their robes, in a void place in the entrance of the gate of Samaria; and all the prophets prophesied before them.

11 And Zedekiah the son of Chenaanah made him horns of iron: and he said, Thus saith the LORD, With these shalt thou push the Syrians, until thou have consumed them.

12 And all the prophets prophesied so, saying, Go up to Ramoth-gilead, and prosper: for the LORD shall deliver *it* into the king's hand.

Micaiah's true prophecy (2 Chr. 18:12-27).

13 And the [k]messenger that was gone to call Micaiah spake unto him, saying, Behold now, the words of the prophets *declare* good unto the king with one mouth: let thy word, I pray thee, be like

B.C. 899.

a 2 Ki. 17:17; Rom. 7:14.

b 1 Ki. 14:10; 2 Ki. 9:8.

c 2 Ki. 10:10.

d 2 Ki. 9:36.

e 1 Ki. 14:11; 16:4.

f Gen. 37:34.

g 2 Ki. 9:25.

h 1 Ki. 15:24; 2 Chr. 18:2.

i Deut. 4:43; Josh. 21:38.

j Heb. *silent from taking it.*

k See vs. 7-9.

B.C. 897.

the word of one of them, and speak *that which is* good.

14 And Micaiah said, *As* the LORD liveth, what the LORD saith unto me, that will I speak.

15 So he came to the king. And the king said unto him, Micaiah, shall we go against Ramoth-gilead to battle, or shall we forbear? And he answered him, Go, and prosper: for the LORD shall deliver *it* into the hand of the king.

16 And the king said unto him, How many times shall I adjure thee that thou tell me nothing but *that which is* true in the name of the LORD?

17 And he said, I saw all Israel scattered upon the hills, as sheep that have not a shepherd: and the LORD said, These have no master: let them return every man to his house in peace.

18 And the king of Israel said unto Jehoshaphat, Did I not tell thee that he would prophesy no good concerning me, but evil?

19 And he said, [a]Hear thou therefore the word of the LORD: [b]I saw the LORD sitting on his throne, [c]and all the host of heaven standing by him on his right hand and on his left.

20 And the LORD said, Who shall [d]persuade Ahab, that he may go up and fall at Ramoth-gilead? And one said on this manner, and another said on that manner.

21 And there came forth a spirit, and stood before the LORD, and said, I will persuade him.

22 And the LORD said unto him, Wherewith? And he said, I will go forth, and I will be a lying spirit in the mouth of all his prophets. And he said, [e]Thou shalt persuade *him*, and prevail also: go forth, and do so.

23 Now therefore, behold, the LORD hath put a lying spirit in the mouth of all these thy prophets, and the LORD hath spoken evil concerning thee.

24 But Zedekiah the son of Chenaanah went near, and smote Micaiah on the cheek, and said, [f]Which way went the Spirit of the LORD from me to speak unto thee?

25 And Micaiah said, Behold, thou shalt see in that day, when thou shalt go into an [g]inner chamber to hide thyself.

26 And the king of Israel said, Take Micaiah, and carry him back unto Amon

a *Parables* (O.T.). vs. 19-23; 2 Ki. 14:9. (Jud. 9:7-15; Zech. 11:7-14.)

b Isa. 6:1; Dan. 7:9.

c Job 1:6; 2:1; Psa. 103:20; Dan. 7:10.

d Heb. or, *entice.*

e Jud. 9:23; Job 12:16; Ezk. 14:9.

f 2 Chr. 18:23.

g Heb. *a chamber in a chamber.* 1 Ki. 20:30.

h Num. 16:29; Deut. 18:20-22.

the governor of the city, and to Joash the king's son;

27 And say, Thus saith the king, Put this *fellow* in the prison, and feed him with bread of affliction and with water of affliction, until I come in peace.

28 And Micaiah said, If thou return at all in peace, [h]the LORD hath not spoken by me. And he said, Hearken, O people, every one of you.

Battle of Ramoth-gilead: defeat and death of Ahab (2 Chr. 18:28-34).

29 So the king of Israel and Jehoshaphat the king of Judah went up to Ramoth-gilead.

30 And the king of Israel said unto Jehoshaphat, I will disguise myself, and enter into the battle; but put thou on thy robes. And the king of Israel disguised himself, and went into the battle.

31 But the king of Syria commanded his thirty and two captains that had rule over his chariots, saying, Fight neither with small nor great, save only with the king of Israel.

32 And it came to pass, when the captains of the chariots saw Jehoshaphat, that they said, Surely it *is* the king of Israel. And they turned aside to fight against him: and Jehoshaphat cried out.

33 And it came to pass, when the captains of the chariots perceived that it *was* not the king of Israel, that they turned back from pursuing him.

34 And a *certain* man drew a bow at a venture, and smote the king of Israel between the joints of the harness: wherefore he said unto the driver of his chariot, Turn thine hand, and carry me out of the host; for I am wounded.

35 And the battle increased that day: and the king was stayed up in his chariot against the Syrians, and died at even: and the blood ran out of the wound into the midst of the chariot.

36 And there went a proclamation throughout the host about the going down of the sun, saying, Every man to his city, and every man to his own country.

37 So the king died, and was brought to Samaria; and they buried the king in Samaria.

38 And *one* washed the chariot in the pool of Samaria; and the dogs licked up

his blood; and they washed his armour;
according [a]unto the word of the LORD
which he spake.
39 Now the rest of the acts of Ahab,
and all that he did, [b]and the ivory house
which he made, and all the cities that he
built, *are* they not written in the book of
the chronicles of the kings of Israel?

Accession of Ahaziah over Israel.

40 So Ahab slept with his fathers; and
Ahaziah his son reigned in his stead.

Accession of Jehoshaphat over Judah (2 Chr. 17:1; 20:31).

41 And [c]Jehoshaphat the son of Asa
began to reign over Judah in the fourth
year of Ahab king of Israel.
42 Jehoshaphat *was* thirty and five
years old when he began to reign; and
he reigned twenty and five years in
Jerusalem. And his mother's name *was*
Azubah the daughter of Shilhi.
43 And he [d]walked in all the ways of
Asa his father; he turned not aside from
it, doing *that which was* right in the eyes
of the LORD: nevertheless [e]the high
places were not taken away; *for* the people
offered and burnt incense yet in the
high places.
44 And [f]Jehoshaphat made [g]peace
with the king of Israel.
45 Now the rest of the acts of Jehoshaphat,
and his might that he shewed, and
how he warred, *are* they not written in
the book of the chronicles of the kings of
Judah?

B.C. 897.

a 1 Ki. 21:19.
b Amos 3:15.
c 2 Chr. 20:31.
d Cf. 2 Chr. 20:32, 33.
e 1 Ki. 14:23; 15:14; 2 Ki. 12:3.
f 2 Chr. 19:2.
g Cf. 2 Chr. 18:1.
h 1 Ki. 14:24; 15:12.
i 1 Ki. 10:22; Cf. 2 Chr. 20:35-37.
j 1 Ki. 9:26.
k 2 Chr. 21:1.
l v. 40.
m 1 Ki. 15:26.
n Jud. 2:11; 1 Ki. 16:31.

46 [h]And the remnant of the sodomites,
which remained in the days of his father
Asa, he took out of the land.
47 *There was* then no king in Edom: a
deputy *was* king.
48 Jehoshaphat made [i]ships of
Tharshish to go to Ophir for gold: but
they went not; for the ships were broken
at [j]Ezion-geber.
49 Then said Ahaziah the son of Ahab
unto Jehoshaphat, Let my servants go
with thy servants in the ships. But
Jehoshaphat would not.

Death of Jehoshaphat: accession of Jehoram over Judah (2 Chr. 21:1).

50 And [k]Jehoshaphat slept with his
fathers, and was buried with his fathers
in the city of David his father: and
Jehoram his son reigned in his stead.

Character of Ahaziah.

51 [l]Ahaziah the son of Ahab began to
reign over Israel in Samaria the seventeenth
year of Jehoshaphat king of Judah,
and reigned two years over Israel.
52 And he did evil in the sight of the
LORD, and [m]walked in the way of his
father, and in the way of his mother, and
in the way of Jeroboam the son of Nebat,
who made Israel to sin:
53 For [n]he served Baal, and worshipped
him, and provoked to anger the
LORD God of Israel, according to all that
his father had done.

THE SECOND BOOK OF THE KINGS

COMMONLY CALLED
THE FOURTH BOOK OF THE KINGS

THIS book continues the history of the kingdoms to the captivities. It includes the translation of Elijah and the ministry of Elisha. During this period Amos and Hosea prophesied in Israel, and Obadiah, Joel, Isaiah, Micah, Nahum, Habakkuk, Zephaniah, and Jeremiah in Judah.

Second Kings is in seven parts: I. The last ministry and translation of Elijah, 1:1–2:11. II. The ministry of Elisha from the translation of Elijah to the anointing of Jehu, 2:12–9:10. III. The reign of Jehu over Israel, 9:11–10:36. IV. The reigns of Athaliah and Jehoash over Judah, 11:1–12:21. V. The reigns of Jehoahaz and Joash over Israel, and the last ministry of Elisha, 13:1-25. VI. From the death of Elisha to the captivity of Israel, 14:1–17:41. VII. From the accession of Hezekiah to the captivity of Judah, 18:1–25:30.

The events recorded in Second Kings cover a period of 308 years (Ussher).

CHAPTER 1.

B.C. 896.

Rebellion of Moab: illness of Ahaziah, king of Israel.

THEN Moab rebelled against Israel after the death of Ahab.

2 And Ahaziah fell down through a lattice in his upper chamber that *was* in Samaria, and was sick: and he sent messengers, and said unto them, Go, enquire of Baal-zebub the god of [a]Ekron whether I shall recover of this disease.

Elijah's message to Ahaziah: Elijah's deliverance.

3 But the [b]angel of the LORD said to Elijah the Tishbite, Arise, go up to meet the messengers of the king of Samaria, and say unto them, *Is it* not because *there is* not a God in Israel, *that* ye go to enquire of Baal-zebub the god of Ekron?

4 Now therefore thus saith the LORD, Thou shalt not come down from that bed on which thou art gone up, but shalt surely die. And Elijah departed.

5 And when the messengers turned back unto him, he said unto them, Why are ye now turned back?

6 And they said unto him, There came a man up to meet us, and said unto us, Go, turn again unto the king that sent you, and say unto him, Thus saith the LORD, *Is it* not because *there is* not a God in Israel, *that* thou sendest to enquire of Baal-zebub the god of Ekron? therefore thou shalt not come down from that bed on which thou art gone up, but shalt surely die.

7 And he said unto them, What manner of man *was he* which came up to meet you, and told you these words?

8 And they answered him, *He was* [c]an hairy man, and girt with a girdle of leather about his loins. And he said, It *is* Elijah the Tishbite.

9 Then the king sent unto him a captain of fifty with his fifty. And he went up to him: and, behold, he sat on the top of an hill. And he spake unto him, Thou man of God, the king hath said, Come down.

10 And Elijah answered and said to the captain of fifty, If I *be* a man of God, then [d]let fire come down from heaven, and consume thee and thy fifty. And there came down fire from heaven, and [e]consumed him and his fifty.

11 Again also he sent unto him another captain of fifty with his fifty. And he answered and said unto him, O man of God, thus hath the king said, Come down quickly.

12 And Elijah answered and said unto them, If I *be* a man of God, let fire come down from heaven, and consume thee and thy fifty. And the fire of God came down from heaven, and consumed him and his fifty.

13 And he sent again a captain of the third fifty with his fifty. And the third captain of fifty went up, and came and fell on his knees before Elijah, and besought him, and said unto him, O man of God, I pray thee, let my life, and the life of these fifty thy servants, be [f]precious in thy sight.

14 Behold, there came fire down from heaven, and burnt up the two captains of the former fifties with their fifties:

---

a 1 Sam. 5:10.
b Heb. 1:4, *note.*
c Zech. 13:4.
d Lk. 9:54.
e *Miracles* (O.T.). vs. 10-12; 2 Ki. 2:7, 8. (Gen. 5:24; Jon. 2:1-10.)
f 1 Sam. 26:21; Psa. 72:14.

therefore let my life now be precious in thy sight.

15 And the [a]angel of the LORD said unto Elijah, Go down with him: be not afraid of him. And he arose, and went down with him unto the king.

16 And he said unto him, Thus saith the LORD, Forasmuch as thou hast sent messengers to enquire of Baal-zebub the god of Ekron, *is it* not because *there is* no God in Israel to enquire of his word? therefore thou shalt not come down off that bed on which thou art gone up, but shalt surely die.

Death of Ahaziah: accession of Jehoram king over Israel.

17 So he died according to the word of the LORD which Elijah had spoken. And Jehoram reigned in his stead in the second year of Jehoram the son of Jehoshaphat king of Judah; because he had no son.

18 Now the rest of the acts of Ahaziah which he did, *are* they not written in the book of the chronicles of the kings of Israel?

CHAPTER 2.

The translation of Elijah.

AND it came to pass, when the LORD would [b]take up Elijah into heaven by a whirlwind, that Elijah went with [c]Elisha from Gilgal.

2 And Elijah said unto Elisha, Tarry here, I pray thee; for the LORD hath sent me to Beth-el. And Elisha said *unto him, As* the LORD liveth, and [d]*as* thy soul liveth, I will not leave thee. So they went down to Beth-el.

3 And the [e]sons of the prophets that *were* at Beth-el came forth to Elisha, and said unto him, Knowest thou that the LORD will take away thy master from thy head to day? And he said, Yea, I know *it*; hold ye your peace.

4 And Elijah said unto him, Elisha, tarry here, I pray thee; for the LORD hath sent me to Jericho. And he said, *As* the LORD liveth, and *as* thy soul liveth, I will not leave thee. So they came to Jericho.

5 And the sons of the prophets that *were* at Jericho came to Elisha, and said unto him, Knowest thou that the LORD will take away thy master from thy head to day? And he answered, Yea, I know *it*; hold ye your peace.

6 And Elijah said unto him, Tarry, I pray thee, here; for the LORD hath sent me to Jordan. And he said, *As* the LORD liveth, and *as* thy soul liveth, I will not leave thee. And they two went on.

7 And fifty men of the sons of the prophets went, and stood to view afar off: and they two stood by Jordan.

8 And Elijah took his mantle, and wrapped *it* together, and smote the waters, and they were [f]divided hither and thither, so that they two went over on dry ground.

9 And it came to pass, when they were gone over, that Elijah said unto Elisha, Ask what I shall do for thee, before I be taken away from thee. And Elisha said, I pray thee, let a double portion of thy [g]spirit be upon me.

10 And he said, Thou hast asked a hard thing: *nevertheless,* if thou see me *when I am* taken from thee, it shall be so unto thee; but if not, it shall not be *so.*

11 And it came to pass, as they still went on, and talked, that, behold, *there appeared* a chariot of fire, and horses of fire, and parted them both asunder; and Elijah [h]went up by a whirlwind into heaven.

The Spirit who was upon Elijah comes upon Elisha.

12 And Elisha saw *it*, and he cried, My father, my father, the chariot of Israel, and the horsemen thereof. And he saw him no more: and he took hold of his own clothes, and rent them in two pieces.

13 He took up also the mantle of Elijah that fell from him, and went back, and stood by the bank of Jordan;

Elisha's faith to use the power.

14 And he took the mantle of Elijah that fell from him, and smote the waters, and said, Where *is* the LORD God of Elijah? and when he also had smitten the waters, they parted hither and thither: and Elisha went over.

15 And when the sons of the prophets which *were* to view at Jericho saw him, they said, The spirit of Elijah doth rest on Elisha. And they came to meet him, and bowed themselves to the ground before him.

B.C. 896.

a Heb. 1:4, *note.*

b Gen. 5:24.

c 1 Ki. 19:21.

d vs. 4, 6; 2 Ki. 4:30; 1 Sam. 1:26.

e vs. 5, 7, 15; 1 Ki. 20:35; 2 Ki. 4:1, 38.

f *Miracles* (O.T.). vs. 7, 8, 14, 21, 22, 24; 2 Ki. 3:16-20. (Gen. 5:24; Jon. 2:1-10.)

g *Holy Spirit.* vs. 9, 15, 16; 1 Chr. 12:18. (Gen. 1:2; Mal. 2:15.)

h Gen. 5:24; Heb. 11:5; 1 Thes. 4:14-17.

The knowledge (vs. 3, 5) of the theological students, and their total lack of faith.

16 And they said unto him, Behold
now, there be with thy servants fifty
strong men; let them go, we pray thee,
and seek thy master: lest peradventure
the [a]Spirit of the LORD hath taken him
up, and cast him upon some mountain,
or into some valley. And he said, Ye shall
not send.
17 And when they urged him till he
was ashamed, he said, Send. They sent
therefore fifty men; and they sought
three days, but found him not.
18 And when they came again to him,
(for he tarried at Jericho,) he said unto
them, Did I not say unto you, Go not?

Elisha's second miracle.

19 And the men of the city said unto
Elisha, Behold, I pray thee, the situation
of this city *is* pleasant, as my lord seeth:
but the water *is* naught, and the ground
barren.
20 And he said, Bring me a new cruse,
and put salt therein. And they brought *it*
to him.
21 And he went forth unto the spring of
the waters, and [b]cast the salt in there, and
said, Thus saith the LORD, I have healed
these waters; there shall not be from
thence any more death or barren *land*.
22 [c]So the waters were healed unto
this day, according to the saying of
Elisha which he spake.

Irreverence cursed.

23 And he went up from thence unto
Beth-el: and as he was going up by the
way, there came forth little children out
of the city, and mocked him, and said
unto him, Go up, thou bald head; go up,
thou bald head.
24 And he turned back, and looked on
them, and cursed them in the name of
the LORD. And there came forth two she
bears out of the wood, and tare forty and
two children of them.
25 And he went from thence to mount
Carmel, and from thence he returned to
Samaria.

CHAPTER 3.

Accession of Jehoram over Israel.

Now [d]Jehoram the son of Ahab began
to reign over Israel in Samaria the
eighteenth year of Jehoshaphat king of
Judah, and reigned twelve years.
2 And he wrought evil in the sight of
the LORD; but not like his father, and like
his mother: for he put away the image of
Baal [e]that his father had made.
3 Nevertheless he cleaved unto [f]the
sins of Jeroboam the son of Nebat, which
made Israel to sin; he departed not
therefrom.

Moab rebels against Israel.

4 And Mesha king of Moab was a
sheepmaster, and rendered unto the king
of Israel an hundred thousand lambs,
and an hundred thousand rams, with
the wool.
5 But it came to pass, when Ahab was
dead, that the king of Moab rebelled
against the king of Israel.
6 And king Jehoram went out of
Samaria the same time, and numbered
all Israel.
7 And he went and sent to
Jehoshaphat the king of Judah, saying,
The king of Moab hath rebelled against
me: wilt thou go with me against Moab
to battle? And he said, I will go up: [g]I *am*
as thou *art*, my people as thy people, *and*
my horses as thy horses.
8 And he said, Which way shall we go
up? And he answered, The way through
the wilderness of Edom.
9 So the king of Israel went, and the
king of Judah, and the king of Edom:
and they fetched a compass of seven
days' journey: and there was no water
for the host, and for the cattle that followed them.

Elisha reproves the alliance of Jehoshaphat with Jehoram.

10 And the king of Israel said, Alas!
that the LORD hath called these three
kings together, to deliver them into the
hand of Moab!
11 But [h]Jehoshaphat said, *Is there* not
here a prophet of the LORD, that we may
enquire of the LORD by him? And one of
the king of Israel's servants answered
and said, Here *is* Elisha the son of
Shaphat, which poured water on the
hands of Elijah.
12 And Jehoshaphat said, The word of
the LORD is with him. So the king of Israel
and Jehoshaphat and the king of Edom
[i]went down to him.
13 And Elisha said unto the king of
Israel, What have I to do with thee?

B.C. 896.

a *Holy Spirit.* vs. 9, 15, 16; 1 Chr. 12:18. (Gen. 1:2; Mal. 2:15.)

b 2 Ki. 4:41; Ex. 15:25.

c *Miracles* (O.T.). vs. 19-22; 2 Ki. 3:16-20. (Gen. 5:24; Jon. 2:1-10.)

d 2 Ki. 1:17.

e 1 Ki. 16:31, 32.

f 1 Ki. 12:28, 31, 32.

g 1 Ki. 22:4.

h 1 Ki. 22:7.

i 2 Ki. 2:25.

[a]get thee to the prophets of thy father, and
to the [b]prophets of thy mother. And the
king of Israel said unto him, Nay: for the
LORD hath called these three kings together, to deliver them into the hand of Moab.
14 And Elisha said, [c]*As* the LORD of
hosts liveth, before whom I stand, surely,
were it not that I regard the presence of
Jehoshaphat the king of Judah, I would
not look toward thee, nor see thee.
15 But now bring me a [d]minstrel. And
it came to pass, when the minstrel
played, that the [e]hand of the LORD came
upon him.

Elisha's promise of water and victory.

16 And he said, Thus saith the LORD,
Make this valley full of ditches.
17 For thus saith the LORD, Ye shall not
see wind, neither shall ye see rain; yet
that valley shall be filled with water, that
ye may drink, both ye, and your cattle,
and your beasts.
18 And this is *but* a light thing in the
sight of the LORD: he will deliver the
Moabites also into your hand.
19 And ye shall smite every fenced
city, and every choice city, and shall fell
every good tree, and stop all wells of
water, and mar every good piece of land
with stones.
20 And it came to pass in the morning,
when the [f]meat-offering was offered,
that, behold, there came [g]water by the
way of Edom, and the country was filled
with water.

Defeat of the Moabites.

21 And when all the Moabites heard
that the kings were come up to fight
against them, they gathered all that were
able to put on armour, and upward, and
stood in the border.
22 And they rose up early in the
morning, and the sun shone upon the
water, and the Moabites saw the water
on the other side *as* red as blood:
23 And they said, This *is* blood: the
kings are surely slain, and they have
smitten one another: now therefore,
Moab, to the spoil.
24 And when they came to the camp
of Israel, the Israelites rose up and smote
the Moabites, so that they fled before
them: but they went forward smiting the
Moabites, even in *their* country.

B.C. 895.

a Jud. 10:14.

b 1 Ki. 18:19.

c 1 Ki. 17:1; 2 Ki. 5:16.

d 1 Sam. 10:5.

e Ezk. 1:3; 3:14, 22; 8:1.

f Lit. *meal.*

g *Miracles* (O.T.). vs. 16-20; 2 Ki. 4:2-7. (Gen. 5:24; Jon. 2:1-10.)

h Psa. 19:9, *note.*

i Lev. 25:39; Neh. 5:2-5.

j *Miracles* (O.T.). vs. 2-7, 32-37, 38-41, 42-44; 2 Ki. 5:10-14. (Gen. 5:24; Jon. 2.1-10.)

25 And they beat down the cities, and
on every good piece of land cast every
man his stone, and filled it; and they
stopped all the wells of water, and felled
all the good trees: only in Kir-haraseth
left they the stones thereof; howbeit the
slingers went about *it*, and smote it.
26 And when the king of Moab saw
that the battle was too sore for him, he
took with him seven hundred men that
drew swords, to break through *even* unto
the king of Edom: but they could not.
27 Then he took his eldest son that
should have reigned in his stead, and
offered him *for* a burnt-offering upon the
wall. And there was great indignation
against Israel: and they departed from
him, and returned to *their own* land.

CHAPTER 4.

The increase of the widow's oil.

NOW there cried a certain woman of
the wives of the sons of the
prophets unto Elisha, saying, Thy servant my husband is dead; and thou
knowest that thy servant did [h]fear the
LORD: and the creditor is come to [i]take
unto him my two sons to be bondmen.
2 And Elisha said unto her, What shall
I do for thee? tell me, what hast thou in
the house? And she said, Thine handmaid hath not any thing in the house,
save a pot of oil.
3 Then he said, Go, borrow thee vessels abroad of all thy neighbours, *even*
empty vessels; borrow not a few.
4 And when thou art come in, thou
shalt shut the door upon thee and upon
thy sons, and shalt pour out into all
those vessels, and thou shalt set aside
that which is full.
5 So she went from him, and shut the
door upon her and upon her sons, who
brought *the vessels* to her; and she
poured out.
6 And it came to pass, when the vessels were full, that she said unto her son,
Bring me yet a vessel. And he said unto
her, *There is* not a vessel more. And the
oil [j]stayed.
7 Then she came and told the man of
God. And he said, Go, sell the oil, and
pay thy debt, and live thou and thy children of the rest.

The "great woman" of Shunem
and her reward.

8 And it fell on a day, that Elisha passed
to [a]Shunem, where *was* a great woman;
and she constrained him to eat bread.
And *so* it was, *that* as oft as he passed by,
he turned in thither to eat bread.
9 And she said unto her husband,
Behold now, I perceive that this *is* an
holy man of God, which passeth by us
continually.
10 Let us make a little chamber, I pray
thee, on the wall; and let us set for him
there a bed, and a table, and a stool, and
a candlestick: and it shall be, when he
cometh to us, that he shall turn in thither.
11 And it fell on a day, that he came
thither, and he turned into the chamber,
and lay there.
12 And he said to Gehazi his servant,
Call this Shunammite. And when he had
called her, she stood before him.
13 And he said unto him, Say now
unto her, Behold, thou hast been careful
for us with all this care; what *is* to be
done for thee? wouldest thou be spoken
for to the king, or to the captain of the
host? And she answered, I dwell among
mine own people.
14 And he said, What then *is* to be
done for her? And Gehazi answered,
Verily she hath no child, and her husband is old.
15 And he said, Call her. And when he
had called her, she stood in the door.
16 And he said, [b]About this season,
according to the time of life, thou shalt
embrace a son. And she said, Nay, my
lord, *thou* man of God, [c]do not lie unto
thine handmaid.
17 And the woman conceived, and bare
a son at that season that Elisha had said
unto her, according to the time of life.

Elisha restores life
to the son of the Shunammite.

18 And when the child was grown, it
fell on a day, that he went out to his
father to the reapers.
19 And he said unto his father, My
head, my head. And he said to a lad,
Carry him to his mother.
20 And when he had taken him, and
brought him to his mother, he sat on her
knees till noon, and *then* died.
21 And she went up, and laid him on
the bed of the man of God, and shut *the*
door upon him, and went out.
22 And she called unto her husband,
and said, Send me, I pray thee, one of
the young men, and one of the asses,
that I may run to the man of God, and
come again.
23 And he said, Wherefore wilt thou go
to him to day? *it is* neither new moon, nor
sabbath. And she said, [d]*It shall be* well.
24 Then she saddled an ass, and said
to her servant, Drive, and go forward;
slack not *thy* riding for me, except I bid
thee.
25 So she went and came unto the
man of God to mount [e]Carmel. And it
came to pass, when the man of God saw
her afar off, that he said to Gehazi his
servant, Behold, *yonder is* that Shunammite:
26 Run now, I pray thee, to meet her,
and say unto her, *Is it* well with thee? *is*
it well with thy husband? *is it* well with
the child? And she answered, *It is* well.
27 And when she came to the man of
God to the hill, she caught him by the
feet: but Gehazi came near to thrust her
away. And the man of God said, Let her
alone; for her soul *is* [f]vexed within her:
and the LORD hath hid *it* from me, and
hath not told me.
28 Then she said, Did I desire a son of
my lord? [g]did I not say, Do not deceive
me?
29 Then he said to Gehazi, [h]Gird up
thy loins, and take my staff in thine
hand, and go thy way: if thou meet any
man, salute him not; and if any salute
thee, answer him not again: and lay my
staff upon the face of the child.
30 And the mother of the child said,
[i]*As* the LORD liveth, and as thy soul
liveth, I will not leave thee. And he
arose, and followed her.
31 And Gehazi passed on before them,
and laid the staff upon the face of the
child; but *there was* neither voice, nor
hearing. Wherefore he went again to
meet him, and told him, saying, The
child is not awaked.
32 And when Elisha was come into the
house, behold, the child was dead, *and*
laid upon his bed.
33 He went in therefore, and shut the
door upon them twain, and prayed unto
the LORD.
34 And he went up, and lay upon the
child, and put his mouth upon his
mouth, and his eyes upon his eyes, and
his hands upon his hands: and he

B.C. 894.

a Josh. 19:18.
b Gen. 18:10, 14.
c v. 28.
d Heb. *peace.*
e 2 Ki. 2:25.
f Heb. *bitter.* 1 Sam. 1:10.
g v. 16.
h 2 Ki. 9:1; 1 Ki. 18:46.
i 2 Ki. 2:2.

stretched himself upon the child; and the flesh of the child waxed warm.

35 Then he returned, and walked in the house to and fro; and went up, and stretched himself upon him: and the child sneezed seven times, and the child [a]opened his eyes.

36 And he called Gehazi, and said, Call this Shunammite. So he called her. And when she was come in unto him, he said, Take up thy son.

37 Then she went in, and fell at his feet, and bowed herself to the ground, and [b]took up her son, and went out.

Elisha heals the noxious pottage.

38 And Elisha came again to [c]Gilgal: and *there was* a dearth in the land; and the sons of the prophets *were* sitting before him: and he said unto his servant, Set on the great pot, and seethe pottage for the sons of the prophets.

39 And one went out into the field to gather herbs, and found a wild vine, and gathered thereof wild gourds his lap full, and came and shred *them* into the pot of pottage: for they knew *them* not.

40 So they poured out for the men to eat. And it came to pass, as they were eating of the pottage, that they cried out, and said, O *thou* man of God, *there is* [d]death in the pot. And they could not eat *thereof*.

41 But he said, Then bring meal. And [e]he cast *it* into the pot; and he said, Pour out for the people, that they may eat. And there was no harm in the pot.

Elisha feeds an hundred men miraculously.

42 And there came a man from [f]Baal-shalisha, and brought the man of God bread of the firstfruits, twenty loaves of barley, and full ears of corn in the husk thereof. And he said, Give unto the people, that they may eat.

43 And his servitor said, [g]What, should I set this before an hundred men? He said again, Give the people, that they may eat: for thus saith the LORD, [h]They shall eat, and shall leave *thereof*.

44 So he set *it* before them, and they did eat, and [i]left *thereof*, according to the word of the LORD.

B.C. 895.

CHAPTER 5.

The healing of Naaman.

NOW Naaman, captain of the host of the king of Syria, was a great man with his master, and honourable, because by him the LORD had given deliverance unto Syria: he was also a mighty man in valour, *but he was* a leper.

2 And the Syrians had gone out by companies, and had brought away captive out of the land of Israel a little maid; and she waited on Naaman's wife.

3 And she said unto her mistress, Would God my lord *were* with the prophet that *is* in Samaria! for he would recover him of his leprosy.

4 And *one* went in, and told his lord, saying, Thus and thus said the maid that *is* of the land of Israel.

5 And the king of Syria said, Go to, go, and I will send a letter unto the king of Israel. And he departed, and [j]took with him ten [k]talents of silver, and six thousand *pieces* of gold, and ten changes of raiment.

6 And he brought the letter to the king of Israel, saying, Now when this letter is come unto thee, behold, I have *therewith* sent Naaman my servant to thee, that thou mayest recover him of his leprosy.

7 And it came to pass, when the king of Israel had read the letter, that he rent his clothes, and said, *Am* I [l]God, to kill and to make alive, that this man doth send unto me to recover a man of his leprosy? wherefore consider, I pray you, and see how he seeketh a quarrel against me.

8 And it was *so*, when Elisha the man of God had heard that the king of Israel had rent his clothes, that he sent to the king, saying, Wherefore hast thou rent thy clothes? let him come now to me, and he shall know that there is a prophet in Israel.

9 So Naaman came with his horses and with his chariot, and stood at the door of the house of Elisha.

10 And Elisha sent a messenger unto him, saying, Go and [m]wash in Jordan seven times, and thy flesh shall come again to thee, and thou shalt be clean.

11 But Naaman was wroth, and went away, and said, Behold, I thought, He

a *Resurrection.* vs. 32-35; Psa. 16:9-11. (Job 19:25; 1 Cor. 15:52.)

b 1 Ki. 17:23; Heb. 11:35.

c 2 Ki. 2:1.

d Ex. 10:17.

e Ex. 15:25; 2 Ki. 2:21.

f 1 Sam. 9:4.

g Lk. 9:13; John 6:9.

h Lk. 9:13; John 6:12.

i Mt. 14:20; 15:37; John 6:13.

j 1 Sam. 9:8.

k One talent = £410, or $1940; also vs. 22, 23.

l Gen. 30:2; Deut. 32:39; 1 Sam. 2:6.

m 2 Ki. 4:41.

B.C. 894.

will surely come out to me, and stand,
and call on the name of the LORD his
God, and strike his hand over the place,
and recover the leper.
12 *Are* not [a]Abana and Pharpar, rivers
of Damascus, better than all the waters
of Israel? may I not wash in them, and
be clean? So he turned and went away in
a rage.
13 And his servants came near, and
spake unto him, and said, My father, *if*
the prophet had bid thee *do some* great
thing, wouldest thou not have done *it*?
how much rather then, when he saith to
thee, Wash, and be clean?
14 Then went he down, and [b]dipped
himself seven times in Jordan, according
to the saying of the man of God: and his
[c]flesh came again like unto the flesh of a
little child, and he was clean.
15 And he returned to the man of God,
he and all his company, and came, and
stood before him: and he said, Behold,
now I know that *there is* [d]no God in all
the earth, but in Israel: now therefore, I
pray thee, take a blessing of thy servant.
16 But he said, [e]*As* the LORD liveth,
before whom I stand, I will receive none.
And he urged him to take *it*; but he
refused.
17 And Naaman said, Shall there not
then, I pray thee, be given to thy servant
two mules' burden of earth? for thy servant will henceforth offer neither burnt-
offering nor sacrifice unto other gods,
but unto the LORD.
18 In this thing the LORD pardon thy
servant, *that* when my master goeth into
the house of Rimmon to worship there,
and he leaneth on my hand, and I bow
myself in the house of Rimmon: when I
bow down myself in the house of
Rimmon, the LORD pardon thy servant in
this thing.
19 And he said unto him, Go in peace.
So he departed from him a little way.

Gehazi's sin and its penalty.

20 But Gehazi, the servant of Elisha the
man of God, said, Behold, my master
hath spared Naaman this Syrian, in not
receiving at his hands that which he
brought: but, *as* the LORD liveth, I will run
after him, and take somewhat of him.
21 So Gehazi followed after Naaman.
And when Naaman saw *him* running
after him, he lighted down from the
chariot to meet him, and said, *Is* all well?
22 And he said, All *is* well. My master
hath sent me, saying, Behold, even now
there be come to me from mount Ephraim
two young men of the sons of the
prophets: give them, I pray thee, a talent
of silver, and two changes of garments.
23 And Naaman said, Be content, take
two talents. And he urged him, and
bound two talents of silver in two bags,
with two changes of garments, and laid
them upon two of his servants; and they
bare *them* before him.
24 And when he came to the tower, he
took *them* from their hand, and
bestowed *them* in the house: and he let
the men go, and they departed.
25 But he went in, and stood before his
master. And Elisha said unto him,
Whence *comest thou*, Gehazi? And he
said, Thy servant went [f]no whither.
26 And he said unto him, Went not
mine heart *with thee*, when the man
turned again from his chariot to meet
thee? *Is it* a time to receive money, and to
receive garments, and oliveyards, and
vineyards, and sheep, and oxen, and
menservants, and maidservants?
27 The leprosy therefore of Naaman
shall [g]cleave unto thee, and unto thy
seed for ever. And he went out from his
presence a [h]leper *as white* as snow.

CHAPTER 6.

Elisha recovers the lost axe.

And the [i]sons of the prophets said
unto Elisha, Behold now, the place
where we dwell with thee is too strait
for us.
2 Let us go, we pray thee, unto Jordan,
and take thence every man a beam, and
let us make us a place there, where we
may dwell. And he answered, Go ye.
3 And one said, Be content, I pray
thee, and go with thy servants. And he
answered, I will go.
4 So he went with them. And when
they came to Jordan, they cut down
wood.
5 But as one was felling a beam, the
axe head fell into the water: and he
cried, and said, Alas, master! for it was
borrowed.
6 And the man of God said, Where fell
it? And he shewed him the place. And

a Or, *Amana*.

b *Miracles* (O.T.). vs. 10-14, 27; 2 Ki. 6:5-7. (Gen. 5:24; Jon. 2:1-10.)

c Job 33:25.

d Dan. 2:47; 3:29; 6:26, 27.

e 2 Ki. 3:14.

f Heb. *not hither or thither.*

g 1 Tim. 6:9.

h 2 Ki. 15:5; Ex. 4:6; Num. 12:10.

i 2 Ki. 4:38.

he cut down a stick, and cast *it* in thither; and the iron did [a]swim.

7 Therefore said he, Take *it* up to thee. And he put out his hand, and took it.

Elisha reveals Ben-hadad's plans.

8 Then the king of Syria warred against Israel, and took counsel with his servants, saying, In such and such a place *shall be* my camp.

9 And the man of God sent unto the king of Israel, saying, Beware that thou pass not such a place; for thither the Syrians are come down.

10 And the king of Israel sent to the place which the man of God told him and warned him of, and saved himself there, not once nor twice.

11 Therefore the heart of the king of Syria was sore troubled for this thing; and he called his servants, and said unto them, Will ye not shew me which of us *is* for the king of Israel?

12 And one of his servants said, None, my lord, O king: but Elisha, the prophet that *is* in Israel, telleth the king of Israel the words that thou speakest in thy bedchamber.

Elisha at Dothan.

13 And he said, Go and spy where he *is*, that I may send and fetch him. And it was told him, saying, Behold, *he is* in [b]Dothan.

14 Therefore sent he thither horses, and chariots, and a great host: and they came by night, and compassed the city about.

15 And when the servant of the man of God was risen early, and gone forth, behold, an host compassed the city both with horses and chariots. And his servant said unto him, Alas, my master! how shall we do?

16 And he answered, Fear not: for [c]they that *be* with us *are* more than they that *be* with them.

17 And Elisha prayed, and [d]said, LORD, I pray thee, open his eyes, that he may see. And the LORD opened the eyes of the young man; and he saw: and, behold, the mountain *was* full of [e]horses and chariots of fire round about Elisha.

Elisha leads the blinded Syrians to Samaria.

18 And when they came down to him, Elisha prayed unto the LORD, and [f]said, Smite this people, I pray thee, with blindness. And he [g]smote them with blindness according to the word of Elisha.

19 And Elisha said unto them, This *is* not the way, neither *is* this the city: follow me, and I will bring you to the man whom ye seek. But he led them to Samaria.

20 And it came to pass, when they were come into Samaria, that Elisha said, LORD, open the eyes of these *men*, that they may see. And the LORD opened their eyes, and they saw; and, behold, *they were* in the midst of Samaria.

21 And the king of Israel said unto Elisha, when he saw them, My father, shall I smite *them*? shall I smite *them*?

22 And he answered, Thou shalt not smite *them*: wouldest thou smite those whom thou hast taken captive with thy sword and with thy bow? set bread and water before them, that they may eat and drink, and go to their master.

23 And he prepared great provision for them: and when they had eaten and drunk, he sent them away, and they went to their master. So the bands of Syria came no more into the land of Israel.

The Syrian siege of Samaria.

24 And it came to pass after this, that Benhadad king of Syria gathered all his host, and went up, and besieged Samaria.

25 And there was a great famine in Samaria: and, behold, they besieged it, until an ass's head was *sold* for fourscore *pieces* of silver, and the fourth part of a [h]cab of dove's dung for five *pieces* of silver.

26 And as the king of Israel was passing by upon the wall, there cried a woman unto him, saying, Help, my lord, O king.

27 And he said, If the LORD do not help thee, whence shall I help thee? out of the barnfloor, or out of the winepress?

28 And the king said unto her, What aileth thee? And she answered, This woman said unto me, Give thy son, that we may eat him to day, and we will eat my son to morrow.

29 So we [i]boiled my son, and did eat him: and I said unto her on the next day, Give thy son, that we may eat him: and she hath hid her son.

30 And it came to pass, when the king heard the words of the woman, that he [j]rent his clothes; and he passed by upon

B.C. 893.

a *Miracles* (O.T.). vs. 5-7, 18-20; 2 Ki. 13:21. (Gen. 5:24; Jon. 2:1-10.)

b Gen. 37:17.

c 2 Chr. 32:7; Psa. 55:18; Rom. 8:31.

d *Bible prayers* (O.T.). 2 Ki. 6:18. (Gen. 15:2; Hab. 3:1-16.)

e 2 Ki. 2:11; Psa. 34:7; 68:17.

f *Bible prayers* (O.T.). 2 Ki. 19:15. (Gen. 15:2; Hab. 3:1-16.)

g Gen. 19:11.

h One cab = 3.84 pts.

i Lev. 26:29; Deut. 28:53, 57.

j 1 Ki. 21:27.

the wall, and the people looked, and,
behold, *he had* sackcloth within upon his
flesh.
31 Then he said, [a]God do so and more
also to me, if the head of Elisha the son
of Shaphat shall stand on him this day.

The king's messenger of vengeance
and the untroubled prophet.

32 But Elisha sat in his house, and the
elders sat with him; and *the king* sent a
man from before him: but ere the messenger came to him, he said to the
elders, See ye how this son of a [b]murder-
er hath sent to take away mine head?
look, when the messenger cometh, shut
the door, and hold him fast at the door:
is not the sound of his master's feet
behind him?
33 And while he yet talked with them,
behold, the messenger came down unto
him: and he said, Behold, this evil *is* of
the LORD; [c]what should I wait for the
LORD any longer?

CHAPTER 7.

Elisha's promise of food
and Jehovah's terror upon the Syrians.

Then Elisha said, Hear ye the word of
the LORD; Thus saith the LORD, To
morrow about this time *shall* a [d]measure
of fine flour *be sold* for a [e]shekel, and two
measures of barley for a shekel, in the
gate of Samaria.
2 Then a lord on whose hand the king
leaned answered the man of God, and
said, Behold, *if* the LORD would make
windows in heaven, might this thing be?
And he said, Behold, thou shalt see *it*
with thine eyes, but shalt not eat thereof.
3 And there were four leprous men [f]at
the entering in of the gate: and they said
one to another, Why sit we here until we
die?
4 If we say, We will enter into the city,
then the famine *is* in the city, and we
shall die there: and if we sit still here, we
die also. Now therefore come, and let us
fall unto the host of the Syrians: if they
save us alive, we shall live; and if they
kill us, we shall but die.
5 And they rose up in the twilight, to
go unto the camp of the Syrians: and
when they were come to the uttermost
part of the camp of Syria, behold, *there
was* no man there.

B.C. 892.

a Ruth 1:17; 1 Ki. 19:2.

b 1 Ki. 18:4.

c Job 2:9.

d One measure = about 4 pecks; also vs. 16, 18.

e One shekel = 2*s*. 9*d*., or 65 cts.; also vs. 16, 18.

f Lev. 13:46.

g 2 Ki. 19:7; Job 15:21; 2 Sam. 5:24.

6 For the Lord had made the host of
the Syrians [g]to hear a noise of chariots,
and a noise of horses, *even* the noise of a
great host: and they said one to another,
Lo, the king of Israel hath hired against
us the kings of the Hittites, and the
kings of the Egyptians, to come upon us.
7 Wherefore they arose and fled in the
twilight, and left their tents, and their
horses, and their asses, even the camp as
it *was*, and fled for their life.
8 And when these lepers came to the
uttermost part of the camp, they went
into one tent, and did eat and drink, and
carried thence silver, and gold, and raiment, and went and hid *it*; and came
again, and entered into another tent, and
carried thence *also*, and went and hid *it*.
9 Then they said one to another, We do
not well: this day *is* a day of good tidings, and we hold our peace: if we tarry
till the morning light, some mischief will
come upon us: now therefore come, that
we may go and tell the king's household.
10 So they came and called unto the
porter of the city: and they told them, saying, We came to the camp of the Syrians,
and, behold, *there was* no man there, neither voice of man, but horses tied, and
asses tied, and the tents as they *were*.
11 And he called the porters; and they
told *it* to the king's house within.
12 And the king arose in the night,
and said unto his servants, I will now
shew you what the Syrians have done to
us. They know that we *be* hungry; therefore are they gone out of the camp to
hide themselves in the field, saying,
When they come out of the city, we shall
catch them alive, and get into the city.
13 And one of his servants answered
and said, Let *some* take, I pray thee, five
of the horses that remain, which are left
in the city, (behold, they *are* as all the
multitude of Israel that are left in it:
behold, *I say*, they *are* even as all the
multitude of the Israelites that are consumed:) and let us send and see.
14 They took therefore two chariot
horses; and the king sent after the host
of the Syrians, saying, Go and see.
15 And they went after them unto
Jordan: and, lo, all the way *was* full of
garments and vessels, which the Syrians

had cast away in their haste. And the messengers returned, and told the king.

Elisha's promise fulfilled.

16 And the people went out, and spoiled the tents of the Syrians. So a measure of fine flour was *sold* for a shekel, and two measures of barley for a shekel, [a]according to the word of the LORD.

17 And the king appointed the lord on whose hand he leaned to have the charge of the gate: and the people trode upon him in the gate, and he died, [b]as the man of God had said, who spake when the king came down to him.

18 And it came to pass as the man of God had spoken to the king, saying, [a]Two measures of barley for a shekel, and a measure of fine flour for a shekel, shall be to morrow about this time in the gate of Samaria:

19 And that lord answered the man of God, and said, Now, behold, *if* the LORD should make windows in heaven, might such a thing be? And he said, Behold, thou shalt see it with thine eyes, but shalt not eat thereof.

20 And so it fell out unto him: for the people trode upon him in the gate, and he died.

CHAPTER 8.

Elisha predicts the seven years' famine.

Then spake Elisha unto the woman, [c]whose son he had restored to life, saying, Arise, and go thou and thine household, and sojourn wheresoever thou canst sojourn: for the LORD [d]hath called for a famine; and it shall also come upon the land seven years.

2 And the woman arose, and did after the saying of the man of God: and she went with her household, and sojourned in the land of the Philistines seven years.

Jehoram restores the Shunammite's land.

3 And it came to pass at the seven years' end, that the woman returned out of the land of the Philistines: and she went forth to cry unto the king for her house and for her land.

4 And the king talked with [e]Gehazi the servant of the man of God, saying, Tell me, I pray thee, all the great things that Elisha hath done.

5 And it came to pass, as he was telling the king how he had restored a dead body to life, that, behold, the woman, whose son he had [c]restored to life, cried to the king for her house and for her land. And Gehazi said, My lord, O king, this *is* the woman, and this *is* her son, whom Elisha restored to life.

6 And when the king asked the woman, she told him. So the king appointed unto her a certain officer, saying, Restore all that *was* hers, and all the fruits of the field since the day that she left the land, even until now.

Elisha Predicts Hazael's Reign Over Syria.

7 And Elisha came to Damascus; and Benhadad the king of Syria was sick; and it was told him, saying, The man of God is come hither.

8 And the king said unto Hazael, Take a present in thine hand, and go, meet the man of God, and enquire of the LORD by him, saying, Shall I recover of this disease?

9 So [f]Hazael went to meet him, and took a present with him, even of every good thing of Damascus, forty camels' burden, and came and stood before him, and said, Thy son Benhadad king of Syria hath sent me to thee, saying, Shall I recover of this disease?

10 And Elisha said unto him, Go, say unto him, Thou mayest certainly recover: howbeit the LORD hath shewed me that he shall surely die.

11 And he settled his countenance stedfastly, until he was ashamed: and the man of God wept.

12 And Hazael said, Why weepeth my lord? And he answered, Because I know [g]the evil that thou wilt do unto the children of Israel: their strong holds wilt thou set on fire, and their young men wilt thou slay with the sword, and [h]wilt dash their children, and rip up their women with child.

13 And Hazael said, But what, [i]*is* thy servant a dog, that he should do this great thing? And Elisha answered, [f]The LORD hath shewed me that thou *shalt be* king over Syria.

14 So he departed from Elisha, and came to his master; who said to him, What said Elisha to thee? And he answered, He told me *that* thou shouldest surely recover.

15 And it came to pass on the morrow, that he took a thick cloth, and dipped *it*

B.C. 892.

a v. 1.
b v. 2; 2 Ki. 6:32.
c 2 Ki. 4:35.
d Psa. 105:16; Hag. 1:11.
e 2 Ki. 5:20, 27.
f 1 Ki. 19:15.
g 2 Ki. 10:32; 12:17; 13:3, 7; Amos 1:3, 4.
h 2 Ki. 15:16; Hos. 13:16; Amos 1:13.
i 1 Sam. 17:43.

in water, and spread *it* on his face, so
that he died: and Hazael reigned in his
stead.

Jehoram co-king with his father
Jehoshaphat over Judah (2 Chr. 21:5).

16 And in the fifth year of Joram the
son of Ahab king of Israel, Jehoshaphat
being then king of Judah, [a]Jehoram the
son of Jehoshaphat king of Judah [b]began
to reign.
17 Thirty and two years old was he
when he began to reign; and he reigned
eight years in Jerusalem.
18 And he walked in the way of the
kings of Israel, as did the house of Ahab:
for the daughter of Ahab was his wife:
and he did evil in the sight of the LORD.
19 Yet the LORD would not destroy
Judah for David his servant's sake, [c]as
he promised him to give him alway a
light, *and* to his children.

The revolt of Edom (2 Chr. 21:8-10).

20 In his days [d]Edom revolted from
under the hand of Judah, and made a
king over themselves.
21 So Joram went over to Zair, and all
the chariots with him: and he rose by
night, and smote the Edomites which
compassed him about, and the captains
of the chariots: and the people fled into
their tents.

The revolt of Libnah (2 Chr. 21:10).

22 Yet Edom revolted from under the
hand of Judah unto this day. Then
[e]Libnah revolted at the same time.
23 And the rest of the acts of Joram,
and all that he did, *are* they not written
in the book of the chronicles of the kings
of Judah?

Death of Jehoram (2 Chr. 21:19, 20).

24 And Joram slept with his fathers,
and was buried with his fathers in the
city of David: and Ahaziah his son
reigned in his stead.

Accession of Ahaziah over Judah
(2 Chr. 22:1, 2).

25 In the twelfth year of Joram the son
of Ahab king of Israel did Ahaziah the son
of Jehoram king of Judah begin to reign.
26 Two and twenty years old *was*
Ahaziah when he began to reign; and he
reigned one year in Jerusalem. And his
mother's name *was* Athaliah, the daughter of Omri king of Israel.
27 And he walked in the way of the
house of Ahab, and did evil in the sight of
the LORD, as *did* the house of Ahab: for he
was the son in law of the house of Ahab.

Ahaziah joins Jehoram in defense of
Ramoth-gilead (2 Chr. 22:5).

28 And he went with Joram the son of
Ahab to the war against Hazael king of
Syria in Ramoth-gilead; and the Syrians
wounded Joram.

Ahaziah visits Jehoram at Jezreel
(2 Chr. 22:6).

29 And king Joram went back to be
healed in Jezreel of the wounds which
the Syrians had given him at Ramah,
when he fought against Hazael king of
Syria. And [f]Ahaziah the son of Jehoram
king of Judah went down to see Joram
the son of Ahab in Jezreel, because he
was sick.

CHAPTER 9.

Jehu anointed king over Israel
at Ramoth-gilead.

And Elisha the prophet called [g]one of
the children of the prophets, and
said unto him, [h]Gird up thy loins, and
take this box of oil in thine hand, and go
to Ramoth-gilead:
2 And when thou comest thither, look
out there Jehu the son of Jehoshaphat
the son of Nimshi, and go in, and make
him arise up from among his brethren,
and carry him to an inner chamber;
3 Then [i]take the box of oil, and pour *it*
on his head, and say, Thus saith the
LORD, I have anointed thee king over
Israel. Then open the door, and flee, and
tarry not.
4 So the young man, *even* the young
man the prophet, went to Ramoth-gilead.
5 And when he came, behold, the captains of the host *were* sitting; and he said,
I have an errand to thee, O captain. And
Jehu said, Unto which of all us? And he
said, To thee, O captain.
6 And he arose, and went into the
house; and he poured the oil on his
head, and said unto him, [j]Thus saith the
LORD God of Israel, I have anointed thee

B.C. 885.

a Called *Joram*, vs. 21, 23, 24.

b Heb. *reigned*, i.e. began to reign in consort with his father.

c 2 Sam. 7:13; 1 Ki. 11:36; 15:4; 2 Chr. 21:7.

d 2 Ki. 3:27; Gen. 27:40; 2 Chr. 21:8-10.

e 2 Chr. 21:10.

f 2 Ki. 9:16; 2 Chr. 22:6, 7.

g 1 Ki. 20:35.

h 2 Ki. 4:29; Jer. 1:17.

i 1 Ki. 19:16.

j 1 Ki. 19:16; 2 Chr. 22:7.

king over the people of the LORD, *even* over Israel.

7 And thou shalt smite the house of Ahab thy master, that I may avenge the blood of my servants the prophets, and the blood of all the servants of the LORD, [a]at the hand of Jezebel.

8 For the whole house of Ahab shall perish: and [b]I will cut off from Ahab him that pisseth against the wall, and him that is shut up and left in Israel:

9 And I will make the house of Ahab like the house of [c]Jeroboam the son of Nebat, and like the house of [d]Baasha the son of Ahijah:

10 [e]And the dogs shall eat Jezebel in the portion of Jezreel, and *there shall be* none to bury *her*. And he opened the door, and fled.

Jehu proclaimed king by the army of Israel.

11 Then Jehu came forth to the servants of his lord: and *one* said unto him, *Is* all well? wherefore came [f]this mad *fellow* to thee? And he said unto them, Ye know the man, and his communication.

12 And they said, *It is* false; tell us now. And he said, Thus and thus spake he to me, saying, Thus saith the LORD, I have anointed thee king over Israel.

13 Then they hasted, and took every man his garment, and put *it* under him on the top of the stairs, and blew with trumpets, saying, Jehu is king.

Jehu slays Jehoram.

14 So Jehu the son of Jehoshaphat the son of Nimshi conspired against Joram. (Now Joram had kept Ramoth-gilead, he and all Israel, because of Hazael king of Syria.

15 But king Joram was returned to be healed in Jezreel of the wounds which the Syrians had given him, when he fought with Hazael king of Syria.) And Jehu said, If it be your minds, *then* let none go forth *nor* escape out of the city to go to tell *it* in Jezreel.

16 So Jehu rode in a chariot, and went to Jezreel; for Joram lay there. And Ahaziah king of Judah was come down to see Joram.

17 And there stood a watchman on the tower in Jezreel, and he spied the company of Jehu as he came, and said, I see a company. And Joram said, Take an horseman, and send to meet them, and let him say, *Is it* peace?

B.C. 884.

a 1 Ki. 18:4; 21:15.

b 1 Ki. 14:10; 21:21; 2 Ki. 10:17.

c 1 Ki. 14:10; 15:29; 21:22.

d 1 Ki. 16:3, 11.

e vs. 35, 36; 1 Ki. 21:23.

f Jer. 29:26; John 10:20; Acts 26:24; 1 Cor. 4:10.

g 2 Chr. 22:7.

h 1 Ki. 21:29.

i 1 Ki. 21:19.

18 So there went one on horseback to meet him, and said, Thus saith the king, *Is it* peace? And Jehu said, What hast thou to do with peace? turn thee behind me. And the watchman told, saying, The messenger came to them, but he cometh not again.

19 Then he sent out a second on horseback, which came to them, and said, Thus saith the king, *Is it* peace? And Jehu answered, What hast thou to do with peace? turn thee behind me.

20 And the watchman told, saying, He came even unto them, and cometh not again: and the driving *is* like the driving of Jehu the son of Nimshi; for he driveth furiously.

21 And Joram said, Make ready. And his chariot was made ready. And [g]Joram king of Israel and Ahaziah king of Judah went out, each in his chariot, and they went out against Jehu, and met him in the portion of Naboth the Jezreelite.

22 And it came to pass, when Joram saw Jehu, that he said, *Is it* peace, Jehu? And he answered, What peace, so long as the whoredoms of thy mother Jezebel and her witchcrafts *are so* many?

23 And Joram turned his hands, and fled, and said to Ahaziah, *There is* treachery, O Ahaziah.

24 And Jehu drew a bow with his full strength, and [g]smote Jehoram between his arms, and the arrow went out at his heart, and he sunk down in his chariot.

25 Then said *Jehu* to Bidkar his captain, Take up, *and* cast him in the portion of the field of Naboth the Jezreelite: for remember how that, when I and thou rode together after Ahab his father, [h]the LORD laid this burden upon him;

26 Surely I have seen yesterday the blood of Naboth, and the blood of his sons, saith the LORD; [i]and I will requite thee in this plat, saith the LORD. Now therefore take *and* cast him into the plat of *ground*, according to the word of the LORD.

Ahaziah slain (2 Chr. 22:9).

27 But when Ahaziah the king of Judah saw *this*, he fled by the way of the garden house. And Jehu followed after him, and said, Smite him also in the chariot. *And they did so* at the going up to

Gur, which *is* by Ibleam. And he fled to
[a]Megiddo, and died there.
28 And his servants carried him in a
chariot to Jerusalem, and buried him in
his sepulchre with his fathers in the city
of David.
29 And in the eleventh year of Joram
the son of Ahab began Ahaziah to reign
over Judah.

The slaying of Jezebel.

30 And when Jehu was come to
Jezreel, Jezebel heard *of it;* [b]and she
painted her face, and tired her head, and
looked out at a window.
31 And as Jehu entered in at the gate,
she said, *Had* Zimri peace, who slew his
master?
32 And he lifted up his face to the
window, and said, Who *is* on my side?
who? And there looked out to him two
or three eunuchs.
33 And he said, Throw her down. So
they threw her down: and *some* of her
blood was sprinkled on the wall, and on
the horses: and he trode her under foot.
34 And when he was come in, he did
eat and drink, and said, Go, see now this
cursed *woman*, and bury her: for [c]she *is* a
king's daughter.
35 And they went to bury her: but they
found no more of her than the skull, and
the feet, and the palms of *her* hands.
36 Wherefore they came again, and
told him. And he said, This *is* the word
of the LORD, which he spake by his servant Elijah the Tishbite, saying, [d]In the
portion of Jezreel shall dogs eat the flesh
of Jezebel:
37 And the carcase of Jezebel shall be
[e]as dung upon the face of the field in the
portion of Jezreel; *so* that they shall not
say, This *is* Jezebel.

CHAPTER 10.

Judgment on the house of Ahab.

And Ahab had seventy sons in
Samaria. And Jehu wrote letters,
and sent to Samaria, unto the rulers of
Jezreel, to the elders, and to [f]them that
brought up Ahab's *children*, saying,
2 Now as soon as this letter cometh to
you, seeing your master's sons *are* with
you, and *there are* with you chariots and
horses, a fenced city also, and armour;
3 Look even out the best and meetest
of your master's sons, and set *him* on his
father's throne, and fight for your master's house.
4 But they were exceedingly afraid,
and said, Behold, two kings stood not
before him: how then shall we stand?
5 And he that *was* over the house, and
he that *was* over the city, the elders also,
and the bringers up *of the children*, sent to
Jehu, saying, We *are* thy servants, and
will do all that thou shalt bid us; we will
not make any king: do thou *that which is*
good in thine eyes.
6 Then he wrote a letter the second
time to them, saying, If ye *be* [g]mine, and
if ye will hearken unto my voice, take ye
the heads of the men your master's sons,
and come to me to Jezreel by to morrow
this time. Now the king's sons, *being* seventy persons, *were* with the great men of
the city, which brought them up.
7 And it came to pass, when the letter
came to them, that they took the king's
sons, and [h]slew seventy persons, and
put their heads in baskets, and sent him
them to Jezreel.
8 And there came a messenger, and
told him, saying, They have brought the
heads of the king's sons. And he said,
Lay ye them in two heaps at the entering
in of the gate until the morning.
9 And it came to pass in the morning,
that he went out, and stood, and said to
all the people, Ye *be* righteous: behold, [i]I
conspired against my master, and slew
him: but who slew all these?
10 Know now that there shall fall unto
the earth nothing of the word of the LORD,
which the LORD [j]spake concerning the
house of Ahab: for the LORD hath done
that which he spake by his servant Elijah.
11 So Jehu slew all that remained of
the house of Ahab in Jezreel, and all his
great men, and his kinsfolks, and his
priests, until he left him none remaining.
12 And he arose and departed, and
came to Samaria. *And* as he *was* at the
shearing house in the way,

The princes of Judah slain (2 Chr. 22:8).

13 Jehu met with the brethren of
Ahaziah king of Judah, and said, Who
are ye? And they answered, We *are* the
brethren of Ahaziah; and we go down to

B.C. 884.

a 2 Chr. 22:9.
b Ezk. 23:40.
c 1 Ki. 16:31.
d 1 Ki. 21:23.
e Psa. 83:10.
f Heb. *nourishers.*
g Heb. *for me.*
h 1 Ki. 21:21.
i 2 Ki. 9:14, 24.
j I Ki. 21:19-24.

salute the children of the king and the children of the queen.

14 And he said, Take them alive. And they took them alive, and slew them at the pit of the shearing house, *even* two and forty men; neither left he any of them.

Jehu spares Jehonadab.

15 And when he was departed thence, he lighted on [a]Jehonadab the son of [b]Rechab *coming* to meet him: and he saluted him, and said to him, Is thine heart right, as my heart *is* with thy heart? And Jehonadab answered, It is. If it be, give *me* thine hand. And he gave *him* his hand; and he took him up to him into the chariot.

16 And he said, Come with me, and see my zeal for the LORD. So they made him ride in his chariot.

17 And when he came to Samaria, he slew all that remained unto Ahab in Samaria, till he had destroyed him, according to the saying of the LORD, which he spake to [c]Elijah.

18 And Jehu gathered all the people together, and said unto them, Ahab served Baal a little; *but* Jehu shall serve him much.

Jehu exterminates Baal worship in Israel.

19 Now therefore call unto me all the [d]prophets of Baal, all his servants, and all his priests; let none be wanting: for I have a great sacrifice *to do* to Baal; whosoever shall be wanting, he shall not live. But Jehu did *it* in subtilty, to the intent that he might destroy the worshippers of Baal.

20 And Jehu said, Proclaim a solemn assembly for Baal. And they proclaimed *it*.

21 And Jehu sent through all Israel: and all the worshippers of Baal came, so that there was not a man left that came not. And they came into [e]the house of Baal; and the house of Baal was full from one end to another.

22 And he said unto him that *was* over the vestry, Bring forth vestments for all the worshippers of Baal. And he brought them forth vestments.

23 And Jehu went, and Jehonadab the son of Rechab, into the house of Baal, and said unto the worshippers of Baal, Search, and look that there be here with you none of the servants of the LORD, but the worshippers of Baal only.

24 And when they went in to offer sacrifices and burnt-offerings, Jehu appointed fourscore men without, and said, *If any of the men whom I have brought into your hands escape, he that letteth him go,* [f]his life *shall be* for the life of him.

25 And it came to pass, as soon as he had made an end of offering the burnt-offering, that Jehu said to the guard and to the captains, Go in, *and* slay them; let none come forth. And they smote them with the edge of the sword; and the guard and the captains cast *them* out, and went to the city of the house of Baal.

26 And they brought forth the images out of the house of Baal, and burned them.

27 And they brake down the image of Baal, and brake down the house of Baal, [g]and made it a draught house unto this day.

28 Thus Jehu destroyed Baal out of Israel.

29 Howbeit *from* the sins of Jeroboam the son of Nebat, who made Israel to sin, Jehu departed not from after them, *to wit,* [h]the golden calves that *were* in Beth-el, and that *were* in Dan.

Four generations promised to Jehu.

30 And the LORD [i]said unto Jehu, Because thou hast done well in executing *that which is* right in mine eyes, *and* hast done unto the house of Ahab according to all that *was* in mine heart, [j]thy children of the fourth *generation* shall sit on the throne of Israel.

31 But Jehu took no heed to walk in the law of the LORD God of Israel with all his heart: for he departed not from the [k]sins of Jeroboam, which made Israel to sin.

Power of Israel diminished.

32 In those days the LORD began to cut Israel short: and Hazael smote them in all the coasts of Israel;

33 From Jordan eastward, all the land of Gilead, the Gadites, and the Reubenites, and the Manassites, from Aroer, which *is* by the river Arnon, even Gilead and Bashan.

Death of Jehu:
accession of Jehoahaz over Israel.

34 Now the rest of the acts of Jehu, and all that he did, and all his might, *are*

B.C. 884.

a Called *Jonadab,* Jer. 35:6, 8, 10, 14, 16, 18, 19.
b 2 Sam. 4:2; 1 Chr. 2:55.
c 1 Ki. 21:21.
d 1 Ki. 22:6.
e 1 Ki. 16:32.
f 1 Ki. 20:39.
g Ezra 6:11; Dan. 2:5; 3:29.
h 1 Ki. 12:28, 29.
i 2 Ki. 9:6, 7.
j v.35; 2 Ki. 13:1, 10; 14:23; 15:8, 12.
k 1 Ki. 14:16.

they not written in the book of the
chronicles of the kings of Israel?
35 And Jehu slept with his fathers: and
they buried him in Samaria. And
Jehoahaz his son reigned in his stead.
36 And the time that Jehu reigned
over Israel in Samaria *was* twenty and
eight years.

CHAPTER 11.

The seed royal of Judah destroyed, save Joash (2 Chr. 22:10-12).

And when [a]Athaliah the [b]mother of
Ahaziah saw that her son was
dead, she arose and destroyed all the
seed royal.
2 But Jehosheba, the daughter of king
Joram, sister of Ahaziah, took Joash the
son of Ahaziah, and stole him from
among the king's sons *which were* slain;
and they hid him, *even* him and his
nurse, in the bedchamber from Athaliah,
so that he was not slain.
3 And he was with her hid in the
house of the LORD six years. And
Athaliah did reign over the land.

Joash becomes king over Judah (2 Chr. 23:1-11).

4 And the seventh [c]year Jehoiada sent
and fetched the rulers over hundreds,
with the captains and the guard, and
brought them to him into the house of
the LORD, and made a covenant with
them, and took an oath of them in the
house of the LORD, and shewed them the
king's son.
5 And he commanded them, saying,
This *is* the thing that ye shall do; A third
part of you that enter in [d]on the sabbath
shall even be keepers of the watch of the
king's house;
6 And a third part *shall be* at the gate of
Sur; and a third part at the gate behind
the guard: so shall ye keep the watch of
the house, that it be not broken down.
7 And two parts of all you that go
forth on the sabbath, even they shall
keep the watch of the house of the LORD
about the king.
8 And ye shall compass the king
round about, every man with his
weapons in his hand: and he that
cometh within the ranges, let him be
slain: and be ye with the king as he
goeth out and as he cometh in.
9 And the [e]captains over the hundreds
did according to all *things* that Jehoiada
the priest commanded: and they took
every man his men that were to come in
on the sabbath, with them that should
go out on the sabbath, and came to
Jehoiada the priest.
10 And to the captains over hundreds
did the priest give king David's spears
and shields, that *were* in the temple of
the LORD.
11 And the guard stood, every man
with his weapons in his hand, round
about the king, from the right corner of
the temple to the left corner of the temple, *along* by the altar and the temple.
12 And he brought forth the king's son,
and put the crown upon him, and *gave
him* the testimony; and they made him
king, and anointed him; and they clapped
their hands, and said, [f]God save the king.

Execution of Athaliah (2 Chr. 23:12-15).

13 And [g]when Athaliah heard the noise
of the guard *and* of the people, she came
to the people into the temple of the LORD.
14 And when she looked, behold, the
king stood by [h]a pillar, as the manner
was, and the princes and the trumpeters
by the king, and all the people of the
land rejoiced, and blew with trumpets:
and Athaliah rent her clothes, and cried,
Treason, Treason.
15 But Jehoiada the priest commanded
the captains of the hundreds, the officers
of the host, and said unto them, Have
her forth without the ranges: and him
that followeth her kill with the sword.
For the priest had said, Let her not be
slain in the house of the LORD.
16 And they laid hands on her; and
she went by the way by the which the
horses came into the king's house: and
there was she slain.

The revival through Jehoiada (2 Chr. 23:16-21).

17 [i]And Jehoiada made a covenant [j]be-
tween the LORD and the king and the people, that they should be the LORD'S people;
between the king also and the people.
18 And all the people of the land went
into the [k]house of Baal, and brake it
down; his altars and his [l]images brake
they in pieces thoroughly, and slew
Mattan the priest of Baal before the
altars. And the priest appointed officers
over the house of the LORD.

B.C. 856.

a 2 Chr. 22:10.
b 2 Ki. 8:26.
c 2 Chr. 23:1.
d 1 Chr. 9:25.
e 2 Chr. 23:8.
f 1 Sam. 10:24.
g 2 Chr. 23:12.
h 2 Ki. 23:3; 2 Chr. 34:31.
i 2 Chr. 23:16.
j 2 Sam. 5:3.
k 2 Ki. 10:26.
l Deut. 12:3; 2 Chr. 23:17.

19 And he took the rulers over hundreds, and the captains, and the guard, and all the people of the land; and they brought down the king from the house of the LORD, and came by the way of the gate of the guard to the king's house. And he sat on the throne of the kings.

20 And all the people of the land rejoiced, and the city was in quiet: and they slew Athaliah with the sword *beside* the king's house.

21 [a]Seven years old *was* Jehoash when he began to reign.

CHAPTER 12.

The reign of Jehoash (Joash) (2 Chr. 24:2).

In the seventh year of Jehu [a]Jehoash began to reign; and forty years reigned he in Jerusalem. And his mother's name *was* Zibiah of Beer-sheba.

2 And Jehoash did *that which was* right in the sight of the LORD all his days wherein Jehoiada the priest instructed him.

3 But the [b]high places were not taken away: the people still sacrificed and burnt incense in the high places.

The faithless priests (2 Chr. 24:4, 5).

4 And Jehoash said to the priests, All the money of the [c]dedicated things that is brought into the house of the LORD, *even* the money of every one that passeth *the account*, the money that every man is set at, *and* all the money that cometh into any man's heart to bring into the house of the LORD,

5 Let the priests take *it* to them, every man of his acquaintance: and let them repair the breaches of the house, wheresoever any breach shall be found.

6 But it was *so, that* in the three and twentieth year of king Jehoash the [d]priests had not repaired the breaches of the house.

7 Then [e]king Jehoash called for Jehoiada the priest, and the *other* priests, and said unto them, Why repair ye not the breaches of the house? now therefore receive no *more* money of your acquaintance, but deliver it for the breaches of the house.

8 And the priests consented to receive no *more* money of the people, neither to repair the breaches of the house.

B.C. 878.

a 2 Chr. 24:1-14.

b 2 Ki. 14:4; 1 Ki. 15:14; 22:43.

c Heb. *holiness*, or *holy things*.

d 2 Chr. 24:5.

e 2 Chr. 24:6.

f 2 Chr. 24:8.

g 2 Chr. 24:14.

h 2 Ki. 22:7.

i Lev. 5:15, 18.

j Lev. 7:7; Num. 18:9.

k 2 Ki. 8:12.

l 2 Chr. 24:23.

m 2 Ki. 18:15, 16; 1 Ki. 15:18.

The temple repaired (2 Chr. 24:8-14).

9 But Jehoiada the priest took a [f]chest, and bored a hole in the lid of it, and set it beside the altar, on the right side as one cometh into the house of the LORD: and the priests that kept the door put therein all the money *that was* brought into the house of the LORD.

10 And it was *so*, when they saw that *there was* much money in the chest, that the king's scribe and the high priest came up, and they put up in bags, and told the money that was found in the house of the LORD.

11 And they gave the money, being told, into the hands of them that did the work, that had the oversight of the house of the LORD: and they laid it out to the carpenters and builders, that wrought upon the house of the LORD,

12 And to masons, and hewers of stone, and to buy timber and hewed stone to repair the breaches of the house of the LORD, and for all that was laid out for the house to repair *it*.

13 Howbeit [g]there were not made for the house of the LORD bowls of silver, snuffers, basons, trumpets, any vessels of gold, or vessels of silver, of the money *that* was brought into the house of the LORD:

14 But they gave that to the workmen, and repaired therewith the house of the LORD.

15 Moreover [h]they reckoned not with the men, into whose hand they delivered the money to be bestowed on workmen: for they dealt faithfully.

16 The [i]trespass money and sin money was not brought into the house of the LORD: [j]it was the priests'.

The Syrians take Gath: Jehoash ransoms Jerusalem by despoiling the temple.

17 Then [k]Hazael king of Syria went up, and fought against Gath, and took it: and [l]Hazael set his face to go up to Jerusalem.

18 And Jehoash king of Judah [m]took all the hallowed things that Jehoshaphat, and Jehoram, and Ahaziah, his fathers, kings of Judah, had dedicated, and his own hallowed things, and all the gold *that was* found in the treasures of

the house of the LORD, and in the king's
house, and sent *it* to Hazael king of Syria:
and he went away from Jerusalem.

Death of Joash: accession of Amaziah
(2 Chr. 24:25-27).

19 And the rest of the acts of Joash,
and all that he did, *are* they not written
in the book of the chronicles of the kings
of Judah?
20 And [a]his servants arose, and made a
conspiracy, and slew Joash in the [b]house
of Millo, which goeth down to Silla.
21 For [c]Jozachar the son of Shimeath,
and Jehozabad the son of Shomer, his
servants, smote him, and he died; and
they buried him with his fathers in the
city of David: and [d]Amaziah his son
reigned in his stead.

CHAPTER 13.

The reign of Jehoahaz over Israel.

In the three and twentieth year of Joash
the son of Ahaziah king of Judah
Jehoahaz the son of Jehu began to reign
over Israel in Samaria, *and reigned* seventeen years.
2 And he did *that which was* evil in the
sight of the LORD, and followed the sins of
Jeroboam the son of Nebat, which made
Israel to sin; he departed not therefrom.
3 And the [e]anger of the LORD was kindled against Israel, and he delivered
them into the hand of [f]Hazael king of
Syria, and into the hand of Benhadad the
son of Hazael, all *their* days.

Johoahaz repents,
but suffers the grove in Samaria.

4 And Jehoahaz [g]besought the LORD,
and the LORD hearkened unto him: for
he [h]saw the oppression of Israel, because
the king of Syria oppressed them.
5 [i](And the LORD gave Israel a saviour,
so that they went out from under the
hand of the Syrians: and the children of
Israel dwelt in their tents, as beforetime.
6 Nevertheless they departed not from
the sins of the house of Jeroboam, who
made Israel sin, *but* walked therein: [j]and
there remained the [k]grove also in
Samaria.)
7 Neither did he leave of the people to
Jehoahaz but fifty horsemen, and ten
chariots, and ten thousand footmen; for
the king of Syria had destroyed them,
and had made them [l]like the dust by
threshing.

B.C. 840.

a 2 Ki. 14:5; 2 Chr. 24:25.
b Or, *Beth-millo.*
c 2 Chr. 24:26.
d 2 Chr. 24:27.
e Jud. 2:14.
f 2 Ki. 8:12.
g Psa. 78:34.
h Ex. 3:7; 2 Ki. 14:26.
i v. 25; 2 Ki. 14:25, 27.
j 1 Ki. 16:33.
k See Deut. 16:21.
l Amos 1:3.
m 2 Ki. 14:15.
n 2 Ki. 14:9.
o 2 Ki. 2:12.
p 1 Ki. 20:26.

Death of Jehoahaz.

8 Now the rest of the acts of Jehoahaz,
and all that he did, and his might, *are*
they not written in the book of the
chronicles of the kings of Israel?
9 And Jehoahaz slept with his fathers;
and they buried him in Samaria: and
Joash his son reigned in his stead.

Accession of Jehoash over Israel.

10 In the thirty and seventh year of
Joash king of Judah began Jehoash the
son of Jehoahaz to reign over Israel in
Samaria, *and reigned* sixteen years.
11 And he did *that which was* evil in
the sight of the LORD; he departed not
from all the sins of Jeroboam the son of
Nebat, who made Israel sin: *but* he
walked therein.

Death of Jehoash (2 Ki. 14:15, 16).

12 [m]And the rest of the acts of Joash,
and all that he did, and [n]his might wherewith he fought against Amaziah king of
Judah, *are* they not written in the book of
the chronicles of the kings of Israel?
13 And Joash slept with his fathers;
and Jeroboam sat upon his throne: and
Joash was buried in Samaria with the
kings of Israel.

Illness of Elisha: visit of Joash.

14 Now Elisha was fallen sick of his
sickness whereof he died. And Joash the
king of Israel came down unto him, and
wept over his face, and said, O my
father, my father, the [o]chariot of Israel,
and the horsemen thereof.
15 And Elisha said unto him, Take
bow and arrows. And he took unto him
bow and arrows.
16 And he said to the king of Israel,
Put thine hand upon the bow. And he
put his hand *upon it*: and Elisha put his
hands upon the king's hands.
17 And he said, Open the window
eastward. And he opened *it*. Then Elisha
said, Shoot. And he shot. And he said,
The arrow of the LORD'S deliverance, and
the arrow of deliverance from Syria: for
thou shalt smite the Syrians in [p]Aphek,
till thou have consumed *them*.

The scant faith of Joash.

18 And he said, Take the arrows. And
he took *them*. And he said unto the king

of Israel, Smite upon the ground. And he smote thrice, and stayed.

19 And the man of God was wroth with him, and said, Thou shouldest have smitten five or six times; then hadst thou smitten Syria till thou hadst consumed *it*: [a]whereas now thou shalt smite Syria *but* thrice.

Death of Elisha: the miracle at his tomb.

20 And Elisha died, and they buried him. And the bands of the Moabites invaded the land at the coming in of the year.

21 And it came to pass, as they were burying a man, that, behold, they spied a band *of men*; and they cast the man into the sepulchre of Elisha: and when the man was let down, and touched the bones of Elisha, he [b]revived, and stood up on his feet.

22 But [c]Hazael king of Syria oppressed Israel all the days of Jehoahaz.

23 [d]And the LORD was gracious unto them, and had compassion on them, and [e]had respect unto them, [f]because of his covenant with Abraham, Isaac, and Jacob, and would not destroy them, neither cast he them from his presence as yet.

24 So Hazael king of Syria died; and Benhadad his son reigned in his stead.

25 And Jehoash the son of Jehoahaz took again out of the hand of Benhadad the son of Hazael the cities, which he had taken out of the hand of Jehoahaz his father by war. [g]Three times did Joash beat him, and recovered the cities of Israel.

CHAPTER 14.

The reign of Amaziah over Judah
(2 Chr. 25:1).

In the second year of Joash son of Jehoahaz king of Israel reigned [h]Amaziah the son of Joash king of Judah.

2 He was twenty and five years old when he began to reign, and reigned twenty and nine years in Jerusalem. And his mother's name *was* Jehoaddan of Jerusalem.

3 And he did *that which was* right in the sight of the LORD, yet not like David his father: he did according to all things as Joash his father did.

4 [i]Howbeit the high places were not taken away: as yet the people did sacrifice and burnt incense on the high places.

5 And it came to pass, as soon as the kingdom was confirmed in his hand, that he slew his servants [j]which had slain the king his father.

6 But the children of the murderers he slew not: according unto that which is written in the book of the law of Moses, wherein the LORD commanded, saying, [k]The fathers shall not be put to death for the children, nor the children be put to death for the fathers; but every man shall be put to death for his own sin.

7 He slew of [l]Edom in the valley of salt ten thousand, and took Selah by war, and called the name of it Joktheel unto this day.

War between Israel and Judah
(2 Chr. 25:17-24).

8 Then Amaziah sent messengers to Jehoash, the son of Jehoahaz son of Jehu, king of Israel, saying, Come, let us look one another in the face.

9 And Jehoash the king of Israel sent to Amaziah king of Judah, saying, [m]The thistle that *was* in Lebanon sent to the cedar that *was* in Lebanon, saying, Give thy daughter to my son to wife: and there passed by a wild beast that *was* in Lebanon, and trode down the thistle.

10 Thou hast indeed smitten Edom, and thine heart hath lifted thee up: glory *of this*, and tarry at home: for why shouldest thou meddle to *thy* hurt, that thou shouldest fall, *even* thou, and Judah with thee?

11 But Amaziah would not hear. Therefore Jehoash king of Israel went up; and he and Amaziah king of Judah looked one another in the face at Beth-shemesh, which *belongeth* to Judah.

12 And Judah was put to the worse before Israel; and they fled every man to their tents.

13 And Jehoash king of Israel took Amaziah king of Judah, the son of Jehoash the son of Ahaziah, at Beth-shemesh, and came to Jerusalem, and brake down the wall of Jerusalem from the gate of Ephraim unto the corner gate, four hundred [n]cubits.

14 And he took all the gold and silver, and all the vessels that were found in the house of the LORD, and in the treasures

B.C. 839.

a v. 25.

b *Miracles* (O.T.). 2 Ki. 19:35. (Gen. 5:24; Jon. 2:1-10.)

c 2 Ki. 8:12.

d 2 Ki. 14:27.

e Ex. 2:24, 25.

f Gen. 17:2-7; Ex. 32.13.

g vs. 18,19.

h 2 Chr. 25:1.

i 2 Ki. 12:3.

j 2 Ki. 12:20.

k Deut. 24:16; Ezk. 18:4, 20.

l See 2 Chr. 25:5-16.

m *Parables* (O.T.). 2 Chr. 25:18. (Jud. 9:7-15; Zech. 11:7-14.)

n One cubit = about 18 in.

of the king's house, and hostages, and returned to Samaria.

(See 2 Ki. 13:12, 13.)

15 Now the rest of the acts of Jehoash which he did, and his might, and how he fought with Amaziah king of Judah, *are* they not written in the book of the chronicles of the kings of Israel?

Jeroboam succeeds Jehoash as king of Israel.

16 And Jehoash slept with his fathers, and was buried in Samaria with the kings of Israel; and Jeroboam his son reigned in his stead.

Death of Amaziah (2 Chr. 25:26-28).

17 And Amaziah the son of Joash king of Judah lived after the death of Jehoash son of Jehoahaz king of Israel fifteen years.
18 And the rest of the acts of Amaziah, *are* they not written in the book of the chronicles of the kings of Judah?
19 Now they made a conspiracy against him in Jerusalem: and he fled to Lachish; but they sent after him to Lachish, and slew him there.
20 And they brought him on horses: and he was buried at Jerusalem with his fathers in the city of David.

Azariah succeeds Amaziah as king of Judah.

21 And all the people of Judah took [a]Azariah, which *was* sixteen years old, and made him king instead of his father Amaziah.
22 He built [b]Elath, and restored it to Judah, after that the king slept with his fathers.

Reign of Jeroboam II. over Israel.

23 In the fifteenth year of Amaziah the son of Joash king of Judah Jeroboam the son of Joash king of Israel began to reign in Samaria, *and reigned* forty and one years.
24 And he did *that which was* evil in the sight of the LORD: he departed not from all the sins of Jeroboam the son of Nebat, who made Israel to sin.
25 He restored the coast of Israel from the entering of Hamath unto the [c]sea of the plain, according to the word of the LORD God of Israel, which he spake by the hand of his servant [d]Jonah, the son of Amittai, the prophet, which *was* of [e]Gath-hepher.
26 For the LORD [f]saw the affliction of Israel, *that it was* very bitter: for [g]*there was* not any shut up, nor any left, nor any helper for Israel.
27 And the LORD said not that he would blot out the name of Israel from under heaven: but he saved them by the hand of Jeroboam the son of Joash.

Death of Jeroboam II.: accession of Zachariah king over Israel.

28 Now the rest of the acts of Jeroboam, and all that he did, and his might, how he warred, and how he recovered Damascus, and Hamath, [h]*which belonged* to Judah, for Israel, *are* they not written in the book of the chronicles of the kings of Israel?
29 And Jeroboam slept with his fathers, *even* with the kings of Israel; and [i]Zachariah his son reigned in his stead.

CHAPTER 15.

Reign of Azariah (Uzziah) over Judah (2 Chr. 26:1-3).

In the twenty and seventh year of Jeroboam king of Israel began Azariah son of Amaziah king of Judah to reign.
2 Sixteen years old was he when he began to reign, and he reigned two and fifty years in Jerusalem. And his mother's name *was* Jecholiah of Jerusalem.
3 And he did *that which was* right in the sight of the LORD, according to all that his father Amaziah had done;
4 [j]Save that the high places were not removed: the people sacrificed and burnt incense still on the high places.
5 And the LORD [k]smote the king, so that he was a leper unto the day of his death, and dwelt in a several house. And Jotham the king's son *was* over the house, judging the people of the land.

Death of Azariah (Uzziah): accession of Jotham.

6 And the rest of the acts of Azariah, and all that he did, *are* they not written in the book of the chronicles of the kings of Judah?
7 So Azariah slept with his fathers; and they [l]buried him with his fathers in

B.C. 826.

a Called *Uzziah*, 2 Chr. 26:1; Isa. 1:1.
b 2 Ki. 16:6-2 Chr. 26:2.
c Deut. 3:17.
d Jon. 1:1.
e Josh. 19:13.
f 2 Ki. 13:4.
g Deut. 32:36.
h 2 Sam. 8:6; 1 Ki. 11:24; 2 Chr. 8:3.
i After an interregnum of 11 years. 2 Ki. 15:8.
j v. 35; 2 Ki. 12:3; 14:4.
k 2 Chr. 26:16-21.
l 2 Chr. 26:23.

the city of David: and Jotham his son reigned in his stead.

Reign of Zachariah over Israel.

8 In the thirty and eighth year of Azariah king of Judah did Zachariah the son of Jeroboam reign over Israel in Samaria six months.

9 And he did *that which was* evil in the sight of the LORD, as his fathers had done: he departed not from the sins of Jeroboam the son of Nebat, who made Israel to sin.

Death of Zachariah: accession of Shallum over Israel.

10 And Shallum the son of Jabesh conspired against him, and [a]smote him before the people, and slew him, and reigned in his stead.

11 And the rest of the acts of Zachariah, behold, they *are* written in the book of the chronicles of the kings of Israel.

12 This *was* the [b]word of the LORD which he spake unto Jehu, saying, Thy sons shall sit on the throne of Israel unto the fourth *generation*. And so it came to pass.

Reign of Shallum: his death.

13 Shallum the son of Jabesh began to reign in the nine and thirtieth year of [c]Uzziah king of Judah; and he reigned a full month in Samaria.

14 For Menahem the son of Gadi went up from [d]Tirzah, and came to Samaria, and smote Shallum the son of Jabesh in Samaria, and slew him, and reigned in his stead.

15 And the rest of the acts of Shallum, and his conspiracy which he made, behold, they *are* written in the book of the chronicles of the kings of Israel.

Reign of Menahem over Israel.

16 Then Menahem smote [e]Tiphsah, and all that *were* therein, and the coasts thereof from Tirzah: because they opened not *to him*, therefore he smote *it; and* all the women therein that were with child he ripped up.

17 In the nine and thirtieth year of Azariah king of Judah began Menahem the son of Gadi to reign over Israel, *and reigned* ten years in Samaria.

18 And he did *that which was* evil in the sight of the LORD: he departed not all his days from the sins of Jeroboam the son of Nebat, who made Israel to sin.

B.C. 758.

a As prophesied, Amos 7:9.

b 2 Ki. 10:30.

c 1 Ki. 14:17; Song 6:4; Mt. 1:8, 9, called *Ozias*, and v. 1, *Azariah*.

d 1 Ki. 14:17.

e 1 Ki. 4:24.

f 1 Chr. 5:26; Isa. 9:1; Hos. 8:9.

g One talent = £410, or $1940.

h One shekel = 2*s*. 9*d*., or 65 cts.

i Isa. 7:1.

j 1 Chr. 5:26; Isa. 9:1.

k 1 Ki. 15:20.

An Assyrian invasion of Israel (1 Chr. 5:26).

19 *And* [f]Pul the king of Assyria came against the land: and Menahem gave Pul a thousand [g]talents of silver, that his hand might be with him to confirm the kingdom in his hand.

20 And Menahem exacted the money of Israel, *even* of all the mighty men of wealth, of each man fifty [h]shekels of silver, to give to the king of Assyria. So the king of Assyria turned back, and stayed not there in the land.

Death of Menahem: accession of Pekahiah over Israel.

21 And the rest of the acts of Menahem, and all that he did, *are* they not written in the book of the chronicles of the kings of Israel?

22 And Menahem slept with his fathers; and Pekahiah his son reigned in his stead.

Death of Pekahiah: accession of Pekah over Israel.

23 In the fiftieth year of Azariah king of Judah Pekahiah the son of Menahem began to reign over Israel in Samaria, *and reigned* two years.

24 And he did *that which was* evil in the sight of the LORD: he departed not from the sins of Jeroboam the son of Nebat, who made Israel to sin.

25 But Pekah the son of Remaliah, a captain of his, conspired against him, and smote him in Samaria, in the palace of the king's house, with Argob and Arieh, and with him fifty men of the Gileadites: and he killed him, and reigned in his room.

26 And the rest of the acts of Pekahiah, and all that he did, behold, they *are* written in the book of the chronicles of the kings of Israel.

Reign of Pekah over Israel: his death.

27 In the two and fiftieth year of Azariah king of Judah [i]Pekah the son of Remaliah began to reign over Israel in Samaria, *and reigned* twenty years.

28 And he did *that which was* evil in the sight of the LORD: he departed not from the sins of Jeroboam the son of Nebat, who made Israel to sin.

29 In the days of Pekah king of Israel came [j]Tiglath-pileser king of Assyria and took [k]Ijon, and Abel-beth-maachah,

and Janoah, and Kedesh, and Hazor, and
Gilead, and Galilee, all the land of
Naphtali, and carried them captive to
Assyria.
30 And Hoshea the son of Elah made a
conspiracy against Pekah the son of
Remaliah, and smote him, and slew him,
and [a]reigned in his stead, in the twentieth year of Jotham the son of Uzziah.
31 And the rest of the acts of Pekah,
and all that he did, behold, they *are* written in the book of the chronicles of the
kings of Israel.

Reign of Jotham over Judah (2 Chr. 23:27).

32 In the second year of Pekah the son
of Remaliah king of Israel began [b]Jotham
the son of Uzziah king of Judah to reign.
33 Five and twenty years old was he
when he began to reign, and he reigned
sixteen years in Jerusalem. And his
mother's name *was* Jerusha, the daughter of Zadok.
34 And he did *that which was* right in
the sight of the LORD: he did according
to all that his father Uzziah had done.
35 [c]Howbeit the high places were not
removed: the people sacrificed and
burned incense still in the high places.
He built the higher gate of the house of
the LORD.
36 Now the rest of the acts of Jotham,
and all that he did, *are* they not written
in the book of the chronicles of the kings
of Judah?
37 In those days the LORD began to
send against Judah [d]Rezin the king of
Syria, and Pekah the son of Remaliah.
38 And Jotham slept with his fathers,
and was buried with his fathers in the
city of David his father: and Ahaz his
son reigned in his stead.

CHAPTER 16.

Reign of Ahaz over Judah (2 Chr. 28:1).

In the seventeenth year of Pekah the
son of Remaliah [e]Ahaz the son of
Jotham king of Judah began to reign.
2 Twenty years old *was* Ahaz when he
began to reign, and reigned sixteen years
in Jerusalem, and did not *that which was*
right in the sight of the LORD his God,
like David his father.
3 But he walked in the way of the kings
of Israel, yea, [f]and made his son to pass
through the fire, according to the [g]abomi-
nations of the heathen, whom the LORD
cast out from before the children of Israel.
4 And he sacrificed and burnt incense
in the high places, and on the hills, and
under every green tree.

Invasion of Judah by Syria and Israel
(2 Chr. 28:5-8).

5 Then Rezin king of Syria and Pekah
son of Remaliah king of Israel came up
to Jerusalem to war: and they besieged
Ahaz, but could not overcome *him*.
6 At that time Rezin king of Syria
recovered Elath to Syria, and drave the
Jews from [i]Elath: and the Syrians came
to Elath, and dwelt there unto this day.

Ahaz seeks the assistance of Assyria
(2 Chr. 28:16-21).

7 So Ahaz sent messengers to [j]Tiglath-
pileser king of Assyria, saying, I *am* thy
servant and thy son: come up, and save
me out of the hand of the king of Syria,
and out of the hand of the king of Israel,
which rise up against me.
8 And Ahaz [k]took the silver and gold
that was found in the house of the LORD,
and in the treasures of the king's house,
and sent *it for* a present to the king of
Assyria.

The Assyrians take Damascus.

9 And the king of Assyria hearkened
unto him: for the king of Assyria went
up against Damascus, and took it, and
carried *the people of* it captive to Kir, and
slew Rezin.
10 And king Ahaz went to Damascus to
meet Tiglath-pileser king of Assyria, and
saw an altar that *was* at Damascus: and
king Ahaz sent to Urijah the priest the
fashion of the altar, and the pattern of it,
according to all the workmanship thereof.
11 And Urijah the priest built an altar
according to all that king Ahaz had sent
from Damascus: so Urijah the priest
made *it* against king Ahaz came from
Damascus.
12 And when the king was come from
Damascus, the king saw the altar: and
the king approached to the altar, and
offered thereon.
13 And he burnt his burnt-offering
and his [l]meat-offering, and poured his
drink-offering, and sprinkled the blood
of his peace-offerings, upon the altar.
14 And he brought also the brasen
altar, which *was* before the LORD, from

B.C. 739.

a 2 Ki. 17:1; Hos. 10:3, 7, 15.
b 2 Chr. 27:1.
c v. 4.
d Isa. 7:1-17.
e 2 Chr. 28:1.
f Lev. 18:21; 2 Chr. 28:3; Psa. 106:37, 38.
g Deut. 12:31.
h i.e. *nations.*
i Heb. *Eloth.*
j Heb. *Tilgath-pilneser*, 1 Chr. 5:26; 2 Chr. 28:20.
k 2 Ki. 12:18; 2 Chr. 28:21.
l Lit. *meal.*

the forefront of the house, from between the altar and the house of the LORD, and put it on the north side of the altar.

15 And king Ahaz commanded Urijah the priest, saying, Upon the great altar burn the morning burnt-offering, and the evening [a]meat-offering, and the king's burnt sacrifice, and his meat-offering, with the burnt-offering of all the people of the land, and their meat-offering, and their drink-offerings; and sprinkle upon it all the blood of the burnt-offering, and all the blood of the sacrifice: and the brasen altar shall be for me to enquire *by*.

16 Thus did Urijah the priest, according to all that king Ahaz commanded.

17 And king Ahaz cut off [b]the borders of the bases, and removed the laver from off them; and took down the [c]sea from off the brasen oxen that *were* under it, and put it upon a pavement of stones.

18 And the covert for the sabbath that they had built in the house, and the king's entry without, turned he from the house of the LORD for the king of Assyria.

Death of Ahaz: accession of Hezekiah
(2 Chr. 28:26, 27).

19 Now the rest of the acts of Ahaz which he did, *are* they not written in the book of the chronicles of the kings of Judah?

20 And Ahaz slept with his fathers, and [d]was buried with his fathers in the city of David: and Hezekiah his son reigned in his stead.

CHAPTER 17.

Reign of Hoshea over Israel.

In the twelfth year of Ahaz king of Judah began [e]Hoshea the son of Elah to reign in Samaria over Israel nine years.

2 And he did *that which was* evil in the sight of the LORD, but not as the kings of Israel that were before him.

Israel becomes tributary to Assyria.

3 Against him came up [f]Shalmaneser king of Assyria; and Hoshea became his servant, and gave him presents.

Israel (the ten tribes)
carried away into Assyria.

4 And the king of Assyria found conspiracy in Hoshea: for he had sent messengers to So king of Egypt, and brought no present to the king of Assyria, as *he had done* year by year: therefore the king of Assyria shut him up, and bound him in prison.

5 Then the king of Assyria came up throughout all the land, and went up to Samaria, and besieged it three years.

6 In the ninth year of Hoshea the king of Assyria took Samaria, and carried [g]Israel away into Assyria, and placed them in Halah and in Habor *by* the river of Gozan, and in the cities of the Medes.

The sins for which Israel
was carried into captivity.

7 For *so* it was, that the children of Israel had [1]sinned against the LORD their God, which had brought them up out of the land of Egypt, from under the hand of Pharaoh king of Egypt, and had feared other gods,

8 And walked in the statutes of the [h]heathen, whom the LORD cast out from before the children of Israel, and of the kings of Israel, which they had made.

9 And the children of Israel did secretly *those* things that *were* not right against the LORD their God, and they built them high places in all their cities, from the tower of the watchmen to the fenced city.

10 And they set them up images and [i]groves in every high hill, and under every green tree:

11 And there they burnt incense in all the high places, as *did* the [h]heathen whom the LORD carried away before them; and wrought wicked things to provoke the LORD to anger:

12 For they served idols, whereof the LORD had said unto them, Ye shall not do this thing.

13 Yet the LORD testified against Israel,

B.C. 740.

a Lit. *meal.*
b 1 Ki. 7:27-29.
c 1 Ki. 7:23, 25.
d 2 Chr. 28:27.
e 2 Ki. 15:30.
f 2 Ki. 18:9.
g *Israel (history).* vs. 6-23; 2 Ki. 24:10-16. (Gen. 12:2, 3; Rom. 11:26.)
h i.e. *nations.*
i See Deut. 16:21.

[1] **(17:7)** Cf. Deut. 28:15-68. From this captivity the ten tribes have never been restored to Palestine. A remnant of Judah returned under Zerubbabel, Ezra, and Nehemiah, and *individuals* out of the ten tribes (called, after the division of Solomon's kingdom, "Israel" in the historical books and Prophets, also "Ephraim" by the latter) went back, but the *national* restoration is yet to be fulfilled. See *Palestinian Covenant,* Deut. 30:1-9; *Kingdom,* 2 Sam. 7:8-17, *refs.*

and against Judah, by all the prophets,
and by all the [a]seers, saying, [b]Turn ye
from your evil ways, and keep my commandments *and* my statutes, according
to all the law which I commanded your
fathers, and which I sent to you by my
servants the prophets.
14 Notwithstanding they would not
hear, but [c]hardened their necks, like to
the neck of their fathers, that did not
believe in the LORD their God.
15 And they [d]rejected his statutes, and
his covenant that he made with their
fathers, and his testimonies which he
testified against them; and they followed
vanity, and [e]became vain, and went after
the [f]heathen that *were* round about them,
concerning whom the LORD had charged
them, that they should not do like them.
16 And they left all the commandments of the LORD their God, and [g]made
them molten images, *even* two calves,
and made a [h]grove, and worshipped all
the host of heaven, and served Baal.
17 And they caused their sons and their
daughters to pass through the fire, and
[i]used divination and enchantments, and
sold themselves to do evil in the sight of
the LORD, to provoke him to anger.
18 Therefore the LORD was very angry
with Israel, and removed them out of his
sight: there was none left [j]but the tribe
of Judah only.
19 Also Judah kept not the commandments of the LORD their God, but walked
in the statutes of Israel which they made.
20 And the LORD rejected all the seed
of Israel, and afflicted them, and [k]deliv-
ered them into the hand of spoilers, until
he had cast them out of his sight.
21 For he rent Israel from the house of
David; and they made Jeroboam the son
of Nebat king: and Jeroboam drave
Israel from following the LORD, and
made them sin a great sin.
22 For the children of Israel walked in
all the sins of Jeroboam which he did;
they departed not from them;
23 Until the LORD removed Israel out
of his sight, [l]as he had said by all his servants the prophets. [m]So was Israel carried away out of their own land to
Assyria unto this day.

B.C. 721.

a 1 Sam. 9:9.
b Jer. 18:11; 25:5; 35:15.
c Deut. 31:27; Prov. 29:1.
d Deut. 32:21; 1 Ki. 16:13.
e Psa. 115:8; Rom. 1:21.
f i.e. *nations.*
g 1 Ki. 12:28.
h See Deut. 16:21.
i Deut. 18:10.
j 1 Ki. 11:13, 32.
k 2 Ki. 13:3; 15:29.
l 1 Ki. 14:16.
m v. 6.
n v. 30.
o Psa. 19:9, *note.*

The king of Assyria repeoples the cities of Israel.

24 And the king of Assyria brought
men from [n]Babylon, and from Cuthah,
and from Ava, and from Hamath, and
from Sepharvaim, and placed *them* in the
cities of Samaria instead of the children
of Israel: and they possessed Samaria,
and dwelt in the cities thereof.
25 And *so* it was at the beginning of
their dwelling there, *that* they [o]feared not
the LORD: therefore the LORD sent lions
among them, which slew *some* of them.
26 Wherefore they spake to the king of
Assyria, saying, The nations which thou
hast removed, and placed in the cities of
Samaria, know not the manner of the
God of the land: therefore he hath sent
lions among them, and, behold, they
slay them, because they know not the
manner of the God of the land.
27 Then the king of Assyria commanded, saying, Carry thither one of the
priests whom ye brought from thence;
and let them go and dwell there, and let
him teach them the manner of the God
of the land.
28 Then one of the priests whom they
had carried away from Samaria came
and dwelt in Beth-el, and taught them
how they should [o]fear the LORD.
29 Howbeit every nation made gods of
their own, and put *them* in the houses of
the high places which the Samaritans
had made, every nation in their cities
wherein they dwelt.
30 And the men of Babylon made
Succoth-benoth, and the men of Cuth
made Nergal, and the men of Hamath
made Ashima,
31 And the Avites made Nibhaz and
Tartak, and the Sepharvites burnt their
children in fire to Adrammelech and
Anammelech, the gods of Sepharvaim.
32 So they [o]feared the LORD, and made
unto themselves of the lowest of them
priests of the high places, which sacrificed
for them in the houses of the high places.
33 They [o]feared the LORD, and served
their own gods, after the manner of the
nations whom they carried away from
thence.
34 Unto this day they do after the former manners: they [o]fear not the LORD,
neither do they after their statutes, or

B.C. 678.

after their ordinances, or after the law and commandment which the LORD commanded the children of Jacob, whom he named Israel;

35 With whom the LORD had made a covenant, and charged them, saying, Ye shall not fear other gods, nor bow yourselves to them, nor serve them, nor sacrifice to them:

36 But the LORD, who brought you up out of the land of Egypt with great power and a stretched out arm, him shall ye [a]fear, and him shall ye worship, and to him shall ye do sacrifice.

37 And the statutes, and the ordinances, and the law, and the commandment, which he wrote for you, ye shall observe to do for evermore; and ye shall not fear other gods.

38 And the covenant that I have made with you ye shall not forget; neither shall ye fear other gods.

39 But the LORD your God ye shall [a]fear; and he shall deliver you out of the hand of all your enemies.

40 Howbeit they did not hearken, but they did after their former manner.

41 So these nations [a]feared the LORD, and served their graven images, both their children, and their children's children: as did their fathers, so do they unto this day.

CHAPTER 18.

Reign of Hezekiah over Judah
(2 Chr. 29:1).

NOW it came to pass in the third year of Hoshea son of Elah king of Israel, *that* Hezekiah the son of Ahaz king of Judah began to reign.

2 Twenty and five years old was he when he began to reign; and he reigned twenty and nine years in Jerusalem. His mother's name also *was* Abi, the daughter of Zachariah.

3 And he did *that which was* right in the sight of the LORD, according to all that David his father did.

Revival under Hezekiah
(2 Chr. 29:3–31:21).

4 He removed the high places, and brake the images, and cut down the [b]groves, and brake in pieces the brasen serpent that Moses had made: for unto those days the children of Israel did burn incense to it: and he called it Nehushtan.

5 He [c]trusted in the LORD God of Israel; so that after him was none like him among all the kings of Judah, nor *any* that were before him.

6 For he clave to the LORD, *and* departed not from following him, but kept his commandments, which the LORD commanded Moses.

7 And the LORD was with him; *and* he prospered whithersoever he went forth: and he rebelled against the king of Assyria, and served him not.

Hezekiah victorious over the Philistines.

8 He smote the Philistines, *even* unto Gaza, and the borders thereof, from the tower of the watchmen to the fenced city.

9 And it came to pass in the fourth year of king Hezekiah, which *was* the seventh year of Hoshea son of Elah king of Israel, *that* Shalmaneser king of Assyria came up against Samaria, and besieged it.

10 And at the end of three years they took it: *even* in the sixth year of Hezekiah, that *is* the ninth year of Hoshea king of Israel, Samaria was taken.

11 And the king of Assyria [d]did carry away Israel unto Assyria, and put them in Halah and in Habor *by* the river of Gozan, and in the cities of the Medes:

12 Because they obeyed not the voice of the LORD their God, but transgressed his covenant, *and* all that Moses the servant of the LORD commanded, and would not hear *them*, nor do *them*.

Sennacherib invades Judah.

13 Now in the fourteenth year of king Hezekiah did Sennacherib king of Assyria come up against all the fenced cities of Judah, and took them.

14 And Hezekiah king of Judah sent to the king of Assyria to Lachish, saying, I have offended; return from me: that which thou puttest on me will I bear. And the king of Assyria appointed unto Hezekiah king of Judah three hundred [e]talents of silver and thirty [f]talents of gold.

15 And Hezekiah [g]gave *him* all the silver that was found in the house of the LORD, and in the treasures of the king's house.

16 At that time did Hezekiah cut off *the gold from* the doors of the temple of the LORD, and *from* the pillars which

a Psa. 19:9, *note.*

b See Deut. 16:21.

c Psa. 2:12, *note.*

d *Times of the Gentiles.* vs. 9, 12; 2 Ki. 25:1-21. (Lk. 21:24; Rev. 16:19.)

e One talent (silver) = £410, or $1940.

f One talent (gold) = £6150, or $29,085.

g 2 Ki. 16:8.

Hezekiah king of Judah had overlaid,
and gave it to the king of Assyria.

Sennacherib seeks to terrify the defenders of Jerusalem (2 Chr. 32:9-19).

17 And the king of Assyria sent Tartan
and Rabsaris and Rab-shakeh from
Lachish to king Hezekiah with a great
host against Jerusalem. And they went
up and came to Jerusalem. And when
they were come up, they came and stood
by the conduit of the upper pool, [a]which
is in the highway of the fuller's field.
18 And when they had called to the
king, there came out to them Eliakim the
son of Hilkiah, which *was* over the
household, and Shebna the scribe, and
Joah the son of Asaph the recorder.
19 And Rab-shakeh said unto them,
Speak ye now to Hezekiah, Thus saith the
great king, the king of Assyria, [b]What
confidence *is* this wherein thou trustest?
20 Thou sayest, (but *they are but* [c]vain
words,) *I have* counsel and strength for
the war. Now on whom dost thou trust,
that thou rebellest against me?
21 [d]Now, behold, thou trustest upon
the staff of this bruised reed, *even* upon
Egypt, on which if a man lean, it will go
into his hand, and pierce it: so *is* Pharaoh
king of Egypt unto all that trust on him.
22 But if ye say unto me, We trust in
the LORD our God: *is* not that he, [e]whose
high places and whose altars Hezekiah
hath taken away, and hath said to Judah
and Jerusalem, Ye shall worship before
this altar in Jerusalem?
23 Now therefore, I pray thee, give
[f]pledges to my lord the king of Assyria,
and I will deliver thee two thousand
horses, if thou be able on thy part to set
riders upon them.
24 How then wilt thou turn away the
face of one captain of the least of my
master's servants, and put thy trust on
Egypt for chariots and for horsemen?
25 Am I now come up without the
LORD against this place to destroy it? The
LORD said to me, Go up against this
land, and destroy it.

The Jewish answer to Rab-shakeh's threats.

26 Then said Eliakim the son of
Hilkiah, and Shebna, and Joah, unto
Rab-shakeh, Speak, I pray thee, to thy
servants in the Syrian language; for we
understand *it*: and talk not with us in the
Jews' language in the ears of the people
that *are* on the wall.

Rab-shakeh's further insolence.

27 But Rab-shakeh said unto them,
Hath my master sent me to thy master,
and to thee, to speak these words? *hath he*
not *sent me* to the men which sit on the
wall, that they may eat their own dung,
and drink their own piss with you?
28 Then Rab-shakeh stood and cried
with a loud voice in the Jews' language,
and spake, saying, Hear the word of the
great king, the king of Assyria:
29 Thus saith the king, [g]Let not
Hezekiah deceive you: for he shall not
be able to deliver you out of his hand:
30 Neither let Hezekiah make you trust
in the LORD, saying, The LORD will surely
deliver us, and this city shall not be delivered into the hand of the king of Assyria.
31 Hearken not to Hezekiah: for thus
saith the king of Assyria, [h]Make *an agreement* with me by a present, and come out
to me, and *then* eat ye every man of his
own vine, and every one of his fig tree,
and drink ye every one the waters of his
cistern:
32 Until I come and take you away to a
land like your own land, [i]a land of corn
and wine, a land of bread and vineyards,
a land of oil olive and of honey, that ye
may live, and not die: and hearken not
unto Hezekiah, when he [j]persuadeth
you, saying, The LORD will deliver us.
33 [k]Hath any of the gods of the
nations delivered at all his land out of
the hand of the king of Assyria?
34 [l]Where *are* the gods of Hamath, and
of Arpad? where *are* the gods of
Sepharvaim, Hena, and [m]Ivah? have they
delivered Samaria out of mine hand?
35 Who *are* they among all the gods of
the countries, that have delivered their
country out of mine hand, [n]that the
LORD should deliver Jerusalem out of
mine hand?
36 But the people held their peace, and
answered him not a word: for the king's
commandment was, saying, Answer him
not.
37 Then came Eliakim the son of
Hilkiah, which *was* over the household,
and Shebna the scribe, and Joah the son
of Asaph the recorder, to Hezekiah [o]with

B.C. 713.

a Isa. 7:3.
b 2 Chr. 32:10; Psa. 118:8-9.
c Heb. *word of the lips.*
d Isa. 30:2-7; Ezk. 29:6, 7.
e v. 4; 2 Chr. 31:1; 32:12.
f Or, *hostages.*
g 2 Chr. 32:15.
h Or, *seek my favour.*
i Deut. 8:7, 8.
j Or, *deceiveth.*
k 2 Ki. 19:12; 2 Chr. 32:14; Isa. 10:9-11.
l 2 Ki. 19:13.
m 2 Ki. 17:24, *Ava.*
n Dan. 3:15.
o Isa. 33:7.

their clothes rent, and told him the words of Rab-shakeh.

CHAPTER 19.

Hezekiah's message to Isaiah.

And [a]it came to pass, when king Hezekiah heard *it*, that he rent his clothes, and covered himself with sackcloth, and went into the house of the LORD.

2 And he sent Eliakim, which *was* over the household, and Shebna the scribe, and the elders of the priests, covered with sackcloth, to [b]Isaiah the prophet the son of Amoz.

3 And they said unto him, Thus saith Hezekiah, This day *is* a day of trouble, and of rebuke, and blasphemy: for the children are come to the birth, and *there is* not strength to bring forth.

4 [c]It may be the LORD thy God will hear all the words of Rab-shakeh, whom the king of Assyria his master hath sent to reproach the living God; and will reprove the words which the LORD thy God hath heard: wherefore lift up *thy* prayer for the remnant that are left.

5 So the servants of king Hezekiah came to Isaiah.

Isaiah's answer.

6 And [d]Isaiah said unto them, Thus shall ye say to your master, Thus saith the LORD, Be not afraid of the words which thou hast heard, with which the [e]servants of the king of Assyria have blasphemed me.

7 Behold, I will send a [f]blast upon him, and he shall hear a rumour, and shall return to his own land; and I will cause him to fall by the sword in his own land.

Sennacherib defies the God of Hezekiah (2 Chr. 32:17).

8 So Rab-shakeh returned, and found the king of Assyria warring against Libnah: for he had heard that he was departed from Lachish.

9 And [g]when he heard say of Tirhakah king of Ethiopia, Behold, he is come out to fight against thee: he sent messengers again unto Hezekiah, saying,

10 Thus shall ye speak to Hezekiah king of Judah, saying, Let not thy God in whom thou [h]trustest deceive thee, saying, Jerusalem shall not be delivered into the hand of the king of Assyria.

11 Behold, thou hast heard what the kings of Assyria have done to all lands, by destroying them utterly: and shalt thou be delivered?

12 Have the gods of the nations delivered them which my fathers have destroyed; *as* Gozan, and Haran, and Rezeph, and the children of Eden which *were* in Thelasar?

13 Where *is* the king of Hamath, and the king of Arpad, and the king of the city of Sepharvaim, of Hena, and Ivah?

Hezekiah's prayer (2 Chr. 32:20).

14 And Hezekiah received the letter of the hand of the messengers, and read it: and Hezekiah went up into the house of the LORD, and spread it before the LORD.

15 And Hezekiah prayed before the LORD, and [i]said, O LORD God of Israel, which dwellest *between* the cherubims, thou art the God, *even* thou alone, of all the kingdoms of the earth; thou hast made heaven and earth.

16 LORD, [j]bow down thine ear, and hear: open, LORD, thine eyes, and see: and hear the words of Sennacherib, which hath sent him to reproach the living God.

17 Of a truth, LORD, the kings of Assyria have destroyed the nations and their lands,

18 And have cast their gods into the fire: for they *were* no gods, but [k]the work of men's hands, wood and stone: therefore they have destroyed them.

19 Now therefore, O LORD our God, I beseech thee, save thou us out of his hand, [l]that all the kingdoms of the earth may know that thou *art* the LORD God, *even* thou only.

Jehovah's answer through Isaiah.

20 Then Isaiah the son of Amoz sent to Hezekiah, saying, Thus saith the LORD God of Israel, [m]*That* which thou hast prayed to me against Sennacherib king of Assyria I have heard.

21 This *is* the word that the LORD hath spoken concerning him; The virgin [n]the daughter of Zion hath despised thee, *and* laughed thee to scorn; the daughter of Jerusalem hath shaken her head at thee.

22 Whom hast thou reproached and blasphemed? and against whom hast thou exalted *thy* voice, and lifted up

B.C. 710.

a Isa. 37:1.
b Lk. 3:4, called *Esaias.*
c 2 Sam. 16:12.
d Isa. 37:6.
e 2 Ki. 18:17.
f vs. 35-37; Jer. 51:1.
g 1 Sam. 23:27.
h Psa. 2:12, *note.*
i *Bible prayers* (O.T.). 2 Ki. 20:3. (Gen. 15:2; Hab. 3:1-16.)
j Psa. 31:2.
k Psa. 115:4; Jer. 10:3.
l Psa. 83:18.
m Isa. 37:21.
n Lam. 2:13.

thine eyes on high? *even* against the Holy *One* of Israel.

23 By thy messengers thou hast reproached the Lord, and hast said, With the multitude of my chariots I am come up to the height of the mountains, to the sides of Lebanon, and will cut down the tall cedar trees thereof, *and* the choice fir trees thereof: and I will enter into the lodgings of his borders, *and into* the forest of his Carmel.

24 I have digged and drunk strange waters, and with the sole of my feet have I dried up all the rivers of besieged places.

25 Hast thou not heard long ago *how* I have done it, *and* of ancient times that I have formed it? now have I brought it to pass, that thou shouldest be to lay waste fenced cities *into* ruinous heaps.

26 Therefore their inhabitants were of small power, they were dismayed and confounded; they were *as* the grass of the field, and *as* the green herb, *as* the grass on the housetops, and *as corn* blasted before it be grown up.

27 But I know thy abode, and thy going out, and thy coming in, and thy rage against me.

28 Because thy rage against me and thy tumult is come up into mine ears, therefore [a]I will put my hook in thy nose, and my bridle in thy lips, and I will turn thee back by the way by which thou camest.

29 And this *shall be* a [b]sign unto thee, Ye shall eat this year such things as grow of themselves, and in the second year that which springeth of the same; and in the third year sow ye, and reap, and plant vineyards, and eat the fruits thereof.

30 And the remnant that is escaped of the house of Judah shall yet again take root downward, and bear fruit upward.

31 For out of Jerusalem shall go forth a remnant, and they that escape out of mount Zion: the zeal of the LORD *of hosts* shall do this.

32 Therefore thus saith the LORD concerning the king of Assyria, He shall not come into this city, nor shoot an arrow there, nor come before it with shield, nor cast a bank against it.

33 By the way that he came, by the same shall he return, and shall not come into this city, saith the LORD.

B.C. 710.

a Job 41:2; Ezk. 29:4; 38:4; Amos 4:2.

b 1 Sam. 2:34; 2 Ki. 20:8, 9; Isa. 7:11-14; Lk. 2:12.

c 2 Ki. 20:6.

d 1 Ki. 11:12, 13.

e 2 Chr. 32:21; Isa. 37:36.

f Heb. 1:4, *note.*

g *Miracles* (O.T.). 2 Ki. 20:9-11. (Gen. 5:24; Jon. 2:1-10.)

h *Bible prayers* (O.T.) 1 Chr. 4:10. (Gen. 15:2; Hab. 3:1-16.)

i See 1 Ki. 8:61.

j 2 Ki. 19:20; Psa. 65:2.

k Psa. 39:12; 56:8.

l 2 Ki. 19:34.

34 For [c]I will defend this city, to save it, for mine own sake, and [d]for my servant David's sake.

Jehovah destroys the Assyrian army (2 Chr. 32:21, 22).

35 And [e]it came to pass that night, that the [f]angel of the LORD went out, and [g]smote in the camp of the Assyrians an hundred fourscore and five thousand: and when they arose early in the morning, behold, they *were* all dead corpses.

Death of Sennacherib (2 Chr. 32:21).

36 So Sennacherib king of Assyria departed, and went and returned, and dwelt at Nineveh.

37 And it came to pass, as he was worshipping in the house of Nisroch his god, that Adrammelech and Sharezer his sons smote him with the sword: and they escaped into the land of Armenia. And Esar-haddon his son reigned in his stead.

CHAPTER 20.

Hezekiah's illness and recovery (2 Chr. 32:24).

In those days was Hezekiah sick unto death. And the prophet Isaiah the son of Amoz came to him, and said unto him, Thus saith the LORD, Set thine house in order; for thou shalt die, and not live.

2 Then he turned his face to the wall, and prayed unto the LORD, saying,

3 I [h]beseech thee, O LORD, remember now how I have walked before thee in truth and with a [i]perfect heart, and have done *that which is* good in thy sight. And Hezekiah wept sore.

4 And it came to pass, afore Isaiah was gone out into the middle court, that the word of the LORD came to him, saying,

5 Turn again, and tell Hezekiah the captain of my people, Thus saith the LORD, the God of David thy father, [j]I have heard thy prayer, I have seen [k]thy tears: behold, I will heal thee: on the third day thou shalt go up unto the house of the LORD.

6 And I will add unto thy days fifteen years; and I will deliver thee and this city out of the hand of the king of Assyria; and [l]I will defend this city for mine own sake, and for my servant David's sake.

7 And Isaiah said, Take a lump of figs.

And they took and laid *it* on the boil, and he recovered.

8 And Hezekiah said unto Isaiah, [a]What *shall be* the sign that the LORD will heal me, and that I shall go up into the house of the LORD the third day?

9 And Isaiah said, [b]This sign shalt thou have of the LORD, that the LORD will do the thing that he hath spoken: shall the shadow go forward ten degrees, or go back ten degrees?

10 And Hezekiah answered, It is a light thing for the shadow to go down ten degrees: nay, but let the shadow return backward ten degrees.

11 And Isaiah the prophet cried unto the LORD: and [c]he brought the shadow ten degrees [d]backward, by which it had gone down in the dial of Ahaz.

Hezekiah imprudently exposes his treasures to men of Babylon (2 Chr. 32:27-31).

12 At that time Berodach-baladan, the son of Baladan, king of Babylon, sent letters and a present unto Hezekiah: for he had heard that Hezekiah had been sick.

13 And [e]Hezekiah hearkened unto them, and shewed them all the house of his precious things, the silver, and the gold, and the spices, and the precious ointment, and *all* the house of his armour, and all that was found in his treasures: there was nothing in his house, nor in all his dominion, that Hezekiah shewed them not.

14 Then came Isaiah the prophet unto king Hezekiah, and said unto him, What said these men? and from whence came they unto thee? And Hezekiah said, They are come from a far country, *even* from Babylon.

15 And he said, What have they seen in thine house? And Hezekiah answered, All *the things* that *are* in mine house have they seen: there is nothing among my treasures that I have not shewed them.

16 And Isaiah said unto Hezekiah, Hear the word of the LORD.

17 Behold, the days come, that all that *is* in thine house, and that which thy fathers have laid up in store unto this day, [f]shall be carried into Babylon: nothing shall be left, saith the LORD.

18 And of thy sons that shall issue from thee, which thou shalt beget, [g]shall they take away; [h]and they shall be eunuchs in the palace of the king of Babylon.

19 Then said Hezekiah unto Isaiah, Good *is* the word of the LORD which thou hast spoken. And he said, *Is it* not *good*, if peace and truth be in my days?

Death of Hezekiah (2 Chr. 32:32, 33).

20 And the rest of the acts of Hezekiah, and all his might, and how he [i]made a pool, and a conduit, and [j]brought water into the city, *are* they not written in the book of the chronicles of the kings of Judah?

21 And [k]Hezekiah slept with his fathers: and Manasseh his son reigned in his stead.

CHAPTER 21.

Accession and reign of Manasseh: his evil ways (2 Chr. 33:1-9).

Manasseh *was* twelve years old when he began to reign, and reigned fifty and five years in Jerusalem. And his mother's name *was* Hephzi-bah.

2 And he did *that which was* evil in the sight of the LORD, after the abominations of the [l]heathen, whom the LORD cast out before the children of Israel.

3 For he built up again the high places which Hezekiah his father had destroyed; and he reared up altars for Baal, and made a [m]grove, as did Ahab king of Israel; and worshipped all the host of heaven, and served them.

4 And he built altars in the house of the LORD, of which the LORD said, In [n]Jerusalem will I put my name.

5 And he built altars for all the host of heaven in the two courts of the house of the LORD.

6 [o]And he made his son pass through the fire, and observed [p]times, and used enchantments, and dealt with familiar spirits and wizards: he wrought much wickedness in the sight of the LORD, to provoke *him* to anger.

7 And he set a graven image of the [m]grove that he had made in the house, of which the LORD said to David, and to Solomon his son, In this house, and in Jerusalem, which I have chosen out of all tribes of Israel, will I put my name for ever:

8 Neither will I make the feet of Israel move any more out of the land which I gave their fathers; only if they will

B.C. 713.

a Jud. 6:17, 37, 39; Isa. 7:11, 14; 38:22.

b Isa. 38:7, 8.

c Josh. 10:12-14; Isa. 38:8.

d *Miracles* (O.T.). vs. 9-11; 2 Chr. 26:16-21. (Gen. 5:24; Jon. 2:1-10.)

e 2 Chr. 32:27, 31.

f 2 Ki. 24:13; 25:13; Jer. 27:21, 22; 52:17.

g 2 Ki. 24:12; 2 Chr. 33:11.

h Fulfilled, Dan. 1:3.

i Neh. 3:16.

j 2 Chr. 32:30.

k 2 Chr. 32:33.

l i.e. *nations*.

m Deut. 16:21.

n 2 Sam. 7:13; 1 Ki. 8:29; 9:3.

o Lev. 18:21; 20:2; 2 Ki. 16:3; 17:17.

p Lev. 19:26; Deut. 18:10; 2 Ki. 17:17.

observe to do according to all that I have
commanded them, and according to all
the law that my servant Moses commanded them.
9 But they hearkened not: and Manasseh seduced them to do more evil than
did the nations whom the LORD
destroyed before the children of Israel.

Jehovah's message concerning Manasseh's idolatries.

10 And the LORD spake by his servants
the prophets, saying,
11 [a]Because Manasseh king of Judah
hath done these abominations, [b]*and* hath
done wickedly above all that the Amorites
did, which *were* before him, and hath
made Judah also to sin with his idols:
12 Therefore thus saith the LORD God of
Israel, Behold, I *am* bringing *such* evil
upon Jerusalem and Judah, that whosoever heareth of it, both [c]his ears shall tingle.
13 And I will stretch over Jerusalem
the [d]line of Samaria, and the plummet of
the house of Ahab: and I will wipe
Jerusalem as *a man* wipeth a dish, wip-
ing *it*, and turning *it* upside down.
14 And I will forsake the remnant of
mine inheritance, and deliver them into
the hand of their enemies; and they shall
become a prey and a spoil to all their
enemies;
15 Because they have done *that which*
was evil in my sight, and have provoked
me to anger, since the day their fathers
came forth out of Egypt, even unto this
day.

Manasseh's continued reign and death (2 Chr. 33:18-20).

16 [e]Moreover Manasseh shed innocent
blood very much, till he had filled
Jerusalem from one end to another;
beside his sin wherewith he made Judah
to sin, in doing *that which was* evil in the
sight of the LORD.
17 Now the [f]rest of the acts of
[g]Manasseh, and all that he did, and his
sin that he sinned, *are* they not written in
the book of the chronicles of the kings of
Judah?
18 And Manasseh slept with his
fathers, and was buried in the garden of
his own house, in the garden of Uzza:
and Amon his son reigned in his stead.

Reign of Amon over Judah (2 Chr. 33:20-23).

19 [h]Amon *was* twenty and two years
old when he began to reign, and he
reigned two years in Jerusalem. And his
mother's name *was* Meshullemeth, the
daughter of Haruz of Jotbah.
20 And he did *that which was* evil in
the sight of the LORD, as his father
Manasseh did.
21 And he walked in all the way that
his father walked in, and served the
idols that his father served, and worshipped them:
22 And he [i]forsook the LORD God of
his fathers, and walked not in the way of
the LORD.

Death of Amon: accession of Josiah (2 Chr. 33:24, 25).

23 [j]And the servants of Amon conspired against him, and slew the king in
his own house.
24 And the people of the land slew all
them that had conspired against king
Amon; and the people of the land made
Josiah his son king in his stead.
25 Now the rest of the acts of Amon
which he did, *are* they not written in the
book of the chronicles of the kings of
Judah?
26 And he was buried in his sepulchre
in the garden of Uzza: and [k]Josiah his
son reigned in his stead.

CHAPTER 22.

Reign of Josiah (2 Chr. 34:1).

Josiah *was* [l]eight years old when he
began to reign, and he reigned thirty
and one years in Jerusalem. And his
mother's name *was* Jedidah, the daughter of Adaiah of [m]Boscath.
2 And he did *that which was* right in
the sight of the LORD, and walked in all
the way of David his father, and [n]turned
not aside to the right hand or to the left.

The repairing of the temple (2 Chr. 34:8-13).

3 [o]And it came to pass in the eighteenth year of king Josiah, *that* the king
sent Shaphan the son of Azaliah, the son
of Meshullam, the scribe, to the house of
the LORD, saying,
4 Go up to Hilkiah the high priest, that
he may sum the silver which is brought
into the house of the LORD, which the
keepers of the door have gathered of the
people:
5 And let them [p]deliver it into the
hand of the doers of the work, that have

B.C. 698.

a 2 Ki. 23:26, 27; 24:3, 4; Jer. 15:4.
b 1 Ki. 21:26.
c 1 Sam. 3:11; Jer. 19:3.
d Isa. 34:11; Lam. 2:8; Amos 7:7, 8.
e 2 Ki. 24:4.
f 2 Chr. 33:11-19.
g 2 Chr. 33:20.
h 2 Chr. 33:21-23.
i Jud. 2:12-13; 1 Ki. 11:33.
j 2 Chr. 33:24, 25.
k Mt. 1:10, called Josias.
l 2 Chr. 34:1.
m Josh. 15:39.
n Deut. 5:32.
o 2 Chr. 34:8.
p 2 Ki. 12:11, 12, 14.

the oversight of the house of the LORD:
and let them give it to the doers of the
work which *is* in the house of the LORD,
to repair the breaches of the house,
6 Unto carpenters, and builders, and
masons, and to buy timber and hewn
stone to repair the house.
7 Howbeit there was no reckoning
made with them of the money that was
delivered into their hand, because they
dealt faithfully.

The law of Moses discovered
(2 Chr. 34:14, 15).

8 And Hilkiah the high priest said
unto Shaphan the scribe, [a]I have found
the book of the law in the house of the
LORD. And Hilkiah gave the book to
Shaphan, and he read it.
9 And Shaphan the scribe came to the
king, and brought the king word again,
and said, Thy servants have gathered
the money that was found in the house,
and have delivered it into the hand of
them that do the work, that have the
oversight of the house of the LORD.
10 And Shaphan the scribe shewed the
king, saying, Hilkiah the priest hath
delivered me a book. And Shaphan read
it before the king.

"By the law is the knowledge of sin"
(2 Chr. 34:16-21).

11 And it came to pass, when the king
had heard the words of the book of the
law, that he rent his clothes.
12 And the king commanded Hilkiah
the priest, and Ahikam the son of
Shaphan, and [b]Achbor the son of
Michaiah, and Shaphan the scribe, and
Asahiah a servant of the king's, saying,
13 Go ye, enquire of the LORD for me,
and for the people, and for all Judah,
concerning the words of this book that is
found: for great *is* the [c]wrath of the LORD
that is kindled against us, because our
fathers have not hearkened unto the
words of this book, to do according unto
all that which is written concerning us.
14 So Hilkiah the priest, and Ahikam,
and Achbor, and Shaphan, and Asahiah,
went unto Huldah the prophetess, the
wife of Shallum the son of [d]Tikvah, the
son of Harhas, keeper of the wardrobe;
(now she dwelt in Jerusalem in the college;) and they communed with her.

B.C. 694.

a Deut. 31:24-26; 2 Chr. 34:14.
b 2 Chr. 34:20.
c Deut. 29:27.
d *Tikvath*, 2 Chr. 34:22.
e Deut. 29:27; Dan. 9:11-14.
f Deut. 29:25-27.
g 2 Chr. 34:26.
h Psa. 51:17; Isa. 57:15.
i 1 Ki. 21:29.
j 2 Chr. 34:29, 30.
k 2 Ki. 22:8.
l 2 Ki. 11:14, 17.

The words of Huldah the prophetess
(2 Chr. 34:22-28).

15 And she said unto them, Thus saith
the LORD God of Israel, Tell the man that
sent you to me,
16 Thus saith the LORD, Behold, [e]I will
bring evil upon this place, and upon the
inhabitants thereof, *even* all the words of
the book which the king of Judah hath
read:
17 [f]Because they have forsaken me, and
have burned incense unto other gods,
that they might provoke me to anger
with all the works of their hands; therefore my wrath shall be kindled against
this place, and shall not be quenched.
18 But to the [g]king of Judah which
sent you to enquire of the LORD, thus
shall ye say to him, Thus saith the LORD
God of Israel, *As touching* the words
which thou hast heard;
19 [h]Because thine heart was tender,
and thou hast [i]humbled thyself before
the LORD, when thou heardest what I
spake against this place, and against the
inhabitants thereof, that they should
become a desolation and a curse, and
hast rent thy clothes, and wept before
me; I also have heard *thee*, saith the LORD.
20 Behold therefore, I will gather thee
unto thy fathers, and thou shalt be gathered into thy grave in peace; and thine
eyes shall not see all the evil which I will
bring upon this place. And they brought
the king word again.

CHAPTER 23.

The law read to the people
(2 Chr. 34:29, 30).

And [j]the king sent, and they gathered
unto him all the elders of Judah
and of Jerusalem.
2 And the king went up into the house
of the LORD, and all the men of Judah
and all the inhabitants of Jerusalem with
him, and the priests, and the prophets,
and all the people, both small and great:
and he read in their ears all the words of
the book of the covenant [k]which was
found in the house of the LORD.

The king's covenant (2 Chr. 34:31, 32).

3 And the king [l]stood by a pillar, and
made a covenant before the LORD, to
walk after the LORD, and to keep his
commandments and his testimonies and

his statutes with all *their* heart and all *their*
soul, to perform the words of this
covenant that were written in this book.
And all the people stood to the covenant.

Josiah's further reformations
(2 Chr. 34:33).

4 And the king commanded Hilkiah
the high priest, and the priests of the second order, and the keepers of the door, to
bring forth out of the temple of the LORD
all the vessels that were made for Baal,
and for the [a]grove, and for all the host of
heaven: and he burned them without
Jerusalem in the fields of Kidron, and carried the ashes of them unto Beth-el.
5 And he put down the idolatrous
priests, whom the kings of Judah had
ordained to burn incense in the high
places in the cities of Judah, and in the
places round about Jerusalem; them also
that burned incense unto Baal, to the
sun, and to the moon, and to the planets,
and [b]to all the host of heaven.
6 And he brought out the [c]grove from
the house of the LORD, without
Jerusalem, unto the brook Kidron, and
burned it at the brook Kidron, and
stamped *it* small to powder, and cast the
powder thereof upon the [d]graves of the
children of the people.
7 And he brake down the houses [e]of
the sodomites, that *were* by the house of
the LORD, [f]where the women wove
hangings for the [c]grove.
8 And he brought all the priests out of
the cities of Judah, and defiled the high
places where the priests had burned
incense, from Geba to Beer-sheba, and
brake down the high places of the gates
that *were* in the entering in of the gate of
Joshua the governor of the city, which
were on a man's left hand at the gate of
the city.
9 [g]Nevertheless the priests of the high
places came not up to the altar of the
LORD in Jerusalem, [h]but they did eat of the
unleavened bread among their brethren.
10 And he defiled Topheth, which *is* in
the [i]valley of the children of Hinnom,
[j]that no man might make his son or his
daughter to pass through the fire to
Molech.
11 And he took away the horses that the
kings of Judah had given to the sun, at the
entering in of the house of the LORD, by
the chamber of Nathan-melech the chamberlain, which *was* in the suburbs, and
burned the chariots of the sun with fire.
12 And the altars that *were* [k]on the top
of the upper chamber of Ahaz, which the
kings of Judah had made, and the altars
which [l]Manasseh had made in the two
courts of the house of the LORD, did the
king beat down, and brake *them* down
from thence, and cast the dust of them
into the brook Kidron.
13 And the high places that *were*
before Jerusalem, which *were* on the
right hand of the mount of corruption,
which [m]Solomon the king of Israel had
builded for [n]Ashtoreth the abomination
of the Zidonians, and for Chemosh the
abomination of the Moabites, and for
Milcom the abomination of the children
of Ammon, did the king defile.
14 And he [o]brake in pieces the images,
and cut down the [c]groves, and filled
their places with the bones of men.
15 Moreover the altar that *was* at Beth-
el, *and* the high place [p]which Jeroboam
the son of Nebat, who made Israel to sin,
had made, both that altar and the high
place he brake down, and burned the
high place, *and* stamped *it* small to powder, and burned the grove.
16 And as Josiah turned himself, he
spied the sepulchres that *were* there in the
mount, and sent, and took the bones out
of the sepulchres, and burned *them* upon
the altar, and polluted it, according to the
[q]word of the LORD which the man of God
proclaimed, who proclaimed these words.
17 Then he said, What title *is* that that
I see? And the men of the city told him,
It is the sepulchre of the man of God,
which came from Judah, and proclaimed
these things that thou hast done against
the altar of Beth-el.
18 And he said, Let him alone; let no
man move his bones. So they let his
bones alone, with the bones of the
[r]prophet that came out of Samaria.
19 And all the houses also of the high
places that *were* [s]in the cities of Samaria,
which the kings of Israel had made to
provoke *the LORD* to anger, Josiah took
away, and did to them according to all
the acts that he had done in Beth-el.

B.C. 624.

a See Deut. 16:21; 2 Ki. 21:3, 7.
b 2 Ki. 21:3; 2 Chr. 34:4.
c See Deut. 16:21, *note*.
d 2 Chr. 34:4.
e 1 Ki. 14:24; 15:12.
f Ezk. 16:16.
g Ezk. 44:10-14.
h 1 Sam. 2:36.
i Josh. 15:8.
j Lev. 18:21; Deut. 18:10; Ezk. 23:37, 39.
k Jer. 19:13; Zeph 1:5.
l 2 Ki. 21:5.
m 1 Ki. 11:5, 7.
n Jud. 2:13, *note*.
o Ex. 23:24; Deut. 7:5, 25.
p 1 Ki. 12:28, 31, 33.
q 1 Ki. 13:2.
r 1 Ki. 13:31.
s 2 Chr. 34:6, 7.

20 And he [a]slew all the priests of the
high places that *were* there upon the
altars, and burned men's bones upon
them, and returned to Jerusalem.

The passover kept (2 Chr. 35:1-19).

21 And the king commanded all the
people, saying, [b]Keep the passover unto
the LORD your God, [c]as *it is* written in
the book of this covenant.
22 Surely there was not holden such a
passover from the days of the judges that
judged Israel, nor in all the days of the
kings of Israel, nor of the kings of Judah;
23 But in the eighteenth year of king
Josiah, *wherein* this passover was holden
to the LORD in Jerusalem.
24 Moreover the *workers with* familiar
spirits, and the wizards, and the images,
and the idols, and all the abominations
that were spied in the land of Judah and
in Jerusalem, did Josiah put away, that
he might perform the words of the law
which were written in the book that
Hilkiah the priest found in the house of
the LORD.
25 And [d]like unto him was there no
king before him, that turned to the LORD
with all his heart, and with all his soul,
and with all his might, according to all
the law of Moses; neither after him arose
there *any* like him.
26 Notwithstanding the LORD turned
not from the fierceness of his great wrath,
wherewith his anger was kindled against
Judah, because of all the provocations
that Manasseh had provoked him withal.
27 And the LORD said, I will remove
Judah also out of my sight, as [e]I have
removed Israel, and will cast off this city
Jerusalem which I have chosen, and the
house of which I said, [f]My name shall be
there.

Death of Josiah (2 Chr. 35:20-27).

28 Now the rest of the acts of Josiah,
and all that he did, *are* they not written
in the book of the chronicles of the kings
of Judah?
29 [g]In his days Pharaoh-nechoh king of
Egypt went up against the king of
Assyria to the river Euphrates: and king
Josiah went against him; and he slew him
at [h]Megiddo, when he [i]had seen him.
30 And his servants carried him in a
chariot dead from Megiddo, and
brought him to Jerusalem, and buried
him in his own sepulchre. [j]And the people of the land took Jehoahaz the son of
Josiah, and anointed him, and made him
king in his father's stead.

Reign and dethronement of Jehoahaz (2 Chr. 36:1, 2).

31 Jehoahaz *was* twenty and three
years old when he began to reign; and
he reigned three months in Jerusalem.
And his mother's name *was* [k]Hamutal,
the daughter of Jeremiah of Libnah.
32 And he did *that which was* evil in
the sight of the LORD, according to all
that his fathers had done.
33 And Pharaoh-nechoh put him in
bands at Riblah in the land of Hamath,
that he might not reign in Jerusalem; and
put the land to a tribute of an hundred
[l]talents of silver, and a [m]talent of gold.

Jehoiakim made king (2 Chr. 36:4, 5).

34 And [n]Pharaoh-nechoh made
Eliakim the son of Josiah king in the
room of Josiah his father, and [o]turned
his name to [p]Jehoiakim, and took
Jehoahaz away: and [q]he came to Egypt,
and died there.
35 And Jehoiakim gave the silver and
the gold to Pharaoh; but he taxed the
land to give the money according to the
commandment of Pharaoh: he exacted
the silver and the gold of the people of
the land, of every one according to his
taxation, to give *it* unto Pharaoh-nechoh.
36 Jehoiakim *was* twenty and five
years old when he began to reign; and
he reigned eleven years in Jerusalem.
And his mother's name *was* Zebudah,
the daughter of Pedaiah of Rumah.
37 And he did *that which was* evil in
the sight of the LORD, according to all
that his fathers had done.

CHAPTER 24.

Jehoiakim tributary to Nebuchadnezzar (2 Chr. 36:6, 7).

In [r]his days Nebuchadnezzar king of
Babylon came up, and Jehoiakim
became his servant three years: then he
turned and rebelled against him.
2 And the LORD sent against him
bands of the Chaldees, and bands of the
Syrians, and bands of the Moabites, and

B.C. 624.

a 1 Ki. 13:2.
b 2 Chr. 35:1.
c Ex. 12:3; Lev. 23:5; Num. 9:2; Deut. 16:2.
d 2 Ki. 18:5.
e 2 Ki. 17:18, 20; 18:11; 21:13.
f I Ki. 8:29; 9:3; 2 Ki. 21:4, 7.
g 2 Chr. 35:20.
h Zech. 12:11.
i 2 Ki. 14:8.
j 2 Chr. 36:1.
k 2 Ki. 24:18.
l One talent (silver) = £410, or $1940.
m One talent (gold) = £6150, or $29,085.
n 2 Chr. 36:4.
o 2 Ki. 24:17.
p Called *Jakim*, Mt. 1:11, marg.
q Jer. 22:11, 12; Ezk. 19:3, 4.
r 2 Chr. 36:6; Jer. 25:1, 9; Dan. 1:1.

bands of the children of Ammon, and sent them against Judah to destroy it, [a]according to the word of the LORD, which he spake by his servants the prophets.

3 Surely at the commandment of the LORD came *this* upon Judah, to remove *them* out of his sight, for the sins of Manasseh, according to all that he did;

4 And also for the innocent blood that he shed: for he filled Jerusalem with innocent blood; which the LORD would not pardon.

5 Now the rest of the acts of Jehoiakim, and all that he did, *are* they not written in the book of the chronicles of the kings of Judah?

Death of Jehoiakim (2 Chr. 36:8): *reign of Jehoiachin* (2 Chr. 36:8, 9).

6 So Jehoiakim slept with his fathers: and Jehoiachin his son reigned in his stead.

7 And the king of Egypt came not again any more out of his land: for the king of Babylon had taken from the river of Egypt unto the river Euphrates all that pertained to the king of Egypt.

8 Jehoiachin *was* [b]eighteen years old when he began to reign, and he reigned in Jerusalem three months. And his mother's name *was* Nehushta, the daughter of Elnathan of Jerusalem.

9 And he did *that which was* evil in the sight of the LORD, according to all that his father had done.

10 At that time the servants of Nebuchadnezzar king of Babylon came up against [c]Jerusalem, and the city was besieged.

The first deportation to Babylon.

11 And Nebuchadnezzar king of Babylon came against the city, and his servants did besiege it.

12 [d]And Jehoiachin the king of Judah went out to the king of Babylon, he, and his mother, and his servants, and his princes, and his officers: and [e]the king of Babylon took him in the eighth year of his reign.

13 And he carried out thence all the treasures of the house of the LORD, and the treasures of the king's house, and [f]cut in pieces all the vessels of gold which Solomon king of Israel had made in the temple of the LORD, [g]as the LORD had said.

14 And [h]he carried away all Jerusalem, and all the princes, and all the mighty men of valour, *even* ten thousand captives, and all the craftsmen and smiths: none remained, save the poorest sort of the people of the land.

15 And he [i]carried away Jehoiachin to Babylon, and the king's mother, and the king's wives, and his officers, and the mighty of the land, *those* carried he into captivity from Jerusalem to Babylon.

16 And all the men of might, *even* seven thousand, and craftsmen and smiths a thousand, all *that were* strong *and* apt for war, even them the king of Babylon brought captive to Babylon.

Zedekiah made king (2 Chr. 36:10-18).

17 And the [j]king of Babylon made Mattaniah his father's brother king in his stead, and [k]changed his name to Zedekiah.

18 [l]Zedekiah *was* twenty and one years old when he began to reign, and he reigned eleven years in Jerusalem. And his mother's name *was* Hamutal, the daughter of Jeremiah of Libnah.

19 And he did *that which was* evil in the sight of the LORD, according to all that Jehoiakim had done.

Zedekiah rebels against Nebuchadnezzar.

20 For through the anger of the LORD it came to pass in Jerusalem and Judah, until he had cast them out from his presence, that Zedekiah rebelled against the king of Babylon.

CHAPTER 25.

Siege of Jerusalem and final deportation (2 Chr. 36:17-20; Jer. 39:8-10).

And it came to pass in the ninth year of his reign, in the [m]tenth month, in the tenth *day* of the month, *that* Nebuchadnezzar king of Babylon came, he, and all his host, against [n]Jerusalem, and pitched against it; and they built forts against it round about.

2 And the city was besieged unto the eleventh year of king Zedekiah.

3 And on the ninth *day* of the [o]*fourth* month the famine prevailed in the city, and there was no bread for the people of the land.

4 [p]And the city was broken up, and all

B.C. 600.

a 2 Ki. 20:17; 21:12-14.

b Cf. 2 Chr. 36:9; see 1 Cor. 10:8, *note.*

c *Israel (history).* vs. 10-16; 2 Ki. 25:1-7. (Gen. 12:2, 3; Rom. 11:26.)

d Jer. 24:1; 29:1, 2; Ezk. 17:12.

e *Nebuchadnezzar's eighth year.* Jer. 25:1.

f See Dan. 5:2, 3.

g Jer. 20:5.

h Jer. 24:1.

i 2 Chr. 36:10; Esth. 2:6; Jer. 22:24.

j Jer. 37:1.

k 2 Ki. 23:34; 2 Chr. 36:4.

l 2 Chr. 36:11; Jer. 37:1; 52:1.

m i.e. *January.*

n *Israel (history).* vs. 1-7; Ezra 1:3-5. (Gen. 12:2, 3; Rom. 11:26.)

o i.e. *July.*

p *Times of the Gentiles.* vs. 1-21; Dan. 2:29-45. (Lk. 21:24; Rev. 16:19.)

the men of war *fled* by night by the way of the gate between two walls, which *is* by the king's garden: (now the Chaldees *were* against the city round about:) and *the king* went the way toward the plain.

5 And the army of the Chaldees pursued after the king, and overtook him in the plains of Jericho: and all his army were scattered from him.

6 So they took the king, and brought him up to the king of Babylon to Riblah; and they gave judgment upon him.

7 And they slew the sons of [a]Zedekiah before his eyes, and put out the eyes of Zedekiah, and bound him with fetters of brass, and carried him to Babylon.

8 And in the [b]fifth month, on the seventh *day* of the month, which *is* the [c]nineteenth year of king Nebuchadnezzar king of Babylon, came Nebuzar-adan, captain of the guard, a servant of the king of Babylon, unto Jerusalem:

9 And he [d]burnt the house of the LORD, and the king's house, and all the houses of Jerusalem, and every great *man's* house burnt he with fire.

10 And all the army of the Chaldees, that *were with* the captain of the guard, [e]brake down the walls of Jerusalem round about.

11 Now the rest of the people *that were* left in the city, and the fugitives that fell away to the king of Babylon, with the remnant of the multitude, did Nebuzar-adan the captain of the guard carry away.

12 But the captain of the guard [f]left of the poor of the land *to be* vinedressers and husbandmen.

13 And the pillars of brass that *were* in the house of the LORD, and the bases, and the brasen sea that *was* in the house of the LORD, did the Chaldees break in pieces, and carried the brass of them to Babylon.

14 And the pots, and the shovels, and the snuffers, and the spoons, and all the vessels of brass wherewith they ministered, took they away.

15 And the firepans, and the bowls, *and* such things as *were* of gold, *in* gold, and of silver, *in* silver, the captain of the guard took away.

16 The two pillars, one sea, and the bases which Solomon had made for the house of the LORD; the brass of all these vessels was without weight.

17 The height of the one pillar *was* eighteen [g]cubits, and the chapiter upon it *was* brass: and the height of the chapiter three cubits; and the wreathen work, and pomegranates upon the chapiter round about, all of brass: and like unto these had the second pillar with wreathen work.

18 And the captain of the guard took Seraiah the chief priest, and Zephaniah the second priest, and the three keepers of the door:

19 And out of the city he took an officer that was set over the men of war, and five men of them that were in the king's presence, which were found in the city, and the principal scribe of the host, which mustered the people of the land, and threescore men of the people of the land *that were* found in the city:

20 And Nebuzar-adan captain of the guard took these, and brought them to the king of Babylon to Riblah:

21 And the king of Babylon smote them, and slew them at Riblah in the land of Hamath. So Judah was carried away out of their land.

Gedaliah made governor of Palestine.

22 [h]And *as for* the people that remained in the land of Judah, whom Nebuchadnezzar king of Babylon had left, even over them he made Gedaliah the son of Ahikam, the son of Shaphan, ruler.

23 And when all the captains of the armies, they and their men, heard that the king of Babylon had made Gedaliah governor, there came to Gedaliah to Mizpah, even Ishmael the son of Nethaniah, and Johanan the son of Careah, and Seraiah the son of Tanhumeth the Netophathite, and Jaazaniah the son of a Maachathite, they and their men.

24 And Gedaliah sware to them, and to their men, and said unto them, Fear not to be the servants of the Chaldees: dwell in the land, and serve the king of Babylon; and it shall be well with you.

Murder of Gedaliah and flight of the people to Egypt.

25 But it came to pass in the [i]seventh month, that Ishmael the son of Nethaniah, the son of Elishama, of the seed royal, came, and ten men with him,

B.C. 588.

a *Kingdom* (O.T.). Psa. 2:1-9. (Gen. 1:26-28; Zech. 12:8.)

b i.e. *August.*

c v. 27; 2 Ki. 24:12.

d 2 Chr. 36:19; Psa. 79:1.

e Neh. 1:3; Jer. 52:14.

f 2 Ki. 24:14; Jer. 39:10; 40:7; 52:16.

g One cubit = about 18 in.

h Jer. 40:5.

i i.e. *October.*

and smote Gedaliah, that he died, and
the Jews and the Chaldees that were
with him at Mizpah.
26 And all the people, both small and
great, and the captains of the armies,
arose, and [a]came to Egypt: for they were
afraid of the Chaldees.

Jehoiachin released.

27 And it came to pass in the seven
and thirtieth year of the captivity of
Jehoiachin king of Judah, in the [b]twelfth
month, on the seven and twentieth *day*
of the month, *that* Evil-merodach king of
Babylon in the year that he began to
reign [c]did lift up the head of Jehoiachin
king of Judah out of prison;
28 And he spake kindly to him, and
set his throne above the throne of the
kings that *were* with him in Babylon;
29 And changed his prison garments:
and he did [d]eat bread continually before
him all the days of his life.
30 And his allowance *was* a continual
allowance given him of the king, a daily
rate for every day, all the days of his life.

B.C. 588.

a Jer. 43:4-7.
b i.e. *March.*
c Gen. 40:13, 20.
d 2 Sam. 9:7.

THE FIRST BOOK OF THE

CHRONICLES

THE two books of Chronicles (like the two books of Kings) are but one book in the Jewish canon. Together they cover the period from the death of Saul to the captivities. They were written probably during the Babylonian captivity, and are distinguished from the two books of the Kings in a fuller account of Judah, and in the omission of many details. The blessing of God's earthly people in connection with the Davidic monarchy is probably the typical significance of these books.

First Chronicles is in three parts: I. Official genealogies, 1:1–9:44. II. From the death of Saul to the accession of David, 10:1–12:40. III. From the accession of David to his death, 13:1–29:30.

Excluding the genealogies (ch. 1–9) the events recorded in First Chronicles cover a period of 41 years (Ussher).

CHAPTER 1.

B.C. 4004.

Adam's line to Noah.

Adam, [a]Sheth, Enosh,
2 Kenan, Mahalaleel, Jered,
3 Henoch, Methuselah, Lamech,
4 [b]Noah, Shem, Ham, and Japheth.

The sons of Japheth.

5 The sons of [c]Japheth; Gomer, and
[d]Magog, and Madai, and Javan, and
Tubal, and Meshech, and Tiras.
6 And the sons of Gomer; Ashchenaz,
and Riphath, and Togarmah.
7 And the sons of Javan; Elishah, and
Tarshish, Kittim, and Dodanim.

The sons of Ham.

8 The sons of [e]Ham; Cush, and Mizraim, Put, and Canaan.
9 And the sons of Cush; Seba, and
Havilah, and Sabta, and Raamah, and
Sabtecha. And the sons of Raamah;
Sheba, and Dedan.
10 And Cush begat [f]Nimrod: he began
to be mighty upon the earth.
11 And Mizraim begat Ludim, and
Anamim, and Lehabim, and Naphtuhim,
12 And Pathrusim, and Casluhim, (of
whom came the Philistines,) and Caphthorim.
13 And [g]Canaan begat Zidon his firstborn, and Heth,
14 The Jebusite also, and the Amorite,
and the Girgashite,
15 And the Hivite, and the Arkite, and
the Sinite,
16 And the Arvadite, and the Zemarite,
and the Hamathite.

The sons of Shem.

17 The sons of [h]Shem; Elam, and
Asshur, and Arphaxad, and Lud, and
Aram, and Uz, and Hul, and Gether, and
Meshech.
18 And Arphaxad begat Shelah, and
Shelah begat Eber.
19 And unto Eber were born two sons:
the name of the one *was* [i]Peleg; because
in his days the earth was divided: and
his brother's name *was* Joktan.
20 And Joktan begat Almodad, and
Sheleph, and Hazarmaveth, and Jerah,
21 Hadoram also, and Uzal, and
Diklah,
22 And Ebal, and Abimael, and Sheba,
23 And Ophir, and Havilah, and
Jobab. All these *were* the sons of Joktan.

Shem's line to Abraham.

24 [j]Shem, Arphaxad, Shelah,
25 Eber, Peleg, Reu,
26 Serug, Nahor, Terah,
27 [k]Abram; the same *is* Abraham.
28 The sons of Abraham; [l]Isaac, and
Ishmael.

Ishmael's sons.

29 These *are* their generations: The
firstborn of Ishmael, Nebaioth; then
Kedar, and Adbeel, and Mibsam,
30 Mishma, and Dumah, Massa,
Hadad, and Tema,
31 Jetur, Naphish, and Kedemah.
These are the sons of Ishmael.

The sons of Keturah.

32 Now the [m]sons of Keturah, Abra-
ham's concubine: she bare Zimran, and
Jokshan, and Medan, and Midian, and
Ishbak, and Shuah. And the sons of
Jokshan; Sheba, and Dedan.
33 And the sons of Midian; Ephah,
and Epher, and Henoch, and Abida, and
Eldaah. All these *are* the sons of Keturah.

a Gen. 4:25, 26; 5:3-4, 6-8.
b Gen. 5:32; 9:26, 27.
c Gen. 10:2, etc.
d Gen. 10:2; Ezk. 38:2, *note:* 39:6; Rev. 20:8.
e Gen. 10:6.
f Gen. 10:8, etc.
g Gen. 10:15.
h Gen. 10:22; 11:10.
i i.e. *division.*
j Lk. 3:36.
k Gen. 17:5.
l Gen. 21:2, 3; 16:11, 15.
m Gen. 25:1, 2.

The sons of Abraham and Isaac.

34 And Abraham begat Isaac. The [a]sons of Isaac; Esau and Israel.

The sons of Esau.

35 The sons of Esau; Eliphaz, Reuel, and Jeush, and Jaalam, and Korah.

36 The sons of Eliphaz; Teman, and Omar, Zephi, and Gatam, Kenaz, and Timna, and Amalek.

37 The sons of Reuel; Nahath, Zerah, Shammah, and Mizzah.

38 And the sons of Seir; Lotan, and Shobal, and Zibeon, and Anah, and Dishon, and Ezer, and Dishan.

39 And the sons of Lotan; Hori, and Homam: and Timna *was* Lotan's sister.

40 The sons of Shobal; Alian, and Manahath, and Ebal, Shephi, and Onam. And the sons of Zibeon; Aiah, and Anah.

41 The sons of Anah; Dishon. And the sons of Dishon; Amram, and Eshban, and Ithran, and Cheran.

42 The sons of Ezer; Bilhan, and Zavan, *and* Jakan. The sons of Dishan; Uz, and Aran.

Early kings of Edom. (Cf. Gen. 36:1-43.)

43 Now these *are* the kings that reigned in the land of Edom before *any* king reigned over the children of Israel; Bela the son of Beor: and the name of his city *was* Dinhabah.

44 And when Bela was dead, Jobab the son of Zerah of Bozrah reigned in his stead.

45 And when Jobab was dead, Husham of the land of the Temanites reigned in his stead.

46 And when Husham was dead, Hadad the son of Bedad, which smote Midian in the field of Moab, reigned in his stead: and the name of his city *was* Avith.

47 And when Hadad was dead, Samlah of Masrekah reigned in his stead.

48 And when Samlah was dead, Shaul of Rehoboth by the river reigned in his stead.

49 And when Shaul was dead, Baal-hanan the son of Achbor reigned in his stead.

50 And when Baal-hanan was dead, Hadad reigned in his stead: and the name of his city *was* Pai; and his wife's name *was* Mehetabel, the daughter of Matred, the daughter of Mezahab.

The dukes of Edom.

51 Hadad died also. And the [b]dukes of Edom were; duke Timnah, duke Aliah, duke Jetheth,

52 Duke Aholibamah, duke Elah, duke Pinon,

53 Duke Kenaz, duke Teman, duke Mibzar,

54 Duke Magdiel, duke Iram. These *are* the dukes of Edom.

CHAPTER 2.

The sons of Jacob (Israel).

These *are* the [c]sons of [d]Israel; Reuben, Simeon, Levi, and Judah, Issachar, and Zebulun,

2 Dan, Joseph, and Benjamin, Naphtali, Gad, and Asher.

The sons of Judah.

3 The sons of Judah; Er, and Onan, and Shelah: *which* three were born unto him of the daughter of Shua the Canaanitess. And Er, the firstborn of Judah, was evil in the sight of the LORD; and he slew him.

4 And Tamar his daughter in law bare him Pharez and Zerah. All the sons of Judah *were* five.

5 The sons of Pharez; Hezron, and Hamul.

6 And the sons of Zerah; Zimri, and Ethan, and Heman, and Calcol, and Dara: five of them in all.

7 And the sons of Carmi; Achar, the troubler of Israel, who transgressed in the thing accursed.

8 And the sons of Ethan; Azariah.

9 The sons also of Hezron, that were born unto him; Jerahmeel, and Ram, and Chelubai.

10 And Ram [e]begat Amminadab; and Amminadab begat Nahshon, [f]prince of the children of Judah;

11 And Nahshon begat Salma, and [g]Salma begat Boaz,

12 And Boaz begat Obed, and Obed begat Jesse,

The posterity of Jesse.

13 And [h]Jesse begat his firstborn Eliab, and Abinadab the second, and [i]Shimma the third,

14 Nethaneel the fourth, Raddai the fifth,

15 Ozem the sixth, David the seventh:

16 Whose sisters *were* Zeruiah, and Abigail. [j]And the sons of Zeruiah; Abishai, and Joab, and Asahel, three.

17 And [k]Abigail bare Amasa: and the

B.C. 4004 to 1056.

a Gen. 25:25, 26.
b R.V. *chiefs.*
c Gen. 29:32; 30:5, etc.; 35:18-22; 46:8, etc.
d See Gen. 32:24-28.
e Ruth 4:19; Mt. 1:4.
f Num. 1:7.
g Ruth 4:21; Mt. 1:5.
h 1 Sam. 16:6.
i Or, *Shammah,* 1 Sam. 16:9.
j 2 Sam. 2:18.
k 2 Sam. 17:25.

father of Amasa *was* Jether the Ishmeelite.

The posterity of Caleb.

18 And Caleb the son of Hezron begat *children* of Azubah *his* wife, and of Jerioth: her sons *are* these; Jesher, and Shobab, and Ardon.

19 And when Azubah was dead, Caleb took unto him Ephrath, which bare him Hur.

20 And Hur begat Uri, and Uri begat Bezaleel.

Posterity of Hezron, father of Caleb, by the daughter of Machir.

21 And afterward Hezron went in to the daughter of Machir the father of Gilead, whom he married when he *was* threescore years old; and she bare him Segub.

22 And Segub begat Jair, who had three and twenty cities in the land of Gilead.

23 And he took Geshur, and Aram, with the towns of Jair, from them, with Kenath, and the towns thereof, *even* threescore cities. All these *belonged to* the sons of Machir the father of Gilead.

24 And after that Hezron was dead in Caleb-ephratah, then [a]Abiah Hezron's wife bare him Ashur the father of Tekoa.

Jerahmeel's posterity.

25 And the sons of Jerahmeel the firstborn of Hezron were, Ram the firstborn, and Bunah, and Oren, and Ozem, *and* Ahijah.

26 Jerahmeel had also another wife, whose name *was* Atarah; she *was* the mother of Onam.

27 And the sons of Ram the firstborn of Jerahmeel were, Maaz, and Jamin, and Eker.

28 And the sons of Onam were, Shammai, and Jada. And the sons of Shammai; Nadab, and Abishur.

29 And the name of the wife of Abishur *was* Abihail, and she bare him Ahban, and Molid.

30 And the sons of Nadab; Seled, and Appaim: but Seled died without children.

31 And the sons of Appaim; Ishi. And the sons of Ishi; Sheshan. And [b]the children of Sheshan; Ahlai.

32 And the sons of Jada the brother of Shammai; Jether, and Jonathan: and Jether died without children.

33 And the sons of Jonathan; Peleth, and Zaza. These were the sons of Jerahmeel.

B.C. 4004 to 1056.

a 1 Chr. 4:5.
b See vs. 34, 35.
c 1 Chr. 11:41.
d Josh. 15:17.
e v. 19.
f I Chr. 4:2.

Sheshan's posterity.

34 Now Sheshan had no sons, but daughters. And Sheshan had a servant, an Egyptian, whose name *was* Jarha.

35 And Sheshan gave his daughter to Jarha his servant to wife; and she bare him Attai.

36 And Attai begat Nathan, and Nathan begat [c]Zabad,

37 And Zabad begat Ephlal, and Ephlal begat Obed,

38 And Obed begat Jehu, and Jehu begat Azariah,

39 And Azariah begat Helez, and Helez begat Eleasah,

40 And Eleasah begat Sisamai, and Sisamai begat Shallum,

41 And Shallum begat Jekamiah, and Jekamiah begat Elishama.

Another branch of Caleb's posterity.

42 Now the sons of Caleb the brother of Jerahmeel *were*, Mesha his firstborn, which *was* the father of Ziph; and the sons of Mareshah the father of Hebron.

43 And the sons of Hebron; Korah, and Tappuah, and Rekem, and Shema.

44 And Shema begat Raham, the father of Jorkoam: and Rekem begat Shammai.

45 And the son of Shammai *was* Maon: and Maon *was* the father of Beth-zur.

46 And Ephah, Caleb's concubine, bare Haran, and Moza, and Gazez: and Haran begat Gazez.

47 And the sons of Jahdai; Regem, and Jotham, and Geshan, and Pelet, and Ephah, and Shaaph.

48 Maachah, Caleb's concubine, bare Sheber, and Tirhanah.

49 She bare also Shaaph the father of Madmannah, Sheva the father of Machbenah, and the father of Gibea: and the daughter of Caleb *was* [d]Achsah.

The posterity of Caleb the son of Hur.

50 These were the sons of Caleb the son of Hur, the firstborn of [e]Ephratah; Shobal the father of Kirjath-jearim,

51 Salma the father of Beth-lehem, Hareph the father of Beth-gader.

52 And Shobal the father of Kirjath-jearim had sons; [f]Haroeh, *and* half of the Manahethites.

53 And the families of Kirjath-jearim; the Ithrites, and the Puhites, and the Shumathites, and the Mishraites; of

them came the Zareathites, and the Eshtaulites.

54 The sons of Salma; Beth-lehem, and the Netophathites, [a]Ataroth, the house of Joab, and half of the Manahethites, the Zorites.

55 And the families of the scribes which dwelt at Jabez; the Tirathites, the Shimeathites, *and* Suchathites. These *are* the [b]Kenites that came of Hemath, the father of the house of [c]Rechab.

CHAPTER 3.

Family of David, born in Hebron.
(2 Sam. 3:2-5; 5:13-16).

Now these were the sons of David, which were born unto him in Hebron; the firstborn [d]Amnon, of Ahinoam the [e]Jezreelitess; the second [f]Daniel, of Abigail the Carmelitess:

2 The third, [g]Absalom the son of Maachah the daughter of Talmai king of Geshur: the fourth, Adonijah the son of Haggith:

3 The fifth, Shephatiah of Abital: the sixth, Ithream by Eglah his wife.

4 *These* six were born unto him in Hebron; and there he reigned seven years and six months: and in Jerusalem he reigned thirty and three years.

5 And these were born unto him in Jerusalem; Shimea, and Shobab, and Nathan, and Solomon, four, of Bath-shua the daughter of Ammiel:

6 Ibhar also, and Elishama, and Eliphelet,

7 And Nogah, and Nepheg, and Japhia,

8 And Elishama, and Eliada, and Eliphelet, [h]nine.

9 *These were* all the sons of David, beside the sons of the concubines, and Tamar their sister.

David's line to Zedekiah.

10 And Solomon's son *was* Rehoboam, Abia his son, Asa his son, Jehoshaphat his son,

11 Joram his son, Ahaziah his son, Joash his son,

12 Amaziah his son, Azariah his son, Jotham his son,

13 Ahaz his son, Hezekiah his son, Manasseh his son,

14 Amon his son, Josiah his son.

15 And the sons of Josiah *were*, the firstborn [i]Johanan, the second [j]Jehoiakim, the third Zedekiah, the fourth Shallum.

16 And the sons of [k]Jehoiakim: Jeconiah his son, Zedekiah his son.

The successors of Jeconiah.

17 And the sons of Jeconiah; Assir, [l]Salathiel his son,

18 Malchiram also, and Pedaiah, and Shenazar, Jecamiah, Hoshama, and Nedabiah.

19 And the sons of Pedaiah *were*, Zerubbabel, and Shimei: and the sons of Zerubbabel; Meshullam, and Hananiah, and Shelomith their sister:

20 And Hashubah, and Ohel, and Berechiah, and Hasadiah, Jushab-hesed, five.

21 And the sons of Hananiah; Pelatiah, and Jesaiah: the sons of Rephaiah, the sons of Arnan, the sons of Obadiah, the sons of Shechaniah.

22 And the sons of Shechaniah; Shemaiah: and the sons of Shemaiah; [m]Hattush, and Igeal, and Bariah, and Neariah, and Shaphat, six.

23 And the sons of Neariah; Elioenai, and Hezekiah, and Azrikam, three.

24 And the sons of Elioenai *were*, Hodaiah, and Eliashib, and Pelaiah, and Akkub, and Johanan, and Dalaiah, and Anani, seven.

CHAPTER 4.

The posterity of Judah
by Caleb the son of Hur.

The sons of Judah; [n]Pharez, Hezron, and Carmi, and Hur, and Shobal.

2 And Reaiah the son of Shobal begat Jahath; and Jahath begat Ahumai, and Lahad. These *are* the families of the Zorathites.

3 And these *were of* the father of Etam; Jezreel, and Ishma, and Idbash: and the name of their sister *was* Hazelelponi:

4 And Penuel the father of Gedor, and Ezer the father of Hushah. These *are* the sons of Hur, the firstborn of Ephratah, the father of Beth-lehem.

Of Ashur, the posthumous son of Hezron.

5 And Ashur the father of Tekoa had two wives, Helah and Naarah.

6 And Naarah bare him Ahuzam, and Hepher, and Temeni, and Haahashtari. These *were* the sons of Naarah.

B.C. 4004 to 1056.

a Or, *Atarites*, or, *crowns of the house of Joab.*
b Jud. 1:16.
c 2 Ki. 10:15; Jer. 35:2.
d 2 Sam. 3:2.
e Josh. 15:56.
f 2 Sam. 3:3.
g 2 Sam. 13:37, *note.*
h See 2 Sam. 5:14-16.
i 2 Ki. 23:30.
j 2 Ki. 23:34.
k Mt. 1:11.
l Heb. *Shealtiel.*
m Ezra 8:2.
n Gen. 38:29; 46:12.

7 And the sons of Helah *were,* Zereth, and Jezoar, and Ethnan.

8 And Coz begat Anub, and Zobebah, and the families of Aharhel the son of Harum.

Of Jabez, and his prayer.

9 And Jabez was more honourable than his brethren: and his mother called his name Jabez, saying, Because I bare him with sorrow.

10 And Jabez [a]called on the God of Israel, saying, Oh that thou wouldest bless me indeed, and enlarge my coast, and that thine hand might be with me, and that thou wouldest keep *me* from evil, that it may not grieve me! And God granted him that which he requested.

11 And Chelub the brother of Shuah begat Mehir, which *was* the father of Eshton.

12 And Eshton begat Beth-rapha, and Paseah, and Tehinnah the father of Ir-nahash. These *are* the men of Rechah.

13 And the sons of Kenaz; [b]Othniel, and Seraiah: and the sons of Othniel; Hathath.

14 And Meonothai begat Ophrah: and Seraiah begat Joab, the father of the [c]valley of Charashim; for they were craftsmen.

15 And the sons of Caleb the son of Jephunneh; Iru, Elah, and Naam: and the sons of Elah, even Kenaz.

16 And the sons of Jehaleleel; Ziph, and Ziphah, Tiria, and Asareel.

17 And the sons of Ezra *were,* Jether, and Mered, and Epher, and Jalon: and she bare Miriam, and Shammai, and Ishbah the father of Eshtemoa.

18 And his wife Jehudijah bare Jered the father of Gedor, and Heber the father of Socho, and Jekuthiel the father of Zanoah. And these *are* the sons of Bithiah the daughter of Pharaoh, which Mered took.

19 And the sons of *his* wife Hodiah the sister of Naham, the father of Keilah the Garmite, and Eshtemoa the Maachathite.

20 And the sons of Shimon *were,* Amnon, and Rinnah, Ben-hanan, and Tilon. And the sons of Ishi *were,* Zoheth, and Ben-zoheth.

The posterity of Shelah.

21 The sons of Shelah [d]the son of Judah *were,* Er the father of Lecah, and Laadah the father of Mareshah, and the families of the house of them that wrought fine linen, of the house of Ashbea,

22 And Jokim, and the men of Chozeba, and Joash, and Saraph, who had the dominion in Moab, and Jashubi-lehem. And *these are* ancient things.

23 These *were* the potters, and those that dwelt among plants and hedges: there they dwelt with the king for his work.

The posterity and cities of Simeon.

24 The sons of Simeon *were,* [e]Nemuel, and Jamin, Jarib, Zerah, *and* Shaul:

25 Shallum his son, Mibsam his son, Mishma his son.

26 And the sons of Mishma; Hamuel his son, Zacchur his son, Shimei his son.

27 And Shimei had sixteen sons and six daughters; but his brethren had not many children, neither did all their family multiply, like to the children of Judah.

28 And they dwelt at [f]Beer-sheba, and Moladah, and Hazar-shual,

29 And at [g]Bilhah, and at Ezem, and at [h]Tolad,

30 And at Bethuel, and at Hormah, and at Ziklag,

31 And at Beth-marcaboth, and Hazar-susim, and at Beth-birei, and at Shaaraim. These *were* their cities unto the reign of David.

32 And their villages *were,* [i]Etam, and Ain, Rimmon, and Tochen, and Ashan, five cities:

33 And all their villages that *were* round about the same cities, unto Baal. These *were* their habitations, and their genealogy.

34 And Meshobab, and Jamlech, and Joshah the son of Amaziah,

35 And Joel, and Jehu the son of Josibiah, the son of Seraiah, the son of Asiel,

36 And Elioenai, and Jaakobah, and Jeshohaiah, and Asaiah, and Adiel, and Jesimiel, and Benaiah,

37 And Ziza the son of Shiphi, the son of Allon, the son of Jedaiah, the son of Shimri, the son of Shemaiah;

38 These mentioned by *their* names *were* princes in their families: and the house of their fathers increased greatly.

The conquest of Gedor and of the Amalekites in Mount Seir.

39 And they went to the entrance of Gedor, *even* unto the east side of the

B.C. 4004 to 1056.

a *Bible prayers* (O.T.). 1 Chr. 29:10-19. (Gen. 15:2; Hab. 3:1-16.)

b Josh. 15:17; Jud. 3:9, 11.

c Neh. 11:35.

d Gen. 38:1, 5; 46:12.

e Or, *Jemuel,* Gen. 46:10; Ex. 6:15; Num. 26:12.

f Josh. 19:2.

g Josh. 19:3.

h Or, *Eltolad,* Josh. 19:4.

i Or, *Ether,* Josh. 19:7.

B.C. 4004 to 1056.

valley, to seek pasture for their flocks.
40 And they found fat pasture and
good, and the land *was* wide, and quiet,
and peaceable; for *they* of Ham had
dwelt there of old.
41 And these written by name came in
the days of Hezekiah king of Judah, and
[a]smote their tents, and the habitations
that were found there, and destroyed
them utterly unto this day, and dwelt in
their rooms: because *there was* pasture
there for their flocks.
42 And *some* of them, *even* of the sons
of Simeon, five hundred men, went to
mount Seir, having for their captains
Pelatiah, and Neariah, and Rephaiah,
and Uzziel, the sons of Ishi.
43 And they smote [b]the rest of the
Amalekites that were escaped, and
dwelt there unto this day.

CHAPTER 5.

The line of Reuben (who lost his birthright) unto the captivity.

Now the sons of Reuben the firstborn
of Israel, (for [c]he *was* the firstborn;
but, forasmuch as he [d]defiled his
father's bed, [e]his birthright was given
unto the sons of Joseph the son of Israel:
and the genealogy is not to be reckoned
after the birthright.
2 For [f]Judah prevailed above his
brethren, and of him *came* the chief ruler;
but the birthright *was* Joseph's:)
3 The sons, *I say*, of [g]Reuben the firstborn of Israel *were*, Hanoch, and Pallu,
Hezron, and Carmi.
4 The sons of Joel; Shemaiah his son,
Gog his son, Shimei his son,
5 Micah his son, Reaia his son, Baal his
son,
6 Beerah his son, whom [h]Tilgath-pil-
neser king of Assyria carried away *captive*: he *was* prince of the Reubenites.
7 And his brethren by their families,
when the genealogy of their generations
was reckoned, *were* the chief, Jeiel, and
Zechariah,
8 And Bela the son of Azaz, the son of
Shema, the son of Joel, who dwelt in
Aroer, even unto Nebo and Baal-meon:

Their habitation and conquest of the Hagarites.

9 And eastward he inhabited unto the
entering in of the wilderness from the
river Euphrates: because their cattle
were multiplied in the land of Gilead.
10 And in the days of Saul they made
war with the [i]Hagarites, who fell by
their hand: and they dwelt in their tents
throughout all the east *land* of Gilead.

The chief men and habitations of Gad.

11 And the children of Gad dwelt over
against them, in the land of [j]Bashan
unto Salchah:
12 Joel the chief, and Shapham the
next, and Jaanai, and Shaphat in Bashan.
13 And their brethren of the house of
their fathers *were*, Michael, and
Meshullam, and Sheba, and Jorai, and
Jachan, and Zia, and Heber, seven.
14 These *are* the children of Abihail the
son of Huri, the son of Jaroah, the son of
Gilead, the son of Michael, the son of
Jeshishai, the son of Jahdo, the son of Buz;
15 Ahi the son of Abdiel, the son of
Guni, chief of the house of their fathers.
16 And they dwelt in Gilead in
Bashan, and in her towns, and in all the
suburbs of [k]Sharon, upon their borders.
17 All these were reckoned by
genealogies in the days of [l]Jotham king
of Judah, and in the days of [m]Jeroboam
king of Israel.

The number and conquests of Reuben, Gad, and the half of Manasseh.

18 The sons of Reuben, and the
Gadites, and half the tribe of Manasseh,
of valiant men, men able to bear buckler
and sword, and to shoot with bow, and
skilful in war, *were* four and forty thousand seven hundred and threescore, that
went out to the war.
19 And they made war with the
Hagarites, with [n]Jetur, and Nephish, and
Nodab.
20 And they were helped against
them, and the Hagarites were delivered
into their hand, and all that *were* with
them: for they cried to God in the battle,
and he was intreated of them; because
they put their [o]trust in him.
21 And they took away their cattle; of
their camels fifty thousand, and of sheep
two hundred and fifty thousand, and of
asses two thousand, and of men an hundred thousand.

a 2 Ki. 18:8.
b 1 Sam. 15:8; 30:17; 2 Sam. 8:12.
c Gen. 29:32; 49:3.
d Gen. 35:22; 49:4.
e Gen. 48:15, 22.
f Gen. 49:8, 10; Psa. 60:7; 108:8.
g Gen. 46:9; Ex. 6:14; Num. 26:5.
h Or, *Tiglath-pileser*, 2 Ki. 15:29; 16:7.
i Gen. 25:12.
j Josh. 13:11, 24.
k 1 Chr. 27:29.
l 2 Ki. 15:5, 32.
m 2 Ki. 14:16, 28.
n Gen. 25:15; 1 Chr. 1:31.
o Psa. 2:12, *note*.

22 For there fell down many slain, because the war *was* of God. And they dwelt in their steads until the captivity.

The habitations and chief men of that half tribe.

23 And the children of the half tribe of Manasseh dwelt in the land: they increased from Bashan unto Baal-hermon and Senir, and unto mount Hermon.

24 And these *were* the heads of the house of their fathers, even Epher, and Ishi, and Eliel, and Azriel, and Jeremiah, and Hodaviah, and Jahdiel, mighty men of valour, famous men, *and* heads of the house of their fathers.

Their captivity for their sins.

25 And they transgressed against the God of their fathers, and went a whoring after the gods of the people of the land, whom God destroyed before them.

26 And the God of Israel stirred up the spirit of Pul king of [a]Assyria, and the spirit of Tilgath-pilneser king of Assyria, and he carried them away, even the Reubenites, and the Gadites, and the half tribe of Manasseh, and brought them unto Halah, and Habor, and Hara, and to the river Gozan, unto this day.

CHAPTER 6.

The sons of Levi.

The sons of Levi; Gershon, Kohath, and Merari.

2 And the sons of Kohath; Amram, Izhar, and Hebron, and Uzziel.

3 And the children of Amram; Aaron, and Moses, and Miriam. The sons also of Aaron; [b]Nadab, and Abihu, Eleazar, and Ithamar.

The line of the priests unto the captivity.

4 Eleazar begat Phinehas, Phinehas begat Abishua,

5 And Abishua begat Bukki, and Bukki begat Uzzi,

6 And Uzzi begat Zerahiah, and Zerahiah begat Meraioth,

7 Meraioth begat Amariah, and Amariah begat Ahitub,

8 And [c]Ahitub begat Zadok, and [d]Zadok begat Ahimaaz,

9 And Ahimaaz begat Azariah, and Azariah begat Johanan,

10 And Johanan begat Azariah, (he *it is* that executed the priest's office in the temple that Solomon built in Jerusalem:)

11 And Azariah begat Amariah, and Amariah begat Ahitub,

12 And Ahitub begat Zadok, and Zadok begat Shallum,

13 And Shallum begat Hilkiah, and Hilkiah begat Azariah,

14 And Azariah begat Seraiah, and Seraiah begat Jehozadak,

15 And Jehozadak went *into captivity*, [e]when the LORD carried away Judah and Jerusalem by the hand of Nebuchadnezzar.

The families of Gershom, Merari, and Kohath.

16 The sons of Levi; [f]Gershom, Kohath, and Merari.

17 And these *be* the names of the sons of Gershom; Libni, and Shimei.

18 And the sons of Kohath *were*, Amram, and Izhar, and Hebron, and Uzziel.

19 The sons of Merari; Mahli, and Mushi. And these *are* the families of the Levites according to their fathers.

20 Of Gershom; Libni his son, Jahath his son, Zimmah his son,

21 [g]Joah his son, [h]Iddo his son, Zerah his son, [i]Jeaterai his son.

22 The sons of Kohath; Amminadab his son, Korah his son, Assir his son,

23 Elkanah his son, and Ebiasaph his son, and Assir his son,

24 Tahath his son, Uriel his son, Uzziah his son, and Shaul his son.

25 And the sons of Elkanah; [j]Amasai, and Ahimoth.

26 *As for* Elkanah: the sons of Elkanah; [k]Zophai his son, and Nahath his son,

27 Eliab his son, Jeroham his son, Elkanah his son.

28 And the sons of Samuel; the firstborn Vashni, and Abiah.

29 The sons of Merari; Mahli, Libni his son, Shimei his son, Uzza his son,

30 Shimea his son, Haggiah his son, Asaiah his son.

31 And these *are they* whom David set over the service of song in the house of the LORD, after that the [l]ark had rest.

32 And they ministered before the dwelling place of the tabernacle of the congregation with singing, until Solomon had built the house of the LORD

B.C. 4004 to 1056.

a Cf. 2 Ki. 15:19.
b Lev. 10:1-2.
c 2 Sam. 8:17.
d 2 Sam. 15:27.
e 2 Ki. 25:18.
f Ex. 6:16.
g Or, *Ethan*, v. 42.
h Or, *Adaiah*, v. 41.
i Or, *Ethni*, v. 41.
j See vs. 35, 36.
k 1 Sam. 1:1.
l 1 Chr. 16:1.

in Jerusalem: and *then* they waited on
their office according to their order.
33 And these *are* they that [a]waited
with their children. Of the sons of the
Kohathites: Heman a singer, the son of
Joel, the son of Shemuel,
34 The son of Elkanah, the son of
Jeroham, the son of Eliel, the son of
Toah,
35 The son of Zuph, the son of
Elkanah, the son of Mahath, the son of
Amasai,
36 The son of Elkanah, the son of Joel,
the son of Azariah, the son of
Zephaniah,
37 The son of Tahath, the son of Assir,
the son of [b]Ebiasaph, the son of Korah,
38 The son of Izhar, the son of Kohath,
the son of Levi, the son of Israel.
39 And his brother Asaph, who stood
on his right hand, *even* Asaph the son of
Berachiah, the son of Shimea,
40 The son of Michael, the son of
Baaseiah, the son of Malchiah,
41 The son of Ethni, the son of Zerah,
the son of Adaiah,
42 The son of Ethan, the son of
Zimmah, the son of Shimei,
43 The son of Jahath, the son of
Gershom, the son of Levi.
44 And their brethren the sons of
Merari *stood* on the left hand: [c]Ethan the
son of [d]Kishi, the son of Abdi, the son of
Malluch,
45 The son of Hashabiah, the son of
Amaziah, the son of Hilkiah,
46 The son of Amzi, the son of Bani,
the son of Shamer,
47 The son of Mahli, the son of Mushi,
the son of Merari, the son of Levi.
48 Their brethren also the Levites *were*
appointed unto all manner of service of
the tabernacle of the house of God.

The office of Aaron and his line unto Ahimaaz.

49 But Aaron and his sons offered
[e]upon the altar of the burnt-offering, and
on the altar of incense, *and were appointed*
for all the work of the *place* most holy,
and to make an [f]atonement for Israel,
according to all that Moses the servant
of God had commanded.
50 And these *are* the sons of Aaron;
Eleazar his son, Phinehas his son,
Abishua his son,
51 Bukki his son, Uzzi his son,
Zerahiah his son,
52 Meraioth his son, Amariah his son,
Ahitub his son,
53 Zadok his son, Ahimaaz his son.

The cities of the priests and Levites.

54 Now [g]these *are* their dwelling places
throughout their castles in their coasts, of
the sons of Aaron, of the families of the
Kohathites: for theirs was the lot.
55 And they gave them Hebron in the
land of Judah, and the suburbs thereof
round about it.
56 But the fields of the city, and the
villages thereof, they gave to Caleb the
son of Jephunneh.
57 And [h]to the sons of Aaron they
gave the cities of Judah, *namely*, Hebron,
the city of refuge, and Libnah with her
suburbs, and Jattir, and Eshtemoa, with
their suburbs,
58 And [i]Hilen with her suburbs, Debir
with her suburbs,
59 And [j]Ashan with her suburbs, and
Beth-shemesh with her suburbs:
60 And out of the tribe of Benjamin;
Geba with her suburbs, and [k]Alemeth
with her suburbs, and Anathoth with
her suburbs. All their cities throughout
their families *were* thirteen cities.
61 And unto the sons of Kohath,
[l]*which were* left of the family of that tribe,
were cities given out of the half tribe,
namely, out of the half *tribe* of Manasseh,
[m]by lot, ten cities.
62 And to the sons of Gershom
throughout their families out of the tribe
of Issachar, and out of the tribe of Asher,
and out of the tribe of Naphtali, and out
of the tribe of Manasseh in Bashan, thirteen cities.
63 Unto the sons of Merari *were given*
by lot, throughout their families, out of
the tribe of Reuben, and out of the tribe
of Gad, and out of the tribe of Zebulun,
[n]twelve cities.
64 And the children of Israel gave to
the Levites *these* cities with their suburbs.
65 And they gave by lot out of the
tribe of the children of Judah, and out of
the tribe of the children of Simeon, and
out of the tribe of the children of
Benjamin, these cities, which are called
by *their* names.
66 And *the* [o]*residue* of the families of
the sons of Kohath had cities of their
coasts out of the tribe of Ephraim.
67 [p]And they gave unto them, *of* the
cities of refuge, Shechem in mount

B.C. 4004 to 1056.

a Heb. *stood.*

b Ex. 6:24.

c Called *Jeduthun*, 1 Chr. 9:16; 25:1, 3, 6.

d Or, *Kushaiah*, 1 Chr. 15:17.

e Lev. 1:9.

f See Ex. 29:33, *note.*

g Josh. 21.

h Josh. 21:13

i Or, *Holon*, Josh. 21:15.

j Or, *Ain*, Josh. 21:16.

k Or, *Almon*, Josh. 21:18.

l v. 66.

m Josh. 21:5.

n Josh. 21:7, 34.

o v. 61.

p Josh. 21:21.

B.C. 4004 to 1056.

Ephraim with her suburbs; *they gave* also Gezer with her suburbs,

68 And [a]Jokmeam with her suburbs, and Beth-horon with her suburbs,

69 And Aijalon with her suburbs, and Gath-rimmon with her suburbs:

70 And out of the half tribe of Manasseh; Aner with her suburbs, and Bileam with her suburbs, for the family of the remnant of the sons of Kohath.

71 Unto the sons of Gershom *were given* out of the family of the half tribe of Manasseh, Golan in Bashan with her suburbs, and Ashtaroth with her suburbs:

72 And out of the tribe of Issachar; Kedesh with her suburbs, Daberath with her suburbs,

73 And Ramoth with her suburbs, and Anem with her suburbs:

74 And out of the tribe of Asher; Mashal with her suburbs, and Abdon with her suburbs,

75 And Hukok with her suburbs, and Rehob with her suburbs:

76 And out of the tribe of Naphtali; Kedesh in Galilee with her suburbs, and Hammon with her suburbs, and Kirjathaim with her suburbs.

77 Unto the rest of the children of Merari *were given* out of the tribe of Zebulun, Rimmon with her suburbs, Tabor with her suburbs:

78 And on the other side Jordan by Jericho, on the east side of Jordan, *were given them* out of the tribe of Reuben, Bezer in the wilderness with her suburbs, and Jahzah with her suburbs,

79 Kedemoth also with her suburbs, and Mephaath with her suburbs:

80 And out of the tribe of Gad; Ramoth in Gilead with her suburbs, and Mahanaim with her suburbs,

81 And Heshbon with her suburbs, and Jazer with her suburbs.

CHAPTER 7.

The sons of Issachar.

Now the sons of Issachar *were,* [b]Tola, and Puah, Jashub, and Shimron, four.

2 And the sons of Tola; Uzzi, and Rephaiah, and Jeriel, and Jahmai, and Jibsam, and Shemuel, heads of their father's house, *to wit,* of Tola: *they were* valiant men of might in their generations; [c]whose number *was* in the days of David two and twenty thousand and six hundred.

3 And the sons of Uzzi; Izrahiah: and the sons of Izrahiah; Michael, and Obadiah, and Joel, Ishiah, five: all of them chief men.

4 And with them, by their generations, after the house of their fathers, *were* bands of soldiers for war, six and thirty thousand *men*: for they had many wives and sons.

5 And their brethren among all the families of Issachar *were* valiant men of might, reckoned in all by their genealogies fourscore and seven thousand.

The sons of Benjamin.

6 *The sons* of [d]Benjamin; Bela, and Becher, and Jediael, three.

7 And the sons of Bela; Ezbon, and Uzzi, and Uzziel, and Jerimoth, and Iri, five; heads of the house of *their* fathers, mighty men of valour; and were reckoned by their genealogies twenty and two thousand and thirty and four.

8 And the sons of Becher; Zemira, and Joash, and Eliezer, and Elioenai, and Omri, and Jerimoth, and Abiah, and Anathoth, and Alameth. All these *are* the sons of Becher.

9 And the number of them, after their genealogy by their generations, heads of the house of their fathers, mighty men of valour, *was* twenty thousand and two hundred.

10 The sons also of Jediael; Bilhan: and the sons of Bilhan; Jeush, and Benjamin, and Ehud, and Chenaanah, and Zethan, and Tharshish, and Ahishahar.

11 All these the sons of Jediael, by the heads of their fathers, mighty men of valour, *were* seventeen thousand and two hundred *soldiers,* fit to go out for war *and* battle.

12 [e]Shuppim also, and Huppim, the children of [f]Ir, *and* Hushim, the sons of [g]Aher.

The sons of Naphtali.

13 The sons of Naphtali; Jahziel, and Guni, and Jezer, and [h]Shallum, the sons of Bilhah.

The sons of Manasseh.

14 The sons of Manasseh; Ashriel, whom she bare: (*but* his concubine the Aramitess bare Machir the father of Gilead:

15 And Machir took to wife *the sister* of Huppim and Shuppim, whose sister's name *was* Maachah;) and the name of the second *was* Zelophehad: and Zelophehad had daughters.

a See Josh. 21:22-35, where many of these cities have other names.

b Gen. 46:13; Num. 26:23.

c 2 Sam. 24:1-9; 1 Chr. 27:1.

d Gen. 46:21; Num. 26:38; 1 Chr. 8:1.

e Num. 26:39; *Shupham* and *Hupham.*

f Or, *Iri,* v. 7.

g Or, *Ahiram,* Num. 26:38.

h Or, *Shillem,* Gen. 46:24.

B.C. 4004 to 1056.

16 And Maachah the wife of Machir bare a son, and she called his name Peresh; and the name of his brother *was* Sheresh; and his sons *were* Ulam and Rakem.

17 And the sons of Ulam; [a]Bedan. These *were* the sons of Gilead, the son of Machir, the son of Manasseh.

18 And his sister Hammoleketh bare Ishod, and [b]Abiezer, and Mahalah.

19 And the sons of Shemida were, Ahian, and Shechem, and Likhi, and Aniam.

The sons of Ephraim.

20 And the [c]sons of Ephraim; Shuthelah, and Bered his son, and Tahath his son, and Eladah his son, and Tahath his son,

21 And Zabad his son, and Shuthelah his son, and Ezer, and Elead, whom the men of Gath *that were* born in *that* land slew, because they came down to take away their cattle.

22 And Ephraim their father mourned many days, and his brethren came to comfort him.

23 And when he went in to his wife, she conceived, and bare a son, and he called his name Beriah, because it went evil with his house.

24 (And his daughter *was* Sherah, who built Beth-horon the nether, and the upper, and Uzzen-sherah.)

25 And Rephah *was* his son, also Resheph, and Telah his son, and Tahan his son,

26 Laadan his son, Ammihud his son, Elishama his son,

27 [d]Non his son, Jehoshua his son.

Ephraim's habitation.

28 And their possessions and habitations *were*, Beth-el and the towns thereof, and eastward [e]Naaran, and westward Gezer, with the towns thereof; Shechem also and the towns thereof, unto Gaza and the towns thereof:

29 And by the borders of the children of [f]Manasseh, Beth-shean and her towns, Taanach and her towns, [g]Megiddo and her towns, Dor and her towns. In these dwelt the children of Joseph the son of Israel.

The sons of Asher.

30 The [h]sons of Asher; Imnah, and Isuah, and Ishuai, and Beriah, and Serah their sister.

31 And the sons of Beriah; Heber, and Malchiel, who *is* the father of Birzavith.

32 And Heber begat Japhlet, and [i]Shomer, and Hotham, and Shua their sister.

33 And the sons of Japhlet; Pasach, and Bimhal, and Ashvath. These *are* the children of Japhlet.

34 And the sons of [j]Shamer; Ahi, and Rohgah, Jehubbah, and Aram.

35 And the sons of his brother Helem; Zophah, and Imna, and Shelesh, and Amal.

36 The sons of Zophah; Suah, and Harnepher, and Shual, and Beri, and Imrah,

37 Bezer, and Hod, and Shamma, and Shilshah, and Ithran, and Beera.

38 And the sons of Jether; Jephunneh, and Pispah, and Ara.

39 And the sons of Ulla; Arah, and Haniel, and Rezia.

40 All these *were* the children of Asher, heads of *their* father's house, choice *and* mighty men of valour, chief of the princes. And the number throughout the genealogy of them that were apt to the war *and* to battle *was* twenty and six thousand men.

CHAPTER 8.

The sons and chief men of Benjamin.

Now Benjamin begat [k]Bela his firstborn, Ashbel the second, and Aharah the third,

2 Nohah the fourth, and Rapha the fifth.

3 And the sons of Bela were, [l]Addar, and Gera, and Abihud,

4 And Abishua, and Naaman, and Ahoah,

5 And Gera, and [m]Shephuphan, and Huram.

6 And these *are* the sons of Ehud: these are the heads of the fathers of the inhabitants of Geba, and they removed them to [n]Manahath:

7 And Naaman, and Ahiah, and Gera, he removed them, and begat Uzza, and Ahihud.

8 And Shaharaim begat *children* in the country of Moab, after he had sent them away; Hushim and Baara *were* his wives.

9 And he begat of Hodesh his wife, Jobab, and Zibia, and Mesha, and Malcham,

10 And Jeuz, and Shachia, and Mirma. These *were* his sons, heads of the fathers.

11 And of Hushim he begat Abitub, and Elpaal.

12 The sons of Elpaal; Eber, and

a 1 Sam. 12:11.
b Num. 26:30.
c Num. 26:35.
d Or, *Nun*, Num. 13:8, 16.
e *Naarath*, Josh. 16:7.
f Josh. 17:7.
g Josh. 17:11.
h Gen. 46:17; Num. 26:44.
i *Shamer*, v. 34.
j *Shomer*, v. 32.
k Gen. 46:21; Num. 26:38; 1 Chr. 7:6.
l Or, *Ard*, Gen. 46:21.
m Or, *Shupham*, Num. 26:39. See 1 Chr. 7:12.
n 1 Chr. 2.52.

B.C. 4004 to 1056.

Misham, and Shamed, who built Ono,
and Lod, with the towns thereof:
13 Beriah also, and [a]Shema, who *were*
heads of the fathers of the inhabitants of
Aijalon, who drove away the inhabitants
of Gath:
14 And Ahio, Shashak, and Jeremoth,
15 And Zebadiah, and Arad, and
Ader,
16 And Michael, and Ispah, and Joha,
the sons of Beriah;
17 And Zebadiah, and Meshullam,
and Hezeki, and Heber,
18 Ishmerai also, and Jezliah, and
Jobab, the sons of Elpaal;
19 And Jakim, and Zichri, and Zabdi,
20 And Elienai, and Zilthai, and Eliel,
21 And Adaiah, and Beraiah, and
Shimrath, the sons of [b]Shimhi;
22 And Ishpan, and Heber, and Eliel,
23 And Abdon, and Zichri, and
Hanan,
24 And Hananiah, and Elam, and
Antothijah,
25 And Iphedeiah, and Penuel, the
sons of Shashak;
26 And Shamsherai, and Shehariah,
and Athaliah,
27 And Jaresiah, and Eliah, and Zichri,
the sons of Jeroham.
28 These *were* heads of the fathers, by
their generations, chief *men*. These dwelt
in Jerusalem.
29 And at Gibeon dwelt the [c]father of
Gibeon; whose [d]wife's name *was*
Maachah:
30 And his firstborn son Abdon, and
Zur, and Kish, and Baal, and Nadab,
31 And Gedor, and Ahio, and [e]Zacher.
32 And Mikloth begat [f]Shimeah. And
these also dwelt with their brethren in
Jerusalem, over against them.

The stock of Saul and Jonathan.

33 And [g]Ner begat Kish, and Kish
begat Saul, and Saul begat Jonathan, and
Malchi-shua, and Abinadab, and [h]Esh-
baal.
34 And the son of Jonathan *was* [i]Merib-
baal; and Merib-baal begat Micah.
35 And the sons of Micah *were*, Pithon,
and Melech, and [j]Tarea, and Ahaz.
36 And Ahaz begat [k]Jehoadah; and
Jehoadah begat Alemeth, and Azmaveth,
and Zimri; and Zimri begat Moza,
37 And Moza begat Binea: [l]Rapha *was*
his son, Eleasah his son, Azel his son:
38 And Azel had six sons, whose
names *are* these, Azrikam, Bocheru, and
Ishmael, and Sheariah, and Obadiah,
and Hanan. All these *were* the sons of
Azel.
39 And the sons of Eshek his brother
were, Ulam his firstborn, Jehush the second, and Eliphelet the third.
40 And the sons of Ulam were mighty
men of valour, archers, and had many
sons, and sons' sons, an hundred and
fifty. All these *are* of the sons of Benjamin.

CHAPTER 9.

The original of Israel's and
Judah's genealogies.

SO [m]all Israel were reckoned by
genealogies; and, behold, they *were*
written in the book of the kings of Israel
and Judah, *who* were carried away to
Babylon for their transgression.

The Israelites.

2 Now the [n]first inhabitants that *dwelt*
in their possessions in their cities *were*,
the Israelites, the priests, Levites, and
the [o]Nethinims.
3 And in Jerusalem dwelt of [p]the children of Judah, and of the children of
Benjamin, and of the children of
Ephraim, and Manasseh;
4 Uthai the son of Ammihud, the son
of Omri, the son of Imri, the son of Bani,
of the children of Pharez the son of
Judah.
5 And of the Shilonites; Asaiah the
firstborn, and his sons.
6 And of the sons of Zerah; Jeuel, and
their brethren, six hundred and ninety.
7 And of the sons of Benjamin; Sallu
the son of Meshullam, the son of
Hodaviah, the son of Hasenuah,
8 And Ibneiah the son of Jeroham, and
Elah the son of Uzzi, the son of Michri,
and Meshullam the son of Shephathiah,
the son of Reuel, the son of Ibnijah;
9 And their brethren, according to
their generations, nine hundred and fifty
and six. All these men *were* chief of the
fathers in the house of their fathers.

a v. 21.
b Or, *Shema*, v. 13.
c Called *Jehiel*, 1 Chr. 9:35.
d 1 Chr. 9:35.
e Or, *Zechariah*, 1 Chr. 9:37.
f Or, *Shimeam*, 1 Chr. 9:38.
g 1 Sam. 14:51.
h Or, *Ishbosheth*, 2 Sam. 2:8.
i Or, *Mephibosheth*, 2 Sam. 4:4; 9:6, 10.
j Or, *Tahrea*, 1 Chr. 9:41.
k *Jarah*, 1 Chr. 9:42.
l *Rephaiah*, 1 Chr. 9:43.
m Ezra 2:59, 62.
n Ezra 2:70; Neh. 7:73.
o Josh. 9:27; Ezra 2:43- 54; 8:20.
p Neh. 11:1, 2.

The priests.

10 And of the [a]priests; Jedaiah, and
Jehoiarib, and Jachin,
11 And [b]Azariah the son of Hilkiah,
the son of Meshullam, the son of Zadok,
the son of Meraioth, the son of Ahitub,
the ruler of the house of God;
12 And Adaiah the son of Jeroham, the
son of Pashur, the son of Malchijah, and
Maasiai the son of Adiel, the son of
Jahzerah, the son of Meshullam, the son
of Meshillemith, the son of Immer;
13 And their brethren, heads of the
house of their fathers, a thousand and
seven hundred and threescore; very
[c]able men for the work of the service of
the house of God.

And the Levites, with Nethinims, who dwelt in Jerusalem.

14 And of the Levites; Shemaiah the
son of Hasshub, the son of Azrikam, the
son of Hashabiah, of the sons of Merari;
15 And Bakbakkar, Heresh, and Galal,
and Mattaniah the son of Micah, the son
of Zichri, the son of Asaph;
16 And Obadiah the son of Shemaiah,
the son of Galal, the son of Jeduthun,
and Berechiah the son of Asa, the son of
Elkanah, that dwelt in the villages of the
Netophathites.
17 And the porters *were*, Shallum, and
Akkub, and Talmon, and Ahiman, and
their brethren: Shallum *was* the chief;
18 Who hitherto *waited* in the king's
gate eastward: they *were* porters in the
companies of the children of Levi.
19 And Shallum the son of Kore, the
son of Ebiasaph, the son of Korah, and
his brethren, of the house of his father,
the Korahites, *were* over the work of the
service, keepers of the [d]gates of the
tabernacle: and their fathers, *being* over
the host of the LORD, *were* keepers of the
entry.
20 And [e]Phinehas the son of Eleazar
was the ruler over them in time past, *and*
the LORD *was* with him.
21 *And* Zechariah the son of
Meshelemiah *was* porter of the door of
the tabernacle of the congregation.
22 All these *which were* chosen to be
porters in the [d]gates *were* two hundred
and twelve. These were reckoned by
their genealogy in their villages, whom
[f]David and Samuel the seer did ordain
in their set office.
23 So they and their children *had* the
oversight of the gates of the house of the
LORD, *namely*, the house of the tabernacle, by wards.
24 In four quarters were the porters,
toward the east, west, north, and south.
25 And their brethren, *which were* in
their villages, *were* to come after [g]seven
days from time to time with them.

The charge of certain Levites.

26 For these Levites, the four chief
porters, were in *their* set office, and were
over the [h]chambers and treasuries of the
house of God.
27 And they lodged round about the
house of God, because the charge *was*
upon them, and the opening thereof
every morning *pertained* to them.
28 And *certain* of them had the charge
of the ministering vessels, that they
should bring them in and out by tale.
29 *Some* of them also *were* appointed to
oversee the vessels, and all the instruments of the sanctuary, and the fine
flour, and the wine, and the oil, and the
frankincense, and the spices.
30 And *some* of the sons of the priests
made the [i]ointment of the spices.
31 And Mattithiah, *one* of the Levites,
who *was* the firstborn of Shallum the
Korahite, had the set [j]office over the
things that were made in the pans.
32 And *other* of their brethren, of the
sons of the [k]Kohathites, *were* over the
[l]shewbread, to prepare *it* every sabbath.
33 And these *are* the [m]singers, chief of
the fathers of the Levites, *who remaining*
in the chambers *were* free: for they were
employed in *that* work day and night.
34 These chief fathers of the Levites
were chief throughout their generations;
these dwelt at Jerusalem.

The stock of Saul and Jonathan.

35 And in Gibeon dwelt the father of
Gibeon, Jehiel, whose wife's name *was*
[n]Maachah:
36 And his firstborn son Abdon, then
Zur, and Kish, and Baal, and Ner, and
Nadab,

B.C. 4004 to 1056.

a Neh. 11:10-14.
b Called *Seraiah*, Neh. 11:11.
c Heb. *strong courageous men.*
d Heb. *thresholds.*
e Cf. Num. 31:6.
f 1 Chr. 26:1, 2.
g 2 Ki. 11:4-7.
h i.e. *storehouses.*
i Ex. 30:22-25.
j Lev. 2:5; 6:21.
k Lev. 24:8.
l Ex. 25:30, *note.*
m 1 Chr. 6:31, 32; 25:1-7.
n 1 Chr. 8:29, etc.

37 And Gedor, and Ahio, and Zechariah, and Mikloth.

38 And Mikloth begat Shimeam. And they also dwelt with their brethren at Jerusalem, over against their brethren.

39 And [a]Ner begat Kish; and Kish begat Saul; and Saul begat Jonathan, and Malchi-shua, and Abinadab, and Esh-baal.

40 And the son of Jonathan *was* Merib-baal: and Merib-baal begat Micah.

41 And the sons of Micah *were*, Pithon, and Melech, and Tahrea, [b]*and Ahaz.*

42 And Ahaz begat Jarah; and Jarah begat Alemeth, and Azmaveth, and Zimri; and Zimri begat Moza;

43 And Moza begat Binea; and Rephaiah his son, Eleasah his son, Azel his son.

44 And Azel had six sons, whose names *are* these, Azrikam, Bocheru, and Ishmael, and Sheariah, and Obadiah, and Hanan: these *were* the sons of Azel.

CHAPTER 10.

Saul's overthrow and death.

Now the Philistines [c]fought against Israel; and the men of Israel fled from before the Philistines, and fell down slain in mount Gilboa.

2 And the Philistines followed hard after Saul, and after his sons; and the Philistines slew Jonathan, and [d]Abinadab, and Malchi-shua, the sons of Saul.

3 And the battle went sore against Saul, and the archers hit him, and he was wounded of the archers.

4 [e]Then said Saul to his armourbearer, Draw thy sword, and thrust me through therewith; lest these uncircumcised come and abuse me. But his armourbearer would not; for he was sore afraid. So Saul took a sword, and fell upon it.

5 And when his armourbearer saw that Saul was dead, he fell likewise on the sword, and died.

6 So Saul died, and his three sons, and all his house died together.

7 And when all the men of Israel that *were* in the valley saw that they fled, and that Saul and his sons were dead, then they forsook their cities, and fled: and the Philistines came and dwelt in them.

B.C. 4004 to 1056.

a 1 Chr. 8:33.

b Added from 1 Chr. 8:35.

c 1 Sam. 31:1, etc.

d Called *Ishui*, 1 Sam. 14:49.

e Cf. 1 Sam. 31:4-7.

f Cf. 1 Sam. 31:9, 10.

B.C. 1056.

g 1 Sam. 31:11-13.

h 1 Sam. 13:13, 14; 15:22-26.

i 1 Sam. 28:7, etc.

j 2 Sam. 5:1, etc.

k 1 Sam. 16:1-13; Psa. 78:70-72.

l Cf. 1 Sam. 16:1-13.

The Philistines triumph over Saul.

8 And it came to pass on the morrow, when the Philistines came to strip the slain, that they found Saul and his sons fallen in mount Gilboa.

9 And when they had stripped him, they [f]took his head, and his armour, and sent into the land of the Philistines round about, to carry tidings unto their idols, and to the people.

10 And they put his armour in the house of their gods, and fastened his head in the temple of Dagon.

The kindness of Jabesh-gilead toward Saul and his sons.

11 And [g]when all Jabesh-gilead heard all that the Philistines had done to Saul,

12 They arose, all the valiant men, and took away the body of Saul, and the bodies of his sons, and brought them to Jabesh, and buried their bones under the oak in Jabesh, and fasted seven days.

Saul's sin for which he lost the kingdom.

13 So Saul died for his [h]transgression which he committed against the LORD, *even* against the word of the LORD, which he kept not, and [i]also for asking *counsel* of *one that had* a familiar spirit, to enquire *of it;*

14 And enquired not of the LORD: therefore he slew him, and turned the kingdom unto David the son of Jesse.

CHAPTER 11.

David becomes king over Israel (2 Sam. 5:1-3).

Then all Israel [j]gathered themselves to David unto Hebron, saying, Behold, *we are* thy bone and thy flesh.

2 And moreover in time past, even when Saul was king, thou *wast* he that leddest out and broughtest in Israel: and the LORD thy [k]God said unto thee, Thou shalt feed my people Israel, and thou shalt be ruler over my people Israel.

3 Therefore came all the elders of Israel to the king to Hebron; and David made a covenant with them in Hebron before the LORD; and they [l]anointed David king over Israel, according to the word of the LORD by Samuel.

B.C. 1047.

Jerusalem made the capital of the united kingdom (2 Sam. 5:6-12).

4 And David and all Israel went to Jerusalem, which *is* [a]Jebus; where the Jebusites *were*, the inhabitants of the land.

5 And the inhabitants of Jebus said to David, Thou shalt not come hither. Nevertheless David took the [b]castle of [1]Zion, which *is* the city of David.

6 And David said, Whosoever smiteth the Jebusites first shall be chief and captain. So Joab the son of Zeruiah went first up, and was chief.

7 And David dwelt in the castle; therefore they called [c]it the city of David.

8 And he built the city round about, even from Millo round about: and Joab repaired the rest of the city.

9 So David waxed greater and greater: for the LORD of hosts *was* with him.

A catalogue of David's mighty men.

10 [d]These also *are* the chief of the mighty men whom David had, who strengthened themselves with him in his kingdom, *and* with all Israel, to make him king, according to the word of the LORD concerning Israel.

11 And this *is* the number of the mighty men whom David had; Jashobeam, an Hachmonite, the chief of the captains: he lifted up his spear against three hundred slain *by him* at one time.

12 And after him *was* Eleazar the son of Dodo, the Ahohite, who *was one* of the three mighties.

13 He was with David at Pasdammim, and there the Philistines were gathered together to battle, where was a parcel of ground full of barley; and the people fled from before the Philistines.

14 And they set themselves in the midst of *that* parcel, and delivered it, and slew the Philistines; and the LORD saved *them* by a great deliverance.

15 Now [e]three of the thirty captains went down to the rock to David, into the cave of Adullam; and the host of the Philistines encamped in the valley of Rephaim.

16 And David *was* then in the hold, and the Philistines' garrison *was* then at Beth-lehem.

17 And David longed, and said, Oh that one would give me drink of the water of the well of Beth-lehem, that *is* at the gate!

18 And the three brake through the host of the Philistines, and drew water out of the well of Beth-lehem, that *was* by the gate, and took *it*, and brought *it* to David: but David would not drink *of* it, but poured it out to the LORD,

19 And said, My God forbid it me, that I should do this thing: shall I drink the blood of these men that have put their lives in jeopardy? for with *the jeopardy of* their lives they brought it. Therefore he would not drink it. These things did these three mightiest.

20 And Abishai the brother of Joab, he was chief of the three: for lifting up his spear against three hundred, he slew *them*, and had a name among the three.

21 Of the three, he was more honourable than the two; for he was their captain: howbeit he attained not to the *first* three.

22 Benaiah the son of Jehoiada, the son of a valiant man of Kabzeel, who had done many acts; he slew two lionlike men of Moab: also he went down and slew a lion in a pit in a snowy day.

23 And he slew an Egyptian, a man of *great* stature, five [f]cubits high; and in the Egyptian's hand *was* a spear like a weaver's beam; and he went down to him with a staff, and plucked the spear out of the Egyptian's hand, and slew him with his own spear.

24 These *things* did Benaiah the son of Jehoiada, and had the name among the three mighties.

25 Behold, he was honourable among the thirty, but attained not to the *first* three: and David set him over his guard.

a Cf. Jud. 1:21; 19:10, 11.

b v. 7.

c See v. 5.

d Cf. 2 Sam. 23:8-39.

e Cf. 2 Sam. 5:18; 1 Chr. 14:9.

f One cubit = about 18 in.

[1] **(11:5)** Heb. *castle.* (1) Zion, the ancient Jebusite stronghold, is the southwest eminence in Jerusalem, called in Scripture the city of David, and associated with the Davidic royalty both historically and prophetically (1 Chr. 11:7; Psa. 2:6; Isa. 2:3). The word is often used of the whole city of Jerusalem considered as the city of God (Psa. 48:2, 3), especially in passages referring to the future kingdom-age (Isa. 1:27; 2:3; 4:1-6; Joel 3:16; Zech. 1:16, 17; 8:3-8; Rom. 11:26). In Heb. 12:22 the word is used symbolically of heaven. (2) In Deut. 4:48 the name is given to a projection or peak of Mount Hermon.

B.C. 1047.

26 Also the valiant men of the armies *were*, Asahel the brother of Joab, Elhanan the son of Dodo of Beth-lehem,

27 Shammoth the Harorite, Helez the Pelonite,

28 Ira the son of Ikkesh the Tekoite, Abi-ezer the Antothite,

29 Sibbecai the Hushathite, Ilai the Ahohite,

30 Maharai the Netophathite, Heled the son of Baanah the Netophathite,

31 Ithai the son of Ribai of Gibeah, *that pertained* to the children of Benjamin, Benaiah the Pirathonite,

32 Hurai of the brooks of Gaash, Abiel the Arbathite,

33 Azmaveth the Baharumite, Eliahba the Shaalbonite,

34 The sons of Hashem the Gizonite, Jonathan the son of Shage the Hararite,

35 Ahiam the son of Sacar the Hararite, Eliphal the son of Ur,

36 Hepher the Mecherathite, Ahijah the Pelonite,

37 Hezro the Carmelite, Naarai the son of Ezbai,

38 Joel the brother of Nathan, Mibhar the son of Haggeri,

39 Zelek the Ammonite, Naharai the Berothite, the armourbearer of Joab the son of Zeruiah,

40 Ira the Ithrite, Gareb the Ithrite,

41 Uriah the Hittite, Zabad the son of Ahlai,

42 Adina the son of Shiza the Reubenite, a captain of the Reubenites, and thirty with him,

43 Hanan the son of Maachah, and Joshaphat the Mithnite,

44 Uzzia the Ashterathite, Shama and Jehiel the sons of Hothan the Aroerite,

45 Jediael the son of Shimri, and Joha his brother, the Tizite,

46 Eliel the Mahavite, and Jeribai, and Joshaviah, the sons of Elnaam, and Ithmah the Moabite,

47 Eliel, and Obed, and Jasiel the Mesobaite.

CHAPTER 12.

The companies that came to David at Ziklag.

(B.C. 1058.)

Now these *are* they that came to David to [a]Ziklag, while he yet kept himself close because of Saul the son of Kish: and they *were* among the mighty men, helpers of the war.

2 *They were* armed with bows, and could use both the right hand and the left [b]in *hurling* stones and *shooting* arrows out of a bow, *even* of Saul's brethren of Benjamin.

3 The chief *was* Ahiezer, then Joash, the sons of Shemaah the Gibeathite; and Jeziel, and Pelet, the sons of Azmaveth; and Berachah, and Jehu the Antothite,

4 And Ismaiah the Gibeonite, a mighty man among the thirty, and over the thirty; and Jeremiah, and Jahaziel, and Johanan, and Josabad the Gederathite,

5 Eluzai, and Jerimoth, and Bealiah, and Shemariah, and Shephatiah the Haruphite,

6 Elkanah, and Jesiah, and Azareel, and Joezer, and Jashobeam, the Korhites,

7 And Joelah, and Zebadiah, the sons of Jeroham of Gedor.

(*In the order of the history* 1 Chr. 12:8-15 *follows* 2 Sam. 5:17; 1 Chr. 14:8.)

8 And of the Gadites there separated themselves unto David into the hold to the wilderness men of might, *and* men of war *fit* for the battle, that could handle shield and buckler, whose faces *were like* the faces of lions, and *were* as swift as the roes upon the mountains;

9 Ezer the first, Obadiah the second, Eliab the third,

10 Mishmannah the fourth, Jeremiah the fifth,

11 Attai the sixth, Eliel the seventh,

12 Johanan the eighth, Elzabad the ninth,

13 Jeremiah the tenth, Machbanai the eleventh.

14 These *were* of the sons of Gad, captains of the host: one of the least *was* over an hundred, and the greatest over a thousand.

15 These *are* they that went over Jordan in the [c]first month, when it had overflown all his banks; and they put to flight all *them* of the valleys, *both* toward the east, and toward the west.

16 And there came of the children of Benjamin and Judah to the hold unto David.

17 And David went out to meet them, and answered and said unto them, If ye be come peaceably unto me to help me, mine heart shall be knit unto you: but if *ye be come* to betray me to mine enemies, seeing *there is* no wrong in mine hands,

a 1 Sam. 27:6.
b Cf. Jud. 20:16.
c i.e. *April*.

B.C. 1058.

the God of our fathers look *thereon*, and rebuke *it*.

18 Then the [a]spirit came upon [b]Amasai, *who was* chief of the captains, *and he said*, Thine *are we*, David, and on thy side, thou son of Jesse: peace, peace *be* unto thee, and peace *be* to thine helpers; for thy God helpeth thee. Then David received them, and made them captains of the band.

19 And there fell *some* of [c]Manasseh to David, when he came with the Philistines against Saul to battle: but they helped them not: for the lords of the Philistines upon advisement sent him away, [d]saying, He will fall to his master Saul to *the jeopardy of* our heads.

20 As he went to Ziklag, there fell to him of Manasseh, Adnah, and Jozabad, and Jediael, and Michael, and Jozabad, and Elihu, and Zilthai, captains of the thousands that *were* of Manasseh.

21 And they [e]helped David against the band *of the rovers*: for they *were* all mighty men of valour, and were captains in the host.

22 For at *that* time day by day there came to David to help him, until *it was* a great host, like the host of God.

The men of Israel who made David king.
(Cf. 2 Sam. 5:1-3.)

23 And these *are* the numbers of the bands *that were* ready armed to the war, *and* came to David [f]to Hebron, to turn the kingdom of Saul to him, [g]according to the word of the LORD.

24 The children of Judah that bare shield and spear *were* six thousand and eight hundred, ready armed to the war.

25 Of the children of Simeon, mighty men of valour for the war, seven thousand and one hundred.

26 Of the children of Levi four thousand and six hundred.

27 And Jehoiada *was* the leader of the Aaronites, and with him *were* three thousand and seven hundred;

28 And [h]Zadok, a young man mighty of valour, and of his father's house twenty and two captains.

29 And of the children of Benjamin, the kindred of Saul, three thousand: for hitherto the greatest part of them had [i]kept the ward of the house of Saul.

30 And of the children of Ephraim twenty thousand and eight hundred, mighty men of valour, famous throughout the house of their fathers.

31 And of the half tribe of Manasseh eighteen thousand, which were expressed by name, to come and make David king.

32 And of the children of Issachar, *which were men* that had understanding of the times, to know what Israel ought to do; the heads of them *were* two hundred; and all their brethren *were* at their commandment.

33 Of Zebulun, such as went forth to battle, expert in war, with all instruments of war, fifty thousand, which could keep rank: *they were* not of double heart.

34 And of Naphtali a thousand captains, and with them with shield and spear thirty and seven thousand.

35 And of the Danites expert in war twenty and eight thousand and six hundred.

36 And of Asher, such as went forth to battle, expert in war, forty thousand.

37 And on the other side of Jordan, of the Reubenites, and the Gadites, and of the half tribe of Manasseh, with all manner of instruments of war for the battle, an hundred and twenty thousand.

38 All these men of war, that could keep rank, came with a [j]perfect heart to Hebron, to make David king over all Israel: and all the rest also of Israel *were* of one heart to make David king.

39 And there they were with David three days, eating and drinking: for their brethren had prepared for them.

40 Moreover they that were nigh them, *even* unto Issachar and Zebulun and Naphtali, brought bread on asses, and on camels, and on mules, and on oxen, *and* meat, meal, cakes of figs, and bunches of raisins, and wine, and oil, and oxen, and sheep abundantly: for *there was* joy in Israel.

CHAPTER 13.

Doing a right thing in the wrong way.

AND David consulted with the captains of thousands and hundreds, *and* with every leader.

2 And [k]David said unto all the congregation of Israel, If *it seem* good unto you, and *that it be* of the LORD our God, let us send abroad unto our brethren every

a *Holy Spirit.* 1 Chr. 28:12. (Gen. 1:2; Mal. 2:15.)
b 2 Sam. 17:25, called *Amasa.*
c 1 Sam. 29:2.
d 1 Sam. 29:4.
e 1 Sam. 30:1-20.
f 2 Sam. 2:1-4; 5:1-3.
g 1 Sam. 16:1-4.
h 2 Sam. 8:17; 1 Chr. 6:8, 53.
i 2 Sam. 2:4-7.
j See 1 Ki. 8:61.
k Cf. 2 Sam. 6:1-10.

where, *that are* left in all the land of Israel, and with them *also* to the priests and Levites *which are* in their cities *and* suburbs, that they may gather themselves unto us:

3 And let us bring again the ark of our God to us: for we enquired not at it in the days of Saul.

4 And all the congregation said that they would do so: for the thing was right in the eyes of all the people.

5 So David gathered all Israel together, from Shihor of Egypt even unto the entering of Hemath, to bring the ark of God from [a]Kirjath-jearim.

6 And David went up, and all Israel, to [b]Baalah, *that is,* to Kirjath-jearim, which *belonged* to Judah, to bring up thence the ark of God the LORD, that [c]dwelleth *between* the cherubims, whose name is called *on it.*

7 And they [d]carried the ark of God in a new cart out of the house of Abinadab: and Uzza and Ahio drave the cart.

8 And David and all Israel played before God with all *their* might, and with singing, and with harps, and with psalteries, and with timbrels, and with cymbals, and with trumpets.

Uzza being smitten, the ark is left at the house of Obed-edom.

9 And when they came unto the threshingfloor of [e]Chidon, Uzza put forth his hand to hold the ark; for the oxen stumbled.

10 And the anger of the LORD was kindled against Uzza, and he smote him, [f]because he put his hand to the ark: and there he died before God.

11 And David was displeased, because the LORD had made a breach upon Uzza: wherefore that place is called [g]Perez-uzza to this day.

12 And David was afraid of God that day, saying, How shall I bring the ark of God *home* to me?

13 So David brought not the ark *home* to himself to the city of David, but carried it aside into the house of Obed-edom the Gittite.

14 And the ark of God [h]remained with the family of Obed-edom in his house three months. And the LORD [i]blessed the house of Obed-edom, and all that he had.

B.C. 1045.

(B.C. 1043.)

a 1 Sam. 6:1-21; 7:1, 2.

b Josh. 15:9, etc.

c Ex. 25:22.

d Cf. Num. 4:15; 1 Chr. 15:2, 15.

e Called *Nachon,* 2 Sam. 6:6.

f See Num. 4:15; cf. 1 Chr. 15:12-15.

g i.e. *the breach of Uzza.*

h 2 Sam. 6:11.

i 1 Chr. 26:4-8.

j 2 Sam. 5:11, 12.

k Called *Eliada,* 2 Sam. 5:16.

l 2 Sam. 5:17-21.

m 2 Sam. 5:22-25.

CHAPTER 14.

The prosperity of King David.

Now [j]Hiram king of Tyre sent messengers to David, and timber of cedars, with masons and carpenters, to build him an house.

2 And David perceived that the LORD had confirmed him king over Israel, for his kingdom was lifted up on high, because of his people Israel.

3 And David took more wives at Jerusalem: and David begat more sons and daughters.

4 Now these *are* the names of *his* children which he had in Jerusalem; Shammua, and Shobab, Nathan, and Solomon,

5 And Ibhar, and Elishua, and Elpalet,

6 And Nogah, and Nepheg, and Japhia,

7 And Elishama, and [k]Beeliada, and Eliphalet.

8 And [l]when the Philistines heard that David was anointed king over all Israel, all the Philistines went up to seek David. And David heard *of it,* and went out against them.

9 And the Philistines came and spread themselves in the valley of Rephaim.

10 And David enquired of God, saying, Shall I go up against the Philistines? and wilt thou deliver them into mine hand? And the LORD said unto him, Go up; for I will deliver them into thine hand.

11 So they came up to Baal-perazim; and David smote them there. Then David said, God hath broken in upon mine enemies by mine hand like the breaking forth of waters: therefore they called the name of that place Baal-perazim.

12 And when they had left their gods there, David gave a commandment, and they were burned with fire.

13 [m]And the Philistines yet again spread themselves abroad in the valley.

14 Therefore David enquired again of God; and God said unto him, Go not up after them; turn away from them, and come upon them over against the mulberry trees.

15 And it shall be, when thou shalt hear a sound of going in the tops of the mulberry trees, *that* then thou shalt go out to battle: for God is gone forth before thee to smite the host of the Philistines.

B.C. 1045.

16 David therefore did as God commanded him: and they smote the host of the Philistines from [a]Gibeon even to Gazer.

17 And the fame of David went out into all lands; and the LORD brought the [b]fear of him upon all nations.

CHAPTER 15.

Doing a right thing in the right way.
(Cf. 1 Chr. 13.)

(B.C. 1042.)

And *David* made him houses in the city of David, and [c]prepared a place for the ark of God, and pitched for it a tent.

2 Then David said, [d]None ought to carry the ark of God but the Levites: for [e]them hath the LORD chosen to carry the ark of God, and to minister unto him for ever.

3 [f]And David gathered all Israel together to Jerusalem, to bring up the ark of the LORD unto his place, which he had prepared for it.

4 And David assembled the children of Aaron, and the Levites:

5 Of the sons of Kohath; Uriel the chief, and his brethren an hundred and twenty:

6 Of the sons of Merari; Asaiah the chief, and his brethren two hundred and twenty:

7 Of the sons of Gershom; Joel the chief, and his brethren an hundred and thirty:

8 Of the sons of Elizaphan; Shemaiah the chief, and his brethren two hundred:

9 Of the sons of Hebron; Eliel the chief, and his brethren fourscore:

10 Of the sons of Uzziel; Amminadab the chief, and his brethren an hundred and twelve.

11 And David called for Zadok and Abiathar the priests, and for the Levites, for Uriel, Asaiah, and Joel, Shemaiah, and Eliel, and Amminadab,

12 And said unto them, Ye *are* the chief of the fathers of the Levites: [g]sanctify yourselves, *both* ye and your brethren, that ye may bring up the ark of the LORD God of Israel unto *the place that* I have prepared for it.

13 For [h]because ye *did it* not at the first, the LORD our God made a breach upon us, for that we sought him not after the due order.

14 So the priests and the Levites sanctified themselves to bring up the ark of the LORD God of Israel.

15 And the children of the Levites bare the ark of God upon their shoulders with the staves thereon, as Moses commanded according to the word of the LORD.

16 And David spake to the chief of the Levites to appoint their brethren *to be* the singers with instruments of musick, psalteries and harps and cymbals, sounding, by lifting up the voice with joy.

17 So the Levites appointed Heman the son of Joel; and of his brethren, Asaph the son of Berechiah; and of the sons of Merari their brethren, Ethan the son of Kushaiah;

18 And with them their brethren of the second *degree*, Zechariah, Ben, and Jaaziel, and Shemiramoth, and Jehiel, and Unni, Eliab, and Benaiah, and Maaseiah, and Mattithiah, and Elipheleh, and Mikneiah, and Obed-edom, and Jeiel, the porters.

19 So the singers, Heman, Asaph, and Ethan, *were appointed* to sound with cymbals of brass;

20 And Zechariah, and [i]Aziel, and Shemiramoth, and Jehiel, and Unni, and Eliab, and Maaseiah, and Benaiah, with psalteries on Alamoth;

21 And Mattithiah, and Elipheleh, and Mikneiah, and Obed-edom, and Jeiel, and Azaziah, with harps on the Sheminith to excel.

22 And Chenaniah, chief of the Levites, *was* for song: he instructed about the song, because he *was* skilful.

23 And Berechiah and Elkanah *were* doorkeepers for the ark.

24 And Shebaniah, and Jehoshaphat, and Nethaneel, and Amasai, and Zechariah, and Benaiah, and Eliezer, the priests, did blow with the trumpets before the ark of God: and [j]Obed-edom and Jehiah *were* doorkeepers for the ark.

David brings up the ark (2 Sam. 6:12-23).

25 [k]So David, and the elders of Israel, and the captains over thousands, went to bring up the ark of the covenant of the LORD out of the house of Obed-edom with joy.

26 And it came to pass, when God helped the Levites that bare the ark of the covenant of the LORD, that they offered seven bullocks and seven rams.

27 And David *was* clothed with a robe of fine linen, and all the Levites that bare the ark, and the singers, and Chenaniah

a Called *Geba*, 2 Sam. 5:25.
b Cf. Deut. 2:25; 11:25; 2 Chr. 20:29.
c 1 Chr. 16:1.
d Cf. 2 Sam. 6:1-11.
e Num. 4:2, 15; Deut. 10:8; 31:9.
f Cf. 2 Chr. 5:3-14.
g i.e. *separate*. Ex. 19:10; 28:41; Lev. 10:3; Josh. 7:13.
h 1 Chr. 13:7-11.
i *Jaaziel*, in v. 18.
j v. 5; 1 Chr. 13:14.
k 1 Ki. 8:1.

B.C. 1042.

the master of the song with the singers: David also *had* upon him an ephod of linen.

28 Thus [a]all Israel brought up the ark of the covenant of the LORD with [b]shouting, and with sound of the cornet, and with trumpets, and with cymbals, making a noise with psalteries and harps.

Michal despises David.

29 And it came to pass, *as* the ark of the covenant of the LORD came to the city of David, that [c]Michal the daughter of Saul looking out at a window saw king David dancing and playing: and she despised him in her heart.

CHAPTER 16.

David's festival sacrifice.

So they brought the [d]ark of God, and set it in the midst of the tent that David had pitched for it: and they offered burnt sacrifices and peace-offerings before God.

2 And when David had made an end of offering the burnt-offerings and the peace-offerings, he blessed the people in the name of the LORD.

3 And he dealt to every one of Israel, both man and woman, to every one a loaf of bread, and a good piece of flesh, and a flagon *of wine.*

David orders a choir.

4 And he appointed *certain* of the Levites to minister before the ark of the LORD, and to [e]record, and to thank and praise the LORD God of Israel:

5 Asaph the chief, and next to him Zechariah, Jeiel, and Shemiramoth, and Jehiel, and Mattithiah, and Eliab, and Benaiah, and Obed-edom: and Jeiel with psalteries and with harps; but Asaph made a sound with cymbals;

6 Benaiah also and Jahaziel the priests with trumpets continually before the ark of the covenant of God.

The psalm of thanksgiving.

7 Then on that day [f]David delivered first *this psalm* to thank the LORD into the hand of Asaph and his brethren.

8 [g]Give thanks unto the LORD, call upon his name, make known his deeds among the people.

9 Sing unto him, sing psalms unto him, talk ye of all his wondrous works.

10 Glory ye in his holy name: let the heart of them rejoice that seek the LORD.

11 Seek the LORD and his strength, seek his face continually.

12 Remember his marvellous works that he hath done, his wonders, and the judgments of his mouth;

13 O ye seed of Israel his servant, ye children of Jacob, his chosen ones.

14 He *is* the LORD our God; his judgments *are* in all the earth.

15 Be ye mindful always of his covenant; the word *which* he commanded to a thousand generations;

16 *Even of the covenant* which he made with [h]Abraham, and of his oath unto Isaac;

17 And hath [i]confirmed the same to Jacob for a law, *and* to Israel *for* an everlasting covenant,

18 Saying, Unto thee will I give the land of Canaan, the lot of your inheritance;

19 When ye were but few, even a few, and strangers in it.

20 And *when* they went from nation to nation, and from *one* kingdom to another people;

21 He suffered no man to do them wrong: yea, he reproved kings for their sakes,

22 *Saying,* Touch not mine anointed, and do my prophets no harm.

23 Sing unto the LORD, all the earth; shew forth from day to day his salvation.

24 Declare his glory among the [j]heathen; his marvellous works among all [k]nations.

25 For great *is* the LORD, and greatly to be praised: he also *is* to be [l]feared above all gods.

26 For all the [m]gods of the people *are* idols: but the LORD made the heavens.

27 Glory and honour *are* in his presence, strength and gladness *are* in his place.

28 Give unto the LORD, ye kindreds of the people, give unto the LORD glory and strength.

29 Give unto the LORD the glory *due* unto his name: bring an offering, and come before him: worship the LORD in the beauty of holiness.

30 Fear before him, all the earth: the world also shall be stable, that it be not moved.

31 Let the heavens be glad, and let the

a 1 Chr. 13:8.

b Num. 23:21; Josh. 6:5, 20; Zech. 4:7; 1 Thes. 4:16.

c 1 Sam. 18:20, 27; 19:11-17; 2 Sam. 3:13, 14; 6:20-23.

d 2 Sam. 6:17-20.

e See titles of Psalms 38 and 70.

f See 2 Sam. 23:1.

g Cf. Psa. 105.

h Gen. 15:18, *note.*

i Gen. 26:3; 28:13; 35:11, 12.

j i.e. *nations.*

k i.e. *peoples.*

l Psa. 19:9, *note.*

m Lev. 19:4; cf. 1 Cor. 8:5-6; 10:20.

earth rejoice: and let *men* say among the
nations, The LORD reigneth.
32 Let the sea roar, and the fulness
thereof: let the fields rejoice, and all that
is therein.
33 Then shall the [a]trees of the wood
sing out at the presence of the LORD,
because he [b]cometh to judge the earth.
34 O give thanks unto the LORD; for *he*
is good; for his mercy *endureth* for ever.
35 And say ye, Save us, O God of our
salvation, and gather us together, and
deliver us from the [c]heathen, that we
may give thanks to thy holy name, *and*
glory in thy praise.
36 Blessed *be* the LORD God of Israel
for ever and ever. And all the people
said, Amen, and praised the LORD.

David appoints ministers, porters, priests, and musicians to attend continually on the ark.

37 So he left there before the [1]ark of
the covenant of the LORD [d]Asaph and his
brethren, to minister before the ark continually, as every day's work required:
38 And [e]Obed-edom with their
brethren, threescore and eight; Obed-edom also the son of Jeduthun and
Hosah *to be* porters:
39 And [f]Zadok the priest, and his
brethren the priests, before the tabernacle of the LORD in the high place that *was*
at Gibeon,
40 To offer burnt-offerings unto the
LORD upon the altar of the burnt-offering
continually morning and evening, and *to*
do according to all that is written in the
law of the LORD, which he commanded
Israel;
41 And with them Heman and
Jeduthun, and the rest that were chosen,
who were expressed by name, to give
thanks to the LORD, because his mercy
endureth for ever;
42 And with them Heman and
Jeduthun with trumpets and cymbals for
those that should make a sound, and
with musical instruments of God. And
the sons of Jeduthun *were* porters.
43 [g]And all the people departed every
man to his house: and David returned to
bless his house.

B.C. 1042.

a Isa. 55:12, 13.

b Joel 3:1-14; Zech. 14:1-4; Mt. 25:31-46.

c i.e. *nations.*

d 1 Chr. 6:39; 15:17; 25:1-9; 2 Chr. 5:12; Ezra 2:41. Writer of Psalms 50, 73, 74, 75, 76, 77, 78, 79, 80, 81, 82, 83.

e 1 Chr. 13:14.

f 2 Sam. 8:17; 15:24-36; 1 Ki. 2:35; 1 Chr. 29:22; Ezra 7:2; Ezk. 40:46.

g 2 Sam. 6:18-21.

h 1 Chr. 14:1.

i Cf. vs. 3, 4; the folly of human opinion in the things of God.

j 1 Sam. 16:11-13.

CHAPTER 17.

David's desire to build the Lord's house (2 Sam. 7:1-3).

Now it came to pass, as David sat in
his house, that David said to
Nathan the prophet, Lo, I dwell in an
house of [h]cedars, but the ark of the
covenant of the LORD *remaineth* under
curtains.
2 Then Nathan [i]said unto David, Do all
that *is* in thine heart; for God *is* with thee.
3 And it came to pass the same night,
that the word of God came to Nathan,
saying,
4 Go and tell David my servant, Thus
saith the LORD, Thou shalt not build me
an house to dwell in:
5 For I have not dwelt in an house
since the day that I brought up Israel
unto this day; but have gone from tent to
tent, and from *one* tabernacle *to another*.
6 Wheresoever I have walked with all
Israel, spake I a word to any of the
judges of Israel, whom I commanded to
feed my people, saying, Why have ye
not built me an house of cedars?

The great Davidic Covenant (2 Sam. 7:4-17, *note*).

7 Now therefore thus shalt thou say
unto my servant David, Thus saith the
LORD of hosts, I took thee [j]from the
sheepcote, *even* [2]from following the
sheep, that thou shouldest be ruler over
my people Israel:
8 And I have been with thee whithersoever thou hast walked, and have cut off
all thine enemies from before thee, and
have made thee a name like the name of
the great men that *are* in the earth.

[1] **(16:37)** It will be understood that the ancient tabernacle was now divided; the ark was brought into "Zion" (1 Chr. 11:5, *note*), while the brazen altar, at least, and probably the vessels of the holy place (Ex. 25:23-40; 37:10-25; 40:22-27) were established in the high place at Gibeon. Asaph and the singers (1 Chr. 6:31-39; 15:16-19; 16:5; 25:6) were "left before the ark" (1 Chr. 16:37), while the priests ministered in Gibeon "before the tabernacle" (1 Chr. 16:39). All this was mere confusion: cf. Heb. 9:1-7. With the construction of the temple the divine order seems to have been restored.

[2] **(17:7)** David is here, as often, a type of his Son after the flesh (Mt. 1:1; Rom. 1:3), Jesus the Shepherd-King. At His first coming He took the shepherd's place, first in death (John 10:11), and now

9 Also I will ordain a place for my people Israel, and will [a]plant them, and they shall dwell in their place, and shall be moved no more; neither shall the children of wickedness waste them any more, as at the beginning,

10 And [b]since the time that I commanded [c]judges *to be* over my people Israel. Moreover I will subdue all thine enemies. Furthermore I tell thee that the LORD will build thee an house.

11 And it shall come to pass, [d]when thy days be expired that thou must go *to be* with thy fathers, that I will raise up [e]thy seed after thee, which shall be of thy sons; and I will establish his kingdom.

12 [f]He shall build me an house, and I will stablish his throne for ever.

13 I will be his father, and he shall be my son: and I will not take my mercy away from him, [g]as I took *it* from *him* that was before thee:

14 But I will settle him in mine house and in my kingdom for ever: and his throne shall be established for evermore.

15 According to all these words, and according to all this vision, so did Nathan speak unto David.

David's worship and prayer (2 Sam. 7:18-29).

16 And David the king came and sat before the LORD, and said, Who *am* I, O LORD God, and what *is* mine house, that thou hast brought me hitherto?

17 And *yet* this was a small thing in thine eyes, O God; for thou hast *also* spoken of thy servant's house for a great while to come, and hast regarded me according to the estate of a man of high degree, O LORD God.

18 What can David *speak* more to thee for the honour of thy servant? for thou knowest thy servant.

19 O LORD, for thy servant's sake, and according to thine own heart, hast thou done all this greatness, in making known all *these* great things.

20 O LORD, *there is* none like thee, neither *is there any* God beside thee, according to all that we have heard with our ears.

21 [h]And what one nation in the earth *is* like thy people Israel, whom God went to [i]redeem *to be* his own people, to make thee a name of greatness and terribleness, by driving out nations from before thy people, whom thou hast [i]redeemed out of Egypt?

22 For thy people Israel didst thou make thine own people for ever; and thou, LORD, becamest their God.

23 Therefore now, LORD, let the thing that thou hast spoken concerning thy servant and concerning his house be established for ever, and do as thou hast said.

24 Let it even be established, that thy name may be magnified for ever, saying, The LORD of hosts *is* the God of Israel, *even* a God to Israel: and *let* the house of David thy servant *be* established before thee.

25 For thou, O my God, hast told thy servant that thou wilt build him an house: therefore thy servant hath found *in his heart* to pray before thee.

26 And now, LORD, thou art God, and hast promised this goodness unto thy servant:

27 Now therefore let it please thee to bless the house of thy servant, that it may be before thee for ever: for thou blessest, O LORD, and *it shall be* blessed for ever.

CHAPTER 18.

The full establishment of David's kingdom (2 Sam. 8:1-18).

Now after this it came to pass, [j]that David smote the Philistines, and subdued them, and took Gath and her towns out of the hand of the Philistines.

2 And he smote [k]Moab; and the Moabites became David's servants, *and* [l]brought gifts.

3 [m]And David smote Hadarezer king of Zobah unto Hamath, as he went to stablish his dominion by the river Euphrates.

4 And David took from him a thousand chariots, and seven thousand horsemen

B.C. 1042.

a Deut. 30:1-9; Isa. 11:11-13; Jer. 16:14-16; 23:5-8; 24:6; Ezk. 37:21-27; Amos 9:14.

b 1 Ki. 2:1; Acts 13:36.

c Or, *as at the beginning, when I set judges over my people*, etc.

d Fulfilled first in Solomon, I Ki. 8:19, 20; and to be fulfilled in Christ, Lk. 1:32, 33; Acts 15:14-16.

e i.e. *Solomon*, 1 Ki. 5:5; 6:12; 8:19, etc. See I Chr. 22:9-13; 28:20.

f Psa. 89:3, 4, 20-37.

g 1 Sam. 15:23-28.

h Deut. 4:6-8, 33-38; Psa. 147:20.

i Ex. 14:30, *note*.

j 2 Sam. 8:1.

k 2 Sam. 8:2; cf. Num. 24: 17; Zeph. 2:9.

l 1 Sam. 10:27.

m 2 Sam. 8:3.

in resurrection power (Heb. 13:20). At His return He will take the place of "ruler over Israel" (Isa 11:10-12; Jer. 23:5-8; Lk. 1:32, 33; Acts 15:14-17). This is the precise order of Psalms 22, 23, 24. In the first the good Shepherd is giving His life for the sheep; in the second He is caring for the sheep; in the third He comes to reign as King of Glory.

and twenty thousand footmen: David also houghed all the chariot *horses*, but reserved of them an hundred chariots.

5 [a]And when the Syrians of Damascus came to help Hadarezer king of Zobah, David slew of the Syrians two and twenty thousand men.

6 Then David put *garrisons* in Syriadamascus; and the Syrians became David's servants, *and* brought gifts. Thus the LORD preserved David whithersoever he went.

7 And David took the shields of gold that were on the servants of Hadarezer, and brought them to Jerusalem.

8 Likewise from [b]Tibhath, and from Chun, cities of Hadarezer, brought David very much brass, wherewith Solomon made the brasen sea, and the pillars, and the vessels of brass.

9 Now when Tou king of Hamath heard how David had smitten all the host of Hadarezer king of Zobah;

10 He sent Hadoram his son to king David, to enquire of his welfare, and to congratulate him, because he had fought against Hadarezer, and smitten him; (for Hadarezer had war with Tou;) and *with him* all manner of [c]vessels of gold and silver and brass.

11 Them also king David dedicated unto the LORD, with the silver and the gold that he brought from all *these* nations; from Edom, and from Moab, and from the children of Ammon, and from the Philistines, and from Amalek.

12 Moreover [d]Abishai the son of Zeruiah slew of the Edomites in the valley of salt eighteen thousand.

13 And he put garrisons in Edom; and all the Edomites became David's servants. Thus the LORD preserved David whithersoever he went.

14 So David reigned over all Israel, and executed judgment and justice among all his people.

15 And [f]Joab the son of Zeruiah *was* over the host; and Jehoshaphat the son of Ahilud, recorder.

16 And Zadok the son of Ahitub, and Abimelech the son of Abiathar, *were* the priests; and Shavsha was scribe;

17 And Benaiah the son of Jehoiada *was* over the Cherethites and the Pelethites; and the sons of David *were* chief about the king.

B.C. 1040.

a 2 Sam. 8:5-7. See 1 Ki. 11:23-25.

b Called *Betah*, and *Berothai*, 2 Sam. 8:8.

c Cf. 2 Sam. 8:10-12.

d Nephew of David, brother to Joab; 2 Sam. 23:18; 1 Chr. 2:16.

e Gen. 27:29-40; Num. 24:18; 2 Sam. 8:14.

f v. 12, *ref.*

g One talent of silver = £410, or $1940.

CHAPTER 19.

The Ammonite-Syrian war
(2 Sam. 10:1-19).
First campaign under Joab.

Now it came to pass after this, that Nahash the king of the children of Ammon died, and his son reigned in his stead.

2 And David said, I will shew kindness unto Hanun the son of Nahash, because his father shewed kindness to me. And David sent messengers to comfort him concerning his father. So the servants of David came into the land of the children of Ammon to Hanun, to comfort him.

3 But the princes of the children of Ammon said to Hanun, Thinkest thou that David doth honour thy father, that he hath sent comforters unto thee? are not his servants come unto thee for to search, and to overthrow, and to spy out the land?

4 Wherefore Hanun took David's servants, and shaved them, and cut off their garments in the midst hard by their buttocks, and sent them away.

5 Then there went *certain*, and told David how the men were served. And he sent to meet them: for the men were greatly ashamed. And the king said, Tarry at Jericho until your beards be grown, and *then* return.

6 And when the children of Ammon saw that they had made themselves odious to David, Hanun and the children of Ammon sent a thousand [g]talents of silver to hire them chariots and horsemen out of Mesopotamia, and out of Syriamaachah, and out of Zobah.

7 So they hired thirty and two thousand chariots, and the king of Maachah and his people; who came and pitched before Medeba. And the children of Ammon gathered themselves together from their cities, and came to battle.

8 And when David heard *of it*, he sent Joab, and all the host of the mighty men.

9 And the children of Ammon came out, and put the battle in array before the gate of the city: and the kings that were come *were* by themselves in the field.

10 Now when Joab saw that the battle

was set against him before and behind, he chose out of all the choice of Israel, and put *them* in array against the Syrians.

11 And the rest of the people he delivered unto the hand of Abishai his brother, and they set *themselves* in array against the children of Ammon.

12 And he said, If the Syrians be too strong for me, then thou shalt help me: but if the children of Ammon be too strong for thee, then I will help thee.

13 Be of good courage, and let us behave ourselves valiantly for our people, and for the cities of our God: and let the LORD do *that which is* good in his sight.

14 So Joab and the people that *were* with him drew nigh before the Syrians unto the battle; and they fled before him.

15 And when the children of Ammon saw that the Syrians were fled, they likewise fled before Abishai his brother, and entered into the city. Then Joab came to Jerusalem.

16 And when the Syrians saw that they were put to the worse before Israel, they sent messengers, and drew forth the Syrians that *were* beyond the river: and Shophach the captain of the host of Hadarezer *went* before them.

Second campaign under David in person.

17 And it was told David; and he gathered all Israel, and passed over Jordan, and came upon them, and set *the battle* in array against them. So when David had put the battle in array against the Syrians, they fought with him.

18 But the Syrians fled before Israel; and David slew of the Syrians seven thousand *men which fought in* chariots, and forty thousand footmen, and killed Shophach the captain of the host.

19 And when the servants of Hadarezer saw that they were put to the worse before Israel, they made peace with David, and became his servants: neither would the Syrians help the children of Ammon any more.

CHAPTER 20.

Joab and David take Rabbah
(2 Sam. 12:26-31).

[a] And it came to pass, that after the year was expired, at the time that kings go out *to battle*, Joab led forth the power of the army, and wasted the country of the children of Ammon, and came and besieged Rabbah. But [b]David tarried at Jerusalem. And Joab smote Rabbah, and destroyed it.

2 And David took the crown of their king from off his head, and found it to weigh a [c]talent of gold, and *there were* precious stones in it; and it was set upon David's head: and he brought also exceeding much spoil out of the city.

3 And he brought out the people that *were* in it, and cut *them* with saws, and with harrows of iron, and with axes. Even so dealt David with all the cities of the children of Ammon. And David and all the people returned to Jerusalem.

War with the Philistines.

4 [d]And it came to pass after this, that there arose war at Gezer with the Philistines; at which time Sibbechai the Hushathite slew Sippai, *that was* of the children of the giant: and they were subdued.

5 And there was war again with the Philistines; and Elhanan the son of Jair slew Lahmi the brother of Goliath the Gittite, whose spear staff *was* like a weaver's beam.

6 And yet again there was war at [e]Gath, where was a man of *great* stature, whose fingers and toes *were* four and twenty, six *on each hand*, and six *on each foot*: and he also was the son of the giant.

7 But when he defied Israel, Jonathan the son of [f]Shimea David's brother slew him.

8 These were born unto the giant in Gath; and they fell by the hand of David, and by the hand of his servants.

CHAPTER 21.

David sins in numbering the people
(2 Sam. 24:1-9).

And [g]Satan stood up against Israel [h]and [i]provoked David to number Israel.

2 And David said to Joab and to the rulers of the people, Go, number Israel from Beer-sheba even to Dan; and [j]bring the number of them to me, that I may know *it*.

Joab's faithful protest.

3 And Joab answered, The LORD make his people an hundred times so many more as they *be*: but, my lord the king, *are* they not all my lord's servants? why

B.C. 1037.

a 2 Sam. 11:1.

b Here should be read 2 Sam. 11:2-12.25, with Psa. 51.

c One talent of gold = £6150, or $29,085.

d 2 Sam. 21:18.

e 2 Sam. 21:20.

f Or, *Shammah*, 1 Sam. 16:9.

g *Satan*, Job 1:6, 7, 8, 9, 12. (Gen. 3:1; Rev. 20:10.)

h 2 Sam. 24:1-9.

i Heb. *enticed*.

j Cf. 1 Chr. 27:23, 24.

[B.C. 1017.

B.C. 1035.]

then doth my lord require this thing?
why will he be a cause of trespass to
Israel?
4 Nevertheless the king's word prevailed against Joab. Wherefore Joab [a]de-
parted, and went throughout all Israel,
and came to Jerusalem.
5 And Joab gave the sum of the number of the people unto David. And all
they of Israel [b]were a thousand thousand
and an hundred thousand men that
drew sword: and Judah *was* four hundred threescore and ten thousand men
that drew sword.
6 But Levi and Benjamin counted he
not among them: for the king's word
was abominable to Joab.
7 And God was displeased with this
thing; therefore he smote Israel.

David chooses his punishment
(2 Sam. 24:10-17).

8 And David said unto God, I have
sinned greatly, because I have done this
thing: but now, I beseech thee, do away
the iniquity of thy servant; for I have
done very foolishly.
9 And the LORD spake unto Gad,
David's [c]seer, saying,
10 Go and tell David, [d]saying, Thus
saith the LORD, I offer thee three *things*:
choose thee one of them, that I may do *it*
unto thee.
11 So Gad came to David, and said unto
him, Thus saith the LORD, Choose thee
12 Either three years' famine; or three
months to be destroyed before thy foes,
while that the sword of thine enemies
overtaketh *thee*; or else three days the
sword of the LORD, even the pestilence,
in the land, and the [e]angel of the LORD
destroying throughout all the coasts of
Israel. Now therefore advise thyself
what word I shall bring again to him
that sent me.
13 And David said unto Gad, I am in a
great strait: let me fall now into the hand
of the LORD; for very great *are* his mercies:
but let me not fall into the hand of man.
14 So the LORD sent pestilence upon
Israel: and there fell of Israel seventy
thousand men.
15 [f]And God sent an [e]angel unto
Jerusalem to destroy it: and as he was
destroying, the LORD beheld, and he
repented him of the evil, and said to the
angel that destroyed, It is enough, stay
now thine hand. And the angel of the
LORD stood by the threshingfloor of
[g]Ornan the Jebusite.
16 And David lifted up his eyes, and
saw the [e]angel of the LORD stand
between the earth and the heaven, having a drawn sword in his hand stretched
out over Jerusalem. Then David and the
elders *of Israel, who were* clothed in sackcloth, fell upon their faces.
17 And David said unto God, *Is it* not I
that commanded the people to be numbered? even I it is that have sinned and
done evil indeed; but *as for* these sheep,
what have they done? let thine hand, I
pray thee, O LORD my God, be on me,
and on my father's house; but not on thy
people, that they should be plagued.

David buys Ornan's threshingfloor
(2 Sam. 24:18-25).

18 Then the [e]angel of the LORD commanded Gad to say to David, that David
should go up, and set up an altar unto
the LORD in the threshingfloor of Ornan
the Jebusite.
19 And David went up at the saying of
Gad, which he spake in the name of the
LORD.
20 And Ornan turned back, and saw
the [e]angel; and his four sons with him
hid themselves. Now Ornan was threshing wheat.
21 And as David came to Ornan, Ornan
looked and saw David, and went out of
the threshingfloor, and bowed himself to
David with *his* face to the ground.
22 Then David said to Ornan, Grant
me the place of *this* threshingfloor, that I
may build an altar therein unto the
LORD: thou shalt grant it me for the full
price: that the plague may be stayed
from the people.
23 And Ornan said unto David, Take *it*
to thee, and let my lord the king do *that*
which is good in his eyes: lo, I give *thee*
the oxen *also* for burnt-offerings, and the
threshing instruments for wood, and the
wheat for the [h]meat-offering; I give it all.
24 And king David said to Ornan,
Nay; but I will verily buy it for the full
price: for I will not take *that* which *is*
thine for the LORD, nor offer burnt-offerings without cost.
25 So David gave to Ornan for the

B.C. 1017.

a Here should be read 2 Sam. 24:4-9.

b Cf. 2 Sam. 24:9, *note*.

c 1 Sam. 9:9; see 2 Ki. 17:13; 1 Chr. 29:29; 2 Chr. 16:7, 10; Isa. 30:9, 10; Amos 7:12, 13.

d 2 Sam. 24:12-14.

e Heb. 1:4, *note*.

f Cf. 2 Sam. 24:16.

g Called *Araunah*, 2 Sam. 24:16, 18-24.

h Lit. *meal*.

place [1]six hundred [a]shekels of gold by weight.

26 And David built there an altar unto the LORD, and offered burnt-offerings and peace-offerings, and called upon the LORD; and he answered him from heaven by fire upon the altar of burnt-offering.

27 And the LORD commanded the [b]angel; and he put up his sword again into the sheath thereof.

28 At that time when David saw that the LORD had answered him in the threshingfloor of Ornan the Jebusite, then he sacrificed there.

29 [c]For the tabernacle of the LORD, which Moses made in the wilderness, and the altar of the burnt-offering, *were* at that season in the high place at Gibeon.

30 But David could not go before it to enquire of God: for he was afraid because of the sword of the angel of the LORD.

CHAPTER 22.

David prepares material for the temple.

Then David said, [d]This *is* the house of the LORD God, and this *is* the altar of the burnt-offering for Israel.

2 And David commanded to gather together the [e]strangers that *were* in the land of Israel; and he set masons to hew wrought stones to build the house of God.

3 And David prepared iron in abundance for the nails for the doors of the gates, and for the joinings; and brass in abundance without weight;

4 Also cedar trees in abundance: for the Zidonians and they of Tyre brought much cedar wood to David.

5 And David [f]said, Solomon my son *is* young and tender, and the house *that is* to be builded for the LORD *must be* exceeding magnifical, of fame and of glory throughout all countries: I will *therefore* now make preparation for it. So David prepared abundantly before his death.

B.C. 1017.

a One shekel (gold) = £2. 1*s*., or $9.69.

b Heb. 1:4, *note*.

c 1 Chr. 16:37, *note*; 1 Ki. 3:4; 2 Chr. 1:3.

d Deut. 12:5-7; 2 Sam. 24:18-25; 1 Chr. 21:18-28; 2 Chr. 3:1.

e 1 Ki. 9:20, 21; 2 Chr. 2:17-18.

f 1 Chr. 29:1, 2.

g 2 Sam. 7:1, 2.

h 1 Chr. 28:3; 2 Sam. 7:5, 13.

i 1 Ki. 4:25.

j 2 Sam. 7:13.

k 1 Ki. 3:9-12.

He instructs Solomon in God's promises, and his duty in building the temple.

6 Then he called for Solomon his son, and charged him to build an house for the LORD God of Israel.

7 And David said to Solomon, My son, as for me, [g]it was in my mind to build an house unto the name of the LORD my God:

8 But the word of the LORD came to me, [h]saying, Thou hast shed blood abundantly, and hast made great wars: thou shalt not build an house unto my name, because thou hast shed much blood upon the earth in my sight.

9 Behold, a son shall be born to thee, who shall be a man of rest; [i]and I will give him rest from all his enemies round about: for his name shall be Solomon, and I will give peace and quietness unto Israel in his days.

10 [j]He shall build an house for my name; and he shall be my son, and I *will be* his father; and I will establish the throne of his kingdom over Israel for ever.

11 Now, my son, the LORD be with thee; and prosper thou, and build the house of the LORD thy God, as he hath said of thee.

12 Only the LORD give thee [k]wisdom and understanding, and give thee charge concerning Israel, that thou mayest keep the law of the LORD thy God.

13 Then shalt thou prosper, if thou takest heed to fulfil the statutes and judgments which the LORD charged Moses with concerning Israel: be strong, and of good courage; dread not, nor be dismayed.

14 Now, behold, in my trouble I have prepared for the house of the LORD an hundred thousand talents of gold, and a thousand thousand talents of silver; and of brass and iron without weight; for it is in abundance: timber also and stone have I prepared; and thou mayest add thereto.

15 Moreover *there are* workmen with thee in abundance, hewers and worker

[1](21:25) A discrepancy has been imagined in the two accounts, 2 Sam. 24:24, and 1 Chr. 21:25. 2 Sam 24:24 records the price of the *threshingfloor* (Heb. *goren*); 1 Chr. 21:25, of the *place* (Heb. *magom,* li "home," 1 Sam. 2:20, same word) or area on which afterward the great temple, with its spaciou courts, was built (2 Chr. 3:1). David gave fifty shekels of silver for the "goren"; six hundred shekels c gold for the "magom."

of stone and timber, and all manner of
cunning men for every manner of work.
16 Of the gold, the silver, and the
brass, and the iron, *there is* no number.
Arise *therefore*, and be doing, and the
LORD be with thee.

The princes are charged to assist Solomon.

17 David also commanded all the
princes of Israel to help Solomon his son,
saying,
18 *Is* not the LORD your God with you?
and hath he *not* given you rest on every
side? for he hath given the inhabitants of
the land into mine hand; and the land is
subdued before the LORD, and before his
people.
19 Now set your heart and your soul
to seek the LORD your God; arise therefore, and build ye the sanctuary of the
LORD God, to [a]bring the ark of the
covenant of the LORD, and the holy vessels of God, into the house that is to be
built to the name of the LORD.

CHAPTER 23.

David in his old age makes Solomon king.

So when David was old and full of
days, he [b]made Solomon his son
king over Israel.

The number and distribution of the Levites.

2 And he gathered together all the
princes of Israel, with the priests and the
Levites.
3 Now the Levites were numbered
from the [c]age of thirty years and upward:
and their number by their polls, man by
man, was thirty and eight thousand.
4 Of which, twenty and four thousand
were to set forward the work of the
house of the LORD; and six thousand
were officers and [d]judges:
5 Moreover four thousand *were*
porters; and four thousand praised the
LORD with the instruments which [e]I
made, *said David*, to praise *therewith*.
6 And David divided them into courses
among the sons of Levi, *namely*, Gershon,
Kohath, and Merari.

The families of the Gershonites.
(Cf. Num. 3:25, 26.)

7 Of the Gershonites *were*, Laadan,
and Shimei.
8 The sons of Laadan; the chief *was*
Jehiel, and Zetham, and Joel, three.
9 The sons of Shimei; Shelomith, and
Haziel, and Haran, three. These *were* the
chief of the fathers of Laadan.
10 And the sons of Shimei *were*,
Jahath, [f]Zina, and Jeush, and Beriah.
These four *were* the sons of Shimei.
11 And Jahath was the chief, and
Zizah the second: but Jeush and Beriah
had not many sons; therefore they were
in one reckoning, according to *their*
father's house.

The sons of Kohath. (Cf. Num. 3:27-31.)

12 The sons of Kohath; Amram, Izhar,
Hebron, and Uzziel, four.
13 The sons of [g]Amram; Aaron and
Moses: and [h]Aaron was separated, that
he should sanctify the most holy things,
he and his sons for ever, to burn incense
before the LORD, to minister unto him,
and to bless in his name for ever.
14 Now *concerning* Moses the man of
God, his sons were named of the tribe of
Levi.
15 The sons of Moses *were*, Gershom,
and Eliezer.
16 Of the sons of Gershom, Shebuel
was the chief.
17 And the sons of Eliezer *were*,
Rehabiah the chief. And Eliezer had
none other sons; but the sons of
Rehabiah were very many.
18 Of the sons of Izhar; Shelomith the
chief.
19 Of the sons of Hebron; Jeriah the
first, Amariah the second, Jahaziel the
third, and Jekameam the fourth.
20 Of the sons of Uzziel; Michah the
first, and Jesiah the second.

The sons of Merari. (Cf. Num. 3:33-37.)

21 The sons of Merari; Mahli, and
Mushi. The sons of Mahli; Eleazar, and
Kish.
22 And Eleazar died, and had no sons,
but daughters: and their [i]brethren the
sons of Kish took them.
23 The sons of Mushi; Mahli, and
Eder, and Jeremoth, three.

The new office of the Levites.
(Cf. Num. 3:5-12.)

24 These *were* the sons of Levi after the
house of their fathers; *even* the chief of
the fathers, as they were counted by
number of names by their polls, that did

B.C. 1017.

a 1 Ki. 8:1-11; 2 Chr. 5:2-14.

b 1 Ki. 1:33-40; 1 Chr. 28:4, 5.

c Num. 4:1-3.

d Deut. 16:18-20.

e Cf. 2 Chr. 29:25-27.

B.C. 1015.]

f Called *Zizah*, v. 11.

g Ex. 6:18, 20.

h Ex. 28:1; Heb. 5:4.

i i.e. *cousins*.

the work for the service of the house of the LORD, from the age of twenty years and upward.

25 For David said, The LORD God of Israel hath given rest unto his people, that they may dwell in Jerusalem for ever:

26 And also unto the Levites; they shall no *more* carry the tabernacle, nor any vessels of it for the service thereof.

27 For by the last words of David the Levites *were* numbered from twenty years old and above:

28 Because their [a]office *was* to wait on the sons of Aaron for the service of the house of the LORD, in the courts, and in the chambers, and in the purifying of all holy things, and the work of the service of the house of God;

29 Both for the [b]shewbread, and for the fine flour for [c]meat-offering, and for the unleavened cakes, and for *that which is baked in* the pan, and for that which is fried, and for all manner of measure and size;

30 And to stand every morning to thank and praise the LORD, and likewise at even;

31 And to offer all burnt sacrifices unto the LORD in the sabbaths, in the new moons, and on the set feasts, by number, according to the order commanded unto them, continually before the LORD:

32 And that they should keep the charge of the tabernacle of the congregation, and the charge of the holy *place*, and the charge of the sons of Aaron their brethren, in the service of the house of the LORD.

CHAPTER 24.

The divisions of the sons of Aaron by lot into four and twenty orders.

NOW *these are* the divisions of the sons of Aaron. The [d]sons of Aaron; Nadab, and Abihu, Eleazar, and Ithamar.

2 [e]But Nadab and Abihu died before their father, and had no children: therefore Eleazar and Ithamar executed the priest's office.

3 And David distributed them, both Zadok of the sons of Eleazar, and Ahimelech of the sons of Ithamar, according to their offices in their service.

4 And there were more chief men found of the sons of Eleazar than of the sons of Ithamar; and *thus* were they divided. Among the sons of Eleazar *there were* sixteen chief men of the house of *their* fathers, and eight among the sons of Ithamar according to the house of their fathers.

The four and twenty orders.

5 Thus were they divided by lot, one sort with another; for the governors of the sanctuary, and governors *of the house* of God, were of the sons of Eleazar, and of the sons of Ithamar.

6 And Shemaiah the son of Nethaneel the scribe, *one* of the Levites, wrote them before the king, and the princes, and Zadok the priest, and Ahimelech the son of Abiathar, and *before* the chief of the fathers of the priests and Levites: one principal household being taken for Eleazar, and *one* taken for Ithamar.

7 Now the first lot came forth to Jehoiarib, the second to Jedaiah,

8 The third to Harim, the fourth to Seorim,

9 The fifth to Malchijah, the sixth to Mijamin,

10 The seventh to Hakkoz, the eighth to [f]Abijah,

11 The ninth to Jeshua, the tenth to Shecaniah,

12 The eleventh to Eliashib, the twelfth to Jakim,

13 The thirteenth to Huppah, the fourteenth to Jeshebeab,

14 The fifteenth to Bilgah, the sixteenth to Immer,

15 The seventeenth to Hezir, the eighteenth to Aphses,

16 The nineteenth to Pethahiah, the twentieth to Jehezekel,

17 The one and twentieth to Jachin, the two and twentieth to Gamul,

18 The three and twentieth to Delaiah, the four and twentieth to Maaziah.

19 These *were* the orderings of them in their service to come into the house of the LORD, according to their manner, under Aaron their father, as the LORD God of Israel had commanded him.

The Kohathites divided.

20 And the rest of the sons of Levi *were these*: Of the sons of Amram; Shubael: of the sons of [g]Shubael; Jehdeiah.

21 Concerning Rehabiah: of the sons of Rehabiah, the first *was* Isshiah.

22 Of the Izharites; Shelomoth: of the sons of Shelomoth; Jahath.

B.C. 1015.

a i.e. their *new* office, since their former office of bearing the tabernacle was ended.

b Ex. 25:30, *note.*

c Lit. *meal.*

d Lev. 10:1-6; Num. 26:60, 61; 1 Chr. 6:3.

e Num. 3:1-4; 26:60, 61.

f Lk. 1:5.

g Called *Shebuel,* 1 Chr. 23:16.

23 And the sons *of Hebron*; Jeriah *the first*, Amariah the second, Jahaziel the third, Jekameam the fourth.

24 *Of* the sons of Uzziel; Michah: of the sons of Michah; Shamir.

25 The brother of Michah *was* Isshiah: of the sons of Isshiah; Zechariah.

And the Merarites divided by lot.

26 The sons of Merari *were* Mahli and Mushi: the sons of Jaaziah; Beno.

27 The sons of Merari by Jaaziah; Beno, and Shoham, and Zaccur, and Ibri.

28 Of Mahli *came* Eleazar, who had no sons.

29 Concerning Kish: the son of Kish *was* Jerahmeel.

30 The sons also of Mushi; Mahli, and Eder, and Jerimoth. These *were* the sons of the Levites after the house of their fathers.

31 These likewise cast lots over against their brethren the sons of Aaron in the presence of David the king, and Zadok, and Ahimelech, and the chief of the fathers of the priests and Levites, even the principal fathers over against their younger brethren.

CHAPTER 25.

The number and offices of the singers.

Moreover David and the captains of the host separated to the service of the sons of Asaph, and of Heman, and of Jeduthun, who should prophesy with harps, with psalteries, and with cymbals: and the number of the workmen according to their service was:

2 Of the sons of Asaph; Zaccur, and Joseph, and Nethaniah, and Asarelah, the sons of Asaph under the hands of Asaph, which prophesied according to the order of the king.

3 Of Jeduthun: the sons of Jeduthun; Gedaliah, and Zeri, and Jeshaiah, Hashabiah, and Mattithiah, six, under the hands of their father Jeduthun, who prophesied with a harp, to give thanks and to praise the LORD.

4 Of Heman: the sons of Heman; Bukkiah, Mattaniah, Uzziel, Shebuel, and Jerimoth, Hananiah, Hanani, Eliathah, Giddalti, and Romamti-ezer, Joshbekashah, Mallothi, Hothir, *and* Mahazioth:

B.C. 1015.

5 All these *were* the sons of Heman the king's seer in the words of God, to lift up the horn. And God gave to Heman fourteen sons and three daughters.

6 All these *were* under the hands of their father for song *in* the house of the LORD, with cymbals, psalteries, and harps, for the service of the house of God, according to the king's order to Asaph, Jeduthun, and Heman.

7 So the number of them, with their brethren that were instructed in the songs of the LORD, *even* all that were cunning, was two hundred fourscore and eight.

Their division by lot into four and twenty orders.

8 And they cast lots, ward against *ward*, as well the small as the great, the teacher as the scholar.

9 Now the first lot came forth for Asaph to Joseph: the second to Gedaliah, who with his brethren and sons *were* twelve:

10 The third to Zaccur, *he*, his sons, and his brethren, *were* twelve:

11 The fourth to Izri, *he*, his sons, and his brethren, *were* twelve:

12 The fifth to Nethaniah, *he*, his sons, and his brethren, *were* twelve:

13 The sixth to Bukkiah, *he*, his sons, and his brethren, *were* twelve:

14 The seventh to Jesharelah, *he*, his sons, and his brethren, *were* twelve:

15 The eighth to Jeshaiah, *he*, his sons, and his brethren, *were* twelve:

16 The ninth to Mattaniah, *he*, his sons, and his brethren, *were* twelve:

17 The tenth to Shimei, *he*, his sons, and his brethren, *were* twelve:

18 The eleventh to Azareel, *he*, his sons, and his brethren, *were* twelve:

19 The twelfth to Hashabiah, *he*, his sons, and his brethren, *were* twelve:

20 The thirteenth to Shubael, *he*, his sons, and his brethren, *were* twelve:

21 The fourteenth to Mattithiah, *he*, his sons, and his brethren, *were* twelve:

22 The fifteenth to Jeremoth, *he*, his sons, and his brethren, *were* twelve:

23 The sixteenth to Hananiah, *he*, his sons, and his brethren, *were* twelve:

24 The seventeenth to Joshbekashah, *he*, his sons, and his brethren, *were* twelve:

25 The eighteenth to Hanani, *he*, his sons, and his brethren, *were* twelve:

26 The nineteenth to Mallothi, *he*, his sons, and his brethren, *were* twelve:

27 The twentieth to Eliathah, *he*, his sons, and his brethren, *were* twelve:

28 The one and twentieth to Hothir, *he*, his sons, and his brethren, *were* twelve:

29 The two and twentieth to Giddalti, *he*, his sons, and his brethren, *were* twelve:

30 The three and twentieth to Mahazioth, *he*, his sons, and his brethren, *were* twelve:

31 The four and twentieth to Romamti-ezer, *he*, his sons, and his brethren, *were* twelve.

CHAPTER 26.

The division of the porters.

Concerning the divisions of the porters: Of the Korhites *was* Meshelemiah the son of Kore, of the sons of Asaph.

B.C. 1015.

2 And the sons of Meshelemiah *were*, Zechariah the firstborn, Jediael the second, Zebadiah the third, Jathniel the fourth,

3 Elam the fifth, Jehohanan the sixth, Elioenai the seventh.

4 Moreover the sons of Obed-edom *were*, Shemaiah the firstborn, Jehozabad the second, Joah the third, and Sacar the fourth, and Nethaneel the fifth,

5 Ammiel the sixth, Issachar the seventh, Peulthai the eighth: for God blessed him.

6 Also unto Shemaiah his son were sons born, that ruled throughout the house of their father: for they *were* mighty men of valour.

7 The sons of Shemaiah; Othni, and Rephael, and Obed, Elzabad, whose brethren *were* strong men, Elihu, and Semachiah.

8 All these of the sons of Obed-edom: they and their sons and their brethren, able men for strength for the service, *were* threescore and two of Obed-edom.

9 And Meshelemiah had sons and brethren, strong men, eighteen.

10 Also Hosah, of the children of Merari, had sons; Simri the chief, (for *though* he was not the firstborn, yet his father made him the chief;)

11 Hilkiah the second, Tebaliah the third, Zechariah the fourth: all the sons and brethren of Hosah *were* thirteen.

12 Among these *were* the divisions of the porters, *even* among the chief men, *having* wards one against another, to minister in the house of the LORD.

The gates assigned by lot.

13 And they cast lots, as well the small as the great, according to the house of their fathers, for every gate.

14 And the lot eastward fell to Shelemiah. Then for Zechariah his son, a wise counsellor, they cast lots; and his lot came out northward.

15 To Obed-edom southward; and to his sons the house of Asuppim.

16 To Shuppim and Hosah *the lot came forth* westward, with the gate Shallecheth, by the causeway of the going up, ward against ward.

17 Eastward *were* six Levites, northward four a day, southward four a day, and toward Asuppim two *and* two.

18 At Parbar westward, four at the causeway, *and* two at Parbar.

19 These *are* the divisions of the porters among the sons of Kore, and among the sons of Merari.

The Levites that had charge of the treasures.

20 And of the Levites, Ahijah *was* over the treasures of the house of God, and over the treasures of the dedicated things.

21 *As concerning* the sons of Laadan, the sons of the Gershonite Laadan, chief fathers, *even* of Laadan the Gershonite, *were* Jehieli.

22 The sons of Jehieli; Zetham, and Joel his brother, *which were* over the treasures of the house of the LORD.

23 Of the Amramites, *and* the Izharites, the Hebronites, *and* the Uzzielites:

24 And Shebuel the son of Gershom, the son of Moses, *was* ruler of the treasures.

25 And his brethren by Eliezer Rehabiah his son, and Jeshaiah his son and Joram his son, and Zichri his son and Shelomith his son.

26 Which Shelomith and his brethren *were* over all the treasures of the dedicated things, which David the king, and the chief fathers, the captains over thousands and hundreds, and the captains of the host, had dedicated.

B.C. 1015.

27 Out of the spoils won in battles did they dedicate to maintain the house of the LORD.

28 And all that Samuel the seer, and Saul the son of Kish, and Abner the son of Ner, and Joab the son of Zeruiah, had dedicated; *and* whosoever had dedicated *any thing, it was* under the hand of Shelomith, and of his brethren.

Officers and judges.

29 Of the Izharites, Chenaniah and his sons *were* for the outward business over Israel, for officers and judges.

30 *And* of the Hebronites, Hashabiah and his brethren, men of valour, a thousand and seven hundred, *were* officers among them of Israel on this side Jordan westward in all the business of the LORD, and in the service of the king.

31 Among the Hebronites *was* Jerijah the chief, *even* among the Hebronites, according to the generations of his fathers. In the fortieth year of the reign of David they were sought for, and there were found among them mighty men of valour at Jazer of Gilead.

32 And his brethren, men of valour, *were* two thousand and seven hundred chief fathers, whom king David made rulers over the Reubenites, the Gadites, and the half tribe of Manasseh, for every matter pertaining to God, and affairs of the king.

CHAPTER 27.

The twelve captains for every several month.

Now the children of Israel after their number, *to wit*, the chief fathers and captains of thousands and hundreds, and their officers that served the king in any matter of the courses, which came in and went out month by month throughout all the months of the year, of every course *were* twenty and four thousand.

2 Over the first course for the [a]first month *was* Jashobeam the son of Zabdiel: and in his course *were* twenty and four thousand.

3 Of the children of Perez *was* the chief of all the captains of the host for the first month.

4 And over the course of the [b]second month *was* Dodai an Ahohite, and of his course *was* Mikloth also the ruler: in his course likewise *were* twenty and four thousand.

5 The third captain of the host for the [c]third month *was* Benaiah the son of Jehoiada, a chief priest: and in his course *were* twenty and four thousand.

6 This *is that* Benaiah, *who was* mighty *among* the thirty, and above the thirty: and in his course *was* Ammizabad his son.

7 The fourth *captain* for the [d]fourth month *was* Asahel the brother of Joab, and Zebadiah his son after him: and in his course *were* twenty and four thousand.

8 The fifth captain for the [e]fifth month *was* Shamhuth the Izrahite: and in his course *were* twenty and four thousand.

9 The sixth *captain* for the [f]sixth month *was* Ira the son of Ikkesh the Tekoite: and in his course *were* twenty and four thousand.

10 The seventh *captain* for the [g]seventh month *was* Helez the Pelonite, of the children of Ephraim: and in his course *were* twenty and four thousand.

11 The eighth *captain* for the [h]eighth month *was* Sibbecai the Hushathite, of the Zarhites: and in his course *were* twenty and four thousand.

12 The ninth *captain* for the [i]ninth month *was* Abi-ezer the Anetothite, of the Benjamites: and in his course *were* twenty and four thousand.

13 The tenth *captain* for the [j]tenth month *was* Maharai the Netophathite, of the Zarhites: and in his course *were* twenty and four thousand.

14 The eleventh *captain* for the [k]eleventh month *was* Benaiah the Pirathonite, of the children of Ephraim: and in his course *were* twenty and four thousand.

15 The twelfth *captain* for the [l]twelfth month *was* Heldai the Netophathite, of Othniel: and in his course *were* twenty and four thousand.

The princes of the twelve tribes.

16 Furthermore over the tribes of Israel: the ruler of the Reubenites *was* Eliezer the son of Zichri: of the Simeonites, Shephatiah the son of Maachah:

17 Of the Levites, Hashabiah the son of Kemuel: of the Aaronites, Zadok:

18 Of Judah, Elihu, *one* of the brethren of David: of Issachar, Omri the son of Michael:

19 Of Zebulun, Ishmaiah the son of

a i.e. *April;* also v. 3.
b i.e. *May.*
c i.e. *June.*
d i.e. *July.*
e i.e. *August.*
f i.e. *September.*
g i.e. *October.*
h i.e. *November.*
i i.e. *December.*
j i.e. *January.*
k i.e. *February.*
l i.e. *March.*

Obadiah: of Naphtali, Jerimoth the son
of Azriel:
20 Of the children of Ephraim, Hoshea
the son of Azaziah: of the half tribe of
Manasseh, Joel the son of Pedaiah:
21 Of the half *tribe* of Manasseh in
Gilead, Iddo the son of Zechariah: of
Benjamin, Jaasiel the son of Abner:
22 Of Dan, Azareel the son of Jeroham.
These *were* the princes of the tribes of
Israel.

The numbering of the people is hindered.

23 But David took not the number of
them from twenty years old and under:
because the LORD had said he would
increase Israel like to the stars of the
heavens.
24 Joab the son of Zeruiah began to
number, but he finished not, because
there fell wrath for it against Israel; neither was the number put in the account
of the chronicles of king David.

David's several officers.

25 And over the king's treasures *was*
Azmaveth the son of Adiel: and over the
storehouses in the fields, in the cities,
and in the villages, and in the castles,
was Jehonathan the son of Uzziah:
26 And over them that did the work of
the field for tillage of the ground *was*
Ezri the son of Chelub:
27 And over the vineyards *was* Shimei
the Ramathite: over the increase of the
vineyards for the wine cellars *was* Zabdi
the Shiphmite:
28 And over the olive trees and the
sycomore trees that *were* in the low
plains *was* Baal-hanan the Gederite: and
over the cellars of oil *was* Joash:
29 And over the herds that fed in
Sharon *was* Shitrai the Sharonite: and
over the herds *that were* in the valleys
was Shaphat the son of Adlai:
30 Over the camels also *was* Obil the
Ishmaelite: and over the asses *was*
Jehdeiah the Meronothite:
31 And over the flocks *was* Jaziz the
Hagerite. All these *were* the rulers of the
substance which *was* king David's.
32 Also Jonathan David's uncle was a
counsellor, a wise man, and a scribe: and
Jehiel the son of Hachmoni *was* with the
king's sons:
33 And Ahithophel *was* the king's

B.C. 1015.

a 1 Chr. 27:16-22.
b 1 Chr. 27:1-15.
c 1 Chr. 27:25-31.
d 1 Chr. 11:10; 2 Sam. 23:8-39.
e 2 Sam. 7:2, and *refs.*
f Psa. 99:5.
g 2 Sam. 7:5, 13.
h 1 Sam. 16:7-13.
i Gen. 49:8, 10; Psa. 60:7.
j 1 Sam. 13:14; Acts 13:22.
k 1 Chr. 22:9.
l 1 Chr. 22:9, 10; 2 Sam. 7:13, 14; 2 Chr. 1:9.

counsellor: and Hushai the Archite *was*
the king's companion:
34 And after Ahithophel *was* Jehoiada
the son of Benaiah, and Abiathar: and
the general of the king's army *was* Joab.

CHAPTER 28.

David in a solemn assembly gives counsel to Israel and to Solomon.

And David assembled all the [a]princes
of Israel, the princes of the tribes,
and the [b]captains of the companies that
ministered to the king by course, and the
captains over the thousands, and captains over the hundreds, and the [c]stew-
ards over all the substance and possession of the king, and of his sons, with the
officers, and with the [d]mighty men, and
with all the valiant men, unto Jerusalem.
2 Then David the king stood up upon
his feet, and said, Hear me, my brethren,
and my people: *As for me,* I *had* in mine
heart [e]to build an house of rest for the
ark of the covenant of the LORD, and for
the [f]footstool of our God, and had made
ready for the building:
3 But God [g]said unto me, Thou shalt
not build an house for my name,
because thou *hast been* a man of war, and
hast shed blood.
4 Howbeit the LORD God of Israel chose
me [h]before all the house of my father to
be king over Israel for ever: for he hath
chosen [i]Judah *to be* the ruler; and of the
house of Judah, the house of my father;
and among the sons of my father he
[j]liked me to make *me* king over all Israel:
5 And of all my sons, (for the LORD hath
given me many sons,) he hath chosen
[k]Solomon my son to sit upon the throne
of the kingdom of the LORD over Israel.
6 [l]And he said unto me, Solomon thy
son, he shall build my house and my
courts: for I have chosen him *to be* my
son, and I will be his father.
7 Moreover I will establish his kingdom for ever, if he be constant to do my
commandments and my judgments, as
at this day.
8 Now therefore in the sight of all
Israel the congregation of the LORD, and
in the audience of our God, keep and
seek for all the commandments of the
LORD your God: that ye may possess this

good land, and leave *it* for an inheritance
for your children after you for ever.
9 And thou, Solomon my son, know
thou the God of thy father, and serve
him with a [a]perfect heart and with a
willing mind: for the LORD searcheth all
hearts, and understandeth all the imaginations of the thoughts: if thou seek him,
he will be found of thee; but if thou forsake him, he will cast thee off for ever.
10 Take heed now; for the LORD hath
chosen thee to build an house for the
sanctuary: be strong, and do *it*.

He gives him patterns for the form,
and gold and silver for the materials.

11 Then David gave to Solomon his
son the pattern of the porch, and of the
houses thereof, and of the treasuries
thereof, and of the upper chambers
thereof, and of the inner parlours thereof, and of the place of the mercy seat,
12 And the pattern of all that he had
by the [b]spirit, of the courts of the house
of the LORD, and of all the chambers
round about, of the treasuries of the
house of God, and of the treasuries of
the dedicated things:
13 Also for the courses of the priests
and the Levites, and for all the work of
the service of the house of the LORD, and
for all the vessels of service in the house
of the LORD.
14 *He gave* of gold by weight for *things*
of gold, for all instruments of all manner
of service; *silver also* for all instruments
of silver by weight, for all instruments of
every kind of service:
15 Even the weight for the candlesticks
of gold, and for their lamps of gold, by
weight for every candlestick, and for the
lamps thereof: and for the candlesticks of
silver by weight, *both* for the candlestick,
and *also* for the lamps thereof, according
to the use of every candlestick.
16 And by weight *he gave* gold for the
tables of [c]shewbread, for every table;
and *likewise* silver for the tables of silver:
17 Also pure gold for the fleshhooks,
and the bowls, and the cups: and for the
golden basons *he gave gold* by weight for
every bason; and *likewise silver* by weight
for every bason of silver:
18 And for the altar of incense refined
gold by weight; and gold for the pattern
of the chariot of the cherubims, that
spread out *their wings*, and covered the
ark of the covenant of the LORD.
19 [d]All *this, said David*, the LORD made
me understand in writing by *his* hand
upon me, *even* all the works of this pattern.

David encourages Solomon
to build the temple.

20 And David said to Solomon his son,
[e]Be strong and of good courage, and do
it: fear not, nor be dismayed: for the
LORD God, *even* my God, *will be* with
thee; [f]he will not fail thee, nor forsake
thee, until thou hast finished all the work
for the service of the house of the LORD.
21 And, behold, the courses of the
priests and the Levites, *even they shall be*
with thee for all the service of the house
of God: and *there shall be* with thee for all
manner of workmanship every willing
skilful man, for any manner of service:
also the princes and all the people *will be*
wholly at thy commandment.

CHAPTER 29.

David exhorts the people.

Furthermore David the king said unto
all the congregation, Solomon my
son, whom alone God hath chosen, *is yet*
[g]young and tender, and the work *is*
great: for the palace *is* not for man, but
for the LORD God.
2 Now I have prepared with all my
might for the house of my God the gold
for *things to be made* of gold, and the silver for *things* of silver, and the brass for
things of brass, the iron for *things* of iron,
and wood for *things* of wood; onyx
stones, and *stones* to be set, glistering
stones, and of divers colours, and all
manner of precious stones, and marble
stones in abundance.
3 Moreover, because I have set my
affection to the house of my God, I have
of mine own proper good, of gold and
silver, *which* I have given to the house of
my God, over and above all that I have
prepared for the holy house,
4 *Even* three thousand [h]talents of gold,
of the gold of Ophir, and seven thousand [i]talents of refined silver, to overlay
the walls of the houses *withal*:

B.C. 1015.

a See 1 Ki. 8:61.
b *Holy Spirit.* 2 Chr. 15:1. (Gen. 1:2; Mal. 2:15.)
c Ex. 25:30, *note.*
d Cf. Ex. 25:40.
e 1 Chr. 22:13; Deut. 31:7, 8; Josh. 1:6-9.
f Cf. Josh. 1:5.
g 1 Chr. 22:5; 1 Ki. 3:7.
h One talent (gold) = £6150, or $29,085.
i One talent (silver) = £410, or $1940; also v. 7.

5 The gold for *things* of gold, and the
silver for *things* of silver, and for all manner of work *to be made* by the hands of
artificers. And who *then* is willing to consecrate his service this day unto the LORD?

The princes and people offer willingly.

6 Then the chief of the fathers and
princes of the tribes of Israel, and the
captains of thousands and of hundreds,
with the rulers of the king's work,
offered willingly,
7 And gave for the service of the
house of God of gold five thousand talents and ten thousand [a]drams, and of
silver ten thousand talents, and of brass
eighteen thousand talents, and one hundred thousand talents of iron.
8 And they with whom *precious* stones
were found gave *them* to the treasure of
the house of the LORD, by the hand of
Jehiel the Gershonite.
9 Then the people rejoiced, for that
they offered [b]willingly, because with
[c]perfect heart they offered willingly to
the LORD: and David the king also
rejoiced with great joy.

David's thanksgiving and prayer.

10 Wherefore David [d]blessed the LORD
before all the congregation: and David
[e]said, Blessed *be* thou, LORD God of
Israel our father, for ever and ever.
11 [f]Thine, O LORD, *is* the greatness,
and the power, and the glory, and the
victory, and the majesty: for all *that is* in
the heaven and in the earth *is thine*; thine
is the kingdom, O LORD, and thou art
exalted as head above all.
12 Both riches and honour *come* of
thee, and thou reignest over all; and in
thine hand *is* power and might; and in
thine hand *it is* to make great, and to
give strength unto all.
13 Now therefore, our God, we thank
thee, and praise thy glorious name.
14 But who *am* I, and what *is* my people, that we should be able to offer so
willingly after this sort? for all things
come of thee, and of thine own have we
given thee.
15 [g]For we *are* strangers before thee,
and sojourners, as *were* all our fathers:
our days on the earth *are* as a shadow,
and *there is* none abiding.
16 O LORD our God, all this store that
we have prepared to build thee an house
for thine holy name *cometh* of thine
hand, and *is* all thine own.
17 I know also, my God, that thou triest
the heart, and hast pleasure in [h]upright-
ness. As for me, in the uprightness of
mine heart I have willingly offered all
these things: and now have I seen with
joy thy people, which are present here, to
offer willingly unto thee.
18 O LORD God of Abraham, Isaac,
and of Israel, our fathers, keep this for
ever in the imagination of the thoughts
of the heart of thy people, and prepare
their heart unto thee:
19 And give unto Solomon my son a
[i]perfect heart, to keep thy commandments, thy testimonies, and thy statutes,
and to do all *these things*, and to build
the palace, *for* the which I have made
provision.

The people, having blessed God and sacrificed, make Solomon king.

20 And David said to all the congregation, Now bless the LORD your God. And
all the congregation blessed the LORD
God of their fathers, and bowed down
their heads, and worshipped the LORD,
and the king.
21 And they sacrificed sacrifices unto
the LORD, and offered burnt-offerings
unto the LORD, on the morrow after that
day, *even* a thousand bullocks, a thousand rams, *and* a thousand lambs, with
their drink-offerings, and sacrifices in
abundance for all Israel:
22 And did eat and drink before the
LORD on that day with great gladness.
And they made Solomon the son of
David king the [j]second time, and anointed *him* unto the LORD *to be* the chief governor, and Zadok *to be* priest.

Accession of Solomon (1 Ki. 2:12).

23 Then Solomon sat on the throne of
the LORD as king instead of David his
father, and prospered; and all Israel
obeyed him.
24 And all the princes, and the mighty
men, and all the sons likewise of king
David, submitted themselves unto
Solomon the king.
25 And the LORD magnified Solomon
exceedingly in the sight of all Israel, and
bestowed upon him *such* royal majesty

B.C. 1015.

a One dram = £1. 1*s*., or $4.97.

b Cf. Ex. 25:2; 2 Cor. 8:12; 9:7.

c See 1 Ki. 8:61.

d Note the order: giving, vs. 3-8; joy, v. 9; blessing, v. 10; prayer, vs. 11-19; worship, v. 20.

e *Bible prayers* (O.T.). 2 Chr. 6:14. (Gen. 15:2; Hab. 3:1-16.)

f Mt. 6:31; 1 Tim. 1:17; Rev. 5:13.

g Psa. 39:12; Heb. 11:13, 14; 1 Pet. 2:11, 12.

h Trans. *a straight way*, Jer. 31:9.

i See 1 Ki. 8:61 *ref.*

j Cf. 1 Sam. 10:1; 1 Ki. 1:32-35.

as had not been on any king before him
in Israel.
26 Thus David the son of Jesse reigned
over all Israel.

Reign and death of David (1 Ki. 2:11, 12).

27 And the time that he reigned over
Israel *was* forty years; seven years
reigned he in [a]Hebron, and thirty and
three *years* reigned he in Jerusalem.
28 [b]And he died in a good old age,
full of days, riches, and honour: and
Solomon his son reigned in his stead.
29 Now the acts of David the king,
first and last, behold, they *are* written in
the book of Samuel the seer, and in the
[c]book of Nathan the prophet, and in the
book of Gad the seer,
30 With all his reign and his might,
and the times that went over him, and
over Israel, and over all the kingdoms of
the countries.

B.C. 1015.

a 2 Sam. 5:5.

b Cf. 1 Sam. 27:1.

c These books have perished.

THE SECOND BOOK OF THE

CHRONICLES

THIS book continues the history begun in First Chronicles. It falls into eighteen divisions, by reigns, from Solomon to the captivities; records the division of the kingdom of David under Jeroboam and Rehoboam, and is marked by an ever growing apostasy, broken temporarily by reformations under Asa, 14–16; Jehoshaphat, 17:1-19; Joash, 24; Hezekiah, 29–32; and Josiah, 34, 35. But the religious state of the people, even at the best, is described in Isaiah 1–5.

The events recorded in Second Chronicles cover a period of 427 years (Ussher).

CHAPTER 1.

B.C. 1015.

Solomon established in his kingdom.

And [a]Solomon the son of David was
strengthened in his kingdom, and
the LORD his God *was* with him, and
[b]magnified him exceedingly.

Solomon sacrifices at Gibeon (1 Ki. 3:4).

2 Then Solomon spake unto all Israel,
to the [c]captains of thousands and of
hundreds, and to the judges, and to
every governor in all Israel, the chief of
the fathers.
3 So Solomon, and all the congregation with him, went to the high place
that *was* at Gibeon; for [d]there was the
tabernacle of the congregation of God,
which Moses the servant of the LORD
had made in the wilderness.
4 But the [e]ark of God had David
brought up from Kirjath-jearim to *the*
place which David had prepared for it: for
he had pitched a tent for it at Jerusalem.
5 Moreover the [f]brasen altar, that
Bezaleel the son of Uri, the son of Hur,
had made, he put before the tabernacle
of the LORD: and Solomon and the congregation sought unto it.
6 And Solomon went up thither to the
brasen altar before the LORD, which *was*
at the tabernacle of the congregation,
and offered a [g]thousand burnt-offerings
upon it.

Solomon's vision of God, and prayer for wisdom (1 Ki. 3:5-15).

7 In that night did God [h]appear unto
Solomon, and said unto him, Ask what I
shall give thee.
8 And Solomon said unto God, Thou
hast shewed great mercy unto David my
father, and hast made me to reign in his
stead.

a 1 Ki. 2:46.
b 1 Chr. 29:23-25.
c 1 Chr. 27:1-34.
d 1 Chr. 16:37, *note.*
e Ex. 25:10-22; 37:1-9; 2 Sam. 6:2-17; 1 Chr. 15:25-16:2.
f Ex. 27:1, 2.
g 1 Ki. 3:4.
h 1 Ki. 3:5-15.
i 2 Sam. 7:8-16.
j Cf. 1 Ki. 10:26-29; 2 Chr. 9:25-28.

9 Now, O LORD God, let thy [i]promise
unto David my father be established: for
thou hast made me king over a people
like the dust of the earth in multitude.
10 Give me now wisdom and knowledge, that I may go out and come in
before this people: for who can judge
this thy people, *that is so* great?
11 And God said to Solomon, Because
this was in thine heart, and thou hast not
asked riches, wealth, or honour, nor the
life of thine enemies, neither yet hast
asked long life; but hast asked wisdom
and knowledge for thyself, that thou
mayest judge my people, over whom I
have made thee king:
12 Wisdom and knowledge *is* granted
unto thee; and I will give thee riches,
and wealth, and honour, such as none of
the kings have had that *have been* before
thee, neither shall there any after thee
have the like.
13 Then Solomon came *from his journey*
to the high place that *was* at Gibeon to
Jerusalem, from before the tabernacle of
the congregation, and reigned over Israel.
14 And [j]Solomon gathered chariots
and horsemen: and he had a thousand
and four hundred chariots, and twelve
thousand horsemen, which he placed in
the chariot cities, and with the king at
Jerusalem.
15 And the king made silver and gold
at Jerusalem *as plenteous* as stones, and
cedar trees made he as the sycomore
trees that *are* in the vale for abundance.
16 And Solomon had horses brought out
of Egypt, and linen yarn: the king's merchants received the linen yarn at a price.

17 And they fetched up, and brought
forth out of Egypt a chariot for six hundred *shekels* of silver, and an horse for an
hundred and fifty: and so brought they
out *horses* for all the kings of the Hittites,
and for the kings of Syria, by their means.

CHAPTER 2.

Solomon prepares to build the temple
(1 Ki. 5:1-18).

And Solomon determined to build an
house for the name of the LORD,
and an house for his kingdom.
2 And [a]Solomon told out threescore
and ten thousand men to bear burdens,
and fourscore thousand to hew in the
mountain, and three thousand and six
hundred to oversee them.
3 And Solomon sent to [b]Huram the
king of Tyre, saying, As thou didst deal
with David my father, and didst send
him cedars to build him an house to
dwell therein, *even so deal with me*.
4 Behold, I build an house to the name
of the LORD my God, to [c]dedicate *it* to
him, *and* to burn before him sweet
incense, and for the continual [d]shew-
bread, and for the burnt-offerings morning and evening, on the sabbaths, and on
the new moons, and on the solemn
feasts of the LORD our God. This *is an*
ordinance for ever to Israel.
5 And the house which I build *is* great:
for great *is* our God above all gods.
6 But who is able to build him an
house, seeing the heaven and heaven of
heavens cannot contain him? who *am* I
then, that I should build him an house,
save only to burn sacrifice before him?
7 Send me now therefore a man cunning to work in gold, and in silver, and
in brass, and in iron, and in purple, and
crimson, and blue, and that can skill to
grave with the cunning men that *are*
with me in Judah and in Jerusalem,
whom David my father did provide.
8 Send me also cedar trees, fir trees,
and algum trees, out of Lebanon: for I
know that thy servants can skill to cut
timber in Lebanon; and, behold, my servants *shall be* with thy servants,
9 Even to prepare me timber in abundance: for the house which I am about to
build *shall be* wonderful great.
10 And, behold, I will give to thy servants, the hewers that cut timber, twenty
thousand [e]measures of beaten wheat,
and twenty thousand measures of barley, and twenty thousand [f]baths of wine,
and twenty thousand baths of oil.
11 Then Huram the king of Tyre
answered in writing, which he sent to
Solomon, Because the LORD hath loved
his people, he hath made thee king over
them.
12 Huram said moreover, Blessed *be*
the LORD God of Israel, that made heav-
en and earth, who hath given to David
the king a wise son, endued with prudence and understanding, that might
build an house for the LORD, and an
house for his kingdom.
13 And now I have sent a cunning
man, endued with understanding, of
Huram my father's,
14 The son of a woman of the daughters of Dan, and his father *was* a man of
Tyre, skilful to work in gold, and in silver, in brass, in iron, in stone, and in timber, in purple, in blue, and in fine linen,
and in crimson; also to grave any manner of graving, and to find out every
device which shall be put to him, with
thy cunning men, and with the cunning
men of my lord David thy father.
15 Now therefore the wheat, and the
barley, the oil, and the wine, which my
lord hath spoken of, let him send unto
his servants:
16 And we will cut wood out of
Lebanon, as much as thou shalt need:
and we will bring it to thee in floats by
sea to Joppa; and thou shalt carry it up
to Jerusalem.
17 And [g]Solomon numbered all the
strangers that *were* in the land of Israel,
after the numbering wherewith David
his father had numbered them; and they
were found an hundred and fifty thousand and three thousand and six hundred.
18 And he set threescore and ten thousand of them *to be* bearers of burdens,
and fourscore thousand *to be* hewers in
the mountain, and three thousand and
six hundred overseers to set the people a
work.

CHAPTER 3.

Solomon begins to build the temple
(1 Ki. 6:1, *note*).

Then Solomon began to build the
house of the LORD at Jerusalem in
mount [h]Moriah, where *the* LORD

B.C. 1015.

a Cf. 1 Ki. 5:13-18.

b Called *Hiram*, 1 Ki. 5:1.

c *Sanctify, holy* (O.T.). 2 Chr. 5:1. (Gen. 2:3; Zech. 8:3.)

d Ex. 25:30, *note*.

e One measure = about 10 bu.

f One bath = about 8 gals.

g Cf. 1 Ki. 5:13-18.

h Gen. 22:2-14; 1 Chr. 21:18-24.

B.C. 1012.

appeared unto David his father, in the place that David had prepared in the threshingfloor of Ornan the Jebusite.

2 And he began to build in the second *day* of the [a]second month, in the fourth year of his reign.

Dimensions and materials of the temple
(1 Ki. 6:2–7:51).

3 Now these *are the things wherein* Solomon was [b]instructed for the building of the house of God. The length by [c]cubits after the first measure *was* threescore cubits, and the breadth twenty cubits.

4 And the [d]porch that *was* in the front *of the house*, the length *of it was* according to the breadth of the house, twenty cubits, and the height *was* an hundred and twenty: and he overlaid it within with pure gold.

5 And the [e]greater house he cieled with fir tree, which he overlaid with fine gold, and set thereon palm trees and chains.

6 And he [f]garnished the house with precious stones for beauty: and the gold *was* gold of Parvaim.

7 He overlaid also the house, the beams, the posts, and the walls thereof, and the doors thereof, with gold; and graved cherubims on the walls.

8 And he made the most holy house, the length whereof *was* according to the breadth of the house, twenty cubits, and the breadth thereof twenty cubits: and he overlaid it with fine gold, *amounting* to six hundred [g]talents.

9 And the weight of the nails *was* fifty shekels of gold. And he overlaid the upper chambers with gold.

10 And in the most holy house he made two cherubims of image work, and [h]overlaid them with gold.

11 And the wings of the cherubims *were* twenty cubits long: one wing *of the one cherub was* five cubits, reaching to the wall of the house: and the other wing *was likewise* five cubits, reaching to the wing of the other cherub.

12 And *one* wing of the other cherub *was* five cubits, reaching to the wall of the house: and the other wing *was* five cubits *also*, joining to the wing of the other cherub.

13 The wings of these cherubims spread themselves forth twenty cubits: and they stood on their feet, and their faces *were* inward.

14 And he made the [i]vail *of* blue, and purple, and crimson, and fine linen, and wrought cherubims thereon.

15 [j]Also he made before the house two pillars of thirty and five cubits high, and the chapiter that *was* on the top of each of them *was* five cubits.

16 And he made chains, *as* in the oracle, and put *them* on the heads of the pillars; and made an hundred pomegranates, and put *them* on the chains.

17 And he reared up the pillars before the temple, one on the right hand, and the other on the left; and called the name of that on the right hand Jachin, and the name of that on the left Boaz.

CHAPTER 4.

The temple, continued.

Moreover he made an [k]altar of brass, twenty [l]cubits the length thereof, and twenty cubits the breadth thereof, and ten cubits the height thereof.

2 Also he made a molten [m]sea of ten cubits from brim to brim, round in compass, and five cubits the height thereof; and a line of thirty cubits did compass it round about.

3 And under it *was* the similitude of oxen, which did compass it round about: ten in a cubit, compassing the sea round about. Two rows of oxen *were* cast, when it was cast.

4 It stood upon twelve oxen, three looking toward the north, and three looking toward the west, and three looking toward the south, and three looking toward the east: and the sea *was set* above upon them, and all their hinder parts *were* inward.

5 And the thickness of it *was* an handbreadth, and the brim of it like the work of the brim of a cup, with flowers of lilies; *and* it received and held three thousand [n]baths.

6 He made also ten lavers, and put five on the right hand, and five on the left, to wash in them: such things as they offered for the burnt-offering they washed in them; but the sea *was* for the [o]priests to wash in.

7 And he made ten [p]candlesticks of gold according to their form, and set *them* in the temple, five on the right hand, and five on the left.

a i.e. *May.*
b 1 Chr. 28:11-18.
c One cubit = about 18 in.; also vs. 8, 11, 12, 13, 15.
d 1 Ki. 6:3.
e 1 Ki. 6:17.
f i.e. *covered.*
g One talent = £6150, or $29,085.
h Cf. Ex. 25:18, 19.
i Ex. 26:31; Mt. 27:51; Heb. 9:3.
j 1 Ki. 7:15-22.
k Cf. Ex. 27:1-8.
l Cubit = about 18 in.; also vs. 2, 3.
m 1 Ki. 7:23; cf. Ex. 30:17-21.
n Bath = about 8 gals.
o Ex. 30:19-21.
p Cf. Ex. 25:31-40.

B.C. 1012.

8 He made also ten [a]tables, and placed *them* in the temple, five on the right side, and five on the left. And he made an hundred basons of gold.

9 Furthermore he made the [b]court of the priests, and the great court, and doors for the court, and overlaid the doors of them with brass.

10 And he set the sea on the right side of the east end, over against the south.

11 And Huram made the pots, and the shovels, and the basons. And Huram finished the work that he was to make for king Solomon for the house of God;

12 *To wit*, the two pillars, and the pommels, and the chapiters *which were* on the top of the two pillars, and the two wreaths to cover the two pommels of the chapiters which *were* on the top of the pillars;

13 And four hundred pomegranates on the two wreaths; two rows of pomegranates on each wreath, to cover the two pommels of the chapiters which *were* upon the pillars.

14 He made also bases, and lavers made he upon the bases;

15 One sea, and twelve oxen under it.

16 The pots also, and the shovels, and the fleshhooks, and all their instruments, did Huram his father make to king Solomon for the house of the LORD of bright brass.

17 In the plain of Jordan did the king cast them, in the clay ground between Succoth and Zeredathah.

18 [c]Thus Solomon made all these vessels in great abundance: for the weight of the brass could not be found out.

19 And Solomon made all the vessels that *were for* the house of God, the golden altar also, and the tables whereon the [d]shewbread *was set*;

20 Moreover the candlesticks with their lamps, that they should burn after the manner before the [e]oracle, of pure gold;

21 And the flowers, and the lamps, and the tongs, *made he of* gold, *and* that perfect gold;

22 And the snuffers, and the basons, and the spoons, and the censers, *of* pure gold: and the entry of the house, the inner doors thereof for the most holy *place*, and the doors of the house of the temple, *were of* gold.

CHAPTER 5.

The ark brought in: the glory fills the house (1 Ki. 8:1-11).

Thus all the work that Solomon made for the house of the LORD was finished: and Solomon brought in *all* the things that David his father had [f]dedicated; and the silver, and the gold, and all the instruments, put he among the treasures of the house of God.

2 [g]Then Solomon assembled the elders of Israel, and all the heads of the tribes, the chief of the fathers of the children of Israel, unto Jerusalem, to bring up the ark of the covenant of the LORD out of the city of David, which *is* Zion.

3 Wherefore all the men of Israel assembled themselves unto the king in the feast which *was* in the [h]seventh month.

4 And all the elders of Israel came; and the Levites took up the ark.

5 And they brought up the ark, and the tabernacle of the congregation, and all the holy vessels that *were* in the tabernacle, these did the priests *and* the Levites bring up.

6 Also king Solomon, and all the congregation of Israel that were assembled unto him before the ark, sacrificed sheep and oxen, which could not be told nor numbered for multitude.

7 And the priests brought in the ark of the covenant of the LORD unto his place, to the oracle of the house, into the most holy *place*, *even* under the wings of the cherubims:

8 For the cherubims spread forth *their* wings over the place of the ark, and the cherubims covered the ark and the staves thereof above.

9 And they drew out the staves *of the ark*, that the ends of the staves were seen from the ark before the oracle; but they were not seen without. And there it is unto this day.

10 *There was* nothing in the ark save the two tables which Moses put *therein* at Horeb, when the LORD made *a covenant* with the children of Israel, when they came out of Egypt.

11 And it came to pass, when the priests were come out of the holy *place*: (for all the priests *that were* present were sanctified, *and* did not *then* wait by course:

12 Also the Levites *which were* the singers, all of them of Asaph, of Heman,

a Cf. Ex. 25:23-30; 1 Ki. 7:4-8.

b The tabernacle had no "court of the priests."

c 1 Ki. 7:47.

d Ex. 25:30, *note.*

e 1 Ki. 6:4, *note.*

f *Sanctify, holy* (O.T.). 2 Chr. 29:5. (Gen. 2.3; Zech. 8.3.)

g 1 Ki. 8:1-11, *note.*

h i.e. *October.*

B.C. 1004.

of Jeduthun, with their sons and their
brethren, *being* arrayed in white linen,
having cymbals and psalteries and
harps, stood at the east end of the altar,
and with them an hundred and twenty
priests sounding with trumpets:)
13 It came even to pass, as the trumpeters and singers *were* as one, to make
one sound to be heard in praising and
thanking the LORD; and when they lifted
up *their* voice with the trumpets and
cymbals and instruments of musick, and
praised the LORD, *saying*, For *he is* good;
for his mercy *endureth* for ever: that *then*
the house was filled with a [a]cloud, *even*
the house of the LORD;
14 So that the priests could not stand
to minister by reason of the cloud: for
the glory of the LORD had filled the
house of God.

CHAPTER 6.

The sermon of Solomon (1 Ki. 8:12-21).

Then [b]said Solomon, The LORD hath
[c]said that he would dwell in the
thick darkness.
2 But I have built an house of habitation for thee, and a place for thy
dwelling for ever.
3 [d]And the king turned his face, and
blessed the whole congregation of Israel:
and all the congregation of Israel stood.
4 And he said, Blessed *be* the LORD
God of Israel, who hath with his hands
fulfilled *that* which he spake with his
mouth to my father David, saying,
5 Since the day that I brought forth my
people out of the land of Egypt I chose
no city among all the tribes of Israel to
build an house in, that my name might
be there; neither chose I any man to be a
ruler over my people Israel:
6 [e]But I have chosen Jerusalem, that
my name might be there; and have chosen [f]David to be over my people Israel.
7 Now it was in the heart of David my
father [g]to build an house for the name of
the LORD God of Israel.
8 But the LORD said to David my
father, Forasmuch as it was in thine heart
to build an house for my name, thou
didst well in that it was in thine heart:
9 Notwithstanding thou shalt not
build the house; but thy son which shall
come forth out of thy loins, he shall
build the house for my name.
10 The LORD therefore hath performed
his word that he hath spoken: for I am
risen up in the room of David my father,
and am set on the throne of Israel, as the
LORD promised, and have built the house
for the name of the LORD God of Israel.
11 And [h]in it have I put the ark,
wherein *is* the covenant of the LORD, that
he made with the children of Israel.

Solomon's prayer of dedication
(1 Ki. 8:22-53).

12 [i]And he stood before the altar of the
LORD in the presence of all the congregation of Israel, and spread forth his hands:
13 For Solomon had made a brasen
scaffold, of five [j]cubits long, and five
cubits broad, and three cubits high, and
had set it in the midst of the court: and
upon it he stood, and kneeled down
upon his knees before all the congregation of Israel, and spread forth his hands
toward heaven,
14 And [k]said, O LORD God of Israel,
[l]*there is* no God like thee in the heaven,
nor in the earth; which keepest covenant,
and *shewest* mercy unto thy servants, that
walk before thee with all their hearts:
15 Thou which hast kept with thy servant David my father that which thou
hast promised him; and spakest with thy
mouth, and hast fulfilled *it* with thine
hand, as *it is* this day.
16 Now therefore, O LORD God of
Israel, keep with thy servant David my
father that which thou hast promised
him, [m]saying, There shall not fail thee a
man in my sight to sit upon the throne of
Israel; yet so that thy children take heed
to their way to walk in my law, as thou
hast walked before me.
17 Now then, O LORD God of Israel, le
thy word be verified, which thou has
spoken unto thy servant David.
18 But will God in very deed dwel
with men on the earth? [n]behold, heaver
and the heaven of heavens cannot con
tain thee; how much less this house
which I have built!
19 Have respect therefore to the
prayer of thy servant, and to his suppli
cation, O LORD my God, to hearken unt

a vs. 11-13; Ex. 40:34, *note.*
b 1 Ki. 8:12-21.
c Ex. 19:9; 20:21.
d 1 Ki. 8:14-21.
e 2 Chr. 12:13; Deut. 12:5-7.
f 1 Sam. 16:7-13; 1 Chr. 28:4.
g 2 Sam. 7:2; 1 Chr. 17:1; Psa. 132:1-5.
h 2 Chr. 5:7, 10.
i 1 Ki. 8:22-61.
j A cubit = about 18 in.
k *Bible prayers* (O.T.). 2 Chr. 14:11. (Gen. 15:2; Hab. 3:1-16.)
l Ex. 15:11; Deut. 4:39.
m 2 Chr. 7:18; 2 Sam. 7:12-16; 1 Ki. 2:4.
n 2 Chr. 2:6; Cf. Isa. 66:1.

the cry and the prayer which thy servant
prayeth before thee:
20 That thine eyes may be open upon
this house day and night, upon the place
whereof thou hast said that thou
wouldest put thy name there; to hearken
unto the prayer which thy servant
prayeth toward this place.
21 Hearken therefore unto the supplications of thy servant, and of thy people
Israel, which they shall make toward
this place: hear thou from thy dwelling
place, *even* from heaven; and when thou
hearest, forgive.
22 If a man sin against his neighbour,
and an oath be laid upon him to make
him swear, and the oath come before
thine altar in this house;
23 Then hear thou from heaven, and
do, and judge thy servants, by requiting
the wicked, by recompensing his way
upon his own head; and by justifying
the righteous, by giving him according
to his righteousness.
24 And if thy people Israel be put to the
worse before the enemy, because they
have sinned against thee; and shall return
and confess thy name, and pray and make
supplication before thee in this house;
25 Then hear thou from the heavens,
and forgive the sin of thy people Israel,
and bring them again unto the land which
thou gavest to them and to their fathers.
26 When the heaven is [a]shut up, and
there is no rain, because they have
sinned against thee; *yet* if they pray
toward this place, and confess thy name,
and turn from their sin, when thou dost
afflict them;
27 Then hear thou from heaven, and
forgive the sin of thy servants, and of
thy people Israel, when thou hast taught
them the good way, wherein they should
walk; and send rain upon thy land,
which thou hast given unto thy people
for an inheritance.
28 If there be dearth in the land, if
there be pestilence, if there be blasting,
or mildew, locusts, or caterpillers; if their
enemies besiege them in the cities of
their land; whatsoever sore or whatsoever sickness *there be*:
29 *Then* what prayer *or* what supplication soever shall be made of any man, or
of all thy people Israel, when every one
shall know his own sore and his own

B.C. 1004.

a Deut. 28:23, 24; 1 Ki. 17:1; 18:45.

b 1 Chr. 28:9; Prov. 21:2; 24:12.

c Psa. 19:9, *note*.

d Prov. 20:9; Eccl. 7:20; Rom. 3:9, 19, 23; 5:12; Gal. 3:10; Jas. 3:2; 1 John 1:8.

e Dan. 6:10.

grief, and shall spread forth his hands in
this house:
30 Then hear thou from heaven thy
dwelling place, and forgive, and render
unto every man according unto all his
ways, whose heart thou knowest; (for
[b]thou only knowest the hearts of the
children of men:)
31 That they may [c]fear thee, to walk in
thy ways, so long as they live in the land
which thou gavest unto our fathers.
32 Moreover concerning the stranger,
which is not of thy people Israel, but is
come from a far country for thy great
name's sake, and thy mighty hand, and
thy stretched out arm; if they come and
pray in this house;
33 Then hear thou from the heavens,
even from thy dwelling place, and do
according to all that the stranger calleth
to thee for; that all people of the earth
may know thy name, and fear thee, as
doth thy people Israel, and may know
that this house which I have built is
called by thy name.
34 If thy people go out to war against
their enemies by the way that thou shalt
send them, and they pray unto thee
toward this city which thou hast chosen,
and the house which I have built for thy
name;
35 Then hear thou from the heavens
their prayer and their supplication, and
maintain their cause.
36 If they sin against thee, (for *there is*
[d]no man which sinneth not,) and thou be
angry with them, and deliver them over
before *their* enemies, and they carry them
away captives unto a land far off or near;
37 Yet *if* they bethink themselves in
the land whither they are carried captive, and turn and pray unto thee in the
land of their captivity, saying, We have
sinned, we have done amiss, and have
dealt wickedly;
38 If they return to thee with all their
heart and with all their soul in the land
of their captivity, whither they have carried them captives, and pray toward
their land, which thou gavest unto their
fathers, and *toward* the [e]city which thou
hast chosen, and toward the house
which I have built for thy name:
39 Then hear thou from the heavens,
even from thy dwelling place, their
prayer and their supplications, and

maintain their cause, and forgive thy people which have sinned against thee.

40 Now, my God, let, I beseech thee, thine eyes be open, and *let* thine ears *be* attent unto the prayer *that is made* in this place.

41 Now therefore [a]arise, O LORD God, into thy resting place, thou, and the ark of thy strength: let thy priests, O LORD God, be clothed with salvation, and let thy saints rejoice in goodness.

42 O LORD God, turn not away the face of thine anointed: remember the [b]mercies of David thy servant.

CHAPTER 7.

The divine acceptance.

Now when Solomon had made an [c]end of praying, the [d]fire came down from heaven, and consumed the burnt-offering and the sacrifices; and the glory of the LORD filled the house.

2 [e]And the priests could not enter into the house of the LORD, because the glory of the LORD had filled the LORD'S house.

3 And when all the children of Israel saw how the fire came down, and the glory of the LORD upon the house, they bowed themselves with their faces to the ground upon the pavement, and worshipped, and praised the LORD, *saying,* [f]For *he is* good; for his mercy *endureth* for ever.

Sacrifice and rejoicing (1 Ki. 8:62-66).

4 Then the king and all the people offered sacrifices before the LORD.

5 And king Solomon offered a sacrifice of twenty and two thousand oxen, and an hundred and twenty thousand sheep: so the king and all the people dedicated the house of God.

6 And the priests waited on their offices: the [g]Levites also with instruments of musick of the LORD, which David the king had made to praise the LORD, because his mercy *endureth* for ever, when David praised by their ministry; and the priests sounded trumpets before them, and all Israel stood.

7 Moreover Solomon [h]hallowed the middle of the court that *was* before the house of the LORD: for there he offered burnt-offerings, and the fat of the peace-offerings, because the brasen altar which Solomon had made was not able to receive the burnt-offerings, and the [i]meat-offerings, and the fat.

8 [j]Also at the same time Solomon kept the feast seven days, and all Israel with him, a very great congregation, from the entering in of Hamath unto the river of Egypt.

9 And in the eighth day they made a solemn assembly: for they kept the dedication of the altar seven days, and the feast seven days.

10 And on the three and twentieth day of the [k]seventh month he sent the people away into their tents, glad and merry in heart for the goodness that the LORD had shewed unto David, and to Solomon, and to Israel his people.

11 Thus Solomon [l]finished the house of the LORD, and the king's house: and all that came into Solomon's heart to make in the house of the LORD, and in his own house, he prosperously effected.

Jehovah appears to Solomon (1 Ki. 9:1-9).

12 And the LORD [m]appeared to Solomon by night, and said unto him, I have heard thy prayer, and have [n]chosen this place to myself for an house of sacrifice.

13 If I [o]shut up heaven that there be no rain, or if I command the locusts to devour the land, or if I send pestilence among my people;

14 If my people, which are called by my name, shall humble themselves, and pray, and seek my face, and turn from their wicked ways; then will I hear from heaven, and will forgive their sin, and will heal their land.

15 Now mine eyes shall be open, and mine ears attent unto the prayer *that is made* in this place.

16 For now have I [p]chosen and sanctified this house, that my name may be there for ever: and mine eyes and mine heart shall be there perpetually.

17 And as for thee, if thou wilt walk before me, as David thy father walked, and do according to all that I have commanded thee, and shalt observe my statutes and my judgments;

18 Then will I stablish the throne of thy kingdom, according as I have covenanted with David thy father,

B.C. 1004.

a Psa. 132:8, 9, 10, 16.
b Psa. 89:49; Isa. 55:3.
c 1 Ki. 8:54.
d Lev. 9:24; Jud. 6:21;1 Ki. 18:38; 1 Chr. 21:26.
e 2 Chr. 5:14.
f Psa. 136:1.
g 1 Chr. 15.16.
h 1 Ki. 8:64.
i Lit. *meal.*
j 1 Ki. 8:65.
k i.e. *October.*
l 1 Ki. 9:1.
m 1 Ki. 9:2.
n Deut. 12:5.
o 2 Chr. 6:26, *refs.*
p 1 Ki. 9:3.

B.C. 1004.

saying, [a]There shall not fail thee a man
to be ruler in Israel.
19 But if ye turn away, and forsake my
statutes and my commandments, which
I have set before you, and shall go and
serve other gods, and worship them;
20 [b]Then will I pluck them up by the
roots out of my land which I have given
them; and this house, which I have sanctified for my name, will I cast out of my
sight, and will make it *to be* a proverb
and a byword among all nations.
21 And [c]this house, which is high,
shall be an astonishment to every one
that passeth by it; so that he shall say,
Why hath the LORD done thus unto this
land, and unto this house?
22 And it shall be answered, Because
they forsook the LORD God of their
fathers, which brought them forth out of
the land of Egypt, and laid hold on other
gods, and worshipped them, and served
them: therefore hath he brought all this
evil upon them.

CHAPTER 8.

The energy and fame of Solomon
(1 Ki. 9:10-28).

And it came to pass [d]at the end of
twenty years, wherein Solomon
had built the house of the LORD, and his
own house,
2 That the cities which Huram had
restored to Solomon, Solomon built
them, and caused the children of Israel
to dwell there.
3 And Solomon went to Hamath-
zobah, and prevailed against it.
4 And he [e]built Tadmor in the wilderness, and all the store cities, which he
built in Hamath.
5 Also he built Beth-horon the upper,
and Beth-horon the nether, fenced cities,
with walls, gates, and bars;
6 And Baalath, and all the store cities
that Solomon had, and all the chariot
cities, and the cities of the horsemen,
and all that Solomon desired to build in
Jerusalem, and in Lebanon, and
throughout all the land of his dominion.
7 *As for* all the people *that were* left [f]of
the Hittites, and the Amorites, and the
Perizzites, and the Hivites, and the
Jebusites, which *were* not of Israel,
8 *But* of their children, who were left
after them in the land, whom the
children of Israel consumed not, them
did Solomon make to pay tribute until
this day.
9 But of the children of Israel did
Solomon make no servants for his work;
but they *were* men of war, and chief of
his captains, and captains of his chariots
and horsemen.
10 And these *were* the [g]chief of king
Solomon's officers, *even* two hundred
and fifty, that bare rule over the people.
11 And Solomon brought up the
[h]daughter of Pharaoh out of the city of
David unto the house that he had built
for her: for he said, My wife shall not
dwell in the house of David king of
Israel, because *the places are* holy, whereunto the ark of the LORD hath come.
12 Then Solomon offered burnt-offerings unto the LORD on the altar of the
LORD, which he had built before the
porch,
13 Even after a certain rate every day,
offering [i]according to the commandment
of Moses, on the sabbaths, and on the
new moons, and on the solemn [j]feasts,
three times in the year, *even* in the feast of
unleavened bread, and in the feast of
weeks, and in the feast of tabernacles.
14 And he appointed, according to the
order of David his father, the [k]courses of
the priests to their service, and the
Levites to their charges, to praise and
minister before the priests, as the duty of
every day required: the porters also by
their courses at every gate: for so had
David the man of God commanded.
15 And they departed not from the
commandment of the king unto the
priests and Levites concerning any matter, or concerning the treasures.
16 Now all the work of Solomon was
prepared unto the day of the foundation
of the house of the LORD, and until it was
finished. *So* the house of the LORD was
perfected.
17 Then went Solomon to [l]Ezion-
geber, and to [m]Eloth, at the sea side in
the land of Edom.
18 And Huram [n]sent him by the
hands of his servants ships, and servants
that had knowledge of the sea; and they
went with the servants of Solomon to
Ophir, and took thence four hundred
and fifty [o]talents of gold, and brought
them to king Solomon.

a 2 Chr. 6:16, *refs.*
b Deut. 28:63-68; 2 Ki. 25:1-7.
c 2 Ki. 25:9.
d 1 Ki. 9:10-14.
e 1 Ki. 9:18.
f Deut. 20:17; Josh. 3:10; Jud. 1:27-35; 2:1-3.
g Cf. 1 Ki. 9:23.
h 1 Ki. 3:1.
i Num. 29:1-39.
j Lev. 23:1-43.
k 1 Chr. 24:1-31.
l 1 Ki. 9:26.
m Called *Elath*, 2 Ki. 14:22.
n 1 Ki. 9:27.
o One talent (gold) = £6150, or $29,085.

CHAPTER 9.

Solomon and the queen of Sheba
(1 Ki. 10:1-13).

And when the [a]queen of Sheba heard of the fame of Solomon, she came to prove Solomon with hard questions at Jerusalem, with a very great company, and camels that bare spices, and gold in abundance, and precious stones: and when she was come to Solomon, she communed with him of all that was in her heart.

2 And Solomon told her all her questions: and there was nothing hid from Solomon which he told her not.

3 And when the queen of Sheba had seen the wisdom of Solomon, and the house that he had built,

4 And the meat of his table, and the sitting of his servants, and the attendance of his ministers, and their apparel; his cupbearers also, and their apparel; and his ascent by which he went up into the house of the LORD; there was no more spirit in her.

5 And she said to the king, *It was a* true report which I heard in mine own land of thine acts, and of thy wisdom:

6 Howbeit I believed not their words, until I came, and mine eyes had seen *it*: and, behold, the one half of the greatness of thy wisdom was not told me: *for* thou exceedest the fame that I heard.

7 Happy *are* thy men, and happy *are* these thy servants, which stand continually before thee, and hear thy wisdom.

8 Blessed be the LORD thy God, which delighted in thee to set thee on his throne, *to be* king for the LORD thy God: because thy God loved Israel, to establish them for ever, therefore made he thee king over them, to do judgment and justice.

9 And she gave the king an hundred and twenty [b]talents of gold, and of spices great abundance, and precious stones: neither was there any such spice as the queen of Sheba gave king Solomon.

10 And the servants also of Huram, and the servants of Solomon, which brought gold from Ophir, brought [c]algum trees and precious stones.

11 And the king made *of* the algum trees terraces to the house of the LORD, and to the king's palace, and harps and psalteries for singers: and there were none such seen before in the land of Judah.

B.C. 992.

a 1 Ki. 10:1-13,

b One talent (gold) = £6150, or $29,085; also v. 13.

c Called *almug*, 1 Ki. 10:11.

12 And king Solomon gave to the queen of Sheba all her desire, whatsoever she asked, beside *that* which she had brought unto the king. So she turned, and went away to her own land, she and her servants.

Solomon's revenue and spendour
(1 Ki. 10:14-29).

13 Now the weight of gold that came to Solomon in one year was six hundred and threescore and six talents of gold;

14 Beside *that which* chapmen and merchants brought. And all the kings of Arabia and governors of the country brought gold and silver to Solomon.

15 And king Solomon made two hundred targets *of* beaten gold: six hundred *shekels* of beaten gold went to one target.

16 And three hundred shields *made he of* beaten gold: three hundred *shekels* of gold went to one shield. And the king put them in the house of the forest of Lebanon.

17 Moreover the king made a great throne of ivory, and overlaid it with pure gold.

18 And *there were* six steps to the throne, with a footstool of gold, *which were* fastened to the throne, and stays on each side of the sitting place, and two lions standing by the stays:

19 And twelve lions stood there on the one side and on the other upon the six steps. There was not the like made in any kingdom.

20 And all the drinking vessels of king Solomon *were of* gold, and all the vessels of the house of the forest of Lebanon *were of* pure gold: none *were of* silver; it was *not* any thing accounted of in the days of Solomon.

21 For the king's ships went to Tarshish with the servants of Huram: every three years once came the ships of Tarshish bringing gold, and silver, ivory, and apes, and peacocks.

22 And king Solomon passed all the kings of the earth in riches and wisdom.

23 And all the kings of the earth sought the presence of Solomon, to hear his wisdom, that God had put in his heart.

24 And they brought every man his present, vessels of silver, and vessels of

gold, and raiment, harness, and spices,
horses, and mules, a rate year by year.
25 And Solomon had four thousand
stalls for horses and chariots, and twelve
thousand horsemen; whom he bestowed
in the chariot cities, and with the king at
Jerusalem.
26 And he reigned over all the kings
from the [a]river even unto the land of the
Philistines, and to the border of Egypt.
27 And the king made [b]silver in
Jerusalem as stones, and cedar trees
made he as the sycomore trees that *are* in
the low plains in abundance.
28 And they [c]brought unto Solomon
horses out of Egypt, and out of all lands.

The death of Solomon (1 Ki. 11:41-43).

29 Now the [d]rest of the acts of
Solomon, first and last, *are* they not written in the book of Nathan the prophet,
and in the prophecy of [e]Ahijah the
Shilonite, and in the visions of Iddo the
seer against Jeroboam the son of Nebat?
30 And Solomon [f]reigned in Jerusalem
over all Israel forty years.
31 And Solomon slept with his fathers,
and he was buried in the city of David
his father: and Rehoboam his son
reigned in his stead.

CHAPTER 10.

Accession and folly of Rehoboam (1 Ki. 12:1-15).

And [g]Rehoboam went to Shechem:
for to Shechem were all Israel come
to make him king.
2 And it came to pass, when
[h]Jeroboam the son of Nebat, who *was* in
Egypt, whither he had [i]fled from the
presence of Solomon the king, heard *it*,
that Jeroboam returned out of Egypt.
3 And they sent and called him. So
Jeroboam and all Israel came and spake
to Rehoboam, saying,
4 [j]Thy father made our yoke grievous:
now therefore ease thou somewhat the
grievous servitude of thy father, and his
heavy yoke that he put upon us, and we
will serve thee.
5 And he [k]said unto them, Come again
unto me after three days. And the people
departed.
6 [l]And king Rehoboam took counsel

B.C. 992.

a *"The river,"* i.e. Euphrates, *to the border of Egypt,* but not to the "river of Egypt." Cf. Gen. 15:18, yet to be fulfilled.
b 1 Ki. 10:27.
c 1 Ki. 10:28.
d 1 Ki. 11:41; 1 Chr. 29:29.
e 1 Ki. 11:29. These books have perished.
f 1 Ki. 11:42, 43.
g 1 Ki. 12:1-15.

B.C. 975.]

h 1 Ki. 11:26-40; 12:3-20; 14:7-20.
i 1 Ki. 11:40.
j 1 Ki. 12:4; cf. Ex. 1:14.
k 1 Ki. 12:5.
l 1 Ki. 12:6.
m 1 Ki. 12:7.
n 1 Ki. 12:8, 9.
o 1 Ki. 12:10, 11.
p 1 Ki. 12:12-14.
q v. 14; Jud. 14:4; 2 Chr. 10:15; 11:4; 22:7; 25:20.

with the old men that had stood before
Solomon his father while he yet lived,
saying, What counsel give ye *me* to
return answer to this people?
7 And they spake unto him, [m]saying,
If thou be kind to this people, and please
them, and speak good words to them,
they will be thy servants for ever.
8 [n]But he forsook the counsel which
the old men gave him, and took counsel
with the young men that were brought
up with him, that stood before him.
9 And he said unto them, What advice
give ye that we may return answer to
this people, which have spoken to me,
saying, Ease somewhat the yoke that thy
father did put upon us?
10 [o]And the young men that were
brought up with him spake unto him,
saying, Thus shalt thou answer the people that spake unto thee, saying, Thy
father made our yoke heavy, but make
thou *it* somewhat lighter for us; thus
shalt thou say unto them, My little *finger*
shall be thicker than my father's loins.
11 For whereas my father put a heavy
yoke upon you, I will put more to your
yoke: my father chastised you with
whips, but I *will chastise you* with scorpions.

Division of the kingdom: accession of Jeroboam over Israel (1 Ki. 12:16-24).

12 So [p]Jeroboam and all the people
came to Rehoboam on the third day, as
the king bade, saying, Come again to me
on the third day.
13 And the king answered them
roughly; and king Rehoboam forsook
the counsel of the old men,
14 And answered them after the
advice of the young men, saying, My
father made your yoke heavy, but I will
add thereto: my father chastised you
with whips, but I *will chastise you* with
scorpions.
15 So the king hearkened not unto the
people: [q]for the cause was of God, that
the LORD might perform his word, which
he spake by the hand of Ahijah the
Shilonite to Jeroboam the son of Nebat.
16 And when all [1]Israel *saw* that the
king would not hearken unto them, the
people answered the king, saying, What

[1] **(10:16)** "Israel," the ten tribes other than Judah and Benjamin, often called "Israel" in distinction from Judah. This division of the kingdom marks an epoch of great importance in the history of the

portion have we in David? and *we have*
none inheritance in the son of Jesse:
every man to your tents, O Israel: *and*
now, David, see to thine own house. So
all Israel went to their tents.
17 But *as for* the children of Israel that
dwelt in the cities of Judah, Rehoboam
reigned over them.
18 Then king Rehoboam sent
Hadoram that *was* over the tribute; and
the children of Israel stoned him with
stones, that he died. But king Rehoboam
made speed to get him up to *his* chariot,
to flee to Jerusalem.
19 And [a]Israel rebelled against the
house of David unto this day.

CHAPTER 11.

Rehoboam returns to Jerusalem.

And [b]when Rehoboam was come to
Jerusalem, he gathered of the
house of Judah and Benjamin an hundred and fourscore thousand chosen
men, which were warriors, to fight
against Israel, that he might bring the
kingdom again to Rehoboam.
2 [c]But the word of the LORD came to
Shemaiah the man of God, saying,
3 Speak unto Rehoboam the son of
Solomon, king of Judah, and to all Israel
in Judah and Benjamin, saying,
4 Thus saith the LORD, Ye shall not go
up, nor fight against your brethren:
return every man to his house: for this
thing is done of me. And they obeyed
the words of the LORD, and returned
from going against Jeroboam.

Rehoboam fortifies his kingdom.

5 And Rehoboam dwelt in Jerusalem,
and built cities for defence in Judah.
6 He built even Bethlehem, and Etam,
and Tekoa,
7 And Beth-zur, and Shoco, and
Adullam,
8 And Gath, and Mareshah, and Ziph,
9 And Adoraim, and Lachish, and
Azekah,
10 And Zorah, and Aijalon, and
Hebron, which *are* in Judah and in
Benjamin fenced cities.
11 And he fortified the strong holds,
and put captains in them, and store of
victual, and of oil and wine.
12 And in every several city *he put*
shields and spears, and made them
exceeding strong, having Judah and
Benjamin on his side.
13 And the priests and the Levites that
were in all Israel resorted to him out of
all their coasts.

Jeroboam rejects the worship of Jehovah.

14 For the Levites left their suburbs
and their possession, and came to Judah
and Jerusalem: for Jeroboam and his
sons had cast them off from executing
the priest's office unto the LORD:
15 And [d]he ordained him priests for
the high [e]places, and for the [f]devils, and
for the calves which he had made.
16 And after them out of all the tribes
of Israel such as set their hearts to seek
the LORD God of Israel came to
Jerusalem, to sacrifice unto the LORD
God of their fathers.
17 So they strengthened the kingdom
of Judah, and made Rehoboam the son
of Solomon strong, three years: for three
years they walked in the way of David
and Solomon.

Rehoboam's family.

18 And Rehoboam took him Mahalath
the daughter of Jerimoth the son of
David to wife, *and* Abihail the daughter
of Eliab the son of Jesse;
19 Which bare him children; Jeush,
and Shamariah, and Zaham.
20 And after her he took [g]Maachah
the daughter of [h]Absalom; which bare
him Abijah, and Attai, and Ziza, and
Shelomith.
21 And Rehoboam loved Maachah the
daughter of Absalom above all his wives
and his concubines: (for he took eighteen
wives, and threescore concubines; and
begat twenty and eight sons, and threescore daughters.)
22 And Rehoboam made [i]Abijah the
son of Maachah the chief, *to be* ruler

B.C. 975.

a 1 Ki. 12:19.
b 1 Ki. 12:21.
c 2 Chr. 12:15.
d i.e. *Jeroboam.*
e Cf. 1 Ki. 12:31.
f Lit. *hairy ones,* i.e. *satyrs,* Isa. 13:21.
g Called *Michaiah,* 2 Chr. 13:2.
h Or, *Abishalom,* 1 Ki. 15:2.
i 2 Chr. 13:1.

nation. Henceforth it is "a kingdom divided against itself" (Mt. 12:25). The two kingdoms are to be reunited in the future kingdom (Isa. 11:10-13; Jer. 23:5, 6; Ezk. 37:15-28). See "Kingdom" (O.T.), Gen. 1:26; Zech. 12:8; (N.T.), Lk. 1:31; 1 Cor. 15:28. "Israel," Gen. 12:2, 3; Rom. 11:26.

among his brethren: for *he thought* to
make him king.
23 And he dealt wisely, and dispersed
of all his children throughout all the countries of Judah and Benjamin, unto every
fenced city: and he gave them victual in
abundance. And he desired many wives.

CHAPTER 12.

Rehoboam's apostasy (1 Ki. 14:21-24).

And it came to pass, when Rehoboam
had established the kingdom, and
had strengthened himself, he [a]forsook the
law of the LORD, and all Israel with him.

Invasion of Shishak (1 Ki. 14:25-28).

2 And it came to pass, *that* in the fifth
year of king Rehoboam Shishak king of
Egypt came up against Jerusalem, because
they had transgressed against the LORD,
3 With twelve hundred chariots, and
threescore thousand horsemen: and the
people *were* without number that came
with him out of Egypt; the [b]Lubims, the
Sukkiims, and the Ethiopians.
4 And he took the fenced cities which
pertained to Judah, and came to Jerusalem.
5 Then came [c]Shemaiah the prophet to
Rehoboam, and *to* the princes of Judah,
that were gathered together to Jerusalem
because of Shishak, and said unto them,
Thus saith the LORD, [d]Ye have forsaken
me, and therefore have I also left you in
the hand of Shishak.
6 [e]Whereupon the princes of Israel
and the king humbled themselves; and
they said, The LORD *is* righteous.
7 And [f]when the LORD saw that they
humbled themselves, the word of the
LORD came to Shemaiah, saying, They
have humbled themselves; *therefore* I will
not destroy them, but I will grant them
some deliverance; and my wrath shall
not be poured out upon Jerusalem by
the hand of Shishak.
8 [g]Nevertheless they shall be his servants; that they may know my service,
and the service of the kingdoms of the
countries.
9 So Shishak king of Egypt came up
against Jerusalem, and [h]took away the
treasures of the house of the LORD, and
the treasures of the king's house; he took
all: he carried away also the shields of
gold which Solomon had made.
10 Instead of which king Rehoboam
made shields of brass, and [i]committed
them to the hands of the chief of the
guard, that kept the entrance of the
king's house.
11 And when the king entered into the
house of the LORD, the guard came and
fetched them, and brought them again
into the guard chamber.
12 And when he humbled himself, the
wrath of the LORD turned from him, that
he would not destroy *him* altogether:
and also in Judah things went well.

Death of Rehoboam(1Ki. 14:31).

13 So king Rehoboam strengthened
himself in Jerusalem, and reigned: for
Rehoboam *was* [j]one and forty years old
when he began to reign, and he reigned
seventeen years in Jerusalem, the city
which the LORD had [k]chosen out of all
the tribes of Israel, to put his name there.
And his mother's name *was* Naamah an
Ammonitess.
14 And he did evil, [l]because he prepared not his heart to seek the LORD.
15 Now the acts of Rehoboam, first
and last, *are* they not written in the book
of Shemaiah the prophet, and of Iddo
the seer concerning genealogies? [m]And
there were wars between Rehoboam and
Jeroboam continually.
16 And Rehoboam slept with his
fathers, and was buried in the city of
David: and [n]Abijah his son reigned in
his stead.

CHAPTER 13.

Accession of Abijah over Judah
(1 Ki. 15:1, 2).

Now in the eighteenth year of king
Jeroboam [o]began Abijah to reign
over Judah.
2 He reigned [p]three years in
Jerusalem. His mother's name also *was*
[q]Michaiah the daughter of Uriel of
Gibeah. And there was war between
Abijah and Jeroboam.

The war between Abijah and Jeroboam
(1 Ki. 15:7).

3 And Abijah set the battle in array
with an army of valiant men of war, *even*
four hundred thousand chosen men:
Jeroboam also set the battle in array
against him with eight hundred

B.C. 974.

a Cf. v. 14.
b 2 Chr. 16:8.
c 2 Chr. 11:2.
d 2 Chr. 15:2.
e 2 Chr. 6:24-25.
f 2 Chr. 6:25.
g Isa. 26:13.
h 1 Ki. 14:25, 26. Cf. 2 Ki. 24:13.
i 2 Sam. 8:8.
j 1 Ki. 14:21.
k 2 Chr. 6:6.
l Cf. 2 Chr. 27:6; 30:19; 1 Sam. 7.3; 1 Chr. 29:18.
m 1 Ki. 14:30.
n Called *Abijam*, 1 Ki. 14:31.
o 1 Ki. 15:1.
p 1 Ki. 15:2.
q Cf. 2 Chr. 11:20. Probably a grandchild of Absalom, called *Abishalom*, 1 Ki. 15:2.

[B.C. 958.

B.C. 957.

thousand chosen men, *being* mighty men of valour.

4 And Abijah stood up upon mount [a]Zemaraim, which *is* in mount Ephraim, and said, Hear me, thou Jeroboam, and all Israel;

5 Ought ye not to know that the LORD God of Israel [b]gave the kingdom over Israel to David for ever, *even* to him and to his sons by a covenant of [c]salt?

6 Yet Jeroboam the son of Nebat, the servant of Solomon the son of David, is risen up, and hath [d]rebelled against his lord.

7 And there are gathered unto him vain men, the children of Belial, and have strengthened themselves against Rehoboam the son of Solomon, when Rehoboam was young and tenderhearted, and could not withstand them.

8 And now ye think to withstand the kingdom of the LORD in the hand of the sons of David; and ye *be* a great multitude, and *there are* with you golden calves, [e]which Jeroboam made you for gods.

9 Have ye not [f]cast out the priests of the LORD, the sons of Aaron, and the Levites, and have made you priests after the manner of the nations of *other* lands? so that whosoever cometh to consecrate himself with a young bullock and seven rams, *the same* may be a priest of *them that are* no gods.

10 But as for us, the LORD *is* our God, and we have not forsaken him; and the priests, which minister unto the LORD, *are* the sons of Aaron, and the Levites *wait* upon *their* business:

11 And they burn unto the LORD every morning and every evening burnt sacrifices and sweet incense: the [g]shewbread also *set they in order* upon the pure table; and the candlestick of gold with the lamps thereof, to burn every evening: for we keep the charge of the LORD our God; but ye have forsaken him.

12 And, behold, God himself *is* with us for *our* captain, and his priests with sounding trumpets to cry alarm against you. O children of Israel, [h]fight ye not against the LORD God of your fathers; for ye shall not prosper.

13 But Jeroboam caused an ambushment to come about behind them: so they were before Judah, and the ambushment *was* behind them.

14 And when Judah looked back, behold, the battle *was* before and behind: and they cried unto the LORD, and the priests sounded with the trumpets.

15 Then the men of Judah gave a shout: and as the men of Judah shouted, it came to pass, that God smote Jeroboam and all Israel before Abijah and Judah.

16 And the children of Israel fled before Judah: and God delivered them into their hand.

17 And Abijah and his people slew them with a great slaughter: so there fell down slain of Israel [i]five hundred thousand chosen men.

18 Thus the children of Israel were brought under at that time, and the children of Judah prevailed, because they relied upon the LORD God of their fathers.

19 And Abijah pursued after Jeroboam, and took cities from him, Beth-el with the towns thereof, and Jeshanah with the towns thereof, and Ephrain with the towns thereof.

Death of Jeroboam (1 Ki. 14:19, 20).

20 Neither did Jeroboam recover strength again in the days of Abijah: and the LORD [j]struck him, and he died.

The family of Abijah.

21 But Abijah waxed mighty, and married fourteen wives, and begat twenty and two sons, and sixteen daughters.

22 And the rest of the acts of Abijah, and his ways, and his sayings, *are* written in the [k]story of the prophet Iddo.

CHAPTER 14.

Death of Abijah (1 Ki. 15:7, 8).
Accession of Asa (1 Ki. 15:8-10).

So Abijah slept with his fathers, and they buried him in the city of David: and Asa his son reigned in his stead. In his days the land was quiet ten years.

2 And Asa did *that which was* good and right in the eyes of the LORD his God:

3 For he took away the altars of the strange *gods*, and the high [l]places, and brake down the images, and cut down the [m]groves:

4 And commanded Judah to seek the LORD God of their fathers, and to do the law and the commandment.

a Josh. 18:22.
b 2 Sam. 7.8-16.
c Num. 18:19.
d 1 Ki. 11:26, etc.
e 1 Ki. 12:28; 14:9; Hos. 8:4-6. Cf. Ex. 32:1-4.
f 2 Chr. 11:13-15.
g Ex. 25:30, *note.*
h Cf. Acts 5:39.
i See 1 Cor. 10:8, *note.*
j 1 Ki. 14:20; cf. Acts 12:23.
k 2 Chr. 12:15.
l Cf. 1 Ki. 3:2, *note,* and 15, 14, *note.*
m See Deut. 16:21; Jud. 3, 7, *note.*

5 Also he took away out of all the cities of Judah the high places and the [a]images: and the kingdom was quiet before him.

6 And he built fenced cities in Judah: for the land had rest, and he had no war in those years; because the LORD had given him rest.

7 Therefore he said unto Judah, Let us build these cities, and make about *them* walls, and towers, gates, and bars, *while* the land *is* yet before us; because we have sought the LORD our God, we have sought *him*, and he hath given us rest on every side. So they built and prospered.

8 And Asa had an army *of men* that bare targets and spears, out of Judah [b]three hundred thousand; and out of Benjamin, that bare shields and drew bows, two hundred and fourscore thousand: all these *were* mighty men of valour.

Asa's victory over Zerah. (See 2 Chr. 16:8).

9 And there came out against them Zerah the Ethiopian with an host of a [b]thousand thousand, and three hundred chariots; and came unto Mareshah.

10 Then Asa went out against him, and they set the battle in array in the valley of Zephathah at Mareshah.

11 And Asa [c]cried unto the LORD his God, and said, LORD, *it is* nothing with thee to help, [d]whether with many, or with them that have no power: help us, O LORD our God; for we rest on thee, and [e]in thy name we go against this multitude. O LORD, thou *art* our God; let not man prevail against thee.

12 So the LORD smote the Ethiopians before Asa, and before Judah; and the Ethiopians fled.

13 And Asa and the people that *were* with him pursued them unto Gerar: and the Ethiopians were overthrown, that they could not recover themselves; for they were destroyed before the LORD, and before his host; and they carried away very much spoil.

14 And they smote all the cities round about Gerar; for the [f]fear of the LORD came upon them: and they spoiled all the cities; for there was exceeding much spoil in them.

15 They smote also the tents of cattle, and carried away sheep and camels in abundance, and returned to Jerusalem.

B.C. 951.

a Heb. *sun gods.*

b See 1 Cor. 10:8, *note.*

c *Bible prayers* (O.T.). 2 Chr. 20:6. (Gen. 15:2; Hab. 3:1-16.)

d 1 Sam. 14:6.

e 1 Sam. 17:45.

f Deut. 11:25; Josh. 2:9; 2 Chr. 17:10.

g *Holy Spirit*, 2 Chr. 20:14. (Gen. 1:2; Mal. 2:15.)

h v. 8.

B.C. 941.]

i 1 Ki. 12:28-33.

j Chapter 14 describes the outward prosperity of the kingdom, and Asa's superficial reformation; chapter 15 the true reformation.

k v. 3.

l i.e. *June.*

m 2 Chr. 14:13-15.

n 2 Chr. 23:16.

CHAPTER 15.

The warning of the Prophet Azariah.

And the [g]Spirit of God came upon Azariah the son of [h]Oded:

2 And he went out to meet Asa, and said unto him, Hear ye me, Asa, and all Judah and Benjamin; The LORD *is* with you, while ye be with him; and if ye seek him, he will be found of you; but if ye forsake him, he will forsake you.

3 Now for a long season [i]Israel *hath been* without the true God, and without a teaching priest, and without law.

4 But when they in their trouble did turn unto the LORD God of Israel, and sought him, he was found of them.

5 And in those times *there was* no peace to him that went out, nor to him that came in, but great vexations *were* upon all the inhabitants of the countries.

6 And nation was destroyed of nation, and city of city: for God did vex them with all adversity.

7 Be ye strong therefore, and let not your hands be weak: for your work shall be rewarded.

The reform under Asa.

8 And [j]when Asa heard these words, and the prophecy of Oded the prophet, he took courage, and put away the abominable idols out of all the land of Judah and Benjamin, and out of the cities which he had taken from mount Ephraim, and renewed the altar of the LORD, that *was* before the porch of the LORD.

9 And he gathered all Judah and Benjamin, and the strangers with them out of Ephraim and Manasseh, and out of Simeon: for they fell to him [k]out of Israel in abundance, when they saw that the LORD his God *was* with him.

10 So they gathered themselves together at Jerusalem in the [l]third month, in the fifteenth year of the reign of Asa.

11 And they offered unto the LORD the same time, of the [m]spoil *which* they had brought, seven hundred oxen and seven thousand sheep.

12 And [n]they entered into a covenant to seek the LORD God of their fathers with all their heart and with all their soul;

13 That whosoever would not seek the

B.C. 941.

LORD God of Israel [a]should be put to
death, whether small or great, whether
man or woman.
14 And they sware unto the LORD with
a loud voice, and with shouting, and
with trumpets, and with cornets.
15 And all Judah rejoiced at the oath:
for they had sworn with all their heart,
and [b]sought him with their whole
desire; and he was found of them: and
the LORD gave them rest round about.
16 And also *concerning* Maachah the
[c]mother of Asa the king, he removed her
from *being* queen, because she had made
an idol in a [d]grove: and Asa cut down
her idol, and stamped *it*, and burnt *it* at
the brook Kidron.
17 But the high places were not taken
away out of [e]Israel: nevertheless the
heart of Asa was [f]perfect all his days.
18 And he brought into the house of
God the things that his father had dedicated, and that he himself had dedicated, silver, and gold, and vessels.
19 And there was no *more* war unto
the five and thirtieth year of the reign of
Asa.

CHAPTER 16.

War between Asa and Baasha
(1 Ki. 15:16-22).

In the six and thirtieth year of the reign
of Asa [g]Baasha king of Israel came up
against Judah, and built Ramah, to the
intent that he might let none go out or
come in [h]to Asa king of Judah.
2 Then Asa brought out silver and
gold out of the treasures of the house of
the LORD and of the king's house, and
sent to Ben-hadad king of Syria, that
dwelt at Damascus, saying,
3 *There is* a league between me and
thee, as *there was* between my father and
thy father: behold, I have sent thee silver
and gold; go, break thy league with
Baasha king of Israel, that he may depart
from me.
4 And Ben-hadad hearkened unto king
Asa, and sent the captains of his armies
against the cities of Israel; and they
smote Ijon, and Dan, and Abel-maim,
and all the store cities of Naphtali.
5 And it came to pass, when Baasha
heard *it*, that he left off building of
Ramah, and let his work cease.
6 Then Asa the king took all Judah;
and they carried away the stones of
Ramah, and the timber thereof, wherewith Baasha was building; and he built
therewith Geba and Mizpah.

Asa rebuked by Hanani.

7 And at that time [i]Hanani the seer
came to Asa king of Judah, and said
unto him, Because thou hast relied on
the king of [j]Syria, and not relied on the
LORD thy God, therefore is the host of
the king of Syria escaped out of thine
hand.
8 Were not [k]the Ethiopians and the
Lubims a huge host, with very many
chariots and horsemen? yet, because
thou didst rely on the LORD, he delivered
them into thine hand.
9 [l]For the eyes of the LORD run to and
fro throughout the whole earth, to shew
himself strong in the behalf of *them*
whose heart *is* [f]perfect toward him.
Herein thou hast done foolishly: therefore from henceforth thou shalt have
wars.

Asa imprisons Hanani.

10 Then Asa was wroth with the seer,
and put him in a [m]prison house; for *he
was* in a rage with him because of this
thing. And Asa oppressed *some* of the
people the same time.
11 And, behold, the [n]acts of Asa, first
and last, lo, they *are* written in the book
of the kings of Judah and Israel.

Asa's illness and death (1 Ki. 15:23, 24).

12 And Asa in the thirty and ninth
year of his reign was diseased in his feet,
until his disease *was* exceeding *great*: yet
in his disease he [o]sought not to the
LORD, but to the physicians.
13 And Asa slept with his fathers, and
died in the one and fortieth year of his
reign.
14 And they buried him in his own
sepulchres, which he had made for himself in the city of David, and laid him in
the bed which was filled with sweet
odours and divers kinds *of spices* prepared by the apothecaries' art: and they
made a very great [p]burning for him.

a Ex. 22:20; Deut. 13:5-10.
b v. 2.
c i.e. grandmother, 1 Ki. 15:13.
d See Deut. 16:21; Jud. 3:7, *note*.
e i.e. the northern or ten-tribe kingdom.
f See 1 Ki. 8:61, *ref*.
g 1 Ki. 15:16-22.
h i.e. none of his subjects. See vs. 5, 6; 2 Chr. 15:9.
i 2 Chr. 19:1, 2; 1 Ki. 16:1.
j vs. 2-4; Jer. 17:5.
k 2 Chr. 14:9.
l Job 34:21, 22; Prov. 5:21; Jer. 16:17; Zech. 4:10.
m Cf. Jer. 32:2, 3; Dan. 6:16, 17; Mt. 14:3.
n 1 Ki. 15:23.
o Cf. 2 Ki. 20:1-5.
p Cf. 2 Chr. 21:18, 19.

CHAPTER 17.

B.C. 914.

Accession of Jehoshaphat (1 Ki. 15:24).

And [a]Jehoshaphat his son reigned in his stead, and strengthened himself against Israel.

2 And he placed forces in all the fenced cities of Judah, and set garrisons in the land of Judah, and in the cities of Ephraim, which [b]Asa his father had taken.

3 And the LORD was with Jehoshaphat, because he walked in the first ways of his [c]father David, and sought not unto Baalim;

4 But sought to the *LORD* God of his father, and walked in his commandments, and not after the doings of [d]Israel.

5 Therefore the LORD stablished the kingdom in his hand; and all Judah [e]brought to Jehoshaphat presents; and he had riches and honour in abundance.

The revival under Jehoshaphat.

6 And his heart was lifted up in the ways of the LORD: moreover he took away the [f]high places and [g]groves out of Judah.

7 Also in the third year of his reign he sent to his princes, *even* to Ben-hail, and to Obadiah, and to Zechariah, and to Nethaneel, and to Michaiah, to teach in the cities of Judah.

8 And with them *he sent* Levites, *even* Shemaiah, and Nethaniah, and Zebadiah, and Asahel, and Shemiramoth, and Jehonathan, and Adonijah, and Tobijah, and Tob-adonijah, Levites; and with them Elishama and Jehoram, priests.

9 And they taught in Judah, and *had* the book of the law of the LORD with them, and went about throughout all the cities of Judah, and taught the people.

Jehoshaphat's growing power.

10 And the fear of the LORD fell upon all the kingdoms of the lands that *were* round about Judah, so that they made no war against Jehoshaphat.

11 Also *some* of the Philistines brought Jehoshaphat presents, and tribute silver; and the Arabians brought him flocks, seven thousand and seven hundred rams, and seven thousand and seven hundred he goats.

12 And Jehoshaphat waxed great exceedingly; and he built in Judah castles, and cities of store.

13 And he had much business in the cities of Judah: and the men of war, mighty men of valour, *were* in Jerusalem.

14 And these *are* the numbers of them according to the house of their fathers: Of Judah, the captains of thousands; Adnah the chief, and with him mighty men of valour [h]three hundred thousand.

15 And next to him *was* Jehohanan the captain, and with him two hundred and fourscore thousand.

16 And next him *was* Amasiah the son of Zichri, who willingly offered himself unto the LORD; and with him two hundred thousand mighty men of valour.

17 And of Benjamin; Eliada a mighty man of valour, and with him armed men with bow and shield two hundred thousand.

18 And next him *was* Jehozabad, and with him an hundred and fourscore thousand ready prepared for the war.

19 These waited on the king, beside *those* whom the king [i]put in the fenced cities throughout all Judah.

CHAPTER 18.

Jehoshaphat's alliance with Ahab (1 Ki. 22:2).

Now Jehoshaphat had [j]riches and honour in abundance, and [k]joined affinity with [l]Ahab.

2 And after *certain* years he [m]went down to Ahab to Samaria. And Ahab killed sheep and oxen for him in abundance, and for the people that *he had* with him, and persuaded him to go up *with him* to Ramoth-gilead.

3 And Ahab king of Israel said unto Jehoshaphat king of Judah, Wilt thou go with me to Ramoth-gilead? And he answered him, I *am* as thou *art*, and my people as thy people; and *we will be* with thee in the war.

The lying prophets of Ahab (1 Ki. 22:5-12).

4 And Jehoshaphat said unto the king of Israel, [n]Enquire, I pray thee, at the word of the LORD to day.

5 Therefore the king of Israel gathered together of prophets four hundred men, and said unto them, Shall we go to Ramoth-gilead to battle, or shall I

a 1 Ki. 15:24; 2 Chr. 20:31.

b 2 Chr. 15:8.

c After the Jewish custom of calling a family, or tribal head, father; e.g. John 8:53.

d i.e. the ten-tribe kingdom.

e 1 Ki. 10:25.

f 1 Ki. 3:2, *note.*

g Deut. 16:21, *ref.;* Jud. 3:7, *note.*

h vs. 15-18; I Cor. 10:8, *note.*

i v. 2.

j 2 Chr. 17:5.

k 2 Chr. 19:1-3; 1 Ki. 22:44.

l See 1 Ki. 16:29; 22:40.

m 1 Ki. 22:2-40.

n 1 Sam. 23:2-9; 2 Sam. 2:1, 2.

B.C. 897.

forbear? And they said, Go up; for God will deliver *it* into the king's hand.

6 But Jehoshaphat said, *Is there* not here a prophet of the LORD besides, that we might enquire of him?

7 And the king of Israel said unto Jehoshaphat, *There is* yet one man, by whom we may enquire of the LORD: but I hate him; for he never prophesied good unto me, but always evil: the same *is* Micaiah the son of Imla. And Jehoshaphat said, Let not the king say so.

8 And the king of Israel called for one *of his* officers, and said, Fetch quickly Micaiah the son of Imla.

9 And the king of Israel and Jehoshaphat king of Judah sat either of them on his throne, clothed in *their* robes, and they sat in a void place at the entering in of the gate of Samaria; and all the prophets prophesied before them.

10 And Zedekiah the son of Chenaanah had made him horns of iron, and said, Thus saith the LORD, With these thou shalt push Syria until they be consumed.

11 And all the prophets prophesied so, saying, Go up to Ramoth-gilead, and prosper: for the LORD shall deliver *it* into the hand of the king.

Micaiah's true prophecy (1 Ki. 22:13-28).

12 And the [a]messenger that went to call Micaiah spake to him, saying, Behold, the words of the prophets *declare* good to the king with one assent; let thy word therefore, I pray thee, be like one of theirs, and speak thou good.

13 And Micaiah said, *As* the LORD liveth, even [b]what my God saith, that will I speak.

14 And when he was come to the king, the king said unto him, Micaiah, shall we go to Ramoth-gilead to battle, or shall I forbear? And he said, Go ye up, and prosper, and they shall be delivered into your hand.

15 And the king said to him, How many times shall I adjure thee that thou say nothing but the truth to me in the name of the LORD?

16 Then he said, I did see all Israel [c]scattered upon the mountains, as sheep that have no shepherd: and the LORD said, These have no master; let them return *therefore* every man to his house in peace.

17 And the king of Israel said to Jehoshaphat, Did I not tell thee *that* he would not prophesy good unto me, but evil?

18 Again he said, Therefore hear the word of the LORD; I saw the LORD sitting upon his throne, and all the host of heaven standing on his right hand and *on* his left.

19 And the LORD said, Who shall entice Ahab king of Israel, that he may go up and fall at Ramoth-gilead? And one spake saying after this manner, and another saying after that manner.

20 Then there came out a spirit, and stood before the LORD, and said, I will entice him. And the LORD said unto him, Wherewith?

21 And he said, I will go out, and be a lying spirit in the mouth of all his prophets. And *the LORD* said, Thou shalt entice *him*, and thou shalt also prevail: go out, and do *even* so.

22 Now therefore, [d]behold, the LORD hath put a lying spirit in the mouth of these thy prophets, and the LORD hath spoken evil against thee.

23 Then Zedekiah the son of Chenaanah came near, and smote Micaiah upon the cheek, and said, Which way went the Spirit of the LORD from me to speak unto thee?

24 And Micaiah said, Behold, thou shalt see on that day when thou shalt go into an inner chamber to hide thyself.

25 Then the king of Israel said, Take ye Micaiah, and carry him back to Amon the governor of the city, and to Joash the king's son;

26 And say, Thus saith the king, [e]Put this *fellow* in the prison, and feed him with bread of affliction and with water of affliction, until I return in peace.

27 And Micaiah said, If thou certainly return in peace, *then* hath not the LORD spoken by me. And he said, Hearken, all ye people.

Battle of Ramoth-gilead: defeat and death of Ahab (1 Ki. 22:29-40).

28 So the king of Israel and Jehoshaphat the king of Judah [f]went up to Ramoth-gilead.

29 And the king of Israel said unto Jehoshaphat, I will disguise myself, and will go to the battle; but put thou on thy robes. So the king of Israel disguised himself; and they went to the battle.

30 Now the king of Syria had

a See vs. 6-8.

b Num. 22:18, 20, 35; 23:12, 26; 24:13.

c Jer. 23:1-8; 31:10.

d Job 12:16, 17; Isa. 19:12-14.

e 2 Chr. 16:10, *refs.*

f 1 Ki. 22:29-40.

commanded the captains of the chariots
that *were* with him, saying, Fight ye not
with small or great, save only with the
king of Israel.
31 And it came to pass, when the captains of the chariots saw Jehoshaphat,
that they said, It *is* the king of Israel.
Therefore they compassed about him to
fight: but Jehoshaphat cried out, and the
LORD helped him; and God moved them
to depart from him.
32 For it came to pass, that, when the
captains of the chariots perceived that it
was not the king of Israel, they turned
back again from pursuing him.
33 And a *certain* man drew a bow at a
venture, and smote the king of Israel
between the joints of the harness: therefore he said to his chariot man, Turn
thine hand, that thou mayest carry me
out of the host; for I am wounded.
34 And the battle increased that day:
howbeit the king of Israel stayed *himself*
up in *his* chariot against the Syrians until
the even: and about the time of the sun
going down he [a]died.

CHAPTER 19.

Jehu rebukes Jehoshaphat's alliance with Ahab.

And Jehoshaphat the king of Judah
returned to his house in peace to
Jerusalem.
2 And Jehu the son of Hanani the seer
went out to meet him, and [b]said to king
Jehoshaphat, Shouldest thou help the
ungodly, and love them that [c]hate the
LORD? therefore *is* wrath upon thee from
before the LORD.
3 Nevertheless there are good things
found in thee, in that thou hast taken
away the [d]groves out of the land, and
hast prepared thine heart to seek God.

Jehoshaphat restores order in worship.

4 And Jehoshaphat dwelt at Jerusalem: and he went out again through
the people from Beer-sheba to mount
Ephraim, and brought them back unto
the LORD God of their fathers.
5 And he set judges in the land
throughout all the fenced cities of Judah,
city by city,
6 And said to the judges, Take heed
what ye do: [e]for ye judge not for man,
but for the LORD, who *is* with you in the
judgment.

B.C. 897.

a 1 Ki. 22:37, 38; cf. Psa. 37:35-36, 38.
b Cf. Isa. 7:1-9; 8:12.
c Psa. 139:21.
d See Deut. 16:21, *refs.*; Jud. 3:7, *note.*
e Lev. 19:15; Deut. 1:17; Psa. 58:1; Isa. 11.3, 4.
f Deut. 32:4; Rom. 9:14.

B.C. 896.]

g Psa. 19:9, *note.*
h See 1 Ki. 8:61, *ref.*
i 1 Chr. 26:30.
j *Bible prayers* (O.T.). 2 Chr. 30:18. (Gen. 15:2; Hab. 3:1-16.)

7 Wherefore now let the fear of the
LORD be upon you; take heed and do *it*:
for *there is* [f]no iniquity with the LORD our
God, nor respect of persons, nor taking
of gifts.
8 Moreover in Jerusalem did
Jehoshaphat set of the Levites, and *of* the
priests, and of the chief of the fathers of
Israel, for the judgment of the LORD, and
for controversies, when they returned to
Jerusalem.
9 And he charged them, saying, Thus
shall ye do in the [g]fear of the LORD, faithfully, and with a [h]perfect heart.
10 And what cause soever shall come
to you of your brethren that dwell in
their cities, between blood and blood,
between law and commandment,
statutes and judgments, ye shall even
warn them that they trespass not against
the LORD, and *so* wrath come upon you,
and upon your brethren: this do, and ye
shall not trespass.
11 And, behold, Amariah the chief
priest *is* over you in all [i]matters of the
LORD; and Zebadiah the son of Ishmael,
the ruler of the house of Judah, for all
the king's matters: also the Levites *shall*
be officers before you. Deal courageous-
ly, and the LORD shall be with the good.

CHAPTER 20.

Judah invaded by Moab.

It came to pass after this also, *that* the
children of Moab, and the children of
Ammon, and with them *other* beside the
Ammonites, came against Jehoshaphat
to battle.
2 Then there came some that told
Jehoshaphat, saying, There cometh a great
multitude against thee from beyond the
sea on this side Syria; and, behold, they *be*
in Hazazon-tamar, which *is* En-gedi.

Jehoshaphat's prayer.

3 And Jehoshaphat feared, and set
himself to seek the LORD, and proclaimed a fast throughout all Judah.
4 And Judah gathered themselves
together, to ask *help* of the LORD: even
out of all the cities of Judah they came to
seek the LORD.
5 And Jehoshaphat stood in the congregation of Judah and Jerusalem, in the
house of the LORD, before the new court,
6 And [j]said, O LORD God of our

fathers, *art* not thou God in heaven? and rulest *not* thou over all the kingdoms of the [a]heathen? and in thine hand *is there not* power and might, so that none is able to withstand thee?

7 *Art* not thou our God, *who* didst drive out the inhabitants of this land before thy people Israel, and [b]gavest it to the seed of Abraham thy friend for ever?

8 And they dwelt therein, and have built thee a sanctuary therein for thy name, saying,

9 If, *when* evil cometh upon us, *as* the sword, judgment, or pestilence, or famine, we stand before this house, and in thy presence, (for thy name *is* in this house,) and cry unto thee in our affliction, then thou wilt hear and help.

10 And now, behold, the children of Ammon and Moab and mount Seir, whom thou wouldest not let Israel invade, when they came out of the land of Egypt, but they turned from them, and destroyed them not;

11 Behold, *I say, how* they reward us, to come to cast us out of thy possession, which thou hast given us to inherit.

12 O our God, wilt thou not judge them? for we have no might against this great company that cometh against us; neither know we what to do: but our eyes *are* upon thee.

13 And all Judah stood before the LORD, with their little ones, their wives, and their children.

Jehovah answers through Jahaziel.

14 Then upon Jahaziel the son of Zechariah, the son of Benaiah, the son of Jeiel, the son of Mattaniah, a Levite of the sons of Asaph, came the [c]Spirit of the LORD in the midst of the congregation;

15 And he said, Hearken ye, all Judah, and ye inhabitants of Jerusalem, and thou king Jehoshaphat, Thus [d]saith the LORD unto you, Be not afraid nor dismayed by reason of this great multitude; [e]for the battle *is* not yours, but God's.

16 To morrow go ye down against them: behold, they come up by the cliff of Ziz; and ye shall find them at the end of the brook, before the wilderness of Jeruel.

17 Ye shall not *need* to fight in this *battle*: set yourselves, stand ye *still*, and see the salvation of the LORD with you, O Judah and Jerusalem: fear not, nor be dismayed; to morrow go out against them: for the LORD *will be* with you.

18 And Jehoshaphat bowed his head with *his* face to the ground: and all Judah and the inhabitants of Jerusalem fell before the LORD, worshipping the LORD.

19 And the Levites, of the children of the Kohathites, and of the children of the Korhites, stood up to praise the LORD God of Israel with a loud voice on high.

The invading armies stricken with death.

20 And they rose early in the morning, and went forth into the wilderness of Tekoa: and as they went forth, Jehoshaphat stood and said, Hear me, O Judah, and ye inhabitants of Jerusalem; Believe in the LORD your God, so shall ye be established; believe his prophets, so shall ye prosper.

21 And when he had consulted with the people, he appointed [f]singers unto the LORD, and that should praise the [g]beauty of holiness, as they went out before the army, and to say, Praise the LORD; [h]for his mercy *endureth* for ever.

22 And when they began to sing and to praise, the LORD set ambushments against the children of Ammon, Moab, and mount Seir, which were come against Judah; and they were smitten.

23 For the children of Ammon and Moab stood up against the inhabitants of mount Seir, utterly to slay and destroy *them*: and when they had made an end of the inhabitants of Seir, [i]every one helped to destroy another.

24 And when Judah came toward the watch tower in the wilderness, they looked unto the multitude, and, behold, they *were* dead bodies fallen to the earth, and none escaped.

25 And when Jehoshaphat and his people came to take away the spoil of them, they found among them in abundance both riches with the dead bodies, and precious jewels, which they stripped off for themselves, more than they could carry away: and they were three days in gathering of the spoil, it was so much.

The triumphant return to Jerusalem.

26 And on the fourth day they assembled themselves in the valley of

B.C. 896.

a i.e. *nations.* Dan. 4:17, 25, 32.

b Gen. 13:14-17.

c *Holy Spirit.* 2 Chr. 24:20. (Gen. 1.2; Mal. 2:15.)

d Deut. 1:29, 30.

e vs. 24, 25; 1 Sam. 17:47; Zech. 14:3.

f Heb. *praisers.* See 1 Chr. 16:29.

g Psa. 29:2; 90:17; 96:9; 110:3.

h Psa. 136:1-26.

i Jud. 7:22; 1 Sam. 14:20.

[a]Berachah; for there they blessed the LORD: therefore the name of the same place was called, The valley of Berachah, unto this day.

B.C. 896.

[B.C. 889.

27 Then they returned, every man of Judah and Jerusalem, and Jehoshaphat in the forefront of them, to go again to Jerusalem with joy; for the LORD had made them to rejoice over their enemies.

28 And they came to Jerusalem [b]with psalteries and harps and trumpets unto the house of the LORD.

29 And the fear of God was on all the kingdoms of *those* countries, when they had heard that the LORD fought against the enemies of Israel.

30 So the realm of Jehoshaphat was quiet: [c]for his God gave him rest round about.

31 And Jehoshaphat [d]reigned over Judah: *he was* thirty and five years old when he began to reign, and he reigned twenty and five years in Jerusalem. And his mother's name *was* Azubah the daughter of Shilhi.

32 And he walked in the way of Asa his father, and departed not from it, doing *that which was* right in the sight of the LORD.

33 Howbeit the [e]high places were not taken away: for as yet the people had not prepared their hearts unto the God of their fathers.

34 Now the rest of the acts of Jehoshaphat, first and last, behold, they *are* written in the book of Jehu the son of Hanani, who *is* mentioned in the book of the kings of Israel.

Jehoshaphat's trading venture with Ahaziah, king of Israel (1 Ki. 22:47-49).

35 And after this did Jehoshaphat king of Judah [f]join himself with Ahaziah king of Israel, [g]who did very wickedly:

36 And he joined himself with him [h]to make ships to go to Tarshish: and they made the ships in Ezion-gaber.

37 Then Eliezer the son of Dodavah of Mareshah prophesied against Jehoshaphat, saying, Because thou hast joined thyself with Ahaziah, the LORD hath broken thy works. And the ships were broken, that they were not able to go to Tarshish.

CHAPTER 21.

Jehoram's reign over Judah after his father's death (2 Ki. 8:16-24).

Now Jehoshaphat [i]slept with his fathers, and was buried with his fathers in the city of David. And [j]Jehoram his son reigned in his stead.

2 And he had brethren the sons of Jehoshaphat, Azariah, and Jehiel, and Zechariah, and Azariah, and Michael, and Shephatiah: all these *were* the sons of Jehoshaphat king of Israel.

3 And their father gave them great gifts of silver, and of gold, and of precious things, with fenced cities in Judah: but the kingdom gave he to Jehoram; because he *was* the firstborn.

4 Now when Jehoram was risen up to the kingdom of his father, he strengthened himself, and slew all his brethren with the sword, and *divers* also of the princes of Israel.

5 Jehoram *was* thirty and two years old when he [k]began to reign, and he reigned eight years in Jerusalem.

6 And he walked in the way of the kings of Israel, like as did the house of Ahab: for he had the daughter of Ahab to wife: and he wrought *that which was* evil in the eyes of the LORD.

7 Howbeit the LORD would not destroy the house of David, because of the [l]covenant that he had made with David, and as he promised to give a light to him and to his sons for ever.

Revolt of Edom (2 Ki. 8:20-22).

8 In his days the Edomites revolted from under the dominion of Judah, and made themselves a king.

9 Then Jehoram went forth with his princes, and all his chariots with him: and he rose up by night, and smote the Edomites which compassed him in, and the captains of the chariots.

Revolt of Libnah (2 Ki. 8:22).

10 So the Edomites revolted from under the hand of Judah unto this day. The same time *also* did Libnah revolt from under his hand; because he had forsaken the LORD God of his fathers.

11 Moreover he made [e]high places in the mountains of Judah, and caused the

a i.e. *blessing.* See also, 1 Chr. 12:3.
b Cf. v. 21.
c Job 34:29.
d 1 Ki. 15:24; 22:41.
e 1 Ki. 3:2, *note.*
f 1 Ki. 22:48, 49.
g 1 Ki. 22:51-53.
h 2 Cor. 6:14-18.
i 1 Ki. 22:50.
j Jehoram reigned for a time as co-king with his father. 2 Ki. 8:16.
k Began, that is, as co-king. v. 1, *ref.* Cf. 2 Chr. 22:2.
l 2 Sam. 7:8-16.

inhabitants of Jerusalem to commit fornication, and compelled Judah *thereto.*

The message of Elijah, written before his translation

12 And there came a writing to him from [a]Elijah the prophet, saying, Thus saith the LORD God of David thy father, Because thou hast not walked in the ways of Jehoshaphat thy father, nor in the ways of Asa king of Judah,
13 But hast walked in the way of the kings of Israel, and hast [b]made Judah and the inhabitants of Jerusalem to go a whoring, [c]like to the whoredoms of the house of Ahab, and also hast [d]slain thy brethren of thy father's house, *which were* better than thyself:
14 Behold, with a great plague will the LORD smite thy people, and thy children, and thy wives, and all thy goods:
15 And thou *shalt have* great sickness [e]by disease of thy bowels, until thy bowels fall out by reason of the sickness day by day.

Invasion of Judah by Arabians and Philistines.

16 Moreover the LORD [f]stirred up against Jehoram the spirit of the Philistines, and of the Arabians, that *were* near the Ethiopians:
17 And they came up into Judah, and brake into it, and carried away all the substance that was found in the king's house, and his [g]sons also, and his wives; so that there was never a son left him, save [h]Jehoahaz, the youngest of his sons.

Jehoram's incurable disease.

18 And after all this the LORD [i]smote him in his bowels with an incurable disease.
19 And it came to pass, that in process of time, after the end of two years, his bowels fell out by reason of his sickness: so he died of sore diseases. And his people made no [j]burning for him, like the burning of his fathers.
20 Thirty and two years old was he when he began to reign, and he reigned in Jerusalem eight years, and departed without being desired. Howbeit they buried him in the city of David, but not in the sepulchres of the kings.

B.C. 889.

[B.C. 885.

a See Elijah's history, 1 Ki. 17:1; 2 Ki. 2:12.
b v. 11.
c 1 Ki. 16:31-34; 2 Ki. 9:22.
d v. 4.
e vs. 18, 19.
f 1 Ki. 11:14-24.
g 2 Chr. 24:7.
h Called *Ahaziah*, 2 Chr. 22:1, and *Azariah*, 2 Chr. 22:6.
i v. 15.
j Cf. 2 Chr. 16:14.
k Cf. 2 Chr. 21:17, where he is called *Jehoahaz.*
l See 2 Ki. 9:22-24.
m 2 Ki. 9:27.

B.C. 885.]

CHAPTER 22.

Accession of Ahaziah over Judah (2 Ki. 8:24-26).

And the inhabitants of Jerusalem made [k]Ahaziah his youngest son king in his stead: for the band of men that came with the Arabians to the camp had slain all the eldest. So Ahaziah the son of Jehoram king of Judah reigned.
2 Forty and two years old *was* Ahaziah when he began to reign, and he reigned one year in Jerusalem. His mother's name also *was* Athaliah the daughter of Omri.
3 He also walked in the ways of the house of Ahab: for his mother was his counsellor to do wickedly.
4 Wherefore he did evil in the sight of the LORD like the house of Ahab: for they were his counsellors after the death of his father to his destruction.

Ahaziah assists Jehoram in the battle of Ramoth-gilead (2 Ki. 8:28).

5 He walked also after their counsel, and went with Jehoram the son of Ahab king of Israel to war against Hazael king of Syria at Ramoth-gilead: and the Syrians smote Joram.

Ahaziah visits Jehoram at Jezreel (2 Ki. 8:29).

6 And he returned to be healed in Jezreel because of the wounds which were given him at Ramah, when he fought with Hazael king of Syria. And Azariah the son of Jehoram king of Judah went down to see Jehoram the son of Ahab at Jezreel, because he was sick.
7 And the [l]destruction of Ahaziah was of God by coming to Joram: for when he was come, he went out with Jehoram against Jehu the son of Nimshi, whom the LORD had anointed to cut off the house of Ahab.

The princes of Judah slain (2 Ki. 10:12-14).

8 And it came to pass, that, when Jehu was executing judgment upon the house of Ahab, and found the princes of Judah, and the sons of the brethren of Ahaziah, that ministered to Ahaziah, he slew them.

Ahaziah slain (2 Ki. 9:27, 28).

9 [m]And he sought Ahaziah: and they caught him, (for he was hid in Samaria,) and brought him to Jehu: and when they

had slain him, they buried him: Because, said they, he *is* the son of Jehoshaphat, who [a]sought the LORD with all his heart. So the house of Ahaziah had no power to keep still the kingdom.

The seed royal of Judah destroyed, save Joash (2 Ki. 11:1-3).

10 But [b]when Athaliah the mother of Ahaziah saw that her son was dead, she arose and destroyed all the seed royal of the house of Judah.

11 But [c]Jehoshabeath, the daughter of the king, took Joash the son of Ahaziah, and stole him from among the king's sons that were slain, and put him and his nurse in a bedchamber. So Jehoshabeath, the daughter of king Jehoram, the wife of Jehoiada the priest, (for she was the sister of Ahaziah,) hid him from Athaliah, so that she slew him not.

12 And he was with them hid in the house of God six years: and Athaliah reigned over the land.

CHAPTER 23.

Joash becomes king over Judah (2 Ki. 11:4-12).

And in the [d]seventh year Jehoiada strengthened himself, and took the captains of hundreds, Azariah the son of Jeroham, and Ishmael the son of Jehohanan, and Azariah the son of Obed, and Maaseiah the son of Adaiah, and Elishaphat the son of Zichri, into covenant with him.

2 And they went about in Judah, and gathered the Levites out of all the cities of Judah, and the chief of the fathers of Israel, and they came to Jerusalem.

3 And all the congregation made a covenant with the king in the house of God. And he said unto them, Behold, the king's son shall reign, as the LORD hath [e]said of the sons of David.

4 This *is* the thing that ye shall do; A third part of you [f]entering on the sabbath, of the priests and of the Levites, *shall be* porters of the doors;

5 And a third part *shall be* at the king's house; and a third part at the gate of the foundation: and all the people *shall be* in the courts of the house of the LORD.

6 But let none come into the house of the LORD, save the priests, and [g]they that minister of the Levites; they shall go in, for they *are* holy: but all the people shall keep the watch of the LORD.

7 And the Levites shall compass the king round about, every man with his weapons in his hand; and whosoever *else* cometh into the house, he shall be put to death: but be ye with the king when he cometh in, and when he goeth out.

8 So the Levites and all Judah did according to all things that Jehoiada the priest had commanded, and took every man his men that were to come in on the sabbath, with them that were to go *out* on the sabbath: for Jehoiada the priest dismissed not the [h]courses.

9 Moreover Jehoiada the priest delivered to the captains of hundreds spears, and bucklers, and shields, that *had been* king David's, which *were* in the house of God.

10 And he set all the people, every man having his weapon in his hand, from the right side of the temple to the left side of the temple, along by the altar and the temple, by the king round about.

11 Then they brought out the king's son, and put upon him the crown, and [i]*gave him* the testimony, and made him king. And Jehoiada and his sons anointed him, and said, God save the king.

Execution of Athaliah (2 Ki. 11:13-16).

12 Now when Athaliah heard the noise of the people running and praising the king, she came to the people into the house of the LORD:

13 And she looked, and, behold, the king stood at his pillar at the entering in, and the princes and the trumpets by the king: and all the people of the land rejoiced, and sounded with trumpets, also the singers with instruments of musick, and [j]such as taught to sing praise. Then Athaliah rent her clothes, and said, Treason, Treason.

14 Then Jehoiada the priest brought out the captains of hundreds that were set over the host, and said unto them, Have her forth of the ranges: and whoso followeth her, let him be slain with the sword. For the priest said, Slay her not in the house of the LORD.

15 So they laid hands on her; and when she was come to the entering [k]of the horse gate by the king's house, they slew her there.

B.C. 884.

a 2 Chr. 17:4; 20:3-4.
b 2 Ki. 11:1.
c 2 Ki. 11:2.
d 2 Ki. 11:4.
e 2 Sam. 7:12; 1 Ki. 2:4; 9:5; 2 Chr. 6:16; 7:18; 21:7.
B.C. 878.]
f 1 Chr. 9:25.
g 1 Chr. 23:28, 32.
h 1 Chr. 24:5-31
i Deut. 17:18.
j 1 Chr. 25:8.
k Neh. 3:28.

The revival through Jehoiada
(2 Ki. 11:17-20).

16 And Jehoiada made a covenant between him, and between all the people, and between the king, that they should be the LORD'S people.

17 Then all the people went to the house of Baal, and brake it down, and brake his altars and his images in pieces, and [a]slew Mattan the priest of Baal before the altars.

18 Also Jehoiada appointed the offices of the house of the LORD by the hand of the priests the Levites, whom David had [b]distributed in the house of the LORD, to offer the burnt-offerings of the LORD, as *it is* written in the [c]law of Moses, with rejoicing and with singing, *as it was ordained* by David.

19 And he set the [d]porters at the gates of the house of the LORD, that none *which was* unclean in any thing should enter in.

20 [e]And he took the captains of hundreds, and the nobles, and the governors of the people, and all the people of the land, and brought down the king from the house of the LORD: and they came through the high gate into the king's house, and set the king upon the throne of the kingdom.

21 And all the people of the land rejoiced: and the city was quiet, after that they had slain Athaliah with the sword.

CHAPTER 24.

Reign of Joash (Jehoash) (2 Ki. 12:1-3).

Joash [f]*was* seven years old when he began to reign, and he reigned forty years in Jerusalem. His mother's name also *was* Zibiah of Beer-sheba.

2 And Joash did *that which was* right in the sight of the LORD all the days of Jehoiada the priest.

3 And Jehoiada took for him two wives; and he begat sons and daughters.

The faithless priests (2 Ki. 12:4-8).

4 And it came to pass after this, *that* Joash was minded to repair the house of the LORD.

5 And he gathered together the priests and the Levites, and said to them, Go out unto the cities of Judah, and [g]gather of all Israel money to repair the house of your God from year to year, and see that ye hasten the matter. Howbeit the Levites hastened *it* not.

6 [h]And the king called for Jehoiada the chief, and said unto him, Why hast thou not required of the Levites to bring in out of Judah and out of Jerusalem the collection, *according to the commandment* of [i]Moses the servant of the LORD, and of the congregation of Israel, for the [j]tabernacle of witness?

7 For the [k]sons of Athaliah, that wicked woman, had broken up the house of God; and also all the dedicated things of the house of the LORD did they bestow upon Baalim.

The temple repaired (2 Ki. 12:9-16).

8 And at the king's commandment [l]they made a chest, and set it without at the gate of the house of the LORD.

9 And they made a proclamation through Judah and Jerusalem, to bring in to the LORD the collection *that* Moses the servant of God *laid* upon Israel in the wilderness.

10 And all the princes and all the people rejoiced, and brought in, and cast into the chest, until they had made an end.

11 Now it came to pass, that at what time the chest was brought unto the king's office by the hand of the Levites, and [m]when they saw that *there was* much money, the king's scribe and the high priest's officer came and emptied the chest, and took it, and carried it to his place again. Thus they did day by day, and gathered money in abundance.

12 And the king and Jehoiada gave it to such as did the work of the service of the house of the LORD, and hired masons and carpenters to repair the house of the LORD, and also such as wrought iron and brass to mend the house of the LORD.

13 So the workmen wrought, and the work was perfected by them, and they set the house of God in his state, and strengthened it.

14 And when they had finished *it*, they brought the rest of the money before the king and Jehoiada, whereof were made vessels for the house of the LORD, *even* vessels to minister, and to offer *withal*, and spoons, and vessels of gold and silver. And they offered burnt-offerings in the house of the LORD continually all the days of Jehoiada.

B.C. 878.

a Deut. 13:9.
b 1 Chr. 23:6, 30, 31; 24:1.
c Num. 28:2.
d 1 Chr. 26.
e 2 Ki. 11:19.
f 2 Ki. 11:21; 12:1.
g 2 Ki. 12.4.
h 2 Ki. 12:7.
i Ex. 30:11-16.
j Num. 1:50; Acts 7:44.
k 2 Chr. 21:17.
l 2 Ki. 12:9.
m 2 Ki. 12:10; cf. Ezra 8:24-30.

Death of Jehoiada the good priest.

B.C. 850.

15 But Jehoiada waxed old, and was
full of days when he died; an hundred
and thirty years old *was he* when he died.
16 And they buried him in the city of
David among the kings, because he had
done good in Israel, both toward God,
and toward his house.

The apostasy of the princes.

17 Now after the death of Jehoiada
came the princes of Judah, and made
obeisance to the king. Then the king
hearkened unto them.
18 And they left the house of the LORD
God of their fathers, and served [a]groves
and idols: and wrath came upon Judah
and Jerusalem for this their trespass.
19 Yet he sent prophets to them, to
bring them again unto the LORD; and
they testified against them: but they
would not give ear.

Zechariah stoned.

20 And the [b]Spirit of God came upon
Zechariah the son of Jehoiada the priest,
which stood above the people, and said
unto them, Thus saith God, Why transgress ye the commandments of the
LORD, that ye cannot prosper? because
ye have forsaken the LORD, he hath also
forsaken you.
21 And they conspired against him,
and stoned him with stones at the commandment of the king in the court of the
house of the LORD.
22 Thus Joash the king remembered
not the kindness which Jehoiada his
father had done to him, but slew his son.
And when he died, he said, The LORD
look upon *it*, and require *it*.

A Syrian invasion: Judah defeated.

23 And it came to pass at the end of
the year, *that* the host of Syria came up
against him: and they came to Judah and
Jerusalem, and destroyed all the princes
of the people from among the people,
and sent all the spoil of them unto the
king of Damascus.
24 For the army of the Syrians came
with a small company of men, and the
LORD delivered a very great host into
their hand, because they had forsaken
the LORD God of their fathers. So they
executed judgment against Joash.

B.C. 839.]

a See Deut. 16:21; Jud. 3:7, *note.*

[B.C. 827.

b *Holy Spirit.* Neh. 9:20, 30. (Gen. 1:2; Mal. 2:15.)

c See 1 Ki. 8:61.

Death of Joash (2 Ki. 12:19-21).

25 And when they were departed
from him, (for they left him in great diseases,) his own servants conspired
against him for the blood of the sons of
Jehoiada the priest, and slew him on his
bed, and he died: and they buried him in
the city of David, but they buried him
not in the sepulchres of the kings.
26 And these are they that conspired
against him; Zabad the son of Shimeath
an Ammonitess, and Jehozabad the son
of Shimrith a Moabitess.
27 Now *concerning* his sons, and the
greatness of the burdens *laid* upon him,
and the repairing of the house of God,
behold, they *are* written in the story of
the book of the kings. And Amaziah his
son reigned in his stead.

CHAPTER 25.

The reign of Amaziah over Judah
(2 Ki. 14:1, 2).

Amaziah *was* twenty and five years
old *when* he began to reign, and he
reigned twenty and nine years in
Jerusalem. And his mother's name *was*
Jehoaddan of Jerusalem.
2 And he did *that which was* right in
the sight of the LORD, but not with a
[c]perfect heart.
3 Now it came to pass, when the kingdom was established to him, that he
slew his servants that had killed the king
his father.
4 But he slew not their children, but
did as *it is* written in the law in the book
of Moses, where the LORD commanded,
saying, The fathers shall not die for the
children, neither shall the children die
for the fathers, but every man shall die
for his own sin.

The expedition against Edom.

5 Moreover Amaziah gathered Judah
together, and made them captains over
thousands, and captains over hundreds,
according to the houses of *their* fathers,
throughout all Judah and Benjamin: and
he numbered them from twenty years
old and above, and found them three
hundred thousand choice *men, able* to go
forth to war, that could handle spear and
shield.
6 He hired also an hundred thousand

mighty men of valour out of Israel for an hundred [a] talents of silver.

B.C. 827.

7 But there came a man of God to him, saying, O king, let not the army of Israel go with thee; for the LORD *is* not with Israel, *to wit, with* all the children of [1]Ephraim.

8 But if thou wilt go, do *it*, be strong for the battle: God shall make thee fall before the enemy: for God hath power to help, and to cast down.

9 And Amaziah said to the man of God, But what shall we do for the hundred talents which I have given to the army of Israel? And the man of God answered, The LORD is able to give thee much more than this.

10 Then Amaziah separated them, *to wit*, the army that was come to him out of Ephraim, to go home again: wherefore their anger was greatly kindled against Judah, and they returned home in great anger.

11 And Amaziah strengthened himself, and led forth his people, and went to the valley of salt, and smote of the children of Seir ten thousand.

12 And *other* ten thousand *left* alive did the children of Judah carry away captive, and brought them unto the top of the rock, and cast them down from the top of the rock, that they all were broken in pieces.

13 But the soldiers of the army which Amaziah sent back, that they should not go with him to battle, fell upon the cities of Judah, from Samaria even unto Beth-horon, and smote three thousand of them, and took much spoil.

14 Now it came to pass, after that Amaziah was come from the slaughter of the Edomites, that he brought the gods of the children of Seir, and set them up *to be* his gods, and bowed down himself before them, and burned incense unto them.

15 Wherefore the anger of the LORD was kindled against Amaziah, and he sent unto him a prophet, which said unto him, Why hast thou sought after the gods of the people, which could not deliver their own people out of thine hand?

16 And it came to pass, as he talked with him, that *the king* said unto him, Art thou made of the king's counsel? forbear; why shouldest thou be smitten? Then the prophet forbare, and said, I know that God hath determined to destroy thee, because thou hast done this, and hast not hearkened unto my counsel.

War between Judah and Israel
(2 Ki. 14:8-14).

[B.C. 826.

17 Then Amaziah king of Judah took advice, and sent to Joash, the son of Jehoahaz, the son of Jehu, king of Israel, saying, Come, let us see one another in the face.

18 And Joash king of Israel sent to Amaziah king of Judah, saying, [b]The thistle that *was* in Lebanon sent to the cedar that *was* in Lebanon, saying, Give thy daughter to my son to wife: and there passed by a wild beast that *was* in Lebanon, and trode down the thistle.

19 Thou sayest, Lo, thou hast smitten the Edomites; and thine heart lifteth thee up to boast: abide now at home; why shouldest thou meddle to *thine* hurt, that thou shouldest fall, *even* thou, and Judah with thee?

20 But Amaziah would not hear; for it *came* of God, that he might deliver them into the hand *of their enemies*, because they sought after the gods of Edom.

21 So Joash the king of Israel went up; and they saw one another in the face, *both* he and Amaziah king of Judah, at Beth-shemesh, which *belongeth* to Judah.

22 And Judah was put to the worse before Israel, and they fled every man to his tent.

23 And Joash the king of Israel took Amaziah king of Judah, the son of Joash, the son of Jehoahaz, at Beth-shemesh, and brought him to Jerusalem, and brake down the wall of Jerusalem from the gate of Ephraim to the corner gate, four hundred [c]cubits.

24 And *he took* all the gold and the silver, and all the vessels that were found in the house of God with Obed-edom, and the treasures of the king's house, the hostages also, and returned to Samaria.

25 And Amaziah the son of Joash king of Judah lived after the death of Joash son of Jehoahaz king of Israel fifteen years.

a One talent (silver) = £410, or $1940; also v. 9.

b *Parables* (O.T.). Isa. 5:1-7. (Jud. 9:7-15; Zech. 11:7-14.)

c One cubit = about 18 in.

[1](25:7) Used in a collective sense for the northern ten-tribe kingdom, called also "Israel."

Death of Amaziah (2 Ki. 14:17-20).

26 Now the rest of the acts of Amaziah, first and last, behold, *are* they not written in the book of the kings of Judah and Israel?

27 Now after the time that Amaziah did turn away from following the LORD they made a conspiracy against him in Jerusalem; and he fled to Lachish: but they sent to Lachish after him, and slew him there.

28 And they brought him upon horses, and buried him with his fathers in the city of Judah.

CHAPTER 26.

Accession of Uzziah (2 Ki. 14:21).

Then all the people of Judah took [a]Uzziah, who *was* sixteen years old, and made him king in the room of his father Amaziah.

2 He built Eloth, and restored it to Judah, after that the king slept with his fathers.

3 Sixteen years old *was* Uzziah when he began to reign, and he reigned fifty and two years in Jerusalem. His mother's name also *was* Jecoliah of Jerusalem.

4 And he did *that which was* right in the sight of the LORD, according to all that his father Amaziah did.

5 And he [b]sought God in the days of Zechariah, who [c]had understanding in the visions of God: and as long as he sought the LORD, God made him to prosper.

Uzziah successful in war: his works and fame.

6 And he went forth and warred against the Philistines, and brake down the wall of Gath, and the wall of Jabneh, and the wall of Ashdod, and built cities about Ashdod, and among the Philistines.

7 And God helped him against [d]the Philistines, and against the Arabians that dwelt in Gur-baal, and the Mehunims.

8 And the Ammonites [e]gave gifts to Uzziah: and his name spread abroad *even* to the entering in of Egypt; for he strengthened *himself* exceedingly.

9 Moreover Uzziah built towers in Jerusalem at the corner gate, and at the valley gate, and at the turning *of the wall*, and fortified them.

B.C. 826.

B.C. 810.]

a 2 Ki. 14:21, 22; 15:1.

b 2 Chr. 24:2.

c Gen. 41:15; Dan. 1:17.

d 2 Chr. 21:16.

e 2 Chr. 17:11; 2 Sam. 8:2.

f Cf. Num. 16:8-10; 1 Sam. 13:9-14.

g 1 Ki. 13:1-4; 2 Ki. 16:12, 13.

h 1 Chr. 6:10.

i Num. 16:40.

j Ex. 30:7, 8.

k *Miracles* (O.T.). vs. 16-21. Dan. 3:19-27. (Gen. 5:24; Jon. 2:1-10.)

10 Also he built towers in the desert, and digged many wells: for he had much cattle, both in the low country, and in the plains: husbandmen *also*, and vine dressers in the mountains, and in Carmel: for he loved husbandry.

11 Moreover Uzziah had an host of fighting men, that went out to war by bands, according to the number of their account by the hand of Jeiel the scribe and Maaseiah the ruler, under the hand of Hananiah, *one* of the king's captains.

12 The whole number of the chief of the fathers of the mighty men of valour *were* two thousand and six hundred.

13 And under their hand *was* an army, three hundred thousand and seven thousand and five hundred, that made war with mighty power, to help the king against the enemy.

14 And Uzziah prepared for them throughout all the host shields, and spears, and helmets, and habergeons, and bows, and slings *to cast* stones.

15 And he made in Jerusalem engines, invented by cunning men, to be on the towers and upon the bulwarks, to shoot arrows and great stones withal. And his name spread far abroad; for he was marvellously helped, till he was strong.

Uzziah's intrusion into the priest's office: his punishment.

16 But when he was strong, his heart was lifted up to *his* destruction: for he [f]transgressed against the LORD his God, and [g]went into the temple of the LORD to burn incense upon the altar of incense.

17 And [h]Azariah the priest went in after him, and with him fourscore priests of the LORD, *that were* valiant men:

18 And they withstood Uzziah the king, and said unto him, *It* [i]*appertaineth* not unto thee, Uzziah, to burn incense unto the LORD, but to the [j]priests the sons of Aaron, that are consecrated to burn incense: go out of the sanctuary; for thou hast trespassed; neither *shall it be* for thine honour from the LORD God.

19 Then Uzziah was wroth, and *had* a censer in his hand to burn incense: and while he was wroth with the priests, the [k]leprosy even rose up in his forehead before the priests in the house of the LORD, from beside the incense altar.

20 And Azariah the chief priest, and all the priests, looked upon him, and, behold, he *was* leprous in his forehead,

and they thrust him out from thence;
yea, himself hasted also to go out,
because the LORD had smitten him.
21 And [a]Uzziah the king was a leper
unto the day of his death, and dwelt in a
[b]several house, *being* a leper; for he was
cut off from the house of the LORD: and
Jotham his son *was* over the king's
house, judging the people of the land.

Death of Uzziah: accession of Jotham over Judah (2 Ki. 15:32).

22 Now the rest of the acts of Uzziah,
first and last, did [c]Isaiah the prophet, the
son of Amoz, write.
23 [d]So Uzziah slept with his fathers,
and they buried him with his fathers in
the field of the burial which *belonged* to
the kings; for they said, He *is* a leper:
and Jotham his son reigned in his stead.

CHAPTER 27.

Reign of Jotham over Judah (2 Ki. 15:32-38).

Jotham [e]*was* twenty and five years old
when he began to reign, and he
reigned sixteen years in Jerusalem. His
mother's name also *was* Jerushah, the
daughter of Zadok.
2 And he did *that which was* right in
the sight of the LORD, according to all
that his father Uzziah did: howbeit he
entered not into the temple of the LORD.
[f]And the people did yet corruptly.
3 He built the high gate of the house
of the LORD, and on the wall of Ophel he
built much.
4 Moreover he built cities in the
mountains of Judah, and in the forests
he built castles and towers.
5 He fought also with the king of the
Ammonites, and prevailed against them.
And the children of Ammon gave him the
same year an hundred [g]talents of silver,
and ten thousand [h]measures of wheat,
and ten thousand of barley. So much did
the children of Ammon pay unto him,
both the second year, and the third.
6 So Jotham became mighty, because
he [i]prepared his ways before the LORD
his God.

Death of Jotham king of Judah (2 Ki. 15:36-38).

7 Now the rest of the acts of Jotham,
and all his wars, and his ways, lo, they
are written in the book of the kings of
Israel and Judah.

B.C. 765.

[B.C. 742.

a 2 Ki. 15:5.
b Lev. 13:46; Num. 5:2.
c Isa. 1:1.
d 2 Ki. 15:7; Isa. 6:1.
e 2 Ki. 15:33.
f 2 Ki. 15:35.

B.C. 758.]

g One talent (silver) = £410, or $1940.
h One measure = about 10 bu.
i Or, *established.*
j 2 Ki. 15:38.
k 2 Ki. 16:2.
l Ex. 34:17; Lev. 19:4.
m 2 Chr. 33:6.
n i.e. *nations.*
o 2 Ki. 16:5, 6.
p 2 Ki. 15:27; Isa. 7:1-17.
q 2 Chr. 11:4.

8 He was five and twenty years old
when he began to reign, and reigned sixteen years in Jerusalem.
9 [j]And Jotham slept with his fathers,
and they buried him in the city of David:
and Ahaz his son reigned in his stead.

CHAPTER 28.

Reign of Ahaz (2 Ki. 16:1).

Ahaz [k]*was* twenty years old when he
began to reign, and he reigned sixteen years in Jerusalem: but he did not
that which was right in the sight of the
LORD, like David his father:
2 For he walked in the ways of the
kings of Israel, and made also [l]molten
images for Baalim.
3 Moreover he burnt incense in the
valley of the son of Hinnom, and burnt
[m]his children in the fire, after the abominations of the [n]heathen whom the LORD
had cast out before the children of Israel.
4 He sacrificed also and burnt incense
in the high places, and on the hills, and
under every green tree.

War between Ahaz and Pekah (2 Ki. 16:5, 6).

5 Wherefore the LORD his God delivered him into the hand of the king of
Syria; and [o]they smote him, and carried
away a great multitude of them captives,
and brought *them* to Damascus. And he
was also delivered into the hand of the
king of Israel, who smote him with a
great slaughter.
6 For [p]Pekah the son of Remaliah slew
in Judah an hundred and twenty thousand in one day, *which were* all valiant
men; because they had forsaken the
LORD God of their fathers.
7 And Zichri, a mighty man of
Ephraim, slew Maaseiah the king's son,
and Azrikam the governor of the house,
and Elkanah *that was* next to the king.
8 And the children of Israel carried
away captive of [q]their brethren two hundred thousand, women, sons, and
daughters, and took also away much
spoil from them, and brought the spoil
to Samaria.

The intercession of Oded.

9 But a prophet of the LORD was there,
whose name *was* Oded: and he went out

B.C. 741.

before the host that came to Samaria,
and said unto them, Behold, [a]because
the LORD God of your fathers was wroth
with Judah, he hath delivered them into
your hand, and ye have slain them in a
rage *that* [b]reacheth up unto heaven.
10 And now ye purpose to keep under
the children of Judah and Jerusalem for
bondmen and bondwomen unto you:
but are there not with you, even with you,
sins against the LORD your God?
11 Now hear me therefore, and deliver
the captives again, which ye have taken
captive of your brethren: for [c]the fierce
wrath of the LORD *is* upon you.
12 Then certain of the heads of the
children of Ephraim, Azariah the son of
Johanan, Berechiah the son of Meshillemoth, and Jehizkiah the son of Shallum,
and Amasa the son of Hadlai, stood up
against them that came from the war,
13 And said unto them, Ye shall not
bring in the captives hither: for whereas
we have offended against the LORD
already, ye intend to add *more* to our sins
and to our trespass: for our trespass is
great, and *there is* fierce wrath against
Israel.
14 So the armed men left the captives
and the spoil before the princes and all
the congregation.
15 And the men [d]which were
expressed by name rose up, and took the
captives, and with the spoil clothed all
that were naked among them, and
arrayed them, and shod them, and [e]gave
them to eat and to drink, and anointed
them, and carried all the feeble of them
upon asses, and brought them to Jericho,
the [f]city of palm trees, to their brethren:
then they returned to Samaria.

Edomite and Philistine invasions of Judah.

16 [g]At that time did king Ahaz send
unto the kings of Assyria to help him.
17 For again the Edomites had come
and smitten Judah, and carried away
captives.
18 The [h]Philistines also had invaded
the cities of the low country, and of the
south of Judah, and had taken Beth-
shemesh, and Ajalon, and Gederoth, and
Shocho with the villages thereof, and
Timnah with the villages thereof, Gimzo
also and the villages thereof: and they
dwelt there.
19 For the LORD brought Judah low
because of Ahaz king of [i]Israel; for he
[j]made Judah naked, and transgressed
sore against the LORD.
20 And [k]Tilgath-pilneser king of
Assyria came unto him, and distressed
him, but strengthened him not.
21 For Ahaz took away a portion *out*
of the house of the LORD, and *out* of the
house of the king, and of the princes,
and gave *it* unto the king of Assyria: but
he helped him not.
22 And in the time of his distress did
he trespass yet more against the LORD:
this *is that* king Ahaz.
23 For he [l]sacrificed unto the gods of
Damascus, which smote him: and he
said, Because the gods of the kings of
Syria help them, *therefore* will I sacrifice to
them, that [m]they may help me. But they
were the ruin of him, and of all Israel.
24 And Ahaz gathered together the
vessels of the house of God, and cut in
pieces the vessels of the house of God,
[n]and shut up the doors of the house of
the LORD, and he made him altars in
every corner of Jerusalem.
25 And in every several city of Judah
he made high places to burn incense
unto other gods, and provoked to anger
the LORD God of his fathers.

Death of Ahaz: accession of Hezekiah
(2 Ki. 16:19, 20).

26 Now [o]the rest of his acts and of all
his ways, first and last, behold, they *are*
written in the book of the kings of Judah
and Israel.
27 And Ahaz slept with his fathers,
and they buried him in the city, *even* in
Jerusalem: but they brought him not into
the sepulchres of the kings of Israel: and
Hezekiah his son reigned in his stead.

CHAPTER 29.

Reign of Hezekiah over Judah
(2 Ki. 18:1. Cf. Isa. 36–39.).

B.C. 726.

HEZEKIAH began to reign *when he was*
five and twenty years old, and he
reigned nine and twenty years in
Jerusalem. And his mother's name *was*
Abijah, the daughter of Zechariah.
2 And he did *that which was* right in

a Psa. 69:26; Isa. 10:5; Ezk. 25:12, 15; 26:2; Zech. 1:15.
b Ezra 9:6; Rev. 18:5.
c Jas. 2:13.
d v. 12.
e 2 Ki. 6:22.
f Deut. 34:3; Jud. 1:16.
g Cf. 2 Ki. 16:7.
h Ezk. 16:27, 57.
i 2 Chr. 21:2.
j Ex. 32:25.
k 2 Ki. 15:29.
l 2 Chr. 25:14.
m Jer. 44:17, 18.
n 2 Chr. 29:3, 7.
o 2 Ki. 16:19, 20.

the sight of the LORD, according to all that David his father had done.

The revival under Hezekiah (2 Ki. 18:3-7).

3 He in the first year of his reign, in the [a]first month, opened the doors of the house of the LORD, and repaired them.

4 And he brought in the priests and the Levites, and gathered them together into the east street,

5 And said unto them, Hear me, ye Levites, [b]sanctify now yourselves, and [c]sanctify the house of the LORD God of your fathers, and carry forth the filthiness out of the holy *place*.

6 For our fathers have trespassed, and done *that which was* evil in the eyes of the LORD our God, and have forsaken him, and have turned away their faces from the habitation of the LORD, and turned *their* backs.

7 Also they have shut up the doors of the porch, and put out the lamps, and have not burned incense nor offered burnt-offerings in the holy *place* unto the God of Israel.

8 Wherefore the [d]wrath of the LORD was upon Judah and Jerusalem, and he hath delivered them to trouble, to astonishment, and to [e]hissing, as ye see with your eyes.

9 For, lo, our fathers have fallen by the sword, and our sons and our daughters and our wives *are* in captivity for this.

10 Now *it is* in mine heart to make a covenant with the LORD God of Israel, that his fierce wrath may turn away from us.

11 My sons, be not now negligent: for the LORD hath chosen you to stand before him, to serve him, and that ye should minister unto him, and burn incense.

12 Then the Levites arose, Mahath the son of Amasai, and Joel the son of Azariah, of the sons of the Kohathites: and of the sons of Merari, Kish the son of Abdi, and Azariah the son of Jehalelel: and of the Gershonites; Joah the son of Zimmah, and Eden the son of Joah:

13 And of the sons of Elizaphan; Shimri, and Jeiel: and of the sons of Asaph; Zechariah, and Mattaniah:

14 And of the sons of Heman; Jehiel, and Shimei: and of the sons of Jeduthun; Shemaiah, and Uzziel.

15 And they gathered their brethren, and sanctified themselves, and came, according to the commandment of the king, by the words of the LORD, to cleanse the house of the LORD.

16 And the priests went into the inner part of the house of the LORD, to cleanse *it*, and brought out all the uncleanness that they found in the temple of the LORD into the court of the house of the LORD. And the Levites took *it*, to carry *it* out abroad into the brook Kidron.

17 Now they began on the first *day* of the [a]first month to sanctify, and on the eighth day of the month came they to the porch of the LORD: so they sanctified the house of the LORD in eight days; and in the sixteenth day of the first month they made an end.

18 Then they went in to Hezekiah the king, and said, We have cleansed all the house of the LORD, and the altar of burnt-offering, with all the vessels thereof, and the [f]shewbread table, with all the vessels thereof.

19 Moreover all the vessels, which king Ahaz in his reign did cast away in his transgression, have we prepared and sanctified, and, behold, they *are* before the altar of the LORD.

The temple worship restored.

20 Then Hezekiah the king rose early, and gathered the rulers of the city, and went up to the house of the LORD.

21 And they brought seven bullocks, and seven rams, and seven lambs, and seven he goats, for a sin-offering for the kingdom, and for the sanctuary, and for Judah. And he commanded the priests the sons of Aaron to offer *them* on the altar of the LORD.

22 So they killed the bullocks, and the priests received the blood, and sprinkled *it* on the altar: likewise, when they had killed the rams, they sprinkled the blood upon the altar: they killed also the lambs, and they sprinkled the blood upon the altar.

23 And they brought forth the he goats *for* the sin-offering before the king and the congregation; and they laid their hands upon them:

24 And the priests killed them, and they made [g]reconciliation with their blood upon the altar, to make an [h]atonement for all Israel: for the king

B.C. 726.

a i.e. *April.*

b Heb. *godesh.*

c *Sanctify, holy* (O.T.). Psa. 2:6. (Gen. 2:3; Zech. 8:3.)

d 2 Chr. 24:18.

e 1 Ki. 9:8; Jer. 18:16; 19:8; 25:9, 18; 29:18.

f Ex. 25:30, *note.*

g Or, *an offering.* See Dan. 9:24, *note.*

h See Ex. 29:33, *note.*

commanded *that* the burnt-offering and the sin-offering *should be made* for all Israel.

25 [a]And he set the Levites in the house of the LORD with cymbals, with psalteries, and with harps, [b]according to the commandment of David, and of [c]Gad the king's seer, and Nathan the prophet: for [d]*so was* the commandment of the LORD by his prophets.

26 And the Levites stood with the instruments of David, and the priests with the trumpets.

27 And Hezekiah commanded to offer the burnt-offering upon the altar. And when the burnt-offering began, [e]the song of the LORD began *also* with the trumpets, and with the instruments *ordained* by David king of Israel.

28 And all the congregation worshipped, and the singers sang, and the trumpeters sounded: *and* all *this continued* until the burnt-offering was finished.

29 And when they had made an end of offering, [f]the king and all that were present with him bowed themselves, and worshipped.

30 Moreover Hezekiah the king and the princes commanded the Levites to sing praise unto the LORD with the words of David, and of Asaph the seer. And they sang praises with gladness, and they bowed their heads and worshipped.

31 Then Hezekiah answered and said, Now ye have consecrated yourselves unto the LORD, come near and bring sacrifices and thank offerings into the house of the LORD. And the congregation brought in sacrifices and [g]thank offerings; and as many as were of a free heart burnt-offerings.

32 And the number of the burnt-offerings, which the congregation brought, was threescore and ten bullocks, an hundred rams, *and* two hundred lambs: all these *were* for a burnt-offering to the LORD.

33 And the consecrated things *were* six hundred oxen and three thousand sheep.

34 But the priests were too few, so that they could not flay all the burnt-offerings: wherefore [h]their brethren the Levites did help them, till the work was ended, and until the *other* priests had sanctified themselves: [i]for the Levites *were* more [j]upright in heart to sanctify themselves than the priests.

35 And also the burnt-offerings *were* in abundance, with the [k]fat of the peace-offerings, and the drink-offerings for *every* burnt-offering. So the service of the house of the LORD was set in order.

36 And Hezekiah rejoiced, and all the people, that God had prepared the people: for the thing was *done* suddenly.

CHAPTER 30.

Preparations for the passover.

And Hezekiah sent to all Israel and Judah, and wrote letters also to Ephraim and Manasseh, that they should come to the house of the LORD at Jerusalem, to keep the passover unto the LORD God of Israel.

2 For the king had taken counsel, and his princes, and all the congregation in Jerusalem, to keep the passover in the [l]second month.

3 For they could not keep it [m]at that time, [n]because the priests had not sanctified themselves sufficiently, neither had the people gathered themselves together to Jerusalem.

4 And the thing pleased the king and all the congregation.

5 So they established a decree to make proclamation throughout all Israel, from Beer-sheba even to Dan, that they should come to keep the passover unto the LORD God of Israel at Jerusalem: for they had not done *it* of a long *time in such sort* as it was written.

6 So the posts went with the letters from the king and his princes throughout all Israel and Judah, and according to the commandment of the king, saying, Ye children of Israel, [o]turn again unto the LORD God of Abraham, Isaac, and Israel, and he will return to the remnant of you, that are escaped out of the hand of the [p]kings of Assyria.

7 And be not ye [q]like your fathers, and like your brethren, which trespassed against the LORD God of their fathers, *who* therefore gave them up to desolation, as ye see.

8 Now be ye not stiffnecked, as your fathers *were, but* yield yourselves unto the LORD, and enter into his sanctuary, which he hath sanctified for ever: and serve the LORD your God, [r]that the fierceness of his wrath may turn away from you.

9 For if ye turn again unto the LORD, your brethren and your children *shall find* [s]compassion before them that lead

B.C. 726.

a 1 Chr. 16:4; 25:6.
b 1 Chr. 23:5; 25:1; 2 Chr. 8:14.
c 2 Sam. 24:11.
d 2 Chr. 30:12.
e 2 Chr. 23:18.
f 2 Chr. 20.18.
g Lev. 7:12.
h 2 Chr. 35:11.
i 2 Chr. 30:3.
j Psa. 7:10.
k Lev. 3:16.
l i.e. *May;* also vs. 13, 15.
m Ex. 12:6, 18.
n 2 Chr. 29:34.
o Jer. 4:1; Joel 2:13.
p 2 Ki. 15:19, 29.
q Ezk. 20:18.
r 2 Chr. 29:10.
s Psa. 106:46.

them captive, so that they shall come
again into this land: for the LORD your
God *is* [a]gracious and merciful, and will
not turn away *his* face from you, if ye
return unto him.
10 So the posts passed from city to city
through the country of Ephraim and
Manasseh even unto Zebulun: but they
[b]laughed them to scorn, and mocked
them.
11 Nevertheless divers of Asher and
Manasseh and of Zebulun humbled
themselves, and came to Jerusalem.
12 Also in Judah the hand of God was
to give them one heart to do the commandment of the king and of the
princes, [c]by the word of the LORD.
13 And there assembled at Jerusalem
much people to keep the feast of unleavened bread in the second month, a very
great congregation.
14 And they arose and took away the
[d]altars that *were* in Jerusalem, and all the
altars for incense took they away, and
cast *them* into the brook Kidron.

The passover kept.

15 Then they killed the passover on
the fourteenth *day* of the second month:
and the priests and the Levites were
[e]ashamed, and sanctified themselves,
and brought in the burnt-offerings into
the house of the LORD.
16 And they stood in their place after
their manner, according to the law of
Moses the man of God: the priests sprinkled the blood, *which they received* of the
hand of the Levites.
17 For *there were* many in the congregation that were not sanctified: therefore
the Levites had the charge of the killing
of the passovers for every one *that was*
not clean, to sanctify *them* unto the LORD.
18 For a multitude of the people, *even*
many of Ephraim, and Manasseh,
Issachar, and Zebulun, had not cleansed
themselves, [f]yet did they eat the
passover otherwise than it was written.
But Hezekiah [g]prayed for them, saying,
The good LORD pardon every one
19 *That* [h]prepareth his heart to seek
God, the LORD God of his fathers,
though *he be* not *cleansed* according to the
purification of the sanctuary.
20 And the LORD hearkened to
Hezekiah, and healed the people.
21 And the children of Israel that were
present at Jerusalem kept [i]the feast of
unleavened bread seven days with great
gladness: and the Levites and the priests
praised the LORD day by day, *singing*
with loud instruments unto the LORD.
22 And Hezekiah spake [j]comfortably
unto all the Levites [k]that taught the good
knowledge of the LORD: and they did eat
throughout the feast seven days, offering
peace-offerings, and [l]making confession
to the LORD God of their fathers.

"Other seven" days kept.

23 And the whole assembly took counsel to keep [m]other seven days: and they
kept *other* seven days with gladness.
24 For Hezekiah king of Judah [n]did
give to the congregation a thousand
bullocks and seven thousand sheep; and
the princes gave to the congregation a
thousand bullocks and ten thousand
sheep: and a great number of priests
[e]sanctified themselves.
25 And all the congregation of Judah,
with the priests and the Levites, and all
the congregation that came out of Israel,
and the strangers that came out of the
land of Israel, and that dwelt in Judah,
rejoiced.
26 So there was great joy in Jerusalem:
for since the time of Solomon the son of
David king of Israel *there was* not the like
in Jerusalem.
27 Then the priests the Levites arose
and blessed the people: and their voice
was heard, and their prayer came *up* to
his holy dwelling place, *even* unto heaven.

CHAPTER 31.

Idols destroyed (2 Ki. 18:4).

NOW when all this was finished, all
Israel that were present went out
to the cities of Judah, and brake the
images in pieces, and cut down the
[o]groves, and threw down the high places
and the altars out of all Judah and
Benjamin, in Ephraim also and Manasseh, until they had utterly destroyed
them all. Then all the children of Israel
returned, every man to his possession,
into their own cities.

Hezekiah's further religious reforms.

2 And Hezekiah appointed [p]the courses
of the priests and the Levites after their
courses, every man according to his

B.C. 726.

a Ex. 34:6.
b 2 Chr. 36:16.
c 2 Chr. 29:25.
d 2 Chr. 28:24.
e 2 Chr. 29:34.
f Ex. 12:43; Num. 9:10.
g *Bible prayers* (O.T.). Ezra 9:6. (Gen. 15:2; Hab. 3:1-16.)
h 2 Chr. 19:3; Ex. 12:15; 13:6.
i 1 Ki. 8:65.
j Heb. *to the heart of all.*
k 2 Chr. 17:9; 2 Chr. 35:3; Deut. 33:10.
l Ezra 10:11.
m 2 Chr. 35:17,18.
n 2 Chr. 29:3-9.
o Jud. 3.7, *note.*
p 1 Chr. 23:6; 24:1.

B.C. 726.

service, the priests and Levites for [a]burnt-
offerings and for peace-offerings, to minister, and to give thanks, and to praise in
the gates of the tents of the LORD.
3 *He appointed* also the king's portion
of his substance for the burnt-offerings,
to wit, for the morning and evening
burnt-offerings, and the burnt-offerings
for the sabbaths, and for the new moons,
and for the set feasts, as *it is* written in
the [b]law of the LORD.
4 Moreover he commanded the people
that dwelt in Jerusalem to give the [c]por-
tion of the priests and the Levites, that
they might be encouraged in the law of
the LORD.
5 And as soon as the commandment
came abroad, the children of Israel
brought in abundance the [d]firstfruits of
corn, wine, and oil, and honey, and of all
the increase of the field; and the tithe of
all *things* brought they in abundantly.
6 And *concerning* the children of Israel
and Judah, that dwelt in the cities of
Judah, they also brought in the tithe of
oxen and sheep, and the [e]tithe of holy
things which were consecrated unto the
LORD their God, and laid *them* by heaps.
7 In the [f]third month they began to lay
the foundation of the heaps, and finished *them* in the [g]seventh month.
8 And when Hezekiah and the princes
came and saw the heaps, they blessed
the LORD, and his people Israel.
9 Then Hezekiah questioned with the
priests and the Levites concerning the
heaps.
10 And Azariah the chief priest of the
house of Zadok answered him, and said,
Since *the people* began to bring the offerings into the house of the LORD, we have
had enough to eat, and have left plenty:
for the LORD hath blessed his people;
and that which is left *is* this great store.
11 Then Hezekiah commanded to prepare chambers in the house of the LORD;
and they prepared *them*,
12 And brought in the offerings and the
tithes and the dedicated *things* faithfully:
over which [h]Cononiah the Levite *was*
ruler, and Shimei his brother *was* the next.
13 And Jehiel, and Azaziah, and
Nahath, and Asahel, and Jerimoth, and
Jozabad, and Eliel, and Ismachiah, and
Mahath, and Benaiah, *were* overseers
under the hand of Cononiah and Shimei
his brother, at the commandment of
Hezekiah the king, and Azariah the ruler
of the house of God.
14 And Kore the son of Imnah the
Levite, the porter toward the east, *was*
over the freewill offerings of God, to distribute the oblations of the LORD, and the
most holy things.
15 And next him *were* Eden, and
Miniamin, and Jeshua, and Shemaiah,
Amariah, and Shecaniah, [i]in the cities of
the priests, in *their* set [j]office, to give to
their brethren by courses, as well to the
great as to the small:
16 Beside their genealogy of males,
from three years old and upward, *even*
unto every one that entereth into the
house of the LORD, his daily portion for
their service in their charges according
to their courses;
17 Both to the genealogy of the priests
by the house of their fathers, and the
Levites from twenty years old and
upward, in their charges by their courses;
18 And to the genealogy of all their little ones, their wives, and their sons, and
their daughters, through all the congregation: for in their set office they sanctified themselves in holiness:
19 Also of the sons of Aaron the priests,
which were [k]in the fields of the suburbs of
their cities, in every several city, the men
that were expressed by name, to give portions to all the males among the priests,
and to all that were reckoned by genealogies among the Levites.
20 And thus did Hezekiah throughout
all Judah, [l]and wrought *that which was*
good and right and truth before the
LORD his God.
21 And in every work that he began in
the service of the house of God, and in
the law, and in the commandments, to
seek his God, he did *it* with all his heart,
and prospered.

CHAPTER 32.

Sennacherib invades Judah
(2 Ki. 18:13–19:37; Isa. 36:1-22).

[B.C. 713.

After these things, and the establishment thereof, [m]Sennacherib king of
Assyria came, and entered into Judah,
and encamped against the fenced cities,
and thought to win them for himself.
2 And when Hezekiah saw that

a 1 Chr. 23:30, 31.
b Num. 28., 29.
c Num. 18:8; Neh. 13:10; Ezk. 44:29.
d Ex. 22:29; Neh. 13:12.
e Lev. 27:30; Deut. 14:28.
f i.e. *June.*
g i.e. *October.*
h Neh. 13:13.
i Josh. 21:9.
j 1 Chr. 9:22, etc.
k Lev. 25:34, 35; Num. 35:1-4.
l 2 Ki. 20:3.
m 2 Ki 18:13.

Sennacherib was come, and that he was
purposed to fight against Jerusalem,
3 He took counsel with his princes and
his mighty men to stop the waters of the
fountains which *were* without the city:
and they did help him.
4 So there was gathered much people
together, who stopped all the fountains,
and the brook that ran through the midst
of the land, saying, Why should the kings
of Assyria come, and find much water?
5 [a]Also he strengthened himself, [b]and
built up all the wall that was broken,
and raised *it* up to the towers, and
another wall without, and repaired
[c]Millo *in* the city of David, and made
darts and shields in abundance.
6 And he set captains of war over the
people, and gathered them together to
him in the street of the gate of the city,
and spake [d]comfortably to them, saying,
7 Be strong and courageous, be not
afraid nor dismayed for the king of
Assyria, nor for all the multitude that *is*
with him: [e]for *there be* more with us than
with him:
8 With him is an [f]arm of flesh; but
with us *is* the LORD our God to help us,
and to fight our battles. And the people
rested themselves upon the words of
Hezekiah king of Judah.

Sennacherib seeks to terrify the inhabitants of Jerusalem (2 Ki. 18:17-25).

9 After this did Sennacherib king of
Assyria send his servants to Jerusalem,
(but he *himself laid siege* against Lachish,
and all his power with him,) unto
Hezekiah king of Judah, and unto all
Judah that *were* at Jerusalem, [g]saying,
10 Thus saith Sennacherib king of
Assyria, Whereon do ye trust, that ye
abide in the siege in Jerusalem?
11 Doth not Hezekiah persuade you to
give over yourselves to die by famine
and by thirst, [g]saying, The LORD our
God shall deliver us out of the hand of
the king of Assyria?
12 Hath not the same Hezekiah [h]taken
away his [i]high places and his altars, and
commanded Judah and Jerusalem, saying, Ye shall worship before one altar,
and burn incense upon it?
13 Know ye not [j]what I and my
fathers have done unto all the people of
other lands? were the gods of the nations
of those lands any ways able to deliver
their lands out of mine hand?
14 Who *was there* among all the gods
of those nations that my fathers utterly
destroyed, that could deliver his people
out of mine hand, that your God should
be able to deliver you out of mine hand?
15 Now therefore let not Hezekiah
deceive you, nor persuade you on this
manner, neither yet believe him: for no
god of any nation or kingdom was able
to deliver his people out of mine hand,
and out of the hand of my fathers: how
much less shall your God deliver you
out of mine hand?
16 And his servants spake yet *more*
against the LORD God, and against his
servant Hezekiah.

Sennacherib defies the God of Hezekiah (2 Ki. 19:9-13).

17 He wrote [k]also letters to rail on the
LORD God of Israel, and to speak against
him, [l]saying, As the gods of the nations
of *other* lands have not delivered their
people out of mine hand, so shall not the
God of Hezekiah deliver his people out
of mine hand.
18 [m]Then they cried with a loud voice
in the Jews' speech unto the people of
Jerusalem that *were* on the wall, to
affright them, and to trouble them; that
they might take the city.
19 And they spake against the God of
Jerusalem, as against the gods of the
people of the earth, *which were* the work
of the hands of man.

Hezekiah's prayer (2 Ki. 19:14-19).

20 [n]And for this *cause* Hezekiah the
king, and the prophet Isaiah the son of
Amoz, prayed and cried to heaven.

Jehovah destroys the Assyrian army (2 Ki. 19:35, 36).

21 And the LORD [o]sent an angel, which
cut off all the mighty men of valour, and
the leaders and captains in the camp of
the king of Assyria. So he returned with
shame of face to his own land. And
[p]when he was come into the house of his
god, they that came forth of his own
bowels slew him there with the sword.

B.C. 713.

a Cf. Isa. 22:1-13, the divine view at this time.
b 2 Chr. 25:22-24.
c 2 Sam. 5:9; 1 Ki. 9:15, 24; 11:27; 2 Ki. 12:20; 1 Chr. 11:8; 2 Chr. 32:5.
d Heb. *to the heart.*
e Rom. 8:31.
f Jer. 17:5.
g 2 Ki. 18:19.
h 2 Ki. 18:22.
i 1 Ki. 3:2, *note.*
j Cf. 2 Ki. 18:29-35.
k 2 Ki. 19:9.
l 2 Ki. 19:12.
m 2 Ki. 18:26-31.
n Cf. Isa. 37:15-20.
o Isa. 37:33-37. See, also, Zech. 14:3.
p Cf. 2 Ki. 19:37.

Hezekiah again prosperous.

22 Thus the LORD saved Hezekiah and the inhabitants of Jerusalem from the hand of Sennacherib the king of Assyria, and from the hand of all *other*, and guided them on every side.

23 And many [a]brought gifts unto the LORD to Jerusalem, and presents to Hezekiah king of Judah: so that he was magnified in the sight of all nations from thenceforth.

Hezekiah's illness and recovery (2 Ki. 20:1-11).

24 In those days Hezekiah was [b]sick to the death, and prayed unto the LORD: and he spake unto him, and he gave him a sign.

25 But Hezekiah rendered not again according to the benefit *done* unto him; for his [c]heart was lifted up: therefore there was [d]wrath upon him, and upon Judah and Jerusalem.

26 Notwithstanding Hezekiah humbled himself for the pride of his heart, *both* he and the inhabitants of Jerusalem, so that the wrath of the LORD came not upon them in the days of Hezekiah.

Hezekiah's wealth.

27 And Hezekiah had exceeding much riches and honour: and he made himself treasuries for silver, and for gold, and for precious stones, and for spices, and for shields, and for all manner of pleasant jewels;

28 Storehouses also for the increase of corn, and wine, and oil; and stalls for all manner of beasts, and cotes for flocks.

29 Moreover he provided him cities, and possessions of flocks and herds in abundance: for God had given him substance very much.

30 This same Hezekiah also [e]stopped the upper watercourse of Gihon, and brought it straight down to the west side of the city of David. And Hezekiah prospered in all his works.

Hezekiah receives an embassy from Babylon (2 Ki. 20:12-19).

31 Howbeit in *the business of* the ambassadors of the princes of Babylon, who sent unto him to enquire of the wonder that was *done* in the land, God left him, to try him, that he might know all *that was* in his heart.

B.C. 710.

- *a* 2 Chr. 17:5; Psa. 45:12.
- *b* 2 Ki. 20:1; Isa. 38:1-22.
- *c* 2 Chr. 26:16; Hab. 2:4.
- *d* 2 Chr. 24:18.
- *e* Isa. 22:9-12.
- *f* Isa. 36-39.
- *g* 2 Ki. 20:21.
- *h* 2 Ki. 21:1.
- *i* 2 Chr. 28:3; Deut. 18:9.
- *j* i.e. *nations.*
- *k* See Deut. 16:21.
- *l* Deut. 17:3.
- *m* 2 Chr. 6:6; 7:16; Deut. 12:11; 1 Ki. 8:29; 9:3.
- *n* 2 Chr. 4:9.
- *o* 2 Chr. 28:3; Lev. 18:21; Deut. 18:10; 2 Ki. 23:10; Ezk. 23:37, 39.
- *p* Deut. 18:10, 11.
- *q* 2 Ki. 21:6.
- *r* 2 Ki. 21:7.
- *s* Psa. 132:14.
- *t* 2 Sam. 7:10.

Death of Hezekiah: accession of Manasseh (2 Ki. 20:20, 21).

32 Now the rest of the acts of Hezekiah, and his goodness, behold, they *are* [f]written in the vision of Isaiah the prophet, the son of Amoz, *and* in the book of the kings of Judah and Israel.

33 And Hezekiah [g]slept with his fathers, and they buried him in the chiefest of the sepulchres of the sons of David: and all Judah and the inhabitants of Jerusalem did him honour at his death. And Manasseh his son reigned in his stead.

CHAPTER 33.

Accession of Manasseh: his evil ways (2 Ki. 21:2-9).

Manasseh [h]*was* twelve years old when he began to reign, and he reigned fifty and five years in Jerusalem:

2 But did *that which was* evil in the sight of the LORD, like unto the [i]abominations of the [j]heathen, whom the LORD had cast out before the children of Israel.

3 For he built again the high places which Hezekiah his father had broken down, and he reared up altars for Baalim, and made [k]groves, and worshipped [l]all the host of heaven, and served them.

4 Also he built altars in the house of the LORD, whereof the LORD had said, [m]In Jerusalem shall my name be for ever.

5 And he built altars for all the host of heaven [n]in the two courts of the house of the LORD.

6 [o]And he caused his children to pass through the fire in the valley of the son of Hinnom: [p]also he observed times, and used enchantments, and used witchcraft, and [q]dealt with a familiar spirit, and with wizards: he wrought much evil in the sight of the LORD, to provoke him to anger.

7 And he [r]set a carved image, the idol which he had made, in the house of God, of which God had said to David and to Solomon his son, In [s]this house, and in Jerusalem, which I have chosen before all the tribes of Israel, will I put my name for ever:

8 [t]Neither will I any more remove the foot of Israel from out of the land which I have appointed for your fathers; so that they will take heed to do all that I have

B.C. 698.

commanded them, according to the whole law and the statutes and the ordinances by the hand of Moses.

9 So Manasseh made Judah and the inhabitants of Jerusalem to err, *and* to do worse than the [a]heathen, whom the LORD had destroyed before the children of Israel.

10 And the LORD spake to Manasseh, and to his people: but they would not hearken.

Manasseh's captivity and restoration.

11 [b]Wherefore the LORD brought upon them the captains of the host of the king of Assyria, which took Manasseh among the thorns, and bound him with fetters, and carried him to Babylon.

12 And when he was in affliction, he besought the LORD his God, and humbled himself greatly before the God of his fathers,

13 And prayed unto him: and he was [c]intreated of him, and heard his supplication, and brought him again to Jerusalem into his kingdom. Then Manasseh knew that the LORD he *was* God.

Manasseh's continued reign, and death (2 Ki. 21:17, 18).

14 Now after this he built a wall without the city of David, on the west side of [d]Gihon, in the valley, even to the entering in at the fish gate, and compassed [e]about Ophel, and raised it up a very great height, and put captains of war in all the fenced cities of Judah.

15 And he took away the [f]strange gods, and the idol out of the house of the LORD, and all the altars that he had built in the mount of the house of the LORD, and in Jerusalem, and cast *them* out of the city.

16 And he repaired the altar of the LORD, and sacrificed thereon peace-offerings and [g]thank offerings, and commanded Judah to serve the LORD God of Israel.

17 [h]Nevertheless the people did sacrifice still in the high places, *yet* unto the LORD their God only.

18 Now the rest of the acts of Manasseh, and his prayer unto his God, and the words of [i]the seers that spake to him in the name of the LORD God of Israel, behold, they *are written* in the book of the kings of Israel.

19 His prayer also, and *how God* was intreated of him, and all his sin, and his trespass, and the places wherein he built high places, and set up [j]groves and graven images, before he was humbled: behold, they *are* written among the sayings of the seers.

20 So [k]Manasseh slept with his fathers, and they buried him in his own house: and Amon his son reigned in his stead.

Reign of Amon (2 Ki. 21:18-22).

21 [l]Amon *was* two and twenty years old when he began to reign, and reigned two years in Jerusalem.

22 But he did *that which was* evil in the sight of the LORD, as did Manasseh his father: for Amon sacrificed unto all the carved images which Manasseh his father had made, and served them;

23 And humbled not himself before the LORD, as Manasseh his father had humbled himself; but Amon trespassed more and more.

Death of Amon: accession of Josiah (2 Ki. 21:23-26).

24 And [m]his servants conspired against him, and slew him in his own house.

25 But the people of the land slew all them that had conspired against king Amon; and the people of the land made Josiah his son king in his stead.

[B.C. 641.

CHAPTER 34.

Reign of Josiah (2 Ki. 22:1–23:30).

Josiah [n]*was* eight years old when he began to reign, and he reigned in Jerusalem one and thirty years.

2 And he did *that which was* right in the sight of the LORD, and walked in the ways of David his father, and declined *neither* to the right hand, nor to the left.

Josiah's early reformations.

3 For in the eighth year of his reign, while he was yet young, he began to [o]seek after the God of David his father: and in the twelfth year he began to [p]purge Judah and Jerusalem [q]from the high places, and the [r]groves, and the carved images, and the molten images.

4 And they brake down the altars of Baalim in his presence; and the images, that *were* on high above them, he cut down; and the [r]groves, and the carved

a i.e. *nations.*
b Deut. 28:36.
c 1 Chr. 5:20; Ezra 8:23.
d 1 Ki. 1:33.
e 2 Chr. 27:3.
f vs. 3, 5, 7.
g Lev. 7:12.
h 2 Chr. 32:12.
i 1 Sam. 9:9.
j See Deut. 16:21.
k 2 Ki. 21:18.
l 2 Ki. 21:19.
m 2 Ki. 21:23, 24.
n 2 Ki. 22:1.
o 2 Chr. 15:2.
p 1 Ki. 13:2.
q 2 Chr. 33:17, 22.
r See Deut. 16:21; Jud. 3:7, *note.*

images, and the molten images, he brake
in pieces, and made dust *of them*, and
[a]strowed *it* upon the graves of them that
had sacrificed unto them.
5 And he [b]burnt the bones of the
priests upon their altars, and cleansed
Judah and Jerusalem.
6 And *so did he* in the cities of
Manasseh, and Ephraim, and Simeon,
even unto Naphtali, with their mattocks
round about.
7 And when he had broken down the
altars and the [c]groves, and had [d]beaten
the graven images into powder, and cut
down all the idols throughout all the
land of Israel, he returned to Jerusalem.

The repairing of the temple (2 Ki. 22:3-7).

8 Now [e]in the eighteenth year of his
reign, when he had purged the land, and
the house, he sent Shaphan the son of
Azaliah, and Maaseiah the governor of
the city, and Joah the son of Joahaz the
recorder, to repair the house of the LORD
his God.
9 And when they came to Hilkiah the
high priest, they delivered [f]the money
that was brought into the house of God,
which the Levites that kept the doors
had gathered of the hand of Manasseh
and Ephraim, and of all the remnant of
Israel, and of all Judah and Benjamin;
and they returned to Jerusalem.
10 And they put *it* in the hand of the
workmen that had the oversight of the
house of the LORD, and they gave it to the
workmen that wrought in the house of
the LORD, to repair and amend the house:
11 Even to the artificers and builders
gave they *it*, to buy hewn stone, and timber for couplings, and to floor the houses
which the kings of Judah had destroyed.
12 And the men did the work faithfully: and the overseers of them *were* Jahath
and Obadiah, the Levites, of the sons of
Merari; and Zechariah and Meshullam,
of the sons of the Kohathites, to set *it* forward; and *other of* the Levites, all that
could skill of instruments of musick.
13 Also *they were* over the bearers of
burdens, and *were* overseers of all that
wrought the work in any manner of service: and [g]of the Levites *there were*
scribes, and officers, and porters.

The law of Moses discovered (2 Ki. 22:8).

14 And when they brought out the
money that was brought into the house
of the LORD, Hilkiah the priest [h]found a
book of the law of the LORD *given* by
Moses.
15 And Hilkiah answered and said to
Shaphan the scribe, I have found the
book of the law in the house of the LORD.
And Hilkiah delivered the book to
Shaphan.
16 And Shaphan carried the book to
the king, and brought the king word
back again, saying, All that was committed to thy servants, they do *it*.
17 And they have [i]gathered together
the money that was found in the house
of the LORD, and have delivered it into
the hand of the overseers, and to the
hand of the workmen.

"By the law is the knowledge of sin" (2 Ki. 22:9-13).

18 Then Shaphan the scribe told the
king, saying, Hilkiah the priest hath
given me a book. And Shaphan [j]read it
before the king.
19 And it came to pass, when the king
had [k]heard the words of the law, that he
rent his clothes.
20 And the king commanded Hilkiah,
and Ahikam the son of Shaphan, and
Abdon the son of Micah, and Shaphan
the scribe, and Asaiah a servant of the
king's, saying,
21 Go, enquire of the LORD for me, and
for them that are left in Israel and in
Judah, concerning the words of the book
that is found: for great *is* the wrath of the
LORD that is poured out upon us,
because our fathers have not kept the
word of the LORD, to do after all that is
written in this book.

The words of Huldah the prophetess (2 Ki. 22:14-20).

22 And Hilkiah, and *they* that the king
had appointed, went to Huldah the
prophetess, the wife of Shallum the son
of [l]Tikvath, the son of Hasrah, keeper of
the wardrobe; (now she dwelt in
Jerusalem in the college:) and they spake
to her to that *effect*.
23 And she answered them, Thus saith
the LORD God of Israel, Tell ye the man
that sent you to me,
24 Thus saith the LORD, Behold, I will
bring evil upon this place, and upon the
inhabitants thereof, *even* all the curses

B.C. 630.

B.C. 624.]

a 2 Ki. 23:6; Ezk. 6:5.

b 1 Ki. 13:2.

c See Deut. 16:21; Jud. 3:7, *note*.

d Deut. 9:21.

e 2 Ki. 22:3.

f See 2 Ki. 12:4.

g 1 Chr. 23:4, 5.

h 2 Ki. 22:8.

i Heb. *poured out*, or *melted*.

j Cf. Neh. 8:1-18.

k Cf. Neh. 8:9, 1.c.

l 2 Ki. 22:14.

that are written in the book which they have read before the king of Judah:

25 Because they have forsaken me, and have burned incense unto other gods, that they might provoke me to anger with all the works of their hands; therefore my wrath shall be poured out upon this place, and shall not be quenched.

26 And as for the king of Judah, who sent you to enquire of the LORD, so shall ye say unto him, Thus saith the LORD God of Israel *concerning* the words which thou hast heard;

27 Because thine heart was tender, and thou didst humble thyself before God, when thou heardest his words against this place, and against the inhabitants thereof, and humbledst thyself before me, and didst rend thy clothes, and weep before me; I have even heard *thee* also, saith the LORD.

28 Behold, I will gather thee to thy fathers, and thou shalt be gathered to thy grave in peace, neither shall thine eyes see all the evil that I will bring upon this place, and upon the inhabitants of the same. So they brought the king word again.

The law read to the people (2 Ki. 23:1, 2).

29 Then the king sent and gathered together all the elders of Judah and Jerusalem.

30 And the king went up into the house of the LORD, and all the men of Judah, and the inhabitants of Jerusalem, and the priests, and the Levites, and all the people, great and small: and he read in their ears all the words of the book of the covenant that was found in the house of the LORD.

The king's covenant (2 Ki 23:3).

31 And the king stood in [a]his place, and made a [b]covenant before the LORD, to walk after the LORD, and to keep his commandments, and his testimonies, and his statutes, with all his heart, and with all his soul, to perform the words of the covenant which are written in this book.

32 And he caused all that were present in Jerusalem and Benjamin to stand *to it*. And the inhabitants of Jerusalem did according to the covenant of God, the God of their fathers.

B.C. 624.

a 2 Ki. 11:14.
b Cf. 2 Chr. 6:13.
c 1 Ki. 11:5.
d Jer. 3:10.
e Ex. 12:6.
f i.e. *April.*
g 2 Chr. 23:18.
h Cf. 2 Chr. 29:5-12.
i Deut. 33:9, 10.
j 2 Chr. 5:7; Ex. 40:20.
k 1 Chr. 9:10.
l 1 Chr. 23–26., incl.
m Cf. Ezra 6:20.
n Cf. 2 Chr. 30:24.

The further reforms of Josiah (2 Ki. 23:4-24).

33 And Josiah took away all the [c]abominations out of all the countries that *pertained* to the children of Israel, and made all that were present in Israel to serve, *even* to serve the LORD their God. [d]*And* all his days they departed not from following the LORD, the God of their fathers.

CHAPTER 35.

The passover kept (2 Ki. 23:21-23).

Moreover Josiah kept a passover unto the LORD in Jerusalem: and they killed the passover on the [e]fourteenth *day* of the [f]first month.

2 And he set the priests in their [g]charges, and [h]encouraged them to the service of the house of the LORD,

3 And said unto the Levites that [i]taught all Israel, which were holy unto the LORD, Put the holy ark in the [j]house which Solomon the son of David king of Israel did build; *it shall* not *be* a burden upon *your* shoulders: serve now the LORD your God, and his people Israel,

4 And prepare *yourselves* [k]by the houses of your fathers, after your courses, according to the [l]writing of David king of Israel, and according to the writing of Solomon his son.

5 And stand in the holy *place* according to the divisions of the families of the fathers of your brethren the people, and *after* the division of the families of the Levites.

6 So [e]kill the passover, and [m]sanctify yourselves, and prepare your brethren, that *they* may do according to the word of the LORD by the hand of Moses.

7 And Josiah [n]gave to the people, of the flock, lambs and kids, all for the passover offerings, for all that were present, to the number of thirty thousand, and three thousand bullocks: these *were* of the king's substance.

8 And his princes gave willingly unto the people, to the priests, and to the Levites: Hilkiah and Zechariah and Jehiel, rulers of the house of God, gave unto the priests for the passover offerings two thousand and six hundred *small cattle*, and three hundred oxen.

9 Conaniah also, and Shemaiah and Nethaneel, his brethren, and Hashabiah

B.C. 623.

and Jeiel and Jozabad, chief of the Levites, gave unto the Levites for passover offerings five thousand *small cattle*, and five hundred oxen.

10 So the service was prepared, and the [a]priests stood in their place, and the [b]Levites in their courses, according to the king's commandment.

11 And they [c]killed the passover, and the priests sprinkled *the blood* from their [d]hands, and the Levites flayed *them*.

12 And they removed the burnt-offerings, that they might give according to the divisions of the families of the people, to offer unto the LORD, as *it is* [e]written in the book of Moses. And so *did they* with the oxen.

13 And they [f]roasted the passover with fire according to the ordinance: but the *other* holy *offerings* sod they in pots, and in caldrons, and in pans, and divided *them* speedily among all the people.

14 And afterward they made ready for themselves, and for the priests: because the priests the sons of Aaron *were busied* in offering of burnt-offerings and the fat until night; therefore the Levites prepared for themselves, and for the priests the sons of Aaron.

15 And the singers the sons of Asaph *were* in their place, [g]according to the commandment of David, and Asaph, and Heman, and Jeduthun the king's seer; and the porters *waited* at every gate; they might not depart from their service; for their brethren the Levites prepared for them.

16 So all the service of the LORD was prepared the same day, to keep the passover, and to offer burnt-offerings upon the altar of the LORD, according to the commandment of king Josiah.

17 And the children of Israel that were present kept the passover at that time, and the [h]feast of unleavened bread seven days.

18 And there was no passover [i]like to that kept in Israel from the days of Samuel the prophet; neither did all the kings of Israel keep such a passover as Josiah kept, and the priests, and the Levites, and all Judah and Israel that were present, and the inhabitants of Jerusalem.

19 In the eighteenth year of the reign of Josiah was this passover kept.

Death of Josiah (2 Ki. 23:28-30).

[B.C. 610.

20 After all this, [j]when Josiah had prepared the temple, Necho king of Egypt came up to fight against Carchemish by Euphrates: and Josiah went out against him.

21 But he sent ambassadors to him, saying, What have I to do with thee, thou king of Judah? *I come* not against thee this day, but against the house wherewith I have war: for God commanded me to make haste: forbear thee from *meddling with* God, who *is* with me, that he destroy thee not.

22 Nevertheless Josiah would not turn his face from him, but disguised himself, that he might fight with him, and hearkened not unto the words of Necho from the mouth of God, and came to fight in the valley of Megiddo.

23 And the archers shot at king Josiah; and the king said to his servants, Have me away; for I am sore wounded.

24 His servants therefore [k]took him out of that chariot, and put him in the second chariot that he had; and they brought him to Jerusalem, and he died, and was buried in *one of* the sepulchres of his fathers. And all Judah and Jerusalem mourned for Josiah.

25 And Jeremiah [l]lamented for Josiah: and all the singing men and the singing women spake of Josiah in their lamentations to this day, and made them an ordinance in Israel: and, behold, they *are* written in the lamentations.

26 Now the rest of the acts of Josiah, and his goodness, according to *that which was* written in the law of the LORD,

27 And his deeds, first and last, behold, they *are* written in the book of the kings of Israel and Judah.

CHAPTER 36.

Reign and dethronement of Jehoahaz (2 Ki. 23:30-33).

[B.C. 610.

Then the people of the land took Jehoahaz the son of Josiah, and made him king in his father's stead in Jerusalem.

2 Jehoahaz *was* twenty and three years old when he began to reign, and he reigned three months in Jerusalem.

3 And the king of Egypt put him down at Jerusalem, and condemned the

a Heb. 9:6.
b 2 Chr. 5:12; 7:6; 8:14, 15; 13:10; 29:25-34.
c v. 6, *ref.*
d Cf. Ex. 12:22.
e Lev. 3:3; Ezra 6:8.
f Ex. 12:8, 9.
g 1 Chr. 25:1-6.
h Ex. 12:15; 1 Cor. 5:8.
i 2 Ki. 23:22, 23.
j 2 Ki. 23:29; Jer. 46:1-12.
k Cf. 2 Ki. 23:29, 30.
l Lam. 4:20.

land in an hundred [a]talents of silver and a [b]talent of gold.

4 And the king of Egypt made Eliakim his brother king over Judah and Jerusalem, and turned his name to Jehoiakim. And Necho took Jehoahaz his brother, and carried him to Egypt.

5 Jehoiakim *was* [c]twenty and five years old when he began to reign, and he reigned eleven years in Jerusalem: and he did *that which was* evil in the sight of the LORD his God.

6 Against him [d]came up Nebuchadnezzar king of Babylon, and bound him in fetters, to carry him to Babylon.

7 Nebuchadnezzar also carried of the vessels of the house of the LORD to Babylon, and put them in his temple at Babylon.

Accession and reign of Jehoiachin
(2 Ki. 24:6-10).

8 Now the rest of the acts of Jehoiakim, and his abominations which he did, and that which was found in him, behold, they *are* written in the book of the kings of Israel and Judah: and Jehoiachin his son reigned in his stead.

9 Jehoiachin *was* [e]eight years old when he began to reign, and he reigned three months and ten days in Jerusalem: and he did *that which was* evil in the sight of the LORD.

10 And when the year was expired, king Nebuchadnezzar sent, and brought him to Babylon, with the goodly vessels of the house of the LORD, and made Zedekiah his brother king over Judah and Jerusalem.

11 Zedekiah *was* one and twenty years old when he began to reign, and reigned eleven years in Jerusalem.

Zedekiah made king (2 Ki. 24:17, 18).

12 And he did *that which was* evil in the sight of the LORD his God, *and* humbled not himself before Jeremiah the prophet *speaking* from the mouth of the LORD.

13 And he also rebelled against king Nebuchadnezzar, who had made him swear by God: but he stiffened his neck, and hardened his heart from turning unto the LORD God of Israel.

14 Moreover all the chief of the priests, and the people, transgressed very much after all the abominations of the heathen; and polluted the house of the LORD which he had hallowed in Jerusalem.

Final deportation:
the captivity of Judah in Babylon
(2 Ki. 25:1-17).

15 And the LORD God of their fathers sent to them by his messengers, rising up betimes, and sending; because he had compassion on his people, and on his dwelling place:

16 But they mocked the messengers of God, and despised his words, and misused his prophets, until the wrath of the LORD arose against his people, till *there was* no remedy.

17 Therefore he brought upon them the king of the Chaldees, who slew their young men with the sword in the house of their sanctuary, and had no compassion upon young man or maiden, old man, or him that stooped for age: he gave *them* all into his hand.

18 And all the vessels of the house of God, great and small, and the treasures of the house of the LORD, and the treasures of the king, and of his princes; all *these* he brought to Babylon.

19 And they burnt the house of God, and brake down the wall of Jerusalem, and burnt all the palaces thereof with fire, and destroyed all the goodly vessels thereof.

20 And them that had escaped from the sword [f]carried he away to Babylon; where they were servants to him and his sons until the reign of the kingdom of Persia:

21 To fulfil the word of the LORD by the [g]mouth of Jeremiah, until the [h]land had enjoyed her sabbaths: *for* as long as she lay desolate she kept sabbath, to fulfil threescore and ten years.

Decree of Cyrus for rebuilding the temple.

22 Now in the first year of Cyrus king of Persia, that the word of the LORD *spoken* by the mouth of Jeremiah might be accomplished, the LORD stirred up the spirit of [i]Cyrus king of Persia, that he made a proclamation throughout all his kingdom, and *put it* also in writing, saying,

23 Thus [j]saith Cyrus king of Persia, All the kingdoms of the earth hath the LORD God of heaven given me; and he hath charged me to build him an house in Jerusalem, which *is* in Judah. Who *is there* among you of all his people? The LORD his God *be* with him, and let him go up.

B.C. 610.

B.C. 607.]

a One talent (silver) = £410, or $1940.

b One talent (gold) = £6150 or $29,085.

c 2 Ki. 23:36, 37.

d 2 Ki. 24:1-6; Jer. 25:1-9; Dan. 1:1; Hab. 1:6. This was the first deportation of Judah. See vs. 15-21, the final deportation.

B.C. 599.]

e Cf. 2 Ki. 24:8.

f Cf. Deut. 28:36, 37.

g Jer. 25:9-12; 27:6-8; 29:10.

h Lev. 26:34-43.

i Ezra 1:1; Isa. 44:28; 4:5, 1; Jer. 25:12; Dan. 9:2.

j Ezra 1:2, 3.

B.C. 593.]

EZRA

EZRA, the first of the post-captivity books (Ezra, Nehemiah, Esther, Haggai, Zechariah, and Malachi), records the return to Palestine under Zerubbabel, by decree of Cyrus, of a Jewish remnant who laid the temple foundations (B.C. 536). Later (B.C. 458) Ezra followed, and restored the law and ritual. But the mass of the nation, and most of the princes, remained by preference in Babylonia and Assyria, where they were prospering. The post-captivity books deal with that feeble remnant which alone had a heart for God.

The book is in two parts: I. From the decree of Cyrus to the dedication of the restored temple, 1:1–6:22. II. The ministry of Ezra, 7:1–10:44.

The events recorded in Ezra cover a period of 80 years (Ussher).

CHAPTER 1.

B.C. 536.

Decree of Cyrus for the restoration of the temple.

NOW in the first year of Cyrus king of Persia, that the [a]word of the LORD by the mouth of Jeremiah might be fulfilled, the LORD stirred up the spirit of [b]Cyrus king of Persia, that he made a proclamation throughout all his kingdom, and *put it* also in writing, saying,

2 Thus saith Cyrus king of Persia, The LORD God of heaven hath [c]given me all the kingdoms of the earth; and he hath [d]charged me to build him an house at Jerusalem, which *is* in Judah.

3 Who *is there* among you of [e]all his people? his God be with him, and let him go up to Jerusalem, which *is* in Judah, and build the house of the LORD God of Israel, ([f]he *is* the God,) which *is* in Jerusalem.

4 And whosoever remaineth in any place where he sojourneth, let the men of his place help him with silver, and with gold, and with goods, and with beasts, beside the freewill offering for the house of God that *is* in Jerusalem.

Preparation for the return of the remnant.

5 Then rose up the chief of the fathers of Judah and Benjamin, and the priests, and the Levites, with all *them* whose spirit God had raised, to go up to build the house of the LORD which *is* in Jerusalem.

6 And all they that *were* about them [g]strengthened their hands with vessels of silver, with gold, with goods, and with beasts, and with precious things, beside all *that* was willingly offered.

7 Also Cyrus the king [h]brought forth the vessels of the house of the LORD, which Nebuchadnezzar had brought forth out of Jerusalem, and had put them in the house of his gods;

8 Even those did Cyrus king of Persia bring forth by the hand of Mithredath the treasurer, and numbered them unto [i]Sheshbazzar, the prince of Judah.

9 And this *is* the number of them: thirty chargers of gold, a thousand chargers of silver, nine and twenty knives,

10 Thirty basons of gold, silver basons of a second *sort* four hundred and ten, *and* other vessels a thousand.

11 All the vessels of gold and of silver *were* five thousand and four hundred. All *these* did Sheshbazzar bring up with *them of* the captivity that were brought up from Babylon unto Jerusalem.

CHAPTER 2.

The returning remnant: (1) *the people.*

NOW [j]these [1]*are* the children of the province that went up out of the captivity, of those which had been carried away, whom [k]Nebuchadnezzar the king of Babylon had carried away unto

a 2 Chr. 36:22, 23; Isa. 44:28; 45:1; Jer. 25:12; 29:10; 33:7-13.

b Isa. 44:28–45:13; Ezra 5:13, 14.

c Cf. Dan. 2:37.

d Isa. 44:28; 45:1-13.

e *Israel (history).* vs. 1-13; Ezra 6:15-18. (Gen. 12:2, 3; Rom. 11:26.)

f Cf. Dan. 6:26.

g i.e. *helped them.*

h Ezra 5:14; 6:5; Dan. 1:2; 5:2, 3.

i v. 11; Ezra 5:14.

j Cf. Neh. 7:6-69.

k 2 Ki. 24:14-16; 2 Chr. 36:19-21.

---

[1](2:1) Probably individuals from all of the tribes returned to Jerusalem under Zerubbabel, Ezra, and Nehemiah, but speaking broadly, the dispersion of the ten tribes (Ephraim—Israel) still continues; nor

Babylon, and came again unto Jerusalem
and Judah, every one unto his city;
2 Which came with [a]Zerubbabel:
Jeshua, Nehemiah, Seraiah, Reelaiah,
Mordecai, Bilshan, Mispar, Bigvai,
Rehum, Baanah. The number of the men
of the people of Israel:
3 The children of Parosh, two thousand an hundred seventy and two.
4 The children of Shephatiah, three hundred seventy and two.
5 The children of Arah, seven hundred seventy and five.
6 The children of Pahath-moab, of the
children of Jeshua *and* Joab, two thousand eight hundred and twelve.
7 The children of Elam, a thousand two hundred fifty and four.
8 The children of Zattu, nine hundred forty and five.
9 The children of Zaccai, seven hundred and threescore.
10 The children of Bani, six hundred forty and two.
11 The children of Bebai, six hundred twenty and three.
12 The children of Azgad, a thousand two hundred twenty and two.
13 The children of Adonikam, six hundred sixty and six.
14 The children of Bigvai, two thousand fifty and six.
15 The children of Adin, four hundred fifty and four.
16 The children of Ater of Hezekiah, ninety and eight.
17 The children of Bezai, three hundred twenty and three.
18 The children of Jorah, an hundred and twelve.
19 The children of Hashum, two hundred twenty and three.
20 The children of Gibbar, ninety and five.
21 The children of Bethlehem, an hundred twenty and three.
22 The men of Netophah, fifty and six.
23 The men of Anathoth, an hundred twenty and eight.
24 The children of Azmaveth, forty and two.
25 The children of Kirjath-arim, Chephirah, and Beeroth, seven hundred and forty and three.
26 The children of Ramah and Gaba, six hundred twenty and one.
27 The men of Michmas, an hundred twenty and two.
28 The men of Bethel and Ai, two hundred twenty and three.
29 The children of Nebo, fifty and two.
30 The children of Magbish, an hundred fifty and six.
31 The children of the other Elam, a thousand two hundred fifty and four.
32 The children of Harim, three hundred and twenty.
33 The children of Lod, Hadid, and Ono, seven hundred twenty and five.
34 The children of Jericho, three hundred forty and five.
35 The children of Senaah, three thousand and six hundred and thirty.

The returning remnant: (2) *the priests.*

36 The priests: the children of Jedaiah, of the house of Jeshua, nine hundred seventy and three.
37 The children of Immer, a thousand fifty and two.
38 The children of Pashur, a thousand two hundred forty and seven.
39 The children of Harim, a thousand and seventeen.

The returning remnant: (3) *the Levites.*

40 The Levites: the children of Jeshua and Kadmiel, of the children of Hodaviah, seventy and four.
41 The singers: the children of Asaph, an hundred twenty and eight.
42 The children of the porters: the children of Shallum, the children of Ater, the children of Talmon, the children of Akkub, the children of Hatita, the children of Shobai, *in* all an hundred thirty and nine.
43 The Nethinims: the children of

B.C. 535.

a Called Zorobabel, Mt. 1:12, 13.

can they now be positively identified. They are, however, preserved distinct from other peoples and are known to God as such, though they themselves, few in number, know Him not (Deut. 28:62; Isa. 11:11-13; Hos. 3:4; 8:8).

The order of the restoration was as follows: (1) The return of the first detachment under Zerubbabel and Jeshua (B.C. 536), Ezra 1–6, and the books of Haggai and Zechariah; (2) the expedition of Ezra (B.C. 458), seventy-eight years later (Ezra 7–10); (3) the commission of Nehemiah (B.C. 444), fourteen years after the expedition of Ezra (Neh. 2:1-5).

B.C. 536.

Ziha, the children of Hasupha, the children of Tabbaoth,

44 The children of Keros, the children of Siaha, the children of Padon,

45 The children of Lebanah, the children of Hagabah, the children of Akkub,

46 The children of Hagab, the children of Shalmai, the children of Hanan,

47 The children of Giddel, the children of Gahar, the children of Reaiah,

48 The children of Rezin, the children of Nekoda, the children of Gazzam,

49 The children of Uzza, the children of Paseah, the children of Besai,

50 The children of Asnah, the children of Mehunim, the children of Nephusim,

51 The children of Bakbuk, the children of Hakupha, the children of Harhur,

52 The children of Bazluth, the children of Mehida, the children of Harsha,

53 The children of Barkos, the children of Sisera, the children of Thamah,

54 The children of Neziah, the children of Hatipha.

The returning remnant:
(4) *descendants of Solomon's servants.*

55 The children of Solomon's servants: the children of Sotai, the children of Sophereth, the children of Peruda,

56 The children of Jaalah, the children of Darkon, the children of Giddel,

57 The children of Shephatiah, the children of Hattil, the children of Pochereth of Zebaim, the children of Ami.

58 All the Nethinims, and the children of Solomon's servants, *were* three hundred ninety and two.

59 And these *were* they which went up from Tel-melah, Tel-harsa, Cherub, Addan, *and* Immer: but they could not shew their father's house, and their seed, whether they *were* of Israel:

60 The children of Delaiah, the children of Tobiah, the children of Nekoda, six hundred fifty and two.

The returning remnant:
(5) *priests whose pedigrees were lost.*

61 And of the children of the priests: the children of Habaiah, the children of Koz, the children of Barzillai; which took a wife of the daughters of Barzillai the Gileadite, and was called after their name:

62 These sought their register *among* those that were reckoned by genealogy, but they were not found: therefore were they, as polluted, put from the priesthood.

63 And the Tirshatha said unto them, that they should not eat of the most holy things, till there stood up a priest with [a]Urim and with Thummim.

The returning remnant:
(6) *the total number.*

64 The whole congregation together *was* forty and two thousand three hundred *and* threescore,

65 Beside their servants and their maids, of whom *there were* seven thousand three hundred thirty and seven: and *there were* among them two hundred singing men and singing women.

The returning remnant:
(7) *their substance and gifts.*

66 Their horses *were* seven hundred thirty and six; their mules, two hundred forty and five;

67 Their camels, four hundred thirty and five; *their* asses, six thousand seven hundred and twenty.

68 [b]And *some* of the chief of the fathers, when they came to the house of the LORD which *is* at Jerusalem, offered freely for the house of God to set it up in his place:

69 They gave after their ability unto the treasure of the work threescore and one thousand [c]drams of gold, and five thousand pound of silver, and one hundred priests' garments.

70 So the priests, and the Levites, and *some* of the people, and the singers, and the porters, and the Nethinims, dwelt in their cities, and all Israel in their cities.

CHAPTER 3.

The altar is set up.

And when the [d]seventh month was come, and the children of Israel *were* in the cities, the people gathered themselves together as one man to Jerusalem.

2 Then stood up Jeshua the son of Jozadak, and his brethren the priests, and Zerubbabel the son of Shealtiel, and his brethren, and builded the altar of the

a See Ex. 28:30, *note.*

b Neh. 7:70.

c One dram = £1.1*s.*, or $4.97.

d i.e. *October;* also v. 6.

God of Israel, to offer burnt-offerings thereon, as *it is* written in the law of Moses the man of God.

3 And they set the altar upon his bases; for fear *was* upon them because of the people of those countries: and they offered burnt-offerings thereon unto the LORD, *even* burnt-offerings morning and evening.

The ancient worship established.

4 They kept also the feast of tabernacles, as *it is* written, and *offered* the daily burnt-offerings by number, according to the custom, as the duty of every day required;

5 And afterward *offered* the continual burnt-offering, both of the new moons, and of all the set feasts of the LORD that were consecrated, and of every one that willingly offered a freewill offering unto the LORD.

6 From the first day of the seventh month began they to offer burnt-offerings unto the LORD. But the foundation of the temple of the LORD was not *yet* laid.

7 They gave money also unto the masons, and to the carpenters; and meat, and drink, and oil, unto them of Zidon, and to them of Tyre, to bring cedar trees from Lebanon to the sea of Joppa, according to the grant that they had of Cyrus king of Persia.

Temple foundations laid in mingled joy and mourning.

8 Now in the second year of their coming unto the house of God at Jerusalem, in the [a]second month, began Zerubbabel the son of Shealtiel, and Jeshua the son of Jozadak, and the remnant of their brethren the priests and the [b]Levites, and all they that were come out of the captivity unto Jerusalem; and appointed the Levites, from twenty years old and upward, to set forward the work of the house of the LORD.

9 Then stood [c]Jeshua *with* his sons and his brethren, Kadmiel and his sons, the sons of Judah, together, to set forward the workmen in the house of God: the sons of Henadad, *with* their sons and their brethren the Levites.

10 And when the builders laid the foundation of the temple of the LORD, they [d]set the priests in their apparel with trumpets, and the Levites the sons of Asaph with cymbals, to praise the LORD, after the ordinance of David king of Israel.

11 And they [e]sang together by course in praising and giving thanks unto the LORD; [f]because *he is* good, for his mercy *endureth* for ever toward Israel. And all the people shouted with a great shout, when they praised the LORD, because the foundation of the house of the LORD was laid.

12 But [g]many of the priests and Levites and chief of the fathers, *who were* ancient men, that had seen the first house, when the foundation of this house was laid before their eyes, wept with a loud voice; and many shouted aloud for joy:

13 So that the people could not discern the noise of the shout of joy from the noise of the weeping of the people: for the people shouted with a loud shout, and the noise was heard afar off.

CHAPTER 4.

Adversaries seek to hinder the work.

Now when the [h]adversaries of Judah and Benjamin heard that the children of the captivity builded the temple unto the LORD God of Israel;

2 Then they came to Zerubbabel, and to the chief of the fathers, and said unto them, Let us build with you: [1]for [i]we seek your God, as ye *do*; and we do sacrifice unto him since the days of Esar-haddon king of Assur, which [j]brought us up hither.

3 But Zerubbabel, and Jeshua, and the rest of the chief of the fathers of Israel, said unto them, [k]Ye have nothing to do with us to build an house unto our God; but we ourselves together will build

B.C. 536.

a i.e. *May.*
b 1 Chr. 23:24-27.
c vs. 2, 8; Ezra 2:2; 4:3; 5:2; Neh. 7:7; 12:1, 7, 10, 26; Hag. 1:1; 2:2-4; Zech. 3:1-9; 6:11.
d 1 Chr. 6:31; 16:4; 25:1.
e Ex. 15:21; 2 Chr. 7:3; Neh. 12:24, 40.
f Psa. 136:1; cf. 2 Chr. 7:3.
g Cf. Hag. 2:3.
h vs. 7-9.
i 2 Ki. 17:32.
j v. 10; 2 Ki. 17:24.
k Cf. Neh. 2:20.

[1](4:2) The people of the land sought to hinder the work in three ways: (1) by seeking to draw the Jews into an unreal union, v. 3 (cf. 2 Ki. 17:32); (2) by "weakening the hands of the people of Judah," v. 4, i.e. by withholding supplies, etc.; and (3) by accusations lodged with Ahasuerus and Darius. The first was by far the most subtle and dangerous. The lives of Ezra and Nehemiah afford many illustrations of true separation. See 2 Cor. 6:14-18; 2 Tim. 2:19-21.

B.C. 534.

unto the LORD God of Israel, [a]as king Cyrus the king of Persia hath commanded us.

4 Then the people of the land weakened the hands of the people of Judah, and troubled them in building,

5 And hired counsellors against them, to frustrate their purpose, all the days of Cyrus king of Persia, even until the reign of [b]Darius king of Persia.

6 And in the reign of [c]Ahasuerus, in the beginning of his reign, wrote they *unto him* an accusation against the inhabitants of Judah and Jerusalem.

7 And in the days of [d]Artaxerxes wrote Bishlam, Mithredath, Tabeel, and the rest of their companions, unto Artaxerxes king of Persia; and the writing of the letter *was* written in the Syrian tongue, and interpreted in the Syrian tongue.

8 Rehum the chancellor and Shimshai the scribe wrote a letter against Jerusalem to Artaxerxes the king in this sort:

9 Then *wrote* Rehum the chancellor, and Shimshai the scribe, and the rest of their companions; the Dinaites, the Apharsathchites, the Tarpelites, the Apharsites, the Archevites, the Babylonians, the Susanchites, the Dehavites, *and* the Elamites,

10 And the rest of the nations whom the great and noble Asnappar brought over, and set in the cities of Samaria, and the rest *that are* on this side the river, and at such a time.

The adversaries' letter to Artaxerxes.

B.C. 522.]

11 This *is* the copy of the letter that they sent unto him, *even* unto Artaxerxes the king; Thy servants the men on this side the river, and at such a time.

12 Be it known unto the king, that the Jews which came up from thee to us are come unto Jerusalem, building the rebellious and the bad city, and have set up the walls *thereof*, and joined the foundations.

13 Be it known now unto the king, that, if this city be builded, and the walls set up *again*, *then* will they not pay toll, tribute, and custom, and *so* thou shalt endamage the revenue of the kings.

14 Now because we have maintenance from *the king's* palace, and it was not meet for us to see the king's dishonour, therefore have we sent and certified the king;

15 That search may be made in the book of the records of thy fathers: so shalt thou find in the book of the records, and know that this city *is* a rebellious city, and hurtful unto kings and provinces, and that they have moved sedition within the same of old time: for which cause was this city destroyed.

16 We certify the king that, if this city be builded *again*, and the walls thereof set up, by this means thou shalt have no portion on this side the river.

Decree of Artaxerxes.

17 *Then* sent the king an answer unto Rehum the chancellor, and *to* Shimshai the scribe, and *to* the rest of their companions that dwell in Samaria, and *unto* the rest beyond the river, Peace, and at such a time.

18 The letter which ye sent unto us hath been plainly read before me.

19 And I commanded, and search hath been made, and it is found that this city of old time hath made insurrection against kings, and *that* rebellion and sedition have been made therein.

20 There have been mighty kings also over Jerusalem, which have [e]ruled over all *countries* [f]beyond the river; and toll, tribute, and custom, was paid unto them.

21 [g]Give ye now commandment to cause these men to cease, and that this city be not builded, until *another* commandment shall be given from me.

22 Take heed now that ye fail not to do this: why should damage grow to the hurt of the kings?

The work suspended.

23 Now when the copy of king Artaxerxes' letter *was* read before Rehum, and Shimshai the scribe, and their companions, they went up in haste to Jerusalem unto the Jews, and made them to cease by force and power.

[B.C. 520.

24 Then ceased the work of the house of God which *is* at Jerusalem. So it ceased unto the second year of the reign of Darius king of Persia.

a See Ezra 1:1-4.

b Ezra 6:1.

c The Cambyses of secular history (529-521 B.C.); not Ahasuerus of Esther, who is the Xerxes of secular history (485 B.C.). See Dan. 5:31, *note.*

d The Artaxerxes of Ezra 4:7 is identical with Ahasuerus of v. 6, i.e. the Cambyses of profane history. The Artaxerxes of Ezra 7:1 is the Longimanus of secular history, B.C. 418. But see Dan. 5:31, *note.*

e 1 Ki. 4:21; 1 Chr. 18:3; Psa. 72:8.

f Gen. 15:18; Josh. 1:4.

CHAPTER 5.

The prophets encourage the prince and the priest: work begun again.

Then the prophets, [a]Haggai the prophet, and [b]Zechariah the son of Iddo, prophesied unto the Jews that *were* in Judah and Jerusalem in the name of the God of Israel, *even* unto them.

2 Then rose up [c]Zerubbabel the son of Shealtiel, and Jeshua the son of Jozadak, and began to build the house of God which *is* at Jerusalem: and with them *were* the prophets of God helping them.

3 At the same time came to them [d]Tatnai, governor on this side the river, and Shethar-boznai, and their companions, and said thus unto them, [e]Who hath commanded you to build this house, and to make up this wall?

4 [f]Then said we unto them after this manner, What are the names of the men that make this building?

5 But [g]the eye of their God was upon the elders of the Jews, that they could not cause them to cease, till the matter came to Darius: and then they returned answer by letter concerning this *matter*.

6 The copy of the letter that Tatnai, governor on this side the river, and Shethar-boznai, and his [h]companions the Apharsachites, which *were* on this side the river, sent unto Darius the king:

The adversaries' letter to Darius.

7 They sent a letter unto him, wherein was written thus; Unto Darius the king, all peace.

8 Be it known unto the king, that we went into the province of Judea, to the house of the great God, which is builded with [i]great stones, and timber is laid in the walls, and this work goeth fast on, and prospereth in their hands.

9 Then asked we those elders, *and* said unto them thus, [j]Who commanded you to build this house, and to make up these walls?

10 We asked their names also, to certify thee, that we might write the names of the men that *were* the chief of them.

11 And thus they returned us answer, saying, We are the servants of the God of heaven and earth, and build the house that was builded these many years ago, which a great king of Israel builded and [k]set up.

B.C. 520.

a Hag. 1:1.
b Zech. 1:1.
c Ezra 3:2.
d v. 6; Ezra 6:6.
e v. 9.
f v. 10.
g See Ezra 7:6, 28; Psa. 33:18.
h Ezra 4:9.

[B.C. 519.

i Chald. *stones of rolling.*
j vs. 3, 4.
k 1 Ki. 6:1.
l 2 Chr. 36:16, 17.
m 2 Ki. 24:2; 25:8, 9, 11.
n Ezra 1:1.
o Hag. 1:14; 2:2, 21.
p Ezra 3:8, 10.
q Ezra 6:15.

[B.C. 519.

r Ezra 6:1, 2.
s Ezra 5:17.

12 But [l]after that our fathers had provoked the God of heaven unto wrath, he gave them into the hand of [m]Nebuchadnezzar the king of Babylon, the Chaldean, who destroyed this house, and carried the people away into Babylon.

13 But in the first year of [n]Cyrus the king of Babylon *the same* king Cyrus made a decree to build this house of God.

14 And the vessels also of gold and silver of the house of God, which Nebuchadnezzar took out of the temple that *was* in Jerusalem, and brought them into the temple of Babylon, those did Cyrus the king take out of the temple of Babylon, and they were delivered unto *one*, [o]whose name *was* Sheshbazzar, whom he had made governor;

15 And said unto him, Take these vessels, go, carry them into the temple that *is* in Jerusalem, and let the house of God be builded in his place.

16 Then came the same Sheshbazzar, *and* [p]laid the foundation of the house of God which *is* in Jerusalem: and since that time even until now hath it been in building, and [q]*yet* it is not finished.

17 Now therefore, if *it seem* good to the king, [r]let there be search made in the king's treasure house, which *is* there at Babylon, whether it be *so*, that a decree was made of Cyrus the king to build this house of God at Jerusalem, and let the king send his pleasure to us concerning this matter.

CHAPTER 6.

Darius confirms the decree of Cyrus.

Then Darius the king made a decree [s]and search was made in the house of the rolls, where the treasures were laid up in Babylon.

2 And there was found at Achmetha in the palace that *is* in the province of the Medes, a roll, and therein *was* a record thus written:

3 In the first year of Cyrus the king *the same* Cyrus the king made a decree *concerning* the house of God at Jerusalem, Let the house be builded, the place where they offered sacrifices, and let the foundations thereof be strongly laid; the

height thereof threescore [a]cubits, *and* the breadth thereof threescore cubits;

4 [b]*With* three rows of great stones, and a row of new timber: and let the expenses be given out of the king's house:

5 And also let the [c]golden and silver vessels of the house of God, which Nebuchadnezzar took forth out of the temple which *is* at Jerusalem, and brought unto Babylon, be restored, and brought again unto the temple which *is* at Jerusalem, *every one* to his place, and place *them* in the house of God.

6 [d]Now *therefore,* Tatnai, governor beyond the river, Shethar-boznai, and [e]your companions the Apharsachites, which *are* beyond the river, be ye far from thence:

7 Let the work of this house of God alone; let the governor of the Jews and the elders of the Jews build this house of God in his place.

8 Moreover I make a decree what ye shall do to the elders of these Jews for the building of this house of God: that of the king's goods, *even* of the tribute beyond the river, forthwith expenses be given unto these men, that they be not hindered.

9 And that which they have need of, both young bullocks, and rams, and lambs, for the burnt-offerings of the God of heaven, wheat, salt, wine, and oil, according to the appointment of the priests which *are* at Jerusalem, let it be given them day by day without fail:

10 [f]That they may offer sacrifices of sweet savours unto the God of heaven, and [g]pray for the life of the king, and of his sons.

11 Also I have made a decree, that whosoever shall alter this word, let timber be pulled down from his house, and being set up, let him be hanged thereon; and [h]let his house be made a dunghill for this.

12 And the God that hath caused [i]his name to dwell there destroy all kings and people, that shall put to their hand to alter *and* to destroy this house of God which *is* at Jerusalem. I Darius have made a decree; let it be done with speed.

13 Then Tatnai, governor on this side the river, Shethar-boznai, and their companions, according to that which Darius the king had sent, so they did speedily.

14 [j]And the elders of the Jews builded, and they prospered through the prophesying of Haggai the prophet and Zechariah the son of Iddo. And they builded, and [1]finished *it,* according to the commandment of the God of Israel, and according to the commandment of [k]Cyrus, and [l]Darius, and [m]Artaxerxes king of Persia.

The restoration temple finished and dedicated.

15 And this [n]house was finished on the third day of the month [o]Adar, which was in the sixth year of the reign of Darius the king.

16 And the children of Israel, the priests, and the Levites, and the rest of the children of the captivity, kept the dedication of this house of God with joy,

17 And offered at the dedication of this house of God an hundred bullocks, two hundred rams, four hundred lambs; and for a sin-offering for all Israel, twelve he goats, according to the number of the tribes of Israel.

18 And they set the priests [p]in their divisions, and the Levites [q]in their courses, for the service of God, which *is* at Jerusalem; as it is written in the book of Moses.

The passover restored.

19 And the children of the captivity kept the passover [r]upon the fourteenth *day* of the [s]first month.

20 For the priests and the Levites were [t]purified together, all of them *were* pure, and killed the passover for all the children of the captivity, and for their brethren the priests, and for themselves.

21 And the children of Israel, which were come again out of captivity, and all such as had [u]separated themselves unto them from the filthiness of the [v]heathen of the land, to seek the LORD God of Israel, did eat,

22 And kept the [w]feast of unleavened

B.C. 519.

a One cubit = about 18 in.
b 1 Ki. 6:36.
c Ezra 1:7, 8; 5:14.
d Ezra 5:3.
e Chald. *their societies.*
f Ezra 7:23; Jer. 29:7.

[B.C. 515.

g 1 Tim. 2:1, 2.
h Dan. 2:5; 3:29.
i 1 Ki. 9:3.
j Ezra 5:1, 2.
k v. 3; Ezra 1:1; 5:13.
l Ezra 4:24; 6:12.
m Ezra 7:1, 11; Neh. 2:1.
n *Israel (history),* vs. 15-18; Neh. 2:1-9. (Gen. 12:2, 3; Rom. 11:26.)
o i.e. *March.*
p 1 Chr. 24:1.
q 1 Chr. 23:6.
r Ex. 12:6.
s i.e. *April.*
t 2 Chr. 30:15.
u *Separation.* Ezra 9:10-12. (Gen. 12:1; 2 Cor. 6:14-17.)
v i.e. *nations.*
w Ex. 12:15; 13:6; 2 Chr. 30:21; 35:17.

[1] **(6:14)** The *worship* of Jehovah was thus re-established in Jerusalem, but the *theocracy* was not restored. The remnant which returned from the Babylonian captivity lived in the land by Gentile sufferance, though doubtless by the providential care of Jehovah, till Messiah came, and was crucified by soldiers of the fourth Gentile world-empire (Rome, Dan. 2:40; 7:7). Soon after (A.D. 70) Rome destroyed the city and temple. See "Times of the Gentiles" (Lk. 21:24; Rev. 16:19).

bread seven days with joy: for the LORD
had made them joyful, and turned the
heart [a]of the king of Assyria unto them,
to strengthen their hands in the work of
the house of God, the God of Israel.

CHAPTER 7.

The expedition of Ezra:
his descent and companions.

NOW after these things, in the reign of
[b]Artaxerxes king of Persia, Ezra
[c]the son of Seraiah, the son of Azariah,
the son of Hilkiah,
2 The son of Shallum, the son of
Zadok, the son of Ahitub,
3 The son of Amariah, the son of
Azariah, the son of Meraioth,
4 The son of Zerahiah, the son of Uzzi,
the son of Bukki,
5 The son of Abishua, the son of
Phinehas, the son of Eleazar, the son of
Aaron the chief priest:
6 This Ezra went up from Babylon;
and he *was* [d]a ready scribe in the law of
Moses, which the LORD God of Israel
had given: and the king granted him all
his request, according to the hand of the
LORD his God upon him.
7 And there went up *some* of the children of Israel, and of the priests, and the
Levites, and the singers, and the porters,
and the Nethinims, unto Jerusalem, in
the seventh year of Artaxerxes the king.
8 And he came to Jerusalem in the
[e]fifth month, which *was* in the seventh
year of the king.
9 For upon the first *day* of the [f]first
month began he to go up from Babylon,
and on the first *day* of the [e]fifth month
came he to Jerusalem, according to the
good hand of his God upon him.
10 For Ezra had prepared his heart to
seek the law of the LORD, and to do *it*, and
[g]to teach in Israel statutes and judgments.

Decree of Artaxerxes in Ezra's behalf.

11 Now this *is* the copy of the letter
that the king Artaxerxes gave unto Ezra
the priest, the scribe, *even* a scribe of the
words of the commandments of the
LORD, and of his statutes to Israel.
12 Artaxerxes, [h]king of kings, unto Ezra
the priest, a scribe of the law of the God of
heaven, perfect *peace*, and at such a time.
13 I make a decree, that all they of the
people of Israel, and *of* his priests and
Levites, in my realm, which are minded
of their own freewill to go up to
Jerusalem, go with thee.
14 Forasmuch as thou art sent of the
king, and of his [i]seven counsellors, to
enquire concerning Judah and Jerusalem, according to the law of thy God
which *is* in thine hand;
15 And to carry the silver and gold,
which the king and his counsellors have
freely offered unto the God of Israel,
whose habitation *is* in Jerusalem,
16 And all the silver and gold that
thou canst find in all the province of
Babylon, with the [j]freewill offering of
the people, and of the priests, offering
willingly for the house of their God
which *is* in Jerusalem:
17 That thou mayest buy speedily
with this money bullocks, rams, lambs,
with their [k]meat-offerings and their
drink-offerings, and offer them upon the
altar of the house of your God which *is*
in Jerusalem.
18 And whatsoever shall seem good to
thee, and to thy brethren, to do with the
rest of the silver and the gold, that do
after the will of your God.
19 The vessels also that are given thee
for the service of the house of thy God,
those deliver thou before the God of
Jerusalem.
20 And whatsoever more shall be needful for the house of thy God, which thou
shalt have occasion to bestow, bestow *it*
out of the king's treasure house.
21 And I, *even* I Artaxerxes the king,
do make a decree to all the treasurers
which *are* beyond the river, that whatsoever Ezra the priest, the scribe of the law
of the God of heaven, shall require of
you, it be done speedily,
22 Unto an hundred [l]talents of silver,
and to an hundred [m]measures of wheat,
and to an hundred [n]baths of wine, and
to an hundred baths of oil, and salt without prescribing *how much*.
23 Whatsoever is commanded by the
God of heaven, let it be diligently done
for the house of the God of heaven: for
why should there be wrath against the
realm of the king and his sons?
24 Also we certify you, that touching
any of the priests and Levites, singers,
porters, Nethinims, or ministers of this

B.C. 515.

B.C. 457.]

a v.6; Ezra 1:1; 2 Ki. 23:29; 2 Chr. 33:11.
b Neh. 2:1.
c 1 Chr. 6:14.
d vs. 11, 12, 21.
e i.e. *August.*
f i.e. *April.*
g vs. 6, 25; Deut. 33:10; Neh. 8:1-8; Mal. 2:7.
h Ezk. 26:7; Dan. 2:37.
i Esth. 1:14.
j 1 Chr. 29:6, 9.
k Lit. *meal.*
l One talent (silver) = £410, or $1940.
m One measure = about 10 bu.
n One bath = about 8 gals.

house of God, it shall not be lawful to impose toll, tribute, or custom, upon them.

25 And thou, Ezra, after the wisdom of thy God, that *is* in thine hand, [a]set magistrates and judges, which may judge all the people that *are* beyond the river, all such as know the laws of thy God; and [b]teach ye them that know *them* not.

26 And whosoever will not do the law of thy God, and the law of the king, let judgment be executed speedily upon him, whether *it be* unto death, or to banishment, or to confiscation of goods, or to imprisonment.

Ezra's thanksgiving.

27 [c]Blessed *be* the LORD God of our fathers, [d]which hath put *such a thing* as this in the king's heart, to beautify the house of the LORD which *is* in Jerusalem:

28 And hath extended mercy unto me before the king, and his counsellors, and before all the king's mighty princes. And I was strengthened as [e]the hand of the LORD my God *was* upon me, and I gathered together out of Israel chief men to go up with me.

CHAPTER 8.

List of Ezra's companions.

These *are* now the chief of their fathers, and *this is* the genealogy of them that went up with me from Babylon, in the reign of Artaxerxes the king.

2 Of the sons of Phinehas; Gershom: of the sons of Ithamar; Daniel: of the sons of David; [f]Hattush.

3 Of the sons of Shechaniah, of the sons of [g]Pharosh; Zechariah: and with him were reckoned by genealogy of the males an hundred and fifty.

4 Of the sons of Pahath-moab; Elihoenai the son of Zerahiah, and with him two hundred males.

5 Of the sons of Shechaniah; the son of Jahaziel, and with him three hundred males.

6 Of the sons also of Adin; Ebed the son of Jonathan, and with him fifty males.

7 And of the sons of Elam; Jeshaiah the son of Athaliah, and with him seventy males.

8 And of the sons of Shephatiah; Zebadiah the son of Michael, and with him fourscore males.

9 Of the sons of Joab; Obadiah the son of Jehiel, and with him two hundred and eighteen males.

10 And of the sons of Shelomith; the son of Josiphiah, and with him an hundred and threescore males.

11 And of the sons of Bebai; Zechariah the son of Bebai, and with him twenty and eight males.

12 And of the sons of Azgad; Johanan the son of Hakkatan, and with him an hundred and ten males.

13 And of the last sons of Adonikam, whose names *are* these, Eliphelet, Jeiel, and Shemaiah, and with them threescore males.

14 Of the sons also of Bigvai; Uthai, and Zabbud, and with them seventy males.

Ezra sends for Levites and Nethinims.

15 And I gathered them together to the river that runneth to Ahava; and there abode we in tents three days: and I viewed the people, and the priests, and found there none of the sons of Levi.

16 Then sent I for Eliezer, for Ariel, for Shemaiah, and for Elnathan, and for Jarib, and for Elnathan, and for Nathan, and for Zechariah, and for Meshullam, chief men; also for Joiarib, and for Elnathan, men of understanding.

17 And I sent them with commandment unto Iddo the chief at the place Casiphia, and I told them what they should say unto Iddo, *and* to his brethren the Nethinims, at the place Casiphia, that they should bring unto us ministers for the house of our God.

18 And by the [h]good hand of our God upon us they [i]brought us a man of understanding, of the sons of Mahli, the son of Levi, the son of Israel; and Sherebiah, with his sons and his brethren, eighteen;

19 And Hashabiah, and with him Jeshaiah of the sons of Merari, his brethren and their sons, twenty;

20 [j]Also of the Nethinims, whom David and the princes had appointed for the service of the Levites, two hundred and twenty Nethinims: all of them were expressed by name.

The fast at the river Ahava.

21 Then I [k]proclaimed a fast there, at the river of Ahava, that we might [l]afflict ourselves before our God, to seek of him a [m]right way for us, and

B.C. 457.

a Ex. 18:21, 22; Deut. 16:18.
b v. 10; 2 Chr. 17:7; Mal. 2:7.
c 1 Chr. 29:10.
d Ezra 6:22.
e See vs. 6, 9; Ezra 5:5; 8:18.
f 1 Chr. 3:22.
g Ezra 2:3.
h Neh. 2:8.
i Neh. 8:7; 9:4, 5.
j See Ezra 2:43.
k 2 Chr. 20:3; Neh. 9:1-2.
l Lev. 16:29; 23:29; Isa. 58:3, 5.
m Psa. 5:8.

for our little ones, and for all our substance.
22 For I was ashamed to require of the
king a band of soldiers and horsemen to
help us against the enemy in the way:
because we had spoken unto the king,
saying, [a]The hand of our God *is* upon all
them for [b]good that seek him; but his
power and his wrath *is* against all them
that forsake him.
23 So we fasted and besought our God
for this: and he was [c]intreated of us.

The treasure committed to twelve priests.

24 Then I separated twelve of the chief
of the priests, Sherebiah, Hashabiah, and
ten of their brethren with them,
25 And weighed unto them the silver,
and the gold, and the vessels, *even* the
offering of the house of our God, which
the king, and his counsellors, and his
lords, and all Israel *there* present, had
offered:
26 I even weighed unto their hand six
hundred and fifty [d]talents of silver, and
silver vessels an hundred talents, *and* of
gold an hundred talents;
27 Also twenty basons of gold, of a
thousand [e]drams; and two vessels of
fine copper, precious as gold.
28 And I said unto them, Ye *are* holy
unto the LORD; the vessels *are* holy also;
and the silver and the gold *are* a freewill
offering unto the LORD God of your
fathers.
29 Watch ye, and keep *them*, until ye
weigh *them* before the chief of the priests
and the Levites, and chief of the fathers
of Israel, at Jerusalem, in the chambers
of the house of the LORD.
30 So took the priests and the Levites
the weight of the silver, and the gold,
and the vessels, to bring *them* to
Jerusalem unto the house of our God.

The arrival of Ezra at Jerusalem.

31 Then we departed from the river of
Ahava on the twelfth *day* of the [f]first
month, to go unto Jerusalem: and the
hand of our God was upon us, and he
delivered us from the hand of the enemy,
and of such as lay in wait by the way.
32 And we [g]came to Jerusalem, and
abode there three days.

B.C. 457.

a Ezra 7:6, 9, 28.

b Psa. 33:18, 19; 34:15, 22.

c 1 Chr. 5:20; 2 Chr. 33:13; Isa. 19:22.

d One talent (silver) = £410, or $1940; (gold) = £6150, or $29,085.

e One dram = £1. 1*s*., or $4.97.

f i.e. *April.*

g Neh. 2:11.

h vs. 26, 30.

i Ezra 6:17.

j Ezra 6:21; Neh. 9:2.

k Deut. 12:30, 31.

l Ex. 34:16; Deut. 7:3; Neh. 13:23.

m Ex. 19:6; 22:31; Deut. 7:6; 14:2.

n Ezra 10:3.

The treasure is brought into the temple.

33 Now on the fourth day was the silver and the gold and the vessels
[h]weighed in the house of our God by the
hand of Meremoth the son of Uriah the
priest; and with him *was* Eleazar the son
of Phinehas; and with them *was* Jozabad
the son of Jeshua, and Noadiah the son
of Binnui, Levites;
34 By number *and* by weight of every
one: and all the weight was written at
that time.
35 *Also* the children of those that had
been carried away, which were come out
of the captivity, [i]offered burnt-offerings
unto the God of Israel, twelve bullocks
for all Israel, ninety and six rams, seventy and seven lambs, twelve he goats *for* a
sin-offering: all *this was* a burnt-offering
unto the LORD.

The king's decree delivered to the governors.

36 And they delivered the king's com-
missions unto the king's lieutenants, and
to the governors on this side the river:
and they furthered the people, and the
house of God.

CHAPTER 9.

The remnant loses its separated position.

Now when these things were done,
the princes came to me, saying,
The people of Israel, and the priests, and
the Levites, have not [j]separated themselves from the people of the lands, [k]*doing* according to their abominations, *even*
of the Canaanites, the Hittites, the
Perizzites, the Jebusites, the Ammonites,
the Moabites, the Egyptians, and the
Amorites.
2 For they have [l]taken of their daughters for themselves, and for their sons: so
that the [m]holy seed have mingled themselves with the people of *those* lands:
yea, the hand of the princes and rulers
hath been chief in this trespass.
3 And when I heard this thing, I rent
my garment and my mantle, and
plucked off the hair of my head and of
my beard, and sat down astonied.
4 Then were assembled unto me every
one that [n]trembled at the words of the
God of Israel, because of the transgression

of those that had been carried away; and I sat astonied until the [a]evening sacrifice.

The prayer and confession of Ezra.

5 And at the evening sacrifice I arose up from my heaviness; and having rent my garment and my mantle, I fell upon my knees, and spread out my hands unto the LORD my God,

6 And [b]said, O my God, I am ashamed and blush to lift up my face to thee, my God: for our iniquities are increased over *our* head, and our trespass is grown up unto the heavens.

7 Since the days of our fathers *have* we *been* in a great trespass unto this day; and for our iniquities have we, our kings, *and* our priests, been delivered into the hand of the kings of the lands, to the sword, to captivity, and to a spoil, and to confusion of face, as *it is* this day.

8 And now for a little space grace hath been *shewed* from the LORD our God, to leave us a remnant to escape, and to give us a nail in his holy place, that our God may lighten our eyes, and give us a little reviving in our bondage.

9 For we *were* bondmen; yet our God hath not forsaken us in our bondage, but hath extended mercy unto us in the sight of the kings of Persia, to give us a reviving, to set up the house of our God, and to repair the desolations thereof, and to give us a wall in Judah and in Jerusalem.

10 And now, O our God, what shall we say after this? for we have forsaken thy commandments,

11 Which thou hast commanded by thy servants the prophets, saying, The land, unto which ye go to possess it, is an unclean land with the filthiness of the people of the lands, with their abominations, which have filled it from one end to another with their uncleanness.

12 Now therefore [c]give not your daughters unto their sons, neither take their daughters unto your sons, nor seek their peace or their wealth for ever: that ye may be strong, and eat the good of the land, and leave *it* for an inheritance to your children for ever.

13 And after all that is come upon us for our evil deeds, and for our great trespass, seeing that thou our God hast punished us less than our iniquities *deserve*, and hast given us *such* deliverance as this;

B.C. 457.

a Ex. 29:39.

b *Bible prayers* (O.T.). Neh. 1:5. (Gen. 15:2; Hab. 3:1-16.)

c *Separation.* vs. 10-12. Ezra 10:10. (Gen. 12.1; 2 Cor. 6.14-17.)

d Deut. 9:8.

e Neh. 9:33; Dan. 9:14.

f 2 Chr. 20:9.

g Neh. 13:23-27.

h 2 Chr. 34:31.

i 1 Chr. 28:10.

j Neh. 5:12.

k Deut. 9:18.

14 Should we again break thy commandments, and join in affinity with the people of these abominations? wouldest not thou be [d]angry with us till thou hadst consumed *us*, so that *there should be* no remnant nor escaping?

15 O LORD God of Israel, [e]thou *art* righteous: for we remain yet escaped, as *it is* this day: behold, we *are* before thee in our trespasses: for we cannot stand before thee because of this.

CHAPTER 10.

Separation restored.

Now when Ezra had prayed, and when he had confessed, weeping and casting himself down [f]before the house of God, there assembled unto him out of Israel a very great congregation of men and women and children: for the people wept very sore.

2 And Shechaniah the son of Jehiel, *one* of the sons of Elam, answered and said unto Ezra, We have [g]trespassed against our God, and have taken strange wives of the people of the land: yet now there is hope in Israel concerning this thing.

3 Now therefore let us make a [h]covenant with our God to put away all the wives, and such as are born of them, according to the counsel of my lord, and of those that tremble at the commandment of our God; and let it be done according to the law.

4 Arise; for *this* matter *belongeth* unto thee: we also *will be* with thee: [i]be of good courage, and do *it*.

5 Then arose Ezra, and made the chief priests, the Levites, and all Israel, [j]to swear that they should do according to this word. And they sware.

6 Then Ezra rose up from before the house of God, and went into the chamber of Johanan the son of Eliashib: and *when* he came thither, he [k]did eat no bread, nor drink water: for he mourned because of the transgression of them that had been carried away.

7 And they made proclamation throughout Judah and Jerusalem unto all the children of the captivity, that they should gather themselves together unto Jerusalem;

8 And that whosoever would not come within three days, according to the counsel of the princes and the elders, all

his substance should be forfeited, and
himself separated from the congregation
of those that had been carried away.
9 Then all the men of Judah and
Benjamin gathered themselves together
unto Jerusalem within three days. It *was*
the [a]ninth month, on the twentieth *day*
of the month; and [b]all the people sat in
the street of the house of God, trembling
because of *this* matter, and for the great
rain.
10 And Ezra the priest stood up, and
said unto them, Ye have transgressed,
and have taken strange wives, to
increase the trespass of Israel.
11 Now therefore make confession
unto the LORD God of your fathers, and
do his pleasure: and [c]separate yourselves from the people of the land, and
from the strange wives.
12 Then all the congregation answered
and said with a loud voice, As thou hast
said, so must we do.
13 But the people *are* many, and *it is* a
time of much rain, and we are not able
to stand without, neither *is this* a work of
one day or two: for we are many that
have transgressed in this thing.
14 Let now our rulers of all the congregation stand, and let all them which
have taken strange wives in our cities
come at appointed times, and with them
the elders of every city, and the judges
thereof, until the fierce wrath of our God
for this matter be turned from us.
15 Only Jonathan the son of Asahel
and Jahaziah the son of Tikvah were
employed about this *matter*: and
Meshullam and Shabbethai the Levite
helped them.
16 And the children of the captivity
did so. And Ezra the priest, *with* certain
chief of the fathers, after the house of
their fathers, and all of them by *their*
names, were separated, and sat down in
the first day of the [d]tenth month to
examine the matter.
17 And they made an end with all the
men that had taken strange wives by the
first day of the [e]first month.
18 And among the sons of the priests
there were found that had taken strange
wives: *namely*, of the sons of Jeshua the
son of Jozadak, and his brethren;
Maaseiah, and Eliezer, and Jarib, and
Gedaliah.
19 And they [f]gave their hands that
they would put away their wives; and
being [g]guilty, *they offered* a ram of the
flock for their trespass.
20 And of the sons of Immer; Hanani,
and Zebadiah.
21 And of the sons of Harim; Maaseiah, and Elijah, and Shemaiah, and
Jehiel, and Uzziah.
22 And of the sons of Pashur; Elioenai,
Maaseiah, Ishmael, Nethaneel, Jozabad,
and Elasah.
23 Also of the Levites; Jozabad, and
Shimei, and Kelaiah, (the same *is* Kelita,)
Pethahiah, Judah, and Eliezer.
24 Of the singers also; Eliashib: and of
the porters; Shallum, and Telem, and Uri.
25 Moreover of Israel: of the sons of
Parosh; Ramiah, and Jeziah, and
Malchiah, and Miamin, and Eleazar, and
Malchijah, and Benaiah.
26 And of the sons of Elam;
Mattaniah, Zechariah, and Jehiel, and
Abdi, and Jeremoth, and Eliah.
27 And of the sons of Zattu; Elioenai,
Eliashib, Mattaniah, and Jeremoth, and
Zabad, and Aziza.
28 Of the sons also of Bebai; Jeho-
hanan, Hananiah, Zabbai, *and* Athlai.
29 And of the sons of Bani; Meshullam, Malluch, and Adaiah, Jashub, and
Sheal, and Ramoth.
30 And of the sons of Pahath-moab;
Adna, and Chelal, Benaiah, Maaseiah,
Mattaniah, Bezaleel, and Binnui, and
Manasseh.
31 And *of* the sons of Harim; Eliezer,
Ishijah, Malchiah, Shemaiah, Shimeon,
32 Benjamin, Malluch, *and* Shemariah.
33 Of the sons of Hashum; Mattenai,
Mattathah, Zabad, Eliphelet, Jeremai,
Manasseh, *and* Shimei.
34 Of the sons of Bani; Maadai,
Amram, and Uel,
35 Benaiah, Bedeiah, Chelluh,
36 Vaniah, Meremoth, Eliashib,
37 Mattaniah, Mattenai, and Jaasau,
38 And Bani, and Binnui, Shimei,
39 And Shelemiah, and Nathan, and
Adaiah,
40 [h]Machnadebai, Shashai, Sharai,
41 Azareel, and Shelemiah, Shemariah,
42 Shallum, Amariah, *and* Joseph.
43 Of the sons of Nebo; Jeiel, Mattithiah, Zabad, Zebina, Jadau, and Joel,
Benaiah.
44 All these had taken strange wives:
and *some* of them had wives by whom
they had children.

B.C. 457.

a i.e. *December.*

b See 1 Sam. 12:18.

c *Separation.* vs. 10-11. Neh. 9:2. (Gen. 12:1; 2 Cor. 6:14-17.)

d i.e. *January.*

e i.e. *April.*

f 2 Ki. 10:15; 1 Chr. 29:24, marg.; 2 Chr. 30:8.

g Lev. 6:4-6.

h Or, *Mabnadebai,* according to some copies.

THE BOOK OF NEHEMIAH

FOURTEEN years after the return of Ezra to Jerusalem, Nehemiah led up a company (B.C. 444) and restored the walls and the civil authority. Of those events this book is the record. It is in eight divisions: I. The journey to Jerusalem, 1:1–2:20. II. The building of the wall, 3:1–6:19. III. The census, 7:1-73. IV. The revival, 8:1–11:36. V. The census of the priests and Levites, 12:1-26. VI. Dedication of the wall, 12:27-43. VII. Restoration of the temple worship, 12:44-47. VIII. The legal order restored, 13:1-31. The moral state of the time is disclosed by the prophet Malachi. This book affords many instances of individual faith acting on the written word (e.g. 1:8, 9; 13:1). It is the principle of 2 Tim. 2.

The events recorded in Nehemiah cover a period of 11 years (Ussher).

CHAPTER 1.

B.C. 446.

Nehemiah learns of the distress of the remnant in Jerusalem.

The words of [a]Nehemiah the son of
Hachaliah. And it came to pass in
the month [b]Chisleu, in the twentieth
year, as I was in [c]Shushan the palace,
2 That Hanani, one of my brethren,
came, he and *certain* men of Judah; and I
asked them concerning the Jews that
had escaped, which were left of the captivity, and concerning Jerusalem.
3 And they said unto me, The remnant
that are left of the captivity there in the
province *are* in great affliction and
reproach: the wall of Jerusalem also *is*
broken down, and the gates thereof are
burned with fire.
4 And it came to pass, when I heard
these words, that I sat down and wept,
and mourned *certain* days, and fasted,
and prayed before the God of heaven,

Nehemiah's prayer.

5 And [d]said, I beseech thee, O LORD
God of heaven, the great and terrible
God, that keepeth covenant and mercy
for them that love him and observe his
commandments:
6 Let thine ear now be attentive, and
thine eyes open, that thou mayest hear
the prayer of thy servant, which I pray
before thee now, day and night, for the
children of Israel thy servants, and confess the sins of the children of Israel,
which we have sinned against thee: both
I and my father's house have sinned.
7 We have dealt very corruptly
against thee, and have not kept the
commandments, nor the statutes, nor
the judgments, which thou commandedst thy servant Moses.
8 Remember, I beseech thee, the word
that thou commandedst thy servant
Moses, [e]saying, *If* ye transgress, I will
scatter you abroad among the nations:
9 But *if* ye turn unto me, and keep my
commandments, and do them; though
there were of you cast out unto the uttermost part of the heaven, *yet* will I gather
them from thence, and will bring them
unto the place that I have chosen to set
my name there.
10 Now these *are* thy servants and thy
people, whom thou hast [f]redeemed by
thy great power, and by thy strong hand.
11 O Lord, I beseech thee, let now
thine ear be attentive to the prayer of thy
servant, and to the prayer of thy servants, who desire to [g]fear thy name: and
prosper, I pray thee, thy servant this day,
and grant him mercy in the sight of this
man. For I was the king's [h]cupbearer.

CHAPTER 2.

Artaxerxes sends Nehemiah to Jerusalem.

And it came to pass in the month
[i]Nisan, in the twentieth year of
[j]Artaxerxes the king, *that* wine *was*
before him: and I took up the wine, and
gave *it* unto the king. Now I had not
been *beforetime* sad in his presence.
2 Wherefore the king said unto me,
Why *is* thy countenance sad, seeing thou
art not sick? this *is* nothing *else* but sorrow of heart. Then I was very sore
afraid,
3 And said unto the king, Let the king
live for ever: why should not my

a Neh. 10:1.
b i.e. *December.*
c Or, *Susa,* ancient capital of Persia.
d *Bible prayers* (O.T.). Neh. 4:4. (Gen. 15:2; Hab. 3:1-16.)
e Deut. 28:63-67; 30:1-5.
f Ex. 14:30, *note.*
g Psa. 19:9, *note.*
h Neh. 2:1; cf. 2 Chr. 9:4.
i i.e. *April.*
j See Ezra 4:6; 7:1.

countenance be sad, [a]when the city, the
place of my fathers' sepulchres, *lieth*
waste, and the gates thereof are consumed with fire?
4 Then the king said unto me, For
what dost thou make request? So I
prayed to the God of heaven.
5 And I said unto the king, If it please
the king, and if thy servant have found
favour in thy sight, that thou wouldest
send me unto Judah, unto the city of my
fathers' sepulchres, that I may build it.
6 And the king said unto me, (the
queen also sitting by him,) For how long
shall thy journey be? and when wilt
thou return? So it pleased the king to
send me; and I set him a [b]time.
7 Moreover I said unto the king, If it
please the king, let letters be given me to
the governors beyond the river, that they
may convey me over till I come into
Judah;
8 And a letter unto Asaph the keeper
of the king's forest, that he may give me
timber to make beams for the gates of
the palace which *appertained* to the
house, and for the wall of the city, and
for the house that I shall enter into. And
the king granted me, according to [c]the
good hand of my God upon me.
9 Then I came to the governors beyond
the river, and gave them the king's letters. Now the king had sent captains of
the army and horsemen with me.
10 When Sanballat the Horonite, and
[1]Tobiah the servant, the Ammonite,
heard *of it*, it grieved them exceedingly
that there was come a man to seek the
welfare of the children of Israel.

Nehemiah views the ruined walls.

11 So I came [d]to Jerusalem, and was
there three days.
12 And I arose in the night, I and some
few men with me; neither told I *any* man
what my God had put in my heart to do
at Jerusalem: neither *was there any* beast
with me, save the beast that I rode upon.
13 And I went out by night by the
[e]gate of the valley, even before the dragon well, and to the dung port, and
viewed the walls of Jerusalem, which
were broken down, and the gates thereof
were consumed with fire.
14 Then I went on to the [f]gate of the
fountain, and to the [g]king's pool: but
there was no place for the beast *that was*
under me to pass.
15 Then went I up in the night by the
[h]brook, and viewed the wall, and turned
back, and entered by the gate of the valley, and *so* returned.
16 And the rulers knew not whither I
went, or what I did; neither had I as yet
told *it* to the Jews, nor to the priests, nor
to the nobles, nor to the rulers, nor to the
rest that did the work.

Nehemiah encourages the people to build the walls.

17 Then said I unto them, Ye see the
distress that we *are* in, how Jerusalem
lieth waste, and the gates thereof are
burned with fire: come, and let us build
up the wall of Jerusalem, that we be no
more a reproach.
18 Then I told them of [i]the hand of my
God which was good upon me; as also
the king's words that he had spoken
unto me. And they said, Let us rise up
and build. So they [j]strengthened their
hands for *this* good *work*.
19 But when Sanballat the Horonite,
and Tobiah the servant, the Ammonite,
and Geshem the Arabian, heard *it*, they
[k]laughed us to scorn, and despised us,
and said, What *is* this thing that ye do?
will ye rebel against the king?
20 Then answered I them, and said
unto them, The God of heaven, he will
prosper us; therefore we his servants will
arise and build: but [l]ye have no portion
nor right, nor memorial, in Jerusalem.

CHAPTER 3.

The builders of the wall.

Then [m]Eliashib the high priest rose up
with his brethren the priests, and
they builded the [n]sheep gate; they sanctified it, and set up the doors of it; even
unto the [o]tower of Meah they sanctified
it, unto the tower of [p]Hananeel.
2 And next unto him builded the men

B.C. 445.

a *Israel (history).* vs. 1-9; Neh. 8:1-8. (Gen. 12:2, 3; Rom. 11:26.)

b Neh. 5:14; 13:6.

c v. 18; 6:9; Ezra 5:5; 7:6, 9, 28.

d Cf. Ezra 8:32.

e 2 Chr. 26:9

f Neh. 3:15.

g Isa. 7:3.

h 2 Sam. 15:23

i v. 8, etc.

j Cf. Ezra 4:4.

k The obstacle of ridicule.

l Cf. Ezra 4:3.

m vs. 20, 21; Neh. 13:4, 7, 28.

n John 5:2, marg. The sheep for sacrifice were brought in here.

o The towers appear to have been on either side the sheep gate.

p Jer. 31:38.

[1] **(2:10)** Two Tobiahs are distinguished by many: (1) "Tobiah the servant, the Ammonite," Neh. 2:10, 19; 4:3, 7; 6:1, 12, 14. (2) A Jew, unable to prove his genealogy. But the reference to the latter (Neh. 7:62) indicates that he was already dead. But one Tobiah, and he the Ammonite, is active in this book.

of Jericho. And next to them builded
Zaccur the son of Imri.
3 But the [a]fish gate did the sons of
Hassenaah build, who *also* laid the beams
thereof, and set up the doors thereof, the
locks thereof, and the bars thereof.
4 And next unto them repaired
Meremoth the son of Urijah, the son of
Koz. And next unto them repaired
Meshullam the son of Berechiah, the son
of Meshezabeel. And next unto them
repaired Zadok the son of Baana.
5 And next unto them the Tekoites
repaired; but their nobles put not their
necks to the work of their Lord.
6 Moreover the old gate repaired
Jehoiada the son of Paseah, and
Meshullam the son of Besodeiah; they
laid the beams thereof, and set up the
doors thereof, and the locks thereof, and
the bars thereof.
7 And next unto them repaired
Melatiah the Gibeonite, and Jadon the
Meronothite, the men of Gibeon, and of
Mizpah, unto the throne of the [b]gover-
nor on this side the [c]river.
8 Next unto him repaired Uzziel the
son of Harhaiah, of the goldsmiths. Next
unto him also repaired Hananiah the son
of *one of* the apothecaries, and they fortified Jerusalem unto the broad wall.
9 And next unto them repaired
Rephaiah the son of Hur, the ruler of the
half part of Jerusalem.
10 And next unto them repaired
Jedaiah the son of Harumaph, even over
against his house. And next unto him
repaired Hattush the son of Hashabniah.
11 Malchijah the son of Harim, and
Hashub the son of Pahath-moab,
repaired the other piece, and the tower
of the furnaces.
12 And next unto him repaired Shallum
the son of Halohesh, the ruler of the half
part of Jerusalem, he and his daughters.
13 The valley gate repaired Hanun,
and the inhabitants of Zanoah; they built
it, and set up the doors thereof, the locks
thereof, and the bars thereof, and a thousand [d]cubits on the wall unto the dung
gate.
14 But the dung gate repaired
Malchiah the son of Rechab, the ruler of
part of Beth-haccerem; he built it, and
set up the doors thereof, the locks thereof, and the bars thereof.
15 But the gate of the fountain repaired
Shallun the son of Col-hozeh, the ruler of
part of Mizpah; he built it, and covered
it, and set up the doors thereof, the locks
thereof, and the bars thereof, and the
wall of the [e]pool of Siloah by the king's
garden, and unto the stairs that go down
from the city of David.
16 After him repaired Nehemiah the
son of Azbuk, the ruler of the half part of
Beth-zur, unto *the place* over against the
sepulchres of David, and to the pool that
was made, and unto the house of the
mighty.
17 After him repaired the Levites,
Rehum the son of Bani. Next unto him
repaired Hashabiah, the ruler of the half
part of Keilah, in his part.
18 After him repaired their brethren,
Bavai the son of Henadad, the ruler of
the half part of Keilah.
19 And next to him repaired Ezer the
son of Jeshua, the ruler of Mizpah,
another piece over against the going up
to the armoury at the turning *of the wall.*
20 After him Baruch the son of Zabbai
earnestly repaired the other piece, from
the turning *of the wall* unto the door of
the house of Eliashib the high priest.
21 After him repaired Meremoth the
son of Urijah the son of Koz another
piece, from the door of the house of
Eliashib even to the end of the house of
Eliashib.
22 And after him repaired the priests,
the men of the plain.
23 After him repaired Benjamin and
Hashub over against their house. After
him repaired Azariah the son of Maaseiah
the son of Ananiah by his house.
24 After him repaired Binnui the son
of Henadad another piece, from the
house of Azariah unto the turning *of the
wall,* even unto the corner.
25 Palal the son of Uzai, over against
the turning *of the wall,* and the tower
which lieth out from the king's high
house, that *was* by the [f]court of the prison.
After him Pedaiah the son of Parosh.
26 Moreover the [g]Nethinims dwelt in
Ophel, unto *the place* over against the
water gate toward the east, and the
tower that lieth out.
27 After them the Tekoites repaired
another piece, over against the great
tower that lieth out, even unto the wall
of [h]Ophel.

B.C. 445.

a Zeph. 1:10.
b Ezra 8:36; cf. Neh. 2:9.
c i.e. Euphrates.
d Cubit = about 18 in.
e Isa. 8:6; John 9:7.
f Jer. 32:2; 37:21.
g i.e. *dedicated* (persons), probably descendants of the Gibeonites (2 Sam. 21:1-3) devoted to the service of the Levites. But see Josh. 9:17-21.
h Trans. *tower,* 2 Ki. 5:24; Cf. 2 Chr. 27:3; 33:14. Perhaps part of the fort called Millo, 1 Ki. 9:15; 2 Chr. 32:5.

28 From above the horse gate repaired
the priests, every one over against his
house.
29 After them repaired Zadok the son
of Immer over against his house. After
him repaired also Shemaiah the son of
Shechaniah, the keeper of the east gate.
30 After him repaired Hananiah the
son of Shelemiah, and Hanun the sixth
son of Zalaph, another piece. After him
repaired Meshullam the son of
Berechiah over against his chamber.
31 After him repaired Malchiah the
goldsmith's son unto the place of the
Nethinims, and of the merchants, over
against the gate Miphkad, and to the
going up of the corner.
32 And between the going up of the
corner unto the sheep gate repaired the
goldsmiths and the merchants.

CHAPTER 4.

Opposition by ridicule.

But it came to pass, that when
[a]Sanballat heard that we builded
the wall, he was wroth, and took great
indignation, and mocked the Jews.
2 And he spake before his brethren
and the army of Samaria, and said, What
do these feeble Jews? will they fortify
themselves? will they sacrifice? will they
make an end in a day? will they revive
the stones out of the heaps of the rubbish which are burned?
3 Now Tobiah the Ammonite *was* by
him, and he said, Even that which they
build, if a fox go up, he shall even break
down their stone wall.

Nehemiah answers by prayer.

4 [b]Hear, O our God; for we are
despised: and [c]turn their reproach upon
their own head, and give them for a prey
in the land of captivity:
5 And cover not their iniquity, and let
not their sin be blotted out from before
thee: for they have provoked *thee* to
anger before the builders.
6 So built we the wall; and all the wall
was joined together unto the half thereof: for the people had a mind to work.

Opposition by anger: the resource of prayer.

7 But it came to pass, *that* when
Sanballat, and Tobiah, and the Arabians,
and the Ammonites, and the Ashdodites,
heard that the walls of Jerusalem were
made up, *and* that the breaches began to
be stopped, then they were very wroth,
8 And conspired all of them together
to come *and* to fight against Jerusalem,
and to hinder it.
9 Nevertheless we made our prayer
unto our God, and set a watch against
them day and night, because of them.

Opposition by discouraged brethren: the resource of faith (vs. 14, 20).

10 And Judah said, The strength of the
bearers of burdens is decayed, and *there*
is much rubbish; so that we are not able
to build the wall.
11 And our adversaries said, They
shall not know, neither see, till we come
in the midst among them, and slay them,
and cause the work to cease.
12 And it came to pass, that when the
Jews which dwelt by them came, they
said unto us ten times, From all places
whence ye shall return unto us *they will*
be upon you.
13 Therefore set I in the lower places
behind the wall, *and* on the higher
places, I even set the people after their
families with their swords, their spears,
and their bows.
14 And I looked, and rose up, and said
unto the nobles, and to the rulers, and to
the rest of the people, Be not ye afraid of
them: remember the Lord, *which is* great
and terrible, and fight for your brethren,
your sons, and your daughters, your
wives, and your houses.
15 And it came to pass, when our enemies heard that it was known unto us,
and God had brought their counsel to
nought, that we returned all of us to the
wall, every one unto his work.
16 And it came to pass from that time
forth, *that* the half of my servants wrought
in the work, and the other half of them
held both the spears, the shields, and the
bows, and the habergeons; and the rulers
were behind all the house of Judah.
17 They which builded on the wall,
and they that bare burdens, with those
that laded, *every one* with one of his
hands wrought in the work, and with
the other *hand* held a weapon.
18 For the builders, every one had his

B.C. 445.

a Neh. 2:10, 19.

b *Bible prayers* (O.T.). Neh. 9:5. (Gen. 15:2; Hab. 3:1-16.)

c Psa. 69:4-7.

B.C. 519.

sword girded by his side, and *so* builded. And he that sounded the trumpet
was by me.
19 And I said unto the nobles, and to
the rulers, and to the rest of the people,
The work *is* great and large, and we are
separated upon the wall, one far from
another.
20 In what place *therefore* ye hear the
sound of the trumpet, resort ye thither
unto us: our God shall fight for us.
21 So we laboured in the work: and half
of them held the spears from the rising of
the morning till the stars appeared.
22 Likewise at the same time said I
unto the people, Let every one with his
servant lodge within Jerusalem, that in
the night they may be a guard to us, and
labour on the day.
23 So neither I, nor my brethren, nor
my servants, nor the men of the guard
which followed me, none of us put off
our clothes, *saving that* every one put
them off for washing.

CHAPTER 5.

Opposition by greed and heartlessness:
the resource of restitution.

And there was a great cry of the
people and of their wives against
their [a]brethren the Jews.
2 For there were that said, We, our
sons, and our daughters, *are* many:
therefore we take up corn *for them*, that
we may eat, and live.
3 *Some* also there were that said, We
have mortgaged our lands, vineyards,
and houses, that we might buy corn,
because of the dearth.
4 There were also that said, We have
borrowed money for the king's tribute,
and that upon our lands and vineyards.
5 Yet now our flesh *is* as the flesh of
our brethren, our children as their children: and, lo, we bring into bondage our
sons and our daughters to be servants,
and *some* of our daughters are brought
unto bondage *already*: neither *is it* in our
power *to redeem them*; for other men
have our lands and vineyards.
6 And I was very angry when I heard
their cry and these words.
7 Then I consulted with myself, and I
rebuked the nobles, and the rulers, and
said unto them, Ye exact usury, every
one of his brother. And I set a great
assembly against them.
8 And I said unto them, We after our
ability have [b]redeemed our brethren the
Jews, which were sold unto the [c]hea-
then; and will ye even sell your
brethren? or shall they be sold unto us?
Then held they their peace, and found
nothing *to answer*.
9 Also I said, It *is* not good that ye do:
ought ye not to walk in the [d]fear of our
God because of the reproach of the [c]hea-
then our enemies?
10 I likewise, *and* my brethren, and my
servants, might exact of them money and
corn: I pray you, let us leave off this usury.
11 Restore, I pray you, to them, even
this day, their lands, their vineyards,
their oliveyards, and their houses, also
the hundredth *part* of the money, and of
the corn, the wine, and the oil, that ye
exact of them.
12 Then said they, We will restore *them*,
and will require nothing of them; so will
we do as thou sayest. Then I called the
priests, and took an oath of them, that
they should do according to this promise.
13 Also I shook my lap, and said, So
God shake out every man from his
house, and from his labour, that performeth not this promise, even thus be
he shaken out, and emptied. And all the
congregation said, Amen, and praised
the LORD. And the people did according
to this promise.

Nehemiah's example of unselfishness.

14 Moreover from the time that I was
appointed to be their governor in the
land of Judah, from the twentieth year
even unto the two and thirtieth year of
Artaxerxes the king, *that is*, twelve years,
I and my brethren have not eaten the
bread of the governor.
15 But the former governors that *had
been* before me were chargeable unto the
people, and had taken of them bread
and wine, beside forty [e]shekels of silver;
yea, even their servants bare rule over
the people: but so did not I, because of
the [d]fear of God.
16 Yea, also I continued in the work of
this wall, neither bought we any land:

a Isa. 5:7, 8.

b Ex. 14:30, *note;* Lev. 25:48.

c i.e. *nations.*

d Psa. 19:9, *note.*

e One shekel – 2*s.* 9*d.*, or 65 cts.

and all my servants *were* gathered thither unto the work.

17 Moreover *there were* at my table an hundred and fifty of the Jews and rulers, beside those that came unto us from among the [a]heathen that *are* about us.

18 Now *that* which was prepared *for me* daily *was* one ox *and* six choice sheep; also fowls were prepared for me, and once in ten days store of all sorts of wine: yet for all this required not I the bread of the governor, because the bondage was heavy upon this people.

19 Think upon me, my God, for good, *according* to all that I have done for this people.

CHAPTER 6.

Opposition by craft:
the resource of manly firmness.

Now it came to pass, when [b]Sanballat, and Tobiah, and [c]Geshem the Arabian, and the rest of our enemies, heard that I had builded the wall, and *that* there was no breach left therein; (though at that time I had not set up the doors upon the gates;)

2 That Sanballat and Geshem sent unto me, saying, Come, let us meet together in *some one of* the villages in the plain of Ono. But they thought to do me mischief.

3 And I sent messengers unto them, saying, I *am* doing a great work, so that I cannot come down: why should the work cease, whilst I leave it, and come down to you?

4 Yet they sent unto me four times after this sort; and I answered them after the same manner.

5 Then sent Sanballat his servant unto me in like manner the fifth time with an open letter in his hand;

6 Wherein *was* written, It is reported among the [a]heathen, and [d]Gashmu saith *it, that* thou and the Jews think to rebel: for which cause thou buildest the wall, that thou mayest be their king, according to these words.

7 And thou hast also appointed prophets to preach of thee at Jerusalem, saying, *There is* a king in Judah: and now shall it be reported to the king according to these words. Come now therefore, and let us take counsel together.

B.C. 445.

a i.e. *nations.*

b Neh. 2:10, 19; 4:1, 7; 13:28.

c Called *Gashmu*, v. 6.

d Called *Geshem*, v. 2.

e Ezra 4:4.

f 2 Cor. 11:26, l.c.

g Neh. 13:29.

h i.e. *September.*

i Neh. 2:10, *note.*

8 Then I sent unto him, saying, There are no such things done as thou sayest, but thou feignest them out of thine own heart.

9 For they all made us afraid, saying, Their [e]hands shall be weakened from the work, that it be not done. Now therefore, *O God*, strengthen my hands.

10 Afterward I came unto the house of Shemaiah the son of Delaiah the son of Mehetabeel, who *was* shut up; and he said, Let us meet together in the house of God, within the temple, and let us shut the doors of the temple: for they will come to slay thee; yea, in the night will they come to slay thee.

11 And I said, Should such a man as I flee? and who *is there*, that, *being* as I *am*, would go into the temple to save his life? I will not go in.

12 And, lo, I perceived that God had not sent him; [f]but that he pronounced this prophecy against me: for Tobiah and Sanballat had hired him.

13 Therefore *was* he hired, that I should be afraid, and do so, and sin, and *that* they might have *matter* for an evil report, that they might reproach me.

14 My God, think thou upon Tobiah and Sanballat [g]according to these their works, and on the prophetess Noadiah, and the rest of the prophets, that would have put me in fear.

The wall is finished.

15 So the wall was finished in the twenty and fifth *day* of *the month* [h]Elul, in fifty and two days.

16 And it came to pass, that when all our enemies heard *thereof*, and all the [a]heathen that *were* about us saw *these things*, they were much cast down in their own eyes: for they perceived that this work was wrought of our God.

17 Moreover in those days the nobles of Judah sent many letters unto [i]Tobiah, and *the letters* of Tobiah came unto them.

18 For *there were* many in Judah sworn unto him, because he *was* the son in law of Shechaniah the son of Arah; and his son Johanan had taken the daughter of Meshullam the son of Berechiah.

19 Also they reported his good deeds before me, and uttered my words to him. *And* Tobiah sent letters to put me in fear.

CHAPTER 7.

Jerusalem given in charge to Hanani and Hananiah.

Now it came to pass, when the wall was built, and I had set up the doors, and the porters and the singers and the Levites were appointed,

2 That I gave my brother Hanani, and Hananiah the ruler of the palace, charge over Jerusalem: for he *was* a faithful man, and [a]feared God above many.

3 And I said unto them, Let not the gates of Jerusalem be opened until the sun be hot; and while they stand by, let them shut the doors, and bar *them*: and appoint watches of the inhabitants of Jerusalem, every one in his watch, and every one *to be* over against his house.

4 Now the city *was* large and great: but the people *were* few therein, and the houses *were* not builded.

Register of the genealogy of the first remnant: the people.

5 And my God put into mine heart to gather together the nobles, and the rulers, and the people, that they might be reckoned by genealogy. And I found a register of the genealogy of them which came up [b]at the first, and found written therein,

6 These *are* the children of the province, that went up out of the captivity, of those that had been carried away, whom Nebuchadnezzar the king of Babylon had carried away, and came again to Jerusalem and to Judah, every one unto his city;

7 Who came with [c]Zerubbabel, Jeshua, Nehemiah, Azariah, Raamiah, Nahamani, Mordecai, Bilshan, Mispereth, Bigvai, Nehum, Baanah. The number, *I say*, of the men of the people of Israel *was this;*

8 The children of Parosh, two thousand an hundred seventy and two.

9 The children of Shephatiah, three hundred seventy and two.

10 The children of Arah, six hundred fifty and two.

11 The children of Pahath-moab, of the children of Jeshua and Joab, two thousand and eight hundred *and* eighteen.

12 The children of Elam, a thousand two hundred fifty and four.

13 The children of Zattu, eight hundred forty and five.

14 The children of Zaccai, seven hundred and threescore.

15 The children of Binnui, six hundred forty and eight.

16 The children of Bebai, six hundred twenty and eight.

17 The children of Azgad, two thousand three hundred twenty and two.

18 The children of Adonikam, six hundred threescore and seven.

19 The children of Bigvai, two thousand threescore and seven.

20 The children of Adin, six hundred fifty and five.

21 The children of Ater of Hezekiah, ninety and eight.

22 The children of Hashum, three hundred twenty and eight.

23 The children of Bezai, three hundred twenty and four.

24 The children of Hariph, an hundred and twelve.

25 The children of Gibeon, ninety and five.

26 The men of Bethlehem and Netophah, an hundred fourscore and eight.

27 The men of Anathoth, an hundred twenty and eight.

28 The men of Beth-azmaveth, forty and two.

29 The men of Kirjath-jearim, Chephirah, and Beeroth, seven hundred forty and three.

30 The men of Ramah and Geba, six hundred twenty and one.

31 The men of Michmas, an hundred and twenty and two.

32 The men of Beth-el and Ai, an hundred twenty and three.

33 The men of the other Nebo, fifty and two.

34 The children of the other Elam, a thousand two hundred fifty and four.

35 The children of Harim, three hundred and twenty.

36 The children of Jericho, three hundred forty and five.

37 The children of Lod, Hadid, and Ono, seven hundred twenty and one.

38 The children of Senaah, three thousand nine hundred and thirty.

Register of the priests of the remnant.

39 The priests: the children of Jedaiah, of the house of Jeshua, nine hundred seventy and three.

40 The children of Immer, a thousand fifty and two.

41 The children of Pashur, a thousand two hundred forty and seven.

B.C. 445.

a Psa. 19:9, *note.*

b Cf. Ezra 2:1-64.

c Called *Zorobabel,* Mt. 1:12, 13.

42 The children of Harim, a thousand
and seventeen.

Register of the Levites of the remnant.

43 The Levites: the children of Jeshua,
of Kadmiel, *and* of the children of
Hodevah, seventy and four.
44 The singers: the children of Asaph,
an hundred forty and eight.
45 The porters: the children of
Shallum, the children of Ater, the children of Talmon, the children of Akkub,
the children of Hatita, the children of
Shobai, an hundred thirty and eight.

Register of the Nethinims of the remnant.

46 The Nethinims: the children of
Ziha, the children of Hashupha, the children of Tabbaoth,
47 The children of Keros, the children
of Sia, the children of Padon,
48 The children of Lebana, the children of Hagaba, the children of Shalmai,
49 The children of Hanan, the children
of Giddel, the children of Gahar,
50 The children of Reaiah, the children
of Rezin, the children of Nekoda,
51 The children of Gazzam, the children of Uzza, the children of Phaseah,
52 The children of Besai, the children
of Meunim, the children of Nephishesim,
53 The children of Bakbuk, the children of Hakupha, the children of
Harhur,
54 The children of Bazlith, the children
of Mehida, the children of Harsha,
55 The children of Barkos, the children
of Sisera, the children of Tamah,
56 The children of Neziah, the children of Hatipha.

Register of the children of Solomon's servants.

57 The children of Solomon's servants:
the children of Sotai, the children of
Sophereth, the children of Perida,
58 The children of Jaala, the children
of Darkon, the children of Giddel,
59 The children of Shephatiah, the children of Hattil, the children of Pochereth
of Zebaim, the children of Amon.
60 All the Nethinims, and the children
of Solomon's servants, *were* three hundred ninety and two.

B.C. 445.

61 And these *were* they which went up
also from Telmelah, Telharesha, Cherub,
Addon, and Immer: but they could not
shew their father's house, nor their seed,
whether they *were* of Israel.
62 The children of Delaiah, the children of Tobiah, the children of Nekoda,
six hundred forty and two.

Register of the priests without pedigree.

63 And of the priests: the children of
Habaiah, the children of Koz, the children of Barzillai, which took *one* of the
daughters of Barzillai the Gileadite to
wife, and was called after their name.
64 These sought their register *among*
those that were reckoned by genealogy,
but it was not found: therefore were
they, as polluted, put from the priesthood.
65 And the [a]Tirshatha said unto them,
that they should not eat of the most holy
things, till there stood *up* a priest with
[b]Urim and Thummim.

Total number of the remnant.

66 The whole congregation together
was forty and two thousand three hundred and threescore,
67 Beside their manservants and their
maidservants, of whom *there were* seven
thousand three hundred thirty and seven:
and they had two hundred forty and five
singing men and singing women.

Their substance and gifts.

68 Their horses, seven hundred thirty
and six: their mules, two hundred forty
and five:
69 *Their* camels, four hundred thirty
and five: six thousand seven hundred
and twenty asses.
70 And some of the chief of the fathers
gave unto the work. The Tirshatha gave
to the treasure a thousand [c]drams of
gold, fifty basons, five hundred and thirty priests' garments.
71 And *some* of the chief of the fathers
gave to the treasure of the work twenty
thousand [c]drams of gold, and two thousand and two hundred pound of silver.
72 And *that* which the rest of the people
gave *was* twenty thousand [c]drams of gold,
and two thousand pound of silver, and
threescore and seven priests' garments.

a i.e. *governor.* Neh. 8:9.
b See Ex. 28:30, *note.*
c One dram = £1. 1s., or $4.97; also vs. 71, 72.

73 So the priests, and the Levites, and the porters, and the singers, and *some* of the people, and the Nethinims, and all Israel, dwelt in their cities; and when the [a]seventh month came, the children of Israel *were* in their cities.

CHAPTER 8.

The law read and explained.

And all the people gathered themselves together as one man into the street that *was* before the water gate; and they spake unto [b]Ezra the scribe to bring the [c]book of the law of Moses, which the LORD had commanded to Israel.

2 And Ezra the priest brought the law before the congregation both of men and women, and all that could hear with understanding, upon the first day of the [a]seventh month.

3 And he read therein before the street that *was* before the water gate from the morning until midday, before the men and the women, and those that could understand; and the ears of all the people *were attentive* unto the book of the law.

4 And Ezra the [d]scribe stood upon a pulpit of wood, which they had made for the purpose; and beside him stood Mattithiah, and Shema, and Anaiah, and Urijah, and Hilkiah, and Maaseiah, on his right hand; and on his left hand, Pedaiah, and Mishael, and Malchiah, and Hashum, and Hashbadana, Zechariah, *and* Meshullam.

5 And Ezra opened the book in the sight of all the people; (for he was above all the people;) and when he opened it, all the people stood up:

6 And Ezra blessed the LORD, the great God. And all the people answered, Amen, Amen, with lifting up their hands: and they bowed their heads, and worshipped the LORD with *their* faces to the ground.

7 Also Jeshua, and Bani, and Sherebiah, Jamin, Akkub, Shabbethai, Hodijah, Maaseiah, Kelita, Azariah, Jozabad, Hanan, Pelaiah, and the Levites, [e]caused the people to understand the law: and the people *stood* in their place.

8 So they read in the book in the law of God distinctly, and gave the sense, and caused *them* to understand the reading.

9 And Nehemiah, which *is* the Tirshatha, and Ezra the priest the scribe, and the Levites that taught the people, said unto all the people, This day *is* holy unto the LORD your God; mourn not, nor weep. For all the people wept, when they heard the words of the law.

10 Then he said unto them, Go your way, eat the fat, and drink the sweet, and send [f]portions unto them for whom nothing is prepared: for *this* day *is* holy unto our Lord: neither be ye sorry; for the joy of the LORD is your strength.

11 So the Levites stilled all the people, saying, Hold your peace, for the day *is* holy; neither be ye grieved.

12 And all the people went their way to eat, and to drink, and to send portions, and to make great mirth, [g]because they had understood the words that were declared unto them.

13 And on the second day were gathered together the chief of the fathers of all the people, the priests, and the Levites, unto Ezra the scribe, even to understand the words of the law.

Feast of tabernacles restored.

14 And they found written in the law which the LORD had commanded by Moses, that the children of Israel should dwell in [h]booths in the feast of the seventh month:

15 And that they should publish and proclaim in all their cities, and in Jerusalem, saying, Go forth unto the mount, and fetch olive branches, and pine branches, and myrtle branches, and palm branches, and branches of thick trees, to make booths, as *it is* [i]written.

16 So the people went forth, and brought *them*, and made themselves booths, every one upon the roof of his house, and in their courts, and in the courts of the house of God, and in the street of the water gate, and in the street of the gate of Ephraim.

17 And all the congregation of them that were come again out of the captivity made booths, and sat under the booths: [1]for since the days of Jeshua the son of Nun unto that day had [j]not the children

B.C. 445.

a i.e. *October;* also Neh. 8:2, 14.

b *Israel (history).* vs.1-8; Psa. 78:1-72. (Gen. 12:2, 3; Rom. 11:26.)

c Cf. 2 Chr. 34:14-16.

d Cf. v. 2.

e Deut. 33:10; Mal. 2:7.

f Deut. 26:11-13; Esth. 9:19, 22; Rev. 11:10.

g vs. 7, 8, 13.

h Lev. 23:34-42.

i Lev. 23:40.

j Cf. Ezra 3:4; 2 Chr. 8:13.

1 **(8:17)** It is not meant that there had not been some formal observance of the feast of tabernacles (cf. 2 Chr. 8:13; Ezra 3:4), but that the people had not dwelt in booths since Joshua's days.

of Israel done so. And there was very great gladness.

18 Also day by day, from the first day unto the last day, he read in the book of the law of God. And they kept the feast seven days; and on the eighth day *was* a solemn assembly, according unto the manner.

CHAPTER 9.

The people fast and repent.

Now in the twenty and fourth day of this [a]month the children of Israel were assembled with fasting, and with sackclothes, and earth upon them.

2 And the seed of Israel [b]separated themselves from all strangers, and stood and confessed their sins, and the iniquities of their fathers.

3 And they stood up in their place, and [c]read in the book of the law of the LORD their God *one* fourth part of the day; and *another* fourth part they confessed, and worshipped the LORD their God.

Confession of the priests and Levites.

4 Then stood up upon the stairs, of the Levites, Jeshua, and Bani, Kadmiel, Shebaniah, Bunni, Sherebiah, Bani, *and* Chenani, and cried with a loud voice unto the LORD their God.

5 Then the Levites, Jeshua, and Kadmiel, Bani, Hashabniah, Sherebiah, Hodijah, Shebaniah, *and* Pethahiah, said, Stand up *and* [d]bless the LORD your God for ever and ever: and blessed be thy glorious name, which is exalted above all blessing and praise.

6 Thou, *even* thou, *art* LORD alone; thou hast made heaven, the heaven of heavens, with all their host, the earth, and all *things* that *are* therein, the seas, and all that *is* therein, and thou preservest them all; and the host of heaven worshippeth thee.

7 Thou *art* the LORD the God, who didst [e]choose Abram, and broughtest him forth out of Ur of the Chaldees, and gavest him the name of Abraham;

8 And foundest his heart [f]faithful before thee, and madest a [g]covenant with him to give the land of the Canaanites, the Hittites, the Amorites, and the Perizzites, and the Jebusites, and the Girgashites, to give *it, I say,* to his seed, and hast [h]performed thy words; for thou *art* righteous:

9 And didst [i]see the affliction of our fathers in Egypt, and heardest their cry by the Red sea;

10 And shewedst [j]signs and wonders upon Pharaoh, and on all his servants, and on all the people of his land: for thou knewest that they dealt proudly against them. So didst thou get thee a name, as *it is* this day.

11 And thou didst [k]divide the sea before them, so that they went through the midst of the sea on the dry land; and their persecutors thou threwest into the deeps, as a stone into the mighty waters.

12 Moreover thou [l]leddest them in the day by a cloudy pillar; and in the night by a pillar of fire, to give them light in the way wherein they should go.

13 Thou [m]camest down also upon mount Sinai, and spakest with them from heaven, and gavest them right judgments, and true laws, good statutes and commandments:

14 And [1]madest known unto them thy holy [n]sabbath, and commandedst them precepts, statutes, and laws, by the hand of Moses thy servant:

15 And [o]gavest them bread from heaven for their hunger, and broughtest forth [p]water for them out of the rock for their thirst, and [q]promisedst them that they should go in to possess the land which thou hadst sworn to give them.

16 But they and our fathers dealt proudly, and hardened their necks, and hearkened not to thy commandments,

17 And refused to obey, neither were mindful of thy wonders that thou didst among them; but hardened their necks, and in their rebellion appointed a captain to return to their bondage: but thou *art* a God ready to pardon, gracious and merciful, slow to anger, and of great kindness, and forsookest them not.

18 Yea, [r]when they had made them a

B.C. 445.

a See Neh. 8:14.

b *Separation.* Neh. 13:3. (Gen. 12:1; 2 Cor. 6:14-17.)

c Neh. 8:7, 8.

d *Bible prayers* (O.T.). Psa. 51. (Gen. 15:2; Hab. 3:1-16.)

e Gen. 11:31; 12:1-3; 17:5.

f Gen. 22:1-3; Jas. 2:21-23.

g Gen. 15:18, *note.*

h Josh. 23:14.

i Ex. 2:25; 3:7.

j Ex. 7-14.

k Ex. 14:20-28.

l Ex. 13:21.

m Ex. 19–24.

n *Sabbath.* vs. 13, 14; Mt. 12:1. (Gen. 2:3; Mt. 12:1.)

o Ex. 16:14-17; John 6:31, etc.

p Num. 20:8; 1 Cor. 10:4.

q Deut. 1:8.

r Ex. 32:1-10.

[1] **(9:14)** This important passage fixes beyond all cavil the time when the sabbath, God's rest (Gen. 2:1-3), was given to man. Cf. Ex. 20:9-11. In Ex. 31:13-17 the sabbath is invested with the character of a sign between Jehovah and Israel. See Mt. 12:1, *note.*

molten calf, and said, This *is* thy God that brought thee up out of Egypt, and had wrought great provocations;

19 Yet thou in thy manifold mercies forsookest them not in the wilderness: the [a]pillar of the cloud departed not from them by day, to lead them in the way; neither the pillar of fire by night, to shew them light, and the way wherein they should go.

20 Thou gavest also thy good [b]spirit to instruct them, and withheldest not thy [c]manna from their mouth, and gavest them water for their thirst.

21 Yea, forty years didst thou sustain them in the wilderness, so *that* they lacked nothing; [d]their clothes waxed not old, and their feet swelled not.

22 Moreover thou gavest them kingdoms and nations, and didst divide them into corners: so they possessed the land of Sihon, and the land of the king of Heshbon, and the land of Og king of Bashan.

23 Their children also multipliedst thou as the stars of heaven, and broughtest them into the land, concerning which thou hadst promised to their fathers, that they should go in to possess *it*.

24 So the children [e]went in and possessed the land, and thou subduedst before them the inhabitants of the land, the Canaanites, and gavest them into their hands, with their kings, and the people of the land, that they might do with them as they would.

25 And they took strong cities, and a fat land, and possessed houses full of all goods, wells digged, vineyards, and oliveyards, and fruit trees in abundance: so they did eat, and were filled, and became fat, and delighted themselves in thy great goodness.

26 Nevertheless they were disobedient, and rebelled against thee, and cast thy law behind their backs, and [f]slew thy prophets which testified against them to turn them to thee, and they wrought great provocations.

27 Therefore thou deliveredst them into the hand of their enemies, who vexed them: and in the time of their trouble, [g]when they cried unto thee, thou heardest *them* from heaven; and according to thy manifold mercies thou gavest them saviours, who saved them out of the hand of their enemies.

B.C. 445.

a Ex. 13:20-23; 1 Cor. 10:1.

b *Holy Spirit.* vs. 20, 30. Job 26:13. (Gen. 1:2; Mal. 2:15.)

c Ex. 16:14-16; John 6:22-60.

d Deut. 29:5.

e Josh. 1:2-4.

f 1 Ki. 18:4; 19:10; Mt. 23:37; Acts 7:52.

g Jud. 2:18.

h 2 Ki. 17:13-18; 2 Chr. 36:11-20.

i Deut. 28:48; Ezra 9:9.

28 But after they had rest, they did evil again before thee: therefore leftest thou them in the hand of their enemies, so that they had the dominion over them: yet when they returned, and cried unto thee, thou heardest *them* from heaven; and many times didst thou deliver them according to thy mercies;

29 And testifiedst against them, that thou mightest bring them again unto thy law: yet they dealt proudly, and hearkened not unto thy commandments, but sinned against thy judgments, (which if a man do, he shall live in them;) and withdrew the shoulder, and hardened their neck, and would not hear.

30 Yet many years didst thou forbear them, and testifiedst against them by thy [b]spirit in thy prophets: yet would they not give ear: [h]therefore gavest thou them into the hand of the people of the lands.

31 Nevertheless for thy great mercies' sake thou didst not utterly consume them, nor forsake them; for thou *art* a gracious and merciful God.

32 Now therefore, our God, the great, the mighty, and the terrible God, who keepest covenant and mercy, let not all the trouble seem little before thee, that hath come upon us, on our kings, on our princes, and on our priests, and on our prophets, and on our fathers, and on all thy people, since the time of the kings of Assyria unto this day.

33 Howbeit thou *art* just in all that is brought upon us; for thou hast done right, but we have done wickedly:

34 Neither have our kings, our princes, our priests, nor our fathers, kept thy law, nor hearkened unto thy commandments and thy testimonies, wherewith thou didst testify against them.

35 For they have not served thee in their kingdom, and in thy great goodness that thou gavest them, and in the large and fat land which thou gavest before them, neither turned they from their wicked works.

36 Behold, we *are* [i]servants this day, and *for* the land that thou gavest unto our fathers to eat the fruit thereof and the good thereof, behold, we *are* servants in it:

37 And it yieldeth much increase unto the kings whom thou hast set over us

B.C. 445.

because of our sins: also they have
dominion over our bodies, and over our
cattle, at their pleasure, and we *are* in
great distress.
38 And because of all this we make a
sure *covenant*, and write *it*; and our
princes, Levites, *and* priests, [a]seal *unto it*.

CHAPTER 10.

The covenant signers: the covenant.

Now those that sealed *were*, Nehemiah, the [b]Tirshatha, the son of
Hachaliah, and Zidkijah,
2 Seraiah, Azariah, Jeremiah,
3 Pashur, Amariah, Malchijah,
4 Hattush, Shebaniah, Malluch,
5 Harim, Meremoth, Obadiah,
6 Daniel, Ginnethon, Baruch,
7 Meshullam, Abijah, Mijamin,
8 Maaziah, Bilgai, Shemaiah: these
were the priests.
9 And the Levites: both Jeshua the son
of Azaniah, Binnui of the sons of
Henadad, Kadmiel;
10 And their brethren, Shebaniah,
Hodijah, Kelita, Pelaiah, Hanan,
11 Micha, Rehob, Hashabiah,
12 Zaccur, Sherebiah, Shebaniah,
13 Hodijah, Bani, Beninu.
14 The chief of the people; Parosh,
Pahath-moab, Elam, Zatthu, Bani,
15 Bunni, Azgad, Bebai,
16 Adonijah, Bigvai, Adin,
17 Ater, Hizkijah, Azzur,
18 Hodijah, Hashum, Bezai,
19 Hariph, Anathoth, Nebai,
20 Magpiash, Meshullam, Hezir,
21 Meshezabeel, Zadok, Jaddua,
22 Pelatiah, Hanan, Anaiah,
23 Hoshea, Hananiah, Hashub,
24 Hallohesh, Pileha, Shobek,
25 Rehum, Hashabnah, Maaseiah,
26 And Ahijah, Hanan, Anan,
27 Malluch, Harim, Baanah.
28 And the rest of the people, the
priests, the Levites, the porters, the
singers, the [c]Nethinims, and all they that
had separated themselves from the people of the lands unto the law of God,
their wives, their sons, and their daughters, every one having knowledge, and
having understanding;
29 They clave to their brethren, their
nobles, and entered into a curse, and
into an oath, to walk in God's law, which
was given by Moses the servant of God,
and to observe and do all the commandments of the LORD our Lord, and his
judgments and his statutes;
30 And that we would not give our
daughters unto the people of the land,
nor take their daughters for our sons:
31 And *if* the people of the land bring
ware or any victuals on the sabbath day
to sell, *that* we would not buy it of them
on the sabbath, or on the holy day: and
that we would leave the seventh year,
and the exaction of every debt.
32 Also we made ordinances for us, to
charge ourselves yearly with the third
part of a [d]shekel for the service of the
house of our God;
33 For the [e]shewbread, and for the
continual [f]meat-offering, and for the continual burnt-offering, of the sabbaths, of
the new moons, for the set feasts, and for
the holy *things*, and for the sin-offerings
to make an [g]atonement for Israel, and *for*
all the work of the house of our God.
34 And we cast the lots among the
priests, the Levites, and the people, for
the wood offering, to bring *it* into the
house of our God, after the houses of
our fathers, at times appointed year by
year, to burn upon the altar of the LORD
our God, as *it is* written in the law:
35 And to bring the [h]firstfruits of our
ground, and the firstfruits of all fruit of
all trees, year by year, unto the house of
the LORD:
36 Also the [i]firstborn of our sons, and
of our cattle, as *it is* written in the law,
and the firstlings of our herds and of our
flocks, to bring to the house of our God,
unto the priests that minister in the
house of our God:
37 And *that* we should bring the firstfruits of our dough, and our offerings,
and the fruit of all manner of trees, of
wine and of oil, unto the priests, to the
chambers of the house of our God; and
the [j]tithes of our ground unto the
Levites, that the same Levites might have
the tithes in all the cities of our tillage.
38 And the priest the son of Aaron
shall be with the Levites, when the
Levites take tithes: and the Levites shall
bring up the tithe of the tithes unto the
house of our God, to the chambers, into
the treasure house.
39 For the children of Israel and the
children of Levi shall bring the offering of
the corn, of the new wine, and the oil,
unto the chambers, where *are* the vessels
of the sanctuary, and the priests that minister, and the porters, and the singers: and
we will not [k]forsake the house of our God.

a Neh. 10:1.
b Neh. 7:65, *ref.*
c Neh. 3:26, *ref.*
d One shekel = 2*s.* 9*d.*, or 65 cts.
e Ex. 25:30, *note.*
f Lit. *meal.*
g See Ex. 29:33, *note.*
h Ex. 23:19; 34:26; Deut. 26:1, 2.
i Ex. 13:1-15; Lev. 27:26, 27.
j Lev. 27:30; Mal. 3:10.
k Heb. 10:25.

CHAPTER 11.

B.C. 445.

The dwellers at Jerusalem.

And the rulers of the people dwelt at Jerusalem: the rest of the people also cast lots, to bring one of ten to dwell in Jerusalem the [a]holy city, and nine parts *to dwell* in *other* cities.

2 And the people blessed all the men, that willingly offered themselves to dwell at Jerusalem.

3 Now these *are* the chief of the province that dwelt in Jerusalem: but in the cities of Judah dwelt every one in his possession in their cities, *to wit*, Israel, the priests, and the Levites, and the [b]Nethinims, and the [c]children of Solomon's servants.

4 And at Jerusalem dwelt *certain* of the children of Judah, and of the children of Benjamin. Of the children of Judah; Athaiah the son of Uzziah, the son of Zechariah, the son of Amariah, the son of Shephatiah, the son of Mahalaleel, of the children of Perez;

5 And Maaseiah the son of Baruch, the son of Col-hozeh, the son of Hazaiah, the son of Adaiah, the son of Joiarib, the son of Zechariah, the son of Shiloni.

6 All the sons of Perez that dwelt at Jerusalem *were* four hundred threescore and eight valiant men.

7 And these *are* the sons of Benjamin; Sallu the son of Meshullam, the son of Joed, the son of Pedaiah, the son of Kolaiah, the son of Maaseiah, the son of Ithiel, the son of Jesaiah.

8 And after him Gabbai, Sallai, nine hundred twenty and eight.

9 And Joel the son of Zichri *was* their overseer: and Judah the son of Senuah *was* second over the city.

10 Of the priests: Jedaiah the son of Joiarib, Jachin.

11 Seraiah the son of Hilkiah, the son of Meshullam, the son of Zadok, the son of Meraioth, the son of Ahitub, *was* the ruler of the house of God.

12 And their brethren that did the work of the house *were* eight hundred twenty and two: and Adaiah the son of Jeroham, the son of Pelaliah, the son of Amzi, the son of Zechariah, the son of Pashur, the son of Malchiah,

13 And his brethren, chief of the fathers, two hundred forty and two: and Amashai the son of Azareel, the son of Ahasai, the son of Meshillemoth, the son of Immer,

14 And their brethren, mighty men of valour, an hundred twenty and eight: and their overseer *was* Zabdiel, the son of *one of* the great men.

15 Also of the Levites: Shemaiah the son of Hashub, the son of Azrikam, the son of Hashabiah, the son of Bunni;

16 And Shabbethai and Jozabad, of the chief of the Levites, *had* the oversight of the outward business of the house of God.

17 And Mattaniah the son of Micha, the son of Zabdi, the son of Asaph, *was* the principal to begin the thanksgiving in prayer: and Bakbukiah the second among his brethren, and Abda the son of Shammua, the son of Galal, the son of Jeduthun.

18 All the Levites in the holy city *were* two hundred fourscore and four.

19 Moreover the porters, Akkub, Talmon, and their brethren that kept the gates, *were* an hundred seventy and two.

The dwellers in the other cities.

20 And the residue of Israel, of the priests, *and* the Levites, *were* in all the cities of Judah, every one in his inheritance.

21 But the [d]Nethinims dwelt in Ophel: and Ziha and Gispa *were* over the Nethinims.

22 The overseer also of the Levites at Jerusalem *was* Uzzi the son of Bani, the son of Hashabiah, the son of Mattaniah, the son of Micha. Of the sons of Asaph, the singers *were* over the business of the house of God.

23 For *it was* the king's commandment concerning them, that a certain portion should be for the singers, due for every day.

24 And Pethahiah the son of Meshezabeel, of the children of Zerah the son of Judah, *was* at the king's hand in all matters concerning the people.

25 And for the villages, with their fields, *some* of the children of Judah dwelt at [e]Kirjath-arba, and *in* the villages thereof, and at Dibon, and *in* the villages thereof, and at Jekabzeel, and *in* the villages thereof,

26 And at Jeshua, and at Moladah, and at Beth-phelet,

27 And at Hazar-shual, and at

a v. 18; Mt. 4:5; 5:35. Cf. Rev. 21:2.

b Neh. 3:26, *ref.*

c See 1 Ki. 9:21.

d Neh. 3:26, *ref.*

e Josh. 14:15.

Beer-sheba, and *in* the villages thereof,

28 And at Ziklag, and at Mekonah, and in the villages thereof,

29 And at En-rimmon, and at Zareah, and at Jarmuth,

30 Zanoah, Adullam, and *in* their villages, at Lachish, and the fields thereof, at Azekah, and *in* the villages thereof. And they dwelt from Beer-sheba unto the valley of Hinnom.

31 The children also of Benjamin from Geba *dwelt* at Michmash, and Aija, and Beth-el, and *in* their villages,

32 *And* at Anathoth, Nob, Ananiah,

33 Hazor, Ramah, Gittaim,

34 Hadid, Zeboim, Neballat,

35 Lod, and Ono, the valley of craftsmen.

36 And of the Levites *were* divisions *in* Judah, *and* in Benjamin.

CHAPTER 12.

The priests and Levites who went up with Zerubbabel.

NOW [a]these *are* the priests and the Levites that went up with [b]Zerubbabel the son of Shealtiel, and Jeshua: Seraiah, Jeremiah, Ezra,

2 Amariah, Malluch, Hattush,

3 Shechaniah, Rehum, Meremoth,

4 Iddo, Ginnetho, Abijah,

5 Miamin, Maadiah, Bilgah,

6 Shemaiah, and Joiarib, Jedaiah,

7 Sallu, Amok, Hilkiah, Jedaiah. These *were* the chief of the priests and of their brethren in the days of Jeshua.

8 Moreover the Levites: Jeshua, Binnui, Kadmiel, Sherebiah, Judah, *and* Mattaniah, *which was* over the thanksgiving, he and his brethren.

9 Also Bakbukiah and Unni, their brethren, *were* over against them in the watches.

Descent of the priests.

10 And Jeshua begat Joiakim, Joiakim also begat Eliashib, and Eliashib begat Joiada,

11 And Joiada begat Jonathan, and Jonathan begat Jaddua.

12 And in the days of Joiakim were priests, the chief of the fathers: of Seraiah, Meraiah; of Jeremiah, Hananiah;

13 Of Ezra, Meshullam; of Amariah, Jehohanan;

14 Of Melicu, Jonathan; of Shebaniah, Joseph;

B.C. 445.

15 Of Harim, Adna; of Meraioth, Helkai;

16 Of Iddo, Zechariah; of Ginnethon, Meshullam;

17 Of Abijah, Zichri; of Miniamin, of Moadiah, Piltai;

18 Of Bilgah, Shammua; of Shemaiah, Jehonathan;

19 And of Joiarib, Mattenai; of Jedaiah, Uzzi;

20 Of Sallai, Kallai; of Amok, Eber;

21 Of Hilkiah, Hashabiah; of Jedaiah, Nethaneel.

The chief Levites.

22 The Levites in the days of Eliashib, Joiada, and Johanan, and Jaddua, *were* recorded chief of the fathers: also the priests, to the reign of Darius the Persian.

23 The sons of Levi, the chief of the fathers, *were* [c]written in the book of the chronicles, even until the days of Johanan the son of Eliashib.

24 And the chief of the Levites: Hashabiah, Sherebiah, and Jeshua the son of Kadmiel, with their brethren over against them, to praise *and* to give thanks, [d]according to the commandment of David the man of God, ward over against ward.

25 Mattaniah, and Bakbukiah, Obadiah, Meshullam, Talmon, Akkub, *were* porters keeping the ward at the thresholds of the gates.

26 These *were* in the days of Joiakim the son of Jeshua, the son of Jozadak, and in the days of Nehemiah the governor, and of Ezra the priest, the scribe.

The dedication of the walls.

27 And at the dedication of the wall of Jerusalem they sought the Levites out of all their places, to bring them to Jerusalem, to keep the dedication with gladness, both with thanksgivings, and with singing, *with* cymbals, psalteries, and with harps.

28 And the sons of the singers gathered themselves together, both out of the plain country round about Jerusalem, and from the villages of Netophathi;

29 Also from the house of Gilgal, and out of the fields of Geba and Azmaveth: for the singers had builded them villages round about Jerusalem.

30 And the priests and the Levites

a Cf. Ezra 2:1-63.

b Called *Zorobabel*, Mt. 1:12, 13.

c 1 Chr. 9:14-32.

d 1 Chr. 23–25.

purified themselves, and purified the
people, and the gates, and the wall.
31 Then I brought up the princes of
Judah upon the wall, and appointed two
great *companies of them that gave* thanks,
whereof one went on the right hand upon
the wall toward the dung gate:
32 And after them went Hoshaiah,
and half of the princes of Judah,
33 And Azariah, Ezra, and Meshullam,
34 Judah, and Benjamin, and Shemaiah, and Jeremiah,
35 And *certain* of the priests' sons with
trumpets; *namely*, Zechariah the son of
Jonathan, the son of Shemaiah, the son
of Mattaniah, the son of Michaiah, the
son of Zaccur, the son of Asaph:
36 And his brethren, Shemaiah, and
Azarael, Milalai, Gilalai, Maai, Nethaneel, and Judah, Hanani, [a]with the musical instruments of David the man of
God, and Ezra the [b]scribe before them.
37 And at the fountain gate, which was
over against them, they went up by the
stairs of the [c]city of David, at the going
up of the wall, above the house of David,
even unto the water gate eastward.
38 And the other *company of them that
gave* thanks went over against *them*, and
I after them, and the half of the people
upon the wall, from beyond the tower of
the furnaces even unto the broad wall;
39 And from above the gate of
Ephraim, and above the old gate, and
above the fish gate, and the tower of
Hananeel, and the tower of Meah, even
unto the sheep gate: and they stood still
in the prison gate.
40 So stood the two *companies of them
that gave* thanks in the house of God, and
I, and the half of the rulers with me:
41 And the priests; Eliakim, Maaseiah,
Miniamin, Michaiah, Elioenai, Zechariah,
and Hananiah, with trumpets;
42 And Maaseiah, and Shemaiah, and
Eleazar, and Uzzi, and Jehohanan, and
Malchijah, and Elam, and Ezer. And the
singers sang loud, with Jezrahiah *their*
overseer.
43 Also that day they offered great sacrifices, and rejoiced: for God had made
them rejoice with great joy: the wives
also and the children rejoiced: so that the
joy of Jerusalem was heard even afar off.

Restoration of the temple order.

44 And at that time were some
appointed over the chambers for the
treasures, for the offerings, for the firstfruits, and for the tithes, to gather into
them out of the fields of the cities the
portions of the law for the priests and
Levites: for Judah rejoiced for the priests
and for the Levites that waited.
45 And both the singers and the
porters kept the ward of their God, and
the ward of the purification, according
to the commandment of David, *and* of
Solomon his son.
46 For [d]in the days of David and
Asaph of old *there were* chief of the
singers, and songs of praise and thanksgiving unto God.
47 And all Israel in the days of
Zerubbabel, and in the days of
Nehemiah, gave the portions of the
singers and the porters, every day his
portion: and they sanctified *holy things*
unto the Levites; and the Levites sanctified *them* unto the children of Aaron.

CHAPTER 13.

The law, and separation.

On that day they read in the [e]book of
Moses in the audience of the people; and therein was found written, that
the Ammonite and the Moabite should
not come into the congregation of God
for ever;
2 Because they met not the children of
Israel with bread and with water, but
hired [f]Balaam against them, that he
should curse them: howbeit our God
turned the curse into a blessing.
3 Now it came to pass, when they had
heard the law, that they [g]separated from
Israel all the [h]mixed multitude.

Cleansing of the temple.

4 And before this, Eliashib the priest,
having the oversight of the chamber of
the house of our God, *was* allied unto
Tobiah:
5 And he had prepared for him a great
chamber, where aforetime they laid the
[i]meat-offerings, the frankincense, and
the vessels, and the tithes of the corn, the
new wine, and the oil, which was commanded *to be given* to the Levites, and
the singers, and the porters; and the
offerings of the priests.

B.C. 445.

a 1 Chr. 23:5.
b v. 26.
c 2 Sam. 5:7-9.
d 1 Chr. 25:1-7; 2 Chr. 29:30.
e Deut. 23:3, 4.
f Num. 22–24.
g *Separation.* John 15:18, 19. (Gen. 12:1; 2 Cor. 6:14-17.)
h Ex. 12:38; 2 Cor. 6:14-18.
i Lit. *meal.*

6 But in all this *time* was not I at Jerusalem: [a]for in the two and thirtieth year of Artaxerxes king of Babylon came I unto the king, and after certain days obtained I leave of the king:

Nehemiah's second visit to Jerusalem.

7 And I came to Jerusalem, and understood of the evil that Eliashib did for [b]Tobiah, in preparing him a chamber in the courts of the house of God.

8 And it grieved me sore: therefore I cast forth all the household stuff of Tobiah out of the chamber.

9 Then I commanded, and they cleansed the chambers: and thither brought I again the vessels of the house of God, with the [c]meat-offering and the frankincense.

The order of God's house.

10 And I perceived that the portions of the Levites had [d]not been given *them*: for the Levites and the singers, that did the work, were fled every one to his field.

11 Then contended I with the rulers, and said, Why is the house of God forsaken? And I gathered them together, and set them in their place.

12 Then brought all Judah the tithe of the corn and the new wine and the oil unto the treasuries.

13 And I made treasurers over the treasuries, Shelemiah the priest, and Zadok the scribe, and of the Levites, Pedaiah: and next to them *was* Hanan the son of Zaccur, the son of Mattaniah: for they were counted faithful, and their office *was* to distribute unto their brethren.

14 Remember me, O my God, concerning this, and wipe not out my good deeds that I have done for the house of my God, and for the offices thereof.

Violation of the sabbath rest.

15 In those days saw I in Judah *some* treading wine presses on the [e]sabbath, and bringing in sheaves, and lading asses; as also wine, grapes, and figs, and all *manner of* burdens, which they brought into Jerusalem on the sabbath day: and I testified *against them* in the day wherein they sold victuals.

16 There dwelt men of Tyre also therein, which brought fish, and all manner of ware, and sold on the sabbath unto the children of Judah, and in Jerusalem.

B.C. 434.

a Neh. 5:14-16.

b Neh. 2:10, *note.*

c v. 5, *ref.*

d Cf. Mal. 3:7-10.

e Ex. 20:10.

f Neh. 12:30.

g Ex. 34:16; Deut. 7:3, 4; Ezra 9:2; Neh. 10:30.

h 1 Ki. 11:1, 2.

i 1 Ki. 11:4-8.

17 Then I contended with the nobles of Judah, and said unto them, What evil thing *is* this that ye do, and profane the sabbath day?

18 Did not your fathers thus, and did not our God bring all this evil upon us, and upon this city? yet ye bring more wrath upon Israel by profaning the sabbath.

19 And it came to pass, that when the gates of Jerusalem began to be dark before the sabbath, I commanded that the gates should be shut, and charged that they should not be opened till after the sabbath: and *some* of my servants set I at the gates, *that* there should no burden be brought in on the sabbath day.

20 So the merchants and sellers of all kind of ware lodged without Jerusalem once or twice.

21 Then I testified against them, and said unto them, Why lodge ye about the wall? if ye do *so* again, I will lay hands on you. From that time forth came they no *more* on the sabbath.

22 And I commanded the Levites that they should cleanse themselves, and [f]*that* they should come *and* keep the gates, to sanctify the sabbath day. Remember me, O my God, *concerning* this also, and spare me according to the greatness of thy mercy.

Intermarriage with other races rebuked.

23 In those days also saw I Jews *that* had [g]married wives of Ashdod, of Ammon, *and* of Moab:

24 And their children spake half in the speech of Ashdod, and could not speak in the Jews' language, but according to the language of each people.

25 And I contended with them, and cursed them, and smote certain of them, and plucked off their hair, and made them swear by God, *saying,* Ye shall not give your daughters unto their sons, nor take their daughters unto your sons, or for yourselves.

26 Did not [h]Solomon king of Israel sin by these things? yet among many nations was there no king like him, who was beloved of his God, and God made him king over all Israel: nevertheless [i]even him did outlandish women cause to sin.

27 Shall we then hearken unto you to

do all this great evil, to transgress
against our God in marrying strange
wives?
28 And *one* of the [a]sons of Joiada, the
son of Eliashib the high priest, *was* son in
law to [b]Sanballat the Horonite: therefore
I chased him from me.
29 Remember them, O my God,
because they have defiled the priesthood, and the covenant [c]of the priesthood, and of the Levites.
30 Thus cleansed I them from all
strangers, and appointed the wards of
the priests and the Levites, every one in
his business;
31 And for the wood offering, at times
appointed, and for the firstfruits.
Remember me, O my God, for good.

B.C. 434.

a Neh. 12:10.

b Neh. 4:1, 7; 6:1, 2.

c Mal. 2:4, 11, 12.

THE BOOK OF ESTHER

THE significance of the Book of Esther is that it testifies to the secret watch care of Jehovah over dispersed Israel. The name of God does not once occur, but in no other book of the Bible is His providence more conspicuous. A mere remnant returned to Jerusalem. The mass of the nation preferred the easy and lucrative life under the Persian rule. But God did not forsake them. What He here does for Judah, He is surely doing for all the covenant people. The book is in seven parts: I. The story of Vashti, 1:1-22. II. Esther made queen, 2:1-23. III. The conspiracy of Haman, 3:1-15. IV. The courage of Esther brings deliverance, 4:1–7:10. V. The vengeance, 8:1–9:19. VI. The feast of Purim, 9:20-32. VII. Epilogue, 10:1-3.

The events recorded in Esther cover a period of 12 years (Ussher).

CHAPTER 1.

B.C. 521.

The story of Vashti.

NOW it came to pass in the days of [a]Ahasuerus, (this *is* Ahasuerus which reigned, from [b]India even unto Ethiopia, [c]*over* an hundred and seven and twenty provinces:)

2 *That* in those days, when the king Ahasuerus [d]sat on the throne of his kingdom, which *was* in [e]Shushan the palace,

3 In the third year of his reign, he [f]made a feast unto all his princes and his servants; the power of Persia and Media, the nobles and princes of the provinces, *being* before him:

4 When he shewed the riches of his glorious kingdom and the honour of his excellent majesty many days, *even* an hundred and fourscore days.

5 And when these days were expired, the king made a feast unto all the people that were present in Shushan the palace, both unto great and small, seven days, in the court of the garden of the king's palace;

6 *Where were* white, green, and blue, *hangings*, fastened with cords of fine linen and purple to silver rings and pillars of marble: the beds *were of* gold and silver, upon a pavement of red, and blue, and white, and black, marble.

7 And they gave *them* drink in vessels of gold, (the vessels being diverse one from another,) and royal wine in abundance, according to the state of the king.

8 And the drinking *was* according to the law; none did compel: for so the king had appointed to all the officers of his house, that they should do according to every man's pleasure.

9 Also Vashti the queen made a feast for the women *in* the royal house which *belonged* to king Ahasuerus.

10 On the seventh day, when the [g]heart of the king was merry with wine, he commanded Mehuman, Biztha, [h]Harbona, Bigtha, and Abagtha, Zethar, and Carcas, the seven [i]chamberlains that served in the presence of Ahasuerus the king,

11 To bring Vashti the queen before the king with the crown royal, to shew the people and the princes her beauty: for she *was* fair to look on.

12 But the queen Vashti refused to come at the king's commandment by *his* chamberlains: therefore was the king very wroth, and his anger burned in him.

13 Then the king said to the wise men, [j]which knew the times, (for so *was* the king's manner toward all that knew law and judgment:

14 And the next unto him *was* Carshena, Shethar, Admatha, Tarshish, Meres, Marsena, *and* Memucan, the [k]seven princes of Persia and Media, [l]which saw the king's face, *and* which sat the first in the kingdom;)

15 What shall we do unto the queen Vashti according to law, because she hath not performed the commandment of the king Ahasuerus by the chamberlains?

16 And Memucan answered before the king and the princes, Vashti the queen hath not done wrong to the king only, but also to all the princes, and to all the people that *are* in all the provinces of the king Ahasuerus.

a Ezra 4:6, marg. *ref.*; Dan. 9:1.
b Esth. 8:9.
c Dan. 6:1.
d 1 Ki. 1:46.
e Neh. 1:1.
f Gen. 40:20.
g 2 Sam. 13:28.
h Esth. 7:9.
i Or, *eunuchs*.
j 1 Chr. 12:32.
k Ezra 7:14.
l 2 Ki. 25:19; Mt. 18:10.

B.C. 519.

17 For *this* deed of the queen shall
come abroad unto all women, so that
they shall despise their husbands in
their eyes, when it shall be reported, The
king Ahasuerus commanded Vashti the
queen to be brought in before him, but
she came not.
18 *Likewise* shall the ladies of Persia
and Media say this day unto all the
king's princes, which have heard of the
deed of the queen. Thus *shall there arise*
too much contempt and wrath.
19 If it please the king, let there go a
royal commandment from him, and let it
be written among the laws of the
Persians and the Medes, that it be not
altered, That Vashti come no more before
king Ahasuerus; and let the king give
her royal estate unto another that is better than she.
20 And when the king's decree which
he shall make shall be published
throughout all his empire, (for it is great,)
all the wives shall give to their husbands
honour, both to great and small.
21 And the saying pleased the king
and the princes; and the king did
according to the word of Memucan:
22 For he sent letters into all the king's
provinces, [a]into every province according to the writing thereof, and to every
people after their language, that every
man should bear rule in his own house,
and that *it* should be published according to the language of every people.

CHAPTER 2.

Esther made queen.

After these things, when the wrath of
king Ahasuerus was appeased, he
remembered Vashti, and what she had
done, and [b]what was decreed against her.
2 Then said the king's servants that
ministered unto him, Let there be fair
young virgins sought for the king:
3 And let the king appoint officers in
all the provinces of his kingdom, that
they may gather together all the fair
young virgins unto Shushan the palace,
to the house of the women, unto the custody of [c]Hege the king's chamberlain,
keeper of the women; and let their
things for purification be given *them*:
4 And let the maiden which pleaseth
the king be queen instead of Vashti. And
the thing pleased the king; and he did so.
5 *Now* in Shushan the palace there was
a certain Jew, whose name *was*
Mordecai, the son of Jair, the son of
Shimei, the son of Kish, a Benjamite;
6 [d]Who had been carried away from
Jerusalem with the captivity which had
been carried away with [e]Jeconiah king
of Judah, whom Nebuchadnezzar the
king of Babylon had carried away.
7 And he brought up Hadassah, that
is, Esther, [f]his uncle's daughter: for she
had neither father nor mother, and the
maid *was* fair and beautiful; whom
Mordecai, when her father and mother
were dead, took for his own daughter.
8 So it came to pass, when the king's
commandment and his decree was heard,
and when many maidens were [g]gathered
together unto Shushan the palace, to the
custody of Hegai, that Esther was
brought also unto the king's house, to the
custody of Hegai, keeper of the women.
9 And the maiden pleased him, and
she obtained kindness of him; and he
speedily gave her her [h]things for purification, with such things as belonged to
her, and seven maidens, *which were* meet
to be given her, out of the king's house:
and he [i]preferred her and her maids unto
the best *place* of the house of the women.
10 [j]Esther had not shewed her people
nor her kindred: for Mordecai had
charged her that she should not shew *it*.
11 And Mordecai walked every day
before the court of the women's house,
to know how Esther did, and what
should become of her.
12 Now when every maid's turn was
come to go in to king Ahasuerus, after
that she had been twelve months,
according to the manner of the women,
(for so were the days of their purifica-
tions accomplished, *to wit*, six months
with oil of myrrh, and six months with
sweet odours, and with *other* things for
the purifying of the women;)
13 Then thus came *every* maiden unto
the king; whatsoever she desired was
given her to go with her out of the house
of the women unto the king's house.

a Esth. 3:12; 8:9.
b Esth. 1:19, 20.
c Or, *Hegai*, v. 8.
d 2 Ki. 24:14, 15; 2 Chr. 36:10, 20; Jer. 24:1.
e Or, *Jehoiachin;* 2 Ki. 24:6.
f v. 15.
g v. 3.
h vs. 3, 12.
i Heb. *he changed her.*
j v. 20.

B.C. 515.

14 In the evening she went, and on the morrow she returned into the second house of the women, to the custody of Shaashgaz, the king's chamberlain, which kept the concubines: she came in unto the king no more, except the king delighted in her, and that she were called by name.

15 Now when the turn of Esther, [a]the daughter of Abihail the uncle of Mordecai, who had taken her for his daughter, was come to go in unto the king, she required nothing but what Hegai the king's chamberlain, the keeper of the women, appointed. And Esther obtained favour in the sight of all them that looked upon her.

16 So Esther was taken unto king Ahasuerus into his house royal in the [b]tenth month, which *is* the month Tebeth, in the seventh year of his reign.

17 And the king loved Esther above all the women, and she obtained grace and favour in his sight more than all the virgins; so that he set the royal crown upon her head, and made her queen instead of Vashti.

18 Then the king [c]made a great feast unto all his princes and his servants, *even* Esther's feast; and he made a [d]release to the provinces, and gave gifts, according to the state of the king.

19 And when the virgins were gathered together the second time, then Mordecai sat in the king's gate.

20 Esther had not *yet* shewed her kindred nor her people; as Mordecai had charged her: for Esther did the commandment of Mordecai, like as when she was brought up with him.

Mordecai saves the king's life.

21 In those days, while Mordecai sat in the king's gate, two of the king's chamberlains, [e]Bigthan and Teresh, of those which kept the door, were wroth, and sought to lay hand on the king Ahasuerus.

22 And the thing was known to Mordecai, [f]who told *it* unto Esther the queen; and Esther certified the king *thereof* in Mordecai's name.

23 And when inquisition was made of the matter, it was found out; therefore they were both hanged on a tree: and it was written [g]in the book of the chronicles before the king.

CHAPTER 3.

The conspiracy of Haman.

After these things did king Ahasuerus promote Haman the son of Hammedatha the [h]Agagite, and advanced him, and set his seat above all the princes that *were* with him.

2 And all the king's servants, that *were* in the king's gate, bowed, and reverenced Haman: for the king had so commanded concerning him. But Mordecai [i]bowed not, nor did *him* reverence.

3 Then the king's servants, which *were* in the king's gate, said unto Mordecai, Why transgressest thou the king's commandment?

4 Now it came to pass, when they spake daily unto him, and he hearkened not unto them, that they told Haman, to see whether Mordecai's matters would stand: for he had told them that he *was* a Jew.

5 And when Haman saw that Mordecai bowed not, nor did him reverence, then was Haman full of wrath.

6 And he thought scorn to lay hands on Mordecai alone; for they had shewed him the people of Mordecai: wherefore Haman [j]sought to destroy all the Jews that *were* throughout the whole kingdom of Ahasuerus, *even* the people of Mordecai.

[B.C. 510

7 In the [k]first month, that *is*, the month Nisan, in the twelfth year of king Ahasuerus, they cast Pur, that *is*, the lot, before Haman from day to day, and from month to month, *to* the [l]twelfth *month*, that *is*, the month Adar.

8 And Haman said unto king Ahasuerus, There is a certain people scattered abroad and dispersed among the people in all the provinces of thy kingdom; and their laws *are* diverse from all people; neither keep they the king's laws: therefore it *is* not for the king's profit to suffer them.

9 If it please the king, let it be written that they may be destroyed: and I will pay ten thousand [m]talents of silver to the hands of those that have the charge of the business, to bring *it* into the king's treasuries.

10 And the king took [n]his ring from his hand, and gave it unto Haman the son of Hammedatha the Agagite, the Jews' [o]enemy.

11 And the king said unto Haman, The

a v. 7.
b i.e. *January.*
c Esth. 1:3.
d Heb. *rest.*
e Or, *Bigthana,* Esth. 6:2.
f Esth. 6:2.
g Esth. 6:1.
h Num. 24:7; 1 Sam. 15:8.
i v. 5.
j Psa. 83:4.
k i.e. *April;* also v. 12.
l i.e. *March;* also v. 13.
m One talent (silver) = £410, or $1940.
n Esth. 8:2, 8.
o Or, *oppressor.* Esth. 7:6.

silver *is* given to thee, the people also, to do with them as it seemeth good to thee.

12 Then were the king's scribes called on the thirteenth day of the first month, and there was written according to all that Haman had commanded unto the king's lieutenants, and to the governors that *were* over every province, and to the rulers of every people of every province [a]according to the writing thereof, and *to* every people after their language; [b]in the name of king Ahasuerus was it written, and sealed with the king's ring.

13 And the letters were [c]sent by posts into all the king's provinces, to destroy, to kill, and to cause to perish, all Jews, both young and old, little children and women, in one day, *even* upon the thirteenth *day* of the twelfth month, which *is* the month Adar, and [d]*to take* the spoil of them for a prey.

14 The copy of the writing for a commandment to be given in every province was published unto all people, that they should be ready against that day.

15 The posts went out, being hastened by the king's commandment, and the decree was given in Shushan the palace. And the king and Haman sat down to drink; but [e]the city Shushan was perplexed.

CHAPTER 4.

Fasting among the Jews.

When Mordecai perceived all that was done, Mordecai [f]rent his clothes, and put on sackcloth with ashes, and went out into the midst of the city, and cried with a loud and a bitter cry;

2 And came even before the king's gate: for none *might* enter into the king's gate clothed with sackcloth.

3 And in every province, whithersoever the king's commandment and his decree came, *there was* great mourning among the Jews, and fasting, and weeping, and wailing; [g]and many lay in sackcloth and ashes.

4 So Esther's maids and her chamberlains came and told *it* her. Then was the queen exceedingly grieved; and she sent raiment to clothe Mordecai, and to take away his sackcloth from him: but he received *it* not.

5 Then called Esther for Hatach, *one* of the king's chamberlains, whom he had appointed to attend upon her, and gave him a commandment to Mordecai, to know what it *was*, and why it *was*.

6 So Hatach went forth to Mordecai unto the street of the city, which *was* before the king's gate.

7 And Mordecai told him of all that had happened unto him, and of [h]the sum of the money that Haman had promised to pay to the king's treasuries for the Jews, to destroy them.

8 Also he gave him the copy of the writing of the decree that was given at Shushan to destroy them, to shew *it* unto Esther, and to declare *it* unto her, and to charge her that she should go in unto the king, to make supplication unto him, and to make request before him for her people.

9 And Hatach came and told Esther the words of Mordecai.

10 Again Esther spake unto Hatach, and gave him commandment unto Mordecai;

11 All the king's servants, and the people of the king's provinces, do know, that whosoever, whether man or woman, shall come unto the king [i]into the inner court, who is not called, [j]*there is* one law of his to put *him* to death, except such [k]to whom the king shall hold out the golden sceptre, that he may live: but I have not been called to come in unto the king these thirty days.

12 And they told to Mordecai Esther's words.

13 Then Mordecai commanded to answer Esther, Think not with thyself that thou shalt escape in the king's house, more than all the Jews.

14 For if thou altogether holdest thy peace at this time, *then* shall there enlargement and deliverance arise to the Jews from another place; but thou and thy father's house shall be destroyed: and who knoweth whether thou art come to the kingdom for *such* a time as this?

15 Then Esther bade *them* return Mordecai *this answer*,

16 Go, gather together all the Jews that are present in Shushan, and fast ye for me, and neither eat nor drink [l]three days, night or day: I also and my maidens will fast likewise; and so will I go in unto the king, which *is* not according to the law: and if I perish, I perish.

B.C. 510.

a Esth. 1:22; 8:9.
b Esth. 8:8, 10; 1 Ki. 21:8.
c Esth. 8:10.
d Esth. 8:11.
e Esth. 8:15.
f 2 Sam. 1:11.
g Heb. *sackcloth and ashes were laid under many.* Isa. 58:5; Dan. 9:3.
h Esth. 3:9.
i Esth. 5:1.
j Dan. 2:9.
k Esth. 5:2; 8:4.
l Esth. 5:1.

17 So Mordecai went his way, and did according to all that Esther had commanded him.

CHAPTER 5.

The courage of Esther.

Now it came to pass on [a]the third day, that Esther put on *her* royal *apparel*, and stood in the inner court of the king's house, over against the king's house: and the king sat upon his royal throne in the royal house, over against the gate of the house.

2 And it was so, when the king saw Esther the queen standing in the court, *that* [b]she obtained favour in his sight: and [c]the king held out to Esther the golden sceptre that *was* in his hand. So Esther drew near, and touched the top of the sceptre.

3 Then said the king unto her, What wilt thou, queen Esther? and what *is* thy request? it shall be even given thee to the half of the kingdom.

4 And Esther answered, If *it seem* good unto the king, let the king and Haman come this day unto the banquet that I have prepared for him.

5 Then the king said, Cause Haman to make haste, that he may do as Esther hath said. So the king and Haman came to the banquet that Esther had prepared.

6 And the king said unto Esther at the banquet of wine, [d]What *is* thy petition? and it shall be granted thee: and what *is* thy request? even to the half of the kingdom it shall be performed.

7 Then answered Esther, and said, My petition and my request *is;*

8 If I have found favour in the sight of the king, and if it please the king to grant my petition, and to perform my request, let the king and Haman come to the banquet that I shall prepare for them, and I will do to morrow as the king hath said.

9 Then went Haman forth that day joyful and with a glad heart: but when Haman saw Mordecai in the king's gate, [e]that he stood not up, nor moved for him, he was full of indignation against Mordecai.

10 Nevertheless Haman refrained himself: and when he came home, he sent and called for his friends, and Zeresh his wife.

B.C. 510.

a Esth. 4:16.
b Prov. 21:1.
c Esth. 4:11; 8:4.
d Esth. 9:12.
e Esth. 3:5.
f Esth. 9:7-10.
g Esth. 3:1.
h One cubit = about 18 in.
i Esth. 7:9.
j Esth. 7:10.
k Heb. *the kings sleep fled away.*
l Esth. 2:21.
m Esth. 5:1.
n Esth. 5:14.

11 And Haman told them of the glory of his riches, and [f]the multitude of his children, and all *the things* wherein the king had promoted him, and how he had [g]advanced him above the princes and servants of the king.

12 Haman said moreover, Yea, Esther the queen did let no man come in with the king unto the banquet that she had prepared but myself; and to morrow am I invited unto her also with the king.

13 Yet all this availeth me nothing, so long as I see Mordecai the Jew sitting at the king's gate.

14 Then said Zeresh his wife and all his friends unto him, Let a gallows be made of fifty [h]cubits high, and to morrow [i]speak thou unto the king that Mordecai may be hanged thereon: then go thou in merrily with the king unto the banquet. And the thing pleased Haman; and he caused the [j]gallows to be made.

CHAPTER 6.

Haman compelled to exalt Mordecai.

On that night [k]could not the king sleep, and he commanded to bring the book of records of the chronicles; and they were read before the king.

2 And it was found written, that Mordecai had told of [l]Bigthana and Teresh, two of the king's chamberlains, the keepers of the door, who sought to lay hand on the king Ahasuerus.

3 And the king said, What honour and dignity hath been done to Mordecai for this? Then said the king's servants that ministered unto him, There is nothing done for him.

4 And the king said, Who *is* in the court? Now Haman was come into [m]the outward court of the king's house, to [n]speak unto the king to hang Mordecai on the gallows that he had prepared for him.

5 And the king's servants said unto him, Behold, Haman standeth in the court. And the king said, Let him come in.

6 So Haman came in. And the king said unto him, What shall be done unto the man whom the king delighteth to honour? Now Haman thought in his heart, To whom would the king delight to do honour more than to myself?

7 And Haman answered the king, For

the man whom the king delighteth to
honour,
8 Let the royal apparel be brought
which the king *useth* to wear, and the
horse that the king rideth upon, and the
crown royal which is set upon his head:
9 And let this apparel and horse be
delivered to the hand of one of the
king's most noble princes, that they may
array the man *withal* whom the king
delighteth to honour, and bring him on
horseback through the street of the city,
and proclaim before him, Thus shall it be
done to the man whom the king
delighteth to honour.
10 Then the king said to Haman, Make
haste, *and* take the apparel and the
horse, as thou hast said, and do even so
to Mordecai the Jew, that sitteth at the
king's gate: let nothing fail of all that
thou hast spoken.
11 Then took Haman the apparel and
the horse, and arrayed Mordecai, and
brought him on horseback through the
street of the city, and proclaimed before
him, Thus shall it be done unto the man
whom the king delighteth to honour.
12 And Mordecai came again to the
king's gate. But Haman [a]hasted to his
house mourning, [b]and having his head
covered.
13 And Haman told Zeresh his wife
and all his friends every *thing* that had
befallen him. Then said his wise men
and Zeresh his wife unto him, If
Mordecai *be* of the seed of the Jews,
before whom thou hast begun to fall,
thou shalt not prevail against him, but
shalt surely fall before him.
14 And while they *were* yet talking
with him, came the king's chamberlains,
and hasted to bring Haman unto [c]the
banquet that Esther had prepared.

CHAPTER 7.

Esther's banquet: Haman hanged.

So the king and Haman came to banquet with Esther the queen.
2 And the king said again unto Esther
on the second day [d]at the banquet of
wine, What *is* thy petition, queen
Esther? and it shall be granted thee: and
what *is* thy request? and it shall be performed, *even* to the half of the kingdom.
3 Then Esther the queen answered and
said, If I have found favour in thy sight,
O king, and if it please the king, let my
life be given me at my petition, and my
people at my request:
4 For we are [e]sold, I and my people, to
be destroyed, to be slain, and to perish.
But if we had been sold for bondmen
and bondwomen, I had held my tongue,
although the enemy could not counter-
vail the king's damage.
5 Then the king Ahasuerus answered
and said unto Esther the queen, Who is
he, and where is he, that durst presume
in his heart to do so?
6 And Esther said, The adversary and
enemy *is* this wicked Haman. Then
Haman was afraid before the king and
the queen.
7 And the king arising from the banquet of wine in his wrath *went* into the
palace garden: and Haman stood up to
make request for his life to Esther the
queen; for he saw that there was evil
determined against him by the king.
8 Then the king returned out of the
palace garden into the place of the banquet of wine; and Haman was fallen
upon [f]the bed whereon Esther *was*. Then
said the king, Will he force the queen
also before me in the house? As the
word went out of the king's mouth, they
covered Haman's face.
9 And Harbonah, one of the chamberlains, said before the king, Behold also,
[g]the gallows fifty [h]cubits high, which
Haman had made for Mordecai, who
had spoken good for the king, standeth
in the house of Haman. Then the king
said, Hang him thereon.
10 So they [i]hanged Haman on the gallows that he had prepared for Mordecai.
Then was the king's wrath pacified.

CHAPTER 8.

The vengeance ordered.

On that day did the king Ahasuerus
give the house of Haman the Jews'
enemy unto Esther the queen. And
Mordecai came before the king; for
Esther had told [j]what he *was* unto her.
2 And the king took off [k]his ring,
which he had taken from Haman, and
gave it unto Mordecai. And Esther set
Mordecai over the house of Haman.
3 And Esther spake yet again before
the king, and fell down at his feet, and
besought him with tears to put away the

B.C. 510.

a 2 Chr. 26:20.
b 2 Sam. 15:30; Jer. 14:3, 4.
c Esth. 5:8.
d Esth. 5:6.
e Esth. 3:9; 4:7; cf. Gen. 37:26-28.
f Esth. 1:6.
g Esth. 5:14; Psa. 7:16; Prov. 11:5, 6.
h One cubit = about 18 in.
i Psa. 37:35, 36; Dan. 6:24.
j Esth. 2:7.
K Esth. 3:10.

mischief of Haman the Agagite, and his device that he had devised against the Jews.

4 Then [a]the king held out the golden sceptre toward Esther. So Esther arose, and stood before the king,

5 And said, If it please the king, and if I have found favour in his sight, and the thing *seem* right before the king, and I *be* pleasing in his eyes, let it be written to reverse the letters devised by Haman the son of Hammedatha the Agagite, which he wrote to destroy the Jews which *are* in all the king's provinces:

6 For how can I endure to see [b]the evil that shall come unto my people? or how can I endure to see the destruction of my kindred?

7 Then the king Ahasuerus said unto Esther the queen and to Mordecai the Jew, Behold, [c]I have given Esther the house of Haman, and him they have hanged upon the gallows, because he laid his hand upon the Jews.

8 Write ye also for the Jews, as it liketh you, in the king's name, and seal *it* with the king's ring: for the writing which is written in the king's name, and sealed with the king's ring, [d]may no man reverse.

9 Then were the king's scribes called at that time in the [e]third month, that *is*, the month Sivan, on the three and twentieth *day* thereof; and it was written according to all that Mordecai commanded unto the Jews, and to the lieutenants, and the deputies and rulers of the provinces which *are* from [f]India unto Ethiopia, an hundred twenty and seven provinces, unto every province [g]according to the writing thereof, and unto every people after their language, and to the Jews according to their writing, and according to their language.

10 [h]And he wrote in the king Ahasuerus' name, and sealed *it* with the king's ring, and sent letters by posts on horseback, *and* riders on mules, camels, *and* young dromedaries:

11 Wherein the king granted the Jews which *were* in every city to gather themselves together, and to stand for their life, to destroy, to slay, and to cause to perish, all the power of the people and province that would assault them, *both* little ones and women, and [i]*to take* the spoil of them for a prey,

12 [j]Upon one day in all the provinces of king Ahasuerus, *namely*, upon the thirteenth *day* of the [k]twelfth month, which *is* the month Adar.

13 The copy of the writing for a commandment to be given in every province *was* published unto all people, and that the Jews should be ready against that day to avenge themselves on their enemies.

14 *So* the posts that rode upon mules *and* camels went out, being hastened and pressed on by the king's commandment. And the decree was given at Shushan the palace.

15 And Mordecai went out from the presence of the king in royal apparel of blue and white, and with a great crown of gold, and with a garment of fine linen and purple: [l]and the city of Shushan rejoiced and was glad.

16 The Jews had [m]light, and gladness, and joy, and honour.

17 And in every province, and in every city, whithersoever the king's commandment and his decree came, the Jews had joy and gladness, a feast and a good day. And many of the people of the land became Jews; [n]for the fear of the Jews fell upon them.

CHAPTER 9.

The vengeance executed.

Now in the [k]twelfth month, that *is*, the month Adar, on the thirteenth day of the same, [o]when the king's commandment and his decree drew near to be put in execution, in the day that the enemies of the Jews hoped to have power over them, (though it was turned to the contrary, that the Jews had rule over them that hated them;)

2 The Jews gathered themselves together in their cities throughout all the provinces of the king Ahasuerus, to lay hand on such as sought their hurt: and no man could withstand them; for the fear of them fell upon all people.

3 And all the rulers of the provinces, and the lieutenants, and the deputies, and officers of the king, helped the Jews, because the fear of Mordecai fell upon them.

4 For Mordecai *was* great in the king's house, and his fame went out

B.C. 510.

a Esth. 4:11; 5:2.
b Esth. 7:4; Neh. 2:3.
c v. 1; Prov. 13:22.
d Esth. 1:19; Dan. 6:8, 12, 15.
e i.e. *June.*
f Esth. 1:1.
g Esth. 1:22; 3:12.
h Esth. 3:12, 13; 1 Ki. 21:8.
i Esth. 9:10, 15, 16.
j Esth. 3:13; 9:1.
k i.e. *March;* also vs. 15, 17, 19, 21, 22.
l Esth. 3:15. Prov. 29:2.
m Psa. 97:11.
n Esth. 9:2; Gen. 35:5; Ex. 15:16; Deut. 2:25; 11:25; 1 Chr. 14:17.
o Esth. 3:13.

throughout all the provinces: for this man
Mordecai waxed greater and greater.
5 Thus the Jews smote all their enemies with the stroke of the sword, and
slaughter, and destruction, and did what
they would unto those that hated them.
6 And in Shushan the palace the Jews
slew and destroyed five hundred men.
7 And Parshandatha, and Dalphon,
and Aspatha,
8 And Poratha, and Adalia, and
Aridatha,
9 And Parmashta, and Arisai, and
Aridai, and Vajezatha,
10 The ten sons of Haman the son of
Hammedatha, the enemy of the Jews,
slew they; [a]but on the spoil laid they not
their hand.
11 On that day the number of those
that were slain in Shushan the palace
was brought before the king.
12 And the king said unto Esther the
queen, The Jews have slain and
destroyed five hundred men in Shushan
the palace, and the ten sons of Haman;
what have they done in the rest of the
king's provinces? [b]now what *is* thy petition? and it shall be granted thee: or
what *is* thy request further? and it shall
be done.
13 Then said Esther, If it please the king,
let it be granted to the Jews which *are* in
Shushan to do to morrow also [c]according
unto this day's decree, and let Haman's
ten sons be hanged upon the gallows.
14 And the king commanded it so to
be done: and the decree was given at
Shushan; and they hanged Haman's ten
sons.
15 For the Jews that *were* in Shushan
[d]gathered themselves together on the
fourteenth day also of the month Adar,
and slew three hundred men at Shushan;
[e]but on the prey they laid not their hand.
16 But the other Jews that *were* in the
king's provinces gathered themselves
together, and stood for their lives, and
had rest from their enemies, and slew of
their foes seventy and five thousand,
[f]but they laid not their hands on the prey,
17 On the thirteenth day of the month
Adar; and on the fourteenth day of the
same rested they, and made it a day of
feasting and gladness.
18 But the Jews that *were* at Shushan
assembled together [g]on the thirteenth *day*
thereof, and on the fourteenth thereof;
and on the fifteenth *day* of the same they
rested, and made it a day of feasting and
gladness.
19 Therefore the Jews of the villages,
that dwelt in the unwalled towns, made
the fourteenth day of the [h]month Adar [i]*a*
day of gladness and feasting, and a good
day, and of [j]sending portions one to
another.

The feast of Purim instituted.

20 And Mordecai wrote these things,
and sent letters unto all the Jews that
were in all the provinces of the king
Ahasuerus, *both* nigh and far,
21 To stablish *this* among them, that
they should keep the fourteenth day of
the month Adar, and the fifteenth day of
the same, yearly,
22 As the days wherein the Jews rested from their enemies, and the month
which was [k]turned unto them from sorrow to joy, and from mourning into a
good day: that they should make them
days of feasting and joy, and of sending
portions one to another, and gifts to the
poor.
23 And the Jews undertook to do as
they had begun, and as Mordecai had
written unto them;
24 Because Haman the son of
Hammedatha, the Agagite, the enemy of
all the Jews, had devised against the
Jews to destroy them, and had cast Pur,
that *is*, the lot, to consume them, and to
destroy them;
25 But when *Esther* came before the
king, he commanded by letters that his
wicked device, which he devised against
the Jews, should [l]return upon his own
head, and that he and his sons should be
hanged on the gallows.
26 Wherefore they called these days
Purim after the name of Pur. Therefore
for all the words of this letter, and *of that*
which they had seen concerning this
matter, and which had come unto them,
27 The Jews ordained, and took upon
them, and upon their seed, and upon all
such [m]as joined themselves unto them,
so as it should not fail, that they would
keep these two days according to their
writing, and according to their *appointed*
time every year;
28 And *that* these days *should be*
remembered and kept throughout every

B.C. 509.

a See Gen. 14:23; Esth. 8:11.
b Esth. 5:6; 7:2.
c Esth. 8:11.
d v. 2; Esth. 8:11.
e v. 10.
f See Esth. 8:11.
g vs. 11, 15.
h i.e. *March;* also vs. 15, 17.
i Deut. 16:11, 14; Esth. 8:16-17.
j v. 22; Neh. 8, 10, 12.
k Psa. 30:11.
l Esth. 7:10; Psa. 7:16.
m Esth. 8:17; Isa. 56:3, 6; Zech. 2:11.

generation, every family, every province,
and every city; and *that* these days of
Purim should not fail from among the
Jews, nor the memorial of them perish
from their seed.
29 Then Esther the queen, [a]the daughter of Abihail, and Mordecai the Jew,
wrote with all authority, to confirm [b]this
second letter of Purim.
30 And he sent the letters unto all the
Jews, to the hundred twenty and seven
provinces of the kingdom of Ahasuerus,
with words of peace and truth,
31 To confirm these days of Purim in
their times *appointed*, according as
Mordecai the Jew and Esther the queen
had enjoined them, and as they had
decreed for themselves and for their seed,
the matters of [c]the fastings and their cry.
32 And the decree of Esther confirmed
these matters of Purim; and it was written in the book.

CHAPTER 10.

Mordecai prime minister.

And the king Ahasuerus laid a tribute
upon the land, and *upon* the [d]isles
of the sea.
2 And all the acts of his power and of
his might, and the declaration of the
greatness of Mordecai, [e]whereunto the
king advanced him, *are* they not written
in the book of the chronicles of the kings
of Media and Persia?
3 For Mordecai the Jew *was* next unto
king Ahasuerus, and great among the
Jews, and accepted of the multitude of his
brethren, [f]seeking the wealth of his people, and speaking peace to all his seed.

B.C. 509.

a Esth. 2:15.
b See v. 20; Esth. 8:10.
c Esth. 4:3, 16.
d i.e. *coasts.*
e Esth. 8:15; 9:4.
f Neh. 2:10; Psa. 122:8, 9.

THE POETICAL BOOKS

THE books classed as poetical are Job, Psalms, Proverbs, Ecclesiastes, Song of Solomon, Lamentations. The term "poetical" is not to be taken as implying fancifulness or unreality, but as relating to form only. They are the books of the human experiences of the people of God under the various exercises of earthly life; but those experiences are, apart from the mere external setting, wrought in them by the Spirit, interpreted to us by the Spirit, and written by holy men of God as they were moved by the Spirit. While this is true of all these books, the Psalms included, the latter have also a prophetic character.

The Hebrew poetic form is peculiar, and demands a word of explanation. Rhythm is not achieved by a repetition of similar sounds, as in rhymed verse; nor by rhythmic accent as in blank verse, but by repetition of ideas. This is called parallelism; e.g.

> "The LORD also will be a refuge for the oppressed,
> A refuge in times of trouble." (Psa. 9:9.)

Parallelism is called *synonymous* when the thought is identical, as in the above instance; *antithetic* when the primary and the secondary ideas are in contrast; e.g.

> "For the LORD knoweth the way of the righteous:
> But the way of the ungodly shall perish" (Psa. 1:6)

and *synthetic* when the thought is developed or enriched by the parallel; e.g.

> "And thou shalt be secure, because there is hope;
> Yea, thou shalt dig about thee, and thou shalt take thy rest in safety."
> (Job 11:18.)

Under this method the Poetical Books are epic, lyric, and dramatic, and supply examples of literary expression unmatched in uninspried literature.

HOW TO USE THE SUBJECT REFERENCES.

THE subject references lead the reader from the first clear mention of a great truth to the last. The first and last references (in parenthesis) are repeated each time, so that wherever a reader comes upon a subject he may recur to the first reference and follow the subject, or turn at once to the Summary at the last reference.

ILLUSTRATION
(at Mark 1:1.)

b Gospel. vs. 1, 14, 15; Mk. 8:35. (Gen. 12:1-3; Rev. 14:6.)

Here *Gospel* is the subject; vs. 1, 14, 15 show where it is at that particular place; Mk. 8:35 is the next reference in the chain, and the references in parenthesis are the first and last.

THE BOOK OF JOB

JOB is in form a dramatic poem. It is probably the oldest of the Bible books, and was certainly written before the giving of the law. It would have been impossible, in a discussion covering the whole field of sin, of the providential government of God, and of man's relation to Him, to avoid all reference to the law if the law had then been known. Job was a veritable personage (Ezk. 14:20; James 5:11), and the events are historical. The book sheds a remarkable light on the philosophic breadth and intellectual culture of the patriarchal age. The problem is, Why do the godly suffer?

Job is in seven parts: I. Prologue, 1:1–2:8. II. Job and his wife, 2:9, 10. III. Job and his three friends, 2:11–31:40. IV. Job and Elihu, 32:1–37:24. V. Jehovah and Job, 38:1–41:34. VI. Job's final answer, 42:1-6. VII. Epilogue, 42:7-17.

The events recorded in Job cover a period of within 1 year.

CHAPTER 1.

Part I. Prologue:

(1) *The character of Job.*

There was a man in the [1]land of [a]Uz,
whose name *was* [b]Job; and that man
was [c]perfect and upright, and one that
[d]feared God, and eschewed evil.

(2) *The family and prosperity of Job.*

2 And there were born unto him seven
sons and three daughters.
3 His substance also was seven thousand sheep, and three thousand camels,
and five hundred yoke of oxen, and five
hundred she asses, and a very great
household; so that this man was the
greatest of all the men of the east.
4 And his sons went and feasted *in*
their houses, every one his day; and sent
and called for their three sisters to eat
and to drink with them.

(3) *The piety of Job and his household.*

5 And it was so, when the days of *their*
feasting were gone about, that Job sent
and sanctified them, and rose up early in
the morning, and offered burnt-offerings
according to the number of them all: for
Job said, It may be that my sons have
sinned, and [e]cursed God in their hearts.
Thus did Job continually.

(4) *Satan's theory: Job was good because prosperous.*

6 Now there was a day when the [f]sons
of God came to present themselves
before the LORD, and [g]Satan came also
among them.
7 And the LORD said unto [h]Satan,
Whence comest thou? Then Satan
answered the LORD, and said, From
going to and fro in the earth, and from
walking up and down in it.
8 And the LORD said unto Satan, [i]Hast
thou considered my servant Job, that
there is none like him in the earth, a [c]per-
fect and an upright man, one that
[d]feareth God, and escheweth evil?
9 Then Satan answered the LORD, and
said, Doth Job [d]fear God for nought?
10 Hast not thou made an hedge about
him, and about his house, and about all
that he hath on every side? thou hast
blessed the work of his hands, and his
substance is increased in the land.
11 But put forth thine hand now, and
touch all that he hath, and he will curse
thee to thy face.
12 And the LORD said unto Satan,
Behold, all that he hath *is* in thy power;
only upon himself put not forth thine
hand. So Satan went forth from the presence of the LORD.

(5) *In the sieve of Satan: mystery of God's permissive will.*
(See "*Satan*," Gen. 3:1; Rev. 20:10.)

13 And there was a day [j]when his

B.C. 1520.

a Gen. 36:28. See Jer. 25:20.

b Ezk. 14:14; Jas. 5:11.

c See 1 Ki. 8:61.

d Psa. 19:9, *note.*

e 1 Ki. 21:10, 13.

f This scene is in heaven. Cf. Job 2:1-7.

g Satan, vs. 7-9, 12; Job 2:1-3, 6, 7. (Gen. 3:1; Rev. 20:10.)

h Heb. *the Adversary.* 1 Chr. 21:1; Rev. 12:9, 10.

i Heb. *hast thou set thy heart on.* Job 2:3.

j Eccl. 9:12.

[1](1:1) A region at the south of Edom, and west of the Arabian desert, extending to Chaldea.

sons and his daughters *were* eating and drinking wine in their eldest brother's house:

14 And there came a messenger unto Job, and said, The oxen were plowing, and the asses feeding beside them:

15 And the Sabeans fell *upon them*, and took them away; yea, they have slain the servants with the edge of the sword; and I only am escaped alone to tell thee.

16 While he *was* yet speaking, there came also another, and said, The fire of God is fallen from heaven, and hath burned up the sheep, and the servants, and consumed them; and I only am escaped alone to tell thee.

17 While he *was* yet speaking, there came also another, and said, The Chaldeans made out three bands, and fell upon the camels, and have carried them away, yea, and slain the servants with the edge of the sword; and I only am escaped alone to tell thee.

18 While he *was* yet speaking, there came also another, and said, [a]Thy sons and thy daughters *were* eating and drinking wine in their eldest brother's house:

19 And, behold, there came a great wind from the wilderness, and smote the four corners of the house, and it fell upon the young men, and they are dead; and I only am escaped alone to tell thee.

20 Then Job arose, and rent his mantle, and shaved his head, and fell down upon the ground, and worshipped,

21 And said, Naked came I out of my mother's womb, and naked shall I return thither: the LORD gave, and the LORD hath taken away; blessed be the name of the LORD.

22 In all this Job sinned not, nor charged God foolishly.

CHAPTER 2.

(6) *Again in Satan's sieve: family, property, health gone.*

Again [b]there was a day when the sons of God came to present themselves before the LORD, and Satan [c]came also among them to present himself before the LORD.

2 And the LORD said unto Satan, From whence comest thou? And [d]Satan answered the LORD, and said, From going to and fro in the earth, and from walking up and down in it.

3 And the LORD said unto Satan, Hast thou considered my servant Job, that *there is* none like him in the earth, a [e]perfect and an upright man, one that [f]feareth God, and escheweth evil? and still he [g]holdeth fast his integrity, although thou movedst me against him, to [h]destroy him without cause.

4 And Satan answered the LORD, and said, Skin for skin, yea, all that a man hath will he give for his life.

5 [i]But put forth thine hand now, and touch his [j]bone and his flesh, and he will curse thee to thy face.

6 [k]And the LORD said unto Satan, Behold, he *is* in thine hand; but save his life.

7 So went Satan forth from the presence of the LORD, and smote Job with sore boils from the sole of his foot unto his crown.

8 And he took him a potsherd to scrape himself withal; and he sat down among the ashes.

Part II. Job and his wife.

9 Then said his wife unto him, Dost thou still retain thine integrity? curse God, and die.

10 But he said unto her, Thou speakest as one of the foolish women speaketh. What? [l]shall we receive good at the hand of God, and shall we not receive evil? In all this did not Job sin with his lips.

Part III. Job and his three friends: scene, the ash heap outside an oriental village.

(1) *The friends arrive.*

11 Now when Job's three friends heard of all this evil that was come upon him, they came every one from his own place; Eliphaz the Temanite, and Bildad the Shuhite, and Zophar the Naamathite: for they had made an appointment together to come to mourn with him and to comfort him.

12 And when they lifted up their eyes afar off, and knew him not, they lifted up their voice, and wept; and they rent every one his mantle, and sprinkled dust upon their heads toward heaven.

13 So they sat down with him upon the ground seven days and seven nights, and none spake a word unto him: for they saw that *his* grief was very great.

B.C. 1520.

[a] vs. 4, 13.
[b] Job 1:6.
[c] *Satan*, vs. 2, 3, 6, 7; Psa. 109:6. (Gen. 3:1; Rev. 20:10.)
[d] Job 1:7.
[e] See 1 Ki. 8:61.
[f] Psa. 19:9, *note*.
[g] Job 27:5, 6.
[h] Heb. *to swallow him up*. Job 9:17.
[i] Job 1:11.
[j] Job 19:20.
[k] Job 1:12.
[l] Job 1:21; Jas. 5:10, 11.

CHAPTER 3.

(2) Job's first discourse:
he tells his misery and despair.

After this opened Job his mouth, and
cursed his day.
2 And Job spake, and said,
3 [a]Let the day perish wherein I was
born, and the night *in which* it was said,
There is a man child conceived.
4 Let that day be darkness; let not God
regard it from above, neither let the light
shine upon it.
5 Let darkness and the [b]shadow of
death stain it; let a cloud dwell upon it;
let the blackness of the day terrify it.
6 *As for* that night, let darkness seize
upon it; let it not be joined unto the days
of the year, let it not come into the number of the months.
7 Lo, let that night be solitary, let no
joyful voice come therein.
8 Let them curse it that curse the day,
who are ready to raise up their mourning.
9 Let the stars of the twilight thereof be
dark; let it look for light, but *have* none;
neither let it see the [c]dawning of the day:
10 Because it shut not up the doors of
my *mother's* womb, nor hid sorrow from
mine eyes.
11 [d]Why died I not from the womb?
why did I *not* give up the ghost when I
came out of the belly?
12 Why did the knees prevent me? or
why the breasts that I should suck?
13 For now should I have lain still and
been quiet, I should have slept: then had
I been at rest,
14 With kings and counsellors of the
earth, [e]which built desolate places for
themselves;
15 Or with princes that had gold, who
filled their houses with silver:
16 Or [f]as an hidden untimely birth I
had not been; as infants *which* never saw
light.
17 There the wicked cease *from* troubling; and there the weary be at rest.
18 *There* the prisoners rest together;
they hear not the voice of the oppressor.
19 The small and great are there; and
the servant *is* free from his master.

B.C. 1520.

a Job 10:18, 19; Jer. 20:14-18.
b Job 10:21, 22.
c Heb. *the eyelids of the morning.* Job 41:18.
d Job 10:18.
e Job 15:28.
f Psa. 58:8.
g Job 39:7.
h Jer. 20:18.
i 1 Sam. 1:10; 2 Ki. 4:27; Prov. 31:6.
j Heb. *wait.* Rev. 9:6.
k Job 19:8; Lam. 3:7.
l Isa. 35:3.
m i.e. *by His anger,* as Isa. 30:33. See Ex. 15:8; Job 1:19; 15:30; Isa. 11:4; 2 Thes. 2:8.

20 [h]Wherefore is light given to him
that is in misery, and life unto the [i]bitter
in soul;
21 Which [j]long for death, but it *cometh*
not; and dig for it more than for hid treasures;
22 Which rejoice exceedingly, *and* are
glad, when they can find the grave?
23 *Why is light given* to a man whose
way is hid, and [k]whom God hath
hedged in?
24 For my sighing cometh before I eat,
and my roarings are poured out like the
waters.
25 For the thing which I greatly feared
is come upon me, and that which I was
afraid of is come unto me.
26 I was not in safety, neither had I rest,
neither was I quiet; yet trouble came.

CHAPTER 4.

(3) First discourse of Eliphaz.

Then [1]Eliphaz the Temanite answered
and said,
2 *If* we assay to commune with thee,
wilt thou be grieved? but who can withhold himself from speaking?
3 Behold, thou hast instructed many,
and thou hast strengthened the weak
hands.
4 Thy words have upholden him that
was falling, and thou [l]hast strengthened
the feeble knees.
5 But now it is come upon thee, and
thou faintest; it toucheth thee, and thou
art troubled.
6 *Is* not *this* thy fear, thy confidence,
thy hope, and the uprightness of thy
ways?
7 Remember, I pray thee, who *ever*
perished, being innocent? or where were
the righteous cut off?
8 Even as I have seen, they that plow
iniquity, and sow wickedness, reap the
same.
9 By the blast of God they perish, and
by the [m]breath of his nostrils are they
consumed.
10 The roaring of the lion, and the
voice of the fierce lion, and the teeth of
the young lions, are broken.

[1] **(4:1)** Eliphaz is a religious dogmatist whose dogmatism rests upon a mysterious and remarkable experience (vs. 12-16). Did a spirit ever pass before *Job's* face? Did *Job's* hair of his flesh ever stand up? Then let him be meek while one so superior as Eliphaz declares the causes of his misfortunes. Eliphaz says many true things (as do the others), and often rises into eloquence, but he remains hard and cruel, a dogmatist who must be heard because of one remarkable experience.

11 The old lion perisheth for lack of prey, and the stout lion's whelps are scattered abroad.

12 Now a thing was [a]secretly brought to me, and mine ear received a little thereof.

13 In thoughts from the visions of the night, when deep sleep falleth on men,

14 Fear came upon me, and trembling, which made all my bones to shake.

15 Then a spirit passed before my face; the hair of my flesh stood up:

16 It stood still, but I could not discern the form thereof: an image *was* before mine eyes, *there was* silence, and I heard a voice, *saying*,

17 Shall mortal man be more just than God? shall a man be more pure than his maker?

18 Behold, he put no [b]trust in his servants; and his [c]angels he charged with folly:

19 How much less *in* them that dwell in houses of clay, whose foundation *is* in the dust, *which* are crushed before the moth?

20 They are destroyed from morning to evening: they perish for ever without any regarding *it*.

21 Doth not their excellency *which is* in them go away? they die, even without wisdom.

CHAPTER 5.

(*First discourse of Eliphaz,* continued.)

Call now, if there be any that will answer thee; and to which of the saints wilt thou turn?

2 For wrath killeth the foolish man, and envy slayeth the silly one.

3 [d]I have seen the foolish taking root: but suddenly I cursed his habitation.

4 [e]His children are far from safety, and they are crushed in the gate, [f]neither *is there* any to deliver *them*.

5 Whose harvest the hungry eateth up, and taketh it even out of the thorns, and the robber swalloweth up their substance.

6 Although affliction cometh not forth of the dust, neither doth trouble spring out of the ground;

7 Yet man is [g]born unto trouble, as the sparks fly upward.

8 I would seek unto God, and unto God would I commit my cause:

9 Which doeth great things and unsearchable; marvellous things without number:

10 [h]Who giveth rain upon the earth, and sendeth waters upon the fields:

11 To set up on high those that be low; that those which mourn may be exalted to safety.

12 He disappointeth the devices of the crafty, so that their hands [i]cannot perform *their* enterprise.

13 He taketh the [j]wise in their own craftiness: and the counsel of the froward is carried headlong.

14 They meet with darkness in the daytime, and grope in the noonday as in the night.

15 But he [k]saveth the poor from the sword, from their mouth, and from the hand of the mighty.

16 [l]So the poor hath hope, and iniquity stoppeth her mouth.

17 [m]Behold, happy *is* the man whom God correcteth: therefore despise not thou the chastening of the Almighty:

18 For he [n]maketh sore, and bindeth up: he woundeth, and his hands make whole.

19 [o]He shall deliver thee in six troubles: yea, in [p]seven there shall no evil touch thee.

20 In [q]famine he shall [r]redeem thee from death: and in war from the power of the sword.

21 [s]Thou shalt be hid from the scourge of the tongue: neither shalt thou be afraid of destruction when it cometh.

22 At destruction and famine thou shalt laugh: [t]neither shalt thou be afraid of the beasts of the earth.

23 For thou shalt be in league with the stones of the field: [u]and the beasts of the field shall be at peace with thee.

24 And thou shalt know that [v]thy tabernacle *shall be* in peace; and thou shalt visit thy habitation, and shalt not sin.

25 Thou shalt know also that thy seed *shall be* great, and thine offspring [w]as the grass of the earth.

26 [x]Thou shalt come to *thy* grave in a full age, like as a shock of corn cometh in in his season.

27 Lo this, we have [y]searched it, so it *is*; hear it, and know thou *it* for thy good.

B.C. 1520.

a Heb. *by stealth.*
b Psa. 2:12, *note.*
c Heb. 1:4, *note.*
d Psa. 37:35, 36; Jer. 12:2, 3.
e Psa. 119:155.
f Psa. 109:12.
g Gen. 3:17-19.
h Job 28:26.
i Or, *cannot perform anything.*
j 1 Cor. 3:19.
k Psa. 35:10.
l 1 Sam. 2:8; Psa. 107:42.
m Psa. 94:12; Prov. 3:11, 12; Heb 12:5; Jas. 1:12; Rev. 3:19.
n Deut. 32:39; 1 Sam. 2:6; Isa. 30:26; Hos. 6:1.
o Psa. 34:19; 91:3; Prov. 24:16; 1 Cor. 10:13.
p Psa. 91:10.
q Psa. 33:19; 37:19.
r Ex. 14:30, *note;* Isa. 59:20, *note.*
s Psa. 31:20.
t Isa. 11:9; 35:9; 65:25; Ezk. 34:25.
u Hos. 2:18.
v Or, *that peace is thy tabernacle.*
w Psa. 72:16.
x Prov. 9:11; 10:27.
y Psa. 111:2.

CHAPTER 6.

(4) *Job's answer to Eliphaz: a touching appeal for pity.*

But Job answered and said,

2 Oh that my grief were throughly weighed, and my calamity laid in the balances together!

3 For now it would be heavier than the sand of the sea: therefore my words are swallowed up.

4 For the arrows of the Almighty *are* within me, the poison whereof drinketh up my spirit: [a]the terrors of God do set themselves in array against me.

5 Doth the wild ass bray when he hath grass? or loweth the ox over his fodder?

6 Can that which is unsavoury be eaten without salt? or is there *any* taste in the white of an egg?

7 The things *that* my soul refused to touch *are* as my sorrowful meat.

8 Oh that I might have my request; and that God would grant *me* the thing that I long for!

9 Even that it would please God to destroy me; that he would let loose his hand, and cut me off!

10 Then should I yet have comfort; yea, I would harden myself in sorrow: let him not spare; for I have not concealed [b]the words of the Holy One.

11 What *is* my strength, that I should hope? and what *is* mine end, that I should prolong my life?

12 *Is* my strength the strength of stones? or *is* my flesh of brass?

13 *Is* not my help in me? and is wisdom driven quite from me?

14 [c]To him that is afflicted pity *should be shewed* from his friend; but he forsaketh the [d]fear of the Almighty.

15 [e]My brethren have dealt deceitfully as a brook, *and* as the stream of brooks they pass away;

16 Which are blackish by reason of the ice, *and* wherein the snow is hid:

17 What time they wax warm, they vanish: when it is hot, they are consumed out of their place.

18 The paths of their way are turned aside; they go to nothing, and perish.

19 The troops of [f]Tema looked, the companies [g]of Sheba waited for them.

20 They were confounded because they had hoped; they came thither, and were ashamed.

21 For now ye are nothing; ye see *my* casting down, and are afraid.

22 Did I say, Bring unto me? or, Give a reward for me of your substance?

23 Or, Deliver me from the enemy's hand? or, [h]Redeem me from the hand of the mighty?

24 Teach me, and I will hold my tongue: and cause me to understand wherein I have erred.

25 How forcible are right words! but what doth your arguing reprove?

26 Do ye imagine to reprove words, and the speeches of one that is desperate, *which are* as wind?

27 Yea, ye overwhelm the fatherless, and ye dig *a pit* for your friend.

28 Now therefore be content, look upon me; for *it is* evident unto you if I lie.

29 [i]Return, I pray you, let it not be iniquity; yea, return again, my righteousness *is* in it.

30 Is there iniquity in my tongue? cannot my taste discern perverse things?

CHAPTER 7.

(*Job's answer to Eliphaz,* continued.)

Is there not [j]an appointed time to man upon earth? *are not* his days also like the days of an hireling?

2 As a servant [k]earnestly desireth the shadow, and as an hireling looketh for *the reward of* his work:

3 So am I made to possess months of vanity, and wearisome nights are appointed to me.

4 [l]When I lie down, I say, When shall I arise, and the night be gone? and I am full of tossings to and fro unto the dawning of the day.

5 My flesh is [m]clothed with worms and clods of dust; my skin is broken, and become loathsome.

6 [n]My days are swifter than a weaver's shuttle, and are spent without hope.

7 O remember that [o]my life *is* wind: mine eye shall no more see good.

8 The eye of him that hath seen me shall see me no *more*: thine eyes *are* upon me, and I *am* not.

9 *As* the cloud is consumed and vanisheth away: so he that goeth down

---

B.C. 1520.

a Psa. 88:15, 16.

b *Inspiration.* Job 32:18. (Ex. 4:15; Rev. 22:19)

c Heb. *to him that melteth.* Prov. 17:17.

d Psa. 19:9, *note.*

e Psa. 38:11; 41:9.

f Gen. 25:15.

g 1 Ki. 10:1; Psa. 72:10; Ezk. 27:22, 23.

h Ex. 14:30, *note;* Isa. 59:20, *note.*

i Job 17:10.

j Job 14:5, 13, 14; Psa. 39:4.

k Heb. *gapeth after.*

l Job 17:12; Deut. 28:67; Psa. 90:5.

m Isa. 14:11.

n Job 9:25; 16:22; 17:11; Psa. 90:5; 102:11; 103:15; 144:4; Isa. 38:12; 40:6; Jas 4:14.

o Psa 78:39; 89:47.

to the [a]grave shall come up no *more.*

10 He shall return no more to his house, neither shall his place know him any more.

11 Therefore I will not refrain my mouth; I will speak in the anguish of my spirit; I will complain in the bitterness of my soul.

12 *Am* I a sea, or a whale, that thou settest a watch over me?

13 When I say, My bed shall comfort me, my couch shall ease my complaint;

14 Then thou scarest me with dreams, and terrifiest me through visions:

15 So that my soul chooseth strangling, *and* death rather than my life.

16 I loathe *it;* I would not live alway: let me alone; for my days *are* vanity.

17 [b]What *is* man, that thou shouldest magnify him? and that thou shouldest set thine heart upon him?

18 And *that* thou shouldest visit him every morning, *and* try him every moment?

19 How long wilt thou not depart from me, nor let me alone till I swallow down my spittle?

20 I have sinned; what shall I do unto thee, O thou preserver of men? why hast thou set me as a mark against thee, so that I am a burden to myself?

21 And why dost thou not pardon my transgression, and take away mine iniquity? for now shall I sleep in the dust; and thou shalt seek me in the morning, but I *shall* not *be.*

CHAPTER 8.

(5) *First discourse of Bildad: he thinks Job a hypocrite.*

Then answered [1]Bildad the Shuhite, and said,

2 How long wilt thou speak these *things?* and *how long shall* the words of thy mouth *be like* a strong wind?

3 [c]Doth God pervert judgment? or doth the Almighty pervert justice?

4 If thy children have sinned against him, and he have cast them away for their transgression;

5 If thou wouldest seek unto God betimes, and make thy supplication to the Almighty;

6 If thou *wert* pure and upright; surely now he would awake for thee, and make the habitation of thy righteousness prosperous.

7 Though thy beginning was small, yet thy latter end should greatly increase.

8 For enquire, I pray thee, of the former age, and prepare thyself to the search of their fathers:

9 (For [d]we *are but of* yesterday, and know nothing, because our days upon earth *are* a shadow:)

10 Shall not they teach thee, *and* tell thee, and utter words out of their heart?

11 Can the rush grow up without mire? can the flag grow without water?

12 Whilst it *is* yet in his greenness, *and* not cut down, it withereth before any *other* herb.

13 So *are* the paths of all that forget God; and the [e]hypocrite's hope shall perish:

14 Whose hope shall be cut off, and whose [f]trust *shall be* a spider's web.

15 He shall lean upon his house, but it shall not stand: he shall hold it fast, but it shall not endure.

16 He *is* green before the sun, and his branch shooteth forth in his garden.

17 His roots are wrapped about the heap, *and* seeth the place of stones.

18 If he destroy him from his place, then *it* shall deny him, *saying,* I have not seen thee.

19 Behold, this *is* the joy of his way, and out of the earth shall others grow.

20 Behold, God will not cast away a perfect *man,* neither will he [g]help the evil doers:

21 Till he fill thy mouth with laughing, and thy lips with rejoicing.

22 They that hate thee shall be [h]clothed with shame; and the dwelling place of the wicked shall come to nought.

CHAPTER 9.

(9) *Job answers Bildad: he is a sinner, and knows not how to be justified—but not a hypocrite.*

Then Job answered and said,

2 I know *it is* so of a truth: but how should [i]man be just with God?

B.C. 1520.

a Heb. *Sheol.* See Hab. 2:5, *note.*

b Psa. 8:4; 144:3; Heb. 2:6.

c Job 34:12, 17; Gen. 18:25; Deut. 32:4; 2 Chr. 19:7; Dan. 9:14; Rom. 3:5.

d Job 7:6; Gen. 47:9; 1 Chr. 29:15; Psa. 39:5; 102:11; 144:4.

e Job 11:20; 18:14; 27:8; Psa. 112:10; Prov. 10:28.

f *Psa. 2:12, note.*

g Heb. *take the ungodly by the hand.*

h Psa. 35:26; 109:29.

i Psa. 143:2; Rom. 3:20. Or, *before God.*

[1](8:1) Bildad is a religious dogmatist of the superficial kind, whose dogmatism rests upon tradition (e.g. 8:8-10) and upon proverbial wisdom and approved pious phrases. These abound in all his

3 If he will contend with him, he cannot answer him one of a thousand.
4 [a]*He is* wise in heart, and mighty in
strength: who hath hardened *himself*
against him, and hath prospered?
5 Which removeth the mountains, and
they know not: which overturneth them
in his anger.
6 [b]Which shaketh the earth out of her
place, and the pillars thereof tremble.
7 Which commandeth the sun, and it
riseth not; and sealeth up the stars.
8 Which alone spreadeth out the heavens, and treadeth upon the waves of the
sea.
9 [c]Which maketh [d]Arcturus, Orion,
and Pleiades, and the chambers of the
south.
10 Which doeth great things past finding out; yea, and wonders without number.
11 Lo, he goeth by me, and I see *him*
not: he passeth on also, but I perceive
him not.
12 Behold, he taketh away, who can
hinder him? who will say unto him,
What dost thou?
13 *If* God will not withdraw his anger,
the proud helpers do stoop under him.
14 How much less shall I answer him,
and choose out my words *to reason* with
him?
15 Whom, though I were righteous, *yet*
would I not answer, *but* I would make
supplication to my judge.
16 If I had called, and he had
answered me; *yet* would I not believe
that he had hearkened unto my voice.
17 For he breaketh me with a tempest,
and multiplieth my wounds [f]without
cause.
18 He will not suffer me to take my
breath, but filleth me with bitterness.
19 If *I speak* of strength, lo, *he is* strong:
and if of judgment, who shall set me a
time *to plead*?
20 If I justify myself, mine own mouth
shall condemn me: *if I say*, I *am* [g]perfect,
it shall also prove me perverse.
21 *Though* I *were* [g]perfect, *yet* would I
not know my soul: I would despise my
life.
22 This *is* one *thing*, therefore I said *it*,
[h]He destroyeth the [g]perfect and the
wicked.
23 If the scourge slay suddenly, he will
laugh at the trial of the innocent.
24 The earth is given into the hand of
the wicked: he covereth the faces of the
judges thereof; if not, where, *and* who *is*
he?
25 Now [i]my days are swifter than a
post: they flee away, they see no good.
26 They are passed away as the [j]swift
ships: as the eagle that hasteth to the
prey.
27 [k]If I say, I will forget my complaint,
I will leave off my heaviness, and comfort *myself*:
28 I am afraid of all my sorrows, I
know that [l]thou wilt not hold me innocent.
29 *If* I be wicked, why then labour I in
vain?
30 [m]If I wash myself with snow water,
and make my hands never so clean;
31 Yet shalt thou plunge me in the
ditch, and mine own clothes shall abhor
me.
32 [n]For *he is* not a man, as I *am*, *that* I
should answer him, *and* we should come
together in judgment.
33 [o]Neither is there any daysman
betwixt us, *that* might lay his hand upon
us both.
34 Let him take his rod away from me,
and let not his fear terrify me:
35 *Then* would I speak, and not fear
him; but *it is* not so with me.

CHAPTER 10.

(*Job's answer to Bildad*, continued.)

My soul is weary of my life; I will
leave my complaint upon myself;
I will speak in the bitterness of my soul.
2 I will say unto God, Do not condemn
me; shew me wherefore thou contendest
with me.
3 *Is it* good unto thee that thou
shouldest oppress, that thou shouldest
despise the work of thine hands, and
shine upon the counsel of the wicked?
4 Hast thou eyes of flesh? [p]or seest
thou as man seeth?
5 *Are* thy days as the days of man? *are*
thy years as man's days,

B.C. 1520.

a Job 36:5.
b Isa. 2:19, 21; Hag. 2:6, 21; Heb. 12:26.
c Job 38:31; Gen. 1:16; Amos 5:8.
d Heb. *Ash, Cesil,* and *Cimah.*
e Job 26:12; Isa. 30:7.
f Job 2:3.
g See 1 Ki. 8:61.
h Eccl. 9:2, 3. Ezk. 21:3; Mt. 5:45.
i Job 7:6, 7.
j Or, *ships of Ebeh.*
k Job 7:13.
l Ex. 20:7.
m Jer. 2:22.
n Isa. 45:9, Jer. 49:19; Rom. 9:20.
o v. 19; 1 Sam. 2:25.
p 1 Sam. 16:7.

discourses. His platitudes are true enough, but then every one knows them (Job 9:1, 2; 13:2), nor do they shed any light on such a problem as Job's.

6 That thou enquirest after mine iniquity, and searchest after my sin?
7 Thou knowest that I am not wicked; and *there is* none that can deliver out of thine hand.
8 [a]Thine hands have made me and fashioned me together round about; yet thou dost destroy me.
9 Remember, I beseech thee, that thou hast made me as the clay; and wilt thou bring me into dust again?
10 Hast thou not poured me out as milk, and curdled me like cheese?
11 Thou hast clothed me with skin and flesh, and hast fenced me with bones and sinews.
12 Thou hast granted me life and favour, and thy visitation hath preserved my spirit.
13 And these *things* hast thou hid in thine heart: I know that this *is* with thee.
14 If I sin, [b]then thou markest me, and thou wilt not acquit me from mine iniquity.
15 If I be wicked, woe unto me; and *if* I be righteous, *yet* will I not lift up my head. *I am* full of confusion; therefore see thou mine affliction;
16 For it increaseth. Thou huntest me as a fierce lion: and again thou shewest thyself marvellous upon me.
17 Thou renewest thy witnesses against me, and increasest thine indignation upon me; changes and war *are* against me.
18 Wherefore then hast thou brought me forth out of the womb? Oh that I had given up the ghost, and no eye had seen me!
19 I should have been as though I had not been; I should have been carried from the womb to the grave.
20 *Are* not my days few? cease *then, and* let me alone, that I may take comfort a little,
21 Before I go *whence* I shall not return, *even* [c]to the land of darkness [d]and the shadow of death;
22 A land of darkness, as darkness *itself; and* of the shadow of death, without any order, and *where* the light *is* as darkness.

CHAPTER 11.

(7) Zophar's first discourse: he thinks Job both hypocrite and liar.

Then answered [1]Zophar the Naamathite, and said,
2 Should not the multitude of words be answered? and should a man full of talk be justified?
3 Should thy lies make men hold their peace? and when thou mockest, shall no man make thee ashamed?
4 For thou hast said, My doctrine *is* pure, and I am clean in thine eyes.
5 But oh that God would speak, and open his lips against thee;
6 And that he would shew thee the secrets of wisdom, that *they are* double to that which is! Know therefore that [e]God exacteth of thee *less* than thine iniquity *deserveth.*
7 [f]Canst thou by searching find out God? canst thou find out the Almighty unto perfection?
8 *It is* as [g]high as heaven; what canst thou do? deeper than hell; what canst thou know?
9 The measure thereof *is* longer than the earth, and broader than the sea.
10 If he cut off, and shut up, or gather together, then who can hinder him?
11 [h]For he knoweth vain men: he seeth wickedness also; will he not then consider *it?*
12 For vain man would be wise, though man be born *like* a wild ass's colt.
13 If thou prepare thine heart, and stretch out thine hands toward him;
14 If iniquity *be* in thine hand, put it far away, and let not wickedness dwell in thy tabernacles.
15 For then shalt thou lift up thy face without spot; yea, thou shalt be stedfast and shalt not fear:
16 Because thou shalt forget *thy* misery, *and* remember *it* as waters *that* pass away:
17 And *thine* age shall be clearer than the noonday; thou shalt shine forth, thou shalt be as the morning.
18 And thou shalt be secure, because there is hope; yea, thou shalt dig *about thee, and* thou shalt take thy rest in safety.
19 Also thou shalt lie down, and none shall make *thee* afraid; yea, many shall make suit unto thee.
20 But [i]the eyes of the wicked shall fail, and they shall not escape, and their hope *shall be* [j]*as* the giving up of the ghost.

B.C. 1520.

a Psa. 119:73.
b Psa. 139:1.
c Psa. 88:12.
d Psa. 23:4.
e Ezra 9:13.
f Eccl. 3:11; Rom. 11:33.
g Heb. *the heights of heaven.*
h Psa. 10:11, 14; 35:22, 94:11.
i Lev. 26:16, Deut. 28:65.
j Or, *a puff of breath.*

[1] **(11:1)** Zophar is a religious dogmatist who assumes to know all about God; what God will do in any given case, why He will do it, and all His thoughts about it. Of all forms of dogmatism this is most irreverent, and least open to reason.

B.C. 1520.

CHAPTER 12.

(8) *Job answers the three:*
he is familiar with their platitudes.

AND Job answered and said,
2 No doubt but ye *are* the people,
and wisdom shall die with you.
3 But I have understanding as well as
you; I *am* not inferior to you: yea, who
knoweth not such things as these?
4 I am *as* one mocked of his neighbour,
[a]who calleth upon God, and he
answereth him: the just upright *man is*
laughed to scorn.
5 [b]He that is ready to slip with *his* feet
is as a lamp despised in the thought of
him that is at ease.
6 The tabernacles of robbers prosper,
and they that provoke God are secure;
into whose hand God bringeth *abundantly.*
7 But ask now the beasts, and they
shall teach thee; and the fowls of the air,
and they shall tell thee:
8 Or speak to the earth, and it shall
teach thee: and the fishes of the sea shall
declare unto thee.
9 Who knoweth not in all these that
the hand of the LORD hath wrought this?
10 [c]In whose hand *is* the soul of every
living thing, and the breath of all
mankind.
11 Doth not the ear try words? and the
mouth taste his meat?
12 With the ancient *is* wisdom; and in
length of days understanding.
13 [d]With him *is* wisdom and strength,
he hath counsel and understanding.
14 Behold, [e]he breaketh down, and it
cannot be built again: he shutteth up a
man, and there can be no opening.
15 Behold, [f]he withholdeth the waters,
and they dry up: [g]also he sendeth them
out, and they overturn the earth.
16 With him *is* strength and wisdom:
the deceived and the deceiver *are* his.
17 He leadeth counsellors away
spoiled, and maketh the judges fools.
18 He looseth the bond of kings, and
girdeth their loins with a girdle.
19 He leadeth princes away spoiled,
and overthroweth the mighty.
20 He removeth away the speech of
the trusty, and taketh away the understanding of the aged.
21 [h]He poureth contempt upon
princes, and weakeneth the strength of
the mighty.
22 [i]He discovereth deep things out of
darkness, and bringeth out to light the
shadow of death.
23 He increaseth the nations, and
destroyeth them: he enlargeth the
nations, and straiteneth them *again.*
24 He taketh away the heart of the
chief of the people of the earth, and
causeth them to wander in a wilderness
where there is no way.
25 They grope in the dark without
light, and he maketh them to stagger
like *a* drunken *man.*

CHAPTER 13.

(*Job's answer,* continued.)

LO, mine eye hath seen all *this,* mine
ear hath heard and understood it.
2 What ye know, *the same* do I know
also: I *am* not inferior unto you.
3 Surely I would speak to the Almighty,
and I desire to reason with God.
4 But ye *are* forgers of lies, ye *are* all
physicians of no value.
5 O that ye would altogether hold your
peace! and it should be your wisdom.
6 Hear now my reasoning, and hearken to the pleadings of my lips.
7 Will ye speak wickedly for God? and
talk deceitfully for him?
8 Will ye accept his person? will ye
contend for God?
9 Is it good that he should search you
out? or as one man mocketh another, do
ye *so* mock him?
10 He will surely reprove you, if ye do
secretly accept persons.
11 Shall not his excellency make you
afraid? and his dread fall upon you?
12 Your remembrances *are* like unto
ashes, your bodies to bodies of clay.
13 Hold your peace, let me alone, that I
may speak, and let come on me what *will.*
14 Wherefore do I take my flesh in my
teeth, and put my life in mine hand?
15 [j]Though he slay me, yet will I trust
in him: but I will maintain mine own
ways before him.
16 He also *shall be* my salvation: for an
hypocrite shall not come before him.
17 Hear diligently my speech, and my
declaration with your ears.

a Psa. 91:15.
b Prov. 14:2.
c Num. 16:22; Dan. 5:23; Acts 17:28.
d i.e. *with God.*
e Job 11:10.
f 1 Ki. 8:35; 17:1.
g Gen. 7:11.
h Psa. 107:40; Dan. 2:21.
i Dan. 2:22; Mt. 10:26; 1 Cor. 4:5.
j Psa. 23:4; Prov. 14:32.

18 Behold now, I have ordered *my*
cause; I know that I shall be justified.
19 Who *is* he *that* will plead with me?
for now, if I hold my tongue, I shall give
up the ghost.
20 Only do not two *things* unto me:
then will I not hide myself from thee.
21 [a]Withdraw thine hand far from me:
and let not thy dread make me afraid.
22 Then call thou, and I will answer:
or let me speak, and answer thou me.
23 How many *are* mine iniquities and
sins? make me to know my transgression and my sin.
24 [b]Wherefore hidest thou thy face,
and holdest me for thine enemy?
25 Wilt thou break a leaf driven to and
fro? and wilt thou pursue the dry stubble?
26 For thou writest bitter things
against me, and makest me to possess
the iniquities of my youth.
27 Thou puttest my feet also in the
stocks, and lookest narrowly unto all my
paths; thou settest a print upon the heels
of my feet.
28 And he, as a rotten thing, consumeth, as a garment that is moth eaten.

CHAPTER 14.

(*Job's answer*, continued.)

Man *that is* born of a woman *is* of few
days, [c]and full of trouble.
2 [d]He cometh forth like a flower, and
is cut down: he fleeth also as a shadow,
and continueth not.
3 And dost thou open thine eyes upon
such an one, and bringest me into judgment with thee?
4 Who can bring a clean *thing* out of
an unclean? not one.
5 Seeing his days *are* determined, the
number of his months *are* with thee,
thou hast appointed his bounds that he
cannot pass;
6 Turn from him, that he may rest, till
he shall accomplish, as an hireling, his
day.
7 For there is hope of a tree, if it be cut
down, that it will sprout again, and that
the tender branch thereof will not cease.
8 Though the root thereof wax old in
the earth, and the stock thereof die in the
ground;
9 *Yet* through the scent of water it will
bud, and bring forth boughs like a plant.
10 But man dieth, and wasteth away:
yea, man giveth up the ghost, and where
is he?
11 *As* the waters fail from the sea, and
the flood decayeth and drieth up:
12 So man lieth down, and riseth not:
[e]till the heavens *be* no more, they shall not
awake, nor be raised out of their sleep.
13 O that thou wouldest hide me in
the [f]grave, that thou wouldest keep me
secret, until thy wrath be past, that thou
wouldest appoint me a set time, and
remember me!
14 If a man die, shall he live *again*? all
the days of my appointed time will I
wait, till my change come.
15 Thou shalt call, and I will answer
thee: thou wilt have a desire to the work
of thine hands.
16 [g]For now thou numberest my steps:
dost thou not watch over my sin?
17 [h]My transgression *is* sealed up in a
bag, and thou sewest up mine iniquity.
18 And surely the mountain falling
cometh to nought, and the rock is
removed out of his place.
19 The waters wear the stones: thou
washest away the things which grow *out*
of the dust of the earth; and thou
destroyest the hope of man.
20 Thou prevailest for ever against
him, and he passeth: thou changest his
countenance, and sendest him away.
21 His sons come to honour, and he
knoweth *it* not; and they are brought
low, but he perceiveth *it* not of them.
22 But his flesh upon him shall have
pain, and his soul within him shall
mourn.

CHAPTER 15.

(9) *Second discourse of Eliphaz: again rests upon superior experience*(v. 8) *and tradition* (v. 10).

Then answered Eliphaz the Temanite,
and said,
2 Should a wise man utter vain knowledge, and fill his belly with the east wind?
3 Should he reason with unprofitable
talk? or with speeches wherewith he can
do no good?
4 Yea, thou castest off fear, and
restrainest prayer before God.
5 For thy mouth uttereth thine iniquity
and thou choosest the tongue of the crafty
6 [i]Thine own mouth condemneth thee

B.C. 1520.

a Psa. 39:10.
b Deut. 32:20; Psa. 13:1; 44:24; 88:14; Isa. 8:17.
c Job 5:7; Eccl. 2:23.
d Job 8:9; Psa. 90:5, 6, 9; 102:11; 103:15; 144:4; Isa. 40:6; Jas. 1:10, 11; 1 Pet. 1:24.
e Psa. 102:25-26; Isa. 51:6; 65:17; 66:22; Acts 3:21; Rom. 8:21; 2 Pet. 3:7, 10, 11; Rev. 20:11; 21:1.
f Heb. *Sheol.* See Hab. 2:5, *note.*
g Job 10:6, 14; 13:27; 31:4; 34:21; Psa. 56:8; 139:1-3; Prov. 5:21; Jer. 32:19.
h Deut. 32:34; Hos. 13:12.
i Job. 9:20; Lk. 19:22.

and not I: yea, thine own lips testify
against thee.
7 *Art* thou the first man *that* was born?
or wast thou made before the hills?
8 Hast thou heard the secret of God?
and dost thou restrain wisdom to thyself?
9 What knowest thou, that we know
not? *what* understandest thou, which *is*
not in us?
10 With us *are* both the grayheaded
and very aged men, much elder than thy
father.
11 *Are* the consolations of God small
with thee? is there any secret thing with
thee?
12 Why doth thine heart carry thee
away? and what do thy eyes wink at,
13 That thou turnest thy spirit against
God, and lettest *such* words go out of thy
mouth?
14 What *is* man, that he should be
clean? and *he which is* born of a woman,
that he should be righteous?
15 Behold, he putteth no [a]trust in his
saints; yea, the heavens are not clean in
his sight.
16 [b]How much more abominable and
filthy *is* man, which drinketh iniquity
like water?
17 I will shew thee, hear me; and that
which I have seen I will declare;
18 Which wise men have told from
their fathers, and have not hid *it*:
19 Unto whom alone the earth was
given, and no stranger passed among
them.
20 The wicked man travaileth with
pain all *his* days, and the number of
years is hidden to the oppressor.
21 [c]A dreadful sound *is* in his ears: in
prosperity the destroyer shall come
upon him.
22 He believeth not that he shall
return out of darkness, and he is waited
for of the sword.
23 He wandereth abroad for bread,
saying, Where *is it*? he knoweth that [d]the
day of darkness is ready at his hand.
24 Trouble and anguish shall make
him afraid; they shall prevail against
him, as a king ready to the battle.
25 For he stretcheth out his hand
against God, and strengtheneth himself
against the Almighty.
26 He runneth upon him, *even* on *his*
neck, upon the thick bosses of his bucklers:

27 [e]Because he covereth his face with
his fatness, and maketh collops of fat on
his flanks.
28 And he dwelleth in desolate cities,
and in houses which no man inhabiteth,
which are ready to become heaps.
29 He shall not be rich, neither shall his
substance continue, neither shall he prolong the perfection thereof upon the earth.
30 He shall not depart out of darkness;
the flame shall dry up his branches, and
[f]by the breath of his mouth shall he go
away.
31 Let not him that is deceived trust in
vanity: for vanity shall be his recompence.
32 It shall be accomplished before his
time, and his branch shall not be green.
33 He shall shake off his unripe grape
as the vine, and shall cast off his flower
as the olive.
34 For the congregation of hypocrites
shall be desolate, and fire shall consume
the tabernacles of bribery.
35 [g]They conceive mischief, and bring
forth vanity, and their belly prepareth
deceit.

CHAPTER 16.

(10) *Job's fourth answer:*
Eliphaz has but heaped up words.

Then Job answered and said,
2 I have heard many such things:
[h]miserable comforters *are* ye all.
3 Shall vain words have an end? or
what emboldeneth thee that thou
answerest?
4 I also could speak as ye *do*: if your
soul were in my soul's stead, I could
heap up words against you, and shake
mine head at you.
5 *But* I would strengthen you with my
mouth, and the moving of my lips
should asswage *your grief*.
6 Though I speak, my grief is not as-
swaged: and *though* I forbear, what am I
eased?
7 But now he hath made me weary:
thou hast made desolate all my company.
8 And thou hast filled me with wrin-
kles, *which* is a witness *against me*: and
my leanness rising up in me beareth witness to my face.
9 He teareth *me* in his wrath, who
hateth me: he gnasheth upon me with
his teeth; mine enemy sharpeneth his
eyes upon me.
10 They have [i]gaped upon me with

B.C. 1520.

a Psa. 2:12, *note.*

b Job 4:19; Psa. 14:3; 53:3.

c Heb. *A sound of fears.*

d Job 18:12.

e Psa. 17:10.

f Job 4:9.

g Psa. 7:14; Isa. 59:4; Hos. 10:13.

h Or, *troublesome.*

i Psa. 22:13; 35:21.

their mouth; they have smitten me upon
the cheek reproachfully; they have gathered themselves together against me.
11 God hath delivered me to the
ungodly, and turned me over into the
hands of the wicked.
12 I was at ease, but he hath broken
me asunder: he hath also taken *me* by
my neck, and shaken me to pieces, and
set me up for his mark.
13 His archers compass me round
about, he cleaveth my reins asunder, and
doth not spare; he poureth out my gall
upon the ground.
14 He breaketh me with breach upon
breach, he runneth upon me like a giant.
15 I have sewed sackcloth upon my
skin, and [a]defiled my horn in the dust.
16 My face is foul with weeping, and
on my eyelids *is* the shadow of death;
17 Not for *any* injustice in mine hands:
also my prayer *is* pure.
18 O earth, cover not thou my blood,
and let my cry have no place.
19 Also now, behold, [b]my witness *is* in
heaven, and my record *is* on high.
20 My friends scorn me: *but* mine eye
poureth out *tears* unto God.
21 [c]O that one might plead for a man
with God, as a man *pleadeth* for his
neighbour!
22 When a few years are come, then I
shall go the way *whence* I shall not return.

CHAPTER 17.

(*Job's fourth answer,* continued.)

My breath is corrupt, my days are
extinct, the graves *are ready* for me.
2 *Are there* not mockers with me? and
doth not mine eye continue in their
provocation?
3 Lay down now, put me in a surety
with thee; [d]who *is* he *that* will strike
hands with me?
4 For thou hast hid their heart from
understanding: therefore shalt thou not
exalt *them*.
5 He that speaketh flattery to *his*
friends, even the eyes of his children
shall fail.
6 He hath made me also a byword of
the people; and aforetime I was as a
tabret.
7 Mine eye also is dim by reason of sorrow, and all my members *are* as a shadow.
8 Upright *men* shall be astonied at this,
and the innocent shall stir up himself
against the hypocrite.
9 The righteous also shall hold on his
way, and he that hath [e]clean hands shall
be stronger and stronger.
10 But as for you all, do ye return, and
come now: for I cannot find *one* wise
man among you.
11 My days are past, my purposes are
broken off, *even* the thoughts of my heart.
12 They change the night into day: the
light *is* short because of darkness.
13 If I wait, the grave *is* mine house: I
have made my bed in the darkness.
14 I have said to corruption, Thou *art*
my father: to the worm, *Thou art* my
mother, and my sister.
15 And where *is* now my hope? as for
my hope, who shall see it?
16 They shall go down to the bars of the
[f]pit, when *our* rest together *is* in the dust.

CHAPTER 18.

(11) *Bildad's second discourse:*
a string of oriental proverbs.

Then answered Bildad the Shuhite,
and said,
2 How long *will it be ere* ye make an
end of words? mark, and afterwards we
will speak.
3 Wherefore are we counted as beasts,
and reputed vile in your sight?
4 He teareth himself in his anger: shall
the earth be forsaken for thee? and shall
the rock be removed out of his place?
5 Yea, [g]the light of the wicked shall be
put out, and the spark of his fire shall
not shine.
6 The light shall be dark in his tabernacle, and [h]his candle shall be put out
with him.
7 The steps of his strength shall be
straitened, and his own counsel shall
cast him down.
8 For he is cast into a net by his own
feet, and he walketh upon a snare.
9 The gin shall take *him* by the heel,
and the robber shall prevail against him.
10 The snare *is* [i]laid for him in the
ground, and a trap for him in the way.

B.C. 1520.

a Job 30:19; Psa. 7:5.
b Job 19:25-27; Rom. 1:9.
c Job 31:35.
d Prov. 6:1; 17:18; 22:26.
e Psa. 24:4.
f Heb. *Sheol.*
g Prov. 13:9; 20:20; 24:20.
h Job 21:17; Psa. 18:28.
i Heb. *hidden.*

B.C. 1520.

11 Terrors shall make him afraid on
every side, and shall drive him to his feet.
12 His strength shall be hungerbitten,
and [a]destruction *shall be* ready at his side.
13 It shall devour the strength of his
skin: *even* the firstborn of death shall
devour his strength.
14 His confidence shall be rooted out
of his tabernacle, and it shall bring him
to the king of terrors.
15 It shall dwell in his tabernacle,
because *it is* none of his: brimstone shall
be scattered upon his habitation.
16 [b]His roots shall be dried up beneath,
and above shall his branch be cut off.
17 His [c]remembrance shall perish
from the earth, and he shall have no
name in the street.
18 He shall be driven from light into
darkness, and chased out of the world.
19 He shall neither have son nor
nephew among his people, nor any
remaining in his dwellings.
20 They that come after *him* shall be
astonied [d]at his day, as they that went
before were affrighted.
21 Surely such *are* the dwellings of the
wicked, and this *is* the place *of him that*
knoweth not God.

CHAPTER 19.

(12) *Job's fifth answer: his sublime faith* (vs. 25-27).

Then Job answered and said,
2 How long will ye vex my soul,
and break me in pieces with words?
3 These ten times have ye reproached
me: ye are not ashamed *that* ye [e]make
yourselves strange to me.
4 And be it indeed *that* I have erred,
mine error remaineth with myself.
5 If indeed ye will magnify *yourselves*
against me, and plead against me my
reproach:
6 Know now that God hath overthrown me, and hath compassed me
with his net.
7 Behold, I cry out of wrong, but I am
not heard: I cry aloud, but *there is* no
judgment.
8 [f]He hath fenced up my way that I
cannot pass, and he hath set darkness in
my paths.
9 [g]He hath stripped me of my glory,
and taken the crown *from* my head.
10 He hath destroyed me on every
side, and I am gone: and mine hope hath
he removed like a tree.
11 He hath also kindled his wrath
against me, and he counteth me unto
him as *one of* his enemies.
12 His troops come together, and raise
up their way against me, and encamp
round about my tabernacle.
13 [h]He hath put my brethren far from
me, and mine acquaintance are verily
estranged from me.
14 My kinsfolk have failed, and my
familiar friends have forgotten me.
15 They that dwell in mine house, and
my maids, count me for a stranger: I am
an alien in their sight.
16 I called my servant, and he gave *me*
no answer; I intreated him with my
mouth.
17 My breath is strange to my wife,
though I intreated for the children's *sake*
of mine own body.
18 Yea, young children despised me; I
arose, and they spake against me.
19 All my inward friends abhorred
me: and they whom I loved are turned
against me.
20 My bone cleaveth to my skin and to
my flesh, and I am escaped with the skin
of my teeth.
21 Have pity upon me, have pity upon
me, O ye my friends; [i]for the hand of
God hath touched me.
22 Why do ye persecute me as God,
and are not satisfied with my flesh?
23 Oh that my words were now written! oh that they were printed in a book!
24 That they were graven with an iron
pen and lead in the rock for ever!
25 For I know *that* my [j]redeemer
liveth, and *that* he shall [k]stand at the latter *day* upon the earth:
26 And *though* after my skin *worms*
destroy this *body*, yet [l]in my flesh shall I
see God:
27 Whom I shall see for myself, and
mine eyes shall behold, and not another;
though my reins be consumed within me.
28 But ye should say, Why persecute
we him, seeing the root of the matter is
found in me?
29 Be ye afraid of the sword: for wrath
bringeth the punishments of the sword,
that ye may know *there is* a judgment.

a Job 15:23.
b Job 29:19.
c Psa. 34:16.
d Psa. 37:13.
e Or, *harden yourselves against me.*
f Job 3:23; Psa. 88:8.
g Psa. 89:44.
h Psa. 31:11; 38:11; 69:8; 88:8, 18.
i Job 1:1; Psa. 38:2
j Heb. *goel, Redemp.* (*Kinsman type*). Isa. 59:20, *note.*
k *Resurrection.* vs. 25-27; Gen. 22:5. (Job 19:25; 1 Cor. 15:52.)
l Psa. 17:15; 1 Cor. 13:12; 1 John 3:2.

B.C. 1520.

CHAPTER 20.

(13) *Zophar's second discourse: tradition and proverb.*

Then answered Zophar the Naamathite, and said,

2 Therefore do my thoughts cause me to answer, and for *this* I make haste.

3 I have heard the check of my reproach, and the spirit of my understanding causeth me to answer.

4 Knowest thou *not* this of old, since man was placed upon earth,

5 That [a]the triumphing of the wicked *is* short, and the joy of the hypocrite *but* for a moment?

6 Though his excellency mount up to the heavens, and his head reach unto the clouds;

7 *Yet* he shall perish for ever like his own dung: they which have seen him shall say, Where *is* he?

8 He shall fly away [b]as a dream, and shall not be found: yea, he shall be chased away as a vision of the night.

9 The eye also *which* saw him shall *see him* no more; neither shall his place any more behold him.

10 His children shall seek to please the poor, and his hands [c]shall restore their goods.

11 His bones are full *of the sin* of his youth, which shall lie down with him in the dust.

12 Though wickedness be sweet in his mouth, *though* he hide it under his tongue;

13 *Though* he spare it, and forsake it not; but keep it still within his mouth:

14 *Yet* his meat in his bowels is turned, *it is* the gall of asps within him.

15 He hath swallowed down riches, and he shall vomit them up again: God shall cast them out of his belly.

16 He shall suck the poison of asps: the viper's tongue shall slay him.

17 He shall not see the rivers, the floods, the brooks of honey and butter.

18 That which he laboured for shall he restore, and shall not swallow *it* down: according to *his* substance *shall* the restitution *be*, and he shall not rejoice *therein*.

19 Because he hath [d]oppressed *and* hath forsaken the poor; *because* he hath violently taken away an house which he builded not;

20 Surely he shall not feel quietness in his belly, he shall not save of that which he desired.

21 There shall none of his meat be left; therefore shall no man look for his goods.

22 In the fulness of his sufficiency he shall be in straits: every hand of the wicked shall come upon him.

23 *When* he is about to fill his belly, *God* shall cast the fury of his wrath upon him, and shall rain *it* upon him while he is eating.

24 He shall flee from the iron weapon, *and* the bow of steel shall strike him through.

25 It is drawn, and cometh out of the body; yea, the glittering sword cometh out of his gall: terrors *are* upon him.

26 All darkness *shall be* hid in his secret places: [e]a fire not blown shall consume him; it shall go ill with him that is left in his tabernacle.

27 The heaven shall reveal his iniquity, and the earth shall rise up against him.

28 The increase of his house shall depart, *and his goods* shall flow away in the day of his wrath.

29 [f]This *is* the portion of a wicked man from God, and the heritage appointed unto him by God.

CHAPTER 21.

(14) *Job's sixth answer: the prosperity of the wicked refutes the view that he is affliced because a secret sinner.*

But Job answered and said,

2 Hear diligently my speech, and let this be your consolations.

3 Suffer me that I may speak; and afte that I have spoken, mock on.

4 As for me, *is* my complaint to man? and if *it were so*, why should not my spirit be troubled?

5 Mark me, and be astonished, and lay *your* hand upon *your* mouth.

6 Even when I remember I am afraid and trembling taketh hold on my flesh.

7 [g]Wherefore do the wicked live become old, yea, are mighty in power?

8 Their seed is established in thei sight with them, and their offspring before their eyes.

9 Their houses *are* safe from fear, [h]neither *is* the rod of God upon them.

10 Their bull gendereth, and faileth

---

a Psa. 37:35, 36.

b Psa. 73:20; 90:5.

c v. 18.

d Heb. *crushed.* Job. 24:2-4; 35:9.

e Psa. 21:9.

f Job 27:13; 31:2, 3.

g Job 12:6; Psa. 17:10, 14; 73:3, 12; Jer. 12:1; Hab. 1:16.

h Psa. 73:5.

not; their cow calveth, and casteth not
her calf.
11 They send forth their little ones like
a flock, and their children dance.
12 They take the timbrel and harp, and
rejoice at the sound of the organ.
13 They spend their days [a]in wealth,
and in a moment go down to the [b]grave.
14 Therefore they say unto God,
Depart from us; for we desire not the
knowledge of thy ways.
15 [c]What *is* the Almighty, that we
should serve him? and [d]what profit
should we have, if we pray unto him?
16 Lo, their good *is* not in their hand:
'the counsel of the wicked is far from me.
17 How oft is the candle of the wicked
put out! and *how oft* cometh their
destruction upon them! [f]God distributeth
sorrows in his anger.
18 They are as stubble before the wind,
and as chaff that the storm [g]carrieth away.
19 God layeth up his [h]iniquity for his
children: he rewardeth him, and he shall
know *it*.
20 His eyes shall see his destruction,
and [i]he shall drink of the wrath of the
Almighty.
21 For what pleasure *hath* he in his
house after him, when the number of his
months is cut off in the midst?
22 [j]Shall *any* teach God knowledge?
eeing he judgeth those that are high.
23 One dieth in his full strength, being
vholly at ease and quiet.
24 His breasts are full of milk, and his
ones are moistened with marrow.
25 And another dieth in the bitterness
f his soul, and never eateth with plea-
ure.
26 They shall lie down alike in the
ust, and the worms shall cover them.
27 Behold, I know your thoughts, and
he devices *which* ye wrongfully imagine
gainst me.
28 For ye say, Where *is* the house of
he prince? and where *are* the [k]dwelling
laces of the wicked?
29 Have ye not asked them that go by
he way? and do ye not know their
okens,
30 That the wicked is reserved to [l]the
ay of destruction? they shall be brought
orth to the day of wrath.
31 Who shall declare his way to his
ice? and who shall repay him *what* he
ath done?
32 Yet shall he be brought to the grave,
and shall remain in the tomb.
33 The clods of the valley shall be
sweet unto him, and every man shall
draw after him, as *there are* innumerable
before him.
34 How then comfort ye me in vain,
seeing in your answers there remaineth
falsehood?

CHAPTER 22.

(15) *Eliphaz' third discourse:*
the old theory—Job has sinned
(vs. 6, 7, 9).

Then Eliphaz the Temanite answered
and said,
2 [m]Can a man be profitable unto God,
as he that is wise may be profitable unto
himself?
3 *Is it* any pleasure to the Almighty,
that thou art righteous? or *is it* gain *to*
him, that thou makest thy ways perfect?
4 Will he reprove thee for fear of thee?
will he enter with thee into judgment?
5 *Is* not thy wickedness great? and
thine iniquities infinite?
6 For thou hast [n]taken a pledge from
thy brother for nought, and stripped the
naked of their clothing.
7 Thou hast not given water to the
weary to drink, and [o]thou hast withholden bread from the hungry.
8 But *as for* the mighty man, he had the
earth; and the honourable man dwelt in it.
9 Thou hast sent widows away empty,
and the arms of the fatherless have been
broken.
10 Therefore snares *are* round about
thee, and sudden fear troubleth thee;
11 Or darkness, *that* thou canst not see;
and abundance of waters cover thee.
12 *Is* not God in the height of heaven?
and behold the height of the stars, how
high they are!
13 And thou sayest, [p]How doth God
know? can he judge through the dark
cloud?
14 [q]Thick clouds *are* a covering to him,
that he seeth not; and he walketh in the
circuit of heaven.
15 Hast thou marked the old way
which wicked men have trodden?
16 Which were cut down out of time,
whose foundation was overflown with a
flood:

B.C. 1520.

a Or, *in mirth.*
b Heb. *Sheol.* See Hab. 2:5, *note.*
c Job 34:9; Ex. 5:2.
d Job 35:3; Mal. 3:14.
e Job 22:18; Psa. 1:1; Prov. 1:10.
f Lk. 12:46.
g Heb. *stealeth away.*
h Heb. *the punishment of his iniquity.*
i Psa. 75:8; Isa. 51:17; Jer. 25:15; Rev. 14:10; 19:15.
j Isa. 40:13; 45:9; Rom. 11:34; 1 Cor. 2:16.
k Heb. *the tent of the tabernacles of the wicked.*
l *Day* (*of destruction*). Isa. 34:1-9. (Job 31:30; Rev. 20:11-15).
m Job 35:7; Psa. 16:2; Lk. 17:10.
n Ex. 22:26, 27; Deut. 24:10.
o Job 31:17; Deut. 15:7; Isa. 58:7; Ezk. 18:7. Mt. 25:42.
p Or, *what.*
q Psa. 139:11, 12.

17 Which said unto God, Depart from us: and what can the Almighty do for them?

18 Yet he filled their houses with good *things*: but the counsel of the wicked is far from me.

19 The righteous see *it*, and are glad: and the innocent laugh them to scorn.

20 Whereas our substance is not cut down, but the remnant of them the fire consumeth.

21 Acquaint now thyself with him, and be at peace: thereby good shall come unto thee.

22 Receive, I pray thee, the law from his mouth, and [a]lay up his words in thine heart.

23 [b]If thou return to the Almighty, thou shalt be built up, thou shalt put away iniquity far from thy tabernacles.

24 Then shalt thou lay up gold as dust, and the *gold* of Ophir as the stones of the brooks.

25 Yea, the Almighty shall be thy defence, and thou shalt have plenty of silver.

26 For then shalt thou have thy delight in the Almighty, and shalt lift up thy face unto God.

27 Thou shalt make thy prayer unto him, and he shall hear thee, and thou shalt pay thy vows.

28 Thou shalt also decree a thing, and it shall be established unto thee: and the light shall shine upon thy ways.

29 When *men* are cast down, then thou shalt say, *There is* lifting up; and he shall save the [c]humble person.

30 He shall deliver the [d]island of the innocent: and it is delivered by the pureness of thine hands.

CHAPTER 23.

(16) *Job's seventh answer: he longs for God.*

Then Job answered and said,

2 Even to day *is* my complaint bitter: my stroke is heavier than my groaning.

3 [e]Oh that I knew where I might find him! *that* I might come *even* to his seat!

4 I would order *my* cause before him, and fill my mouth with arguments.

5 I would know the words *which* he would answer me, and understand what he would say unto me.

6 [f]Will he plead against me with *his* great power? No; but he would put *strength* in me.

B.C. 1520.

a Job 5:11; Psa. 119:11.

b Job 8:5, 6; 11:13, 14.

c Prov. 29:23; Jas. 4:6; 1 Pet. 5:5. Heb. *him that hath low eyes.*

d i.e. *coast.*

e Job 13:3; 16:21.

f Isa. 27:4, 8; 57:16.

g Job 9:11.

h Psa. 139:1, 2, 3.

i Psa. 17:3; 66:10; Jas. 1:2.

j Acts 1:7.

7 There the righteous might dispute with him; so should I be delivered for ever from my judge.

8 [g]Behold, I go forward, but he *is* not *there*; and backward, but I cannot perceive him:

9 On the left hand, where he doth work, but I cannot behold *him*: he hideth himself on the right hand, that I cannot see *him*:

10 But [h]he knoweth the way that I take: [i]*when* he hath tried me, I shall come forth as gold.

11 My foot hath held his steps, his way have I kept, and not declined.

12 Neither have I gone back from the commandment of his lips; I have esteemed the words of his mouth more than my necessary *food*.

13 But he *is* in one *mind*, and who can turn him? and *what* his soul desireth, even *that* he doeth.

14 For he performeth *the thing that is* appointed for me: and many such *things are* with him.

15 Therefore am I troubled at his presence: when I consider, I am afraid of him.

16 For God maketh my heart soft, and the Almighty troubleth me:

17 Because I was not cut off before the darkness, *neither* hath he covered the darkness from my face.

CHAPTER 24.

(*Job's seventh answer,* continued.)

Why, seeing [j]times are not hidden from the Almighty, do they that know him not see his days?

2 *Some* remove the landmarks; they violently take away flocks, and feed *thereof.*

3 They drive away the ass of the fatherless, they take the widow's ox for a pledge.

4 They turn the needy out of the way: the poor of the earth hide themselves together.

5 Behold, *as* wild asses in the desert, go they forth to their work; rising betimes for a prey: the wilderness *yieldeth* food for them *and* for *their* children.

6 They reap *every one* his corn in the field: and they gather the vintage of the wicked.

7 They cause the naked to lodge without clothing, that *they have* no covering in the cold.

B.C. 1520.

8 They are wet with the showers of the mountains, and [a]embrace the rock for want of a shelter.

9 They pluck the fatherless from the breast, and take a pledge of the poor.

10 They cause *him* to go naked without clothing, and they take away the sheaf *from* the hungry;

11 *Which* make oil within their walls, *and* tread *their* winepresses, and suffer thirst.

12 Men groan from out of the city, and the soul of the wounded crieth out: yet God layeth not folly *to them.*

13 They are of those that rebel against the light; they know not the ways thereof, nor abide in the paths thereof.

14 The murderer rising with the light killeth the poor and needy, and in the night is as a thief.

15 The [b]eye also of the adulterer waiteth for the twilight, saying, No eye shall see me: and disguiseth *his* face.

16 In the dark they dig through houses, *which* they had marked for themselves in the daytime: they know not the light.

17 For the morning *is* to them even as the shadow of death: if *one* know *them, they are in* the terrors of the shadow of death.

18 He *is* swift as the waters; their portion is cursed in the earth: he beholdeth not the way of the vineyards.

19 Drought and heat consume the snow waters: *so doth* the [c]grave *those which* have sinned.

20 The womb shall forget him; the worm shall feed sweetly on him; [d]he shall be no more remembered; and wickedness shall be broken as a tree.

21 He evil entreateth the barren *that* beareth not: and doeth not good to the widow.

22 He draweth also the mighty with his power: he riseth up, and no *man* is sure of life.

23 *Though* it be given him *to be* in safety, whereon he resteth; [e]yet his eyes *are* upon their ways.

24 They are exalted for a little while, but are gone and brought low; they are taken out of the way as all *other,* and cut off as the tops of the ears of corn.

25 And if *it be* not *so* now, who will make me a liar, and make my speech nothing worth?

a Lam. 4:5.

b Prov. 7:9.

c Heb. *Sheol.* See Hab. 2:5, *note.*

d Prov. 10:7.

e Psa. 11:4; Prov. 15:3.

f Jas. 1:17.

g Job 4:17; 15:14; Psa. 130:3; 143:2.

h Psa. 22:6.

i Psa. 139:8, 11; Prov. 15:11; Heb. 4:13. Heb. *Sheol.*

j Job 38:8; Psa. 33:7; 104:9; Prov. 8:29; Jer. 5:22.

k *Holy Spirit.* Job 33:4. (Gen. 1:2; Mal. 2:15.)

CHAPTER 25.

(17) *Bildad's third discourse: sententious sayings.*

Then answered Bildad the Shuhite, and said,

2 Dominion and fear *are* with him, he maketh peace in his high places.

3 Is there any number of his armies? and upon whom doth not his [f]light arise?

4 [g]How then can man be justified with God? or how can he be clean *that is* born of a woman?

5 Behold even to the moon, and it shineth not; yea, the stars are not pure in his sight.

6 How much less man, *that is* a [h]worm? and the son of man, *which is* a worm?

CHAPTER 26.

(18) *Job's eighth answer: Bildad's view leads to despair. Job's faith in God.*

But Job answered and said,

2 How hast thou helped *him that is* without power? *how* savest thou the arm *that hath* no strength?

3 How hast thou counselled *him that hath* no wisdom? and *how* hast thou plentifully declared the thing as it is?

4 To whom hast thou uttered words? and whose spirit came from thee?

5 Dead *things* are formed from under the waters, and the inhabitants thereof.

6 [i]Hell *is* naked before him, and destruction hath no covering.

7 He stretcheth out the north over the empty place, *and* hangeth the earth upon nothing.

8 He bindeth up the waters in his thick clouds; and the cloud is not rent under them.

9 He holdeth back the face of his throne, *and* spreadeth his cloud upon it.

10 [j]He hath compassed the waters with bounds, until the day and night come to an end.

11 The pillars of heaven tremble and are astonished at his reproof.

12 He divideth the sea with his power, and by his understanding he smiteth through the proud.

13 By his [k]spirit he hath garnished the heavens; his hand hath formed the crooked serpent.

14 Lo, these *are* parts of his ways: but how little a portion is heard of him? but

the thunder of his power who can understand?

CHAPTER 27.

(*Job's eighth answer,* continued.)

Moreover Job continued his parable, and said,

2 *As* God liveth, *who* hath taken away my judgment; and the Almighty, *who* hath [a]vexed my soul;

3 All the while my breath *is* in me, and the [b]spirit of God *is* in my nostrils;

4 My lips shall not speak wickedness, nor my tongue utter deceit.

5 God forbid that I should justify you: till I die I will not remove mine integrity from me.

6 My righteousness I hold fast, and will not let it go: my heart shall not reproach *me* so long as I live.

7 Let mine enemy be as the wicked, and he that riseth up against me as the unrighteous.

8 [c]For what *is* the hope of the hypocrite, though he hath gained, when God taketh away his soul?

9 Will God hear his cry when trouble cometh upon him?

10 Will he delight himself in the Almighty? will he always call upon God?

11 I will teach you by the hand of God: *that* which *is* with the Almighty will I not conceal.

12 Behold, all ye yourselves have seen *it;* why then are ye thus altogether vain?

13 This *is* the portion of a wicked man with God, and the heritage of oppressors, *which* they shall receive of the Almighty.

14 If his children be multiplied, *it is* for the sword: and his offspring shall not be satisfied with bread.

15 Those that remain of him shall be buried in death: and his widows shall not weep.

16 Though he heap up silver as the dust, and prepare raiment as the clay;

17 He may prepare *it,* [d]but the just shall put *it* on, and the innocent shall divide the silver.

18 He buildeth his house as a moth, and as a booth *that* the keeper maketh.

19 The rich man shall lie down, but he shall not be gathered: he openeth his eyes, and he *is* not.

20 [e]Terrors take hold on him as waters, a tempest stealeth him away in the night.

21 The east wind carrieth him away, and he departeth: and as a storm hurleth him out of his place.

22 For *God* shall cast upon him, and not spare: he would fain flee out of his hand.

23 *Men* shall clap their hands at him, and shall hiss him out of his place.

CHAPTER 28.

(*Job's eighth answer,* continued.)

Surely there is a [f]vein for the silver, and a place for gold *where* they fine *it.*

2 Iron is taken out of the earth, and brass *is* molten *out of* the stone.

3 He setteth an end to darkness, and searcheth out all perfection: the stones of darkness, and the shadow of death.

4 The flood breaketh out from the inhabitant; *even the waters* forgotten of the foot: they are dried up, they are gone away from men.

5 *As for* the earth, out of it cometh bread: and under it is turned up as it were fire.

6 The stones of it *are* the place of sapphires: and it hath dust of gold.

7 *There is* a path which no fowl knoweth, and which the vulture's eye hath not seen:

8 The lion's whelps have not trodden it, nor the fierce lion passed by it.

9 He putteth forth his hand upon the rock; he overturneth the mountains by the roots.

10 He cutteth out rivers among the rocks; and his eye seeth every precious thing.

11 He bindeth the floods [g]from overflowing; and *the thing that is* hid bringeth he forth to light.

12 But [h]where shall wisdom be found? and where *is* the place of understanding?

13 Man knoweth not the [i]price thereof; neither is it found in the land of the living.

14 The depth saith, It *is* not in me: and the sea saith, *It is* not with me.

15 It cannot be gotten for gold, neither shall silver be weighed *for* the price thereof.

16 It cannot be valued with the gold of Ophir, with the precious onyx, or the sapphire.

17 The gold and the crystal cannot equal it: and the exchange of it *shall not be for* jewels of fine gold.

18 No mention shall be made of coral

B.C. 1520.

a Heb. *made my soul bitter.*

b Gen. 2:7; cf. Job 32:8; 33:4.

c Mt. 16:26; Lk. 12:20.

d Prov. 28:8; Eccl. 2:26.

e Job 18:11.

f Or, *a mine.*

g Heb. *from weeping.*

h v. 20; Eccl. 7:24.

i Prov. 3:15.

or of pearls: for the price of wisdom *is*
above rubies.
19 The topaz of Ethiopia shall not
equal it, neither shall it be valued with
pure gold.
20 [a]Whence then cometh wisdom? and
where *is* the place of understanding?
21 Seeing it is hid from the eyes of all
living, and kept close from the fowls of
the air.
22 [b]Destruction and death say, We have
heard the fame thereof with our ears.
23 God understandeth the way thereof, and he knoweth the place thereof.
24 For he looketh to the ends of the
earth, *and* seeth under the whole heaven;
25 [c]To make the weight for the winds;
and he weigheth the waters by measure.
26 When he made a decree for the
rain, and a way for the lightning of the
thunder:
27 Then did he see it, and declare it; he
prepared it, yea, and searched it out.
28 And unto man he said, Behold, the
[d]fear of the Lord, that *is* wisdom; and to
depart from evil *is* understanding.

CHAPTER 29.

(*Job's eighth answer,* continued.
He answers the false charges of Eliphaz,
Job 22:6-9.)

Moreover Job continued his parable,
and said,
2 Oh that I were as *in* months past, as
in the days *when* God preserved me;
3 When his candle shined upon my
head, *and when* by his light I walked
through darkness;
4 As I was in the days of my youth,
when [e]the secret of God *was* upon my
tabernacle;
5 When the Almighty *was* yet with me,
when my children *were* about me;
6 When I washed my steps with butter,
and the rock poured me out rivers of oil;
7 When I went out to the gate through
the city, *when* I prepared my seat in the
street!
8 The young men saw me, and hid
themselves: and the aged arose, *and*
stood up.
9 The princes refrained talking, and
laid *their* hand on their mouth.
10 The nobles held their peace, and
their tongue cleaved to the roof of their
mouth.

B.C. 1520.

a v. 12.

b v. 14.

c Psa. 135:7.

d Psa. 19:9, *note.*

e Psa. 25:14.

f *Righteousness (garment).* Psa. 132:9. (Gen. 3:21; Rev. 19:8.)

11 When the ear heard *me,* then it
blessed me; and when the eye saw *me,* it
gave witness to me:
12 Because I delivered the poor that
cried, and the fatherless, and *him that had*
none to help him.
13 The blessing of him that was ready
to perish came upon me: and I caused
the widow's heart to sing for joy.
14 I put on [f]righteousness, and it
clothed me: my judgment *was* as a robe
and a diadem.
15 I was eyes to the blind, and feet *was*
I to the lame.
16 I *was* a father to the poor: and the
cause *which* I knew not I searched out.
17 And I brake the jaws of the wicked,
and plucked the spoil out of his teeth.
18 Then I said, I shall die in my nest,
and I shall multiply *my* days as the sand.
19 My root *was* spread out by the
waters, and the dew lay all night upon
my branch.
20 My glory *was* fresh in me, and my
bow was renewed in my hand.
21 Unto me *men* gave ear, and waited,
and kept silence at my counsel.
22 After my words they spake not
again; and my speech dropped upon
them.
23 And they waited for me as for the
rain; and they opened their mouth wide
as for the latter rain.
24 *If* I laughed on them, they believed
it not; and the light of my countenance
they cast not down.
25 I chose out their way, and sat chief,
and dwelt as a king in the army, as one
that comforteth the mourners.

CHAPTER 30.

(*Job's eighth answer,* continued.)

But now *they that are* younger than I
have me in derision, whose fathers I
would have disdained to have set with
the dogs of my flock.
2 Yea, whereto *might* the strength of
their hands *profit* me, in whom old age
was perished?
3 For want and famine *they were*
solitary; fleeing into the wilderness in
former time desolate and waste.
4 Who cut up mallows by the

bushes, and juniper roots *for* their meat.

5 They were driven forth from among *men*, (they cried after them as *after* a thief;)

6 To dwell in the clifts of the valleys, *in* caves of the earth, and *in* the rocks.

7 Among the bushes they brayed; under the nettles they were gathered together.

8 *They were* children of fools, yea, children of base men: they were viler than the earth.

9 [a]And now am I their song, yea, I am their byword.

10 They abhor me, they flee far from me, and spare not [b]to spit in my face.

11 Because he hath [c]loosed my cord, and afflicted me, they have also let loose the bridle before me.

12 Upon *my* right *hand* rise the youth; [d]they push away my feet, and they raise up against me the ways of their destruction.

13 They mar my path, they set forward my calamity, they have no helper.

14 They came *upon me* as a wide breaking in *of waters*: in the desolation they rolled themselves *upon me*.

15 Terrors are turned upon me: they pursue my soul as the wind: and my welfare passeth away as a cloud.

16 [e]And now my soul is poured out upon me; the days of affliction have taken hold upon me.

17 My bones are pierced in me in the night season: and my sinews take no rest.

18 By the great force *of my disease* is my garment changed: it bindeth me about as the collar of my coat.

19 He hath cast me into the mire, and I am become like dust and ashes.

20 I cry unto thee, and thou dost not hear me: I stand up, and thou regardest me *not*.

21 Thou art become cruel to me: with thy strong hand thou opposest thyself against me.

22 Thou liftest me up to the wind; thou causest me to ride *upon it*, and dissolvest my substance.

23 For I know *that* thou wilt bring me *to* death, and *to* the house [f]appointed for all living.

24 Howbeit he will not stretch out *his* hand to the grave, though they cry in his destruction.

B.C. 1520.

a Job 17:6; Psa. 35:15; 69:12; Lam. 3:14, 63.

b Num. 12:14; Deut. 25:9; Isa. 50:6; Mt. 26:67; 27:30.

c See Job 12:18.

d Job 19:12.

e Psa. 42:4.

f Heb. 9:27.

g Jer. 8:15.

h Psa. 38:6; 42:9; 43:2.

i Psa. 102:6; Mic. 1:8.

j Psa. 119:83; Lam. 4:8; 5:10.

k Psa. 102:3.

l Heb. *Let him weigh me in balances of justice.*

m Lev. 26:16; Deut. 28:30, 38.

n 2 Sam. 12:11; Jer. 8:10.

o Gen. 38:24; Lev. 20:10; Deut. 22:22; see v. 28.

p Psa. 44.21.

25 Did not I weep for him that was in trouble? was *not* my soul grieved for the poor?

26 [g]When I looked for good, then evil came *unto me*: and when I waited for light, there came darkness.

27 My bowels boiled, and rested not: the days of affliction prevented me.

28 [h]I went mourning without the sun: I stood up, *and* I cried in the congregation.

29 [i]I am a brother to dragons, and a companion to owls.

30 [j]My skin is black upon me, and [k]my bones are burned with heat.

31 My harp also is *turned* to mourning, and my organ into the voice of them that weep.

CHAPTER 31.

(*Job's eighth answer,* continued.)

I made a covenant with mine eyes; why then should I think upon a maid?

2 For what portion of God *is there* from above? and *what* inheritance of the Almighty from on high?

3 *Is* not destruction to the wicked? and a strange *punishment* to the workers of iniquity?

4 Doth not he see my ways, and count all my steps?

5 If I have walked with vanity, or if my foot hath hasted to deceit;

6 [l]Let me be weighed in an even balance, that God may know mine integrity.

7 If my step hath turned out of the way, and mine heart walked after mine eyes, and if any blot hath cleaved to mine hands;

8 [m]*Then* let me sow, and let another eat; yea, let my offspring be rooted out.

9 If mine heart have been deceived by a woman, or *if* I have laid wait at my neighbour's door;

10 *Then* let my wife grind unto [n]another, and let others bow down upon her.

11 For this *is* an heinous crime; yea, [o]it *is* an iniquity *to be punished by* the judges.

12 For it *is* a fire *that* consumeth to destruction, and would root out all mine increase.

13 If I did despise the cause of my manservant or of my maidservant, when they contended with me;

14 What then shall I do [p]when God

riseth up? and when he visiteth, what shall I answer him?

15 [a]Did not he that made me in the womb make him? and did not one fashion us in the womb?

16 If I have withheld the poor from *their* desire, or have caused the eyes of the widow to fail;

17 Or have eaten my morsel myself alone, and the fatherless hath not eaten thereof;

18 (For from my youth he was brought up with me, as *with* a father, and I have guided her from my mother's womb;)

19 If I have seen any perish for want of clothing, or any poor without covering;

20 If his loins have not [b]blessed me, and *if* he were *not* warmed with the fleece of my sheep;

21 If I have lifted up my hand [c]against the fatherless, when I saw my help in the gate:

22 *Then* let mine arm fall from my shoulder blade, and mine arm be broken from the bone.

23 For [d]destruction *from* God *was* a ter-ror to me, and by reason of his highness I could not endure.

24 If I have made gold my hope, or have said to the fine gold, *Thou art* my confidence;

25 If I rejoiced because my wealth *was* great, and because mine hand had gotten much;

26 If I beheld the sun when it shined, or the moon walking *in* brightness;

27 And my heart hath been secretly enticed, or my mouth hath kissed my hand:

28 This also *were* an iniquity *to be punished by* the judge: for I should have denied the God *that is* above.

29 If I rejoiced at the destruction of him that hated me, or lifted up myself when evil found him:

B.C. 1520.

a Job 34:19; Prov. 14:31; 22:2; Mal. 2:10.

b Deut. 24:13.

c Job 22:9.

d Isa. 13:6; Joel 1:15.

e Job 19:7; 33:6.

f 1 Ki. 21:19.

g Job 6:29; 31:6; 33:9.

h Gen. 22:21.

30 Neither have I suffered my mouth to sin by wishing a curse to his soul.

31 If the men of my tabernacle said not, Oh that we had of his flesh! we cannot be satisfied.

32 The stranger did not lodge in the street: *but* I opened my doors to the traveller.

33 If I covered my transgressions as Adam, by hiding mine iniquity in my bosom:

34 Did I fear a great multitude, or did the contempt of families terrify me, that I kept silence, *and* went not out of the door?

35 [e]Oh that one would hear me! behold, my desire *is, that* the Almighty would answer me, and *that* mine adversary had written a book.

36 Surely I would take it upon my shoulder, *and* bind it *as* a crown to me.

37 I would declare unto him the number of my steps; as a prince would I go near unto him.

38 If my land cry against me, or that the furrows likewise thereof complain;

39 If I have eaten the fruits thereof without money, [f]or have caused the owners thereof to lose their life:

40 Let thistles grow instead of wheat, and cockle instead of barley. The words of Job are ended.

CHAPTER 32.

Part IV. Job and Elihu.

[1]SO these three men ceased to answer Job, because he *was* [g]righteous in his own eyes.

(1) *Elihu's discourse.*

2 Then was kindled the wrath of [2]Elihu the son of Barachel the [h]Buzite, of the kindred of Ram: against Job was his

[1](32:1) Despite minor differences, Eliphaz, Bildad, and Zophar have one view of the problem of Job's afflictions. He is a hypocrite. Outwardly good, he is, they hold, really a bad man. Otherwise, according to their conception of God, Job's sufferings would be unjust. Job, though himself the sufferer, will not so accuse the justice of God, and his self-defence is complete. Before God he is guilty, helpless, and undone, and there is no daysman (9.). Later, his faith is rewarded by a revelation of a coming Redeemer, and of the resurrection (19.). But Eliphaz, Bildad, and Zophar are sinners also as before God, and yet they are not afflicted. Job refutes the theory of the three that he is a secret sinner as against the common moralities, but the real problem, Why are the righteous afflicted? remains. It is solved in the last chapter.

[2](32:2) Elihu has a far juster and more spiritual conception of the problem than Eliphaz, Bildad, and Zophar because he has an infinitely higher conception of God. The God of Eliphaz and the others, great though they perceive Him to be in His works, becomes in their thought petty and exacting in

wrath kindled, because he justified
[a]himself rather than God.
3 Also against his three friends was
his wrath kindled, because they had
found no answer, and *yet* had condemned Job.
4 Now Elihu had waited till Job had
spoken, because they *were* elder than he.
5 When Elihu saw that *there was* no
answer in the mouth of *these* three men,
then his wrath was kindled.
6 And Elihu the son of Barachel the
Buzite answered and said, I *am* young,
and [b]ye *are* very old; wherefore I was
afraid, and durst not shew you mine
opinion.
7 I said, Days should speak, and multitude of years should teach wisdom.
8 But *there is* a spirit in man: and the
[c]inspiration of the Almighty giveth them
understanding.
9 Great men are not *always* wise: neither do the aged understand judgment.
10 Therefore I said, Hearken to me; I
also will shew mine opinion.
11 Behold, I waited for your words; I
gave ear to your reasons, whilst ye
searched out what to say.
12 Yea, I attended unto you, and,
behold, *there was* none of you that convinced Job, *or* that answered his words:
13 [d]Lest ye should say, We have found
out wisdom: God thrusteth him down,
not man.
14 Now he hath not directed *his* words
against me: neither will I answer him
with your speeches.
15 They were amazed, they answered
no more: they left off speaking.
16 When I had waited, (for they spake
not, but stood still, *and* answered no
more;)
17 *I said*, I will answer also my part, I
also will shew mine opinion.
18 For I am full of matter, the spirit
within me [e]constraineth me.
19 Behold, my belly *is* as wine *which*
hath no vent; it is ready to burst like new
bottles.
20 I will speak, that I may be refreshed:
I will open my lips and answer.

B.C. 1520.

a Heb. *his soul.*

b Job 15:10.

c Job 35:11; 38:36; 1 Ki. 3:12; 4:29; Prov. 2:6; Eccl. 2:26; Dan. 1:17; 2:21; Mt. 11:25; Jas. 1:5.

d Jer. 9:23; 1 Cor. 1:29.

e *Inspiration.* Psa. 68:11. (Ex. 4:15; Rev. 22:19.)

f *Holy Spirit.* Psa. 51:11, 12. (Gen. 1:2; Mal. 2:15.)

g Gen. 2:7.

h Job 9:17; 10:7; 11:4; 16:17; 23:10, 11; 27:5; 29:14; 31:1.

21 Let me not, I pray you, accept any
man's person, neither let me give flattering titles unto man.
22 For I know not to give flattering
titles; *in so doing* my maker would soon
take me away.

CHAPTER 33.

(*Elihu's discourse*, continued.)

Wherefore, Job, I pray thee, hear my
speeches, and hearken to all my
words.
2 Behold, now I have opened my
mouth, my tongue hath spoken in my
mouth.
3 My words *shall be of* the uprightness
of my heart: and my lips shall utter
knowledge clearly.
4 The [f]Spirit of God [g]hath made me,
and the breath of the Almighty hath
given me life.
5 If thou canst answer me, set *thy*
words in order before me, stand up.
6 Behold, I *am* according to thy wish in
God's stead: I also am formed out of the
clay.
7 Behold, my terror shall not make
thee afraid, neither shall my hand be
heavy upon thee.
8 Surely thou hast spoken in mine
hearing, and I have heard the voice of
thy words, *saying*,
9 [h]I am clean without transgression, I
am innocent; neither *is there* iniquity in
me.
10 Behold, he findeth occasions against
me, he counteth me for his enemy,
11 He putteth my feet in the stocks, he
marketh all my paths.
12 Behold, *in* this thou art not just: I
will answer thee, that God is greater
than man.
13 Why dost thou strive against him?
for he giveth not account of any of his
matters.
14 For God speaketh once, yea twice,
yet man perceiveth it not.
15 In a dream, in a vision of the night,
when deep sleep falleth upon men, in
slumberings upon the bed;

His relations with mankind. It is the fatal misconception of all religious externalists and moralizers. Their God is always a small God. Elihu's account of God is noble and true, and it is noteworthy that at the last Jehovah does not class him with Eliphaz, Bildad, and Zophar (cf. Job 42:7); but he is still a dogmatist, and his eloquent discourse is marred by self-assertiveness (e.g. 32:8, 9; 33:3). Jehovah's judgment of Elihu is that he darkened counsel by words (38:2); the very charge that Elihu had brought against Job (34:35; 35:16). Furthermore, the discourse of Jehovah is wholly free from the accusations of Job with which even Elihu's lofty discourse abounds.

16 Then he openeth the ears of men, and sealeth their instruction,

17 That he may withdraw man *from his* purpose, and hide pride from man.

18 He keepeth back his soul from the pit, and his life from perishing by the sword.

19 He is chastened also with pain upon his bed, and the multitude of his bones with strong *pain*:

20 [a]So that his life abhorreth bread, and his soul dainty meat.

21 His flesh is consumed away, that it cannot be seen; and his bones *that* were not seen stick out.

22 Yea, his soul draweth near unto the grave, and his life to the destroyers.

23 If there be a messenger with him, an interpreter, one among a thousand, to shew unto man his uprightness:

24 Then he is gracious unto him, and saith, Deliver him from going down to the pit: I have found a [b]ransom.

25 His flesh shall be fresher than a child's: he shall return to the days of his youth:

26 He shall pray unto God, and he will be favourable unto him: and he shall see his face with joy: for he will render unto man his righteousness.

27 He looketh upon men, and *if any* say, I have sinned, and perverted *that which was* right, and it profited me not;

28 He will deliver his soul from going into the pit, and his life shall see the light.

29 Lo, all these *things* worketh God oftentimes with man,

30 To bring back his soul from the pit, to be enlightened with the light of the living.

31 Mark well, O Job, hearken unto me: hold thy peace, and I will speak.

32 If thou hast any thing to say, answer me: speak, for I desire to justify thee.

33 If not, hearken unto me: hold thy peace, and I shall teach thee wisdom.

CHAPTER 34.

(*Elihu's discourse*, continued.)

Furthermore Elihu answered and said,

2 Hear my words, O ye wise *men*; and give ear unto me, ye that have knowledge.

3 [d]For the ear trieth words, as the mouth tasteth meat.

4 Let us choose to us judgment: let us know among ourselves what *is* good.

5 For Job hath said, [e]I am righteous: and God hath taken away my judgment.

6 Should I lie against my right? my wound *is* incurable without transgression.

7 What man *is* like Job, *who* drinketh up scorning like water?

8 Which goeth in company with the workers of iniquity, and walketh with wicked men.

9 For he hath said, It profiteth a man nothing that he should delight himself with God.

10 Therefore hearken unto me, ye men of understanding: [f]far be it from God, *that he should do* wickedness; and *from* the Almighty, *that he should commit* iniquity.

11 For the work of a man shall he render unto him, and cause every man to find according to *his* ways.

12 Yea, surely God will not do wickedly, neither will the Almighty pervert judgment.

13 Who hath given him a charge over the earth? or who hath disposed the whole world?

14 If he set his heart upon man, *if* he [g]gather unto himself his spirit and his breath;

15 [h]All flesh shall perish together, and man shall turn again unto dust.

16 If now *thou hast* understanding, hear this: hearken to the voice of my words.

17 Shall even he that hateth right govern? and wilt thou condemn him that is most just?

18 *Is it fit* to say to a king, *Thou art* wicked? *and* to princes, *Ye are* ungodly?

19 *How much less to him* that accepteth not the persons of princes, nor regardeth the rich more than the poor? [i]for they all *are* the work of his hands.

20 In a moment shall they die, and the people shall be troubled at midnight, and pass away: and the mighty shall be taken away without hand.

21 [j]For his eyes *are* upon the ways of man, and he seeth all his goings.

22 *There is* no darkness, nor shadow of death, where the workers of iniquity may hide themselves.

23 For he will not lay upon man more *than right*; that he should enter into judgment with God.

B.C. 1520.

a Psa. 107:18.

b Or, *an atonement.*

c 2 Sam. 12:13; Prov. 28:13; Lk. 15:21; 1 John 1:9.

d Job 6:30; 12:11.

e Job 33:9.

f Job 8:3; 36:23; Gen. 18:25; Deut. 32:4; 2 Chr. 19:7; Psa. 92:15; Rom. 9:14.

g Psa. 104:29.

h Gen. 3:19; Eccl. 12:7.

i Job 31:15.

j Job 31:4; 2 Chr. 16:9; Psa. 34:15; Prov. 5:21; 15:3; Jer. 16:17; 32:19.

24 [a]He shall break in pieces mighty
men without number, and set others in
their stead.
25 Therefore he knoweth their works,
and he overturneth *them* in the night, so
that they are destroyed.
26 He striketh them as wicked men in
the open sight of others;
27 [b]Because they turned back from him,
and would not consider any of his ways:
28 So that they [c]cause the cry of the
poor to come unto him, [d]and he heareth
the cry of the afflicted.
29 When he giveth quietness, who
then can make trouble? and when he
hideth *his* face, who then can behold
him? whether *it be done* against a nation,
or against a man only:
30 That the hypocrite reign not, lest
the people be ensnared.
31 Surely it is meet to be said unto
God, I have borne *chastisement*, I will not
offend *any more*:
32 *That which* I see not teach thou me:
if I have done iniquity, I will do no more.
33 *Should it be* according to thy mind?
he will recompense it, whether thou
refuse, or whether thou choose; and not
I: therefore speak what thou knowest.
34 Let men of understanding tell me,
and let a wise man hearken unto me.
35 Job hath spoken without knowledge,
and his words *were* without wisdom.
36 My [e]desire *is that* Job may be tried
unto the end because of *his* answers for
wicked men.
37 For he addeth rebellion unto his
sin, he clappeth *his hands* among us, and
multiplieth his words against God.

CHAPTER 35.

(*Elihu's discourse*, continued.)

Elihu spake moreover, and said,
2 Thinkest thou this to be right, *that*
thou saidst, My righteousness *is* more
than God's?
3 For [f]thou saidst, What advantage
will it be unto thee? *and*, What profit
shall I have, *if I be cleansed* from my sin?
4 I will answer thee, and [g]thy companions with thee.
5 [h]Look unto the heavens, and see;
and behold the clouds *which* are higher
than thou.
6 If thou sinnest, what doest thou

B.C. 1520.

a Dan. 2:21.
b 1 Sam. 15:11.
c Job 35:9; Jas. 5:4.
d Ex. 22:23.
e Or, *My father, let Job be tried.*
f Job 21:15; 34:9.
g Job 34:8.
h Job 22:12
i Isa. 51:13.
j Psa. 42:8; 77:6; 149:5; Acts 16:25.
k Job 9:4; 12:13, 16; 37:23; Psa. 99:4.
l Psa. 107:10.

against him? or *if* thy transgressions be
multiplied, what doest thou unto him?
7 If thou be righteous, what givest thou
him? or what receiveth he of thine hand?
8 Thy wickedness *may hurt* a man as
thou *art*; and thy righteousness *may profit* the son of man.
9 By reason of the multitude of
oppressions they make *the oppressed* to
cry: they cry out by reason of the arm of
the mighty.
10 But none saith, [i]Where *is* God my
maker, [j]who giveth songs in the night;
11 Who teacheth us more than the
beasts of the earth, and maketh us wiser
than the fowls of heaven?
12 There they cry, but none giveth
answer, because of the pride of evil men.
13 Surely God will not hear vanity,
neither will the Almighty regard it.
14 Although thou sayest thou shalt
not see him, *yet* judgment *is* before him;
therefore trust thou in him.
15 But now, because *it is* not *so*, he
hath visited in his anger; yet he knoweth
it not in great extremity:
16 Therefore doth Job open his mouth
in vain; he multiplieth words without
knowledge.

CHAPTER 36.

(*Elihu's discourse*, continued.)

Elihu also proceeded, and said,
2 Suffer me a little, and I will shew
thee that *I have* yet to speak on God's
behalf.
3 I will fetch my knowledge from afar,
and will ascribe righteousness to my
Maker.
4 For truly my words *shall* not *be* false:
he that is perfect in knowledge *is* with
thee.
5 Behold, God *is* mighty, and despiseth
not *any*: [k]*he is* mighty in strength *and*
wisdom.
6 He preserveth not the life of the
wicked: but giveth right to the poor.
7 He withdraweth not his eyes from
the righteous: but with kings *are they* on
the throne; yea, he doth establish them
for ever, and they are exalted.
8 And [l]if *they be* bound in fetters, *and*
be holden in cords of affliction;
9 Then he sheweth them their work

and their transgressions that they have
exceeded.
10 [a]He openeth also their ear to discipline, and commandeth that they return
from iniquity.
11 If they obey and serve *him*, they
shall spend their days in prosperity, and
their years in pleasures.
12 But if they obey not, they shall perish by the sword, and they shall die
without knowledge.
13 But the hypocrites in heart [b]heap
up wrath: they cry not when he bindeth
them.
14 They die in youth, and their life *is*
among the unclean.
15 He delivereth the poor in his affliction, and openeth their ears in oppression.
16 Even so would he have removed
thee out of the strait [c]*into* a broad place,
where *there is* no straitness; and that
which should be set on thy table *should*
be full of fatness.
17 But thou hast fulfilled the judgment
of the wicked: judgment and justice take
hold *on thee*.
18 Because *there is* wrath, *beware* lest
he take thee away with *his* stroke: then a
great ransom cannot deliver thee.
19 Will he esteem thy riches? *no*, not
gold, nor all the forces of strength.
20 Desire not the night, when people
are cut off in their place.
21 Take heed, regard not iniquity: for
[d]this hast thou chosen rather than affliction.
22 Behold, God exalteth by his power:
who teacheth like him?
23 Who hath enjoined him his way? or
who can say, Thou hast wrought iniquity?
24 Remember that thou magnify his
work, which men behold.
25 Every man may see it; man may
behold *it* afar off.
26 Behold, God *is* great, and we [e]know
him not, neither can the number of his
years be searched out.
27 For he maketh small the drops of
water: they pour down rain according to
the vapour thereof:
28 Which the clouds do drop *and* distil
upon man abundantly.
29 Also can *any* understand the
spreadings of the clouds, *or* the noise of
his tabernacle?
30 Behold, he spreadeth his light upon
it, and covereth the bottom of the sea.

B.C. 1520.

a Job 33:16.
b Rom. 2:5.
c Psa. 18:19; 31:8; 118:5.
d See Heb. 11:24-26.
e 1 Cor. 13:12.
f Psa. 147:8.
g Job 5:9; 9:10; 36:26; Rev. 15:3.
h Psa. 147:16, 17.
i Psa. 109:27.
j Psa. 104:22.
k Job 38:29, 30; Psa. 147:17, 18.
l Psa. 148:8.
m Job 36:27-32; Ex. 9:18, 23; 1 Sam. 12:18, 19; Ezra 10:9.
n Psa. 111:2.

31 For by them judgeth he the people;
he giveth meat in abundance.
32 With [f]clouds he covereth the light;
and commandeth it *not to shine* by *the*
cloud that cometh betwixt.
33 The noise thereof sheweth concerning it, the cattle also concerning the
vapour.

CHAPTER 37.

(*Elihu's discourse,* continued.)

At this also my heart trembleth, and
is moved out of his place.
2 Hear attentively the noise of his
voice, and the sound *that* goeth out of
his mouth.
3 He directeth it under the whole
heaven, and his lightning unto the ends
of the earth.
4 After it a voice roareth: he thundereth with the voice of his excellency;
and he will not stay them when his voice
is heard.
5 God thundereth marvellously with
his voice; [g]great things doeth he, which
we cannot comprehend.
6 [h]For he saith to the snow, Be thou *on*
the earth; likewise to the small rain, and
to the great rain of his strength.
7 He sealeth up the hand of every
man; [i]that all men may know his work.
8 Then the beasts [j]go into dens, and
remain in their places.
9 Out of the south cometh the whirlwind: and cold out of the north.
10 [k]By the breath of God frost is given:
and the breadth of the waters is straitened.
11 Also by watering he wearieth the
thick cloud: he scattereth his bright
cloud:
12 And it is turned round about by his
counsels: [l]that they may do whatsoever
he commandeth them upon the face of
the world in the earth.
13 [m]He causeth it to come, whether for
correction, or for his land, or for mercy.
14 Hearken unto this, O Job: stand
still, and [n]consider the wondrous works
of God.
15 Dost thou know when God disposed them, and caused the light of his
cloud to shine?
16 Dost thou know the balancings of

the clouds, the wondrous works of him
which is perfect in knowledge?
17 How thy garments *are* warm, when
he quieteth the earth by the south *wind*?
18 Hast thou with him [a]spread out the
sky, *which is* strong, *and* as a molten looking glass?
19 Teach us what we shall say unto
him; *for* we cannot order *our speech* by
reason of darkness.
20 Shall it be told him that I speak? if a
man speak, surely he shall be swallowed
up.
21 And now *men* see not the bright
light which *is* in the clouds: but the wind
passeth, and cleanseth them.
22 Fair weather cometh out of the
north: with God *is* terrible majesty.
23 *Touching* the Almighty, [b]we cannot
find him out: *he is* excellent in power,
and in judgment, and in plenty of justice: he will not afflict.
24 Men do therefore [c]fear him: he
respecteth not any *that are* wise of heart.

CHAPTER 38.

Part V. Jehovah and Job.

Then the LORD [1]answered Job [d]out of
the whirlwind, and said,
2 [e]Who *is* this that darkeneth counsel
by words without knowledge?
3 Gird up now thy loins like a man; for I
will demand of thee, and answer thou me.
4 [f]Where wast thou when I laid the
foundations of the earth? declare, if thou
hast understanding.
5 Who hath laid the measures thereof,
if thou knowest? or who hath stretched
the line upon it?
6 Whereupon are the foundations
thereof fastened? or who laid the corner
stone thereof;
7 When the morning stars sang together, and all the [g]sons of God shouted for
joy?
8 [h]Or *who* shut up the sea with doors,
when it brake forth, *as if* it had issued
out of the womb?
9 When I made the cloud the garment
thereof, and thick darkness a swaddling-
band for it,
10 And brake up for it my decreed
place, and set bars and doors,
11 And said, Hitherto shalt thou come,
but no further: and here shall [i]thy proud
waves be stayed?
12 Hast thou [j]commanded the morning since thy days; *and* caused the
dayspring to know his place;
13 That it might take hold of the ends
of the earth, that the wicked might be
shaken out of it?
14 It is turned as clay *to* the seal; and
they stand as a garment.
15 And from the wicked their light is
withholden, and the high arm shall be
broken.
16 [k]Hast thou entered into the springs
of the sea? or hast thou walked in the
search of the depth?
17 [l]Have the gates of death been
opened unto thee? or hast thou seen the
doors of the shadow of death?
18 Hast thou perceived the breadth of
the earth? declare if thou knowest it all.
19 Where *is* the way *where* light
dwelleth? and *as for* darkness, where *is*
the place thereof,
20 That thou shouldest take it to the
bound thereof, and that thou shouldest
know the paths *to* the house thereof?
21 Knowest thou *it*, because thou wast
then born? or *because* the number of thy
days *is* great?
22 [m]Hast thou entered into the treasures of the snow? or hast thou seen the
treasures of the hail,
23 [n]Which I have reserved against the
time of trouble, against the day of battle
and war?
24 By what way is the light parted,
which scattereth the east wind upon the
earth?
25 Who hath divided a watercourse
for the overflowing of waters, or a way
for the lightning of thunder;
26 To cause it to rain on the earth,
where no man *is; on* the wilderness,
wherein *there is* no man;
27 To satisfy the desolate and waste
ground; and to cause the bud of the tender herb to spring forth?
28 [o]Hath the rain a father? or who
hath begotten the drops of dew?

B.C. 1520.

a Gen. 1:6; Isa. 44:24.
b 1 Tim. 6:16.
c Mt. 10:28.
d So Ex. 19:16, 18; 1 Ki. 19:11; Ezk. 1:4; Nah. 1:3.
e Job 34:35; 42:3.
f Psa. 104:5; Prov. 8:29; 30:4.
g Heb. 1:4, *note.*
h Gen. 1:9; Psa. 33:7; 104:9; Prov. 8:29; Jer. 5:22.
i Psa. 89:9; 93:4.
j Psa. 74:16; 148:5.
k Psa. 77:19.
l Psa. 9:13.
m Psa. 147:16.
n Ex. 9:18; Josh. 10:11; Isa. 30:30; Ezk. 13:11, 13; Rev. 16:21.
o Psa. 147:8; Jer. 14:22.

[1] **(38:1)** The words of Jehovah have the effect of bringing Job consciously into His presence (Job 42:5). Hitherto the discussions have been about God, but He has been conceived of as absent. Now Job and the LORD are face to face, It is noteworthy that Job does not answer Elihu. Despite his harsh judgment he has spoken so truly about God that Job remains silent. Job 38:1 might be paraphrased, "Then Jehovah answered *for* [or on behalf of] Job."

29 Out of whose womb came the ice?
[a]and the hoary frost of heaven, who hath
gendered it?
30 The waters are hid as *with* a stone,
and the face of the deep is frozen.
31 Canst thou bind the sweet influ-
ences of [b]Pleiades, or loose the bands of
Orion?
32 Canst thou bring forth Mazzaroth
in his season? or canst thou guide
Arcturus with his sons?
33 Knowest thou [c]the ordinances of
heaven? canst thou set the dominion
thereof in the earth?
34 Canst thou lift up thy voice to the
clouds, that abundance of waters may
cover thee?
35 Canst thou send lightnings, that
they may go, and say unto thee, Here we
are?
36 Who hath put wisdom in the
inward parts? or who hath given understanding to the heart?
37 Who can number the clouds in wisdom? or who can stay the bottles of
heaven,
38 When the dust groweth into hardness, and the clods cleave fast together?
39 [d]Wilt thou hunt the prey for the
lion? or fill the appetite of the young
lions,
40 When they couch in *their* dens, *and*
abide in the covert to lie in wait?
41 [e]Who provideth for the raven his
food? when his young ones cry unto
God, they wander for lack of meat.

CHAPTER 39.

(*Jehovah and Job*, continued.)

Knowest thou the time when the wild
goats of the rock bring forth? *or*
canst thou mark when the hinds do
calve?
2 Canst thou number the months *that*
they fulfil? or knowest thou the time
when they bring forth?
3 They bow themselves, they bring
forth their young ones, they cast out
their sorrows.
4 Their young ones are in good liking,
they grow up with corn; they go forth,
and return not unto them.
5 Who hath sent out the wild ass free?
or who hath loosed the bands of the
wild ass?
6 [f]Whose house I have made the
wilderness, and the [g]barren land his
dwellings.

B.C. 1520.

a Psa. 147:16.

b Or, *the seven stars.* Job 9:9; Amos 5:8.

c Psa. 148:6; Jer. 31:35.

d Psa. 104:21; 145:15.

e Psa. 147:9; Mt. 6:26.

f Job 24:5; Jer. 2:24; Hos. 8:9.

g Heb. *salt places.*

h Num. 23:22; Deut. 33:17.

i Lam. 4:3.

j Jer. 49:16; Oba. 4.

7 He scorneth the multitude of the city,
neither regardeth he the crying of the
driver.
8 The range of the mountains *is* his
pasture, and he searcheth after every
green thing.
9 [h]Will the unicorn be willing to serve
thee, or abide by thy crib?
10 Canst thou bind the unicorn with
his band in the furrow? or will he harrow the valleys after thee?
11 Wilt thou trust him, because his
strength *is* great? or wilt thou leave thy
labour to him?
12 Wilt thou believe him, that he will
bring home thy seed, and gather *it into*
thy barn?
13 *Gavest thou* the goodly wings unto
the peacocks? or wings and feathers
unto the ostrich?
14 Which leaveth her eggs in the earth,
and warmeth them in dust,
15 And forgetteth that the foot may
crush them, or that the wild beast may
break them.
16 She is [i]hardened against her young
ones, as though *they were* not hers: her
labour is in vain without fear;
17 Because God hath deprived her of
wisdom, neither hath he imparted to her
understanding.
18 What time she lifteth up herself on
high, she scorneth the horse and his
rider.
19 Hast thou given the horse strength?
hast thou clothed his neck with thunder?
20 Canst thou make him afraid as a
grasshopper? the glory of his nostrils *is*
terrible.
21 He paweth in the valley, and
rejoiceth in *his* strength: he goeth on to
meet the armed men.
22 He mocketh at fear, and is not
affrighted; neither turneth he back from
the sword.
23 The quiver rattleth against him, the
glittering spear and the shield.
24 He swalloweth the ground with
fierceness and rage: neither believeth he
that *it is* the sound of the trumpet.
25 He saith among the trumpets, Ha,
ha; and he smelleth the battle afar off,
the thunder of the captains, and the
shouting.
26 Doth the hawk fly by thy wisdom,
and stretch her wings toward the south?
27 Doth the eagle [j]mount up at thy
command, and make her nest on high?
28 She dwelleth and abideth on the

rock, upon the crag of the rock, and the strong place.

29 From thence she seeketh the prey, *and* her eyes behold afar off.

30 Her young ones also suck up blood: and where the slain *are*, there *is* she.

CHAPTER 40.

(*Jehovah and Job,* continued.)

Moreover the LORD answered Job, and said,

2 Shall he that contendeth with the Almighty instruct *him*? he that reproveth God, let him answer it.

3 Then Job answered the LORD, and said,

4 [a]Behold, I am vile; what shall I answer thee? I will lay mine hand upon my mouth.

5 Once have I spoken; but I will not answer: yea, twice; but I will proceed no further.

6 Then [b]answered the LORD unto Job out of the whirlwind, and said,

7 Gird up thy loins now like a man: I will demand of thee, and declare thou unto me.

8 Wilt thou also disannul my judgment? wilt thou condemn me, that thou mayest be righteous?

9 Hast thou an arm like God? or canst thou thunder with a voice like him?

10 Deck thyself now *with* majesty and excellency; and array thyself with glory and beauty.

11 Cast abroad the rage of thy wrath: and behold every one *that is* proud, and abase him.

12 Look on every one *that is* [c]proud, *and* bring him low; and tread down the wicked in their place.

13 Hide them in the dust together; *and* bind their faces in secret.

14 Then will I also confess unto thee that thine own right hand can save thee.

15 Behold now [d]behemoth, which I made with thee; he eateth grass as an ox.

16 Lo now, his strength *is* in his loins, and his force *is* in the navel of his belly.

17 He moveth his tail like a cedar: the sinews of his stones are wrapped together.

18 His bones *are as* strong pieces of brass; his bones *are* like bars of iron.

19 He *is* the chief of the ways of God: he that made him can make his sword to approach *unto him*.

20 Surely the mountains [e]bring him forth food, where all the beasts of the field play.

21 He lieth under the shady trees, in the covert of the reed, and fens.

22 The shady trees cover him *with* their shadow; the willows of the brook compass him about.

23 Behold, he drinketh up a river, *and* hasteth not: he trusteth that he can draw up Jordan into his mouth.

24 He taketh it with his eyes: *his* nose pierceth through snares.

CHAPTER 41.

(*Jehovah and Job,* continued.)

Canst thou draw out leviathan with an hook? or his tongue with a cord *which* thou lettest down?

2 Canst thou put an hook into his nose? or bore his jaw through with a thorn?

3 Will he make many supplications unto thee? will he speak soft *words* unto thee?

4 Will he make a covenant with thee? wilt thou take him for a servant for ever?

5 Wilt thou play with him as *with* a bird? or wilt thou bind him for thy maidens?

6 Shall the companions make a banquet of him? shall they part him among the merchants?

7 Canst thou fill his skin with barbed irons? or his head with fish spears?

8 Lay thine hand upon him, remember the battle, do no more.

9 Behold, the hope of him is in vain: shall not *one* be cast down even at the sight of him?

10 None *is so* fierce that dare stir him up: who then is able to stand before me?

11 Who hath prevented me, that I should repay *him? whatsoever is* under the whole heaven is [f]mine.

12 I will not conceal his parts, nor his power, nor his comely proportion.

13 Who can discover the face of his garment? *or* who can come *to him* with his double bridle?

14 Who can open the doors of his face? his teeth *are* terrible round about.

15 *His* scales *are his* pride, shut up together *as with* a close seal.

B.C. 1520.

a Job 42:6; Ezra 9:6; Psa. 51:4.

b Job 38:1.

c Isa. 2:12; Dan. 4:37.

d Or, *the elephant,* as some think.

e Psa. 104:14.

f Deut. 10:14; Rom. 11:35.

16 One is so near to another, that no
air can come between them.
17 They are joined one to another, they
stick together, that they cannot be sundered.
18 By his neesings a light doth shine,
and his eyes *are* like the eyelids of the
morning.
19 Out of his mouth go burning
lamps, *and* sparks of fire leap out.
20 Out of his nostrils goeth smoke, as
out of a seething pot or caldron.
21 His breath kindleth coals, and a
flame goeth out of his mouth.
22 In his neck remaineth strength, and
[a]sorrow is turned into joy before him.
23 The flakes of his flesh are joined
together: they are firm in themselves;
they cannot be moved.
24 His heart is as firm as a stone; yea,
as hard as a piece of the nether *millstone*.
25 When he raiseth up himself, the
mighty are afraid: by reason of breakings they purify themselves.
26 The sword of him that layeth at him
cannot hold: the spear, the dart, nor the
[b]habergeon.
27 He esteemeth iron as straw, *and*
brass as rotten wood.
28 The arrow cannot make him flee:
slingstones are turned with him into
stubble.
29 Darts are counted as stubble: he
laugheth at the shaking of a spear.
30 [c]Sharp stones *are* under him: he
spreadeth sharp pointed things upon the
mire.
31 He maketh the deep to boil like a
pot: he maketh the sea like a pot of ointment.
32 He maketh a path to shine after him;
one would think the deep *to be* hoary.
33 Upon earth there is not his like,
[d]who is made without fear.
34 He beholdeth all high *things*: he *is* a
king over all the children of pride.

B.C. 1520.

a Heb. *sorrow rejoiceth.*

b Or, *breastplate.*

c Heb. *sharp pieces of potsherd.*

d Or, *who behave themselves without fear.*

e Zech. 8:14, *note.*

f Num. 23:1.

g Psa. 14:7; 85:1-3; 126:1.

h See Job 19:13.

CHAPTER 42.

Part VI. Job's self-judgment.

Then Job answered the LORD, and
said,
2 I know that thou canst do every
thing, and *that* no thought can be withholden from thee.
3 Who *is* he that hideth counsel without knowledge? therefore have I uttered
that I understood not; things too wonderful for me, which I knew not.
4 Hear, I beseech thee, and I will
speak: I will demand of thee, and
declare thou unto me.
5 I have heard of thee by the hearing
of the ear: but now mine eye seeth thee.
6 [1]Wherefore I abhor *myself*, and [e]repent in dust and ashes.

Part VII. Epilogue:
Job vindicated and honoured.

7 And it was *so*, that after the LORD
had spoken these words unto Job, the
LORD said to Eliphaz the Temanite, My
wrath is kindled against thee, and
against thy two friends: for ye have not
spoken of me *the thing that is* right, as my
servant Job *hath*.
8 Therefore take unto you now [f]seven
bullocks and seven rams, and go to my
servant Job, and offer up for yourselves
a burnt-offering; and my servant Job
shall pray for you: for him will I accept:
lest I deal with you *after your* folly, in
that ye have not spoken of me *the thing
which is* right, like my servant Job.
9 So Eliphaz the Temanite and Bildad
the Shuhite *and* Zophar the Naamathite
went, and did according as the LORD commanded them: the LORD also accepted Job.
10 [g]And the LORD turned the captivity
of Job, when he prayed for his friends:
also the LORD gave Job twice as much as
he had before.
11 Then came there unto him [h]all his
brethren, and all his sisters, and all they

[1]**(42:6)** The problem, of which the book of Job is the profound discussion, finds here its solution. Brought into the presence of God, Job is revealed to himself. In no sense a hypocrite, but godly and possessing a faith which all his afflictions could not shake, Job was yet self-righteous and lacking in humility. Chapter 29 fully discloses this. But in the presence of God he anticipates, as it were, the experience of Paul (Phil. 3:4-9), and the problem is solved. *The godly are afflicted that they may be brought to self-knowledge and self-judgment.* Such afflictions are not penal for their sins, but remedial and purifying. The book of Job affords a sublime illustration of the truth announced in 1 Cor. 11:31, 32, and Heb. 12:7-11. Best of all, such self-knowledge and self-judgment is the prelude to greater fruitfulness (vs. 7-17; John 15:2). Cf. Josh. 5:13, 14; Ezk. 1:28; 2:1-3; Dan. 10:5-11; Rev. 1:17-19.

that had been of his acquaintance before,
and did eat bread with him in his house:
and they bemoaned him, and comforted
him over all the evil that the LORD had
brought upon him: every man also gave
him a piece of money, and every one an
earring of gold.
12 So the LORD blessed [a]the latter end
of Job more than his beginning: for he
had [b]fourteen thousand sheep, and six
thousand camels, and a thousand yoke
of oxen, and a thousand she asses.
13 [c]He had also seven sons and three
daughters.
14 And he called the name of the first,
Jemima; and the name of the second,
Kezia; and the name of the third, Keren-happuch.
15 And in all the land were no women
found *so* fair as the daughters of Job: and
their father gave them inheritance
among their brethren.
16 After this [d]lived Job an hundred
and forty years, and saw his sons, and
his sons' sons, *even* four generations.
17 So Job died, *being* old and [e]full of
days.

B.C. 1520.

a Job 8:7; Jas. 5:11.
b Job 1:3.
c Job 1:2.
d Job 5:26; Prov. 3:16.
e Gen. 25:8.

THE BOOK OF PSALMS

THE simplest description of the five books of Psalms is that they were the inspired prayer-and-praise book of Israel. They are revelations of truth, not abstractly, but in the terms of human experience. The truth revealed is wrought into the emotions, desires, and sufferings of the people of God by the circumstances through which they pass. But those circumstances are such as to constitute an anticipation of analogous conditions through which Christ in His incarnation, and the Jewish remnant in the tribulation (Isa. 10:21, *refs.*), should pass; so that many Psalms are prophetic of the sufferings, the faith, and the victory of both. Psalms 22 and 60 are examples. The former—the holy of holies of the Bible—reveals all that was in the mind of Christ when He uttered the desolate cry, "My God, My God, why hast Thou forsaken Me?" The latter is an anticipation of what will be in the heart of Israel when she shall turn to Jehovah again (Deut. 30:1, 2). Other Psalms are directly prophetic of "the sufferings of Christ, and the glories which should follow" (Luke 24:25-27, 44). Psa. 2 is a notable instance, presenting Jehovah's Anointed as rejected and crucified (vs. 1-3; Acts 4:24-28), but afterward set as King in Zion.

The great themes of the Psalms are, Christ, Jehovah, the Law, Creation, the future of Israel, and the exercises of the renewed heart in suffering, in joy, in perplexity. The promises of the Psalms are primarily Jewish, and suited to a people under the law, but are spiritually true in Christian experience also, in the sense that they disclose the mind of God, and the exercises of His heart toward those who are perplexed, afflicted, or cast down.

The imprecatory Psalms are the cry of the oppressed in Israel for *justice*—a cry appropriate and right in the earthly people of God, and based upon a distinct promise in the Abrahamic Covenant (Gen. 15:18, *refs.*); but a cry unsuited to the church, a heavenly people who have taken their place with a rejected and crucified Christ (Luke 9:52-55).

The Psalms are in five books, each ending in a doxology: I. Psalms 1–41. II. Psalms 42–72. III. Psalms 73–89. IV. Psalms 90–106. V. Psalms 107–150.

BOOK I

PSALM 1.

Psalm of the two ways: introductory to entire Psalter.

Blessed *is* the man that walketh not in the counsel of the ungodly, nor standeth in the way of sinners, nor sitteth in the seat of the scornful.

2 But his delight *is* in the [a]law of the LORD; and in his law doth he meditate day and night.

3 And he shall be like a tree planted by the rivers of water, that bringeth forth his fruit in his season; his leaf also shall not wither; and whatsoever he doeth shall prosper.

4 The ungodly *are* not so: but *are* like the chaff which the wind driveth away.

5 Therefore the ungodly shall not stand in the judgment, nor sinners in the congregation of the righteous.

6 For the LORD knoweth the way of the righteous: but the way of the ungodly shall perish.

PSALM 2.

Psalm of the King: (1) *rejected;* (2) *established;* (3) *reigning over the nations.*

Why [b]do the heathen rage, and the people imagine [c]a vain thing?

2 The kings of the earth set themselves, and the [d]rulers take counsel together, against the LORD, and against his [e]anointed, *saying,*

3 Let us break their bands asunder, and cast away their cords from us.

4 He that sitteth in the heavens shall laugh: the Lord shall have them in derision.

5 Then shall he speak unto them

a *Law (of Moses).* Psa. 19:7, 8. (Ex. 19:1; Gal. 3:1-29.)

b *Kingdom* (O.T.). vs. 1-9; Psa. 16:8-11. (Gen. 1:26; Zech. 12:8.)

c *Sacrifice (prophetic).* vs. 1-3; Psa. 22:1-18. (Gen. 4:4; Heb. 10:18.)

d Mt. 12:14; 26:3, 4, 47, 57, 59-66; 27:1, 2, 11-14; Mk. 3:6; 11:18; Lk. 6:11; John 5:16, 18; 8:40, 59; 10.

e *Christ (First Advent).* Psa. 16:10. (Gen. 3:15; Acts 1:9.)

in his wrath, and [a]vex them in his sore
displeasure.
6 Yet have I set my [1]king upon my
[bc]holy hill of Zion.
7 I will declare the decree: the LORD
hath said unto me, [d]Thou *art* my Son;
this day have I begotten thee.
8 Ask of me, and I shall give *thee* the
heathen *for* thine inheritance, and the
uttermost parts of the earth *for* thy possession.
9 [e]Thou shalt break them with a rod of
iron; thou shalt [f]dash them in pieces like
a potter's vessel.
10 Be wise now therefore, O ye kings:
be instructed, ye judges of the earth.
11 Serve the LORD with [g]fear, and
rejoice with trembling.
12 Kiss the Son, lest he be angry, and
ye perish *from* the way, when his wrath
is kindled but a little. Blessed *are* all they
that [h]put their [2]trust in him.

PSALM 3.

A Psalm of David,
when he fled from Absalom his son.

LORD, how are they increased that
trouble me! many *are* they that rise
up against me.
2 Many *there be* which say of my soul,
There is no help for him in God. Selah.
3 But thou, O LORD, *art* a shield for me;
my glory, and the lifter up of mine head.
4 I cried unto the LORD with my voice,
and he heard me out of his holy hill.
Selah.

a *Tribulation (the great).* Jer. 30:4-7. (Psa. 2:5; Rev. 7:14.)

b Heb. *qodesh.*

c *Sanctify, holy* (O.T.). Psa. 20:2. (Gen. 2:3; Zech. 8:3.)

d Acts 13:33; Heb. 1:5; 5:5.

e *Christ (Second Advent).* Psa. 24:1-10. (Deut. 30:3; Acts 1:9-11.)

f *Day (of Jehovah).* v. 9; Rev. 6:15-17. (Isa. 2:10-22; Rev. 19:11-21.)

g Psa. 19:9, *note.*

h *Faith.* Psa. 28:7. (Gen. 3:20; Heb. 11:39.)

i Eph. 4:26.

j Psa. 2:12, *note.*

5 I laid me down and slept; I awaked;
for the LORD sustained me.
6 I will not be afraid of ten thousands
of people, that have set *themselves*
against me round about.
7 Arise, O LORD; save me, O my God:
for thou hast smitten all mine enemies
upon the cheek bone; thou hast broken
the teeth of the ungodly.
8 Salvation *belongeth* unto the LORD:
thy blessing *is* upon thy people. Selah.

PSALM 4.

To the chief Musician on [3]Neginoth,
A Psalm of David.

HEAR me when I call, O God of my
righteousness: thou hast enlarged
me *when I was* in distress; have mercy
upon me, and hear my prayer.
2 O ye sons of men, how long *will ye*
turn my glory into shame? *how long* will
ye love vanity, *and* seek after leasing?
Selah.
3 But know that the LORD hath set
apart him that is godly for himself: the
LORD will hear when I call unto him.
4 Stand in awe, [i]and sin not: commune
with your own heart upon your bed,
and be still. Selah.
5 Offer the sacrifices of righteousness,
and put your [j]trust in the LORD.
6 *There be* many that say, Who

[1] **(2:6)** The second Psalm gives the *order* of the establishment of the kingdom. It is in six parts: (1) The rage of the Gentiles, the vain imagination of "the people" (Jews), and the antagonism of rulers against Jehovah's anointed (vs. 1-3). The inspired interpretation of this is in Acts 4:25-28, which asserts its fulfilment in the crucifixion of Christ. (2) The derision of Jehovah (v. 4) that men should suppose it possible to set aside His covenant (2 Sam. 7:8-17), and oath (Psa. 89:34-37). (3) The vexation (v. 5) fulfilled, *first* in the destruction of Jerusalem, A.D. 70; and in the final dispersion of the Jews at that time; and to be fulfilled more completely in the tribulation (Mt. 24:29) which immediately precedes the return of the King (Mt. 24:30). (4) The establishment of the rejected King upon Zion (v. 6). (5) The subjection of the earth to the King's rule (vs. 7-9); and (6) the present appeal to the world-powers (vs. 10-12). See Psa. 8, next in order of the Messianic Psalms. (Note. Psalms 2; 8; 16; 22; 23; 24; 40; 41; 45; 68; 69; 72; 89; 102; 110; 118, are classed as Messianic. It is not questioned that many other Psalms also refer to Christ.)

[2] **(2:12)** Trust is the characteristic O. T. word for the N. T. "faith," "believe." It occurs 152 times in the O. T., and is the rendering of Heb. words signifying *to take refuge* (e.g. Ruth 2:12); *to lean on* (e.g. Psa. 56:3); *to roll on* (e.g. Psa. 22:8); *to stay upon* (e.g. Job 35:14).

[3] **(4, inscription)** Neginoth: stringed instruments mentioned in connection with Psalms 3; 5; 53; 54; 60; 66; 75, where it seems clear that the musical directions now appearing as titles of Psalms 4; 6; 54; 55; 61; 67; and 76, were anciently appended to the preceding Psalms.

will shew us *any* good? LORD, [a]lift thou
up the light of thy countenance upon us.
7 Thou hast put [b]gladness in my heart,
more than in the time *that* their corn and
their wine increased.
8 [c]I will both lay me down in peace,
and sleep: for thou, LORD, [d]only makest
me dwell in safety.

PSALM 5.

To the chief Musician upon [1]Nehiloth,
A Psalm of David.

Give ear to my words, O LORD, consider my meditation.
2 Hearken unto the voice of my cry,
my King, and my God: for unto thee will
I pray.
3 My voice shalt thou hear in the morning, O LORD; in the morning will I direct
my prayer unto thee, and will look up.
4 For thou *art* not a God that hath
pleasure in wickedness: neither shall evil
dwell with thee.
5 [e]The foolish shall not stand in thy
sight: thou hatest all workers of iniquity.
6 Thou shalt destroy them that speak
leasing: the LORD will abhor the bloody
and deceitful man.
7 But as for me, I will come *into* thy
house in the multitude of thy mercy: *and*
in thy [f]fear will I worship toward thy
holy temple.
8 Lead me, O LORD, in thy righteousness because of mine enemies; make thy
way straight before my face.
9 For *there is* no faithfulness in their
mouth; their inward part *is* very wickedness; [g]their throat *is* an open sepulchre;
they flatter with their tongue.
10 Destroy thou them, O God; let them
fall by their own counsels; cast them out
in the multitude of their transgressions;
for they have rebelled against thee.
11 But let all those that put their [h]trust
in thee rejoice: let them ever shout for joy,
because thou defendest them: let them
also that love thy name be joyful in thee.
12 For thou, LORD, wilt bless the righteous; with favour wilt thou compass
him as *with* a shield.

a Num. 6:26; Psa. 80:3, 7, 19; 119:135.
b Isa. 9.3.
c Job 11:18, 19; Psa. 3:5.
d Lev. 25:18, 19; 26:5; Deut. 12:10.
e Hab. 1:13.
f Psa. 19:9, *note.*
g Rom. 3:13.
h Psa. 2:12, *note.*
i *Stringed instruments.*
j *The word means "the eighth"—in music an octave.*
k Mt. 7:23.
l *Shiggaion = praise.*
m Psa. 31:15.
n Heb. *not a deliverer.*
o 2 Sam. 16:7, 8.
p Psa. 94:2.

PSALM 6.

To the chief Musician on [i]Neginoth upon
[j]Sheminith, A Psalm of David.

O LORD, rebuke me not in thine anger,
neither chasten me in thy hot displeasure.
2 Have mercy upon me, O LORD; for I
am weak: O LORD, heal me; for my bones
are vexed.
3 My soul is also sore vexed: but thou,
O LORD, how long?
4 Return, O LORD, deliver my soul: oh
save me for thy mercies' sake.
5 For in death *there is* no remembrance
of thee: in the grave who shall give thee
thanks?
6 I am weary with my groaning; all
the night make I my bed to swim; I
water my couch with my tears.
7 Mine eye is consumed because of
grief; it waxeth old because of all mine
enemies.
8 Depart from me, all ye workers of
[k]iniquity; for the LORD hath heard the
voice of my weeping.
9 The LORD hath heard my supplication; the LORD will receive my prayer.
10 Let all mine enemies be ashamed
and sore vexed: let them return *and* be
ashamed suddenly.

PSALM 7.

[l]Shiggaion of David, which he sang
unto the LORD, concerning the words
of Cush the Benjamite.

O LORD my God, in thee do I put my
[h]trust: [m]save me from all them that
persecute me, and deliver me:
2 Lest he tear my soul like a lion, rending *it* in pieces, while *there is* [n]none to
deliver.
3 O LORD my God, [o]if I have done this;
if there be iniquity in my hands;
4 If I have rewarded evil unto him that
was at peace with me; (yea, I have delivered him that without cause is mine
enemy:)
5 Let the enemy persecute my soul,
and take *it*; yea, let him tread down my
life upon the earth, and lay mine honour
in the dust. Selah.
6 Arise, O LORD, in thine anger,
[p]lift up thyself because of the rage

[1]**(5, inscription)** Nehiloth is not a musical instrument, but means "inheritance," and indicates the character of the Psalm. The righteous are the Lord's inheritance.

of mine enemies: and awake for me *to* the
judgment *that* thou hast commanded.
7 So shall the congregation of the people compass thee about: for their sakes
therefore return thou on high.
8 The LORD shall judge the people:
judge me, O LORD, [a]according to my
righteousness, and according to mine
integrity *that is* in me.
9 Oh let the wickedness of the wicked
come to an end; but establish the just: for
the righteous God trieth the hearts and
reins.
10 My [b]defence *is* of God, which
saveth the upright in heart.
11 God judgeth the righteous, and
God is angry *with the wicked* every day.
12 If he turn not, he will whet his
sword; he hath bent his bow, and made
it ready.
13 He hath also prepared for him the
instruments of death; he ordaineth his
arrows against the persecutors.
14 Behold, he travaileth with iniquity,
and hath conceived mischief, and
brought forth falsehood.
15 He made a pit, and digged it, and is
fallen into the ditch *which* he made.
16 His mischief shall return upon his
own head, and his violent dealing shall
come down upon his own pate.
17 I will praise the LORD according to
his righteousness: and will sing praise to
the name of the LORD most high.

PSALM 8.

To the chief Musician upon [1]Gittith,
A Psalm of David.

O LORD our Lord, how excellent *is* thy
name in all the earth! who hast set
thy glory above the heavens.
2 Out of the mouth of babes and
[c]sucklings hast thou ordained strength
because of thine enemies, that thou
mightest still the enemy and the
avenger.
3 When I consider thy heavens, the
work of thy fingers, the moon and the
stars, which thou hast ordained;
4 What is [d]man, that thou art mindful
of him? and the son of man, that thou
visitest him?
5 [2]For thou hast made him a little
lower than the [e]angels, and hast
crowned him with glory and honour.
6 Thou madest him to have dominion
over the works of thy hands; thou hast
put [f]all *things* under his feet:
7 All sheep and oxen, yea, and the
beasts of the field;
8 The fowl of the air, and the fish of
the sea, *and whatsoever* passeth through
the paths of the seas.
9 O LORD our Lord, how excellent *is*
thy name in all the earth!

PSALM 9.

To the chief Musician upon
[3]Muth-labben, A Psalm of David.

I will praise *thee*, O LORD, with my
whole heart; I will shew forth all thy
marvellous works.
2 I will be glad and rejoice in thee: I
will sing praise to thy name, O thou
most High.
3 When mine enemies are turned back,
they shall fall and perish at thy presence.
4 For thou hast maintained my right
and my cause; thou satest in the throne
judging right.
5 Thou hast rebuked the [g]heathen,

a Psa. 18:20; 35:24.
b Heb. *my buckler is upon God.*
c Mt. 21:16; cf. 1 Cor. 1:26-31.
d Job 7:17-18; Heb. 2:6-8.
e Heb. 1:4, *note.*
f 1 Cor. 15:27.
g i.e. *nations.*

[1] **(8, inscription)** *Gittith* = "winepress," and so, of the harvest, in the sense of judgment (Isa. 63:3; Rev. 19:15). Psalm 7, to which the title of Psalm 8 properly belongs, is a Psalm of judgment.

[2] **(8:5)** In Psa. 2 Christ was presented as Jehovah's Son and King, rejected and crucified but yet to reign in Zion. In Psa. 8, while His deity is fully recognized (v. 1; Psa. 110 with Mt. 22:41-46), He is seen as Son of man (vs. 4-6) who, "made for a little [while] lower than the angels," is to have dominion over the redeemed creation (Heb. 2:6-11). The authority here is racial and Adamic, rather than purely divine as in Psa. 2, or Davidic as in Psa. 89. That which the first man lost, the second man and "last Adam" more than regained. Heb. 2:6-11, in connection with Psa. 8, and Rom. 8:17-21, show that the "many sons" whom He is bringing to glory, are joint heirs with Him in both the royal right of Psa. 2. and the human right of Heb. 2. See Psa. 16, next in order of the Messianic Psalms.

[3] **(9, inscription)** *Muth-labben,* "death of the son," is not a musical instrument but the title of the Psalm. Possibly connected with 2 Sam. 12:20.

thou hast destroyed the wicked, thou hast put out their name for ever and ever.

6 O thou enemy, destructions are come to a perpetual end: and thou hast destroyed cities; their memorial is perished with them.

7 [a]But the LORD shall endure for ever: he hath prepared his throne for judgment.

8 [b]And he shall judge the world in righteousness, he shall minister judgment to the people in uprightness.

9 [c]The LORD also will be a refuge for the oppressed, a refuge in times of trouble.

10 And they that know thy name will put their [d]trust in thee: for thou, LORD, hast not forsaken them that seek thee.

11 Sing praises to the LORD, which dwelleth in Zion: declare among the people his doings.

12 [e]When he maketh inquisition for blood, he remembereth them: he forgetteth not the cry of the [f]humble.

13 Have mercy upon me, O LORD; consider my trouble *which I suffer* of them that hate me, thou that liftest me up from the gates of death:

14 That I may shew forth all thy praise in the gates of the daughter of Zion: [g]I will rejoice in thy salvation.

15 The [h]heathen are sunk down in the pit *that* they made: in the net which they hid is their own foot taken.

16 The LORD is known *by* the judgment *which* he executeth: the wicked is snared in the work of his own hands. [i]Higgaion. Selah.

17 The wicked shall be turned into hell, *and* all the nations that forget God.

18 For the needy shall not alway be forgotten: the expectation of the poor shall *not* perish for ever.

19 Arise, O LORD; let not man prevail: let the [h]heathen be judged in thy sight.

20 Put them in fear, O LORD: *that* the nations may know themselves *to be but* men. Selah.

PSALM 10.

Why standest thou afar off, O LORD? *why* hidest thou *thyself* in times of trouble?

2 The wicked in *his* pride doth persecute the poor: let them be taken in the devices that they have imagined.

3 For the wicked boasteth of his heart's desire, and blesseth the covetous, *whom* the LORD abhorreth.

4 The wicked, through the pride of his countenance, will not seek *after God*: God *is* not in all his thoughts.

5 His ways are always grievous; thy judgments *are* far above out of his sight: *as for* all his enemies, he puffeth at them.

6 He hath said in his heart, I shall not be moved: for *I shall* never *be* in adversity.

7 His mouth is full of [j]cursing and deceit and fraud: under his tongue *is* mischief and vanity.

8 He sitteth in the lurking places of the villages: in the secret places doth he murder the innocent: his eyes [k]are privily set against the poor.

9 He lieth in wait secretly as a lion in his den: he lieth in wait to catch the poor: he doth catch the poor, when he draweth him into his net.

10 He croucheth, *and* humbleth himself, that the poor may fall [l]by his strong ones.

11 He hath said in his heart, God hath forgotten: he hideth his face; he will never see *it*.

12 Arise, O LORD; O God, [m]lift up thine hand: forget not the humble.

13 Wherefore doth the wicked contemn God? he hath said in his heart, Thou wilt not require *it*.

14 Thou hast seen *it*; for thou beholdest mischief and spite, to requite *it* with thy hand: the poor committeth himself unto thee; [n]thou art the helper of the fatherless.

15 Break thou the arm of the wicked and the evil *man*: seek out his wickedness *till* thou find none.

16 The LORD *is* King for ever and ever: the [h]heathen are perished out of his land.

17 LORD, thou hast heard the desire of the humble: thou wilt prepare their heart, thou wilt cause thine ear to hear:

18 To judge the fatherless and the oppressed, that the man of the earth may no more oppress.

a Psa. 102:12, 26; Heb. 1:11.
b Psa. 96:13; 98:9; Acts 17:31.
c Psa. 32:7; 37:39; 46:1; 91:2.
d Psa. 2:12, *note.*
e Gen. 9:5; cf. 1 Ki. 21:17-19.
f Or, *afflicted.*
g Psa. 13:5; 20:5; 35:9.
h i.e. *nations.*
i *Meditation.*
j Rom. 3:14.
k Heb. *hide themselves.*
l Or, *into his strong parts.*
m Mic. 5:9.
n Psa. 68:5; Hos. 14:3.

PSALM 11.

To the chief Musician,
A Psalm of David.

In the LORD put I my [a]trust: how say ye to my soul, Flee *as* a bird to your mountain?

2 For, lo, the wicked bend *their* bow, they make ready their arrow upon the string, that they may [b]privily shoot at the upright in heart.

3 [c]If the foundations be destroyed, what can the righteous do?

4 The LORD *is* in his holy temple, the LORD'S [d]throne *is* in heaven: his eyes behold, his eyelids try, the children of men.

5 The LORD [e]trieth the righteous: but the wicked and him that loveth violence his soul hateth.

6 Upon the wicked he shall rain [f]snares, fire and brimstone, and an horrible tempest: [g]*this shall be* the portion of their cup.

7 For the righteous LORD loveth righteousness; his countenance doth behold the upright.

PSALM 12.

To the chief Musician upon [h]Sheminith,
A Psalm of David.

Help, LORD; for the godly man ceaseth; for the faithful fail from among the children of men.

2 They speak vanity every one with his neighbour: *with* flattering lips *and* with a double heart do they speak.

3 The LORD shall cut off all flattering lips, *and* [i]the tongue that speaketh proud things:

4 Who have said, With our tongue will we prevail; our lips *are* our own: who *is* lord over us?

5 For the oppression of the poor, for the sighing of the needy, now will I arise, saith the LORD; I will set *him* in safety *from him that* [j]puffeth at him.

6 The words of the LORD *are* [k]pure words: *as* silver tried in a furnace of earth, purified seven times.

7 Thou shalt keep them, O LORD, thou shalt preserve them from this generation for ever.

8 The wicked walk on every side, when the vilest men are exalted.

a Psa. 2:12, *note.*
b Heb. *in darkness.*
c Psa. 82:5.
d Psa. 2:4; Isa. 66:1; Mt. 5:34; 23:22; Acts 7:49; Rev. 4:2.
e Gen. 22:1; Jas. 1:12.
f Or, *quick burning coals.*
g See Gen. 43:34; 1 Sam. 9:23; Psa. 75:8.
h See Psa. 6, title.
i Psa. 17:10; 1 Sam. 2:3; Dan. 7:8, 25.
j Or, *would ensnare him.*
k Psa. 18:30; 119:140; Prov. 30:5.
l v. 3; Rom. 3:10.
m Rom. 3:11.
n Rom. 3:12.
o Jer. 10:25; Amos 8:4; Mic. 3:3.
p Psa. 53:6; Rom. 11:25-27.

PSALM 13.

To the chief Musician,
A Psalm of David.

How long wilt thou forget me, O LORD? for ever? how long wilt thou hide thy face from me?

2 How long shall I take counsel in my soul, *having* sorrow in my heart daily? how long shall mine enemy be exalted over me?

3 Consider *and* hear me, O LORD my God: lighten mine eyes, lest I sleep the *sleep of* death;

4 Lest mine enemy say, I have prevailed against him; *and* those that trouble me rejoice when I am moved.

5 But I have [a]trusted in thy mercy; my heart shall rejoice in thy salvation.

6 I will sing unto the LORD, because he hath dealt bountifully with me.

PSALM 14.

To the chief Musician,
A Psalm of David.

The fool hath said in his heart, *There is* no God. [l]They are corrupt, they have done abominable works, *there is* none that doeth good.

2 The LORD looked down from heaven upon the children of men, to see if there were any that did [m]understand, *and* seek God.

3 [n]They are all gone aside, they are *all* together become filthy: *there is* none that doeth good, no, not one.

4 Have all the workers of iniquity no knowledge? [o]who eat up my people *as* they eat bread, and call not upon the LORD.

5 There were they in great fear: for God *is* in the generation of the righteous.

6 Ye have shamed the counsel of the poor, because the LORD *is* his refuge.

7 [p]Oh that the salvation of Israel *were come* out of Zion! when the LORD bringeth back the captivity of his people, Jacob shall rejoice, *and* Israel shall be glad.

PSALM 15.

A Psalm of David.

LORD, who shall abide in thy tabernacle? who shall dwell in thy holy hill?

2 He that walketh uprightly, and worketh righteousness, and speaketh the truth in his heart.

3 *He that* backbiteth not with his tongue, nor doeth evil to his neighbour, nor taketh up a reproach against his neighbour.

4 In whose eyes a vile person is contemned; but he honoureth them that [a]fear the LORD. *He that* sweareth to *his own* hurt, and changeth not.

5 *He that* putteth not out his money to usury, nor taketh reward against the innocent. He that doeth these *things* shall never be moved.

PSALM 16.

[1]Michtam of David.

Preserve me, O God: for in thee do I put my [b]trust.

2 *O my soul*, thou hast said unto the LORD, Thou *art* my Lord: my goodness *extendeth* not to thee;

3 *But* to the saints that *are* in the earth, and *to* the excellent, in whom *is* all my delight.

4 Their sorrows shall be multiplied *that* hasten *after* another *god*: their drink offerings of blood will I not offer, nor take up their names into my lips.

5 The LORD *is* the portion of mine inheritance and of my cup: thou maintainest my lot.

6 The lines are fallen unto me in pleasant *places*; yea, I have a goodly heritage.

7 I will bless the LORD, who hath given me counsel: my reins also instruct me in the night seasons.

8 I have set the LORD always before me: because *he is* at my right hand, I shall not be moved.

9 [c]Therefore my heart is glad, and my glory rejoiceth: [2]my flesh also shall rest in [d]hope.

10 For thou wilt not [e]leave [f]my soul in [g]hell; neither wilt thou suffer thine Holy One to see corruption.

11 Thou wilt shew me the path of life: in thy presence *is* fulness of joy; at thy right hand *there are* pleasures for evermore.

a Psa. 19:9, *note*.

b Psa. 2:12, *note*.

c *Kingdom* (O.T.). vs. 8-11; Psa. 72:1-20. (Gen. 1:26; Zech. 12:8.)

d *Resurrection*. vs. 9-11; Isa. 26:19. (Job 19:25; 1 Cor. 15:52.)

e vs. 8-11; Acts 2:25-28; 13:35.

f *Christ (First Advent)*. Psa. 22:1-18. (Gen. 3:15; Acts 1:9.)

g *Sheol*. See Hab. 2:5, *note*.

h i.e. *earth*.

PSALM 17.

A Prayer of David.

Hear the right, O LORD, attend unto my cry, give ear unto my prayer, *that goeth* not out of feigned lips.

2 Let my sentence come forth from thy presence; let thine eyes behold the things that are equal.

3 Thou hast proved mine heart; thou hast visited *me* in the night; thou hast tried me, *and* shalt find nothing; I am purposed *that* my mouth shall not transgress.

4 Concerning the works of men, by the word of thy lips I have kept *me from* the paths of the destroyer.

5 Hold up my goings in thy paths, *that* my footsteps slip not.

6 I have called upon thee, for thou wilt hear me, O God: incline thine ear unto me, *and hear* my speech.

7 Shew thy marvellous lovingkindness, O thou that savest by thy right hand them which put their [b]trust *in thee* from those that rise up *against them*.

8 Keep me as the apple of the eye, hide me under the shadow of thy wings,

9 From the wicked that oppress me, *from* my deadly enemies, *who* compass me about.

10 They are inclosed in their own fat: with their mouth they speak proudly.

11 They have now compassed us in our steps: they have set their eyes bowing down to the earth;

12 Like as a lion *that* is greedy of his prey, and as it were a young lion lurking in secret places.

13 Arise, O LORD, disappoint him, cast him down: deliver my soul from the wicked, *which is* thy sword:

14 From men *which are* thy hand, O LORD, from men of the [h]world, *which have* their portion in *this* life, and whose belly thou fillest with thy hid *treasure*: they are full of children, and leave the rest of their *substance* to their babes.

15 As for me, I will behold thy face in

[1] **(16, inscription)** *Michtam*, "a prayer," or "meditation." See Psa. 56; 57; 58; 59; 60.

[2] **(16:9)** The 16th Psalm is a prediction of the resurrection of the King. As a prophet David understood that, not at His first advent, but at some time subsequent to His death and resurrection Messiah would assume the Davidic throne. See Acts 2:25-31, with Lk. 1:32, 33, and Acts 15:13-17. See "Davidic Covenant," 2 Sam. 7:14, *refs.*; "Kingdom (O. T.)," Zech. 12:8. See Psa. 22, next in order of the Messianic Psalms.

righteousness: I shall be satisfied, when I
awake, with thy likeness.

PSALM 18.

To the chief Musician, *A Psalm* of David,
the servant of the LORD, who spake unto
the LORD the words of this song in the
day *that* the LORD delivered him from the
hand of all his enemies, and from the
hand of Saul: And he said,

[a]1 I will love thee, O LORD, my strength.
2 The LORD *is* my rock, and my
fortress, and my deliverer; my God, my
strength, [b]in whom I will trust; my buckler, and the horn of my salvation, *and* my
high tower.
3 I will call upon the LORD, [c]*who is*
worthy to be praised: so shall I be saved
from mine enemies.
4 [d]The sorrows of death compassed
me, and the floods of [e]ungodly men
made me afraid.
5 The sorrows of [f]hell compassed me
about: the snares of death prevented me.
6 In my distress I called upon the
LORD, and cried unto my God: he heard
my voice out of his temple, and my cry
came before him, *even* into his ears.
7 [g]Then the earth shook and trembled;
the foundations also of the hills moved
and were shaken, because he was wroth.
8 There went up a smoke [h]out of his
nostrils, and fire out of his mouth
devoured: coals were kindled by it.
9 [i]He bowed the heavens also, and
came down: and darkness *was* under his
feet.
10 [j]And he rode upon a cherub, and
did fly: yea, he did fly upon the wings of
the wind.
11 He made darkness his secret place;
[k]his pavilion round about him *were* dark
waters *and* thick clouds of the skies.
12 [l]At the brightness *that was* before
him his thick clouds passed, hail *stones*
and coals of fire.
13 The LORD also thundered in the
heavens, and the Highest gave [m]his
voice; hail *stones* and coals of fire.
14 [n]Yea, he sent out his arrows, and
scattered them; and he shot out lightnings, and discomfited them.
15 Then the channels of waters were
seen, and the foundations of the world

a Psa. 144:1.
b Heb. 2:13.
c Rev. 5:12.
d Psa. 116:3.
e Heb. *Belial.*
f *Sheol.* See Hab. 2:5, *note.*
g Mt. 27:45-51.
h Heb. *by his.*
i Psa. 144:5.
j Psa. 99:1
k Psa. 97:2.
l Psa. 97:3.
m Psa. 29:3-9.
n Psa. 144:6; Josh. 10:10; Isa. 30:30.
o Psa. 144:7.
p Psa. 31:8; 118:5.
q 1 Sam. 26:23.
r Job 18:6; 29:3; Psa. 119:105.
s Psa. 12:6; 119:140; Prov. 30:5.
t Psa.2.12, *note.*
u 2 Sam. 2:18; Hab. 3:19.
v Deut. 32:13; 33:29.

were discovered at thy rebuke, O LORD,
at the blast of the breath of thy nostrils.
16 [o]He sent from above, he took me,
he drew me out of many waters.
17 He delivered me from my strong
enemy, and from them which hated me:
for they were too strong for me.
18 They prevented me in the day of
my calamity: but the LORD was my stay.
19 [p]He brought me forth also into a
large place; he delivered me, because he
delighted in me.
20 The LORD rewarded me according
to my righteousness; according to the
cleanness of my hands hath he recompensed me.
21 For I have kept the ways of the
LORD, and have not wickedly departed
from my God.
22 For all his judgments *were* before
me, and I did not put away his statutes
from me.
23 I was also upright before him, and I
kept myself from mine iniquity.
24 [q]Therefore hath the LORD recompensed me according to my righteousness, according to the cleanness of my
hands in his eyesight.
25 With the merciful thou wilt shew
thyself merciful; with an upright man
thou wilt shew thyself upright;
26 With the pure thou wilt shew thyself pure; and with the froward thou wilt
shew thyself froward.
27 For thou wilt save the afflicted people; but wilt bring down high looks.
28 [r]For thou wilt light my candle: the
LORD my God will enlighten my darkness.
29 For by thee I have run through a
troop; and by my God have I leaped
over a wall.
30 *As for* God, his way *is* perfect: [s]the
word of the LORD is tried: he *is* a buckler
to all those that [t]trust in him.
31 For who *is* God save the LORD? or
who *is* a rock save our God?
32 *It is* God that girdeth me with
strength, and maketh my way perfect.
33 [u]He maketh my feet like hinds' *feet*,
and [v]setteth me upon my high places.
34 He teacheth my hands to war, so that
a bow of steel is broken by mine arms.

35 Thou hast also given me the shield of thy salvation: and thy right hand hath holden me up, and thy gentleness hath made me great.

36 Thou hast enlarged my steps under me, that my feet did not slip.

37 I have pursued mine enemies, and overtaken them: neither did I turn again till they were consumed.

38 I have wounded them that they were not able to rise: they are fallen under my feet.

39 For thou hast girded me with strength unto the battle: thou hast [a]subdued under me those that rose up against me.

40 Thou hast also given me the necks of mine enemies; that I might destroy them that hate me.

41 They cried, but *there was* none to save *them: even* unto the LORD, but he answered them not.

42 Then did I beat them small as the dust before the wind: I did [b]cast them out as the dirt in the streets.

43 Thou hast delivered me from the strivings of the people; *and* thou hast made me the head of the [c]heathen: a [d]people *whom* I have not known shall serve me.

44 As soon as they hear of me, they shall obey me: the strangers shall submit themselves unto me.

45 The strangers shall fade away, and be afraid out of their close places.

46 The LORD liveth; and blessed *be* my rock; and let the God of my salvation be exalted.

47 *It is* God that avengeth me, and subdueth the people under me.

48 He delivereth me from mine enemies: yea, thou liftest me up above those that rise up against me: thou hast delivered me from the violent man.

49 Therefore will I give [e]thanks unto thee, O LORD, among the [c]heathen, and sing praises unto thy name.

50 Great deliverance giveth he to his king; and sheweth mercy to his anointed, to David, and to his seed for evermore.

PSALM 19.

To the chief Musician,
A Psalm of David.

The heavens declare the glory of God; and the firmament sheweth his handywork.

2 Day unto day uttereth speech, and night unto night sheweth knowledge.

3 *There is* no speech nor language, *where* their voice is not heard.

4 [f]Their line is gone out through all the earth, and their words to the end of the world. In them hath he set a tabernacle for the sun,

5 Which *is* as a bridegroom coming out of his chamber, *and* [g]rejoiceth as a strong man to run a race.

6 His going forth *is* from the end of the heaven, and his circuit unto the ends of it: and there is nothing hid from the heat thereof.

7 The [h]law of the LORD *is* perfect, converting the soul: the testimony of the LORD *is* sure, making wise the simple.

8 The statutes of the LORD *are* right, rejoicing the heart: [i]the commandment of the LORD *is* pure, enlightening the eyes.

9 The [1]fear of the LORD *is* clean, enduring for ever: the judgments of the LORD *are* true *and* righteous altogether.

10 More to be desired *are they* than gold, [j]yea, than much fine gold: sweeter also than honey and the honeycomb.

11 Moreover by them is thy servant warned: *and* in keeping of them *there is* great reward.

12 Who can understand *his* errors? [k]cleanse thou me from secret *faults*.

13 Keep back thy servant also from presumptuous *sins*; [l]let them not have dominion over me: then shall I be upright, and I shall be innocent from the great transgression.

14 [m]Let the words of my mouth, and the meditation of my heart, be acceptable in thy sight, O LORD, my [n]strength, and my [o]redeemer.

PSALM 20.

To the chief Musician,
A Psalm of David.

The LORD hear thee in the day of trouble; the name of the God of Jacob [p]defend thee;

2 Send thee help from the [q]sanctuary, and strengthen thee out of Zion;

3 Remember all thy offerings, and accept thy burnt sacrifice; Selah.

4 Grant thee according to thine own heart, and fulfil all thy counsel.

a Heb. *caused to bow.*
b Zech. 10:5.
c i.e. *nations.*
d Isa. 52:15; 55:5.
e 2 Sam. 22:50; Rom. 15:9.
f Cited in Rom. 10:18.
g Eccl. 1:5.
h *Law (of Moses).* vs. 7, 8; Psa. 37:31, (Ex. 19:1; Gal. 3:1-29.)
i Psa. 12:6.
j Psa. 119:72, 127; Prov. 8:10, 11, 19.
k Lev. 4:2.
l Psa. 119:133; Rom. 6:12, 14.
m Psa. 51:15.
n Heb. *my rock.*
o Heb. *goel, Redemp. (Kinsman type).* Isa. 59:20, *note.*
p Heb. *set thee on an high place.*
q Heb. *qodesh* (tr. "holy," v. 6).

1 (19:9) The "fear of the Lord," a phrase of the O.T. piety, meaning *reverential trust*, with *hatred of evil*.

5 We will rejoice in thy salvation, and in the name of our God we will set up *our* banners: the LORD fulfil all thy petitions.

6 Now know I that the LORD saveth his anointed; he will hear him [a]from his [b]holy heaven with the saving strength of his right hand.

7 Some *trust* in chariots, and some in horses: [c]but we will remember the name of the LORD our God.

8 They are brought down and fallen: but we are risen, and stand upright.

9 Save, LORD: let the king hear us when we call.

PSALM 21.

To the chief Musician,
A Psalm of David.

The king shall joy in thy strength, O LORD; and in thy salvation how greatly shall he rejoice!

2 Thou hast given him his heart's desire, and hast not withholden the request of his lips. Selah.

3 For thou preventest him with the blessings of goodness: thou settest a crown of pure gold on his head.

4 [d]He asked life of thee, *and* thou gavest *it* him, *even* length of days for ever and ever.

5 His glory *is* great in thy salvation: honour and majesty hast thou laid upon him.

6 For thou hast made him most blessed for ever: [e]thou hast made him exceeding glad with thy countenance.

7 For the king [f]trusteth in the LORD, and through the mercy of the most High he shall not be moved.

8 Thine hand shall find out all thine enemies: thy right hand shall find out those that hate thee.

a Heb. *from the heaven of his holiness.*

b *Sanctify, holy* (O.T.). Psa. 89:20. (Gen. 2:3; Zech. 8:3.)

c 2 Chr. 32:8.

d Psa. 61:5, 6.

e Psa. 16:11; 45:7.

f Psa. 2:12, *note.*

g Mt. 27:46; Mk. 15:34.

h *Sacrifice (prophetic).* vs. 1-18; Isa. 52:14. (Gen. 4:4; Heb. 10:18.)

i *Christ (First Advent).* vs. 1-18; Isa. 7:13, 14. (Gen. 3:15; Acts 1:9.)

j vs. 7, 8, 11-13; Psa. 109:25; Mt. 27:39-44.

9 Thou shalt make them as a fiery oven in the time of thine anger: the LORD shall swallow them up in his wrath, and the fire shall devour them.

10 Their fruit shalt thou destroy from the earth, and their seed from among the children of men.

11 For they intended evil against thee: they imagined a mischievous device, *which* they are not able *to perform.*

12 Therefore shalt thou make them turn their back, *when* thou shalt make ready *thine arrows* upon thy strings against the face of them.

13 Be thou exalted, LORD, in thine own strength: *so* will we sing and praise thy power.

PSALM 22.

To the chief Musician upon
[1]Aijeleth Shahar, A Psalm of David.

[2]My [g]God, [h]my God, why hast thou forsaken [i]me? *why art thou so* far from helping me, *and from* the words of my roaring?

2 O my God, I cry in the daytime, but thou hearest not; and in the night season, and am not silent.

3 But thou *art* holy, *O thou* that inhabitest the praises of Israel.

4 Our fathers trusted in thee: they [f]trusted, and thou didst deliver them.

5 They cried unto thee, and were delivered: they trusted in thee, and were not confounded.

6 But I *am* a worm, and no man; a reproach of men, and [j]despised of the people.

7 [3]All they that see me laugh me to scorn: they shoot out the lip, they shake the head, *saying,*

[1]**(22, inscription)** Or, *Ay-ys-leth Shachar,* "hind of the morning," a title, not a musical instrument.

[2]**(22:1)** Psalms 22, 23, and 24. form a trilogy. In Psalm 22. the *good* Shepherd gives His life for the sheep (John 10:11); in Psalm 23 the *great* Shepherd, "brought again from the dead through the blood of the everlasting covenant" (Heb. 13:20), tenderly cares for the sheep; in Psalm 24 the *chief* Shepherd appears as King of glory to own and reward the sheep (1 Pet. 5:4).

[3]**(22:7)** Psalm 22 is a graphic picture of death by crucifixion. The bones (of the hands, arms, shoulders, and pelvis) out of joint (v. 14); the profuse perspiration caused by intense suffering (v. 14); the action of the heart affected (v. 14) strength exhausted, and extreme thirst (v. 15); the hands and feet pierced (v. 16); partial nudity with the hurt to modesty (v. 17), are all incidental to that mode of death. The accompanying circumstances are precisely those fulfilled in the crucifixion of Christ. The desolate cry of verse 1 (Mt. 27:46); the periods of light and darkness of verse 2 (Mt. 27:45); the contumely of verses 6-8, 12, 13 (Mt. 27:39-43); the casting lots of verse 18 (Mt. 27:35), all were literally fulfilled. When it is remembered that crucifixion was a Roman, not Jewish, form of execution, the proof of inspiration is irresistible.

8 He [a]trusted on the LORD *that* he
would deliver him: let him deliver him,
seeing he delighted in him.
9 [b]But thou *art* he that took me out of
the womb: thou [c]didst make me hope
when I was upon my mother's breasts.
10 I was cast upon thee from the
womb: thou *art* my God from my
mother's belly.
11 Be not far from me; for trouble *is*
near; for *there is* none to help.
12 [d]Many bulls have compassed me:
strong *bulls* of Bashan have beset me
round.
13 [e]They gaped upon me *with* their
mouths, *as* a ravening and a roaring lion.
14 I am poured out like water, and all
my bones are out of joint: my heart is
like wax; it is melted in the midst of my
bowels.
15 My strength is dried up like a potsherd; and my tongue cleaveth to my
jaws; and thou hast brought me into the
dust of death.
16 [f]For dogs have compassed me: the
assembly of the wicked have inclosed me:
[g]they pierced my hands and my feet.
17 I may tell all my bones: they look
and stare upon me.
18 They part my garments among
them, and [h]cast lots upon my vesture.
19 But be not thou far from me, O LORD:
O my strength, haste thee to help me.
20 Deliver my soul from the sword;
my darling from the power of the dog.
21 Save me from the lion's mouth: for
thou hast heard me from the horns of
the unicorns.
22 [1]I will declare thy name unto my
[i]brethren: in the midst of the congregation will I praise thee.
23 Ye that [j]fear the LORD, praise him;
all ye the seed of Jacob, glorify him; and
fear him, all ye the seed of Israel.
24 For he hath not despised nor
abhorred the affliction of the afflicted;
neither hath he hid his face from him;
but when he cried unto him, he heard.
25 My praise *shall be* of thee in the
great congregation: I will pay my vows
before them that [j]fear him.
26 The meek shall eat and be satisfied:
they shall praise the LORD that seek him:
your heart shall live for ever.
27 All the ends of the world shall
remember and turn unto the LORD: and
all the kindreds of the nations shall worship before thee.
28 [2]For the kingdom *is* the LORD'S: and
he *is* the governor among the nations.
29 All *they that be* fat upon earth shall
eat and worship: all they that go down
to the dust shall bow before him: and
none can keep alive his own soul.
30 A seed shall serve him; it shall be
accounted to the Lord for a generation.
31 They shall come, and shall declare
his righteousness unto a people that
shall be born, that he hath done *this*.

PSALM 23.

A Psalm of David.

The LORD *is* [k]my shepherd; [l]I shall not
want.
2 [m]He maketh me to lie down in green
pastures: he leadeth me beside the [n]still
waters.
3 He restoreth my soul: [o]he leadeth me
in the paths of righteousness for his
name's sake.
4 Yea, though I walk through the valley of [p]the shadow of death, [q]I will fear
no evil: [r]for thou *art* with me; thy rod
and thy staff they comfort me.
5 [s]Thou preparest a table before me in
the presence of mine enemies: thou
[t]anointest my head with oil; my cup
runneth over.
6 Surely goodness and mercy shall follow me all the days of my life: and I will
dwell in the house of the LORD for ever.

PSALM 24.

A Psalm of David.

The [u]earth *is* the LORD'S, and the fulness thereof; the world, and they
that dwell therein.

a Mt. 27:43.
b Psa. 71:6.
c Or, *keptest me in safety.*
d Psa. 68:30; Deut. 32:14; Ezk. 39:18; Amos 4:1.
e Job 16:10.
f Rev. 22:15.
g Isa. 53:7; cf. John 20:20-25.
h Mt. 27:35; Mk. 15:24; Lk. 23:34; John 19:23, 24.
i Heb. 2:12.
j Psa. 19:9, *note.*
k Isa. 40:11; Jer. 23:4; Ezk. 34:11, 12, 23; John 10:11; 1 Pet. 2:25; Rev. 7:17.
l Phil. 4:19.
m Ezk. 34:14, Heb. *pastures of tender grass.*
n Heb. *waters of quietness.* Rev. 7:17.
o Psa. 5:8; 31:3; Prov. 8:20.
p Job 3:5; 10:21, 22; 24:17; Psa. 44:19.
q Psa. 3:6; 27:1; 118:6.
r Isa. 43:2.
s Psa. 104:15.
t Heb. *makest fat.* Psa. 92:10.
u 1 Cor. 10:26.

[1]**(22:22)** At verse 22 the Psalm breaks from crucifixion to resurrection; fulfilled in the "Go to my brethren," etc., of John 20:17. The risen Christ declares to His brethren the name, "Father."

[2]**(22:28)** Cf. v. 30. The kingdom is Jehovah's. In verse 30 Adonai is in view as ruling on behalf of Jehovah. See Psa. 110, with Mt. 22:42-45. The great end and object of the rule of Adonai (Lord) is the restoration of the kingdom to Jehovah (LORD). See 1 Cor. 15:23, 24. See "Names of Deity," Gen. 2:4, *note;* Gen. 15:2, *note.*

2 For he hath founded it upon the seas, and established it upon the floods.

3 [1]Who shall ascend into the hill of the LORD? or who shall stand in his holy place?

4 He that hath clean hands, and a pure heart; who hath not lifted up his soul unto vanity, nor sworn deceitfully.

5 He shall receive the blessing from the LORD, and righteousness from the God of his salvation.

6 This *is* the generation of them that seek him, that seek thy face, O Jacob. Selah.

7 Lift up your heads, O ye gates; and be ye lift up, ye everlasting doors; and the King of glory shall come in.

8 Who *is* this King of glory? The LORD strong and mighty, the LORD mighty in battle.

9 Lift up your heads, O ye gates; even lift *them* up, ye everlasting doors; and the King of glory shall come in.

10 Who is this [a]King of glory? The LORD of hosts, he *is* the King of glory. Selah.

PSALM 25.

A Psalm of David.

Unto thee, O LORD, do I lift up my soul.

2 O my God, I [b]trust in thee: let me not be ashamed, [c]let not mine enemies triumph over me.

3 Yea, let none that wait on thee be ashamed: let them be ashamed which transgress without cause.

4 [d]Shew me thy ways, O LORD; teach me thy paths.

5 Lead me in thy truth, and teach me: for thou *art* the God of my salvation; on thee do I wait all the day.

6 Remember, O LORD, [e]thy tender mercies and thy lovingkindnesses; for they *have been* ever of old.

7 Remember not [f]the sins of my youth, nor my transgressions: [g]according to thy mercy remember thou me for thy goodness' sake, O LORD.

8 Good and upright *is* the LORD: therefore will he teach sinners in the way.

9 The meek will he guide in judgment: and the meek will he teach his way.

10 All the paths of the LORD *are* mercy and truth unto such as keep his covenant and his testimonies.

11 [h]For thy name's sake, O LORD, pardon mine iniquity; [i]for it *is* great.

12 What man *is* he that [j]feareth the LORD? him shall he teach in the way *that* he shall choose.

13 His soul [k]shall dwell at ease; and his seed shall inherit the earth.

14 [l]The secret of the LORD *is* with them that fear him; and he will shew them his covenant.

15 Mine eyes *are* ever toward the LORD; for he [m]shall pluck my feet out of the net.

16 Turn thee unto me, and have mercy upon me; for I *am* desolate and afflicted.

17 The troubles of my heart are enlarged: *O* bring thou me out of my distresses.

18 Look upon mine affliction and my pain; and forgive all my sins.

19 Consider mine enemies; for they are many; and they hate me with cruel hatred.

20 O keep my soul, and deliver me: let me not be ashamed; for I put my [b]trust in thee.

21 Let integrity and uprightness preserve me; for I wait on thee.

22 [n]Redeem Israel, O God, out of all his troubles.

PSALM 26.

A Psalm of David.

Judge me, O LORD; for I have walked in mine integrity: I have [b]trusted also in the LORD; *therefore* I shall not slide.

2 Examine me, O LORD, and prove me; try my reins and my heart.

3 For thy lovingkindness *is* before mine eyes: and I have walked in thy truth.

4 I have not sat with vain persons, neither will I go in with dissemblers.

5 I have hated the congregation of evil doers; and will not sit with the wicked.

6 I will wash mine hands in innocency:

a *Christ (Second Advent).* Psa. 50:1-5. (Deut. 30:3; Acts 1:9-11.)
b Psa. 2:12, *note.*
c Psa. 13:4.
d Ex. 33:13; Psa. 5:8; 27:11; 86:11; 119:10; 143:8, 10.
e Psa. 103:17; 106:1; 107:1; Isa. 63:15; Jer. 33:11.
f Job 13:26; 20:11; Jer. 3:25.
g Psa. 51:1.
h Psa. 31:3; 79:9; 109:21; 143:11.
i See Rom. 5:20.
j Psa.19:9, *note.*
k Heb. *shall lodge in goodness.*
l Prov. 3:32; see John 7:17; 15:15.
m Heb. *bring forth.*
n Ex. 14:30, *note;* Isa. 59:20, *note.*

[1]**(24:3)** The order is: (1) the declaration of title, "The earth is the LORD'S" (vs. 1, 2). (2) Who shall rule the earth? (vs. 3-6). It is a question of *worthiness,* and no one is worthy but the Lamb. Cf. Dan. 7:13, 14; Rev. 5:3-10; Mt. 25:31. (3) The King of glory takes the throne of earth (vs. 7-10). See Psa. 40, next in order of the Messianic Psalms.

so will I compass thine altar, O LORD:

7 That I may publish with the voice of thanksgiving, and tell of all thy wondrous works.

8 LORD, I have loved the habitation of thy house, and the place where thine honour dwelleth.

9 Gather not my soul with sinners, nor my life with bloody men:

10 In whose hands *is* mischief, and their right hand is full of bribes.

11 But as for me, I will walk in mine integrity: [a]redeem me, and be merciful unto me.

12 My foot standeth in an even place: in the congregations will I bless the LORD.

PSALM 27.

A Psalm of David.

The LORD *is* [b]my light and my salvation; whom shall I fear? [c]the LORD *is* the strength of my life; of whom shall I be afraid?

2 When the wicked, *even* mine enemies and my foes, came upon me to eat up my flesh, they stumbled and fell.

3 [d]Though an host should encamp against me, my heart shall not fear: though war should rise against me, in this *will* I *be* confident.

4 [e]One *thing* have I desired of the LORD, that will I seek after; that I may [f]dwell in the house of the LORD all the days of my life, to behold the beauty of the LORD, and to enquire in his temple.

5 [g]For in the time of trouble he shall hide me in his pavilion: in the secret of his tabernacle shall he hide me; [h]he shall set me up upon a rock.

6 And now shall mine head be lifted up above mine enemies round about me: therefore will I offer in his tabernacle sacrifices of joy; I will sing, yea, I will sing praises unto the LORD.

7 Hear, O LORD, *when* I cry with my voice: have mercy also upon me, and answer me.

8 [i]*When thou saidst,* Seek ye my face; my heart said unto thee, Thy face, LORD, will I seek.

9 [j]Hide not thy face *far* from me; put not thy servant away in anger: thou hast been my help; leave me not, neither forsake me, O God of my salvation.

10 When my father and my mother forsake me, then the LORD [k]will take me up.

11 [l]Teach me thy way, O LORD, and lead me in a plain path, because of [m]mine enemies.

12 Deliver me not over unto the will of mine enemies: [n]for false witnesses are risen up against me, and such as breathe out cruelty.

13 *I had fainted,* unless I had believed to see the goodness of the LORD in the land of the living.

14 [o]Wait on the LORD: be of good courage, and he shall strengthen thine heart: wait, I say, on the LORD.

PSALM 28.

A Psalm of David.

Unto thee will I cry, O LORD my rock; be not silent to me: lest, *if* thou be silent to me, I become like them that go down into the pit.

2 Hear the voice of my supplications, when I cry unto thee, when I lift up my hands [p]toward thy holy oracle.

3 Draw me not away with the wicked, and with the workers of iniquity, which speak peace to their neighbours, but mischief *is* in their hearts.

4 [q]Give them according to their deeds, and according to the wickedness of their endeavours: give them after the work of their hands; render to them their desert.

5 Because they regard not the works of the LORD, nor the operation of his hands, he shall destroy them, and not build them up.

6 Blessed *be* the LORD, because he hath heard the voice of my supplications.

7 The LORD *is* my strength and my shield; my heart [r]trusted in him, and I am helped: therefore my heart greatly rejoiceth; and with my song will I praise him.

8 The LORD *is* their strength, and he *is* the saving strength of his anointed.

9 Save thy people, and bless thine inheritance: feed them also, and lift them up for ever.

PSALM 29.

A Psalm of David.

Give unto the LORD, O ye mighty, give unto the LORD glory and strength.

2 Give unto the LORD the glory due

a Ex. 14:30, *note;* Isa. 59:20, *note.*
b Psa. 84:11; Isa. 60:19, 20; Mic. 7:8.
c Psa. 62:2, 6; 118:14, 21; Isa. 12:2.
d Psa. 3:6.
e Psa. 26:8.
f Psa. 65:4; Lk. 2:37.
g Psa. 31:20; 83:3; 91:1; Isa. 4:6.
h Psa. 40:2.
i Or, *My heart said unto thee, Let my face seek thy face.*
j Psa. 69:17; 143:7.
k Heb. *will gather me.* Isa. 40:11.
l Psa. 25:4; 86:11; 119:33.
m Heb. *those which observe me.*
n Psa. 35:11; 1 Sam. 22:9; 2 Sam. 16:7, 8; Mt. 26:60.
o Psa. 31:24; 62:1, 5; 130:5; Isa. 25:9; Hab. 2:3.
p Psa. 138:2.
q 2 Tim. 4:14; Rev.18:6.
r *Faith.* Psa. 32:10. (Gen. 3:20; Heb. 11:39.)

unto his name; worship the LORD in the beauty of holiness.

3 The voice of the LORD *is* upon the waters: the God of glory thundereth: the LORD *is* upon many waters.

4 The voice of the LORD *is* powerful; the voice of the LORD *is* full of majesty.

5 The voice of the LORD breaketh the cedars; yea, the LORD breaketh the cedars of Lebanon.

6 He maketh them also to skip like a calf; Lebanon and Sirion like a young unicorn.

7 The voice of the LORD divideth the flames of fire.

8 The voice of the LORD shaketh the wilderness; the LORD shaketh the wilderness of Kadesh.

9 The voice of the LORD maketh the hinds to calve, and discovereth the forests: and in his temple doth every one speak of *his* glory.

10 [a]The LORD sitteth upon the flood; yea, [b]the LORD sitteth King for ever.

11 [c]The LORD will give strength unto his people; the LORD will bless his people with peace.

PSALM 30.

A Psalm *and* Song *at* the dedication of the house of David.

I will extol thee, O LORD; for thou hast lifted me up, and hast not made my foes to rejoice over me.

2 O LORD my God, I cried unto thee, [d]and thou hast healed me.

3 O LORD, thou hast brought up my soul from the [e]grave: thou hast kept me alive, that I should not go down to the pit.

4 [f]Sing unto the LORD, O ye saints of his, and give thanks at the remembrance of his holiness.

5 [g]For his anger *endureth but* a moment; in his favour *is* life: weeping may endure [h]for a night, [i]but joy *cometh* in the morning.

6 And in my prosperity I said, I shall never be moved.

7 LORD, by thy favour thou hast [j]made my mountain to stand strong: thou didst hide thy face, *and* I was troubled.

8 I cried to thee, O LORD; and unto the LORD I made supplication.

9 What profit *is there* in my blood, when I go down to the pit? Shall the dust praise thee? shall it declare thy truth?

10 Hear, O LORD, and have mercy upon me: LORD, be thou my helper.

a Gen. 6:17; Job 38:8, 25.
b Psa. 10:16.
c Psa. 28:8.
d Psa. 6:2; 103:3.
e Heb. *Sheol.* See Hab. 2:5, *note.*
f Psa.97:12; 1 Chr. 16:4.
g Psa. 103:9; Isa. 26:20; 54:7, 8; 2 Cor. 4:17.
h Heb. *in the evening.*
i Heb. *singing.*
j Heb. *settled strength for my mountain.*
k 2 Sam. 6:14; Isa. 61:3; Jer. 31:4.
l i.e. *my tongue,* or *my soul.* See Gen. 49:6; Psa. 16:9; 57:8.
m Psa. 2:12, *note.*
n Lk. 23:46.
o Ex. 14:30, *note;* Isa. 59, 20, *note.*
p Psa. 4:1; 18:19.
q Job 19:13; Psa. 38:11; 88:8, 18.

11 [k]Thou hast turned for me my mourning into dancing: thou hast put off my sackcloth, and girded me with gladness;

12 To the end that [l]*my* glory may sing praise to thee, and not be silent. O LORD my God, I will give thanks unto thee for ever.

PSALM 31.

To the chief Musician, A Psalm of David.

In thee, O LORD, do I put my [m]trust; let me never be ashamed: deliver me in thy righteousness.

2 Bow down thine ear to me; deliver me speedily: be thou my strong rock, for an house of defence to save me.

3 For thou *art* my rock and my fortress; therefore for thy name's sake lead me, and guide me.

4 Pull me out of the net that they have laid privily for me: for thou *art* my strength.

5 Into thine [n]hand I commit my spirit: thou hast [o]redeemed me, O LORD God of truth.

6 I have hated them that regard lying vanities: but I trust in the LORD.

7 I will be glad and rejoice in thy mercy: for thou hast considered my trouble; thou hast known my soul in adversities;

8 And hast not shut me up into the hand of the enemy: [p]thou hast set my feet in a large room.

9 Have mercy upon me, O LORD, for I am in trouble: mine eye is consumed with grief, *yea,* my soul and my belly.

10 For my life is spent with grief, and my years with sighing: my strength faileth because of mine iniquity, and my bones are consumed.

11 I was a reproach among all mine enemies, but [q]especially among my neighbours, and a fear to mine acquaintance: they that did see me without fled from me.

12 I am forgotten as a dead man out of mind: I am like a broken vessel.

13 For I have heard the slander of many: fear *was* on every side: while they took counsel together against me, they devised to take away my life.

14 But I trusted in thee, O LORD: I said, Thou *art* my God.

15 My times *are* in thy hand: deliver
me from the hand of mine enemies, and
from them that persecute me.
16 Make thy face to shine upon thy
servant: save me for thy mercies' sake.
17 Let me not be ashamed, O LORD; for
I have called upon thee: let the wicked
be ashamed, *and* let them be silent in the
[p]grave.
18 Let the lying lips be put to silence;
which speak grievous things proudly and
contemptuously against the righteous.
19 *Oh* how great *is* thy goodness, which
thou hast laid up for them that [a]fear thee;
which thou hast wrought for them that
trust in thee before the sons of men!
20 [b]Thou shalt hide them in the secret
of thy presence from the pride of man:
thou shalt keep them secretly in a pavilion from the strife of tongues.
21 Blessed *be* the LORD: for he hath
shewed me his marvellous kindness in a
strong city.
22 For I said in my haste, I am cut off
from before thine eyes: nevertheless
thou heardest the voice of my supplications when I cried unto thee.
23 O love the LORD, all ye his saints: *for*
the LORD preserveth the faithful, and
plentifully rewardeth the proud doer.
24 Be of good courage, and he shall
strengthen your heart, all ye that hope in
the LORD.

PSALM 32.

A Psalm of David, [c]Maschil.

Blessed *is he whose* transgression *is* forgiven, *whose* sin *is* covered.
2 Blessed *is* the man unto whom the
LORD [d]imputeth not iniquity, and in
whose spirit *there is* no guile.
3 When I kept silence, my bones waxed
old through my roaring all the day long.
4 For day and night thy hand was
heavy upon me: my moisture is turned
into the drought of summer. Selah.
5 I acknowledged my sin unto thee,
and mine iniquity have I not hid. I said, I
will confess my transgressions unto the
LORD; and thou [e]forgavest the iniquity of
my sin. Selah.
6 For this shall every one that is godly
pray unto thee in a time when thou
mayest be found: surely in the floods of
great waters they shall not come nigh
unto him.
7 Thou *art* my hiding place; thou shalt
preserve me from trouble; thou shalt
compass me about with songs of deliverance. Selah.
8 I will instruct thee and teach thee in
the way which thou shalt go: I will
guide thee with mine eye.
9 Be ye not as the horse, *or* as the mule,
which have no understanding: whose
mouth must be held in with bit and bridle, lest they come near unto thee.
10 Many sorrows *shall be* to the
wicked: but he that [f]trusteth in the LORD,
mercy shall compass him about.
11 Be glad in the LORD, and rejoice, ye
righteous: and shout for joy, all *ye that
are* upright in heart.

PSALM 33.

[g]Rejoice in the LORD, O ye righteous:
for praise is comely for the upright.
2 Praise the LORD with harp: sing unto
him with the psaltery *and* an instrument
of ten strings.
3 Sing unto him a new song; play skilfully with a loud noise.
4 For the word of the LORD *is* right;
and all his works *are done* in truth.
5 He loveth righteousness and judgment: [h]the earth is full of the goodness
of the LORD.
6 [i]By the word of the LORD were the
heavens made; [j]and all the host of them
[k]by the breath of his mouth.
7 [l]He gathereth the waters of the sea
together as an heap: he layeth up the
depth in storehouses.
8 Let all the earth [a]fear the LORD: let all
the inhabitants of the world stand in
awe of him.
9 [m]For he spake, and it was *done*; he
commanded, and it stood fast.
10 [n]The LORD bringeth the counsel of
the [o]heathen to nought: he maketh the
devices of the people of none effect.
11 The counsel of the LORD standeth
for ever, the thoughts of his heart to all
generations.
12 Blessed *is* the nation whose
God *is* the LORD; *and* the people

a Psa. 19:9, *note.*
b Psa. 27:5; 32:7.
c *Maschil, "instruction."*
d *Imputation.* vs. 1, 2; Lk. 22:37. (Lev. 25:50; Jas. 2:23.)
e *Forgiveness.* Psa. 99:8. (Lev. 4:20; Mt. 26:28.)
f *Faith.* Psa. 37:3-5. (Gen. 3:20; Heb. 11:39.)
g Psa. 32:11; 97:12.
h Psa. 119:64.
i Gen. 1:6, 7; Heb. 11:3; 2 Pet. 3:5.
j Gen. 2:1.
k Job 26:13.
l Gen. 1:9; Job 26:10; 38:8.
m Gen. 1:3; Psa. 148:5.
n Isa. 8:10; 19:3.
o i.e. *nations.*
p Heb. *Sheol.* See Hab. 2:5, *note.*

whom he hath [a]chosen for his own inheritance.

13 The LORD looketh from heaven; he beholdeth all the sons of men.

14 From the place of his habitation he looketh upon all the inhabitants of the earth.

15 He fashioneth their hearts alike; he considereth all their works.

16 There is no king saved by the multitude of an host: a mighty man is not delivered by much strength.

17 An horse *is* a vain thing for safety: neither shall he deliver *any* by his great strength.

18 Behold, the eye of the LORD *is* upon them that [b]fear him, upon them that hope in his mercy;

19 To deliver their soul from death, and to keep them alive in famine.

20 Our soul waiteth for the LORD: he *is* our help and our shield.

21 For our heart shall rejoice in him, because we have [c]trusted in his holy name.

22 Let thy mercy, O LORD, be upon us, according as we hope in thee.

PSALM 34.

A Psalm of David, when he changed his behaviour before Abimelech; who drove him away, and he departed.

I will bless the LORD at all times: his praise *shall* continually *be* in my mouth.

2 My soul shall make her boast in the LORD: the humble shall hear *thereof*, and be glad.

3 O magnify the LORD with me, and let us exalt his name together.

4 [d]I sought the LORD, and he heard me, and delivered me from all my fears.

5 They looked unto him, and were lightened: and their faces were not ashamed.

6 This poor man cried, and the LORD heard *him*, and saved him out of all his troubles.

7 [e]The angel of the LORD encampeth round about them that fear him, and delivereth them.

8 O taste and see that the LORD *is* good: blessed *is* the man *that* [c]trusteth in him.

9 O [b]fear the LORD, ye his saints: for *there is* no want to them that [b]fear him.

10 The young lions do lack, and suffer hunger: but they that seek the LORD shall not want any good *thing*.

11 Come, ye children, hearken unto me: I will teach you the [b]fear of the LORD.

12 What man *is he that* [f]desireth life, *and* loveth *many* days, that he may see good?

13 Keep thy tongue from evil, and thy lips from speaking guile.

14 Depart from evil, and do good; seek peace, and pursue it.

15 The eyes of the LORD *are* upon the righteous, and his ears *are open* unto their cry.

16 The face of the LORD *is* against them that do evil, to cut off the remembrance of them from the earth.

17 *The righteous* cry, and the LORD heareth, and delivereth them out of all their troubles.

18 The LORD *is* nigh unto them that are of a broken heart; and saveth such as be of a contrite spirit.

19 Many *are* the afflictions of the righteous: but the LORD delivereth him out of them all.

20 [g]He keepeth all his bones: not one of them is broken.

21 Evil shall slay the wicked: and they that hate the righteous shall be desolate.

22 The LORD [h]redeemeth the soul of his servants: and none of them that [c]trust in him shall be desolate.

PSALM 35.

A Psalm of David.

Plead *my cause*, O LORD, with them that strive with me: fight against them that fight against me.

2 [i]Take hold of shield and buckler, and stand up for mine help.

3 Draw out also the spear, and stop *the way* against them that persecute me: say unto my soul, I *am* thy salvation.

4 [j]Let them be confounded and put to shame that seek after my soul: let them be [k]turned back and brought to confusion that devise my hurt.

5 Let them be as chaff before the wind: and let the [e]angel of the LORD chase *them*.

6 Let their way be dark and slippery: and let the [e]angel of the LORD persecute them.

7 For without cause have they hid for me their net *in* a pit, *which* without cause they have digged for my soul.

8 Let [l]destruction come upon him at unawares; and let his net that he hath

a *Election (corporate).* Psa. 105:43. (Deut. 7:6; 1 Pet. 1:2.)

b Psa. 19:9, *note.*

c Psa. 2:12, *note.*

d Mt. 7:7; Lk. 11:9.

e Heb. 1:4, *note.*

f vs. 12-16; 1 Pet. 3:10-12.

g Ex. 12:46; John 19:36.

h Ex. 14:30, *note;* Isa. 59:20, *note.*

i Isa. 42:13; cf. Psa. 44:26.

j v. 26; Psa. 40:14, 15; 70:2, 3.

k Psa. 129:5.

l I Thes. 5:3.

hid catch himself: into that very destruction let him fall.

9 And my soul shall be joyful in the LORD: it shall rejoice in his salvation.

10 [a]All my bones shall say, LORD, [b]who *is* like unto thee, which deliverest the poor from him that is too strong for him, yea, the poor and the needy from him that spoileth him?

11 [c]False witnesses did rise up; they laid to my charge *things* that I knew not.

12 They rewarded me evil for good *to* the spoiling of my soul.

13 But as for me, [d]when they were sick, my clothing *was* sackcloth: I humbled my soul with fasting; [e]and my prayer returned into mine own bosom.

14 I [f]behaved myself as though *he had been* my friend *or* brother: I bowed down heavily, as one that mourneth *for his* mother.

15 But in mine adversity they rejoiced, and gathered themselves together: *yea,* the abjects gathered themselves together against me, and I knew *it* not; they did tear *me*, and ceased not:

16 With hypocritical mockers in feasts, they gnashed upon me with their teeth.

17 Lord, how long wilt thou [g]look on? rescue my soul from their destructions, my [h]darling from the lions.

18 I will give thee thanks in the great congregation: I will praise thee among much people.

19 [i]Let not them that are mine enemies wrongfully rejoice over me: *neither* let them wink with the eye that hate me without a cause.

20 For they speak not peace: but they devise deceitful matters against *them that are* quiet in the land.

21 Yea, they opened their mouth wide against me, *and* said, Aha, aha, our eye hath seen *it*.

22 *This* thou hast seen, O LORD: keep not silence: O Lord, be not far from me.

23 Stir up thyself, and awake to my judgment, *even* unto my cause, my God and my Lord.

24 Judge me, O LORD my God, [j]according to thy righteousness; and let them not rejoice over me.

25 Let them not say in their hearts, Ah, so would we have it: let them not say, We have swallowed him up.

26 Let them be ashamed and brought to confusion together that rejoice at mine hurt: let them be clothed with shame and dishonour that magnify *themselves* against me.

27 [k]Let them shout for joy, and be glad, that favour my righteous cause: yea, let them say continually, Let the LORD be magnified, which hath pleasure in the prosperity of his servant.

28 And my tongue shall speak of thy righteousness *and* of thy praise all the day long.

PSALM 36.

To the chief Musician, *A Psalm* of David the servant of the LORD.

The transgression of the wicked saith within my heart, *that there is* [l]no fear of God before his eyes.

2 For he flattereth himself in his own eyes, until his iniquity be found to be hateful.

3 The words of his mouth *are* iniquity and deceit: he hath left off to be wise, *and* to do good.

4 He deviseth mischief upon his bed; he setteth himself in a way *that is* not good; he abhorreth not evil.

5 Thy mercy, O LORD, *is* in the heavens; *and* thy faithfulness *reacheth* unto the clouds.

6 Thy righteousness *is* like the great mountains; thy judgments *are* a great deep: O LORD, thou preservest man and beast.

7 How excellent *is* thy lovingkindness, O God! therefore the children of men put their [m]trust under the shadow of thy wings.

8 They shall be [n]abundantly satisfied with the fatness of thy house; and thou shalt make them drink of the river of thy pleasures.

9 [o]For with thee *is* the fountain of life: in thy light shall we see light.

10 [p]O continue thy lovingkindness unto them that know thee; and thy righteousness to the upright in heart.

11 Let not the foot of pride come against me, and let not the hand of the wicked remove me.

12 There are the workers of iniquity fallen: they are cast down, and shall not be able to rise.

a Psa. 51:8.
b Ex. 15:11; Psa. 71:19; Mic. 7:18.
c Heb. *witnesses of wrong.*
d Job 30:25; Psa. 69:10, 11.
e Mt. 10:13; Lk. 10:6.
f Heb. *walked.*
g Hab. 1:13.
h Heb. *my only one.* Psa. 22:20.
i Psa. 69:4; 109:3; 119:161; Lam. 3:52; John 15:25.
j 2 Thes. 1:6.
k Rev. 16:5-7; 18:20.
l Rom 3:18.
m Psa. 2:12, *note.*
n Heb. *watered.* Psa. 65:4.
o Jer. 2:13; John 4:10, 14.
p Heb. *draw out at length.*

PSALM 37.

A Psalm of David.

Fret [a]not thyself because of evildoers, neither be thou envious against the workers of iniquity.

2 For they shall soon be cut down like the grass, and wither as the green herb.

3 [b]Trust in the LORD, and do good; *so* shalt thou dwell in the land, and verily thou shalt be fed.

4 [c]Delight thyself also in the LORD; and he shall give thee the desires of thine heart.

5 [d]Commit thy way unto the LORD; trust also in him; and he shall bring *it* to pass.

6 [e]And he shall bring forth thy righteousness as the light, and thy judgment as the noonday.

7 [f]Rest in the LORD, and wait patiently for him: [g]fret not thyself because of him who prospereth in his way, because of the man who bringeth wicked devices to pass.

8 Cease from anger, and forsake wrath: [h]fret not thyself in any wise to do evil.

9 For evildoers shall be cut off: but those that wait upon the LORD, they shall inherit the earth.

10 For [i]yet a little while, and the wicked *shall* not *be*: yea, thou shalt diligently consider his place, and it *shall* not *be*.

11 [j]But the meek shall inherit the earth; and shall delight themselves in the abundance of peace.

12 The wicked plotteth against the just, and gnasheth upon him with his teeth.

13 The Lord shall laugh at him: for he seeth that his day is coming.

14 The wicked have drawn out the sword, and have bent their bow, to cast down the poor and needy, *and* to slay such as be of upright conversation.

15 [k]Their sword shall enter into their own heart, and their bows shall be broken.

16 [l]A little that a righteous man hath *is* better than the riches of many wicked.

17 For the arms of the wicked shall be broken: but the LORD upholdeth the righteous.

18 The LORD knoweth the days of the upright: and their inheritance shall be for ever.

19 They shall not be ashamed in the evil time: and in the days of famine they shall be satisfied.

20 But the wicked shall perish, and the enemies of the LORD *shall be* as [m]the fat of lambs: they shall consume; into smoke shall they consume away.

21 The wicked borroweth, and payeth not again: but the righteous sheweth mercy, and giveth.

22 For *such as be* blessed of him shall inherit the earth; and *they that be* cursed of him shall be cut off.

23 The steps of a *good* man are ordered by the LORD: and he delighteth in his way.

24 Though he fall, he shall not be utterly cast down: for the LORD upholdeth *him with* his hand.

25 I have been young, and *now* am old; yet have I not seen the righteous forsaken, nor his seed begging bread.

26 *He is* ever merciful, and lendeth; and his seed *is* blessed.

27 Depart from evil, and do good; and dwell for evermore.

28 For the LORD loveth judgment, and forsaketh not his saints; they are preserved for ever: but the seed of the wicked shall be cut off.

29 The righteous shall inherit the land, and dwell therein for ever.

30 The mouth of the righteous speaketh wisdom, and his tongue talketh of judgment.

31 [n]The law of his God *is* in his heart; none of his steps shall slide.

32 The wicked watcheth the righteous, and seeketh to slay him.

33 The LORD will not leave him in his hand, nor condemn him when he is judged.

34 [o]Wait on the LORD, and keep his way, and he shall exalt thee to inherit the land: when the wicked are cut off, thou shalt see *it*.

35 I have seen the wicked in great power, and spreading himself like [p]a green bay tree.

36 Yet he passed away, and, lo, he *was* not: yea, I sought him, but he could not be found.

37 Mark the [q]perfect *man*, and behold the upright: for the end of *that* man *is* peace.

38 But the transgressors shall be destroyed together: the end of the wicked shall be cut off.

39 But the salvation of the righteous *is* of the LORD: *he is* their strength in the time of trouble.

40 And the LORD shall help them, and deliver them: he shall deliver them from the wicked, and save them, because they [r]trust in him.

a v. 7; Psa. 73:3; Prov. 23:17; 24:19.

b *Faith.* Psa. 84:12. (Gen. 3:20; Heb. 11:39.

c Isa. 58:14.

d Heb. *roll thy way upon the Lord.*

e Job 11:17; Mic. 7:9.

f Heb. *be silent to the Lord.* Psa. 62:1.

g vs. 1, 8; Jer. 12:1.

h Psa. 73:3; Eph. 4:26.

i Heb. 10:36, 37.

j Mt. 5:5.

k 1 Sam. 17:50, 51.

l Prov. 15:16; 16:8; 1 Tim. 6:6.

m Heb. *the preciousness of lambs.*

n *Law (of Moses).* Psa. 40:8. (Ex. 19:1; Gal. 3:1-29.)

o v. 9; Psa. 27:14; Prov. 20:22.

p Or, *a green tree that groweth in his own soil.*

q See 1 Ki. 8:61.

r Psa. 2:12, *note.*

PSALM 38.

A Psalm of David,
to bring to remembrance.

O LORD, rebuke me not in thy wrath: neither chasten me in thy hot displeasure.
2 For thine arrows stick fast in me, and thy hand presseth me sore.
3 *There is* no soundness in my flesh because of thine anger; neither *is there any* [a]rest in my bones because of my sin.
4 For mine iniquities are gone over mine head: as an heavy burden they are too heavy for me.
5 My wounds stink *and* are corrupt because of my foolishness.
6 I am troubled; I am bowed down greatly; I go mourning all the day long.
7 For my loins are filled with a loathsome *disease*: and *there is* no soundness in my flesh.
8 I am feeble and sore broken: I have roared by reason of the disquietness of my heart.
9 Lord, all my desire *is* before thee; and my groaning is not hid from thee.
10 My heart panteth, my strength faileth me: as for the light of mine eyes, it also is gone from me.
11 My lovers and my friends stand aloof from my sore; [b]and my kinsmen stand afar off.
12 They also that seek after my life lay snares *for me*: and they that seek my hurt speak mischievous things, and imagine deceits all the day long.
13 But I, as a deaf *man*, heard not; and I *was* as a dumb man *that* openeth not his mouth.
14 Thus I was as a man that heareth not, and in whose mouth *are* no reproofs.
15 For in thee, O LORD, do I hope: thou wilt [d]hear, O Lord my God.
16 For I said, *Hear me*, lest *otherwise* they should rejoice over me: when my foot slippeth, they magnify *themselves* against me.
17 [e]For I *am* ready to halt, and my sorrow *is* continually before me.
18 For I will declare mine iniquity; [f]I will be sorry for my sin.
19 But mine enemies *are* lively, *and* they are strong: and they that hate me wrongfully are multiplied.
20 They also that render evil for good are mine adversaries; [g]because I follow *the thing that* good *is*.
21 Forsake me not, O LORD: O my God, [h]be not far from me.
22 Make haste to help me, O Lord my salvation.

PSALM 39.

To the chief Musician, *even* to [1]Jeduthun, A Psalm of David.

I said, I will take heed to my ways, that I sin not with my tongue: I will [i]keep my mouth with a bridle, while the wicked is before me.
2 I was dumb with silence, I held my peace, *even* from good; and my sorrow was stirred.
3 My heart was hot within me, while I was musing [j]the fire burned: *then* spake I with my tongue,
4 LORD, [k]make me to know mine end, and the measure of my days, what it *is*; *that* I may know [l]how frail I *am*.
5 Behold, thou hast made my days *as* an handbreadth; and mine age *is* as nothing before thee: verily every man at his best state *is* altogether vanity. Selah.
6 Surely every man walketh in [m]a vain shew: surely they are disquieted in vain: he heapeth up *riches*, and knoweth not who shall gather them.
7 And now, Lord, what wait I for? [n]my hope *is* in thee.
8 Deliver me from all my transgressions: make me not the reproach of the foolish.
9 I was dumb, I opened not my mouth; because thou didst *it*.
10 [o]Remove thy stroke away from me: I am consumed by the blow of thine hand.
11 When thou with rebukes dost correct man for iniquity, thou makest his beauty to consume away like a moth: surely every man *is* vanity. Selah.
12 Hear my prayer, O LORD, and give ear unto my cry; hold not thy peace at my tears: [p]for I *am* a stranger with thee, *and* a sojourner, as all my fathers *were*.
13 O spare me, that I may recover strength, before I go hence, and be no more.

a Heb. *peace*, or *health*.
b Lk. 23:49.
c 2 Sam. 16:7, 8.
d Or, *answer*.
e Psa. 51:3.
f 2 Cor. 7:9, 10.
g See 1 Pet. 3:14; 1 John 3:12.
h Psa. 35:22.
i Heb. *a bridle*, or *muzzle for my mouth*.
j Jer. 20:9.
k Psa. 90:12; 119:84.
l Or, *what time I have here*.
m Heb. *an image*. 1 Cor. 7:31; Jas. 4:14.
n Psa. 38:15.
o Job 9:34; 13:21.
p Lev. 25:23; 1 Chr. 29:15; Psa. 119:19; 2 Cor. 5:6; Heb. 11:13; 1 Pet. 1.17; 2:11.

[1] **(39, inscription)** Jeduthun, a Levite, chief singer and instructor. See 1 Chr. 9:16; 16:38, 41, 42; 25:1, 3, 6; 2 Chr. 5:12; 35:15; Neh. 11:17. He is mentioned in Psalms 39, 62, 77. Jeduthun was first called Ethan.

PSALM 40.

To the chief Musician,
A Psalm of David.

[1]I waited patiently for the LORD; and he inclined unto me, and heard my cry.

2 He brought me up also out of [a]an horrible pit, out of the miry clay, and set my feet upon a rock, *and* established my goings.

3 And he hath put a new song in my mouth, *even* praise unto our God: many shall see *it*, and [b]fear, and shall trust in the LORD.

4 Blessed *is* that man that maketh the LORD his [c]trust, and respecteth not the proud, nor such as turn aside to lies.

5 Many, O LORD my God, *are* thy wonderful works *which* thou hast done, and thy thoughts *which are* to us-ward: they cannot be reckoned up in order unto thee: *if* I would declare and speak *of them*, they are more than can be numbered.

6 [d]Sacrifice and offering thou didst not desire; mine ears hast thou opened: burnt offering and sin offering hast thou not required.

7 Then said I, Lo, I come: in the volume of the book *it is* written of me,

8 I delight to do thy [e]will, O my God: yea, [f]thy law *is* within my heart.

9 I have preached righteousness in the great congregation: lo, I have not refrained my lips, O LORD, thou knowest.

10 [g]I have not hid thy righteousness within my heart; I have declared thy faithfulness and thy salvation: I have not concealed thy lovingkindness and thy truth from the great congregation.

11 Withhold not thou thy tender mercies from me, O LORD: let thy lovingkindness and thy truth continually preserve me.

12 For innumerable evils have compassed me about: mine iniquities have taken hold upon me, so that I am not able to look up; they are more than the hairs of mine head: therefore my heart faileth me.

a Heb. *a pit of noise.*
b Psa. 19:9, *note.*
c Psa. 2:12, *note.*
d vs. 6-8; Heb. 10:5-9.
e vs. 7, 8; Mt. 26:39; John 4:34; 6:38; Heb. 10:7.
f *Law (of Moses).* Psa. 78:9, 10. (Ex. 19:1; Gal. 3:1-29.)
g Acts 20:20, 27.
h 1 Pet. 5:7.
i Prov. 14:21; or, *the weak,* or *sick.*
j Psa. 6:2; 147:3; 2 Chr. 30:20.
k Heb. *a thing of Belial.*
l Psa. 55:12-14; Mt. 26:14-16, 21-25, 47-50; Mk. 14:10, 11, 18-21, 43-45; Lk. 22:3-6, 21-23, 47, 48; John 13:18, 21-30; 18:3; Acts 1:16-17.

13 Be pleased, O LORD, to deliver me: O LORD, make haste to help me.

14 Let them be ashamed and confounded together that seek after my soul to destroy it; let them be driven backward and put to shame that wish me evil.

15 Let them be desolate for a reward of their shame that say unto me, Aha, aha.

16 Let all those that seek thee rejoice and be glad in thee: let such as love thy salvation say continually, The LORD be magnified.

17 But I *am* poor and needy; [h]*yet* the Lord thinketh upon me: thou *art* my help and my deliverer; make no tarrying, O my God.

PSALM 41.

To the chief Musician,
A Psalm of David.

Blessed [i]*is* he that considereth the poor: the LORD will deliver him in time of trouble.

2 The LORD will preserve him, and keep him alive; *and* he shall be blessed upon the earth: and thou wilt not deliver him unto the will of his enemies.

3 The LORD will strengthen him upon the bed of languishing: thou wilt make all his bed in his sickness.

4 I said, LORD, be merciful unto me: [j]heal my soul; for I have sinned against thee.

5 Mine enemies speak evil of me, When shall he die, and his name perish?

6 And if he come to see *me*, he speaketh vanity: his heart gathereth iniquity to itself; *when* he goeth abroad, he telleth *it*.

7 All that hate me whisper together against me: against me do they devise my hurt.

8 [k]An evil disease, *say they*, cleaveth fast unto him: and *now* that he lieth he shall rise up no more.

9 [2]Yea, mine own familiar friend, in whom I [c]trusted, which did eat of my [l]bread, hath lifted up *his* heel against me.

[1] **(40:1)** The 40th Psalm speaks of Messiah, Jehovah's Servant, obedient unto death. The Psalm begins with the joy of Christ in resurrection (vs. 1, 2). He has been in the horrible pit of the grave, but has been brought up. Verses 3-5 are His resurrection testimony, His "new song." Verses 6 and 7 are retrospective. When sacrifice and offering had become abominable because of the wickedness of the people (Isa. 1:10-15), then the obedient Servant came to make the pure offering (vs. 7-17; Heb. 10:5-17 . See Psalm 41, next in order of the. Messianic Psalms.

[2] **(41:9)** Psalm 41. is the Psalm of the betrayal of the Son of man, as Jesus Himself taught (John 13:18-19). See Psa. 45, next in order of the Messianic Psalms.

10 But thou, O LORD, be merciful unto me, and raise me up, that I may requite them.

11 By this I know that thou favourest me, because mine enemy doth not triumph over me.

12 And as for me, thou upholdest me in mine integrity, and [a]settest me before thy face for ever.

13 [b]Blessed *be* the LORD God of Israel from everlasting, and to everlasting. Amen, and Amen.

BOOK II

PSALM 42.

To the chief Musician,
[c]Maschil, for the sons of Korah.

As the hart panteth after the water brooks, so panteth my soul after thee, O God.

2 [d]My soul thirsteth for God, [e]for the living God: when shall I come and appear before God?

3 [f]My tears have been my meat day and night, while [g]they continually say unto me, Where *is* thy God?

4 When I remember these *things*, I pour out my soul in me: for I had gone with the multitude, I went with them to the house of God, with the voice of joy and praise, with a multitude that kept holyday.

5 Why art thou [h]cast down, O my soul? and *why* art thou disquieted in me? hope thou in God: for I shall yet [j]praise him *for* the help of his countenance.

6 O my God, my soul is cast down within me: therefore will I remember thee from the land of Jordan, and of the Hermonites, from the hill [k]Mizar.

7 Deep calleth unto deep at the noise of thy waterspouts: all thy waves and thy billows are gone over me.

8 *Yet* the LORD will [l]command his lovingkindness in the daytime, and [m]in the night his song *shall be* with me, *and* my prayer unto the God of my life.

9 I will say unto God my rock, Why hast thou forgotten me? why go I mourning because of the oppression of the enemy?

10 *As* with a sword in my bones, mine enemies reproach me; [n]while they say daily unto me, Where *is* thy God?

11 [o]Why art thou cast down, O my soul? and why art thou disquieted within me? hope thou in God: for I shall yet praise him, *who is* the health of my countenance, and my God.

PSALM 43.

Judge me, O God, and plead my cause against an ungodly nation: O deliver me from the deceitful and unjust man.

2 For thou *art* the God of my strength: why dost thou cast me off? why go I mourning because of the oppression of the enemy?

3 O send out thy light and thy truth: let them lead me; let them bring me unto thy holy hill, and to thy tabernacles.

4 Then will I go unto the altar of God, unto God my [p]exceeding joy: yea, upon the harp will I praise thee, O God my God.

5 [q]Why art thou cast down, O my soul? and why art thou disquieted within me? hope in God: for I shall yet praise him, *who is* the health of my countenance, and my God.

PSALM 44.

To the chief Musician
for the sons of Korah, [c]Maschil.

We have heard with our ears, O God, [r]our fathers have told us, *what* work thou didst in their days, in the times of old.

2 *How* thou didst drive out the [s]heathen with thy hand, and plantedst them; *how* thou didst afflict the people, and cast them out.

3 [t]For they got not the land in possession by their own sword, neither did their own arm save them: but thy right hand, and thine arm, and the light of thy countenance, [u]because thou hadst a favour unto them.

4 Thou art my King, O God: command deliverances for Jacob.

5 Through thee [v]will we push down our enemies: through thy name will we tread them under that rise up against us.

6 For I will not [w]trust in my bow, neither shall my sword save me.

a Psa. 34:15; Job 36:7.
b Psa. 106:48.
c *Maschil, "instruction."*
d Psa. 63:1; 84:2; John 7:37.
e 1 Thes. 1:9.
f Psa. 80:5; 102:9.
g v. 10; Psa. 79:10; 115:2.
h Heb. *bowed down.*
i Lam. 3:24.
j Or, *give thanks.*
k Or, *the little hill.* Psa. 133:3.
l Psa. 133:3; Lev. 25:21; Deut. 28:8.
m Psa. 32:7; 63:6; 149:5; Job 35:10.
n v. 3; Joel 2:17; Mic. 7:10.
o v. 5; Psa. 43:5.
p Heb. *the gladness of my joy.*
q Psa. 42:5, 11.
r Psa. 78:3; Ex. 12:26, 27.
s i.e. *nations.*
t Deut. 8:17; Josh. 24:12.
u Deut. 4:37; 7:7, 8.
v Dan. 8:4.
w Psa. 2:12, *note.*

7 But thou hast saved us from our enemies, and hast put them to shame that
hated us.
8 [a]In God we boast all the day long,
and praise thy name for ever. Selah.
9 But thou hast cast off, and put us to
shame; and goest not forth with our
armies.
10 Thou makest us to turn back from
the enemy: and they which hate us spoil
for themselves.
11 [b]Thou hast given us like sheep
appointed for meat; and hast scattered us
among the [c]heathen.
12 Thou sellest thy people [d]for
nought, and dost not increase *thy wealth*
by their price.
13 [e]Thou makest us a reproach to our
neighbours, a scorn and a derision to
them that are round about us.
14 Thou makest us a byword among
the [c]heathen, a shaking of the head
among the people.
15 My confusion *is* continually before
me, and the shame of my face hath covered me,
16 For the voice of him that reproacheth and blasphemeth; by reason of the
enemy and avenger.
17 All this is come upon us; yet have
we not forgotten thee, neither have we
dealt falsely in thy covenant.
18 Our heart is not turned back, neither
have our steps declined from thy way;
19 Though thou hast sore broken us in
the place of dragons, and covered us
with the shadow of death.
20 If we have forgotten the name of
our God, or stretched out our hands to a
strange god;
21 [f]Shall not God search this out? for
he knoweth the secrets of the heart.
22 Yea, [b]for thy sake are we killed all
the day long; we are counted as sheep
for the slaughter.
23 Awake, why sleepest thou, O Lord?
arise, cast *us* not off for ever.
24 Wherefore hidest thou thy face, *and*
forgettest our affliction and our oppression?
25 [g]For our soul is bowed down to the
dust: our belly cleaveth unto the earth.
26 Arise [h]for our help, and [i]redeem us
for thy mercies' sake.

PSALM 45.

To the chief Musician upon
[1]Shoshannim, for the sons of Korah,
Maschil, A Song of loves.

My heart is inditing a good matter: I
speak of the things which I have
made touching the [2]king: my tongue *is*
the pen of a ready writer.
2 Thou art fairer than the children of
men: [j]grace is poured into thy lips:
therefore God hath blessed thee for ever.
3 Gird thy sword upon *thy* thigh, O
most mighty, with thy glory and thy
majesty.
4 And in thy majesty ride prosperously because of truth and meekness *and*
righteousness; and thy right hand shall
teach thee terrible things.
5 Thine arrows *are* sharp in the heart
of the king's enemies; *whereby* the people
fall under thee.
6 [k]Thy throne, O God, *is* for ever and
ever: the sceptre of thy kingdom *is* a
right sceptre.
7 Thou lovest righteousness, and
hatest wickedness: therefore God, thy
God, hath anointed thee with [l]the oil of
gladness above thy fellows.
8 [m]All thy garments *smell* of myrrh
and aloes, *and* cassia, out of the ivory

a Psa. 34:2; Jer. 9:24; Rom. 2:17.
b Rom. 8:36.
c i.e. *nations.*
d Heb. *without riches.*
e Psa. 79:4; 80:6; Deut. 28:37.
f Psa. 139:1; Job 31:14; Jer. 17:10.
g Psa. 119:25.
h Heb. *a help for us.*
i Ex. 14:30, *note;* Isa. 59:20, *note.*
j Lk. 4:22.
k Psa. 93:2; Heb. 1:8.
l Psa. 21:6; Heb. 1:8, 9.
m Song 1:3, 12-13.

[1]**(45, inscription)** *Shoshannim,* "lilies," and so, the spring; the Shoshannim Psalms were probably connected with the Passover season, and hence reminders of redemption out of bondage, and of the origins of Israel.

[2]**(45:1)** This great Psalm of the King, with Psalms 46–47, obviously looks forward to the advent in glory. The reference in Heb. 1:8, 9 is not so much to the anointing as an event (Mt. 3:16, 17) as to the permanent state of the King. Cf. Isa. 11:1, 2. The divisions are: (1) The supreme beauty of the King (vs. 1, 2); (2) the coming of the King in glory (vs. 3-5. Cf. Rev. 19:11-21); (3) the deity of the King and the character of His reign (vs. 6, 7; Heb. 1:8, 9; Isa. 11:1-5); (4) as associated with Him in earthly rule, the queen is presented (vs. 9-13), and in that relation the King is not called Elohim (Gen. 1:1, *note*), as in verse 6, but Adonai, the husband name of Deity (Gen. 15:1, *note*); (5) the virgin companions of the queen, who would seem to be the Jewish remnant (Rom. 11:5, *note:* Rev. 14:1-4), are next seen (vs. 14-15); and (6) the Psalm closes with a reference to the earthly fame of the King (vs. 16, 17). See Psa. 68 next in order of the Messianic Psalms.

palaces, whereby they have made thee glad.

9 [a]Kings' daughters *were* among thy honourable women: [b]upon thy right hand did stand the queen in gold of Ophir.

10 Hearken, O daughter, and consider, and incline thine ear; [c]forget also thine own people, and thy father's house;

11 So shall the king greatly desire thy beauty: [d]for he *is* thy Lord; and worship thou him.

12 And the daughter of Tyre *shall be there* with a gift; *even* the rich among the people shall intreat [e]thy favour.

13 [f]The king's daughter *is* all glorious within: her clothing *is* of wrought gold.

14 [g]She shall be brought unto the king in raiment of needlework: the virgins her companions that follow her shall be brought unto thee.

15 With gladness and rejoicing shall they be brought: they shall enter into the king's palace.

16 Instead of thy fathers shall be thy children, whom thou mayest make princes in all the earth.

17 [h]I will make thy name to be remembered in all generations: therefore shall the people praise thee for ever and ever.

PSALM 46.

To the chief Musician for the sons of Korah, A Song upon [1] Alamoth.

God *is* our [i]refuge and strength, [j]a very present help in trouble.

2 Therefore will not we fear, though the earth be removed, and though the mountains be carried into the [k]midst of the sea;

3 *Though* the waters thereof roar *and* be troubled, *though* the mountains shake with the swelling thereof. Selah.

4 [l]*There is* a river, the streams whereof shall make glad [m]the city of God, the holy *place* of the tabernacles of the most High.

5 God *is* [n]in the midst of her; she shall not be moved: God shall help her, *and that* right early.

6 The [o]heathen raged, the kingdoms were moved: he uttered his voice, the earth melted.

7 [p]The LORD of hosts *is* with us; the God of Jacob *is* [q]our refuge. Selah.

8 Come, behold the works of the LORD, what desolations he hath made in the earth.

9 [r]He maketh wars to cease unto the end of the earth; [s]he breaketh the bow, and cutteth the spear in sunder; [t]he burneth the chariot in the fire.

10 Be still, and know that I *am* God: I will be exalted among the [o]heathen, I will be exalted in the earth.

11 The LORD of hosts *is* with us; the God of Jacob *is* our refuge. Selah.

PSALM 47.

To the chief Musician, A Psalm for the sons of Korah.

O clap your hands, all ye people; shout unto God with the voice of triumph.

2 For the LORD most high [u]*is* terrible; [v]*he is* a great King over all the earth.

3 [w]He shall subdue the people under us, and the nations under our feet.

4 He shall choose [x]our inheritance for us, the excellency of Jacob whom he loved. Selah.

5 [y]God is gone up with a shout, the LORD with the sound of a trumpet.

6 Sing praises to God, sing praises: sing praises unto our King, sing praises.

7 For [z]God *is* the King of all the earth: sing ye praises with understanding.

8 God reigneth over the [o]heathen: God sitteth upon the throne of his holiness.

9 The princes of the people are gathered together, [aa]*even* the people of the God of Abraham: [bb]for the shields of the earth *belong* unto God: he is greatly exalted.

PSALM 48

A Song *and* Psalm for the sons of Korah.

Great *is* the LORD, and greatly to be praised in [cc]the city of our God, *in* the mountain of his holiness.

2 Beautiful for situation, the joy of the whole earth, *is* mount Zion, *on* the sides

a Song 6:8.
b See 1 Ki. 2:19.
c See Deut. 21:13.
d Psa. 95:6; Isa. 54:5.
e Heb. *thy face.*
f Rev. 19:7, 8.
g Song 1:4.
h Mal. 1:11.
i Psa. 62:7, 8; 91:2; 142:5.
j Deut. 4:7; Psa. 145:18.
k Heb. *the heart of the seas.*
l See Ezk. 47:1-12.
m Psa. 48:1, 8; Isa. 60:14.
n Deut. 23:14; Isa. 12:6; Ezk. 43:7; Hos. 11:9; Joel 2:27; Zeph. 3:15; Zech. 2:5, 10, 11; 8:3.
o i.e. *nations.*
p v. 11; Num. 14:9; 2 Chr. 13:12.
q Heb. *an high place for us.* Psa. 9:9.
r Isa. 2:4.
s Psa. 76:3.
t Ezk. 39:9.
u Psa. 76:12; Deut. 7:21; Neh. 1:5.
v Mal. 1:14.
w Psa. 18:47.
x 1 Pet. 1:4.
y Psa. 68:24, 25.
z Zech. 14:9.
aa Rom. 4:11, 12.
bb Psa. 89:18.
cc Psa. 46:4; 87:3.

[1] **(46, inscription)** *Alamoth,* "soprano," from *almah,* a virgin. Some have thought the *alamoth,* "virgins," were a temple choir, singing antiphonally to the *sheminith,* or male choir. See Psa. 6, title, *note.* But *contra,* see 1 Chr. 15:20.

of the north, [a]the city of the great King.

3 God is known in her palaces for a refuge.

4 For, lo, the kings were assembled, they passed by together.

5 They saw *it, and* so they marvelled; they were troubled, *and* hasted away.

6 Fear took hold upon them there, *and* pain, as of a woman in travail.

7 [b]Thou breakest the ships of Tarshish with an east wind.

8 As we have heard, so have we seen [c]in the city of the LORD of hosts, in the city of our God: [d]God will establish it for ever. Selah.

9 We have thought of thy lovingkindness, O God, in the midst of thy temple.

10 According to thy name, O God, so *is* thy praise unto the ends of the earth: thy right hand is full of righteousness.

11 Let mount Zion rejoice, let the daughters of Judah be glad, because of thy judgments.

12 Walk about Zion, and go round about her: tell the towers thereof.

13 [e]Mark ye well her bulwarks, consider her palaces; that ye may tell *it* to the generation following.

14 For this God *is* our God for ever and ever: [f]he will be our guide *even* unto death.

PSALM 49.

To the chief Musician,
A Psalm for the sons of Korah.

Hear this, all *ye* people; give ear, all *ye* inhabitants of the [g]world:

2 Both low and high, rich and poor, together.

3 My mouth shall speak of wisdom; and the meditation of my heart *shall be* of understanding.

4 I will incline mine ear to a parable: I will open my dark saying upon the harp.

5 Wherefore should I fear in the days of evil, *when* the iniquity of my heels shall compass me about?

6 They that [h]trust in their wealth, and boast themselves in the multitude of their riches;

7 None *of them* can by any means [i]redeem his brother, nor give to God a ransom for him:

8 (For the [i]redemption of their soul *is* precious, and it ceaseth for ever:)

9 That he should still live for ever, *and* not see corruption.

10 For he seeth *that* wise men die, likewise the fool and the brutish person perish, and leave their wealth to others.

11 Their inward thought *is, that* their houses *shall continue* for ever, *and* their dwelling places to all generations; they call *their* lands after their own names.

12 Nevertheless man *being* in honour abideth not: he is like the beasts *that* perish.

13 This their way *is* their folly: yet their posterity approve their sayings. Selah.

14 Like sheep they are laid in the [j]grave; death shall feed on them; and the upright shall have dominion over them in the morning; and their beauty shall consume in the grave from their dwelling.

15 But God will [i]redeem my soul from the power of the [j]grave: for he shall receive me. Selah.

16 Be not thou afraid when one is made rich, when the glory of his house is increased;

17 For when he dieth he shall carry nothing away: his glory shall not descend after him.

18 Though while he lived he blessed his soul: and *men* will praise thee, when thou doest well to thyself.

19 He shall go to the generation of his fathers; they shall never see light.

20 Man *that is* in honour, and understandeth not, is like the beasts *that* perish.

PSALM 50.

A Psalm of Asaph.

The mighty God, *even* the LORD, hath spoken, and called the earth from the rising of the sun unto the going down thereof.

2 Out of Zion, the perfection of beauty, God hath shined.

3 Our God shall [k]come, and shall not keep silence: [l]a fire shall [m]devour before him, and it shall be very tempestuous round about him.

4 He shall call to the heavens from above, and to the earth, that he may judge his people.

5 Gather my saints together unto me; those that have made a covenant with me by sacrifice.

6 And the [n]heavens shall declare his righteousness: for God *is* judge himself. Selah.

7 Hear, O my people, and I will speak; O Israel, and I will testify against thee: [o]I *am* God, *even* thy God.

8 I will not reprove thee for thy

a Psa. 46:4; Mt. 5:35.

b Ezk.27.26.

c vs .1, 2.

d Isa. 2:2; Mic. 4:1.

e Heb. *set your heart to her bulwarks.*

f Isa. 58:11.

g i.e. *earth.*

h Psa. 2:12, *note.*

i Ex. 14:30, *note;* Isa. 59:20, *note.*

j Heb. *Sheol.* See Hab. 2:5, *note.*

k *Christ (Second Advent).* Psa. 96:10-13. (Deut. 30:3; Acts 1:9-11.)

l *Judgments (the seven).* vs. 3, 4, 22; Ezk. 20:33-44. (2 Sam. 7:14; Rev. 22:12.)

m Lev. 10:2; Num. 16:35; Dan. 7:10.

n Psa. 97:6.

o Ex. 20:2.

sacrifices or thy burnt offerings, *to have*
been continually before me.
9 I will [a]take no bullock out of thy
house, *nor* he goats out of thy folds.
10 For every beast of the forest *is* mine,
and the cattle upon a thousand hills.
11 I know all the fowls of the mountains: and the wild beasts of the field *are*
mine.
12 If I were hungry, I would not tell
thee: [b]for the world *is* mine, and the fulness thereof.
13 Will I eat the flesh of bulls, or drink
the blood of goats?
14 [c]Offer unto God thanksgiving; and
pay thy vows unto the most High:
15 And [d]call upon me in the day of
trouble: I will deliver thee, and thou
shalt glorify me.
16 But unto the wicked God saith,
What hast thou to do to declare my
statutes, or *that* thou shouldest take my
covenant in thy mouth?
17 Seeing thou hatest instruction, and
castest my words behind thee.
18 When thou sawest a thief, then
thou [f]consentedst with him, and hast
been [g]partaker with adulterers.
19 Thou givest thy mouth to evil, and
thy tongue frameth deceit.
20 Thou sittest *and* speakest against
thy brother; thou slanderest thine own
mother's son.
21 These *things* hast thou done, and I
kept silence; [h]thou thoughtest that I was
altogether *such an one* as thyself: [i]*but* I
will reprove thee, and set *them* in order
before thine eyes.
22 Now consider this, ye that forget

a vs. 9-16.
b Psa. 24:1; Ex. 19:5; Deut. 10:14; Job 41:11; 1 Cor. 10:26.
c Hos. 14:2; Heb. 13:15.
d Psa. 91:15; 107:6, 13; Job 22:27; Zech. 13:9.
e Neh. 9:26.
f Rom. 1:32.
g 1 Tim. 5:22.
h See Rom. 2:4.
i Psa. 90:8.
j vs. 3, 4.
k *Bible prayers* (O.T.). Isa. 37:15. (Gen. 15:2; Hab. 3:1-16.)
l Rom. 3:4.
m Psa. 58:3; Job 14:4; John 3:6; Rom. 5:12; Eph. 2:3.
n Job 14:4.
o Heb. *warm me.*
p Lev. 14:4, 6, 49; Num. 19:18; Heb. 9:19.
q Isa. 1:18.
r Mt. 5:4.
s Acts 15:9; Eph. 2:10.

God, lest I [j]tear *you* in pieces, and *there*
be none to deliver.
23 Whoso offereth praise glorifieth me:
and to him that ordereth *his* conversation
aright will I shew the salvation of God.

PSALM 51.

To the chief Musician,
A Psalm of David, when Nathan
the prophet came unto him,
after he had gone in to Bath-sheba.

[1]Have [k]mercy upon me, O God, according to thy lovingkindness: according
unto the multitude of thy tender mercies
blot out my transgressions.
2 Wash me throughly from mine iniquity, and cleanse me from my sin.
3 For I acknowledge my transgressions: and my sin *is* ever before me.
4 Against thee, thee only, have I
sinned, and done *this* evil in thy sight:
that thou mightest be [l]justified when
thou speakest, *and* be clear when thou
judgest.
5 [m]Behold, I was shapen in iniquity;
and [n]in sin did my mother [o]conceive me.
6 Behold, thou desirest truth in the
inward parts: and in the hidden *part*
thou shalt make me to know wisdom.
7 [p]Purge me with [2]hyssop, and I shall
be clean: wash me, and I shall be [q]whiter
than snow.
8 Make me to hear joy and gladness;
that the bones *which* thou hast broken
[r]may rejoice.
9 Hide thy face from my sins, and blot
out all mine iniquities.
10 [s]Create in me a clean heart, O

[1](51:1) This Psalm must ever be, in its successive steps, the mould of the experience of a sinning saint who comes back to full communion and service. The steps are: (1) sin thoroughly judged before God (vs. 1-6); (2) forgiveness and cleansing through the blood (v. 7, f.c.); (3) cleansing (v. 7, l.c. to 10. Cf. John 13:4-10; Eph. 5:26; 1 John 1:9); (4) Spirit-filled for joy and power (vs. 11, 12); (5) service (v. 13); (6) worship (vs. 14-17); (7) the restored saint in fellowship with God, not about self, but about the blessing of Zion. Personally, it was David's pathway to restored communion after his sin with Bathsheba. Dispensationally, it will be the pathway of returning Israel (Deut. 30:1-10, *refs.*).

[2](51:7) Hyssop was the little shrub (1 Ki. 4:33) with which the blood and water of purification were applied (Lev. 14:1-7; Num. 19:1-19).

Cleansing in Scripture is twofold: (1) Of a sinner from the guilt of sin; the blood ("hyssop") aspect; (2) of a saint from the defilement of sin—the water ("wash me") aspect. Under grace the sinner *is* purged by blood when he believes (Mt. 26:28; Heb. 1:3; 9:12; 10:14). Both aspects of cleansing, by blood and by water, are brought out in John 13:10, and Eph. 5:25, 26: "He that is bathed needeth not save to wash his feet"; "Christ loved the church and gave Himself for it [redemption by blood, "hyssop," the bath"] that He might sanctify and cleanse it with the washing of water by the word": answering to the "wash me" of verse 7.

God; and renew a right spirit within me.

11 Cast me not away from thy presence; and [1]take not thy holy [a]spirit from me.

12 Restore unto me the joy of thy salvation; and uphold me *with thy* [b]free spirit.

13 *Then* will I teach transgressors thy ways; and sinners shall be converted unto thee.

14 Deliver me from bloodguiltiness, O God, thou God of my salvation: *and* my tongue shall sing aloud of thy righteousness.

15 O Lord, open thou my lips; and my mouth shall shew forth thy praise.

16 For thou desirest not sacrifice; else would I give *it*: thou delightest not in burnt offering.

17 [c]The sacrifices of God *are* a broken spirit: a broken and a contrite heart, O God, thou wilt not despise.

18 Do good in thy good pleasure unto Zion: build thou the walls of Jerusalem.

19 Then shalt thou be pleased with the [d]sacrifices of righteousness, with burnt offering and whole burnt offering: then shall they offer bullocks upon thine altar.

PSALM 52.

To the chief Musician, [e]Maschil, *A Psalm* of David, when Doeg the Edomite came and told Saul, and said unto him, David is come to the house of Ahimelech.

Why boastest thou thyself in mischief, O mighty man? the goodness of God *endureth* continually.

2 Thy tongue deviseth mischiefs; like a sharp razor, working deceitfully.

3 Thou lovest evil more than good; *and* lying rather than to speak righteousness. Selah.

4 Thou lovest all devouring words, O *thou* deceitful tongue.

5 God shall likewise [f]destroy thee for ever, he shall take thee away, and pluck thee out of *thy* dwelling place, and root thee out of the land of the living. Selah.

6 The righteous also shall see, and fear, and shall laugh at him:

7 Lo, *this is* the man *that* made not God his strength; but [g]trusted in the abundance of his riches, *and* strengthened himself in his wickedness.

8 But I *am* like a green olive tree in the house of God: I trust in the mercy of God for ever and ever.

9 I will praise thee for ever, because thou hast done *it*: and I will wait on thy name; for *it is* good before thy saints.

PSALM 53.

To the chief Musician upon [h]Mahalath, [e]Maschil, *A Psalm* of David.

The [i]fool hath said in his heart, *There is* no God. Corrupt are they, and have done abominable iniquity: [j]*there is* none that doeth good.

2 God looked down from heaven upon the children of men, to see if there were *any* that did understand, that did [k]seek God.

3 Every one of them is gone back: they are altogether become filthy; *there is* none that doeth good, no, not one.

4 Have the workers of iniquity no knowledge? who eat up my people *as* they eat bread: they have not called upon God.

5 [l]There were they in great fear, *where* no fear was: for God hath scattered the bones of him that encampeth *against* thee: thou hast put *them* to shame, because God hath despised them.

6 [m]Oh that the salvation of Israel *were come* out of Zion! When God bringeth back the captivity of his people, Jacob shall rejoice, *and* Israel shall be glad.

PSALM 54.

To the chief Musician on [n]Neginoth, [e]Maschil, *A Psalm* of David, when the [o]Ziphims came and said to Saul, Doth not David hide himself with us?

Save me, O God, by thy name, and judge me by thy strength.

2 Hear my prayer, O God; give ear to the words of my mouth.

3 For strangers are risen up against me, and oppressors seek after my soul: they have not set God before them. Selah.

4 Behold, God *is* mine helper: the

a *Holy Spirit.* vs. 11, 12; Psa. 139:7. (Gen. 1:2; Mal. 2.15.)

b 2 Cor. 3:17.

c Psa. 34:18; Isa. 57:15; 66:2.

d Psa. 4:5; Mal. 3:3.

e *Maschil, "instruction."*

f Heb. *beat thee down.*

g Psa. 2:12, *note.*

h *Mahalath,* aparently a temple choir.

i Psa. 10:4; 14:1.

j Rom. 3:10-12.

k 2 Chr. 15:2; 19:3.

l Lev. 26:17, 36; Prov. 28:1.

m Psa. 14:7.

n *Neginoth,* stringed instruments.

o Or, *Ziphites.* Cf. 1 Sam. 23:19.

[1]**(51:11)** No believer of this dispensation, aware of the promise of His abiding (John 14:16), should pray, "take not Thy Holy Spirit from me" (Eph. 4:30); but, while Christian *position* is not found here, Christian *experience* in essence is.

Lord *is* with them that uphold my soul.

5 He shall reward evil unto mine [a]enemies: cut them off in thy truth.

6 I will freely sacrifice unto thee: I will praise thy name, O LORD; for *it is* good.

7 For he hath delivered me out of all trouble: [b]and mine eye hath seen *his desire* upon mine enemies.

PSALM 55.

To the chief Musician on [c]Neginoth, [d]Maschil, *A Psalm* of David.

Give ear to my prayer, O God; and hide not thyself from my supplication.

2 Attend unto me, and hear me: I mourn in my complaint, and make a noise;

3 Because of the voice of the enemy, because of the oppression of the wicked: for they cast iniquity upon me, and in wrath they hate me.

4 My heart is sore pained within me: and the terrors of death are fallen upon me.

5 Fearfulness and trembling are come upon me, and horror hath [e]overwhelmed me.

6 And I said, Oh that I had wings like a dove! *for then* would I fly away, and be at rest.

7 Lo, *then* would I wander far off, *and* remain in the wilderness. Selah.

8 I would hasten my escape from the windy storm *and* tempest.

9 Destroy, O Lord, *and* divide their tongues: for I have seen violence and strife in the city.

10 Day and night they go about it upon the walls thereof: mischief also and sorrow *are* in the midst of it.

11 Wickedness *is* in the midst thereof: deceit and guile depart not from her streets.

12 [f]For *it was* not an enemy *that* reproached me; then I could have borne it: neither *was it* he that hated me *that* did [g]magnify *himself* against me; then I would have hid myself from him:

13 But *it was* thou, a man mine equal, my guide, and mine [h]acquaintance.

14 We took sweet counsel together, and walked unto the house of God in company.

15 Let death seize upon them, *and* let them go down quick into [i]hell: for wickedness *is* in their dwellings, *and* among them.

16 As for me, I will call upon God; and the LORD shall save me.

17 Evening, and morning, and at noon, will I pray, and cry aloud: and he shall hear my voice.

18 He hath delivered my soul in peace from the battle *that was* against me: [j]for there were many with me.

19 God shall hear, and afflict them, [k]even he that abideth of old. Selah. Because they have no changes, therefore they fear not God.

20 [l]He hath put forth his hands against such as [m]be at peace with him: [n]he hath broken his covenant.

21 [o]*The words* of his mouth were smoother than butter, but war *was* in his heart: his words were softer than oil, yet *were* they drawn swords.

22 [p]Cast thy burden upon the LORD, and he shall sustain thee: [q]he shall never suffer the righteous to be moved.

23 But thou, O God, shalt bring them down into the pit of destruction: bloody and deceitful men shall not live out half their days; but I will trust in thee.

PSALM 56.

To the chief Musician upon [r]Jonath-elem-rechokim, [s]Michtam of David, when the Philistines took him in Gath.

[t]Be merciful unto me, O God: for man would swallow me up; he fighting daily oppresseth me.

2 Mine enemies would daily swallow *me* up: for *they be* many that fight against me, O thou most High.

3 What time I am afraid, I will [u]trust in thee.

4 In God I will praise his word, in God I have put my trust; [v]I will not fear what flesh can do unto me.

5 Every day they wrest my words: all their thoughts *are* against me for evil.

6 They gather themselves together, they hide themselves, they mark my steps, when they wait for my soul.

7 Shall they escape by iniquity? in *thine* anger cast down the people, O God.

a Heb. *those that observe me.*

b Psa. 59:10; 92:11.

c i.e. stringed instruments.

d i.e. *instruction.*

e Heb. *covered me.*

f Psa. 41:9.

g Psa. 35:26; 38:16.

h Psa. 41:9; Jer. 9:4.

i Or, *the grave.*

j 2 Chr. 32:7, 8.

k Deut. 33:27.

l Acts 12:1.

m Psa. 7:4.

n Heb. *he hath profaned.*

o Psa. 28:3; 57:4; 62:4; 64:3; Prov. 5:3, 4; 12:18.

p Psa. 37:5; Mt. 6:25; Lk. 12:22; 1 Pet. 5:7.

q Psa. 37:24.

r Meaning, "the cry of the dove of distant terebinth trees."

s *Michtam, a prayer.*

t Psa. 57:1.

u Psa. 2:12, *note.*

v Psa. 118:6; Isa. 31:3; Heb. 13:6.

8 Thou tellest my wanderings: put thou my tears into thy bottle: [a]*are they* not in thy book?
9 When I cry *unto thee*, then shall mine enemies turn back: this I know; for [b]God *is* for me.
10 In God will I praise *his* word: in the LORD will I praise *his* word.
11 In God have I put my trust: I will not be afraid what man can do unto me.
12 Thy vows *are* upon me, O God: I will render praises unto thee.
13 [c]For thou hast delivered my soul from death: *wilt* not *thou deliver* my feet from falling, that I may walk before God in the light of the living?

PSALM 57.

To the chief Musician, [d]Al-taschith, [e]Michtam of David, when he fled from Saul in the cave.

Be merciful unto me, O God, be merciful unto me: for my soul [f]trusteth in thee: [g]yea, in the shadow of thy wings will I make my refuge, [h]until *these* calamities be overpast.
2 I will cry unto God most high; unto God that performeth *all things* for me.
3 [i]He shall send from heaven, and save me *from* the reproach of him that would swallow me up. Selah. God shall send forth his mercy and his truth.
4 My soul *is* among lions: *and* I lie *even among* them that are set on fire, *even* the sons of men, whose teeth *are* spears and arrows, and their tongue a sharp sword.
5 Be thou exalted, O God, above the heavens; *let* thy glory *be* above all the earth.
6 They have prepared a net for my steps; my soul is bowed down: they have digged a pit before me, into the midst whereof they are fallen *themselves*. Selah.
7 My heart is fixed, O God, my heart is fixed: I will sing and give praise.
8 Awake up, my glory; awake, psaltery and harp: I *myself* will awake early.
9 I will praise thee, O Lord, among the people: I will sing unto thee among the nations.
10 For thy mercy *is* great unto the heavens, and thy truth unto the clouds.
11 Be thou exalted, O God, above the heavens: *let* thy glory *be* above all the earth.

PSALM 58.

To the chief Musician, [d]Al-taschith, [e]Michtam of David.

Do ye indeed speak righteousness, O congregation? do ye judge uprightly, O ye sons of men?
2 Yea, in heart ye work wickedness; ye weigh the violence of your hands in the earth.
3 The wicked are estranged from the womb: they go astray as soon as they be born, speaking lies.
4 Their poison *is* like the poison of a serpent: *they are* like the deaf adder *that* stoppeth her ear;
5 Which will not hearken to the voice of charmers, charming never so wisely.
6 Break their teeth, O God, in their mouth: break out the great teeth of the young lions, O LORD.
7 [j]Let them melt away as waters *which* run continually: *when* he bendeth *his bow to shoot* his arrows, let them be as cut in pieces.
8 As a snail *which* melteth, let *every one of them* pass away: *like* the untimely birth of a woman, *that* they may not see the sun.
9 Before your pots can feel the thorns, he shall take them away as with a whirlwind, [k]both living, and in *his* wrath.
10 The righteous shall rejoice when he seeth the vengeance: [l]he shall wash his feet in the blood of the wicked.
11 So that a man shall say, Verily *there is* a reward for the righteous: verily he is a God that judgeth in the earth.

PSALM 59.

To the chief Musician, [d]Al-taschith, [e]Michtam of David; when Saul sent, and they watched the house to kill him.

Deliver me from mine enemies, O my God: defend me from them that rise up against me.
2 Deliver me from the workers of iniquity, and save me from bloody men.
3 For, lo, they lie in wait for my soul: the mighty are gathered against me; [m]not *for* my transgression, nor *for* my sin, O LORD.
4 They run and prepare themselves without *my* fault: awake to help me, and behold.
5 Thou therefore, O LORD God of hosts, the God of Israel, awake to visit all the [n]heathen:

a Psa. 118:6; Mal. 3:16.
b Rom. 8:31.
c Psa. 116:8.
d *Al-taschith, destroy not.*
e *Michtam, a prayer.*
f Psa. 2:12, *note.*
g Psa. 17:8; 63:7.
h Isa. 26:20.
i Psa. 144:5, 7.
j Psa. 112:10; Josh. 7:5.
k Heb. *as living as wrath.*
l Psa. 68:23.
m 1 Sam. 24:11.
n i.e. *nations.*

be not merciful to any wicked transgressors. Selah.

6 They return at evening: they make a noise like a dog, and go round about the city.

7 Behold, they belch out with their mouth: swords *are* in their lips: for who, *say they*, doth hear?

8 But thou, O LORD, shalt laugh at them; thou shalt have all the [a]heathen in derision.

9 *Because of* his strength will I wait upon thee: for God *is* [b]my defence.

10 The God of my mercy shall prevent me: God shall let [c]me see *my desire* upon mine enemies.

11 Slay them not, lest my people forget: scatter them by thy power; and bring them down, O Lord our shield.

12 *For* the sin of their mouth *and* the words of their lips let them even be taken in their pride: and for cursing and lying *which* they speak.

13 [d]Consume *them* in wrath, consume *them*, that they *may* not *be*: and [e]let them know that God ruleth in Jacob unto the ends of the earth. Selah.

14 And at evening let them return; *and* let them make a noise like a dog, and go round about the city.

15 Let them wander up and down for meat, and grudge if they be not satisfied.

16 But I will sing of thy power; yea, I will sing aloud of thy mercy in the morning: for thou hast been my defence and refuge in the day of my trouble.

17 Unto thee, O my strength, will I sing: for God *is* my defence, *and* the God of my mercy.

PSALM 60.

To the chief Musician upon [f]Shushan-eduth, [g]Michtam of David, to teach; [h]when he strove with Aram-naharaim and with Aram-zobah, when Joab returned, and smote of Edom in the valley of salt twelve thousand.

O God, thou hast cast us off, thou hast scattered us, thou hast been displeased; O turn thyself to us again.

2 Thou hast made the earth to tremble; thou hast broken it: heal the breaches thereof; for it shaketh.

3 [i]Thou hast shewed thy people hard things: [j]thou hast made us to drink the wine of astonishment.

4 Thou hast given a banner to them that [k]fear thee, that it may be displayed because of the truth. Selah.

5 [l]That thy beloved may be delivered; save *with* thy right hand, and hear me.

6 God hath spoken in his holiness; I will rejoice, I will [m]divide [n]Shechem, and mete out the valley [o]of Succoth.

7 Gilead *is* mine, and Manasseh *is* mine; [p]Ephraim also *is* the strength of mine head; [q]Judah *is* my lawgiver;

8 [r]Moab *is* my washpot; [s]over Edom will I cast out my shoe: [t]Philistia, triumph thou because of me.

9 Who will bring me *into* the strong city? who will lead me into Edom?

10 *Wilt* not thou, O God, *which* hadst cast us off? and *thou*, O God, *which* didst not go out with our armies?

11 Give us help from trouble: [u]for vain *is* the [v]help of man.

12 Through God we shall do valiantly: for he *it is that* shall tread down our enemies.

PSALM 61.

To the chief Musician upon [w]Neginah, *A Psalm* of David.

Hear my cry, O God; attend unto my prayer.

2 From the end of the earth will I cry unto thee, when my heart is overwhelmed: lead me to the rock *that* is higher than I.

3 For thou hast been a shelter for me, *and* a strong tower from the enemy.

4 I will abide in thy tabernacle for ever: I will [x]trust in the covert of thy wings. Selah.

5 For thou, O God, hast heard my vows: thou hast given *me* the heritage of those that fear thy name.

6 Thou wilt prolong the king's life: *and* his years as many generations.

7 He shall abide before God for ever: O prepare mercy and truth, *which* may preserve him.

8 So will I sing praise unto thy name for ever, that I may daily perform my vows.

---

a i.e. *nations.*
b Heb. *my high place.*
c Psa. 54:7; 92:11; 112:8.
d Psa. 7:9.
e Psa. 83:18.
f *Shushaneduth, the lily of speech.*
g *Michtam, a prayer.*
h 2 Sam. 8:3-13.
i Psa. 71:20.
j Isa. 51:17, 22; Jer. 25:15.
k Psa. 19:9, *note.*
l vs. 5-12 are identical with Psa. 108:6-13.
m Josh. 1:6.
n Gen. 12.6.
o Josh. 13:27.
p See Deut. 33:17.
q Gen. 49:10.
r 2 Sam. 8:2.
s 2 Sam. 8:14; Psa.108:9.
t 2 Sam. 8:1.
u Psa. 118:8; 146:3.
v Heb. *salvation.*
w Or, *Neginoth, stringed instruments.*
x Psa. 2:12, *note.*

PSALM 62.

To the chief Musician, to [a]Jeduthun,
A Psalm of David.

Truly my soul [b]waiteth upon God: from him *cometh* my salvation.

2 He only *is* my rock and my salvation; *he is* my [c]defence; I shall not be greatly moved.

3 How long will ye imagine mischief against a man? ye shall be slain all of you: as a bowing wall *shall ye be, and as* a tottering fence.

4 They only consult to cast *him* down from his excellency: they delight in lies: they bless with their mouth, but they curse inwardly. Selah.

5 My soul, wait thou only upon God; for my expectation *is* from him.

6 He only *is* my rock and my salvation: *he is* my defence; I shall not be moved.

7 In God *is* my salvation and my glory: the rock of my strength, *and* my refuge, *is* in God.

8 [d]Trust in him at all times; ye people, [e]pour out your heart before him: God *is* a refuge for us. Selah.

9 Surely men of low degree *are* vanity, *and* men of high degree *are* a lie: to be laid in the balance, they *are* altogether *lighter* than vanity.

10 Trust not in oppression, and become not vain in robbery: if riches increase, set not your heart *upon them.*

11 God hath spoken once; twice have I heard this; that power *belongeth* unto God.

12 Also unto thee, O Lord, *belongeth* mercy: for thou renderest to every man according to his work.

PSALM 63.

A Psalm of David, when he was
in the wilderness of Judah.

O God, thou *art* my God; early will I seek thee: [f]my soul thirsteth for thee, my flesh longeth for thee in a dry and thirsty land, where no water is;

2 To see thy power and thy glory, so *as* I have seen thee in the sanctuary.

3 [g]Because thy lovingkindness *is* better than life, my lips shall praise thee.

4 Thus will I bless thee while I live: I will lift up my hands in thy name.

5 My soul shall be satisfied as *with* marrow and fatness; and my mouth shall praise *thee* with joyful lips:

6 When [h]I remember thee upon my bed, *and* meditate on thee in the *night* watches.

7 Because thou hast been my help, therefore in the shadow of thy wings will I rejoice.

8 My soul followeth hard after thee: thy right hand upholdeth me.

9 But those *that* seek my soul, to destroy *it*, shall go into the lower parts of the earth.

10 They shall fall by the sword: they shall be a portion for foxes.

11 But the king shall rejoice in God; every one that sweareth by him shall glory: but the mouth of them that speak lies shall be stopped.

PSALM 64.

To the chief Musician,
A Psalm of David.

Hear my voice, O God, in my prayer: preserve my life from fear of the enemy.

2 Hide me from the secret counsel of the wicked; from the insurrection of the workers of iniquity:

3 Who whet their tongue like a sword, *and* bend *their bows to shoot* their arrows, *even* bitter words:

4 That they may shoot in secret at the [i]perfect: suddenly do they shoot at him, and fear not.

5 They encourage themselves *in* an evil matter: they commune of laying snares privily; they say, Who shall see them?

6 They search out iniquities; [j]they accomplish a diligent search: both the inward *thought* of every one *of them*, and the heart, *is* deep.

7 But God shall shoot at them *with* an arrow; suddenly shall they be wounded.

8 So they shall make their own tongue to fall upon themselves: all that see them shall flee away.

9 And all men shall fear, and shall declare the work of God; for they shall wisely consider of his doing.

10 [k]The righteous shall be glad in the LORD, and shall [d]trust in him; and all the upright in heart shall glory.

a See Psa. 39, title, *note.*

b Heb. *is silent.* Psa. 65:1.

c Heb. *high place.*

d Psa. 2:12, *note.*

e Psa. 42:4; 1 Sam. 1:15; Lam.2:19.

f Psa. 42:2; 84:2; 143:6; Mt. 5:6.

g Psa. 30.5.

h Psa. 42:8; 119:55; 149:5.

i See 1 Ki. 8:61.

j Or, *we are consumed by that which they have thoroughly searched.*

k Psa. 32:11; 58:10; 68:3.

PSALM 65.

To the chief Musician,
A Psalm *and* Song of David.

Praise waiteth for thee, O God, in
Sion: and unto thee shall the vow be
performed.
2 O thou that hearest prayer, [a]unto
thee shall all flesh come.
3 Iniquities prevail against me: *as for*
our transgressions, thou shalt [b]purge
them away.
4 Blessed *is the man whom* thou choosest, and causest to approach *unto thee,*
that he may dwell in thy courts: [c]we
shall be satisfied with the goodness of
thy house, *even* of thy holy temple.
5 *By* terrible things in righteousness
wilt thou answer us, O God of our salvation; *who art* the confidence of all the
ends of the earth, and of them that are
afar off *upon* the sea:
6 Which by his strength setteth fast the
mountains; *being* girded with power:
7 Which stilleth the noise of the seas,
the noise of their waves, and the tumult
of the people.
8 They also that dwell in the uttermost
parts are afraid at thy tokens: thou makest the outgoings of the morning and
evening to rejoice.
9 Thou [d]visitest the earth, and waterest it: thou greatly enrichest it [e]with the
river of God, *which* is full of water: thou
preparest them corn, when thou hast so
provided for it.
10 Thou waterest the ridges thereof
abundantly: thou settlest the furrows
thereof: [f]thou makest it soft with showers: thou blessest the springing thereof.
11 Thou crownest the year with thy
goodness; and thy paths drop fatness.
12 They drop *upon* the pastures of the
wilderness: and the little hills rejoice on
every side.
13 The pastures are clothed with
flocks; the valleys also are covered over
with corn; they shout for joy, they also
sing.

PSALM 66.

To the chief Musician, A Song *or* Psalm.

Make a joyful noise unto God, all ye
lands:
2 Sing forth the honour of his name:
make his praise glorious.
3 Say unto God, How [g]terrible *art thou*
in thy works! [h]through the greatness of
thy power shall thine enemies submit
themselves unto thee.
4 All the earth shall worship thee, and
shall sing unto thee; they shall sing *to*
thy name. Selah.
5 Come and see the works of God: *he*
is terrible *in his* doing toward the children of men.
6 [i]He turned the sea into dry *land*:
[j]they went through the flood on foot:
there did we rejoice in him.
7 He ruleth by his power for ever; his
eyes behold the nations: let not the rebellious exalt themselves. Selah.
8 O bless our God, ye people, and
make the voice of his praise to be heard:
9 Which [k]holdeth our soul in life, and
suffereth not our feet to be moved.
10 For thou, O God, hast proved us:
[l]thou hast tried us, as silver is tried.
11 Thou broughtest us into the net;
thou laidst affliction upon our loins.
12 Thou hast caused men to ride over
our heads; we went through fire and
through water: but thou broughtest us
out into a wealthy *place*.
13 [m]I will go into thy house with burnt
offerings: I will pay thee my vows,
14 Which my lips have uttered, and
my mouth hath spoken, when I was in
trouble.
15 I will offer unto thee burnt sacrifices of fatlings, with the incense of
rams; I will offer bullocks with goats.
Selah.
16 Come *and* hear, all ye that [n]fear
God, and I will declare what he hath
done for my soul.
17 I cried unto him with my mouth,
and he was extolled with my tongue.
18 [o]If I regard iniquity in my heart, the
Lord will not hear *me*:
19 *But* verily God hath heard *me*; he
hath attended to the voice of my prayer.
20 Blessed *be* God, which hath not
turned away my prayer, nor his mercy
from me.

a Isa. 66:23.
b Psa. 51:2; 79:9; Isa. 6:7; Heb.9:14; 1 John 1:7, 9.
c Psa. 36:8.
d Deut. 11:12.
e Psa. 46:4.
f Heb. *thou dissolvest it.*
g Psa. 65:5.
h Psa. 18:44.
i Ex. 14:21.
j Josh. 3:14, 16.
k Heb. *putteth.*
l Zech. 13:9; 1 Pet. 1:6, 7.
m Psa. 100:4; 116:14, 17-19.
n Psa. 19:9, *note.*
o Job 27:9; Prov.15:29; 28:9; Isa. 1:15; John 9:31; Jas. 4:3.

PSALM 67.

To the chief Musician on [a]Neginoth,
A Psalm *or* Song.

God be merciful unto us, and bless us; *and* cause his face to shine upon us; Selah.

2 That thy way may be known upon earth, thy saving health among all nations.

3 Let the people praise thee, O God; let all the people praise thee.

4 O let the nations be glad and sing for joy: [b]for thou shalt judge the people righteously, and [c]govern the nations upon earth. Selah.

5 Let the people praise thee, O God; let all the people praise thee.

6 [d]*Then* shall the earth yield her increase; *and* God, *even* our own God, shall bless us.

7 God shall bless us; and all the ends of the earth shall [e]fear him.

PSALM 68.

To the chief Musician,
A Psalm *or* Song of David.

[1]Let God arise, let his enemies be scattered: let them also that hate him flee before him.

2 As smoke is driven away, *so* drive *them* away: [f]as wax melteth before the fire, *so* let the wicked perish at the presence of God.

3 But [g]let the righteous be glad; let them rejoice before God: yea, let them exceedingly rejoice.

4 Sing unto God, sing praises to his name: [h]extol him that rideth upon the heavens [i]by his name JAH, and rejoice before him.

5 [j]A father of the fatherless, and a judge of the widows, *is* God in his holy habitation.

6 [k]God setteth the solitary in families: [l]he bringeth out those which are bound with chains: but the rebellious dwell in a dry *land*.

7 O God, when thou wentest forth before thy people, when thou didst march through the wilderness; Selah:

8 The earth shook, the heavens also dropped at the presence of God: *even* Sinai itself *was moved* at the presence of God, the God of Israel.

9 Thou, O God, didst send a plentiful rain, whereby thou didst confirm thine inheritance, when it was weary.

10 Thy congregation hath dwelt therein: [m]thou, O God, hast prepared of thy goodness for the poor.

11 The Lord gave the [n]word: great *was* the company of those that published *it*.

12 Kings of armies did flee apace: and she that tarried at home divided the spoil.

13 Though ye have lien among the pots, *yet shall ye be as* the wings of a dove covered with silver, and her feathers with yellow gold.

14 When the Almighty scattered kings in it, it was *white* as snow in Salmon.

15 The hill of God *is as* the hill of Bashan; an high hill *as* the hill of Bashan.

16 Why leap ye, ye high hills? *this is* the hill *which* God desireth to dwell in; yea, the LORD will dwell *in it* for ever.

17 The chariots of God *are* twenty thousand, *even* thousands of [o]angels: the Lord *is* among them, *as in* Sinai, in the holy *place*.

18 Thou hast ascended on high, thou hast led captivity [p]captive: thou hast received [q]gifts for men; yea, *for* the rebellious also, that the LORD God might dwell *among them*.

19 Blessed *be* the Lord, *who* daily loadeth us *with benefits, even* the God of our salvation. Selah.

20 *He that is* our God *is* the God of salvation; and unto GOD the Lord *belong* the issues from death.

21 But God shall wound the head of his enemies, *and* the hairy scalp of such an one as goeth on still in his trespasses.

22 The Lord said, I will bring [r]again from Bashan, I will bring *my people* again from the depths of the sea:

23 That thy foot may be dipped in the blood of *thine* enemies, *and* the tongue of thy dogs in the same.

a *Neginoth,* stringed instruments.
b Psa. 96:10, 13; 98:9.
c Heb. *lead.*
d Lev. 26:4; Psa. 85:12; Ezk. 34:27.
e Psa. 19:9, *note.*
f Psa. 97:5; Mic. 1:4.
g Psa. 32:11; 58:10; 64:10.
h v. 33; Deut. 33:26.
i Ex. 6:3.
j Psa. 10:14, 18; 146:9.
k 1 Sam. 2:5; Psa. 113:9.
l Psa. 107:10, 14; 146:7; Acts 12:7.
m Deut. 26:5-9; Psa. 74:19.
n *Inspiration.* Isa. 6:5-9. (Ex. 4:15; Rev. 22:19.)
o Heb. 1:4, *note.*
p Eph. 4:8.
q Acts 2:4, 33; 10:44-46; 1 Cor. 12:4-11; Eph. 4:7-12.
r Deut. 30:1-9.

[1] **(68:1)** The entire Psalm is pervaded by the joy of Israel in the kingdom, but a stricter order of events begins with verse 18. This is quoted (Eph. 4:7-16) of Christ's ascension ministry. Verses 21-2[illegible] refer to the regathering of Israel, and the destruction of the Beast and his armies. (See "Beast," Dan. 7:[illegible] Rev. 19:20; "Armageddon," Rev. 16:16; Rev. 19:17-19, *note.*) Verses 24-35 are descriptive of full and universal kingdom blessing. (See "Kingdom" (O.T.), Gen. 1:26; Zech. 12:8.) See Psalm 69, next in order of the Messianic Psalms.

24 They have seen thy goings, O God;
even the goings of my God, my King, in
the sanctuary.
25 The singers went before, the players
on instruments *followed* after; among *them*
were the damsels playing with timbrels.
26 Bless ye God in the congregations,
even the Lord, [a]from the fountain of Israel.
27 There *is* [b]little Benjamin *with* their
ruler, the princes of Judah *and* their
council, the princes of Zebulun, *and* the
princes of Naphtali.
28 Thy God hath commanded thy
strength: strengthen, O God, that which
thou hast wrought for us.
29 Because of thy temple at Jerusalem
shall kings bring presents unto thee.
30 Rebuke the company of spearmen,
the multitude of the bulls, with the
calves of the people, *till every one* submit
himself with pieces of silver: scatter thou
the people *that* delight in war.
31 Princes shall come out of Egypt;
Ethiopia shall soon stretch out her hands
unto God.
32 Sing unto God, ye kingdoms of the
earth; O sing praises unto the Lord; Selah:
33 To him that rideth upon the heavens of heavens, *which were* of old; lo, he
doth send out his voice, *and that* a
mighty voice.
34 Ascribe ye strength unto God: his
excellency *is* over Israel, and his strength
is in the clouds.
35 O God, *thou art* terrible out of thy
holy places: the God of Israel *is* he that
giveth strength and power unto *his* people. Blessed *be* God.

PSALM 69.

To the chief Musician upon
[c]Shoshannim, *A Psalm* of David.

Save [1]me, O God; for the waters are
come in unto *my* soul.
2 I sink in deep mire, where *there is* no
standing: I am come into deep waters,
where the floods overflow me.
3 I am weary of my crying: my throat
is dried: mine eyes fail while I wait for
my God.
4 [d]They that hate me without a cause
are more than the hairs of mine head:
they that would destroy me, *being* mine
enemies wrongfully, are mighty: then I
restored *that* which I took not away.
5 O God, thou knowest my foolishness; and my sins are not hid from thee.
6 Let not them that wait on thee, O
Lord GOD of hosts, be ashamed for my
sake: let not those that seek thee be confounded for my sake, O God of Israel.
7 Because for thy sake I have borne
reproach; shame hath covered my face.
8 [e]I am become a stranger unto my
brethren, and an alien unto my mother's
children.
9 [f]For the zeal of thine house hath
eaten me up; and the [g]reproaches of
them that reproached thee are fallen
upon me.
10 When I wept, *and chastened* my soul
with fasting, that was to my reproach.
11 I made sackcloth also my garment;
and I became a proverb to them.
12 They that sit in the gate speak
against me; and I *was* the song of the
drunkards.
13 But as for me, my prayer *is* unto
thee, O LORD, *in* an acceptable time: O
God, in the multitude of thy mercy hear
me, in the truth of thy salvation.
14 Deliver me out of the mire, and let
me not sink: let me be delivered from
them that hate me, and out of the deep
waters.
15 Let not the waterflood overflow me,
neither let the deep swallow me up, and
let not the pit shut her mouth upon me.
16 Hear me, O LORD; for thy lovingkindness *is* good: turn unto me
according to the multitude of thy tender
mercies.
17 And hide not thy face from thy servant; for I am in trouble: hear me speedily.

a Or, *ye that are of the fountain of Israel*
b 1 Sam. 9:21.
c See Psa. 45, title, *note.*
d Psa. 35:19; John 15:25.
e John 7:3-5.
f John 2:17.
g Rom.15:3.

[1] **(69:1)** The N.T. quotations from, and references to, this Psalm indicate in what way it adumbrates Christ. It is the Psalm of His humiliation and rejection (vs. 4, 7, 8, 10-12). Verses 14-20 may well describe the exercises of His holy soul in Gethsemane (Mt. 26:36-45); while verse 21 is a direct reference to the cross (Mt. 27:34, 48; John 19:28). The imprecatory verses (22-28) are connected (Rom. 11:9, 10) with the present judicial blindness of Israel, verse 25 having special reference to Judas (Acts 1:20), who is thus made typical of his generation, which shared his guilt. See Psalm 72, next in order of the Messianic Psalms.

18 Draw nigh unto my soul, *and* [a]redeem it: deliver me because of mine enemies.

19 Thou hast known my reproach, and my shame, and my dishonour: mine adversaries *are* all before thee.

20 Reproach hath broken my heart; and I am full of heaviness: and I looked *for some* to take pity, but *there was* none; and for comforters, but I found none.

21 They gave me also gall for my meat; [b]and in my thirst they gave me vinegar to drink.

22 [c]Let their table become a snare before them: and *that which should have been* for *their* welfare, *let it become* a trap.

23 Let their eyes be darkened, that they see not; and make their loins continually to shake.

24 Pour out thine indignation upon them, and let thy wrathful anger take hold of them.

25 Let their habitation be [d]desolate; *and* let none dwell in their tents.

26 For they persecute *him* whom thou hast smitten; and they talk to the grief of those whom thou hast wounded.

27 Add iniquity unto their iniquity: and let them not come into thy righteousness.

28 Let them [e]be blotted out of the book of the living, and not be written with the righteous.

29 But I *am* poor and sorrowful: let thy salvation, O God, set me up on high.

30 I will praise the name of God with a song, and will magnify him with thanksgiving.

31 [f]*This* also shall please the LORD better than an ox *or* bullock that hath horns and hoofs.

32 [g]The humble shall see *this, and* be glad: and [h]your heart shall live that seek God.

33 For the LORD heareth the poor, and despiseth not his prisoners.

34 Let the heaven and earth praise him, the seas, and every thing that [i]moveth therein.

35 [j]For God will save Zion, and will build the cities of Judah: that they may dwell there, and have it in possession.

36 The seed also of his servants shall inherit it: and they that love his name shall dwell therein.

PSALM 70.

To the chief Musician, *A Psalm* of David, to bring to remembrance.

Make haste, O God, to deliver me; make haste [k]to help me, O LORD.

2 Let them be ashamed and confounded that seek after my soul: let them be turned backward, and put to confusion, that desire my hurt.

3 [l]Let them be turned back for a reward of their shame that say, Aha, aha.

4 Let all those that seek thee rejoice and be glad in thee: and let such as love thy salvation say continually, Let God be magnified.

5 [m]But I *am* poor and needy: [n]make haste unto me, O God: thou *art* my help and my deliverer; O LORD, make no tarrying.

PSALM 71.

In thee, O LORD, do I put my [o]trust: le me never be put to confusion.

2 Deliver me in thy righteousness, anc cause me to escape: incline thine ea unto me, and save me.

3 [p]Be thou my strong habitation whereunto I may continually resort: thou hast given commandment to save me; fo thou *art* my rock and my fortress.

4 Deliver me, O my God, out of th hand of the wicked, out of the hand o the unrighteous and cruel man.

5 For thou *art* my hope, O Lord GOD *thou art* my [o]trust from my youth.

6 By thee have I been holden up fron the womb: thou art he that took me ou of my mother's bowels: my praise *sha be* continually of thee.

7 [q]I am as a wonder unto many; bu thou *art* my strong refuge.

8 Let my mouth be filled *with* th praise *and with* thy honour all the day.

9 Cast me not off in the time of old age forsake me not when my strength faileth.

10 For mine enemies speak agains me; and they that lay wait for my sou take counsel together,

11 Saying, God hath forsaken hir persecute and take him; for *there is* non to deliver *him*.

12 [r]O God, be not far from me: O m God, make haste for my help.

13 Let them be confounded *and* cor sumed that are adversaries to my sou let them be covered *with* reproach an dishonour that seek my hurt.

a Heb. *goel, Redemp. (Kinsman type).* Isa. 59:20, *note.*
b Mt. 27:34, 48.
c Rom. 11:9, 10.
d Mt. 23:38; Acts 1:20.
e Ex. 32:32; Phil. 4:3; Rev. 3:5; 13:8.
f Psa. 50:13, 14, 23.
g Psa. 34:2.
h Psa. 22:26.
i Heb. *creepeth.*
j Psa. 51:18; Isa. 44:26.
k Heb. *to my help.*
l Psa. 40:15.
m Psa. 40:17; 72:12-13.
n Psa. 141:1.
o Psa. 2:12, *note.*
p Heb. *be thou to me for a rock of habitation.*
q Isa. 8:18; Zech. 3:8; 1 Cor. 4:9.
r Psa. 22:11, 19; 35:22; 38:21, 22.

14 But I will hope continually, and will yet praise thee more and more.

15 My mouth shall shew forth thy righteousness *and* thy salvation all the day; for I know not the numbers *thereof.*

16 I will go in the strength of the Lord GOD: I will make mention of thy righteousness, *even* of thine only.

17 O God, thou hast taught me from my youth: and hitherto have I declared thy wondrous works.

18 [a]Now also when I am old and grayheaded, O God, forsake me not; until I have shewed thy strength unto *this* generation, *and* thy power to every one *that* is to come.

19 [b]Thy righteousness also, O God, *is* very high, who hast done great things: O God, who *is* like unto thee!

20 *Thou,* which hast shewed me great and sore troubles, shalt quicken me again, and shalt bring me up again from the depths of the earth.

21 Thou shalt increase my greatness, and comfort me on every side.

22 I will also praise thee with the psaltery, *even* thy truth, O my God: unto thee will I sing with the harp, O thou Holy One of Israel.

23 My lips shall greatly rejoice when I sing unto thee; and my soul, which thou hast [c]redeemed.

24 My tongue also shall talk of thy righteousness all the day long: for they are confounded, for they are brought unto shame, that seek my hurt.

PSALM 72.

A Psalm for Solomon.

Give the [d]king thy judgments, O God, and thy righteousness unto the king's son.

2 He shall judge thy people with righteousness, and thy poor with judgment.

3 The mountains shall bring peace to the people, and the little hills, by righteousness.

4 He shall judge the poor of the people, he shall save the children of the needy, and shall break in pieces the oppressor.

5 They shall [e]fear thee as long as the sun and moon endure, throughout all generations.

6 He shall come down like rain upon the mown grass: as showers *that* water the earth.

7 In his days shall the righteous flourish; and abundance of peace so long as the moon endureth.

8 He shall have dominion also from sea to sea, and from the river unto the ends of the earth.

9 They that dwell in the wilderness shall bow before him; and his enemies shall lick the dust.

10 The kings of Tarshish and of the [f]isles shall bring presents: the kings of Sheba and Seba shall offer gifts.

11 Yea, all kings shall fall down before him: all nations shall serve him.

12 For he shall deliver the needy when he crieth; the poor also, and *him* that hath no helper.

13 He shall spare the poor and needy, and shall save the souls of the needy.

14 He shall [g]redeem their soul from deceit and violence: and precious shall their blood be in his sight.

15 And he shall live, and to him shall be given of the gold of Sheba: prayer also shall be made for him continually; *and* daily shall he be praised.

16 There shall be an handful of corn in the earth upon the top of the mountains; the fruit thereof shall shake like Lebanon: [h]and *they* of the city shall flourish like grass of the earth.

17 [i]His name [j]shall endure for ever: [k]his name shall be continued as long as the sun: and *men* shall be blessed in him: all nations shall call him blessed.

18 Blessed *be* the LORD God, the God of Israel, who only doeth wondrous things.

19 And blessed *be* his glorious name for ever: [l]and let the whole earth be filled *with* his glory; Amen, and Amen.

20 The prayers of David the son of Jesse are [m]ended.

a Heb. *unto old age and grey hairs.*
b Psa. 57:10.
c Ex. 14:30, *note;* Isa. 59:20, *note.*
d *Kingdom* (O.T.). vs. 1-20; Psa. 89:3, 4, 21, 28-36. (Gen. 1:26; Zech. 12:8.)
e Psa. 19:9, *note.*
f i.e. *coasts.*
g Heb. *goel, Redemp. (Kinsman type).* Isa. 59:20, *note.*
h 1 Ki. 4:20.
i Psa. 89:36.
j Heb. *shall be.*
k Heb. *shall be as a son to continue his father's name for ever.*
l Num. 14:21; Zech. 14:9.
m Lit. *to be ended,* i.e. in complete answer. 2 Sam. 23:1-4.

[1] **(72:1)** The Psalm as a whole forms a complete vision of Messiah's kingdom so far as the O.T. revelation extended. All David's prayers will find their fruition in the kingdom (v. 20; 2 Sam. 23:1-4). Verse 1 refers to the investiture of the King's Son with the kingdom, of which investiture the formal description is given in Dan. 7:13, 14; Rev. 5:5-10. Verses 2-7, 12-14 give the character of the kingdom. (Cf. Isa. 11:3-9.) The emphatic word is righteousness. The Sermon on the Mount describes the kingdom

BOOK III

PSALM 73.

A Psalm of Asaph.

Truly God *is* good to Israel, *even* to such as are of a clean heart.

2 But as for me, my feet were almost gone; my steps had well nigh slipped.

3 For I was envious at the foolish, *when* I saw the prosperity of the wicked.

4 For *there are* no bands in their death: but their strength *is* firm.

5 They *are* not in trouble *as other* men; neither are they plagued [a]like *other* men.

6 Therefore pride compasseth them about as a chain; violence covereth them *as* a garment.

7 Their eyes stand out with fatness: they have more than heart could wish.

8 They are corrupt, and speak wickedly *concerning* oppression: [b]they speak loftily.

9 They set their mouth [c]against the heavens, and their tongue walketh through the earth.

10 Therefore his people return hither: and waters of a full *cup* are wrung out to them.

11 And they say, [d]How doth God know? and is there knowledge in the most High?

12 Behold, these *are* the ungodly, who prosper [e]in the world; they increase *in* riches.

13 Verily [f]I have cleansed my heart *in* vain, and washed my hands in innocency.

14 For all the day long have I been plagued, and chastened every morning.

15 If I say, I will speak thus; behold, I should offend *against* the generation of thy children.

16 When I thought to know this, it *was* too painful for me;

17 Until I went into the sanctuary of God; *then* understood I their end.

18 Surely thou didst set them in slippery places: thou castedst them down into destruction.

19 How are they *brought* into desolation, as in a moment! they are utterly consumed with terrors.

20 As a dream when *one* awaketh; *so,* O Lord, when thou awakest, thou shalt despise their image.

21 Thus my heart was grieved, and I was pricked in my reins.

22 So foolish *was* I, and ignorant: I was *as* a beast before thee.

23 Nevertheless I *am* continually with thee: thou hast holden *me* by my right hand.

24 Thou shalt guide me with thy counsel, and afterward receive me *to* glory.

25 Whom have I in heaven *but thee?* and *there is* none upon earth *that* I desire beside thee.

26 My flesh and my heart faileth: *but* God *is* the strength of my heart, and my portion for ever.

27 For, lo, they that are far from thee shall perish: thou hast destroyed all them that go a whoring from thee.

28 But *it is* good for me to draw near to God: I have put my [g]trust in the Lord GOD, that I may declare all thy works.

PSALM 74.

[h]Maschil of Asaph.

O God, why hast thou cast *us* off for ever? *why* doth thine anger smoke against the sheep of thy pasture?

2 Remember thy congregation, *which* thou hast purchased of old; the rod of thine inheritance, *which* thou hast [i]redeemed; this mount Zion, wherein thou hast dwelt.

3 Lift up thy feet unto the perpetual desolations; *even* all *that* the enemy hath done wickedly in the sanctuary.

4 [j]Thine enemies roar in the midst of thy congregations; [k]they set up their ensigns *for* signs.

a Heb. *with.*
b 2 Pet. 2:18; Jude 16.
c Rev. 13:6.
d Job 22:13; Psa. 10:11; 94:7.
e Or, *continually.*
f Mal. 3:14.
g Psa. 2:12, *note.*
h *Maschil, instruction.*
i Heb. *goel, Redemp. (Kinsman type).* Isa. 59:20, *note.*
j Lam. 2:7.
k Dan. 6:2 7.

righteousness. Verses 8-11 speak of the universality of the kingdom. Verse 16 hints at the means by which universal blessing is to be brought in. Converted Israel will be the "handful of corn" (Amos 9:9) as the King Himself in death and resurrection was the single grain, the "corn of wheat" (John 12:24). "To the Jew first" is the order alike of Church and kingdom (Rom. 1:16; Acts 13:46; 15:16, 17). It is through restored Israel that the kingdom is to be extended over the earth (Zech. 8:13, 20-23). See Psa 89, the next in order of the Messianic Psalms.

5 *A man* was famous according as he had lifted up axes upon the thick trees.

6 But now they break down the carved work thereof at once with axes and hammers.

7 [a]They have cast fire into thy sanctuary, they have defiled *by casting down* the dwelling place of thy name to the ground.

8 They said in their hearts, Let us destroy them together: they have burned up all the synagogues of God in the land.

9 We see not our signs: *there is* no [b]more any prophet: neither *is there* among us any that knoweth how long.

10 O God, how long shall the adversary reproach? shall the enemy blaspheme thy name for ever?

11 Why withdrawest thou thy hand, even thy right hand? pluck *it* out of thy bosom.

12 For [c]God *is* my King of old, working salvation in the midst of the earth.

13 Thou didst [d]divide the sea by thy strength: thou brakest the heads of the dragons in the waters.

14 Thou brakest the heads of leviathan in pieces, *and* gavest him *to be* meat to the people inhabiting the wilderness.

15 [e]Thou didst cleave the fountain and the flood: [f]thou driedst up mighty rivers.

16 The day *is* thine, the night also *is* thine: [g]thou hast prepared the light and the sun.

17 Thou hast [h]set all the borders of the earth: [i]thou hast made summer and winter.

18 Remember this, *that* the enemy hath reproached, O LORD, and *that* the foolish people have blasphemed thy name.

19 O deliver not the soul [j]of thy turtledove unto the multitude *of the wicked*: forget not the congregation of thy poor for ever.

20 [k]Have respect unto the covenant: for the dark places of the earth are full of the habitations of cruelty.

21 O let not the oppressed return ashamed: let the poor and needy praise thy name.

22 Arise, O God, plead thine own cause: remember how the foolish man reproacheth thee daily.

23 Forget not the voice of thine enemies: the tumult of those that rise up against thee [l]increaseth continually.

PSALM 75.

To the chief Musician, [m]Al-taschith, A Psalm *or* Song of Asaph.

Unto thee, O God, do we give thanks, *unto thee* do we give thanks: for *that* thy name is near thy wondrous works declare.

2 When I shall receive the congregation I will judge uprightly.

3 The earth and all the inhabitants thereof are dissolved: I bear up the pillars of it. Selah.

4 I said unto the fools, Deal not foolishly: and to the wicked, [n]Lift not up the horn:

5 Lift not up your horn on high: speak *not with* a stiff neck.

6 For promotion *cometh* neither from the east, nor from the west, nor from the south.

7 But God *is* the judge: he putteth down one, and setteth up another.

8 For [o]in the hand of the LORD *there is* a cup, and the wine is red; it is full of mixture; and he poureth out of the same: but the dregs thereof, all the wicked of the earth shall wring *them* out, *and* drink *them*.

9 But I will declare for ever; I will sing praises to the God of Jacob.

10 [p]All the horns of the wicked also will I cut off; [q]*but* the horns of the righteous shall be exalted.

PSALM 76.

To the chief Musician on [r]Neginoth, A Psalm *or* Song of Asaph.

[s]In Judah *is* God known: his name *is* great in Israel.

2 In Salem also is his tabernacle, and his dwelling place in Zion.

3 There brake he the arrows of the bow, the shield, and the sword, and the battle. Selah.

4 Thou *art* more glorious *and* excellent than the mountains of prey.

5 The stouthearted are spoiled, they have slept their sleep: and none of the men of might have found their hands.

6 [t]At thy rebuke, O God of Jacob, both the chariot and horse are cast into a dead sleep.

7 Thou, *even* thou, *art* to be feared: and who may stand in thy sight when once thou art angry?

8 Thou didst cause judgment to be heard from heaven; the earth feared, and was still,

9 When God arose to judgment, to

a Heb. *they have sent thy sanctuary into the fire.*

b 1 Sam. 3:1; Amos 8:11.

c Psa. 44:4.

d Heb. *break.*

e Ex. 17:5, 6; Num. 20:11; Psa. 105:41; Isa. 48:21.

f Josh. 3:13.

g Gen. 1:14.

h Acts 17:26.

i Gen.8:22.

j Song 2:14.

k Gen. 17:7, 8; Lev. 26:44, 45.

l Heb. *ascendeth.* Jon. 1:2.

m *Al-taschith, destroy not.*

n 1 Sam. 2:3; Zech. 1:21.

o Psa. 60:3; Job 21:20; Jer. 25:15; Rev. 14:10; 16:19.

p Psa. 101:8; Jer. 48:25.

q Psa. 89:17; 148:14.

r *Neginoth, stringed instruments.*

s Psa. 48:1.

t Ex. 15:1, 21; Ezk. 39:20; Nah. 2:13; Zech.12:4.

save all the meek of the earth. Selah.

10 Surely the wrath of man shall praise thee: the remainder of wrath shalt thou restrain.

11 Vow, and pay unto the LORD your God: let all that be round about him bring presents unto him that ought to be feared.

12 He shall cut off the spirit of princes: *he is* terrible to the kings of the earth.

PSALM 77.

To the chief Musician, to [a]Jeduthun,
A Psalm of Asaph.

I cried unto God with my voice, *even* unto God with my voice; and he gave ear unto me.

2 In the day of my trouble I sought the Lord: my sore ran in the night, and ceased not: my soul refused to be comforted.

3 I remembered God, and was troubled: I complained, and my spirit was overwhelmed. Selah.

4 Thou holdest mine eyes waking: I am so troubled that I cannot speak.

5 I have considered the days of old, the years of ancient times.

6 I call to remembrance my song in the night: I commune with mine own heart: and my spirit made diligent search.

7 Will the Lord cast off for ever? and will he be favourable no more?

8 Is his mercy clean gone for ever? doth *his* promise fail for evermore?

9 Hath God forgotten to be gracious? hath he in anger shut up his tender mercies? Selah.

10 And I said, This *is* my infirmity: *but I will remember* the years of the right hand of the most High.

11 I will remember the works of the LORD: surely I will remember thy wonders of old.

12 I will meditate also of all thy work, and talk of thy doings.

13 Thy way, O God, *is* in the sanctuary: who *is so* great a God as *our* God?

14 Thou *art* the God that doest wonders: thou hast declared thy strength among the people.

15 Thou hast with *thine* arm [b]redeemed thy people, the sons of Jacob and Joseph. Selah.

16 The waters saw thee, O God, the waters saw thee; they were afraid: the depths also were troubled.

17 The clouds poured out water: the skies sent out a sound: thine arrows also went abroad.

18 The voice of thy thunder *was* in the heaven: the lightnings lightened the world: the earth trembled and shook.

19 Thy way *is* in the sea, and thy path in the great waters, and thy footsteps are not known.

20 Thou leddest thy people like a flock by the hand of Moses and Aaron.

PSALM 78.

[c]Maschil of Asaph.

Give ear, O my people, *to* my law: incline your ears to the words of my [d]mouth.

2 I will open my mouth in a [e]parable: I will utter dark sayings of old:

3 Which we have heard and known, and our fathers have told us.

4 We will not hide *them* from their children, shewing to the generation to come the praises of the LORD, and his strength, and his wonderful works that he hath done.

5 [f]For he established a testimony in Jacob, and appointed a law in Israel, which he commanded our fathers, [g]that they should make them known to their children:

6 That the generation to come might know *them, even* the children *which* should be born; *who* should arise and declare *them* to their children:

7 That they might set their hope in God, and not forget the works of God, but keep his commandments:

8 And might not be as their fathers, a stubborn and rebellious generation; a generation [h]*that* set not their heart aright, and whose spirit was not stedfast with God.

9 The children of Ephraim, *being* armed, *and* carrying bows, turned back in the day of battle.

10 [i]They kept not the covenant of God, and refused to walk in his [j]law;

11 And forgat his works, and his wonders that he had shewed them.

12 Marvellous things did he in the sight of their fathers, in the land of Egypt, *in* the field of Zoan.

13 He divided the sea, and caused them to pass through; and he made the waters to stand as an heap.

14 In the daytime also he led them with a cloud, and all the night with a light of fire.

15 He clave the rocks in the

a See Psa. 39, title, *note.*

b Heb. *goel, Redemp. (Kinsman type).* Isa. 59:20, *note.*

c *Maschil, instruction.*

d *Israel (history).* vs. 1-72; Psa.106:1-46. (Gen. 12:2, 3; Rom. 11:26.)

e Mt.13:35.

f Psa. 147:19.

g Deut. 4:9; 6:7; 11:19.

h Heb. *that prepared not their heart.*

i 2 Ki. 17:15.

j *Law (of Moses).* vs. 9, 10; Psa. 119:1-176. (Ex. 19:1; Gal. 3:1-29.)

wilderness, and gave *them* drink as *out of*
the great depths.
16 He brought streams also out of the
rock, and caused waters to run down
like rivers.
17 And they sinned yet more against
him by provoking the most High in the
wilderness.
18 And they [a]tempted God in their
heart by asking meat for their lust.
19 Yea, they spake against God; they
said, Can God furnish a table in the
wilderness?
20 Behold, he smote the rock, that the
waters gushed out, and the streams
overflowed; can he give bread also? can
he provide flesh for his people?
21 Therefore the LORD heard *this*, and
was wroth: so a fire was kindled against
Jacob, and anger also came up against
Israel;
22 Because they believed not in God,
and [b]trusted not in his salvation:
23 Though he had commanded the
clouds from above, and opened the
doors of heaven,
24 And had rained down manna upon
them to eat, and had given them of the
corn of [c]heaven.
25 Man did eat [d]angels' food: he sent
them meat to the full.
26 [e]He caused an east wind to blow in
the heaven: and by his power he
brought in the south wind.
27 He rained flesh also upon them as
dust, and feathered fowls like as the
sand of the sea:
28 And he let *it* fall in the midst of their
camp, round about their habitations.
29 [f]So they did eat, and were well
filled: for he gave them their own desire;
30 They were not estranged from their
lust. [g]But while their meat *was* yet in
their mouths,
31 The wrath of God came upon them,
and slew the fattest of them, and smote
down the chosen *men* of Israel.
32 For all this they sinned still, and
believed not for his wondrous works.
33 Therefore their days did he consume
in vanity, and their years in trouble.
34 [h]When he slew them, then they
sought him: and they returned and
enquired early after God.
35 And they remembered that God
was their rock, and the high God their
redeemer.
36 Nevertheless they did [j]flatter him
with their mouth, and they lied unto
him with their tongues.
37 For their heart was not right with
him, neither were they stedfast in his
covenant.
38 [k]But he, *being* full of compassion,
forgave *their* iniquity, and destroyed *them*
not: yea, many a time turned he his anger
away, and did not stir up all his wrath.
39 [l]For he remembered that they *were*
but flesh; [m]a wind that passeth away,
and cometh not again.
40 How oft did they provoke him in the
wilderness, *and* grieve him in the desert!
41 Yea, [n]they turned back and tempted
God, and limited the Holy One of Israel.
42 They remembered not his hand, *nor*
the day when he delivered them from
the enemy.
43 How he had wrought his signs in
Egypt, and his wonders in the field of
Zoan:
44 And had turned their rivers into
blood; and their floods, that they could
not drink.
45 He sent divers sorts of flies among
them, which devoured them; and frogs,
which destroyed them.
46 He gave also their increase unto the
caterpiller, and their labour unto the
locust.
47 He destroyed their vines with hail,
and their sycomore trees with frost.
48 He gave up their cattle also to the
hail, and their flocks to hot thunderbolts.
49 He cast upon them the fierceness of
his anger, wrath, and indignation, and
trouble, by sending evil angels *among*
them.
50 He made a way to his anger; he
spared not their soul from death, but
gave their life over to the pestilence;
51 And smote all the firstborn in
Egypt; the chief of *their* strength in the
tabernacles of Ham:
52 But made his own people to go
forth like sheep, and guided them in the
wilderness like a flock.
53 And he led them on safely, so that
they feared not: but the sea overwhelmed their enemies.
54 And he brought them to the border
of his sanctuary, *even to* this mountain,
which his right hand had purchased.
55 He cast out the [o]heathen also before
them, and [p]divided them an inheritance

a *Temptation.* vs. 18, 41, 56; Psa. 95:9. (Gen. 3:1; Jas. 1:2.)
b Psa. 2:12, *note.*
c John 6:31.
d Heb. 1:4, *note.*
e Num.11:31.
f Num. 11:20.
g Num. 11:33.
h Hos. 5:15.
i Ex. 15:13; Deut. 7:8; Isa. 41:14; 44:6; 63:9.
j Ex. 24:7-8; Ezk. 33:31.
k Num. 14:18, 20.
l Psa. 103:14, 16.
m Job 7:7, 16; Jas. 4:14.
n Num. 14:22; Deut. 6:16.
o i.e. *nations.*
p Psa. 136:21; Josh. 13:7; 19:51.

by line, and made the tribes of Israel to
dwell in their tents.
56 [a]Yet they tempted and provoked
the most high God, and kept not his testimonies:
57 But [b]turned back, and dealt
unfaithfully like their fathers: they were
turned aside like a deceitful bow.
58 For they provoked him to anger
with their [c]high places, and moved him
to jealousy with their graven images.
59 When God heard *this*, he was
wroth, and greatly abhorred Israel:
60 [d]So that he forsook the tabernacle
of Shiloh, the tent *which* he placed
among men;
61 And delivered his strength into
captivity, and his glory into the enemy's
hand.
62 [e]He gave his people over also unto
the sword; and was wroth with his
inheritance.
63 The fire consumed their young
men; and [f]their maidens were not given
to marriage.
64 Their priests fell by the sword; and
their widows made no lamentation.
65 Then the Lord awaked as one out of
sleep, *and* like a mighty man that
shouteth by reason of wine.
66 And he smote his enemies in the
hinder parts: he put them to a perpetual
reproach.
67 Moreover he refused the tabernacle
of Joseph, and chose not the tribe of
Ephraim:
68 But chose the tribe of Judah, the
mount Zion [g]which he loved.
69 And he built his sanctuary like high
palaces, like the earth which he hath
established for ever.
70 [h]He chose David also his servant,
and took him from the sheepfolds:
71 From following the ewes great with
young he brought him [i]to feed Jacob his
people, and Israel his inheritance.
72 So he fed them according to the [j]in-
tegrity of his heart; and guided them by
the skilfulness of his hands.

PSALM 79.

A Psalm of Asaph.

O God, the [k]heathen are come into
thine inheritance; thy holy temple
have they defiled; [l]they have laid
Jerusalem on heaps.
2 The dead bodies of thy servants
have they given *to be* meat unto the
fowls of the heaven, the flesh of thy
saints unto the beasts of the earth.
3 Their blood have they shed like
water round about Jerusalem; and *there*
was none to bury *them*.
4 [m]We are become a reproach to our
neighbours, a scorn and derision to them
that are round about us.
5 How long, LORD? wilt thou be angry
for ever? shall thy jealousy burn like fire?
6 Pour out thy wrath upon the [k]hea-
then that have [n]not known thee, and
upon the kingdoms that have not called
upon thy name.
7 For they have devoured Jacob, and
laid waste his dwelling place.
8 O remember not against us former
iniquities: let thy tender mercies speedily
prevent us: for we are brought very low.
9 Help us, O God of our salvation, for
the glory of thy name: and deliver us,
and purge away our sins, [o]for thy
name's sake.
10 Wherefore should the [k]heathen say,
Where *is* their God? let him be known
among the [k]heathen in our sight *by* the
revenging of the blood of thy servants
which is shed.
11 Let the sighing of the prisoner come
before thee; according to the greatness of
thy power preserve thou those that are
appointed to die;
12 And render unto our neighbours
sevenfold into their bosom their
reproach, wherewith they have
reproached thee, O Lord.
13 So [p]we thy people and sheep of thy
pasture will give thee thanks for ever
we will shew forth thy praise to all gen
erations.

PSALM 80.

To the chief Musician upon
[q]Shoshannim-eduth, A Psalm of Asaph.

Give ear, O Shepherd of Israel, [r]thou
that leadest Joseph like a flock
thou that dwellest *between* the cheru
bims, shine forth.
2 Before Ephraim and Benjamin and
Manasseh stir up thy strength, and come
and save us.
3 Turn us again, O God, and [s]cause
thy face to shine; and we shall be saved.
4 O LORD God of hosts, how long wilt
thou be angry against the prayer of thy
people?
5 [t]Thou feedest them with the bread of

a Jud. 2:11, 12.
b v. 41; Ezk. 20:27, 28; Hos. 7:16.
c Deut. 12:2, 4; 1 Ki. 11:7; 12:31.
d 1 Sam. 4:11; Jer. 7:12, 14; 26:6, 9.
e 1 Sam. 4:10.
f Jer. 7:34; 16:9; 25:10.
g Psa. 87:2.
h 1 Sam. 16:11, 12; 2 Sam. 7:8.
i 2 Sam. 5:2; 1 Chr.11:2.
j 1 Ki. 9:4.
k i.e. *nations*.
l 2 Ki. 25:9, 10; 2 Chr. 36:19; Mic. 3:12.
m Psa. 44:13; 80:6.
n Isa. 45:4, 5; 2 Thes. 1:8.
o Jer. 14:7, 21.
p Psa. 74:1; 95:7; 100:3.
q See Psa. 45, title, *note*.
r Ex. 25:20, 22; 1 Sam. 4:4; 2 Sam. 6:2; Psa. 99:1.
s Psa. 4:6; 67:1; Num. 6:25.
t Psa. 42:3; 102:9; Isa. 30:20.

tears; and givest them tears to drink in great measure.

6 Thou makest us a strife unto our neighbours: and our enemies laugh among themselves.

7 Turn us again, O God of hosts, and cause thy face to shine; and we shall be saved.

8 Thou hast brought a [a]vine out of Egypt: thou hast cast out the [b]heathen, and planted it.

9 Thou preparedst *room* before it, and didst cause it to take deep root, and it filled the land.

10 The hills were covered with the shadow of it, and the boughs thereof *were like* the goodly cedars.

11 She sent out her boughs unto the sea, and her branches unto the river.

12 Why hast thou *then* broken down her hedges, so that all they which pass by the way do pluck her?

13 The boar out of the wood doth waste it, and the wild beast of the field doth devour it.

14 Return, we beseech thee, O God of hosts: [c]look down from heaven, and behold, and visit this vine;

15 And the vineyard which thy right hand hath planted, and the branch *that* thou madest strong [d]for thyself.

16 *It is* burned with fire, *it is* cut down: they perish at the rebuke of thy countenance.

17 Let thy hand be upon the man of thy right hand, upon the son of man *whom* thou madest strong for thyself.

18 So will not we go back from thee: quicken us, and we will call upon thy name.

19 Turn us again, O LORD God of hosts, cause thy face to shine; and we shall be saved.

PSALM 81.

To the chief Musician upon [e]Gittith, *A Psalm* of Asaph.

Sing aloud unto God our strength: make a joyful noise unto the God of Jacob.

2 Take a psalm, and bring hither the timbrel, the pleasant harp with the psaltery.

3 Blow up the trumpet in the new moon, in the time appointed, on our solemn feast day.

4 For [f]this *was* a statute for Israel, *and* a law of the God of Jacob.

5 This he ordained in Joseph *for* a testimony, when he went out through the land of Egypt: *where* I heard a language *that* I understood not.

6 I removed his shoulder from the burden: his hands were delivered from the pots.

7 [g]Thou calledst in trouble, and I delivered thee; [h]I answered thee in the secret place of thunder: I [i]proved thee at the waters of Meribah. Selah.

8 Hear, O my people, and I will testify unto thee: O Israel, if thou wilt hearken unto me;

9 There shall [j]no strange god be in thee; neither shalt thou worship any strange god.

10 [k]I *am* the LORD thy God, which brought thee out of the land of Egypt: open thy mouth wide, and I will fill it.

11 But my people would not hearken to my voice; and Israel would none of me.

12 [l]So I gave them up unto their own hearts' lust: *and* they walked in their own counsels.

13 [m]Oh that my people had hearkened unto me, *and* Israel had walked in my ways!

14 I should soon have subdued their enemies, and turned my hand against their adversaries.

15 The haters of the LORD should have submitted themselves unto him: but their time should have endured for ever.

16 He should have fed them also with the finest of the wheat: and with honey out of the rock should I have satisfied thee.

PSALM 82.

A Psalm of Asaph.

God [n]standeth in the congregation of the mighty; he judgeth among the gods.

2 How long will ye judge unjustly, and accept the persons of the wicked? Selah.

3 Defend the poor and fatherless: do justice to the afflicted and needy.

4 Deliver the poor and needy: rid *them* out of the hand of the wicked.

5 They know not, neither will they understand; they walk on in darkness: all the foundations of the earth are out of course.

6 I have said, [o]Ye *are* gods; and all of you *are* children of the most High.

a Isa. 5:1, 7; Jer. 2:21; Ezk. 15:6; 17:6; 19:10.
b i.e. *nations.*
c Isa. 63:15.
d Isa. 49:5.
e See Psa. 8, title, *note.*
f Lev. 23:24; Num. 10:10.
g Ex. 2:23; 14:10; Psa. 50:15.
h Ex. 19:19.
i Ex. 17:6, 7; Num. 20:13.
j Deut. 32:12; Isa. 43:12.
k Ex. 20:2.
l Acts 7:42; 14:16; Rom. 1:24-26.
m Deut. 5:29; 10:12, 13; 32:29; Isa. 48:18.
n 2 Chr. 19:6; Eccl. 5:8.
o John 10:34.

7 But ye shall die like men, and fall
like one of the princes.
8 [a]Arise, O God, judge the earth: [b]for
thou shalt inherit all nations.

PSALM 83.

A Song *or* Psalm of Asaph.

KEEP not thou silence, O God: hold
not thy peace, and be not still, O
God.
2 For, lo, [c]thine enemies make a
tumult: and they that hate thee have lifted up the head.
3 They have taken crafty counsel
against thy people, and consulted
against thy hidden ones.
4 They have said, Come, and [d]let us
cut them off from *being* a nation; that the
name of Israel may be no more in
remembrance.
5 For they have consulted together
with one [e]consent: they are confederate
against thee:
6 The tabernacles of Edom, and the
Ishmaelites; of Moab, and the
Hagarenes;
7 Gebal, and Ammon, and Amalek; the
Philistines with the inhabitants of Tyre;
8 Assur also is joined with them: they
have [f]holpen the children of Lot. Selah.
9 Do unto them as *unto* the
[g]Midianites; as *to* [h]Sisera, as *to* Jabin, at
the brook of Kison:
10 *Which* perished at Endor: they
became *as* dung for the earth.
11 Make their nobles like [i]Oreb, and
like Zeeb: yea, all their princes as
[j]Zebah, and as Zalmunna:
12 Who said, Let us take to ourselves
the houses of God in possession.
13 O my God, make them like a wheel;
as the stubble before the wind.
14 As the fire burneth a wood, and as
the flame setteth the mountains on fire;
15 So persecute them with thy tempest,
and make them afraid with thy storm.
16 Fill their faces with shame; that
they may seek thy name, O LORD.
17 Let them be confounded and troubled for ever; yea, let them be put to
shame, and perish:
18 That *men* may know that thou,
whose [k]name alone *is* JEHOVAH, *art* the
most high over all the earth.

PSALM 84.

To the chief Musician upon [l]Gittith,
A Psalm for the sons of Korah.

HOW [m]amiable *are* thy tabernacles, O
LORD of hosts!
2 [n]My soul longeth, yea, even faintet
for the courts of the LORD: my heart an
my flesh crieth out for the living God.
3 Yea, the sparrow hath found a
house, and the swallow a nest for her
self, where she may lay her young, *eve*
thine altars, O LORD of hosts, my King
and my God.
4 Blessed *are* they that dwell in th
house: they will be still praising thee
Selah.
5 Blessed *is* the man whose strength *i*
in thee; in whose heart *are* the ways o
them.
6 *Who* passing through the valley o
[o]Baca make it a well; the rain also fillet
the pools.
7 They go from strength to strength
every one of them in Zion appearet
before God.
8 O LORD God of hosts, hear m
prayer: give ear, O God of Jacob. Selah.
9 Behold, [p]O God our shield, and loo
upon the face of thine anointed.
10 For a day in thy courts *is* bette
than a thousand. [q]I had rather be a door
keeper in the house of my God, than t
dwell in the tents of wickedness.
11 For the LORD God *is* a sun an
shield: the LORD will give grace an
glory: [r]no good *thing* will he withhol
from them that walk uprightly.
12 O LORD of hosts, blessed *is* the ma
that [s]trusteth in thee.

PSALM 85.

To the chief Musician,
A Psalm for the sons of Korah.

LORD, thou hast been favourable unt
thy land: thou hast [t]brought bac
the captivity of Jacob.
2 Thou hast forgiven the iniquity o
thy people, thou hast covered all thei
sin. Selah.
3 Thou hast taken away all thy wrath
thou hast turned *thyself* from the fierce
ness of thine anger.
4 Turn us, O God of our salvation, an
cause thine anger toward us to cease.

a Mic. 7:2, 7.
b Psa. 2:8; Rev. 11:15.
c Psa. 2:1; Acts 4:25.
d See Esth. 3:6, 9; Jer. 11:19; 31:36.
e Heb. *heart.*
f Heb. *they have been an arm to the children of Lot.*
g Num. 31:7; Jud. 7:22.
h Jud. 4:15, 24; 5:21.
i Jud. 7:25.
j Jud. 8, 12, 21.
k Ex. 6:3.
l See Psa. 8, title, *note.*
m Psa. 27:4.
n Psa. 42:1, 2; 63:1; 73:26; 119:20.
o Or, *weeping.* Not a literal valley, but any place of tears. Cf. Psa. 23:4.
p Gen. 15:1.
q Heb. *I would choose rather to sit at the threshold.*
r Psa. 34:9, 10.
s *Faith.* Psa. 125:1. (Gen. 3:20; Heb. 11:39.)
t Psa. 14:7; Ezra 1:11; 2:1; Jer. 30:18; 31:23; Ezk. 39:25; Joel 3:1.

5 Wilt thou be angry with us for ever?
wilt thou draw out thine anger to all
generations?
6 Wilt thou not revive us again: that
thy people may rejoice in thee?
7 Shew us thy mercy, O LORD, and
grant us thy salvation.
8 I will hear what God the LORD will
speak: for he will speak peace unto his
people, and to his saints: but let them
not turn again to folly.
9 Surely his salvation *is* nigh them that
[a]fear him; that glory may dwell in our
land.
10 Mercy and truth are met together;
[b]righteousness and peace have kissed
each other.
11 Truth shall spring out of the earth;
and righteousness shall look down from
heaven.
12 Yea, the LORD shall give *that which is*
good; and our land shall yield her
increase.
13 Righteousness shall go before him;
and shall set *us* in the way of his steps.

PSALM 86.

A Prayer of David.

Bow down thine ear, O LORD, hear me:
for I *am* poor and needy.
2 Preserve my soul; for I *am* holy: O
thou my God, save thy servant that
[c]trusteth in thee.
3 Be merciful unto me, O Lord: for I
cry unto thee daily.
4 Rejoice the soul of thy servant: [d]for
unto thee, O Lord, do I lift up my soul.
5 [e]For thou, Lord, *art* good, and ready
to forgive; and plenteous in mercy unto
all them that call upon thee.
6 Give ear, O LORD, unto my prayer;
and attend to the voice of my supplications.
7 In the day of my trouble I will call
upon thee: for thou wilt answer me.
8 [f]Among the gods *there is* none like
unto thee, O Lord; neither *are there any*
works like unto thy works.
9 All nations whom thou hast made
shall come and worship before thee, O
Lord; and shall glorify thy name.
10 For thou *art* great, and doest wondrous things: thou *art* God alone.
11 Teach me thy way, O LORD; I will
walk in thy truth: unite my heart to [a]fear
thy name.
12 I will praise thee, O Lord my God,
with all my heart: and I will glorify thy
name for evermore.
13 For great *is* thy mercy toward me:
and thou hast delivered my soul from
the lowest [g]hell.
14 O God, the proud are risen against
me, and the assemblies of violent *men*
have sought after my soul; and have not
set thee before them.
15 [h]But thou, O Lord, *art* a God full of
compassion, and gracious, longsuffering, and plenteous in mercy and truth.
16 O turn unto me, and have mercy
upon me; give thy strength unto thy servant, and save the son of thine handmaid.
17 Shew me a token for good; that
they which hate me may see *it*, and be
ashamed: because thou, LORD, hast
holpen me, and comforted me.

PSALM 87.

A Psalm *or* Song for the sons of Korah.

His foundation *is* in the holy mountains.
2 The LORD loveth the gates of Zion
more than all the dwellings of Jacob.
3 Glorious things are spoken of thee,
O city of God. Selah.
4 I will make mention of [i]Rahab and
Babylon to them that know me: behold
Philistia, and Tyre, with Ethiopia; this
man was born there.
5 And of Zion it shall be said, This and
that man was born in her: and the highest himself shall establish her.
6 The LORD shall count, when he
[j]writeth up the people, *that* this *man* was
born there. Selah.
7 As well the singers as the players on
instruments *shall be there*: all my springs
are in thee.

PSALM 88.

A Song *or* Psalm for the sons of Korah,
to the chief Musician
upon [k]Mahalath Leannoth,
[l]Maschil of Heman the Ezrahite.

O LORD God of my salvation, I have
[m]cried day *and* night before thee:
2 Let my prayer come before thee:
incline thine ear unto my cry;
3 For my soul is full of troubles:

a Psa. 19:9, *note.*
b Psa. 72:3; Isa. 32:17; Lk. 2:14.
c Psa. 2:12, *note.*
d Psa. 25:1; 143:8.
e v. 15; Psa. 130:7; 145:9; Joel 2:13.
f Ex. 15:11; Psa. 89:6; cf. 1 Cor. 8:5-6.
g Heb. *Sheol.* See Hab. 2:5, *note.*
h v. 5; Psa. 103:8; 111:4; 130:4, 7; 145:8; Ex. 34:6; Num. 14:18; Neh. 9:17; Joel 2:13.
i Psa. 89:10; Isa. 51:9.
j Ezk. 13:9.
k Or, *M'hôloth,* meaning *dancing with glad noises.*
l *Maschil, instruction.*
m Lk. 18:7.

and my life draweth nigh unto the [a]grave.

4 [b]I am counted with them that go down into the pit: [c]I am as a man *that hath* no strength:

5 Free among the dead, like the slain that lie in the grave, whom thou rememberest no more: and they are cut off from thy hand.

6 Thou hast laid me in the lowest pit, in darkness, in the deeps.

7 Thy wrath lieth hard upon me, and [d]thou hast afflicted *me* with all thy waves. Selah.

8 [e]Thou hast put away mine acquaintance far from me; thou hast made me an abomination unto them: [f]*I am* shut up, and I cannot come forth.

9 Mine eye mourneth by reason of affliction: [g]LORD, I have called daily upon thee, I have stretched out my hands unto thee.

10 Wilt thou shew wonders to the dead? shall the [h]dead arise *and* praise thee? Selah.

11 Shall thy lovingkindness be declared in the grave? *or* thy faithfulness in destruction?

12 Shall thy wonders be known in the dark? and thy righteousness in the land of forgetfulness?

13 But unto thee have I cried, O LORD; and in the morning shall my prayer prevent thee.

14 LORD, why castest thou off my soul? [i]*why* hidest thou thy face from me?

15 I *am* afflicted and ready to die from *my* youth up: *while* I suffer thy terrors I am distracted.

16 Thy fierce wrath goeth over me; thy terrors have cut me off.

17 They came round about me daily like water; they compassed me about together.

18 [j]Lover and friend hast thou put far from me, *and* mine acquaintance into darkness.

PSALM 89.

[k]Maschil of Ethan the Ezrahite.

I will sing of the mercies of the LORD for ever: with my mouth will I make known thy faithfulness to all generations.

2 For I have said, Mercy shall be built up for ever: thy faithfulness shalt thou establish in the very heavens.

3 I have made a [l]covenant with my chosen, I have [m]sworn unto David my servant,

4 Thy seed will I establish for ever, and build up thy throne [n]to all generations. Selah.

5 And the heavens shall praise thy wonders, O LORD: thy faithfulness also in the congregation of the saints.

6 [o]For who in the heaven can be compared unto the LORD? *who* among the sons of the mighty can be likened unto the LORD?

7 God is greatly to be feared in the assembly of the saints, and to be had in reverence of all *them that are* about him.

8 O LORD God of hosts, who *is* a strong LORD [p]like unto thee? or to thy faithfulness round about thee?

9 [q]Thou rulest the raging of the sea: when the waves thereof arise, thou stillest them.

10 [r]Thou hast broken [s]Rahab in pieces, as one that is slain; thou hast scattered thine enemies with thy strong arm.

11 The heavens *are* thine, the earth also *is* thine: *as for* the world and the fulness thereof, thou hast founded them.

12 The north and the south thou hast created them: [t]Tabor and [u]Hermon shall rejoice in thy name.

13 Thou hast a [v]mighty arm: strong is thy hand, *and* high is thy right hand.

14 Justice and judgment *are* the habitation of thy throne: mercy and truth shall go before thy face.

15 Blessed *is* the people that know the [w]joyful sound: they shall walk, O LORD, in the light of thy countenance.

16 In thy name shall they rejoice all the day: and in thy righteousness shall they be exalted.

17 For thou *art* the glory of their strength: [x]and in thy favour our horn shall be exalted.

18 For the LORD *is* our defence; and the Holy One of Israel *is* our king.

19 Then thou spakest in vision to thy holy one, and saidst, I have laid help upon *one that is* mighty; I have exalted *one* [y]chosen out of the people.

20 I have found David my [z]servant; with my [aa]holy [bb]oil have I anointed him:

21 With whom my hand shall be established: mine arm also shall strengthen him.

22 The enemy shall not exact upon

a Heb. *Sheol.* See Hab. 2:5, *note.*
b Psa. 28:1.
c Psa. 31:12.
d Psa. 42:7.
e Psa. 31:11; 142:4; Job 19:13, 19.
f Lam. 3:7.
g Psa. 86:3.
h Eccl. 9:10, *note.*
i Mt. 27:46; Mk. 15:34.
j Psa. 31:11; 38:11; Job 19:13.
k *Maschil, instruction.*
l *Kingdom* (O.T.). vs. 3, 4, 20, 21, 28-36; Isa. 1:25, 26. (Gen. 1:26; Zech. 12:8.)
m 2 Sam. 7:11; 1 Chr. 17:10. See Jer. 30:9; Ezk. 34:23; Hos. 3:5.
n v. 1; Lk. 1:32, 33.
o Psa. 40:5; 71:19; 86:8; 113:5.
p Psa. 35:10; 71:19; Ex. 15:11; 1 Sam. 2:2.
q Psa. 65:7; 93:3, 4; 107:29.
r Psa. 87:4; Ex. 14:26-28; Isa. 30:7; 51:9.
s Or, *Egypt.*
t Josh. 19:22.
u Josh. 12:1.
v Heb. *an arm with might.*
w Psa. 98:6; Num. 10:10; 23:21.
x v. 24; Psa. 75:10; 92:10; 132:17.
y v. 3; 1 Ki. 11:34.
z Acts 13:22.
aa Heb. *qodesh.*
bb *Sanctify, holy* (O.T.). Jer. 1:5. (Gen. 2:3; Zech. 8:3.)

him; nor the son of wickedness afflict
him.
23 And I will beat down his foes
before his face, and plague them that
hate him.
24 But my faithfulness and my mercy
shall be with him: and in my name shall
his horn be exalted.
25 I will set his hand also in the sea,
and his right hand in the rivers.
26 He shall cry unto me, Thou *art* my
father, my God, and the rock of my salvation.
27 Also I will make him *my* firstborn,
higher [1]than the kings of the earth.
28 My mercy will I keep for him for
evermore, and my covenant shall stand
fast with him.
29 His seed also will I make *to endure*
for ever, and his throne as the days of
heaven.
30 If his children forsake my law, and
walk not in my judgments;
31 If they break my statutes, and keep
not my commandments;
32 Then will I visit their transgression
with the rod, and their iniquity with
stripes.
33 Nevertheless my lovingkindness
will I not utterly take from him, nor suffer my faithfulness to fail.
34 My covenant will I not break, nor
alter the thing that is gone out of my
lips.
35 Once have I sworn by my holiness
that I will not lie unto David.
36 His seed shall endure for ever, and
his throne as the sun before me.
37 It shall be established for ever as
the moon, and *as* a faithful witness in
heaven. Selah.
38 But thou hast cast off and abhorred,
thou hast been wroth with thine anointed.
39 Thou hast made void the covenant
of thy servant: thou hast profaned his
crown *by casting it* to the ground.
40 Thou hast broken down all his
hedges; thou hast brought his strong
holds to ruin.
41 All that pass by the way spoil him:
he is a reproach to his neighbours.
42 Thou hast set up the right hand of
his adversaries; thou hast made all his
enemies to rejoice.
43 Thou hast also turned the edge of
his sword, and hast not made him to
stand in the battle.
44 Thou hast made his glory to cease,
and cast his throne down to the ground.
45 The days of his youth hast thou
shortened: thou hast covered him with
shame. Selah.
46 How long, LORD? wilt thou hide
thyself for ever? shall thy wrath burn
like fire?
47 Remember how short my time is:
wherefore hast thou made all men in
vain?
48 What man *is he that* liveth, and shall
not see death? shall he deliver his soul
from the hand of the [a]grave? Selah.
49 Lord, where *are* thy former lovingkindnesses, *which* thou swarest unto
David in thy truth?
50 Remember, Lord, the reproach of
thy servants; *how* I do bear in my bosom
the reproach of all the mighty people;
51 Wherewith thine enemies have
reproached, O LORD; wherewith they
have reproached the footsteps of thine
anointed.
52 [b]Blessed *be* the LORD for evermore.
Amen, and Amen.

a Heb. *Sheol.* See Hab. 2:5, *note.*

b Psa. 41:13; 72:19.

[1] **(89:27)** The eighty-ninth Psalm is at once the confirmation and exposition of the Davidic Covenant (2 Sam. 7:9-14). That the covenant itself looks far beyond David and Solomon is sure from verse 27. "Higher than the kings of the earth" can only refer to Immanuel (Isa. 7:13-15; 9:6, 7; Mic. 5:2). The Psalm is in four parts: (1) The covenant, though springing from the lovingkindness of Jehovah, yet rests upon His oath (vs. 1-4). (2) Jehovah is glorified for His power and goodness in connection with the covenant (vs. 5-18). (3) The response of Jehovah (vs. 19-37). This is in two parts: *(a)*, it confirms the covenant (vs. 19-29), but, *(b)*, warns that disobedience in the royal posterity of David will be punished with chastening (vs. 30-32). Historically this chastening began in the division of the Davidic kingdom (1 Ki. 11:26-36; 12:16-20) and culminated in the captivities and that subordination of Israel to the Gentiles which still continues. See "Gentiles, times of" (Lk. 21:24; Rev. 16:14). (4) The plea of the Remnant (Isa. 1:9; Rom. 11:5) who urge the severity and long continuance of the chastening (vs. 38-52). See Psa. 102, next in order of the Messianic Psalms.

BOOK IV

PSALM 90.

A Prayer of Moses the man of God.

Lord, [a]thou hast been our dwelling
place in all generations.
2 [b]Before the mountains were brought
forth, or ever thou hadst formed the
earth and the world, even from everlasting to everlasting, thou *art* God.
3 Thou turnest man to destruction;
and sayest, [c]Return, ye children of men.
4 [d]For a thousand years in thy sight
are but as yesterday when it is past, and
as a watch in the night.
5 Thou carriest them away as with a
flood; they are *as* a sleep: in the morning
[e]*they are* like grass *which* groweth up.
6 In the morning it flourisheth, and
groweth up; in the evening it is cut
down, and withereth.
7 For we are consumed by thine anger,
and by thy wrath are we troubled.
8 [f]Thou hast set our iniquities before
thee, [g]our secret *sins* in the light of thy
countenance.
9 For all our days are passed away in
thy wrath: we spend our years as a tale
that is told.
10 The days of our years *are* threescore
years and ten; and if by reason of
strength *they be* fourscore years, yet *is*
their strength labour and sorrow; for it is
soon cut off, and we fly away.
11 Who knoweth the power of thine
anger? even according to thy fear, *so is*
thy wrath.
12 [h]So teach *us* to number our days,
that we may apply *our* hearts unto wisdom.
13 Return, O LORD, how long? and let
it [i]repent thee concerning thy servants.
14 O satisfy us early with thy mercy;
that we may rejoice and be glad all our
days.
15 Make us glad according to the days
wherein thou hast afflicted us, *and* the
years *wherein* we have seen evil.
16 Let thy work appear unto thy servants, and thy glory unto their children.
17 [j]And let the beauty of the LORD our
God be upon us: and [k]establish thou the
work of our hands upon us; yea, the
work of our hands establish thou it.

a Deut. 33:27; Ezk. 11:16.
b Prov. 8:25, 26.
c Gen. 3:19; Eccl. 12:7.
d 2 Pet. 3:8.
e Psa. 103:15; Isa. 40:6.
f Psa. 50:21; Jer. 16:17.
g Psa. 19:12.
h Isa. 39:4.
i Zech. 8:14, *note.*
j Psa. 27:4.
k Isa. 26:12.
l Psa. 27:5; 31:20; 32:7.
m Psa. 2:12, *note.*
n Psa. 124:7.
o Psa. 17:8; 57:1; 61:4.
p Psa. 112:7; 121:7; Job 5:19; Prov. 3:23, 24; Isa. 43:2.
q Psa. 37:34; Mal. 1:5.
r Psa. 71:3; 90:1.
s Prov. 12:21.
t Psa. 34:7; 71:3; Mt. 4:6; Lk. 4:10, 11; Heb. 1:14.
u Heb. 1:4, *note.*
v Mt. 4:6; Lk. 4:10, 11.
w Or, *asp.*
x Psa. 9:10.
y Psa. 50:15.
z Isa. 43:2.

PSALM 91.

He [l]that dwelleth in the secret place
of the most High shall abide under
the shadow of the Almighty.
2 I will say of the LORD, *He is* my
refuge and my fortress: my God; in him
will I [m]trust.
3 Surely [n]he shall deliver thee from
the snare of the fowler, *and* from the noisome pestilence.
4 [o]He shall cover thee with his feathers, and under his wings shalt thou
[m]trust: his truth *shall be thy* shield and
buckler.
5 [p]Thou shalt not be afraid for the terror by night; *nor* for the arrow *that* flieth
by day;
6 *Nor* for the pestilence *that* walketh in
darkness; *nor* for the destruction *that*
wasteth at noonday.
7 A thousand shall fall at thy side, and
ten thousand at thy right hand; *but* it
shall not come nigh thee.
8 Only [q]with thine eyes shalt thou
behold and see the reward of the
wicked.
9 Because thou hast made the LORD,
which is my refuge, *even* the most High,
[r]thy habitation;
10 [s]There shall no evil befall thee, neither shall any plague come nigh thy
dwelling.
11 [t]For he shall give his [u]angels charge
over thee, to keep thee in all thy ways.
12 They shall bear thee up in *their*
hands, [v]lest thou dash thy foot against a
stone.
13 Thou shalt tread upon the lion and
[w]adder: the young lion and the dragon
shalt thou trample under feet.
14 Because he hath set his love upon
me, therefore will I deliver him: I will set
him on high, because he hath [x]known
my name.
15 [y]He shall call upon me, and I will
answer him: [z]I *will be* with him in trouble; I will deliver him, and honour him.
16 With long life will I satisfy him, and
shew him my salvation.

PSALM 92.

A Psalm *or* Song for the sabbath day.

It *is a* [a]good *thing* to give thanks unto
the LORD, and to sing praises unto thy
name, O most High:
2 [b]To shew forth thy lovingkindness in
the morning, and thy faithfulness [c]every
night,
3 Upon an instrument of ten strings,
and upon the psaltery; upon the harp
with a solemn sound.
4 For thou, LORD, hast made me glad
through thy work: I will triumph in the
works of thy hands.
5 [d]O LORD, how great are thy works!
and [e]thy thoughts are very deep.
6 A brutish man knoweth not; neither
doth a fool understand this.
7 When [f]the wicked spring as the
grass, and when all the workers of iniquity do flourish; *it is* that they shall be
destroyed for ever:
8 But thou, LORD, *art most* high for
evermore.
9 For, lo, thine enemies, O LORD, for,
lo, thine enemies shall perish; all the
workers of iniquity shall be scattered.
10 [g]But my horn shalt thou exalt like
the horn of an unicorn: I shall be [h]anoint-
ed with fresh oil.
11 [i]Mine eye also shall see *my desire* on
mine enemies, *and* mine ears shall hear
my desire of the wicked that rise up
against me.
12 [j]The righteous shall flourish like
the palm tree: he shall grow like a cedar
in Lebanon.
13 Those that be planted in the house
of the LORD shall flourish in the courts of
our God.
14 They shall still bring forth fruit in
old age; they shall be fat and [k]flourishing;
15 To shew that the LORD *is* upright: *he
is* my rock, and [l]*there is* no unrighteousness in him.

PSALM 93.

The LORD reigneth, he is clothed with
majesty; the LORD is clothed with
strength, *wherewith* he hath girded himself: [m]the world also is stablished, that it
cannot be moved.
2 Thy throne *is* established of old: thou
art from everlasting.
3 The floods have lifted up, O LORD,
the floods have lifted up their voice; the
floods lift up their waves.
4 The LORD on high *is* mightier than
the noise of many waters, *yea, than* the
mighty waves of the sea.
5 Thy testimonies are very sure: holiness becometh thine house, O LORD, for
ever.

PSALM 94.

O LORD [n]God, to whom vengeance
belongeth; O God, to whom
vengeance belongeth, [o]shew thyself.
2 Lift up thyself, thou judge of the
earth: render a reward to the proud.
3 LORD, how long shall the wicked,
how long shall the wicked triumph?
4 *How long* shall they [p]utter *and* speak
hard things? *and* all the workers of iniquity boast themselves?
5 They break in pieces thy people, O
LORD, and afflict thine heritage.
6 They slay the widow and the
stranger, and murder the fatherless.
7 Yet they say, The LORD shall not see,
neither shall the God of Jacob regard *it*.
8 Understand, ye brutish among the
people: and *ye* fools, when will ye be
wise?
9 [q]He that planted the ear, shall he not
hear? he that formed the eye, shall he
not see?
10 He that chastiseth the [r]heathen,
shall not he correct? he that teacheth
man knowledge, *shall not he know*?
11 The LORD [s]knoweth the thoughts of
man, that they *are* vanity.
12 Blessed *is* the man whom thou
chastenest, O LORD, and teachest him out
of thy law;
13 That thou mayest give him rest
from the days of adversity, until the pit
be digged for the wicked.
14 For the LORD will not cast off his
people, neither will he forsake his inheritance.
15 But judgment shall return unto
righteousness: and all the upright in
heart shall follow it.
16 Who will rise up for me against the
evildoers? *or* who will stand up for me
against the workers of iniquity?
17 Unless the LORD *had been* my help,
my soul had almost dwelt in silence.
18 When I said, My foot slippeth; thy
mercy, O LORD, held me up.

a Psa. 147:1.
b Psa. 89:1.
c Heb. *in the nights.*
d Psa. 40:5; 139:17.
e Isa. 28:29; Rom. 11:33, 34.
f Psa. 37:1, 2, 35, 38; Job 12:6; 21:7; Jer. 12:1, 2; Mal. 3:15.
g Psa. 89:17, 24.
h Psa. 23:5.
i Psa. 54:7; 59:10; 112:8.
j Psa. 52:8; Isa. 65:22; Hos. 14:5, 6.
k Heb. *green.*
l Rom. 9:14.
m Psa. 96:10.
n Heb. *God of revenges.*
o Heb. *shine forth.*
p Psa. 31:18; Jude 15.
q Ex. 4:11; Prov. 20:12.
r i.e. *nations.*
s 1 Cor. 3:20.

19 In the multitude of my thoughts within me thy comforts delight my soul.

20 Shall the throne of iniquity have fellowship with thee, which frameth mischief by a law?

21 They gather themselves together against the soul of the righteous, and condemn the innocent blood.

22 But the LORD is my defence; and my God *is* the rock of my refuge.

23 And he shall bring upon them their own iniquity, and shall cut them off in their own wickedness; *yea*, the LORD our God shall cut them off.

PSALM 95.

O come, let us sing unto the LORD: let us make a joyful noise to the rock of our salvation.

2 Let us come before his presence with thanksgiving, and make a joyful noise unto him with psalms.

3 For the LORD *is* a great God, and a great King above all gods.

4 In his hand *are* the deep places of the earth: the strength of the hills *is* his also.

5 The sea *is* his, and he made it: and his hands formed the dry *land*.

6 O come, let us worship and bow down: let us kneel before the LORD our maker.

7 For he *is* our God; and we *are* the people of his pasture, and the sheep of his hand. [a]To day if ye will hear his voice,

8 Harden not your heart, as in the provocation, *and* as *in* the day of temptation in the wilderness:

9 When your fathers [b]tempted me, proved me, and saw my work.

10 Forty years long was I grieved with *this* generation, and said, It *is* a people that do err in their heart, and they have not known my ways:

11 Unto whom I [c]sware in my wrath that they should not enter into my rest.

PSALM 96.

O sing unto the LORD a new song: sing unto the LORD, all the earth.

2 Sing unto the LORD, bless his name; shew forth his salvation from day to day.

3 Declare his glory among the [d]heathen, his wonders among all people.

4 For the LORD *is* great, and greatly to be praised: he *is* to be [e]feared above all gods.

5 For [f]all the gods of the nations *are* idols: [g]but the LORD made the heavens.

6 Honour and majesty *are* before him: strength and beauty *are* in his sanctuary.

7 Give unto the LORD, O ye kindreds of the people, give unto the LORD glory and strength.

8 Give unto the LORD the glory [h]*due unto* his name: bring an offering, and come into his courts.

9 O worship the LORD [i]in the beauty of holiness: fear before him, all the earth.

10 Say among the [d]heathen *that* [j]the LORD reigneth: the world also shall be established that it shall not be moved: he shall judge the people righteously.

11 Let the heavens rejoice, and let the earth be glad; let the sea roar, and the fulness thereof.

12 Let the field be joyful, and all that *is* therein: then shall all the trees of the wood rejoice

13 Before the LORD: for he [k]cometh, for he cometh to judge the earth: he shall judge the world with righteousness, and the people with his truth.

PSALM 97.

The LORD reigneth; let the earth rejoice; let the multitude of [l]isles be glad *thereof*.

2 Clouds and darkness *are* round about him: righteousness and judgment *are* the habitation of his throne.

3 A fire goeth before him, and burneth up his enemies round about.

4 His lightnings enlightened the world: the earth saw, and trembled.

5 The hills melted like wax at the presence of the LORD, at the presence of the Lord of the whole earth.

6 The heavens declare his righteousness, and all the people see his glory.

7 Confounded be all they that serve graven images, that boast themselves of idols: [m]worship him, all *ye* gods.

8 Zion heard, and was glad; and the daughters of Judah rejoiced because of thy judgments, O LORD.

9 For thou, LORD, *art* high above all the earth: [n]thou art exalted far above all gods.

10 Ye that love the LORD, hate evil:

a vs. 7-11; Heb. 3:7-11.
b *Temptation.* Psa. 106:14. (Gen. 3:1; Jas. 1:2.)
c Heb. 4:3.
d i.e. *nations.*
e Psa. 19:9, *note.*
f See Jer. 10:11, 12.
g Psa. 115:15; Isa. 42:5; Jer. 10:12.
h Heb. *of his name.*
i Or, *in the glorious sanctuary.*
j Psa. 93:1; 97:1; Rev. 11:15; 19:6.
k *Christ (Second Advent).* Psa. 110:1. (Deut. 30:3; Acts 1:9-11.)
l i.e. *coasts.*
m Heb. 1:6.
n Psa. 95:3; 96:4; Ex. 18:11.

[a]he preserveth the souls of his saints; he delivereth them out of the hand of the wicked.

11 Light is sown for the righteous, and gladness for the upright in heart.

12 Rejoice in the LORD, ye righteous; and give thanks at the remembrance of his holiness.

PSALM 98.

A Psalm.

O [b]sing unto the LORD a new song; for [c]he hath done marvellous things: his right hand, and his holy arm, hath gotten him the victory.

2 [d]The LORD hath made known his salvation: his righteousness hath he openly shewed in the sight of the [e]heathen.

3 He hath remembered his mercy and his truth toward the house of Israel: [f]all the ends of the earth have seen the salvation of our God.

4 Make a joyful noise unto the LORD, all the earth: make a loud noise, and rejoice, and sing praise.

5 Sing unto the LORD with the harp; with the harp, and the voice of a psalm.

6 With trumpets and sound of cornet make a joyful noise before the LORD, the King.

7 Let the sea roar, and the fulness thereof; the world, and they that dwell therein.

8 Let the floods clap *their* hands: let the hills be joyful together

9 Before the LORD; [g]for he cometh to judge the earth: with righteousness shall he judge the world, and the people with equity.

PSALM 99.

The LORD reigneth; let the people tremble: [h]he sitteth *between* the cherubims; let the earth be moved.

2 The LORD *is* great in Zion; and he *is* high above all the people.

3 Let them praise [i]thy great and terrible name; *for* it *is* holy.

4 The king's strength also loveth judgment; thou dost establish equity, thou executest judgment and righteousness in Jacob.

5 Exalt ye the LORD our God, and worship at his footstool; *for* he *is* holy.

6 Moses and Aaron among his priests, and Samuel among them that call upon his name; they called upon the LORD, and he answered them.

7 He spake unto them in the cloudy pillar: they kept his testimonies, and the ordinance *that* he gave them.

8 Thou answeredst them, O LORD our God: thou wast a God that [j]forgavest them, though thou tookest vengeance of their inventions.

9 Exalt the LORD our God, and worship at his holy hill; for the LORD our God *is* holy.

PSALM 100.

A Psalm of praise.

Make a joyful noise unto the LORD, all ye lands.

2 Serve the LORD with gladness: come before his presence with singing.

3 Know ye that the LORD he *is* God: [k]*it is* he *that* hath made us, and not we ourselves; [l]*we are* his people, and the sheep of his pasture.

4 [m]Enter into his gates with thanksgiving, *and* into his courts with praise: be thankful unto him, *and* bless his name.

5 For the LORD *is* good; his mercy *is* everlasting; and his truth *endureth* [n]to all generations.

PSALM 101.

A Psalm of David.

I will sing of mercy and judgment: unto thee, O LORD, will I sing.

2 I will behave myself wisely in a [o]perfect way. O when wilt thou come unto me? I will walk within my house with a perfect heart.

3 I will set no wicked thing before mine eyes: I hate the work of them that turn aside; *it* shall not cleave to me.

4 A froward heart shall depart from me: I will not know a wicked *person*.

5 Whoso privily slandereth his neighbour, him will I cut off: him that hath an high look and a proud heart will not I suffer.

6 Mine eyes *shall be* upon the faithful of the land, that they may dwell with me: he that walketh in a perfect way, he shall serve me.

7 He that worketh deceit shall not dwell within my house: he that telleth lies shall not tarry in my sight.

8 I will [p]early destroy all the wicked of

a Psa. 31:23; 37:28; 145:20; Prov. 2:8.
b Psa. 33:3; 96:1; Isa. 42:10.
c Ex. 15:11; Psa. 77:14; 86:10; 105:5; 136:4; 139:14.
d Isa. 52:10; Lk. 2:30, 31.
e i.e. *nations.*
f Isa. 49:6; 52:10; Lk. 2:30, 31; 3:6; Acts 13:47; 28:28.
g Psa. 96:10, 13.
h Psa. 80:1; Ex. 25:22.
i Deut. 28:58; Rev. 15:4.
j *Forgiveness.* Psa. 103:12. (Lev. 4:20; Mt. 26:28.)
k Psa. 119:73; 139:13; 149:2; Eph. 2:10.
l Psa. 95:7; Ezk. 34:30, 31.
m Psa. 66:13; 116:17-19.
n Heb. *to generation and generation.*
o See 1 Ki. 8:61; also v. 6.
p Psa. 75:10; Jer. 21:12.

the land; that I may cut off all wicked
doers [a]from the city of the LORD.

PSALM 102.

A Prayer of the afflicted, when he is overwhelmed, and poureth out his complaint before the LORD.

Hear [1]my prayer, O LORD, and let my
cry come unto thee.
2 [b]Hide not thy face from me in the
day *when* I am in trouble; incline thine
ear unto me: in the day *when* I call
answer me speedily.
3 For my days are consumed like
smoke, and my bones are burned as an
hearth.
4 My heart is smitten, and withered like
grass; so that I forget to eat my bread.
5 By reason of the voice of my groaning
my bones cleave to my skin.
6 I am like a pelican of the wilderness:
I am like an owl of the desert.
7 I watch, and am as a sparrow alone
upon the house top.
8 Mine enemies reproach me all the
day; *and* they that are mad against me
are sworn against me.
9 For I have eaten ashes like bread,
and mingled my drink with weeping,
10 Because of thine indignation and
thy wrath: for thou hast lifted me up,
and cast me down.
11 My days *are* like a shadow that
declineth; and I am withered like grass.
12 But thou, O LORD, shalt endure for
ever; and thy remembrance unto all generations.
13 Thou shalt arise, *and* have mercy
upon Zion: for the time to favour her,
yea, the set time, is come.
14 For thy servants take pleasure in
her stones, and favour the dust thereof.
15 So the [c]heathen shall [d]fear the
name of the LORD, and all the kings of
the earth thy glory.
16 When the LORD shall build up Zion,
he shall appear in his glory.
17 [e]He will regard the prayer of the
destitute, and not despise their prayer.
18 This shall be written for the generation
to come: and the people which shall
be created shall praise the LORD.
19 For he hath looked down from the
height of his sanctuary; from heaven did
the LORD behold the earth;
20 [f]To hear the groaning of the prisoner;
to loose [g]those that are appointed to
death;
21 To declare the name of the LORD in
Zion, and his praise in Jerusalem;
22 When the people are gathered
together, and the kingdoms, to serve the
LORD.
23 He weakened my strength in the
way; he shortened my days.
24 I said, O my God, take me not away
in the midst of my days: thy years *are*
throughout all generations.
25 Of old hast thou laid the [h]foundation
of the earth: and the heavens *are* the
work of thy hands.
26 They shall perish, but [i]thou shalt
endure: yea, all of them shall wax old
like a garment; as a vesture shalt thou
change them, and they shall be changed:
27 [j]But thou *art* the same, and thy
years shall have no end.
28 The children of thy servants shall
continue, and their seed shall be established
before thee.

PSALM 103.

A Psalm of David.

Bless the LORD, O my soul: and all that
is within me, *bless* his holy name.
2 Bless the LORD, O my soul, and forget
not all his benefits:
3 Who [k]forgiveth all thine iniquities;
who [l]healeth all thy diseases;
4 Who [m]redeemeth thy life from
destruction; who crowneth thee with
lovingkindness and tender mercies;
5 Who satisfieth thy mouth with good
things; [n]*so that* thy youth is renewed like
the eagle's.
6 The LORD executeth righteousness
and judgment for all that are oppressed.
7 He made known his ways unto
Moses, his acts unto the children of Israel.

a Psa. 48:2, 8.
b Psa. 27:9; 69:17.
c i.e. *nations.*
d Psa. 19:9, *note.*
e Neh. 1:6, 11; 2:8.
f Psa. 79:11.
g Heb. *the children of death.*
h vs. 25-27; Heb. 1:10-12.
i Isa. 34:4; 51:6; 65:17; 66:22; Rom. 8:20; 2 Pet. 3:7, 10-12.
j Mal. 3:6; Heb. 13:8; Jas. 1:17.
k Psa. 130:8; Isa. 33:24; Mt. 9:2, 6; Mk. 2:5, 10, 11; Lk. 7:47.
l Ex. 15:26; Psa. 147:3; Isa. 53:5; Jer. 17:14.
m Heb. *goel, Redemp. (Kinsman type).* Isa. 59:20, *note.*
n Isa. 40:31.

[1] **(102:1)** The reference of verses 25-27 to Christ (Heb. 1:10-12) assures us that in the preceding verses of Psalm 102 we have, prophetically, the exercises of His holy soul in the days of His humiliation and rejection. See Psa. 110, next in order of the Messianic Psalms.

8 [a]The LORD *is* merciful and gracious, slow to anger, and plenteous in mercy.

9 [b]He will not always chide: neither will he keep *his anger* for ever.

10 He hath not dealt with us after our sins; nor rewarded us according to our iniquities.

11 For as the heaven is high above the earth, *so* great is his mercy toward them that [c]fear him.

12 As far as the east is from the west, *so* far hath he [d]removed [1]our transgressions from us.

13 Like as a father pitieth *his* children, *so* the LORD pitieth them that fear him.

14 For he knoweth our frame; he remembereth that we *are* dust.

15 *As for* man, his days *are* as grass: as a flower of the field, so he flourisheth.

16 For the wind passeth over it, and it is gone; and the place thereof shall know it no more.

17 But the mercy of the LORD *is* from everlasting to everlasting upon them that fear him, and his righteousness unto children's children;

18 To such as keep his covenant, and to those that remember his commandments to do them.

19 The LORD hath prepared his throne in the heavens; and his kingdom ruleth over all.

20 Bless the LORD, ye his [e]angels, that excel in strength, that do his commandments, hearkening unto the voice of his word.

21 Bless ye the LORD, all *ye* his hosts; *ye* ministers of his, that do his pleasure.

22 Bless the LORD, all his works in all places of his dominion: bless the LORD, O my soul.

PSALM 104.

Bless the LORD, O my soul. O LORD my God, thou art very great; thou art clothed with honour and majesty.

2 Who coverest *thyself* with light as *with* a garment: who stretchest out the heavens like a curtain:

3 Who layeth the beams of his chambers in the waters: who maketh the clouds his chariot: who walketh upon the wings of the wind:

4 Who maketh his [e]angels [f]spirits; his ministers a flaming fire:

5 *Who* laid the foundations of the earth, *that* it should not be removed for ever.

6 Thou coveredst it with the deep as *with* a garment: the waters stood above the mountains.

7 At thy rebuke they fled; at the voice of thy thunder they hasted away.

8 They go up by the mountains; they go down by the valleys unto the place which thou hast founded for them.

9 [g]Thou hast set a bound that they may not pass over; [h]that they turn not again to cover the earth.

10 He sendeth the springs into the valleys, *which* run among the hills.

11 They give drink to every beast of the field: the wild asses quench their thirst.

12 By them shall the fowls of the heaven have their habitation, *which* sing among the branches.

13 [i]He watereth the hills from his chambers: the earth is satisfied with the fruit of thy works.

14 He causeth the grass to grow for the cattle, and herb for the service of man: that he may bring forth food out of the earth;

15 And [j]wine *that* maketh glad the heart of man, *and* oil to make *his* face to shine, and bread *which* strengtheneth man's heart.

16 The trees of the LORD are full *of sap*; the cedars of Lebanon, [k]which he hath planted;

17 Where the birds make their nests: *as for* the stork, the fir trees *are* her house.

18 The high hills *are* a refuge for the wild goats; *and* the rocks for the conies.

19 [l]He appointed the moon for seasons: [m]the sun knoweth his going down.

20 [n]Thou makest darkness, and it is night: wherein all the beasts of the forest do creep *forth*.

21 [o]The young lions roar after their prey, and seek their meat from God.

22 The sun ariseth, they gather themselves together, and lay them down in their dens.

a Psa. 86.15; Ex. 34:6, 7; Num. 14:18; Deut. 5:10; Neh. 9:17; Jer. 32:18.

b Psa. 30:5; Isa. 57:15; Jer. 3:5; Mic. 7:18.

c Also v. 13; Psa. 19:9, *note*.

d *Forgiveness*. Jer. 31:34. (Lev. 4:20; Mt. 26:28.)

e Heb. 1:4, *note*.

f Heb. 1:7.

g Psa. 33:7; Job 26:10; Jer. 5:22.

h Gen. 9:11, 15.

i Psa. 147:8.

j Jud. 9:13; Psa. 23:5; Prov. 31:6.

k Num. 24:6.

l Gen. 1:14.

m Job 38:12

n Isa. 45:7.

o Job 38:39; Joel 1:20.

1 **(103:12)** Three Hebrew words are trans. forgive, forgiven: *kaphar*, to cover; *nasa*, to lift away; *salach*, to send away (cf. Lev. 16:21, 22), the fundamental O.T. idea of forgiveness being not the remission of penalty, but the separation of the sinner from his sin. Psa. 103:12 expresses this.

23 Man goeth forth unto [a]his work and to his labour until the evening.

24 O LORD, how manifold are thy works! in wisdom hast thou made them all: the earth is full of thy riches.

25 *So is* this great and wide sea, wherein *are* things creeping innumerable, both small and great beasts.

26 There go the ships: *there is* that leviathan, *whom* thou hast made to play therein.

27 [b]These wait all upon thee; that thou mayest give *them* their meat in due season.

28 *That* thou givest them they gather: thou openest thine hand, they are filled with good.

29 Thou hidest thy face, they are troubled: thou takest away their breath, they die, and return to their dust.

30 [c]Thou sendest forth thy spirit, they are created: and thou renewest the face of the earth.

31 The glory of the LORD shall endure for ever: the LORD shall rejoice in his works.

32 He looketh on the earth, and it [d]trembleth: he toucheth the hills, and they smoke.

33 I will sing unto the LORD as long as I live: I will sing praise to my God while I have my being.

34 My meditation of him shall be sweet: I will be glad in the LORD.

35 Let the sinners be consumed out of the earth, and let the wicked be no more. Bless thou the LORD, O my soul. Praise ye the LORD.

PSALM 105.

O [e]give thanks unto the LORD; call upon his name: make known his deeds among the people.

2 Sing unto him, sing psalms unto him: talk ye of all his wondrous works.

3 Glory ye in his holy name: let the heart of them rejoice that seek the LORD.

4 Seek the LORD, and his strength: [f]seek his face evermore.

5 [g]Remember his marvellous works that he hath done; his wonders, and the judgments of his mouth;

6 O ye seed of Abraham his servant, ye children of Jacob his chosen.

7 He *is* the LORD our God: [h]his judgments *are* in all the earth.

8 He hath [i]remembered his covenant for ever, the word *which* he commanded to a thousand generations.

9 [j]Which *covenant* he made with Abraham, and his oath unto Isaac;

10 And confirmed the same unto Jacob for a law, *and* to Israel *for* an everlasting covenant:

11 Saying, [k]Unto thee will I give the land of Canaan, the [l]lot of your inheritance:

12 [m]When they were *but* a few men in number; yea, very few, and [n]strangers in it.

13 When they went from one nation to another, from *one* kingdom to another people;

14 [o]He suffered no man to do them wrong: yea, he reproved kings for their sakes;

15 *Saying*, Touch not mine anointed, and do my prophets no harm.

16 Moreover he called for a famine upon the land: he brake the whole staff of bread.

17 He sent a man before them, *even* Joseph, *who* was sold for a servant:

18 Whose feet they hurt with fetters: he was laid in iron:

19 Until the time that his word came: the word of the LORD tried him.

20 The king sent and loosed him; *even* the ruler of the people, and let him go free.

21 He made him lord of his house, and ruler of all his substance:

22 To bind his princes at his pleasure; and teach his senators wisdom.

23 Israel also came into Egypt; and Jacob sojourned in the land of Ham.

24 And he [p]increased his people greatly; and made them stronger than their enemies.

25 [q]He turned their heart to hate his people, to deal subtilly with his servants.

26 [r]He sent Moses his servant; *and* Aaron whom he had chosen.

27 [s]They shewed his signs among them, and wonders in the land of Ham.

28 He sent darkness, and made it dark; and they rebelled not against his word.

29 [t]He turned their waters into blood, and slew their fish.

30 Their land brought forth frogs in abundance, in the chambers of their kings.

31 He spake, and there came

a Gen. 3:19.
b Psa. 136:25; 145:15; 147.9; cf. Mt. 6:26-30.
c Isa. 32:15; Ezk. 37:9.
d Hab. 3:10.
e 1 Chr. 16:8-36; Isa. 12:4.
f Psa. 27:8.
g Psa. 77:11.
h Isa. 26:9.
i Lk. 1:72.
j Gen. 17:2; 22:16; 26:3; 28:13; 35:11; Lk. 1:73; Heb. 6:17.
k Gen. 13:15; 15:18.
l Heb. *the cord.*
m Gen. 34:30; Deut. 7:7; 26:5.
n Heb. 11:9.
o Gen. 35:5.
p Ex. 1:7.
q Ex. 1:8.
r Ex. 3:10; 4:12, 14; Num. 16:5; 17:5.
s Ex. 7–12.; Psa. 78:43.
t Ex. 7:20; Psa. 78:44.

divers sorts of flies, *and* lice in all their
coasts.
32 He gave them hail for rain, *and*
flaming fire in their land.
33 He smote their vines also and their
fig trees; and brake the trees of their
coasts.
34 He spake, and the locusts came, and
caterpillers, and that without number,
35 And did eat up all the herbs in their
land, and devoured the fruit of their
ground.
36 He smote also all the firstborn in
their land, the chief of all their strength.
37 [a]He brought them forth also with
silver and gold: and *there was* not one
feeble *person* among their tribes.
38 Egypt was glad when they departed: for the fear of them fell upon them.
39 [b]He spread a cloud for a covering;
and fire to give light in the night.
40 *The people* asked, and he brought
quails, and satisfied them with the bread
of heaven.
41 He opened the rock, and the waters
gushed out; they ran in the dry places
like a river.
42 For he remembered his holy
promise, *and* Abraham his servant.
43 And he brought forth his people
with joy, *and* his [c]chosen with gladness:
44 And gave them the lands of the
[d]heathen: and they inherited the labour
of the people;
45 That they might observe his
statutes, and keep his laws. Praise ye the
LORD.

PSALM 106.

Praise ye the LORD. O give thanks unto
the LORD; for *he is* good: for his
mercy *endureth* for ever.
2 Who can utter the mighty acts of the
LORD? *who* can shew forth all his praise?
3 Blessed *are* they that keep judgment,
and he that doeth righteousness at all
times.
4 Remember me, O LORD, with the
favour [e]*that thou bearest unto* thy people:
O visit me with thy salvation;
5 That I may see the good of thy [f]cho-
sen, that I may rejoice in the gladness of
thy nation, that I may glory with thine
inheritance.
6 [g]We have sinned with our fathers,
we have committed iniquity, we have
done wickedly.
7 Our fathers understood not thy wonders in Egypt; they remembered not the
multitude of thy mercies; but provoked
him at the sea, [h]*even* at the Red sea.
8 Nevertheless he saved them [i]for his
name's sake, [j]that he might make his
mighty power to be known.
9 [k]He rebuked the Red sea also, and it
was dried up: [l]so he led them through
the depths, as through the wilderness.
10 [m]And he saved them from the hand
of him that hated *them*, and [n]redeemed
them from the hand of the enemy.
11 And the waters covered their enemies: there was not one of them left.
12 Then believed they his words; they
sang his praise.
13 They soon forgat his works; they
waited not for his counsel:
14 But lusted exceedingly in the wilderness, and [o]tempted God in the desert.
15 And he gave them their request;
but [p]sent leanness into their soul.
16 [q]They envied Moses also in the
camp, *and* Aaron the saint of the LORD.
17 [r]The earth opened and swallowed
up Dathan, and covered the company of
Abiram.
18 And a fire was kindled in their company; the flame burned up the wicked.
19 [s]They made a calf in Horeb, and
worshipped the molten image.
20 [t]Thus they changed their glory into
the similitude of an ox that eateth grass.
21 They forgat God their saviour,
which had done great things in Egypt;
22 Wondrous works in the land of
Ham, *and* terrible things by the Red sea.
23 Therefore he said that he would
destroy them, had not Moses his chosen
stood before him in the breach, to turn
away his wrath, lest he should destroy
them.
24 Yea, they despised the pleasant
land, [u]they believed not his word:
25 [v]But murmured in their tents, *and*
hearkened not unto the voice of the
LORD.
26 [w]Therefore he lifted up his hand
against them, to overthrow them in the
wilderness:

a Ex. 12:35.
b Ex. 13:21; Neh. 9:12.
c *Election (corporate)*. Psa. 106:5. (Deut. 7:6; 1 Pet. 1:2.)
d i.e. *nations*.
e *Israel (history)*. vs. 1-45; Isa. 1:24-26. (Gen. 12:2, 3; Rom. 11:26.)
f *Election (corporate)*. Isa. 43:20. (Deut. 7:6; 1 Pet. 1:2.)
g Lev. 26:40; 1 Ki. 8:47; Dan. 9:5.
h Ex. 14:11, 12.
i Ezk. 20:14.
j Ex. 9:16.
k Ex. 14:21; Psa. 18:15; Nah. 1:4.
l Isa. 63:11-14.
m Ex. 14:30.
n Heb. *goel*, *Redemp. (Kinsman type)*. Isa. 59:20, *note*.
o *Temptation*. Isa. 7:12. (Gen. 3:1; Jas. 1:2.)
p Isa. 10:16.
q Num. 16:3.
r Num. 16:31, 32; Deut. 11:6.
s Ex. 32:4.
t Jer. 2:11; Rom. 1:23.
u Heb. 3:18.
v Num. 14:2, 27.
w Psa. 95:11; Num. 14:28; Ezk. 20:15; Heb. 3:11, 18.

27 [a]To overthrow their seed also among the nations, and to scatter them in the lands.

28 They joined themselves also unto Baal-peor, and ate the sacrifices of the dead.

29 Thus they provoked *him* to anger with their inventions: and the plague brake in upon them.

30 [b]Then stood up Phinehas, and executed judgment: and *so* the plague was stayed.

31 And that was counted unto him [c]for righteousness unto all generations for evermore.

32 [d]They angered *him* also at the waters of strife, [e]so that it went ill with Moses for their sakes:

33 [f]Because they provoked his spirit, so that he spake unadvisedly with his lips.

34 [g]They did not destroy the nations, concerning whom the LORD commanded them:

35 But were mingled among the [h]heathen, and learned their works.

36 And they served their idols: which were a snare unto them.

37 Yea, they sacrificed their sons and their daughters unto [i]devils,

38 And shed innocent blood, *even* the blood of their sons and of their daughters, whom they sacrificed unto the idols of Canaan: and the land was polluted with blood.

39 Thus were they defiled with their own works, and went a whoring with their own inventions.

40 Therefore was the wrath of the LORD kindled against his people, insomuch that he abhorred his own inheritance.

41 And he gave them into the hand of the [h]heathen; and they that hated them ruled over them.

42 Their enemies also oppressed them, and they were brought into subjection under their hand.

43 [j]Many times did he deliver them; but they provoked *him* with their counsel, and were brought low for their iniquity.

44 Nevertheless he regarded their affliction, when he heard their cry:

45 And he remembered for them his covenant, and [k]repented according to the multitude of his mercies.

46 [l]He made them also to be pitied of all those that carried them captives.

47 [m]Save us, O LORD our God, and gather us from among the [h]heathen, to give thanks unto thy holy name, *and* to triumph in thy praise.

48 [n]Blessed *be* the LORD God of Israel from everlasting to everlasting: and let all the people say, Amen. Praise ye the LORD.

a Psa. 44:11; Lev. 26.33; Ezk. 20:23.
b Num. 25:7, 8.
c Num. 25:11-13.
d Psa. 81:7; Num. 20:3-13.
e Num. 20:12; Deut. 1:37; 3:26.
f Num. 20:10.
g Deut. 7:2, 16; Jud. 2:2.
h i.e. *nations.*
i Lit. *spoilers, destroyers.*
j Jud. 2:16; Neh. 9:27.
k Zech. 8:14, note.
l Ezra 9:9; Jer. 42:12.
m 1 Chr. 16:35, 36.
n Psa. 41:13.

BOOK V

PSALM 107.

O give thanks unto the LORD, for *he is* good: for his mercy *endureth* for ever.

2 Let the [o]redeemed of the LORD say *so*, whom he hath redeemed from the hand of the enemy;

3 And [p]gathered them out of the lands, from the east, and from the west, from the north, and from the south.

4 [q]They wandered in the wilderness in a solitary way; they found no city to dwell in.

5 Hungry and thirsty, their soul fainted in them.

6 [r]Then they cried unto the LORD in their trouble, *and* he delivered them out of their distresses.

7 And he led them forth [s]by the right way, that they might go to a city of habitation.

8 Oh that *men* would praise the LORD *for* his goodness, and *for* his wonderful works to the children of men!

9 [t]For he satisfieth the longing soul, and filleth the hungry soul with goodness.

10 [u]Such as sit in darkness and in the shadow of death, *being* bound in affliction and iron;

11 [v]Because they rebelled against the words of God, and contemned the counsel of the most High:

12 Therefore he brought down their heart with labour; they fell down, and *there was* none to help.

13 Then they cried unto the LORD in their trouble, *and* he saved them out of their distresses.

14 He brought them out of darkness and the shadow of death, and brake [w]their bands in sunder.

15 Oh that *men* would praise the LORD *for* his goodness, and *for* his wonderful works to the children of men!

16 For he hath broken the gates of

o Heb. *goel, Redemp. (Kinsman type).* Isa. 59:20, *note.*
p Psa. 106:47; Isa. 43:5, 6; Jer. 29:14; 31:8, 10; Ezk. 39:27, 28.
q v. 40; Deut. 32:10.
r vs. 13, 19, 28; Psa. 50:15; Hos. 5:15.
s Ezra 8:21.
t Psa. 34:10; Lk. 1:53.
u Lk. 1:79.
v Lam. 3:42.
w Psa. 68:6; 146:7; Acts 12:7; 16:26.

brass, and cut the bars of iron in
sunder.
17 Fools because of their transgression, and because of their iniquities, are
afflicted.
18 Their soul abhorreth all manner of
meat; and they draw near unto the gates
of death.
19 Then they cry unto the LORD in
their trouble, *and* he saveth them out of
their distresses.
20 [a]He sent his word, and healed
them, and delivered *them* from their
destructions.
21 Oh that *men* would praise the LORD
for his goodness, and *for* his wonderful
works to the children of men!
22 [b]And let them sacrifice the sacrifices of thanksgiving, and declare his
works with rejoicing.
23 They that go down to the sea in
ships, that do business in great waters;
24 These see the works of the LORD,
and his wonders in the deep.
25 For he commandeth, and [c]raiseth
the stormy wind, which lifteth up the
waves thereof.
26 They mount up to the heaven, they
go down again to the depths: their soul
is melted because of trouble.
27 They reel to and fro, and stagger
like a drunken man, and are [d]at their
wits' end.
28 Then they cry unto the LORD in
their trouble, and he bringeth them out
of their distresses.
29 [e]He maketh the storm a calm, so
that the waves thereof are still.
30 Then are they glad because they be
quiet; so he bringeth them unto their
desired haven.
31 Oh that *men* would praise the LORD
for his goodness, and *for* his wonderful
works to the children of men!
32 Let them exalt him also in the congregation of the people, and praise him
in the assembly of the elders.
33 [f]He turneth rivers into a wilderness, and the watersprings into dry
ground;
34 [g]A fruitful land into barrenness, for
the wickedness of them that dwell therein.
35 [h]He turneth the wilderness into a
standing water, and dry ground into
watersprings.
36 And there he maketh the hungry to

a 2 Ki. 20:4, 5; Psa. 147:15, 18; Mt. 8:8.

b Lev. 7:12; Psa. 50:14; 116:17; Heb. 13:15.

c Heb. *maketh to stand;* Jon. 1:4.

d Heb. *all their wisdom is swallowed up.*

e Psa. 89:9; Mt. 8:26.

f 1 Ki. 17:1, 7.

g Gen. 13:10; 14:3; 19:25.

h Psa. 114:8; Isa. 41:18.

i Gen. 12:2; 17:16, 20.

j Job 12.21, 24.

k 1 Sam. 2:8; Psa. 113:7, 8.

l Psa. 64:9; Jer. 9:12; Hos. 14:9.

m Vs. 6-13 are identical with Psa. 60:5-12.

n Gen. 49:10.

dwell, that they may prepare a city for
habitation;
37 And sow the fields, and plant vineyards, which may yield fruits of increase.
38 [i]He blesseth them also, so that they
are multiplied greatly; and suffereth not
their cattle to decrease.
39 Again, they are minished and
brought low through oppression, affliction, and sorrow.
40 [j]He poureth contempt upon
princes, and causeth them to wander in
the wilderness, *where there is* no way.
41 [k]Yet setteth he the poor on high
from affliction, and maketh *him* families
like a flock.
42 The righteous shall see *it*, and rejoice:
and all iniquity shall stop her mouth.
43 [l]Whoso *is* wise, and will observe
these *things*, even they shall understand
the lovingkindness of the LORD.

PSALM 108.

A Song *or* Psalm of David.

O God, my heart is fixed; I will sing
and give praise, even with my glory.
2 Awake, psaltery and harp: I *myself*
will awake early.
3 I will praise thee, O LORD, among the
people: and I will sing praises unto thee
among the nations.
4 For thy mercy *is* great above the
heavens: and thy truth *reacheth* unto the
clouds.
5 Be thou exalted, O God, above the
heavens: and thy glory above all the
earth;
6 [m]That thy beloved may be delivered:
save *with* thy right hand, and answer me.
7 God hath spoken in his holiness; I
will rejoice, I will divide Shechem, and
mete out the valley of Succoth.
8 Gilead *is* mine; Manasseh *is* mine;
Ephraim also *is* the strength of mine
head; [n]Judah *is* my lawgiver;
9 Moab *is* my washpot; over Edom
will I cast out my shoe; over Philistia
will I triumph.
10 Who will bring me into the strong
city? who will lead me into Edom?
11 *Wilt* not *thou*, O God, *who* hast cast
us off? and wilt not thou, O God, go
forth with our hosts?
12 Give us help from trouble: for vain
is the help of man.

13 [a]Through God we shall do valiantly: for he *it is that* shall tread down our
enemies.

PSALM 109.

To the chief Musician,
A Psalm of David.

Hold not thy peace, O God of my
praise;
2 For the mouth of the wicked and the
mouth of the deceitful are [b]opened
against me: they have spoken against me
with a [c]lying tongue.
3 They compassed me about also with
words of hatred; and fought against me
[d]without a cause.
4 For my love they are my adversaries:
but I *give myself unto* prayer.
5 And they have rewarded me evil for
good, and hatred for my love.
6 Set thou a wicked man over him:
and let [e]Satan stand at his right hand.
7 When he shall be judged, let him be
condemned: and let his prayer become
sin.
8 Let his days be few; [f]*and* let another
take his office.
9 Let his children be fatherless, and his
wife a widow.
10 Let his children be continually
vagabonds, and beg: let them seek *their
bread* also out of their desolate places.
11 Let the extortioner catch all that he
hath; and let the strangers spoil his labour.
12 Let there be none to extend mercy
unto him: neither let there be any to
favour his fatherless children.
13 Let his posterity be cut off; *and* in
the generation following let their name
be blotted out.
14 Let the iniquity of his fathers be
remembered with the LORD; and let not
the sin of his mother be blotted out.
15 Let them be before the LORD continually, that he may cut off the memory of
them from the earth.
16 Because that he remembered not to
shew mercy, but persecuted the poor
and needy man, that he might even slay
the broken in heart.
17 As he loved cursing, so let it come
unto him: as he delighted not in blessing, so let it be far from him.
18 As he clothed himself with cursing
like as with his garment, so let it come
into his bowels like water, and like oil
into his bones.
19 Let it be unto him as the garment
which covereth him, and for a girdle
wherewith he is girded continually.
20 *Let* this *be* the reward of mine
adversaries from the LORD, and of them
that speak evil against my soul.
21 But do thou for me, O GOD the
Lord, for thy name's sake: because thy
mercy *is* good, deliver thou me.
22 For I *am* poor and needy, and my
heart is wounded within me.
23 I am gone like the shadow when it
declineth: I am tossed up and down as
the locust.
24 My knees are weak through fasting;
and my flesh faileth of fatness.
25 I became also a reproach unto
them: *when* they looked upon me they
[g]shaked their heads.
26 Help me, O LORD my God: O save
me according to thy mercy:
27 That they may know that this *is* thy
hand; *that* thou, LORD, hast done it.
28 Let them curse, but bless thou:
when they arise, let them be ashamed;
but let thy servant rejoice.
29 Let mine adversaries be clothed
with shame, and let them cover themselves with their own confusion, as with
a mantle.
30 I will greatly praise the LORD with
my mouth; yea, I will praise him among
the multitude.
31 For he shall stand at the right hand
of the poor, to save *him* from those that
condemn his soul.

PSALM 110.

A Psalm of David.

[1]The LORD said unto my Lord, Sit
thou at my right [h]hand, [i]until I
make thine enemies thy [j]footstool.
2 The LORD shall send the rod of thy
strength [k]out of Zion: rule thou in the
midst of thine enemies.
3 Thy people *shall be* willing in the day
of thy power, in the beauties of holiness

a Psa. 60:12; cf. Phil. 4:13.
b Heb. *have opened themselves.*
c Psa. 27:12; Mt. 26:59-62; Lk. 23:1-5.
d Psa. 35:7; 69:4; John 15:25.
e *Satan.* Isa. 14:12-14. (Gen. 3:1; Rev. 20:10.)
f Acts 1:20.
g Mt. 27:39.
h See Mt. 22:44; Mk. 12:36; Lk. 20:42, 43; Acts 2:34, 35; Heb. 1:13; 10:12, 13.
i *Christ (Second Advent).* Isa. 9:7. (Deut. 30:3; Acts 1:9-11.)
j 1 Cor. 15:25.
k Rom. 11:26, 27.

[1]**(110:1)** The importance of Psalm 110 is attested by the remarkable prominence given to it in the New Testament. (1) It affirms the deity of Jesus, thus answering those who deny the full divine meaning of His N.T. title of "Lord" (v. 1; Mt. 22:41-45; Mk. 12:35-37; Lk. 20:41-44; Acts 2:34, 35;

from the womb of the morning: thou
hast the dew of thy youth.
4 The LORD hath sworn, and will not
[a]repent, Thou *art* a priest for ever after
the order of [b]Melchizedek.
5 The Lord at thy right hand shall
strike through kings in the day of his
wrath.
6 He shall judge among the [c]heathen,
he shall fill *the places* with the dead bodies; he shall wound the heads over many
countries.
7 He shall drink of the brook in the
way: therefore shall he lift up the head.

PSALM 111.

Praise ye the LORD. I will praise the
LORD with *my* whole heart, in the
assembly of the upright, and *in* the congregation.
2 The works of the LORD *are* great,
sought out of all them that have pleasure
therein.
3 His work *is* honourable and glorious: and his righteousness endureth for
ever.
4 He hath made his wonderful works
to be remembered: the LORD *is* gracious
and full of compassion.
5 He hath given meat unto them that
[d]fear him: he will ever be mindful of his
covenant.
6 He hath shewed his people the
power of his works, that he may give
them the heritage of the heathen.
7 The works of his hands *are* verity
and judgment; all his commandments
are sure.
8 They stand fast for ever and ever,
and are done in truth and uprightness.
9 He sent [e]redemption unto his people: he hath commanded his covenant
for ever: holy and reverend *is* his name.
10 The [f]fear of the LORD *is* the beginning of wisdom: a good understanding
have all they that do *his commandments*:
his praise endureth for ever.

PSALM 112.

Praise ye the LORD. [g]Blessed *is* the
man *that* feareth the LORD, *that*
delighteth greatly in his commandments.
2 [h]His seed shall be mighty upon
earth: the generation of the upright shall
be blessed.
3 Wealth and riches *shall be* in his
house: and his righteousness endureth
for ever.
4 [i]Unto the upright there ariseth light
in the darkness: *he is* gracious, and full
of compassion, and righteous.
5 [j]A good man sheweth favour, and
lendeth: he will guide his affairs [k]with
discretion.
6 Surely he shall not be moved for
ever: [l]the righteous shall be in everlasting remembrance.
7 He shall not be afraid of evil tidings:
his heart is fixed, [m]trusting in the LORD.
8 His heart *is* established, he shall not
be afraid, until he see *his desire* upon his
enemies.
9 He hath [n]dispersed, he hath given to
the poor; his righteousness endureth for
ever; his horn shall be exalted with honour.
10 The wicked shall see *it*, and be
grieved; he shall gnash with his teeth,
and melt away: the desire of the wicked
shall perish.

PSALM 113.

Praise ye the LORD. Praise, O ye servants of the LORD, praise the name
of the LORD.
2 [o]Blessed be the name of the LORD
from this time forth and for evermore.
3 [p]From the rising of the sun unto

a Zech. 8:14, *note.*
b See Heb. 5:6; 6:20; 7:21.
c i.e. *nations;* also Psa. 111:6.
d Psa. 19:9, *note.*
e Ex. 14:30, *note;* Isa. 59:20, *note.*
f Psa. 112:1; also Psa. 19:9, *note.*
g Psa. 128:1.
h Psa. 25:13; 37:26; 102:28.
i Psa. 97:11; Job 11:17.
j Psa. 37:26; Lk. 6:35.
k Eph. 5:15; Col. 4:5.
l Prov. 10:7.
m Psa. 2:12, *note.*
n 2 Cor. 9:9.
o Dan. 2:20.
p Isa. 59:19; Mal. 1:11.

Heb. 1:13; 10:12, 13). (2) This Psalm announces the eternal priesthood of Messiah—one of the most important statements of Scripture (v. 4; Gen. 14:18, *note;* Heb. 5:6, *note;* 7:1-28; 1 Tim. 2:5, 6; John 14:6). (3) Historically, the Psalm begins with the ascension of Christ (v. 1; John 20:17; Acts 7:56; Rev. 3:21). (4) Prophetically, the Psalm looks on *(a)* to the time when Christ will appear as the Rod of Jehovah's strength, the Deliverer out of Zion (Rom. 11:25-27), and the conversion of Israel (v. 3; Joel 2:27; Zech. 13:9. See Deut. 30:1-9, *note*); and *(b)* to the judgment upon the Gentile powers which precedes the setting up of the kingdom (vs. 5, 6; Joel 3:9-17; Zech. 14:1-4; Rev. 19:11-21). See "Armageddon" (Rev. 16:14; 19:17, *note*); "Israel" (Gen. 12:2, 3; Rom. 11:26, *note*); "Kingdom" (Zech. 12:8, *note;* 1 Cor. 15:28, *note*). See Psa. 2, *note,* first, and Psa. 118, last in order of the Messianic Psalms.

the going down of the same the LORD'S name *is* to be praised.

4 The LORD *is* high above all nations, *and* [a]his glory above the heavens.

5 Who *is* like unto the LORD our God, who dwelleth on high,

6 [b]Who humbleth *himself* to behold *the things that are* in heaven, and in the earth!

7 [c]He raiseth up the poor out of the dust, *and* lifteth the needy out of the dunghill;

8 [d]That he may set *him* with princes, *even* with the princes of his people.

9 He maketh the barren woman to keep house, *and to be* a joyful mother of children. Praise ye the LORD.

PSALM 114.

When Israel went out of Egypt, the house of Jacob [e]from a people of strange language;

2 [f]Judah was his sanctuary, *and* Israel his dominion.

3 [g]The sea saw *it*, and fled: [h]Jordan was driven back.

4 The mountains skipped like rams, *and* the little hills like lambs.

5 [i]What *ailed* thee, O thou sea, that thou fleddest? thou Jordan, *that* thou wast driven back?

6 Ye mountains, *that* ye skipped like rams; *and* ye little hills, like lambs?

7 Tremble, thou earth, at the presence of the Lord, at the presence of the God of Jacob;

8 [j]Which turned the rock *into* a standing water, the flint into a fountain of waters.

PSALM 115.

[k]Not unto us, O LORD, not unto us, but unto thy name give glory, for thy mercy, *and* for thy truth's sake.

2 Wherefore should the [l]heathen say, Where *is* now their God?

3 [m]But our God *is* in the heavens: he hath done whatsoever he hath pleased.

4 Their idols *are* silver and gold, the work of men's hands.

5 They have mouths, but they speak not: eyes have they, but they see not:

6 They have ears, but they hear not: noses have they, but they smell not:

7 They have hands, but they handle not: feet have they, but they walk not: neither speak they through their throat.

8 They that make them are like unto them; *so is* every one that trusteth in them.

9 O Israel, [n]trust thou in the LORD: he *is* their help and their shield.

10 O house of Aaron, trust in the LORD: he *is* their help and their shield.

11 Ye that [o]fear the LORD, trust in the LORD: he *is* their help and their shield.

12 The LORD hath been mindful of us: he will bless *us*; he will bless the house of Israel; he will bless the house of Aaron.

13 [p]He will bless them that fear the LORD, *both* small and great.

14 The LORD shall increase you more and more, you and your children.

15 Ye *are* blessed of the LORD which made heaven and earth.

16 The heaven, *even* the heavens, *are* the LORD'S: but the earth hath he given to the children of men.

17 The [q]dead praise not the LORD, neither any that go down into silence.

18 But we will bless the LORD from this time forth and for evermore. Praise the LORD.

PSALM 116.

I love the LORD, because he hath heard my voice *and* my supplications.

2 Because he hath inclined his ear unto me, therefore will I call upon *him* as long as I live.

3 [r]The sorrows of death compassed me, and the pains of [s]hell [t]gat hold upon me: I found trouble and sorrow.

4 Then called I upon the name of the LORD; O LORD, I beseech thee, deliver my soul.

5 Gracious *is* the LORD, and [u]righteous; yea, our God *is* merciful.

6 The LORD preserveth the simple: I was brought low, and he helped me.

7 [v]Return unto thy rest, O my soul; [w]for the LORD hath dealt bountifully with thee.

8 [x]For thou hast delivered my soul from death, mine eyes from tears, *and* my feet from falling.

9 I will walk before the LORD in the land of the living.

a Psa. 8:1.
b Psa. 11:4; 138:6; Isa. 57:15.
c 1 Sam. 2:8; Psa. 107:41.
d Job 36:7.
e Psa. 81:5.
f Ex. 6:7; 19:6; 25:8; 29:45, 46; Deut. 27:9.
g Psa. 77:16; Ex. 14:21.
h Josh. 3:13-16.
i Hab. 3:8.
j Psa. 107:35; Ex. 17:6; Num. 20:11.
k See Isa. 48:11; Ezk. 36:32.
l i.e. *nations.*
m Psa. 135:6; 1 Chr. 16:26; Dan. 4:35.
n Also v. 11; Psa. 2:12, *note.*
o Also v. 13; Psa. 19:9, *note.*
p Psa. 128:1, 4.
q Eccl. 9:5, *note.*
r Psa. 18:4-6.
s Heb. *Sheol.* See Hab. 2:5, *note.*
t Heb. *found me.*
u Psa. 119:137; 145:17; Ezra 9:15; Neh. 9:8.
v Jer. 6:16; Mt. 11:29.
w Psa. 13:6; 119:17.
x Psa. 56:13.

10 I believed, [a]therefore have I spoken:
I was greatly afflicted:
11 I said in my haste, All men *are* liars.
12 What shall I render unto the LORD
for all his benefits toward me?
13 I will take the cup of salvation, and
call upon the name of the LORD.
14 I will pay my vows unto the LORD
now in the presence of all his people.
15 [b]Precious in the sight of the LORD *is*
the death of his saints.
16 O LORD, truly I *am* thy servant; I *am*
thy servant, *and* the son of thine handmaid: thou hast loosed my bonds.
17 [c]I will offer to thee the sacrifice of
thanksgiving, and will call upon the
name of the LORD.
18 I will pay my vows unto the LORD
now in the presence of all his people,
19 In the courts of the LORD'S house, in
the midst of thee, O Jerusalem. Praise ye
the LORD.

PSALM 117.

O [d]praise the LORD, all ye nations:
praise him, all ye people.
2 For his merciful kindness is great
toward us: and the truth of the LORD
endureth for ever. Praise ye the LORD.

PSALM 118.

O give thanks unto the LORD; for *he is*
good: because his mercy *endureth*
for ever.
2 Let Israel now say, that his mercy
endureth for ever.
3 Let the house of Aaron now say, that
his mercy *endureth* for ever.
4 Let them now that [e]fear the LORD
say, that his mercy *endureth* for ever.
5 I called upon the LORD in distress:
the LORD answered me, *and set me* in a
large place.
6 The [f]LORD *is* on my side; I will not
fear: what can man do unto me?
7 The LORD taketh my part with them
that help me: therefore shall I see *my
desire* upon them that hate me.
8 *It is* better to trust in the LORD than
to put confidence in man.
9 *It is* better to [g]trust in the LORD than
to put confidence in princes.
10 All nations compassed me about:
but in the name of the LORD will I
destroy them.
11 [h]They compassed me about; yea,
they compassed me about: but in the
name of the LORD I will destroy them.
12 They compassed me about like
[i]bees; they are quenched as the fire of
thorns: for in the name of the LORD I will
destroy them.
13 Thou hast thrust sore at me that I
might fall: but the LORD helped me.
14 [j]The LORD *is* my strength and song,
and is become my salvation.
15 The voice of rejoicing and salvation
is in the tabernacles of the righteous: the
right hand of the LORD doeth valiantly.
16 The right hand of the LORD is exalted: the right hand of the LORD doeth
valiantly.
17 [k]I shall not die, but live, and declare
the works of the LORD.
18 The LORD [l]hath chastened me sore:
but he hath not given me over unto death.
19 Open to me the gates of righteousness: I will go into them, *and* I will praise
the LORD:
20 [m]This gate of the LORD, [n]into which
the righteous shall enter.
21 I will praise thee: for thou hast
heard me, and art become my salvation.
22 [1]The [o]stone *which* the builders
refused is become the head *stone* of the
corner.
23 [p]This is the LORD'S doing; it *is* marvellous in our eyes.
24 This *is* the day *which* the LORD hath
made; we will rejoice and be glad in it.
25 Save now, I beseech thee, O LORD: O
LORD, I beseech thee, send now prosperity.
26 Blessed *be* he that cometh in the
name of the [q]LORD: we have blessed you
out of the house of the LORD.
27 God *is* the LORD, which hath
shewed us light: bind the sacrifice with
cords, *even* unto the horns of the altar.
28 Thou *art* my God, and I will praise
thee: *thou art* my God, I will exalt thee.

a 2 Cor. 4:13.
b Psa. 72:14.
c Psa. 50:14; 107:22; Lev, 7:12.
d Rom. 15:11.
e Psa. 19:9, *note.*
f Heb. 13:6.
g Psa. 2:12, *note.*
h Psa. 88:17.
i Deut. 1:44.
j Ex. 15:2; Isa. 12:2.
k Psa. 6:5; Hab. 1:12.
l 2 Cor. 6:9.
m Psa. 24:7.
n Isa. 35:8; Rev. 21:27; 22:14, 15.
o *Christ (as Stone).* Isa. 8:14. (Ex. 17:6; 1 Pet. 2:8.)
p Heb. *This is from the Lord.*
q Mt. 21:9; 23:39; Mk. 11:9; Lk. 13:35; 19:38; John 12:13.

[1] **(118:22)** See "Christ (as Stone)," Ex. 17:6; 1 Pet. 2:8, *note.* Psa. 118 looks beyond the rejection of the Stone (Christ) to His final exaltation in the kingdom (v. 22). See Psa. 2, first of the Messianic Psalms.

29 [1]O give thanks unto the LORD; for *he is* good: for his mercy *endureth* for ever.

PSALM 119.

א ALEPH.

Blessed *are* the undefiled in the way, who walk [a]in the law of the LORD.

2 Blessed *are* they that keep his testimonies, *and that* seek him with the whole heart.

3 [b]They also do no iniquity: they walk in his ways.

4 Thou hast commanded *us* to keep thy precepts diligently.

5 O that my ways were directed to keep thy statutes!

6 Then shall I not be ashamed, when I have respect unto all thy commandments.

7 I will praise thee with uprightness of heart, when I shall have learned thy righteous judgments.

8 I will keep thy statutes: O forsake me not utterly.

ב BETH.

9 Wherewithal shall a young man cleanse his way? by taking heed *thereto* according to thy word.

10 [c]With my whole heart have I sought thee: O let me not wander from thy commandments.

11 Thy word have I hid in mine heart, that I might not sin against thee.

12 Blessed *art* thou, O LORD: teach me thy statutes.

13 With my lips have I declared all the judgments of thy mouth.

14 I have rejoiced in the way of thy testimonies, as *much as* in all riches.

15 I will meditate in thy precepts, and have respect unto thy ways.

16 I will delight myself in thy statutes: I will not forget thy word.

ג GIMEL.

17 [d]Deal bountifully with thy servant, *that* I may live, and keep thy word.

18 Open thou mine eyes, that I may behold wondrous things out of thy law.

19 [e]I *am* a stranger in the earth: hide not thy commandments from me.

20 My soul breaketh for the longing *that it hath* unto thy judgments at all times.

21 Thou hast rebuked the proud *that are* cursed, which do err from thy commandments.

22 [f]Remove from me reproach and contempt; for I have kept thy testimonies.

23 Princes also did sit *and* speak against me: *but* thy servant did meditate in thy statutes.

24 Thy testimonies also *are* my delight *and* my counsellors.

ד DALETH.

25 [g]My soul cleaveth unto the dust: [h]quicken thou me according to thy word.

26 I have declared my ways, and thou heardest me: teach me thy statutes.

27 Make me to understand the way of thy precepts: [i]so shall I talk of thy wondrous works.

28 My soul [j]melteth for heaviness: strengthen thou me according unto thy word.

29 Remove from me the way of

a *Law (of Moses).* vs. 1-176; Isa. 1:10-14. (Ex. 19:1; Gal. 3:1-29.)
b 1 John 3:9; 5:18.
c 2 Chr. 15:15.
d Psa. 116:7.
e Psa. 39:12; Gen. 47:9; 1 Chr. 29:15; 2 Cor. 5:6; Heb. 11:13.
f Psa. 39:8.
g Psa. 44:25.
h v. 40; Psa. 143:11.
i Psa. 145:5, 6.
j Heb. *droppeth.*

[1]**(118:29)** The Messianic Psalms: Summary. That the Psalms contain a testimony to Christ our Lord Himself affirmed (Lk. 24:44, etc.); and the N.T. quotations from the Psalter point unerringly to those Psalms which have the Messianic character. A close spiritual and prophetic character as surely identifies others. Christ is seen in the Psalms (1) in two general characters, as *suffering* (e.g. Psa. 22), and as entering into His kingdom *glory* (e.g. Psa. 2; 24. Cf. Lk. 24:25-27).

(2) Christ is seen in His *person (a)* as Son of God (Psa. 2:7), and very God (Psa. 45:6, 7; 102:25; 110:1); *(b)* as Son of man (Psa. 8:4-6); *(c)* as Son of David (Psa. 89:3, 4, 27, 29).

(3) Christ is seen in His *offices (a)* as Prophet (Psa. 22:22, 25; 40:9, 10); *(b)* as Priest (Psa. 110:4); and *(c)* as King (e.g. Psa. 2, 24).

(4) Christ is seen in His varied work. As Priest He offers Himself in sacrifice (Psa. 22; 40:6, with Heb. 10:5-12), and, in resurrection, as the Priest-Shepherd, ever living to make intercession (Psa. 23, with Heb. 7:21-25; 13:20). As Prophet He proclaims the name of Jehovah as Father (Psa. 22:22, with John 20:17). As King He fulfils the Davidic Covenant (Psa. 89) and restores alike the dominion of man over creation (Psa. 8:4-8; Rom. 8:17-21); and of the Father over all (1 Cor. 15:25-28).

(5) The Messianic Psalms give, also, the inner thoughts, the exercises of soul, of Christ in His earthy experiences. (See, e.g., Psa. 16:8-11; 22:1-21; 40:1-17.)

lying: and grant me thy law graciously.
30 I have chosen the way of truth: thy
judgments have I laid *before me*.
31 I have stuck unto thy testimonies:
O LORD, put me not to shame.
32 I will run the way of thy commandments, when thou shalt [a]enlarge my
heart.

ה HE.

33 Teach me, O LORD, the way of thy
statutes; and I shall keep it *unto* the end.
34 [b]Give me understanding, and I
shall keep thy law; yea, I shall observe it
with *my* whole heart.
35 Make me to go in the path of thy
commandments; for therein do I delight.
36 Incline my heart unto thy testimonies, and not to [c]covetousness.
37 Turn away mine eyes from beholding vanity; *and* quicken thou me in thy
way.
38 Stablish thy word unto thy servant,
who *is devoted* to thy [d]fear.
39 Turn away my reproach which I
fear: for thy judgments *are* good.
40 Behold, I have longed after thy precepts: quicken me in thy righteousness.

ו VAU.

41 Let thy mercies come also unto me,
O LORD, *even* thy salvation, according to
thy word.
42 So shall I have wherewith to
answer him that reproacheth me: for I
[e]trust in thy word.
43 And take not the word of truth
utterly out of my mouth; for I have
hoped in thy judgments.
44 So shall I keep thy law continually
for ever and ever.
45 And I will walk at liberty: for I seek
thy precepts.
46 [f]I will speak of thy testimonies also
before kings, and will not be ashamed.
47 And I will delight myself in thy
commandments, which I have loved.
48 My hands also will I lift up unto
thy commandments, which I have loved;
and I will meditate in thy statutes.

ז ZAIN.

49 Remember the word unto thy servant, upon which thou hast caused me
to hope.
50 [g]This *is* my comfort in my affliction: for thy word hath quickened me.
51 The proud have had me greatly [h]in
derision: *yet* have I not declined from
thy law.
52 I remembered thy judgments of
old, O LORD; and have comforted myself.
53 [i]Horror hath taken hold upon me
because of the wicked that forsake thy
law.
54 Thy statutes have been my songs in
the house of my pilgrimage.
55 I have remembered thy name, O
LORD, in the night, and have kept thy law.
56 This I had, because I kept thy precepts.

ח CHETH.

57 [j]*Thou art* my portion, O LORD: I
have said that I would keep thy words.
58 I intreated thy [k]favour with *my*
whole heart: be merciful unto me
according to thy word.
59 [l]I thought on my ways, and turned
my feet unto thy testimonies.
60 I made haste, and delayed not to
keep thy commandments.
61 The bands of the wicked have
robbed me: *but* I have not forgotten thy
law.
62 At midnight I will rise to give
thanks unto thee because of thy righteous judgments.
63 I *am* a companion of all *them* that
[m]fear thee, and of them that keep thy
precepts.
64 The earth, O LORD, is full of thy
mercy: teach me thy statutes.

ט TETH.

65 Thou hast dealt well with thy servant, O LORD, according unto thy word.
66 Teach me good judgment and
knowledge: for I have believed thy commandments.
67 Before I was afflicted I went astray:
but now have I kept thy word.
68 Thou *art* good, and doest good;
teach me thy statutes.
69 The proud have forged a lie against
me: *but* I will keep thy precepts with *my*
whole heart.
70 Their heart is as fat as grease; *but* I
delight in thy law.
71 *It is* good for me that I have been
afflicted; that I might learn thy statutes.
72 The law of thy mouth *is* better unto
me than thousands of gold and silver.

a 1 Ki. 4:29; Isa. 60:5; 2 Cor. 6:11.
b v. 73; Prov. 2:6; Jas. 1:5.
c Ezk. 33:31; Mk. 7:21, 22; Lk. 12:15; I Tim. 6:10; Heb. 13:5.
d Psa. 19:9, *note*.
e Psa. 2:12, *note*.
f Psa. 138:1; Mt. 10:18, 19; Acts 26:1-2.
g Rom. 15:4.
h Jer. 20:7.
i Ezra 9:3; Neh. 13:25.
j Psa. 16:5; Jer. 10:16; Lam. 3:24.
k Heb. *face*. Job 11:19.
l Lk. 15:17, 18.
m Also v. 74. Psa. 19:9, *note*.

י JOD.

73 Thy hands have made me and fashioned me: give me understanding, that I may learn thy commandments.
74 They that fear thee will be glad when they see me; because I have hoped in thy word.
75 I know, O LORD, that thy judgments *are* right, and [a]*that* thou in faithfulness hast afflicted me.
76 Let, I pray thee, thy merciful kindness be for my comfort, according to thy word unto thy servant.
77 Let thy tender mercies come unto me, that I may live: [b]for thy law *is* my delight.
78 Let the proud be ashamed; for they dealt perversely with me without a cause: *but* I will meditate in thy precepts.
79 Let those that fear thee turn unto me, and those that have known thy testimonies.
80 Let my heart be sound in thy statutes; that I be not ashamed.

כ CAPH.

81 [c]My soul fainteth for thy salvation: *but* I hope in thy word.
82 Mine eyes fail for thy word, saying, When wilt thou comfort me?
83 [d]For I am become like a bottle in the smoke; *yet* do I not forget thy statutes.
84 How many *are* the days of thy servant? [e]when wilt thou execute judgment on them that persecute me?
85 The proud have digged pits for me, which *are* not after thy law.
86 All thy commandments *are* faithful: [f]they persecute me wrongfully; help thou me.
87 They had almost consumed me upon earth; but I forsook not thy precepts.
88 Quicken me after thy lovingkindness; so shall I keep the testimony of thy mouth.

ל LAMED.

89 [g]For ever, O LORD, thy word is settled in heaven.
90 Thy faithfulness *is* unto all generations: thou hast established the earth, and it [h]abideth.
91 They continue this day according to thine ordinances: for all *are* thy servants.
92 Unless thy law *had been* my delights, I should then have perished in mine affliction.
93 I will never forget thy precepts: for with them thou hast quickened me.
94 I *am* thine, save me; for I have sought thy precepts.
95 The wicked have waited for me to destroy me: *but* I will consider thy testimonies.
96 I [i]have seen an end of all perfection: *but* thy commandment *is* exceeding broad.

מ MEM.

97 O how love I thy law! [j]it *is* my meditation all the day.
98 Thou through thy commandments hast made me wiser than mine enemies: for they *are* ever with me.
99 I have more understanding than all my teachers: [k]for thy testimonies *are* my meditation.
100 I understand more than the ancients, because I keep thy precepts.
101 [l]I have refrained my feet from every evil way, that I might keep thy word.
102 I have not departed from thy judgments: for thou hast taught me.
103 [m]How sweet are thy words unto my taste! *yea, sweeter* than honey to my mouth!
104 Through thy precepts I get understanding: therefore I hate every false way.

נ NUN.

105 [n]Thy word *is* a lamp unto my feet, and a light unto my path.
106 [o]I have sworn, and I will perform *it*, that I will keep thy righteous judgments.
107 I am afflicted very much: quicken me, O LORD, according unto thy word.
108 Accept, I beseech thee, [p]the freewill offerings of my mouth, O LORD, and teach me thy judgments.
109 My soul *is* continually in my hand: yet do I not forget thy law.
110 The wicked have laid a snare for me: yet I erred not from thy precepts.
111 [q]Thy testimonies have I taken as an heritage for ever: for they *are* the rejoicing of my heart.
112 I have inclined mine heart to perform thy statutes alway, *even unto* the end.

ס SAMECH.

113 I hate *vain* thoughts: but thy law do I love.
114 [r]Thou *art* my hiding place and my shield: I hope in thy word.

a Heb. 12:10.
b vs. 24, 47, 174.
c Psa. 73:26; 84:2.
d Job 30:30.
e Rev. 6:10.
f Psa. 35:19; 38:19.
g Psa. 89:2; Mt. 24:34, 35; 1 Pet. 1:25.
h Heb. *standeth.*
i Rom. 3:10-19.
j Psa. 1:2.
k 2 Tim. 3:15.
l Prov. 1:15.
m Psa. 19:10; Prov. 8:11.
n Prov. 6:23.
o Neh. 10.29.
p Hos. 14:2; Heb. 13:15.
q Deut. 33:4.
r Psa. 32:7; 91:1.

115 [a]Depart from me, ye evildoers: for I
will keep the commandments of my God.
116 Uphold me according unto thy
word, that I may live: [b]and let me not be
ashamed of my hope.
117 Hold thou me up, and I shall be
safe: and I will have respect unto thy
statutes continually.
118 Thou hast trodden down all them
that err from thy statutes: for their deceit
is falsehood.
119 Thou puttest away all the wicked
of the earth [c]*like* dross: therefore I love
thy testimonies.
120 [d]My flesh trembleth for fear of
thee; and I am afraid of thy judgments.

ע AIN.

121 I have done judgment and justice:
leave me not to mine oppressors.
122 [e]Be surety for thy servant for good:
let not the proud oppress me.
123 Mine eyes fail for thy salvation,
and for the word of thy righteousness.
124 Deal with thy servant according
unto thy mercy, and [f]teach me thy
statutes.
125 I *am* thy servant; give me understanding, that I may know thy testimonies.
126 *It is* time for *thee*, LORD, to work: *for*
they have made void thy law.
127 [g]Therefore I love thy commandments above gold; yea, above fine gold.
128 Therefore I esteem all *thy* precepts
concerning all *things to be* right; *and* I hate
every false way.

פ PE.

129 Thy testimonies *are* wonderful:
therefore doth my soul keep them.
130 The entrance of thy words giveth
light; [h]it giveth understanding unto the
simple.
131 I opened my mouth, and panted:
for I longed for thy commandments.
132 [i]Look thou upon me, and be [j]mer-
ciful unto me, as thou usest to do unto
those that love thy name.
133 Order my steps in thy word: and let
not any iniquity have dominion over me.
134 [k]Deliver me from the oppression of
man: so will I keep thy precepts.
135 [l]Make thy face to shine upon thy
servant; and teach me thy statutes.

a Psa. 6:8; 139:19; Mt. 7:23.
b Psa. 25:2; Rom. 5:5; 9:33; 10:11.
c Ezk. 22:18.
d Hab. 3:16.
e Heb. 7:22.
f v. 12.
g v. 72; Psa. 19:10; Prov. 8:11.
h Psa. 19:7; Prov. 1:4.
i Psa. 106:4.
j Psa. 51:1.
k Lk. 1:74.
l Psa. 4:6.
m Jer. 9:1; 14:17. See Ezk. 9:4.
n Heb. *righteousness*
o *faithfulness.*
p Heb. *tried*, or *refined.*
q v. 151; Psa. 19:9; John 17:17.
r Psa. 5:3; 88:13; 130:6.
s Psa. 63:1, 6.
t Psa. 145:18.
u Lk. 21:33.
v Lam. 5:1.
w Heb. *goel*, *Redemp. (Kinsman type).* Isa. 59:20, *note.*

136 [m]Rivers of waters run down mine
eyes, because they keep not thy law.

צ TZADDI.

137 [n]Righteous *art* thou, O LORD, and
upright *are* thy judgments.
138 Thy testimonies *that* thou hast commanded *are* [o]righteous and very faithful.
139 My zeal hath consumed me,
because mine enemies have forgotten
thy words.
140 Thy word *is* very [p]pure: therefore
thy servant loveth it.
141 I *am* small and despised: *yet* do not
I forget thy precepts.
142 Thy righteousness *is* an everlasting
righteousness, and [q]thy law *is* the truth.
143 Trouble and anguish have taken
hold on me: *yet* thy commandments *are*
my delights.
144 The righteousness of thy testimonies *is* everlasting: give me understanding, and I shall live.

ק KOPH.

145 I cried with *my* whole heart; hear
me, O LORD: I will keep thy statutes.
146 I cried unto thee; save me, and I
shall keep thy testimonies.
147 [r]I prevented the dawning of the
morning, and cried: I hoped in thy word.
148 [s]Mine eyes prevent the *night*
watches, that I might meditate in thy
word.
149 Hear my voice according unto thy
lovingkindness: O LORD, quicken me
according to thy judgment.
150 They draw nigh that follow after
mischief: they are far from thy law.
151 [t]Thou *art* near, O LORD; and all thy
commandments *are* truth.
152 Concerning thy testimonies, I have
known of old [u]that thou hast founded
them for ever.

ר RESH.

153 [v]Consider mine affliction, and
deliver me: for I do not forget thy law.
154 Plead my cause, and [w]deliver me:
quicken me according to thy word.
155 Salvation *is* far from the wicked:
for they seek not thy statutes.
156 Great *are* thy tender mercies, O

LORD: quicken me according to thy judgments.

157 Many *are* my persecutors and mine enemies; *yet* do I not [a]decline from thy testimonies.

158 I beheld the transgressors, and was grieved; because they kept not thy word.

159 Consider how I love thy precepts: quicken me, O LORD, according to thy lovingkindness.

160 Thy word *is* true *from* the beginning: and every one of thy righteous judgments *endureth* for ever.

ש SCHIN.

161 [b]Princes have persecuted me without a cause: but my heart standeth in awe of thy word.

162 I rejoice at thy word, as one that findeth great spoil.

163 I hate and abhor lying: *but* thy law do I love.

164 Seven times a day do I praise thee because of thy righteous judgments.

165 [c]Great peace have they which love thy law: [d]and nothing shall offend them.

166 LORD, [e]I have hoped for thy salvation, and done thy commandments.

167 My soul hath kept thy testimonies; and I love them exceedingly.

168 I have kept thy precepts and thy testimonies: for all my ways *are* before thee.

ת TAU.

169 Let my cry come near before thee, O LORD: [f]give me understanding according to thy word.

170 Let my supplication come before thee: deliver me according to thy word.

171 My lips shall utter praise, when thou hast taught me thy statutes.

172 My tongue shall speak of thy word: for all thy commandments *are* righteousness.

173 Let thine hand help me; for [g]I have chosen thy precepts.

174 I have longed for thy salvation, O LORD; and thy law *is* my delight.

175 Let my soul live, and it shall praise thee; and let thy judgments help me.

176 [h]I have gone astray like a lost sheep; seek thy servant; for I do not forget thy commandments.

PSALM 120.

A Song of [1]degrees.

In my distress I cried unto the LORD, and he heard me.

2 Deliver my soul, O LORD, from lying lips, *and* from a deceitful tongue.

3 What shall be given unto thee? or what shall be done unto thee, thou false tongue?

4 Sharp arrows of the mighty, with coals of juniper.

5 Woe is me, that I sojourn in [i]Mesech, [j]*that* I dwell in the tents of Kedar!

6 My soul hath long dwelt with him that hateth peace.

7 I *am for* peace: but when I speak, they *are* for war.

PSALM 121.

A Song of [1]degrees.

I [k]will lift up mine eyes unto the hills, from whence cometh my help.

2 [l]My help *cometh* from the LORD, which made heaven and earth.

3 [m]He will not suffer thy foot to be moved: [n]he that keepeth thee will not slumber.

4 Behold, he that keepeth Israel shall neither slumber nor sleep.

5 The LORD *is* thy keeper: the LORD *is* [o]thy shade [p]upon thy right hand.

6 [q]The sun shall not smite thee by day, nor the moon by night.

7 The LORD shall preserve thee from all evil: he shall [r]preserve thy soul.

8 The LORD shall [s]preserve thy going out and thy coming in from this time forth, and even for evermore.

PSALM 122.

A Song of [1]degrees of David.

I was glad when they said unto me, [t]Let us go into the house of the LORD.

2 Our feet shall stand within thy gates, O Jerusalem.

3 Jerusalem is builded as a city that is [u]compact together:

4 [v]Whither the tribes go up, the tribes of the LORD, unto the testimony of Israel, to give thanks unto the name of the LORD.

a v. 51; Psa. 44:18.
b v. 23; 1 Sam. 24:11, 14; 26:18.
c Prov. 3:2; Isa. 32:17.
d Heb. *they shall have no stumbling block.*
e v. 174; Gen. 49:18.
f v. 144.
g Josh. 24:22; Prov. 1:29; Lk. 10:42.
h Isa. 53.6; Lk. 15:4; 1 Pet. 2:25.
i Gen. 10.2; Ezk. 27:13.
j Gen. 25:13; Jer. 49:28, 29.
k Or, *Shall I lift up mine eyes to the hills? whence should my help come? My help cometh from the LORD.*
l See Jer. 3:23.
m 1 Sam. 2:9; Prov. 3:23, 26.
n Psa. 127:1; Isa. 27:3.
o Isa. 25:4.
p Psa. 16:8; 109:31.
q Psa. 91:5; Isa. 49:10; Rev. 7:16.
r Psa. 41:2; 97:10; 145:20.
s Deut. 28:6; Prov. 2:8; 3:6.
t Isa. 2:3; Zech. 8:21.
u See 2 Sam. 5:9.
v Ex. 23:17; Deut. 16:16.

[1] **(120–134, inscriptions)** Literally, "of ascents." Perhaps chanted by the people as they went up to Jerusalem to the feasts. See, e.g. Psa. 122:1, 2.

5 [a]For there are set thrones of judgment, the thrones of the house of David.

6 Pray for the peace of Jerusalem: they shall prosper that love thee.

7 Peace be within thy walls, *and* prosperity within thy palaces.

8 For my brethren and companions' sakes, I will now say, Peace *be* within thee.

9 Because of the house of the LORD our God I will seek thy good.

PSALM 123.

A Song of [b]degrees.

Unto thee lift I up mine eyes, O thou that dwellest in the heavens.

2 Behold, as the eyes of servants *look* unto the hand of their masters, *and* as the eyes of a maiden unto the hand of her mistress; so our eyes *wait* upon the LORD our God, until that he have mercy upon us.

3 Have mercy upon us, O LORD, have mercy upon us: for we are exceedingly filled with contempt.

4 Our soul is exceedingly filled with the scorning of those that are at ease, *and* with the contempt of the proud.

PSALM 124.

A Song of [b]degrees of David.

If *it had not been* the LORD who was on our side, now may Israel say;

2 If *it had not been* the LORD who was on our side, when men rose up against us:

3 [c]Then they had swallowed us up quick, when their wrath was kindled against us:

4 Then the waters had overwhelmed us, the stream had gone over our soul:

5 Then the proud waters had gone over our soul.

6 Blessed *be* the LORD, who hath not given us *as* a prey to their teeth.

7 [d]Our soul is escaped as a bird out of the snare of the fowlers: the snare is broken, and we are escaped.

8 Our help *is* in the name of the LORD, who made heaven and earth.

PSALM 125.

A Song of [b]degrees.

They that [e]trust in the LORD *shall be* as mount Zion, *which* cannot be removed, *but* abideth for ever.

2 *As* the mountains *are* round about Jerusalem, so the LORD *is* round about his people from henceforth even for ever.

3 For [f]the rod of the wicked shall not rest upon the lot of the righteous; lest the righteous put forth their hands unto iniquity.

4 Do good, O LORD, unto *those that be* good, and to *them that are* upright in their hearts.

5 As for such as turn aside unto their crooked ways, the LORD shall lead them forth with the workers of iniquity: *but* peace *shall be* upon Israel.

PSALM 126.

A Song of [b]degrees.

[g]When the LORD turned again the captivity of Zion, [h]we were like them that dream.

2 Then was our mouth filled with laughter, and our tongue with singing: then said they among the [i]heathen, The LORD hath done great things for them.

3 The LORD hath done great things for us; *whereof* we are glad.

4 Turn again our captivity, O LORD, as the streams in the south.

5 [j]They that sow in tears shall reap in [k]joy.

6 He that goeth forth and weepeth, bearing precious seed, shall doubtless come again with rejoicing, bringing his sheaves *with him*.

PSALM 127.

A Song of [b]degrees for Solomon.

Except the LORD build the house, they labour in vain that build it: [l]except the LORD keep the city, the watchman waketh *but* in vain.

2 *It is* vain for you to rise up early, to sit up late, [m]to eat the bread of sorrows: *for* so he giveth his beloved sleep.

3 Lo, [n]children *are* an heritage of the LORD: *and* [o]the fruit of the womb *is his* reward.

4 As arrows *are* in the hand of a mighty man; so *are* children of the youth.

5 Happy *is* the man that hath his quiver full of them: they shall not be ashamed, but they shall speak with the enemies in the gate.

a Deut. 17:8; 2 Chr. 19:8.
b See Psa. 120, title, *note.*
c Psa. 56:1, 2; 57:3; Prov. 1:12.
d Psa. 91:3; Prov. 6:5.
e *Faith.* Jon. 3:5. (Gen. 3:20; Heb. 11:39.)
f Or, *the sceptre.* Cf. Prov. 22:8; Isa. 14:5.
g Psa. 53:6; 85:1; Hos. 6:11.
h Joel 3:1; Acts 12:9.
i i.e. *nations.*
j See Jer. 31:9.
k Or, *singing.* Cp. Neh. 12:43
l Psa. 121:1-5.
m Gen. 3:17-19.
n Gen. 33:5; 48:4; Josh. 24:3, 4.
o Deut. 28:4.

PSALM 128.

A Song of [a]degrees.

Blessed *is* every one that [b]feareth the LORD; that walketh in his ways.

2 For thou shalt eat the labour of thine hands: happy *shalt* thou *be*, and *it shall be* well with thee.

3 Thy wife *shall be* [c]as a fruitful vine by the sides of thine house: thy children [d]like olive plants round about thy table.

4 Behold, that thus shall the man be blessed that feareth the LORD.

5 The LORD shall bless thee out of Zion: and thou shalt see the good of Jerusalem all the days of thy life.

6 Yea, [e]thou shalt see thy children's children, *and* peace upon Israel.

PSALM 129.

A Song of [a]degrees.

Many a time have they afflicted me [f]from my youth, may Israel now say:

2 Many a time have they afflicted me from my youth: yet they have not prevailed against me.

3 The plowers plowed upon my back: they made long their furrows.

4 The LORD *is* righteous: he hath cut asunder the cords of the wicked.

5 Let them all be confounded and turned back that hate Zion.

6 Let them be [g]as the grass *upon* the housetops, which withereth afore it groweth up:

7 Wherewith the mower filleth not his hand; nor he that bindeth sheaves his bosom.

8 Neither do they which go by say, The blessing of the LORD *be* upon you: we bless you in the name of the LORD.

PSALM 130.

A Song of [a]degrees.

Out of the depths have I cried unto thee, O LORD.

2 Lord, hear my voice: let thine ears be attentive to the voice of my supplications.

3 If thou, LORD, shouldest mark iniquities, O Lord, who shall stand?

4 But *there is* forgiveness with thee, that thou mayest be [b]feared.

5 I wait for the LORD, my soul doth wait, and in his word do I hope.

6 [h]My soul *waiteth* for the Lord more than they that watch for the morning: *I say, more than* they that watch for the morning.

7 Let Israel hope in the LORD: for with the LORD [i]*there is* mercy, and with him *is* plenteous [j]redemption.

8 And he shall redeem Israel from all his iniquities.

PSALM 131.

A Song of [a]degrees of David.

LORD, my heart is not haughty, nor mine eyes lofty: neither do I exercise myself in great matters, or in things too high for me.

2 Surely I have behaved and quieted myself, as a child that is weaned of his mother: my soul *is* even as a weaned child.

3 Let Israel hope in the LORD from henceforth and for ever.

PSALM 132.

A Song of [a]degrees.

LORD, remember David, *and* all his afflictions:

2 How he sware unto the LORD, *and* vowed unto the mighty *God* of Jacob;

3 Surely I will not come into the tabernacle of my house, nor go up into my bed;

4 I will not give sleep to mine eyes, *or* slumber to mine eyelids,

5 [k]Until I find out a place for the LORD, an habitation for the mighty *God* of Jacob.

6 Lo, we heard of it at Ephratah: we found it in the fields of the wood.

7 [l]We will go into his tabernacles: we will worship at his footstool.

8 Arise, O LORD, into thy rest; thou, and the ark of thy strength.

9 Let thy priests be clothed with [m]righteousness; and let thy saints shout for joy.

10 For thy servant David's sake turn not away the face of thine anointed.

11 [n]The LORD hath sworn *in* truth unto David; he will not turn from it; [o]Of the fruit of thy body will I set upon thy throne.

12 If thy children will keep my covenant and my testimony that I shall teach them, their children shall also sit upon thy throne for evermore.

---

a See Psa. 120, title, *note.*
b Psa. 19:9, *note.*
c Ezk. 19:10.
d Psa. 52:8; 144:12.
e Gen. 50:23; Job 42:16.
f Ezk. 23:3; Hos. 2:15; 11:1.
g Psa. 37:2.
h Psa. 63:6; 119:147.
i Psa. 86:5, 15; Isa. 55:7.
j Ex. 14:30, *note;* Isa. 59:20, *note.*
k Acts 7:46.
l Psa. 122:1, 2.
m Righteousness (garment). Isa. 11:5. (Gen. 3:21; Rev. 19:8.)
n Psa. 89:3, 4, 33; 110.4.
o 2 Sam. 7:12; 1 Ki. 8:25; 2 Chr. 6:16; Lk. 1:69; Acts 2:30.

13 [a]For the LORD hath chosen Zion; he
hath desired *it* for his habitation.
14 [b]This *is* my rest for ever: here will I
dwell; for I have desired it.
15 I will abundantly bless her provision: I will satisfy her poor with bread.
16 [c]I will also clothe her priests with
salvation: [d]and her saints shall shout
aloud for joy.
17 [e]There will I make the horn of
David to bud: [f]I have ordained a lamp
for mine anointed.
18 His enemies will [g]I clothe with
shame: but upon himself shall his crown
flourish.

PSALM 133.

A Song of [h]degrees of David.

Behold, how good and how pleasant *it*
is [i]for brethren to dwell together in
unity!
2 *It is* like the precious ointment upon
the head, that ran down upon the beard,
even Aaron's beard: that went down to
the skirts of his garments;
3 [j]As the dew of Hermon, *and as the*
dew that descended upon the mountains
of Zion: for [k]there the LORD commanded
the blessing, *even* life for evermore.

PSALM 134.

A Song of [h]degrees.

Behold, bless ye the LORD, all *ye* servants of the LORD, which by night
stand in the house of the LORD.
2 Lift up your hands *in* the sanctuary,
and bless the LORD.
3 The LORD that made heaven and
earth bless thee out of Zion.

PSALM 135.

Praise ye the LORD. Praise ye the name
of the LORD; praise *him*, O ye servants of the LORD.
2 Ye that stand in the house of the LORD,
in the courts of the house of our God,
3 Praise the LORD; [m]for the LORD *is*
good: sing praises unto his name; for *it is*
pleasant.
4 [n]For the LORD hath chosen Jacob
unto himself, *and* Israel for his peculiar
treasure.
5 [o]For I know that the LORD *is* great,
and *that* our Lord *is* above all gods.

6 [p]Whatsoever the LORD pleased, *that*
did he in heaven, and in earth, in the
seas, and all deep places.
7 He causeth the vapours to ascend
from the ends of the earth; [q]he maketh
lightnings for the rain; he bringeth the
wind out of [r]his treasuries.
8 [s]Who smote the firstborn of Egypt,
both of man and beast.
9 [t]*Who* sent tokens and wonders into
the midst of thee, O Egypt, upon
Pharaoh, and upon all his servants.
10 Who smote great nations, and slew
mighty kings;
11 Sihon king of the Amorites, and Og
king of Bashan, [u]and all the kingdoms of
Canaan:
12 [v]And gave their land *for* an heritage, an heritage unto Israel his people.
13 [w]Thy name, O LORD, *endureth* for
ever; *and* thy memorial, O LORD,
throughout all generations.
14 For the LORD will judge his people,
and he will [x]repent himself concerning
his servants.
15 The idols of the [y]heathen *are* silver
and gold, the work of men's hands.
16 They have mouths, but they speak
not; eyes have they, but they see not;
17 They have ears, but they hear not;
neither is there *any* breath in their
mouths.
18 They that make them are like unto
them: *so is* every one that trusteth in them.
19 Bless the LORD, O house of Israel:
bless the LORD, O house of Aaron:
20 Bless the LORD, O house of Levi: ye
that [z]fear the LORD, bless the LORD.
21 Blessed be the LORD out of Zion,
which dwelleth at Jerusalem. Praise ye
the LORD.

PSALM 136.

O give thanks unto the LORD; for *he is*
good: [aa]for his mercy *endureth* for
ever.
2 O give thanks unto [bb]the God of
gods: for his mercy *endureth* for ever.
3 O give thanks to the Lord of lords:
for his mercy *endureth* for ever.
4 To him who alone doeth great wonders: for his mercy *endureth* for ever.
5 [cc]To him that by wisdom made the

a Psa. 48:1, 2.
b Psa. 68:16.
c v. 9; Psa. 132:9; 149:4; 2 Chr. 6:41.
d 1 Sam. 4:5.
e Ezk. 29:21; Lk. 1:69.
f See 1 Ki. 11:36; 15:4; 2 Chr. 21:7.
g Psa. 35:26; 109:29.
h See Psa. 120, title, *note.*
i Gen. 13:8; Heb. 13:1.
j Deut. 4:48.
k Lev. 25:21; Deut. 28:8; Psa. 42:8.
l Psa. 92:13; 96:8; 116:19.
m Psa. 119:68.
n Ex. 19:5; Deut. 7:6, 7; 10:15.
o Psa. 95:3.
p Psa. 115:3.
q Job 28:25, 26; 38:24; Zech. 10:1.
r Job 38:22.
s Psa. 78:51; 136:10; Ex. 12:12, 29.
t Ex. 7.—14.
u Josh. 12:7.
v Psa. 78:55; 136:21, 22.
w Psa. 102:12; Ex. 3:15.
x Zech. 8:14, *note.*
y i.e. *nations.*
z Psa. 19:9, *note.*
aa 1 Chr. 16:34, 41; 2 Chr. 20:21.
bb Deut. 10:17.
cc Gen. 1:1, 6; Prov. 3:19; Jer. 51:15.

heavens: for his mercy *endureth* for ever.
6 [a]To him that stretched out the earth
above the waters: for his mercy *endureth*
for ever.
7 [b]To him that made great lights: for
his mercy *endureth* for ever:
8 [c]The sun to rule by day: for his
mercy *endureth* for ever:
9 The moon and stars to rule by night:
for his mercy *endureth* for ever.
10 [d]To him that smote Egypt in their
firstborn: for his mercy *endureth* for ever:
11 [e]And brought out Israel from
among them: for his mercy *endureth* for
ever:
12 [f]With a strong hand, and with a
stretched out arm: for his mercy *endureth*
for ever.
13 [g]To him which divided the Red sea
into parts: for his mercy *endureth* for
ever:
14 And made Israel to pass through
the midst of it: for his mercy *endureth* for
ever:
15 [h]But overthrew Pharaoh and his
host in the Red sea: for his mercy
endureth for ever.
16 To him which led his people
through the wilderness: for his mercy
endureth for ever.
17 [i]To him which smote great kings:
for his mercy *endureth* for ever:
18 [j]And slew famous kings: for his
mercy *endureth* for ever:
19 [k]Sihon king of the Amorites: for his
mercy *endureth* for ever:
20 [l]And Og the king of Bashan: for his
mercy *endureth* for ever:
21 [m]And gave their land for an heritage: for his mercy *endureth* for ever:
22 *Even* an heritage unto Israel his servant: for his mercy *endureth* for ever.
23 [n]Who remembered us in our low
estate: for his mercy *endureth* for ever:
24 And hath [o]redeemed us from our
enemies: for his mercy *endureth* for ever.
25 [p]Who giveth food to all flesh: for
his mercy *endureth* for ever.
26 O give thanks unto the God of
heaven: for his mercy *endureth* for ever.

PSALM 137.

By the rivers of Babylon, there we sat
down, yea, we wept, when we
remembered Zion.
2 We hanged our harps upon the willows in the midst thereof.
3 For there they that carried us away
captive required of us [q]a song; and they
that wasted us *required of us* mirth,
saying, Sing us *one* of the songs of Zion.
4 How shall we sing the LORD'S song
in a strange land?
5 If I forget thee, O Jerusalem, let my
right hand forget *her cunning*.
6 If I do not remember thee, let my
[r]tongue cleave to the roof of my mouth; if
I prefer not Jerusalem above my chief joy.
7 Remember, O LORD, the children of
[s]Edom in the day of Jerusalem; who
said, Rase *it,* rase *it, even* to the foundation thereof.
8 O daughter of Babylon, [t]who art to
be destroyed; happy *shall he be,* that
rewardeth thee as thou hast served us.
9 Happy *shall he be,* that taketh and
dasheth thy little ones against the stones.

PSALM 138.

A Psalm of David.

I will praise thee with my whole heart:
before the gods will I sing praise unto
thee.
2 I will worship toward thy holy temple, and praise thy name for thy lovingkindness and for thy truth: for thou
hast magnified thy word above all thy
name.
3 In the day when I cried thou
answeredst me, *and* strengthenedst me
with strength in my soul.
4 [u]All the kings of the earth shall
praise thee, O LORD, when they hear the
words of thy mouth.
5 Yea, they shall sing in the ways of the
LORD: for great *is* the glory of the LORD.
6 Though the LORD *be* high, yet [v]hath
he respect unto the lowly: but the proud
he knoweth afar off.
7 [w]Though I walk in the midst of trouble, thou wilt revive me: thou shalt
stretch forth thine hand against the
wrath of mine enemies, and thy right
hand shall save me.
8 [x]The LORD will perfect *that which*
concerneth me: thy mercy, O LORD,
endureth for ever: forsake not the works
of thine own hands.

a Gen. 1:9; Psa. 24:2; Jer. 10:12.
b Gen. 1:14.
c Gen. 1:16.
d Psa. 135:8; Ex. 12:29.
e Ex. 12:51; 13:3, 17.
f Ex. 6:6.
g Psa. 78:13; Ex. 14:21, 22.
h Psa. 135:9; Ex. 14:27.
i Psa. 135:10, 11.
j Deut. 29:7.
k Num. 21:21.
l Num. 21:33.
m Psa. 135:12; Josh. 12:1.
n Psa. 113:7; Gen. 8:1; Deut. 32:36.
o Ex. 14:30, *note;* Isa. 59:20, *note.*
p Psa. 104:27; 145:15; 147:9.
q Heb. *the words of a song.*
r Ezk. 3:26.
s Jer. 49:7; Lam. 4:22; Ezk. 25:12; Oba. 10; Gen. 36:1, *note.*
t Isa. 13:1, 6; 47:1; Jer. 25:12; 50:2.
u Psa. 102:15, 22.
v Prov. 3:34; Jas. 4:6; 1 Pet. 5:5.
w Psa. 23:3, 4.
x Psa. 57:2; Phil. 1:6.

PSALM 139.

To the chief Musician,
A Psalm of David.

O LORD, thou hast searched me, and known *me.*

2 [a]Thou knowest my downsitting and mine uprising, thou [b]understandest my thought afar off.

3 Thou compassest my path and my lying down, and art acquainted *with* all my ways.

4 For *there is* not a word in my tongue, *but,* lo, O LORD, [c]thou knowest it altogether.

5 Thou hast beset me behind and before, and laid thine hand upon me.

6 [d]*Such* knowledge *is* too wonderful for me; it is high, I cannot *attain* unto it.

7 [e]Whither shall I go from thy [f]spirit? or whither shall I flee from thy presence?

8 If I ascend up into heaven, thou *art* there: if I make my bed in [g]hell, behold, thou *art there.*

9 *If* I take the wings of the morning, *and* dwell in the uttermost parts of the sea;

10 Even there shall thy hand lead me, and thy right hand shall hold me.

11 If I say, Surely the darkness shall cover me; even the night shall be light about me.

12 Yea, [h]the darkness hideth not from thee; but the night shineth as the day: the darkness and the light *are* both alike *to thee.*

13 For thou hast possessed my reins: thou hast covered me in my mother's womb.

14 I will praise thee; for I am fearfully *and* wonderfully made: marvellous *are* thy works; and *that* my soul knoweth right well.

15 [i]My substance was not hid from thee, when I was made in secret, *and* curiously wrought in the lowest parts of the earth.

16 Thine eyes did see my substance, yet being unperfect; and in thy book all *my members* were written, *which* in continuance were fashioned, when *as yet there was* none of them.

17 [j]How precious also are thy thoughts unto me, O God! how great is the sum of them!

18 *If* I should count them, they are more in number than the sand: when I awake, I am still with thee.

19 [k]Surely thou wilt slay the wicked, O God: depart from me therefore, ye bloody men.

20 For they [l]speak against thee wickedly, *and* thine enemies take *thy name* in vain.

21 Do not I hate them, O LORD, that hate thee? and am not I grieved with those that rise up against thee?

22 I hate them with perfect hatred: I count them mine enemies.

23 [m]Search me, O God, and know my heart: try me, and know my thoughts:

24 And see if *there be any* wicked way in me, [n]and lead me in the way everlasting.

PSALM 140.

To the chief Musician,
A Psalm of David.

Deliver me, O LORD, from the evil man: [o]preserve me from the violent man;

2 Which imagine mischiefs in *their* heart; continually are they gathered together *for* war.

3 They have sharpened their tongues like a serpent; adders' poison *is* under their [p]lips. Selah.

4 Keep me, O LORD, from the hands of the wicked; preserve me from the violent man; who have purposed to overthrow my goings.

5 [q]The proud have hid a snare for me, and cords; they have spread a net by the wayside; they have set gins for me. Selah.

6 I said unto the LORD, Thou *art* my God: hear the voice of my supplications, O LORD.

7 O GOD the Lord, the strength of my salvation, thou hast covered my head in the day of battle.

8 Grant not, O LORD, the desires of the wicked: further not his wicked device; [r]*lest* they exalt themselves. Selah.

9 *As for* the head of those that compass me about, let the mischief of their own lips cover them.

10 Let burning coals fall upon them: let them be cast into the fire; into deep pits, that they rise not up again.

11 Let not an evil speaker be established in the earth: evil shall hunt the violent man to overthrow *him.*

12 I know [s]that the LORD will maintain the cause of the afflicted, *and* the right of the poor.

a 2 Ki. 19:27.
b Mt. 9:4; John 2:24, 25.
c Heb. 4:13.
d Psa. 40:5; 131:1; Job 42:3.
e Jer. 23:24; Amos 9:2-4; Jon. 1:3.
f *Holy Spirit.* Isa. 4:4. (Gen. 1:2; Mal. 2:15.)
g Heb. *Sheol.* See Hab. 2:5, *note.*
h Job 26:6; 34:22; Dan. 2:22; Heb. 4:13.
i Job 10:8, 9; Eccl. 11:5.
j Psa. 40:5.
k Isa. 11:4.
l Jude 15.
m Psa. 26:2; Job 31:6.
n Psa. 5:8; 143:10.
o Heb. *man of violences.*
p Psa. 58:4; Rom. 3:13.
q Psa. 35:7; 57:6; 119:110; 141:9; Jer. 18:22.
r Deut. 32:27.
s Psa. 9:4; 1 Ki. 8:45.

13 Surely the righteous shall give thanks unto thy name: the upright shall dwell in thy presence.

PSALM 141.

A Psalm of David.

LORD, I cry unto thee: make haste unto me; give ear unto my voice, when I cry unto thee.

2 Let my prayer be set forth before thee [a]*as* incense; *and* [b]the lifting up of my hands *as* the evening sacrifice.

3 Set a watch, O LORD, before my mouth; keep the door of my lips.

4 Incline not my heart to *any* evil thing, to practise wicked works with men that work iniquity: and let me not eat of their dainties.

5 [c]Let the righteous smite me; *it shall be* a kindness: and let him reprove me; *it shall be* an excellent oil, *which* shall not break my head: for yet my prayer also *shall be* in their calamities.

6 When their judges are overthrown in stony places, they shall hear my words; for they are sweet.

7 [d]Our bones are scattered at the grave's mouth, as when one cutteth and cleaveth *wood* upon the earth.

8 [e]But mine eyes *are* unto thee, O GOD the Lord: in thee is my [f]trust; leave not my soul [g]destitute.

9 Keep me from the snares *which* they have laid for me, and the gins of the workers of iniquity.

10 Let the wicked fall into their own nets, whilst that I withal [h]escape.

PSALM 142.

[i]Maschil of David;
A Prayer when he was in the cave.

I cried unto the LORD with my voice; with my voice unto the LORD did I make my supplication.

2 I poured out my complaint before him; I shewed before him my trouble.

3 [j]When my spirit was overwhelmed within me, then thou knewest my path. In the way wherein I walked have they privily laid a snare for me.

4 I looked on *my* right hand, and beheld, but *there was* no man that would know me: refuge failed me; [k]no man cared for my soul.

5 I cried unto thee, O LORD: I said, Thou *art* my refuge *and* my portion in the land of the living.

a Rev. 8:3.
b Psa. 134:2; 1 Tim. 2:8.
c Prov. 9:8; 19:25; 25:12; Gal. 6:1.
d 2 Cor. 1:9.
e Psa. 25:15; 123:1, 2; 2 Chr. 20:12.
f Psa. 2:12, *note.*
g Heb. *make not my soul bare.*
h Heb. *pass over.*
i *Maschil, instruction.*
j Psa. 143:4.
k Heb. *no man sought after my soul.*
l Psa. 34:2.
m Psa. 130:3; Ex. 34:7; Job 4:17; 9:2; 15:14; 25:4; Eccl. 7:20; Rom. 3:20; Gal. 2:16.
n Psa. 77:3; 142:3.
o Psa. 77:5, 10, 11.
p Psa. 5:8.
q Heb. *hide me with thee.*
r Neh. 9:20.
s Isa. 26:10.

6 Attend unto my cry; for I am brought very low: deliver me from my persecutors; for they are stronger than I.

7 Bring my soul out of prison, that I may praise thy name: [l]the righteous shall compass me about; for thou shalt deal bountifully with me.

PSALM 143.

A Psalm of David.

Hear my prayer, O LORD, give ear to my supplications: in thy faithfulness answer me, *and* in thy righteousness.

2 And enter not into judgment with thy servant: [m]for in thy sight shall no man living be justified.

3 For the enemy hath persecuted my soul; he hath smitten my life down to the ground; he hath made me to dwell in darkness, as those that have been long dead.

4 [n]Therefore is my spirit overwhelmed within me; my heart within me is desolate.

5 [o]I remember the days of old; I meditate on all thy works; I muse on the work of thy hands.

6 I stretch forth my hands unto thee: my soul *thirsteth* after thee, as a thirsty land. Selah.

7 Hear me speedily, O LORD: my spirit faileth: hide not thy face from me, lest I be like unto them that go down into the pit.

8 Cause me to hear thy lovingkindness in the morning; for in thee do I trust: [p]cause me to know the way wherein I should walk; for I lift up my soul unto thee.

9 Deliver me, O LORD, from mine enemies: I [q]flee unto thee to hide me.

10 Teach me to do thy will; for thou *art* my God: [r]thy spirit *is* good; lead me into [s]the land of uprightness.

11 Quicken me, O LORD, for thy name's sake: for thy righteousness' sake bring my soul out of trouble.

12 And of thy mercy cut off mine enemies, and destroy all them that afflict my soul: for I *am* thy servant.

PSALM 144.

A Psalm of David.

Blessed *be* the LORD my strength, which teacheth my hands to war, *and* my fingers to fight:

2 My goodness, and my fortress; my

high tower, and my deliverer; my shield,
and *he* in whom I trust; who subdueth
my people under me.
3 LORD, [a]what *is* man, that thou takest
knowledge of him! *or* the son of man,
that thou makest account of him!
4 Man is like to vanity: [b]his days *are* as
a shadow that passeth away.
5 [c]Bow thy heavens, O LORD, and
come down: touch the mountains, and
they shall smoke.
6 Cast forth lightning, and scatter
them: shoot out thine arrows, and
destroy them.
7 Send thine hand from above; rid me,
and deliver me out of great waters,
[d]from the hand of strange children;
8 Whose mouth speaketh vanity, and
their right hand *is* a right hand of falsehood.
9 I will sing [e]a new song unto thee, O
God: upon a psaltery *and* an instrument
of ten strings will I sing praises unto
thee.
10 *It is he* that giveth salvation unto
kings: who delivereth David his servant
from the hurtful sword.
11 Rid me, and deliver me from the
hand of strange children, whose mouth
speaketh vanity, and their right hand *is* a
right hand of falsehood:
12 That our sons *may be* as plants
grown up in their youth; *that* our daughters *may be* as corner stones, polished
after the similitude of a palace:
13 *That* our garners *may be* full, affording all manner of store: *that* our sheep
may bring forth thousands and ten thousands in our streets:
14 *That* our oxen *may be* strong to
labour; *that there be* no breaking in, nor
going out; that *there be* no complaining
in our streets.
15 [f]Happy *is that* people, that is in
such a case: *yea,* happy *is that* people,
whose God *is* the LORD.

PSALM 145.

David's *Psalm* of praise.

I will extol thee, my God, O king; and I
will bless thy name for ever and ever.
2 Every day will I bless thee; and I will
praise thy name for ever and ever.
3 [g]Great *is* the LORD, and greatly to be
praised; and [h]his greatness *is* unsearchable.

a Psa. 8:4; Job 7:17; Heb. 2:6.
b Job 8:9; Psa. 102:11.
c Psa. 18:9; Isa. 64:1.
d Psa. 54:3; Mal. 2:11.
e Psa. 33:2, 3; 40:3.
f Deut. 33:29; Psa. 33:12; 65:4; 146:5.
g Psa. 96:4; 147:5.
h Job 5:9; 9:10; Rom. 11:33.
i Psa. 86:5, 15; 103:8; Ex. 34:6, 7; Num. 14:18.
j Psa. 100:5; Nah. 1:7.
k Psa. 146:10; 1 Tim. 1:17.
l Heb. *a kingdom of all ages.*
m Deut. 4:7.
n John 4:24.
o Psa. 19:9, *note.*
p Psa. 31:23; 97:10.
q Psa. 103:1.
r Psa. 2:12, *note.*

4 One generation shall praise thy
works to another, and shall declare thy
mighty acts.
5 I will speak of the glorious honour of
thy majesty, and of thy wondrous works.
6 And *men* shall speak of the might of
thy terrible acts: and I will declare thy
greatness.
7 They shall abundantly utter the
memory of thy great goodness, and shall
sing of thy righteousness.
8 The LORD [i]*is* gracious, and full of compassion; slow to anger, and of great mercy.
9 The LORD [j]*is* good to all: and his tender mercies *are* over all his works.
10 All thy works shall praise thee, O
LORD; and thy saints shall bless thee.
11 They shall speak of the glory of thy
kingdom, and talk of thy power;
12 To make known to the sons of men
his mighty acts, and the glorious majesty
of his kingdom.
13 [k]Thy kingdom *is* an [l]everlasting
kingdom, and thy dominion *endureth*
throughout all generations.
14 The LORD upholdeth all that fall,
and raiseth up all *those that be* bowed
down.
15 The eyes of all wait upon thee; and
thou givest them their meat in due season.
16 Thou openest thine hand, and satis-
fiest the desire of every living thing.
17 The LORD *is* righteous in all his
ways, and holy in all his works.
18 The LORD [m]*is* nigh unto all them
that call upon him, to all that call upon
him [n]in truth.
19 He will fulfil the desire of them that
[o]fear him: he also will hear their cry, and
will save them.
20 The LORD [p]preserveth all them that
love him: but all the wicked will he
destroy.
21 My mouth shall speak the praise of
the LORD: and let all flesh bless his holy
name for ever and ever.

PSALM 146.

Praise ye the LORD. [q]Praise the LORD,
O my soul.
2 While I live will I praise the LORD: I
will sing praises unto my God while I
have any being.
3 Put not your [r]trust in princes,

nor in the son of man, in whom *there is* no help.

4 His breath goeth forth, he returneth to his earth; in that very day [a]his thoughts perish.

5 [b]Happy *is he* that *hath* the God of Jacob for his help, whose hope *is* in the LORD his God:

6 [c]Which made heaven, and earth, the sea, and all that therein *is*: which keepeth truth for ever:

7 Which executeth judgment for the oppressed: [d]which giveth food to the hungry. [e]The LORD looseth the prisoners:

8 [f]The LORD openeth *the eyes of* the blind: the LORD [g]raiseth them that are bowed down: the LORD loveth the righteous:

9 The LORD [h]preserveth the strangers; he relieveth the fatherless and widow: [i]but the way of the wicked he turneth upside down.

10 The LORD [j]shall reign for ever, *even* thy God, O Zion, unto all generations. Praise ye the LORD.

PSALM 147.

Praise ye the LORD: for *it is* good to sing praises unto our God; for *it is* pleasant; *and* praise is comely.

2 The LORD doth build up Jerusalem: [k]he gathereth together the outcasts of Israel.

3 He [l]healeth the broken in heart, and bindeth up their [m]wounds.

4 He [n]telleth the number of the stars; he calleth them all by *their* names.

5 Great *is* our Lord, and of great power: [o]his understanding *is* infinite.

6 The LORD [p]lifteth up the meek: he casteth the wicked down to the ground.

7 Sing unto the LORD with thanksgiving; sing praise upon the harp unto our God:

8 [q]Who covereth the heaven with clouds, who prepareth rain for the earth, who maketh grass to grow upon the mountains.

9 He [r]giveth to the beast his food, *and* to the young ravens which cry.

10 He delighteth not in the strength of the horse: he taketh not pleasure in the legs of a man.

11 The LORD taketh pleasure in them that [s]fear him, in those that hope in his mercy.

12 Praise the LORD, O Jerusalem; praise thy God, O Zion.

13 For he hath strengthened the bars of thy gates; he hath blessed thy children within thee.

14 He maketh peace *in* thy borders, *and* filleth thee with the finest of the wheat.

15 He sendeth forth his commandment *upon* earth: his word runneth very swiftly.

16 He giveth snow like wool: he scattereth the hoarfrost like ashes.

17 He casteth forth his ice like morsels: who can stand before his cold?

18 He sendeth out his word, and melteth them: he causeth his wind to blow, *and* the waters flow.

19 [t]He sheweth his word unto Jacob, [u]his statutes and his judgments unto Israel.

20 [v]He hath not dealt so with any nation: and *as for his* judgments, they have not known them. Praise ye the LORD.

PSALM 148.

Praise ye the LORD. Praise ye the LORD from the heavens: praise him in the heights.

2 Praise ye him, all his [w]angels: praise ye him, all his hosts.

3 Praise ye him, sun and moon: praise him, all ye stars of light.

4 Praise him, ye heavens of heavens, and ye waters that *be* above the heavens.

5 Let them praise the name of the LORD: for he commanded, and they were created.

6 He hath also stablished them for ever and ever: he hath made a decree which shall not pass.

7 Praise the LORD from the earth, [x]ye dragons, and all deeps:

8 Fire, and hail; snow, and vapour; stormy wind fulfilling his word:

9 Mountains, and all hills; fruitful trees, and all cedars:

10 Beasts, and all cattle; creeping things, and flying fowl:

11 Kings of the earth, and all people; princes, and all judges of the earth:

12 Both young men, and maidens; old men, and children:

13 Let them praise the name of the LORD: for [y]his name alone is [z]excellent; his glory *is* above the earth and heaven.

14 [aa]He also exalteth the horn of his people, [bb]the praise of all his saints; *even* of the children of Israel, a [cc]people near unto him. Praise ye the LORD.

a See 1 Cor. 2:6.
b Psa. 144:15; Jer. 17:7.
c Gen. 1:1; Acts 4:24; Rev. 14:7.
d Psa. 107:9.
e Psa. 68:6; 107:10, 14.
f Mt. 9:30; John 9:7, 32.
g Psa. 145:14; 147:6; Lk. 13:13.
h Psa. 68:5; Deut. 10:18.
i Psa. 147:6.
j Psa. 10:16; 145:13; Ex. 15:18; Rev. 11:15.
k Deut. 30:3.
l Psa. 51:17; Isa. 57:15; 61:1; Lk. 4:18.
m Heb. *griefs.*
n Gen. 15:5; Isa. 40:26.
o Isa. 40:28.
p Psa. 146:8, 9.
q Psa. 104:13, 14; Job 38:26, 27.
r Psa. 104:27, 28; 136:25; 145:15; Job 38:41.
s Psa. 19:9, *note.*
t Psa. 76:1; 78:5; 103:7; Deut. 33:2-4.
u Mal. 4:4.
v See Deut. 4:32-34; Rom. 3:1, 2.
w Heb. 1:4, *note.*
x Isa. 43:20.
y Psa. 8:1.
z Heb. *exalted.*
aa Psa. 75:10.
bb Psa. 149:9.
cc Eph. 2:17.

PSALM 149.

Praise ye the LORD. Sing unto the LORD
a new song, *and* his praise in the
congregation of saints.
2 Let Israel rejoice in him that made
him: let the children of Zion be joyful in
their [a]King.
3 Let them praise his name in the
dance: let them sing praises unto him
with the timbrel and harp.
4 For the LORD [b]taketh pleasure in his
people: [c]he will beautify the meek with
salvation.
5 Let the saints be joyful in glory: let
them [d]sing aloud upon their beds.
6 *Let* the high *praises* of God *be* [e]in
their mouth, and [f]a twoedged sword in
their hand;
7 To execute vengeance upon the [g]hea-
then, *and* punishments upon the people;
8 To bind their kings with chains, and
their nobles with fetters of iron;
9 To [h]execute upon them the judgment
written: [i]this honour have all his saints.
Praise ye the LORD.

PSALM 150.

Praise ye the LORD. Praise God in his
sanctuary: praise him in the firmament of his power.
2 [j]Praise him for his mighty acts:
praise him according to his excellent
[k]greatness.
3 Praise him with the sound of the
trumpet: praise him with the psaltery
and harp.
4 Praise him with the timbrel and
dance: praise him with stringed instruments and organs.
5 Praise him upon the loud cymbals:
praise him upon the high sounding cymbals.
6 Let every thing that hath breath
praise the LORD. Praise ye the LORD.

a Zech. 9:9; Mt. 21:5.
b Psa. 35:27.
c Psa. 132:16.
d Job 35:10.
e Heb. *in their throat.*
f Heb. 4:12; Rev. 1:16.
g i.e. *nations.*
h Deut. 7:1, 2.
i Psa. 148:14.
j Psa. 145:5, 6.
k Deut. 3:24.

THE PROVERBS

THIS collection of sentientious sayings is divine wisdom applied to the earthly conditions of the people of God. That the Proverbs were Solomon's (1:1) implies no more than that he gathered into orderly arrangement sayings already current amongst the people, the wisdom of the Spirit, perhaps through many centuries (Eccl. 12:9). Chapters 25–29 were current in Hezekiah's time (25:1). Chapters 30 and 31 are by Agur and Lemuel.

The book is in six parts: I. To sons, 1–7. II. The praise of wisdom, 8–9. III. The folly of sin, 10–19. IV. Warnings and instructions, 20–29. V. The words of Agur, 30. VI. The words of King Lemuel, 31.

CHAPTER 1.

B.C. 1000.

Part I. Instruction and exhortation to sons.

The [a]proverbs of Solomon the son of David, king of Israel;

2 To know wisdom and instruction; to perceive the words of understanding;

3 To receive the instruction of wisdom, justice, and judgment, and equity;

4 To give subtilty to the [b]simple, to the young man knowledge and [c]discretion.

5 [d]A wise *man* will hear, and will increase learning; and a man of understanding shall attain unto wise counsels:

6 To understand a proverb, and the interpretation; the words of the wise, and their [e]dark sayings.

7 The [f]fear of the LORD *is* the beginning of knowledge: *but* fools despise wisdom and instruction.

8 My son, hear the instruction of thy father, and forsake not the law of thy mother:

9 [g]For they *shall be* an [h]ornament of grace unto thy head, and chains about thy neck.

10 My son, if sinners entice thee, [i]consent thou not.

11 If they say, Come with us, let us lay wait for blood, let us lurk privily for the innocent without cause:

12 Let us swallow them up alive as the [j]grave; and whole, [k]as those that go down into the pit:

13 We shall find all precious substance, we shall fill our houses with spoil:

14 Cast in thy lot among us; let us all have one purse:

15 My son, walk not thou in the way with them; refrain thy foot from their path:

16 [l]For their feet run to evil, and make haste to shed blood.

17 Surely in vain the net is spread in the sight of any bird.

18 And they lay wait for their *own* blood; they lurk privily for their *own* lives.

19 [m]So *are* the ways of every one that is greedy of gain; *which* taketh away the life of the owners thereof.

20 [n]Wisdom crieth without; she uttereth her voice in the streets:

21 She crieth in the chief place of concourse, in the openings of the gates: in the city she uttereth her words, *saying*,

22 How long, ye simple ones, will ye love simplicity? and the scorners delight in their scorning, and fools hate knowledge?

23 Turn you at my reproof: behold, [o]I will pour out my spirit unto you, I will make known my words unto you.

24 [p]Because I have called, and ye refused; I have stretched out my hand, and no man regarded;

25 But ye have set at nought all my counsel, and would none of my reproof:

26 I also will laugh at your calamity; I will mock when your fear cometh;

27 When your fear cometh as desolation, and your destruction cometh as a whirlwind; when distress and anguish cometh upon you.

28 [q]Then shall they call upon me, but I will not answer; they shall seek me early, but they shall not find me:

29 For that they hated knowledge, and did not choose the fear of the LORD:

a Prov. 10:1; 25:1; 1 Ki. 4:32; Eccl. 12:9.
b Prov. 9:4.
c Or, *advisment.*
d Prov. 9:9.
e Psa. 78:2.
f Also v. 29. Psa. 19:9, *note.*
g Prov. 3:22.
h Heb. *an adding.*
i Gen. 39:7-8; Psa. 1:1; Eph. 5:11.
j Heb. *Sheol.* See Hab. 2:5, *note.*
k Psa. 28:1; 143:7.
l Isa. 59:7; Rom. 3:15.
m Prov. 15:27; 1 Tim. 6:10.
n Prov. 8:1; 9:3; John 7:37.
o Joel 2:28.
p Isa. 65:12; 66:4; Jer. 7:13; Zech. 7:11.
q Job 27:9; 35:12; Isa. 1:15; Jer. 11:11; 14:12; Ezk. 8:18; Mic. 3:4; Zech. 7:13; Jas. 4:3.

30 They would none of my counsel: they despised all my reproof.
31 Therefore shall they eat of the fruit of their own way, and be filled with their own devices.
32 For the turning away of the simple shall slay them, and the prosperity of fools shall destroy them.
33 But whoso hearkeneth unto me shall dwell safely, and [a]shall be quiet from fear of evil.

CHAPTER 2.

(*To sons*, continued.)

My son, if thou wilt receive my words, and [b]hide my commandments with thee;
2 So that thou incline thine ear unto wisdom, *and* apply thine heart to understanding;
3 Yea, if thou criest after knowledge, *and* liftest up thy voice for understanding;
4 If thou seekest her as silver, and searchest for her as *for* hid treasures;
5 Then shalt thou understand the [c]fear of the LORD, and find the knowledge of God.
6 For the LORD giveth wisdom: out of his mouth *cometh* knowledge and understanding.
7 He layeth up sound wisdom for the righteous: [d]*he is* a buckler to them that walk uprightly.
8 He keepeth the paths of judgment, and [e]preserveth the way of his saints.
9 Then shalt thou understand righteousness, and judgment, and equity; *yea*, every good path.
10 When wisdom entereth into thine heart, and knowledge is pleasant unto thy soul;
11 Discretion shall preserve thee, understanding shall keep thee:
12 To deliver thee from the way of the evil *man*, from the man that speaketh froward things;
13 Who leave the paths of uprightness, to walk in the ways of darkness;
14 [f]Who rejoice to do evil, *and* delight in the frowardness of the wicked;
15 Whose ways *are* crooked, and *they* froward in their paths:
16 To deliver thee from the strange woman, *even* from the stranger *which* flattereth with her words;
17 Which forsaketh the guide of her youth, and forgetteth the covenant of her God.

B.C. 1000.

a Psa. 112:7.
b Prov. 4:21; 7:1.
c Also Prov. 3:7; Psa. 19:9, *note.*
d Prov. 30:5; Psa. 84:11.
e 1 Sam. 2:9; Psa. 66:9.
f Prov. 10:23; Jer. 11:15; Rom. 1:32.
g See 1 Ki. 8:61, *note.*
h Prov. 6:21; 7:3; Ex. 13:9; Deut. 6.8.
i Jer. 17:1; 2 Cor. 3:3.
j Psa. 2:12, *note.*
k Jer. 9:23.
l 1 Chr. 28:9.
m Heb. *medicine.*
n Ex. 22:29; 23:19; 34:26; Deut. 26:2; Mal. 3:10; Lk. 14:13.
o Deut. 28:8.
p vs. 11, 12; Job 5:17; Psa. 94:12; Heb. 12:5, 6; Rev. 3:19.
q Job 28:13

18 For her house inclineth unto death, and her paths unto the dead.
19 None that go unto her return again, neither take they hold of the paths of life.
20 That thou mayest walk in the way of good *men*, and keep the paths of the righteous.
21 For the upright shall dwell in the land, and the [g]perfect shall remain in it.
22 But the wicked shall be cut off from the earth, and the transgressors shall be rooted out of it.

CHAPTER 3.

(*To sons*, continued.)

My son, forget not my law; but let thine heart keep my commandments:
2 For length of days, and long life, and peace, shall they add to thee.
3 Let not mercy and truth forsake thee: [h]bind them about thy neck; [i]write them upon the table of thine heart:
4 So shalt thou find favour and good understanding in the sight of God and man.
5 [j]Trust in the LORD with all thine heart; and [k]lean not unto thine own understanding.
6 [l]In all thy ways acknowledge him, and he shall direct thy paths.
7 Be not wise in thine own eyes: fear the LORD, and depart from evil.
8 It shall be [m]health to thy navel, and marrow to thy bones.
9 [n]Honour the LORD with thy substance, and with the firstfruits of all thine increase:
10 [o]So shall thy barns be filled with plenty, and thy presses shall burst out with new wine.
11 [p]My son, despise not the chastening of the LORD; neither be weary of his correction:
12 For whom the LORD loveth he correcteth; even as a father the son *in whom* he delighteth.
13 Happy *is* the man *that* findeth wisdom, and the man *that* getteth understanding.
14 For the merchandise of it *is* better than the merchandise of silver, and the gain thereof than fine gold.
15 [q]She *is* more precious than rubies: and all the things thou canst desire are not to be compared unto her.
16 Length of days *is* in her right

hand; [a]*and* in her left hand riches and honour.

17 Her ways *are* ways of pleasantness, and all her paths *are* peace.

18 She *is* a tree of life to them that lay hold upon her: and happy *is every one* that retaineth her.

19 The LORD by wisdom hath founded the earth; by understanding hath he established the heavens.

20 By his knowledge the depths are broken up, and the clouds drop down the dew.

21 My son, let not them depart from thine eyes: keep sound wisdom and discretion:

22 So shall they be life unto thy soul, and grace to thy neck.

23 [b]Then shalt thou walk in thy way safely, and thy foot shall not stumble.

24 When thou liest down, thou shalt not be afraid: yea, thou shalt lie down, and thy sleep shall be sweet.

25 Be not afraid of sudden fear, neither of the desolation of the wicked, when it cometh.

26 For the LORD shall be thy confidence, and shall keep thy foot from being taken.

27 [c]Withhold not good from them to whom it is due, when it is in the power of thine hand to do *it*.

28 [d]Say not unto thy neighbour, Go, and come again, and to morrow I will give; when thou hast it by thee.

29 Devise not evil against thy neighbour, seeing he dwelleth securely by thee.

30 [e]Strive not with a man without cause, if he have done thee no harm.

31 [f]Envy thou not the [g]oppressor, and choose none of his ways.

32 For the froward *is* abomination to the LORD: [h]but his secret *is* with the righteous.

33 The [i]curse of the LORD *is* in the house of the wicked: [j]but he blesseth the habitation of the just.

34 Surely he scorneth the scorners: but he giveth [k]grace unto the lowly.

35 The wise shall inherit glory: but shame shall be the promotion of fools.

CHAPTER 4.

(*To sons,* continued.)

Hear, [l]ye children, the instruction of a father, and attend to know understanding.

2 For I give you good doctrine, forsake ye not my law.

3 For I was my father's son, tender and only *beloved* in the sight of my mother.

4 [m]He taught me also, and said unto me, Let thine heart retain my words: keep my commandments, and live.

5 Get wisdom, get understanding: forget *it* not; neither decline from the words of my mouth.

6 Forsake her not, and she shall preserve thee: [n]love her, and she shall keep thee.

7 [o]Wisdom *is* the principal thing; *therefore* get wisdom: and with all thy getting get understanding.

8 [p]Exalt her, and she shall promote thee: she shall bring thee to honour, when thou dost embrace her.

9 She shall give to thine head an ornament of grace: [q]a crown of glory shall she deliver to thee.

10 Hear, O my son, and receive my sayings; and the years of thy life shall be many.

11 I have taught thee in the way of wisdom; I have led thee in right paths.

12 When thou goest, thy steps shall not be straitened; and when thou runnest, thou shalt not stumble.

13 Take fast hold of instruction; let *her* not go: keep her; for she *is* thy life.

14 Enter not into the path of the wicked, and go not in the way of evil *men*.

15 Avoid it, pass not by it, turn from it, and pass away.

16 For they sleep not, except they have done mischief; and their sleep is taken away, unless they cause *some* to fall.

17 For they eat the bread of wickedness, and drink the wine of violence.

18 [r]But the path of the just [s]*is* as the shining light, that shineth more and more unto the perfect day.

19 [t]The way of the wicked *is* as darkness: they know not at what they stumble.

20 My son, attend to my words; incline thine ear unto my sayings.

21 Let them not depart from thine eyes; keep them in the midst of thine heart.

22 For they *are* life unto those that find them, and health to all their flesh.

23 Keep thy heart with all diligence

B.C. 1000.

a Prov. 8:18; 1 Tim. 4:8.
b Prov. 10:9; Psa. 37:24; 91:11, 12.
c Rom. 13:7; Gal. 6:10.
d Lev. 19:13; Deut. 24:15.
e Rom. 12:18.
f Prov. 24:1; Psa. 37:1; 73:3.
g Heb. *a man of violence.*
h Psa. 25:14; cf. Dan. 2:19.
i Lev. 26:14; Psa. 37:22; Zech. 5:4; Mal. 2:2.
j Psa. 1:3.
k Jas. 4:6; 1 Pet. 5:5.
l Prov. 1:8; Psa. 34:11.
m 1 Chr. 28:9; Eph. 6:4.
n 2 Thes. 2:10.
o Prov. 3:13, 14.
p 1 Sam. 2:30.
q Or, *she shall compass thee with a crown of glory.*
r Mt. 5:14; Phil. 2:15.
s 2 Sam. 23:4.
t 1 Sam. 2:9; Job 18:5, 6; Isa. 59:9, 10; Jer. 23:12; John 12:35.

for out of it *are* the issues of life.

24 Put away from thee a froward mouth, and perverse lips put far from thee.

25 Let thine eyes look right on, and let thine eyelids look straight before thee.

26 Ponder the path of thy feet, and [a]let all thy ways be established.

27 Turn not to the right hand nor to the left: remove thy foot from evil.

CHAPTER 5.

(*To sons*, continued.)

My son, attend unto my wisdom, *and* bow thine ear to my understanding:

2 That thou mayest regard discretion, and *that* thy lips [b]may keep knowledge.

3 For the lips of a strange woman drop *as* an honeycomb, and her mouth *is* [c]smoother than oil:

4 But her end is [d]bitter as wormwood, sharp as a twoedged sword.

5 Her feet go down to death; [e]her steps take hold on [f]hell.

6 Lest thou shouldest ponder the path of life, her ways are moveable, *that* thou canst not know *them*.

7 Hear me now therefore, O ye children, and depart not from the words of my mouth.

8 Remove thy way far from her, and come not nigh the door of her house:

9 Lest thou give thine honour unto others, and thy years unto the cruel:

10 Lest strangers be filled with [g]thy wealth; and thy labours *be* in the house of a stranger;

11 And thou mourn at the last, when thy flesh and thy body are consumed,

12 And say, How have I hated instruction, and my heart despised reproof;

13 And have not obeyed the voice of my teachers, nor inclined mine ear to them that instructed me!

14 I was almost in all evil in the midst of the congregation and assembly.

15 Drink waters out of thine own cistern, and running waters out of thine own well.

16 Let thy fountains be dispersed abroad, *and* rivers of waters in the streets.

17 Let them be only thine own, and not strangers' with thee.

18 Let thy fountain be blessed: and rejoice [h]with the wife of thy youth.

B.C. 1000.

a Or, *all thy ways shall be ordered aright.*
b Mal. 2.7.
c Psa. 55:21.
d Eccl. 7:26.
e Prov. 7:27.
f Heb. *Sheol.* See Hab. 2:5, *note.*
g Heb. *thy strength.*
h Mal. 2:14.
i Song 2:9; 4:5; 7:3.
j Heb. *err thou always in her love.*
k Prov. 15:3; 2 Chr. 16:9; Job 31:4; 34:21; Jer. 16:17; 32:19; Hos. 7:2; Heb. 4:13.
l Or, *so shalt thou prevail with thy friend.*
m Job 12:7.
n Prov. 24:33, 34.
o Prov. 10:4; 13:4; 20:4.
p Heb. *casteth forth.*

19 [i]*Let her be as* the loving hind and pleasant roe; let her breasts satisfy thee at all times; and [j]be thou ravished always with her love.

20 And why wilt thou, my son, be ravished with a strange woman, and embrace the bosom of a stranger?

21 [k]For the ways of man *are* before the eyes of the LORD, and he pondereth all his goings.

22 His own iniquities shall take the wicked himself, and he shall be holden with the cords of his sins.

23 He shall die without instruction; and in the greatness of his folly he shall go astray.

CHAPTER 6.

(*To sons*, continued.)

My son, if thou be surety for thy friend, *if* thou hast stricken thy hand with a stranger,

2 Thou art snared with the words of thy mouth, thou art taken with the words of thy mouth.

3 Do this now, my son, and deliver thyself, when thou art come into the hand of thy friend; go, humble thyself, and [l]make sure thy friend.

4 Give not sleep to thine eyes, nor slumber to thine eyelids.

5 Deliver thyself as a roe from the hand *of the hunter*, and as a bird from the hand of the fowler.

6 [m]Go to the ant, thou sluggard; consider her ways, and be wise:

7 Which having no guide, overseer, or ruler,

8 Provideth her meat in the summer, *and* gathereth her food in the harvest.

9 [n]How long wilt thou sleep, O sluggard? when wilt thou arise out of thy sleep?

10 *Yet* a little sleep, a little slumber, a little folding of the hands to sleep:

11 [o]So shall thy poverty come as one that travelleth, and thy want as an armed man.

12 A naughty person, a wicked man, walketh with a froward mouth.

13 He winketh with his eyes, he speaketh with his feet, he teacheth with his fingers;

14 Frowardness *is* in his heart, he deviseth mischief continually; he [p]soweth discord.

15 Therefore shall his calamity come suddenly; suddenly shall he be broken without remedy.

16 These six *things* doth the LORD hate: yea, seven *are* an abomination unto him:

17 A proud look, [a]a lying tongue, and hands that shed innocent blood,

18 An heart that deviseth wicked imaginations, [b]feet that be swift in running to mischief,

19 [c]A false witness *that* speaketh lies, and he that soweth discord among brethren.

20 My son, [d]keep thy father's commandment, and forsake not the law of thy mother:

21 [e]Bind them continually upon thine heart, *and* tie them about thy neck.

22 [f]When thou goest, it shall lead thee; when thou sleepest, it shall keep thee; and *when* thou awakest, it shall talk with thee.

23 [g]For the commandment *is* a lamp; and the law *is* light; and reproofs of instruction *are* the way of life:

24 To keep thee from the evil woman, from the flattery of the tongue of a strange woman.

25 [h]Lust not after her beauty in thine heart; neither let her take thee with her eyelids.

26 For by means of a whorish woman *a man is brought* to a piece of bread: and the adulteress will [i]hunt for the precious life.

27 Can a man take fire in his bosom, and his clothes not be burned?

28 Can one go upon hot coals, and his feet not be burned?

29 So he that goeth in to his neighbour's wife; whosoever toucheth her shall not be innocent.

30 *Men* do not despise a thief, if he steal to satisfy his soul when he is hungry;

31 But *if* he be found, [j]he shall restore sevenfold; he shall give all the substance of his house.

32 *But* whoso committeth adultery with a woman lacketh understanding: he *that* doeth it destroyeth his own soul.

33 A wound and dishonour shall he get; and his reproach shall not be wiped away.

34 For jealousy *is* the rage of a man: therefore he will not spare in the day of vengeance.

35 He will not regard any ransom; neither will he rest content, though thou givest many gifts.

B.C. 1000.

a Psa. 120:2, 3; cf. Acts 5:1-10.

b Isa. 59:7; Rom. 3:15.

c Prov. 19:5, 9; Psa. 27:12.

d Prov. 1:8; Eph. 6:1.

e Prov. 3:3; 7:3.

f Prov. 3:23, 24.

g Psa. 19:8; 119:105.

h Mt. 5:28.

i Ezk. 13:18.

j Ex. 22:1, 4.

k Prov. 4:4; Lev. 18:5; Isa. 55:3.

l Deut. 6:8.

m Job 24:15.

n I Tim. 5:13; Tit. 2:5.

o Psa. 12:2.

p Heb. *suddenly*.

CHAPTER 7.

(*To sons*, concluded.)

My son, keep my words, and lay up my commandments with thee.

2 [k]Keep my commandments, and live; and my law as the apple of thine eye.

3 [l]Bind them upon thy fingers, write them upon the table of thine heart.

4 Say unto wisdom, Thou *art* my sister; and call understanding *thy* kinswoman:

5 That they may keep thee from the strange woman, from the stranger *which* flattereth with her words.

6 For at the window of my house I looked through my casement,

7 And beheld among the simple ones, I discerned among the youths, a young man void of understanding,

8 Passing through the street near her corner; and he went the way to her house,

9 [m]In the twilight, in the evening, in the black and dark night:

10 And, behold, there met him a woman *with* the attire of an harlot, and subtil of heart.

11 (She *is* loud and stubborn; [n]her feet abide not in her house:

12 Now *is she* without, now in the streets, and lieth in wait at every corner.)

13 So she caught him, and kissed him, *and* with an impudent face said unto him,

14 *I have* peace-offerings with me; this day have I payed my vows.

15 Therefore came I forth to meet thee, diligently to seek thy face, and I have found thee.

16 I have decked my bed with coverings of tapestry, with carved *works*, with fine linen of Egypt.

17 I have perfumed my bed with myrrh, aloes, and cinnamon.

18 Come, let us take our fill of love until the morning: let us solace ourselves with loves.

19 For the goodman *is* not at home, he is gone a long journey:

20 He hath taken a bag of money with him, *and* will come home at the day appointed.

21 With her much fair speech she caused him to yield, [o]with the flattering of her lips she forced him.

22 He goeth after her [p]straightway, as an ox goeth to the slaughter, or as a fool to the correction of the stocks;

B.C. 1000.

23 Till a dart strike through his liver; [a]as a bird hasteth to the snare, and knoweth not that it *is* for his life.

24 Hearken unto me now therefore, O ye children, and attend to the words of my mouth.

25 Let not thine heart decline to her ways, go not astray in her paths.

26 For she hath cast down many wounded: yea, [b]many strong *men* have been slain by her.

27 Her house *is* the way to [c]hell, going down to the chambers of death.

CHAPTER 8.

Part II. In praise of wisdom.

Doth not wisdom cry? and understanding put forth her voice?

2 She standeth in the top of high places, by the way in the places of the paths.

3 She crieth at the gates, at the entry of the city, at the coming in at the doors.

4 Unto you, O men, I call; and my voice *is* to the sons of man.

5 O ye simple, understand wisdom: and, ye fools, be ye of an understanding heart.

6 Hear; for I will speak of excellent things; and the opening of my lips *shall be* right things.

7 For my mouth shall speak truth; and wickedness *is* [d]an abomination to my lips.

8 All the words of my mouth *are* in righteousness; *there is* nothing froward or perverse in them.

9 They *are* all plain to him that understandeth, and right to them that find knowledge.

10 Receive my instruction, and not silver; and knowledge rather than choice gold.

11 [e]For wisdom *is* better than rubies; and all the things that may be desired are not to be compared to it.

12 I wisdom dwell with prudence, and find out knowledge of witty inventions.

13 [f]The fear of the LORD *is* to hate evil: pride, and arrogancy, and the evil way, and the froward mouth, do I hate.

14 Counsel *is* mine, and sound wisdom: I *am* understanding; I have strength.

15 [g]By me kings reign, and princes decree justice.

16 By me princes rule, and nobles, *even* all the judges of the earth.

17 [h]I love them that love me; and [i]those that seek me early shall find me.

18 [j]Riches and honour *are* with me; *yea*, durable riches and righteousness.

19 My fruit *is* better than gold, yea, than fine gold; and my revenue than choice silver.

20 I lead in the way of righteousness, in the midst of the paths of judgment:

21 That I may cause those that love me to inherit substance; and I will fill their treasures.

22 [k]The LORD possessed [1]me in the beginning of his way, before his works of old.

23 [l]I was set up from everlasting, from the beginning, or ever the earth was.

24 When *there were* no depths, I was brought forth; when *there were* no fountains abounding with water.

25 [m]Before the mountains were settled, before the hills was I brought forth:

26 While as yet he had not made the earth, nor the fields, nor the highest part of the dust of the world.

27 When he prepared the heavens, I *was* there: when he set a compass upon the face of the depth:

28 When he established the clouds above: when he strengthened the fountains of the deep:

29 [n]When he gave to the sea his decree, that the waters should not pass his commandment: [o]when he appointed the foundations of the earth:

30 [p]Then I was by him, *as* one brought up *with him*: [q]and I was daily *his* delight, rejoicing always before him;

31 Rejoicing in the habitable part of his earth; and [r]my delights *were* with the sons of men.

32 Now therefore hearken unto me, O ye children: for [s]blessed *are they that* keep my ways.

33 Hear instruction, and be wise, and refuse it not.

34 Blessed *is* the man that heareth me, watching daily at my gates, waiting at the posts of my doors.

a Eccl. 9:12.
b Neh. 13:26.
c Heb. *Sheol.* See Hab. 2:5, *note.*
d Heb. *the abomination of my lips.* Prov. 3:14, 15; 4:5, 7; 16:16.
e Job 28:15; Psa. 19:10; 119:127.
f Psa. 19:9, *note.*
g Dan. 2:21; Rom. 13:1.
h 1 Sam. 2:30; Psa. 91:14; John 14:21.
i Jas. 1:5.
j Prov. 3:16; Mt. 6:33.
k Prov. 3:19; John 1:1.
l Psa. 2:6.
m Job 15:7, 8.
n Gen. 1:9, 10; Job 38:10, 11; Psa. 33:7; 104:9; Jer. 5:22.
o Job 38:4.
p John 1:1, 2, 18.
q Mt. 3:17; Col. 1:13.
r Psa. 16:3.
s Psa. 119:1, 2; 128:1, 2; Lk. 11:28.

[1] **(8:22)** That wisdom is more than the personification of an attribute of God, or of the will of God as best for man, but is a distinct adumbration of Christ, is sure to the devout mind. Prov. 8:22-36, with John 1:1-3; Col. 1:17, can refer to nothing less than the Eternal Son of God.

35 For whoso findeth me findeth life, and shall obtain favour of the LORD.

36 But he that sinneth against me wrongeth his own soul: all they that hate me love death.

CHAPTER 9.

(*The praise of wisdom,* continued.)

Wisdom hath [a]builded her house, she hath hewn out her seven pillars:

2 [b]She hath killed her beasts; she hath mingled her wine; she hath also furnished her table.

3 She hath sent forth her maidens: she crieth upon the highest places of the city,

4 Whoso *is* simple, let him turn in hither: *as for* him that wanteth understanding, she saith to him,

5 [c]Come, eat of my bread, and drink of the wine *which* I have mingled.

6 Forsake the foolish, and live; and go in the way of understanding.

7 He that reproveth a scorner getteth to himself shame: and he that rebuketh a wicked *man getteth* himself a blot.

8 [d]Reprove not a scorner, lest he hate thee: [e]rebuke a wise man, and he will love thee.

9 Give *instruction* to a wise *man,* and he will be yet wiser: teach a just *man,* and he will increase in learning.

10 The [f]fear of the LORD *is* the beginning of wisdom: and the knowledge of the holy *is* understanding.

11 For by me thy days shall be multiplied, and the years of thy life shall be increased.

12 [g]If thou be wise, thou shalt be wise for thyself: but *if* thou scornest, thou alone shalt bear *it.*

13 A foolish woman *is* clamorous: *she is* simple, and knoweth nothing.

14 For she sitteth at the door of her house, on a seat in the high places of the city,

15 To call passengers who go right on their ways:

16 Whoso *is* simple, let him turn in hither: and *as for* him that wanteth understanding, she saith to him,

B.C. 1000.

a Mt. 16:18; Eph. 2:20-22; 1 Pet. 2:5.

b Mt. 22:4.

c v. 2; Song 5:1; Isa. 55:1; John 6:27.

d Mt. 7:6.

e Psa. 141:5.

f Psa. 19:9, *note.*

g Prov. 16:26; Job 35:6, 7.

h Prov. 20:17.

i Prov. 2:18; 7:27.

j Heb. *Sheol.* See Hab. 2:5, *note.*

k Prov. 15:20; 17:21, 25; 19:13; 29:3, 15.

l Psa. 10:14; 34:9, 10; 37:25.

m Prov. 12:24; 13:4; 21:5.

n v. 11; Esth. 7:8.

o Psa. 112:6; Eccl. 8:10.

p Heb. *a fool of lips.*

q 1 Cor. 13:7.

r Prov. 18:11; Job 31:24; Psa. 52:7; 1 Tim. 6:17.

17 [h]Stolen waters are sweet, and bread *eaten* in secret is pleasant.

18 But he knoweth not that the [i]dead *are* there; *and that* her guests *are* in the depths of [j]hell.

CHAPTER 10.

Part III. The folly of wickedness; the wisdom of righteousness.

The proverbs of Solomon. [k]A wise son maketh a glad father: but a [1]foolish son *is* the heaviness of his mother.

2 Treasures of wickedness profit nothing: but righteousness delivereth from death.

3 [l]The LORD will not suffer the soul of the righteous to famish: but he casteth away the substance of the wicked.

4 He becometh poor that dealeth *with* a slack hand: [m]but the hand of the diligent maketh rich.

5 He that gathereth in summer *is* a wise son: *but* he that sleepeth in harvest *is* a son that causeth shame.

6 Blessings *are* upon the head of the just: [n]but violence covereth the mouth of the wicked.

7 [o]The memory of the just *is* blessed: but the name of the wicked shall rot.

8 The wise in heart will receive commandments: but [p]a prating fool shall fall.

9 He that walketh uprightly walketh surely: but he that perverteth his ways shall be known.

10 He that winketh with the eye causeth sorrow: but a prating fool shall fall.

11 The mouth of a righteous *man is* a well of life: but violence covereth the mouth of the wicked.

12 Hatred stirreth up strifes: but [q]love covereth all sins.

13 In the lips of him that hath understanding wisdom is found: but a rod *is* for the back of him that is void of understanding.

14 Wise *men* lay up knowledge: but the mouth of the foolish *is* near destruction.

15 [r]The rich man's wealth *is* his strong

1(10:1) A "fool" in Scripture is never a mentally deficient person, but rather one arrogant and self-sufficient; one who orders his life as if there were no God. See, for illustration, Lk. 12:16-20. The rich man was not mentally deficient, but he was a "fool" because he supposed that his soul could live on the things in the barn, giving no thought to his eternal wellbeing.

city: the destruction of the poor *is* their poverty.

16 The labour of the righteous *tendeth* to life: the fruit of the wicked to sin.

17 He *is in* the way of life that keepeth instruction: but he that refuseth reproof erreth.

18 He that hideth hatred *with* lying lips, and he that uttereth a slander, *is* a fool.

19 In the multitude of words there wanteth not sin: [a]but he that refraineth his lips *is* wise.

20 The tongue of the just *is as* choice silver: the heart of the wicked *is* little worth.

21 The lips of the righteous feed many: but fools die for want of wisdom.

22 [b]The blessing of the LORD, it maketh rich, and he addeth no sorrow with it.

23 *It is* as sport to a fool to do mischief: but a man of understanding hath wisdom.

24 The fear of the wicked, it shall come upon him: [c]but the desire of the righteous shall be granted.

25 As the whirlwind passeth, so *is* the wicked no *more*: [d]but the righteous *is* an everlasting foundation.

26 As vinegar to the teeth, and as smoke to the eyes, so *is* the sluggard to them that send him.

27 [e]The fear of the LORD prolongeth days: but the years of the wicked shall be shortened.

28 The hope of the righteous *shall be* gladness: but the expectation of the wicked shall perish.

29 The way of the LORD *is* strength to the upright: but destruction *shall be* to the workers of iniquity.

30 [f]The righteous shall never be removed: but the wicked shall not inhabit the earth.

31 The mouth of the just bringeth forth wisdom: but the froward tongue shall be cut out.

32 The lips of the righteous know what is acceptable: but the mouth of the wicked *speaketh* frowardness.

CHAPTER 11.

(*The contrast of righteousness and wickedness,* continued.)

[g]A false balance *is* abomination to the LORD: but a just weight *is* his delight.

2 *When* pride cometh, then cometh shame: but with the lowly *is* wisdom.

3 The integrity of the upright shall guide them: but the perverseness of transgressors shall destroy them.

4 [h]Riches profit not in the day of wrath: but righteousness delivereth from death.

5 The righteousness of the [i]perfect shall direct his way: but the wicked shall fall by his own wickedness.

6 The righteousness of the upright shall deliver them: but transgressors shall be taken in *their own* naughtiness.

7 When a wicked man dieth, *his* expectation shall perish: and the hope of unjust *men* perisheth.

8 The righteous is delivered out of trouble, and the wicked cometh in his stead.

9 An hypocrite with *his* mouth destroyeth his neighbour: but through knowledge shall the just be delivered.

10 When it goeth well with the righteous, the city rejoiceth: and when the wicked perish, *there is* shouting.

11 By the blessing of the upright the city is exalted: but it is overthrown by the mouth of the wicked.

12 He that is void of wisdom despiseth his neighbour: but a man of understanding holdeth his peace.

13 A talebearer revealeth secrets: but he that is of a faithful spirit concealeth the matter.

14 Where no counsel *is,* the people fall: but in the multitude of counsellors *there is* safety.

15 He that is surety for a stranger shall smart *for it*: and he that hateth suretiship is sure.

16 A gracious woman retaineth honour: and strong *men* retain riches.

17 The merciful man doeth good to his own soul: but *he that is* cruel troubleth his own flesh.

18 The wicked worketh a deceitful work: but to him [j]that soweth righteousness *shall be* a sure reward.

19 As righteousness *tendeth* to life: so he that pursueth evil *pursueth it* to his own death.

20 They that are of a froward heart *are* abomination to the LORD: but *such as are* upright in *their* way *are* his delight.

21 *Though* hand *join* in hand, the wicked shall not be unpunished:

B.C. 1000.

a Jas. 3:2.

b Gen. 24:35; 26:12; Psa. 37:22.

c Psa. 145:19; Mt. 5:6; 1 John 5:14, 15.

d v. 30; Psa. 15:5; Mt. 7:24, 25.

e Psa. 19:9, *note.*

f Psa. 37:22, 29; 125:1.

g Prov. 16:11; 20:10, 23; Lev. 19:35, 36; Deut. 25:13-16.

h Prov. 10:2; Ezk. 7:19; Zeph. 1:18.

i See 1 Ki. 8:61, *note.*

j Hos. 10:12; Gal. 6:8, 9; Jas. 3:18.

but [a]the seed of the righteous shall be delivered.

22 *As* a jewel of gold in a swine's snout, *so is* a fair woman which is without discretion.

23 The desire of the righteous *is* only good: *but* the expectation of the wicked *is* wrath.

24 There is that scattereth, and yet increaseth; and *there is* that withholdeth more than is meet, but *it tendeth* to poverty.

25 [b]The liberal soul shall be made fat: and he that watereth shall be watered also himself.

26 [c]He that withholdeth corn, the people shall curse him: but blessing *shall be* upon the head of him that selleth *it*.

27 He that diligently seeketh good procureth favour: but he that seeketh mischief, it shall come unto him.

28 He that [d]trusteth in his riches shall fall: but [e]the righteous shall flourish as a branch.

29 He that troubleth his own house shall inherit the wind: and the fool *shall be* servant to the wise of heart.

30 The fruit of the righteous *is* a tree of life; and [f]he that winneth souls *is* wise.

31 Behold, the righteous shall be recompensed in the earth: much more the wicked and the sinner.

CHAPTER 12.

(*The contrast of righteousness and wickedness,* continued.)

Whoso loveth instruction loveth knowledge: but he that hateth reproof *is* brutish.

2 A good *man* obtaineth favour of the LORD: but a man of wicked devices will he condemn.

3 A man shall not be established by wickedness: but the root of the righteous shall not be moved.

4 A [g]virtuous woman *is* a crown to her husband: but she that maketh ashamed *is* as rottenness in his bones.

5 The thoughts of the righteous *are* right: *but* the counsels of the wicked *are* deceit.

6 The words of the wicked *are* to lie in wait for blood: but the mouth of the upright shall deliver them.

7 [h]The wicked are overthrown, and *are* not: but the house of the righteous shall stand.

8 A man shall be commended according to his wisdom: but he that is of a perverse heart shall be despised.

9 *He that is* despised, and hath a servant, *is* better than he that honoureth himself, and lacketh bread.

10 [i]A righteous *man* regardeth the life of his beast: but the tender mercies of the wicked *are* cruel.

11 [j]He that tilleth his land shall be satisfied with bread: but he that followeth vain *persons is* void of understanding.

12 The wicked desireth the net of evil *men*: but the root of the righteous yieldeth *fruit*.

13 The wicked is snared by the transgression of *his* lips: but the just shall come out of trouble.

14 A man shall be satisfied with good by the fruit of *his* mouth: and the recompence of a man's hands shall be rendered unto him.

15 [k]The way of a fool *is* right in his own eyes: but he that hearkeneth unto counsel *is* wise.

16 A fool's wrath is presently known: but a prudent *man* covereth shame.

17 *He that* speaketh truth sheweth forth righteousness: but a false witness deceit.

18 There is that speaketh like the piercings of a sword: but the tongue of the wise *is* health.

19 The lip of truth shall be established for ever: but [l]a lying tongue *is* but for a moment.

20 Deceit *is* in the heart of them that imagine evil: but to the counsellors of peace *is* joy.

21 There shall no evil happen to the just: but the wicked shall be filled with mischief.

22 [m]Lying lips *are* abomination to the LORD: but they that deal truly *are* his delight.

23 A prudent man concealeth knowledge: but the heart of fools proclaimeth foolishness.

24 [n]The hand of the diligent shall bear rule: but the slothful shall be under tribute.

25 [o]Heaviness in the heart of man maketh it stoop: [p]but a good word maketh it glad.

26 The righteous *is* more excellent than his neighbour: but the way of the wicked seduceth them.

27 The slothful *man* roasteth not that which he took in hunting: but the substance of a diligent man *is* precious.

28 In the way of righteousness *is* life; and *in* the pathway *thereof there is* no death.

B.C. 1000.

a Psa. 112:2; Prov. 14:26.

b 2 Cor. 9:6-10.

c Amos 8:5, 6.

d Psa. 2:12, *note.*

e Psa. 1:3; 52:8; 92:12; Jer. 17:8.

f Dan. 12:3; 1 Cor. 9:19; Jas. 5:20.

g Prov. 31:23; 1 Cor. 11:7.

h Psa. 37:36, 37; Prov. 11:21; Mt. 7:24-27.

i Deut. 25:4.

j Gen. 3:19.

k Prov. 3:7; Lk. 18:11.

l Prov. 19:9; Psa. 52:5.

m Prov. 6:17; 11:20; Rev. 22:15.

n Prov. 10:4.

o Prov. 15:13.

p Isa. 50:4.

CHAPTER 13.

(*The contrast of righteousness and wickedness,* continued.)

A wise son *heareth* his father's instruction: but [a]a scorner heareth not rebuke.

2 A man shall eat good by the fruit of *his* mouth: but the soul of the transgressors *shall eat* violence.

3 He that keepeth his mouth keepeth his life: *but* he that openeth wide his lips shall have destruction.

4 [b]The soul of the sluggard desireth, and *hath* nothing: but the soul of the diligent shall be made fat.

5 A righteous *man* hateth lying: but a wicked *man* is loathsome, and cometh to shame.

6 [c]Righteousness keepeth *him that is* upright in the way: but wickedness overthroweth the sinner.

7 [d]There is that maketh himself rich, yet *hath* nothing: *there is* that maketh himself poor, yet *hath* great riches.

8 The ransom of a man's life *are* his riches: but the poor heareth not rebuke.

9 The light of the righteous rejoiceth: [e]but the [f]lamp of the wicked shall be put out.

10 Only by pride cometh contention: but with the well advised *is* wisdom.

11 Wealth *gotten* by vanity shall be diminished: but he that gathereth [g]by labour shall increase.

12 Hope deferred maketh the heart sick: but *when* the desire cometh, *it is* a tree of life.

13 Whoso despiseth the word shall be destroyed: but he that feareth the commandment shall be rewarded.

14 The law of the wise *is* a fountain of life, to depart from the snares of death.

15 Good understanding giveth favour: but the way of transgressors *is* hard.

16 Every prudent *man* dealeth with knowledge: but a fool [h]layeth open *his* folly.

17 A wicked messenger falleth into mischief: but a faithful ambassador *is* health.

18 Poverty and shame *shall be to* him that refuseth instruction: but he that regardeth reproof shall be honoured.

19 The desire accomplished is sweet to the soul: but *it is* abomination to fools to depart from evil.

20 He that walketh with wise *men* shall be wise: but a companion of fools shall be destroyed.

B.C. 1000.

a 1 Sam. 2:25.
b Prov. 10:4.
c Prov. 11.3, 5, 6.
d Prov. 12:9.
e Prov. 24:20; Job 18:5, 6; 21:17.
f Or, *candle.*
g Heb. *with the hand.*
h Heb. *spreadeth.*
i Prov. 28:8; Job 27:16, 17; Eccl. 2:26.
j Prov. 19:18; 22:15; 23:13; 29:15,17.
k Psa. 19:9, *note.*
l Prov. 10:23.
m Heb. *the bitterness of his soul.*
n Rom. 6:21.

21 Evil pursueth sinners: but to the righteous good shall be repayed.

22 A good *man* leaveth an inheritance to his children's children: and the [i]wealth of the sinner *is* laid up for the just.

23 Much food *is in* the tillage of the poor: but there is *that is* destroyed for want of judgment.

24 [j]He that spareth his rod hateth his son: but he that loveth him chasteneth him betimes.

25 The righteous eateth to the satisfying of his soul: but the belly of the wicked shall want.

CHAPTER 14.

(*The contrast of goodness and evil,* continued.)

Every wise woman buildeth her house: but the foolish plucketh it down with her hands.

2 He that walketh in his uprightness [k]feareth the LORD: but *he that is* perverse in his ways despiseth him.

3 In the mouth of the foolish *is* a rod of pride: but the lips of the wise shall preserve them.

4 Where no oxen *are*, the crib *is* clean: but much increase *is* by the strength of the ox.

5 A faithful witness will not lie: but a false witness will utter lies.

6 A scorner seeketh wisdom, and *findeth it* not: but knowledge *is* easy unto him that understandeth.

7 Go from the presence of a foolish man, when thou perceivest not *in him* the lips of knowledge.

8 The wisdom of the prudent *is* to understand his way: but the folly of fools *is* deceit.

9 [l]Fools make a mock at sin: but among the righteous *there is* favour.

10 [m]The heart knoweth his own bitterness; and a stranger doth not intermeddle with his joy.

11 The house of the wicked shall be overthrown: but the tabernacle of the upright shall flourish.

12 There is a way which seemeth right unto a man, but [n]the end thereof *are* the ways of death.

13 Even in laughter the heart is sorrowful; and the end of that mirth *is* heaviness.

14 The backslider in heart shall be

[a]filled with his own ways: and a good man *shall be satisfied* from himself.

15 The simple believeth every word: but the prudent *man* looketh well to his going.

16 A wise *man* feareth, and departeth from evil: but the fool rageth, and is confident.

17 *He that is* soon angry dealeth foolishly: and a man of wicked devices is hated.

18 The simple inherit folly: but the prudent are crowned with knowledge.

19 The evil bow before the good; and the wicked at the gates of the righteous.

20 The poor is hated even of his own neighbour: [b]but the rich *hath* many friends.

21 He that despiseth his neighbour sinneth: but he that hath mercy on the poor, happy *is* he.

22 Do they not err that devise evil? but mercy and truth *shall be* to them that devise good.

23 In all labour there is profit: but the talk of the lips *tendeth* only to penury.

24 The crown of the wise *is* their riches: *but* the foolishness of fools *is* folly.

25 A true witness delivereth souls: but a deceitful *witness* speaketh lies.

26 In the [c]fear of the LORD *is* strong confidence: and his children shall have a place of refuge.

27 The [d]fear of the LORD *is* a fountain of life, to depart from the snares of death.

28 In the multitude of people *is* the king's honour: but in the want of people *is* the destruction of the prince.

29 [e]*He that is* slow to wrath *is* of great understanding: but *he that is* hasty of spirit exalteth folly.

30 A sound heart *is* the life of the flesh: but envy the rottenness of the bones.

31 [f]He that oppresseth the poor reproacheth his Maker: but he that honoureth him hath mercy on the poor.

32 The wicked is driven away in his wickedness: but the righteous hath hope in his death.

33 Wisdom resteth in the heart of him that hath understanding: but *that which is* in the midst of fools is made known.

34 Righteousness exalteth a nation: but sin *is* a reproach to any people.

35 [g]The king's favour *is* toward a wise servant: but his wrath is *against* him that causeth shame.

CHAPTER 15.

(*The contrast of goodness and evil, continued.*)

A [h]soft answer turneth away wrath: [i]but grievous words stir up anger.

2 The tongue of the wise useth knowledge aright: but the mouth of fools [j]poureth out foolishness.

3 [k]The eyes of the LORD *are* in every place, beholding the evil and the good.

4 A wholesome tongue *is* a tree of life: but perverseness therein *is* a breach in the spirit.

5 A fool despiseth his father's instruction: but he that regardeth reproof is prudent.

6 In the house of the righteous *is* much treasure: but in the revenues of the wicked is trouble.

7 The lips of the wise disperse knowledge: but the heart of the foolish *doeth* not so.

8 [l]The sacrifice of the wicked *is* an abomination to the LORD: but the prayer of the upright *is* his delight.

9 The way of the wicked *is* an abomination unto the LORD: but he loveth him that followeth after righteousness.

10 Correction *is* grievous unto him that forsaketh the way: *and* he that hateth reproof shall die.

11 [m]Hell and destruction *are* before the LORD: how much more then the hearts of the children of men?

12 A scorner loveth not one that reproveth him: neither will he go unto the wise.

13 [n]A merry heart maketh a cheerful countenance: but by sorrow of the heart the spirit is broken.

14 The heart of him that hath understanding seeketh knowledge: but the mouth of fools feedeth on foolishness.

15 All the days of the afflicted *are* evil: but he that is of a merry heart *hath* a continual feast.

16 [o]Better *is* little with the fear of the LORD than great treasure and trouble therewith.

17 [p]Better *is* a dinner of herbs where love is, than a stalled ox and hatred therewith.

18 A wrathful man stirreth up strife: but *he that is* slow to anger appeaseth strife.

B.C. 1000.

a Prov. 1:31; 12:14.

b Heb. *many are the lovers of the rich.*

c Also, Prov. 15:16; Psa. 19:9, *note.*

d Prov. 13:14.

e Prov. 16:32; Jas. 1:19.

f Prov. 17:5; Mt. 25:40-45.

g Mt. 24:45, 47.

h Prov. 25:15; Jud. 8:1-3.

i 1 Sam. 25:10; 1 Ki. 12:13-16.

j Heb. *belcheth.*

k Prov. 5:21; Job 34:21; Jer. 16:17; 32:19; Heb. 4:13.

l Prov. 21:27; 28:9; Isa. 1:11; 61:8; 66:3; Jer. 6:20; 7:22; Amos 5:22.

m Heb. *Sheol.* See Hab. 2:5, *note.* Job 26:6; Psa. 139:8.

n Prov. 17:22.

o Prov. 16:8; Psa. 37:16; 1 Tim. 6:6.

p Prov. 17:1.

19 The way of the slothful *man is* as an
hedge of thorns: but the way of the
righteous *is* made plain.
20 A wise son maketh a glad father:
but a foolish man despiseth his mother.
21 Folly *is* joy to *him that is* destitute of
wisdom: [a]but a man of understanding
walketh uprightly.
22 Without counsel purposes are disappointed: but in the multitude of counsellors they are established.
23 A man hath joy by the answer of his
mouth: and a word *spoken* in due season,
how good *is it*!
24 [b]The way of life *is* above to the
wise, that he may depart from [c]hell
beneath.
25 The LORD will destroy the house of
the proud: but he will establish the border of the widow.
26 The thoughts of the wicked *are* an
abomination to the LORD: but *the words*
of the pure *are* pleasant words.
27 [d]He that is greedy of gain troubleth
his own house; but he that hateth gifts
shall live.
28 The heart of the righteous [e]studieth
to answer: but the mouth of the wicked
poureth out evil things.
29 The LORD *is* far from the wicked: but
he heareth the prayer of the righteous.
30 The light of the eyes rejoiceth the
heart: *and* a good report maketh the
bones fat.
31 The ear that heareth the reproof of
life abideth among the wise.
32 He that refuseth instruction
despiseth his own soul: but he that
heareth reproof getteth understanding.
33 The [f]fear of the LORD *is* the instruction of wisdom; and before honour *is*
humility.

CHAPTER 16.

(*The contrast of goodness and evil,*
continued.)

The preparations of the heart in man,
and the answer of the tongue, *is*
from the LORD.
2 All the ways of a man *are* clean in his
own eyes; but the LORD [g]weigheth the
spirits.
3 [h]Commit thy works unto the LORD,
and thy thoughts shall be established.
4 [i]The LORD hath made all *things* for
himself: [j]yea, even the wicked for the
day of evil.
5 [k]Every one *that is* proud in heart *is*
an abomination to the LORD: *though* hand
join in hand, he shall not be unpunished.
6 By mercy and truth iniquity is
purged: and by the fear of the LORD *men*
depart from evil.
7 When a man's ways please the LORD,
he maketh even his enemies to be at
peace with him.
8 [l]Better *is* a little with righteousness
than great revenues without right.
9 A man's heart deviseth his way:
[m]but the LORD directeth his steps.
10 [n]A divine sentence *is* in the lips of
the king: his mouth transgresseth not in
judgment.
11 A just weight and balance *are* the
LORD'S: all the weights of the bag *are* his
work.
12 *It is* an abomination to kings to
commit wickedness: for the throne is
established by righteousness.
13 Righteous lips *are* the delight of
kings; and they love him that speaketh
right.
14 The wrath of a king *is as* messengers
of death: but a wise man will pacify it.
15 In the light of the king's countenance *is* life; and his favour *is* as [o]a cloud
of the latter rain.
16 [p]How much better *is it* to get wisdom than gold! and to get understanding rather to be chosen than silver!
17 The highway of the upright *is* to
depart from evil: he that keepeth his
way preserveth his soul.
18 Pride *goeth* before destruction, and
an haughty spirit before a fall.
19 Better *it is to be* of an humble spirit
with the lowly, than to divide the spoil
with the proud.
20 He that handleth a matter wisely
shall find good: and whoso [q]trusteth in
the LORD, happy *is* he.
21 The wise in heart shall be called
prudent: and the sweetness of the lips
increaseth learning.
22 Understanding *is* a wellspring of
life unto him that hath it: but the instruction of fools *is* folly.
23 The heart of the wise teacheth his
mouth, and addeth learning to his lips.
24 Pleasant words *are as* an honeycomb, sweet to the soul, and health to
the bones.
25 There is a way that seemeth right
unto a man, but the end thereof *are* the
ways of death.
26 He that laboureth laboureth

B.C. 1000.

a Eph. 5:15.
b Phil. 3:20; Col. 3:1, 2.
c Heb. *Sheol.* See Hab. 2:5, *note.*
d Isa. 5:8; Jer. 17:11.
e 1 Pet. 3:15.
f Psa .19:9, *note.*
g 1 Sam. 16:7.
h Heb. *roll.*
i Isa. 43:7; Rom. 11:36.
j Job 21:30; Rom. 9:22.
k Prov. 6:17; 8:13.
l Prov. 15:16; Psa. 37:16.
m Prov. 20:24; Psa. 37:23; Jer. 10:23.
n Heb. *divination.*
o Job 29:23; Zech. 10:1.
p Prov. 8:11, 19.
q Psa. 2:12, *note.*

B.C. 1000.

for himself; for his mouth craveth it of him.

27 An ungodly man diggeth up evil: and in his lips *there is* as a burning fire.

28 A froward man soweth strife: and [a]a whisperer separateth chief friends.

29 A violent man enticeth his neighbour, and leadeth him into the way *that is* not good.

30 He shutteth his eyes to devise froward things: moving his lips he bringeth evil to pass.

31 [b]The hoary head *is* a crown of glory, *if* it be found in the way of righteousness.

32 *He that is* slow to anger *is* better than the mighty; and he that ruleth his spirit than he that taketh a city.

33 The lot is cast into the lap; but the whole disposing thereof *is* of the LORD.

CHAPTER 17.

(*The contrast of goodness and evil,* continued.)

Better *is* a dry morsel, and quietness therewith, than an [c]house full of sacrifices *with* strife.

2 A wise servant shall have rule over a son that causeth shame, and shall have part of the inheritance among the brethren.

3 [d]The fining pot *is* for silver, and the furnace for gold: but the LORD trieth the hearts.

4 A wicked doer giveth heed to false lips; *and* a liar giveth ear to a naughty tongue.

5 [e]Whoso mocketh the poor reproacheth his Maker: [f]*and* he that is glad at calamities shall not be [g]unpunished.

6 [h]Children's children *are* the crown of old men; and the glory of children *are* their fathers.

7 Excellent speech becometh not a fool: much less do lying lips a prince.

8 A gift *is as* a precious stone in the eyes of him that hath it: whithersoever it turneth, it prospereth.

9 He that covereth a transgression seeketh love; but he that repeateth a matter separateth *very* friends.

10 A reproof entereth more into a wise man than an hundred stripes into a fool.

11 An evil *man* seeketh only rebellion: therefore a cruel messenger shall be sent against him.

12 [i]Let a bear robbed of her whelps meet a man, rather than a fool in his folly.

13 [j]Whoso rewardeth evil for good, evil shall not depart from his house.

14 The beginning of strife *is as* when one letteth out water: therefore leave off contention, before it be meddled with.

15 [k]He that justifieth the wicked, and he that condemneth the just, even they both *are* abomination to the LORD.

16 Wherefore *is there* a price in the hand of a fool to get wisdom, seeing *he hath* no heart *to it*?

17 A friend loveth at all times, and a brother is born for adversity.

18 A man void of understanding striketh hands, *and* becometh surety in the presence of his friend.

19 He loveth transgression that loveth strife: *and* he that exalteth his gate seeketh destruction.

20 He that hath a froward heart findeth no good: [l]and he that hath a perverse tongue falleth into mischief.

21 He that begetteth a fool *doeth it* to his sorrow: and the father of a fool hath no joy.

22 [m]A merry heart doeth good *like* a medicine: but a broken spirit drieth the bones.

23 A wicked *man* taketh a gift out of the bosom to pervert the ways of judgment.

24 Wisdom *is* before him that hath understanding; but the eyes of a fool *are* in the ends of the earth.

25 [n]A foolish son *is* a grief to his father, and bitterness to her that bare him.

26 Also to punish the just *is* not good, *nor* to strike princes for equity.

27 [o]He that hath knowledge spareth his words: *and* a man of understanding is of an excellent spirit.

28 Even a fool, when he holdeth his peace, is counted wise: *and* he that shutteth his lips *is esteemed* a man of understanding.

CHAPTER 18.

(*The contrast of goodness and evil,* continued.)

Through desire a man, having separated himself, seeketh *and* intermeddleth with all wisdom.

2 A fool hath no delight in understanding, but that his heart may discover itself

a Prov. 17:9.
b Prov. 20:29.
c i.e. *feasting.*
d Prov. 27:21; Psa. 26:2; Jer. 17:10; Mal. 3:3.
e Prov. 14:31.
f Job 31:29; Oba. 12; 1 Cor. 13:6.
g Heb. *held innocent.*
h Psa. 127:3; 128:3.
i Hos. 13:8.
j Psa. 109:4, 5; Jer. 18:20. See also Rom. 12:17; 1 Thes. 5:15; 1 Pet. 3:9.
k Prov. 24:24; Ex. 23:7; Isa. 5:23.
l Jas. 3:8.
m Prov. 12:25; 15:13, 15.
n v. 21; Prov. 10:1; 15:20; 19:13.
o Jas. 1:19.

3 When the wicked cometh, *then* cometh also contempt, and with ignominy reproach.

4 The words of a man's mouth *are as* deep waters, *and* the wellspring of wisdom *as* a flowing brook.

5 *It is* not good to accept the person of the wicked, to overthrow the righteous in judgment.

6 A fool's lips enter into contention, and his mouth calleth for strokes.

7 A fool's mouth *is* his destruction, and his lips *are* the snare of his soul.

8 The words of a [a]talebearer *are* as [b]wounds, and they go down into the innermost parts of the belly.

9 He also that is slothful in his work is brother to him that is a great waster.

10 [c]The name of the LORD *is* a strong tower: the righteous runneth into it, and is safe.

11 The rich man's wealth *is* his strong city, and as an high wall in his own conceit.

12 Before destruction the heart of man is haughty, and before honour *is* humility.

13 He that answereth a matter [d]before he heareth *it*, it *is* folly and shame unto him.

14 The spirit of a man will sustain his infirmity; but a wounded spirit who can bear?

15 The heart of the prudent getteth knowledge; and the ear of the wise seeketh knowledge.

16 [e]A man's gift maketh room for him, and bringeth him before great men.

17 *He that is* first in his own cause *seemeth* just; but his neighbour cometh and searcheth him.

18 The lot causeth contentions to cease, and parteth between the mighty.

19 A brother offended *is harder to be won* than a strong city: and *their* contentions *are* like the bars of a castle.

20 A man's belly shall be satisfied with the fruit of his mouth; *and* with the increase of his lips shall he be filled.

21 [f]Death and life *are* in the power of the tongue: and they that love it shall eat the fruit thereof.

22 [g]*Whoso* findeth a wife findeth a good *thing*, and obtaineth favour of the LORD.

23 The poor useth intreaties; but the rich answereth [h]roughly.

24 A man *that hath* friends must shew himself friendly: and [i]there is a friend *that* sticketh closer than a brother.

CHAPTER 19.

(*The contrast of goodness and evil, continued.*)

Better *is* the poor that walketh in his integrity, than *he that is* perverse in his lips, and is a fool.

2 Also, *that* the soul *be* without knowledge, *it is* not good; and he that hasteth with *his* feet sinneth.

3 The foolishness of man perverteth his way: and his heart fretteth against the LORD.

4 [j]Wealth maketh many friends; but the poor is separated from his neighbour.

5 [k]A false witness shall not be unpunished, and *he that* speaketh lies shall not escape.

6 Many will intreat the favour of the prince: and [l]every man *is* a friend to him that giveth gifts.

7 All the brethren of the poor do hate him: how much more do his friends go far from him? he pursueth *them with* words, *yet* they *are* wanting *to him*.

8 He that getteth wisdom loveth his own soul: he that keepeth understanding shall find good.

9 A false witness shall not be unpunished, and *he that* speaketh lies shall perish.

10 Delight is not seemly for a fool; much less for a servant to have rule over princes.

11 The discretion of a man deferreth his anger; and *it is* his glory to pass over a transgression.

12 The king's wrath *is* as the roaring of a lion; but his favour *is* [m]as dew upon the grass.

13 A foolish son *is* the calamity of his father: and the contentions of a wife *are* a continual dropping.

14 House and riches *are* the inheritance of fathers: and [n]a prudent wife *is* from the LORD.

15 Slothfulness casteth into a deep sleep; and an idle soul shall suffer hunger.

16 [o]He that keepeth the commandment keepeth his own soul; *but* he that despiseth his ways shall die.

17 [p]He that hath pity upon the poor lendeth unto the LORD; and that which he hath given will he pay him again.

18 Chasten thy son while there is

B.C. 1000.

a Or, *whisperer.*

b Or, *like as when men are wounded.*

c 2 Sam. 22:3, 51; Psa. 18:2; 61:3, 4; 91:2; 144:2.

d John 7:51.

e Prov. 17:8; 21:14; Gen. 32:20; 1 Sam. 25:27.

f Mt. 12:37.

g Prov. 19:14; 31:10.

h Jas. 2:3.

i Prov. 17:17.

j Prov. 14:20.

k v. 9; Prov. 6:19; 21:28; Ez. 23:1; Deut. 19:16, 19.

l Prov. 17:8; 18:16; 21:14.

m Hos. 14:5.

n Prov. 18:22.

o Lk. 10:28; 11:28.

p Prov. 28:27; Eccl. 11:1; Mt. 10:42; 25:40; 2 Cor. 9:6-8; Heb. 6:10.

B.C. 1000.

hope, and let not thy soul spare for his crying.

19 A man of great wrath shall suffer punishment: for if thou deliver *him*, yet thou must do it again.

20 Hear counsel, and receive instruction, that thou mayest be wise in thy latter end.

21 [a]*There are* many devices in a man's heart; nevertheless the counsel of the LORD, that shall stand.

22 The desire of a man *is* his kindness: and a poor man *is* better than a liar.

23 [b]The fear of the LORD *tendeth* to life: and *he that hath it* shall abide satisfied; he shall not be visited with evil.

24 A slothful *man* hideth his hand in *his* bosom, and will not so much as bring it to his mouth again.

25 Smite a scorner, and the simple [c]will beware: and reprove one that hath understanding, *and* he will understand knowledge.

26 He that wasteth *his* father, *and* chaseth away *his* mother, *is* a son that causeth shame, and bringeth reproach.

27 Cease, my son, to hear the instruction *that causeth* to err from the words of knowledge.

28 An ungodly witness scorneth judgment: and the mouth of the wicked devoureth iniquity.

29 Judgments are prepared for scorners, and stripes for the back of fools.

CHAPTER 20.

Part IV. Warnings and instructions.

Wine [d]*is* a mocker, strong drink *is* raging: and whosoever is deceived thereby is not wise.

2 The fear of a king *is* as the roaring of a lion: *whoso* provoketh him to anger sinneth *against* his own soul.

3 *It is* an honour for a man to cease from strife: but every fool will be meddling.

4 The sluggard will not plow by reason of the cold; *therefore* shall he beg in harvest, and *have* nothing.

5 [e]Counsel in the heart of man *is like* deep water; but a man of understanding will draw it out.

6 [f]Most men will proclaim every one his own goodness: but a faithful man who can find?

7 [g]The just *man* walketh in his integrity: his children *are* blessed after him.

8 A king that sitteth in the throne of judgment scattereth away all evil with his eyes.

9 [h]Who can say, I have made my heart clean, I am pure from my sin?

10 [i]Divers weights, *and* [j]divers measures, both of them *are* alike abomination to the LORD.

11 Even a child is known by his doings, whether his work *be* pure, and whether *it be* right.

12 The hearing ear, and the seeing eye, the LORD hath made even both of them.

13 Love not sleep, lest thou come to poverty; open thine eyes, *and* thou shalt be satisfied with bread.

14 *It is* naught, *it is* naught, saith the buyer: but when he is gone his way, then he boasteth.

15 There is gold, and a multitude of rubies: [k]but the lips of knowledge *are* a precious jewel.

16 Take his garment that is surety *for* a stranger: and take a pledge of him for a strange woman.

17 Bread of deceit *is* sweet to a man; but afterwards his mouth shall be filled with gravel.

18 *Every* purpose is established by counsel: and with good advice make war.

19 He that goeth about *as* a talebearer revealeth secrets: therefore meddle not with him [l]that flattereth with his lips.

20 [m]Whoso curseth his father or his mother, [n]his lamp shall be put out in obscure darkness.

21 [o]An inheritance *may be* gotten hastily at the beginning; [p]but the end thereof shall not be blessed.

22 [q]Say not thou, I will recompense evil; *but* [r]wait on the LORD, and he shall save thee.

23 Divers weights *are* an abomination unto the LORD; and a false balance *is* not good.

24 Man's goings *are* of the LORD; how can a man then understand his own way?

25 *It is* a snare to the man *who* devoureth *that which is* holy, and after vows to make enquiry.

26 A wise king scattereth the wicked, and bringeth the wheel over them.

27 [s]The spirit of man *is* the candle of the LORD, searching all the inward parts of the belly.

28 Mercy and truth preserve the king: and his throne is upholden by mercy.

29 The glory of young men *is* their

---

a Prov. 16:1, 9; Job 23:13; Psa. 33:10, 11; Isa. 14:26, 27; 46:10; Acts 5:39; Heb. 6:17.

b Psa. 19:9, *note.*

c Heb. *will be cunning.*

d Prov. 23:29-35; Gen. 9:21; Isa. 28:7; Hos. 4:11.

e Prov. 18:4.

f Prov. 25:14; Mt. 6:2; Lk. 18:11.

g 2 Cor. 1:12.

h 1 Ki. 8:46; 2 Chr. 6:36; Job 9:30; 14:4; Psa. 51:5; Eccl. 7:20; 1 John 1:8.

i v. 23; Prov. 11:1; 16:11; Deut. 25:13; Mic. 6:10, 11. Heb. *a stone and a stone.*

j Heb. *an ephah and an ephah.*

k Prov. 3:15; 8:11; Job 28:12, 16-19.

l Rom. 16:18.

m Ex. 21:17; Lev. 20:9; Mt. 15:4.

n Prov. 24:20; Job 18:5, 6.

o Prov. 28:20.

p Hab. 2:6.

q Prov. 17:13; 24:29; Deut. 32:35; Rom. 12:17, 19; 1 Thes. 5:15; 1 Pet. 3:9.

r 2 Sam. 16:12.

s 1 Cor. 2:11.

28 [a]He that *hath* no rule over his own spirit *is like* a city *that is* broken down, *and* without walls.

CHAPTER 26.

(*Warnings and instructions,* continued.)

As snow in summer, and [b]as rain in harvest, so honour is not seemly for a fool.

2 As the bird by wandering, as the swallow by flying, [c]so the curse causeless shall not come.

3 A whip for the horse, a bridle for the ass, and a rod for the fool's back.

4 Answer not a fool according to his folly, lest thou also be like unto him.

5 [d]Answer a fool according to his folly, lest he be wise in his own conceit.

6 He that sendeth a message by the hand of a fool cutteth off the feet, *and* drinketh damage.

7 The legs of the lame are not equal: so *is* a parable in the mouth of fools.

8 As he that bindeth a stone in a sling, so *is* he that giveth honour to a fool.

9 *As* a thorn goeth up into the hand of a drunkard, so *is* a parable in the mouth of fools.

10 The great *God* that formed all *things* both rewardeth the fool, and rewardeth transgressors.

11 As a [e]dog returneth to his vomit, *so* a fool returneth to his folly.

12 [f]Seest thou a man wise in his own conceit? *there is* more hope of a fool than of him.

13 The slothful *man* saith, *There is* a lion in the way; a lion *is* in the streets.

14 *As* the door turneth upon his hinges, so *doth* the slothful upon his bed.

15 [g]The slothful hideth his hand in *his* bosom; it grieveth him to bring it again to his mouth.

16 The sluggard *is* wiser in his own conceit than seven men that can render a reason.

17 He that passeth by, *and* meddleth with strife *belonging* not to him, *is like* one that taketh a dog by the ears.

18 As a mad *man* who casteth firebrands, arrows, and death,

19 So *is* the man *that* deceiveth his neighbour, and saith, [h]Am not I in sport?

20 Where no wood is, *there* the fire goeth out: so where *there is* no talebearer, the strife ceaseth.

21 [i]*As* coals *are* to burning coals, and wood to fire; so *is* a contentious man to kindle strife.

22 The words of a talebearer *are* as wounds, and they go down into the innermost parts of the belly.

23 Burning lips and a wicked heart *are like* a potsherd covered with silver dross.

24 He that hateth dissembleth with his lips, and layeth up deceit within him;

25 When he speaketh fair, believe him not: for *there are* seven abominations in his heart.

26 *Whose* hatred is covered by deceit, his wickedness shall be shewed before the *whole* congregation.

27 [j]Whoso diggeth a pit shall fall therein: and he that rolleth a stone, it will return upon him.

28 A lying tongue hateth *those that are* afflicted by it; and a flattering mouth worketh ruin.

CHAPTER 27.

(*Warnings and instructions,* continued.)

Boast [k]not thyself of to morrow; for thou knowest not what a day may bring forth.

2 [l]Let another man praise thee, and not thine own mouth; a stranger, and not thine own lips.

3 A stone *is* heavy, and the sand weighty; but a fool's wrath *is* heavier than them both.

4 [m]Wrath *is* cruel, and anger *is* outrageous; [n]but who *is* able to stand before envy?

5 [o]Open rebuke *is* better than secret love.

6 Faithful *are* the wounds of a friend; but the kisses of an enemy *are* deceitful.

7 The full soul loatheth an honeycomb; but to the hungry soul every bitter thing is sweet.

8 As a bird that wandereth from her nest, so *is* a man that wandereth from his place.

9 Ointment and perfume rejoice the heart: so *doth* the sweetness of a man's friend [p]by hearty counsel.

10 Thine own friend, and thy father's friend, forsake not; neither go into thy brother's house in the day of thy calamity: *for* better *is* a neighbour *that is* near than a brother far off.

11 [q]My son, be wise, and make my

B.C. 700.

a Prov. 16:32.
b 1 Sam. 12:17.
c Num. 23:8.
d Mt. 16:1-4; 21:24-27.
e 2 Pet. 2:22.
f Prov. 29:20; Lk. 18:11; Rom. 12:16; Rev. 3:17.
g Prov. 19:24.
h Eph. 5:4.
i Prov. 15:18; 29:22.
j Prov. 28:10; Psa. 7:15, 16; 9:15; 10:2; 57:6; Eccl. 10:8.
k Lk. 12:19, 20; Jas. 4:13.
l Prov. 25:27.
m Heb. *wrath is cruelty and anger an overflowing.*
n 1 John 3:12.
o Prov. 28:23; Gal. 2:14.
p Heb. *from the counsel of the soul.*
q Prov. 10:1; 23:15, 24.

heart glad, that I may answer him that reproacheth me.

12 A prudent *man* foreseeth the evil, *and* hideth himself; *but* the simple pass on, *and* are punished.

13 Take his garment that is surety for a stranger, and take a pledge of him for a strange woman.

14 He that blesseth his friend with a loud voice, rising early in the morning, it shall be counted a curse to him.

15 [a]A continual dropping in a very rainy day and a contentious woman are alike.

16 Whosoever hideth her hideth the wind, and the ointment of his right hand, *which* bewrayeth *itself*.

17 Iron sharpeneth iron; so a man sharpeneth the countenance of his friend.

18 [b]Whoso keepeth the fig tree shall eat the fruit thereof: so he that waiteth on his master shall be honoured.

19 As in water face *answereth* to face, so the heart of man to man.

20 [c]Hell and destruction are never full; so the eyes of man are [d]never satisfied.

21 *As* the fining pot for silver, and the furnace for gold; so *is* a man to his praise.

22 Though thou shouldest bray a fool in a mortar among wheat with a pestle, *yet* will not his foolishness depart from him.

23 Be thou diligent to know the state of thy flocks, *and* look well to thy herds.

24 For riches *are* not for ever: and doth the crown *endure* to every generation?

25 [e]The hay appeareth, and the tender grass sheweth itself, and herbs of the mountains are gathered.

26 The lambs *are* for thy clothing, and the goats *are* the price of the field.

27 And *thou shalt have* goats' milk enough for thy food, for the food of thy household, and *for* the maintenance for thy maidens.

CHAPTER 28.

(*Warnings and instructions,* continued.)

The [f]wicked flee when no man pursueth: but the righteous are bold as a lion.

2 For the transgression of a land many *are* the princes thereof: but by a man of understanding *and* knowledge the state *thereof* shall be prolonged.

3 [g]A poor man that oppresseth the poor *is like* a sweeping rain which leaveth no food.

4 They that forsake the law praise the wicked: [h]but such as keep the law contend with them.

5 Evil men understand not judgment: but [i]they that seek the LORD understand all *things*.

6 Better *is* the poor that walketh in his uprightness, than *he that is* perverse *in his* ways, though he *be* rich.

7 Whoso keepeth the law *is* a wise son: but he that is a companion of riotous *men* shameth his father.

8 [j]He that by usury and unjust gain increaseth his substance, he shall gather it for him that will pity the poor.

9 [k]He that turneth away his ear from hearing the law, [l]even his prayer *shall be* abomination.

10 Whoso causeth the righteous to go astray in an evil way, he shall fall himself into his own pit: but the upright shall have good *things* in possession.

11 The rich man *is* wise in his own conceit; but the poor that hath understanding searcheth him out.

12 When righteous *men* do rejoice, *there is* great glory: but when the wicked rise, a man is hidden.

13 [m]He that covereth his sins shall not prosper: but whoso confesseth and forsaketh *them* shall have mercy.

14 Happy *is* the man that feareth alway: but he that hardeneth his heart shall fall into mischief.

15 [n]*As* a roaring lion, and a ranging bear; *so is* a wicked ruler over the poor people.

16 The prince that wanteth understanding *is* also a great oppressor: *but* he that hateth covetousness shall prolong *his* days.

17 A man that doeth violence to the blood of *any* person shall flee to the pit; let no man stay him.

18 Whoso walketh uprightly shall be saved: but *he that is* perverse *in his* ways shall fall at once.

19 He that tilleth his land shall have plenty of bread: but he that followeth after vain *persons* shall have poverty enough.

20 A faithful man shall abound with blessings: [o]but he that maketh haste to be rich shall not be innocent.

21 To have respect of persons *is* not

B.C. 700.

a Prov. 19:13.
b 1 Cor. 9:7-13.
c Prov. 30:16; Hab. 2:5. Heb. *Sheol.* See Hab. 2:5, *note.*
d Heb. *not.*
e Psa. 104:14.
f Lev. 26:17, 36; Psa. 53:5.
g Mt. 18:28.
h 1 Ki. 18:18, 21; Mt. 3:7; 14:4; Eph. 5:11.
i John 7:17; 1 Cor. 2:15; 1 John 2:20, 27.
j Prov. 13:22; Job 27:16, 17; Eccl. 2:26.
k Zech. 7:11.
l Prov. 15:8; Psa. 66:18; 109:7.
m Psa. 32:3, 5; 1 John 1:8-10.
n 1 Pet. 5:8.
o v. 22; Prov. 13:11; 20:21; 23:4; 1 Tim. 6:9.

B.C. 700.

good: for for a piece of bread *that* man
will transgress.
22 He that hasteth to be rich *hath* an
evil eye, and considereth not that poverty shall come upon him.
23 He that rebuketh a man afterwards
shall find more favour than he that flattereth with the tongue.
24 Whoso robbeth his father or his
mother, and saith, *It is* no transgression;
the same *is* the companion of a destroyer.
25 He that is of a proud heart stirreth
up strife: but he that putteth his [a]trust in
the LORD shall be made fat.
26 He that trusteth in his own heart is
a fool: but whoso walketh wisely, he
shall be delivered.
27 [b]He that giveth unto the poor shall
not lack: but he that hideth his eyes shall
have many a curse.
28 When the wicked rise, men hide
themselves: but when they perish, the
righteous increase.

CHAPTER 29.

(*Warnings and instructions*, continued.)

He, that being often reproved hardeneth *his* neck, shall suddenly be
destroyed, and that without remedy.
2 When the righteous are in authority,
the people rejoice: but when the wicked
beareth rule, the people mourn.
3 Whoso loveth wisdom rejoiceth his
father: but he that keepeth company
with harlots spendeth *his* substance.
4 The king by judgment establisheth
the land: but he that receiveth gifts overthroweth it.
5 A man that flattereth his neighbour
spreadeth a net for his feet.
6 In the transgression of an evil man
there is a snare: but the righteous doth
sing and rejoice.
7 [c]The righteous considereth the cause
of the poor: *but* the wicked regardeth not
to know *it*.
8 Scornful men bring a city into a
snare: but wise *men* turn away wrath.
9 *If* a wise man contendeth with a foolish man, whether he rage or laugh, *there*
is no rest.
10 [d]The bloodthirsty hate the upright:
but the just seek his soul.
11 A fool uttereth all his mind: but a
wise *man* keepeth it in till afterwards.
12 If a ruler hearken to lies, all his servants *are* wicked.
13 The poor and the deceitful man
meet together: the LORD lighteneth both
their eyes.
14 The king that faithfully judgeth the
poor, his throne shall be established for
ever.
15 The rod and reproof give wisdom:
but a child left *to himself* bringeth his
mother to shame.
16 When the wicked are multiplied,
transgression increaseth: [e]but the righteous shall see their fall.
17 Correct thy son, and he shall give
thee rest; yea, he shall give delight unto
thy soul.
18 [f]Where *there is* no vision, the people
perish: but he that keepeth the law,
happy *is* he.
19 A servant will not be corrected by
words: for though he understand he will
not answer.
20 Seest thou a man *that is* hasty in his
words? [g]*there is* more hope of a fool than
of him.
21 He that delicately bringeth up his
servant from a child shall have him
become *his* son at the length.
22 An angry man stirreth up strife,
and a furious man aboundeth in transgression.
23 [h]A man's pride shall bring him low:
but honour shall uphold the humble in
spirit.
24 Whoso is partner with a thief
hateth his own soul: he heareth cursing,
and bewrayeth *it* not.
25 The fear of man bringeth a snare:
but whoso putteth his trust in the LORD
shall be safe.
26 Many seek the ruler's favour; but
every man's judgment *cometh* from the
LORD.
27 An unjust man *is* an abomination to
the just: and *he that is* upright in the way
is abomination to the wicked.

CHAPTER 30.

Part V. The words of Agur.

The [i]words of Agur the son of Jakeh,
even the prophecy: the man spake
unto Ithiel, even unto Ithiel and Ucal,
2 Surely I *am* more brutish than *any*
man, and have not the understanding of
a man.
3 I neither learned wisdom, nor have
the knowledge of the holy.
4 [j]Who hath ascended up into heaven,
or descended? who hath gathered the
wind in his fists? who hath bound the

a Psa. 2:12, *note;* also Prov. 29:25.
b Prov. 19:17; 22:9; Deut. 15:7.
c Job 29:16; 31:13; Psa. 41:1.
d Gen. 4:5, 8; 1 John 3:12.
e Psa. 37:36; 58:10; 91:8; 92:11.
f 1 Sam. 3:1; Amos 8:11, 12.
g Prov. 26:12.
h Prov. 15:33; 18:12; Isa. 66:2; Dan. 4:30; Mt. 23:12; Lk. 14:11; 18:14; Acts 12:23; Jas. 4:6, 10; 1 Pet. 5:5.
i Prov. 31:1.
j John 3:13.

waters in a garment? who hath established all the ends of the earth? what *is* his name, and what *is* his son's name, if thou canst tell?

5 [a]Every word of God *is* [b]pure: he *is* a [c]shield unto them that put their [d]trust in him.

6 Add thou not unto his words, lest he reprove thee, and thou be found a liar.

7 Two *things* have I required of thee; deny me *them* not before I die:

8 Remove far from me vanity and lies: give me neither poverty nor riches; feed me with food convenient for me:

9 [e]Lest I be full, and deny *thee*, and say, Who *is* the LORD? or lest I be poor, and steal, and take the name of my God *in vain*.

10 [f]Accuse not a servant unto his master, lest he curse thee, and thou be found guilty.

11 *There is* a generation *that* curseth their father, and doth not bless their mother.

12 *There is* a generation *that are* pure in their own eyes, and *yet* is not washed from their filthiness.

13 *There is* a generation, O how lofty are their eyes! and their eyelids are lifted up.

14 *There is* a generation, whose teeth *are as* swords, and their jaw teeth *as* knives, [g]to devour the poor from off the earth, and the needy from *among* men.

15 The horseleach hath two daughters, *crying*, Give, give. There are three *things that* are never satisfied, *yea*, four *things* say not, *It is* enough:

16 The [h]grave; and the barren womb; the earth *that* is not filled with water; and the fire *that* saith not, *It is* enough.

17 [i]The eye *that* mocketh at *his* father, and despiseth to obey *his* mother, the ravens of the valley shall pick it out, and the young eagles shall eat it.

18 There be three *things which* are too wonderful for me, yea, four which I know not:

19 The way of an eagle in the air; the way of a serpent upon a rock; the way of a ship in the midst of the sea; and the way of a man with a maid.

20 Such *is* the way of an adulterous woman; she eateth, and wipeth her mouth, and saith, I have done no wickedness.

B.C. 700.

a Psa. 12:6; 18:30; 19:8; 119:140.

b Heb. *purified.*

c Psa. 18:30; 84:11; 115:9-11.

d Psa. 2:12, *note.*

e Deut. 8:12-14, 17; 31:20; 32:15; Neh. 9:25, 26; Job 31:24; Hos. 13:6.

f Heb. *hurt not with thy tongue.*

g Psa. 14:4; Amos 8:4.

h Heb. *Sheol.* See Hab. 2:5, *note.*

i Prov. 20:20; 23:22; Gen. 9:22; Lev. 20:9.

j Heb. *made wise.*

k Prov. 6:6.

[B.C. 1015.

l Psa. 104:18.

m Job 21:5; 40:4.

n Eccl. 10:17; Hos. 4:11.

o Heb. *bitter of soul.* 1 Sam. 1:10.

21 For three *things* the earth is disquieted, and for four *which* it cannot bear:

22 For a servant when he reigneth; and a fool when he is filled with meat;

23 For an odious *woman* when she is married; and an handmaid that is heir to her mistress.

24 There be four *things which are* little upon the earth, but they *are* [j]exceeding wise:

25 [k]The ants *are* a people not strong, yet they prepare their meat in the summer;

26 [l]The conies *are but* a feeble folk, yet make they their houses in the rocks;

27 The locusts have no king, yet go they forth all of them by bands;

28 The spider taketh hold with her hands, and is in kings' palaces.

29 There be three *things* which go well, yea, four are comely in going:

30 A lion *which is* strongest among beasts, and turneth not away for any;

31 A greyhound; an he goat also; and a king, against whom *there is* no rising up.

32 If thou hast done foolishly in lifting up thyself, or if thou hast thought evil, [m]lay thine hand upon thy mouth.

33 Surely the churning of milk bringeth forth butter, and the wringing of the nose bringeth forth blood: so the forcing of wrath bringeth forth strife.

CHAPTER 31.

Part VI. The words of King Lemuel.

The words of king Lemuel, the prophecy that his mother taught him.

2 What, my son? and what, the son of my womb? and what, the son of my vows?

3 Give not thy strength unto women, nor thy ways to that which destroyeth kings.

4 [n]*It is* not for kings, O Lemuel, *it is* not for kings to drink wine; nor for princes strong drink:

5 Lest they drink, and forget the law, and pervert the judgment of any of the afflicted.

6 Give strong drink unto him that is ready to perish, and wine unto those that be of [o]heavy hearts.

7 Let him drink, and forget his

poverty, and remember his misery no more.

8 [a]Open thy mouth for the dumb [b]in the cause of all such as are appointed to destruction.

9 Open thy mouth, [c]judge righteously, and [d]plead the cause of the poor and needy.

10 Who can find a virtuous woman? for her price *is* far above rubies.

11 The heart of her husband doth safely [e]trust in her, so that he shall have no need of spoil.

12 She will do him good and not evil all the days of her life.

13 She seeketh wool, and flax, and worketh willingly with her hands.

14 She is like the merchants' ships; she bringeth her food from afar.

15 [f]She riseth also while it is yet night, and [g]giveth meat to her household, and a portion to her maidens.

16 She considereth a field, and buyeth it: with the fruit of her hands she planteth a vineyard.

17 She girdeth her loins with strength, and strengtheneth her arms.

18 She [h]perceiveth that her merchandise *is* good: her candle goeth not out by night.

19 She layeth her hands to the spindle, and her hands hold the distaff.

20 She [i]stretcheth out her hand to the poor; yea, she reacheth forth her hands to the needy.

21 She is not afraid of the snow for her household: for all her household *are* clothed with scarlet.

22 She maketh herself coverings of tapestry; her clothing *is* silk and purple.

23 [j]Her husband is known in the gates, when he sitteth among the elders of the land.

24 She maketh fine linen, and selleth *it*; and delivereth girdles unto the merchant.

25 Strength and honour *are* her clothing; and she shall rejoice in time to come.

26 She openeth her mouth with wisdom; and in her tongue *is* the law of kindness.

27 She looketh well to the ways of her household, and eateth not the bread of idleness.

28 Her children arise up, and call her blessed; her husband *also*, and he praiseth her.

29 Many daughters [k]have done virtuously, but thou excellest them all.

30 Favour *is* deceitful, and beauty *is* vain: *but* a woman *that* [l]feareth the LORD, she shall be praised.

31 Give her of the fruit of her hands; and let her own works praise her in the gates.

B.C. 1015.

a Job 29:15, 16.

b 1 Sam. 19:4; Esth. 4:16.

c Lev. 19:15; Deut. 1:16.

d Job 29:12; Isa. 1:17; Jer. 22:16.

e Psa. 2:12, *note.*

f Rom. 12:11.

g Lk. 12:42.

h Heb. *tasteth.*

i Eph. 4:28; Heb. 13:16.

j Prov. 12:4.

k Or, *have gotten riches.*

l Psa. 19:9, *note.*

ECCLESIASTES

OR, THE PREACHER

THIS is the book of man "under the sun," reasoning about life; it is the best man can do, with the knowledge that there is a holy God, and that He will bring everything into judgment. The key phrases are "under the sun"; "I perceived"; "I said in my heart." Inspiration sets down accurately what passes, but the conclusions and reasonings are, after all, man's. That those conclusions are just in declaring it "vanity," in view of judgment, to devote life to earthly things, is surely true; but the "conclusion" (12:13) is legal, the best that man apart from redemption can do, and does not anticipate the Gospel. Ecclesiastes is in five parts: I. Theme, 1:1-3. II. Theme proved, 1:4–3:22. III. Theme unfolded in the light of human sufferings, hypocrisies, uncertainties, poverty and riches, 4:1–10:20. IV. The best thing possible to the natural man apart from God, 11:1–12:12. V. The best thing possible to man under the law, 12:13, 14.

CHAPTER 1.

B.C. 977.

Part I. The theme: All is vanity.

The words of the Preacher, the son of
David, king in Jerusalem.
2 [1]Vanity of vanities, saith the
Preacher, vanity of vanities; [a]all *is* vanity.
3 [b]What profit hath a man of all his
labour which he taketh under the sun?

Part II. The theme proved:
(1) *by the transitoriness of all things.*

4 *One* generation passeth away, and
another generation cometh: but [c]the earth
abideth for ever.
5 The sun also ariseth, and the sun
goeth down, and [d]hasteth to his place
where he arose.
6 [e]The wind goeth toward the south,
and turneth about unto the north; it
whirleth about continually, and the wind
returneth again according to his circuits.
7 All the rivers run into the sea; yet the
sea *is* not full; unto the place from
whence the rivers come, thither they
return again.
8 All things *are* full of labour; man
cannot utter *it*: [f]the eye is not satisfied
with seeing, nor the ear filled with hearing.
9 [g]The thing that hath been, it *is that*
which shall be; and that which is done *is*
that which shall be done: and *there is* no
new *thing* under the sun.
10 Is there *any* thing whereof it may be
said, See, this *is* new? it hath been
already of old time, which was before
us.
11 *There is* no remembrance of former
things; neither shall there be *any* remembrance of *things* that are to come with
those that shall come after.

(The proof, continued: (2) *evil remains despite power, widsom, and knowledge.)*

12 I the Preacher was king over Israel
in Jerusalem.
13 And I gave my heart to seek and
search out by wisdom concerning all
things that are done under heaven: [h]this
sore travail hath God given to the sons
of man to be exercised therewith.
14 I have seen all the works that are
done under the sun; and, behold, all *is*
vanity and vexation of spirit.
15 *That which is* crooked cannot be
made straight: and that which is wanting cannot be numbered.
16 I communed with mine own heart,
saying, Lo, I am come to great estate,
and have gotten more wisdom than all
they that have been before me in Jerusalem: yea, my heart had great experience of wisdom and knowledge.
17 [i]And I gave my heart to know wisdom, and to know madness and folly: I
perceived that this also is vexation of
spirit.

a Psa. 39:5-6; Rom. 8:20.
b Eccl. 2:22; 3:9.
c Psa. 104:5; 119:90.
d Heb. *panteth.*
e John 3:8.
f Prov. 27:20.
g Eccl. 3:15.
h Gen. 3:19; Eccl. 3:10.
i Eccl. 2:3, 12; 7:23, 25; 1 Thes. 5:21.

1 (1:2) "Vanity," in Ecclesiastes, and usually in Scripture, means, not foolish pride, but the emptiness in final result of all life apart from God. It is to be born, to toil, to suffer, to experience some transitory joy, which is as nothing in view of eternity, to leave it all, and to die. See Rom. 8:20-22.

B.C. 977.

18 For in much wisdom *is* much grief: and he that increaseth knowledge increaseth sorrow.

CHAPTER 2.

(The proof, continued:
(3) *pleasure ends in emptiness.)*

I [a]said in mine heart, Go to now, I will prove thee with mirth, therefore enjoy pleasure: and, behold, this also *is* vanity.

2 I said of laughter, *It is* mad: and of mirth, What doeth it?

3 I sought in mine heart [b]to give myself unto wine, yet acquainting mine heart with wisdom; and to lay hold on folly, till I might see what *was* that good for the sons of men, which they should do under the heaven all the days of their life.

(The proof, continued: (4) *riches and great works give no enduring satisfaction.)*

4 I made me great works; I builded me houses; I planted me vineyards:

5 I made me gardens and orchards, and I planted trees in them of all *kind of* fruits:

6 I made me pools of water, to water therewith the wood that bringeth forth trees:

7 I got *me* servants and maidens, and had servants born in my house; also I had great possessions of great and small cattle above all that were in Jerusalem before me:

8 [c]I gathered me also silver and gold, and the peculiar treasure of kings and of the provinces: I gat me men singers and women singers, and the delights of the sons of men, *as* musical instruments, and that of all sorts.

9 [d]So I was great, and increased more than all that were before me in Jerusalem: also my wisdom remained with me.

10 And whatsoever mine eyes desired I kept not from them, I withheld not my heart from any joy; for my heart rejoiced in all my labour: and [e]this was my portion of all my labour.

11 Then I looked on all the works that my hands had wrought, and on the labour that I had laboured to do: and, behold, all *was* [f]vanity and vexation of spirit, and *there was* no profit under the sun.

(The proof, continued: (5) *wisdom is better than folly, but both have an end.)*

12 And I turned myself to behold wisdom, and [g]madness, and folly: for what *can* the man *do* that cometh after the king? *even* that which hath been already done.

13 Then I saw that wisdom excelleth folly, as far as light excelleth darkness.

14 [h]The wise man's eyes *are* in his head; but the fool walketh in darkness: and I myself perceived also that [i]one event happeneth to them all.

15 Then said I in my heart, As it happeneth to the fool, so it happeneth even to me; and why was I then more wise? Then I said in my heart, that this also *is* vanity.

16 For *there is* no remembrance of the wise more than of the fool for ever; seeing that which now *is* in the days to come shall all be forgotten. And how dieth the wise *man*? as the fool.

17 Therefore I hated life; because the work that is wrought under the sun *is* grievous unto me: for all *is* vanity and vexation of spirit.

18 Yea, I hated all my labour which I had taken under the sun: because [j]I should leave it unto the man that shall be after me.

19 And who knoweth whether he shall be a wise *man* or a fool? yet shall he have rule over all my labour wherein I have laboured, and wherein I have shewed myself wise under the sun. This *is* also vanity.

20 Therefore I went about to cause my heart to despair of all the labour which I took under the sun.

21 For there is a man whose labour *is* in wisdom, and in knowledge, and in equity; yet to a man that hath not laboured therein shall he leave it *for* his portion. This also *is* vanity and a great evil.

22 [k]For what hath man of all his labour, and of the vexation of his heart, wherein he hath laboured under the sun?

23 For all his days *are* sorrows, and his travail grief; yea, his heart taketh not rest in the night. This is also vanity.

24 *There is* nothing better for a man, *than* that he should eat and drink, and *that* he [l]should make his soul enjoy good

a Lk. 12:19.
b Heb. *to draw my flesh with wine.*
c 1 Ki. 9:28; 10:10, 14, 21.
d Eccl. 1:16.
e Eccl. 3:22; 5:18; 9:9.
f Eccl. 1:2, 14.
g Eccl. 1:17; 7:25.
h Eccl. 8:1; Prov. 17:24.
i Eccl. 9:2, 3; Psa. 49:10.
j Psa. 49:10.
k Eccl. 1:3; 3:9.
l Or, *delight his senses.*

in his labour. This also I saw, that it *was* from the hand of God.

25 For who can eat, or who else can hasten *hereunto*, more than I?

26 For *God* giveth to a man that *is* good [a]in his sight wisdom, and knowledge, and joy: but to the sinner he giveth travail, to gather and to heap up, that [b]he may give to *him that is* good before God. This also *is* vanity and vexation of spirit.

CHAPTER 3.

(The proof, continued:
(6) *the weary round of life.)*

To every *thing there is* a season, and a time to every purpose under the heaven:

2 A time to be born, and [c]a time to die; a time to plant, and a time to pluck up *that which is* planted;

3 A time to kill, and a time to heal; a time to break down, and a time to build up;

4 A time to weep, and a time to laugh; a time to mourn, and a time to dance;

5 A time to cast away stones, and a time to gather stones together; a time to embrace, and [d]a time to refrain from embracing;

6 A time to get, and a time to lose; a time to keep, and a time to cast away;

7 A time to rend, and a time to sew; [e]a time to keep silence, and a time to speak;

8 A time to love, and a time to [f]hate; a time of war, and a time of peace.

9 What profit hath he that worketh in that wherein he laboureth?

10 I have seen the travail, which God hath given to the sons of men to be exercised in it.

11 He hath made every *thing* beautiful in his time: also he hath set the [g]world in their heart, so that no man can find out the work that God maketh from the beginning to the end.

12 I know that *there is* no good in them, but for *a man* to rejoice, and to do good in his life.

13 And also that every man should eat and drink, and enjoy the good of all his labour, it *is* the gift of God.

14 I know that, whatsoever God doeth, it shall be for ever: [h]nothing can be put to it, nor any thing taken from it: and God doeth *it*, that *men* should [i]fear before him.

B.C. 977.

a Heb. *before Him.* Gen. 7:1; Lk. 1:6.

b Job 27:16, 17; Prov. 28:8.

c Heb. 9:27.

d Joel 2:16; 1 Cor. 7:5.

e Amos 5:13.

f Prov. 13:5; Lk. 14:26.

g i.e. *ages.*

h Jas. 1:17.

i Psa. 19:9, *note.*

j Rom. 2:6-8; 2 Cor. 5:10; 2 Thes. 1:6, 7.

k Eccl. 2:16; Psa. 49:12, 20; 73:22.

l Gen. 3:19.

m Heb. *of the sons of man.*

n Eccl. 3:16; 5:8.

o Heb. *hand.*

p Heb. *all the rightness of work.*

q Heb. *this is the envy of a man from his neighbour.*

15 That which hath been is now; and that which is to be hath already been; and God requireth that which is past.

16 And moreover I saw under the sun the place of judgment, *that* wickedness *was* there; and the place of righteousness, *that* iniquity *was* there.

17 I said in mine heart, [j]God shall judge the righteous and the wicked: for *there is* a time there for every purpose and for every work.

18 I said in mine heart concerning the estate of the sons of men, that God might manifest them, and that they might see that they themselves are beasts.

19 [k]For that which befalleth the sons of men befalleth beasts; even one thing befalleth them: as the one dieth, so dieth the other; yea, they have all one breath; so that a man hath no preeminence above a beast: for all *is* vanity.

20 All go unto one place; [l]all are of the dust, and all turn to dust again.

21 Who knoweth the spirit [m]of man that goeth upward, and the spirit of the beast that goeth downward to the earth?

22 Wherefore I perceive that *there is* nothing better, than that a man should rejoice in his own works; for that *is* his portion: for who shall bring him to see what shall be after him?

CHAPTER 4.

Part III. The theme unfolded: (1) *in view of the oppressions and iniquities of life.*

So I returned, and considered all the [n]oppressions that are done under the sun: and behold the tears of *such as were* oppressed, and they had no comforter; and on the [o]side of their oppressors *there was* power; but they had no comforter.

2 Wherefore I praised the dead which are already dead more than the living which are yet alive.

3 Yea, better *is he* than both they, which hath not yet been, who hath not seen the evil work that is done under the sun.

4 Again, I considered all travail, and [p]every right work, that [q]for this a man is envied of his neighbour. This *is* also vanity and vexation of spirit.

5 The fool foldeth his hands together, and eateth his own flesh.

6 [a]Better *is* an handful *with* quietness, than both the hands full *with* travail and vexation of spirit.

7 Then I returned, and I saw vanity under the sun.

8 There is one *alone*, and *there is* not a second; yea, he hath neither child nor brother: yet *is there* no end of all his labour; neither is his [b]eye satisfied with riches; [c]neither *saith he*, For whom do I labour, and bereave my soul of good? This *is* also vanity, yea, it *is* a sore travail.

9 Two *are* better than one; because they have a good reward for their labour.

10 For if they fall, the one will lift up his fellow: but woe to him *that is* alone when he falleth; for *he hath* not another to help him up.

11 Again, if two lie together, then they have heat: but how can one be warm *alone*?

12 And if one prevail against him, two shall withstand him; and a threefold cord is not quickly broken.

13 Better *is* a poor and a wise child than an old and foolish king, who will no more be admonished.

14 For out of prison he cometh to reign; whereas also *he that is* born in his kingdom becometh poor.

15 I considered all the living which walk under the sun, with the second child that shall stand up in his stead.

16 *There is* no end of all the people, *even* of all that have been before them: they also that come after shall not rejoice in him. Surely this also *is* vanity and vexation of spirit.

CHAPTER 5.

(The unfolding, continued:
(2) *in view of riches and poverty.)*

Keep [d]thy foot when thou goest to the house of God, and be more ready to hear, [e]than to give the sacrifice of fools: for they consider not that they do evil.

2 Be not rash with thy mouth, and let not thine heart be hasty to utter *any* thing before God: for God *is* in heaven, and thou upon earth: therefore let thy words [f]be few.

3 For a dream cometh through the multitude of business; and a fool's voice *is known* by multitude of words.

4 [g]When thou vowest a vow unto God, defer not to pay it; for *he hath* no pleasure in fools: [h]pay that which thou hast vowed.

5 [i]Better *is it* that thou shouldest not vow, than that thou shouldest vow and not pay.

6 Suffer not thy mouth to cause thy flesh to sin; [j]neither say thou before the [k]angel, that it *was* an error: wherefore should God be angry at thy voice, and destroy the work of thine hands?

7 For in the multitude of dreams and many words *there are* also *divers* vanities: but [l]fear thou God.

8 If thou seest the oppression of the poor, and violent perverting of judgment and justice in a province, marvel not at the matter: for *he that is* higher than the highest regardeth; and *there be* higher than they.

9 Moreover the profit of the earth is for all: the king *himself* is served by the field.

10 He that loveth silver shall not be satisfied with silver; nor he that loveth abundance with increase: this *is* also vanity.

11 When goods increase, they are increased that eat them: and what good *is there* to the owners thereof, saving the beholding *of them* with their eyes?

12 The sleep of a labouring man *is* sweet, whether he eat little or much: but the abundance of the rich will not suffer him to sleep.

13 There is a sore evil *which* I have seen under the sun, *namely*, riches kept for the owners thereof to their hurt.

14 But those riches perish by evil travail: and he begetteth a son, and *there is* nothing in his hand.

15 [m]As he came forth of his mother's womb, naked shall he return to go as he came, and shall take nothing of his labour, which he may carry away in his hand.

16 And this also *is* a sore evil, *that* in all points as he came, so shall he go: and what profit hath he [n]that hath laboured for the wind?

17 All his days also he eateth in darkness, and *he hath* much sorrow and wrath with his sickness.

18 Behold *that* which I have seen: [o]*it is* good and comely *for one* to eat and to drink, and to enjoy the good of all his labour that he taketh under the sun all the days of his life, which God giveth him: for it *is* his portion.

19 [p]Every man also to whom God hath given riches and wealth, and hath given

B.C. 977.

a Prov. 15:16, 17; 16:8.

b Prov. 27:20; 1 John 2:16.

c Psa. 39:6.

d Ex. 3:5.

e 1 Sam. 15:22; Psa. 50:8; Prov. 15:8; 21:27; Hos. 6:6.

f Prov. 10:19; Mt. 6:7.

g Num. 30:2; Deut. 23:21-23; Psa. 50:14; 76:11.

h Psa. 66:13, 14.

i Prov. 20:25; Acts 5:4.

j 1 Cor. 11:10.

k Heb. 1:4, *note*.

l Psa. 19:9, *note*.

m Job 1:21; Psa. 49:17; 1 Tim. 6:7.

n Prov. 11:29.

o Eccl. 2:24; 3:12, 13; 9:7; 11:9; 1 Tim. 6:17.

p Eccl. 2:24; 3:13; 6:.2.

him power to eat thereof, and to take his
portion, and to rejoice in his labour; this
is the gift of God.
20 For he shall not much remember
the days of his life; because God
answereth *him* in the joy of his heart.

CHAPTER 6.

(*The unfolding,* continued:
(3) *in view of man's inevitable end.*)

There is an evil which I have seen
under the sun, and it *is* common
among men:
2 A man to whom God hath given
riches, wealth, and honour, [a]so that he
wanteth nothing for his soul of all that
he desireth, [b]yet God giveth him not
power to eat thereof, but a stranger
eateth it: this *is* vanity, and it *is* an evil
disease.
3 If a man beget an hundred *children,*
and live many years, so that the days of
his years be many, and his soul be not
filled with good, and [c]also *that* he have
no burial; I say, *that* an untimely birth *is*
better than he.
4 For he cometh in with vanity, and
departeth in darkness, and his name
shall be covered with darkness.
5 Moreover he hath not seen the sun,
nor known *any thing*: this hath more rest
than the other.
6 Yea, though he live a thousand years
twice *told,* yet hath he seen no good: do
not all go to one place?
7 [d]All the labour of man *is* for his
mouth, and yet the [e]appetite is not filled.
8 For what hath the wise more than
the fool? what hath the poor, that
knoweth to walk before the living?
9 Better *is* the sight of the eyes [f]than
the wandering of the desire: this *is* also
vanity and vexation of spirit.
10 That which hath been is named
already, and it is known that it *is* man:
[g]neither may he contend with him that
is mightier than he.
11 Seeing there be many things that
increase vanity, what *is* man the better?
12 For who knoweth what *is* good for
man in *this* life, all the days of his vain
life which he spendeth [h]as a shadow? for
who can tell a man what shall be after
him under the sun?

CHAPTER 7.

(*The unfolding,* continued:
(4) *in view of the incurable evil of man.*)

A [i]good name *is* better than precious
ointment; and the day of death
than the day of one's birth.
2 *It is* better to go to the house of
mourning, than to go to the house of
feasting: for that *is* the end of all men;
and the living will lay *it* to his heart.
3 Sorrow *is* better than laughter: [j]for
by the sadness of the countenance the
heart is made better.
4 The heart of the wise *is* in the house
of mourning; but the heart of fools *is* in
the house of mirth.
5 [k]*It is* better to hear the rebuke of the
wise, than for a man to hear the song of
fools.
6 For as the crackling of thorns under
a pot, so *is* the laughter of the fool: this
also *is* vanity.
7 Surely oppression maketh a wise
man mad; [l]and a gift destroyeth the
heart.
8 Better *is* the end of a thing than the
beginning thereof: *and* the [m]patient in
spirit *is* better than the proud in spirit.
9 [n]Be not hasty in thy spirit to be
angry: for anger resteth in the bosom of
fools.
10 Say not thou, What is *the cause* that
the former days were better than these?
for thou dost not enquire wisely concerning this.
11 Wisdom *is* [o]good with an inheritance: and *by it there is* profit to them that
see the sun.
12 For wisdom *is* a defence, *and*
money *is* a defence: but the excellency of
knowledge *is, that* wisdom giveth life to
them that have it.
13 Consider the work of God: for who
can make *that* straight, which he hath
made crooked?
14 In the day of prosperity be joyful,
but in the day of adversity consider:
God also hath set the one over against
the other, to the end that man should
find nothing after him.
15 All *things* have I seen in the days of
my vanity: there is a just *man* that perisheth in his righteousness, and there is a
wicked *man* that prolongeth *his life* in his
wickedness.
16 [p]Be not righteous over much;
neither make thyself over wise: why

B.C. 977.

a Job 21:9; Psa. 17:14; 73:7.

b Lk. 12:20; cf. Eccl. 5:13.

c 2 Ki. 9:35; Isa. 14:19, 20; Jer. 22:19.

d Prov. 16:26.

e Heb. *soul.*

f Heb. *than the walking of the soul.*

g Job 9:32; Isa. 45:9; Jer. 49:19.

h Psa. 102:11; 109:23; 144:4; Jas. 4:14.

i Prov. 15:30; 22:1.

j 2 Cor. 7:10.

k See Psa. 141:5; Prov. 13:18; 15:31, 32.

l Ex. 23:8; Deut. 16:19.

m Prov. 14:29.

n Prov. 14:17; 16:32; Jas. 1:19.

o Or, *as good as an inheritance, yea, better too.*

p vs. 16, 17. Natural wisdom: be moderately religious and moderately wicked.

shouldest thou destroy thyself?

17 Be not over much wicked, neither be thou foolish: why shouldest thou die before thy time?

18 *It is* good that thou shouldest take hold of this; yea, also from this withdraw not thine hand: for he that feareth God shall come forth of them all.

19 Wisdom strengtheneth the wise more than ten mighty *men* which are in the city.

20 For *there is* not a [a]just [b]man upon earth, that doeth good, and sinneth not.

21 Also take no heed unto all words that are spoken; lest thou hear thy servant curse thee:

22 For oftentimes also thine own heart knoweth that thou thyself likewise hast cursed others.

23 All this have I proved by wisdom: I said, I will be wise; but it *was* far from me.

24 [c]That which is far off, and [d]exceeding deep, who can find it out?

25 I applied mine heart to know, and to search, and to seek out wisdom, and the reason *of things,* and to know the wickedness of folly, even of foolishness *and* madness:

26 And I find more bitter than death the woman, whose heart *is* snares and nets, *and* her hands *as* bands: whoso pleaseth God shall escape from her; but the sinner shall be taken by her.

27 Behold, this have I found, saith the preacher, *counting* one by one, to find out the account:

28 Which yet my soul seeketh, but I find not: one man among a thousand have I found; but a woman among all those have I not found.

29 Lo, this only have I found, that God hath made man upright; but they have sought out many inventions.

CHAPTER 8.

(The unfolding, continued: (5) *in view of the mystery of the divine providences.)*

Who *is* as the wise *man*? and who knoweth the interpretation of a thing? [e]a man's wisdom maketh his face to shine, and the [f]boldness of his face shall be changed.

2 I *counsel thee* to keep the king's commandment, and [g]*that* in regard of the oath of God.

3 Be not hasty to go out of his sight: stand not in an evil thing; for he doeth whatsoever pleaseth him.

4 Where the word of a king *is, there is* power: and [h]who may say unto him, What doest thou?

5 Whoso keepeth the commandment [i]shall feel no evil thing: and a wise man's heart discerneth both time and judgment.

6 Because to every purpose there is time and judgment, therefore the misery of man *is* great upon him.

7 [j]For he knoweth not that which shall be: for who can tell him when it shall be?

8 *There is* no man that hath power [k]over the spirit to retain the spirit; neither *hath he* power in the day of death: and *there is* no discharge in *that* war; neither shall wickedness deliver those that are given to it.

9 All this have I seen, and applied my heart unto every work that is done under the sun: *there is* a time wherein one man ruleth over another to his own hurt.

10 And so I saw the wicked buried, who had come and gone from the place of the holy, and they were forgotten in the city where they had so done: this *is* also vanity.

11 Because sentence against an evil work is not executed speedily, therefore the heart of the sons of men is fully set in them to do evil.

12 [l]Though a sinner do evil an hundred times, and his *days* be prolonged, yet surely I know that [m]it shall be well with them that [n]fear God, which fear before him:

13 But it shall not be well with the wicked, neither shall he prolong *his* days, *which are* as a shadow; because he feareth not before God.

14 There is a vanity which is done upon the earth; that there be just *men,* unto whom it happeneth according to the work of the wicked; again, there be wicked *men,* to whom it happeneth according to the work of the righteous: I said that this also *is* vanity.

15 Then I commended mirth, because a man hath no better thing under the sun, than to eat, and to drink, and to be merry: for that shall abide with him of his labour the days of his life, which God giveth him under the sun.

16 When I applied mine heart to know wisdom, and to see the business that is done upon the earth: (for also *there is that*

B.C. 977.

a *Righteousness.* Isa. 26:7. (Gen. 6:9; Lk. 2:25.)

b 1 Ki. 8:46; 2 Chr. 6:36; Prov. 20:9; Rom. 3:23; 1 John 1:8.

c Job 28:12, 20; 1 Tim. 6:16.

d Rom. 11:33.

e Prov. 4:8, 9; 17:24.

f Heb. *strength.*

g 1 Chr. 29:24; Ezk. 17:18; Rom. 13:5.

h Job 34:18.

i Heb. *shall know.*

j Eccl. 6:12; 9:12; 10:14; Prov. 24:22.

k Job 14:5.

l Isa. 65:20; Rom. 2:5.

m Psa. 37:11, 18, 19; Prov. 1:32, 33; Isa. 3:10, 11; Mt. 25:34, 41.

n Psa. 19:9, *note.*

B.C. 977.

neither day nor night seeth sleep with his eyes:)

17 Then I beheld all the work of God, that [a]a man cannot find out the work that is done under the sun: because though a man labour to seek *it* out, yet he shall not find *it*; yea further; though a wise *man* think to know *it*, [b]yet shall he not be able to find *it*.

CHAPTER 9

(The unfolding, continued: (6) *in view of the world's wrong standard of values.)*

For all this I considered in my heart even to declare all this, that the righteous, and the wise, and their works, *are* in the hand of God: no man knoweth either love or hatred *by* all *that is* before them.

2 [c]All *things come* alike to all: *there is* one event to the righteous, and to the wicked; to the good and to the clean, and to the unclean; to him that sacrificeth, and to him that sacrificeth not: as *is* the good, so *is* the sinner; *and* he that sweareth, as *he* that feareth an oath.

3 This *is* an evil among all *things* that are done under the sun, that *there is* one event unto all: yea, also the heart of the sons of men is full of evil, and madness *is* in their heart while they live, and after that *they go* to the dead.

4 For to him that is joined to all the living there is hope: for a living dog is better than a dead lion.

5 For the living know that they shall die: but the dead know not any thing, neither have they any more a reward; for the memory of them is forgotten.

6 Also their love, and their hatred, and their envy, is now perished; neither have they any more a portion for ever in any *thing* that is done under the sun.

7 Go thy way, [d]eat thy bread with joy, and drink thy wine with a merry heart; for God now accepteth thy works.

8 Let thy garments be always white; and let thy head lack no ointment.

9 [e]Live joyfully with the wife whom thou lovest all the days of the life of thy vanity, which he hath given thee under the sun, all the days of thy vanity: [f]for that *is* thy portion in *this* life, and in thy labour which thou takest under the sun.

10 Whatsoever thy hand findeth to do, do *it* with thy might; [1]for *there is* no work, nor device, nor knowledge, nor wisdom, in the [g]grave, whither thou goest.

11 I returned, and [h]saw under the sun, that the race *is* not to the swift, nor the battle to the strong, neither yet bread to the wise, nor yet riches to men of understanding, nor yet favour to men of skill; but time and chance happeneth to them all.

12 For man also knoweth not his time: as the fishes that are taken in an evil net, and as the birds that are caught in the snare; so *are* the sons of men [i]snared in an evil time, when it falleth suddenly upon them.

13 This wisdom have I seen also under the sun, and it *seemed* great unto me:

14 [j]*There was* a little city, and few men within it; and there came a great king against it, and besieged it, and built great bulwarks against it:

15 Now there was found in it a poor wise man, and he by his wisdom delivered the city; yet no man remembered that same poor man.

16 Then said I, Wisdom *is* better than strength: nevertheless [k]the poor man's wisdom *is* despised, and his words are not heard.

17 The words of wise *men are* heard in quiet more than the cry of him that ruleth among fools.

18 Wisdom *is* better than weapons of war: but [l]one sinner destroyeth much good.

a Eccl. 3:11; Job 5:9; Rom. 11:33.
b Job. 9:1, 10; Psa. 73:16.
c Job 21:7; Psa. 73:3, 12, 13; Mal. 3:15.
d Eccl. 8:15.
e Heb. *see,* or *enjoy life.*
f Eccl. 2:10, 24; 3:13, 22; 5:18.
g Heb. *Sheol.* See Hab. 2:5, *note.*
h Jer. 9:23; Amos 2:14, 15.
i Prov. 29:6; Lk. 12:20, 39; 17:26; 1 Thes. 5:3.
j See 2 Sam. 20:16, 22.
k Mk. 6:2, 3.
l Josh. 7:1, 11, 12.

1(9:10) Verse 10 is no more a divine revelation concerning the state of the dead than any other conclusion of "the Preacher" (Eccl. 1:1) is such a revelation. Reasoning from the standpoint of man "under the sun," the natural man can see no difference between a dead man and a dead lion (v. 4). A living dog is better than either. No one would quote verse 2 as a divine revelation. These reasonings of man apart from divine revelation are set down by inspiration just as the words of Satan (Gen. 3:4; Job 2:4, 5, etc.) are so set down. But that life and consciousness continue between death and resurrection is directly affirmed in Scripture (Isa. 14:9-11; Mt. 22:32; Mk. 9:43-48; Lk. 16:19-31; John 11:26; 2 Cor. 5:6-8; Phil. 1:21-23; Rev. 6:9-11).

CHAPTER 10.

(The unfolding, continued:
(7) *in view of the anarchy of the world.)*

Dead flies cause the ointment of the
apothecary to send forth a stinking
savour: *so doth* a little folly him that is in
reputation for wisdom *and* honour.
2 A wise man's heart *is* at his right
hand; but a fool's heart at his left.
3 Yea also, when he that is a fool
walketh by the way, [a]his wisdom faileth
him, and [b]he saith to every one *that* he *is* a
fool.
4 If the spirit of the ruler rise up
against thee, leave not thy place; for
[c]yielding pacifieth great offences.
5 There is an evil *which* I have seen
under the sun, as an error *which* proceedeth from the ruler:
6 Folly is set in great dignity, and the
rich sit in low place.
7 I have seen servants upon horses,
and princes walking as servants upon
the earth.
8 [d]He that diggeth a pit shall fall into
it; and whoso breaketh an hedge, a serpent shall bite him.
9 Whoso removeth stones shall be hurt
therewith; *and* he that cleaveth wood
shall be endangered thereby.
10 If the iron be blunt, and he do not
whet the edge, then must he put to more
strength: but wisdom *is* profitable to
direct.
11 Surely the serpent will bite [e]without
enchantment; and a babbler is no better.
12 The words of a wise man's mouth
are gracious; but the lips of a fool will
swallow up himself.
13 The beginning of the words of his
mouth *is* foolishness: and the end of his
talk *is* mischievous madness.
14 A fool also is full of words: a man
cannot tell what shall be; and what shall
be after him, who can tell him?
15 The labour of the foolish wearieth
every one of them, because he knoweth
not how to go to the city.
16 [f]Woe to thee, O land, when thy
king *is* a child, and thy princes eat in the
morning!
17 Blessed *art* thou, O land, when thy
king *is* the son of nobles, and [g]thy
princes eat in due season, for strength,
and not for drunkenness!
18 By much slothfulness the building
decayeth; and through idleness of the
hands the house droppeth through.
19 A feast is made for laughter, and
[h]wine maketh merry: but money
answereth all *things.*
20 [i]Curse not the king, no not in thy
thought; and curse not the rich in thy
bedchamber: for a bird of the air shall
carry the voice, and that which hath
wings shall tell the matter.

CHAPTER 11.

Part IV. The best thing possible
to the natural man.

Cast thy bread [j]upon the waters: [k]for
thou shalt find it after many days.
2 [l]Give a portion to seven, and also to
eight; for thou knowest not what evil
shall be upon the earth.
3 If the clouds be full of rain, they
empty *themselves* upon the earth: and if
the tree fall toward the south, or toward
the north, in the place where the tree
falleth, there it shall be.
4 He that observeth the wind shall not
sow; and he that regardeth the clouds
shall not reap.
5 As [m]thou knowest not what *is* the
way of the spirit, [n]*nor* how the bones *do*
grow in the womb of her that is with
child: even so thou knowest not the
works of God who maketh all.
6 In the morning sow thy seed, and in
the evening withhold not thine hand: for
thou knowest not whether [o]shall prosper, either this or that, or whether they
both *shall be* alike good.
7 Truly the light *is* sweet, and a pleasant
thing it is for the eyes [p]to behold the sun:
8 But if a man live many years, *and*
rejoice in them all; yet let him remember
the days of darkness; for they shall be
many. All that cometh *is* vanity.
9 Rejoice, O young man, in thy youth;
and let thy heart cheer thee in the days of
thy youth, and [q]walk in the ways of
thine heart, and in the sight of thine eyes:
but know thou, that for all these *things*
[r]God will bring thee into judgment.
10 Therefore remove sorrow from thy
heart, and [s]put away evil from thy flesh:
for childhood and youth *are* vanity.

B.C. 977.

a Heb. *his heart.*
b Prov. 13:16; 18:2.
c 1 Sam. 25:24; Prov. 25:15.
d Psa. 7:15; Prov. 26:27.
e Psa. 58:4, 5; Jer. 8:17.
f Isa. 3:4, 5, 12; 5:11.
g Prov. 31:4.
h Psa. 104:15.
i Ex. 22:28; Acts 23:5.
j Isa. 32:20.
k Deut. 15:10; Prov. 19:17; Mt. 10:42; 2 Cor. 9:8; Gal. 6:9, 10; Heb. 6:10.
l Psa. 112:9; Lk. 6:30; 1 Tim. 6:18, 19.
m John 3:8.
n Psa. 139:14, 15.
o Heb. *shall be right.*
p Eccl. 7:11.
q Num. 15:39.
r Eccl. 12:14; Rom. 2:6-11.
s 2 Cor. 7:1; 2 Tim. 2:22.

B.C. 977.

CHAPTER 12.

(The best thing possible to the natural man.)

Remember [a]now thy Creator in the days of thy youth, while the evil days come not, nor the years draw nigh, [b]when thou shalt say, I have no pleasure in them;

2 While the sun, or the light, or the moon, or the stars, be not darkened, nor the clouds return after the rain:

3 In the day when the keepers of the house shall tremble, and the strong men shall bow themselves, and the grinders cease because they are few, and those that look out of the windows be darkened,

4 And the doors shall be shut in the streets, when the sound of the grinding is low, and he shall rise up at the voice of the bird, and all the [c]daughters of musick shall be brought low;

5 Also *when* they shall be afraid of *that which is* high, and fears *shall be* in the way, and the almond tree shall flourish, and the grasshopper shall be a burden, and desire shall fail: because man goeth to [d]his long home, and the [e]mourners go about the streets:

6 Or ever the silver cord be loosed, or the golden bowl be broken, or the pitcher be broken at the fountain, or the wheel broken at the cistern.

7 [f]Then shall the dust return to the earth as it was: and [g]the spirit shall return unto God [h]who gave it.

8 Vanity of vanities, saith the preacher; all *is* vanity.

9 And moreover, because the preacher was wise, he still taught the people knowledge; yea, he gave good heed, and sought out, *and* [i]set in order many proverbs.

10 The preacher sought to find out acceptable words: and *that which was* written *was* upright, *even* words of truth.

11 The words of the wise *are* as goads, and as nails fastened *by* the masters of assemblies, *which* are given from one shepherd.

12 And further, by these, my son, be admonished: of making many books *there is* no end; and much study *is* a weariness of the flesh.

Part V. The best thing possible to man under the law.

13 Let us hear the conclusion of the whole matter: [j]Fear God, and keep his commandments: for this *is* the whole *duty* of man.

14 For [k]God shall bring every work into judgment, with every secret thing, whether *it be* good, or whether *it be* evil.

a Prov. 22:6; Lam. 3:27.

b See 2 Sam. 19:35.

c 2 Sam. 19:35.

d Job 17:13.

e Jer. 9:17.

f Gen. 3:19; Job 34:15; Psa. 90:3.

g Eccl. 3:21.

h Num. 16:22; 27:16; Job 34:14; Isa. 57:16; Zech. 12:1.

i 1 Ki. 4:32.

j Deut. 6:2; 10:12; Psa. 19:9, *note.*

k Eccl. 11:9; Mt. 12:36; Acts 17:30, 31; Rom. 2:16; 14:10-12; 1 Cor. 4:5; 2 Cor. 5:10.

THE SONG OF SOLOMON

NOWHERE in Scripture does the unspiritual mind tread upon ground so mysterious and incomprehensible as in this book, while the saintliest men and women of the ages have found it a source of pure and exquisite delight. That the love of the divine Bridegroom should follow all the analogies of the marriage relation seems evil only to minds so ascetic that marital desire itself seems to them unholy.

The interpretation is twofold: Primarily, the book is the expression of pure marital love as ordained of God in creation, and the vindication of that love as against both asceticism and lust—the two profanations of the holiness of marriage. The secondary and larger interpretation is of Christ, the Son and His heavenly bride, the Church (2 Cor. 11:1-4, *refs.*).

In this sense the book has six divisions: I. The bride seen in restful communion with the Bridegroom, 1:1–2:7. II. A lapse and restoration, 2:8–3:5. III. Joy of fellowship, 3:6–5:1. IV. Separation of interest—the bride satisfied, the Bridegroom toiling for others, 5:2-5. V. The bride seeking and witnessing, 5:6–6:3. VI. Unbroken communion, 6:4–8:14.

CHAPTER 1.

B.C. 1014.

Part I. The bride and Bridegroom in joyful [1]*communion* (to 2:7).

The [a]song of songs, which *is* Solomon's.

2 Let him kiss me with the kisses of his mouth: [b]for thy love *is* better than wine.

3 Because of the savour of thy good ointments thy name *is as* ointment poured forth, therefore do the virgins love thee.

4 [c]Draw me, [d]we will run after thee: the king [e]hath brought me into his chambers: we will be glad and rejoice in thee, we will remember thy love more than wine: the upright love thee.

5 I *am* black, but comely, O ye daughters of Jerusalem, as the tents of Kedar, as the curtains of Solomon.

6 Look not upon me, because I *am* black, because the sun hath looked upon me: my mother's children were angry with me; they made me the keeper of the vineyards; *but* mine own vineyard have I not kept.

7 Tell me, O thou whom my soul loveth, where thou feedest, where thou makest *thy flock* to rest at noon: for why should I be [f]as one that turneth aside by the flocks of thy companions?

8 If thou know not, O thou fairest among women, go thy way forth by the footsteps of the flock, and feed thy kids beside the shepherds' tents.

9 I have compared thee, [g]O my love, to a company of horses in Pharaoh's chariots.

10 [h]Thy cheeks are comely with rows *of jewels*, thy neck with chains *of gold*.

11 We will make thee borders of gold with studs of silver.

12 While the king *sitteth* at his table, my spikenard sendeth forth the smell thereof.

13 A bundle of myrrh *is* my well-beloved unto me; he shall lie all night betwixt my breasts.

14 My beloved *is* unto me *as* a cluster of [i]camphire in the vineyards of En-gedi.

15 [j]Behold, thou *art* fair, my love; behold, thou *art* fair; thou *hast* doves' eyes.

16 Behold, thou *art* fair, my beloved, yea, pleasant: also our bed *is* green.

17 The beams of our house *are* cedar, *and* our rafters of fir.

CHAPTER 2.

I *am* the rose of Sharon, *and* the lily of the valleys.

a 1 Ki. 4:32.

b Song 4:10.

c Hos. 11:4; John 6:44; 12:32.

d Phil. 3:12-14.

e Psa. 45:14, 15; John 14:2; Eph. 2:6.

f Or, *as one that is veiled.*

g Song 2:2, 10, 13; 4:1, 7; 5:2; 6:4; John 15:14, 15.

h Ezk. 16:11-13.

i Or, *cypress.* Song 4:13.

j Song 4:1; 5:12.

[1]**(1, heading)** It is most comforting to see that all these tender thoughts of Christ are for His bride in her unperfected state. The varied exercises of her heart are part of that inner discipline suggested by Eph. 5:25-27.

B.C. 1014.

2 As the lily among thorns, [1]so *is* my
love among the daughters.
3 As the apple tree among the trees of
the wood, so *is* my beloved among the
sons. I sat down under his shadow with
great delight, and [a]his fruit *was* sweet to
my taste.
4 He brought me to the banqueting
house, and his banner over me *was* love.
5 Stay me with flagons, comfort me
with apples: for I *am* sick of love.
6 [b]His left hand *is* under my head, and
his right hand doth embrace me.
7 [c]I charge you, O ye daughters of
Jerusalem, by the roes, and by the hinds
of the field, that ye stir not up, nor
awake *my* love, till he please.

Part II. A lapse and restoration (to 3:5).

8 The voice of my beloved! behold, he
cometh leaping upon the mountains,
skipping upon the hills.
9 My beloved is like a roe or a young
hart: behold, he standeth behind [2]our
wall, he looketh forth at the windows,
[d]shewing himself through the lattice.
10 My beloved spake, and said unto
me, Rise up, my love, my fair one, and
come away.
11 For, lo, the winter is past, the rain is
over *and* gone;
12 The flowers appear on the earth;
the time of the singing *of birds* is come,
and the voice of the turtle is heard in our
land;
13 The fig tree putteth forth her green
figs, and the vines *with* the tender grape
give a *good* smell. [e]Arise, my love, my
fair one, and come away.
14 O my [3]dove, *that art* in the clefts of
the rock, in the secret [f]*places* of the stairs,
let me see thy countenance, let me hear
thy voice; for sweet *is* thy voice, and thy
countenance *is* comely.
15 Take us [g]the foxes, the little foxes,
that spoil the vines: for our vines *have*
tender grapes.
16 [h]My beloved *is* mine, and I *am* his:
he feedeth among the lilies.
17 [i]Until the day break, and the shadows flee away, turn, my beloved, and be
thou [j]like a roe or a young hart upon the
mountains of Bether.

CHAPTER 3.

By [k]night on my bed I sought him
whom my soul loveth: I sought
him, but I found him not.
2 I will rise now, and go about the city
in the streets, and in the broad ways I
will seek him whom my soul loveth: I
sought him, but I found him not.
3 [l]The watchmen that go about the
city found me: *to whom I said,* Saw ye
him whom my soul loveth?
4 *It was* but a little that I passed from
them, but I found him whom my soul
loveth: I held him, and would not let
him go, until I had brought him into my
mother's house, and into the chamber of
her that conceived me.
5 [m]I charge you, O ye daughters of
Jerusalem, by the roes, and by the hinds
of the field, that ye stir not up, nor
awake *my* love, till he please.

Part III. Happy communion (to 5:1):
the bride speaks.

6 [n]Who *is* this that cometh out of the
wilderness like pillars of smoke, perfumed with myrrh and frankincense,
with all powders of the merchant?
7 Behold his bed, which *is* Solomon's;
threescore valiant men *are* about it, of
the valiant of Israel.

a Song 4:16; cf. Rev. 22:1, 2.
b Song 8:3.
c Song 3:5; 8:4.
d Heb. *flourishing.*
e v. 10.
f Omit *places.*
g Psa. 80:13; Ezk. 13:4; Lk. 13:32.
h Song 6:3; 7:10.
i Song 4:6.
j v. 9; Song 8:14.
k Isa. 26:9.
l Song 5:7.
m Song 2:7; 8:4.
n Song 8:5.

[1] **(2:2)** How poor are the similes of the bride as compared with those of the Bridegroom. To Him she is a "lily among *thorns*"; she can only say that He is "as the apple tree among the trees of the wood."

[2] **(2:9)** "*Our* wall." The bride had returned to her own home: the Bridegroom seeks her.

[3] **(2:14)** There is a beautiful order here. First we have what the bride is as seen in Christ, "My dove." In herself most faulty; in Him "blameless and harmless" (Phil. 2:15), the very character of the dove. Then the bride's place of *safety*, "in the clefts of the rock"—hidden, so to speak, in the wounds of Christ. Thirdly, her *privilege*. "Stairs" speaks of access. It is not "secret *places*,' as in A.V., but "the secret of the stairs"—the way and privilege of access to His presence (Eph. 2:18; Col. 3:1; Heb. 10:19-22). Fourthly, the order of approach: she is to come near before she speaks, "Let Me see thy countenance," then "Let Me hear thy voice." Lastly, now that she is near and has spoken, He speaks a tender word of admonition: "Take us the foxes," etc.

8 They all hold swords, *being* expert in war: every man *hath* his sword upon his thigh because of fear in the night.

9 King Solomon made himself a chariot of the wood of Lebanon.

10 He made the pillars thereof *of* silver, the bottom thereof *of* gold, the covering of it *of* purple, the midst thereof being paved *with* love, for the daughters of Jerusalem.

11 Go forth, O ye daughters of Zion, and behold king Solomon with the crown wherewith his mother crowned him in the day of his espousals, and in the day of the gladness of his heart.

CHAPTER 4.

The Bridegroom speaks.

Behold, [a]thou *art* fair, my love; behold, thou *art* fair; thou *hast* doves' eyes within thy locks: thy hair *is* as a [b]flock of goats, that appear from mount Gilead.

2 [c]Thy teeth *are* like a flock *of sheep that are even* shorn, which came up from the washing; whereof every one bear twins, and none *is* barren among them.

3 Thy lips *are* like a thread of scarlet, and thy speech *is* comely: thy [d]temples *are* like a piece of a pomegranate within thy locks.

4 [e]Thy neck *is* like the tower of David builded for an [f]armoury, whereon there hang a thousand bucklers, all shields of mighty men.

5 [g]Thy two breasts *are* like two young roes that are twins, which feed among the lilies.

6 [h]Until the day [i]break, and the shadows flee away, I will get me to the mountain of myrrh, and to the hill of frankincense.

7 [j]Thou *art* all fair, my love; *there is* no spot in thee.

8 Come with me from Lebanon, *my* spouse, with me from Lebanon: look from the top of Amana, from the top of Shenir [k]and Hermon, from the lions' dens, from the mountains of the leopards.

B.C. 1014.

a Song 1:15; 5:12.
b Song 6:5.
c Song 6:6.
d Song 6:7.
e Song 7:4.
f Neh. 3:19.
g Song 7:3. See Prov. 5:19.
h Song 2:17.
i Heb. *breathe.*
j Eph. 5:27.
k Deut. 3:9.
l Or, *taken away my heart.*
m Song 5:1; Prov. 24:13, 14.
n Gen. 27:27; Hos. 14:6, 7.
o Heb. *barred.*
p John 4:10; 7:38.
q Song 5:1.
r Song 4:16.
s Song 4:11.

9 Thou hast [l]ravished my heart, my [1]sister, *my* spouse; thou hast ravished my heart with one of thine eyes, with one chain of thy neck.

10 How fair is thy love, my sister, *my* spouse! how much better is thy love than wine! and the smell of thine ointments than all spices!

11 Thy lips, O *my* spouse, drop *as* the honeycomb: [m]honey and milk *are* under thy tongue; and the smell of thy garments *is* [n]like the smell of Lebanon.

12 A garden [o]inclosed *is* my sister, *my* spouse; a spring shut up, a fountain sealed.

13 Thy plants *are* an orchard of pomegranates, with pleasant fruits; camphire, with spikenard,

14 Spikenard and saffron; calamus and cinnamon, with all trees of frankincense; myrrh and aloes, with all the chief spices:

15 A fountain of gardens, [p]a well of living waters, and streams from Lebanon.

The bride speaks.

16 Awake, O north wind; and come, thou south; blow upon my garden, *that* the spices thereof may flow out. [q]Let my beloved come into his garden, and eat his pleasant fruits.

CHAPTER 5.

The Bridegroom replies.

I [r]am come into my garden, my sister, *my* spouse: I have gathered my myrrh with my spice; [s]I have eaten my honeycomb with my honey; I have drunk my wine with my milk: eat, O friends; drink, yea, drink abundantly, O beloved.

Part IV. A separation of interest: the bride speaks (to v. 5).

2 I [2]sleep, but my heart waketh: *it is* the voice of my beloved that knocketh,

[1] **(4:9)** The word "sister" here is of infinitely delicate significance, intimating the very whiteness of purity in the midst of an ardour which is, like the shekinah, aglow but unspeakably holy. Sin has almost deprived us of the capacity even to stand with unshod feet before this burning bush.

[2] **(5:2)** The bride is satisfied with her washed feet while the Bridegroom, His "head filled with dew," and His "locks with the drops of the night," is toiling for others. See Lk. 6:12; 14:21-23. The state of the bride is not one of sin, but of neglect of service. She is preoccupied with the graces and perfections which she has in Christ through the Spirit (1 Cor. 12:4-11; Gal. 5:22, 23). It is mysticism, unbalanced by the activities of the Christian warfare. Her feet are washed, her hands drop with sweet-smelling myrrh; but He has gone on, and now she must seek Him (cf. Lk. 2:44, 45).

saying, Open to me, my sister, my love,
my dove, my undefiled: for my head is
filled with dew, *and* my locks with the
drops of the night.
3 I have put off my coat; how shall I
put it on? I have washed my feet; how
shall I defile them?
4 My beloved put in his hand by the
hole *of the door*, and my bowels were
moved for him.
5 I rose up to open to my beloved; and
my hands dropped *with* myrrh, and my
fingers *with* sweet smelling myrrh, upon
the handles of the lock.

Part V. The seeking bride (to 6:3).

6 I opened to my beloved; but my
beloved had withdrawn himself, *and*
was gone: my soul failed when he spake:
I sought [1]him, but I could not find him; I
called him, but he gave me no answer.
7 [a]The watchmen that went about the
city found me, they smote me, they
wounded me; the keepers of the walls
took away my veil from me.
8 I charge you, O daughters of
Jerusalem, if ye find my beloved, that ye
tell him, that I *am* sick of love.

The daughters of Jerusalem speak.

9 What *is* thy beloved more than *another*
beloved, [b]O thou fairest among women?
what *is* thy beloved more than *another*
beloved, that thou dost so charge us?

The bride answers.

10 My beloved *is* white and ruddy, the
[c]chiefest among ten thousand.
11 His head *is as* the most fine gold,
his locks *are* bushy, *and* black as a raven.
12 [d]His eyes *are* as *the eyes* of doves by
the rivers of waters, washed with milk,
and [e]fitly set.
13 His cheeks *are* as a bed of spices, *as*
sweet flowers: his lips *like* lilies, dropping sweet smelling myrrh.
14 His hands *are as* gold rings set with
the beryl: his belly *is as* bright ivory
overlaid *with* sapphires.
15 His legs *are as* pillars of marble, set
upon sockets of fine gold: his countenance
is as Lebanon, excellent as the cedars.

B.C. 1014.

a Song 3:3.
b Song 1:8.
c Heb. *a standard bearer.*
d Song 1:15; 4:1.
e Heb. *sitting in fulness;* i.e. fitly placed, and set as a precious stone in the foil of a ring.
f Song 1:8; 5:9.
g Song 2:16; 7:10.
h Song 4:1.
i Song 4:2.
j Song 4:3.
k v. 4.
l Song 7:12.

16 His mouth *is* most sweet: yea, he *is*
altogether lovely. This *is* my beloved,
and this *is* my friend, O daughters of
Jerusalem.

CHAPTER 6.

The daughters of Jerusalem speak.

Whither is thy beloved gone, [f]O thou
fairest among women? whither is
thy beloved turned aside? that [2]we may
seek him with thee.

The bride answers.

2 My beloved is gone down into his
garden, to the beds of spices, to feed in
the gardens, and to gather lilies.
3 [g]I *am* my beloved's, and my beloved
is mine: he feedeth among the lilies.

Part VI. Unbroken communion
(to the end): *the Bridegroom speaks.*

4 Thou *art* beautiful, O my love, as
Tirzah, comely as Jerusalem, terrible as
an army with banners.
5 Turn away thine eyes from me, for
they have overcome me: thy hair *is* [h]as a
flock of goats that appear from Gilead.
6 [i]Thy teeth *are* as a flock of sheep
which go up from the washing, whereof
every one beareth twins, and *there is* not
one barren among them.
7 [j]As a piece of a pomegranate *are* thy
temples within thy locks.
8 There are threescore queens, and
fourscore concubines, and virgins without number.
9 My dove, my undefiled is *but* one;
she *is* the *only* one of her mother, she *is*
the choice *one* of her that bare her. The
daughters saw her, and blessed her; *yea*,
the queens and the concubines, and they
praised her.
10 Who *is* she *that* looketh forth as the
morning, fair as the moon, clear as the
sun, [k]*and* terrible as *an army* with banners?
11 I went down into the garden of nuts
to see the fruits of the valley, *and* [l]to see
whether the vine flourished, *and* the
pomegranates budded.

[1] **(5:6)** Observe, it is now the Bridegroom Himself who occupies her heart, not His gifts—myrrh and washed feet (John 13:2-9).

[2] **(6:1)** So soon as the bride witnesses to the Bridegroom's own personal loveliness, a desire is awakened in the daughters of Jerusalem to seek Him.

B.C. 1014.

12 Or ever I was aware, my soul [a]made
me *like* the chariots of Amminadib.
13 Return, return, O Shulamite; return,
return, that we may look upon thee.
What will ye see in the Shulamite? As it
were the company [b]of two armies.

CHAPTER 7.

How beautiful are thy feet with
shoes, [c]O prince's daughter! the
joints of thy thighs *are* like jewels, the
work of the hands of a cunning workman.
2 Thy navel *is like* a round goblet, *which*
wanteth not [d]liquor: thy belly *is like* an
heap of wheat set about with lilies.
3 Thy two breasts *are* like two young
roes *that are* twins.
4 Thy neck *is* as a tower of ivory; thine
eyes *like* the fishpools in Heshbon, by the
gate of Bath-rabbim: thy nose *is* as the
tower of Lebanon which looketh toward
Damascus.
5 Thine head upon thee *is* like
[e]Carmel, and the hair of thine head like
purple; the king *is* [f]held in the galleries.
6 How fair and how pleasant art thou,
O love, for delights!
7 This thy stature is like to a palm tree,
and thy breasts to clusters *of grapes*.
8 I said, I will go up to the palm tree, I
will take hold of the boughs thereof: now
also thy breasts shall be as clusters of the
vine, and the smell of thy nose like apples;
9 And the roof of thy mouth like the
best wine for my beloved, that goeth
down sweetly, causing the lips [g]of those
that are asleep to speak.

The bride speaks.

10 I *am* my beloved's, and [h]his desire
is toward me.
11 Come, my beloved, let us go forth
into the field; let us lodge in the villages.
12 Let us get up early to the vineyards;
let us see if the vine flourish, *whether* the
tender grape appear, *and* the pomegranates bud forth: there will I give thee my
loves.
13 The [i]mandrakes give a smell, and
at our gates [j]*are* all manner of pleasant
fruits, new and old, *which* I have laid up
for thee, O my beloved.

CHAPTER 8.

O that thou *wert* as my brother, that
sucked the breasts of my mother!
when I should find thee without, I would
kiss thee; yea, I should not be despised.
2 I would lead thee, *and* bring thee into
my mother's house, *who* would instruct
me: I would cause thee to drink of spiced
wine of the juice of my pomegranate.
3 His left hand *should be* under my
head, and his right hand should
embrace me.
4 [k]I charge you, O daughters of
Jerusalem, that ye stir not up, nor awake
my love, until he please.

The Bridegroom speaks.

5 Who *is* this that cometh up from the
wilderness, leaning upon her beloved? I
raised thee up under the apple tree: there
thy mother brought thee forth: there she
brought thee forth *that* bare thee.
6 [l]Set me as a seal upon thine heart, as
a seal upon thine arm: for love *is* strong
as death; [m]jealousy *is* cruel as the [n]grave:
the coals thereof *are* coals of fire, *which*
hath a most vehement flame.
7 Many waters cannot quench love, neither can the floods drown it: if *a* man
would give all the substance of his house
for love, it would utterly be contemned.

The bride speaks.

8 [o]We have a little sister, and she hath
no breasts: what shall we do for our sister
in the day when she shall be spoken for?

The Bridegroom speaks.

9 If she *be* a wall, we will build upon
her a palace of silver: and if she *be* a door,
we will inclose her with boards of cedar.

The bride speaks.

10 I *am* a wall, and my breasts like
towers: then was I in his eyes as one that
found [p]favour.
11 Solomon had a vineyard at Baal-
hamon; [q]he let out the vineyard unto
keepers; every one for the fruit thereof
was to bring a thousand *pieces* of silver.
12 My vineyard, which *is* mine, *is*
before me: thou, O Solomon, *must have* a
thousand, and those that keep the fruit
thereof two hundred.
13 Thou that dwellest in the gardens,
the companions hearken to thy voice:
cause me to hear *it*.
14 [r]Make haste, my beloved, and be
thou like to a roe or to a young hart
upon the mountains of spices.

a Or, *set me on the chariots of my willing people.*
b Or, *of Mahanaim.* Gen. 32:2.
c Psa. 45:13.
d Heb. *mixture.*
e Or, *crimson.*
f Heb. *bound.*
g Or, *of the ancient.*
h Psa. 45:11.
i Gen. 30:14.
j Mt. 13:52.
k Song 2:7; 3:5.
l Isa. 49:16; Jer. 22:24; Hag. 2:23.
m Prov. 6:34-35.
n Heb. *Sheol.* See Hab. 2:5, *note.*
o The reference here is obscure.
p Heb. *peace.*
q Mt. 21:33.
r See Rev. 22:17, 20.

HOW TO USE THE SUBJECT REFERENCES.

THE subject references lead the reader from the first clear mention of a great truth to the last. The first and last references (in parenthesis) are repeated each time, so that wherever a reader comes upon a subject he may recur to the first reference and follow the subject, or turn at once to the Summary at the last reference.

ILLUSTRATION
(at Mark 1:1.)

b Gospel. vs. 1,
14, 15; Mk. 8:35.
(Gen. 12:1-3;
Rev. 14:6.)

Here *Gospel* is the subject; vs. 1, 14, 15 show where it is at that particular place; Mk. 8:35 is the next reference in the chain, and the references in parenthesis are the first and last.

THE PROPHETICAL BOOKS.

PROPHETS were men raised up of God in times of declension and apostasy in Israel. They were primarily revivalists and patriots, speaking on behalf of God to the heart and conscience of the nation. The prophetic messages have a twofold character: first, that which was local and for the prophet's time; secondly, that which was predictive of the divine purpose in the future. Often the prediction springs immediately from the local circumstance (e.g. Isa. 7:1-11 with vs. 12-14).

It is necessary to keep this Israelitish character of the prophet in mind. Usually his predictive, equally with his local and immediate ministry, is not didactic and abstract, but has in view the covenant people, their sin and failure, and their glorious future. The Gentile is mentioned as used for the chastisement of Israel, as judged therefor, but also as sharing the grace that is yet to be shown toward Israel. The Church, corporately, is not in the vision of the O.T. prophet (Eph. 3:1-6). The future blessing of Israel as a nation rests upon the Palestinian Covenant of restoration and conversion (Deut. 30:1-9, *refs.*), and the Davidic Covenant of the Kingship of the Messiah, David's Son (2 Sam. 7:8-17, *refs.*), and this gives to predictive prophecy its Messianic character. The exaltation of Israel is secured in the kingdom, and the kingdom takes its power to bless from the Person of the King, David's Son, but also "Immanuel."

But as the King is also Son of Abraham (Mt. 1:1), the promised Redeemer, and as redemption is only through the sacrifice of Christ, so Messianic prophecy of necessity presents Christ in a twofold character—a suffering Messiah (e.g. Isa. 53), and a reigning Messiah (e.g. Isa. 11). This duality, suffering and glory, weakness and power, involved a mystery which perplexed the prophets (1 Pet. 1:10-12; Lk. 24:26, 27).

The solution of that mystery lies, as the New Testament makes clear, in the two advents—the first advent to redemption through suffering; the second advent to the kingdom in glory, when the national promises to Israel will be fulfilled (Mt. 1:21-23; Lk. 2:28-35; 24:46-48, with Lk. 1:31-33, 68-75; Mt. 2:2, 6; 19:27, 28; Acts 2:30-32; 15:14-16). The prophets indeed describe the advent in two forms which could not be contemporaneous (e.g. Zech. 9:9; *contra,* 14:1-9), but to them it was not revealed that between the advent to suffering, and the advent to glory, would be accomplished certain "mysteries of the kingdom" (Mt. 13:11-16), nor that, consequent upon Messiah's rejection, the New Testament Church would be called out. These were, to them, "mysteries hid in God" (Eph. 3:1-10).

Speaking broadly, then, *predictive* prophecy is occupied with the fulfilment of the Palestinian and Davidic Covenants; the Abrahamic Covenant having also its place.

Gentile powers are mentioned as connected with Israel, but prophecy, save in Daniel, Obadiah, Jonah, and Nahum, is not *occupied* with Gentile world-history. Daniel, as will be seen, has a distinctive character.

The predictions of the restoration from the Babylonian captivity at the end of seventy years, must be distinguished from those of the restoration from the present world-wide dispersion. The context is always clear. The Palestinian Covenant (Deut. 28:1–30:9) is the mould of predictive prophecy in its larger sense—national disobedience, world-wide dispersion, repentance, the return of the Lord, the regathering of Israel and establishment of the kingdom, the conversion and blessing of Israel, and the judgment of Israel's oppressors.

The true division of the prophets is into *pre-exilic,* viz., in Judah: Isaiah, Jeremiah (extending into the exile), Joel, Obadiah, Micah, Nahum, Habakkuk, Zephaniah. In Israel: Hosea, Amos, and Jonah. *Exilic,* Ezekiel and Daniel, both of Judah, but prophesying to the whole nation. *Post-exilic,* all of Judah: Haggai, Zechariah, and Malachi. The division into major and minor prophetic writings, based upon the mere bulk of the books, is unhistoric and non-chronological.

The keys which unlock the meanings of prophecy are: the *two advents of Messiah,* the advent to suffer (Gen. 3:15; Acts 1:9), and the advent to reign (Deut. 30:3; Acts 1:9-11); the doctrine of the *Remnant* (Isa. 10:20, *refs.*), the doctrine of the *day of the* LORD (Isa. 2:10-22; Rev. 19:11-21), and the doctrine of the *Kingdom* (O.T., Gen. 1:26-28; Zech. 12:8, *note;* N.T., Lk. 1:31-33; 1 Cor. 15:28, *note*). The pivotal chapters, taking prophecy as a whole, are, Deut. 28, 29, 30; Psa. 2; Dan. 2, 7.

The whole scope of prophecy must be taken into account in determining the meaning of any particular passage (2 Pet. 1:20). Hence the importance of first mastering the great themes above indicated, which, in this edition of the Scriptures, may readily be done by tracing through the body of the prophetic writings the subjects mentioned in the preceding paragraph. The detail of the "time of the end," upon which all prophecy converges, will be more clearly understood if to those subjects the student adds the *Beast* (Dan. 7:8; Rev. 19:20), and *Armageddon* (Rev. 16:14; 19:17, *note*).

CHRONOLOGICAL ORDER OF THE PROPHETS,

ACCORDING TO USSHER.

I. Prophets Before the Exile.

(1) To Nineveh.

Jonah, 862 B.C.

(2) To the 10 tribes "Israel."

Amos, 787 B.C.
Hosea, 785–725 B.C.
Obadiah, 887 B.C.
Joel, 800 B.C.

(3) To Judah.

Isaiah, 760–698 B.C.
Micah, 750–710 B.C.
Nahum, 713 B.C.
Habakkuk, 626 B.C.
Zephaniah, 630 B.C.
Jeremiah, 629–588 B.C.

II. Prophets During the Exile.

Ezekiel, 595–574 B.C.
Daniel, 607–534 B.C.

III. Prophets After the Exile.

Haggai, 520 B.C.
Zechariah, 520–518 B.C.
Malachi, 397 B.C.

THE BOOK OF THE PROPHET
ISAIAH

ISAIAH is justly accounted the chief of the writing prophets. He has the more comprehensive testimony and is distinctively the prophet of redemption. Nowhere else in the Scriptures written under the law have we so clear a view of grace. The New Testament Church does not appear (Eph. 3:3-10), but Messiah in His Person and sufferings, and the blessing of the Gentiles through Him, are in full vision.

Apart from his testimony to his own time, which includes warnings of coming judgments upon the great nations of that day, the predictive messages of Isaiah cover seven great themes: I. Israel in exile and divine judgment upon Israel's oppressors. II. The return from Babylon. III. The manifestation of Messiah in humiliation (e.g. chap. 53). IV. The blessing of the Gentiles. V. The manifestation of Messiah in judgment ("the day of vengeance of our God"). VI. The reign of David's righteous Branch in the kingdom-age. VII. The new heavens and the new earth.

Isaiah is in two chief divisions: I. Looking toward the captivities, 1:1–39:8. Key verses, 1:1, 2. II. Looking beyond the captivities, 40:1–66:24. Key verses, 40:1, 2. These chief divisions fall into subdivisions, as indicated in the text.

The events recorded in Isaiah cover a period of 62 years (Ussher).

PART I. LOOKING TOWARD THE CAPTIVITIES: CHAPTERS 1–39

CHAPTER 1.

Jehovah's case against Judah (vs. 1-24).

The [a]vision of Isaiah the son of Amoz,
which he saw concerning Judah and
Jerusalem in the days [b]of Uzziah,
Jotham, Ahaz, *and* Hezekiah, kings of
Judah.
2 [1]Hear, [c]O heavens, and give ear, O
earth: for the LORD hath spoken, I have
nourished and brought up [d]children,
and they have rebelled against me.
3 The ox knoweth his owner, and the
ass his master's crib: *but* Israel [e]doth not
know, my people doth not consider.
4 Ah sinful nation, a people laden
with iniquity, a [f]seed of evildoers, children that are corrupters: they have forsaken the LORD, they have provoked the
Holy One of Israel unto anger, they are
gone away backward.
5 [g]Why should ye be stricken any
more? ye will revolt more and more: the
whole head is sick, and the whole heart
faint.
6 From the sole of the foot even unto
the head *there is* no soundness in it; *but*
wounds, and bruises, and putrifying
sores: they have not been closed, neither
bound up, neither mollified with ointment.
7 [h]Your country *is* desolate, your cities
are burned with fire: your land, strangers
devour it in your presence, and *it is* desolate, as overthrown by strangers.
8 And the daughter of Zion is left as a
cottage in a vineyard, as a lodge in a garden of cucumbers, as a besieged city.
9 Except the LORD of hosts had left
unto us a very small [i]remnant, we
should have been as [j]Sodom, *and* we
should have been like unto Gomorrah.
10 Hear the word of the LORD, ye
rulers of [k]Sodom; give ear unto the [l]law
of our God, ye people of Gomorrah.
11 To what purpose *is* the multitude of
your sacrifices unto me? saith the LORD: I
am full of the burnt-offerings of rams,
and the fat of fed beasts; and I delight
not in the blood of bullocks, or of lambs,
or of he goats.
12 When ye come to appear before

B.C. 760.

a Num. 12:6.
b 2 Chr. 26–32.
c Deut. 32:1; Jer. 2:12; 6:19; 22:29; Ezk. 36:4; Mic. 1:2; 6:1, 2.
d Gal. 4:1-4.
e Jer. 9:3, 6.
f Isa. 57:3, 4; Mt. 3:7.
g Isa. 9:13; Jer. 2:30; 5:3.
h Deut. 28:51, 52.
i *Remnant.* Isa. 10:20. (Isa. 1:9; Rom. 11:5.)
j Rom. 9:29.
k i.e. Jerusalem. v. 9; Rev. 11:8.
l *Law (of Moses).* vs. 10-18; Isa. 5:24, 25. (Ex. 19:1; Gal. 3:1-29.)

[1] **(1:2)** The chapter, down to verse 23, states the case of Jehovah against Judah. Chastening, according to Deut. 28, 29, had been visited upon Israel in the land (vs. 5-8), and now the time of expulsion from the land is near. But just here Jehovah renews the promise of the Palestinian Covenant of future restoration and exaltation (Isa. 1:26, 27; 2:1-4).

me, who hath required this at your hand, to tread my courts?

13 [a]Bring no more vain oblations; incense is an abomination unto me; the new moons and sabbaths, the calling of assemblies, I cannot away with; *it is* iniquity, even the solemn meeting.

14 Your new moons and your appointed feasts my soul hateth: they are a trouble unto me; I am weary to bear *them*.

15 And when ye spread forth your hands, I will hide mine eyes from you: yea, when ye make many prayers, I will not hear: your hands are full of blood.

16 Wash you, make you clean; put away the evil of your doings from before mine eyes; cease to do evil;

17 Learn to do well; seek judgment, relieve the oppressed, judge the fatherless, plead for the widow.

18 Come now, and let us reason together, saith the LORD: though your sins be as scarlet, they shall be as white as snow; though they be red like crimson, they shall be as wool.

19 If ye be willing and obedient, ye shall eat the good of the land:

20 But if ye refuse and rebel, ye shall be devoured with the sword: for the mouth of the LORD hath spoken *it*.

21 How is the faithful city become an harlot! it was full of judgment; righteousness lodged in it; but now murderers.

22 Thy silver is become dross, thy wine mixed with water:

23 Thy princes *are* rebellious, and companions of thieves: every one loveth gifts, and followeth after rewards: they judge not the fatherless, neither doth the cause of the widow come unto them.

24 Therefore saith the Lord, the LORD of hosts, the mighty One of Israel, Ah, I will ease me of mine adversaries, and avenge me of mine enemies:

Mingled warning and promise.

25 And I will turn my hand upon [b]thee, and purely [c]purge away thy dross, and take away all thy tin:

26 And I will restore [1]thy judges as at the first, and thy counsellors as at the beginning: afterward thou shalt be called, The city of righteousness, the faithful city.

27 Zion shall be redeemed with judgment, and her converts with righteousness.

28 And the destruction of the transgressors and of the sinners *shall be* together, and they that forsake the LORD shall be consumed.

29 For they shall be ashamed of the oaks which ye have desired, and ye shall be confounded for the gardens that ye have chosen.

30 For ye shall be as an oak whose leaf fadeth, and as a garden that hath no water.

31 And the strong shall be as tow, and the maker of it as a spark, and they shall both burn together, and none shall quench *them*.

CHAPTER 2.

The promise for the last days.

The word that Isaiah the son of Amoz saw concerning [d]Judah and Jerusalem.

2 And it shall come to [e]pass in the last days, *that* the [2]mountain of the LORD'S house shall be established in the top of the mountains, and shall be exalted above the hills; and all nations shall flow unto it.

3 [f]And many people shall go and say, Come ye, and let us go up to the mountain of the LORD, to the house of the God of Jacob; and he will teach us of his ways, and we will walk in his paths: for out of Zion shall go forth the law, and the word of the LORD from Jerusalem.

4 And he shall judge among the nations, and shall rebuke many people: and they shall beat their swords into plowshares, and their spears into pruninghooks: nation shall not lift up sword against nation, neither shall they learn war any more.

5 O house of Jacob, come ye, and let us walk in the light of the LORD.

Chastisement before blessing (2:6–3:26).

6 Therefore thou hast forsaken thy people the house of Jacob, because they be replenished from the

B.C. 760.

a vs. 11-17; 2 Cor. 8:1, *note*.

b Israel (prophecies). vs. 24-26; Isa. 2:1-4. (Gen. 12:2, 3; Rom. 11:26.)

c Kingdom (O.T.). vs. 25, 26; Isa. 2:1-4. (Gen. 1:26-28; Zech. 12:8.)

d Kingdom (O.T.). vs. 1-4; Isa. 4:1-6. (Gen. 1:26; Zech. 12:8.)

e Israel (prophecies). vs. 1-4; Isa. 9:6, 7. (Gen. 12:2, 3; Rom. 11:26.)

f Jer. 50:5; Zech. 8:21-23; 14:16-21.

[1] **(1:26)** Under the kingdom the ancient method of administering the theocratic government over *Israel* is to be restored. Cf. Jud. 2:18; Mt. 19:28.

[2] **(2:2)** A mountain, in Scripture symbolism, means a kingdom (Dan. 2:35; Rev. 13:1, with Rev. 17:9-11).

east, and *are* soothsayers like the Philistines, and they please themselves in the children of strangers.

7 Their land also is full of silver and gold, neither *is there any* end of their treasures; their land is also full of horses, neither *is there any* end of their chariots:

8 Their land also is full of idols; they worship the work of their own hands, that which their own fingers have made:

9 And the mean man boweth down, and the great man humbleth himself: therefore forgive them not.

10 Enter into the rock, and hide thee in the dust, for fear of the LORD, and for the glory of his majesty.

11 The lofty looks of man shall be humbled, and the haughtiness of men shall be bowed down, and the LORD alone shall be exalted in that day.

12 [a]For the day of the LORD of hosts *shall be* upon every *one that is* proud and lofty, and upon every *one that is* lifted up; and he shall be brought low:

13 And [b]upon all the cedars of Lebanon, *that are* high and lifted up, and upon all the oaks of Bashan,

14 And upon all the high mountains, and upon all the hills *that are* lifted up,

15 And upon every high tower, and upon every fenced wall,

16 And [c]upon all the ships of Tarshish, and upon all [d]pleasant pictures.

17 And the loftiness of man shall be bowed down, and the haughtiness of men shall be made low: and the LORD alone shall be exalted in that day.

18 And the idols he shall utterly abolish.

19 And they shall go into [e]the holes of the rocks, and into the caves of the earth, [f]for fear of the LORD, and for the glory of his majesty, when he ariseth to [g]shake terribly the earth.

20 In that day a man shall cast his idols of silver, and his idols of gold, which they made *each one* for himself to worship, to the moles and to the bats;

21 [h]To go into the clefts of the rocks, and into the tops of the ragged rocks, for fear of the LORD, and for the glory of his majesty, when he ariseth to shake terribly the earth.

22 [i]Cease ye from man, whose breath

B.C. 760.

a *Day (of Jehovah).* vs. 10-22; Isa. 4:1-6. (Isa. 2:10-22; Rev. 19:11-21.)

b Isa. 14:8; 37.24; Ezk. 31:3-18; Zech. 11:1, 2.

c 1 Ki. 10:22.

d Heb. *pictures of desire.*

e v. 10; Hos. 10:8; Lk. 23:30; Rev. 6:16; 9:6.

f 2 Thes. 1:9.

g Isa. 30:32; Hag. 2:6, 21; Heb. 12:26.

h v. 19.

i Psa. 146:3; Jer. 17:5.

j Jer. 37:21; 38:9.

k See 2 Ki. 24:14.

l Eccl. 10:16.

m Heb. *binder up.*

n Mic. 3:12.

o Gen. 13:13; 18:20, 21; 19:5.

p Eccl. 8:12.

q Psa. 11:6; Eccl. 8:13.

r Mic. 6:2.

is in his nostrils: for wherein is he to be accounted of?

CHAPTER 3.

For, behold, the Lord, the LORD of hosts, [j]doth take away from Jerusalem and from Judah the stay and the staff, the whole stay of bread, and the whole stay of water,

2 [k]The mighty man, and the man of war, the judge, and the prophet, and the prudent, and the ancient,

3 The captain of fifty, and the honourable man, and the counsellor, and the cunning artificer, and the eloquent orator.

4 And I will give [l]children *to be* their princes, and babes shall rule over them.

5 And the people shall be oppressed, every one by another, and every one by his neighbour: the child shall behave himself proudly against the ancient, and the base against the honourable.

6 When a man shall take hold of his brother of the house of his father, *saying*, Thou hast clothing, be thou our ruler, and *let* this ruin *be* under thy hand:

7 In that day shall he swear, saying, I will not be [m]an healer; for in my house *is* neither bread nor clothing: make me not a ruler of the people.

8 For [n]Jerusalem is ruined, and Judah is fallen: because their tongue and their doings *are* against the LORD, to provoke the eyes of his glory.

9 The shew of their countenance doth witness against them; and they declare their sin as [o]Sodom, they hide *it* not. Woe unto their soul! for they have rewarded evil unto themselves.

10 Say ye to the righteous, [p]that *it shall be* well *with him*: for they shall eat the fruit of their doings.

11 Woe unto the wicked! [q]*it shall be* ill *with him*: for the reward of his hands shall be given him.

12 *As for* my people, children *are* their oppressors, and women rule over them. O my people, they which lead thee cause *thee* to err, and destroy the way of thy paths.

13 The LORD standeth up [r]to plead, and standeth to judge the people.

14 The LORD will enter into judgment with the ancients of his people, and the princes thereof: for ye

B.C. 760.

have eaten up [a]the vineyard; the spoil of the poor *is* in your houses.

15 What mean ye *that* ye [b]beat my people to pieces, and grind the faces of the poor? saith the Lord GOD of hosts.

16 Moreover the LORD saith, Because the daughters of Zion are haughty, and walk with stretched forth necks and wanton eyes, walking and mincing *as* they go, and making a tinkling with their feet:

17 Therefore the Lord will smite with a [c]scab the crown of the head of the daughters of Zion, and the LORD will [d]discover their secret parts.

18 In that day the Lord will take away the bravery of *their* tinkling ornaments *about their feet*, and *their* cauls, and *their* round tires like the moon,

19 The chains, and the bracelets, and the mufflers,

20 The bonnets, and the ornaments of the legs, and the headbands, and the tablets, and the earrings,

21 The rings, and nose jewels,

22 The changeable suits of apparel, and the mantles, and the wimples, and the crisping pins,

23 The glasses, and the fine linen, and the hoods, and the vails.

24 And it shall come to pass, *that* instead of sweet smell there shall be stink; and instead of a girdle a rent; and instead of well set hair [e]baldness; and instead of a stomacher a girding of sackcloth; *and* burning instead of beauty.

25 Thy men shall fall by the sword, and thy mighty in the war.

26 [f]And her gates shall lament and mourn; and she *being* desolate [g]shall sit upon the ground.

CHAPTER 4.

The vision of the future kingdom.
(vs. 1-6. Cf. Isa. 11:1-16.)

And in that [h]day seven women shall take hold of one man, saying, We will eat our own bread, and wear our own apparel: only let us be called by thy name, to take away our reproach.

2 [i]In that day shall the [1]branch of the LORD be beautiful and glorious, and the fruit of the earth *shall be* excellent and comely for them that are escaped of Israel.

3 And it shall come to pass, *that he that is* left in Zion, and *he that* remaineth in Jerusalem, shall be called holy, *even* every one that is written among the living in Jerusalem:

4 When the Lord shall have washed away the filth of the daughters of Zion, and shall have purged the blood of Jerusalem from the midst thereof by the [j]spirit of judgment, and by the spirit of burning.

5 And the LORD will create upon every dwelling place of mount Zion, and upon her assemblies, a cloud and smoke by day, and the shining of a flaming fire by night: for upon all the glory *shall be* a defence.

6 And there shall be a tabernacle for a shadow in the daytime from the heat, and for a place of refuge, and for a covert from storm and from rain.

CHAPTER 5.

Parable of Jehovah's vineyard.
(Cf. Mt. 21:33-44.)

Now will I sing to my wellbeloved a song of my beloved touching his [k]vineyard. My wellbeloved hath a vineyard in a very fruitful hill:

2 And he fenced it, and gathered out the stones thereof, and planted it with the choicest vine, and built a tower in the midst of it, and also made a winepress therein: and he looked that it should bring forth grapes, and it brought forth wild grapes.

3 And now, O inhabitants of Jerusalem, and men of Judah, judge, I pray you, betwixt me and my vineyard.

4 What could have been done more to my vineyard, that I have not done in it? wherefore, when I looked that it should

a Isa. 5:7; Mt. 21:33.
b Isa. 58:4; Mic. 3:2, 3.
c Deut. 28:27.
d Heb. *make naked.*
e Isa. 22:12; Mic. 1:16.
f Jer. 14:2; Lam. 1:4.
g Lam. 2:10.
h *Kingdom* (O.T.). vs. 1-6; Isa. 7:14. (Gen. 1:26; Zech. 12:8.)
i *Day (of Jehovah).* vs. 1-6; Isa. 11:10-13. (Isa. 2:10-22; Rev. 19:11-21.)
j *Holy Spirit.* Isa. 11:2. (Gen. 1:2; Mal. 2:15.)
k *Parables* (O.T.). vs. 1-7; Jer. 13:1-11. (Jud. 9:7-15; Zech. 11:7-14.)

[1]**(4:2)** A name of Christ, used in a fourfold way: (1) "The Branch of Jehovah" (Isa. 4:2), that is, the "Immanuel" character of Christ (Isa. 7:14) to be fully manifested to restored and converted Israel after His return in divine glory (Mt. 25:31); (2) the "Branch of David" (Isa. 11:1; Jer. 23:5; 33:15), that is, the Messiah, "of the seed of David according to the flesh" (Rom. 1:3), revealed in His earthly glory as King of kings, and Lord of lords; (3) Jehovah's "Servant, the Branch" (Zech. 3:8), Messiah's humiliation and obedience unto death according to Isa. 52:13-15; 53:1-12; Phil. 2:5-8; (4) the "man whose name is the Branch"

bring forth grapes, brought it forth wild
grapes?
5 And now go to; I will tell you what I
will do to my vineyard: I will take away
the hedge thereof, and it shall be eaten
up; *and* break down the wall thereof, and
it shall be trodden down:
6 And I will lay it waste: it shall not be
pruned, nor digged; but there shall come
up briers and thorns: I will also command
the clouds that they rain no rain upon it.
7 For the vineyard of the LORD of hosts
is the house of Israel, and the men of
Judah his pleasant plant: and he looked
for judgment, but behold oppression; for
righteousness, but behold a cry.

The six woes upon Israel.

8 Woe unto them that join house to
house, *that* lay field to field, till *there be*
no place, that they may be placed alone
in the midst of the earth!
9 In mine ears *said* the LORD of hosts, Of
a truth many houses shall be desolate,
even great and fair, without inhabitant.
10 Yea, ten acres of vineyard shall
yield one [a]bath, and the seed of an
[b]homer shall yield an [c]ephah.
11 Woe unto them that rise up early in
the morning, *that* they may follow strong
drink; that continue until night, *till* wine
inflame them!
12 And the harp, and the viol, the
tabret, and pipe, and wine, are in their
feasts: but they regard not the work of
the LORD, neither consider the operation
of his hands.
13 [d]Therefore my people are gone into
captivity, because *they have* no knowledge:
and their honourable men *are* famished,
and their multitude dried up with thirst.
14 Therefore [e]hell hath enlarged herself, and opened her mouth without
measure: and their glory, and their multitude, and their pomp, and he that
rejoiceth, shall descend into it.
15 And the mean man shall be
brought down, and the mighty man
shall be humbled, and the eyes of the
lofty shall be humbled:
16 But the LORD of hosts shall be exalted in judgment, and God that is holy
shall be sanctified in righteousness.
17 Then shall the lambs feed after their
manner, and the waste places of the [f]fat
ones shall strangers eat.
18 Woe unto them that draw iniquity
with cords of vanity, and sin as it were
with a cart rope:
19 [g]That say, Let him make speed, *and*
hasten his work, that we may see *it*: and
let the counsel of the Holy One of Israel
draw nigh and come, that we may know
it!
20 Woe unto them that call evil good,
and good evil; that put darkness for
light, and light for darkness; that put bitter for sweet, and sweet for bitter!
21 Woe unto *them that are* [h]wise in
their own eyes, and prudent in their
own sight!
22 Woe unto *them that are* mighty to
drink wine, and men of strength to mingle strong drink:
23 Which [i]justify the wicked for
reward, and take away the righteousness of the righteous from him!
24 Therefore as the fire devoureth the
stubble, and the flame consumeth the
chaff, *so* their [j]root shall be as rottenness,
and their blossom shall go up as dust:
because they have cast away the [k]law of
the LORD of hosts, and despised the
word of the Holy One of Israel.
25 Therefore is the anger of the LORD
kindled against his people, and he hath
stretched forth his hand against them,
and hath smitten them: and the hills did
tremble, and their carcases *were* torn in
the midst of the streets. [l]For all this his
anger is not turned away, but his hand *is*
stretched out still.
26 And [m]he will lift up an ensign to the
nations from far, and will hiss unto them
[n]from the end of the earth: and, behold,
[o]they shall come with speed swiftly:
27 None shall be weary nor stumble
among them; none shall slumber nor
sleep; neither [p]shall the girdle of their
loins be loosed, nor the latchet of their
shoes be broken:
28 Whose arrows *are* sharp, and all
their bows bent, their horses' hoofs shall
be counted like flint, and their wheels
like a whirlwind:
29 Their roaring *shall be* like a lion,

B.C. 760.

a One bath = about 8 gals.

b One homer = about 86 gals.

c One ephah = 1 bu. 3 pts.

d Hos. 4:6.

e Heb. *Sheol.* See Hab. 2:5, *note.*

f Isa. 10:16.

g Jer. 17:15; 2 Pet. 3:3, 4.

h Prov. 3:7; Rom. 1:22; 12:16.

i Prov. 17:15; 24:24; Isa. 1:23.

j Job 18.16; Hos. 9:16; Amos 2:9.

k *Law (of Moses).* vs. 24, 25; Jer. 9:13-16. (Ex. 19:1; Gal. 3:1-29.)

l Isa. 9:12, 17, 21; 10:4; Lev. 26:14.

m Isa. 11:12.

n Zech. 10:8.

o Joel 2:7.

p Dan. 5:6.

(Zech. 6:12, 13), that is, His character as Son of man, the "last Adam," the "second Man" (1 Cor. 15:45-47), reigning, as Priest-King, over the earth in the dominion given to and lost by the first Adam. Matthew is the Gospel of the "Branch of David"; Mark of "Jehovah's Servant, the Branch"; Luke of "the man whose name is the Branch"; John of "the Branch of Jehovah."

they shall roar like young lions: yea, they shall roar, and lay hold of the prey, and shall carry *it* away safe, and none shall deliver *it*.

30 And in that day they shall roar against them like the roaring of the sea: and if *one* [a]look unto the land, behold darkness *and* sorrow, and the light is darkened in the heavens thereof.

CHAPTER 6.

Isaiah's transforming vision.
(Cf. Josh. 5:13, 14; Job 42:5, 6; Ezk. 1:28; Dan. 10:5-11; Rev. 1:12-19.)

In the year that [b]king Uzziah died I [c]saw also the Lord sitting upon a throne, high and lifted up, and his train filled the temple.

2 Above it stood the [1]seraphims: each one had six wings; with [d]twain he covered his face, and with twain he covered his feet, and with twain he did fly.

3 And one cried unto another, and said, Holy, holy, holy, *is* the LORD of hosts: the whole earth *is* full of his glory.

4 And the posts of the door moved at the voice of him that cried, and [e]the house was filled with smoke.

The effect of the vision.

5 Then said I, Woe *is* me! for I am undone; because I *am* a man of unclean lips, and I dwell in the midst of a people of unclean lips: [f]for mine eyes have seen the King, the LORD of hosts.

The cleansing fire.

6 Then flew one of the seraphims unto me, having a live coal in his hand, *which* he had taken with the tongs from off the altar:

7 And he laid *it* upon my mouth, and said, Lo, this hath touched thy lips; and thine iniquity is taken away, and thy sin purged.

B.C. 758.

a Isa. 8:22; Jer. 4:23; Lam. 3:2; Ezk. 32:7, 8.

b 2 Ki. 15:7.

c 1 Ki. 22:19; John 12:41, Rev. 4:2.

d Ezk. 1:11.

e Ex. 40:34; 1 Ki. 8:10.

f *Inspiration.* vs. 5-9; Isa. 8:1. (Ex. 4:15; Rev. 22:19.)

g vs. 9, 10; Mt. 13:14, 15; Mk. 4:12; Lk. 8:10; John 12:40; Acts 28:26, 27; 2 Cor. 3:14, 15.

[B.C. 742.

8 Also I heard the voice of the Lord, saying, Whom shall I send, and who will go for us? Then said I, Here *am* I; send me.

Isaiah's new commission. (Cf. Mt. 13:14.)

9 And he said, Go, and [g]tell this people, Hear ye indeed, but understand not; and see ye indeed, but perceive not.

10 Make the heart of this people fat, and make their ears heavy, and shut their eyes; lest they see with their eyes, and hear with their ears, and understand with their heart, and convert, and be healed.

11 Then said I, Lord, how long? And he answered, Until the cities be wasted without inhabitant, and the houses without man, and the land be utterly desolate,

12 And the LORD have removed men far away, and *there be* a great forsaking in the midst of the land.

13 But yet in it *shall be* [2]a tenth, and *it* shall [3]return, and shall be eaten: as a teil tree, and as an oak, whose substance *is* in them, when they cast *their leaves: so* the holy seed *shall be* the substance thereof.

CHAPTER 7.

Under the reign of Ahaz
(Isa. 7:1–14:32. Cf. 2 Chr. 28:1-27):
The evil confederacy of Rezin and Pekah.

And it came to pass in the days of Ahaz the son of Jotham, the son of Uzziah, king of Judah, *that* Rezin the king of Syria, and Pekah the son of Remaliah, king of Israel, went up toward Jerusalem to war against it, but could not prevail against it.

2 And it was told the house of David, saying, Syria is confederate with [4]Ephraim. And his heart was moved, and the heart of his people, as the trees of the wood are moved with the wind.

3 Then said the LORD unto Isaiah, Go

[1] **(6:2)** Heb. *Burners.* The word occurs only here. Cf. Ezk. 1:5, *note.* The Seraphim are, in many respects, in contrast with the Cherubim, though both are expressive of the divine holiness, which demands that the *sinner* shall have access to the divine presence only through a sacrifice which really vindicates the righteousness of God (Rom. 3:24-26, *notes*), and that the *saint* shall be cleansed before serving. Gen. 3:22-24 illustrates the first; Isa. 6:1-8 the second. The Cherubim may be said to have to do with the altar, the Seraphim with the laver. See Psa. 51:7, *note;* John 13:10, *note.* The Seraphim appear to be actual angelic beings.

[2] **(6:13)** See "Remnant," Rom. 11:5, *note.*

[3] **(6:13)** See Isa. 8:18, *note.*

[4] **(7:2)** In the prophetic books "Ephraim" and "Israel" are the collective names of the ten tribes who, under Jeroboam, established the northern kingdom, subsequently called Samaria (1 Ki. 16:24).

forth now to meet Ahaz, thou, and [a]Shear-jashub thy son, at the end of the conduit of the upper pool in the highway of the fuller's field;

4 And say unto him, Take heed, and be quiet; fear not, neither be fainthearted for the two tails of these smoking firebrands, for the fierce anger of Rezin with Syria, and of the son of Remaliah.

5 Because Syria, Ephraim, and the son of Remaliah, have taken evil counsel against thee, saying,

6 Let us go up against Judah, and vex it, and let us make a breach therein for us, and set a king in the midst of it, *even* the son of Tabeal:

7 Thus saith the Lord GOD, It shall not stand, neither shall it come to pass.

8 For the head of Syria *is* Damascus, and the head of Damascus *is* Rezin; and within threescore and five years shall Ephraim be broken, that it be not a people.

9 And the head of Ephraim *is* Samaria, and the head of Samaria *is* Remaliah's son. If ye will not believe, surely ye shall not be established.

The great sign: Immanuel, the virgin's son.

10 Moreover the LORD spake again unto Ahaz, saying,

11 Ask thee a sign of the LORD thy God; ask it either in the depth, or in the height above.

12 But Ahaz said, I will not ask, neither will I [b]tempt the LORD.

13 And he said, Hear [1]ye now, O house of David; *Is it* a small thing for you to weary men, but will ye weary my God also?

14 Therefore the Lord himself shall give you a sign; Behold, a virgin shall [c]conceive, and bear a [d]son, and shall [e]call his name [f]Immanuel.

15 [2]Butter and honey shall he eat, that he may know to refuse the evil, and choose the good.

16 For before the child shall know to refuse the evil, and choose the good, the land that thou abhorrest shall be forsaken of both her kings.

Prediction of an impending invasion of Judah. (Cf. 2 Chr. 28:1-20.)

17 [g]The LORD shall bring upon thee, and upon thy people, and upon thy father's house, days that have not come, from the day that [h]Ephraim departed from Judah; *even* the king of Assyria.

18 And it shall come to pass in that day, *that* the LORD shall hiss for the fly that *is* in the uttermost part of the rivers of Egypt, and for the bee that *is* in the land of Assyria.

19 And they shall come, and shall rest all of them in the desolate valleys, and in the [i]holes of the rocks, and upon all thorns, and upon all bushes.

20 In the same day shall the Lord shave with a [j]razor that is hired, *namely*, by them beyond the river, by the king of Assyria, the head, and the hair of the feet: and it shall also consume the beard.

21 And it shall come to pass in that day, *that* a man shall nourish a young cow, and two sheep;

22 And it shall come to pass, for the abundance of milk *that* they shall give he shall eat butter: for butter and honey shall every one eat that is left in the land.

23 And it shall come to pass in that day, *that* every place shall be, where there were a thousand vines at a thousand silverlings, it shall *even* be for briers and thorns.

24 With arrows and with bows shall *men* come thither; because all the land shall become briers and thorns.

25 And *on* all hills that shall be digged with the mattock, there shall not come thither the fear of briers and thorns: but it shall be for the sending forth of oxen, and for the treading of lesser cattle.

B.C. 742.

a Meaning, *a remnant shall return.* Cf. Isa. 8:3

b *Temptation.* Mal. 3:15. (Gen. 3:1; Jas. 1:2.)

c Mt. 1:23.

d *Christ (First Advent).* Isa. 9:6. (Gen. 3:15; Acts 1:9.)

e *Kingdom* (O.T.). Isa. 9:6, 7. (Gen. 1:26; Zech. 12:8.)

f i.e. *God with us.*

g 2 Chr. 28:19.

h 1 Ki. 12:16.

i Isa. 2:19; Jer. 16:16.

j 2 Ki. 16:7, 8; 2 Chr. 28:20, 21; see Ezk. 5:1.

and were (B.C. 722) sent into an exile which still continues (2 Ki. 17:1-6). They are distinguished as "the outcasts of Israel" from "the dispersed of Judah" (Isa. 11:12). "Hidden" in the world (Mt. 13:44) they, with Judah, are yet to be restored to Palestine and made one nation again (Jer. 23:5-8; Ezk. 37:11-24).

[1] **(7:13)** The prophecy is not addressed to the faithless Ahaz, but to the whole "house of David." The objection that such a far-off event as the birth of Christ could be no "sign" to Ahaz, is, therefore, puerile. It was a continuing prophecy addressed to the Davidic family, and accounts at once for the instant assent of Mary (Lk. 1:38).

[2] **(7:15)** Indicating the plainness and simplicity of the life in which the young Immanuel should be brought up.

CHAPTER 8.

Prediction of the Assyrian invasion.

Moreover the LORD said unto me, Take thee a great roll, and [a]write in it with a man's pen concerning [b]Maher-shalal-hash-baz.

2 And I took unto me faithful witnesses to record, Uriah the priest, and Zechariah the son of Jeberechiah.

3 And I went unto the prophetess; and she conceived, and bare a son. Then said the LORD to me, Call his name [b]Maher-shalal-hash-baz.

4 For before the child shall have knowledge to cry, My father, and my mother, the riches of Damascus and the spoil of Samaria shall be taken away before the king of Assyria.

5 The LORD spake also unto me again, saying,

6 Forasmuch as this people refuseth the waters of [c]Shiloah that go softly, and rejoice in [d]Rezin and Remaliah's son;

7 Now therefore, behold, the Lord bringeth up upon them the waters of the river, strong and many, *even* the king of Assyria, and all his glory: and he shall come up over all his channels, and go over all his banks:

8 And he shall pass through Judah; he shall overflow and go over, [e]he shall reach *even* to the neck; and the stretching out of his wings shall fill the breadth of thy land, O [f]Immanuel.

9 Associate yourselves, O ye people, and ye shall be broken in pieces; and give ear, all ye of far countries: gird yourselves, and ye shall be broken in pieces; gird yourselves, and ye shall be broken in pieces.

10 Take counsel together, and it shall come to nought; speak the word, and it shall not stand: [g]for God *is* with us.

11 For the LORD spake thus to me with a strong hand, and instructed me that I should not walk in the way of this people, saying,

12 Say ye not, A [1]confederacy, to all *them to* whom this people shall say, A confederacy; [h]neither fear ye their fear, nor be afraid.

13 [i]Sanctify the LORD of hosts himself; and *let* him *be* your fear, and *let* him *be* your dread.

14 And he shall be for a sanctuary; but for a [j]stone of stumbling and for a rock of offence to both the houses of Israel, for a gin and for a snare to the inhabitants of Jerusalem.

15 And many among them shall stumble, and fall, and be broken, and be snared, and be taken.

16 Bind up the testimony, seal the law among my disciples.

17 And I will wait upon the LORD, that hideth his face from the house of Jacob, and I will look for [k]him.

18 Behold, I and the children whom the LORD hath given me [l]*are* for [2]signs and for wonders in Israel from the LORD of hosts, which dwelleth in mount Zion.

19 And when they shall say unto you, Seek unto them that have familiar spirits, and unto wizards that peep, and that mutter: should not a people seek unto their God? for the living to the dead?

20 To the law and to the testimony: if they speak not according to this word, *it is* because *there is* no light in them.

21 And they shall pass through it, hardly bestead and hungry: and it shall come to pass, that when they shall be hungry, they shall fret themselves, and curse their king and their God, and look upward.

22 And they shall look unto the earth; and behold trouble and darkness, dimness of anguish; and *they shall be* driven to darkness.

CHAPTER 9.

A divine child Israel's only hope.

Nevertheless the dimness *shall* not *be* such as *was* in her vexation, when at the first he lightly afflicted the land of Zebulun and the land of Naphtali, and afterward did more grievously afflict *her by* the way of the sea, beyond Jordan, in Galilee of the nations.

B.C. 742.

a *Inspiration.* Isa. 30:8. (Ex. 4:15; Rev. 22:19.)

b i.e. *haste ye, haste ye to the spoil.* Cf. Isa. 7:3.

c Neh. 3:15; John 9:7.

d Isa. 7:1-9.

e Isa. 30:28.

f Isa. 7:14; Mt. 1:23; Gal. 3:16.

g Isa. 7:14; Acts 5:38, 39; Rom. 8:31.

h 1 Pet. 3:14, 15.

i Num. 20:12.

j *Christ (as Stone).* Isa. 28:16. (Ex. 17:6; 1 Pet. 2:8.)

k Cited in Heb. 2:13 from Septuagint Version.

l Heb. 2:13.

[1] **(8:12)** The reference is to the attempt to terrify Judah by the confederacy between Syria and Samaria (Isa. 7:1, 2).

[2] **(8:18)** The primary application here is to the two sons of Isaiah, Maher-shalal-hash-baz = "haste ye, haste ye to the spoil," a "sign" of the coming judgment of the captivity of Judah; Shear-jashub = "a remnant shall return" a "sign" of the return of a remnant of Judah at the end of the seventy years (Jer 25:11, 12; Dan. 9:2). The larger and final reference is to our Lord (Heb. 2:13, 14).

2 [a]The people that walked in darkness
have seen a great light: they that dwell
in the land of the shadow of death, upon
them hath the light shined.
3 Thou hast multiplied the nation, *and*
[b]not increased the joy: they joy before
thee according to the joy in harvest, *and*
as *men* rejoice when they divide the spoil.
4 For thou hast broken the yoke of his
burden, and the staff of his shoulder, the
rod of his oppressor, as in the day of
Midian.
5 For every battle of the warrior *is*
with confused noise, and garments
rolled in blood; but *this* shall be with
burning *and* fuel of fire.
6 For unto us a [c]child is [d]born, unto us
a [e]son is given: and the government
shall be upon his [f]shoulder: and his
name shall be called Wonderful,
Counsellor, The mighty God, The everlasting Father, The Prince of Peace.
7 Of the increase of *his* government
and peace *there shall be* no end, upon the
[f]throne [1]of David, and upon his kingdom, [g]to order it, and to establish it with
judgment and with justice from henceforth even for ever. The zeal of the LORD
of hosts will perform this.

The vision of the stretched-out hand: the unavailing chastisement.

8 The Lord sent a word into [h]Jacob,
and it hath lighted upon Israel.
9 And all the people shall know, *even*
Ephraim and the inhabitant of Samaria,
that say in the pride and stoutness of
heart,
10 The bricks are fallen down, but we
will build with hewn stones: the syco-
mores are cut down, but we will change
them into cedars.
11 Therefore the LORD shall set up the
adversaries of Rezin against him, and
join his enemies together;
12 The Syrians before, and the
Philistines behind; and they shall devour
Israel with open mouth. [2]For all this his
anger is not turned away, but his hand *is*
stretched out still.
13 For the people turneth not unto
him that smiteth them, neither do they
seek the LORD of hosts.
14 Therefore the LORD will cut off from
Israel head and tail, branch and rush, [i]in
one day.
15 The ancient and honourable, he *is*
the head; and the prophet that teacheth
lies, he *is* the tail.
16 For the leaders of this people cause
them to err; and *they that are* led of them
are [j]destroyed.
17 Therefore the Lord shall have no
joy in their young men, neither shall
have mercy on their fatherless and widows: for every one *is* an hypocrite and
an evildoer, and every mouth speaketh
folly. For all this his anger is not turned
away, but his hand *is* stretched out still.
18 For wickedness [k]burneth as the fire:
it shall devour the briers and thorns, and
shall kindle in the thickets of the forest,
and they shall mount up *like* the lifting
up of smoke.
19 Through the wrath of the LORD of
hosts is the land darkened, and the people shall be as the fuel of the fire: [l]no
man shall spare his brother.
20 And he shall snatch on the right
hand, and be hungry; and he shall eat on
the left hand, and they shall not be satisfied: they shall eat every man the flesh of
his own arm:
21 Manasseh, Ephraim; and Ephraim,
Manasseh: *and* they together *shall be*
against Judah. For all this his anger is
not turned away, but his hand *is*
stretched out still.

CHAPTER 10.

Woe unto them that decree unrighteous decrees, and that write
grievousness *which* they have prescribed;
2 To turn aside the needy from judgment, and to take away the right from
the poor of my people, that widows may
be their prey, and *that* they may rob the
fatherless!
3 And what will ye do in [m]the day of

B.C. 740.

a vs. 1, 2; Mt. 4:15, 16.

b Omit, *not.* Isaiah complains that despite the wickedness of the northern kingdom her afflictions are light, her prosperity great.

c Lk. 2:7; John 3:16; 1 John 4:9.

d *Christ (First Advent).* Isa. 28:16. (Gen. 3:15; Acts 1:9.)

e *Kingdom* (O.T.). vs. 6, 7; Isa. 11:1-12. (Gen. 1:26; Zech. 12:8.)

f *Israel (prophecies)*. vs. 6, 7; Isa. 11:1-13. (Gen. 12:2, 3; Rom. 11:26.)

g *Christ (Second Advent).* Isa. 11:10-12. (Deut. 30:3; Acts 1:9-11.)

h Gen. 32:28, *note.*

i Isa. 10:17; Mal. 4:1; Rev. 18:8.

j Heb. *swallowed up.*

k Isa. 10:17; Mal. 4:1.

l Mic. 7:2, 6.

m Hos. 9:7; Lk. 19:44.

[1] **(9:7)** The "throne of David" is a phrase as definite, historically, as "throne of the Caesars," and as little admits of "spiritualizing" (Lk. 1:32, 33). See "Kingdom (O.T.)," Zech. 12:8; "Davidic Covenant," 2 Sam. 7:8-17, *note;* Acts 15:14-16.

[2] **(9:12)** See vs. 17, 21, and Isa. 5:25; 10:4. The context explains. Jehovah's hand is outstretched still because His chastisement is followed by no amendment on the part of Israel.

visitation, and in the desolation *which*
shall come from far? to whom will ye
flee for help? and where will ye leave
your glory?
4 Without me they shall bow down
under the prisoners, and they shall fall
under the slain. [a]For all this his anger is
not turned away, but his hand *is*
stretched out still.

Predicted judgment on Assyria,
God's rod on Samaria.

5 O [b]Assyrian, the rod of mine anger,
and the staff in their hand is mine indignation.
6 I will send him against an hypocritical nation, and against the people of my
wrath will I [c]give him a charge, to take
the spoil, and to take the prey, and to
tread them down like the mire of the
streets.
7 [d]Howbeit he meaneth not so, neither
doth his heart think so; but *it is* in his
heart to destroy and cut off nations not a
few.
8 For he saith, *Are* not my princes altogether kings?
9 *Is* not [e]Calno as Carchemish? *is* not
Hamath as Arpad? *is* not Samaria as
Damascus?
10 As my hand hath found the kingdoms of the idols, and whose graven
images did excel them of Jerusalem and
of Samaria;
11 Shall I not, as I have done unto
Samaria and her idols, so do to
Jerusalem and her idols?
12 Wherefore it shall come to pass, *that*
[1]when the Lord hath performed his
whole work [f]upon mount Zion and on
Jerusalem, [g]I will punish the fruit of the
stout heart of the king of Assyria, and
the glory of his high looks.
13 [h]For he saith, By the strength of my
hand I have done *it*, and by my wisdom;
for I am prudent: and I have removed
the bounds of the people, and have
robbed their treasures, and I have put
down the inhabitants like a valiant *man*:
14 And my hand hath found as a nest
the riches of the people: and as one gathereth eggs *that are* left, have I gathered
all the earth; and there was none that
moved the wing, or opened the mouth,
or peeped.
15 Shall [i]the axe boast itself against
him that heweth therewith? *or* shall the
saw magnify itself against him that
shaketh it? as if the rod should shake
itself against them that lift it up, *or* as if
the staff should lift up *itself, as if it were*
no wood.
16 Therefore shall the Lord, the Lord
of hosts, send among his fat ones leanness; and under his glory he shall kindle
a burning like the burning of a fire.
17 And the light of Israel shall be for a
fire, and his Holy One for a flame: and it
shall burn and devour his thorns and his
briers in one day;
18 And shall consume the glory of his
forest, and of his fruitful field, both soul
and body: and they shall be as when a
standardbearer fainteth.
19 And the rest of the trees of his forest shall be few, that a child may write
them.

The vision of the Jewish remnant
in the great tribulation.

20 And it shall come to pass in [2]that
day, *that* the [j]remnant of Israel, and such
as are escaped of the house of Jacob,
shall no more again stay upon him that
smote them; but shall stay upon the
LORD, the Holy One of Israel, in truth.
21 The remnant shall return, *even* the
remnant of Jacob, unto the mighty God.
22 For [k]though thy people Israel be as
the sand of the sea, *yet* a remnant of
them shall return: the consumption
decreed shall overflow with righteousness.
23 For the Lord GOD of hosts shall
make a consumption, even determined,
in the midst of all the land.

B.C. 713.

a Isa. 5:25; 9:12, 17, 21.
b Heb. *Asshur.*
c Jer. 34:22.
d Gen. 50:20; Mic. 4:12.
e Amos 6:2.
f 2 Ki. 19:31.
g Jer. 50:18; cf. 2 Ki. 19:35-37.
h Isa. 37:24; Ezk. 28:4; Dan. 4:30.
i Jer. 51:20.
j *Remnant.* vs. 20-22; Isa. 11:11. (Isa. 1:9; Rom. 11:5.)
k vs. 22, 23; Rom. 9:27, 28.

1 (10:12) A permanent method in the divine government of the earth. Israel is always the centre of the divine counsels earthward (Deut. 32:8). The Gentile nations are permitted to afflict Israel in chastisement for her national sins, but invariably and inevitably retribution falls upon them. (See Gen. 15:13, 14; Deut. 30:5-7; Isa. 14:1, 2; Joel 3:1-8; Mic. 5:7-9; Mt. 25:31-40.)

2 (10:20) "That day": often the equivalent of "the day of the LORD" (Isa. 2:10-22; Rev. 19:11-21). The prophecy here passes from the general to the particular, from historic and fulfilled judgments upon Assyria to the final destruction of *all* Gentile world-power at the return of the Lord in glory. (See "Armageddon," Rev. 16:14; 19:21; "Times of the Gentiles," Luke 21:24; Rev. 16:19; "The great tribulation," Psa. 2:5; Rev. 7:14, and Isa. 13:19, *note.*)

24 Therefore thus saith the Lord GOD of hosts, O my people that dwellest in Zion, be not afraid of the Assyrian: he shall smite thee with a rod, and shall lift up his staff against thee, after the manner of Egypt.
25 For yet a very little while, and the indignation shall cease, and mine anger in their destruction.
26 And the LORD of hosts shall stir up a scourge for him according to the slaughter of Midian at the rock of Oreb: and *as* his rod *was* upon the sea, so shall he lift it up after the manner of Egypt.
27 And it shall come to pass in that [a]day, *that* his burden shall be taken away from off thy shoulder, and his yoke from off thy neck, and the yoke shall be destroyed because of the anointing.

The approach of the Gentile hosts to the battle of Armageddon (Rev. 16:14; 19:11).

28 He is come to Aiath, he is passed to Migron; at Michmash he hath laid up his carriages:
29 They are gone over the passage: they have taken up their lodging at Geba; Ramah is afraid; Gibeah of Saul is fled.
30 Lift up thy voice, O daughter of Gallim: cause it to be heard unto Laish, O poor Anathoth.
31 Madmenah is removed; the inhabitants of Gebim gather themselves to flee.
32 As yet shall he remain at Nob that day: he shall shake his hand *against* the mount of the daughter of Zion, the hill of Jerusalem.
33 Behold, the Lord, the LORD of hosts, shall lop the bough with terror: and the high ones of stature *shall be* hewn down, and the haughty shall be humbled.
34 And he shall cut down the thickets of the forest with iron, and Lebanon shall fall by a mighty one.

CHAPTER 11.

[1]*The Davidic kingdom set up:*
(1) *The King's ancestry.* (Cf. Mt. 1:1.)

1 And there shall [2]come forth a [b]rod out of the stem of [c]Jesse, and a [d]Branch shall grow out of his roots:

(2) *The source of the King's power: the sevenfold Spirit.* (Cf. Rev. 1:4.)

2 And the [e]spirit of the LORD shall rest upon him, the spirit of wisdom and understanding, the spirit of counsel and might, the spirit of knowledge and of the [f]fear of the LORD;

(3) *The character of his reign.*

3 And shall make him of quick understanding in the [f]fear of the LORD: and he shall not judge after the sight of his eyes, neither reprove after the hearing of his ears:
4 But [g]with righteousness shall he judge the poor, and reprove with equity for the meek of the earth: and he shall smite the earth with the rod of his mouth, and with the breath of his lips shall he slay the wicked.
5 And righteousness shall be the [h]girdle of his loins, and faithfulness the girdle of his reins.

(4) *The quality of the kingdom.*

6 The [i]wolf also shall dwell with the lamb, and the leopard shall lie down with the kid; and the calf and the young lion and the fatling together; and a little child shall lead them.
7 And the cow and the bear shall feed; their young ones shall lie down together:

B.C. 713.

a *Armageddon (battle of).* vs. 27-34; Isa. 24:21-23. (Rev. 16:14; 19:21.)
b *Kingdom* (O.T.). vs. 1-12; Isa. 24:23. (Gen. 1:26; Zech. 12:8.)
c *Israel (prophecies).* vs. 1-13; Isa. 60:1-12. (Gen. 12:2, 3; Rom. 11:26.)
d Isa. 4:2, *note.*
e *Holy Spirit.* Isa. 32:15. (Gen. 1:2; Mal. 2:15.)
f Psa. 19:9, *note.*
g Psa. 72:2, 4; Rev. 19:11.
h *Righteousness (garment).* Isa. 59:17. (Gen. 3:21; Rev. 19:8.)
i Isa. 65:25; Ezk. 34:25; Hos. 2:18.

[1]**(11:1, heading)** The order of events in Isa. 10, 11, is noteworthy. Isa. 10 gives the distress of the Remnant in Palestine in the great tribulation (Psa. 2:5; Rev. 7:14), and the approach and destruction of the Gentile hosts under the Beast (Dan. 7:8; Rev. 19:20). Isa. 11 immediately follows with its glorious picture of the kingdom-age. Precisely the same order is found in Rev. 19, 20. (See "Kingdom," O.T., Gen. 1:26-28; Zech. 12:8; N.T., Lk. 1:31-33; 1 Cor. 15:28. Also Mt. 3:2, *note;* 6:33, *note.*)

That nothing of this occurred at the first coming of Christ is evident from a comparison of the history of the times of Christ with this and all the other parallel prophecies. So far from regathering dispersed Israel and establishing peace in the earth, His crucifixion was soon followed (A.D. 70) by the destruction of Jerusalem, and the utter scattering of the Palestinian Jews amongst the nations.

[2]**(11:1)** This chapter is a prophetic picture of the glory of the future kingdom. This is the kingdom announced by John Baptist as "at hand." It was then rejected, but will be set up when David's Son returns in glory (Lk. 1:31, 32; Acts 15:15, 16).

and the lion shall eat straw like the ox.
8 And the sucking child shall play on
the hole of the asp, and the weaned child
shall put his hand on the cockatrice' den.

(5) *The extent of the kingdom.*

9 They shall not hurt nor destroy in all
my holy mountain: [a]for the earth shall
be full of the knowledge of the LORD, as
the waters cover the sea.

(6) *How the kingdom will be set up.*

10 And in that day there shall be [b]a root
of Jesse, which shall stand for [c]an ensign
of the people; to it shall the Gentiles seek:
and his rest shall be glorious.
11 And it shall come to pass in that
day, *that* the Lord shall set his hand again
the second time to [d]recover the [e]remnant
of his people, which shall be left, from
Assyria, and from Egypt, and from
Pathros, and from Cush, and from Elam,
and from Shinar, and from Hamath, and
from the [f]islands of the sea.
12 And he shall set up an ensign for
the nations, and shall assemble the outcasts of Israel, and gather together the
dispersed of Judah from the four corners
of the earth.
13 The envy also of Ephraim shall
depart, and the adversaries of Judah
shall be cut off: Ephraim shall not envy
Judah, and Judah shall not vex Ephraim.
14 But they shall fly upon the shoulders of the Philistines toward the west;
they shall spoil them of the east together: they shall lay their hand upon Edom
and Moab; and the children of Ammon
shall obey them.
15 And the LORD [g]shall utterly destroy
the tongue of the Egyptian sea; and with
his mighty wind shall he shake his hand
over the river, and shall smite it in the
seven streams, and make *men* go over
dryshod.
16 And there shall be an highway for
the remnant of his people, which shall
be left, from Assyria; like as it was to
Israel in the day that he came up out of
the land of Egypt.

B.C. 713.

a Cf. Hab. 2:14, *note.*

b Rom. 15:12.

c *Day (of Jehovah).* vs. 10-13; Isa. 13:9-16. (Isa. 2:10-22; Rev. 19:11-21.)

d *Christ (Second Advent).* vs. 10-12; Jer. 23:5, 6. (Deut. 30:3 Acts 1:9-11.)

e *Remnant.* vs. 11-13, 16; Isa. 24:13, 15. (Isa. 1:9; Rom. 11:5.)

f i.e. *coasts.*

g Zech. 10:11.

h Psa. 2:12, *note.*

i John 4:10, 14; 7:37, 38.

j Isa. 54:1; Zeph. 3:14.

CHAPTER 12.

(7) *The worship of the kingdom.*

And in that day thou shalt say, O
LORD, I will praise thee: though
thou wast angry with me, thine anger is
turned away, and thou comfortedst me.
2 Behold, God *is* my salvation; I will
[h]trust, and not be afraid: for the LORD
JEHOVAH *is* my strength and *my* song;
he also is become my salvation.
3 Therefore with joy shall ye draw
[i]water out of the wells of salvation.
4 And in that day shall ye say, Praise
the LORD, call upon his name, declare his
doings among the people, make mention
that his name is exalted.
5 Sing unto the LORD; for he hath done
excellent things: this *is* known in all the
earth.
6 [j]Cry out and shout, thou inhabitant
of Zion: for great *is* the Holy One of
Israel in the midst of thee.

CHAPTER 13.

The burden of Babylon: a prophecy to be fulfilled in the day of the LORD
(Isa. 2:10-22; Rev. 19:11-21), Chapters
13, 14: (1) *The Gentile nations,* vs. 1-11.

The [1]burden of [2]Babylon, which
Isaiah the son of Amoz did see.
2 Lift ye up a banner upon the high
mountain, exalt the voice unto them,
shake the hand, that they may go into
the gates of the nobles.
3 I have commanded my sanctified
ones, I have also called my mighty ones
for mine anger, *even* them that rejoice in
my highness.
4 The noise of a multitude in the

[1] **(13:1)** A "burden," Heb. *massa* = a heavy, weighty thing, is a message, or oracle concerning Babylon, Assyria, Jerusalem, etc. It is "heavy" because the wrath of God is in it, and grievous for the prophet to declare.

[2] **(13:1)** The *city,* Babylon, is not in view here, as the immediate context shows. It is important to note the significance of the name when used symbolically. "Babylon" is the Greek form: invariably in the O.T. Hebrew the word is simply Babel, the meaning of which is *confusion,* and in this sense the word is used symbolically. (1) In the prophets, when the actual city is not meant, the reference is to the "confusion" into which the whole social order of the world has fallen under Gentile world-domination. (See "Times of the Gentiles," Lk. 21:24; Rev. 16:14.) Isa. 13:4 gives the divine view of the welter of warring Gentile

mountains, like as of a great people; a
tumultuous noise of the kingdoms of
nations gathered together: the LORD of
hosts mustereth the host of the battle.
5 They come from a far country, from
the end of heaven, *even* the LORD, and
the weapons of his indignation, to
destroy the whole land.
6 Howl ye; for the [a]day of the LORD *is*
at hand; it shall come as a destruction
from the Almighty.
7 Therefore shall all hands be faint,
and every man's heart shall melt:
8 And they shall be afraid: pangs and
sorrows shall take hold of them; they
shall be in pain as a woman that travaileth: they shall be amazed one at
another; their faces *shall be as* flames.
9 Behold, [b]the day of the LORD cometh,
cruel both with wrath and fierce anger,
to lay the land desolate: and he shall
destroy the sinners thereof out of it.
10 For the stars of heaven and the constellations thereof shall not give their
light: [c]the sun shall be darkened in his
going forth, and the moon shall not
cause her light to shine.
11 And I will punish the world for
their evil, and the wicked for their iniquity; and I will cause the arrogancy of the
proud to cease, and will lay low the
haughtiness of the terrible.

B.C. 713.

a *Day (of Jehovah).* vs. 9-16; Isa. 24:21-23. (Isa. 2:10-22; Rev. 19:11-21.)

b Mal. 4:1.

c Isa. 24:21-23; Ezk. 32:7; Joel 2:31; 3:15; Mt. 24:29; Mk. 13:24; Lk. 21:25.

d Isa. 34:4; Hag. 2:6.

e Jer. 50:16; 51:9.

f Psa. 137:9; Nah. 3:10; Zech. 14:2.

g Isa. 21:2; Jer. 51:11, 28; Dan. 5:28, 31.

h See Isa. 13:1, *note.*

(2) *The Jewish remnant* (Isa. 1:9;
Rom. 11:5) *in the great tribulation*
(Psa. 2:5; Rev. 7:14). (Cf. Zech. 14:1, 2.)
12 I will make a man more precious
than fine gold; even a man than the
golden wedge of Ophir.
13 [d]Therefore I will shake the heavens,
and the earth shall remove out of her
place, in the wrath of the LORD of hosts,
and in the day of his fierce anger.
14 And it shall be as the chased roe,
and as a sheep that no man taketh up:
[e]they shall every man turn to his own
people, and flee every one into his own
land.
15 Every one that is found shall be
thrust through; and every one that is
joined *unto them* shall fall by the sword.
16 Their [f]children also shall be dashed
to pieces before their eyes; their houses
shall be spoiled, and their wives ravished.

(3) *The destruction of "Babylon."*

17 [g]Behold, I will stir up the Medes
against them, which shall not regard silver; and *as for* gold, they shall not
delight in it.
18 *Their* bows also shall dash the
young men to pieces; and they shall
have no pity on the fruit of the womb;
their eye shall not spare children.
19 [1]And [h]Babylon, the glory of

powers. The *divine* order is given in Isa. 11. Israel in her own land, the centre of the divine government of the world and channel of the divine blessing; and the Gentiles blessed in association with Israel. Anything else is, politically, mere "Babel." (2) In Rev. 14:8-11; 16:19 the Gentile world-system is in view in connection with Armageddon (Rev. 16:14; 19:21), while in Rev. 17 the reference is to apostate Christianity, destroyed by the nations (Rev. 17:16) headed up under the Beast (Dan. 7:8; Rev. 19:20) and false prophet. In Isaiah the political Babylon is in view, literally as to the then existing city, and symbolically as to the times of the Gentiles. In the Revelation both the symbolical-political and symbolical-religious Babylon are in view, for there both are alike under the tyranny of the Beast. Religious Babylon is destroyed by political Babylon (Rev. 17:16); political Babylon by the appearing of the Lord (Rev. 19:19-21). That Babylon the *city* is not to be rebuilt is clear from Isa. 13:19-22; Jer. 51:24-26, 62-64. By political Babylon is meant the Gentile world-system. (See "World," John 7:7; Rev. 13:8.) It may be added that, in Scripture symbolism, Egypt stands for the world as such; Babylon for the world of corrupt power and corrupted religion; Nineveh for the pride, the haughty glory of the world.

[1] **(13:19)** Verses 12-16 look forward to the apocalyptic judgments (Rev. 6–13). Verses 17-22 have a near and far view. They predict the destruction of the literal Babylon then existing; with the further statement that, once destroyed, Babylon should never be rebuilt (cf. Jer. 51:61-64). All of this has been literally fulfilled. But the place of this prediction in a great prophetic strain which looks forward to the destruction of both politico-Babylon and ecclesio-Babylon in the time of the Beast shows that the destruction of the actual Babylon typifies the greater destruction yet to come upon the mystical Babylons. Cf. v. 1, *note.*

kingdoms, the beauty of the Chaldees' excellency, shall be as when God overthrew Sodom and Gomorrah.

20 [a]It shall never be inhabited, neither shall it be dwelt in from generation to generation: neither shall the Arabian pitch tent there; neither shall the shepherds make their fold there.

21 But wild beasts of the desert shall lie there; and their houses shall be full of doleful creatures; and owls shall dwell there, and satyrs shall dance there.

22 And the wild beasts of the islands shall cry in their desolate houses, and dragons in *their* pleasant palaces: [b]and her time *is* near to come, and her days shall not be prolonged.

CHAPTER 14.

(4) *The kingdom set up: Israel restored and exalted.* (See *"Kingdom,* O.T.," Gen. 1:26-28; Zech. 12:8, *note;* N.T., Lk. 1:31-33; 1 Cor. 15:28.)

For the LORD will have mercy on Jacob, and will [c]yet choose Israel, and set them in their own land: and the strangers shall be joined with them, and they shall cleave to the house of Jacob.

2 And the people shall take them, and bring them to their place: and the house of Israel shall possess them in the land of the LORD for servants and handmaids: and they shall take them captives, whose captives they were; and they shall rule over their oppressors.

3 And it shall come to pass in the day that the LORD shall give thee rest from thy sorrow, and from thy fear, and from the hard bondage wherein thou wast made to serve,

4 That thou [d]shalt take up this proverb against the king of Babylon, and say, How hath the oppressor ceased! the golden city ceased!

5 The LORD hath broken the staff of the wicked, *and* the sceptre of the rulers.

6 He who smote the people in wrath with a continual stroke, he that ruled the nations in anger, is persecuted, *and* none hindereth.

B.C. 712.

a Jer. 50:3, 39; 51:29, 62.

b Jer. 51:33.

c Zech. 1:17; 2:12.

d Isa. 13:19; Hab. 2:6.

e Isa. 55:12; Ezk. 31:16.

f Heb. *Sheol;* also v. 15. See Hab. 2:5, *note.*

g Heb. *Sheol.* See Hab. 2:5, *note.*

h Lk. 10:18; Rev. 12:8, 9.

i *Satan.* vs. 12-14; Ezk. 28:12-15. (Gen. 3:1; Rev. 20:10.)

j See v. 9.

(5) *The joy of the kingdom.*

7 The whole earth is at rest, *and* is quiet: they break forth into singing.

8 [e]Yea, the fir trees rejoice at thee, *and* the cedars of Lebanon, *saying,* Since thou art laid down, no feller is come up against us.

The "Beast" in hell (Dan. 7:8; Rev. 19:20).

9 [f]Hell from beneath is moved for thee to meet *thee* at thy coming: it stirreth up the dead for thee, *even* all the chief ones of the earth; it hath raised up from their thrones all the kings of the nations.

10 All they shall speak and say unto thee, Art thou also become weak as we? art thou become like unto us?

11 Thy pomp is brought down to the [g]grave, *and* the noise of thy viols: the worm is spread under thee, and the worms cover thee.

Satan, the real prince of this world, and organizer of "Babylon" (Isa. 13:1, *note*), *addressed through his tool, the "Beast."*

12 How art thou fallen from heaven, [h]O Lucifer, [1]son of the [i]morning! *how* art thou cut down to the ground, which didst weaken the nations!

13 For thou hast said in thine heart, I will ascend into heaven, I will exalt my throne above the stars of God: I will sit also upon the mount of the congregation, in the sides of the north:

14 I will ascend above the heights of the clouds; I will be like the most High.

15 Yet thou shalt be brought down to [j]hell, to the sides of the pit.

16 They that see thee shall narrowly look upon thee, *and* consider thee, *saying, Is* this the man that made the earth to tremble, that did shake kingdoms;

17 *That* made the world as a wilderness, and destroyed the cities thereof; *that* opened not the house of his prisoners?

[1] **(14:12)** Verses 12-14 evidently refer to Satan, who, as prince of this world-system (see "World," John 7:7; Rev. 13:8, *note*), is the real though unseen ruler of the successive world-powers, Tyre, Babylon, Medo-Persia, Greece, Rome, etc. (see Ezk. 28:12-14). Lucifer, "day-star," can be none other than Satan. This tremendous passage marks the beginning of sin in the universe. When Lucifer said, "I will," sin began. See Rev. 20:10, *note.* See other instances of addressing Satan through another, Gen. 3:15; Mt. 16:22, 23.

B.C. 712.

Judgment of "Babylon."
(Cf. Rev. 18:1-24; 18:2, *note.*)

18 All the kings of the nations, *even* all
of them, lie in glory, every one in his
own house.
19 But thou art cast out of thy grave
like an abominable branch, *and as* the
raiment of those that are slain, thrust
through with a sword, that go down to
the stones of the pit; as a carcase trodden
under feet.
20 Thou shalt not be joined with them
in burial, because thou hast destroyed
thy land, *and* slain thy people: the seed
of evildoers shall never be renowned.
21 Prepare slaughter for his children
for the iniquity of their fathers; that they
do not rise, nor possess the land, nor fill
the face of the world with cities.
22 For I will rise up against them, saith
the LORD of hosts, and cut off from
[a]Babylon the name, and remnant, and
son, and nephew, saith the LORD.
23 [b]I will also make it a possession for
the bittern, and pools of water: and I will
sweep it with the besom of destruction,
saith the LORD of hosts.
24 The LORD of hosts hath sworn, saying, Surely as I have thought, so shall it
come to pass; and as I have purposed, *so*
shall it stand:
25 That I will break the Assyrian in my
land, and upon my mountains tread him
under foot: then shall his yoke depart
from off them, and his burden depart
from off their shoulders.
26 This *is* the purpose that is purposed
upon the [1]whole earth: and this *is* the
hand that is stretched out upon all the
nations.
27 For the LORD of hosts hath purposed, and who shall disannul *it*? and
his hand *is* stretched out, and who shall
turn it back?

The burden of Palestina:
worse oppressors than Ahaz yet to come.

28 In the year that king Ahaz died was
this [c]burden.
29 Rejoice not thou, whole Palestina,
because the rod of [d]him that smote thee
is broken: for out of the serpent's root
shall [e]come forth a cockatrice, and his
fruit *shall be* a fiery flying serpent.
30 And the firstborn of the poor shall
feed, and the needy shall lie down in
safety: and I will kill thy root with
famine, and he shall slay thy remnant.
31 Howl, O gate; cry, O city; thou,
whole Palestina, *art* dissolved: for there
shall come from the north a smoke, and
none *shall be* alone in his appointed times.
32 What shall *one* then answer the
messengers of the nation? That the LORD
hath founded Zion, and the poor of his
people shall [f]trust in it.

CHAPTER 15.

The burden of Moab:
(1) *the destruction* (vs. 1-9).

The [c]burden of [2]Moab. Because in the
night Ar of Moab is laid waste, *and*
brought to silence; because in the night
Kir of Moab is laid waste, *and* brought to
silence;
2 He is gone up to Bajith, and to
Dibon, the high places, to weep: Moab
shall howl over Nebo, and over Medeba:
[g]on all their heads *shall be* baldness, *and*
every beard cut off.
3 In their streets they shall gird themselves with sackcloth: [h]on the tops of
their houses, and in their streets, every
one shall howl, weeping abundantly.
4 And Heshbon shall cry, and Elealeh:
their voice shall be heard *even* unto
Jahaz: therefore the armed soldiers of
Moab shall cry out; his life shall be
grievous unto him.

a See Isa. 13:1, *note.*
b Isa. 34:11; Zeph. 2:14.
c Isa. 13:1, *note.*
d i.e. Ahaz.
e The descendants of Ahaz.
f Psa. 2:12, *note.*
g See Lev. 21:5; Isa. 3:24; 22:12; Jer. 47:5; 48:1, 37, 38; Ezk. 7:18.
h Jer. 48:38.

[1]**(14:26)** This universality is significant and marks the whole passage as referring, not merely to a near judgment upon Assyria, but in a yet larger sense to the final crash of the present world-system at the end of the age. (See "Times of the Gentiles," Luke 21:24; Rev. 16:14; Dan. 2:44, 45; "Armageddon," Rev. 16:14; 19:17.) No other such universal catastrophe on the nations is known to Scripture.

[2]**(15:1)** This "burden" had a precursive fulfilment in Sennacherib's invasion, B.C. 704, three years after the prediction (Isa. 16:14), but the words have a breadth of meaning which includes also the final world-battle. (See Rev. 19:17, *note.*) Isa. 16:1-5, which is a continuation of this "burden," shows the "tabernacle of David" set up, the next event in order after the destruction of the Beast and his armies. Cf. the order in Isa. 10:28-34, and 11:1-10; also Acts 15:14-17; Rev. 19:17-21, and 20:1-4.

5 [a]My heart shall cry out for Moab; his
fugitives *shall flee* unto Zoar, an heifer of
three years old: for by the mounting up
of Luhith with weeping shall they go it
up; for in the way of Horonaim they
shall raise up a cry of destruction.
6 For the waters [b]of Nimrim shall be
desolate: for the hay is withered away,
the grass faileth, there is no green thing.
7 Therefore the abundance they have
gotten, and that which they have laid
up, shall they carry away to the [c]brook
of the willows.
8 For the cry is gone round about the
borders of Moab; the howling thereof
unto Eglaim, and the howling thereof
unto Beer-elim.
9 For the waters of Dimon shall be full
of blood: for I will bring more upon
Dimon, [d]lions upon him that escapeth of
Moab, and upon the remnant of the land.

CHAPTER 16.

(2) The women of Moab anticipate the Davidic kingdom.

Send ye the lamb to the ruler of the
land [e]from [f]Sela to the wilderness,
unto the mount of the daughter of Zion.
2 For it shall be, *that*, as a wandering
bird cast out of the nest, *so* the daughters
of Moab shall be at the fords of [g]Arnon.
3 Take counsel, execute judgment;
make thy shadow as the night in the
midst of the noonday; hide the outcasts;
bewray not him that wandereth.
4 Let mine outcasts dwell with thee,
Moab; be thou a covert to them from the
face of the spoiler: for the extortioner is
at an end, the spoiler ceaseth, the oppressors are consumed out of the land.
5 And in mercy shall the throne be
established: and he shall sit upon it in
truth in the [h]tabernacle of David, judging, and seeking judgment, and hasting
righteousness.

(3) They lament the pride of Moab.

6 We have heard of the pride of Moab;
he is very proud: *even* of his haughtiness,
and his pride, and his wrath: *but* his lies
shall not *be* so.
7 Therefore shall Moab howl for
Moab, every one shall howl: for the
foundations of Kir-hareseth shall ye
mourn; surely *they are* stricken.
8 For the fields of Heshbon languish,
and the vine of Sibmah: the lords of the
[i]heathen have broken down the principal plants thereof, they are come *even*
unto Jazer, they wandered *through* the
wilderness: her branches are stretched
out, they are gone over the sea.
9 Therefore [j]I will bewail with the
weeping of Jazer the vine of Sibmah: I
will water thee with my tears, O
Heshbon, and Elealeh: for the shouting
for thy summer fruits and for thy harvest is fallen.
10 And [k]gladness is taken away, and
joy out of the plentiful field; and in the
vineyards there shall be no singing, neither shall there be shouting: the treaders
shall tread out no wine in *their* presses; I
have made *their vintage* shouting to cease.
11 Wherefore [l]my bowels shall sound
like an harp for Moab, and mine inward
parts for Kir-haresh.
12 And it shall come to pass, when it is
seen that Moab is weary on the high
place, that he shall come to his sanctuary
to pray; but he shall not prevail.

(4) A first fulfilment within three years (Isa. 15:1, *note*).

13 This *is* the word that the LORD hath
spoken concerning Moab since that time.
14 But now the LORD hath spoken,
saying, Within three years, as the years
of an hireling, and the glory of Moab
shall be contemned, with all that great
multitude; and the remnant *shall be* very
small *and* feeble.

CHAPTER 17.

The burden of Damascus.

The [1]burden of Damascus. Behold,
[m]Damascus is taken away from
being a city, and it shall be a ruinous
heap.
2 The cities of Aroer *are* forsaken: they
shall be for flocks, which shall lie down,
and [n]none shall make *them* afraid.
3 The fortress also shall cease from
Ephraim, and the kingdom from

B.C. 726.

a Isa. 16:11; Jer. 48:31.
b Num. 32:3, 36.
c Or, *valley of the Arabians.*
d 2 Ki. 17:25.
e 2 Ki. 14:7.
f Or, *Petra:* Heb. *a rock.*
g Num. 21:13.
h See Acts 15:13-17, *note.*
i i.e. *nations.*
j Jer. 48.32.
k Isa. 24:8; Jer. 48:33.
l Isa. 15:5; 63:15; Jer. 48:36.
m 2 Ki. 16:9; Jer. 49:23; Amos 1:3; Zech. 9:1.
n Jer. 7:33.

[1] **(17:1)** As in the burden of Moab, there was doubtless a near fulfilment in Sennacherib's approaching invasion, but verses 12-14 as evidently look forward to the final invasion and battle ("Armageddon," Rev. 16:14; 19:17, *note.*) Cf. Isa. 10:26-34.)

Damascus, and the remnant of Syria:
they shall be as the glory of the children
of Israel, saith the LORD of hosts.
4 And in that day it shall come to pass,
that the glory of Jacob shall be made
thin, and the fatness of his flesh shall
wax lean.
5 [a]And it shall be as when the harvestman gathereth the corn, and reapeth the
ears with his arm; and it shall be as he
that gathereth ears in the valley of
Rephaim.
6 Yet gleaning grapes shall be left in it,
as the shaking of an olive tree, two *or*
three berries in the top of the uppermost
bough, four *or* five in the outmost fruitful branches thereof, saith the LORD God
of Israel.
7 At that day shall a man [b]look to his
Maker, and his eyes shall have respect to
the Holy One of Israel.
8 And he shall not look to the altars,
the work of his hands, neither shall
respect *that* which his fingers have
made, either the [c]groves, or the images.
9 In that day shall his strong cities be
as a forsaken bough, and an uppermost
branch, which they left because of the
children of Israel: and there shall be desolation.
10 Because thou hast forgotten the
God of thy salvation, and hast not been
mindful of the rock of thy strength,
therefore shalt thou plant pleasant
plants, and shalt set it with strange slips:
11 In the day shalt thou make thy
plant to grow, and in the morning shalt
thou make thy seed to flourish: *but* the
harvest *shall be* a heap in the day of grief
and of desperate sorrow.
12 Woe to the multitude of many people, *which* make a noise like the noise of
the seas; and to the rushing of nations,
that make a rushing like the rushing of
mighty waters!
13 The nations shall rush like the rushing of many waters: [d]but *God* shall
rebuke them, and they shall flee far off,
and [e]shall be chased as the chaff of the
mountains before the wind, and like a
rolling thing before the whirlwind.
14 And behold at eveningtide trouble;
and before the morning he *is* not. This *is*
the portion of them that spoil us, and the
lot of them that rob us.

B.C. 741.

a Jer. 51:33.

b Mic. 7:7.

c Deut. 16:21.

d Isa 37:29-38.

e Psa. 83:13; Hos. 13:3.

f Isa. 20:4, 5; Ezk. 30:4, 5, 9; Zeph. 2:12; 3:10.

g Cf. Isa. 5:26; 11:10-12.

h Isa. 14:1-3; 66:20; Mic. 4:1-8.

i Isa. 13:1, *note.*

j Ex. 12:12; Jer. 43:12.

CHAPTER 18.

The woe of the land beyond the rivers of Ethiopia, in the day of the regathering of Israel.
(See *"Israel,"* Gen. 12:2, 3; Rom. 11:26.)

Woe [f]to the land shadowing with
wings, which *is* beyond the rivers
of Ethiopia:
2 [1]That sendeth ambassadors by the
sea, even in vessels of bulrushes upon the
waters, *saying,* Go, ye swift messengers,
to a nation scattered and peeled, to a people terrible from their beginning hitherto;
a nation meted out and trodden down,
whose land the rivers have spoiled!
3 All ye inhabitants of the world, and
dwellers on the earth, see ye, when he
[g]lifteth up an ensign on the mountains;
and when he bloweth a trumpet, hear ye.
4 For so the LORD said unto me, I will
take my rest, and I will consider in my
dwelling place like a clear heat upon
herbs, *and* like a cloud of dew in the heat
of harvest.
5 For afore the harvest, when the bud
is perfect, and the sour grape is ripening
in the flower, he shall both cut off the
sprigs with pruning hooks, and take
away *and* cut down the branches.
6 They shall be left together unto the
fowls of the mountains, and to the beasts
of the earth: and the fowls shall summer
upon them, and all the beasts of the
earth shall winter upon them.
7 In that time [h]shall the present be
brought unto the LORD of hosts of a people scattered and peeled, and from a
people terrible from their beginning
hitherto; a nation meted out and trodden
under foot, whose land the rivers have
spoiled, to the place of the name of the
LORD of hosts, the mount Zion.

CHAPTER 19.

The burden of Egypt. Looks forward through desolations to kingdom blessing with Israel. (See *"Kingdom, O.T.,"* Zech. 12:8, *note.*)

The [i]burden of Egypt. Behold, the
LORD rideth upon a swift cloud, and
shall come into Egypt: and the [j]idols of
Egypt shall be moved at his presence,

[1]**(18:2)** The local reference is evidently to an embassy from Egypt, resulting in the alliance denounced in Isa. 30, 31; Jer. 37:7-11.

and the heart of Egypt shall melt in the
midst of it.
2 And I will [a]set the Egyptians against
the Egyptians: and they shall fight every
one against his brother, and every one
against his neighbour; city against city,
and kingdom against kingdom.
3 And the spirit of Egypt shall fail in
the midst thereof; and I will destroy the
counsel thereof: and they shall seek to
the idols, and to the charmers, and to
them that have familiar spirits, and to
the wizards.
4 And the Egyptians will I give over
[b]into the hand of a cruel lord; and a
fierce king shall rule over them, saith the
Lord, the LORD of hosts.
5 [c]And the waters shall fail from the
sea, and the river shall be wasted and
dried up.
6 And they shall turn the rivers far
away; *and* the brooks of defence shall be
emptied and dried up: the reeds and
flags shall wither.
7 The paper reeds by the brooks, by
the mouth of the brooks, and every thing
sown by the brooks, shall wither, be
driven away, and be no *more*.
8 The fishers also shall mourn, and all
they that cast angle into the brooks shall
lament, and they that spread nets upon
the waters shall languish.
9 Moreover they that work in fine flax,
and they that weave networks, shall be
confounded.
10 And they shall be broken in the
purposes thereof, all that make sluices
and ponds for fish.
11 Surely the princes of Zoan *are* fools,
the counsel of the wise counsellors of
Pharaoh is become brutish: how say ye
unto Pharaoh, I *am* the son of the wise,
the son of ancient kings?
12 Where *are* they? where *are* thy wise
men? and let them tell thee now, and let
them know what the LORD of hosts hath
purposed upon Egypt.
13 The princes of Zoan are become
fools, [d]the princes of Noph are deceived;
they have also seduced Egypt, *even they
that are* the stay of the tribes thereof.
14 The LORD hath mingled a perverse
spirit in the midst thereof: and they have
caused Egypt to err in every work thereof,
as a drunken *man* staggereth in his vomit.
15 Neither shall there be *any* work for
Egypt, which the head or tail, branch or
rush, may do.

B.C. 714.

a Jud. 7:22; 1 Sam. 14:16, 20; 2 Chr. 20:23.

b Isa. 20:4; Jer. 46:26; Ezk. 29:19.

c Jer. 51:36; Ezk. 30:12.

d Jer. 2:16.

e Jer. 51:30; Nah. 3:13.

f Zeph. 3:9.

g 2 Ki. 18:17.

16 In that day shall Egypt [e]be like unto
women: and it shall be afraid and fear
because of the shaking of the hand of the
LORD of hosts, which he shaketh over it.
17 And the land of Judah shall be a
terror unto Egypt, every one that maketh
mention thereof shall be afraid in himself, because of the counsel of the LORD
of hosts, which he hath determined
against it.
18 In that day shall five cities in the
land of Egypt [f]speak the language of
Canaan, and swear to the LORD of hosts;
one shall be called, The city of destruction.
19 In that day shall there be an altar to
the LORD in the midst of the land of
Egypt, and a pillar at the border thereof
to the LORD.
20 And it shall be for a sign and for a
witness unto the LORD of hosts in the
land of Egypt: for they shall cry unto the
LORD because of the oppressors, and he
shall send them a saviour, and a great
one, and he shall deliver them.
21 And the LORD shall be known to
Egypt, and the Egyptians shall know the
LORD in that day, and shall do sacrifice
and oblation; yea, they shall vow a vow
unto the LORD, and perform *it*.
22 And the LORD shall smite Egypt: he
shall smite and heal *it*: and they shall
return *even* to the LORD, and he shall be
intreated of them, and shall heal them.
23 In that day shall there be a highway
out of Egypt to Assyria, and the Assyrian
shall come into Egypt, and the Egyptian
into Assyria, and the Egyptians shall
serve with the Assyrians.
24 In that day shall Israel be the third
with Egypt and with Assyria, *even* a
blessing in the midst of the land:
25 Whom the LORD of hosts shall bless,
saying, Blessed *be* Egypt my people, and
Assyria the work of my hands, and
Israel mine inheritance.

CHAPTER 20.

A prophecy that Assyria will waste Egypt and Ethiopia.

In the year that [g]Tartan came unto
Ashdod, (when Sargon the king of
Assyria sent him,) and fought against
Ashdod, and took it;
2 At the same time spake the LORD by

B.C. 714.

Isaiah the son of Amoz, saying, Go and
loose the [a]sackcloth from off thy loins,
and put off thy shoe from thy foot. And
he did so, [b]walking naked and barefoot.
3 And the LORD said, Like as my servant Isaiah hath walked naked and barefoot three years *for* a sign and wonder
upon Egypt and upon Ethiopia;
4 So shall the king of Assyria lead
away the Egyptians prisoners, and the
Ethiopians captives, young and old,
naked and barefoot, [c]even with *their* buttocks uncovered, to the shame of Egypt.
5 [d]And they shall be afraid and
ashamed of Ethiopia their expectation,
and of Egypt their glory.
6 And the inhabitant of this [e]isle shall
say in that day, Behold, such *is* our
expectation, whither we flee for help to
be delivered from the king of Assyria:
and how shall we escape?

CHAPTER 21.

The four burdens, anticipating Sennacherib's invasion (2 Ki. 18:13):

(1) *The burden of the desert.*

The [f]burden of the desert of the sea.
As [g]whirlwinds in the south pass
through; *so* it cometh from the desert,
from a terrible land.
2 A grievous vision is declared unto
me; the treacherous dealer dealeth
treacherously, and the spoiler spoileth.
[h]Go up, O Elam: besiege, O Media; all
the sighing thereof have I made to cease.
3 Therefore are my loins filled with
pain: pangs have taken hold upon me, as
the pangs of a woman that travaileth: I
was bowed down at the hearing *of it*; I
was dismayed at the seeing *of it*.
4 My heart panted, fearfulness
affrighted me: [i]the night of my pleasure
hath he turned into fear unto me.
5 Prepare the table, watch in the
watchtower, eat, drink: arise, ye princes,
and anoint the shield.
6 For thus hath the Lord said unto me,
Go, set a watchman, let him declare
what he seeth.
7 And he saw a chariot *with* a couple
of horsemen, a chariot of asses, *and* a
chariot of camels; and he hearkened diligently with much heed:
8 And he cried, A lion: My lord, I
stand continually upon the watchtower
in the daytime, and I am set in my ward
whole nights:
9 And, behold, here cometh a chariot
of men, *with* a couple of horsemen. And
he answered and said, [j]Babylon is fallen,
is fallen; and all the graven images of
her gods he hath broken unto the
ground.
10 O my threshing, and the corn of my
floor: that which I have heard of the
LORD of hosts, the God of Israel, have I
declared unto you.

(2) *The burden of Dumah.*

11 The [f]burden of [k]Dumah. He calleth
to me out of Seir, Watchman, what of the
night? Watchman, what of the night?
12 The watchman said, The morning
cometh, and also the night: if ye will
enquire, enquire ye: return, come.

(3) *The burden upon Arabia.*

13 The [f]burden upon Arabia. In the
forest in Arabia shall ye lodge, O ye
travelling companies [l]of Dedanim.
14 The inhabitants of the land of Tema
brought water to him that was thirsty,
they prevented with their bread him that
fled.
15 For they fled from the swords, from
the drawn sword, and from the bent
bow, and from the grievousness of war.
16 For thus hath the Lord said unto
me, Within a year, according to the years
of an hireling, and all the glory of Kedar
shall fail:
17 And the residue of the number of
archers, the mighty men of the children
of Kedar, shall be diminished: for the
LORD God of Israel hath spoken *it*.

CHAPTER 22.

(4) *The burden of the valley of vision.*

The [f]burden of the valley of vision.
What aileth thee now, that thou art
wholly gone up to the housetops?
2 Thou that art full of stirs, a tumultuous city, a joyous city: thy slain *men are*
not slain with the sword, nor dead in
battle.
3 All thy rulers are fled together, they
are bound by the archers: all that are

a Zech. 13:4.
b 1 Sam. 19:24; Mic. 1:8, 11.
c Isa. 3:17; 2 Sam. 10:4; Jer. 13:22, 26; Mic. 1:11.
d 2 Ki. 18:21; Isa. 30:3-7; 36:6.
e i.e. *coast.*
f Isa. 13:1, *note.*
g Zech. 9:14.
h Isa. 13:17; Jer. 49:34.
i Deut. 28:67.
j Jer. 51:8; Rev. 14:8; 18:2.
k 1 Chr. 1:30; Jer. 49:7, 8; Ezk. 35:2; Oba. 1.
l 1 Chr. 1:9, 32.

found in thee are bound together, *which*
have fled from far.
4 Therefore said I, Look away from
me; [a]I will weep bitterly, labour not to
comfort me, because of the spoiling of
the daughter of my people.
5 For *it is* a day of trouble, and of
treading down, and of perplexity [b]by the
Lord GOD of hosts in the valley of vision,
breaking down the walls, and of crying
to the mountains.
6 And Elam bare the quiver with chariots of men *and* horsemen, and [c]Kir
uncovered the shield.
7 And it shall come to pass, *that* thy
choicest valleys shall be full of chariots,
and the horsemen shall set themselves in
array at the gate.
8 And he discovered the covering of
Judah, and thou didst look in that day to
the armour of the house of the forest.
9 Ye have seen also the breaches of the
city of David, that they are many: and ye
gathered together the [d]waters of the
lower pool.
10 And ye have numbered the houses
of Jerusalem, and the houses have ye
broken down to fortify the wall.
11 [e]Ye made also a ditch between the
two walls for the water of the old pool:
but ye have not looked unto the maker
thereof, neither had respect unto him
that fashioned it long ago.
12 And in that day did the Lord GOD
of hosts [f]call to weeping, and to mourning, and to [g]baldness, and to girding
with sackcloth:
13 And behold joy and gladness, slaying oxen, and killing sheep, eating flesh,
and drinking wine: [h]let us eat and drink;
for to morrow we shall die.
14 And it was revealed in mine ears by
the LORD of hosts, Surely this iniquity
[i]shall not be purged from you till ye die,
saith the Lord GOD of hosts.
15 Thus saith the Lord GOD of hosts,
Go, get thee unto this treasurer, *even* unto
[j]Shebna, which *is* over the house, *and say*,
16 What hast thou here? and whom
hast thou here, that thou hast hewed
thee out a sepulchre here, *as* he that
heweth him out a sepulchre on high, *and*
that graveth an habitation for himself in
a rock?

B.C. 712.

a Jer. 4:19; 9:1; Lk. 19:41.

b Lam. 1:5; 2:2.

c Isa. 15:1.

d 2 Ki. 20:20; 2 Chr. 32:4, 5, 30.

e Neh. 3:16.

f Joel 1:13.

g Isa. 15:2; Ezra 9:3; Mic. 1:16.

h Isa. 56:12; 1 Cor. 15:32.

i 1 Sam. 3:14; Ezk. 24:13.

j vs. 15-19. A foreigner and court favourite displaced as treasurer by Eliakim. Isa. 36:3; 37:2.

k Esth. 7:8.

l 2 Ki. 18:18.

m Here the prophecy looks forward to Christ. Rev. 3:7.

n Isa. 13:1, *note*.

o i.e. *coast*.

17 Behold, the LORD will carry thee
away with a mighty captivity, and [k]will
surely cover thee.
18 He will surely violently turn and
toss thee *like* a ball into a large country:
there shalt thou die, and there the chariots of thy glory *shall be* the shame of thy
lord's house.
19 And I will drive thee from thy station, and from thy state shall he pull
thee down.
20 And it shall come to pass in that
day, that I will call my servant [l]Eliakim
the son of Hilkiah:
21 And I will clothe him with thy robe,
and strengthen him with thy girdle, and
I will commit thy government into his
hand: and he shall be a father to the
inhabitants of Jerusalem, and to the
house of Judah.
22 And the key of the house of David
will I lay upon his shoulder; so he shall
[m]open, and none shall shut; and he shall
shut, and none shall open.
23 And I will fasten him *as* a nail in a
sure place; and he shall be for a glorious
throne to his father's house.
24 And they shall hang upon him all
the glory of his father's house, the offspring and the issue, all vessels of small
quantity, from the vessels of cups, even
to all the vessels of flagons.
25 In that day, saith the LORD of hosts,
shall the nail that is fastened in the sure
place be removed, and be cut down, and
fall; and the burden that *was* upon it shall
be cut off: for the LORD hath spoken *it*.

CHAPTER 23.

The burden of Tyre: desolations preceding the final deliverance of Israel.

The [n]burden of Tyre. Howl, ye ships
of Tarshish; for it is laid waste, so that
there is no house, no entering in: from the
land of Chittim it is revealed to them.
2 Be still, ye inhabitants of the [o]isle;
thou whom the merchants of Zidon, that
pass over the sea, have replenished.
3 And by great waters the seed of
Sihor, the harvest of the river, *is* her revenue; and she is a mart of nations.
4 Be thou ashamed, O Zidon: for the
sea hath spoken, *even* the strength of the
sea, saying, I travail not, nor bring forth

children, neither do I nourish up young
men, *nor* bring up virgins.
5 As at the report concerning Egypt, *so*
shall they be sorely pained at the report
of Tyre.
6 Pass ye over to Tarshish; howl, ye
inhabitants of the [a]isle.
7 *Is* this your joyous *city*, whose antiquity *is* of ancient days? her own feet
shall carry her afar off to sojourn.
8 Who hath taken this counsel against
Tyre, [b]the crowning *city*, whose merchants *are* princes, whose traffickers *are*
the honourable of the earth?
9 The LORD of hosts hath purposed it,
to stain the pride of all glory, *and* to
bring into contempt all the honourable
of the earth.
10 Pass through thy land as a river, O
daughter of Tarshish: *there is* no more
strength.
11 He stretched out his hand over the
sea, he shook the kingdoms: the LORD
hath given a commandment against the
merchant *city*, to destroy the strong
holds thereof.
12 And he said, [c]Thou shalt no more
rejoice, O thou oppressed virgin, daughter of Zidon: arise, pass over to Chittim;
there also shalt thou have no rest.
13 Behold the land of the Chaldeans;
this people was not, *till* the Assyrian
founded it for them that dwell in the
wilderness: they set up the towers thereof, they raised up the palaces thereof;
and he brought it to ruin.
14 [d]Howl, ye ships of Tarshish: for
your strength is laid waste.
15 And it shall come to pass in that
day, that Tyre shall be forgotten seventy
years, according to the days of one king:
after the end of seventy years shall Tyre
sing as an harlot.
16 Take an harp, go about the city,
thou harlot that hast been forgotten;
make sweet melody, sing many songs,
that thou mayest be remembered.
17 And it shall come to pass after the
end of seventy years, that the LORD will
visit Tyre, and she shall turn to her hire,
and shall commit fornication with all the
kingdoms of the world upon the face of
the earth.
18 And her merchandise and her hire
[e]shall be holiness to the LORD: it shall not
be treasured nor laid up; for her merchandise shall be for them that dwell
before the LORD, to eat sufficiently, and
for durable clothing.

CHAPTER 24.

Looking through troubles to the kingdom-age (v. 23).

Behold, the LORD [f]maketh the earth
empty, and maketh it waste, and
turneth it upside down, and scattereth
abroad the inhabitants thereof.
2 And it shall be, as with the people,
so with the priest; as with the servant, so
with his master; as with the maid, so with
her mistress; as with the buyer, so with
the seller; as with the lender, so with the
borrower; as with the taker of usury, so
with the giver of usury to him.
3 The land shall be utterly emptied,
and utterly spoiled: for the LORD hath
spoken this word.
4 The earth mourneth *and* fadeth
away, the world languisheth *and* fadeth
away, the haughty people of the earth do
languish.
5 [g]The earth also is defiled under the
inhabitants thereof; because they have
transgressed the laws, changed the ordinance, broken the everlasting covenant.
6 Therefore hath [h]the curse devoured
the earth, and they that dwell therein are
desolate: therefore the inhabitants of the
earth are burned, and few men left.
7 [i]The new wine mourneth, the vine
languisheth, all the merryhearted do sigh.
8 The mirth of tabrets ceaseth, the
noise of them that rejoice endeth, the joy
of the harp ceaseth.
9 They shall not drink wine with a
song; strong drink shall be bitter to them
that drink it.
10 The city of confusion is broken
down: every house is shut up, that no
man may come in.
11 *There is* a crying for wine in the
streets; all joy is darkened, the mirth of
the land is gone.
12 In the city is left desolation, and the
gate is smitten with destruction.

The Jewish remnant.

13 When thus it shall be in the midst of
the land [j]among the people, *there shall be*
as the shaking of an olive tree, *and* as the
gleaning grapes when the vintage is done.
14 They shall lift up their voice, they

B.C. 715.

a i.e. *coast.*

b See Ezk. 28:2, 12.

c Rev. 18:22.

d Ezk. 27:25, 30.

e Zech. 14:20, 21.

f See Gen. 1:2, *note* 3; Jer. 4:23, *note.*

g Gen. 3:17; Num. 35:33.

h Mal. 4:6.

i Isa. 16:8, 9; Joel 1:10, 12.

j *Remnant.* Isa. 37:32. (Isa. 1:9; Rom. 11:5.)

shall sing for the majesty of the LORD, they shall cry aloud from the sea.

15 Wherefore glorify ye the LORD in the fires, *even* the [a]name of the LORD God of Israel in the [b]isles of the sea.

The great tribulation (Psa. 2:5; Rev. 7:14).

16 From the uttermost part of the earth have we heard songs, *even* glory to the righteous. But I said, My leanness, my leanness, woe unto me! the treacherous dealers have dealt treacherously; yea, the treacherous dealers have dealt very treacherously.

17 [c]Fear, and the pit, and the snare, *are* upon thee, O inhabitant of the earth.

18 And it shall come to pass, *that* he who fleeth from the noise of the fear shall fall into the pit; and he that cometh up out of the midst of the pit shall be taken in the snare: for the windows from on high are open, and the foundations of the earth do shake.

19 The earth is utterly broken down, the earth is clean dissolved, the earth is moved exceedingly.

20 The earth shall reel to and fro like a drunkard, and shall be removed like a cottage; and the transgression thereof shall be heavy upon it; and it shall fall, and not rise again.

Destruction of Gentile world-power.
(See "*Kingdom,* O.T.," Gen. 1:26; Zech. 12:8, *note.*)

21 And it shall come to pass [d]in that day, *that* the LORD shall [e]punish the host of the high ones *that are* on high, and the kings of the earth upon the earth.

The first resurrection: the kingdom-age begun.

22 And they shall be gathered together, *as* prisoners are gathered in the pit, and shall be shut up in the prison, and after many days shall they be visited.

23 Then the moon shall be confounded, and the sun ashamed, when the LORD of hosts shall [f]reign in mount Zion, and in Jerusalem, and before his ancients gloriously.

CHAPTER 25.

Triumphs of the kingdom-age.

O LORD, thou *art* my God; I will exalt thee, I will praise thy name; for thou hast done wonderful *things; thy* counsels of old *are* faithfulness *and* truth.

2 For thou hast made of a city an heap; *of* a defenced city a ruin: a palace of strangers to be no city; it shall never be built.

3 Therefore shall the strong people glorify thee, the city of the terrible nations shall fear thee.

4 For thou hast been a strength to the poor, a strength to the needy in his distress, a refuge from the storm, a shadow from the heat, when the blast of the terrible ones *is* as a storm *against* the wall.

5 Thou shalt bring down the noise of strangers, as the heat in a dry place; *even* the heat with the shadow of a cloud: the branch of the terrible ones shall be brought low.

6 And in this mountain shall the LORD of hosts make unto all people a feast of fat things, a feast of wines on the lees, of fat things full of marrow, of wines on the lees well refined.

7 And he will destroy in this mountain the face of the covering cast over all people, and the vail that is spread over all nations.

8 He will [g]swallow up death in victory; and the Lord GOD will [h]wipe away tears from off all faces; and the rebuke of his people shall he take away from off all the earth: for the LORD hath spoken *it.*

9 And it shall be said in that day, Lo, this *is* our God; [i]we have waited for him, and he will save us: this *is* the LORD; we have waited for him, we will be glad and rejoice in his salvation.

10 For in this mountain shall the hand of the LORD rest, and Moab shall be trodden down under him, even as straw is trodden down for the dunghill.

11 And he shall spread forth his hands in the midst of them, as he that swimmeth spreadeth forth *his hands* to swim: and he shall bring down their pride together with the spoils of their hands.

12 And the fortress of the high fort of thy walls shall he bring down, lay low, *and* bring to the ground, *even* to the dust.

CHAPTER 26.

The worship and testimony of restored and converted Israel.

[j]In that day shall this song be sung in the land of Judah; We have a strong city; [k]salvation

B.C. 712.

a Mal. 1:11.

b i.e. *coasts.* Isa. 42:4.

c See 1 Ki. 19:17; Jer. 48:43; Amos 5:19.

d *Day (of Jehovah).* vs. 21-23; Isa. 26:20, 21. (Isa. 2:10-22; Rev. 19:11-21.)

e *Armageddon (battle of).* Isa. 26:20, 21. (Rev. 16:14; 19:11-21.)

f *Kingdom* (O.T.). Isa. 32:1, 2, 14-18. (Gen. 1:26; Zech. 12:8.)

g Hos. 13:14; 1 Cor. 15:54; Rev. 20:14; 21:4.

h Rev. 7:17; 21:4.

i Gen. 49:18; Tit. 2:13.

j Isa. 2:11.

k Isa. 60:18.

will *God* appoint *for* walls and bulwarks.
2 Open ye the gates, that the righteous
nation which keepeth the truth may
enter in.
3 Thou wilt keep *him* in perfect peace,
whose mind *is* stayed *on thee*: because he
[a]trusteth in thee.
4 Trust ye in the LORD for ever: for in
the LORD JEHOVAH *is* [b]everlasting
strength:
5 For he bringeth down them that
dwell on high; the lofty city, he layeth it
low; he layeth it low, *even* to the ground;
he bringeth it *even* to the dust.
6 The foot shall tread it down, *even* the
feet of the poor, *and* the steps of the
needy.
7 The way of the just *is* [c]uprightness:
thou, most upright, dost weigh the path
of the just.
8 Yea, in the way of thy judgments, O
LORD, have we waited for thee; the
desire of *our* soul *is* to thy name, and to
the remembrance of thee.
9 With my soul have I desired thee in
the night; yea, with my spirit within me
will I seek thee early: for when thy judgments *are* in the earth, the inhabitants of
the world will learn righteousness.
10 Let favour be shewed to the
wicked, *yet* will he not learn righteousness: in the land of uprightness will he
deal unjustly, and will not behold the
majesty of the LORD.
11 LORD, *when* thy hand is lifted up,
they will not see: *but* they shall see, and
be ashamed for *their* envy at the people;
yea, the fire of thine enemies shall
devour them.
12 LORD, thou wilt ordain peace for us:
for thou also hast wrought all our works
in us.
13 O LORD our God, *other* lords beside
thee have had dominion over us: *but* by
thee only will we make mention of thy
name.
14 *They are* dead, they shall not live; *they*
are deceased, they shall not rise: therefore
hast thou visited and destroyed them, and
made all their memory to perish.

B.C. 712.

a Psa. 2:12, *note.*

b Heb. *the rock of ages.* Deut. 32:4.

c *Righteousness.* Ezk. 18:5-9. (Gen. 6:9; Lk. 2:25.)

d Hos. 5:15.

e *Resurrection.* Dan. 12:2, 13. (Job 19:25; 1 Cor. 15:52.)

f *Day (of Jehovah).* vs. 20, 21; Isa. 34:1-8. (Isa. 2:10-22; Rev. 19:11-21.)

g *Armageddon (battle of).* Isa. 34:1-8. (Rev. 16:14; 19:11-21.)

15 Thou hast increased the nation, O
LORD, thou hast increased the nation:
thou art glorified: thou hadst removed *it*
far *unto* all the ends of the earth.
16 LORD, [d]in trouble have they visited
thee, they poured out a prayer *when* thy
chastening *was* upon them.
17 Like as a woman with child, *that*
draweth near the time of her delivery, is
in pain, *and* crieth out in her pangs; so
have we been in thy sight, O LORD.
18 We have been with child, we have
been in pain, we have as it were brought
forth wind; we have not wrought any
deliverance in the earth; neither have the
inhabitants of the world fallen.
19 [e]Thy dead [1]*men* shall live, *together*
with my dead body shall they arise.
Awake and sing, ye that dwell in dust:
for thy dew *is as* the dew of herbs, and
the earth shall cast out the dead.

Retrospect: order of events in establishing the kingdom.

(1) *The Gentile world-power destroyed.*

20 Come, my people, enter thou into
thy chambers, and shut thy doors about
thee: hide thyself as it were for a little
moment, until the [f]indignation be overpast.
21 For, behold, the LORD cometh out of
his place to [g]punish the inhabitants of
the earth for their iniquity: the earth also
shall disclose her blood, and shall no
more cover her slain.

CHAPTER 27.

In that day the LORD with his sore and
great and strong sword shall punish
leviathan the piercing serpent, even
leviathan that crooked serpent; and he
shall slay the dragon that *is* in the sea.
2 In that day sing ye unto her, A vineyard of red wine.
3 I the LORD do keep it; I will water it
every moment: lest *any* hurt it, I will
keep it night and day.
4 Fury *is* not in me: who would set the

[1] **(26:19)** Eliminate the supplied words, *men*, and, *together with.* "Body" is in the plural, "bodies." Verses 19-21, with chapter 27, constitute Jehovah's answer to the plaint of Israel, verses 11-18. Verse 19 should read: "Thy dead shall live: my dead bodies shall rise" (i.e. the dead bodies of Jehovah's people). The restoration and re-establishment of Israel as a nation is also spoken of as a resurrection (Ezk. 37:1-11), and many hold that no more than this is meant in Isa. 26:19. But since the first resurrection is unto participation in the kingdom (Rev. 20:4-6), it seems the better view that both meanings are here.

briers *and* thorns against me in battle? I would go through them, I would burn them together.

5 Or let him take hold of my strength, *that* he may make peace with me; *and* he shall make peace with me.

6 He shall cause them that come of Jacob to take root: Israel shall blossom and bud, and fill the face of the world with fruit.

7 Hath he smitten him, as he smote those that smote him? *or* is he slain according to the slaughter of them that are slain by him?

8 In measure, when it shooteth forth, thou wilt debate with it: he stayeth his rough wind in the day of the east wind.

9 By this therefore shall the iniquity of Jacob be purged; and this *is* all the fruit to take away his sin; when he maketh all the stones of the altar as chalkstones that are beaten in sunder, the [a]groves and images shall not stand up.

10 Yet the defenced city *shall be* desolate, *and* the habitation forsaken, and left like a wilderness: there shall the calf feed, and there shall he lie down, and consume the branches thereof.

11 When the boughs thereof are withered, they shall be broken off: the women come, *and* set them on fire: for it *is* a people of no understanding: therefore he that made them will not have mercy on them, and he that formed them will shew them no favour.

(2) *Israel regathered.*

12 And it shall come to pass in that day, *that* the LORD shall beat off from the channel of the river unto the stream of Egypt, and ye shall be gathered one by one, O ye children of Israel.

13 And it shall come to pass in that day, *that* the great trumpet shall be blown, and they shall come which were ready to perish in the land of Assyria, and the outcasts in the land of Egypt, and shall worship the LORD in the holy mount at Jerusalem.

CHAPTER 28.

The woe of Ephraim. Prediction of the Assyrian captivity of Ephraim
(2 Ki. 17:3-18).

Woe to the crown of pride, to the drunkards of [b]Ephraim, whose glorious beauty *is* a fading flower, which *are* on the head of the fat valleys of them that are overcome with wine!

2 Behold, the Lord hath a mighty and strong one, [c]*which* as a tempest of hail *and* a destroying storm, as a flood of mighty waters overflowing, shall cast down to the earth with the hand.

3 The crown of pride, the drunkards of Ephraim, shall be trodden under feet:

4 And the glorious beauty, which *is* on the head of the fat valley, shall be a fading flower, *and* as the hasty fruit before the summer; which *when* he that looketh upon it seeth, while it is yet in his hand he eateth it up.

5 In that day shall the LORD of hosts be for a crown of glory, and for a diadem of beauty, unto the residue of his people,

6 And for a spirit of judgment to him that sitteth in judgment, and for strength to them that turn the battle to the gate.

7 But they also [d]have erred through wine, and through strong drink are out of the way; the priest and the prophet have erred through strong drink, they are swallowed up of wine, they are out of the way through strong drink; they err in vision, they stumble *in* judgment.

8 For all tables are full of vomit *and* filthiness, *so that there is* no place *clean.*

9 Whom shall he teach knowledge? and whom shall he make to understand doctrine? *them that are* weaned from the milk, *and* drawn from the breasts.

10 For precept *must be* upon precept, precept upon precept; line upon line, line upon line; here a little, *and* there a little:

11 For with stammering lips and another tongue will he speak to this people.

12 To whom he said, This *is* the rest *wherewith* ye may cause the weary to rest; and this *is* the refreshing: yet they would not hear.

13 But the word of the LORD was unto them precept upon precept, precept upon precept; line upon line, line upon line; here a little, *and* there a little; that they might go, and fall backward, and be broken, and snared, and taken.

The fate of Ephraim a warning to Judah.

14 Wherefore hear the word of the

B.C. 712.

a Deut. 16:21.
b See Isa. 7:2, *note.*
c Isa. 30:30; Ezk. 13:11.
d Prov. 20:1; Hos. 4:11.

LORD, ye scornful men, that rule this people which *is* in Jerusalem.

15 Because ye have said, We have made a covenant with death, and with [a]hell are we at agreement; when the overflowing scourge shall pass through, it shall not come unto us: for we have made lies our refuge, and under falsehood have we hid ourselves:

16 Therefore thus saith the Lord GOD, Behold, I lay in Zion for a foundation a [b]stone, a tried [c]stone, a precious corner *stone,* a sure foundation: he that believeth shall not make haste.

17 Judgment also will I lay to the line, and righteousness to the plummet: and the hail shall sweep away the refuge of lies, and the waters shall overflow the hiding place.

18 And your covenant with death shall be disannulled, and your agreement with [d]hell shall not stand; when the overflowing scourge shall pass through, then ye shall be trodden down by it.

19 From the time that it goeth forth it shall take you: for morning by morning shall it pass over, by day and by night: and it shall be a vexation only *to* understand the report.

20 For the bed is shorter than that *a man* can stretch himself *on it*: and the covering narrower than that he can wrap himself *in it*.

21 For the LORD shall rise up as *in* mount [e]Perazim, he shall be wroth as *in* the valley of [f]Gibeon, that he may do his work, his strange work; and bring to pass his act, his strange act.

22 Now therefore be ye not mockers, lest your bands be made strong: for I have heard from the Lord GOD of hosts a consumption, even determined upon the whole earth.

23 Give ye ear, and hear my voice; hearken, and hear my speech.

24 Doth the plowman plow all day to sow? doth he open and break the clods of his ground?

25 When he hath made plain the face thereof, doth he not cast abroad the fitches, and scatter the cummin, and cast in the principal wheat and the appointed barley and the rie in their place?

26 For his God doth instruct him to discretion, *and* doth teach him.

27 For the fitches are not threshed with a threshing instrument, neither is a cart wheel turned about upon the cummin; but the fitches are beaten out with a staff, and the cummin with a rod.

28 Bread *corn* is bruised; because he will not ever be threshing it, nor break *it with* the wheel of his cart, nor bruise it *with* his horsemen.

29 This also cometh forth from the LORD of hosts, [g]*which* is wonderful in counsel, *and* excellent in working.

CHAPTER 29.

Warnings to Judah and Jerusalem of impending discipline
(Chapters 29, 30, 31): (1) *The discipline.*

Woe to [h]Ariel, to Ariel, the city *where* David dwelt! add ye year to year; let them kill sacrifices.

2 Yet I will distress Ariel, and there shall be heaviness and sorrow: and it shall be unto me as Ariel.

3 [1]And I will camp against thee round about, and will lay siege against thee with a mount, and I will raise forts against thee.

4 And thou shalt be brought down, *and* shalt speak out of the ground, and thy speech shall be low out of the dust, and thy voice shall be, as of one that hath a familiar spirit, out of the ground, and thy speech shall whisper out of the dust.

5 Moreover the multitude of thy strangers shall be like small dust, and the multitude of the terrible ones *shall be* [i]as chaff that passeth away: yea, it

B.C. 725.

a Heb. *Sheol.* See Hab. 2:5, *note.*

b *Christ (as Stone).* Dan. 2:34. (Ex. 17:6; 1 Pet. 2:8.)

c *Christ (First Advent).* Isa. 42:1-3. (Gen. 3:15; Acts 1:9.)

d See v. 15.

e 2 Sam. 5:20; 1 Chr. 14:11.

f Josh. 10:10, 12; 2 Sam. 5:25; 1 Chr. 14-16.

g Psa. 92:5; Isa. 9:6; Jer. 32:19.

h *"Lion of God"* = *Jerusalem.*

i Isa. 17:13; Job 21:18.

[1] **(29:3)** Here, as often in prophecy, and especially in Isaiah, the near and far horizons blend. The near view is of Sennacherib's invasion and the destruction of the Assyrian host by the angel of the LORD (Isa. 36, 37); the far view is that of the final gathering of the Gentile hosts against Jerusalem at the end of the great tribulation (Psa. 2.5; Rev. 7:14), when a still greater deliverance will be wrought. (See "Times of the Gentiles," Lk. 21:24; Rev. 16:14.) The same remark applies also to Isa. 28:14-18, where there is a near reference to the Egyptian alliance ("we have made a covenant," etc.), while the reference to the stone (v. 16) carries the meaning forward to the end-time, and the covenant of unbelieving Israel with the Beast (Dan. 9:27).

shall be at an instant suddenly.

6 Thou shalt be visited of the LORD of hosts with thunder, and with [a]earthquake, and great noise, with storm and tempest, and the flame of devouring fire.

7 And the multitude of all the nations that fight against Ariel, even all that fight against her and her munition, and that distress her, shall be as a dream of a night vision.

8 It shall even be as when an hungry *man* dreameth, and, behold, he eateth; but he awaketh, and his soul is empty: or as when a thirsty man dreameth, and, behold, he drinketh; but he awaketh, and, behold, *he is* faint, and his soul hath appetite: so shall the multitude of all the nations be, that fight against mount Zion.

(2) *The reasons for the discipline.*

9 Stay yourselves, and wonder; cry ye out, and cry: they are drunken, but not with wine; they stagger, but not with strong drink.

10 For the LORD hath poured out upon you the spirit of deep [b]sleep, and hath closed your eyes: the prophets and your rulers, the seers hath he covered.

11 And the vision of all is become unto you as the words of a book that is sealed, which *men* deliver to one that is learned, saying, Read this, I pray thee: and he saith, I cannot; for it *is* sealed:

12 And the book is delivered to him that is not learned, saying, Read this, I pray thee: and he saith, I am not learned.

13 Wherefore the Lord said, Forasmuch as this people draw near *me* with their mouth, [c]and with their lips do honour me, but have removed their heart far from me, and their fear toward me is taught by the precept of men:

14 Therefore, behold, I will proceed to do a [d]marvellous work among this people, *even* a marvellous work and a wonder: for the [e]wisdom of their wise *men* shall perish, and the understanding of their prudent *men* shall be hid.

15 Woe unto them that seek deep to hide their counsel from the LORD, and their works are in the dark, and they say, Who seeth us? and who knoweth us?

16 Surely your turning of things upside down shall be esteemed as the potter's clay: for shall the work say of him that made it, He made me not? or shall the thing framed say of him that framed it, He had no understanding?

(3) *Blessing after deliverance* (Isa. 37:33-36): *type of blessing in the kingdom after Rev.* 19:19-21.

17 *Is* it not yet a very little while, and Lebanon shall be turned into a fruitful field, and the fruitful field shall be esteemed as a forest?

18 And in that day shall the deaf hear the words of the book, and the eyes of the blind shall see out of obscurity, and out of darkness.

19 The meek also shall increase *their* joy in the LORD, and the poor among men shall rejoice in the Holy One of Israel.

20 For the terrible one is brought to nought, and the scorner is consumed, and all that watch for iniquity are cut off:

21 That make a man an offender for a word, and lay a snare for him that reproveth in the gate, and turn aside the just for a thing of nought.

22 Therefore thus saith the LORD, who [f]redeemed Abraham, concerning the house of Jacob, Jacob shall not now be ashamed, neither shall his face now wax pale.

23 But when he seeth his children, the work of mine hands, in the midst of him, they shall sanctify my name, and sanctify the Holy One of Jacob, and shall fear the God of Israel.

24 They also that erred in spirit shall come to understanding, and they that murmured shall learn doctrine.

CHAPTER 30.

(4) *Warnings against an alliance with Egypt against Sennacherib.*

WOE to the rebellious children, saith the LORD, that take counsel, but not of me; and that cover with a covering, but not of my spirit, [g]that they may add sin to sin:

2 That walk to go down into Egypt, and [h]have not asked at my mouth; to strengthen themselves in the strength of Pharaoh, and to trust in the shadow of Egypt!

3 Therefore shall the strength of Pharaoh be your shame, and the [i]trust in the shadow of Egypt *your* confusion.

B.C. 712.

a Zech. 14:4; Rev. 16:18-19.

b Rom. 11:8.

c Ezk. 33:31; Mt. 15:8, 9; Mk. 7:6, 7.

d Hab. 1:5.

e Jer. 49:7; Oba. 8; 1 Cor. 1:19.

f Ex. 14:30, *note;* Isa. 59:20, *note.*

g Deut. 29:19.

h Num. 27:21; Josh. 9:14; 1 Ki. 22:7; Jer. 21:2; 42:2, 3, 20.

i Psa. 2:12, *note.*

4 For his princes were at Zoan, and his ambassadors came to Hanes.

5 They were all ashamed of a people *that* could not profit them, nor be an help nor profit, but a shame, and also a reproach.

6 The [a]burden of the beasts of the south: into the land of trouble and anguish, from whence *come* the young and old lion, the viper and fiery flying serpent, they will carry their riches upon the shoulders of young asses, and their treasures upon the bunches of camels, to a people *that* shall not profit *them*.

7 For the Egyptians shall help in vain, and to no purpose: therefore have I cried concerning this, Their strength *is* to sit still.

8 Now go, [b]write it before them in a table, and note it in a book, that it may be for the time to come for ever and ever:

9 That this *is* a rebellious people, lying children, children *that* will not hear the law of the LORD:

10 Which say to the seers, See not; and to the prophets, Prophesy not unto us right things, speak unto us smooth things, prophesy deceits:

11 Get you out of the way, turn aside out of the path, cause the Holy One of Israel to cease from before us.

12 Wherefore thus saith the Holy One of Israel, Because ye despise this word, and [c]trust in oppression and perverseness, and stay thereon:

13 Therefore this iniquity shall be to you as a breach ready to fall, swelling out in a high wall, whose breaking cometh suddenly at an instant.

14 And he shall break it as the breaking of the potters' vessel that is broken in pieces; he shall not spare: so that there shall not be found in the bursting of it a sherd to take fire from the hearth, or to take water *withal* out of the pit.

(5) Exhortation to turn to the LORD for help against Sennacherib: foreshadowing of kingdom blessing.

15 For thus saith the Lord GOD, the Holy One of Israel; In returning and rest shall ye be saved; in quietness and in confidence shall be your strength: [d]and ye would not.

16 But ye said, No; for we will flee upon horses; therefore shall ye flee: and, We will ride upon the swift; therefore shall they that pursue you be swift.

17 [e]One thousand *shall flee* at the rebuke of one; at the rebuke of five shall ye flee: till ye be left as a beacon upon the top of a mountain, and as an ensign on an hill.

18 And therefore will the LORD wait, that he may be gracious unto you, and therefore will he be exalted, that he may have mercy upon you: for the LORD *is* a God of judgment: [f]blessed *are* all they that wait for him.

19 For the people shall dwell in Zion at Jerusalem: thou shalt weep no more: he will be very gracious unto thee at the voice of thy cry; when he shall hear it, he will answer thee.

20 And *though* the Lord give you the bread of adversity, and the water of affliction, yet shall not thy teachers be removed into a corner any more, but thine eyes shall see thy teachers:

21 And thine ears shall hear a word behind thee, saying, This *is* the way, walk ye in it, when ye turn to the right hand, and when ye turn to the left.

22 Ye shall defile also the covering of thy graven images of silver, and the ornament of thy molten images of gold: thou shalt cast them away as a menstruous cloth; thou shalt say unto it, Get thee hence.

23 [g]Then shall he give the rain of thy seed, that thou shalt sow the ground withal; and bread of the increase of the earth, and it shall be fat and plenteous: in that day shall thy cattle feed in large pastures.

24 The oxen likewise and the young asses that ear the ground shall eat clean provender, which hath been winnowed with the shovel and with the fan.

25 And there shall be upon every high mountain, and upon every high hill, rivers *and* streams of waters in the day of the great slaughter, when the towers fall.

26 Moreover the light of the moon shall be as the light of the sun, and the light of the sun shall be sevenfold, as the light of seven days, in the day that the LORD bindeth up the breach of his people, and healeth the stroke of their wound.

B.C. 713.

a Isa. 13:1, *note*.

b *Inspiration*. Isa. 59:21. (Ex. 4:15; Rev. 22:19.)

c Psalm 2:12, *note*.

d Mt. 23:37.

e Lev. 26:8; Deut. 28:25; 32:30; Josh. 23:10.

f Psa. 2:12; 34:8; Prov. 16:20; Jer. 17:7.

g Mt. 6:33; 1 Tim. 4:8.

27 [1]Behold, the name of the LORD cometh from far, burning *with* his anger, and the burden *thereof is* heavy: his lips are full of indignation, and his tongue as a devouring fire:

28 And [a]his breath, as an overflowing stream, shall reach to the midst of the neck, to sift the nations with the sieve of vanity: and *there shall be* a bridle in the jaws of the people, causing *them* to err.

29 Ye shall have a song, as in the night *when* a holy solemnity is kept; and gladness of heart, as when one goeth with a pipe to come into the mountain of the LORD, to the [b]mighty One of Israel.

30 And the LORD shall cause [c]his glorious voice to be heard, and shall shew the lighting down of his arm, with the indignation of *his* anger, and *with* the flame of a devouring fire, *with* scattering, and tempest, and hailstones.

31 For through the voice of the LORD shall the Assyrian be beaten down, *which* smote with a rod.

32 And *in* every place where the grounded staff shall pass, which the LORD shall lay upon him, *it* shall be with tabrets and harps: and in battles of shaking will he fight with it.

33 For [d]Tophet *is* ordained of old; yea, for the king it is prepared; he hath made *it* deep *and* large: the pile thereof *is* fire and much wood; the breath of the LORD, like a stream of brimstone, doth kindle it.

CHAPTER 31.

(6) Judah again warned against the Egyptian alliance: Jehovah will defend Jerusalem.

Woe to them that go down to Egypt for help; and stay on horses, and [e]trust in chariots, because *they are* many; and in horsemen, because they are very strong; but they look not unto the Holy One of Israel, [f]neither seek the LORD!

2 Yet he also *is* wise, and will bring evil, and will not call back his words: but will arise against the house of the evildoers, and against the help of them that work iniquity.

3 Now the Egyptians *are* men, and not God; and their horses flesh, and not spirit. When the LORD shall stretch out his hand, both he that helpeth shall fall, and he that is holpen shall fall down, and they all shall fail together.

4 For thus hath the LORD spoken unto me, [g]Like as the lion and the young lion roaring on his prey, when a multitude of shepherds is called forth against him, *he* will not be afraid of their voice, nor abase himself for the noise of them: so shall the LORD of hosts come down to fight for mount Zion, and for the hill thereof.

5 [h]As birds flying, so will the LORD of hosts defend Jerusalem; defending also he will deliver *it; and* passing over he will preserve *it*.

6 Turn ye unto *him from* whom the children of Israel have [i]deeply revolted.

7 For in that day every man shall cast away his idols of silver, and his idols of gold, which your own hands have made unto you *for* a sin.

8 Then shall the Assyrian [j]fall with the sword, not of a mighty man; and the sword, not of a mean man, shall devour him: but he shall flee from the sword, and his young men shall be discomfited.

9 And he shall pass over to his strong hold for fear, and his princes shall be afraid of the ensign, saith the LORD, whose fire *is* in Zion, and his furnace in Jerusalem.

CHAPTER 32.

Promise and warning: tribulation: the King-Deliverer (Chapters 32–35).

Behold, a [2]king shall [k]reign in righteousness, and princes shall rule in judgment.

2 And a man shall be as an hiding place from the wind, and a covert from

B.C. 713.

a Isa. 11:4; 2 Thes. 2:8.

b Heb. *Rock.* Deut. 32:4.

c Heb. *the glory of his voice.*

d Jer. 7:31; 19:6; 2 Ki. 23:10. Historically a place in the valley of Hinnom where human sacrifices were offered. The word means "place of fire." The symbolic reference is to the lake of fire and the doom of the Beast (Rev. 19:20).

e Psa. 2:12, *note.*

f Dan. 9:13; Hos. 7:7.

g Hos. 11:10; Amos 3:8.

h Deut. 32:11; Psa. 91:4.

i Hos. 9:9.

j See 2 Ki. 19:35, 36; Isa. 37:36.

k *Kingdom* (O.T.). vs. 1, 2, 14-18; Isa. 33:17-22. (Gen. 1:26; Zech. 12:8.)

[1] **(30:27)** The imagery of verses 27, 28 is cumulative. Judah is making an alliance with Egypt when she might be in league with Him whose judgment upon the world-powers will be like a terrible thunder-tempest (v. 27), turning streams into torrents neck-deep (v. 28, f.c.); who will sift the nations in their own sieve of vanity (or "destruction"), and put His bridle into the jaws of the peoples.

[2] **(32:1)** See Isa. 29:3, *note.* In chapters 32–35 the same blended meanings of near and far fulfilments are found. The near view is still of Sennacherib's invasion, the far view of the day of the LORD (Isa. 2:10-22; Rev. 19:11-21), and the kingdom blessing to follow.

the tempest; as rivers of water in a dry place, as the shadow of a great rock in a weary land.

3 And the eyes of them that see shall not be dim, and the ears of them that hear shall hearken.

4 The heart also of the rash shall understand knowledge, and the tongue of the stammerers shall be ready to speak plainly.

5 The vile person shall be no more called liberal, nor the churl said *to be* bountiful.

6 For the vile person will speak villany, and his heart will work iniquity, to practise hypocrisy, and to utter error against the LORD, to make empty the soul of the hungry, and he will cause the drink of the thirsty to fail.

7 The instruments also of the churl *are* evil: he deviseth wicked devices to destroy the poor with lying words, even when the needy speaketh right.

8 But the liberal deviseth liberal things; and by liberal things shall he stand.

9 Rise up, ye women that are at ease; hear my voice, ye careless daughters; give ear unto my speech.

10 Many days and years shall ye be troubled, ye careless women: for the vintage shall fail, the gathering shall not come.

11 Tremble, ye women that are at ease; be troubled, ye careless ones: strip you, and make you bare, and gird *sackcloth* upon *your* loins.

12 They shall lament for the teats, for the pleasant fields, for the fruitful vine.

13 Upon the land of my people shall come up thorns *and* briers; yea, upon all the houses of joy *in* the joyous city:

14 Because the palaces shall be forsaken; the multitude of the city shall be left; the forts and towers shall be for dens for ever, a joy of wild asses, a pasture of flocks;

15 Until the [a]spirit be poured upon us from on high, and the wilderness be a fruitful field, and the fruitful field be counted for a forest.

16 Then judgment shall dwell in the wilderness, and righteousness remain in the fruitful field.

17 And the work of righteousness shall be peace; and the effect of righteousness quietness and [b]assurance for ever.

18 And my people shall dwell in a peaceable habitation, and in sure dwellings, and in quiet resting places;

19 When it shall hail, coming down on the forest; and the city shall be low in a low place.

20 Blessed *are* ye that sow beside all waters, that send forth *thither* the feet of the ox and the ass.

CHAPTER 33.

(*Promise and warning*, continued.)

Woe to thee [c]that spoilest, and thou *wast* not spoiled; and dealest treacherously, and they dealt not treacherously with thee! when thou shalt cease to spoil, thou shalt be spoiled; *and* when thou shalt make an end to deal treacherously, they shall deal treacherously with thee.

2 O LORD, be gracious unto us; we have waited for thee: be thou their arm every morning, our salvation also in the time of trouble.

3 At the noise of the tumult the people fled; at the lifting up of thyself the nations were scattered.

4 And your spoil shall be gathered *like* the gathering of the caterpiller: as the running to and fro of locusts shall he run upon them.

5 [d]The LORD is exalted; for he dwelleth on high: he hath filled Zion with judgment and righteousness.

6 And wisdom and knowledge shall be the stability of thy times, *and* strength of salvation: the [e]fear of the LORD *is* his treasure.

7 Behold, their valiant ones shall cry without: the [f]ambassadors of peace shall weep bitterly.

8 The highways lie waste, the wayfaring man ceaseth: he hath broken the covenant, [g]he hath despised the cities, he regardeth no man.

9 The earth mourneth *and* languisheth: Lebanon is ashamed *and* hewn down: Sharon is like a wilderness; and Bashan and Carmel shake off *their fruits*.

10 Now will I rise, saith the LORD; now will I be exalted; now will I lift up myself.

11 Ye shall conceive chaff, ye shall bring forth stubble: your breath, *as* fire, shall devour you.

12 And the people shall be *as* the burnings of lime: *as* thorns cut up shall they be burned in the fire.

13 Hear, ye *that are* far off, what I have done; and, ye *that are* near, acknowledge my might.

B.C. 713.

a *Holy Spirit.* Isa. 40:7, 13. (Gen. 1:2; Mal. 2:15.)

b *Assurance.* John 10:10-14, 28, 29. (Isa. 32:17; Jude 1.)

c Isa. 21:2; Hab. 2:8.

d Psa. 97:9.

e Psa. 19:9, *note.*

f 2 Ki. 18:18, 37.

g 2 Ki. 18:13-17.

14 The sinners in Zion are afraid; fearfulness hath surprised the hypocrites. Who among us shall dwell with the devouring fire? who among us shall dwell with everlasting burnings?

15 He that walketh righteously, and speaketh uprightly; he that despiseth the gain of oppressions, that shaketh his hands from holding of bribes, that stoppeth his ears from hearing of blood, and shutteth his eyes from seeing evil;

16 He shall dwell on high: his place of defence *shall be* the munitions of rocks: bread shall be given him; his waters *shall be* sure.

17 Thine eyes shall [a]see the king in his beauty: they shall behold the land that is very far off.

18 Thine heart shall meditate terror. Where *is* the scribe? where *is* the receiver? where *is* he that counted the towers?

19 Thou shalt not see a fierce people, a people of a deeper speech than thou canst perceive; of a stammering tongue, *that thou canst* not understand.

20 Look upon Zion, the city of our solemnities: thine eyes shall see Jerusalem a quiet habitation, a tabernacle *that* shall not be taken down; not one of the stakes thereof shall ever be removed, neither shall any of the cords thereof be broken.

21 But there the glorious LORD *will be* unto us a place of broad rivers *and* streams; wherein shall go no galley with oars, neither shall gallant ship pass thereby.

22 For the LORD *is* our judge, the LORD *is* our lawgiver, the LORD *is* our king; he will save us.

23 Thy tacklings are loosed; they could not well strengthen their mast, they could not spread the sail: then is the prey of a great spoil divided; the lame take the prey.

24 And the inhabitant shall not say, I am sick: the people that dwell therein *shall be* forgiven *their* iniquity.

CHAPTER 34.

The day of the LORD: Armageddon.

Come near, ye nations, to hear; and hearken, ye people: let the earth hear, and all that is therein; the world, and all things that come forth of it.

2 For the [b]indignation of the LORD *is* upon all nations, and *his* fury upon all their armies: [c]he hath utterly destroyed them, he hath delivered them to the slaughter.

3 Their slain also shall be cast out, and their stink shall come up out of their carcases, and the mountains shall be melted with their blood.

4 And all the host of heaven shall be dissolved, and the heavens shall be rolled together as a scroll: and all their host shall fall down, as the leaf falleth off from the vine, and as a falling *fig* from the fig tree.

5 For my sword shall be bathed in heaven: behold, it shall come down upon [d]Idumea, and upon the people of my curse, to judgment.

6 The sword of the LORD is filled with blood, it is made fat with fatness, *and* with the blood of lambs and goats, with the fat of the kidneys of rams: for the LORD hath a sacrifice in Bozrah, and a great slaughter in the land of Idumea.

7 And the unicorns shall come down with them, and the bullocks with the bulls; and their land shall be soaked with blood, and their dust made fat with fatness.

8 [e]For *it is* the day of the LORD'S vengeance, *and* the year of recompences for the controversy of Zion.

9 And [f]the streams thereof shall be turned into pitch, and the dust thereof into brimstone, and the land thereof shall become burning pitch.

10 It shall not be quenched night nor day; [g]the smoke thereof shall go up for ever: from generation to generation it shall lie waste; none shall pass through it for ever and ever.

11 [h]But the cormorant and the bittern shall possess it; the owl also and the raven shall dwell in it: and he shall stretch out upon it the line of confusion, and the stones of emptiness.

12 They shall call the nobles thereof to the kingdom, but none *shall be* there, and all her princes shall be nothing.

13 And thorns shall come up in her palaces, nettles and brambles in the fortresses thereof: and it shall be an habitation of dragons, *and* a court for owls.

14 The wild beasts of the desert shall also meet with the wild beasts of the island, and the satyr shall cry to his fellow; the screech owl also shall rest there, and find for herself a place of rest.

B.C. 713.

a *Kingdom* (O.T.). vs. 17-22; Isa. 35:1-10. (Gen. 1:26; Zech. 12:8.)

b *Day (of destruction).* vs. 1-9; Isa. 61:2. (Job 21:30; Rev. 20:11-15.)

c *Armageddon (battle of).* vs. 1-8; Isa. 63:1-6. (Rev. 16:14; 19:11-21.)

d vs. 1-8; Gen. 36:1, *note.*

e *Day (of Jehovah).* vs. 1-8; Isa. 63:1-6. (Isa. 2:10-22; Rev. 19:11-21.)

f Deut. 29:23.

g Rev. 14:11; 18:18; 19:3.

h Isa. 14:23; Zeph. 2:14; Rev. 18:2.

15 There shall the great owl make her nest, and lay, and hatch, and gather under her shadow: there shall the vultures also be gathered, every one with her mate.

16 Seek ye out of the book of the LORD, and read: no one of these shall fail, none shall want her mate: for my mouth it hath commanded, and his spirit it hath gathered them.

17 And he hath cast the lot for them, and his hand hath divided it unto them by line: they shall possess it for ever, from generation to generation shall they dwell therein.

CHAPTER 35.

Kingdom blessing: the regathering of Israel.

The wilderness and the solitary place shall be glad for [a]them; and the desert shall rejoice, and blossom as the rose.

2 It shall blossom abundantly, and rejoice even with joy and singing: the glory of Lebanon shall be given unto it, the excellency of Carmel and Sharon, they shall see the glory of the LORD, *and* the excellency of our God.

3 Strengthen ye the weak [b]hands, and confirm the feeble knees.

4 Say to them *that are* of a fearful heart, Be strong, fear not: behold, your God will come *with* vengeance, *even* God *with* a recompence; he will come and save you.

5 Then the eyes of the blind shall be opened, and the ears of the deaf shall be unstopped.

6 Then shall the lame *man* leap as an hart, and the tongue of the dumb sing: for in the wilderness shall waters break out, and streams in the desert.

7 And the parched ground shall become a pool, and the thirsty land springs of water: in the habitation of dragons, where each lay, *shall be* grass with reeds and rushes.

8 And an highway shall be there, and a way, and it shall be called The way of holiness; [c]the unclean shall not pass over it; but it *shall be* for those: the wayfaring men, though fools, shall not err *therein*.

9 No [d]lion shall be there, nor *any* ravenous beast shall go up thereon, it shall not be found there; but the [e]redeemed shall walk *there*:

10 And the ransomed of the LORD shall return, and come to Zion with songs and everlasting joy upon their heads: they shall obtain joy and gladness, and sorrow and sighing shall flee away.

B.C. 713.

a *Kingdom* (O.T.). vs. 1-10. Isa. 40:9-11. (Gen. 1:26; Zech. 12:8.)

b Job 4:3, 4; Heb. 12:12.

c Isa. 52:1; Joel 3:17; Rev. 21:27.

d Isa. 11:9; Lev. 26:6; Ezk. 34:25.

e Heb. *goel*, *Redemp.* *(Kinsman type).* Isa. 59:20, *note.*

f Psa. 2:12, *note.*

CHAPTER 36.

Sennacherib's invasion and Jehovah's deliverance (Chapters 36, 37): (1) *The invasion.*

Now it came to pass in the fourteenth year of king Hezekiah, *that* Sennacherib king of Assyria came up against all the defenced cities of Judah, and took them.

2 And the king of Assyria sent Rabshakeh from Lachish to Jerusalem unto king Hezekiah with a great army. And he stood by the conduit of the upper pool in the highway of the fuller's field.

3 Then came forth unto him Eliakim, Hilkiah's son, which was over the house, and Shebna the scribe, and Joah, Asaph's son, the recorder.

(2) *The threats of Rabshakeh.*

4 And Rabshakeh said unto them, Say ye now to Hezekiah, Thus saith the great king, the king of Assyria, What confidence *is* this wherein thou trustest?

5 I say, *sayest thou*, (but *they are but* vain words) *I have* counsel and strength for war: now on whom dost thou [f]trust, that thou rebellest against me?

6 Lo, thou trustest in the staff of this broken reed, on Egypt; whereon if a man lean, it will go into his hand, and pierce it: so *is* Pharaoh king of Egypt to all that trust in him.

7 But if thou say to me, We trust in the LORD our God: *is it* not he, whose high places and whose altars Hezekiah hath taken away, and said to Judah and to Jerusalem, Ye shall worship before this altar?

8 Now therefore give pledges, I pray thee, to my master the king of Assyria, and I will give thee two thousand horses, if thou be able on thy part to set riders upon them.

9 How then wilt thou turn away the face of one captain of the least of my master's servants, and put thy trust on Egypt for chariots and for horsemen?

10 And am I now come up without the LORD against this land to destroy it? the LORD said unto me, Go up against this land, and destroy it.

11 Then said Eliakim and Shebna and

Joah unto Rabshakeh, Speak, I pray thee, unto thy servants in the Syrian language; for we understand *it*: and speak not to us in the Jews' language, in the ears of the people that *are* on the wall.

12 But Rabshakeh said, Hath my master sent me to thy master and to thee to speak these words? *hath he* not *sent me* to the men that sit upon the wall, that they may eat their own dung, and drink their own piss with you?

13 Then Rabshakeh stood, and cried with a loud voice in the Jews' language, and said, Hear ye the words of the great king, the king of Assyria.

14 Thus saith the king, Let not Hezekiah deceive you: for he shall not be able to deliver you.

15 Neither let Hezekiah make you trust in the LORD, saying, The LORD will surely deliver us: this city shall not be delivered into the hand of the king of Assyria.

16 Hearken not to Hezekiah: for thus saith the king of Assyria, Make *an agreement* with me *by* a present, and come out to me: [a]and eat ye every one of his vine, and every one of his fig tree, and drink ye every one the waters of his own cistern;

17 Until I come and take you away to a land like your own land, a land of corn and wine, a land of bread and vineyards.

18 *Beware* lest Hezekiah persuade you, saying, The LORD will deliver us. Hath any of the gods of the nations delivered his land out of the hand of the king of Assyria?

19 Where *are* the gods of Hamath and Arphad? where *are* the gods of Sepharvaim? and have they delivered Samaria out of my hand?

20 Who *are they* among all the gods of these lands, that have delivered their land out of my hand, that the LORD should deliver Jerusalem out of my hand?

21 But they held their peace, and answered him not a word: for the king's commandment was, saying, Answer him not.

(3) *Rabshakeh's threats told to Hezekiah.*

22 Then came Eliakim, the son of Hilkiah, that *was* over the household, and Shebna the scribe, and Joah, the son of Asaph, the recorder, to Hezekiah with *their* clothes rent, and told him the words of Rabshakeh.

B.C. 710.

a Zech. 3:10.

b 2 Ki. 19:1.

c Or, *provocation.*

d Heb. *found.*

e Or, *put a spirit into him.*

f Psa. 2:12, *note.*

CHAPTER 37.

And [b]it came to pass, when king Hezekiah heard *it*, that he rent his clothes, and covered himself with sackcloth, and went into the house of the LORD.

2 And he sent Eliakim, who *was* over the household, and Shebna the scribe, and the elders of the priests covered with sackcloth, unto Isaiah the prophet the son of Amoz.

3 And they said unto him, Thus saith Hezekiah, This day *is* a day of trouble, and of rebuke, and of [c]blasphemy: for the children are come to the birth, and *there is* not strength to bring forth.

4 It may be the LORD thy God will hear the words of Rabshakeh, whom the king of Assyria his master hath sent to reproach the living God, and will reprove the words which the LORD thy God hath heard: wherefore lift up *thy* prayer for the remnant that is [d]left.

(4) *Message of Jehovah by Isaiah.*

5 So the servants of king Hezekiah came to Isaiah.

6 And Isaiah said unto them, Thus shall ye say unto your master, Thus saith the LORD, Be not afraid of the words that thou hast heard, wherewith the servants of the king of Assyria have blasphemed me.

7 Behold, I will [e]send a blast upon him, and he shall hear a rumour, and return to his own land; and I will cause him to fall by the sword in his own land.

(5) *Sennacherib's message to Hezekiah.*

8 So Rabshakeh returned, and found the king of Assyria warring against Libnah: for he had heard that he was departed from Lachish.

9 And he heard say concerning Tirhakah king of Ethiopia, He is come forth to make war with thee. And when he heard *it*, he sent messengers to Hezekiah, saying,

10 Thus shall ye speak to Hezekiah king of Judah, saying, Let not thy God, in whom thou [f]trustest, deceive thee, saying, Jerusalem shall not be given into the hand of the king of Assyria.

11 Behold, thou hast heard what the kings of Assyria have done to all lands

by destroying them utterly; and shalt thou be delivered?
12 Have the gods of the nations delivered them which my fathers have destroyed, *as* Gozan, and Haran, and Rezeph, and the children of Eden which *were* in Telassar?
13 Where *is* the king of Hamath, and the king of Arphad, and the king of the city of Sepharvaim, Hena, and Ivah?

(6) *Hezekiah's prayer.*

14 And Hezekiah received the letter from the hand of the messengers, and read it: and Hezekiah went up unto the house of the LORD, and spread it before the LORD.
15 And Hezekiah [a]prayed unto the LORD, saying,
16 O LORD of hosts, God of Israel, that dwellest *between* the cherubims, thou *art* the God, *even* thou alone, of all the kingdoms of the earth: thou hast made heaven and earth.
17 [b]Incline thine ear, O LORD, and hear; open thine eyes, O LORD, and see: and hear all the words of Sennacherib, which hath sent to reproach the living God.
18 Of a truth, LORD, the kings of Assyria have laid waste all the nations, and their countries,
19 And have cast their gods into the fire: for they *were* no gods, but the work of men's hands, wood and stone: therefore they have destroyed them.
20 Now therefore, O LORD our God, save us from his hand, that all the kingdoms of the earth may know that thou *art* the LORD, *even* thou only.

(7) *Jehovah's answer by Isaiah.*

21 Then Isaiah the son of Amoz sent unto Hezekiah, saying, Thus saith the LORD God of Israel, Whereas thou hast prayed to me against Sennacherib king of Assyria:
22 This *is* the word which the LORD hath spoken concerning him; The virgin, the daughter of Zion, hath despised thee, *and* laughed thee to scorn; the daughter of Jerusalem hath shaken her head at thee.
23 Whom hast thou reproached and blasphemed? and against whom hast thou exalted *thy* voice, and lifted up thine eyes on high? *even* against the Holy One of Israel.

B.C. 710.

a *Bible prayers* (O.T.). Isa. 38:3. (Gen. 15:2; Hab. 3:1-16.)

b Dan. 9:18.

c Heb. *by the hand of thy servants.*

d Or, *fenced and closed.*

e Heb. *short of hand.*

f Or, *sitting.*

g Isa. 30:28; Ezk. 38:4.

h *Remnant.* Isa. 46:3. (Isa. 1:9; Rom. 11:5.)

i Isa. 9:7; 2 Ki. 19:31.

24 [c]By thy servants hast thou reproached the Lord, and hast said, By the multitude of my chariots am I come up to the height of the mountains, to the sides of Lebanon; and I will cut down the tall cedars thereof, *and* the choice fir trees thereof: and I will enter into the height of his border, *and* the forest of his Carmel.
25 I have digged, and drunk water; and with the sole of my feet have I dried up all the rivers of the [d]besieged places.
26 Hast thou not heard long ago, *how* I have done it; *and* of ancient times, that I have formed it? now have I brought it to pass, that thou shouldest be to lay waste defenced cities *into* ruinous heaps.
27 Therefore their inhabitants *were* [e]of small power, they were dismayed and confounded: they were *as* the grass of the field, and *as* the green herb, *as* the grass on the housetops, and *as corn* blasted before it be grown up.
28 But I know thy [f]abode, and thy going out, and thy coming in, and thy rage against me.
29 Because thy rage against me, and thy tumult, is come up into mine ears, therefore [g]will I put my hook in thy nose, and my bridle in thy lips, and I will turn thee back by the way by which thou camest.
30 And this *shall be* a sign unto thee, Ye shall eat *this* year such as groweth of itself; and the second year that which springeth of the same: and in the third year sow ye, and reap, and plant vineyards, and eat the fruit thereof.
31 And the remnant that is escaped of the house of Judah shall again take root downward, and bear fruit upward:
32 For out of Jerusalem shall go forth a [h]remnant, and they that escape out of mount Zion: [i]the zeal of the LORD of hosts shall do this.
33 Therefore thus saith the LORD concerning the king of Assyria, He shall not come into this city, nor shoot an arrow there, nor come before it with shields, nor cast a bank against it.
34 By the way that he came, by the same shall he return, and shall not come into this city, saith the LORD.
35 For I will defend this city to save it for mine own sake, and for my servant David's sake.

(8) *Destruction of the Assyrian host.*
(Cf. Isa. 10:12.)

36 Then the [a]angel of the LORD went
forth, and smote in the camp of the
Assyrians a hundred and fourscore and
five thousand: and when they arose
early in the morning, behold, they *were*
all dead corpses.
37 So Sennacherib king of Assyria
departed, and went and returned, and
dwelt at Nineveh.
38 And it came to pass, as he was worshipping in the house of Nisroch his god,
that Adrammelech and Sharezer his sons
smote him with the sword; and they
escaped into the land of Armenia: and
Esar-haddon his son reigned in his stead.

CHAPTER 38.

Hezekiah's sickness and recovery.

In those days was Hezekiah sick unto
death. And Isaiah the prophet the son
of Amoz came unto him, and said unto
him, Thus saith the LORD, Set thine house
in order: for thou shalt die, and not live.
2 Then Hezekiah turned his face
toward the wall, and prayed unto the
LORD,
3 And said, Remember now, O LORD, I
[b]beseech thee, how I have walked before
thee in truth and with a [c]perfect heart,
and have done *that which is* good in thy
sight. And Hezekiah wept sore.
4 Then came the word of the LORD to
Isaiah, saying,
5 Go, and say to Hezekiah, Thus saith
the LORD, the God of David thy father, I
have heard thy prayer, I have seen thy
tears: behold, I will add unto thy days
fifteen years.
6 And I will deliver thee and this city
out of the hand of the king of Assyria:
and I will defend this city.
7 And this *shall be* a sign unto thee
from the LORD, that the LORD will do this
thing that he hath spoken;
8 Behold, I will bring again the shadow of the degrees, which is gone down
in the sun dial of Ahaz, ten degrees
backward. So the sun returned ten
degrees, by which degrees it was gone
down.
9 The writing of Hezekiah king of
Judah, when he had been sick, and was
recovered of his sickness:
10 I said in the cutting off of my days,
I shall go to the gates of the [d]grave: I am
deprived of the residue of my years.

B.C. 710.

a Heb. 1:4, *note.*

b *Bible prayers* (O.T.). Jer. 14:7. (Gen. 15:2; Hab. 3:1-16.)

c 1 Ki. 8:61.

d Heb. *Sheol.* See Hab. 2:5, *note.*

e *Forgiveness.* Isa. 44:22. (Lev. 4:20; Mt. 26:28.)

f Eccl. 9:5, *note.*

g 2 Ki. 20:7.

h 2 Ki. 20:8.

11 I said, I shall not see the LORD, *even*
the LORD, in the land of the living: I shall
behold man no more with the inhabitants of the world.
12 Mine age is departed, and is
removed from me as a shepherd's tent: I
have cut off like a weaver my life: he
will cut me off with pining sickness:
from day *even* to night wilt thou make
an end of me.
13 I reckoned till morning, *that*, as a
lion, so will he break all my bones: from
day *even* to night wilt thou make an end
of me.
14 Like a crane *or* a swallow, so did I
chatter: I did mourn as a dove: mine
eyes fail *with looking* upward: O LORD, I
am oppressed; undertake for me.
15 What shall I say? he hath both spoken unto me, and himself hath done *it*: I
shall go softly all my years in the bitterness of my soul.
16 O Lord, by these *things men* live,
and in all these *things is* the life of my
spirit: so wilt thou recover me, and make
me to live.
17 Behold, for peace I had great bitterness: but thou hast in love to my soul
delivered it from the pit of corruption: for
thou hast cast all my sins behind thy
[e]back.
18 For the [d]grave cannot praise thee,
[f]death can *not* celebrate thee: they that
go down into the pit cannot hope for thy
truth.
19 The living, the living, he shall
praise thee, as I *do* this day: the father to
the children shall make known thy truth.
20 The LORD *was ready* to save me:
therefore we will sing my songs to the
stringed instruments all the days of our
life in the house of the LORD.
21 For [g]Isaiah had said, Let them take
a lump of figs, and lay *it* for a plaister
upon the boil, and he shall recover.
22 [h]Hezekiah also had said, What *is*
the sign that I shall go up to the house of
the LORD?

CHAPTER 39.

Hezekiah's folly: the Babylonian captivity of Judah foretold. (Cf. 2 Ki. 24, 25)

At that time Merodach-baladan, the
son of Baladan, king of Babylon,
sent letters and a present to Hezekiah:

for he had heard that he had been sick, and was recovered.

2 And Hezekiah was glad of them, and shewed them the house of his precious things, the silver, and the gold, and the spices, and the precious ointment, and all the house of his armour, and all that was found in his treasures: there was nothing in his house, nor in all his dominion, that Hezekiah shewed them not.

3 Then came Isaiah the prophet unto king Hezekiah, and said unto him, What said these men? and from whence came they unto thee? And Hezekiah said, They are come from a far country unto me, *even* from Babylon.

4 Then said he, What have they seen in thine house? And Hezekiah answered, All that *is* in mine house have they seen: there is nothing among my treasures that I have not shewed them.

5 Then said Isaiah to Hezekiah, Hear the word of the LORD of hosts:

6 Behold, the days come, that all that *is* in thine house, and *that* which thy fathers have laid up in store until this day, shall be carried to Babylon: nothing shall be left, saith the LORD.

7 And of thy [a]sons that shall issue from thee, which thou shalt beget, shall they take away; and they shall be eunuchs in the palace of the king of Babylon.

8 Then said Hezekiah to Isaiah, Good *is* the word of the LORD which thou hast spoken. He said moreover, For there shall be peace and truth in my days.

B.C. 712.

a Dan. 1:3, 4.

PART II. LOOKING BEYOND THE CAPTIVITIES: CHAPTERS 40–66

CHAPTER 40.

The prophet's new message.

[1]Comfort ye, comfort ye my people, saith your God.

2 Speak ye comfortably to Jerusalem, and cry unto her, that her warfare is accomplished, that her iniquity is pardoned: for she hath received of the LORD'S hand double for all her sins.

The mission of John the Baptist
(Cf. Mt. 3:3.)

3 [b]The voice of him that crieth in the wilderness, Prepare ye the way of the LORD, make straight in the desert a highway for our God.

4 Every valley shall be exalted, and every mountain and hill shall be made low: and the crooked shall be made straight, and the rough places plain:

5 And the glory of the LORD shall be revealed, and all flesh shall see *it* together: for the mouth of the LORD hath spoken *it*.

The greatness of God and man's weakness
(Isa. 40:6–41:29).

6 The voice said, Cry. And he said, What shall I cry? [c]All flesh *is* grass, and all the goodliness thereof *is* as the flower of the field:

7 The grass withereth, the flower fadeth: because the [d]spirit of the LORD bloweth upon it: surely the people *is* grass.

8 The grass withereth, the flower fadeth: but the word of our God shall stand for ever.

9 O Zion, that bringest good tidings, get thee up into the high mountain; O [e]Jerusalem, that bringest good tidings, lift up thy voice with strength; lift *it* up,

B.C. 712.

b vs. 3-5; Mt. 3:3; Mk. 1:3; Lk. 3:4-6; John 1:23.

c vs. 6-8; Jas. 1:10; 1 Pet. 1:24, 25.

d *Holy Spirit.* vs. 7, 13; Isa. 42:1. (Gen. 1:2; Mal. 2:15.)

e *Kingdom* (O.T.). vs. 9-11; Isa. 62:10-12. (Gen. 1:26; Zech. 12:8.)

[1] **(40:1)** The first two verses of Isa. 40 give the key-note of the second part of the prophecy of Isaiah. The great theme of this section is Jesus Christ in His sufferings, and the glory that shall follow in the Davidic kingdom. (See "Christ in O.T.," *sufferings*, Gen. 4:4; Heb. 10:18; *glory*, 2 Sam. 7:8-15; Zech. 12:8.) Since Israel is to be regathered, converted, and made the centre of the new social order when the kingdom is set up, this part of Isaiah appropriately contains glowing prophecies concerning those events. The full view of the redemptive sufferings of Christ (e.g. Isa. 53) leads to the evangelic strain so prominent in this part of Isaiah (e.g. 44:22, 23; 55:1-3).

The change in style, about which so much has been said, is no more remarkable than the change of theme. A prophet who was also a patriot would not write of the sins and coming captivity of his people in the same exultant and joyous style which he would use to describe their redemption, blessing, and power. In John 12:37-44 quotations from Isaiah 53 and 6 are both ascribed to Isaiah.

be not afraid; say unto the cities of Judah, Behold your God!

10 Behold, the Lord GOD will come with strong *hand*, and his arm shall rule for him: behold, his reward *is* with him, and his work before him.

11 He shall feed his flock like a [a]shepherd: he shall gather the lambs with his arm, and carry *them* in his bosom, *and* shall gently lead those that are with young.

12 Who hath measured the waters in the hollow of his hand, and meted out heaven with the span, and comprehended the dust of the earth in a measure, and weighed the mountains in scales, and the hills in a balance?

13 Who hath [b]directed the Spirit of the LORD, or *being* his counsellor hath taught him?

14 With whom took he counsel, and *who* instructed him, and taught him in the path of judgment, and taught him knowledge, and shewed to him the way of understanding?

15 Behold, the nations *are* as a drop of a bucket, and are counted as the small dust of the balance: behold, he taketh up the [c]isles as a very little thing.

16 And Lebanon *is* not sufficient to burn, nor the beasts thereof sufficient for a burnt-offering.

17 All nations before him *are* as [d]nothing; and they are counted to him less than nothing, and vanity.

18 To whom then will ye [e]liken God? or what likeness will ye compare unto him?

19 The workman melteth a graven image, and the goldsmith spreadeth it over with gold, and casteth silver chains.

20 He that *is* so impoverished that he hath no oblation chooseth a tree *that* will not rot; he seeketh unto him a cunning workman to prepare a graven image, *that* shall not be moved.

21 [f]Have ye not known? have ye not heard? hath it not been told you from the beginning? have ye not understood from the foundations of the earth?

22 *It is* he that sitteth upon the [g]circle of the earth, and the inhabitants thereof *are* as grasshoppers; that stretcheth out the heavens as a curtain, and spreadeth them out as a tent to dwell in:

23 That bringeth the princes to nothing; he maketh the judges of the earth as vanity.

24 Yea, they shall not be planted; yea, they shall not be sown: yea, their stock shall not take root in the earth: and he shall also blow upon them, and they shall wither, and the whirlwind shall take them away as stubble.

25 [h]To whom then will ye liken me, or shall I be equal? saith the Holy One.

26 Lift up your eyes on high, and behold who hath created these *things*, that bringeth out their host by number: [i]he calleth them all by names by the greatness of his might, for that *he is* strong in power; not one faileth.

27 Why sayest thou, O Jacob, and speakest, O Israel, My way is hid from the LORD, and my judgment is passed over from my God?

28 Hast thou not known? hast thou not heard, *that* the everlasting God, the LORD, the Creator of the ends of the earth, fainteth not, neither is weary? *there is* no searching of his understanding.

29 He giveth power to the faint; and to *them that have* no might he increaseth strength.

30 Even the youths shall faint and be weary, and the young men shall utterly fall:

31 But they that wait upon the LORD [j]shall renew *their* strength; they shall mount up with wings as eagles; they shall run, and not be weary; *and* they shall walk, and not faint.

CHAPTER 41.

(*The greatness of God and the weakness of man*, continued.)

Keep silence before me, O [c]islands; and let the people renew *their* strength: let them come near; then let them speak: let us come near together to judgment.

2 Who raised up [1]the righteous *man*

B.C. 712.

a Cf. John 10:11, 14-16; Heb. 13:20; 1 Pet. 2:25; 5:4.

b Rom. 11:34; 1 Cor. 2:16.

c i.e. *coasts.*

d Dan. 4:35.

e v. 25; Isa. 46:5; Acts 17:29.

f Psa 19:1; Acts 14:17; Rom. 1:19, 20.

g A remarkable reference to the sphericity of the earth. See also Isa. 42:5; 44:24; 51:13; Job 9:8; Psa. 104:2; Jer. 10:12.

h v. 18; Deut. 4:15.

i Psa. 147:4.

j Psa. 103:5.

[1] **(41:2)** The reference here seems to be to Cyrus, whose victories and rapid growth in power are here ascribed to the providence of God. Verses 5-7 describe the effect upon the nations of the rise of the Persian power. They heartened each other, and made (v. 7) new idols. At verse 8 the prophet addresses Israel. Since it was their God who raised up Cyrus, they should expect good, not evil, from him (vs. 8-20). Verses 21-24 form a contemptuous challenge to the idols in whom the nations are trusting.

from the east, called him to his foot, gave the nations before him, and made *him* rule over kings? he gave *them* as the dust to his sword, *and* as driven stubble to his bow.

3 He pursued them, *and* passed safely; *even* by the way *that* he had not gone with his feet.

4 Who hath wrought and done *it*, calling the generations from the beginning? I the LORD, the first, and with the last; I *am* he.

5 The [a]isles saw *it*, and feared; the ends of the earth were afraid, drew near, and came.

6 They helped every one his neighbour; and *every one* said to his brother, Be of good courage.

7 So the carpenter encouraged the goldsmith, *and* he that smootheth *with* the hammer him that smote the anvil, saying, It *is* ready for the sodering: and he fastened it with nails, *that* it should not be moved.

8 But thou, Israel, *art* my [1]servant, Jacob whom I have chosen, the seed of Abraham my friend.

9 *Thou* whom I have taken from the ends of the earth, and called thee from the chief men thereof, and said unto thee, Thou *art* my servant; I have chosen thee, and not cast thee away.

10 Fear thou not; for I *am* with thee: be not dismayed; for I *am* thy God: I will strengthen thee; yea, I will help thee; yea, I will uphold thee with the right hand of my righteousness.

11 Behold, all they that were incensed against thee shall be ashamed and confounded: they shall be as nothing; and they that strive with thee shall perish.

12 Thou shalt seek them, and shalt not find them, *even* them that contended with thee: they that war against thee shall be as nothing, and as a thing of nought.

13 For I the LORD thy God will hold thy right hand, saying unto thee, Fear not; I will help thee.

14 Fear not, thou worm Jacob, *and* ye men of Israel; I will help thee, saith the LORD, and thy [b]redeemer, the Holy One of Israel.

15 Behold, I will make thee a new sharp threshing instrument having teeth: thou shalt thresh the mountains, and beat *them* small, and shalt make the hills as chaff.

16 Thou shalt fan them, and the wind shall carry them away, and the whirlwind shall scatter them: and thou shalt rejoice in the LORD, *and* shalt glory in the Holy One of Israel.

17 *When* the poor and needy seek water, and *there is* none, *and* their tongue faileth for thirst, I the LORD will hear them, I the God of Israel will not forsake them.

18 I will open rivers in high places, and fountains in the midst of the valleys: I will make the wilderness a pool of water, and the dry land springs of water.

19 I will plant in the wilderness the cedar, the [c]shittah tree, and the myrtle, and the oil tree; I will set in the desert the fir tree, *and* the pine, and the box tree together:

20 That they may see, and know, and consider, and understand together, that the hand of the LORD hath done this, and the Holy One of Israel hath created it.

21 Produce your cause, saith the LORD; bring forth your strong *reasons*, saith the King of Jacob.

22 Let them bring *them* forth, and shew us what shall happen: let them shew the former things, what they *be*, that we may [d]consider them, and know the latter end of them; or declare us things for to come.

23 Shew the things that are to come hereafter, that we may know that ye *are* gods: yea, do good, or do evil, that we may be dismayed, and behold *it* together.

24 Behold, [e]ye *are* of nothing, and your work of nought: an abomination *is he that* chooseth you.

25 I have raised up *one* from the north, and he shall come: from the rising of the sun shall he call upon my name: and he shall come upon princes as *upon* morter, and as the potter treadeth clay.

B.C. 712.

a i.e. *coasts.*

b Heb. *goel, Redemp. (Kinsman type).* Isa. 59:20, *note.*

c i.e. *acacia.*

d Heb. *set our heart upon them.*

e Isa. 44:9; Psa. 115:8; Rom. 3:10-20; 1 Cor. 8:4.

[1] **(41:8)** Three servants of Jehovah are mentioned in Isaiah: (1) David (Isa. 37:35); (2) Israel the nation (Isa. 41:8-16; 43:1-10; 44:1-8, 21; 45:4; 48:20); (3) Messiah (42:1-12; 49, entire chapter, but note especially verses 5-7, where the Servant Christ restores the servant nation; 50:4-6; 52:13-15; 53:1-12). Israel the nation was a faithless servant, but restored and converted will yet thresh mountains. Against the Servant Christ no charge of unfaithfulness or failure is brought. See Isa. 42:1, *note.*

26 Who hath declared from the beginning, that we may know? and beforetime, that we may say, *He is* righteous? yea, *there is* none that sheweth, yea, *there is* none that declareth, yea, *there is* none that heareth your words.

27 The first *shall say* to Zion, Behold, behold them: and I will give to Jerusalem one that bringeth good [a]tidings.

28 For I beheld, and *there was* no man; even among them, and *there was* no counsellor, that, when I asked of them, could answer a word.

29 Behold, they *are* all vanity; their works *are* nothing: their molten images *are* wind and confusion.

CHAPTER 42.

Christ, the Servant of Jehovah (Mt. 12:18-21. Cf. Phil. 2:5-8).

Behold my [1]servant, whom I uphold; mine elect, *in whom* my soul delighteth; I have put my [b]spirit upon him: he shall bring forth judgment to the Gentiles.

2 He shall not cry, nor lift up, nor cause his voice to be heard in the street.

3 [c]A bruised reed shall he not break, and [d]the smoking flax shall he not quench: he shall bring forth judgment unto truth.

4 He shall not fail nor be discouraged, till he have set judgment in the earth: and the [e]isles shall wait for his law.

5 Thus saith God the LORD, he that created the heavens, and stretched them out; he that spread forth the earth, and that which cometh out of it; he that giveth breath unto the people upon it, and spirit to them that walk therein:

6 I the LORD have called thee in righteousness, and will hold thine hand, and will keep thee, and give thee for a covenant of the people, [2]for a light of the [f]Gentiles;

7 To open the blind eyes, to bring out the prisoners from the prison, *and* them that sit in darkness out of the prison house.

Israel, chosen, sinning, chastened, restored (Isa. 42:8–44:27).

8 I *am* the LORD: that *is* my name: and my glory will I not give to another, neither my praise to graven images.

9 Behold, the [g]former things are come to pass, and new things do I declare: before they spring forth I tell you of them.

10 Sing unto the LORD a new song, *and* his praise from the end of the earth, ye that go down to the sea, and all that is therein; the [e]isles, and the inhabitants thereof.

11 Let the wilderness and the cities thereof lift up *their voice,* the villages *that* Kedar doth inhabit: let the inhabitants of the rock sing, let them shout from the top of the mountains.

12 Let them give glory unto the LORD, and declare his praise in the [e]islands.

(1) *The chastening of Israel.*

13 The LORD shall go forth as a mighty man, he shall stir up jealousy like a man of war: he shall cry, yea, roar; he shall prevail against his enemies.

14 I have long time holden my peace; I have been still, *and* refrained myself: *now* will I cry like a travailing woman; I will destroy and devour at once.

15 I will make waste mountains and hills, and dry up all their herbs; and I will make the rivers [e]islands, and I will dry up the pools.

16 And I will bring the blind by a way *that* they knew not; I will lead them in paths *that* they have not known: I will

B.C. 712.

a *Gospel.* Isa. 52:7. (Gen. 12:1-3; Rev. 14:6.)

b *Holy Spirit.* Isa. 44:3. (Gen. 1:2; Mal. 2:15.)

c *Christ (First Advent).* vs. 1-7; Isa. 49:1-6. (Gen. 3:15; Acts 1:9.)

d Mt. 12:18-21.

e i.e. *coasts.*

f Isa. 49:6; 60:3; Mt. 4:16; Lk. 2:32; Acts 13:47, 48; Rom. 9:24-30; 10:19, 20; 11:11, 12; 15:9-12.

g i.e. Isaiah's prediction of Sennacherib's invasion and its results, Isa. 10. and 37. See also Isa. 41:21-23; 43:8-12; 44:7; 48:3, 5, 16. This appeal of the prophet to the fulfilment of his former predictions strongly confirms the unity of the book.

[1] **(42:1)** There is a twofold account of the Coming Servant: (1) He is represented as weak, despised, rejected, slain; (2) and also as a mighty conqueror, taking vengeance on the nations and restoring Israel (e.g. 40:10; 63:1-4). The former class of passages relate to the first advent, and are fulfilled; the latter to the second advent, and are unfulfilled.

[2] **(42:6)** The prophets connect the Gentiles with Christ in a threefold way: (1) as the Light He brings *salvation* to the Gentiles (Lk. 2:32; Acts 13:47, 48); (2) as the "Root of Jesse" He is to reign over the Gentiles in His kingdom (Isa. 11:10; Rom. 15:12). He *saves* the Gentiles, which is the distinctive feature of this present age (Rom. 11:17-24; Eph. 2:11, 12). He *reigns* over the Gentiles in the kingdom-age, to follow this. See "Kingdom (O.T.)," Gen. 1:26-28; Zech. 12:8. (3) Believing Gentiles in the present age, together with believing Jews, constitute "the church which is His body" (Eph. 1:23). See Eph. 3:6, *note.*

make darkness light before them, and crooked things straight. These things will I do unto them, and not forsake them.

17 They shall be turned back, they shall be greatly ashamed, that trust in graven images, that say to the molten images, Ye *are* our gods.

18 Hear, ye deaf; and look, ye blind, that ye may see.

19 Who *is* blind, but my servant? or deaf, as my messenger *that* I sent? who *is* blind as *he that is* perfect, and blind as the LORD'S servant?

20 Seeing many things, but thou observest not; opening the ears, but he heareth not.

21 The LORD is well pleased for his righteousness' sake; he will magnify the law, and make *it* honourable.

22 But this *is* a people robbed and spoiled; *they are* all of them snared in holes, and they are hid in prison houses: they are for a prey, and none delivereth; for a spoil, and none saith, Restore.

23 Who among you will give ear to this? *who* will hearken and hear for the time to come?

24 Who gave Jacob for a spoil, and Israel to the robbers? did not the LORD, he against whom we have sinned? for they would not walk in his ways, neither were they obedient unto his law.

25 Therefore he hath poured upon him the fury of his anger, and the strength of battle: and it hath set him on fire round about, yet he knew not; and it burned him, yet he laid *it* not to heart.

CHAPTER 43.

(2) *The chosen nation redeemed, and restored.*

But now thus saith the LORD that created thee, O Jacob, and he that formed thee, O Israel, Fear not: for I have [a]redeemed thee, I have called *thee* by thy name; thou *art* mine.

2 When thou passest through the waters, I *will be* with thee; and through the rivers, they shall not overflow thee: [b]when thou walkest through the fire, thou shalt not be burned; neither shall the flame kindle upon thee.

3 For I *am* the LORD thy God, the Holy One of Israel, thy Saviour: [c]I gave Egypt *for* thy ransom, Ethiopia and Seba for thee.

4 Since thou wast precious in my sight, thou hast been honourable, and I have loved thee: therefore will I give men for thee, and people for thy life.

5 [d]Fear not: for I *am* with thee: I will bring thy seed from the east, and gather thee from the west;

6 I will say to the north, Give up; and to the south, Keep not back: bring my sons from far, and my daughters from the ends of the earth;

7 *Even* every one that is [e]called by my name: for [f]I have created him for my glory, I have formed him; yea, I have made him.

8 Bring forth the blind people that have eyes, and the deaf that have ears.

9 Let all the nations be gathered together, and let the people be assembled: who among them can declare this, and shew us former things? let them bring forth their witnesses, that they may be justified: or let them hear, and say, *It is* truth.

10 [g]Ye *are* my witnesses, saith the LORD, and my servant whom I have chosen: that ye may know and believe me, and understand that I *am* he: [h]before me there was no God formed, neither shall there be after me.

11 [i]I, *even* I, *am* the LORD; and beside me *there is* no saviour.

12 I have declared, and have saved, and I have shewed, when *there was* no strange *god* among you: therefore ye *are* my witnesses, saith the LORD, that I *am* God.

13 Yea, before the day *was* I *am* he; and *there is* none that can deliver out of my hand: I will work, and who shall let it?

14 Thus saith the LORD, your redeemer, the Holy One of Israel; For your sake I have sent to Babylon, and have brought down all their nobles, and the Chaldeans, whose cry *is* in the ships.

15 I *am* the LORD, your Holy One, the creator of Israel, your King.

16 Thus saith the LORD, which maketh a way in the sea, and a path in the mighty waters;

17 Which bringeth forth the chariot and horse, the army and the power; they shall lie down together, they shall not rise: they are extinct, they are quenched as tow.

B.C. 712.

a Heb. *goel, Redemp. (Kinsman type).* Isa. 59:20, *note.*

b Psa. 66:12; Dan. 3:25-27.

c Prov. 11:8; 21:18; cf. 1 Tim. 2:6.

d Isa. 41:10, 14; 44:2; Jer. 30:10, 11; 46:27, 28.

e Isa. 63:19; Jas. 2:7.

f Isa. 29:23; Psa. 100:3; John 3:3-5; 2 Cor. 5:17; Eph. 2:10.

g Isa. 44:8.

h Isa. 41:4; 44:6.

i Isa. 45:21; Hos. 13:4.

18 Remember ye not the former things, neither consider the things of old.

19 Behold, I will do a new thing; now it shall spring forth; shall ye not know it? I will even make a way in the wilderness, *and* rivers in the desert.

20 The beast of the field shall honour me, the dragons and the owls: because I give waters in the wilderness, *and* rivers in the desert, to give drink to my people, my [a]chosen.

21 This people have I formed for myself; they shall shew forth my praise.

22 But thou hast not called upon me, O Jacob; but thou hast been weary of me, O Israel.

23 Thou hast not brought me the small cattle of thy burnt-offerings; neither hast thou honoured me with thy sacrifices. I have not caused thee to serve with an offering, nor wearied thee with incense.

24 Thou hast bought me no sweet cane with money, neither hast thou filled me with the fat of thy sacrifices: but thou hast made me to serve with thy sins, thou hast wearied me with thine iniquities.

25 I, *even* I, *am* he that [b]blotteth out thy transgressions [c]for mine own sake, [d]and will not remember thy sins.

26 Put me in remembrance: let us plead together: declare thou, that thou mayest be justified.

27 Thy first father hath sinned, and thy [e]teachers have transgressed against me.

28 Therefore I have profaned the princes of the sanctuary, [f]and have given Jacob to the curse, and Israel to reproaches.

CHAPTER 44.

(3) *The promise of the Spirit: the folly of idolatry.*

Yet now hear, O Jacob my servant; and Israel, whom I have chosen:

2 Thus saith the LORD that made thee, and formed thee from the womb, *which* will help thee; Fear not, O Jacob, my servant; and thou, [g]Jesurun, whom I have chosen.

3 For I will [h]pour water upon him that is thirsty, and floods upon the dry ground: I will pour my [i]spirit upon thy seed, and my blessing upon thine offspring:

4 And they shall spring up *as* among the grass, as willows by the water courses.

5 One shall say, I *am* the LORD'S; and another shall call *himself* by the name of Jacob; and another shall subscribe *with* his hand unto the LORD, and surname *himself* by the name of Israel.

6 Thus saith the LORD the King of Israel, and his [j]redeemer the LORD of hosts; [k]I *am* the first, and I *am* the last; and beside me *there is* no God.

7 And who, as I, shall call, and shall declare it, and set it in order for me, since I appointed the ancient people? and the things that are coming, and shall come, let them shew unto them.

8 Fear ye not, neither be afraid: have not I told thee from that time, and have declared *it*? [l]ye *are* even my witnesses. Is there a God beside me? yea, *there is* no God; I know not *any*.

9 They that make a graven image *are* all of them vanity; and their delectable things shall not profit; and they *are* their own witnesses; they see not, nor know; that they may be ashamed.

10 Who hath formed a god, or molten a graven image *that* is profitable for nothing?

11 Behold, all his fellows shall be ashamed: and the workmen, they *are* of men: let them all be gathered together, let them stand up; *yet* they shall fear, *and* they shall be ashamed together.

12 The smith with the tongs both worketh in the coals, and fashioneth it with hammers, and worketh it with the strength of his arms: yea, he is hungry, and his strength faileth: he drinketh no water, and is faint.

13 The carpenter stretcheth out *his* rule; he marketh it out with a line; he fitteth it with planes, and he marketh it out with the compass, and maketh it after the figure of a man, according to the beauty of a man; that it may remain in the house.

14 He heweth him down cedars, and taketh the cypress and the oak, which he strengtheneth for himself among the trees of the forest: he planteth an ash, and the rain doth nourish *it*.

15 Then shall it be for a man to burn: for he will take thereof, and warm himself; yea, he kindleth *it*, and baketh bread; yea, he maketh a god, and

B.C. 712.

a *Election (corporate).* Mk. 13:20. (Deut. 7:6; 1 Pet. 1:2.)

b Isa. 44:22; 48:9; Jer. 50:20; Acts 3:19.

c Ezk. 36:22.

d Isa. 1:18; Jer. 31:34.

e Heb. *interpreters.* Mal. 2:7, 8.

f Psa. 79:4; Jer. 24:9; Dan. 9:11; Zech. 8:13.

g i.e. *upright.* Symbolical name of Israel. Deut. 32:15; 33:5, 26.

h Isa. 35:7; Joel 2:28; John 7:38; Acts 2:18.

i *Holy Spirit.* Isa. 59:19, 21. (Gen. 1:2; Mal. 2:15.)

j Heb. *goel, Redemp. (Kinsman type).* Isa. 59:20, *note.*

k Isa. 41:4; 48:12; Rev. 1:8, 17; 22:13.

l Isa. 43:10, 12.

worshippeth *it*; he maketh it a graven image, and falleth down thereto.

16 He burneth part thereof in the fire; with part thereof he eateth flesh; he roasteth roast, and is satisfied: yea, he warmeth *himself*, and saith, Aha, I am warm, I have seen the fire:

17 And the residue thereof he maketh a god, *even* his graven image: he falleth down unto it, and worshippeth *it*, and prayeth unto it, and saith, Deliver me; for thou *art* my god.

18 They have not known nor understood: for he hath shut their eyes, that they cannot see; *and* their hearts, that they cannot understand.

19 And none considereth in his heart, neither *is there* knowledge nor understanding to say, I have burned part of it in the fire; yea, also I have baked bread upon the coals thereof; I have roasted flesh, and eaten *it*: and shall I make the residue thereof an abomination? shall I fall down to the stock of a tree?

20 He feedeth on ashes: a deceived heart hath turned him aside, that he cannot deliver his soul, nor say, *Is there* not a lie in my right hand?

21 Remember these, O Jacob and Israel; for thou *art* my servant: I have formed thee; thou *art* my servant: O Israel, thou shalt not be forgotten of me.

22 I have blotted out, as a thick cloud, thy transgressions, and, as a cloud, thy sins: [a]return unto me; for I have [b]redeemed thee.

23 Sing, O ye heavens; for the LORD hath done *it*: shout, ye lower parts of the earth: break forth into singing, ye mountains, O forest, and every tree therein: for the LORD hath [b]redeemed Jacob, and glorified himself in Israel.

24 Thus saith the LORD, thy [b]redeemer, and he that formed thee from the womb, I *am* the LORD that maketh all *things*; that stretcheth forth the heavens alone; that spreadeth abroad the earth by myself;

25 That frustrateth the tokens of the liars, and maketh diviners mad; that turneth wise *men* backward, and maketh their knowledge foolish;

26 That confirmeth the word of his servant, and performeth the counsel of his messengers; that saith to Jerusalem, Thou shalt be inhabited; and to the cities of Judah, Ye shall be built, and I will raise up the decayed places thereof:

27 [c]That saith to the deep, Be dry, and I will dry up thy rivers:

The prophecy concerning Cyrus, and the restoration under Ezra and Nehemiah.

28 That saith of [1]Cyrus, *He is* my shepherd, and shall perform all my pleasure: even saying to Jerusalem, Thou shalt be built; and to the temple, Thy foundation shall be laid.

CHAPTER 45.

Thus saith the LORD to his [2]anointed, to Cyrus, whose right hand I have holden, to subdue nations before him; and I will loose the loins of kings, to open before him the two leaved gates; and the gates shall not be shut;

2 I will go before thee, [d]and make the crooked places straight: [e]I will break in pieces the gates of brass, and cut in sunder the bars of iron:

3 And I will give thee the treasures of darkness, and hidden riches of secret places, [f]that thou mayest know that I, the LORD, which call *thee* by thy name, *am* the God of Israel.

4 For Jacob my servant's sake, and Israel mine elect, I have even called thee by thy name: I have surnamed thee, though thou hast [g]not known me.

Israel reminded that safety and salvation are to be found only in Jehovah.

5 [h]I *am* the LORD, and *there is* none else,

B.C. 712.

a *Forgiveness*. Mt. 6:12, 14, 15. (Lev. 4:20; Mt. 26:28.)

b Heb. *goel, Redemp. (Kinsman type)*. Isa. 59:20, *note*.

c Jer. 50:38; 51:36.

d Isa. 40:4.

e Psa. 107:16.

f Isa. 41:23.

g Jud. 2:10; 1 Thes. 4:5.

h Isa. 44:8; 46:9; Deut. 4:35, 39; 32:39.

[1] **(44:28)** Cf. 1 Ki. 13:2, where Josiah was mentioned by name three hundred years before his birth.

[2] **(45:1)** The only instance where the word is applied to a Gentile. Nebuchadnezzar is called the "servant" of Jehovah (Jer. 25:9; 27:6; 43:10). This, with the designation "My shepherd" (Isa. 44:28), also a Messianic title, marks Cyrus as that startling exception, a Gentile type of Christ. The points are: (1) both are irresistible conquerors of Israel's enemies (Isa. 45:1; Rev. 19:19-21); (2) both are restorers of the holy city (Isa. 44:28; Zech. 14:1-11); (3) through both is the name of the one true God glorified (Isa. 45:6; 1 Cor. 15:28).

there is no God beside me: I girded thee,
though thou hast not known me:
6 [a]That they may know from the rising
of the sun, and from the west, that *there*
is none beside me. I *am* the LORD, and
there is none else.
7 I form the light, and create darkness:
I make peace, and [b]create [1]evil: I the
LORD do all these *things*.
8 Drop down, ye heavens, from above,
and let the skies pour down righteousness: let the earth open, and let them
bring forth salvation, and let righteousness spring up together; I the LORD have
created it.
9 Woe unto him that striveth with his
Maker! *Let* the potsherd *strive* with the
potsherds of the earth. [c]Shall the clay say
to him that fashioneth it, What makest
thou? or thy work, He hath no hands?
10 Woe unto him that saith unto *his*
father, What begettest thou? or to the
woman, What hast thou brought forth?
11 Thus saith the LORD, the Holy One
of Israel, and his Maker, Ask me of
things to come concerning [d]my sons,
and concerning the work of my hands
command ye me.
12 I have made the earth, and created
man upon it: I, *even* my hands, have
stretched out the heavens, and all their
host have I commanded.
13 I have raised him up in righteousness, and I will direct all his ways: he
shall build my city, and he shall let go
my captives, not for price nor reward,
saith the LORD of hosts.
14 Thus saith the LORD, [e]The labour of
Egypt, and merchandise of Ethiopia and
of the Sabeans, men of stature, shall
come over unto thee, and they shall be
thine: they shall come after thee; in
chains they shall come over, and they
shall fall down unto thee, they shall
make supplication unto thee, *saying*,
Surely God *is* in thee; and *there is* none
else, *there is* no God.
15 Verily thou *art* a God that hidest
thyself, O God of Israel, the Saviour.
16 They shall be ashamed, and also confounded, all of them: they shall go to confusion together *that are* makers of idols.

B.C. 712.

a Isa. 37:20; Psa. 102:15; Mal. 1:11.

b Amos 3:6.

c Isa. 29:16; Jer. 18:6; Rom. 9:20.

d Jer. 31:9.

e Psa. 68:31; 72:10, 11; Isa. 49.23; 60:9, 10, 14, 16; Zech. 8:22, 23.

f v. 25; Isa. 26:4; Rom. 11:26.

g Psa. 22:27; 65:5; cf. Num 21:8-9.

h Gen. 22:16; Heb. 6:13.

i Rom. 14:11; Phil. 2:10.

17 [f]But Israel shall be saved in the
LORD with an everlasting salvation: ye
shall not be ashamed nor confounded
world without end.
18 For thus saith the LORD that created
the heavens; God himself that formed
the earth and made it; he hath established it, he created it not in vain, he
formed it to be inhabited: I *am* the LORD;
and *there is* none else.
19 I have not spoken in secret, in a
dark place of the earth: I said not unto
the seed of Jacob, Seek ye me in vain: I
the LORD speak righteousness, I declare
things that are right.
20 Assemble yourselves and come;
draw near together, ye *that are* escaped of
the nations: they have no knowledge that
set up the wood of their graven image,
and pray unto a god *that* cannot save.
21 Tell ye, and bring *them* near; yea, let
them take counsel together: who hath
declared this from ancient time? *who*
hath told it from that time? *have* not I the
LORD? and *there is* no God else beside
me; a just God and a Saviour; *there is*
none beside me.
22 [g]Look unto me, and be ye saved, all
the ends of the earth: for I *am* God, and
there is none else.
23 [h]I have sworn by myself, the word is
gone out of my mouth *in* righteousness,
and shall not return, That unto me [i]every
knee shall bow, every tongue shall swear.
24 Surely, shall *one* say, in the LORD
have I righteousness and strength: *even*
to him shall *men* come; and all that are
incensed against him shall be ashamed.
25 In the LORD shall all the seed of
Israel be justified, and shall glory.

CHAPTER 46.

Israel exhorted to remember the power of Jehovah, and the powerlessness of idols.

Bel boweth down, Nebo stoopeth,
their idols were upon the beasts,
and upon the cattle: your carriages *were*
heavy loaden; *they are* a burden to the
weary *beast*.
2 They stoop, they bow down together;

[1](45:7) Heb. *ra*, translated "sorrow," "wretchedness," "adversity," "afflictions," "calamities," but never translated *sin*. God created evil only in the sense that He made sorrow, wretchedness, etc., to be the sure fruits of sin.

they could not deliver the burden, [a]but themselves are gone into captivity.

3 Hearken unto me, O house of Jacob, and all the [b]remnant of the house of Israel, which are borne *by me* from the belly, which are carried from the womb:

4 And *even* to *your* old age I *am* he; and *even* to hoar hairs will I carry *you*: I have made, and I will bear; even I will carry, and will deliver *you*.

5 To whom will ye liken me, and make *me* equal, and compare me, that we may be like?

6 They lavish gold out of the bag, and weigh silver in the balance, *and* hire a goldsmith; and he maketh it a god: they fall down, yea, they worship.

7 They bear him upon the shoulder, they carry him, and set him in his place, and he standeth; from his place shall he not remove: yea, *one* shall cry unto him, yet can he not answer, nor save him out of his trouble.

8 Remember this, and shew yourselves men: bring *it* again to mind, O ye transgressors.

9 [c]Remember the former things of old: for I *am* God, and *there is* none else; *I am* God, and *there is* none like me,

10 Declaring the end from the beginning, and from ancient times *the things* that are not *yet* done, saying, [d]My counsel shall stand, and I will do all my pleasure:

11 Calling a ravenous bird from the east, the man [e]that executeth my counsel from a far country: yea, I have spoken *it*, I will also bring it to pass; I have purposed *it*, I will also do it.

12 Hearken unto me, ye [f]stouthearted, that *are* far from righteousness:

13 I bring near my righteousness; it shall not be far off, and my salvation shall not tarry: and I will place salvation in Zion for Israel my glory.

CHAPTER 47.

Judgment upon Babylon.

Come down, and sit in the dust, O virgin daughter of Babylon, sit on the ground: *there is* no throne, O daughter of the Chaldeans: for thou shalt no more be called tender and delicate.

2 Take the millstones, and grind meal: uncover thy locks, make bare the leg, uncover the thigh, pass over the rivers.

3 Thy nakedness shall be uncovered, yea, thy shame shall be seen: I will take vengeance, and I will not meet *thee as* a man.

4 *As for* our [g]redeemer, the LORD of hosts *is* his name, the Holy One of Israel.

5 Sit thou silent, and get thee into darkness, O daughter of the Chaldeans: for thou shalt no more be called, The lady of kingdoms.

6 [h]I was wroth with my people, I have polluted mine inheritance, and given them into thine hand: thou didst shew them no mercy; upon the ancient hast thou very heavily laid thy yoke.

7 And thou saidst, I shall be a lady for ever: *so* that thou didst not lay these *things* to thy heart, neither didst remember the latter end of it.

8 Therefore hear now this, *thou that art* given to pleasures, that dwellest carelessly, that sayest in thine heart, I *am*, and none else beside me; I shall not sit *as* a widow, neither shall I know the loss of children:

9 But these two *things* shall come to thee in a moment in one day, the loss of children, and widowhood: they shall come upon thee in their perfection for the multitude of thy sorceries, *and* for the great abundance of thine enchantments.

10 For thou hast [i]trusted in thy wickedness: thou hast said, None seeth me. Thy wisdom and thy knowledge, it hath perverted thee; and thou hast said in thine heart, I *am*, and none else beside me.

11 Therefore shall evil come upon thee; thou shalt not know from whence it riseth: and mischief shall fall upon thee; thou shalt not be able to put it off: and [j]desolation shall come upon thee suddenly, *which* thou shalt not know.

12 Stand now with thine enchantments, and with the multitude of thy sorceries, wherein thou hast laboured from thy youth; if so be thou shalt be able to profit, if so be thou mayest prevail.

13 Thou art wearied in the multitude of thy counsels. [k]Let now the astrologers, the stargazers, the monthly prognosticators, stand up, and save thee from *these things* that shall come upon thee.

14 Behold, they shall be [l]as stubble; the fire shall burn them; they shall not deliver [m]themselves from the power of

B.C. 712.

a Jer. 48:7.

b *Remnant*. Jer. 15:11-21. (Isa. 1:9; Rom. 11:5.)

c Deut. 32:7.

d Psa. 33:11; Prov. 19:21; 21:30; Isa. 14:24; Acts 5:39; Heb. 6:17.

e Isa. 44:28; 45:15.

f Psa. 76:5.

g Heb. *goel, Redemp. (Kinsman type).* Isa. 59:20, *note*.

h 2 Sam. 24:14; 2 Chr. 28:9; Zech. 1:15.

i Psa. 2:12, *note*.

j 1 Thes. 5:3.

k Isa. 44:25; Dan. 2:2.

l Nah. 1:10; Mal. 4:1.

m Heb. *their souls*.

the flame: *there shall* not *be* a coal to warm at, *nor* fire to sit before it.

15 Thus shall they be unto thee with whom thou hast laboured, *even* thy merchants, from thy youth: they shall wander every one to his quarter; none shall save thee.

CHAPTER 48.

Israel to be restored under the Holy One, Jehovah's servant (Isa. 48:1–52:15):

(1) *Israel reminded of the promises.*

Hear ye this, O house of Jacob, which are called by the name of Israel, and are come forth out of the waters of Judah, which swear by the name of the LORD, and make mention of the God of Israel, *but* [a]not in truth, nor in righteousness.

2 For they call themselves of the holy city, and [b]stay themselves upon the God of Israel; The LORD of hosts *is* his name.

3 I have declared the former things from the beginning; and they went forth out of my mouth, and I shewed them; I did *them* suddenly, and they came to pass.

4 Because I knew that thou *art* [c]obstinate, and thy neck *is* an iron sinew, and thy brow brass;

5 I have even from the beginning declared *it* to thee; before it came to pass I shewed *it* thee: lest thou shouldest say, Mine idol hath done them, and my graven image, and my molten image, hath commanded them.

6 Thou hast heard, see all this; and will not ye declare *it*? I have shewed thee new things from this time, even hidden things, and thou didst not know them.

7 They are created now, and not from the beginning; even before the day when thou heardest them not; lest thou shouldest say, Behold, I knew them.

8 Yea, thou heardest not; yea, thou knewest not; yea, from that time *that* thine ear was not opened: for I knew that thou wouldest deal very treacherously, and wast called a transgressor from the womb.

9 [d]For my name's sake will I defer mine anger, and for my praise will I refrain for thee, that I cut thee not off.

10 [e]Behold, I have refined thee, but not with silver; I have chosen thee in the furnace of affliction.

11 [f]For mine own sake, *even* for mine own sake, will I do *it*: for how should *my name* be polluted? and I will not give my glory unto another.

12 Hearken unto me, O Jacob and Israel, my called; I *am* he; I [g]*am* the first, I also *am* the last.

13 Mine hand also hath laid the foundation of the earth, and my right hand hath spanned the heavens: *when* I call unto them, they stand up together.

14 All ye, assemble yourselves, and hear; which among them hath declared these *things*? The LORD hath loved him: he will do his pleasure on Babylon, and his arm *shall be on* the Chaldeans.

15 I, *even* I, have spoken; yea, I have called him: I have brought him, and he shall make his way prosperous.

16 Come ye near unto me, hear ye this; I have not spoken in secret from the beginning; from the time that it was, there *am* I: and now [h]the Lord GOD, and his Spirit, hath sent me.

17 Thus saith the LORD, thy [i]Redeemer, the Holy One of Israel; I *am* the LORD thy God which teacheth thee to profit, which leadeth thee by the way *that* thou shouldest go.

18 O that thou hadst hearkened to my commandments! then had thy peace been as a river, and thy righteousness as the waves of the sea:

19 Thy seed also had been as the sand, and the offspring of thy bowels like the gravel thereof; his name should not have been cut off nor destroyed from before me.

20 Go ye forth of Babylon, flee ye from the Chaldeans, with a voice of singing declare ye, tell this, utter it *even* to the end of the earth; say ye, The LORD hath [i]redeemed his servant Jacob.

21 And they thirsted not *when* he led them through the deserts: he caused the waters to flow out of the rock for them: he clave the rock also, and the waters gushed out.

22 *There is* no peace, saith the LORD, unto the wicked.

CHAPTER 49.

(2) *The Holy One, Israel's Redeemer.*

Listen, O [j]isles, unto me; and hearken, ye people, from far; The LORD hath called [k]me from the womb; from the

B.C. 712.

a Jer. 4:2; 5:2.

b Mic. 3:11; Rom. 2:17.

c Heb. *hard.*

d v. 11; Isa. 43:25; Psa. 79:9; 106:8; Ezk. 20:9, 14, 22, 44.

e Psa. 66:10.

f v. 9.

g Isa. 41:4; 44:6; Rev. 1:17; 22:13.

h Isa. 61:1; Zech. 2:8, 9, 11.

i Heb. *goel, Redemp. (Kinsman type).* Isa. 59:20, *note.*

j i.e. *coasts.*

k *Christ (First Advent).* vs. 1-6; Isa. 50:5, 6. (Gen. 3:15; Acts 1:9.)

bowels of my mother hath he made mention of my name.

2 And he hath made my mouth like a sharp sword; in the shadow of his hand hath he hid me, and made me a polished shaft; in his quiver hath he hid me;

3 And said unto me, Thou *art* my servant, O Israel, in whom I will be glorified.

4 Then I said, I have laboured in vain, I have spent my strength for nought, and in vain: *yet* surely my judgment *is* with the LORD, and my work with my God.

5 And now, saith the LORD that formed me from the womb *to be* his servant, to bring Jacob again to him, Though Israel be not gathered, yet shall I be glorious in the eyes of the LORD, and my God shall be my strength.

6 And he said, It is a light thing that thou shouldest be my servant to raise up the tribes of Jacob, and to restore the preserved of Israel: I will also give thee for a light to the [a]Gentiles, that thou mayest be my salvation unto the end of the earth.

7 Thus saith the LORD, [b]the Redeemer of Israel, *and* his Holy One, to him whom man despiseth, to him whom the nation abhorreth, to a servant of rulers, Kings shall see and arise, princes also shall worship, because of the LORD that is faithful, *and* the Holy One of Israel, and he shall choose thee.

(3) [1]*Israel to be preserved and restored.*

8 Thus saith the LORD, [c]In an acceptable time have I heard thee, and in a day of salvation have I helped thee: and I will preserve thee, and give thee for a covenant of the people, to establish the earth, to cause to inherit the desolate heritages;

9 [d]That thou mayest say to the prisoners, Go forth; to them that *are* in darkness, Shew yourselves. They shall feed in the ways, and their pastures *shall be* in all high places.

10 [e]They shall not hunger nor thirst; [f]neither shall the heat nor sun smite them: for he that hath mercy on them [g]shall lead them, even by the springs of water shall he guide them.

11 [h]And I will make all my mountains a way, and my highways shall be exalted.

B.C. 712.

a See Isa. 42:6, and *note.*

b Heb. *goel, Redemp. (Kinsman type).* Isa. 59:20, *note.*

c 2 Cor. 6:2.

d Isa. 61:1; cf. Mt. 13:44.

e Rev. 7:16.

f Psa. 121:6.

g Psa. 23:2; Isa. 48:17.

h Isa. 40:4.

i Isa. 45:5, 6.

j Psa. 103:13; Mal. 3:17; Mt. 7:11.

k Rom. 11:29.

l Ex. 13:9; Song 8:6.

12 Behold, [i]these shall come from far: and, lo, these from the north and from the west; and these from the land of [2]Sinim.

13 Sing, O heavens; and be joyful, O earth; and break forth into singing, O mountains: for the LORD hath comforted his people, and will have mercy upon his afflicted.

14 But Zion said, The LORD hath forsaken me, and my Lord hath forgotten me.

15 [j]Can a woman forget her sucking child, that she should not have compassion on the son of her womb? yea, they may forget, [k]yet will I not forget thee.

16 Behold, [l]I have graven thee upon the palms of *my* hands; thy walls *are* continually before me.

17 Thy children shall make haste; thy destroyers and they that made thee waste shall go forth of thee.

18 Lift up thine eyes round about, and behold: all these gather themselves together, *and* come to thee. *As* I live, saith the LORD, thou shalt surely clothe thee with them all, as with an ornament, and bind them *on thee,* as a bride *doeth.*

19 For thy waste and thy desolate places, and the land of thy destruction, shall even now be too narrow by reason of the inhabitants, and they that swallowed thee up shall be far away.

20 The children which thou shalt have, after thou hast lost the other, shall say again in thine ears, The place *is* too strait for me: give place to me that I may dwell.

21 Then shalt thou say in thine heart, Who hath begotten me these, seeing I have lost my children, and am desolate, a captive, and removing to and fro? and who hath brought up these? Behold, I was left alone; these, where *had* they *been*?

(4) *Judgment on Israel's oppressors* (Gen. 12:3; 15:14).

22 Thus saith the Lord GOD, Behold, I will lift up mine hand to the Gentiles, and set up my standard to the people: and they shall bring thy sons in *their*

[1] **(49:8, heading)** The Lord Jesus and the believing remnant of Israel are here joined. What is said is true of both.

[2] **(49:12)** The word is supposed to refer to a people of the far East, perhaps the Chinese.

arms, and thy daughters shall be carried upon *their* shoulders.

23 And kings shall be thy nursing fathers, and their queens thy nursing mothers: they shall bow down to thee with *their* face toward the earth, and lick up the dust of thy feet; and thou shalt know that I *am* the LORD: [a]for they shall not be ashamed that wait for me.

24 Shall the prey be taken from the mighty, or the lawful captive delivered?

25 But thus saith the LORD, Even the captives of the mighty shall be taken away, and the prey of the terrible shall be delivered: for I will contend with him that contendeth with thee, and I will save thy children.

26 And I will feed them that oppress thee with their own flesh; and they shall be drunken with their own blood, as with sweet wine: and all flesh [b]shall know that I the LORD *am* thy Saviour and thy [c]Redeemer, the mighty One of Jacob.

CHAPTER 50.

(5) *The humiliation of the Holy One.*

Thus saith the LORD, Where *is* [d]the bill of your mother's divorcement, whom I have put away? or which of my [e]creditors *is it* to whom I have sold you? Behold, for your iniquities have ye sold yourselves, and for your transgressions is your mother put away.

2 Wherefore, when I came, *was there* no man? when I called, *was there* none to answer? Is my hand shortened at all, that it cannot [f]redeem? or have I no power to deliver? behold, [g]at my rebuke I dry up the sea, I make the rivers a wilderness: their fish stinketh, because *there is* no water, and dieth for thirst.

3 I clothe the heavens with blackness, and I make sackcloth their covering.

4 [h]The Lord GOD hath given me the tongue of the learned, that I should know how to speak a word in season to *him that is* weary: he wakeneth morning by morning, he wakeneth mine ear to hear as the learned.

5 The Lord GOD hath [i]opened mine ear, and I was not rebellious, neither turned away back.

6 [j]I gave my back to the smiters, and my cheeks to them that plucked off the hair: [k]I hid not my face from [l]shame and spitting.

7 For the Lord GOD will help me; therefore shall I not be confounded: therefore [m]have I set my face like a flint, and I know that I shall not be ashamed.

8 [n]*He is* near that justifieth me; who will contend with me? let us stand together: who *is* mine adversary? let him come near to me.

9 Behold, the Lord GOD will help me; who *is* he *that* shall condemn me? lo, [o]they all shall wax old as a garment; the moth shall eat them up.

10 Who *is* among you that [p]feareth the LORD, that obeyeth the voice of his servant, that walketh *in* darkness, and hath no light? [q]let him trust in the name of the LORD, and stay upon his God.

11 Behold, all ye that kindle a fire, that compass *yourselves* about with sparks: walk in the light of your fire, and in the sparks *that* ye have kindled. This shall ye have of mine hand; ye shall lie down in sorrow.

CHAPTER 51.

(6) *Israel to be redeemed: oppressors punished.*

Hearken to me, ye that follow after righteousness, ye that seek the LORD: look unto the rock *whence* ye are hewn, and to the hole of the pit *whence* ye are digged.

2 [r]Look unto Abraham your father, and unto Sarah *that* bare you: for I called him alone, and blessed him, and increased him.

3 For the LORD [s]shall comfort Zion: he will comfort all her waste places; and he will make her wilderness like Eden, and [t]her desert like the garden of the LORD; joy and gladness shall be found therein, thanksgiving, and the voice of melody.

4 Hearken unto me, my people; and give ear unto me, O my nation: for a law shall proceed from me, and I will make my judgment to rest for a light of the people.

5 My righteousness *is* near; my salvation is gone forth, and mine arms shall judge the people; the [u]isles shall wait upon me, and on mine arm shall they trust.

6 Lift up your eyes to the heavens, and look upon the earth beneath: for the

---

B.C. 712.

a Psa. 34:22; Rom. 5:5; 9:33; 10:11.

b Psa. 9:16.

c Heb. *goel, Redemp. (Kinsman type)*. Isa. 59:20, *note.*

d Deut. 24:1; Jer. 3:8; Hos. 2:2.

e See 2 Ki. 4:1; Mt. 18:25.

f Ex. 14:30, *note;* Isa. 59:20, *note.*

g Psa. 106:9; Nah. 1:4.

h Ex. 4:11.

i Mt. 26:39; John 14:31; Phil. 2:8; Heb. 10:5.

j Mt. 26:67; 27:26; John 18:22.

k *Christ (First Advent).* vs. 4-7; Isa. 52:13-15. (Gen. 3:15; Acts 1:9.)

l Mt. 26:67; 27:30; Mk. 14:65; 15:19.

m Ezk. 3:8, 9.

n Rom. 8:32-34.

o Isa. 51:6, 8; Job 13:28; Psa. 102:26.

p Psa. 19:9, *note.*

q 2 Chr. 20:20; Psa. 20:7.

r Rom. 4:1, 16; Heb. 11:11.

s Isa. 40:1; 52:9; Psa. 102:13.

t Gen. 13:10; Joel 2:3.

u i.e. *coasts.*

heavens shall vanish away like smoke,
and [a]the earth shall wax old like a garment, and they that dwell therein shall
die in like manner: but my salvation
shall be for ever, and my righteousness
shall not be abolished.
7 Hearken unto me, ye that know righteousness, the people in whose heart *is* my
law; fear ye not the reproach of men, neither be ye afraid of their revilings.
8 For the moth shall eat them up like a
garment, and the worm shall eat them
like wool: but my righteousness shall be
for ever, and my salvation from generation to generation.
9 Awake, awake, put on strength, O
arm of the LORD; awake, as in the ancient
days, in the generations of old. [b]*Art* thou
not it that hath cut Rahab, *and* wounded
the dragon?
10 *Art* thou not it which hath dried the
sea, the waters of the great deep; that
hath made the depths of the sea a way
for the [c]ransomed to pass over?
11 Therefore the redeemed of the LORD
shall return, and come with singing unto
Zion; and everlasting joy *shall be* upon
their head: they shall obtain gladness
and joy; *and* sorrow and mourning shall
flee away.
12 I, *even* I, *am* he [d]that comforteth you:
who *art* thou, that thou shouldest be
afraid of a man *that* shall die, and of the
son of man *which* shall be made *as* grass;
13 And forgettest the LORD thy maker,
that hath stretched forth the heavens,
and laid the foundations of the earth;
and hast feared continually every day
because of the fury of the oppressor, as if
he were ready to destroy? and where *is*
the fury of the oppressor?
14 The captive exile hasteneth that he
may be loosed, and that he should not die
in the pit, nor that his bread should fail.
15 But I *am* the LORD thy God, that
divided the sea, whose waves roared:
The LORD of hosts *is* his name.
16 [e]And I have put my words in thy
mouth, and I have covered thee in the
shadow of mine hand, that I may plant
the heavens, and lay the foundations of
the earth, and say unto Zion, Thou *art*
my people.
17 Awake, awake, stand up, O
Jerusalem, which hast drunk at the hand
of the LORD the cup of his fury; thou hast
drunken the dregs of the cup of trembling, *and* wrung *them* out.
18 *There is* none to guide her among all
the sons *whom* she hath brought forth;
neither *is there any* that taketh her by the
hand of all the sons *that* she hath
brought up.
19 These two *things* are come unto thee;
who shall be sorry for thee? desolation,
and destruction, and the famine, and the
sword: by whom shall I comfort thee?
20 Thy sons have fainted, they lie at
the head of all the streets, as a wild bull
in a net: they are full of the fury of the
LORD, the rebuke of thy God.
21 Therefore hear now this, thou
afflicted, and drunken, but not with
wine:
22 Thus saith thy Lord the LORD, and
thy God [f]*that* pleadeth the cause of his
people, Behold, I have taken out of thine
hand the cup of trembling, *even* the
dregs of the cup of my fury; thou shalt
no more drink it again:
23 [g]But I will put it into the hand of
them that afflict thee; which have said to
thy soul, Bow down, that we may go
over: and thou hast laid thy body as the
ground, and as the street, to them that
went over.

CHAPTER 52.

(7) *Vision of Jerusalem in the kingdom-age.*

Awake, awake; put on thy strength, O
Zion; put on thy beautiful garments, O Jerusalem, the holy city: for
henceforth there shall no more come into
thee the uncircumcised and the unclean.
2 Shake thyself from the dust; arise,
and sit down, O Jerusalem: loose thyself
from the bands of thy neck, O captive
daughter of Zion.
3 For thus saith the LORD, Ye have sold
yourselves for nought; and ye shall be
[c]redeemed without money.
4 For thus saith the Lord GOD, My
people went down aforetime into Egypt
to sojourn there; and the Assyrian
oppressed them without cause.
5 Now therefore, what have I here,
saith the LORD, that my people is taken
away for nought? they that rule over
them make them to howl, saith the

B.C. 712.

a Isa. 50:9; Heb. 1:10-12.

b The ref. is to Egypt (Isa. 30:7) at the Exodus.

c Heb. *goel*, *Redemp.* *(Kinsman type).* Isa. 59:20, *note.*

d v. 3; 2 Cor. 1:3.

e Deut. 18:18; Isa. 59:21; John 3:34.

f Jer. 50:34.

g Jer. 25:17, 26, 28; Zech. 12:2.

LORD; and my name continually every
day *is* [a]blasphemed.
6 Therefore my people shall know my
name: therefore *they shall know* in that day
that I *am* he that doth speak: behold, *it is* I.
7 How beautiful upon the mountains
are the [b]feet of him that bringeth good
[c]tidings, that publisheth peace; that
bringeth good tidings of good, that publisheth salvation; that saith unto Zion,
Thy God reigneth!
8 Thy watchmen shall lift up the voice;
with the voice together shall they sing:
for they shall see eye to eye, when the
LORD shall bring again Zion.
9 Break forth into joy, sing together, ye
waste places of Jerusalem: for the LORD
hath comforted his people, he hath
redeemed Jerusalem.
10 The LORD hath made bare his holy
arm in the eyes of all the nations; and all
the ends of the earth shall see the salvation of our God.
11 Depart ye, depart ye, go ye out
from thence, touch no unclean *thing*; go
ye out of the midst of her; be ye [d]clean,
that bear the vessels of the LORD.
12 [e]For ye shall not go out with haste,
nor go by flight: [f]for the LORD will go
before you; and the God of Israel *will be*
your [g]rereward.

(8) *Jehovah's Servant,*
marred and afterward exalted.

13 Behold, my servant shall deal pru-
dently, he shall be exalted and extolled,
and be very high.
14 As many were astonied at thee; his
visage was [1]so [h]marred more than any
man, and his form more than the sons of
men:
15 So shall [i]he sprinkle many nations;
the kings shall shut their mouths at him:
for *that* which had not been told them
shall they [j]see; and *that* which they had
not heard shall they consider.

CHAPTER 53.

The vicarious sacrifice of Christ,
Jehovah's Servant.

[k]Who hath believed our report? and
[l]to whom is the arm of the LORD
revealed?
2 For he shall grow up before him as a
tender plant, and as a root out of a dry
ground: he hath no form nor comeliness;
and when we shall see him, *there is* no
beauty that we should desire him.
3 [m]He is despised and rejected of men;
a man of sorrows, and acquainted with
grief: and we hid as it were *our* faces
from him; he was despised, and we
esteemed him not.
4 Surely he hath borne our griefs, and
[n]carried our sorrows: yet we did esteem
him stricken, smitten of God, and afflicted.
5 But he *was* wounded for our transgressions, *he was* bruised for our iniquities: the chastisement of our peace *was*
upon him; and with his stripes we are
healed.
6 All we like sheep have gone astray;
we have turned every one to his own
way; and the LORD hath laid on him the
iniquity of us all.
7 He was oppressed, and he was
afflicted, yet he opened not his mouth:
he is brought as a lamb to the slaughter,
and as a sheep before her shearers is
dumb, [o]so he openeth not his mouth.
8 [p]He was taken from prison and from
judgment: and who shall declare his
generation? for he was cut off out of the
land of the living: for the transgression
of my people was he stricken.
9 And he made his grave with the
wicked, and [q]with the rich in his death;
because he had done no violence, [r]nei-
ther *was any* deceit in his mouth.
10 Yet it pleased the LORD to bruise
him; he hath put *him* to grief: when thou
shalt make his soul an offering for sin,
he shall see *his* seed, he shall prolong *his*
days, and the pleasure of the LORD shall
prosper in his hand.
11 He shall see of the travail of his
soul, *and* shall be satisfied: by his knowledge shall my righteous servant [s]justify
many; for he shall bear their iniquities.
12 Therefore will I divide him *a portion*
with the great, and he shall divide the
spoil with the strong; because he [t]hath
poured out his soul unto death: and [u]he
was numbered with the transgressors;

B.C. 712.

a Rom. 2:24.

b Isa. 60:13, 14; Psa. 22:16; Nah. 1:15; Zech. 14:4; Lk. 7:38; Rom. 10:15; Rev. 1:15, 17.

c *Gospel.* Isa. 61:1-3. (Gen. 12:1-3; Rev. 14:6.)

d 2 Cor. 6:17.

e *Contra,* Ex. 12:33, 39.

f Mic. 2:13.

g Cf. Ex. 14:19.

h *Sacrifice (prophetic).* Isa. 53:1-12. (Gen. 4:4; Heb. 10:18.)

i *Christ (First Advent).* Isa. 53:1-12. (Gen. 3:15; Acts 1:9.)

j Rom. 15:21.

k John 12:38; Rom. 10:16.

l *Sacrifice (prophetic).* vs. 1-12; Dan. 9:26. (Gen. 4:4; Heb. 10:18.)

m Mt. 27:30, 31.

n Mt. 8:17; 1 Pet. 2:24.

o Mt. 26:62, 63; 27:12-14; Mk. 15:3-5; Lk. 23:9; John 19:9; Acts 8:32, 33.

p Mt. 27:11-26; Lk. 23:1-25.

q Mt. 27:57-60.

r 1 Pet. 2:22.

s Acts 13:38, 39; Rom. 5:15, 18.

t Isa. 50:6; Rom. 3:25.

u Mt. 27:38; Mk. 15:28; Lk. 22:37.

[1]**(52:14)** The literal rendering is terrible: "So marred from the form of man was His aspect that His appearance was not that of a son of man"—i.e. not human—the effect of the brutalities described in Mt. 26:67, 68; 27:27-30.

and [a]he bare the sin of many, and made
intercession [b]for the transgressors.

CHAPTER 54.

Israel the restored wife of Jehovah.
(Cf. Hos. 2:1-23.)

Sing, O barren, [c]thou *that* didst not
bear; break forth into singing, and
cry aloud, thou *that* didst not [d]travail
with child: for more *are* the children of
the desolate than the children of the
married wife, saith the LORD.
2 Enlarge the place of thy tent, and let
them stretch forth the curtains of thine
habitations: spare not, lengthen thy
cords, and strengthen thy stakes;
3 For thou shalt break forth on the
right hand and on the left; and thy seed
shall inherit the Gentiles, and make the
desolate cities to be inhabited.
4 Fear not; for thou shalt not be
ashamed: neither be thou confounded;
for thou shalt not be put to shame: for
thou shalt forget the shame of thy youth,
and shalt not remember the reproach of
thy widowhood any more.
5 For thy Maker *is* thine [e]husband; the
LORD of hosts *is* his name; and thy
Redeemer the Holy One of Israel; The
God of the whole earth shall he be called.
6 For the LORD hath called thee as a
woman forsaken and grieved in spirit,
and a wife of youth, when thou wast
refused, saith thy God.
7 For a small moment have I forsaken
thee; but with great mercies will I gather
thee.
8 In a little wrath I hid my face from
thee for a moment; but with everlasting
kindness will I have mercy on thee, saith
the LORD thy Redeemer.
9 For this *is as* the waters of Noah unto
me: for *as* I have sworn that the [f]waters
of Noah should no more go over the
earth; so have I sworn that I would not
be wroth with thee, nor rebuke thee.
10 For the mountains shall depart, and
the hills be removed; but my kindness
shall not depart from thee, neither shall
the covenant of my peace be removed,
saith the LORD that hath mercy on thee.

Security and blessing of restored Israel.
(Cf. Deut. 30:1-9, *note.*)

11 O thou afflicted, tossed with
tempest, *and* not comforted, behold, I
will lay thy stones with fair colours, and
lay thy foundations with sapphires.
12 And I will make thy windows of
agates, and thy gates of carbuncles, and
all thy borders of pleasant stones.
13 And all thy [g]children *shall be* taught
of the LORD; and great *shall be* the peace
of thy children.
14 In righteousness shalt thou be established:
thou shalt be far from oppression;
for thou shalt not fear: and from terror;
for it shall not come near thee.
15 Behold, they shall surely gather
together, *but* not by me: whosoever shall
gather together against thee shall fall for
thy sake.
16 Behold, I have created the smith that
bloweth the coals in the fire, and that
bringeth forth an instrument for his work;
and I have created the waster to destroy.
17 No weapon that is formed against
thee shall prosper; and every tongue *that*
shall rise against thee in judgment thou
shalt condemn. This *is* the heritage of the
servants of the LORD, and their righteousness
is of me, saith the LORD.

CHAPTER 55.

The everlasting salvation.

Ho, [h]every one that thirsteth, come ye
to the waters, and he that hath no
money; [i]come ye, buy, and eat; yea,
come, buy wine and milk without
money and without price.
2 Wherefore do ye spend money for
that which is not bread? and your labour
for *that which* satisfieth not? hearken diligently
unto me, and eat ye *that which is*
good, and let your soul delight itself in
fatness.
3 Incline your ear, and come unto me:
hear, and your soul shall live; and I will
make an everlasting covenant with you,
even the sure mercies of [j]David.
4 Behold, I have given him *for* a witness
to the people, a leader and commander
to the people.
5 Behold, [k]thou shalt call a nation *that*
thou knowest not, and nations *that* knew
not thee shall run unto thee because of
the LORD thy God, and for the Holy One
of Israel; for he hath glorified thee.
6 [l]Seek ye the LORD while he may be

B.C. 712.

a *Christ (First Advent).* Isa. 61:1. (Gen. 3:15; Acts 1:9.)

b Lk. 23:34.

c Gal. 4:27.

d Mic. 5:1, *note.*

e *Wife (of Jehovah).* Jer. 31:32. (Isa. 54:5; Hos. 2:1-23.)

f Isa. 55:11; Gen. 8:21; 9:11; Jer. 31:35, 36.

g John 6:45; 1 Cor. 2:10; 1 Thes. 4:9; 1 John 2:20.

h John 4:14; 7:37; Rev. 21:6; 22:17.

i Rev. 3:18.

j 2 Sam. 7:8; Psa. 89:28; Acts 13:34.

k Isa. 52:15; Eph. 2:11, 12.

l Psa. 32:6; Mt. 5:25; 25:11; John 7:34; 8:21; 2 Cor. 6:1, 2.

B.C. 712.

found, call ye upon him while he is near:

7 Let the wicked forsake his way, and the unrighteous man [a]his thoughts: and let him return unto the LORD, and he will have mercy upon him; and to our God, for [b]he will abundantly pardon.

8 [c]For my thoughts *are* not your thoughts, neither *are* your ways my ways, saith the LORD.

9 For *as* the heavens are higher than the earth, so are my ways higher than your ways, and my thoughts than your thoughts.

10 For as the rain cometh down, and the snow from heaven, and returneth not thither, but watereth the earth, and maketh it bring forth and bud, that it may give seed to the sower, and bread to the eater:

11 So shall my word be that goeth forth out of my mouth: it shall not return unto me void, but it shall accomplish that which I please, and it shall prosper *in the thing* whereto I sent it.

12 For ye shall go out with joy, and be led forth with peace: the mountains and the hills shall break forth before you into singing, and all the trees of the field shall clap *their* hands.

13 [d]Instead of the thorn shall come up the fir tree, and instead of the brier shall come up the myrtle tree: and it shall be to the LORD for a name, for an everlasting sign *that* shall not be cut off.

CHAPTER 56.

Ethical instructions.

Thus saith the LORD, Keep ye judgment, and do justice: [e]for my salvation *is* near to come, and my righteousness to be revealed.

2 Blessed *is* the man *that* doeth this, and the son of man *that* layeth hold on it; that keepeth the sabbath from polluting it, and keepeth his hand from doing any evil.

3 Neither let the son of the stranger, that hath joined himself to the LORD, speak, saying, The LORD hath utterly separated me from his people: neither let the eunuch say, Behold, I *am* a dry tree.

4 For thus saith the LORD unto the eunuchs that keep my sabbaths, and choose *the things* that please me, and take hold of my covenant;

5 Even unto them will I give in mine house and within my walls a place and a name better than of sons and of daughters: I will give them an everlasting name, that shall not be cut off.

6 Also the sons of the stranger, that join themselves to the LORD, to serve him, and to love the name of the LORD, to be his servants, every one that keepeth the sabbath from polluting it, and taketh hold of my covenant;

7 Even them will I bring to my holy mountain, and make them joyful in my [f]house of prayer: [g]their burnt-offerings and their sacrifices *shall be* accepted upon mine altar; for mine [f]house shall be called an house of prayer for all people.

8 The Lord GOD [h]which gathereth the outcasts of Israel saith, Yet will I gather *others* to him, beside those that are gathered unto him.

9 All ye beasts of the field, come to devour, *yea*, all ye beasts in the forest.

10 His watchmen *are* blind: they are all ignorant, they *are* all dumb dogs, they cannot bark; sleeping, lying down, loving to slumber.

11 Yea, *they are* greedy dogs *which* can never have enough, and they *are* shepherds *that* cannot understand: they all look to their own way, every one for his gain, from his quarter.

12 Come ye, *say they*, I will fetch wine, and we will fill ourselves with strong drink; and [i]to morrow shall be as this day, *and* much more abundant.

CHAPTER 57.

(*Ethical instructions*, continued.)

The righteous perisheth, and no man layeth *it* to heart: and merciful men *are* taken away, none considering that the righteous is taken away from the evil *to come*.

2 He shall enter into peace: they shall rest in their beds, *each one* walking *in* his uprightness.

3 But draw near hither, ye sons of the sorceress, the seed of the adulterer and the whore.

4 Against whom do ye sport yourselves? against whom make ye a wide mouth, *and* draw out the tongue? *are* ye not children of transgression, a seed of falsehood,

5 Enflaming yourselves with idols under every green tree, slaying the children in the valleys under the clifts of the rocks?

a Zech. 8:17.

b Heb. *he will multiply to pardon.*

c 2 Sam. 7:19.

d Isa. 41:19.

e Isa. 46:13; Mt. 3:2; 4:17; Rom. 13:11, 12.

f Mt. 21:13; Mk. 11:17; Lk. 19:46.

g Rom. 12:1; Heb. 13:15; 1 Pet. 2:5.

h Isa. 11:12; Psa. 147:2.

i Psa. 10:6; Prov. 23:35; Isa. 22:13; Lk. 12:19; 1 Cor. 15:32.

6 Among the smooth *stones* of the
stream *is* thy portion; they, they *are* thy lot:
even to them hast thou poured a drink-
offering, thou hast offered a [a]meat-offer-
ing. Should I receive comfort in these?
7 Upon a lofty and high mountain hast
thou set thy bed: even thither wentest
thou up to offer sacrifice.
8 Behind the doors also and the posts
hast thou set up thy remembrance: for
thou hast discovered *thyself to another*
than me, and art gone up; thou hast
enlarged thy bed, and made thee *a*
covenant with them; thou lovedst their
bed where thou sawest *it*.
9 And thou wentest to the king with
ointment, and didst increase thy per-
fumes, and didst send thy messengers
far off, and didst debase *thyself even* unto
[b]hell.
10 Thou art wearied in the greatness
of thy way; *yet* saidst thou not, There is
no hope: thou hast found the life of thine
hand; therefore thou wast not grieved.
11 And of whom hast thou been afraid
or feared, that thou hast lied, and hast
not remembered me, nor laid *it* to thy
heart? [c]have not I held my peace even of
old, and thou fearest me not?
12 I will declare thy righteousness, and
thy works; for they shall not profit thee.
13 When thou criest, let thy companies
deliver thee; but the wind shall carry
them all away; vanity shall take *them*:
but he that putteth his [d]trust in me shall
possess the land, and shall inherit my
holy mountain;
14 And shall say, Cast ye up, cast ye
up, prepare the way, take up the stumblingblock out of the way of my people.
15 For thus saith the high and lofty
One that inhabiteth eternity, [e]whose
name *is* Holy; [f]I dwell in the high and
holy *place*, with him also *that is* of a contrite and humble spirit, to revive the
spirit of the humble, and to revive the
heart of the contrite ones.
16 [g]For I will not contend for ever, neither will I be always wroth: for the spirit
should fail before me, and the souls
which I have made.
17 For the iniquity of his [h]covetous-
ness was I wroth, and smote him: I hid
me, and was wroth, and he went on
frowardly in the way of his heart.

B.C. 698.

a Lit. *meal.*

b Heb. *Sheol.* See Hab. 2:5, *note.*

c Psa. 50:21; Eccl. 8:11.

d Psa. 2:12, *note.*

e Job 6:10; Lk. 1:49.

f Psa. 68:4; Zech. 2:13.

g Psa. 85:5; 103:9; Mic. 7:18.

h Jer. 6:13.

i Jer. 3:22.

j Heb. 13:15.

k Acts 2:39; Eph. 2:17.

l Job 15:20; Prov. 4:16.

m 1 Ki. 21:9, 12, 13.

n Zech. 7:5.

o Lk. 4:18, 19.

p Neh. 5:10-12.

q Jer. 34:9.

r Ezk. 18:7, 16; Mt. 25:35.

s Job 31:19.

t Gen. 29:14; Neh. 5:5.

18 I have seen his ways, and [i]will heal
him: I will lead him also, and restore
comforts unto him and to his mourners.
19 I create the [j]fruit of the lips; Peace,
peace to *him that is* far off, and [k]to *him that*
is near, saith the LORD; and I will heal him.
20 [l]But the wicked *are* like the troubled sea, when it cannot rest, whose
waters cast up mire and dirt.
21 *There is* no peace, saith my God, to
the wicked.

CHAPTER 58.

(*Ethical instructions*, continued.)

Cry aloud, spare not, lift up thy voice
like a trumpet, and shew my people their transgression, and the house of
Jacob their sins.
2 Yet they seek me daily, and delight
to know my ways, as a nation that did
righteousness, and forsook not the ordinance of their God: they ask of me the
ordinances of justice; they take delight in
approaching to God.
3 Wherefore have we fasted, *say they*,
and thou seest not? *wherefore* have we
afflicted our soul, and thou takest no
knowledge? Behold, in the day of your
fast ye find pleasure, and exact all your
labours.
4 [m]Behold, ye fast for strife and debate,
and to smite with the fist of wickedness:
ye shall not fast as *ye do this* day, to make
your voice to be heard on high.
5 Is it [n]such a fast that I have chosen?
a day for a man to afflict his soul? *is it* to
bow down his head as a bulrush, and to
spread sackcloth and ashes *under him*?
wilt thou call this a fast, and an acceptable day to the LORD?
6 *Is* not this the fast that I have chosen? to [o]loose the bands of wickedness,
to [p]undo the heavy burdens, and [q]to let
the oppressed go free, and that ye break
every yoke?
7 *Is it* not to [r]deal thy bread to the
hungry, and that thou bring the poor
that are cast out to thy house? [s]when
thou seest the naked, that thou cover
him; and that thou hide not thyself
[t]from thine own flesh?
8 Then shall thy light break forth
as the morning, and thine health
shall spring forth speedily: and thy
righteousness shall go before thee;

[a]the glory of the LORD shall be thy rereward.

9 Then shalt thou call, and the LORD shall answer; thou shalt cry, and he shall say, Here I *am*. If thou take away from the midst of thee the yoke, the putting forth of the finger, and speaking vanity;

10 And *if* thou draw out thy soul to the hungry, and satisfy the afflicted soul; then shall thy light rise in obscurity, and thy darkness *be* as the noonday:

11 And the LORD shall guide thee continually, and satisfy thy soul in drought, and make fat thy bones: and thou shalt be like a watered garden, and like a spring of water, whose waters fail not.

12 And *they that shall be* of thee shall build the old waste places: thou shalt raise up the foundations of many generations; and thou shalt be called, The repairer of the breach, The restorer of paths to dwell in.

13 If thou turn away thy foot from the sabbath, *from* doing thy pleasure on my holy day; and call the sabbath a delight, the holy of the LORD, honourable; and shalt honour him, not doing thine own ways, nor finding thine own pleasure, nor speaking *thine own* words:

14 Then shalt thou delight thyself in the LORD; and I will cause thee to ride upon the high places of the earth, and feed thee with the heritage of Jacob thy father: for the mouth of the LORD hath spoken *it*.

CHAPTER 59.

(*Ethical instructions,* continued.)

Behold, the LORD'S hand is not shortened, that it cannot save; neither his ear heavy, that it cannot hear:

2 But your iniquities have separated between you and your God, and your sins have hid *his* face from you, that he will not hear.

3 For your hands are defiled with blood, and your fingers with iniquity; your lips have spoken lies, your tongue hath muttered perverseness.

4 None calleth for justice, nor *any* pleadeth for truth: they [b]trust in vanity, and speak lies; they conceive mischief, and bring forth iniquity.

5 They hatch cockatrice' eggs, and weave the spider's web: he that eateth of their eggs dieth, and that which is crushed breaketh out into a viper.

B.C. 698.

a Isa. 52:12; Ex. 14:19.

b Psa. 2:12, *note.*

c Rom. 3:15.

d vs. 7, 8; Rom. 3:16, 17.

e *Righteousness (garment).* Isa. 61:10. (Gen. 3:21; Rev. 19:8.)

6 Their webs shall not become garments, neither shall they cover themselves with their works: their works *are* works of iniquity, and the act of violence *is* in their hands.

7 Their feet run to [c]evil, and they make haste to shed innocent blood: their thoughts *are* thoughts of iniquity; wasting and [d]destruction *are* in their paths.

8 The way of peace they know not; and *there is* no judgment in their goings: they have made them crooked paths: whosoever goeth therein shall not know peace.

9 Therefore is judgment far from us, neither doth justice overtake us: we wait for light, but behold obscurity; for brightness, *but* we walk in darkness.

10 We grope for the wall like the blind, and we grope as if *we had* no eyes: we stumble at noonday as in the night; *we are* in desolate places as dead *men*.

11 We roar all like bears, and mourn sore like doves: we look for judgment, but *there is* none; for salvation, *but* it is far off from us.

12 For our transgressions are multiplied before thee, and our sins testify against us: for our transgressions *are* with us; and *as for* our iniquities, we know them;

13 In transgressing and lying against the LORD, and departing away from our God, speaking oppression and revolt, conceiving and uttering from the heart words of falsehood.

14 And judgment is turned away backward, and justice standeth afar off: for truth is fallen in the street, and equity cannot enter.

15 Yea, truth faileth; and he *that* departeth from evil maketh himself a prey: and the LORD saw *it*, and it displeased him that *there was* no judgment.

16 And he saw that *there was* no man, and wondered that *there was* no intercessor: therefore his arm brought salvation unto him; and his righteousness, it sustained him.

17 For he put on [e]righteousness as a breastplate, and an helmet of salvation upon his head; and he put on the garments of vengeance *for* clothing, and was clad with zeal as a cloke.

18 According to *their* deeds, accordingly he will repay, fury to his adversaries

recompence to his enemies; to the
[a]islands he will repay recompence.
19 So shall they [b]fear the name of the
LORD from the west, and his glory from
the rising of the sun. When the enemy
shall come in like a flood, the [c]Spirit of the
LORD shall lift up a standard against him.

The Deliverer out of Zion.
(Cf. Rom. 11:23-29.)

20 [1]And the Redeemer shall [2]come to
[d]Zion, and unto them that turn from
transgression in Jacob, saith the LORD.
21 As for me, this *is* my covenant with
them, saith the LORD; My [c]spirit that *is*
upon thee, and my [e]words which I have
put in thy mouth, shall not depart out of
thy mouth, nor out of the mouth of thy
seed, nor out of the mouth of thy seed's
seed, saith the LORD, from henceforth
and for ever.

CHAPTER 60.

(*The Deliverer out of Zion,* continued.)

Arise, shine; for thy light is come, and
the glory of the LORD is [f]risen upon
thee.
2 For, behold, the darkness shall cover
the earth, and gross darkness the people:
but the LORD shall arise upon thee, and
his glory shall be seen upon thee.
3 And the Gentiles shall come to thy
[g]light, and kings to the brightness of thy
rising.
4 Lift up thine eyes round about, and
see: all they gather themselves together,
they come to thee: thy sons shall come
from far, and thy daughters shall be
nursed at *thy* side.
5 Then thou shalt see, and flow
together, and thine heart shall fear, and
be enlarged; because [h]the abundance of
the sea shall be converted unto thee, the
forces of the Gentiles shall come unto
thee.
6 The multitude of camels shall cover
thee, the dromedaries of Midian and
[i]Ephah; all they from Sheba shall come:
they shall bring gold and incense; and
they shall shew forth the praises of the
LORD.
7 All the flocks of [j]Kedar shall be gathered together unto thee, the rams of
Nebaioth shall minister unto thee: they
shall come up with acceptance on mine
altar, and [k]I will glorify the house of my
glory.
8 Who *are* these *that* fly as a cloud, and
as the doves to their windows?
9 Surely the [a]isles shall wait for me,
and the ships of Tarshish first, to bring
thy sons from far, their silver and their
gold with them, unto the name of the
LORD thy God, and to the Holy One of
Israel, because he hath glorified thee.
10 And the sons of strangers shall
build up thy walls, and their kings shall
minister unto thee: for in my wrath I
smote thee, but in my favour have I had
mercy on thee.
11 Therefore thy gates shall be open
continually; they shall not be shut day
nor night; that *men* may bring unto thee
the forces of the Gentiles, and *that* their
kings *may be* brought.
12 For the nation and kingdom that
will not serve thee shall perish; yea, *those*
nations shall be utterly wasted.
13 The glory of Lebanon shall come
unto thee, the fir tree, the pine tree, and
the box together, to beautify the place of
my sanctuary; and I will make the place
of my [l]feet glorious.
14 The sons also of them that afflicted
thee shall come bending unto thee; and
all they that despised thee shall bow
themselves down at the soles of thy
[l]feet; and they shall call thee, The city of

B.C. 698.

a i.e. *coasts.*
b Psa. 19.9, note.
c *Holy Spirit.* Isa. 61:1. (Gen. 1:2; Mal. 2:15.)
d vs. 20, 21; Rom. 11:26, 27.
e *Inspiration.* vs. 19, 21; Jer. 1:9. (Ex. 4:15; Rev. 22:19.)
f *Israel (prophecies).* vs. 1-12; Jer. 23:3-8. (Gen. 12:2, 3; Rom. 11:26.)
g See Isa. 42:6, and *note.*
h Rom. 11:25-27.
i Gen. 25:4.
j Gen. 25:13.
k Hag. 2:7, 9.
l Isa. 52:7.

[1] **(59:20)** Redemption: Kinsman type, summary. The *goel,* or Kinsman-Redeemer, is a beautiful type of Christ.

(1) The kinsman redemption was of *persons,* and an *inheritance* (Lev. 25:48; 25:25; Gal. 4:5; Eph. 1:7, 11, 14).

(2) The Redeemer must be a kinsman (Lev. 25:48, 49; Ruth 3:12, 13; Gal. 4:4; Heb. 2:14, 15).

(3) The Redeemer must be able to redeem (Ruth 4:4-6; Jer. 50:34; John 10:11, 18).

(4) Redemption is effected by the *goel* paying the just demand in full (Lev. 25:27; 1 Pet. 1:18, 19; Gal. 3:13). See Ex. 14:30, *note;* Rom. 3:24, *note.*

[2] **(59:20)** The *time* when the "Redeemer shall come to Zion" is fixed, relatively, by Rom. 11:23-29 as following the completion of the Gentile Church. That is also the order of the great dispensational passage, Acts 15:14-17. In both, the return of the Lord to Zion follows the outcalling of the Church.

the LORD, The Zion of the Holy One of
Israel.
15 Whereas thou hast been forsaken
and hated, so that no man went through
thee, I will make thee an eternal excellency, a joy of many generations.
16 Thou shalt also suck the milk of the
Gentiles, and shalt suck the breast of
kings: and thou shalt know that I the
LORD *am* thy Saviour and thy [a]Redeemer,
the mighty One of Jacob.
17 For brass I will bring gold, and for
iron I will bring silver, and for wood
brass, and for stones iron: I will also
make thy officers peace, and thine exac-
tors righteousness.
18 Violence shall no more be heard in
thy land, wasting nor destruction within
thy borders; but thou shalt call thy walls
Salvation, and thy gates Praise.
19 The [b]sun shall be no more thy light
by day; neither for brightness shall the
moon give light unto thee: but the LORD
shall be unto thee an everlasting light,
and [c]thy God thy glory.
20 [d]Thy sun shall no more go down;
neither shall thy moon withdraw itself:
for the LORD shall be thine everlasting
light, and the days of thy mourning shall
be ended.
21 [e]Thy people also *shall be* all righteous: [f]they shall inherit the land for ever,
the [g]branch of my planting, the work of
my hands, that I may be glorified.
22 A [h]little one shall become a thousand, and a small one a strong nation: I
the LORD will hasten it in his time.

CHAPTER 61.

The two advents in one view.

The [i]Spirit of the Lord GOD *is* [j]upon
[k]me; because the LORD hath [l]anoint-
ed me to preach good [m]tidings unto the
meek; he hath sent me to bind up the
brokenhearted, to proclaim liberty to the
captives, and the opening of the prison
to *them that are* bound;

B.C. 698.

a Heb. *goel, Redemp. (Kinsman type).* Isa. 59:20, *note.*

b Rev. 21:23; 22:5.

c Zech. 2:5.

d See Amos 8:9.

e Isa. 52:1; Rev. 21:27.

f Psa. 37:11, 22; Mt. 5:5.

g Isa. 61:3; Mt. 15:15.

h Isa. 29:23; 45:11; Eph. 2:10.

i *Holy Spirit.* Isa. 63:10. (Gen. 1:2; Mal. 2:15.)

j Lk. 4:18, 19.

k *Christ (First Advent).* Dan. 9:25, 26. (Gen. 3:15; Acts 1:9.)

l Lk. 7:22; Acts 10:38.

m *Gospel.* vs. 1-3. Mt. 3:1, 2. (Gen. 12:1-3; Rev. 14:6.)

n *Day (of destruction).* Isa. 63:1-6. (Job 21:30; Rev. 20:11-15.)

o *Covenant (New).* Jer. 31:31-34. (Isa. 61:8; Heb. 8:8-12.)

p *Righteousness (garment).* Isa. 64:6. (Gen. 3:21; Rev. 19:8.)

2 To proclaim the acceptable [1]year of
the LORD, and the [n]day of vengeance of
our God; to comfort all that mourn;

Kingdom peace and blessing after the day of vengeance anticipated (Isa. 61:3–65:24): (1) *The restoration of Israel* (extends to Isa. 62:12).

3 To appoint unto them that mourn in
Zion, to give unto them beauty for
ashes, the oil of joy for mourning, the
garment of praise for the spirit of heaviness; that they might be called trees of
righteousness, the planting of the LORD,
that he might be glorified.
4 And they shall build the old wastes,
they shall raise up the former desolations, and they shall repair the waste
cities, the desolations of many generations.
5 And strangers shall stand and feed
your flocks, and the sons of the alien
shall be your plowmen and your vinedressers.
6 But ye shall be named the Priests of
the LORD: *men* shall call you the
Ministers of our God: ye shall eat the
riches of the Gentiles, and in their glory
shall ye boast yourselves.
7 For your shame *ye shall have* double;
and *for* confusion they shall rejoice in
their portion: therefore in their land they
shall possess the double: everlasting joy
shall be unto them.
8 For I the LORD love judgment, I hate
robbery for burnt-offering; and I will
direct their work in truth, and I will make
an everlasting [o]covenant with them.
9 And their seed shall be known
among the Gentiles, and their offspring
among the people: all that see them shall
acknowledge them, that they *are* the
seed *which* the LORD hath blessed.
10 I will greatly rejoice in the LORD,
my soul shall be joyful in my God; for he
hath clothed me with the garments of
salvation, he hath covered me with the
[p]robe of righteousness, as a bridegroom

1 (61:2) Observe that Jesus suspended the reading of this passage in the synagogue at Nazareth (Lk 4:16-21) at the comma in the middle of Isa. 61:2. The first advent, therefore, opened the day of *grace* "the acceptable year of Jehovah," but does not fulfil the day of *vengeance*. That will be taken up when Messiah returns (2 Thes. 1:7-10). Cf. Isa. 34:8; 35:4-10. The last verse, taken with the 4th, gives the historic connection: the vengeance precedes the regathering of Israel, and synchronizes with the day of the LORD (Isa. 2:10-22; Rev. 19:11-21; also Isa. 63:1-6).

decketh *himself* with ornaments, and as a bride adorneth *herself* with her jewels.

11 For as the earth bringeth forth her bud, and as the garden causeth the things that are sown in it to spring forth; so the Lord GOD will cause righteousness and praise to spring forth before all the nations.

CHAPTER 62.

(*Restoration of Israel,* continued.)

For Zion's sake will I not hold my peace, and for Jerusalem's sake I will not rest, until the righteousness thereof go forth as brightness, and the salvation thereof as a lamp *that* burneth.

2 And the Gentiles shall see thy righteousness, and all kings thy glory: and [a]thou shalt be called by a new name, which the mouth of the LORD shall name.

3 Thou shalt also be [b]a crown of glory in the hand of the LORD, and a royal diadem in the hand of thy God.

4 [c]Thou shalt no more be termed Forsaken; neither shall thy land any more be termed Desolate: but thou shalt be called [d]Hephzi-bah, and thy land [e]Beulah: for the LORD delighteth in thee, and thy land shall be married.

5 For *as* a young man marrieth a virgin, *so* shall thy sons marry thee: and *as* the bridegroom rejoiceth over the bride, *so* shall thy God rejoice over thee.

6 [f]I have set watchmen upon thy walls, O Jerusalem, *which* shall never hold their peace day nor night: ye that make mention of the LORD, keep not silence,

7 And give him no rest, till he establish, and till he make Jerusalem a praise in the earth.

8 The LORD hath sworn by his right hand, and by the arm of his strength, Surely I will no more give thy corn *to be* meat for thine enemies; and the sons of the stranger shall not drink thy wine, for the which thou hast laboured:

9 But they that have gathered it shall eat it, and praise the LORD; and they that have brought it together shall drink it in the courts of my holiness.

10 Go through, go through the gates; prepare ye the way of the people; cast up, cast up the highway; gather out the stones; lift up a [g]standard for the people.

11 Behold, the LORD hath proclaimed unto the end of the world, [h]Say ye to the daughter of Zion, Behold, thy salvation cometh; behold, his reward *is* with him, and his work before him.

12 And they shall call them, The holy people, The [i]redeemed of the LORD: and thou shalt be called, Sought out, A city not forsaken.

CHAPTER 63.

(2) *The day of vengeance.*
(Cf. Isa 2:10-22; Rev. 19:11-21.)

[j]Who *is* this that cometh from Edom, with dyed garments from Bozrah? this *that is* glorious in his apparel, travelling in the greatness of his strength? I that speak in righteousness, mighty to save.

2 Wherefore *art thou* red in thine apparel, and thy garments like him that treadeth in the winefat?

3 I have trodden the winepress alone; and of the people *there was* none with me: for I will [k]tread them in mine anger, and trample them in my fury; and their blood shall be sprinkled upon my garments, and I will stain all my raiment.

4 For the [l]day of vengeance *is* in mine heart, and the year of my [i]redeemed is come.

5 And I looked, and *there was* none to help; and I wondered that *there was* none to uphold: therefore mine own arm brought salvation unto me; and my fury, it upheld me.

6 And I will tread down the people in mine anger, and make them drunk in my fury, and I will bring down their strength to the earth.

Fear and hope of the Remnant (Isa. 1:9; Rom 11:5) *in the day of vengeance.*

7 I will mention the lovingkindnesses of the LORD, *and* the praises of the LORD, according to all that the LORD hath bestowed on us, and the great goodness toward the house of Israel, which he hath bestowed on them according to his mercies, and according to the multitude of his lovingkindnesses.

8 For he said, Surely they *are* my people, children *that* will not lie: so he was their Saviour.

9 In all their affliction he was afflicted,

B.C. 698.

a vs. 4:12; Isa. 65:15; cf. Rev. 2:17.

b Zech. 9:16.

c Hos. 1:10; 1 Pet. 2:10.

d i.e. *My delight is in her.*

e i.e. *Married.* Cf. Isa. 54:5.

f Ezk. 3:17; 33:7.

g *Kingdom* (O.T.). vs. 10-12; Isa. 65:25. (Gen. 1:26; Zech. 12:8.)

h Mt. 21:5; John 12:15.

i Heb. *goel, Redemp. (Kinsman type).* Isa. 59:20, *note.*

j *Day (of Jehovah).* vs. 1-6; Isa. 66:15-24. (Isa. 2:10-22; Rev. 19:11-21.)

k See Gen. 36:1, *note.* Also *Armageddon (battle of).* vs. 1-6; Isa. 66:15, 16. (Rev. 16:14; 19:11-21.)

l *Day (of destruction).* Mt. 25:31-46. (Job 21:30; Rev. 20:11-15.)

and the [a]angel of his presence saved them: in his love and in his pity he [b]redeemed them; and he bare them, and carried them all the days of old.

10 But they rebelled, and [c]vexed his [d]holy Spirit: therefore he was turned to be their enemy, *and* he fought against them.

11 Then he remembered the days of old, Moses, *and* his people, *saying*, Where *is* he that brought them up out of the sea with the shepherd of his flock? where *is* he that put his holy Spirit within him?

12 That led *them* by the right hand of Moses with his glorious arm, dividing the water before them, to make himself an everlasting name?

13 That led them through the deep, as an horse in the wilderness, *that* they should not stumble?

14 As a beast goeth down into the valley, the Spirit of the LORD caused him to rest: so didst thou lead thy people, to make thyself a glorious name.

15 Look down from heaven, and behold from the habitation of thy holiness and of thy glory: where *is* thy zeal and thy strength, the sounding of thy bowels and of thy mercies toward me? are they restrained?

16 Doubtless thou *art* our [1]father, though Abraham be ignorant of us, and Israel acknowledge us not: thou, O LORD, *art* our father, our [b]redeemer; thy name *is* from everlasting.

17 O LORD, why hast thou made us to err from thy ways, *and* hardened our heart from thy [e]fear? Return for thy servants' sake, the tribes of thine inheritance.

18 The people of thy holiness have possessed *it* but a little while: our adversaries have trodden down thy sanctuary.

19 We are *thine*: thou never barest rule over them; they were not called by thy name.

CHAPTER 64.

(*Fear and hope of the Remnant, continued.*)

Oh that thou wouldest rend the heavens, that thou wouldest come down, that the mountains might flow down at thy presence,

2 As *when* the melting fire burneth, the fire causeth the waters to boil, to make thy name known to thine adversaries, *that* the nations may tremble at thy presence!

3 When thou didst terrible things *which* we looked not for, thou camest down, the mountains flowed down at thy presence.

4 For since the beginning of the world *men* have not heard, nor perceived by the ear, neither hath the eye seen, O God, beside thee, [f]*what* he hath prepared for him that waiteth for him.

5 Thou meetest him that rejoiceth and worketh righteousness, *those that* remember thee in thy ways: behold, thou art wroth; for we have sinned: in those is continuance, and we shall be saved.

6 But we are all as an unclean *thing*, and all [g]our righteousnesses *are* as filthy rags; and we all do fade as a leaf; and our iniquities, like the wind, have taken us away.

7 And *there is* none that calleth upon thy name, that stirreth up himself to take hold of thee: for thou hast hid thy face from us, and hast consumed us, because of our iniquities.

8 But now, O LORD, thou *art* our [2]father, we *are* the clay, and thou [h]our potter; and we all *are* the work of thy hand.

9 Be not wroth very sore, O LORD, neither remember iniquity for ever: behold, see, we beseech thee, we *are* all thy people.

10 Thy holy cities are a wilderness, Zion is a wilderness, Jerusalem a desolation.

11 Our holy and our beautiful house, where our fathers praised thee, is

B.C. 698.

a Heb. 1:4, *note.*

b Heb. *goel, Redemp. (Kinsman type).* Isa. 59:20, *note.*

c i.e. *grieved.*

d *Holy Spirit.* Ezk. 2:2. (Gen. 1:2; Mal. 2:15.)

e Psa. 19:9, *note.*

f Or, *who hath worked for him, who hath waited for him.* Cf. Isa. 65:17; John 14:2; 1 Cor. 2:9; Rev. 21:1.

g *Righteousness (garment).* Rom. 3:22. (Gen. 3:21; Rev. 19:8.)

h Isa. 29:16; 45:9; Jer. 18:6; Rom. 9:20, 21.

[1]**(63:16)** Cf. Isa. 1:2; 64:8. Israel, collectively, the national Israel, recognizes God as the national Father (cf. Ex. 4:22, 23). Doubtless the believing Israelite was born anew (cf. John 3:3, 5 with Lk. 13:28), but the O.T. Scriptures show no trace of the consciousness of personal sonship. The explanation is given in Gal. 4:1-7. The Israelite, though a child, "differed nothing from a servant." The Spirit, as the "Spirit of His Son," could not be given to impart the consciousness of sonship until redemption had been accomplished (Gal. 4:4-6). See "Adoption" (Rom. 8:15; Eph. 1:5).

[2]**(64:8)** Here the reference is to relationship through creation, rather than through faith, as in Acts 17:28, 29, *note.*

burned up with fire: and all our pleasant
things are laid waste.
12 Wilt thou refrain thyself for these
things, O LORD? wilt thou hold thy peace,
and afflict us very sore?

CHAPTER 65.

The answer of Jehovah to the Remnant.

I am sought of *them that* asked not *for*
me; I am found of *them that* sought me
[a]not: I said, Behold me, behold me, unto
a nation *that* was not called by my name.
2 [b]I have spread out my hands all the
day unto a rebellious people, which
walketh in a way *that was* not good, after
their own thoughts;
3 A people [c]that provoketh me to
anger continually to my face; that sacrificeth in gardens, and burneth incense
upon altars of brick;
4 [d]Which remain among the graves,
and lodge in the monuments, which eat
swine's flesh, and broth of abominable
things is in their vessels;
5 Which say, Stand by thyself, come
not near to me; for I am holier than thou.
These *are* a smoke in my nose, a fire that
burneth all the day.
6 Behold, *it is* written before me: I will
not keep silence, but will recompense,
even recompense into their bosom,
7 Your iniquities, and [e]the iniquities of
your fathers together, saith the LORD,
[f]which have burned incense upon the
mountains, and [g]blasphemed me upon
the hills: therefore will I measure their
former work into their bosom.
8 Thus saith the LORD, As the new
wine is found in the cluster, and *one*
saith, Destroy it not; for a blessing *is* in
it: so will I do for my servants' sakes,
that I may not destroy them all.
9 And I will bring forth a seed out of
Jacob, and out of Judah an inheritor of my
mountains: and mine [h]elect shall inherit
it, and my servants shall dwell there.
10 And [i]Sharon shall be a fold of
flocks, and the [j]valley of Achor a place
for the herds to lie down in, for my people that have sought me.
11 But ye *are* they that forsake the LORD,
that forget my holy mountain, that prepare a table for that troop, and that furnish the drink-offering unto that number.
12 Therefore will I number you to the
sword, and ye shall all bow down to the
slaughter: because when I called, ye did
not answer; when I spake, ye did not
hear; but did evil before mine eyes, and
did choose *that* wherein I delighted not.
13 Therefore thus saith the Lord GOD,
Behold, my servants shall eat, but ye
shall be hungry: behold, my servants
shall drink, but ye shall be thirsty:
behold, my servants shall rejoice, but ye
shall be ashamed:
14 Behold, my servants shall sing for
joy of heart, but ye shall cry for sorrow
of heart, and shall howl for vexation of
spirit.
15 And ye shall leave your name [k]for a
curse unto my chosen: for the Lord GOD
shall slay thee, and [l]call his servants by
another name:
16 That he who blesseth himself in the
earth shall bless himself in the God of
truth; and he that sweareth in the earth
shall swear by the God of truth; because
the former troubles are forgotten, and
because they are hid from mine eyes.

The eternal blessing of Israel in the new earth. (Cf. Rev. 21, 22.)

17 For, [1]behold, I [m]create new heavens
and a new earth: and the former shall
not be remembered, nor come into mind.
18 But be ye glad and rejoice for ever
in that which I create: for, behold, I create
Jerusalem a rejoicing, and her people a
joy.
19 And I will rejoice in Jerusalem, and
joy in my people: and [n]the voice of
weeping shall be no more heard in her,
nor the voice of crying.
20 There shall be no more thence an
infant of days, nor an old man that hath
not filled his days: for the child shall die
an hundred years old; but the sinner
being an hundred years old shall be
accursed.
21 [o]And they shall build houses, and
inhabit *them*; and they shall plant vineyards, and eat the fruit of them.

B.C. 698.

a Rom. 10:20.
b Rom. 10:21.
c Deut. 32:21.
d Isa. 66:17; Lev. 11:7.
e Ex. 20:5.
f Ezk. 18:6.
g Isa. 57:7; Ezk. 20:27, 28.
h vs. 15, 22; Mt. 24:22; Rom. 11:5, 7.
i Isa. 33:9; 35:2.
j Josh. 7:24, 26; Hos. 2:15.
k Jer. 29:22; Zech. 8:13.
l Isa. 62:2; Acts 11:26.
m Isa. 51:16; 66:22; 2 Pet. 3:13; Rev. 21:1.
n Isa. 35:10; 51:11; Rev. 7:17; 21:4.
o Isa. 61:9.

1(65:17) Verse 17 looks beyond the kingdom-age to the new heavens and the new earth (see *refs.* at "create"), but verses 18-25 describe the kingdom-age itself. Longevity is restored, but death, the "last enemy" 1 Cor. 15:26), is not destroyed till after Satan's rebellion at the end of the thousand years (Rev. 20:7-14).

B.C. 698.

22 They shall not build, and another inhabit; they shall not plant, and another eat: for as the days of a tree *are* the days of my people, and mine elect shall long enjoy the work of their hands.

23 They shall not labour in vain, nor bring forth for trouble; [a]for they *are* the seed of the blessed of the LORD, and their offspring with them.

24 And it shall come to pass, that before they call, I will answer; and while they are yet speaking, I will hear.

25 The wolf and the lamb shall feed together, and the lion shall eat straw like the bullock: and dust *shall be* the serpent's meat. [a]They shall not hurt nor destroy in all my holy mountain, saith the LORD.

CHAPTER 66.

Kingdom blessing, continued.

Thus saith the LORD, The [b]heaven *is* my throne, and the earth *is* my footstool: where *is* the house that ye build unto me? and where *is* the place of my rest?

2 For all those *things* hath mine hand made, and all those *things* have been, saith the LORD: but to this *man* will I look, [c]*even* to *him that is* poor and of a contrite spirit, and trembleth at my word.

3 He that killeth an ox *is as if* he slew a man; he that sacrificeth a lamb, *as if* he cut off a dog's neck; he that offereth an oblation, as *if he offered* swine's blood; he that burneth incense, *as if* he blessed an idol. Yea, they have chosen their own ways, and their soul delighteth in their abominations.

4 I also will choose their delusions, and will bring their fears upon them; because when I called, none did answer; when I spake, they did not hear: but they did evil before mine eyes, and chose *that* in which I delighted not.

5 Hear the word of the LORD, ye that tremble at his word; Your brethren that hated you, that cast you out for my name's sake, said, Let the LORD be glorified: but [d]he shall appear to your joy, and they shall be ashamed.

6 A voice of noise from the city, a voice from the temple, a voice of the LORD that rendereth recompence to his enemies.

7 Before she [e]travailed, she brought forth; before her pain came, she was delivered of a man child.

8 Who hath heard such a thing? who hath seen such things? Shall the earth be made to bring forth in one day? *or* shall a nation be born at once? for as soon as Zion travailed, she brought forth her children.

9 Shall I bring to the birth, and not cause to bring forth? saith the LORD: shall I cause to bring forth, and shut *the womb*? saith thy God.

10 Rejoice ye with Jerusalem, and be glad with her, all ye that love her: rejoice for joy with her, all ye that mourn for her:

11 That ye may suck, and be satisfied with the breasts of her consolations; that ye may milk out, and be delighted with the abundance of her glory.

12 For thus saith the LORD, Behold, [f]I will extend peace to her like a river, and the glory of the Gentiles like a flowing stream: then shall ye suck, ye shall be borne upon *her* sides, and be dandled upon *her* knees.

13 As one whom his mother comforteth, so will I comfort you; and ye shall be comforted in Jerusalem.

14 And when ye see *this*, your heart shall rejoice, and [g]your bones shall flourish like an herb: and the hand of the LORD shall be known toward his servants, and *his* indignation toward his enemies.

15 For, behold, the [h]LORD will come with fire, and with his chariots like a whirlwind, to [i]render his anger with fury, and his rebuke with flames of fire.

16 For by fire and by his [j]sword will the LORD plead with all flesh: and the slain of the LORD shall be many.

17 They that sanctify themselves, and purify themselves in the gardens behind one *tree* in the midst, eating swine's flesh, and the abomination, and the mouse, shall be consumed together, saith the LORD.

18 For I *know* their works and their thoughts: it shall come, that I will gather all nations and tongues; and they shall come, and see my glory.

19 And I will set a sign among them, and I will send those that escape of them unto the nations, *to* Tarshish, Pul, and Lud, that draw the bow, *to* Tubal, and Javan, *to* the [k]isles afar off, that have not

a Kingdom (O.T.). vs. 18-25; Jer. 16:12-16. (Gen. 1:26; Zech. 12:8.)

b vs. 1, 2; Acts 7:49, 50; 17:24.

c Psa. 34:18; 51:17; Isa. 57:15.

d 2 Thes. 1:10; Tit. 2:13.

e vs. 7, 8; Mic. 5:1, *note.*

f Isa. 48:18; 60:5.

g See Ezk. 37:1.

h Isa. 9:5; 2 Thes. 1:8.

i Day (of Jehovah). vs. 15-24; Jer. 25:29-38. (Isa. 2:10-22; Rev. 19:11-21.)

j Armageddon (battle of). vs. 15, 16; Jer. 25:29-33. (Rev. 16:14; 19:11-21.)

k i.e. *coasts.*

heard my fame, neither have seen my
glory; [a]and they shall declare my glory
among the Gentiles.
20 And they shall bring all your
brethren [b]*for* an offering unto the LORD
out of all nations upon horses, and in
chariots, and in litters, and upon mules,
and upon swift beasts, to my holy
mountain Jerusalem, saith the LORD, as
the children of Israel bring an offering in
a clean vessel into the house of the LORD.
21 And I will also take of them for
priests *and* for Levites, saith the LORD.
22 For [c]as the new heavens and the
new earth, which I will make, shall
remain before me, saith the LORD, so
shall your seed and your name remain.
23 And it shall come to pass, [d]*that*
from one new moon to another, and
from one sabbath to another, shall all
flesh come to worship before me, saith
the LORD.
24 And they shall go forth, and look
upon the carcases of the men that have
transgressed against me: for [e]their worm
shall not die, neither shall their fire be
quenched; and they shall be an abhorring unto all flesh.

B.C. 698.

a Mal. 1:11.

b Isa. 18:7.

c Isa. 65:17; 2 Pet. 3:13; Rev. 21:1.

d Zech. 14:17-21.

e Mk. 9:44.

THE BOOK OF THE PROPHET
JEREMIAH

JEREMIAH began his ministry in the 13th year of Josiah, about 60 years after Isaiah's death. Zephaniah and Habakkuk were contemporaries of his earlier ministry, Daniel of his later. After the death of Josiah, the kingdom of Judah hastened to its end in the Babylonian captivity. Jeremiah remained in the land ministering to the poor Remnant (2 Ki. 24:14) until they went into Egypt, whither he followed them, and where he died, early in the 70 years' captivity. Jeremiah, prophesying before and during the exile of Judah, connects the pre-exile prophets with Ezekiel and Daniel, prophets of the exile.

Jeremiah's vision includes: the Babylonian captivity; the return after 70 years; the world-wide dispersion; the final regathering; the kingdom-age; the day of judgment on the Gentile powers, and the Remnant.

Jeremiah is in six chief divisions: I. From the prophet's call to his message to the first captives, 1:1–29:32. II. Prophecies and events not chronological, 30:1–36:32. III. From the accession to the captivity of Zedekiah, 37:1–39:18. IV. Jeremiah's prophecies in the land after the final captivity of Judah, 40:1–42:22. V. The prophet in Egypt, 43:1–44:30. VI. Miscellaneous prophecies, 45:1–52:34.

The events recorded in Jeremiah cover a period of 41 years (Ussher).

PART I. FROM THE CALL OF JEREMIAH TO HIS MESSAGE TO THE FIRST CAPTIVES: CHAPTERS 1–29

CHAPTER 1.

Introduction.

The words of Jeremiah the son of
Hilkiah, of the priests that *were* in
Anathoth in the land of Benjamin:
2 To whom the word of the LORD came
in the days of Josiah the son of Amon
king of Judah, in the thirteenth year of
his reign.
3 It came also in the days of Jehoiakim
the son of Josiah king of Judah, unto the
end of the eleventh year of Zedekiah the
son of Josiah king of Judah, unto the carrying away of Jerusalem captive in the
[a]fifth month.

The prophet's call and enduement.

4 Then the word of the LORD came
unto me, saying,
5 Before I formed thee in the belly I
knew thee; and before thou camest forth
out of the womb I [b]sanctified thee, *and* I
ordained thee a prophet unto the
nations.
6 Then said I, Ah, Lord GOD! behold, I
cannot speak: for I *am* a child.
7 But the LORD said unto me, Say not, I
am a child: for thou shalt go to all that I
shall send thee, and whatsoever I command thee thou shalt speak.

B.C. 629.

a i.e. *August.*

b *Sanctify, holy* (O.T.). Dan. 4:13, 23. (Gen. 2:3; Zech. 8:3.)

c Ex. 3:12; Deut. 31:6, 8; Josh. 1:5; Jer. 15:20; Acts 26:17; Heb. 13:6.

d *Inspiration.* Jer. 30:2. (Ex. 4:15; Rev. 22:19.)

e Num. 17:8, *note.*

f Ezk. 11:3, 7; 24:3-14.

g Jer. 5:15; 6:22; 10:22; 25:9.

8 Be not afraid of their faces: for I [c]*am*
with thee to deliver thee, saith the LORD.
9 Then the LORD put forth his hand,
and touched my mouth. And the LORD
said unto me, Behold, I have put my
[d]words in thy mouth.
10 See, I have this day set thee over
the nations and over the kingdoms, to
root out, and to pull down, and to
destroy, and to throw down, to build,
and to plant.

The sign of the almond rod and seething pot.

11 Moreover the word of the LORD
came unto me, saying, Jeremiah, what
seest thou? And I said, I see a [e]rod of an
almond tree.
12 Then said the LORD unto me, Thou
hast well seen: for I will hasten my word
to perform it.
13 And the word of the LORD came
unto me the second time, saying, What
seest thou? And I said, I see [f]a seething
pot; and the face thereof *is* toward the
north.
14 Then the LORD said unto me, Out of
the north an evil shall break forth upon
all the inhabitants of the land.
15 For, lo, I will [g]call all the families of the kingdoms of the north

saith the LORD; and they shall come, and
they shall set every one his throne at the
entering of the gates of Jerusalem, and
against all the walls thereof round about,
and against all the cities of Judah.
16 And I will utter my judgments
against them touching all their wickedness, [a]who have forsaken me, and have
burned incense unto other gods, and worshipped the works of their own hands.
17 Thou therefore gird up thy loins,
and arise, and speak unto them all that I
command thee: be not dismayed at their
faces, lest I confound thee before them.
18 For, behold, I have made thee this
day [b]a defenced city, and an iron pillar,
and brasen walls against the whole land,
against the kings of Judah, against the
princes thereof, against the priests thereof, and against the people of the land.
19 And they shall fight against thee;
but they shall not prevail against thee;
for I *am* with thee, saith the LORD, to
deliver thee.

CHAPTER 2.

First message to backslidden Judah
(Jer. 2:1–3:5).

Moreover the [1]word of the LORD
came to me, saying,
2 Go and cry in the ears of Jerusalem,
saying, Thus saith the LORD; I remember
thee, the kindness of [c]thy youth, the love
of thine espousals, when [d]thou wentest
after me in the wilderness, in a land *that
was* not sown.
3 [e]Israel *was* holiness unto the LORD,
and the firstfruits of his increase: all that
devour him shall offend; evil shall come
upon them, saith the LORD.
4 Hear ye the word of the LORD, O
house of Jacob, and all the families of the
house of Israel:
5 Thus saith the LORD, [f]What iniquity
have your fathers found in me, that they
are gone far from me, and have walked
after vanity, and are become vain?
6 Neither said they, Where *is* the LORD
that [g]brought us up out of the land of
Egypt, that led us through the wilderness, through a land of deserts and of
pits, through a land of drought, and of
the shadow of death, through a land that
no man passed through, and where no
man dwelt?
7 And I brought you into [h]a plentiful
country, to eat the fruit thereof and the
goodness thereof; but when ye entered,
ye defiled my land, and made mine heritage an abomination.
8 The priests said not, Where *is* the
LORD? and they that handle the law
knew me not: the pastors also transgressed against me, and the prophets
prophesied by Baal, and walked after
things that do not profit.
9 Wherefore [i]I will yet plead with you,
saith the LORD, and with your children's
children will I plead.
10 For pass over the [j]isles of Chittim,
and see; and send unto Kedar, and consider diligently, and see if there be such
a thing.
11 Hath a nation changed *their* gods,
which *are* yet no gods? but my people
have changed their glory for *that which*
doth not profit.
12 Be astonished, O ye heavens, at
this, and be horribly afraid, be ye very
desolate, saith the LORD.
13 For my people have committed two
evils; they have forsaken me the [k]foun-
tain of living waters, *and* hewed them
out cisterns, broken cisterns, that can
hold no water.
14 *Is* Israel a servant? *is* he a homeborn
slave? why is he spoiled?
15 The young lions roared upon him,
and yelled, and they made his land waste:
his cities are burned without inhabitant.
16 Also the children of Noph and
[l]Tahapanes have broken the crown of
thy head.
17 Hast thou not procured this unto
thyself, in that thou hast forsaken the
LORD thy God, [m]when he led thee by the
way?
18 And now what hast thou to do in
the way of Egypt, to drink the waters of
[n]Sihor? or what hast thou to do in the
way of Assyria, to drink the waters of
the river?
19 Thine own wickedness shall

B.C. 629.

a Deut. 28:20; Jer. 17:13.
b Isa. 50:7; Jer. 6:27; 15:20.
c Ezk. 16:8, 22, 60; 23:3, 8, 19; Hos. 2:15.
d Deut. 2:7.
e Ex. 19:5, 6.
f Isa. 5:4; Mic. 6:3.
g Isa. 63:9, 11, 13; Hos. 13:4.
h Or, *the land of Carmel.* Num. 13:27; 14:7, 8; Deut. 8:7-9.
i Ezk. 20:35, 36; Mic. 6:2.
j i.e. *coasts.*
k Psa. 36:9; Jer. 17:13; 18:14; John 4:14.
l Jer. 43:7-9.
m Deut. 32:10.
n Josh. 13:3.

[1] **(2:1)** The general character of the first message from Jehovah to Judah by Jeremiah is threefold: (1) He reminds Israel of the days of blessing and deliverance, e.g. 2:1-7; (2) He reproaches them with forsaking Him, e.g. 2:13; (3) He accuses them of choosing other, and impotent, gods, e.g. 2:10-12, 26-28. All these messages are to be thought of as inspired sermons, spoken to the people and subsequently written. Cf. Jer. 36:1-32.

correct thee, and thy backslidings shall
reprove thee: know therefore and see
that *it is* an evil *thing* and bitter, that
thou hast forsaken the LORD thy God,
and that my fear *is* not in thee, saith the
Lord GOD of hosts.
20 For of old time I have broken thy
yoke, *and* burst thy bands; and [a]thou
saidst, I will not transgress; when [b]upon
every high hill and under every green
tree thou wanderest, playing the harlot.
21 Yet I had planted thee a noble vine,
wholly a right seed: how then art thou
turned into [c]the degenerate plant of a
strange vine unto me?
22 For though thou wash thee with
nitre, and take thee much soap, *yet*
[d]thine iniquity is marked before me,
saith the Lord GOD.
23 How canst thou say, I am not polluted, I have not gone after Baalim? see
thy way in the valley, know what thou
hast done: *thou art* a swift dromedary
traversing her ways;
24 A wild ass used to the wilderness,
that snuffeth up the wind at her pleasure; in her occasion who can turn her
away? all they that seek her will not
weary themselves; in her month they
shall find her.
25 Withhold thy foot from being
unshod, and thy throat from thirst: but
thou saidst, There is no hope: no; for I
have loved strangers, and after them
will I go.
26 As the thief is ashamed when he is
found, so is the house of Israel ashamed;
they, their kings, their princes, and their
priests, and their prophets,
27 Saying to a stock, Thou *art* my
father; and to a stone, Thou hast brought
me forth: for they have turned *their* back
unto me, and not *their* face: but in the
time of their trouble they will say, Arise,
and save us.
28 But [e]where *are* thy gods that thou
hast made thee? let them arise, if they
can save thee in the time of thy trouble:
for *according to* the number of thy cities
are thy gods, O Judah.
29 [f]Wherefore will ye plead with me?
ye all have transgressed against me,
saith the LORD.
30 In vain have I smitten your children; they received no correction: your
own sword hath [g]devoured your
prophets, like a destroying lion.
31 O generation, see ye the word of
the LORD. Have I been a wilderness unto
Israel? a land of darkness? wherefore say
my people, We are lords; we will come
no more unto thee?
32 Can a maid forget her ornaments, *or*
a bride her attire? yet my people [h]have
forgotten me days without number.
33 Why trimmest thou thy way to seek
love? therefore hast thou also taught the
wicked ones thy ways.
34 Also in thy skirts is found the blood
of the souls of the poor innocents: I have
not found it by secret search, but upon
all these.
35 Yet thou sayest, Because I am innocent, surely his anger shall turn from me.
Behold, I will plead with thee, because
thou sayest, I have not sinned.
36 [i]Why gaddest thou about so much
to change thy way? thou also shalt be
ashamed of Egypt, as thou wast
ashamed of Assyria.
37 Yea, thou shalt go forth from him,
and thine hands upon thine head: for the
LORD hath rejected thy confidences, and
thou shalt not prosper in them.

CHAPTER 3.

(*First message*, continued.)

They say, If a man put away his wife,
and she go from him, and become
another man's, shall he return unto her
again? shall not that land be greatly polluted? but [j]thou hast played the harlot
with many lovers; yet return again to
me, saith the LORD.
2 Lift up thine eyes unto the high
places, and see where thou hast not been
lien with. In the ways hast thou sat for
them, as the Arabian in the wilderness;
and thou hast polluted the land with thy
whoredoms and with thy wickedness.
3 Therefore the [k]showers have been
withholden, and there hath been no latter rain; and thou hadst a whore's forehead, thou refusedst to be ashamed.
4 Wilt thou not from this time cry unto
me, My father, thou *art* the guide [l]of my
youth?
5 Will he reserve *his anger* for ever?
will he keep *it* to the end? Behold, thou
hast spoken and done evil things as thou
couldest.

B.C. 629.

a Ex. 19:8; Josh. 24:18; Jud. 10:16; 1 Sam. 12:10.
b Isa. 57:5, 7; Jer. 3:6; cf. Deut. 12:2.
c Deut. 32:32; Isa. 1:21; 5:4.
d Deut. 32:34; Job 14:17; Hos. 13:12.
e Deut. 32:37; Jud. 10:14.
f vs. 23, 35.
g 2 Chr. 36:16; Neh. 9:26; Mt. 23:29; Acts 7:52; 1 Thes. 2:15.
h Psa. 106:21; Hos. 8:14; Jer. 13:25.
i v.18; Jer. 31:22; Hos. 5:13; 12:1.
j Jer. 2:20; Ezk. 16:26, 28, 29.
k Lev. 26:19; Deut. 28:23, 24; Jer. 9:12; 14:4.
l Jer. 2:2; Hos. 2:15.

The second message to backslidden Judah (Jer. 3:6–6:30).

6 The LORD [1]said also unto me in the days of Josiah the king, Hast thou seen *that* which backsliding [2]Israel hath done? she is gone up upon every high mountain and under every green tree, and there hath played the harlot.

7 And I said after she had done all these *things*, Turn thou unto me. But she returned not. And her treacherous [a]sister Judah saw *it*.

8 And I saw, when for all the causes whereby backsliding Israel committed adultery I had put her away, and given her a bill of divorce; yet her treacherous sister Judah feared not, but went and played the harlot also.

9 And it came to pass through the lightness of her whoredom, that she defiled the land, and committed adultery with stones and with stocks.

10 And yet for all this her treacherous sister Judah hath not turned unto me [b]with her whole heart, but feignedly, saith the LORD.

11 And the LORD said unto me, The backsliding Israel hath justified herself more than treacherous Judah.

12 Go and proclaim these words toward the north, and say, Return, thou backsliding Israel, saith the LORD; *and* I will not cause mine anger to fall upon you: for I *am* merciful, saith the LORD, *and* I will not keep *anger* for ever.

13 [c]Only acknowledge thine iniquity, that thou hast transgressed against the LORD thy God, and hast scattered thy ways to the strangers under every green tree, and ye have not obeyed my voice, saith the LORD.

14 Turn, O backsliding children, saith the LORD; for I am [d]married unto you: and I will take you one of a city, and two of a family, and I will bring you to Zion:

15 And I will give you [e]pastors according to mine heart, which shall [f]feed you with knowledge and understanding.

16 And it shall come to pass, when ye be multiplied and increased in the land, in those days, saith the LORD, they shall say no more, The ark of the covenant of the LORD: neither shall it come to mind: neither shall they remember it; neither shall they visit *it*; neither shall *that* be done any more.

17 At that time they shall call Jerusalem the throne of the LORD; and all the nations shall be gathered unto it, [g]to the name of the LORD, to Jerusalem: neither shall they walk any more after the imagination of their evil heart.

18 In those days [h]the house of Judah shall walk with the house of Israel, and they shall come together out of the land of the north to the land that I have given for an inheritance unto your fathers.

19 But I said, How shall I put thee among the children, and give thee a pleasant land, a goodly heritage of the hosts of nations? and I said, Thou shalt call me, [i]My father; and shalt not turn away from me.

20 Surely *as* a wife treacherously departeth from her husband, so have ye dealt treacherously with me, O house of Israel, saith the LORD.

21 A voice was heard upon the high places, weeping *and* supplications of the children of Israel: for they have perverted their way, *and* they have forgotten the LORD their God.

22 Return, ye backsliding children, *and* [j]I will heal your backslidings. Behold, we come unto thee; for thou *art* the LORD our God.

23 Truly in vain *is salvation hoped for* from the hills, *and from* the multitude of mountains: [k]truly in the LORD our God *is* the salvation of Israel.

24 For shame hath devoured the labour of our fathers from our youth; their flocks and their herds, their sons and their daughters.

B.C. 612.

a Ezk. 16:46; 23:2, 4.
b 2 Chr. 34:33; Hos. 7:14.
c Lev. 26:40; Deut. 30:1, 2; Prov. 28:13.
d Jer. 31:32; Hos. 2:19, 20.
e Jer. 23:4; Ezk. 34:23; Eph. 4:11.
f Acts 20:28.
g Isa. 60:9.
h Isa. 11:13; Ezk. 37:16-22; Hos. 1:11.
i Isa. 63:16.
j Hos. 6:1; 14:4.
k Psa. 3:8.

[1]**(3:6)** The general character of the second message to Judah is: (1) of reproach that the example of Jehovah's chastening of the northern kingdom (2 Ki. 17:1-18) had produced no effect upon Judah, e.g. 3:6-10; (2) of warning of a like chastisement impending over Judah, e.g. vs. 15-17; (3) of touching appeals to return to Jehovah, e.g. 3:12-14; and (4) of promises of final national restoration and blessing, e.g. 3:16-18.

[2]**(3:6)** "Israel" and "Ephraim": names by which the northern kingdom (the ten tribes) is usually called in the prophets. When by "Israel" the whole nation is meant, it will appear from the context.

25 We lie down in our shame, and our confusion covereth us: [a]for we have sinned against the LORD our God, we and our fathers, from our youth even unto this day, and have not obeyed the voice of the LORD our God.

CHAPTER 4.

(*Second message*, continued.)

If thou wilt return, O Israel, saith the LORD, [b]return unto me: and if thou wilt put away thine abominations out of my sight, then shalt thou not remove.

2 And thou shalt swear, The LORD liveth, in truth, in judgment, and in righteousness; and the nations shall bless themselves in him, and in him shall they glory.

3 For thus saith the LORD to the men of Judah and Jerusalem, [c]Break up your fallow ground, and sow not among thorns.

4 [d]Circumcise yourselves to the LORD, and take away the foreskins of your heart, ye men of Judah and inhabitants of Jerusalem: lest my fury come forth like fire, and burn that none can quench *it*, because of the evil of your doings.

5 Declare ye in Judah, and publish in Jerusalem; and say, Blow ye the trumpet in the land: cry, gather together, and say, Assemble yourselves, and let us go into the defenced cities.

6 Set up the standard toward Zion: retire, stay not: for I will bring evil from the [e]north, and a great destruction.

7 The lion is come up from his thicket, and the destroyer of the Gentiles is on his way; he is gone forth from his place to make thy land desolate; *and* thy cities shall be laid waste, without an inhabitant.

8 For this [f]gird you with sackcloth, lament and howl: for the fierce anger of the LORD is not turned back from us.

9 And it shall come to pass at that day, saith the LORD, *that* the heart of the king shall perish, and the heart of the princes; and the priests shall be astonished, and the prophets shall wonder.

10 Then said I, Ah, Lord GOD! [g]surely thou hast greatly deceived this people and Jerusalem, saying, Ye shall have peace; whereas the sword reacheth unto the soul.

B.C. 612.

a Ezra 9:7.

b Jer. 3:1, 22; Joel 2:12.

c Hos. 10:12.

d Deut. 10:16; 30:6; Jer. 9:26; Rom. 2:28, 29; Col. 2:11.

e Jer. 1:13-15; 6:1, 22.

f Isa. 22:12; Jer. 6:26.

g Ezk. 14:9; 2 Thes. 2:11.

h Jer. 51:1; Ezk. 17:10; Hos. 13:15.

i Isa. 5:28.

j Deut. 28:49; Lam. 4:19; Hos. 8:1; Hab. 1:8.

k Isa. 1:16; Jas. 4:8.

l Ezk. 7:26.

11 At that time shall it be said to this people and to Jerusalem, [h]A dry wind of the high places in the wilderness toward the daughter of my people, not to fan, nor to cleanse,

12 *Even* a full wind from those *places* shall come unto me: now also will I give sentence against them.

13 Behold, he shall come up as clouds, and his [i]chariots *shall be* as a whirlwind: his [j]horses are swifter than eagles. Woe unto us! for we are spoiled.

14 O Jerusalem, [k]wash thine heart from wickedness, that thou mayest be saved. How long shall thy vain thoughts lodge within thee?

15 For a voice declareth from Dan, and publisheth affliction from mount Ephraim.

16 Make ye mention to the nations; behold, publish against Jerusalem, *that* watchers come from a far country, and give out their voice against the cities of Judah.

17 As keepers of a field, are they against her round about; because she hath been rebellious against me, saith the LORD.

18 Thy way and thy doings have procured these *things* unto thee; this *is* thy wickedness, because it is bitter, because it reacheth unto thine heart.

19 My bowels, my bowels! I am pained at my very heart; my heart maketh a noise in me; I cannot hold my peace because thou hast heard, O my soul, the sound of the trumpet, the alarm of war.

20 [l]Destruction upon destruction is cried; for the whole land is spoiled: suddenly are my tents spoiled, *and* my curtains in a moment.

21 How long shall I see the standard *and* hear the sound of the trumpet?

22 For my people *is* foolish, they have not known me; they *are* sottish children and they have none understanding: they *are* wise to do evil, but to do good they have no knowledge.

23 I beheld the earth, and, lo, *it* [1]*was* without form, and void; and the heavens, and they *had* no light.

[1] **(4:23)** Cf. Gen. 1:2. "Without form and void" describes the condition of the earth as the result of the judgment (vs. 24-26; Isa. 24:1) which overthrew the primal order of Gen. 1:1.

24 [a]I beheld the mountains, and, lo,
they trembled, and all the hills moved
lightly.
25 I beheld, and, lo, *there was* no man,
and all the birds of the heavens were fled.
26 I beheld, and, lo, the fruitful place
was a wilderness, and all the cities thereof were broken down at the presence of
the LORD, *and* by his fierce anger.
27 For thus hath the LORD said, The
whole land shall be desolate; yet will I
not make a full end.
28 For this shall the earth mourn, and
the heavens above be black: because I
have spoken *it*, I have purposed *it*, and
will not [b]repent, neither will I turn back
from it.
29 The whole city shall flee for the
noise of the horsemen and bowmen;
they shall go into thickets, and climb up
upon the rocks: every city *shall be* forsak-
en, and not a man dwell therein.
30 And *when* thou *art* spoiled, what wilt
thou do? Though thou clothest thyself
with crimson, though thou deckest thee
with ornaments of gold, though [c]thou
rentest thy face with painting, in vain
shalt thou make thyself fair; *thy* lovers
will despise thee, they will seek thy life.
31 For I have heard a voice as of a
woman in travail, *and* the anguish as of
her that bringeth forth her first child, the
voice of the daughter of Zion, *that*
bewaileth herself, *that* spreadeth her
hands, *saying*, Woe *is* me now! for my
soul is wearied because of murderers.

CHAPTER 5.

(*Second message*, continued.)

Run ye to and fro through the streets
of Jerusalem, and see now, and
know, and seek in the broad places
thereof, if ye can find a man, if there be
any that executeth judgment, that
seeketh the truth; and I will pardon it.
2 And [d]though they say, The LORD
liveth; surely they swear falsely.
3 O LORD, *are* not [e]thine eyes upon the
truth? thou hast stricken them, but they
have not grieved; thou hast consumed
them, *but* they have [f]refused to receive
correction: they have made their faces
harder than a rock; they have refused to
return.
4 Therefore I said, Surely these *are*
poor; they are foolish: for they know not
the way of the LORD, *nor* the judgment of
their God.
5 I will get me unto the great men, and
will speak unto them; for [g]they have
known the way of the LORD, *and* the
judgment of their God: but these have
altogether broken the yoke, *and* burst the
bonds.
6 Wherefore a lion out of the forest
shall slay them, *and* a wolf of the
evenings shall spoil them, a leopard shall
watch over their cities: every one that
goeth out thence shall be torn in pieces:
because their transgressions are many,
and their backslidings are increased.
7 How shall I pardon thee for this? thy
children have forsaken me, and [h]sworn
by *them that* [i]*are* no gods: when I had fed
them to the full, they then committed
adultery, and assembled themselves by
troops in the harlots' houses.
8 [j]They were *as* fed horses in the
morning: every one neighed after his
neighbour's wife.
9 Shall I not visit for these *things*? saith
the LORD: and shall not my soul be
avenged on such a nation as this?
10 Go ye up upon her walls, and
destroy; but make not a full end: take
away her battlements; for they *are* not
the LORD'S.
11 For the house of Israel and the
house of Judah have dealt very treacherously against me, saith the LORD.
12 [k]They have belied the LORD, and
said, *It is* not he; neither shall evil come
upon us; neither shall we see sword nor
famine:
13 And the prophets shall become
wind, and the word *is* not in them: thus
shall it be done unto them.
14 Wherefore thus saith the LORD God
of hosts, Because ye speak this word,
behold, I will make my words in thy
mouth fire, and this people wood, and it
shall devour them.
15 Lo, [l]I will bring a nation upon you
from far, O house of Israel, saith the
LORD: it *is* a mighty nation, it *is* an
ancient nation, a nation whose language
thou knowest not, neither understandest
what they say.
16 Their quiver *is* as an open sepulchre, they *are* all mighty men.
17 And they shall eat up [m]thine harvest, and thy bread, *which* thy sons and
thy daughters should eat: they shall eat

B.C. 612.

a Isa. 5:25; Ezk. 38:20.
b Zech. 8:14, *note*.
c 2 Ki. 9:30; Ezk. 23:40.
d Tit. 1:16.
e 2 Chr. 16:9.
f Jer. 7:28; Zeph. 3:2.
g Mic. 3:1.
h Josh. 23:7; Zeph. 1:5.
i Deut. 32:21; Gal. 4:8.
j Ezk. 22:11.
k 2 Chr. 36:16.
l Deut. 28:49; Isa. 5:26; Jer. 1:15; 6:22.
m Lev. 26:16; Deut. 28:31, 33.

up thy flocks and thine herds: they shall eat up thy vines and thy fig trees: they shall impoverish thy fenced cities, wherein thou [a]trustedst, with the sword.

18 Nevertheless in those days, saith the LORD, I will not make a full end with you.

19 And it shall come to pass, when ye shall say, [b]Wherefore doeth the LORD our God all these *things* unto us? then shalt thou answer them, Like as ye have forsaken me, and served strange gods in your land, so shall ye serve strangers in a land *that is* not yours.

20 Declare this in the house of Jacob, and publish it in Judah, saying,

21 Hear now this, [c]O foolish people, and without understanding; which have eyes, and see not; which have ears, and hear not:

22 Fear ye not me? saith the LORD: will ye not tremble at my presence, which have placed the sand *for* the bound of the sea by a perpetual decree, that it cannot pass it: and though the waves thereof toss themselves, yet can they not prevail; though they roar, yet can they not pass over it?

23 But this people hath a revolting and a rebellious heart; they are revolted and gone.

24 Neither say they in their heart, Let us now [d]fear the LORD our God, [e]that giveth rain, both the [f]former and the latter, in his season: he reserveth unto us the appointed weeks of the harvest.

25 Your iniquities have turned away these *things*, and your sins have withholden good *things* from you.

26 For among my people are found wicked *men*: they lay wait, as he that setteth snares; they set a trap, they catch men.

27 As a cage is full of birds, so *are* their houses full of deceit: therefore they are become great, and waxen rich.

28 They are waxen fat, they shine: yea, they overpass the deeds of the wicked: they judge not the cause, the cause of the fatherless, yet they prosper; and the right of the needy do they not judge.

29 [g]Shall I not visit for these *things*? saith the LORD: shall not my soul be avenged on such a nation as this?

30 A wonderful and [h]horrible thing is committed in the land;

B.C. 612.

a Psa. 2:12, *note*.

b Deut. 29:24; 1 Ki. 9:8, 9; Jer. 13:22; 16:10.

c Isa. 6:9; Ezk. 12:2; Mt. 13:14; John 12:40; Acts 28:26; Rom. 11:8.

d Psa. 19:9, *note*.

e Psa. 147:8; Jer. 14:22; Mt. 5:45; Acts 14:17.

f Deut. 11:14; Joel 2:23.

g v. 9; Mal. 3:5.

h Jer. 23:14; Hos. 6:10; 2 Tim. 4:3.

i Neh. 3:14.

j 2 Ki. 25:1, 4; Jer. 4:17.

k Jer. 51:27; Joel 3:9.

l Ezk. 23:18; Hos. 9:12.

m Ex. 6:12; Jer. 7:26; Acts 7:51.

n Jer. 20:9.

31 The prophets prophesy falsely, and the priests bear rule by their means; and my people love *to have it* so: and what will ye do in the end thereof?

CHAPTER 6.

(*Second message,* continued.)

O ye children of Benjamin, gather yourselves to flee out of the midst of Jerusalem, and blow the trumpet in Tekoa, and set up a sign of fire in [i]Bethhaccerem: for evil appeareth out of the north, and great destruction.

2 I have likened the daughter of Zion to a comely and delicate *woman*.

3 The shepherds with their flocks shall come unto her; [j]they shall pitch *their* tents against her round about; they shall feed every one in his place.

4 [k]Prepare ye war against her; arise, and let us go up at noon. Woe unto us! for the day goeth away, for the shadows of the evening are stretched out.

5 Arise, and let us go by night, and let us destroy her palaces.

6 For thus hath the LORD of hosts said, Hew ye down trees, and cast a mount against Jerusalem: this *is* the city to be visited; she *is* wholly oppression in the midst of her.

7 As a fountain casteth out her waters, so she casteth out her wickedness: violence and spoil is heard in her; before me continually *is* grief and wounds.

8 Be thou instructed, O Jerusalem, [l]lest my soul depart from thee; lest I make thee desolate, a land not inhabited.

9 Thus saith the LORD of hosts, They shall throughly glean the remnant of Israel as a vine: turn back thine hand as a grapegatherer into the baskets.

10 To whom shall I speak, and give warning, that they may hear? behold, [m]their ear *is* uncircumcised, and they cannot hearken: behold, the word of the LORD is unto them a reproach; they have no delight in it.

11 Therefore I am full of the fury of the LORD; [n]I am weary with holding in: I will pour it out upon the children abroad, and upon the assembly of young men together: for even the husband with

the wife shall be taken, the aged with *him that is* full of days.

12 And [a]their houses shall be turned unto others, *with their* fields and wives together: for I will stretch out my hand upon the inhabitants of the land, saith the LORD.

13 For from the least of them even unto the greatest of them every one *is* given to [b]covetousness; and from the prophet even unto the priest every one dealeth falsely.

14 They have healed also the [c]hurt *of the daughter* of my people slightly, saying, Peace, peace; when *there is* no peace.

15 Were they ashamed when they had committed abomination? nay, they were not at all ashamed, neither could they blush: therefore they shall fall among them that fall: at the time *that* I visit them they shall be cast down, saith the LORD.

16 Thus saith the LORD, Stand ye in the ways, and see, and ask for the [d]old paths, where *is* the good way, and walk therein, and ye shall find rest for your souls. But they said, We will not walk *therein.*

17 Also I set watchmen over you, *saying,* [e]Hearken to the sound of the trumpet. But they said, We will not hearken.

18 Therefore hear, ye nations, and know, O congregation, what *is* among them.

19 [f]Hear, O earth: behold, I will bring evil upon this people, *even* [g]the fruit of their thoughts, because they have not hearkened unto my words, nor to my law, but rejected it.

20 [h]To what purpose cometh there to me incense from Sheba, and the sweet cane from a far country? your burnt-offerings *are* not acceptable, nor your sacrifices sweet unto me.

21 Therefore thus saith the LORD, Behold, I will lay stumblingblocks before this people, and the fathers and the sons together shall fall upon them; the neighbour and his friend shall perish.

22 Thus saith the LORD, Behold, a people cometh from [i]the north country, and a great nation shall be raised from the sides of the earth.

23 They shall lay hold on bow and spear; they *are* cruel, and have no mercy; their voice roareth like the sea; and they ride upon horses, set in array as men for war against thee, O daughter of Zion.

24 We have heard the fame thereof: our hands wax feeble: anguish hath taken hold of us, *and* pain, as of a woman in travail.

25 Go not forth into the field, nor walk by the way; for the sword of the enemy *and* fear *is* on every side.

26 O daughter of my people, gird *thee* with sackcloth, and [j]wallow thyself in ashes: make thee mourning, *as for* an only son, most bitter lamentation: for the spoiler shall suddenly come upon us.

27 I have set thee *for* a tower *and* a fortress among my people, that thou mayest know and try their way.

28 They *are* all grievous revolters, walking with slanders: *they are* brass and iron; they *are* all corrupters.

29 The bellows are burned, the lead is consumed of the fire; the founder melteth in vain: for the wicked are not plucked away.

30 [k]Reprobate silver shall *men* call them, because the LORD hath rejected them.

CHAPTER 7.

The message in the gate of the LORD'S house (Jer. 7:1–10:25).

The [1]word that came to Jeremiah from the LORD, saying,

2 Stand in the gate of the LORD'S house, and proclaim there this word, and say, Hear the word of the LORD, all *ye of* Judah, that enter in at these gates to worship the LORD.

3 Thus saith the LORD of hosts, the God of Israel, Amend your ways and your doings, and I will cause you to dwell in this place.

4 [l]Trust ye not in lying words, saying, The temple of the LORD, The temple of the LORD, The temple of the LORD, *are* these.

5 For if ye throughly amend your ways and your doings; if ye throughly execute judgment between a man and his neighbour;

6 *If* ye oppress not the stranger, the fatherless, and the widow, and shed not

B.C. 612.

a Deut. 28:30; Jer. 8:10.

b Isa. 56:11; Jer. 8:10; 23:11; Mic. 3:5, 11.

c Heb. *bruise,* or *breach.*

d Jer. 18:15.

e Isa. 8:20; Mal. 4:4; Lk. 16:29.

f Isa. 1:2.

g Prov. 1:31.

h Psa. 40:6; 50:7-9; Isa. 1:11; 66:3; Amos 5:21; Mic. 6:6.

[B.C. 600.

i Jer. 1:15; 5:15; 10:22; 50:41-43.

j Jer. 25:34; Mic. 1:10.

k Or, *refuse silver.*

l Mic. 3:11.

1 (7:1) The general character of the message in the temple gate is, like the first and second messages, one of rebuke, warning, and exhortation, but this message is addressed more to such in Judah as still maintain outwardly the worship of Jehovah; it is a message to *religious* Judah, e.g. 7:2, 9, 10; 8:10, 11.

innocent blood in this place, [a]neither
walk after other gods to your hurt:
7 Then will I cause you to dwell in this
place, in the land that I gave to your
fathers, for ever and ever.
8 Behold, ye [b]trust in lying words, that
cannot profit.
9 Will ye steal, murder, and commit
adultery, and swear falsely, and burn
incense unto Baal, and walk after other
gods whom ye know not;
10 And come and stand before me in
this house, which is called by my name,
and say, We are delivered to do all these
abominations?
11 Is this house, [c]which is called by
my name, become a den of robbers in
your eyes? Behold, even I have seen *it*,
saith the LORD.
12 But go ye now unto [d]my place
which *was* in Shiloh, where I set my
name at the first, and see what I did to it
for the wickedness of my people Israel.
13 And now, because ye have done all
these works, saith the LORD, and I spake
unto you, rising up early and speaking,
but ye heard not; and I called you, but
ye answered not;
14 Therefore will I do unto *this* house,
which is called by my name, wherein ye
trust, and unto the place which I gave to
you and to your fathers, as I have done
to [e]Shiloh.
15 And I will cast you out of my sight,
as I have cast out all your brethren, *even*
the whole seed of Ephraim.
16 Therefore [f]pray not thou for this
people, neither lift up cry nor prayer for
them, neither make intercession to me:
for I will not hear thee.
17 Seest thou not what they do in the
cities of Judah and in the streets of
Jerusalem?
18 The children gather wood, and the
fathers kindle the fire, and the women
knead *their* dough, to make cakes to the
queen of heaven, and to pour out drink-
offerings unto other gods, that they may
provoke me to anger.
19 [g]Do they provoke me to anger? saith
the LORD: *do they* not *provoke* themselves
to the confusion of their own faces?
20 Therefore thus saith the Lord GOD;
Behold, mine anger and my fury shall be

B.C. 600.

a Deut. 6:14, 15; 8:19; 11:28; 13:10.

b Psa. 2:12, *note*.

c Mt. 21:13; Mk. 11:17; Lk. 19:46.

d Josh. 18:1; Jud. 18:31.

e 1 Sam. 4:10, 11; Psa. 78:60; Jer. 26:6.

f Jer. 11:14; 14:11.

g Deut. 32:16, 21.

h Isa. 1:11; Jer. 6:20; Amos 5:21; Hos. 8:13.

i 1 Sam. 15:22; Psa. 51:16, 17; Hos. 6:6.

j Ex. 15:26; Deut. 6:3; Jer. 11:4, 7.

k Ex. 19:5; Lev. 26:12.

l Psa. 81:11; Jer. 11:8.

m Deut. 29:19; Psa. 81:12.

n 2 Chr. 36:15; Jer. 25:4; 29:19.

o Ezk. 2:7.

p Job 1:20; Isa. 15:2; Jer. 16:6; 48:37; Mic. 1:16.

q 2 Ki. 21:4, 7; 2 Chr. 33:4, 7; Jer. 23:11; 32:34; Ezk. 7:20.

poured out upon this place, upon man,
and upon beast, and upon the trees of
the field, and upon the fruit of the
ground; and it shall burn, and shall not
be quenched.
21 Thus saith the LORD of hosts, the
God of Israel; [h]Put your burnt-offerings
unto your sacrifices, and eat flesh.
22 [i]For I spake not unto your fathers,
[1]nor commanded them in the day that I
brought them out of the land of Egypt,
concerning burnt-offerings or sacrifices:
23 But this thing commanded I them,
saying, [j]Obey my voice, and I [k]will be
your God, and ye shall be my people:
and walk ye in all the ways that I have
commanded you, that it may be well
unto you.
24 [l]But they hearkened not, nor inclined
their ear, but [m]walked in the counsels *and*
in the imagination of their evil heart, and
went backward, and not forward.
25 Since the day that your fathers
came forth out of the land of Egypt unto
this day I have even sent unto you [n]all
my servants the prophets, daily rising
up early and sending *them*:
26 Yet they hearkened not unto me,
nor inclined their ear, but hardened their
neck: they did worse than their fathers.
27 [o]Therefore thou shalt speak all
these words unto them; but they will not
hearken to thee: thou shalt also call unto
them; but they will not answer thee.
28 But thou shalt say unto them, This
is a nation that obeyeth not the voice of
the LORD their God, nor receiveth correction: truth is perished, and is cut off
from their mouth.
29 [p]Cut off thine hair, *O Jerusalem*, and
cast *it* away, and take up a lamentation
on high places; for the LORD hath rejected
and forsaken the generation of his wrath.
30 For the children of Judah have done
evil in my sight, saith the LORD: [q]they
have set their abominations in the house
which is called by my name, to pollute it.
31 And they have built the high places
of Tophet, which *is* in the valley of the son
of Hinnom, to burn their sons and their
daughters in the fire; which I commanded
them not, neither came it into my heart.

[1]**(7:22)** Cf. Ex. 20:4, *note* 2, the threefold giving of the law. The command concerning burnt-offerings and sacrifices was not given to the people till they had broken the decalogue, the law of obedience.

B.C. 600.

32 Therefore, behold, the days come, saith the LORD, that it shall no more be called Tophet, nor the valley of the son of Hinnom, but the valley of slaughter: for they shall bury in Tophet, till there be no place.

33 And the [a]carcases of this people shall be meat for the fowls of the heaven, and for the beasts of the earth; and none shall fray *them* away.

34 Then will I cause to cease from the cities of Judah, and from the streets of Jerusalem, the voice of mirth, and the voice of gladness, the voice of the bridegroom, and the voice of the bride: [b]for the land shall be desolate.

CHAPTER 8.

(*The message in the temple gate, continued.*)

At that time, saith the LORD, they shall bring out the bones of the kings of Judah, and the bones of his princes, and the bones of the priests, and the bones of the prophets, and the bones of the inhabitants of Jerusalem, out of their graves:

2 And they shall spread them before the sun, and the moon, and all the host of heaven, whom they have loved, and whom they have served, and after whom they have walked, and whom they have sought, and whom they have worshipped: they shall not be gathered, nor be buried; they shall be for dung upon the face of the earth.

3 [c]And death shall be chosen rather than life by all the residue of them that remain of this evil family, which remain in all the places whither I have driven them, saith the LORD of hosts.

4 Moreover thou shalt say unto them, Thus saith the LORD; Shall they fall, and not arise? shall he turn away, and not return?

5 Why *then* is this people of Jerusalem slidden back by a perpetual backsliding? they hold fast deceit, they refuse to return.

6 [d]I hearkened and heard, *but* they spake not aright: no man [e]repented him of his wickedness, saying, What have I done? every one turned to his course, as the horse rusheth into the battle.

7 Yea, [f]the stork in the heaven knoweth her appointed times; and the [g]turtle and the crane and the swallow observe the time of their coming; but my people know not the judgment of the LORD.

8 How do ye say, [h]We *are* wise, and the law of the LORD *is* with us? Lo, certainly in vain made he *it*; the pen of the scribes *is* in vain.

9 The wise *men* are ashamed, they are dismayed and taken: lo, they have rejected the word of the LORD; and what wisdom *is* in them?

10 Therefore [i]will I give their wives unto others, *and* their fields to them that shall inherit *them*: for every one from the least even unto the greatest is given to covetousness, from the prophet even unto the priest every one dealeth falsely.

11 For they have healed the hurt of the daughter of my people slightly, saying, [j]Peace, peace; when *there is* no peace.

12 Were they ashamed when they had committed abomination? nay, they were not at all ashamed, neither could they blush: therefore shall they fall among them that fall: in the time of their visitation they shall be cast down, saith the LORD.

13 I will surely consume them, saith the LORD: *there shall be* no grapes on the vine, nor figs on the fig tree, and the leaf shall fade; and *the things that* I have given them shall pass away from them.

14 Why do we sit still? assemble yourselves, and let us enter into the defenced cities, and let us be silent there: for the LORD our God hath put us to silence, and given us water of gall to drink, because we have sinned against the LORD.

15 We [k]looked for peace, but no good *came; and* for a time of health, and behold trouble!

16 The snorting of his horses was heard from Dan: the whole land trembled at the sound of the neighing of his strong ones; for they are come, and have devoured the land, and all that is in it; the city, and those that dwell therein.

17 For, behold, I will send serpents, cockatrices, among you, which *will* not *be* charmed, and they shall bite you, saith the LORD.

18 *When* I would comfort myself against sorrow, my heart *is* faint in me.

19 Behold the voice of the cry of the daughter of my people because of them that dwell in a far country: *Is* not the LORD in Zion? *is* not her king in her?

a 2 Ki. 23:10; Jer. 19:11; Ezk. 6:5. Fulfilled in part in all the destructions of Jerusalem, but with a final look toward Rev. 19:17-21.

b Lev. 26:33; Isa. 1:7; 3:26.

c Job 3:21, 22; 7:15, 16; Rev. 9:6.

d 2 Pet. 3:9.

e Zech. 8:14, *note*.

f Isa. 1:3.

g Song 2:12.

h Rom. 2:17.

i Deut. 28:30; Jer. 6:12; Amos 5:11; Zeph. 1:13.

j Ezk. 13:10.

k Jer. 14:19.

Why have they provoked me to anger
with their graven images, *and* with
strange vanities?
20 The harvest is past, the summer is
ended, and we are not saved.
21 For the hurt of the daughter of my
people am I hurt; I am black; astonishment hath taken hold on me.
22 [a]*Is there* no balm in Gilead; *is there*
no physician there? why then is not the
health of the daughter of my people
recovered?

CHAPTER 9.

(*The message in the temple gate,*
continued.)

Oh that my head were waters, and
mine eyes a fountain of tears, that I
might weep day and night for the slain
of the daughter of my people!
2 Oh that I had in the wilderness a
lodging place of wayfaring men; that I
might leave my people, and go from
them! for they *be* all adulterers, an
assembly of treacherous men.
3 And they bend their tongues *like*
their bow *for* lies: but they are not
valiant for the truth upon the earth; for
they proceed from evil to evil, and they
[b]know not me, saith the LORD.
4 Take ye heed every one of his neighbour, and [c]trust ye not in any brother: for
every brother will utterly supplant, and
every neighbour will walk with slanders.
5 And they will deceive every one his
neighbour, and will not speak the truth:
they have taught their tongue to speak
lies, *and* weary themselves to commit
iniquity.
6 Thine habitation *is* in the midst of
deceit; through deceit they refuse to
know me, saith the LORD.
7 Therefore thus saith the LORD of
hosts, Behold, [d]I will melt them, and try
them; for how shall I do for the daughter
of my people?
8 Their tongue *is as* an arrow shot out;
it speaketh deceit: *one* speaketh peaceably to his neighbour with his mouth,
but in heart he layeth his wait.
9 [e]Shall I not visit them for these
things? saith the LORD: shall not my soul
be avenged on such a nation as this?
10 For the mountains will I take up a
weeping and wailing, and for the habitations of the wilderness a lamentation,
because they are burned up, so that none
can pass through *them*; neither can *men*
hear the voice of the cattle; both the fowl
of the heavens and the beast are fled;
they are gone.
11 [f]And I will make Jerusalem heaps,
and a den of dragons; and I will make
the cities of Judah desolate, without an
inhabitant.
12 Who *is* the wise man, that may
understand this? and *who is he* to whom
the mouth of the LORD hath spoken, that
he may declare it, for what the land perisheth *and* is burned up like a wilderness, that none passeth through?
13 And the LORD saith, Because they
have forsaken my [g]law which I set
before them, and have not obeyed my
voice, neither walked therein;
14 But have [h]walked after the imagination of their own heart, and after Baalim,
[i]which their fathers taught them:
15 Therefore thus saith the LORD of
hosts, the God of Israel; Behold, I will feed
them, *even* this people, with wormwood,
and give them water of gall to drink.
16 I will [j]scatter them also among the
[k]heathen, whom neither they nor their
fathers have known: and I will send a
sword after them, till I have consumed
them.
17 Thus saith the LORD of hosts,
Consider ye, and call for the mourning
women, that they may come; and send
for cunning *women*, that they may come:
18 And let them make haste, and take
up a wailing for us, that our eyes may
run down with tears, and our eyelids
gush out with waters.
19 For a voice of wailing is heard out
of Zion, How are we spoiled! we are
greatly confounded, because we have
forsaken the land, because our dwellings
have cast *us* out.
20 Yet hear the word of the LORD, O ye
women, and let your ear receive the
word of his mouth, and teach your
daughters wailing, and every one her
neighbour lamentation.
21 For death is come up into our windows, *and* is entered into our palaces, to
cut off the children from without, *and*
the young men from the streets.
22 Speak, Thus saith the LORD, Even
the carcases of men shall fall as dung
upon the open field, and as the handful

B.C. 600.

a Gen. 37:25; 43:11; Jer. 46:11; 51:8.

b 1 Sam. 2:12; Hos. 4:1.

c Psa. 2:12, *note.*

d Isa. 1:25; Mal. 3:3.

e Jer. 5:9, 29.

f Isa. 25:2.

g *Law (of Moses).* vs. 13-16; Ezk. 22:26. (Ex. 19:1; Gal. 3:1-29.)

h Jer. 3:17; 7:24.

i Gal. 1:14.

j Lev. 26:33; Deut. 28:64.

k i.e. *nations.*

after the harvestman, and none shall gather *them*.

23 Thus saith the LORD, Let not the wise *man* glory in his wisdom, neither let the mighty *man* glory in his might, let not the rich *man* glory in his riches:

24 But let him that [a]glorieth glory in this, that he understandeth and knoweth me, that I *am* the LORD which exercise lovingkindness, judgment, and righteousness, in the earth: [b]for in these *things* I delight, saith the LORD.

25 Behold, the days come, saith the LORD, that I will punish all *them which are* circumcised with the uncircumcised;

26 Egypt, and Judah, and Edom, and the children of Ammon, and Moab, and all *that are* in the utmost corners, that dwell in the wilderness: for all *these* nations *are* [c]uncircumcised, and all the house of Israel *are* uncircumcised in the heart.

CHAPTER 10.

(*The message in the temple gate,* concluded.)

Hear ye the word which the LORD speaketh unto you, O house of Israel:

2 Thus saith the LORD, Learn not the way of the [d]heathen, and be not dismayed at the signs of heaven; for the heathen are dismayed at them.

3 For the customs of the people *are* vain: for *one* cutteth a tree out of the forest, the work of the hands of the workman, with the axe.

4 They deck it with silver and with gold; they fasten it with nails and with hammers, that it move not.

5 They *are* upright as the palm tree, but speak not: they must needs be borne, because they cannot go. Be not afraid of them; for they cannot do evil, neither also *is it* in them to do good.

6 Forasmuch as *there is* none like unto thee, O LORD; thou *art* great, and thy name *is* great in might.

7 Who would not [e]fear thee, O King of nations? for to thee doth it appertain: forasmuch as among all the wise *men* of the nations, and in all their kingdoms, *there is* none like unto thee.

8 But they are altogether brutish and foolish: the stock *is* a doctrine of vanities.

9 Silver spread into plates is brought from Tarshish, and [f]gold from Uphaz, the work of the workman, and of the hands of the founder: blue and purple *is* their clothing: they *are* all the work of cunning *men*.

10 But the LORD *is* the [g]true God, he *is* [h]the living God, and an [i]everlasting king: at his wrath the earth shall tremble, and the nations shall not be able to abide his indignation.

11 Thus shall ye say unto them, The gods that have not made the heavens and the earth, *even* they shall perish from the earth, and from under these heavens.

12 [j]He hath made the earth by his power, [k]he hath established the world by his wisdom, and [l]hath stretched out the heavens by his discretion.

13 When he uttereth his voice, *there is* a multitude of waters in the heavens, and [m]he causeth the vapours to ascend from the ends of the earth; he maketh lightnings with rain, and bringeth forth the wind out of his treasures.

14 Every man is brutish in *his* knowledge: every founder is confounded by the graven image: for his molten image *is* falsehood, and *there is* no breath in them.

15 They *are* vanity, *and* the work of errors: in the time of their visitation they shall perish.

16 The portion of Jacob *is* not like them: for he *is* the former of all *things*; and [n]Israel *is* the rod of his inheritance: The LORD of hosts *is* his name.

17 Gather up thy wares out of the land, O inhabitant of the fortress.

18 For thus saith the LORD, Behold, I will sling out the inhabitants of the land at this once, and will distress them, that they may find *it so*.

19 Woe is me for my hurt! my wound is grievous: but I said, Truly this *is* a grief, and I must bear it.

20 My tabernacle is spoiled, and all my cords are broken: my children are gone forth of me, and they *are* not: *there is* none to stretch forth my tent any more, and to set up my curtains.

21 For the pastors are become brutish, and have not sought the LORD: therefore they shall not prosper, and all their flocks shall be scattered.

22 Behold, the noise of the bruit is

B.C. 600.

a 1 Cor. 1:31; 2 Cor. 10:17.
b Mic. 6:8; 7:18.
c Lev. 26:41; Ezk. 44:7; Rom. 2:28, 29.
d i.e. *nations*.
e Psa. 19:9, *note*.
f Dan. 10:5.
g Heb. *God of truth*. Psa. 31:5.
h 1 Tim. 6:17.
i Heb. *King of Eternity*.
j Gen. 1:1, 6, 7; Psa. 136:5, 6; Jer. 51:15.
k Psa. 93:1.
l Job 9:8; Psa. 104:2; Isa. 40:22.
m Psa. 135:7.
n Deut. 32:9; Psa. 74:2.

come, and a great commotion out of the
north country, to make the cities of
Judah desolate, *and* a den of dragons.
23 O LORD, I know that [a]the way of
man *is* not in himself: *it is* not in man
that walketh to direct his steps.
24 O LORD, [b]correct me, but with judgment; not in thine anger, lest thou bring
me to nothing.
25 Pour out thy fury upon the [c]hea-
then that know thee not, and upon the
families that call not on thy name: for
they have eaten up Jacob, and devoured
him, and consumed him, and have made
his habitation desolate.

CHAPTER 11.

The message on the broken covenant
(Jer. 11:1–12:17).

The [1]word that came to Jeremiah from
the LORD, saying,
2 Hear ye the words of this covenant,
and speak unto the men of Judah, and to
the inhabitants of Jerusalem;
3 And say thou unto them, Thus saith
the LORD God of Israel; [d]Cursed *be* the
man that obeyeth not the words of this
covenant,
4 Which I commanded your fathers in
the day *that* I brought them forth out of
the land of Egypt, from the [e]iron furnace, saying, [f]Obey my voice, and do
them, according to all which I command
you: so shall ye be my people, and I will
be your God:
5 That I may perform [g]the oath which
I have sworn unto your fathers, to give
them a land flowing with milk and
honey, as *it is* this day. Then answered I,
and said, [h]So be it, O LORD.
6 Then the LORD said unto me,
Proclaim all these words in the cities of
Judah, and in the streets of Jerusalem,
saying, Hear ye the words of this
covenant, [i]and do them.
7 For I earnestly protested unto your
fathers in the day *that* I brought them up
out of the land of Egypt, *even* unto this
day, rising early and protesting, saying,
Obey my voice.
8 Yet they obeyed not, nor inclined
their ear, but walked every one in the
imagination of their evil heart: therefore
I will bring upon them all the words of
this covenant, which I commanded *them*
to do; but they did *them* not.
9 And the LORD said unto me, A conspiracy is found among the men of Judah,
and among the inhabitants of Jerusalem.
10 They are turned back to the iniquities of their forefathers, which refused to
hear my words; and they went after other
gods to serve them: the house of Israel
and the house of Judah have broken my
covenant which I made with their fathers.
11 Therefore thus saith the LORD,
Behold, I will bring evil upon them,
which they shall not be able to escape;
[j]and though they shall cry unto me, I
will not hearken unto them.
12 Then shall the cities of Judah and
inhabitants of Jerusalem go, and cry
unto the gods unto whom they offer
incense: but they shall not save them at
all in the time of their [k]trouble.
13 For *according to* the number of thy
cities were thy gods, O Judah; and
according to the number of the streets of
Jerusalem have ye set up altars to *that*
shameful thing, *even* altars to burn
incense unto Baal.
14 Therefore [l]pray not thou for this
people, neither lift up a cry or prayer for
them: for I will not hear *them* in the time
that they cry unto me for their trouble.
15 What hath my beloved to do in
mine house, *seeing* she hath wrought
lewdness with many, and the [m]holy
flesh is passed from thee? when thou
doest evil, then thou rejoicest.
16 The LORD called thy name, [n]A
green olive tree, fair, *and* of goodly fruit:
with the noise of a great tumult he hath
kindled fire upon it, and the branches of
it are broken.
17 For the LORD of hosts, that planted
thee, hath pronounced evil against thee,
for the evil of the house of Israel and of
the house of Judah, which they have
done against themselves to provoke me

B.C. 600.

a Prov. 16:1; 20:24.

b Psa. 6:1; 38:1; Jer. 30:11.

c i.e. *nations.*

d Deut. 27:26; Gal. 3:10.

e Deut. 4:20; 1 Ki. 8:51.

f Lev. 26:3, 12; Jer. 7:23.

B.C. 608.]

g Deut. 7:12, 13; Psa. 105:9, 10.

h Heb. *Amen.*

i Rom. 2:13; Jas. 1:22.

j Psa. 18:41; Prov. 1:28; Isa. 1:15; Jer. 14:12; Ezk. 8:18; Mic. 3:4; Zech. 7:13.

k Heb. *evil.*

l Ex. 32:10; Jer. 7:16; 14:11; 1 John 5:16.

m Hag. 2:12. i.e. to what purpose the "holy flesh" of sacrifices? Its efficacy is "passed from thee" who rejoicest in evil. Cf. Isa. 1:13-15.

n Psa. 52:8; Rom. 11:17.

[1] **(11:1)** This, like the other messages, is made up of rebuke, exhortation, and warning, but in this instance these are based upon the violation of the Palestinian Covenant (Deut. 28:1 to 30:1-9, *note*). The Assyrian and Babylonian Captivities of Israel and of Judah were the execution of the warning, Deut. 28:63-68.

to anger in offering incense unto Baal.

18 And the LORD hath given me knowledge *of it*, and I know *it*: then thou shewedst me their doings.

19 But I *was* like a lamb *or* an ox *that* is brought to the slaughter; and I knew not that they had devised devices against me, *saying*, Let us destroy the tree with the fruit thereof, and let us cut him off from the land of the living, that his name may be no more remembered.

20 But, O LORD of hosts, that judgest righteously, that [a]triest the reins and the heart, let me see thy vengeance on them: for unto thee have I revealed my cause.

21 Therefore thus saith the LORD of the men of Anathoth, that seek thy life, saying, [b]Prophesy not in the name of the LORD, that thou die not by our hand:

22 Therefore thus saith the LORD of hosts, Behold, I will punish them: the young men shall die by the sword; their sons and their daughters shall die by famine:

23 And there shall be no remnant of them: for I will bring evil upon the men of Anathoth, *even* [c]the year of their visitation.

CHAPTER 12.

(*The message on the broken covenant*, concluded.)

Righteous [d]*art* thou, O LORD, when I plead with thee: yet let me talk with thee of *thy* judgments: [e]Wherefore doth the way of the wicked prosper? *wherefore* are all they happy that deal very treacherously?

2 Thou hast planted them, yea, they have taken root: they grow, yea, they bring forth fruit: [f]thou *art* near in their mouth, and far from their reins.

3 But thou, O LORD, knowest me: thou hast seen me, and tried mine heart toward thee: pull them out like sheep for the slaughter, and prepare them for the day of slaughter.

4 How long shall [g]the land mourn, and the herbs of every field wither, for the wickedness of them that dwell therein? the beasts are consumed, and the birds; because they said, He shall not see our last end.

5 If thou hast run with the footmen, and they have wearied thee, then how canst thou contend with horses? and *if* in the land of peace, *wherein* thou trustedst, *they wearied thee*, then how wilt thou do in the [h]swelling of Jordan?

6 For even thy brethren, and the house of thy father, even they have dealt treacherously with thee; yea, they have called a multitude after thee: believe them not, though they speak fair words unto thee.

7 I have forsaken mine house, I have left mine heritage; I have given the dearly beloved of my soul into the hand of her enemies.

8 Mine heritage is unto me as a lion in the forest; it [i]crieth out against me: therefore have I hated it.

9 Mine heritage *is* unto me *as* a speckled bird, the birds round about *are* against her; come ye, assemble all the beasts of the field, come to devour.

10 Many pastors have destroyed my vineyard, they have trodden my portion under foot, they have made my pleasant portion a desolate wilderness.

11 They have made it desolate, *and being* desolate it mourneth unto me; the whole land is made desolate, because no man layeth *it* to heart.

12 The spoilers are come upon all high places through the wilderness: for the sword of the LORD shall devour from the *one* end of the land even to the *other* end of the land: no flesh shall have peace.

13 [j]They have sown wheat, but shall reap thorns: they have put themselves to pain, *but* shall not profit: and they shall be ashamed of your revenues because of the fierce anger of the LORD.

14 Thus saith the LORD against all mine evil neighbours, that [k]touch the inheritance which I have caused my people Israel to inherit; Behold, I will pluck them out of their land, and pluck out the house of Judah from among them.

15 And it shall come to pass, after that I have plucked them out I will return, and have compassion on them, and will bring them again, every man to his heritage, and every man to his land.

16 And it shall come to pass, if they will diligently learn the ways of my people, to swear by my name, The LORD liveth; as they taught my people to swear by Baal; then shall they be [l]built in the midst of my people.

B.C. 608.

a 1 Sam. 16:7; 1 Chr. 28:9; Psa. 7:9; Jer. 17:10; 20:12; Rev. 2:23.

b Isa. 30:10; Amos 2:12; 7:13, 16; Mic. 2:6.

c Jer. 23:12; 46:21; 48:44; 50:27; Lk. 19:44.

d Psa, 51:4.

e Job 12:6; 21:7; Psa. 37:1, 35; 73:3; Jer. 5:28; Hab. 1:4; Mal 3:15.

f Isa. 29:13; Mt. 15:8; Mk. 7:6.

g Jer. 23:10; Hos. 4:3.

h i.e. under such a test as in Jer. 49:19; 50:44; Josh. 3:15; 1 Chr. 12:15.

i Or, *yelleth*.

j Lev. 26:16; Deut. 28:38; Mic. 6:15; Hag. 1:6.

k Zech. 2:8.

l Eph. 2:20, 21; 1 Pet. 2:5.

17 But if they will not [a]obey, I will utterly pluck up and destroy that nation, saith the LORD.

CHAPTER 13.

The sign of the linen girdle (vs. 1-27).

Thus saith the LORD unto me, [b]Go and get thee a linen [c]girdle, and put it upon thy loins, and put it not in water.

2 So I got a girdle according to the word of the LORD, and put *it* on my loins.

3 And the word of the LORD came unto me the second time, saying,

4 Take the girdle that thou hast got, which *is* upon thy loins, and arise, go to Euphrates, and hide it there in a hole of the rock.

5 So I went, and hid it by Euphrates, as the LORD commanded me.

6 And it came to pass after many days, that the LORD said unto me, Arise, go to Euphrates, and take the girdle from thence, which I commanded thee to hide there.

7 Then I went to Euphrates, and digged, and took the girdle from the place where I had hid it: and, behold, the girdle was marred, it was profitable for nothing.

8 Then the word of the LORD came unto me, saying,

9 Thus saith the LORD, After this manner [d]will I mar the pride of Judah, and the great pride of Jerusalem.

10 This evil people, which refuse to hear my words, which [e]walk in the imagination of their heart, and walk after other gods, to serve them, and to worship them, shall even be as this girdle, which is good for nothing.

11 For as the girdle cleaveth to the loins of a man, so have I caused to cleave unto me the whole house of Israel and the whole house of Judah, saith the LORD; that [f]they might be unto me for a people, and for a name, and for a praise, and for a glory: but they would not hear.

12 Therefore thou shalt speak unto them this word; Thus saith the LORD God of Israel, Every bottle shall be filled with wine: and they shall say unto thee, Do we not certainly know that every bottle shall be filled with wine?

13 Then shalt thou say unto them, Thus saith the LORD, Behold, I will fill all the inhabitants of this land, even the kings that sit upon David's throne, and the priests, and the prophets, and all the inhabitants of Jerusalem, [g]with drunkenness.

14 And I will dash them one against another, even the fathers and the sons together, saith the LORD: I will not pity, nor spare, nor have mercy, but destroy them.

15 Hear ye, and give ear; be not proud: for the LORD hath spoken.

16 [h]Give glory to the LORD your God, before he cause [i]darkness, and before your feet stumble upon the dark mountains, and, while ye look for light, he turn it into the shadow of death, *and* make *it* gross darkness.

17 But if ye will not hear it, my soul shall weep in secret places for *your* pride; and mine eye shall weep sore, and run down with tears, because the LORD'S flock is carried away captive.

18 Say unto the king and to the queen, Humble yourselves, sit down: for your principalities shall come down, *even* the crown of your glory.

19 The cities of the south shall be shut up, and none shall open *them*: Judah shall be carried away captive all of it, it shall be wholly carried away captive.

20 Lift up your eyes, and behold them that come from the north: where *is* the flock *that* was given thee, thy beautiful flock?

21 What wilt thou say when he shall punish thee? for thou hast taught them *to be* captains, *and* as chief over thee: shall not sorrows take thee, as a woman in travail?

22 And if thou say in thine heart, [j]Wherefore come these things upon me? For the greatness of thine iniquity are thy skirts discovered, *and* thy heels made bare.

23 Can the Ethiopian change his skin, or the leopard his spots? *then* may ye also do good, that are accustomed to do evil.

24 Therefore will I scatter them [k]as the stubble that passeth away by the wind of the wilderness.

25 This *is* thy lot, the portion of thy measures from me, saith the LORD; because thou hast forgotten me, and [l]trusted in falsehood.

26 Therefore will I discover thy skirts upon thy face, that thy shame may appear.

27 I have seen thine adulteries, and

B.C. 602.

a Isa. 60:12.
b See vs. 9-11.
c *Parables* (O.T.) vs. 1-11; Jer. 18:1-6. (Jud. 9:7-15; Zech. 11:7-14.)
d Lev. 20:19.
e Jer. 9:14; 11:8; 16:12.
f Ex. 19:5.
g Isa. 51:17, 21; 63:6; Jer. 25:27; 51:7.
h Josh. 7:19.
i Isa. 5:30; 8:22; Amos 8:9.
j Jer. 5:19; 16:10.
k Psa. 1:4; Hos. 13:3.
l Psa. 2:12, *note.*

thy neighings, the lewdness of thy whoredom, *and* thine abominations on the hills in the fields. Woe unto thee, O Jerusalem! wilt thou not be made clean? when *shall it* once *be*?

CHAPTER 14.

The message on the drought
(Jer. 14:1–15:21).

The word of the LORD that came to Jeremiah concerning the [1] dearth.

2 Judah mourneth, and the gates thereof languish; they are black unto the ground; and the cry of Jerusalem is gone up.

3 And their nobles have sent their little ones to the waters: they came to the pits, *and* found no water; they returned with their vessels empty; they were ashamed and confounded, and covered their heads.

4 Because the ground is chapt, for there was no rain in the earth, the plowmen were ashamed, they covered their heads.

5 Yea, the hind also calved in the field, and forsook *it*, because there was no grass.

6 And the wild asses did stand in the high places, they snuffed up the wind like dragons; their eyes did fail, because *there was* no grass.

7 O [a] LORD, though our iniquities testify against us, do thou *it* for thy name's sake: for our backslidings are many; we have sinned against thee.

8 [b] O the hope of Israel, the saviour thereof in time of trouble, why shouldest thou be as a stranger in the land, and as a wayfaring man *that* turneth aside to tarry for a night?

9 Why shouldest thou be as a man astonied, as a mighty man [c] *that* cannot save? yet thou, O LORD, [d] *art* in the midst of us, and we are called by thy name; leave us not.

10 Thus saith the LORD unto this people, [e] Thus have they loved to wander, they have not refrained their feet, therefore the LORD doth not accept them; he will now remember their iniquity, and visit their sins.

B.C. 602.

B.C. 601.]

a *Bible prayers* (O.T.). Ezk. 9:8. (Gen. 15:2; Hab. 3:1-16.)

b Jer. 17:13.

c Isa. 59:1.

d Ex. 29:45, 46; Lev. 26:11, 12.

e See Jer. 2:23-25.

f Ex. 32:10; Jer. 7:16; 11:14.

g Prov. 1:28; Isa. 1:15; 58:3; Jer. 11:11; Ezk. 8:18; Mic. 3:4; Zech. 7:13.

h 1 Thes. 5:2, 3.

i Psa. 79:3.

j Ezk. 7:15.

11 Then said the LORD unto me, [f] Pray not for this people for *their* good.

12 [g] When they fast, I will not hear their cry; and when they offer burnt-offering and an oblation, I will not accept them: but I will consume them by the sword, and by the famine, and by the pestilence.

13 Then said I, Ah, Lord GOD! behold, the prophets say unto them, Ye shall not see the sword, neither shall ye have famine; but I will give you assured [h] peace in this place.

14 Then the LORD said unto me, The prophets prophesy lies in my name: I sent them not, neither have I commanded them, neither spake unto them: they prophesy unto you a false vision and divination, and a thing of nought, and the deceit of their heart.

15 Therefore thus saith the LORD concerning the prophets that prophesy in my name, and I sent them not, yet they say, Sword and famine shall not be in this land; By sword and famine shall those prophets be consumed.

16 And the people to whom they prophesy shall be cast out in the streets of Jerusalem because of the famine and the sword; [i] and they shall have none to bury them, them, their wives, nor their sons, nor their daughters: for I will pour their wickedness upon them.

17 Therefore thou shalt say this word unto them; Let mine eyes run down with tears night and day, and let them not cease: for the virgin daughter of my people is broken with a great breach, with a very grievous blow.

18 If I go forth into [j] the field, then behold the slain with the sword! and if I enter into the city, then behold them that are sick with famine! yea, both the prophet and the priest go about into a land that they know not.

19 Hast thou utterly rejected Judah? hath thy soul lothed Zion? why hast thou smitten us, and *there is* no healing for us? we looked for peace, and *there is* no good; and for the time of healing, and behold trouble!

20 We acknowledge, O LORD, our

1 (14:1) The significance of a drought at this time was very great. It was one of the signs predicted in the Palestinian Covenant (Deut. 28:23, 24), and already fulfilled in part in the reign of Ahab (1 Ki. 17:1, etc.). As that sign had been followed, even though after a long interval, by the Assyrian captivity of the northern kingdom, it should have been received by Judah as a most solemn warning.

wickedness, *and* the iniquity of our
fathers: [a]for we have sinned against
thee.
21 Do not abhor *us*, for thy name's
sake, do not disgrace the throne of thy
glory: remember, break not thy covenant
with us.
22 Are there *any* among [b]the vanities
of the Gentiles that can cause rain? or
can the heavens give showers? *art* not
thou he, O LORD our God? therefore we
will wait upon thee: for thou hast made
all these *things*.

CHAPTER 15.

(*The message on the drought*, concluded.)

THEN said the LORD unto me, Though
[c]Moses and [d]Samuel stood before
me, *yet* my mind *could* not *be* toward this
people: cast *them* out of my sight, and let
them go forth.
2 And it shall come to pass, if they say
unto thee, Whither shall we go forth?
then thou shalt tell them, Thus saith the
LORD; [e]Such as *are* for death, to death;
and such as *are* for the sword, to the
sword; and such as *are* for the famine, to
the famine; and such as *are* for the captivity, to the captivity.
3 And I will [f]appoint over them four
kinds, saith the LORD: the sword to slay,
and the dogs to tear, and the fowls of the
heaven, and the beasts of the earth, to
devour and destroy.
4 And I will cause them to be [g]removed into all kingdoms of the earth,
because of Manasseh the son of
Hezekiah king of Judah, for *that* which
he did in Jerusalem.
5 For [h]who shall have pity upon thee, O
Jerusalem? or who shall bemoan thee? or
who shall go aside to ask how thou doest?
6 Thou hast forsaken me, saith the
LORD, thou art gone backward: therefore
will I stretch out my hand against thee,
and destroy thee; [i]I am weary with [j]repenting.
7 And I will fan them with a fan in the
gates of the land; I will bereave *them* of
children, I will destroy my people, *since*
[k]they return not from their ways.
8 Their widows are increased to me
above the sand of the seas: I have
brought upon them against the mother
of the young men a spoiler at noonday: I
have caused *him* to fall upon it suddenly,
and terrors upon the city.
9 [l]She that hath borne seven languisheth: she hath given up the ghost;
her sun is gone down while *it was* yet
day: she hath been ashamed and confounded: and the residue of them will I
deliver to the sword before their enemies, saith the LORD.
10 Woe is me, my mother, that thou
hast borne me a man of strife and a man
of contention to the whole earth! I have
neither lent on usury, nor men have lent
to me on usury; *yet* every one of them
doth curse me.
11 The LORD [1]said, Verily it shall be
well with thy remnant; verily I will cause
the enemy to entreat thee *well* in the time
of evil and in the time of affliction.
12 Shall iron break the northern iron
and the steel?
13 Thy substance and thy treasures will
I give to the spoil without price, and *that*
for all thy sins, even in all thy borders.
14 And I will make *thee* to pass with
thine enemies [m]into a land *which* thou
knowest not: for a fire is kindled in mine
anger, *which* shall burn upon you.
15 O LORD, thou knowest: remember
me, and visit me, and revenge me of my
persecutors; take me not away in thy
longsuffering: know that for thy sake I
have suffered rebuke.
16 Thy words were found, and I did
[n]eat them; and thy word was unto me the
joy and rejoicing of mine heart: for I am
called by thy name, O LORD God of hosts.
17 I sat not in the assembly of the
mockers, nor rejoiced; I sat alone
because of thy hand: for thou hast filled
me with indignation.
18 Why is my pain perpetual, and my
wound incurable, *which* refuseth to be

B.C. 601.

a Psa. 106:6; Dan. 9:8.
b Deut. 32:21.
c Ex. 32:11, 12; Psa. 99:6.
d 1 Sam. 7:9.
e Jer. 43:11; Ezk. 5:2, 12; Zech. 11:9.
f Lev. 26:16.
g Deut. 28:25; 2 Ki. 21:1-18; 23:26, 27; 24:3, 4.
h Isa. 51:19.
i Hos. 13:14.
j Zech. 8:14, *note*.
k Isa. 9:13; Jer. 5:3; Amos 4:10, 11.
l 1 Sam. 2:5.
m Jer. 16:13; 17:4.
n Ezk. 3:1, 3; Rev. 10:9, 10.

[1] **(15:11)** The Remnant, of whom Jeremiah was the representative, are carefully distinguished from the unbelieving mass of the people. The coming captivity, which they must share, for they too have sinned (v. 13), though Jehovah's judgment upon the nation, will be but a purifying chastisement to them, and they receive a special promise (v. 11). Verses 15-18 give the answer of the Remnant to verses 11-14. Two things characterize the believing Remnant always—loyalty to the word of God, and separation from those who mock at that word (vs. 16, 17. Cf. Rev. 3:8-10).

healed? wilt thou be altogether unto me as a liar, *and as* waters *that* fail?

19 Therefore thus saith the LORD, [a]If thou return, then will I bring thee again, *and* thou shalt stand before me: and if thou [b]take forth the precious from the vile, thou shalt be as my mouth: let them return unto thee; but return not thou unto them.

20 And I will make thee unto this people a fenced brasen wall: and they shall fight against thee, but they shall not prevail against thee: for I *am* with thee to save thee and to deliver thee, saith the LORD.

21 And I will deliver [c]thee out of the hand of the wicked, and I will [d]redeem thee out of the hand of the terrible.

CHAPTER 16.

The sign of the unmarried prophet
(Jer. 16:1–17:18).

The word of the LORD came also unto me, [1]saying,

2 Thou shalt not take thee a wife, neither shalt thou have sons or daughters in this place.

3 For thus saith the LORD concerning the sons and concerning the daughters that are born in this place, and concerning their mothers that bare them, and concerning their fathers that begat them in this land;

4 They shall die of grievous deaths; they shall not be lamented; neither shall they be buried; *but* they shall be as dung upon the face of the earth: and they shall be consumed by the sword, and by famine; and their [e]carcases shall be meat for the fowls of heaven, and for the beasts of the earth.

5 For thus saith the LORD, Enter not into the house of mourning, neither go to lament nor bemoan them: for I have taken away my peace from this people, saith the LORD, *even* lovingkindness and mercies.

6 Both the great and the small shall die in this land: they shall not be buried, neither shall *men* lament for them, nor [f]cut themselves, nor [g]make themselves bald for them:

B.C. 601.

a Zech. 3:7.
b Ezk. 22:26; 44:23.
c *Remnant.* vs. 11-21; Jer. 23:3-8. (Isa. 1:9; Rom. 11:5.)
d Ex. 14:30, *note;* Isa. 59:20, *note.*
e Psa. 79:2; Jer. 7:33; 34:20.
f Lev. 19:28; Deut. 14:1; Jer. 41:5; 47:5.
g Isa. 22:12; Jer. 7:29.
h Isa. 24:7, 8; Jer. 7:34; 25:10; Ezk. 26:13; Hos. 2:11; Rev. 18:23.
i Deut. 29:24; Jer. 5:19; 13:22; 22:8.
j Deut. 29:25; Jer. 22:9.
k *Kingdom* (O.T.). vs. 12:16; Jer. 23:5-8. (Gen. 1:26; Zech. 12:8.)
l Deut. 4:26-28; 28:36, 63-65.
m Isa. 11:11, 12; 43:18; Jer. 23:7, 8; Ezk. 37:21-25.
n Jer. 24:6; 30:3; 32:37.
o Amos 4:2; Hab. 1:15.

7 Neither shall *men* tear *themselves* for them in mourning, to comfort them for the dead; neither shall *men* give them the cup of consolation to drink for their father or for their mother.

8 Thou shalt not also go into the house of feasting, to sit with them to eat and to drink.

9 For thus saith the LORD of hosts, the God of Israel; Behold, [h]I will cause to cease out of this place in your eyes, and in your days, the voice of mirth, and the voice of gladness, the voice of the bridegroom, and the voice of the bride.

10 And it shall come to pass, when thou shalt shew this people all these words, and they shall say unto thee, [i]Wherefore hath the LORD pronounced all this great evil against us? or what *is* our iniquity? or what *is* our sin that we have committed against the LORD our God?

11 Then shalt thou say unto them, [j]Because your fathers have forsaken me, saith the LORD, and have walked after other gods, and have served them, and have worshipped them, and have forsaken me, and have not kept my law;

12 And ye have done worse than your fathers; for, behold, [k]ye walk every one after the imagination of his evil heart, that they may not hearken unto me:

13 [l]Therefore will I cast you out of this land into a land that ye know not, *neither* ye nor your fathers; and there shall ye serve other gods day and night; where I will not shew you favour.

14 Therefore, behold, the [m]days come, saith the LORD, that it shall no more be said, The LORD liveth, that brought up the children of Israel out of the land of Egypt;

15 But, The LORD liveth, that brought up the children of Israel from the land of the north, and from all the lands whither he had driven them: [n]and I will bring them again into their land that I gave unto their fathers.

16 Behold, I will send for many [o]fishers, saith the LORD, and they shall fish them; and after will I send for many hunters, and they shall hunt them from

[1] **(16:1)** The sign of the unmarried prophet is interpreted by the context. The whole social life of Judah was about to be disrupted and cease from the land. But note the promises of verses 14-16; Jer. 17:7, 8.

B.C. 601.

every mountain, and from every hill, and out of the holes of the rocks.

17 [a]For mine eyes *are* upon all their ways: they are not hid from my face, neither is their iniquity hid from mine eyes.

18 And first I will recompense their iniquity and their sin [b]double; [c]because they have defiled my land, they have filled mine inheritance with the carcases of their detestable and abominable things.

19 O LORD, my strength, and my fortress, and my refuge in the day of affliction, the Gentiles shall come unto thee from the ends of the earth, and shall say, Surely our fathers have inherited lies, vanity, and *things* wherein *there is* no profit.

20 Shall a man make gods unto himself, and they *are* no gods?

21 Therefore, behold, I will this once cause them to know, I will cause them to know mine hand and my might; and they shall know that [d]my name *is* The LORD.

CHAPTER 17.

(*The sign of the unmarried prophet, concluded.*)

The sin of Judah *is* written with [e]a pen of iron, *and* with the point of a diamond: *it is* [f]graven upon the table of their heart, and upon the horns of your altars;

2 Whilst their children remember their altars and their [g]groves by the green trees upon the high hills.

3 O my mountain in the field, I will give thy substance *and* all thy treasures to the spoil, *and* thy high places for sin, throughout all thy borders.

4 And thou, even thyself, shalt discontinue from thine heritage that I gave thee; and I will cause thee to serve thine enemies in the land which thou knowest not: for ye have kindled a fire in mine anger, *which* shall burn for ever.

5 Thus saith the LORD; Cursed *be* the man that [h]trusteth in man, and maketh flesh his arm, and whose heart departeth from the LORD.

6 For he shall be like the heath in the desert, and shall not see when good cometh; but shall inhabit the parched places in the wilderness, *in* a salt land and not inhabited.

7 [i]Blessed *is* the man that trusteth in the LORD, and whose hope the LORD is.

8 For he shall be [j]as a tree planted by the waters, and *that* spreadeth out her roots by the river, and shall not see when heat cometh, but her leaf shall be green; and shall not be careful in the year of drought, neither shall cease from yielding fruit.

9 The heart *is* deceitful above all *things*, and desperately wicked: who can know it?

10 I the LORD [k]search the heart, *I* try the reins, even to give every man according to his ways, *and* according to the fruit of his doings.

11 *As* the partridge sitteth *on eggs*, and hatcheth *them* not; *so* he that getteth riches, and not by right, shall leave them in the midst of his days, and at his end shall be a fool.

12 A glorious high throne from the beginning *is* the place of our sanctuary.

13 O LORD, [l]the hope of Israel, [m]all that forsake thee shall be ashamed, *and* they that depart from me shall be [n]written in the earth, because they have forsaken the LORD, the fountain of living waters.

14 Heal me, O LORD, and I shall be healed; save me, and I shall be saved: for thou *art* my praise.

15 Behold, they say unto me, [o]Where *is* the word of the LORD? let it come now.

16 As for me, I have not hastened from *being* a pastor to follow thee: neither have I desired the woeful day; thou knowest: that which came out of my lips was *right* before thee.

17 Be not a terror unto me: thou *art* my hope in the day of evil.

18 Let them be confounded that persecute me, but let not me be confounded: let them be dismayed, but let not me be dismayed: bring upon them the day of evil, and destroy them with double destruction.

The message in the gates concerning the sabbath.

19 Thus said the LORD unto me; Go and stand in the gate of the children of the people, whereby the kings of Judah come in, and by the which they go out, and in all the gates of Jerusalem;

20 And say unto them, Hear ye the word of the LORD, ye kings of Judah, and all Judah, and all the inhabitants of Jerusalem, that enter in by these gates:

21 Thus saith the LORD; [p]Take heed to yourselves, and bear no burden on the sabbath day, nor bring *it* in by the gates of Jerusalem;

a Job 34:21; Prov. 5:21; 15:3; Jer. 32:19.
b Isa. 40:2; Jer. 17:18.
c Ezk. 43:7, 9.
d Or, *JEHOVAH*. Psa. 83:18.
e Job 19:24.
f Prov. 3:3; 2 Cor. 3:3.
g Deut. 16:21.
h Psa. 2:12, *note*.
i Psa. 2:12; 34:8; 125:1; 146:5; Prov. 16:20; Isa. 30:18.
j Job 8:16; Psa. 1:3.
k 1 Sam. 16:7; 1 Chr. 28:9; Psa. 7:9; 139:23, 24; Prov. 17:3; Jer. 11:20; 20:12; Rom. 8:27; Rev. 2:23.
l Jer. 14:8.
m Psa. 73:27; Isa. 1:28.
n See Lk. 10:20.
o Isa. 5:19; Ezk. 12:22; 2 Pet. 3:4.
p Num. 15:32; Neh. 13:19.

22 Neither carry forth a burden out of your houses on the sabbath day, neither do ye any work, but hallow ye the sabbath day, as I commanded your fathers.

23 [a]But they obeyed not, neither inclined their ear, but made their neck stiff, that they might not hear, nor receive instruction.

24 And it shall come to pass, if ye diligently hearken unto me, saith the LORD, to bring in no burden through the gates of this city on the sabbath day, but hallow the sabbath day, to do no work therein;

25 Then shall there enter into the gates of this city kings and princes sitting upon the throne of David, riding in chariots and on horses, they, and their princes, the men of Judah, and the inhabitants of Jerusalem: and this city shall remain for ever.

26 And they shall come from the cities of Judah, and from the places about Jerusalem, and from the land of Benjamin, and from [b]the plain, and from the mountains, and from the [b]south, bringing burnt-offerings, and sacrifices, and [c]meat-offerings, and incense, and bringing sacrifices of praise, unto the house of the LORD.

27 But if ye will not hearken unto me to hallow the sabbath day, and not to bear a burden, even entering in at the gates of Jerusalem on the sabbath day; then will I kindle a fire in the gates thereof, and it shall devour the palaces of Jerusalem, and it shall not be quenched.

CHAPTER 18.

The sign of the potter's house
(Jer. 18:1–19:13).

The [1]word which came to Jeremiah from the LORD, [d]saying,

2 Arise, and go down to the potter's house, and there I will cause thee to hear my words.

3 Then I went down to the potter's house, and, behold, he wrought a work on the wheels.

4 And the vessel that he made of clay was marred in the hand of the potter: so he made it again another vessel, as seemed good to the potter to make *it*.

5 Then the word of the LORD came to me, saying,

6 O house of Israel, [e]cannot I do with you as this potter? saith the LORD. Behold, [f]as the clay *is* in the potter's hand, so *are* ye in mine hand, O house of Israel.

7 *At what* instant I shall speak concerning a nation, and concerning a kingdom, to pluck up, and to pull down, and to destroy *it*;

8 If that nation, against whom I have pronounced, turn from their evil, I will [g]repent of the evil that I thought to do unto them.

9 And *at what* instant I shall speak concerning a nation, and concerning a kingdom, to build and to plant *it*;

10 If it do evil in my sight, that it obey not my voice, then I will repent of the good, wherewith I said I would benefit them.

11 Now therefore go to, speak to the men of Judah, and to the inhabitants of Jerusalem, saying, Thus saith the LORD; Behold, I frame evil against you, and devise a device against you: return ye now every one from his evil way, and make your ways and your doings good.

12 And they said, There is no hope: but we will walk after our own devices, and we will every one do the imagination of his evil heart.

13 Therefore thus saith the LORD; Ask ye now among the [h]heathen, who hath heard such things: the virgin of Israel hath done a very horrible thing.

14 Will *a man* leave the snow of Lebanon *which cometh* from the rock of the field? *or* shall the cold flowing waters that come from another place be forsaken?

15 Because my people hath [i]forgotten me, they have burned incense to vanity, and they have caused them to stumble in their ways *from* the ancient paths, to walk in paths, *in* a way not cast up;

16 To make their land [j]desolate, *and* a perpetual [k]hissing; every one that passeth thereby shall be astonished, and wag his head.

17 [l]I will scatter them as with an east wind before the enemy; [m]I will shew them the back, and not the face, in the day of their calamity.

18 Then said they, Come, and let us devise devices against Jeremiah; [n]for the law shall not perish from the priest, nor

B.C. 601.

a Jer. 7:24, 26; 11:10.
b Zech. 7:7.
c Lit. *meal.*
d *Parables* (O.T.). vs. 1-6; Jer. 24:1-10. (Jud. 9:7-15; Zech. 11:7-14.)
e Isa. 45:9; Rom. 9:20, 21.
f Isa. 64:8.
g Zech. 8:14, *note.*
h i.e. *nations.*
i Jer. 2:13, 32; 3:21; 13:25; 17:13.
j Jer. 19:8; 49:13; 50:13.
k 1 Ki. 9:8; Lam. 2:15; Mic. 6:16.
l Jer. 13:24.
m See Jer. 2:27.
n Lev. 10:11; Mal. 2:7; John 7:48, 49.

[1] **(18:1)** Israel (the whole nation) a vessel marred in the Potter's hand, is the key to this prophetic strain. But Jehovah will make "it again another vessel" (v. 4).

B.C. 605.

counsel from the wise, nor the word
from the prophet. Come, and let us
smite him with the tongue, and let us
not give heed to any of his words.
19 Give heed to me, O LORD, and hearken to the voice of them that contend
with me.
20 Shall evil be recompensed for
good? for they have digged a pit for my
soul. Remember that I stood before thee
to speak good for them, *and* to turn
away thy wrath from them.
21 Therefore deliver up their children
to the famine, and pour out their *blood*
by the force of the sword; and let their
wives be bereaved of their children, and
be widows; and let their men be put to
death; *let* their young men *be* slain by the
sword in battle.
22 Let a cry be heard from their houses,
when thou shalt bring a troop suddenly
upon them: for they have digged a pit to
take me, and hid snares for my feet.
23 Yet, LORD, thou knowest all their
counsel against me to slay *me*: forgive
not their iniquity, neither blot out their
sin from thy sight, but let them be overthrown before thee; deal *thus* with them
in the time of thine anger.

CHAPTER 19.

(*The sign of the potter's house,*
concluded.)

Thus saith the LORD, Go and get a potter's earthen bottle, and *take* of the
ancients of the people, and of the
ancients of the priests;
2 And go forth unto the [a]valley of the
son of Hinnom, which *is* by the entry of
the east gate, and proclaim there the
words that I shall tell thee,
3 And say, Hear ye the word of the
LORD, O kings of Judah, and inhabitants
of Jerusalem; Thus saith the LORD of
hosts, the God of Israel; Behold, I will
bring evil upon this place, the which
whosoever heareth, his ears shall [b]tingle.
4 [c]Because they have forsaken me, and
have estranged this place, and have
burned incense in it unto other gods,
whom neither they nor their fathers
have known, nor the kings of Judah, and
have filled this place with the blood of
innocents;
5 They have built also the high places
of Baal, to burn their sons with fire *for*
burnt-offerings unto Baal, which I commanded not, nor spake *it*, neither came *it*
into my mind:
6 Therefore, behold, the days come,
saith the LORD, that this place shall no
more be called Tophet, [d]nor The valley
of the son of Hinnom, but The valley of
slaughter.
7 And I will make void the counsel of
Judah and Jerusalem in this place; and [e]I
will cause them to fall by the sword
before their enemies, and by the hands of
them that seek their lives: and their carcases will I give to be meat for the fowls of
the heaven, and for the beasts of the earth.
8 And I will make this city desolate,
and an hissing; every one that passeth
thereby shall be astonished and hiss
because of all the plagues thereof.
9 And I will cause them to eat the flesh
of their sons and the [f]flesh of their daughters, and they shall eat every one the flesh
of his friend in the siege and straitness,
wherewith their enemies, and they that
seek their lives, shall straiten them.
10 Then shalt thou break the bottle in
the sight of the men that go with thee,
11 And shalt say unto them, Thus saith
the LORD of hosts; [g]Even so will I break
this people and this city, as *one* breaketh
a potter's vessel, that cannot be made
whole again: and they shall bury *them* in
Tophet, till *there be* no place to bury.
12 Thus will I do unto this place, saith
the LORD, and to the inhabitants thereof,
and *even* make this city as Tophet:
13 And the houses of Jerusalem, and
the houses of the kings of Judah, shall be
defiled as the place of Tophet, because of
all the houses upon whose [h]roofs they
have burned incense unto all the host of
heaven, and have poured out drink-
offerings unto other gods.

Parenthetic: Jeremiah's first persecution
(Jer. 19:14–20:18. Cf. Jer. 32:2).

14 Then came Jeremiah from Tophet,
whither the LORD had sent him to prophesy; and he stood in the court of the
LORD'S house; and said to all the people,
15 Thus saith the LORD of hosts, the
God of Israel; Behold, I will bring upon
this city and upon all her towns all the

a Josh. 15:8; 2 Ki. 23:10; Jer. 7:31.
b 1 Sam. 3:11; 2 Ki. 21:12.
c Deut. 28:20; Isa. 65:11; Jer. 2:13, 17, 19; 15:6; 17:13.
d Josh. 15:8.
e Lev. 26:17; Deut. 28:25.
f Lev. 26:29; Deut. 28:53; Isa. 9:20; Lam. 4:10.
g Psa. 2:9; Isa. 30:14; Lam. 4:2.
h 2 Ki. 23:12; Jer. 32:29; Zeph. 1:5.

B.C. 605.

evil that I have pronounced against it, because they have hardened their necks, that they might not hear my words.

CHAPTER 20.

Now Pashur the son of Immer the priest, who *was* also chief governor in the house of the LORD, heard that Jeremiah prophesied these things.

2 Then Pashur smote Jeremiah the prophet, and put him in the stocks that *were* in the high gate of Benjamin, which *was* by the house of the LORD.

3 And it came to pass on the morrow, that Pashur brought forth Jeremiah out of the stocks. Then said Jeremiah unto him, The LORD hath not called thy name Pashur, but [a]Magor-missabib.

4 For thus saith the LORD, Behold, I will make thee a terror to thyself, and to all thy friends: and they shall fall by the sword of their enemies, and thine eyes shall behold *it*: and I will give all Judah into the hand of the king of Babylon, and he shall carry them captive into Babylon, and shall slay them with the sword.

5 Moreover [b]I will deliver all the strength of this city, and all the labours thereof, and all the precious things thereof, and all the treasures of the kings of Judah will I give into the hand of their enemies, which shall spoil them, and take them, and carry them to Babylon.

6 And thou, Pashur, and all that dwell in thine house shall go into captivity: and thou shalt come to Babylon, and there thou shalt die, and shalt be buried there, thou, and all thy friends, to whom thou hast prophesied lies.

7 O LORD, thou hast deceived me, and I was deceived: thou art stronger than I, and hast prevailed: I am in derision daily, every one mocketh me.

8 For since I spake, I cried out, I cried violence and spoil; because the word of the LORD was made a reproach unto me, and a derision, daily.

9 Then I said, I will not make mention of him, nor speak any more in his name. But *his word* was in mine heart [c]as a burning fire shut up in my bones, and I was weary with forbearing, and [d]I could not *stay*.

10 For I heard the defaming of many, fear on every side. Report, *say they*, and we will report it. [e]All my familiars watched for my halting, *saying*, Peradventure he will be enticed, and we shall prevail against him, and we shall take our revenge on him.

11 But the LORD *is* with me as a mighty terrible one: therefore my persecutors shall stumble, and they shall not prevail: they shall be greatly ashamed; for they shall not prosper: *their* everlasting confusion shall never be forgotten.

12 But, O LORD of hosts, that [f]triest the righteous, *and* seest the reins and the heart, let me see thy vengeance on them: for unto thee have I opened my cause.

13 Sing unto the LORD, praise ye the LORD: for [g]he hath delivered the soul of the poor from the hand of evildoers.

14 Cursed *be* the day wherein I was born: let not the day wherein my mother bare me be blessed.

15 Cursed *be* the man who brought tidings to my father, saying, A man child is born unto thee; making him very glad.

16 And let that man be as the cities which the LORD overthrew, and [h]repented not: and let him hear the cry in the morning, and the shouting at noontide;

17 Because he slew me not from the womb; or that my mother might have been my grave, and her womb *to be* always great *with me*.

18 Wherefore came I forth out of the womb to see labour and sorrow, that my days should be consumed with shame?

CHAPTER 21.

The message to King Zedekiah (Jer. 21:1–22:30). *The Babylonian captivity foretold.* (Cf. 2 Ki. 25:1-11.)

The word which came unto Jeremiah from the LORD, when [i]king Zedekiah sent unto him Pashur the son of Melchiah, and [j]Zephaniah the son of Maaseiah the priest, saying,

2 Enquire, I pray thee, of the LORD for us; for Nebuchadrezzar king of Babylon maketh war against us; if so be that the LORD will deal with us according to all his wondrous works, that he may go up from us.

a i.e. Terror on every side.

b 2 Ki. 20:17; 24:12-16; 25:13.

c Job 32:18, 19; Psa. 39:3.

d Job 32:18; Acts 18:5.

e Heb. *every man of my peace.*

f Jer. 11:20; 17:10.

g Psa. 35:9, 10; 109:30, 31.

h Zech. 8:14, *note.*

i 2 Ki. 24:17.

j 2 Ki. 25:18; Jer. 29:25; 37:3.

3 Then said Jeremiah unto them, Thus shall ye say to Zedekiah:

4 Thus saith the LORD God of Israel; Behold, I will turn back the weapons of war that *are* in your hands, wherewith ye fight against the king of Babylon, and *against* the Chaldeans, which besiege you without the walls, and I will assemble them into the midst of this city.

5 And I myself will fight against you with [a]an outstretched hand and with a strong arm, even in anger, and in fury, and in great wrath.

6 And I will smite the inhabitants of this city, both man and beast: they shall die of a great pestilence.

7 And afterward, saith the LORD, I will deliver Zedekiah king of Judah, and his servants, and the people, and such as are left in this city from the pestilence, from the sword, and from the famine, into the hand of Nebuchadrezzar king of Babylon, and into the hand of their enemies, and into the hand of those that seek their life: and he shall smite them with the edge of the sword; [b]he shall not spare them, neither have pity, nor have mercy.

8 And unto this people thou shalt say, Thus saith the LORD; Behold, [c]I set before you the way of life, and the way of death.

9 He that abideth in this city shall die by the sword, and by the famine, and by the pestilence: but he that goeth out, and falleth to the Chaldeans that besiege you, he shall live, and [d]his life shall be unto him for a prey.

10 For I have set my face against this city for evil, and not for good, saith the LORD: it shall be given into the hand of the king of Babylon, and he shall burn it with fire.

11 And touching the house of the king of Judah, *say*, Hear ye the word of the LORD;

12 O house of David, thus saith the LORD; Execute judgment in the morning, and deliver *him that is* spoiled out of the hand of the oppressor, lest my fury go out like fire, and burn that none can quench *it*, because of the evil of your doings.

13 Behold, [e]I *am* against thee, O inhabitant of the valley, *and* rock of the plain, saith the LORD; which say, Who shall come down against us? or who shall enter into our habitations?

14 But I will [f]punish you according to the [g]fruit of your doings, saith the LORD: and I will kindle a fire in the forest thereof, and it shall devour all things round about it.

CHAPTER 22.

(*The message to Zedekiah*, concluded.)

Thus saith the LORD; Go down to the house of the king of Judah, and speak there this word,

2 And say, [h]Hear the word of the LORD, O king of Judah, that sittest upon the throne of David, thou, and thy servants, and thy people that enter in by these gates:

3 Thus saith the LORD; [i]Execute ye judgment and righteousness, and deliver the spoiled out of the hand of the oppressor: and do no wrong, do no violence to the stranger, the fatherless, nor the widow, neither shed innocent blood in this place.

4 For if ye do this thing indeed, [j]then shall there enter in by the gates of this house kings sitting upon the throne of David, riding in chariots and on horses, he, and his servants, and his people.

5 But if ye will not hear these words, [k]I swear by myself, saith the LORD, that this house shall become a desolation.

6 For thus saith the LORD unto the king's house of Judah; Thou *art* Gilead unto me, *and* the head of Lebanon: *yet* surely I will make thee a wilderness, *and* cities *which* are not inhabited.

7 And I will prepare destroyers against thee, every one with his weapons: and they shall cut down thy choice cedars, and cast *them* into the fire.

8 And many nations shall pass by this city, and they shall say every man to his neighbour, [l]Wherefore hath the LORD done thus unto this great city?

9 Then they shall answer, [m]Because they have forsaken the covenant of the LORD their God, and worshipped other gods, and served them.

10 Weep ye not for [n]the dead, neither bemoan him: *but* weep sore for him that goeth away: for he shall return no more, nor see his native country.

11 For thus saith the LORD touching [o]Shallum the son of Josiah king of Judah, which reigned instead of Josiah his father, which went forth out of this

B.C. 589.

a Ex. 6:6.
b Deut. 28:50; 2 Chr. 36:17.
c Deut. 30:19.
d Or, *his life shall be that of one hunted.* Jer. 39:18.
e Ezk. 13:8.
f Heb. *visit upon.*
g Prov. 1:31; Isa. 3:10, 11.
h Jer. 17:20.
i Jer. 21:12.
j Jer. 17:25.
k Heb. 6:13, 17.
l Deut. 29:24, 25; 1 Ki. 9:8, 9.
m 2 Ki. 22:17; 2 Chr. 34:25.
n 2 Ki. 22:20.
o 1 Chr. 3:15, with 2 Ki. 23:30.

place; He shall not return thither any more:
12 But he shall die in the place whither they have led him captive, and shall see this land no more.
13 Woe unto him that buildeth his house by unrighteousness, and his chambers by wrong; [a]*that* useth his neighbour's service without wages, and giveth him not for his work;
14 That saith, I will build me a wide house and large chambers, and cutteth him out windows; and *it is* cieled with cedar, and painted with vermilion.
15 Shalt thou reign, because thou closest *thyself* in cedar? did not thy father eat and drink, and do judgment and justice, *and* then *it was* well with him?
16 He judged the cause of the poor and needy; then *it was* well *with him: was* not this to know me? saith the LORD.
17 But thine eyes and thine heart *are* not but for thy covetousness, and for to shed innocent blood, and for oppression, and for violence, to do *it*.
18 Therefore thus saith the LORD concerning Jehoiakim the son of Josiah king of Judah; They shall not lament for him, *saying*, Ah my brother! or, Ah sister! they shall not lament for him, *saying*, Ah lord! or, Ah his glory!
19 He shall be buried with the burial of an ass, drawn and cast forth beyond the gates of Jerusalem.
20 Go up to Lebanon, and cry; and lift up thy voice in Bashan, and cry from the passages: for all thy lovers are destroyed.
21 I spake unto thee in thy prosperity; *but* thou saidst, I will not hear. This *hath been* thy manner from thy youth, that thou obeyedst not my voice.
22 The wind shall eat up all thy pastors, and thy lovers shall go into captivity: surely then shalt thou be ashamed and confounded for all thy wickedness.
23 O inhabitant of Lebanon, that makest thy nest in the cedars, how gracious shalt thou be when pangs come upon thee, the pain as of a woman in travail!
24 *As* I live, saith the LORD, though [b]Coniah the son of Jehoiakim king of Judah were the signet upon my right hand, yet would I pluck thee thence;
25 And I will give thee into the hand of them that seek thy life, and into the hand *of them* whose face thou fearest, even into the hand of Nebuchadrezzar king of Babylon, and into the hand of the Chaldeans.
26 And I will cast thee out, and thy mother that bare thee, into another country, where ye were not born; and there shall ye die.
27 But to the land whereunto they desire to return, thither shall they not return.
28 *Is* this man Coniah a despised broken idol? *is he* a vessel wherein *is* no pleasure? wherefore are they cast out, he and his seed, and are cast into a land which they know not?
29 O earth, earth, earth, hear the word of the LORD.
30 Thus saith the LORD, Write ye this man childless, a man *that* shall not prosper in his days: [c]for no man of his seed shall prosper, sitting upon the throne of David, and ruling any more in Judah.

CHAPTER 23.

The future [1]restoration and conversion of Israel: message against the faithless shepherds (vs. 1-40).

Woe be unto the pastors that destroy and scatter the sheep of my pasture! saith the LORD.
2 Therefore thus saith the LORD God of Israel against the pastors that feed my people; Ye have scattered my flock, and driven them away, and have not visited them: behold, I will visit upon you the evil of your doings, saith the LORD.
3 And I will gather the [d]remnant of my [e]flock out of all countries whither I

B.C. 609.

a Lev. 19:13; Deut. 24:14, 15; Mal. 3:10; Jas. 5:4.

b Contracted from Jeconiah, 1 Chr. 3:16.

c Jer. 36:30.

d *Remnant.* vs. 3-8; Jer. 31:7-14. (Isa. 1:9; Rom. 11:5.)

e *Israel (prophecies).* vs. 3-8; Jer. 30:1-9. (Gen. 12:2, 3; Rom. 11:26.)

[1] **(23, heading)** This final restoration is shown to be accomplished after a period of unexampled tribulation (Jer. 30:3-10), and in connection with the manifestation of David's righteous Branch (v. 5), who is also Jehovah-tsidkenu (v. 6). The restoration here foretold is not to be confounded with the return of a feeble remnant of Judah under Ezra, Nehemiah, and Zerubbabel at the end of the 70 years (Jer. 29:10). At His first advent Christ, David's righteous Branch (Lk. 1:31-33), did not "execute justice and judgment in the earth," but was crowned with thorns and crucified. Neither was Israel the nation restored, nor did the Jewish people say, "The Lord our righteousness." Cf. Rom. 10:3. The prophecy is yet to be fulfilled (Acts 15:14-17).

have driven them, and will bring them again to their folds; and they shall be fruitful and increase.

4 And I will set up shepherds over them which shall feed them: and they shall fear no more, nor be dismayed, neither shall they be lacking, saith the LORD.

5 Behold, the days come, saith the LORD, that I will raise unto David a righteous [a]Branch, and a [b]King shall reign and prosper, and shall execute judgment and justice in the earth.

6 [c]In his days Judah shall be saved, and Israel shall dwell safely: and this *is* his name whereby he shall be called, [d]THE LORD OUR RIGHTEOUSNESS.

7 Therefore, behold, the days come, saith the LORD, that they shall no more say, The LORD liveth, which brought up the children of Israel out of the land of Egypt;

8 But, The LORD liveth, which brought up and which led the seed of the house of Israel out of the north country, and [e]from all countries whither I had driven them; and they shall dwell in their own land.

9 Mine heart within me is broken because of the prophets; all my bones shake; I am like a drunken man, and like a man whom wine hath overcome, because of the LORD, and because of the words of his holiness.

10 For the land is full of adulterers; for because of swearing the land mourneth; the pleasant places of the wilderness are dried up, and their course is evil, and their force *is* not right.

11 For both prophet and priest are profane; yea, in my house have I found their wickedness, saith the LORD.

12 Wherefore their way shall be unto them as slippery *ways* in the darkness: they shall be driven on, and fall therein: for I will bring evil upon them, *even* the year of their visitation, saith the LORD.

13 And I have seen folly in the prophets of Samaria; they prophesied in Baal, and caused my people Israel to err.

14 I have seen also in the prophets of Jerusalem an horrible thing: they commit adultery, and walk in lies: they strengthen also the hands of evildoers, that none doth return from his wickedness: they are all of them unto me [f]as Sodom, and the inhabitants thereof as Gomorrah.

15 Therefore thus saith the LORD of hosts concerning the prophets; Behold, I will feed them with wormwood, and make them drink the water of gall: for from the prophets of Jerusalem is profaneness gone forth into all the land.

16 Thus saith the LORD of hosts, Hearken not unto the words of the prophets that prophesy unto you: they make you vain: [g]they speak a vision of their own heart, *and* not out of the mouth of the LORD.

17 They say still unto them that despise me, The LORD hath said, Ye shall have peace; and they say unto every one that walketh after the imagination of his own heart, No evil shall come upon you.

18 For [h]who hath stood in the counsel of the LORD, and hath perceived and heard his word? who hath marked his word, and heard *it*?

19 Behold, a whirlwind of the LORD is gone forth in fury, even a grievous whirlwind: it shall fall grievously upon the head of the wicked.

20 [i]The anger of the LORD shall not return, until he have executed, and till he have performed the thoughts of his heart: [j]in the latter days ye shall consider it perfectly.

21 [k]I have not sent these prophets, yet they ran: I have not spoken to them, yet they prophesied.

22 But if they had stood in my counsel, and had caused my people to hear my words, then they should have turned them from their evil way, and from the evil of their doings.

23 *Am* I a God at hand, saith the LORD, and not a God afar off?

24 [l]Can any hide himself in secret places that I shall not see him? saith the LORD. [m]Do not I fill heaven and earth? saith the LORD.

25 I have heard what the prophets said, that prophesy lies in my name, saying, I have dreamed, I have dreamed.

26 How long shall *this* be in the heart of the prophets that prophesy lies? yea, *they are* prophets of the deceit of their own heart;

27 Which think to cause my people to forget my name by their dreams which they tell every man to his neighbour, as their fathers have forgotten my name for Baal.

B.C. 599.

a Isa. 4:2, *note.*

b *Kingdom* (O.T.). vs. 5-8; Jer. 30:7-9. (Gen. 1:26; Zech. 12:8.)

c *Christ (Second Advent).* vs. 5, 6; Ezk. 37:21, 22. (Deut. 30:3; Acts 1:9-11.)

d Heb. *Jehovah-tsidkenu.*

e v. 3; Isa. 43:5, 6.

f Deut. 32:32; Isa. 1:9, 10.

g v. 21; Jer. 14:14.

h Job 15:8; 1 Cor. 2:16.

i Jer. 30:24.

j Gen. 49:1.

k Jer. 14:14; 27:15; 29:9.

l Psa. 139:7; Amos 9:2, 3.

m 1 Ki. 8:27; Psa. 139:8.

28 The prophet that hath a dream, let him tell a dream; and he that hath my word, let him speak my word faithfully. What *is* the chaff to the wheat? saith the LORD.

29 *Is* not my word like as a fire? saith the LORD; and like a hammer *that* breaketh the rock in pieces?

30 Therefore, behold, [a]I *am* against the prophets, saith the LORD, that steal my words every one from his neighbour.

31 Behold, I *am* against the prophets, saith the LORD, that use their tongues, and say, He saith.

32 Behold, I *am* against them that prophesy false dreams, saith the LORD, and do tell them, and cause my people to err by their lies, and by [b]their lightness; yet I sent them not, nor commanded them: therefore they shall not profit this people at all, saith the LORD.

33 And when this people, or the prophet, or a priest, shall ask thee, saying, [c]What *is* the burden of the LORD? thou shalt then say unto them, What burden? I will even forsake you, saith the LORD.

34 And *as for* the prophet, and the priest, and the people, that shall say, The burden of the LORD, I will even punish that man and his house.

35 Thus shall ye say every one to his neighbour, and every one to his brother, What hath the LORD answered? and, What hath the LORD spoken?

36 And the burden of the LORD shall ye mention no more: for every man's word shall be his burden; for ye have perverted the words of the living God, of the LORD of hosts our God.

37 Thus shalt thou say to the prophet, What hath the LORD answered thee? and, What hath the LORD spoken?

38 But since ye say, The burden of the LORD; therefore thus saith the LORD; Because ye say this word, The burden of the LORD, and I have sent unto you, saying, Ye shall not say, The burden of the LORD;

39 Therefore, behold, I, even I, [d]will utterly forget you, and I will forsake you, and the city that I gave you and your fathers, *and cast you* out of my presence:

40 And I will bring an everlasting reproach upon you, and a perpetual shame, which shall not be forgotten.

B.C. 599.

a Deut. 18:20; Jer. 14:14, 15.

b Zeph. 3:4.

c Mal. 1:1.

d Hos. 4:6.

e Jer. 23:39, 40.

f *Parables* (O.T.). vs. 1-10; Jer. 27:1-7. (Jud. 9:7-15; Zech. 11:7-14.)

g 2 Ki. 24:12; 2 Chr. 36:10.

h Jer. 12:15; 29:10.

i Deut. 30:6; Ezk. 11:19; 36:26, 27.

j Jer. 30:22; 31:33; 32:38.

k Deut. 28:25, 37; 1 Ki. 9:7; 2 Chr. 7:20; Jer. 15:4; 29:18; 34:17.

CHAPTER 24.

The sign of the figs (vs. 1-3). *Judah yet to be restored,* [e]*but not they of the second deportation* (vs. 4-10).

The LORD shewed me, and, behold, [f]two baskets of figs *were* set before the temple of the LORD, after that Nebuchadrezzar [g]king of Babylon had carried away captive Jeconiah the son of Jehoiakim king of Judah, and the princes of Judah, with the carpenters and smiths, from Jerusalem, and had brought them to Babylon.

2 One basket *had* very good figs, *even* like the figs *that are* first ripe: and the other basket *had* very naughty figs, which could not be eaten, they were so bad.

3 Then said the LORD unto me, What seest thou, Jeremiah? And I said, Figs; the good figs, very good; and the evil, very evil, that cannot be eaten, they are so evil.

4 Again the word of the LORD came unto me, saying,

5 Thus saith the LORD, the God of Israel; Like these good figs, so will I acknowledge them that are carried away captive of Judah, whom I have sent out of this place into the land of the Chaldeans for *their* good.

6 For I will set mine eyes upon them for good, and [h]I will bring them again to this land: and I will build them, and not pull *them* down; and I will plant them, and not pluck *them* up.

7 And I will give them [i]an heart to know me, that I *am* the LORD: and they shall be [j]my people, and I will be their God: for they shall return unto me with their whole heart.

8 And as the evil figs, which cannot be eaten, they are so evil; surely thus saith the LORD, So will I give Zedekiah the king of Judah, and his princes, and the residue of Jerusalem, that remain in this land, and them that dwell in the land of Egypt:

9 And [k]I will deliver them to be removed into all the kingdoms of the earth for *their* hurt, *to be* a reproach and a proverb, a taunt and a curse, in all places whither I shall drive them.

10 And I will send the sword, the famine, and the pestilence, among them, till they be consumed from off the land that I gave unto them and to their fathers.

CHAPTER 25.

Prophecy of the seventy years' captivity
(vs. 1-14. Cf. Dan. 9:2).

The word that came to Jeremiah concerning all the people of Judah [a]in
the fourth year of Jehoiakim the son of
Josiah king of Judah, that *was* the first
year of Nebuchadrezzar king of Babylon;
2 The which Jeremiah the prophet
spake unto all the people of Judah, and to
all the inhabitants of Jerusalem, saying,
3 From the thirteenth year of Josiah the
son of Amon king of Judah, even unto this
day, that *is* the three and twentieth year,
the word of the LORD hath come unto me,
and I have spoken unto you, rising early
and speaking; but ye have not hearkened.
4 And the LORD hath sent unto you all
his servants the prophets, rising early
and sending *them*; but ye have not hearkened, nor inclined your ear to hear.
5 They said, [b]Turn ye again now every
one from his evil way, and from the evil
of your doings, and dwell in the land
that the LORD hath given unto you and
to your fathers for ever and ever:
6 And go not after other gods to serve
them, and to worship them, and provoke me not to anger with the works of
your hands; and I will do you no hurt.
7 Yet ye have not hearkened unto me,
saith the LORD; that ye might [c]provoke
me to anger with the works of your
hands to your own hurt.
8 Therefore thus saith the LORD of
hosts; Because ye have not heard my
words,
9 Behold, I will send and take all the
families of the north, saith the LORD, and
Nebuchadrezzar the king of Babylon, [d]my
servant, and will bring them against this
land, and against the inhabitants thereof,
and against all these nations round about,
and will utterly destroy them, and make
them an astonishment, and an hissing,
and perpetual desolations.

B.C. 607.

a Jer. 36:1.
b 2 Ki. 17:13; Jer. 18:11; 35:15; Jon. 3:8.
c Deut. 32:21; Jer. 7:19; 32:30.
d Isa. 44:28; 45:1; Jer. 27:6; 43:10.
e Isa. 13:19; 14:23; 21:1; 47:1; Jer. 50:3, 13, 23, 39, 40, 45; 51:25, 26.
f Job 21:20; Psa. 75:8; Isa. 51:17; Rev. 14:10.
g Jer. 51:7; Ezk. 23:34; Nah. 3:11.

10 Moreover I will take from them the
voice of mirth, and the voice of gladness,
the voice of the bridegroom, and the
voice of the bride, the sound of the millstones, and the light of the candle.
11 And this whole land shall be a desolation, *and* an astonishment; and these
nations shall serve the king of Babylon
[1]seventy years.
12 And it shall come to pass, when
seventy years are accomplished, *that* I
will punish the king of Babylon, and that
nation, saith the LORD, for their iniquity,
[e]and the land of the Chaldeans, and will
make it perpetual desolations.
13 And I will bring upon that land all
my words which I have pronounced
against it, *even* all that is written in this
book, which Jeremiah hath prophesied
against all the nations.
14 For many nations and great kings
shall serve themselves of them also: and
I will recompense them according to
their deeds, and according to the works
of their own hands.

The sign of the wine cup of fury
(vs. 15-38).

15 For thus saith the LORD God of
Israel unto me; Take the [f]wine cup of
this fury at my hand, and cause all the
nations, to whom I send thee, to drink it.
16 And [g]they shall drink, and be
moved, and be mad, because of the
sword that I will send among them.
17 Then took I the cup at the LORD'S
hand, and made all the nations to drink,
unto whom the LORD had sent me:
18 *To wit*, Jerusalem, and the cities of
Judah, and the kings thereof, and the
princes thereof, to make them a desolation, an astonishment, an hissing, and a
curse; as *it is* this day;
19 Pharaoh king of Egypt, and his servants, and his princes, and all his people;

[1] **(25:11)** Cf. Lev. 26:33-35; 2 Chr. 36:21; Dan. 9:2. The 70 years may be reckoned to begin with the first deportation of Judah to Babylon (2 Ki. 24:10-15), B.C. 604 according to the Assyrian Eponym Canon, or B.C. 606 according to Ussher; or, from the final deportation (2 Ki. 25; 2 Chr. 36:17-20; Jer. 39:8-10), B.C. 586 (Assyr. Ep. Canon), or B.C. 588 (Ussher). In the first case the 70 years extend to the decree of Cyrus for the return (Ezra 1:1-3), B.C. 534 (Assyr. Ep. Canon), or B.C. 536 (Ussher). In the second case the 70 years terminate B.C. 516 (Assyr. Ep. Canon) with the completion of the temple. The latter is the more probable reckoning in the light of Dan. 9:25.

B.C. 606.

20 And all the mingled people, and all the kings of the land of Uz, and all the kings of the land of the Philistines, and Ashkelon, and Azzah, and Ekron, and the remnant of Ashdod,

21 Edom, and Moab, and the children of Ammon,

22 And all the kings of Tyrus, and all the kings of Zidon, and the kings of the [a]isles which *are* beyond the sea,

23 Dedan, and Tema, and Buz, and all *that are* in the utmost corners,

24 And all the kings of Arabia, and all the kings of the mingled people that dwell in the desert,

25 And all the kings of Zimri, and all the kings of Elam, and all the kings of the Medes,

26 And all the kings of the north, far and near, one with another, and all the kingdoms of the world, which *are* upon the face of the earth: and the king of [b]Sheshach shall drink after them.

27 Therefore thou shalt say unto them, Thus saith the LORD of hosts, the God of Israel; Drink ye, and be drunken, and spue, and fall, and rise no more, because of the sword which I will send among you.

28 And it shall be, if they refuse to take the cup at thine hand to drink, then shalt thou say unto them, Thus saith the LORD of hosts; Ye shall certainly drink.

29 For, lo, I begin to bring evil on the city which is called by my name, and should ye be utterly unpunished? Ye shall not be unpunished: for [c]I will call for a [d]sword upon [1]all the inhabitants of the earth, saith the LORD of hosts.

30 Therefore prophesy thou against them all these words, and say unto them, The LORD shall roar from on high, and utter his voice from his holy habitation; he shall mightily [e]roar upon his habitation; he shall give a shout, as they that tread *the grapes*, against all the inhabitants of the earth.

31 A noise shall come *even* to the ends of the earth; for the LORD hath a [f]controversy with the nations, [g]he will plead with all flesh; he will give them *that are* wicked to the sword, saith the LORD.

32 Thus saith the LORD of hosts, Behold, evil shall go forth from nation to nation, and a great whirlwind shall be raised up from the coasts of the earth.

33 [h]And the slain of the LORD shall be at that day from *one* end of the earth even unto the *other* end of the earth: they shall not be lamented, neither gathered, nor buried; they shall be dung upon the ground.

34 Howl, ye shepherds, and cry; and wallow yourselves *in the ashes*, ye principal of the flock: for the days of your slaughter and of your dispersions are accomplished; and ye shall fall like a pleasant vessel.

35 And the shepherds shall have no way to flee, nor the principal of the flock to escape.

36 A voice of the cry of the shepherds, and an howling of the principal of the flock, *shall be heard*: for the LORD hath spoiled their pasture.

37 And the peaceable habitations are cut down because of the fierce anger of the LORD.

38 He hath forsaken his covert, as the lion: for their land is desolate because of the fierceness of the oppressor, and because of his fierce anger.

CHAPTER 26.

The message in the temple court (vs. 1-19). (Cf. Jer. 7:1, *note.*)

In the beginning of the reign of Jehoiakim the son of Josiah king of Judah came this word from the LORD, saying,

2 Thus saith the LORD; Stand in the court of the LORD'S house, and speak unto all the cities of Judah, which come to worship in the LORD'S house, [i]all the words that I command thee to speak unto them; diminish not a word:

3 If so be they will hearken, and turn every man from his evil way, that I may [j]repent me of the evil, which I purpose to do unto them because of the evil of their doings.

4 And thou shalt say unto them, Thus saith the LORD; If ye will not hearken to me, to walk in my law, which I have set before you,

a i.e. *coasts.*

b A name for Babylon. Jer. 51:41.

c *Day (of Jehovah).* vs. 29-38; Ezk. 30:3. (Isa. 2:10-22; Rev. 19:11-21.)

d *Armageddon (battle of).* vs. 29-33; Ezk. 38:1—39:16. (Rev. 16:14; 19:11-21.)

e Isa. 42:13; Joel 3:16; Amos 1:2.

f Hos. 4:1; Mic. 6:2.

g Isa. 66:16; Joel 3:2.

h Isa. 66:16.

i Ezk. 3:10; Mt. 28:20.

j Zech. 8:14, *note.*

1 (25:29) The scope of this great prophecy cannot be limited to the invasion of Nebuchadnezzar. If Jehovah does not spare His own city, should the Gentile nations imagine that there is no judgment for them? The prophecy leaps to the very end of this age. (See "Day of the LORD," Isa. 2:10-22; Rev. 19:11-21; "Armageddon," Rev. 16:14; 19:11-21.)

5 To hearken to the words of my servants the prophets, whom I sent unto you, both rising up early, and sending *them*, but ye have not hearkened;

6 Then will I make this house like [a]Shiloh, and will make this city a curse to all the nations of the earth.

7 So the priests and the prophets and all the people heard Jeremiah speaking these words in the house of the LORD.

8 Now it came to pass, when Jeremiah had made an end of speaking all that the LORD had commanded *him* to speak unto all the people, that the priests and the prophets and all the people took him, saying, Thou shalt surely die.

9 Why hast thou prophesied in the name of the LORD, saying, This house shall be like Shiloh, and this city shall be desolate without an inhabitant? And all the people were gathered against Jeremiah in the house of the LORD.

10 When the princes of Judah heard these things, then they came up from the king's house unto the house of the LORD, and sat down in the entry of the new gate of the LORD'S *house*.

11 Then spake the priests and the prophets unto the princes and to all the people, saying, This man *is* worthy to die; for he hath prophesied against this city, as ye have heard with your ears.

12 Then spake Jeremiah unto all the princes and to all the people, saying, The LORD sent me to prophesy against this house and against this city all the words that ye have heard.

13 Therefore now amend your ways and your doings, and obey the voice of the LORD your God; and the LORD will [b]repent him of the evil that he hath pronounced against you.

14 As for me, behold, I *am* in your hand: do with me as seemeth good and meet unto you.

15 But know ye for certain, that if ye put me to death, ye shall surely bring innocent blood upon yourselves, and upon this city, and upon the inhabitants thereof: for of a truth the LORD hath sent me unto you to speak all these words in your ears.

16 Then said the princes and all the people unto the priests and to the prophets; This man *is* not worthy to die: for he hath spoken to us in the name of the LORD our God.

B.C. 609.

a 1 Sam. 4:10, 11; Psa. 78:60; Jer. 7:12, 14.

b Zech. 8:14, *note.*

c Mic. 1:1.

d Mic. 3:12.

e Psa. 19:9, *note.*

f 2 Ki. 22:12, 14; Jer. 39:14.

g *Parables* (O.T.). vs. 1-7; Ezk. 17:1-14. (Jud. 9:7-15; Zech. 11:7-14.)

17 Then rose up certain of the elders of the land, and spake to all the assembly of the people, saying,

18 [c]Micah the Morasthite prophesied in the days of Hezekiah king of Judah, and spake to all the people of Judah, saying, Thus saith the LORD of hosts; [d]Zion shall be plowed *like* a field, and Jerusalem shall become heaps, and the mountain of the house as the high places of a forest.

19 Did Hezekiah king of Judah and all Judah put him at all to death? did he not [e]fear the LORD, and besought the LORD, and the LORD [b]repented him of the evil which he had pronounced against them? Thus might we procure great evil against our souls.

Martyrdom of Urijah (vs. 20-24).

20 And there was also a man that prophesied in the name of the LORD, Urijah the son of Shemaiah of Kirjath-jearim, who prophesied against this city and against this land according to all the words of Jeremiah:

21 And when Jehoiakim the king, with all his mighty men, and all the princes, heard his words, the king sought to put him to death: but when Urijah heard it, he was afraid, and fled, and went into Egypt;

22 And Jehoiakim the king sent men into Egypt, *namely*, Elnathan the son of Achbor, and *certain* men with him into Egypt.

23 And they fetched forth Urijah out of Egypt, and brought him unto Jehoiakim the king; who slew him with the sword, and cast his dead body into the graves of the common people.

24 Nevertheless [f]the hand of Ahikam the son of Shaphan was with Jeremiah, that they should not give him into the hand of the people to put him to death.

CHAPTER 27.

The sign of the yokes (vs. 1-11):
to surrounding Gentile kings.

In the beginning of the reign of Jehoiakim the son of Josiah king of Judah came this word unto Jeremiah from the LORD, [g]saying,

2 Thus saith the LORD to me; Make thee bonds and yokes, and put them upon thy neck,

3 And send them to the king of Edom, and to the king of Moab, and to the king

of the Ammonites, and to the king of
Tyrus, and to the king of Zidon, by the
hand of the messengers which come to
Jerusalem unto Zedekiah king of Judah;
4 And command them to say unto
their masters, Thus saith the LORD of
hosts, the God of Israel; Thus shall ye
say unto your masters;
5 I have made the earth, the man and
the beast that *are* upon the ground, by
my great power and by my outstretched
arm, and have given it unto whom it
seemed meet unto me.
6 And now have I given all these lands
into the hand of Nebuchadnezzar the
king of Babylon, [a]my servant; and the
beasts of the field have I given him also
to serve him.
7 And all nations shall serve him, and
his son, and his son's son, [b]until the very
time of his land come: and then many
nations and great kings shall serve
themselves of him.
8 And it shall come to pass, *that* the
nation and kingdom which will not
serve the same Nebuchadnezzar the
king of Babylon, and that will not put
their neck under the yoke of the king of
Babylon, that nation will I punish, saith
the LORD, with the sword, and with the
famine, and with the pestilence, until I
have consumed them by his hand.
9 Therefore hearken not ye to your
prophets, nor to your diviners, nor to
your dreamers, nor to your enchanters,
nor to your sorcerers, which speak unto
you, saying, Ye shall not serve the king
of Babylon:
10 For they prophesy a lie unto you, to
remove you far from your land; and that
I should drive you out, and ye should
perish.
11 But the nations that bring their neck
under the yoke of the king of Babylon,
and serve him, those will I let remain
still in their own land, saith the LORD;
and they shall till it, and dwell therein.

(The sign of the yokes, continued:
to King Zedekiah.)

12 I spake also to Zedekiah king of
Judah according to all these words, saying, Bring your necks under the yoke of
the king of Babylon, and serve him and
his people, and live.
13 Why will ye die, thou and thy people, by the sword, by the famine, and by
the pestilence, as the LORD hath spoken

B.C. 598.

a Jer. 25:9; 43:10; Ezk. 29:18, 20.

b Jer. 25:12; 50:27; Dan. 5:26.

c 2 Chr. 36:7, 10; Jer. 28:3; Dan. 1:2.

d 2 Ki. 25:13; Jer. 52:17, 20, 21.

e 2 Ki. 24:14, 15; Jer. 24:1.

f 2 Ki. 25:13; 2 Chr. 36:18.

g 2 Chr. 36:21; Jer. 29:10; 32:5.

h Ezra 1:7; 7:19.

against the nation that will not serve the
king of Babylon?
14 Therefore hearken not unto the
words of the prophets that speak unto
you, saying, Ye shall not serve the king of
Babylon: for they prophesy a lie unto you.
15 For I have not sent them, saith the
LORD, yet they prophesy a lie in my
name; that I might drive you out, and
that ye might perish, ye, and the
prophets that prophesy unto you.
16 Also I spake to the priests and to all
this people, saying, Thus saith the LORD;
Hearken not to the words of your
prophets that prophesy unto you, saying, [c]Behold, the vessels of the LORD'S
house shall now shortly be brought
again from Babylon: for they prophesy a
lie unto you.
17 Hearken not unto them; serve the
king of Babylon, and live: wherefore
should this city be laid waste?
18 But if they *be* prophets, and if the
word of the LORD be with them, let them
now make intercession to the LORD of
hosts, that the vessels which are left in
the house of the LORD, and *in* the house
of the king of Judah, and at Jerusalem,
go not to Babylon.
19 For thus saith the LORD of hosts
concerning the pillars, and [d]concerning
the sea, and concerning the bases, and
concerning the residue of the vessels
that remain in this city,
20 Which Nebuchadnezzar king of
Babylon took not, when he carried away
[e]captive Jeconiah the son of Jehoiakim
king of Judah from Jerusalem to Babylon,
and all the nobles of Judah and Jerusalem;
21 Yea, thus saith the LORD of hosts,
the God of Israel, concerning the vessels
that remain *in* the house of the LORD,
and *in* the house of the king of Judah
and of Jerusalem;
22 They shall [f]be carried to Babylon,
and there shall they be until the day that
[g]I visit them, saith the LORD; then [h]will I
bring them up, and restore them to this
place.

CHAPTER 28.

(Sign of the yokes, continued: *the false
prophecy and death of Hananiah.)*

And it came to pass the same year, in
the beginning of the reign of
Zedekiah king of Judah, in the fourth

year, *and* in the [a]fifth month, *that* Hananiah the son of Azur the prophet, which *was* of Gibeon, spake unto me in the house of the LORD, in the presence of the priests and of all the people, saying,

2 Thus speaketh the LORD of hosts, the God of Israel, saying, I have broken [b]the yoke of the king of Babylon.

3 Within two full years will I bring again into this place all the vessels of the LORD'S house, that Nebuchadnezzar king of Babylon took away from this place, and carried them to Babylon:

4 And I will bring again to this place Jeconiah the son of Jehoiakim king of Judah, with all the captives of Judah, that went into Babylon, saith the LORD: for I will break the yoke of the king of Babylon.

5 Then the prophet Jeremiah said unto the prophet Hananiah in the presence of the priests, and in the presence of all the people that stood in the house of the LORD,

6 Even the prophet Jeremiah said, [c]Amen: the LORD do so: the LORD perform thy words which thou hast prophesied, to bring again the vessels of the LORD'S house, and all that is carried away captive, from Babylon into this place.

7 Nevertheless hear thou now this word that I speak in thine ears, and in the ears of all the people;

8 The prophets that have been before me and before thee of old prophesied both against many countries, and against great kingdoms, of war, and of evil, and of pestilence.

9 [d]The prophet which prophesieth of peace, when the word of the prophet shall come to pass, *then* shall the prophet be known, that the LORD hath truly sent him.

10 Then Hananiah the prophet took the yoke from off the prophet Jeremiah's neck, and brake it.

11 And Hananiah spake in the presence of all the people, saying, Thus saith the LORD; Even so will I break the yoke of Nebuchadnezzar king of Babylon [e]from the neck of all nations within the space of two full years. And the prophet Jeremiah went his way.

12 Then the word of the LORD came unto Jeremiah *the prophet*, after that Hananiah the prophet had broken [f]the yoke from off the neck of the prophet Jeremiah, saying,

13 Go and tell Hananiah, saying, Thus saith the LORD; Thou hast broken the yokes of wood; but thou shalt make for them yokes of iron.

14 For thus saith the LORD of hosts, the God of Israel; [g]I have put a yoke of iron upon the neck of all these nations, that they may serve Nebuchadnezzar king of Babylon; and they shall serve him: and I have given him the beasts of the field also.

15 Then said the prophet Jeremiah unto Hananiah the prophet, Hear now, Hananiah; The LORD hath not sent thee; [h]but thou makest this people to [i]trust in a lie.

16 Therefore thus saith the LORD; Behold, I will cast thee from off the face of the earth: this year thou shalt die, because thou hast taught rebellion against the LORD.

17 So Hananiah the prophet died the same year in the [j]seventh month.

CHAPTER 29.

The message to the Jews of the first captivity (vs. 1-32).

NOW these *are* the words of the letter that Jeremiah the prophet sent from Jerusalem unto the residue of the elders which were [1]carried away captives, and to the priests, and to the prophets, and to all the people whom Nebuchadnezzar had carried away captive from Jerusalem to Babylon;

2 (After that [k]Jeconiah the king, and the queen, and the eunuchs, the princes of Judah and Jerusalem, and the carpenters, and the smiths, were departed from Jerusalem;)

3 By the hand of Elasah the son of Shaphan, and Gemariah the son of Hilkiah, (whom Zedekiah king of Judah sent unto Babylon to Nebuchadnezzar king of Babylon) saying,

4 Thus saith the LORD of hosts, the God of Israel, unto all that are carried away captives, whom I have caused to be carried away from Jerusalem unto Babylon;

5 Build ye houses, and dwell *in them*;

B.C. 596.

a i.e. *August.*
b Jer. 27:12.
c 1 Ki. 1:36.
d Deut. 18:22.
e Jer. 27:7.
f Jer. 27:2.
g Deut. 28:48; Jer. 27:7.
h Jer. 29:31; Ezk. 13:22.
i Psa. 2:12, *note.*
j i.e. *October.*
k 2 Ki. 24:12; Jer. 22:26.

[1] **(29:1)** Cf. 2 Ki. 24:10-16. The complete captivity of Judah came eleven years later (2 Ki. 25:1-7).

and plant gardens, and eat the fruit of them;

6 Take ye wives, and beget sons and daughters; and take wives for your sons, and give your daughters to husbands, that they may bear sons and daughters; that ye may be increased there, and not diminished.

7 And seek the peace of the city whither I have caused you to be carried away captives, [a]and pray unto the LORD for it: for in the peace thereof shall ye have peace.

8 For thus saith the LORD of hosts, the God of Israel; Let not your prophets and your diviners, that *be* in the midst of you, [b]deceive you, neither hearken to your dreams which ye cause to be dreamed.

9 For they prophesy falsely unto you in my name: I have not sent them, saith the LORD.

10 For thus saith the LORD, That [c]after seventy years be accomplished at Babylon I will visit you, and perform my good word toward you, in causing you to return to this place.

11 For I know the thoughts that I think toward you, saith the LORD, thoughts of peace, and not of evil, to give you an expected end.

12 [d]Then shall ye call upon me, and ye shall go and pray unto me, and I will hearken unto you.

13 And [e]ye shall seek me, and find *me*, when ye shall search for me with all your heart.

14 [f]And I will be found of you, saith the LORD: and I will turn away your captivity, and [g]I will gather you from all the nations, and from all the places whither I have driven you, saith the LORD; and I will bring you again into the place whence I caused you to be carried away captive.

15 Because ye have said, The LORD hath raised us up prophets in Babylon;

16 *Know* that thus saith the LORD of the king that sitteth upon the throne of David, and of all the people that dwelleth in this city, *and* of your brethren that are not gone forth with you into captivity;

17 Thus saith the LORD of hosts; Behold, I will send upon them the sword, the famine, and the pestilence, and will make them like vile figs, that cannot be eaten, they are so evil.

B.C. 599.

a Ezra 6:10; 1 Tim. 2:2.

b Jer. 14:14; 23:21; 27:14, 15; Eph. 5:6.

c 2 Chr. 36:21, 22; Ezra 1:1; Jer. 25:12; 27:22; Dan. 9:2.

d Dan. 9:3.

e Lev. 26:39, 40, 42; Deut. 30:1-3.

f Deut. 4:7; Psa. 32:6; 46:1; Isa. 55:6.

g Jer. 23:3, 8; 30:3; 32:37.

h Deut. 28:25; 2 Chr. 29:8; Jer. 15:4; 24:9; 34:17.

i See Gen. 48:20; Isa. 65:15.

j Dan. 3:6.

k 2 Ki. 25:18; Jer. 21:1.

l 2 Ki. 9:11; Acts 26:24.

18 And I will persecute them with the sword, with the famine, and with the pestilence, and [h]will deliver them to be removed to all the kingdoms of the earth, to be a curse, and an astonishment, and an hissing, and a reproach, among all the nations whither I have driven them:

19 Because they have not hearkened to my words, saith the LORD, which I sent unto them by my servants the prophets, rising up early and sending *them*; but ye would not hear, saith the LORD.

20 Hear ye therefore the word of the LORD, all ye of the captivity, whom I have sent from Jerusalem to Babylon:

21 Thus saith the LORD of hosts, the God of Israel, of Ahab the son of Kolaiah, and of Zedekiah the son of Maaseiah, which prophesy a lie unto you in my name; Behold, I will deliver them into the hand of Nebuchadrezzar king of Babylon; and he shall slay them before your eyes;

22 And [i]of them shall be taken up a curse by all the captivity of Judah which *are* in Babylon, saying, The LORD make thee like Zedekiah and like [j]Ahab, whom the king of Babylon roasted in the fire;

23 Because they have committed villany in Israel, and have committed adultery with their neighbours' wives, and have spoken lying words in my name, which I have not commanded them; even I know, and *am* a witness, saith the LORD.

24 *Thus* shalt thou also speak to Shemaiah the Nehelamite, saying,

25 Thus speaketh the LORD of hosts, the God of Israel, saying, Because thou hast sent letters in thy name unto all the people that *are* at Jerusalem, and [k]to Zephaniah the son of Maaseiah the priest, and to all the priests, saying,

26 The LORD hath made thee priest in the stead of Jehoiada the priest, that ye should be officers in the house of the LORD, for every man *that is* [l]mad, and maketh himself a prophet, that thou shouldest put him in prison, and in the stocks.

27 Now therefore why hast thou not reproved Jeremiah of Anathoth, which maketh himself a prophet to you?

28 For therefore he sent unto us *in* Babylon, saying, This *captivity is* long: build ye houses, and dwell *in them*; and plant gardens, and eat the fruit of them.

B.C. 606.

29 And Zephaniah the priest read
this letter in the ears of Jeremiah the
prophet.
30 Then came the word of the LORD
unto Jeremiah, saying,
31 Send to all them of the captivity,
saying, Thus saith the LORD concerning
Shemaiah the Nehelamite; Because that
Shemaiah hath prophesied unto you,
and I sent him not, and he caused you to
trust in a lie:
32 Therefore thus saith the LORD;
Behold, I will punish Shemaiah the Nehelamite, and his seed: he shall not have a
man to dwell among this people; neither
shall he behold the good that I will do for
my people, saith the LORD; because he
hath taught rebellion against the LORD.

PART II. PROPHECIES NOT CHRONOLOGICAL: CHAPTERS 30–36

CHAPTER 30.

Jeremiah's first writing.
(Cf. Jer. 36:1-23, 28.) *Summary of Israel in the tribulation* (Jer. 30:1–31:40).

The [1]word that came to Jeremiah from
the LORD, saying,
2 Thus speaketh the LORD God of
Israel, saying, [2]Write thee all the [a]words
that I have spoken unto thee in a book.
3 For, lo, the days come, saith the
LORD, that [b]I will bring again the captivity of my people Israel and Judah, saith
the LORD: and I will cause them to return
to the land that I gave to their fathers,
and they shall possess it.
4 And these *are* the words that the
LORD spake concerning Israel and concerning Judah.
5 For thus saith the LORD; We have
heard a voice of trembling, of fear, and
not of peace.
6 Ask ye now, and see whether a man
doth [c]travail with child? wherefore do I
see every man with his hands on his
loins, as a woman in travail, and all faces
are turned into paleness?
7 Alas! for [d]that day *is* great, so that
none *is* like it: it *is* even the time of Jacob's
trouble; but he shall be saved out of it.
8 For it shall come to pass in that day,
saith the LORD of hosts, *that* I will break
his yoke from off thy neck, and will
burst thy bonds, and strangers shall no
more serve themselves of him:
9 [e]But they shall serve the LORD their
God, and [f]David their king, whom I will
raise up unto them.
10 Therefore fear thou not, O my servant Jacob, saith the LORD; neither be
dismayed, O Israel: for, lo, I will save
thee from afar, and thy seed from the
[g]land of their captivity; and Jacob shall
return, and shall be in rest, and be quiet,
and none shall make *him* afraid.
11 For I *am* with thee, saith the LORD, to
save thee: [h]though I make a full end of all
nations whither I have scattered thee, yet
will I not make a full end of thee: but I
will correct thee in measure, and will not
leave thee altogether unpunished.
12 For thus saith the LORD, [i]Thy bruise
is incurable, *and* thy wound *is* grievous.
13 *There is* none to plead thy cause,
that thou mayest be bound up: thou hast
no healing medicines.
14 All thy lovers have forgotten thee;
they seek thee not; for I have wounded
thee with the wound of an enemy, with
the chastisement of a cruel one, for the
multitude of thine iniquity; *because* thy
sins were increased.
15 Why criest thou for thine affliction?
thy sorrow *is* incurable for the multitude
of thine iniquity: *because* thy sins were

a *Inspiration.* Jer. 36:1-32. (Ex. 4:15; Rev. 22:19.)

b *Israel (prophecies).* vs. 1-9; Jer. 31:7-14, 31-40. (Gen. 12:2, 3; Rom. 11:26.)

c Mic. 5:1, *note.*

d *Tribulation (the great).* vs. 4-7; Dan. 12:1. (Psa. 2:5; Rev. 7:14.)

e *Kingdom* (O.T.). vs. 7-9; Jer. 33:14-17. (Gen. 1:26; Zech. 12:8.)

f Isa. 55:3, 4; Ezk. 34:23; 37:24; Hos. 3:5.

g Jer. 3:18.

h Amos 9:8.

i 2 Chr. 36:16; Jer. 15:18.

[1] **(30:1)** The writings of Jeremiah in Chapters 30–36 cannot with certainty be arranged in consecutive order. Certain dates are mentioned (e.g. 32:1; 33:1; 34:1, 8; 35:1), but retrospectively. The narrative, so far as Jeremiah gives a narrative, is resumed at 37:1. These chapters constitute a kind of summary of prophecy concerning Israel as a nation, looking on especially to the last days, the day of the LORD, and the kingdom-age to follow. If the marginal references are carefully followed the order will become clear. But these prophecies are interspersed with much historical matter concerning Jeremiah and his time.

[2] **(30:2)** Three "writings" by Jeremiah are to be distinguished: (1) 30:1–31:40. This is impersonal—a general prophecy, and probably the earliest. (2) 1:1–36:23, destroyed by Jehoiakim. (3) The destroyed writing re-written (36:27), doubtless the writing preserved to us.

increased, I have done these things unto thee.

16 Therefore all they that devour thee [a]shall be devoured; and all thine adversaries, every one of them, shall go into captivity; and they that spoil thee shall be a spoil, and all that prey upon thee will I give for a prey.

17 [b]For I will restore health unto thee, and I will heal thee of thy wounds, saith the LORD; because they called thee an Outcast, *saying*, This *is* Zion, whom no man seeketh after.

18 Thus saith the LORD; Behold, I will bring again the captivity of Jacob's tents, and have mercy on his dwellingplaces; and the city shall be builded upon her own heap, and the palace shall remain after the manner thereof.

19 And out of them shall proceed thanksgiving and the voice of them that make merry: and I will multiply them, and they shall not be few; I will also glorify them, and they shall not be small.

20 Their children also shall be as aforetime, and their congregation shall be established before me, and I will punish all that oppress them.

21 And their nobles shall be of themselves, and their governor shall proceed from the midst of them; and I will cause him to draw near, and he shall approach unto me: for who *is* this that engaged his heart to approach unto me? saith the LORD.

22 And ye shall be [c]my people, and I will be your God.

23 Behold, the whirlwind of the LORD goeth forth with fury, a continuing whirlwind: it shall fall with pain upon the head of the wicked.

24 The fierce anger of the LORD shall not return, until he have done *it*, and until he have performed the intents of his heart: in the latter days ye shall consider it.

CHAPTER 31.

Summary: Israel in the last days.

At the same time, saith the LORD, will I be the God of all the families of Israel, and they shall be my people.

2 Thus saith the LORD, The people *which were* left of the sword found grace in the wilderness; *even* Israel, when I went to cause him to rest.

3 The LORD hath appeared of old unto me, *saying*, Yea, I have loved thee with an everlasting love: therefore with lovingkindness have I drawn thee.

4 Again I will build thee, and thou shalt be built, O virgin of Israel: thou shalt again be adorned with thy tabrets, and shalt go forth in the dances of them that make merry.

5 Thou shalt yet plant vines upon the mountains of Samaria: the planters shall plant, and shall eat *them* as common things.

6 For there shall be a day, *that* the watchmen upon the mount Ephraim shall cry, Arise ye, and let us go up to Zion unto the LORD our God.

7 For thus saith the LORD; Sing with gladness for Jacob, and shout among the chief of the nations: publish ye, praise ye, and say, O LORD, save thy people, the [d]remnant of [e]Israel.

8 Behold, I will bring them from the north country, and gather them from the coasts of the earth, *and* with them the blind and the lame, the woman with child and her that travaileth with child together: a great company shall return thither.

9 They shall come with weeping, and with supplications will I lead them: I will cause them to walk by the rivers of waters in a straight way, wherein they shall not stumble: for I am a father to Israel, and Ephraim *is* my firstborn.

10 Hear the word of the LORD, O ye nations, and declare *it* in the [f]isles afar off, and say, He that scattered Israel will gather him, and keep him, as a shepherd *doth* his flock.

11 For the LORD hath [g]redeemed Jacob, and [h]ransomed him from the hand of *him that was* stronger than he.

12 Therefore they shall come and sing in the height of Zion, and shall flow together to the goodness of the LORD, for wheat, and for wine, and for oil, and for the young of the flock and of the herd: and their soul shall be as a watered garden; and they shall not sorrow any more at all.

13 Then shall the virgin rejoice in the dance, both young men and old together: for I will turn their mourning into joy, and will comfort them, and make them rejoice from their sorrow.

14 And I will satiate the soul of the priests with fatness, and my people shall

B.C. 606.

a Ex. 23:22; Isa. 33:1; 41:11; Jer. 10:25.

b Jer. 33:6.

c Jer. 24:7; 31:1, 33; 32:38; Ezk. 11:20; 36:28; 37:27.

d *Remnant.* vs. 7-14; Ezk. 6:8. (Isa. 1:9; Rom. 11:5.)

e *Israel (prophecies).* vs. 7-14, 31-40; Ezk. 36:22-38. (Gen. 12:2, 3; Rom. 11:26.)

f i.e. *coasts.*

g Ex. 14:30, *note;* Isa. 59:20, *note.*

h Heb. *goel, Redemp. (Kinsman type).* Isa. 59:20, *note.*

be satisfied with my goodness, saith the
LORD.
15 Thus saith the LORD; A voice was
heard in Ramah, lamentation, *and* bitter
weeping; Rahel [a]weeping for her children refused to be comforted for her
children, because they *were* not.
16 Thus saith the LORD; Refrain thy
voice from weeping, and thine eyes from
tears: for thy work shall be rewarded,
saith the LORD; and they shall come
again from the land of the enemy.
17 And there is hope in thine end,
saith the LORD, that thy children shall
come again to their own border.
18 I have surely heard Ephraim
bemoaning himself *thus*; Thou hast chastised me, and I was chastised, as a bullock unaccustomed *to the yoke*: turn thou
me, and I shall be turned; for thou *art*
the LORD my God.
19 Surely after that I was turned, I [b]re-
pented; and after that I was instructed, I
smote upon *my* thigh: I was ashamed,
yea, even confounded, because I did
bear the reproach of my youth.
20 *Is* Ephraim my dear son? *is he* a
pleasant child? for since I spake against
him, I do earnestly remember him still:
therefore my bowels are troubled for
him; I will surely have mercy upon him,
saith the LORD.
21 Set thee up waymarks, make thee
high heaps: set thine heart toward the
highway, *even* the way *which* thou wentest: turn again, O virgin of Israel, turn
again to these thy cities.
22 How long wilt thou go about, O
thou backsliding daughter? for the LORD
hath created a new thing in the earth, A
woman shall compass a man.
23 Thus saith the LORD of hosts, the
God of Israel; As yet they shall use this
speech in the land of Judah and in the
cities thereof, when I shall bring again
their captivity; The LORD bless thee, O
habitation of justice, *and* mountain of
holiness.
24 And there shall dwell in Judah
itself, and in all the cities thereof together, husbandmen, and they *that* go forth
with flocks.
25 For I have satiated the weary soul,
and I have replenished every sorrowful
soul.

B.C. 606.

a Mt. 2:18.

b Zech. 8:14, *note.*

c vs. 31-34; Heb. 8:8-12.

d *Covenant* (New). vs. 31-34; Jer. 32:37-40. (Isa. 61:8; Heb. 8:8-12.)

e *Wife (of Jehovah).* Hos. 2:1-23. (Isa. 54:5; Hos. 2:1-23.)

f vs. 33, 34; Heb. 10:16, 17.

g *Forgiveness.* Isa. 38:17. (Lev. 4:20; Mt. 26:28.)

h Psa. 148:6; Isa. 54:9, 10; Jer. 33:20.

i Jer. 33:22.

26 Upon this I awaked, and beheld;
and my sleep was sweet unto me.
27 Behold, the days come, saith the
LORD, that I will sow the house of Israel
and the house of Judah with the seed of
man, and with the seed of beast.
28 And it shall come to pass, *that* like
as I have watched over them, to pluck
up, and to break down, and to throw
down, and to destroy, and to afflict; so
will I watch over them, to build, and to
plant, saith the LORD.
29 In those days they shall say no more,
The fathers have eaten a sour grape, and
the children's teeth are set on edge.
30 But every one shall die for his own
iniquity: every man that eateth the sour
grape, his teeth shall be set on edge.
31 [c]Behold, the days come, saith the
LORD, that I will make a new [d]covenant
with the house of Israel, and with the
house of Judah:
32 Not according to the covenant that I
made with their fathers in the day *that* I
took them by the hand to bring them out
of the land of Egypt; which my covenant
they brake, although I was an [e]husband
unto them, saith the LORD:
33 But this *shall be* the covenant that I
will make with the house of Israel; After
those days, saith the LORD, I will put my
[f]law in their inward parts, and write it in
their hearts; and will be their God, and
they shall be my people.
34 And they shall teach no more every
man his neighbour, and every man his
brother, saying, Know the LORD: for they
shall all know me, from the least of them
unto the greatest of them, saith the LORD:
for I will [g]forgive their iniquity, and I
will remember their sin no more.
35 Thus saith the LORD, which giveth
the sun for a light by day, *and* the ordinances of the moon and of the stars for a
light by night, which divideth the sea
when the waves thereof roar; The LORD
of hosts *is* his name:
36 [h]If those ordinances depart from
before me, saith the LORD, *then* the seed
of Israel also shall cease from being a
nation before me for ever.
37 Thus saith the LORD; [i]If heaven
above can be measured, and the foundations of the earth searched out beneath, I

B.C. 606.

will also cast off all the seed of Israel for all that they have done, saith the LORD.

38 Behold, the days come, saith the LORD, that the city shall be built to the LORD [a]from the tower of Hananeel unto the gate of the corner.

39 And [b]the measuring line shall yet go forth over against it upon the hill Gareb, and shall compass about to Goath.

40 And the whole valley of the dead bodies, and of the ashes, and all the fields unto the brook of Kidron, [c]unto the corner of the horse gate toward the east, [d]*shall be* holy unto the LORD; it shall not be plucked up, nor thrown down any more for ever.

CHAPTER 32.

The sign of the field of Hanameel: Jeremiah's second persecution.
(Cf. Jer. 20:1-18; 37:11, *note.*)

The word that came to Jeremiah from the LORD [e]in the tenth year of Zedekiah king of Judah, which *was* the eighteenth year of Nebuchadrezzar.

2 For then the king of Babylon's army besieged Jerusalem: and Jeremiah the prophet was shut up in the court of the prison, which *was* in the king of Judah's house.

3 For Zedekiah king of Judah had shut him up, saying, Wherefore dost thou prophesy, and say, Thus saith the LORD, Behold, I will give this city into the hand of the king of Babylon, and he shall take it;

4 And Zedekiah king of Judah shall not escape out of the hand of the Chaldeans, but shall surely be delivered into the hand of the king of Babylon, and shall speak with him mouth to mouth, and his eyes shall behold his eyes;

5 And he shall lead Zedekiah to Babylon, and there shall he be until I visit him, saith the LORD: though ye fight with the Chaldeans, ye shall not prosper.

6 And Jeremiah said, The word of the LORD came unto me, saying,

7 Behold, Hanameel the son of Shallum thine uncle shall come unto thee, saying, Buy thee my field that *is* in Anathoth: for [f]the right of redemption *is* thine to buy *it.*

8 So Hanameel mine uncle's son came to me in the court of the prison according to the word of the LORD, and said unto me, Buy my field, I pray thee, that *is* in Anathoth, which *is* in the country of Benjamin: for the right of inheritance *is* thine, and the redemption *is* thine; buy *it* for thyself. Then I knew that this *was* the word of the LORD.

9 And I [1]bought the field of Hanameel my uncle's son, that *was* in Anathoth, and weighed him the money, *even* seventeen [g]shekels of silver.

10 And I subscribed the evidence, and sealed *it,* and took witnesses, and weighed *him* the money in the balances.

11 So I took the evidence of the purchase, *both* that which was sealed *according* to the law and custom, and that which was open:

12 And I gave the evidence of the purchase unto Baruch the son of Neriah, the son of Maaseiah, in the sight of Hanameel mine uncle's *son,* and in the presence of the [h]witnesses that subscribed the book of the purchase, before all the Jews that sat in the court of the prison.

13 And I charged Baruch before them, saying,

14 Thus saith the LORD of hosts, the God of Israel; Take these evidences, this evidence of the purchase, both which is sealed, and this evidence which is open; and put them in an earthen vessel, that they may continue many days.

15 For thus saith the LORD of hosts, the God of Israel; Houses and fields and vineyards shall be possessed again in this land.

A prayer of Jeremiah.

16 Now when I had delivered the evidence of the purchase unto Baruch the son of Neriah, I [i]prayed unto the LORD, saying,

17 Ah Lord GOD! behold, [j]thou hast made the heaven and the earth by thy great power and stretched out arm, *and* [k]there is nothing too hard for thee:

18 Thou shewest [l]lovingkindness unto thousands, and recompensest the iniquity of the fathers into the bosom of their children after them: the Great, the Mighty God, the LORD of hosts, *is* his name,

a Neh. 3:1; Zech. 14:10.
b Ezk. 40:8; Zech. 2:1.
c 2 Chr. 23:15; Neh. 3:28.
d Joel 3:17.
e 2 Ki. 25:1, 2; Jer. 39:1.
f Lev. 25:24, 25, 32; Ruth 4:4.
g One shekel = 2*s.* 9*d.*, or 65 cts.
h See Isa. 8:2.
i See *Bible prayers* (O.T.). Gen. 15:2.
j 2 Ki. 19:15.
k Gen. 18:14; Lk. 1:37.
l Ex. 20:6; 34:7; Deut. 5:9, 10.

[1](32:9) A (1) sign of Jeremiah's faith in his own predictions of the restoration of Judah (v. 15), for the field was then occupied by the Babylonian army; and (2) a sign to Judah of that coming restoration.

19 Great in counsel, and mighty in
work: for [a]thine eyes *are* open upon all
the ways of the sons of men: to give
every one according to his ways, and
according to the fruit of his doings:
20 Which hast set signs and wonders
in the land of Egypt, *even* unto this day,
and in Israel, and among *other* men; and
hast made thee [b]a name, as at this day;
21 And [c]hast brought forth thy people
Israel out of the land of Egypt with
signs, and with wonders, and with a
strong hand, and with a stretched out
arm, and with great terror;
22 And hast given them this land,
which thou didst swear to their fathers
to give them, a [d]land flowing with milk
and honey;
23 And they came in, and possessed it;
but they obeyed not thy voice, neither
walked in thy law; they have done nothing of all that thou commandedst them
to do: therefore thou hast caused all this
evil to come upon them:
24 Behold the [e]mounts, they are come
unto the city to take it; and the city is
given into the hand of the Chaldeans,
that fight against it, because of the
sword, and of the famine, and of the
pestilence: and what thou hast spoken is
come to pass; and, behold, thou seest *it*.
25 And thou hast said unto me, O
Lord GOD, Buy thee the field for money,
and take witnesses; for the city is given
into the hand of the Chaldeans.

The answer of Jehovah.

26 Then came the word of the LORD
unto Jeremiah, saying,
27 Behold, I *am* the LORD, the [f]God of all
flesh: is there any thing too hard for me?
28 Therefore thus saith the LORD;
Behold, I will give this city into the hand
of the Chaldeans, and into the hand of
Nebuchadrezzar king of Babylon, and he
shall take it:
29 And the Chaldeans, that fight
against this city, shall come and set fire
on this city, and burn it with the houses,
upon whose roofs they have offered
incense unto Baal, and poured out
drink-offerings unto other gods, to provoke me to anger.
30 For the children of Israel and the
children of Judah have only done evil
before me from their youth: for the children of Israel have only provoked me to
anger with the work of their hands, saith
the LORD.
31 For this city hath been to me *as* a
provocation of mine anger and of my
fury from the day that they built it even
unto this day; [g]that I should remove it
from before my face,
32 Because of all the evil of the children of Israel and of the children of
Judah, which they have done to provoke
me to anger, [h]they, their kings, their
princes, their priests, and their prophets,
and the men of Judah, and the inhabitants of Jerusalem.
33 And they have turned unto me the
back, and not the face: though I taught
them, rising up early and teaching *them*,
yet they have not hearkened to receive
instruction.
34 But they set their abominations in
the house, which is called by my name,
to defile it.
35 And they built the high places of
Baal, which *are* in the valley of the son of
Hinnom, to cause their sons and their
daughters to pass through *the fire* unto
[i]Molech; which I commanded them not,
neither came it into my mind, that they
should do this abomination, to cause
Judah to sin.
36 And now therefore thus saith the
LORD, the God of Israel, concerning this
city, whereof ye say, It shall be delivered
into the hand of the king of Babylon by
the sword, and by the famine, and by
the pestilence;
37 Behold, [j]I will gather them out of
all countries, whither I have driven them
in mine anger, and in my fury, and in
great wrath; and I will bring them again
unto this place, and I will cause them to
dwell safely:
38 And [k]they shall be my people, and I
will be their God:
39 And I will [l]give them one heart,
and one way, that they may fear me for
ever, for the good of them, and of their
children after them:
40 And I will make an [m]everlasting
covenant with them, that I will not turn
away from them, to do them good; but I
will put my [n]fear in their hearts, that
they shall not depart from me.
41 Yea, I will [o]rejoice over them to do
them good, and I will [p]plant them in this
land assuredly with my whole heart and
with my whole soul.

B.C. 590.

a Job 34:21; Psa. 33:13; Prov. 5:21; Jer. 16:17.

b Ex. 9:16; 1 Chr. 17:21; Isa. 63:12; Dan. 9:15.

c Ex. 6:6; 2 Sam. 7:23; 1 Chr. 17:21; Psa. 136:11, 12.

d Ex. 3:8, 17; Jer. 11:5.

e Or, *engines of shot.*

f Num. 16:22.

g 2 Ki. 23:27.

h Isa. 1:4, 6; Dan. 9:8.

i Lev. 18:21; 1 Ki. 11:33.

j Deut. 30:3; Jer. 23:3; 29:14; 31:10; Ezk. 37:21.

k Jer. 24:7; 30:22; 31:33.

l Jer. 24:7; Ezk. 11:19, 20.

m *Covenant* (New). vs. 37-40; Jer. 50:4, 5. (Isa. 61:8; Heb. 8:8-12.)

n Psa. 19:9, *note.*

o Deut. 30:9; Zeph. 3:17.

p Jer. 24:6; 31:28; Amos 9:15.

42 For thus saith the LORD; [a]Like as I
have brought all this great evil upon this
people, so will I bring upon them all the
good that I have promised them.
43 And fields shall be bought in this
land, whereof ye say, *It is* desolate without man or beast; it is given into the
hand of the Chaldeans.
44 Men shall buy fields for money, and
subscribe evidences, and seal *them*, and
take witnesses [b]in the land of Benjamin,
and in the places about Jerusalem, and
in the cities of Judah, and in the cities of
the mountains, and in the cities of the
valley, and in the cities of the south: for
[c]I will cause their captivity to return,
saith the LORD.

CHAPTER 33.

The great prophecy concerning the Davidic Kingdom. (Cf. 2 Sam. 7:8-16.)

MOREOVER the word of the LORD came
unto Jeremiah the second time,
[d]while he was yet shut up in the court of
the prison, saying,
2 Thus saith the LORD the maker thereof, the LORD that formed it, to establish
it; the LORD *is* his name;
3 [e]Call unto me, and I will answer
thee, and shew thee great and mighty
things, which thou knowest not.
4 For thus saith the LORD, the God of
Israel, concerning the houses of this city,
and concerning the houses of the kings
of Judah, which are thrown down by the
mounts, and by the sword;
5 They come to fight with the
Chaldeans, but *it is* to fill them with the
dead bodies of men, whom I have slain
in mine anger and in my fury, and for all
whose wickedness I have hid my face
from this city.
6 Behold, I will bring it health and
cure, and I will cure them, and will
reveal unto them the abundance of
peace and truth.
7 [f]And I will cause the captivity of
Judah and the captivity of Israel to return,
and will build them, as at the first.
8 And I will [g]cleanse them from all
their iniquity, whereby they have sinned
against me; and I will pardon all their
iniquities, whereby they have sinned,
and whereby they have transgressed
against me.
9 And it shall be to me a name of joy, a
praise and an honour before all the
nations of the earth, which shall hear all
the good that I do unto them: and they
shall fear and tremble for all the goodness and for all the prosperity that I procure unto it.
10 Thus saith the LORD; Again there
shall be heard in this place, which ye say
shall be desolate without man and without beast, *even* in the cities of Judah, and
in the streets of Jerusalem, that are desolate, without man, and without inhabitant, and without beast,
11 [h]The voice of joy, and the voice of
gladness, the voice of the bridegroom,
and the voice of the bride, the voice of
them that shall say, Praise the LORD of
hosts: for the LORD *is* good; for his mercy
endureth for ever: *and* of them that shall
bring the sacrifice of praise into the
house of the LORD. For I will cause to
return the captivity of the land, as at the
first, saith the LORD.
12 Thus saith the LORD of hosts; [i]Again
in this place, which is desolate without
man and without beast, and in all the
cities thereof, shall be an habitation of
shepherds causing *their* flocks to lie down.
13 In the cities of the mountains, in the
cities of the vale, and in the cities of the
south, and in the land of Benjamin, and
in the places about Jerusalem, and in the
cities of Judah, shall the flocks pass
again under the hands of him that telleth
them, saith the LORD.
14 Behold, the days come, saith the
LORD, that I will [j]perform that good thing
which I have promised unto the house of
Israel and to the house of Judah.
15 [1]In those days, and at that time, will
I cause the [k]Branch of righteousness to
grow up unto David; and he shall execute
judgment and righteousness in the land.
16 In those days shall Judah be saved,
and Jerusalem shall dwell safely: and
this *is the name* wherewith she shall be
called, [l]The LORD our righteousness.
17 For thus saith the LORD; David shall
never [m]want a man to sit upon the
throne of the house of Israel;

B.C. 590.

a Jer. 31:28.
b Jer. 17:26.
c Jer. 33:7, 11, 26.
d Cf. Jer. 37:11, *note.*
e Psa. 91:15; Jer. 29:12.
f v. 11; Jer. 30:3; 32:44.
g Ezk. 36:25; Zech. 13:1; Heb. 9:13, 14.
h Jer. 7:34; 16:9; 25:10; Rev. 18:23.
i Isa. 65:10; Jer. 31:24; 50:19.
j *Kingdom* (O.T.). vs. 14-17; Ezk. 11:14-20. (Gen. 1:26; Zech. 12:8.)
k Isa. 4:2, *note.*
l Heb. *Jehovah-tsidkenu.*
m 2 Sam. 7:16; 1 Ki. 2:4; Psa. 89:29, 36; Lk. 1:32, 33.

1 (33:15) See "Davidic Covenant" (2 Sam. 7:8-17, *note*); "Kingdom (O.T.)" (Gen. 1:26; Zech. 12:8, *note*); "Kingdom (N.T.)" (Lk. 1:31-33; 1 Cor. 15:28).

18 Neither shall the priests the Levites
want a man before me to offer burnt-
offerings, and to kindle [a]meat-offerings,
and to do sacrifice continually.
19 And the word of the LORD came
unto Jeremiah, saying,
20 Thus saith the LORD; If ye can break
my covenant of the day, and my covenant
of the night, and that there should not be
day and night in their season;
21 *Then* may also my covenant be broken with David my servant, that he
should not have a son to reign upon his
throne; and with the Levites the priests,
my ministers.
22 As the host of heaven cannot be
numbered, neither the sand of the sea
measured: so will I multiply the seed of
David my servant, and the Levites that
minister unto me.
23 Moreover the word of the LORD
came to Jeremiah, saying,
24 Considerest thou not what this people have spoken, saying, The two families which the LORD hath chosen, he hath
even cast them off? thus they have
despised my people, that they should be
no more a nation before them.
25 Thus saith the LORD; [b]If my
covenant *be* not with day and night, *and*
if I have not appointed the ordinances of
heaven and earth;
26 [c]Then will I cast away the seed of
Jacob, and David my servant, *so* that I
will not take *any* of his seed *to be* rulers
over the seed of Abraham, Isaac, and
Jacob: for I will cause their captivity to
return, and have mercy on them.

CHAPTER 34.

The message to Zedekiah concerning his coming captivity. (Cf. 2 Ki. 25:1-7.)

The word which came unto Jeremiah
from the LORD, [d]when Nebuchadnezzar king of Babylon, and all his army,
and all the kingdoms of the earth of his
dominion, and all the people, fought
against Jerusalem, and against all the
cities thereof, saying,
2 Thus saith the LORD, the God of
Israel; Go and speak to Zedekiah king of
Judah, and tell him, Thus saith the LORD;
Behold, I will give this city into the hand
of the king of Babylon, and he shall burn
it with fire:
3 And thou shalt not escape out of his
hand, but shalt surely be taken, and delivered into his hand; and thine eyes shall
behold the eyes of the king of Babylon,
and he shall speak with thee mouth to
mouth, and thou shalt go to Babylon.
4 Yet hear the word of the LORD, O
Zedekiah king of Judah; Thus saith the
LORD of thee, Thou shalt not die by the
sword:
5 *But* thou shalt die in peace: and with
the burnings of thy fathers, the former
kings which were before thee, so shall
they burn *odours* for thee; and they will
lament thee, *saying*, Ah lord! for I have
pronounced the word, saith the LORD.
6 Then Jeremiah the prophet spake all
these words unto Zedekiah king of
Judah in Jerusalem,
7 When the king of Babylon's army
fought against Jerusalem, and against all
the cities of Judah that were left, against
Lachish, and against Azekah: for [e]these
defenced cities remained of the cities of
Judah.

Zedekiah's ineffectual decree (vs. 8-22).

8 *This is* the word that came unto
Jeremiah from the LORD, after that the
king Zedekiah had made a covenant
with all the people which *were* at
Jerusalem, to proclaim liberty unto them;
9 That every man should let his
manservant, and every man his maidservant, *being* an Hebrew or an Hebrewess,
go free; that none should serve himself
of them, *to wit*, of a Jew his brother.
10 Now when all the princes, and all
the people, which had entered into the
covenant, heard that every one should
let his manservant, and every one his
maidservant, go free, that none should
serve themselves of them any more, then
they obeyed, and let *them* go.
11 But afterward they turned, and
caused the servants and the handmaids,
whom they had let go free, to return,
and brought them into subjection for
servants and for handmaids.
12 Therefore the word of the LORD
came to Jeremiah from the LORD, saying,
13 Thus saith the LORD, the God of
Israel; I made a covenant with your
fathers in the day that I brought them

B.C. 590.

a Lit. *meal*

b v. 20; Gen. 8:22.

c Jer. 31:37.

d 2 Ki. 25:1; Jer. 39:1; 52:4.

e 2 Ki. 18:13; 19:8; 2 Chr. 11:5, 9.

forth out of the land of Egypt, out of the house of bondmen, saying,

14 At the end of [a]seven years let ye go every man his brother an Hebrew, which hath been sold unto thee; and when he hath served thee six years, thou shalt let him go free from thee: but your fathers hearkened not unto me, neither inclined their ear.

15 And ye were now turned, and had done right in my sight, in proclaiming liberty every man to his neighbour; and ye had made a covenant before me in the house which is called by my name:

16 But ye turned and polluted my name, and caused every man his servant, and every man his handmaid, whom ye had set at liberty at their pleasure, to return, and brought them into subjection, to be unto you for servants and for handmaids.

17 Therefore thus saith the LORD; Ye have not hearkened unto me, in proclaiming liberty, every one to his brother, and every man to his neighbour: behold, [b]I proclaim a liberty for you, saith the LORD, to the sword, to the pestilence, and to the famine; and I will make you to be removed into all the kingdoms of the earth.

18 And I will give the men that have transgressed my covenant, which have not performed the words of the covenant which they had made before me, [c]when they cut the calf in twain, and passed between the parts thereof,

19 The princes of Judah, and the princes of Jerusalem, the eunuchs, and the priests, and all the people of the land, which passed between the parts of the calf;

20 I will even give them into the hand of their enemies, and into the hand of them that seek their life: and their dead bodies shall be for meat unto the fowls of the heaven, and to the beasts of the earth.

21 And Zedekiah king of Judah and his princes will I give into the hand of their enemies, and into the hand of them that seek their life, and into the hand of the king of Babylon's army, which are gone up from you.

22 Behold, I will command, saith the LORD, and cause them to return to this city; and they shall fight against it, and take it, and burn it with fire: and [d]I will make the cities of Judah a desolation without an inhabitant.

B.C. 590.

a Ex. 21:2; Deut. 15:12.

b Mt. 7:2; Gal. 6:7; Jas. 2:13.

c Gen. 15:10, 17.

d Jer. 9:11; 44:2, 6.

e 2 Sam. 4:2.

f 2 Ki. 12:9; 25:18; 1 Chr. 9:18, 19.

g Ex. 20:12; Eph. 6:2, 3.

CHAPTER 35.

The obedience of the Rechabites in the reign of Jehoiakim. (Cf. 2 Ki. 23:36–24:5.)

The word which came unto Jeremiah from the LORD in the days of Jehoiakim the son of Josiah king of Judah, saying,

2 Go unto the house of the [e]Rechabites, and speak unto them, and bring them into the house of the LORD, into one of the chambers, and give them wine to drink.

3 Then I took Jaazaniah the son of Jeremiah, the son of Habaziniah, and his brethren, and all his sons, and the whole house of the Rechabites;

4 And I brought them into the house of the LORD, into the chamber of the sons of Hanan, the son of Igdaliah, a man of God, which *was* by the chamber of the princes, which *was* above the chamber of Maaseiah the son of Shallum, [f]the keeper of the door:

5 And I set before the sons of the house of the Rechabites pots full of wine, and cups, and I said unto them, Drink ye wine.

6 But they said, We will drink no wine: for Jonadab the son of Rechab our father commanded us, saying, Ye shall drink no wine, *neither ye*, nor your sons for ever:

7 Neither shall ye build house, nor sow seed, nor plant vineyard, nor have *any*: but all your days ye shall dwell in tents; [g]that ye may live many days in the land where ye *be* strangers.

8 Thus have we obeyed the voice of Jonadab the son of Rechab our father in all that he hath charged us, to drink no wine all our days, we, our wives, our sons, nor our daughters;

9 Nor to build houses for us to dwell in: neither have we vineyard, nor field, nor seed:

10 But we have dwelt in tents, and have obeyed, and done according to all that Jonadab our father commanded us.

11 But it came to pass, when Nebuchadrezzar king of Babylon came up into the land, that we said, Come, and let us go to Jerusalem for fear of the army of the Chaldeans, and for fear of the army of the Syrians: so we dwell at Jerusalem.

12 Then came the word of the LORD unto Jeremiah, saying,

13 Thus saith the LORD of hosts, the God of Israel; Go and tell the men of

Judah and the inhabitants of Jerusalem, Will ye not receive instruction to hearken to my words? saith the LORD.

14 The words of Jonadab the son of Rechab, that he commanded his sons not to drink wine, are performed; for unto this day they drink none, but obey their father's commandment: [a]notwithstanding I have spoken unto you, [b]rising early and speaking; but ye hearkened not unto me.

15 I have sent also unto you all my servants the prophets, rising up early and sending *them*, saying, Return ye now every man from his evil way, and amend your doings, and go not after other gods to serve them, and ye shall dwell in the land which I have given to you and to your fathers: but ye have not inclined your ear, nor hearkened unto me.

16 Because the sons of Jonadab the son of Rechab have performed the commandment of their father, which he commanded them; but this people hath not hearkened unto me:

17 Therefore thus saith the LORD God of hosts, the God of Israel; Behold, I will bring upon Judah and upon all the inhabitants of Jerusalem all the evil that I have pronounced against them: [c]because I have spoken unto them, but they have not heard; and I have called unto them, but they have not answered.

18 And Jeremiah said unto the house of the Rechabites, Thus saith the LORD of hosts, the God of Israel; Because ye have obeyed the commandment of Jonadab your father, and kept all his precepts, and done according unto all that he hath commanded you:

19 Therefore thus saith the LORD of hosts, the God of Israel; Jonadab the son of Rechab shall not want a man to stand before me for ever.

CHAPTER 36.

Jeremiah's writing in the days of Jehoiakim. (Cf. vs. 27-32; Jer. 30:2.)

And it came to pass in the fourth year of [d]Jehoiakim the son of Josiah king of Judah, *that* this [e]word came unto Jeremiah from the LORD, saying,

2 Take thee [f]a roll of a book, and write therein all the words that I have spoken unto thee against Israel, and against Judah, and against all the nations, from the day I spake unto thee, from the days of Josiah, even unto this day.

3 It may be that the house of Judah will hear all the evil which I purpose to do unto them; that they may [g]return every man from his evil way; that I may forgive their iniquity and their sin.

4 Then Jeremiah called [h]Baruch the son of Neriah: and Baruch wrote from the mouth of Jeremiah all the words of the LORD, which he had spoken unto him, upon a roll of a book.

5 And Jeremiah commanded Baruch, saying, I *am* shut up; I cannot go into the house of the LORD:

6 Therefore go thou, and read in the roll, which thou hast written from my mouth, the words of the LORD in the ears of the people in the LORD'S house upon the [i]fasting day: and also thou shalt read them in the ears of all Judah that come out of their cities.

7 It may be they will present their supplication before the LORD, and will return every one from his evil way: for great *is* the anger and the fury that the LORD hath pronounced against this people.

8 And Baruch the son of Neriah did according to all that Jeremiah the prophet commanded him, reading in the book the words of the LORD in the LORD'S house.

9 And it came to pass in the fifth year of Jehoiakim the son of Josiah king of Judah, in the [j]ninth month, *that* they proclaimed a fast before the LORD to all the people in Jerusalem, and to all the people that came from the cities of Judah unto Jerusalem.

10 Then read Baruch in the book the words of Jeremiah in the house of the LORD, in the chamber of Gemariah the son of Shaphan the scribe, in the higher court, at the entry of the new gate of the LORD'S house, in the ears of all the people.

11 When Michaiah the son of Gemariah the son of Shaphan, had heard out of the book all the words of the LORD,

12 Then he went down into the king's house, into the scribe's chamber: and, lo all the princes sat there, *even* Elishama the scribe, and Delaiah the son of Shemaiah and Elnathan the son of Achbor, and Gemariah the son of Shaphan, and Zedekiah the son of Hananiah, and all the princes.

B.C. 607.

a 2 Chr. 36:15.
b Jer. 7:13; 25:3.
c Prov. 1:24; Isa. 65:12; 66:4; Jer. 7:13.
d 2 Ki. 23:34-37.
e *Inspiration.* vs. 1-32; Jer. 45:1, 2. (Ex. 4:15; Rev. 22:19.)
f Isa. 8:1; Ezk. 2:9; Zech. 5:1.
g Jer. 18:8; Jon. 3:8.
h Jer. 32:12; 45:1.
i Lev. 16:29; 23:27-32; Acts 27:9.
j i.e. *December.*

B.C. 606.

13 Then Michaiah declared unto them all the words that he had heard, when Baruch read the book in the ears of the people.

14 Therefore all the princes sent Jehudi the son of Nethaniah, the son of Shelemiah, the son of Cushi, unto Baruch, saying, Take in thine hand the roll wherein thou hast read in the ears of the people, and come. So Baruch the son of Neriah took the roll in his hand, and came unto them.

15 And they said unto him, Sit down now, and read it in our ears. So Baruch read *it* in their ears.

16 Now it came to pass, when they had heard all the words, they were afraid both one and other, and said unto Baruch, We will surely tell the king of all these words.

17 And they asked Baruch, saying, Tell us now, How didst thou write all these words at his mouth?

18 Then Baruch answered them, He pronounced all these words unto me with his mouth, and I wrote *them* with ink in the book.

19 Then said the princes unto Baruch, Go, hide thee, thou and Jeremiah; and let no man know where ye be.

20 And they went in to the king into the court, but they laid up the roll in the chamber of Elishama the scribe, and told all the words in the ears of the king.

21 So the king sent Jehudi to fetch the roll: and he took it out of Elishama the scribe's chamber. And Jehudi read it in the ears of the king, and in the ears of all the princes which stood beside the king.

22 Now the king sat in the winterhouse in the [a]ninth month: and *there was a fire* on the hearth burning before him.

23 And it came to pass, *that* when Jehudi had read three or four leaves, he cut it with the penknife, and cast *it* into the fire that *was* on the hearth, until all the roll was consumed in the fire that *was* on the hearth.

24 Yet they were not afraid, nor [b]rent their garments, *neither* the king, nor any of his servants that heard all these words.

25 Nevertheless Elnathan and Delaiah and Gemariah had made intercession to the king that he would not burn the roll: but he would not hear them.

26 But the king commanded Jerahmeel the son of Hammelech, and Seraiah the son of Azriel, and Shelemiah the son of Abdeel, to take Baruch the scribe and Jeremiah the prophet: but the LORD hid them.

The destroyed roll rewritten.
(Cf. Jer. 30:2, *note.*)

27 Then the word of the LORD came to Jeremiah, after that the king had burned the roll, and the words which Baruch wrote at the mouth of Jeremiah, saying,

28 Take thee again another roll, and write in it all the former words that were in the first roll, which Jehoiakim the king of Judah hath burned.

29 And thou shalt say to Jehoiakim king of Judah, Thus saith the LORD; Thou hast burned this roll, saying, Why hast thou written therein, saying, The king of Babylon shall certainly come and destroy this land, and shall cause to cease from thence man and beast?

30 Therefore thus saith the LORD of Jehoiakim king of Judah; [c]He shall have none to sit upon the throne of David: and his dead body shall be [d]cast out in the day to the heat, and in the night to the frost.

31 And I will punish him and his seed and his servants for their iniquity; and I will bring upon them, and upon the inhabitants of Jerusalem, and upon the men of Judah, all the evil that I have pronounced against them; but they hearkened not.

32 Then took Jeremiah another roll, and gave it to Baruch the scribe, the son of Neriah; who wrote therein from the mouth of Jeremiah all the words of the book which Jehoiakim king of Judah had burned in the fire: and there were added besides unto them many like words.

a i.e. *December.*
b 2 Ki. 22:11; Isa. 36:22; 37:1.
c Jer. 22:30.
d Jer. 22:19.

PART III. FROM THE ACCESSION TO THE CAPTIVITY OF ZEDEKIAH: CHAPTERS 37–39

B.C. 599

CHAPTER 37.

Jeremiah's imprisonment in the days of Zedekiah. (Cf. v. 11, *note.*)

And king [e]Zedekiah the son of Josiah reigned instead of Coniah the son of Jehoiakim, whom Nebuchadrezzar king of Babylon made king in the land of Judah.

2 [f]But neither he, nor his servants, nor the people of the land, did hearken unto the words of the LORD, which he spake by the prophet Jeremiah.

e 2 Ki. 24:17; 2 Chr. 36:10; Jer. 22:24.
f 2 Chr. 36:12, 14.

B.C. 599.

3 And Zedekiah the king sent Jehucal
the son of Shelemiah and Zephaniah the
son of Maaseiah the priest to the prophet
Jeremiah, saying, Pray now unto the
LORD our God for us.
4 Now Jeremiah came in and went out
among the people: for they had not put
him into prison.
5 Then [a]Pharaoh's army was come
forth out of Egypt: and when the
Chaldeans that besieged Jerusalem
heard tidings of them, they departed
from Jerusalem.
6 Then came the word of the LORD
unto the prophet Jeremiah, saying,
7 Thus saith the LORD, the God of
Israel; Thus shall ye say to the king of
Judah, that sent you unto me to enquire
of me; Behold, Pharaoh's army, which is
come forth to help you, shall return to
Egypt into their own land.
8 [b]And the Chaldeans shall come
again, and fight against this city, and
take it, and burn it with fire.
9 Thus saith the LORD; Deceive not
yourselves, saying, The Chaldeans shall
surely depart from us: for they shall not
depart.
10 For though ye had smitten the
whole army of the Chaldeans that fight
against you, and there remained *but*
wounded men among them, *yet* should
they rise up every man in his tent, and
burn this city with fire.
11 And it came to [1]pass, that when the
army of the Chaldeans was broken up
from Jerusalem for fear of Pharaoh's
army,
12 Then Jeremiah went forth out of
Jerusalem to go into the land of
Benjamin, to separate himself thence in
the midst of the people.
13 And when he was in the gate of
Benjamin, a captain of the ward *was*
there, whose name *was* Irijah, the son of
Shelemiah, the son of Hananiah; and he
took Jeremiah the prophet, saying, Thou
fallest away to the Chaldeans.
14 Then said Jeremiah, *It is* false; I fall
not away to the Chaldeans. But he hearkened not to him: so Irijah took Jeremiah,
and brought him to the princes.
15 Wherefore the princes were wroth
with Jeremiah, and smote him, [c]and put
him in prison in the house of Jonathan the
scribe: for they had made that the prison.
16 When Jeremiah was entered into the
dungeon, and into the cabins, and
Jeremiah had remained there many days;
17 Then Zedekiah the king sent, and
took him out: and the king asked him
secretly in his house, and said, Is there *any*
word from the LORD? And Jeremiah said,
There is: for, said he, thou shalt be delivered into the hand of the king of Babylon.
18 Moreover Jeremiah said unto king
Zedekiah, What have I offended against
thee, or against thy servants, or against
this people, that ye have put me in
prison?
19 Where *are* now your prophets
which prophesied unto you, saying, The
king of Babylon shall not come against
you, nor against this land?
20 Therefore hear now, I pray thee, O
my lord the king: let my supplication, I
pray thee, be accepted before thee; that
thou cause me not to return to the house
of Jonathan the scribe, lest I die there.
21 Then Zedekiah the king commanded
that they should commit Jeremiah [d]into
the court of the prison, and that they
should give him daily a piece of bread out
of the bakers' street, [e]until all the bread in
the city were spent. Thus Jeremiah
remained in the court of the prison.

CHAPTER 38.

(*Jeremiah's imprisonment*, continued.)

Then Shephatiah the son of Mattan,
and Gedaliah the son of Pashur, and
Jucal the son of Shelemiah, and Pashur
the son of Malchiah, heard the words
that Jeremiah had spoken unto all the
people, saying,
2 Thus saith the LORD, He that
remaineth in this city shall die by the

a See 2 Ki. 24:7; Ezk. 17:15.
b Jer. 34:22.
c Jer. 38:26.
d Jer. 32:2; 38:13, 28.
e Jer. 38:9; 52:6.

[1] **(37:11)** Five phases of Jeremiah's prison experiences are recorded: (1) He is arrested in the gate and committed to a dungeon on the false charge of treason (Jer. 37:11-15); (2) he is released from the dungeon, but restrained to the court of the prison; (3) he is imprisoned in the miry dungeon of Malchiah (Jer. 38:1-6); (4) he is again released from the dungeon and kept in the prison court (Jer. 38:13-28) until the capture of the city; (5) carried in chains from the city by Nebuzar-adan, captain of the guard, he is finally released at Ramah (Jer. 40:1-4).

sword, by the famine, and by the pestilence: but he that goeth forth to the Chaldeans shall live; for he shall have his life for a prey, and shall live.

3 Thus saith the LORD, [a]This city shall
surely be given into the hand of the king of Babylon's army, which shall take it.

4 Therefore the princes said unto the
king, We beseech thee, [b]let this man be put to death: for thus he weakeneth the hands of the men of war that remain in this city, and the hands of all the people, in speaking such words unto them: for this man seeketh not the welfare of this people, but the hurt.

5 Then Zedekiah the king said, Behold,
he *is* in your hand: for the king *is* not *he that* can do *any* thing against you.

6 [c]Then took they Jeremiah, and cast
him into the dungeon of Malchiah the son of Hammelech, that *was* in the court of the prison: and they let down Jeremiah with cords. And in the dungeon *there was* no water, but mire: so Jeremiah sunk in the mire.

7 [d]Now when Ebed-melech the
Ethiopian, one of the eunuchs which was in the king's house, heard that they had put Jeremiah in the dungeon; the king then sitting in the gate of Benjamin;

8 Ebed-melech went forth out of the
king's house, and spake to the king, saying,

9 My lord the king, these men have
done evil in all that they have done to Jeremiah the prophet, whom they have cast into the dungeon; and he is like to die for hunger in the place where he is: for *there is* no more bread in the city.

10 Then the king commanded Ebed-
melech the Ethiopian, saying, Take from hence thirty men with thee, and take up Jeremiah the prophet out of the dungeon, before he die.

11 So Ebed-melech took the men with
him, and went into the house of the king under the treasury, and took thence old cast clouts and old rotten rags, and let them down by cords into the dungeon to Jeremiah.

12 And Ebed-melech the Ethiopian
said unto Jeremiah, Put now *these* old cast clouts and rotten rags under thine armholes under the cords. And Jeremiah did so.

13 So they drew up Jeremiah with
cords, and took him up out of the dungeon: and Jeremiah remained in the court of the prison.

14 Then Zedekiah the king sent, and
took Jeremiah the prophet unto him into the third entry that *is* in the house of the LORD: and the king said unto Jeremiah, I will ask thee a thing; hide nothing from me.

15 Then Jeremiah said unto Zedekiah,
If I declare *it* unto thee, wilt thou not surely put me to death? and if I give thee counsel, wilt thou not hearken unto me?

16 So Zedekiah the king sware secretly
unto Jeremiah, saying, *As* the LORD liveth, [e]that made us this soul, I will not put thee to death, neither will I give thee into the hand of these men that seek thy life.

17 Then said Jeremiah unto Zedekiah,
Thus saith the LORD, the God of hosts, the God of Israel; If thou wilt assuredly [f]go forth unto the king of Babylon's princes, then thy soul shall live, and this city shall not be burned with fire; and thou shalt live, and thine house:

18 But if thou wilt not go forth to the
king of Babylon's princes, then shall this city be given into the hand of the Chaldeans, and they shall burn it with fire, and thou shalt not escape out of their hand.

19 And Zedekiah the king said unto
Jeremiah, I am afraid of the Jews that are fallen to the Chaldeans, lest they deliver me into their hand, and they mock me.

20 But Jeremiah said, They shall not
deliver *thee*. Obey, I beseech thee, the voice of the LORD, which I speak unto thee: so it shall be well unto thee, and thy soul shall live.

21 But if thou refuse to go forth, this *is*
the word that the LORD hath shewed me:

22 And, behold, all the women that
are left in the king of Judah's house *shall be* brought forth to the king of Babylon's princes, and those *women* shall say, Thy friends have set thee on, and have prevailed against thee: thy feet are sunk in the mire, *and* they are turned away back.

23 So they shall bring out all thy wives
and [g]thy children to the Chaldeans: and [h]thou shalt not escape out of their hand, but shalt be taken by the hand of the king of Babylon: and thou shalt cause this city to be burned with fire.

24 Then said Zedekiah unto Jeremiah,

B.C. 589.

a Jer. 21:10; 32:3.

b See Jer. 26:11. The fundamental reason why the prophetic warnings of the Old and New Testaments are unwelcome to an unreasoning optimism.

c Jer. 37:11, *note.*

d Jer. 39:16.

e Isa. 57:16.

f 2 Ki. 24:12.

g Jer. 39:6; 41:10.

h v. 18.

Let no man know of these words, and thou shalt not die.

25 But if the princes hear that I have talked with thee, and they come unto thee, and say unto thee, Declare unto us now what thou hast said unto the king, hide it not from us, and we will not put thee to death; also what the king said unto thee:

26 Then thou shalt say unto them, I [a]presented my supplication before the king, that he would not cause me to return [b]to Jonathan's house, to die there.

27 Then came all the princes unto Jeremiah, and asked him: and he told them according to all these words that the king had commanded. So they left off speaking with him; for the matter was not perceived.

28 So [c]Jeremiah abode in the court of the prison until the day that Jerusalem was taken: and he was *there* when Jerusalem was taken.

CHAPTER 39.

The final captivity of Judah. (Cf. 2 Ki. 25:1-7; 2 Chr. 36:17-21; Jer. 52:4-17.)

In the [d]ninth year of Zedekiah king of Judah, in the [e]tenth month, came Nebuchadrezzar king of Babylon and all his army against Jerusalem, and they besieged it.

2 *And* in the eleventh year of Zedekiah, in the [f]fourth month, the ninth *day* of the month, the city was broken up.

3 And all the princes of the king of Babylon came in, and sat in the middle gate, *even* Nergal-sharezer, Samgar-nebo, Sarsechim, Rab-saris, Nergal-sharezer, Rab-mag, with all the residue of the princes of the king of Babylon.

4 [g]And it came to pass, *that* when Zedekiah the king of Judah saw them, and all the men of war, then they fled, and went forth out of the city by night, by the way of the king's garden, by the gate betwixt the two walls: and he went out the way of the plain.

5 But the Chaldeans' army pursued after them, and [h]overtook Zedekiah in the plains of Jericho: and when they had taken him, they brought him up to Nebuchadnezzar king of Babylon to [i]Riblah in the land of Hamath, where he gave judgment upon him.

6 Then the king of Babylon slew the sons of Zedekiah in Riblah before his eyes: also the king of Babylon slew all the nobles of Judah.

7 Moreover he put out Zedekiah's [j]eyes, and bound him with chains, to carry him to [1]Babylon.

8 And the [k]Chaldeans burned the king's house, and the houses of the people, with fire, and brake down the walls of Jerusalem.

9 Then Nebuzar-adan the captain of the guard carried away captive into Babylon the remnant of the people that remained in the city, and those that fell away, that fell to him, with the rest of the people that remained.

10 But Nebuzar-adan the captain of the guard left of the poor of the people, which had nothing, in the land of Judah, and gave them vineyards and fields at the same time.

11 Now Nebuchadrezzar king of Babylon gave charge concerning Jeremiah to Nebuzar-adan the captain of the guard, saying,

12 Take him, and look well to him, and do him no harm; but do unto him even as he shall say unto thee.

13 So Nebuzar-adan the captain of the guard sent, and Nebushasban, Rab-saris, and Nergal-sharezer, Rab-mag, and all the king of Babylon's princes;

14 Even they sent, and took Jeremiah out of the court of the prison, and committed him unto Gedaliah the son of Ahikam the son of Shaphan, that he should carry him home: so he dwelt among the people.

15 Now the word of the LORD came unto Jeremiah, while he was shut up in the court of the prison, saying,

16 Go and speak to Ebed-melech the Ethiopian, saying, Thus saith the LORD of hosts, the God of Israel; Behold, [l]I will bring my words upon this city for evil, and not for good; and they shall be

B.C. 589.

a Jer. 37:20.
b Jer. 37:15.
c Jer. 37:21; 39:14.
d 2 Ki. 25:1-4.
e i.e. *January.*
f i.e. *July.*
g 2 Ki. 25:4; Jer. 52:7.
h Jer. 32:4; 38:18, 23.
i 2 Ki. 23:33.
j Jer. 32:4; Ezk. 12:13.
k 2 Ki. 25:9; Jer. 38:18; 52:13.
l Dan. 9:12.

[1] **(39:7)** Here began the "times of the Gentiles," the mark of which is that Jerusalem is "trodden down of the Gentiles," i.e. under Gentile overlordship. This has been true from the time of Nebuchadnezzar to this day. See "Times of the Gentiles" (Lk. 21:24, *note;* Rev. 16:19, *note*).

accomplished in that day before thee.

17 But I will deliver thee in that day, saith the LORD: and thou shalt not be given into the hand of the men of whom thou *art* afraid.

18 For I will surely deliver thee, and thou shalt not fall by the sword, but thy life shall be for a prey unto thee: [a]because thou hast put thy [b]trust in me, saith the LORD.

B.C. 588.

a 1 Chr. 5:20; Psa. 37:40.

b Psa. 2:12, *note*.

PART IV. JEREMIAH'S PROPHECIES AMONGST THE REMNANT IN THE LAND, AFTER THE CAPTIVITY OF ZEDEKIAH: CHAPTERS 40–42

CHAPTER 40.

The word that came to Jeremiah from the LORD, [c]after that Nebuzar-adan the captain of the guard had let him go from Ramah, when he had taken him being bound in chains among all that were carried away captive of Jerusalem and Judah, which were carried away captive unto Babylon.

2 And the captain of the guard took Jeremiah, and said unto him, The LORD thy God hath pronounced this evil upon this place.

3 Now the LORD hath brought *it*, and done according as he hath said: [d]because ye have sinned against the LORD, and have not obeyed his voice, therefore this thing is come upon you.

4 And now, behold, I loose thee this day from the chains which *were* upon thine hand. If it seem good unto thee to come with me into Babylon, come; and I will look well unto thee: but if it seem ill unto thee to come with me into Babylon, forbear: behold, [e]all the land *is* before thee: whither it seemeth good and convenient for thee to go, thither go.

5 Now while he was not yet gone back, *he said*, Go back also to Gedaliah the son of Ahikam the son of Shaphan, [f]whom the king of Babylon hath made governor over the cities of Judah, and dwell with him among the people: or go wheresoever it seemeth convenient unto thee to go. So the captain of the guard gave him victuals and a reward, and let him go.

6 Then went Jeremiah unto Gedaliah the son of Ahikam to [g]Mizpah; and dwelt with him among the people that were left in the land.

7 [h]Now when all the captains of the forces which *were* in the fields, *even* they and their men, heard that the king of Babylon had made Gedaliah the son of Ahikam governor in the land, and had committed unto him men, and women, and children, and of the poor of the land, of them that were not carried away captive to Babylon;

8 Then they came to Gedaliah to Mizpah, even Ishmael the son of Nethaniah, and Johanan and Jonathan the sons of Kareah, and Seraiah the son of Tanhumeth, and the sons of Ephai the Netophathite, and Jezaniah the son of a Maachathite, they and their men.

9 And Gedaliah the son of Ahikam the son of Shaphan sware unto them and to their men, saying, Fear not to serve the Chaldeans: dwell in the land, and serve the king of Babylon, and it shall be well with you.

10 As for me, behold, I will dwell at Mizpah to serve the Chaldeans, which will come unto us: but ye, gather ye wine, and summer fruits, and oil, and put *them* in your vessels, and dwell in your cities that ye have taken.

11 Likewise when all the Jews that *were* in Moab, and among the Ammonites, and in Edom, and that *were* in all the countries, heard that the king of Babylon had left a remnant of Judah, and that he had set over them Gedaliah the son of Ahikam the son of Shaphan;

12 Even all the Jews returned out of all places whither they were driven, and came to the land of Judah, to Gedaliah, unto Mizpah, and gathered wine and summer fruits very much.

13 Moreover Johanan the son of Kareah, and all the captains of the forces that *were* in the fields, came to Gedaliah to Mizpah,

14 And said unto him, Dost thou certainly know that [i]Baalis the king of the Ammonites hath sent Ishmael the son of Nethaniah to slay thee? But Gedaliah the son of Ahikam believed them not.

15 Then Johanan the son of Kareah spake to Gedaliah in Mizpah secretly, saying, Let me go, I pray thee, and I will

B.C. 588.

c Jer. 39:14.

d Deut. 29:24, 25; Dan. 9:11.

e Gen. 20:15.

f 2 Ki. 25:22.

g Jud. 20:1.

h 2 Ki. 25:23.

i Jer. 41:10.

slay Ishmael the son of Nethaniah, and no man shall know *it*: wherefore should he slay thee, that all the Jews which are gathered unto thee should be scattered, and the remnant in Judah perish?

16 But Gedaliah the son of Ahikam said unto Johanan the son of Kareah, Thou shalt not do this thing: for thou speakest falsely of Ishmael.

CHAPTER 41.

(*Jeremiah's prophecies to the remnant in the land,* continued.)

Now it came to pass in the [a]seventh month, [b]*that* Ishmael the son of Nethaniah the son of Elishama, of the seed royal, and the princes of the king, even ten men with him, came unto Gedaliah the son of Ahikam to Mizpah; and there they did eat bread together in Mizpah.

2 Then arose Ishmael the son of Nethaniah, and the ten men that were with him, and [c]smote Gedaliah the son of Ahikam the son of Shaphan with the sword, and slew him, whom the king of Babylon had made governor over the land.

3 Ishmael also slew all the Jews that were with him, *even* with Gedaliah, at Mizpah, and the Chaldeans that were found there, *and* the men of war.

4 And it came to pass the second day after he had slain Gedaliah, and no man knew *it,*

5 That there came certain from Shechem, from Shiloh, and from Samaria, *even* fourscore men, having their beards shaven, and their clothes rent, and having cut themselves, with offerings and incense in their hand, to bring *them* to [d]the house of the LORD.

6 And Ishmael the son of Nethaniah went forth from Mizpah to meet them, weeping all along as he went: and it came to pass, as he met them, he said unto them, Come to Gedaliah the son of Ahikam.

7 And it was *so,* when they came into the midst of the city, that Ishmael the son of Nethaniah slew them, *and cast them* into the midst of the pit, he, and the men that *were* with him.

8 But ten men were found among them that said unto Ishmael, Slay us not: for we have treasures in the field, of wheat, and of barley, and of oil, and of honey. So he forbare, and slew them not among their brethren.

9 Now the pit wherein Ishmael had cast all the dead bodies of the men, whom he had slain because of Gedaliah, *was* it [e]which Asa the king had made for fear of Baasha king of Israel: *and* Ishmael the son of Nethaniah filled it with *them that were* slain.

10 Then Ishmael carried away captive all the residue of the people that *were* in Mizpah, *even* the king's daughters, and all the people that remained in Mizpah, whom Nebuzar-adan the captain of the guard had committed to Gedaliah the son of Ahikam: and Ishmael the son of Nethaniah carried them away captive, and departed to go over to the [f]Ammonites.

11 But when Johanan the son of Kareah, and all the captains of the forces that *were* with him, heard of all the evil that Ishmael the son of Nethaniah had done,

12 Then they took all the men, and went to fight with Ishmael the son of Nethaniah, and found him by [g]the great waters that *are* in Gibeon.

13 Now it came to pass, *that* when all the people which *were* with Ishmael saw Johanan the son of Kareah, and all the captains of the forces that *were* with him, then they were glad.

14 So all the people that Ishmael had carried away captive from Mizpah cast about and returned, and went unto Johanan the son of Kareah.

15 But Ishmael the son of Nethaniah escaped from Johanan with eight men, and went to the Ammonites.

16 Then took Johanan the son of Kareah, and all the captains of the forces that *were* with him, all the remnant of the people whom he had recovered from Ishmael the son of Nethaniah, from Mizpah, after *that* he had slain Gedaliah the son of Ahikam, *even* mighty men of war, and the women, and the children, and the eunuchs, whom he had brought again from Gibeon:

17 And they departed, and dwelt in the habitation of [h]Chimham, which is by Beth-lehem, to go to enter into Egypt,

18 Because of the Chaldeans: for they were afraid of them, because Ishmael the son of Nethaniah had slain Gedaliah the

B.C. 588.

a i.e. *October.*
b 2 Ki. 25:25; Jer. 40:8.
c 2 Ki. 25:25.
d See 1 Sam. 1:7; 2 Ki. 25:9.
e 1 Ki. 15:22; 2 Chr. 16:6.
f Jer. 40:14.
g 2 Sam. 2:13.
h 2 Sam. 19:37, 38.

son of Ahikam, whom the king of
Babylon made governor in the land.

CHAPTER 42.

Then all the captains of the forces, and
[a]Johanan the son of Kareah, and
Jezaniah the son of Hoshaiah, and all the
people from the least even unto the
greatest, came near,
2 And said unto Jeremiah the prophet,
Let, we beseech thee, our supplication be
accepted before thee, and [b]pray for us
unto the LORD thy God, *even* for all this
remnant; (for we are left *but* a few of
many, as thine eyes do behold us:)
3 That the LORD thy God may shew us
[c]the way wherein we may walk, and the
thing that we may do.
4 Then Jeremiah the prophet said unto
them, I have heard *you*; behold, I will
pray unto the LORD your God according
to your words; and it shall come to pass,
that [d]whatsoever thing the LORD shall
answer you, I will declare *it* unto you; I
will [e]keep nothing back from you.
5 Then they said to Jeremiah, [f]The
LORD be a true and faithful witness
between us, if we do not even according
to all things for the which the LORD thy
God shall send thee to us.
6 Whether *it be* good, or whether *it be*
evil, we will obey the voice of the LORD
our God, to whom we send thee; [g]that it
may be well with us, when we obey the
voice of the LORD our God.
7 And it came to pass after ten days,
that the word of the LORD came unto
Jeremiah.
8 Then called he Johanan the son of
Kareah, and all the captains of the forces
which *were* with him, and all the people
from the least even to the greatest,
9 And said unto them, Thus saith the
LORD, the God of Israel, unto whom ye
sent me to present your supplication
before him;
10 If ye will still abide in this land,
then will I build you, and not pull *you*
down, and I will plant you, and not
pluck *you* up: for I [h]repent me of the evil
that I have done unto you.
11 Be not afraid of the king of Babylon,
of whom ye are afraid; be not afraid of
him, saith the LORD: for I *am* with you to
save you, and to deliver you from his
hand.

B.C. 588.

a Jer. 40:8, 13; 41:11
b 1 Sam. 7:8; 12:19; Isa. 37:4; Jas. 5:16.
c Ezra 8:21.
d 1 Ki. 22:14.
e 1 Sam. 3:18; Acts 20:20.
f Gen. 31:50.
g Deut. 6:3; Jer. 7:23.
h Zech. 8:14, *note.*
i Deut. 17:16; Jer. 44:12-14.
j Lk. 9:51.
k Ezk. 11:8.
l See Jer. 44:14, 28.
m Jer. 18:16; 24:9; 26:6; 29:18; 44:12; Zech. 8:13.
n Deut. 17:16.
o v. 17; Ezk. 6:11.

12 And I will shew mercies unto you,
that he may have mercy upon you, and
cause you to return to your own land.
13 But if ye say, We will not dwell in
this land, neither obey the voice of the
LORD your God,
14 Saying, No; but we will go into the
land of Egypt, where we shall see no
war, nor hear the sound of the trumpet,
nor have hunger of bread; and there will
we dwell:
15 And now therefore hear the word
of the LORD, ye remnant of Judah; Thus
saith the LORD of hosts, the God of Israel;
If ye [i]wholly set your [j]faces to enter into
Egypt, and go to sojourn there;
16 Then it shall come to pass, *that* the
sword, [k]which ye feared, shall overtake
you there in the land of Egypt, and the
famine, whereof ye were afraid, shall
follow close after you there in Egypt;
and there ye shall die.
17 So shall it be with all the men that
set their faces to go into Egypt to sojourn
there; they shall die by the sword, by the
famine, and by the pestilence: and [l]none
of them shall remain or escape from the
evil that I will bring upon them.
18 For thus saith the LORD of hosts, the
God of Israel; As mine anger and my
fury hath been poured forth upon the
inhabitants of Jerusalem; so shall my
fury be poured forth upon you, when ye
shall enter into Egypt: and ye shall be an
[m]execration, and an astonishment, and a
curse, and a reproach; and ye shall see
this place no more.
19 The LORD hath said concerning you,
O ye remnant of Judah; [n]Go ye not into
Egypt: know certainly that I have
admonished you this day.
20 For ye dissembled in your hearts,
when ye sent me unto the LORD your
God, saying, Pray for us unto the LORD
our God; and according unto all that the
LORD our God shall say, so declare unto
us, and we will do *it*.
21 And *now* I have this day declared *it*
to you; but ye have not obeyed the voice
of the LORD your God, nor any *thing* for
the which he hath sent me unto you.
22 Now therefore know certainly that
[o]ye shall die by the sword, by the
famine, and by the pestilence, in the
place whither ye desire to go *and* to
sojourn.

PART V. JEREMIAH'S MINISTRY IN EGYPT: CHAPTERS 43, 44

B.C. 588.

CHAPTER 43.

Jeremiah carried to Tahpanhes in Egypt.

And it came to pass, *that* when
Jeremiah had made an end of
speaking unto all the people all the
words of the LORD their God, for which
the LORD their God had sent him to
them, *even* all these words,
2 Then [a]spake Azariah the son of
Hoshaiah, and Johanan the son of
Kareah, and all the proud men, saying
unto Jeremiah, Thou speakest falsely:
the LORD our God hath not sent thee to
say, Go not into Egypt to sojourn there:
3 But Baruch the son of Neriah setteth
thee on against us, for to deliver us into
the hand of the Chaldeans, that they
might put us to death, and carry us
away captives into Babylon.
4 So Johanan the son of Kareah, and
all the captains of the forces, and all the
people, obeyed not the voice of the
LORD, to dwell in the land of Judah.
5 But Johanan the son of Kareah, and
all the captains of the forces, took [b]all the
remnant of Judah, that were returned
from all nations, whither they had been
driven, to dwell in the land of Judah;
6 *Even* men, and women, and children,
and [c]the king's daughters, [d]and every
person that Nebuzar-adan the captain of
the guard had left with Gedaliah the son
of Ahikam the son of Shaphan, and
Jeremiah the prophet, and Baruch the
son of Neriah.
7 So they came into the land of Egypt:
for they obeyed not the voice of the
LORD: thus came they *even* to [e]Tahpan-
hes.

The sign of the hidden stones.

8 Then came the word of the LORD
unto Jeremiah in Tahpanhes, saying,
9 Take great stones in thine hand, and
hide them in the clay in the brickkiln,
which *is* at the entry of Pharaoh's house
in Tahpanhes, in the sight of the men of
Judah;
10 And say unto them, Thus saith the
LORD of hosts, the God of Israel; Behold,
I will send and take Nebuchadrezzar the
king of Babylon, [f]my servant, and will
set his throne upon these stones that I
have hid; and he shall spread his royal
pavilion over them.
11 And when he cometh, he shall
smite the land of Egypt, *and deliver* [g]such
as are for death to death; and such *as are*
for captivity to captivity; and such *as are*
for the sword to the sword.
12 And I will kindle a fire in the houses of the gods of Egypt; and he shall
burn them, and carry them away captives: and he shall array himself with the
land of Egypt, as a shepherd putteth on
his garment; and he shall go forth from
thence in peace.
13 He shall break also the images of
Beth-shemesh, that *is* in the land of
Egypt; and the houses of the gods of the
Egyptians shall he burn with fire.

CHAPTER 44.

The message to the Jews in Egypt.

The word that came to Jeremiah concerning all the Jews which dwell in
the land of Egypt, which dwell at
Migdol, and at Tahpanhes, and at Noph,
and in the country of Pathros, saying,
2 Thus saith the LORD of hosts, the
God of Israel; Ye have seen all the evil
that I have brought upon Jerusalem, and
upon all the cities of Judah; and, behold,
this day they *are* a [h]desolation, and no
man dwelleth therein,
3 Because of their wickedness which
they have committed to provoke me to
anger, in that they went to burn incense,
and to [i]serve other gods, whom they knew
not, *neither* they, ye, nor your fathers.
4 Howbeit [j]I sent unto you all my servants the prophets, rising early and
sending *them*, saying, Oh, do not this
abominable thing that I hate.
5 But they hearkened not, nor inclined
their ear to turn from their wickedness,
to burn no incense unto other gods.
6 Wherefore my fury and mine anger
was poured forth, and was kindled in
the cities of Judah and in the streets of
Jerusalem; and they are wasted *and* desolate, as at this day.
7 Therefore now thus saith the LORD,
the God of hosts, the God of Israel;
Wherefore commit ye *this* great evil
[k]against your souls, to cut off from you

a Jer. 42:1.
b Jer. 40:11, 12.
c Jer. 41:10.
d Jer. 39:10; 40:7.
e Jer. 2:16; 44:1. Called *Hanes*, Isa. 30:4.
f Jer. 25:9; 27:6. See Ezk. 29:18, 20.
g Jer. 15:2; Zech. 11:9.
h Jer. 9:11; 34:22.
i Deut. 13:6; 32:17.
j 2 Chr. 36:15; Jer. 7:25; 25:4; 26:5; 29:19.
k Num. 16:38; Jer. 7:19.

man and woman, child and suckling, out of Judah, to leave you none to remain;

8 In that ye provoke me unto wrath with the works of your hands, burning incense unto other gods in the land of Egypt, whither ye be gone to dwell, that ye might cut yourselves off, and that ye might be a curse and a reproach among all the nations of the earth?

9 Have ye forgotten the wickedness of your fathers, and the wickedness of the kings of Judah, and the wickedness of their wives, and your own wickedness, and the wickedness of your wives, which they have committed in the land of Judah, and in the streets of Jerusalem?

10 They are not humbled *even* unto this day, neither have they [a]feared, nor walked in my law, nor in my statutes, that I set before you and before your fathers.

11 Therefore thus saith the LORD of hosts, the God of Israel; Behold, I [b]will set my face against you for evil, and to cut off all Judah.

12 And I will take the remnant of Judah, that have set their faces to go into the land of Egypt to sojourn there, and [c]they shall all be consumed, *and* fall in the land of Egypt; they shall *even* be consumed by the sword *and* by the famine: they shall die, from the least even unto the greatest, by the sword and by the famine: and [d]they shall be an execration, *and* an astonishment, and a curse, and a reproach.

13 For [e]I will punish them that dwell in the land of Egypt, as I have punished Jerusalem, by the sword, by the famine, and by the pestilence:

14 So that none of the remnant of Judah, which are gone into the land of Egypt to sojourn there, shall escape or remain, that they should return into the land of Judah, to the which they have a desire to return to dwell there: for none shall return but such as shall escape.

15 Then all the men which knew that their wives had burned incense unto other gods, and all the women that stood by, a great multitude, even all the people that dwelt in the land of Egypt, in Pathros, answered Jeremiah, saying,

16 *As for* the word that thou hast spoken unto us in the name of the LORD, we will not hearken unto thee.

17 But we will certainly do [f]whatsoever thing goeth forth out of our own mouth, to burn incense unto the [g]queen of heaven, and to pour out drink-offerings unto her, as we have done, we, and our fathers, our kings, and our princes, in the cities of Judah, and in the streets of Jerusalem: for *then* had we plenty of victuals, and were well, and saw no evil.

18 But since we left off to burn incense to the queen of heaven, and to pour out drink-offerings unto her, we have wanted all *things*, and have been consumed by the sword and by the famine.

19 And when we burned incense to the queen of heaven, and poured out drink-offerings unto her, did we make her cakes to worship her, and pour out drink-offerings unto her, without our men?

20 Then Jeremiah said unto all the people, to the men, and to the women, and to all the people which had given him *that* answer, saying,

21 The incense that ye burned in the cities of Judah, and in the streets of Jerusalem, ye, and your fathers, your kings, and your princes, and the people of the land, did not the LORD remember them, and came it *not* into his mind?

22 So that the LORD could no longer bear, because of the evil of your doings, *and* because of the abominations which ye have committed; therefore is your land a desolation, and an astonishment, and a curse, without an inhabitant, as at this day.

23 Because ye have burned incense, and because ye have sinned against the LORD, and have not obeyed the voice of the LORD, nor walked in his law, nor in his statutes, nor in his testimonies; therefore this evil is happened unto you, as at this day.

24 Moreover Jeremiah said unto all the people, and to all the women, Hear the word of the LORD, all Judah that *are* in the land of Egypt:

25 Thus saith the LORD of hosts, the God of Israel, saying; Ye and your wives have both spoken with your mouths, and fulfilled with your hand, saying, We will surely perform our vows that we have vowed, to burn incense to the queen of heaven, and to pour out drink-offerings unto her: ye will surely

B.C. 587.

a Psa. 19:9, *note*.

b Lev. 17:10; 20:5, 6; Jer. 21:10; Amos 9:4.

c Jer. 42:15-17, 22.

d Jer. 42:18.

e Jer. 43:11.

f See v. 25; Num. 30:12, 14; Deut. 23:23; Jud. 11, 36.

g See Jud. 2:13, *note*.

B.C. 587.

accomplish your vows, and surely perform your vows.

26 Therefore hear ye the word of the LORD, all Judah that dwell in the land of Egypt; Behold, [a]I have sworn by my great name, saith the LORD, that [b]my name shall no more be named in the mouth of any man of Judah in all the land of Egypt, saying, The Lord GOD liveth.

27 Behold, [c]I will watch over them for evil, and not for good: and all the men of Judah that *are* in the land of Egypt shall be consumed by the sword and by the famine, until there be an end of them.

28 [d]Yet a small number that escape the sword shall return out of the land of Egypt into the land of Judah, and all the remnant of Judah, that are gone into the land of Egypt to sojourn there, shall know whose words shall stand, mine, or theirs.

29 And this *shall be* a sign unto you, saith the LORD, that I will punish you in this place, that ye may know that my words shall [e]surely stand against you for evil:

30 Thus saith the LORD; Behold, I will give [f]Pharaoh-hophra king of Egypt into the hand of his enemies, and into the hand of them that seek his life; as I gave Zedekiah king of Judah into the hand of Nebuchadrezzar king of Babylon, his enemy, and that sought his life.

a Heb. 6:13.
b Ezk. 20:39.
c Jer. 31:28.
d v. 14; Isa. 27:13.
e Psa. 33:11.
f Jer. 46:25, 26; Ezk. 29:3; 30:21.

PART VI. MISCELLANEOUS PROPHECIES: CHAPTERS 45–52

B.C. 607.

CHAPTER 45.

A message to Baruch in the days of Jehoiakim.
(Cf. 2 Ki. 23:34–25:6; Jer. 36:1-32.)

The word that Jeremiah the prophet spake unto Baruch the son of Neriah, when he had written these words in a book at the mouth of Jeremiah, in the fourth year of Jehoiakim the son of Josiah king of Judah, saying,

2 [g]Thus saith the LORD, the God of Israel, unto thee, O Baruch;

3 Thou didst say, Woe is me now! for the LORD hath added grief to my sorrow; I fainted in my sighing, and I find no rest.

4 Thus shalt thou say unto him, The LORD saith thus; Behold, *that* which I have built will I break down, and that which I have planted I will pluck up, even this whole land.

5 And seekest thou great things for thyself? seek *them* not: for, behold, I will bring evil upon all flesh, saith the LORD: but thy life will I give unto thee [h]for a prey in all places whither thou goest.

CHAPTER 46.

Prophecies against Gentile powers
(Jer. 46:1–51:64).

The word of the LORD which came to Jeremiah the prophet against the [1]Gentiles;

(1) *Against Egypt.*

2 Against Egypt, [i]against the army of Pharaoh-necho king of Egypt, which was by the river Euphrates in Carchemish, which Nebuchadrezzar king of Babylon smote in the fourth year of Jehoiakim the son of Josiah king of Judah.

3 Order ye the buckler and shield, and draw near to battle.

4 Harness the horses; and get up, ye horsemen, and stand forth with *your* helmets; furbish the spears, *and* put on the brigandines.

5 Wherefore have I seen them dismayed *and* turned away back? and their mighty ones are beaten down, and are fled apace, and look not back: *for* fear *was* round about, saith the LORD.

6 Let not the swift flee away, nor the mighty man escape; [j]they shall stumble, and fall toward the north by the river Euphrates.

7 Who *is* this *that* cometh up [k]as a flood, whose waters are moved as the rivers?

8 Egypt riseth up like a flood, and *his* waters are moved like the rivers; and he saith, I will go up, *and* will cover the earth; I will destroy the city and the inhabitants thereof.

9 Come up, ye horses; and rage, ye chariots; and let the mighty men come forth; the Ethiopians and the Libyans

g *Inspiration.* vs. 1, 2; Ezk. 2:2. (Ex. 4:15; Rev. 22:19.)
h Jer. 21:9; 38:2; 39:18.
i 2 Ki. 23:29; 2 Chr. 35:20.
j Dan. 11:19.
k Isa. 8:7, 8; Jer. 47:2; Dan. 11:22.

1 **(46:1)** A near and a far fulfilment of these prophecies against Gentile powers are to be distinguished. In Chapter 46 the near vision is of a Babylonian invasion of Egypt, but verses 27, 28 look forward to the judgment of the nations (Mt. 25:32, *note*) after Armageddon (Rev. 16:14; Rev. 19:17, *note*).

that handle the shield; and the Lydians,
that handle *and* bend the bow.
10 For this *is* the [a]day of the Lord GOD
of hosts, a day of vengeance, that he may
avenge him of his adversaries: and the
sword shall devour, and it shall be satiate
and made drunk with their blood: for the
Lord GOD of hosts hath a sacrifice in the
north country by the river Euphrates.
11 Go up into Gilead, and take balm,
O virgin, the daughter of Egypt: in vain
shalt thou use many medicines; *for* thou
shalt not be cured.
12 The nations have heard of thy
shame, and thy cry hath filled the land:
for the mighty man hath stumbled
against the mighty, *and* they are fallen
both together.
13 The word that the LORD spake to
Jeremiah the prophet, how Nebuchadrezzar king of Babylon should come *and*
[b]smite the land of Egypt.
14 Declare ye in Egypt, and publish in
Migdol, and publish in Noph and in
Tahpanhes: say ye, Stand fast, and prepare thee; for the sword shall devour
round about thee.
15 Why are thy valiant *men* swept
away? they stood not, because the LORD
did drive them.
16 He made many to fall, yea, one fell
upon another: and they said, Arise, and
let us go again to our own people, and to
the land of our nativity, from the
oppressing sword.
17 They did cry there, Pharaoh king of
Egypt *is but* a noise; he hath passed the
ime appointed.
18 *As* I live, saith the King, [c]whose
name *is* the LORD of hosts, Surely as
Tabor *is* among the mountains, and as
Carmel by the sea, *so* shall he come.
19 O thou daughter dwelling in Egypt,
furnish thyself to go into captivity: for
Noph shall be waste and desolate without an inhabitant.
20 Egypt *is like* a very fair heifer, *but*
destruction cometh; it cometh [d]out of the
north.
21 Also her hired men *are* in the midst
of her like fatted bullocks; for they also
are turned back, *and* are fled away
together: they did not stand, because the
lay of their calamity was come upon
hem, *and* the time of their visitation.

B.C. 607.

a See *Day (of Jehovah)*. Isa. 2:10-22.

b Isa. 19:1; Jer. 43:10, 11; Ezk. 29.

c Isa. 47:4; 48:2.

d vs. 6, 10; Jer. 1:14; 47:2.

e Isa. 10:34.

f Ezk. 30:14-16; Nah. 3:8.

g Psa. 2:12, *note*.

h Jer. 44:30; Ezk. 32:11.

i Ezk. 29:11, 13, 14.

j Isa. 41:13, 14; 43:5; 44:2; Jer. 30:10, 11.

k Isa. 8:7; Jer. 46:7, 8.

22 The voice thereof shall go like a serpent; for they shall march with an army,
and come against her with axes, as hewers of wood.
23 They shall [e]cut down her forest,
saith the LORD, though it cannot be
searched; because they are more than the
grasshoppers, and *are* innumerable.
24 The daughter of Egypt shall be confounded; she shall be delivered into the
hand of the people of the north.
25 The LORD of hosts, the God of Israel,
saith; Behold, I will punish the multitude
of [f]No, and Pharaoh, and Egypt, with
their gods, and their kings; even
Pharaoh, and *all* them that [g]trust in him:
26 [h]And I will deliver them into the
hand of those that seek their lives, and
into the hand of Nebuchadrezzar king of
Babylon, and into the hand of his servants: and [i]afterward it shall be inhabited, as in the days of old, saith the LORD.
27 But [j]fear not thou, O my servant
Jacob, and be not dismayed, O Israel: for,
behold, I will save thee from afar off, and
thy seed from the land of their captivity;
and Jacob shall return, and be in rest and
at ease, and none shall make *him* afraid.
28 Fear thou not, O Jacob my servant,
saith the LORD: for I *am* with thee; for I
will make a full end of all the nations
whither I have driven thee: but I will not
make a full end of thee, but correct thee
in measure; yet will I not leave thee
wholly unpunished.

CHAPTER 47.

(2) *Against Philistia, Tyre, etc.*

The word of the LORD that came to
Jeremiah the prophet against the
Philistines, before that Pharaoh smote
Gaza.
2 Thus saith the LORD; Behold, [k]waters
rise up out of the north, and shall be an
overflowing flood, and shall overflow
the land, and all that is therein; the city,
and them that dwell therein: then the
men shall cry, and all the inhabitants of
the land shall howl.
3 At the noise of the stamping of the
hoofs of his strong *horses*, at the rushing
of his chariots, *and at* the rumbling of his

nd the deliverance of Israel ("Israel," Gen. 12:2, 3; Rom. 11:26, *note*). Jer. 50:4-7 also looks forward to
he last days.

wheels, the fathers shall not look back to *their* children for feebleness of hands;

4 Because of the day that cometh to spoil all the Philistines, *and* to cut off from Tyrus and Zidon every helper that remaineth: for the LORD will spoil the Philistines, the [a]remnant of the country of Caphtor.

5 [b]Baldness is come upon Gaza; Ashkelon is cut off *with* the remnant of their valley: how long wilt thou cut thyself?

6 O thou [c]sword of the LORD, how long *will it be* ere thou be quiet? put up thyself into thy scabbard, rest, and be still.

7 How can it be quiet, seeing the LORD hath given it [d]a charge against Ashkelon, and against the sea shore? there hath he appointed it.

CHAPTER 48.

(3) *Against Moab.*

Against Moab thus saith the LORD of hosts, the God of Israel; Woe unto [e]Nebo! for it is spoiled: [f]Kiriathaim is confounded *and* taken: Misgab is confounded and dismayed.

2 *There shall be* no more praise of Moab: in Heshbon they have devised evil against it; come, and let us cut it off from *being* a nation. Also thou shalt be cut down, O Madmen; the sword shall pursue thee.

3 A voice of crying *shall be* from Horonaim, spoiling and great destruction.

4 Moab is destroyed; her little ones have caused a cry to be heard.

5 For in the going up of Luhith continual weeping shall go up; for in the going down of Horonaim the enemies have heard a cry of destruction.

6 Flee, save your lives, and be like the heath in the wilderness.

7 For because thou hast [g]trusted in thy works and in thy treasures, thou shalt also be taken: and [h]Chemosh shall go forth into captivity *with* his priests and his princes together.

8 And the spoiler shall come upon every city, and no city shall escape: the valley also shall perish, and the plain shall be destroyed, as the LORD hath spoken.

9 Give wings unto Moab, that it may flee and get away: for the cities thereof shall be desolate, without any to dwell therein.

10 Cursed *be* he that doeth the work of the LORD [i]deceitfully, and cursed *be* he that keepeth back his sword from blood.

11 Moab hath been at ease from his youth, and he hath [j]settled on his lees, and hath not been emptied from vessel to vessel, neither hath he gone into captivity: therefore his taste remained in him, and his scent is not changed.

12 Therefore, behold, the days come, saith the LORD, that I will send unto him wanderers, that shall cause him to wander, and shall empty his vessels, and break their bottles.

13 And Moab shall be ashamed of [k]Chemosh, as the house of Israel [l]was ashamed of [m]Beth-el their confidence.

14 How say ye, We *are* mighty and strong men for the war?

15 Moab is spoiled, and gone up *out of* her cities, and his chosen young men are gone down to the slaughter, saith the King, whose name *is* the LORD of hosts.

16 The calamity of Moab *is* near to come, and his affliction hasteth fast.

17 All ye that are about him, bemoan him; and all ye that know his name, say, How is the strong staff broken, *and* the beautiful rod!

18 Thou daughter that dost inhabit [n]Dibon, come down from *thy* glory, and sit in thirst; for the spoiler of Moab shall come upon thee, *and* he shall destroy thy strong holds.

19 O inhabitant of [o]Aroer, stand by the way, and espy; ask him that fleeth, and her that escapeth, *and* say, What is done?

20 Moab is confounded; for it is broken down: howl and cry; tell ye it in Arnon, that Moab is spoiled,

21 And judgment is come upon the plain country; upon Holon, and upon Jahazah, and upon Mephaath,

22 And upon Dibon, and upon Nebo, and upon Beth-diblathaim,

23 And upon Kiriathaim, and upon Beth-gamul, and upon Beth-meon,

24 And upon [p]Kerioth, and upon Bozrah, and upon all the cities of the land of Moab, far or near.

25 The horn of Moab is cut off, and his arm is broken, saith the LORD.

26 Make ye him drunken: for he magnified *himself* against the LORD: Moab

B.C. 600.

a Ezk. 25:16; Amos 1:8; 9:7.
b Amos 1:7; Mic. 1:16; Zeph. 2:4; Zech. 9:5.
c Deut. 32:41; Ezk. 21:3-5.
d Ezk. 14:17.
e Num. 32:38; 33:47; Isa. 15:2.
f Num. 32:37.
g Psa. 2:12, *note.*
h Num. 21:29; Jud. 11:24. See Isa. 46:1, 2; Jer. 43:12.
i Or, *negligently.*
j Zeph. 1:12.
k Jud. 11:24; 1 Ki. 11:7.
l Hos. 10:6.
m 1 Ki. 12:29.
n Num. 21:30; Isa. 15:2.
o Deut. 2:36.
p v. 41; Amos 2:2.

also shall wallow in his vomit, and he
also shall be in derision.
27 For was not Israel a derision unto
thee? was he found among thieves? for
since thou spakest of him, thou
skippedst for joy.
28 O ye that dwell in Moab, leave the
cities, and dwell in the rock, and be like
the [a]dove *that* maketh her nest in the
sides of the hole's mouth.
29 We have heard the [b]pride of Moab,
(he is exceeding proud) his loftiness, and
his arrogancy, and his pride, and the
haughtiness of his heart.
30 I know his wrath, saith the LORD;
but *it shall* not *be* so; his lies shall not so
effect *it*.
31 Therefore will I howl for Moab, and
I will cry out for all Moab; *mine heart*
shall mourn for the men of Kir-heres.
32 O vine of Sibmah, I will weep for
thee with the weeping of Jazer: thy plants
are gone over the sea, they reach *even* to
the sea of Jazer: the spoiler is fallen upon
thy summer fruits and upon thy vintage.
33 And joy and gladness is taken from
the plentiful field, and from the land of
Moab; and I have caused wine to fail
from the winepresses: none shall tread
with shouting; *their* shouting *shall be* no
shouting.
34 [c]From the cry of Heshbon *even* unto
Elealeh, *and even* unto Jahaz, have they
uttered their voice, from Zoar *even* unto
Horonaim, *as* an heifer of three years
old: for the waters also of Nimrim shall
be desolate.
35 Moreover I will cause to cease in
Moab, saith the LORD, him that offereth
in the high places, and him that burneth
incense to his gods.
36 Therefore mine heart shall sound
for Moab like pipes, and mine heart
shall sound like pipes for the men of Kir-
heres: because the riches *that* he hath
gotten are perished.
37 For every head *shall be* bald, and
every beard clipped: upon all the hands
shall be cuttings, and upon the loins sackcloth.
38 *There shall be* lamentation generally
upon all the housetops of Moab, and in
the streets thereof: for [d]I have broken
Moab like a vessel wherein *is* no pleasure, saith the LORD.
39 They shall howl, *saying*, How is it
broken down! how hath Moab turned

B.C. 600.

a Song 2:14.

b Isa. 16:6.

c Isa. 15:4-6.

d Jer. 22:28.

e Deut. 28:49; Jer. 49:22; Dan. 7:4; Hos. 8:1; Hab. 1:8.

f Num. 21:28.

g Num. 24:17.

h Amos 1:13.

i Ezk. 25:5; Amos 1:14.

the back with shame! so shall Moab be a
derision and a dismaying to all them
about him.
40 For thus saith the LORD; Behold, [e]he
shall fly as an eagle, and shall spread his
wings over Moab.
41 Kerioth is taken, and the strong
holds are surprised, and the mighty
men's hearts in Moab at that day shall be
as the heart of a woman in her pangs.
42 And Moab shall be destroyed from
being a people, because he hath magnified *himself* against the LORD.
43 Fear, and the pit, and the snare,
shall be upon thee, O inhabitant of Moab,
saith the LORD.
44 He that fleeth from the fear shall fall
into the pit; and he that getteth up out of
the pit shall be taken in the snare: for I
will bring upon it, *even* upon Moab, the
year of their visitation, saith the LORD.
45 They that fled stood under the
shadow of Heshbon because of the force:
but a [f]fire shall come forth out of
Heshbon, and a flame from the midst of
Sihon, and [g]shall devour the corner of
Moab, and the crown of the head of the
tumultuous ones.
46 Woe be unto thee, O Moab! the people of Chemosh perisheth: for thy sons
are taken captives, and thy daughters
captives.
47 Yet will I bring again the captivity
of Moab in the latter days, saith the
LORD. Thus far *is* the judgment of Moab.

CHAPTER 49.

(4) *Against the Ammonites and their cities.*

Concerning the Ammonites, thus
saith the LORD; Hath Israel no sons?
hath he no heir? why *then* doth their
king inherit Gad, and his people dwell
in his cities?
2 [h]Therefore, behold, the days come,
saith the LORD, that I will cause an alarm
of war to be heard in [i]Rabbah of the
Ammonites; and it shall be a desolate
heap, and her daughters shall be burned
with fire: then shall Israel be heir unto
them that were his heirs, saith the LORD.
3 Howl, O Heshbon, for Ai is spoiled:
cry, ye daughters of Rabbah, gird you
with sackcloth; lament, and run to and
fro by the hedges; for their king shall go
into captivity, *and* his priests and his
princes together.

4 Wherefore gloriest thou in the valleys, thy flowing valley, O backsliding
daughter? that trusted in her treasures,
saying, Who shall come unto me?
5 Behold, I will bring a fear upon thee,
saith the Lord GOD of hosts, from all
those that be about thee; and ye shall be
driven out every man right forth; and
none shall gather up him that wandereth.
6 And [a]afterward I will bring again
the captivity of the children of Ammon,
saith the LORD.

(5) *Against Edom.*

7 [b]Concerning Edom, thus saith the
LORD of hosts; *Is* wisdom no more in
Teman? is counsel perished from the
prudent? is their wisdom vanished?
8 Flee ye, turn back, dwell deep, O
inhabitants of [c]Dedan; for I will bring
the calamity of Esau upon him, the time
that I will visit him.
9 If grapegatherers come to thee,
would they not leave *some* gleaning
grapes? if thieves by night, they will
destroy till they have enough.
10 [d]But I have made Esau bare, I have
uncovered his secret places, and he shall
not be able to hide himself: his seed is
spoiled, and his brethren, and his neighbours, and he *is* not.
11 Leave thy fatherless children, I will
preserve *them* alive; and let thy widows
[e]trust in me.
12 For thus saith the LORD; Behold,
they whose judgment *was* not to drink of
the cup have assuredly drunken; and *art*
thou he *that* shall altogether go unpunished? thou shalt not go unpunished,
but thou shalt surely drink *of it*.
13 For I have sworn by myself, saith
the LORD, that [f]Bozrah shall become a
desolation, a reproach, a waste, and a
curse; and all the cities thereof shall be
perpetual wastes.
14 I have heard a rumour from the
LORD, and an ambassador is sent unto the
[g]heathen, *saying*, Gather ye together, and
come against her, and rise up to the battle.
15 For, lo, I will make thee small among
the heathen, *and* despised among men.
16 Thy terribleness hath deceived
thee, *and* the pride of thine heart, O thou
that dwellest in the clefts of the rock,
that holdest the height of the hill: though
thou shouldest make thy nest as high as
the eagle, I will bring thee down from
thence, saith the LORD.
17 Also [h]Edom shall be a desolation:
every one that goeth by it shall be astonished, and shall hiss at all the plagues
thereof.
18 [i]As in the overthrow of Sodom and
Gomorrah and the neighbour *cities*
thereof, saith the LORD, no man shall
abide there, neither shall a son of man
dwell in it.
19 Behold, he shall come up like a lion
from the swelling of Jordan against the
habitation of the strong: but I will suddenly make him run away from her: and
who *is* a chosen *man, that* I may appoint
over her? for who *is* like me? and who
will appoint me the time? and who *is*
that shepherd that will stand before me?
20 Therefore hear the counsel of the
LORD, that he hath taken against Edom;
and his purposes, that he hath purposed
against the inhabitants of Teman: Surely
the least of the flock shall draw them
out: surely he shall make their habitations desolate with them.
21 The earth is moved at the noise of
their fall, at the cry the noise thereof was
heard in the [j]Red sea.
22 Behold, he shall come up and fly as
the eagle, and spread his wings over
Bozrah: and at that day shall the heart of
the mighty men of Edom be as the heart
of a woman in her pangs.

(6) *Against Damascus.*

23 [k]Concerning Damascus. Hamath is
confounded, and Arpad: for they have
heard evil tidings: they are fainthearted;
there is sorrow on the sea; it cannot be
quiet.
24 Damascus is waxed feeble, *and*
turneth herself to flee, and fear hath
seized on *her*: anguish and sorrows have
taken her, as a woman in travail.
25 How is the city of praise not left,
the city of my joy!
26 Therefore [l]her young men shall fall
in her streets, and all the men of war
shall be cut off in that day, saith the
LORD of hosts.
27 And I will kindle a fire in the wall
of Damascus, and it shall consume the
palaces of Ben-hadad.

B.C. 600.

a v. 39; Jer. 48:47.
b Ezk. 25:12; Amos 1:11.
c Jer. 25:23.
d Mal. 1:3.
e Psa. 2:12, *note.*
f Isa. 34:6; 63:1.
g i.e. *nations*
h vs. 14-22; Gen. 36:1, *note.*
i Gen. 19:25; Deut. 29:23; Jer. 50:40; Amos 4:11.
j Heb. *weedy sea.*
k Isa. 17:1; 37:13; Amos 1:3; Zech. 9:1, 2.
l Jer. 50:30; 51:4.

(7) *Against Kedar
and the kingdoms of Hazor.*

28 Concerning Kedar, and concerning
the kingdoms of Hazor, which Nebuchadrezzar king of Babylon shall smite, thus
saith the LORD; Arise ye, go up to Kedar,
and spoil the men of the east.
29 Their tents and their flocks shall
they take away: they shall take to themselves their curtains, and all their vessels, and their camels; and they shall cry
unto them, Fear *is* on every side.
30 Flee, get you far off, dwell deep, O
ye inhabitants of Hazor, saith the LORD;
for Nebuchadrezzar king of Babylon
hath taken counsel against you, and hath
conceived a purpose against you.
31 Arise, get you up unto [a]the wealthy
nation, that dwelleth without care, saith
the LORD, which have neither gates nor
bars, [b]*which* dwell alone.
32 And their camels shall be a booty,
and the multitude of their cattle a spoil:
and I will [c]scatter into all winds them
that are in the utmost corners; and I will
bring their calamity from all sides thereof, saith the LORD.
33 And Hazor [d]shall be a dwelling for
dragons, *and* a desolation for ever: there
shall no man abide there, nor *any* son of
man dwell in it.

(8) *Against Elam.*

34 The word of the LORD that came to
Jeremiah the prophet against Elam in the
beginning of the reign of Zedekiah king
of Judah, saying,
35 Thus saith the LORD of hosts;
Behold, I will break the bow of Elam, the
chief of their might.
36 And upon Elam will I bring the four
winds from the four quarters of heaven,
and will scatter them toward all those
winds; and there shall be no nation whither the outcasts of Elam shall not come.
37 For I will cause Elam to be dismayed before their enemies, and before
them that seek their life: and I will bring
evil upon them, *even* my fierce anger,
saith the LORD; and I will send the sword
after them, till I have consumed them:
38 And I will set my throne in Elam,
and will destroy from thence the king
and the princes, saith the LORD.
39 But it shall come to pass in the
latter days, *that* I will bring again the
captivity of Elam, saith the LORD.

CHAPTER 50.

(9) *Against Babylon and Chaldea.*

The word that the LORD spake against
Babylon *and* against the land of the
Chaldeans by Jeremiah the prophet.
2 Declare ye among the nations, and
publish, and set up a standard; publish,
and conceal not: say, Babylon is taken,
Bel is confounded, Merodach is broken
in pieces; her idols are confounded, her
images are broken in pieces.
3 For [e]out of the north there cometh
up a nation against her, which shall
make her land desolate, and none shall
dwell therein: they shall remove, they
shall depart, both man and beast.
4 In those days, and in that time, saith
the LORD, the children of Israel shall
come, they and the children of Judah
together, going and weeping: they shall
go, and seek the LORD their God.
5 They shall ask the way to Zion with
their faces thitherward, *saying*, Come,
and let us join ourselves to the LORD in a
perpetual [f]covenant *that* shall not be forgotten.
6 My people hath been [g]lost sheep:
their shepherds have caused them to go
astray, they have turned them away *on*
the mountains: they have gone from
mountain to hill, they have forgotten
their restingplace.
7 All that found them have devoured
them: and their adversaries said, We
offend not, because they have sinned
against the LORD, the habitation of justice,
even the LORD, the hope of their fathers.
8 Remove out of the midst of Babylon,
and go forth out of the land of the
Chaldeans, and be as the he goats before
the flocks.
9 For, lo, [h]I will raise and cause to
come up against Babylon an assembly of
great nations from the north country:
and they shall [i]set themselves in array
against her; from thence she shall be
taken: their arrows *shall be* as of a mighty
expert man; [j]none shall return in vain.
10 And Chaldea shall be a spoil: all that
spoil her shall be satisfied, saith the LORD.
11 Because ye were glad, because ye

B.C. 600.

a Ezk. 38:11.
b Num. 23:9; Deut. 33:28; Mic. 7:14.
c v. 36; Ezk. 5:10.
d Jer. 9:11; 10:22; Mal. 1:3.
e Isa. 13:17, 18, 20; vs. 39, 40.
f *Covenant (New).* vs. 4, 5; Mt. 26:28. (Isa. 61:8; Heb. 8:8-12.)
g v. 17; Isa. 53:6; 1 Pet. 2:25.
h vs. 3, 41; Jer. 51:27.
i vs. 14, 29.
j 2 Sam. 1:22.

rejoiced, O ye destroyers of mine heritage, because ye are grown fat as the heifer at grass, and bellow as bulls;

12 Your mother shall be sore confounded; she that bare you shall be ashamed: behold, the hindermost of the nations *shall be* a wilderness, a dry land, and a desert.

13 Because of the wrath of the LORD it shall not be inhabited, but it shall be wholly desolate: [a]every one that goeth by Babylon shall be astonished, and hiss at all her plagues.

14 Put yourselves in array against Babylon round about: all ye that bend the bow, shoot at her, spare no arrows: for she hath sinned against the LORD.

15 Shout against her round about: she hath given her hand: her foundations are fallen, her walls are thrown down: for [b]it *is* the vengeance of the LORD: take vengeance upon her; as she hath done, do unto her.

16 Cut off the sower from Babylon, and him that handleth the sickle in the time of harvest: for fear of the oppressing sword they shall turn every one to his people, and they shall flee every one to his own land.

17 Israel *is* [c]a scattered sheep; the lions have driven *him* away: first the king of Assyria hath devoured him; and last this [d]Nebuchadrezzar king of Babylon hath broken his bones.

18 Therefore thus saith the LORD of hosts, the God of Israel; Behold, I will punish the king of Babylon and his land, as I have punished the king of Assyria.

19 And I will bring Israel again to his habitation, and he shall feed on Carmel and Bashan, and his soul shall be satisfied upon mount Ephraim and Gilead.

20 In those days, and in that time, saith the LORD, the [e]iniquity of Israel shall be sought for, and *there shall be* none; and the sins of Judah, and they shall not be found: for I will pardon them [f]whom I reserve.

21 Go up against the land of Merathaim, *even* against it, and against the inhabitants of [g]Pekod: waste and utterly destroy after them, saith the LORD, and do according to all that I have commanded thee.

22 A sound of battle *is* in the land, and of great destruction.

23 How is the hammer of the whole earth cut asunder and broken! how is Babylon become a desolation among the nations!

24 I have laid a snare for thee, and thou art also taken, O Babylon, and thou wast not aware: thou art found, and also caught, because thou hast striven against the LORD.

25 The LORD hath opened his armoury, and hath brought forth the weapons of his indignation: for this *is* the work of the Lord GOD of hosts in the land of the Chaldeans.

26 Come against her from the utmost border, open her storehouses: cast her up as heaps, and destroy her utterly: let nothing of her be left.

27 Slay all her bullocks; let them go down to the slaughter: woe unto them! for their day is come, the time of their visitation.

28 The voice of them that flee and escape out of the land of Babylon, to declare in Zion the vengeance of the LORD our God, the vengeance of his temple.

29 Call together the archers against Babylon: all ye that bend the bow, camp against it round about; let none thereof escape: recompense her according to her work; according to all that she hath done, do unto her: for she hath been [h]proud against the LORD, against the Holy One of Israel.

30 Therefore shall her young men fall in the streets, and all her men of war shall be cut off in that day, saith the LORD.

31 Behold, I *am* against thee, *O thou* most proud, saith the Lord GOD of hosts: for thy day is come, the time *that* I will visit thee.

32 And the most proud shall stumble and fall, and none shall raise him up: and I will kindle a fire in his cities, and it shall devour all round about him.

33 Thus saith the LORD of hosts; The children of Israel and the children of Judah *were* oppressed together: and all that took them captives held them fast; they refused to let them go.

34 Their [i]Redeemer *is* strong; the LORD of hosts *is* his name: he shall throughly plead their cause, that he may give rest to the land, and disquiet the inhabitants of Babylon.

35 A sword *is* upon the Chaldeans, saith the LORD, and upon the inhabitants

B.C. 595.

a Jer. 49:17.
b Jer. 51:6, 11.
c v. 6.
d 2 Ki. 24:10, 14.
e Jer. 31:34.
f Isa. 1:9.
g Ezk. 23:23.
h Isa. 47:10.
i Heb, *goel, Redemp. (Kinsman type).* Isa. 59:20, *note.*

of Babylon, and upon her princes, and upon her wise *men*.

36 A sword *is* upon the liars; and they shall dote: a sword *is* upon her mighty men; and they shall be dismayed.

37 A sword *is* upon their horses, and upon their chariots, and upon all the mingled people that *are* in the midst of her; and they shall become as women: a sword *is* upon her treasures; and they shall be robbed.

38 A drought *is* upon her waters; and they shall be dried up: for it *is* the land of graven images, and they are mad upon *their* idols.

39 Therefore the wild beasts of the desert with the wild beasts of the [a]islands shall dwell *there*, and the owls shall dwell therein: and it shall be no more inhabited for ever; neither shall it be dwelt in from generation to generation.

40 [b]As God overthrew Sodom and Gomorrah and the neighbour *cities* thereof, saith the LORD; *so* shall no man abide there, neither shall any son of man dwell therein.

41 Behold, a people shall come from the north, and a great nation, and many kings shall be raised up from the coasts of the earth.

42 They shall hold the bow and the lance: they *are* cruel, and will not shew mercy: their voice shall roar like the sea, and they shall ride upon horses, *every one* put in array, like a man to the battle, against thee, O daughter of Babylon.

43 The king of Babylon hath heard the report of them, and his hands waxed feeble: anguish took hold of him, *and* pangs as of a woman in travail.

44 Behold, he shall come up like a lion from the swelling of Jordan unto the habitation of the strong: but I will make them suddenly run away from her: and who *is* a chosen *man, that* I may appoint over her? for who *is* like me? and who will appoint me the time? and who *is* that [c]shepherd that will stand before me?

45 Therefore hear ye the counsel of the LORD, that he hath taken against Babylon; and his purposes, that he hath purposed against the land of the Chaldeans: Surely the least of the flock shall draw them out: surely he shall make *their* habitation desolate with them.

46 At the noise of the taking of Babylon the earth is moved, and the cry is heard among the nations.

CHAPTER 51.

(*The prophecy against Babylon,* continued.)

Thus saith the LORD; Behold, I will raise up against Babylon, and against them that dwell in the midst of them that rise up against me, a destroying wind;

2 And will send unto Babylon fanners, that shall fan her, and shall empty her land: for [d]in the day of trouble they shall be against her round about.

3 Against *him that* bendeth let the archer bend his bow, and against *him that* lifteth himself up in his brigandine: and spare ye not her young men; destroy ye utterly all her host.

4 Thus the slain shall fall in the land of the Chaldeans, and *they that are* thrust through in her streets.

5 For Israel *hath* not *been* forsaken, nor Judah of his God, of the LORD of hosts; though their land was filled with sin against the Holy One of Israel.

6 [e]Flee out of the midst of Babylon, and deliver every man his soul: be not cut off in her iniquity; for this *is* the time of the LORD'S vengeance; he will render unto her a recompence.

7 [f]Babylon *hath been* a golden cup in the LORD'S hand, that made all the earth drunken: the [g]nations have drunken of her wine; therefore the nations are mad.

8 Babylon is suddenly [h]fallen and destroyed: howl for her; take balm for her pain, if so be she may be healed.

9 We would have healed Babylon, but she is not healed: forsake her, and let us go every one into his own country: for her judgment reacheth unto heaven, and is lifted up *even* to the skies.

10 The LORD [i]hath brought forth our righteousness: come, and let us declare in Zion the work of the LORD our God.

11 Make bright the arrows; gather the shields: the [j]LORD hath raised up the spirit of the kings of the Medes: for his device *is* against Babylon, to destroy it; because it *is* [k]the vengeance of the LORD, the vengeance of his temple.

B.C. 595.

a i.e. *coasts.*

b Gen. 19:25; Isa. 13:19; Jer. 49:18; 51:26.

c Job 41:10; Jer. 49:19.

d Jer. 50:14.

e Jer. 50:8; Rev. 18:4.

f Rev. 17:4.

g Rev. 14:8.

h Isa. 21:9; Rev. 14:8; 18:2.

i Psa. 37:6.

j Isa. 13:17.

k Jer. 50:28.

12 [a]Set up the standard upon the walls of Babylon, make the watch strong, set up the watchmen, prepare the ambushes: for the LORD hath both devised and done that which he spake against the inhabitants of Babylon.
13 O thou that dwellest upon many waters, abundant in treasures, thine end is come, *and* the measure of thy covetousness.
14 The LORD of hosts hath sworn by himself, *saying*, Surely I will fill thee with men, as with caterpillers; and they shall lift up a shout against thee.
15 He hath made the earth by his power, he hath established the world by his wisdom, and [b]hath stretched out the heaven by his understanding.
16 When he uttereth *his* voice, *there is* a multitude of waters in the heavens; and he causeth the vapours to ascend from the ends of the earth: he maketh lightnings with rain, and bringeth forth the wind out of his treasures.
17 Every man is brutish by *his* knowledge; every founder is confounded by the graven image: for his molten image *is* falsehood, and *there is* no breath in them.
18 They *are* vanity, the work of errors: in the time of their visitation they shall perish.
19 The portion of Jacob *is* not like them; for he *is* the former of all things: and *Israel is* the rod of his inheritance: the LORD of hosts *is* his name.
20 Thou *art* my battle axe *and* weapons of war: for with thee will I break in pieces the nations, and with thee will I destroy kingdoms;
21 And with thee will I break in pieces the horse and his rider; and with thee will I break in pieces the chariot and his rider;
22 With thee also will I break in pieces man and woman; and with thee will I break in pieces old and young; and with thee will I break in pieces the young man and the maid;
23 I will also break in pieces with thee the shepherd and his flock; and with thee will I break in pieces the husbandman and his yoke of oxen; and with thee will I break in pieces captains and rulers.
24 And [c]I will render unto Babylon and to all the inhabitants of Chaldea all their evil that they have done in Zion in your sight, saith the LORD.

B.C. 595.

a Nah. 2:1; 3:14.
b Job 9:8; Psa. 104:2; Isa. 40:22.
c Jer. 50:15, 29.
d Isa. 13:1, *note;* Zech. 4:7.
e Jer. 50:40.
f Jer. 50:24.

25 Behold, I *am* against thee, [d]O destroying mountain, saith the LORD, which destroyest all the earth: and I will stretch out mine hand upon thee, and roll thee down from the rocks, and will make thee a burnt mountain.
26 And they shall not take of thee a stone for a corner, nor a stone for foundations; but [e]thou shalt be desolate for ever, saith the LORD.
27 Set ye up a standard in the land, blow the trumpet among the nations, prepare the nations against her, call together against her the kingdoms of Ararat, Minni, and Ashchenaz; appoint a captain against her; cause the horses to come up as the rough caterpillers.
28 Prepare against her the nations with the kings of the Medes, the captains thereof, and all the rulers thereof, and all the land of his dominion.
29 And the land shall tremble and sorrow: for every purpose of the LORD shall be performed against Babylon, to make the land of Babylon a desolation without an inhabitant.
30 The mighty men of Babylon have forborn to fight, they have remained in *their* holds: their might hath failed; they became as women: they have burned her dwellingplaces; her bars are broken.
31 [f]One post shall run to meet another, and one messenger to meet another, to shew the king of Babylon that his city is taken at *one* end,
32 And that the passages are stopped, and the reeds they have burned with fire, and the men of war are affrighted.
33 For thus saith the LORD of hosts, the God of Israel; The daughter of Babylon *is* like a threshingfloor, *it is* time to thresh her: yet a little while, and the time of her harvest shall come.
34 Nebuchadrezzar the king of Babylon hath devoured me, he hath crushed me, he hath made me an empty vessel, he hath swallowed me up like a dragon, he hath filled his belly with my delicates, he hath cast me out.
35 The violence done to me and to my flesh *be* upon Babylon, shall the inhabitant of Zion say; and my blood upon the inhabitants of Chaldea, shall Jerusalem say.

36 Therefore thus saith the LORD;
Behold, [a]I will plead thy cause, and take
vengeance for thee; and I will dry up her
sea, and make her springs dry.
37 [b]And Babylon shall become heaps,
a dwellingplace for dragons, an astonishment, and an hissing, without an
inhabitant.
38 They shall roar together like lions:
they shall yell as lions' whelps.
39 In their heat I will make their feasts,
and I will make them drunken, that they
may rejoice, and sleep a perpetual sleep,
and not wake, saith the LORD.
40 I will bring them down like lambs
to the slaughter, like rams with he goats.
41 How is [c]Sheshach taken! and how
is [d]the praise of the whole earth surprised! how is Babylon become an astonishment among the nations!
42 [e]The sea is come up upon Babylon:
she is covered with the multitude of the
waves thereof.
43 [f]Her cities are a desolation, a dry
land, and a wilderness, a land wherein
no man dwelleth, neither doth *any* son of
man pass thereby.
44 And I will punish Bel in Babylon,
and I will bring forth out of his mouth
that which he hath swallowed up: and
the nations shall not flow together any
more unto him: yea, the wall of Babylon
shall fall.
45 [g]My people, go ye out of the midst
of her, and deliver ye every man his soul
from the fierce anger of the LORD.
46 And lest your heart faint, and ye
fear for the rumour that shall be heard in
the land; a rumour shall both come *one*
year, and after that in *another* year *shall*
come a rumour, and violence in the land,
ruler against ruler.
47 Therefore, behold, the days come,
that I will do judgment upon the graven
images of Babylon: and her whole land
shall be confounded, and all her slain
shall fall in the midst of her.
48 [h]Then the heaven and the earth,
and all that *is* therein, shall sing for
Babylon: for the spoilers shall come unto
her from the north, saith the LORD.
49 As Babylon *hath caused* the slain of
Israel to fall, so at Babylon shall fall the
slain of all the earth.
50 Ye that have escaped the sword, go
away, stand not still: remember the LORD
afar off, and let Jerusalem come into
your mind.
51 We are confounded, because we
have heard reproach: shame hath covered our faces: for strangers are come
into the sanctuaries of the LORD'S house.
52 Wherefore, behold, the days come,
saith the LORD, that I will do judgment
upon her graven images: and through all
her land the wounded shall groan.
53 [i]Though Babylon should mount up
to heaven, and though she should fortify
the height of her strength, *yet* from me
shall spoilers come unto her, saith the
LORD.
54 A sound of a cry *cometh* from
Babylon, and great destruction from the
land of the Chaldeans:
55 Because the LORD hath spoiled
Babylon, and destroyed out of her the
great voice; when her waves do roar like
great waters, a noise of their voice is
uttered:
56 Because the spoiler is come upon
her, *even* upon Babylon, and her mighty
men are taken, every one of their bows is
broken: [j]for the LORD God of recompences shall surely requite.
57 And I will make drunk her princes,
and her wise *men*, her captains, and her
rulers, and her mighty men: and they
shall sleep a perpetual sleep, and not
wake, saith [k]the King, whose name *is* the
LORD of hosts.
58 Thus saith the LORD of hosts; The
broad walls of Babylon shall be utterly
broken, and her high gates shall be
burned with fire; and the people shall
labour in vain, and the folk in the fire,
and they shall be weary.
59 The word which Jeremiah the
prophet commanded Seraiah the son of
Neriah, the son of Maaseiah, when he
went with Zedekiah the king of Judah
into Babylon in the fourth year of his
reign. And *this* Seraiah *was* a quiet prince.
60 So Jeremiah wrote in a book all the
evil that should come upon Babylon,
even all these words that are written
against Babylon.
61 And Jeremiah said to Seraiah,
When thou comest to Babylon, and shalt
see, and shalt read all these words;
62 Then shalt thou say, O LORD, thou
hast spoken against this place, to cut it
off, that none shall remain in it, neither

B.C. 595.

a Jer. 50:34.
b Isa. 13:22; Jer. 50:39; Rev. 18:2.
c Jer. 25:26.
d Isa. 13:19; Jer. 49:25; Dan. 4:30.
e See Isa. 8:7, 8.
f Jer. 50:39, 40.
g v. 6; Jer. 50:8; Rev. 18:4.
h Isa. 44:23; 49:13; Rev. 18:20.
i Jer. 49:16; Amos 9:2; Oba. 4.
j v. 24; Jer. 50:29; Psa. 94:1.
k Jer. 46:18; 48:15.

man nor beast, but that it shall be desolate for ever.
63 And it shall be, when thou hast made an end of reading this book, [a]*that* thou shalt bind a stone to it, and cast it into the midst of Euphrates:
64 And thou shalt say, Thus shall Babylon sink, and shall not rise from the evil that I will bring upon her: and they shall be weary. Thus far *are* the words of Jeremiah.

CHAPTER 52.

A retrospect: the overthrow and captivity of Judah. (Cf. Jer. 39:1-10.)

Zedekiah [b]*was* one and twenty years old when he began to reign, and he reigned eleven years in Jerusalem. And his mother's name *was* Hamutal the daughter of Jeremiah of Libnah.
2 And he did *that which was* evil in the eyes of the LORD, according to all that Jehoiakim had done.
3 For through the anger of the LORD it came to pass in Jerusalem and Judah, till he had cast them out from his presence, that Zedekiah rebelled against the king of Babylon.
4 And it came to pass in the [c]ninth year of his reign, in the [d]tenth month, in the tenth *day* of the month, *that* Nebuchadrezzar king of Babylon came, he and all his army, against Jerusalem, and pitched against it, and built forts against it round about.
5 So the city was besieged unto the eleventh year of king Zedekiah.
6 And in the [e]fourth month, in the ninth *day* of the month, the famine was sore in the city, so that there was no bread for the people of the land.
7 Then the city was broken up, and all the men of war fled, and went forth out of the city by night by the way of the gate between the two walls, which *was* by the king's garden; (now the Chaldeans *were* by the city round about:) and they went by the way of the plain.
8 But the army of the Chaldeans pursued after the king, and overtook Zedekiah in the plains of Jericho; and all his army was scattered from him.
9 [f]Then they took the king, and carried him up unto the king of Babylon to

B.C. 595.

a Rev. 18:21.
b 2 Ki. 24:18.
c 2 Ki. 25:1-27; Jer. 39:1; Zech. 8:19.
d i.e. *January.*
e i.e. *July.*
f Jer. 32:4.
g Ezk. 12:13.
h i.e. *August.*
i Jer. 39:9.
j See 1 Ki. 7:15, 23, 27.
k Ex. 27:3; 2 Ki. 25:14-16.
l 1 Ki. 7:47.
m 1 Ki. 7:15; 2 Ki. 25:17; 2 Chr. 3:15.

Riblah in the land of Hamath; where he gave judgment upon him.
10 And the king of Babylon slew the sons of Zedekiah before his eyes: he slew also all the princes of Judah in Riblah.
11 [g]Then he put out the eyes of Zedekiah; and the king of Babylon bound him in chains, and carried him to Babylon, and put him in prison till the day of his death.
12 Now in the [h]fifth month, in the tenth *day* of the month, which *was* the nineteenth year of Nebuchadrezzar king of Babylon, came [i]Nebuzar-adan, captain of the guard, *which* served the king of Babylon, into Jerusalem,
13 And burned the house of the LORD, and the king's house; and all the houses of Jerusalem, and all the houses of the great *men*, burned he with fire:
14 And all the army of the Chaldeans, that *were* with the captain of the guard, brake down all the walls of Jerusalem round about.
15 Then [i]Nebuzar-adan the captain of the guard carried away captive *certain* of the poor of the people, and the residue of the people that remained in the city, and those that fell away, that fell to the king of Babylon, and the rest of the multitude.
16 But Nebuzar-adan the captain of the guard left *certain* of the poor of the land for vinedressers and for husbandmen.
17 [j]Also the pillars of brass that *were* in the house of the LORD, and the bases, and the brasen sea that *was* in the house of the LORD, the Chaldeans brake, and carried all the brass of them to Babylon.
18 [k]The caldrons also, and the shovels, and the snuffers, and the bowls, and the spoons, and all the vessels of brass wherewith they ministered, took they away.
19 And the basons, and the firepans, and the bowls, and the caldrons, and the candlesticks, and the spoons, and the cups; *that* which *was* of gold *in* gold, and *that* which *was* of silver *in* silver, took the captain of the guard away.
20 The two pillars, one sea, and twelve brasen bulls that *were* under the bases, which king Solomon had made in the house of the LORD: [l]the brass of all these vessels was without weight.
21 And *concerning* [m]the pillars, the height of one pillar *was* eighteen

B.C. 588.

[a]cubits; and a fillet of twelve cubits did compass it; and the thickness thereof *was* four fingers: *it was* hollow.

22 And a chapiter of brass *was* upon it; and the height of one chapiter *was* five cubits, with network and pomegranates upon the chapiters round about, all *of* brass. The second pillar also and the pomegranates *were* like unto these.

23 And there were ninety and six pomegranates on a side; *and* [b]all the pomegranates upon the network *were* an hundred round about.

24 And the captain of the guard took [c]Seraiah the chief priest, and [d]Zephaniah the second priest, and the three keepers of the door:

25 He took also out of the city an eunuch, which had the charge of the men of war; and seven men of them that were near the king's person, which were found in the city; and the principal scribe of the host, who mustered the people of the land; and threescore men of the people of the land, that were found in the midst of the city.

26 So Nebuzar-adan the captain of the guard took them, and brought them to the king of Babylon to Riblah.

27 And the king of Babylon smote them, and put them to death in Riblah in the land of Hamath. Thus Judah was carried away captive out of his own land.

28 [e]This *is* the people whom Nebuchadrezzar carried away captive: in the [f]seventh year [g]three thousand Jews and three and twenty:

29 In the eighteenth year of Nebuchadrezzar he carried away captive from Jerusalem eight hundred thirty and two persons:

30 In the three and twentieth year of Nebuchadrezzar Nebuzar-adan the captain of the guard carried away captive of the Jews seven hundred forty and five persons: all the persons *were* four thousand and six hundred.

The latter days of Jehoiachin.
(Cf. 2 Ki. 25:27-30.)

31 [h]And it came to pass in the seven and thirtieth year of the captivity of Jehoiachin king of Judah, in the [i]twelfth month, in the five and twentieth *day* of the month, *that* Evil-merodach king of Babylon in the *first* year of his reign [j]lifted up the head of Jehoiachin king of Judah, and brought him forth out of prison,

32 And spake kindly unto him, and set his throne above the throne of the kings that *were* with him in Babylon,

33 And changed his prison garments: and [k]he did continually eat bread before him all the days of his life.

34 And *for* his diet, there was a continual diet given him of the king of Babylon, every day a portion until the day of his death, all the days of his life.

a One cubit = about 18 in.; also v. 22.
b See 1 Ki. 7:20.
c 2 Ki. 25:18.
d Jer. 21:1; 29:25.
e 2 Ki. 24:2; cf. Ezra 2:1-65; Neh. 7:6-67; Dan. 1:1-7.
f See 2 Ki. 24:12.
g 2 Ki. 24:14.
h 2 Ki. 25:27-30.
i i.e. *March.*
j Gen. 40:13-20.
k 2 Sam. 9:13.

THE
LAMENTATIONS OF JEREMIAH

THE touching significance of this book lies in the fact that it is the disclosure of the love and sorrow of Jehovah for the very people whom He is chastening—a sorrow wrought by the Spirit in the heart of Jeremiah (Jer. 13:17; Mt. 23:36, 38; Rom. 9:1-5).

The chapters indicate the analysis, viz., five lamentations.

CHAPTER 1.

The first lamentation.

HOW doth the city sit solitary, *that was*
full of people! [a]*how* is she become
as a widow! she *that was* great among
the nations, *and* [b]princess among the
provinces, *how* is she become tributary!
2 She weepeth sore in the night, and
her tears *are* on her cheeks: among all
her lovers she hath none to comfort *her*:
all her friends have dealt treacherously
with her, they are become her enemies.
3 [c]Judah is gone into captivity because
of affliction, and because of great servitude: she dwelleth among the [d]heathen,
she findeth no rest: all her persecutors
overtook her between the straits.
4 The ways of Zion do mourn, because
none come to the solemn feasts: all her
gates are desolate: her priests sigh, her
virgins are afflicted, and she *is* in bitterness.
5 Her adversaries are the chief, her
enemies prosper; for the LORD hath
afflicted her [e]for the multitude of her
transgressions: her children are gone
into captivity before the enemy.
6 And from the daughter of Zion all
her beauty is departed: her princes are
become like harts *that* find no pasture,
and they are gone without strength
before the pursuer.
7 Jerusalem remembered in the days
of her affliction and of her miseries all
her pleasant things that she had in the
days of old, when her people fell into
the hand of the enemy, and none did
help her: the adversaries saw her, *and*
did mock at her sabbaths.
8 [f]Jerusalem hath grievously sinned;
therefore she is removed: all that honoured her despise her, because they have
seen her nakedness: yea, she sigheth,
and turneth backward.
9 Her filthiness *is* in her skirts; she
remembereth not her last end; therefore
she came down wonderfully: she had no
comforter. O LORD, behold my affliction:
for the enemy hath magnified *himself*.
10 The adversary hath spread out his
hand upon all her pleasant things: for
she hath seen *that* the [d]heathen entered
[g]into her sanctuary, whom thou didst
command *that* they should not enter into
thy congregation.
11 All her people sigh, they seek bread;
they have given their pleasant things for
meat to relieve the soul: see, O LORD, and
consider; for I am become vile.
12 *Is it* nothing to you, all ye that pass
by? behold, and see [h]if there be any sorrow like unto my sorrow, which is done
unto me, wherewith the LORD hath
afflicted *me* in the day of his fierce anger.
13 From above hath he sent fire into
my bones, and it prevaileth against
them: [i]he hath spread a net for my feet,
he hath turned me back: he hath made
me desolate *and* faint all the day.
14 [j]The yoke of my transgressions is
bound by his hand: they are wreathed,
and come up upon my neck: he hath
made my strength to fall, the Lord hath
delivered me into *their* hands, *from whom*
I am not able to rise up.
15 The Lord hath trodden under foot
all my mighty *men* in the midst of me: he
hath called an assembly against me to
crush my young men: [k]the Lord hath
trodden the virgin, the daughter of
Judah, *as* in a winepress.
16 For these *things* I weep; mine
eye, mine eye runneth down
with water, because the comforter
that should relieve my soul is far from

B.C. 588.

a Isa. 47:7-9.
b Ezra 4:20.
c Jer. 52:27.
d i.e. *nations.*
e Jer. 30:14, 15; 52:28; Dan. 9:7, 16.
f 1 Ki. 8:46.
g Jer. 51:51.
h Dan. 9:12.
i Ezk. 12:13; 17:20.
j Deut. 28:48.
k Isa. 63:3; Rev. 14:19, 20; 19:15.

me: my children are desolate, because the enemy prevailed.

17 Zion spreadeth forth her hands, *and there is* none to comfort her: the LORD hath commanded concerning Jacob, *that* his adversaries *should be* round about him: Jerusalem is as a menstruous woman among them.

18 The LORD is righteous; for I have rebelled against his commandment: hear, I pray you, all people, and behold my sorrow: my virgins and my young men are gone into captivity.

19 I called for my lovers, *but* they deceived me: my priests and mine elders gave up the ghost in the city, while they sought their meat to relieve their souls.

20 Behold, O LORD; for I *am* in distress: my bowels are troubled; mine heart is turned within me; for I have grievously rebelled: [a]abroad the sword bereaveth, at home *there is* as death.

21 They have heard that I sigh: *there is* none to comfort me: all mine enemies have heard of my trouble; they are glad that thou hast done *it*: thou wilt bring [b]the day *that* thou hast called, and they shall be like unto me.

22 Let all their wickedness come before thee; and do unto them, as thou hast done unto me for all my transgressions: for my sighs *are* many, and my heart *is* faint.

CHAPTER 2.

The second lamentation.

How hath the Lord covered the daughter of Zion with a cloud in his anger, [c]*and* cast down from heaven unto the earth the beauty of Israel, and remembered not his footstool in the day of his anger!

2 The Lord hath swallowed up all the habitations of Jacob, [d]and hath not pitied: he hath thrown down in his wrath the strong holds of the daughter of Judah; he hath brought *them* down to the ground: he hath polluted the kingdom and the princes thereof.

3 He hath cut off in *his* fierce anger all the horn of Israel: he hath drawn back his right hand from before the enemy, and he burned against Jacob like a flaming fire, *which* devoureth round about.

4 [e]He hath bent his bow like an enemy: he stood with his right hand as an adversary, and slew all *that were* pleasant to the eye in the tabernacle of the daughter of Zion: he poured out his fury like fire.

5 The Lord was as an enemy: he hath swallowed up Israel, [f]he hath swallowed up all her palaces: he hath destroyed his strong holds, and hath increased in the daughter of Judah mourning and lamentation.

6 And he hath violently [g]taken away his tabernacle, as *if it were of* a garden: he hath destroyed his places of the assembly: the LORD hath caused the solemn feasts and sabbaths to be forgotten in Zion, and hath despised in the indignation of his anger the king and the priest.

7 The Lord hath cast off his altar, he hath abhorred his sanctuary, he hath given up into the hand of the enemy the walls of her palaces; they have made a noise in the house of the LORD, as in the day of a solemn feast.

8 The LORD hath purposed to destroy the wall of the daughter of Zion: [h]he hath stretched out a line, he hath not withdrawn his hand from destroying: therefore he made the rampart and the wall to lament; they languished together.

9 Her gates are sunk into the ground; he hath destroyed and broken her bars: [i]her king and her princes *are* among the Gentiles: the law *is* no *more*; her prophets also find no vision from the LORD.

10 The elders of the daughter of Zion sit upon the ground, *and* keep silence: they have cast up dust upon their heads; they have girded themselves with sackcloth: the virgins of Jerusalem hang down their heads to the ground.

11 [j]Mine eyes do fail with tears, my bowels are troubled, my liver is poured upon the earth, for the destruction of the daughter of my people; because the children and the sucklings swoon in the streets of the city.

12 They say to their mothers, Where *is* corn and wine? when they swooned as the wounded in the streets of the city, when their soul was poured out into their mothers' bosom.

13 [k]What thing shall I take to witness for thee? what thing shall I liken to thee, O daughter of Jerusalem? what shall I equal to thee, that I may comfort thee, O

B.C. 588.

a Deut. 32:25; Ezk. 7:15.

b Isa. 13.; Jer. 46.

c Mt. 11:23.

d vs. 17, 21; Lam. 3:43.

e Isa. 63:10.

f 2 Ki. 25:9; Jer. 52:13.

g Psa. 80:12; 89:40; Isa. 5:5; Jer 7:14.

h 2 Ki. 21:13; Isa. 34:11.

i Deut. 28:36; 2 Ki. 24:15; 25:7; Lam. 1:3; 4:20.

j Psa. 6:7; Lam. 3:48.

k Dan. 9:12; Lam. 1:12.

virgin daughter of Zion? for thy breach
is great like the sea: who can heal thee?
14 Thy prophets have seen vain and
foolish things for thee: and they have not
discovered thine iniquity, to turn away
thy captivity; but have seen for thee false
burdens and causes of banishment.
15 [a]All that pass by clap *their* hands at
thee; they hiss and wag their head at the
daughter of Jerusalem, *saying, Is* this the
city that *men* call The perfection of beauty, The joy of the whole earth?
16 All thine enemies have opened
their mouth against thee: they hiss and
gnash the teeth: they say, We have swallowed *her* up: certainly this *is* the day
that we looked for; we have found, we
have seen *it*.
17 [b]The LORD hath done *that* which he
had devised; he hath fulfilled his word
that he had commanded in the days of
old: he hath thrown down, and hath not
pitied: and he hath caused *thine* enemy
to rejoice over thee, he hath set up the
horn of thine adversaries.
18 Their heart cried unto the Lord, O
wall of the daughter of Zion, [c]let tears
run down like a river day and night:
give thyself no rest; let not the apple of
thine eye cease.
19 Arise, cry out in the night: in the
beginning of the watches [d]pour out thine
heart like water before the face of the
Lord: lift up thy hands toward him for
the life of thy young children, that faint
for hunger in the top of every street.
20 Behold, O LORD, and consider to
whom thou hast done this. [e]Shall the
women eat their fruit, *and* children of a
[f]span long? shall the priest and the
prophet be slain in the sanctuary of the
Lord?
21 The young and the old lie on the
ground in the streets: my virgins and my
young men are fallen by the sword; thou
hast slain *them* in the day of thine anger;
thou hast killed, *and* not pitied.
22 Thou hast called as in a solemn day
my terrors round about, so that in the
day of the LORD'S anger none escaped
nor remained: those that I have swaddled and brought up hath mine enemy
consumed.

[1]CHAPTER 3.

The third lamentation.

I *am* the man *that* hath seen affliction by
the rod of his wrath.
2 He hath led me, and brought *me into*
darkness, but not *into* light.
3 Surely against me is he turned; he
turneth his hand *against me* all the day.
4 [g]My flesh and my skin hath he made
old; he hath broken my bones.
5 He hath builded against me, and
compassed *me* with gall and travail.
6 [h]He hath set me in dark places, as
they that be dead of old.
7 [i]He hath hedged me about, that I
cannot get out: he hath made my chain
heavy.
8 [j]Also when I cry and shout, he shutteth out my prayer.
9 He hath inclosed my ways with hewn
stone, he hath made my paths crooked.
10 He *was* unto me *as* a bear lying in
wait, *and as* a lion in secret places.
11 He hath turned aside my ways, and
pulled me in pieces: he hath made me
desolate.
12 [k]He hath bent his bow, and set me
as a mark for the arrow.
13 He hath caused the arrows of his
quiver to enter into my reins.
14 I was a derision to all my people;
and their song all the day.
15 [l]He hath filled me with bitterness, he
hath made me drunken with wormwood.
16 He hath also broken my teeth with
gravel stones, he hath covered me with
ashes.
17 And thou hast removed my soul far
off from peace: I forgat prosperity.
18 And I said, My strength and my
hope is perished from the LORD:
19 Remembering mine affliction and
my misery, the wormwood and the gall.
20 My soul hath *them* still in remembrance, and is humbled in me.

B.C. 588.

a 1 Ki. 9:8; Jer. 18:16; Nah. 3:19..
b Lev. 26:16; Deut. 28:15.
c Jer. 14:17; Lam. 1:16.
d Psa. 62:8.
e Lev. 26:29; Deut. 28:53; Jer. 19:9; Lam. 4:10; Ezk. 5:10.
f About 9 in.
g Job 16:8.
h Psa. 88:5, 6; 143:3.
i Job 3:23; 19:8; Hos. 2:6.
j Job 30:20; Psa. 22.2.
k Job 7:20; 16:12; Psa. 38:2.
l Jer. 9:15.

[1]**(3:1, heading)** The literary form of Lamentations is necessarily obscured in the translation. It is an acrostic dirge, the lines arranged in couplets or triplets, each of which begins with a letter of the Hebrew alphabet. In the third Lament, which consists of sixty-six stanzas instead of twenty-two, each *line* of each triplet begins with the same letter, so that the entire sixty-six verses are required to give the twenty-two letters of the alphabet. Thus verses 1-3 of our version form but three lines of the original, each line beginning with A, etc.

21 This I recall to my mind, therefore have I hope.
22 [a]*It is of* the LORD'S mercies that we are not consumed, because his compassions fail not.
23 [b]*They are* new every morning: great *is* thy faithfulness.
24 The LORD *is* [c]my portion, saith my soul; therefore will I hope in him.
25 The LORD *is* good unto them that [d]wait for him, to the soul *that* seeketh him.
26 *It is* good that *a man* should both hope and quietly wait for the salvation of the LORD.
27 *It is* good for a man that he bear the yoke in his youth.
28 He sitteth alone and keepeth silence, because he hath borne *it* upon him.
29 He putteth his mouth in the dust; if so be there may be hope.
30 He giveth *his* cheek to him that [e]smiteth him: he is filled full with reproach.
31 [f]For the Lord will not cast off for ever:
32 But though he cause grief, yet will he have compassion according to the multitude of his mercies.
33 [g]For he doth not afflict willingly nor grieve the children of men.
34 To crush under his feet all the prisoners of the earth,
35 To turn aside the right of a man before the face of the most High,
36 To subvert a man in his cause, [h]the Lord approveth not.
37 Who *is* he *that* saith, and it cometh to pass, *when* the Lord commandeth *it* not?
38 Out of the mouth of the most High proceedeth [i]not evil and good?
39 Wherefore doth a living man complain, a man for the punishment of his sins?
40 Let us search and try our ways, and turn again to the LORD.
41 Let us lift up our heart with *our* hands unto God in the heavens.
42 We have transgressed and have rebelled: thou hast not pardoned.
43 Thou hast covered with anger, and persecuted us: thou hast slain, thou hast not pitied.
44 Thou hast covered thyself with a cloud, that *our* prayer should not pass through.

B.C. 588.

a Mal. 3:6.
b Isa. 33:2.
c Psa. 16:5; 73:26; 119:57; Jer. 10:16.
d Psa. 130:6; Isa. 30:18; Mic. 7:7.
e Mt. 27:30; Mk. 15:19; Lk. 22:63; John 18:22.
f Psa. 77:7; 94:14; Isa. 54:7-10.
g Ezk. 33:11; Heb. 12:10.
h Heb. 1:13.
i Jas. 3:10, 11.
j 1 Cor. 4:13.
k Isa. 63:15.
l Psa. 130:1; Jon. 2:2.
m Jas. 4:8.
n Heb. *goel, Redemp. (Kinsman type).* Isa. 59:20, *note.*
o Psa. 28:4; Jer. 11:20; 2 Tim. 4:14.

45 [j]Thou hast made us *as* the offscouring and refuse in the midst of the people.
46 All our enemies have opened their mouths against us.
47 Fear and a snare is come upon us, desolation and destruction.
48 Mine eye runneth down with rivers of water for the destruction of the daughter of my people.
49 Mine eye trickleth down, and ceaseth not, without any intermission,
50 [k]Till the LORD look down, and behold from heaven.
51 Mine eye affecteth mine heart because of all the daughters of my city.
52 Mine enemies chased me sore, like a bird, without cause.
53 They have cut off my life in the dungeon, and cast a stone upon me.
54 Waters flowed over mine head; *then* I said, I am cut off.
55 [l]I called upon thy name, O LORD, out of the low dungeon.
56 Thou hast heard my voice: hide not thine ear at my breathing, at my cry.
57 [m]Thou drewest near in the day *that* I called upon thee: thou saidst, Fear not.
58 O Lord, thou hast pleaded the causes of my soul; thou hast [n]redeemed my life.
59 O LORD, thou hast seen my wrong: judge thou my cause.
60 Thou hast seen all their vengeance *and* all their imaginations against me.
61 Thou hast heard their reproach, O LORD, *and* all their imaginations against me;
62 The lips of those that rose up against me, and their device against me all the day.
63 Behold their sitting down, and their rising up; I *am* their musick.
64 [o]Render unto them a recompence, O LORD, according to the work of their hands.
65 Give them sorrow of heart, thy curse unto them.
66 Persecute and destroy them in anger from under the heavens of the LORD.

CHAPTER 4.

The fourth lamentation.

How is the gold become dim! *how* is the most fine gold changed! the stones of the sanctuary are poured out in the top of every street.

B.C. 588.

2 The precious sons of Zion, comparable to fine gold, how are they esteemed as [a]earthen pitchers, the work of the hands of the potter!

3 Even the sea monsters draw out the breast, they give suck to their young ones: the daughter of my people *is become* cruel, like the ostriches in the wilderness.

4 The tongue of the sucking child cleaveth to the roof of his mouth for thirst: the young children ask bread, *and* no man breaketh *it* unto them.

5 They that did feed delicately are desolate in the streets: they that were brought up in scarlet embrace dunghills.

6 For the punishment of the iniquity of the daughter of my people is greater than the punishment of the sin of Sodom, [b]that was overthrown as in a moment, and no hands stayed on her.

7 Her Nazarites were purer than snow, they were whiter than milk, they were more ruddy in body than rubies, their polishing *was* of sapphire:

8 Their visage is blacker than a coal; they are not known in the streets: their skin cleaveth to their bones; it is withered, it is become like a stick.

9 *They that be* slain with the sword are better than *they that be* slain with hunger: for these pine away, stricken through for *want of* the fruits of the field.

10 The hands of the pitiful women have sodden their own children: they were their meat in the destruction of the daughter of my people.

11 The LORD hath accomplished his fury; [c]he hath poured out his fierce anger, and [d]hath kindled a fire in Zion, and it hath devoured the foundations thereof.

12 The kings of the earth, and all the inhabitants of the world, would not have believed that the adversary and the enemy should have entered into the gates of Jerusalem.

13 [e]For the sins of her prophets, *and* the iniquities of her priests, that have shed the blood of the just in the midst of her,

14 They have wandered *as* blind *men* in the streets, they have polluted themselves with blood, so that men could not touch their garments.

15 They cried unto them, Depart ye; *it is* unclean; depart, depart, touch not: when they fled away and wandered, they said among the [f]heathen, They shall no more sojourn *there*.

16 The anger of the LORD hath divided them; he will no more regard them: they respected not the persons of the priests, they favoured not the elders.

17 As for us, our eyes as yet failed for our vain help: in our watching we have watched for a nation *that* could not save *us*.

18 They hunt our steps, that we cannot go in our streets: [g]our end is near, our days are fulfilled; for our end is come.

19 Our persecutors are swifter than the eagles of the heaven: they pursued us upon the mountains, they laid wait for us in the wilderness.

20 The breath of our nostrils, the anointed of the LORD, was taken in their pits, of whom we said, Under his shadow we shall live among the [f]heathen.

21 [h]Rejoice and be glad, O daughter of Edom, that dwellest in the land of Uz; the cup also shall pass through unto thee: thou shalt be drunken, and shalt make thyself naked.

22 The punishment of thine iniquity is accomplished, O daughter of Zion; he will no more carry thee away into captivity: [i]he will visit thine iniquity, O daughter of Edom; he will discover thy sins.

CHAPTER 5.

The fifth lamentation.

Remember, O LORD, what is come upon us: consider, and behold our reproach.

2 [j]Our inheritance is turned to strangers, our houses to aliens.

3 We are orphans and fatherless, our mothers *are* as widows.

4 We have drunken our water for money; our wood is sold unto us.

5 [k]Our necks *are* under persecution: we labour, *and* have no rest.

6 We have given the hand *to* the Egyptians, *and to* the Assyrians, to be satisfied with bread.

7 Our fathers have sinned, *and are* not; and we have borne their iniquities.

8 Servants have ruled over us: *there is* none that doth deliver *us* out of their hand.

9 We gat our bread with *the peril of*

a Isa. 30:14; Jer. 19:11; 2 Cor. 4:7.
b Gen. 19:24-25.
c Jer. 7:20.
d Deut. 32:22; Jer. 21:14.
e Jer. 5:31; 6:13; 14:14; 23:11, 21; Ezk. 22:26, 28; Zeph. 3:4.
f i.e. *nations*.
g Ezk. 7:2, 3, 6; Amos 8:2.
h Eccl. 11:9.
i Psa. 137:7.
j Psa. 79:1.
k Deut. 28:48; Jer. 28:14.

our lives because of the sword of the wilderness.
10 Our skin was black like an oven because of the terrible famine.
11 [a]They ravished the women in Zion, *and* the maids in the cities of Judah.
12 Princes are hanged up by their hand: the faces of elders were not honoured.
13 [b]They took the young men to grind, and the children fell under the wood.
14 The elders have ceased from the gate, the young men from their musick.
15 The joy of our heart is ceased; our dance is turned into mourning.
16 The crown is fallen *from* our head: woe unto us, that we have sinned!
17 For this our heart is faint; for these *things* our eyes are dim.
18 Because of the mountain of Zion, which is desolate, the foxes walk upon it.
19 [c]Thou, O LORD, remainest for ever; thy throne from generation to generation.
20 Wherefore dost thou forget us for ever, *and* forsake us so long time?
21 [d]Turn thou us unto thee, O LORD, and we shall be turned; renew our days as of old.
22 But thou hast utterly rejected us; thou art very wroth against us.

B.C. 588.

a Isa. 13:16; Zech. 14:2.

b Jud. 16:21.

c Psa. 9:7; 10:16; 29:10; 90:2; 102:12; 145:13; Hab. 1:12.

d Psa. 80:3, 7, 19; Jer. 31:18.

THE BOOK OF THE PROPHET
EZEKIEL

EZEKIEL was carried away to Babylon between the first and final deportations of Judah (2 Ki. 24:11-16), Like Daniel and the Apostle John, he prophesied out of the land, and his prophecy, like theirs, follows the method of symbol and vision. Unlike the pre-exilic prophets, whose ministry was primarily to either Judah or the ten-tribe kingdom, Ezekiel is the voice of Jehovah to "the whole house of Israel."

Speaking broadly, the purpose of his ministry is to keep before the generation born in exile the national sins which had brought Israel so low (e.g. Ezk. 14:23); to sustain the faith of the exiles by predictions of national restoration, of the execution of justice upon their oppressors, and of national glory under the Davidic monarchy.

Ezekiel is in seven great prophetic strains indicated by the expression, "The hand of the LORD was upon me" (Ezk. 1:3; 3:14, 22; 8:1; 33:22; 37:1; 40:1). The minor divisions are indicated by the formula, "And the word of the LORD came unto me." These divisions are indicated in the text.

The events recorded in Ezekiel cover a period of 21 years (Ussher).

PART I. EZEKIEL'S PREPARATION AND COMMISSION (SEE v. 3): CHAPTERS 1:1–3:9.

CHAPTER 1.

B.C. 595.

(1) *Introduction.*

NOW it came to pass in the thirtieth
year, in the [a]fourth *month*, in the
fifth *day* of the month, as I *was* among
the captives [b]by the river of Chebar, *that*
the heavens were opened, and I saw
visions of God.

(2) *The vision of the glory.*

2 In the fifth *day* of the month, which
was the fifth year of king Jehoiachin's
captivity,
3 The word of the LORD came expressly unto Ezekiel the priest, the son of
Buzi, in the land of the Chaldeans by the
river Chebar; and the [c]hand of the LORD
was there upon him.
4 And I looked, and, behold, a whirlwind came out of the north, a great
cloud, and a fire infolding itself, and a
brightness *was* about it, and out of the
midst thereof as the colour of amber, out
of the midst of the fire.
5 Also out of the midst thereof *came*
the likeness of four [1]living creatures.
And this *was* their appearance; they had
the likeness of a man.
6 And every one had four faces, and
every one had four wings.
7 And their feet *were* straight feet; and
the sole of their feet *was* like the sole of a
calf's foot: and they sparkled like the
colour of burnished brass.
8 And *they had* the hands of a man
under their wings on their four sides;
and they four had their faces and their
wings.
9 Their wings *were* joined one to
another; they turned not when they

a i.e. *July* "of the thirtieth year of Ezekiel's age."

b v. 3; Ezk. 3:15, 23; 10:15.

c Ezk. 3:14, 22; 8:1; 33:22; 37:1; 40:1; 1 Ki. 18:46; 2 Ki. 3:15.

[1] **(1:5)** The "living creatures" are identical with the Cherubim. The subject is somewhat obscure, but from the position of the Cherubim at the gate of Eden, upon the cover of the ark of the covenant, and in Rev. 4, it is clearly gathered that they have to do with the vindication of the holiness of God as against the presumptuous pride of sinful man who, despite his sin, would "put forth his hand, and take also of the tree of life" (Gen. 3:22-24). Upon the ark of the covenant, of one substance with the mercy-seat, they saw the sprinkled blood which, in type, spake of the perfect maintenance of the divine righteousness by the sacrifice of Christ (Ex. 25:17-20; Rom. 3:24-26, *notes*). The living creatures (or Cherubim) appear to be actual beings of the angelic order. Cf. Isa. 6:2, *note.* The Cherubim or living creatures are not identical with the Seraphim (Isa. 6:2-7). They appear to have to do with the holiness of God as outraged by *sin;* the Seraphim with *uncleanness* in the people of God. The passage in Ezekiel is highly figurative, but the effect was the revelation to the prophet of the Shekinah glory of the LORD. Such revelations are connected invariably with new blessing and service. Cf. Ex. 3:2-10; Isa. 6:1-10; Dan. 10:5-14; Rev. 1:12-19.

went; they went every one straight
forward.
10 As for the [a]likeness of their faces,
they four [b]had the face of a man, and [c]the
face of a lion, on the right side: [d]and they
four had the face of an ox on the left side;
[e]they four also had the face of an eagle.
11 Thus *were* their faces: and their
wings *were* stretched upward; two *wings*
of every one *were* joined one to another,
and two covered their bodies.
12 And they went every one straight
forward: [f]whither the spirit was to go,
they went; *and* they turned not when
they went.
13 As for the likeness of the living creatures, their appearance *was* like burning
coals of fire, *and* like the appearance of
lamps: it went up and down among the
living creatures; and the fire was bright,
and out of the fire went forth lightning.
14 And the living creatures [g]ran and
returned as the appearance of a flash of
lightning.
15 Now as I beheld the living creatures,
behold one wheel upon the earth by the
living creatures, with his four faces.
16 The appearance of the wheels and
their work *was* [h]like unto the colour of a
beryl: and they four had one likeness: and
their appearance and their work *was* as it
were a wheel in the middle of a wheel.
17 When they went, they went upon
their four sides: *and* they turned not
when they went.
18 As for their rings, they were so high
that they were dreadful; and their rings
[i]*were* full of eyes round about them four.
19 And when the living creatures went,
the wheels went by them: and when the
living creatures were lifted up from the
earth, the wheels were lifted up.
20 Whithersoever the spirit was to go,
they went, thither *was their* spirit to go;
and the wheels were lifted up over
against them: for the spirit of the living
creature *was* in the wheels.
21 When those went, *these* went; and
when those stood, *these* stood; and when

B.C. 595.

a Cf. Rev. 4:7.
b Num. 2:3, 10, 18, 25.
c Num. 2:3.
d Num. 2:18.
e Num. 2:25.
f v. 20.
g Zech. 4:10.
h Dan. 10:6.
i Ezk. 10:12; Zech. 4:10.
j Ezk. 43:2; Dan. 10:6; Rev. 1:15.
k Job 37:4, 5; Psa. 29:3, 4; 68:33.
l Ex. 24:10.
m Rev. 4:3; 10:1.
n Ezk. 3:23; Dan. 8:17; Acts 9:4; Rev. 1:17.
o Dan. 10:11.

those were lifted up from the earth, the
wheels were lifted up over against them:
for the spirit of the living creature *was* in
the wheels.
22 And the likeness of the firmament
upon the heads of the living creature *was*
as the colour of the terrible crystal,
stretched forth over their heads above.
23 And under the firmament *were* their
wings straight, the one toward the other:
every one had two, which covered on
this side, and every one had two, which
covered on that side, their bodies.
24 And when they went, I heard the
noise of their wings, [j]like the noise of
great waters, [k]as the voice of the
Almighty, the voice of speech, as the
noise of an host: when they stood, they
let down their wings.
25 And there was a voice from the firmament that *was* over their heads, when
they stood, *and* had let down their wings.
26 And above the firmament that *was*
over their heads *was* the likeness of a
throne, [l]as the appearance of a sapphire
stone: and upon the likeness of the
throne *was* the likeness as the appearance of a man above upon it.
27 And I saw as the colour of amber,
as the appearance of fire round about
within it, from the appearance of his
loins even upward, and from the
appearance of his loins even downward,
I saw as it were the appearance of fire,
and it had brightness round about.
28 [m]As the appearance of the bow that
is in the cloud in the day of rain, so *was*
the appearance of the brightness round
about. This *was* the appearance of the
likeness of the glory of the LORD. And
when I saw *it*, [n]I fell upon my face, and I
heard a voice of one that spake.

CHAPTER 2.

(3) *The filling with the Spirit.*

And he said unto me, [1]Son of man,
[o]stand upon thy feet, and I will
speak unto thee.

[1](2:1) "Son of man," used by our Lord of Himself seventy-nine times, is used by Jehovah ninety-one times when addressing Ezekiel. (1) In the case of our Lord the meaning is clear: it is His racial name as the representative Man in the sense of 1 Cor. 15:45-47. The same thought, implying transcendence of mere Judaism, is involved in the phrase when applied to Ezekiel. Israel had forgotten her mission (Gen. 11:10, *note;* Ezk. 5:5-8). Now, in her captivity, Jehovah will not forsake His people, but He will remind them that they are but a small part of the race for whom He also cares. Hence the emphasis upon the word "man."

2 And the [a]spirit entered into me when he [b]spake unto me, and set me upon my feet, that I heard him that spake unto me.

(4) *The prophet commissioned.*

3 And he said unto me, Son of man, I send thee to the children of Israel, to a rebellious nation that hath rebelled against me: they and their fathers have transgressed against me, *even* unto this very day.

4 For *they are* impudent children and stiffhearted. I do send thee unto them; and thou shalt say unto them, Thus saith the Lord GOD.

5 And they, whether they will hear, or whether they will forbear, (for they *are* a rebellious house,) yet shall know that there hath been a prophet among them.

6 And thou, son of man, be not afraid of them, neither be afraid of their words, though briers and thorns *be* with thee, and thou dost dwell among scorpions: be not afraid of their words, nor be dismayed at their looks, though they *be* a rebellious house.

7 And thou shalt speak my words unto them, whether they will hear, or whether they will forbear: for they *are* most rebellious.

8 But thou, son of man, hear what I say unto thee; Be not thou rebellious like that rebellious house: open thy mouth, and eat that I give thee.

9 And when I looked, behold, an hand *was* sent unto me; and, lo, a roll of a book *was* therein;

10 And he spread it before me; and it *was* written within and without: and *there was* written therein lamentations, and mourning, and woe.

B.C. 595.

a *Holy Spirit.* Ezk. 3:12, 14, 24. (Gen. 1:2; Mal. 2:15.)

b *Inspiration.* Amos 3:7. (Ex. 4:15; Rev. 22:19.)

c Cf. Ezk. 2:10 and Rev. 10:9. Whatever its message, the word of God is sweet to faith because it *is* the word of God.

d Isa. 50:7; Jer. 1:18; 15:20; Mic. 3:8.

CHAPTER 3.

(*The prophet's commission,* continued, ends v. 21.)

Moreover he said unto me, Son of man, eat that thou findest; eat this roll, and go speak unto the house of Israel.

2 So I opened my mouth, and he caused me to eat that roll.

3 And he said unto me, Son of man, cause thy belly to eat, and fill thy bowels with this roll that I give thee. Then did I [c]eat *it;* and it was in my mouth as honey for sweetness.

4 And he said unto me, Son of man, go, get thee unto the house of Israel, and speak with my words unto them.

5 For thou *art* not sent to a people of a strange speech and of an hard language, *but* to the house of Israel;

6 Not to many people of a strange speech and of an hard language, whose words thou canst not understand. Surely, had I sent thee to them, they would have hearkened unto thee.

7 But the house of Israel will not hearken unto thee; for they will not hearken unto me: for all the house of Israel *are* impudent and hardhearted.

8 Behold, I have made thy face strong against their faces, and thy forehead strong against their foreheads.

9 [d]As an adamant harder than flint have I made thy forehead: fear them not, neither be dismayed at their looks, though they *be* a rebellious house.

PART II. THE PROPHET'S COMMISSION AS A WATCHMAN (SEE v. 17): CHAPTER 3:10-21.

10 Moreover he said unto me, Son of man, all my words that I shall speak unto thee receive in thine heart, and hear with thine ears.

11 And go, get thee to them of the captivity, unto the children of thy people, and speak unto them, and tell them, Thus saith the Lord GOD; whether they will hear, or whether they will forbear.

12 Then [e]the spirit took me up, and I heard behind me a voice of a great rushing, *saying,* Blessed *be* the glory of the LORD from his place.

e *Holy Spirit.* vs. 12, 14, 24; Ezk. 8:3. (Gen. 1:2; Mal. 2:15.)

The Cherubim "had the likeness of a *man*" (Ezk. 1:5); and when the prophet beheld the throne of God, he saw "the likeness as the appearance of a *man* above upon it" (Ezk. 1:26). See Mt. 8:20, *note;* Rev. 1:12, 13.

(2) As used of Ezekiel, the expression indicates, not what the prophet is in himself, but what he is to God: a son of man *(a)* chosen, *(b)* endued with the Spirit, and *(c)* sent of God. All this is true also of Christ who was, furthermore, the representative man—the head of regenerate humanity.

B.C. 595.

13 *I heard* also the noise of the wings of the living creatures that touched one another, and the noise of the wheels over against them, and a noise of a great rushing.

14 So the spirit lifted me up, and took me away, and I went in bitterness, in the heat of my spirit; but the [a]hand of the LORD was strong upon me.

15 Then I came to them of the captivity at Tel-abib, that dwelt by the river of Chebar, and I sat where they sat, and remained there astonished among them seven days.

16 And it came to pass at the end of seven days, that the word of the LORD came unto me, saying,

17 Son of man, I have made thee a [b]watchman unto the house of Israel: therefore hear the word at my mouth, and give them warning from me.

18 When I say unto the wicked, Thou shalt surely die; and thou givest him not warning, nor speakest to warn the wicked from his wicked way, to save his life; the same wicked *man* [c]shall die in his iniquity; but his blood will I require at thine hand.

19 Yet if thou warn the wicked, and he turn not from his wickedness, nor from his wicked way, he shall die in his iniquity; [d]but thou hast delivered thy soul.

20 Again, When a righteous *man* doth turn from his righteousness, and commit iniquity, and I lay a stumblingblock before him, he shall die: because thou hast not given him warning, he shall die in his sin, and his righteousness which he hath done shall not be remembered; but his blood will I require at thine hand.

21 Nevertheless if thou warn the righteous *man*, that the righteous sin not, and he doth not sin, he shall surely live, because he is warned; also thou hast delivered thy soul.

a 2 Ki. 3:15; Ezk. 1:3; 8:1; 37:1.
b Isa. 52:8; 56:10; 62:6; Jer. 6:17; cf. Isa. 56:10.
c Ezk. 33:6; John 8:21, 24.
d Isa. 49:4, 5; Acts 20:26.

PART III. EZEKIEL'S SECOND VISION OF THE GLORY, AND THE RESULT IN SERVICE: CHAPTERS 3:22–7:27.

22 And the hand of the LORD was there upon me; and he said unto me, Arise, go forth into the plain, and I will there talk with thee.

23 Then I arose, and went forth into the plain: and, behold, the glory of the LORD stood there, as the glory which I saw by the river of Chebar: and I fell on my face.

(1) *Ezekiel again filled with the Spirit* (cf. Acts 2:4; 4:31): *his dumbness.*

24 Then the spirit entered into me, and set me upon my feet, and spake with me, and said unto me, Go, shut thyself within thine house.

25 But thou, O son of man, behold, they shall put bands upon thee, and shall bind thee with them, and thou shalt not go out among them:

26 And I will make thy tongue cleave to the roof of thy mouth, that thou shalt be [e]dumb, and shalt not be to them a reprover: for they *are* a rebellious house.

27 [f]But when I speak with thee, I will open thy mouth, and thou shalt say unto them, Thus saith the Lord GOD; He that heareth, let him hear; and he that forbeareth, let him forbear: for they *are* a rebellious house.

CHAPTER 4.

(2) *The sign of the tile: symbolic actions.*

Thou also, son of man, [1]take thee a tile, and lay it before thee, and pourtray upon it the city, *even* Jerusalem:

2 And lay siege against it, and build a fort against it, and cast a mount against it; set the camp also against it, and set *battering* rams against it round about.

3 Moreover take thou unto thee an iron pan, and set it *for* a wall of iron between thee and the city: and set thy face against it, and it shall be besieged, and thou shalt lay siege against it. [g]This *shall be* a sign to the house of Israel.

4 Lie thou also upon thy left side, and lay the iniquity of the house of Israel upon it: *according* to the number of the

e Cf. Ezk. 24:27; 29:21.
f Ezk. 24:27; 33:22.
g Ezk. 12:6, 11; 24:24, 27.

[1] **(4:1)** The symbolic actions during the prophet's dumbness were testimonies to the past wickedness and chastisement of the house of Israel (the whole nation), and prophetic of a coming siege. They are therefore intermediate between the siege of 2 Ki. 24:10-16, at which time Ezekiel was carried to Babylon, and the siege of 2 Ki. 25:1-11, eleven years later.

days that thou shalt lie upon it thou shalt
bear their iniquity.
5 For I have laid upon thee the years
of their iniquity, according to the number of the days, three hundred and ninety days: so shalt thou bear the iniquity of
the house of Israel.
6 And when thou hast accomplished
them, lie again on thy right side, and
thou shalt bear the iniquity of the house
of Judah forty days: I have appointed
thee each day for a year.
7 Therefore thou shalt set thy face
toward the siege of Jerusalem, and thine
arm *shall be* uncovered, and thou shalt
prophesy against it.
8 And, behold, I will lay bands upon
thee, and thou shalt not turn thee from
one side to another, till thou hast ended
the days of thy siege.
9 Take thou also unto thee wheat, and
barley, and beans, and lentiles, and millet, and fitches, and put them in one vessel, and make thee bread thereof, *according* to the number of the days that thou
shalt lie upon thy side, three hundred
and ninety days shalt thou eat thereof.
10 And thy meat which thou shalt eat
shall be by weight, twenty shekels a day:
from time to time shalt thou eat it.
11 Thou shalt drink also water by
measure, the sixth part of an [a]hin: from
time to time shalt thou drink.
12 And thou shalt eat it *as* barley
cakes, and thou shalt bake it with dung
that cometh out of man, in their sight.
13 And the LORD said, Even thus [b]shall
the children of Israel eat their defiled
bread among the Gentiles, whither I will
drive them.
14 Then said I, [c]Ah Lord GOD! behold,
my soul hath not been polluted: for from
my youth up even till now have I not
eaten of that which dieth of itself, or is
torn in pieces; neither came there abominable flesh into my mouth.
15 Then he said unto me, Lo, I have
given thee cow's dung for man's dung,
and thou shalt prepare thy bread therewith.
16 Moreover he said unto me, Son of
man, behold, I will break [d]the staff of
bread in Jerusalem: and they shall eat
bread by weight, and with care; and they
shall drink water by measure, and with
astonishment:

B.C. 595.

a One hin = about 6 qts.

b Hos. 9:3.

c Acts 10:14.

d Lev. 26:26; Psa. 105:16; Isa. 3:1; Ezk. 5:16; 14:13.

e See Lev. 21:5; Isa. 7:20; Ezk. 44:20.

f Jer. 40:6; 52:16.

g Lam. 4:6; Dan. 9:12; Amos 3:2.

17 That they may want bread and
water, and be astonied one with another,
and consume away for their iniquity.

CHAPTER 5.

(3) *The sign of the sharp knife:*
i.e. *famine, pestilence, the sword.*

And thou, son of man, take thee a
sharp knife, take thee a barber's
razor, and [e]cause *it* to pass upon thine
head and upon thy beard: then take thee
balances to weigh, and divide the *hair*.
2 Thou shalt burn with fire a third part
in the midst of the city, when the days of
the siege are fulfilled: and thou shalt
take a third part, *and* smite about it with
a knife: and a third part thou shalt scatter in the wind; and I will draw out a
sword after them.
3 [f]Thou shalt also take thereof a few in
number, and bind them in thy skirts.
4 Then take of them again, and cast
them into the midst of the fire, and burn
them in the fire; *for* thereof shall a fire
come forth into all the house of Israel.
5 Thus saith the Lord GOD; This *is*
Jerusalem: I have set it in the midst of
the nations and countries *that are* round
about her.
6 And she hath changed my judgments
into wickedness more than the nations,
and my statutes more than the countries
that *are* round about her: for they have
refused my judgments and my statutes,
they have not walked in them.
7 Therefore thus saith the Lord GOD;
Because ye multiplied more than the
nations that *are* round about you, *and*
have not walked in my statutes, neither
have kept my judgments, neither have
done according to the judgments of the
nations that *are* round about you;
8 Therefore thus saith the Lord GOD;
Behold, I, even I, *am* against thee, and
will execute judgments in the midst of
thee in the sight of the nations.
9 [g]And I will do in thee that which I
have not done, and whereunto I will not
do any more the like, because of all thine
abominations.
10 Therefore the fathers shall eat the
sons in the midst of thee, and the sons
shall eat their fathers; and I will execute
judgments in thee, and the whole

B.C. 594.

remnant of thee will I [a]scatter into all the winds.

11 Wherefore, *as* I live, saith the Lord GOD; Surely, because thou hast defiled my sanctuary with all thy detestable things, and with all thine abominations, therefore will I also diminish *thee;* [b]neither shall mine eye spare, neither will I have any pity.

12 A third part of thee shall die with the pestilence, and with famine shall they be consumed in the midst of thee: and a third part shall fall by the sword round about thee; and I [c]will scatter a third part into all the winds, and I will draw out a sword after them.

13 Thus shall mine anger be accomplished, and I will cause my fury to rest upon them, and I will be comforted: [d]and they shall know that I the LORD have spoken *it* in my zeal, when I have accomplished my fury in them.

14 Moreover [e]I will make thee waste, and a reproach among the nations that *are* round about thee, in the sight of all that pass by.

15 So it shall be a [f]reproach and a taunt, an instruction and an astonishment unto the nations that *are* round about thee, when I shall execute judgments in thee in anger and in fury and in furious rebukes. I the LORD have spoken *it*.

16 When I shall send upon them the evil arrows of famine, which shall be for *their* destruction, *and* which I will send to destroy you: and I will increase the famine upon you, and will break your staff of bread:

17 So will I send upon you famine and evil beasts, and they shall bereave thee; and pestilence and blood shall pass through thee; and I will bring the sword upon thee. I the LORD have spoken *it*.

CHAPTER 6.

(4) *The message against the mountains of Israel.*

And the word of the LORD came unto me, saying,

2 Son of man, set thy face toward the mountains of Israel, and prophesy against them,

3 And say, Ye mountains of Israel, hear the word of the Lord GOD; Thus saith the Lord GOD to the mountains, and to the hills, to the rivers, and to the valleys; Behold, I, *even* I, will bring a sword upon you, and [g]I will destroy your high places.

4 And your altars shall be desolate, and your images shall be broken: and [g]I will cast down your slain *men* before your idols.

5 And I will lay the dead carcases of the children of Israel before their idols; and I will scatter your bones round about your altars.

6 In all your dwellingplaces the cities shall be laid waste, and the high places shall be desolate; that your altars may be laid waste and made desolate, and your idols may be broken and cease, and your images may be cut down, and your works may be abolished.

7 And the slain shall fall in the midst of you, and ye shall know that I *am* the LORD.

(5) *A remnant to be spared.*

8 Yet will I leave a [h]remnant, that ye may have *some* that shall escape the sword among the nations, when ye shall be scattered through the countries.

9 And they that escape of you shall remember me among the nations whither they shall be carried captives, because I am broken with their whorish heart, which hath departed from me, and with their eyes, which go a whoring after their idols: and they shall lothe themselves for the evils which they have committed in all their abominations.

10 And they shall know that I *am* the LORD, *and that* I have not said in vain that I would do this evil unto them.

(6) *Desolation upon the land.*

11 Thus saith the Lord GOD; [i]Smite with thine hand, and stamp with thy foot, and say, Alas for all the evil abominations of the house of Israel! [j]for they shall fall by the sword, by the famine, and by the pestilence.

12 He that is far off shall die of the pestilence; and he that is near shall fall by the sword; and he that remaineth and is besieged shall die by the famine: [k]thus will I accomplish my fury upon them.

13 Then shall ye know that I *am* the LORD, when their slain *men* shall be among their idols round about their altars, [l]upon every high hill, [m]in all the tops of the mountains, and [n]under every green tree, and under every thick oak,

a v. 12; Ezk. 12:14; Lev. 26:33; Deut. 28:64; Zech. 2:6.
b Ezk. 7:4, 9; 8:18; 9:10.
c vs. 2, 10; Ezk. 6:8; Jer. 9:16.
d Ezk. 36:6; 38:19.
e Lev. 26:31, 32; Neh. 2:17.
f Deut. 28:37; 1 Ki. 9:7; Psa. 79:4; Jer. 24:9; Lam. 2:15.
g Lev. 26:30.
h *Remnant.* vs. 8:11-14; Ezk. 9:4. (Isa. 1:9; Rom. 11:5.)
i Ezk. 21:14.
j Ezk. 5:12.
k Ezk. 5:13.
l Jer. 2:20; 3:6.
m Hos. 4:13.
n Isa. 57:5.

the place where they did offer sweet
savour to all their idols.
14 So will I stretch out my hand upon
them, and make the land desolate, yea,
more desolate than the wilderness
toward [a]Diblath, in all their habitations:
and they shall know that I *am* the LORD.

CHAPTER 7.

(*Part III.*, concluded.)

Moreover the word of the LORD came
unto me, saying,
2 Also, thou son of man, thus saith the
Lord GOD unto the land of Israel; [b]An
end, the end is come upon the four corners of the land.
3 Now *is* the end *come* upon thee, and
I will send mine anger upon thee, and
will judge thee according to thy ways,
and will recompense upon thee all thine
abominations.
4 [c]And mine eye shall not spare thee,
neither will I have pity: but I will recompense thy ways upon thee, and thine
abominations shall be in the midst of thee:
[d]and ye shall know that I *am* the LORD.
5 Thus saith the Lord GOD; An evil, an
only evil, behold, is come.
6 An end is come, the end is come: it
watcheth for thee; behold, it is come.
7 The morning is come unto thee, O
thou that dwellest in the land: the [e]time is
come, the day of trouble *is* near, and not
the sounding again of the mountains.
8 Now will I shortly pour out my fury
upon thee, and accomplish mine anger
upon thee: and I will judge thee according to thy ways, and will recompense
thee for all thine abominations.
9 And mine eye shall not spare, neither will I have pity: I will recompense
thee according to thy ways and thine
abominations *that* are in the midst of
thee; and ye shall know that I *am* the
LORD that smiteth.
10 Behold the day, behold, it is come:
the morning is gone forth; the rod hath
blossomed, pride hath budded.
11 Violence is risen up into a rod of
wickedness: none of them *shall remain*, nor
of their multitude, nor of any of theirs:
neither *shall there be* wailing for them.
12 [f]The time is come, the day draweth
near: let not the buyer rejoice, nor the
seller mourn: for wrath *is* upon all the
multitude thereof.
13 For the seller shall not return to that
which is sold, although they were yet
alive: for the vision *is* touching the
whole multitude thereof, *which* shall not
return; neither shall any strengthen himself in the iniquity of his life.
14 They have blown the trumpet, even
to make all ready; but none goeth to the
battle: for my wrath *is* upon all the multitude thereof.
15 [g]The sword *is* without, and the
pestilence and the famine within: he that
is in the field shall die with the sword;
and he that *is* in the city, famine and
pestilence shall devour him.
16 But they that escape of them shall
escape, and shall be on the mountains
like doves of the valleys, all of them
mourning, every one for his iniquity.
17 [h]All hands shall be feeble, and all
knees shall be weak *as* water.
18 [i]They shall also gird *themselves* with
sackcloth, and horror shall cover them;
and shame *shall be* upon all faces, and
baldness upon all their heads.
19 They shall cast their silver in the
streets, and their gold shall be removed:
[j]their silver and their gold shall not be able
to deliver them in the day of the wrath of
the LORD: they shall not satisfy their souls,
neither fill their bowels: because it is the
stumblingblock of their iniquity.
20 As for the beauty of his ornament,
he set it in majesty: but they made the
images of their abominations *and* of their
detestable things therein: therefore have
I set it far from them.
21 And I will give it into the hands of
the strangers for a prey, and to the
wicked of the earth for a spoil; and they
shall pollute it.
22 My face will I turn also from them,
and they shall pollute my secret *place*:
for the robbers shall enter into it, and
defile it.
23 Make a chain: for the land is full of
bloody crimes, and the city is full of violence.
24 Wherefore I will bring the worst of
the [k]heathen, and they shall possess
their houses: I will also make the pomp
of the strong to cease; and their holy
places shall be defiled.
25 Destruction cometh; and they

B.C. 594.

a Num. 33:46; Jer. 48:22.

b vs. 3, 6; Amos 8:2; Mt. 24:6, 13, 14.

c v. 9; Ezk. 5:11; 8:18; 9:10.

d v. 27; Ezk. 6:7; 12:20.

e v. 12; Zeph. 1:14, 15.

f v. 7.

g Ezk. 5:12; Lam. 1:20.

h Ezk. 21:7; Isa. 13:7; Jer. 6:24.

i Isa. 3:24; 15:2, 3; Jer. 48:37; Amos 8:10.

j Prov. 11:4; Zeph. 1:18.

k i.e. *nations*.

shall seek peace, and *there shall be* none.
26 Mischief shall come upon mischief,
and rumour shall be upon rumour; [a]then
shall they seek a vision of the prophet;
but the law shall perish from the priest,
and counsel from the ancients.
27 The king shall mourn, and the
prince shall be clothed with desolation,
and the hands of the people of the land
shall be troubled: I will do unto them
after their way, and according to their
deserts will I judge them; and they shall
know that I *am* the LORD.

B.C. 594.

a Ezk. 20:1, 3; Psa. 74:9; Lam. 2:9.

PART IV. GENERAL THEME: JEHOVAH JUSTIFIED IN SENDING HIS PEOPLE INTO CAPTIVITY: CHAPTERS 8:1–33:20; KEY VERSE, 33:20.

CHAPTER 8.

And it came to pass in the [b]sixth year,
in the sixth *month,* in the fifth *day* of
the month, *as* I sat in mine house, and the
elders of Judah sat before me, that the
hand of the Lord GOD fell there upon me.

Third vision of the glory.
(Cf. Ezk. 1:1; 3:12, 22.)

2 Then I beheld, and lo a likeness as
the appearance of fire: from the appearance of his loins even downward, fire;
and from his loins even upward, as the
appearance of brightness, as the colour
of amber.
3 And he put forth the form of an
hand, and took me by a lock of mine
head; and the [c]spirit [d]lifted me up
between the earth and the heaven, and
brought me in the [1]visions of God to
Jerusalem, to the door of the inner gate
that looketh toward the north; [e]where
was the seat of the image of jealousy,
[f]which provoketh to jealousy.
4 And, behold, the glory of the God of
Israel *was* there, according to the vision
that I [g]saw in the plain.

Former profanations of the temple.

5 Then said he unto me, [2]Son of man,
lift up thine eyes now the way toward
the north. So I lifted up mine eyes the
way toward the north, and behold
northward at the gate of the altar this
image of jealousy in the entry.
6 He said furthermore unto me, Son of
man, seest thou what they do? *even* the
great abominations that the house of
Israel committeth here, that I should go
far off from my sanctuary? but turn thee
yet again, *and* thou shalt see greater
abominations.
7 And he brought me to the door of
the court; and when I looked, behold a
hole in the wall.
8 Then said he unto me, Son of man,
dig now in the wall: and when I had
digged in the wall, behold a door.
9 And he said unto me, Go in, and
behold the wicked abominations that
they do here.
10 So I went in and saw; and behold
every form of creeping things, and
abominable beasts, and all the idols of
the house of Israel, pourtrayed upon the
wall round about.
11 And there stood before them seventy men of the ancients of the house of
Israel, and in the midst of them stood
Jaazaniah the son of Shaphan, with
every man his censer in his hand; and a
thick cloud of incense went up.
12 Then said he unto me, Son of man,

b i.e. *September.*

c *Holy Spirit.* Ezk. 10:17. (Gen. 1:2; Mal. 2:15.)

d Acts 8:39; cf. 2 Cor. 12:2-4.

e Ezk. 5:11; Jer. 7:30; 32:34.

f Deut. 32:16, 21.

g Ezk. 1:28; 3:22, 23.

[1] **(8:3)** Visions, that is, of former profanations of the temple, and of the wickedness because of which Israel was then in Babylon, shown the prophet that he might justify to the new generation born in Assyria and Babylonia during the captivity, the righteousness of God in the present national chastening. The visions are retrospective; Israel had done these things, hence the captivities. This strain continues to Ezk. 33:20. It is the divine view of the national sinfulness and apostasy, revealed to Ezekiel in a series of visions so vivid that though the prophet was by the river Chebar (Ezk. 1:1, 3; 3:23; 10:15, 20, 22; 43:3) it was as if he were transported back to Jerusalem, and to the time when these things were occurring. These visions of the sinfulness of Israel are interspersed with promises of restoration and blessing which are yet to be fulfilled. See "Israel" (Gen. 12:2, 3; Rom. 11:26). Also "Kingdom, (O.T.)" (Gen. 1:26-28; Zech. 12:8).

[2] **(8:5)** The combined purport of the four visions of profanation in Chapter 8 is idolatry set up in the entire temple, even in the holy of holies (vs. 10, 11); women given over to phallic cults (v. 14); and nature-worship (v. 16).

hast thou seen what the ancients of the house of Israel do in the dark, every man in the chambers of his imagery? for they say, The LORD seeth us not; the LORD hath forsaken the earth.

13 He said also unto me, Turn thee yet again, *and* thou shalt see greater abominations that they do.

14 Then he brought me to the door of the gate of the LORD'S house which *was* toward the north; and, behold, there sat women weeping for [a]Tammuz.

15 Then said he unto me, Hast thou seen *this*, O son of man? turn thee yet again, *and* thou shalt see greater abominations than these.

16 And he brought me into the inner court of the LORD'S house, and, behold, at the door of the temple of the LORD, [b]between the porch and the altar, *were* about five and twenty men, with their backs toward the temple of the LORD, and their faces toward the east; and they worshipped the [c]sun toward the east.

17 Then he said unto me, Hast thou seen *this*, O son of man? Is it a light thing to the house of Judah that they commit the abominations which they commit here? for they have filled the land with violence, and have returned to provoke me to anger: and, lo, they put the branch to their nose.

18 Therefore will I also deal in fury: mine eye shall not spare, neither will I have pity: and though they [d]cry in mine ears with a loud voice, *yet* will I not hear them.

CHAPTER 9.

The vision of the slaying in Jerusalem.

HE cried also in mine ears with a loud voice, saying, Cause them that have charge over the city to draw near, even every man *with* his destroying weapon in his hand.

2 And, behold, six men came from the way of the higher gate, which lieth toward the north, and every man a slaughter weapon in his hand; and one man among them *was* clothed with linen, with a writer's inkhorn by his side: and they went in, and stood beside the brasen altar.

3 [e]And the glory of the God of Israel was [1]gone up from the cherub, whereupon he was, to the threshold of the house. And he called to the man clothed with linen, which *had* the writer's inkhorn by his side;

4 And the LORD said unto him, [f]Go through the midst of the city, through the midst of Jerusalem, and [g]set a mark upon the foreheads of the men that sigh and that cry for all the abominations that be done in the midst thereof.

5 And to the others he said in mine hearing, Go ye after him through the city, and smite: let not your eye spare, neither have ye pity:

6 [h]Slay utterly old *and* young, both maids, and little children, and women: but come not near any man upon whom *is* the mark; and [i]begin at my sanctuary. Then they began at the ancient men which *were* before the house.

7 And he said unto them, Defile the house, and fill the courts with the slain: go ye forth. And they went forth, and slew in the city.

8 And it came to pass, while they were slaying them, and I was left, that I fell upon my face, and cried, and [j]said, Ah Lord GOD! wilt thou destroy all the residue of Israel in thy pouring out of thy fury upon Jerusalem?

9 Then said he unto me, The iniquity of the house of Israel and Judah *is* exceeding great, and [k]the land is full of blood, and the city full of perverseness: for they say, The LORD hath forsaken the earth, and the LORD seeth not.

10 And as for me also, mine eye shall not spare, neither will I have pity, *but* I will recompense their way upon their head.

11 And, behold, the man clothed with linen, which *had* the inkhorn by his side, reported the matter, saying, I have done as thou hast commanded me.

B.C. 594.

a i.e. the Greek Adonis.

b Joel 2:17.

c Deut. 4:19; 2 Ki. 23:5, 11; Job 31:26; Jer. 44:17.

d Prov. 1:28; Isa. 1:15; Jer. 11:11; 14:12; Mic. 3:4; Zech. 7:13.

e See Ezk. 3:23; 8:4; 10:4,18; 11:22, 23.

f Ex. 12:7; Rev. 7:3; 9:4; 13:16, 17; 20:4.

g *Remnant.* Ezk. 11:16-21. (Isa. 1:9; Rom. 11:5.)

h 2 Chr. 36:17.

i 1 Pet. 4:17.

j *Bible prayers* (O.T.). Dan. 9:4. (Gen. 15:2; Hab. 3:1-16.)

k Ezk. 8:17; 2 Ki. 21:16.

1(9:3) It is noteworthy that to Ezekiel the *priest* was given the vision of the glory of the LORD (1) departing from the Cherubim to the threshold of the temple (Ezk. 9:3; 10:4); (2) from the threshold (Ezk. 10:18); (3) from temple and city to the mountain on the East of Jerusalem (Olivet, Ezk. 11:23); and (4) returning to the millennial temple to abide (Ezk. 43:2-5).

CHAPTER 10.

The vision of altar fire scattered over Jerusalem.

Then I looked, and, behold, in the firmament that was above the head of the cherubims there appeared over them as it were a sapphire stone, as the appearance of the likeness of a throne.

2 [a]And he spake unto the man clothed with linen, and said, Go in between the wheels, *even* under the cherub, and fill [b]thine hand with coals of fire from between the cherubims, and [c]scatter *them* over the city. And he went in in my sight.

3 Now the cherubims stood on the right side of the house, when the man went in; and the cloud filled the inner court.

4 Then the glory of the LORD went up from the cherub, *and stood* over the threshold of the house; and [d]the house was filled with the cloud, and the court was full of the brightness of the LORD'S glory.

5 And the sound of the cherubims' wings was heard *even* to the outer court, [e]as the voice of the Almighty God when he speaketh.

6 And it came to pass, *that* when he had commanded the man clothed with linen, saying, Take fire from between the wheels, from between the cherubims; then he went in, and stood beside the wheels.

7 And *one* cherub stretched forth his hand from between the cherubims unto the fire that *was* between the cherubims, and took *thereof*, and put *it* into the hands of *him that was* clothed with linen: who took *it*, and went out.

Description of the cherubim.

8 And there appeared in the cherubims the form of a man's hand under their wings.

9 And when I looked, behold the four wheels by the cherubims, one wheel by one cherub, and another wheel by another cherub: and the appearance of the wheels *was* as the colour of a beryl stone.

10 And *as for* their appearances, they four had one likeness, as if a wheel had been in the midst of a wheel.

11 [f]When they went, they went upon their four sides; they turned not as they went, but to the place whither the head looked they followed it; they turned not as they went.

12 And their whole [g]body, and their backs, and their hands, and their wings, and the wheels, *were* full of eyes round about, *even* the wheels that they four had.

13 As for the wheels, it was cried unto them in my hearing, O wheel.

14 And every one had four faces: the first face *was* the face of a cherub, and the second face *was* the face of a man, and the third the face of a lion, and the fourth the face of an eagle.

15 And the cherubims were lifted up. [h]This *is* the living creature that I saw by the river of Chebar.

16 And when the cherubims went, the wheels went by them: and when the cherubims lifted up their wings to mount up from the earth, the same wheels also turned not from beside them.

17 When they stood, *these* stood; and when they were lifted up, *these* lifted up themselves *also*: for the [i]spirit of the living creature *was* in them.

18 Then the glory of the LORD [j]departed from off the threshold of the house, and stood over the cherubims.

19 And the cherubims lifted up their wings, and mounted up from the earth in my sight: when they went out, the wheels also *were* beside them, and *every one* stood at the door of the east gate of the LORD'S house; and the glory of the God of Israel *was* over them above.

20 [k]This *is* the living creature that I saw under the God of Israel by the river of Chebar; and I knew that they *were* the cherubims.

21 Every one had four faces apiece, and every one four wings; and the likeness of the hands of a man *was* under their wings.

22 And the likeness of their faces *was* the same faces which I saw by the river of Chebar, their appearances and themselves: they went every one straight forward.

CHAPTER 11.

Vision of wrath against the lying princes.

Moreover [l]the spirit lifted me up, and brought me unto the east gate of the LORD'S house, which looketh eastward: and behold at the door of the gate

B.C. 594.

a Ezk. 9:2, 3; Dan. 10:5.

b Heb. *the hollow of thine hand.*

c See Rev. 8:5.

d Ezk. 43:5; 1 Ki. 8:10, 11.

e Psa. 29:3.

f Ezk. 1:17.

g Heb. *flesh.*

h Ezk. 1:5.

i *Holy Spirit.* Ezk. 36:27. (Gen. 1:2; Mal. 2:15.)

j Hos. 9:12.

k Ezk. 1:22; 10:15.

l v. 24; Ezk. 3:12, 14; 8:3.

five and twenty men; among whom I
saw Jaazaniah the son of Azur, and
Pelatiah the son of Benaiah, princes of
the people.
2 Then said he unto me, Son of man,
these *are* the men that devise mischief,
and give wicked counsel in this city:
3 Which say, *It is* not near; let us build
houses: this *city is* the caldron, and we *be*
the flesh.
4 Therefore prophesy against them,
prophesy, O son of man.
5 And [a]the Spirit of the LORD fell upon
me, and said unto me, Speak; Thus saith
the LORD; Thus have ye said, O house of
Israel: for I know the things that come
into your mind, *every one of* them.
6 Ye have multiplied your slain in this
city, and ye have filled the streets thereof
with the slain.
7 Therefore thus saith the Lord GOD;
[b]Your slain whom ye have laid in the
midst of it, they *are* the flesh, and this
city is the caldron: but I will bring you
forth out of the midst of it.
8 Ye have feared the sword; and I will
bring a sword upon you, saith the Lord
GOD.
9 And I will bring you out of the midst
thereof, and deliver you into the hands
of strangers, and will execute judgments
among you.
10 [c]Ye shall fall by the sword; I will
judge you in the border of Israel; and ye
shall know that I *am* the LORD.
11 This *city* shall not be your caldron,
neither shall ye be the flesh in the midst
thereof; *but* I will judge you in the border of Israel:
12 And ye shall know that I *am* the
LORD: for ye have not walked in my
statutes, neither executed my judgments,
but have done after the manners of the
[d]heathen that *are* round about you.
13 And it came to pass, when I prophesied, that Pelatiah the son of Benaiah
died. Then fell I down upon my face,
and cried with a loud voice, and said,
Ah Lord GOD! wilt thou make a full end
of the remnant of Israel?

The promise to spare the remnant.

14 Again the word of the LORD came
unto me, saying,
15 Son of man, thy brethren, *even* thy
brethren, the men of thy kindred, and
[e]all the house of Israel wholly, *are* they
unto whom the inhabitants of Jerusalem
have said, Get you far from the LORD:
unto us is this land given in possession.
16 Therefore say, Thus saith the Lord
GOD; Although I have cast them far off
among the [d]heathen, and although I have
[f]scattered them among the countries, [g]yet
will I be to them as a little sanctuary in
the countries where they shall come.

Israel to be restored to the land and converted.

17 Therefore say, Thus saith the Lord
GOD; I will even [h]gather you from the
people, and assemble you out of the
countries where ye have been scattered,
and I will give you the land of Israel.
18 And they shall come thither, and
they shall take away all the detestable
things thereof and all the abominations
thereof from thence.
19 And [i]I will give them one heart, and
[j]I will put a new spirit within you; and I
will take the stony heart out of their flesh,
and will give them an heart of flesh:
20 That they may walk in my statutes,
and keep mine ordinances, and do them:
and [k]they shall be my people, and I will
be their God.
21 But *as for them* whose heart walketh
after the heart of their detestable things
and their abominations, I will recompense their way upon their own heads,
saith the Lord GOD.

Vision of the departure of the glory from Jerusalem (Cf. 1 Ki. 8:5-11; Ezra 3:12; Ezk. 43:2-5.)

22 Then did the cherubims lift up their
wings, and the wheels beside them; and
the glory of the God of Israel *was* over
them above.
23 [l]And the glory of the LORD went up
from the midst of the city, and stood
upon the mountain which *is* on the east
side of the city.
24 Afterwards the spirit took me up,
and brought me in a vision by the Spirit
of God into Chaldea, to them of the captivity. So the vision that I had seen went
up from me.
25 Then I spake unto them of the captivity all the things that the LORD had
shewed me.

CHAPTER 12.

Vision of the prophet as a sign (v. 11).

The word of the LORD also came unto
me, saying,
2 Son of man, thou dwellest in the

B.C. 594.

a Ezk. 2:2; 3:24.
b Ezk. 24:3, 6, 10,11; Mic. 3:3.
c 2 Ki. 25:19-21; Jer. 39:6; 52:10.
d i.e. *nations*.
e *Kingdom* (O.T.). vs. 14-20; Ezk. 20:33-44. (Gen. 1:26; Zech. 12:8.)
f *Remnant.* vs. 16-21; Joel 2:32. (Isa. 1:9; Rom. 11:5.)
g Psa. 90:1; 91:9; Isa. 8:14.
h Ezk. 28:25; 34:13; 36:24; Jer. 24:6.
i Ezk. 36:26; Jer. 32:39; Zeph. 3:9.
j Ezk. 18:31; Psa. 51:10; Jer. 31:33; 32:39.
k Ezk. 14:11; 36:28; 37:27; Jer. 24:7.
l Ezk. 8:4; 9:3; 10:4, 18; 43:4.

midst of a rebellious house, which have
eyes to see, and see not; they have ears
to hear, and hear not: for they *are* a rebellious house.
3 Therefore, thou son of man, prepare
thee stuff for removing, and remove by
day in their sight; and thou shalt remove
from thy place to another place in their
sight: it may be they will consider,
though they *be* a rebellious house.
4 Then shalt thou bring forth thy stuff
by day in their sight, as stuff for removing: and thou shalt go forth at even in
their sight, as they that go forth into captivity.
5 Dig thou through the wall in their
sight, and carry out thereby.
6 In their sight shalt thou bear *it* upon
thy shoulders, *and* carry *it* forth in the
twilight: thou shalt cover thy face, that
thou see not the ground: [a]for I have set
thee *for* a sign unto the house of Israel.
7 And I did so as I was commanded: I
brought forth my stuff by day, as stuff
for captivity, and in the even I digged
through the wall with mine hand; I
brought *it* forth in the twilight, *and* I bare
it upon *my* shoulder in their sight.
8 And in the morning came the word
of the LORD unto me, saying,
9 Son of man, hath not the house of
Israel, the rebellious house, said unto
thee, What doest thou?
10 Say thou unto them, Thus saith the
Lord GOD; This [b]burden *concerneth* the
prince in Jerusalem, and all the house of
Israel that *are* among them.
11 Say, I *am* your sign: like as I have
done, so shall it be done unto them: they
shall remove *and* go into captivity.
12 And the [c]prince that *is* among them
shall bear upon *his* shoulder in the twilight, and shall go forth: they shall dig
through the wall to carry out thereby: he
shall cover his face, that he see not the
ground with *his* eyes.
13 My net also will I spread upon him,
[d]and he shall be taken in my snare: and I
will bring him to Babylon *to* the land of
the Chaldeans; yet shall he not see it,
though he shall die there.
14 And [e]I will scatter toward every
wind all that *are* about him to help him,
and all his bands; and I will draw out
the sword after them.

B.C. 594.

a v. 11; Ezk. 4:3; 24:24; Isa. 8:18.

b Isa. 13:1, *note.*

c Jer. 39:4; 52:7.

d Jer. 32:4, 5.

e Ezk. 5:10; 2 Ki. 25:4, 5.

f vs. 16, 20; Ezk. 6:7, 14; 11:10; Psa. 9:16.

g i.e. *nations.*

h v. 27; Ezk. 11:3; 2 Pet. 3:4.

i Joel 2:1; Zeph. 1:14.

j Isa. 55:11; Ezk. 12:28; Dan. 9:12; Lk. 21:33.

15 [f]And they shall know that I *am* the
LORD, when I shall scatter them among
the nations, and disperse them in the
countries.
16 But I will leave a few men of them
from the sword, from the famine, and
from the pestilence; that they may
declare all their abominations among the
[g]heathen whither they come; and they
shall know that I *am* the LORD.

The full captivity near at hand.
(Cf. 2 Ki. 25:1-10.)

17 Moreover the word of the LORD
came to me, saying,
18 Son of man, eat thy bread with
quaking, and drink thy water with trembling and with carefulness;
19 And say unto the people of the land,
Thus saith the Lord GOD of the inhabitants of Jerusalem, *and* of the land of
Israel; They shall eat their bread with
carefulness, and drink their water with
astonishment, that her land may be desolate from all that is therein, because of the
violence of all them that dwell therein.
20 And the cities that are inhabited
shall be laid waste, and the land shall be
desolate; and ye shall know that I *am* the
LORD.
21 And the word of the LORD came
unto me, saying,
22 Son of man, what *is* that proverb
that ye have in the land of Israel, saying,
[h]The days are prolonged, and every
vision faileth?
23 Tell them therefore, Thus saith the
Lord GOD; I will make this proverb to
cease, and they shall no more use it as a
proverb in Israel; but say unto them,
[i]The days are at hand, and the effect of
every vision.
24 For there shall be no more any vain
vision nor flattering divination within
the house of Israel.
25 For I *am* the LORD: I will speak, and
[j]the word that I shall speak shall come to
pass; it shall be no more prolonged: [1]for
in your days, O rebellious house, will I
say the word, and will perform it, saith
the Lord GOD.
26 Again the word of the LORD came
to me, saying,
27 Son of man, behold, *they of* the

[1]**(12:25)** It must constantly be remembered that though the prophet was in Babylonia he prophesies as if in the land, and during the eleven years' interval between the first and the final deportation. See Ezk. 8:3, *note.*

house of Israel say, The vision that he seeth *is* [a]for many days *to come*, and he prophesieth of the times *that are* far off.

28 Therefore say unto them, Thus saith the Lord GOD; There shall none of my words be prolonged any more, but the word which I have spoken shall be done, saith the Lord GOD.

CHAPTER 13.

The message against the lying prophets.

And the word of the LORD came unto me, saying,

2 Son of man, prophesy against the prophets of Israel that prophesy, and say thou unto them that prophesy out of their own hearts, Hear ye the word of the LORD;

3 Thus saith the Lord GOD; Woe unto the foolish prophets, that follow their own spirit, and have seen nothing!

4 O Israel, thy prophets are like the foxes in the deserts.

5 [b]Ye have not gone up into the gaps, neither made up the hedge for the house of Israel to stand in the battle in the day of the LORD.

6 They have seen vanity and lying divination, saying, The LORD saith: and the LORD hath not sent them: and they have made *others* to hope that they would confirm the word.

7 Have ye not seen a vain vision, and have ye not spoken a lying divination, whereas ye say, The LORD saith *it*; albeit I have not spoken?

8 Therefore thus saith the Lord GOD; Because ye have spoken vanity, and seen lies, therefore, behold, I *am* against you, saith the Lord GOD.

9 And mine hand shall be upon the prophets that see vanity, and that divine lies: they shall not be in the assembly of my people, [c]neither shall they be written in the writing of the house of Israel, neither shall they enter into the land of Israel; and ye shall know that I *am* the Lord GOD.

10 Because, even because they have seduced my people, saying, Peace; and *there was* no peace; and one built up a wall, and, lo, others [d]daubed it with untempered *morter*:

11 Say unto them which daub *it* with untempered *morter*, that it shall fall: [e]there shall be an overflowing shower; and ye, O great hailstones, shall fall; and a stormy wind shall rend *it*.

12 Lo, when the wall is fallen, shall it not be said unto you, Where *is* the daubing wherewith ye have daubed *it*?

13 Therefore thus saith the Lord GOD; I will even rend *it* with a stormy wind in my fury; and there shall be an overflowing shower in mine anger, and great hailstones in *my* fury to consume *it*.

14 So will I break down the wall that ye have daubed with untempered *morter*, and bring it down to the ground, so that the foundation thereof shall be discovered, and it shall fall, and ye shall be consumed in the midst thereof: and [f]ye shall know that I *am* the LORD.

15 Thus will I accomplish my wrath upon the wall, and upon them that have daubed it with untempered *morter*, and will say unto you, The wall *is* no *more*, neither they that daubed it;

16 *To wit*, the prophets of Israel which prophesy concerning Jerusalem, and which [g]see visions of peace for her, and *there is* no peace, saith the Lord GOD.

17 Likewise, thou son of man, set thy face against the daughters of thy people, which prophesy out of their own heart; and prophesy thou against them,

18 And say, Thus saith the Lord GOD; Woe to the *women* that sew pillows to all armholes, and make kerchiefs upon the head of every stature to hunt souls! [h]Will ye hunt the souls of my people, and will ye save the souls alive *that come* unto you?

19 And will ye pollute me among my people [i]for handfuls of barley and for pieces of bread, to slay the souls that should not die, and to save the souls alive that should not live, by your lying to my people that hear *your* lies?

20 Wherefore thus saith the Lord GOD; Behold, I *am* against your pillows, wherewith ye there hunt the souls to make *them* fly, and I will tear them from your arms, and will let the souls go, *even* the souls that ye hunt to make *them* fly.

21 Your kerchiefs also will I tear, and deliver my people out of your hand, and they shall be no more in your hand to be hunted; and ye shall know that I *am* the LORD.

B.C. 594.

a 2 Pet. 3:4.
b Ezk. 22:30; Psa. 106:23, 30.
c Ezra 2:59, 62; Neh. 7:5; Psa. 69:28.
d Ezk. 22:28.
e Ezk. 38:22.
f vs. 9, 21, 23; Ezk. 14:8.
g Jer. 6:14; 28:9.
h 2 Pet. 2:14.
i See Prov. 28:21; Mic. 3:5.

22 Because with lies ye have made the
heart of the righteous sad, whom I have
not made sad; and [a]strengthened the
hands of the wicked, that he should not
return from his wicked way, by promising him life:
23 Therefore [b]ye shall see no more
vanity, nor divine divinations: for I will
deliver my people out of your hand: and
ye shall know that I *am* the LORD.

CHAPTER 14.

The vision of the elders of Israel.

Then [c]came certain of the elders of
Israel unto me, and sat before me.
2 And the word of the LORD came unto
me, saying,
3 Son of man, these men have set up
their idols in their heart, and put the
stumblingblock of their iniquity before
their face: [d]should I be enquired of at all
by them?
4 Therefore speak unto them, and say
unto them, Thus saith the Lord GOD;
Every man of the house of Israel that setteth up his idols in his heart, and putteth
the stumblingblock of his iniquity before
his face, and cometh to the prophet; I the
LORD will answer him that cometh
according to the multitude of his idols;
5 That I may take the house of Israel in
their own heart, because they are all
estranged from me through their idols.
6 Therefore say unto the house of
Israel, Thus saith the Lord GOD; Repent,
and turn *yourselves* from your idols; and
turn away your faces from all your
abominations.
7 For every one of the house of Israel,
or of the stranger that sojourneth in
Israel, which separateth himself from me,
and setteth up his idols in his heart, and
putteth the stumblingblock of his iniquity
before his face, and cometh to a prophet
to enquire of him concerning me; I the
LORD will answer him by myself:
8 [e]And I will set my face against that
man, and [f]will make him a sign and a
proverb, and I will cut him off from the
midst of my people; and ye shall know
that I *am* the LORD.
9 And if the prophet be deceived
when he hath spoken a thing, I the LORD
have [g]deceived that prophet, and I will
stretch out my hand upon him, and will

B.C. 594.

a Jer. 23:14.

b v. 6; Ezk. 12:24; Mic. 3:6.

c Ezk. 8:1; 20:1; 33:31.

d 2 Ki. 3:13; Ezk. 20:31.

e Ezk. 15:7; Lev. 17:10; 20:3, 5, 6; Jer. 44:11.

f Ezk. 5:15; Num. 26:10; Deut. 28:37.

g 1 Ki. 22:23; Job 12:16; Jer. 4:10; 2 Thes. 2:11.

h 2 Pet. 2:15.

i Important contemporaneous testimony to the character and historicity of Daniel who was yet living. Cf. Jer. 15:1; Ezk. 14:16, 18, 20. See Jer. 7:16; 11:14; 14:11.

j Ezk. 25:13; Zeph. 1:3.

k Ezk. 38:22; 2 Sam. 24:15.

destroy him from the midst of my people Israel.
10 And they shall bear the punishment of their iniquity: the punishment of
the prophet shall be even as the punishment of him that seeketh *unto him;*
11 That the house of Israel may [h]go no
more astray from me, neither be polluted
any more with all their transgressions;
but that they may be my people, and I
may be their God, saith the Lord GOD.

Jerusalem on no account to be spared.

12 The word of the LORD came again
to me, saying,
13 Son of man, when the land sinneth
against me by trespassing grievously,
then will I stretch out mine hand upon
it, and will break the staff of the bread
thereof, and will send famine upon it,
and will cut off man and beast from it:
14 [i]Though these three men, Noah,
Daniel, and Job, were in it, they should
deliver *but* their own souls by their
righteousness, saith the Lord GOD.
15 If I cause noisome beasts to pass
through the land, and they spoil it, so
that it be desolate, that no man may pass
through because of the beasts:
16 *Though* these three men *were* in it, *as*
I live, saith the Lord GOD, they shall
deliver neither sons nor daughters; they
only shall be delivered, but the land
shall be desolate.
17 Or *if* I bring a sword upon that
land, and say, Sword, go through the
land; so that I [j]cut off man and beast
from it:
18 Though these three men *were* in it,
as I live, saith the Lord GOD, they shall
deliver neither sons nor daughters, but
they only shall be delivered themselves.
19 Or *if* I send a [k]pestilence into that
land, and pour out my fury upon it in
blood, to cut off from it man and beast:
20 Though Noah, Daniel, and Job, *were*
in it, *as* I live, saith the Lord GOD, they
shall deliver neither son nor daughter;
they shall *but* deliver their own souls by
their righteousness.
21 For thus saith the Lord GOD; How
much more when I send my four sore
judgments upon Jerusalem, the sword,
and the famine, and the noisome beast,

and the pestilence, to cut off from it man
and beast?
22 Yet, behold, therein shall be left a
remnant that shall be brought forth, *both*
sons and daughters: behold, they shall
come forth unto you, and ye shall see
their way and their doings: and ye shall
be comforted concerning the evil that I
have brought upon Jerusalem, *even* concerning all that I have brought upon it.
23 And they shall comfort you, when
ye see their ways and their doings: and
ye shall know that I have not done
[a]without cause all that I have done in it,
saith the Lord GOD.

CHAPTER 15.

The vision of the burning vine.
(Cf. Isa. 5:1-24.)

And the word of the LORD came unto
me, saying,
2 Son of man, What is the [b]vine tree
more than any tree, *or than* a branch
which is among the trees of the forest?
3 Shall wood be taken thereof to do
any work? or will *men* take a pin of it to
hang any vessel thereon?
4 Behold, it is cast into the fire for fuel;
the fire devoureth both the ends of it,
and the midst of it is burned. Is it meet
for *any* work?
5 Behold, when it was whole, it was
meet for no work: how much less shall it
be meet yet for *any* work, when the fire
hath devoured it, and it is burned?
6 Therefore thus saith the Lord GOD; As
the vine tree among the trees of the forest,
which I have given to the fire for fuel, so
will I give the inhabitants of Jerusalem.
7 And [c]I will set my face against them;
they shall go out from *one* fire, and
another fire shall devour them; and ye
shall know that I *am* the LORD, when I set
my face against them.
8 And I will make the land desolate,
because they have committed a trespass,
saith the Lord GOD.

CHAPTER 16.

The harlotry of Jerusalem.

Again the word of the LORD came
unto me, saying,
2 Son of man, cause Jerusalem to
know her abominations,
3 And say, Thus saith the Lord GOD
unto Jerusalem; Thy birth and thy nativity *is* of the land of Canaan; thy father *was*
an Amorite, and thy mother an Hittite.
4 And *as for* thy nativity, [d]in the day
thou wast born thy navel was not cut,
neither wast thou washed in water to
supple *thee*; thou wast not salted at all,
nor swaddled at all.
5 None eye pitied thee, to do any of
these unto thee, to have compassion
upon thee; but thou wast cast out in the
open field, to the lothing of thy person,
in the day that thou wast born.
6 And when I passed by thee, and saw
thee polluted in thine own blood, I said
unto thee *when thou wast* in thy blood,
Live; yea, I said unto thee *when thou wast*
in thy blood, Live.
7 I have caused thee to multiply as the
bud of the field, and thou hast increased
and waxen great, and thou art come to
excellent ornaments: *thy* breasts are fashioned, and thine hair is grown, whereas
thou *wast* naked and bare.
8 Now when I passed by thee, and
looked upon thee, behold, thy time *was*
the time of love; and I spread my skirt
over thee, and covered thy nakedness:
yea, I sware unto thee, and entered into
a covenant with thee, saith the Lord
GOD, and [e]thou becamest mine.
9 Then washed I thee with water; yea,
I throughly washed away thy blood
from thee, and I anointed thee with oil.
10 I clothed thee also with broidered
work, and shod thee with badgers' skin,
and I girded thee about with fine linen,
and I covered thee with silk.
11 I decked thee also with ornaments,
and I put bracelets upon thy hands, and
a chain on thy neck.
12 And I put a jewel on thy [f]forehead,
and earrings in thine ears, and a beautiful crown upon thine head.
13 Thus wast thou decked with gold
and silver; and thy raiment *was of* fine
linen, and silk, and broidered work;
thou didst eat fine flour, and honey, and
oil: and thou wast exceeding beautiful,
and thou didst prosper into a kingdom.
14 And thy renown went forth among
the [g]heathen for thy beauty: for it *was*
perfect through my comeliness, which I
had put upon thee, saith the Lord GOD.
15 But thou didst [h]trust [i]in thine

B.C. 594.

a Jer. 22:8, 9.
b Cf. Isa. 5:1-7; John 15:6.
c Ezk. 14:8; Lev. 17:10.
d Hos. 2:3.
e Ex. 19:5; Jer. 2:2.
f Heb. *nose.* See Isa. 3:21.
g i.e. *nations.*
h Psa. 2:12, *note.*
i See Deut. 32:15; Jer. 7:4; Mic. 3:11.

B.C. 594.

own beauty, and [a]playedst the harlot because of thy renown, and pouredst out thy fornications on every one that passed by; his it was.

16 And of thy garments thou didst take, and deckedst thy high places with divers colours, and playedst the harlot thereupon: *the like things* shall not come, neither shall it be *so*.

17 Thou hast also taken thy fair jewels of my gold and of my silver, which I had given thee, and madest to thyself images of men, and didst commit whoredom with them,

18 And tookest thy broidered garments, and coveredst them: and thou hast set mine oil and mine incense before them.

19 My meat also which I gave thee, fine flour, and oil, and honey, *wherewith* I fed thee, thou hast even set it before them for a sweet savour: and *thus* it was, saith the Lord GOD.

20 Moreover thou hast taken thy sons and thy daughters, whom thou hast borne unto me, and these hast thou sacrificed unto them to be devoured. *Is this* of thy whoredoms a small matter,

21 That thou hast slain my children, and delivered them to cause them to pass through *the fire* for them?

22 And in all thine abominations and thy whoredoms thou hast not remembered the days of thy [b]youth, when thou wast naked and bare, *and* wast polluted in thy blood.

23 And it came to pass after all thy wickedness, (woe, woe unto thee! saith the Lord GOD;)

24 *That* thou hast also built unto thee an eminent place, and [c]hast made thee an high place in every street.

25 Thou hast built thy high place at every head of the way, and hast made thy beauty to be abhorred, and hast opened thy feet to every one that passed by, and multiplied thy whoredoms.

26 Thou hast also committed fornication with the Egyptians thy neighbours, great of flesh; and hast increased thy whoredoms, to provoke me to anger.

27 Behold, therefore I have stretched out my hand over thee, and have diminished thine ordinary *food*, and delivered thee unto the will of them that hate thee, the daughters of the Philistines, which are ashamed of thy lewd way.

28 [d]Thou hast played the whore also with the Assyrians, because thou wast unsatiable; yea, thou hast played the harlot with them, and yet couldest not be satisfied.

29 Thou hast moreover multiplied thy fornication in the land of Canaan unto Chaldea; and yet thou wast not satisfied herewith.

30 How weak is thine heart, saith the Lord GOD, seeing thou doest all these *things*, the work of an imperious whorish woman;

31 In that thou buildest thine eminent place in the head of every way, and makest thine high place in every street; and hast not been as an harlot, in that thou scornest hire;

32 *But as* a wife that committeth adultery, *which* taketh strangers instead of her husband!

33 They give gifts to all whores: but thou givest thy gifts to all thy lovers, and hirest them, that they may come unto thee on every side for thy whoredom.

34 And the contrary is in thee from *other* women in thy whoredoms, whereas none followeth thee to commit whoredoms: and in that thou givest a reward, and no reward is given unto thee, therefore thou art contrary.

35 Wherefore, O harlot, hear the word of the LORD:

36 Thus saith the Lord GOD; Because thy filthiness was poured out, and thy nakedness discovered through thy whoredoms with thy lovers, and with all the idols of thy abominations, and by the blood of thy children, which thou didst give unto them;

37 Behold, therefore I will gather all thy lovers, with whom thou hast taken pleasure, and all *them* that thou hast loved, with all *them* that thou hast hated; I will even gather them round about against thee, and will discover thy nakedness unto them, that they may see all thy nakedness.

38 And I will judge thee, [e]as women that break wedlock and shed blood are judged; and I will give thee blood in fury and jealousy.

39 And I will also give thee into their hand, and they shall throw down thine eminent place, and shall break down thy high places: they shall strip thee also of thy clothes, and shall take thy fair jewels, and leave thee naked and bare.

a Ezk. 23:3, 8, 11-20; Isa. 1:21; 57:8; Jer. 2:20; 3:2, 6, 20; Hos. 1:2.

b vs. 43, 60; Jer. 2:2; Hos. 11:1.

c Isa. 57:5, 7; Jer. 2:20; 3:2.

d Ezk. 23:12; 2 Ki. 16:7, 10; 2 Chr. 28:20; Jer. 2:18, 36.

e Ezk. 23:45; Lev. 20:10; Deut. 22:22.

40 They shall also bring up a company
against thee, and they shall stone thee
with stones, and thrust thee through
with their swords.
41 And [a]they shall burn thine houses
with fire, and execute judgments upon
thee in the sight of many women: and I
will cause thee to cease from playing the
harlot, and thou also shalt give no hire
any more.
42 So will I make my fury toward thee
to rest, and my jealousy shall depart
from thee, and I will be quiet, and will
be no more angry.
43 Because thou hast not remembered
the days of thy youth, but hast fretted
me in all these *things*; behold, therefore
[b]I also will recompense thy way upon
thine head, saith the Lord GOD: and thou
shalt not commit this lewdness above all
thine abominations.
44 Behold, every one that useth
proverbs shall use *this* proverb against
thee, saying, As *is* the mother, *so is* her
daughter.
45 Thou *art* thy mother's daughter,
that lotheth her husband and her children; and thou *art* the sister of thy sisters, which lothed their husbands and
their children: your mother *was* an
Hittite, and your father an Amorite.
46 And thine elder sister *is* Samaria,
she and her daughters that dwell at thy
left hand: and thy younger sister, that
dwelleth at thy right hand, *is* Sodom and
her daughters.
47 Yet hast thou not walked after their
ways, nor done after their abominations:
but, as *if that were* a very little *thing*, thou
wast corrupted more than they in all thy
ways.
48 *As* I live, saith the Lord GOD,
[c]Sodom thy sister hath not done, she nor
her daughters, as thou hast done, thou
and thy daughters.
49 Behold, this was the iniquity of thy
sister Sodom, pride, fulness of bread, and
abundance of idleness was in her and in
her daughters, neither did she strengthen
the hand of the poor and needy.
50 And they were haughty, and [d]com-
mitted abomination before me: therefore
I took them away as I saw *good*.
51 Neither hath Samaria committed
half of thy sins; but thou hast multiplied
thine abominations more than they, and
hast justified thy sisters in all thine
abominations which thou hast done.
52 Thou also, which hast judged thy
sisters, bear thine own shame for thy
sins that thou hast committed more
abominable than they: they are more
righteous than thou: yea, be thou confounded also, and bear thy shame, in
that thou hast justified thy sisters.
53 [e]When I shall bring again their captivity, the captivity of Sodom and her
daughters, and the captivity of Samaria
and her daughters, then *will I bring again*
the captivity of thy captives in the midst
of them:
54 That thou mayest bear thine own
shame, and mayest be confounded in all
that thou hast done, in that thou art a
comfort unto them.
55 When thy sisters, Sodom and her
daughters, shall return to their former
estate, and Samaria and her daughters
shall return to their former estate, then
thou and thy daughters shall return to
your former estate.
56 For thy sister Sodom was not mentioned by thy mouth in the day of thy
pride,
57 Before thy wickedness was discovered, as at the time of *thy* [f]reproach of the
daughters of Syria, and all *that are* round
about her, the daughters of the Philistines,
which despise thee round about.
58 Thou hast borne thy lewdness and
thine abominations, saith the LORD.
59 For thus saith the Lord GOD; I will
even deal with thee as thou hast done,
which hast despised the oath in breaking
the covenant.

The promise of future blessing under the Palestinian Covenant (Deut. 30:1-10, *note*) *and the New Covenant* (Heb. 8:8-12, *note*).

60 Nevertheless [g]I will remember my
covenant with thee in the days of thy
youth, and I will establish unto thee [h]an
everlasting covenant.
61 Then thou shalt remember thy
ways, and be ashamed, when thou shalt
receive thy sisters, thine elder and thy
younger: and I will give them unto thee
for daughters, but not by thy covenant.
62 And [i]I will establish my covenant
with thee; and thou shalt know that I *am*
the LORD:
63 That thou mayest remember, and
be confounded, and never open thy

B.C. 594.

a Deut. 13:16; 2 Ki. 25:9; Jer. 39:8; 52:13.
b Ezk. 9:10; 11:21; 22:31.
c Mt. 10:15; 11:24.
d Gen. 13:13; 18:20; 19:5.
e See vs. 60, 61; Isa. 1:9.
f 2 Ki. 16:5; 2 Chr. 28:18.
g Psa. 106:45.
h Jer. 32:40; 50:5.
i Hos. 2:19, 20.

mouth any more because of thy shame,
when I am pacified toward thee for all
that thou hast done, saith the Lord GOD.

CHAPTER 17.

The parable of the great eagle.

And the word of the LORD came unto
me, [a]saying,
2 Son of man, put forth a riddle, and
speak a parable unto the house of Israel;
3 And say, Thus saith the Lord GOD; A
great eagle with great wings, long-
winged, full of feathers, which had
divers colours, came unto Lebanon, and
took the highest branch of the cedar:
4 He cropped off the top of his young
twigs, and carried it into a land of traffick; he set it in a city of merchants.
5 He took also of the seed of the land,
and planted it in a fruitful field; he
placed *it* by great waters, *and* set it *as* a
willow tree.
6 And it grew, and became a spreading vine of low stature, whose branches
turned toward him, and the roots thereof
were under him: so it became a vine,
and brought forth branches, and shot
forth sprigs.
7 There was also another great eagle
with great wings and many feathers:
and, behold, this vine did bend her roots
toward him, and shot forth her branches
toward him, that he might water it by
the furrows of her plantation.
8 It was planted in a good soil by great
waters, that it might bring forth branches, and that it might bear fruit, that it
might be a goodly vine.
9 Say thou, Thus saith the Lord GOD;
Shall it prosper? [b]shall he not pull up the
roots thereof, and cut off the fruit thereof, that it wither? it shall wither in all the
leaves of her spring, even without great
power or many people to pluck it up by
the roots thereof.
10 Yea, behold, *being* planted, shall it
prosper? [c]shall it not utterly wither,
when the east wind toucheth it? it shall
wither in the furrows where it grew.

The rebellion of Zedekiah and its results.
(Cf. 2 Ki. 24:17-20; 25:1-10.)

11 Moreover the word of the LORD
came unto me, saying,
12 Say now to the rebellious house,
Know ye not what these *things mean*? tell
them, Behold, [d]the king of Babylon is
come to Jerusalem, and hath taken the
king thereof, and the princes thereof,
and led them with him to Babylon;
13 [e]And hath taken of the king's seed,
and made a covenant with him, and
hath taken an oath of him: he hath also
taken the mighty of the land:
14 That the kingdom might be base,
that it might not lift itself up, *but* that by
keeping of his covenant it might stand.
15 But he rebelled against him in sending his ambassadors into Egypt, that
they might give him horses and much
people. [f]Shall he prosper? shall he
escape that doeth such *things*? or shall he
break the covenant, and be delivered?
16 *As* I live, saith the Lord GOD, surely
in the place *where* the king *dwelleth* that
made him king, whose oath he despised,
and whose covenant he brake, *even* with
him in the midst of Babylon he shall die.
17 [g]Neither shall Pharaoh with *his*
mighty army and great company make
for him in the war, [h]by casting up
mounts, and building forts, to cut off
many persons:
18 Seeing he despised the oath by
breaking the covenant, when, lo, he had
[i]given his hand, and hath done all these
things, he shall not escape.
19 Therefore thus saith the Lord GOD;
As I live, surely mine oath that he hath
despised, and my covenant that he hath
broken, even it will I recompense upon
his own head.
20 And I will spread my net upon
him, and he shall be taken in my snare,
and I will bring him to Babylon, and will
plead with him there for his trespass
that he hath trespassed against me.
21 And all his fugitives with all his
bands shall fall by the sword, and they
that remain shall be scattered toward all
winds: and ye shall know that I the LORD
have spoken *it*.
22 Thus saith the Lord GOD; I will also
take of the highest [j]branch of the high
cedar, and will set *it*; I will crop off from
the top of his young twigs [k]a tender one,
and will plant *it* upon an high mountain
and eminent:
23 [l]In the mountain of the height
of Israel will I plant it: and it shall

B.C. 594.

a *Parables* (O.T.). vs. 1-14; Ezk. 19:1-14. (Jud. 9:7-15; Zech. 11:7-14.)

b 2 Ki. 25:7.

c Ezk. 19:12; Hos. 13:15.

d v. 3; 2 Ki. 24:11-16.

e 2 Ki. 24:17.

f Deut. 17:16; Isa. 31:1, 3; 36:6, 9.

g Jer. 37:7; Ezk. 29:6.

h Ezk. 4:2; Jer. 52:4.

i 1 Chr. 29:24; Lam. 5:6.

j Isa. 11:1; Jer. 23:5; Zech. 3:8.

k Isa. 53:2.

l Ezk. 20:40; Isa. 2:2, 3; Mic. 4:1.

bring forth boughs, and bear fruit, and be a goodly cedar: and [a]under it shall dwell all fowl of every wing; in the shadow of the branches thereof shall they dwell.

24 And all the trees of the field shall know that I the LORD have brought down the high tree, have exalted the low tree, have dried up the green tree, and have made the dry tree to flourish: I the LORD have spoken and have done *it*.

CHAPTER 18.

Ethical instructions for Israel in captivity.

The word of the LORD came unto me again, saying,

2 What mean ye, that ye use this proverb concerning the land of Israel, saying, The fathers have eaten sour grapes, and the children's teeth are set on edge?

3 *As* I live, saith the Lord GOD, ye shall not have *occasion* any more to use this proverb in Israel.

4 Behold, all souls are mine; as the soul of the father, so also the soul of the son is mine: [b]the soul that sinneth, it shall die.

5 But if a man be [c]just, and do that which is lawful and right,

6 *And* hath not eaten upon the mountains, neither hath lifted up his eyes to the idols of the house of Israel, neither hath defiled his neighbour's wife, neither hath come near to a menstruous woman,

7 And hath not oppressed any, *but* hath restored to the debtor his [d]pledge, hath spoiled none by violence, hath given his bread to the hungry, and hath covered the naked with a garment;

8 He *that* hath not given forth upon [e]usury, neither hath taken any increase, *that* hath withdrawn his hand from iniquity, hath executed true judgment between man and man,

9 Hath walked in my statutes, and hath kept my judgments, to deal truly; he *is* just, he shall surely [f]live, saith the Lord GOD.

10 If he beget a son *that is* a robber, a [g]shedder of blood, and *that* doeth the like to *any* one of these *things*,

11 And that doeth not any of those *duties*, but even hath eaten upon the mountains, and defiled his neighbour's wife,

12 Hath oppressed the poor and needy, hath spoiled by violence, hath not restored the pledge, and hath lifted up his eyes to the idols, hath committed abomination,

13 Hath given forth upon usury, and hath taken increase: shall he then live? he shall not live: he hath done all these abominations; he shall surely die; [h]his blood shall be upon him.

14 Now, lo, *if* he beget a son, that seeth all his father's sins which he hath done, and considereth, and doeth not such like,

15 *That* hath not eaten upon the mountains, neither hath lifted up his eyes to the idols of the house of Israel, hath not defiled his neighbour's wife,

16 Neither hath oppressed any, hath not withholden the pledge, neither hath spoiled by violence, *but* hath given his bread to the hungry, and hath covered the naked with a garment,

17 *That* hath taken off his hand from the poor, *that* hath not received usury nor increase, hath executed my judgments, hath walked in my statutes; he shall not die for the iniquity of his father, he shall surely live.

18 *As for* his father, because he cruelly oppressed, spoiled his brother by violence, and did *that* which *is* not good among his people, lo, even he shall die in his iniquity.

19 Yet say ye, Why? [i]doth not the son bear the iniquity of the father? When the son hath done that which is lawful and right, *and* hath kept all my statutes, and hath done them, he shall surely live.

20 [j]The soul that sinneth, it shall die. [k]The son shall not bear the iniquity of the father, neither shall the father bear the iniquity of the son: the [l]righteousness of the righteous shall be upon him, and the [m]wickedness of the wicked shall be upon him.

21 But [n]if the wicked will turn from all his sins that he hath committed, and keep all my statutes, and do that which is lawful and right, he shall surely live, he shall not die.

22 All his transgressions that he hath committed, they shall not be mentioned unto him: in his righteousness that he hath done he shall live.

23 [o]Have I any pleasure at all that the wicked should die? saith the Lord GOD

B.C. 594.

a Ezk. 31:6; Dan. 4:12.
b v. 20; Rom. 6:23.
c *Righteousness.* vs. 5-9; Hab. 2:4. (Gen. 6:9; Lk. 2:25.)
d Ex. 22:26; Deut. 24:12, 13.
e Ex. 22:25; Lev. 25:36, 37; Deut. 23:19; Neh. 5:7; Psa. 15:5.
f Ezk. 20:11; Amos 5:4.
g Gen. 9:6; Ex. 21:12; Num. 35:31.
h Ezk. 3:18; 33:4; Lev. 20:9, 11, 12, 13, 16, 27; Acts 18:6.
i Ex. 20:5; Deut. 5:9; 2 Ki. 23:26; 24:3, 4.
j v. 4.
k Deut. 24:16; 2 Ki. 14:6; 2 Chr. 25:4; Jer. 31:29, 30.
l Isa. 3:10, 11.
m Rom. 2:9.
n v. 27; Ezk. 33:12, 19.
o v. 32; Ezk. 33:11; 1 Tim. 2:4; 2 Pet. 3:9.

and not that he should return from his
ways, and live?
24 But when the righteous turneth
away from his righteousness, and committeth iniquity, *and* doeth according to
all the abominations that the wicked *man*
doeth, shall he live? All his righteousness that he hath done shall not be mentioned: in his trespass that he hath trespassed, and in his sin that he hath
sinned, in them shall he die.
25 Yet ye say, [a]The way of the Lord is
not equal. Hear now, O house of Israel;
Is not my way equal? are not your ways
unequal?
26 When a righteous *man* turneth away
from his righteousness, and committeth
iniquity, and dieth in them; for his iniquity that he hath done shall he die.
27 Again, when the wicked *man* turneth
away from his wickedness that he hath
committed, and doeth that which is lawful and right, he shall save his soul alive.
28 Because he considereth, and turneth away from all his transgressions that
he hath committed, he shall surely live,
he shall not die.
29 Yet saith the house of Israel, The
way of the Lord is not equal. O house of
Israel, are not my ways equal? are not
your ways unequal?
30 Therefore I will judge you, O house
of Israel, every one according to his
ways, saith the Lord GOD. [b]Repent, and
turn *yourselves* from all your transgressions; so iniquity shall not be your ruin.
31 [c]Cast away from you all your transgressions, whereby ye have transgressed; and make you a [d]new heart and
a new spirit: for why will ye die, O
house of Israel?
32 [e]For I have no pleasure in the death
of him that dieth, saith the Lord GOD:
wherefore turn *yourselves*, and live ye.

CHAPTER 19.

Lamentation for the princes of Israel.

MOREOVER take thou up a [f]lamenta-
tion for the princes of Israel,
2 And say, What *is* thy mother? A
lioness: she lay down among lions, she
nourished her whelps among young
lions.
3 And she brought up one of her
whelps: [g]it became a young lion, and it
learned to catch the prey; it devoured
men.
4 The nations also heard of him; he
was taken in their pit, and they brought
him with chains unto the land of [h]Egypt.
5 Now when she saw that she had
waited, *and* her hope was lost, then she
took [i]another of her whelps, *and* made
him a young lion.
6 And he went up and down among the
lions, he became a young lion, and learned
to catch the prey, *and* devoured men.
7 And he knew their desolate palaces,
and he laid waste their cities; and the
land was desolate, and the fulness thereof, by the noise of his roaring.
8 [j]Then the nations set against him on
every side from the provinces, and
spread their net over him: he was taken
in their pit.
9 [k]And they put him in ward in
chains, and brought him to the king of
Babylon: they brought him into holds,
that his voice should no more be heard
upon the mountains of Israel.
10 Thy mother *is* like a vine in thy
blood, planted by the waters: she was
fruitful and full of branches by reason of
many waters.
11 And she had strong rods for the
sceptres of them that bare rule, and her
stature was exalted among the thick
branches, and she appeared in her height
with the multitude of her branches.
12 But she was plucked up in fury, she
was cast down to the ground, and the
east wind dried up her fruit: her strong
rods were broken and withered; the fire
consumed them.
13 And now she *is* planted in the
wilderness, in a dry and thirsty ground.
14 And [l]fire is gone out of a rod of her
branches, *which* hath devoured her fruit,
so that she hath no strong rod *to be* a
sceptre to rule. This *is* a lamentation, and
shall be for a lamentation.

CHAPTER 20.

Jehovah vindicated in the chastisement of Israel.

AND it came to pass in the seventh
year, in the [m]fifth *month*, the tenth
day of the month, *that* certain of the
elders of Israel came to enquire of the
LORD, and sat before me.

B.C. 594.

a v. 29; Ezk. 33:17, 20.
b Mt. 3:2; Rev. 2:5.
c Isa. 1:16; Eph. 4:22, 23.
d Ezk. 11:19; 36:26; Jer. 32:39.
e v. 23; Ezk. 33:11; Lam. 3:33; 2 Pet. 3:9.
f *Parables* (O.T.). vs. 1-14; Ezk. 23:1-17. (Jud. 9:7-15; Zech. 11:7-14.)
g v. 6; 2 Ki. 23:31, 32.
h 2 Ki. 23:33; 2 Chr. 36:4; Jer. 22:11, 12.
i 2 Ki. 23:34.
j 2 Ki. 24:2.
k 2 Chr. 36:6; Jer. 52:11.
l Jud. 9:15; 2 Ki. 24:20.
m i.e. *August.*

2 Then came the word of the LORD unto me, saying,

3 Son of man, speak unto the elders of Israel, and say unto them, Thus saith the Lord GOD; Are ye come to enquire of me? *As* I live, saith the Lord GOD, I will not be enquired of by you.

4 Wilt thou judge them, son of man, wilt thou judge *them*? cause them to know the abominations of their fathers:

5 And say unto them, Thus saith the Lord GOD; In the day when I chose Israel, and lifted up mine hand unto the seed of the house of Jacob, and made myself known unto them in the land of Egypt, when I lifted up mine hand unto them, saying, I *am* the LORD your God;

6 In the day *that* I lifted up mine hand unto them, [a]to bring them forth of the land of Egypt into a land that I had espied for them, flowing with milk and honey, [b]which *is* the glory of all lands:

7 Then said I unto them, Cast ye away every man the abominations of his eyes, and defile not yourselves with the [c]idols of Egypt: I *am* the LORD your God.

8 But they rebelled against me, and would not hearken unto me: they did not every man cast away the abominations of their eyes, neither did they forsake the idols of Egypt: then I said, I will pour out my fury upon them, to accomplish my anger against them in the midst of the land of Egypt.

9 [d]But I wrought for my name's sake, that it should not be polluted before the [e]heathen, among whom they *were*, in whose sight I made myself known unto them, in bringing them forth out of the land of Egypt.

10 Wherefore I caused them to go forth out of the land of Egypt, and brought them into the wilderness.

11 [f]And I gave them my statutes, and shewed them my judgments, which *if* a man do, he shall even live in them.

12 Moreover also I gave them my [g]sabbaths, to be a sign between me and them, that they might know that I *am* the LORD that sanctify them.

13 But the house of Israel rebelled against me in the wilderness: they walked not in my statutes, and they despised my judgments, which *if* a man do, he shall even live in them; and my sabbaths they greatly polluted: then I said, I would pour out my fury upon them in the wilderness, to consume them.

14 But I wrought for my name's sake, that it should not be polluted before the [e]heathen, in whose sight I brought them out.

15 [h]Yet also I lifted up my hand unto them in the wilderness, that I would not bring them into the land which I had given *them*, flowing with milk and honey, which *is* the glory of all lands;

16 Because they despised my judgments, and walked not in my statutes, but polluted my sabbaths: [i]for their heart went after their idols.

17 Nevertheless mine eye spared them from destroying them, neither did I make an end of them in the wilderness.

18 But I said unto their children in the wilderness, Walk ye not in the statutes of your fathers, neither observe their judgments, nor defile yourselves with their idols:

19 I *am* the LORD your God; walk in my statutes, and keep my judgments, and do them;

20 And [j]hallow my sabbaths; and they shall be a sign between me and you, that ye may know that I *am* the LORD your God.

21 Notwithstanding [k]the children rebelled against me: they walked not in my statutes, neither kept my judgments to do them, which *if* a man do, he shall even live in them; they polluted my sabbaths: then I said, I would pour out my fury upon them, to accomplish my anger against them in the wilderness.

22 Nevertheless I withdrew mine hand, and wrought for my name's sake, that it should not be polluted in the sight of the [e]heathen, in whose sight I brought them forth.

23 I lifted up mine hand unto them also in the wilderness, that I would [l]scatter them among the [e]heathen, and disperse them through the countries;

24 Because they had not executed my judgments, but had despised my statutes, and had polluted my sabbaths, and their eyes were after their fathers' idols.

25 Wherefore [m]I gave them also statutes *that were* not good, and judgments whereby they should not live;

26 And I polluted them in their own gifts, in that they caused to pass through *the fire* all that openeth the womb, that I

B.C. 593.

a Ex. 3:8, 17; Deut. 8:7-9; Jer. 32:22.

b v. 15. Psa. 48:2; Dan. 8:9; 11:16, 41; Zech. 7:14.

c Lev. 17:7; 18:3; Deut. 29:16-18; Josh. 24:14.

d vs. 14, 22; Ezk. 36:21, 22; Ex. 32:12; Num. 14:13; Deut. 9:28.

e i.e. *nations.*

f Deut. 4:8; Neh. 9:13, 14; Psa. 147:19, 20.

g Ex. 20:8; 31:13; 35:2; Deut. 5:12; Neh. 9:14.

h Num. 14:28; Psa. 95:11; 106:26.

i Num. 15:39; Psa. 78:37; Amos 5:25, 26; Acts 7:42, 43.

j v. 12; Jer. 17:22.

k Num. 25:1, 2; Deut. 9:23, 24; 31:27.

l Lev. 26:33; Deut. 28:64; Psa. 106:27; Jer. 15:4.

m See v. 39; Psa. 81:12; Rom. 1:24; 2 Thes. 2:11.

might make them desolate, to the end that they might know that I *am* the LORD.

27 Therefore, son of man, speak unto the house of Israel, and say unto them, Thus saith the Lord GOD; Yet in this your fathers have blasphemed me, in that they have committed a trespass against me.

28 *For* when I had brought them into the land, *for* the which I lifted up mine hand to give it to them, then they saw every high hill, and all the thick trees, and they offered there their sacrifices, and there they presented the provocation of their offering: there also they made their sweet savour, and poured out there their drink-offerings.

29 Then I said unto them, What *is* the high place whereunto ye go? And the name thereof is called Bamah unto this day.

30 Wherefore say unto the house of Israel, Thus saith the Lord GOD; Are ye polluted after the manner of your fathers? and commit ye whoredom after their abominations?

31 For when ye offer your gifts, when ye make your sons to pass through the fire, ye pollute yourselves with all your idols, even unto this day: and shall I be enquired of by you, O house of Israel? *As* I live, saith the Lord GOD, I will not be enquired of by you.

32 And that which cometh into your mind shall not be at all, that ye say, We will be as the [a]heathen, as the families of the countries, to serve wood and stone.

The future judgment of Israel.

33 *As* I live, saith the Lord GOD, surely with a mighty hand, and with a stretched out arm, and with fury poured out, [b]will I rule [c]over you:

34 And I will bring you out from the people, and will gather you out of the countries wherein ye are scattered, with a mighty hand, and with a stretched out arm, and with fury poured out.

35 And I will bring you into the wilderness of the people, and there will I plead with you face to face.

36 [d]Like as I pleaded with your fathers in the wilderness of the land of Egypt, so will I plead with you, saith the Lord GOD.

37 And I will cause you to [e]pass under the [1]rod, and I will bring you into the bond of the covenant:

38 And I will purge out from among you the rebels, and them that transgress against me: I will bring them forth out of the country where they sojourn, and they shall not enter into the land of Israel: and ye shall know that I *am* the LORD.

39 As for you, O house of Israel, thus saith the Lord GOD; [f]Go ye, serve ye every one his idols, and hereafter *also*, if ye will not hearken unto me: but pollute ye my holy name no more with your gifts, and with your idols.

40 For in mine holy mountain, in the mountain of the height of Israel, saith the Lord GOD, there shall all the house of Israel, all of them in the land, serve me: [g]there will I accept them, and there will I require your offerings, and the firstfruits of your oblations, with all your holy things.

41 I will accept you with your sweet savour, when I bring you out from the people, and gather you out of the countries wherein ye have been scattered; and I will be sanctified in you before the [a]heathen.

42 And ye shall know that I *am* the LORD, [h]when I shall bring you into the land of Israel, into the country *for* the which I lifted up mine hand to give it to your fathers.

43 And there shall ye remember your ways, and all your doings, wherein ye have been defiled; and [i]ye shall lothe yourselves in your own sight for all your evils that ye have committed.

44 And ye shall know that I *am* the LORD, when I have wrought with you for my name's sake, not according to your wicked ways, nor according to your corrupt doings, O ye house of Israel, saith the Lord GOD.

The parable of the forest of the south field.

45 Moreover the word of the LORD came unto me, saying,

B.C. 593.

a i.e. *nations.*

b *Judgments (the seven).* vs. 33-44. Dan. 7:22. (2 Sam. 7:14; Rev. 22:12.)

c *Kingdom* (O.T.). vs. 33-44; Ezk. 34:11-15, 22-25. (Gen. 1:26; Zech. 12:8.)

d See Num. 14:21, 22, 23, 28, 29.

e Lev. 27:32; Jer. 33:13.

f Jud. 10:14; Psa. 81:12; Amos 4:4.

g Isa. 56:7; 60:7; Ezk. 43:27; Zech. 8:20; Mal. 3:4; Rom. 12:1.

h Ezk. 11:17; 34:13; 36:24.

i Lev. 26:39; Ezk. 6:9; Hos. 5:15.

[1] **(20:37)** The passage is a prophecy of the future judgment upon Israel, regathered from all nations (see "Israel," Isa. 1:24-26, *refs.*) into the old wilderness of the wanderings (v. 35). The issue of this judgment determines who of Israel in that day shall enter the land for kingdom blessing (Psa. 50:1-7; Ezk. 20:33-44; Mal. 3:2-5; 4:1, 2); see other judgments, John 12:31, *note;* 1 Cor. 11:31, *note;* 2 Cor. 5:10, *note;* Mt. 25:32, *note;* Jude 6, *note;* Rev. 20:12, *note.*

46 Son of man, set thy face toward the
south, and drop *thy word* toward the
south, and prophesy against the forest of
the south field;
47 And say to the forest of the south,
Hear the word of the LORD; Thus saith
the Lord GOD; Behold, I will kindle a fire
in thee, and it shall devour every green
tree in thee, and every dry tree: the flaming flame shall not be quenched, and all
faces from the south to the north shall be
burned therein.
48 And all flesh shall see that I the LORD
have kindled it: it shall not be quenched.
49 Then said I, Ah Lord GOD! they say
of me, Doth he not speak parables?

CHAPTER 21.

The parable of the sighing prophet.

And the word of the LORD came unto
me, saying,
2 Son of man, set thy face toward
Jerusalem, and [a]drop *thy word* toward
the holy places, and prophesy against
the land of Israel,
3 And say to the land of Israel, Thus
saith the LORD; Behold, I *am* against thee,
and will draw forth my sword out of his
sheath, and will cut off from thee the
righteous and the wicked.
4 Seeing then that I will cut off from
thee the righteous and the wicked, therefore shall my sword go forth out of his
sheath against all flesh from the south to
the north:
5 That all flesh may know that I the
LORD have drawn forth my sword out of
his sheath: it shall not return any more.
6 Sigh therefore, thou son of man,
with the breaking of *thy* loins; and with
bitterness sigh before their eyes.
7 And it shall be, when they say unto
thee, Wherefore sighest thou? that thou
shalt answer, For the tidings; because it
cometh: and every heart shall melt, and
all hands shall be feeble, and every spirit
shall faint, and all knees shall be weak *as*
water: behold, it cometh, and shall be
brought to pass, saith the Lord GOD.

The parable of the sword of God.

8 Again the word of the LORD came
unto me, saying,
9 Son of man, prophesy, and say, Thus
saith the LORD; Say, [b]A sword, a sword is
sharpened, and also furbished:
10 It is sharpened to make a sore
slaughter; it is furbished that it may glit-
ter: should we then make mirth? it con-
temneth the rod of my son, *as* every tree.
11 And he hath given it to be furbished, that it may be handled: this
sword is sharpened, and it is furbished,
to give it into the hand of the slayer.
12 Cry and howl, son of man: for it
shall be upon my people, it *shall be* upon
all the princes of Israel: terrors by reason
of the sword shall be upon my people:
smite therefore upon *thy* thigh.
13 Because *it is* a trial, and what if *the
sword* contemn even the rod? it shall be
no *more*, saith the Lord GOD.
14 Thou therefore, son of man, prophesy, and smite *thine* hands together, and
let the sword be doubled the third time,
the sword of the slain: it *is* the sword of
the great *men that are* slain, which
entereth into their privy chambers.
15 I have set the point of the sword
against all their gates, that *their* heart
may faint, and *their* ruins be multiplied:
ah! *it is* made bright, *it is* wrapped up for
the slaughter.
16 Go thee one way or other, *either* on
the right hand, *or* on the left, whithersoever thy face *is* set.
17 I will also [c]smite mine hands
together, and I will cause my fury to rest:
I the LORD have said *it*.

No king till Messiah comes to reign
(vs. 26, 27; Acts 15:14-17).

18 The word of the LORD came unto
me again, saying,
19 Also, thou son of man, appoint thee
two ways, that the sword of the king of
Babylon may come: both twain shall
come forth out of one land: and choose
thou a place, choose *it* at the head of the
way to the city.
20 Appoint a way, that the sword may
come to [d]Rabbath of the Ammonites,
and to Judah in Jerusalem the defenced.
21 For the king of Babylon stood at the
parting of the way, at the head of the
two ways, to use divination: he made *his*
arrows bright, he consulted with images,
he looked in the liver.

B.C. 593.

a Deut. 32:2; Amos 7:16; Mic. 2:6, 11.

b vs. 15, 28; Deut. 32:41.

c v. 14; Ezk. 22:13.

d Ezk. 25:5; Jer. 49:2; Amos 1:14.

22 At his right hand was the divination for Jerusalem, to appoint captains, to open the mouth in the slaughter, to lift up the voice with shouting, to appoint *battering* rams against the gates, to cast a mount, *and* to build a fort.

23 And it shall be unto them as a false divination in their sight, to them that have sworn oaths: but he will call to remembrance the iniquity, that they may be taken.

24 Therefore thus saith the Lord GOD; Because ye have made your iniquity to be remembered, in that your transgressions are discovered, so that in all your doings your sins do appear; because, *I say*, that ye are come to remembrance, ye shall be taken with the hand.

25 And thou, [a]profane wicked prince of Israel, whose day is come, when iniquity *shall have* an end,

26 Thus saith the Lord GOD; Remove the diadem, and take off the crown: this *shall* not *be* the same: exalt *him that is* low, and abase *him that is* high.

27 I will overturn, overturn, overturn, it: [b]and it shall be no *more*, until he come whose right it is; and I will give it *him*.

28 And thou, son of man, prophesy and say, Thus saith the Lord GOD [c]concerning the Ammonites, and concerning their reproach; even say thou, The sword, the sword *is* drawn: for the slaughter *it is* furbished, to consume because of the glittering:

29 Whiles they see vanity unto thee, whiles they divine a lie unto thee, to bring thee upon the necks of *them that are* slain, of the wicked, [d]whose day is come, when their iniquity *shall have* an end.

30 Shall I cause *it* to return into his sheath? [e]I will judge thee in the place where thou wast created, [f]in the land of thy nativity.

31 And I will pour out mine indignation upon thee, I will blow against thee in the fire of my wrath, and deliver thee into the hand of brutish men, *and* skilful to destroy.

32 Thou shalt be for fuel to the fire; thy blood shall be in the midst of the land; thou shalt be no *more* remembered: for I the LORD have spoken *it*.

CHAPTER 22.

The sins of Israel enumerated.

Moreover the word of the LORD came unto me, saying,

2 Now, thou son of man, wilt thou judge, wilt thou judge the bloody city? yea, thou shalt shew her all her abominations.

3 Then say thou, Thus saith the Lord GOD, The city sheddeth blood in the midst of it, that her time may come, and maketh idols against herself to defile herself.

4 Thou art become guilty in thy blood that thou hast [g]shed; and hast defiled thyself in thine idols which thou hast made; and thou hast caused thy days to draw near, and art come *even* unto thy years: [h]therefore have I made thee a reproach unto the [i]heathen, and a mocking to all countries.

5 *Those that be* near, and *those that be* far from thee, shall mock thee, *which art* infamous *and* much vexed.

6 Behold, [j]the princes of Israel, every one were in thee to their power to shed blood.

7 In thee have they [k]set light by father and mother: in the midst of thee have they dealt by oppression with the stranger: in thee have they vexed the fatherless and the widow.

8 Thou hast despised mine holy things, and hast profaned my sabbaths.

9 In thee are men that carry tales to shed blood: and in thee they eat upon the mountains: in the midst of thee they commit lewdness.

10 In thee have they discovered their fathers' nakedness: in thee have they humbled her that was [l]set apart for pollution.

11 And one hath committed abomination with his neighbour's wife; and another hath lewdly defiled his daughter in law; and another in thee hath humbled his sister, his father's daughter.

12 In thee [m]have they taken gifts to shed blood; thou hast taken usury and increase, and thou hast greedily gained of thy neighbours by extortion, and [n]hast forgotten me, saith the Lord GOD.

13 Behold, therefore I have smitten mine hand at thy dishonest gain which thou hast made, and at thy blood which hath been in the midst of thee.

14 Can thine heart endure, or can thine hands be strong, in the days that I shall deal with thee? I the LORD have spoken *it*, and will do *it*.

15 And I will scatter thee among the [i]heathen, and disperse thee in the

B.C. 593.

a Ezk. 12:10; 17:19; 2 Chr. 36:13; Jer. 52:2.

b v. 13; Gen. 49:10; Lk. 1:32, 33; John 1:49.

c Ezk. 25:2, 3, 6; Jer. 49:1; Zeph. 2:8-10.

d v. 25; Job 18:20; Psa. 37:13.

e Gen. 15:14.

f Ezk. 16:3

g 2 Ki. 21:16.

h Ezk. 5:14; Deut. 28:37; 1 Ki. 9:7; Dan. 9:16.

i i.e. *nations*.

j Isa. 1:23; Mic. 3:1-3; Zeph. 3:3.

k Deut. 27:16.

l Ezk. 18:6; Lev. 18:19; 20:18.

m Ex. 23:8; Deut. 16:19; 27:25.

n Ezk. 23:35; Deut. 32:18; Jer. 3:21.

countries, and will consume thy filthiness out of thee.

16 And thou shalt take thine inheritance in thyself in the sight of the [a]heathen, and thou shalt know that I *am* the LORD.

The parable of the dross in the furnace.

17 And the word of the LORD came unto me, saying,

18 Son of man, [b]the house of Israel is to me become dross: all they *are* brass, and tin, and iron, and lead, in the midst of the furnace; they are *even* the dross of silver.

19 Therefore thus saith the Lord GOD; Because ye are all become dross, behold, therefore I will gather you into the midst of Jerusalem.

20 *As* they gather silver, and brass, and iron, and lead, and tin, into the midst of the furnace, to blow the fire upon it, to melt *it*; so will I gather *you* in mine anger and in my fury, and I will leave *you there*, and melt you.

21 Yea, I will gather you, and [c]blow upon you in the fire of my wrath, and ye shall be melted in the midst thereof.

22 As silver is melted in the midst of the furnace, so shall ye be melted in the midst thereof; and ye shall know that I the LORD have [d]poured out my fury upon you.

Sins of the priests, princes, prophets, and people.

23 And the word of the LORD came unto me, saying,

24 Son of man, say unto her, Thou *art* the land that is not cleansed, nor rained upon in the day of indignation.

25 *There is* a conspiracy of her prophets in the midst thereof, like a roaring lion ravening the prey; they have devoured souls; [e]they have taken the treasure and precious things; they have made her many widows in the midst thereof.

26 Her priests have violated my [f]law, and have [g]profaned mine holy things: they have put no difference between the holy and profane, neither have they shewed *difference* between the unclean and the clean, and have hid their eyes from my sabbaths, and I am profaned among them.

27 [h]Her princes in the midst thereof *are* like wolves ravening the prey, to shed blood, *and* to destroy souls, to get dishonest gain.

B.C. 593.

a i.e. *nations.*

b Psa. 119:119; Isa. 1:22; Jer. 6:28.

c Ezk. 22:20-22.

d v. 31; Ezk. 20:8, 33.

e Mic. 3:11; Zeph. 3:3, 4.

f *Law (of Moses).* Dan. 9:8-13. (Ex. 19:1; Gal. 3:1-29.)

g Lev. 22:2; 1 Sam. 2:29.

h v. 6; Isa. 1:23; Mic. 3:2, 3, 9-11; Zeph. 3:3.

i Psa. 106:23.

j *Parables.* (O.T.). vs. 1-17; Ezk. 24:3, 6. (Jud. 9:7-15; Zech. 11:7-14.)

k Ezk. 16:8, 20.

28 And her prophets have daubed them with untempered *morter*, seeing vanity, and divining lies unto them, saying, Thus saith the Lord GOD, when the LORD hath not spoken.

29 The people of the land have used oppression, and exercised robbery, and have vexed the poor and needy: yea, they have oppressed the stranger wrongfully.

30 And I sought for a man among them, that should make up the hedge, and [i]stand in the gap before me for the land, that I should not destroy it: but I found none.

31 Therefore have I poured out mine indignation upon them; I have consumed them with the fire of my wrath: their own way have I recompensed upon their heads, saith the Lord GOD.

CHAPTER 23.

The parable of Aholah and Aholibah.

The word of the LORD came again unto me, [j]saying,

2 Son of man, there were two women, the daughters of one mother:

3 And they committed whoredoms in Egypt; they committed whoredoms in their youth: there were their breasts pressed, and there they bruised the teats of their virginity.

4 And the names of them *were* Aholah the elder, and Aholibah her sister: and [k]they were mine, and they bare sons and daughters. Thus *were* their names; Samaria *is* Aholah, and Jerusalem Aholibah.

5 And Aholah played the harlot when she was mine; and she doted on her lovers, on the Assyrians *her* neighbours,

6 *Which were* clothed with blue, captains and rulers, all of them desirable young men, horsemen riding upon horses.

7 Thus she committed her whoredoms with them, with all them *that were* the chosen men of Assyria, and with all on whom she doted: with all their idols she defiled herself.

8 Neither left she her whoredoms *brought* from Egypt: for in her youth they lay with her, and they bruised the breasts of her virginity, and poured their whoredom upon her.

B.C. 593.

9 Wherefore I have delivered her into the hand of her lovers, into the hand of the [a]Assyrians, upon whom she doted.

10 These discovered her nakedness: they took her sons and her daughters, and slew her with the sword: and she became famous among women; for they had executed judgment upon her.

11 And when her sister Aholibah saw *this*, she was more corrupt in her inordinate love than she, and in her whoredoms more than her sister in *her* whoredoms.

12 She doted upon the Assyrians *her* neighbours, captains and rulers clothed most gorgeously, horsemen riding upon horses, all of them desirable young men.

13 Then I saw that she was defiled, *that* they *took* both one way,

14 And *that* she increased her whoredoms: for when she saw men pourtrayed upon the wall, the images of the Chaldeans pourtrayed with vermilion,

15 Girded with girdles upon their loins, exceeding in dyed attire upon their heads, all of them princes to look to, after the manner of the Babylonians of Chaldea, the land of their nativity:

16 [b]And as soon as she saw them with her eyes, she doted upon them, and sent messengers unto them into Chaldea.

17 And the Babylonians came to her into the bed of love, and they defiled her with their whoredom, and she was polluted with them, and her mind was alienated from them.

18 So she discovered her whoredoms, and discovered her nakedness: then [c]my mind was alienated from her, like as my mind was alienated from her sister.

19 Yet she multiplied her whoredoms, in calling to remembrance the days of her youth, wherein she had played the harlot in the land of Egypt.

20 For she doted upon their paramours, whose flesh *is as* the flesh of asses, and whose issue *is like* the issue of horses.

21 Thus thou calledst to remembrance the lewdness of thy youth, in bruising thy teats by the Egyptians for the paps of thy youth.

22 Therefore, O Aholibah, thus saith the Lord GOD; [d]Behold, I will raise up thy lovers against thee, from whom thy mind is alienated, and I will bring them against thee on every side;

23 The Babylonians, and all the Chaldeans, [e]Pekod, and Shoa, and Koa, *and* all the Assyrians with them: all of them desirable young men, captains and rulers, great lords and renowned, all of them riding upon horses.

24 And they shall come against thee with chariots, wagons, and wheels, and with an assembly of people, *which* shall set against thee buckler and shield and helmet round about: and I will set judgment before them, and they shall judge thee according to their judgments.

25 And I will set my jealousy against thee, and they shall deal furiously with thee: they shall take away thy nose and thine ears; and thy remnant shall fall by the sword: they shall take thy sons and thy daughters; and thy residue shall be devoured by the fire.

26 They shall also [f]strip thee out of thy clothes, and take away thy fair jewels.

27 Thus will I make thy lewdness to cease from thee, and thy whoredom *brought* from the land of Egypt: so that thou shalt not lift up thine eyes unto them, nor remember Egypt any more.

28 For thus saith the Lord GOD; Behold, I will deliver thee into the hand *of them* [g]whom thou hatest, into the hand *of them* [h]from whom thy mind is alienated:

29 And they shall deal with thee hatefully, and shall take away all thy labour, and shall leave thee naked and bare: and the nakedness of thy whoredoms shall be discovered, both thy lewdness and thy whoredoms.

30 I will do these *things* unto thee, because thou hast gone a whoring after the [i]heathen, *and* because thou art polluted with their idols.

31 Thou hast walked in the way of thy sister; therefore will I give her [j]cup into thine hand.

32 Thus saith the Lord GOD; Thou shalt drink of thy sister's cup deep and large: thou shalt be laughed to scorn and had in derision; it containeth much.

33 Thou shalt be filled with drunkenness and sorrow, with the cup of astonishment and desolation, with the cup of thy sister Samaria.

a 2 Ki. 17:3-6, 23; 18:9-11.
b 2 Ki. 24:1.
c Jer. 6:8.
d v. 28; Ezk. 16:37-41.
e Jer. 50:21.
f Ezk. 16:39.
g Ezk. 16:37.
h v. 17.
i i.e. *nations*.
j Jer. 25:15.

34 Thou shalt even [a]drink it and suck *it* out, and thou shalt break the sherds thereof, and pluck off thine own breasts: for I have spoken *it*, saith the Lord GOD.

35 Therefore thus saith the Lord GOD; Because thou [b]hast forgotten me, and cast me behind thy back, therefore bear thou also thy lewdness and thy whoredoms.

36 The LORD said moreover unto me; Son of man, wilt thou judge Aholah and Aholibah? yea, declare unto them their abominations;

37 That they have committed adultery, and blood *is* in their hands, and with their idols have they committed adultery, and have also caused their sons, [c]whom they bare unto me, to pass for them through *the fire*, to devour *them*.

38 Moreover this they have done unto me: they have defiled my sanctuary in the same day, and have profaned my sabbaths.

39 For when they had slain their children to their idols, then they came the same day into my sanctuary to profane it; and, lo, [d]thus have they done in the midst of mine house.

40 And furthermore, that ye have sent for men to come from far, unto whom a messenger *was* sent; and, lo, they came: for whom thou didst wash thyself, [e]paintedst thy eyes, and deckedst thyself with ornaments,

41 And satest upon a stately bed, and a table prepared before it, [f]whereupon thou hast set mine incense and mine oil.

42 And a voice of a multitude being at ease *was* with her: and with the men of the common sort *were* brought Sabeans from the wilderness, which put bracelets upon their hands, and beautiful crowns upon their heads.

43 Then said I unto *her that was* old in adulteries, Will they now commit whoredoms with her, and she *with them*?

44 Yet they went in unto her, as they go in unto a woman that playeth the harlot: so went they in unto Aholah and unto Aholibah, the lewd women.

45 And the righteous men, they shall judge them after the manner of adulteresses, and after the manner of women that shed blood; because they *are* adulteresses, and blood *is* in their hands.

46 For thus saith the Lord GOD; I will bring up a company upon them, and will give them to be removed and spoiled.

47 And the company shall stone them with stones, and dispatch them with their swords; [g]they shall slay their sons and their daughters, and burn up their houses with fire.

48 Thus will I cause lewdness to cease out of the land, [h]that all women may be taught not to do after your lewdness.

49 And they shall recompense your lewdness upon you, and ye shall bear the sins of your idols: and ye shall know that I *am* the Lord GOD.

CHAPTER 24.

The parable of the boiling pot.

Again in the ninth year, in the [i]tenth month, in the tenth *day* of the month, the word of the LORD came unto me, saying,

2 Son of man, write thee the name of the day, *even* of this same day: the king of Babylon set himself against Jerusalem this same day.

3 And utter a [j]parable unto the rebellious house, and say unto them, Thus saith the Lord GOD; Set on a pot, set *it* on, and also pour water into it:

4 Gather the pieces thereof into it, *even* every good piece, the thigh, and the shoulder; fill *it* with the choice bones.

5 Take the choice of the flock, and burn also the bones under it, *and* make it boil well, and let them seethe the bones of it therein.

6 Wherefore thus saith the Lord GOD; [k]Woe to the bloody city, to the pot whose scum *is* therein, and whose scum is not gone out of it! bring it out piece by piece; let no [l]lot fall upon it.

7 For her blood is in the midst of her; she set it upon the top of a rock; [m]she poured it not upon the ground, to cover it with dust;

8 That it might cause fury to come up to take vengeance; I have set her blood upon the top of a rock, that it should not be covered.

9 Therefore thus saith the Lord GOD; [n]Woe to the bloody city! I will even make the pile for fire great.

10 Heap on wood, kindle the fire, consume the flesh, and spice it well, and let the bones be burned.

11 Then set it empty upon the coals

B.C. 593.

a Psa. 75:8; Isa. 51:17.
b Ezk. 22:12; Jer. 2:32; 3:21; 13:25.
c Ezk. 16:20, 21, 36, 45; 20:26, 31.
d 2 Ki. 21:4.
e 2 Ki. 9:30; Jer. 4:30.
f Ezk. 16:18, 19; Prov. 7:17; Hos. 2:8.
g Ezk. 24:21; 2 Chr. 36:17, 19.
h Deut. 13:11; 2 Pet. 2:6.
i i.e. *January*.
j *Parables* (O.T.). vs. 3-6; Ezk. 31:3-14. (Jud. 9:7-15; Zech. 11:7-14.)
k v. 9; Ezk. 22:3; 23:37.
l See 2 Sam. 8:2; Joel 3:3; Oba. 11; Nab. 3:10.
m Lev. 17:13; Deut. 12:16, 24.
n v. 6; Nah. 3:1; Hab. 2:12.

thereof, that the brass of it may be hot, and may burn, and *that* the filthiness of it may be molten in it, *that* the scum of it may be consumed.

12 She hath wearied *herself* with lies, and her great scum went not forth out of her: her scum *shall be* in the fire.

13 In thy filthiness *is* lewdness: because I have purged thee, and thou wast not purged, thou shalt not be purged from thy filthiness any more, [a]till I have caused my fury to rest upon thee.

14 [b]I the LORD have spoken *it*: it shall come to pass, and I will do *it*; I will not go back, neither will I spare, neither will I [c]repent; according to thy ways, and according to thy doings, shall they judge thee, saith the Lord GOD.

Ezekiel again made a sign to Israel.
(Cf. Ezk. 12:11.)

15 Also the word of the LORD came unto me, saying,

16 Son of man, behold, I take away from thee the desire of thine eyes with a stroke: yet neither shalt thou mourn nor weep, neither shall thy tears run down.

17 Forbear to cry, make no mourning for the dead, bind the tire of thine head upon thee, and [d]put on thy shoes upon thy feet, and cover not *thy* lips, and eat not the bread of men.

18 So I spake unto the people in the morning: and at even my wife died; and I did in the morning as I was commanded.

19 And the people said unto me, [e]Wilt thou not tell us what these *things are* to us, that thou doest *so*?

20 Then I answered them, The word of the LORD came unto me, saying,

21 Speak unto the house of Israel, Thus saith the Lord GOD; Behold, I will profane my sanctuary, the excellency of your strength, the desire of your eyes, and that which your soul pitieth; and your sons and your daughters whom ye have left shall fall by the sword.

22 And ye shall do as I have done: ye shall not cover *your* lips, nor eat the bread of men.

23 And your tires *shall be* upon your heads, and your shoes upon your feet: ye shall not mourn nor weep; [f]but ye shall pine away for your iniquities, and mourn one toward another.

24 Thus [g]Ezekiel is unto you a sign: according to all that he hath done shall ye do: and when this cometh, ye shall know that I *am* the Lord GOD.

25 Also, thou son of man, *shall it* not *be* in the day when I take from them their strength, the joy of their glory, the desire of their eyes, and that whereupon they set their minds, their sons and their daughters,

26 *That* he that escapeth in that day shall come unto thee, to cause *thee* to hear *it* with *thine* ears?

27 In that day shall thy mouth be opened to him which is escaped, and thou shalt speak, and be no more dumb: and [h]thou shalt be a sign unto them; and they shall know that I *am* the LORD.

CHAPTER 25.

The prophecy against the Ammonites.

The word of the LORD came again unto me, saying,

2 Son of man, set thy face [i]against the Ammonites, and prophesy against them;

3 And say unto the Ammonites, Hear the word of the Lord GOD; Thus saith the Lord GOD; [j]Because thou saidst, Aha, against my sanctuary, when it was profaned; and against the land of Israel, when it was desolate; and against the house of Judah, when they went into captivity;

4 Behold, therefore I will deliver thee to the men of the east for a possession, and they shall set their palaces in thee, and make their dwellings in thee: they shall eat thy fruit, and they shall drink thy milk.

5 And I will make Rabbah a stable for camels, and the Ammonites a couching-place for flocks: and ye shall know that I *am* the LORD.

6 For thus saith the Lord GOD; [k]Because thou hast clapped *thine* hands, and stamped with the feet, and rejoiced in heart with all thy despite against the land of Israel;

7 Behold, therefore I will stretch out mine hand upon thee, and will deliver thee for a spoil to the [l]heathen; and I will cut thee off from the people, and I will cause thee to perish out of the countries: I will destroy thee; and thou shalt know that I *am* the LORD.

B.C. 590.

a Ezk. 5:13; 8:18; 16:42.

b 1 Sam. 15:29.

c Zech. 8:14, *note.*

d 2 Sam. 15:30.

e Ezk. 12:9; 37:18.

f Ezk. 33:10; Lev. 26:39.

g Ezk. 4:3; 12:6, 11; Isa. 20:3.

h v. 24.

i Ezk. 21:28; Jer. 49:1; Amos 1:13; Zeph. 2:9.

j Jer. 33:24; Ezk. 26:2; Prov. 17:5.

k Job 27:23; Lam. 2:15; Zeph. 2:15.

l i.e. *nations.*

The coming judgment upon Moab.

8 [1]Thus saith the Lord GOD; Because
that Moab and Seir do say, Behold, the
house of Judah *is* like unto all the [a]hea-
then;
9 Therefore, behold, I will open the
side of Moab from the cities, from his
cities *which are* on his frontiers, the glory
of the country, Beth-jeshimoth, Baal-
meon, and Kiriathaim,
10 Unto the men of the east with the
Ammonites, and will give them in possession, that the Ammonites may not be
remembered among the nations.
11 And I will execute judgments upon
Moab; and they shall know that I *am* the
LORD.

The coming judgment upon Edom.

12 Thus saith the Lord GOD; [b]Because
that [c]Edom hath dealt against the house
of Judah by taking vengeance, and hath
greatly offended, and revenged himself
upon them;
13 Therefore thus saith the Lord GOD; I
will also stretch out mine hand upon
Edom, and will cut off man and beast
from it; and I will make it desolate from
Teman; and they of Dedan shall fall by
the sword.
14 And I will lay my vengeance upon
Edom by the hand of my people Israel:
and they shall do in Edom according to
mine anger and according to my fury;
and they shall know my vengeance,
saith the Lord GOD.

The coming judgment upon Philistia.

15 Thus saith the Lord GOD; Because
the [d]Philistines have dealt by revenge,
and have taken vengeance with a despiteful heart, to destroy *it* for the old hatred;
16 Therefore thus saith the Lord GOD;
Behold, I will stretch out mine hand
upon the Philistines, and I will cut off
the Cherethims, and destroy the remnant of the sea coast.
17 And I will execute great vengeance
upon them with furious rebukes; and
they shall know that I *am* the LORD, when
I shall lay my vengeance upon them.

CHAPTER 26.

The coming judgment upon Tyre.

AND it came to pass in the eleventh
year, in the first *day* of the month,
that the word of the LORD came unto me,
saying,
2 Son of man, [e]because that Tyrus hath
said against Jerusalem, Aha, she is broken *that was* the gates of the people: she
is turned unto me: I shall be replenished,
now she is laid waste:
3 Therefore thus saith the Lord GOD;
Behold, I *am* against thee, O Tyrus, and
will cause many nations to come up
against thee, as the sea causeth his
waves to come up.
4 And they shall destroy the walls of
Tyrus, and break down her towers: I will
also scrape her dust from her, and make
her like the top of a rock.
5 It shall be *a place for* the spreading of
nets in the midst of the sea: for I have
spoken *it*, saith the Lord GOD: and it
shall become a spoil to the nations.
6 And her daughters which *are* in the
field shall be slain by the sword; and
they shall know that I *am* the LORD.
7 For thus saith the Lord GOD; Behold,
I will bring upon Tyrus Nebuchadrezzar
king of Babylon, [f]a king of kings, from
the north, with horses, and with chariots, and with horsemen, and companies,
and much people.
8 He shall slay with the sword thy
daughters in the field: and he shall make
a fort against thee, and cast a mount
against thee, and lift up the buckler
against thee.
9 And he shall set engines of war
against thy walls, and with his axes he
shall break down thy towers.
10 By reason of the abundance of his
horses their dust shall cover thee: thy
walls shall shake at the noise of the
horsemen, and of the wheels, and of the
chariots, when he shall enter into thy

B.C. 590.

a i.e. *nations.*

b Ezk. 35:2; 2 Chr. 28:17; Psa. 137:7; Jer. 49:7, 8; Amos 1:11; Oba. 10.

c vs. 12-14; Gen. 36:1, *note.*

d 2 Chr. 28:18.

e Isa. 23; Jer. 25:22; 47:4; Amos 1:9; Zech. 9:2.

f Ezra 7:12; Dan. 2:37.

[1] **(25:8)** The prophecies upon Gentile powers (extending to Ezk. 32:32) have doubtless had partial fulfilments of which history and the present condition of those cities and countries bear witness, but the mention of the day of Jehovah (Ezk. 30:3) makes it evident that a fulfilment in the final sense is still future. See "Day of Jehovah." (Isa. 2:10-22; Rev. 19:21, *note*). Also "Armageddon" (Rev. 16:14; 19:17, *note*). Those countries are once more to be the battle-ground of the nations.

gates, as men enter into a city wherein is made a breach.

11 With the hoofs of his horses shall he tread down all thy streets: he shall slay thy people by the sword, and thy strong garrisons shall go down to the ground.

12 And they shall make a spoil of thy riches, and make a prey of thy merchandise: and they shall break down thy walls, and destroy thy pleasant houses: and they shall lay thy stones and thy timber and thy dust in the midst of the water.

13 [a]And I will cause the noise of thy songs to cease; and the sound of thy harps shall be no more heard.

14 And I will make thee like the top of a rock: thou shalt be *a place* to spread nets upon; thou shalt be built no more: for I the LORD have spoken *it*, saith the Lord GOD.

15 Thus saith the Lord GOD to Tyrus; Shall not the [b]isles shake at the sound of thy fall, when the wounded cry, when the slaughter is made in the midst of thee?

16 Then all the [c]princes of the sea shall come down from their thrones, and lay away their robes, and put off their broidered garments: they shall clothe themselves with trembling; they shall sit upon the ground, and [d]shall tremble at *every* moment, and [e]be astonished at thee.

17 And they shall take up a lamentation for thee, and say to thee, How art thou destroyed, *that wast* inhabited of seafaring men, the renowned city, which wast strong in the sea, she and her inhabitants, which cause their terror *to be* on all that haunt it!

18 Now shall the [b]isles tremble in the day of thy fall; yea, the isles that *are* in the sea shall be troubled at thy departure.

19 For thus saith the Lord GOD; When I shall make thee a desolate city, like the cities that are not inhabited; when I shall bring up the deep upon thee, and great waters shall cover thee;

20 When I shall bring thee down [f]with them that descend into the pit, with the people of old time, and shall set thee in the low parts of the earth, in places desolate of old, with them that go down to the pit, that thou be not inhabited; and I shall set glory in the land of the living;

21 I will make thee a terror, and thou *shalt be* no *more*: [g]though thou be sought for, yet shalt thou never be found again, saith the Lord GOD.

B.C. 588.

a Isa. 14:11; 24:8; Jer. 7:34; 16:9; 25:10.
b i.e. *coasts.* Isa. 41:5.
c Isa. 23:8.
d Ezk. 32:10.
e Ezk. 27:35.
f Ezk. 32:18, 24.
g Psa. 37:36.
h Ezk. 28:2.
i Ezk. 28:12.
j Psa. 83:7.
k Ezk. 30:5; 38:5; Jer. 46:9.
l Gen. 10:4; 2 Cor. 20:36.
m Ezk. 38:6; Gen. 10:3.

CHAPTER 27.

The lamentation for Tyre.
(Cf. Rev. 18:1-24.)

The word of the LORD came again unto me, saying,

2 Now, thou son of man, take up a lamentation for Tyrus;

3 And say unto Tyrus, [h]O thou that art situate at the entry of the sea, *which art* a merchant of the people for many isles, Thus saith the Lord GOD; O Tyrus, thou hast said, [i]I *am* of perfect beauty.

4 Thy borders *are* in the midst of the seas, thy builders have perfected thy beauty.

5 They have made all thy *ship* boards of fir trees of Senir: they have taken cedars from Lebanon to make masts for thee.

6 *Of* the oaks of Bashan have they made thine oars; the company of the Ashurites have made thy benches *of* ivory, *brought* out of the [b]isles of Chittim.

7 Fine linen with broidered work from Egypt was that which thou spreadest forth to be thy sail; blue and purple from the isles of Elishah was that which covered thee.

8 The inhabitants of Zidon and Arvad were thy mariners: thy wise *men*, O Tyrus, *that* were in thee, were thy pilots.

9 The ancients of [j]Gebal and the wise *men* thereof were in thee thy calkers: all the ships of the sea with their mariners were in thee to occupy thy merchandise.

10 They of Persia and of Lud and of [k]Phut were in thine army, thy men of war: they hanged the shield and helmet in thee; they set forth thy comeliness.

11 The men of Arvad with thine army *were* upon thy walls round about, and the Gammadims were in thy towers: they hanged their shields upon thy walls round about; they have made thy beauty perfect.

12 [l]Tarshish *was* thy merchant by reason of the multitude of all *kind of* riches; with silver, iron, tin, and lead, they traded in thy fairs.

13 Javan, Tubal, and Meshech, they *were* thy merchants: they traded the persons of men and vessels of brass in thy market.

14 They of the house of [m]Togarmah

traded in thy fairs with horses and horsemen and mules.

15 The men of [a]Dedan *were* thy merchants; many [b]isles *were* the merchandise of thine hand: they brought thee *for* a present horns of ivory and ebony.

16 Syria *was* thy merchant by reason of the multitude of the wares of thy making: they occupied in thy fairs with emeralds, purple, and broidered work, and fine linen, and coral, and agate.

17 Judah, and the land of Israel, they *were* thy merchants: they traded in thy market [c]wheat of Minnith, and Pannag, and honey, and oil, and balm.

18 Damascus *was* thy merchant in the multitude of the wares of thy making, for the multitude of all riches; in the wine of Helbon, and white wool.

19 Dan also and Javan going to and fro occupied in thy fairs: bright iron, cassia, and calamus, were in thy market.

20 Dedan *was* thy merchant in precious clothes for chariots.

21 Arabia, and all the princes of Kedar, they occupied with thee in lambs, and rams, and goats: in these *were they* thy merchants.

22 The merchants of Sheba and Raamah, they *were* thy merchants: they occupied in thy fairs with chief of all spices, and with all precious stones, and gold.

23 [d]Haran, and Canneh, and Eden, the merchants of [e]Sheba, Asshur, *and* Chilmad, *were* thy merchants.

24 These *were* thy merchants in all sorts *of things*, in blue clothes, and broidered work, and in chests of rich apparel, bound with cords, and made of cedar, among thy merchandise.

25 The ships of Tarshish did sing of thee in thy market: and thou wast replenished, and made very glorious in the midst of the seas.

26 Thy rowers have brought thee into great waters: the east wind hath broken thee in the midst of the seas.

27 Thy riches, and thy fairs, thy merchandise, thy mariners, and thy pilots, thy calkers, and the occupiers of thy merchandise, and all thy men of war, that *are* in thee, and in all thy company which *is* in the midst of thee, shall fall into the midst of the seas in the day of thy ruin.

28 The suburbs shall shake at the sound of the cry of thy pilots.

B.C. 588.

a Gen. 10:7.

b i.e. *coasts.*

c 1 Ki. 5:9, 11; Ezra 3:7; Acts 12:20.

d Gen. 11:31; 2 Ki. 19:12.

e Gen. 25:3.

f Rev. 18:18.

g v. 9.

h Ezk. 27:3, 4; 2 Thes. 2:3-10.

29 And all that handle the oar, the mariners, *and* all the pilots of the sea, shall come down from their ships, they shall stand upon the land;

30 And shall cause their voice to be heard against thee, and shall cry bitterly, and shall cast up dust upon their heads, they shall wallow themselves in the ashes:

31 And they shall make themselves utterly bald for thee, and gird them with sackcloth, and they shall weep for thee with bitterness of heart *and* bitter wailing.

32 And in their wailing they shall take up a lamentation for thee, and lament over thee, *saying*, [f]What *city is* like Tyrus, like the destroyed in the midst of the sea?

33 When thy wares went forth out of the seas, thou filledst many people; thou didst enrich the kings of the earth with the multitude of thy riches and of thy merchandise.

34 In the time *when* thou shalt be broken by the seas in the depths of the waters thy merchandise and all thy company in the midst of thee shall fall.

35 All the inhabitants of the [b]isles shall be astonished at thee, and their kings shall be sore afraid, they shall be troubled in *their* countenance.

36 The merchants among the people shall hiss at thee; thou shalt be a terror, and never *shalt be* any more.

CHAPTER 28.

The rebuke of the king of Tyre.

The word of the LORD came again unto me, saying,

2 Son of man, say unto the prince of Tyrus, Thus saith the Lord GOD; [g]Because thine heart *is* lifted up, and thou hast said, I *am* a [h]God, I sit *in* the seat of God, in the midst of the seas; yet thou *art* a man, and not God, though thou set thine heart as the heart of God:

3 Behold, thou *art* wiser than Daniel; there is no secret that they can hide from thee:

4 With thy wisdom and with thine understanding thou hast gotten thee riches, and hast gotten gold and silver into thy treasures:

5 By thy great wisdom *and* by thy traffick hast thou increased thy riches, and thine heart is lifted up because of thy riches:

6 Therefore thus saith the Lord GOD; [a]Because thou hast set thine heart as the heart of God;

7 Behold, therefore I will bring strangers upon thee, the terrible of the nations: and they shall draw their swords against the beauty of thy wisdom, and they shall defile thy brightness.

8 They shall bring thee down to the pit, and thou shalt die the deaths of *them that are* slain in the midst of the seas.

9 Wilt thou yet say before him that slayeth thee, I *am* God? but thou *shalt be* a man, and no God, in the hand of him that slayeth thee.

10 Thou shalt die the deaths of the uncircumcised by the hand of strangers: for I have spoken *it*, saith the Lord GOD.

11 Moreover the word of the LORD came unto me, saying,

12 Son of man, take up a lamentation upon the king of Tyrus, and say unto him, Thus saith the Lord GOD; [1]Thou [b]sealest up the sum, full of wisdom, and [c]perfect in beauty.

13 Thou hast been in Eden the garden of God; every precious stone *was* thy covering, the sardius, topaz, and the diamond, the beryl, the onyx, and the jasper, the sapphire, the emerald, and the carbuncle, and gold: the workmanship of thy tabrets and of thy pipes was prepared in thee in the day that thou wast created.

14 Thou *art* the anointed [d]cherub that covereth; and I have set thee *so*: thou wast upon the holy mountain of God; thou hast walked up and down in the midst of the stones of fire.

15 Thou *wast* perfect in thy ways from the day that thou wast created, till iniquity was found in thee.

16 By the multitude of thy merchandise they have filled the midst of thee with violence, and thou hast sinned: therefore I will cast thee as profane out of the mountain of God: and I will destroy thee, O covering cherub, from the midst of the stones of fire.

17 Thine heart was lifted up because of thy beauty, thou hast corrupted thy wisdom by reason of thy brightness: I will cast thee to the ground, I will lay thee before kings, that they may behold thee.

18 Thou hast defiled thy sanctuaries by the multitude of thine iniquities, by the iniquity of thy traffick; therefore will I bring forth a fire from the midst of thee, it shall devour thee, and I will bring thee to ashes upon the earth in the sight of all them that behold thee.

19 All they that know thee among the people shall be astonished at thee: [e]thou shalt be a terror, and never *shalt* thou *be* any more.

The judgment of Zidon.

20 Again the word of the LORD came unto me, saying,

21 Son of man, set thy face against Zidon, and prophesy against it,

22 And say, Thus saith the Lord GOD; [f]Behold, I *am* against thee, O Zidon; and I will be glorified in the midst of thee: and they shall know that I *am* the LORD, when I shall have executed judgments in her, and shall be sanctified in her.

23 [g]For I will send into her pestilence, and blood into her streets; and the wounded shall be judged in the midst of her by the sword upon her on every side; and they shall know that I *am* the LORD.

24 And there shall be no more [h]a pricking brier unto the house of Israel, nor *any* grieving thorn of all *that are* round about them, that despised them; and they shall know that I *am* the Lord GOD.

The future regathering of Israel.

25 Thus saith the Lord GOD; When I shall have [i]gathered the house of Israel from the people among whom they are scattered, and shall be sanctified in them in the sight of the [j]heathen, then shall they dwell in their land that I have given to my servant Jacob.

26 And they shall [k]dwell safely

B.C. 588.

a *The Beast.* vs. 2-8; Mt. 24:15. (Dan. 7:8; Rev. 19:20.)

b Ezk. 27:3; 28:2.

c *Satan.* vs. 12-15; Zech. 3:1, 2. (Gen. 3:1; Rev. 20:10.)

d See v. 16. Ex. 25:20.

e Ezk. 26:21; 27:36.

f Ezk. 39:13; Ex. 14:4, 17.

g Jer. 47:4; Ezk. 38:22.

h Num. 33:55; Josh. 23:13.

i Ezk. 11:17; 20:41; 34:13; 37:21; Isa. 11:12.

j i.e. *nations.*

k Ezk. 36:28; Jer. 23:6.

[1]**(28:12)** Here (vs. 12-15), as in Isa. 14:12, the language goes beyond the king of Tyre to Satan, inspirer and unseen ruler of all such pomp and pride as that of Tyre. Instances of thus indirectly addressing Satan are: Gen. 3:14, 15; Mt. 16:23. The unfallen state of Satan is here described; his fall in Isa. 14:12-14. (See Rev. 20:10, *note.*) But there is more. The vision is not of Satan in his own person, but of Satan fulfilling himself in and through an earthly king who arrogates to himself divine honours, so that the prince of Tyrus foreshadows the Beast (Dan. 7:8; Rev. 19:20).

therein, and shall build houses, and plant vineyards; yea, they shall dwell with confidence, when I have executed judgments upon all those that despise them round about them; and they shall know that I *am* the LORD their God.

CHAPTER 29.

The prophecy against Egypt.

In the tenth year, in the [a]tenth *month*, in the twelfth *day* of the month, the word of the LORD came unto me, saying,

2 Son of man, set thy face against Pharaoh king of Egypt, and prophesy against him, and against all Egypt:

3 Speak, and say, Thus saith the Lord GOD; [b]Behold, I *am* against thee, Pharaoh king of Egypt, the great [c]dragon that lieth in the midst of his rivers, which hath said, My river *is* mine own, and I have made *it* for myself.

4 But [d]I will put hooks in thy jaws, and I will cause the fish of thy rivers to stick unto thy scales, and I will bring thee up out of the midst of thy rivers, and all the fish of thy rivers shall stick unto thy scales.

5 And I will leave thee *thrown* into the wilderness, thee and all the fish of thy rivers: thou shalt fall upon the open fields; thou shalt not be brought together, [e]nor gathered: I have given thee for meat to the beasts of the field and to the fowls of the heaven.

6 And all the inhabitants of Egypt shall know that I *am* the LORD, because they have been [f]a staff of reed to the house of Israel.

7 When they took hold of thee by thy hand, thou didst break, and rend all their shoulder: and when they leaned upon thee, thou brakest, and madest all their loins to be at a stand.

8 Therefore thus saith the Lord GOD; Behold, I will bring a sword upon thee, and cut off man and beast out of thee.

9 And the land of Egypt shall be desolate and waste; and they shall know that I *am* the LORD: because he hath said, The river *is* mine, and I have made *it*.

10 Behold, therefore I *am* against thee, and against thy rivers, and I will make the land of Egypt utterly waste *and* desolate, [g]from the tower of Syene even unto the border of Ethiopia.

B.C. 588.

a i.e. *January.*

b v.10; Ezk. 28:22;. Jer. 44:30.

c Ezk. 32:2; Psa. 74:13, 14; Isa. 27:1; 51:9.

d Ezk. 38:4; Isa. 37:29.

e Jer. 8:2; 16:4; 25:33.

f 2 Ki. 18:21; Isa. 36:6.

g Or, *from Migdol to Syene.* Ex. 14:2; Jer. 44:1.

h i.e. *April.*

i Ezk. 26:7, 8; Jer. 27:6.

j Psa. 132:17.

11 No foot of man shall pass through it, nor foot of beast shall pass through it, neither shall it be inhabited forty years.

12 And I will make the land of Egypt desolate in the midst of the countries *that are* desolate, and her cities among the cities *that are* laid waste shall be desolate forty years: and I will scatter the Egyptians among the nations, and will disperse them through the countries.

13 Yet thus saith the Lord GOD; At the end of forty years will I gather the Egyptians from the people whither they were scattered:

14 And I will bring again the captivity of Egypt, and will cause them to return *into* the land of Pathros, into the land of their habitation; and they shall be there a base kingdom.

15 It shall be the basest of the kingdoms; neither shall it exalt itself any more above the nations: for I will diminish them, that they shall no more rule over the nations.

16 And it shall be no more the confidence of the house of Israel, which bringeth *their* iniquity to remembrance, when they shall look after them: but they shall know that I *am* the Lord GOD.

17 And it came to pass in the seven and twentieth year, in the [h]first *month*, in the first *day* of the month, the word of the LORD came unto me, saying,

18 Son of man, [i]Nebuchadrezzar king of Babylon caused his army to serve a great service against Tyrus: every head *was* made bald, and every shoulder *was* peeled: yet had he no wages, nor his army, for Tyrus, for the service that he had served against it:

19 Therefore thus saith the Lord GOD; Behold, I will give the land of Egypt unto Nebuchadrezzar king of Babylon; and he shall take her multitude, and take her spoil, and take her prey; and it shall be the wages for his army.

20 I have given him the land of Egypt *for* his labour wherewith he served against it, because they wrought for me, saith the Lord GOD.

21 In that day [j]will I cause the horn of the house of Israel to bud forth, and I will give thee the opening of the mouth in the midst of them; and they shall know that I *am* the LORD.

B.C. 572.

CHAPTER 30.

Egypt in the day of Jehovah.

The word of the LORD came again unto
me, saying,
2 Son of man, prophesy and say, Thus
saith the Lord GOD; Howl ye, Woe worth
the day!
3 For [a]the day *is* near, even the [b]day of
the LORD *is* near, a cloudy day; it shall be
the time of the [c]heathen.
4 And the sword shall come upon
Egypt, and great pain shall be in Ethiopia,
when the slain shall fall in Egypt, and
they shall take away her multitude, and
her foundations shall be broken down.
5 Ethiopia, and Libya, and Lydia, and
all the mingled people, and Chub, and
the men of the land that is in league,
shall fall with them by the sword.
6 Thus saith the LORD; They also that
uphold Egypt shall fall; and the pride of
her power shall come down: from the
tower of Syene shall they fall in it by the
sword, saith the Lord GOD.
7 And [d]they shall be desolate in the
midst of the countries *that are* desolate,
and her cities shall be in the midst of the
cities *that are* wasted.
8 And they shall know that I *am* the
LORD, when I have set a fire in Egypt, and
when all her helpers shall be destroyed.
9 In that day shall messengers go forth
from me in ships to make the careless
Ethiopians afraid, and great pain shall
come upon them, as in the day of Egypt:
for, lo, it cometh.
10 Thus saith the Lord GOD; I will also
make the multitude of Egypt to cease by
the hand of Nebuchadrezzar king of
Babylon.
11 He and his people with him, the
terrible of the nations, shall be brought
to destroy the land: and they shall draw
their swords against Egypt, and fill the
land with the slain.
12 [e]And I will make the rivers dry, and
sell the land into the hand of the wicked:
and I will make the land waste, and all
that is therein, by the hand of strangers:
I the LORD have spoken *it*.
13 Thus saith the Lord GOD; I will also
[f]destroy the idols, and I will cause *their*
images to cease out of Noph; and [g]there
shall be no more a prince of the land of
Egypt: and I will put a fear in the land of
Egypt.
14 And I will make [h]Pathros desolate,
and will set fire in Zoan, and will execute judgments in No.
15 And I will pour my fury upon Sin,
the strength of Egypt; and I will cut off
the multitude of No.
16 And I will set fire in Egypt: Sin
shall have great pain, and No shall be
rent asunder, and Noph *shall have* distresses daily.
17 The young men of Aven and of Pi-
beseth shall fall by the sword: and these
cities shall go into captivity.
18 At [i]Tehaphnehes also the day shall
be darkened, when I shall break there
the yokes of Egypt: and the pomp of her
strength shall cease in her: as for her, a
cloud shall cover her, and her daughters
shall go into captivity.
19 Thus will I execute judgments in
Egypt: and they shall know that I *am* the
LORD.

Jehovah against Pharaoh in the war with Babylon.

20 And it came to pass in the eleventh
year, in the [j]first *month*, in the seventh
day of the month, *that* the word of the
LORD came unto me, saying,
21 Son of man, I have broken the arm
of Pharaoh king of Egypt; and, lo, it shall
not be bound up to be healed, to put a
roller to bind it, to make it strong to hold
the sword.
22 Therefore thus saith the Lord GOD;
Behold, I *am* against Pharaoh king of
Egypt, and will break his arms, the strong,
and that which was broken; and I will
cause the sword to fall out of his hand.
23 [k]And I will scatter the Egyptians
among the nations, and will disperse
them through the countries.
24 And I will strengthen the arms of
the king of Babylon, and put my sword
in his hand: but I will break Pharaoh's
arms, and he shall groan before him with
the groanings of a deadly wounded *man*.
25 But I will strengthen the arms of the
king of Babylon, and the arms of
Pharaoh shall fall down; and [l]they shall
know that I *am* the LORD, when I shall
put my sword into the hand of the king
of Babylon, and he shall stretch it out
upon the land of Egypt.
26 And I will scatter the Egyptians

a Ezk. 7:7, 12; Joel 2:1; Zeph. 1:7.
b *Day (of Jehovah).* Joel 1:15. (Isa. 2:10-22; Rev. 19:11-21.)
c i.e. *nations.*
d Ezk. 29:12.
e Isa. 19:5, 6; cf. Ezk. 29:3, 9.
f Isa. 19:1; Jer. 43:12; 46:25; Zech. 13:2.
g Zech. 10:11.
h Ezk. 29:14.
i Jer. 2:16.
j i.e. *April.*
k v. 26; Ezk. 29:12.
l Psa. 9:16.

among the nations, and disperse them
among the countries; and they shall
know that I *am* the LORD.

CHAPTER 31.

The prophecy against Pharaoh.

And it came to pass in the eleventh
year, in the [a]third *month*, in the first
day of the month, *that* the word of the
LORD came unto me, saying,
2 Son of man, speak unto Pharaoh
king of Egypt, and to his multitude;
Whom art thou like in thy greatness?
3 [b]Behold, the Assyrian *was* a [c]cedar in
Lebanon with fair branches, and with a
shadowing shroud, and of an high
stature; and his top was among the thick
boughs.
4 [d]The waters made him great, the
deep set him up on high with her rivers
running round about his plants, and sent
out her little rivers unto all the trees of
the field.
5 Therefore his height was exalted
above all the trees of the field, and his
boughs were multiplied, and his branches became long because of the multitude
of waters, when he shot forth.
6 All the fowls of heaven made their
nests in his boughs, and under his
branches did all the beasts of the field
bring forth their young, and under his
shadow dwelt all great nations.
7 Thus was he fair in his greatness, in
the length of his branches: for his root
was by great waters.
8 The cedars in the [e]garden of God
could not hide him: the fir trees were not
like his boughs, and the chesnut trees
were not like his branches; nor any tree
in the garden of God was like unto him
in his beauty.
9 I have made him fair by the multitude of his branches: so that all the trees
of Eden, that *were* in the garden of God,
envied him.
10 Therefore thus saith the Lord GOD;
Because thou hast lifted up thyself in
height, and he hath shot up his top
among the thick boughs, and his heart is
lifted up in his height;
11 I have therefore delivered him into
the hand of the mighty one of the [f]hea-
then; he shall surely deal with him: I
have driven him out for his wickedness.

B.C. 588.

a i.e. *June.*

b *Parables* (O.T.). vs. 3-14; Ezk. 37:1-14. (Jud. 9:7-15; Zech. 11:7-14.)

c Ezk. 17:23, 24; Dan. 4:4-37; Rev. 7:1.

d Jer. 51:36.

e Ezk. 28:13; Gen. 2:8; 13:10.

f i.e. *nations.*

g Ezk. 32:4; Isa. 18:6.

h Ezk. 32:18.

i Heb. *Sheol.* See Hab. 2:5, *note.*

j Isa. 14:15.

k Ezk. 32:31.

l Ezk. 28:10; 32:19, 21, 24.

m i.e. *March;* also v. 17.

12 And strangers, the terrible of the
nations, have cut him off, and have left
him: upon the mountains and in all the
valleys his branches are fallen, and his
boughs are broken by all the rivers of the
land; and all the people of the earth are
gone down from his shadow, and have
left him.
13 [g]Upon his ruin shall all the fowls of
the heaven remain, and all the beasts of
the field shall be upon his branches:
14 To the end that none of all the trees
by the waters exalt themselves for their
height, neither shoot up their top among
the thick boughs, neither their trees
stand up in their height, all that drink
water: for they are all delivered unto
death, [h]to the nether parts of the earth,
in the midst of the children of men, with
them that go down to the pit.
15 Thus saith the Lord GOD; In the day
when he went down to the [i]grave I
caused a mourning: I covered the deep
for him, and I restrained the floods thereof, and the great waters were stayed: and
I caused Lebanon to mourn for him, and
all the trees of the field fainted for him.
16 I made the nations to shake at the
sound of his fall, when I [j]cast him down
to [i]hell with them that descend into the
pit: and all the trees of Eden, the choice
and best of Lebanon, all that drink
water, [k]shall be comforted in the nether
parts of the earth.
17 They also went down into hell with
him unto *them that be* slain with the
sword; and *they that were* his arm, *that*
dwelt under his shadow in the midst of
the [f]heathen.
18 To whom art thou thus like in glory
and in greatness among the trees of
Eden? yet shalt thou be brought down
with the trees of Eden unto the nether
parts of the earth: [l]thou shalt lie in the
midst of the uncircumcised with *them that
be* slain by the sword. This *is* Pharaoh and
all his multitude, saith the Lord GOD.

CHAPTER 32.

The lamentation for Pharaoh.

And it came to pass in the twelfth
year, in the [m]twelfth month, in the
first *day* of the month, *that* the word of
the LORD came unto me, saying,

2 Son of man, take up a lamentation for Pharaoh king of Egypt, and say unto him, Thou art like a young lion of the nations, and thou *art* as a whale in the seas: and thou camest forth with thy rivers, and troubledst the waters with thy feet, and fouledst their rivers.

3 Thus saith the Lord GOD; I will therefore spread out my net over thee with a company of many people; and they shall bring thee up in my net.

4 Then [a]will I leave thee upon the land, I will cast thee forth upon the open field, and will cause all the fowls of the heaven to remain upon thee, and I will fill the beasts of the whole earth with thee.

5 And I will lay thy flesh upon the mountains, and fill the valleys with thy height.

6 I will also water with thy blood the land wherein thou swimmest, *even* to the mountains; and the rivers shall be full of thee.

7 And when I shall put thee out, [b]I will cover the heaven, and make the stars thereof dark; I will cover the sun with a cloud, and the moon shall not give her light.

8 All the bright lights of heaven will I make dark over thee, and set darkness upon thy land, saith the Lord GOD.

9 I will also vex the hearts of many people, when I shall bring thy destruction among the nations, into the countries which thou hast not known.

10 Yea, I will make many people amazed at thee, and their kings shall be horribly afraid for thee, when I shall brandish my sword before them; and they shall tremble at *every* moment, every man for his own life, in the day of thy fall.

11 For [c]thus saith the Lord GOD; The sword of the king of Babylon shall come upon thee.

12 By the swords of the mighty will I cause thy multitude to fall, the terrible of the nations, all of them: and they shall spoil the pomp of Egypt, and all the multitude thereof shall be destroyed.

13 I will destroy also all the beasts thereof from beside the great waters; neither shall the foot of man trouble them any more, nor the hoofs of beasts trouble them.

14 Then will I make their waters deep, and cause their rivers to run like oil, saith the Lord GOD.

B.C. 587.

a Ezk. 29:5.

b Isa. 13:10; Joel 2:31; 3:15; Amos 8:9; Mt. 24:29; Rev. 6:12, 13.

c Ezk. 30:4; Jer. 46:26.

d v. 2; Ezk. 2:10; 26:17; 2 Sam. 1:17; 2 Chr. 35:25.

e Ezk. 31:2, 18.

f v. 27; Isa. 1:31; 14:9, 10.

g v. 27. Heb. *Sheol.* See Hab. 2:5, *note.*

h Isa. 14:15.

i Jer. 49:34.

15 When I shall make the land of Egypt desolate, and the country shall be destitute of that whereof it was full, when I shall smite all them that dwell therein, then shall they know that I *am* the LORD.

16 [d]This *is* the lamentation wherewith they shall lament her: the daughters of the nations shall lament her: they shall lament for her, *even* for Egypt, and for all her multitude, saith the Lord GOD.

Lamentation for Egypt.

17 It came to pass also in the twelfth year, in the fifteenth *day* of the month, *that* the word of the LORD came unto me, saying,

18 Son of man, wail for the multitude of Egypt, and cast them down, *even* her, and the daughters of the famous nations, unto the nether parts of the earth, with them that go down into the pit.

19 [e]Whom dost thou pass in beauty? go down, and be thou laid with the uncircumcised.

20 They shall fall in the midst of *them that are* slain by the sword: she is delivered to the sword: draw her and all her multitudes.

21 [f]The strong among the mighty shall speak to him out of the midst of [g]hell with them that help him: they are gone down, they lie uncircumcised, slain by the sword.

22 Asshur *is* there and all her company: his graves *are* about him: all of them slain, fallen by the sword:

23 [h]Whose graves are set in the sides of the pit, and her company is round about her grave: all of them slain, fallen by the sword, which caused terror in the land of the living.

24 There *is* [i]Elam and all her multitude round about her grave, all of them slain, fallen by the sword, which are gone down uncircumcised into the nether parts of the earth, which caused their terror in the land of the living; yet have they borne their shame with them that go down to the pit.

25 They have set her a bed in the midst of the slain with all her multitude: her graves *are* round about him: all of them uncircumcised, slain by the sword: though their terror was caused in the land of the living, yet have they borne their shame with them that go down to the pit: he is put in the midst of *them that be* slain.

B.C. 587.

26 There *is* [a]Meshech, Tubal, and all her multitude: her graves *are* round about him: all of them uncircumcised, slain by the sword, though they caused their terror in the land of the living.

27 And they shall not lie with the mighty *that are* fallen of the uncircumcised, which are gone down to hell with their weapons of war: and they have laid their swords under their heads, but their iniquities shall be upon their bones, though *they were* the terror of the mighty in the land of the living.

28 Yea, thou shalt be broken in the midst of the uncircumcised, and shalt lie with *them that are* slain with the sword.

29 There *is* [b]Edom, her kings, and all her princes, which with their might are laid by *them that were* slain by the sword: they shall lie with the uncircumcised, and with them that go down to the pit.

30 [c]There *be* the princes of the north, all of them, and all the Zidonians, which are gone down with the slain; with their terror they are ashamed of their might; and they lie uncircumcised with *them that be* slain by the sword, and bear their shame with them that go down to the pit.

31 Pharaoh shall see them, and shall be [d]comforted over all his multitude, *even* Pharaoh and all his army slain by the sword, saith the Lord GOD.

32 For I have caused my terror in the land of the living: and he shall be laid in the midst of the uncircumcised with *them that are* slain with the sword, *even* Pharaoh and all his multitude, saith the Lord GOD.

CHAPTER 33.

Ethical instructions for the captivity.

Again the word of the LORD came unto me, saying,

2 Son of man, speak to the children of thy people, and say unto them, When I bring the sword upon a land, if the people of the land take a man of their coasts, and set him for their [e]watchman:

3 If when he seeth the sword come upon the land, he blow the trumpet, and warn the people;

4 Then [f]whosoever heareth the sound of the trumpet, and taketh not warning; if the sword come, and take him away, his blood shall be upon his own head.

5 He heard the sound of the trumpet, and took not warning; his blood shall be upon him. But he that taketh warning shall deliver his soul.

6 But if the watchman see the sword come, and blow not the trumpet, and the people be not warned; if the sword come, and take *any* person from among them, he is taken away in his iniquity; but his blood will I require at the watchman's hand.

7 [g]So thou, O son of man, I have set thee a watchman unto the house of Israel; therefore thou shalt hear the word at my mouth, and warn them from me.

8 When I say unto the wicked, O wicked *man*, thou shalt surely die; if thou dost not speak to warn the wicked from his way, that wicked *man* shall die in his iniquity; but his blood will I require at thine hand.

9 Nevertheless, if thou warn the wicked of his way to turn from it; if he do not turn from his way, he shall die in his iniquity; but thou hast delivered thy soul.

10 Therefore, O thou son of man, speak unto the house of Israel; Thus ye speak, saying, If our transgressions and our sins *be* upon us, and we pine away in them, how should we then live?

11 Say unto them, *As* I live, saith the Lord GOD, [h]I have no pleasure in the death of the wicked; but that the wicked turn from his way and live: turn ye, turn ye from your evil ways; for [i]why will ye die, O house of Israel?

12 Therefore, thou son of man, say unto the children of thy people, The [j]righteousness of the righteous shall not deliver him in the day of his transgression: as for the wickedness of the wicked, he shall not fall thereby in the day that he turneth from his wickedness; neither shall the righteous be able to live for his *righteousness* in the day that he sinneth.

13 When I shall say to the righteous, *that* he shall surely live; [k]if he trust to his own righteousness, and commit iniquity, all his righteousnesses shall not be remembered; but for his iniquity that he hath committed, he shall die for it.

14 Again, when I say unto the wicked, Thou shalt surely die; if he turn from his

a Ezk. 27:13; 38:2; Gen. 10:2.

b Ezk. 25:12.

c Ezk. 38:6, 15; 39:2.

d Ezk. 31:16.

e 2 Sam. 18:24, 25; 2 Ki. 9:17; Hos. 9:8.

f Ezk. 3:17.

g The nation having failed in corporate responsibility, the appeal is now to individual loyalty. Cf. 2 Tim. 2:1-26.

h Ezk. 18:23, 32; 2 Sam. 14:14; 2 Pet. 3:9.

i Ezk. 18:31.

j Ezk. 3:20; 18:24, 26, 27.

k Ezk. 3:20; 18:24.

sin, and do that which is lawful and
right;
15 *If* the wicked [a]restore the pledge,
[b]give again that he had robbed, walk in
the statutes of life, without committing
iniquity; he shall surely live, he shall not
die.
16 None of his sins that he hath committed shall be mentioned unto him: he
hath done that which is lawful and right;
he shall surely live.

B.C. 587.

a Ezk. 18:7.

b Ex. 22:1-4; Lev. 6:2, 4, 5; Num. 5:6, 7; Lk. 19:8.

c v. 17; Ezk. 18:25, 29.

17 Yet the children of thy people say,
The way of the Lord is not equal: but as
for them, their way is not equal.
18 When the righteous turneth from
his righteousness, and committeth iniquity, he shall even die thereby.
19 But if the wicked turn from his
wickedness, and do that which is lawful
and right, he shall live thereby.
20 Yet ye say, [c]The way of the Lord is
not equal. O ye house of Israel, I will
judge you every one after his ways.

PART V. GENERAL THEME: THE FUTURE KINGDOM OF THE SON OF DAVID: CHAPTERS 33:21–36:38.

21 And it came to pass in the twelfth
year of our captivity, in the [d]tenth *month*,
in the fifth *day* of the month, *that* one
that had escaped out of Jerusalem came
unto me, saying, The city is smitten.
22 Now the hand of the LORD was
upon me in the evening, afore he that
was escaped came; and had opened my
mouth, until he came to me in the morning; and my mouth was opened, and I
was no more dumb.

Hearers of the word, but not doers.

23 Then the word of the LORD came
unto me, saying,
24 Son of man, they that inhabit those
wastes of the land of Israel speak, saying, [e]Abraham was one, and he inherited the land: [f]but we *are* many; the land is
given us for inheritance.
25 Wherefore say unto them, Thus
saith the Lord GOD; Ye eat with the
blood, and lift up your eyes toward your
idols, and shed blood: and shall ye possess the land?
26 Ye stand upon your sword, ye work
abomination, and ye defile every one his
neighbour's wife: and shall ye possess
the land?
27 Say thou thus unto them, Thus
saith the Lord GOD; *As* I live, surely they
that *are* in the wastes shall fall by the
sword, and him that *is* in the open field
will I give to the beasts to be devoured,
and they that *be* in the forts and in the
caves shall die of the pestilence.
28 [g]For I will lay the land most desolate, and the pomp of her strength shall
cease; and the mountains of Israel shall
be desolate, that none shall pass through.

d i.e. *January*.

e Isa. 51:2; Mt. 3:9; Acts 7:5.

f Mic. 3:11; Mt. 3:9; John 8:39.

g Ezk. 36:34, 35; Jer. 44:2, 6, 22.

h Ezk. 8:1.

i Psa. 78:36, 37; Isa. 29:13.

j 1 Sam. 3:20.

k Ezk. 2:5.

l Jer. 23:1; Zech. 11:17.

m Isa. 56:11; Zech. 11:16.

n Ezk. 33:25, 26; Mic. 3:1-3; Zech. 11:5.

29 Then shall they know that I *am* the
LORD, when I have laid the land most
desolate because of all their abominations which they have committed.
30 Also, thou son of man, the children
of thy people still are talking against
thee by the walls and in the doors of the
houses, and speak one to another, every
one to his brother, saying, Come, I pray
you, and hear what is the word that
cometh forth from the LORD.
31 And they come unto thee as the
people cometh, and [h]they sit before thee
as my people, and they hear thy words,
but they will not do them: [i]for with their
mouth they shew much love, *but* their
heart goeth after their covetousness.
32 And, lo, thou *art* unto them as a
very lovely song of one that hath a
pleasant voice, and can play well on an
instrument: for they hear thy words, but
they do them not.
33 [j]And when this cometh to pass, (lo,
it will come,) then [k]shall they know that
a prophet hath been among them.

CHAPTER 34.

Message to the faithless shepherds of Israel.

And the word of the LORD came unto
me, saying,
2 Son of man, prophesy against the
shepherds of Israel, prophesy, and say
unto them, Thus saith the Lord GOD unto
the shepherds; [l]Woe *be* to the shepherds
of Israel that do feed themselves! should
not the shepherds feed the flocks?
3 [m]Ye eat the fat, and ye clothe you
with the wool, ye [n]kill them that are fed:
but ye feed not the flock.

4 The [a]diseased have ye not strengthened, neither have ye healed that which was sick, neither have ye bound up *that which was* broken, neither have ye brought again that which was driven away, neither have ye [b]sought that which was lost; but with [c]force and with cruelty have ye ruled them.

5 And they were scattered, because *there is* no shepherd: [d]and they became meat to all the beasts of the field, when they were scattered.

6 My sheep wandered through all the mountains, and upon every high hill: yea, my flock was scattered upon all the face of the earth, and none did search or seek *after them.*

7 Therefore, ye shepherds, hear the word of the LORD;

8 *As* I live, saith the Lord GOD, surely because my flock became a prey, and my flock became meat to every beast of the field, because *there was* no shepherd, neither did my shepherds search for my flock, but the shepherds fed themselves, and fed not my flock;

9 Therefore, O ye shepherds, hear the word of the LORD;

10 Thus saith the Lord GOD; Behold, I *am* against the shepherds; and I will [e]require my flock at their hand, and cause them to cease from feeding the flock; neither shall the shepherds feed themselves any more; for I will deliver my flock from their mouth, that they may not be meat for them.

Israel to be restored:
the Davidic kingdom to be set up.

11 For thus saith the Lord GOD; Behold, I, *even* I, will both search my sheep, [f]and seek them out.

12 As a shepherd seeketh out his flock in the day that he is among his sheep *that are* scattered; so will I seek out my sheep, and will deliver them out of all places where they have been scattered in the cloudy and dark day.

13 And [g]I will bring them out from the people, and gather them from the countries, and will bring them to their own land, and feed them upon the mountains of Israel by the rivers, and in all the inhabited places of the country.

14 I will feed them in a good pasture, and upon the high mountains of Israel shall their fold be: there shall they lie in a good fold, and *in* a fat pasture shall they feed upon the mountains of Israel.

15 I will feed my flock, and I will cause them to lie down, saith the Lord GOD.

16 I [h]will seek that which was lost, and bring again that which was driven away, and will bind up *that which was* broken, and will strengthen that which was sick: but I will destroy the fat and the strong; I will feed them with judgment.

17 And *as for* you, O my flock, thus saith the Lord GOD; Behold, I judge between cattle and cattle, between the rams and the he goats.

18 *Seemeth it* a small thing unto you to have eaten up the good pasture, but ye must tread down with your feet the residue of your pastures? and to have drunk of the deep waters, but ye must foul the residue with your feet?

19 And *as for* my flock, they eat that which ye have trodden with your feet; and they drink that which ye have fouled with your feet.

20 Therefore thus saith the Lord GOD unto them; Behold, I, *even* I, will judge between the fat cattle and between the lean cattle.

21 Because ye have thrust with side and with shoulder, and pushed all the diseased with your horns, till ye have scattered them abroad;

22 Therefore will I save my flock, and they shall no more be a prey; and I will judge between cattle and cattle.

23 And I will set up [i]one shepherd over them, and he shall feed them, *even* my servant David; he shall feed them, and he shall be their shepherd.

24 [j]And I the LORD will be their God, and my servant David a prince among them; I the LORD have spoken *it.*

25 [k]And I will make with them a covenant of peace, and [l]will cause the evil beasts to cease out of the land: and they shall dwell safely in the wilderness, and sleep in the woods.

26 And I will make them and the places round about my hill [m]a blessing; and I will cause the shower to come down in his season; there shall be showers of blessing.

27 And the tree of the field shall yield her fruit, and the earth shall yield her increase, and they shall be safe in their land, and shall know that I *am* the LORD,

B.C. 587.

a v. 16; Zech. 11:16.
b Lk. 15:4.
c 1 Pet. 5:3.
d v. 8; Isa. 56:9; Jer. 12:9.
e Ezk. 3:18; Heb. 13:17.
f *Kingdom* (O.T.). vs. 11-15, 22-25; Ezk. 37:21-28. (Gen. 1:26; Zech. 12:8.)
g Ezk. 28:25; 36:24; 37:21, 22; Isa. 65:9, 10; Jer. 23:3.
h v. 4; Isa. 40:11; Mic. 4:6; Mt. 18:11; Mk. 2:17; Lk. 5:32.
i Isa. 11:1-5, 10; 40:11; Jer. 23:4, 5; John 10:11; Heb. 13:20; 1 Pet. 2:25; 5:4.
j v. 30; Ezk. 37:27; Ex. 29:45.
k Ezk. 37:26.
l Lev. 26:6; Isa. 11:6-9; 35:9; Hos 2:18.
m Gen. 12:2; Isa. 19:24; Zech. 8:13.

when I have [a]broken the bands of their
yoke, and delivered them out of the hand
of those that served themselves of them.
28 And they shall no more be a [1]prey to
the [b]heathen, neither shall the beast of the
land devour them; but [c]they shall dwell
safely, and none shall make *them* afraid.
29 And I will raise up for them a plant
of renown, and they shall be no more consumed with hunger in the land, neither
bear the shame of the [b]heathen any more.
30 Thus shall they know that I the
LORD their God *am* with them, and *that*
they, *even* the house of Israel, *are* my people, saith the Lord GOD.
31 And ye my flock, the flock of my
pasture, *are* men, *and* I *am* your God,
saith the Lord GOD.

CHAPTER 35.

The prophecy against Mount Seir.

Moreover the word of the LORD came
unto me, saying,
2 Son of man, set thy face against
[d]mount Seir, and prophesy against it,
3 And say unto it, Thus saith the Lord
GOD; Behold, O mount Seir, I *am* against
thee, and I will stretch out mine hand
against thee, and I will make thee most
desolate.
4 I will lay thy cities waste, and thou
shalt be desolate, and thou shalt know
that I *am* the LORD.
5 [e]Because thou hast had a perpetual
hatred, and hast shed *the blood of* the
children of Israel by the force of the
sword in the time of their calamity, in
the time *that their* iniquity *had* an end:
6 Therefore, *as* I live, saith the Lord
GOD, I will prepare thee unto blood, and
blood shall pursue thee: sith thou hast
not hated blood, even blood shall pursue
thee.
7 Thus will I make mount Seir most
desolate, and cut off from it him that
passeth out and him that returneth.
8 And I will fill his mountains with his
slain *men*: in thy hills, and in thy valleys,
and in all thy rivers, shall they fall that
are slain with the sword.

B.C. 587.

a Lev. 26:13; Jer. 2:20.

b i.e. *nations.*

c v. 25; Jer. 30:10; 46:27.

d Deut. 2:5; Joel 3:19.

e Ezk. 25:12; Oba. 10.

f v. 4; Ezk. 25:13; Jer. 49:17, 18; Mal. 1:3, 4.

g Isa. 65:13, 14.

h Ezk. 35:12; 36:4-7; Oba. 12, 15.

9 [f]I will make thee perpetual desolations, and thy cities shall not return: and
ye shall know that I *am* the LORD.
10 Because thou hast said, These two
nations and these two countries shall be
mine, and we will possess it; whereas
the LORD was there:
11 Therefore, *as* I live, saith the Lord
GOD, I will even do according to thine
anger, and according to thine envy which
thou hast used out of thy hatred against
them; and I will make myself known
among them, when I have judged thee.
12 And thou shalt know that I *am* the
LORD, *and that* I have heard all thy blasphemies which thou hast spoken against
the mountains of Israel, saying, They are
laid desolate, they are given us to consume.
13 Thus with your mouth ye have
boasted against me, and have multiplied
your words against me: I have heard
them.
14 Thus saith the Lord GOD; [g]When
the whole earth rejoiceth, I will make
thee desolate.
15 [h]As thou didst rejoice at the inheritance of the house of Israel, because it
was desolate, so will I do unto thee: thou
shalt be desolate, O mount Seir, and all
Idumea, *even* all of it: and they shall
know that I *am* the LORD.

[2]CHAPTER 36.

Message to the mountains of Israel:
the restoration predicted.

Also, thou son of man, prophesy unto
the mountains of Israel, and say, Ye
mountains of Israel, hear the word of the
LORD:
2 Thus saith the Lord GOD; Because
the enemy hath said against you, Aha,
even the ancient high places are ours in
possession:
3 Therefore prophesy and say, Thus
saith the Lord GOD; Because they have
made *you* desolate, and swallowed you

[1] **(34:28)** The whole passage (vs. 23-30) speaks of a restoration yet future, for the remnant which returned after the 70 years, and their posterity, were continually under the Gentile yoke, until, in A.D. 70, they were finally driven from the land into a dispersion which still continues.

[2] **(36, heading)** A beautiful order is discernible in this and the succeeding prophecies: (1) Restoration of the land (36:1-15); (2) of the people (36:16–37:28); (3) judgment on Israel's enemies (38:1–39:24). Afterward follows that which concerns the worship of Jehovah that He may dwell amongst His people.

up on every side, that ye might be a possession unto the residue of the [a]heathen,
and [b]ye are taken up in the lips of talk-
ers, and *are* an infamy of the people:
4 Therefore, ye mountains of Israel,
hear the word of the Lord GOD; Thus
saith the Lord GOD to the mountains, and
to the hills, to the rivers, and to the valleys, to the desolate wastes, and to the
cities that are forsaken, which became a
prey and derision to the residue of the
[a]heathen that *are* round about;
5 Therefore thus saith the Lord GOD;
Surely in the fire of my jealousy have I
spoken against the residue of the [a]hea-
then, and against all Idumea, which have
appointed my land into their possession
with the joy of all *their* heart, with
despiteful minds, to cast it out for a prey.
6 Prophesy therefore concerning the
land of Israel, and say unto the mountains, and to the hills, to the rivers, and
to the valleys, Thus saith the Lord GOD;
Behold, I have spoken in my jealousy
and in my fury, because ye have [c]borne
the shame of the [a]heathen:
7 Therefore thus saith the Lord GOD; I
have lifted up mine hand, Surely the
[a]heathen that *are* about you, they shall
bear their shame.
8 But ye, O mountains of Israel, ye
shall shoot forth your branches, and
yield your fruit to my people of Israel;
for they are at hand to come.
9 For, behold, I *am* for you, and I will
turn unto you, and ye shall be tilled and
sown:
10 And I will multiply men upon you,
all the house of Israel, *even* all of it: and
the cities shall be inhabited, and the
wastes shall be builded:
11 And I will multiply upon you man
and beast; and they shall increase and
bring fruit: and I will settle you after
your old estates, and will do better *unto
you* than at your beginnings: and ye
shall know that I *am* the LORD.
12 Yea, I will cause men to walk upon
you, *even* my people Israel; and [d]they
shall possess thee, and thou shalt be
their inheritance, and thou shalt no more
henceforth [e]bereave them *of men.*
13 Thus saith the Lord GOD; Because
they say unto you, Thou *land* devourest
up men, and hast bereaved thy nations;
14 Therefore thou shalt devour men

B.C. 587.

a i.e. *nations.*

b Deut. 28:37; 1 Ki. 9:7; Lam. 2:15; Dan. 9:16.

c v. 15; Ezk. 34:29; Psa. 123:3, 4.

d Oba. 17.

e See Jer. 15:7.

f Lev. 18:25, 27, 28; Jer. 2:7.

g Isa. 52:5; Rom. 2:24.

h *Israel (prophecies).* vs. 22-38; Ezk. 37:21-28. (Gen. 12:2, 3; Rom. 11:26.)

i Ezk. 20:41; 28:22; 38:23.

j Isa. 52:15; Heb. 10:22.

no more, neither bereave thy nations any
more, saith the Lord GOD.
15 Neither will I cause *men* to hear in
thee the shame of the [a]heathen any
more, neither shalt thou bear the
reproach of the people any more, neither
shalt thou cause thy nations to fall any
more, saith the Lord GOD.

The past sins of Israel:
her future restoration and conversion.

16 Moreover the word of the LORD
came unto me, saying,
17 Son of man, when the house of
Israel dwelt in their own land, [f]they
defiled it by their own way and by their
doings: their way was before me as the
uncleanness of a removed woman.
18 Wherefore I poured my fury upon
them for the blood that they had shed
upon the land, and for their idols *wherewith* they had polluted it:
19 And I scattered them among the
[a]heathen, and they were dispersed
through the countries: according to their
way and according to their doings I
judged them.
20 And when they entered unto the
[a]heathen, whither they went, they [g]pro-
faned my holy name, when they said to
them, These *are* the people of the LORD,
and are gone forth out of his land.
21 But I had pity for mine holy name,
which the house of Israel had profaned
among the [a]heathen, whither they went.
22 Therefore say unto the house of
Israel, Thus saith the Lord GOD; I do not
this for your sakes, [h]O house of Israel,
but for mine holy name's sake, which ye
have profaned among the [a]heathen,
whither ye went.
23 And I will sanctify my great name,
which was profaned among the [a]hea-
then, which ye have profaned in the
midst of them; and the [a]heathen shall
know that I *am* the LORD, saith the Lord
GOD, when I shall be [i]sanctified in you
before their eyes.
24 For I will take you from among the
[a]heathen, and gather you out of all
countries, and will bring you into your
own land.
25 [j]Then will I sprinkle clean water
upon you, and ye shall be clean: from all

your filthiness, and from all your idols,
will I cleanse you.
26 [a]A new heart also will I give you,
and a new spirit will I put within you:
and I will take away the stony heart out
of your flesh, and I will give you an
heart of flesh.
27 And I will put my [b]spirit within
you, and cause you to walk in my
statutes, and ye shall keep my judgments, and do *them*.
28 [c]And ye shall dwell in the land that
I gave to your fathers; and [d]ye shall be
my people, and I will be your God.
29 [e]I will also save you from all your
uncleannesses: and I will call for the
corn, and will increase it, and lay no
famine upon you.
30 And I will multiply the fruit of the
tree, and the increase of the field, that ye
shall receive no more reproach of famine
among the [f]heathen.
31 Then shall ye remember your own
evil ways, and your doings that *were* not
good, and [g]shall lothe yourselves in
your own sight for your iniquities and
for your abominations.
32 [h]Not for your sakes do I *this*, saith
the Lord GOD, be it known unto you: be
ashamed and confounded for your own
ways, O house of Israel.
33 Thus saith the Lord GOD; In the day
that I shall have cleansed you from all
your iniquities I will also cause *you* to
dwell in the cities, and the wastes shall
be builded.
34 And the desolate land shall be
tilled, whereas it lay desolate in the sight
of all that passed by.
35 And they shall say, This land that
was desolate is become like the [i]garden
of Eden; and the waste and desolate and
ruined cities *are become* fenced, *and* are
inhabited.
36 Then the [f]heathen that are left
round about you shall know that I the
LORD build the ruined *places, and* plant
that that was desolate: I the LORD have
spoken *it*, and I will do *it*.
37 Thus saith the Lord GOD; [j]I will yet
for this be enquired of by the house of
Israel, to do *it* for them; I will increase
them with men like a flock.
38 As the holy flock, as the flock of
Jerusalem in her solemn feasts; so shall
the waste cities be filled with flocks of
men: and they shall know that I *am* the
LORD.

B.C. 587.

a Ezk. 11:19; Jer. 32:39.

b *Holy Spirit.* Ezk. 37:1, 14. (Gen. 1:2; Mal. 2:15.)

c Ezk. 28:25; 37:25.

d Ezk. 11:20; 37:27; Jer. 30:22.

e Mt. 1:21; Rom. 11:26.

f i.e. *nations.*

g Ezk. 6, 9; 20:43.

h v. 22; Deut. 9:5.

i Ezk. 28:13; Isa. 51:3; Joel 2:3.

j See Ezk. 14:3; 20:3, 31.

PART VI. GENERAL THEME: RESTORATION OF ISRAEL; THE DAVIDIC KINGDOM; JUDGMENT ON THE NATIONS: CHAPTERS 37:1–39:29.

CHAPTER 37.

The vision of the valley of dry bones.

The hand of the LORD was upon me,
and [k]carried me out in the [l]spirit of
the LORD, and set me down in the midst
of the valley which *was* full of [1]bones,
2 And caused me to pass by them
round about: and, behold, *there were* very
many in the open valley; and, lo, *they
were* very dry.
3 And he said unto me, Son of man,
can these bones live? And I answered, O
Lord GOD, thou knowest.
4 Again he said unto me, Prophesy
upon these bones, and say unto them, O
ye dry bones, hear the word of the LORD.
5 Thus saith the Lord GOD unto these
bones; Behold, I will cause breath to
enter into you, and ye shall live:
6 And I will lay sinews upon you, and
will bring up flesh upon you, and cover
you with skin, and put breath in you,

B.C. 587.

k *Parables* (O.T.). vs. 1-14; Ezk. 37:16-22. (Jud. 9:7-15; Zech. 11:7-14.)

l *Holy Spirit.* vs. 1, 14; Ezk. 39:29. (Gen. 1:2; Mal. 2:15.)

[1] **(37:1)** Having announced (Ezk. 36:24-38) the restoration of the nation, Jehovah now gives in vision and symbol the method of its accomplishment. Verse 11 gives the clue." The "bones" are the whole house of Israel who shall then be living. The "graves" are the nations where they dwell. The order of procedure is: (1) the bringing of the people out (v. 12); (2) the bringing of them in (v. 12); (3) their conversion (v. 13); (4) the filling with the Spirit (v. 14). The symbol follows. The two sticks are Judah and the ten tribes; united, they are one nation (vs. 19-21). Then follows (vs. 21-27) the plain declaration as to Jehovah's purpose, and verse 28 implies that then Jehovah will become known to the Gentiles in a marked way. This is also the order of Acts 15:16, 17, and the two passages strongly indicate the time of full Gentile conversion. See also Isa. 11:10.

and ye shall live; and ye shall know that I *am* the LORD.

7 So I prophesied as I was commanded: and as I prophesied, there was a noise, and behold a shaking, and the bones came together, bone to his bone.

8 And when I beheld, lo, the sinews and the flesh came up upon them, and the skin covered them above: but *there was* no breath in them.

9 Then said he unto me, Prophesy unto the wind, prophesy, son of man, and say to the wind, Thus saith the Lord GOD; Come from the four winds, O breath, and breathe upon these slain, that they may live.

10 So I prophesied as he commanded me, and the breath came into them, and they lived, and stood up upon their feet, an exceeding great army.

The vision explained.

11 Then he said unto me, Son of man, these bones are the whole house of Israel: behold, they say, Our bones are dried, and our hope is lost: we are cut off for our parts.

12 Therefore prophesy and say unto them, Thus saith the Lord GOD; Behold, O my people, I will open your graves, and cause you to come up out of your graves, and bring you into the land of Israel.

13 And ye shall know that I *am* the LORD, when I have opened your graves, O my people, and brought you up out of your graves,

14 And shall put my spirit in you, and ye shall live, and I shall place you in your own land: then shall ye know that I the LORD have spoken *it*, and performed *it*, saith the LORD.

The sign of the two sticks.

15 The word of the LORD came again unto me, saying,

16 Moreover, thou son of man, take thee one [a]stick, and write upon it, For Judah, and for the children of Israel his companions: then take another stick, and write upon it, For Joseph, the stick of Ephraim, and *for* all the house of Israel his companions:

17 And join them one to another into one stick; and they shall become one in thine hand.

18 And when the children of thy people shall speak unto thee, saying, Wilt thou not shew us what thou *meanest* by these?

B.C. 587.

a *Parables* (O.T.). vs. 16-22; Zech. 6:9-15. (Jud. 9:7-15; Zech. 11:7-14.)

b *Israel (prophecies)*. vs. 21-28; Ezk. 39:25, 29. (Gen. 12:2, 3; Rom. 11:26.)

c i.e. *nations*.

d *Kingdom* (O.T.). vs. 21-28; Dan. 2:34-45. (Gen. 1:26; Zech. 12:8.)

e Christ *(Second Advent)*. Dan. 7:13, 14. (Deut. 30:3; Acts 1:9-11.)

f Isa. 40:11; Jer. 23:5; 30:9; Ezk. 34:23, 24; Hos. 3:5; Lk. 1:32.

g Isa. 60:21; Joel 3:20; Amos 9:15.

h v. 24; Psa. 89:3-4; John 12:34.

i Ezk. 34:25; Psa. 89:3; Isa. 55:3; Jer. 32:40.

19 Say unto them, Thus saith the Lord GOD; Behold, I will take the stick of Joseph, which *is* in the hand of Ephraim, and the tribes of Israel his fellows, and will put them with him, *even* with the stick of Judah, and make them one stick, and they shall be one in mine hand.

20 And the sticks whereon thou writest shall be in thine hand before their eyes.

21 And say unto them, Thus saith the Lord GOD; Behold, I will take the [b]children of Israel from among the [c]heathen, whither they be gone, and will gather them on every side, and [d]bring them into their own land:

22 And I will make them one nation in the land upon the mountains of Israel; and one [e]king shall be king to them all: and they shall be no more two nations, neither shall they be divided into two kingdoms any more at all:

23 Neither shall they defile themselves any more with their idols, nor with their detestable things, nor with any of their transgressions: but I will save them out of all their dwellingplaces, wherein they have sinned, and will cleanse them: so shall they be my people, and I will be their God.

24 And [f]David my servant *shall be* king over them; and they all shall have one shepherd: they shall also walk in my judgments, and observe my statutes, and do them.

25 And they shall dwell in the land that I have given unto Jacob my servant, wherein your fathers have dwelt; and they shall dwell therein, *even* they, and their children, and their children's children [g]for ever: and [h]my servant David *shall be* their prince for ever.

26 Moreover I will make a [i]covenant of peace with them; it shall be an everlasting covenant with them: and I will place them, and multiply them, and will set my sanctuary in the midst of them for evermore.

27 My tabernacle also shall be with them: yea, I will be their God, and they shall be my people.

28 And the [c]heathen shall know that I the LORD do sanctify Israel, when my sanctuary shall be in the midst of them for evermore.

CHAPTER 38.

The prophecy against Gog.

And the word of the LORD came unto
me, saying,
2 Son of man, set thy face against
[1]Gog, the land of Magog, the chief
prince of Meshech and Tubal, and
prophesy against him,
3 And say, Thus saith the Lord GOD;
Behold, I *am* against thee, O [a]Gog, the
chief prince of Meshech and Tubal:
4 And I will turn thee back, and put
hooks into thy jaws, and I will bring thee
forth, and all thine army, horses and
horsemen, all of them clothed with all
sorts *of armour, even* a great company
with bucklers and shields, all of them
handling swords:
5 Persia, Ethiopia, and Libya with
them; all of them with shield and helmet:
6 Gomer, and all his bands; the house
of Togarmah of the north quarters, and
all his bands: *and* many people with thee.
7 Be thou prepared, and prepare for
thyself, thou, and all thy company that
are assembled unto thee, and be thou a
guard unto them.
8 After many days thou shalt be visited: in the latter years thou shalt come
into the land *that is* brought back from
the sword, *and is* gathered out of many
people, against the mountains of Israel,
which have been always waste: but it is
brought forth out of the nations, and
they shall dwell safely all of them.
9 Thou shalt ascend and come like a
storm, thou shalt be like a cloud to cover
the land, thou, and all thy bands, and
many people with thee.
10 Thus saith the Lord GOD; It shall
also come to pass, *that* at the same time
shall things come into thy mind, and
thou shalt think an evil thought:
11 And thou shalt say, I will go up to
the land of unwalled villages; I will go to
them that are at rest, that dwell safely, all
of them dwelling without walls, and
having neither bars nor gates,
12 To take a spoil, and to take a prey; to
turn thine hand upon the desolate places
that are now inhabited, and upon the people *that are* gathered out of the nations,
which have gotten cattle and goods, that
dwell in the midst of the land.
13 Sheba, and Dedan, and the merchants of Tarshish, with all the young
lions thereof, shall say unto thee, Art
thou come to take a spoil? hast thou
gathered thy company to take a prey? to
carry away silver and gold, to take away
cattle and goods, to take a great spoil?
14 Therefore, son of man, prophesy
and say unto [a]Gog, Thus saith the Lord
GOD; In that day when my people of
Israel dwelleth safely, shalt thou not
know *it*?
15 And thou shalt come from thy
place out of the north parts, thou, and
many people with thee, all of them riding upon horses, a great company, and a
mighty army:
16 And thou shalt come up against my
people of Israel, as a cloud to cover the
land; it shall be in the latter days, and I
will bring thee against my land, that the
[b]heathen may know me, when I shall be
sanctified in thee, O [a]Gog, before their
eyes.
17 Thus saith the Lord GOD; *Art* thou
he of whom I have spoken in old time by
my servants the prophets of Israel, which
prophesied in those days *many* years that
I would bring thee against them?
18 And it shall come to pass at the
same time when [a]Gog shall come against
the land of Israel, saith the Lord GOD, *that*
my fury shall come up in my face.
19 For in my jealousy *and* in the
fire of my wrath have I spoken,

B.C. 587.

a v. 2, note

b i.e. nations.

[1] **(38:2)** That the primary reference is to the northern (European) powers, headed up by Russia, all agree. The whole passage should be read in connection with Zech. 12:1-4; 14:1-9; Mt. 24:14-30; Rev. 14:14-20; 19:17-21. "Gog" is the prince, "Magog," his land. The reference to Meshech and Tubal (Moscow and Tobolsk) is a clear mark of identification. Russia and the northern powers have been the latest persecutors of dispersed Israel, and it is congruous both with divine justice and with the covenants (e.g. Gen. 15:18, *note;* Deut. 30:3, *note*) that destruction should fall at the climax of the last mad attempt to exterminate the remnant of Israel in Jerusalem. The whole prophecy belongs to the yet future "day of Jehovah" (Isa. 2:10-22; Rev. 19:11-21), and to the battle of Armageddon (Rev. 16:14; 19:19, *note*), but includes also the final revolt of the nations at the close of the kingdom-age (Rev. 20:7-9).

[a]Surely in that day there shall be a great shaking in the land of Israel;

20 So that the fishes of the sea, and the fowls of the heaven, and the beasts of the field, and all creeping things that creep upon the earth, and all the men that *are* upon the face of the earth, shall shake at my presence, [b]and the mountains shall be thrown down, and the steep places shall fall, and every wall shall fall to the ground.

21 And I will call for a [c]sword against him throughout all my mountains, saith the Lord GOD: [d]every man's sword shall be against his brother.

22 And I will plead against him with pestilence and with blood; and I will rain upon him, and upon his bands, and upon the many people that *are* with him, an overflowing rain, and great hailstones, fire, and brimstone.

23 Thus will I magnify myself, and sanctify myself; [e]and I will be known in the eyes of many nations, and they shall know that I *am* the LORD.

CHAPTER 39.

(*The prophecy against Gog,* continued.)

Therefore, thou son of man, prophesy against [f]Gog, and say, Thus saith the Lord GOD; Behold, I *am* against thee, O Gog, the chief prince of Meshech and Tubal:

2 And I will turn thee back, and leave but the sixth part of thee, and will cause thee to come up from the north parts, and will bring thee upon the mountains of Israel:

3 And I will smite thy bow out of thy left hand, and will cause thine arrows to fall out of thy right hand.

4 Thou shalt fall upon the mountains of Israel, thou, and all thy bands, and the people that *is* with thee: I will give thee unto the ravenous birds of every sort, and *to* the beasts of the field to be devoured.

5 Thou shalt fall upon the open field: for I have spoken *it*, saith the Lord GOD.

6 And [g]I will send a fire on Magog, and among them that dwell carelessly in the [h]isles: and they shall know that I *am* the LORD.

7 So will I make my holy name known in the midst of my people Israel; and I will not *let them* pollute my holy name any more: and the [i]heathen shall know that I *am* the LORD, the Holy One in Israel.

B.C. 587.

a Hag. 2:6, 7; Rev. 16:18.

b Jer. 4:24; Nah. 1:5, 6

c *Armageddon (battle of).* vs. 1-23; and Ezk. 39:1-16; Joel 2:1-11. (Rev. 16:14; 19:11-21.)

d Jud. 7:22; 1 Sam. 14:20.

e v. 16; Ezk. 37:28; 39:7; Psa. 9:16.

f Ezk. 38:2, *note.*

g Ezk. 38:22; Amos 1:4.

h i.e. *coasts.*

i i.e. *nations.*

j Rev. 16:17; 21:6.

k Isa. 14:2.

l i.e. *The multitude.*

m *Armageddon,* Rev. 19:17.

n Zeph. 1:7.

8 [j]Behold, it is come, and it is done, saith the Lord GOD; [c]this *is* the day whereof I have spoken.

9 And they that dwell in the cities of Israel shall go forth, and shall set on fire and burn the weapons, both the shields and the bucklers, the bows and the arrows, and the handstaves, and the spears, and they shall burn them with fire seven years:

10 So that they shall take no wood out of the field, neither cut down *any* out of the forests; for they shall burn the weapons with fire: [k]and they shall spoil those that spoiled them, and rob those that robbed them, saith the Lord GOD.

11 And it shall come to pass in that day, *that* I will give unto Gog a place there of graves in Israel, the valley of the passengers on the east of the sea: and it shall stop the *noses* of the passengers: and there shall they bury Gog and all his multitude: and they shall call *it* The valley of Hamon-gog.

12 And seven months shall the house of Israel be burying of them, that they may cleanse the land.

13 Yea, all the people of the land shall bury *them*; and it shall be to them a renown the day that I shall be glorified, saith the Lord GOD.

14 And they shall sever out men of continual employment, passing through the land to bury with the passengers those that remain upon the face of the earth, to cleanse it: after the end of seven months shall they search.

15 And the passengers *that* pass through the land, when *any* seeth a man's bone, then shall he set up a sign by it, till the buriers have buried it in the valley of Hamon-gog.

16 And also the name of the city *shall be* [l]Hamonah. Thus shall they cleanse the land.

17 And, thou son of man, thus saith the Lord GOD; [m]Speak unto every feathered fowl, and to every beast of the field, [n]Assemble yourselves, and come; gather yourselves on every side to my sacrifice that I do sacrifice for you, *even* a great sacrifice upon the mountains of Israel, that ye may eat flesh, and drink blood.

18 Ye shall eat the flesh of the mighty, and drink the blood of the princes of the

earth, of rams, of lambs, and of goats, of
bullocks, all of them [a]fatlings of Bashan.
19 And ye shall eat fat till ye be full, and
drink blood till ye be drunken, of my sacrifice which I have sacrificed for you.
20 Thus ye shall be filled at my table
with horses and chariots, with mighty
men, and with all men of war, saith the
Lord GOD.
21 [b]And I will set my glory among the
[c]heathen, and all the heathen shall see
my judgment that I have executed, and
my hand that I have laid upon them.
22 So the house of Israel shall know
that I *am* the LORD their God from that
day and forward.
23 And the [c]heathen [d]shall know that
the house of Israel went into captivity for
their iniquity: because they trespassed
against me, therefore [e]hid I my face from
them, and gave them into the hand of
their enemies: so fell they all by the sword.
24 According to their uncleanness and
according to their transgressions have I
done unto them, and hid my face from
them.

Vision of restored and converted Israel.

25 Therefore thus saith the Lord GOD;
[f]Now will I bring again the captivity of
Jacob, and have mercy upon [g]the whole
house of Israel, and will be jealous for
my holy name;
26 After that they have borne their
shame, and all their trespasses whereby
they have trespassed against me, when
they dwelt safely in their land, and none
made *them* afraid.
27 [h]When I have brought them again
from the people, and gathered them out
of their enemies' lands, and am sanctified
in them in the sight of many nations;
28 [i]Then shall they know that I *am* the
LORD their God, which caused them to
be led into captivity among the [c]hea-
then: but I have gathered them unto
their own land, and have left none of
them any more there.
29 Neither will I hide my face any
more from them: for I have poured out
my [j]spirit upon the house of Israel, saith
the Lord GOD.

B.C. 587.

a Deut. 32:14; Psa. 22:12.
b Ezk. 38:16, 23.
c i.e. *nations*.
d Ezk. 36:18-20, 23.
e Deut. 31:17; Isa. 59:2.
f *Israel (prophecies)*. Hos. 3:4, 5. (Gen. 12:2, 3; Rom. 11:26.)
g Ezk. 20:40; Hos. 1:11.
h Ezk. 28:25, 26.
i Ezk. 34:30; v. 22.
j *Holy Spirit*. Ezk. 43:5. (Gen. 1:2; Mal. 2:15.)

PART VII. GENERAL THEME: ISRAEL IN THE LAND DURING THE KINGDOM-AGE: CHAPTERS 40:1–48:35.

CHAPTER 40.

Vision of the man with the measuring reed.

In the five and twentieth year of our
captivity, in the beginning of the year,
in the tenth *day* of the month, in the fourteenth year after that the city was smitten,
in the selfsame day the hand of the LORD
was upon me, and brought me thither.
2 In the visions of God brought he me
into the land of Israel, and set me upon a
very high mountain, by which *was* as the
frame of a city on the south.
3 And he brought me thither, and,
behold, *there was* a [k]man, whose appearance *was* like the appearance of brass,
with a line of flax in his hand, and a measuring [l]reed; and he stood in the gate.
4 And the man said unto me, Son of
man, behold with thine eyes, and hear
with thine ears, and set thine heart upon
all that I shall shew thee; for to the intent
that I might shew *them* unto thee *art*
thou brought hither: declare all that thou
seest to the house of Israel.

Vision of the future temple.

5 And behold a wall on the outside of
the house round about, and in the man's
hand a measuring reed of six [m]cubits
long by the cubit and an hand breadth:
so he measured the breadth of the building, one reed; and the height, one reed.
6 Then came he unto the gate which
looketh toward the east, and went up
the stairs thereof, and measured the
threshold of the gate, *which was* one reed
broad; and the other threshold *of the gate,*
which was one reed broad.
7 And *every* little chamber *was* one reed
long, and one reed broad; and between
the little chambers *were* five cubits; and
the threshold of the gate by the porch of
the gate within *was* one reed.
8 He measured also the porch of the
gate within, one reed.
9 Then measured he the porch of the
gate, eight cubits; and the posts thereof,
two cubits; and the porch of the gate *was*
inward.

B.C. 574.

k *The theophanies*. Dan. 8:15. (Gen. 12:7; Rev. 1:9.)
l One reed = about 10 ft.; also vs. 5-8.
m One cubit = about 18 in.

10 And the little chambers of the gate eastward *were* three on this side, and three on that side; they three *were* of one measure: and the posts had one measure on this side and on that side.

11 And he measured the breadth of the entry of the gate, ten cubits; *and* the length of the gate, thirteen cubits.

12 The space also before the little chambers *was* one cubit *on this side*, and the space *was* one cubit on that side: and the little chambers *were* six cubits on this side, and six cubits on that side.

13 He measured then the gate from the roof of *one* little chamber to the roof of another: the breadth *was* five and twenty cubits, door against door.

14 He made also posts of threescore cubits, even unto the post of the court round about the gate.

15 And from the face of the gate of the entrance unto the face of the porch of the inner gate *were* fifty cubits.

16 And *there were* [a]narrow windows to the little chambers, and to their posts within the gate round about, and likewise to the arches: and windows *were* round about inward: and upon *each* post *were* palm trees.

17 Then brought he me into the [b]outward court, and, lo, *there were* [c]chambers, and a pavement made for the court round about: [d]thirty chambers *were* upon the pavement.

18 And the pavement by the side of the gates over against the length of the gates *was* the lower pavement.

19 Then he measured the breadth from the forefront of the lower gate unto the forefront of the inner court without, an hundred cubits eastward and northward.

20 And the gate of the outward court that looked toward the north, he measured the length thereof, and the breadth thereof.

21 And the little chambers thereof *were* three on this side and three on that side; and the posts thereof and the arches thereof were after the measure of the first gate: the length thereof *was* fifty cubits, and the breadth five and twenty cubits.

22 And their windows, and their arches, and their palm trees, *were* after the measure of the gate that looketh toward the east; and they went up unto it by seven steps; and the arches thereof *were* before them.

B.C. 574.

a 1 Ki. 6:4.

b Ezk. 42:1; Rev. 11:2.

c 1 Ki. 6:5.

d Ezk. 45:5.

e See vs. 21, 25, 33, 36.

23 And the gate of the inner court *was* over against the gate toward the north, and toward the east; and he measured from gate to gate an hundred cubits.

24 After that he brought me toward the south, and behold a gate toward the south: and he measured the posts thereof and the arches thereof according to these measures.

25 And *there were* windows in it and in the arches thereof round about, like those windows: the length *was* fifty cubits, and the breadth five and twenty cubits.

26 And *there were* seven steps to go up to it, and the arches thereof *were* before them: and it had palm trees, one on this side, and another on that side, upon the posts thereof.

27 And *there was* a gate in the inner court toward the south: and he measured from gate to gate toward the south an hundred cubits.

28 And he brought me to the inner court by the south gate: and he measured the south gate according to these measures;

29 And the little chambers thereof, and the posts thereof, and the arches thereof, according to these measures: and *there were* windows in it and in the arches thereof round about: *it was* fifty cubits long, and [e]five and twenty cubits broad.

30 And the arches round about *were* five and twenty cubits long, and five cubits broad.

31 And the arches thereof *were* toward the utter court; and palm trees *were* upon the posts thereof: and the going up to it *had* eight steps.

32 And he brought me into the inner court toward the east: and he measured the gate according to these measures.

33 And the little chambers thereof, and the posts thereof, and the arches thereof, *were* according to these measures: and *there were* windows therein and in the arches thereof round about: *it was* fifty cubits long, and five and twenty cubits broad.

34 And the arches thereof *were* toward the outward court; and palm trees *were* upon the posts thereof, on this side, and on that side: and the going up to it *had* eight steps.

35 And he brought me to the north

B.C. 574.

gate, and measured *it* according to these measures;

36 The little chambers thereof, the posts thereof, and the arches thereof, and the windows to it round about: the length *was* fifty cubits, and the breadth five and twenty cubits.

37 And the posts thereof *were* toward the utter court; and palm trees *were* upon the posts thereof, on this side, and on that side: and the going up to it *had* eight steps.

38 And the chambers and the entries thereof *were* by the posts of the gates, where they washed the burnt-offering.

39 And in the porch of the gate *were* two tables on this side, and two tables on that side, to slay thereon the burnt-offering and the [a]sin-offering and the [b]trespass-offering.

40 And at the side without, [c]as one goeth up to the entry of the north gate, *were* two tables; and on the other side, which *was* at the porch of the gate, *were* two tables.

41 Four tables *were* on this side, and four tables on that side, by the side of the gate; eight tables, whereupon they slew *their sacrifices*.

42 And the four tables *were* of hewn stone for the burnt-offering, of a cubit and an half long, and a cubit and an half broad, and one cubit high: whereupon also they laid the instruments wherewith they slew the burnt-offering and the sacrifice.

43 And within *were* [d]hooks, an hand broad, fastened round about: and upon the tables *was* the flesh of the offering.

The chambers of the singers and priests.

44 And without the inner gate *were* the chambers of the singers in the inner court, which *was* at the side of the north gate; and their prospect *was* toward the south: one at the side of the east gate *having* the prospect toward the north.

45 And he said unto me, This chamber, whose prospect *is* toward the south, *is* for the priests, the [e]keepers of the charge of the house.

46 And the chamber whose prospect *is* toward the north *is* for the priests, the keepers of the charge of the altar: these *are* the sons of [f]Zadok among the sons of Levi, which come near to the LORD to minister unto him.

47 So he measured the court, an hundred cubits long, and an hundred cubits broad, foursquare; and the altar *that was* before the house.

The porch of the temple.

48 And he brought me to the porch of the house, and measured *each* post of the porch, five cubits on this side, and five cubits on that side: and the breadth of the gate *was* three cubits on this side, and three cubits on that side.

49 The length of the porch *was* twenty cubits, and the breadth eleven cubits; and *he brought me* by the steps whereby they went up to it: and *there were* pillars by the posts, one on this side, and another on that side.

CHAPTER 41.

Description of the temple.

Afterward he brought me to the temple, and measured the posts, six cubits broad on the one side, and six cubits broad on the other side, *which was* the breadth of the tabernacle.

2 And the breadth of the door *was* ten cubits; and the sides of the door *were* five cubits on the one side, and five cubits on the other side: and he measured the length thereof, forty cubits: and the breadth, twenty cubits.

3 Then went he inward, and measured the post of the door, two cubits; and the door, six cubits; and the breadth of the door, seven cubits.

4 So [g]he measured the length thereof, twenty cubits; and the breadth, twenty cubits, before the temple: and he said unto me, This *is* the most holy *place*.

5 After he measured the wall of the house, six [h]cubits; and the breadth of *every* side chamber, four cubits, round about the house on every side.

6 And the side chambers *were* three, one over another, and thirty in order; and they entered into the wall which *was* of the house for the side chambers round about, that they might have hold, but they had not hold in the wall of the house.

7 And [i]*there was* an enlarging, and a winding about still upward to the side chambers: for the winding about of the house went still upward round about the house: therefore the breadth of the house

a Lev. 4:2, 3.

b Lev. 5:6; 6:6; 7:1.

c Or, *at the step.*

d Or, *endirons*, or, the two hearth-stones.

e Lev. 8:35; Num. 3:27, 28, 32, 38; 18:5 ; 1 Chr. 9:23; 2 Chr. 13:11; Psa. 134:1.

f Ezk. 43:19; 44:15, 16; 1 Ki. 2:35.

g 1 Ki. 6:20; 2 Chr. 3:8.

h One cubit = about 18 in.

i 1 Ki. 6:8.

was still upward, and so increased *from* the lowest *chamber* to the highest by the midst.

8 I saw also the height of the house round about: the foundations of the side chambers *were* a full [a]reed of six great cubits.

9 The thickness of the wall, which *was* for the side chamber without, *was* five cubits: and *that* which *was* left *was* the place of the side chambers that *were* within.

10 And between the chambers *was* the wideness of twenty cubits round about the house on every side.

11 And the doors of the side chambers *were* toward *the place that was* left, one door toward the north, and another door toward the south: and the breadth of the place that was left *was* five cubits round about.

12 Now the building that *was* before the separate place at the end toward the west *was* seventy cubits broad; and the wall of the building *was* five cubits thick round about, and the length thereof ninety cubits.

13 So he measured the house, an hundred cubits long; and the separate place, and the building, with the walls thereof, an hundred cubits long;

14 Also the breadth of the face of the house, and of the separate place toward the east, an hundred cubits.

15 And he measured the length of the building over against the separate place which *was* behind it, and the galleries thereof on the one side and on the other side, an hundred cubits, with the inner temple, and the porches of the court;

16 The door posts, and the narrow windows, and the galleries round about on their three stories, over against the door, cieled with wood round about, and from the ground up to the windows, and the windows *were* covered;

17 To that above the door, even unto the inner house, and without, and by all the wall round about within and without, by measure.

18 And *it was* made [b]with cherubims and palm trees, so that a palm tree *was* between a cherub and a cherub; and *every* cherub had two faces;

19 So that the face of a man *was* toward the palm tree on the one side, and the face of a young lion toward the palm tree on the other side: *it was* made through all the house round about.

20 From the ground unto above the door *were* cherubims and palm trees made, and *on* the wall of the temple.

21 The posts of the temple *were* squared, *and* the face of the sanctuary; the appearance *of the one* as the appearance *of the other*.

22 [c]The altar of wood *was* three cubits high, and the length thereof two cubits; and the corners thereof, and the length thereof, and the walls thereof, *were* of wood: and he said unto me, This *is* the table that *is* before the LORD.

23 [d]And the temple and the sanctuary had two doors.

24 And the doors had two leaves apiece, two turning leaves; two *leaves* for the one door, and two leaves for the other *door*.

25 And *there were* made on them, on the doors of the temple, cherubims and palm trees, like as *were* made upon the walls; and *there were* thick planks upon the face of the porch without.

26 And *there were* narrow windows and palm trees on the one side and on the other side, on the sides of the porch, and *upon* the side chambers of the house, and thick planks.

CHAPTER 42.

(*Description of the temple,* continued.)

Then he brought me forth into the utter court, the way toward the north: and he brought me into the [e]chamber that *was* over against the separate place, and which *was* before the building toward the north.

2 Before the length of an hundred [f]cubits *was* the north door, and the breadth *was* fifty cubits.

3 Over against the twenty *cubits* which *were* for the inner court, and over against the pavement which *was* for the utter court, *was* gallery against gallery in three *stories*.

4 And before the chambers *was* a walk of ten cubits breadth inward, a way of one cubit; and their doors toward the north.

5 Now the upper chambers *were* shorter: for the galleries were higher than these, than the lower, and than the middlemost of the building.

6 For they *were* in three *stories*, but had

B.C. 574.

a One reed = about 10 ft.

b 1 Ki. 6:29.

c Ex. 30:1; 1 Ki. 6:20.

d 1 Ki. 6:31-35.

e Ezk. 41:12, 15.

f One cubit = about 18 in. also vs. 4, 7, 8.

not pillars as the pillars of the courts:
therefore *the building* was straitened
more than the lowest and the middlemost from the ground.
7 And the wall that *was* without over
against the chambers, toward the utter
court on the forepart of the chambers,
the length thereof *was* fifty cubits.
8 For the length of the chambers that
were in the utter court *was* fifty cubits:
and, lo, before the temple *were* an hundred cubits.
9 And from under these chambers *was*
the entry on the east side, as one goeth
into them from the utter court.
10 The chambers *were* in the thickness
of the wall of the court toward the east,
over against the separate place, and over
against the building.
11 And the way before them *was* like
the appearance of the chambers which
were toward the north, as long as they,
and as broad as they: and all their goings
out *were* both according to their fashions,
and according to their doors.
12 And according to the doors of the
chambers that *were* toward the south *was*
a door in the head of the way, *even* the
way directly before the wall toward the
east, as one entereth into them.
13 Then said he unto me, The north
chambers *and* the south chambers,
which *are* before the separate place, they
be holy chambers, where the priests that
approach unto the LORD [a]shall eat the
most holy things: there shall they lay the
most holy things, and the [b]meat-offer-
ing, and the sin-offering, and the trespass-offering; for the place *is* holy.
14 When the priests enter therein, then
shall they not go out of the holy *place*
into the utter court, but there they shall
lay their garments wherein they minister; for they *are* holy; and shall put on
other garments, and shall approach to
those things which *are* for the people.
15 Now when he had made an end of
measuring the inner house, he brought
me forth toward the gate whose
prospect *is* toward the east, and measured it round about.
16 He measured the east side with the
measuring [c]reed, five hundred reeds,
with the measuring reed round about.
17 He measured the north side, five
hundred reeds, with the measuring reed
round about.

B.C. 574.

a Lev. 6:16, 26; 24:9.

b Lit. *meal.* Lev. 2:3, 10; 6:14,17, 25, 29; 7:1; 10:13, 14; Num. 18:9, 10.

c A reed = about 10 ft.; also vs. 17-19.

d Ezk. 11:23.

e Ezk. 1:24; Rev. 1:15; 14:2; 19:1, 6.

f Ezk. 10:4; Rev. 18:1.

g Ezk. 11:23.

h *Holy Spirit.* Joel 2:28, 29. (Gen. 1:2; Mal. 2:15.)

i Ezk. 44:4; 1 Ki. 8:10, 11.

j See *Kingdom* (O.T.). Gen. 1:26-28; Zech. 12:8. (N.T.) Lk. 1:31-33; 1 Cor. 15:28.

18 He measured the south side, five
hundred reeds, with the measuring reed.
19 He turned about to the west side,
and measured five hundred reeds with
the measuring reed.
20 He measured it by the four sides: it
had a wall round about, five hundred
reeds long, and five hundred broad, to
make a separation between the sanctuary and the profane place.

CHAPTER 43.

(*Description of the temple,* continued.)

Afterward he brought me to the gate,
even the gate that looketh toward
the east:

Vision of the glory of the Lord filling the temple.

2 [d]And, behold, the glory of the God of
Israel came from the way of the east: and
[e]his voice *was* like a noise of many waters:
[f]and the earth shined with his glory.
3 And *it was* according to the appearance of the vision which I saw, *even*
according to the vision that I saw when I
came to destroy the city: and the visions
were like the vision that I saw by the
river Chebar; and I fell upon my face.
4 [g]And the glory of the LORD came
into the house by the way of the gate
whose prospect *is* toward the east.
5 So the [h]spirit took me up, and
brought me into the inner court; and,
behold, [i]the glory of the LORD filled the
house.
6 And I heard *him* speaking unto me
out of the house; and the man stood by
me.

The place of the throne of the future kingdom.

7 And he said unto me, Son of man,
the [j]place of my throne, and the place of
the soles of my feet, where I will dwell
in the midst of the children of Israel for
ever, and my holy name, shall the house
of Israel no more defile, *neither* they, nor
their kings, by their whoredom, nor by
the carcases of their kings in their high
places.
8 In their setting of their threshold by
my thresholds, and their post by my
posts, and the wall between me and
them, they have even defiled my holy

name by their abominations that they have committed: wherefore I have consumed them in mine anger.

9 Now let them put away their whoredom, and the carcases of their kings, far from me, and I will dwell in the midst of them for ever.

10 Thou son of man, shew the house to the house of Israel, that they may be ashamed of their iniquities: and let them measure the pattern.

11 And if they be ashamed of all that they have done, shew them the form of the house, and the fashion thereof, and the goings out thereof, and the comings in thereof, and all the forms thereof, and all the ordinances thereof, and all the forms thereof, and all the laws thereof: and write *it* in their sight, that they may keep the whole form thereof, and all the ordinances thereof, and do them.

12 This *is* the law of the house; Upon the top of the mountain the whole limit thereof round about *shall be* most holy. Behold, this *is* the law of the house.

The measure of the altar.

13 And these *are* the measures of the altar after the [a]cubits: The cubit *is* a cubit and an hand breadth; even the bottom *shall be* a cubit, and the breadth a cubit, and the border thereof by the edge thereof round about *shall be* a [b]span: and this *shall be* the higher place of the altar.

14 And from the bottom *upon* the ground *even* to the lower settle *shall be* two cubits, and the breadth one cubit; and from the lesser settle *even* to the greater settle *shall be* four cubits, and the breadth *one* cubit.

15 So the altar *shall be* four cubits; and from the altar and upward *shall be* four horns.

16 And the altar *shall be* twelve *cubits* long, twelve broad, square in the four squares thereof.

17 And the settle *shall be* fourteen *cubits* long and fourteen broad in the four squares thereof; and the border about it *shall be* half a cubit; and the bottom thereof *shall be* a cubit about; and his stairs shall look toward the east.

B.C. 574.

a One cubit = 18 in.; also vs. 14-17.

b One span = about 9 in.

c Lev. 1:5.

d Ezk. 44:15.

e Ezk. 45:18, 19; Ex. 29:10-12; Lev. 8:14, 15.

f Ex. 29:14.

g Heb. 13:11.

h Lev. 2:13.

i Ex. 29:35, 36; Lev. 8:33.

j Lev. 9:1.

18 And he said unto me, Son of man, thus saith the Lord GOD; These *are* the ordinances of the altar in the day when they shall make it, to offer burnt-offerings thereon, and to [c]sprinkle blood thereon.

The offerings.

19 [1]And thou shalt give to the [d]priests the Levites that be of the seed of Zadok, which approach unto me, to minister unto me, saith the Lord GOD, a [e]young bullock for a sin-offering.

20 And thou shalt take of the blood thereof, and put *it* on the four horns of it, and on the four corners of the settle, and upon the border round about: thus shalt thou cleanse and purge it.

21 Thou shalt take the bullock also of the sin-offering, and he [f]shall burn it in the appointed place of the house, [g]without the sanctuary.

22 And on the second day thou shalt offer a kid of the goats without blemish for a sin-offering; and they shall cleanse the altar, as they did cleanse *it* with the bullock.

23 When thou hast made an end of cleansing *it*, thou shalt offer a young bullock without blemish, and a ram out of the flock without blemish.

24 And thou shalt offer them before the LORD, [h]and the priests shall cast salt upon them, and they shall offer them up *for* a burnt-offering unto the LORD.

25 [i]Seven days shalt thou prepare every day a goat *for* a sin-offering: they shall also prepare a young bullock, and a ram out of the flock, without blemish.

26 Seven days shall they purge the altar and purify it; and they shall consecrate themselves.

27 [j]And when these days are expired, it shall be, *that* upon the eighth day, and *so* forward, the priests shall make your burnt-offerings upon the altar, and your peace-offerings; and I will accept you, saith the Lord GOD.

CHAPTER 44.

The gate for the prince.

Then he brought me back the way of the gate of the outward sanctuary

[1] **(43:19)** Doubtless these offerings will be memorial, looking back to the cross, as the offerings under the old covenant were anticipatory, looking forward to the cross. In neither case have animal sacrifices power to put away sin (Heb. 10:4; Rom. 3:25).

which looketh toward the east; and it
was shut.
2 Then said the LORD unto me; This
gate shall be shut, it shall not be opened,
and no man shall enter in by it; because
the LORD, the God of Israel, hath entered
in by it, therefore it shall be shut.
3 *It is* for the prince; the prince, he
shall sit in it to [a]eat bread before the
LORD; [b]he shall enter by the way of the
porch of *that* gate, and shall go out by
the way of the same.

The glory fills the house.

4 Then brought he me the way of the
north gate before the house: and I
looked, and, behold, [c]the glory of the
LORD filled the house of the LORD: and I
fell upon my face.
5 And the LORD said unto me, Son of
man, mark well, and behold with thine
eyes, and hear with thine ears all that I
say unto thee concerning all the ordinances of the house of the LORD, and all
the laws thereof; and mark well the
entering in of the house, with every
going forth of the sanctuary.
6 And thou shalt say to the rebellious,
even to the house of Israel, Thus saith the
Lord GOD; O ye house of Israel, [d]let it
suffice you of all your abominations,
7 In that [e]ye have brought *into my sanctuary* strangers, uncircumcised in heart,
and uncircumcised in flesh, to be in my
sanctuary, to pollute it, *even* my house,
when ye offer my bread, the fat and the
blood, and they have broken my covenant
because of all your abominations.
8 And ye have not kept the charge of
mine holy things: but ye have set keepers of my charge in my sanctuary for
yourselves.

The priests of the future temple.

9 Thus saith the Lord GOD; No
stranger, uncircumcised in heart, nor
uncircumcised in flesh, shall enter into
my sanctuary, of any stranger that *is*
among the children of Israel.
10 [f]And the Levites that are gone
away far from me, when Israel went
astray, which went astray away from me
after their idols; they shall even bear
their iniquity.
11 Yet they shall be ministers in my
sanctuary, *having* charge at the gates of
the house, and ministering to the house:
they shall slay the burnt-offering and the
sacrifice for the people, and they shall
stand before them to minister unto them.
12 Because they ministered unto them
before their idols, and caused the house
of Israel to fall into iniquity; therefore
have I [g]lifted up mine hand against
them, saith the Lord GOD, and they shall
bear their iniquity.
13 [h]And they shall not come near unto
me, to do the office of a priest unto me,
nor to come near to any of my holy
things, in the most holy *place*: but they
shall bear their shame, and their abominations which they have committed.
14 But I will make them [i]keepers of
the charge of the house, for all the service thereof, and for all that shall be
done therein.
15 But the priests the Levites, the [j]sons
of Zadok, that kept the charge of my
sanctuary when the children of Israel
went astray from me, they shall come
near to me to minister unto me, and they
[k]shall stand before me to offer unto me
the fat and the blood, saith the Lord GOD:
16 They shall enter into my sanctuary,
and they shall come near to my table, to
minister unto me, and they shall keep
my charge.
17 And it shall come to pass, *that*
when they enter in at the gates of the
inner court, [l]they shall be clothed with
linen garments; and no wool shall come
upon them, whiles they minister in the
gates of the inner court, and within.
18 [m]They shall have linen bonnets
upon their heads, and shall have linen
breeches upon their loins; they shall not
gird *themselves* with any thing that
causeth sweat.
19 And when they go forth into the
utter court, *even* into the utter court to the
people, they shall put off their garments
wherein they ministered, and lay them in
the holy chambers, and they shall put on
other garments; and they shall [n]not sanctify the people with their garments.
20 Neither shall they shave their
heads, nor suffer their locks to grow
long; they shall only poll their heads.
21 Neither shall any priest drink wine,
when they enter into the inner court.
22 Neither shall they take for their
wives a [o]widow, nor her that is put
away: but they shall take maidens of the
seed of the house of Israel, or a widow
that had a priest before.

B.C. 574.

a Gen. 31:54; 1 Cor. 10:18.
b Ezk. 46:2, 8.
c Ezk. 3:23; 43:5.
d Ezk. 45:9; 1 Pet. 4:3.
e v. 9; Ezk. 43:8; Acts 21:28.
f See 2 Ki. 23:8; 2 Chr. 29:4, 5.
g Psa. 106:26.
h Num. 18:3; 2 Ki. 23:9.
i Num. 18:4; 1 Chr. 23:28, 32.
j 1 Sam. 2:35; 2 Sam. 8:17; 15:24-29; 20:25.
k Deut. 10:8.
l Ex. 28:39, 40, 43; 39:27, 28.
m Ex. 28:40, 42; 39:28.
n Ezk. 46:20; Lev. 6:27; Mt. 23:17, 19.
o Lev. 21:7, 13, 14.

B.C. 574.

23 And they shall [a]teach my people *the difference* between the holy and profane, and cause them to discern between the unclean and the clean.

24 And in [b]controversy they shall stand in judgment; *and* they shall judge it according to my judgments: and they shall keep my laws and my statutes in all mine assemblies; and they shall hallow my sabbaths.

25 And they shall come at no dead person to defile themselves: but for father, or for mother, or for son, or for daughter, for brother, or for sister that hath had no husband, they may defile themselves.

26 And after he is cleansed, they shall reckon unto him seven days.

27 And in the day that he goeth into the sanctuary, unto the inner court, to minister in the sanctuary, he shall offer his sin-offering, saith the Lord GOD.

28 And it shall be unto them for an inheritance: [c]I *am* their inheritance: and ye shall give them no possession in Israel: I *am* their possession.

29 They shall eat the [d]meat-offering, and the sin-offering, and the trespass-offering; and every dedicated thing in Israel shall be theirs.

30 [e]And the first of all the firstfruits of all *things*, and every oblation of all, of every *sort* of your oblations, shall be the priest's: ye shall also give unto the priest the first of your dough, that he may cause the blessing to rest in thine house.

31 The priests shall not eat of any thing that is dead of itself, or torn, whether it be fowl or beast.

CHAPTER 45.

The Lord's portion of the land.

Moreover, when ye shall divide by lot the land for inheritance, ye shall offer an oblation unto the LORD, an holy portion of the land: the length *shall be* the length of five and twenty thousand *reeds*, and the breadth *shall be* ten thousand. This *shall be* holy in all the borders thereof round about.

2 Of this there shall be for the sanctuary five hundred *in length*, with five hundred *in breadth*, square round about; and fifty [f]cubits round about for the suburbs thereof.

3 And of this measure shalt thou measure the length of five and twenty thousand, and the breadth of ten thousand: and in it shall be the sanctuary *and* the most holy *place*.

4 The holy *portion* of the land shall be for the priests the ministers of the sanctuary, which shall come near to minister unto the LORD: and it shall be a place for their houses, and an holy place for the sanctuary.

5 And the five and twenty thousand of length, and the ten thousand of breadth, shall also the Levites, the ministers of the house, have for themselves, for a possession for twenty chambers.

6 And ye shall appoint the possession of the city five thousand broad, and five and twenty thousand long, over against the oblation of the holy *portion*: it shall be for the whole house of Israel.

The portion for the prince.

7 And a *portion shall be* for the prince on the one side and on the other side of the oblation of the holy *portion*, and of the possession of the city, before the oblation of the holy *portion*, and before the possession of the city, from the west side westward, and from the east side eastward: and the length *shall be* over against one of the portions, from the west border unto the east border.

8 In the land shall be his possession in Israel: and my princes shall no more oppress my people; and *the rest of* the land shall they give to the house of Israel according to their tribes.

9 Thus saith the Lord GOD; Let it suffice you, O princes of Israel: remove violence and spoil, and execute judgment and justice, take away your exactions from my people, saith the Lord GOD.

10 Ye shall have just balances, and a just [g]ephah, and a just [h]bath.

11 The ephah and the bath shall be of one measure, that the bath may contain the tenth part of an [i]homer, and the ephah the tenth part of an homer: the measure thereof shall be after the homer.

12 And the [j]shekel *shall be* twenty [k]gerahs: twenty shekels, five and twenty shekels, fifteen shekels, shall be your [l]maneh.

13 This *is* the oblation that ye shall offer; the sixth part of an ephah of an homer of wheat, and ye shall give the

a Ezk. 22:26; Lev. 10:10, 11; Mal. 2:7.

b Deut. 17;8; 2 Chr. 19:8-10.

c Num. 18:20; Deut. 10:9; 18, 1, 2; Josh. 13:14, 33.

d Lit. *meal.*

e Ex. 13:2; Num. 3:13.

f One cubit = about 18 in.

g One ephah = 1 bu. 3 pts.; also vs. 10, 11, 13, 24.

h One bath = about 8 gals.; also vs. 11, 14.

i One homer = about 86 gals.; also vs. 11, 14.

j One shekel = 2*s.* 9*d.*, or 65 cts.

k One gerah = 11.2 grains.

l One maneh = one sixtieth of a talent.

sixth part of an ephah of an homer of barley:

14 Concerning the ordinance of oil, the bath of oil, *ye shall offer* the tenth part of a bath out of the [a]cor, *which is* an homer of ten baths; for ten baths *are* an homer:

15 And one lamb out of the flock, out of two hundred, out of the fat pastures of Israel; for a [b]meat-offering, and for a burnt-offering, and for peace-offerings, to make [c]reconciliation for them, saith the Lord GOD.

16 All the people of the land shall give this oblation for the prince in Israel.

17 And it shall be the prince's part *to give* burnt-offerings, and meat-offerings, and drink-offerings, in the feasts, and in the new moons, and in the sabbaths, in all solemnities of the house of Israel: he shall prepare the sin-offering, and the meat-offering, and the burnt-offering, and the peace-offerings, to make [c]reconciliation for the house of Israel.

18 Thus saith the Lord GOD; In the [d]first *month*, in the first *day* of the month, thou shalt take a young bullock without blemish, and cleanse the sanctuary:

19 And the priest shall take of the blood of the sin-offering, and put *it* upon the posts of the house, and upon the four corners of the settle of the altar, and upon the posts of the gate of the inner court.

20 And so thou shalt do the seventh *day* of the month for every one that erreth, and for *him that is* simple: so shall ye [c]reconcile the house.

21 [e]In the first *month*, in the fourteenth day of the month, ye shall have the passover, a feast of seven days; unleavened bread shall be eaten.

22 And upon that day shall the prince prepare for himself and for all the people of the land a [f]bullock *for* a sin-offering.

23 And seven days of the feast he shall prepare a burnt-offering to the LORD, seven bullocks and seven rams without blemish daily the seven days; and a kid of the goats daily *for* a sin-offering.

24 And he shall prepare a [b]meat-offering of an [g]ephah for a bullock, and an ephah for a ram, and an [h]hin of oil for an ephah.

25 In the [i]seventh *month*, in the fifteenth day of the month, shall he do the like in the feast of the seven days, according to the sin-offering, according to the burnt-offering, and according to the [b]meat-offering, and according to the oil.

CHAPTER 46.

The worship of the prince and the people.

Thus saith the Lord GOD; The gate of the inner court that looketh toward the east shall be shut the six working days; but on the sabbath it shall be opened, and in the day of the new moon it shall be opened.

2 And the prince shall enter by the way of the porch of *that* gate without, and shall stand by the post of the gate, and the priests shall prepare his burnt-offering and his peace-offerings, and he shall worship at the threshold of the gate: then he shall go forth; but the gate shall not be shut until the evening.

3 Likewise the people of the land shall worship at the door of this gate before the LORD in the sabbaths and in the new moons.

4 And the burnt-offering that the prince shall offer unto the LORD in the sabbath day *shall be* six lambs without blemish, and a ram without blemish.

5 And the [b]meat-offering *shall be* an ephah for a ram, and the meat-offering for the lambs as he shall be able to give, and an [h]hin of oil to an ephah.

6 And in the day of the new moon *it shall be* a young bullock without blemish, and six lambs, and a ram: they shall be without blemish.

7 And he shall prepare a [b]meat-offering, an ephah for a bullock, and an ephah for a ram, and for the lambs according as his hand shall attain unto, and an [h]hin of oil to an ephah.

8 And when the prince shall enter, he shall go in by the way of the porch of *that* gate, and he shall go forth by the way thereof.

9 But when the people of the land shall come before the LORD in the solemn feasts, he that entereth in by the way of the north gate to worship shall go out by the way of the south gate; and he that entereth by the way of the south gate shall go forth by the way of the north gate: he shall not return by the way of the gate whereby he came in, but shall go forth over against it.

10 And the prince in the midst of

B.C. 574.

a One cor = about 86 gals.

b Lit. *meal;* also v. 17.

c Heb. *kaphar, atone.* See Dan. 9:24, *note.*

d i.e. *April;* also v. 21.

e Ex. 12:18; Num. 9:2, 3; 28:16, 17; Deut. 16:1.

f Lev. 4:14.

g One ephah = 1 bu. 3 pts.; also Ezk. 46:5, 7, 11, 14.

h 1 hin = about 6 qts.

i i.e. *October.*

them, when they go in, shall go in; and
when they go forth, shall go forth.
11 And in the feasts and in the solemnities the [a]meat-offering shall be an
ephah to a bullock, and an ephah to a
ram, and to the lambs as he is able to
give, and an [b]hin of oil to an ephah.
12 Now when the prince shall prepare
a voluntary burnt-offering or peace-
offerings voluntarily unto the LORD, *one*
shall then open him the gate that looketh
toward the east, and he shall prepare his
burnt-offering and his peace-offerings,
as he did on the sabbath day: then he
shall go forth; and after his going forth
one shall shut the gate.
13 Thou shalt daily prepare a burnt-
offering unto the LORD *of* a lamb of the
first year without blemish: thou shalt
prepare it every morning.
14 And thou shalt prepare a [a]meat-
offering for it every morning, the sixth
part of an ephah, and the third part of an
[b]hin of oil, to temper with the fine flour;
a meat-offering continually by a perpetual ordinance unto the LORD.
15 Thus shall they prepare the lamb,
and the [a]meat-offering, and the oil, every
morning *for* a continual burnt-offering.
16 Thus saith the Lord GOD; If the
prince give a gift unto any of his sons,
the inheritance thereof shall be his sons';
it *shall be* their possession by inheritance.
17 But if he give a gift of his inheritance to one of his servants, then it shall
be his to [c]the year of liberty; after it shall
return to the prince: but his inheritance
shall be his sons' for them.
18 Moreover [d]the prince shall not take
of the people's inheritance by oppression,
to thrust them out of their possession; *but*
he shall give his sons inheritance out of
his own possession: that my people be not
scattered every man from his possession.

The place for boiling the offerings.

19 After he brought me through the
entry, which *was* at the side of the gate,
into the holy chambers of the priests,
which looked toward the north: and,
behold, there *was* a place on the two
sides westward.
20 Then said he unto me, This *is* the
place where the priests shall [e]boil the
trespass-offering and the sin-offering,
where they shall [f]bake the [a]meat-offer-
ing; that they bear *them* not out into the
utter court, to sanctify the people.
21 Then he brought me forth into the
utter court, and caused me to pass by
the four corners of the court; and,
behold, in every corner of the court *there*
was a court.
22 In the four corners of the court *there*
were courts joined of forty *cubits* long
and thirty broad: these four corners *were*
of one measure.
23 And *there was* a row *of building*
round about in them, round about them
four, and *it was* made with boiling places
under the rows round about.
24 Then said he unto me, These *are* the
places of them that boil, where the ministers of the house shall boil the sacrifice
of the people.

CHAPTER 47.

The river of the sanctuary.
(Cf. Zech. 14:8, 9; Rev. 22:1, 2.)

Afterward he brought me again unto
the door of the house; and, behold,
[g]waters issued out from under the
threshold of the house eastward: for the
forefront of the house *stood toward* the
east, and the waters came down from
under from the right side of the house,
at the south *side* of the altar.
2 Then brought he me out of the way of
the gate northward, and led me about the
way without unto the utter gate by the
way that looketh eastward; and, behold,
there ran out waters on the right side.
3 And when the [h]man that had the
line in his hand went forth eastward, he
measured a thousand [i]cubits, and he
brought me through the waters; the
waters *were* to the ankles.
4 Again he measured a thousand, and
brought me through the waters; the
waters *were* to the knees. Again he measured a thousand, and brought me
through; the waters *were* to the loins.
5 Afterward he measured a thousand;
and it was a river that I could not pass
over: for the waters were risen, waters to
swim in, a river that could not be passed
over.
6 And he said unto me, Son of man,
hast thou seen *this*? Then he brought me,
and caused me to return to the brink of
the river.

B.C. 574.

a Lit. *meal.*

b One hin = about 6 qts.

c Lev. 25:10.

d Ezk. 45:8; cf. Isa. 11:3-4.

e 2 Chr. 35:13.

f Lev. 2:4, 5, 7.

g Joel 3:18; Zech. 13:1; 14:8; Rev. 22:1.

h Ezk. 40:3.

i One cubit = about 18 in.

7 Now when I had returned, behold, at the bank of the river *were* very many [a]trees on the one side and on the other.

8 Then said he unto me, These waters issue out toward the east country, and go down into the desert, and go into the sea: *which being* brought forth into the sea, the waters shall be healed.

9 And it shall come to pass, *that* every thing that liveth, which moveth, whithersoever the [b]rivers shall come, shall live: and there shall be a very great multitude of fish, because these waters shall come thither: for they shall be healed; and every thing shall live whither the river cometh.

10 And it shall come to pass, *that* the fishers shall stand upon it from En-gedi even unto En-eglaim; they shall be a *place* to spread forth nets; their fish shall be according to their kinds, as the fish [c]of the great sea, exceeding many.

11 But the miry places thereof and the marishes thereof shall not be healed; they shall be given to salt.

12 And by the river upon the bank thereof, on this side and on that side, shall grow all trees for meat, [d]whose leaf shall not fade, neither shall the fruit thereof be consumed: it shall bring forth new fruit according to his months, because their waters they issued out of the sanctuary: and the fruit thereof shall be for meat, and the leaf thereof for medicine.

The borders of the land.
(Cf. Gen. 15:18-21.)

13 Thus saith the Lord GOD; This *shall be* the border, whereby ye shall inherit the land according to the twelve tribes of Israel: [e]Joseph *shall have two* portions.

14 And ye shall inherit it, one as well as another: *concerning* the which I [f]lifted up mine hand to give it unto your fathers: and this land shall fall unto you for inheritance.

15 And this *shall be* the border of the land toward the north side, from the great sea, [g]the way of Hethlon, as men go to [h]Zedad;

16 [h]Hamath, [i]Berothah, Sibraim, which is between the border of Damascus and the border of Hamath; Hazar-hatticon, which *is* by the coast of Hauran.

17 And the border from the sea shall be [j]Hazar-enan, the border of Damascus, and the north northward, and the border of Hamath. And *this is* the north side.

B.C. 574.

a v. 12; Rev. 22:2.
b Heb. *two rivers.*
c Ezk. 48:28; Num. 34:6; Josh. 23:4.
d Job 8:16; Psa. 1:3; Jer. 17:8.
e Ezk. 48:4, 5; Gen. 48:5; 1 Chr. 5:1.
f Ezk. 20:5, 6, 28, 42; Gen. 12:7; 13:15; 15:7; 17:8; 26:3; 28:13.
g Ezk. 48:1.
h Num. 34:8.
i 2 Sam. 8:8.
j Ezk. 48:1; Num. 34:9.
k Ezk. 48:28; Num. 20:13; Deut. 32:51; Psa. 81:7.
l Cf. Eph. 3:6; Rev. 7:9, 10.
m Rom. 10:12; Gal. 3:28; Col. 3:11.
n Ezk. 47:15.

18 And the east side ye shall measure from Hauran, and from Damascus, and from Gilead, and from the land of Israel *by* Jordan, from the border unto the east sea. And *this is* the east side.

19 And the south side southward, from Tamar *even* to [k]the waters of strife *in* Kadesh, the river to the great sea. And *this is* the south side southward.

20 The west side also *shall be* the great sea from the border, till a man come over against Hamath. This *is* the west side.

21 So shall ye divide this land unto you according to the tribes of Israel.

22 And it shall come to pass, *that* ye shall divide it by lot for an inheritance unto you, [l]and to the strangers that sojourn among you, which shall beget children among you: and [m]they shall be unto you as born in the country among the children of Israel; they shall have inheritance with you among the tribes of Israel.

23 And it shall come to pass, *that* in what tribe the stranger sojourneth, there shall ye give *him* his inheritance, saith the Lord GOD.

CHAPTER 48.

The division of the land.
(Cf. Josh. 13:1–19:51.)

Now these *are* the names of the tribes. [n]From the north end to the coast of the way of Hethlon, as one goeth to Hamath, Hazar-enan, the border of Damascus northward, to the coast of Hamath; for these are his sides east *and* west; a *portion for* Dan.

2 And by the border of Dan, from the east side unto the west side, a *portion for* Asher.

3 And by the border of Asher, from the east side even unto the west side, a *portion for* Naphtali.

4 And by the border of Naphtali, from the east side unto the west side, a *portion for* Manasseh.

5 And by the border of Manasseh, from the east side unto the west side, a *portion for* Ephraim.

6 And by the border of Ephraim, from the east side even unto the west side, a *portion for* Reuben.

7 And by the border of Reuben, from the east side unto the west side, a *portion for* Judah.

8 And by the border of Judah, from the east side unto the west side, shall be [a]the offering which ye shall offer of five and twenty thousand *reeds in* breadth, and *in* length as one of the *other* parts, from the east side unto the west side: and the sanctuary shall be in the midst of it.

9 The oblation that ye shall offer unto the LORD *shall be* of five and twenty thousand in length, and of ten thousand in breadth.

For the priests and Levites.

10 And for them, *even* for the priests, shall be *this* holy oblation; toward the north five and twenty thousand *in length*, and toward the west ten thousand in breadth, and toward the east ten thousand in breadth, and toward the south five and twenty thousand in length: and the sanctuary of the LORD shall be in the midst thereof.

11 [b]*It shall be* for the priests that are sanctified of the sons of Zadok; which have kept my charge, which went not astray when the children of Israel went astray, [c]as the Levites went astray.

12 And *this* oblation of the land that is offered shall be unto them a thing most holy by the border of the Levites.

13 And over against the border of the priests the Levites *shall have* five and twenty thousand in length, and ten thousand in breadth: all the length *shall be* five and twenty thousand, and the breadth ten thousand.

14 [d]And they shall not sell of it, neither exchange, nor alienate the firstfruits of the land: for *it is* holy unto the LORD.

15 And the five thousand, that are left in the breadth over against the five and twenty thousand, shall be a [e]profane *place* for the city, for dwelling, and for suburbs: and the city shall be in the midst thereof.

16 And these *shall be* the measures thereof; the north side four thousand and five hundred, and the south side four thousand and five hundred, and on the east side four thousand and five hundred, and the west side four thousand and five hundred.

17 And the suburbs of the city shall be toward the north two hundred and fifty, and toward the south two hundred and fifty, and toward the east two hundred and fifty, and toward the west two hundred and fifty.

B.C. 574.

a Ezk. 45:1-6.
b Ezk. 40:46; 44:15.
c Ezk. 44:10.
d Lev. 27:10, 28, 33.
e Ezk. 42:20.
f Ezk. 45:7.
g vs. 8, 10.
h Heb. *one portion.*
i Ezk. 47:19.
j Heb. *Meribah-Kadesh.*
k Ezk. 47:14, 21, 22.

18 And the residue in length over against the oblation of the holy *portion shall be* ten thousand eastward, and ten thousand westward: and it shall be over against the oblation of the holy *portion*; and the increase thereof shall be for food unto them that serve the city.

19 And they that serve the city shall serve it out of all the tribes of Israel.

20 All the oblation *shall be* five and twenty thousand by five and twenty thousand: ye shall offer the holy oblation foursquare, with the possession of the city.

The portion for the prince.

21 [f]And the residue *shall be* for the prince, on the one side and on the other of the holy oblation, and of the possession of the city, over against the five and twenty thousand of the oblation toward the east border, and westward over against the five and twenty thousand toward the west border, over against the portions for the prince: and it shall be the holy oblation; [g]and the sanctuary of the house *shall be* in the midst thereof.

22 Moreover from the possession of the Levites, and from the possession of the city, *being* in the midst *of that* which is the prince's, between the border of Judah and the border of Benjamin, shall be for the prince.

23 As for the rest of the tribes, from the east side unto the west side, Benjamin *shall have* a [h]*portion.*

24 And by the border of Benjamin, from the east side unto the west side, Simeon *shall have* a *portion.*

25 And by the border of Simeon, from the east side unto the west side, Issachar a *portion.*

26 And by the border of Issachar, from the east side unto the west side, Zebulun a *portion.*

27 And by the border of Zebulun, from the east side unto the west side, Gad a *portion.*

28 And by the border of Gad, at the south side southward, the border shall be even from Tamar *unto* the [i]waters of [j]strife *in* Kadesh, *and* to the river toward the great sea.

29 [k]This *is* the land which ye shall divide by lot unto the tribes of Israel for inheritance, and these *are* their portions, saith the Lord GOD.

The city and its gates. (Cf. Rev. 21:10-27.)

30 And these *are* the goings out of the
city on the north side, four thousand and
five hundred measures.

31 [a]And the gates of the city *shall be*
after the names of the tribes of Israel:
three gates northward; one gate of Reuben, one gate of Judah, one gate of Levi.

32 And at the east side four thousand
and five hundred: and three gates; and
one gate of Joseph, one gate of Benjamin,
one gate of Dan.

33 And at the south side four thousand and five hundred measures: and
three gates; one gate of Simeon, one gate
of Issachar, one gate of Zebulun.

34 At the west side four thousand and
five hundred, *with* their three gates; one
gate of Gad, one gate of Asher, one gate
of Naphtali.

35 *It was* round about eighteen thousand *measures*: [b]and the name of the
city from *that* day *shall be*, [c]The LORD *is*
there.

B.C. 574.

a Rev. 21:12.

b Heb. *Jehovah-shammah.* See Ex. 17:15; Jud. 6:24.

c Jer. 3:17; Joel 3:21; Zech. 2:10; Rev. 21:3; 22:3.

THE BOOK OF DANIEL

DANIEL, like Ezekiel, was a Jewish captive in Babylon. He was of royal or princely descent (1:3). For his rank and comeliness he was trained for palace service. In the polluted atmosphere of an oriental court he lived a life of singular piety and usefulness. His long life extended from Nebuchadnezzar to Cyrus. He was a contemporary of Jeremiah, Ezekiel (14:20), Joshua, the high priest of the restoration, Ezra, and Zerubbabel.

Daniel is the indispensable introduction to New Testament prophecy, the themes of which are, the apostasy of the Church, the manifestation of the man of sin, the great tribulation, the return of the Lord, the resurrections and the judgments. These, except the first, are Daniel's themes also.

But Daniel is distinctively the prophet of the "times of the Gentiles" (Lk. 21:24, *refs.*). His vision sweeps the whole course of Gentile world-rule to its end in catastrophe, and to the setting up of the Messianic kingdom.

Daniel is in four broad divisions: I. Introduction. The personal history of Daniel from the conquest of Jerusalem to the second year of Nebuchadnezzar, 1:1-21. II. The visions of Nebuchadnezzar and their results, 2:1–4:37. III. The personal history of Daniel under Belshazzar and Darius, 5:1–6:28. IV. The visions of Daniel, 7:1–12:13.

The events recorded in Daniel cover a period of 73 years (Ussher).

CHAPTER 1.

Part I. Introduction:
the personal history of Daniel (vs. 1-21).

In the third year of the reign of
[a]Jehoiakim king of Judah came
Nebuchadnezzar king of Babylon unto
Jerusalem, and besieged it.
2 And the Lord gave Jehoiakim king of
Judah into his hand, with part of the
[b]vessels of the house of God: which he
carried into the land of Shinar to the
house of his god; and he brought the vessels into the treasure house of his god.
3 And the king spake unto Ashpenaz
the master of his eunuchs, that he should
bring *certain* of the children of Israel, and
of the [c]king's seed, and of the princes;
4 Children in whom *was* no blemish,
but well favoured, and skilful in all wisdom, and cunning in knowledge, and
understanding science, and such as *had*
ability in them to stand in the king's
palace, and whom they might teach the
learning and the tongue of the
Chaldeans.
5 And the king appointed them a daily
provision of the king's meat, and of the
wine which he drank: so nourishing
them three years, that at the end thereof
they might stand before the king.
6 Now among these were of the children of Judah, Daniel, Hananiah,
Mishael, and Azariah:

B.C. 607.

a 2 Ki. 24:1, 2; 2 Chr. 36:5-7; Jer. 25:1; 52:12-30. Daniel was deported 8 years before Ezekiel.

b Dan. 5:1-3; 2 Chr. 36:5-7; Jer. 27:19, 20.

c Foretold, 2 Ki. 20:18; Isa. 39:7.

d i.e. *the king's leader*, or *attendant.* Dan. 2:26; 4:8, 9, 18, 19; 5:12. Identical in meaning with Belshazzar.

e Cf. Num. 6:1-4; 1 Cor. 10:21.

f Gen. 39:21; Prov. 16:7; Acts 7:10.

g Or, *sadder.*

7 Unto whom the prince of the
eunuchs gave names: for he gave unto
Daniel *the name* of [d]Belteshazzar; and to
Hananiah, of Shadrach; and to Mishael,
of Meshach; and to Azariah, of Abed-
nego.
8 But Daniel purposed in his heart that
he would not defile himself with the
portion of the king's meat, nor with the
[e]wine which he drank: therefore he
requested of the prince of the eunuchs
that he might not defile himself.
9 Now God had [f]brought Daniel into
favour and tender love with the prince
of the eunuchs.
10 And the prince of the eunuchs said
unto Daniel, I fear my lord the king, who
hath appointed your meat and your
drink: for why should he see your faces
[g]worse liking than the children which
are of your sort? then shall ye make *me*
endanger my head to the king.
11 Then said Daniel to Melzar, whom
the prince of the eunuchs had set over
Daniel, Hananiah, Mishael, and Azariah,
12 Prove thy servants, I beseech thee,
ten days; and let them give us pulse to
eat, and water to drink.
13 Then let our countenances be
looked upon before thee, and the countenance of the children that eat of the
portion of the king's meat: and as thou
seest, deal with thy servants.
14 So he consented to them in

this matter, and proved them ten days.
15 And at the end of ten days their countenances appeared fairer and fatter in flesh than all the children which did eat the portion of the king's meat.
16 Thus Melzar took away the portion of their meat, and the wine that they should drink; and gave them pulse.
17 As for these four children, God [a]gave them [b]knowledge and skill in all learning and wisdom: and Daniel had understanding in all visions and dreams.
18 Now at the end of the days that the king had said he should bring them in, then the prince of the eunuchs brought them in before Nebuchadnezzar.
19 And the king communed with them; and among them all was found none like Daniel, Hananiah, Mishael, and Azariah: therefore stood they before the king.
20 And in all matters of [c]wisdom *and* understanding, that the king enquired of them, he found them ten times better than all the magicians *and* astrologers that *were* in all his realm.
21 And Daniel [d]continued *even* unto the first year of king Cyrus.

CHAPTER 2.

Part II. The visions of Nebuchadnezzar and their results (Dan. 2:1–4:37). (1) *The forgotten dream: failure of the magi.*

And in the second year of the reign of Nebuchadnezzar Nebuchadnezzar dreamed dreams, wherewith his spirit was troubled, and his sleep brake from him.
2 Then the king commanded to call the magicians, and the astrologers, and the sorcerers, and the [e]Chaldeans, for to shew the king his dreams. So they came and stood before the king.
3 And the king said unto them, I have dreamed a dream, and my spirit was troubled to know the dream.
4 Then spake the Chaldeans to the king in [1]Syriack, O king, live for ever: tell thy servants the dream, and we will shew the interpretation.
5 The king answered and said to the Chaldeans, The thing is gone from me: if ye will not make known unto me the dream, with the interpretation thereof, ye shall be cut in pieces, and your houses shall be made a dunghill.
6 But if ye shew the dream, and the interpretation thereof, ye shall receive of me gifts and rewards and great honour: therefore shew me the dream, and the interpretation thereof.
7 They answered again and said, Let the king tell his servants the dream, and we will shew the interpretation of it.
8 The king answered and said, I know of certainty that ye would gain the time, because ye see the thing is gone from me.
9 But if ye will not make known unto me the dream, *there is but* one decree for you: for ye have prepared lying and corrupt words to speak before me, till the time be changed: therefore tell me the dream, and I shall know that ye can shew me the interpretation thereof.
10 The Chaldeans answered before the king, and said, There is not a man upon the earth that can

B.C. 606.

a v. 20; 2 Chr. 1:10-12; Lk. 21:15; Jas. 1:5-7.

b Acts 7:22.

c Heb. *wisdom of understanding.*

d i.e. to see the return of the remnant of Judah at the end of the 70 years (Jer. 25:11, 12; 29:10). Daniel actually lived beyond the first year of Cyrus. Dan. 10:1.

e i.e. the men having the ancient wisdom; the learned; Chaldeans *par excellence* (v. 13, "wise").

[1] **(2:4)** From Dan. 2:4 to 7:28 the Book of Daniel is written in Aramaic, the ancient language of Syria, and substantially identical with Chaldaic, the language of ancient Babylonia. Upon this fact, together with the occurrence of fifteen Persian, and three Greek words, has been based an argument against the historicity of Daniel, and in favour of a date after the conquest of Palestine by Alexander (B.C. 332). It has, however, seemed, with some modern exceptions, to the Hebrew and Christian scholarship of the ages an unanswerable proof rather of the Danielic authorship of the book that, living from boyhood in a land the language of which was Chaldaic, a great part of his writing should be in that tongue. It has often been pointed out that the Chaldaic of Daniel is of high antiquity, as is shown by comparison with that of the Targums. The few words of Persian and Greek in like manner confirm the writer's residence at a court constantly visited by emissaries from those peoples. It is noteworthy that the Aramaic section is precisely that part of Daniel which most concerned the peoples amongst whom he lived, and to whom a prophecy written in Hebrew would have been unintelligible. The language returns to Hebrew in the predictive portions which have to do with the future of Israel. "The Hebrew of Daniel is closely related to that of Ezekiel."—*Delitzsch.*

shew the king's matter: therefore *there is*
no king, lord, nor ruler, *that* asked such
things at any magician, or astrologer, or
Chaldean.
11 And *it is* a rare thing that the king
requireth, and there is none other that
can shew it before the king, except the
gods, whose dwelling is not with flesh.
12 For this cause the king was angry
and very furious, and commanded to
destroy all the wise *men* of Babylon.
13 And the decree went forth that the
wise *men* should be slain; and they
sought Daniel and his fellows to be slain.

(2) *The prayer for wisdom.*

14 Then Daniel answered with counsel
and wisdom to Arioch the [a]captain of
the king's guard, which was gone forth
to slay the wise *men* of Babylon:
15 He answered and said to Arioch the
king's captain, Why *is* the decree *so*
hasty from the king? Then Arioch made
the thing known to Daniel.
16 Then Daniel went in, and desired of
the king that he would give him time,
and that he would shew the king the
interpretation.
17 Then Daniel went to his house, and
made the thing known to Hananiah,
Mishael, and Azariah, his companions:
18 That they would desire mercies of
the God [b]of heaven concerning this
secret; that Daniel and his fellows
should not perish with the rest of the
wise *men* of Babylon.

(3) *The secret revealed to Daniel.*

19 Then was the secret revealed unto
Daniel in a night vision. Then Daniel
blessed the God of heaven.
20 Daniel answered and said, Blessed
be the name of God for ever and ever:
for wisdom and might are his:
21 And he [c]changeth the times and the
seasons: [d]he removeth kings, and setteth
up kings: he giveth wisdom unto the
wise, and knowledge to them that know
understanding:
22 He [e]revealeth the deep and secret
things: he knoweth what *is* in the darkness, and the light dwelleth with him.

B.C. 603.

a Or. *executioner* (v. 24).

b Lit. *of the heavens.* vs. 19, 28, 37, 44; Dan. 4:37; 5:23.

c Cf. Dan. 7:25.

d Dan. 4:35.

e Gen. 41:45, marg.; Dan. 4:9; Job 15:8; Psa. 25:14; Prov. 3:32; Mt. 6:6.

f v. 14.

g v. 22.

h *Times (of the Gentiles).* vs. 29-45. Rev. 16:19. (Lk. 21:24; Rev. 16:19.)

23 I thank thee, and praise thee, O
thou God of my fathers, who hast given
me wisdom and might, and hast made
known unto me now what we desired of
thee: for thou hast *now* made known
unto us the king's matter.
24 Therefore Daniel went in unto
[f]Arioch, whom the king had ordained to
destroy the wise *men* of Babylon: he
went and said thus unto him; Destroy
not the wise *men* of Babylon: bring me in
before the king, and I will shew unto the
king the interpretation.
25 Then Arioch brought in Daniel
before the king in haste, and said thus
unto him, I have found a man of the captives of Judah, that will make known
unto the king the interpretation.
26 The king answered and said to
Daniel, whose name *was* Belteshazzar,
Art thou able to make known unto me
the dream which I have seen, and the
interpretation thereof?
27 Daniel answered in the presence of
the king, and said, The secret which the
king hath demanded cannot the wise
men, the astrologers, the magicians, the
soothsayers, shew unto the king;
28 But there is a God in heaven that [g]re-
vealeth secrets, and maketh known to the
king Nebuchadnezzar what shall be in the
latter days. Thy dream, and the visions of
thy head upon thy bed, are these;
29 As for thee, O king, thy thoughts
came *into thy mind* upon thy bed, [h]what
should come to pass hereafter: and he
that revealeth secrets maketh known to
thee what shall come to pass.
30 But as for me, this secret is not
revealed to me for *any* wisdom that I
have more than any living, but for *their*
sakes that shall make known the interpretation to the king, and that thou
mightest know the thoughts of thy heart.

(4) *The forgotten dream recovered.*

31 Thou, O king, sawest, and behold a
great [1]image. This great image, whose
brightness *was* excellent, stood before
thee; and the form thereof *was* terrible.
32 This image's head *was* of fine

[1](2:31) The monarchy-vision. Nebuchadnezzar's dream, as interpreted by Daniel, gives the course and end of "the times of the Gentiles" (Lk. 21:24; Rev. 16:19, *note*), that is, of Gentile world-empire. The four metals composing the image are explained as symbolizing (vs. 38-40) four empires, not necessarily possessing the inhabited earth, but able to do so (v. 38), and fulfilled in Babylon, Media-Persia

B.C. 603.

gold, his breast and his arms of silver,
his belly and his [a]thighs of brass,
33 His legs of iron, his feet part of iron
and part of clay.
34 Thou sawest till that a [b]stone was
cut out without hands, which smote the
image upon his feet *that were* of iron and
clay, and brake them to pieces.
35 [c]Then was the iron, the clay, the
brass, the silver, and the gold, broken to
pieces together, and became like the
[d]chaff of the summer threshingfloors;
and the wind carried them away, that no
place was found for them: [e]and the stone
that smote the image became a great
[f]mountain, and filled the whole earth.

(5) *The interpretation.*

36 This *is* the dream; and we will tell
the interpretation thereof before the
king.

(a) The first world-empire: Babylon under Nebuchadnezzar. (Cf. Dan. 7:4.)

37 Thou, O king, *art* a king of kings:
for the God of heaven hath given thee a
kingdom, power, and strength, and
glory.
38 And [g]wheresoever the children of
men dwell, the beasts of the field and
the fowls of the heaven hath he given
into thine hand, and hath made thee
ruler over them all. Thou *art* this head of
gold.

(b) The second world-empire: Media-Persia. (Cf. Dan. 7:5.)

(c) The third world-empire: Greece. (Cf. Dan. 7:6.)

39 And after thee shall arise another
kingdom inferior to thee, and another
third kingdom of brass, which shall bear
rule over all the earth.

(d) The fourth world-empire: Rome. (Cf. Dan. 7:7.)

40 [h]And the fourth kingdom shall be
strong as iron: forasmuch as iron
breaketh in pieces and subdueth all
things: and as iron that breaketh all
these, shall it break in pieces and bruise.
41 And whereas thou sawest the feet
and toes, part of potters' clay, and part of
iron, the kingdom shall be divided; [1]but
there shall be in it of the strength of the
iron, forasmuch as thou sawest the iron
mixed with [i]miry clay.
42 And *as* the [j]toes of the feet *were*
part of iron, and part of clay, *so* the

a Or, *sides.*

b *Christ (as Stone).* vs. 34, 35, 44, 45; Zech. 4:7. (Ex. 17:6; 1 Pet. 2:8.)

c Dan. 7:23-27. See Rev. 19:17-21. See "Armageddon" (Rev. 16:14; 19:17).

d Psa. 1:4; Mt. 3:12.

e *Kingdom* (O.T.). vs. 34-45; Dan. 7:1-27. (Gen. 1:26-28; Zech. 12:8.)

f A mountain is one of the biblical symbols of a kingdom. Isa. 2:2, *note.*

g This is universal dominion. It was never fully realized, but power was given for it.

h Dan. 7:7, 23.

i Lit. *brittle.*

j Dan. 7:24.

Greece (under Alexander), and Rome. The latter power is seen divided, first into two (the legs), fulfilled in the Eastern and Western Roman empires, and then into ten (the toes) (see Dan. 7:26, *note*). As a whole, the image gives the imposing outward greatness and splendour of the Gentile world-power.

The smiting Stone (2:34, 35) destroys the Gentile world-system (in its final form) by a sudden and irremediable blow, not by the gradual processes of conversion and assimilation; and then, and not before, does the Stone become a mountain which fills "the whole earth." (Cf. Dan. 7:26, 27.) Such a destruction of the Gentile monarchy-system did not occur at the first advent of Christ. On the contrary, He was put to death by the sentence of an officer of the fourth empire, which was then at the zenith of its power. Since the crucifixion the Roman empire has followed the course marked out in the vision, but Gentile world-dominion still continues, and the crushing blow is still suspended. The detail of the end-time is given in Dan. 7:1-28, and Rev. 13–19. It is important to see (1) that Gentile world-power is to end in a sudden catastrophic judgment (see "Armageddon," Rev. 16:14; 19:21); (2) that it is immediately followed by the kingdom of heaven, and that the God of the heavens does not set up His kingdom till after the destruction of the Gentile world-system. It is noteworthy that Gentile world-dominion begins and ends with a great image (Dan. 2:31; Rev. 13:14, 15).

[1] **(2:41)** From the "head of gold" (v. 38) to the "iron" of the "fourth kingdom" (Rome) there is deterioration in fineness, but increase of strength (v. 40). Then comes the deterioration of the "fourth kingdom" in that very quality, strength. (1) Deterioration by division: The kingdom is divided into two, the legs (Eastern and Western empires), and these are again divided into kingdoms, the number of which when the Stone smites the image will be ten (toes, v. 42; cf. Dan. 7:23, 24). (2) Deterioration by admixture; the iron of the Roman *imperium* mixed with the clay of the popular will, fickle and easily moulded. This is precisely what has come to pass in the constitutional monarchies which, with the Republic of France and the despotism of Turkey, cover the sphere of ancient Roman rule.

B.C. 603.

kingdom shall be partly strong, and partly [a]broken.

43 And whereas thou sawest iron mixed with [b]miry clay, they shall mingle themselves with the seed of men: but they shall not cleave one to another, even as iron is not mixed with clay.

(e) The final world-empire: the kingdom of heaven. (See Mt. 3:2, *note*.)

44 [1]And in the days of these kings shall the God of heaven set up a [c]kingdom, which shall never be destroyed: and the kingdom shall not be left to other people, *but* it shall break in pieces and consume all these kingdoms, and it shall stand for ever.

45 Forasmuch as thou sawest that the [d]stone was cut out of the mountain without hands, and that it brake in pieces the iron, the brass, the clay, the silver, and the gold; the great God hath made known to the king what shall come to pass hereafter: and the dream *is* certain, and the interpretation thereof sure.

(6) *The promotion of Daniel.*

46 [e]Then the king Nebuchadnezzar fell upon his face, and worshipped Daniel, and commanded that they should offer an oblation and sweet odours unto him.

47 The king answered unto Daniel, and said, Of a truth *it is*, that your God *is* a God of gods, and a Lord of kings, and a [f]revealer of secrets, seeing thou couldest reveal this secret.

48 [g]Then the king made Daniel a great man, and gave him many great gifts, and made him ruler over the whole province of Babylon, and chief of the governors over all the wise *men* of Babylon.

49 Then Daniel requested of the king, and he set Shadrach, Meshach, and Abed-nego, over the affairs of the province of Babylon: but [h]Daniel *sat* in the gate of the king.

CHAPTER 3.

The pride of Nebuchadnezzar and his punishment: (1) *the image of gold.*

Nebuchadnezzar the king made an [2][i]image of gold, whose height *was* threescore cubits, *and* the breadth thereof six cubits: he set it up in the plain of Dura, in the province of Babylon.

2 Then Nebuchadnezzar the king sent to gather together the princes, the governors, and the captains, the judges, the treasurers, the counsellors, the sheriffs, and all the rulers of the provinces, to come to the dedication of the image which Nebuchadnezzar the king had set up.

3 Then the princes, the governors, and captains, the judges, the treasurers, the counsellors, the sheriffs, and all the rulers of the provinces, were gathered together unto the dedication of the image that Nebuchadnezzar the king had set up; and they stood before the image that Nebuchadnezzar had set up.

4 Then an herald cried aloud, To you it is commanded, O people, nations, and languages,

5 *That* at what time ye hear the sound of the cornet, flute, harp, sackbut, psaltery, dulcimer, and all kinds of musick, ye fall down and worship the golden image that Nebuchadnezzar the king hath set up:

6 And whoso falleth not down and worshippeth shall the same hour be cast into the midst of a burning fiery furnace

a Or, *brittle.*

b Or, *baked,* i.e. *brittle.*

c Dan. 7:14, 27; Lk. 1:32, 33, *refs.*

d v. 34, *refs.*

e Cf. vs. 27, 28, 30; Acts. 10:25.

f v. 22, *refs.*

g Prov. 14:35; 21:1.

h Cf. Gen. 19:1, Lot the compromiser with Daniel the inflexible.

i Cf. Rev. 13:14, 15.

[1] **(2:44)** The passage fixes authoritatively the *time* relative to other predicted events, when the kingdom of the heavens will be set up. It will be "in the days of these kings," i.e. the days of the ten kings (cf. Dan. 7:24-27) symbolized by the toes of the image. That condition did not exist at the advent of Messiah, nor was it even possible until the dissolution of the Roman empire, and the rise of the present national world-system. See "Kingdom (O.T.)" (Gen. 1:26; Zech. 12:8); "Kingdom (N.T.)" (Lk. 1:31-33; 1 Cor. 15:28); Mt. 3:2, *note* (defining "kingdom of heaven"). Verse 45 repeats the *method* by which the kingdom will be set up. (Cf. v. 31, *note;* Psa. 2:5 with Psa. 2:6; Zech. 14:1-8 with Zech. 14:9.)

[2] **(3:1)** The attempt of this great king of Babylon to unify the religions of his empire by self-deification will be repeated by the beast, the last head of the Gentile world-dominion (Rev. 13:11-15). See "Beast, the" (Dan. 7:8; Rev. 19:20). It has repeatedly characterized Gentile authority in the earth, e.g. Dan. 6:7; Acts 12:22, and the later Roman emperors.

7 Therefore at that time, when all the people heard the sound of the cornet, flute, harp, sackbut, psaltery, and all kinds of musick, all the people, the nations, and the languages, fell down *and* worshipped the golden image that Nebuchadnezzar the king had set up.

(2) *The three Jews refuse to worship the image.*

8 Wherefore at that time certain [a]Chaldeans came near, and accused the Jews.

9 They spake and said to the king Nebuchadnezzar, O king, live for ever.

10 Thou, O king, hast made a decree, that every man that shall hear the sound of the cornet, flute, harp, sackbut, psaltery, and dulcimer, and all kinds of musick, shall fall down and worship the golden image:

11 And whoso falleth not down and worshippeth, *that* he should be cast into the midst of a burning fiery furnace.

12 There are certain Jews [b]whom thou hast set over the affairs of the province of Babylon, Shadrach, Meshach, and Abed-nego; these men, O king, have not regarded thee: they serve not thy gods, nor worship the golden image which thou hast set up.

13 Then Nebuchadnezzar in *his* rage and fury commanded to bring Shadrach, Meshach, and Abed-nego. Then they brought these men before the king.

14 Nebuchadnezzar spake and said unto them, *Is it* true, O Shadrach, Meshach, and Abed-nego, do not ye serve my gods, nor worship the golden image which I have set up?

15 Now if ye be ready that at what time ye hear the sound of the cornet, flute, harp, sackbut, psaltery, and dulcimer, and all kinds of musick, ye fall down and worship the image which I have made; *well*: but if ye worship not, ye shall be cast the same hour into the midst of a burning fiery furnace; and who *is* that God that shall deliver you out of my hands?

16 Shadrach, Meshach, and Abed-nego, answered and said to the king, O Nebuchadnezzar, we *are* not careful to answer thee in this matter.

17 If it be *so*, our [c]God whom we serve is able to deliver us from the burning fiery furnace, [1]and he will deliver *us* out of thine hand, O king.

18 But if not, be it known unto thee, O king, that [d]we will not serve thy gods, nor [e]worship the golden image which thou hast set up.

(3) *The harmless furnace.*

19 Then was Nebuchadnezzar full of fury, and the form of his visage was changed against Shadrach, Meshach, and Abed-nego: *therefore* he spake, and commanded that they should heat the furnace one seven times more than it was wont to be heated.

20 And he commanded the most mighty men that *were* in his army to bind Shadrach, Meshach, and Abed-nego, *and* to cast *them* into the burning fiery furnace.

21 Then these men were bound in their coats, their hosen, and their hats, and their *other* garments, and were cast into the midst of the burning fiery furnace.

22 Therefore because the king's commandment was urgent, and the furnace exceeding hot, the flame of the fire slew those men that took up Shadrach, Meshach, and Abed-nego.

23 And these three men, Shadrach, Meshach, and Abed-nego, fell down bound into the midst of the burning fiery furnace.

24 Then Nebuchadnezzar the king was astonied, and rose up in haste, *and* spake, and said unto his counsellors, Did not we cast three men bound into the midst of the fire? They answered and said unto the king, True, O king.

25 He answered and said, Lo, I see four men loose, walking in the midst of the fire, and they have [f]no hurt; and the [g]form of the fourth is like [h]the Son of God.

(4) *The convinced king.*

26 Then Nebuchadnezzar came near to the mouth of the burning fiery furnace, *and* spake, and said, Shadrach, Meshach, and Abed-nego, ye servants [i]of the most high God, come forth, and come *hither*. Then Shadrach, Meshach,

B.C. 580.

a Cf. the conduct of Daniel, Dan 2:24.
b Dan. 2:49.
c Cf. Dan. 6:19-22; Isa. 51:12-13; Jer. 30:7-9.
d Job 13:15; Acts 4:19.
e Ex. 20:3-5; Lev. 19:4.
f Isa. 43:2.
g Phil. 2:6-8.
h Or, *a Son of God.*
i Cf. Dan. 4:2, 3, 17, 34, 35.

[1] **(3:17)** The three Jews, faithful to God while the nation of Israel far from their land bear no testimony, are a fit type of the Jewish remnant in the last days (Isa. 1:9; Rom. 11:5), who will be faithful in the furnace of the great tribulation (Psa. 2:5; Rev. 7:14).

and Abed-nego, [a]came forth of the midst of the fire.

27 And the princes, governors, and captains, and the king's counsellors, being gathered together, saw these men, upon whose bodies the fire had no power, nor was an hair of their head singed, neither were their coats changed, nor the smell of fire had passed on them.

28 *Then* Nebuchadnezzar spake, and said, Blessed *be* the God of Shadrach, Meshach, and Abed-nego, who hath sent his [b]angel, and delivered his servants that trusted in him, and have changed the king's word, and yielded their bodies, that they might not serve nor worship any god, except their own God.

(5) *The decree of Nebuchadnezzar.*

29 Therefore I make a decree, That every people, nation, and language, which speak any thing amiss against the God of Shadrach, Meshach, and Abed-nego, shall be cut in pieces, and their houses shall be made a dunghill: because there is no other God that can deliver after this sort.

30 Then the king promoted Shadrach, Meshach, and Abed-nego, in the province of Babylon.

CHAPTER 4.

(6) *The king's proclamation.*

Nebuchadnezzar the king, [c]unto all people, nations, and languages, that [1]dwell in all the earth; Peace be multiplied unto you.

2 I thought it good to shew the signs and wonders that the high God hath wrought toward me.

3 How great *are* his signs! and how mighty *are* his wonders! his kingdom *is* an [d]everlasting kingdom, and his dominion *is* from generation to generation.

(7) *The tree vision of Nebuchadnezzar.*

4 I Nebuchadnezzar was at rest in mine house, and flourishing in my palace:

5 I saw a dream which made me afraid, and the thoughts upon my bed and the visions of my head troubled me.

B.C. 580.

a *Miracles* (O.T.). vs. 19-27; Dan. 6:16-23. (Gen. 5:24; Jon. 2:1-10.)

b Heb. 1:4, *note.*

c Cf. Dan. 2:37, 38; 3:29.

d 2 Sam. 7:16; Psa. 89:35-37; Dan. 7:13, 14; Lk. 1:31-33.

e Cf. Dan. 2:1, 2.

f Symbol of a great king. (Ezk. 31:1-14.) See v. 22.

g vs. 17, 23; plural in 17.

h *Sanctify, holy* (O.T.). Joel 1:14. (Gen. 2:3; Zech. 8:3.)

i Cf. Mt. 3:10; 7:19; Lk. 13:6-10.

j The number of completeness.

6 Therefore made I a decree [e]to bring in all the wise *men* of Babylon before me, that they might make known unto me the interpretation of the dream.

7 Then came in the magicians, the astrologers, the Chaldeans, and the soothsayers: and I told the dream before them; but they did not make known unto me the interpretation thereof.

8 But at the last Daniel came in before me, whose name *was* Belteshazzar, according to the name of my god, and in whom *is* the spirit of the holy gods: and before him I told the dream, *saying,*

9 O Belteshazzar, master of the magicians, because I know that the spirit of the holy gods *is* in thee, and no secret troubleth thee, tell me the visions of my dream that I have seen, and the interpretation thereof.

10 Thus *were* the visions of mine head in my bed; I saw, and behold a [f]tree in the midst of the earth, and the height thereof *was* great.

11 The tree grew, and was strong, and the height thereof reached unto heaven, and the sight thereof to the end of all the earth:

12 The leaves thereof *were* fair, and the fruit thereof much, and in it *was* meat for all: the beasts of the field had shadow under it, and the fowls of the heaven dwelt in the boughs thereof, and all flesh was fed of it.

13 I saw in the visions of my head upon my bed, and, behold, a [g]watcher and an [h]holy one came down from heaven;

14 He cried aloud, and said thus, [i]Hew down the tree, and cut off his branches, shake off his leaves, and scatter his fruit: let the beasts get away from under it, and the fowls from his branches:

15 Nevertheless leave the stump of his roots in the earth, even with a band of iron and brass, in the tender grass of the field; and let it be wet with the dew of heaven, and *let* his portion *be* with the beasts in the grass of the earth:

16 Let his heart be changed from man's, and let a beast's heart be given unto him; and let [j]seven times pass over him.

[1] **(4:1)** Nebuchadnezzar, first of the Gentile world-kings in whom the times of the Gentiles (Lk. 21:24; Rev. 16:14) began, perfectly comprehended the universality of the sway committed to him (Dan. 2:37, 38); as also did Cyrus (Ezra 1:2). That they did not actually subject the known earth to their sway is true, but they might have done so. The earth lay in their power.

B.C. 570.

17 This matter *is* by the decree of the watchers, and the demand by the word of the holy ones: to the intent [a]that the living may know [b]that the most High ruleth in the kingdom of men, and giveth it to whomsoever he will, and setteth up over it the basest of men.

18 This dream I king Nebuchadnezzar have seen. Now thou, O Belteshazzar, declare the interpretation thereof, forasmuch as all the wise *men* of my kingdom are not able to make known unto me the interpretation: but thou *art* able; for the spirit of the holy gods *is* in thee.

(8) *The tree vision interpreted.*

19 Then Daniel, whose name *was* Belteshazzar, was astonied for one hour, and his thoughts troubled him. The king spake, and said, Belteshazzar, let not the dream, or the interpretation thereof, trouble thee. Belteshazzar answered and said, My lord, [c]the dream *be* to them that hate thee, and the interpretation thereof to thine enemies.

20 The tree that thou sawest, which grew, and was strong, whose height reached unto the heaven, and the sight thereof to all the earth;

21 Whose leaves *were* fair, and the fruit thereof much, and in it *was* meat for all; under which the beasts of the field dwelt, and upon whose branches the fowls of the heaven had their habitation:

22 It *is* thou, O king, that art grown and become strong: for thy greatness is grown, and reacheth unto heaven, and thy dominion to the end of the earth.

23 And whereas the king saw a watcher and an holy one coming down from heaven, and saying, Hew the tree down, and destroy it; yet leave the stump of the roots thereof in the earth, even with a band of iron and brass, in the tender grass of the field; and let it be wet with the dew of heaven, and *let* his portion *be* with the beasts of the field, till seven times pass over him;

24 This *is* the interpretation, O king, and this *is* the decree of the most High, which is come upon my lord the king:

25 That they shall drive thee from men, and thy dwelling shall be with the beasts of the field, and they shall make thee to eat grass as oxen, and they shall wet thee with the dew of heaven, and seven times shall pass over thee, [d]till thou know that the most High ruleth in the kingdom of men, and giveth it to whomsoever he will.

26 And whereas they commanded to leave the stump of the tree roots; thy kingdom shall be sure unto thee, after that thou shalt have known that the heavens do rule.

27 Wherefore, O king, let my counsel be acceptable unto thee, and [e]break off thy sins by righteousness, and thine iniquities by shewing mercy to the poor; if it may be a lengthening of thy tranquillity.

(9) *The tree vision fulfilled: restoration of Nebuchadnezzar.*

28 All this came upon the king Nebuchadnezzar.

29 At the end of twelve months he walked in the palace of the kingdom of Babylon.

30 The king spake, and said, Is not this great Babylon, that [f]I have built for the house of the kingdom by the might of my power, and for the honour of my majesty?

31 [g]While the word *was* in the king's mouth, there fell a voice from heaven, *saying,* [h]O king Nebuchadnezzar, to thee it is spoken; The kingdom is departed from thee.

32 And they shall drive thee from men, and thy dwelling *shall be* with the beasts of the field: they shall make thee to eat grass as oxen, and seven times shall pass over thee, until thou know that the most High ruleth in the kingdom of men, and giveth it to whomsoever he will.

33 The same hour was the thing fulfilled upon Nebuchadnezzar: and he was driven from men, and did eat grass as oxen, and his body was wet with the dew of heaven, till his hairs were grown like eagles' *feathers,* and his nails like birds' *claws.*

34 And at the end of the days I Nebuchadnezzar lifted up mine eyes unto heaven, and mine understanding returned unto me, and [1]I blessed the most High, and I praised and honoured

a Psa. 9:16; 83:18.
b vs. 25, 32; Dan. 2:21; 5:21.
c See 2 Sam. 18:32; Jer. 29:7.
d The discipline was effective. Cf. v. 30 with v. 37.
e Isa. 55:7; Rom. 2:9-11.
f Cf. v. 37.
g 1 Thes. 5:3.
h Cf. Lk. 12:19, 20.

[1] **(4:34)** A progress may be traced in Nebuchadnezzar's apprehension of the true God. (1) "God is a God of gods [one amongst the national or tribal gods, but greater than they], and a Lord [Adonai = Master] of kings, and a revealer of secrets" (Dan. 2:47). (2) He is still a Hebrew deity, but Master of

him that liveth for ever, whose dominion
is [a]an everlasting dominion, and his kingdom *is* from generation to generation:
35 And all the inhabitants of the earth
are reputed as nothing: and he doeth
according to his will in the army of
heaven, and *among* the inhabitants of the
earth: and none can stay his hand, or say
unto him, What doest thou?
36 At the same time my reason
returned unto me; and for the glory of
my kingdom, mine honour and brightness returned unto me; and my counsellors and my lords sought unto me; and I
was established in my kingdom, and
excellent majesty was added unto me.
37 Now I Nebuchadnezzar praise and
extol and honour the King of heaven, all
whose works *are* truth, and his ways
judgment: [b]and those that walk in pride
he is able to abase.

CHAPTER 5.

Part III. The personal history of Daniel under Belshazzar and Darius (Dan. 5:1–6:28). *The pride of Belshazzar and his downfall.*

Belshazzar the king made a great feast
to a thousand of his lords, and
drank wine before the thousand.
2 Belshazzar, whiles he tasted the
wine, commanded to bring the golden
and silver vessels which his [c]father
Nebuchadnezzar had taken out of the
temple which *was* in Jerusalem; that the
king, and his princes, his wives, and his
concubines, might drink therein.
3 Then they brought the golden vessels
that were taken out of the temple of the
house of God which *was* at Jerusalem;
and the king, and his princes, his wives,
and his concubines, drank in them.
4 They drank wine, and praised the
gods of gold, and of silver, of brass, of
iron, of wood, and of stone.

(1) *The writing on the wall.*

5 [d]In the same hour came forth fingers
of a man's hand, and wrote over against
the candlestick upon the plaister of the
wall of the king's palace: and the king
saw the part of the hand that wrote.
6 Then the king's countenance was
changed, [e]and his thoughts troubled
him, so that the joints of his loins were
loosed, and his knees smote one against
another.
7 The king cried aloud to bring in the
[f]astrologers, the Chaldeans, and the
soothsayers. *And* the king spake, and
said to the wise *men* of Babylon,
Whosoever shall read this writing, and
shew me the interpretation thereof, shall
be clothed with scarlet, and *have* a chain
of gold about his neck, and shall be the
third ruler in the kingdom.
8 Then came in all the king's wise *men*:
but they could not read the writing, nor
make known to the king the interpretation thereof.
9 Then was king Belshazzar greatly
troubled, and his [g]countenance was
changed in him, and his lords were
astonied.
10 *Now* the queen, by reason of the
words of the king and his lords, came
into the banquet house: *and* the queen
spake and said, O king, live for ever: let
not thy thoughts trouble thee, nor let thy
countenance be changed:
11 There is a man in thy kingdom, in
whom *is* the spirit of the holy gods; and
in the days of [h]thy father light and
understanding and wisdom, like the
wisdom of the gods, was found in him;
whom the king Nebuchadnezzar thy
father, the king, *I say*, thy father, made
master of the magicians, astrologers,
Chaldeans, *and* soothsayers;
12 Forasmuch as an excellent spirit,
and knowledge, and understanding,
interpreting of dreams, and shewing of
hard sentences, and dissolving of
[i]doubts, were found in the same Daniel,
whom the king named Belteshazzar:
now let Daniel be called, and he will
shew the interpretation.
13 Then was Daniel brought in before
the king. *And* the king spake and said
unto Daniel, *Art* thou that Daniel, which
art of the children of the captivity of
Judah, whom the king [h]my father
brought out of Jewry?
14 I have even heard of thee, that the
spirit of the gods *is* in thee, and *that* ligh

B.C. 563.

a Dan. 2:44; 7:14; Psa. 10:16; Mic. 4:7; Lk. 1:33.

b Dan. 5:20; Ex. 18:11.

c Nebuchadnezzar was "father" of Belshazzar in the biblical sense that David is called "father" of Jesus (Lk. 1:32). B. was probably a grandson.

d Lk. 12:19, 20; 1 Thes 5:2, 3.

e Cf. Isa. 21:1-4.

f Isa. 47:13.

g Chald. *brightnesses*. v. 6.

h Or, *grandfather*. v. 2.

i Chald. *knots*.

angels, and a God who responds to faith (Dan. 3:28). (3) Here (Dan. 4:34, 35) the king rises into true apprehension of God. Cf. Darius, Dan. 6:25-27.

and understanding and excellent wisdom is found in thee.
15 And now the wise *men,* the
astrologers, have been brought in before
me, that they should read this writing,
and make known unto me the interpretation thereof: but they could not shew
the interpretation of the thing:
16 And I have heard of thee, that thou
canst make interpretations, and dissolve
doubts: now if thou canst read the writing, and make known to me the interpretation thereof, thou shalt be clothed
with scarlet, and *have* a chain of gold
about thy neck, and shalt be the third
ruler in the kingdom.

(2) *The writing interpreted.*

17 Then Daniel answered and said
before the king, Let thy gifts be to thyself, and give thy rewards to another; yet
I will read the writing unto the king, and
make known to him the interpretation.
18 O thou king, the most high [a]God
gave Nebuchadnezzar thy father a kingdom, and majesty, and glory, and honour:
19 And for the majesty that he gave
him, all people, nations, and languages,
trembled and feared before him: whom
he would he slew; and whom he would
he kept alive; and whom he would he
set up; and whom he would he put
down.
20 But when his heart was lifted up,
and his mind hardened in pride, he was
deposed from his kingly throne, and
they took his glory from him:
21 And he was driven from the sons of
men; and his heart was made like the
beasts, and his dwelling *was* with the
wild asses: they fed him with grass like
oxen, and his body was wet with the
dew of heaven; till he knew that the
most high God ruled in the kingdom of
men, and *that* he appointeth over it
whomsoever he will.
22 And thou his son, O Belshazzar,
hast not humbled thine heart, though
thou knewest all this;
23 But hast [b]lifted up thyself against
the Lord of heaven; and they have
brought the [c]vessels of his house before
thee, and thou, and thy lords, thy wives,
and thy concubines, have drunk wine in
them; and thou hast praised the gods of
silver, and gold, of brass, iron, wood,
and stone, which see not, nor hear, nor
know: [d]and the God in whose hand thy
breath *is,* and whose *are* all thy ways,
hast thou not glorified:
24 Then was the part of the hand sent
from him; and this writing was written.
25 And this *is* the writing that was
written, MENE, MENE, TEKEL,
UPHARSIN.
26 This *is* the interpretation of the
thing: MENE; God hath numbered thy
kingdom, and finished it.
27 TEKEL; Thou art weighed in the
balances, and art found wanting.
28 PERES; Thy kingdom is divided,
and [e]given to the Medes and Persians.
29 Then commanded Belshazzar, and
they clothed Daniel with scarlet, and *put*
a chain of gold about his neck, and made
a proclamation concerning him, that he
should be the third ruler in the kingdom.
30 In that night was Belshazzar the
king of the Chaldeans slain.
31 And [1]Darius the Median took the
kingdom, *being* about threescore and
two years old.

B.C. 538.

a Jer. 27:5-7; Dan. 2:37, 38.

b Num. 14:41; Job 9:4.

c Ex. 40:9; Num. 18:3; Isa. 52:11; Heb. 9:21.

d Rom. 1:21; 3:23.

e Foretold, Isa. 21:2. Cf. v. 31, and Dan. 9:1.

[1] **(5:31)** The biblical order of the monarchs of Daniel's time, and of the period of the captivity and restoration of Judah, is as follows:

(1) Nebuchadnezzar (B.C. 604-561) with whom the captivity of Judah and the "times of the Gentiles" (Lk. 21:24, *note;* Rev. 16:19, *note*) began, and who established the first of the four world-monarchies (Dan. 2:37, 38; 7:4).

(2) Belshazzar (prob. B.C. 556), the Bel-shar-uzzar of the inscriptions, grandson of Nebuchadnezzar, and son of the victorious general Nabonidus. Belshazzar seems to have reigned as viceroy.

(3) Darius the Mede (Dan. 5:31; 6:1-27; 9:1). Concerning this Darius secular history awaits further discoveries, as formerly in the case of Belshazzar. He has been conjectured to be identical with Gobryas, a Persian general. This Darius was "the son of Ahasuerus, of the seed of the Medes, which was made king over the realm of the Chaldeans" (Dan. 9:1). "Ahasuerus," more a title than a name, the equivalent of the modern "Majesty," is used in Scripture of at least four personages, and is Persian rather than Median. That Darius the Mede was the "son" (or grandson) of an Ahasuerus proves no more than that

CHAPTER 6.

B.C. 538.

History of Daniel to the accession of Cyrus.

It pleased Darius to set [a]over the kingdom an hundred and twenty princes, which should be over the whole kingdom;

2 And over these three presidents; of whom Daniel *was* first: that the princes might give accounts unto them, and the king should have no damage.

3 Then this Daniel was preferred above the presidents and princes, because an excellent spirit *was* in him; and the king thought to set him over the whole realm.

(1) *The decree of Darius.*

4 Then the presidents and princes sought to find occasion against Daniel concerning the kingdom; but they could find none occasion nor fault; forasmuch as he *was* faithful, neither was there any error or fault found in him.

5 Then said these men, [b]We shall not find any occasion against this Daniel, except we find *it* against him concerning the law of his God.

6 Then these presidents and princes assembled together to the king, and said thus unto him, King Darius, live for ever.

7 All the presidents of the kingdom, the governors, and the princes, the counsellors, and the captains, have consulted together to establish a royal statute, and to make a firm decree, that whosoever shall ask a petition of any God or man for thirty days, [c]save of thee, O king, he shall be cast into the den of lions.

8 Now, O king, establish the decree, and sign the writing, that it be not changed, [d]according to the law of the Medes and Persians, which altereth not.

9 Wherefore king Darius signed the writing and the decree.

(2) *The steadfastness of Daniel.*

10 Now when Daniel [e]knew that the writing was signed, he went into his house; and his windows being open in his chamber [f]toward Jerusalem, he kneeled upon his knees three times a day, and prayed, and gave thanks before his God, as he did aforetime.

11 Then these men assembled, and found Daniel praying and making supplication before his God.

12 Then they came near, and spake before the king concerning the king's decree; Hast thou not signed a decree, that every man that shall ask *a petition* of any God or man within thirty days, save of thee, O king, shall be cast into the den of lions? The king answered and said, The thing *is* true, according to the law of the Medes and Persians, which altereth not.

13 Then answered they and said before the king, That Daniel, which *is* [g]of the children of the captivity of Judah, regardeth not thee, O king, nor the decree that thou hast signed, but maketh his petition three times a day.

14 Then the king, when he heard *these* words, was sore displeased with himself, and set *his* heart on Daniel to deliver him: and he [h]laboured till the going down of the sun to deliver him.

15 Then these men assembled unto the king, and said unto the king, Know, O king, that the law of the Medes and Persians *is*, That no decree nor statute which the king establisheth may be changed.

(3) *Daniel cast into the lions' den.*

16 Then the king commanded, and they brought Daniel, and cast *him* into the den of lions. *Now* the king spake and said unto Daniel, Thy God whom thou servest continually, he will [i]deliver thee.

17 And a stone was brought, and laid upon the mouth of the den; and the king sealed it with his own signet, and with the signet of his lords; that the purpose might not be changed concerning Daniel.

a Cf. Esth. 1:1.
b Acts 24:13-21; 1 Pet. 4:12-16.
c Rev. 13:15.
d Esth. 1:19.
e Acts 20:22-24.
f 1 Ki. 8:29, 30, 46-48; Psa. 5:7; Jon. 2:4.
g Dan. 5:13.
h Psa. 49:7.
i Psa. 34:7, 19; 37:39, 40; 50:15; Mt. 27:43; Col. 1:13; 1 Thes. 1:10; 2 Pet. 2:9.

he was, probably through his mother, of the seed royal not only of Media, but also of Persia. There is but one Darius in Daniel. (See Dan. 9:1.)

(4) Cyrus, with whose rise to power came fully into existence the Medo-Persian, second of the world-empires (Dan. 2:39; 7:5). In Daniel's vision of this empire in "the third year of the reign of King Belshazzar" (Dan. 8:1-4) the Median power of Darius is seen as the lesser of the two horns of the ram, the Persian power of Cyrus, under whom the Medo-Persian power was consolidated, as the "higher" horn which "came up last." Under Cyrus, who was prophetically named more than a century before his birth (Isa. 44:28–45:1-4), the return to Palestine of the Jewish remnant began (Ezra 1:1-4). See Dan 11:2, marg. *ref.*

(4) *The delivering God.*

18 Then the king went to his palace, and passed the night fasting: neither were instruments of musick brought before him: and his sleep went from him.

19 Then the [a]king arose very early in the morning, and went in haste unto the den of lions.

20 And when he came to the den, he cried with a lamentable voice unto Daniel: *and* the king spake and said to Daniel, O Daniel, servant of the living God, is thy God, whom thou servest continually, able to deliver thee from the lions?

21 Then said Daniel unto the king, O king, live for ever.

22 My God hath [b]sent his [c]angel, and hath shut the lions' mouths, that they have not hurt me: forasmuch as before him innocency was found in me; and also before thee, O king, have I done no hurt.

23 Then was the king exceeding glad for him, and commanded that they should take Daniel up out of the den. So Daniel was taken up out of the den, and no manner of hurt was found upon him, because he believed in his God.

24 And the king commanded, and they brought those men which had accused Daniel, and they cast *them* into the den of lions, them, their children, and their wives; and the lions had the mastery of them, and brake all their bones in pieces or ever they came at the bottom of the den.

(5) *The decree of Darius.*

25 Then king Darius wrote [d]unto all people, nations, and languages, that dwell in all the earth; Peace be multiplied unto you.

26 I make a decree, [e]That in every dominion of my kingdom men tremble and fear before the God of Daniel: for he *is* the living God, and stedfast for ever, and his kingdom *that* which shall not be destroyed, and his dominion *shall be even* unto the end.

27 He delivereth and rescueth, and he worketh signs and wonders in heaven and in earth, who hath delivered Daniel from the power of the lions.

28 So this Daniel prospered in the reign of Darius, and in the reign of Cyrus the Persian.

B.C. 537.

a Cf. Dan. 3:17, 24.

b *Miracles* (O.T.). vs. 16-23; Jon. 2:1-10. (Gen. 5:24; Jon. 2:1-10)

c Heb. 1:4, *note.*

d Dan. 4:1, *note.*

e Cf. Dan. 2:47; 3:28, 29; 4:1-3, 34, 35.

f Cf. Rev. 1:19.

g *Times (of the Gentiles).* vs. 1-27; Rev. 16:19. (Lk. 21:24; Rev. 16:19.)

h Cf. v. 17.

i Jer. 4:7 with Jer. 25:9.

j Ezk. 17:3 with Ezk. 17:12.

k Dan. 4:16, 34.

l A reference to the threefold dominion of the second empire, Media, Persia, Babylonia.

m i.e. Lydia, Babylonia, Egypt, etc.

n Swiftness of Alexander's conquests.

o Cf. Dan. 8:22.

p A horn symbolizes a king. Cf. Rev. 17:12.

CHAPTER 7.

Part IV. The visions of Daniel (Dan. 7:1–12:13). *The beast vision of Daniel.*

In the first year of Belshazzar king of Babylon Daniel had a dream and visions of his head upon his bed: [f]then he wrote the dream, *and* told the sum of the matters.

2 Daniel spake and said, [g]I saw in my vision by night, and, behold, the four winds of the heaven strove upon the [1]great sea.

3 And [h]four great beasts came up from the sea, diverse one from another.

(1) *The world-empire of Nebuchadnezzar.* (Cf. Dan. 2:37, 38.)

4 The first *was* like a [i]lion, and had [j]eagle's wings: I beheld till the wings thereof were plucked, and it was lifted up from the earth, and made stand upon the feet as a man, and a [k]man's heart was given to it.

(2) *The world-empire of Media-Persia.* (Cf. Dan. 2:39.)

5 And behold another beast, a second, like to a bear, and it raised up itself on one side, and *it had* [l]three ribs in the mouth of it between the teeth of it: and they said thus unto it, Arise, [m]devour much flesh.

(3) *The world-empire of Greece under Alexander.* (Cf. Dan. 2:39; 8:20-22; 10:20; 11:2-4.)

6 After this I beheld, and lo another, like a [n]leopard, which had upon the back of it four wings of a fowl; the beast had also [o]four heads; and dominion was given to it.

(4) *The Roman world-empire.* (Cf. vs. 23, 24; Dan. 2:40-43.)

7 After this I saw in the night visions, and behold a fourth beast, dreadful and terrible, and strong exceedingly; and it had great iron teeth: it devoured and brake in pieces, and stamped the residue with the feet of it: and it *was* diverse from all the beasts that *were* before it; and it had ten [p]horns.

(5) *The ten kings* (vs. 24) *and the "little horn"* (vs. 24-27). See v. 14, *note.*

8 I considered the horns, and, behold,

[1](7:2) The "sea" in Scripture imagery stands for the populace, the mere unorganized mass of mankind (Mt. 13:47; Rev. 13:1).

there came up among them another [1a]little horn, before whom there were three of the first horns plucked up by the roots: and, behold, in this horn *were* eyes like the eyes of man, and a mouth speaking great things.

(6) *The vision of the coming of the Son of man in glory.* (Cf. Mt. 24:27-30; 25:31-34; Rev. 19:11-21.)

9 I beheld till the thrones were [b]cast down, and the Ancient of days did sit, whose garment *was* white as snow, and the hair of his head like the pure wool: his [c]throne *was like* the fiery flame, *and* his wheels *as* burning fire.

10 A fiery stream issued and came forth from before him: thousand thousands ministered unto him, and ten thousand times ten thousand stood before him: the judgment was set, and the books were opened.

11 I beheld then because of the voice of the great words which the horn spake: I beheld *even* till the beast was slain, and his body destroyed, and given to the burning flame.

12 As concerning the rest of the beasts, they had their dominion taken away: yet their lives were prolonged for a season and time.

Scene in heaven before the coming of the Son of man in vs. 9-12.

13 I [d]saw in the night visions, and, behold, *one* like the Son of man came with the clouds of heaven, and came to the Ancient of days, [2]and they brought him near before him.

14 And there was given [3]him dominion, and glory, and a kingdom, that all people, nations, and languages, should serve him: his [e]dominion *is* an everlasting dominion, which shall not pass away, and his kingdom *that* which shall not be destroyed.

(7) *The interpretation of the beast vision.*

15 I Daniel was grieved in my spirit in the midst of *my* body, and the visions of my head troubled me.

16 I came near unto one of them that stood by, and asked him the truth of all this. So he told me, and made me know the interpretation of the things.

17 These great [4]beasts, which are four, *are* four kings, *which* shall arise out of the earth.

B.C. 555.

a *The Beast.* vs. 20-26. (Dan. 7:8; Rev. 19:20.)

b *placed.*

c *Kingdom* (O.T.). vs. 9, 13, 14; Hos. 3:4, 5. (Gen. 1:26; Zech. 12:8.)

d Cf. Rev. 5:6-10.

e *Christ (Second Advent).* vs. 13, 14; Hos. 3:4, 5. (Deut. 30:3; Acts 1:9-11.)

[1] **(7:8)** The vision is of the end of Gentile world-dominion. The former Roman empire (the iron kingdom of Dan. 2:33-35, 40-44; 7:7) will have ten horns (i.e. kings, Rev. 17:12), corresponding to the ten toes of the image. As Daniel considers this vision of the ten kings, there rises up amongst them a "little horn" (king), who subdues three of the ten kings so completely that the separate identity of their kingdoms is destroyed. Seven kings of the ten are left, and the "little horn." He is the "king of fierce countenance" typified by that other "king of fierce countenance," Antiochus Epiphanes, Dan. 8:23-25; the "prince that shall come" of Dan. 9:26, 27; the "king" of Dan. 11:36-45; the "abomination" of Dan. 12:11 and Mt. 24:15; the "man of sin" of 2 Thes. 2:4-8, and the "Beast" of Rev. 13:4-10. See "Beast" (Dan. 7:8; Rev. 19:20).

[2] **(7:13)** This scene is identical with that of Rev. 5:6-10. There the ascription of praise of the "kings and priests" (cf. v. 18, *ref. a*) ends with the words, "and we shall reign on the earth." Rev. 6 opens the "vexing" of Psa. 2:5, introductory to setting the king on Zion (Psa. 2:6; Rev. 20:4). The vision (Dan. 7:9-14) reverses the order of events as they will be fulfilled. Verse 13 describes the scene in heaven (cf. Rev. 5:6-10) which, in fulfilment, precedes the events which Daniel sees in vision in vs. 9-12. The historic order will be: (1) The investiture of the Son of man with the kingdom (Dan. 7:13, 14; Rev. 5:6-10). (2) The "vexing" of Psa. 2:5, fully described in Mt. 24:21, 22; Rev. 6–18. (3) The return of the Son of man in glory to deliver the "smiting" blow of Dan. 2:45 (Dan. 7:9-11; Rev. 19:11-21). (4) The judgment of the nations and the setting up of the kingdom (Dan. 7:10, 26, 27; Mt. 25:31-46; Rev. 20:1-6).

[3] **(7:14)** Dan. 7:3, 14 is identical with Rev. 5:1-7, and antedates the fulfilment of Dan. 2:34, 35. Dan. 7:13, 14 and Rev. 5:1-7 describe the investiture of the Son of man and Son of David with the kingdom authority, while Dan. 2:34, 35 describes the crushing blow (*Armageddon*, Rev. 16:14, *refs.*) which destroys Gentile world-power, thus clearing the way for the actual setting up of the kingdom of heaven. Dan. 2:34, 35 and Rev. 19:19-21 are the same event.

[4] **(7:17)** The monarchy vision of Nebuchadnezzar (Dan. 2) covers the same historic order as the beast vision of Daniel, but with this difference: Nebuchadnezzar saw the imposing outward power and

18 But the [a]saints of the most High shall take the kingdom, and possess the kingdom for ever, even for ever and ever.

19 Then I would [b]know the truth of the fourth beast, which was diverse from all the others, exceeding dreadful, whose teeth *were of* iron, and his nails *of* brass; *which* devoured, brake in pieces, and stamped the residue with his feet;

20 And of the ten horns that *were* in his head, and *of* the other which came up, and before whom three fell; even *of* that [c]horn that had eyes, and a mouth that spake very great things, whose look *was* more stout than his fellows.

21 I beheld, and the same horn made war with the saints, and prevailed against them;

22 Until the Ancient of days came, and [d]judgment was given to the saints of the most High; and the time came that the saints possessed the kingdom.

23 Thus he said, The fourth beast shall be the fourth kingdom upon earth, which shall be diverse from all kingdoms, and shall devour the whole earth, and shall tread it down, and break it in pieces.

24 And the [e]ten horns out of this kingdom *are* ten kings *that* shall arise: and [f]another shall rise after them; and he shall be diverse from the first, and he shall subdue three kings.

25 And he [g]shall speak *great* words against the most High, and shall wear out the saints of the most High, and think to change times and laws: and they shall be given into his hand until a time and times and the dividing of time.

26 But the [h]judgment shall sit, [1]and they shall take away his dominion, to consume and to destroy *it* unto the end.

27 And the kingdom and dominion, and the greatness of the kingdom under the whole heaven, shall be given to the people of the saints of the most High, whose kingdom *is* an [i]everlasting kingdom, and all dominions shall serve and obey him.

28 Hitherto *is* the end of the matter. As for me Daniel, my cogitations much troubled me, and my countenance changed in me: but I kept the matter in my heart.

CHAPTER 8.

The ram and rough goat vision.
(Dan. 8:1-27). (1) *The vision.*

In the [j]third year of the reign of king Belshazzar a [2]vision appeared unto me, *even unto* me Daniel, after that which appeared unto me at the first.

2 And I saw in a vision; and it came to pass, when I saw, that I *was* at Shushan *in* the palace, which *is* in the province of Elam; and I saw in a vision, and I was by the river of Ulai.

3 Then I lifted up mine eyes, and saw, and, behold, there stood before the river a [k]ram which had *two* horns: and the *two*

B.C. 555.

a vs. 18, 22, 25, 27. That church saints will also share in the rule seems clear from Acts 16:17; Rom. 8:17; 2 Tim. 2:10-12; 1 Pet. 2:9; Rev. 1:6; 3:21; 5:10; 20:4-6.

b See *note* 4, p. 910.

c The Beast. vs. 20-26. Dan. 8:19-25. (Dan. 7:8; Rev. 19:20.)

d Judgments (the seven). Joel 3:1-14. (2 Sam. 7:14; Rev. 22:12.)

e Rev. 13:1.

f v. 8.

g Rev. 13:1-6.

h See Dan. 2:35, *ref. c.*

i Dan. 4:3, *ref. d.*

j About B.C. 530.

k v. 20.

splendour of the "times of the Gentiles" (Lk. 21:24; Rev. 16:19), while Daniel saw the true character of Gentile world-government as rapacious and warlike, established and maintained by force. It is remarkable that the heraldic insignia of the Gentile nations are all beasts or birds of prey.

[1] **(7:26)** The end of Gentile world-power. (1) In the beast vision of Daniel 7 the fourth beast (v. 7) is declared to be "the fourth kingdom," i.e. the Roman empire, the "iron" kingdom of Dan. 2. The "ten horns" upon the fourth beast (Roman empire), v. 7, are declared to be "ten kings that shall arise" (v. 24) answering to the ten toes of the image vision of Dan. 2. The ten kingdoms, covering the regions formerly ruled by Rome, will constitute, therefore, the form in which the fourth or Roman empire will exist when the whole fabric of Gentile world-domination is smitten by the "stone cut out without hands" = Christ (Dan. 2:44, 45; 7:9). (2) But Daniel sees a "little horn" rise up and subdue three of the ten kings (vs. 24-26). His distinguishing mark is hatred of God and of the saints. He is not to be confounded with the "little horn" of Dan. 8—a prophecy fulfilled in Antiochus Epiphanes (Dan. 8:9, *note*). In Rev. 13 additional particulars of the "little horn" of Dan. 7 are given (Rev. 13:1, *note*).

[2] **(8:1)** The eighth chapter gives details concerning the second and third world-kingdoms the silver and brass kingdoms of Dan. 2; the bear and leopard kingdoms of Dan. 7, viz., the Medo-Persian and Macedonian kingdoms of history. At the time of this vision (Dan. 8:1) the first monarchy was nearing its end. Belshazzar was the last king of that monarchy.

horns *were* high; but one *was* higher than
the other, and the higher came up last.
4 I saw the ram pushing westward,
and northward, and southward; so that
no beasts might stand before him, neither *was there any* that could deliver out
of his hand; but he did according to his
will, and became great.
5 And as I was considering, behold, an
he [a]goat came from the west on the face
of the whole earth, and touched not the
ground: and the goat *had* a notable horn
between his eyes.
6 And he came to the ram that had *two*
horns, which I had seen standing before
the river, and ran unto him in the fury of
his power.
7 And I saw him come close unto the
ram, and he was moved with choler
against him, and smote the ram, and
brake his two horns: and there was no
power in the ram to stand before him, but
he cast him down to the ground, and
stamped upon him: and there was none
that could deliver the ram out of his hand.
8 Therefore the he goat waxed very
great: and when he was strong, the
[a]great horn was broken; and for it came
up [b]four notable ones toward the four
winds of heaven.
9 And out of [c]one of them came forth
a [1]little horn, which waxed exceeding
great, toward the south, and toward the
east, and toward the pleasant *land*.
10 [2]And it waxed great, *even* to the
host of heaven; and it cast down *some* of
the host and of the stars to the ground,
and stamped upon them.
11 Yea, he magnified *himself* even to
the prince of the host, and by him the
daily *sacrifice* was taken away, and the
place of his sanctuary was cast down.
12 And an host was given *him* against
the [d]daily *sacrifice* by reason of transgression, and it cast down the truth to
the ground; and it practised, and prospered.
13 Then I heard one [e]saint speaking,
and another saint said unto that certain
saint which spake, How long *shall be* the
vision *concerning* the daily *sacrifice*, and
the transgression of [3]desolation, to give
both the sanctuary and the host to be
trodden under foot?
14 And he said unto me, Unto two
thousand and three hundred days; then
shall the sanctuary be cleansed.

(2) *The vision interpreted.*

15 And it came to pass, when I, *even* I
Daniel, had seen the vision, and sought
for the meaning, then, behold, there
stood before me as the appearance of a
[f]man.
16 And I heard a man's voice between

B.C. 553.

a v. 21.

b v. 22; Dan 7:6; 11:4.

c Antiochus Epiphanes came out of Syria, one of the "four notable" kingdoms into which Alexander's empire was divided.

d Cf. Dan. 9:27, where the. Beast comes into view.

e Or, *holy one, idem.* Dan. 4:13, 17.

f *The theophanies.* Dan. 10:18. (Gen. 12:7; Rev. 1:9.)

[1] **(8:9)** The "little horn" here is a prophecy fulfilled in Antiochus Epiphanes, B.C. 175, who profaned the temple and terribly persecuted the Jews. He is not to be confounded with the "little horn" of Dan. 7 who is yet to come, and who will dominate the earth during the great tribulation. See "The Beast," Dan. 7:8; Rev. 19:20, *notes*, and "The great tribulation," Psa. 2:5; Rev. 7:14, *note*. But Antiochus is a remarkable type of the Beast, the terrible "little horn" of the last days. Verses 24, 25 go beyond Antiochus and evidently refer to the "little horn" of Daniel 7. Both Antiochus and the Beast, but the Beast pre-eminently, are in view in verses 24, 25. That the "little horn" of Dan. 7 cannot be the little horn of Dan. 8:9-13, 23, is evident. The former comes up among the *ten* horns into which the *fourth* empire (Roman) is to be divided; the little horn of Dan. 8 comes out of one of the *four* kingdoms into which the *third* (Grecian) empire was divided (v. 23), and in "the latter time" of the four kingdoms (vs. 22, 23). This was historically true of Antiochus Epiphanes. They are alike in hatred of the Jews and of God, and in profaning the temple. Cf. 7:25 (the Beast) with 8:10-12 (Antiochus).

[2] **(8:10)** This passage (vs. 10-14) is confessedly the most difficult in prophecy, a difficulty increased by the present state of the text. Historically this was fulfilled in and by Antiochus Epiphanes, but in a more intense and final sense Antiochus but adumbrates the awful blasphemy of the "little horn" of Dan. 7:8, 24, 25; 9:27; 11:36-45; 12:11. In Daniel 8:10-14 the actions of both "little horns" blend.

[3] **(8:13)** Seven times in Daniel the "desolation" is spoken of: (1) Of the sanctuary, 8:13, fulfilled by Antiochus Epiphanes, B.C. 175-170. (2) Of the sanctuary, 9:17, the condition in Daniel's time, when the Jews were in exile and the sanctuary desolate. (3) Generally, of the land, 9:18, also referring to Daniel's time. (4) Of the sanctuary, 9:26, fulfilled A.D. 70, in the destruction of city and temple after the cutting

the banks of Ulai, which called, and said, [a]Gabriel, make this *man* to understand the vision.

17 So he came near where I stood: and when he came, I was afraid, and fell upon my face: but he said unto me, Understand, O son of man: for at the time of the end *shall be* the vision.

18 Now as he was speaking with me, I was in a deep sleep on my face toward the ground: but he touched me, and set me upright.

19 And he [b]said, Behold, I will make thee know what shall be in the last end of the indignation: for at the time appointed the [1]end *shall be.*

20 The [c]ram which thou sawest having *two* horns *are* the kings of Media and Persia.

21 And the rough goat *is* the king of Grecia: and the great horn that *is* between his eyes *is* the [d]first king.

22 Now that being broken, whereas four stood up for it, [e]four kingdoms shall stand up out of the nation, but not in his power.

23 And in the latter time of their kingdom, when the transgressors are come to the full, a [f]king of fierce countenance, and understanding dark sentences, shall stand up.

24 And his power shall be mighty, but not by his own power: and he shall destroy wonderfully, and shall prosper, and practise, and shall destroy the mighty and the holy people.

25 And through [g]his policy also he shall cause craft to prosper in his hand; and he shall magnify *himself* in his heart, and by peace shall destroy many: he shall [h]also stand up against the Prince of princes; but he shall be broken without hand.

26 And the vision of the evening and the morning which was told *is* true: wherefore shut thou up the vision; for it *shall be* for many days.

27 And I Daniel fainted, and was sick *certain* days; afterward I rose up, and did the king's business; and I was astonished at the vision, but none understood *it.*

B.C. 553.

a Dan. 9:21; Lk. 1:19, 26.

b v. 20.

c vs. 3, 4. The "higher" horn which "came up last" is Cyrus, the other "Darius the Mede."

d i.e. Alexander the Great.

e The four empires into which Alexander's empire was divided about B.C. 300; Greece, Asia Minor, including Syria, Egypt the East.

f i.e. Antiochus Epiphanes who arose out of Syria, one of the "four kingdoms," B.C. 170.

g *The Beast.* vs. 24, 25; Dan. 9:26, 27. (Dan. 7:8; Rev. 19:20.)

h Rev. 19:19, 20.

i Cf. Jer. 25:11, 12, *note.*

j *Bible prayers* (O.T.). Jon. 2:2. (Gen. 15:2; Hab. 3:1-16.)

CHAPTER 9.

Vision of the seventy weeks (vs. 1-27).

In the first year of Darius the son of Ahasuerus, of the seed of the Medes, which was made king over the realm of the Chaldeans;

2 In the first year of his reign I Daniel understood by books the number of the years, whereof the word of the LORD came to Jeremiah the prophet, that he would accomplish [i]seventy years in the desolations of Jerusalem.

(1) *Daniel's prayer and confession.*

3 And I set my face unto the Lord God, to seek by prayer and supplications, with fasting, and sackcloth, and ashes:

4 And I [j]prayed unto the LORD my God, and made my confession, and said, O Lord, the great and dreadful God, keeping the covenant and mercy to them that love him, and to them that keep his commandments;

5 We have sinned, and have committed iniquity, and have done wickedly, and have rebelled, even by departing from thy precepts and from thy judgments:

6 Neither have we hearkened unto thy servants the prophets, which spake in thy name to our kings, our princes, and our fathers, and to all the people of the land.

7 O Lord, righteousness *belongeth* unto thee, but unto us confusion of faces, as at this day; to the men of Judah, and to the inhabitants of Jerusalem, and unto all Israel, *that are* near, and *that are* far off, through all the countries whither thou hast driven them, because of their trespass that they have trespassed against thee.

8 O Lord, to us *belongeth* confusion of face, to our kings, to our princes, and to our fathers, because we have sinned against thee.

9 To the Lord our God *belong*

off of Messiah (Lk. 21:20). (5, 6, 7) Of the sanctuary, by the Beast, 9:27; 11:31; 12:11. (Cf. Mt. 24:15; Mk. 13:14; 2 Thes. 2:3, 8-12; Rev. 13:14, 15.)

[1]**(8:19)** Two "ends" are in view here: (1) historically, the end of the third, or Grecian empire of Alexander out of one of the divisions of which the little horn of verse 9 (Antiochus) arose; (2) prophetically, the end of the times of the Gentiles (Lk. 21:24; Rev. 16:14), when the "little horn" of Dan. 7:8, 24-26, the Beast, will arise—Daniel's *final* time of the end (Dan. 12:4, *note*).

B.C. 538.

mercies and forgivenesses, though we have rebelled against him;

10 Neither have we obeyed the voice of the LORD our God, to walk in his laws, which he set before us by his servants the prophets.

11 Yea, all Israel have transgressed thy law, even by departing, that they might not obey thy voice; therefore the curse is poured upon us, and the oath that *is* written in the [a]law of Moses the servant of God, because we have sinned against him.

12 And he hath confirmed his words, which he spake against us, and against our judges that judged us, by bringing upon us a great evil: for under the whole heaven hath not been done as hath been done upon Jerusalem.

13 As *it is* written in the law of Moses, all this evil is come upon us: yet made we not our prayer before the LORD our God, that we might turn from our iniquities, and understand thy truth.

14 Therefore hath the LORD watched upon the evil, and brought it upon us: for the LORD our God *is* righteous in all his works which he doeth: for we obeyed not his voice.

15 And now, O Lord our God, that hast brought thy people forth out of the land of Egypt with a mighty hand, and hast gotten thee renown, as at this day; we have sinned, we have done wickedly.

16 O Lord, according to all thy righteousness, I beseech thee, let thine anger and thy fury be turned away from thy city Jerusalem, thy holy mountain: because for our sins, and for the iniquities of our fathers, Jerusalem and thy people *are become* a reproach to all *that are* about us.

17 Now therefore, O our God, hear the prayer of thy servant, and his supplications, and cause thy face to shine upon thy sanctuary that is desolate, for the Lord's sake.

18 O my God, incline thine ear, and hear; open thine eyes, and behold our desolations, and the city which is called by thy name: for we do not present our supplications before thee for our righteousnesses, but for thy great mercies.

19 O Lord, hear; O Lord, forgive; O Lord, hearken and do; defer not, for thine own sake, O my God: for thy city and thy people are called by thy name.

(2) *The seventy weeks of years.*

20 And whiles I *was* speaking, and praying, and confessing my sin and the sin of my people Israel, and presenting my supplication before the LORD my God for the holy mountain of my God;

21 Yea, whiles I *was* speaking in prayer, even the man [b]Gabriel, whom I had seen in the vision at the beginning, being caused to fly swiftly, touched me about the time of the evening oblation.

22 And he informed *me*, and talked with me, and said, O Daniel, I am now come forth to give thee skill and understanding.

23 At the beginning of thy supplications the commandment came forth, and I am come to shew *thee*; for thou *art* greatly beloved: therefore understand the matter, and consider the vision.

24 Seventy [1]weeks are determined upon [c]thy people and upon thy holy

a *Law (of Moses).* vs. 8-13; Mt. 5:17, 18. (Ex. 19:1; Gal. 3:1-29.).

b Dan. 8:16; Lk. 1:19, 26.

c Cf. Hos. 1:9. The Jews, rejected, are "thy people," i.e. Daniel's, not Jehovah's, though yet to be restored.

[1] **(9:24)** These are "weeks" or, more accurately, sevens of years; seventy weeks of seven years each. Within these "weeks" the national chastisement must be ended and the nation re-established in everlasting righteousness (v. 24). The seventy weeks are divided into seven = 49 years; sixty-two = 434 years; one = 7 years (vs. 25-27). In the seven weeks = 49 years, Jerusalem was to be rebuilt in "troublous times." This was fulfilled, as Ezra and Nehemiah record. Sixty-two weeks = 434 years, thereafter Messiah was to come (v. 25). This was fulfilled in the birth and manifestation of Christ. Verse 26 is obviously an indeterminate period. The date of the crucifixion is not fixed. It is only said to be "after" the threescore and two weeks. It is the first event in verse 26. The second event is the destruction of the city, fulfilled A.D. 70. Then, "unto the end," a period not fixed, but which has already lasted nearly 2000 years. To Daniel was revealed only that wars and desolations should continue (cf. Mt. 24:6-14). The N.T reveals, that which was hidden from the O.T. prophets (Mt. 13:11-17; Eph. 3:1-10), that during this period should be accomplished the mysteries of the kingdom of Heaven (Mt. 13:1-50), and the outcalling of the Church (Mt. 16:18; Rom. 11:25). When the Church-age will end, and the seventieth week begin, is nowhere revealed. Its duration can be but seven years. To make it more violates the principle of interpretation already confirmed by fulfillment. Verse 27 deals with the last week. The "he" of verse 27 is the

city, to finish the transgression, and to
make an end of sins, and to [1]make [a]rec-
onciliation for iniquity, and to bring in
everlasting righteousness, and to seal up
the vision and prophecy, and to anoint
the most Holy.
25 Know therefore and understand,
that [2]from the going forth of the commandment to restore and to build
Jerusalem unto the Messiah the Prince
shall be seven weeks, and threescore and
two weeks: the street shall be built
again, and the wall, even in troublous
times.
26 And after threescore and two
weeks shall [b]Messiah be [c]cut off, but
[d]not for himself: and the people of the
[e]prince that shall come shall destroy the
city and the sanctuary; and the end
thereof *shall be* with a flood, and unto the
[f]end of the war desolations are determined.
27 And he shall confirm the covenant
with many for one week: and in the
midst of the week he shall cause the sacrifice and the oblation to cease, and for
the overspreading of [3]abominations he
shall make *it* desolate, even until the
consummation, and that determined
shall be poured upon the [g]desolate.

CHAPTER 10.

The vision of the glory of God.

In the third year of Cyrus king of Persia
a [h]thing was revealed unto Daniel,
whose [i]name was called Belteshazzar;
[j]and the thing *was* true, but the time
appointed *was* [k]long: and he understood
the thing, and had understanding of the
vision.
2 In those days I Daniel was mourning
three full weeks.
3 I ate no pleasant bread, neither came
flesh nor wine in my mouth, neither did
I anoint myself at all, till three whole
weeks were fulfilled.
4 And in the four and twentieth day of
the [l]first month, as I was by the side of
the great river, which *is* Hiddekel;
5 Then I lifted up mine eyes, and
looked, and behold a certain man

B.C. 538.

a Heb. *kaphar, atonement.* See v. 24, *note;* Ex. 29:33, *note.*

b *Christ (First Advent).* Hos. 2:23. (Gen. 3:15; Acts 1:9.)

c *Sacrifice. (prophetic).* Zech. 13:6, 7. (Gen. 4:4; Heb. 10:18.)

d Lit. *shall have nothing.* Nothing, that is, which rightly was His.

e *The Beast.* vs. 26, 27; Dan. 11:36-45. (Dan. 7:8; Rev. 19:20.)

f Lit. *unto the end wars and desolations are determined.* Cf. Mt. 24:6-14.

g Lit. *desolator.*

h Or, *word.*

i Dan. 1:7.

j Dan. 8:26; Rev. 19:9.

k Heb. *great.*

l i.e. *April.*

"prince that shall come" of verse 26, whose people (Rome) destroyed the temple, A.D. 70. He is the same with the "little horn" of chapter 7. He will covenant with the Jews to restore their temple sacrifices for one week (seven years), but in the middle of that time he will break the covenant and fulfil Dan. 12:11; 2 Thes. 2:3, 4. Between the sixty-ninth week, after which Messiah was cut off, and the seventieth week, within which the "little horn" of Dan. 7 will run his awful course, intervenes this entire Church-age. Verse 27 deals with the last three and a half years of the seven, which are identical with the "great tribulation" (Mt. 24:15-28); "time of trouble" (Dan. 12:1); "hour of temptation" (Rev. 3:10). (See "Tribulation," Psa. 2:5; Rev. 7:14.)

[1] **(9:24)** There is no word in the O.T. properly rendered *reconcile.* In A.V. the English word is found in 1 Sam. 29:4; 2 Chr. 29:24; Lev. 6:30; 8:15; 16:20; Ezk. 45:15, 17, 20; Dan. 9:24, but always improperly; atonement is invariably the meaning. Reconciliation is a N.T. doctrine (Rom. 5:10; Col. 1:21, *note*).

[2] **(9:25)** Three decrees concerning Jerusalem are recorded, that of Cyrus, B.C. 536 (Ussher), for the restoration of the "house of the LORD God of Israel" (2 Chr. 36:22, 23; Ezra 1:1-3); that of Darius (Ezra 6:3-8, B.C. 521-486), and that of Artaxerxes in his seventh year (Ezra 7:7, say, B.C. 458). Artaxerxes in his twentieth year, B.C. 444 (Hales, Jahn), 446 (A.V.), 454 (Ussher, Hengstenberg), gave permission for the rebuilding of the "city," i.e. "Jerusalem" (Neh. 2:1-8). The latter decree is, obviously, that from which the "seven weeks" (49 years) run, unless by "the commandment to restore," etc., is meant the *divine* decree (Dan. 9:23). In the present state of biblical chronology the date of the decree of Artaxerxes cannot be unanswerably fixed farther than to say that it was issued between 454 and 444 B.C. In either case we are brought to the time of Christ. Prophetic time is invariably so near as to give full warning, so indeterminate as to give no satisfaction to mere curiosity (cf. Mt. 24:36; Acts 1:7). The 434 years reckon, of course, from the end of the seven weeks, so that the whole time from "the going forth of the commandment to restore," etc., "unto the Messiah" is sixty-nine weeks of years, or 483 years.

[3] **(9:27)** Cf. Mt. 24:15. The expression occurs three times in Daniel. In Dan. 9:27 and 12:11 the reference is to the "Beast," "man of sin"; (2 Thes. 2:3, 4), and is identical with Mt. 24:15. In Dan. 11:31 the reference is to the act of Antiochus Epiphanes, the prototype of the man of sin, who sacrificed a sow upon the altar, and entered the holy of holies.

clothed in linen, whose [a]loins *were* girded with fine gold of Uphaz:

6 [b]His body also *was* like the [c]beryl, and his face as the appearance of lightning, and his eyes as lamps of fire, and his arms and his feet like in colour to polished brass, and the voice of his words like the voice of a multitude.

7 And I Daniel alone saw the vision: for the men that were with me saw not the vision; but a great quaking fell upon them, so that they fled to hide themselves.

8 Therefore I was left alone, and saw this great vision, and there [d]remained no strength in me: for my comeliness was turned in me into corruption, and I retained no strength.

9 Yet heard I the voice of his words: and when I heard the voice of his words, then was I in a deep sleep on my face, and my face toward the ground.

10 [e]And, behold, an hand touched me, which set me upon my knees and *upon* the palms of my hands.

11 And he said unto me, O Daniel, a man greatly beloved, understand the words that I speak unto thee, and stand upright: for unto thee am I now sent. And when he had spoken this word unto me, I stood trembling.

12 Then said he unto me, Fear not, Daniel: for from the first day that thou didst set thine heart to understand, and to chasten thyself before thy God, thy words were heard, and I am come for thy words.

13 But the [f]prince of the kingdom of Persia withstood me one and twenty days: but, lo, [g]Michael, one of the chief princes, came to help me; and I remained there with the kings of Persia.

14 Now I am come to make thee understand what shall befall thy people in the latter days: for yet the vision *is* for *many* days.

B.C. 534.

a Cf. Rev. 1:13.

b *The theophanies.* Rev. 1:9. (Gen. 12:7; Rev. 1:9.)

c *Chrysolite.* Cf. Ezk. 1:16.

d Cf. Ex. 3:2-10; Isa. 6:1-10; Rev. 1:12-19.

e vs. 10-15 introduce an angel. The theophany begins again at v. 16.

f v. 20. The intimation is clear that as the holy angels are sent forth in behalf of the heirs of salvation, so demons are concerned in behalf of the world-system of Satan. (John 7:7; Rev. 13:8.)

g v. 21; Dan. 12:1; Jude 9; Rev. 12:7.

h Ahasuerus (Ezra 4:6); Artaxerxes (Ezra 4:7); and Darius called "Hystaspes" (Ezra 4:24).

i Xerxes, who invaded Greece B.C. 483-480.

15 And when he had spoken such words unto me, I set my face toward the ground, and I became dumb.

16 And, behold, *one* like the similitude of the sons of men touched my lips: then I opened my mouth, and spake, and said unto him that stood before me, O my lord, by the vision my sorrows are turned upon me, and I have retained no strength.

17 For how can the servant of this my lord talk with this my lord? for as for me, straightway there remained no strength in me, neither is there breath left in me.

18 Then there came again and touched me *one* like the appearance of a man, and he strengthened me,

19 And said, O man greatly beloved, fear not: peace *be* unto thee, be strong, yea, be strong. And when he had spoken unto me, I was strengthened, and said, Let my lord speak; for thou hast strengthened me.

20 Then said he, Knowest thou wherefore I come unto thee? and now will I return to fight with the prince of Persia: and when I am gone forth, lo, the prince of Grecia shall come.

21 But I will shew thee that which is noted in the scripture of truth: and *there is* none that holdeth with me in these things, but Michael your prince.

CHAPTER 11.

From Darius to the man of sin
(2 Thes. 2:3, 4), Dan. 11:1–12:13.

ALSO I in the first year of Darius the Mede, *even* I, stood to confirm and to strengthen him.

2 And now will I shew thee the truth.
[1]Behold, there shall stand up yet [h]three kings in Persia; and the [i]fourth shall be far richer than *they* all: and by his strength

[1](11:2) The spirit of prophecy here returns to that which more immediately concerned Daniel and his royal masters—the near future of the empire in which he was so great a personage. Four kings were yet to follow in Media-Persia. Then will come Alexander the "mighty king" of Grecia (v. 3). The division of Alexander's empire into four parts (v. 4) as already predicted (Dan. 8:22) is foretold. The troublous course of affairs in two parts of the disintegrated Alexandrian empire, Syria and Egypt, is then traced down to verse 20. Here Antiochus Epiphanes, the "little horn" of Chapter 8, occupies the vision down to verse 36. His pollution of the sanctuary is again mentioned. (Cf. Dan. 8:9, *note.*) From verse 36 the interpretation is of the final "little horn" (Dan. 7:8, 24-26). See Dan. 11:35, *note.*

through his riches he shall stir up all against the realm of Grecia.

3 And a mighty [a]king shall stand up, that shall rule with great dominion, and do according to his will.

4 And when he shall stand up, his kingdom shall be broken, and shall be divided toward the four winds of heaven; and not to his posterity, nor according to his dominion which he ruled: for his kingdom shall be plucked up, even for others beside those.

5 And the king of the [b]south shall be strong, and *one* of [c]his princes; and [d]he shall be strong above him, and have dominion; his dominion *shall be* a great dominion.

6 And in the end of years [e]they shall join themselves together; for the king's daughter of the south shall come to the king of the north to make an agreement: but she shall not retain the power of the arm; neither shall he stand, nor his arm: but she shall be given up, and they that brought her, and he that begat her, and he that strengthened her in *these* times.

7 But out of a [f]branch of her roots shall *one* stand up in his estate, which shall come with an army, and shall enter into the fortress of the king of the north, and shall deal against them, and shall prevail:

8 And shall also carry captives into Egypt their gods, with their princes, *and* with their precious vessels of silver and of gold; and he shall continue *more* years than the king of the north.

9 So the king of the south shall come into *his* kingdom, and shall return into his own land.

10 [g]But his sons shall be stirred up, and shall assemble a multitude of great forces: and *one* shall certainly come, and overflow, and pass through: then shall he return, and be stirred up, *even* to his fortress.

11 And the king of the south shall be moved with choler, and shall come forth and fight with him, *even* with the king of the north: and he shall set forth a great multitude; but the multitude shall be given into his hand.

12 *And* when he hath taken away the multitude, his heart shall be lifted up; and he shall cast down *many* ten thousands: but he shall not be strengthened *by it*.

13 For the king of the north shall return, and shall set forth a multitude greater than the former, and shall certainly come after certain years with a great army and with much riches.

14 And in those times there shall many stand up against the king of the south: also the robbers of thy people shall exalt themselves to establish the vision; but they shall fall.

15 So the [h]king of the north shall come, and cast up a mount, and take the most fenced cities: and the arms of the south shall not withstand, neither his chosen people, neither *shall there be any* strength to withstand.

16 But he that cometh against him shall do according to his own will, and none shall stand before him: and he shall stand in the glorious land, which by his hand shall be consumed.

17 He shall also set his face to enter with the strength of his whole kingdom, and upright ones with him; thus shall he do: and he shall give him the [i]daughter of women, corrupting her: but she shall not stand *on his side*, neither be for him.

18 After this shall he turn his face unto the [j]isles, and shall take many: but a [k]prince for his own behalf shall cause the reproach offered by him to cease; without his own reproach he shall cause *it* to turn upon him.

19 Then he shall turn his face toward the fort of his own land: but he shall stumble and fall, and not be found.

20 Then shall stand up in his estate [l]a raiser of taxes *in* the glory of the kingdom: but within few days he shall be destroyed, neither in anger, nor in battle.

The "little horn" of Dan. 8.:
Antiochus Epiphanes (to v. 35).
(See Dan. 11:2, *note*.)

21 And in his estate shall stand up a vile person, to whom they shall not give the honour of the kingdom: but he shall come in peaceably, and obtain the kingdom by flatteries.

22 And with the arms of a flood shall they be overflown from before him, and shall be broken; yea, also the prince of the covenant.

23 And after the league *made* with him he shall work deceitfully: for he shall come up, and shall become strong with a small people.

B.C. 534.

a Alexander the Great, B.C. 332. See Dan. 8:5-8, 21-26.

b i.e. "south" of Palestine Egypt is meant.

c i.e. One of Alexander' s princes; historically Ptolemy Lagidae.

d Not the "king of the south" (Ptolemy Lagidae, to whom Egypt was given), but the "king of the north" (v.6), Seleucus, to whom Syria was given.

e i.e. the descendants and successors of Ptolemy Lagidae and Seleucus, not those very personages. The prediction was fulfilled in the marriage of Berenice, daughter of Ptolemy Philadelphus, to Antiochus Theos, third king of Syria, B.C. 285-247.

f Ptolemy Euergetes, brother of Berenice, who invaded Syria as described in vs. 7-9.

g vs. 10-19, prophetic foreview of the wars of Egypt and Syria, Palestine (v.17) the battleground, B.C. 284-175.

h Antiochus the Great, B.C. 198.

i Probably a reference to the marriage of Cleopatra to an Egyptian king, Ptolemy Philometor.

j i.e. of Greece. Isa. 66:9.

k i.e. Historically one of the Scipios: the power of Rome felt in the East for the first time.

l A reference to the tribute exacted of the son of Antiochus the Great by the Romans.

24 He shall enter peaceably even upon the fattest places of the province; and he shall do *that* which his fathers have not done, nor his fathers' fathers; he shall scatter among them the prey, and spoil, and riches: *yea*, and he shall forecast his devices against the strong holds, even for a time.

25 And he shall stir up his power and his courage against the king of the [a]south with a great army; and the king of the south shall be stirred up to battle with a very great and mighty army; but he shall not stand: for they shall forecast devices against him.

26 Yea, they that feed of the portion of his meat shall destroy him, and his army shall overflow: and many shall fall down slain.

27 And both these kings' hearts *shall be* to do mischief, and they shall speak lies at one table; but it shall not prosper: for yet the end *shall be* at the time appointed.

28 Then shall he return into his land with great riches; and his heart *shall be* against the holy covenant; and he shall do *exploits*, and return to his own land.

29 At the time appointed he shall return, and [b]come toward the south; but it shall not be as the former, or as the latter.

30 For the ships of Chittim shall come against him: therefore he shall be grieved, and return, and have indignation against the holy covenant: so shall he do; he shall even return, and have intelligence with them that forsake the holy covenant.

31 And arms shall stand on his part, and they shall pollute the sanctuary of strength, and shall take away the daily *sacrifice*, and they shall place the [c]abomination that maketh desolate.

32 And such as do wickedly against the covenant shall he corrupt by flatteries: but the people that do know their God shall be [d]strong, and do *exploits*.

33 And they that understand among the people shall instruct many: yet they shall fall by the sword, and by flame, by captivity, and by spoil, *many* days.

34 Now when they shall fall, they shall be holpen with a little help: but many shall cleave to them with flatteries.

35 And *some* of them of understanding shall fall, to try them, and to purge, and to make *them* white, *even* to the [1]time of the end: because *it is* yet for a time appointed.

The end-time. The "little horn" of Dan. 7.
(See Dan. 11:2, *note.*)

36 And the king shall do according to his will; and [e]he shall exalt himself, and magnify himself above every god, and shall speak marvellous things against the God of gods, and shall prosper till

B.C. 534.

a Egypt.

b Antiochus Epiphanes' second expedition against Egypt. Stopped by the mandate of Rome (v. 30), he turns against the Jews.

c This is historic—the act of Antiochus Epiphanes. Mt. 24:15 refers to Dan. 12:11. See Dan. 9:27, *note.*

d e.g. the Maccabees. B.C. 168 and following.

e *The Beast.* vs. 36-45; Dan. 12:11. (Dan. 7:8; Rev. 19:20.)

[1]**(11:35)** Here the prophetic foreview, having traced the history of the two parts of Alexander's empire which had to do with Palestine and the Jews, viz. Syria and Egypt, to the time of Antiochus Epiphanes, and having described his career, overleaps the centuries to "the time of the end," when he of whom Antiochus Epiphanes was a type, the "little horn" of Dan. 7:8, the "Beast out of the sea" of Rev. 13:4-10, shall appear (cf. Dan. 7:8, *note*). Prophecy does not concern itself with history as such, but only with history as it affects Israel and the Holy Land. Antiochus Epiphanes was insignificant as compared with historical personages whom the Bible does not mention, but he scourged the covenant people and defiled God's altar, thus coming into prophetic light. From verse 36 the "little horn" of Dan. 7:8, 24-26 fills the scene. His prosperity lasts until "the indignation" (the "time of trouble" of Dan. 12:1 and Mt. 24:21) is accomplished (v. 36). This is parallel with Rev. 17:10-14; 19:19-21. Verses 37-45 supply details not mentioned in the N.T. The expression "God of his fathers" (v. 37) has been held to indicate that the "king" is an apostate Jew, but this does not accord with Dan. 9:26, which was fulfilled by the Gentile armies of Rome. The "little horn" is an apostate, but from Christianity, not Judaism (cf. 1 John 2:18, 19). Verses 38-45 describe his career. Substituting "the god of forces" (i.e. forces of nature) for the true God (vs. 38, 39), he soon presents himself as that god (cf. 2 Thes. 2:3, 4). While his career lasts he is an irresistible conqueror (vs. 40-44). He establishes his palace in Jerusalem, probably at the time of his supreme act of blasphemous impiety (Dan. 9:27; 12:11; Mt. 24:15; 2 Thes. 2:4). From this time begins the great tribulation (Dan. 12:1; Mt. 24:21) which runs its course during the last half of Daniel's seventieth week, viz., three and one half years (Dan. 7:25; 12:7, 11; Rev. 13:5). See Rev. 19:20, *note.*

the indignation be accomplished: for
that that is determined shall be done.
37 Neither shall he regard the God of
his fathers, nor the desire of women, nor
regard any god: for he shall magnify
himself above all.
38 But in his estate shall he honour the
God of forces: and a god whom his
fathers knew not shall he honour with
gold, and silver, and with precious
stones, and pleasant things.
39 Thus shall he do in the most strong
holds with a strange god, whom he shall
acknowledge *and* increase with glory:
and he shall cause them to rule over
many, and shall divide the land for gain.
40 And at the time of the end shall the
king of the south push at him: and the
king of the north shall come against him
like a whirlwind, with chariots, and with
horsemen, and with many ships; and he
shall enter into the countries, and shall
overflow and pass over.
41 He shall enter also into the glorious
land, and many *countries* shall be overthrown: but these shall escape out of his
hand, *even* Edom, and Moab, and the
chief of the children of Ammon.
42 He shall stretch forth his hand also
upon the countries: and the land of
Egypt shall not escape.
43 But he shall have power over the
treasures of gold and of silver, and over
all the precious things of Egypt: and the
Libyans and the Ethiopians *shall be* at his
steps.
44 But tidings out of the east and out
of the north shall trouble him: therefore
he shall go forth with great fury to
destroy, and utterly to make away many.
45 And he shall plant the tabernacles of
his [a]palace between the seas in the glorious holy mountain; yet he shall come to
his end, and none shall help him.

CHAPTER 12.

The great tribulation (Psa. 2:5; Rev. 7:14).
(See Dan. 11:35, *note.*)

And at that time shall Michael stand
up, the great prince which standeth
for the children of [1]thy people: and there
shall be a time of trouble, [b]such as never
was since there was a nation *even* to that
same time: and at that time thy people
shall be delivered, every one that shall be
found written in the book.

The Resurrections (Job 19:25;
1 Cor. 15:52). (See Dan. 11:35, *note.*)

2 And many of them that sleep in the
dust of the earth shall [c]awake, some to
everlasting life, and some to shame *and*
everlasting contempt.
3 And they that be wise shall shine [d]as
the brightness of the firmament; and
they that turn many to righteousness as
the stars for ever and ever.

The last message to Daniel.

4 But thou, O Daniel, shut up the
words, and seal the book, *even* to the
time of the [2]end: many shall run to and
fro, and knowledge shall be increased.
5 Then I Daniel looked, and, behold,
there stood other two, the one on this
side of the bank of the river, and the
other on that side of the bank of the river.
6 And *one* said to the man clothed in
linen, which *was* upon the waters of the
river, How long *shall it be to* the end of
these wonders?
7 And I heard the man clothed in
linen, which *was* upon the waters of the
river, when he held up his right hand

B.C. 534.

a See Dan. 11:2, *note.*

b *Tribulation (the great).* Mt. 24:21, 22. (Psa. 2:5; Rev. 7:14.)

c *Resurrection.* vs. 2, 13; Hos. 13:14. (Job 19:25; 1 Cor. 15:52.)

d *Rewards.* Mt. 5:12. (Dan. 12:3; 1 Cor. 3:14.)

[1] **(12:1)** That is, Daniel's people, the Jews. Cf. Dan. 9:15, 16, 20, 24; 10:14.

[2] **(12:4)** The "time of the end" in Daniel. The expression, or its equivalent, "in the end," occurs, Dan. 8:17-19; 9:26; 11:35, 40, 45; 12:4, 6, 9. Summary: (1) The time of the end in Daniel begins with the violation by "the prince that shall come" (i.e. "little horn," "man of sin," "Beast") of his covenant with the Jews for the restoration of the temple and sacrifice (Dan. 9:27), and his presentation of himself as God (Dan. 9:27; 11:36-38; Mt. 24:15; 2 Thes. 2:4; Rev. 13:4-6), and ends with his destruction by the appearing of the LORD in glory (2 Thes. 2:8; Rev. 19:19, 20). (2) The duration of the "time of the end" is three and one half years, coinciding with the last half of the seventieth week of Daniel (Dan. 7:25; 12:7; Rev. 13:5). (3) This "time of the end" is the "time of Jacob's trouble" (Jer. 30:7); "a time of trouble such as never was since there was a nation" (Dan. 12:1); "great tribulation such as was not from the beginning of the world . . . nor ever shall be" (Mt. 24:21). The N.T., especially the Book of the Revelation, adds many details.

and his left hand unto heaven, and
sware by him that liveth for ever that *it*
shall be for a time, times, and an half; and
when he shall have accomplished to
scatter the power of the holy people, all
these *things* shall be finished.
8 And I heard, but I understood not:
then said I, O my Lord, what *shall be* the
end of these *things*?
9 And he said, Go thy way, Daniel: for
the words *are* closed up and sealed till
the time of the end.
10 [a]Many shall be purified, and made
white, and tried; but the wicked shall do
wickedly: and none of the wicked shall
understand; but the wise shall understand.
11 And from the time *that* the daily
sacrifice shall be taken away, and the
[b]abomination [c]that maketh desolate set
up, *there shall be* a thousand two hundred
and ninety days.
12 Blessed *is* he that waiteth, and
cometh to the [1]thousand three hundred
and five and thirty days.
13 But go thou thy way till the end *be*:
for thou shalt rest, and stand in thy lot at
the end of the [d]days.

B.C. 534.

a A prophecy describing the moral state of the world from Daniel's day to the time of the end. Cf. Mt. 13:24-30, 36-43, 47-49.

b See Dan. 9:27, *note*.

c *The Beast*. Ezk. 28:2-8. (Dan. 7:8; Rev. 19:20.)

d i.e. of the 1260, 1290, and 1335 days.

[1]**(12:12)** Three periods of "days" date from the "abomination" (i.e. the blasphemous assumption of diety by the Beast, v. 11; Mt. 24:15; 2 Thes. 2:4): (1) Twelve hundred and sixty days to the destruction of the Beast (Dan. 7:25; 12:7; Rev. 13:5; 19:19, 20). This is also the duration of the great tribulation (cf. Dan. 12:4, *note*). (2) Dating from the same event is a period of 1290 days, an addition of thirty days (Dan. 12:11). (3) Again forty-five days are added, and with them the promise of verse 12. No account is directly given of that which occupies the interval of seventy-five days between the end of the tribulation and the full blessing of verse 12. It is suggested that the explanation may be found in the prophetic descriptions of the events following the battle of Armageddon (Rev. 16:14; 19:21). The Beast is destroyed, and Gentile world-dominion ended, by the smiting of the "Stone cut out without hands" at the end of the 1260 days, but the scene is, so to speak, filled with the debris of the image which the "wind" must carry away before full blessing comes in (Dan. 2:35).

HOSEA

HOSEA was a contemporary of Amos in Israel, and of Isaiah and Micah in Judah, and his ministry continued after the first, or Assyrian, captivity of the northern kingdom (2 Ki. 15:29). His style is abrupt, metaphorical, and figurative.

Israel is Jehovah's adulterous wife, repudiated, but ultimately to be purified and restored. This is Hosea's distinctive message, which may be summed up in his two words, Lo-ammi, "not my people," and Ammi, "my people." Israel is not merely apostate and sinful—that is said also; but her sin takes its character from the exalted relationship into which she has been brought.

The book is in three parts: I. The dishonoured wife, 1:1–3:5. II. The sinful people, 4:1–13:8. III. The ultimate blessing and glory of Israel, 13:9–14:9.

The events recorded in Hosea cover a period of 60 years (Ussher).

CHAPTER 1.

Part I. Israel Jehovah's dishonoured wife, repudiated but to be restored
(Hos. 1:1–3:5).

The word of the LORD that came unto
Hosea, the son of Beeri, in the days
of Uzziah, Jotham, Ahaz, *and* Hezekiah,
kings of Judah, and in the days of
Jeroboam the son of Joash, king of Israel.

(1) *The symbolic marriage: the birth of Jezreel.*

2 The beginning of the word of the
LORD by Hosea. And the LORD said to
Hosea, Go, take unto thee a wife of
whoredoms and children of whoredoms:
[a]for the land hath committed great
whoredom, *departing* from the LORD.
3 So he went and took Gomer the
daughter of Diblaim; which conceived,
and bare him a son.
4 And the LORD said unto him, Call his
name Jezreel; for yet a little *while*, and I
will avenge the blood of [b]Jezreel upon
the house of Jehu, and will cause to
cease the kingdom of the house of Israel.
5 And it shall come to pass at that day,
that I will break the bow of Israel in the
valley of Jezreel.

(2) *The birth of Lo-ruhamah.*

6 And she conceived again, and bare a
daughter. And *God* said unto him, Call
her name [c]Lo-ruhamah: for I will no
more have mercy upon the house of
Israel; but I will utterly take them away.
7 [d]But I will have mercy upon the
house of Judah, and will save them by
the LORD their God, and will not save
them by bow, nor by sword, nor by battle, by horses, nor by horsemen.

(3) *The birth of Lo-ammi.*

8 Now when she had weaned Lo-
ruhamah, she conceived, and bare a son.
9 Then said *God*, Call his name [e]Lo-
ammi: for ye *are* not [1]my people, and I
will not be your *God*.

(4) *The future blessing and restoration of Israel.*

10 Yet the number of the children of
[2]Israel shall be as the sand of the sea,
which cannot be measured nor numbered; and it shall come to pass, *that* in
the place where it was said unto them,
Ye *are* not my [f]people, *there* it shall be
said unto them, *Ye are* the sons of the living God.
11 Then shall the children of Judah
and the children of Israel be gathered
together, and appoint themselves one
head, and they shall come up out of the
land: for great *shall be* the day of Jezreel.

B.C. 785.

a Deut. 31:16; Psa. 73:27; Jer. 2:13; Ezk. 16:1-59; 23:3.

b 2 Ki. 10:1-14.

c i.e. *unpitied.*

d 2 Ki. 19:35.

e i.e. *not my people.*

f Rom. 9:25, 26.

[1] **(1:9)** "My people" is an expression used in the O.T. exclusively of Israel the nation. It is never used of the patriarchs, Abraham, Isaac, and Jacob. See Mt. 2:6.

[2] **(1:10)** "Israel" in Hosea means the ten tribes forming the northern kingdom as distinguished from "Judah" (the tribes of Judah and Benjamin) forming the southern kingdom which adhered to the Davidic family. (See 1 Ki. 12:1-21.) The promise of verse 10 awaits fulfilment. See "Israel" (Gen. 12:2, 3; Rom. 11:26).

CHAPTER 2.

(5) *The chastisement of adulterous Israel.* (Cf. 2 Ki. 17:1-18.)

Say ye unto your brethren, [a]Ammi; and to your sisters, [b]Ruhamah.

2 Plead with your mother, plead: for [1]she *is* not my [c]wife, neither *am* I her husband: let her therefore put away her whoredoms out of her sight, and her adulteries from between her breasts;

3 [d]Lest I strip her naked, and set her as in the day that she was born, and make her as a wilderness, and set her like a dry land, and slay her with thirst.

4 And I will not have mercy upon her children; for they *be* the children of whoredoms.

5 For their mother hath played the harlot: she that conceived them hath done shamefully: for she said, I will go after my lovers, that give *me* my bread and my water, my wool and my flax, mine oil and my drink.

6 Therefore, [e]behold, I will hedge up thy way with thorns, and make a wall, that she shall not find her paths.

7 And she shall follow after her lovers, but she shall not overtake them; and she shall seek them, but shall not find *them*: then shall she say, I will go and return to my first husband; for then *was it* better with me than now.

8 For she did not know that I gave her corn, and wine, and oil, and multiplied her silver and gold, *which* they prepared for Baal.

9 Therefore will I return, and take away my corn in the time thereof, and my wine in the season thereof, and will recover my wool and my flax *given* to cover her nakedness.

10 And now will I discover her lewdness in the sight of her lovers, and none shall deliver her out of mine hand.

11 I will also cause all her mirth to cease, her feast days, her new moons, and her sabbaths, and all her solemn feasts.

12 And I will destroy her vines and her fig trees, whereof she hath said, These *are* my rewards that my lovers have given me: and I will make them a forest, and the beasts of the field shall eat them.

13 And I will visit upon her the days of Baalim, wherein she burned incense to them, and she decked herself with her earrings and her jewels, and she went after her lovers, and forgat me, saith the LORD.

(6) *Israel, the adulterous wife, to be restored.*

14 Therefore, behold, I will allure her, and bring her into the wilderness, and speak comfortably unto her.

15 And I will give her her vineyards from thence, and the valley of [f]Achor for a door of hope: and she shall sing there, as in the days of her youth, and as in the day when she came up out of the land of Egypt.

16 And it shall be at that day, saith the LORD, *that* thou shalt call me [g]Ishi; and shalt call me no more [h]Baali.

17 For I will take away the names of Baalim out of her mouth, and they shall no more be remembered by their name.

18 And in that day will I make a covenant for them with the beasts of the field, and with the fowls of heaven, and *with* the creeping things of the ground: and I will break the bow and the sword and the battle out of the earth, and will make them to lie down safely.

19 And I will betroth thee unto me for ever; yea, I will betroth thee unto me in righteousness, and in judgment, and in lovingkindness, and in mercies.

20 I will even betroth thee unto me in faithfulness: and thou shalt know the LORD.

21 And it shall come to pass in that day, I will hear, saith the

B.C. 785.

a i.e. *my people.*

b i.e. *having obtained pity.*

c *Wife of Jehovah.* vs. 1-23. (Isa. 54:5; Hos. 2:1-23.)

d Jer. 13:22, 26; Ezk. 16:37, 39.

e Job 3:23; 19:8; Lam. 3:7, 9.

f i.e. *trouble.* Josh. 7:26; Isa. 65:10.

g i.e. *my husband.*

h i.e. *my lord.*

[1] **(2:2)** That Israel is the wife of Jehovah (see vs. 16-23), now disowned but yet to be restored, is the clear teaching of the passages. This relationship is not to be confounded with that of the Church to Christ (John 3:29, *refs.*). In the mystery of the Divine tri-unity both are true. The N.T. speaks of the Church as a virgin espoused to one husband (2 Cor. 11:1, 2); which could never be said of an adulterous wife, restored in grace. Israel is, then, to be the restored and forgiven wife of Jehovah, the Church the virgin wife of the Lamb (John 3:29; Rev. 19:6-8); Israel Jehovah's earthly wife (Hos. 2:23); the Church the Lamb's heavenly bride (Rev. 19:7).

LORD, I will hear the heavens, and they
shall hear the earth;

22 And the earth shall hear the corn,
and the wine, and the oil; and they shall
hear Jezreel.

23 And I will sow her unto me in the
earth; and I will have mercy upon her
that had not obtained mercy; and I will
say to *them which were* not my [a]people,
Thou *art* my people; and [b]they shall say,
Thou art my God.

CHAPTER 3.

(7) *The undying love of Jehovah:*
the future Davidic kingdom.

Then said the LORD unto me, Go yet,
love a woman beloved of *her* friend,
yet an adulteress, according to the love
of the LORD toward the children of Israel,
who look to other gods, and love flagons
of wine.

2 So I bought her to me for fifteen
pieces of silver, and *for* an [c]homer of barley, and an half homer of barley:

3 And I said unto her, Thou shalt
abide for me many days; thou shalt not
play the harlot, and thou shalt not be for
another man: so *will* I also *be* for thee.

4 For the children of Israel shall abide
many days [d]without a [e]king, and without a prince, and without a sacrifice, and
without an image, and without an
ephod, and *without* teraphim:

5 Afterward shall the children of Israel
[f]return, and seek the LORD their God,
and David their [g]king; and shall fear the
LORD and his goodness in the latter days.

CHAPTER 4.

Part II. The sinful people
(Hos. 4:1–13:8). (1) *The general charge.*

Hear the word of the LORD, ye chil
dren of Israel: for the LORD hath [h]a
controversy with the inhabitants of the
land, because *there is* no truth, nor mercy,
nor knowledge of God in the land.

2 By swearing, and lying, and killing,
and stealing, and committing adultery,
they break out, and blood toucheth
blood.

3 [i]Therefore shall the land mourn, and
every one that dwelleth therein shall
languish, with the beasts of the field,
and with the fowls of heaven; yea, the
fishes of the sea also shall be taken away.

4 Yet let no man strive, nor reprove
another: for thy people *are* as they that
strive with the priest.

5 Therefore shalt thou fall in the day,
and the prophet also shall fall with thee in
the night, and I will destroy thy mother.

(2) *The wilful ignorance of Israel.*

6 [j]My people are destroyed for lack of
knowledge: because thou hast rejected
knowledge, I will also reject thee, that
thou shalt be no priest to me: seeing
thou hast forgotten the law of thy God, I
will also forget thy children.

7 As they were increased, so they
sinned against me: [k]*therefore* will I
change their glory into shame.

8 They eat up the sin of my people,
and they set their heart on their iniquity.

9 And there shall be, [l]like people, like
priest: and I will punish them for their
ways, and reward them their doings.

10 [m]For they shall eat, and not have
enough: they shall commit whoredom,
and shall not increase: because they have
left off to take heed to the LORD.

11 Whoredom and wine and new wine
take away the heart.

(3) *The idolatry of Israel.*

12 My people ask counsel at their
stocks, and their staff declareth unto
them: for the spirit of whoredoms hath
caused *them* to err, and they have gone a
whoring from under their God.

13 [n]They sacrifice upon the tops of the
mountains, and burn incense upon the
hills, under oaks and poplars and elms,
because the shadow thereof *is* good:
[o]therefore your daughters shall commit
whoredom, and your spouses shall commit adultery.

14 I will not punish your daughters
when they commit whoredom, nor your
spouses when they commit adultery: for
themselves are separated with whores,
and they sacrifice with harlots: therefore
the people *that* doth not understand
shall fall.

15 Though thou, Israel, play the harlot, *yet* let not Judah offend; and come

---

B.C. 785.

a Zech. 13:9; Rom. 9:25, 26; Eph. 2:11-22; 1 Pet. 2:10.

b *Christ (First Advent).* Mic. 5:2. (Gen. 3:15; Acts 1:9.)

c One homer = about 86 gals.

d *Kingdom* (O.T.). vs. 4, 5; Joel 3:16-20. (Gen. 1:26; Zech. 12:8.)

e John 19:15.

f *Israel (prophecies).* vs. 4, 5. Joel 3:1-8, 15-20. (Gen. 12:2, 3; Rom. 11:26.)

g *Christ (Second Advent).* vs. 4, 5; Mic. 4:7. (Deut. 30:3; Acts 1:9-11.)

h Hos. 12:2; Isa. 1:18; 3:13, 14; Jer. 25:31; Mic. 6:2.

i Jer. 4:28; 12:4; Amos 5:16; 8:8.

j Isa. 5:13.

k 1 Sam. 2:30; Mal. 2:9; Phil. 3:19.

l 2 Tim. 4:3, 4.

m Lev. 26:26; Mic. 6:14; Hag. 1:6.

n Isa. 1:29; 57:5, 7; Ezk. 6:13; 20:28.

o Amos 7:17; Rom. 1:28.

not ye unto Gilgal, neither go ye up to Beth-aven, nor swear, The LORD liveth.

16 [a]For Israel slideth back as a backsliding heifer: now the LORD will feed them as a lamb in a large place.

17 Ephraim *is* joined to idols: [b]let him alone.

18 Their drink is sour: they have committed whoredom continually: her rulers *with* shame do love, Give ye.

19 The wind hath bound her up in her wings, and they shall be ashamed because of their sacrifices.

CHAPTER 5.

(4) *The withdrawn face of Jehovah.*

Hear ye this, O priests; and hearken, ye house of Israel; and give ye ear, O house of the king; for judgment *is* toward you, because ye have been a snare on Mizpah, and a net spread upon Tabor.

2 And the revolters are profound to make slaughter, though I *have been* a rebuker of them all.

3 I know Ephraim, and Israel is not hid from me: for now, O Ephraim, thou committest whoredom, *and* Israel is defiled.

4 They will not frame their doings to turn unto their God: for the spirit of whoredoms *is* in the midst of them, and they have not known the LORD.

5 And [c]the pride of Israel doth testify to his face: therefore shall Israel and Ephraim fall in their iniquity; Judah also shall fall with them.

6 [d]They shall go with their flocks and with their herds to seek the LORD; but they shall not find *him*; he hath withdrawn himself from them.

7 They have dealt treacherously against the LORD: for they have begotten strange children: now shall a month devour them with their portions.

8 [e]Blow ye the cornet in Gibeah, *and* the trumpet in Ramah: [f]cry aloud *at* Beth-aven, [g]after thee, O Benjamin.

9 Ephraim shall be desolate in the day of rebuke: among the tribes of Israel have I made known that which shall surely be.

10 The princes of Judah were like them that [h]remove the bound: *therefore* I will pour out my wrath upon them like water.

11 Ephraim *is* [i]oppressed *and* broken in judgment, because he willingly walked after the commandment.

12 Therefore *will* I *be* unto Ephraim as a moth, and to the house of Judah [j]as rottenness.

13 When Ephraim saw his sickness, and Judah *saw* [k]his wound, then went Ephraim to the Assyrian, and sent to king Jareb: yet could he not heal you, nor cure you of your wound.

14 For [l]I *will be* unto Ephraim as a lion, and as a young lion to the house of Judah: I, *even* I, will tear and go away; I will take away, and none shall rescue *him*.

15 I will go *and* return to my place, till they acknowledge their offence, and seek my face: in their affliction they will seek me early.

CHAPTER 6.

(5) *The voice of the remnant in the last days.*

(Cf. *"Remnant,"* Isa. 1:9; Rom. 11:5.)

Come, and let us return unto the LORD: for he hath torn, and he will heal us; he hath smitten, and he will bind us up.

2 After two days will he revive us: in the third day he will raise us up, and we shall live in his sight.

3 Then shall we know, *if* we follow on to know the LORD: his going forth is prepared as the morning; and he shall come unto us as the rain, as the latter *and* former rain unto the earth.

(6) *The response of Jehovah.*

4 [m]O Ephraim, what shall I do unto thee? O Judah, what shall I do unto thee? for your goodness *is* as a morning cloud, and as the early dew it goeth away.

5 Therefore have I hewed *them* by the prophets; I have slain them by the words of my mouth: and thy judgments *are as* the light *that* goeth forth.

6 For I desired [n]mercy, and not sacrifice; and the knowledge of God more than burnt-offerings.

7 But they like men have transgressed the covenant: there have they dealt treacherously against me.

8 Gilead *is* a city of them that work iniquity, *and is* polluted with blood.

B.C. 780.

a Jer. 3:6; 7:24; 8:5; Zech. 7:11.

b Mt. 15:14.

c Hos. 7:10.

d Prov. 1:28; Isa. 1:15; Jer. 11:11; Ezk. 8:18; Mic. 3:4; John 7:34.

e Hos. 8:1; Joel 2:1.

f Hos. 4:15; Josh. 7:2.

g Jud. 5:14.

h Deut. 19:14; 27:17.

i Deut. 28:33.

j Prov. 12:4.

k Jer. 30:12.

l Hos. 13:7, 8; Lam. 3:10.

m Hos. 11:8.

n Mt. 9:13; 12:7.

B.C. 780.

9 And as troops of robbers wait for a man, *so* the company of priests murder in the way by consent: for they commit lewdness.

10 I have seen an horrible thing in the house of Israel: there *is* the whoredom of Ephraim, Israel is defiled.

11 Also, O Judah, he hath set an harvest for thee, when I returned the captivity of my people.

CHAPTER 7.

(*Response of Jehovah,* continued. Begins Hos. 6:4.)

When I would have healed Israel, then the iniquity of Ephraim was discovered, and the wickedness of Samaria: for they commit falsehood; and the thief cometh in, *and* the troop of robbers spoileth without.

2 And they consider not in their hearts *that* I remember all their wickedness: now their own doings have beset them about; they are before my face.

3 They make the king glad with their wickedness, and the princes with their lies.

4 They *are* all adulterers, as an oven heated by the baker, *who* ceaseth from raising after he hath kneaded the dough, until it be leavened.

5 In the day of our king the princes have made *him* sick with bottles of wine; he stretched out his hand with scorners.

6 For they have made ready their heart like an oven, whiles they lie in wait: their baker sleepeth all the night; in the morning it burneth as a flaming fire.

7 They are all hot as an oven, and have devoured their judges; all their kings are fallen: [a]*there is* none among them that calleth unto me.

8 Ephraim, he hath mixed himself among the people; Ephraim is a cake not turned.

9 Strangers have devoured his strength, and he knoweth *it* not: yea, gray hairs are here and there upon him, yet he knoweth not.

10 And the pride of Israel testifieth to his face: and they do not return to the LORD their God, nor seek him for all this.

11 [b]Ephraim also is like a silly dove without heart: they call to Egypt, they go to Assyria.

12 When they shall go, [c]I will spread my net upon them; I will bring them down as the fowls of the heaven; I will chastise them, as their congregation hath heard.

13 Woe unto them! for they have fled from me: destruction unto them! because they have transgressed against me: though I have [d]redeemed them, yet they have spoken lies against me.

14 [e]And they have not cried unto me with their heart, when they howled upon their beds: they assemble themselves for corn and wine, *and* they rebel against me.

15 Though I have bound *and* strengthened their arms, yet do they imagine mischief against me.

16 They return, *but* not to the most High: they are like a deceitful bow: their princes shall fall by the sword for the rage of their tongue: this *shall be* their derision in the land of Egypt.

CHAPTER 8.

(*Response of Jehovah,* continued. Begins Hos. 6:4.)

Set the trumpet to thy mouth. *He shall come* as an eagle against the house of the LORD, because they have transgressed my covenant, and trespassed against my law.

2 [f]Israel shall cry unto me, My God, we know thee.

3 Israel hath cast off *the thing that is* good: the enemy shall pursue him.

4 They have set up kings, but not by me: they have made princes, and I knew *it* not: of their silver and their gold have they made them idols, that they may be cut off.

5 Thy calf, O Samaria, hath cast *thee* off; mine anger is kindled against them: how long *will it be* ere they attain to innocency?

6 For from Israel *was* it also: the workman made it; therefore it *is* not God: but the calf of Samaria shall be broken in pieces.

7 [g]For they have sown the wind, and they shall reap the whirlwind: it hath no stalk: the bud shall yield no meal: if so be it yield, the strangers shall swallow it up.

8 Israel is swallowed up: now shall they be among the Gentiles as a vessel wherein *is* no pleasure.

9 For they are gone up to Assyria, a wild ass alone by himself: Ephraim hath hired lovers.

a Isa. 64:7.
b Hos. 11:11.
c Ezk. 12:13.
d Ex. 14:30, *note;* Isa. 59:20, *note.*
e Job 35:9, 10; Psa. 78:36; Jer. 3:10; Zech. 7:5.
f Hos. 5:15; Psa. 78:34.
g Hos. 10:12, 13; Prov. 22:8.

B.C. 760.

10 Yea, though they have hired among the nations, now will I gather them, and they shall sorrow a little for the burden of the king of princes.

11 Because Ephraim hath made many altars to sin, altars shall be unto him to sin.

12 I have written to him [a]the great things of my law, *but* they were counted as a strange thing.

13 They sacrifice flesh *for* the sacrifices of mine offerings, and eat *it; but* the LORD accepteth them not; [b]now will he remember their iniquity, and visit their sins: they shall return to Egypt.

14 [c]For Israel hath forgotten his Maker, and buildeth temples; and Judah hath multiplied fenced cities: but I will send a fire upon his cities, and it shall devour the palaces thereof.

CHAPTER 9.

(*Response of Jehovah,* continued.
Begins Hos. 6:4.)

Rejoice not, O Israel, for joy, as *other* people: for thou hast gone a whoring from thy God, thou hast loved a reward upon every cornfloor.

2 The floor and the winepress shall not feed them, and the new wine shall fail in her.

3 They shall not dwell [d]in the LORD'S land; [e]but Ephraim shall return to Egypt, and [f]they shall eat unclean *things* in Assyria.

4 They shall not offer wine *offerings* to the LORD, neither shall they be pleasing unto him: their sacrifices *shall be* unto them as the bread of mourners; all that eat thereof shall be polluted: for their bread for their soul shall not come into the house of the LORD.

5 What will ye do in the solemn day, and in the day of the feast of the LORD?

6 For, lo, they are gone because of destruction: Egypt shall gather them up, Memphis shall bury them: the pleasant *places* for their silver, [g]nettles shall possess them: thorns *shall be* in their tabernacles.

7 The days of visitation are come, the days of recompence are come; Israel shall know *it*: the prophet *is* a fool, the spiritual man *is* mad, for the multitude of thine iniquity, and the great hatred.

8 The [h]watchman of Ephraim *was* with my God: *but* the prophet *is* a snare of a fowler in all his ways, *and* hatred in the house of his God.

9 They have deeply corrupted *themselves,* as in the days of Gibeah: *therefore* he will remember their iniquity, he will visit their sins.

10 I found Israel like grapes in the wilderness; I saw your fathers as the [i]firstripe in the fig tree at her first time: *but* they went to [j]Baal-peor, and separated themselves unto *that* shame; and *their* abominations were according as they loved.

11 *As for* Ephraim, their glory shall fly away like a bird, from the birth, and from the womb, and from the conception.

12 Though they bring up their children, yet will I bereave them, *that there shall* not *be* a man *left*: yea, woe also to them when I depart from them!

13 Ephraim, as I saw Tyrus, *is* planted in a pleasant place: but Ephraim shall bring forth his children to the murderer.

14 Give them, O LORD: what wilt thou give? give them a miscarrying womb and dry breasts.

15 All their wickedness *is* in Gilgal: for there I hated them: for the wickedness of their doings I will drive them out of mine house, I will love them no more: all their princes *are* revolters.

16 Ephraim is smitten, their root is dried up, they shall bear no fruit: yea, though they bring forth, yet will I slay *even* the beloved *fruit* of their womb.

17 My God will [k]cast them away, because they did not hearken unto him: and they shall be [l]wanderers among the nations.

CHAPTER 10.

(*Response of Jehovah,* continued.
Begins Hos. 6:4.)

Israel *is* an empty vine, he bringeth forth [m]fruit unto himself: according to the multitude of his fruit he hath increased the altars; according to the goodness of his land they have made goodly images.

2 Their heart is divided; now shall they be found faulty: he shall break down their altars, he shall spoil their images.

3 For now they shall say, We have no

a Deut. 4:6-8; Psa. 119:18; 147:19, 20.
b Hos. 9:9; Amos 8:7.
c Deut. 32:18.
d Lev. 25:23; Jer. 2:7; 16:18.
e Hos. 8:13; 11:5.
f Ezk. 4:13; Dan. 1:8.
g Hos. 10:8; Isa. 5:6; 32:13; 34:13.
h Jer. 6:17; 31:6; Ezk. 3:17; 33:7.
i Isa. 28:4; Mic. 7:1.
j Num. 25:3; Psa. 106:28.
k 1 Ki. 18:21; Zech. 10:6; Mt. 6:24.
l Lev. 26:33.
m Cf. Hos. 14:8.

king, because we feared not the LORD;
what then should a king do to us?
4 They have spoken words, swearing
falsely in making a covenant: thus judgment springeth up as hemlock in the furrows of the field.
5 The inhabitants of Samaria shall fear
because of [a]the calves of Beth-aven: for
the people thereof shall mourn over it,
and the priests thereof *that* rejoiced on it,
[b]for the glory thereof, because it is
departed from it.
6 It shall be also carried unto Assyria
for a present to king Jareb: Ephraim shall
receive shame, and Israel shall be
ashamed of his own counsel.
7 *As for* Samaria, her king is cut off as
the foam upon the water.
8 The high places also of Aven, the sin
of Israel, shall be destroyed: the thorn and
the thistle shall come up on their altars;
and they shall say to the mountains,
[c]Cover us; and to the hills, Fall on us.
9 O Israel, thou hast sinned from the
days of Gibeah: there they stood: [d]the
battle in Gibeah against the children of
iniquity did not overtake them.
10 *It is* in my desire that I should chastise them; and the people shall be gathered against them, when they shall bind
themselves in their two furrows.
11 And Ephraim *is as* [e]an heifer *that is*
taught, *and* loveth to tread out *the corn*;
but I passed over upon her fair neck: I
will make Ephraim to ride; Judah shall
plow, *and* Jacob shall break his clods.
12 Sow to yourselves in righteousness,
reap in mercy; [f]break up your fallow
ground: for *it is* time to seek the LORD,
till he come and rain righteousness upon
you.
13 Ye have plowed wickedness, ye have
reaped iniquity; ye have eaten the fruit of
lies: because thou didst [g]trust in thy way,
in the multitude of thy mighty men.
14 Therefore shall a tumult arise
among thy people, and all thy fortresses
shall be spoiled, as Shalman spoiled
[h]Beth-arbel in the day of battle: the
mother was dashed in pieces upon *her*
children.
15 So shall Beth-el do unto you because
of your great wickedness: in a morning
shall the king of Israel utterly be cut off.

B.C. 740.

a Hos. 8:5, 6; 1 Ki. 12:28, 29.
b Hos. 9:11.
c Lk. 23:30.
d See Jud. 20.
e Jer. 50:11; Mic. 4:13.
f Jer. 4:3.
g Psa. 2:12, *note.*
h 2 Ki. 18:34; 19:13.
i Mt. 2:15.
j Lev. 26:13.
k i.e. to Jehovah.
l Gen. 14:8; 19:24, 25; Deut. 29:23; Amos 4:11.
m Zech. 8:14, *note.*
n Hos. 8:7.

CHAPTER 11.

(*Response of Jehovah*, continued.
Begins Hos. 6:4.)

When Israel *was* a child, then I loved
him, and called [i]my son out of
Egypt.
2 *As* they called them, so they went
from them: they sacrificed unto Baalim,
and burned incense to graven images.
3 I taught Ephraim also to go, taking
them by their arms; but they knew not
that I healed them.
4 I drew them with cords of a man,
with bands of love: and [j]I was to them as
they that take off the yoke on their jaws,
and I laid meat unto them.
5 He shall not return into the land of
Egypt, but the Assyrian shall be his king,
because they refused to [k]return.
6 And the sword shall abide on his
cities, and shall consume his branches,
and devour *them*, because of their own
counsels.
7 And my people are bent to backsliding from me: though they called them to
the most High, none at all would exalt
him.
8 How shall I give thee up, Ephraim?
how shall I deliver thee, Israel? how shall I
make thee as [l]Admah? *how* shall I set thee
as Zeboim? mine heart is turned within
me, my [m]repentings are kindled together.
9 I will not execute the fierceness of
mine anger, I will not return to destroy
Ephraim: for I *am* God, and not man; the
Holy One in the midst of thee: and I will
not enter into the city.
10 They shall walk after the LORD: he
shall roar like a lion: when he shall roar,
then the children shall tremble from the
west.
11 They shall tremble as a bird out of
Egypt, and as a dove out of the land of
Assyria: and I will place them in their
houses, saith the LORD.
12 Ephraim compasseth me about
with lies, and the house of Israel with
deceit: but Judah yet ruleth with God,
and is faithful with the saints.

CHAPTER 12.

(*Response of Jehovah*, continued.
Begins Hos. 6:4.)

Ephraim [n]feedeth on wind, and followeth after the east wind: he daily
increaseth lies and desolation; and they

do make a covenant with the Assyrians,
and oil is carried into Egypt.
2 [a]The LORD hath also a controversy
with Judah, and will punish Jacob
according to his ways; according to his
doings will he recompense him.
3 He took his brother [b]by the heel in
the womb, and by his strength he [c]had
power with God:
4 Yea, he had power over the [d]angel,
and prevailed: he wept, and made supplication unto him: he found him in
[e]Beth-el, and there he spake with us;
5 Even the LORD God of hosts; the
LORD *is* his [f]memorial.
6 Therefore [g]turn thou to thy God:
keep mercy and judgment, and wait on
thy God continually.
7 *He is* a merchant, the balances of
deceit *are* in his hand: he loveth to
oppress.
8 And Ephraim said, Yet I am become
rich, I have found me out substance: *in*
all my labours they shall find none iniquity in me that *were* sin.
9 And I *that am* the LORD thy God from
the land of Egypt will yet make thee to
dwell in tabernacles, as in the days of
the solemn feast.
10 [h]I have also spoken by the
prophets, and I have multiplied visions,
and used similitudes, by the ministry of
the prophets.
11 *Is there* iniquity *in* Gilead? surely
they are vanity: they sacrifice bullocks in
Gilgal; yea, their altars *are* as heaps in
the furrows of the fields.
12 And Jacob [i]fled into the country of
Syria, and [j]Israel served for a wife, and
for a wife he kept *sheep*.
13 And [k]by a prophet the LORD
brought Israel out of Egypt, and by a
prophet was he preserved.
14 Ephraim provoked *him* to anger
most bitterly: therefore shall he leave his
blood upon him, and his reproach shall
his Lord return unto him.

CHAPTER 13.

(*Response of Jehovah,* concluded.
Begins Hos. 6:4.)

WHEN Ephraim spake trembling, he
exalted himself in Israel; but
[l]when he offended in Baal, he died.
2 And now they sin more and more,
and have made them molten images of
their silver, *and* idols according to their
own understanding, all of it the work of
the craftsmen: they say of them, Let the
men that sacrifice kiss the calves.
3 Therefore they shall be as the morning cloud, and as the early dew that passeth away, as the chaff *that* is driven with
the whirlwind out of the floor, and as
the smoke out of the chimney.
4 Yet I *am* the LORD thy God from the
land of Egypt, and thou shalt know no
god but me: for *there is* no saviour beside
me.
5 I did know thee in the wilderness, in
the land of great drought.
6 According to their pasture, so were
they filled; they were filled, and their
heart was exalted; therefore have they
forgotten me.
7 Therefore I will be unto them as a
lion: as a leopard by the way will I
observe *them*:
8 I will meet them [m]as a bear *that is*
bereaved *of her whelps*, and will rend the
caul of their heart, and there will I
devour them like a lion: the wild beast
shall tear them.

Part III. [1]*The ultimate blessing of Israel in the kingdom* (Hos. 13:9—14:9).

9 O Israel, thou hast destroyed thyself;
but in me *is* thine help.
10 I will be thy king: where *is any other*
that may save thee in all thy cities? and
thy judges of whom thou saidst, Give
me a king and princes?
11 I gave thee a king in mine anger,
and took *him* away in my wrath.
12 The iniquity of Ephraim *is* bound
up; his sin *is* hid.
13 The sorrows of a travailing woman
shall come upon him: he *is* an unwise
son; for he should not stay long in *the
place of* the breaking forth of children.
14 I will ransom them from the power
of the [n]grave; I will [o]redeem them from
[p]death: O death, I will be thy plagues;
[q]O grave, I will be thy destruction:
repentance shall be hid from mine eyes.
15 Though he be fruitful among *his*
brethren, an east wind shall come, the
wind of the LORD shall come up from the
wilderness, and his spring shall become

B.C. 725.

a Hos. 4:1; Mic. 6:2.
b Gen. 25:26.
c Gen. 32:24-28.
d Heb. 1:4, *note.*
e Gen. 28:12, 19; 35:9, 10, 15.
f Ex. 3:15.
g Hos. 14:1; Mic. 6:8.
h 2 Ki. 17:13.
i Gen. 28:5; Deut. 26:5.
j Gen. 29:20, 28.
k Ex. 12:50, 51; 13:3; Psa. 77:20; Isa. 63:11; Mic. 6:4.
l Hos. 11:2; 2 Ki. 17:16, 18.
m 2 Sam. 17:8; Prov. 17:12.
n *Resurrection.* Mt. 9:23-25. (Job 19:25; 1 Cor. 15:52.)
o Heb. *goel, Redemp. (Kinsman type).* Isa. 59:20, *note.*
p 1 Cor. 15:55.
q Heb. *Sheol,* also in preceding clause. See Hab. 2:5, *note.*

[1]**(13:9, heading)** The response of Jehovah continues to the end, but at verse 9 changes to entreaty and promise.

dry, and his fountain shall be dried up: he shall spoil the treasure of all pleasant vessels.

16 Samaria shall become desolate; [a]for she hath rebelled against her God: they shall fall by the sword: their infants shall be dashed in pieces, and their women with child shall be ripped up.

CHAPTER 14.

O Israel, [b]return unto the LORD thy God; for thou hast fallen by thine iniquity.

2 Take with you words, and turn to the LORD: say unto him, Take away all iniquity, and receive *us* graciously: so will we render the calves of our lips.

3 Asshur shall not save us; we will not ride upon horses: neither will we say any more to the work of our hands, *Ye are* our gods: for in thee the fatherless findeth mercy.

4 [c]I will heal their backsliding, [d]I will love them freely: for mine anger is turned away from him.

5 [e]I will be as the dew unto Israel: he shall grow as the lily, and cast forth his roots as Lebanon.

6 His branches shall spread, and [f]his beauty shall be as the olive tree, and his smell as Lebanon.

7 They that dwell under his shadow shall return; they shall revive *as* the corn, and grow as the vine: the scent thereof *shall be* as the wine of Lebanon.

8 Ephraim *shall say*, What have I to do any more with idols? I have heard *him*, and observed him: I *am* like a green fir tree. [g]From me is thy fruit found.

9 Who *is* wise, and he shall understand these *things*? prudent, and he shall know them? for the ways of the LORD *are* right, and the just shall walk in them: but the transgressors shall fall therein.

B.C. 725.

a 2 Ki. 18:12.

b Hos. 12:6; Joel 2:13.

c Hos. 11:7; Jer. 5:6; 14:7.

d Eph. 1:6.

e Job 29:19; Prov. 19:12.

f Psa. 52:8; 128:3.

g John 15:4. Cf. Hos. 10:1. See Jas. 1:17.

JOEL

JOEL, a prophet of Judah, probably exercised his ministry during the reign of Joash (2 Chr. 22 to 24). In his youth he may have known Elijah, and he certainly was a contemporary of Elisha. The plagues of insects, which were the token of the divine chastening, give occasion for the unveiling of the coming "day of the LORD" (Isa. 2:12, *refs.*), in its two aspects of judgment on the Gentiles and blessing for Israel.

Joel is in three chief parts: I. The plague of insects, 1:1-20. II. The day of the LORD, 2:1–3:8. III. Retrospect of the day of the LORD, and full kingdom blessing, 3:9-21.

B.C. 800.

CHAPTER 1.

Part I. The plague of insects (vs. 1-20).

(1) *Introduction* (vs. 1-3).

The word of the LORD that came to Joel the son of Pethuel.

2 Hear this, ye old men, and give ear, all ye inhabitants of the land. Hath this been in your days, or even in the days of your fathers?

3 Tell ye your children of it, and *let* your children *tell* their children, and their children another generation.

(2) *Desolation of the land.*

4 That which the [1]palmerworm hath left hath the locust eaten; and that which the locust hath left hath the cankerworm eaten; and that which the cankerworm hath left hath the caterpiller eaten.

5 Awake, ye drunkards, and weep; and howl, all ye drinkers of wine, because of the new wine; for it is cut off from your mouth.

6 For a nation is come up upon my land, strong, and without number, whose teeth *are* the teeth of a lion, and he hath the cheek teeth of a great lion.

7 He hath laid my vine waste, and barked my fig tree: he hath made it clean bare, and cast *it* away; the branches thereof are made white.

8 Lament like a virgin girded with sackcloth for the husband of her youth.

9 The [a]meat-offering and the drink-offering is cut off from the

a Lit. *meal*

[1] **(1:4)** The palmerworm, locust, etc., are thought to be different forms, at different stages of development, of one insect. The essential fact is that, according to the usual method of the Spirit in prophecy, some local circumstance is shown to be of spiritual significance, and is made the occasion of a far-reaching prophecy (e.g. Isa. 7:1-14, where the Syrian invasion and the unbelief of Ahaz give occasion to the great prophecy of verse 14). Here in Joel a plague of devouring insects is shown to have spiritual significance (Joel 1:13, 14), and is made the occasion of the prophecy of the day of the LORD, not yet fulfilled (Isa. 2:12. *refs.*). This is more developed in Joel 2, where the literal locusts are left behind, and the future day of Jehovah fills the scene.

The whole picture is of the end-time of this present age, of the "times of the Gentiles" (Lk. 21:24; Rev. 16:14); of the battle of Armageddon (Rev. 16:14; 19:11-21); of the regathering of Israel (Rom 11:26, *note*), and of kingdom blessing. It is remarkable that Joel, coming at the very beginning of written prophecy (B.C. 836), gives the fullest view of the consummation of all written prophecy.

The order of events is: (1) The invasion of Palestine from the north by Gentile world-powers headed up under the Beast and false prophet (Joel 2:1-10; "Armageddon," Rev. 16:14, *refs.*); (2) the Lord's army and destruction of the invaders (Joel 2:11; Rev. 19:11-21); (3) the repentance of Judah in the land (Joel 2:12-17; Deut. 30:1-9, *note*); (4) the answer of Jehovah (Joel 2:18-27); (5) the effusion of the Spirit in the (Jewish) "last days" (Joel 2:28, 29); (6) the return of the Lord in glory and the setting up of the kingdom (Joel 2:30-32; Acts 15:15-17) by the regathering of the nation and the judgment of the nations (Joel 3:1-16); (7) full and permanent kingdom blessing (Joel 3:17-21; Zech. 14:1-21; Mt. 25:32, *note*).

house of the LORD; the priests, the LORD'S ministers, mourn.

10 The field is wasted, the land mourneth; for the corn is wasted: the new wine is dried up, the oil languisheth.

11 Be ye ashamed, O ye husbandmen; howl, O ye vinedressers, for the wheat and for the barley; because the harvest of the field is perished.

12 The vine is dried up, and the fig tree languisheth; the pomegranate tree, the palm tree also, and the apple tree, *even* all the trees of the field, are withered: because joy is withered away from the sons of men.

13 Gird yourselves, and lament, ye priests: howl, ye ministers of the altar: come, lie all night in sackcloth, ye ministers of my God: for the [a]meat-offering and the drink-offering is withholden from the house of your God.

14 [b]Sanctify ye a fast, call a solemn assembly, gather the elders *and* all the inhabitants of the land *into* the house of the LORD your God, and cry unto the LORD,

The plague of insects:
(3) *A type of the day of the Lord.*

15 Alas for the day! [c]for the day of the LORD *is* at hand, and as a destruction from the Almighty shall it come.

16 Is not the meat cut off before our eyes, *yea,* joy and gladness from the house of our God?

17 The seed is rotten under their clods, the garners are laid desolate, the barns are broken down; for the corn is withered.

18 How do the beasts groan! the herds of cattle are perplexed, because they have no pasture; yea, the flocks of sheep are made desolate.

19 O LORD, to thee will I cry: for the fire hath devoured the pastures of the wilderness, and the flame hath burned all the trees of the field.

20 The beasts of the field cry also unto thee: for the rivers of waters are dried up, and the fire hath devoured the pastures of the wilderness.

B.C. 800.

a Lit. *meal.*

b *Sanctify, holy* (O.T.). Zech. 8:3. (Gen. 2:3; Zech. 8:3.)

c *Day (of Jehovah).* Joel 2:1-11, 28-32 (Isa. 2:10-22; Rev. 19:11-21.)

d *Day (of Jehovah).* vs. 1-11, 28-32; Joel 3:9-21. (Isa. 2:10-22; Rev. 19:11-21.)

e Gen. 2:8; 13:10; Isa. 51:3.

f Joel 3:16; Jer. 25:30; Amos 1:2.

g *Armageddon (battle of).* vs. 1-11, 20; Joel 3:9-13. (Rev. 16:14; 19:11-21.)

CHAPTER 2.

Part II. The day of the LORD: (1) *The invading host from the north preparatory to Armageddon* (Rev. 16:14, *refs.*).

BLOW ye the trumpet in Zion, and sound an alarm in my holy mountain: let all the inhabitants of the land tremble: for the day of the LORD [d]cometh, for *it is* nigh at hand;

2 A day of darkness and of gloominess, a day of clouds and of thick darkness, as the morning spread upon the mountains: a great people and a strong; there hath not been ever the like, neither shall be any more after it, *even* to the years of many generations.

3 A fire devoureth before them; and behind them a flame burneth: the land *is* [e]as the garden of Eden before them, and behind them a desolate wilderness; yea, and nothing shall escape them.

4 The appearance of them *is* as the appearance of horses; and as horsemen, so shall they run.

5 Like the noise of chariots on the tops of mountains shall they leap, like the noise of a flame of fire that devoureth the stubble, as a strong people set in battle array.

6 Before their face the people shall be much pained: all faces shall gather blackness.

7 They shall run like mighty men; they shall climb the wall like men of war; and they shall march every one on his ways, and they shall not break their ranks:

8 Neither shall one thrust another; they shall walk every one in his path: and *when* they fall upon the sword, they shall not be wounded.

9 They shall run to and fro in the city; they shall run upon the wall, they shall climb up upon the houses; they shall enter in at the windows like a thief.

10 The earth shall quake before them; the heavens shall tremble: the sun and the moon shall be dark, and the stars shall withdraw their shining:

(2) *The Lord's army at Armageddon* (Rev. 19:11-21).

11 And the LORD [f]shall utter his voice before [1]his [g]army: for his

[1] **(2:11)** To verse 10 inclusive the invading army is described; at verse 11 Jehovah's army. This "army" is described, Rev. 19:11-18. The call to repentance is based upon the Lord's promise of deliverance, vs. 12-17. At verses 18-20 we have the deliverance (v. 20; see "Armageddon," Rev. 16:14, *refs.*), and kingdom blessing

camp *is* very great: for *he is* strong that
executeth his word: [a]for the day of the
LORD *is* great and very terrible; and who
can abide it?

(3) *Repentance of the Jews who are in the land.*

12 Therefore also now, saith the LORD,
turn [b]ye *even* to me with all your heart,
and with fasting, and with weeping, and
with mourning:
13 And rend your heart, and not your
garments, and turn unto the LORD your
God: for he *is* gracious and merciful,
slow to anger, and of great kindness, and
[c]repenteth him of the evil.
14 Who knoweth *if* he will return and
[c]repent, and leave a blessing behind
him; *even* a [d]meat-offering and a drink-
offering unto the LORD your God?
15 Blow the trumpet in Zion, sanctify
a fast, call a solemn assembly:
16 Gather the people, sanctify the congregation, assemble the elders, gather the
children, and those that suck the breasts:
let the bridegroom go forth of his chamber, and the bride out of her closet.
17 Let the priests, the ministers of the
LORD, weep between the porch and the
altar, and let them say, Spare thy people,
O LORD, and give not thine heritage to
reproach, that the [e]heathen should rule
over them: wherefore should they say
among the people, Where *is* their God?

(4) *The LORD's response (a) in promise of deliverance.*

18 Then will the LORD be jealous for
his land, and pity his people.
19 Yea, the LORD will answer and say
unto his people, Behold, I will send you
corn, and wine, and oil, and ye shall be
satisfied therewith: and I will no more
make you a reproach among the [e]heathen:
20 But I will remove far off from you
the northern *army*, and will drive him into
a land barren and desolate, with his face
toward the east sea, and his hinder part
toward the utmost sea, and his stink shall
come up, and his ill savour shall come up,
because he hath done great things.

B.C. 800.

a Jer. 30:7; Amos 5:18; Zeph. 1:15.

b Deut. 4:29; Jer. 4:1; Ezk. 33:11; Hos. 12:6; 14:1.

c Zech. 8:14, *note*.

d Lit. *meal*.

e i.e. *nations*.

f *Holy Spirit*. vs. 28, 29; Mic. 2:7. (Gen. 1:2; Mal. 2:15.)

g vs. 28-32; Acts 2:17-21.

21 Fear not, O land; be glad and
rejoice: for the LORD will do great things.
22 Be not afraid, ye beasts of the field:
for the pastures of the wilderness do
spring, for the tree beareth her fruit, the
fig tree and the vine do yield their
strength.
23 Be glad then, ye children of Zion,
and rejoice in the LORD your God: for he
hath given you the former rain moderately, and he will cause to come down
for you the rain, the former rain, and the
latter rain in the first *month*.
24 And the floors shall be full of
wheat, and the fats shall overflow with
wine and oil.
25 And I will restore to you the years
that the locust hath eaten, the cankerworm, and the caterpiller, and the
palmerworm, my great army which I
sent among you.
26 And ye shall eat in plenty, and be
satisfied, and praise the name of the
LORD your God, that hath dealt wondrously with you: and my people shall
never be ashamed.
27 And ye shall know that I *am* in the
midst of Israel, and *that* I *am* the LORD
your God, and none else: and my people
shall never be ashamed.

(b) The promise of the Spirit.

28 And it shall come to pass [1]after-
ward, *that* I will pour out my [f]spirit
upon all [g]flesh; and your sons and your
daughters shall prophesy, your old men
shall dream dreams, your young men
shall see visions:
29 And also upon the servants and
upon the handmaids in those days will I
pour out my spirit.

(5) *The signs preceding the second advent and the day of the LORD*. (Cf. Isa. 13:9, 10; 24:21-23; Ezk. 32:7-10; Mt. 24:29, 30.)

30 And I will shew wonders in the
heavens and in the earth, blood, and fire,
and pillars of smoke.
31 The sun shall be turned into darkness, and the moon into blood, before

in verses 21-27. Verses 28-32 give the outpouring of the Spirit, and verses 29-32 the cosmical signs preceding the day of the LORD. See Rev. 19:11-21, *note*.

[1]**(2:28)** Cf. Acts 2:17, which gives a specific interpretation of "afterward" (Heb. *ache-rith* = "latter," "last"). "Afterward" in Joel 2:28 means "in the last days" (Gr. *eschatos*), and has a partial and continuous fulfilment during the "last days" which began with the first advent of Christ (Heb. 1:2); but the greater fulfilment awaits the "last days" as applied to Israel. See Acts 2:17, *note*, for phrase, "the last days."

the great and the terrible day of the LORD come.

32 And it shall come to pass, *that* [a]whosoever shall call on the name of the LORD shall be delivered: for in mount Zion and in Jerusalem shall be deliverance, as the LORD hath said, and in the [b]remnant whom the LORD shall call.

CHAPTER 3.

(6) *The restoration of Israel.*
(Cf. Isa. 11:10-12; Jer. 23:5-8;
Ezk. 37:21-28; Acts 15:15-17.)

For, behold, in those days, [c]and in that time, [d]when I shall bring again the captivity of Judah and Jerusalem,

(7) *The judgment of the Gentile nations after Armageddon.* (See Mt. 25:32, *note.*)

2 I will also gather all nations, and will bring them down into the valley of Jehoshaphat, and will plead with them there for my people and *for* my heritage Israel, whom they have scattered among the nations, and parted my land.

3 And they have cast lots for my people; and have given a boy for an harlot, and sold a girl for wine, that they might drink.

4 Yea, and what have ye to do with me, O Tyre, and Zidon, and all the coasts of Palestine? will ye render me a recompence? and if ye recompense me, swiftly *and* speedily will I return your recompence upon your own head;

5 Because ye have taken my silver and my gold, and have carried into your temples my goodly pleasant things:

6 The children also of Judah and the children of Jerusalem have ye sold unto the Grecians, that ye might remove them far from their border.

7 Behold, I will raise them out of the place whither ye have sold them, and will return your recompence upon your own head:

8 And I will sell your sons and your daughters into the hand of the children of Judah, and they shall sell them to the Sabeans, to a people far off: for the LORD hath spoken *it*.

Part III. (1) *Retrospect:*
the day of the LORD.

9 [e]Proclaim ye this among the Gentiles; [1]Prepare [f]war, wake up the mighty men, let all the men of war draw near; let them come up:

10 Beat your plowshares into swords, and your pruninghooks into spears: let the weak say, I *am* strong.

11 Assemble yourselves, and come, all ye [g]heathen, and gather yourselves together round about: thither cause thy mighty ones to come down, O LORD.

12 Let the [g]heathen be wakened, and come up to the valley of Jehoshaphat: for there will I sit to judge all the heathen round about.

13 Put ye in the sickle, for the harvest is ripe: come, get you down; for the press is full, the fats overflow; for their wickedness *is* great.

14 Multitudes, multitudes in the valley of decision: for the day of the LORD *is* near in the valley of decision.

15 The sun and the moon shall be darkened, and the stars shall withdraw their shining.

16 The LORD also shall roar out of Zion, and utter his voice from [h]Jerusalem; and the heavens and the earth shall shake: but the LORD *will be* the hope of his people, and the strength of the children of Israel.

(2) *Full kingdom blessing.*
(Zech. 12:8, *note.*)

17 So shall ye know that I *am* the LORD your God dwelling in Zion, [i]my holy mountain: then shall Jerusalem be holy, and there shall [j]no strangers pass through her any more.

18 And it shall come to pass in that day, *that* the mountains shall drop down new wine, and the hills shall flow with milk, and all the rivers of Judah shall flow with waters, [k]and a fountain shall come forth of the house of the LORD, and shall water the valley of Shittim.

19 Egypt shall be a desolation, and Edom shall be a desolate wilderness, for the violence *against* the children of Judah, because they have shed innocent blood in their land.

20 But Judah shall [l]dwell for ever, and Jerusalem from generation to generation.

21 For I will cleanse their blood *that* I have not cleansed: for the LORD dwelleth in Zion.

B.C. 800.

a Rom. 10:13.

b *Remnant.* Amos 5:15. (Isa. 1:9; Rom. 11:5.)

c *Judgments (the seven).* vs. 1-14; Mt. 13:40-42. (2 Sam. 7:14; Rev. 22:12.)

d *Israel (prophecies).* vs. 1-8, 15-20; Zech. 10:6-12. (Gen. 12:2, 3; Rom. 11:26.)

e *Day (of Jehovah).* vs. 9-21; Amos 5.18-20. (Isa. 2:10-22; Rev. 19:11-21.)

f Armageddon (battle of). vs. 9-13; Oba. 15. (Rev. 16:14; 19:11-21.)

g i.e. *nations.*

h *Kingdom* (O.T.) vs. 16-20; Amos 9:11-15. (Gen. 1:26; Zech. 12:8.)

i Dan. 11:45; Oba. 16; Zech. 8:3.

j Isa. 35:8; 52:1; Nah. 1:15; Zech. 14:21; Rev. 21:27.

k Psa. 46:4; Ezk. 47:1; Zech. 14:8; Rev. 22:1.

l Amos 9:15.

[1] **(3:9)** Verses 9-14 refer to Armageddon; verses 15, 16 are parallel with Joel 2:30-32. From verses 9 to 16 we have a *résumé* of Joel 2:9-32.

AMOS

AMOS, a Jew, but prophesying (B.C. 776–763) in the northern kingdom (1:1; 7:14, 15), exercised his ministry during the reign of Jeroboam II, an able but idolatrous king who brought his kingdom to the zenith of its power. Nothing could seem more improbable than the fulfilment of Amos' warnings; yet within fifty years the kingdom was utterly destroyed. The vision of Amos is, however, wider than the northern kingdom, including the whole "house of Jacob."

Amos is in four parts: I. Judgments on the cities surrounding Palestine, 1:1–2:3. II. Judgments on Judah and Israel, 2:4-16. III. Jehovah's controversy with "the whole family" of Jacob, 3:1–9:10. IV. The future glory of the Davidic kingdom, 9:11-15.

CHAPTER 1.

Part I. Judgments on surrounding peoples (Amos 1:1–2:3).

THE words of Amos, who was among
the [a]herdmen of Tekoa, which he
saw concerning Israel in the days of
[b]Uzziah king of Judah, and in the days
of Jeroboam the son of Joash king of
Israel, two years before the [c]earthquake.
2 And he said, The LORD will [1]roar
from Zion, and utter his voice from
Jerusalem; and the habitations of the
shepherds shall mourn, and the top of
Carmel shall wither.
3 Thus saith the LORD; For three transgressions of [d]Damascus, and for four, I
will not turn away *the punishment* thereof; because they have threshed Gilead
with threshing instruments of iron:
4 But I will send a fire into the house
of [e]Hazael, which shall devour the
palaces of [f]Ben-hadad.
5 I will [g]break also the bar of
Damascus, and cut off the inhabitant
from the plain of Aven, and him that
holdeth the sceptre from the house of
Eden: and the people of Syria shall go
into captivity unto Kir, saith the LORD.
6 Thus saith the LORD; For three transgressions of [h]Gaza, and for four, I will
not turn away *the punishment* thereof;
because they carried away captive the
whole captivity, to deliver *them* up to
Edom:

B.C. 787.

a Amos 7:14.

b 2 Ki. 15:1-7; (marg.); 2 Chr. 26:1-23; Isa. 1:1; Hos. 1:1.

c Cf. Isa. 42:13; Jer. 25:30; Joel 3:16; Zech. 14:5.

d Isa. 7:8; 17:1.

e Jer. 49:27.

f 1 Ki. 20:1; 2 Ki. 6:24.

g Isa. 8:4; Jer. 51:30; 2 Ki. 14:28.

h Isa. 8:4; Jer. 47:1, 5; Zeph. 2:4.

7 But I will send a fire on the wall of
Gaza, which shall devour the palaces
thereof:
8 And I will cut off the inhabitant from
Ashdod, and him that holdeth the sceptre from Ashkelon, and I will turn mine
hand against Ekron: and the remnant of
the Philistines shall perish, saith the
Lord GOD.
9 Thus saith the LORD; For three transgressions of Tyrus, and for four, I will
not turn away *the punishment* thereof;
because they delivered up the whole
captivity to Edom, and remembered not
the brotherly covenant:
10 But I will send a fire on the wall of
Tyrus, which shall devour the palaces
thereof.
11 Thus saith the LORD; For three
transgressions of Edom, and for four, I
will not turn away *the punishment* thereof; because he did pursue his brother
with the sword, and did cast off all pity,
and his anger did tear perpetually, and
he kept his wrath for ever:
12 But I will send a fire upon Teman,
which shall devour the palaces of
Bozrah.
13 Thus saith the LORD; For three
transgressions of the children of
Ammon, and for four, I will not turn
away *the punishment* thereof; because
they have ripped up the women with
child of Gilead, that they might enlarge
their border:

[1] **(1:2)** "Roar," etc. Cf. Isa. 42:13; Jer. 25:30-33; Hos. 11:10, 11; Joel 3:16. It will be found that wherever the phrase occurs it is connected with the destruction of Gentile dominion (see "Times of the Gentiles," Lk. 21:24; Rev. 16:19, *note*), and the blessing of Israel in the kingdom. Without doubt a near fulfilment upon Syria occurred (2 Ki. 14:28), but the expression, "the LORD will roar," looks forward to a vaster fulfilment. See Joel 1:4, *note*.

B.C. 787.

14 But I will kindle a fire in the wall of Rabbah, and it shall devour the palaces thereof, with shouting in the day of battle, with a tempest in the day of the whirlwind:

15 And their king shall go into captivity, he and his princes together, saith the LORD.

CHAPTER 2.

(*Judgments on surrounding peoples, continued.*)

Thus saith the LORD; [a]For three transgressions of Moab, and for four, I will not turn away *the punishment* thereof; because he burned the bones of the king of Edom into lime:

2 But I will send a fire upon Moab, and it shall devour the palaces of Kerioth: and Moab shall die with tumult, with shouting, *and* with the sound of the trumpet:

3 And I will cut off the judge from the midst thereof, and will slay all the princes thereof with him, saith the LORD.

Part. II. Judgments on Judah and Israel (vs. 4-16).

4 Thus saith the LORD; [1]For three transgressions of [b]Judah, and for four, I will not turn away *the punishment* thereof; because they have despised the law of the LORD, and have not kept his commandments, and their lies caused them to err, after the which their fathers have walked:

5 But I will send a fire upon Judah, and it shall devour the palaces of Jerusalem.

6 Thus saith the LORD; For three transgressions of [c]Israel, and for four, I will not turn away *the punishment* thereof; because they sold the righteous for silver, and the poor for a pair of shoes;

7 That pant after the dust of the earth on the head of the poor, and turn aside the way of the meek: and a man and his father will go in unto the *same* maid, to profane my holy name:

8 And they lay *themselves* down upon clothes laid to pledge by every altar, and they drink the wine of the condemned *in* the house of their god.

9 Yet destroyed I the Amorite before them, whose height *was* like the height of the cedars, and he *was* strong as the oaks; yet I destroyed his fruit from above, and his roots from beneath.

10 Also I brought you up from the land of Egypt, and led you forty years through the wilderness, to possess the land of the Amorite.

11 And I raised up of your sons for prophets, and of your young men for [d]Nazarites. *Is it* not even thus, O ye children of Israel? saith the LORD.

12 But ye gave the Nazarites wine to drink; and commanded the prophets, saying, Prophesy not.

13 Behold, I am pressed under you, as a cart is pressed *that is* full of sheaves.

14 Therefore the flight shall perish from the swift, and the strong shall not strengthen his force, neither shall the mighty deliver himself:

15 Neither shall he stand that handleth the bow; and *he that is* swift of foot shall not deliver *himself*: neither shall he that rideth the horse deliver himself.

16 And *he that is* courageous among the mighty shall flee away naked in that day, saith the LORD.

CHAPTER 3.

Part III. Jehovah's controversy with "the whole family" of Jacob (Amos 3:1–9:10).

Hear this word that the LORD hath spoken against you, O children of Israel, against the [2]whole family which I brought up from the land of Egypt, saying,

2 You only have I known of all the families of the earth: [3]therefore

a Ezk. 25:8, 9.

b Amos 3:2; 2 Ki. 17:19; Hos. 12:2.

c Cf. Jud. 2:17-20; 2 Ki. 22:11-17.

d Num. 6:1-8.

[1] **(2:4)** The judgments on Judah and Israel were fulfilled as to Judah in the 70 years' captivity; as to Israel (the northern kingdom) in the world-wide dispersion which still continues.

[2] **(3:1)** The language here, and the expression "house of Jacob," v. 13, evidently gives the prophecy a wider application than to "Israel," the ten-tribe northern kingdom, though the judgment was, in the event, executed first upon the northern kingdom (2 Ki. 17:18-23).

[3] **(3:2)** It is noteworthy that Jehovah's controversy with the Gentile cities which hated Israel is brief: "I will send a fire." But Israel had been brought into the place of privilege and so of responsibility, and the LORD'S indictment is detailed and unsparing. Cf. Mt. 11:23; Lk. 12:47, 48.

I will punish you for all your iniquities.
3 Can two walk together, except they
be agreed?
4 Will a lion roar in the forest, when he
hath no prey? will a young lion cry out
of his den, if he have taken nothing?
5 Can a bird fall in a snare upon the
earth, where no gin *is* for him? shall *one*
take up a snare from the earth, and have
taken nothing at all?
6 Shall a trumpet be blown in the city,
and the people not be afraid? shall there
be evil in a city, [a]and the LORD hath not
done *it*?
7 Surely the Lord GOD will do nothing,
but he revealeth his secret unto his servants the [b]prophets.
8 The lion hath roared, who will not
fear? the Lord GOD hath spoken, [c]who
can but prophesy?
9 Publish in the palaces at Ashdod,
and in the palaces in the land of Egypt,
and say, Assemble yourselves upon the
mountains of Samaria, and behold the
great tumults in the midst thereof, and
the oppressed in the midst thereof.
10 For they know not to do right, saith
the LORD, who store up violence and
robbery in their palaces.
11 Therefore thus saith the Lord GOD;
An adversary *there shall be* even round
about the land; and he shall bring down
thy strength from thee, and thy palaces
shall be spoiled.
12 Thus saith the LORD; As the shepherd taketh out of the mouth of the lion
two legs, or a piece of an ear; so shall the
children of Israel be taken out that dwell
in Samaria in the corner of a bed, and in
Damascus *in* a couch.
13 Hear ye, and testify in the house of
Jacob, saith the Lord GOD, the God of
hosts,
14 That in the day that I shall visit the
transgressions of Israel upon him I will
also visit the altars of Beth-el: and the
horns of the altar shall be cut off, and fall
to the ground.
15 And I will smite the winter house
with the summer house; and the houses
of ivory shall perish, and the great
houses shall have an end, saith the LORD.

B.C. 787.

a Or, *and shall not the Lord do somewhat?*

b *Inspiration.* Mic. 3:8. (Ex. 4:15; Rev. 22:19.)

c Jer. 20:9; Acts 4:20; 5:20, 29; 1 Cor. 9:16.

d Psa. 22:12; Ezk. 39:18.

e Psa. 89:35.

f See Lev. 7:13, *note.*

g *Leaven.* Mt. 16:6, 11, 12. (Gen. 19:3; Mt. 13:33.)

h i.e. *freewill.*

i vs. 8, 9; Isa. 26:11; Jer. 5:3; Hag. 2:17.

CHAPTER 4.

The very sacrifices at Beth-el were the scorn of Jehovah.

Hear this word, [d]ye kine of Bashan,
that *are* in the mountain of
Samaria, which oppress the poor, which
crush the needy, which say to their masters, Bring, and let us drink.
2 [e]The Lord GOD hath sworn by his
holiness, that, lo, the days shall come
upon you, that he will take you away
with hooks, and your posterity with
fishhooks.
3 And ye shall go out at the breaches,
every *cow at that which is* before her; and
ye shall cast *them* into the palace, saith
the LORD.
4 Come to [1]Beth-el, and transgress; at
Gilgal multiply transgression; and bring
your sacrifices every morning, *and* your
tithes after three years:
5 And offer a sacrifice of [f]thanksgiving
with [g]leaven, and proclaim *and* publish
the free [h]offerings: for this liketh you, O
ye children of Israel, saith the Lord GOD.

Israel reminded of Jehovah's chastenings.

6 And I also have given you cleanness
of teeth in all your cities, and want of
bread in all your places: [i]yet have ye not
returned unto me, saith the LORD.
7 And also I have withholden the rain
from you, when *there were* yet three
months to the harvest: and I caused it to
rain upon one city, and caused it not to
rain upon another city: one piece was
rained upon, and the piece whereupon it
rained not withered.
8 So two *or* three cities wandered unto
one city, to drink water; but they were
not satisfied: yet have ye not returned
unto me, saith the LORD.
9 I have smitten you with blasting and
mildew: when your gardens and your
vineyards and your fig trees and your
olive trees increased, the palmerworm
devoured *them*: yet have ye not returned
unto me, saith the LORD.
10 I have sent among you the pestilence after the manner of Egypt: your
young men have I slain with the sword,

[1] **(4:4)** Cf. 1 Ki. 12:25-33. *Any* altar at Beth-el, after the establishment of Jehovah's worship at Jerusalem, was of necessity divisive and schismatic (Deut. 12:4-14). Cf. John 4:21-24; Mt. 18:20; Heb. 13:10-14.

B.C. 787.

and have taken away your horses; and I have made the stink of your camps to come up unto your nostrils: yet have ye not returned unto me, saith the LORD.

11 I have overthrown *some* of you, [a]as God overthrew Sodom and Gomorrah, and ye were as a firebrand plucked out of the burning: yet have ye not returned unto me, saith the LORD.

12 Therefore thus will I do unto thee, O Israel: *and* because I will do this unto thee, [b]prepare to meet thy God, O Israel.

13 For, lo, he that formeth the mountains, and createth the wind, and [c]declareth unto man what *is* his thought, that maketh the morning darkness, and treadeth upon the high places of the earth, The LORD, The God of hosts, *is* his name.

CHAPTER 5.

Jehovah's lamentation over Israel.

Hear ye this word which I take up against you, *even* a lamentation, O house of Israel.

2 The virgin of Israel is fallen; she shall no more rise: she is forsaken upon her land; *there is* none to raise her up.

3 For thus saith the Lord GOD; The city that went out *by* a thousand shall leave an hundred, and that which went forth *by* an hundred shall leave ten, to the house of Israel.

4 For thus saith the LORD unto the house of Israel, [d]Seek ye me, and ye shall live:

5 But seek not Beth-el, nor enter into Gilgal, and pass not to Beer-sheba: for Gilgal shall surely go into captivity, and [e]Beth-el shall come to nought.

6 Seek the LORD, and ye shall live; lest he break out like fire in the house of Joseph, and devour *it*, and *there be* none to quench *it* in Beth-el.

7 Ye who turn judgment to wormwood, and leave off righteousness in the earth,

8 [f]*Seek him* that maketh the seven stars and Orion, and turneth the shadow of death into the morning, and maketh the day dark with night: that calleth for the waters of the sea, and poureth them out upon the face of the earth: The LORD *is* his name:

9 That strengtheneth the spoiled against the strong, so that the spoiled shall come against the fortress.

10 They hate him that rebuketh in the gate, and they abhor him that speaketh uprightly.

11 Forasmuch therefore as your treading *is* upon the poor, and ye take from him burdens of wheat: [g]ye have built houses of hewn stone, but ye shall not dwell in them; ye have planted pleasant vineyards, but ye shall not drink wine of them.

12 For I know your manifold transgressions and your mighty sins: they afflict the just, they take a bribe, and they turn aside the poor in the gate *from their right*.

13 Therefore the prudent shall keep silence in that time; for it *is* an evil time.

14 Seek good, and not evil, that ye may live: and so the LORD, the God of hosts, shall be with you, as ye have spoken.

15 Hate the evil, and love the good, and establish judgment in the gate: [h]it may be that the LORD God of hosts will be gracious unto the [i]remnant of Joseph.

The day of the LORD.

16 Therefore the LORD, the God of hosts, the Lord, saith thus; Wailing *shall be* in all streets; and they shall say in all the highways, Alas! alas! and they shall call the husbandman to mourning, and such as are skilful of lamentation to wailing.

17 And in all vineyards *shall be* wailing: for I will pass through thee, saith the LORD.

18 Woe unto you that desire the day of the LORD! to what end *is* it for you? the [j]day of the LORD *is* darkness, and not light.

19 As if a man did flee from a lion, and a bear met him; or went into the house, and leaned his hand on the wall, and a serpent bit him.

20 *Shall* not the day of the LORD *be* darkness, and not light? even very dark, and no brightness in it?

Worship without righteousness Jehovah's abomination.

21 I hate, I despise your feast days, and I will not smell in your solemn assemblies.

22 Though ye offer me burnt-offerings and your [k]meat-offerings, I will not accept *them*: neither will I regard the peace-offerings of your fat beasts.

23 Take thou away from me the noise

a Gen. 19:24, 25; Isa. 13:19; Jer. 49:18.

b See Ezk. 13:5; 22:30; Lk. 14:31, 32.

c Psa. 139:2; Dan. 2:28.

d v. 6; 2 Chr. 15:2; Jer. 29:13.

e Hos. 4:15; 10:8.

f Job 9:9; 38:31.

g Deut. 28:30, 38, 39; Mic. 6:15; Zeph. 1:13; Hag. 1:6.

h 2 Ki. 19:4; Joel 2:14.

i *Remnant.* Mic. 2:12, 13. (Isa. 1:9; Rom. 11:5.)

j *Day (of Jehovah).* vs. 18-20; Oba. 15-21. (Isa. 2:10-22; Rev. 19:11-21.)

k Lit. *meal.*

B.C. 787.

of thy songs; for I will not hear the
melody of thy viols.
24 But let judgment run down as
waters, and righteousness as a mighty
stream.
25 Have ye offered unto me [a]sacrifices
and offerings in the wilderness forty
years, O house of Israel?
26 But ye have borne the tabernacle
[b]of your Moloch and Chiun your
images, the star of your god, which ye
made to yourselves.
27 Therefore will I cause you to go into
captivity beyond Damascus, saith the
LORD, whose name *is* The God of hosts.

CHAPTER 6.

Woe to those at ease in a day of unrighteousness.

Woe [c]to them *that are* at ease in Zion,
and [d]trust in the mountain of
Samaria, *which are* named chief of the
nations, to whom the house of Israel
came!
2 Pass ye unto [e]Calneh, and see; and
from thence go ye to [f]Hamath the great:
then go down to Gath of the Philistines:
be they better than these kingdoms? or
their border greater than your border?
3 Ye that put far away the evil day, and
cause the seat of violence to come near;
4 That lie upon beds of ivory, and
stretch themselves upon their couches,
and eat the lambs out of the flock, and
the calves out of the midst of the stall;
5 That chant to the sound of the viol,
and invent to themselves instruments of
musick, [g]like David;
6 That drink wine in bowls, and
anoint themselves with the chief ointments: [h]but they are not grieved for the
affliction of Joseph.
7 Therefore now shall they go captive
with the first that go captive, and the
banquet of them that stretched themselves shall be removed.
8 [i]The Lord GOD hath sworn by himself, saith the LORD the God of hosts, [j]I
abhor the excellency of Jacob, and hate
his palaces: therefore will I deliver up
the city with all that is therein.
9 And it shall come to pass, if there
remain ten men in one house, that they
shall die.
10 And a man's uncle shall take him
up, and he that burneth him, to bring
out the bones out of the house, and shall
say unto him that *is* by the sides of the
house, *Is there* yet *any* with thee? and he
shall say, No. Then shall he say, Hold thy
tongue: for we may not make mention of
the name of the LORD.
11 For, behold, the LORD commandeth,
and he will smite the great house with
breaches, and the little house with clefts.
12 Shall horses run upon the rock? will
one plow *there* with oxen? for ye have
turned judgment into gall, and the fruit
of righteousness into hemlock:
13 Ye which rejoice in a thing of
nought, which say, Have we not taken to
us horns by our own strength?
14 But, behold, I will raise up against
you a nation, O house of Israel, saith the
LORD the God of hosts; and they shall
afflict you from the entering in of
Hemath unto the river of the wilderness.

CHAPTER 7.

The prophet's intercession to prevail no longer.

Thus hath the Lord GOD shewed unto
me; and, behold, he formed grasshoppers in the beginning of the shooting
up of the latter growth; and, lo, *it was* the
latter growth after the king's mowings.
2 And it came to pass, *that* when they
had made an end of eating the grass of
the land, then I said, O Lord GOD, forgive, I beseech thee: by whom shall
Jacob arise? for he *is* small.
3 The LORD [k]repented for this: It shall
not be, saith the LORD.
4 Thus hath the Lord GOD shewed
unto me: and, behold, the Lord GOD
called to contend by fire, and it devoured
the great deep, and did eat up a part.
5 Then said I, O Lord GOD, cease, I
beseech thee: by whom shall Jacob arise?
for he *is* small.
6 The LORD [k]repented for this: This
also shall not be, saith the Lord GOD.
7 Thus he shewed me: and, behold, the
Lord stood upon a wall *made* by a
plumbline, with a plumbline in his hand.
8 And the LORD said unto me, Amos,
what seest thou? And I said, A
[l]plumbline. Then said the Lord, Behold,
I will set a [m]plumbline in the midst of

a vs. 25-27; Deut. 32:17-19; Acts 7:42, 43.
b 1 Ki. 11:33.
c Lk. 6:24.
d Psa. 2:12, *note.*
e Isa. 10:9.
f 2 Ki. 18:34.
g 1 Chr. 23:5.
h Gen. 49:23.
i Jer. 51:14; Heb. 6:13, 17.
j Amos 8:7; Psa. 47:4; Ezk. 24:21.
k Zech. 8:14, *note.*
l Isa. 28:17; 34:11; Lam. 2:8
m Symbol of judgment according to righteousness.

B.C. 787.

my people Israel: I will not again pass by
them any more:
9 And the high places of Isaac shall be
desolate, and the sanctuaries of Israel
shall be laid waste; and I will rise against
the house of Jeroboam with the sword.

The priest of Beth-el
charges Amos before the king.

10 Then [a]Amaziah the priest of Beth-el
sent to Jeroboam king of Israel, saying,
Amos hath conspired against thee in the
midst of the house of Israel: the land is
not able to bear all his words.
11 For thus Amos saith, Jeroboam shall
die by the sword, and Israel shall surely
be led away captive out of their own land.
12 Also Amaziah said unto Amos, O
thou seer, go, flee thee away into the
land of Judah, and there eat bread, and
prophesy there:
13 But prophesy not again any more at
Beth-el: for it *is* the king's chapel, and it
is the king's court.

The answer of Amos.

14 Then answered Amos, and said to
Amaziah, I *was* no prophet, neither *was* I
a prophet's son; but I *was* an herdman,
and a gatherer of sycomore fruit:
15 And the LORD took me as I followed the flock, and the LORD said unto
me, Go, prophesy unto my people Israel.
16 Now therefore hear thou the word
of the LORD: Thou sayest, Prophesy not
against Israel, and drop not *thy word*
against the house of Isaac.
17 Therefore thus saith the LORD; Thy
wife shall be an harlot in the city, and
thy sons and thy daughters shall fall by
the sword, and thy land shall be divided
by line; and thou shalt die in a polluted
land: and Israel shall surely go into captivity forth of his land.

CHAPTER 8.

The basket of summer fruit:
Israel soon to perish.

Thus hath the Lord GOD shewed unto
me: and behold a basket of summer
fruit.
2 And he said, Amos, what seest thou?
And I said, A [b]basket of [c]summer fruit.
Then said the LORD unto me, The end is
come upon my people of Israel; I will
not again pass by them any more.
3 And the songs of the temple shall be
howlings in that day, saith the Lord GOD:
there shall be many dead bodies in every
place; they shall cast *them* forth with
silence.

Jehovah's full case against Israel.

4 Hear this, O ye that swallow up the
needy, even to make the poor of the land
to fail,
5 Saying, When will the new moon be
gone, that we may sell corn? and the sabbath, that we may set forth wheat, making
the [d]ephah small, and the shekel great,
and falsifying the balances by deceit?
6 That we may buy the poor for silver,
and the needy for a pair of shoes; *yea*,
and sell the refuse of the wheat?
7 The LORD hath sworn by the excellency of Jacob, Surely I will never forget
any of their works.
8 Shall not the land tremble for this,
and every one mourn that dwelleth
therein? and it shall rise up wholly as a
flood; and it shall be cast out and
drowned, as *by* the flood of Egypt.
9 And it shall come to pass in that day,
saith the Lord GOD, that I will cause the
sun to go down at noon, and I will dark-
en the earth in the clear day:
10 And I will turn your feasts into
mourning, and all your songs into
lamentation; and I will bring up sackcloth upon all loins, and baldness upon
every head; and I will make it as the
mourning of an only *son*, and the end
thereof as a bitter day.
11 Behold, the days come, saith the
Lord GOD, that I will send a famine in
the land, not a famine of bread, nor a
thirst for water, [e]but of hearing the
words of the LORD:
12 And they shall wander from sea to
sea, and from the north even to the east,
they shall run to and fro to seek the
word of the LORD, and shall not find *it*.
13 In that day shall the fair virgins and
young men faint for thirst.
14 They that swear by the sin of
Samaria, and say, Thy god, O Dan,
liveth; and, The [f]manner of Beer-sheba
liveth; even they shall fall, and never rise
up again.

a 1 Ki. 12:31, 32.
b Cf. Jer. 24:1-3.
c i.e. *soon to perish.*
d One ephah = 1 bu. 3 pts.
e Cf. 1 Sam. 28:6; 2 Chr. 15:3, 4; Ezk. 7:26; Mic. 3:6, 7.
f Heb. *ways.* See Acts 9:2; 18:25; 19:9, 23; 24:14.

CHAPTER 9.

The final prophecy of dispersion.
(Cf. v. 9; Deut. 28:63-68.)

I saw the Lord [1]standing upon the altar: and he said, Smite the lintel of the door, that the posts may shake: and cut them in the head, all of them; and I will slay the last of them with the sword: he that fleeth of them shall not flee away, and he that escapeth of them shall not be delivered.

2 [a]Though they dig into [b]hell, thence shall mine hand take them; [c]though they climb up to heaven, thence will I bring them down:

3 And though they hide themselves in the top of Carmel, I will search and take them out thence; and though they be hid from my sight in the bottom of the sea, thence will I command the serpent, and he shall bite them:

4 And though they go into captivity before their enemies, thence will I command the sword, and it shall slay them: and I will set mine eyes upon them for evil, and not for good.

5 And the Lord GOD of hosts *is* he that toucheth the land, and it shall melt, and all that dwell therein shall mourn: and it shall rise up wholly like a flood; and shall be drowned, as *by* the flood of Egypt.

6 *It is* he that buildeth his stories in the heaven, and hath founded his troop in the earth; he that calleth for the waters of the sea, and poureth them out upon the face of the earth: The LORD *is* his name.

7 *Are* ye not as children of the Ethiopians unto me, O children of Israel? saith the LORD. Have not I brought up Israel out of the land of Egypt? and the Philistines from Caphtor, and the Syrians from Kir?

8 Behold, the eyes of the Lord GOD *are* upon the sinful kingdom, and I will destroy it from off the face of the earth; saving that I will not utterly destroy the house of Jacob, saith the LORD.

9 For, lo, I will command, and I will [d]sift the house of Israel among all nations, like as *corn* is sifted in a sieve, yet shall not the least grain fall upon the earth.

10 All the sinners of my people shall die by the sword, which say, The evil shall not overtake nor prevent us.

Part IV. Future kingdom blessing:
(1) *The LORD's return and the re-establishment of the Davidic monarchy.*

11 In that [e]day will I raise up the tabernacle of [f]David that is fallen, and close up the breaches thereof; and I will raise up his ruins, and I will build it as in the days of old:

12 That they may possess the remnant of Edom, and of all the [g]heathen, which are called by my name, saith the LORD that doeth this.

(2) *Full kingdom blessing of restored Israel.*

13 Behold, the days come, saith the LORD, that the plowman shall overtake the reaper, and the treader of grapes him that soweth seed; and the mountains shall drop sweet wine, and all the hills shall melt.

14 And I will bring again the captivity of my people of Israel, and they shall build the waste cities, and inhabit *them*; and they shall plant vineyards, and drink the wine thereof; they shall also make gardens, and eat the fruit of them.

15 And I will plant them upon their land, [h]and they shall no more be pulled up out of their land which I have given them, saith the LORD thy God.

B.C. 787.

a Psa. 139:8.
b Heb. *Sheol.* See Hab. 2:5, *note.*
c Job 20:6; Jer. 51:53; Oba. 4; Mt. 11:23.
d See Psa. 72:1, *note.*
e vs. 11, 12; Acts 15:16, 17.
f *Kingdom* (O.T.). vs. 11-15; Mic. 4:1-3. (Gen. 1:26; Zech. 12:8.)
g i.e. *nations.*
h Isa. 60:21; Jer. 32:41; Ezk. 34:28; Joel 3:20.

[1] **(9:1)** The position of the Lord (Adonai) is significant. The altar speaks properly of mercy because of judgment executed upon an interposed sacrifice, but when altar and sacrifice are despised the altar becomes a place of judgment. Cf. John 12:31.

OBADIAH

INTERNAL evidence seems to fix the date of Obadiah's ministry in the reign of the bloody Athaliah (2 Ki. 8:16-26). If this be true, and if the ministry of Joel was during the reign of Joash, then Obadiah is chronologically first of the writing prophets, and first to use the formula, "the day of the LORD." (Cf. Joel 1:4, *note.*)

The book is in four parts: I. Edom's humiliation, vs. 1-9. II. The crowning sin of Edom, vs. 10-14. III. The future visitation of Edom in the day of the LORD, vs. 15, 16 (Isa. 34, 63:1-6). IV. The inclusion of Edom in the future kingdom, vs. 17-21 (Num. 24:17-19).

Part I. The humiliation of Edom.

THE vision of Obadiah. Thus saith the Lord GOD [a]concerning Edom; We have heard a rumour from the LORD, and an ambassador is sent among the [b]heathen, Arise ye, and let us rise up against her in battle.

2 Behold, I have made thee small among the [b]heathen: thou art greatly despised.

3 The pride of thine heart hath deceived thee, thou that dwellest in the clefts of the rock, whose habitation *is* high; that saith in his heart, Who shall bring me down to the ground?

4 Though thou exalt *thyself* as the eagle, and though thou set thy nest among the stars, thence will I bring thee down, saith the LORD.

5 If thieves came to thee, if robbers by night, (how art thou cut off!) would they not have stolen till they had enough? if the grapegatherers came to thee, would they not leave *some* grapes?

6 How are *the things* of Esau searched out! *how* are his hidden things sought up!

7 All the men of thy confederacy have brought thee *even* to the border: the men that were at peace with thee have deceived thee, *and* prevailed against thee; *they that eat* thy bread have laid a wound under thee: *there is* none understanding in him.

8 Shall I not in that day, saith the LORD, even destroy the wise *men* out of [c]Edom, and understanding out of the mount of Esau?

9 And thy mighty *men*, O [d]Teman, shall be dismayed, to the end that every one of the mount of Esau may be cut off by slaughter.

B.C. 887.

a Psa. 137:7; Isa. 34:1-15; 63:1-6; Jer. 49:7-22; Ezk. 25:12-13.

b i.e. *nations.*

c Gen. 36:1, *note.*

d Gen. 36:11; 1 Chr. 1:45; Job 2:11; Jer. 49:7, 20.

e *Day (of Jehovah).* vs. 15-21; Zeph. 1:15-18. (Isa. 2:10-22; Rev. 19:11-21.)

f *Armageddon (battle of).* Zeph. 3:8. (Rev. 16:14; 19:11-21.)

Part II. The great sin of Edom. (Cf. Num. 20:14-21; Psa. 137:7; Ezk. 35:5.)

10 For *thy* violence against thy brother Jacob shame shall cover thee, and thou shalt be cut off for ever.

11 In the day that thou stoodest on the other side, in the day that the strangers carried away captive his forces, and foreigners entered into his gates, and cast lots upon Jerusalem, even thou *wast* as one of them.

12 But thou shouldest not have looked on the day of thy brother in the day that he became a stranger; neither shouldest thou have rejoiced over the children of Judah in the day of their destruction; neither shouldest thou have spoken proudly in the day of distress.

13 Thou shouldest not have entered into the gate of my people in the day of their calamity; yea, thou shouldest not have looked on their affliction in the day of their calamity, nor have laid *hands* on their substance in the day of their calamity;

14 Neither shouldest thou have stood in the crossway, to cut off those of his that did escape; neither shouldest thou have delivered up those of his that did remain in the day of distress.

Part III. Edom in the day of the LORD.

15 For the [e]day of the LORD *is* near [f]upon all the [b]heathen: as thou hast done, it shall be done unto thee: thy reward shall return upon thine own head.

16 For as ye have drunk upon my holy mountain, *so* shall all the [b]heathen drink continually, yea,

they shall drink, and they shall swallow
down, and they shall be as though they
had not been.

Part IV. Edom to be included
in the kingdom.

17 [a]But upon mount Zion shall be
deliverance, and there shall be holiness;
and the house of Jacob shall possess
their possessions.
18 [b]And the house of Jacob shall be a
fire, and the house of Joseph a flame,
and the house of Esau for stubble, and
they shall kindle in them, and devour
them; and there shall not be *any* remaining of the house of Esau; for the LORD
hath spoken *it*.

19 And *they of* the south [c]shall possess
the mount of Esau; and [d]*they of* the plain
the Philistines: and they shall possess
the fields of Ephraim, and the fields of
Samaria: and Benjamin *shall possess*
Gilead.
20 And the captivity of this host of the
children of Israel *shall possess* that of the
Canaanites, *even* unto Zarephath; and
the captivity of Jerusalem, which *is* in
Sepharad, shall possess the cities of the
south.
21 And saviours shall come up on
mount Zion to judge the mount of Esau;
and the [e]kingdom shall be the LORD'S.

a Joel 2:32.
b Ezk. 25:14; Dan. 11:41.
c Isa. 11:14; Amos 9:12.
d Zeph. 2:7.
e See *Kingdom*, Zech. 12:8, *note;* 1 Cor. 15:28, *note.*

JONAH

THE historical character of the man Jonah is vouched for by Jesus Christ (Mt. 12:39-41), as also that his preservation in the great fish was a "sign" or type of our Lord's own entombment and resurrection. Both are miraculous and both are equally credible. 2 Ki. 14:25 records the fulfilment of a prophecy by Jonah. The man himself was a bigoted Jew, unwilling to testify to a Gentile city, and angry that God had spared it. Typically he foreshadows the nation of Israel out of its own land; a trouble to the Gentiles, yet witnessing to them; cast out by them, but miraculously preserved; in their future deepest distress calling upon Jehovah-Saviour, and finding deliverance, and then becoming missionaries to the Gentiles (Zech. 8:7-23). He typifies Christ as the sent One, raised from the dead, and carrying salvation to the Gentiles. The chapter divisions indicate the analysis of Jonah.

CHAPTER 1.

B.C. 862.

The prophet's first commission.

NOW the word of the LORD came unto Jonah the son of Amittai, saying,

2 Arise, go to [a]Nineveh, that [b]great city, and cry against it; for their wickedness is come up before me.

The prophet's flight from Jehovah; the great storm.

3 But Jonah rose up to flee unto Tarshish from the presence of the LORD, and went down to Joppa; and he found a ship going to Tarshish: so he paid the fare thereof, and went down into it, to go with them unto Tarshish [c]from the presence of the LORD.

4 But the LORD sent out a great wind into the sea, and there was a mighty tempest in the sea, so that the ship was like to be broken.

5 Then the mariners were afraid, and cried every man unto his god, and cast forth the wares that *were* in the ship into the sea, to lighten *it* of them. But Jonah was gone down into the sides of the ship; and he lay, and was fast asleep.

6 So the shipmaster came to him, and said unto him, What meanest thou, O sleeper? arise, call upon thy God, if so be that God will think upon us, that we perish not.

7 And they said every one to his fellow, Come, and let us cast lots, that we may know for whose cause this evil *is* upon us. So they cast lots, and the lot fell upon Jonah.

8 Then said they unto him, Tell us, we pray thee, for whose cause this evil *is* upon us; What *is* thine occupation? and whence comest thou? what *is* thy country? and of what people *art* thou?

9 And he said unto them, I *am* an Hebrew; and I [d]fear the LORD, the God of heaven, [e]which hath made the sea and the dry *land*.

10 Then were the men exceedingly afraid, and said unto him, Why hast thou done this? For the men knew that he fled from the presence of the LORD, because he had told them.

11 Then said they unto him, What shall we do unto thee, that the sea may be calm unto us? for the sea wrought, and was tempestuous.

The prophet swallowed by the great fish.

12 And he said unto them, Take me up, and cast me forth into the sea; so shall the sea be calm unto you: for I know that for my sake this great tempest *is* upon you.

13 Nevertheless the men rowed hard to bring *it* to the land; but they could not: for the sea wrought, and was tempestuous against them.

14 Wherefore they cried unto the LORD, and said, We beseech thee, O LORD, we beseech thee, let us not perish for this man's life, and lay not upon us innocent blood: for thou, O LORD, hast done as it pleased thee.

15 So they took up Jonah, and cast him forth into the sea: and the sea ceased from her raging.

16 Then the men [d]feared the LORD exceedingly, and offered a sacrifice unto the LORD, and made vows.

a Isa. 37:37; Nah. 1:1, *note.*
b Jon. 3:2, 3; 4:11; Gen. 10:11, 12.
c Gen. 4:16; Job 1:12; 2:7.
d Psa. 19:9, *note.*
e Psa. 146:6; Acts 17:24.

17 Now the LORD had [a]prepared a
[1]great fish to swallow up Jonah. And
Jonah was in the belly of the fish three
days and three nights.

CHAPTER 2.

The prophet's prayer; Jehovah's answer.

Then Jonah [b]prayed unto the LORD his
God out of the fish's belly,
2 And said, [c]I cried by reason of mine
affliction unto the LORD, and he heard
me; out of the belly of [d]hell cried I, *and*
thou heardest my voice.
3 For thou hadst cast me into the deep,
in the midst of the seas; and the floods
compassed me about: [e]all thy billows
and thy waves passed over me.
4 [f]Then I said, I am cast out of thy
sight; yet I will look again toward thy
holy temple.
5 [g]The waters compassed me about,
even to the soul: the depth closed me
round about, the weeds were wrapped
about my head.
6 I went down to the bottoms of the
mountains; the earth with her bars *was*
about me for ever: yet hast thou brought
up my life from corruption, O LORD my
God.
7 When my soul fainted within me I
remembered the LORD: and my prayer
came in unto thee, into thine holy temple.
8 They that observe lying vanities forsake their own mercy.
9 But I will sacrifice unto thee with the
voice of thanksgiving; I will pay *that* that
I have vowed. Salvation *is* of the LORD.
10 And the LORD [h]spake unto the fish,
and it vomited out Jonah upon the dry
land.

CHAPTER 3.

The prophet's second commission;
his obedience; the repentance of Nineveh.

And the word of the LORD came unto
Jonah the second time, saying,
2 Arise, go unto [i]Nineveh, that great
city, and preach unto it the preaching
that I bid thee.
3 So Jonah arose, and went unto
Nineveh, according to the word of the
LORD. Now Nineveh was an exceeding
great city of three days' journey.
4 And Jonah began to enter into the
city a day's journey, and he cried, and
said, Yet forty days, and Nineveh shall
be overthrown.
5 So the people of Nineveh [j]believed
God, and proclaimed a fast, and put on
sackcloth, from the greatest of them even
to the least of them.
6 For word came unto the king of
Nineveh, and he arose from his throne,
and he laid his robe from him, and covered *him* with sackcloth, and sat in ashes.
7 And he caused *it* to be proclaimed
and published through Nineveh by the
decree of the king and his nobles, saying, Let neither man nor beast, herd nor
flock, taste any thing: let them not feed,
nor drink water:
8 But let man and beast be covered
with sackcloth, and cry mightily unto
God: yea, let them turn every one from
his evil way, and from the violence that
is in their hands.
9 Who can tell *if* God will turn and
[k]repent, and turn away from his fierce
anger, that we perish not?
10 And God saw their works, that they
turned from their evil way; and God
[k]repented of the evil, that he had said that
he would do unto them; and he did *it* not.

CHAPTER 4.

The prophet's displeasure;
the sheltering gourd.

But it displeased Jonah exceedingly,
and he was very angry.
2 And he prayed unto the LORD, and
said, I pray thee, O LORD, *was* not this my
saying, when I was yet in my country?
Therefore I fled before unto Tarshish: for
I knew that thou *art* a [l]gracious God, and
merciful, slow to anger, and of great
kindness, and [k]repentest thee of the evil.
3 Therefore now, O LORD, take, I

B.C. 862.

a Four prepared things. Jon. 4:6, 7, 8.

b *Bible prayers* (O.T.). Hab. 3:1-16.

c Psa. 18:4-6; 120:1; 130:1; 142:1; Lam. 3:55, 56.

d Heb. *Sheol*. See Hab. 2:5, *note*.

e Psa. 42:7.

f Psa. 31:22.

g Psa. 69:1; Lam. 3:54.

h *Miracles* (O.T.). vs. 1-10. (Gen. 5:24.)

i Nah. 1:1, *note*.

j *Faith*. Hab. 2:4. (Gen. 3:20; Heb. 11:39.)

k Zech. 8:14, *note*.

l Ex. 34:6; Psa. 86:5; Joel 2:13.

[1] **(1:17)** No miracle of Scripture has called forth so much unbelief. The issue is not between the doubter and this ancient record, but between the doubter and the Lord Jesus Christ (Mt. 12:39, 40). Science, "falsely so called" (1 Tim. 6:20), failing to take account of the fact that it deals only with the outward phenomena of a fallen race, and of an earth under a curse (Gen. 3:17-19), is intolerant of miracle. To faith, and to true science, miracle is what might be expected of divine love, interposing for good in a physically and morally disordered universe (Rom. 8:19-23).

beseech thee, my life from me; for *it is* better for me to die than to live.
4 Then said the LORD, Doest thou well to be angry?
5 So Jonah went out of the city, and sat on the east side of the city, and there made him a booth, and sat under it in the shadow, till he might see what would become of the city.
6 And the LORD God [a]prepared a gourd, and made *it* to come up over Jonah, that it might be a shadow over his head, to deliver him from his grief. So Jonah was exceeding glad of the gourd.
7 But God prepared a worm when the morning rose the next day, and it smote the gourd that it withered.
8 And it came to pass, when the sun did arise, that God prepared a vehement east wind; and the sun beat upon the head of Jonah, that he [1]fainted, and wished in himself to die, and said, *It is* better for me to die than to live.
9 And God said to Jonah, Doest thou well to be angry for the gourd? And he said, I do well to be angry, *even* unto death.
10 Then said the LORD, Thou hast had pity on the gourd, for the which thou hast not laboured, neither madest it grow; which came up in a night, and perished in a night:
11 And should not I spare [b]Nineveh, that great city, wherein are more than sixscore thousand persons that cannot discern between their right hand and their left hand; and *also* much cattle?

B.C. 862.

a Four prepared things. Jon. 1:17; 4:6, 7, 8.

b Nah. 1:1, *note.*

[1] **(4:8)** Cf. 1 Ki. 19:4-8. Taken as a lesson in service we have in Jonah a servant, (1) *disobedient,* Chapter 1:1-11; (2) *afflicted,* Chapter 1:12-17; (3) *praying,* Chapter 2:1-9; (4) *delivered,* Chapter 2:10; (5) *recommissioned,* Chapter 3:1-3; (6) *powerful,* Chapter 3:4-9; (7) *perplexed and fainting but not forsaken,* Chapter 4:1-11.

MICAH

MICAH, a contemporary of Isaiah, prophesied during the reigns of Jotham, Ahaz, and Hezekiah over Judah, and of Pekahiah, Pekah, and Hoshea over Israel (2 Ki. 15:23-30; 17:1-6). He was a prophet in Judah (Jer. 26:17-19), but the book called by his name chiefly concerns Samaria.

Micah falls into three prophetic strains, each beginning, "Hear": I. 1:1–2:13. II. 3:1–5:15. III. 6:1–7:20.

The events recorded in Micah cover a period of 40 years (Ussher).

CHAPTER 1.

B.C. 750.

Part I. (1) *The case of Jehovah against the "house of Israel"* (Mic. 1:1–2:13).

The word of the LORD that came to
[a]Micah the Morasthite in the days
of [b]Jotham, Ahaz, *and* Hezekiah, kings of
Judah, which he saw concerning
Samaria and Jerusalem.
2 Hear, all ye people; hearken, O earth,
and all that therein is: and let the Lord
GOD be witness against you, the Lord
from his holy temple.
3 For, behold, the LORD [c]cometh forth
out of his place, and will come down, and
tread upon [d]the high places of the earth.
4 And the mountains shall be molten
under him, and the valleys shall be cleft,
as wax before the fire, *and* as the waters
that are poured down a steep place.
5 For the transgression of Jacob *is* all
this, and for the sins of the house of
Israel. What *is* the transgression of
Jacob? *is it* not Samaria? and what *are* the
high places of Judah? *are they* not
Jerusalem?
6 [1]Therefore I will make Samaria [e]as
an heap of the field, *and* as plantings of a
vineyard: and I will pour down the
stones thereof into the valley, and I will
discover the foundations thereof.
7 And all the graven images thereof
shall be beaten to pieces, and all the
[f]hires thereof shall be burned with the
fire, and all the idols thereof will I lay
desolate: for she gathered *it* of the hire of
an harlot, and they shall return to the
hire of an harlot.
8 Therefore I will wail and howl, I will
go stripped and naked: [g]I will make a
wailing like the dragons, and mourning
as the owls.
9 For her wound *is* incurable; for it is
come unto Judah; he is come unto the
gate of my people, *even* to Jerusalem.
10 Declare ye *it* not at Gath, weep ye
not at all: in the house of Aphrah roll
thyself in the dust.
11 Pass ye away, thou inhabitant of
Saphir, having thy shame naked: the
inhabitant of Zaanan came not forth in
the mourning of Beth-ezel; he shall
receive of you his standing.
12 For the inhabitant of Maroth waited
carefully for good: but [h]evil came down
from the LORD unto the gate of Jerusalem.
13 O thou inhabitant of Lachish, bind
the chariot to the swift beast: she *is* the
beginning of the sin to the daughter of
Zion: for the transgressions of Israel
were found in thee.
14 Therefore shalt thou give presents
to Moresheth-gath: the houses of
[i]Achzib *shall be* a lie to the kings of
Israel.
15 Yet will I bring an heir unto thee, O
inhabitant of Mareshah: he shall come
unto [j]Adullam the glory of Israel.
16 Make thee bald, and poll thee for
thy delicate children; enlarge thy baldness as the eagle; for they are gone into
captivity from thee.

CHAPTER 2.

(*Jehovah against Israel,* continued).

Woe to them that devise iniquity,
and work evil upon their beds!
when the morning is light, they practise
it, because it is in the power of their
hand.

a Jer. 26:18.
b 2 Ki. 15:1-5, 7, 32-38; 2 Chr. 27:1-9; Isa. 1:1.
c Isa. 63:1; Zech. 14:3, 4; Mal. 4:2, 3; Mt. 24:27-30; 2 Thes. 2:8; Rev. 1:7; 19:11-21.
d Deut. 32:13; 33:29; Amos 4:13.
e Mic. 3:12; 2 Ki. 19:25.
f Hos. 2:5, 12.
g Job 30:29; Psa. 102:6.
h Amos 3:6.
i Josh. 15:44.
j 2 Chr. 11:7.

[1] **(1:6)** In verses 6-16 the Assyrian invasion is described. Cf. 2 Ki. 17:1-18. This is the local circumstance which gives rise to the prophecy of the greater invasion in the last days (Mic. 4:9-13), and of the Lord's deliverance at Armageddon (Rev. 16:14; 19:17).

2 And they covet fields, and take *them* by violence; and houses, and take *them* away: so they oppress a man and his house, even a man and his heritage.

3 Therefore thus saith the LORD; Behold, against [a]this family do I devise an evil, from which ye shall not remove your necks; neither shall ye go haughtily: [b]for this time *is* evil.

4 In that day shall *one* take up a parable against you, and lament with a doleful lamentation, *and* say, We be utterly spoiled: he hath changed the portion of my people: how hath he removed *it* from me! turning away he hath divided our fields.

5 Therefore thou shalt have none that shall cast a cord by lot in the congregation of the LORD.

6 Prophesy ye not, *say they to them that* prophesy: they shall not prophesy to them, *that* they shall not take shame.

7 O *thou that art* named the house of Jacob, is the [c]spirit of the LORD straitened? *are* these his doings? do not my words do good to him that walketh uprightly?

8 Even of late my people is risen up as an enemy: ye pull off the robe with the garment from them that pass by securely as men averse from war.

9 The women of my people have ye cast out from their pleasant houses; from their children have ye taken away my glory for ever.

10 Arise ye, and depart; for this *is* not *your* rest: because it is polluted, it shall destroy *you*, even with a sore destruction.

11 If a man walking in the spirit and falsehood do lie, *saying*, I will prophesy unto thee of wine and of strong drink; he shall even be the prophet of this people.

(2) *The promise to the remnant.*

12 I will surely assemble, O Jacob, all of thee; I will surely gather the [d]remnant of Israel; I will put them together as the sheep of Bozrah, as the flock in the midst of their fold: they shall make great noise by reason of *the multitude of* men.

13 The breaker is come up before them: they have broken up, and have passed through the gate, and are gone out by it: and their king shall pass before them, and the LORD on the head of them.

B.C. 730.

a Ex. 20:5; Jer. 8:3.

b Amos 5:13; Eph. 5:16.

c *Holy Spirit.* Mic. 3:8. (Gen. 1:2; Mal. 2:15.)

d *Remnant.* vs. 12, 13; Mic. 4:1-7. (Isa. 1:9; Rom. 11:5.)

e *Inspiration.* Hab. 2:2. (Ex. 4:15; Rev. 22:19.)

f *Holy Spirit.* Zech. 4:6. (Gen. 1:2; Mal. 2:15.)

g Prediction of the destruction of Jerusalem, fulfilled A.D. 70. Cf. Dan. 9:26.

CHAPTER 3.

Part II. (Mic. 3:1–5:15.)

(1) *The coming judgment of the captivities.*

And I said, Hear, I pray you, O heads of Jacob, and ye princes of the house of Israel; *Is it* not for you to know judgment?

2 Who hate the good, and love the evil; who pluck off their skin from off them, and their flesh from off their bones;

3 Who also eat the flesh of my people, and flay their skin from off them; and they break their bones, and chop them in pieces, as for the pot, and as flesh within the caldron.

4 Then shall they cry unto the LORD, but he will not hear them: he will even hide his face from them at that time, as they have behaved themselves ill in their doings.

5 Thus saith the LORD concerning the prophets that make my people err, that bite with their teeth, and cry, Peace; and he that putteth not into their mouths, they even prepare war against him.

6 Therefore night *shall be* unto you, that ye shall not have a vision; and it shall be dark unto you, that ye shall not divine; and the sun shall go down over the prophets, and the day shall be dark over them.

7 Then shall the seers be ashamed, and the diviners confounded: yea, they shall all cover their lips; for *there is* no answer of God.

8 But truly I am full of [e]power by the [f]spirit of the LORD, and of judgment, and of might, to declare unto Jacob his transgression, and to Israel his sin.

9 Hear this, I pray you, ye heads of the house of Jacob, and princes of the house of Israel, that abhor judgment, and pervert all equity.

10 They build up Zion with blood, and Jerusalem with iniquity.

11 The heads thereof judge for reward, and the priests thereof teach for hire, and the prophets thereof divine for money: yet will they lean upon the LORD, and say, *Is* not the LORD among us? none evil can come upon us.

12 [g]Therefore shall Zion for your sake be plowed *as* a field, and Jerusalem shall become heaps, and the mountain of the house as the high places of the forest.

CHAPTER 4.

(2) The future kingdom of Messiah:
(a) the kingdom to be supreme.

But in the last days it shall come to pass, *that* the [1]mountain of the house of the LORD shall be established in the [a]top of the mountains, and [b]it shall be exalted above the hills; and people shall flow unto it.

(b) The kingdom to be universal.

2 And many nations shall come, and say, Come, and let us go up to the mountain of the LORD, and to the house of the God of Jacob; and he will teach us of his ways, and we will walk in his paths: for the law shall go forth of Zion, and the word of the LORD from Jerusalem.

(c) The kingdom to be peaceful.

3 And he shall judge among many people, and rebuke strong nations afar off; and they shall beat their swords into plowshares, and their spears into pruninghooks: nation shall not lift up a sword against nation, neither shall they learn war any more.

(d) The kingdom to secure universal prosperity.

4 But they shall sit every man under his vine and under his fig tree; and none shall make *them* afraid: for the mouth of the LORD of hosts hath spoken *it*.

5 For [c]all people will walk every one in the name of his god, and we will walk in the name of the LORD our God for ever and ever.

(e) Israel to be regathered.

6 In that day, saith the LORD, will I assemble her that halteth, and I will gather her that is driven out, and her that I have afflicted;

7 And I will make her that halted a remnant, and her that was cast far off a strong nation: and [d]the LORD shall reign over them in mount Zion from henceforth, even for ever.

8 And thou, O tower of the flock, the strong hold of the daughter of Zion, unto thee shall it come, even the first dominion; the kingdom shall come to the daughter of Jerusalem.

(f) The intervening Babylonian captivity.

9 Now why dost thou cry out aloud? *is there* no king in thee? is thy counsellor perished? for pangs have taken thee as a woman in travail.

10 Be in pain, and labour to bring forth, O daughter of Zion, like a woman in travail: for now shalt thou go forth out of the city, and thou shalt dwell in the field, and thou shalt go *even* to Babylon; there shalt thou be delivered; there the LORD shall [e]redeem thee from the hand of thine enemies.

(g) How the kingdom is set up: the gathering of the Gentile nations against Jerusalem, and battle of Armageddon (Rev. 16:14; 19:17, *note*).

11 Now also many nations are gathered against thee, that say, Let her be defiled, and let our eye look upon Zion.

12 But they know not the thoughts of the LORD, neither understand they his counsel: for he shall gather them as the sheaves into the floor.

13 [f]Arise and thresh, O daughter of Zion: for I will make thine horn iron, and I will make thy hoofs brass: and thou shalt beat in pieces many people: and I will consecrate their gain unto the LORD, and their substance unto the Lord of the whole earth.

CHAPTER 5.

Parenthesis: the birth and rejection of the King. (Cf. Mt. 2:1-6; 27:24, 25, 37.)

[2]Now gather thyself in troops, O daughter of troops: he hath laid siege against us: they shall [g]smite the judge of Israel with a rod upon the cheek.

2 But thou, Beth-lehem Ephratah, *though* thou be little among the

B.C. 710.

a *Kingdom* (O.T.). vs. 1-3; Mic. 5:2. (Gen. 1:26; Zech. 12:8.)

b *Remnant.* vs. 1-7; Mic. 5:3-9. (Isa. 1:9; Rom. 11:5.)

c Lit. *all the peoples do now walk in the name of their god, but shall walk in the name of Jehovah our Elohim for ever.*

d *Christ (Second Advent).* Zech. 2:10-12. (Deut. 30:3; Acts 1:9-11.)

e Heb. *goel, Redemp. (Kinsman type).* Isa. 59:20, *note.*

f Zech. 12:1-8; 14:14.

g Cf. Mt. 26:67; 27:30.

[1] **(4:1)** General predictions concerning the kingdom. In Scripture a mountain is the symbol of a great earth power (Dan. 2:35); hills, of smaller powers. The prediction asserts (1) the ultimate establishment of the kingdom, with Jerusalem for the capital (v. 1); (2) the universality of the future kingdom (v. 2); (3) its character—peace (v. 3); (4) its effect—prosperity (v. 4). Cf. Isa. 2:1-5; 11:1-12.

[2] **(5:1)** The "word of the LORD that came to Micah" (Mic. 1:1), having described the future kingdom (Mic. 4:1-8), and glanced at the Babylonian captivities (Mic. 4:9-10), goes forward into the last days to refer to the great battle (see "Armageddon," Rev. 16:14; 19:17, *note*), which immediately precedes the

thousands of Judah, *yet* [a]out of [b]thee
shall he come forth unto me *that is* to be
[c]ruler in Israel; whose goings forth *have*
been from of old, from [1]everlasting.

Interval between the rejection and return of the King. End of parenthesis.

3 Therefore will he give them up, until
the time *that* she which travaileth hath
brought forth: then the [d]remnant of his
brethren shall return unto the children of
Israel.

In the kingdom-age.

4 And he shall stand and feed in the
strength of the LORD, in the majesty of
the name of the LORD his God; and they
shall abide: for now [e]shall he be great
unto the ends of the earth.
5 And this *man* shall be the peace,
when the Assyrian shall come into our
land: and when he shall tread in our
palaces, then shall we raise against him
seven shepherds, and eight principal
men.
6 And they shall waste the land of
Assyria with the sword, and the [f]land of
Nimrod in the entrances thereof: thus
shall he deliver *us* from the Assyrian,
when he cometh into our land, and
when he treadeth within our borders.
7 And the [2]remnant of Jacob shall be
in the midst of many people [g]as a dew
from the LORD, as the showers upon the
grass, that tarrieth not for man, nor waiteth for the sons of men.
8 And the remnant of Jacob shall be
among the Gentiles in the midst of many
people as a lion among the beasts of the
forest, as a young lion among the flocks
of sheep: who, if he go through, both
treadeth down, and teareth in pieces,
and none can deliver.
9 Thine hand shall be lifted up upon
thine adversaries, and all thine enemies
shall be cut off.
10 [h]And it shall come to pass in that
day, saith the LORD, that I will cut off thy
horses out of the midst of thee, and I will
destroy thy chariots:
11 And I will cut off the cities of thy
land, and throw down all thy strong
holds:
12 And I will cut off witchcrafts out of
thine hand; and thou shalt have no *more*
soothsayers:
13 Thy graven images also will I cut
off, and thy standing images out of the
midst of thee; and thou shalt no more
worship the work of thine hands.
14 And I will pluck up thy [i]groves out
of the midst of thee: so will I destroy thy
cities.
15 And I will execute vengeance in
anger and fury upon the [j]heathen, such
as they have not heard.

CHAPTER 6.

Part III. (Mic. 6:1–7:20.) (1) *The LORD'S past and present controversy with Israel.*

Hear ye now what the LORD saith;
Arise, contend thou before the

B.C. 710.

a Mt. 2:5-12; Lk. 2:4, 11; John 7:42.

b *Christ (First Advent).* Hag. 2:7. (Gen. 3:15; Acts 1:9.)

c *Kingdom* (O.T.). Zeph. 3:13-20. (Gen. 1:26; Zech. 12:8.)

d *Remnant.* vs. 3-9; Mic. 7:18. (Isa. 1:9; Rom. 11:5.)

e Psa. 72:8; Isa. 52:13; Zech. 9:10; Lk. 1:32.

f Gen. 10:8-12.

g Deut. 32:2; Psa. 72:6; 110:3.

h Zech. 9:10.

i Deut. 16:21.

j i.e. *nations.*

setting up of the Messianic kingdom (see "Kingdom (O.T.)," Gen. 1:26; Zech. 12:8, *note;* also, "Kingdom (N.T.)," Lk. 1:31-33; 1 Cor. 15:28).

Mic. 5:1, 2 forms a parenthesis in which the "word of the LORD" goes back from the time of the great battle (yet future) to the birth and rejection of the King, Messiah-Christ (Mt. 27:24, 25, 37). This is followed by the statement that He will "give them up until the time that she which travaileth hath brought forth" (v. 3). There is a twofold "travail" of Israel: (1) that which brings forth the "man child" (Christ) (Rev. 12:1, 2); and (2) that which, in the last days, brings forth a believing "remnant" out of the still dispersed and unbelieving nation (v. 3; Jer. 30:6-14; Mic. 4:10). Both aspects are combined in Isa. 66. In verse 7 we have the "man child" (Christ) of Rev. 12:1, 2; in verses 8-24 the remnant, established in kingdom blessing. The meaning of Mic. 5:3 is that, from the rejection of Christ at His first coming Jehovah will give Israel up till the believing remnant appears; *then* He stands and feeds in His proper strength as Jehovah (v. 4); He is the defence of His people as in Mic. 4:3, 11-13, and afterward the remnant go as missionaries to Israel and to all the world (vs. 7, 8; Zech. 8:23).

[1] **(5:2)** Cf. Isa. 7:13, 14; 9:6, 7. The "child" was born in Bethlehem, but the "Son" was "from everlasting."

[2] **(5:7)** The ministry of the Jewish remnant (Isa. 1:9; Rom. 11:5, *note*) has a twofold aspect, "a dew from the LORD"; "a lion among the beasts." Turning to the Lord in the great tribulation (Psa. 2:5; Rev. 7:14, *note*), the remnant takes up the beautiful gospel of the kingdom (Rev. 14:6, *note*) and proclaims it under awful

mountains, and let the hills hear thy voice.

2 Hear ye, O mountains, the LORD'S controversy, and ye strong foundations of the earth: for the LORD hath a controversy with his people, and he will plead with Israel.

3 O my people, what have I done unto thee? and wherein have I wearied thee? testify against me.

4 For I brought thee up out of the land of Egypt, and [a]redeemed thee out of the house of servants; and I sent before thee Moses, Aaron, and Miriam.

5 O my people, remember now what [b]Balak king of Moab consulted, and what Balaam the son of Beor answered him from Shittim unto Gilgal; that ye may know the righteousness of the LORD.

6 Wherewith shall I come before the LORD, *and* bow myself before the high God? shall I come before him with burnt-offerings, with calves of a year old?

7 Will the LORD be pleased with thousands of rams, *or* with ten thousands of rivers of oil? shall I give my firstborn *for* my transgression, the fruit of my body *for* the sin of my soul?

8 [c]He hath shewed thee, O man, what *is* good; and what doth the LORD require of thee, but [d]to do justly, and to love mercy, and to walk humbly with thy God?

9 The LORD'S voice crieth unto the city, and *the man of* wisdom shall see thy name: hear ye the rod, and who hath appointed it.

10 Are there yet the treasures of wickedness in the house of the wicked, and the scant measure *that is* abominable?

11 Shall I count *them* pure with the wicked balances, and with the bag of deceitful weights?

12 For the rich men thereof are full of violence, and the inhabitants thereof have spoken lies, and their tongue *is* deceitful in their mouth.

13 Therefore also will I make *thee* sick in smiting thee, in making *thee* desolate because of thy sins.

14 Thou shalt eat, but not be satisfied; and thy casting down *shall be* in the midst of thee; and thou shalt take hold, but shalt not deliver; and *that* which thou deliverest will I give up to the sword.

15 [e]Thou shalt sow, but thou shalt not reap; thou shalt tread the olives, but thou shalt not anoint thee with oil; and sweet wine, but shalt not drink wine.

16 For the statutes of [f]Omri are kept, and all the works of the house of [g]Ahab, and ye walk in their counsels; that I should make thee a desolation, and the inhabitants thereof an hissing: therefore ye shall bear the reproach of my people.

B.C. 710.

a Ex. 14:30, *note;* Isa. 59:20, *note.*

b Num. 23:7-10, 18-24; 24:3-9, 15-24.

c Deut. 10:12; 1 Sam. 15:22; Hos. 6:6; 12:6.

d Gen. 18:19; Isa. 1:17.

e Deut. 28:38-40; Amos 5:11; Zeph. 1:13; Hag. 1:6.

f 1 Ki. 16:25, 26.

g 1 Ki. 16:30; 21:25, 26; 2 Ki. 21:3.

h Psa. 2:12, *note.*

CHAPTER 7.

Woe is me! for I am as when they have gathered the summer fruits, as the grapegleanings of the vintage: *there is* no cluster to eat: my soul desired the firstripe fruit.

2 The good *man* is perished out of the earth: and *there is* none upright among men: they all lie in wait for blood; they hunt every man his brother with a net.

3 That they may do evil with both hands earnestly, the prince asketh, and the judge *asketh* for a reward; and the great *man,* he uttereth his mischievous desire: so they wrap it up.

4 The best of them *is* as a brier: the most upright *is sharper* than a thorn hedge: the day of thy watchmen *and* thy visitation cometh; now shall be their perplexity.

5 [h]Trust ye not in a friend, put ye not confidence in a guide: keep the doors of thy mouth from her that lieth in thy bosom.

6 For the son dishonoureth the father, the daughter riseth up against her mother, the daughter in law against her mother in law; a man's enemies *are* the men of his own house.

persecution "unto all nations, for a witness" (Mt. 24:14). The result is seen in Rev. 7:4-14. This is the "dew" aspect, and is followed by the "day of the LORD" (Isa. 2:10-22; Rev. 19:11-21), in the morning of which the kingdom is set up in power. Again there is a world-wide preaching to Jew and Gentile, but now it is the word that the King is on His holy hill of Zion (Psa. 2), and the unrepentant will be broken with His rod of iron (Psa. 2:6-9). The preaching is given in Psa. 2:10-12. This is the "lion" aspect of the remnant's testimony (Rev. 2:26-28). The full kingdom-age of blessing follows the "rod of iron" aspect.

(2) *The voice of the remnant in the last days.*

7 [1]Therefore I will look unto the LORD;
I will wait for the God of my salvation:
my God will hear me.
8 Rejoice not against me, O mine
enemy: when I fall, I shall arise; when I
sit in darkness, the LORD *shall be* a light
unto me.
9 I will bear the indignation of the
LORD, because I have sinned against
him, until he plead my cause, and execute judgment for me: he will bring me
forth to the light, *and* I shall behold [a]his
righteousness.
10 Then *she that is* mine enemy shall
see *it*, and shame shall cover her which
said unto me, Where is the LORD thy
God? mine eyes shall behold her: now
shall she be trodden down as the mire of
the streets.
11 *In* the day that thy [b]walls are to be
built, *in* that day shall the decree be far
removed.
12 *In* that day *also* he shall come even
to thee from Assyria, and *from* the fortified cities, and from the fortress even to
the river, and from sea to sea, and *from*
mountain to mountain.
13 Notwithstanding the land shall be
desolate because of them that dwell
therein, for the fruit of their doings.
14 Feed thy people with thy rod, the
flock of thine heritage, which dwell soli-
tarily *in* the wood, in the midst of
Carmel: let them feed *in* Bashan and
Gilead, as in the days of old.
15 [c]According to the days of thy coming out of the land of Egypt will I shew
unto him marvellous *things*.
16 The nations shall see and be confounded at all their might: they shall lay
their hand upon *their* mouth, their ears
shall be deaf.
17 They shall [d]lick the dust like a serpent, they shall move out of their holes
like worms of the earth: [e]they shall be
afraid of the LORD our God, and shall
fear because of thee.
18 Who *is* a God like unto thee, that
pardoneth iniquity, and passeth by the
transgression of the [f]remnant of his heritage? he retaineth not his anger for ever,
because he delighteth *in* mercy.
19 He will turn again, he will have
compassion upon us; he will subdue our
iniquities; and thou wilt cast all their
sins into the depths of the sea.
20 Thou wilt perform the truth to
Jacob, *and* the mercy to Abraham, which
thou hast sworn unto our fathers from
the days of old.

B.C. 710.

a Rom. 10:1-4; 11:23-27.
b Amos 9:11.
c Psa. 78:12.
d Psa. 72:9; Isa. 49:23.
e Jer. 33:9.
f *Remnant.* Zeph. 2:1-3, 7-9. (Isa. 1:9; Rom. 11:5.)

[1]**(7:7)** Mic. 7:7-20 is, primarily, the confession and intercession of the prophet, who identifies himself with Israel. Cf. Dan. 9:3-19. Intercession was a test of the prophetic office (Jer. 27:18; Gen. 20:7). But Micah's prayer voices also the heart exercise of the remnant in the last days. Such is prophecy, an intermingling of the near and the far. (Cf. Psa. 22:1; Mt. 27:46.)

NAHUM

NAHUM prophesied during the reign of Hezekiah, probably about one hundred and fifty years after Jonah. He has but one subject—the destruction of Nineveh. According to Diodorus Siculus, the city was destroyed nearly a century later, precisely as here predicted. The prophecy is one continuous strain which does not yield to analysis. The moral theme is: the holiness of Jehovah which must deal with sin in judgment.

CHAPTER 1.

The holiness of Jehovah.

THE [a]burden of [1]Nineveh. The book of
the vision of Nahum the Elkoshite.
2 [2]God *is* jealous, and the LORD
revengeth; the LORD revengeth, and *is*
furious; the LORD will take vengeance on
his adversaries, and he reserveth *wrath*
for his enemies.
3 [b]The LORD *is* slow to anger, and great
in power, and will not at all acquit *the
wicked*: [c]the LORD *hath* his way in the
whirlwind and in the storm, and the
clouds *are* the dust of his feet.
4 He rebuketh the sea, and maketh it
dry, and drieth up all the rivers: Bashan
languisheth, and Carmel, and the flower
of Lebanon languisheth.
5 The mountains quake at him, and
the hills melt, and the earth is burned at
his presence, yea, the world, and all that
dwell therein.
6 [d]Who can stand before his indignation? and who can abide in the fierceness of his anger? his fury is poured out
like fire, and the rocks are thrown down
by him.
7 The LORD *is* [e]good, a strong hold in
the day of trouble; and [f]he knoweth
them that trust in him.
8 But with an overrunning flood he
will make an utter end of the place
thereof, and darkness shall pursue his
enemies.
9 What do ye imagine against the
LORD? he will make an utter end: affliction shall not rise up the second time.
10 For while *they be* folden together *as*
thorns, and while they are drunken *as*
drunkards, they shall be devoured as
stubble fully dry.

B.C. 713.

a Isa. 13:1, *note.*

b Ex. 34:6, 7; Neh. 9:17; Psa. 103:8; Jon. 4:2.

c Psa. 18:7-15; 97:2; Hab. 3:5, 11, 12.

d Mal. 3:2.

e Psa. 25:8; 37:39, 40; 100:5; Jer. 33:11; Lam. 3:25.

f Psa. 1:6; 2 Tim. 2:19; Psa. 2:12, *note.*

1 **(1:1)** Nineveh stands in Scripture as the representative of apostate *religious* Gentiledom, as Babylon represents the confusion into which the Gentile *political* world-system has fallen (Dan. 2:41-43). See Isa. 13:1, *note.* Under the preaching of Jonah, B.C. 862, the city and king had turned to God (*Elohim*), Jon. 3:3-10. But in the time of Nahum, more than a century later, the city had wholly apostatized from God. It is this which distinguishes Nineveh from all the other ancient Gentile cities, and which makes her the suited symbol of the present religious Gentile world-system in the last days. Morally, Nineveh is described in Rom. 1:21-23. The chief deity of apostate Nineveh was the bull-god, with the face of a man and the wings of a bird: "an image made like to corruptible man, and to birds, and four-footed beasts."

The message of Nahum, uttered about one hundred years before the destruction of Nineveh, is therefore, not a call to repentance, but an unrelieved warning of judgment: "He will make an utter end: affliction shall not rise up the second time," v. 9; see, also, Nah. 3:10. For there is no remedy for *apostasy* but utter judgment, and a new beginning. Cf. Isa. 1:4, 5, 24-28; Heb. 6:4-8; Prov. 29:1. It is the way of God; *apostasy* is punished by catastrophic destruction. Of this the flood and the destruction of Nineveh are witnesses. The coming destruction of apostate Christendom is foreshadowed by these (Cf. Dan. 2:34, 35; Lk. 17:26, 27; Rev. 19:17-21.)

2 **(1:2)** The great ethical lesson of Nahum is that the character of God makes Him not only "slow to anger," and "a stronghold to them that trust Him," but also one who "will not at all acquit the wicked." He can be "just, and the justifier of him which believeth in Jesus" (Rom. 3:26), but only because His holy law has been vindicated in the cross.

11 There is *one* come out of thee, that
imagineth evil against the LORD, a
wicked counsellor.
12 Thus saith the LORD; Though *they be*
quiet, and likewise many, yet thus shall
they be cut down, when he shall pass
through. Though I have afflicted thee, I
will afflict thee no more.
13 For now will I break his yoke from
off thee, and will burst thy bonds in sunder.
14 And the LORD hath given a commandment concerning thee, *that* no
more of thy name be sown: out of the
house of thy gods will I cut off the
graven image and the molten image: I
will make thy grave; for thou art vile.

The future evangel.

15 Behold upon the mountains the
[a]feet of him that bringeth good tidings,
that publisheth peace! O Judah, keep thy
solemn feasts, perform thy vows: for the
wicked shall no more pass through thee;
he is utterly cut off.

CHAPTER 2.

The battle in the streets.

He that dasheth in pieces is come up
before thy face: keep the munition,
watch the way, make *thy* loins strong,
fortify *thy* power mightily.
2 [b]For the LORD hath turned away the
excellency of Jacob, as the excellency of
Israel: for the emptiers have emptied
them out, and marred their vine branches.
3 The shield of his mighty men is
made red, the valiant men *are* in scarlet:
the chariots *shall be* with flaming torches
in the day of his preparation, and the fir
trees shall be terribly shaken.
4 The chariots shall rage in the streets,
they shall justle one against another in
the broad ways: they shall seem like
torches, they shall run like the lightnings.
5 He shall recount his worthies: they
shall stumble in their walk; they shall
make haste to the wall thereof, and the
defence shall be prepared.
6 The gates of the rivers shall be
opened, and the palace shall be dissolved.
7 And Huzzab shall be led away captive, she shall be brought up, and her
maids shall lead *her* as with the voice of
doves, tabering upon their breasts.
8 But Nineveh *is* of old like a pool of
water: yet they shall flee away. Stand,
stand, *shall they cry*; but none shall look
back.
9 Take ye the spoil of silver, take the
spoil of gold: for *there is* none end of the
store *and* glory out of all the pleasant
furniture.
10 She is empty, and void, and waste:
and the heart melteth, and the knees
smite together, and much pain *is* in all
loins, and the faces of them all gather
blackness.
11 Where *is* the dwelling of the [c]lions,
and the feedingplace of the young lions,
where the lion, *even* the old lion, walked,
and the lion's whelp, and none made
them afraid?
12 The lion did tear in pieces enough
for his whelps, and strangled for his
lionesses, and filled his holes with prey,
and his dens with ravin.
13 [d]Behold, I *am* against thee, saith the
LORD of hosts, and I will burn her chariots in the smoke, and the sword shall
devour thy young lions: and I will cut off
thy prey from the earth, and the voice of
thy messengers shall no more be heard.

CHAPTER 3.

As Nineveh sowed, so must she reap.

Woe to [e]the bloody city! it *is* all full
of lies *and* robbery; the prey
departeth not;
2 The noise of a whip, and the noise of
the rattling of the wheels, and of the
pransing horses, and of the jumping
chariots.
3 The horseman lifteth up both the
bright sword and the glittering spear:
and *there is* a multitude of slain, and a
great number of carcases; and *there is*
none end of *their* corpses; they stumble
upon their corpses:
4 Because of the multitude of the
whoredoms of the wellfavoured harlot,
the [f]mistress of witchcrafts, that selleth
nations through her whoredoms, and
families through her witchcrafts.
5 Behold, I *am* against thee, saith the
LORD of hosts; and I will discover thy
skirts upon thy face, and I will shew the
nations thy nakedness, and the kingdoms thy shame.
6 And I will cast abominable filth
upon thee, and make thee vile, and will
set thee as a gazingstock.

B.C. 713.

a Isa. 52:7; Rom. 10:15.
b Isa. 10:12; Jer. 25:29.
c Job 4:10, 11; Ezk. 19:2, 7.
d Nah. 3:5; Ezk. 29:3; 38:3; 39:1.
e Ezk. 22:2, 3; 24:6, 9; Hab. 2:12.
f Isa. 47:9, 12; Rev. 18:2, 3.

7 And it shall come to pass, *that* all
they that look upon thee shall flee from
thee, and say, [a]Nineveh is laid waste:
who will bemoan her? whence shall I
seek comforters for thee?

8 Art thou better than populous [b]No,
that was situate among the rivers, *that*
had the waters round about it, whose
rampart *was* the sea, *and* her wall *was*
from the sea?

9 Ethiopia and Egypt *were* her strength,
and *it was* infinite; Put and Lubim were
thy helpers.

10 Yet *was* she carried away, she went
into captivity: her young children also
were dashed in pieces at the top of all
the streets: and they cast lots for her
honourable men, and all her great men
were bound in chains.

11 Thou also shalt be drunken: thou
shalt be hid, thou also shalt seek
strength because of the enemy.

12 All thy strong holds *shall be like* [c]fig
trees with the firstripe figs: if they be
shaken, they shall even fall into the
mouth of the eater.

13 Behold, thy people in the midst of
thee *are* women: the gates of thy land
shall be set wide open unto thine enemies: the fire shall devour thy bars.

14 Draw thee waters for the siege, fortify thy strong holds: go into clay, and tread
the morter, make strong the brickkiln.

15 There shall the fire devour thee; the
sword shall cut thee off, it shall eat thee
up like the [d]cankerworm: make thyself
many as the cankerworm, make thyself
many as the locusts.

16 Thou hast multiplied thy [e]mer-
chants above the stars of heaven: the
cankerworm spoileth, and flieth away.

17 Thy crowned *are* as the locusts, and
thy captains as the great grasshoppers,
which camp in the hedges in the cold
day, *but* when the sun ariseth they flee
away, and their place is not known
where they *are*.

18 Thy shepherds slumber, O king of
Assyria: thy nobles shall dwell *in the*
dust: thy people is scattered upon the
mountains, and no man gathereth *them*.

19 *There is* no healing of thy bruise; thy
wound is grievous: [f]all that hear the
bruit of thee shall clap the hands over
thee: for upon whom hath not thy
wickedness passed continually?

B.C. 713.

a Nah. 1:1, *note*.

b Or, *No-Amon*. Jer. 46:25; Ezk. 30:15, 16.

c Rev. 6:12, 13.

d Joel 1:4.

e Cf. Rev. 18:7-19.

f Job. 27:23; Lam. 2:15; Zeph. 2:15. See Isa. 14:8.

HABAKKUK

IT seems most probable that Habakkuk prophesied in the latter years of Josiah. Of the prophet himself nothing is known. To him the character of Jehovah was revealed in terms of the highest spirituality. He alone of the prophets was more concerned that the holiness of Jehovah should be vindicated than that Israel should escape chastisement. Written just upon the eve of the captivity, Habakkuk was God's testimony to Himself as against both idolatry and pantheism.

The book is in five parts: I. Habakkuk's perplexity in view of the sins of Israel and the silence of God, 1:1-4. Historically this was the time of Jehovah's forbearance because of Josiah's repentance (2 Ki. 22:18-20). II. The answer of Jehovah to the prophet's perplexity, 1:5-11. III. The prophet, thus answered, utters the testimony to Jehovah, 1:12-17; but he will watch for further answers, 2:1. IV. To the watching prophet comes the response of the "vision," 2:2-20. V. All ends in Habakkuk's sublime Psalm of the Kingdom.

As a whole the Book of Habakkuk raises and answers the question of God's consistency with Himself in view of permitted evil. The prophet thought that the holiness of God forbade him to go on with evil Israel. The answer of Jehovah announces a Chaldean invasion (1:6), and a world-wide dispersion (1:5). But Jehovah is not mere wrath; "He delighteth in mercy" (Mic. 7:18), and introduces into His answers to the perplexed prophet the great promises, 1:5; 2:3, 4, 14, 20.

CHAPTER 1.

Part I. Prayer of Habakkuk: evil in dispersed Israel. (Cf. Deut. 28:64-67.)

The [a]burden which Habakkuk the
prophet did see.
2 O LORD, how long shall I cry, and
thou wilt not hear! *even* cry out unto thee
of violence, and thou wilt not save!
3 Why dost thou shew me iniquity,
and cause *me* to behold grievance? for
spoiling and violence *are* before me: and
there are *that* raise up strife and contention.
4 Therefore the law is slacked, and
judgment doth never go forth: for the
wicked doth compass about the righteous; therefore wrong judgment proceedeth.

Part II. Voice of Jehovah to Israel "among the nations."

5 Behold ye among the [b]heathen, and
regard, and wonder marvellously: [1]for I
will [c]work a work in your days, *which* ye
will not believe, though it be told *you*.
6 For, lo, I raise up the Chaldeans, *that*
bitter and hasty nation, which shall
march through the breadth of the land,
to possess the dwellingplaces *that are* not
theirs.
7 They *are* terrible and dreadful: their
judgment and their dignity shall proceed of themselves.
8 Their horses also are swifter than the
leopards, and are more fierce than the
evening wolves: and their horsemen
shall spread themselves, and their horsemen shall come from far; they shall fly
as the eagle *that* hasteth to eat.
9 They shall come all for violence:
their faces shall sup up *as* the east wind,
and they shall gather the captivity as the
sand.
10 And they shall scoff at the kings,
and the princes shall be a scorn unto
them: they shall deride every strong
hold; for they shall heap dust, and take
it.
11 Then shall *his* mind change, and he
shall pass over, and offend, *imputing* this
his power unto his god.

Part III. Habakkuk's testimony to Jehovah (extends to Hab. 2:1).

12 *Art* thou not from everlasting,

B.C. 626.

a Isa. 13:1, *note*.

b i.e. *nations*.

c Acts 13:41.

[1](1:5) Verse 5 anticipates the dispersion "among the nations" (cf. Deut. 28:64-67). While Israel as a nation is thus dispersed, Jehovah will "work a work" which Israel "will not believe." Acts 13:37-41 interprets this prediction of the redemptive work of Christ. It is significant that Paul quotes this to Jews of the dispersion in the synagogue at Antioch.

O LORD my God, mine Holy One? we shall not die. O LORD, thou hast ordained them for judgment; and, O mighty God, thou hast established them for correction.

13 *Thou art* of purer eyes than to behold evil, and canst not look on iniquity: wherefore lookest thou upon them that deal treacherously, *and* holdest thy tongue when the wicked devoureth *the man that is* more righteous than he?

14 And makest men as the fishes of the sea, as the creeping things, *that have* no ruler over them?

15 They take up all of them with the angle, they catch them in their net, and gather them in their drag: therefore they rejoice and are glad.

16 Therefore they sacrifice unto their net, and burn incense unto their drag; because by them their portion *is* fat, and their meat plenteous.

17 Shall they therefore empty their net, and not spare continually to slay the nations?

CHAPTER 2.

I will stand upon my watch, and set me upon the tower, and will watch to see what he will say unto me, and what I shall answer when I am reproved.

B.C. 626.

a Inspiration. Zech. 7:7. (Ex. 4:15; Rev. 22:19.)

b vs. 3, 4. Heb. 10:37, 38.

c Righteousness. Mal. 3:18. (Gen. 6:9; Lk. 2:25.)

d Rom. 1:17; Gal. 3:11; Heb. 10:38.

e Faith. Mt. 8:10. (Gen. 3:20; Heb. 11:39.)

f Mic. 2:4.

Part IV. Jehovah's response to Habakkuk's testimony: the "vision."

2 And the LORD answered me, and said, [a]Write the vision, and make *it* plain upon tables, that he may [1]run that readeth it.

3 For the vision *is* yet for an [2]appointed time, but at the end it shall speak, and not lie: though it [b]tarry, wait for it; because it will surely come, it will not tarry.

4 Behold, his soul *which* is lifted up is not [c]upright in him: but the [d]just shall live by his [e]faith.

5 Yea also, because he transgresseth by wine, *he is* a proud man, neither keepeth at home, who enlargeth his desire as [3]hell, and *is* as death, and cannot be satisfied, but gathereth unto him all nations, and heapeth unto him all people:

6 Shall not all these [f]take up a parable against him, and a taunting proverb against him, and say, Woe to him that increaseth *that which is* not his! how long? and to him that ladeth himself with thick clay!

7 Shall they not rise up suddenly that shall bite thee, and awake that shall vex

[1] **(2:2)** Not, as usually quoted, "that he that runneth may read," but, "that he may run that readeth"; i.e. as a messenger of the "vision." Cf. Zech. 2:4, 5.

[2] **(2:3)** To the watching prophet comes the response of the "vision" (vs. 2-20). Three elements are to be distinguished: (1) The moral judgment of Jehovah upon the evils practised by dispersed Israel (vs. 5-13, 15-19). (2) The future purpose of God that, "the earth shall be filled with the knowledge of the glory of Jehovah, as the waters cover the sea" (v. 14). That this revelation awaits the return of the Lord in glory is shown *(a)* by the parallel passage in Isa. 11:9-12; and *(b)* by the quotation of verse 3 in Heb. 10:37, 38, where the "it" of the "vision" becomes "he" and refers to the return of the Lord. It is *then*, after the "vision" is fulfilled, that "the knowledge of the glory," etc., shall fill the earth. But (3) meantime, "the just shall live by his faith." This great evangelic word is applied to Jew and Gentile in Rom. 1:17; to the Gentiles in Gal. 3:11-14; and to Hebrews (especially) in Heb. 10:38. This opening of life to faith alone, makes possible not only the salvation of the Gentiles during the dispersion of Israel "among the nations" (Hab. 1:5; Gal. 3:11-14), but also makes possible a believing remnant in Israel while the nation, as such, is in blindness and unbelief (Rom. 11:1-5, *note*), with neither priesthood nor temple, and consequently unable to keep the ordinances of the law. Such is Jehovah! In disciplinary government His ancient Israel is cast out of the land and judicially blinded (2 Cor. 3:12-15), but in covenanted mercy the individual Jew may resort to the simple faith of Abraham (Gen. 15:6; Rom. 4:1-5) and be saved. But this does not set aside the Palestinian (Deut. 30:1-9, *refs.*) and Davidic (2 Sam. 7:8-16, *refs.*) Covenants, for "the earth shall be filled," etc. (v. 14), and Jehovah will again be in His temple (v. 20). Cf. Rom. 11:25-27.

[3] **(2:5)** *Sheol* is, in the O.T., the place to which the dead go. (1) Often, therefore, it is spoken of as the equivalent of the grave, merely, where all human activities cease; the *terminus* toward which all human life moves (e.g. Gen. 42:38, *grave;* Job 14:13, *grave;* Psa. 88:3, *grave*). (2) To the man "under the sun," the natural man, who of necessity judges from appearances, *sheol* seems no *more* than the grave—the end and total cessation, not only of the activities of life, but of life itself (Eccl. 9:5, 10).

thee, and thou shalt be for booties unto them?

8 [a]Because thou hast spoiled many nations, all the remnant of the people shall spoil thee; because of men's blood, and *for* the violence of the land, of the city, and of all that dwell therein.

9 Woe to him that coveteth an evil covetousness to his house, that he may [b]set his nest on high, that he may be delivered from the power of evil!

10 Thou hast consulted shame to thy house by cutting off many people, and hast sinned *against* thy soul.

11 For the stone shall cry out of the wall, and the beam out of the timber shall answer it.

12 Woe to him that buildeth a town [c]with blood, and stablisheth a city by iniquity!

13 Behold, [d]*is it* not of the LORD of hosts that the people shall labour in the very fire, and the people shall weary themselves for very vanity?

14 [1]For the earth shall be filled with the [e]knowledge of the glory of the LORD, as the waters cover the sea.

15 Woe unto him that giveth his neighbour drink, that puttest thy bottle to *him*, and makest *him* drunken also, that thou mayest look on their nakedness!

16 Thou art filled with shame for glory: drink thou also, and let thy foreskin be uncovered: the cup of the LORD'S right hand shall be turned unto thee, and shameful spewing *shall be* on thy glory.

17 For the violence of Lebanon shall cover thee, and the spoil of beasts, *which* made them afraid, because of men's blood, and for the violence of the land, of the city, and of all that dwell therein.

18 What profiteth the graven image that the maker thereof hath graven it; the molten image, and a [f]teacher of lies, that the maker of his work [g]trusteth therein, to make dumb idols?

19 Woe unto him that saith to the wood, Awake; to the dumb stone, Arise, it shall teach! Behold, it *is* laid over with gold and silver, and *there is* no breath at all in the midst of it.

20 [h]But the LORD *is* in his holy temple: let all the earth keep silence before him.

CHAPTER 3.

Part V. Habakkuk's answer of faith.

A [2][i]prayer of Habakkuk the prophet upon Shigionoth.

2 O LORD, I have heard thy speech, *and* was afraid: O LORD, revive thy work in the midst of the years, in the midst of the years make known; in wrath remember mercy.

3 God came from Teman, and the [j]Holy One from mount Paran. Selah. His glory covered the heavens, and the earth was full of his praise.

4 And *his* brightness was as the light; he had horns *coming* out of his hand: and there *was* the hiding of his power.

5 Before him went the pestilence, and burning coals went forth at his feet.

B.C. 626.

a Isa. 33:1; Jer. 27:7.

b Jer. 49:16; Oba. 4.

c Jer. 22:13; Ezk. 24:9; Mic. 3:10; Nah. 3:1.

d Or, *it is not of the LORD*, etc., i.e. though permitted in His providence, not His plan. Cf. Mic. 4:2-4.

e Isa. 11:9.

f Jer. 10:8, 14; Zech. 10:2.

g Psa. 2:12, *note.*

h Zeph. 1:7; Zech. 2:13.

i *Bible prayers* (O.T.). Gen. 15:2.

j Deut. 33:2; Jud. 5:4; Psa. 68:7.

(3) But Scripture reveals *sheol* as a place of sorrow (2 Sam. 22:6; Psa. 18:5; 116:3), into which the wicked are turned (Psa. 9:17), and where they are fully conscious (Isa. 14:9-17; Ezk. 32:21; see, especially, Jon. 2:2; what the belly of the great fish was to Jonah that *sheol* is to those who are therein). The *sheol* of the O.T. and *hades* of the N.T. (Lk. 16:23, *note*) are identical.

1 **(2:14)** Cf. Isa. 11:9, which fixes the *time* when "the earth," etc. It is when David's righteous Branch has set up the kingdom. (See "Kingdom (O.T.)," 2 Sam. 7:9; Zech. 12:8; also, "Kingdom (N.T.)," Lk. 1:31-33; 1 Cor. 15:28.) Habakkuk's phrase marks an advance on that of Isaiah. In the latter it is "the knowledge of the LORD." That, in a certain sense, is being diffused now; but in Habakkuk it is "the knowledge of the *glory* of the LORD," and that cannot be till He is manifested in glory (Mt. 24:30; 25:31; Lk. 9:26; 2 Thes. 1:7; 2:8; Jude 14). The transfiguration was a foreview of this (Lk. 9:26-29).

2 **(3:1)** Prayer in the O.T. is in contrast with prayer in the N.T. in two respects: (1) In the former the basis of prayer is a covenant of God, or an appeal to his revealed character as merciful, gracious, etc. In the latter the basis is relationship: "When ye pray, say, Our Father" (Mt. 6:9). (2) A comparison, e.g. of the prayers of Moses and Paul, will show that one was praying for an earthly people whose dangers and blessings were earthly; the other for a heavenly people whose dangers and blessings were spiritual.

6 He stood, and measured the earth: he beheld, and drove asunder the nations; and the everlasting mountains were scattered, the perpetual hills did bow: his ways *are* everlasting.

7 I saw the tents of [a]Cushan in affliction: *and* the curtains of the land of Midian did tremble.

8 Was the LORD displeased against the rivers? *was* thine anger against the rivers? *was* thy wrath against the sea, [b]that thou didst ride upon thine horses *and* thy chariots of salvation?

9 Thy bow was made quite naked, *according* to the oaths of the tribes, *even thy* word. Selah. Thou didst cleave the earth with rivers.

10 [c]The mountains saw thee, *and* they trembled: the overflowing of the water passed by: the deep uttered his voice, [d]*and* lifted up his hands on high.

11 [e]The sun *and* moon stood still in their habitation: [f]at the light of thine arrows they went, *and* at the shining of thy glittering spear.

12 Thou didst march through the land in indignation, thou didst thresh the [g]heathen in anger.

13 Thou wentest forth for the salvation of thy people, *even* for salvation with thine anointed; thou woundedst the head out of the house of the wicked, by discovering the foundation unto the neck. Selah.

14 Thou didst strike through with his staves the head of his villages: they came out as a whirlwind to scatter me: their rejoicing *was* as to devour the poor secretly.

15 [h]Thou didst walk through the sea with thine horses, *through* the heap of great waters.

16 When I heard, my belly trembled; my lips quivered at the voice: rottenness entered into my bones, and I trembled in myself, that I might rest in the day of trouble: when he cometh up unto the people, he will invade them with his troops.

17 [i]Although the fig tree shall not blossom, neither *shall* fruit *be* in the vines; the labour of the olive shall fail, and the fields shall yield no meat; the flock shall be cut off from the fold, and *there shall be* no herd in the stalls:

18 Yet I will [j]rejoice in the LORD, I will joy in the God of my salvation.

19 The LORD God *is* [k]my strength, and he will make my feet like [l]hinds' *feet*, and he will make me to [m]walk upon mine high places. To the chief singer on my stringed instruments.

B.C. 626.

a Or, *Ethiopia.*

b v. 15; Deut. 33:26, 27; Psa. 68:4; 104:3.

c Ex. 19:16, 18; Jud. 5:4, 5; Psa. 68:8; 77:18; 114:4.

d Ex. 14:22; Josh. 3:16.

e Josh. 10:12, 13.

f Or, *thine arrows walked in the light,* etc.

g i.e. *nations.*

h v. 8; Psa. 77:19.

i i.e. despite the afflictions of Israel in dispersion, the prophet will rejoice because of the Lord, as yet to return to His temple.

j Isa. 41:16; 61:10.

k Psa. 23:1; 27:1.

l 2 Sam. 22:34; Psa. 18:33.

m Deut. 32:13; 33:29.

ZEPHANIAH

THIS prophet, a contemporary of Jeremiah, exercised his ministry during the reign of Josiah. It was a time of revival (2 Ki. 22), but the captivity was impending, nevertheless, and Zephaniah points out the moral state which, despite the superficial revival under Josiah (Jer. 2:11-13), made it inevitable.

Zephaniah is in four parts: I. The coming invasion of Nebuchadnezzar a figure of the day of the LORD, 1:1–2:3. II. Predictions of judgment on certain peoples, 2:4-15. III. The moral state of Israel for which the captivity was to come, 3:1-7. IV. The judgment of the nations followed by kingdom blessing under Messiah, 3:8-20.

CHAPTER 1.

Part I. The coming judgment on Judah a figure of the future day of the LORD (Zeph. 1:1–2:3).

The word of the LORD which came
unto Zephaniah the son of Cushi,
the son of Gedaliah, the son of Amariah,
the son of Hizkiah, in the days of [a]Josiah
the son of Amon, king of Judah.
2 I will utterly consume all *things* from
off the land, saith the LORD.
3 I will consume man and beast; I will
consume the fowls of the heaven, and
the fishes of the sea, and the stumblingblocks with the wicked; and I will cut off
man from off the land, saith the LORD.
4 I will also stretch out mine hand
upon Judah, and upon all the inhabitants of Jerusalem; and I will cut off the
remnant of Baal from this place, *and* the
name of the [b]Chemarims with the
priests;
5 And them that worship the [c]host of
heaven upon the housetops; and them
that worship *and* that swear by the LORD,
and that swear by [d]Malcham;
6 And them that are turned back from
the LORD; and *those* that have not sought
the LORD, nor enquired for him.
7 Hold thy peace at the presence of the
Lord GOD: [1]for the [e]day of the LORD *is* at
hand: for the LORD hath prepared a sacrifice, he hath bid his guests.
8 And it shall come to pass in the day
of the LORD'S sacrifice, that I will punish
the princes, and the king's children, and
all such as are clothed with strange
apparel.
9 In the same day also will I punish all
those that leap on the threshold, which
fill their masters' houses with violence
and deceit.
10 And it shall come to pass in that
day, saith the LORD, *that there shall be* the
noise of a cry from the fish gate, and an
howling from the second, and a great
crashing from the hills.
11 Howl, ye inhabitants of [f]Maktesh,
for all the merchant people are cut
down; all they that bear silver are cut
off.
12 And it shall come to pass at that
time, *that* I will search Jerusalem with
candles, and punish the men that are
[g]settled on their lees: that say in their
heart, The LORD will not do good, neither will he do evil.
13 Therefore their goods shall become
a booty, and their houses a desolation:
they shall also build houses, but not
inhabit *them*; and they shall plant vineyards, but not drink the wine thereof.
14 [h]The great day of the LORD *is* near,
it is near, and hasteth greatly, *even* the
voice of the day of the LORD: the mighty
man shall cry there bitterly.
15 [i]That day *is* a day of wrath, a
day of trouble and distress, a day
of wasteness and desolation, a day
of darkness and gloominess, a
day of clouds and thick darkness,

B.C. 630.

a 2 Ki. 22:1–23:30; 2 Chr. 34:1-33; Jer. 1:2; 22:11.

b i.e. *idolatrous priests*. Cf. 2 Ki. 23:5.

c 2 Ki. 23:12; Jer. 19:13.

d An idol of the Ammonites, same as *Molech*, or *Milcom*.

e *Day (of Jehovah)*. vs. 7-18; Zech. 12:1-14. (Isa. 2:10-22; Rev. 19:11-21)

f Lit. *The Mortar*, a depression in Jerusalem where the bazaars were.

g Jer. 48:11; Amos 6:1.

h Joel 2:1, 11.

i v. 2; Isa. 22:5; Jer. 30:7; Joel 2:2, 11; Amos 5:18.

[1] **(1:7)** As in the other Prophets, the approaching invasion of Nebuchadnezzar is treated as an adumbration of the true day of the LORD in which all earth-judgments will culminate, to be followed by the restoration and blessing of Israel and the nations in the kingdom. See "Day of the LORD" (Isa. 2:10-22; Rev. 19:11-21); "Israel" (Gen. 12:2, 3; Rom. 11:26). Cf. Joel 1, 2.

B.C. 630.

16 A day of the trumpet and alarm against the fenced cities, and against the high towers.

17 And I will bring distress upon men, that they shall walk like blind men, because they have sinned against the LORD: and their blood shall be poured out as dust, and their flesh as the dung.

18 [a]Neither their silver nor their gold shall be able to deliver them in the day of the LORD'S wrath; but the whole land shall be devoured by the fire of his jealousy: for he shall make even a speedy riddance of all them that dwell in the land.

CHAPTER 2.

The call to the remnant
(Isa. 1:9; Rom. 11:5),
in the day of judgment on the nations.

Gather yourselves together, yea, gather together, O nation not [b]desired;

2 Before the decree bring forth, *before* the day pass as the chaff, before the fierce anger of the LORD come upon you, before the day of the LORD'S anger come upon you.

3 Seek ye the LORD, all ye meek of the earth, which have wrought his judgment; seek righteousness, seek meekness: it may be ye shall be hid in the day of the LORD'S anger.

Part II. Judgments on certain nations.

4 For Gaza shall be forsaken, and Ashkelon a desolation: they shall drive out Ashdod at the noon day, and Ekron shall be rooted up.

5 Woe unto the inhabitants of the sea coast, the nation of the Cherethites! the word of the LORD *is* against you; O Canaan, the land of the Philistines, I will even destroy thee, that there shall be no inhabitant.

6 And the sea coast shall be dwellings *and* cottages for shepherds, and folds for flocks.

7 And the coast shall be for the [c]remnant of the house of Judah; they shall feed thereupon: in the houses of Ashkelon shall they lie down in the evening: for the LORD their God shall visit them, [d]and turn away their captivity.

8 I have heard the reproach of Moab, and the revilings of the children of Ammon, whereby they have reproached my people, and magnified *themselves* against their border.

9 Therefore *as* I live, saith the LORD of hosts, the God of Israel, Surely Moab shall be as Sodom, and the children of Ammon as Gomorrah, *even* the breeding of nettles, and saltpits, and a perpetual desolation: the residue of my people shall spoil them, and the remnant of my people shall possess them.

10 This shall they have for their pride, because they have reproached and magnified *themselves* against the people of the LORD of hosts.

11 The LORD *will be* terrible unto them: for he will famish all the gods of the earth; and *men* shall worship him, every one from his place, *even* all the [e]isles of the [f]heathen.

12 Ye Ethiopians also, ye *shall be* slain by my sword.

13 And he will stretch out his hand against the north, and destroy [g]Assyria; and will make [h]Nineveh a desolation, *and* dry like a wilderness.

14 And flocks shall lie down in the midst of her, all the beasts of the nations: both the cormorant and the bittern shall lodge in the upper lintels of it; *their* voice shall sing in the windows; desolation *shall be* in the thresholds: for he shall uncover the cedar work.

15 This *is* the rejoicing city that dwelt carelessly, that said in her heart, I *am*, and *there is* none beside me: how is she become a desolation, a place for beasts to lie down in! every one that passeth by her shall hiss, *and* wag his hand.

CHAPTER 3.

Part III. The moral state of Jerusalem in the prophet's time.
(Cf. Isa. 3:1-26; Jer. 6:1-15.)

Woe to her that is filthy and polluted, to the oppressing city!

2 She obeyed not the voice; she received not correction; she [i]trusted not in the LORD; she drew not near to her God.

3 Her princes within her *are* roaring lions; her judges *are* evening wolves; they gnaw not the bones till the morrow.

4 Her prophets *are* light *and* treacherous persons: her priests have polluted

a Prov. 11:4; Ezk. 7:19.

b Lit. *that hath not shame.* Cf. Jer. 3:3.

c *Remnant.* vs. 1-3, 7-9; Zeph. 3:13-20. (Isa. 1:9; Rom. 11:5.)

d Or, *bring again.* Cf. Zeph. 3:19, 20; Deut. 30:1-9; Isa. 11:11; Jer. 23:5-8.

e i.e. *coasts.*

f i.e. *nations.*

g Isa. 10:12; Ezk. 31:3; Nah. 1:1; 2:10; 3:15, 18.

h Nah. 1:1, *note.*

i Psa. 2:12, *note.*

the sanctuary, they have done violence
to the law.
5 The just LORD *is* in the midst thereof;
he will not do iniquity: every morning
doth he bring his judgment to light, he
faileth not; but the unjust knoweth no
shame.
6 I have cut off the nations: their towers are desolate; I made their streets
waste, that none passeth by: their cities
are destroyed, so that there is no man,
that there is none inhabitant.
7 I said, Surely thou wilt [a]fear me,
thou wilt receive instruction; so their
dwelling should not be cut off, howsoever I punished them: but they rose early,
and corrupted all their doings.

Part IV. (1) *The judgment of the nations.*
(Cf. Zech. 14:1-21; Mt. 25:32, *note.*)

8 Therefore wait ye upon me, saith the
LORD, until the day that I rise up to the
prey: for my determination *is* to gather
the nations, that I may assemble the
kingdoms, [b]to pour upon them mine
indignation, *even* all my fierce anger: for
all the earth shall be devoured with the
fire of my jealousy.
9 For [1]then will I turn to the [c]people a
pure language, that they may all call
upon the name of the LORD, to serve him
with one consent.
10 From beyond the rivers of Ethiopia
my suppliants, *even* the daughter of my
dispersed, shall bring mine offering.
11 In that day shalt thou not be
ashamed for all thy doings, wherein
thou hast transgressed against me: for
then I will take away out of the midst of
thee them that [d]rejoice in thy pride, and
thou shalt no more be haughty [e]because
of my holy mountain.

B.C. 630.

a Psa. 19:9, *note.*

b *Armageddon.* Zech. 12:1-9. (Rev. 16:14; 19:11-21)

c Lit. *the peoples,* i.e. *Gentiles.*

d Isa. 2:12; Jer. 7:4; Mic. 3:11; Mt. 3:9.

e Heb. *in my holy name.*

f Psa. 2:12, *note.*

g *Remnant.* vs. 13-20; Hag. 1:14. (Isa. 1:9; Rom. 11:5.)

h *Kingdom* (O.T.). vs. 13-20; Zech. 6:12, 13. (Gen. 1:26; Zech. 12:8.)

i Isa. 35:3, 4.

j Deut. 30:9; Isa. 62:5; 65:19; Jer. 32:41.

k Isa. 11:12; 27:12; 56:8; Ezk. 28:25; 34:13; 37:21; Amos 9:14.

12 I will also leave in the midst of thee
an afflicted and poor people, and they
shall [f]trust in the name of the LORD.
13 The [g]remnant of Israel shall not do
iniquity, nor speak lies; neither shall a
deceitful tongue be found in their
mouth: for they shall feed and lie down,
and none shall make *them* afraid.

(2) *The kingdom blessing of Israel.*

14 Sing, O daughter of Zion; shout, O
Israel; be glad and rejoice with all the
heart, O daughter of Jerusalem.
15 The LORD hath taken away thy
judgments, he hath cast out thine
enemy: the [h]king of Israel, *even* the LORD,
is in [2]the midst of thee: thou shalt not
see evil any more.
16 In that day [i]it shall be said to
Jerusalem, Fear thou not: *and to* Zion, Let
not thine hands be slack.
17 The LORD thy God in the midst of
thee *is* mighty; he will save, [j]he will
rejoice over thee with joy; he will rest in
his love, he will joy over thee with
singing.
18 I will gather *them that are* sorrowful
for the solemn assembly, *who* are of thee,
to whom the reproach of it *was* a burden.
19 Behold, at that time I will undo all
that afflict thee: and I will save her that
halteth, and gather her that was driven
out; and I will get them praise and fame
in every land where they have been put
to shame.
20 At that time [k]will I bring you *again,*
even in the time that I gather you: for I
will make you a name and a praise
among all people of the earth, when I
turn back your captivity before your
eyes, saith the LORD.

[1] **(3:9)** In Zephaniah the conversion of "the peoples" is stated out of the usual prophetic order, in which the blessing of Israel and the setting up of the kingdom precedes the conversion of the Gentiles. See Zech. 12:1, *note,* and Zech. 12:8, *note.* But the passage gives clear testimony as to when the conversion of the nations will occur. It is *after* the smiting of the nations. Cf. Isa. 11:9 with context; Dan. 2:34, 35; Psa. 2:5-8; Acts 15:15-17; Rev. 19:19–20:6.

[2] **(3:15)** That this, and all like passages in the Prophets (see "Kingdom (O.T.)," Gen. 1:26; Zech. 12:8), cannot refer to anything which occurred at the first coming of Christ is clear from the context. The precise reverse was true. See Isa. 11:1, *note.*

HAGGAI

HAGGAI was a prophet of the restored remnant after the 70 years' captivity. The circumstances are detailed in Ezra and Nehemiah. To hearten, rebuke, and instruct that feeble and divided remnant was the task of Haggai, Zechariah, and Malachi. The *theme* of Haggai is the unfinished temple, and his *mission* to admonish and encourage the builders.

The divisions of the book are marked by the formula, "came the word of the LORD by Haggai": I. The event which drew out the prophecy, 1:1, 2. II. The divine displeasure because of the interrupted work, 1:3-15. III. The temples—Solomon's, the restoration temple, and the kingdom-age temple, 2:1-9. IV. Uncleanness and chastening, 2:10-19. V. The final victory, 2:20-23 (see Rev. 19:17-20; 14:19, 20; Zech. 14:1-3).

CHAPTER 1.

Part I. The occasion and theme of the prophecy (v. 2, l.c).

In the [a]second year of Darius the king, in the [b]sixth month, in the first day of the month, came the word of the LORD by [c]Haggai the prophet unto [d]Zerubbabel the son of Shealtiel, governor of Judah, and to [e]Joshua the son of Josedech, the high priest, saying,

2 Thus speaketh the LORD of hosts, saying, This people say, The time is not come, the time that the LORD'S house should be built.

Part II. (1) *Jehovah's chastening because of the interrupted work.*

3 Then came the word of the LORD by Haggai the prophet, saying,

4 *Is it* time for you, O ye, to dwell in your cieled houses, and this house *lie* waste?

5 Now therefore thus saith the LORD of hosts; Consider your ways.

6 Ye have sown much, and bring in little; ye eat, but ye have not enough; ye drink, but ye are not filled with drink; ye clothe you, but there is none warm; and he that earneth wages earneth wages *to put it* into a bag with holes.

7 Thus saith the LORD of hosts; Consider your ways.

8 Go up to the mountain, and bring wood, and build the house; and I will take pleasure in it, and I will be glorified, saith the LORD.

9 Ye looked for much, and, lo, *it came* to little; and when ye brought *it* home, I did blow upon it. Why? saith the LORD of hosts. Because of mine house that *is* waste, and ye run every man unto his own house.

10 Therefore the heaven over you is stayed from dew, and the earth is stayed *from* her fruit.

11 And I called for a drought upon the land, and upon the mountains, and upon the corn, and upon the new wine, and upon the oil, and upon *that* which the ground bringeth forth, and upon men, and upon cattle, and upon all the labour of the hands.

(2) *The work recommenced.*

12 Then Zerubbabel the son of Shealtiel, and Joshua the son of Josedech, the high priest, with all the remnant of the people, obeyed the voice of the LORD their God, and the words of Haggai the prophet, as the LORD their God had sent him, and the people did [f]fear before the LORD.

13 Then spake Haggai the LORD'S messenger in the LORD'S message unto the people, saying, I *am* with you, saith the LORD.

14 And the LORD stirred up the spirit of Zerubbabel the son of Shealtiel, governor of Judah, and the spirit of Joshua the son of Josedech, the high priest, and the spirit of all the [g]remnant of the people; and they came and did work in the house of the LORD of hosts, their God,

15 In the four and twentieth day of the sixth month, in the second year of Darius the king.

B.C. 520

a Hag. 2:10; Ezra 4:24; Zech. 1:1, 7.

b i.e. *September;* also v. 15.

c Ezra 5:1; 6:14.

d 1 Chr. 3:19; Ezra 2:2; Neh. 7:7; Zech. 4:6; Mt. 1:12, 13.

e Ezra 3:2; Neh. 12:1; Zech. 3:1-5; 6:11, 12.

f Psa. 19:9, *note.*

g *Remnant.* Zech. 8:6-12. (Isa. 1:9; Rom. 11:5.)

CHAPTER 2.

B.C. 520.

Part III. The temples.

In the [a]seventh *month,* in the one and
twentyeth *day* of the month, came the
word of the LORD by the prophet
Haggai, saying,
2 Speak now to Zerubbabel the son of
Shealtiel, governor of Judah, and to
Joshua the son of Josedech, the high priest,
and to the residue of the people, saying,
3 [b]Who *is* left among you that saw this
[1]house in her first glory? and how do ye
see it now? *is it* not in your eyes in comparison of it as nothing?
4 Yet now be strong, O Zerubbabel,
saith the LORD; and be strong, O Joshua,
son of Josedech, the high priest; and be
strong, all ye people of the land, saith
the LORD, and work: for I *am* with you,
saith the LORD of hosts:
5 *According to* the word that I
covenanted with you when ye came out
of Egypt, so my spirit remaineth among
you: fear ye not.
6 For thus saith the LORD of hosts; [c]Yet
once, it *is* a little while, and I will shake
the heavens, and the earth, and the sea,
and the dry *land;*
7 And I will shake all nations, and the
[d]desire of all nations shall come: and I
will fill this house with glory, saith the
LORD of hosts.
8 The silver *is* mine, and the gold *is*
mine, saith the LORD of hosts.
9 The [e]glory of this latter [2]house shall
be greater than of the former, saith the
LORD of hosts: and in this place will I
give peace, saith the LORD of hosts.

Part IV. The chastening of the LORD for the impurity of the priests, and delay of the people. (vs. 15-19).

10 In the four and twentieth *day* of the
ninth *month,* in the second year of
Darius, came the word of the LORD by
Haggai the prophet, saying,
11 Thus saith the LORD of hosts; Ask
now the priests *concerning* the law, saying,
12 If one bear holy flesh in the skirt of
his garment, and with his skirt do touch
bread, or pottage, or wine, or oil, or any
meat, shall it be holy? And the priests
answered and said, No.
13 Then said Haggai, If *one that is*
unclean by a dead body touch any of
these, shall it be unclean? And the priests
answered and said, It shall be unclean.
14 Then answered Haggai, and said,
So *is* this people, and so *is* this nation
before me, saith the LORD; and so *is*
every work of their hands; and that
which they offer there *is* unclean.
15 And now, I pray you, consider from
this day and upward, from before a
stone was laid upon a stone in the temple of the LORD:
16 Since those *days* were, when *one*
came to an heap of twenty *measures,*
there were *but* ten: when *one* came to the
pressfat for to draw out fifty *vessels* out
of the press, there were *but* twenty.
17 I smote you with blasting and with
mildew and with hail in all the labours
of your hands; yet ye *turned* not to me,
saith the LORD.
18 Consider now from this day and
upward, from the four and twentieth
day of the ninth *month, even* from the
day that the foundation of the LORD'S
temple was laid, consider *it.*
19 Is the seed yet in the barn? yea, as
yet the vine, and the fig tree, and the
pomegranate, and the olive tree, hath
not brought forth: from this day will I
bless *you.*

a i.e. *October.*
b Cf. Ezra 3:12-13.
c Heb. 12:26.
d *Christ (First Advent).* Zech. 9:9. (Gen. 3:15; Acts 1:9.)
e Or, *the future glory of this house shall be greater than the former.*

[1] **(2:3)** The prophet calls the old men who remembered Solomon's temple to witness to the new generation how greatly that structure exceeded the present in magnificence; and he then utters a prophecy (vs. 7-9) which can only refer to the future kingdom temple described by Ezekiel. It is certain that the restoration temple and all subsequent structures, including Herod's, were far inferior in costliness and splendour to Solomon's. The present period is described in Hos. 3:4, 5. Verse 6 is quoted in Heb. 12:26, 27. Verse 7: "I will shake all nations," refers to the great tribulation and is followed by the coming of Christ in glory, as in Mt. 24:29, 30. "The desire of all nations" is Christ. See Mal. 3:1, *note.*

[2] **(2:9)** In a sense all the temples (i.e. Solomon's; Ezra's; Herod's; that which will be used by the unbelieving Jews under covenant with the Beast [Dan. 9:27; Mt. 24:15; 2 Thes. 2:3, 4]; and Ezekiel's future kingdom temple [Ezk. 40–47]), are treated as one "house"—the "house of the LORD," since they all profess to be that. For that reason Christ purified the temple of His day, erected though it was by an Idumean usurper to please the Jews (Mt. 21:12, 13).

Part V. The future destruction of Gentile power.

20 And again the word of the LORD
came unto Haggai in the four and twentieth *day* of the month, saying,
21 Speak to Zerubbabel, [a]governor of
Judah, saying, I will shake the heavens
and the earth;
22 And I will [b]overthrow the throne of
kingdoms, and I will destroy the strength
of the kingdoms of the [c]heathen; and I
will overthrow the chariots, and those
that ride in them; and the horses and
their riders shall come down, every one
by the sword of his brother.
23 In that day, saith the LORD of hosts,
will I take thee, O Zerubbabel, my servant, the son of Shealtiel, saith the LORD,
[d]and will make thee as a signet: for [e]I
have chosen thee, saith the LORD of
hosts.

B.C. 520

a Hag. 1:1-14; Ezra 5:1-3; Zech. 4:6-10.

b Dan. 2:34, 35, 44, 45; Rev. 19:11-21.

c i.e. *nations.*

d Song 8:6; Jer. 22:24.

e Isa. 42:1; 43:10.

ZECHARIAH

ZECHARIAH, like Haggai, was a prophet to the remnant which returned after the 70 years. There is much of symbol in Zechariah, but these difficult passages are readily interpreted in the light of the whole body of related prophecy. The great Messianic passages are, upon comparison with the other prophecies of the kingdom, perfectly clear. Both advents of Christ are in Zechariah's prophecy (Zech. 9:9 with Mt. 21:1-11 and Zech. 14:3, 4). More than Haggai or Malachi, Zechariah gives the mind of God about the Gentile world-powers surrounding the restored remnant. He has given them their authority (Dan. 2:37-40), and will hold them to account; the test, as always, being their treatment of Israel. See Gen. 15:18, *note* 3, clause 6; Zech. 2:8.

Zechariah, therefore, falls into three broad divisions: I. Symbolic visions in the light of the Messianic hope, 1:1–6:15. II. The mission from Babylon, 7, 8. III. Messiah in rejection and afterwards in power, 9–14.

CHAPTER 1.

Part I. Symbolic visions in the light of the Messianic hope (Zech. 1:1–6:15): *the people warned.*

In the [a]eighth month, in the second
year of [b]Darius, came the word of the
LORD unto [c]Zechariah, the son of
Berechiah, the son of [d]Iddo the prophet,
saying,
2 The LORD hath been sore displeased
with your fathers.
3 Therefore say thou unto them, Thus
saith the LORD of hosts; Turn ye unto me,
saith the LORD of hosts, and I will turn
unto you, saith the LORD of hosts.
4 Be ye not as your fathers, unto
whom the [e]former prophets have cried,
saying, Thus saith the LORD of hosts;
Turn ye now from your evil ways, and
from your evil doings: but they did not
hear, nor hearken unto me, saith the
LORD.
5 Your fathers, where *are* they? and the
prophets, do they live for ever?
6 But my words and my statutes,
which I commanded my servants the
prophets, did they not take hold of your
fathers? and they returned and said,
Like as the LORD of hosts thought to do
unto us, according to our ways, and
according to our doings, so hath he dealt
with us.

The ten visions:

(1) *the rider on the red horse.*

7 Upon the four and twentieth day of
the eleventh month, which *is* the month
[f]Sebat, in the second year of Darius,
came the word of the LORD unto
Zechariah, the son of Berechiah, the son
of Iddo the prophet, saying,
8 I [1]saw by night, and behold a man
riding upon a [g]red horse, and he stood
among the myrtle trees that *were* in the
bottom; and behind him *were there* red
horses, speckled, and white.

B.C. 520.

a i.e. *November.*

b v. 7; Zech. 7:1; Ezra 4:24; 6:15; Hag. 1:1.

c Ezra 5:1.

d Neh. 12:4, 16.

e Zech. 7:7; 2 Chr. 24:19.

f i.e. *February.*

g Cf. Rev. 6:4. The whole Gentile period is characterized by the red horse, i.e. "sword." Dan. 9:26; Mt. 24:6, 7.

[1] **(1:8)** The "man" (v. 8) is the "my lord," "the angel that talked with me" (v. 9), and "the angel of the LORD" (vs. 10, 11). The "man" "stood among the myrtle trees" (v. 8). The prophet addresses him as "my lord" (cf. Gen. 19:2), but when the "man" answers he perceives that he has addressed an angel—"the angel that talked with me" (v. 9). In verse 10 the being of the vision is again "the man that stood among the myrtle trees." In verse 11 he is called "the angel of the LORD)," and to him the (riders on the) "red horses, speckled and white" say: "We have walked to and fro," etc. Then (v. 12) "the angel of the LORD (i.e. the "man," "my lord," "the angel that talked with me") intercedes for the land against a world at ease. The date of the intercession was at the end of the 70 years' captivity of Judah.

Taken as a whole (vs. 8-17), Zechariah's first vision reveals Judah in dispersion; Jerusalem under adverse possession; and the Gentile nations at rest about it. This condition still continues, and Jehovah's answer to the intercession of the angel sweeps on to the end-time of Gentile domination, when "the LORD shall yet comfort Zion," etc. (vs. 16, 17; Isa. 40:1-5). See "Kingdom (O.T.)" (Gen. 1:26; Zech. 12:8, *note*).

The first vision explained.

9 Then said I, O my lord, what *are*
these? And the [a]angel that talked with
me said unto me, I will shew thee what
these *be.*
10 And the man that stood among the
myrtle trees answered and said, These
are they whom the LORD hath sent to
walk to and fro through the earth.
11 And they answered the [a]angel of
the LORD that stood among the myrtle
trees, and said, We have walked to and
fro through the earth, and, behold, all
the earth sitteth still, and is at rest.

Jehovah displeased with the nations.

12 Then the [a]angel of the LORD
answered and said, O LORD of hosts,
how long wilt thou not have mercy on
Jerusalem and on the cities of Judah,
against which thou hast had indignation
these threescore and ten years?
13 And the LORD answered the [a]angel
that talked with me *with* good words *and*
comfortable words.
14 So the [a]angel that communed with
me said unto me, Cry thou, saying, Thus
saith the LORD of hosts; I am jealous for
Jerusalem and for Zion with a great jealousy.
15 And I am very sore displeased with
the [b]heathen *that are* at ease: for I was
but a little displeased, and they helped
forward the affliction.
16 Therefore thus saith the LORD; I am
returned to Jerusalem with mercies: my
house shall be built in it, saith the LORD
of hosts, and a line shall be stretched
forth upon Jerusalem.
17 Cry yet, saying, Thus saith the
LORD of hosts; My cities through prosperity shall yet be spread abroad; and
the LORD shall yet comfort Zion, and
shall yet choose Jerusalem.

B.C. 519.

a Heb. 1:4, *note.*

b i.e. nations.

c Or, carvers, or smiths.

The ten visions: (2) *the four horns.*

18 [1]Then lifted I up mine eyes, and
saw, and behold four horns.
19 And I said unto the [a]angel that
talked with me, What *be* these? And he
answered me, These *are* the horns which
have scattered Judah, Israel, and
Jerusalem.

The ten visions: (3) *the four carpenters.*

20 [2]And the LORD shewed me four
[c]carpenters.
21 Then said I, What come these to
do? And he spake, saying, These *are* the
horns which have scattered Judah, so
that no man did lift up his head: but
these are come to fray them, to cast out
the horns of the Gentiles, which lifted up
their horn over the land of Judah to scatter it.

CHAPTER 2.

The ten visions:

(4) *the man with the measuring line.*

I lifted up mine eyes [3]again, and
looked, and behold a man with a
measuring line in his hand.
2 Then said I, Whither goest thou?
And he said unto me, To measure
Jerusalem, to see what *is* the breadth
thereof, and what *is* the length thereof.
3 And, behold, the [a]angel that talked
with me went forth, and another angel
went out to meet him,

[1] **(1:18)** A "horn" is the symbol of a Gentile king (Dan. 7:24; Rev. 17:12), and the vision is of the four world-empires (Dan. 2:36-44; 7:3-7) which have "scattered Judah, Israel, and Jerusalem" (v. 19).

[2] **(1:20)** The word *charash,* trans. "carpenter," is lit. *carver, engraver.* Verse 21 makes it plain that, whatever the four carvers may be, they are used to "fray," or carve away (Heb. *charad*) in the sense of diminishing, enfeebling, the great Gentile world-powers. They may stand for Jehovah's "four sore judgments," the sword, famine, evil beasts, and pestilence (Ezk. 14:21), the four horses of Rev. 6.

[3] **(2:1)** As in Zech. 1:8-11, the "man" of verse 1 is "the angel that talked with me" of verse 3. The measuring-line (or reed) is used by Ezekiel (Ezk. 40:3, 5) as a symbol of preparation for rebuilding the city and temple in the kingdom-age. Here also it has that meaning, as the context (vs. 4-13) shows. The subject of the vision is the restoration of nation and. city. In no sense has this prophecy been fulfilled. The order is: (1) The LORD in glory in Jerusalem, v. 5 (cf. Mt. 24:29, 30); (2) the restoration of Israel, v. 6; (3) the judgment of Jehovah upon the nations, v. 8, "*after* the glory" (Mt. 25:31, 32); (4) the full blessing of the earth in the kingdom, vs. 10-13. See "Kingdom (O.T.)" (Gen. 1:26; Zech. 12:8, *note.* "Israel," Gen. 12:2; Rom. 11:26).

Jerusalem in the kingdom-age.

4 And said unto him, Run, speak to this young man, saying, Jerusalem shall be inhabited *as* towns without walls for the multitude of men and cattle therein:

5 For I, saith the LORD, will be unto her a wall of fire round about, and will be the glory in the midst of her.

6 Ho, ho, *come forth,* and flee from the land of the north, saith the LORD: for I have spread you abroad as the four winds of the heaven, saith the LORD.

7 Deliver thyself, O Zion, that dwellest *with* the daughter of Babylon.

8 For thus saith the LORD of hosts; After the glory hath he sent me unto the nations which spoiled you: for he that toucheth you toucheth the apple of his eye.

9 For, behold, I will shake mine hand upon them, and they shall be a spoil to their servants: and ye shall know that the LORD of hosts hath sent me.

10 Sing and rejoice, O daughter of Zion: for, lo, I come, and I will dwell in the midst of thee, saith the LORD.

11 And many nations shall be joined to the LORD in that day, and shall be my people: and I will dwell in the midst of thee, and thou shalt know that the LORD of hosts hath sent me unto thee.

12 And the LORD shall inherit Judah his portion in the holy land, and shall choose [a]Jerusalem again.

13 Be silent, O all flesh, before the LORD: for he is raised up out of his holy habitation.

CHAPTER 3.

The ten visions: (5) *Joshua the high priest.*

And he shewed me [1]Joshua the high priest standing before the [b]angel of the LORD, and [c]Satan standing at his right hand to [d]resist him.

2 And the LORD said unto Satan, The LORD rebuke thee, O Satan; even the LORD that hath chosen Jerusalem rebuke thee: *is* not this a brand plucked out of the fire?

3 Now Joshua was [e]clothed with filthy garments, and stood before the [b]angel.

4 And he answered and spake unto those that stood before him, saying, Take away the filthy garments from him. And unto him he said, Behold, I have caused thine iniquity to pass from thee, and I will [f]clothe thee with change of raiment.

5 And I said, Let them set a fair mitre upon his head. So they set a fair mitre upon his head, and clothed him with garments. And the [b]angel of the LORD stood by.

6 And the [b]angel of the LORD protested unto Joshua, saying,

7 Thus saith the LORD of hosts; If thou wilt walk in my ways, and if thou wilt keep my charge, then thou shalt also judge my house, and shalt also keep my courts, and I will give thee places to walk among these that stand by.

The ten visions:
(6) *Jehovah's Servant the BRANCH.*

8 [g]Hear now, O Joshua the high priest, thou, and thy fellows that sit before thee: for they *are* men wondered at: for, behold, I will bring forth my servant the [g]BRANCH.

9 For behold the [h]stone that I have laid before Joshua; upon one stone *shall be* [i]seven eyes: behold, I will engrave the graving thereof, saith the LORD of hosts, and I will remove the iniquity of that land in one day.

10 In [2]that day, saith the LORD of hosts, shall ye call every man his neighbour under the [j]vine and under the fig tree.

B.C. 519.

a *Christ (Second Advent).* Zech. 6:12, 13. (Deut. 30:3; Acts 1:9-11.)

b Heb. 1:4, *note.*

c *Satan.* vs. 1, 2; Mt. 4:1, 8, 10, 11. (Gen. 3:1; Rev. 20:10.)

d Job 1:6; Rev. 12:10.

e Isa. 64:6; *contra,* Phil. 3:1-9.

f Gen. 3:21, *refs.*

g Isa. 4:2, *note.*

h See 1 Pet. 2:8, *note.*

i Zech. 4:10, l.c. Cf. Rev. 5:6.

j Mic. 4:1-6.

[1] **(3:1)** The fifth vision discloses: (1) The change from self-righteousness to the righteousness of God (Rom. 3:22, *note*), of which Paul's experience, Phil. 3:1-9, is the illustration, as it is also the foreshadowing of the conversion of Israel. (2) In type, the preparation of Israel for receiving Jehovah's "BRANCH" (Isa. 4:2, *note*). The refusal of the Jews to abandon self-righteousness for the righteousness of God blinded them to the presence of the BRANCH in their midst at His first advent (Rom. 10:1-4; 11:7, 8). Cf. Zech. 6:12-15, which speaks of the manifestation of the BRANCH in glory (v. 13) as the Priest-King, when Israel will receive Him. See Heb. 5:6, *note.*

[2] **(3:10)** Verse 10 marks the time of fulfilment as in the future kingdom. It speaks of a security which Israel has never known since the captivity, nor will know till the kingdom comes. (Cf. Isa. 11:1-9.)

CHAPTER 4.

The ten visions: (7) the golden candlestick, and the two olive trees.

And the [a]angel [b]that talked with me came again, and waked me, as a man that is wakened out of his sleep,

2 And said unto me, What seest thou? [1]And I said, I have looked, and behold a candlestick all *of* gold, with a bowl upon the top of it, and his seven lamps thereon, and [c]seven pipes to the seven lamps, which *are* upon the top thereof:

3 And [d]two olive trees by it, one upon the right *side* of the bowl, and the other upon the left *side* thereof.

4 So I answered and spake to the angel that talked with me, saying, What *are* these, my lord?

5 Then the angel that talked with me answered and said unto me, Knowest thou not what these be? And I said, No, my lord.

6 Then he answered and spake unto me, saying, This *is* the word of the LORD unto Zerubbabel, saying, Not by might, nor by power, but by my [e]spirit, saith the LORD of hosts.

7 Who *art* thou, O great mountain? before Zerubbabel *thou shalt become* a plain: and he shall bring forth the [f]headstone *thereof with* shoutings, *crying*, Grace, grace unto it.

Zerubbabel to finish the restoration temple.

8 Moreover the word of the LORD came unto me, saying,

9 The hands of Zerubbabel have laid the foundation of this house; his hands shall also finish it; and thou shalt know that the LORD of hosts hath sent me unto you.

B.C. 519.

a Heb. 1:4, *note.*

b Zech. 1:8, *note.*

c Cf. v. 12.

d Rev. 11:3, 4.

e *Holy Spirit.* Zech. 12:10. (Gen. 1:2; Mal. 2:15.)

f *Christ (as Stone).* Mt. 7:24, 25. (Ex. 17:6; 1 Pet. 2:8.)

g Zech 3:9, *refs.*

h Cf. v. 2.

i One cubit = about 18 in.

j Lit. *land,* i.e. Palestine.

10 For who hath despised the day of small things? for they shall rejoice, and shall see the plummet in the hand of Zerubbabel *with* those seven; they *are* the [g]eyes of the LORD, which run to and fro through the whole earth.

The olive trees explained.
(Cf. Rev. 11:3, 4.)

11 Then answered I, and said unto him, What *are* these two olive trees upon the right *side* of the candlestick and upon the left *side* thereof?

12 And I answered again, and said unto him, What *be these* two olive branches which through the [h]two golden pipes empty the golden *oil* out of themselves?

13 And he answered me and said, Knowest thou not what these *be*? And I said, No, my lord.

14 Then said he, These *are* the two anointed ones, that stand by the Lord of the whole earth.

CHAPTER 5.

The ten visions: (8) the flying roll.

Then I turned, and lifted up mine eyes, and looked, and behold a [2]flying roll.

2 And he said unto me, What seest thou? And I answered, I see a flying roll; the length thereof *is* twenty [i]cubits, and the breadth thereof ten cubits.

3 Then said he unto me, This *is* the curse that goeth forth over the face of the whole [j]earth: for every one that stealeth shall be cut off *as* on this side according to it; and every one that sweareth shall be cut off *as* on that side according to it.

[1] **(4:2)** The vision of the candlestick and olive trees (lit. *trees of oil*) is, as we know, from Rev. 11:3-12, a prophecy to be fulfilled in the last days of the present age. That which marks the ministry of the "two witnesses" (Rev. 11:3, 4) is *power.* (Cf. Zech. 4:6.) In measure this power would rest upon Zerubbabel, who, having begun the restoration temple of Zechariah's time, would finish it (v. 9) laying the "headstone" amid the shoutings of the people. The whole scene forms a precursive fulfilment of the ministry of the two witnesses of Rev. 11 and of the coming of the true "headstone," Prince Messiah, of whom prince Zerubbabel is a type. Oil is a uniform symbol of the Spirit (Acts 2:4, *note*). Joshua and Zerubbabel were doubtless the two olive trees for that day, as the two witnesses of Rev. 11 may, in turn, but point to Christ as Priest-King in the kingdom-age (Zech. 6:12, 13).

[2] **(5:1)** A "roll," in Scripture symbolism, means the written word whether of God or man (Ezra 6:2; Jer. 36:2, 4, 6, etc.; Ezk. 3:1-3, etc.). Zechariah's eighth vision is of the rebuke of sin by the word of God. The two sins mentioned really transgress both tables of the law. To steal is to set aside our neighbor's right; to swear is to set aside God's claim to reverence. As always the law can only curse (v. 3; Gal. 3:10-14).

4 I will bring it forth, saith the LORD of
hosts, and it shall enter into the house of
the thief, and into the house of him that
sweareth falsely by my name: and it
shall remain in the midst of his house,
and shall consume it with the timber
thereof and the stones thereof.

The ten visions: (9) the ephah.

5 Then the angel that talked with me
went forth, and said unto me, Lift up
now thine eyes, and see what *is* this that
goeth forth.
6 And I said, [1]What *is* it? And he said,
This *is* an [a]ephah that goeth forth. He
said moreover, This *is* their resemblance
through all the [b]earth.
7 And, behold, there was lifted up a
talent of lead: and this *is* a woman that
sitteth in the midst of the ephah.
8 And he said, This *is* wickedness.
And he cast it into the midst of the
ephah; and he cast the weight of lead
upon the mouth thereof.
9 Then lifted I up mine eyes, and
looked, and, behold, there came out two
women, and the wind *was* in their
wings; for they had wings like the wings
of a stork: and they lifted up the ephah
between the earth and the heaven.
10 Then said I to the [c]angel that talked
with me, Whither do these bear the
ephah?
11 And he said unto me, To build it an
house in the land of [d]Shinar: and it shall
be established, and set there upon her
own base.

B.C. 519.

a One ephah = 1 bu. 3 pts.; also vs. 7-10.

b Lit. *land,* i.e. Palestine.

c Heb. 1:4, *note.*

d i.e. *Babylonia.* Dan. 1:2.

CHAPTER 6.

The ten visions: (10) the four chariots.

And I turned, and lifted up mine
eyes, and looked, and, behold,
there came [2]four chariots out from
between two mountains; and the mountains *were* mountains of brass.
2 In the first chariot *were* red horses;
and in the second chariot black horses;
3 And in the third chariot white horses;
and in the fourth chariot grisled and bay
horses.
4 Then I answered and said unto the
[c]angel that talked with me, What *are*
these, my lord?
5 And the [c]angel answered and said
unto me, These *are* the four spirits of the
heavens, which go forth from standing
before the Lord of all the earth.
6 The black horses which *are* therein
go forth into the north country; and the
white go forth after them; and the

[1] **(5:6)** In the vision of the ephah local and prophetic elements are to be distinguished. The elements are: an ephah or measure; a woman in the ephah; a sealing weight upon the mouth of the ephah confining the woman, and the stork-winged women whose only function is to bear the ephah and woman away into Babylonia (Shinar). The thing thus symbolized was "through all the land" (v. 6).

Symbolically, a "measure" (or "cup") stands for something which has come to the full, so that God must judge it (2 Sam. 8:2; Jer. 51:13; Hab. 3:6, 7; Mt. 7:2; 23:32). A woman, *in the bad ethical sense,* is always a symbol of that which, *religiously,* is out of its place. The "woman" in Mt. 13:33 is dealing with *doctrine,* a sphere forbidden to her (1 Tim. 2:12). In Thyatira a woman is suffered to teach (Rev. 2:20). The Babylon phase of the apostate church is symbolized by an unchaste woman, sodden with the greed and luxury of commercialism (Rev. 17:1-6; 18:3, 11-20).

The local application of Zechariah's ninth vision is, therefore, evident. The Jews then in the land had been in captivity in Babylon. Outwardly they had put away idolatry, but they had learned in Babylon that insatiate greed of gain (Neh. 5:1-9; Mal. 3:8), that intense commercial spirit which had been foreign to Israel as a pastoral people, but which was thenceforward to characterize them through the ages. These things were out of place in God's people and land. Symbolically He judged them as belonging to Babylon and sent them there to build a temple—they could have no part in His. The "woman" was to be "set *there* upon her *own* base" (v. 11). It was Jehovah's moral judgment upon Babylonism in His own land and people.

Prophetically, the application to the Babylon of the Revelation is obvious. The professing Gentile church at that time condoning every iniquity of the rich, doctrinally a mere "confusion," as the name indicates, and corrupted to the core by commercialism, wealth, and luxury, falls under the judgment of God (Rev. 18).

[2] **(6:1)** The interpretation of the tenth vision must be governed by the authoritative declaration of verse 5. That which is symbolized by the four chariots with their horses is not the four world-empires

grisled go forth toward the south country.
7 And the bay went forth, and sought
to go that they might walk to and fro
through the earth: and he said, Get you
hence, walk to and fro through the earth.
So they walked to and fro through the
earth.
8 Then cried he upon me, and spake
unto me, saying, Behold, these that go
toward the north country have quieted
my spirit in the north country.

The symbolic crowning of Joshua.

9 And the word of the LORD came unto
me, [a]saying,
10 Take of *them of* the captivity, *even* of
Heldai, of Tobijah, and of Jedaiah, which
are come from Babylon, and come thou
the same day, and go into the house of
Josiah the son of Zephaniah;
11 Then take silver and gold, and
make [1]crowns, and set *them* upon the
head of Joshua the son of Josedech, the
high priest;
12 And speak unto him, saying, Thus
speaketh the LORD of hosts, saying,
Behold the man whose name *is* The
[b]BRANCH; and he shall grow up out of
his place, and he shall build the temple
of the LORD:
13 Even he shall build the temple of
the LORD; and he shall bear the glory,
and shall sit and rule upon his [c]throne;
and he shall be a priest upon his [d]throne:
and the counsel of peace shall be
between them both.
14 And the crowns shall be to Helem,
and to Tobijah, and to Jedaiah, and to
Hen the son of Zephaniah, for a memorial in the temple of the LORD.
15 And they *that are* far off shall come
and build in the temple of the LORD, and
ye shall know that the LORD of hosts
hath sent me unto you. And *this* shall
come to pass, if ye will diligently obey
the voice of the LORD your God.

CHAPTER 7.

Part II. (Zech. 7:1–8:23.) *The mission from Babylon: the question of the fasts.*

And it came to pass in the fourth year
of king Darius, *that* the word of the
LORD came unto Zechariah in the fourth
day of the ninth month, *even* in [e]Chisleu;
2 When [2]they had sent unto the house
of God Sherezer and Regem-melech, and
their men, to pray before the LORD,
3 *And* to speak unto the priests which
were in the house of the LORD of hosts,
and to the prophets, saying, Should I
weep in the [f]fifth month, separating
myself, as I have done these so many
years?

B.C. 519.

a *Parables* (O.T.). vs. 9-15; Zech. 11:7-14. (Jud. 9:7-15; Zech. 11:7-14.)

b Isa. 4:2, *note.*

c *Kingdom* (O.T.). vs. 12, 13; Zech. 14:16-21. (Gen. 1:26; Zech. 12:8.)

d *Christ (Second Advent).* Zech. 12:10. (Deut. 30:3; Acts 1:9-11.)

e i.e. *December.*

f i.e. *August.*

of Daniel, but "the four spirits of heaven which go forth from standing before the Lord of all the earth" (v. 5). These "spirits" are angels (Lk. 1:19; Heb. 1:14), and are most naturally interpreted of the four angel's of Rev. 7:1-3; 9:14, 15. These have also a ministry earthward, and of like nature with the '"spirits" of Zech. 6:1-8, viz. judgment. The symbol (chariots and horses) is in perfect harmony with this. Always in Scripture symbolism they stand for the power of God earthward in judgment (Jer. 46:9, 10; Joel 2:3-11; Nah. 3:1-7). The vision, then, speaks of the LORD'S judgments upon the Gentile nations north and south in the day of the LORD (Isa. 2:10-22; Rev. 19:11-21).

[1]**(6:11)** Following the earth-judgments symbolized in the horsed chariots (Zech. 6:1-8) comes the manifestation of Christ in His kingdom glory (vs. 9-15). This is the invariable prophetic order: first the judgments of the day of the LORD (Isa. 2:10-22; Rev. 19:11-21), then the kingdom (cf. Psa. 2:5 with Psa. 2:6; Isa. 3:24-26 with 4:2-6; 10:33, 34 with 11:1-10; Rev. 19:19-21 with 20:4-6). This is set forth symbolically by the crowning of Joshua, which was not a vision, but actually done (cf. Isa. 8:3, 4; Ezk. 37:16-22). The fulfilment in the BRANCH will infinitely transcend the symbol. He "shall bear the glory" (v. 13; Mt. 16:27; 24:30; 25:31) as the Priest-King on His own throne (vs. 12, 13; Heb. 7:1-3). Christ is now a Priest, but still in the holiest within the veil (Lev. 16:15; Heb. 9:11-14, 24), and seated on the Father's throne (Rev. 3:21). He has not yet come out to take His own throne (Heb. 9:28). The crowns made for the symbolical crowning of Joshua were to be laid up in the temple as a memorial to keep alive this larger hope of Israel.

[2]**(7:2)** "They," i.e. of the captivity in Babylon. The mission of these Jews of the captivity concerned a fast day instituted by the Jews in commemoration of the destruction of Jerusalem, wholly of their own will, and without warrant from the word of God. In the beginning there was doubtless sincere contrition in the observance of the day; now it had become a mere ceremonial. The Jews of the dispersion

The answer of Jehovah:
(1) *their fast was a mere form; they should have heeded the prophets.*

4 Then came the word of the LORD of hosts unto me, saying,
5 Speak unto all the people of the land, and to the priests, saying, When ye fasted and mourned in the fifth and seventh *month*, even those seventy years, did ye at all fast unto me, *even* to me?
6 And when ye did eat, and when ye did drink, did not ye [a]eat *for yourselves*, and drink *for yourselves*?
7 *Should ye* not *hear* the [b]words which the LORD hath cried by the former prophets, when Jerusalem was inhabited and in prosperity, and the cities thereof round about her, when *men* inhabited the south and the plain?

(2) *Why their prayers were not answered.*

8 And the word of the LORD came unto Zechariah, saying,
9 Thus speaketh the LORD of hosts, saying, Execute true judgment, and shew mercy and compassions every man to his brother:
10 And oppress not the widow, nor the fatherless, the stranger, nor the poor; and let none of you imagine evil against his brother in your heart.
11 But they refused to hearken, and pulled away the shoulder, and stopped their ears, that they should not hear.
12 Yea, they made their hearts *as* an adamant stone, lest they should hear the law, and the words which the LORD of hosts hath sent in his spirit by the former prophets: therefore came a great wrath from the LORD of hosts.
13 Therefore it is come to pass, *that* as he cried, and they would not hear; so they cried, and I would not hear, saith the LORD of hosts:
14 But I scattered them with a whirlwind among all the nations whom they knew not. Thus the land was desolate after them, that no man passed through nor returned: for they laid the pleasant land desolate.

B.C. 518.

a Cf. 1 Cor. 10:31; 11:20-22.

b *Inspiration.* Mt. 4:4, 7, 10. (Ex. 4:15. Rev. 22:19.)

c *Sanctify, holy* (O.T.). Gen. 2:3.

CHAPTER 8.

(3) *Jehovah's unchanged purpose to bless Israel in the kingdom.*

Again the word of the LORD of hosts came *to me*, saying,
2 Thus saith the LORD of hosts; I was jealous for Zion with great jealousy, and I was jealous for her with great fury.
3 Thus saith the LORD; I am returned unto Zion, and will dwell in the midst of Jerusalem: and Jerusalem shall be called a city of truth; and the mountain of the LORD of hosts the [1c]holy mountain.
4 Thus saith the LORD of hosts; There shall yet old men and old women dwell in the streets of Jerusalem, and every man with his staff in his hand for very age.
5 And the streets of the city shall be

would be rid of it, but seek authority from the priests. The whole matter, like much in modem pseudo-Christianity, was extra-Biblical, formal, and futile. Jehovah takes the occasion to send a divine message to the dispersion. That message is in five parts: (1) Their fast was a mere religious form; they should rather have given heed to the "former prophets" (vs. 4-7; cf. Isa. 1:12; Mt. 15:1-10); (2) they are told why their 70 years' prayer has not been answered (vs. 8-14; cf. Psa. 66:18; Isa. 1:14-17); (3) the unchanged purpose of Jehovah, and the blessing of Israel in the kingdom (Zech. 8:1-8; cf. a like order in Isa. 1:24-31 with 2:1-4); (4) the messengers of the captivity are exhorted to hear the prophets of "these days," i.e. Haggai, Zechariah, and Malachi, and to do justly; then all their fasts and feasts will become gladness and joy (8:9-19); (5) they are assured that Jerusalem is yet to be the religious centre of the earth (8:20-23; cf. Isa. 2:1-3; Zech. 14:16-21).

[1] **(8:3)** Holiness, Sanctification, Summary: In the O.T. the words consecration, dedication, sanctification, and holiness are various renderings of one Hebrew word, are used of *persons* and of *things*, and have an identical meaning, i.e. set apart for God. Only when used of God himself (e.g. Lev. 11:45), or of the holy angels (e.g. Dan. 4:13), is any inward moral quality *necessarily* implied. Doubtless a priest or other person set apart to the service of God, whose whole will and desire went with his setting apart, experienced progressively an inner detachment from evil; but that aspect is distinctively of the N.T., not of the O.T. See Mt. 4:5.

full of boys and girls playing in the
streets thereof.
6 Thus saith the LORD of hosts; If it be
marvellous in the eyes of the [a]remnant
of this people in [1]these days, should it
also be marvellous in mine eyes? saith
the LORD of hosts.
7 Thus saith the LORD of hosts; Behold,
I will save my people from the east
country, and from the west country;
8 And I will bring them, and they shall
dwell in the midst of Jerusalem: [b]and
they shall be my people, and I will be
their God, in truth and in righteousness.

(4) *The people to heed the restoration prophets*, i.e. *Haggai and Zechariah.*

9 Thus saith the LORD of hosts; Let
your hands be strong, ye that hear in
these days these words by the mouth of
[c]the prophets, which *were* in the day *that*
the foundation of the house of the LORD
of hosts was laid, that the temple might
be built.
10 For before these days there was no
hire for man, nor any hire for beast; neither *was there any* peace to him that went
out or came in because of the affliction:
for I set all men every one against his
neighbour.
11 But now I *will* not *be* unto the
[d]residue of this people as in the former
days, saith the LORD of hosts.
12 For the seed *shall be* prosperous; the
vine shall give her fruit, and the ground
shall give her increase, and the heavens
shall give their dew; and I will cause the
remnant of this people to possess all
these *things*.
13 And it shall come to pass, *that* as ye
were a curse among the [e]heathen, O
house of Judah, and house of Israel; so
will I save you, and [f]ye shall be a blessing: fear not, *but* let your hands be strong.
14 For thus saith the LORD of hosts; As
I thought to punish you, when your
fathers provoked me to wrath, saith the
LORD of hosts, and I [2]repented not:
15 So again have I thought in these
days to do well unto Jerusalem and to
the house of Judah: fear ye not.
16 These *are* the things that ye shall
do; [g]Speak ye every man the truth to his
neighbour; execute the judgment of
truth and peace in your gates:
17 And let none of you imagine evil in
your hearts against his neighbour; and
love no false oath: for all these *are things*
that I hate, saith the LORD.
18 And the word of the LORD of hosts
came unto me, saying,
19 Thus saith the LORD of hosts; The
fast of the [h]fourth *month*, and the fast of
the [i]fifth, and the fast of the [j]seventh,
and the fast of the [k]tenth, shall be to the
house of Judah joy and gladness, and
cheerful feasts; therefore love the truth
and peace.

(5) *Jerusalem yet to be the religious centre of the earth.*

20 Thus saith the LORD of hosts; *It shall*
yet *come to pass*, that there shall come
people, and the inhabitants of many
cities:
21 And the inhabitants of one *city* shall
go to another, saying, Let us go speedily
to pray before the LORD, and to seek the
LORD of hosts: I will go also.
22 Yea, many people and strong
nations shall come to seek the LORD of
hosts in Jerusalem, and to pray before
the LORD.
23 Thus saith the LORD of hosts; In
[3]those days *it shall come to pass*, that ten
men shall take hold out of all languages
of the nations, even shall take hold of the
skirt of him that is a Jew, saying, We will

B.C. 518.

a *Remnant.* vs. 6-8, 11, 12; Zech. 11:7. (Isa. 1:9; Rom. 11:5.)

b Zech. 13:9; Jer. 30:22; 31:1, 33.

c Ezra 5:1, 2; Hag. 2:4.

d Or, *remnant.*

e i.e. *nations.*

f Gen. 12:2; Ruth 4:11, 12; Isa. 19:24, 25; Zeph. 3:20; Hag. 2:19.

g Eph. 4:25.

h i.e. *July.*

i i.e. *August.*

j i.e. *October.*

k i.e. *January.*

[1] **(8:6)** The "remnant" in verses 6, 11, 12 refers to the remnant of Judah which returned from Babylon, and among whom Zechariah was prophesying. See Rom. 11:5, *note.*

[2] **(8:14)** Repentance (O.T.), Summary: In the O.T., repentance is the English word used to translate the Heb. *nacham,* to be "eased" or "comforted." It is used of both God and man. Notwithstanding the literal meaning of *nacham,* it is evident, from a study of all the passages, that the sacred writers use it in the sense of *metanoia* in the N.T.—a change of mind. See Mt. 3:2; Acts 17:30, *note.* As in the N.T., such change of mind is often accompanied by contrition and self-judgment. When applied to God the word is used *phenomenally* according to O.T. custom. God *seems* to change His mind. The phenomena are such as, in the case of a man, would indicate a change of mind.

[3] **(8:23)** i.e. in the days when Jerusalem has been made the centre of earth's worship. Verse 23

go with you: for we have heard *that* God *is* with you.

CHAPTER 9.

Part III. (Zech. 9:1–14:21.)
Burden upon cities surrounding Palestine.
(See v. 8, *note.*)

The [a]burden of the word of the LORD in the land of Hadrach, and Damascus *shall be* the rest thereof: when the eyes of man, as of all the tribes of Israel, *shall be* toward the LORD.

2 And Hamath also shall border thereby; Tyrus, and Zidon, though it be very wise.

3 And Tyrus did build herself a strong hold, and heaped up silver as the dust, and fine gold as the mire of the streets.

4 Behold, [b]the Lord will cast her out, and he will smite her power in the sea; and she shall be devoured with fire.

5 Ashkelon shall see *it*, and fear; Gaza also *shall see it*, and be very sorrowful, and Ekron; for her expectation shall be ashamed; and the king shall perish from Gaza, and Ashkelon shall not be inhabited.

6 And a bastard shall dwell [c]in Ashdod, and I will cut off the pride of the Philistines.

7 And I will take away his blood out of his mouth, and his abominations from between his teeth: but he that remaineth, even he, *shall be* for our God, and he shall be as a governor in Judah, and Ekron as a Jebusite.

8 And I will encamp about mine house because of the army, [1]because of him that passeth by, and because of him that returneth: and no oppressor shall pass through them any more: for now have I seen with mine eyes.

Presentation of Christ as King at His first advent.

9 Rejoice greatly, O daughter of Zion; shout, O daughter of Jerusalem: [2]behold, thy [d]King cometh unto thee: [e]he *is* just, and having salvation; lowly, and riding upon an ass, and upon a colt the foal of an ass.

The future deliverance of Judah and Ephraim, and the world-wide kingdom.

10 [3]And I will cut off the chariot from Ephraim, and the horse from Jerusalem, and the battle bow shall be cut off: and he shall speak peace unto the [f]heathen: and his dominion *shall be* from sea *even* to sea, and from the river *even* to the ends of the earth.

11 As for thee also, by the blood of thy covenant I have sent forth thy [g]prisoners out of the pit wherein *is* no water.

12 Turn you to the [h]strong hold, ye prisoners of hope: even to day do I declare *that* I will render double unto thee;

13 [i]When I have bent Judah for me, filled the bow with Ephraim, [j]and raised up thy sons, O Zion, against thy sons, O Greece, and made thee as the sword of a mighty man.

14 And the LORD shall be seen over them, and his arrow shall go forth as the lightning: and the Lord GOD shall blow the trumpet, and shall go with whirlwinds of the south.

15 The LORD of hosts shall defend them; and they shall devour, and subdue [k]with sling stones; and they shall drink, *and* make a noise as through wine; and they shall be filled like bowls, *and* as the corners of the altar.

B.C. 487.

a Isa. 13:1, *note.*
b Isa. 23:1.
c Amos 1:8.
d Mt. 21:1-10; Mk. 11:1-10; Lk. 19:29-40; John 12:12-15.
e *Christ (First Advent).* Zech. 11:11-13. (Gen. 3:15; Acts 1:9.)
f i.e. *nations.*
g Cf. Isa. 24:17-23. vs. 21, 23 fix the *time* as the day of the LORD. Rev. 19:11-21.
h Jer. 16:19. See context from v. 14.
i Or, *For I have,* etc.
j Or, *I will raise up,* etc.
k Or, *the,* not *with.*

explains: the Jew (see "Remnant," Isa. 1:9; Rom. 11:5) will then be the missionary, and to the very "nations" now called "Christian"!

1 (9:8) There seems to be a reference here to the advance and return of Alexander (v. 13) after the battle of Issus, who subdued the cities mentioned in verses 1-6, and afterward returned to Greece without harming Jerusalem. But the greater meaning converges on the yet future last days (Acts 2:17, *note*), as the last clause of verse 8 shows, for many oppressors *have* passed through Jerusalem since the days of Alexander.

2 (9:9) The events following this manifestation of Christ as King are recorded in the Gospels. The real faith of the multitude who cried, "Hosanna" is given in Mt. 21:11; and so little was Jesus deceived by His apparent reception as King, that He wept over Jerusalem and announced its impending destruction (fulfilled A.D. 70; Lk. 19:38-44). The same multitude soon cried, "Crucify Him."

3 (9:10) Having introduced the King in verse 9, verse 10 and the verses which follow look forward to the end-time and kingdom. Except in verse 9, this present age is not seen in Zechariah.

16 And the LORD their God shall save them in that day as the flock of his people: for they *shall be as* the stones of a crown, lifted up as an ensign upon his land.

17 For how great *is* his goodness, and how great *is* his beauty! corn shall make the young men cheerful, and new wine the maids.

CHAPTER 10.

The future strengthening of Judah and Ephraim.

Ask ye of the LORD rain in the time of the [1]latter rain; *so* the LORD shall make bright clouds, and give them showers of rain, to every one grass in the field.

2 For the idols have spoken vanity, and the diviners have seen a lie, and have told false dreams; they comfort in vain: therefore they went their way as a flock, they were troubled, because *there was* no shepherd.

3 Mine anger was kindled against the shepherds, and I punished the goats: for the LORD of hosts hath visited his flock the house of Judah, and hath made them as his goodly horse in the [a]battle.

4 Out of him [2]came forth the corner, out of him the nail, out of him the battle bow, out of him every oppressor together.

5 And they shall be as mighty *men*, which tread down *their enemies* in the mire of the streets in the battle: and they shall fight, because the LORD *is* with them, and the riders on horses shall be confounded.

6 And I will strengthen the house of Judah, and I will save the house of Joseph, and I will bring them again to place them; for I have mercy upon them: and [b]they shall be as though I had not cast them off: for I *am* the LORD their God, and will hear them.

7 And *they of* Ephraim shall be like a mighty *man*, and their heart shall rejoice as through wine: yea, their children shall see *it*, and be glad; their heart shall rejoice in the LORD.

8 I will hiss for them, and gather them; for I have [c]redeemed them: and they shall increase as they have increased.

The dispersion and regathering of Israel in one view.

9 And I will sow them among the people: and they shall remember me in far countries; and they shall live with their children, and turn again.

10 I will bring them again also out of the land of Egypt, and gather them out of Assyria; and I will bring them into the land of Gilead and Lebanon; and *place* shall not be found for them.

11 And he shall pass through the sea with affliction, and shall smite the waves in the sea, and all the deeps of the river shall dry up: and the pride of Assyria shall be brought down, and the sceptre of Egypt shall depart away.

12 And I will strengthen them in the LORD; and they shall walk up and down in his name, saith the LORD.

CHAPTER 11.

The first advent and rejection of Messiah, and the result: the wrath.

Open thy doors, O Lebanon, that the fire may devour thy cedars.

2 Howl, fir tree; for the cedar is fallen; because the mighty are spoiled: howl, O ye oaks of Bashan; for the forest of the vintage is come down.

3 *There is* a voice of the howling of the shepherds; for their glory is spoiled: a voice of the roaring of

B.C. 487.

a See *Armageddon.* (Rev. 16:14; 19:17.)

b *Israel (prophecies).* vs. 6-12. Mt. 24:31. (Gen. 12:2, 3; Rom. 11:26.)

c Ex. 14:30, *note;* Isa. 59:20, *note.*

1(10:1) Cf. Hos. 6:3; Joel 2:23-32; Zech. 12:10. There is both a physical and spiritual meaning: Rain as of old will be restored to Palestine, but, also, there will be a mighty effusion of the Spirit upon restored Israel.

2(10:4) The tense is future: "From him [Judah] shall be the cornerstone (Ex. 17:6; 1 Pet. 2:8, *note*), from him the nail (Isa. 22:23, 24), from him the battle-bow," etc. The whole scene is of the events which group about the deliverance of the Jews in Palestine in the time of the northern invasion under the "Beast" (Dan. 7:8; Rev. 19:20, and "Armageddon," Rev. 16:14; 19:17). The final deliverance is wholly effected by the return of the LORD (Rev. 19:11-21), but previously He strengthens the hard-pressed Israelites (Mic. 4:13; Zech. 9:13-15; 10:5-7; 12:2-6; 14:14). That there may have been a precursive fulfilment in the Maccabean victories can neither be affirmed nor denied from Scripture.

young lions; for the pride of Jordan is
spoiled.
4 Thus saith the LORD my God; Feed
the flock of the slaughter;
5 Whose possessors slay them, and
hold themselves not guilty: and they
that sell them say, Blessed *be* the LORD;
for I am rich: and their own shepherds
pity them not.
6 For I will no more pity the inhabitants of the land, saith the LORD: but, lo, I
will deliver the men every one into his
neighbour's hand, and into the hand of
his king: and they shall smite the land,
and out of their hand I will not deliver
them.

The cause of the wrath, the rejection of Messiah.

7 And I will feed the flock of slaughter, *even* you, O [a]poor of the flock. And I
took unto me [1]two [b]staves; [2]the one I
called Beauty, and the other I called
Bands; and I fed the flock.
8 Three shepherds also I cut off in one
month; and my soul lothed them, and
their soul also abhorred me.
9 Then said I, I will not feed you: that
that dieth, let it die; and that that is to be
cut off, let it be cut off; and let the rest
eat every one the flesh of another.
10 And I took my staff, *even* Beauty,
and cut it asunder, that I might break my
covenant which I had made with all the
people.
11 And it was broken in that day: and
so the [3]poor of the flock that waited
upon me knew that it *was* the word of
the LORD.
12 And I said unto them, If ye think
good, give *me* my price; and if not, forbear. [c]So they weighed for my price thirty *pieces* of silver.
13 And the LORD said unto me, Cast it
unto the potter: a goodly price that I was
prised at of them. And I took the [d]thirty
pieces of silver, and cast them to the potter in the house of the LORD.
14 Then I cut asunder mine other staff,
even Bands, that I might break the brotherhood between Judah and Israel.

The Beast and his judgment.

15 [4]And the LORD said unto me, [e]Take
unto thee yet the instruments of a foolish
shepherd.
16 For, lo, I will raise up a shepherd in
the land, *which* shall not visit those that
be [f]cut off, neither shall seek the young
one, nor heal that that is broken, nor
feed that that standeth still: but he shall
eat the flesh of the fat, and tear their
claws in pieces.
17 [g]Woe to the idol shepherd that
leaveth the flock! the sword *shall be* upon
his arm, and upon his right eye: his arm

B.C. 487.

a *Remnant.* vs. 7, 11; Mal. 3:16-18. (Isa. 1:9; Rom. 11:5.)

b *Parables* (O.T.). vs. 7-14. (Jud. 9:7-15.)

c Mt. 26:15; 27:9,10.

d *Christ (First Advent).* vs. 11-13; Zech. 13:7. (Gen. 3:15; Acts 1:9.)

e Ezk. 34:2-4.

f Or, *hidden.*

g Jer. 23:1; Ezk. 34:2; John 10:12, 13.

[1] **(11:7)** The scene belongs to the first advent. Beauty and Bands—literally "graciousness and union"; the first signifying God's attitude toward His people Israel, in sending His Son (Mt. 21:37); the second, His purpose to reunite Judah and Ephraim (Ezk. 37:15-22). Christ, at His first advent, came with grace (John 1:17) to offer union (Mt. 4:17), and was sold for thirty pieces of silver (Zech. 11:12, 13). "Beauty" (i.e. *graciousness*) was "cut in sunder" (vs. 10, 11), signifying that Judah was abandoned to the destruction foretold in verses 1-6, and fulfilled A.D. 70. After the betrayal of the Lord for thirty pieces of silver (vs. 12, 13) "Bands" (i.e. *union*) was broken (v. 14), signifying the abandonment, *for the time,* of the purpose to reunite Judah and Israel. The order of Zech. 11 is, (1) the wrath against the land (vs. 1-6), fulfilled in the destruction of Jerusalem after the rejection of Christ (Lk. 19:41-44); (2) the cause of that wrath in the sale and rejection of Christ (vs. 7-14); (3) the rise of the "idol shepherd," the Beast (Dan. 7:8; Rev. 19:20), and his destruction (vs. 15-17).

[2] **(11:7)** The O.T. Parables: Summary. A parable is a similitude used to teach or enforce a truth. The O.T. parables fall into three classes: (1) The story-parable, of which Jud. 9:7-15 is an instance; (2) parabolic discourses; e.g. Isa. 5:1-7; (3) parabolic actions; e.g. Ezk. 37:16-22.

[3] **(11:11)** The "poor of the flock": i.e. the "remnant according to the election of grace" (Rom. 11:5); those Jews who did not wait for the manifestation of Christ in glory, but believed on Him at His first coming, and since. Of them it is said that they "waited upon Me," and "knew." Neither the Gentiles nor the Gentile church, corporately, are in view: only the believers out of *Israel* during this age. The church, corporately, is not in O.T. prophecy (Eph. 3:8-10).

[4] **(11:15)** The reference to the Beast is obvious; no other personage of prophecy in any sense meets the description. He who came in His Father's name was rejected: the alternative is one who comes in his own name (John 5:43; Rev. 13:4-8).

shall be clean dried up, and his right eye shall be utterly darkened.

CHAPTER 12.

The siege of Jerusalem by the Beast and his armies. (Cf. Rev. 19:19-21.)

The [1]burden of the word of the LORD for Israel, saith the LORD, which stretcheth forth the heavens, and layeth the foundation of the earth, and formeth the spirit of man within him.

2 [a]Behold, I will make Jerusalem a cup of trembling unto all the people round about, when they shall be in the [b]siege both against Judah *and* against Jerusalem.

3 And in that day will I make Jerusalem a burdensome stone for all people: all that burden themselves with it shall be cut in pieces, though all the people of the earth be gathered together against it.

The siege: Judah strengthened; the Lord's deliverance.

4 In that day, saith the LORD, I will smite every horse with astonishment, and his rider with madness: and I will open mine eyes upon the house of Judah, and will smite every horse of the people with blindness.

5 And the governors of Judah shall say in their heart, The inhabitants of Jerusalem *shall be* my strength in the LORD of hosts their God.

6 [c]In that day will I make the governors of Judah like an hearth of fire among the wood, and like a torch of fire in a sheaf; and they shall devour all the people round about, on the right hand and on the left: and Jerusalem shall be inhabited [d]again in her own place, *even* in Jerusalem.

7 The LORD also shall save the tents of Judah first, that the glory of the house of David and the glory of the inhabitants of Jerusalem do not magnify *themselves* against Judah.

8 In that day shall the LORD defend the inhabitants of Jerusalem; and he that is feeble among them at that day shall be as David; and the house of [2]David *shall be* as God, as the [e]angel of the LORD before them.

9 And it shall come to pass in that day, *that* I will seek to destroy

B.C. 487.

a *Day (of Jehovah).* vs. 1-14; Zech. 13:1-6. (Isa. 2:10-22; Rev. 19:11-21.)

b *Armageddon (battle of).* vs. 1-9; Zech. 14:1-5. (Rev. 16:14; 19:11-21)

c Cf. Zech. 9:13-15; 10:5-7; 12:2-6; 14:14.

d *Kingdom* (O.T.). vs. 6-8; Gen. 1:26; see *note.*

e Heb. 1:4, *note.*

[1](12:1) Zech. 12–14 form one prophecy the general theme of which is the return of the Lord and the establishment of the kingdom. The *order* is: (1)The siege of Jerusalem preceding the battle of Armageddon (vs. 1-3); (2) the battle itself (vs. 4-9); (3) the "latter rain" in the pouring out of the Spirit and the personal revelation of Christ to the family of David and the remnant in Jerusalem, not merely as the glorious Deliverer, but as the One whom Israel pierced and has long rejected (v. 10); (4) the godly sorrow which follows that revelation (vs. 11-14); (5) the cleansing fountain (Zech. 13:1) then to be *effectually* "opened" to Israel.

[2](12:8) Kingdom in O.T., Summary:

I. Dominion over the earth before the call of Abraham.

(1) Dominion over creation was given to the first man and woman (Gen. 1:26, 28). Through the fall this dominion was lost, Satan becoming "prince of this world" (Mt. 4:8-10; John 14:30).

(2) After the flood, the principle of human government was established under the covenant with Noah (Gen. 9:1, *note*). Biblically this is still the charter of all Gentile government.

II. The Theocracy in Israel. The call of Abraham involved, with much else, the creation of a distinctive people through whom great purposes of God toward the race might be worked out (see "Israel" Gen. 12:1-3; Rom. 11:26, *summary*). Among these purposes is the establishment of a universal kingdom. The order of the development of the Divine rule in Israel is:

(1) The mediatorship of Moses (Ex. 3:1-10; 19:9; 24:12).

(2) The leadership of Joshua (Josh. 1:1-5).

(3) The institution of Judges (Jud. 2:16-18)

(4) The popular rejection of the Theocracy, and choice of a king—Saul (1 Sam. 8:1-7; 9:12-17).

III. The Davidic kingdom.

(1) The divine choice of David (1 Sam. 16:1-13).

(2) The giving of the Davidic Covenant (2 Sam. 7:8-16; Psa. 89:3, 4, 20, 21, 28-37).

all the nations that come against
Jerusalem.

The Spirit poured out: the pierced
One revealed to the delivered remnant.

10 And I will pour upon the house of
David, and upon the inhabitants of Jerusalem, the [a]spirit of grace and of supplications: and they shall look upon me
[b]whom they have [c]pierced, and they
shall mourn for him, as one mourneth
for *his* only *son*, and shall be in bitterness
for him, as one that is in bitterness for *his*
firstborn.

The repentance of the remnant.

11 In that day shall there be a great
mourning in Jerusalem, as the mourning
of Hadadrimmon in the valley of
Megiddon.
12 And the land shall mourn, every
family apart; the family of the house of
David apart, and their wives apart; the
family of the house of Nathan apart, and
their wives apart;
13 The family of the house of Levi
apart, and their wives apart; the family
of Shimei apart, and their wives apart;
14 All the families that remain, every
family apart, and their wives apart.

B.C. 487.

a Holy Spirit. Mal. 2:15. (Gen. 1:2; Mal. 2:15.)

b John 19:37; Rev. 1:7.

c Christ (Second Advent). Zech. 13:6. (Deut. 30:3; Acts 1:9-11.)

d Day (of Jehovah). vs. 1-6; Zech. 14:1-21. (Isa. 2:10-22; Rev. 19:11-21.)

CHAPTER 13.

The repentant remnant pointed to the cross.

In that [d]day there shall be a fountain
opened to the house of David and to
the inhabitants of Jerusalem for sin and
for uncleanness.

Idols and false prophets cease
(Isa. 2:18; 10:11).

2 And it shall come to pass in that day,
saith the LORD of hosts, *that* I will cut off
the names of the idols out of the land,
and they shall no more be remembered:
and also I will cause the prophets and
the unclean spirit to pass out of the land.
3 And it shall come to pass, *that* when
any shall yet prophesy, then his father

(3) The exposition of the Davidic Covenant by the prophets (Isa. 1:25, 26 to Zech. 12:6-8. See marg. Isa. 1:25, "Kingdom" and *refs.*). The kingdom as described by the prophets is:

(a) Davidic, to be established under an heir of David, who is to be born of a virgin, therefore truly man, but also "Immanuel," "the mighty God, the everlasting Father, the Prince of Peace" (Isa. 7:13, 14; 9:6, 7; 11:1; Jer. 23:5; Ezk. 34:23; 37:24; Hos. 3:4, 5).

(b) A kingdom heavenly in origin, principle, and authority (Dan. 2:34, 35, 44, 45), but set up on the earth, with Jerusalem as the capital (Isa. 2:2-4; 4:3, 5; 24:23; 33:20; 62:1-7; Jer. 23:5; 31:38-40; Joel 3:1, 16, 17).

(c) The kingdom is to be established first over regathered, restored, and converted Israel, and is then to become universal (Psa. 2:6-8; 24; 22; Isa. 1:2, 3; 11:1, 10-13; 60:12; Jer. 23:5-8; 30:7-11; Ezk. 20:33-40; 37:21-25; Zech. 9:10; 14:16-19).

(d) The *moral* characteristics of the kingdom are to be righteousness and peace. The meek, not the proud, will inherit the earth; longevity will be greatly increased; the knowledge of the LORD will be universal; beast ferocity will be removed; absolute equity will be enforced; and outbreaking sin visited with instant judgment; while the enormous majority of earth's inhabitants will be saved (Isa. 11:4, 6-9; 65:20; Psa. 2:9; Isa. 26:9; Zech. 14:16-21). The N.T. (Rev. 20:1-5) adds a detail of immense significance—the removal of Satan from the scene. It is impossible to conceive to what heights of spiritual, intellectual, and physical perfection humanity will attain in this, its coming age of righteousness and peace (Isa. 11:4-9; Psa. 72:1-10).

(e) The kingdom is to be established by power, not persuasion, and is to follow divine judgment upon the Gentile world-powers (Psa. 2:4-9; Isa. 9:7; Dan. 2:35, 44, 45; 7:26, 27; Zech. 14:1-19). See Zech. 6:11, *note.*

(f) The restoration of Israel and the establishment of the kingdom are connected with an advent of the Lord, yet future (Deut. 30:3-5; Psa. 2:1-9; Zech. 14:4).

(g) The chastisement reserved for disobedience in the house of David (2 Sam. 7:14; Psa. 89:30-33) fell in the captivities and world-wide dispersion, since which time, though a remnant returned under prince Zerubbabel, Jerusalem has been under the overlordship of Gentiles. But the Davidic Covenant has not been abrogated (Psa. 89:33-37), but is yet to be fulfilled (Acts 15:14-17).

and his mother that begat him shall say unto him, Thou shalt not live; for thou speakest lies in the name of the LORD: and his father and his mother that begat him shall thrust him through when he prophesieth.

4 And it shall come to pass in that day, *that* the prophets shall be ashamed every one of his vision, when he hath prophesied; neither shall they wear a rough garment to deceive:

5 But he shall say, I *am* no prophet, I *am* an husbandman; for man taught me to keep cattle from my youth.

The preaching to Israel after the return of the LORD.

6 And *one* shall say unto [a]him, What *are* these [b]wounds in thine [c]hands? Then he shall answer, *Those* with which I was wounded *in* the house of my friends.

7 Awake, O sword, against my shepherd, and against the man *that is* my fellow, saith the LORD of hosts: [d]smite the [e]shepherd, and the sheep shall be scattered: and I will turn mine hand upon the little ones.

Résumé: *Result of the Gentile invasion under the Beast.*

8 [1]And it shall come to pass, *that* in all the land, saith the LORD, two parts therein shall be cut off *and* die; but the third shall be left therein.

9 And I will bring the third part through the fire, and will refine them as silver is refined, and will try them as gold is tried: they shall call on my name, and I will hear them: I will say, It *is* my people: and they shall say, The LORD *is* my God.

B.C. 487.

a *Christ (Second Advent).* Zech. 14:4. (Deut. 30:3; Acts 1:9-11.)

b Psa. 22:16.

c *Sacrifice (prophetic).* Mt. 26:28. (Gen. 4:4; Heb. 10:18.)

d *Christ (First Advent).* Mal. 3:1, 2. (Gen. 3:15; Acts 1:9.)

e Mt. 26:31, 67; Mk. 14:27, 65; 15:19.

f *Day (of Jehovah).* vs. 1-21; Mal. 4:1-6. (Isa. 2:10-22; Rev. 19:11-21.)

g *Armageddon (battle of).* vs. 1-5; Mt. 24:27, 28. (Rev. 16:14; 19:11-21.)

h Isa. 52:7.

i *Christ (Second Advent).* Mt. 19:28. (Deut. 30:3; Acts 1:9-11.)

j Amos 1:1.

CHAPTER 14.

Summary of events at the return of the LORD in glory: (1) *Armageddon.*

Behold, the [f]day of the LORD cometh, and thy spoil shall be divided in the midst of thee.

2 For I will gather all nations against Jerusalem to battle; and the city shall be taken, and the houses rifled, and the women ravished; and half of the city shall go forth into captivity, and the residue of the people shall not be cut off from the city.

3 Then shall the LORD go forth, and [g]fight against those nations, as when he fought in the day of battle.

(2) *The visible return in glory: physical changes in Palestine* (vs. 4, 10).

4 And his [h]feet [i]shall stand in that day upon the mount of Olives, which *is* before Jerusalem on the east, [2]and the mount of Olives shall cleave in the midst thereof toward the east and toward the west, *and there shall be* a very great valley; and half of the mountain shall remove toward the north, and half of it toward the south.

5 And ye shall flee *to* the valley of the mountains; for the valley of the mountains shall reach unto Azal: yea, ye shall flee, like as ye fled from before the [j]earthquake in the days of Uzziah king of Judah: and the LORD my God shall come, *and* all the saints with thee.

6 And it shall come to pass in that day, *that* the light shall not be clear, *nor* dark:

7 But it shall be one day which shall be known to the LORD, not day, nor night:

[1]**(13:8)** Zech. 13 now returns to the subject of Zech. 12:10. Verses 8, 9 refer to the sufferings of the remnant (Isa. 1:9; Rom. 11:5) *preceding* the great battle. Zech. 14 is a recapitulation of the whole matter. The order is: (1) The gathering of the nations, v. 2 (see "Armageddon," Rev. 16:14; 19:11, *note*); (2) the deliverance, v. 3; (3) the return of Christ to the Mount of Olives, and the physical change of the scene, vs. 4-8; (4) the setting up of the kingdom, and full earthly blessing, vs. 9-21.

[2]**(14:4)** Verse 5 implies that the cleavage of the Mount of Olives is due to an earthquake, and this is confirmed by Isa. 29:6; Rev. 16:19. In both passages the context, as in Zech. 14 (see vs. 1-3) associates the earthquake with the Gentile invasion under the Beast (Dan. 7:8; Rev. 19:20). Surely, in a land seamed by seismic disturbances it should not be difficult to believe that another earthquake might cleave the little hill called the Mount of Olives. Not one of the associated events of Zech. 14 occurred at the first coming of Christ, closely associated though He then was with the Mount of Olives.

but it shall come to pass, *that* at evening time it shall be light.

(3) *The river of the sanctuary.*
(Cf. Ezk. 47:1-12; Rev. 22:1, 2.)

8 And it shall be in that day, *that* living waters shall go out from Jerusalem; half of them toward the former sea, and half of them toward the hinder sea: in summer and in winter shall it be.

(4) *The kingdom set up on the earth.*

9 And the LORD shall be king over all the [1]earth: in that day shall there be one LORD, and his name one.

10 All the land shall be turned as a plain from Geba to Rimmon south of Jerusalem: and it shall be lifted up, and inhabited in her place, from Benjamin's gate unto the place of the first gate, unto the corner gate, and *from* the tower of Hananeel unto the king's winepresses.

11 And *men* shall dwell in it, and there shall be no more utter destruction; but Jerusalem shall be safely inhabited.

12 And this shall be the plague wherewith the LORD will smite all the people that have fought against Jerusalem; Their flesh shall consume away while they stand upon their feet, and their eyes shall consume away in their holes, and their tongue shall consume away in their mouth.

13 And it shall come to pass in that day, *that* a great tumult from the LORD shall be among them; and they shall lay hold every one on the hand of his neighbour, and his hand shall rise up against the hand of his neighbour.

14 And Judah also shall fight at Jerusalem; and the wealth of all the [a]heathen round about shall be gathered together, gold, and silver, and apparel, in great abundance.

15 And so shall be the plague of the horse, of the mule, of the camel, and of the ass, and of all the beasts that shall be in these tents, as this plague.

(5) *The worship and spirituality of the kingdom.*

16 And it shall come to pass, *that* every one that is left of all the nations which came against Jerusalem shall even go up from year to year to worship the [b]King, the LORD of hosts, and to keep the feast of tabernacles.

17 And it shall be, *that* whoso will not come up of *all* the families of the earth unto Jerusalem to worship the King, the LORD of hosts, even upon them shall be no rain.

18 And if the family of Egypt go not up, and come not, that *have* no *rain*; there shall be the plague, wherewith the LORD will smite the heathen that come not up to keep the feast of tabernacles.

19 This shall be the punishment of Egypt, and the punishment of all nations that come not up to keep the feast of tabernacles.

20 In that day shall there be upon the [c]bells of the horses, [d]HOLINESS UNTO THE LORD; and the pots in the LORD'S house shall be like the bowls before the altar.

21 Yea, every pot in Jerusalem and in Judah shall be holiness unto the LORD of hosts: and all they that sacrifice shall come and take of them, and seethe therein: and in that day there shall be no more the [e]Canaanite in [f]the house of the LORD of hosts.

B.C. 487.

a i.e. *nations.*

b *Kingdom* (O.T.). vs. 16-21; Zech. 12:6-8. (Gen. 1:26; Zech. 12:8.)

c Or, *bridles.*

d Isa. 23:18; Jer. 2:3.

e Isa. 35:8; Ezk. 44:9; Joel 3:17; Rev. 21:27; 22:15.

f Eph. 2:19-22.

[1] **(14:9)** The final answer to the prayer of Mt. 6:10. Cf. Dan. 2:44, 45; 7:24-27. See "Kingdom (N.T.)" (Lk. 1:31-33; 1 Cor. 15:28).

MALACHI

MALACHI, "my messenger," the last of the prophets to the restored remnant after the 70 years' captivity, probably prophesied in the time of confusion during Nehemiah's absence (Neh. 13:6). The burden of his message is, the love of Jehovah, the sins of the priests and of the people, and the day of the LORD. Malachi, like Zechariah, sees both advents, and predicts two forerunners (Mal. 3:1 and 4:5, 6). As a whole, Malachi gives the moral judgment of God on the remnant restored by His grace under Ezra and Nehemiah. He had established His house among them, but their worship was formal and insincere.

The book is in four natural divisions: I. The love of God for Israel, 1:1-5. II. The sins of the priests rebuked, 1:6–2:9. III. The sins of the people rebuked, 2:10–3:18. IV. The day of the LORD, 4:1-6.

CHAPTER 1.

Part I. The love of God for Israel (vs. 1-5).

The burden of the word of the LORD to
Israel by Malachi.
2 I have [a]loved you, saith the LORD.
Yet ye say, Wherein hast thou loved us?
Was not Esau Jacob's brother? saith the
LORD: yet I loved [b]Jacob,
3 And I hated Esau, and laid his
mountains and his heritage waste for the
dragons of the wilderness.
4 Whereas [c]Edom saith, We are
impoverished, but we will return and
build the desolate places; thus saith the
LORD of hosts, They shall build, but I
will throw down; and they shall call
them, The border of wickedness, and,
The people against whom the LORD hath
indignation for ever.
5 And your eyes shall see, and ye shall
say, [d]The LORD will be magnified from
the border of Israel.

Part II. The sins of the restoration priests (Mal. 1:6–2:9).

6 A son [e]honoureth *his* father, and a
servant his master: [1]if then I *be* a [f]father,
where *is* mine honour? and if I *be* a master, where *is* my fear? saith the LORD of
hosts unto you, O priests, that despise
my name. And ye say, Wherein have we
despised thy name?
7 Ye offer polluted bread upon mine
altar; and ye say, Wherein have we
polluted thee? In that ye say, The table of
the LORD *is* contemptible.
8 And if ye offer the blind for sacrifice,
is it not evil? and if ye offer the lame and
sick, *is it* not evil? offer it now unto thy
governor; will he be pleased with thee,
or accept thy person? saith the LORD of
hosts.
9 And now, I pray you, beseech God
that he will be gracious unto us: this
hath been by your means: will he regard
your persons? saith the LORD of hosts.
10 [g]Who *is there* even among you that
would shut the doors *for nought*? neither
do ye kindle *fire* on mine altar for
nought. I have no pleasure in you, saith
the LORD of hosts, neither will I accept
an offering at your hand.
11 [h]For from the rising of the sun even
unto the going down of the same my
name *shall be* great among the Gentiles;
and in every place incense *shall be*
offered unto my name, and a pure offering: for my name *shall be* great among
the [i]heathen, saith the LORD of hosts.
12 But ye have profaned it, in that ye
say, The table of the LORD *is* polluted;
and the fruit thereof, *even* his meat, *is*
contemptible.
13 Ye said also, Behold, what a weariness *is it*! and ye have snuffed at it, saith
the LORD of hosts; and ye brought *that
which was* torn, and the lame, and the
sick; thus ye brought an offering: should
I accept this of your hand? saith the
LORD.

B.C. 397.

a Deut. 4:37; 7:7, 8.
b Rom. 9:13.
c i.e. Esau's descendants. See Gen. 25:30.
d Mic. 5:4.
e Ex. 20:12; Mt. 15:4-8; Eph. 6:2-3.
f Isa. 63:16; 64:8; Jer. 31:9.
g Or, *I would that one among you would shut the doors* [of the temple] *that no more vain fire should kindle on mine altar.* Cf. Isa. 1:11-15.
h i.e. So it *would* have been had Israel been true. Isa. 45:5, 6. So it shall be despite Israel's failure.
i i.e. *nations.*

[1] **(1:6)** Cf. Isa. 63:16, *note.* The relationship here is national, not personal (Jer. 3:18, 19); here, apparently, the Jews were calling Jehovah "Father," but yielding Him no filial obedience. See John 8:37-39; Rom. 9:1-8.

14 But cursed *be* the deceiver, which
hath in his flock a male, and voweth,
and sacrificeth unto the Lord a [a]corrupt
thing: for I *am* a great King, saith the
LORD of hosts, and my name *is* dreadful
among the heathen.

CHAPTER 2.

(*The message to the priests,* continued.)

And now, O ye priests, this commandment *is* for you.
2 If ye will not hear, and if ye will not
lay *it* to heart, to give glory unto my
name, saith the LORD of hosts, I will even
send a curse upon you, and I will [b]curse
your blessings: yea, I have cursed them
already, because ye do not lay *it* to heart.
3 Behold, I will corrupt your seed, and
spread dung upon your faces, *even* the
dung of your solemn feasts; and *one*
shall take you away with it.
4 And ye shall know that I have sent
this commandment unto you, that my
covenant might be with Levi, saith the
LORD of hosts.
5 My [c]covenant was with him of life
and peace; and I gave them to him *for*
the fear wherewith he feared me, and
was afraid before my name.
6 The law of truth was in his mouth,
and iniquity was not found in his lips:
he walked with me in peace and equity,
and did turn many away from iniquity.
7 For the priest's lips should keep
knowledge, and they should seek the
law at his mouth: for he *is* the messenger
of the LORD of hosts.
8 But ye are departed out of the way;
ye have caused many to stumble at the
law; ye have corrupted the covenant of
Levi, saith the LORD of hosts.
9 Therefore have I also made you contemptible and base before all the people,
according as ye have not kept my ways,
but have been partial in the law.

Part III. (Mal. 2:10–3:18.) *The sins of the people:* (1) *sins against brotherhood.*

10 [d]Have we not all one father? hath
not one God created us? why do we deal
treacherously every man against his
brother, by profaning the covenant of
our fathers?

(2) *Sins against God in the family.*

11 Judah hath dealt treacherously, and
an abomination is committed in Israel
and in Jerusalem; for Judah hath profaned the holiness of the LORD which he
loved, and hath married the daughter of
a strange god.
12 The LORD will cut off the man that
doeth this, the master and the scholar,
out of the tabernacles of Jacob, and him
that offereth an offering unto the LORD of
hosts.
13 And this have ye done again, covering the altar of the LORD with tears,
with weeping, and with crying out, insomuch that he regardeth not the offering
any more, or receiveth *it* with good will
at your hand.
14 Yet ye say, Wherefore? Because the
LORD hath been witness between thee
and the wife of thy youth, against whom
thou hast dealt treacherously: yet *is* she
thy companion, and the wife of thy
covenant.
15 And did not he make one? Yet had
he the [e]residue of the [1][f]spirit. And
wherefore one? That he might seek a
godly seed. Therefore take heed to your
spirit, and let none deal treacherously
against the wife of his youth.
16 For the LORD, the God of Israel,

B.C. 397.

a Lev. 22:18-20.

b Cf. Deut. 28:3-14 with vs. 15-35. Israel's *distinctive* blessings should turn to curses.

c Num. 25:10-13; Deut. 33:8-9.

d Cf. Acts 17:24-29. In both instances the reference is to creation, not the new birth.

e *Deity (names of).* Mal. 3:18. (Gen. 1:1; Mal. 3:18.)

f *Holy Spirit.* (Gen. 1:2.)

[1] **(2:15)** Summary of the O.T. doctrine of the Holy Spirit: (1) The personality and Deity of the Holy Spirit appear from the *attributes* ascribed to Him, and from His *works.* (2) He is revealed as sharing the work of creation and therefore *omnipotent* (Gen. 1:2; Job 26:13; 33:4; Psa. 104:30); as *omnipresent* (Psa. 139:7); as *striving with men* (Gen. 6:3); as *enlightening* (Job 32:8); enduing with *constructive skill* (Ex. 28:3; 31:3); giving *physical strength* (Jud. 14:6, 19); *executive ability* and *wisdom* (Jud. 3:10; 6:34; 11:29; 13:25),; enabling men to receive and utter *divine revelations* (Num. 11:25; 2 Sam. 23:2); and, generally, as *empowering* the servants of God (Psa. 51:12; Joel 2:28; Mic. 3:8; Zech. 4:6). (3) He is called *holy* (Psa. 51:11); *good* (Psa. 143:10); the Spirit of *judgment and burning* (Isa. 4:4); of *Jehovah,* of *wisdom, understanding, counsel, might, good, knowledge, the fear of the LORD* (Isa. 11:2), and of *grace* and *supplications* (Zech. 12:10). (4) In the O.T. the Spirit acts in free sovereignty, coming upon men and even upon a dumb beast as He will, nor are conditions set forth (as in the N.T.)

saith that he hateth putting away: for *one* covereth violence with his garment, saith the LORD of hosts: therefore take heed to your spirit, that ye deal not treacherously.

(3) *The sin of insincere religious profession.*

17 Ye have wearied the LORD with
your words. Yet ye say, Wherein have
we wearied *him*? When ye say, Every
one that doeth evil *is* good in the sight of
the LORD, and he delighteth in them; or,
Where *is* the God of judgment?

CHAPTER 3.

Parenthesis: The mission of John the Baptist and coming of the Lord foretold (vs. 1-6).

Behold, I will send [a]my messenger,
and [b]he shall prepare the way
before me: and the [1]Lord, whom ye seek,
shall suddenly come to his temple, even
the messenger of the covenant, whom ye
delight in: behold, he shall come, saith
the LORD of hosts.
2 But who may abide [c]the day of his
coming? and [d]who shall stand when he
appeareth? for [e]he *is* like a refiner's fire,
and like fullers' soap:
3 And [f]he shall sit *as* a refiner and
purifier of silver: and he shall purify the
sons of Levi, and purge them as gold
and silver, that they may [g]offer unto the
LORD an offering in righteousness.
4 Then shall the offering of Judah and
Jerusalem be pleasant unto the LORD, as
in the days of old, and as in former
years.
5 And I will come near to you to judgment;
and I will be a swift witness
against the sorcerers, and against the
adulterers, [h]and against false swearers,
and against those that oppress the
hireling in *his* wages, the widow, and the
fatherless, and that turn aside the
stranger *from his right*, and fear not me,
saith the LORD of hosts.
6 For I *am* the LORD, [i]I change not;
therefore ye sons of Jacob are not consumed.

Part III. resumed:
The people have robbed God.

7 Even from the days of your fathers
ye are gone away from mine ordinances,
and have not kept *them*. [j]Return unto
me, and I will return unto you, saith the
LORD of hosts. But ye said, Wherein shall
we return?
8 Will a man rob God? Yet ye have
robbed me. But ye say, Wherein have we
robbed thee? [k]In tithes and offerings.
9 Ye *are* cursed with a curse: for ye
have robbed me, *even* this whole nation.
10 [l]Bring ye all the tithes into the
storehouse, that there may be meat in
mine house, and prove me now herewith,
saith the LORD of hosts, if I will not
open you the windows of heaven, and
pour you out a blessing, that *there shall*
not *be room* enough *to receive it*.
11 And I will rebuke the devourer for
your sakes, and he shall not destroy the
fruits of your ground; neither shall your
vine cast her fruit before the time in the
field, saith the LORD of hosts.
12 And all nations shall call you
blessed: for ye shall be a delightsome
land, saith the LORD of hosts.
13 Your words have been stout
against me, saith the LORD. Yet ye say,

B.C. 397.

a Mt. 11:10; Mk. 1:2; Lk. 7:27.
b *Christ (First Advent)*. Mt. 1:1, 23. (Gen. 3:15; Acts 1:9.)
c Jer. 10:10; Mal. 4:1.
d Rev. 6:17.
e Isa. 4:4; Mt. 3:10-12.
f Isa. 1:25; Zech. 13:9.
g 1 Pet. 2:5.
h Zech. 5:4; Jas. 5:4, 12.
i Num. 23:19; Rom. 11:29; Jas. 1:17.
j Zech. 1:3.
k Neh. 13:10, 12.
l Prov. 3:9, 10; 1 Chr. 26:20; 2 Chr. 31:11; Neh. 10:38; 13:12.

by complying with which any one may receive the Spirit. The indwelling of every believer by the abiding Spirit is a N.T. blessing consequent upon the death and resurrection of Christ (John 7:39; 16:7; Acts 2:33; Gal. 3:1-6). (5) The O.T. contains predictions of a future pouring out of the Spirit upon Israel (Ezk. 37:14; 39:29), and upon "all flesh" (Joel 2:28, 29). The expectation of Israel, therefore, was twofold—of the coming of Messiah-Immanuel, and of such an effusion of the Spirit as the prophets described. See Mt. 1:18, *refs.*

[1] **(3:1)** The f.c. of verse 1 is quoted of John the Baptist (Mt. 11:10; Mk. 1:2; Lk. 7:27), but the second clause, "the Lord whom ye seek," etc., is *nowhere quoted* in the N.T. The reason is obvious: in everything save the fact of Christ's first advent, the latter clause awaits fulfilment (Hab. 2:20). Verses 2-5 speak of judgment, not of grace. Malachi, in common with other O.T. prophets, saw both advents of Messiah blended in one horizon, but did not see the separating interval described in Mt. 13 consequent upon the rejection of the King (Mt. 13:16, 17). Still less was the Church-age in his vision (Eph. 3:3-6; Col. 1:25-27). "My messenger" (v. 1) is John the Baptist; the "messenger of the covenant" is Christ in both of His advents, but with especial reference to the events which are to follow His return.

What have we spoken *so much* against
thee?
14 Ye have said, It *is* vain to serve God:
and what profit *is it* that we have kept
his ordinance, and that we have walked
mournfully before the LORD of hosts?
15 And now we call the proud happy;
yea, they that work wickedness are set
up; yea, *they that* [a]tempt God are even
delivered.

The faithful remnant.

16 Then [b]they that [c]feared the LORD
spake often one to another: and the LORD
hearkened, and heard *it*, and a book of
remembrance was written before him for
them that feared the LORD, and that
thought upon his name.
17 And they shall be mine, saith the
LORD of hosts, in that day when I make up
my jewels; and I will spare them, as a man
spareth his own son that serveth him.
18 Then shall ye return, and discern
between the [d]righteous and the wicked,
between him that serveth [1e]God and him
that serveth him not.

CHAPTER 4.

Part IV. The day of the LORD.

For, behold, the day [f]cometh, that shall
burn as an oven; and all the proud,
yea, and all that do wickedly, shall be
stubble: and the day that cometh shall
burn them up, saith the LORD of hosts, that
it shall leave them neither root nor branch.

The second coming of Christ.

2 But unto you that [c]fear my name
shall the [g]Sun of righteousness arise

B.C. 397.

a *Temptation.* Mt. 4:1, 3, 7. (Gen. 3:1; Jas. 1:2.)

b *Remnant.* vs. 16-18. Rom. 9:25-29. (Isa. 1:9; Rom. 11:5.)

c Psa. 19:9, *note.*

d *Righteousness.* Lk. 1:6. (Gen. 6:9; Lk. 2:25.)

e *Deity (names of).* (Gen. 1:1.)

f *Day of Jehovah.* vs. 1-6; Mt. 24:29-31. (Isa. 2:10-22; Rev. 19:11-21.)

g See Gen. 1:16, *note.*

[1] **(3:18)** Summary of the O.T. revelation of Deity: God is revealed in the O.T. (1) through His names, as follows:

CLASS.	ENGLISH FORM.	HEBREW EQUIVALENT.
Primary	God LORD Lord	El, Elah, or Elohim (Gen. 1:1, *note*) Jehovah (Gen. 2:4, *note*) Adon or Adonai (Gen. 15:2, *note*)
Compound (with El = God)	Almighty God Most High, or most high God everlasting God	El Shaddai (Gen. 17:1, *note*) El Elyon (Gen. 14:14, *note*) El Olam (Gen. 21:33, *note*)
Compound (with Jehovah = LORD)	LORD God Lord GOD LORD of hosts	Jehovah Elohim (Gen. 2:4, *note*) Adonai Jehovah (Gen. 15:2, *note*) Jehovah Sabaoth (1 Sam. 1:3, *note*)

The Trinity is *suggested* by the three times repeated groups of threes. This is not an arbitrary arrangement, but inheres in the O.T. itself.

This revelation of God by His names is invariably made in connection with some particular need of His people, and there can be no need of man to which these names do not answer as showing that man's true resource is in God. Even human failure and sin but evoke new and fuller revelations of the divine fulness.

(2) The O.T. Scriptures reveal the existence of a Supreme Being, the Creator of the universe and of man, the Source of all life and of all intelligence, who is to be worshipped and served by men and angels. This Supreme Being is One, but, in some sense not fully revealed in the O.T., is a unity in plurality. This is shown by the plural name, *Elohim*, by the use of the plural pronoun in the interrelation of Deity as evidenced in Gen. 1:26; 3:22; Psa. 110:1; and Isa. 6:8. That this plurality is really a Trinity is intimated in the three primary names of Deity, and in the threefold ascription of the Seraphim in Isa. 6:3. That the interrelation of Deity is that of Father and Son is directly asserted in Psa. 2:7 (with Heb. 1:5); and the Spirit is distinctly recognized in His personality, and to Him are ascribed all the divine attributes (e.g. Gen. 1:2; Num. 11:25; 24:2; Jud. 3:10; 6:34; 11:29; 13:25; 14:6, 19; 15:14; 2 Sam. 23:2; Job 26:13; 33:4; Psa. 106:33; 139:7; Isa. 40:7; 59:19; 63:10. See Mal. 2:15, *note*). (3) The future incarnation is *intimated* in the theophanies, or appearances of God in human form (e.g. Gen. 18:1, 13, 17-22; 32:24-30), and *distinctly* predicted in the promises connected with redemption (e.g. Gen. 3:15) and with the Davidic Covenant (e.g. Isa. 7:13, 14;

with healing in his wings; and ye shall go forth, and grow up as calves of the stall.

3 And ye shall tread down the wicked; for they shall be ashes under the soles of your feet in the day that I shall do *this*, saith the LORD of hosts.

4 Remember ye the law of Moses my servant, which I commanded unto him in Horeb for all Israel, *with* the statutes and judgments.

B.C. 397.

a Lk. 1:17.

Elijah to come again before the day of the LORD. (Cf. Rev. 11:3-6.)

5 Behold, I will send you Elijah the prophet before the coming of the great and dreadful day of the LORD:

6 And he [a]shall turn the heart of the fathers to the children, and the heart of the children to their fathers, lest I come and smite the earth with a curse.

9:6, 7; Jer. 23:5, 6). The revelation of Deity in the N.T. so illuminates that of the O.T. that the latter is seen to be, from Genesis to Malachi, the foreshadowing of the coming incarnation of God in Jesus the Christ. In promise, covenant, type, and prophecy, the O.T. points forward to Him. (4) The revelation of God to man is one of authority and of redemption. He requires righteousness from man, but saves the unrighteous through sacrifice; and in His redemptive dealings with man all the divine persons and attributes are brought into manifestation. The O.T. reveals the justice of God equally with His mercy, but never in opposition to His mercy. The flood, e.g., was an unspeakable mercy to unborn generations. From Genesis to Malachi He is revealed as the seeking God who has no pleasure in the death of the wicked, and who heaps up before the sinner every possible motive to persuade to faith and obedience. (5) In the experience of the O.T. men of faith their God inspires reverence but never slavish fear; and they exhaust the resources of language to express their love and adoration in view of His lovingkindness and tender mercy. This adoring love of His saints is the triumphant answer to those who pretend to find the O.T. revelation of God cruel and repellent. It is in harmony, not contrast, with the N.T. revelation of God in Christ. (6) Those passages which attribute to God bodily parts and human emotions (e.g. Ex. 33:11, 20; Deut. 29:20; 2 Chr. 16:9; Gen. 6:6, 7; Jer. 15:6) are metaphorical and mean that in the infinite being of God exists that which answers to these things—eyes, a hand, feet, etc.; and the jealousy and anger attributed to Him are the emotions of perfect Love in view of the havoc of sin. (7) In the O.T. revelation there is a true sense in which, wholly apart from sin or infirmity, God is like His creature man (Gen. 1:27), and the supreme and perfect revelation of God, toward which the O.T. points, is a revelation in and through a perfect Man.

FROM MALACHI TO MATTHEW.

THE close of the Old Testament canon left Israel in two great divisions. The mass of the nation were dispersed throughout the Persian Empire, more as colonists than captives. A remnant, chiefly of the tribe of Judah, with Zerubbabel, a prince of the Davidic family, and the survivors of the priests and Levites, had returned to the land under the permissive decrees of Cyrus and his successors (Dan. 5:31, *note;* 9:25, *note*), and had established again the temple worship. Upon this remnant the interest of the student of Scripture centres; and this interest concerns both their political and religious history.

I. Politically, the fortunes of the Palestinian Jews followed, with one exception—the Maccabean revolt—the history of the Gentile world-empires foretold by Daniel (Dan. 2, 7).

(1) The Persian rule continued about one hundred years after the close of the O.T. canon, and seems to have been mild and tolerant, allowing to the high priest, along with his religious functions, a measure of civil power, but under the overlordship of the governors of Syria. The sources of the history of the Jewish remnant during the Persian period were purely legendary when Josephus wrote. During this period the rival worship of Samaria (John 4:19, 20) was established.

Palestine suffered much from the constant wars between Persia and Egypt, lying as it did "between the anvil and the hammer."

(2) In 333 B.C. Syria fell under the power of the third of the world-empires, the Græco-Macedonian of Alexander. That conqueror, as Josephus relates, was induced to treat the Jews with much favour; but, upon the breaking up of his empire, Judæa again fell between the hammer and the anvil of Syria and Egypt, falling first under the power of Syria, but later under Egypt as ruled by the Ptolemaic kings. During this period (B.C. 320–198) great numbers of Jews were established in Egypt, and the Septuagint translation of the O.T. was made (B.C. 285).

(3) In B.C. 198 Judaea was conquered by Antiochus the Great, and annexed to Syria. At this time the division of the land into the five provinces familiar to readers of the Gospels, Galilee, Samaria, Judaea (often collectively called *Judaea*), Trachonitis and Peraea, was made. The Jews at first were permitted to live under their own laws under the high priest and a council. About B.C. 180 the land became the dowry of Cleopatra, a Syrian princess married to Ptolemy Philometor, king of Egypt, but on the death of Cleopatra was reclaimed by Antiochus Epiphanes (the "little horn" of Dan. 8:9, *note*), after a bloody battle. In 170 B.C., Antiochus, after repeated interferences with the temple and priesthood, plundered Jerusalem, profaned the temple, and enslaved great numbers of the inhabitants. December 25, B.C. 168, Antiochus offered a sow upon the great altar, and erected an altar to Jupiter. This is the "desolation" of Dan. 8:13, type of the final "abomination of desolation" of Mt. 24:15. The temple worship was forbidden, and the people compelled to eat swine's flesh.

(4) The excesses of Antiochus provoked the revolt of the Maccabees, one of the most heroic pages of history. Mattathias, the first of the Maccabees, a priest of great sanctity and energy of character, began the revolt. He did little more than to gather a band of godly and determined Jews pledged to free the nation and restore the ancient worship, and was succeeded by his son Judas, known in history as Maccabaeus, from the Hebrew word for hammer. He was assisted by four brothers of whom Simon is best known.

In B.C. 165 Judas regained possession of Jerusalem, purified and rededicated the temple, an event celebrated in the Jewish Feast of the Dedication. The struggle with Antiochus and his successor continued. Judas was slain in battle, his brother Jonathan succeeding. In him the civil and priestly authority were united (B.C. 143). Under Jonathan, his brother Simon, and his nephew John Hyrcanus, the Hasmonean line of priest-rulers was established, under sufferance of other powers. They possessed none of the Maccabean virtues.

(5) A civil war followed, which was terminated by the Roman conquest of Judea and Jerusalem by Pompey (B.C. 63), who left Hyrcanus, the last of the Hasmoneans, a nominal sovereignty, Antipater, an Idumean, wielding the actual power. B.C. 47 Antipater was made procurator of Judaea by Julius Caesar, and appointed his son, Herod, governor of Galilee. After the murder of

Caesar disorder ensued in Judaea, and Herod fled to Rome. There he was appointed (B.C. 40) king of the Jews, and returning, he conciliated the people by his marriage (B.C. 38) with Mariamne, the beautiful grand-daughter of Hyrcanus, and appointed her brother, the Maccabean Aristobulus III, high priest. Herod was king when Jesus Christ was born.

II. The religious history of the Jews during the long period from Malachi (B.C. 397) to Christ followed, as to outer ceremonial, the high-priestly office, and the temple worship, the course of the troublous political history, and is of scant interest.

Of greater moment are the efforts and means by which the real faith of Israel was kept alive and nurtured.

(1) The tendency to idolatry seems to have been destroyed by the Jews' experience and observation of it during the captivity. Deprived of temple and priest, and of the possibility of continuing a ceremonial worship, the Jewish people were thrown back upon that which was fundamental in their faith, the revelation of God as One, the Creator, to be conceived of as having made man in His own image, and therefore as having such analogies to the nature and life of man as to be comprehensible by man, while remaining the Eternal Spirit, God. This conception of God, enforced by the mighty ministries of the pre-exilic and exilic prophets, finally prevailed over all idolatrous conceptions, and this ministry was continued amongst the returned remnant by Haggai, Zechariah, and Malachi. The high ethics of the older prophets, their stern rebuke of mere formalism, and their glowing prophecies of the ultimate restoration of Israel in national and religious supremacy under Messiah, were all repeated by the three prophets of the restoration.

The problem was to keep alive this exalted ideal in the midst of outward persecutions and sordid and disgraceful divisions within.

(2) The organic means to this end was the synagogue, an institution which formed no part of the biblical order of the national life. Its origin is obscure. Probably, during the captivity, the Jews, deprived of the temple and its rites, met on the Sabbath day for prayer. This would give opportunity for the reading of the Scriptures. Such meetings would require some order of procedure, and some authority for the restraint of disorder. The synagogue doubtless grew out of the necessities of the situation in which the Jews were placed, but it served the purpose of maintaining familiarity with the inspired writings, and upon these the spiritual life of the true Israel (see Rom. 9:6, *note*) was nourished.

(3) But during this period, also, was created that mass of tradition, comment and interpretation, known as Mishna, Gemara (forming the Talmud), Halachoth, Midrashim and Kabbala, so superposed upon the Law that obedience was transferred from the Law itself to the traditional interpretation.

(4) During this period also rose the two great sects known to the Gospel narratives as Pharisees and Sadducees. (See Mt. 3:7, *notes* 2, 3.) The Herodians were a party rather than a sect.

Amongst such a people, governed, under the suzerainty of Rome, by an Idumean usurper, rent by bitter and unspiritual religious controversies, and maintaining an elaborate religious ritual, appeared Jesus, the Son and Christ of God.

The Scofield® Study Bible

THE NEW TESTAMENT

AUTHORIZED KING JAMES VERSION

With a new system of connected topical references to all the greater themes of Scripture, with annotations, revised marginal renderings, summaries, definitions, chronology, and index, to which are added, helps at hard places, explanations of seeming discrepancies, and a new system of paragraphs

EDITED BY

REV. C. I. SCOFIELD, D.D.

CONSULTING EDITORS

REV. HENRY G. WESTON, D.D., LL.D.,
President Crozer Theological Seminary.

REV. JAMES M. GRAY, D.D.,
President Moody Bible Institute.

REV. WILLIAM J. ERDMAN, D.D.,
Author "The Gospel of John," etc., etc.

REV. ARTHUR T. PIERSON, D.D.,
Author, Editor, Teacher.

REV. W. G. MOOREHEAD, D.D.,
President Xenia (U.P.) Theological Seminary.

REV. ELMORE HARRIS, D.D.,
President Toronto Bible Institute.

REV. ARNO C. GAEBELEIN, D.D.,
Author "Harmony of Prophetic Word," etc., etc.

REV. WILLIAM I. PETTINGILL, D.D.,
Author, Editor, Teacher.

New and Improved Edition

NEW YORK
OXFORD UNIVERSITY PRESS

THE FOUR GOSPELS.

THE four Gospels record the eternal being, human ancestry, birth, death, resurrection, and ascension of Jesus the Christ, Son of God, and Son of Man. They record also a selection from the incidents of His life, and from His words and works. Taken together, they set forth, not a biography but a Personality.

These two facts, that we have in the four Gospels a complete Personality, but not a complete biography, indicate the spirit and intent in which we should approach them. What is important is that through these narratives we should come to see and know Him whom they reveal. It is of relatively small importance that we should be able to piece together out of these confessedly incomplete records (John 21:25) a connected story of His life. For some adequate reason—perhaps lest we should be too much occupied with "Christ after the flesh"—it did not please God to cause to be written a biography of His Son. The twenty-nine formative years are passed over in a silence which is broken but once, and that in but twelve brief verses of Luke's Gospel. It may be well to respect the divine reticencies.

But the four Gospels, though designedly incomplete as a story, are divinely perfect as a revelation. We may not through them know everything that He did, but we may know the Doer. In four great characters, each of which completes the other three, we have Jesus Christ Himself. The Evangelists never describe Christ—they set Him forth. They tell us almost nothing of what they thought about Him, they let Him speak and act for Himself.

This is the essential respect in which these narratives differ from mere biography or portraiture. "The words that I speak unto you, they are spirit, and they are life." The student in whom dwells an ungrieved Spirit finds here the living Christ.

The distinctive part which each Evangelist bears in this presentation of the living Christ is briefly noted in separate Introductions, but it may be profitable to add certain general suggestions.

I. The Old Testament is a divinely provided Introduction to the New; and whoever comes to the study of the four Gospels with a mind saturated with the Old Testament foreview of the Christ, His person, work, and kingdom, will find them open books.

For the Gospels are woven of Old Testament quotation, allusion, and type. The very first verse of the New Testament drives the thoughtful reader back to the Old; and the risen Christ sent His disciples to the ancient oracles for an explanation of His sufferings and glory (Lk. 24:27, 44, 45). One of His last ministries was the opening of their understandings to understand the Old Testament.

Therefore, in approaching the study of the Gospels the mind should be freed, so far as possible, from mere theological concepts and presuppositions. Especially is it necessary to exclude the notion—a legacy in Protestant thought from post-apostolic and Roman Catholic theology—that the Church is the true Israel, and that the Old Testament foreview of the kingdom is fulfilled in the Church.

Do not, therefore, assume interpretations to be true because familiar. Do not assume that "the throne of David" (Lk. 1:32) is synonymous with "My Father's throne" (Rev. 3:21), or that "the house of Jacob" (Lk. 1:33) is the Church composed both of Jew and Gentile.

II. The mission of Jesus was, *primarily,* to the Jews (Mt. 10:5, 6; 15:23-25; John 1:11). He was "made under the law" (Gal. 4:4), and was "a minister of the circumcision for the truth of God, to confirm the promises made unto the fathers" (Rom. 15:8), and to fulfil the law that grace might flow out.

Expect, therefore, a strong legal and Jewish colouring up to the cross (e.g. Mt. 5:17-19; 6:12; cf. Eph. 4:32; Mt. 10:5, 6; 15:22-28; Mk. 1:44; Mt. 23:2, etc.) The Sermon on the Mount is law, not grace, for it demands as the condition of blessing (Mt. 5:3-9) that perfect character which grace, through divine power, creates (Gal.5:22, 23).

III. The *doctrines* of grace are to be sought in the Epistles, not in the Gospels; but those doctrines rest back upon the death and resurrection of Christ, and upon the great germ-truths to which He gave utterance, and of which the Epistles are the unfolding. Furthermore, the only perfect example of perfect grace is the Christ of the Gospels.

IV. The Gospels do not unfold the doctrine of the Church. The word occurs in Matthew only. After His rejection as King and Saviour by the Jews, our Lord, announcing a mystery until that moment "hid in God" (Eph. 3:3-10), said, "I will build my church" (Mt. 16:16, 18). It was, therefore, yet future; but His personal ministry had gathered out the believers who were, on the day of Pentecost, by the baptism with the Spirit, made the first members of "the church which is his body" (1 Cor. 12:12, 13; Eph. 1:23).

The Gospels present a group of Jewish disciples, associated on earth with a Messiah in humiliation; the Epistles a Church which is the body of Christ in glory, associated with Him in the heavenlies, co-heirs with Him of the Father, co-rulers with Him over the coming kingdom, and, as to the earth, pilgrims and strangers (1 Cor. 12:12, 13; Eph. 1:3-14, 20-23; 2:4-6; 1 Pet. 2:11).

V. The Gospels present Christ in His three offices of Prophet, Priest, and King.

As *Prophet* His ministry does not differ in kind from that of the Old Testament prophets. It is the dignity of His Person which makes Him the unique Prophet. Of old, God spoke through the prophets; now He speaks in the Son (Heb. 1:1, 2). The old prophet was a voice from God; the Son is God Himself (Deut. 18:18, 19).

The prophet in any dispensation is God's messenger to His people, first to establish truth, and, secondly, when they are in declension and apostasy to call them back to truth. His message, therefore, is, usually, one of rebuke and appeal. Only when these fall on deaf ears does he become a foreteller of things to come. In this, too, Christ is at one with the other prophets. His predictive ministry follows His rejection as King.

The sphere and character of Christ's *Kingly* office are defined in the Davidic Covenant (2 Sam. 7:8-16, and *refs.*), as interpreted by the prophets, and confirmed by the New Testament. The latter in no way abrogates or modifies either the Davidic Covenant or its prophetic interpretation. It adds details which were not in the prophet's vision. The Sermon on the Mount is an elaboration of the idea of "righteousness" as the predominant characteristic of the Messianic kingdom (Isa. 11:2-5; Jer. 23:5, 6; 33:14-16). The Old Testament prophet was perplexed by seeing in one horizon, so to speak, the suffering and the glory of Messiah (1 Pet. 1:10, 11). The New Testament shows that these are separated by the present church-age, and points forward to the Lord's return as the time when the Davidic Covenant of blessing through power will be fulfilled (Lk. 1:30-33; Acts 2:29-36; 15:14-17); just as the Abrahamic Covenant of blessing through suffering was fulfilled at His first coming (Acts 3:25; Gal. 3:6-14).

Christ is never called King of the Church. "The King" is indeed one of the divine titles, and the Church in her worship joins Israel in exalting "the king, eternal, immortal, invisible" (Psa. 10:16; 1 Tim. 1:17). But the Church is to reign with Him. The Holy Spirit is now calling out, not the subjects, but the co-heirs and co-rulers of the kingdom (2 Tim. 2:11, 12; Rev. 1:6; 3:21; 5:10; Rom. 8:15-18; 1 Cor. 6:2, 3).

Christ's *Priestly* office is the complement of His prophetic office. The prophet is God's representative with the people; the priest is the people's representative with God. Because they are sinful he must be a sacrificer; because they are needy he must be a compassionate intercessor (Heb. 5:1, 2; 8:1-3). So Christ, on the cross, entered upon His high-priestly work, offering Himself without spot unto God (Heb. 9:14), as now He compassionates His people in an ever-living intercession (Heb. 7:25). Of that intercession John 17 is the pattern.

VI. Distinguish, in the Gospels, *interpretation* from *moral application*. Much in the Gospels which belongs in strictness of interpretation to the Jew or the kingdom, is yet such a revelation of the mind of God, and so based on eternal principles, as to have a moral application to the people of God whatever their position dispensationally. It is always true that the "pure in heart" are happy because they "see God," and that "woe" is the portion of religious formalists whether under law or grace.

VII. Especial emphasis rests upon that to which all four Gospels bear a united testimony. That united testimony is sevenfold:

1. In all alike is revealed the one unique Personality. The one Jesus is King in Matthew, Servant in Mark, Man in Luke, and God in John. But not only so: for Matthew's King is also Servant, Man, and God; and Mark's Servant is also King, and Man, and God; Luke's Man is also King, and Servant, and God; and John's eternal Son is also King, and Servant, and Man.

The pen is a different pen; the incidents in which He is seen are sometimes different incidents; the distinctive character in which He is presented is a different character; but He is always the same Christ. That fact alone would mark these books as inspired.

2. All the Evangelists record the ministry of John the Baptist.

3. All record the feeding of the five thousand.

4. All record Christ's offer of Himself as King, according to Micah.

5. All record the betrayal by Judas; the denial by Peter; the trial, crucifixion, and literal resurrection of Christ. And this record is so made as to testify that the death of Christ was the supreme business which brought Him into the world; that all which precedes that death is but preparation for it; and that from it flow all the blessings which God ever has or ever will bestow upon man.

6. All record the resurrection ministry of Christ; a ministry which reveals Him as unchanged by the tremendous event of His passion, but a ministry keyed to a new note of universality, and of power.

7. All point forward to His second coming.

HOW TO USE THE SUBJECT REFERENCES.

THE subject references lead the reader from the first clear mention of a great truth to the last. The first and last references (in parenthesis) are repeated each time, so that wherever a reader comes upon a subject he may recur to the first reference and follow the subject, or turn at once to the Summary at the last reference.

ILLUSTRATION
(at Mark 1:1.)

b Gospel. vs. 1,
14, 15; Mk. 8:35.
(Gen. 12:1-3;
Rev. 14:6.)

Here *Gospel* is the subject; vs. 1, 14, 15 show where it is at that particular place; Mk. 8:35 is the next reference in the chain, and the references in parenthesis are the first and last.

THE GOSPEL ACCORDING TO

ST. MATTHEW

WRITER. The writer of the first Gospel, as all agree, was Matthew, called also Levi, a Jew of Galilee who had taken service as a tax-gatherer under the Roman oppressor. He was, therefore, one of the hated and ill-reputed publicans.

The date of Matthew has been much discussed, but no convincing reason has been given for discrediting the traditional date of A.D. 37.

Theme. The scope and purpose of the book are indicated in the first verse. Matthew is the "book of the generation of Jesus Christ, the Son of David, the Son of Abraham" (Mt. 1:1). This connects Him at once with two of the most important of the Old Testament covenants: the Davidic Covenant of kingship, and the Abrahamic Covenant of promise (2 Sam. 7:8-16; Gen. 15:18).

Of Jesus Christ in that twofold character, then, Matthew writes. Following the order indicated in the first verse, he writes first of the King, the Son of David; then of the Son of Abraham, obedient unto death, according to the Isaac type (Gen. 22:1-18; Heb. 11:17-19).

But the prominent character of Christ in Matthew is that of the covenanted King, David's "righteous Branch" (Jer. 23:5; 33:15). Matthew records His genealogy; His birth in Bethlehem the city of David, according to Micah (5:2); the ministry of His forerunner according to Malachi (3:1); the ministry of the King Himself; His rejection by Israel; and His predictions of His second coming in power and great glory.

Only then (Mt. 26–28) does Matthew turn to the earlier covenant, and record the sacrificial death of the Son of Abraham.

This determines the purpose and structure of Matthew. It is peculiarly the Gospel for Israel; and, as flowing from the death of Christ, a Gospel for the whole world.

Matthew falls into three principal divisions:

I. The manifestation to Israel and rejection of Jesus Christ the Son of David, born King of the Jews, 1:1–25:46. The subdivisions of this part are: (1) The official genealogy and birth of the King, 1:1-25; (2) the infancy and obscurity of the King, 2:1-23; (3) the kingdom "at hand," 3:1–12:50 (the order of events of this subdivision is indicated in the text); (4) the mysteries of the kingdom, 13:1-52; (5) the ministry of the rejected King, 13:53–23:39; (6) the promise of the King to return in power and glory, 24:1–25:46.

II. The sacrifice and resurrection of Jesus Christ, the Son of Abraham, 26:1–28:8.

III. The risen Lord in ministry to His own, 28:9-20.

The events recorded in Matthew cover a period of 38 years (Ussher).

CHAPTER 1.

The book of the generation of Jesus
Christ, the son of David, the son of
Abraham.
2 Abraham begat Isaac; and Isaac
begat Jacob; and Jacob begat [a]Judas and
his brethren;
3 And Judas begat [b]Phares and Zara of
Thamar; and Phares begat Esrom; and
Esrom begat Aram;
4 And Aram begat Aminadab; and
Aminadab begat Naasson; and Naasson
begat Salmon;
5 And Salmon begat [c]Booz of Rachab;
and Booz begat Obed of Ruth; and Obed
begat Jesse;
6 And Jesse begat David the king; and

a *Judah*, Gen. 29:35.
b *Pharez*, Gen. 38:24-30.
c *Boaz*, 1 Chr. 2:11.
d *Uriah*, 2 Sam. 11:3.
e *Rehoboam*, 1 Ki. 11:43.
f *Abijah*, 2 Chr. 11:20.
g *Jehoshaphat*, 1 Chr. 3:10.
h *Uzziah*, 2 Ki. 15:13. Called also *Azariah*, 2 Chr. 22:6.
i *Ahaz*, 2 Ki. 15:38.
j *Josiah*, 1 Ki. 13:2.

David the king begat Solomon of her
that had been the wife of [d]Urias;
7 And Solomon begat [e]Roboam; and
Roboam begat [f]Abia; and Abia begat
Asa;
8 And Asa begat [g]Josaphat; and
Josaphat begat Joram; and Joram begat
[h]Ozias;
9 And Ozias begat Joatham; and
Joatham begat [i]Achaz; and Achaz begat
Ezekias;
10 And Ezekias begat Manasses; and
Manasses begat Amon; and Amon begat
[j]Josias;
11 And Josias begat Jechonias and his
brethren, about the time they were carried away to Babylon:
12 And after they were brought to

Babylon, Jechonias begat Salathiel; and
Salathiel begat [a]Zorobabel;
13 And Zorobabel begat Abiud; and
Abiud begat Eliakim; and Eliakim begat
Azor;
14 And Azor begat Sadoc; and Sadoc
begat Achim; and Achim begat Eliud;
15 And Eliud begat Eleazar; and
Eleazar begat Matthan; and Matthan
begat Jacob;
16 And Jacob begat Joseph the husband of [1]Mary, [2]of whom was born
Jesus, who is called [3]Christ.
17 So all the generations from Abraham
to David *are* fourteen generations; and
from David until the carrying away into
Babylon *are* fourteen generations; and
from the carrying away into Babylon
unto Christ *are* fourteen generations.

Conception and birth of Jesus
(Lk. 1:26-35; 2:1-7; John 1:1, 2, 14).

18 [b]Now the birth of Jesus Christ was
on this wise: When as his mother Mary
was espoused to Joseph, before they
came together, she was found with child
of the [c]Holy Ghost.
19 Then Joseph her husband, being a
just *man*, and not willing to make her a
publick example, was minded to put her
away privily.

a *Zerubbabel*, 1 Chr. 3:19; Ezra 2:2.
b *Christ (First Advent).* Mt. 2:1-6. (Gen. 3:15; Acts 1:9.)
c *Holy Spirit.* (N.T.). vs. 18-20; Mt. 3:11-16. (Mt. 1:18; Acts 2:4.)
d Gr. *an angel.*
e Rom. 1:16, *note.*
f Rom. 3:23, *note.*
g Isa. 7:14. Lit. *by the Lord through the prophet.*
h Lit. *the virgin.*
i Heb. 1:4, *note.*
j The Gr. form of the Heb. *Jehoshua*, meaning Saviour.
k Lk. 2:4-7.

20 But while he thought on these
things, behold, [d]the angel of the Lord
appeared unto him in a dream, saying,
Joseph, thou son of David, fear not to
take unto thee Mary thy wife: for that
which is conceived in her is of the Holy
Ghost.
21 And she shall bring forth a son, and
thou shalt call his name JESUS: for he
shall [e]save his people from their [f]sins.
22 Now all this was done, that it might
be fulfilled which was spoken [g]of the
Lord by the prophet, saying,
23 Behold, [h]a virgin shall be with
child, and shall bring forth a son, and
they shall call his name Emmanuel,
which being interpreted is, God with us.
24 Then Joseph being raised from
sleep did as the [i]angel of the Lord had
bidden him, and took unto him his wife:
25 And knew her not till she had
brought forth her firstborn son: and he
called his name [j]JESUS.

CHAPTER 2

Visit of the Magi.

NOW when Jesus was [k]born in
Bethlehem of Judaea in the
days of [4]Herod the king, behold, there

[1] **(1:16)** Six Marys are to be distinguished in the N.T.: (1) Mary the mother of Jesus; always clearly identified by the context. (2) Mary Magdalene, a woman of Magdala, "out of whom went seven demons" (Lk. 8:2). She is never mentioned apart from the identifying word "Magdalene." (3) The mother of James (called "the less," Mk. 15:40) and Joses, the apostles. A comparison of John 19:25, Mt. 27:56, and Mk. 15:40 establishes the inference that this Mary, the mother of James the less, and of Joses, was the wife of Alphaeus (called also Cleophas, John 19:25), and a sister of Mary the mother of Jesus. Except in Mt. 27:61, and 28:1, where she is called "the other Mary" (i.e. "other" than her sister, Mary the Virgin); and John 19:25, where she is called "of Cleophas," she is mentioned only in connection with one or both of her sons. (4) Mary of Bethany, sister of Martha and Lazarus, mentioned by name only in Lk. 10:39, 42; John 11:1, 2, 19, 20, 28, 31, 32, 45; 12:3, but referred to in Mt. 26:7; Mk. 14:3-9. (5) The mother of John Mark and sister of Barnabas (Acts 12:12). (6) A helper of Paul in Rome (Rom. 16:6).

[2] **(1:16)** The changed expression here is important. It is no longer, "who begat," but, "Mary, of whom was born Jesus." Jesus was not "begotten" of natural generation.

[3] **(1:16)** Christ (*Christos* = anointed), the Greek form of the Hebrew "Messiah" (Dan. 9:25, 26), is the official name of our Lord, as Jesus is His human name (Lk. 1:31; 2:21). The name, or title, "Christ," connects Him with the entire O.T. foreview (Zech. 12:8, *note*) of a coming Prophet (Deut. 18:15-19), Priest (Psa. 110:4), and King (2 Sam. 7:7-10). As these were typically anointed with oil (1 Ki. 19:16; Ex. 29:7; 1 Sam. 16:13), so Jesus was anointed with the Holy Spirit (Mt. 3:16; Mk. 1:10, 11; Lk. 3:21, 22; John 1:32, 33), thus becoming officially "the Christ."

[4] **(2:1)** Called Herod the Great, son of Antipater, an Idumean (see Gen. 36:1, *note*), and Cypros, an Arabian woman. Antipater was appointed Procurator of Judaea by Julius Caesar, B.C. 47. At the age of fifteen Herod was appointed to the government of Galilee. B.C. 40 the Roman senate made him king of Judaea. An able, strong, and cruel man, he increased greatly the splendour of Jerusalem, erecting the temple which was the centre of Jewish worship in the time of our Lord.

came wise men from the east to Jerusalem,

2 Saying, Where is he that is born [1a]King of the Jews? for we have seen his star in the east, and are come to worship him.

3 When Herod the king had heard *these things*, he was troubled, and all Jerusalem with him.

4 And when he had gathered all the chief priests and [2]scribes of the people together, he demanded of them where [b]Christ should be born.

5 And they said unto him, In Bethlehem of Judaea: [c]for thus it is written by the prophet,

6 And thou Bethlehem, *in* the land of Juda, art not the least among the princes of Juda: for out of thee shall come a Governor, that shall [d]rule my people Israel.

7 Then Herod, when he had privily called the wise men, enquired of them diligently what time the [e]star appeared.

8 And he sent them to Bethlehem, and said, Go and search diligently for the young child; and when ye have found *him*, bring me word again, that I may come and worship him also.

9 When they had heard the king, they departed; and, lo, the star, which they saw in the east, went before them, till it came and stood over where the young child was.

10 When they saw the star, they rejoiced with exceeding great joy.

11 And when they were come into the house, they saw the young child with Mary his mother, and fell down, and worshipped him: and when they had opened their treasures, they presented unto him gifts; gold, and frankincense, and myrrh.

12 And being warned of God in a dream that they should not return to Herod, they departed into their own country another way.

The flight into Egypt.

13 And when they were departed, behold, [f]the angel of the Lord appeareth to Joseph in a dream, saying, Arise, and take the young child and his mother, and flee into Egypt, and be thou there until I bring thee word: for Herod will seek the young child to destroy him.

14 When he arose, he took the young child and his mother by night, and departed into Egypt:

15 And was there until the death of Herod: that it might be fulfilled which was spoken [g]of the Lord by the prophet, saying, [3]Out of [h]Egypt have I called my son.

Herod's slaughter of the innocents.

16 Then Herod, when he saw that he was mocked of the wise men, was exceeding wroth, and sent forth, and slew all the children that were in Bethlehem, and in all the coasts thereof, from two years old and under, according to the time which he had diligently enquired of the wise men.

17 Then was fulfilled that which

B.C. 4.

a *Kingdom* (N.T.). Mt. 2:6. (Lk. 1:31-33; 1 Cor. 15:24.)

b Lit. *the Christ.*

c *Christ (First Advent).* Mt. 4:15, 16. (Gen. 3:15; Acts 1:9.)

d *Kingdom* (N.T.). Mt. 3:2. (Lk. 1:31-33; 1 Cor. 15:28.)

e Num. 24:17.

f Lit. *an angel.*

g Isa. 7:14. Lit. *by the Lord through the prophet.*

h Hos. 11:1.

[1] **(2:2)** "The King" is one of the divine titles (Psa. 10:16), and so used in the *worship* of the Church (1 Tim. 1:17), but Christ is never called "King of the Church." He is "King of the Jews" (Mt. 2:2) and Lord and "Head of the Church" (Eph. 1:22, 23). See "Church" (Mt. 16:18; Heb. 12:23).

[2] **(2:4)** Gr. *grammateis*, "writer." Heb. *sopherim*, "to write," "set in order," "count." The scribes were so called because it was their office to make copies of the Scriptures; to classify and teach the precepts of the oral law (see "Pharisees," Mt. 3:7, *note*), and to keep careful count of every letter in the O.T. writings. Such an office was necessary in a religion of law and precept, and was an O.T. function (2 Sam. 8:17; 20:25; 1 Ki. 4:3; Jer. 8:8; 36:10, 12, 26). To this legitimate work the scribes added a record of rabbinical decisions on questions of ritual (Halachoth); the new code resulting from those decisions (Mishna); the Hebrew sacred legends (Gemara, forming with the Mishna the Talmud); commentaries on the O.T. (Midrashim); reasonings upon these (Hagada); and, finally, mystical interpretations which found in Scripture meanings other than the grammatical, lexical, and obvious ones (the Kabbala); not unlike the allegorical method of Origen, or the modern Protestant "spiritualizing" interpretation. In our Lord's time, to receive this mass of writing superposed upon the Scriptures was to be orthodox; to return to the Scriptures themselves was heterodoxy—our Lord's most serious offence.

[3] **(2:15)** The words quoted are in Hos. 11:1, and the passage illustrates the truth that prophetic utterances often have a latent and deeper meaning than at first appears. Israel, nationally, was a "son" (Ex. 4:22), but Christ was the greater "Son." See Rom. 9:4, 5; Isa. 41:8, with Isa. 42:1-4; 52:13, 14, where the servant-nation and the Servant-Son are both in view.

was spoken by Jeremy the prophet,
saying,
18 [a]In Rama was there a voice heard,
lamentation, and weeping, and great
mourning, Rachel weeping *for* her children, and would not be comforted,
because they are not.

The return from Egypt to Nazareth.
(Cf. Lk. 2:39, 40.)

19 But when Herod was dead, behold,
an [b]angel of the Lord appeareth in a
dream to Joseph in Egypt,
20 Saying, Arise, and take the young
child and his mother, and go into the
land of Israel: for they are dead which
sought the young child's life.
21 And he arose, and took the young
child and his mother, and came into the
land of Israel.
22 But when he heard that [c]Archelaus
did reign in Judaea in the room of his
father Herod, he was afraid to go thither:
notwithstanding, being warned of God
in a dream, he turned aside into the
parts of Galilee:
23 And he came and dwelt in a city
called Nazareth: that it might be fulfilled
which was spoken by the prophets, [d]He
shall be called a Nazarene.

CHAPTER 3

Ministry of John the Baptist (Mk. 1:3-8;
Lk. 3:2-17; John 1:6-8, 19-28).

In those days came John the Baptist,
preaching in the wilderness of Judaea,
2 And [e]saying, [f]Repent ye: for [g]the
[1]kingdom of heaven is [h]at hand.
3 For this is he that was spoken of by
the prophet Esaias, saying, The voice of
one crying in the wilderness, Prepare ye
the way of the [i]Lord, make his paths
straight.
4 And the same John had his raiment
of camel's hair, and a leathern girdle
about his loins; and his meat was locusts
and wild honey.
5 Then went out to him Jerusalem, and
all Judaea, and all the region round
about Jordan,
6 And were baptized of him in Jordan,
confessing their [j]sins.
7 But when he saw many of the
[2]Pharisees and [3]Sadducees come to his

B.C. 3.

a Jer. 31:15.

b Heb. 1:4, *note.*

c Son of Herod the Great (Mt. 2:1) and Malthace, a Samaritan woman. Deposed A.D. 6.

d Probably referring to Isa. 11:1, where Christ is spoken of as *"a netzer* (or, *'rod')* *out of the stem of Jesse."*

e See Acts 17:30, *note.*

f *Repentance.* vs. 2, 8, 11; Mt. 4:17. (Mt. 3:2; Acts 17:30.)

g *Kingdom* (N.T.). Mt. 4:17. (Lk. 1:31-33; 1 Cor. 15:24.)

h *Gospel.* vs. 1, 2; Mt. 4:23. (Gen. 12:1-3; Rev. 14:6.)

i *Jehovah.* Isa. 40:3.

j *Sin.* Rom. 3:23, *note.*

[1](3:2) (1) The phrase, kingdom of heaven (lit. of the heavens), is peculiar to Matthew and signifies the Messianic earth rule of Jesus Christ, the Son of David. It is called the kingdom of the heavens because it is the rule of the heavens over the earth (Mt. 6:10). The phrase is derived from Daniel, where it is defined (Dan. 2:34-36, 44; 7:23-27) as the kingdom which "the God of heaven" will set up after the destruction by "the stone cut out without hands" of the Gentile world-system. It is the kingdom covenanted to David's seed (2 Sam. 7:7-10, *refs.*); described in the prophets (Zech. 12:8, *note*); and confirmed to Jesus the Christ, the Son of Mary, through the angel Gabriel (Lk. 1:32, 33).

(2) The kingdom of heaven has three aspects in Matthew: *(a)* "at hand" from the beginning of the ministry of John the Baptist (Mt. 3:2) to the virtual rejection of the King, and the announcement of the new brotherhood (Mt. 12:46-50); *(b)* in seven "mysteries of the kingdom of heaven," to be fulfilled during the present age (Mt. 13:1-52), to which are to be added the parables of the kingdom of heaven which were spoken after those of Mt. 13, and which have to do with the sphere of Christian profession during this age, *(c)* the prophetic aspect—the kingdom to be set up after the return of the King in glory (Mt. 24:29–25:46; Lk. 19:12-19; Acts 15:14-17). See "Kingdom (N.T.)" (Lk. 1:33; 1 Cor. 15:28). Cf. "Kingdom of God," Mt. 6:33, *note.*

[2](3:7) So called from a Heb. word meaning "separate." After the ministry of the post-exilic prophets ceased, godly men called "Chasidim" (saints) arose who sought to keep alive reverence for the law amongst the descendants of the Jews who returned from the Babylonian captivity. This movement degenerated into the Pharisaism of our Lord's day—a letter-strictness which overlaid the law with traditional interpretations held to have been communicated by Jehovah to Moses as oral explanations of equal authority with the law itself (cf. Mt. 15:2, 3; Mk. 7:8-13; Gal. 1:14).

The Pharisees were strictly a sect. A member was "chaber" (i.e. "knit together," Jud. 20:11), and took an obligation to remain true to the principles of Pharisaism. They were correct, moral, zealous, and self-denying, but self-righteous (Lk. 18:9), and destitute of the sense of sin and need (Lk. 7:39). They were the foremost persecutors of Jesus Christ and the objects of His unsparing denunciation (e.g. Mt. 23:13-29; Lk. 11:42, 43).

[3](3:7) Not strictly a sect, but rather those amongst the Jews who denied the existence of angels or other spirits, and all miracles, especially the resurrection. They were the religious rationalists of the

baptism, he said unto them, O [a]genera-
tion of vipers, who hath warned you to
flee from the wrath to come?
8 Bring forth therefore fruits meet for
[b]repentance:
9 And think not to say within yourselves, We have Abraham to *our* father:
for I say unto you, that God is able of
these stones to raise up children unto
Abraham.
10 And now also the axe is laid unto
the root of the trees: therefore every tree
which bringeth not forth good fruit is
hewn down, and cast into the fire.
11 I indeed baptize you with water
unto repentance: but he that cometh
after me is mightier than I, whose shoes
I am not worthy to bear: he shall baptize
you with the [c]Holy Ghost, and *with* fire:
12 Whose fan *is* in his hand, and he
will throughly purge his floor, and gather his wheat into the garner; but he will
burn up the chaff with unquenchable
fire.

Baptism of Jesus (Mk. 1:9-11;
Lk. 3:21, 22; cf. John 1:31-34).

13 Then cometh Jesus from Galilee to
Jordan unto John, to be baptized of him.
14 But John [d]forbad him, saying, I
have need to be baptized of thee, and
comest thou to me?

A.D. 27.

a Lit. *progeny.*
b *Repentance.* vs. 2, 8, 11; Mt. 4:17. (Mt. 3:2; Acts 17:30.)
c *Holy Spirit.* vs. 11, 16; Mt. 4:1. (Mt. 1:18; Acts 2:4.)
d *would have hindered.*
e 1 John 3:7, *note.*
f Lit. *This is my Son—the Beloved.* Mt. 17:5; Mk. 9:7; Lk. 9:35. Cf. Isa. 42:1; Eph. 1:3-6.
g *Holy Spirit.* Mt. 10:20. (Mt. 1:18; Acts 2:4.)
h *Temptation.* vs. 1, 3, 7; Mt. 6:13. (Gen. 3:1; Jas. 1:14.)
i *Satan.* Gr. *diabolos,* accuser. vs. 1, 5, 8, 10, 11; Mt. 12:26. (Gen. 3:1; Rev. 20:10.)
j Deut. 8:3.
k *Inspiration.* vs. 4, 7, 10; Mt. 5:18. (Ex. 4:15; Rev. 22:19.)
l *Jehovah.* Deut. 8:3.

15 And Jesus answering said unto
him, [1]Suffer *it to be so* now: for thus it
becometh us to fulfil all [e]righteousness.
Then he suffered him.
16 And [2]Jesus, when he was baptized,
went up straightway out of the water:
and, lo, the heavens were opened unto
him, and he saw the Spirit of God
descending like a dove, and lighting
upon him:
17 And lo a voice from heaven, saying,
[f]This is my beloved Son, in whom I am
well pleased.

CHAPTER 4.

The temptation of Jesus
(Mk. 1:12, 13; Lk. 4:1-13; cf. Gen. 3:6).

[3]Then was Jesus led up of the [g]spirit
into the wilderness to be [h]tempted
of the [i]devil.
2 And when he had fasted forty days
and forty nights, he was afterward an
hungred.
3 And when the tempter came to him,
he said, If thou be the Son of God, command that these stones be made bread.
4 But he answered and said, It is written, [j]Man shall not live by bread alone,
but by [k]every word that proceedeth out
of the mouth of [l]God.

time (Mk. 12:18-23; Acts 5:15-17; 23:8), and strongly entrenched in the Sanhedrin and priesthood (Acts 4:1; 5:17). They are identified with no affirmative doctrine, but were mere deniers of the supernatural.

[1] **(3:15)** Why one who needed no repentance should insist upon receiving a rite which signified confession (v. 6) and repentance (v. 11) is nowhere directly explained. It may be suggested: (1) That Jesus was now to receive His anointing with the Holy Spirit (v. 16) unto His threefold office of Prophet, Priest, and King. In the Levitical order (Ex. 29:4-7) the high priest was first washed, then anointed. While Christ's priestly work did not begin till He "offered Himself without spot to God" (Heb. 9:14), and His full manifestation as the King-Priest after the order of Melchisedek awaits the kingdom (Gen. 14:18, *note*), yet He was then *anointed,* once for all. (2) But John's baptism was the voice of God to Israel, and the believing remnant responded (v. 5). It was an act of righteousness on the part of Him who had become, as to the flesh, an Israelite, to take His place with this believing remnant.

[2] **(3:16)** For the first time the Trinity, foreshadowed in many ways in the O.T., is fully manifested. The Spirit descends upon the Son, and at the same moment the Father's voice is heard from heaven.

[3] **(4:1)** The temptation of Christ, the "last Adam" (1 Cor. 15:45), is best understood when contrasted with that of "the first man Adam." Adam was tempted in his place of lord of creation, a lordship with but one reservation, the knowledge of good and evil (Gen. 1:26; 2:16, 17). Through the woman he was tempted to add that also to his dominion. Falling, he lost all. But Christ had taken the place of a lowly Servant, acting only from and in obedience to the Father (Phil. 2:5-8; John 5:19; 6:57; 8:28, 54. Cf. Isa. 41:8, *note*), that He might redeem a fallen race and a creation under the curse (Gen. 3:17-19; Rom. 8:19-23). Satan's one object in the threefold temptation was to induce Christ to act from Himself, in independency of His Father. The first two temptations were a challenge to Christ from the god of this

5 Then the devil taketh him up into
the [1a]holy city, and setteth him on a pinnacle of the temple,
6 And saith unto him, If thou be the
Son of God, cast thyself down: for it is
written, He shall give his [b]angels charge
concerning thee: [c]and in *their* hands they
shall bear thee up, lest at any time thou
dash thy foot against a stone.
7 Jesus said unto him, It is written
again, Thou shalt not tempt the [d]Lord
thy God.
8 Again, the devil taketh him up into
an exceeding high mountain, and
sheweth him all the kingdoms of the
[2]world, and the glory of them;
9 And saith unto him, All these things
will I give thee, if thou wilt fall down
and worship me.
10 Then saith Jesus unto him, Get thee
hence, Satan: for it is written, Thou shalt
worship the [e]Lord thy God, and him
only shalt thou serve.
11 Then the devil leaveth him, and,
behold, [b]angels came and ministered
unto him.

Jesus comes to Capernaum, and begins his public ministry Mk. 1:14; Lk. 4:14, 15).

12 Now when Jesus had heard that
John was cast into prison, he departed
into Galilee;

A.D. 27.

a *Sanctify, holy (things)* (N.T.). Mt. 7:6. (Mt. 4:5; Rev. 22:11.)

b Heb. 1:4, *note.*

c Psa. 91:11, 12.

d *Jehovah.* Deut. 6:16.

e *Jehovah.* Deut. 6:13; 10:20.

f *Christ (First Advent).* Mt. 12:18-21. (Gen. 3:15; Acts 1:9.)

g Isa. 42:6, 7.

h Isa. 9:1, 2.

i *Repentance.* Mt. 9:13. (Mt. 3:2; Acts 17:30.)

j *Kingdom* (N.T.). Mt. 5:2, 35, and *note.*. (Lk. 1:31-33; 1 Cor. 15:24.)

k Mt. 3:2, *note.*

l Peter and John were already disciples (John 1:35-42). This is a call to service.

13 And leaving Nazareth, he came and
dwelt in Capernaum, which is upon the
sea coast, in the borders of Zabulon and
Nephthalim:
14 That it might be fulfilled which was
spoken by Esaias the prophet, saying,
15 The land of Zabulon, and the land
of Nephthalim, *by* the way of the sea,
beyond Jordan, Galilee of the [f]Gentiles;
16 The people which sat in darkness
saw great [g]light; [h]and to them which sat
in the region and shadow of death light
is sprung up.
17 From that time Jesus began to
preach, and to say, [i]Repent: for the
[j]kingdom of heaven [k]is [3]at hand.

The call of Peter and Andrew to service (Mk.1:16-20; cf. Lk. 5:2-11.

18 And Jesus, walking by the sea of
Galilee, saw [l]two brethren, Simon called
Peter, and Andrew his brother, casting a
net into the sea: for they were fishers.
19 And he saith unto them, Follow me,
and I will make you fishers of men.
20 And they straightway left *their* nets,
and followed him.

The call of James and John, sons of Zebedee.

21 And going on from thence, he saw

world to prove Himself indeed the Son of God (vs. 3, 6). The third was the offer of the usurping prince of this world to divest himself of that which rightfully belonged to Christ as Son of man and Son of David, on the condition that He accept the sceptre on Satan's world-principles (cf. John 18:36; Rev. 13:8, *note*). Christ defeated Satan by a means open to His humblest follower, the intelligent use of the word of God (vs. 4, 7). In his second temptation Satan also used Scripture, but a promise available only to one in the path of obedience. The scene gives emphasis to the vital importance of "rightly dividing the word of truth" (2 Tim. 2:15).

[1] **(4:5)** In the N.T. one Greek word, *hagios,* in its various forms, is rendered, "holy," "holiness," "sanctify," "sanctified," "sanctification." Like the Heb. *qodesh,* it signifies "set apart for God." The important references follow Mt. 4:5, *marg.*

[2] **(4:8)** The Greek word *kosmos* means "order," "arrangement," and so, with the Greeks, "beauty"; for order and arrangement in the sense of *system* are at the bottom of the Greek conception of beauty.

When used in the N.T. of humanity, the "world" of men, it is *organized* humanity—humanity in families, tribes, nations—which is meant. The word for chaotic, unorganized humanity—the mere mass of men—is *thalassa,* the "sea" of men (e.g. Rev. 13:1). For "world" (*kosmos*) in the bad ethical sense, see John 7:7, *refs.*

[3] **(4:17)** "At hand" is never a positive affirmation that the person or thing said to be "at hand" will immediately appear, but only that no known or predicted event must intervene. When Christ appeared to the Jewish people, the next thing, in the order of revelation as it then stood, should have been the setting up of the Davidic kingdom. In the knowledge of God, not yet disclosed, lay the rejection of the kingdom (and King), the long period of the mystery-form of the kingdom, the world-wide preaching of the cross, and the out-calling of the Church. But this was as yet locked up in the secret counsels of God (Mt. 13:11, 17; Eph. 3:3-10).

other two brethren, [1]James *the son* of
Zebedee, and John his brother, in a [a]ship
with Zebedee their father, mending their
nets; and he called them.
22 And they immediately left the ship
and their father, and followed him.
23 And Jesus went about all Galilee,
teaching in their synagogues, and
preaching the [b]gospel of the [c]kingdom,
and healing all manner of sickness and
all manner of disease among the people.
24 And his fame went throughout all
Syria: and they [d]brought unto him all
sick people that were taken with divers
diseases and torments, and those which
were [e]possessed with devils, and those
which were lunatick, and those that had
the palsy; and he healed them.
25 And there followed him great [f]multitudes of people from Galilee, and *from*
Decapolis, and *from* Jerusalem, and *from*
Judaea, and *from* beyond Jordan.

CHAPTER 5

The sermon on the mount.
(Cf. Lk. 6:20-49.)

The beatitudes. (Cf. Lk. 6:20-23.)

And seeing the multitudes, he [g]went
up into a mountain: and when he
was set, his disciples came unto him:
2 [2]And he opened his mouth, and
taught them, [h]saying,
3 [i]Blessed *are* the poor in spirit: for
theirs is the kingdom of heaven.
4 Blessed *are* they that mourn: for they
shall be comforted.
5 Blessed *are* the meek: for they shall
inherit the earth.
6 Blessed *are* they which do [j]hunger
and thirst after righteousness: for they
shall be filled.
7 Blessed *are* the merciful: for they
shall obtain mercy.
8 Blessed *are* the pure in heart: for they
shall see God.
9 Blessed *are* the peacemakers: for they
shall be called the children of God.
10 Blessed *are* they which are persecuted for righteousness' sake: for theirs is
the [k]kingdom of heaven.
11 Blessed are ye, when *men* shall
revile you, and persecute *you*, and shall
say all manner of evil against you falsely, for my sake.
12 Rejoice, and be exceeding glad: for
great *is* your [l]reward in heaven: for so
persecuted they the prophets which
were before you.

Similitudes of the believer.
(Cf. Mk. 4:21-23; Lk. 8:16-18.)

13 Ye are the [m]salt of the earth: but if
the salt have lost his savour, wherewith
shall it be salted? it is thenceforth good
for nothing, but to be cast out, and to be
trodden under foot of men.
14 Ye are the light of the [n]world. A city
that is set on an hill cannot be hid.
15 Neither do men light a candle, and
put it under a bushel, but on a

A.D. 31.

a *boat.*

b *Gospel.* Mt. 9:35. (Gen. 12:1-3; Rev. 14:6.)

c Mt. 3:2, *note.*

d Mk. 1:32, 33; Lk. 4:40.

e Gr. *daimonizomai, demonized;* Mt. 7:22, *note.*

f Mt. 5:1; Mk. 3:7, 8; Mt. 8:1, 18.

g Cf. Mt. 17:1; 8:1; 14:23.

h The beatific character, unattainable by effort, is wrought in the believer by the Spirit (Gal. 5:22, 23).

i Psa. 1:1; 32:1; 119:1.

j Isa. 55:1; Lk. 1:53; 15:17.

k Mt. 3:2, *note.*

l *Rewards.* Mt. 6:1-4. (Dan. 12:3; 1 Cor. 3:14.)

m *Parables* (N.T.). vs. 13-16; Mt. 7:24-27. (Mt. 5:13-16; Lk. 21:29-31.)

n *kosmos* (Mt. 4:8), = mankind.

[1] **(4:21)** Two persons are called by this name in the N.T.: (1) James the son of Zebedee, an apostle (Mt. 10:2), and the brother of the Apostle John, apart from whom he is never mentioned, and with whom, together with Peter, he was admitted to the especial intimacy of our Lord (Mt. 17:1; Mk. 5:37; 9:2; 14:33). He was martyred by Herod (Acts 12:2). (2) A son of Alphaeus (or Cleopas) and of Mary the sister of Mary the mother of Jesus (see Mt. 1:16, *note*), and brother of Joses (Mk. 15:40). He was, therefore, a cousin of the Lord Jesus. He is called James "the less" (Mk. 15:40; lit. *little,* i.e. of shorter stature than James the son of Zebedee). He was an apostle (Mt. 10:3). It has been conjectured that "Lebbaeus, whose surname was Thaddaeus" (Mt. 10:3) was identical with the Judas of Lk. 6:16, who is there called "of [i.e. 'son' or 'brother' as it has been variously translated] James." A Juda is mentioned with a James and Joses and Simon in Mk. 6:3 as "brother" of our Lord (see Mt. 13:55, *marg.*). The Gospels mention no other James who could be called the brother of the Lord Jesus, but James the less was certainly the son of Alphaeus and Mary the sister of our Lord's mother. The conclusion seems, therefore, most probable that Mt. 10:3; 13:55; Mk. 3:18; 6:3; Lk. 6:15; Acts 1:13; 12:17; 15:13; 21:18; Gal. 1:19; 2:9, 12; and Jas. 1:1 refer to James the less, son of Alphaeus and Mary, and cousin, or, according to Jewish usage, "brother" of the Lord Jesus. He was the author of the Epistle of James.

[2] **(5:2)** Having announced the kingdom of heaven as "at hand," the King, in Mt 5–7, declares the *principles* of the kingdom. The Sermon on the Mount has a twofold application: (1) Literally to the kingdom.

candlestick; and it giveth light unto all that are in the house.

16 Let your light so shine before men, that they may see your good works, and glorify your Father which is in heaven.

Relation of Christ to the law.

17 Think not that I am come to destroy the law, or the prophets: [1]I am not come to destroy, but to fulfil.

18 For verily I say unto you, Till heaven and earth pass, [a]one jot or one tittle shall in no wise pass from [b]the law, till all be fulfilled.

19 Whosoever therefore shall break one of these least commandments, and shall teach men so, he shall be called the least in the kingdom of heaven: but whosoever shall do and teach *them*, the same shall be called great in the kingdom of heaven.

A.D. 31.

a *Inspiration.* vs. 17, 18; Mt. 10:14. (Ex. 4:15; Rev. 22:19.)

b *Law of Moses.* Mt. 22:36-39. (Ex. 19:1; Gal. 3:1-29.)

c Cf. Lk. 18:11, 12; Rom. 3:20; Phil. 3:5-7.

d *Righteousness.* vs. 6. 10, 20; Rom. 10:10, *note.*

e Ex. 20:13.

20 For I say unto you, That except your righteousness shall [c]exceed *the* [d]*righteousness* of the scribes and Pharisees, ye shall in no case enter into the kingdom of heaven.

21 Ye have heard that it was said by them of old time, [e]Thou shalt not kill; and whosoever shall kill shall be in danger of the judgment:

22 But I say unto you, That whosoever is angry with his brother without a cause shall be in danger of the judgment: and whosoever shall say to his brother, Raca, shall be in danger of the council: but whosoever shall say, Thou fool, shall be in danger of [2]hell fire.

23 Therefore if thou bring thy gift to the altar, and there rememberest that thy brother hath ought against thee;

24 Leave there thy gift before the altar, and go thy way; first be reconciled to

In this sense it gives the divine constitution for the righteous government of the earth. Whenever the kingdom of heaven is established on earth it will be according to that constitution, which may be regarded as an explanation of the word "righteousness" as used by the prophets in describing the kingdom (e.g. Isa. 11:4, 5; 32:1; Dan. 9:24). In this sense the Sermon on the Mount is pure law, and transfers the offence from the overt act to the motive (Mt. 5:21, 22, 27, 28). Here lies the deeper reason why the Jews rejected the kingdom. They had reduced "righteousness" to mere ceremonialism, and the Old Testament idea of the kingdom to a mere affair of outward splendour and power. They were never rebuked for expecting a visible and powerful kingdom, but the words of the prophets should have prepared them to expect also that only the poor in spirit and the meek could share in it (e.g. Isa. 11:4). The seventy-second Psalm, which was universally received by them as a description of the kingdom, was full of this. For these reasons the Sermon on the Mount in its primary application gives neither the privilege nor the duty of the Church. These are found in the Epistles. Under the law of the kingdom, for example, no one may hope for forgiveness who has not first forgiven (Mt. 6:12, 14, 15). Under grace the Christian is exhorted to forgive because he is already forgiven (Eph. 4:30-32).

(2) But there is a beautiful moral application to the Christian. It always remains true that the poor in spirit, rather than the proud, are blessed, and those who mourn because of their sins, and who are meek in the consciousness of them, will hunger and thirst after righteousness, and hungering will be filled. The merciful *are* "blessed," the pure in heart do "see God." These principles fundamentally reappear in the teaching of the Epistles.

[1] **(5:17)** Christ's relation to the law of Moses may be thus summarized: (1) He was made under the law (Gal. 4:4); (2) He lived in perfect obedience to the law (John 8:46; Mt. 17:5; 1 Pet. 2:21-23); (3) He was a minister of the law to the Jews, clearing it from rabbinical sophistries, enforcing it in all its pitiless severity upon those who professed to obey it (e.g. Lk. 10:25-37), but confirming the promises made to the fathers under the Mosaic Covenant (Rom. 15:8); (4) He fulfilled the types of the law by His holy life and sacrificial death (Heb. 9:11-26); (5) He bore, vicariously, the curse of the law that the Abrahamic Covenant might avail all who believe (Gal. 3:13, 14); (6) He brought out by His redemption all who believe from the place of servants under the law into the place of sons (Gal. 4:1-7); (7) He mediated by His blood the New Covenant of assurance and grace in which all believers stand (Rom. 5:2; Heb. 8:6-13), so establishing the "law of Christ" (Gal. 6:2; *refs.*) with its precepts of higher exaltation made possible by the indwelling Spirit.

[2] **(5:22)** Gr. *Geenna* = Gehenna, the place in the valley of Hinnom where, anciently, human sacrifices were offered (2 Chr. 33:6; Jer. 7:31). The word occurs, Mt. 5:22, 29, 30; 10:28; 18:9; 23:15, 33; Mk. 9:43, 45, 47; Lk. 12:5; Jas. 3:6. In every instance except the last the word comes from the lips of Jesus Christ in

thy brother, and then come and offer thy
gift.
25 Agree with thine [a]adversary quickly,
whiles thou art in the way with him; lest
at any time the adversary deliver thee to
the judge, and the judge deliver thee to
the officer, and thou be cast into prison.
26 Verily I say unto thee, Thou shalt
by no means come out thence, till thou
hast [b]paid the uttermost [c]farthing.
27 Ye have heard that it was said by
them of old time, [d]Thou shalt not commit adultery:
28 But I say unto you, That whosoever
[e]looketh on a woman to lust after her
hath committed adultery with her
already in his heart.
29 And if thy right eye [f]offend thee,
pluck it out, and cast *it* from thee: for it
is profitable for thee that one of thy
members should perish, and not *that* thy
whole body should be cast into hell.
30 And if thy right hand [f]offend thee,
cut it off, and cast *it* from thee: for it is
profitable for thee that one of thy members should perish, and not *that* thy
whole body should be cast into hell.

Jesus and divorce. (Cf. Mt. 19:3-11;
Mk. 10:2-12; 1 Cor. 7:1-15.)

31 It hath been said, Whosoever shall
put away his wife, let him give her a
[g]writing of divorcement:
32 But I say unto you, That whosoever
shall put away his wife, saving for the
cause of fornication, [h]causeth her to commit adultery: and whosoever shall marry
her that is divorced committeth adultery.
33 Again, ye have heard that it hath
been said by them of old time, [i]Thou
shalt not forswear thyself, but shalt perform unto the [j]Lord thine oaths:
34 But I say unto you, [k]Swear not at all;
neither by heaven; for it is God's throne:
35 Nor by the earth; for it is his footstool: neither by Jerusalem; for it is the
city [l]of the [m]great King.
36 Neither shalt thou swear by thy

A.D. 31.

a Lk. 12:58, 59. Cf. Prov. 25:8-9; Lam. 2:4, 5.
b Cf. Isa. 40:2 with Ruth 1:21, 22.
c One fourth of a cent.
d Ex. 20:14.
e Job 31:1; 2 Sam. 11:2-5; Jas. 1:14, 15; Mt. 15:19.
f Lit. *is causing thee to offend.*
g Gen. 2:23, 24; Deut. 24:1; Jer. 3:1.
h Mt. 19:3-9; Mk. 10:2-12; Lk. 16:18; 1 Cor. 7:10, 11; 8:12.
i Lev. 19:12.
j *Jehovah.* Deut. 23:23.
k Cf. Mt. 26:63; 2 Cor. 2:17; 1 Thes. 2:5.
l *Kingdom* (N.T.). Mt. 6:10. (Lk. 1:31-33; 1 Cor. 15:24.)
m Psa. 48:2.
n Or, *the evil one.*
o Ex. 21:24; Lev. 24:20; Deut. 19:21.
p Deut. 15:7-11; Lk. 6:30:34; 1 Tim. 6:18.
q Lev. 19:18; Deut. 23:3-6.
r *pray for.*
s Acts 14:17; Psa. 65:9-13; Lk. 12:16, 17.
t *tax-gatherers.*
u Or, *righteous acts.* The word refers to religious externalities. These may be seen of men, but that must not be the motive.
v *Rewards.* vs. 1-4; Mt. 10:41, 42. (Dan. 12:3; 1 Cor. 3:14.)

head, because thou canst not make one
hair white or black.
37 But let your communication be,
Yea, yea; Nay, nay: for whatsoever is
more than these cometh of [n]evil.
38 Ye have heard that it hath been
said, An [o]eye for an eye, and a tooth for
a tooth:
39 But I say unto you, That ye resist not
evil: but whosoever shall smite thee on
thy right cheek, turn to him the other also.
40 And if any man will sue thee at the
law, and take away thy coat, let him
have *thy* cloke also.
41 And whosoever shall compel thee
to go a mile, go with him twain.
42 [p]Give to him that asketh thee, and
from him that would borrow of thee
turn not thou away.
43 Ye have heard that it hath been
said, [q]Thou shalt love thy neighbour,
and hate thine enemy.
44 But I say unto you, Love your enemies, [r]bless them that curse you, do
good to them that hate you, and pray for
them which despitefully use you, and
persecute you;
45 That ye may be the children of your
Father which is in heaven: for he
[s]maketh his sun to rise on the evil and
on the good, and sendeth rain on the just
and on the unjust.
46 For if ye love them which love you,
what reward have ye? do not even the
[t]publicans the same?
47 And if ye salute your brethren only,
what do ye more *than others*? do not
even the publicans so?
48 Be ye therefore [1]perfect, even as
your Father which is in heaven is perfect.

CHAPTER 6.

Sermon on the mount, continued:
mere externalism in religion condemned.

Take heed that ye do not your [u]alms
before men, to be seen of them: otherwise ye have no [v]reward of your
Father which is in heaven.

most solemn warning of the consequences of sin. He describes it as the place where "their" worm never dies and of fire never to be quenched. The expression is identical in meaning with "lake of fire" (Rev. 19:20; 20:10, 14, 15). See "Death, the second" (John 8:24; Rev. 21:8); also Lk. 16:23, *note.*

[1] **(5:48)** The word implies full development, growth into maturity of godliness, not sinless perfection. See Eph. 4:12, 13. In this passage the Father's kindness, not His sinlessness, is the point in question. Cf. Lk. 6:35, 36.

2 Therefore when thou doest *thine* alms, do not sound a trumpet before thee, as the hypocrites do in the synagogues and in the streets, that they may have glory of men. Verily I say unto you, They have their [a]reward.

3 But when thou doest alms, let not thy [b]left hand know what thy right hand doeth:

4 That thine alms may be in secret: and thy [c]Father which seeth in secret himself shall reward thee openly.

5 And when thou prayest, thou shalt not be as the hypocrites *are*: for they love to pray standing in the synagogues and in the corners of the streets, that they may be seen of men. Verily I say unto you, They have their [d]reward.

6 But thou, when thou [e]prayest, enter into thy closet, and when thou hast shut thy door, pray to thy Father which is in secret; and thy Father which seeth in secret shall reward thee openly.

7 But when ye pray, use not [f]vain repetitions, as the [g]heathen *do*: for they think that they shall be heard for their much speaking.

The new revelation concerning prayer.
(See Lk. 11:1-13, *note.*)

8 Be not ye therefore like unto them: for your Father [h]knoweth what things ye have need of, before ye ask him.

9 After this [i]manner therefore [j]pray ye: [k]Our Father which art in heaven, Hallowed be thy [l]name.

10 Thy [m]kingdom [n]come. Thy will be done in earth, as *it is* in heaven.

11 Give us this day our daily bread.

12 And [o]forgive us our [p]debts, as [1]we forgive our debtors.

13 And lead us not into [q]temptation, but deliver us from evil: For thine is the kingdom, and the power, and the glory, for ever. Amen.

14 For if ye forgive men their trespasses, your heavenly Father will also forgive you:

15 But if ye forgive not men their trespasses, neither [r]will your Father forgive your trespasses.

Externalism again rebuked.

16 Moreover when ye [s]fast, be not, as the hypocrites, of a sad countenance: for they disfigure their faces, that they may appear unto men to fast. Verily I say unto you, They have their [d]reward.

17 But thou, when thou fastest, [t]anoint thine head, and wash thy face;

18 That thou appear not unto men to fast, but unto thy Father which is in secret: and thy Father, which seeth in secret, shall reward thee openly.

The kingdom law of riches.

19 Lay not up for yourselves [u]treasures upon earth, where moth and rust doth corrupt, and where thieves break through and steal:

20 But lay up for yourselves treasures in heaven, where neither moth nor rust doth corrupt, and where thieves do not break through nor steal:

21 For where your treasure is, there will your heart be also.

22 The [v]light of the body is the eye: if therefore thine eye be single, thy whole body shall be full of light.

23 But if thine eye be evil, thy whole body shall be full of darkness. If therefore the light that is in thee be darkness, how great *is* that darkness!

24 No man can serve [w]two masters: for either he will hate the one, and love the other; or else he will hold to the one, and despise the other. Ye cannot serve God and mammon.

The cure of anxiety:
trust in the Father's care.

25 Therefore I say unto you, [x]Take no thought for your life, what ye shall eat, or what ye shall drink; nor yet for your body, what ye shall put on. Is not the life more than meat, and the body than raiment?

26 Behold the fowls of the air: for they sow not, neither do they reap, nor gather into barns; yet your heavenly Father feedeth them. Are ye not much better than they?

27 Which of you by taking thought can add one [y]cubit unto his stature?

28 And why take ye thought for raiment? Consider the lilies of the field,

A.D. 31.

a i.e. the reward they have sought.
b Mt. 8:4.
c Lk. 14:12-14; Phil. 4:17-19; 2 Tim. 1:16-18.
d i.e. the praise of men.
e Mt. 23:5-7, 14; Mk. 12:38-40; Lk. 18:10-12; 20:46, 47.
f Cf. 1 Ki. 18:26-39; Mt. 26:39-44; 2 Cor. 12:8, 9.
g i.e. *Gentiles.*
h Rom. 8:26, 27.
i Lk. 11:1-4; John 16:24; Eph. 6:18; Jude 20.
j *Bible prayers* (N.T.). Mt. 8:2. (Mt. 6:9; Rev. 22:20.)
k Mt. 5:9, 16.
l Mal. 1:11.
m *Kingdom* (N.T.). Mt. 11:27-30. (Lk. 1:31-33; 1 Cor. 15:24.)
n Mt. 3:2, *note.*
o *Forgiveness.* vs. 12, 14, 15; Mt. 9:2, 5, 6. (Lev. 4:20; Mt. 26:28.)
p *Sin.* Rom. 3:23, *note.*
q *Temptation.* Mt. 16:1. (Gen. 3:1; Jas. 1:14.)
r Cf. Mt. 18:21-35; Jas. 2:13.
s Cf. Isa. 58:3-7; Lk. 18:12.
t Dan. 1:12-16. Cf. Prov. 14:10; 2 Cor. 6:10.
u Prov. 23:4; 1 Tim. 6:6-11.
v Or, *lamp.*
w Lk. 16:13. Cf. 1 Ki. 18:21; 2 Ki. 17:41; Rev. 3:15, 16.
x v. 31; Lk. 12:22-31; Heb. 13:5, 6; Phil. 3:18, 19; 4:6, 7.
y About 18 in.

[1]**(6:12)** This is legal ground. Cf. Eph. 4:32, which is grace. Under law forgiveness is conditioned upon a like spirit in us; under grace we are forgiven for Christ's sake, and exhorted to forgive because we have been forgiven. See Mt. 18:32; 26:28, *note.*

how they grow; they toil not, neither do
they spin:
29 And yet I say unto you, That even
Solomon in all his glory was not arrayed
like one of these.
30 Wherefore, if God so clothe the
grass of the field, which to day is, and to
morrow is cast into the oven, *shall he* not
much more *clothe* you, O ye of little
faith?
31 Therefore [a]take no thought, saying,
What shall we eat? or, What shall we
drink? or, Wherewithal shall we be
clothed?
32 (For after all these things do the
Gentiles seek:) for [b]your heavenly Father
knoweth that ye have need of all these
things.
33 But seek ye first the kingdom of
[1]God, and his righteousness; and all
these things shall be added unto you.
34 Take therefore no thought for the
[c]morrow: for the morrow shall take
thought for the things of itself. Sufficient
unto the day *is* the evil thereof.

CHAPTER 7.

Sermon on the mount, continued:
judgment of others forbidden.

Judge [d]not, that ye [e]be not judged.
2 For with what judgment ye judge,
ye shall be judged: and with what measure ye mete, it shall be measured to you
again.
3 And why beholdest thou the [f]mote
that is in thy brother's eye, but considerest not the beam that is in thine own
eye?
4 Or how wilt thou say to thy brother,
Let me pull out the mote out of thine
eye; and, behold, a beam *is* in thine own
eye?
5 Thou hypocrite, [g]first cast out the
beam out of thine own eye; and then
shalt thou see clearly to cast out the
mote out of thy brother's eye.
6 Give not that which is [h]holy unto the
dogs, neither cast ye your pearls before
swine, lest they trample them under
their feet, and turn again and rend you.

Encouragements to pray.
(See Lk. 11:1-13, *note.*)

7 Ask, and it shall be [i]given you; seek,
and ye shall find; knock, and it shall be
opened unto you:
8 For every one that asketh receiveth;
and he that seeketh findeth; and to him
that knocketh it shall be opened.
9 Or what man is there of you, whom
if his son ask bread, will he give him a
stone?
10 Or if he ask a fish, will he give him
a serpent?
11 If ye then, being evil, know how to
give good gifts unto your children, how
[j]much more shall your Father which is
in heaven give good things to them that
ask him?

A.D. 31.

a Or, *have no anxiety.* v. 34.
b v. 8; Ex. 3:7; Deut. 2:7; Psa. 103:14; Mk. 6:38; Lk. 12:29, 30.
c Jas. 4:13, 14.
d In the sense of condemnation.
e Lk. 6:37; Rom. 14:4, 10, 13; 1 Cor. 4:3-5; 5:12.
f Lk. 6:41, 42; Rom. 2:1, 21; 1 Cor. 10:12; Gal. 6:1.
g Cf. 2 Chr. 28:10; Mt. 5:23, 24; John 8:7.
h *Sanctify, holy (things)* (N.T.). Mt. 23:17, 19. (Mt. 4:5; Rev. 22:11.)
i Mt. 21:22; Lk. 11:9-13; 18:1; John 15:7; Jas. 1:5.
j Psa. 84:11; Lk. 11:13; Jas. 1:17.

[1] **(6:33)** The kingdom of God is to be distinguished from the kingdom of heaven (Mt. 3:2, *note*) in five respects: (1) The kingdom of God is universal, including all moral intelligences willingly subject to the will of God, whether angels, the Church, or saints of past or future dispensations (Lk. 13:28, 29; Heb. 12:22, 23); while the kingdom of heaven is Messianic, mediatorial, and Davidic, and has for its object the establishment of the kingdom of God in the earth (Mt. 3:2, *note;* 1 Cor. 15:24, 25). (2) The kingdom of God is entered only by the new birth (John 3:3, 5-7); the kingdom of heaven, during this age, is the sphere of a profession which may be real or false (Mt. 13:3, *note;* 25:1, 11, 12). (3) Since the kingdom of heaven is the earthly sphere of the universal kingdom of God, the two have almost all things in common. For this reason many parables and other teachings are spoken of the kingdom of heaven in Matthew, and of the kingdom of God in Mark and Luke. It is the omissions which are significant. The parables of the wheat and tares, and of the net (Mt. 13:24-30, 36-43, 47-50) are not spoken of the kingdom of God. In that kingdom there are neither tares nor bad fish. But the parable of the leaven (Mt. 13:33) is spoken of the kingdom of God also, for, alas, even the true doctrines of the kingdom are leavened with the errors of which the Pharisees, Sadducees, and the Herodians were the representatives. (See Mt. 13:33, *note.*) (4) The kingdom of God "comes not with outward show" (Lk. 17:20), but is chiefly that which is inward and spiritual (Rom. 14:17); while the kingdom of heaven is organic, and is to be manifested in glory on the earth. (See "Kingdom (O.T.)," Zech. 12:8, *note;* (N.T.), Lk. 1:31-33; 1 Cor. 15:24, *note;* Mt. 17:2, *note.*) (5) The kingdom of heaven merges into the kingdom of God when Christ, having "put all enemies under His feet," "shall have delivered up the kingdom to God, even the Father" (1 Cor. 15:24-28). Cf. Mt. 3:2, *note.*

Summary of O.T. righteousness.

12 Therefore all things [a]whatsoever ye would that men should do to you, do ye even so to them: for this is the law and the prophets.

The two ways. (Cf. Psa. 1.)

13 Enter ye in at the [b]strait gate: for wide *is* the gate, and broad *is* the way, that leadeth to destruction, and many there be which go in thereat:

14 Because strait *is* the gate, and narrow *is* the way, which leadeth unto [c]life, and few there be that find it.

Warning against false teachers: the test.

15 Beware of [d]false prophets, which come to you in sheep's clothing, but inwardly they are ravening wolves.

16 Ye shall know them by their fruits. Do men gather grapes of thorns, or figs of thistles?

17 Even so every good tree bringeth forth good fruit; but a corrupt tree bringeth forth evil fruit.

18 A good tree cannot bring forth evil fruit, neither *can* a corrupt tree bring forth good fruit.

19 Every tree that bringeth not forth good fruit is [e]hewn down, and cast into the fire.

20 Wherefore by their fruits ye shall know them.

The danger of profession without faith.

21 Not every one that [f]saith unto me, Lord, Lord, shall enter into the [g]kingdom of heaven; but he that doeth the will of my Father which is in heaven.

22 Many will say to me in that day, Lord, Lord, have we not prophesied in thy name? and in thy name have cast out [1h]devils? and in thy name done many wonderful works?

23 And then will I profess unto them, I never knew you: [i]depart from me, ye that [j]work [k]iniquity.

The two foundations. (Cf. Lk. 6:47-49.)

24 Therefore whosoever heareth these sayings of mine, and doeth them, I will [l]liken him unto a wise man, which built his house upon a [m]rock:

25 And the rain descended, and the floods came, and the winds blew, and beat upon that house; and it fell not: for it was founded upon a rock.

26 And every one that heareth these sayings of mine, and doeth them not, shall be likened unto a foolish man, which built his house upon the sand:

27 And the rain descended, and the floods came, and the winds blew, and

A.D. 31.

a Mt. 5:7; 18:23-25; Lk. 6:31.
b *narrow.* Mk. 10:23-27; Lk. 13:24; John 10:7, 9.
c *Life (eternal).* Mt. 18:8, 9. (Mt. 7:14; Rev. 22:19.)
d Deut. 13:1-5; Rev. 13:11-17; 19:20.
e Mt. 3:10; 25:41-46; John 15:2, 6.
f Isa. 29:13; Ezk. 33:31; Lk. 6:46; 2 Tim. 3:5.
g Mt. 3:2, *note.*
h *demons.* Cf. Lk. 10:17-20.
i Mt. 25:41; Psa. 6:8; Rev. 20:11, 14.
j *Sin.* Rom. 3:23, *note.*
k *lawlessness.*
l *Parables* (N.T.). vs. 24-27; Mt. 9:16. (Mt. 5:13-16; Lk. 21:29-31.)
m *Christ (as Stone).* vs. 24, 25; Mt. 21:42-44. (Ex. 17:6; 1 Pet. 2:8.)

1 **(7:22)** Devils, lit. demons. To the reality and personality of demons the N.T. Scriptures bear abundant testimony. As to their origin nothing is clearly revealed, but they are not to be confounded with the angels mentioned in 2 Pet. 2:4; Jude 6. Summary: Demons are spirits (Mt. 12:43, 45); are Satan's emissaries (Mt. 12:26, 27; 25:41); and so numerous as to make Satan's power practically ubiquitous (Mk. 5:9). They are capable of entering and controlling both men and beasts (Mk. 5:8, 11-13). and earnestly seek embodiment, without which, apparently, they are powerless for evil (Mt. 12:43, 44; Mk. 5:10-12). Demon influence and demon possession are discriminated in the N.T. Instances of the latter are Mt. 4:24; 8:16, 28, 33; 9:32: 12:22; Mk. 1:32; 5:15, 16, 18; Lk. 8:36; Acts 8:7; 16:16. They are unclean, sullen, violent, and malicious (Mt. 8:28; 9:33; 10:1; 12:43; Mk. 1:23; 5:3-5; 9:17, 20; Lk. 6:18; 9:39). They know Jesus Christ as Most High God, and recognize His supreme authority (Mt. 8:31, 32; Mk. 1:24; Acts 19:15; Jas. 2:19). They know their eternal fate to be one of torment (Mt. 8:29; Lk. 8:31). They inflict physical maladies (Mt. 12:22; 17:15-18; Lk. 13:16), but mental *disease* is to be distinguished from the disorder of mind due to demoniacal control. Demon influence may manifest itself in religious asceticism and formalism (1 Tim. 4:1-3), degenerating into uncleanness (2 Pet. 2:10-12). The sign of demon influence in religion is departing from the faith, i.e. the body of revealed truth in the Scriptures (1 Tim. 4:1). The demons maintain especially a conflict with believers who would be spiritual (Eph. 6:12; 1 Tim. 4:1-3). All unbelievers are open to demon possession (Eph. 2:2). The believer's resources are, prayer and bodily control (Mt. 17:21), "the whole armour of God" (Eph. 6:13-18). Exorcism in the name of Jesus Christ (Acts 16:18) was practised for demon possession. One of the awful features of the apocalyptic judgments in which this age will end is an irruption of demons out of the abyss (Rev. 9:1-11).

beat upon that house; and it fell: and
great was the fall of it.
28 And it came to pass, when Jesus
had ended these sayings, the people
were [a]astonished at his [b]doctrine:
29 For he taught them as *one* having
authority, and not as the scribes.

CHAPTER 8.

Jesus heals a leper
(Mk. 1:40; Lk. 5:12-14).

When he was come down from the
mountain, great multitudes followed him.
2 And, [1]behold, there came a [c]leper
and worshipped him, [d]saying, [2]Lord, if
thou wilt, thou canst make me clean.
3 And Jesus put forth *his* hand, and
touched him, saying, I will; be thou
clean. And immediately his [e]leprosy was
cleansed.
4 And Jesus saith unto him, See thou
tell no man; but go thy way, shew thyself
to the priest, and offer the [f]gift that Moses
commanded, for a testimony unto them.

Jesus heals the centurion's servant
(Lk. 7:1-10).

5 And when Jesus was entered into
Capernaum, there came unto him a
[g]centurion, beseeching him,
6 And saying, Lord, my servant lieth
at home sick of the palsy, grievously tormented.
7 And Jesus saith unto him, I will
come and heal him.
8 The centurion answered and said,
Lord, I am not worthy that thou
shouldest come under my roof: but
speak the word only, and my servant
shall be healed.
9 For I am a man under [h]authority,
having soldiers under me: and I say to
this *man*, Go, and he goeth; and to
another, Come, and he cometh; and to
my servant, Do this, and he doeth *it*.
10 When Jesus heard *it*, he marvelled,
and said to them that followed, Verily I
say unto you, I have not found so great
[i]faith, no, not in Israel.
11 And I say unto you, That many
shall come from the east and west, and
shall sit down with Abraham, and Isaac,
and Jacob, in the kingdom of [j]heaven.
12 But the children of the kingdom shall
be cast out into outer darkness: there shall
be weeping and gnashing of teeth.
13 And Jesus said unto the centurion,
Go thy way; and [k]as thou hast believed,
so be it done unto thee. And his servant
was healed in the selfsame hour.

Jesus heals Peter's wife's mother
(Mk. 1:29-34; Lk. 4:38-41).

14 And when Jesus was come into
Peter's house, he saw his wife's mother
laid, and sick of a fever.
15 And he [l]touched her hand, and the
fever left her: and she arose, and [m]minis-
tered unto [n]them.
16 When the even was come, they
brought unto him many that were [o]pos-
sessed with devils: and he cast out the
spirits with [p]*his* word, and healed all
that were sick:
17 That it might be [q]fulfilled which
was spoken by Esaias the prophet, [r]say-
ing, Himself [s]took our infirmities, and
bare *our* sicknesses.
18 Now when Jesus saw great multitudes about him, he gave commandment
to depart unto the other side.

Professed disciples tested (Lk. 9:57-62).

19 And a certain scribe came, and said

A.D. 31.

a Mt. 13:54; Mk. 1:22; Lk. 4:32.
b Or, *teaching*.
c Lev. 13:1-46; 2 Ki. 5:1-14; Mk. 1:40-45; Lk. 5:12-15.
d *Bible prayers* (N.T.). Mt. 8:25. (Mt. 6:9; Rev. 22:20.)
e *Miracles* (N.T.). vs. 2, 3, 5-17, 24-27, 28-32; Mt. 9:2-8. (Mt. 8:2, 3; Acts 28:8, 9.)
f Lev. 14:4-32; Deut. 24:8; Rom. 3:21 with Mt. 5:17.
g A Roman commander of 100 men.
h Cf. Mk. 1:27; Lk. 9:1.
i *Faith*. Mt. 9:2. (Gen. 3:20; Heb. 11:39.)
j Mt. 3:2, *note*.
k Mt. 9:22, 28, 29; Lk. 7:50; 8:48, 50.
l v. 3.
m Lk. 8:2, 3.
n *unto him*.
o Gr. *daimonizomai, demonized*. Mt. 7:22, *note*.
p Lit. *a word*.
q Mt. 1:22; Isa. 53:4.
r Isa. 53:4.
s 2 Cor. 5:21; 1 Pet. 2:24.

[1] **(8:2)** The King, having in Chapters 5–7 declared the principles of the kingdom, makes proof, in Chapters 8, 9, of His power to banish from the earth the consequences of sin, and to control the elements of nature.

[2] **(8:2)** Gr. *kurios*. The first occurrence of the word as applied to Jesus with His evident sanction. In itself the word means "master," and is so used of mere human relationships in, e.g., Mt. 6:24; 15:27; Mk. 13:35; Eph. 6:9. Both uses, divine and human, are brought together in Col. 4:1. It is the Gr. equivalent of the Heb. Adonai (see Gen. 15:2, *note*), and is so used by Jesus Christ in Mt. 22:43-45. In the N.T. the distinctive uses of *kurios* (Lord) are: (1) As the N.T. translation of the Heb. Jehovah (LORD), e.g. Mt. 1:20, 22; 2:15; 3:3; 4:7, 10; 11:25; 21:9; Mk. 12:29, 30; Lk. 1:68; 2:9. (2) Jesus Himself so uses *kurios*, e.g. Mt. 4:7, 10; 11:25; Mk. 12:11, etc. (3) But the great use of *kurios* is as the divine title of Jesus, the Christ. In this sense it occurs in the N.T. 663 times. That the intent is to identify Jesus Christ with the O.T. Deity is evident from Mt. 3:3; 12:8; 21:9 (Psa. 118:26); 22:43-45; Lk. 1:43; John 8:58; 14:8-10; 20:28; Acts 9:5; 13:33 (Psa. 2). See John 20:28, *note*.

unto him, Master, I will follow thee whithersoever thou goest.

20 And Jesus [a]saith unto him, The foxes have holes, and the birds of the air *have* nests; but the [1]Son of man hath not where to lay *his* head.

21 And another of his disciples said unto him, Lord, suffer me first to go and bury my father.

22 But Jesus said unto him, Follow me; and [b]let the [c]dead bury their dead.

Jesus stills the waves
(Mk. 4:36-41; Lk. 8:22-25).

23 And when he was entered into a ship, his disciples followed him.

24 And, behold, there arose a great tempest in the sea, insomuch that the ship was covered with the waves: but he was asleep.

25 And his disciples came to *him,* and awoke him, [d]saying, Lord, save us: we perish.

26 And he saith unto them, Why are ye fearful, O ye of [e]little faith? Then he arose, and rebuked the winds and the sea; and there was a great calm.

27 But the men marvelled, saying, What manner of man is this, that even the winds and the sea obey him!

Jesus casts out demons at Gadara
(Mk. 5:1-21; Lk. 8:26-40).

28 And when he was come to the other side into the country of the [f]Gergesenes, there met him two [g]possessed with [h]devils, coming out of the tombs, exceeding fierce, so that no man might pass by that way.

29 And, behold, they cried out, saying, [i]What have we to do with thee, Jesus, thou Son of God? art thou come hither to [j]torment us before the time?

30 And there was a good way off from them an herd of many swine feeding.

31 So the [k]devils besought him, saying, If thou cast us out, suffer us to go away into the [l]herd of swine.

32 And he said unto them, Go. And when they were come out, they went into the herd of swine: and, behold, the whole herd of swine ran violently down a steep place into the sea, and perished in the waters.

33 And they that kept them fled, and went their ways into the city, and told every thing, and what was befallen to the [g]possessed of the devils.

34 And, behold, the whole city came out to meet Jesus: and when they saw him, they besought *him* that he would [m]depart out of their coasts.

CHAPTER 9.

Jesus returns to Capernaum: heals the palsied man (Mk. 2:3-12; Lk. 5:18-26).

And he entered into a ship, and passed over, and came into his [n]own city.

2 And, behold, they [o]brought to him a man sick of the palsy, lying on a bed: and Jesus seeing their [p]faith said unto the sick of the palsy; Son, be of good cheer; thy sins be [q]forgiven thee.

3 And, behold, certain of the scribes said within themselves, This *man* blasphemeth.

4 And Jesus knowing their thoughts said, Wherefore think ye evil in your hearts?

5 For whether is easier, to [r]say, *Thy* [s]*sins be forgiven thee;* or to say, Arise, and walk?

6 But that ye may know that the [t]Son of man hath [u]power on earth to forgive

A.D. 31.

a Cf. vs. 21, 22; Mt. 10:36; John 6:68, 69.
b Or, *leave the dead to bury their own dead.*
c *Death (spiritual).* Lk. 15:24. (Gen. 2:17; Eph. 2:5.)
d *Bible prayers* (N.T.). Mt. 9:18. (Mt. 6:9; Rev. 22:20.)
e Mt. 17:20; Mk. 16:17, 18.
f *Gadarenes.*
g Gr. *daimonizomai, demonized.* Mt. 7:22, *note.*
h *demons.*
i Lk. 5:8; Acts 1:25; 24:25.
j Cf. Mt. 25:41 with Rev. 19:20.
k *demons.* Mt. 7:22, *note.*
l Mt. 7:6; Lk. 15:15, 16.
m v. 29; Lk. 4:29; Acts 16:39.
n Mt. 4:13; 11:23.
o Mk. 2:1-12; Lk. 5:17-26.
p *Faith.* Mt. 9:22. (Gen. 3:20; Heb. 11:39.)
q *Forgiveness.* vs. 2, 5, 6; Mt. 12:31, 32. (Lev. 4:20; Mt. 26:28.)
r Mt. 8:8; Mk. 1:27; Rom. 10:8-13.
s *Sin.* Rom. 3:23, *note.*
t See Mt. 8:20, *note.*
u Mt. 21:23-27; John 3:35; 5:27; Acts 2:36; 4:7-12.

1 (8:20) Cf. Ezk. 2:1, *note.* Our Lord thus designates Himself about eighty times. It is His racial name as the representative Man, in the sense of 1 Cor. 15:45-47; as Son of David is distinctively His Jewish name, and Son of God His divine name. Our Lord constantly uses this term as implying that His mission (e.g. Mt. 11:19; Lk. 19:10), His death and resurrection (e.g. Mt. 12:40; 20:18; 26:2), and His second coming (e.g. Mt. 24:37-44; Lk. 12:40), transcended in scope and result all merely Jewish limitations. When Nathanael confesses Him as "King of Israel," our Lord's answer is, "Thou shalt see greater things . . . the angels of God ascending and descending upon the Son of man." When His messengers are cast out by the Jews His thought leaps forward to the time when the Son of man shall come, not then to Israel only but to the race (Mt. 10:5, 6 with v. 23). It is in this name, also, that universal judgment is committed to Him (John 5:22, 27). It is also a name indicating that in Him is fulfilled the O.T. foreview of blessing through a coming man (Gen. 1:26, *note;* 3:15; 12:3; Psa. 8:4; 80:17; Isa. 7:14; 9:6, 7; 32:2; Zech. 13:7).

[a]sins, (then saith he to the sick of the
palsy,) Arise, take up thy bed, and go
unto thine house.
7 [b]And he arose, and departed to his
house.
8 But when the multitudes saw *it*, they
[c]marvelled, and glorified God, which
had given such power unto men.

The call of Matthew
(Mk. 2:14; Lk. 5:27-29).

9 And as Jesus passed forth from
thence, he saw a man, named Matthew,
sitting at the receipt of custom: and he
saith unto him, [d]Follow me. And he
arose, and followed him.

Jesus answers the Pharisees
(Mk. 2:15-20; Lk. 5:29-35).

10 And it came to pass, as Jesus sat at
meat in the house, behold, many publicans and sinners [e]came and sat down
with him and his disciples.
11 And when the [f]Pharisees saw *it*, they
said unto his disciples, [g]Why eateth your
Master with publicans and [a]sinners?
12 But when Jesus heard *that*, he said
unto them, They that be [h]whole need not
a physician, but they that are sick.
13 But go ye and learn what *that*
meaneth, [i]I will have mercy, and not sacrifice: for I am not come to call the [j]right-
eous, but sinners to [k]repentance.
14 Then came to him the disciples of
John, saying, Why do we and the
Pharisees fast oft, but thy disciples fast
not?
15 And Jesus said unto them, Can the
children of the bridechamber mourn, as
long as the [l]bridegroom is with them?
but the days will come, when the bridegroom shall be taken from them, and
then shall they fast.

Parables of the garment and bottles
(Mk. 2:21, 22; Lk. 5:36-39).

16 No man putteth a piece of new
[m]cloth unto an old garment, for that
which is put in to fill it up taketh from
the garment, and the rent is made worse.
17 Neither do men put new wine into
old [n]bottles: else the bottles break, and
the wine runneth out, and the bottles
perish: but they put new wine into new
bottles, and both are preserved.

Jesus heals the woman with an issue of blood, and raises the daughter of a ruler (Jairus) (Mk. 5:22-43; Lk. 8:41-56).

18 While he spake these things unto
them, behold, there came a [o]certain ruler,
and worshipped him, [p]saying, My daughter is even now dead: but come and lay
thy hand upon her, and she shall live.
19 And Jesus arose, and followed him,
and *so did* his disciples.
20 And, behold, a woman, which was
diseased with an issue of blood twelve
years, came behind *him*, and [q]touched
the hem of his garment:
21 For she said within herself, If I may
but touch his garment, I shall be whole.
22 But Jesus turned him about, and
when he saw her, he said, Daughter, be
of good comfort; thy [r]faith hath made
thee whole. And the woman was made
whole from that hour.
23 And when Jesus came into the
ruler's house, and saw the minstrels and
the people making a noise,
24 He said unto them, Give place: for
the maid is not dead, but [s]sleepeth. And
they laughed him to scorn.
25 But when the people were put
forth, he went in, and [t]took her by the
hand, and the maid [u]arose.
26 And the fame hereof went abroad
into all that land.

Two blind men healed: a demon cast out.

27 And when Jesus departed thence,
two blind men followed him, crying,
and [v]saying, [w]*Thou* Son of David, have
mercy on us.
28 And when he was come into the
house, the blind men came to him: and
Jesus saith unto them, Believe ye that I
am able to do this? They said unto him,
Yea, Lord.
29 Then touched he their eyes, saying,
According to your [x]faith be it unto you.
30 And their eyes were opened; and
Jesus straitly charged them, saying, See
that no man know *it*.
31 But they, when they were departed,
spread abroad his fame in all that country.
32 As they went out, behold, they
brought to him a dumb man [y]possessed
with a [z]devil.
33 And when the [z]devil was cast out,
the dumb spake: and the multitudes

A.D. 31.

a *Sin.* Rom. 3:23, *note.*
b *Miracles* (N.T.). vs. 2-8, 18, 20-22, 23-25, 27-30, 32-35; Mt. 12:10-13. (Mt. 8:2, 3; Acts 28:8, 9.)
c Mt. 8:27; Acts 2:43; 5:11.
d Mt. 4:18-22.
e Mt. 4:13; 11:23.
f v. 3; Lk. 7:39.
g Mt. 11:19.
h Lk. 18:9-14; John 9:39-41.
i Hos. 6:6.
j Rom. 10:10, *note.*
k *Repentance.* Mt. 11:20. (Mt. 3:2; Acts 17:30.)
l Mk. 2:19, 20; Lk. 5:34, 35; John 3:29; Eph. 5:28-32; Rev. 19:6-9.
m *Parables* (N.T.). vs. 16, 17; Mt. 13:3-9. (Mt. 5:13-16; Lk. 21:29-31.)
n *wine-skins.*
o Mk. 5:22-43; Lk. 8:41-56.
p *Bible prayers* (N.T.). Mt. 9:27. (Mt. 6:9; Rev. 22:20.)
q Mt. 8:3.
r *Faith.* Mt. 9:29. (Gen. 3:20; Heb. 11:39.)
s John 11:11-14; 1 Thes. 4:13, 14.
t Mt. 8:3, 15; Rom. 6:10 with Eph. 2:5, 6.
u *Resurrection.* vs. 23-25; Mt. 10:8. (Job 19:25; 1 Cor. 15:52.)
v *Bible prayers* (N.T.). Mt. 11:25, 26. (Mt. 6:9; Rev. 22:20.)
w Mt. 15:22; Lk. 18:38, 39.
x *Faith.* Mt. 17:20-22. (Gen. 3:20; Heb. 11:39.)
y Gr. *daimonizomai, demonized.* Mt. 7:22, *note.*
z *demon.* See Mt. 7:22, *note.*

marvelled, saying, It was never so seen in Israel.

34 But the Pharisees said, He casteth out [a]devils through the prince of the devils.

Jesus preaches and heals in Galilee
(Mk. 6:5, 6).

35 And Jesus went about all the cities and villages, teaching in their synagogues, and preaching the [b]gospel of the kingdom, and healing every sickness and every disease among the people.

36 But when he saw the multitudes, he was moved with compassion on them, because they fainted, and were scattered abroad, as sheep having no shepherd.

37 Then saith he unto his disciples, The harvest truly *is* plenteous, but the labourers *are* few;

38 Pray ye therefore the Lord of the harvest, that he will send forth labourers into his harvest.

CHAPTER 10.

The twelve instructed and sent forth
(Mk. 6:7-13; Lk. 9:1-6).

And when he had called unto *him* his [c]twelve disciples, he gave them [d]power *against* unclean spirits, to cast them out, and to heal all manner of sickness and all manner of disease.

2 Now the [e]names of the twelve [1]apostles are these; The first, Simon, who is called Peter, and Andrew his brother; [f]James *the son* of Zebedee, and John his brother;

3 Philip, and Bartholomew; Thomas, and Matthew the publican; James *the son* of Alphaeus, and Lebbaeus, whose surname was Thaddaeus;

4 Simon the Canaanite, and Judas Iscariot, who also betrayed him.

5 These twelve Jesus sent forth, and commanded them, saying, Go not into the way of the [g]Gentiles, and into *any* city of the Samaritans enter ye not:

6 But go rather to the [h]lost sheep of the house of Israel.

7 And as ye go, preach, saying, The [i]kingdom of heaven is at hand.

8 [j]Heal the sick, cleanse the lepers, [k]raise the dead, cast out [a]devils: freely ye have received, freely give.

9 [2]Provide neither gold, nor silver, nor brass in your purses,

10 Nor scrip for *your* journey, neither two coats, neither shoes, nor yet staves: for the [l]workman is worthy of his meat.

A.D. 31.

a *demons.* See Mt. 7:22, *note.*

b *Gospel.* Mt. 11:5. (Gen. 12:1-3; Rev. 14:6.)

c Mk. 3:13-19; Lk. 6:12-16.

d Mk. 6:7-12; Lk. 9:1-6.

e Mk. 3:13-19; Lk. 6:12-16; Acts 1:13.

f Mt. 4:21, *note.*

g The kingdom was promised to the Jews. Gentiles could be blessed only through Christ crucified and risen. Cf. John 12:20-24.

h Gr. *apollumi.* John 3:16, *note;* Mt. 15:24, 26; Acts 13:46.

i Mt. 3:2; 4:17.

j v. 1; 2 Cor. 12:12.

k *Resurrection.* Mt. 17:3. (Job 19:25; 1 Cor. 15:52.)

l Lk. 10:7; 1 Cor. 9:4-15; 1 Tim. 5:18.

[1]**(10:2)** The word apostle, = "one sent forth," is used of our Lord (Heb. 3:1). Elsewhere it is used of the twelve who were called to that office by our Lord during His earth ministry; of Paul, called to the apostleship by the risen and ascended Lord, and of Barnabas (Acts 14:14), specially designated by the Holy Spirit (Acts 13:2). Of Matthias, chosen by lot by the eleven to take the place of Judas Iscariot (Acts 1:16-26), it is said: "And he was numbered with the eleven" (Acts 1:26). See Acts 1:26.

The "signs of an apostle" were: (1) They were chosen directly by the Lord Himself, or, as in the case of Barnabas, by the Holy Spirit (Mt. 10:1, 2; Mk. 3:13, 14; Lk. 6:13; Acts 9:6, 15; 13:2; 22:10, 14, 15; Rom. 1:1). (2) They were endued with sign gifts, miraculous powers which were the divine credentials of their office (Mt. 10:1; Acts 5:15, 16; 16:16-18; 28:8, 9). (3) Their relation to the kingdom was that of heralds, announcing, to Israel only (Mt. 10:5, 6), the kingdom as at hand (Mt. 4:17, *note*), and manifesting kingdom powers (Mt. 10:7, 8). (4) To one of them, Peter, the keys of the kingdom of heaven, viewed as the sphere of Christian profession, as in Mt. 13, were given (Mt. 16:19). (5) Their future relation to the kingdom will be that of judges over the twelve tribes (Mt. 19:28). (6) Consequent upon the rejection of the kingdom, and the revelation of the mystery hid in God (Mt. 16:18; Eph. 3:1-12), the Church, the apostolic office was invested with a new enduement, the baptism with the Holy Spirit (Acts 2:1-4); a new power, that of imparting the Spirit to Jewish-Christian believers; a new relation, that of foundation stones of the new temple (Eph. 2:20-22); and a new function, that of preaching the glad tidings of salvation through a crucified and risen Lord to Jew and Gentile alike. (7) The indispensable qualification of an apostle was that he should have been an eye-witness of the resurrection (Acts 1:22; 1 Cor. 9:1).

[2]**(10:9)** Cf. Mk. 6:8, 9; Lk. 9:3. The central thought here, urgency, must be kept in mind. The emphasis is upon "provide." Time is not to be taken to search for additional staves or shoes. The disciples were to go in their ordinary sandals, with such staff as they might have, or with none. Cf. Paul, Rom. 1:15.

11 And into whatsoever city or town ye shall enter, enquire who in it is worthy; and there abide till ye go thence.

12 And when ye come into an house, salute it.

13 And if the house be worthy, let your peace come upon it: but if it be not worthy, let your peace return to you.

14 And whosoever shall not receive you, [a]nor hear your words, when ye depart out of that house or city, [b]shake off the dust of your feet.

15 Verily I say unto you, It shall be more [c]tolerable for the land of Sodom and Gomorrha [d]in the day of judgment, than for that city.

16 Behold, I [1]send you forth as [e]sheep in the midst of wolves: be ye therefore wise as [f]serpents, and harmless as [g]doves.

17 But [h]beware of men: for they will deliver you up to the councils, and they will scourge you in their synagogues;

18 And ye shall be brought before governors and kings for my sake, for a testimony against them and the Gentiles.

19 But when they deliver you up, [i]take no thought how or what ye shall speak: [j]for it shall be given you in that same hour what ye shall speak.

20 For it is not ye that speak, but the [k]Spirit of your Father which speaketh in you.

21 And the brother shall deliver up the brother to death, and the father the child: and the children shall rise up against *their* parents, and cause them to be put to death.

22 And ye shall be hated of all *men* for my name's sake: but he that [l]endureth to the end shall be saved.

23 But when they persecute you in this city, flee ye into another: for verily I say unto you, Ye shall not have [m]gone over the cities of Israel, till the [n]Son of man be come.

24 [o]The disciple is not above *his* master, nor the servant above his lord.

25 It is enough for the disciple that he be as his master, and the servant as his lord. If they have called the [p]master of the house [q]Beelzebub, how much more *shall they call* them of his household?

26 Fear them not therefore: for there is [r]nothing covered, that shall not be revealed; and hid, that shall not be known.

27 What I tell you in darkness, *that* [s]speak ye in light: and what ye hear in the ear, *that* preach ye upon the housetops.

28 And fear not them which kill the body, but are not able to kill the soul: but rather fear [t]him which is able to destroy both soul and body in [u]hell.

29 Are not two [v]sparrows sold for a [w]farthing? and one of them shall not fall on the ground without your Father.

30 But the very [x]hairs of your head are all numbered.

31 Fear ye not therefore, ye are of more value than many sparrows.

32 Whosoever therefore shall [y]confess me before men, him will I confess also before my Father which is in heaven.

33 But whosoever shall deny me before men, him will I also [z]deny before my Father which is in heaven.

34 Think not that I am come to send [2]peace on earth: I came not to send peace, but a sword.

35 For I am come to set a man at [aa]variance against his father, and the daughter

A.D. 31.

a *Inspiration.* Mt. 11:13. (Ex. 4:15; Rev. 22:19.)
b Lk. 10:10-12; Acts 13:51.
c Mt. 11:22.
d *Day of judgment.* Mt. 11:22. (Mt. 10:15; Rev. 20:11.)
e Mt. 7:15; Lk. 10:3.
f Cf. 2 Cor. 12:16; Col. 4:5.
g Phil. 2:14-16.
h 1 Pet. 3:13, 14.
i Mk. 13:11-13; Lk. 12:11, 12; 21:14-19.
j An instruction to martyrs, not to preachers.
k *Holy Spirit.* Mt. 12:18, 28, 32. (Mt. 1:18; Acts 2:4.)
l Mt. 24:13.
m Mt. 24:4-30.
n See Mt. 8:20, *note.*
o John 15:19-21.
p John 8:48 with Acts 2:13.
q *Beelzebul,* title of a heathen deity.
r Mk. 4:22; Lk. 12:2, 3; 1 Cor. 4 5.
s Acts 5:20; Col. 1:23.
t 2 Cor. 5:11.
u Mt. 5:22, *note.*
v Lk. 12:4-7.
w 1-4 penny, or 1-2 cent.
x Lk. 21:18; Acts 27:34.
y Psa. 119:46; Lk. 12:8; Rev. 3:8.
z Mt. 7:23; Lk. 12:9.
aa Mic. 7:6; John 9:18-23.

[1] **(10:16)** The scope of verses 16-23 reaches beyond the personal ministry of the twelve covering in a general sense the sphere of service during the present age. Verse 23 has in view the preaching of the remnant (Isa. 1:9; Rom. 11:5, *note*) in the tribulation (Psa. 2:5; Rev. 7:14, *note*), and immediately preceding the return of Christ in glory (Deut. 30:3; Acts 1:9-11, *note*). The remnant then will not have gone over the cities of Israel till the Lord comes.

[2] **(10:34)** Cf. John 14:27. Peace is spoken of in Scripture in three ways: (1) "Peace with God" (Rom. 5:1); this is the work of Christ into which the individual enters by faith (Eph. 2:14-17; Rom. 5:1). (2) "The peace of God" (Phil. 4:7); inward peace, the state of soul of that believer who, having entered into peace with God through faith in Christ, has also committed to God through prayer and supplication with thanksgiving all his anxieties (Lk. 7:50; Phil. 4:6). (3) Peace "on earth" (Lk. 2:14; Psa. 72:7; 85:10; Isa. 9:6, 7; 11:1-12); the universal prevalency of peace in the earth under the kingdom. Mt. 10:34 was Christ's warning that the truth which He was proclaiming would not bring in the kingdom-age of peace, but conflict rather. (Cf. John 14:27.)

against her mother, and the daughter in law against her mother in law.

36 And a man's foes *shall be* they of his own household.

37 He that loveth father or mother more than me is not worthy of me: and he that loveth son or daughter more than me is not [a]worthy of me.

38 And he that taketh not his cross, and followeth after me, is not worthy of me.

39 He that findeth his life shall lose it: and he that loseth his life for my sake shall find it.

40 [b]He that receiveth you receiveth me, and he that receiveth me receiveth him that sent me.

41 He that receiveth a prophet in the name of a prophet shall receive a prophet's [c]reward; and he that receiveth a [d]righteous man in the name of a righteous man shall receive a righteous man's reward.

42 And whosoever shall give to drink unto one of these little ones a [e]cup of cold *water* only in the name of a disciple, verily I say unto you, he shall in no wise lose his reward.

CHAPTER 11.

And it came to pass, when Jesus had made an end of commanding his twelve disciples, he departed thence to teach and to preach in their cities.

John the Baptist sends disciples to question Jesus (Lk. 7:18-35).

2 Now when [f]John had heard in the prison the works of Christ, he sent two of his disciples,

3 And said unto him, Art thou he that should come, or do we look for another?

4 Jesus answered and said unto them, Go and shew John again those things which ye do hear and see:

5 The [g]blind [h]receive their sight, and the lame walk, the lepers are cleansed, and the deaf hear, the dead are raised up, and the poor have the [i]gospel preached to them.

6 And [j]blessed is *he*, whosoever shall not [k]be offended in me.

7 And as they departed, Jesus began to say unto the multitudes concerning John, [l]What went ye out into the wilderness to see? A reed shaken with the wind?

8 But what went ye out for to see? A man clothed in soft raiment? behold, they that wear soft *clothing* are in kings' houses.

9 But what went ye out for to see? A prophet? yea, I say unto you, and more than a prophet.

10 For this is *he*, of whom it is written, [m]Behold, I send my messenger before thy face, which shall prepare thy way before thee.

11 Verily I say unto you, Among them that are born of women there hath not risen a greater than John the Baptist: notwithstanding he that is [n]least in the [o]kingdom of heaven is [1]greater than he.

12 And from the days of John the Baptist until now the kingdom of heaven [p]suffereth [2]violence, and the violent take it by force.

13 [q]For all the prophets and the law prophesied until John.

14 And if ye will receive *it*, [r]this is [s]Elias, which was for to come.

15 He that hath ears to hear, let him hear.

16 But whereunto shall I liken this generation? It is like unto children sitting in the markets, and calling unto their fellows,

17 And saying, We have piped unto you, and ye have not danced; we have mourned unto you, and ye have not lamented.

18 For John came neither eating nor drinking, and they say, He hath a [t]devil.

19 The [u]Son of man came [v]eating and drinking, and they say, Behold a man

A.D. 31.

a Deut. 33:9; Lk. 14:26; 2 Cor. 5:16.
b Mt. 25:40, 45; Acts 9:4.
c *Rewards.* vs. 41, 42; Mt. 16:27. (Dan. 12:3; 1 Cor. 3:14.)
d *Righteousness.* Rom. 10:10, *note.*
e 1 Ki. 18:4; Lk. 21:1-4.
f Mt. 4:12; 14:3.
g Mt. 9:27.
h Isa. 35:4-6.
i *Gospel.* Mt. 24:14. (Gen. 12:1-3; Rev. 14:6.)
j In prison, the King rejected, John's faith wavers; the Lord exhorts and encourages His servant. Cf. John 15:20; Isa. 42:3.
k *find cause of offence.*
l Lk. 7:24-30.
m Isa. 40:3; Mal. 3:1.
n Eph. 3:4-10; Heb. 11:40; 1 Pet. 1:10-12.
o Mt. 3:2, *note.*
p Lk. 5:19, 20; 16:16.
q *Inspiration,* Mt. 12:3-5, 40. (Ex. 4:15; Rev. 22:19.)
r See Mt. 17:10, *note.*
s Mt. 17:12; Mal. 4:5.
t *demon.* See Mt. 7:22, *note.*
u See Mt. 8:20, *note.*
v Lk. 5:29-32; 7:36; John 2:1-11.

[1] **(11:11)** Positionally greater, not morally. John Baptist was as great, morally, as any man "born of woman," but as to the *kingdom* he but announced it at hand. The kingdom did not then come, but was rejected, and John was martyred, and the King presently crucified. The least in the kingdom when it is set up in glory (see "Kingdom (N.T.)," Lk. 1:31-33; 1 Cor. 15:24) will be in the fullness of power and glory. It is not heaven which is in question, but Messiah's kingdom. (See Mt. 3:2, *note;* 6:33, *note.*)

[2] **(11:12)** It has been much disputed whether the "violence" here is external, as *against* the kingdom in the persons of John the Baptist and Jesus; or that, considering the opposition of the scribes and Pharisees, only the violently resolute would press into it. Both things are true. The King and His herald suffered violence, and this is the primary and greater meaning, but also, some were resolutely becoming disciples. (Cf. Lk. 16:16.)

gluttonous, and a winebibber, a friend of
publicans and [a]sinners. But wisdom is
justified of her children.

Jesus, rejected, predicts judgment.

20 [1]Then began he to upbraid the
cities wherein most of his mighty works
were done, because they [b]repented not:
21 Woe unto thee, Chorazin! woe unto
thee, Bethsaida! for if the mighty works,
which were done in you, had been done
in Tyre and Sidon, they would have
repented long ago in sackcloth and
ashes.
22 But I say unto you, It shall be more
tolerable for Tyre and Sidon at the [c]day
of judgment, than for you.
23 And thou, Capernaum, which art
exalted unto heaven, shalt be brought
down to [d]hell: for if the mighty works,
which have been done in thee, had been
done in Sodom, it would have remained
until this day.
24 But I say unto you, That it shall be
more tolerable for the land of Sodom in
the day of judgment, than for thee.
25 At that time Jesus answered and
[e]said, I thank thee, O Father, Lord of
heaven and earth, because thou hast [f]hid
these things from the wise and prudent,
and hast revealed them unto babes.
26 Even so, Father: for so it seemed
good in thy sight.
27 [g]All things are delivered unto me of
my Father: and no man knoweth the
Son, but the Father; neither knoweth any
man the Father, save the Son, and *he* to
whomsoever the Son will reveal *him*.

The new message of Jesus:
not the kingdom, but personal discipleship.

28 [2]Come unto [h]me, all *ye* that labour
and are heavy laden, and I will give you
rest.
29 Take my yoke upon you, and learn
of me; for [i]I am meek and lowly in heart:
and ye shall find rest unto your souls.
30 For my yoke *is* easy, and my burden is light.

CHAPTER 12.

Jesus declares himself Lord of the sabbath
(Mk. 2:23-28; Lk. 6:1-5).

At that time Jesus went on the [3j]sab-
bath day through the corn; and his
disciples were an hungred, and began to
pluck the ears of corn, and to eat.

A.D. 31.

a *Sin*, Rom. 3:23, *note.*

b *Repentance.* vs. 20, 21; Mt. 12:41. (Mt. 3:2; Acts 17:30.)

c *Day of judgment.* Mt. 12:35, 41, 42. (Mt. 10:15; Rev. 20:11.)

d Lk. 16:23, *note.*

e *Bible prayers* (N.T.). Mt. 15:22. (Mt. 6:9; Rev. 22:20.)

f Psa. 8:2; Lk. 10:21; 1 Cor. 1:19-31.

g *Kingdom* (N.T.). Mt. 12:3, *note.* (Lk. 1:31-33; 1 Cor. 15:24.)

h John 1:38, 39; 6:35, 37.

i Phil. 2:5-8; 1 Cor. 3:18; 1 John 3:2.

j *Sabbath.* (Gen. 2:3.)

[1] **(11:20)** The kingdom of heaven announced as "at hand" by John the Baptist, by the King Himself, and by the twelve, and attested by mighty works, has been *morally* rejected. The places chosen for the testing of the nation, Chorazin, Bethsaida, etc., having rejected both John and Jesus, the rejected King now speaks of judgment. The final official rejection is later (Mt. 27:31-37).

[2] **(11:28)** The new message of Jesus. The rejected King now turns from the rejecting *nation* and offers, not the *kingdom*, but *rest* and *service* to such in the nation as are conscious of need. It is a pivotal point in the ministry of Jesus.

[3] **(12:1)** (1) The sabbath ("cessation") appears in Scripture as the day of God's rest in the finished work of creation (Gen. 2:2, 3). For 2500 years of human life absolutely no mention is made of it. Then the sabbath was revealed (Ex. 16:23; Neh. 9:13, 14); made a part of the law (Ex. 20:8-11); and invested with the character of a "sign" between Jehovah and Israel, and a perpetual reminder to Israel of their separation to God (Ex. 31:13-17). It was observed by complete rest (Ex. 35:2, 3), and by Jehovah's express order a man was put to death for gathering sticks on the sabbath day (Num. 15:32-36). Apart from maintaining the continued burnt-offering (Num. 28:9), and its connection with the annual feasts (Ex. 12:16; Lev. 23:3, 8; Num. 28:25), the seventh-day sabbath was never made a day of sacrifice, worship, or any manner of religious service. It was simply and only a day of complete rest for man and beast, a humane provision for man's needs. In Christ's words, "The sabbath was made for man, and not man for the sabbath" (Mk. 2:27). (2) Our Lord found the observance of the day encrusted with rabbinical evasions (Mt. 12:2) and restrictions, wholly unknown to the law, so that He was Himself held to be a sabbath-breaker by the religious authorities of the time. The sabbath will be again observed during the kingdom-age (Isa. 66:23). (3) The Christian first day perpetuates in the dispensation of grace the principle that one-seventh of the time is especially sacred, but in all other respects is in contrast with the sabbath. One is the seventh day, the other the first. The sabbath commemorates God's creation rest, the first day Christ's resurrection. On the seventh day God rested, on the first day Christ

2 But when the Pharisees saw *it*, they said unto him, Behold, thy disciples do that which is not lawful to do upon the sabbath day.

3 But he said unto them, Have ye not [a]read [1]what [b]David did, when he was an hungred, and they that were with him;

4 How he entered into the house of God, and did eat the [c]shewbread, which was not lawful for him to eat, neither for them which were with him, but only for the priests?

5 Or have ye not read in the law, how that on the sabbath days the [d]priests in the temple profane the sabbath, and are blameless?

6 But I say unto you, That in this place is *one* [e]greater than the temple.

7 But if ye had known what *this* meaneth, I will have [f]mercy, and not sacrifice, ye would not have condemned the guiltless.

8 For the [g]Son of man is Lord even of the sabbath day.

The healing of the withered hand on the sabbath (Mk. 3:1-6; Lk. 6:6-11).

9 And when he was departed thence, he went into their synagogue:

10 And, behold, there was a man which had *his* hand withered. And they asked him, saying, Is it lawful to heal on the sabbath days? that they might accuse him.

11 And he said unto them, What man shall there be among you, that shall have one sheep, and if it fall into a pit on the sabbath day, will he not lay hold on it, and lift *it* out?

12 How much then is a man better than a sheep? Wherefore it is lawful to do well on the sabbath days.

13 Then saith he to the man, Stretch forth thine hand. And he stretched *it* forth; and [h]it was restored whole, like as the other.

14 Then the Pharisees went out, and held a council against him, how they might [i]destroy him.

Jesus and the multitudes (at the sea of Tiberias) (Mk. 3:7-12).

15 But when Jesus knew *it*, he withdrew himself from thence: and great multitudes followed him, and he healed them all;

16 And charged them that they should not make him known:

17 That it might be fulfilled which was spoken by Esaias the prophet, saying,

18 Behold my [j]servant, whom I have chosen; my beloved, in whom my soul is well pleased: I will put my [k]spirit upon him, and he shall shew judgment to the [2]Gentiles.

19 He shall not strive, nor cry; neither shall any man hear his voice in the streets.

20 A bruised reed shall he not break, and smoking flax shall he not quench, till he send forth judgment unto victory.

21 And in his name shall the Gentiles [m]trust.

A demoniac healed: the Pharisees blaspheme (Mk. 3:22-30; Lk. 11:14-23).

22 Then was brought unto him one [n]possessed with a devil, blind, and dumb: and he healed him, insomuch that the blind and dumb both spake and saw.

23 And all the people were amazed, and said, Is not this the [o]son of David?

24 But when the Pharisees heard *it*, they said, This *fellow* doth not cast out [p]devils, but by [q]Beelzebub the prince of the devils.

25 And Jesus knew their thoughts, and said unto them, Every kingdom divided

A.D. 31.

a *Inspiration.* vs. 3-5, 40; Mt. 19:4-8. (Ex. 4:15; Rev. 22:19.)

b *Kingdom* (N.T.). Mt. 12:38-45. (Lk. 1:31-33; 1 Cor. 15:24.)

c Ex. 25:30, *note.*

d Num. 28:9, 10.

e 2 Chr. 6:18; Isa. 66:1, 2.

f 1 Sam. 15:22; Hos. 6:6; Mic. 6:6-8.

g See Mt. 8:20.

h *Miracles* (N.T.). vs. 10-13, 22; Mt. 14:19-21. (Mt. 8:2, 3; Acts 28:8, 9.)

i Psa. 2:2.

j vs. 18-21; Isa. 42:1-4.

k *Holy Spirit.* vs. 18, 28, 32; Mt. 22:43. (Mt. 1:18; Acts 2:4.)

l *Christ (First Advent).* Mt. 21:1-5. (Gen. 3:15; Acts 1:9.)

m *i.e. hope.*

n Gr. *daimonizomai, demonized.* Mt. 7:22, *note.*

o Mt. 9:27; 21:9.

p demons. Mt. 7:22, *note.*

q Mt. 9:34; Mk. 3:22, 30; Lk. 11:14, 20.

was ceaselessly active. The sabbath commemorates a finished creation, the first day a finished redemption. The sabbath was a day of legal obligation, the first day one of voluntary worship and service. The sabbath is mentioned in the Acts only in connection with the Jews, and in the rest of the N.T. but twice (Col. 2:16; Heb. 4:4). In these passages the seventh-day sabbath is explained to be to the Christian not a day to be observed, but a type of the present rest into which he enters when "he also ceases from his own works" and trusts Christ.

[1] **(12:3)** Jesus' action (Mt. 12:1-7) is highly significant. "What David did" refers to the time of his rejection and persecution by Saul (1 Sam. 21:6). Jesus here is not so much the rejected *Saviour* as the rejected *King;* hence the reference to David.

[2] **(12:18)** This too is most significant. The rejected King of Israel will turn to the Gentiles (cf. Mt. 10:5-6). In *fulfilment* this awaited the *official* rejection, crucifixion, and resurrection of Christ, and the final rejection of the risen Christ (Lk. 24:46, 47; Acts 9:15; 13:46; 28:25-28; Rom. 11:11).

against itself is brought to desolation;
and every city or house divided against
itself shall not stand:
26 And if [a]Satan cast out Satan, he is
divided against himself; how shall then
his kingdom stand?
27 And if I by Beelzebub cast out devils, by whom do your [b]children cast *them*
out? therefore they shall be your judges.
28 But if I cast out devils by the Spirit
of God, then the kingdom of God is
come unto you.
29 Or else how can one enter into a
strong man's house, and spoil his goods,
except he first bind the strong man? and
then he will spoil his house.
30 He that is not with me is against
me; and he that gathereth not with me
scattereth abroad.

The unpardonable sin: ascribing to Satan the works of the Spirit (Mk. 3:29, 30).

31 Wherefore I say unto you, All manner of [c]sin and blasphemy shall be [d]for-
given unto men: but the [e]blasphemy
against the *Holy* Ghost shall not be forgiven unto men.
32 And whosoever speaketh a word
against the Son of man, it shall be [d]for-
given him: but whosoever speaketh
against the Holy Ghost, it shall not be
forgiven him, neither in this [f]world, neither in the *world* to come.

Destiny in words.

33 Either make the [g]tree good, and his
fruit good; or else make the tree corrupt,
and his fruit corrupt: for [h]the tree is
known by *his* fruit.
34 O [i]generation of vipers, how can
ye, being evil, speak good things? for
out of the abundance of the heart the
mouth speaketh.
35 A good man out of the good treasure of the heart bringeth forth good
things: and an evil man out of the evil
treasure bringeth forth evil things.
36 But I say unto you, That every idle
word that men shall speak, they shall give
account thereof in the [j]day of judgment.

A.D. 31.

a *Satan*, vs. 26, 27; Mt. 13:39. (Gen. 3:1; Rev. 20:10.)
b Lk. 9:49, 50; 10:17; Acts 19:13-16.
c *Sin.* Rom. 3:23, *note.*
d *Forgiveness.* vs. 31, 32; Mt. 18:21, 27, 32, 35. (Lev. 4:20; Mt. 26:28.)
e Ascribing to Satan the work of the Holy Spirit. Cf. vs. 24, 32, 40.
f i.e. *age.*
g Mt. 7:17, 18; Lk. 6:43-44.
h Jas. 3:12.
i *Progeny.* Mt. 3:7; 23:33.
j *Day of judgment.* vs. 36, 41, 42; Mk. 6:11. (Mt. 10:15; Rev. 20:11.)
k Mt. 16:1-4; Mk. 8:11; cf. John 2:18-22.
l *Kingdom* (N.T.). Mt. 12:46-50. (Lk. 1:31-33; 1 Cor. 15:24.)
m Jon. 1:17.
n Jon. 3:5-9; Lk. 11:32; see Nah. 1:1, *note.*
o *Repentance.* Mk. 1:4. (Mt. 3:2; Acts 17:30.)
p 2 Chr. 9:1-12.
q Lk. 11:24-26.
r Cf. Mt. 24:34, *note.*

37 For by thy words thou shalt be justified, and by thy words thou shalt be
condemned.

The sign of the prophet Jonas: Jesus foretells his death and resurrection (Lk. 11:29-44).

38 Then certain of the scribes and of
the Pharisees answered, saying, Master,
we would see a [k]sign from thee.
39 But he answered and said unto
them, An evil and adulterous [l]genera-
tion seeketh after a sign; and there shall
no sign be given to it, but the sign of the
prophet Jonas:
40 For as [m]Jonas was three days and
three nights in the whale's belly; so shall
the Son of man be three days and three
nights in the heart of the earth.
41 [1]The men of [n]Nineveh shall rise in
judgment with this generation, and shall
condemn it: because they [o]repented at
the preaching of Jonas; and, behold, a
greater than Jonas *is* here.
42 [p]The queen of the south shall rise
up in the judgment with this generation,
and shall condemn it: for she came from
the uttermost parts of the earth to hear
the wisdom of Solomon; and, behold, a
greater than Solomon *is* here.

The worthlessness of self-reformation (Lk. 11:24-26).

43 [q]When the unclean spirit is gone
out of a man, he walketh through dry
places, seeking rest, and findeth none.
44 Then he saith, I will return into my
house from whence I came out; and
when he is come, he findeth *it* empty,
swept, and garnished.
45 Then goeth he, and taketh with
himself seven other spirits more wicked
than himself, and they enter in and
dwell there: and the last *state* of that man
is worse than the first. Even so shall it be
also unto this wicked [r]generation.

The new relationships (Mk. 3:31-35; Lk. 8:19-21).

46 [2]While he yet talked to the people,
behold, *his* mother and his brethren

[1]**(12:41)** Again the rejected King announces judgment (cf. Mt. 11:20-24). Israel, in the midst of the Pharisaic revival of outward religious strictness, was like a man out of whom a demon had "gone," i.e. of his own volition. He would come back and find an empty house, etc. The personal application is to a mere self-cleansed moralist.

[2]**(12:46)** Rejected by Israel, His "kinsmen according to the flesh" (cf. Rom. 9:3), our Lord intimates

stood without, desiring to speak with him.

47 Then one said unto him, Behold, [a]thy mother and thy brethren stand without, desiring to speak with thee.

48 But he answered and said unto him that told him, Who is my mother? and who are my brethren?

49 And he stretched forth his hand toward his disciples, and said, Behold my mother and my brethren!

50 For [b]whosoever shall do the will of my Father which is in heaven, the same is my brother, and sister, and mother.

CHAPTER 13.

The mysteries of the kingdom of heaven: (1) *the sower* (Mk. 4:1-20; Lk. 8:4-15).

The same day went Jesus out of the house, and sat by the sea side.

2 And great multitudes were gathered together unto him, so that he went into a ship, and sat; and the whole multitude stood on the shore.

3 And he [1]spake many things unto them in [c]parables, saying, Behold, a [2]sower went forth to sow;

4 And when he sowed, some *seeds* fell by the way side, and the fowls came and devoured them up:

5 Some fell upon stony places, where they had not much earth: and forthwith they sprung up, because they had no deepness of earth:

6 And when the sun was up, they were scorched; and because they had no root, they withered away.

7 And some fell among thorns; and the thorns sprung up, and choked them:

8 But other fell into good ground, and brought forth fruit, some an hundredfold, some sixtyfold, some thirtyfold.

9 Who hath ears to hear, let him hear.

10 And the disciples came, and said unto him, Why speakest thou unto them in parables?

11 He answered and said unto them, Because it is given unto you to know the [3][d]mysteries of the [e]kingdom of heaven, but to them it is not given.

12 For whosoever hath, to him shall be given, and he shall have more abundance: but whosoever hath not, from him shall be taken away even that he hath.

13 Therefore speak I to them in parables: [f]because they seeing see not; and hearing they hear not, neither do they understand.

A.D. 31.

a Mk. 3:31-35; Lk. 8:19-21.

b *Kingdom* (N.T.). Mt. 13:1-50. (Lk. 1:31-33; 1 Cor. 15:24.)

c *Parables* (N.T.). vs. 3-9, 18-23, 24-30, 36-43, 31, 32, 33, 44, 45, 46, 47-50; Mt. 18:12-14. (Mt. 5:13-16; Lk. 21:29-31.

d Mk. 4:10, 11; Lk. 8:9, 10.

e Mt. 3:2, *note.*

f John 7:16, 17; 8:43.

the formation of the new family of faith which, overstepping mere racial claims, receives "whosoever" will be His disciple (vs. 49, 50. Cf. John 6:28, 29).

[1] **(13:3)** The seven parables of Mt. 13, called by our Lord "mysteries of the kingdom of heaven" (v. 11), taken together, describe the result of the presence of the Gospel in the world during the present age, that is, the time of seed-sowing which began with our Lord's personal ministry, and ends with the "harvest" (vs. 40-43). Briefly, that result is the mingled tares and wheat, good fish and bad, in the sphere of Christian profession. It is Christendom.

[2] **(13:3)** The figure marks a new beginning. To labour in God's *vineyard* (Israel, Isa. 5:1-7) is one thing to go forth sowing the seed of the word in a field which is the *world,* quite another (cf. Mt. 10:5). One-fourth of the seed takes permanent root, but the result is "wheat" (v. 25; 1 Pet. 1:23), or "children of the kingdom" (v. 38). This parable (vs. 3-9, 18-23) is treated throughout as foundational to the mysteries of the kingdom of heaven. It is interpreted by our Lord Himself.

[3] **(13:11)** A "mystery" in Scripture is a previously hidden truth, now divinely revealed, but in which a supernatural element still remains despite the revelation. The greater mysteries are: (1) The mysteries of the kingdom of heaven (Mt. 13:3-50); (2) the mystery of Israel's blindness during this age (Rom. 11:25, with context); (3) the mystery of the translation of living saints at the end of this age (1 Cor. 15:51, 52; 1 Thes. 4:14-17); (4) the mystery of the N.T. church as one body composed of Jew and Gentile (Eph. 3:1-11; Rom. 16:25; Eph. 6:19; Col. 4:3); (5) the mystery of the church as the bride of Christ (Eph. 5:28-32); (6) the mystery of the inliving Christ (Gal. 2:20; Col. 1:26, 27); (7) the "mystery of God even Christ," i.e. Christ as the incarnate fullness of the Godhead embodied, in whom all the divine wisdom for man subsists (Col. 2:2, 9; 1 Cor. 2:7); (8) the mystery of the processes by which godlikeness is restored to man (1 Tim. 3:16); (9) the mystery of iniquity (2 Thes. 2:7; Mt. 13:33); (10) the mystery of the seven stars (Rev. 1:20); (11) the mystery of Babylon (Rev. 17:5, 7).

14 And in them is fulfilled the [a]prophecy of Esaias, which saith, By hearing ye shall hear, and shall not understand; and seeing ye shall see, and shall not perceive:
15 For this people's heart is waxed gross, and *their* ears are dull of hearing, and their eyes they have closed; lest at any time they should see with *their* eyes, and hear with *their* ears, and should understand with *their* heart, and should be [b]converted, and I should heal them.
16 But [c]blessed *are* your eyes, for they see: and your ears, for they hear.
17 For verily I say unto you, That many [1]prophets and [d]righteous *men* have desired to see *those things* which ye see, and have not seen *them;* and to hear *those things* which ye hear, and have not heard *them.*
18 Hear ye therefore the parable of the sower.
19 When any one heareth the word of the [e]kingdom, and understandeth *it* not, then cometh the wicked *one,* and catcheth away that which was sown in his heart. This is he which received seed by the way side.
20 But he that received the seed into stony places, the same is he that heareth the word, and [f]anon with joy receiveth it;
21 Yet hath he not root in himself, but dureth for a while: for when [g]tribulation or persecution ariseth because of the word, by and by he is offended.
22 He also that received seed among the thorns is he that heareth the word; and the care of this [h]world, and the deceitfulness of riches, choke the word, and he becometh unfruitful.
23 But [i]he that received seed into the good ground is he that heareth the word, and understandeth *it;* which also beareth [j]fruit, and bringeth forth, some an hundredfold, some sixty, some thirty.

Second mystery, the tares among the wheat (vs. 24-30, 36-43).

24 [2]Another parable put he forth unto them, saying, [e]The kingdom of heaven is likened unto a man which sowed [k]good seed in his field:
25 But while men slept, his enemy came and sowed [l]tares among the wheat, and went his way.
26 But when the blade was sprung up, and brought forth fruit, then appeared the tares also.
27 So the servants of the householder came and said unto him, Sir, didst not thou sow good seed in thy field? from whence then hath it tares?
28 He said unto them, An enemy hath done this. The servants said unto him,

A.D. 31.

a Isa. 6:9, 10; Mk. 4:12; Lk. 8:10; John 12:39-41.
b i.e. *turn again.*
c Lk. 8:11-15; 10:23, 24.
d *Righteousness.* Rom. 10:10, *note.*
e Mt. 3:2, *note.*
f *at once.*
g Cf. Heb. 6:4-6 with 10:34; Acts 14:22.
h i.e. *age.*
i Lk. 8:15.
j John 15:5; Phil. 1:11; Col. 1:6.
k 2 Tim. 3:15-17; 1 Pet. 1:23; 1 John 3:9.
l Acts 20:29, 30.

[1] **(13:17)** The O.T. prophets saw in one blended vision the rejection and crucifixion of the King (see "Christ, sacrifice," Gen. 4:4; Heb. 10:18, note), and also His glory as David's Son (Zech. 12:8, note), but "what manner of *time* the Spirit of Christ which was in them did signify when it testified beforehand the sufferings of Christ and the glory that should follow," was not revealed to them—only that the vision was not for themselves (1 Pet. 1:10-12). That revelation Christ makes in these parables. A period of time is to intervene between His sufferings and His glory. That interval is occupied with the "mysteries of the kingdom of heaven" here described.

[2] **(13:24)** This parable (vs. 24-30) is also interpreted by our Lord (vs. 36-43). Here the "good seed" is not the "word," as in the first parable (vs. 19, 23), but rather that which the word has produced (1 Pet. 1:23), viz.: the children of the kingdom. These are, providentially (v. 37), "sown," i.e. scattered, here and there in the "field" of the "world" (v. 38). The "world" here is both geographical and ethnic—the earth-world, and also the world of men. The wheat of God at once becomes the scene of Satan's activity. Where children of the kingdom are gathered, there "among the wheat" (vs. 25, 38, 39), Satan "sows" "children of the wicked one," who profess to be children of the kingdom, and in outward ways are so like the true children that only the angels may, in the end, be trusted to separate them (vs. 28-30, 40-43). So great is Satan's power of deception that the tares often really suppose themselves to be children of the kingdom (Mt. 7:21-23). Many other parables and exhortations have this mingled condition in view (e.g. Mt. 22:11-14; 25:1-13, 14-30; Lk. 18:10-14; Heb. 6:4-9). Indeed, it characterizes Matthew from Chapter 13 to the end. The parable of the wheat and tares is not a description of the world, but of that which professes to be the kingdom. Mere unbelievers are never called children of the devil, but only *religious* unbelievers are so called (cf. v. 38; John 8:38-44; Mt. 23:15).

Wilt thou then that we go and gather
them up?
29 But he said, Nay; lest while ye gather up the tares, ye root up also the wheat
with them.
30 Let [a]both grow together until the
harvest: and in the time of harvest I will
say to the reapers, [1]Gather ye together
first the tares, and bind them in bundles
to burn them: but gather the wheat into
my barn.

Third mystery, the grain of mustard seed (Mk. 4:30-32).

31 [2]Another parable put he forth unto
them, saying, The [b]kingdom of heaven is
like to a grain of [c]mustard seed, which a
man took, and sowed in his field:
32 Which indeed is the least of all
seeds: but when it is grown, it is the
greatest among herbs, and becometh a
[d]tree, so that the birds of the air come
and lodge in the branches thereof.

Fourth mystery, the leaven (Lk. 13:20,21).

33 [3]Another parable spake he unto
them; The kingdom of heaven is like
unto [4e]leaven, which a woman took, and
[f]hid in [g]three measures of meal, till the
[h]whole was leavened.
34 All these things spake Jesus unto
the multitude in parables; and without a
parable spake he not unto them:
35 That it might be [i]fulfilled which
was spoken by the prophet, saying, I
will open my mouth in parables; I will

A.D. 31.

a Phil. 3:18, 19; 2 Thes. 3:6; 2 Tim. 2:19.

b Mt. 3:2, *note.*

c Mk. 4:30-32; Lk. 13:18, 19; Acts 1:15.

d Ezk. 17:22-24; 31:3-9; cf. Dan. 4:20-22.

e *Leaven* (Gen. 19:3.)

f v. 25; Gal. 2:4; 3:1.

g Num. 15:8, 9; John 6:32-35.

h 1 Cor. 5:6; 15:33; Gal. 5:6-9.

i Psa. 78:2.

[1] **(13:30)** The gathering of the tares into bundles for burning does not imply immediate judgment. At the end of this age (v. 40) the tares are set apart for burning, but first the wheat is gathered into the barn (John 14:3; 1 Thes. 4:14-17).

[2] **(13:31)** The parable of the Mustard Seed prefigures the rapid but unsubstantial growth of the mystery form of the kingdom from an insignificant beginning (Acts 1:15; 2:41; 1 Cor. 1:26) to a great place in the earth. The figure of the fowls finding shelter in the branches is drawn from Dan. 4:20-22. How insecure was such a refuge the context in Daniel shows.

[3] **(13:33)** That interpretation of the parable of the Leaven (v. 33) which makes (with variation as to details) the leaven to be the Gospel, introduced into the world ("three measures of meal") by the church, and working subtly until the world is converted ("till the whole was leavened") is open to fatal objection: (1) It does violence to the unvarying symbolical meaning of leaven, and especially to the meaning fixed by our Lord Himself (Mt. 16:6-12; Mk. 8:15: See "Leaven," Gen. 19:3; Mt. 13:33, *note*). (2) The implication of a converted world in this age ("till the whole was leavened"), is explicitly contradicted by our Lord's interpretation of the parables of the Wheat and Tares, and of the Net. Our Lord presents a picture of a partly converted kingdom in an unconverted world; of good fish and bad in the very kingdom-net itself. (3) The method of the extension of the kingdom is given in the first parable. It is by sowing seed, not by mingling leaven. The symbols have, in Scripture, a meaning fixed by inspired usage. Leaven is the principle of corruption working subtly; is invariably used in a bad sense (see "Leaven," Gen. 19:3, *refs.*), and is defined by our Lord as evil doctrine (Mt. 16:11, 12; Mk. 8:15). Meal, on the contrary, was used in one of the sweet-savour offerings (Lev. 2:1-3), and was food for the priests (Lev. 6:15-17). A woman, in the bad ethical sense, always symbolizes something out of place *religiously* (see Zech. 5:6, *note*). In Thyatira it was a woman teaching (cf. Rev. 2:20 with Rev. 17:1-6). Interpreting the parable by these familiar symbols, it constitutes a warning that the true doctrine given for the nourishment of the children of the kingdom (Mt. 4:4; 1 Tim. 4:6; 1 Pet. 2:2), would be mingled with corrupt and corrupting false doctrine, and that officially, by the apostate church itself (1 Tim. 4:1-3; 2 Tim. 2:17, 18; 4:3, 4; 2 Pet. 2:1-3).

[4] **(13:33)** Summary: (1) Leaven, as a symbolic or typical substance, is always mentioned in the O.T. in an evil sense (Gen. 19:3, *refs.*). (2) The use of the word in the N.T. explains its symbolic meaning. It is "malice and wickedness," as contrasted with "sincerity and truth" (1 Cor. 5:6-8). It is evil doctrine (Mt. 16:12) in its threefold form of Pharisaism, Sadduceeism, and Herodianism (Mt. 16:6; Mk. 8:15). The leaven of the Pharisees was externalism in religion (Mt. 23:14, 16, 23-28); of the Sadducees, scepticism as to the supernatural and as to the Scriptures (Mt. 22:23, 29); of the Herodians, worldliness—a Herod party amongst the Jews (Mt. 22:16-21; Mk. 3:6). (3) The use of the word in Mt. 13:33 is congruous with its universal meaning.

utter things which have been kept secret
from the foundation of the [a]world.

The second mystery explained.

36 Then Jesus sent the multitude away,
and went into the house: and his disciples came unto him, saying, [b]Declare
unto us the parable of the tares of the
field.
37 He answered and said unto them,
He that soweth the good seed is the Son
of man;
38 The field is the [c]world; the good
seed are the children of the [d]kingdom;
but the tares are the children of the
wicked *one*;
39 The enemy that sowed them is the
[e]devil; the harvest is the [f]end of the
world; and the reapers are the [g]angels.
40 As therefore the tares are gathered
and burned in the fire; so shall it be in
the [f]end of this world.
41 The [h]Son of man shall send forth
his [g]angels, and they shall [i]gather out of
his [d]kingdom all things that offend, and
[j]them which do [k]iniquity;
42 And shall cast them into a furnace
of fire: there shall be wailing and [l]gnash-
ing of teeth.
43 [1]Then shall the [m]righteous shine
forth as the sun in the kingdom of their
Father. [n]Who hath ears to hear, let him
hear.

Fifth mystery, the hid treasure.

44 Again, the [d]kingdom of heaven is
like unto [o]treasure [2]hid in a field; the
which when a man hath found, he
hideth, and for joy thereof goeth and
[p]selleth all that he hath, and buyeth that
field.

Sixth mystery, the pearl.

45 Again, the [d]kingdom of heaven is
like unto a merchant man, seeking goodly [3]pearls:
46 Who, when he had found [q]one
pearl of great price, went and sold all
that he had, and bought it.

Seventh mystery, the drag-net.

47 Again, [4]the kingdom of [d]heaven is
like unto a net, that was cast into the sea,
and gathered of every kind:
48 Which, when it was full, they drew

A.D. 31.

a i.e. *earth.*
b Mk. 4:13, 33, 34.
c *kosmos* (Mt. 4:8), = mankind.
d Mt. 3:2, *note.*
e *Satan.* Gr. *diabolos, accuser.* Mt. 16:23. (Gen. 3:1; Rev. 20:10.)
f *consummation of the age.* Mt. 24:3.
g Heb. 1:4, *note.*
h See Mt. 8:20, *note.*
i Lk. 17:26-37.
j *Sin.* Rom. 3:23, *note.*
k i.e. *lawlessness.*
l *Judgments (the seven).* Mt. 16:27. (2 Sam. 7:14; Rev. 20:12.)
m Rom. 10:10, *note.* Col. 3:4; 2 Thes. 1:5-10.
n v. 15; Acts 28:26; Rev. 2:7.
o Ex. 19:5; Deut. 4:20.
p Isa. 53:4-10; Psa. 22:1; 2 Cor. 8:9.
q Eph. 5:25-27; Rev. 21:21.

[1] **(13:43)** The kingdom does not become the kingdom of the "Father" until Christ, having "put all enemies under His feet," including the last enemy, death, has "delivered up the kingdom to God, *even the Father*" (1 Cor. 15:24-28; Rev. 20:2). There is triumph over death at the first resurrection (1 Cor. 15:54, 55), but death, "the last enemy," is not *destroyed* till the end of the millennium (Rev. 20:14).

[2] **(13:44)** The interpretation of the parable of the treasure, which makes the buyer of the field to be a sinner who is seeking Christ, has no warrant in the parable itself. The field is defined (v. 38) to be the world. The seeking sinner does not buy, but forsakes, the world to win Christ. Furthermore, the sinner has nothing to sell, nor is Christ for sale, nor is He hidden in a field, nor, having found Christ, does the sinner hide Him again (cf. Mk. 7:24; Acts 4:20). At every point the interpretation breaks down.

Our Lord is the buyer at the awful cost of His blood (1 Pet. 1:18), and Israel, especially Ephraim (Jer. 31:5-12, 18-20), the lost tribes hidden in "the field," the world (v. 38), is the treasure (Ex. 19:5; Psa. 135:4). Again, as in the separation of tares and wheat, the angels are used (Mt. 24:31; Jer. 16:16). The divine Merchantman buys the field (world) for the sake of the treasure (v. 44; Rom. 11:28), beloved for the fathers' sakes, and yet to be restored and saved. The note of joy (v. 44) is also that of the prophets in view of Israel's restoration (Deut. 30:9; Isa. 49:13; 52:1-3; 62:4-7; 65:18, 19). (See "Israel," Gen. 11:10; Rom. 11:26.)

[3] **(13:45)** The true Church, "one body" formed by the Holy Spirit (1 Cor. 12:12, 13). As Israel is the hid treasure, so the Church is the pearl of great cost. Covering the same period of time as the mysteries of the kingdom, is the mystery of the Church (Rom. 16:25, 26; Eph. 3:3-10; 5:32). Of the true Church a pearl is a perfect symbol: (1) A pearl is one, a perfect symbol of unity (1 Cor. 10:17; 12:12, 13; Eph. 4:4-6). (2) A pearl is formed by accretion, and that not mechanically, but vitally, through a living one, as Christ adds to the Church (Acts 2:41, 47; 5:14; 11:24; Eph. 2:21; Col. 2:19). (3) Christ, having given Himself for the pearl, is now preparing it for presentation to Himself (Eph. 5:25-27). The kingdom is not the Church, but the true children of the kingdom during the fulfilment of these mysteries, baptized by one Spirit into one body (1 Cor. 12:12, 13), compose the true Church, the pearl.

[4] **(13:47)** The parable of the Net (Gr. *drag-net*) presents another view from that of the wheat and tares

to shore, and sat down, and [a]gathered
the good into vessels, but cast the bad
away.
49 So shall it be at the [b]end of the
world: the angels shall come forth, and
sever the wicked from among the just,
50 And shall cast them into the [c]fur-
nace of fire: there shall be wailing and
gnashing of [d]teeth.
51 Jesus saith unto them, Have ye
understood all these things? They say
unto him, Yea, Lord.
52 Then said he unto them, Therefore
every scribe *which is* instructed unto the
kingdom of heaven is like unto a man *that
is* an householder, which bringeth forth
out of his treasure *things* new and old.

Jesus returns to Nazareth: again rejected (Mk. 6:1-6; cf. Lk. 4:16-32).

53 And it came to pass, *that* when
Jesus had finished these parables, he
departed thence.
54 And when he was come into his
own country, he taught them in their synagogue, insomuch that they were [e]aston-
ished, and said, Whence hath this *man*
this wisdom, and *these* mighty works?
55 Is not this the [f]carpenter's son? is
not his mother called Mary? and his
brethren, [g]James, and Joses, and Simon,
and Judas?
56 And his sisters, are they not all with
us? Whence then hath this *man* all these
things?
57 And they were offended in him.
But Jesus said unto them, A prophet is
not without honour, save in his own
country, and in his own house.
58 And he did not many mighty
works there [h]because of their unbelief.

CHAPTER 14.

Herod's troubled conscience. Murder of John the Baptist. (Mk. 6:14-29; Lk. 9:7-9).

At that time [i]Herod the tetrarch heard
of the fame of Jesus,
2 And said unto his servants, This is
John the Baptist; he is risen from the
dead; and therefore mighty works do
shew forth themselves in him.
3 For [j]Herod had laid hold on John, and
bound him, and put *him* in prison for
[k]Herodias' sake, his brother Philip's wife.
4 For John said unto him, It is not lawful for thee to have her.
5 And when he would have put him
to death, he feared the multitude,
because they counted him as a prophet.
6 But when Herod's birthday was
kept, the daughter of Herodias danced
before them, and pleased Herod.
7 Whereupon he promised with an
oath to give her whatsoever she would
ask.
8 And she, being before instructed of
her mother, said, Give me here John
Baptist's head in a charger.
9 And the king was [l]sorry: nevertheless for the oath's sake, and them which
sat with him at meat, he commanded *it*
to be given *her*.
10 And he sent, and beheaded John in
the prison.
11 And his head was brought in a
charger, and given to the damsel: and
she brought *it* to her mother.
12 And his disciples came, and took

A.D. 32.

a Mt. 24:31; 25:31-46.
b *Consummation of the age.* Mt. 24:3.
c v. 42; Rev. 19:20.
d *Kingdom* (N.T.). vs. 1-50; Mt. 15:21-28. (Lk. 1:31-33; 1 Cor. 15:24.)
e John 7:15.
f John 6:42; 7:41, 48, 52.
g Son of Alphaeus, Mt. 4:21, *note.*
h Mk. 6:5, 6; John 5:44, 46, 47.
i Called Antipas; son of Herod the Great (Mt. 2:1, *note*) and Malthace, a Samaritan woman; brother of Archelaus (Mt. 2:22). *Mar.* (1) a daughter of King Aretas; (2) Herodias, wife of his half-brother, Philip.
j vs. 1, 6.
k See Lk. 3:1, *refs.*
l Prov. 29:25; Lk. 18:23; Acts 7:52.

of the mysteries of the kingdom as the sphere of profession, but with this difference: there Satan was the active agent; here the admixture is more the result of the tendency of a movement to gather to itself that which is not really of it. The kingdom of heaven is like a net which, cast into the sea of humanity, gathers of every kind, good and bad. And these remain together *in the net* (v. 49), and not merely in the sea, until the end of the age. It is not even a converted net, much less a converted sea. Infinite violence has been done to sound exegesis by the notion that the world is to be converted *in this age.* Against that notion stands our Lord's own interpretation of the Parables of the Sower, the Wheat and Tares, and the Net.

Such, then, is the mystery form of the kingdom (see Mt. 3:2, *note;* 6:33, *note*). It is the sphere of Christian profession during this age. It is a mingled body of true and false, wheat and tares, good and bad. It is defiled by formalism, doubt, and worldliness. But within it Christ sees the true children of the true kingdom who, at the end, are to "shine forth as the sun." In the great field, the world, He sees the redeemed of all ages, but especially His hidden Israel, yet to be restored and blessed. Also, in this form of the kingdom, so unlike that which is to be, He sees the Church, His body and bride, and for joy He sells all that He has (2 Cor. 8:9) and buys the field, the treasure, and the pearl.

up the body, and buried it, and went and [a]told Jesus.

13 When Jesus heard *of it,* he [b]departed thence by [c]ship into a desert place apart: and when the people had heard *thereof,* they followed him on foot out of the cities.

14 And Jesus went forth, and saw a great multitude, and was moved with [d]compassion toward them, and he healed their sick.

The five thousand fed (Mk. 6:32-44; Lk. 9:10-17; John 6:1-14).

15 And when it was evening, his disciples came to him, saying, This is a desert place, and the time is now past; send the multitude away, that they may go into the villages, and buy themselves victuals.

16 But Jesus said unto them, They need not depart; [e]give ye them to eat.

17 And they say unto him, We have here but five loaves, and two fishes.

18 He said, [f]Bring them hither to me.

19 And he commanded the multitude to sit down on the grass, and took the [g]five loaves, and the two fishes, and looking up to heaven, he [h]blessed, and brake, and gave the loaves to *his* disciples, and the disciples to the multitude.

20 [i]And they did all eat, and were filled: and they took up of the fragments that [j]remained twelve baskets full.

21 And they that had eaten were about five thousand men, beside women and children.

Jesus walks on the water: Peter's little faith (Mk. 6:45-56; John 6:15-21).

22 And straightway Jesus constrained his disciples to get into a ship, and to go before him unto the other side, while he sent the multitudes away.

23 And when he had sent the multitudes away, he went up into a [k]mountain apart to pray: and when the evening was come, he was there alone.

24 But the ship was now in the midst of the sea, [l]tossed with waves: for the wind was contrary.

25 And in the fourth watch of the night Jesus went unto them, walking on the sea.

26 And when the disciples saw him walking on the sea, they were [m]troubled, saying, It is a spirit; and they cried out for fear.

A.D. 32.

a John 1:35-37; 11:21.
b Mt. 12:15; Mk. 6:32-46.
c *boat.*
d Mt. 9:36.
e Mt. 10:8; 2 Cor. 4:5, 6.
f Mt. 28:18.
g John 6:1-14.
h John 6:23; 11:41, 42; 1 Cor. 11:24.
i *Miracles* (N.T.). vs. 19-21, 24-33, 35, 36; Mt. 15:21-28. (Mt. 8:2, 3; Acts 28:8, 9.)
j 2 Ki. 4:1-7, 42-44; Mt. 15:27.
k Mk. 6:46; Lk. 5:16.
l Mk. 6:47-52; John 6:16-21.
m Lk. 24:36-40; John 14:27; 16:33.
n John 14:27; 16:33.
o Lk. 8:24, 25.
p Mt. 8:25.
q Mt. 8:26.
r Mt. 16:16; 27:54; Psa. 46:10; John 1:49.
s Mk. 5:24, 34.
t Mt. 23:16-18; Mk. 7:1-23.
u Mt. 23:23; John 18:28; *contra,* Rom. 3:31.
v Ex. 20:12; Jer. 35:18, 19.
w Ex. 21:17.
x *surely die.* See Lev. 20:9; Deut. 27:16; Prov. 30:17. Cf. 1 Tim. 5:4-8.
y i.e. dedicated to God. Mt. 5:23, 24. See Mk. 7:11, *ref.*

27 But straightway Jesus spake unto them, saying, [n]Be of good cheer; it is I; be not afraid.

28 And Peter answered him and said, Lord, if it be thou, bid me come unto thee on the water.

29 And he said, Come. And when Peter was come down out of the ship, he walked on the water, to go to Jesus.

30 But when he saw the [o]wind boisterous, he was afraid; and beginning to sink, [p]he cried, saying, Lord, save me.

31 And immediately Jesus stretched forth *his* hand, and caught him, and said unto him, O thou of [q]little faith, wherefore didst thou doubt?

32 And when they were come into the ship, the wind ceased.

33 Then they that were in the ship came and worshipped him, saying, Of a truth thou art the [r]Son of God.

34 And when they were gone over, they came into the land of Gennesaret.

35 And when the men of that place had knowledge of him, they sent out into all that country round about, and brought unto him all that were diseased;

36 And besought him that they might only [s]touch the hem of his garment: and as many as touched were made perfectly whole.

CHAPTER 15.

Jesus rebukes scribes and Pharisees (Mk. 7:1-23).

Then came to Jesus scribes and Pharisees, which were of Jerusalem, saying,

2 Why do thy disciples transgress the [t]tradition of the elders? for they wash not their hands when they eat bread.

3 But he answered and said unto them, Why do ye also transgress the [u]commandment of God by your tradition?

4 For God commanded, saying, [v]Honour thy father and mother: and, [w]He that curseth father or mother, let him [x]die the death.

5 But ye say, Whosoever shall say to *his* father or *his* mother, *It is* a [y]gift, by whatsoever thou mightest be profited by me;

6 And honour not his father or his mother, *he shall be free.* Thus have ye

made the commandment of God of none effect by your tradition.

7 *Ye* hypocrites, well did [a]Esaias prophesy of you, saying,

8 This people draweth nigh unto me with their [b]mouth, and honoureth me with *their* lips; but their heart is far from me.

9 But in vain they do worship me, teaching *for* doctrines the commandments of men.

10 And he called the multitude, and said unto them, Hear, and understand:

11 [c]Not that which goeth into the mouth defileth a man; but that which [d]cometh out of the mouth, this defileth a man.

12 Then came his disciples, and said unto him, Knowest thou that the Pharisees were offended, after they heard this saying?

13 But he answered and said, Every plant, which my heavenly Father hath not planted, shall be [e]rooted up.

14 Let them alone: they be blind leaders of the blind. And if the blind lead the blind, both shall fall into the ditch.

15 Then answered Peter and said unto him, Declare unto us this parable.

16 And Jesus said, Are ye also [f]yet without understanding?

17 Do not ye yet understand, that whatsoever entereth in at the mouth goeth into the belly, and is cast out into the draught?

18 But those things which proceed out of the mouth come forth from the [g]heart; and they defile the man.

19 For out of the heart proceed [h]evil thoughts, murders, adulteries, fornications, thefts, false witness, blasphemies:

20 These are *the things* which defile a man: but to eat with unwashen hands defileth not a man.

The Syrophenician woman's daughter healed (Mk. 7:24-30).

21 Then Jesus went thence, and [1]departed into the coasts of Tyre and Sidon.

22 And, behold, a woman of Canaan came out of the same coasts, and [i]cried unto him, saying, Have mercy on me, O Lord, *thou* [j]son of David; my daughter is grievously vexed with a devil.

23 But he answered her not a word. And his disciples came and besought him, saying, Send her away; for she crieth after us.

24 But he answered and said, I am not sent but unto the [k]lost sheep of the house of Israel.

25 Then came she and worshipped him, saying, Lord, [l]help me.

26 But he answered and said, It is not meet to take the children's bread, and to cast *it* to [m]dogs.

27 And she said, Truth, Lord: yet the [n]dogs eat of the crumbs which fall from their masters' table.

28 [o]Then Jesus answered and said unto her, O woman, [p]great *is* thy faith: be it unto thee even [q]as thou wilt. And her daughter was made [r]whole from that very hour.

The multitudes healed. (Cf. Mk. 7:31-37.)

29 And Jesus departed from thence, and came nigh unto the sea of Galilee; and went up into a mountain, and sat down there.

30 And great multitudes came unto him, having with them *those that were* lame, blind, dumb, maimed, and many others, and [s]cast them down at Jesus' feet; and he healed them:

31 Insomuch that the multitude wondered, when they saw the dumb to speak, the maimed to be whole, the lame to walk, and the blind to see: and they [t]glorified the God of Israel.

The four thousand fed (Mk. 8:1-9).

32 Then Jesus called his disciples *unto him*, and said, I have [u]compassion on the multitude, because they continue with me now three days, and have nothing to eat: and I will not send them away fasting, lest they faint in the way.

33 And his disciples say unto him, Whence should we have so much bread in the wilderness, as to fill so great a multitude?

34 And Jesus saith unto them, How

A.D. 32.

a Isa. 29:13; Ezk. 33:31.
b vs. 8, 9; Isa. 29:13.
c Rom. 14:14-23; Col. 2:20, 23.
d Jer. 17:9, 10; Rom. 3:10-18; Tit. 1:15.
e Mt. 5:20; Acts 15:10.
f Or, *even yet.*
g Gen. 6:5; Jer. 17:9, 10; Jas. 3:10-12.
h Prov. 6:14; Gal. 5:19-21.
i *Bible prayers* (N.T.). Mt. 26:39. (Mt. 6:9; Rev. 22:20.)
j Mt. 1:1; 22:41, 42; Psa. 132:11.
k Gr. *apollumi.* John 3:16, *note.*
l Psa. 145:18.
m Mt. 7:6; John 4:22.
n Lit. *little dogs.*
o *Kingdom* (N.T.). vs. 21-28; Mt. 16:20, 21. (Lk. 1:31-33; 1 Cor. 15:24.)
p Lk. 7:7, 9; cf. Mk. 6:6. Faith honours God, knowing that he is faithful; cf. 1 John 5:10.
q Mt. 9:27-29; 21:21, 22.
r *Miracles* (N.T.). vs. 21-28, 32-39; Mt. 17:14-18. (Mt. 8:2, 3; Acts 28:8, 9.)
s Mk. 7:25; Lk. 7:38; 8:41; 10:39.
t Mt. 11:20-24; Lk. 5:25, 26; 19:37, 38.
u Mt. 9:36-38; Mk. 8:1-9.

1 (15:21) For the first time the rejected Son of David ministers to a Gentile. It is a precursive fulfilment of Mt. 12:18. Addressed by a Gentile as Son of David, He makes no reply, for a Gentile has no claim upon Him in that character (see Mt. 2:2, *note;* Eph. 2:12). Addressing Him as "Lord," she obtained an immediate answer. See Rom. 10:12, 13.

many loaves have ye? And they said, [a]Seven, and a few little fishes.

35 And he commanded the multitude to sit down on the ground.

36 And he took the seven loaves and the fishes, and gave thanks, and brake *them*, and gave to his disciples, and the disciples to the multitude.

37 And they did all eat, and were filled: and they took up of the broken *meat* that was left [b]seven baskets full.

38 And they that did eat were [c]four thousand men, beside women and children.

39 And he sent away the multitude, and took ship, and came into the coasts of Magdala.

CHAPTER 16.

Jesus rebukes the blind Pharisees (Mk. 8:10-12).

The Pharisees also with the Sadducees came, and [d]tempting desired him that he would shew them [e]a sign from heaven.

2 He answered and said unto them, When it is [f]evening, ye say, *It will be* fair weather: for the sky is red.

3 And in the morning, *It will be* foul weather to day: for the sky is red and lowring. O *ye* hypocrites, ye can discern the face of the sky; but can ye not *discern* the signs of the times?

4 A [g]wicked and adulterous generation seeketh after a sign; and there shall no sign be given unto it, but the sign of the prophet Jonas. And he left them, and departed.

5 And when his disciples were come to the other side, they had forgotten to take bread.

Jesus interprets the symbol of leaven (Mk. 8:13-21).

6 Then Jesus said unto them, Take heed and beware of the [h]leaven of the Pharisees and of the Sadducees.

7 And they reasoned among themselves, saying, *It is* because we have taken no bread.

8 *Which* when Jesus perceived, he said unto them, O ye of little faith, why reason ye among yourselves, because ye have brought no bread?

9 Do ye not [i]yet understand, neither remember the five loaves of the five thousand, and how many baskets ye took up?

10 Neither the seven loaves of the four thousand, and how many [j]baskets ye took up?

11 How is it that ye do not understand that I spake *it* not to you concerning bread, that ye should beware of the [k]leaven of the Pharisees and of the Sadducees?

12 Then understood they how that he bade *them* not beware of the leaven of bread, but of the doctrine of the Pharisees and of the Sadducees.

Peter's confession. (Cf. Mk. 8:27-30; Lk. 9:18-21; John 6:68, 69.)

13 When Jesus came into the coasts of [l]Caesarea Philippi, he asked his disciples, saying, Whom do men say that I the [m]Son of man am?

14 And they said, Some *say that thou art* John the Baptist: some, Elias; and others, Jeremias, or one of the prophets.

15 He saith unto them, But whom say [n]ye that I am?

16 And Simon Peter answered and said, Thou art the [o]Christ, the Son of the living God.

First mention of the church.

17 And Jesus answered and said unto him, [p]Blessed art thou, Simon [q]Bar-jona: for [r]flesh and blood hath not revealed *it* unto thee, but my Father which is in heaven.

18 And I say also unto thee, That thou art [1]Peter, and upon this rock I will build my [2s]church; and the gates of [t]hell shall not prevail against it.

A.D. 32.

a v. 37; Mt. 14:17.
b Mt. 14:20.
c Mt. 14:21.
d *Temptation.* Mt. 19:3. (Gen. 3:1; Jas. 1:14.)
e Mt. 12:38-41; Mk. 8:10-13.
f Lk. 12:54-57.
g Mt. 21:23-27.
h *Leaven.* vs. 6, 11, 12; Lk. 12:1. (Gen. 19:3; Mt. 13:33.)
i John 12:37.
j A different Gr. word from that translated "baskets" in v. 9.
k Gal. 1:6-9; Col. 2:4, 18.
l Mk. 8:27-33; Lk. 9:18-22.
m Also vs. 27, 28. See Mt. 8:20, *note.*
n John 6:67.
o Mt. 14:33; John 6:69; 11:27; Acts 9:20.
p Mt. 11:27; 1 John 4:15; 5:1, 5; John 1:12, 13.
q *Son of Jonas.*
r John 6:63.
s *Church (the true).* Acts 2:47. (Mt. 16:18; Heb. 12:23.)
t Gr. *hades.* Lk. 16:23, *note.*

[1] **(16:18)** There is in the Greek a play upon the words, "thou art Peter [*petros*—literally 'a little rock'], and upon this rock [*Petra*] I will build my church." He does not promise to build His church upon Peter, but upon Himself, as Peter himself is careful to tell us (1 Pet. 2:4-9).

[2] **(16:18)** Gr. *ecclesia* (*ek* = "out of," *kaleo* = "to call"), an assembly of called-out ones. The word is used of any assembly, the word itself implies no more, as, e.g., the town-meeting at Ephesus (Acts 19:39), and Israel, called out of Egypt and assembled in the wilderness (Acts 7:38). Israel was a true "church," but not in any sense the N.T. church—the only point of similarity being that both were "called out" and by the same God. All else is contrast. See Acts 7:38, *note;* Heb. 12:23, *note.*

19 And I will give unto thee the [1]keys of the [a]kingdom of heaven: and whatsoever thou shalt bind on earth shall be bound in heaven: and whatsoever thou shalt loose on earth shall be loosed in heaven.

20 Then [2b]charged he his disciples that they should tell no man that he was [c]Jesus the Christ.

Christ foretells his death and resurrection (Mk. 8:31-38; Lk. 9:22-27).

21 From that time forth began Jesus to shew unto his disciples, how that he must go unto Jerusalem, and [d]suffer many things of the elders and chief priests and scribes, and be killed, and be raised again the third day.

22 Then Peter took him, and began to [e]rebuke him, saying, Be it far from thee, Lord: this shall not be unto thee.

23 But he turned, and said unto Peter, Get thee behind me, [f]Satan: thou art an [g]offence unto me: for thou savourest not the things that be of God, but those that be of men.

24 Then said Jesus unto his disciples, If any *man* will come after me, let him deny himself, and take up his [h]cross, and follow me.

25 For whosoever will save his life shall lose it: and whosoever will lose his life for my sake shall find it.

26 For what is a man [i]profited, if he shall gain the whole [j]world, and lose his own soul? or what shall a man give in exchange for his soul?

A.D. 32.

- a Mt. 3:2, *note.*
- b *Kingdom* (N.T.). vs. 20, 21; Mt. 16:28. (Lk. 1:31-33; 1 Cor. 15:28.)
- c Omit "Jesus."
- d Mt. 17:12.
- e v. 16; John 13:36-38.
- f *Satan,* Mt. 25:41. (Gen. 3:1; Rev. 20:10.)
- g Gal. 1:8; John 18:10, 11.
- h Mk. 8:34-38; Lk. 9:23-26; 2 Cor. 4:10, 11.
- i Mk. 8:36, 37; Lk. 12:20, 21; Jas. 5:1-6.
- j i.e. *kosmos* = world-system.
- k *Rewards.* Mk. 9:41. (Dan. 12:3; 1 Cor. 3:14.)
- l *Judgments (the seven).* Mt. 25:31-46. (2 Sam. 7:14; Rev. 20:12.)
- m *Kingdom* (N.T.). Mt. 17:1-3. (Lk. 1:31-33; 1 Cor. 15:24.)
- n Mk. 9:2-10; Lk. 9:27-36.
- o See Mt. 4:21, *note.*
- p Rev. 1:13-16; Heb. 2:9; 2 Cor. 4:6.
- q *Resurrection.* Mt. 22:23, 28-31. (Job 19:25; 1 Cor. 15:52.)
- r *Kingdom* (N.T.). vs. 1-3; Mt. 19:27, 28. (Lk. 1:31-33; 1 Cor. 15:28.)
- s Mt. 3:17; 1 Pet. 1:21.

27 For the Son of man shall come in the glory of his Father with his angels; and then he shall [k]reward every man [l]according to his works.

The transfiguration: a picture of the future kingdom (Mk. 9:2-13; Lk. 9:28-36).

28 Verily I say unto you, There be some standing here, which shall not taste of death, till they see the Son of man coming in [a]his [m]kingdom.

CHAPTER 17.

And [n]after six days Jesus taketh Peter, [o]James, and John his brother, and bringeth them up into an high mountain apart,

2 And [3]was [p]transfigured before them: and his face did shine as the sun, and his raiment was white as the light.

3 And, behold, there appeared unto them [q]Moses and Elias talking with [r]him.

4 Then answered Peter, and said unto Jesus, Lord, it is good for us to be here: if thou wilt, let us make here three tabernacles; one for thee, and one for Moses, and one for Elias.

5 While he yet spake, behold, a bright cloud overshadowed them: and behold a voice out of the cloud, which said, This is my beloved [s]Son, in whom I am well pleased; hear ye him.

6 And when the disciples heard *it,* they fell on their face, and were sore afraid.

7 And Jesus came and touched them, and said, Arise, and be not afraid.

[1] **(16:19)** Not the keys of the church, but of the kingdom of heaven in the sense of Mt. 13, i.e. the sphere of Christian profession. A key is a badge of power or authority (cf. Isa. 22:22; Rev. 3:7). The apostolic history explains and limits this trust, for it was Peter who opened the door of Christian opportunity to Israel on the day of Pentecost (Acts 2:38-42), and to Gentiles in the house of Cornelius (Acts 10:34-46). There was no assumption by Peter of any other authority (Acts 15:7-11). In the council James, not Peter, seems to have presided (Acts 15:19; cf. Gal. 2:11-15). Peter claimed no more for himself than to be an apostle by gift (1 Pet. 1:1), and an elder by office (1 Pet. 5:1).

The power of binding and loosing was shared (Mt. 18:18; John 20:23) by the other disciples. That it did not involve the determination of the eternal destiny of souls is clear from Rev. 1:18. The keys of death and the place of departed spirits are held by Christ alone.

[2] **(16:20)** The disciples had been proclaiming Jesus as the Christ, i.e. the covenanted King of a kingdom promised to the Jews, and "at hand." The church, on the contrary, must be built upon testimony to Him as crucified, risen from the dead, ascended, and made "Head over all things to the church" (Eph. 1:20-23). The former testimony was ended, the new testimony was not yet ready, because the blood of the new covenant had not yet been shed, but our Lord begins to speak of His death and resurrection (v. 21). It is a turning-point of immense significance.

[3] **(17:2)** The transfiguration scene contains, in miniature, all the elements of the future kingdom in manifestation: (1) The Lord, not in humiliation, but in glory (v. 2). (2) Moses, glorified, representative

8 And when they had lifted up their
eyes, they saw no man, save Jesus only.
9 And as they came down from the
mountain, Jesus charged them, saying,
Tell the vision to no man, until the [a]Son
of man be risen again from the dead.
10 And his disciples asked him, saying, [1]Why then say the scribes that Elias
must first come?
11 And Jesus answered and said unto
them, [b]Elias truly shall first come, and
restore all things.
12 But I say unto you, That Elias is
come already, and they knew him not,
but have done unto him whatsoever
they listed. Likewise shall also the Son of
man suffer of them.
13 Then the disciples understood that
he spake unto them of John the Baptist.

The powerless disciples: the mighty Christ (Mk. 9:14-29; Lk. 9:37-43).

14 And [c]when they were come to the
multitude, there came to him a *certain*
man, kneeling down to him, and saying,
15 Lord, have mercy on my son: for he
is lunatick, and sore vexed: for ofttimes
he falleth into the fire, and oft into the
water.
16 And I brought him to thy disciples,
and they could not cure him.
17 Then Jesus answered and said, O
faithless and perverse generation, how
long shall I be with you? how long shall
I suffer you? bring him hither to [d]me.
18 And Jesus rebuked the [e]devil; and
he departed out of him: and [f]the child
was cured from that very hour.
19 Then came the disciples to Jesus
apart, and said, Why could not we cast
him out?

A.D. 32.

a Also vs. 12, 22. See Mt. 8:20, *note.*
b Mt. 11:14; Lk. 1:17; Mal. 4:5; Mk. 9:11-13.
c Mk. 9:14-29; Lk. 9:37-42; Psa. 72:4-6.
d Mt. 14:18; John 15:5; Phil. 4:13.
e *demon.* Mt. 7:22, *note.*
f *Miracles* (N.T.). vs. 14-18, 24-27; Mt. 20:30-34. (Mt. 8:2, 3; Acts 28:8, 9.)
g Lit. *little faith.* Mt. 16:8; 21:21; Lk. 17:6.
h *Faith.* Mk. 9:23. (Gen. 3:20; Heb. 11:39.)
i The two best MSS. omit v. 21.
j Acts 13:2, 3; 2 Cor. 12:9.
k Mt. 16:21; Mk. 9:30-32; Lk. 9:43-45; Acts 2:23.
l *anticipated.*
m Isa. 60:10-17; 49:22, 23.

20 And Jesus said unto them, Because
of your [g]unbelief: for verily I say unto
you, If ye have [h]faith as a grain of mustard seed, ye shall say unto this mountain, Remove hence to yonder place; and
it shall remove; and nothing shall be
impossible unto you.
21 [i]Howbeit this kind goeth not out
but by [j]prayer and fasting.

Jesus again foretells his death and resurrection (Mk. 9:30-32; Lk. 9:43-45).

22 And while they abode in Galilee,
Jesus said unto them, The Son of man
shall be [k]betrayed into the hands of men:
23 And they shall kill him, and the
third day he shall be raised again. And
they were exceeding sorry.

The miracle of the tribute money. (Cf. Mk. 12:13.)

24 And when they were come to
Capernaum, they that received tribute
money came to Peter, and said, Doth not
your master pay tribute?
25 He saith, Yes. And when he was
come into the house, Jesus [l]prevented
him, saying, What thinkest thou, Simon?
of whom do the kings of the earth take
custom or tribute? of their own children,
or of [m]strangers?
26 Peter saith unto him, Of strangers.
Jesus saith unto him, Then are the children free.
27 Notwithstanding, lest we should
offend them, go thou to the sea, and cast
an hook, and take up the fish that first
cometh up; and when thou hast opened
his mouth, thou shalt find a piece of

of the redeemed who have passed through death into the kingdom (Mt. 13:43; cf. Lk. 9:30, 31). (3) Elijah, glorified, representative of the redeemed who have entered the kingdom by translation (1 Cor. 15:50-53; 1 Thes. 4:14-17). (4) Peter, James, and John, not glorified, representatives (for the moment) of Israel in the flesh in the future kingdom (Ezk. 37:21-27). (5) The multitude at the foot of the mountain (v. 14), representative of the nations who are to be brought into the kingdom after it is established over Israel (Isa. 11:10-12, etc.).

[1] **(17:10)** Cf. Mt. 11:14; Mk. 9:11, 12, 13; Lk. 1:17; Mal. 3:1; 4:5, 6. All the passages must be construed together. (1) Christ confirms the specific and still unfulfilled prophecy of Mal. 4:5, 6: "Elias shall truly first come and restore all things." Here, as in Malachi, the prediction fulfilled in John the Baptist, and that yet to be fulfilled in Elijah, are kept distinct. (2) But John the Baptist had come already, and with a ministry so completely in the spirit and power of Elijah's future ministry (Lk. 1:17) that in an adumbrative and typical sense it could be said: "Elias is come already." Cf. Mt. 10:40; Phm. 12, 17, where the same thought of identification, while yet preserving personal distinction, occurs (cf. John 1:27).

money: that take, and give unto them for
me and thee.

CHAPTER 18.

The sermon on the child-text
(Mk. 9:33-37; Lk. 9:46-48).

At the same time came the disciples
unto Jesus, saying, [a]Who is the
greatest in the [b]kingdom of heaven?
2 And Jesus called a little [c]child unto
him, and set him in the midst of them,
3 And said, Verily I say unto you,
Except ye be converted, and become as
little children, ye shall not enter into the
kingdom of heaven.
4 Whosoever therefore shall humble
himself as this little child, the same is
greatest in the kingdom of heaven.
5 And whoso shall receive one such
little child in my name receiveth me.
6 But whoso shall [d]offend one of these
little ones which believe in me, it were
better for him that a millstone were
hanged about his neck, and *that* he were
drowned in the depth of the sea.
7 Woe unto the [e]world because of
offences! for it must needs be that
offences come; but woe to that man by
whom the offence cometh!
8 Wherefore [f]if thy hand or thy foot
offend thee, cut them off, and cast *them*
from thee: it is better for thee to enter
into [g]life halt or maimed, rather than
having two hands or two feet to be cast
into [h]everlasting fire.
9 And if thine eye offend thee, pluck it
out, and cast *it* from thee: it is better for
thee to enter into life with one eye,
rather than having two eyes to be cast
into [i]hell fire.
10 Take heed that ye despise not one of
these little ones; for I say unto you, That
in heaven their [j]angels do always behold
the face of my Father which is in heaven.

The lost sheep: the seeking Lord.
(Cf. Lk. 15:3-7.)

11 For the [k]Son of man is come to
[l]save that which was [m]lost.
12 How think ye? [n]if a man have an
[o]hundred sheep, and one of them be
gone astray, doth he not leave the ninety
and nine, and goeth into the mountains,
and seeketh that which is gone astray?
13 And if so be that he find it, verily I
say unto you, he rejoiceth more of that
sheep, than of the ninety and nine which
went not astray.
14 Even so it is not the will of your
Father which is in heaven, that one of
these little ones should perish.

Discipline in the future church.

15 Moreover if thy [p]brother shall [q]tres-
pass against thee, go and tell him his fault
between thee and him alone: if he shall
hear thee, thou hast gained thy brother.
16 But if he will not hear *thee, then* take
with thee one or two more, that in the
mouth of [r]two or three witnesses every
word may be established.
17 And if he shall neglect to hear them,
tell *it* unto the [s]church: but if he neglect
to hear the church, let him be unto thee
as an [t]heathen man and a publican.
18 Verily I say unto you, Whatsoever
ye shall [u]bind on earth shall be bound in
heaven: and whatsoever ye shall loose
on earth shall be loosed in heaven.
19 Again I say unto you, That if two of
you shall [v]agree on earth as touching any
thing that they shall ask, it shall be done
for them of my Father which is in heaven.

The simplest form of a local church.

20 For [w]where two or three are gathered together in my name, there am I in
the midst of them.

The law of forgiveness (Lk. 17:3, 4).

21 Then came Peter to him, and said,
Lord, how [x]oft shall my brother [y]sin
against me, and I [z]forgive him? till seven
times?
22 Jesus saith unto him, I say not unto
thee, Until seven times: but, Until [aa]sev-
enty times seven.
23 Therefore is the [b]kingdom of heav-
en likened unto a certain king, which
would [bb]take account of his servants.
24 And when he had begun to reckon,
one was brought unto him, which owed
him ten thousand talents.
25 But forasmuch as he had [cc]not to
pay, his lord commanded him to be sold,
and his wife, and children, and all that
he had, and payment to be made.
26 The servant therefore fell down
and worshipped him, saying, Lord, have

A.D. 32.

a Lk. 9:46-48.
b Mt. 3:2, *note.*
c Lk. 18:14-17; Psa. 131:2.
d *cause to stumble.* Mk. 9:42; Lk. 17:1, 2.
e *kosmos* = mankind. Mt. 4:8, *note.*
f Mt. 5:29, 30; Mk. 9:43-48.
g *Life (eternal).* vs. 8, 9. Mt. 19:16-29. (Mt. 7:14; Rev. 22:19.)
h The Greek has *the* before "everlasting."
i Gr. *gehenna.* Mt. 5:22, *note.*
j Heb. 1:4, *note.*
k See Mt. 8:20, *note.*
l Rom. 1:16, *note.*
m Gr. *apollumi.* John 3:16, *note.*
n *Parables* (N.T.). vs. 12-14, 23-35; Mt. 20:1-16. (Mt. 5:13-16; Lk. 21:29-31.)
o Lk. 15:4-7.
p Lk. 17:3, 4; Gal. 6:1, 2; Eph. 4:30-32.
q *Sin.* Rom. 3:23, *note.*
r Mt. 18:19.
s Or, *assembly.* 1Cor. 5:3-5; 6:1, 5.
t *the Gentile and the tax-gatherer.* Cf. 1 Cor. 5:9-13.
u Mt. 16:19; John 20:22, 23.
v 1 Pet. 3:7.
w Acts 20:7; 1 Cor. 14:26.
x Cf. v. 15. Lk. 17:4.
y Rom. 3:23, *note.*
z *Forgiveness.* vs. 21, 27, 32, 35; Mk. 2:5-10. (Lev. 4:20; Mt. 26:28.)
aa Psa. 78:40.
bb Or, *make settlement with.*
cc Rom. 3:19, 20; 5:8.

patience with me, and I [a]will pay thee
all.
27 Then the lord of that servant was
moved with compassion, and loosed
him, and [b]forgave him the debt.
28 But the same servant went out, and
found one of his fellowservants, which
owed him an hundred [c]pence: and he
laid hands on him, and took *him* by the
throat, saying, Pay me that thou owest.
29 And his fellowservant fell down at
his feet, and besought him, saying, Have
patience with me, and I will pay thee all.
30 And he [d]would not: but went and
cast him into prison, till he should pay
the debt.
31 So when his fellowservants saw
what was done, they were very sorry,
and came and told unto their lord all
that was done.
32 Then his lord, after that he had
called him, said unto him, O thou
wicked servant, [e]I forgave thee all that
debt, because thou desiredst me:
33 Shouldest not thou also have had
compassion on thy fellowservant, even
as I had pity on thee?
34 And his lord was wroth, and delivered him to the [f]tormentors, till he
should pay all that was due unto him.
35 So likewise shall my heavenly
Father do also unto you, if ye from your
hearts forgive not every one his brother
their trespasses.

CHAPTER 19.

Jesus again in Judæa.

And it came to pass, *that* when Jesus
had finished these sayings, he [g]de-
parted from Galilee, and came into the
coasts of Judaea beyond Jordan;
2 And great multitudes followed him;
and he [h]healed them there.

Christ and divorce. (Cf. Mt. 5:31, 32; Mk. 10:1-12; Lk. 16:18; 1 Cor. 7:10-15.)

3 The Pharisees also came unto him,
[i]tempting him, and saying unto him, [j]Is
it lawful for a man to put away his wife
for every cause?
4 And he answered and said unto
them, [k]Have ye not read, [l]that he which
made *them* at the beginning made them
male and female,
5 And said, For this cause shall a man
leave father and mother, and shall cleave
to his wife: and [m]they twain shall be one
flesh?
6 Wherefore they are no more twain,
but one flesh. What therefore God hath
joined together, let not man put asunder.
7 They say unto him, Why did [n]Moses
then command to give a writing of
divorcement, and to put her away?
8 He saith unto them, [o]Moses because
of the [p]hardness of your hearts suffered
you to put away your wives: but from
the beginning it was not so.
9 And I say unto you, [q]Whosoever shall
put away his wife, except *it be* for fornication, and shall marry another, committeth
adultery: and whoso marrieth her which
is put away doth commit adultery.
10 His disciples say unto him, If the
case of the man be so with *his* wife, it is
not good to marry.
11 But he said unto them, [r]All *men*
cannot receive this saying, save *they* to
whom it is given.
12 For there are some eunuchs, which
were so born from *their* mother's womb:
and there are some eunuchs, which were
made eunuchs of men: and there be
eunuchs, which have [s]made themselves
eunuchs for the [t]kingdom of heaven's
sake. He that is able to receive *it*, let him
receive *it*.

Jesus receives and blesses little children (Mk. 10:13-16; Lk. 18:15-17).

13 Then were there brought unto him
little children, that he should put *his*
hands on them, and pray: and the disciples rebuked them.
14 But Jesus said, Suffer little children,
and forbid them not, to come unto me:
for [u]of such is the [t]kingdom of heaven.
15 And he laid *his* hands on them, and
departed thence.

The rich young ruler (Mk. 10:17-30; Lk. 18:18-30; cf. Lk. 10:25-30).

16 And, behold, one came and said
unto him, Good Master, what good thing
shall I do, that I may have [v]eternal life?
17 And he said unto him, Why callest
thou me good? *there is* none good but
one, *that is*, God: but if thou wilt enter
into life, [w]keep the commandments.
18 He saith unto him, Which? Jesus

A.D. 33.

a Lk. 15:19; Ezk. 18:21.
b Eph. 1:7.
c *denarius* = 7 1-2 pence; 15 cents.
d Eph. 4:31, 32; Col. 3:12, 13.
e Lk. 7:41-43.
f The ground of law, of exact justice. Cf. grace, Rom. 3:23, 24; Eph. 4:30; also John 1:17, *note*.
g Mk. 10:1-12; John 10:40. See also Mt. 7:28.
h Mt. 4:23; 12:15; Mk. 7:23-25.
i *Temptation*. Mt. 22:18. (Gen. 3:1; Jas. 1:14.)
j Mt. 5:31; 1 Cor. 7:10-16.
k Gen. 1:27; 2:23, 24. The passage is significant as Jesus' confirmation of the Genesis narrative of creation.
l *Inspiration*. vs. 4-8; Mt. 22:31, 32. (Ex. 4:15; Rev. 22:19.)
m Gen. 2:23; Eph. 5:29-32; 1 Cor. 6:16.
n Deut. 24:1-4.
o Thus confirming the Mosaic authorship of Deut.
p Rom. 8:3; Heb. 3:15; 7:18, 19.
q Mt. 5:32; Lk. 16:18; 1 Cor. 7:10, 11. But see v. 11; 1 Cor. 7:7. Cf. John 16:12.
r John 16:12.
s 1 Cor. 7:7, 8. Cf. 1 Tim. 4:1-3.
t Mt. 3:2, *note*.
u Mt. 18:3; 1 Pet. 2:2.
v *Life (eternal)*. vs. 16, 17, 29. Mt. 25:46. (Mt. 7:14; Rev. 22:19.)
w Lk. 10:25-28. Cf. Rom. 3:19; 10:1-4.

said, [a]Thou shalt do no murder, Thou shalt not commit adultery, Thou shalt not steal, Thou shalt not bear false witness,

19 [b]Honour thy father and *thy* mother: and, [c]Thou shalt love thy neighbour as thyself.

20 The young man saith unto him, All these things have I [d]kept from my youth up: what lack I yet?

21 Jesus said unto him, If thou wilt be [e]perfect, go *and* sell that thou hast, and give to the poor, and thou shalt have treasure in heaven: and come *and* follow me.

22 But when the young man heard that saying, he went away sorrowful: for he had great possessions.

23 Then said Jesus unto his disciples, Verily I say unto you, That a [f]rich man shall hardly enter into the [g]kingdom of heaven.

24 And again I say unto you, It is easier for a camel to go through the eye of a needle, than for a rich man to enter into the kingdom of God.

25 When his disciples heard *it*, they were exceedingly amazed, saying, Who then can be [h]saved?

26 But Jesus beheld *them*, and said unto them, With men this is [i]impossible; but with God all things are possible.

The apostles' future place in the kingdom.

27 Then answered Peter and said unto him, Behold, we have forsaken all, and followed thee; what shall we have therefore?

28 And Jesus said unto them, Verily I say unto you, That ye which have followed me, in the [1]regeneration [j]when the Son of man shall sit in the [kl]throne of his glory, ye also shall sit upon twelve thrones, [2]judging the twelve tribes of Israel.

29 And [m]every one that hath forsaken houses, or brethren, or sisters, or father, or mother, or wife, or children, or lands, for my name's sake, shall receive an hundredfold, and shall inherit everlasting life.

A.D. 33.

a Ex. 20:13.
b Ex. 20:12; Eph. 6:1, 20.
c Lev. 19:18; Lk. 10:29-37; Rom. 13:9.
d Phil. 3:6, 7; *contra* vs. 7-9.
e See Mt. 5:48, *note*.
f Mk. 10:23-27; Lk. 18:24-27; Jas. 5:1-3; cf. Jas. 2:5.
g Mt. 3:2, *note*.
h Rom. 1:16, *note*. Cf. Mt. 13:3-9.
i Gen. 18:14; Ex. 14:13; Jer. 32:17; Mk. 10:27.
j *Christ (Second Advent)*. Mt. 23:39. (Deut. 30:3; Acts 1:9-11.)
k See Mt. 25:31; Rev. 3:21. Cf. Lk. 1:31-33.
l *Kingdom* (N.T.). vs. 27, 28. Mt. 21:1-11. (Lk. 1:31-33; 1 Cor. 15:24.)
m Mk. 10:29; Lk. 18:29. Cf. Heb. 11:36-40; 1 Pet. 1:3-5.
n Mt. 21:31.
o *Parables* (N.T.). vs. 1-16; Mt. 21:28-32. (Mt. 5:13-16; Lk. 21:29-31.)
p Isa. 5:7; Mt. 21:28-33; John 15:1-5. Cf. Mt. 28:19, *note*.
q Lk. 14:21; Mt. 21:43.
r Mk. 13:34; John 9:4; 1 Cor. 12:7-11.
s 2 Cor. 5:10.
t 1 Cor. 3:14, *note*; 9:24; 2 Tim. 4:7, 8.
u Rom. 14:10, 11.
v Lk. 17:7-10; 1 Cor. 9:16, 17.

30 [n]But many *that are* first shall be last; and the last *shall be* first.

CHAPTER 20.

Parable of the labourers in the vineyard.

For the kingdom of heaven is [o]like unto a man *that is* an householder, which went out early in the morning to hire labourers into his [p]vineyard.

2 And when he had agreed with the labourers for a penny a day, he sent them into his vineyard.

3 And he went out about the third hour, and saw [q]others standing idle in the marketplace,

4 And said unto them; Go ye also into the vineyard, and whatsoever is right I will give you. And they went their way.

5 Again he went out about the sixth and ninth hour, and did likewise.

6 And about the eleventh hour he went out, and found others standing idle, and saith unto them, [r]Why stand ye here all the day idle?

7 They say unto him, Because no man hath hired us. He saith unto them, Go ye also into the vineyard; and whatsoever is right, *that* shall ye receive.

8 So when [s]even was come, the lord of the vineyard saith unto his steward, Call the labourers, and give them *their* hire, beginning from the last unto the first.

9 And when they came that *were hired* about the eleventh hour, they [t]received every man a penny.

10 But when the first came, they supposed that they should have received more; and they likewise received every man a penny.

11 And when they had received *it*, they [u]murmured against the goodman of the house,

12 Saying, These last have wrought *but* one hour, and thou hast made them [v]equal unto us, which have borne the burden and heat of the day.

13 But he answered one of them, and

1 (19:28) Gr. *palingenesia* = "re-creation," "making new." The word occurs once again, in Tit. 3:5. There it refers to the new birth of a believing person; here to the re-creation of the social order, and renewal of the earth (Isa. 1:6-9; Rom. 8:19-23) when the kingdom shall come. (See "Kingdom (O.T.)," Zech. 12:8, *note*; 1 Cor. 15:24, *note*.)

2 (19:28) Disclosing how the promise (Isa. 1:26) will be fulfilled when the kingdom is set up. The kingdom will be administered over Israel through the apostles, according to the ancient theocratic judgeship (Jud. 2:18).

said, Friend, I do thee no wrong: didst not thou agree with me for a penny?

14 Take *that* thine *is*, and go thy way: I will give unto this last, even as unto thee.

15 Is it not lawful for me to do [a]what I will with mine own? Is thine eye evil, because I am good?

16 So the [b]last shall be first, and the first last: for many be called, but few chosen.

Jesus again foretells his death and resurrection (Mk. 10:32-34; Lk. 18:31-34. See Mt. 12:38-42; 16:21-28; 17:22, 23).

17 And Jesus going up to Jerusalem took the twelve disciples apart in the way, and said unto them,

18 [c]Behold, we go up to Jerusalem; and the [d]Son of man shall be betrayed unto the chief priests and unto the scribes, and they shall condemn him to death,

19 And shall deliver him to the [e]Gentiles to [f]mock, and to [g]scourge, and to [h]crucify *him*: and the third day he shall [i]rise again.

James and John, through their mother, make an ambitious request (Mk. 10:35-45).

20 Then came to him the [j]mother of Zebedee's children with her sons, worshipping *him*, and desiring a certain thing of him.

21 And he said unto her, What wilt thou? She saith unto him, Grant that these my [k]two sons may sit, the one on thy right hand, and the other on the left, in thy [l]kingdom.

22 But Jesus answered and said, Ye know not what ye ask. Are ye able to drink of the [m]cup that I shall drink of, and to be baptized with the baptism that I am baptized with? They say unto him, We are able.

23 And he saith unto them, Ye shall drink indeed of my cup, and be baptized with the baptism that I am baptized with: but to sit on my right hand, and on my left, is not mine to give, but *it shall be given to them* for whom it is prepared of my Father.

A.D. 33.

a Rom. 9:20, 21.
b Mt. 19:30; 22:14, *refs.*
c Mt. 16:21.
d Mt. 26:47-57.
e Mt. 27:1.
f Mt. 26:67, 68.
g Mt. 27:26.
h Mt. 27:35.
i Mt. 28:5, 6.
j Cf. Mk. 10:35-37.
k Cf. Rev. 3:21, 22.
l Mt. 3:2, *note.*
m Mt. 26:39; 27:46; Lk. 22:41, 42; John 18:11; Isa. 53:4-6; 2 Cor. 5:21; Gal. 3:13; 1 Pet. 2:24; 3:18.
n Lk. 22:23-27.
o Mt. 23:11; 1 Pet. 5:3.
p *servant.* 1 Cor. 9:19-22.
q *bond servant.*
r Mt. 8:20, *note.* Phil. 2:7.
s Isa. 53:10, 11; Mt. 20:22, "cup," *refs.;* Ex. 14:30, *note;* Isa. 59:20, *note;* Rom. 3:24, *note.*
t Cf. Mk. 10:46-52; Lk. 18:35-43.
u 2 Sam. 7:14-17; Psa. 89:3-5, 19-37; Isa. 11:10-12; Ezk. 37:21-25; Mt. 1:1; Lk. 1:31, 32; Acts 15:14-17.
v Mt. 15:28; John 5:6.
w Mt. 9:36; 14:14; 15:32; 18:27; 20:34.
x *Miracles* (N.T.). vs. 30-34; Mt. 21:17-22. (Mt. 8:2, 3; Acts 28:8, 9.)
y vs. 1-9; Zech. 9:9. Cf. Zech. 14:4-9. The two advents are in striking contrast.

24 And when the ten heard *it*, they were moved with [n]indignation against the two brethren.

25 But Jesus called them *unto him*, and said, Ye know that the princes of the Gentiles exercise dominion over them, and they that are great exercise authority upon them.

26 But it shall [o]not be so among you: but whosoever will be great among you, let him be your [p]minister;

27 And whosoever will be chief among you, let him be your [q]servant:

28 Even as the [r]Son of man came not to be ministered unto, but to minister, and to give his life a [s]ransom for many.

The healing of two blind men
(Mk. 10:46-52. Cf. Lk. 18:35-43).

29 And as they [t]departed from Jericho, a great multitude followed him.

30 And, behold, [1]two blind men sitting by the way side, when they heard that Jesus passed by, cried out, saying, Have mercy on us, O Lord, *thou* [u]son of David.

31 And the multitude rebuked them, because they should hold their peace: but they cried the more, saying, Have mercy on us, O Lord, *thou* Son of David.

32 And Jesus stood still, and called them, and said, [v]What will ye that I shall do unto you?

33 They say unto him, Lord, that our eyes may be opened.

34 So Jesus had [w]compassion *on them*, and touched their eyes: and [x]immediately their eyes received sight, and they followed him.

CHAPTER 21.

The King's public offer of himself as King
(Zech. 9:9; Mk. 11:1-10;
Lk. 19:29-38; John 12:12-19).

And when they drew [y]nigh unto Jerusalem, and were come to

1 **(20:30)** A discrepancy has been imagined between this account and those in Mk. 10:46; Lk. 18:35. Matthew and Mark obviously refer to a work of healing as Jesus *departed* from Jericho. Bartimaeus, the active one of the two, the one who cried, "Jesus, thou Son of David," is specifically mentioned by Mark. Of the other one of the "two," we know nothing. The healing described by Luke (18:35) occurred before Jesus entered Jericho. As to the form of appeal, "Son of David" (cf. Mt. 9:27; 15:22; 21:9), Jesus must have been so addressed constantly. The narratives therefore supplement, but in no wise contradict each other.

Bethphage, unto the mount of Olives, then sent Jesus two disciples,

2 Saying unto them, Go into the village over against you, and straightway ye shall find an ass tied, and a colt with her: loose *them*, and bring *them* unto me.

3 And if any *man* say ought unto you, ye shall say, The Lord hath [a]need of them; and straightway he will send them.

4 All this was done, that it might be [1]fulfilled which was spoken by the prophet, saying,

5 Tell ye the daughter of Sion, [b]Behold, thy [c]King cometh unto thee, meek, and sitting upon an ass, and a colt the foal of an ass.

6 And the disciples went, and did as Jesus commanded them,

7 And brought the ass, and the colt, and put on them their clothes, and they set *him* thereon.

8 And a very great multitude spread their garments in the way; others cut down branches from the trees, and strawed *them* in the way.

9 And the multitudes that went before, and that followed, cried, saying, [d]Hosanna to the son of David: Blessed *is* he that cometh in the name of the [e]Lord; Hosanna in the highest.

10 And when he was come into Jerusalem, all the city was moved, saying, Who is this?

11 And the [f]multitude said, This is Jesus the prophet of Nazareth of Galilee.

Jesus' second purification of the temple
(Mk. 11:15-18; Lk. 19:45-47.
Cf. John 2:13-16).

12 And Jesus went into the temple of God, and [g]cast out all them that sold and bought in the temple, and overthrew the tables of the moneychangers, and the seats of them that sold doves,

13 And said unto them, It is written, [h]My house shall be called the house of prayer; but [i]ye have made it a den of thieves.

14 And the [j]blind and the lame came to him in the temple; and he healed them.

15 And when the chief priests and scribes saw the wonderful things that he did, and the children crying in the temple, and saying, [f]Hosanna to the [k]son of David; they were sore displeased,

A.D. 33.

a Psa. 50:10.
b *Christ (First Advent).* Mt. 21:42. (Gen. 3:15; Acts 1:9.)
c *Kingdom* (N.T.). vs. 1-11; Mt. 21:33-43. (Lk. 1:31-33; 1 Cor. 15:24.)
d Cf. Mt. 27:22; Psa. 118:26.
e i.e. *Jehovah.*
f Cf. v. 9.
g Lk. 19:45; Mk. 11:15-18. Cf. John 2:13-25, which introduced, as this cleansing closed, the offer of Christ to Israel as King.
h Isa. 56:7.
i Jer. 7:11.
j Cf. Lk. 14:21; Acts 3:1-10.
k See Mt. 20:30, *refs.*
l Psa. 8:2.
m John 11:54.
n John 11:1, 2; Lk. 10:39-42. Cf. Mk. 11:1-11; Lk. 19:29-35; John 12:1-8. With no other place is the human Christ so tenderly associated, while it also was the place of manifestation of His divine power (John 11:43, 44).
o John 4:6; Mk. 11:12-14.
p Lit. *a solitary fig tree.* Lk. 13:6-9. The withered fig tree is a parabolic miracle concerning Israel (Lk. 13:6-9). Cf. Mt. 24:32, 33; a prophecy that Israel shall again bud.
q *Miracles* (N.T.). vs. 18-22; Mk. 1:23-26. (Mt. 8:2, 3; Acts 28:8, 9.)
r Mt. 17:20; Mk. 11:23; Lk. 17:6; 1 Cor. 13:2.
s Mt. 7:7-11; John 15:7; 1 John 5:14, 15.
t Mk. 11:27-33; Lk. 20:1-8.
u John 1:19-28.
v Cf. v. 46. See Prov. 29:25.

16 And said unto him, Hearest thou what these say? And Jesus saith unto them, Yea; have ye never read, [l]Out of the mouth of babes and sucklings thou hast perfected praise?

17 And he [m]left them, and went out of the city into [n]Bethany; and he lodged there.

The barren fig tree cursed
(Mk. 11:12-14, 20-24).

18 Now in the morning as he returned into the city, he [o]hungered.

19 And when he saw a [p]fig tree in the way, he came to it, and found nothing thereon, but leaves only, and said unto it, Let no fruit grow on thee henceforward for ever. And presently the fig tree [q]withered away.

20 And when the disciples saw *it*, they marvelled, saying, How soon is the fig tree withered away!

21 Jesus answered and said unto them, Verily I say unto you, If ye have [r]faith, and doubt not, ye shall not only do this *which is done* to the fig tree, but also if ye shall say unto this mountain, Be thou removed, and be thou cast into the sea; it shall be done.

22 And [s]all things, whatsoever ye shall ask in prayer, believing, ye shall receive.

Jesus' authority questioned
(Mk. 11:27-33; Lk. 20:1-8).

23 And when he was come into the temple, the chief priests and the elders of the people came unto him as he was teaching, and said, By what [t]authority doest thou these things? and who gave thee this authority?

24 And Jesus answered and said unto them, I also will ask you one thing, which if ye tell me, I in like wise will tell you by what authority I do these things.

25 The [u]baptism of John, whence was it? from heaven, or of men? And they reasoned with themselves, saying, If we shall say, From heaven; he will say unto us, Why did ye not then believe him?

26 But if we shall say, Of men; we [v]fear the people; for all hold John as a prophet.

27 And they answered Jesus, and said, We cannot tell. And he said unto them,

[1](21:4) The King's final and official offer of Himself according to Zech. 9:9. Acclaimed by an unthinking multitude whose real belief is expressed in verse 11, but with no welcome from the official

[a]Neither tell I you by what authority I do these things.

Parable of the two sons.

28 But what think ye? [b]A *certain* man had two sons; and he came to the first, and said, Son, go work to day in my [c]vineyard.

29 He answered and said, I will not: but afterward he [d]repented, and went.

30 And he came to the second, and said likewise. And he answered and said, I *go*, sir: and went [e]not.

31 Whether of them twain did the will of *his* father? **They say unto him, The first. Jesus saith unto them,** Verily I say unto you, That the publicans and the harlots go into the kingdom of God before you.

32 For John came unto you in the way of [f]righteousness, and ye believed him not: but the publicans and the harlots [g]believed him: and ye, when ye had seen *it*, repented not afterward, that ye might believe him.

Parable of the householder demanding fruit from his vineyard (Mk. 12:1-9; Lk. 20:9-19. Cf. Isa. 5:1-7).

33 Hear another parable: There was a certain householder, which planted a [c]vineyard, and hedged it round about, and digged a winepress in it, and built a tower, and let it out to [h]husbandmen, and went into a far country:

34 And when the [i]time of the fruit drew near, he sent his servants to the husbandmen, that they might receive the fruits of it.

35 And the husbandmen took his servants, and beat one, and killed another, and stoned another.

36 Again, he sent other servants more than the first: and they did unto them likewise.

37 But last of all he sent unto them his [j]son, saying, They will reverence my son.

38 But when the husbandmen saw the son, they said among themselves, This is the [k]heir; come, let us kill him, and let us seize on his inheritance.

39 And they caught him, and cast *him* out of the vineyard, and slew *him*.

40 When the lord therefore of the vineyard cometh, what will he do unto those husbandmen?

41 [l]**They say unto him, He will miserably destroy those wicked men, and will let out *his* vineyard unto other husbandmen, which shall render him the fruits in their seasons.**

42 **Jesus saith unto them,** Did ye never [m]read in the scriptures, The [n]stone which the builders [o]rejected, the same is become the head of the corner: this is the [p]Lord's doing, and it is marvellous in our eyes?

43 Therefore say I unto [q]you, The [1r]kingdom of God shall be taken from you, and given to a nation bringing forth the fruits thereof.

44 [s]And whosoever shall fall on this [2]stone shall be broken: but on whomsoever it shall fall, it will grind him to powder.

45 **And when the chief priests and Pharisees had heard his parables, they perceived that he spake of them.**

46 **But when they sought to lay hands on him, they [t]feared the multitude, because they took him for a prophet.**

CHAPTER 22.

Parable of the marriage feast (Lk. 14:16-24).

And Jesus answered and spake unto them again by [u]parables, and said,

2 The [v]kingdom of heaven is [w]like unto a certain king, which made a marriage for his son,

3 And sent forth his servants to call them that were bidden to the wedding: and they would not come.

4 Again, he sent forth other servants, saying, Tell them which are bidden, Behold, I have prepared my dinner: my oxen and *my* fatlings *are* killed, and all things *are* ready: come unto the marriage.

5 But they made light of *it*, and went their ways, one to his farm, another to his merchandise:

A.D. 33.

a Cf. v. 32. See Mt. 3:3.
b *Parables* (N.T.). vs. 28-32; Mt. 21:33-43; 22:2-14. (Mt. 5:13-16; Lk. 21:29-31.)
c See Mt. 20:1, "vineyard," *refs.*
d Cf. Lk. 15:20, the other perfect illustration of repentance. See Acts 17:30, *note.*
e Mt. 7:21-23; 15:8.
f See Rom. 10:10, "righteousness," *note.*
g Lk. 3:12, 13.
h Mt. 23:2; John 15:1; Jas. 5:7, 8.
i Mk. 11:13.
j John 3:16; Heb. 1:2.
k Heb. 1:2; Rom. 8:16, 17.
l Cf. 2 Sam. 12:5-9.
m Psa. 118:22, 23.
n *Christ (as Stone).* vs. 42-44; Acts 4:11. (Ex. 17:6; 1 Pet. 2:8.)
o *Christ (First Advent).* Mt. 26:31. (Gen. 3:15; Acts 1:9.)
p *Jehovah.* Psa. 118:23.
q i.e. national Israel, the barren vine. (vs. 33-41.) Cf. Isa. 5:1-7.
r *Kingdom* (N.T.). vs. 33-43; Mt. 23:37-39. (Lk. 1:31-33; 1 Cor. 15:24.)
s Or, *Whosoever falls on this stone shall be crushed together* [i.e. the Jews, Isa. 8:14; Rom. 9:32, 33; 1 Cor. 1:23] *but on whomsoever it may fall, he will be scattered as dust* (Gr. *"winnowed,"* i.e. the Gentile nations, Dan. 2:34, 35, 45, *note*).
t Mt. 14:5; 21:26, 46; Mk. 11:18, 32.
u Mt. 13:13, 14.
v Mt. 3:2, *note.*
w *Parables* (N.T.). vs. 2-14; Mt. 24:32, 33. (Mt. 5:13-16; Lk. 21:29-31.)

representatives of the nation, He was soon to hear the multitude shout: "Crucify Him."

[1] **(21:43)** Note that Matthew here as in verse 31 uses the larger word, kingdom of God. (Cf. Mt. 6:33, *note.*) The kingdom of heaven (Mt. 3:2, *note;* 1 Cor. 15:24, summary) will yet be set up. Meantime the kingdom of God and His righteousness is taken from Israel nationally and given to the Gentiles (Rom. 9:30-33).

[2] **(21:44)** Christ as the "Stone" is revealed in a threefold way: (1) To *Israel* Christ, coming not as a

6 And the remnant took his servants, and entreated *them* spitefully, and slew *them*.

7 But when the king heard *thereof*, he was wroth: and he sent forth his armies, and destroyed those murderers, and [a]burned up their city.

8 Then saith he to his servants, The wedding is ready, but they which were bidden were not worthy.

9 [b]Go ye therefore into the highways, and as many as ye shall find, bid to the marriage.

10 So those servants went out into the [c]highways, and gathered together all as many as they found, [d]both bad and good: and the wedding was furnished with guests.

11 And when the king came in to see the guests, he saw there a man which had not on a wedding garment:

12 And he saith unto him, Friend, how camest thou in hither not having a [e]wedding garment? And he was [f]speechless.

13 Then said the king to the servants, Bind him hand and foot, and take him away, and cast *him* into [g]outer darkness; there shall be weeping and gnashing of teeth.

14 For [h]many are called, but few *are* chosen.

Jesus answers the Herodians
(Mk. 12:13-17; Lk. 20:20-26).

15 [i]Then went the Pharisees, and took counsel how they might entangle him in *his* talk.

16 And they sent out unto him their disciples with the [j]Herodians, saying, Master, we know that thou art true, and teachest the way of God in truth, neither carest thou for any *man*: for thou regardest not the person of men.

17 Tell us therefore, What thinkest thou? Is it lawful to give [k]tribute unto Caesar, or not?

18 But Jesus perceived their wickedness, and said, Why [l]tempt ye me, *ye* hypocrites?

19 Shew me the tribute money. And they brought unto him a penny.

20 And he saith unto them, Whose *is* this image and superscription?

21 They say unto him, Cæsar's. Then saith he unto them, [m]Render therefore unto Cæsar the things which are Cæsar's; and unto [n]God the things that are God's.

22 When they had heard *these words*, they marvelled, and left him, and went their way.

Jesus answers the Sadducees
(Mk. 12:18-27; Lk. 20:27-38).

23 The same day came to him the Sadducees, which say that there is no [o]resurrection, and asked him,

24 Saying, Master, Moses said, [p]If a man die, having no children, his brother shall marry his wife, and raise up seed unto his brother.

25 [q]Now there were with us seven brethren: and the first, when he had married a wife, deceased, and, having no issue, left his wife unto his brother:

26 Likewise the second also, and the third, unto the seventh.

27 And last of all the woman died also.

28 Therefore in the resurrection whose wife shall she be of the seven? for they all had her.

29 Jesus answered and said unto them, [r]Ye do err, not knowing the scriptures, nor the power of God.

30 For in the [s]resurrection they neither marry, nor are given in marriage, but are [t]as the angels of God in heaven.

31 But as touching the resurrection of the dead, have ye not read [u]that which was spoken unto you by God, saying,

32 [v]I am the God of Abraham, and the God of Isaac, and the God of Jacob? God is not the God of the dead, but of the living.

33 And when the multitude heard *this*, they were astonished at his doctrine.

Jesus answers the Pharisees
(Mk. 12:28-34. Cf. Lk. 10:25-28).

34 But when the Pharisees had heard that he had put the Sadducees to silence, they were gathered together.

A.D. 33.

a Fulfilled as to Jerusalem A.D. 70. Lk. 21:20-24.
b The world-wide call. Mt. 28:16-20; Rev. 22:17.
c Acts 28:28; cf. Rom. 10:18.
d Mt. 13:47.
e Rom. 10:1-3; *contra*, Phil. 3:7-9.
f Rom. 3:19.
g Mt. 13:40-43, 49, 50.
h Mt. 20:16; Isa. 65:2; Mt. 23:37; Rom. 8:30.
i In the different classes, vs. 15-40, Jesus meets representatives of all Israel, Pharisees, Sadducees, Herodians (Mt. 3:7, *note*). For them, silenced but unrepentant, no message is left but "woe" (Mt. 23).
j Cf. Mk. 3:6; 8:15.
k Cf. Mt. 17:24-27.
l *Temptation.* Mt. 26:41. (Gen. 3:1; Jas. 1:14.)
m 1 Pet. 2:13-17.
n 1 Cor. 3:23; 12:27; 2 Cor. 6:15.
o *Resurrection.* vs. 23:28-31; Mt. 27:52, 53. (Job 19:25; 1 Cor. 15:52.)
p Deut. 25:5.
q 1 Tim. 1:4; 4:7; 6:4; 2 Tim. 2:24-26.
r Or, *ye deceive yourselves*, etc. Jesus' answer gives the three incapacities of the rationalist: self-deception (Rom. 1:21, 22); ignorance of the spiritual content of Scripture (Acts 13:27); disbelief in the intervention of divine power (2 Pet. 3:5-9).
s Mt. 27:52, 53.
t Heb. 1:4, *note*.
u *Inspiration.* vs. 31, 32; Mt. 24; 15, 37-39. (Ex. 4:15; Rev. 22:19.)
v Ex. 3:6.

splendid monarch but in the form of a servant, is a stumbling-stone and rock of offence (Isa. 8:14, 15; Rom. 9:32, 33; 1 Cor. 1:23; 1 Pet. 2:8); (2) to the *church*, Christ is the foundation-stone and the head of the corner (1 Cor. 3:11; Eph. 2:20-22; 1 Pet. 2:4, 5); (3) to the Gentile world-powers (see "Gentiles," Lk. 21:24; Rev. 16:19) He is to be the smiting-stone of destruction (Dan. 2:34). Israel stumbled *over* Christ; the church is built *upon* Christ; Gentile world-dominion will be broken *by* Christ. (See "Armageddon," Rev. 16:14; 19:19.)

35 Then one of them, *which was* a [1a]lawyer, asked *him a question*, tempting him, and saying,
36 Master, which *is* the [b]great commandment in the [c]law?
37 Jesus said unto him, Thou shalt [d]love the [e]Lord thy God with all thy heart, and with all thy soul, and with all thy mind.
38 This is the first and great commandment.
39 And the second *is* like unto it, [f]Thou shalt love thy neighbour as thyself.
40 On these two commandments hang [g]all the law and the prophets.

Jesus questions the Pharisees
(Mk 12:35-37; Lk. 20:41-44).

41 While the Pharisees were gathered together, Jesus [h]asked them,
42 Saying, What think ye of Christ? whose son is he? They say unto him, *The Son* of David.
43 He saith unto them, How then doth David [i]in [j]spirit call him Lord, saying,
44 [k]The LORD said unto my Lord, Sit thou on my right hand, till I make thine enemies thy footstool?
45 If David then call him Lord, how is he his son?
46 And no man was able to answer him a word, neither durst any *man* from that day forth ask him any more *questions*.

CHAPTER 23.

The marks of a Pharisee
(Mk. 12:38-40; Lk. 20:45-47).

Then spake Jesus to the multitude, and to his disciples,
2 Saying, The scribes and the Pharisees [l]sit in Moses' seat:
3 All therefore whatsoever they bid you observe, *that* observe and do; but do not ye after their works: for they say, and do not.
4 For [m]they bind heavy burdens and grievous to be borne, and lay *them* on men's shoulders; but they *themselves* will not move them with one of their fingers.
5 But all their works they do for to [n]be seen of men: they make broad their [o]phylacteries, and enlarge the borders of their garments,
6 And love the uppermost rooms at feasts, and the chief seats in the synagogues,

A.D. 33.

a Cf. Lk. 10:25.
b Cf. Mt. 5:17-48; Lk. 10:27.
c *Law (of Moses).* vs. 36-39. Lk. 1:6. (Ex. 19:1; Gal. 3:1-29.)
d Deut. 6:5; Rom. 3:19; Gal. 3:10.
e *Jehovah.* Deut. 6:5.
f Lev. 19:18. Cf. Lk. 10:29-37; Rom. 7:14, 15.
g Mt. 7:12; Rom. 13:8-10.
h Cf. Mt. 21:24; John 19:7. Jesus' question is not personal but doctrinal: "Whose son is the Messiah?" Cf. Acts 2:25-36; Rom. 1:3, 4.
i Lit. *in the spirit.* Cf. Mk. 12:36; Acts 2:30.
j *Holy Spirit.* Mt. 28:19. (Mt. 1:18; Acts 2:4.)
k Psa. 110:1.
l Cf. Ezra 7:6, 25, 26. Jesus' disciples were to honour the law, but not the hypocritical teachers of it.
m Cf. Mt. 11:29, 30; Acts 15:10; Gal. 5:1; Col. 2:16.
n Mt. 6:1, 2, 5, 16.
o Passages of Scripture enclosed in a small case, bound upon arm or forehead, Deut. 6:8.
p Gr. *teacher.*
q i.e. authoritative teacher.
r Lit. *Neither may ye be called leaders, because your leader is Christ.*
s The best MSS. omit v. 14.
t *condemnation.*
u Acts 2:10.
v *Gehenna.* Mt. 5:22, *note.*
w Mt. 15:14; Mal. 2:8.
x Or, *bound;* also v. 18, "guilty."
y *Sanctify, holy (things).* vs. 17-19; Mt. 27:53. (Mt. 4:5; Rev. 22:11.)

7 And greetings in the markets, and to be called of men, Rabbi, Rabbi.
8 But be not ye called Rabbi: for one is your [p]Master, *even* Christ; and all ye are brethren.
9 And call no *man* your [q]father upon the earth: for one is your Father, which is in heaven.
10 [r]Neither be ye called masters: for one is your Master, *even* Christ.
11 But he that is greatest among you shall be your servant.
12 And whosoever shall exalt himself shall be abased; and he that shall humble himself shall be exalted.

Jesus denounces woe upon the Pharisees
(Mk. 12:38-40; Lk. 20:47).

13 But woe unto you, scribes and Pharisees, hypocrites! for ye shut up the kingdom of heaven against men: for ye neither go in *yourselves*, neither suffer ye them that are entering to go in.
14 [s]Woe unto you, scribes and Pharisees, hypocrites! for ye devour widows' houses, and for a pretence make long prayer: therefore ye shall receive the greater [t]damnation.
15 Woe unto you, scribes and Pharisees, hypocrites! for ye [u]compass sea and land to make one proselyte, and when he is made, ye make him twofold more the child of [v]hell than yourselves.
16 Woe unto you, *ye* [w]blind guides, which say, Whosoever shall swear by the temple, it is nothing; but whosoever shall swear by the gold of the temple, he is a [x]debtor!
17 *Ye* fools and blind: for whether is greater, the gold, or the temple that [y]sanctifieth the gold?
18 And, Whosoever shall swear by the altar, it is nothing; but whosoever sweareth by the gift that is upon it, he is guilty.
19 *Ye* fools and blind: for whether *is* greater, the gift, or the altar that sanctifieth the gift?
20 Whoso therefore shall swear by the altar, sweareth by it, and by all things thereon.
21 And whoso shall swear by the temple, sweareth by it, and by him that dwelleth therein.

[1] **(22:35)** Gr. *nomikos*, "of the law"; occurs also, Lk. 7:30; 10:25; 11:45, 46, 52; 14:3; Tit. 3:13. Except in the last instance, "lawyer" is another name for "scribe" (Mt. 2:4, *note*). In Tit. 3:13 the term has the modern meaning.

22 And he that shall swear by heaven, sweareth by the throne of God, and by him that sitteth thereon.

23 Woe unto you, scribes and Pharisees, hypocrites! for ye pay [a]tithe of mint and anise and cummin, and have omitted the [b]weightier *matters* of the law, judgment, mercy, and faith: these ought ye to have done, and not to leave the other undone.

24 *Ye* blind guides, which strain [c]at a gnat, and swallow a camel.

25 Woe unto you, scribes and Pharisees, hypocrites! for ye make clean the [d]outside of the cup and of the platter, but within they are full of extortion and excess.

26 *Thou* blind Pharisee, cleanse first that *which is* within the cup and platter, that the outside of them may be clean also.

27 Woe unto you, scribes and Pharisees, hypocrites! for ye are like unto [e]whited sepulchres, which indeed appear beautiful outward, but are within full of dead *men's* bones, and of all uncleanness.

28 Even so ye also outwardly appear righteous unto men, but within ye are full of hypocrisy and [f]iniquity.

29 Woe unto you, scribes and Pharisees, hypocrites! because ye [g]build the tombs of the prophets, and garnish the sepulchres of the righteous,

30 And say, If we had been in the days of our fathers, we would not have been partakers with them in the blood of the prophets.

31 Wherefore ye be witnesses unto yourselves, that ye are the [h]children of them which killed the prophets.

32 Fill ye up then the measure of your fathers.

33 *Ye* serpents, *ye* generation of vipers, how can ye escape the [i]damnation of [j]hell?

34 Wherefore, behold, I [k]send unto you prophets, and wise men, and scribes: and *some* of them ye shall [l]kill and crucify; and *some* of them shall ye scourge in your synagogues, and persecute *them* from city to city:

A.D. 33.

a Lk. 11:42; 18:12.
b 1 Sam. 15:22; Isa. 1:11-17.
c *strain out.*
d Mk. 7:4, 8, 9; Lk. 11:39, 40.
e Lk. 11:44; Acts 23:3; Phil. 3:4-6.
f Lit. *Lawlessness.* Rom. 3:23, *note.*
g Dan. 9:5-8; Lk. 11:47, 48.
h Acts 7:51, 52.
i *condemnation.*
j v. 15, *ref.*
k The Jews' treatment of the apostles is proved, vs. 31-33.
l John 16:2; Acts 5:40; 7:54-60.
m Rev. 18:24.
n Jesus' confirmation of Gen. 4:8-10. Cf. Heb. 12:24.
o 2 Chr. 24:20-22.
p Rev. 18:21-24. It is the way also of history: judgment falls upon one generation for the sins of centuries. The prediction was fulfilled in the destruction of Jerusalem, A.D. 70.
q Lk. 13:34, 35; 19:41, 42.
r Mt. 11:28-30; John 10:30.
s *Kingdom* (N.T.). vs. 37-39. Mt. 24:29-51. (Lk. 1:31-33; 1 Cor. 15:24.)
t *Christ (Second Advent).* Mt. 24:27-30. (Deut. 30:3; Acts 1:9-11.)
u Jesus leaves that which He abandons to judgment. See Mk. 8:21, 23, *note,* in the light of Mt. 11:21, 22. Cf. Rev. 18:4.
v 1 Ki. 9:7-9; Psa. 79:1; Isa. 64:11; Lk. 19:44.
w Mk. 13:3-37; Lk. 21:7-37.
x Lk. 17:20-37.
y v. 30; 2 Pet. 3:4.
z *Consummation of the age.*

35 That upon you may come [m]all the righteous blood shed upon the earth, from the blood of righteous [n]Abel unto the blood of [o]Zacharias son of Barachias, whom ye slew between the temple and the altar.

36 Verily I say unto you, All these things shall [p]come upon this generation.

The lament over Jerusalem (Lk. 13:34, 35).

37 O [q]Jerusalem, Jerusalem, *thou* that killest the prophets, and stonest them which are sent unto thee, how often would [r]I have gathered thy children together, even as a hen gathereth her chickens under *her* wings, and ye would not!

38 Behold, your house is left unto you desolate.

39 For I say unto you, Ye shall not see me henceforth, [1s]till ye shall say, [t]Blessed *is* he that cometh in the name of the Lord.

CHAPTER 24.

The Olivet discourse: (1) *destruction of the temple foretold* (Mk. 13:1, 2; Lk. 21:5, 6).

And Jesus went out, and [u]departed from the temple: and his disciples came to *him* for to shew him the buildings of the temple.

2 And Jesus said unto them, See ye not all these things? verily I say unto you, [v]There shall not be left here one stone upon another, that shall not be thrown down.

The Olivet discourse: (2) *the threefold question* (Mk. 13:3, 4; Lk. 21:7).

3 And [w]as he sat upon the mount of Olives, the disciples came unto him privately, saying, [2]Tell us, [x]when shall these things be? and what *shall be* the sign of thy [y]coming, and of the [z]end of the world?

The Olivet discourse: (3) *the course of this age* (Mk. 13:5-13; Lk. 21:3-19).

4 And Jesus answered and said unto

[1] **(23:39)** The three "untils" of Israel's blessing: (1) Israel must say, "Blessed is He" (Mt. 23:39; cf. Rom. 10:3, 4). (2) Gentile world-power must run its course (Lk. 21:24; Dan. 2:34, 35). (3) The elect number of the Gentiles must be brought in. *Then* "the Deliverer shall come out of Zion," etc. (Rom. 11:25-27).

[2] **(24:3)** Mt. 24 with Lk. 21:20-24 answers the threefold question. The order is as follows: "When shall these things be?"—i.e. destruction of the temple and city. Answer, Lk. 21:20-24. Second and third

them, Take heed that no man deceive
you.
5 For [a]many shall come in my name,
saying, I am Christ; and shall deceive
many.
6 And ye shall hear of [b]wars and
rumours of wars: see that ye be not troubled: for all *these things* must come to
pass, but the end is not yet.
7 For [c]nation shall rise against nation,
and kingdom against kingdom: and
there shall be [d]famines, and pestilences,
and [e]earthquakes, in divers places.
8 All these *are* the beginning of sorrows.
9 Then shall they [f]deliver you up to be
afflicted, and shall kill you: and ye shall
be hated of all nations for my name's
sake.
10 And then shall [g]many be offended,
and shall betray one another, and shall
hate one another.
11 And many [h]false prophets shall
rise, and shall deceive many.
12 And because [ij]iniquity shall abound,
the love of many shall wax [k]cold.
13 But he that shall endure unto the
end, the same shall be saved.
14 And this [l]gospel of the [m]kingdom
shall be preached in all the [n]world for a
witness unto all nations; and then shall
the end come.

A.D. 33.

a v. 24; John 5:43; 1 John 2:18.
b Rev. 6:2-4.
c Hag. 2:22.
d Rev. 6:5, 6.
e Rev. 6:12.
f Mt. 10:17, 18; Rev. 2:10.
g Dan. 12:10.
h 2 Pet. 2:1; Rev. 13:11; 19:20.
i i. e. *lawlessness.*
j *Sin.* Rom. 3:23, *note.*
k 2 Thes. 2:3, 4; 2 Tim. 3:1.
l *Gospel.* Mt. 26:13. (Gen. 12:1-3; Rev. 14:6.)
m Mt. 3:2, *note.*
n *oikoumene = inhabited earth.* (Lk. 2:1.)
o *The Beast.* John 5:43. (Dan. 7:8; Rev. 19:20.)
p *Inspiration.* vs. 15, 37-39; Mt. 26:54. (Ex. 4:15; Rev. 22:19.)
q Dan. 9:27; 11:31; 12:11.
r *Tribulation (the great).* vs. 21, 22; Rev. 3:10. (Psa. 2:5; Rev. 7:14.)
s i.e. *earth.*
t Isa. 65:8, 9; Dan. 9:27; Zech. 13:8, 9; Rev. 12:6-17.

The Olivet discourse: (4) *the great tribulation* (Mk. 13:14-23).

15 When ye therefore shall see the
[o]abomination of desolation, [p]spoken of
by [q]Daniel the prophet, stand in the holy
place, (whoso readeth, let him understand:)
16 [1]Then let them which be in Judaea
flee into the mountains:
17 Let him which is on the housetop
not come down to take any thing out of
his house:
18 Neither let him which is in the field
return back to take his clothes.
19 And woe unto them that are with
child, and to them that give suck in
those days!
20 But pray ye that your flight be not
in the winter, neither on the sabbath day:
21 For then shall be [r]great tribulation,
such as was not since the beginning of the
[s]world to this time, no, nor ever shall be.
22 And except those days should be
[t]shortened, there should no flesh be
saved: but for the elect's sake those days
shall be shortened.
23 Then if any man shall say unto you,
Lo, here *is* Christ, or there; believe *it* not.
24 For there shall arise false Christs,
and false prophets, and shall shew great

questions: "And what shall be the sign of thy coming, and of the end of the age?" Answer, Mt. 24:4-33. Verses 4 to 14 have a double interpretation: They give (1) the character of the age—wars, international conflicts, famines, pestilences, persecutions, and false Christs (cf. Dan. 9:26). This is not the description of a converted world. (2) But the same answer (vs. 4-14) applies in a specific way to the *end* of the age, viz. Daniel's seventieth week (Dan. 9:24-27, *note* 2). All that has characterized the *age* gathers into awful intensity at the *end.* Verse 14 has specific reference to the proclamation of the good news that the kingdom is again "at hand" by the Jewish remnant (Isa. 1:9; Rev. 14:6, 7; Rom. 11:5, *note*). Verse 15 gives the sign of the abomination (Dan. 9:27, *note*)—the "man of sin," or "Beast" (2 Thes. 2:3-8; Dan. 9:27; 12:11; Rev. 13:4-7).

This introduces the great tribulation (Psa. 2:5; Rev. 7:14, *note*), which runs its awful course of three and a half years, culminating in the battle of Rev. 19:19-21, *note,* at which time Christ becomes the smiting Stone of Dan. 2:34. The *detail* of this period (vs. 15-28) is: (1) The abomination in the holy place (v. 15); (2) the warning (vs. 16-20) to believing Jews who will then be in Jerusalem; (3) the great tribulation, with renewed warning as to false Christs (vs. 21-26); (4) the sudden smiting of the Gentile world-power (vs. 27, 28); (5) the glorious appearing of the Lord, visible to all nations, and the regathering of Israel (vs. 29-31); (6) the sign of the fig-tree (vs. 32, 33); (7) warnings, applicable to this present age over which these events are ever impending (vs. 34-51; Phil. 4:5). Careful study of Dan. 2, 7, 9, and Rev. 13 will make the interpretation clear. See, also, "Remnant" (Isa. 1:9; Rom. 11:5).

[1]**(24:16)** Cf. Lk. 21:20-24. The passage in Luke refers in express terms to a destruction of Jerusalem which was fulfilled by Titus, A.D. 70; the passage in Matthew to a future crisis in Jerusalem after the manifestation of the "abomination." See "Beast" (Dan. 7:8; Rev. 19:20); and "Armageddon" (Rev. 16:14; 19:17). As the circumstances in both cases will be similar, so are the warnings. In the former case Jerusalem was destroyed; in the latter it will be delivered by divine interposition.

signs and wonders; insomuch that, if *it were* possible, they shall deceive the very elect.

25 Behold, I have told you before.

26 Wherefore if they shall say unto you, Behold, he is in the desert; go not forth: behold, *he is* in the secret chambers; believe *it* not.

The Olivet discourse:
(5) *the return of the King in glory*
(Mk. 13:24-37; Lk. 21:25-36).

27 For as the [a]lightning cometh out of the east, and shineth even unto the west; [b]so shall also the coming of the [c]Son of man be.

28 For wheresoever the [d]carcase is, there will the eagles be gathered together.

29 Immediately after the tribulation of [e]those days shall the sun be darkened, and the moon shall not give her light, and the stars shall fall from heaven, and the powers of the heavens shall be shaken:

30 And then shall appear the sign of the Son of man in heaven: and then shall all the tribes of the earth mourn, and they shall see [f]the Son of man coming in the clouds of heaven with power and great glory.

31 And he shall [g]send his [h]angels with a great sound of a trumpet, and they [i]shall gather together his elect from the four winds, from one end of heaven to the other.

Parable of the fig tree
(Mk. 13:28, 29; Lk. 21:29-31).

32 Now learn a [j]parable of the fig tree; When his branch is yet tender, and putteth forth leaves, ye know that summer *is* nigh:

33 So likewise ye, when ye shall [k]see all these things, know that [l]it is near, *even* at the doors.

34 Verily I say unto you, [1m]This generation shall not pass, till all these things be fulfilled.

35 [n]Heaven and earth shall pass away, but my words shall not pass away.

36 But of that day and hour [o]knoweth no *man*, no, not the [h]angels of heaven, but my Father only.

37 But as the [p]days of Noe *were*, so shall also the coming of the Son of man be.

38 For as in the days that were before the flood they were eating and drinking, marrying and giving in marriage, until the day that Noe entered into the ark,

39 And knew not until the flood came, and took them all away; [q]so shall also the coming of the Son of man be.

40 Then shall two be in the field; the one shall be taken, and the other left.

41 Two *women shall be* grinding at the mill; the one shall be taken, and the other left.

42 [r]Watch therefore: for ye know not [s]what hour your Lord doth come.

43 But know this, that if the goodman of the house had known in what watch the thief would come, he would have watched, and would not have suffered his house to be broken up.

44 Therefore be ye also [t]ready: for in such an hour as ye think not the Son of man cometh.

45 Who then is a [u]faithful and wise servant, whom his lord hath made ruler over his household, [v]to give them meat in due season?

46 Blessed *is* that servant, whom his lord when he cometh shall find so doing.

47 Verily I say unto you, That he shall make him ruler over all his goods.

48 But and if that evil servant shall say in his heart, [w]My lord delayeth his coming;

49 And shall begin to smite *his* fellowservants, and to eat and drink with the drunken;

50 The lord of that servant shall [x]come in a day when he looketh not for *him*, and in an hour that he is not aware of,

51 And shall cut him asunder, and appoint *him* his portion with the [y]hypocrites: there shall be weeping and gnashing of teeth.

A.D. 33.

a Isa. 30:30; 1 Thes. 5:1-3.
b Gen. 7:11; Lk. 17:26, 27; 1 Thes. 5:3; 2 Pet. 2:5; 3:6.
c Also vs. 37, 39, 44. See Mt. 8:20, *note.*
d *Armageddon (battle of).* Rev. 19:17. (Rev. 16:14; 19:21.)
e *Day of Jehovah.* vs. 29-31; Mt. 25:31-46. (Isa. 2:10-22; Rev. 19:11-21.)
f *Christ (Second Advent).* Mt. 24:36-50. (Deut. 30:3; Acts 1:9-11.)
g Psa. 50:4, 5; Mt. 13:41.
h Heb. 1:4, *note.*
i *Israel (prophecies).* Lk. 1:31-33. (Gen. 12:2,3; Rom. 11:26.)
j *Parables* (N.T.). vs. 32, 33; Mt. 25:1-13. (Mt. 5:13-16; Lk. 21:29-31.)
k v. 15; 1 Thes. 5:1-5.
l Or, *he.*
m Mt. 12:45; 23:35, 36.
n Psa. 119:89, 160; 138:2; Isa. 51:6; Mt. 5:18; 1 Pet. 1:23, 25.
o vs. 42, 44; Acts 1:7.
p Gen. 6:5-8; 1 Pet. 3:20.
q *Christ (Second Advent).* vs. 36-50; Mt. 25:31-46. (Deut. 30:3; Acts 1:9-11.)
r Mt. 25:13; Rev. 3:3.
s *on what day.*
t Mt. 25:10; Lk. 12:35-40, 43; 21:34-36.
u Lk. 12:42-46; 1 Cor. 4:2. It is *faithfulness,* not ability, in the Lord's service that is first approved by Him.
v John 21:15; 1 Pet. 5:2.
w Heb. 10:37; 2 Pet. 3:4, 9; Rev. 22:7, 12, 20.
x *Kingdom* (N.T.). vs. 29-51; Mt. 25:31-46. (Lk. 1:31-33; 1 Cor. 15:24.)
y Mt. 7:21-23; 25:3, 11, 12; 2 Pet. 2:20-22.

1 (24:34) Gr. *genea,* the primary definition of which is, "race, kind, family, stock, breed." (So all lexicons.) That the word is used in this sense here is sure because none of "these things," i.e. the worldwide preaching of the kingdom, the great tribulation, the return of the Lord in visible glory, and the regathering of the elect, occurred at the destruction of Jerusalem by Titus, A.D. 70. The promise is, therefore, that the generation—nation, or family of Israel—will be preserved unto "these things"; a promise wonderfully fulfilled to this day.

CHAPTER 25.

The Olivet discourse:
(6) *the Lord's return tests the real state of the kingdom in mystery.*

Then [1]shall the kingdom of [a]heaven be [b]likened unto ten [2]virgins, which took their lamps, and went forth to meet the bridegroom.

2 And five of them were [c]wise, and five *were* [d]foolish.

3 They that *were* foolish took their lamps, and took no oil with them:

4 But the wise took oil in their vessels with their lamps.

5 While the bridegroom tarried, they all slumbered and slept.

6 And at midnight there was a cry made, Behold, the bridegroom cometh; go ye out to meet him.

7 Then all those virgins arose, and trimmed their lamps.

8 And the foolish said unto the wise, Give us of your oil; for our lamps are [e]gone out.

9 But the wise answered, saying, *Not so*; lest there be not enough for us and you: but go ye rather to them that sell, and buy for yourselves.

10 And while they went to buy, the bridegroom came; and they that were [f]ready went in with him to the marriage: and the door was shut.

11 Afterward came also the other virgins, saying, Lord, Lord, [g]open to us.

12 But he answered and said, Verily I say unto you, I know you not.

13 Watch therefore, for ye [h]know neither the day nor the hour wherein the [i]Son of man cometh.

The Olivet discourse:
(7) *the Lord's return tests the servants.*

14 For [j]*the kingdom of heaven is* as a man travelling into a far country, *who* called his own servants, and delivered unto them his [k]goods.

15 And unto one he gave five talents, to another two, and to another one; to every man [l]according to his several ability; and straightway took his journey.

16 Then he that had received the five talents went and [m]traded with the same, and made *them* other five talents.

17 And likewise he that *had received* two, he also gained other two.

18 But he that had received one went and digged in the earth, and [n]hid his lord's money.

19 After a long time the lord of those servants cometh, and [o]reckoneth with them.

20 And so he that had received five talents came and brought other five talents, saying, Lord, thou deliveredst unto me five talents: behold, I have gained beside them five talents more.

21 His lord said unto him, [p]Well done, *thou* good and faithful servant: thou hast been [q]faithful over a few things, I will make thee ruler over many things: enter thou into the joy of thy lord.

22 He also that had received two talents came and said, Lord, thou deliveredst unto me two talents: behold, I have gained two other talents beside them.

23 His lord said unto him, [r]Well done, good and faithful servant; thou hast been faithful over a few things, I will make thee ruler over many things: enter thou into the [s]joy of thy lord.

24 Then he which had received the one talent came and said, Lord, I knew thee that thou art an [t]hard man, reaping where thou hast not sown, and gathering where thou hast not strawed:

25 And I was afraid, and went and hid thy talent in the earth: lo, *there* thou hast *that is* thine.

26 His lord answered and said unto him, *Thou* [u]wicked and slothful servant,

A.D. 33.

- *a* Mt. 3:2, *note*.
- *b* *Parables* (N.T.). vs. 1-13, 14-30; Mk. 2:21. (Mt. 5:13-16; Lk. 21:29-31.)
- *c* Mt. 7:24, 25; Deut. 32:29.
- *d* Mt. 7:26, 27; 22:11; Lk. 12:20, 21.
- *e* *going out*.
- *f* Mt. 24:44; Col. 1:12-14.
- *g* Lk. 13:25-30.
- *h* Mt. 24:36, 42.
- *i* Also v. 31; Mt. 8:20, *note*.
- *j* Omit the italicised words.
- *k* Lk. 19:12-27; 1 Tim. 6:20.
- *l* Lk. 12:48; Rom. 12:6-8; 1 Cor. 12:7.
- *m* Eph. 5:16; 1 Tim. 4:12-13; 2 Pet. 1:5-8.
- *n* Prov. 26:15; 1 Pet. 4:10; 2 Pet. 1:9-12.
- *o* Rom. 14:10-12; 2 Cor. 5:10.
- *p* The Lord's commendation may be earned by the weakest of His servants; it is given for *faithful* service.
- *q* Lk. 16:10-12; 1 Cor. 4:2; 2 Tim. 4:7, 8.
- *r* The same commendation is gained by the servant with two talents as by him with five: he was equally *faithful* though his gift was less.
- *s* Psa. 16:11; Zeph. 3:17; John 15:10, 11; Heb. 12:1, 2.
- *t* Mt. 20:11, 12; Mal. 1:13. Cf. 1 John 5:3.
- *u* Mt. 22:12, 13; 24:48-50.

[1] **(25:1)** This part of the Olivet discourse goes beyond the "sign" questions of the disciples (Mt. 24:3), and presents our Lord's return in three aspects: (1) As testing profession, vs. 1-13; (2) as testing service, vs. 14-30; (3) as testing the Gentile nations, vs. 31-46.

[2] **(25:1)** The kingdom of heaven here is the sphere of profession, as in Mt. 13. All alike have lamps, but two facts fix the real status of the foolish virgins: They "took no oil, and the Lord said, "I know you not." Oil is the symbol of the Holy Spirit, and "If any man have not the spirit of Christ, he is none of his" (Rom. 8:9). Nor could the Lord say to any believer, however unspiritual, "I know you not."

thou knewest that I reap where I sowed not, and gather where I have not strawed:

27 Thou oughtest therefore to have put my money to the exchangers, and *then* at my coming I should have received mine own with usury.

28 Take therefore the talent from him, and give *it* unto him which hath ten talents.

29 For unto [a]every one that hath shall be given, and he shall have abundance: but from him that hath not shall be taken away even [b]that which he hath.

30 And [c]cast ye the unprofitable servant into [d]outer darkness: there shall be weeping and gnashing of teeth.

The Olivet discourse:
(8) *the Lord's return tests the Gentile nations.* (Cf. Joel 3:11-16.)

31 When the Son of man shall [e]come in his glory, and all the [f]holy [g]angels with him, [h]then shall he sit upon the throne of his glory:

32 [1]And before him shall be [i]gathered all nations: and he shall separate them one from another, as a shepherd divideth *his* sheep from the goats:

33 And he shall set the [j]sheep on his right hand, but the [k]goats on the left.

34 Then shall the King say unto them on his right hand, Come, ye blessed of my Father, inherit the [l]kingdom prepared for you from the foundation of the [m]world:

35 For I was an [n]hungred, and ye gave me meat: I was thirsty, and ye gave me drink: I was a stranger, and ye took me in:

36 Naked, and ye clothed me: I was sick, and ye visited me: I was in prison, and ye came unto me.

37 Then shall the [o]righteous answer him, saying, Lord, when saw we thee an hungred, and fed *thee*? or thirsty, and gave *thee* drink?

38 When saw we thee a stranger, and took *thee* in? or naked, and clothed *thee*?

39 Or when saw we thee sick, or in prison, and came unto thee?

40 And the King shall answer and say unto them, Verily I say unto you, Inasmuch as ye have done *it* unto one of the [p]least of these my brethren, ye have done *it* unto me.

41 Then shall he say also unto them on the left hand, [q]Depart from me, ye cursed, into everlasting fire, prepared for the [r]devil and his [g]angels:

42 For I was an [s]hungred, and ye gave me no meat: I was thirsty, and ye gave me no drink:

43 I was a stranger, and ye took me not in: naked, and ye clothed me not: sick, and in prison, and ye visited me not.

44 Then shall they also answer him, saying, Lord, when saw we thee an hungred, or athirst, or a stranger, or naked, or sick, or in prison, and did not minister unto thee?

45 Then shall he answer them, saying, Verily I say unto you, [t]Inasmuch as ye did *it* not to one of the least of these, ye did *it* not to me.

46 [u]And these shall go away [v]into everlasting [w]punishment: but the [o]righteous into [x]life eternal.

CHAPTER 26.

The Jewish authorities consult to put Jesus to death (Mk. 14:1, 2; Lk. 22:1, 2).

And it came to pass, when Jesus had finished all these sayings, he said unto his disciples,

2 Ye know that after two days is *the feast of* the passover, and the Son of man is betrayed to be crucified.

3 Then assembled together the chief priests, and the scribes, and the elders of the people, unto the palace of the high priest, who was called Caiaphas,

A.D. 33.

a Mt. 13:12; Lk. 19:26; John 15:2.
b Lk. 8:18, last clause.
c Mt. 7:21-23.
d *the outer darkness.*
e *Christ (Second Advent).* Mk. 13:24-27. (Deut. 30:3; Acts 1:9-11.)
f *Sanctify, holy (persons)* (N.T.). Mk. 6:20. (Mt. 4:5; Rev. 22:11.)
g Heb. 1:4, *note.*
h *Day of Jehovah.* vs. 31-46; Acts 2:19, 20. (Isa. 2:10-22; Rev. 19:11-21.)
i Psa. 96:13; John 5:28, 29; Rev. 20:11-15.
j Psa. 79:13; 100:3; Ezk. 20:38; 34:17, 22, 31; John 10:11.
k Zech. 10:3.
l Mt. 3:2, *note.*
m *i.e. earth.*
n Mt. 10:40; Heb. 11:37, 38.
o Rom. 10:10, *note.*
p Mt. 10:40-42; Acts 9:2, 4, 5.
q Mt. 7:23.
r *Satan, Gr. diabolos, accuser.* Mk. 1:13. (Gen. 3:1; Rev. 20:10.)
s vs. 35, 40, 45, *refs.*
t Prov. 14:31; Zech. 2:8.
u *Kingdom* (N.T.). vs. 31-46; Acts 1:6, 7. (Lk. 1:31-33; 1 Cor. 15:24.)
v *Judgments (the seven).* Lk. 14:14. (2 Sam. 7:14; Rev. 20:12.) "Eternal" and "everlasting" are the same word.
w *Day of destruction.* 2 Thes. 1:7-10. (Job 21:30; Rev. 20:11-15.)
x *Life (eternal).* Lk. 10:25. (Mt. 7:14; Rev. 22:19.)

[1] **(25:32)** This judgment is to be distinguished from the judgment of the great white throne. Here there is no resurrection; the persons judged are living nations; no books are opened; three classes are present, sheep, goats, brethren; the time is at the return of Christ (v. 31); and the scene is on the earth. All these particulars are in contrast with Rev. 20:11-15. The test in this judgment is the treatment accorded by the nations to those whom Christ here calls "my brethren." These "brethren" are the Jewish Remnant who will have preached the Gospel of the kingdom to all nations during the tribulation. See "Remnant" (Isa. 1:9; Rom. 11:5). The test in Rev. 20:11-15, is the possession of eternal life. See, for the other six judgments, John 12:31, *note;* 1 Cor. 11:31, *note;* 2 Cor. 5:10, *note;* Ezk. 20:37, *note;* Jude 6, *note;* Rev. 20:12, *note.*

4 And [a]consulted that they might take Jesus by subtilty, and kill *him*.

5 But they said, Not on the feast *day*, lest there be an [b]uproar among the people.

Jesus anointed by Mary of Bethany
(Mk. 14:3-9; John 12:1-8).

6 Now when Jesus was in [c]Bethany, in the house of Simon the [d]leper,

7 There came unto him a [e]woman having an alabaster box of very precious ointment, and poured it on his [1]head, as he sat *at meat*.

8 But when his disciples saw *it*, they had indignation, saying, To what purpose *is* this waste?

9 For this ointment might have been sold for much, and given to the poor.

10 When Jesus understood *it*, he said unto them, Why trouble ye the woman? for she hath wrought a good work upon me.

11 For ye have the poor always with you; but [f]me ye have not always.

12 For in that she hath poured this ointment on my body, she did *it* [g]for my [h]burial.

13 Verily I say unto you, Wheresoever this [i]gospel shall be preached in the whole [j]world, *there* shall also this, that this woman hath done, be told for a memorial of her.

Judas Iscariot sells the Lord
(Mk. 14:10, 11; Lk. 22:3-6).

14 Then one of the twelve, called Judas Iscariot, went unto the chief priests,

15 And said *unto them*, What will ye give me, and I will deliver him unto you? And they covenanted with him for [k]thirty pieces of silver.

16 And from that time he sought opportunity to betray him.

A.D. 33.

a John 11:47; Acts 4:25-28.
b Mt. 21:26; Mk. 14:2.
c Mk. 14:3; John 12:1-8.
d Mt. 8:2; Mk. 16:9; Lk. 15:2.
e i.e. Mary of Bethany.
f Lk. 5:34, 35; John 16:28.
g Supply *to prepare me.*
h Mt. 16:21-23; Mk. 16:1.
i *Gospel.* Mk. 1:1, 14, 15. (Gen. 12:1-3; Rev. 14:6.)
j i.e. *earth.*
k Zech. 11:12, 13.
l Lk. 9:51; John 8:20; 16:32.
m John 6:70, 71; 13:21.
n Psa. 41:9; 55:12-14; John 13:18, 26.
o Mk. 9:12; Lk. 24:25-27, 44-46; John 19:28.
p John 17:12; Acts 1:25.

The preparation of the passover
(Mk. 14:12-16; Lk. 22:7-13).

17 Now the first *day* of the *feast of* unleavened bread the disciples came to Jesus, saying unto him, Where wilt thou that we prepare for thee to eat the passover?

18 And he said, Go into the city to such a man, and say unto him, The Master saith, [l]My time is at hand; I will keep the passover at thy house with my disciples.

19 And the disciples did as Jesus had appointed them; and they made ready the passover.

The last passover (Mk. 14:17-21;
Lk. 22:14-20, 24-30).

20 Now when the even was come, he [2]sat down with the twelve.

(Here read John 13:2-30.)

21 And as they did eat, he said, Verily I say unto you, that one of you shall [m]betray me.

22 And they were exceeding sorrowful, and began every one of them to say unto him, Lord, is it I?

23 And he answered and said, He that [n]dippeth *his* hand with me in the dish, the same shall betray me.

24 The Son of man goeth as it is [o]written of him: but woe unto that man by whom the Son of man is betrayed! [p]it had been good for that man if he had not been born.

25 Then Judas, which betrayed him, answered and said, Master, is it I? He said unto him, Thou hast said.

Jesus institutes the Lord's Supper (Mk. 14:22-25; Lk. 22:17-20; 1 Cor. 11:23-25).

26 And as they were eating, Jesus

[1] **(26:7)** No contradiction of John 12:3 is implied. The ordinary anointing of hospitality and honour was of the feet (Lk. 7:38) *and* head (Lk. 7:46). But Mary of Bethany, who alone of our Lord's disciples had comprehended His thrice repeated announcement of His coming death and resurrection, invested the anointing with the deeper meaning of the preparation of His body for burying. Mary of Bethany was not among the women who went to the sepulchre with intent to embalm the body of Jesus.

[2] **(26:20)** The order of events on the night of the Passover supper appears to have been: (1) The taking by our Lord and the disciples of their places at the table; (2) the contention who should be greatest; (3) the feet-washing; (4) the identification of Judas as the traitor; (5) the withdrawal of Judas; (6) the institution of the supper; (7) the words of Jesus while still in the room (Mt. 26:26-29; Lk. 22:35-38; John 13:31-35; 14:1-31); (8) the words of Jesus between the room and the garden (Mt. 26:31-35; Mk. 14:26-31; John 15, 16, 17); it seems probable that the high-priestly prayer (John 17) was uttered after they reached the garden; (9) the agony in the garden; (10) the betrayal and arrest; (11) Jesus before Caiaphas; Peter's denial.

[a]took bread, and [b]blessed *it*, and brake *it*, and gave *it* to the disciples, and said, Take, eat; this is my [c]body.

27 And he took the cup, and gave thanks, and gave *it* to them, saying, Drink ye all of it;

28 For this is my [d]blood of the [e]new [f]testament, which is shed for many for the [1g]remission of [h]sins.

29 But I say unto you, I will not drink henceforth of this fruit of the vine, until that day when I drink it new with you in my Father's [i]kingdom.

(Here read John 14:1-31.)

Jesus foretells Peter's denial (Mk. 14:26-31; Lk. 22:31-34; John 13:36-38).

30 And when they had sung an [j]hymn, they went out into the mount of Olives.

(Here read John 15, 16, 17)

31 Then saith Jesus unto them, [k]All ye shall be offended because of me this night: for it is written, I will [l]smite the [m]shepherd, and the sheep of the flock shall be scattered abroad.

32 But after I am risen again, I will go before you into Galilee.

33 Peter answered and said unto him, Though [n]all *men* shall be offended because of thee, *yet* will I never be offended.

34 Jesus said unto him, Verily I say unto thee, That this night, before the [o]cock crow, thou shalt deny me thrice.

35 Peter said unto him, Though I should die with thee, yet will I not deny thee. Likewise also said all the disciples.

Jesus' agony in the Garden

(Mk. 14:32-42; Lk. 22:39-46; John 18:1).

36 Then [p]cometh Jesus with them unto a place called Gethsemane, and saith unto the disciples, Sit ye here, while I go and pray yonder.

37 And he took with him Peter and the two sons of Zebedee, and began to be [q]sorrowful and very heavy.

38 Then saith he unto them, My soul is exceeding sorrowful, even unto death: tarry ye here, and watch with me.

The first prayer

(Mk. 14:35; Lk. 22:41, 42).

39 And he went a little further, and fell on his face, and [r]prayed, saying, O my Father, if it be possible, let this [2s]cup pass from me: nevertheless not as I will, [t]but as thou *wilt*.

The sleeping disciples

(Mk. 14:37, 38, 40; Lk. 22:45, 46).

40 And he cometh unto the disciples, and findeth them asleep, and saith unto Peter, What, could ye not watch with me one hour?

41 Watch and pray, that ye enter not into [u]temptation: [v]the spirit indeed *is* willing, but the flesh *is* weak.

A.D. 33.

a Mk. 14:22-25; Lk. 22:19, 20.
b 1 Cor. 10:16.
c 1 Cor. 11:23-29; 1 Pet. 2:24.
d *Sacrifice (of Christ)*. John 1:29. (Gen. 4:4; Heb. 10:18.)
e *Covenant (new)*. Mk. 14:24. (Isa. 61:8; Heb. 8:8-12.)
f *covenant.*
g *Forgiveness.* (Lev. 4:20.)
h *Sin.* Rom. 3:23, *note.*
i Mt. 3:2, *note.*
j Mk. 14:26.
k Mk. 14:27.
l Zech. 13:7.
m *Christ (First Advent)*. Mt. 27:9, 10. (Gen. 3:15; Acts 1:9.)
n Mk. 14:29-31; Lk. 22:31-34; John 13:36-38.
o Mk. 13:35; John 18:27.
p Mk. 14:32-42; Lk. 22:40-46; John 18:1.
q Isa. 53:3; Lam. 1:12; John 12:27.
r *Bible prayers (N.T.)*. Mt. 27:46. (Mt. 6:9; Rev. 22:20.)
s Gen. 22:6-8; Heb. 5:7.
t Psa. 40:8.
u *Temptation*. Lk. 8:13. (Gen. 3:1; Jas. 1:2.)
v Psa. 103:14-16; Rom. 7:15; 8:23; Gal. 5:17.

[1] **(26:28)** Forgiveness. Summary: The Greek word translated "remission" in Mt. 26:28; Acts 10:43; Heb. 9:22, is elsewhere rendered "forgiveness." It means, to send off, or away. And this, throughout Scripture, is the one fundamental meaning of forgiveness—to separate the sin from the sinner. Distinction must be made between divine and human forgiveness: (1) Human forgiveness means the remission of penalty. In the Old Testament and the New, in type and fulfilment, the divine forgiveness follows the *execution* of the penalty. "The priest shall make an atonement for his sin that he hath committed, and it shall be forgiven him" (Lev. 4:35). "This is my blood of the new covenant, which is shed for many for the remission [sending away, forgiveness] of sins" (v. 28). "Without shedding of blood there is no remission" (Heb. 9:22). See "Sacrifice" (Gen. 4:4; Heb. 10:18, *note*). The sin of the justified *believer* interrupts his fellowship, and is forgiven upon confession, but always on the ground of Christ's propitiating sacrifice (1 John 1:6-9; 2:2). (2) Human forgiveness rests upon and results from the divine forgiveness. In many passages this is assumed rather than stated, but the principle is declared in Eph. 4:32; Mt. 18:32, 33.

[2] **(26:39)** The "cup" must be interpreted by our Lord's own use of that symbol in speaking of His approaching sacrificial death (Mt. 20:22; John 18:11). In view of John 10:17, 18, He could have been in no fear of an unwilling death. The value of the account of the agony in the Garden is in the evidence it affords that He knew fully what the agony of the cross would mean when His soul was made an offering for sin (Isa. 53:10) in the hiding of the Father's face. Knowing the cost to the utmost, He voluntarily paid it.

The second prayer (Mk. 14:39; Lk. 22:44).

42 He went away again the second time, and prayed, saying,O my Father, if this cup may not pass away from me, except I drink it, thy will be done.

43 And he came and found them asleep again: for their eyes were heavy.

The third prayer (Mk. 14:41).

44 And he left them, and went away again, and prayed the third time, saying the same words.

45 Then cometh he to his disciples, and saith unto them,[a]Sleep on now, and take *your* rest: behold, the hour is at hand, and the Son of man is betrayed into the hands of [b]sinners.

46 Rise, let us be going: behold, he is at hand that doth betray me.

The betrayal and arrest of Jesus (Mk. 14:43-50; Lk. 22:47-53; John 18:3-11).

47 And [c]while he yet spake, lo, Judas, one of the twelve, came, and with him a great multitude with swords and staves, from the chief priests and elders of the people.

48 Now he that betrayed him gave them a sign, saying, Whomsoever I shall [d]kiss, that same is he: hold him fast.

49 And forthwith he came to Jesus, and said, Hail, master; and [e]kissed him.

50 And Jesus said unto him,[f]Friend, wherefore art thou come? Then came they, and laid hands on Jesus, and took him.

51 And, behold, one of them which were with Jesus stretched out *his* hand, and [g]drew his sword, and struck a servant of the high priest's, and smote off his ear.

52 Then said Jesus unto him,Put up again thy sword into his place: for all they that take the sword shall perish with the sword.

53 Thinkest thou that I cannot now pray to my Father, and he shall presently give me more than [h]twelve legions of [i]angels?

54 But how then shall the [j]scriptures be [k]fulfilled, that thus it must be?

55 In that same hour said Jesus to the multitudes,[l]Are ye come out as against a thief with swords and staves for to take me? I sat daily with you teaching in the temple, and ye laid no hold on me.

56 But all this was done, that the scriptures of the prophets might be fulfilled. Then all the disciples [m]forsook him, and fled.

Jesus brought before Caiaphas and the Sanhedrin

(Mk. 14:53-65. Cf. John 18:12, 19-24).

57 And they that had laid hold on Jesus [1]led *him* away to [n]Caiaphas the high priest, where the scribes and the elders were assembled.

58 But [o]Peter followed him afar off unto the high priest's [p]palace, and went in, and sat with the [q]servants, to see the end.

59 Now the chief priests, and elders, and all the council, sought [r]false witness against Jesus, to put him to death;

60 But found none: yea, though many false witnesses came, *yet* found they none. At the last came two false witnesses,

61 And said, This *fellow* said, I am able to [s]destroy the temple of God, and to build it in three days.

62 And the high priest arose, and said unto him, Answerest thou nothing? what *is it which* these witness against thee?

63 But Jesus [t]held his peace. And the high priest answered and said unto him, I [u]adjure thee by the living God, that thou tell us whether thou be the Christ, the Son of God.

64 Jesus saith unto him, Thou hast

A.D. 33.

a Psa. 69:20; John 2:25.
b *Sin.* Rom. 3:23, *note.*
c Mk. 14:43; Lk. 22:47; John 18:3; Acts 1:16.
d v. 50; Psa. 55:13; Mk. 14:44, 45; Lk. 22:48.
e 2 Sam. 20:9; Psa. 55:13.
f Gr. *Hetaire, comrade.* Perhaps the most touching thing in the Bible. The Lord does not disown Judas.
g Mk. 14:47; Lk. 22:49-51; John 18:10, 11.
h 2 Ki. 6:17; Lk. 2:13, 14.
i Heb. 1:4, *note.*
j v. 24; John 19:28; Acts 13:29.
k *Inspiration.* Mt. 28:19, 20. (Ex. 4:15; Rev. 22:19.)
l Mk. 14:48, 49; Lk. 22:52, 53.
m Mk. 14:50. Cf. 2 Tim. 4:16.
n Mk. 14:53; Lk. 22:54; John 18:12-14.
o Mk. 14:54; John 18:15, 16.
p *court.*
q *officers.*
r Psa. 35:11; Mk. 14:55-60.
s Mt. 27:40; John 2:19-22.
t Isa. 53:7.
u Mk. 14:61-64; Lk. 22:69-71.

[1] **(26:57)** A comparison of the narratives gives the following order of events on the crucifixion day: (1) Early in the morning Jesus is brought before Caiaphas and the Sanhedrin. He is condemned and mocked (Mt. 26:57-68; Mk. 14:55-65; Lk. 22:63-71; John 18:19-24). (2) The Sanhedrin lead Jesus to Pilate (Mt. 27:1, 2, 11-14; Mk. 15:1-5; Lk. 23:1-5; John 18:28-38). (3) Pilate sends Jesus to Herod (Lk. 23:6-12; John 19:4). (4) Jesus is again brought before Pilate, who releases Barabbas and delivers Jesus to be crucified (Mt. 27:15-26; Mk. 15:6-15: Lk. 23:13-25; John 18:39, 40; 19:4-16). (5) Jesus is crowned with thorns, and mocked (Mt. 27:26-30; Mk. 15:15-20; John 19:1-3). (6) Suicide of Judas (Mt. 27:3-10). (7) Led forth to be crucified, the cross is laid upon Simon: Jesus discourses to the women (Mt. 27:31, 32; Mk. 15:20-23; Lk. 23:26-33; John 19:16, 17). For the order of events at the crucifixion see Mt. 27:33, *note.*

said: nevertheless I say unto you, Hereafter shall ye see the Son of man [a]sitting on the right hand of power, and [b]coming in the clouds of heaven.

65 Then the high priest rent his clothes, saying, He hath spoken blasphemy; what further need have we of witnesses? behold, now ye have heard his [c]blasphemy.

66 What think ye? They answered and said, He is guilty of death.

67 Then did they [d]spit in his face, and buffeted him; and others [e]smote *him* with the palms of their hands,

68 Saying, Prophesy unto us, thou Christ, Who is he that smote thee?

Peter denies the Lord (Mk. 14:66-72; Lk. 22:55-62; John 18:15-18, 25-27).

69 Now Peter [f]sat without in the palace: and a damsel came unto him, saying, Thou also wast with Jesus of Galilee.

70 But he denied before *them* all, saying, I know not what thou sayest.

71 And when he was gone out into the porch, another [1]*maid* saw him, and said unto them that were there, This *fellow* was also with Jesus of Nazareth.

72 And again he denied with an oath, I do not know the man.

73 And after a while came unto *him* they that stood by, and said to Peter, Surely thou also art *one* of them; for thy [g]speech bewrayeth thee.

74 Then began he to [h]curse and to swear, *saying*, I know not the man. And immediately the [i]cock crew.

75 And Peter remembered the word of Jesus, which said unto him, Before the cock crow, thou shalt deny me thrice. And he went out, and wept bitterly.

CHAPTER 27.

The Sanhedrin deliver Jesus to Pilate (Mk. 15:1; Lk. 23:1; John 18:28).

When the morning was come, all the chief priests and elders of the people took counsel against Jesus to put him to death:

2 And when they had bound him, they led *him* away, and [j]delivered him to Pontius Pilate the governor.

Judas' unavailing remorse. (Cf. Acts 1:16-19.)

3 Then Judas, which had betrayed him, when he saw that he was condemned, repented himself, and brought again the [k]thirty pieces of silver to the chief priests and elders,

4 Saying, I have [l]sinned in that I have betrayed the innocent blood. And they said, What *is that* to us? see thou *to that*.

5 And he cast down the pieces of silver in the temple, and departed, and went and [m]hanged himself.

6 And the chief priests took the silver pieces, and said, It is not lawful for to put them into the treasury, because it is the price of blood.

7 And they took counsel, and bought with them the potter's field, to bury strangers in.

8 Wherefore that field was called, The field of blood, unto this day.

9 Then was [n]fulfilled that which was spoken by [2]Jeremy the prophet, saying, And they took the [o]thirty pieces of silver, the price of him that was valued, whom they of the children of Israel did value;

10 And gave them for the potter's field, as the [p]Lord appointed me.

Jesus interrogated by Pilate (Mk. 15:2-5; Lk. 23:2, 3; John 18:29-38).

11 And Jesus stood before the governor: and the governor [q]asked him, saying, Art thou the King of the Jews? And Jesus said unto him, [r]Thou sayest.

12 And when he was accused of the chief priests and elders, he answered [s]nothing.

13 Then said Pilate unto him, Hearest thou not how many things they witness against thee?

14 And he answered him to never a word; insomuch that the governor marvelled greatly.

A.D. 33.

a Psa. 110:1; Mk. 14:62; Acts 7:55, 56.
b Dan. 7:13, 14; Mt. 24:30; Rev. 1:7.
c John 10:31-36.
d Isa. 50:6; 52:14; Mk. 14:65; Lk. 22:63-65; John 18:22, 23.
e Mic. 5:1; John 19:3.
f Mk. 14:66-72; Lk. 22:55-62; John 18:15-18, 25-27.
g Acts 2:7.
h *Contra*, Mt. 16:16, 17.
i v. 34.
j Mk. 15:1; Lk. 23:1; John 18:28.
k Zech. 11:12, 13.
l *Sin.* Rom. 3:23, *note.*
m 1 Sam. 31:4; 2 Sam. 17:23.
n Lk. 24:27, 44.
o *Christ (First Advent).* Mt. 27:34, 35. (Gen. 3:15; Acts 1:9.)
p *Jehovah.* Zech. 11:12, 13.
q Mk. 15:2-5; Lk. 23:3.
r John 18:33-37; 1 Tim. 6:13.
s Isa. 53:7.

[1] **(26:71)** Cf. v. 69; Mk. 14:69; Lk. 22:58; John 18:25. A discrepancy has been imagined in these accounts. Let it be remembered that an excited crowd had gathered, and that Peter was interrogated in two places: "With the servants" (Mt. 26:58) where the first charge was made (v. 69); "the porch" where a great number of people would be gathered, and where the second and third interrogations were made by "another maid" and by the crowd, i.e. "they" (vs. 71, 73; John 18:25).

[2] **(27:9)** The allusion is to Jeremiah 18:1-4; 19:1-3, but more distinctly to Zech. 11:12, 13.

Jesus or Barabbas? (Mk. 15:6-15; Lk. 23:13-25; cf. John 18:38-40).

15 Now at *that* feast the governor was
[a]wont to release unto the people a prisoner, whom they would.
16 And they had then a notable prisoner, called Barabbas.
17 Therefore when they were gathered
together, Pilate said unto them, Whom
will ye that I release unto you? Barabbas,
or Jesus which is called Christ?
18 For he knew that for [b]envy they
had delivered him.
19 When he was set down on the judgment seat, his wife sent unto him, saying,
Have thou nothing to do with that just
man: for I have suffered many things this
day in a [c]dream because of him.
20 But the chief priests and elders persuaded the multitude that they should
ask Barabbas, and destroy Jesus.
21 The governor answered and said
unto them, Whether of the twain will ye
that I release unto you? They said,
[d]Barabbas.
22 Pilate saith unto them, What shall I
do then with Jesus which is called
Christ? *They* all say unto him, Let him be
[e]crucified.
23 And the governor said, Why, what
evil hath he done? But they cried out the
more, saying, Let him be crucified.
24 When Pilate saw that he could prevail nothing, but *that* rather a tumult
was made, he took [f]water, and washed
his hands before the multitude, saying, I
am innocent of the blood of this just person: see ye *to it*.
25 Then answered all the people, and
said, [g]His blood *be* on us, and on our
children.

Barabbas released (Mk. 15:15; Lk. 23:24, 25).

26 Then released he Barabbas unto
them: and when he had [h]scourged Jesus,
he delivered *him* to be crucified.

The King crowned with thorns, and led away to crucifixion (Mk. 15:16-23; Lk. 23:26-32; John 19:16, 17).

27 Then the soldiers of the governor
[i]took Jesus into the common hall, and
gathered unto him the whole band *of soldiers*.
28 And they [j]stripped him, and put on
him a [k]scarlet robe.
29 And when they had platted a crown
of [l]thorns, they put *it* upon his head, and
a [m]reed in his right hand: and they
bowed the knee before him, and mocked
him, saying, Hail, King of the Jews!
30 And they [n]spit upon him, and took
the reed, and [o]smote him on the head.
31 And after that they had mocked
him, they took the robe off from him,
and put his own raiment on him, and
led him away to crucify *him*.
32 And as they came out, they found a
man of Cyrene, Simon by name: him
they compelled to [p]bear his cross.

The crucifixion (Mk. 15:22-32; Lk. 23:33-43; John 19:17-24).

33 [1]And when they were come unto a
place called Golgotha, that is to say, [q]a
[r]place of a skull,
34 They gave him [s]vinegar to drink
mingled with gall: and when he had
tasted *thereof*, he would not drink.

The law fulfilled in Christ (Mt. 5:17, 18; Gal. 3:11-14).

35 And they crucified him, and parted
his garments, casting lots: that it might
be [t]fulfilled which was spoken by the
prophet, [u]They parted my garments
among them, and upon my vesture did
they cast lots.
36 And sitting down they watched
him there;

A.D. 33.

a Mk. 15:6-15; Lk. 23:17-25; John 18:39, 40.
b Mt. 21:38; John 15:22-25. Cf. Gen. 37:11; Dan. 3:8-12.
c Gen. 31:29.
d John 5:43; Acts 3:14.
e Lk. 23:21.
f Deut. 21:6.
g Gen. 4:10; Mt. 23:35; Acts 5:28.
h John 19:1
i Isa. 53:8.
j Mk. 15:16-20; John 19:2, 3.
k Lk. 23:11. Cf. Psa. 69:19
l Gen. 3:18; Gal. 3:13.
m Isa. 36:6.
n vs. 30, 31; Psa. 22:6; Isa. 50:6; 53:3; Zech. 13:7.
o Mt. 26:67.
p Mk. 15:21; Lk. 23:26; 2 Cor. 4:10.
q *the place*, etc.
r Mk. 15:22; Lk. 23:33; John 19:17.
s Psa. 69:21; Mk. 15:23; Lk. 23:36.
t *Christ (First Advent).* Mt. 27:50. (Gen. 3:15; Acts 1:9.)
u Psa. 22:18; Mk. 15:24; Lk. 23:34; John 19:23, 24.

[1]**(27:33)** The order of events at the crucifixion: (1) The arrival at Golgotha (Mt. 27:33; Mk. 15:22; Lk. 23:33; John 19:17). (2) The offer of the stupefying drink refused (Mt. 27:34; Mk. 15:23). (3) Jesus is crucified between two thieves (Mt. 27:35-38; Mk. 15:24-28; Lk. 23:33-38; John 19:18-24). (4) He utters the first cry from the cross, "Father, forgive," etc. (Lk. 23:34). (5) The soldiers part His garments (Mt. 27:35; Mk. 15:24; Lk. 23:34; John 19:23). (6) The Jews mock Jesus (Mt. 27:39-44; Mk. 15:29-32; Lk. 23:35-38). (7) The thieves rail on Him, but one repents and believes (Mt. 27:44; Mk. 15:32; Lk. 23:39-43). (8) The second cry from the cross, "To-day shalt thou be with me," etc. (Lk. 23:43). (9) The third cry, "Woman, behold thy son" (John 19:26, 27). (10) The darkness (Mt. 27:45; Mk. 15:33; Lk. 23:44). (11) The fourth cry, "My God," etc. (Mt. 27:46, 47; Mk. 15:34-36). (12) The fifth cry, "I thirst" (John 19:28). (13) The sixth cry,

37 And set up over his head his accusation written, [1]THIS IS JESUS THE KING OF THE JEWS.

38 Then were there two thieves [a]crucified with him, one on the right hand, and another on the left.

39 And they that passed by reviled him, [b]wagging their heads,

40 And saying, Thou that destroyest the temple, and buildest *it* in three days, save thyself. If thou be the Son of God, come down from the cross.

41 Likewise also the chief priests mocking *him*, with the scribes and elders, said,

42 He [c]saved others; himself he cannot save. If he be the King of Israel, let him now come down from the cross, and we will [d]believe him.

43 He [e]trusted in [f]God; let him deliver him now, if he will have him: for he said, I am the Son of God.

44 The thieves also, which were crucified with him, [g]cast the same in his teeth.

The death of Jesus Christ (Mk. 15:33-41; Lk. 23:44-49; John 19:30-37).

45 Now from the sixth hour there was [h]darkness over all the land unto the ninth hour.

46 And about the ninth hour Jesus cried with a loud voice, [i]saying, Eli, Eli, lama sabachthani? that is to say, My [j]God, my God, [k]why hast thou forsaken me?

47 Some of them that stood there, when they heard *that*, said, This *man* calleth for Elias.

48 And straightway one of them ran, and took a spunge, and filled *it* with [l]vinegar, and put *it* on a reed, and gave him to drink.

49 The rest said, Let be, let us see whether Elias will come to save him.

50 Jesus, when he had cried again with a loud voice, [2m]yielded up the [n]ghost.

The Dispensation of Law ends. (See John 1:17, *note;* Heb. 9:3-8; 10:19, 20.)

51 And, behold, the [3o]veil of the temple was rent in twain from the top to the bottom; and the earth did quake, and the rocks rent;

52 And the [4]graves were opened; and many bodies of the saints which slept [p]arose,

53 And came out of the graves after his resurrection, and went into the [q]holy city, and appeared unto many.

54 Now when the centurion, and they that were with him, watching Jesus, saw the earthquake, and those things that

A.D. 33.

a Isa. 53:12.
b Psa. 22:7, 8, 11-13; 109:25.
c Lk. 15:2; John 3:14, 15; Heb. 9:22.
d *believe on.*
e Psa. 22:8.
f *Jehovah.* Psa. 22:8.
g Mk. 15:32; Lk. 23:39-43.
h Mk. 15:33; Lk. 23:44.
i *Bible prayers (N.T.).* Mk. 10:47. (Mt. 6:9; Rev. 22:20.)
j *God.* Psa. 22:1; 88:14.
k Psa. 22:3 gives the answer to this significant and terrible cry.
l Psa. 69:21.
m Mk. 15:37; Lk. 23:46; John 10:18; 19:30; 1 Cor. 15:3.
n *Christ (First Advent).* Mt. 28:5, 6. (Gen. 3:15; Acts 1:9.)
o Lev. 16:2, 11-14; Mk. 15:38; Lk. 23:45; Heb. 9:7, 8, 11, 12; 10:19, 20.
p *Resurrection.* vs. 52, 53; Mt. 28:1-6. (Job 19:25; 1 Cor. 15:52.)
q *Sanctify, holy (things)* (N.T.). Acts 6:13. (Mt. 4:5; Rev. 22:11.)

"It is finished" (John 19:30). (14) The seventh cry, "Father, into thy hands," etc. (Lk. 23:46). (15) Our Lord dismisses His spirit (Mt. 27:50; Mk. 15:37; Lk. 23:46; John 19:30).

[1] **(27:37)** Cf. Mk. 15:26; Lk. 23:38; John 19:19. These accounts supplement, but do not contradict each other. No one of the Evangelists quotes the entire inscription. All have "The King of the Jews." Luke adds to this the further words, "This is", Matthew quotes the name, "Jesus"; whilst John gives the additional words "of Nazareth." The narratives combined give the entire inscription; "This is [Matthew, Luke] Jesus [Matthew, John] of Nazareth [John] the King of the Jews"

[2] **(27:50)** Literally, "dismissed His spirit." The Gr. implies an act of the will. This expression, taken with Mk. 15:37; Lk. 23:46; John 19:30, differentiates the death of Christ from all other physical death. He died by His own volition when He could say of His redemptive work, "It is finished." "No man taketh it from me, but I lay it down of myself" (John 10:18).

[3] **(27:51)** The veil which was rent was the veil which divided the holy place into which the priests entered from the holy of holies into which only the high priest might enter on the day of atonement (Ex. 26:31, *note;* Lev. 16:1-30). The rending of that veil, which was a type of the human body of Christ (Heb. 10:20) signified that a "new and living way" was opened for all believers into the very presence of God with no other sacrifice or priesthood save Christ's (cf. Heb. 9:1-8; 10:19-22).

[4] **(27:52)** That these bodies returned to their graves is not said and may not be inferred. The wave-sheaf (Lev. 23:10-12) typifies the resurrection of Christ, but a sheaf implies plurality. It was a single "corn of wheat" that fell into the ground in the crucifixion and entombment of Christ (John 12:24); it was a sheaf which came forth in resurrection. The inference is that these saints, with the spirits of "just men made perfect" (Heb. 12:23) from Paradise, went with Jesus (Eph. 4:8-10) into heaven.

were done, they feared greatly, saying,
[a]Truly this was the Son of God.
55 And many women were there
beholding afar off, which followed Jesus
from Galilee, ministering unto him:
56 Among which was Mary Magdalene, and Mary the mother of [b]James
and Joses, and the mother of Zebedee's
children.

The entombment of Christ (Mk. 15:42-47; Lk. 23:50-56; John 19:38-42).

57 When the even was come, there
came a rich man of Arimathæa, named
Joseph, who also himself was Jesus' disciple:
58 He went to Pilate, and begged the
body of Jesus. Then Pilate commanded
the body to be delivered.
59 And when Joseph had taken the
body, he wrapped it in a clean linen cloth,
60 And laid it in [c]his own new tomb,
which he had hewn out in the rock: and
he rolled a great stone to the door of the
sepulchre, and departed.
61 And there was Mary Magdalene,
and the [d]other Mary, sitting over against
the sepulchre.

The sepulchre sealed and guarded.

62 Now the next day, that followed the
day of the preparation, the chief priests
and Pharisees came together unto Pilate,
63 Saying, Sir, we remember that that
deceiver said, while he was yet alive,
[e]After three days I will rise again.
64 Command therefore that the sepulchre be made sure until the third day,
lest his disciples come by night, and
steal him away, and say unto the people,
He is risen from the dead: so the last
error shall be worse than the first.
65 Pilate said unto them, Ye have a
watch: go your way, make *it* as sure as
ye can.
66 So they went, and made the sepulchre sure, sealing the stone, and setting a
watch.

A.D. 33.

a Mk. 15:39-41; Lk. 23:47-49; Acts 8:37.
b Son of Alphæus. Mt. 4:21, *note.*
c Isa. 53:9.
d Supposed to be Mary the mother of James and Joses.
e Mt. 16:21; 17:23; 20:19; 26:61; Mk. 8:31; 10:34; Lk. 9:22; 18:33; 24:6, 7; John 2:19.
f Lit. *end of the sabbaths.* The sabbaths end, the first day comes. Mt. 12:1 *note;* John 20:19; Acts 20:7; 1 Cor. 16:2; Rev. 1:10.
g *an angel,* etc.
h Heb. 1:4, *note.*
i Cf. Dan. 10:6; Rev. 10:1.
j Acts 17:31; Rev. 1:17.
k Mk. 16:6; 2 Tim. 1:7; Rom. 8:15.
l *Christ (First Advent).* Acts 1:9. (Gen. 3:15; Acts 1:9.)
m *Resurrection.* vs. 1-6; Mk. 5:41. (Job 19:25; 1 Cor. 15:52.)
n Lit. *O joy!*

CHAPTER 28.

The resurrection of Jesus Christ, and events of that day (Mk. 16:1-14; Lk. 24:1-49; John 20:1-23.)

[1]In the [f]end of the sabbath, as it began
to dawn toward the first *day* of the
week, came Mary Magdalene and the
[d]other Mary to see the sepulchre.
2 And, behold, there was a great earthquake: for [g]the [h]angel of the Lord
descended from heaven, and came and
rolled back the stone from the door, and
sat upon it.
3 [i]His countenance was like lightning,
and his raiment white as snow:
4 And for fear of him the keepers did
shake, and became as [j]dead *men.*
5 And the [h]angel answered and said
unto the women, [k]Fear not ye: for I know
that ye seek Jesus, which was crucified.
6 He is not here: for [l]he is [m]risen, as he
said. Come, see the place where the Lord
lay.
7 And go quickly, and tell his disciples
that he is risen from the dead; and,
behold, he goeth before you into Galilee;
there shall ye see him: lo, I have told you.
8 And they departed quickly from the
sepulchre with fear and great joy; and
did run to bring his disciples word.
9 And as they went to tell his disciples, behold, [2]Jesus met them, saying,
[n]All hail. And they came and held him
by the feet, and worshipped him.
10 Then said Jesus unto them, Be not

[1] **(28:1)** The order of *events,* combining the four narratives, is as follows: Three women, Mary Magdalene, and Mary the mother of James, and Salome, start for the sepulchre, followed by other women bearing spices. The three find the stone rolled away, and Mary Magdalene goes to tell the disciples (Lk. 23:55-24:9; John 20:1, 2) Mary, the mother of James and Joses, draws nearer the tomb and sees the angel of the Lord (Mt. 28:2). She goes back to meet the other women following with the spices. Meanwhile Peter and John, warned by Mary Magdalene, arrive, look in, and go away (John 20:3-10). Mary Magdalene returns weeping, sees the two angels and then Jesus (John 20:11-18), and goes as He bade her to tell the disciples. Mary (mother of James and Joses), meanwhile, has met the women with the spices and, returning with them, they see the *two* angels (Lk. 24:4, 5; Mk. 16:5). They also receive the angelic message, and, going to seek the disciples, are met by Jesus (Mt. 28:8-10).

[2] **(28:9)** The order of our Lord's *appearances* would seem to be: On the day of His resurrection: (1) To Mary Magdalene (John 20:14-18). (2) To the women returning from the tomb with the angelic

afraid: go tell my [a]brethren that they go
into Galilee, and there shall they see me.

11 Now when they were going,
behold, some of the watch came into the
city, and shewed unto the chief priests
all the things that were done.

12 And when they were assembled
with the elders, and had taken counsel,
they gave large [b]money unto the soldiers,

13 Saying, Say ye, His disciples came
by night, and stole him *away* while we
slept.

14 And if this come to the governor's
ears, we will [c]persuade him, and secure
you.

15 So they took the money, and did as
they were taught: and this saying is
commonly reported among the Jews
until this day.

A.D. 33.

a John 20:17; Heb. 2:11, 12.
b Mt. 27:4.
c Cf. Acts 12:19.
d John 20:24-29; 1 Cor. 15:5, 6.
e John 5:22; 17:2; Eph. 1:22.
f Or, *disciple.* Mk. 16:15, 16; Lk. 24:47, 48; Acts 1:8.
g Acts 2:38, 41.
h Or, *unto.*
i *Holy Spirit.* Mk. 1:8, 10, 12. (Mt. 1:18; Acts 2:4.)
j *Inspiration.* vs. 19, 20; Mk. 1:44. (Ex. 4:15; Rev. 22:19.)
k Acts 4:31; 23:11.
l *consummation of the age.*

Jesus in Galilee: the great commission (Mk. 16:15-18).

16 Then the eleven disciples went
away into Galilee, into a mountain
where Jesus had appointed them.

17 And when they saw him, they worshipped him: but [d]some doubted.

18 And Jesus came and spake unto
them, saying, [e]All power is given unto
me in heaven and in earth.

19 [1]Go ye therefore, and [f]teach all
nations, [g]baptizing them [h]in the [2]name
of the Father, and of the Son, and of the
[i]Holy Ghost:

20 Teaching them to observe all things
[j]whatsoever I have commanded you:
and, lo, I am [k]with you alway, *even* unto
the [l]end of the world. Amen.

message (Mt. 28:8-10). (3) To Peter, probably in the afternoon (Lk. 24:34; 1 Cor. 15:5). (4) To the Emmaus disciples toward evening (Lk. 24:13-31). (5) To the apostles, except Thomas (Lk. 24:36-43; John 20:19-24). Eight days afterward: (1) To the apostles, Thomas being present (John 20:24-29). In Galilee: (1) To the seven by the Lake of Tiberias (John 21:1-23). (2) On a mountain, to the apostles and five hundred brethren (1 Cor. 15:6). At Jerusalem and Bethany again: (1) To James (1 Cor. 15:7). (2) To the eleven (Mt. 28:16-20; Mk. 16:14-20; Lk. 24:33-53; Acts 1:3-12). To Paul: (1) Near Damascus (Acts 9:3-6; 1 Cor. 15:8). (2) In the temple (Acts 22:17-21; 23:11). To Stephen, outside Jerusalem (Acts 7:55). To John on Patmos (Rev. 1:10-19).

[1] **(28:19)** With the death and resurrection of Jesus Christ begins the "dispensation of the grace of God" (Eph. 3:2), which is defined as "his kindness toward us through Christ Jesus"; and, "the gift of God: not of works, lest any man should boast" (Eph. 2:7-9). Under grace God freely gives to the believing sinner eternal life (Rom. 6:23); accounts to him a perfect righteousness (Rom. 3:21, 22; 4:4, 5); and accords to him a perfect position (Eph. 1:6). The predicted results of this sixth testing of man are: (1) The salvation of all who believe (Acts 16:31); (2) judgment upon an unbelieving world and an apostate church (Mt. 25:31-46; 2 Thes. 1:7-10; 1 Pet. 4:17, 18; Rev. 3:15, 16).

(1) Man's state at the beginning of the dispensation of grace (Rom. 3:19; Gal. 3:22; Eph. 2:11, 12). (2) Man's responsibility under grace (John 1:11, 12; 3:36; 6:28, 29). (3) His predicted failure (Mt. 24:37-39; Lk. 18:8; 19:12-14). (4) The judgment (2 Thes. 2:7-12).

[2] **(28:19)** The word is in the singular, the "name," not names. Father, Son, and Holy Spirit is the final name of the one true God. It affirms: (1) That God is one. (2) That He subsists in a personality which is threefold, indicated by *relationship* as Father and Son; by a *mode of being* as Spirit; and by the *different parts* taken by the Godhead in manifestation and in the work of redemption, e.g. John 3:5, 6 (Spirit), 16, 17 (Father and Son). In Mt. 3:16, 17; Mk. 1:10, 11; Lk. 3:21, 22, the three persons are in manifestation together. (3) The conjunction in one name of the Three affirms equality and oneness of substance. See O.T. Names of God: Gen. 1:1, *note;* 2:4, *note;* 14:18, *note;* 15:2, *note;* 17:1, *note;* 21:33, *note;* 1 Sam. 1:3, *note;* Mal. 3:18, Summary. See "Lord," Mt. 8:2, *note;* "Word" (*Logos*), John 1:1, *note;* "Holy Spirit," Acts 2:4, Summary. See "Christ, Deity of," John 20:28, *note.*

THE GOSPEL ACCORDING TO
ST. MARK

WRITER. The writer of the second Gospel, Mark, called also John, was the son of one of the New Testament Marys, and nephew of Barnabas. He was an associate of the apostles, and is mentioned in the writings of Paul and of Luke (Acts 12:12, 25; 15:37, 39; Col. 4:10; 2 Tim. 4:11; Phm. 24).

The date of Mark has been variously placed between A.D. 57 and 63.

Theme. The scope and purpose of the book are evident from its contents. In it Jesus is seen as the mighty Worker, rather than as the unique Teacher. It is the Gospel of Jehovah's "Servant the Branch" (Zech. 3:8), as Matthew is the Gospel of the "Branch . . . unto David" (Jer. 33:15).

Everywhere the servant character of the incarnate Son is manifest. The key-verse is 10:45, "For even the Son of man came not to be ministered unto, but to minister." The characteristic word is "straightway," a servant's word. There is no genealogy, for who gives the genealogy of a servant? The distinctive character of Christ in Mark is that set forth in Phil. 2:6-8.

But this lowly Servant, who emptied Himself of the "form of God," "and was found in fashion as a man," was, nevertheless, "the mighty God" (Isa. 9:6), as Mark distinctly declares (1:1), and therefore mighty works accompanied and authenticated His ministry. As befits a Servant-Gospel, Mark is characteristically a Gospel of deeds, rather than of words.

The best preparation of heart for the study of Mark is the prayerful reading of Isa. 42:1-21; 50:4-11; 52:13–53:12; Zech. 3:8; Phil. 2:5-8.

Mark is in five principal divisions: I. The manifestation of the Servant-Son, 1:1-11. II. The Servant-Son tested as to His fidelity, 1:12, 13. III. The Servant-Son at work, 1:14–13:37. IV. The Servant-Son "obedient unto death," 14:1–15:47. V. The ministry of the risen Servant-Son, now exalted to all authority, 16:1-20.

The events recorded in this book cover a period of 7 years.

CHAPTER 1.

The ministry of John the Baptist (Mt. 3:1-11; Lk. 3:1-16; John 1:6-8, 19-28).

The [a]beginning of the [b]gospel of Jesus
Christ, the Son of God;
2 As it is written in the prophets,
[c]Behold, I send my messenger before thy
face, which shall prepare thy way before
thee.
3 The [d]voice of one crying in the
wilderness, Prepare ye the way of the
[e]Lord, make his paths straight.
4 John did baptize in the wilderness,
and preach the baptism of [f]repentance
for the remission of [g]sins.
5 And there went out unto him all the
land of Judæa, and they of Jerusalem,
and were all baptized of him in the river
of Jordan, confessing their [g]sins.
6 And John was [h]clothed with camel's
hair, and with a girdle of a skin about his
loins; and he did eat locusts and wild
honey;
7 And preached, saying, There
[i]cometh one mightier than I after me, the
latchet of whose shoes I am not worthy
to stoop down and unloose.

A.D. 26.

a Mt. 1:1; Lk. 1:1, 5; John 1:1.
b *Gospel.* vs. 1, 14, 15; Mk. 8:35. (Gen. 12:1-3; Rev. 14:6.)

[A.D. 27.

c Mal. 3:1; Mt. 11:10; Lk. 1:76; 7:27.
d Isa. 40:3; Mt. 3:3; Lk. 3:4; John 1:23.
e *Jehovah.* Isa. 40.3.
f *Repentance.* Mk. 2:17. (Mt. 3:2; Acts 17:30.)
g *Sins.* Rom. 3:23, *note.*
h Mt. 3:4; 11:8, 9.
i Mt. 3:11; Lk. 3:16; John 1:15, 26, 33.
j *Holy Spirit.* vs. 8, 10, 12; Mk. 3:29. (Mt. 1:18; Acts 2:4.)
k Mt. 3:13.
l Lev. 8:12; Psa. 89:20; Ezek. 1:1; Mt. 3:16, 17; Lk. 3:21, 22; Acts 10:38.
m *Straightway.*
n Mt. 4:1; Lk. 4:1.
o *Satan.* Mk. 3:23, 26. (Gen. 3:1; Rev. 20:10.)

8 I indeed have baptized you with
water: but he shall baptize you with the
[j]Holy Ghost.

The baptism of Jesus
(Mt. 3:13-17; Lk. 3:21, 22).

9 And it [k]came to pass in those days,
that Jesus came from Nazareth of
Galilee, and was baptized of John in
Jordan.
10 And straightway coming up out of
the water, he saw the [l]heavens opened,
and the Spirit like a dove descending
upon him:
11 And there came a voice from heav-
en, *saying,* Thou art my beloved Son, in
whom I am well pleased.

The temptation of Jesus
(Mt. 4:1-11; Lk. 4:1-13).

12 And [m]immediately the Spirit [n]driv-
eth him into the wilderness.
13 And he was there in the wilderness
forty days, tempted of [o]Satan; and was
with the wild beasts; and the angels
ministered unto him.

The first Galilean ministry
(Mt. 4:12-17; Lk. 4:14).

14 Now after that John was put in prison, Jesus came into Galilee, preaching the gospel of the [a]kingdom of God,

15 And saying, The time is fulfilled, and the kingdom of God is at hand: repent ye, and believe the gospel.

The call of Peter and Andrew (Mt. 4:18-22; Lk. 5:10, 11. Cf. John 1:35-42).

16 Now as he walked by the sea of Galilee, he saw Simon and Andrew his brother casting a net into the sea: for they were fishers.

17 And Jesus said unto them, Come ye after me, and I will make you to become [b]fishers of men.

18 And straightway they forsook their nets, and followed him.

19 And when he had gone a little further thence, he saw [c]James the *son* of Zebedee, and John his brother, who also were in the [d]ship mending their nets.

20 And straightway he called them: and they left their father Zebedee in the ship with the hired servants, and went after him.

Jesus casts out demons in Capernaum
(Lk. 4:31-37).

21 And they went into Capernaum; and straightway on the sabbath day he entered into the [e]synagogue, and taught.

22 And they were [f]astonished at his doctrine: for he taught them as one that had authority, and not as the scribes.

23 And there was in their synagogue a man with an [g]unclean spirit; and he cried out,

24 Saying, Let *us* alone; what have we to do with thee, [h]thou Jesus of Nazareth? art thou come to destroy us? I [i]know thee who thou art, the Holy One of God.

25 And Jesus rebuked him, saying, Hold thy peace, and come out of him.

26 And when the unclean spirit had torn him, and cried with a loud voice, [j]he came out of him.

27 And they were all amazed, insomuch that they questioned among themselves, saying, What thing is this? what new doctrine *is* this? for with authority commandeth he even the unclean spirits, and they do obey him.

28 And [k]immediately his fame spread abroad throughout all the region round about Galilee.

Simon's wife's mother healed of a fever
(Mt. 8:14, 15; Lk. 4:38, 39).

29 And [k]forthwith, when they were come out of the synagogue, they entered into the house of Simon and Andrew, with James and John.

30 But Simon's wife's [l]mother lay sick of a fever, and anon they tell him of her.

31 And he came and took her by the hand, and lifted her up; and [k]immediately the fever left her, and she [m]ministered unto them.

Demons cast out: many healed
(Mt. 8:16, 17; Lk. 4:40, 41).

32 And at [n]even, when the sun did set, they brought unto him [o]all that were diseased, and them that were possessed with [p]devils.

33 And all the city was gathered together at the door.

34 And he healed many that were sick of divers diseases, and cast out many [p]devils; and [q]suffered not the devils to speak, because they knew him.

Jesus prays: a preaching tour in Galilee
(Lk. 4:42-44).

35 And in the morning, [r]rising up a great while before day, he went out, and departed into a solitary place, and there prayed.

36 And Simon and they that were with him followed after him.

37 And when they had found him, they said unto him, All *men* seek for thee.

38 And he said unto them, Let us go into the next towns, that I may preach there also: for [s]therefore came I forth.

39 And he preached in their synagogues throughout all Galilee, and cast out [p]devils.

A leper healed (Mt. 8:2-4; Lk. 5:12-14).

40 And there came a [t]leper to him, beseeching him, and kneeling down to him, and saying unto him, If thou wilt, thou canst make me clean.

41 And Jesus, moved with compassion, put forth *his* hand, and touched him, and saith unto him, [u]I will; be thou clean.

42 And as soon as he had spoken, [k]immediately the leprosy departed from him, and he was cleansed.

43 And he straitly charged him, and forthwith sent him away;

A.D. 31.

a See Mt. 6:33, *note.*
b Mt. 13:47-50; Lk. 5:10, 11.
c Mt. 4:21, 22.
d *boat.*
e Mt. 4:13, 23; Lk. 4:31.
f Mt. 7:28, 29.
g Lk. 4:33-37; Rev. 16:13.
h Lit. *Jesus, Nazarene!*
i v. 34; Jas. 2:19.
j *Miracles* (N.T.). vs. 23-26, 30, 31, 32-34, 39, 40-42; Mk. 2:3-12. (Mt. 8:2, 3; Acts 28:8, 9.)
k *straightway.*
l Mt. 8:14, 15; Lk. 4:38, 39.
m Mt. 27:55; Phm. 13.
n Mt. 8:16, 17; Lk. 4:40, 41; John 8:12
o Mt. 11:4, 5; Lk. 9:11.
p *demons.* Mt. 7:22, *note.*
q vs. 24, 25; Mk. 3:12; Acts 16,17, 18.
r Lk. 4:42-44; 5:16.
s Isa. 61:1, 2; Mt. 10:5, 6.
t Lev. 13:44-46; Isa. 1:5, 6; Mt. 8:2-4; Lk. 5:12-14.
u John 6:37.

44 And saith unto him, [a]See thou say nothing to any man: but go thy way, shew thyself to the priest, and offer for thy cleansing [b]those things which [c]Moses commanded, for a testimony unto them.

45 But he went out, and began to publish *it* much, and to blaze abroad the matter, insomuch that Jesus could no more openly enter into the city, but was without in [d]desert places: and they came to him from every quarter.

CHAPTER 2.

The palsied man healed
(Mt. 9:1-8; Lk. 5:18-26).

AND again he entered into Capernaum after *some* days; and it was noised that he was in the house.

2 And straightway many were gathered together, insomuch that there was no room to receive *them*, no, not so much as about the door: and he preached the word unto them.

3 And they come unto him, bringing one sick of the [e]palsy, which was borne of four.

4 And when they could not come nigh unto him for the press, they uncovered the roof where he was: and when they had [f]broken *it* up, they let down the bed wherein the sick of the palsy lay.

5 When Jesus saw their faith, he said unto the sick of the palsy, Son, thy [g]sins be [h]forgiven thee.

6 But there were certain of the scribes sitting there, and reasoning in their hearts,

7 Why doth this *man* thus speak blasphemies? who can forgive sins but [i]God only?

8 And [j]immediately when Jesus [k]perceived in his spirit that they so reasoned within themselves, he said unto them, Why reason ye these things in your hearts?

9 Whether is it easier [l]to say to the sick of the palsy, *Thy* [g]sins be forgiven thee; or to say, Arise, and take up thy bed, and walk?

10 But that ye may know that the [m]Son of man hath power on earth to forgive sins, (he saith to the sick of the palsy,)

11 I say unto thee, Arise, and take up thy bed, and go thy way into thine house.

12 [n]And [j]immediately he arose, took up the bed, and went forth before them all; insomuch that they were all amazed, and [o]glorified God, saying, We never saw it on this fashion.

The call of Levi (Matthew)
(Mt. 9:9-13; Lk. 5:27-32).

13 And he went forth again by the sea side; and all the multitude resorted unto him, and he taught them.

14 And as he [p]passed by, he saw Levi the *son* of Alphæus sitting at the receipt of custom, and said unto him, Follow me. And he arose and followed him.

15 And it came to pass, that, as Jesus sat at meat in his house, many publicans and [g]sinners sat also together with Jesus and his disciples: for there were many, and they followed him.

16 And when the scribes and Pharisees saw him eat with publicans and [g]sinners, they said unto his disciples, How is it that he eateth and drinketh with publicans and sinners?

17 When Jesus heard *it*, he saith unto them, They that are [q]whole have no need of the physician, but they that are sick: I came not to call the righteous, but sinners to [r]repentance.

18 And the disciples of John and of the Pharisees [s]used to fast: and they come and say unto him, Why do the disciples of John and of the Pharisees fast, but thy disciples fast not?

19 And Jesus said unto them, Can the children of the bridechamber fast, while the [t]bridegroom is with them? as long as they have the bridegroom with them, they cannot fast.

20 But the days will come, when the bridegroom shall be [u]taken away from them, and then shall they fast in those days.

Parable of the cloth and the bottles
(Cf. Mt. 9:16, 17; Lk. 5:36-39.)

21 No man also [v]seweth a piece of new cloth on an old garment: else the new piece that filled it up taketh away from the old, and the rent is made worse.

22 And [w]no man putteth new wine into old [x]bottles: else the new wine doth burst the bottles, and the wine is spilled, and the bottles will be [y]marred: but new wine must be put into new bottles.

A.D. 31.

a Mk. 5:43.
b *Inspiration.* Mk. 7:8-13. (Ex. 4:15; Rev. 22:19.)
c Lev. 14:2-20.
d Isa. 35:1; Mk. 6:31, 32.
e Isa. 40:29; Mt. 9:2-8; Lk. 5:18-26; Acts. 9:33.
f Mt. 15:23-28; Lk. 18:39.
g *Sin.* Rom. 3:23, *note.*
h *Forgiveness.* Lk. 7:47-49. (Lev. 4:20; Mt. 26:28.)
i Isa. 43:25; John 1:1, 14 with John 8:11.
j *straightway.*
k Mt. 9:4; John 2:25.
l Psa. 33:6, 9; Mk. 1:27; Lk. 4:32.
m Mt. 8:20, *note.*
n *Miracles* (N.T.). vs. 3, 12; Mk. 3:1-5. (Mt. 8:2, 3; Acts 28:8, 9.)
o Mt. 15:31; Phil. 2:11.
p Mt. 9:9-13; Lk. 5:27-32.
q Mt. 18:11; Lk. 19:7, 10; 1 Tim. 1:15.
r *Repentance.* Mk. 6:12. (Mt. 3:2; Acts 17:30.)
s Mt. 6:16-18; 9:14-17; Lk. 5:33-39.
t John 3:29.
u John 16:6, 20, 22.
v *Parables* (N.T.). vs. 21-22, Mk. 4:3-20. (Mt. 5:13-16; Lk. 21:29-31.)
w Gal. 3:1-3.
x *wine-skins.*
y Gr. *apollumi.* John 3:16, *note.*

Jesus Lord of the sabbath
(Mt. 12:1-8; Lk. 6:1-5).

23 And it came to pass, that he [a]went through the corn fields on the sabbath day; and his disciples began, as they went, to pluck the ears of corn.

24 And the Pharisees said unto him, Behold, why do they on the sabbath day that which is not lawful?

25 And he said unto them, Have ye never read what [b]David did, when he had need, and was an hungred, he, and they that were with him?

26 How he went into the house of God in the days of Abiathar the high priest, and did eat the [c]shewbread, which is not lawful to eat but for the [d]priests, and gave also to them which were with him?

27 And he said unto them, The [e]sabbath was made for man, and not man for the sabbath:

28 Therefore the [f]Son of man is Lord also of the sabbath.

CHAPTER 3.

Jesus heals the withered hand on the sabbath (Mt. 12:10-14; Lk. 6:6-11).

And he entered again into the synagogue; and there was a man there which had a [g]withered hand.

2 And they watched him, whether he would heal him on the sabbath day; that they might accuse him.

3 And he saith unto the man which had the withered hand, Stand forth.

4 And he saith unto them, Is it lawful to do [h]good on the sabbath days, or to do evil? to save life, or to kill? But they held their peace.

5 And when he had looked round about on them with [i]anger, being grieved for the hardness of their hearts, he saith unto the man, [j]Stretch forth thine hand. And he stretched *it* out: and his hand was [k]restored whole as the other.

The multitudes healed
(Mt. 12:15, 16; Lk. 6:17-19).

6 And the Pharisees went forth, and straightway took [l]counsel with the Herodians against him, how they might destroy him.

7 But Jesus withdrew himself with his disciples to the sea: and a great [m]multitude from Galilee followed him, and from Judæa,

A.D. 31.

a Mt. 12:1-8; Lk. 6:1-5.
b 1 Sam. 21:1-6; Mt. 12:9-13; Lk. 6:6-10.
c Ex. 25:30, *note.*
d Lev. 24:5-9.
e Lk. 14:5.
f Mt. 12:8; John 5:16-18.
g Mt. 12:9-13; Lk. 6:6-10.
h Lk. 14:3.
i Mt. 23:13.
j John 4:50; Rom. 4:19-25.
k *Miracles* (N.T.). vs. 1-5, 10; Mk. 4:37-41. (Mt. 8:2, 3; Acts 28:8, 9.)
l Psa. 109:4, 5; Mt. 12:14; Lk. 6:11.
m Mt. 12:15; Lk. 6:17-19.
n Mt. 14:36; Mk. 6:56; Lk. 6:19.
o Mt. 12:16; Mk. 1:25, 34; Lk. 4:41.
p Mt. 10:1-4; Lk. 6:13-16; 9:1; John 15:16. Cf. Rev. 21:14 with Eph. 2:20.
q See Mt. 4:21, *note.*
r v. 31; John 7:5; 8:48; Acts 26:24.
s Mt. 9:34; 10:25; 12:24; Lk. 11:14, 15; John 10:20.
t *demons.*
u *Satan.* vs. 22, 23, 26; Mk. 4:15. (Gen. 3:1; Rev. 20:10.)

8 And from Jerusalem, and from Idumaea, and *from* beyond Jordan; and they about Tyre and Sidon, a great multitude, when they had heard what great things he did, came unto him.

9 And he spake to his disciples, that a small ship should wait on him because of the multitude, lest they should throng him.

10 For he had healed many; insomuch that they pressed upon him for to [n]touch him, as many as had plagues.

11 And unclean spirits, when they saw him, fell down before him, and cried, saying, Thou art the Son of God.

12 And he straitly [o]charged them that they should not make him known.

The twelve chosen
(Mt. 10:1-4; Lk. 6:12-16).

13 And he goeth up into a mountain, and [p]calleth *unto him* whom he would: and they came unto him.

14 And he ordained twelve, that they should be with him, and that he might send them forth to preach,

15 And to have power to heal sicknesses, and to cast out devils:

16 And Simon he surnamed Peter;

17 And [q]James the *son* of Zebedee, and John the brother of James; and he surnamed them Boanerges, which is, The sons of thunder:

18 And Andrew, and Philip, and Bartholomew, and Matthew, and Thomas, and James the *son* of Alphaeus, and Thaddaeus, and Simon the Canaanite,

19 And Judas Iscariot, which also betrayed him: and they went into an house.

20 And the multitude cometh together again, so that they could not so much as eat bread.

21 And when his [r]friends heard *of it*, they went out to lay hold on him: for they said, He is beside himself.

The unpardonable sin
(Mt. 12:24-29; Lk. 11:14-20).

22 And the scribes which came down from Jerusalem said, He hath [s]Beelzebub, and by the prince of the devils casteth he out [t]devils.

23 And he called them *unto him*, and said unto them in parables, [u]How can Satan cast out Satan?

24 And if a kingdom be divided

against itself, that kingdom cannot
stand.
25 And if a house be divided against
itself, that house cannot stand.
26 And if [a]Satan rise up against himself, and be divided, he cannot stand,
but hath an end.
27 No man can enter into a [b]strong
man's house, and spoil his goods, except
he will first [c]bind the strong man; and
then he will spoil his house.
28 Verily I say unto you, All [d]sins shall
be forgiven unto the sons of men, and
blasphemies wherewith soever they
shall blaspheme:
29 But he that shall [e]blaspheme against
the [f]Holy Ghost hath never forgiveness,
but is [g]in danger of eternal damnation:
30 [h]Because they said, He hath an
unclean spirit.

The new relationships
(Mt. 12:46-50; Lk. 8:19-21).

31 There came then his [i]brethren and
his mother, and, standing without, sent
unto him, calling him.
32 And the multitude sat about him,
and they said unto him, Behold, thy
mother and thy brethren without seek
for thee.
33 And he answered them, saying,
Who is my mother, or my brethren?
34 And he looked round about on
them which sat about him, and said,
Behold my mother and my brethren!
35 For whosoever shall do the [j]will of
God, the same is my brother, and my sister, and mother.

CHAPTER 4.

The parable of the sower
(Mt. 13:1-23; Lk. 8:4-15).

And he began again to teach by the
[k]sea side: and there was gathered
unto him a great multitude, so that he
entered into a ship, and sat in the sea;
and the whole multitude was by the sea
on the land.
2 And he taught them many things by
parables, and said unto them in his doctrine,
3 Hearken; Behold, there went out a
[l]sower to sow:
4 And it came to pass, as he sowed,
some fell by the way side, and the [m]fowls
of the air came and devoured it up.
5 And some fell on stony ground,
where it had not much earth; and immediately it sprang up, because it had no
depth of earth:
6 But when the sun was up, it was
scorched; and because it had no root, it
withered away.
7 And some fell among thorns, and
the thorns grew up, and choked it, and it
yielded no fruit.
8 And other fell on good ground, and
did yield fruit that sprang up and
increased; and brought forth, some thirty,
and some sixty, and some an hundred.
9 **And he said unto them,** He that hath
[n]ears to hear, let him hear.
10 **And when he was alone, they that
were about him with the twelve asked of
him the parable.**
11 **And he said unto them,** Unto you it
is given to know the [o]mystery of the kingdom of God: but unto them that are without, all *these* things are done in parables:
12 That [p]seeing they may see, and not
perceive; and hearing they may hear,
and not understand; lest at any time
they should [q]be converted, and *their*
[d]sins should be forgiven them.

The parable of the sower explained
(Mt. 13:18-23; Lk. 8:11-15).

13 **And he said unto them,** Know ye
not this parable? and how then will ye
know all parables?
14 The sower soweth the word.
15 And these are they by the way side,
where the word is sown; but when they
have heard, [r]Satan cometh immediately,
and taketh away the word that was
sown in their hearts.
16 And these are they likewise which
are sown on stony ground; who, when
they have heard the word, immediately
receive it with gladness;
17 And have no root in themselves,
and so endure but for a time: afterward,
when [s]affliction or persecution ariseth
for the word's sake, immediately they
are offended.
18 And these are they which are sown
among thorns; such as hear the word,
19 And the [t]cares of this [u]world, and
the deceitfulness of riches, and the lusts
of other things entering in, choke the
word, and it becometh unfruitful.
20 And these are they which are sown
on good ground; such as hear the word,
and [v]receive *it*, and bring forth fruit,

A.D. 31.

a Mt. 12:25-28; Lk. 11:16-20.
b Psa. 35:10; Mt. 12:29; Lk. 11:21, 22; 13:16.
c Heb. 2:14, 15; 1 John 3:8.
d *Sin.* Rom. 3:23, *note.*
e Mt. 12:31, 32; Lk. 12:10; 1 John 1:7. Cf. Eph. 4:30 with Eph. 1:13, 14.
f *Holy Spirit.* Mk. 12:36. (Mt. 1:18; Acts 2:4.)
g *is bound by an eternal sin.*
h Isa. 5:20; 1 Cor. 12:3; 1 Pet. 4:4, 5.
i Mt. 12:46-50; Mk. 6:3; Lk. 8:19-21.
j Psa. 16:2, 3; John 20:17; Rom. 8:17; Heb. 2:11, 12.
k Isa. 60:5; Mt. 13:1, 2; Lk. 8:4.
l *Parables* (N.T.). vs. 3-20, 21-23, 26-29, 30-32; Mk. 12:1-11. (Mt. 5:13-16; Lk. 21:29-31.)
m v. 15.
n Mt. 11:15; Rev. 2:7.
o Mt. 13:11, *note.*
p Isa. 6:9, 10; Rom. 8:5-7; 1 Cor. 2:14.
q i.e. *turn again.*
r *Satan.* Mk. 8:33. (Gen. 3:1; Rev. 20:10.)
s vs. 5, 6 with Prov. 28:14; Psa. 51:17.
t Cf. v. 7 with Prov. 22:5; 1 Tim. 6:9, 10.
u *age.*
v v. 8 with Jer. 4:3, 4; Hos. 10:12; 1 Thes. 2:13.

some thirtyfold, some sixty, and some an
hundred.

Parable of the candle.
(Cf. Mt. 5:15, 16; Lk. 8:16; 11:33.)

21 And he said unto them, Is a candle
brought to be put under a [a]bushel, or
under a [b]bed? and not to be set on a candlestick?
22 [c]For there is nothing hid, which
shall not be [d]manifested; neither was
any thing kept secret, but that it should
come abroad.
23 If any man have ears to hear, let
him hear.
24 And he said unto them, Take [e]heed
what ye hear: with what measure ye
mete, it shall be measured to you: and
unto you that hear shall more be given.
25 For he that hath, to him shall be
given: and he that hath not, from him
shall be taken even that which he hath.

The unconscious growth.

26 And he said, So is the [f]kingdom of
God, as if a man should cast [g]seed into
the ground;
27 And should sleep, and rise night
and day, and the seed should spring and
grow up, he knoweth not how.
28 For the [h]earth bringeth forth fruit of
herself; first the blade, then the ear, after
that the full corn in the ear.
29 But when the fruit is brought forth,
immediately he putteth in the sickle,
because the [i]harvest is come.

Parable of the mustard seed
(Mt. 13:31, 32, *note*; Lk. 13:18, 19).

30 And he said, Whereunto shall we
liken the kingdom of God? or with what
comparison shall we compare it?
31 *It is* like a grain of [j]mustard seed,
which, when it is sown in the earth, is
less than all the seeds that be in the earth:
32 But when it is sown, it groweth up,
and becometh greater than all herbs, and
shooteth out great branches; so that the
[k]fowls of the air may lodge under the
shadow of it.
33 And with [l]many such parables
spake he the word unto them, as they
were able to hear *it*.
34 But without a parable spake he not
unto them: and when they were alone,
he expounded all things to his disciples.

Jesus stills the storm
(Mt. 8:23-27; Lk. 8:22-25).

35 And the same day, when the even
was come, he saith unto them, Let us
pass over unto the [m]other side.
36 And when they had sent away the
multitude, they took him even as he was
in the ship. And there were also with
him other little ships.
37 And there arose a great storm of
wind, and the waves beat into the ship,
so that it was now [n]full.
38 And he was in the hinder part of
the ship, [o]asleep on a pillow: and they
awake him, and say unto him, Master,
[p]carest thou not that we perish?
39 And he arose, and rebuked the
wind, and said unto the sea, [q]Peace, be
still. And the wind [r]ceased, and there
was a great calm.
40 And he said unto them, Why are ye
so fearful? how is it that ye have no [s]faith?
41 And they feared exceedingly, and
said one to another, [t]What manner of
man is this, that even the wind and the
sea obey him?

CHAPTER 5.

The maniac of Gadara
(Mt. 8:28-34; Lk. 8:26-37).

And they [u]came over unto the other
side of the sea, into the country of
the Gadarenes.
2 And when he was come out of the
ship, immediately there met him out of
the tombs a man with an [v]unclean spirit,
3 Who had *his* dwelling among the
tombs; and no man could bind him, no,
not with chains:
4 Because that he had been [w]often
bound with fetters and chains, and the
chains had been plucked asunder by
him, and the fetters broken in pieces:
neither could any *man* tame him.
5 And always, night and day, he was
in the [x]mountains, and in the [y]tombs,
crying, and cutting himself with stones.
6 But when he saw Jesus afar off, he
ran and worshipped him,
7 And cried with a loud voice, and
said, [z]What have I to do with thee, Jesus,
thou Son of the most high God? I adjure
thee by God, that thou torment me not.
8 For he said unto him, Come out of
the man, *thou* unclean spirit.

A.D. 31.

a Mt. 5:15; Lk. 8:16; 11:33.
b Prov. 19:15; Eph. 5:14.
c *For nothing is hidden except unto manifestation, nor a secret thing done that shall not be exposed.* Cf. Rev. 20:12; *contra,* Rom. 4:6; Heb. 10:16-17.
d Mt. 10:26; Phil. 2:15, 16.
e Jas. 1:19; Acts 16:14.
f See Mt. 6:33, *note.*
g Mt. 13:24-30, 36-43.
h 1 Cor. 3:6, 7.
i Rev. 14:14-16; cf. Isa. 51:11.
j Mt. 13:31, 32; Lk. 13:18, 19; Acts 1:15 with Acts 2:41; Ex. 12:38.
k v. 4 with Dan. 4:20-22.
l Mt. 13:34, 35.
m Mt. 8:18; Lk. 8:22.
n *being filled.*
o Mt. 8:23-27; Lk. 6:12; 8:23-25.
p Psa. 44:23; Lk. 10:40.
q Psa. 65:7; 89:9; 107:29.
r *Miracles* (N.T.). vs. 37-41; Mk. 5:1-13. (Mt. 8:2, 3; Acts 28:8, 9.)
s Mt. 14:31, 32; Mk. 16:14.
t Mt. 14:33.
u Mt. 8:28-34; Lk. 8:26-36.
v Mk. 7:25; Rev. 16:13, 14.
w v. 26; Mk. 3:27. Cf. Rom. 3:20 with Rom. 8:7.
x Jer. 13:16.
y Prov. 21:16.
z Mk. 1:24.

9 And he asked him, What *is* thy name? And he answered, saying, My name *is* Legion: for we are [a]many.

10 And he besought him much that he would not send them away out of the country.

11 Now there was there nigh unto the mountains a great herd of swine feeding.

12 And all the devils besought him, saying, Send us into the swine, that we may enter into them.

13 And forthwith Jesus gave them leave. [b]And the unclean spirits went out, and entered into the [c]swine: and the herd ran violently down a steep place into the sea, (they were about two thousand;) and were choked in the sea.

14 And they that fed the swine fled, and told *it* in the city, and in the country. And they went out to see what it was that was done.

15 And they come to Jesus, and see him that was possessed with the devil, and had the legion, [d]sitting, and clothed, and in his right mind: and they were afraid.

16 And they that saw *it* told them how it befell to him that was possessed with the devil, and *also* concerning the swine.

17 And they began to pray him to [e]depart out of their [f]coasts.

18 And when he was come into the ship, he that had been possessed with the devil prayed him that he might be [g]with him.

19 Howbeit Jesus suffered him not, but saith unto him, Go home to thy friends, and [h]tell them how great things the Lord hath done for thee, and hath had compassion on thee.

20 And he departed, and began to publish in Decapolis how great things Jesus had done for him: and all *men* did marvel.

Jesus heals the woman with an issue of blood, and raises the daughter of Jairus
(Mt. 9:18-26; Lk. 8:41-56).

21 And when Jesus was passed over again by ship unto the other side, much people gathered unto him: and he was nigh unto the sea.

22 And, behold, there cometh one of the rulers of the synagogue, [i]Jairus by name; and when he saw him, he fell at his feet,

23 And besought him greatly, saying, My little daughter lieth at the point of death: *I pray thee,* come and lay thy hands on her, that she may be healed; and she shall live.

24 And *Jesus* went with him; and much people followed him, and thronged him.

25 And a certain [j]woman, which had an issue of blood [k]twelve years,

26 And had suffered many things of many physicians, and had [l]spent all that she had, and was nothing bettered, but rather grew worse,

27 When she had heard of Jesus, came in the press behind, and [m]touched his garment.

28 For she said, If I may touch but his clothes, I shall be whole.

29 And straightway the fountain of her blood was dried up; and she felt in *her* body that she was healed of that plague.

30 And Jesus, immediately [n]knowing in himself that [o]virtue had gone out of him, turned him about in the press, and said, Who touched my clothes?

31 And his disciples said unto him, Thou seest the multitude [p]thronging thee, and sayest thou, Who touched me?

32 And he looked round about to see her that had done this thing.

33 But the woman fearing and trembling, knowing what was done in her, came and [q]fell down before him, and told him all the truth.

34 And he said unto her, Daughter, thy [r]faith hath made thee whole; go in peace, and be whole of thy plague.

35 While he yet spake, there came from the ruler of the synagogue's *house certain* which said, Thy daughter is dead: why troublest thou the Master any further?

36 [s]As soon as Jesus heard the word that was spoken, he saith unto the ruler of the synagogue, [t]Be not afraid, only believe.

37 And he suffered no man to follow him, save Peter, and [u]James, and John the brother of James.

38 And he cometh to the house of the ruler of the synagogue, and seeth the tumult, and them that wept and wailed greatly.

39 And when he was come in, he saith unto them, Why make ye this ado, and weep? the damsel is not dead, but [v]sleepeth.

40 And they laughed him to scorn. But when he had [w]put them all out, he taketh the father and the mother of the damsel, and them that were with him, and entereth in where the damsel was lying.

A.D. 31.

a Mk. 16:9. See Mt. 7:22, *note.*

b *Miracles* (N.T.). vs. 1-13; 22-24, 35-42, 25-34; Mk. 6:13. (Mt. 8:2, 3; Acts 28:8, 9.)

c Lk. 15:15.

d Mt. 11:28-30; Lk. 10:39.

e Ex. 20:18; Mt. 8:34; Lk. 8:37; Acts 16:39.

f *borders.*

g Lk. 8:38; Rom. 5:2.

h Lk. 8:39; Acts 26:19, 20; Mk. 1:44 with John 1:11.

i Mt. 9:1, 18, 19, 23-26; Lk. 8:41, 42, 49-56.

j Mt. 9:20-22; Lk. 8:43-48. Cf. Lev. 15:25-31 with Mt. 15:19.

k v. 42.

l Lk. 10:31, 32; Rom. 5:6; 10:2, 3.

m Mt. 14:35, 36; Rom. 4:5.

n John 2:25.

o Gr. *dynamin, power.* Cf. Lk. 6:19; 8:46.

p Lk. 13:26, 27 with Rom. 9:6; 10:16-18.

q Rom. 10:9, 10. Cf. Lk. 17:14-19.

r Mk. 10:52; Gal. 2:16.

s *But Jesus, overhearing that word, said to the synagogue-ruler, Fear not, simply have faith.* Cf. Lk. 7:50.

t Mt. 14:27. Cf. Isa. 43:1.

u See Mt. 4:21, *note.*

v John 11:11-14, 25; 1 Cor. 15:55-57.

w Acts 9:40; 1 Ki. 17:19; Mt. 26:56; 27:46.

41 And he took the damsel by the [a]hand, and said unto her, Talitha cumi; which is, being interpreted, Damsel, I say unto thee, [b]arise.

42 And straightway the damsel arose, and [c]walked; for she was *of the age* of twelve years. And they were [d]astonished with a great astonishment.

43 And he [e]charged them straitly that no man should know it; and commanded that something should be given her to [f]eat.

CHAPTER 6.

Jesus again at Nazareth
(Mt. 13:54-58. See Lk. 4:16, *note*).

And he went out from thence, and came into his own country; and his disciples follow him.

2 And when the sabbath day was come, he began to teach in the synagogue: and many hearing *him* were astonished, saying, From [g]whence hath this *man* these things? and what wisdom *is* this which is given unto him, that even such mighty works are wrought by his hands?

3 Is not this the [h]carpenter, the son of Mary, the brother of James, and Joses, and of Juda, and Simon? and are not his sisters here with us? And they were [i]offended at him.

4 But Jesus said unto them, [j]A prophet is not without honour, but in his own country, and among his own kin, and in his own house.

5 And he [k]could there do no mighty work, save that he laid his hands upon a few sick folk, and [l]healed *them*.

6 And he [m]marvelled because of their unbelief. And he went round about the villages, teaching.

The twelve sent out to preach and heal
(Mt. 10:1-42; Lk. 9:1-6).

7 And he called *unto him* the twelve, and began to [n]send them forth by two and two; and gave them power over unclean spirits;

8 And commanded them that they should [o]take nothing for *their* journey, save a staff only; no [p]scrip, no bread, no money in *their* [q]purse:

9 But *be* [r]shod with sandals; and not put on two coats.

10 And he said unto them, In what place soever ye enter into an house, there abide till ye depart from that place.

11 And whosoever shall not receive you, nor hear you, when ye depart thence, [s]shake off the dust under your feet for a testimony against them. Verily I say unto you, It shall be more tolerable for Sodom and Gomorrha in [t]the day of judgment, than for that city.

12 And they went out, and preached that men should [u]repent.

13 And they [v]cast out many devils, and [w]anointed with oil many that were sick, and healed *them*.

Herod's troubled conscience: murder of John the Baptist (Mt. 14:1-14; Lk. 9:7-9).

14 And king [x]Herod heard *of him*; (for his name was spread abroad:) and he said, That John the Baptist was [y]risen from the dead, and therefore mighty works do shew forth themselves in him.

15 Others said, That it is [z]Elias. And others said, That it is a prophet, or as one of the prophets.

16 But when Herod heard *thereof*, he said, It is John, whom I beheaded: he is risen from the dead.

17 For Herod himself had sent forth and [aa]laid hold upon John, and bound him in prison for Herodias' sake, his brother Philip's wife: for he had married her.

18 For John [bb]had said unto Herod, It is not [cc]lawful for thee to have thy brother's wife.

19 Therefore Herodias had a quarrel against him, and would have killed him; but she could not:

20 For Herod [dd]feared John, knowing that he was a just man and an [ee]holy, [ff]and observed him; and when he heard him, he did many things, and heard him [gg]gladly.

21 And when a convenient day was come, that Herod on his birthday made a supper to his lords, high captains, and [hh]chief *estates* of Galilee;

22 And when the daughter of the said Herodias came in, and danced, and pleased Herod and them that sat with him, the king said unto the damsel, Ask of me whatsoever thou wilt, and I will give *it* thee.

23 And he sware unto her, Whatsoever thou shalt ask of me, I will give *it* thee, unto the half of my kingdom.

24 And she went forth, and said unto her mother, What shall I ask? And she said, The head of John the Baptist.

25 And she came in straightway with haste unto the king, and asked, saying, I

A.D. 31.

a Acts 3:6, 7; Rev. 1:17, 18.
b *Resurrection.* vs. 41; Mk. 16:1-6. (Job 19:25; 1 Cor. 15:52.)
c Rom. 6:4.
d Mk. 1:27; cf. John 12:12, 13, 17, 18.
e Mk. 3:12.
f 1 Pet. 2:2; cf. Col. 3:1; Heb. 5:14.
g John 6:42; 7:15; Acts 2:7-11; 4:13.
h Lk. 2:51, 52 with Phil. 2:7, 8; Acts 18:3 with John 13:16.
i Mt. 11:6; 1 Pet. 2:7, 8.
j John 7:5; 4:44; Acts 22:17-23.
k Mk. 9:23; 5:17; Lk. 13:34.
l MK. 7:24, 25.
m Mt. 8:10-12; Isa. 59:16.
n Mt. 10:1; Mk. 3:13, 14; Lk. 9:1-6; Mt. 28:19, 20.
o Cf. Mt. 10, 9, *note.*
p *provision-bag.*
q *belt.*
r Eph. 6:15.
s Lk. 10:10, 11; Acts 13:51; 18:6; 28:24-29.
t *Day of judgment.* Lk. 10:14. (Mt. 10:15; Rev. 20:11.)
u *Repentance.* Lk. 3:3, 8. (Mt. 3:2; Acts 17:30.)
v *Miracles* (N.T.). vs. 13, 35-44, 48-51, 56; Mk. 7:24-30. (Mt. 8:2, 3; Acts 28:8, 9.)
w Jas. 5:14.
x Son of the Herod of our Lord's nativity; also vs. 16, 17, 18, 20, 21, 22. See Mt. 14:1, *refs.*
y Acts 17:31.
z Mt. 16:14; Mk. 8:28; cf. John 1:21.
aa Lk. 3:19, 20.
bb *kept saying.*
cc Lev. 18:16.
dd Acts 24:24, 25; 2 Cor. 7:10.
ee *Sanctify, holy (persons)* (N.T.). Mk. 8:38. (Mt. 4:5; Rev. 22:11.)
ff *kept him safely, and, hearing him, did many things, hearing him gladly.*
gg Mt. 13:5, 20; cf. Acts 2:41.
hh *principal persons.*

will that thou give me [a]by and by in a
charger the head of John the Baptist.
26 And the king was exceeding [b]sorry;
yet for his oath's sake, and for their sakes
which sat with him, he would not reject
her.
27 And immediately the king sent [c]an
executioner, and commanded his head
to be brought: and he went and beheaded him in the prison,
28 And brought his head in a charger,
and gave it to the damsel: and the
damsel gave it to her mother.
29 And when his disciples [d]heard *of it,*
[e]they came and took up his corpse, and
laid it in a tomb.

Return of the apostles from their first preaching tour (Lk. 9:10).

30 And the apostles [f]gathered themselves together unto Jesus, and told him
all things, both what they had done, and
what they had taught.
31 And he said unto them, Come ye
yourselves [g]apart into a desert place,
and rest a while: for there were many
coming and going, and they had no
leisure so much as to eat.

The five thousand fed (Mt. 14:13-21; Lk. 9:10-17; John 6:5-13).

32 And they departed into a desert
place [h]by ship privately.
33 And the people saw them departing, and many knew him, and ran afoot
thither out of all cities, and outwent
them, and came together unto him.
34 And Jesus, when he came out, saw
much people, and was moved with [i]com-
passion toward them, because they were
as sheep not having a shepherd: and he
began to [j]teach them many things.
35 And when the day was now far
spent, his disciples came unto him, and
said, This is a desert place, and now the
time *is* far passed:
36 [k]Send them away, that they may go
into the country round about, and into
the villages, and buy themselves bread:
for they have nothing to eat.
37 He answered and said unto them,
Give ye them to eat. And they say unto
him, Shall we go and buy two hundred
pennyworth of bread, and give them to
eat?
38 He saith unto them, [m]How many
loaves have ye? go and see. And when
they knew, they say, Five, and two fishes.

A.D. 32.

a *straightway.*
b Mt. 27:3, 4.
c *a guard.*
d John 1 35-37; 3:29, 30.
e Cf. Mt. 14:12.
f Mt. 14:13, 14; Lk. 9:10.
g Mt. 12:15.
h *by boat secretly.*
i Mt. 9:36-38.
j Lk. 9:11.
k Mt. 14:15-21; Lk. 9:12-17; John 6:5-17.
l Mt. 10:8; John 6:5-17.
m 2 Ki. 4:2; 1 Cor. 14:19.
n Mk. 8:6.
o Psa. 16:1 with John 11:41, 42.
p 2 Chr. 31:10; Mal. 3:10; cf. Psa. 132:15.
q 2 Ki. 4:42-44; Eph. 3:20.
r Mt. 14:22-27; John 6:15-21.
s Mk. 1:35; Rom. 8:34.
t Mt. 24:7, 9; John 16:5, 6, 20, 33.
u Psa. 77:19; Mt. 24:30; Jas. 5:8.
v Lk. 24:37.
w Isa. 25:9; 2 Thes. 1:7.
x Psa. 46:9, 11; 107:29; Mt. 8:26.
y Mk. 8:17-21.
z Lk. 8:40; John 4:45.

39 And he commanded them to make
all [n]sit down by companies upon the
green grass.
40 And they sat down in ranks, by
hundreds, and by fifties.
41 And when he had taken the five
loaves and the two fishes, he looked up
to heaven, and [o]blessed, and brake the
loaves, and gave *them* to his disciples to
set before them; and the two fishes
divided he among them all.
42 And they did all eat, and were
[p]filled.
43 And they took up [q]twelve baskets
full of the fragments, and of the fishes.
44 And they that did eat of the loaves
were about five thousand men.

Jesus walks on the sea (Mt. 14:22-32; John 6:15-21).

45 And straightway he [r]constrained his
disciples to get into the ship, and to go to
the other side before unto Bethsaida,
while he sent away the people.
46 And when he had sent them away,
he [s]departed into a mountain to pray.
47 And when even was come, the ship
was in the midst of the sea, and he alone
on the land.
48 And he saw them [t]toiling in rowing;
for the wind was contrary unto them: and
about the fourth watch of the night he
cometh unto them, [u]walking upon the
sea, and would have passed by them.
49 But when they saw him walking
upon the sea, they [v]supposed it had
been a spirit, and cried out:
50 For they all saw him, and were
troubled. And immediately he talked
with them, and saith unto them, [w]Be of
good cheer: it is I; be not afraid.
51 And he went up unto them into the
ship; and the [x]wind ceased: and they
were sore amazed in themselves beyond
measure, and wondered.
52 For they [y]considered not *the miracle*
of the loaves: for their heart was hardened.

Jesus heals at Gennesaret (Mt. 14:34-36).

53 And when they had passed over,
they came into the land of Gennesaret,
and drew to the shore.
54 And when they were come out of
the ship, straightway they [z]knew him,

55 And ran through that whole region round about, and began to carry about in beds those that were sick, where they heard he was.

56 And whithersoever he entered, into villages, or cities, or country, they laid the sick in the streets, and besought him that they might [a]touch if it were but the border of his garment: and as many as touched him were made whole.

CHAPTER 7.

The Pharisees rebuked (Mt. 15:1-20).

Then came together unto him the Pharisees, and certain of the scribes, which came from Jerusalem.

2 And when they saw some of his disciples [b]eat bread with defiled, that is to say, with unwashen, hands, they found fault.

3 For the Pharisees, and all the Jews, except they wash *their* hands oft, eat not, holding the [c]tradition of the elders.

4 And *when they come* from the market, except they wash, they eat not. And many other things there be, which they have received to hold, *as* the washing of cups, and pots, brasen vessels, and of tables.

5 Then the Pharisees and scribes asked him, Why walk not thy disciples according to the [d]tradition of the elders, but eat bread with unwashen hands?

6 He answered and said unto them, Well hath [e]Esaias prophesied of you hypocrites, as it is written, This people honoureth me with *their* lips, but their heart is far from me.

7 Howbeit in vain do they worship me, teaching [f]*for* doctrines the commandments of men.

8 For laying aside [g]the commandment of God, ye hold the tradition of men, *as* the washing of pots and cups: and many other such like things ye do.

9 And he said unto them, Full well ye reject the commandment of God, that ye may keep your own tradition.

10 For [h]Moses said, Honour thy father and thy mother; and, Whoso curseth father or mother, [i]let him die the death:

11 But ye say, If a man shall say to his father or mother, *It is* Corban, that is to say, [j]a gift, by whatsoever thou mightest be profited by me; *he shall be free*.

12 And ye [k]suffer him no more to do ought for his father or his mother;

13 Making the word of God of none effect through your tradition, which ye have delivered: and many such like things do ye.

14 And when he had called all the people *unto him*, he said unto them, Hearken unto me every one *of you*, and understand:

15 There is [l]nothing from without a man, that entering into him can defile him: but the things which come out of him, those are they that defile the man.

16 If any man have ears to hear, let him hear.

17 And when he was entered into the house from the people, his disciples asked him concerning the parable.

18 And he saith unto them, Are ye so without understanding also? Do ye not perceive, that whatsoever thing from without entereth into the man, *it* cannot defile him;

19 [m]Because it entereth not into his heart, but into the belly, and goeth out into the draught, purging all meats?

20 And he said, That which cometh out of the man, that defileth the man.

21 For from within, [n]out of the heart of men, proceed evil thoughts, adulteries, fornications, murders,

22 Thefts, covetousness, wickedness, deceit, lasciviousness, an evil eye, blasphemy, pride, foolishness:

23 All these evil things come from within, and defile the man.

Jesus and the Syrophenician woman (Mt. 15:21-28).

24 And from thence he arose, and went into the [o]borders of Tyre and Sidon, and entered into an house, and would have no man know *it*: but he [p]could not be hid.

25 For a *certain* woman, whose young daughter had an unclean spirit, heard of him, and came and fell at his feet:

26 The woman was a [q]Greek, a Syrophenician by nation; and she besought him that he would cast forth the [r]devil out of her daughter.

27 But Jesus said unto her, Let the [s]children first be filled: for it is not mee

A.D. 32.

a Mk. 5:27, 28.

b Mt. 15:1-9.

c Col. 2:8; Gal. 1:14; 1 Pet. 1:18; cf. Col. 2:20-23.

d i.e. the so-called "oral law" alleged to have been handed down from Moses; really a traditional interpretation of the written law. Cf. v. 7, *ref.*

e Isa. 29:13; Ezk. 33:31; Amos 4:4, 5.

f *as authoritative the precepts of men.* Cf. v. 5. See "Pharisees," Mt. 3:7, *note.* Cf. Col. 2:8, 16, 18, 20, 23.

g *inspiration.* vs. 8-13; Mk. 10:4-9, 19. (Ex. 4:15; Rev. 22:19.)

h Ex. 20:12; 21:17; Lev. 20:9; Deut. 21:18-21.

i *shall surely die.* Ex. 21:17; Lev. 20:9; Deut. 21:18-21.

j Or, *I have dedicated to God that which would relieve your need;* [12] *No longer do you permit him to use it for his father or mother.* Cf. Mt. 15:5, 6.

k 1 Tim. 5:8; Eph. 4:28.

l Mt. 15:10-20; Rom. 14:14; 1 Tim. 4:4.

m *Because it does not enter into the heart of him, but into the bowels is passed—purifying all the food.*

n Mt. 12:34, 35; cf. Gen. 6:5; Psa. 45:1; Jas. 3:10-12.

o Mt. 15:21-28.

p Mk. 2:1, 2; John 4:4-7.

q See Mt. 15:21, *note.*

r *demon.*

s Mt. 8:11, 12; 10:5, 6; John 4:22.

to take the children's bread, and to [a]cast
it unto the dogs.
28 [b]And she answered and said unto
him, Yes, Lord: yet the dogs under the
table eat of the children's crumbs.
29 And he said unto her, For [c]this saying go thy way; the devil is gone out of
thy daughter.
30 And when she was come to her
house, [d]she found the devil gone out,
and her daughter [e]laid upon the bed.

A deaf and dumb man healed
(Mt. 15:29-31).

31 And again, departing from the
coasts of Tyre and Sidon, he [f]came unto
the sea of Galilee, through the midst of
the coasts of Decapolis.
32 And they bring unto him one that
was [g]deaf, and had an impediment in
his speech; and they beseech him to put
his hand upon him.
33 And he took him [h]aside from the
multitude, and put his fingers into his
ears, and he [i]spit, and touched his tongue;
34 And looking up to heaven, he
[j]sighed, and saith unto him, Ephphatha,
that is, Be opened.
35 And straightway his [k]ears were
opened, and the string of his tongue was
loosed, and he spake plain.
36 And he charged them that they
should tell no man: but the more he
[l]charged them, so much the more a great
deal they published *it*;
37 And were beyond measure [m]aston-
ished, saying, He hath done all things
well: he maketh both the deaf to hear,
and the dumb to speak.

CHAPTER 8.

The four thousand fed (Mt. 15:32-39).

In those days the multitude being very
great, and having [n]nothing to eat,
Jesus called his disciples *unto him*, and
saith unto them,
2 I have compassion on the multitude,
because they have now been with me
three days, and have nothing to eat:
3 And if I send them away fasting to
their own houses, they will [o]faint by the
way: for divers of them came from far.
4 And his disciples answered him,
From [p]whence can a man satisfy these
men with bread here in the wilderness?

A.D. 32.

a Acts 13:46, 47; Col. 1:27.
b *She, however, answered, saying, True Lord! and yet the little dogs under the table eat from the children's crumbs.* Rom. 11:24; Eph. 2:11-22.
c Lk. 18:14.
d *Miracles* (N.T.). vs. 24-30, 31-37; Mk. 8:1-9. (Mt. 8:2, 3; Acts 28:8, 9.)
e Mk. 5:15.
f Mt. 15:29.
g Isa. 29:18; 35:5.
h Mk. 5:37.
i Mk. 8:23; John 9:6.
j Lk. 19:41; John 11:33, 35, 38.
k Job 33:16; 36:10, 15, 16.
l Mk. 1:43, 44; 5:43.
m Lk. 5:26.
n Mt. 15:32-38; Mk. 6:34-44; Lk. 9:12.
o Psa. 107:4, 5; Mt. 9:36.
p 2 Ki. 7:1, 2; Psa. 78:19, 20.
q Jud. 7:3, 4; 2 Chr. 14:11.
r *Miracles* (N.T.). vs. 1-9, 22-25; Mk. 9:17-29. (Mt. 8:2, 3; Acts 28:8, 9.)
s Psa. 132:15.
t Mt. 15:39.
u Mt. 12:38-40; 16:1-4; John 6:30, 31.
v Mt. 21:23-27; Lk. 16:30, 31.
w See Mt. 13:33, *note*.
x See Mt. 14:1, *ref.*
y Psa. 115:5, 6, 8.
z Mk. 6:35-44.
aa vs. 1-9.

5 And he asked them, How many
loaves have ye? And they said, Seven.
6 And he commanded the people to sit
down on the ground: and he took the
seven loaves, and gave thanks, and
brake, and gave to his disciples to set
before *them*; and they did set *them* before
the people.
7 And they had a [q]few small fishes:
and he blessed, and commanded to set
them also before *them*.
8 So they did eat, and [r]were [s]filled:
and they took up of the broken *meat* that
was left seven baskets.
9 And they that had eaten were about
four thousand: and he sent them away.

The Pharisees ask a sign: the meaning of
leaven explained (Mt. 16:1-12).

10 And straightway he [t]entered into a
ship with his disciples, and came into
the parts of Dalmanutha.
11 And the Pharisees came forth, and
began to question with him, seeking of
him a [u]sign from heaven, tempting him.
12 And he sighed deeply in his spirit,
and saith, Why doth this generation seek
after a sign? verily I say unto you, There
shall [v]no sign be given unto this generation.
13 And he left them, and entering into
the ship again departed to the other side.
14 Now *the disciples* had forgotten to
take bread, neither had they in the ship
with them more than one loaf.
15 And he charged them, saying, Take
heed, beware of the [w]leaven of the
Pharisees, and *of* the leaven of [x]Herod.
16 And they reasoned among themselves, saying, *It is* because we have no
bread.
17 And when Jesus knew *it*, he saith
unto them, Why reason ye, because ye
have no bread? perceive ye not yet, neither understand? have ye your heart yet
hardened?
18 Having [y]eyes, see ye not? and having ears, hear ye not? and do ye not
remember?
19 When I brake the [z]five loaves
among five thousand, how many baskets full of fragments took ye up? They
say unto him, Twelve.
20 And when the [aa]seven among four
thousand, how many baskets full of

fragments took ye up? And they said, Seven.

21 And he said unto them, How is it that ye do not understand?

The blind man healed outside Bethsaida.

22 And he cometh to Bethsaida; and they bring a [a]blind man unto him, and besought him to touch him.

23 [1]And he took the blind man by the hand, and led him [b]out of the town; and when he had spit on his eyes, and put his hands upon him, he asked him if he saw ought.

24 And he looked up, and said, I see men as [c]trees, walking.

25 After that he put *his* hands again upon his eyes, and made him look up: and he was restored, and saw every man [d]clearly.

26 And he sent him away to his house, saying, [e]Neither go into the town, nor tell *it* to any in the town.

Peter's confession of faith
(Mt. 16:13-16; Lk. 9:18-20).

27 And Jesus [f]went out, and his disciples, into the towns of Cæsarea Philippi: and by the way he asked his disciples, saying unto them, [g]Whom do men say that I am?

28 And they answered, John the Baptist: but some *say*, Elias; and others, One of the prophets.

29 And he saith unto them, But whom say ye that I am? And Peter answereth and saith unto him, [h]Thou art the Christ.

30 And he charged them that they should tell no man of him.

31 And he began to teach them, that the [i]Son of man must suffer many things, and be rejected of the elders, and *of* the chief priests, and scribes, and be killed, and after three days rise again.

32 And he spake that saying openly. And Peter took him, and began to [j]rebuke him.

33 But when he had turned about and looked on his disciples, he rebuked Peter, saying, [k]Get thee behind me, [l]Satan: for [m]thou savourest not the things that be of God, but the things that be of men.

The true use of life: value of a soul
(Mt. 16:24-27; Lk. 9:23-26).

34 And when he had called the people *unto him* with his disciples also, he said unto them, [n]Whosoever will come after me, let him deny himself, and take up his cross, and follow me.

35 For [o]whosoever will save his life shall lose it; but whosoever shall lose his life for my sake and the [p]gospel's, the same shall save it.

36 For [q]what shall it profit a man, if he shall gain the whole [r]world, and lose his own soul?

37 Or what shall a man give in exchange for his soul?

38 Whosoever therefore shall be [s]ashamed of me and of my words in this adulterous and [t]sinful generation; of him also shall the Son of man be ashamed, when he cometh in the glory of his Father with the [u]holy [v]angels.

CHAPTER 9.

The transfiguration
(Mt. 17:1-8; Lk. 9:28-36).

And he said unto them, Verily I say unto you, That there be some of them that stand here, which shall not taste of death, till they have [w]seen the [x]kingdom of God come with power.

2 And after six days Jesus taketh *with him* Peter, and [y]James, and John, and leadeth them up into an high mountain apart by themselves: and he was [z]transfigured before them.

3 And his raiment became shining, exceeding white as snow; so as no fuller on earth can white them.

4 And there appeared unto them Elias with Moses: and they were talking with Jesus.

5 And Peter answered and said to Jesus, Master, it is good for us to be here: and let us make [aa]three tabernacles; one for thee, and one for Moses, and one for Elias.

6 For he [bb]wist not what to say; for they were sore afraid.

7 And there was a [cc]cloud that overshadowed them: and a voice came out of

A.D. 32.

a Isa. 42:16, 18.
b Mk. 7:33; John 9:35-38
c Acts 18:24-28; Phil. 1:10.
d 1 Pet. 2:9; 1 John 2:27; Rev. 3:18.
e v. 30; Mk. 7:36.
f Mt. 16:13-20; Lk. 9:18-21
g Mt. 22:42-46.
h 1 Cor. 12:3; 1 John 1:2, 3; 5:1; cf. John 1:49.
i Mt. 8:20, *note;* 16:21-28; Mk. 9:31; Lk. 9:22-27; cf. Lk. 24:6.
j v. 29; John 21:18, 19; 2 Pet. 1:14, 15.
k Mt. 4:10; Gal. 1:8, 9.
l *Satan.* Lk. 4:8. (Gen. 3:1; Rev. 20:10.)
m i.e. thou art thinking man's thoughts, not the thoughts of God. *Contra,* Mt. 16:17.
n Mt. 16:24-28; Lk. 9:23-27; 14:27; Phil. 3:7-10.
o Lk. 17:33; John 12:24-26; Rom. 6:1-7.
p *Gospel.* Mk. 10:29. (Gen. 12:1-3; Rev. 14:6.)
q Psa. 49:6-8; Jas. 5:1-3.
r i.e. *earth.*
s Mt. 10:32, 33; John 5:44; 12:42, 43; Rom. 1:16; 2 Tim. 1:7-9; Phil. 1:20, 21.
t *Sin.* Rom. 3:23, *note.*
u *Sanctify, holy (persons)* (N.T.). Lk. 1:35. (Mt. 4:5; Rev. 22:11.)
v Heb. 1:4, *note.*
w Cf. Mt. 17:2, *note;* 2 Pet. 1:16-18.
x See Mt. 6:33, *note.*
y See Mt. 4:21, *note.*
z Phil. 2:9, 10; Heb. 2:9; Rev. 1:13-16.
aa Mk. 8:28, 29; Phil. 2:9; Heb. 3:5, 6.
bb Mt. 20:20-23; Acts 4:11, 12.
cc Ex. 40:34; Acts 1:9; Rev. 1:7.

[1] **(8:23)** Our Lord's action here is most significant. Having abandoned Bethsaida to judgment (Mt. 11:21-24), He would neither heal in that village, nor permit further testimony to be borne there (v. 26). The probation of Bethsaida as a community was ended, but He would still show mercy to individuals. Cf. Rev. 3:20. Christ is outside the door of that church, but "If any man hear My voice," etc.

the cloud, saying, [a]This is my beloved
Son: hear him.
8 And suddenly, when they had looked
round about, they saw [b]no man any
more, save Jesus only with themselves.
9 And as they came down from the
mountain, he [c]charged them that they
should tell no man what things they had
seen, till the Son of man were [d]risen
from the dead.
10 And they kept that saying with
themselves, questioning one with another what the rising from the dead should
mean.
11 And they asked him, saying, Why
say the scribes that [e]Elias must first come?
12 And he answered and told them,
Elias verily cometh first, and restoreth
all things; and how it is written of the
Son of man, that he must suffer many
things, and be set at nought.
13 But I say unto you, [f]That Elias is
indeed come, and they have done unto
him whatsoever they listed, as it is written of him.

The impotent disciples: the mighty Christ
(Mt. 17:14-21; Lk. 9:37-42).

14 And when he came to *his* disciples,
he saw a [g]great multitude about them,
and the scribes questioning with them.
15 And straightway all the people,
when they beheld him, were greatly
[h]amazed, and running to *him* saluted him.
16 And he asked the scribes, What
question ye with them?
17 And one of the multitude answered
and said, Master, I have brought unto
thee my son, which hath a [i]dumb spirit;
18 And wheresoever he taketh him, he
teareth him: and he foameth, and
gnasheth with his teeth, and pineth away:
and I spake to thy disciples that they
should cast him out; and they [j]could not.
19 He answereth him, and saith, O
[k]faithless generation, how long shall I be
with you? how long shall I suffer you?
bring him unto me.
20 And they brought him unto him:
and [l]when he saw him, straightway the
spirit tare him; and he fell on the
ground, and wallowed foaming.
21 And he asked his father, How long
is it ago since this came unto him? And
he said, Of a child.
22 And ofttimes it hath cast him into
the fire, and into the waters, to destroy
him: but [m]if thou canst do any thing,
have compassion on us, and help us.
23 Jesus said unto him, If thou canst
[n]believe, [o]all things *are* possible to him
that believeth.
24 And straightway the father of the
child cried out, and said with tears, Lord,
I believe; [p]help thou mine unbelief.
25 When Jesus saw that the people
came running together, he rebuked the
foul spirit, saying unto him, *Thou* dumb
and deaf spirit, [q]I charge thee, come out
of him, and enter [r]no more into him.
26 And *the spirit* cried, and rent him
sore, and came out of him: and he was
as one dead; insomuch that many said,
He is dead.
27 [s]But Jesus took him by the hand,
[t]and lifted him up; and he arose.
28 And when he was come into the
house, his disciples asked him privately,
Why could not we cast him out?
29 And he said unto them, [u]This kind
can come forth by nothing, but by
prayer and fasting.

Jesus foretells his death and resurrection
(Mt. 17:22, 23; Lk. 9:43-45).

30 And they departed thence, and
passed through Galilee; and he would
not that any man should [v]know *it*.
31 For he taught his disciples, and said
unto them, [w]The Son of man is delivered
into the hands of men, and they shall kill
him; and after that he is killed, he shall
rise the third day.
32 But they [x]understood not that saying, and were afraid to ask him.

The dispute who should be greatest
(Mt. 18:1-6; Lk. 9:46-48).

33 And he [y]came to Capernaum: and
being in the house he asked them, What
was it that ye disputed among yourselves by the way?
34 But they held their peace: for by the
way they had disputed among themselves, who *should be* the [z]greatest.
35 And he sat down, and called the
twelve, and saith unto them, If any man
desire to be [aa]first, *the same* shall be last
of all, and servant of all.
36 And he took a [bb]child, and set him
in the midst of them: and when he had

A.D. 32.

a Mk. 1:11.
b John 3:30; 6:68; Col. 3:11.
c Mt. 17:9-13; Mk. 8:30.
d Mt. 20:19; 26:61; 27:63; Mk. 8:31; Acts 2:32.
e Mal. 4:5, 6. See Mt. 17:10, *note.*
f Mt. 11:14; Lk. 1:17.
g Mt. 17:14-18; Lk. 9:37-42; Rev. 19:11-21.
h Mk. 10:32; cf. Ex. 34:29, 30.
i Mt. 12:22.
j Mk. 6:7; cf. vs. 28, 29.
k John 4:48; 14:12.
l Rev. 12:12.
m Mk. 1:40.
n *Faith.* Mk. 10:46-52. (Gen. 3:20; Heb. 11:39.)
o Mt. 9:28, 29; Mk. 11:22, 23.
p Cf. Eph. 2:8 with John 6:44.
q Mk. 1:25-27.
r Mt. 12:43-45.
s *But Jesus, grasping his hand, raised him, and he stood erect.* Cf. Acts 3:7.
t *Miracles* (N.T.). vs. 17-29; Mk. 10:46-52. (Mt. 8:2, 3; Acts 28:8, 9.)
u 1 Ki. 18:42-45; Acts 13:2. The two best MSS. omit "and fasting." Cf. Mt. 17:21.
v Mk. 7:24.
w Mk. 8:31; Mt. 8:20, *note.*
x Cf. John 16:12, 13 with John 1:5.
y Mt. 18:1-5; Lk. 9:46-48; 22:24-27.
z Lk. 22:24; Phil. 2:3.
aa 1 Cor. 15:9.
bb Mk. 10:13-16; 1 Cor. 3:18, 19.

taken him in his arms, he said unto them,

37 Whosoever shall [a]receive one of such children in my name, receiveth me: and whosoever shall receive me, receiveth not me, but him that sent me.

The rebuke of sectarianism (Lk. 9:49, 50).

38 And John answered him, saying, Master, we saw one [b]casting out devils in thy name, and he followeth not us: and we forbad him, because he followeth not us.

39 But Jesus said, Forbid him not: for there is no man which shall do a [c]miracle in my name, that can lightly speak evil of me.

40 For he that is not [d]against us is on our part.

41 For whosoever shall give you a [e]cup of water to drink in my name, because ye belong to Christ, verily I say unto you, he shall not lose his [f]reward.

Jesus' solemn warning of hell.

42 And whosoever shall [g]offend one of *these* little ones that believe in me, it is better for him that a millstone were hanged about his neck, and he were cast into the sea.

43 And if thy [h]hand offend thee, cut it off: it is better for thee to enter into life maimed, than having two hands to go into [i]hell, into the fire that never shall be quenched:

44 Where their worm [j]dieth not, and the fire is not quenched.

45 And if thy foot offend thee, cut it off: it is better for thee to enter halt into life, than having two feet to be cast into [i]hell, into the fire that [k]never shall be quenched:

46 Where their worm dieth not, and the fire is not quenched.

47 And if thine eye offend thee, pluck it out: it is better for thee to enter into the kingdom of God with one eye, than having two eyes to be cast into [i]hell fire:

48 Where their [l]worm dieth not, and the fire is not quenched.

49 For every one shall be [m]salted with fire, and every sacrifice shall be salted with salt.

50 Salt *is* good: but if the salt have [n]lost his saltness, wherewith will ye season it? Have salt in yourselves, and have [o]peace one with another.

A.D. 32-33.

a Mt. 10:40; John 13:20.
b Lk. 9:49, 50; cf. Num. 11:26-29.
c *work of power upon my name, who will find it possible soon* [after] *to revile me.*
d Mt. 12:30; 1 John 2:18, 19; 4:1-6.
e Mt. 10:42; 25:40; Heb. 6:10; 2 Tim. 1:16-18.
f *Rewards.* Lk. 6:23, 35. (Dan. 12:3; 1 Cor. 3:14.)
g *cause to stumble.* Mt. 18:6; Lk. 17:1, 2; Rom. 14:15-23; 1 Cor. 8:7-13.
h Mt. 5:29, 30; 18:8, 9; Gal. 2:20 with Col. 3:5-11.
i *gehenna.* Mt. 5:22, *note.*
j Isa. 66:24.
k 2 Thes. 1:8, 9; Rev. 19:20; 20:10, 14, 15.
l Lk. 16:22-26; cf. Jer. 8:20.
m Lev. 2:13; Mt. 3:11; Lk. 12:49.
n Mt. 5:13; 2 Tim. 3:5; Rev. 3:1.
o Col. 4:6; Gal. 5:15.
p Mt. 19:1, 2; John 10:40.
q Mt. 5:17-20; Lk. 10:26.
r Deut. 24:1-4; Mt. 5:31.
s *Inspiration.* vs. 4-9, 19. Mk. 12:26, 36. (Ex. 4:15; Rev. 22:19.)
t *God.* Gen. 1:27.
u Gen. 2:21-25; Mal. 2:14, 15; 1 Cor. 6:16; Eph. 5:31, 32.
v Gen. 2:24.
w Lk. 16:18; 1 Cor. 7:10.
x *little.* Cf. v. 16.
y *moved with indignation.*
z *to be coming unto me; be not hindering them.*
aa Lit. *and folding them in his arms, he was blessing* [them], *putting hands upon them.*

CHAPTER 10.

Jesus' law of divorce (Cf. Mt. 5:31, 32; 19:1-9; Lk. 16:18; 1 Cor. 7:10-15.)

And he arose from thence, and cometh into the [p]coasts of Judæa by the farther side of Jordan: and the people resort unto him again; and, as he was wont, he taught them again.

2 And the Pharisees came to him, and asked him, Is it lawful for a man to put away *his* wife? tempting him.

3 And he answered and said unto them, What did [q]Moses command you?

4 And they said, Moses [r]suffered to write a bill of divorcement, and to put *her* away.

5 And Jesus answered and said unto them, For the hardness of your heart [s]he wrote you this precept.

6 But from the beginning of the creation [t]God made them male and female.

7 For this cause shall a man [u]leave his father and mother, and cleave to his wife;

8 And [v]they twain shall be one flesh: so then they are no more twain, but one flesh.

9 What therefore God hath joined together, let not man put asunder.

10 And in the house his disciples asked him again of the same *matter*.

11 And he saith unto them, [w]Whosoever shall put away his wife, and marry another, committeth adultery against her.

12 And if a woman shall put away her husband, and be married to another, she committeth adultery.

Jesus blesses little children (Mt. 19:13-15; Lk. 18:15-17).

13 And they brought [x]young children to him, that he should touch them: and *his* disciples rebuked those that brought *them*.

14 But when Jesus saw *it*, he was [y]much displeased, and said unto them, Suffer the little children [z]to come unto me, and forbid them not: for of such is the kingdom of God.

15 Verily I say unto you, Whosoever shall not receive the kingdom of God as a little child, he shall not enter therein.

16 [aa]And he took them up in his arms,

put *his* hands upon them, and [1]blessed
them.

The rich young ruler (Mt. 19:16-30;
Lk. 18:18-30. Cf. Lk. 10:25).

17 [a]And when he was gone forth into
the way, there came one running, and
kneeled to him, and asked him, Good
[b]Master, what shall I do that I may
inherit eternal life?
18 And Jesus said unto him, [c]Why
callest thou me good? *there is* none good
but one, *that is,* God.
19 Thou knowest the [d]command-
ments, Do not commit adultery, Do not
kill, Do not steal, Do not bear false witness, Defraud not, Honour thy father
and mother.
20 And he answered and said unto
him, Master, all these have I observed
from my youth.
21 Then Jesus beholding him loved
him, and said unto him, One thing thou
lackest: go thy way, sell whatsoever thou
hast, and give to the poor, and thou shalt
have [e]treasure in heaven: and come, take
up the cross, and follow me.
22 And he was sad at that saying, and
went away grieved: for he had great
possessions.

The warning against riches.

23 [f]And Jesus looked round about,
and saith unto his disciples, How hardly
shall they that have riches enter into the
kingdom of God!
24 And the disciples were [g]astonished
at his words. But Jesus answereth again,
and saith unto them, Children, how hard
is it for them that [h]trust in riches to enter
into the kingdom of God!
25 It is easier for a camel to go through
the [i]eye of a needle, than for a rich man
to enter into the kingdom of God.
26 And they were astonished out of
measure, saying among themselves,
Who then can be saved?
27 And Jesus looking upon them saith,
With men *it is* impossible, but not with
God: for with God all things are possible.
28 [j]Then Peter began to say unto him,
Lo, we have left all, and have followed
thee.
29 And Jesus answered and said, Verily
I say unto you, There is no man that hath
left house, or brethren, or sisters, or

A.D. 33.

- *a* Mt. 19:16; Lk. 18:18.
- *b* *Teacher.*
- *c* Par., Believing Me to be but a human teacher, why callest thou Me "good," etc.
- *d* Ex. 20:12-16; Deut. 5:16-20.
- *e* Mt. 6:19, 20; 19:21; Lk. 12:33; 16:11.
- *f* Mt. 19:23; Lk. 18:24.
- *g* Or, *amazed,* i.e. as Jews: knowing that temporal prosperity was to the Jew as such, a token of divine favour. e. g. Deut. 28:1-12.
- *h* Psa. 52:7; 62:10; Prov. 11:28; 1 Tim. 6:17.
- *i* It has been thought the reference here was to a postern door set in a gate of Jerusalem.
- *j* Cf. Mt. 19:27-30, *note.*
- *k* *Gospel.* Mk. 13:10. (Gen. 12:1-3; Rev. 14:6.)
- *l* Mt. 8:14; 9:10; 26:6; Lk. 5:29; John 14:2.
- *m* Mt. 12:48-50.
- *n* *age.*
- *o* Mk. 8:31; 9:31; Lk. 9:22; 18:31.
- *p* Cf. Mk. 8:31; 9:12.
- *q* See Mt. 8:20, *note.*
- *r* Mt. 26:67; 27:30; Mk. 14:65; cf. Mt. 16:20-22; Mk. 9:30-32.
- *s* Cf. Mt. 19:28.
- *t* Cf. Mt. 20:22
- *u* Cf. Acts 12:2; Rev. 1:9.
- *v* Lk. 12:50.
- *w* Cf. Mt. 13:11; 20:23.
- *x* Cf. Lk. 22:25-27.

father, or mother, or wife, or children, or
lands, for my sake, and the [k]gospel's,
30 But he shall receive an hundredfold
now in this time, [l]houses, and
[m]brethren, and sisters, and mothers, and
children, and lands, with persecutions;
and in the [n]world to come eternal life.
31 But many *that are* first shall be last;
and the last first.

*Jesus again foretells his death and
resurrection* (Mt. 20:17-19; Lk. 18:31-33).

32 And they were in the way going up
to Jerusalem; and Jesus went before them:
and they were amazed; and as they followed, they were afraid. [o]And he took
again the twelve, and began to tell them
what things should happen unto him,
33 *Saying,* Behold, we go up to
Jerusalem; [p]and the [q]Son of man shall be
delivered unto the chief priests, and
unto the scribes; and they shall condemn
him to death, and shall deliver him to
the Gentiles:
34 And they [r]shall mock him, and
shall scourge him, and shall spit upon
him, and shall kill him: and the third
day he shall rise again.

The desire of James and John to be first
(Mt. 20:20-28).

35 And James and John, the sons of
Zebedee, come unto him, saying, Master,
we would that thou shouldest do for us
whatsoever we shall desire.
36 And he said unto them, What
would ye that I should do for you?
37 They said unto him, [s]Grant unto us
that we may sit, one on thy right hand,
and the other on thy left hand, in thy
glory.
38 But Jesus said unto them, Ye know
not what ye ask: [t]can ye drink of the cup
that I drink of? and be baptized with the
baptism that I am baptized with?
39 And they said unto him, We can.
[u]And Jesus said unto them, Ye shall
indeed drink of the cup that I drink of;
and with the [v]baptism that I am baptized withal shall ye be baptized:
40 But to sit on my right hand and on
my left hand is not mine to give; [w]but *it
shall be given to them* for whom it is prepared.
41 [x]And when the ten heard *it,* they

[1] **(10:16)** In Hebrew custom, a father's act. (Cf. Gen. 27:38.) "He had no children that He might adopt all children."—*Bengel.*

began to be much displeased with James
and John.
42 But Jesus called them *to him*, and
saith unto them, Ye know that they
which are accounted to rule over the
Gentiles exercise lordship over them;
and their great ones exercise authority
upon them.
43 But so shall it not be among you:
[a]but whosoever will be great among
you, shall be your minister:
44 And whosoever of you will be the
chiefest, shall be servant of all.
45 For even the Son of man came not
to be ministered unto, but to minister,
and to give his [b]life a ransom for many.

Bartimæus receives his sight
(Mt. 20:29-34. Cf. Lk. 18:35-43).

46 [c]And they came to Jericho: and as
he went out of Jericho with his disciples
and a great number of people, blind
Bartimæus, the son of Timæus, sat by
the highway side begging.
47 [d]And when he heard that it was
Jesus of Nazareth, he began to cry out,
and say, Jesus, *thou* Son of David, have
mercy on me.
48 And many charged him that he
should hold his peace: but he cried the
more a great deal, *Thou* Son of David,
have mercy on me.
49 [e]And Jesus stood still, and commanded him to be called. And they call
the blind man, saying unto him, [f]Be of
good comfort, rise; he calleth thee.
50 And he, casting away his garment,
rose, and came to Jesus.
51 And Jesus answered and said unto
him, What wilt thou that I should do
unto thee? The blind man said unto him,
[g]Lord, that I might receive my sight.
52 And Jesus said unto him, Go thy
way; thy [h]faith hath made thee whole.
And [i]immediately he received his sight,
and followed Jesus in the way.

CHAPTER 11.

The official presentation of Jesus as King
(Zech. 9:9; Mt. 21:1-9;
Lk. 19:29-38; John 12:12-19).

And when they came nigh to
Jerusalem, unto [j]Bethphage and
[k]Bethany, at the mount of Olives, he
sendeth forth two of his disciples,
2 And saith unto them, Go your way
into the village over against you: and as
soon as ye be entered into it, ye shall
find a colt tied, whereon never man sat;
loose him, and bring *him*.
3 And if any man say unto you, Why
do ye this? say ye that the Lord hath
need of him; and straightway he will
send him hither.
4 And they went their way, and found
the colt tied by the door without in a
place where two ways met; and they
loose him.
5 And certain of them that stood there
said unto them, What do ye, loosing the
colt?
6 And they said unto them even as
Jesus had commanded: and they let
them go.
7 And they brought the colt to Jesus,
and cast their garments on him; and he
sat upon him.
8 And many spread their garments in
the way: and others cut down branches
off the trees, and strawed *them* in the way.
9 And they that went before, and they
that followed, cried, saying, Hosanna;
Blessed *is* he that cometh in the name of
the Lord:
10 Blessed *be* the [l]kingdom of our
father David, that cometh in the name of
the Lord: Hosanna in the highest.
11 And Jesus entered into Jerusalem,
and into the temple: and when he had
looked round about upon all things, and
now the [m]eventide was come, he went
out unto Bethany with the twelve.

The barren fig tree (Mt. 21:19-21).

12 [n]And on the morrow, when they
were come from Bethany, he was hungry:
13 And seeing a [o]fig tree afar off having [p]leaves, he came, if haply he might
find any thing thereon: and when he
came to it, he found nothing but leaves;
for the time of figs was not *yet*.
14 [q]And Jesus answered and said unto
it, [r]No man eat fruit of thee hereafter for
ever. And his disciples heard *it*.

Jesus purifies the temple (Mt. 21:12-16;
Lk. 19:45-47. Cf. John 2:13-16).

15 And they come to Jerusalem: and
Jesus went into the temple, and began to
cast out them that sold and bought in
the temple, and overthrew the tables of
the moneychangers, and the seats of
them that sold doves;
16 And would not suffer that any man

A.D. 33.

a Mk. 9:35; Mt. 20:26.
b Or, *soul.* (Cf. Isa. 53:10, 12.) Gr. *psuche,* the soul, or the essential life, not, as commonly, *zoe,* the active life.
c Cf. Mt. 20:30, *note.*
d *Bible prayers* (N.T.). Lk. 11:2. (Mt. 6:9; Rev. 22:20.)
e *And, coming to a stand, Jesus said, Call him!*
f Cf. Mt. 9:2.
g Gr. *Rabboni, my Master,* a term of reverent love. Cf. John 20:16.
h *Faith.* Lk. 7:50. (Gen. 3:20; Heb. 11:39.)
i *Miracles* (N.T.). vs. 46-52; Mk. 11:12-14. (Mt. 8:2, 3; Acts 28:8, 9.)
j Meaning, *house of unripe figs* (see vs. 12, 20), probably so called after the fig tree was cursed.
k See Mt. 21:17.
l Mt. 3:2, *note.*
m Mk. 11:19, *ref.*
n Mt. 21:18-22.
o Cf. Lk. 13:6-11; Jer. 24:1-6.
p Fig trees which have retained their leaves through the winter usually have figs also. It was still too early for new leaves or fruit.
q *Miracles* (N.T.). vs. 12-14; Lk. 4:33-36. (Mt. 8:2, 3; Acts 28:8, 9.)
r See vs. 20-25; Mt. 23:37-39.

should carry *any* vessel through the temple.

17 And he taught, saying unto them, Is it not written, [a]My house shall be called of all nations the house of prayer? [b]but ye have made it a den of thieves.

18 And the scribes and chief priests heard *it*, and [c]sought how they might destroy [d]him: for they feared him, because all the people was [e]astonished at his doctrine.

19 And [f]when even was come, he went out of the city.

20 And in the morning, as they passed by, they saw the fig tree dried up from the roots.

21 And Peter calling to remembrance saith unto him, Master, behold, the fig tree which thou cursedst is withered away.

The prayer of faith. (Cf. Jas. 5:15.)

22 And Jesus answering saith unto them, [g]Have faith in God.

23 For verily I say unto you, That [h]whosoever shall say unto this mountain, Be thou removed, and be thou cast into the sea; and shall not doubt in his heart, but shall believe that those things which he saith shall come to pass; he shall have whatsoever he saith.

24 Therefore I say unto you, What things soever ye desire, when ye pray, believe that ye receive *them*, and ye shall have *them*.

25 And when ye stand praying, forgive, if ye have ought against any: that your Father also which is in heaven may forgive you your trespasses.

26 But [i]if ye do not forgive, neither will your Father which is in heaven forgive your trespasses.

Jesus' authority questioned
(Mt. 21:23-27; Lk. 20:1-8).

27 And they come again to Jerusalem: and as he was walking in the temple, there come to him the chief priests, and the scribes, and the elders,

28 And say unto him, By what authority doest thou these things? and who gave thee this authority to do these things?

29 And Jesus answered and said unto them, I will also ask of you one question, and answer me, and I will tell you by what authority I do these things.

30 [j]The baptism of John, was *it* from heaven, or of men? answer me.

31 And they reasoned with themselves, saying, If we shall say, From heaven; he will say, Why then did ye not believe him?

32 But if we shall say, Of men; they feared the people: for all *men* counted John, that he was a prophet indeed.

33 And they answered and said unto Jesus, We cannot tell. And Jesus answering saith unto them, Neither do I tell you by what authority I do these things.

CHAPTER 12.

Parable of the householder demanding fruit from his vineyard (Mt. 21:33-46; Lk. 20:9-19. Cf. Isa. 5:1-7).

And he began to speak unto [k]them by [l]parables. A *certain* man planted a [m]vineyard, and set an hedge about *it*, and digged *a place for* the winefat, and built a tower, and let it out to husbandmen, and went into a far country.

2 And at the season he [n]sent to the husbandmen a servant, that he might receive from the husbandmen of the fruit of the vineyard.

3 And they caught *him*, and beat him, and sent *him* away empty.

4 And again he sent unto them another servant; and at him they cast stones, and wounded *him* in the head, and sent *him* away shamefully handled.

5 And again he sent another; and him they killed, and many others; beating some, and killing some.

6 Having yet therefore one [o]son, his wellbeloved, he sent him also last unto them, saying, They will reverence my son.

7 But those husbandmen said among themselves, This is the heir; come, let us kill him, and the inheritance shall be ours.

8 And they took him, and killed *him*, and cast *him* out of the vineyard.

9 What shall therefore the lord of the vineyard do? he will come and [p]destroy the husbandmen, and will give the vineyard unto others.

10 And have ye not read this scripture; [q]The stone which the builders rejected is become the head of the corner:

11 This was the [r]Lord's doing, and it is marvellous in our eyes?

12 And they [s]sought to lay hold on him, but feared the people: for they knew that he had spoken the parable

A.D. 33.

a Isa. 56:7.

b Jer. 7:11.

c Mt. 21:45, 46; Lk. 19:47, 48.

d Psa. 2:2.

e Mt. 7:28; Mk. 1:22.

f *whenever*, i.e. every day when evening came.

g *Have the faith of God;* i.e. the faith which God gives. Cf. 1 Cor. 12:9; Eph. 2:8.

h Mt. 17:20; Lk. 11:1, *note*; 17:6; John 14:13, 14.

i Mt. 6:12, *note*. Verse 26 is omitted from the best MSS.

j Lk. 7:24-35.

k Cf. Mt. 13:10-15.

l *Parables* (N.T.). vs. 1-11; Mk. 13:28, 29. (Mt. 5:13-16; Lk. 21:29-31.)

m Israel. Isa. 5:1-7. Israel was not fruitless, but brought forth only wild grapes. Cf. John 3:6; Hos. 10:1; *contra*, Hos. 14:8.

n vs. 2-5, the prophets and John the Baptist.

o Jesus Himself. Cf. Heb. 1:1-3.

p Fulfilled in the destruction of Jerusalem, A.D. 70 Cf. Lk. 21:20-24.

q Psa. 118:22, 23; cf. 1 Pet. 2:8, *note*.

r *Jehovah*. vs. 10, 11; Psa. 118:22, 23.

s John 7:30.

against them: and they left him, and went their way.

The question of tribute
(Mt. 22:15-22; Lk. 20:19-26).

13 And they [a]send unto him certain of the Pharisees and of the Herodians, to catch him in *his* words.

14 And when they were come, they say unto him, Master, we know that thou art true, and carest for no man: for thou regardest not the person of men, but teachest the way of God in truth: [b]Is it lawful to give tribute to Cæsar, [c]or not?

15 Shall we give, or shall we not give? But he, knowing their hypocrisy, said unto them, Why tempt ye me? bring me a [d]penny, that I may see *it*.

16 And they brought *it*. And he saith unto them, Whose *is* this image and superscription? And they said unto him, Cæsar's.

17 And Jesus answering said unto them, [e]Render to Cæsar the things that are Cæsar's, and to [f]God the things that are God's. And they marvelled at him.

Jesus answers the Sadducees
(Mt. 22:23-33; Lk. 20:27-38).

18 Then come unto him the [g]Sadducees, which say there is no resurrection; and they asked him, saying,

19 Master, [h]Moses wrote unto us, If a man's brother die, and leave *his* wife *behind him*, and leave no children, that his [i]brother should take his wife, and raise up seed unto his brother.

20 Now there were seven brethren: and the first took a wife, and dying left no seed.

21 And the second took her, and died, neither left he any seed: and the third likewise.

22 And the seven had her, and left no seed: last of all the woman died also.

23 In the resurrection therefore, when they shall rise, whose wife shall she be of them? for the seven had her to wife.

24 And Jesus answering [j]said unto them, Do ye not therefore err, because ye know not the scriptures, neither the power of God?

25 For [k]when they shall rise [l]from the dead, they neither marry, nor are given in marriage; but are as the [m]angels which are in heaven.

26 And as touching the dead, that they rise: have ye not [n]read in the book of Moses, how in the bush God [o]spake unto him, saying, I *am* the [p]God of Abraham, and the [p]God of Isaac, and the [p]God of Jacob?

27 He is not the God of the dead, but the God of the living: ye therefore do greatly err.

The great commandments
(Mt. 22:34-40; cf. Lk. 10:25-37).

28 And one of the scribes came, and having heard them reasoning together, and perceiving that he had answered them well, asked him, Which is the first commandment of all?

29 And Jesus answered him, The first of all the commandments *is*, Hear, O Israel; The Lord our God is one [q]Lord:

30 And thou shalt love the Lord thy God with all thy heart, and with all thy soul, and with all thy mind, and with all thy strength: this *is* the first commandment.

31 And the second *is* like, *namely* this, [r]Thou shalt love thy neighbour as thyself. There is none other commandment greater than these.

32 And the scribe said unto him, Well, Master, thou hast said the truth: for there is one God; and there is none other but he:

33 And to love him with all the heart, and with all the understanding, and with all the soul, and with all the strength, and to love *his* neighbour as himself, is more than all whole burnt offerings and sacrifices.

34 And when Jesus saw that he answered [s]discreetly, he said unto him, Thou art not [t]far from the kingdom of God. And no man after that durst ask him *any question*.

Jesus questions the Pharisees
(Mt. 22:41-46; Lk. 20:41-44).

35 And Jesus answered and said, while he taught in the temple, How say the scribes that Christ is the [u]Son of David?

36 [v]For David himself said by the [w]Holy Ghost, The [x]LORD said to my [y]Lord, Sit thou on my right hand, till I make thine enemies thy footstool.

37 David therefore himself calleth him Lord; and whence is he *then* his son? And the common people heard him gladly.

38 And he said unto them in his doctrine, Beware of the scribes, which love

A.D. 33.

a Mt. 22:15.
b Deut. 7:2, 6.
c Lk. 23:2.
d *denarius.* Cf. Mt. 18:28, *refs.*
e Mt. 17:25-27; Rom. 13:7; 1 Pet. 2:17; cf. Acts 2:39.
f Eccl. 5:4, 5; Mal. 1:6.
g Mt. 3:7, *note;* 22, 23, *ref.*
h Deut. 25:5.
i Ruth 1:11, 12.
j Mt. 22:29, *ref.*
k Cf. Mt. 22:30.
l Lit. *from amongst;* cf. Phil. 3:11. Here it is the first resurrection, 1 Cor. 15:52, *note.*
m Heb. 1:4, *note.*
n Jesus affirms the historic truth and inspiration of Ex. 3.
o *Inspiration.* vs. 26, 36; Mk. 12:36. (Ex. 4:15; Rev. 22:19.)
p *Elohim.* Ex. 3:6.
q *Jehovah.* Deut. 6:4.
r Lev. 19:18.
s *with intelligence.*
t i.e. not far in knowledge. He knew the very law which utterly condemns the best man—its true office. Rom. 3:19; 10:3-5; Gal. 3:10, 22-24.
u i.e. David's Son only. Cf. Rom. 1:3, 4.
v *Inspiration.* (Jesus affirms the inspiration and Davidic authorship of Psa. 110.) v. 36; Lk. 1:3. (Ex. 4:15; Rev. 22:19.)
w *Holy Spirit.* Mk. 13:11. (Mt. 1:18; Acts 2:4.)
x *Jehovah.*
y *Adonai,* Psa. 110:1.

to go in long clothing, and *love* salutations in the marketplaces,
39 And the chief seats in the synagogues, and the uppermost rooms at
feasts:
40 Which devour widows' houses,
and for a pretence make long prayers:
these shall receive greater [a]damnation.

Jesus and the widow's mite (Lk. 21:1-4).

41 And Jesus sat over against the treasury, and beheld how the people cast
money into the treasury: and many that
were rich cast in much.
42 And there came a certain poor
widow, and she threw in two [b]mites,
which make a [c]farthing.
43 And he called *unto him* his disciples, and saith unto them, Verily I say
unto you, That this poor widow hath
cast more in, than all they which have
cast into the treasury:
44 For all *they* did cast in of their abundance; but she of her want did cast in all
that she had, *even* all her living.

CHAPTER 13.

The Olivet discourse: the disciple's questions. (Cf. Mt. 24, 25; Lk. 21.)

And as he went out of the temple, one
of his disciples saith unto him,
Master, see what manner of stones and
what buildings *are here*!
2 [d]And Jesus answering said unto
him, Seest thou these great buildings?
there shall not be left one stone upon
another, that shall not be thrown down.
3 And as he sat upon the mount of
Olives over against the temple, Peter
and James and John and Andrew asked
him privately,
4 Tell us, when shall these things be?
and what *shall be* the sign when all these
things shall be fulfilled?

The Olivet discourse: the course of this age.

5 And Jesus answering them began to
say, Take heed lest any *man* [e]deceive you:
6 For many shall come in my name,
saying, I am *Christ*; and shall deceive
many.
7 And when ye shall hear of wars and
rumours of wars, [f]be ye not troubled: for
such things must needs be; but the end
shall not *be* yet.
8 For nation shall rise against nation,
and kingdom against kingdom: and
there shall be earthquakes in divers
places, and there shall be famines and
troubles: these *are* the beginnings of
[g]sorrows.
9 But take heed to yourselves: for they
shall [h]deliver you up to councils; and in
the synagogues ye shall be beaten: and
ye shall be brought before rulers and
kings for my sake, for a testimony
against them.
10 [i]And the [j]gospel must first be published among all nations.
11 But when they shall lead *you*, and
deliver you up, [k]take no thought beforehand what ye shall speak, neither do ye
premeditate: but whatsoever shall be
given you in that hour, that speak ye: for
it is not ye that speak, [l]but the [m]Holy
Ghost.
12 Now the [n]brother shall betray the
brother to death, and the father the son;
and children shall rise up against *their*
parents, and shall cause them to be put
to death.
13 And ye shall be hated of all *men* for
my name's sake: but he that shall endure
unto the [o]end, the same shall be [p]saved.

The great tribulation (Mt. 24:15). See "Tribulation" (Psa. 2:5; Rev. 7:14).

14 But [q]when ye shall see the abomination of desolation, spoken of by
Daniel the prophet, standing where [r]it
ought not, (let him that readeth understand,) [s]then let them that be in Judæa
flee to the mountains:
15 And let him that is on the housetop
not go down into the house, neither enter
therein, to take any thing out of his house:
16 And let him that is in the field not
turn back again for to take up his garment.
17 But woe to them that are with child,
and to them that give suck in those days!
18 And pray ye that your flight be not
in the winter.
19 For *in* those days shall be [t]affliction,
such as was not from the beginning of
the creation which God created unto this
time, neither shall be.
20 And except that the Lord had shortened those days, no flesh should be

A.D. 33.

a i.e. *condemnation.*
b One mite = 1-4 farthing or 1-8 cent.
c One farthing here = 1-4 cent.
d See Mt. 24:3, *note* on the Olivet discourse.
e Cf. 2 Thes. 2:1-3.
f *be ye not surprised, for it must so be, but not then is the end;* i.e. vs. 7, 8 describe the age, not the end only.
g *birthpangs.* Answering to the "seals." (Rev. 6.) The death-agony of this age is the birth-agony of the next.
h Mt. 10:17; Acts 5:18; 12:1-4; 25:15.
i Cf. Mt. 24:14. *"Gospel of the Kingdom."* See Rev. 14:6, *note.*
j *Gospel.* Mk. 14:9. (Gen. 12:1-3; Rev. 14:6.)
k *be not anxious.*
l Acts 4:8, 31.
m *Holy Spirit.* Lk. 1:15, 17, 35, 41, 67, 80. (Mt. 1:18; Acts 2:4.)
n Cf. Mic. 7:6.
o Not the end of the believer's life, but the end of the great tribulation.
p In the sense of Rev. 13:8; 20:4.
q See "Beast." (Dan. 7:8; Rev. 19:20.)
r Or, *he.* Cf. 2 Thes. 2:4; Rev. 13:6, 14, 16; Dan. 11:36; 12:11.
s Cf. Lk. 21:20-24, which is a prophecy fulfilled in the destruction of Jerusalem, A.D. 70, when the Christians escaped, and which foreshadowed the more terrible day here described. See "Great Tribulation," Psa. 2:5; Rev. 7:14.
t *tribulation.* Cf. Mt. 24:21. See "Tribulation." (Psa. 2:5; Rev. 7:14.)

saved: but for the [a]elect's sake, whom he
hath chosen, he hath shortened the days.
21 And then if any man shall say to
you, Lo, here *is* Christ; or, lo, *he is* there;
believe *him* not:
22 For false Christs and false prophets
shall rise, and shall shew signs and wonders, to seduce, if *it were* possible, even
the elect.
23 But take ye heed: behold, I have
foretold you all things.

The Lord's return in glory (Mt. 24:27-31).

24 But in those days, after that tribulation, the sun shall be darkened, and the
moon shall not give her light,
25 And the stars of heaven shall fall,
and the powers that are in heaven shall
be shaken.
26 And then shall they see the [b]Son of
man coming in the clouds with great
power and glory.
27 And then shall he send his [c]angels,
and shall gather together his elect from
the four winds, from the uttermost part of
the earth to the uttermost part of heaven.

Parable of the fig tree.
(Cf. Mt. 24:32, 33; Lk. 21:29-31.)

28 Now learn a [d]parable of the fig tree;
When her branch is yet tender, and putteth forth leaves, ye know that summer
is near:
29 So ye in like manner, when ye shall
see these things come to pass, know that
it is nigh, *even* at the doors.
30 Verily I say unto you, that this generation shall not pass, till all these things
be done.
31 Heaven and earth shall pass away:
but my words shall not pass away.
32 But of that day and *that* hour
knoweth no man, no, not the [c]angels
which are in heaven, neither the Son, but
the Father.
33 Take ye heed, watch and pray: for
ye know not when the time is.

Watchfulness in view
of the return of the Lord.

34 *For the Son of man is* as a man taking
a far journey, who left his house, and
gave authority to his servants, and to
[e]every man his work, and commanded
the porter to watch.
35 Watch ye therefore: for ye know not
when the master of the house cometh, at
even, or at midnight, or at the cockcrow-
ing, or in the morning:
36 Lest coming suddenly he find you
sleeping.
37 And what I say unto you I say unto
all, [f]Watch.

CHAPTER 14.

The plot to put Jesus to death
(Mt. 26:2-5; Lk. 22:1, 2).

After two days was *the feast of* the
passover, and of unleavened bread:
and the chief priests and the scribes
sought how they might take him by
craft, and put *him* to death.
2 But they said, Not on the feast *day*,
lest there be an uproar of the people.

Jesus anointed by Mary of Bethany
(Mt. 26:6-13; John 12:1-8).

3 [g]And being in Bethany in the house
of Simon the leper, as he sat at meat,
there came a [h]woman having an
alabaster box of ointment of spikenard
very precious; and she brake the box,
and poured *it* on his [i]head.
4 And there were some that had indignation within themselves, and said, Why
was this waste of the ointment made?
5 For it might have been sold for more
than three hundred [j]pence, and have
been given to the poor. And they murmured against her.
6 And Jesus said, Let her alone; why
trouble ye her? she hath wrought a good
work on me.
7 [k]For ye have the poor with you
always, and whensoever ye will ye may
do them good: but me ye have not
always.
8 She hath done what she could: she is
come aforehand to [l]anoint my body to
the burying.
9 Verily I say unto you, [m]Wheresoever
this [n]gospel shall be preached throughout the whole [o]world, *this* also that she
hath done shall be spoken of for a
memorial of her.

Judas covenants to betray Jesus
(Mt. 26:14-16; Lk. 22:3-6).

10 And [p]Judas Iscariot, one of the
twelve, went unto the chief priests, to
betray him unto them.
11 And when they heard *it*, they were
glad, and promised to give him money.
And he sought how he might conveniently betray him.

A.D. 33.

a *Election (corporate).* Acts 13:17. (Deut. 7:6; 1 Pet. 1:2.)

b *Christ (second advent).* Lk. 12:35-40. (Deut. 30:3; Acts 1:9-11.) See Mt. 8:20, *note.*

c Heb. 1:4, *note.*

d *Parables* (N.T.). vs. 28, 29, 34-37; Lk. 5:36, 37. (Mt. 5:13-16; Lk. 21:29-31.)

e Mt. 25:14.

f Mt. 24:42; 25:13; 1 Pet. 1:13.

g Mt. 21:17; 26:6; Lk. 7:37; John 12:1.

h Mary of Bethany.

i See Mt. 26:7, *note.*

j Gr. *denarion.* A denarius was = 8 1-2 d., 17 cents.

k Deut. 15:11; Mt. 26:11; John 12:8.

l Cf. John 19:40.

m Mt. 26:13.

n *Gospel.* Mk. 16:15. (Gen. 12:1-3; Rev. 14:6.)

o i.e. *earth.*

p Psa. 41:9; 55:12-14; Mt. 10:2-4.

The preparation of the passover
(Mt. 26:17-19; Lk. 22:7-13).

12 And the [a]first day of unleavened
bread, when they [b]killed the passover,
his disciples said unto him, Where wilt
thou that we go and prepare that thou
mayest eat the passover?
13 And he sendeth forth two of his disciples, and saith unto them, Go ye into
the city, and there shall meet you a man
bearing a pitcher of water: follow him.
14 And wheresoever he shall go in,
say ye to the goodman of the house, The
[c]Master saith, Where is the guestchamber, where I shall eat the passover with
my disciples?
15 And he will shew you a large upper
room furnished *and* prepared: there
make ready for us.
16 And his disciples went forth, and
came into the city, and [d]found as he had
said unto them: and they made ready
the passover.

The last passover (Mt. 26:20-24;
Lk. 22:14, 21-23; John 13:18, 19).

17 [e]And in the evening he cometh
with the twelve.
18 And as they sat and did eat, Jesus
said, Verily I say unto you, One of you
which [f]eateth with me shall betray me.
19 And they began to be sorrowful,
and to say unto him one by one, *Is* it I?
and another *said, Is* it I?
20 And he answered and said unto
them, *It is* one of the twelve, that dip-
peth with me in the dish.
21 [g]The Son of man indeed goeth, as it
is written of him: but woe to that man by
whom the Son of man is betrayed! [h]good
were it for that man if he had never been
born.

Jesus institutes the Lord's Supper (Mt.
26:26-29; Lk. 22:17-20; 1 Cor. 11:23-26).

22 And as they did eat, Jesus took
bread, and blessed, and [i]brake *it*, and
gave to them, and said, Take, [j]eat: this is
my body.
23 And he took the cup, and [k]when he
had given thanks, he gave *it* to them:
and they all drank of it.
24 And he said unto them, [l]This is my
blood of the [m]new [n]testament, which is
shed for many.
25 Verily I say unto you, I will drink
no more of the fruit of the vine, until
that day that I drink it new in the kingdom of God.

Peter's denial foretold (Mt. 26:31-35;
Lk. 22:31-34; John 13:36-38).

26 And when they had sung an
[p]hymn, they went out into the mount of
Olives.
27 And Jesus saith unto them, All ye
shall be offended because of me this
night: for it is [q]written, I will smite the
shepherd, and the sheep shall be scattered.
28 [r]But after that I am risen, I will go
before you into Galilee.
29 But [s]Peter said unto him, Although
all shall be offended, yet *will* not I.
30 And Jesus saith unto him, Verily I
say unto thee, That this day, *even* in this
night, before the cock crow twice, thou
shalt deny me thrice.
31 But he spake the more vehemently,
If I should die with thee, I will not deny
thee in any wise. [t]Likewise also said
they all.

The agony in the garden. (Cf. Mt. 26:36-
46; Lk. 22:39-46; John 18:1.)

32 And they came to a place which was
named Gethsemane: and he saith to his
disciples, Sit ye here, while I shall pray.
33 And he [u]taketh with him Peter and
James and John, and began to be sore
amazed, and to be very heavy;
34 And saith unto them, My [v]soul is
exceeding sorrowful unto death: tarry ye
here, and watch.

The first prayer.
(Cf. Mt. 26:39; Lk. 22:41, 42.)

35 And he went forward a little, and fell
on the ground, and prayed that, if it were
possible, the hour might pass from him.
36 And he said, Abba, Father, all
things *are* possible unto thee; take away
this [w]cup from me: [x]nevertheless not
what I will, but what thou wilt.
37 And he cometh, and findeth them
sleeping, and saith unto Peter, Simon,
sleepest thou? couldest not thou watch
one hour?
38 [y]Watch ye and pray, lest ye enter
into temptation. The spirit truly *is* ready,
but the [z]flesh *is* weak.

The second prayer.
(Cf. Mt. 26:42; Lk. 22:44.)

39 And again he went away, and
prayed, and spake the same words.

A.D. 33.

a Ex. 12:8.
b *sacrificed.*
c John 13:13.
d John 16:4.
e For the order of events on the night of the last passover, see Mt. 26:20, *note.*
f Psa. 41:9.
g Cf. Acts 2:23; Rom. 9:19-23.
h Mt. 18:6.
i Lk. 24:30.
j 1 Cor. 10:15, 16; 11:23, 24; 1 Pet. 2:24.
k 1 Cor. 11:24, 25.
l Lev. 17:11; 1 Cor. 10:16; Heb. 9:14-22.
m *Covenant (new).* Lk. 22:20. (Isa. 61:8; Heb. 8:8-12.)
n *covenant.*
o Isa. 25:6-9; Ezk. 34:23, 24; 37:21-28; Joel 3:17-20; Amos 9:13-15.
p Or, *psalm.* Cf. Neh. 8:10; Psa. 47:6, 7; 150:1-6.
q Zech. 13:7.
r Mk. 16:7.
s Mt. 26:33; Lk. 22:31; John 13:36.
t Cf. v. 50.
u Mt. 17:1; 26:37; Mk. 5:37; 9:2; 13:3; Lk. 8:51; 9:28; 22:8; John 18:15.
v Isa. 53:4-6; Mt. 27:46; John 12:27.
w Mt. 26:39, *note* on the meaning of the cup.
x John 4:34.
y Lk. 21:36; Eph. 5:18.
z Rom. 7:18, 21-24; Jude 23, *note.*

40 And when he returned, he found them asleep again, (for their eyes were heavy,) neither wist they what to answer him.

The third prayer. (Cf. Mt. 26:44.)

41 And he cometh the third time, and saith unto them, Sleep on now, and take *your* rest: it is enough, the [a]hour is come; behold, the Son of man is betrayed into the hands of [b]sinners.
42 Rise up, let us go; lo, he that betrayeth me is at hand.

The betrayal and arrest of Jesus (Mt. 26:47-56; Lk. 22:47-53; John 18:3-11).

43 And immediately, while he yet spake, cometh [c]Judas, one of the twelve, and with him a great [d]multitude with swords and staves, from the chief priests and the scribes and the elders.
44 And he that betrayed him had given them a token, saying, Whomsoever I shall kiss, that same is he; take him, and lead *him* away safely.
45 [e]And as soon as he was come, he goeth straightway to him, and saith, [f]Master, master; and kissed him.
46 And they laid their hands on him, and took him.

Peter smites with the sword and follows afar off. Jesus forsaken by all (Mt. 26:51-56).

47 And one of them that stood by drew a sword, and smote a servant of the high priest, and cut off his ear.
48 And Jesus answered and said unto them, Are ye come out, as against a thief, with swords and *with* staves to take me?
49 I was daily with you in the temple teaching, and ye took me not: but the scriptures must be fulfilled.
50 And they [g]all forsook him, and fled.
51 And there followed him a certain young man, having a linen cloth cast about *his* naked *body*; and the young men laid hold on him:
52 And he left the linen cloth, and fled from them naked.

Jesus is brought before the high priest and Sanhedrin (Mt. 26:57-68; John 18:12-14, 19-24).

53 [h]And they [i]led Jesus away to the high priest: and with him were assembled all the chief priests and the elders and the scribes.

A.D. 33.

a John 17:1.
b *Sin.* Rom. 3:23, *note.*
c v. 10.
d Psa. 3:1.
e *And, coming, instantly stepping forward to him, he said, Rabbi, rabbi! and eagerly kissed him.*
f Never once in the Gospel record does Judas Iscariot call Jesus *Lord.* He was the first Arian amongst the professed followers of Jesus. No one can in reality say that Jesus is Lord, but by the Holy Ghost (1 Cor. 12:3), but it is possible to use the term as an empty formality without believing the Lordship of Christ; Mt. 7:21; 25:11, 12.
g Cf. v. 31.
h Mt. 26:57, *note* on order of events on the day of the crucifixion.
i John 18:13.
j See v. 68; Mt. 26:3.
k *court.*
l John 2:19; Mt. 26:61; Mk. 15:29.
m Mt. 26:63; Lk. 22:67.
n Isa. 53:7.
o Psa. 110:1; Rev. 3:21; Mt. 24:30, 31; 25:31; Lk. 1:31-33.
p Num. 14:6, 7; Acts 14:13, 14.
q John 10:33.
r Isa. 50:6; 52:14, *note;* cf. Rev. 20:11.
s Mt. 26:68; Lk. 22:64.
t Lit. *with heavy blows take him.*

54 And Peter followed him afar off, [j]even into the [k]palace of the high priest: and he sat with the servants, and warmed himself at the fire.
55 And the chief priests and all the council sought for witness against Jesus to put him to death; and found none.
56 For many bare false witness against him, but their witness agreed not together.
57 And there arose certain, and bare false witness against him, saying,
58 We heard him [l]say, I will destroy this temple that is made with hands, and within three days I will build another made without hands.
59 But neither so did their witness agree together.
60 And the high priest stood up in the midst, and asked Jesus, saying, Answerest thou nothing? what *is it which* these witness against thee?
61 [m]But he held his peace, and [n]answered nothing. Again the high priest asked him, and said unto him, Art thou the Christ, the Son of the Blessed?
62 And Jesus said, I am: and ye shall see the Son of man [o]sitting on the right hand of power, and coming in the clouds of heaven.
63 Then the high priest [p]rent his clothes, and saith, What need we any further witnesses?
64 Ye have heard the [q]blasphemy: what think ye? And they all condemned him to be guilty of death.
65 And some began to [r]spit on him, and to cover his face, and to buffet him, and to say unto him, [s]Prophesy: and the servants [t]did strike him with the palms of their hands.

Peter denies his Lord (Mt. 26:69-75; Lk. 22:56-62; John 18:16-18, 25-27).

66 And as Peter was beneath in the palace, there cometh one of the maids of the high priest:
67 And when she saw Peter warming himself, she looked upon him, and said, And thou also wast with Jesus of Nazareth.
68 But he denied, saying, I know not, neither understand I what thou sayest. And he went out into the porch; and the cock crew.

69 And a maid saw him again, and began to say to them that stood by, This is *one* of them.

70 And he denied it again. And a little after, they that stood by said again to Peter, Surely thou art *one* of them: for thou art a Galilaean, and thy speech agreeth *thereto*.

71 But he began to curse and to swear, *saying*, I know not this man of whom ye speak.

72 And the second time the cock crew. And Peter called to mind the word that Jesus said unto him, Before the cock crow twice, thou shalt deny me thrice. [a]And when he thought thereon, he wept.

CHAPTER 15.

Jesus sent before Pilate (Mt. 27:1, 2, 11-15; Lk. 23:1-7, 13-18; John 18:28-40; 19:1-16).

And straightway in the morning the chief priests held a [b]consultation with the elders and scribes and the whole council, and bound Jesus, and carried *him* away, and delivered *him* to Pilate.

2 And Pilate [c]asked him, Art thou the King of the Jews? And he answering said unto him, Thou sayest *it*.

3 And the chief priests accused him of many things: but he answered nothing.

4 And Pilate asked him again, saying, [d]Answerest thou nothing? behold how many things they witness against thee.

5 [e]But Jesus yet answered nothing; so that Pilate marvelled.

6 Now at *that* feast he released unto them one prisoner, whomsoever they desired.

Not Jesus but Barabbas (Mt. 27:16-26; Lk. 23:16-25; John 18:40).

7 And there was *one* named Barabbas, *which lay* bound with them that had made insurrection with him, who had committed murder in the insurrection.

8 And the multitude crying aloud began to desire *him to do* as he had ever done unto them.

9 But Pilate answered them, saying, Will ye that I release unto you the King of the Jews?

10 For he knew that the chief priests had delivered him for [f]envy.

11 But the chief priests moved the people, that he should rather [g]release Barabbas unto them.

12 And Pilate answered and said again unto them, What will ye then that I shall do *unto him* whom ye call the [h]King of the Jews?

13 And they cried out again, Crucify him.

14 Then Pilate said unto them, Why, [i]what evil hath he done? And they cried out the more exceedingly, Crucify him.

15 And *so* Pilate, willing to content the people, released Barabbas unto them, and delivered Jesus, when he had scourged *him*, to be [j]crucified.

Jesus crowned with thorns (Mt. 27:27-31).

16 And the soldiers led him away into [k]the hall, called Prætorium; and they call together the whole band.

17 And they clothed him with purple, and [l]platted a crown of [m]thorns, and put it about his *head*,

18 And began to salute him, [n]Hail, King of the Jews!

19 [o]And they [p]smote him on the head with a reed, and did spit upon him, and bowing *their* knees worshipped him.

20 And when they had mocked him, they took off the purple from him, and put his own clothes on him, and led him out to crucify him.

21 [q]And they compel one Simon a Cyrenian, who passed by, coming out of the country, the father of Alexander and [r]Rufus, to bear his cross.

22 [s]And they bring him unto the place Golgotha, which is, being interpreted, The place of a skull.

23 And they gave him to [t]drink wine mingled with myrrh: [u]but he received *it* not.

Jesus crucified (Mt. 27:33-56; Lk. 23:33-49; John 19:17-37).

24 [v]And when they had crucified him, they [w]parted his garments, [x]casting lots upon them, what every man should take.

25 And it was the [y]third hour, and they crucified him.

26 And the [z]superscription of his accusation was written over, THE KING OF THE JEWS.

27 And with him they crucify two thieves; the one on his right hand, and the other on his left.

28 [aa]And the scripture was fulfilled,

A.D. 33.

a Lit. *having thought thereon was weeping.*
b Psa. 2:2; Mt. 27:1; Lk. 23:1; John 18:28; Acts 2:23; 4:27.
c Mt. 27:27-32.
d Cf. John 19:10.
e Isa. 53:7.
f See Mt. 5:22; 21:38; John 12:19.
g Acts 3:14.
h Psa. 2:6; Jer. 23:5; Lk. 1:31-33; Acts 5:31; 15:14-17.
i Isa. 53:9.
j Isa. 53:8.
k Or, *the court which is the judgment-hall.*
l *plaited.*
m Gen. 3:17, 18; cf. 2 Cor. 5:21; Gal. 3:13.
n *Joy to thee! King of the Jews!*
o *And they were striking him on the head with a reed and spitting on him.*
p Isa. 50:6; Zech. 13:7.
q Mt. 27:32; Lk. 23:26.
r It is possible that this may be the same Rufus mentioned in Rom. 16:13.
s Mt. 27:33-44; Lk. 23:33-43; John 19:17-24.
t The stupefying drink usually given to those crucified.
u Cf. John 18:11.
v For order of events at the crucifixion, see Mt. 27:33, *note.*
w Psa. 22:18.
x Cf. John 19:24.
y Cf. John 19:14. John uses the Roman Mark the Hebrew computation of time.
z See Mt. 27:37, *note.*
aa Isa. 53:9, 12; Lk. 22:37.

which saith, And he was numbered with the transgressors.

29 [a]And they that passed by railed on him, wagging their heads, and saying, [b]Ah, thou that destroyest the temple, and buildest *it* in three days,

30 Save thyself, and come down from the cross.

31 Likewise also the chief priests [c]mocking said among themselves with the scribes, [d]He saved others; himself he cannot save.

32 Let Christ the King of Israel descend now from the cross, that we may [e]see and believe. [f]And they that were crucified with him reviled him.

33 And when the sixth hour was come, there was darkness over the whole land until the ninth hour.

34 And at the ninth hour Jesus cried with a loud voice, [g]saying, Eloi, Eloi, lama sabachthani? which is, being interpreted, My God, my God, why hast thou forsaken me?

35 And some of them that stood by, when they heard *it*, said, Behold, he calleth Elias.

36 And one ran and filled a spunge full of vinegar, and put *it* on a reed, and [h]gave him to drink, saying, Let alone; let us see whether Elias will come to take him down.

37 And Jesus cried with a loud voice, and [i]gave up the ghost.

38 And the [j]veil of the temple was rent in twain from the [k]top to the bottom.

39 And when the centurion, which stood over against him, saw that he so cried out, and gave up the ghost, he said, Truly this man was the Son of God.

40 There were also women looking on afar off: among whom was Mary Magdalene, and Mary the mother of James the less and of Joses, and Salome;

41 (Who also, when he was in Galilee, followed him, and ministered unto him;) and many other women which came up with him unto Jerusalem.

The entombment (Mt. 27:57-61; Lk. 23:50-56; John 19:38-42).

42 And now when the even was come, because it was the preparation, that is, the day before the sabbath,

43 [l]Joseph of Arimathaea, an honourable counsellor, which also waited for the kingdom of God, came, and went in boldly unto Pilate, and craved the body of Jesus.

44 And Pilate marvelled if he were already dead: and calling *unto him* the centurion, he asked him whether he had been any while dead.

45 And when he knew *it* of the centurion, he gave the body to Joseph.

46 And he bought fine linen, and took him down, and wrapped him in the linen, and [m]laid him in a sepulchre which was hewn out of a rock, and rolled a stone unto the door of the sepulchre.

47 And Mary Magdalene and [n]Mary *the mother* of Joses beheld where he was laid.

CHAPTER 16.

The resurrection of Jesus Christ and the events of that day (Mt. 28:1-15; Lk. 24:1-49; John 20:1-23).

And [o]when the sabbath was past, Mary Magdalene, and [n]Mary the *mother* of James, and Salome, had bought sweet spices, that they might come and anoint him.

2 [1]And very early in the morning the first *day* of the week, they came unto the sepulchre at the rising of the sun.

3 And they said among themselves, [p]Who shall roll us away the stone from the door of the sepulchre?

4 And when they looked, they saw that the stone was rolled away: for it was very great.

5 And entering into the sepulchre, they saw a young man sitting on the right side, clothed in a long white garment; and they were affrighted.

6 And he saith unto them, Be not affrighted: [q]Ye seek Jesus of Nazareth, which was crucified: he is [r]risen; he is not here: behold the place where they laid him.

7 But go your way, tell his disciples and Peter that he goeth before you into Galilee: there shall ye see him, [s]as he said unto you.

8 And they went out quickly, and fled from the sepulchre; for they trembled

A.D. 33.

- *a* Psa. 22:6, 7; 109:25.
- *b* John 2:19, 20, 21.
- *c* Psa. 35:16; Isa. 28:22; Jer. 23:1-6; Mt. 3:7; 23:33; Lk. 18:32.
- *d* Lk. 7:14; John 11:43. Cf. John 3:14, 15 with Heb. 9:22.
- *e* Cf. John 20:29. Also Lk. 16:31; Acts 6:7; Rom. 3:3; 2 Tim. 2:13; 1 Pet. 1:8.
- *f* Cf. Mt. 27:44; Lk. 23:39, 40.
- *g* Psa. 22:1. Cf. Psa. 88:14.
- *h* Psa. 69:21.
- *i* See Mt. 27:50, *note*.
- *j* Ex. 26:31-33; Lev. 16:1, 2; Heb. 9:6, 8; 10:14-22.
- *k* God rent it down; it was rent from the top. Christ having made atonement and glorified God, the way into the holiest was now made manifest. Cf. Heb. 9:8, 24; 10:19-22.
- *l* Mt. 27:57-59; Lk. 23:50; John 19:38.
- *m* Isa. 53:9.
- *n* See Mt. 1:16, *note*.
- *o* Mt. 28:1; Lk. 24:1; John 20:1.
- *p* Mt. 28:2. Cf. Ex. 14:13-16.
- *q* *Jesus ye seek—the Nazarene, the crucified. He arose! He is not here!* The tone is of triumph. Cf. Psa. 2:4.
- *r* Lk. 7:11-15; Psa. 16:8-11; 22:24; 71:20; Isa. 26:19.
- *s* Mk. 14:28.

[1]**(16:2)** For the order of events on the day of the resurrection, and for the order of our Lord's appearances after His resurrection, see Mt. 28:1, 9, *notes* 1 and 2.

and were amazed: neither said they any
thing to any *man*; for they were afraid.
9 [1]Now when *Jesus* was risen early the
first *day* of the week, he [a]appeared first
to Mary Magdalene, out of whom he
had cast seven devils.
10 *And* she went and told them that
had been with him, as they mourned
and wept.
11 And they, when they had heard that
he was alive, and had been seen of her,
believed not.
12 After that he [b]appeared in another
form unto two of them, as they walked,
and went into the country.
13 And they went and told *it* unto the
residue: neither believed they them.
14 Afterward he appeared unto the
[2]eleven as they sat at meat, and upbraided them with their unbelief and hardness of heart, because they believed not
them which had seen him after he was
risen.

A.D. 33.

a See Mt. 28:9, *note.*
b Lk. 24:13-35.
c i.e. *earth.*
d *Gospel.* Lk. 2:10, 11. (Gen. 12:1-3; Rev. 14:6.)
e Rom. 1:16, *note.*
f i.e. *condemned.*
g Acts 4:29-31; 5:12.
h Acts 16:18.
i Acts 2:4.
j Acts 28:3-6.
k 2 Ki. 4:39-41.
l Acts 9:32-35.
m Lk. 24:50-53; Acts 1:9; Eph. 4:8-10.
n Acts 3:13; Heb. 2:4.

15 And he said unto them, Go ye into
all the [c]world, and preach the [d]gospel to
every creature.
16 He that believeth and is baptized
shall be [e]saved; but he that believeth not
shall be [f]damned.
17 And these [g]signs shall follow them
that believe; In my name shall they cast
out [h]devils; they shall speak with [i]new
tongues;
18 They shall take up [j]serpents; and if
they drink any [k]deadly thing, it shall not
hurt them; they shall lay hands on the
[l]sick, and they shall recover.

The ascension (Lk. 24:50-53; Acts 1:6-11).

19 So then after the Lord had spoken
unto them, he was [m]received up into
heaven, and sat on the right hand of
God.
20 And they went forth, and preached
every where, the Lord [n]working with
them, and confirming the word with
signs following. Amen.

[1]**(16:9)** The passage from verse 9 to the end is not found in the two most ancient manuscripts, the Sinaitic and Vatican, and others have it with partial omissions and variations. But it is quoted by Irenaeus and Hippolytus in the second or third century.

[2]**(16:14)** A collective term, equivalent to "The Sanhedrin," "The Commons," not necessarily implying that eleven persons were present. See Lk. 24:33; 1 Cor. 15:5; and cf. Mt. 28:16 where "eleven *disciples*" implies a definite number of persons.

THE GOSPEL ACCORDING TO

St. LUKE

WRITER. The writer of the third Gospel is called by Paul "the beloved physician" (Col. 4:14); and, as we learn from the Acts, was Paul's frequent companion. He was of Jewish ancestry, but his correct Greek marks him as a Jew of the dispersion. Tradition says that he was a Jew of Antioch, as Paul was of Tarsus.

Date. The date of Luke falls between A.D. 63 and 68.

Theme. Luke is the Gospel of the human-divine One, as John is of the divine-human One. The key-phrase is "Son of man," and the key-verse (19:10), "For the Son of man is come to seek and to save that which was lost." In harmony with this intent, Luke relates those things concerning Jesus which demonstrate how entirely human He was. His genealogy is traced to Adam, and the most detailed account is given of His mother, and of His infancy and boyhood. The parables peculiar to Luke have distinctively the human and the seeking note. But Luke is careful to guard the Deity and Kingship of Jesus Christ (Lk. 1:32-35). Luke, then, is the Gospel of "the man whose name *is* The BRANCH" (Zech. 6:12)

Luke has seven chief divisions: I. The Evangelist's Introduction, 1:1-4. II. The human relationships of Jesus, 1:5–2:52. III. The baptism, ancestry, and testing of Jesus, 3:1–4:13. IV. The ministry of the Son of man as Prophet-King in Galilee, 4:14–9:50. V. The journey of the Son of man from Galilee to Jerusalem, 9:51–19:44. VI. The final offer of the Son of man as King to Israel, His rejection and sacrifice, 19:45–23:56. VII. The resurrection, resurrection ministry, and ascension of the Son of man, 24:1-53.

The events recorded in this book cover a period of 39 years.

CHAPTER 1.

Introduction.

Forasmuch as many have taken in hand to set forth in order a declaration of those things which are most surely believed among us,

2 Even as they delivered them unto us, which from the beginning [a]were eyewitnesses, and ministers of [b]the word;

3 It seemed good to me also, [c]having had perfect [d]understanding of all things [1]from the very first, to write unto thee [e]in order, most excellent [f]Theophilus,

4 That thou mightest know the certainty of those things, wherein thou hast been instructed.

Birth of John the Baptist foretold.

5 There was in the days of [g]Herod, the king of Judæa, a certain priest named Zacharias, of the course of Abia: and his [h]wife *was* of the daughters of Aaron, and her name *was* Elisabeth.

6 And they were both [i]righteous before God, walking in all the [j]commandments and ordinances of the Lord blameless.

7 And they had no child, because that Elisabeth was barren, and they both were *now* well stricken in years.

8 And it came to pass, that while he executed the priest's office before God in the order of his course,

9 According to the custom of the priest's office, his lot was to burn incense when he went into the temple of the Lord.

10 And the whole multitude of the people were praying without at the time of incense.

11 And there appeared unto him an angel of the Lord standing on the right side of the altar of incense.

12 And when Zacharias saw *him*,

B.C. 7.

a John 15:27; Acts 1:3; 10:39; Heb. 2:3; 1 Pet. 5:1; 2 Pet. 1:16; 1 John 1:1.
b Rom. 15:16; Eph. 3:7, 8.
c *Inspiration.* Lk. 4:17-21, 27. (Ex. 4:15; Rev. 22:19.)
d Gr. *parakolouthekoti,* lit. *followed alongside of;* or, *closely traced.*
e The words "in order" are emphatic, indicating Luke's purpose to reduce to order the Gospel story.
f Acts 1:1.
g Herod the Great. Cf. Mt. 2:1, *note.*
h 1 Chr. 24:1, 10.
i *Righteousness.* Lk. 2:25. (Gen. 6:9; Lk. 2:25.)
j *Law (of Moses).* Lk. 10:25-37. (Ex. 19:1; Gal. 3:1-29.)

[1] **(1:3)** "From the very first": Gr. *anothen,* "from above." So translated in John 3:31; 19:11; Jas. 1:17; 3:15, 17. In no other place is *anothen* translated "from the very first." The use by Luke of *anothen* is an affirmation that his knowledge of these things, derived from those who had been eye-witnesses from the beginning (Lk. 1:2), was confirmed by revelation. In like manner Paul had doubtless heard from the eleven the story of the institution of the Lord's Supper, but he also had it by revelation from the Lord (cf. 1 Cor. 11:23), and his writing, like Luke's "*anothen*" knowledge, thus became first-hand, not traditional, merely.

he was troubled, and fear fell upon him.

13 But the [a]angel said unto him, Fear not, Zacharias: for thy [b]prayer is heard; and thy wife Elisabeth shall bear thee a son, and thou shalt call his name John.

14 And thou shalt have joy and gladness; and many shall rejoice at his birth.

15 For he shall be [c]great in the sight of the Lord, and shall drink neither wine nor strong drink; and he shall be filled with the [d]Holy Ghost, [e]even from his mother's womb.

16 And many of the children of Israel shall he turn to the Lord their God.

17 And he [f]shall go before him in the [g]spirit and power of Elias, to turn the hearts of the fathers to the children, and the disobedient to the wisdom of the just; to make ready a [h]people prepared for the Lord.

18 And Zacharias said unto the angel, Whereby shall I know this? for I am an old man, and my wife well stricken in years.

19 And the [a]angel answering said unto him, I am [i]Gabriel, that stand in the presence of God; and am [j]sent to speak unto thee, and to shew thee these glad tidings.

20 And, behold, thou shalt be dumb, and not able to speak, until the day that these things shall be performed, because thou believest not my words, which shall be fulfilled in their season.

21 And the people waited for Zacharias, and marvelled that he tarried so long in the temple.

22 And when he came out, he could not speak unto them: and they perceived that he had seen a vision in the temple: for he beckoned unto them, and remained speechless.

23 And it came to pass, that, as soon as the days of his ministration were accomplished, he departed to his own house.

24 And after those days his wife Elisabeth conceived, and hid herself five months, saying,

25 Thus hath the Lord dealt with me in the days wherein he looked on *me*, to [k]take away my reproach among men.

The annunciation.

26 And in the [l]sixth month the [a]angel Gabriel was sent from God unto a city of Galilee, named Nazareth,

27 To a [m]virgin espoused to a man whose name was Joseph, of the house of David; and the virgin's name *was* Mary.

28 And the [a]angel came in unto her, and said, Hail, *thou that art* [n]highly favoured, the Lord *is* with thee: blessed *art* thou among women.

29 And when she saw *him*, she was troubled at his saying, and cast in her mind what manner of salutation this should be.

30 And the [a]angel said unto her, Fear not, Mary: for thou hast found favour with God.

31 And, behold, [o]thou shalt conceive in thy womb, and bring forth a son, and shalt call his name JESUS.

32 He shall be [p]great, and shall be called the [q]Son of the Highest: and the Lord God shall give unto him the [r]throne of his [s]father David:

33 And [t]he shall reign over the house of Jacob for ever; and [u]of his [v]kingdom there shall be no end.

34 Then said Mary unto the angel, How shall this be, seeing I know not a man?

35 And the angel answered and said unto her, The Holy Ghost shall come upon thee, [w]and the power of the Highest shall overshadow thee: therefore also that [x]holy thing which shall be born of thee shall be called the [y]Son of God.

36 And, behold, thy cousin Elisabeth, she hath also conceived a son in her old age: and this is the sixth month with her, who was called barren.

37 For [z]with God nothing shall be impossible.

38 And Mary said, Behold the handmaid of the Lord; be it unto me according to thy word. And the angel departed from her.

Mary visits Elisabeth.

39 And Mary arose in those days, and went into the hill country with haste, into a city of Juda;

40 And entered into the house of Zacharias, and saluted Elisabeth.

41 And it came to pass, that, when Elisabeth heard the salutation of Mary, the babe leaped in her womb; and Elisabeth was filled with the Holy Ghost:

42 And she spake out with a loud

B.C. 7.

a Heb. 1:4, *note.*
b Gen. 25:21; 1 Sam. 1:20.
c Lk. 7:24-28.
d *Holy Spirit.* vs. 15, 17, 35, 41, 67, 80; Lk. 2:25, 26, 27, 40. (Mt. 1:18; Acts 2:4.)
e Jer. 1:5.
f Mal. 4:5: See Mt. 17:10, *note.*
g 1 Ki. 21:20; 2 Ki. 1:8; Mt. 3:4; 7:12.
h 1 Pet. 2:9.
i i.e. *Man of God.* Cf. Psa. 103:20; Dan. 8:16.
j Lk. 7:27.
k Gen. 30:23; 1 Sam. 1:6.
l also v. 36.
m Mt. 1:18.
n Or, *graciously accepted,* or, *much graced.*
o Isa. 7:14; Mt. 1:21.
p Phil. 2:9, 11.
q v. 35.
r Isa. 9:6, 7.
s Lk. 3:23, 31; Mt. 1:1.
t *Israel (prophecies).* vs. 31-33; Lk. 21:20-24. (Gen. 12:2, 3; Rom. 11:26.)
u Dan. 7:14, 27; Rev. 11:15.
v *Kingdom* (N.T.). vs. 31-33; Mt. 2:2. (Lk. 1:31-33; 1 Cor. 15:24.)
w vs. 26-35; Isa. 7:14.
x *Sanctify, holy (persons)* (N.T.). vs. 35-49, 70; Lk. 2:23. (Mt. 4:5; Rev. 22:11.)
y Acts 5:31; Rom. 1:3, 4; Heb. 1:1, 8.
z Mt. 19:26; Rom. 4:21.

voice, and said, Blessed *art* thou among women, and blessed *is* the fruit of thy womb.

43 And whence *is* this to me, that the mother of my [a]Lord should come to me?

44 For, lo, as soon as the voice of thy salutation sounded in mine ears, the babe leaped in my womb for joy.

45 And blessed *is* she [b]that believed: for there shall be a performance of those things which were told her from the Lord.

The magnificat. (Cf. 1 Sam. 2:1-10.)

46 And Mary said, [c]My soul doth magnify the Lord,

47 And my spirit hath rejoiced in God my [d]Saviour.

48 For he hath regarded the low estate of his handmaiden: for, behold, from henceforth all generations shall call me blessed.

49 For he that is mighty hath done to me great things; and [e]holy *is* his name.

50 And his [f]mercy *is* on them that fear him from generation to generation.

51 He hath shewed strength with his arm; he hath scattered the proud in the imagination of their hearts.

52 He hath put down the mighty from *their* seats, and exalted them of low degree.

53 He hath filled the hungry with good things; and the rich he hath sent empty away.

54 He hath holpen his servant Israel, in remembrance of *his* mercy;

55 As he [g]spake to our fathers, to Abraham, and to his seed for ever.

56 And Mary abode with her about three months, and returned to her own house.

Birth of John the Baptist.

57 Now Elisabeth's full time came that she should be delivered; and she brought forth a son.

58 And her neighbours and her cousins heard how the Lord had shewed great mercy upon her; and they rejoiced with her.

59 And it came to pass, that on the eighth day they came to [h]circumcise the child; and they called him Zacharias, after the name of his father.

60 And his mother answered and said, Not *so;* but he shall be called John.

61 And they said unto her, There is none of thy kindred that is called by this name.

62 And they made signs to his father, how he would have him called.

63 And he asked for a writing table, and wrote, saying, His name is [i]John. And they marvelled all.

64 And his [j]mouth was opened immediately, and his tongue *loosed,* and he spake, and praised God.

65 And fear came on all that dwelt round about them: and all these sayings were noised abroad throughout all the hill country of Judæa.

66 And all they that heard *them* laid *them* up in their hearts, saying, What manner of child shall this be! And the hand of the Lord was with him.

67 And his father Zacharias was filled with the Holy Ghost, and prophesied, saying,

68 Blessed *be* the [k]Lord God of Israel; for he hath visited and [l]redeemed his people,

69 And hath raised up an [d]horn of salvation for us in the [m]house of his servant David;

70 As he spake [n]by the mouth of his holy prophets, which have been since the world began:

71 That we should be [d]saved from our enemies, and from the hand of all that hate us;

72 To perform the mercy *promised* to our fathers, and to remember his holy covenant;

73 The [o]oath which he sware to our father Abraham,

74 That he would grant unto us, that we being delivered out of the hand of our enemies might [p]serve him without fear,

75 In holiness and righteousness before him, all the days of our life.

76 And thou, child, shalt be called the prophet of the Highest: for thou shalt go before the face of the Lord to prepare his ways;

77 To give knowledge of salvation unto his people by the remission of their [q]sins,

78 Through the tender mercy of our God; whereby the [r]dayspring from on high hath visited us,

79 To give light to them that sit in darkness and *in* the shadow of [s]death, to guide our feet into the way of peace.

80 And the child grew, and waxed

B.C. 7.

a John 13:13.
b v. 38.
c 1 Sam. 2:1; Psa. 34:2,3.
d Rom. 1:16, *note.*
e Psa. 111:9; Rev. 4:8.
f Gen. 17:7; Ex. 20:5, 6; Psa. 103:17.
g Gen. 17:19.
h Gen. 17:12.
i v. 13.
j v. 20.
k *Jehovah.* Psa. 106:48.
l Rom. 3:24, *note.*
m Lk. 3:23, 31, Mt. 1:1, 6, 16.
n Gen. 3:15; 12:3; 49:10; Jer. 23:5, 6; Dan. 9:24.
o Gen. 22:16.
p Rom. 6:22.
q *Sin.* Rom. 3:23, *note.*
r Or, *sunrising,* or, *branch.* Isa. 11:1; Zech. 3:8; 6:12.
s vs. 76-79; Mal. 3:1.

B.C. 6.]

strong in spirit, and was in the deserts
till the day of his shewing unto Israel.

CHAPTER 2.

The birth of Jesus
(Mt. 1:18-25; 2:1; cf. John 1:14).

And it came to pass in those days,
that there went out a decree from
Cæsar Augustus, that all the [1a]world
should be taxed.
2 (*And* this taxing was first made
when Cyrenius was governor of Syria.)
3 And all went to be taxed, every one
into his own city.
4 And Joseph also went up from
Galilee, out of the city of Nazareth, into
Judæa, unto the city of David, which is
called [b]Bethlehem; (because he was of
the house and lineage of David:)
5 To be taxed with Mary his espoused
wife, being great with child.
6 And so it was, that, while they were
there, the days were accomplished that
she should be delivered.
7 And [c]she brought forth her firstborn
son, and wrapped him in swaddling
clothes, and laid him in a manger; because
there was no room for them in the inn.

Adoration of the shepherds.

8 And there were in the same country
shepherds abiding in the field, keeping
watch over their flock by night.
9 And, lo, the [d]angel of the Lord came
upon them, and the glory of the Lord
shone round about them: and they were
sore afraid.
10 And the angel said unto them, Fear
not: for, behold, I bring you good [e]tidings
of great joy, which shall be to all people.
11 For unto you is born this day in the
city of David a [f]Saviour, which is Christ
the Lord.
12 And this *shall be* a sign unto you; Ye
shall find the babe wrapped in swaddling clothes, lying in a manger.
13 And suddenly there was with the
[d]angel a multitude of the heavenly host
praising God, and saying,
14 Glory to God in the highest, and
[g]on earth peace, [h]good will toward men.
15 And it came to pass, as the [d]angels
were gone away from them into heaven,
the shepherds said one to another, Let us
now go even unto Bethlehem, and see
this thing which is come to pass, which
the Lord hath made known unto us.
16 And they came with haste, and
found Mary, and Joseph, and the babe
lying in a manger.
17 And when they had seen *it*, they
made known abroad the saying which
was told them concerning this child.
18 And all they that heard *it* wondered
at those things which were told them by
the shepherds.
19 But Mary kept all these things, and
pondered *them* in her heart.
20 And the shepherds returned, glorifying and praising God for all the things
that they had heard and seen, as it was
told unto them.

Circumcision of Jesus. (Cf. Lk. 1:59.)

21 And when eight days were accomplished [i]for the circumcising of the child,
his name was called [j]JESUS, which was
so named of the [d]angel before he was
conceived in the womb.
22 And when the [k]days of her purification according to the law of Moses
were accomplished, they brought him to
Jerusalem, to present *him* to the Lord;
23 (As it is written in the law of the
[l]Lord, [m]Every male that openeth the
womb shall be called holy to the Lord;)
24 And to offer a sacrifice according to
that which is said in the law of the Lord,
A [n]pair of turtledoves, or two young
pigeons.

Adoration and prophecy of Simeon.

25 And, behold, there was a man in
Jerusalem, whose name *was* Simeon; and
the same man *was* [2o]just and devout,
waiting for the consolation of Israel: and
the Holy Ghost was upon him.
26 And it was revealed unto him by
the [p]Holy Ghost, that he should not see

B.C. 5.

a *oikoumene* = *inhabited earth.*
b Mic. 5:2; 1 Sam. 17:12.
c Mt. 1:25; Isa. 7:14.
d Heb. 1:4, *note.*
e *Gospel.* vs. 10:11; Lk. 4:18. (Gen. 12:1-3; Rev. 14:6.)
f Rom. 1:16, *note.*
g Cf. Mt. 10:34, *note.*
h 2 Cor. 5:18, 20; Eph. 2:14, 18.
i Lev. 12:3; Gal. 4:4, 5; 5:3.
j Lk. 1:31; Mt. 1:21.
k *Sanctify, holy (persons)* Lk. 9:26. (Mt. 4:5; Rev. 22:11.)
l *Jehovah.* Ex. 13:2, 12.
m Ex. 13:12, 16; Num. 3:13; 8:17.
n Lev. 12:8.
o *Righteousness.* (Gen. 6:9.)
p *Holy Spirit.* vs. 25, 26, 27, 40; Lk. 3:16, 22. (Mt. 1:18; Acts 2:4.)

1 (2:1) Gr. *oikoumene* = "inhabited earth." This passage is noteworthy as defining the usual N.T. use of *oikoumene* as the sphere of Roman rule at its greatest extent, that is, of the great Gentile world-monarchies (Dan. 2, 7). That part of the earth is therefore peculiarly the sphere of prophecy.

2 (2:25) The O.T. righteousness. Summary: In the O.T. "righteous" and "just" are English words used

death, before he had seen the Lord's Christ.

27 And he came by the Spirit into the temple: and when the parents brought in the child Jesus, to do for him after the custom of the law,

28 Then took he him up in his arms, and blessed God, and said,

29 Lord, now lettest thou thy servant depart [a]in peace, according to thy word:

30 For mine eyes have seen thy [b]salvation,

31 Which thou hast prepared before the face of all people;

32 A light to lighten the [c]Gentiles, and the glory of thy people Israel.

33 And Joseph and his mother marvelled at those things which were spoken of him.

34 And Simeon blessed them, and said unto Mary his mother, Behold, this *child* is set for the [d]fall and rising again of many in Israel; and for a sign which shall be spoken against;

35 (Yea, a [e]sword shall pierce through thy own soul also,) [f]that the thoughts of many hearts may be revealed.

Adoration of Anna.

36 And there was one Anna, a prophetess, the daughter of Phanuel, of the tribe of Aser: she was of a great age, and had lived with an husband seven years from her virginity;

37 And she *was* a widow of about fourscore and four years, which departed not from the temple, but served *God* with fastings and [g]prayers night and day.

38 And she coming in that instant gave thanks likewise unto the Lord, and spake of him to all them that looked for [h]redemption in Jerusalem.

Return to Nazareth: the silent years.

39 And when they had performed all things according to the law of the Lord, they returned into Galilee, to their own city [i]Nazareth.

B.C. 4.

a Isa. 57:1, 2; Rev. 14:13.
b Rom. 1:16, *note.*
c Isa. 42:6, 7.
d Isa. 8:14; Rom. 9:32, 33; 1 Cor. 1:23, 24; 2 Cor. 2:16; 1 Pet. 2:7.
e John 19:25.
f 1 Cor. 11:19; 1 John 2:19.
g 1 Tim. 5:5.
h Rom. 3:24, *note.*
i Mt. 2:23.
j Ex. 23:15; Deut. 16:1.
k John 9:4.
l Isa. 11:2, 3; Col. 2:2, 3.

40 And the child grew, and waxed strong in spirit, filled with wisdom: and the grace of God was upon him.

Jesus and his parents at the passover.

41 Now his parents went to Jerusalem [j]every year at the feast of the passover.

42 And when he was twelve years old, they went up to Jerusalem after the custom of the feast.

43 And when they had fulfilled the days, as they returned, the child Jesus tarried behind in Jerusalem; and Joseph and his mother knew not *of it.*

44 But they, supposing him to have been in the company, went a day's journey; and they sought him among *their* kinsfolk and acquaintance.

45 And when they found him not, they turned back again to Jerusalem, seeking him.

46 And it came to pass, that after three days they found him in the temple, sitting in the midst of the doctors, both hearing them, and asking them questions.

47 And all that heard him were astonished at his understanding and answers.

48 And when they saw him, they were amazed: and his mother said unto him, Son, why hast thou thus dealt with us? behold, thy father and I have sought thee sorrowing.

49 And he said unto them, How is it that ye sought me? wist ye not that I must be [k]about my Father's business?

50 And they understood not the saying which he spake unto them.

51 And he went down with them, and came to Nazareth, and was subject unto them: but his mother kept all these sayings in her heart.

52 And Jesus increased in [l]wisdom and stature, and in favour with God and man.

to translate the Hebrew words *yasher,* "upright"; *tsadiq,* "just"; *tsidkah,* "righteous." In all of these words but one idea inheres: the righteous, or just, man is so called, because he is *right with God;* and he is right with God because he has walked "in all the commandments and ordinances of the Lord blameless" (Lk. 1:6; Rom. 10:5; Phil. 3:6). The O.T. righteous man was not sinless (Eccl. 7:20), but one who, for his sins, resorted to the ordinances, and offered in faith the required sacrifice (e.g. Lev. 4:27-35). Cf. "Righteousness (N.T.)," Rom. 10:10, *note,* and Paul's contrast, Phil. 3:4-9.

CHAPTER 3.

The ministry of John the Baptist (Mt. 3:1-12; Mk. 1:1-8; John 1:6-8, 15-36).

Now in the fifteenth year of the reign
of Tiberius Cæsar, Pontius Pilate
being governor of Judæa, and [a]Herod
being tetrarch of Galilee, and his brother
Philip tetrarch of Ituraea and of the
region of Trachonitis, and Lysanias the
tetrarch of Abilene,
2 [b]Annas and Caiaphas being the high
priests, the word of God came unto John
the son of Zacharias in the wilderness.
3 [c]And he came into all the country
about Jordan, preaching the baptism of
[d]repentance for the remission of [e]sins;
4 As it is written in the book of the
words of Esaias the [f]prophet, saying,
The voice of one crying in the wilderness, Prepare ye the way of the [g]Lord,
make his paths straight.
5 Every valley shall be filled, and
every mountain and hill shall be brought
low; and the crooked shall be made
straight, and the rough ways *shall be*
made smooth;
6 [h]And all flesh shall see the [i]salvation
of God.
7 Then said he to the multitude that
came forth to be baptized of him, O
[j]generation of vipers, who hath warned
you to flee from the wrath to come?
8 Bring forth therefore fruits worthy of
[k]repentance, and begin not to say within
yourselves, [l]We have Abraham to *our*
father: for I say unto you, That God is
able of these stones to raise up children
unto Abraham.
9 And now also the axe is laid unto
the root of the trees: [m]every tree therefore which bringeth not forth good fruit
is hewn down, and cast into the fire.
10 And the people asked him, saying,
[n]What shall we do then?
11 He answereth and saith unto them,
[o]He that hath two [p]coats, let him impart
to him that hath none; and he that hath
meat, let him do likewise.
12 Then came also [q]publicans to be
baptized, and said unto him, Master,
what shall we do?
13 And he said unto them, Exact no
more than that which is appointed you.
14 And the soldiers likewise demanded of him, saying, And what shall we
do? And he said unto them, Do violence
to no man, neither accuse *any* falsely;
and be [r]content with your [s]wages.
15 And as the people were [t]in expectation, and all men mused in their hearts of
John, whether he were the Christ, or not;
16 John answered, saying unto *them*
all, I indeed [u]baptize you with water;
but one mightier than I cometh, the
latchet of whose shoes I am not worthy
to unloose: he shall baptize you with the
[v]Holy Ghost and with fire:
17 Whose fan *is* in his hand, and he
will throughly purge his floor, and will
[w]gather the wheat into his garner; but
the chaff he will burn with fire
unquenchable.
18 And many other things in his
exhortation preached he unto the people.
19 But [x]Herod the tetrarch, being
reproved by him for Herodias his
brother Philip's wife, and for all the evils
which Herod had done,
20 Added yet this above all, that he
shut up [y]John in prison.

The baptism of Jesus
(Mt. 3:13-17; Mk. 1:9-11).

21 Now when all the people were baptized, it came to pass, that [z]Jesus also
being baptized, and praying, the heaven
was opened,
22 And the [aa]Holy Ghost descended in
a bodily shape like a dove upon him,
and a voice came from heaven, which
said, [bb]Thou art my beloved Son; in thee
I am well pleased.

The genealogy of Mary, mother of Jesus.

23 And Jesus himself began to be
about thirty years of age, being (as was
supposed) the son of Joseph, which was
the [1]*son* of Heli,
24 Which was *the son* of Matthat, which
was *the son* of Levi, which was *the son* of

A.D. 26.

- a Also v. 19: See Mt. 14:1, *ref.*
- b John 11:49; 18:13; Acts 4:6.
- c Mt. 3:1; Mk. 1:4.
- d *Repentance.* vs. 3, 8. (Mt. 3:2; Acts 17:30.)
- e *Sin.* Rom. 3:23, *note.*
- f Isa. 40:3-5.
- g *Jehovah.* vs. 4-6: See Isa. 40:3-5.
- h Lk. 2:30; Psa. 98:2; Isa. 52:10; Rom. 10:12, 18.
- i vs. 4-6: Isa. 52:10. See Isa. 40:3-5.
- j Mt. 12:34.
- k *Repentance.* vs. 3, 8; Lk. 5:32. (Mt. 3:2; Acts 17:30.)
- l Rom. 9:6, 8; Gal. 3:29; 6:15.
- m Lk. 13:5-9; Rev. 21:8.
- n Acts 2:37, 38; 16:30.
- o 1 John 3:17.
- p Jas. 2:15, 17.
- q Lk. 7:29; Mt. 21:32.
- r Phil. 4:11; 1 Tim. 6:8.
- s Or, *allowance.*
- t Or, *in suspense.*
- u 1 Pet. 3:21.
- v *Holy Spirit.* vs. 16, 22; Lk. 4:1. (Mt. 1:18; Acts 2:4.)
- w Mt. 13:30.
- x Mt. 14:1, *ref.*
- y Mt. 11:2.
- z Mt. 3:13-15.
- aa *Holy Spirit.* Lk. 4:1, 14, 18. (Mt. 1:18; Acts 2:4.)
- bb Lit. *This is my Son, the beloved, in whom I delighted.* Cf. John 1:1, 2; 8:29; Mt. 17:5.

[1](3:23) In Matthew, where unquestionably we have the genealogy of Joseph, we are told (1:16) that Joseph was the son of Jacob. In what sense, then, could he be called in Luke "the son of Heli"? He could not be by natural generation the son both of Jacob and of Heli. But in Luke it is not said that Heli *begat* Joseph, so that the natural explanation is that Joseph was the son-in-law of Heli, who was,

Melchi, which was *the son* of Janna,
which was *the son* of Joseph,
25 Which was *the son* of Mattathias,
which was *the son* of Amos, which was
the son of Naum, which was *the son* of
Esli, which was *the son* of Nagge,
26 Which was *the son* of Maath, which
was *the son* of Mattathias, which was *the*
son of Semei, which was *the son* of
Joseph, which was *the son* of Juda,
27 Which was *the son* of Joanna, which
was *the son* of Rhesa, which was *the son*
of Zorobabel, which was *the son* of
Salathiel, which was *the son* of Neri,
28 Which was *the son* of Melchi, which
was *the son* of Addi, which was *the son* of
Cosam, which was *the son* of Elmodam,
which was *the son* of Er,
29 Which was *the son* of Jose, which
was *the son* of Eliezer, which was *the son*
of Jorim, which was *the son* of Matthat,
which was *the son* of Levi,
30 Which was *the son* of Simeon,
which was *the son* of Juda, which was *the*
son of Joseph, which was *the son* of
Jonan, which was *the son* of Eliakim,
31 Which was *the son* of Melea, which
was *the son* of Menan, which was *the son*
of Mattatha, which was *the son* of
Nathan, which was *the son* of David,
32 Which was *the son* of Jesse, which
was *the son* of Obed, which was *the son*
of Booz, which was *the son* of Salmon,
which was *the son* of Naasson,
33 Which was *the son* of Aminadab,
which was *the son* of Aram, which was
the son of Esrom, which was *the son* of
Phares, which was *the son* of Juda,
34 Which was *the son* of Jacob, which
was *the son* of Isaac, which was *the son* of
Abraham, which was *the son* of Thara,
which was *the son* of Nachor,
35 Which was *the son* of Saruch, which
was *the son* of Ragau, which was *the son*
of Phalec, which was *the son* of Heber,
which was *the son* of Sala,
36 Which was *the son* of Cainan, which
was *the son* of [a]Arphaxad, which was *the*
son of Sem, which was *the son* of Noe,
which was *the son* of Lamech,
37 Which was *the son* of Mathusala,
which was *the son* of Enoch, which was
the son of Jared, which was *the son* of
Maleleel, which was *the son* of Cainan,
38 Which was *the son* of Enos, which
was *the son* of Seth, which was *the son* of
Adam, which was *the son* of God.

CHAPTER 4.

The temptation of Christ
(Mt. 4:1-11; Mk. 1:12, 13).

And Jesus being full of the [b]Holy
Ghost returned from Jordan, and
was led by the Spirit into the wilderness,
2 Being forty days [c]tempted of the
devil. And in those days he did eat nothing: and when they were ended, he
afterward hungered.
3 And the devil said unto him, If thou
be the Son of God, [d]command this stone
that it be made bread.
4 And Jesus answered him, saying, It
is written, That man shall not live by
bread alone, but by every word of [e]God.
5 And the devil, taking him up into an
high mountain, shewed unto him all the
kingdoms of the [f]world in a moment of
time.
6 And the devil said unto him, All this
power will I give thee, and the glory of
them: for that is [g]delivered unto me; and
to whomsoever I will I give it.
7 If thou therefore wilt worship me, all
shall be thine.
8 And Jesus answered and said unto
him, Get thee behind me, [h]Satan: for it is
written, [i]Thou shalt worship the [j]Lord
thy God, and him only shalt thou serve.
9 And he brought him to Jerusalem,
and set him on a pinnacle of the temple,
and said unto him, If thou be the Son of
God, cast thyself down from hence:
10 For it is written, [k]He shall give his
[l]angels charge over thee, [m]to keep thee:
11 And in *their* hands they shall bear

A.D. 26.

a *Arphaxad.* Gen. 10:22.
b *Holy Spirit.* vs. 1, 14, 18; Lk. 11:13. (Mt. 1:18; Acts 2:4.)
c See Mt. 4:1, *note.*
d Lk. 9:12-17.
e *Jehovah.* Deut. 8:3.
f *Oikoumene = inhabited earth* (Lk. 2:1).
g John 12:31; 14:30; 2 Cor. 4:4.
h *Satan.* Lk. 8:12. (Gen. 3:1; Rev. 20:10.)
i Deut. 6:13; 10:20.
j *Jehovah.* Deut. 6:13.
k Psa. 91:11, 12.
l Heb. 1:4, *note.*
m After Satan's failure to tempt the Lord away from the Word, he seeks to tempt Him by it: He however *mis*quotes by the omission of "*in all thy ways*" (Psa. 91:11). The Lord's "ways" were those marked out for Him in perfect dependence upon His Father's will; cf. Heb. 10:7, 9:

like himself, a descendant of David. That he should in that case be called "*son* of Heli" ("son" is not in the Greek, but rightly supplied by the translators) would be in accord with Jewish usage (cf. 1 Sam. 24:16). The conclusion is therefore inevitable that in Luke we have Mary's genealogy; and Joseph was "*son* of Heli" because espoused to Heli's daughter. The genealogy in Luke is Mary's, whose father, Heli, was descended from David.

thee up, lest at any time thou dash thy foot against a stone.

12 And Jesus answering said unto him, It is said, [a]Thou shalt not tempt the [b]Lord thy God.

13 And when the devil had ended all the temptation, he departed from him for a season.

Jesus returns to Galilee
(Mt. 4:12-16; Mk. 1:14).

14 And Jesus returned in the [c]power of the Spirit into Galilee: and there went out a [d]fame of him through all the region round about.

15 And he taught in their synagogues, being glorified of all.

Jesus in the synagogue at Nazareth.

16 And he [1]came to [e]Nazareth, where he had been brought up: and, as his custom was, [f]he went into the synagogue on the sabbath day, and stood up for to read.

17 And there was delivered unto him the book of the prophet Esaias. And when he had opened the book, he found the place [g]where it was written,

18 The Spirit of the [h]Lord *is* upon me, because he hath anointed me to preach the [i]gospel to the poor; he hath sent me to heal the brokenhearted, to preach deliverance to the captives, and recovering of sight to the blind, to set at liberty them that are bruised,

19 To preach the [2]acceptable year of the [j]Lord.

20 And he closed the book, and he gave *it* again to the minister, and sat down. And the eyes of all them that were in the synagogue were fastened on him.

21 And he began to say unto them, This day is this scripture fulfilled in your ears.

22 And all bare him witness, and wondered at the [k]gracious words which proceeded out of his mouth. And they said, [l]Is not this Joseph's son?

23 And he said unto them, Ye will surely say unto me this proverb, Physician, heal thyself: whatsoever we have heard done in Capernaum, do also here in thy country.

24 And he said, Verily I say unto you, [m]No prophet is accepted in his own country.

25 But I tell you of a truth, many widows were in Israel in the [n]days of Elias, when the heaven was shut up three years and six months, when great famine was throughout all the land;

26 But unto none of them was Elias sent, save unto Sarepta, *a city* of Sidon, unto a woman *that was* a widow.

27 And many lepers were in Israel in the time of Eliseus the prophet; and none of them was cleansed, [o]saving Naaman the Syrian.

28 And all they in the synagogue, when they heard these things, were filled with wrath,

29 [p]And rose up, and thrust him out of the city, and led him unto the brow of the hill whereon their city was built, that they might cast him down headlong.

30 But he passing through the midst of them went his way,

Jesus goes to Capernaum, and casts out demons (Mk. 1:23-26).

31 And came down to Capernaum, a city of Galilee, and taught them on the sabbath days.

32 And they were astonished at his doctrine: for [q]his word was with power.

33 And in the [r]synagogue there was a man, which had a spirit of an [s]unclean devil, and cried out with a loud voice,

34 Saying, Let *us* alone; what have we to do with thee, *thou* Jesus of Nazareth? art thou come to destroy us? I know thee who thou art; the Holy One of God.

35 And Jesus rebuked him, saying, Hold thy peace, and come out of him. And when the devil had thrown him in the midst, [t]he came out of him, and hurt him not.

36 And they were all amazed, and spake among themselves, saying, [u]What a word *is* this! for with authority and power he commandeth the unclean spirits, and they come out.

37 And the [v]fame of him went out

A.D. 27.

a Deut. 6:16.
b *Jehovah.* Deut. 6:16.
c v. 1; Mt. 4:12.
d Mt. 4:24.
e Mt. 13:54.
f v. 15; Mk. 1:21; John 18:20.
g *Inspiration.* vs. 17-21, 27; Lk. 10:16. (Ex. 4:15; Rev. 22:19.)
h *Adonai Jehovah.* Isa. 61:1-2.
i *Gospel.* Lk. 7:22. (Gen. 12:1-3; Rev. 14:6.)
j *Jehovah.* Isa. 61:1, 2.
k Psa. 45:2; John 7:46.
l Mt. 13:55.
m John 4:44.
n 1 Ki. 17:9; 18:1.
o 2 Ki. 5:1, 14.
p John 8:37, 59; 10:31, 39.
q John 8:26, 28, 38, 47; 12:49; cf. Lk. 8:25; v. 36.
r Mk. 1:23.
s Cf. v. 34, l.c.
t *Miracles* (N.T.). vs. 33-36, 38-40, 41; Lk. 5:3-8. (Mt. 8:2, 3; Acts 28:8, 9.)
u v. 32; Lk. 8:25; John 8:26.
v vs. 14, 15; Mk. 1:28, 45:

1 (4:16) Our Lord visited Nazareth twice after beginning His public ministry. See Mt. 13:54-58; Mk. 6:1-6.

2 (4:19) A comparison with the passage quoted, Isa. 61:1, 2, affords an instance of the exquisite accuracy of Scripture. Jesus stopped at, "the acceptable year of the Lord," which is connected with the first advent and the dispensation of grace (Gen. 3:15; Acts 1:11, *note*); "the day of vengeance of our God" belongs to the second advent (Deut. 30:3; Acts 1:11, *note*) and judgment.

into every place of the country round about.

Jesus heals Peter's wife's mother, and many others (Mt. 8:14-17; Mk. 1:29-38).

38 And he arose out of the synagogue, and entered into Simon's house. And [a]Simon's wife's mother was taken with a great fever; and they besought him for her.

39 And he stood over her, and rebuked the fever; and it left her: and immediately she arose and [b]ministered unto them.

40 Now when the [c]sun was setting, all they that had any sick with divers diseases brought them unto him; and he laid his hands on every one of them, and healed them.

41 And devils also came out of many, crying out, and saying, Thou art Christ the Son of God. [d]And he rebuking *them* suffered them not to speak: for they knew that he was Christ.

42 And when it was day, he departed and went into a desert place: and the people sought him, and came unto him, and stayed him, that he should not depart from them.

43 And he said unto them, I must preach the kingdom of God to other cities also: [e]for therefore am I sent.

44 And he preached in the synagogues of Galilee.

CHAPTER 5.

The miraculous draught of fishes.
(Cf. John 21:6-8.)

And it came to pass, that, as the people pressed upon him to hear the word of God, he stood by the [f]lake of Gennesaret,

2 And saw two ships standing by the lake: but the fishermen were gone out of them, and were washing *their* nets.

3 And he entered into one of the ships, which was Simon's, and prayed him that he would thrust out a little from the land. And he sat down, and [g]taught the people out of the ship.

4 Now when he had left speaking, he said unto Simon, Launch out into the deep, and [h]let down your nets for a draught.

5 And Simon answering said unto him, Master, we have [i]toiled all the night, and have taken nothing: nevertheless [j]at thy word I will let down the net.

6 And when they had this done, they [k]inclosed a great multitude of fishes: and their net brake.

7 And they beckoned unto *their* partners, which were in the other ship, that they should come and help them. And they came, and filled both the ships, so that they [l]began to sink.

8 When Simon Peter saw *it*, [m]he fell down at Jesus' knees, saying, Depart from me; for I am a [n]sinful man, O Lord.

9 For he was astonished, and all that were with him, at the draught of the fishes which they had taken:

10 And so *was* also James, and John, the sons of Zebedee, which were partners with Simon. And Jesus said unto Simon, [o]Fear not; from henceforth thou shalt catch men.

11 And when they had brought their ships to land, they [p]forsook all, and followed him.

Jesus heals a leper
(Mt. 8:2-4; Mk. 1:40-44).

12 And it came to pass, when he was in a certain city, behold a man full of [q]leprosy: who seeing Jesus fell on *his* face, and besought him, saying, Lord, [r]if thou wilt, thou canst make me clean.

13 And he put forth *his* hand, and touched him, saying, I will: be thou clean. And immediately the leprosy departed from him.

14 And he charged him to tell no man: but go, and shew thyself to the priest, and offer for thy [s]cleansing, according as Moses commanded, for a testimony unto them.

15 But so much the more went there a fame abroad of him: and great multitudes came together to hear, and to be healed by him of their infirmities.

16 And he withdrew himself into the wilderness, [t]and prayed.

A paralytic healed
(Mt. 9:2-8; Mk. 2:1-12).

17 And it came to pass on a certain day, as he was teaching, that there were Pharisees and doctors of the law sitting by, which were come out of every town of Galilee, and Judæa, and Jerusalem: and the power of the Lord was *present* to heal them.

18 And, behold, men brought in a bed a man which was taken with a palsy:

A.D. 30.

a Mt. 8:14; Mk. 1:29.
b Lk. 8:2, 3.
c Mt. 8:16, 17; Mk. 1:32-34.
d Mk. 1:34.
e Mt. 10:7; Mk. 1:38.
f Mt. 4:18.
g Mt. 13:2.
h John 21:6.
i John 21:3.
j Psa. 33:9; Mt. 8:8.
k *Miracles* (N.T.). vs. 3-8, 12-15, 18-26; Lk. 6:6-10. (Mt. 8:2, 3; Acts 28:8, 9.)
l v. 6.
m John 21:7.
n *Sin.* Rom. 3:23, *note.*
o Mt. 4:19; cf. Mt. 8:26.
p Mt. 4:22; 19:27; Mk. 8:34, 35; 10:28-31, 52; Lk. 9:23, 59-62; John 12:26; 14:15.
q Lev. 13:14; Mt. 8:2-4; Mk. 1:40-45.
r The leper, knowing the Lord's power to heal, seems to question His willingness.
s Lev. 14:4.
t Mt. 14:23; Mk. 6:46; Lk. 11:1.

and they sought *means* to bring him in, and to lay *him* before him.

19 And when they could not find by what *way* they might bring him in [a]because of the multitude, they went upon the housetop, and let him down through the tiling with *his* couch into the midst [b]before Jesus.

20 And when he saw [c]their faith, he said unto him, Man, thy [d]sins are forgiven thee.

21 And the scribes and the Pharisees began to reason, saying, Who is this which speaketh [e]blasphemies? [f]Who can forgive sins, but God alone?

22 But when Jesus perceived their thoughts, he answering said unto them, What reason ye in your hearts?

23 Whether is easier, to say, Thy sins be forgiven thee; or to say, Rise up and walk?

24 But that ye may [g]know that the Son of man hath power upon earth to forgive sins, (he said unto the sick of the palsy,) [h]I say unto thee, Arise, and take up thy couch, and go into thine house.

25 And immediately he rose up before them, and took up that whereon he lay, and departed to his own house, [i]glorifying God.

26 And they were all amazed, and they [j]glorified God, and were filled with fear, saying, We have seen strange things to day.

The call of Matthew
(Mt. 9:9; Mk. 2:13, 14).

27 And after these things he went forth, and saw a publican, named Levi, sitting at the receipt of custom: and he said unto him, [k]Follow me.

28 And he left all, rose up, and followed him.

29 And Levi made him a [l]great feast in his own house: and there was a great company of publicans and of others that sat down with them.

Jesus answers the scribes and Pharisees
(Mt. 9:10-17; Mk. 2:16-22).

30 But their scribes and Pharisees murmured against his disciples, saying, [m]Why do ye eat and drink with publicans and [n]sinners?

31 And Jesus answering said unto them, They that are whole need not a physician; but they that are sick.

32 I came not to call the righteous, but [o]sinners to [p]repentance.

33 And they said unto him, Why do the [q]disciples of John fast often, and make prayers, and likewise *the disciples* of the Pharisees; but [r]thine eat and drink?

34 And he said unto them, Can ye make the children of the bridechamber fast, while [s]the bridegroom is with them?

35 But the days will come, when the [t]bridegroom shall be taken away from them, and then shall they fast in those days.

Parables of the garment and bottles
(Mt. 9:16, 17; Mk. 2:21, 22).

36 And he spake also a [u]parable unto them; No man putteth a piece of a new garment upon an old; if otherwise, then both the new maketh a rent, and the piece that was *taken* out of the new agreeth not with the old.

37 And no man putteth new wine into old [v]bottles; else the new wine will burst the bottles, and be spilled, and the bottles shall perish.

38 But new wine must be put into new bottles; and both are preserved.

39 No man also having drunk old *wine* straightway desireth new: for he saith, The old is better.

CHAPTER 6.

Jesus and the sabbath
(Mt. 12:1-8; Mk. 2:23-28).

And it came to pass on the second sabbath after the first, that he went through the corn fields; and his disciples plucked the ears of corn, and did eat, rubbing *them* in *their* hands.

2 And certain of the Pharisees said unto them, Why do ye that which is not [w]lawful to do on the sabbath days?

3 And Jesus answering them said, Have ye not read so much as this, what [x]David did, when himself was an hungred, and they which were with him;

4 How he went into the house of God, and did take and eat the [y]shewbread, and gave also to them that were with him; which it is not lawful to eat but for the priests alone?

5 And he said unto them, [z]That the Son of man is Lord also of the sabbath.

A.D. 31.

a v. 15; Mt. 13:2.
b Mt. 15:30; 17:17.
c Mk. 2:5.
d *Sin:* Rom. 3:23, *note.*
e John 10:33; Mt. 26:65.
f Lk. 7:49; John 9:31.
g Acts 2:22.
h Psa. 33:9; Mt. 28:18; Lk. 7:14.
i Lk. 17:15,18; Acts 3:8.
j Lk. 7:16.
k Mt. 4:22; 19 27; Mk. 8:34, 35; 10:28, 52; Lk. 5:11; 9:23, 59-62; John 12:26, 14:15; 21:19, 22.
l Mt. 9:10; Mk. 2:15.
m Lk. 7:34; 15:2.
n *Sin.* Rom. 3:23, *note.*
o Rom. 5:6, 8; 1 Tim. 1:15.
p *Repentance.* Lk. 10:13. (Mt. 3:2; Acts 17:30.)
q Lk. 7:33.
r Lk. 7:34.
s John 3:29.
t John 16:6, 20, 22.
u *Parables* (N.T.): vs. 36, 37-39; Lk. 6:39-47. (Mt. 5:13-16; Lk. 21:29-31.)
v i.e. *wineskins.*
w Lk. 14:1-6.
x 1 Sam. 21:6.
y Ex. 25:30, *note.*
z Mt. 12:8; Mk. 2:28:

The withered hand healed
(Mt. 12:9-14; Mk. 3:1-6).

6 And it came to pass also on another sabbath, that he [a]entered into the synagogue and taught: and there was a man whose right hand was withered.

7 And the scribes and Pharisees watched him, whether he would heal on the sabbath day; that they might find an [b]accusation against him.

8 But he [c]knew their thoughts, and said to the man which had the withered hand, Rise up, and stand forth in the midst. And he arose and stood forth.

9 Then said Jesus unto them, I will ask you one thing; [d]Is it lawful on the sabbath days to do good, or to do evil? to save life, or to destroy *it*?

10 And looking round about upon them all, he said unto the man, Stretch forth thy hand. And he did so: [e]and his hand was restored whole as the other.

11 And they were filled with [f]madness; [g]and communed one with another what they might do to Jesus.

The twelve chosen
(Mt. 10:2-4; Mk. 3:13-19).

12 And it came to pass in those days, that he went out into a [h]mountain to pray, and continued all night in prayer to God.

13 And when it was day, he called *unto him* his disciples: and of them he [i]chose twelve, whom also he named apostles;

14 Simon, (whom he also named Peter,) and Andrew his brother, James and John, Philip and Bartholomew,

15 Matthew and Thomas, James the *son* of Alphæus, and Simon called Zelotes,

16 And Judas *the brother* of James, and Judas Iscariot, which also was the traitor.

17 And he came down with them, and stood in the plain, and the company of his disciples, and a great [j]multitude of people out of all Judæa and Jerusalem, and from the sea coast of Tyre and Sidon, which came to hear him, and to be healed of their diseases;

18 And they that were vexed with unclean spirits: and they were healed.

19 And the whole multitude sought to [k]touch him: for there went [l]virtue out of him, and healed *them* all.

The beatitudes. (Mt. 5:3-12).

20 And he lifted up his eyes on his disciples, and said, Blessed *be ye* poor: for yours is the kingdom of God.

21 Blessed *are ye* that hunger now: for ye shall be filled. Blessed *are ye* that weep now: for ye shall laugh.

22 Blessed are ye, when men shall hate you, and when they shall separate you *from their company*, and shall reproach *you*, and cast out your name as evil, for the Son of man's sake.

23 Rejoice ye in that day, and leap for joy: for, behold, your reward *is* great in heaven: for in the like manner did their fathers unto the prophets.

24 But woe unto you that are rich! for [m]ye have received your consolation.

25 Woe unto you that are full! for ye shall hunger. Woe unto you that laugh now! for ye shall mourn and weep.

26 Woe unto you, when all men shall speak well of you! for so did their fathers to the false prophets.

27 But I say unto you which hear, [n]Love your enemies, do good to them which hate you,

28 [o]Bless them that curse you, and [p]pray for them which despitefully use you.

29 And unto him that smiteth thee on the *one* cheek offer also the other; and him that [q]taketh away thy cloke forbid not *to take thy* coat also.

30 [r]Give to every man that asketh of thee; and of him that taketh away thy goods ask *them* not again.

31 And as ye would that men should do to you, do ye also to them likewise.

32 For if ye love them which love you, what thank have ye? for [s]sinners also [t]love those that love them.

33 And if ye do good to them which do good to you, what thank have ye? for sinners also do even the same.

34 And if ye lend *to them* of whom ye hope to receive, what thank have ye? for sinners also lend to sinners, to receive as much again.

35 But love ye your enemies, and

a Mk. 1:21; Lk. 4:15, 16; John 18:20.
b Lk. 20:20.
c John 2:25; cf. 1 Sam. 16:7.
d Mk. 3:4.
e *Miracles* (N.T.). vs. 6-10; Lk. 7:1-10. (Mt. 8:2, 3; Acts 28:8, 9.)
f Psa. 2:2.
g Mk. 3:6.
h Mt. 14:23; John 8:1.
i *Election (personal).* John 15:16. (Deut. 7:6; 1 Pet. 1:2.)
j Mt. 4:25; Mk. 3:7, 8.
k Mt. 14:36; Mk. 5:27, 28; Lk. 8:44-47.
l Lk. 8:46.
m Lk. 16:25.
n Rom. 12:20.
o Rom. 12:14.
p Lk. 23:34; Acts 7:60.
q Rom. 13:10.
r 1 John 3:17.
s *Sin.* Rom. 3:23, *note.*
t Mt. 5:46, 47.

[a]do good, and lend, hoping for nothing
again; and your [b]reward shall be great,
and ye shall be the children of the
Highest: [c]for he is kind unto the
unthankful and *to* the evil.
36 [d]Be ye therefore merciful, as your
Father also is merciful.
37 [e]Judge not, and ye shall not be
judged: condemn not, and ye shall not
be condemned: [f]forgive, and ye shall be
forgiven:
38 [g]Give, and it shall be given unto
you; good measure, pressed down, and
shaken together, and running over, shall
men give into your bosom. [h]For with the
same measure that ye mete withal it
shall be measured to you again.
39 And he spake a [i]parable unto them,
[j]Can the blind lead the blind? shall they
not both fall into the ditch?
40 [k]The disciple is not above his master: but every one that is perfect shall be
as his master.
41 And why [l]beholdest thou the mote
that is in thy brother's eye, but perceivest
not the beam that is in thine own eye?
42 Either how canst thou say to thy
brother, Brother, let me pull out the mote
that is in thine eye, when thou thyself
beholdest not the beam that is in thine
own eye? Thou hypocrite, cast out [m]first
the beam out of thine own eye, and then
shalt thou see clearly to pull out the
mote that is in thy brother's eye.
43 For a [n]good tree bringeth not forth
corrupt fruit; neither doth a corrupt tree
bring forth good fruit.
44 [o]For every tree is known by his own
fruit. For of thorns men do not gather figs,
nor of a bramble bush gather they grapes.
45 A good man out of the good treasure of his heart bringeth forth that
which is good; and an evil man out of
the evil treasure of his heart bringeth
forth that which is evil: for of the abundance of the heart [p]his mouth speaketh.
46 And why call ye me, [q]Lord, Lord,
and do not the things which I say?

Parable of the house built on the rock (Mt. 7:24-27).

47 Whosoever cometh to me, and
heareth my sayings, and [r]doeth them, I
will shew you to whom he is like:
48 [s]He is like a man which built an
house, and digged [t]deep, and laid the
foundation on a [u]rock: and when the

A.D. 31.

a Heb. 13:16.
b *Rewards.* 1 Cor. 3:8. (Dan. 12:3; 1 Cor. 3:14.)
c Mt. 5:45.
d Eph. 4:32; 1 Pet. 3:9.
e Rom. 14:4; 1 Cor. 4:5.
f Mt. 18:21, 22, 35.
g Prov. 28:27; 2 Cor. 8:1, *note.*
h *Law (of Christ).* vs. 27-38; John 13:34. (Gal. 6:2; 2 John 5.)
i *Parables* (N.T.). vs. 39, 47-49. (Mt. 5:13-16; Lk. 21:29-31)
j Mt. 15:14; 23:16.
k Mt. 10:24; John 15:20.
l Mt. 7:3.
m Gal. 6:4.
n Mt. 7:17:18; 12:33; Jas. 3:12.
o Mt. 12:33, 34.
p Prov. 15:2, 28; 16:23; 18:21; Jas. 3:10.
q Mt 25:11, 12; Lk. 13:25; cf. 1 Cor. 12:3.
r Mt. 7:24-27; John 14:21; Jas. 1:22-25.
s *Parables* (N.T.). vs. 47-49; Lk. 7:41-48. (Mt. 5:13-16; Lk. 21:29-31.)
t Mt. 13:5.
u 1 Cor. 3:11.
v Psa. 32:6.
w 1 John 2:17.
x Prov. 1:29-31.
y Mt. 8:5-13.
z Acts 10:22.
aa Psa. 33:9; 107:20, Lk. 4:36; John 5:24; 11:43.
bb Mt. 15:28.
cc *Miracles* (N.T.) vs. 1-10, 11-15, 21, 22; Lk. 8:22-25. (Mt. 8:2, 3; Acts 28:8, 9.)

[v]flood arose, the stream beat vehemently
upon that house, and [w]could not shake
it: for it was founded upon a rock.
49 But he that heareth, and doeth not,
is like a man that without a foundation
built an house upon the earth; against
which the stream did beat vehemently,
and immediately it fell; and the [x]ruin of
that house was great.

CHAPTER 7.

The centurion's servant healed (Mt. 8:5-13).

NOW when he had ended all his sayings in the audience of the people,
he entered into Capernaum.
2 And a certain [y]centurion's servant,
who was dear unto him, was sick, and
ready to die.
3 And when he heard of Jesus, he sent
unto him the elders of the Jews, beseeching him that he would come and heal his
servant.
4 And when they came to Jesus, they
besought him instantly, saying, That he
was [z]worthy for whom he should do this:
5 For he loveth our nation, and he
hath built us a synagogue.
6 Then Jesus went with them. And
when he was now not far from the
house, the centurion sent friends to him,
saying unto him, Lord, trouble not thyself: for I am not worthy that thou
shouldest enter under my roof:
7 Wherefore neither thought I myself
worthy to come unto thee: but [aa]say in a
word, and my servant shall be healed.
8 For I also am a man set under
authority, having under me soldiers, and
I say unto one, Go, and he goeth; and to
another, Come, and he cometh; and to
my servant, Do this, and he doeth *it.*
9 When Jesus heard these things, he
[bb]marvelled at him, and turned him
about, and said unto the people that followed him, I say unto you, I have not
found so great faith, no, not in Israel.
10 And they that were sent, returning
to the house, found the servant [cc]whole
that had been sick.

The widow's son raised.

11 And it came to pass the day after,
that he went into a city called Nain; and
many of his disciples went with him,
and much people.
12 Now when he came nigh to the

gate of the city, behold, there was a dead
man carried out, the only son of his
mother, and she was a widow: and
much people of the city was with her.
13 And when the Lord saw her, he had
compassion on her, and said unto her,
[a]Weep not.
14 And he came and touched the bier:
and they that bare *him* stood still. And he
said, Young man, I say unto thee, Arise.
15 And [b]he that was dead [c]sat up, and
began to speak. And he delivered him to
his mother.
16 And there came a fear on all: and
they [d]glorified God, saying, That a great
prophet is risen up among us; and, [e]That
God hath visited his people.
17 And this rumour of him went forth
throughout all Judæa, and throughout
all the region round about.
18 And the disciples of John [f]shewed
him of all these things.

John the Baptist sends disciples to question Jesus (Mt. 11:2-6).

19 And John calling *unto him* two of
his disciples sent *them* to Jesus, saying,
Art thou he that should come? or look
we for another?
20 When the men were come unto
him, they said, John Baptist hath sent us
unto thee, saying, Art thou he that
should come? or look we for another?
21 And in that same hour he cured
many of *their* infirmities and plagues,
and of evil spirits; and unto many *that*
were blind he gave sight.
22 Then Jesus answering said unto
them, Go your way, and [g]tell John what
things ye have seen and heard; how that
the blind see, the lame walk, the lepers are
cleansed, the deaf hear, the [h]dead are
raised, to the poor the [i]gospel is preached.
23 And [j]blessed is *he*, whosoever shall
not be offended in me.

Jesus' testimony to John the Baptist (Mt. 11:7-15).

24 And when the messengers of John
[k]were departed, he began to speak unto
the people concerning John, What went
ye out into the [l]wilderness for to see?
[m]A reed shaken with the wind?
25 But what went ye out for to see? A
man clothed in [n]soft raiment? Behold,
they which are gorgeously apparelled,
and live delicately, are in kings' courts.
26 But what went ye out for to see? A
prophet? Yea, I say unto you, and much
more than a prophet.
27 This is *he*, of whom it is written,
[o]Behold, I send my messenger before thy
face, which shall prepare thy way before
thee.
28 For I say unto you, Among those
that are born of women there is not a
greater prophet than John the Baptist:
but [p]he that is least in the kingdom of
God is greater than he.
29 And all the people that heard *him*,
and the publicans, justified God, being
[q]baptized with the baptism of John.

Jesus exposes the unreason of unbelief (Mt. 11:16-19).

30 But the [r]Pharisees and lawyers
rejected the counsel of God against
themselves, being not baptized of him.
31 And the Lord said, Whereunto then
shall I liken the men of this generation?
and to what are they like?
32 They are like unto children sitting
in the marketplace, and calling one to
another, and saying, We have piped unto
you, and ye have not danced; we have
mourned to you, and ye have not wept.
33 For John the Baptist came [s]neither
eating bread nor drinking wine; and ye
say, He hath a devil.
34 The Son of man is come [t]eating and
drinking; and ye say, Behold a gluttonous man, and a winebibber, a friend
of publicans and [u]sinners!
35 But [v]wisdom is justified of all her
children.

Jesus in the Pharisee's house.

36 And one of the [w]Pharisees desired
him that he would eat with him. And he
went into the Pharisee's house, and sat
down to meat.
37 And, behold, a woman in the city,
which was a [x]sinner, when she knew that
Jesus sat at meat in the Pharisee's house,
brought an [y]alabaster box of ointment,
38 And stood at his [z]feet behind *him*
weeping, and began to wash his feet
with tears, and did wipe *them* with the
[aa]hairs of her head, and kissed his feet,
and anointed *them* with the ointment.
39 Now when the Pharisee which had
bidden him saw *it*, he spake within

A.D. 31.

a Lk. 8:52; John 11:35.
b Mt. 11:5; Lk. 8:54, 55; John 11:44.
c *Resurrection.* vs. 11-15; Lk. 14:13, 14. (Job 19:25; 1 Cor. 15:52.)
d Lk. 5:26.
e Lk. 1:68.
f Mt. 11:2.
g v. 21; Isa. 61:1-3.
h vs. 14, 15.
i *Gospel.* Lk. 9:6. (Gen. 12:1-3; Rev. 14:6.)
j Mt. 16:17; 1 Pet. 2:8.
k Having gently removed His servant's doubt, the Lord bears witness to him before others: He knows when to reprove, and where, and when, to praise.
l Mt. 3:1.
m Mt. 11:7-11.
n Mt. 3:4; Mk. 1:6.
o Mal. 3:1.
p See Mt. 11:11.
q Mt. 3:6, 11; 21:32; Lk. 3:12.
r Mt. 21:23-25.
s Lk. 1:15.
t v. 36; Lk. 15:2.
u *Sin:* Rom. 3: 23, *note.*
v 1 Cor. 1:21-24.
w Lk. 14:1.
x i.e. in the sense of unchaste.
y Mk. 14 3.
z Isa. 52:7.
aa 1 Cor. 11:15.

himself, saying, [a]This man, if he were a
prophet, would have known who and
what manner of woman *this is* that
toucheth him: for she is a sinner.
40 And Jesus answering said unto
him, Simon, I have somewhat to say
unto thee. And he saith, Master, say on.

Parable of the creditor and two debtors.

41 [b]There was a certain creditor which
had two debtors: the one owed five hundred pence, and the other fifty.
42 And when they had nothing to pay,
he [c]frankly forgave them both. Tell me
therefore, which of them will love him
most?
43 Simon answered and said, I suppose that *he,* to whom he forgave most.
And he said unto him, Thou hast rightly
judged.
44 And he turned to the woman, and
said unto [1]Simon, Seest thou this
woman? I entered into thine house, thou
gavest me no water for my feet: but she
hath washed my feet with tears, and
wiped *them* with the hairs of her head.
45 Thou gavest me no kiss: but this
woman since the time I came in hath not
ceased to kiss my feet.
46 [d]My head with oil thou didst not
anoint: but this woman hath anointed
my feet with ointment.
47 Wherefore I say unto thee, Her sins,
which are many, are [e]forgiven; for she
loved much: but to whom little is forgiv-
en, *the same* loveth little.
48 And he said unto her, Thy sins are
forgiven.
49 And they that sat at meat with him
began to say within themselves, [f]Who is
this that forgiveth sins also?
50 And he said to the woman, Thy
[g]faith hath saved thee; go in peace.

CHAPTER 8.

Jesus preaches and heals in Galilee.

And it came to pass afterward, that he
went [h]throughout every city and
village, preaching and shewing the glad
tidings of the kingdom of God: and the
twelve *were* with him,
2 And [i]certain women, which had
been healed of evil spirits and infirmities, Mary called Magdalene, out of
whom went seven devils,
3 And Joanna the wife of Chuza
[j]Herod's steward, and Susanna, and
many others, which ministered unto him
of their substance.

Parable of the sower
(Mt. 13:1-23; Mk. 4:1-20).

4 And when much people were gathered together, and were come to him out
of every city, he spake by a [k]parable:
5 A [l]sower went out to sow his seed:
and as he sowed, some fell by the way
side; and it was trodden down, and the
fowls of the air devoured it.
6 And some fell upon a rock; and as
soon as it was sprung up, it withered
away, because it lacked moisture.
7 And some fell among thorns; and the
thorns sprang up with it, and choked it.
8 And other fell on good ground, and
sprang up, and bare fruit an hundredfold. And when he had said these things,
he cried, [m]He that hath ears to hear, let
him hear.
9 And his disciples asked him, saying,
What might this parable be?
10 And he said, Unto you it is given to
know the [n]mysteries of the kingdom of
God: but to others in parables; that [o]see-
ing they might not see, and hearing they
might not understand.
11 Now the parable is this: The seed is
the [p]word of God.
12 Those by the way side are they that
hear; then cometh the [q]devil, and taketh
away the word out of their [r]hearts, lest
they should believe and be [s]saved.
13 They on the rock *are they,* which,
when they hear, receive the word with
joy; and these have no root, which for a
while believe, and in time of [t]temptation
fall away.

A.D. 31.

a Lk. 15:2; 19:7.
b *Parables* (N.T.). vs. 41-48; Lk. 8:4-15. (Mt. 5:13-16; Lk. 21:29-31.)
c Psa. 32:1-5; Rom. 5:15, 16; Eph. 1:7.
d Psa. 23:5.
e *Forgiveness.* vs. 47-49; Lk. 17:3, 4. (Lev. 4:20; Mt. 26:28.)
f Mt. 9:3-6.
g *Faith.* Lk. 8:50. (Gen. 3:20; Heb. 11:39.)
h Mk. 1:38.
i Mt. 27:55.
j Mt. 14:1, *refs.*
k *Parables* (N.T.). vs. 4-15, 16-18; Lk. 10:30-37. (Mt. 5:13-16; Lk. 21:29-31.)
l Mt. 13:3-8; Mk. 4:3-8.
m Mt. 11:15; 13:9; Mk. 4:9; Rev. 2:7.
n Mt. 13:11, *note.*
o Isa. 6:9, 10; Acts 28:26, 27.
p 1 Pet. 1:23.
q *Satan.* Lk. 10:18. (Gen. 3:1; Rev. 20:10.)
r Cf. v. 15.
s Rom. 1:16, *note.*
t *Temptation.* Lk. 10:25. (Gen. 3:1; Jas. 1:14.)

[1] **(7:44)** See Jas. 2:14-26. When Jesus would justify the woman in the eyes of *Simon,* He points to her *works,* for only through her works could Simon see the proof of her faith; but when He would send the *woman* away in peace, He points to her *faith,* not her works. See Tit. 2:14; 3:4-8. His own works can never be to the believer his own ground of assurance which must rest upon the work of Christ (cf. Mt. 7:22, 23). See "Assurance" (Isa. 32:17; Jude 1).

14 And that which fell among thorns are they, which, when they have heard, go forth, and are choked with cares and [a]riches and pleasures of *this* life, and bring no fruit to perfection.

15 But that on the good ground are they, which in an [b]honest and good heart, having [c]heard the word, keep *it*, and bring forth fruit with [d]patience.

Parable of the lighted candle
(Mt. 5:15, 16; Mk. 4:21-23; Lk. 11:33).

16 No man, when he hath lighted a [e]candle, covereth it with a vessel, or putteth *it* under a bed; but setteth *it* on a candlestick, that they which enter in may [f]see the light.

17 For [g]nothing is secret, that shall not be made manifest; neither *any thing* hid, that shall not be known and come abroad.

18 [h]Take heed therefore how ye hear: for whosoever hath, to him shall be given; and whosoever hath not, from him shall be taken even that which he seemeth to have.

The new relationships
(Mt. 12:46-50; Mk. 3:31-35).

19 Then came to him *his* [i]mother and his brethren, and could not come at him for the press.

20 And it was told him *by certain* which said, Thy mother and thy brethren stand without, desiring to see thee.

21 And he answered and said unto them, My mother and my brethren are these which [j]hear the word of God, and do it.

Jesus stills the waves
(Mt. 8:23-27; Mk. 4:36-41).

22 Now it came to pass on a certain day, that [k]he went into a ship with his disciples: and he said unto them, Let us go over unto the other side of the lake. And they launched forth.

23 But as they sailed he [l]fell asleep: and there came down a storm of wind on the lake; and they were filled *with water*, and were in jeopardy.

24 And they came to him, and awoke him, saying, Master, master, we perish. Then he arose, and rebuked the wind and the raging of the water: and they [m]ceased, and there was a calm.

25 And he said unto them, [n]Where is your faith? And they being afraid wondered, saying one to another, [o]What manner of man is this! for he commandeth even the winds and water, and they obey him.

Demons cast out of the maniac of Gadara
(Mt. 8:28-34; Mk. 5:1-17).

26 And they arrived at the country of the Gadarenes, which is over against Galilee.

27 And when he went forth to land, there met him out of the city a certain man, which had [p]devils long time, and [q]ware no clothes, neither abode in *any* house, but in the [r]tombs.

28 When he saw Jesus, he cried out, and fell down before him, and with a loud voice said, [s]What have I to do with thee, Jesus, *thou* Son of God [t]most high? I beseech thee, torment me not.

29 (For he had commanded the unclean spirit to come out of the man. For oftentimes it had caught him: and he was kept bound with chains and in fetters; and he [u]brake the bands, and was driven of the devil into the wilderness.)

30 And Jesus asked him, saying, [v]What is thy name? And he said, Legion: because many devils were entered into him.

31 And they besought him that he would not command them to go out into the [w]deep.

32 And there was there an herd of many swine feeding on the mountain: and they besought him that he would suffer them to enter into them. And he suffered them.

33 Then went the devils out of the man, and entered into the [x]swine: and the herd ran violently down a steep place into the lake, and were choked.

34 When they that fed *them* saw what was done, they fled, and went and told *it* in the city and in the country.

35 Then they went out to see what was done; and came to Jesus, and found the man, out of whom the devils were departed, [y]sitting at the feet of Jesus, [z]clothed, and [aa]in his right mind: and they were afraid.

36 They also which saw *it* told them by what means he that was possessed of the devils was healed.

37 Then the whole multitude of the country of the Gadarenes round about [bb]besought him to [cc]depart from them; for they were taken with great fear: and he went up into the ship, and returned back again.

A.D. 31.

a 1 Tim. 6:9, 10; 2 Tim. 4:10.
b Psa. 32:2, 5.
c Jas. 1:22.
d Rom. 2:7; Heb. 10:36; Jas. 5:7, 8.
e Mt. 5:14; Mk. 4:21; Lk. 11:33.
f 2 Cor. 3:2; Phil. 2:15, 16.
g Mt 10:26; Lk. 12:2; 1 Cor. 4:5; 2 Cor. 5:10.
h Mt. 13:12; 25:29; Mk. 4:24, 25.
i Mt. 12:46-50; Mk. 3:31-35.
j Mt. 25:40; 1 John 2:5.
k Mt. 8:23; Mk. 4:35-41.
l Mt. 8:24; Mk. 4:38.
m *Miracles* (N.T.). vs. 22-25, 26-33, 41, 42, 43-48, 49-56; Lk. 9:12-17. (Mt. 8:2, 3; Acts 28:8, 9.)
n Lk. 9:41; cf. Mt. 8:10.
o Lk. 5:26.
p Mt. 8:28.
q Gen. 3:7-11.
r Prov. 21:16.
s Mk. 1:23, 24; Jas. 2:19.
t Gen. 14:19.
u Rom. 8:7.
v Gen. 32:27; 1 John 1:9.
w Rev. 20:1-3.
x Lk. 15:15; 2 Pet. 2:22.
y Mt. 11:28; see v. 41, *refs.*
z Phil. 3:9.
aa 2 Tim. 1:7.
bb Unconscious of their own need, the Gadarenes beseech the Lord to depart—His power terrifies and condemns them; whilst he whose need has been met beseeches Him that he may follow Him.
cc Acts 16:39.

38 Now the man out of whom the devils were departed [a]besought him that he might be with him: but Jesus sent him away, saying,

39 [b]Return to thine own house, and shew how great things God hath done unto thee. And he went his way, and published throughout the whole city how great things Jesus had done unto him.

A woman healed: Jairus' daughter raised
(Mt. 9:18-26; Mk. 5:22-43).

40 And it came to pass, that, when Jesus was returned, the people *gladly* received him: for they were all waiting for him.

41 And, behold, there came a man named [c]Jairus, and he was a [d]ruler of the synagogue: and he [e]fell down at Jesus' feet, and besought him that he would come into his house:

42 For he had one only [f]daughter, about twelve years of age, and she [g]lay a dying. But as he went the people thronged him.

43 And a woman having an [h]issue of blood twelve years, which had [i]spent all her living upon physicians, neither could be healed of any,

44 Came behind *him*, and [j]touched the border of his garment: and immediately her issue of blood stanched.

45 And Jesus said, Who touched me? When all denied, Peter and they that were with him said, Master, the multitude [k]throng thee and press *thee*, and sayest thou, Who touched me?

46 And Jesus said, Somebody hath touched me: for I perceive that [l]virtue is gone out of me.

47 And when the woman saw that she was not hid, she came trembling, and falling down before him, she [m]declared unto him before all the people for what cause she had touched him, and how she was healed immediately.

48 And he said unto her, Daughter, be of good comfort: [n]thy faith hath made thee whole; [o]go in peace.

49 While he yet spake, there cometh one from the ruler of the synagogue's *house*, saying to him, Thy daughter is [p]dead; trouble not the Master.

50 But when Jesus heard *it*, he answered him, saying, [q]Fear not: [r]believe only, and she shall be made whole.

51 And when he came into the house, he [s]suffered no man to go in, save Peter, and James, and John, and the father and the mother of the maiden.

52 And all wept, and bewailed her: but he said, Weep not; she is not dead, but [t]sleepeth.

53 And they laughed him to scorn, knowing that she was dead.

54 And he put them all out, and took her by the [u]hand, and called, saying, [v]Maid, [w]arise.

55 And her spirit came again, and she arose straightway: and he commanded to [x]give her meat.

56 And her parents were astonished: but [y]he charged them that they should tell no man what was done.

CHAPTER 9.

The twelve sent forth to preach
(Mt. 10:1-42. Cf. Mk. 6:7-13).

Then he called his [z]twelve disciples together, and gave them power and authority over all devils, and to cure diseases.

2 And he sent them to preach the kingdom of God, and to heal the sick.

3 And he said unto them, [aa]Take [bb]nothing for *your* journey, neither staves, nor scrip, neither bread, neither money; neither have two coats apiece.

4 And whatsoever house ye enter into, there abide, and thence depart.

5 And whosoever will not [cc]receive you, when ye go out of that city, shake off the very dust from your feet for a testimony against them.

6 And they departed, and went through the towns, preaching the [dd]gospel, and healing every where.

7 Now [ee]Herod the tetrarch heard of all that was done by him: and he was perplexed, because that it was said of some, that John was risen from the dead;

8 And of some, that Elias had appeared; and of others, that one of the old prophets was risen again.

9 And Herod said, John have I beheaded: but who is this, of whom I hear such things? [ff]And he desired to see him.

The apostles return: the five thousand fed (Mt. 14:13-21; Mk. 6:30-44; John 6:1-14).

10 And the apostles, when they were [gg]returned, told him all that they had done. And he took them, and

A.D. 31.

a Lk. 18:43; Phil. 1:23, 24.
b Lk. 5:14-15; cf. Mt. 11:20 with John 4:48; Acts 4:20.
c Mt. 9:18, 26; Mk. 5:22.
d John 7:48.
e Mt. 28:9; Mk. 7:25; Lk. 7:38; 8:35; 10:39; 17:16; John 11:32.
f Isa. 37:22; Lk. 9:38.
g Lk. 7:2; John 11:3.
h Lev. 15:19.
i Rom. 10:3; Gal. 3:21.
j Lk. 5:13; Rom. 4:4, 5.
k Mt. 11:20; Lk. 13:25.
l Mt. 15:28; Lk. 5:17.
m Rom. 10:10.
n Lk. 7:50.
o John 8:11.
p John 11:21; cf. Ezk. 37:11, 12.
q John 11:39, 40.
r *Faith.* Lk. 17:5, 6. (Gen. 3:20; Heb. 11:39.)
s Mt. 26:37; Mk. 13:3; Lk. 9:28.
t John 11:11-14.
u Mk. 1:31; cf. Heb. 2:14-16.
v Or, *Child.*
w Lk. 7:14; John 11:43; cf. John 5:25, 28.
x 1 Pet. 2:2.
y Mt. 8:4; 9:30; Mk. 5:43.
z Mt. 10:1; Mk. 6:7.
aa Cf. Mt. 10:9, *note.*
bb Lk. 10:4; 22:35; 3 John 5-8; 1 Cor. 9:7, 14.
cc John 13:20; Acts 13:51.
dd *Gospel.* Lk. 20:1. (Gen. 12:1-3; Rev. 14:6.)
ee Also v. 9. See Mt. 14:1, *ref.*
ff Lk. 23:8.
gg Mk. 6:30.

[a]went aside privately into a desert place
belonging to the city called Bethsaida.
11 And the people, when they knew *it*,
followed him: and he received them,
and [b]spake unto them of the kingdom of
God, and healed them that had [c]need of
healing.
12 And when the day began to wear
away, then came the twelve, and said
unto him, [d]Send the multitude away, that
they may go into the towns and country
round about, and lodge, and get victuals:
for we are here in a desert place.
13 But he said unto them, Give ye
them to eat. And they said, We have no
more but [e]five loaves and two fishes;
except we should go and buy meat for
all this people.
14 For they were about five thousand
men. And he said to his disciples, Make
them [f]sit down by fifties in a company.
15 And they did so, and made them
all sit down.
16 Then he took the five loaves and
the two fishes, and looking up to heav-
en, he [g]blessed them, and brake, and
gave to the disciples to set before the
multitude.
17 And they did eat, and [h]were all
filled: and there was taken up of [i]frag-
ments that remained to them twelve baskets.

Peter's confession of Christ
(Mt. 16:13-20; Mk. 27-30).

18 And it came to pass, as he was
alone [j]praying, his disciples were with
him: and he asked them, saying, [k]Whom
say the people that I am?
19 They answering said, John the
Baptist; but some *say*, Elias; and others
say, that one of the old prophets is risen
again.
20 He said unto them, But whom say
ye that I am? [l]Peter answering said, The
Christ of God.
21 And he straitly charged them, and
commanded *them* to tell no man that
thing;

Jesus foretells his death and resurrection
(Mt. 16:21; Mk. 8:31).

22 Saying, The Son of man must suffer
many things, and be rejected of the
elders and chief priests and scribes, and
be slain, and be [m]raised the third day.

The test of discipleship
(Mt. 16:22-28; Mk. 8:32-38).

23 And he said to *them* all, [n]If any *man*
will come after me, let him deny himself,
and take up his cross daily, and follow
me.
24 For whosoever will [o]save his life
shall lose it: but whosoever will lose his
life for my sake, the same shall save it.
25 For what is a man [p]advantaged, if
he gain the whole [q]world, and lose himself, or be cast away?
26 For whosoever shall be [r]ashamed
of me and of my words, of him shall the
Son of man be [s]ashamed, when he shall
[t]come in his own glory, and *in his*
Father's, and of the [u]holy [v]angels.

The transfiguration
(Mt. 17:1-8; Mk. 9:2-8).

27 But I tell you of a truth, there be
[w]some standing here, which shall not
taste of death, till they see the kingdom
of God.
28 [x]And it came to pass about an eight
days after these sayings, he took Peter
and John and James, and went up into a
mountain to pray.
29 And as he [y]prayed, the [z]fashion of
his countenance was altered, and his raiment *was* white *and* glistering.
30 And, behold, there talked with him
[aa]two men, which were Moses and Elias:
31 Who appeared in glory, and spake
of his [bb]decease which he should accomplish at Jerusalem.
32 But Peter and they that were with
him were heavy with [cc]sleep: and when
they were awake, they saw his glory,
and the two men that stood with him.
33 And it came to pass, as they departed from him, Peter said unto Jesus,
Master, it is good for us to be here: and
let us make [dd]three tabernacles; one for
thee, and one for Moses, and one for
Elias: [ee]not knowing what he said.
34 While he thus spake, there came a
[ff]cloud, and overshadowed them: and
they feared as they entered into the cloud.
35 And there came a voice out of the
cloud, saying, [gg]This is my beloved Son:
hear him.
36 And when the voice was past, Jesus
was found alone. And they [hh]kept *it*
close, and told no man in those days any
of those things which they had seen.

A.D. 32.

a Mt. 12:15; 14:13, 14.
b Lk. 4:43.
c Lk. 4:40; Rom. 5:20. Wherever there is need acknowledged the Lord is ready to meet it. Men might have put the bodily need of healing first, since that is keenly felt. Spiritual need is often the greatest where there is the least consciousness of it; cf. Rev. 3:17.
d Mt. 14:15-21; Mk. 6:35-44; John 6:5-13.
e 1 Cor. 1:27, 28.
f Rom. 4:5.
g Prov. 10:22; Lk. 22:19; 24:30.
h *Miracles* (N.T.). vs. 12-17, 37-42; Lk. 11:14. (Mt. 8:2, 3; Acts 28:8, 9.)
i 2 Ki. 4:42-44; Eph. 3:18, 19.
j vs. 28, 29; Lk. 3:21; 5:16; 6:12; 11:1; 22:40-46; 23:34.
k Mt. 16:13-20; Mk. 8:27-30.
l John 6:68.
m Lk. 24:6, 7, 46.
n Mt. 10:38; 16:24-28; Mk. 8:34-38; cf. Phil. 3:10.
o John 12:25, 26; Acts 20:24.
p Lk. 12:15-21; 16:19-31.
q i.e. *earth.*
r Mt. 10:32, 33; Rom. 1:16.
s Heb. 11:16.
t Mt. 25:31.
u *Sanctify, holy (persons)* (N.T.). John 10:36. (Mt. 4:5; Rev. 22:11.)
v Heb. 1:4, *note.*
w 2 Pet. 1:16-18.
x See Mt. 17:2, *note* on the transfiguration.
y v. 18.
z 2 Cor. 4:6; Heb. 2:9.
aa Mt. 18:16.
bb Or, *departure.*
cc Lk. 22:45, 46.
dd *Contra*, vs. 19, 20.
ee Mt. 20:21, 22; John 14:8-11.
ff Ex. 13:21; Acts 1:9.
gg Mt. 3:17; Lk. 3:22; John 5:36, 37; 12:28-30.
hh v. 21; Mt. 17:9.

The powerless disciples. Demon cast out of a child (Mt. 17:14-21; Mk. 9:14-29).

37 And it came to pass, that on the
next day, when they were [a]come down
from the hill, much people met him.
38 And, behold, a man of the company
cried out, saying, Master, I beseech thee,
look upon my son: for he is mine [b]only
child.
39 And, lo, a [c]spirit taketh him, and he
suddenly crieth out; and it teareth him
that he foameth again, and bruising him
hardly departeth from him.
40 And I besought thy [d]disciples to
cast him out; and they could not.
41 And Jesus answering said, O [e]faith-
less and perverse generation, how long
shall I be with you, and suffer you?
Bring thy son hither.
42 And as he was [f]yet a coming, the
devil threw him down, and tare *him*.
And Jesus rebuked the unclean spirit,
and healed the child, and delivered him
again to his father.
43 And they were all amazed at [g]the
mighty power of God. But while they
wondered every one at all things which
Jesus did, he said unto his disciples,

Jesus again foretells his death (Mt. 17:22, 23; Mk. 9:30-32).

44 Let these sayings [h]sink down into
your ears: for the Son of man shall be
delivered into the hands of men.
45 But they understood not this saying, and it was hid from them, that they
perceived it not: and they feared to ask
him of that saying.

The sermon on the child (Mt. 18:1-5; Mk. 9:33-37).

46 Then there arose a [i]reasoning
among them, which of them should be
greatest.
47 And Jesus, [j]perceiving the thought
of their heart, took a [k]child, and set him
by him,
48 And said unto them, [l]Whosoever
shall receive this child in my name
receiveth me: and whosoever shall
receive me receiveth him that sent me:
for he that is [m]least among you all, the
same shall be great.

The rebuke of sectarianism (Mk. 9:38-40).

49 And John answered and said,
Master, we saw one casting out devils in
thy name; and we forbad him, because
he [n]followeth not with us.
50 And Jesus said unto him, Forbid
him not: for [o]he that is not against us is
for us.

The new spirit of grace: final departure from Galilee. (Cf. John 7:2-10.)

51 And it came to pass, when the time
was come that he should be received up,
he [p]stedfastly set his face to go to
Jerusalem,
52 And sent messengers before his face:
and they went, and entered into a village
of the Samaritans, to make ready for him.
53 And [q]they did not receive him,
because his face was as though he would
go to Jerusalem.
54 And when his disciples James and
John saw *this*, they said, Lord, wilt thou
that we command [r]fire to come down
from heaven, and consume them, even
as Elias did?
55 But he turned, and rebuked them,
and said, Ye know not what manner of
spirit ye are of.
56 For the [s]Son of man is not come to
destroy men's lives, but to save *them*.
And they went to another village.

Another test of discipleship (Mt. 8:18-22).

57 And it came to pass, that, as they
went in the way, a [t]certain *man* said unto
him, Lord, I will follow thee whithersoever thou goest.
58 And Jesus said unto him, Foxes
have holes, and birds of the air *have*
[u]nests; but the Son of man [v]hath not
where to lay *his* head.
59 And he said unto another, [w]Follow
me. But he said, Lord, suffer me first to
go and [x]bury my father.
60 Jesus said unto him, Let the dead
bury their dead: but go thou and preach
the kingdom of God.
61 And another also said, Lord, I will
follow thee; but let me first go [y]bid them
farewell, which are at home at my house.
62 And Jesus said unto him, No man,
having put his hand to the [z]plough, and
looking back, is fit for the kingdom of
God.

A.D. 32.

a Mt. 17:14; Mk. 9:14.
b Gen. 22:2; Lk. 7:12; cf. John 3:16.
c Mt. 15:22; Lk. 8:27.
d v. 1.
e John 14:12.
f Lk. 8:49.
g Or, *the majesty of God.* 2 Pet. 1:16.
h v. 31; Mt. 17:22.
i Mt. 18:1-6; Mk. 9:33-37; Lk. 22:24-27.
j John 2:24, 25.
k *little child.* Lk. 18:17.
l Mt. 10:40; 18:5; Mk. 9:37; John 12:44; 13:20.
m 1 Cor. 15:9; Phil. 2:3-11; Eph. 3:8.
n Num. 11:26-30; Mk. 9:38-40; 1 Cor. 3:5.
o Mt. 10:42; Lk. 11:23; Phil. 1:15-18.
p Isa. 50:7; Mt. 26:53, 54, Heb. 12:2.
q John 4:5, 9.
r v. 30; 2 Ki. 1:10, 12.
s Lk. 19:10; John 12:47.
t v. 23; Mt. 8:19, 20.
u Or, *roosting-places.*
v Lk. 2:7; 8:23; 1 Cor. 4:11.
w Mt. 8:22.
x Mt. 8:21; Lk. 18:28-30.
y 1 Ki. 19:20, 21.
z Acts 15:37, 38; 2 Tim. 4:10, 11.

CHAPTER 10.

The seventy sent before him.
(Cf. Mt. 10:1-42.)

After these things the Lord appointed other seventy also, and sent them two and two before his face into every city and place, whither he himself would come.

2 Therefore said he unto [a]them, The harvest truly *is* great, but [b]the labourers *are* few: pray ye therefore the Lord of the harvest, that he would send forth labourers into his harvest.

3 [c]Go your ways: behold, I send you forth as lambs among wolves.

4 [d]Carry neither purse, nor scrip, nor shoes: and [e]salute no man by the way.

5 And into whatsoever house ye enter, first say, Peace *be* to this house.

6 And if the [f]son of peace be there, your peace shall rest upon it: if not, it shall [g]turn to you again.

7 And in the same house remain, eating and drinking such things as they give: [h]for the labourer is worthy of his hire. Go not from house to house.

8 And into whatsoever city ye enter, and they receive you, eat such things as are set before you:

9 And heal the sick that are therein, and say unto them, [i]The kingdom of God is come nigh unto you.

10 But into whatsoever city ye enter, and they receive you not, go your ways out into the streets of the same, and say,

11 Even the very dust of your city, which cleaveth on us, we do wipe off against you: notwithstanding be ye sure of this, that the kingdom of God is come nigh unto you.

12 But I say unto you, that [j]it shall be more tolerable in that day for Sodom, than for that city.

Jesus denounces judgment on the cities (Mt. 11:20-24).

13 [k]Woe unto thee, Chorazin! woe unto thee, Bethsaida! for if the mighty works had been done in Tyre and Sidon, which have been done in you, they had a great while ago [l]repented, sitting in sackcloth and ashes.

14 But it shall be more tolerable for Tyre and Sidon [m]at the judgment, than for you.

15 And thou, Capernaum, [n]which art exalted to heaven, shalt be thrust down to hell.

16 He that [o]heareth you [p]heareth me; and he that despiseth you despiseth me; and he that despiseth me despiseth him that sent me.

17 And the seventy returned again with joy, saying, Lord, even the devils are subject unto us through thy name.

18 And he said unto them, I beheld [q]Satan as [r]lightning fall from heaven.

19 Behold, I give unto you power to tread on [s]serpents and scorpions, and over all the power of the enemy: and nothing shall by any means hurt you.

20 Notwithstanding in this rejoice not, that the spirits are subject unto you; but rather rejoice, because your names are written in heaven.

21 In that hour Jesus rejoiced in [t]spirit, and said, I thank thee, O Father, Lord of heaven and earth, that thou hast hid these things from the wise and prudent, and hast revealed them unto babes: even so, Father; for so it seemed good in thy sight.

22 All things [u]are delivered to me of my Father: and no man knoweth who the Son is, but the Father; and who the Father is, but the Son, and *he* to whom the Son will reveal *him*.

23 And he turned him unto *his* disciples, and said privately, [v]Blessed *are* the eyes which see the things that ye see:

24 For I tell you, that [w]many prophets and kings have desired to see those things which ye see, and have not seen *them*; and to hear those things which ye hear, and have not heard *them*.

A lawyer questions Jesus.
(Cf. Mt. 22:34-40; Mk. 12:28-34.)

25 And, behold, a certain lawyer stood up, and [x]tempted him, saying, Master, what shall I do to inherit [y]eternal life?

26 He said unto him, What is written in the [z]law? how readest thou?

27 And he answering said, Thou shalt love the [aa]Lord thy God with all thy heart, and with all thy soul, and with all thy strength, and with all thy mind; and thy neighbour as thyself.

28 And he said unto him, Thou hast answered right: this do, and thou shalt live.

A.D. 32.

a John 4:35.
b 1 Cor. 3:9.
c See Mt. 10:16, *note.* The same remark is applicable here.
d Lk. 9:3; 22:35; 1 Cor. 9:7.
e Gen. 24:33, 56; 2 Ki. 4:29.
f Isa. 57:21.
g Psa. 35:13.
h 1 Cor. 9:4, 14.
i Mt. 3:2.
j Lk. 12:47; Heb. 2:3; 10:26, 31.
k See Mt. 11:20, *note;* Mk. 8:23, *note.*
l *Repentance.* Lk. 11:32. (Mt. 3:2; Acts 17:30.)
m *Day of Judgment.* Lk. 11:31, 32. (Mt. 10:15; Rev. 20:11.)
n Isa. 14:13, 15.
o John 13:20.
p *Inspiration.* Lk. 11:49-51. (Ex. 4:15; Rev. 22:19.)
q *Satan.* Lk. 11:18, 19. (Gen. 3:1; Rev. 20:10.)
r Isa. 14:12-19; Rev. 12:8, 9.
s Gen. 3:15; Mt. 13:39; Mk. 16:18; Acts 28:5; Rom. 16:20.
t *the spirit.* Many have, *Spirit.*
u Mt. 28:18; John 3:35; Eph. 1:20, 23; Heb. 2:8.
v Mt. 13:16.
w John 8:56.
x *Temptation.* Lk. 11:16. (Gen. 3:1; Jas. 1:14.)
y *Life (eternal).* Lk. 12:15. (Mt. 7:14; Rev. 22:19.)
z *Law (of Moses).* vs. 25-37; John 1:17. (Ex. 19:1; Gal. 3:1-29.)
aa *Jehovah.* Deut. 6:5; Lev. 19:18.

29 But he, willing to [a]justify himself, said unto Jesus, And who is my [b]neighbour?

Parable of the good Samaritan.

30 And Jesus answering said, [c]A certain *man* went down from Jerusalem to Jericho, and fell among thieves, which stripped him of his raiment, and wounded *him*, and departed, leaving *him* half dead.

31 And by chance there came down a certain priest that way: and when he saw him, he passed by on the other side.

32 And likewise a Levite, when he was at the place, came and looked *on him*, and passed by on the other side.

33 But a certain [d]Samaritan, as he journeyed, came where he was: and when he saw him, he had compassion *on him*,

34 And went to *him*, and bound up his wounds, pouring in oil and wine, and set him on his own beast, and brought him to an inn, and took care of him.

35 And on the morrow when he departed, he took out two [e]pence, and gave *them* to the host, and said unto him, Take care of him; and whatsoever thou spendest more, when I come again, I will repay thee.

36 Which now of these three, thinkest thou, was neighbour unto him that fell among the thieves?

37 And he said, He that shewed [f]mercy on him. Then said Jesus unto him, Go, and do thou likewise.

A.D. 32.

a Lk. 16:15; Rom. 4:2; Gal. 3:11.
b Mt. 5:43.
c *Parables* (N.T.). vs. 30-37; Lk. 11:5-10. (Mt. 5:13-16; Lk. 21:29-31.)
d John 4:9.
e The Roman penny is the eighth part of an ounce, which at five shillings the ounce is seven pence half penny, or 15 cents.
f Prov. 14:21; Mic. 6:8.
g John 11:1; 12:2, 3.
h Lk. 8:35; Acts 22:3.
i Lk. 21:34; Mk. 4:19; 1 Cor. 7:32, 35.
j Lk. 18:22; Psa. 27:4; 73:25; Mk. 8:36.
k *Bible prayers.* (N.T.). Lk. 15:18, 19. (Mt. 6:9; Rev. 22:20.)
l Mt. 6:9.
m Mt. 3:2, *note.*
n Or, *for the day.*

Martha and Mary in contrast.

38 Now it came to pass, as they went, that he entered into a certain village: and a certain woman named Martha [g]received him into her house.

39 And she had a sister called Mary, which also [h]sat at Jesus' feet, and heard his word.

40 But Martha was cumbered about much serving, and came to him, and said, Lord, dost thou not care that my sister hath left me to serve alone? bid her therefore that she help me.

41 And Jesus answered and said unto her, Martha, Martha, thou [i]art careful and troubled about many things:

42 But one [j]thing is needful: and Mary hath chosen that good part, which shall not be taken away from her.

CHAPTER 11.

Jesus' doctrine of prayer.

And it came to pass, that, as he was [k]praying in a certain place, when he ceased, one of his disciples said unto him, Lord, [1]teach us to pray, as John also taught his disciples.

2 And he said unto them, When ye [k]pray, say, [l]Our Father which art in heaven, Hallowed be thy name. [m]Thy kingdom come. Thy will be done, as in heaven, so in earth.

3 Give us [n]day by day our daily bread.

[1] **(11:1)** This is the central N.T. passage on prayer. In the Sermon on the Mount Christ had announced the new basis of prayer, viz.: relationship (Mt. 6:9, 28-32). The believer is a child of God through the new birth (John 3:3, *note*). The clear revelation of this fact at once establishes the reasonableness of prayer; a reasonableness against which the argument from the apparent uniformity of natural law shatters itself. God is more than a Creator, bringing a universe into being, and establishing laws for it; more than a decree-maker determining future events by an eternal fiat. Above all this is the divine family for whom the universe with its laws exists (Col. 1:16-20; Heb. 1:2; 2:10, 11; Rom. 8:17): "When *ye* pray, say, Our Father." What God habitually does in the material universe concerns the reverent investigator of that universe. What He may do in His own family concerns Him, and them and is matter for divine promise and revelation. Science, which deals only with natural phenomena, cannot intrude there (1 Cor. 2:9).

Christ's law of prayer may be thus summarized: (1) He grounds prayer upon relationship, and reveals God as freely charging Himself with all the responsibilities, as His heart glows with all the affections of a Father toward all who believe on Jesus Christ (Mt. 6:25-32; 7:9-11). Prayer, therefore, is a child's petition to an all-wise, all-loving, and all-powerful, Father-God. (2) In the so-called Lord's prayer Christ gives an incomparable model for all prayer. It teaches that right prayer begins with worship; puts the interest of the kingdom before merely personal interest; accepts beforehand the Father's will, whether to grant or withhold, and petitions for present need, leaving the future to the Father's care and love. Used as a *form*, the Lord's prayer is, dispensationally, upon legal, not church ground;

4 And [a]forgive us our [b]sins; for we also forgive every one that is indebted to us. And lead us not into temptation; but deliver us from evil.

Parable of the importunate friend.

5 And he said unto them, [c]Which of you shall have a friend, and shall go unto him at midnight, and say unto him, Friend, lend me three loaves;

6 For a friend of mine in his journey is come to me, and I have nothing to set before him?

7 And he from within shall answer and say, Trouble me not: the door is now shut, and my children are with me in bed; I cannot rise and give thee.

8 I say unto you, Though he will not rise and give him, because he is his friend, yet because of his [d]importunity he will rise and give him as many as he needeth.

9 And I say unto you, [e]Ask, and it shall be given you; [f]seek, and ye shall find; [g]knock, and it shall be opened unto you.

10 For every one that asketh receiveth; and he that seeketh findeth; and to him that knocketh it shall be opened.

Parable of the fatherhood.

11 If a son shall ask bread of any of you that is a father, will he give him a stone? or if *he ask* a fish, will he for a fish give him a serpent?

12 Or if he shall ask an egg, will he offer him a scorpion?

13 If ye then, being evil, know how to give good gifts unto your children: how much more shall *your* heavenly Father [1]give the [h]Holy Spirit to them that ask him?

A.D. 33.

a Mt. 6:12, *note.*

b *Sin.* Rom. 3:23, *note.*

c *Parables* (N.T.). vs. 5-10, 11-13, 33-36; Lk. 12:16-21. (Mt. 5:13-16; Lk. 21:29-31.)

d Lk. 18:1-8.

e Mt. 7:7; 21:22; John 15:7; Jas. 1:5; 1 John 3:22.

f Isa. 55:6.

g Lk. 13:25.

h *Holy Spirit.* Lk. 12:10, 12. (Mt. 1:18; Acts 2:4.)

i *demon.*

j *Miracles* (N.T.). Lk. 13:11-13. (Mt. 8:2, 3; Acts 28:8, 9.)

k *Beelzebul;* so vs. 18, 19.

l *Temptation.* Lk. 22:28. (Gen. 3:1; Jas. 1:14.)

m *Satan.* Lk. 13:16. (Gen. 3:1; Rev. 20:10.)

n Mt. 3:2.

o Isa. 53:12; Col. 2:15; Heb. 2:14, 15; Rev. 20:2, 3.

p Mt. 6:24.

q See Mt. 12:43.

Jesus charged with casting out demons by Beelzebub (Mt. 12:22-37).

14 And he was casting out a [i]devil, and it was dumb. And it came to pass, when the devil was gone out, the dumb [j]spake; and the people wondered.

15 But some of them said, He casteth out devils through [k]Beelzebub the chief of the devils.

16 And others, [l]tempting *him*, sought of him a sign from heaven.

17 But he, knowing their thoughts, said unto them, Every kingdom divided against itself is brought to desolation; and a house *divided* against a house falleth.

18 If [m]Satan also be divided against himself, how shall his kingdom stand? because ye say that I cast out devils through Beelzebub.

19 And if I by Beelzebub cast out devils, by whom do your sons cast *them* out? therefore shall they be your judges.

20 But if I with the finger of God cast out devils, no doubt [n]the kingdom of God is come upon you.

21 When a strong man armed keepeth his palace, his goods are in peace:

22 But when a [o]stronger than he shall come upon him, and overcome him, he taketh from him all his armour wherein he trusted, and divideth his spoils.

23 He that is not with me is [p]against me: and he that gathereth not with me scattereth.

Worthlessness of self-reformation (Mt. 12:43-45).

24 [q]When the unclean spirit is gone out of a man, he walketh through dry places, seeking rest; and finding none,

it is not a prayer in the name of Christ (cf. John 14:13, 14; 16:24); and it makes human forgiveness, as under the law it must, the condition of divine forgiveness; an order which grace exactly reverses (cf. Eph. 4:32). (3) Prayer is to be definite (vs. 5, 6), and, (4) importunate, that is, undiscouraged by delayed answers.

[1]**(11:13)** It is evident that none of the disciples, with the possible exception of Mary of Bethany, asked for the Spirit in the faith of this promise. It was a new and staggering thing to a Jew that, in advance of the fulfilment of Joel 2:28, 29, all might receive the Spirit. Mary alone of the disciples understood Christ's repeated declaration concerning His own death and resurrection (John 12:3-7). Save Mary, not one of the disciples but Peter, and he only in the great confession (Mt. 16:16), manifested a spark of spiritual intelligence till after the resurrection of Christ and the impartation of the Spirit (John 20:22; Acts 2:1-4). To go back to the promise of Lk. 11:13, is to forget Pentecost, and to ignore the truth that now every believer has the indwelling Spirit (Rom. 8:9, 15; 1 Cor. 6:19; Gal. 4:6; 1 John 2:20, 27). See Acts 2:4, *note.*

he saith, I will return unto my house
whence I came out.
25 And when he cometh, he findeth *it*
[a]swept and garnished.
26 Then goeth he, and taketh *to him*
seven other spirits more wicked than
himself; and they enter in, and dwell
there: and the last *state* of that man is
[b]worse than the first.
27 And it came to pass, as he spake
these things, a certain woman of the company lifted up her voice, and said unto
him, [c]Blessed *is* the womb that bare thee,
and the paps which thou hast sucked.
28 But he said, Yea rather, [d]blessed *are*
they that hear the word of God, and
keep it.

The sign of Jonas (Mt. 12:39-42).

29 And when the people were gathered thick together, he began to say, This
is an evil generation: they seek a sign;
and [e]there shall no sign be given it, but
the sign of Jonas the prophet.
30 For as [f]Jonas was a sign unto the
Ninevites, so shall also [g]the Son of man
be to this generation.
31 The queen of the south shall rise up
in the judgment with the men of this
generation, and condemn them: for she
came from the utmost parts of the earth
to hear the wisdom of Solomon; and,
behold, a greater than Solomon *is* here.
32 The men of Nineve shall rise up [h]in
the judgment with this generation, and
shall condemn it: for they [i]repented at
the preaching of Jonas; and, behold, a
greater than Jonas *is* here.

Parable of the lighted candle
(Mt. 5:15, 16; Mk. 4:21, 22. Cf. Lk. 8:16).

33 No man, when he hath lighted a
[j]candle, putteth *it* in a secret place, neither
under a bushel, but on a candlestick, that
they which come in may see the light.
34 The [k]light of the body is the eye:
therefore when thine eye is single, thy
whole body also is full of light; but
when *thine eye* is evil, thy body also *is*
full of darkness.
35 Take heed therefore that the light
which is in thee be not darkness.
36 If thy whole body therefore *be* full
of light, having no part dark, the whole
shall be full of light, as when the bright
[l]shining of a candle doth give thee light.
37 And as he spake, a certain Pharisee
besought him to dine with him: and he
went in, and sat down to meat.
38 And [m]when the Pharisee saw *it*, he
marvelled that he had not first washed
before dinner.

Jesus denounces woes upon
the Pharisees. (Cf. Mt. 23:13-35.)

39 And the Lord said unto him, Now
do ye Pharisees make clean the outside
of the cup and the platter; but your
inward part is full of ravening and
wickedness.
40 *Ye* fools, did not he that made that
which is without make that which is
within also?
41 But rather give alms of such things
as ye have; and, behold, all things are
clean unto you.
42 But [n]woe unto you, Pharisees! for
ye tithe mint and rue and all manner of
herbs, and [o]pass over judgment and the
love of God: these ought ye to have
done, and not to leave the other undone.
43 Woe unto you, Pharisees! [p]for ye
love the uppermost seats in the synagogues, and greetings in the markets.
44 Woe unto you, scribes and
Pharisees, hypocrites! for ye are as
[q]graves which appear not, and the men
that walk over *them* are not aware *of them*.

Jesus denounces woes upon the lawyers.

45 Then answered one of the [r]lawyers,
and said unto him, Master, thus saying
thou reproachest us also.
46 And he said, Woe unto you also, *ye*
lawyers! for ye [s]lade men with burdens
grievous to be borne, and ye yourselves
touch not the burdens with one of your
fingers.
47 Woe unto you! for ye build the
sepulchres of the prophets, and your
fathers killed them.
48 Truly ye bear witness that ye allow
the deeds of your fathers: for they
indeed killed [t]them, and ye build their
sepulchres.
49 Therefore also said the wisdom of
God, I will send them prophets and
apostles, and *some* of them they shall
slay and persecute:
50 That the blood of all the prophets,
which was shed from the foundation of
the [u]world, may be [v]required of this
generation;

A.D. 33.

a 1 Cor. 3:16; Eph. 3:16, 17; 5:18.
b John 5:14; Heb. 6:4, 8; 10:26, 29; 2 Pet. 2:20.
c Lk. 1:28, 48.
d Lk. 8:21; Psa. 119:1, 2; Mt. 7:21.
e Mt. 12:40; Mk. 8:11.
f Jon. 1:17.
g Mt. 8:20, *note*.
h *Day of Judgment.* vs. 31, 32; John 5:22, 27, 30. (Mt. 10:15; Rev. 20:11.)
i *Repentance.* Lk. 13:3. (Mt. 3:2; Acts 17:30.)
j Cf. Lk. 8:16; Mt. 5:15; Mk. 4:21.
k Mt. 6:22, 23.
l Prov. 4:18; 20:27.
m Mk. 7:3.
n Mt. 23:23.
o Mic. 6:7, 8.
p Mt. 23:6; Mk. 12:38.
q Psa. 5:9.
r Mt. 22:35, *note*.
s Mk. 7:7, 8.
t Heb. 11:35.
u i.e. *earth*.
v Ex. 20:5; Jer. 51:56.

51 From the blood of [a]Abel unto the blood of [b]Zacharias, which perished between the altar and the [c]temple: verily I say unto you, It shall be required of this generation.

52 Woe unto you, lawyers! for ye have taken away the key of knowledge: [d]ye entered not in yourselves, and them that were entering in ye hindered.

53 And as he said these things unto them, the scribes and the Pharisees began to urge *him* vehemently, and to [e]provoke him to speak of many things:

54 Laying wait for him, and seeking to catch something out of his mouth, that they might accuse him.

CHAPTER 12.

Jesus warns of the leaven of the Pharisees. (Cf. Mk. 8:14-21.)

In [f]the mean time, when there were gathered together an innumerable multitude of people, insomuch that they trode one upon another, he began to say unto his disciples first of all, Beware ye of the [g]leaven of the Pharisees, which is [h]hypocrisy.

2 For [i]there is nothing covered, that shall not be revealed; neither hid, that shall not be known.

3 Therefore whatsoever ye have spoken in darkness shall be heard in the light; and that which ye have spoken in the ear in closets shall be proclaimed upon the housetops.

4 And I say unto [j]you my friends, Be not afraid of them that kill the body, and after that have no more that they can do.

5 But I will forewarn you whom ye shall fear: Fear him, which after he hath killed hath power to cast into [k]hell; yea, I say unto you, Fear him.

6 Are not five sparrows sold for two [l]farthings, and not one of them is forgotten before God?

7 But even the very hairs of your head are all numbered. Fear not therefore: ye are of more value than many sparrows.

8 Also I say unto you, Whosoever shall confess me before men, him shall the [m]Son of man also confess before the [n]angels of God:

9 But he that denieth me before men shall be denied before the angels of God.

10 And whosoever shall speak a word against the [m]Son of man, it shall be forgiven him: but unto him that blasphemeth against the [o]Holy Ghost it shall not be forgiven.

11 And when they bring you unto the synagogues, and *unto* magistrates, and powers, [p]take ye no thought how or what thing ye shall answer, or what ye shall say:

12 For the [o]Holy Ghost shall teach you in the same hour what ye ought to say.

13 And one of the company said unto him, Master, speak to my brother, that he divide the inheritance with me.

14 And he said unto him, [q]Man, who made me a judge or a divider over you?

15 And he said unto them, Take heed, and beware of covetousness: for a man's [r]life consisteth not in the abundance of the things which he possesseth.

Parable of the rich fool.

16 And he spake a [s]parable unto them, saying, The ground of a certain rich man brought forth plentifully:

17 And he thought within himself, saying, What shall I do, because I have no room where to bestow my fruits?

18 And he said, This will [t]I do: I will pull down my barns, and build greater; and there will I bestow all my fruits and my goods.

19 And I will say to my soul, [u]Soul, thou hast much goods laid up for many years; take thine ease, [v]eat, drink, *and* be merry.

20 But God said unto him, *Thou* fool, this night [w]thy soul shall be required of thee: then whose shall those things be, which thou hast provided?

21 So *is* he that layeth up treasure for himself, and is not [x]rich toward God.

22 [y]And he said unto his disciples, Therefore I say unto you, [z]Take no thought for your life, what ye shall eat; neither for the body, what ye shall put on.

23 The life is more than meat, and the [aa]body *is more* than raiment.

24 Consider the ravens: for they neither sow nor reap; which neither have storehouse nor barn; and God feedeth them: how much more are ye better than the fowls?

25 And which of you with taking thought can add to his stature one [bb]cubit?

26 If ye then be not able to do that

A.D. 33.

a Gen. 4:8.
b 2 Chr. 24:20, 21.
c *Inspiration.* vs. 49-51. Lk. 16:29-31. (Ex. 4:15; Rev. 22:19.)
d Mal. 2:7; Mk. 7:13.
e 1 Cor. 13:5.
f Mt. 16:6.
g *Leaven.* Lk. 13:21. (Gen. 19:3; Mt. 13:33.)
h Lk. 11:39.
i Mt. 10:26; 1 Cor. 4:5.
j Psa. 49:16.
k Mt. 5:22, *note.*
l Two farthings here = 1 cent.
m Mt. 8:20, *note.*
n Heb. 1:4, *note.*
o *Holy Spirit.* vs. 10, 12; John 1:32, 33. (Mt. 1:18; Acts 2:4.)
p Lk. 21:14, 15; Mt. 10:19.
q John 18:36.
r *Life (eternal).* John 1:4. (Mt. 7:14; Rev. 22:19.)
s *Parables* (N.T.). vs. 16-21, 35-40, 42-48; Lk. 13:6-9. Mt. 5:13-16; Lk. 21:29-31.)
t Jas. 4:15.
u Psa. 49:15, 16.
v Eccl. 11:9; Jas. 5:1, 5.
w Psa. 52:5, 7; Jas. 4:14.
x Hab. 2:9.
y Cf. Mt. 6:25-33.
z Mt. 6:25; Phil. 4:6.
aa Psa. 139:14.
bb One cubit = about 18 in.

thing which is least, why take ye
thought for the rest?
27 Consider the lilies how they grow:
they toil not, they spin not; and yet I say
unto you, that Solomon in all his glory
was not arrayed like one of these.
28 If then God so clothe the grass,
which is to day in the field, and to morrow is cast into the oven; how much more
will he clothe you, O ye of little faith?
29 And seek not ye what ye shall eat,
or what ye shall drink, neither be ye of
doubtful mind.
30 For all these things do the nations
of the [a]world seek after: and your Father
knoweth that ye have need of these
[b]things.
31 But [c]rather seek ye the kingdom of
God; and all these things shall be added
unto you.
32 Fear not, little flock; for it is your
Father's good pleasure to give you the
[d]kingdom.
33 [e]Sell that ye have, and give alms;
provide yourselves bags which wax not
old, a treasure in the heavens that faileth
not, where no thief approacheth, neither
moth corrupteth.
34 [f]For where your treasure is, there
will your heart be also.

Parable and warnings connected with the second coming (Mt. 24:37–25:30).

35 [g]Let your loins be girded about,
and *your* lights burning;
36 And ye yourselves like unto men
that wait for their lord, when he will
return from the wedding; that when he
cometh and knocketh, they may open
unto him immediately.
37 Blessed *are* those servants, whom the
lord when he cometh shall find watching:
verily I say unto you, that he shall gird
himself, and [h]make them to sit down to
meat, and will come forth and serve them.
38 And if he shall come in the second
watch, or come in the third watch, and
find *them* so, blessed are those servants.
39 And [i]this know, that if the goodman of the house had known what hour
the [j]thief would come, he would have
watched, and not have suffered his
house to be broken through.
40 Be ye therefore ready also: for the
[k]Son of man [l]cometh at an hour when ye
think not.
41 Then Peter said unto him, Lord,
speakest thou this parable unto us, or
even to all?

Parable of the steward and his servants.

42 And the Lord said, Who then is that
faithful and wise [m]steward, whom *his*
lord shall make ruler over his household, to give *them their* portion of meat
in due season?
43 Blessed *is* that servant, whom his
lord when he cometh shall find so doing.
44 Of a truth I say unto you, that he
will make him [n]ruler over all that he
hath.
45 But and if that servant say in his
heart, My lord [o]delayeth his coming;
and shall begin to beat the menservants
and maidens, and to eat and drink, and
to be drunken;
46 The lord of that servant will come in
a [p]day when he looketh not for *him*, and
at an hour when he is not aware, and
will [q]cut him in sunder, and will appoint
him his portion with the unbelievers.
47 And that servant, [r]which knew his
lord's will, and prepared not *himself*, neither did according to his will, shall be
beaten with many *stripes*.
48 But [s]he that knew not, and did
commit things worthy of stripes, shall be
beaten with few *stripes*. [t]For unto whomsoever much is given, of him shall be
much required: and to whom men have
committed much, of him they will ask
the more.

Christ a divider of men.

49 I am come to send [u]fire on the
earth; and what will I, if it be already
kindled?
50 But I have a [v]baptism to be baptized with; and how am I straitened till it
be accomplished!
51 [w]Suppose ye that I am come to give
peace on earth? I tell you, Nay; but
rather division:
52 For from henceforth there shall be
five in one house divided, three against
two, and two against three.
53 The [x]father shall be divided against
the son, and the son against the father;
the mother against the daughter, and the
daughter against the mother; the mother
in law against her daughter in law, and
the daughter in law against her mother
in law.
54 And he said also to the people,
[y]When ye see a cloud rise out of the

A.D. 33.

a i.e. *earth.*
b Psa. 23:1.
c Mt. 6:33.
d Mt. 3:2; *note.*
e Mt. 19:21; Acts 2:44-45; 4:34, 35.
f Col. 3:1, 3.
g Eph. 6:14.
h v. 33; 1 Tim. 6:18; Jas. 2:5.
i Mt. 24:43.
j 1 Thes. 5:2.
k Mt. 8:20, *note.*
l *Christ (Second Advent).* vs. 35-40; Lk. 17:24-36. (Deut. 30:3; Acts 1:9-11.)
m 1 Cor. 4:2.
n Rev. 3:21.
o Eccl. 8:11; 2 Pet. 3:3, 4.
p 1 Thes. 5:3.
q Or, *cut him off.*
r Jas. 4:17.
s Acts 17:30.
t Lev. 5:17; John 15:22; 1 Tim. 1:13.
u v. 51.
v Mt. 20:18, 22; Mk. 10:38, 39.
w Mt. 10:34.
x Mic. 7:6.
y Mt. 16:2.

west, straightway ye say, There cometh a shower; and so it is.

55 And when *ye see* the south wind blow, ye say, There will be heat; and it cometh to pass.

56 *Ye* hypocrites, ye can discern the face of the sky and of the earth; [a]but how is it that ye do not discern this time?

57 Yea, and why even of yourselves judge ye not what is right?

58 [b]When thou goest with thine adversary to the magistrate, [c]*as thou art* in the way, give diligence that thou mayest be delivered from him; lest he hale thee to the judge, and the judge deliver thee to the officer, and the officer cast thee into prison.

59 I tell thee, thou shalt not depart thence, till thou hast paid the very last [d]mite.

CHAPTER 13.

Men are not to judge, but repent.

There were present at that season some that told him of the [e]Galilæans, whose blood Pilate had mingled with their sacrifices.

2 And Jesus answering said unto them, Suppose ye that these Galilæans were [f]sinners above all the Galilæans, because they suffered such things?

3 I tell you, Nay: but, except ye [g]repent, ye shall all likewise perish.

4 Or those eighteen, upon whom the tower in Siloam fell, and slew them, think ye that they were [f]sinners above all men that dwelt in Jerusalem?

5 I tell you, Nay: but, except ye [g]repent, ye shall all likewise perish.

Parable of the barren fig tree.
(Cf. Isa. 5:1-7; Mt. 21:18-20.)

6 He spake also this [h]parable; A certain *man* had a fig tree planted in his vineyard; and he came and sought fruit thereon, and found none.

7 Then said he unto the dresser of his vineyard, Behold, these three years I come seeking fruit on this fig tree, and find none: cut it [i]down; why cumbereth it the ground?

8 And he answering said unto him, Lord, let it alone this year also, till I shall dig about it, and dung *it*:

9 And if it bear fruit, *well*: and if not, *then* after that [j]thou shalt cut it down.

The woman loosed from her infirmity.

10 And he was teaching in one of the synagogues on the sabbath.

11 And, behold, there was a woman which had a spirit of infirmity eighteen years, and was bowed together, and could in no wise lift up *herself*.

12 And when Jesus saw her, he called *her to him*, and said unto her, Woman, thou art loosed from thine infirmity.

13 And he laid *his* hands on her: and [k]immediately she was made straight, and glorified God.

14 And the ruler of the synagogue answered with indignation, because that Jesus had [l]healed on the sabbath day, and said unto the people, [m]There are six days in which men ought to work: in them therefore come and be healed, and not on the sabbath day.

15 The Lord then answered him, and said, *Thou* hypocrite, [n]doth not each one of you on the sabbath loose his ox or *his* ass from the stall, and lead *him* away to watering?

16 And ought not this woman, being a [o]daughter of Abraham, whom [p]Satan hath bound, lo, these eighteen years, be loosed from this bond on the sabbath day?

17 And when he had said these things, all his adversaries were [q]ashamed: and all the people rejoiced for all the glorious things that were done by him.

Parable of the mustard seed
(Mt. 13:31, 32, *note*; Mk. 4:30-32).

18 Then said he, [r]Unto what is the kingdom of God like? and whereunto shall I resemble it?

19 It is like a grain of mustard seed, which a man took, and cast into his garden; and it grew, and [s]waxed a great tree; and the fowls of the air lodged in the branches of it.

Parable of the leaven (Mt. 13:33, *note*).

20 And again he said, Whereunto shall I liken the kingdom of God?

21 It is like [t]leaven, which a woman took and hid in three measures of meal, till the whole was leavened.

Teachings on the way to Jerusalem.

22 And he went through the cities and

A.D. 33.

a Mt. 16:3.
b Mt. 5:25.
c Isa. 55:6.
d One mite = 1-4 farthing or 1-8 cent.
e Acts 5:37.
f *Sin.* Rom. 3:23, *note.*
g *Repentance.* Lk. 15:7. (Mt. 3:2; Acts 17:30.)
h *Parables* (N.T.). vs. 6-9, 18, 19, 20, 21; Lk. 14:16-24. (Mt. 5:13-16; Lk. 21:29-31.)
i Ex. 32:10, 14.
j John 15:2.
k *Miracles* (N.T.). vs. 11-13; Lk. 14:1-14. (Mt. 8:2, 3; Acts 28:8, 9.)
l Lk. 6:7, 9; 14:3, 6; Mt. 12:10; Mk. 3:2, 4; John 5:16.
m Ex. 20:9.
n Prov. 11:9; Mt. 7:5; 23:13, 28.
o Lk. 19:9; Rom. 4:11, 12.
p *Satan.* Lk. 22:3, 31. (Gen. 3:1; Rev. 20:10.)
q Isa. 45:24; 1 Pet. 3:16.
r Mt. 13:31; Mk. 4:30.
s Isa. 2:2, 4.
t *Leaven.* 1 Cor. 5:6-8. (Gen. 19:3; Mt. 13:33.)

villages, teaching, and journeying toward Jerusalem.

23 Then said one unto him, Lord, are there [a]few that be [b]saved? And he said unto them,

24 [c]Strive to enter in at the [d]strait gate: for many, I say unto you, will seek to enter in, and shall not be able.

25 When [e]once the master of the house is risen up, and hath [f]shut to the door, and ye begin to stand without, and to knock at the door, saying, Lord, Lord, open unto us; and he shall answer and say unto you, I know you not whence ye are:

26 Then shall ye begin to say, We have eaten and drunk in thy presence, and thou hast taught in our streets.

27 But [g]he shall say, I tell you, I know you not whence ye are; depart from me, all ye [h]workers of iniquity.

28 There shall be weeping and gnashing of teeth, when ye shall see Abraham, and Isaac, and Jacob, and all the prophets, in the kingdom of God, and you *yourselves* thrust out.

29 And [i]they shall come from the east, and *from* the west, and from the north, and *from* the south, and shall sit down in the kingdom of God.

30 And, behold, [j]there are last which shall be first, and there are first which shall be last.

31 The same day there came certain of the Pharisees, saying unto him, Get thee out, and depart hence: for [k]Herod will kill thee.

32 And he said unto them, Go ye, and tell that fox, Behold, I cast out devils, and I do cures to day and to morrow, and the third *day* I shall be [l]perfected.

33 Nevertheless I must walk to day, and to morrow, and the *day* following: for it cannot be that a prophet perish out of Jerusalem.

Jesus' lament over Jerusalem
(Mt. 23:37-39. Cf. Lk. 19:41-44).

34 O [m]Jerusalem, Jerusalem, which killest the prophets, and stonest them that are sent unto thee; how often would [n]I have [o]gathered thy children together, as a hen *doth gather* her brood under *her* wings, and ye would not!

35 Behold, your house is left unto you desolate: and verily I say unto you, Ye shall not see me, [p]until *the time* come

A.D. 33.

a Mt. 7:14; 20:16; Rev. 7:9.
b Rom. 1:16, *note.*
c Mt. 7:13, 14.
d Mt. 7:13; 16:24; Lk. 9:23; 14:33; 1 Pet. 3:20.
e Psa. 32:6; Isa. 55:6.
f Mt. 25:10; Rev. 22:11.
g Psa. 5:4, 5; Mt. 7:21, 23; 25:12, 41.
h Psa. 101:4, 8.
i Rev. 7:9, 10.
j Mt. 19:30; 21:31, 32; Rom. 9:30, 33.
k See Mt. 14:1, *ref.*
l John 17:4, 5; 19:30; Heb. 2:10; 5:8, 9.
m Mt. 23:37.
n John 10:30.
o Deut. 32:11, 12; Psa. 91:4.
p See Mt. 23:39, *note.*
q *Jehovah.* Psa. 118:26.
r *Miracles* (N.T.). vs. 1-4; Lk. 17:11-19. (Mt. 8:2, 3; Acts 28:8, 9.)
s Prov. 15:33; Jas. 4:6.
t Isa. 57:15; Mt. 5:3.
u Neh. 8:10, 12.
v Mt. 25:34, 40.

when ye shall say, Blessed *is* he that cometh in the name of the [q]Lord.

CHAPTER 14.

Jesus heals on the sabbath.

And it came to pass, as he went into the house of one of the chief Pharisees to eat bread on the sabbath day, that they watched him.

2 And, behold, there was a certain man before him which had the dropsy.

3 And Jesus answering spake unto the lawyers and Pharisees, saying, Is it lawful to heal on the sabbath day?

4 And they held their peace. And he took *him*, and [r]healed him, and let him go;

5 And answered them, saying, Which of you shall have an ass or an ox fallen into a pit, and will not straightway pull him out on the sabbath day?

6 And they could not answer him again to these things.

Parable of the ambitious guest.

7 And he put forth a parable to those which were bidden, when he marked how they chose out the chief rooms; saying unto them,

8 When thou art bidden of any *man* to a wedding, sit not down in the highest room; lest a more honourable man than thou be bidden of him;

9 And he that bade thee and him come and say to thee, Give this man place; and thou begin with shame to take the lowest room.

10 But when thou art bidden, go and sit down in the lowest room; that when he that bade thee cometh, he may say unto thee, Friend, go up higher: then shalt thou have worship in the presence of them that sit at meat with thee.

11 For whosoever [s]exalteth himself shall be abased; and he that [t]humbleth himself shall be exalted.

12 Then said he also to him that bade him, When thou makest a dinner or a supper, call not thy friends, nor thy brethren, neither thy kinsmen, nor *thy* rich neighbours; lest they also bid thee again, and a recompence be made thee.

13 But when thou makest a feast, call the [u]poor, the maimed, the lame, the blind:

14 And [v]thou shalt be blessed; for they

cannot recompense thee: for thou shalt be [a]recompensed at the [b]resurrection of the just.

15 And when one of them that sat at meat with him heard these things, he said unto him, Blessed *is* he that shall eat bread in the [c]kingdom of God.

Parable of the great supper.
(Cf. Mt. 22:1-14.)

16 Then said he unto him, [d]A certain man made a great supper, and bade many:

17 And [e]sent his servant at supper time to say to them that were bidden, Come; for all things are now ready.

18 [f]And they all with one *consent* began to make excuse. The first said unto him, I have bought a piece of ground, and I must needs go and see it: I pray thee have me excused.

19 And another said, I have bought five yoke of oxen, and I go to prove them: I pray thee have me excused.

20 And another said, I have married a wife, and therefore I cannot come.

21 So that servant came, and shewed his lord these things. Then the master of the house being angry said to his servant, Go out quickly into the [g]streets and lanes of the city, and bring in hither the [h]poor, and the maimed, and the [i]halt, and the blind.

22 And the servant said, Lord, it is done as thou hast commanded, and [j]yet there is room.

23 And the lord said unto the servant, Go out into the highways and hedges, and [k]compel *them* to come in, that my house may be filled.

24 For I say unto you, That [l]none of those men which were bidden shall taste of my supper.

Discipleship again tested.
(Cf. Mt. 10:37-39.)

25 And there went great multitudes with him: and he turned, and said unto them,

26 If any *man* come to me, and [1m]hate not his father, and mother, and wife, and children, and brethren, and sisters, yea, and his own life also, he cannot be my disciple.

A.D. 33.

a *Judgment. (the seven).* John 5:22, 24, R.V. (2 Sam. 7:14; Rev. 20:12.)

b *Resurrection.* John 2:19-22. (Job 19:25; 1 Cor. 15:52.)

c Mt. 6:33, *note.*

d *Parables* (N.T.). vs. 16-24, 28-30, 31-33; Lk. 15:3-7. (Mt. 5:13-16; Lk. 21:29-31.)

e Lk. 10:1, 6; Mt. 3:1, 3; 10:1-15.

f Isa. 30:15; Mt. 23:37; 13:14, 15; John 5:40.

g Rev. 22:17.

h 1 Sam. 2:8; Mt. 5:3; Mk. 12:37; Jas. 2:5.

i Isa. 35:6.

j Psa. 130:7.

k Psa. 110:3.

l Prov. 1:24, 28; Mt. 21:43; Heb. 12:25.

m Mt. 10:37; Acts. 14:22.

n Lk. 9:23; Mt. 16:24; Mk. 8:34, 35; 2 Tim. 3:12.

o Heb. 6:11.

p Prov. 20:18.

q Phil. 3:7, 8.

r Mt. 5:13; Mt. 9:50; Col. 4:6.

s John 15:6.

t Mt. 9:10, 11.

u *Sin.* Rom. 3:23, *note.*

v *Parables* (N.T.). vs. 3-7, 8-10, 11-32. Lk. 16:1-13. (Mt. 5:13-16; Lk. 21:29-31.)

w Mt. 18:12.

27 And [n]whosoever doth not bear his cross, and come after me, cannot be my disciple.

Parable of the tower.

28 For which of you, intending to build a tower, sitteth not down first, and counteth the cost, whether he have *sufficient* to finish *it*?

29 Lest haply, after he hath laid the foundation, and is not able to finish *it*, all that behold *it* begin to mock him,

30 Saying, This man began to build, and was not able to [o]finish.

Parable of the king going to war.

31 Or what king, going to make war against another king, sitteth not down first, and [p]consulteth whether he be able with ten thousand to meet him that cometh against him with twenty thousand?

32 Or else, while the other is yet a great way off, he sendeth an ambassage, and desireth conditions of peace.

33 So likewise, whosoever he be of you that forsaketh not [q]all that he hath, he cannot be my disciple.

Parable of the savourless salt.
(Cf. Mt. 5:13; Mk. 9:50.)

34 [r]Salt *is* good: but if the salt have lost his savour, wherewith shall it be seasoned?

35 It is neither fit for the land, nor yet for the dunghill; *but* [s]men cast it out. He that hath ears to hear, let him hear.

CHAPTER 15.

The murmuring Pharisees.

Then drew [t]near unto him all the publicans and [u]sinners for to hear him.

2 And the Pharisees and scribes murmured, saying, This man receiveth [u]sinners, and eateth with them.

Parable of the lost sheep.
(Cf. Mt. 18:12-14.)

3 And he spake this [v]parable unto them, saying,

4 What [w]man of you, having an hundred sheep, if he lose one of them, doth not leave the ninety and nine in the

[1] **(14:26)** All terms which define the emotions or affections are *comparative.* Natural affection is to be, as compared with the believer's devotedness to Christ, as if it were hate. See Mt. 12:47-50, where Christ illustrates this principle in His own person. But in the Lord the natural affections are sanctified and lifted to the level of the divine love (cf. John 19:26, 27; Eph. 5:25-28).

wilderness, and go after that which is
[a]lost, until he find it?
5 And when he hath found *it*, he
layeth *it* on his shoulders, rejoicing.
6 And when he cometh home, he calleth together *his* friends and neighbours,
saying unto them, Rejoice with me; for I
have found my [b]sheep which was lost.
7 I say unto you, that likewise joy shall
be in heaven over one sinner that [c]re-
penteth, more than over ninety and nine
just persons, which need no [c]repentance.

Parable of the lost coin.

8 Either what woman having ten
[d]pieces of silver, if she lose one piece,
doth not light a candle, and sweep the
house, and seek diligently till she find *it*?
9 And when she hath found *it*, she
calleth *her* friends and *her* neighbours
together, saying, Rejoice with me; for I
have found the piece which I had lost.
10 Likewise, I say unto you, [e]there is
joy in the presence of the [f]angels of God
over one [g]sinner that repenteth.

Parable of the lost son.

11 And he said, A certain man had two
sons:

(The departure.)

12 And the younger of them said to *his*
father, Father, give me the portion of
goods that falleth *to me*. And he divided
unto them *his* living.
13 And not many days after the
younger son gathered all together, and
took his journey into a far country, and
there wasted his substance with riotous
living.

(The misery of the far country.)

14 And when he had spent all, there
arose a mighty famine in that land; and
he began to be in want.
15 And he went and joined himself to
a citizen of that country; and he sent him
into his fields to feed swine.
16 And he would fain have filled his
belly with the husks that the swine did
eat: and no man gave unto him.

(The repentance.)

17 And when he came to himself, he
said, How many hired servants of my
father's have bread enough and to spare,
and I perish with hunger!

A.D. 33.

a Gr. *apollumi*. John 3:16, *note*.

b Psa. 119:176; 1 Pet. 2:25.

c *Repentance*. Lk. 16:30. (Mt. 3:2; Acts 17:30.)

d *drachma*, here translated *a piece of silver*, is the eighth part of an ounce, and is equal to the Roman penny. See Mt. 18:28.

e Ezk. 18:23; Acts 11:18.

f Heb. 1:4, *note*.

g Sin. Rom. 3:23, *note*.

h Lk. 18:11.

i *Bible prayers (N.T.)*. Lk. 17:5. (Mt. 6:9; Rev. 22:20.)

j Psa. 51:4.

k Zech. 3:3-5.

l *Death (spiritual)*. John 5:24. (Gen. 2:17; Eph. 2:5.)

m Lk. 18:11.

18 I [h]will arise and go to my father,
and will [i]say unto him, Father, I have
[g]sinned against heaven, and before thee,
19 And am no more worthy to be
called thy son: make me as one of thy
hired servants.

(The return and the father.)

20 And he arose, and came to his father.
But when he was yet a great way off, his
father saw him, and had compassion, and
ran, and fell on his neck, and kissed him.
21 And the son said unto him, Father, I
have [g]sinned against [j]heaven, and in thy
sight, and am no more worthy to be
called thy son.
22 But the father said to his servants,
[k]Bring forth the best robe, and put *it* on
him; and put a ring on his hand, and
shoes on *his* feet:

(The rejoicing.)

23 And bring hither the fatted calf,
and kill *it*; and let us eat, and be merry:
24 For this my son was [l]dead, and is
alive again; he was lost, and is found.
And they began to be merry.

(The Pharisee.)

25 Now his elder son was in the field:
and as he came and drew nigh to the
house, he heard musick and dancing.
26 And he called one of the servants,
and asked what these things meant.
27 And he said unto him, Thy brother
is come; and thy father hath killed the
fatted calf, because he hath received him
safe and sound.
28 And he was angry, and would not
go in: therefore came his father out, and
intreated him.
29 And he answering said to *his* father,
Lo, these many years do [m]I serve thee,
neither transgressed I at any time thy
commandment: and yet thou never
gavest me a kid, that I might make
merry with my friends:
30 But as soon as this thy son was
come, which hath devoured thy living
with harlots, thou hast killed for him the
fatted calf.
31 And he said unto him, Son, thou art
ever with me, and all that I have is thine.
32 It was meet that we should make
merry, and be glad: for this thy brother
was dead, and is alive again; and was
lost, and is found.

CHAPTER 16.

Parable of the unjust steward.

And he said also unto his disciples, [a]There was a certain rich man, which had a steward; and the same was accused unto him that he had wasted his goods.

2 And he called him, and said unto him, How is it that I hear this of thee? give an account of thy stewardship; for thou mayest be no longer steward.

3 Then the steward said within himself, What shall I do? for my lord taketh away from me the stewardship: I cannot dig; to beg I am ashamed.

4 I am resolved what to do, that, when I am put out of the stewardship, they may receive me into their houses.

5 So he called every one of his lord's debtors *unto him*, and said unto the first, How much owest thou unto my lord?

6 And he said, An hundred [b]measures of oil. And he said unto him, Take thy bill, and sit down quickly, and write fifty.

7 Then said he to another, And how much owest thou? And he said, An hundred [c]measures of wheat. And he said unto him, Take thy bill, and write fourscore.

8 And the lord commended the unjust steward, because he had done wisely: for the children of this world are in their generation wiser than the [d]children of light.

9 And I say unto you, [e]Make to yourselves friends of the [f]mammon of [g]unrighteousness; that, when ye [h]fail, they may receive you into everlasting habitations.

10 He that is faithful in that which is least is faithful also in much: and he that is unjust in the least is unjust also in much.

11 If therefore ye have not been faithful in the unrighteous mammon, who will commit to your trust [i]the true *riches*?

12 And if ye have not been faithful in that which is [j]another man's, who shall give you that which is [k]your own?

13 [l]No servant can serve two masters: for either he will hate the one, and love the other; or else he will hold to the one, and despise the other. [m]Ye cannot serve God and mammon.

Jesus answers the Pharisees.

14 And the Pharisees also, who were covetous, heard all these things: and they derided him.

15 And he said unto them, Ye are they which justify [n]yourselves before men; but [o]God knoweth your hearts: for that which is highly esteemed [p]among men is abomination in the sight of God.

16 The law and the prophets *were* until John: since that time [q]the kingdom of God is preached, and every man presseth into it.

17 And it is easier for heaven and earth to pass, than one tittle of the law to fail.

Jesus and divorce. (Cf. Mt. 5:31, 32; 19:3-11; Mk. 10:2-12; 1 Cor. 7:1-15.)

18 Whosoever [r]putteth away his wife, and marrieth another, committeth adultery: and whosoever marrieth her that is put away from *her* husband committeth adultery.

The rich man and Lazarus.

19 [s]There was a certain rich man, which was clothed in purple and fine linen, and fared sumptuously every day:

20 And there was a certain beggar named Lazarus, which was laid at his gate, full of sores,

21 And desiring to be fed with the crumbs which fell from the rich man's table: moreover the dogs came and licked his sores.

22 And it came to pass, that the beggar died, and was carried by the [t]angels into [u]Abraham's bosom: the [v]rich man also [w]died, and was buried;

23 [x]And in [1]hell he lift up his eyes, being in torments, and seeth Abraham afar off, and Lazarus in his bosom.

24 And he cried and said, Father Abraham, have mercy on me, and send

A.D. 33.

- a *Parables* (N.T.). vs. 1-13; Lk. 17:7-10. (Mt. 5:13-16; Lk. 21:29-31.)
- b One measure = about 8 1-2 gals. See Ezk. 45:10, 14.
- c One measure = about 10 bu.
- d John 12:36; Eph. 5:8.
- e 1 Tim. 6:18, 19.
- f Or, *riches*.
- g Lk. 12:15; Prov. 22:16; Jer. 17:11; Mk. 10:24; Jas. 5:1, 4.
- h Psa. 73:26.
- i 2 Cor. 6:10; Eph. 1:18; 1 Tim. 6:17.
- j Lk. 19:13.
- k 1 Pet. 1:4.
- l Josh. 24:15.
- m Gal. 1:10; 2 Tim. 4:10; Jas. 4:4.
- n Rom. 4:2; Gal. 3:11.
- o 1 Sam. 16:7; Jer. 17:10.
- p Psa. 10:3; Prov. 16:5; Mal. 3:15; Tit. 1:16.
- q See Mt. 11:12, *note*.
- r Mt. 5:32.
- s vs. 19-31 are not said to be a parable. Rich men and beggars are common; there is no reason why Jesus may not have had in mind a particular case. *In no parable is an individual named.*
- t Heb. 1:4, *note*.
- u Mt. 8:11.
- v Prov. 14:32.
- w *Death (physical).* vs. 22, 23; John 11:11-14. (Gen. 3:19; Heb. 9:27.)
- x Rev. 14:10, 11.

[1]**(16:23)** Gr. *hades*, "the unseen world," is revealed as the place of departed human spirits between death and resurrection. The word occurs, Mt. 11:23; 16:18; Lk. 10:15; Acts 2:27, 31; Rev. 1:18; 6:8; 20:13, 14, and is the equivalent of the O.T. *sheol* (Hab. 2:5, *note*). The Septuagint invariably renders *sheol* by *hades*.

Summary: (1) *Hades before the ascension of Christ*. The passages in which the word occurs make it clear that hades was formerly in two divisions, the abodes respectively of the saved and of the lost. The former was called "paradise" and "Abraham's bosom." Both designations were Talmudic, but

Lazarus, that he may dip the tip of his
finger in water, and cool my tongue; for
I am tormented in this [a]flame.
25 But Abraham said, Son, remember
that thou in thy [b]lifetime receivedst thy
good things, and likewise Lazarus evil
things: but now he is comforted, and
thou art tormented.
26 And beside all this, between us and
you there is a great gulf fixed: so that
they which would pass from hence to
you cannot; neither can they pass to us,
that *would come* from thence.
27 Then he said, I pray thee therefore,
father, that thou wouldest send him to
my father's house:
28 For I have five brethren; that he
may testify unto them, lest they also
come into this place of torment.
29 Abraham saith unto him, They
have Moses and the prophets; let them
hear [c]them.
30 And he said, Nay, father Abraham:
but if one went unto them from the
dead, they will [d]repent.
31 And he said unto him, [c]If they hear
not Moses and the prophets, neither will
they be persuaded, though one rose
from the dead.

CHAPTER 17.

An instruction in forgiveness.
(Cf. Mt. 18:7, 15.)

Then said he unto the disciples, [e]It is
impossible but that offences will
come: but woe *unto him*, through whom
they come!
2 It were better for him that a millstone were hanged about his neck, and
he cast into the sea, than that he should
offend one of these little ones.
3 Take heed to yourselves: If thy
brother [f]trespass against thee, rebuke
him; and if he [g]repent, [h]forgive him.
4 And if he [f]trespass against thee
seven times in a day, and seven times in
a day turn again to thee, saying, I [g]re-
pent; thou shalt [i]forgive him.
5 And the apostles [j]said unto the Lord,
Increase our faith.
6 And the Lord said, If ye had [k]faith as
a grain of mustard seed, ye might say
unto this sycamine tree, Be thou plucked
up by the root, and be thou planted in
the sea; and it should obey you.

A parable of service.

7 But [l]which of you, having a servant
plowing or feeding cattle, will say unto
him by and by, when he is come from
the field, Go and sit down to meat?
8 And will not rather say unto him,
Make ready wherewith I may sup, and
gird thyself, and serve me, till I have
eaten and drunken; and afterward thou
shalt eat and drink?
9 Doth he thank that servant because
he did the things that were commanded
him? I trow not.
10 So likewise ye, when ye shall have
done all those things which are commanded you, say, We [m]are unprofitable
servants: we have done that which was
our duty to do.

Ten lepers healed

11 And it came to pass, as he went to
Jerusalem, that he passed through the
midst of Samaria and Galilee.

A.D. 33.

a Mk. 9:42-48.
b Lk. 6:24; Job 21:13; Psa. 73:12.
c *Inspiration.* vs. 29-31; Lk. 17:27, 29, 32. (Ex. 4:15; Rev. 22:19.)
d *Repentance.* Lk. 17:3, 4. (Mt. 3:2; Acts 17:30.)
e Mt. 12:35; 1 Cor. 11:19; Gal. 5:19, 21.
f *Sin.* Rom. 3:23, *note.*
g *Repentance.* Lk. 24:47. (Mt. 3:2; Acts 17:30.)
h Rom. 12:21; 1 Cor. 6:6, 8.
i *Forgiveness.* vs. 3, 4; Lk. 23:34. (Lev. 4:20; Mt. 26:28.)
j *Bible prayers* (N.T.). Lk. 17:13. (Mt. 6:9; Rev. 22:20.)
k *Faith.* John 1:12. (Gen. 3:20; Heb. 11:39.)
l *Parables* (N.T.). vs. 7-10; Lk. 18:1-8. (Mt. 5:13-16; Lk. 21:29-31.)
m 1 Chr. 29:14; Psa. 16:2, 3; Isa. 64:6; 1 Cor. 9:16, 17.

adopted by Christ in Lk. 16:22; 23:43. The blessed dead were with Abraham, they were conscious and were "comforted" (Lk. 16:25). The believing malefactor was to be, that day, with Christ in "paradise." The lost were separated from the saved by a "great gulf fixed" (Lk. 16:26). The representative man of the lost who are now in hades is the rich man of Lk. 16:19-31. He was alive, conscious, in the full exercise of his faculties, memory, etc., and in torment.

(2) *Hades since the ascension of Christ.* So far as the unsaved dead are concerned, no change of their place or condition is revealed in Scripture. At the judgment of the great white throne, hades will give them up, they will be judged, and will pass into the lake of fire (Rev. 20:13, 14). But a change has taken place which affects paradise. Paul was "caught up to the third heaven . . . into paradise" (2 Cor. 12:1-4). Paradise, therefore, is now in the immediate presence of God. It is believed that Eph. 4:8-10 indicates the time of the change. "When he ascended up on high he led a multitude of captives." It is immediately added that He had previously "descended first into the lower parts of the earth," i.e. the paradise division of hades. During the present church-age the saved who died are "absent from the body, at home with the Lord." The wicked dead in hades, and the righteous dead "at home with the Lord," alike await the resurrection (Job 19:25; 1 Cor. 15:52). See Mt. 5:22, *note.*

12 And as he entered into a certain village, there met him ten men that were lepers, which stood afar off:

13 And they lifted up *their* voices, and [a]said, Jesus, Master, have mercy on us.

14 And when he saw *them*, he said unto them, Go shew yourselves unto the priests. And it came to pass, that, as they went, they were cleansed.

15 And one of them, when he saw that he was healed, turned back, and with a loud voice glorified God,

16 And fell down on *his* face at his feet, giving him thanks: and he was a Samaritan.

17 And Jesus answering said, Were there not ten cleansed? but where *are* the nine?

18 There are not found that returned to give glory to God, save this stranger.

19 And he said unto him, Arise, go thy way: thy faith [b]hath made thee whole.

The kingdom in its spiritual aspect.
(Cf. Lk. 19:11, 12.)

20 And when he was demanded of the Pharisees, when the kingdom of God should come, he answered them and said, The kingdom of God cometh not with [c]observation:

21 Neither shall they say, Lo here! or, lo there! for, behold, [d]the kingdom of God is [1e]within you.

Jesus foretells his second coming
(Deut. 30:3; Acts 1:9-11, *note*).

22 And he said unto the disciples, The days will come, when ye shall desire to see one of the days of the [f]Son of man, and ye shall not see *it*.

23 [g]And they shall say to you, See here; or, see there: go not after *them*, nor follow *them*.

24 For as the lightning, that lighteneth out of the one *part* under heaven, shineth unto the other *part* under heaven; so shall also the Son of man be in his day.

25 But first must he suffer many things, and be rejected of this generation.

26 And as it was in the days of Noe, [h]so shall it be also in the days of the [f]Son of man.

27 They did eat, they drank, they married wives, they were given in marriage, until the day that Noe entered into the ark, and the flood came, and destroyed them all.

28 Likewise also as it was in the days of Lot; they did eat, they drank, they bought, they sold, they planted, they builded;

29 But the same day that Lot went out of Sodom it rained fire and brimstone from heaven, and destroyed *them* all.

30 Even [i]thus shall it be in the day when the [f]Son of man is revealed.

31 In that day, he which shall be upon the housetop, and his stuff in the house, let him not come down to take it away: and he that is in the field, let him likewise not return back.

32 [j]Remember Lot's wife.

33 Whosoever shall seek to save his life shall lose it; and whosoever shall lose his life shall preserve it.

34 I tell you, [k]in that night there shall be two *men* in one bed; the one shall be taken, and the other shall be left.

35 Two *women* shall be grinding together; the one shall be taken, and the other left.

36 Two *men* shall be in the field; the one shall be taken, and the other left.

37 And they answered and said unto him, Where, Lord? And he said unto them, [2]Wheresoever the body *is*, [l]thither will the eagles be gathered together.

CHAPTER 18.

Parable of the unjust judge.

And he spake a [m]parable unto them *to this end*, that men ought always to pray, and not to faint;

A.D. 33.

a *Bible prayers* (N.T.). Lk. 18:11, (Mt. 6:9; Rev. 22:20.)

b *Miracles* (N.T.). vs. 11-19; Lk. 18:35-43. (Mt. 8:2, 3; Acts 28:8, 9.)

c Or, *outward show.*

d Rom. 14:17.

e *in the midst of.*

f Mt. 8:20, *note.*

g Lk. 21:8; Mt. 24, 23; Mk. 13:21.

h vs. 26, 27; Gen. 7:11; Mt. 24:37; 1 Thes. 5:3; 2 Pet. 2:5; 3:6.

i *Christ (Second Advent)* vs. 24-36; Lk. 18:8. (Deut. 30:3; Acts 1:9-11.)

j *Inspiration.* vs. 27, 29, 32; Lk. 20:37. (Ex. 4:15; Rev. 22:19.)

k Mt. 24:40.

l 2 Ki. 21:14; Job 39:30; Isa. 10:6; Jer. 4:6, 7; Mt. 24:28.

m *Parables* (N.T.) vs. 1-8, 9-14; Lk. 19:11-27. (Mt. 5:13-16; Lk. 21:29-31.)

[1] **(17:21)** Gr. *entos* = "in the midst." It could not be said of a self-righteous, Christ-rejecting Pharisee, that the kingdom of God, as to its spiritual content, was within him. Our Lord's whole answer, designedly enigmatic to the Pharisees (cf. Mt. 13:10-13), has a dispensational meaning. The kingdom in its outward form, as covenanted to David (2 Sam. 7:8-17) and described by the prophets (Zech, 12:8, *note*), had been rejected by the Jews; so that, during this present age, it would not "come with observation" (lit. "outward show") but in the hearts of men. (cf. Lk. 19:11, 12; Acts 1:6-8, *note;* Rom. 14:17). Meantime, the kingdom was actually "in the midst" of the Pharisees in the persons of the King and His disciples. Ultimately the kingdom of heaven *will* come, with outward show. (See v. 24.)

[2] **(17:37)** See "Armageddon" (Rev. 16:14; 19:17, *note*).

2 Saying, There was in a city a judge, which feared not God, neither regarded man:

3 And there was a widow in that city; and she came unto him, saying, Avenge me of mine adversary.

4 And he would not for a while: but afterward he said within himself, Though I fear not God, nor regard man;

5 Yet because this widow troubleth me, I will avenge her, lest by her continual coming she weary me.

6 And the Lord said, Hear what the unjust judge saith.

7 And shall not God [a]avenge his own elect, which cry day and night unto him, though he bear long with them?

8 I tell you that he will avenge them speedily. Nevertheless when the [b]Son of man [c]cometh, shall he find [1d]faith on the earth?

Parable of the Pharisee and the publican.

9 And he spake this parable unto certain which trusted in themselves that they were [e]righteous, and despised others:

10 Two men went up into the temple to pray; the one a Pharisee, and the other a publican.

11 The Pharisee stood and [f]prayed thus with himself, God, I thank thee, that I am not as other men *are*, extortioners, unjust, adulterers, or even as this publican.

12 I fast twice in the week, I give tithes of all that I possess.

13 And the publican, standing afar off, would not lift up so much as *his* eyes unto heaven, but smote upon his breast, [g]saying, God be [2h]merciful to me a [i]sinner.

14 I tell you, this man went down to his house [j]justified *rather* than the other: for every one that exalteth himself shall be abased; and he that humbleth himself shall be exalted.

Jesus blesses little children
(Mt. 19:13-15; Mk. 10:13-16).

15 [k]And they brought unto him also infants, that he would touch them: but when *his* disciples saw *it*, they rebuked them.

16 But Jesus called them *unto him*, and said, Suffer little children to come unto me, and forbid them not: for of [l]such is the kingdom of God.

17 Verily I say unto you, Whosoever shall not receive the kingdom of God as a little child [m]shall in no wise enter therein.

The rich young ruler
(Mt. 19:16-30; Mk. 10:17-31).

18 [n]And a certain ruler asked him, saying, Good Master, what shall I do to inherit eternal life?

19 And Jesus said unto him, Why callest thou me good? none *is* good, save [o]one, *that is*, God.

20 Thou knowest the [p]commandments, Do not commit adultery, Do not kill, Do not steal, Do not bear false witness, Honour thy father and thy mother.

21 And he said, All [q]these have I kept from my youth up.

22 Now when Jesus heard these things, he said unto him, [r]Yet lackest thou one thing: sell all that thou hast, and distribute unto the poor, and thou shalt have treasure in heaven: and come, follow me.

23 And when he heard this, [s]he was very sorrowful: for he was very rich.

24 And when Jesus saw that he was very sorrowful, he said, [t]How hardly shall they that have riches enter into the kingdom of God!

25 For it is easier for a camel to go through a needle's eye, than for a rich man to enter into the kingdom of God.

26 And they that heard *it* said, Who then can be [u]saved?

27 And he said, The [v]things which are impossible with men are possible with God.

28 Then Peter said, Lo, we have [w]left all, and followed thee.

29 And he said unto them, Verily I say unto you, There is no man that hath [x]left house, or parents, or brethren, or wife,

A.D. 33.

a Rev. 6:10.
b Mt. 8:20, *note.*
c *Christ (Second Advent).* Lk. 21:25-28. (Deut. 30:3; Acts 1:9-11.)
d *Apostasy.* 2 Thes. 2:1-12. (Lk. 18:8; 2 Tim 3:1-8.)
e Rom. 10:3, *note.*
f *Bible prayers (N.T.).* Lk. 18:13. (Mt. 6:9; Rev. 22:20.)
g *Bible prayers (N.T.).* Lk. 23:34. (Mt. 6:9; Rev. 22:20.)
h i.e. *propitiated.*
i *Sin.* Rom. 3:23, note.
j *Justification.* vs. 10-14; Acts 13:39 (Lk. 18:14; Rom. 3:28.)
k Mt. 19:13; Mk. 10:13.
l Mt. 18:3; 1 Pet. 2:2.
m Psa. 131:2.
n Lk. 10:25, 37; Mt. 19:16; Mk. 10:17; Rom. 6:22, 23; 1 John 5:11, 13.
o Psa. 86:5; 119:68.
p Ex. 20:3-17.
q Gal. 3:24; Phil. 3:6.
r Jas. 2:10.
s Ezk. 33:31; Mt. 6:24; 13:22; Eph. 5:5.
t Psa. 62:10; Mk. 10:24; 1 Tim. 6:9, 10.
u Rom. 1:16, *note.*
v Gen. 18:14; Job 42:2.
w Phil. 3:8.
x 1 Cor. 2:9, 10.

1 (18:8) The reference is not to personal faith, but to belief in the whole body of revealed truth. (Cf. Rom. 1:5; 1 Cor. 16:13; 2 Cor. 13:5; Col. 1:23; 2:7; Tit. 1:13; Jude 3. See "Apostasy," above, in *marg.* of Lk. 18:8; 2 Tim. 3:1, *note.*)

2 (18:13) Gr. *hilaskomai,* used in the Septuagint and N.T. in connection with the mercy-seat (Ex. 25:17, 18, 21; Heb. 9:5). As an instructed Jew the publican is thinking, not of mere mercy, but of the blood-sprinkled mercy-seat (Lev. 16:5, *note;* "Propitiation," Rom. 3:25, *note*). His prayer might be paraphrased, "Be toward me as thou art when thou lookest upon the atoning blood." The Bible knows nothing of divine forgiveness apart from sacrifice (see Mt. 26:28, *note*).

or children, for the kingdom of God's
sake,
30 Who shall not receive [a]manifold
more in this present time, and in the
[b]world to come life everlasting.

Jesus again foretells his death and resurrection (Mt. 20:17-19; Mk. 10:32-34).

31 Then he took *unto him* the twelve,
and said unto them, Behold, we go up to
Jerusalem, and [c]all things that are written by the prophets concerning the [d]Son
of man shall be accomplished.
32 For he shall be [e]delivered unto the
Gentiles, and shall be mocked, and spitefully entreated, and spitted on:
33 And they shall scourge *him*, and
put him to death: and the third day he
shall rise again.
34 And they understood none of these
things: and this saying was hid from
them, neither knew they the things
which were spoken.

A blind man healed near Jericho.
(Cf. Mt. 20:29-34; Mk. 10:46-52.)

35 And it [f]came to pass, that as he was
come nigh unto Jericho, a certain [g]blind
man sat by the way side begging:
36 And hearing the multitude pass by,
he asked what it meant.
37 And they told him, that Jesus of
Nazareth passeth by.
38 And he cried, saying, Jesus, *thou*
Son of David, have mercy on me.
39 And they which went before
rebuked him, that he should hold his
peace: but he cried [h]so much the more,
Thou Son of David, have mercy on me.
40 And Jesus stood, and commanded
him to be brought unto him: and when
he was come near, he asked him,
41 Saying, What wilt thou that I shall
do unto thee? And he said, Lord, that I
may receive my sight.
42 And Jesus said unto him, Receive
thy sight: thy faith hath [i]saved thee.
43 And immediately he [j]received his
sight, and followed him, glorifying God:
and all the people, when they saw *it*,
gave praise unto God.

CHAPTER 19.

Conversion of Zacchæus.

AND *Jesus* entered and passed
through Jericho.
2 And, behold, *there was* a man named
Zacchæus, which was the chief among
the publicans, and he was rich.
3 And he sought to see Jesus who he
was; and could not for the press, because
he was little of stature.
4 And he ran before, and climbed up
into a sycomore tree to see him: for he
was to pass that *way*.
5 And when Jesus came to the place,
he looked up, and saw him, and said
unto him, Zacchæus, make haste, and
come down; for to day I must [k]abide at
thy house.
6 And he made haste, and came down,
and received him joyfully.
7 And when they saw *it*, they all murmured, saying, [l]That he was gone to be
guest with a man that is a sinner.
8 And Zacchæus stood, and said unto
the Lord; Behold, Lord, the half of my
goods I give to the [m]poor; and if I have
taken any thing from any man by false
accusation, I [n]restore *him* fourfold.
9 And Jesus said unto him, This day is
[o]salvation come to this house, forso-
much as he also is a son of Abraham.
10 For the [p]Son of man is come to seek
and to save that which was lost.

Parable of the ten pounds:
the postponed kingdom. (See Lk. 17:21,
note; Acts 1:6-8, *note*.)

11 And as they heard these things, he
added and spake a [q]parable, because he
was nigh to Jerusalem, and [r]because
they thought that the kingdom of God
should immediately appear.
12 He said therefore, [s]A certain nobleman went into a far country to receive
for himself a kingdom, and to return.
13 And he called his ten servants, and
delivered them ten [t]pounds, and said
unto them, [u]Occupy till I come.
14 But his citizens hated him, and sent
a message after him, saying, We will not
have this *man* to reign over us.
15 And it came to pass, that when he
was returned, having received the

A.D. 33.

a John 16:33; Phil. 4:7.
b i.e. *age*.
c Psa. 22; Isa. 53.
d Mt. 8:20, *note*.
e Lk. 23:1; Mt. 17:22.
f Mt. 20:29; Mk. 10:46.
g Mt. 20:30, *note*.
h Jer. 29:13; Lk. 18:1; Col. 4:2.
i Rom. 1:16 *note*.
j Miracles (N.T.). vs. 35-43; Lk. 22:50, 51. (Mt. 8:2, 3; Acts 28:8, 9.)
k John 14:23.
l Mt. 9:11, 13.
m Psa. 41:1.
n Ex. 22:1.
o Rom. 1:16, *note*.
p Mt. 8:20, *note*.
q *Parables* (N.T.). vs. 11-27; Lk. 20:9-18. (Mt. 5:13-16; Lk. 21:29-31.)
r Acts 1:6.
s Mt. 25:14; Mk. 13:34.
t *mina*, here translated a pound, is 12 ounces and a half.
u 1 Pet. 4:10, 11.

kingdom, then he commanded these servants to be called unto him, to whom he
had given the [a]money, that he might
know how much every man had gained
by trading.
16 Then came the first, saying, Lord,
thy pound hath gained ten pounds.
17 And he said unto him, Well, thou
good servant: because thou hast been
faithful in a very little, have thou authority over ten cities.
18 And the second came, saying, Lord,
thy pound hath gained five pounds.
19 And he said likewise to him, Be
thou also over five cities.
20 And another came, saying, Lord,
behold, *here is* thy pound, which I have
kept laid up in a napkin:
21 For I [b]feared thee, because thou art
an austere man: thou takest up that thou
layedst not down, and reapest that thou
didst not sow.
22 And he saith unto him, [c]Out of
thine own mouth will I judge thee, *thou*
wicked servant. Thou knewest that I was
an austere man, taking up that I laid not
down, and reaping that I did not sow:
23 Wherefore then gavest not thou my
money into the bank, that at my coming
I might have required mine own with
usury?
24 And he said unto them that stood
by, Take from him the pound, and give *it*
to him that hath ten pounds.
25 (And they said unto him, Lord, he
hath ten pounds.)
26 For I say unto you, [d]That unto
every one which hath shall be given; and
from him that hath not, even that he
hath shall be taken away from him.
27 But those mine [e]enemies, which
would not that I should reign over them,
bring hither, and slay *them* before me.

[f]*The triumphal entry* (Mt. 21:1-9; Mk. 11:1-10; John 12:12-19).

28 And when he had thus spoken, he
went before, ascending up to Jerusalem.
29 And [g]it came to pass, when he was
come nigh to Bethphage and Bethany, at
the mount called *the mount* of Olives, he
sent two of his disciples,
30 Saying, Go ye into the village over
against *you;* in the which at your entering
ye shall find a colt tied, whereon yet never
man sat: loose him, and bring *him hither.*

A.D. 33.

a *silver;* also v. 23.
b Rom. 8:15; 2 Tim. 1:6, 7; Jas. 2:19.
c 2 Sam. 1:16; Job 15:6; Mt. 12:37; Rom. 3:19.
d Lk. 8;18; Mt. 13:12; Mk. 4:25.
e 1 Cor. 15:25; Heb. 10:13; Rev. 19:11, 21.
f Mt. 21:4, *note.*
g Mt. 21:1; Mk. 11:1; John 12:14.
h Zech. 9:9.
i Psa. 118:26.
j Lk. 2:14; Rom. 5:1; Eph. 2:14.
k Lk. 2:14.
l John 11:35.
m Lk. 13:34.
n Deut. 5:29; Psa. 95:7, 8; Heb. 3:13.
o Lk. 1:77, 79; Isa. 48:18; Acts 10:36; Rom. 5:1.
p Mic. 3:12; Mt. 23:37.
q Lk. 1:68; Isa. 55:6; John 12:35; 2 Cor. 6:1, 2.
r Mt. 21:12; Mk. 11:15.

31 And if any man ask you, Why do
ye loose *him?* thus shall ye say unto him,
Because the Lord hath need of him.
32 And they that were sent went their
way, and found even as he had said unto
them.
33 And as they were loosing the colt,
the owners thereof said unto them, Why
loose ye the colt?
34 And they said, The Lord hath need
of him.
35 And they brought him to Jesus: and
they cast their garments upon the colt,
and they [h]set Jesus thereon.
36 And as he went, they spread their
clothes in the way.
37 And when he was come nigh, even
now at the descent of the mount of
Olives, the whole multitude of the disciples began to rejoice and praise God
with a loud voice for all the mighty
works that they had seen;
38 Saying, [i]Blessed *be* the King that
cometh in the name of the Lord: [j]peace
in heaven, and [k]glory in the highest.
39 And some of the Pharisees from
among the multitude said unto him,
Master, rebuke thy disciples.
40 And he answered and said unto
them, I tell you that, if these should hold
their peace, the stones would immediately cry out.

Jesus weeps over Jerusalem. (Cf. Lk. 13:34, 35.)

41 And when he was come near, he
beheld the city, and [l]wept over it,
42 Saying, [m]If thou hadst known, even
thou, at least in this [n]thy day, the things
which [o]*belong* unto thy peace! but now
they are hid from thine eyes.
43 For the days shall come upon thee,
that thine enemies shall cast a trench
about thee, and compass thee round,
and keep thee in on every side,
44 [p]And shall lay thee even with the
ground, and thy children within thee;
and they shall not leave in thee one
stone upon another; because thou
knewest not [q]the time of thy visitation.

Second purification of the temple (Mt. 21:12-16; Mk. 11:15-18. Cf. John 2:13-17).

45 And [r]he went into the temple, and
began to cast out them that sold therein,
and them that bought;

46 Saying unto them, It is written, My house is the [a]house of prayer: but ye have made it a [b]den of thieves.

47 And he taught daily in the temple. But the chief priests and the scribes and the chief of the people sought to destroy him,

48 And could not find what they might do: for all the people [c]were very attentive to hear him.

CHAPTER 20.

Jesus' authority questioned (Mt. 21:23-27; Mk. 11:27-33).

And [d]it came to pass, *that* on one of those days, as he taught the people in the temple, and preached the [e]gospel, the chief priests and the scribes came upon *him* with the elders,

2 And spake unto him, saying, Tell us, [f]by what authority doest thou these things? or who is he that gave thee this authority?

3 And he answered and said unto them, I will also ask you one thing; and answer me:

4 The baptism of John, was it from heaven, or of men?

5 And they reasoned with themselves, saying, If we shall say, From heaven; he will say, Why then believed ye him not?

6 But and if we say, Of men; all the people will stone us: for they [g]be persuaded that John was a prophet.

7 And they answered, that they could not tell whence *it was*.

8 And Jesus said unto them, Neither tell I you by what authority I do these things.

Parable of the vineyard (Mt. 21:33-46; Mk. 12:1-12. Cf. Isa. 5:1-7).

9 Then began he to speak to the people this [h]parable; A [i]certain man planted a [j]vineyard, and let it forth to husbandmen, and went into a far country for a long time.

10 And at the season he [k]sent a servant to the husbandmen, that they should give him of the [l]fruit of the vineyard: but the husbandmen beat him, and sent *him* away empty.

11 And again he sent another servant: and they beat him also, and entreated *him* shamefully, and sent *him* away empty.

12 And again he sent a third: and they wounded him also, and cast *him* out.

A.D. 33.

a Isa. 56:7.
b Jer. 7:11.
c Or, *hanged on him.*
d Mt. 21:23; Mk. 11:27.
e *Gospel.* Lk. 24:47. (Gen. 12:1-3; Rev. 14:6.)
f Acts. 4:7, 10.
g Mt. 3:5, 6; Mk. 6:20.
h *Parables* (N.T.). vs. 9-18; Lk. 21:29-31. (Mt. 5:13; Lk. 21:29-31.)
i Mt. 21:33; Mk. 12:1.
j Isa. 5:1, 7.
k 2 Ki. 17:13.
l John 15:1, 8.
m Heb. 1:1, 2.
n Heb. 1:2.
o Mt. 27:21, 25.
p Acts 2:23; 4:25, 27.
q Prov. 1:24, 31; Dan. 9:26.
r Rom. 11:11.
s Psa. 118:22, 23. See Mt. 21:44, *note.*
t Dan. 2:34, 35.
u John 7:30.
v Mt. 18:28.
w Mt. 17:25, 27; Rom. 13:7.
x 1 Pet. 2:13, 17.
y Col. 4:6.

13 Then said the lord of the vineyard, What shall I do? I will [m]send my beloved son: it may be they will reverence *him* when they see him.

14 But when the husbandmen saw him, they reasoned among themselves, saying, [n]This is the heir: come, [o]let us kill him, that the inheritance may be ours.

15 So they [p]cast him out of the vineyard, and killed *him*. What therefore shall the lord of the vineyard do unto them?

16 He shall come and [q]destroy these husbandmen, and shall give the vineyard to [r]others. And when they heard *it*, they said, God forbid.

17 And he beheld them, and said, What is this then that is written, The [s]stone which the builders rejected, the same is become the head of the corner?

18 Whosoever shall fall upon that stone shall be broken; [t]but on whomsoever it shall fall, it will grind him to powder.

Question of the tribute-money (Mt. 22:15-22; Mk. 12:13-17).

19 And the chief priests and the scribes the same hour [u]sought to lay hands on him; and they feared the people: for they perceived that he had spoken this parable against them.

20 And they watched *him*, and sent forth spies, which should feign themselves just men, that they might take hold of his words, that so they might deliver him unto the power and authority of the governor.

21 And they asked him, saying, Master, we know that thou sayest and teachest rightly, neither acceptest thou the person *of any*, but teachest the way of God truly:

22 Is it lawful for us to give tribute unto Cæsar, or no?

23 But he perceived their craftiness, and said unto them, Why tempt ye me?

24 Shew me a [v]penny. Whose image and superscription hath it? They answered and said, Cæsar's.

25 And he said unto them, [w]Render therefore unto Cæsar the things which be Cæsar's, and unto [x]God the things which be God's.

26 And they could not take hold of his words before the people: and they [y]marvelled at his answer, and held their peace.

Jesus answers the Sadducees about the resurrection (Mt. 22:23-33; Mk. 12:18-27).

27 [a]Then came to *him* certain of the [b]Sadducees, which deny that there is any resurrection; and they asked him,

28 Saying, Master, [c]Moses wrote unto us, If any man's brother die, having a wife, and he die without children, that his brother should take his wife, and raise up seed unto his brother.

29 There were therefore seven brethren: and the first took a wife, and died without children.

30 And the second took her to wife, and he died childless.

31 And the third took her; and in like manner the seven also: and they left no children, and died.

32 Last of all the woman died also.

33 Therefore in the resurrection whose wife of them is she? for seven had her to wife.

34 And Jesus answering said unto them, The children of this [d]world marry, and are given in marriage:

35 But they which shall be accounted [e]worthy to obtain that [d]world, and the resurrection from the dead, neither marry, nor are given in marriage:

36 Neither can they die any more: for they are equal unto the [f]angels; and are the children of God, being the children of the resurrection.

37 Now that the dead are raised, [g]even Moses shewed at the bush, when he calleth the Lord the [h]God of Abraham, and the God of Isaac, and the God of Jacob.

38 For he is not a God of the dead, but of the living: for all live unto him.

Jesus questions the scribes (Mt. 22:41-46; Mk. 12:35-37).

39 Then certain of the scribes answering said, Master, thou hast well said.

40 And after that they durst not ask him any *question at all*.

41 [i]And he said unto them, How say they that Christ is David's son?

42 And David himself saith in the book of Psalms, [j]The LORD said unto my [k]Lord, Sit thou on my right hand,

43 Till I make thine enemies thy footstool.

44 David therefore calleth him Lord, [l]how is he then his son?

45 Then in the audience of all the people he said unto his disciples,

46 [m]Beware of the scribes, which desire to walk in long robes, and [n]love greetings in the markets, and the [o]highest seats in the synagogues, and the chief rooms at feasts;

47 Which [p]devour widows' houses, and for a shew make long prayers: the same shall receive [q]greater [r]damnation.

CHAPTER 21.

The widow's mite: Jesus' estimate of giving (Mk. 12:41-44).

And he looked up, and saw the [s]rich men casting their gifts into the treasury.

2 And he saw also a certain poor [t]widow casting in thither two [u]mites.

3 And he said, Of a truth I say unto you, that [v]this poor widow hath cast in more than they all:

4 For all these have of their abundance cast in unto the offerings of God: but she of her penury hath cast in [w]all the living that she had.

The Olivet discourse. (Cf. Mt. 24, 25; Mk. 13).

5 And as some spake of the [x]temple, how it was adorned with goodly stones and gifts, he said,

6 *As for* these things which ye behold, the days will come, in the which there shall not be left one [y]stone upon another, that shall not be thrown down.

The disciples' question. (Cf. Mt. 24:3.)

7 And they asked him, saying, Master, but when shall these things be? and what sign *will there be* when these things shall come to pass?

The course of this age. (Cf. Mt. 24:4-14.)

8 [z]And he said, Take heed that ye be not [aa]deceived: for many shall come in my name, saying, I am *Christ*; and the time draweth near: go ye not therefore after them.

9 But when ye shall hear of [bb]wars and commotions, be not terrified: for these things must first come to pass; but the end *is* not [cc]by and by.

10 Then said he unto them, [dd]Nation

A.D. 33.

a Mt. 22:23; Mk. 12:18.
b Acts 4: 1-2; 23:6, 8.
c Deut. 25:5, 6,
d i.e. *age.*
e Lk. 21:36; Rev. 3:4.
f Heb. 1:4, *note.*
g *Inspiration.* Lk. 24:25-27, 44, 45. (Ex. 4:15; Rev. 22:19.)
h *Elohim.* Ex. 3:6.
i Mt. 22:42, 45; Mk. 12:35.
j vs. 42, 43; Psa. 110:1.
k *Adonai.* Psa. 110:1.
l Acts 2:34; 13:22, 23; Rom. 1:3; 9:5.
m Mt. 23:1, Lk. 12:1.
n Lk. 11:43.
o Lk. 14:7.
p Mt. 23:14.
q Lk. 10:12-14.
r i.e. *condemnation.*
s Mk. 12:41-44; Lk. 6:24; 12:16-21; 16:19-31; 18:23-27; 19:2-10.
t Lk. 18:3; 2 Cor. 6:10.
u One mite = 1-4 farthing, or 1-8 cent.
v 2 Cor. 8:12.
w Cf. Lk. 18:12; 2 Cor. 5:14, 15.
x Mt. 24:1; Mk. 13:1; John 2:19-21.
y Lk. 19:44.
z Mt. 24:3, *note* on the Olivet discourse.
aa 2 Cor. 11:13-15; 2 Thes. 2:3; 2 Tim. 3:13.
bb 2 Chr. 15:5, 6; Mt. 24:6, 7; Mk. 13:7.
cc i.e. *come yet.*
dd Hag. 2:21, 22; Zech. 14:2, 3; Rev. 6:4.

shall rise against nation, and kingdom
against kingdom:
11 And great [a]earthquakes shall be in
divers places, and famines, and pestilences; and fearful sights and great signs
shall there be from heaven.
12 But before all these, they shall [b]lay
their hands on you, and persecute *you*,
delivering *you* up to the synagogues,
and into [c]prisons, being brought before
kings and rulers [d]for my name's sake.
13 And it shall turn to you for [e]a testimony.
14 Settle *it* therefore in your hearts, not
to [f]meditate before what ye shall
answer:
15 For I will give you a mouth and
wisdom, [g]which all your adversaries
shall not be able to gainsay nor resist.
16 And [h]ye shall be betrayed both by
parents, and brethren, and kinsfolks,
and friends; and [i]*some* of you shall they
cause to be put to death.
17 And ye shall be [j]hated of all *men* for
my name's sake.
18 But there shall not an [k]hair of your
head perish.
19 In your [l]patience possess ye your
souls.

The destruction of Jerusalem foretold.

20 And [1]when ye shall see [m]Jerusalem
compassed with armies, then know that
the desolation thereof is nigh.
21 Then let them which are in Judæa
flee to the mountains; and let them
which are in the midst of it depart out;
and let not them that are in the countries
enter thereinto.
22 For these be the days of vengeance,
that [n]all things which are written may be
fulfilled.
23 But woe unto them that are with
child, and to them that give suck, in
those days! for there shall be great distress in the land, and wrath upon this
people.
24 And they shall fall by the edge of
the sword, and shall be led away captive
into all nations: and Jerusalem shall be
[2]trodden down of the Gentiles, until the
[o]times of the Gentiles be fulfilled.

The return of the Lord in glory.
(Cf. Mt. 24:29-31.)

25 And there shall be [p]signs in the
sun, and in the moon, and in the stars;
and upon the earth distress of nations,
with perplexity; the sea and the waves
roaring;
26 [q]Men's hearts failing them for fear,
and for looking after those things which
are coming on the [r]earth: for the [s]pow-
ers of heaven shall be shaken.
27 And then shall they see the [t]Son of
man [u]coming [v]in a cloud with power
and great glory.
28 And when these things begin to
come to pass, then look up, and lift up
your heads; for your [w]redemption
draweth nigh.

Parable of the fig tree
(Mt. 24:32, 33; Mk. 13:28, 29).

29 And he spake to them a [x]parable;
Behold the fig tree, and all the trees;
30 When they now shoot forth, ye see
and know of your own selves that summer is now nigh at hand.
31 So likewise ye, when ye see these
things come to pass, know ye that the
[y]kingdom of God is nigh at hand.
32 Verily I say unto you, This generation shall not pass away, till all be fulfilled.
33 [z]Heaven and earth shall pass away:
but my words shall not pass away.

A.D. 33.

a Rev. 6:5, 6, 12.
b Mt. 10:16-22; John 16:2; 1 Pet. 4, 12-14.
c Acts 4:3; 5:18; 12:4; 16:24.
d 1 Pet. 2:13.
e Phil. 1:12, 13, 28; 2 Thes. 1:4, 5.
f Mt. 10:19; Mk. 13;11; Lk. 12:11.
g Acts 6:10.
h Mic. 7:6; Mk. 13:12.
i Acts 7:59; 12:2.
j Mt. 10:22; John 7:7.
k Mt. 10:30.
l Heb. 10:36.
m *Israel (prophecies).* Acts 2:29-32. (Gen. 12:2, 3; Rom. 11:26.)
n Hos. 9:7; Isa. 65:12-15.
o *Times of the Gentiles.* vs. 20-24; Deut. 28:28-68. (Lk. 21:24; Rev. 16:19.)
p Isa. 13:9, 10, 13; Mt. 24:29; Mk. 13:24; 2 Pet. 3:10, 12.
q Lk. 23:30; Rev. 6:12-17.
r *oikoumene = inhabited earth.*
s Mt. 24:20.
t Mt. 8:20, *note.*
u *Christ (Second Advent).* vs. 25-28; Lk. 24:25, 26. (Deut. 30:3; Acts 1:9-11.)
v Mt. 24:29-31; Mk. 13:24-27; 2 Thes. 1:7-10; Rev. 1:7-10.
w Rom. 3:24, *note;* 8:19, 23.
x *Parables* (N.T.). vs. 29-31. (Mt. 5:13-16; Lk. 21:29-31.)
y Heb. 10:37; Jas. 5:8, 9.
z Isa. 40:8; 51:6; Mt. 24:35; Heb. 1:11; 1 Pet. 1:23, 25.

[1]**(21:20)** Verses 20, 24 are not included in the report of the Olivet discourse as given by Matthew and Mark. Two sieges of Jerusalem are in view in that discourse. Luke 21:20-24 refers to the siege by Titus, A.D. 70, when the city was taken, and verse 24 literally fulfilled. But that siege and its horrors but adumbrate the final siege at the end of this age, in which the "great tribulation" culminates. At that time the city will be taken, but delivered by the glorious appearing of the Lord (Rev. 19:11-21). The references in Mt. 24:15-28; Mk. 13:14-26 are to the final tribulation siege; Lk. 21:20-24 to the destruction of Jerusalem by Titus. In Luke the sign is the compassing of Jerusalem by armies (Lk. 21:20); in Matthew (24:15) and Mark (13:14) the sign is the abomination in the holy place. (2 Thes. 2:4).

[2]**(21:24)** The "times of the Gentiles" began with the captivity of Judah under Nebuchadnezzar (2 Chr. 36:1-21), since which time Jerusalem has been under Gentile overlordship.

Warnings in view of the Lord's return.
(Cf. Mt. 24:34-51; Mk. 13:30-37.)

34 And [a]take heed to yourselves, lest
at any time your hearts be overcharged
with surfeiting, and drunkenness, and
[b]cares of this life, and *so* that day come
upon you unawares.
35 For [c]as a snare shall it come on all
them that dwell on the face of the whole
earth.
36 [d]Watch ye therefore, and [e]pray
always, that ye may be accounted worthy to [f]escape all these things that shall
come to pass, and to [g]stand before the
Son of man.
37 And in [h]the day time he was teaching in the temple; and [i]at night he went
out, and abode in the mount that is
called *the mount* of Olives.
38 And all the people came early in
the morning to him in the temple, for to
hear him.

CHAPTER 22.

Judas covenants to betray Jesus
(Mt. 26:2, 14, 15; Mk. 14:1, 2, 10, 11).

Now the feast of unleavened bread
drew nigh, which is called the
Passover.
2 And the [j]chief priests and scribes
sought how they might kill him; for they
[k]feared the people.
3 Then entered [l]Satan into Judas surnamed Iscariot, being of the number of
the twelve.
4 And he went his way, and communed
with the chief priests and captains, how
he might betray him unto them.
5 And they were glad, and [m]covenant-
ed to give him money.
6 And he promised, and sought
opportunity to [n]betray him unto them in
the absence of the multitude.

Preparation of the passover
(Mt. 26:17-19; Mk. 14:12-16).

7 Then came the day of unleavened
bread, when the [o]passover must be killed.
8 And he sent Peter and John, saying,
Go and prepare us the passover, that we
may eat.
9 And they said unto him, Where wilt
thou that we prepare?
10 And he said unto them, Behold,
when ye are entered into the city, there
shall a man meet you, bearing a [p]pitcher
of water; follow him into the house
where he entereth in.
11 And ye shall say unto the goodman
of the house, The Master saith unto thee,
Where is the guestchamber, where I shall
eat the passover with my disciples?
12 And he shall shew you a large
upper room furnished: there make
ready.
13 And they went, and found as he
had said unto them: and they made
ready the passover.

The last passover. (Cf. Mt. 26:20;
Mk. 14:17; John 13.)

14 [1]And when the hour was come, he
sat down, and the twelve apostles with
him.
15 And he said unto them, [q]With
desire I have desired to eat this passover
with you before I suffer:
16 For I say unto you, I [r]will not any
more eat thereof, until it be fulfilled in
the kingdom of God.
17 And he took the [s]cup, and gave
thanks, and said, Take this, and divide *it*
among yourselves:
18 For I say unto you, I will not drink
of the fruit of the vine, [t]until the kingdom of God shall come.

The Lord's supper instituted
(Mt. 26:26-29; Mk. 14:22-25).

19 And he took bread, and gave
thanks, and brake *it*, and gave unto them,
saying, This is my body which is given
for you: [u]this do in remembrance of me.
20 Likewise also the cup after supper,
saying, [v]This cup *is* the [w]new [x]testament
in my blood, which is shed for you.

Jesus announces his betrayal (Mt. 26:21-
25; Mk. 14:18-21; John 13:18-30).

21 [y]But, behold, the hand of him that
betrayeth me *is* with me on the table.
22 And truly the [z]Son of man goeth,
[aa]as it was determined: but woe unto
that man by whom he is betrayed!
23 And they [bb]began to enquire among
themselves, which of them it was that
should do this thing.

The strife which should be greatest.
(Cf. Mt. 20:25-28; Mk. 10:42-45.)

24 And there was also a [cc]strife among

A.D. 33.

a Rom. 13:13; 1 Thes. 5:6; 1 Pet. 4:7.
b Lk. 14:18-20; 17:28.
c 1 Thes. 5:2-3; 2 Pet. 3:10; Rev. 3:3; 16:15.
d Mt. 24:42; 25:13; Mk. 13:33.
e Lk. 18:1.
f Lk. 17:33-37; Rev. 7:3.
g Psa. 1:5; Eph. 6:13.
h John 8:1, 2.
i Lk. 22:39.
j Psa. 2:2; John 11:47; Acts 4:27.
k Lk. 19:48; 20:19.
l Mt. 26:14; Mk. 14:10; John 13:2, 27.
m Zech. 11:12; John 12:6.
n vs. 3-6, 21, 23, 47, 48; Psa. 41:9.
o Ex. 12:6.
p 1 Sam. 10:3; John 2:6-10.
q Heb. 9:11, 12, 26 with Heb. 10:1-9; 1 Cor. 5:7.
r v. 30; Mt. 8:11.
s v. 20.
t Mt. 26:29; Mk. 14:25.
u 1 Cor. 11:24.
v 1 Cor. 10:16.
w *Covenant (new).* Heb. 8:8-12. (Isa. 61:8; Heb. 8:8-12.)
x i.e. *covenant.*
y Psa. 41:9; John 13:21.
z Mt. 8:20, *note.*
aa Acts 2:23; 4:28.
bb Mt. 26:22; John 13:22, 25.
cc Mk. 9:34; Lk. 9:46.

[1] **(22:14)** For order of events on the night of the last passover, see Mt. 26:20, *note.*

them, which of them should be accounted the greatest.

25 And he said unto them, The kings of the Gentiles exercise lordship over them; and they that exercise authority upon them are called benefactors.

26 [a]But ye *shall* not *be* so: [b]but he that is greatest among you, let him be as the younger; and he that is chief, as he that doth serve.

27 For [c]whether *is* greater, he that sitteth at meat, or he that serveth? *is* not he that sitteth at meat? but I am among you as he that [d]serveth.

The apostles' place in the future kingdom (Mt. 19:28. Cf. Rev. 3:21).

28 Ye are they which have continued with me in my [e]temptations.

29 [f]And I appoint unto you a [g]kingdom, as my Father hath appointed unto me;

30 That ye [h]may eat and drink at my table in my [g]kingdom, and [i]sit on thrones judging the twelve tribes of Israel.

Jesus predicts Peter's denial (Mt. 26:33-35; Mk. 14:29-31).

31 And the Lord said, Simon, Simon, behold, [j]Satan [k]hath desired *to have* you, that he may sift *you* as [l]wheat:

32 [m]But I have prayed for thee, that thy faith fail not: and when thou [n]art converted, [o]strengthen thy brethren.

33 And he said unto him, Lord, I am ready to go with thee, both into prison, and to death.

34 And he said, I tell thee, Peter, the cock shall not crow this day, before that thou shalt thrice deny that thou knowest me.

The disciples warned of coming conflicts.

35 And he said unto them, [p]When I sent you without purse, and scrip, and shoes, lacked ye any thing? And they said, Nothing.

36 Then said he unto them, But now, he that hath a purse, let him take *it*, and likewise *his* scrip: and he that hath no sword, let him sell his garment, and buy one.

37 For I say unto you, that this that is written must yet be accomplished in me, And he was [q]reckoned [r]among the transgressors: for the things concerning me have an end.

38 And they said, Lord, behold, here *are* two swords. And he said unto them, It is enough.

Jesus in the garden (Mt. 26:36-46; Mk. 14:32-42; John 18:1).

39 And he came out, and [s]went, as he was wont, to the mount of Olives; and his disciples also followed him.

40 And when he was at the place, he said unto them, Pray that ye enter not into temptation.

41 And he was withdrawn from them about a stone's cast, and kneeled down, and prayed,

42 Saying, Father, if thou be willing, remove this [t]cup from me: nevertheless not my will, but thine, be done.

43 And there appeared an [u]angel unto him from heaven, strengthening him.

44 And being in an agony he prayed more earnestly: and his sweat was as it were great drops of blood falling down to the ground.

45 And when he rose up from prayer, and was come to his disciples, he found them [v]sleeping for sorrow,

46 And said unto them, Why sleep ye? rise and pray, lest ye enter into temptation.

Jesus betrayed by Judas; restores a severed ear (Mt. 26:47-56; Mk. 14:43-50; John 18:3-11).

47 And while he yet spake, behold a multitude, and he that was called Judas, one of the twelve, went before them, and drew near unto Jesus to kiss him.

48 But Jesus said unto him, Judas, betrayest thou the [w]Son of man with a kiss?

49 When they which were about him saw what would follow, they said unto him, Lord, shall we smite with the sword?

50 And [x]one of them smote the servant of the high priest, and cut off his right ear.

51 And Jesus answered and said, Suffer ye thus far. And he touched his ear, and [y]healed him.

52 Then Jesus said unto the chief priests, and captains of the temple, and the elders, which were come to him, Be ye come out, as against a [z]thief, with swords and staves?

53 When I was daily with you in the temple, ye stretched forth no hands against me: but [aa]this is your hour, and the power of darkness.

A.D. 33.

a Mt. 20:26; 1 Pet. 5:3.
b Lk. 9:48.
c Lk. 12:37.
d John 13:13-17; 1 Cor. 9:19; Phil. 2:7.
e *Temptation.* Acts 5:9. (Gen. 3:1; Jas. 1:14.)
f Mt. 24:47; Lk. 12:32; 2 Cor. 1:7; 2 Tim. 2:12.
g Mt. 3:2, *note.*
h Mt. 8:11; Lk. 14:15; Rev. 19:9.
i Mt. 19:28; cf. 1 Cor. 6:2; Rev. 3:21.
j *Satan.* vs. 3:31; John 8:44. (Gen. 3:1; Rev. 20:10.)
k 1 Pet. 5:8.
l Peter was the wheat, his self-confidence the chaff. Cf. Mt. 13:30; John 5:24; 10:28; Rom. 6:1, 2; 1 John 1:8; 2:1.
m John 17:9, 11, 15; Rom. 8:27; Heb. 7:25; 1 John 2:1.
n *hast turned back again.*
o John 21:15-17; 1 Pet. 5:12; 2 Pet. 1:10-15.
p Mt. 10:9; Lk. 9:3; 10:4.
q *Imputation.* vs. 24, 37; Rom. 4:24. (Lev. 25:50; Jas. 2:23.)
r Isa. 53:12; Mk. 15:28.
s Lk. 21:37.
t See Mt. 26:39, *note.*
u Heb. 1:4, *note.*
v Peter was sleeping while his Master was praying (v. 45); resisting while his Master was submitting (vs. 49-51); he followed afar off; sat down amongst his Lord's enemies; and denied his Lord, the faith, and the brotherhood.
w Mt. 8:20, *note.*
x Mt. 26:51; Mk. 14:47; John 18:10.
y *Miracles* (N.T.). vs. 50, 51; John 2:1-10. (Mt. 8:2, 3; Acts 28:8, 9.)
z v. 37; Lk. 23:32.
aa John 12:27; 14:30.

Jesus arrested: Peter's denial (Mt. 26:57, 69-75; Mk. 14:53, 54, 66-72; John 18:12, 15-18, 25-27).

54 Then took they him, and led *him*, and brought him into the high priest's house. And Peter followed [a]afar off.

55 And when they had kindled a fire in the midst of the hall, and were set down together, Peter sat down [b]among them.

56 But a certain maid beheld him as he sat by the fire, and earnestly looked upon him, and said, This man was also with him.

57 And he [c]denied him, saying, Woman, I know him not.

58 And after a little while another saw him, and said, Thou art also of them. And Peter said, Man, I am not.

59 And about the space of one hour after another confidently affirmed, saying, Of a truth this *fellow* also was with him: for he is a [d]Galilæan.

60 And Peter said, Man, I know not what thou sayest. And immediately, while he yet spake, the cock crew.

61 And the Lord turned, and [e]looked upon Peter. And Peter remembered the word of the Lord, [f]how he had said unto him, Before the cock crow, thou shalt deny me thrice.

62 And Peter went out, and [g]wept bitterly.

Jesus buffeted (Mt. 26:67, 68; Mk. 14:65; John 18:22, 23),

63 And the men that held Jesus [h]mocked him, and [i]smote *him*.

64 And when they had blindfolded him, they [j]struck him on the face, and asked him, saying, Prophesy, who is it that smote thee?

65 And many other things blasphemously spake they against him.

Jesus before the Sanhedrin (Mt. 26:59-68; Mk. 14:55-65; John 18:19-24).

66 [k]And as soon as it was day, the [l]elders of the people and the chief priests and the scribes came together, and led him into their council, saying,

67 Art thou the Christ? tell us. And he said unto them, If I tell you, ye will not believe:

68 And if I also ask *you*, ye will not answer me, nor let *me* go.

69 [m]Hereafter shall the [n]Son of man sit on the right hand of the power of God.

70 Then said they all, Art thou then

A.D. 33.

a Cf. Mk. 14:50; John 13:23; 21:19.
b Gen. 12:11; Jas. 4:4.
c v. 34.
d Acts 1:11; 2:7.
e Cf. Psa. 32:8.
f v. 34.
g 2 Cor. 7:10, 11.
h Psa. 69:12.
i Isa. 50:6.
j Zech. 13:7.
k For order of events on the day of the crucifixion, see Mt. 26:57, *note.*
l Acts 4:26; 22:5.
m Acts 7:55, 56 with Rev. 1:7; Heb. 1:3.
n Mt. 8:20, *note.*
o John 10:30.
p Mk. 14:55-59.
q Mt. 17:27; 22:21; Mk. 12:17.
r vs. 1-5; Psa. 27:12.
s John 18:33-36; 19:12.
t vs. 14, 22; 1 Pet. 2:22.
u Cf. John 6:15; Lk. 14:25-27.
v Lk. 4:14.
w Also vs. 8, 11, 12, 15. See Mt. 14:1, *ref;* Lk. 3:1.
x Lk. 9:9.
y Mt. 14:1; Mk. 6:14.
z John 19:9.
aa Isa. 53:3.
bb Acts 4:27; cf. Prov. 1:10-16.

the Son of God? And he said unto them, Ye say that [o]I am.

71 And they said, What [p]need we any further witness? for we ourselves have heard of his own mouth.

CHAPTER 23.

Jesus before Pilate (Mt. 27:2, 11-14; Mk. 15:1-5; John 18:28-38).

And the whole multitude of them arose, and led him unto Pilate.

2 And they began to accuse him, saying, We found this *fellow* perverting the nation, and forbidding to give [q]tribute to Cæsar, saying that he himself is [r]Christ a [s]King.

3 And Pilate asked him, saying, Art thou the King of the Jews? And he answered him and said, Thou sayest *it.*

4 Then said Pilate to the chief priests and *to* the people, [t]I find no fault in this man.

5 And they were the more fierce, saying, [u]He stirreth up the people, teaching throughout all Jewry, beginning from [v]Galilee to this place.

Jesus sent before Herod.

6 When Pilate heard of Galilee, he asked whether the man were a Galilæan.

7 And as soon as he knew that he belonged unto [w]Herod's jurisdiction, he sent him to Herod, who himself also was at Jerusalem at that time.

8 And when Herod saw Jesus, he was exceeding glad: for he was [x]desirous to see him of a long *season*, because he had [y]heard many things of him; and he hoped to have seen some miracle done by him.

9 Then he questioned with him in many words; but he answered him [z]nothing.

10 And the chief priests and scribes stood and vehemently accused him.

11 [aa]And Herod with his men of war set him at nought, and mocked *him*, and arrayed him in a gorgeous robe, and sent him again to Pilate.

12 And the same day [bb]Pilate and Herod were made friends together: for before they were at enmity between themselves.

Jesus again before Pilate: Barabbas released, Jesus condemned (Mt. 27:15-26; Mk. 15:6-15; John 18:39, 40).

13 And Pilate, when he had called

together the chief priests and the rulers and the people,

14 Said unto them, [a]Ye have brought this man unto me, as one that perverteth the people: and, behold, I, having examined *him* before you, have found no [b]fault in this man touching those things whereof ye accuse him:

15 No, nor yet Herod: for I sent you to him; and, lo, nothing worthy of death is done unto him.

16 [c]I will therefore chastise him, and release *him.*

17 ([d]For of necessity he must release one unto them at the feast.)

18 And [e]they cried out all at once, saying, Away with this *man,* and release unto us Barabbas:

19 (Who for a certain sedition made in the city, and for murder, was cast into prison.)

20 Pilate therefore, [f]willing to release Jesus, spake again to them.

21 But they cried, saying, [g]Crucify *him,* crucify him.

22 And he said unto them the third time, Why, what evil hath he done? I have found no cause of death in him: I will therefore chastise him, and let *him* go.

23 And they were instant with loud voices, requiring that he might be crucified. And the [h]voices of them and of the chief priests prevailed.

24 And Pilate gave sentence that it should be as they required.

25 [i]And he released unto them him that for sedition and murder was cast into prison, whom they had desired; but he [j]delivered Jesus to their will.

26 And as they led him away, they laid hold upon one [k]Simon, a Cyrenian, coming out of the country, and on him they laid the cross, that he might bear *it* after Jesus.

The crucifixion (Mt. 27:33-38; Mk. 15:22-28; John 19:17-19).

27 And there [l]followed him a great company of people, and of women, which also bewailed and lamented him.

28 But Jesus turning unto them said, Daughters of Jerusalem, [m]weep not for me, but weep for yourselves, and for your children.

29 For, behold, the days are coming, in the which they shall say, [n]Blessed *are* the barren, and the wombs that never bare, and the paps which never gave suck.

30 Then shall they begin to say to the mountains, [o]Fall on us; and to the hills, Cover us.

31 For if they do these things in a [p]green tree, what shall be done in the [q]dry?

32 And there were also two other, [r]malefactors, led with him to be put to death.

33 [1]And when they were come to the place, which is called [s]Calvary, there they crucified him, and the malefactors, one on the right hand, and the other on the left.

34 Then [t]said Jesus, [u]Father, [v]forgive them; for they know not what they do. And [w]they parted his raiment, and cast lots.

35 And the [2x]people stood beholding. And the rulers also with them [y]derided *him,* saying, He saved others; let him save himself, if he be Christ, the chosen of God.

36 And the soldiers also mocked him, coming to him, and offering him vinegar,

37 And saying, If thou be the king of the Jews, save thyself.

38 And a [z]superscription also was written over him in letters of Greek, and Latin, and Hebrew, THIS IS THE KING OF THE JEWS.

The repentant thief.
(Cf. Mt. 27:44; Mk. 15:32.)

39 And one of the malefactors which were hanged railed on him, saying, If thou be Christ, save thyself and us.

40 But the other answering rebuked him, saying, Dost not thou fear God, seeing thou art in the same condemnation?

41 And we indeed [aa]justly; for we receive the due reward of our deeds: but this man [bb]hath done nothing amiss.

A.D. 33.

a vs. 1,2.
b v. 4; cf. Dan. 6:4.
c Mt. 27:26; John 19:1.
d Mt. 27;15; Mk. 15:6; John 18:39.
e Acts 3:14.
f John 19:8,12.
g Psa. 69:20; John 19:15.
h Ex. 23:2.
i vs. 1-25; Isa. 53:8.
j Acts 4:27, 28.
k Cf. Mt. 27:31, 32; Mk. 15:20-23.
l Lk. 8:1-3.
m Lk. 19:41.
n Mt. 24:19; Lk. 21:23.
o Hos. 10:8; Rev. 6:16, 17.
p Psa. 1:3; 1 Pet. 4:17.
q Mt. 21:19; Jude 12.
r Isa. 53:12.
s Or, *The Skull.*
t *Bible prayers* (N.T.). Lk. 23:42. (Mt. 6:9; Rev. 22:20.)
u Isa. 53:12.
v *Forgiveness.* Acts 13:38, 39. (Lev. 4:20; Mt. 26:28.)
w Psa. 22:18.
x Psa. 22:17; Zech. 12:10.
y Psa. 22:6-8; 69:12, 21; Mt. 27:39-43; Mk. 15:29-32.
z Mt. 27:37; Mk. 15:26; John 19:19.
aa Lk. 18:13.
bb 2 Cor. 5:21; Heb. 7:26; 1 Pet. 2:22.

[1]**(23:33)** For order of events at the crucifixion, see Mt. 27:33, *note.*

[2]**(23:35)** Jesus crucified is the true touchstone revealing what the world is: "The people stood beholding" in stolid indifference; the rulers, who wanted religion, but without a divine Christ crucified for their sins, "reviled"; the brutal amongst them mocked or railed; the conscious sinner prayed; the covetous sat down before the cross and played their sordid game. The cross is the judgment of this world (John 12:31).

42 And he [a]said unto Jesus, Lord,
remember me when thou comest into
thy [b]kingdom.
43 And Jesus said unto him, [c]Verily I
say unto thee, To day shalt thou be with
me in paradise.
44 And it was about the sixth hour,
and there was a darkness over all the
earth until the ninth hour.
45 And the sun was darkened, and the
[d]veil of the temple was rent in the midst.

Jesus dismisses his spirit
(Mt. 27:50; Mk. 15:37; John 19:30).

46 And when Jesus had cried with a
loud voice, [e]he said, Father, [f]into thy
hands I commend my spirit: and having
said thus, he [1]gave up the ghost.
47 Now when the [g]centurion saw
what was done, he glorified God, saying, Certainly this was a [h]righteous man.
48 And all the people that came
together to that sight, beholding the
things which were done, [i]smote their
breasts, and returned.
49 And all his acquaintance, and the
women that followed him from Galilee,
stood afar off, beholding these things.

The entombment (Mt. 27:57-61;
Mk. 15:42-47; John 19:38-42).

50 And, behold, *there was* a man
named Joseph, a counsellor; *and he was* a
good man, and a just:
51 (The same had not consented to the
counsel and deed of them;) *he was* of
Arimathæa, a city of the Jews: [j]who also
himself waited for the kingdom of God.
52 This *man* went unto Pilate, and
begged the body of Jesus.
53 And he took it down, and wrapped
it in linen, and [k]laid it in a sepulchre that
was hewn in stone, [l]wherein never man
before was laid.
54 And that day was the [m]preparation,
and the sabbath drew on.
55 And the [n]women also, which came
with him from Galilee, followed after,
and beheld the sepulchre, and how his
body was laid.
56 And they returned, and [o]prepared
spices and ointments; and rested the
sabbath day [p]according to the commandment.

A.D. 33.

a *Bible prayers* (N.T.). Lk. 23:46. (Mt. 6:9; Rev. 22:20.)
b Mt. 3:2, *note.*
c As to "paradise," cf. Lk. 16:23, *note.* One thief was saved, that none need despair; but only one, that none should presume.
d Mt. 27:51; Mk. 15:38; Heb. 9:3-8, 11, 12; 10:19-22.
e *Bible prayers* (N.T.). John 4:15. (Mt. 6:9; Rev. 22:20.)
f Psa. 31:5; cf. Acts 7:59; 1 Pet 2:23.
g Mt. 27:54; John 7:45, 46.
h Rom. 10:10, *note.*
i Zech 12:10; Rev. 1:7.
j Mk. 15:43; Lk. 2:25, 38.
k Isa. 53:9.
l Acts 2:24-31.
m Mt. 27:62.
n Lk. 8:2.
o Mk. 16:1.
p Ex. 20:10.
q Lk. 23:56; cf. Mt. 26:12; Mk. 14:8; John 12:7.
r John 10:18; 11:38, 39.
s v. 23; Mk. 16:5.
t John 20:12; Acts 1:10.
u Or, *him that liveth.* Rev. 1:18.
v Mt. 16:21; 17:23; Mk. 8:31; 9:31; Lk. 9:22.
w Mt. 8:20, *note.*
x *Sin.* Rom. 3:23, *note.*
y *Resurrection.* vs. 1-7; Acts 2:25-32. (Job 19:25; 1 Cor. 15:52.)
z John 2:22.
aa Lk. 8:3.
bb v. 25; Mk. 16:11.
cc v. 34; Lk. 9:20; John 20:3, 6.
dd Mk. 16:12, 13.
ee One furlong = 582 ft.

CHAPTER 24.

The resurrection of Jesus Christ
(Mt. 28:1-6; Mk. 16:1-8; John 20:1-17).

NOW [2]upon the first *day* of the week,
very early in the morning, they
came unto the sepulchre, [q]bringing the
spices which they had prepared, and
certain *others* with them.
2 And they found the [r]stone rolled
away from the sepulchre.
3 And they entered in, and [s]found not
the body of the Lord Jesus.
4 And it came to pass, as they were
much perplexed thereabout, behold, [t]two
men stood by them in shining garments:
5 And as they were afraid, and bowed
down *their* faces to the earth, they said
unto them, Why seek ye the [u]living
among the dead?
6 He is not here, but is risen: remember [v]how he spake unto you when he
was yet in Galilee,
7 Saying, The [w]Son of man must be
delivered into the hands of [x]sinful men,
and be crucified, and the third day [y]rise
again.
8 And they [z]remembered his words,
9 And returned from the sepulchre,
and told all these things unto the eleven,
and to all the rest.
10 It was Mary Magdalene, and
[aa]Joanna, and Mary *the mother* of James,
and other *women that were* with them,
which told these things unto the apostles.
11 And [bb]their words seemed to them
as idle tales, and they believed them not.
12 Then arose [cc]Peter, and ran unto the
sepulchre; and stooping down, he
beheld the linen clothes laid by themselves, and departed, wondering in himself at that which was come to pass.

Ministry of the risen Christ:
(1) *to the Emmaus disciples.*

13 [3]And, behold, [dd]two of them went
that same day to a village called
Emmaus, which was from Jerusalem
about threescore [ee]furlongs.
14 And they talked together of all
these things which had happened.
15 And it came to pass, that, while
they communed *together* and reasoned,

[1] **(23:46)** See Mt. 27:50, *note.*
[2] **(24:1)** For order of events at the resurrection, see Mt. 28:1, *note.*
[3] **(24:13)** For order of our Lord's appearances after His resurrection, see Mt. 28:9, *note.*

Jesus himself drew near, and went with
them.
16 But their [a]eyes were holden that
they should not know him.
17 And he said unto them, What manner of communications *are* these that ye
have one to another, as ye walk, and are
sad?
18 And the one of them, whose name
was [b]Cleopas, answering said unto him,
Art thou only a stranger in Jerusalem,
and hast not known the things which are
come to pass there in these days?
19 And he said unto them, What
things? And they said unto him,
Concerning Jesus of Nazareth, which
was a [c]prophet mighty in deed and
word before God and all the people:
20 [d]And how the chief priests and our
rulers delivered him to be condemned to
death, and have crucified him.
21 But we [e]trusted that it had been he
which should have [f]redeemed Israel:
and beside all this, to day is the third
day since these things were done.
22 Yea, and [g]certain women also of
our company made us astonished,
which were early at the sepulchre;
23 And when they found not his body,
they came, saying, that they had also
seen a vision of [h]angels, which said that
he was alive.
24 And [i]certain of them which were
with us went to the sepulchre, and
found *it* even so as the women had said:
but him they saw not.
25 Then he said unto them, O fools,
and slow of heart to believe [j]all that the
[k]prophets have spoken:
26 [l]Ought not Christ to have suffered
these things, and to [m]enter into his glory?
27 And [n]beginning at Moses and all
the prophets, he expounded unto them
in all the scriptures the things concerning [o]himself.
28 And they drew nigh unto the village, whither they went: and he made as
though he would have gone further.
29 But they [p]constrained him, saying,
Abide with us: for it is toward evening,
and the day is far spent. And he went in
to tarry with them.
30 And it came to pass, as he sat at
meat with them, he [q]took bread, and
blessed *it*, and brake, and gave to them.
31 And their [r]eyes were opened, and
they knew him; and he vanished out of
their sight.
32 And they said one to another, Did
not our [s]heart burn within us, while he
talked with us by the way, and while he
opened to us the scriptures?
33 And they rose up the same hour,
and returned to Jerusalem, and found
the [t]eleven gathered together, and them
that were with them,
34 Saying, The Lord is risen indeed,
and [u]hath appeared to Simon.
35 And they told what things *were*
done in the way, and how he was known
of them in breaking of bread.

(2) *To the ten.* (Cf. Mt. 28:16-17;
Mk. 16:14; John 20:19-23.)

36 And as they thus spake, Jesus himself [v]stood in the midst of them, and
saith unto them, Peace *be* unto you.
37 But they were terrified and affrighted, and supposed that they had seen [w]a
spirit.
38 And he said unto them, Why are ye
troubled? and why do thoughts arise in
your hearts?
39 Behold my [x]hands and my feet,
that it is I myself: [y]handle me, and see;
for a [z]spirit hath not flesh and bones, as
ye see me have.
40 And when he had thus spoken, he
shewed them *his* hands and *his* feet.
41 And while they yet [aa]believed not
for joy, and wondered, he said unto
them, Have ye here [bb]any meat?
42 And they gave him a piece of a
broiled fish, and of an honeycomb.
43 And he took *it*, and did eat before
them.
44 And he said unto them, These *are*
the words which I spake unto you, while
I was yet with you, that all things must
be fulfilled, which were written in the
law of Moses, and *in* the prophets, and
in the [cc]psalms, concerning me.
45 Then opened he their understanding, that they might understand the
[dd]scriptures,

The commission to evangelize
(Mt. 28:18-20; Mk. 16:15-18; Acts 1:8).

46 And said unto them, Thus it is written, and thus it behoved Christ to suffer,
and to rise from the dead the third day:
47 And that [ee]repentance and [ff]remis-
sion of [gg]sins should be preached in his

A.D. 33.

a John 20:14; 21:4; cf. 2 Cor. 3:18.
b John 19:25.
c Mt. 21:11; Lk. 9:19; Acts 2:22; 7:22.
d Lk. 23:1; Acts 13:27, 28.
e Mt. 3:2, *note.*
f Rom. 3:24, *note.*
g vs. 9, 10; Mt. 28:8; Mk. 16:10; John 20:18.
h Heb. 1:4, *note.*
i v. 12.
j *Inspiration.* vs. 25, 27, 44, 45; John 3:14. (Ex. 4:15; Rev. 22:19.)
k Acts 3:24.
l Heb. 2:9, 10; 1 Pet. 1:10-12.
m *Christ (Second Advent).* vs. 25, 26; John 14:2, 3. (Deut. 30:3; Acts 1:9-11.).
n v. 45.
o Rom, 1:3; Rev. 19:10.
p Gen. 18:1-8; John 14:23.
q Lk. 9:16; 22:19.
r Psa. 119:18; Gal. 1:16; 1 John 3:2.
s 1 Pet. 1:8; John 20:29-31.
t See Mk. 16:14, *note.*
u 1 Cor. 15:5.
v Mk. 16:14; John 20:19, 21, 26.
w Mk. 6:49.
x Cf. Zech. 13:6; 1 John 1:1.
y John 20:20, 27.
z 1 Cor. 15:20, 50.
aa Gen. 45:26; Acts 12:14.
bb Acts 10:40; 41.
cc See Psa. 118:29, Summary.
dd John 16:13; Acts 16:14.
ee *Repentance.* Acts 2:38. (Mt. 3:2; Acts 17:30.)
ff *Gospel.* Acts 8:25. (Gen. 12:1-3; Rev. 14:6.)
gg *Sin.* Rom. 3:23, *note.*

name among all nations, beginning at
Jerusalem.
48 And [a]ye are witnesses of these
things.

The ascension of Jesus Christ
(Mk. 16:19, 20; Acts 1:9-11).

49 And, behold, I send the [b]promise of
my Father [c]upon you: but tarry ye in the
city of Jerusalem, until ye be endued
with power from on high.

A.D. 33.

a Acts 1:21, 22; 2:32; 1 Cor. 15:4-9,
b John 14:16, 17; Acts 1:8.
c Acts 2:4, *note.*
d *until they were opposite Bethany.*
e 2 Ki. 2:11; Acts 1:9; 7:55, 56; Rev. 3:21; cf. Acts 1:10, 11.
f Acts 2:46; 5:42.

50 And he led them out [d]as far as to
Bethany, and he lifted up his hands, and
blessed them.
51 And it came to pass, [1]while he
blessed them, he was [e]parted from them,
and carried up into [2]heaven.
52 And they worshipped him, and
returned to Jerusalem with great joy:
53 And were continually in the [f]temple, praising and blessing God. Amen.

[1] **(24:51) The attitude of our Lord here characterizes this age. It is one of grace; an ascended Lord is blessing a believing people with spiritual blessings. The Jewish age was marked by temporal blessings as the reward of an obedient people (Deut. 28:1-15). In the kingdom-age spiritual and temporal blessings unite.**

[2] **(24:51) The Scriptures distinguish three heavens: *first,* the lower heavens, or the region of the clouds; *secondly,* the second or planetary heavens; and, *thirdly,* the heaven of heavens, the abode of God.**

THE GOSPEL ACCORDING TO
ST. JOHN

WRITER. The fourth Gospel was written by the Apostle John (John 21:24). This has been questioned on critical grounds, but on the same grounds and with equal scholarship, the early date and Johanean authorship have been maintained.

Date. The date of John's Gospel falls between A.D. 85 and 90. Probably the latter.

Theme. This is indicated both in the Prologue (1:1-14), and in the last verse of the Gospel proper (20:31), and is: The incarnation of the eternal Word, and Son of God, Himself God, in Jesus the Christ, (1) to reveal God in the terms of a human life; (2) that as many as believe on Him as "the Christ, the Son of God" (20:31) may have eternal life. The prominent words are, "believed" and "life."

The book is in seven natural divisions: I. Prologue: The eternal Word incarnate in Jesus the Christ, 1:1-14. II. The witness of John the Baptist, 1:15-34. III. The public ministry of Christ, 1:35–12:50. IV. The private ministry of Christ to His own, 13:1–17:26. V. The sacrifice of Christ, 18:1–19:42. VI. The manifestation of Christ in resurrection, 20:1-31. VII. Epilogue: Christ the Master of life and service, 21:1-25.

The events recorded in this book cover a period of 7 years.

CHAPTER 1.

The deity of Jesus Christ.
(Cf. Heb. 1:5-13.)

In the beginning was the [1a]Word, and the Word was with [b]God, and the Word was [c]God.

2 The same was in the beginning with God.

His pre-incarnation work. (Cf. Heb. 1:2.)

3 [d]All things were made by him; and without him was not any thing made that was made.

4 In him was [e]life; and the life was the light of men.

5 And the light shineth in darkness; and the darkness [f]comprehended it not.

Ministry of John Baptist. (See vs. 29-34. Cf. Mt. 3:1-17; Mk. 1:1-11; Lk. 3:1-23.)

6 There was a [g]man sent from God, whose name *was* John.

7 The same came for a [h]witness, to bear witness of the Light, that all *men* through him might believe.

8 [i]He was not that Light, but *was sent* to bear witness of that Light.

Jesus Christ the true Light.
(Cf. John 8:12; 9:5; 12:46.)

9 *That* was the true [j]Light, which lighteth every man that cometh into the [k]world.

10 He was in the [k]world, and the world was made by him, and the world knew him not.

The two classes: sons and unbelievers.
(Cf. 1 John 3:1, 2; 5:11, 12.)

11 [l]He came unto his own, and his own received him not.

12 But as many as received him, to them gave he [m]power to become the sons of God, *even* to them that [n]believe on his name:

13 Which were born, not of blood, nor of the will of the [o]flesh, nor of the will of man, but of God.

The incarnation. (Cf. Mt. 1:18-23; Lk. 1:30-35; Rom. 1:3, 4.)

14 And the [p]Word was made flesh, and dwelt among us, (and we beheld his glory, the glory as of the only begotten of the Father,) full of grace and truth.

A.D. 26.

a Rev. 19:13.
b John 17:5.
c Heb. 1:8, 13; 1 John 5:20.
d Eph. 3:9.
e *Life (eternal).* John 3:15, 16, 36. (Mt. 7:14; Rev. 22:19.)
f Or, *apprehended;* lit. *laid not hold of it.*
g Mal. 3:1; Lk. 3:2, 3.
h John 3:26-36.
i Acts 19:4.
j Isa. 49:6.
k *kosmos* (Mt. 4:8) = mankind.
l i.e. He came unto his own things, and his own people received him not.
m Or, *authority.*
n *Faith.* John 3:15, 16, 18, 36. (Gen. 3:20; Heb. 11:39.)
o Flesh. John 3:6. (John 1:13; Jude 23.)
p 1 Tim. 3:16.

[1]**(1:1)** Gr. *Logos* (Aram. *Memra,* used in the Targums, or Heb. paraphrases, for God). The Greek term means, (1) a thought or concept; (2) the expression or utterance of that thought. As a designation of Christ, therefore, *Logos* is peculiarly felicitous because, (1) in Him are embodied all the treasures of the divine wisdom, the collective "thought" of God (1 Cor. 1:24; Eph. 3:11; Col. 2:2, 3); and, (2) He is, from eternity, but especially in His incarnation, the utterance or expression of the Person, and "thought" of Deity (John 1:3-5, 9, 14-18; 14:9-11; Col. 2:9). In the Being, Person, and work of Christ, Deity is told out.

The witness of John Baptist.
(Cf. Mt. 3:1-17; Mk. 1:1-11; Lk. 3:1-18.)

A.D. 26.

15 John bare [a]witness of him, and cried, saying, This was he of whom I spake, He that cometh after me is preferred before me: for he was before me.

16 And of his fulness have all we received, and grace for grace.

17 For the [b]law was given by Moses, *but* [1c]grace and truth came by Jesus Christ.

18 No man hath [2]seen God at any time; the only begotten Son, which is in the bosom of the Father, he hath [d]declared *him*.

19 And [e]this is the record of John, when the Jews sent priests and Levites from Jerusalem to ask him, Who art thou?

20 And he confessed, and denied not; but confessed, I am not the Christ.

21 And they asked him, What then? Art thou Elias? And he saith, I am not. Art thou that [f]prophet? And he answered, No.

22 Then said they unto him, Who art thou? that we may give an answer to them that sent us. What sayest thou of thyself?

23 [g]He said, I *am* the voice of one crying in the wilderness, Make straight the way of the [h]Lord, as said the [i]prophet Esaias.

24 And they which were sent were of the Pharisees.

25 And they asked him, and said unto him, Why baptizest thou then, if thou be not that Christ, nor Elias, neither that prophet?

26 John answered them, saying, I baptize with water: but there standeth one among you, whom ye know not;

27 He it is, who coming after me is preferred before me, whose shoe's latchet I am not worthy to unloose.

28 These things were done in [j]Bethabara beyond Jordan, where John was baptizing.

29 The next day John seeth Jesus coming unto him, and saith, Behold the [k]Lamb of God, which taketh away the [l]sin of the world.

30 This is he of whom I said, After me cometh a man which is preferred before me: for he was before me.

31 And I knew him not: but that he should be made manifest to Israel, therefore am I come baptizing with water.

32 And John bare record, saying, I saw the [m]Spirit descending from heaven like a dove, and it abode upon him.

33 And I knew him not: but he that sent me to baptize with water, the same said unto me, Upon whom thou shalt see the Spirit descending, and remaining on him, the same is he which baptizeth with the Holy Ghost.

34 And I saw, and bare record that this is the Son of God.

a vs. 6-8, 15; Mal. 3:1.
b *Law, (of Moses).* John 7:19. (Ex. 19:1; Gal. 3:1-29.)
c *Grace (in salvation).* (Rom. 3:24.)
d Lit. *led him forth,* i.e. into full revelation. John 14:9.
e Lk. 3:15.
f Deut. 18:15; John 6:14.
g Mt. 3:3.
h *Jehovah.* Isa. 40:3.
i Isa. 40:3.
j *Bethany.*
k *Sacrifice (of Christ).* John 6:33-35. (Gen. 4:4; Heb. 10:18.)
l *Sin.* Rom. 3:23, *note.*
m *Holy Spirit.* vs. 32, 33; John 3:5, 6, 8, 34. (Mt. 1:18; Acts 2:4.)

[1] **(1:17)** Grace. Summary: (1) Grace is "the kindness and love of God our Saviour toward man . . . not by works of righteousness which we have done" (Tit; 3:4, 5), It is, therefore, constantly set in contrast to law, under which God demands righteousness from man, as, under grace, he gives righteousness to man (Rom. 3:21, 22; 8:4; Phil. 3:9). Law is connected with Moses and works; grace with Christ and faith (John 1:17; Rom. 10:4-10). Law blesses the good; grace saves the bad (Ex. 19:5; Eph. 2:1-9). Law demands that blessings be earned; grace is a free gift (Deut. 28:1-6; Eph. 2:8; Rom. 4:4, 5).

(2) As a dispensation, grace begins with the death and resurrection of Christ (Rom. 3:24-26; 4:24, 25). The point of testing is no longer legal obedience as the condition of salvation, but acceptance or rejection of Christ, with good works as a fruit of salvation (John 1:12, 13; 3:36; Mt. 21:37; 22:42; John 15:22, 25; Heb. 1:2; 1 John 5:10-12). The *immediate result* of this testing was the rejection of Christ by the Jews, and His crucifixion by Jew and Gentile (Acts 4:27). The *predicted end* of the testing of man under grace is the apostasy of the professing church (see "Apostasy," 2 Tim. 3:1-8, *note*), and the resultant apocalyptic judgments.

(3) Grace has a twofold manifestation: in *salvation* (Rom. 3:24, *refs.*), and in the *walk* and *service* of the saved (Rom. 6:15, *refs.*). See, for the other six dispensations: *Innocence*, Gen. 1:28; *Conscience*, Gen. 3:23; *Human Government*, Gen. 8:21; *Promise*, Gen. 12:1; *Law*, Ex. 19:8; *Kingdom*, Eph. 1:10.

[2] **(1:18)** Cf. Gen. 32:30; Ex. 24:10; 33:18; Jud. 6:22; 13:22; Rev. 22:4. The divine essence, God, in His own triune Person, no human being in the flesh has seen. But God, veiled in angelic form, and especially as incarnate in Jesus Christ, has been seen of men (Gen. 18:2, 22; John 14:8, 9).

The public ministry of Jesus Christ (John 1:35-12:50).

35 Again the next day after John stood, and two of his disciples;

36 And looking upon Jesus as he walked, he saith, Behold the Lamb of God!

37 And the two disciples heard him speak, and [a]they followed Jesus.

38 Then Jesus turned, and saw them following, and saith unto them, What seek ye? They said unto him, Rabbi, (which is to say, being interpreted, Master,) where dwellest thou?

39 He saith unto them, [b]Come and see. They came and saw where he dwelt, and abode with him that day: for it was about [c]the tenth hour.

40 One of the two which heard John *speak*, and followed him, was Andrew, Simon Peter's brother.

41 He first findeth his own brother Simon, and saith unto him, We have found the Messias, which is, being interpreted, [d]the Christ.

42 And he brought him to Jesus. And when Jesus beheld him, he said, Thou art Simon the son of Jona: thou shalt be called Cephas, which is by interpretation, A stone.

43 The day following Jesus would go forth into Galilee, and findeth Philip, and saith unto him, Follow me.

44 Now Philip was of Bethsaida, the city of Andrew and Peter.

45 Philip findeth Nathanael, and saith unto him, We have found him, of whom [e]Moses in the law, and the prophets, did write, [f]Jesus of Nazareth, the son of Joseph.

46 And Nathanael said unto him, Can there any good thing come out of Nazareth? Philip saith unto him, Come and see.

47 Jesus saw Nathanael coming to him, and saith of him, [g]Behold an Israelite indeed, in whom is no guile!

48 Nathanael saith unto him, Whence knowest thou me? Jesus answered and said unto him, Before that Philip called thee, when thou wast under the fig tree, I [h]saw thee.

49 Nathanael answered and saith unto him, Rabbi, [i]thou art the Son of God; thou art the [j]King of Israel.

50 Jesus answered and said unto him, Because I said unto thee, I saw thee under the fig tree, believest thou? thou shalt see greater things than these.

51 And he saith unto him, Verily, verily, I say unto you, Hereafter ye shall see heaven open, and the [k]angels of God ascending and descending upon the Son of man.

CHAPTER 2.

The marriage at Cana: the first miracle.

And the third day there was a marriage in Cana of Galilee; and the mother of Jesus was there:

2 And both Jesus was called, and his disciples, to the [l]marriage.

3 And when they wanted wine, the mother of Jesus saith unto him, They have no wine.

4 Jesus saith unto her, [m]Woman, what have I to [n]do with thee? mine [o]hour is not yet come.

5 His mother saith unto the servants, Whatsoever he saith unto you, do *it*.

6 And there were set there six waterpots of stone, after the manner of the [p]purifying of the Jews, containing two or three [q]firkins apiece.

7 Jesus saith unto them, Fill the waterpots with water. And they filled them up to the brim.

8 And he saith unto them, Draw out now, and bear unto the governor of the feast. And they bare *it*.

9 When the ruler of the feast had tasted the water that was [r]made wine, and knew not whence it was: (but the servants which drew the water knew;) the governor of the feast called the bridegroom,

10 And saith unto him, Every man at the beginning doth set forth good wine; and when men have well drunk, then that which is worse: *but* thou hast kept the good wine until now.

11 This beginning of miracles did Jesus in Cana of Galilee, and manifested forth his glory; and his disciples believed on him.

12 After this he went down to Capernaum, he, and his mother, and his brethren, and his disciples: and they continued there not many days.

The first passover (vs. 13, 23; cf. John 6:4; 11:55): *first purification of the temple.* (Cf. Mt. 21:12, 13; Mk. 11:15-17; Lk. 19:45, 46.)

13 And the Jews' [s]passover was at

A.D. 30.

a Cf. Mk. 1:16-20; Lk. 5:1-11.

b The call to discipleship. Cf. Mt. 4:18-22, the call to service.

c That was two hours before night.

d Or, *the anointed.*

e Lk. 24:27.

f Deut. 18:15.

g Rom. 2:28, 29.

h Psa. 139:1.

i John 5:17.

j Mt. 21:4, 5; 27:11.

k Heb. 1:4, *note.*

l Heb. 13:4.

m John 19:26; 20:13.

n Lk. 2:49.

o Isa. 30:18.

p Mt. 15:2; Lk. 11:39.

q One firkin = about 9 gals.

r *Miracles* (N.T.). vs. 1-10; John 4:46-54. (Mt. 8:2, 3; Acts 28:8, 9.)

s Ex. 12:14.

hand, and [a]Jesus went up to Jerusalem,
14 And [b]found in the [c]temple those
that sold [d]oxen and sheep and doves,
and the changers of [e]money sitting:
15 And when he had made a scourge
of small cords, he drove them all out of
the temple, and the sheep, and the oxen;
and poured out the changers' money,
and overthrew the tables;
16 And said unto them that sold
doves, Take these things hence; make
not my Father's house an house of merchandise.
17 And his disciples remembered that
it was written, The [f]zeal of thine house
hath eaten me up.
18 Then answered the Jews and said
unto him, What [g]sign shewest thou unto
us, seeing that thou doest these things?
19 Jesus answered and said unto them,
[h]Destroy this temple, and in three days I
will raise it up.
20 Then said the Jews, Forty and six
years was this temple in building, and
wilt thou rear it up in three days?
21 But he spake of the [i]temple of his
body.
22 When therefore he was [j]risen from
the dead, his disciples remembered that
he had said this unto them; and they
believed the scripture, and the word
which Jesus had said.
23 Now when he was in Jerusalem at
the passover, in the feast *day*, many
believed in his name, when they saw the
miracles which he did.
24 But Jesus did not commit himself
unto them, because he [k]knew all *men*,
25 And needed not that any should
testify of man: for he knew what was in
man.

CHAPTER 3.

Jesus and Nicodemus: the new birth.
(Cf. v. 3, *note.*)

There was a man of the Pharisees,
named [l]Nicodemus, a ruler of the
Jews:
2 The same came to Jesus by night,
and said unto him, Rabbi, we know that
thou art a teacher come from God: for no
man can do these miracles that thou
doest, except [m]God be with him.
3 Jesus answered and said unto him,
Verily, verily, I say unto thee, [n]Except a
man be [1]born [o]again, he cannot see the
kingdom of God.
4 Nicodemus saith unto him, How can
a man be born when he is old? can he
enter the second time into his mother's
womb, and be born?
5 Jesus answered, Verily, verily, I say
unto thee, Except a man be born of [p]wa-
ter and *of* the Spirit, he cannot enter into
the kingdom of God.
6 That which is born of the flesh is
[q]flesh; and that which is born of the
Spirit is spirit.
7 Marvel not that I said unto thee, Ye
must be born again.
8 The wind bloweth where it listeth,
and thou hearest the sound thereof, but
canst not tell whence it cometh, and
whither it goeth: [r]so is every one that is
born of the Spirit.
9 Nicodemus answered and said unto
him, How can these things be?
10 Jesus answered and said unto him,
Art thou [s]a master of Israel, and knowest not these things?
11 Verily, verily, I say unto thee, We
speak that we do know, and testify that
we have seen; and ye receive not our
witness.
12 If I have told you [t]earthly things,
and ye believe not, how shall ye believe,
if I tell you *of* [u]heavenly things?
13 And no man hath ascended up to
heaven, but he that came down from
heaven, *even* the [v]Son of man which is in
heaven.
14 And [w]as Moses lifted up the serpent in the wilderness, even so must the
Son of man be lifted up:
15 That whosoever believeth in him
should not perish, but have eternal life.
16 For God so loved the [x]world,
that he gave his only begotten
[y]Son, that whosoever believeth in

A.D. 30.

a John 5:1; 6:4; 11:55.
b Mt. 21:12; Mk. 11:15; Lk. 19:45.
c Mal. 3:1; Rev. 11:2.
d Lev. 22:19.
e Ex. 30:12.
f Psa. 69:9.
g John 6:30; Mt. 12:38; 21:23.
h Mt. 26:61; 27:40.
i Eph. 2:21, 22; Col. 2:9.
j *Resurrection.* vs. 19-23; John 5:25-29. (Job 19:25; 1 Cor. 15:52.)
k 1 Sam. 16:7; Rev. 2:23.
l John 7:50, 51; 19:39.
m Acts 10:38.
n John 1:13; Gal. 6:15; Eph. 2:10; Tit. 3:5; Jas. 1:18; 1 Pet. 1:23.
o Or, *from above.*
p Ezk. 36:25; Mk. 16:16; Acts 2:38; Tit. 3:5, 6; 1 Pet. 3:21.
q *Flesh.* John 6:63. (John 1:13; Jude 23.)
r Rom. 9:15, 18.
s Lit. *Art thou the teacher of Israel,* etc.
t vs. 3, 5, 8; Heb. 5:11, 12.
u 1 Tim. 3:16; 1 John 5:7.
v See Mt. 8:20, *note.*
w *Inspiration.* John 5:46, 47. (Ex. 4:15; Rev. 22:19.)
x *kosmos* (Mt. 4:8) = mankind.
y Isa. 9:6.

[1] **(3:3)** *Regeneration:* (1) The *necessity* of the new birth grows out of the incapacity of the natural man to "see" or "enter into" the kingdom of God. However gifted, moral, or refined, the natural man is absolutely blind to spiritual truth, and impotent to enter the kingdom; for he can neither obey, understand, nor please" God (John 3:3, 5, 6; Psa. 51:5; Jer. 17:9; Mk. 7:21-23; 1 Cor. 2:14; Rom. 8:7, 8; Eph. 2:3. See Mt. 6:33, *note*). (2) The new birth is not a reformation of the old nature (Rom. 6:6, *note*), but a

him should not [1]perish, but have everlasting life.

17 For God sent not his Son into the [a]world to [b]condemn the world; but that the world through him might be [c]saved.

18 [d]He that believeth on him is not condemned: but he that believeth not is condemned already, because he hath not believed in the name of the only begotten Son of God.

19 And this is the condemnation, that light is come into the [a]world, and men loved darkness rather than light, because their deeds were evil.

20 For every one that doeth evil hateth the light, neither cometh to the light, lest his deeds should be [e]reproved.

21 But he that [f]doeth truth cometh to the light, that his deeds may be made manifest, that they are [g]wrought in God.

Last testimony of John Baptist.

22 After these things came Jesus and his disciples into the land of Judæa; and there he tarried with them, and [h]baptized.

23 And John also was baptizing in Ænon near to Salim, because there was much water there: and they [i]came, and were baptized.

24 For John [j]was not yet cast into prison.

25 Then there arose a question between *some* of John's disciples and the Jews about [k]purifying.

26 And they came unto John, and said unto him, Rabbi, he that was with thee beyond Jordan, to whom thou barest witness, behold, the same baptizeth, and all *men* come to him.

27 John answered and said, A [l]man can receive nothing, except it be given him from heaven.

28 Ye yourselves bear me witness, that I said, I am not the Christ, but that [m]I am sent before him.

29 He that hath the bride is the [n]bridegroom: but the friend of the bridegroom, which standeth and heareth him, rejoiceth greatly because of the bridegroom's voice: this my joy therefore is fulfilled.

30 [o]He must increase, but I *must* decrease.

A.D. 30.

a kosmos (Mt. 4:8) = mankind.
b Or, *judge*, and so in vs. 18, 19; cf. John 15:22-24.
c Rom. 1:16, *note*.
d John 6:40, 47; Rom. 8:1.
e Or, *discovered*.
f Psa. 119:105; 139:23.
g John 15:4, 5; 1 Cor. 15:10.
h John 4:2.
i Mt. 3:5, 6.
j Mt. 14:3.
k Num. 19:7; Heb. 9:9, 14; 1 Pet. 3:21.
l Rom. 12:5, 8; 1 Cor. 3:6; Heb. 5:4; 1 Pet. 4:10, 11.
m Mal. 3:1.
n *Bride (of Christ)*. Rom. 7:4. (John 3:29; Rev. 19:6-8.)
o Isa. 9:7.
p John 15:15.
q Isa. 55:4, 11; 1 John 5:10.
r John 7:16.
s *Holy Spirit*. vs. 5, 6, 8, 34; John 4:23, 24. (Mt. 1:18; Acts 2:4.)
t *Faith*. vs. 15, 16, 18, 36; John 5:24, 44. (Gen. 3:20; Heb. 11:39.)
u *Life (Eternal)*. vs. 15, 16, 36; John 4:14, 36. (Mt. 7:14; Rev. 22:19.)
v Gal. 3:10; 1 Thes. 1:10.
w Gen. 33:19.

Declarative statement concerning Jesus Christ.

31 He that cometh from above is above all: he that is of the earth is earthly, and speaketh of the earth: he that cometh from heaven is above all.

32 And what [p]he hath seen and heard, that he testifieth; and no man receiveth his testimony.

33 He that hath received his testimony hath [q]set to his seal that God is true.

34 For [r]he whom God hath sent speaketh the words of God: for God giveth not the [s]Spirit by measure *unto him*.

35 The Father loveth the Son, and hath given all things into his hand.

36 He that [t]believeth on the Son [u]hath everlasting life: and he that believeth not the Son shall not see life; but the [v]wrath of God abideth on him.

CHAPTER 4.

Jesus departs into Galilee.

When therefore the Lord knew how the Pharisees had heard that Jesus made and baptized more disciples than John,

2 (Though Jesus himself baptized not, but his disciples,)

3 He left Judæa, and departed again into Galilee.

4 And he must needs go through Samaria.

5 Then cometh he to a city of Samaria, which is called Sychar, near to the parcel of ground that Jacob [w]gave to his son Joseph.

Jesus and the Samaritan woman.

6 Now Jacob's well was there. Jesus therefore, being wearied with *his* journey, sat thus on the well: *and* it was about the sixth hour.

creative act of the Holy Spirit (John 3:5; 1:12, 13; 2 Cor. 5:17; Eph. 2:10; 4:24). (3) The condition of the new birth is faith in Christ crucified (John 3:14, 15; 1:12, 13; Gal. 3:24). (4) Through the new birth the believer becomes a partaker of the divine nature and of the life of Christ Himself (Gal. 2:20; Eph. 2:10; 4:24; Col. 1:27; 1 Pet. 1:23-25; 2 Pet. 1:4; 1 John 5:10-12).

1 **(3:16)** Gr. *apollumi*, trans. "marred," Mk. 2:22; "lost," Mt. 10:6; 15:24; 18:11; Lk. 15:4, 6, 32. In no N.T. instance does it signify cessation of existence or of consciousness. It is the condition of every non-believer.

A.D. 30.

7 There cometh a woman of Samaria to draw water: Jesus saith unto her, Give me to drink.

8 (For his disciples were gone away unto the city to buy meat.)

9 Then saith the woman of Samaria unto him, How is it that thou, being a Jew, askest drink of me, which am a woman of Samaria? for the Jews have no [a]dealings with the Samaritans.

10 Jesus answered and said unto her, If thou knewest the gift of God, and who it is that saith to thee, Give me to drink; thou wouldest have asked of him, and he would have given thee living water.

11 The woman saith unto him, Sir, thou hast nothing to draw with, and the well is deep: from whence then hast thou that living water?

12 Art thou greater than our father Jacob, which gave us the well, and drank thereof himself, and his children, and his cattle?

13 Jesus answered and said unto her, Whosoever drinketh of this [b]water shall thirst again:

The indwelling Spirit. (Cf. John 7:37-39.)

14 But whosoever drinketh of the water that I shall give him shall never thirst; but the water that I shall give him shall [c]be in him a well of water springing up into [d]everlasting life.

15 The woman [e]saith unto him, Sir, give me this water, that I thirst not, neither come hither to draw.

16 Jesus saith unto her, Go, call thy husband, and come hither.

17 The woman answered and said, I have no husband. Jesus said unto her, Thou hast well said, I have no husband:

18 For thou hast had five husbands; and he whom thou now hast is not thy husband: in that saidst thou truly.

19 The woman saith unto him, Sir, I perceive that thou art a prophet.

20 Our fathers worshipped in this [f]mountain; and ye say, that in [g]Jerusalem is the place where men ought to worship.

21 Jesus saith unto her, Woman, believe me, the hour cometh, when ye shall neither in this mountain, nor yet at Jerusalem, worship the Father.

22 Ye worship ye know not what: we know what we worship: for [h]salvation is of the Jews.

23 But the hour cometh, and now is, when the [i]true worshippers shall worship the Father in [j]spirit and in truth: for the Father seeketh such to worship him.

24 [k]God *is* a [l]Spirit: and they that worship him must worship *him* in spirit and in truth.

25 The woman saith unto him, I know that Messias cometh, which is called Christ: when he is come, he will [m]tell us all things.

26 Jesus saith unto her, I that speak unto thee am *he.*

27 And upon this came his disciples, and marvelled [n]that he talked with the woman: yet no man said, What seekest thou? or, Why talkest thou with her?

28 The woman then left her waterpot, and went her way into the city, and saith to the men,

29 Come, see a man, which told me all things that ever I did: is not this the Christ?

30 Then they went out of the city, and came unto him.

31 In the mean while his disciples prayed him, saying, Master, eat.

32 But he said unto them, I have meat to eat that ye know not of.

33 Therefore said the disciples one to another, Hath any man brought him *ought* to eat?

34 Jesus saith unto them, My meat is to do the [o]will of him that sent me, and to [p]finish his work.

35 Say not ye, There are yet four months, and *then* cometh harvest? behold, I say unto you, Lift up your eyes, and look on the fields; for they are white already to harvest.

36 And he that reapeth receiveth wages, and gathereth [q]fruit unto life eternal: that [r]both he that soweth and he that reapeth may rejoice together.

37 And herein is that saying true, One [s]soweth, and another reapeth.

38 I sent you to reap that whereon ye bestowed no labour: [t]other men laboured, and ye are entered into their labours.

39 And many of the Samaritans of that city believed on him for the saying of the woman, which testified, He told me all that ever I did.

Jesus and the Samaritans.

40 So when the Samaritans were come unto him, they besought him that he would tarry with them: and he abode there two days.

41 And many more believed because of his own word;

a Acts 10:28.
b *Christ (as Stone).* vs. 13, 14; John 7:37-39. (Ex. 17:6; 1 Pet. 2:8.)
c Or, *become.*
d *Life (eternal).* vs. 14, 36; John 5:24-40. (Mt. 7:14; Rev. 22:19.)
e *Bible prayers.* John 4:49. (Mt. 6:9; Rev. 22:20.)
f Gen. 12:6-8; 33:18; Jud. 9:7.
g Deut. 12:5; 1 Ki. 9:3.
h Rom. 1:16, *note.*
i Or, *real.*
j That the Holy Spirit is meant is clear from v. 24.
k Cf. John 1:18, *note.*
l *Holy Spirit.* John 6:63. (Mt. 1:18; Acts 2:4.)
m Deut. 18:15.
n *that he was talking with a woman.*
o Psa. 40:8.
p *complete.* Cf. John 17:4.
q Rom. 6:22.
r 1 Cor. 3:5, 9; 1 Thes. 2:19.
s Mic. 6:15.
t Jer. 44:4; 1 Pet. 1:12.

A.D. 30.

42 And said unto the woman, Now we
believe, not because of thy saying: for
we have heard *him* ourselves, and know
that this is indeed the Christ, the
[a]Saviour of the [b]world.
43 Now after two days he departed
thence, and went into Galilee.
44 For Jesus himself testified, [c]that a
prophet hath no honour in his own
country.
45 Then when he was come into
Galilee, the Galilæans received him, having [d]seen all the things that he did at
Jerusalem at the feast: [e]for they also
went unto the feast.

The nobleman's son healed.

46 So Jesus came again into Cana of
Galilee, where he [f]made the water wine.
And there was a certain [g]nobleman,
whose son was sick at Capernaum.
47 When he heard that Jesus was come
out of Judæa into Galilee, he went unto
him, and besought him that he would
come down, and heal his son: for he was
at the point of death.
48 Then said Jesus unto him, Except
ye see signs and wonders, ye will not
believe.
49 The nobleman [h]saith unto him, Sir,
come down ere my child die.
50 Jesus saith unto him, [i]Go thy way;
thy son liveth. And the man believed the
word that Jesus had spoken unto him,
and he went his way.
51 And as he was now going down,
his servants met him, and told *him*, saying, Thy son liveth.
52 Then enquired he of them the hour
when he began to amend. And they said
unto him, Yesterday at the seventh hour
the [j]fever left him.
53 So the father knew that *it was* at the
same hour, in the which Jesus said unto
him, Thy son liveth: and himself
believed, and his whole house.
54 This *is* again the second miracle *that*
Jesus did, when he was come out of
Judæa into Galilee.

CHAPTER 5.

The feast (Pentecost?): the pool of Bethesda, and healing.

After this there was a [k]feast of the
Jews; and Jesus went up to
Jerusalem.
2 Now there is at Jerusalem by the
sheep [l]*market* a pool, which is called in
the Hebrew tongue Bethesda, having
five porches.
3 In these lay a great multitude of
impotent folk, of blind, halt, withered,
[m]waiting for the moving of the water.
4 For an [n]angel went down at a certain
season into the pool, and troubled the
water: whosoever then first after the
troubling of the water stepped in was
made whole of whatsoever disease he
had.
5 And a certain man was there, which
had an infirmity thirty and eight years.
6 When Jesus saw him lie, [o]and knew
that he had been now a long time *in that*
case, he saith unto him, [p]Wilt thou be
made whole?
7 The impotent man answered him,
Sir, I have no man, when the water is
troubled, to put me into the pool: but
while I am coming, another steppeth
down before me.
8 Jesus saith unto him, Rise, take up
thy bed, and walk.
9 And immediately the man was made
[q]whole, and took up his bed, and
walked: and on the same day was the
sabbath.
10 The Jews therefore said unto him
that was cured, It is the [r]sabbath day: it
is not lawful for thee to carry *thy* bed.
11 He answered them, He that made
me whole, the same said unto me, Take
up thy bed, and walk.
12 Then asked they him, What man is
that which said unto thee, Take up thy
bed, and walk?
13 And he that was healed wist not
who it was: for Jesus had [s]conveyed
himself away, a multitude being in *that*
place.
14 Afterward Jesus findeth him in the
temple, and said unto him, Behold, thou
art made whole: [t]sin no more, lest a
worse thing come unto thee.
15 The man departed, and told the
Jews that it was Jesus, which had made
him whole.
16 And therefore did the Jews persecute Jesus, and sought to [u]slay him,
because he had done these things on the
sabbath day.
17 But Jesus answered them, My
Father worketh hitherto, and I work.
18 Therefore the Jews sought the more
to [u]kill him, because he not only had
broken the sabbath, but said also that
God was [v]his Father, [w]making himself
equal with God.

a Rom. 1:16, *note.*
b *kosmos* (Mt. 4:8) = mankind.
c Mt. 13:57; Mk. 6:4; Lk. 4:24.
d John 2:13, 23.
e Deut. 16:16.
f John 2:1, 11.
g Or, *courtier*, or, *ruler.*
h *Bible prayers* (N.T.). John 11:41, 42. (Mt. 6:9; Rev. 22:20.)
i Mt. 8:13; Mk. 7:29, 30.
j *Miracles* (N.T.). vs. 46-54; John 5:1-9. (Mt. 8:2, 3; Acts 28:8, 9.)
k John 2:13; Lev. 23:2; Deut. 16:16.
l Or, *gate.* Neh. 3:1; 12:39.
m The Sinai MS. omits "waiting for the moving of the water." and all of v. 4.
n Heb. 1:4, *note.*
o Psa. 142:3.
p v. 40.
q *Miracles* (N.T.). vs. 1-9; John 6:5-14. (Mt. 8:2, 3; Acts 28:8, 9.)
r Jer. 17:21; Mt. 12:2.
s Lk. 4:30.
t *Sin.* Rom. 3:23, *note.*
u Psa. 2:2.
v Gr. *patera idion, his own Father.* The Jews understood perfectly that Jesus was claiming to be God. Cf. John 10:33.
w John 10:30, 33; Phil. 2:6.

19 **Then answered Jesus and said unto them,** Verily, verily, I say unto you, The Son can do nothing of himself, but what he seeth the Father [a]do: for what things soever he doeth, these also doeth the Son likewise.

20 [b]For the Father loveth the Son, and sheweth him all things that himself doeth: and he will shew him greater works than these, that ye may marvel.

21 For [c]as the Father raiseth up the dead, and quickeneth *them;* [d]even so the Son quickeneth whom he will.

22 For the Father judgeth no man, but hath committed all [e]judgment unto the Son:

23 That all *men* should honour the Son, even as they honour the Father. He that honoureth not the Son honoureth not the Father which hath sent him.

24 Verily, verily, I say unto you, He that heareth my word, and believeth on him that sent me, [f]hath everlasting life, and shall not come into [g]condemnation; but is passed from [h]death unto life.

25 Verily, verily, I say unto you, The hour is coming, and now is, when the [i]dead shall hear the voice of the Son of God: and they that hear shall live.

26 For [j]as the Father hath life in himself; so hath he given to the Son to have [k]life in himself;

27 And hath given him authority to execute judgment also, because he is the Son of man.

The two resurrections. (See v. 29, *marg.*)

28 Marvel not at this: for the hour is coming, in the which all that are in the graves shall hear his voice,

29 And shall come forth; they that have done good, unto the [l]resurrection of life; and they that have done evil, unto the resurrection of [m]damnation.

30 I can of mine own self do nothing: as I hear, I [e]judge: and my judgment is just; because I seek not mine own will, but the will of the Father which hath sent me.

31 If I bear [1]witness of myself, my witness is not true.

A.D. 31.

a Lit. *doing.*
b Mt. 3:17.
c 1 Ki. 17:21; Rom. 8:11.
d John 11:25; Lk. 8:54; Col. 2:13.
e *Day of judgment.* vs. 22, 27, 30; Acts 17:31. (Mt. 10:15; Rev. 20:11.)
f *Life (eternal).* vs. 24-40; John 6:27-68. (Mt. 7:14; Rev. 22:19.)
g *Judgments (the seven).* John 19:16-18. (2 Sam. 7:14; Rev. 20:12.)
h *Death (spiritual).* Eph. 4:18, 19. (Gen. 2:17; Eph. 2:5.)
i v. 28; Eph. 2:1.
j Psa. 36:9.
k John 1:4; 14:6; 1 Cor. 15:45.
l *Resurrection.* vs. 25-29; John 6:39, 40. (Job 19:25; 1 Cor. 15:52.)
m i.e. *condemnation.*
n v. 37; Acts 10:43.
o Rom. 1:16, *note.*
p Mt. 5:16; Phil. 2:15, 16.
q *complete.*
r Cf. John 1:18, *note.*
s Or, *Ye search.*
t *The Beast.* 2 Thes. 2:3-8. (Dan. 7:8; Rev. 19:20.)
u i.e. *hope.*
v *Inspiration.* vs. 46, 47; John 6:31, 32, 45, 49, 63. (Ex. 4:15; Rev. 22:19.)
w *Faith.* vs. 24, 44, 46; John 6:29, 35, 47. (Gen. 3:20; Heb. 11:39.)

32 There is [n]another that beareth witness of me; and I know that the witness which he witnesseth of me is true.

The fourfold witness to Jesus:
(1) *John Baptist.*

33 Ye sent unto John, and he bare witness unto the truth.

34 But I receive not testimony from man: but these things I say, that ye might be [o]saved.

35 He was a burning and a shining [p]light: and ye were willing for a season to rejoice in his light.

(2) *The works.*

36 But I have greater witness than *that* of John: for the works which the Father hath given me to [q]finish, the same works that I do, bear witness of me, that the Father hath sent me.

(3) *The Father* (Mt. 3:17).

37 And the Father himself, which hath sent me, hath borne witness of me. Ye have neither heard his voice at any time, nor [r]seen his shape.

38 And ye have not his word abiding in you: for whom he hath sent, him ye believe not.

(4) *The Scriptures.* (Cf. Lk. 24:27, 44-46.)

39 [s]Search the scriptures; for in them ye think ye have eternal life: and they are they which testify of me.

40 And ye will not come to me, that ye might have [f]life.

41 I receive not honour from men.

42 But I know you, that ye have not the love of God in you.

43 I am come in my Father's name, and ye receive me not: if [t]another shall come in his own name, him ye will receive.

44 How can ye believe, which receive honour one of another, and seek not the honour that *cometh* from God only?

45 Do not think that I will accuse you to the Father: there is *one* that accuseth you, *even* Moses, in whom ye [u]trust.

46 For had ye believed Moses, ye would have believed me: [v]for he wrote [w]of me.

[1]**(5:31)** Cf. John 8:14. In John 5:31 our Lord, defending His Messianic claims before Jews who denied those claims, accepts the biblical rule of evidence, which required "two witnesses" (John 8:17; Num. 35:30; Deut. 17:6). A paraphrase of verse 31 would be: "If I bear witness of myself [ye will say] my witness is not true." Cf. John 8:14.

47 But if ye believe not his writings, how shall ye believe my words?

CHAPTER 6.

Feeding the five thousand (Mt. 14:13-21; Mk. 6:32-44; Lk. 9:10-17).

After these things Jesus went over the sea of Galilee, which is *the sea* of Tiberias.

2 And a great multitude followed him, because they saw his miracles which he did on them that were diseased.

3 And Jesus went up into a mountain, and there he sat with his disciples.

4 And the [a]passover, a feast of the Jews, was nigh.

5 When Jesus then lifted up *his* eyes, and saw a great company come unto him, he saith unto Philip, Whence shall we buy bread, that these may eat?

6 And this he said to prove him: for he himself knew what he would do.

7 Philip answered him, [b]Two hundred pennyworth of bread is not sufficient for them, that every one of them may take a little.

8 One of his disciples, Andrew, Simon Peter's brother, saith unto him,

9 There is a lad here, which hath five barley loaves, and two small fishes: but what are they among so many?

10 And Jesus said, Make the men sit down. Now there was much grass in the place. So the men sat down, in number about five thousand.

11 And Jesus took the loaves; and when he had [c]given thanks, he distributed to the disciples, and the disciples to them that were set down; and likewise of the fishes as much as they would.

12 When they were filled, he said unto his disciples, Gather up the fragments that remain, that nothing be lost.

13 Therefore they gathered *them* together, and filled twelve baskets with the fragments of the five barley loaves, which remained over and above unto them that had eaten.

14 Then those men, when they had seen the [d]miracle that Jesus did, said, This is of a truth [e]that prophet that should come into the [f]world.

A.D. 31.

a Cf. John 2:13; 11:55.
b Num. 11:21, 22.
c 1 Sam. 9:13; Mt. 26:26; 1 Cor. 10:31; 1 Tim. 4:4, 5.
d *Miracles* (N.T.): vs. 5-14, 16-21; John 9:1-7. (Mt. 8:2, 3; Acts 28:8, 9.)
e Gen. 49:10; Deut. 18:15, 18.
f *kosmos* (Mt. 4:8) = mankind.
g John 18:36.
h Mt. 14:23; Mk. 6:47.
i One furlong = 582 ft.
j Isa. 43:1, 2.
k v. 11.
l *boats.*
m Isa. 55:2; Mt. 6:19, 34; Phil. 2:13; Col. 3:1, 2.
n vs. 54, 58; Jer. 15:16.
o Mt. 8:20, *note.*
p Eph. 2:8, 9.
q Psa. 2:7; Isa. 42:1; Acts 2:22; 2 Pet. 1:17.

Jesus walks upon the sea (Mt. 14:22-36; Mk. 6:45-56).

15 When Jesus therefore perceived that they would come and take him by force, to make him a [g]king, he departed again into a mountain himself alone.

16 [h]And when even was *now* come, his disciples went down unto the sea,

17 And entered into a ship, and went over the sea toward Capernaum. And it was now dark, and Jesus was not come to them.

18 And the sea arose by reason of a great wind that blew.

19 So when they had rowed about five and twenty or thirty [i]furlongs, they see Jesus walking on the sea, and drawing nigh unto the ship: and they were afraid.

20 But he saith unto them, [j]It is I; be not afraid.

21 Then they willingly received him into the ship: and immediately the ship was at the land whither they went.

The great discourse on the bread of life.

22 The day following, when the people which stood on the other side of the sea saw that there was none other boat there, save that one whereinto his disciples were entered, and that Jesus went not with his disciples into the boat, but *that* his disciples were gone away alone;

23 (Howbeit there came other boats from Tiberias nigh unto [k]the place where they did eat bread, after that the Lord had given thanks:)

24 When the people therefore saw that Jesus was not there, neither his disciples, they also took [l]shipping, and came to Capernaum, seeking for Jesus.

25 And when they had found him on the other side of the sea, they said unto him, Rabbi, when camest thou hither?

26 Jesus answered them and said, Verily, verily, I say unto you, Ye seek me, not because ye saw the miracles, but because ye did eat of the loaves, and were filled.

27 [m]Labour not for the meat which perisheth, but for [n]that meat which endureth unto everlasting life, which the [o]Son of man shall [p]give unto you: [q]for him hath God the Father sealed.

28 Then said they unto him, What

shall we do, that we might work the
works of God?
29 Jesus answered and said unto them,
This is the work of God, that ye [a]believe
on him whom he hath sent.
30 They said therefore unto him, What
[b]sign shewest thou then, that we may see,
and believe thee? what dost thou work?
31 Our fathers did eat manna in the
desert; [c]as it is written, He gave them
[d]bread from heaven to eat.
32 Then Jesus said unto them, Verily,
verily, I say unto you, Moses gave you
not that bread from heaven; but [e]my
Father giveth you the true bread from
heaven.
33 For the bread of God [f]is he which
cometh down from heaven, and [g]giveth
life unto the [h]world.
34 Then said they unto him, Lord,
evermore give us this bread.
35 And Jesus said unto them, I am the
bread of life: he that cometh to me shall
never hunger; and [i]he that [a]believeth on
me shall never thirst.
36 But I said unto you, That [j]ye also
have seen me, and believe not.
37 [k]All that the Father giveth me shall
come to me; and [l]him that cometh to me
I will in no wise cast out.
38 For I came down from heaven, not
to do mine own will, [m]but the will of
him that sent me.
39 And this is the Father's will which
hath sent me, that of all which he hath
given me I should lose nothing, but
should raise it up again at the last day.
40 And this is the will of him that sent
me, [n]that every one which seeth the Son,
and believeth on him, may have everlasting life: and I will [o]raise him up at
the last day.
41 The Jews then murmured at him,
because he said, I am the bread which
came down from heaven.
42 And they said, [p]Is not this Jesus,
the son of Joseph, whose father and
mother we know? how is it then that he
saith, I came down from heaven?
43 Jesus therefore answered and said
unto them, Murmur not among yourselves.
44 No man can [q]come to me, except the
Father which hath sent me [r]draw him:
and I will raise him up at the last day.
45 It is written in the prophets, And
they shall be all taught of [s]God. Every
man therefore that hath heard, and hath
learned of the Father, cometh unto me.
46 Not that any man hath seen the
Father, save he which is of [t]God, he hath
seen the Father.
47 Verily, verily, I say unto [u]you, He
that believeth on me hath everlasting life.
48 I [v]am that bread of life.
49 Your fathers did eat manna in the
wilderness, and are dead.
50 This is the bread which cometh
down from heaven, that a man may eat
thereof, and not die.
51 I am the living bread which came
down from heaven: if any man eat of
this bread, he shall live for ever: and the
bread that I will give is my flesh, which I
will give for the [w]life of the [x]world.
52 The Jews therefore strove among
themselves, saying, How can this man
give us *his* flesh to eat?
53 Then Jesus said unto them, Verily,
verily, I say unto you, Except ye eat the
flesh of the Son of man, and drink his
blood, ye have no life in you.
54 [y]Whoso eateth my flesh, and drinketh my blood, hath eternal life; and I will
raise him up at the last day.
55 For my flesh is meat indeed, and
my blood is drink indeed.
56 He that eateth my flesh, and drinketh my blood, dwelleth in me, and I in
him.
57 As the living Father hath sent me,
and I live by the Father: so he that eateth
me, even he shall live by me.
58 This is that bread which came
down from heaven: not as your fathers
did eat manna, and are dead: he that
eateth of this bread shall live for ever.
59 These things said he in the synagogue, as he taught in Capernaum.

Discipleship tested by doctrine.
(Cf. Mt. 8:19-22; 10:36.)

60 Many therefore of his disciples,
when they had heard *this*, said, This is
an hard saying; who can hear it?
61 When Jesus knew in himself that
his disciples murmured at it, he said
unto them, Doth this offend you?
62 *What* and if ye shall see the Son of
man [z]ascend up where he was before?

A.D. 31.

a *Faith.* vs. 29, 35, 47; John 7:38, 39. (Gen. 3:20; Heb. 11:39.)
b Mt. 12:38.
c *Inspiration.* vs. 31, 32, 45, 49, 63; John 7:21-23. (Ex. 4:15; Rev. 22:19.)
d Neh. 9:15; cf. Psa. 78:24; 105:40.
e John 3:13, 16.
f vs. 48, 58.
g *Sacrifice (of Christ).* John 12:24. (Gen. 4:4; Heb. 10:18.)
h *kosmos* (Mt. 4:8) = mankind.
i John 5:40; Isa. 55:1, 2; Rev. 7:16.
j John 10:26.
k v. 45; John 17:2.
l Isa. 1:18; 55:1, 7; Mt. 11:28; Lk. 23:42, 43; 1 Tim. 1:15; Heb. 4:15, 16; 7:25; Rev. 22:17.
m John 4:34; 5:30; Psa. 40, 7, 8; Mt. 26:39.
n vs. 47, 54; John 3:15, 16.
o *Resurrection.* vs. 39, 40; John 11:11-14, 23-25, 42-44. (Job 19:25; 1 Cor. 15:52.)
p Mt. 13:55.
q v. 37.
r Eph. 2:8, 9; Phil. 1:29; 2:12, 13.
s *Jehovah.* Isa. 54:13.
t Lk. 10:22.
u v. 40.
v vs. 33, 35; Gal. 2:20; Col. 3:3, 4.
w John 3:16; Lk. 19:10.
x *kosmos* (Mt. 4:8) = mankind.
y v. 40.
z Mk. 16:19; Acts 1:9.

63 It is the [a]spirit that quickeneth; the [b]flesh profiteth nothing: the words that I speak unto you, *they* are spirit, and *they* are life.

64 But there are some of you that believe not. For Jesus knew from the beginning who they were that believed not, and who should betray him.

65 And he said, Therefore said I unto you, that no man can come unto me, except it were given unto him of my Father.

66 From that *time* many of his disciples went [c]back, and walked no more with him.

Peter's confession of faith. (Cf. Mt. 16:13-20; Mk. 8:27-30; Lk. 9:18-21.)

67 Then said Jesus unto the twelve, Will ye also go away?

68 Then Simon Peter answered him, Lord, to whom shall we go? thou hast the words of [d]eternal life.

69 And [e]we believe and are sure that thou art that Christ, the Son of the living God.

70 Jesus answered them, Have not I chosen you twelve, and one of you is a [f]devil?

71 He spake of Judas Iscariot *the son* of Simon: for he it was that should betray him, being one of the twelve.

CHAPTER 7.

Jesus urged to go to the feast of tabernacles. (Cf. Lk. 9:51-62.)

After these things Jesus walked in Galilee: for he would not walk in Jewry, because the Jews sought to kill him.

2 Now the Jews' [g]feast of tabernacles was at hand.

3 His brethren therefore said unto him, Depart hence, and go into Judæa, that thy disciples also may see the works that thou doest.

4 For *there is* no man *that* doeth any thing in secret, and he himself seeketh to be known openly. If thou do these things, shew thyself to the [h]world.

5 For [i]neither did his brethren believe in him.

6 Then Jesus said unto them, [j]My time is not yet come: but your time is alway ready.

7 The [k]world cannot hate you; but me it hateth, because I testify of it, that the works thereof are evil.

8 Go ye up unto this feast: I go not up yet unto this feast; for my time is not yet full come.

9 When he had said these words unto them, he abode *still* in Galilee.

Final departure from Galilee.

10 But when his brethren were gone up, then went he also up unto the feast, not openly, but as it were in secret.

11 Then the Jews sought him at the feast, and said, Where is he?

12 And [l]there was much murmuring among the people concerning him: for some said, He is a good man: others said, Nay; but he deceiveth the people.

13 Howbeit no man spake openly of him for [m]fear of the Jews.

Jesus at the feast of tabernacles.

14 Now about the midst of the feast Jesus went up into the temple, and taught.

15 And the Jews marvelled, saying, How knoweth this man letters, having never learned?

16 Jesus answered them, and said, My doctrine is not mine, but [n]his that sent me.

17 If any man [o]will do his will, he shall know of the doctrine, whether it be of God, or *whether* I speak of myself.

18 He [p]that speaketh of himself seeketh his own glory: but he that seeketh his glory that sent him, the same is true, and no unrighteousness is in him.

19 Did not Moses give you the [q]law, and *yet* none of you keepeth the law? Why go ye about to kill me?

20 The people answered and said, Thou hast a [r]devil: who goeth about to kill thee?

21 Jesus answered and said unto them, I have done one work, and ye all marvel.

22 Moses therefore gave unto you circumcision; (not because it is of Moses, [s]but of the fathers;) and ye on the sabbath day circumcise a man.

23 If a man on the sabbath day receive circumcision, [t]that the law of Moses should not be broken; are ye angry at me, because I have made a man every whit whole on the sabbath day?

24 Judge not according to the appearance, but judge [u]righteous judgment.

25 Then said some of them of Jerusalem, Is not this he, whom they seek to kill?

A.D. 32.

a *Holy Spirit.* John 7:39. (Mt. 1:18; Acts 2:4.)

b *Flesh.* John 8:15. (John 1:13; Jude 23.)

c 1 John 2:19.

d *Life (eternal).* vs. 27-68; John 8:12. (Mt. 7:14; Rev. 22:19.)

e Or, *we have believed and come to understand that thou art the Holy One of God.*

f Gr. *diabolos, adversary,* usually trans. *Satan.* Cf. Rev. 20:10, *note;* see John 13:27.

g Lev. 23:34; Neh. 8:14, 18.

h *kosmos* (Mt. 4:8) = mankind.

i vs. 3-5; Psa. 69:8.

j John 17:1; Lk. 9:51.

k *kosmos* = world-system. John 8:23. (John 7:7; Rev. 13:8.)

l John 9:16.

m John 9:22.

n Deut. 18:15, 18, 19.

o *willeth to do.*

p John 8:50; Phil. 2:3, 8.

q *Law (of Moses).* Acts 13:39. (Ex. 19:1; Gal. 3:1-29.)

r *demon.* Mt. 7:22, *note.*

s Gen. 17:10: Mt. 12:1, *note.*

t *Inspiration.* vs. 21-23. John 8:40, 47, 56. (Ex. 4:15; Rev. 22:19.)

u 1 John 3:7, *note.*

26 But, lo, he speaketh boldly, and they
say nothing unto him. [a]Do the rulers
know indeed that this is the very Christ?
27 [b]Howbeit we know this man
whence he is: but when Christ cometh,
no man knoweth whence he is.
28 Then cried Jesus in the temple as he
taught, saying, Ye both know me, and ye
know whence I am: and [c]I am not come
of myself, but he that sent me is true,
whom ye know not.
29 But I know him: for I am from him,
and he hath sent me.
30 Then they sought to take him: but
no man laid hands on him, because his
hour was not yet come.
31 And many of the people believed
on him, and said, When Christ cometh,
will he do more miracles than these
which this *man* hath done?
32 The Pharisees heard that the people
murmured such things concerning him;
and the Pharisees and the chief priests
sent officers to take him.
33 Then said Jesus unto them, Yet a little while am I with you, and *then* I go
unto him that sent me.
34 Ye shall seek me, and shall not find
me: and where I am, *thither* ye cannot
come.
35 Then said the Jews among themselves, Whither will he go, that we shall
not find him? will he go unto the [d]dis-
persed among the Gentiles, and teach
the Gentiles?
36 What *manner of* saying is this that
he said, Ye shall seek me, and shall not
find *me*: and where I am, *thither* ye cannot come?

The greatest prophecy concerning the Holy Spirit for power
(Acts 2:2-4. Cf. John 4:14).

37 In the [e]last day, that great *day* of the
feast, Jesus stood and cried, saying, If
any man [f]thirst, let him come unto me,
and drink.
38 He that [g]believeth on me, as the
scripture hath said, out of his belly shall
flow rivers of living water.
39 (But this spake he of the [h]Spirit,
which they that believe on him should
receive: for the Holy Ghost was not yet
given; because that Jesus was not yet
[i]glorified.)

The people divided in opinion.

40 Many of the people therefore, when
they heard this saying, said, Of a truth
this is the [j]Prophet.
41 Others said, This is [k]the Christ. But
some said, [l]Shall Christ come out of
Galilee?
42 Hath not the scripture said, [m]That
Christ cometh of the seed of David, and
out of the town of [n]Bethlehem, where
David was?
43 So there was a division among the
people because of him.
44 And some of them would have taken
him; but no man laid hands on him.
45 Then came the officers to the chief
priests and Pharisees; and they said unto
them, Why have ye not brought him?
46 The officers answered, [o]Never man
spake like this man.
47 Then answered them the Pharisees,
Are ye also deceived?
48 Have any of the rulers or of the
Pharisees believed on him?
49 But this people who knoweth not
the law are cursed.
50 Nicodemus saith unto them, ([p]he
that came to Jesus by night, being one of
them,)
51 Doth our law judge *any* man, before
it hear him, and know what he doeth?
52 They answered and said unto him,
Art thou also of Galilee? Search, and look:
for out of Galilee ariseth no prophet.
53 [1]And every man went unto his own
house.

CHAPTER 8.

The woman taken in adultery.

Jesus went unto the mount of Olives.
2 And early in the morning he came
again into the temple, and all the people
came unto him; and he sat down, and
taught them.
3 And the scribes and Pharisees

A.D. 32.

a v. 48; John 12:42.
b Mt. 13:55.
c John 6:38; Ex. 23:21.
d Jas. 1:1.
e Lev. 23:36.
f *Christ (as Stone).* vs. 37-39; Psa. 118:22. (Ex. 17:6; 1 Pet. 2:8.)
g *Faith.* vs. 38, 39; John 8:24. (Gen. 3:20; Heb. 11:39.)
h *Holy Spirit.* John 14:17, 26. (Mt. 1:18; Acts 2:4.) See Acts 2:4, Summary.
i John 13:31; 17:5; Acts 3:13.
j John 6:14; Deut. 18:15, 18.
k John 4:42; 6:69.
l v. 52; John 1:46.
m 2 Sam. 7:12; Psa. 132:11; Jer. 23:5.
n Mic. 5:2; Lk. 2:4.
o Mt. 13:54, 56; Lk. 4:22.
p John 3:2.

[1] **(7:53)** John 7:53–8:1-11 is not found in some of the most ancient manuscripts. Augustine declares that it was stricken from many copies of the sacred story because of a prudish fear that it might teach immorality! But the immediate context (vs. 12-46), beginning with Christ's declaration, "I am the light of the world," seems clearly to have its occasion in the conviction wrought in the hearts of the Pharisees as recorded in verse 9; as, also, it explains the peculiar virulence of the Pharisees' words (v. 41).

brought unto him a woman taken in adultery; and when they had set her in the midst,

4 They say unto him, Master, this woman was taken in adultery, in the very act.

5 Now [a]Moses in the law commanded us, that such should be stoned: but what sayest thou?

6 This they said, tempting him, that they [b]might have to accuse him. But Jesus stooped down, and with *his* finger wrote on the ground, *as though he heard them not*.

7 So when they continued asking him, he lifted up himself, and said unto them, He that is without [c]sin among you, [d]let him first cast a stone at her.

8 And again he stooped down, and wrote on the ground.

9 And they which heard *it*, being convicted by *their own* conscience, went out one by one, beginning at the eldest, *even* unto the last: and Jesus was left alone, and the woman standing in the midst.

10 When Jesus had lifted up himself, and saw none but the woman, he said unto her, Woman, where are those thine accusers? hath no man [e]condemned thee?

11 She said, No man, Lord. And Jesus said unto her, Neither do I condemn thee: go, and [f]sin no more.

Discourse after the feast: Jesus the light of the world. (Cf. John 1:9.)

12 Then spake Jesus again unto them, saying, [g]I am the light of the [h]world: he that followeth me shall not walk in darkness, but shall have the light of [i]life.

13 The Pharisees therefore said unto him, Thou bearest record of thyself; thy record is not true.

14 Jesus answered and said unto them, [j]Though I bear record of myself, *yet* my record is true: for I know whence I came, and whither I go; but ye cannot tell whence I come, and whither I go.

15 Ye judge after the [k]flesh; I judge no man.

16 And yet if I judge, my judgment is true: for I am not alone, but I and the Father that sent me.

17 It is also [l]written in your law, that the testimony of two men is true.

18 I am one that bear witness of myself, and the Father that sent me beareth witness of me.

A.D. 32.

a Lev. 20:10; Deut. 22:22.
b John 18:31.
c *Sin.* Rom. 3:23, *note.*
d Mt. 7:1, 5.
e Lk. 12:14.
f John 5:14.
g Isa. 9:2; Mal. 4:2; 2 Tim. 1:10.
h *kosmos* (Mt. 4:8) = mankind.
i *Life (eternal).* John 10:10, 28. (Mt. 7:14; Rev. 22:19.)
j Cf. John 5:31.
k *Flesh.* Rom. 7:5-25. (John 1:13; Jude 23.)
l Deut. 19:15.
m John 17:25.
n John 14:7, 9.
o *kosmos* = world-system. John 12:25, 31. (John 7:7; Rev. 13:8.)
p *Death (the second).* vs. 21, 24; Rev. 2:11 (John 8:21, 24; Rev. 21:8.)
q *Faith.* John 10:26. (Gen. 3:20; Heb. 11:39.)
r *kosmos* (Mt. 4:8) = mankind.
s Mt. 8:20, *note.*
t Deut. 18:15, 18, 19.
u Rom. 8:15, 17.

19 Then said they unto him, Where is thy Father? Jesus answered, [m]Ye neither know me, nor my Father: [n]if ye had known me, ye should have known my Father also.

20 These words spake Jesus in the treasury, as he taught in the temple: and no man laid hands on him; for his hour was not yet come.

21 Then said Jesus again unto them, I go my way, and ye shall seek me, and shall die in your [c]sins: whither I go, ye cannot come.

22 Then said the Jews, Will he kill himself? because he saith, Whither I go, ye cannot come.

23 And he said unto them, Ye are from beneath; I am from above: ye are of this world; I am not of this [o]world.

24 I said therefore unto you, that ye shall [p]die in your [c]sins: for if ye [q]believe not that I am *he*, ye shall die in your sins.

25 Then said they unto him, Who art thou? And Jesus saith unto them, Even *the same* that I said unto you from the beginning.

26 I have many things to say and to judge of you: but he that sent me is true; and I speak to the [r]world those things which I have heard of him.

27 They understood not that he spake to them of the Father.

28 Then said Jesus unto them, When ye have lifted up the [s]Son of man, then shall ye know that I am *he*, and *that* [t]I do nothing of myself; but as my Father hath taught me, I speak these things.

29 And he that sent me is with me: the Father hath not left me alone; for I do always those things that please him.

30 As he spake these words, many believed on him.

31 Then said Jesus to those Jews which believed on him, If ye continue in my word, *then* are ye my disciples indeed;

32 And ye shall know the truth, and the truth shall make you free.

33 They answered him, We be Abraham's seed, and were never in bondage to any man: how sayest thou, Ye shall be made free?

34 Jesus answered them, Verily, verily, I say unto you, Whosoever committeth [c]sin is the servant of sin.

35 And the servant abideth not in the house for ever: *but* the Son [u]abideth ever.

36 If the Son therefore shall make you free, ye shall be free indeed.

37 I know that ye are [1]Abraham's seed; but ye seek to kill me, because my word hath no place in you.

38 [a]I speak that which I have seen with my Father: and ye do that which ye have seen with your father.

39 They answered and said unto him, Abraham is our father. Jesus saith unto them, If ye were Abraham's children, ye would do the works of Abraham.

40 But now ye seek to kill me, a man that hath told you the truth, [b]which I have heard of God: this did not Abraham.

41 Ye do the deeds of your father. **Then said they to him, We be not born of fornication; we have one Father, *even* God.**

42 Jesus said unto them, If God were your Father, ye would love me: for I proceeded forth and came from God; neither came I of myself, but [c]he sent me.

43 [d]Why do ye not understand my speech? *even* because ye cannot hear my word.

44 Ye are of *your* father [e]the [f]devil, and the lusts of your father ye will do. He was a murderer from the beginning, and [g]abode not in the truth, because there is no truth in him. When he speaketh a lie, he speaketh of his own: for he is a [h]liar, and the father of it.

45 And because [i]I tell *you* the truth, ye believe me not.

46 Which of you convinceth me of [j]sin? And if I say the truth, why do ye not believe me?

47 He that is of God [k]heareth God's words: ye therefore hear *them* not, because ye are not of God.

48 Then answered the Jews, and said unto him, Say we not well that thou art a [l]Samaritan, and [m]hast a [n]devil?

49 Jesus answered, I have not a [n]devil; [o]but I honour my Father, and ye do dishonour me.

50 And I [p]seek not mine own glory: there is one that seeketh and judgeth.

51 Verily, verily, I say unto you, [q]If a man keep my saying, he shall never see death.

52 Then said the Jews unto him, Now we know that thou hast a [n]devil. [r]Abraham is dead, and the prophets; and thou sayest, If a man keep my saying, he shall never taste of death.

53 Art thou [s]greater than our father Abraham, which is dead? and the prophets are dead: whom makest thou thyself?

54 Jesus answered, [t]If I honour myself, my honour is nothing: [u]it is my Father that honoureth me; of whom ye say, that he is your God:

55 Yet [v]ye have not known him; but I know him: and if I should say, I know him not, I shall be a liar like unto you: but I know him, and [w]keep his saying.

56 Your father Abraham [x]rejoiced to see my day: and [y]he saw *it*, and was glad.

57 Then said the Jews unto him, Thou art not yet fifty years old, and hast thou seen Abraham?

58 Jesus said unto them, Verily, verily, I say unto you, Before Abraham was, [z]I am.

59 Then [aa]took they up stones to cast at him: but Jesus hid himself, and went out of the temple, [bb]going through the midst of them, and so passed by.

CHAPTER 9.

The man born blind is healed.

And as *Jesus* passed by, he saw a man which was blind from *his* birth.

2 And his disciples asked him, saying, Master, [cc]who did [j]sin, this man, or his parents, that he was born blind?

3 Jesus answered, Neither hath this man [j]sinned, nor his parents: but [dd]that the works of God should be made manifest in him.

4 [ee]I must work the works of him that sent me, while it is [ff]day: the night cometh, when no man can work.

5 As long as I am in the [gg]world, I am [hh]the light of the world.

6 When he had thus spoken, [ii]he spat on the ground, and made clay of the spittle, and he anointed

A.D. 32.

- *a* John 14:10, 24
- *b* *Inspiration.* vs. 40, 47, 56; John 12:48. (Ex. 4:15; Rev. 22:19.)
- *c* Gal. 4:4.
- *d* John 7:17; 1 Cor. 2:14.
- *e* *diabolos.* Rev. 20:10, *note.*
- *f* *Satan.* John 13:2, 27. (Gen. 3:1; Rev. 20:10.)
- *g* Ezk. 28:12-17; 1 John 3:8; Jude 5.
- *h* Gen. 3:4, 13; 2 Cor. 11:3; Rev. 12:9.
- *i* 2 Thes. 2:11, 12.
- *j* *Sin.* Rom. 3:23, *note.*
- *k* Lk. 8:15; John 6:37, 44; 10:26; 1 John 4:6.
- *l* John 4:9; Lk. 10:33.
- *m* v. 52; John 7:20; 10:20.
- *n* *demon.* Mt. 7:20, *note.*
- *o* John 5:41; 12:28.
- *p* v. 54; John 7:18; . Phil. 2:6-8.
- *q* John 5:24; 11:26; 14:23, 24.
- *r* Zech 1:5; Heb. 11:13.
- *s* John 4:12; Heb. 3:3.
- *t* John 5:31.
- *u* v. 50; John 5:31, 41; 16:14; 17:1; Acts 3:13.
- *v* v. 19; John 7:28, 29.
- *w* v. 29; John 15:10.
- *x* Lk. 10:24.
- *y* Heb. 11:13.
- *z* Ex. 3:14; Isa. 43:13; John 17:5, 24; Col. 1:17; Rev. 1:8.
- *aa* John 10:31, 39; 11:8.
- *bb* Lk. 4:30.
- *cc* v. 34.
- *dd* John 11:4.
- *ee* John 4:34; 5:19, 36; 11:9; 12:35; 17:4.
- *ff* John 11:9, 10.
- *gg* *kosmos* (Mt. 4:8) = mankind.
- *hh* John 1:5, 9; 3:19; 8:12; 12:35, 46.
- *ii* Mk. 7:33; 8:23.

[1](8:37) Cf. v. 39. The contrast, "I know that ye are Abraham's seed"—"If ye were Abraham's children," is that between the natural and the spiritual posterity of Abraham. The Israelitish people and Ishmaelites are the former; all who are "of like precious faith with Abraham," whether Jews or Gentiles, are the latter (Rom. 9:6-8; Gal. 3:6-14. See "Abrahamic Covenant," Gen. 15:18, *note*).

the eyes of the blind man with the clay,

7 And said unto him, Go, wash in the [a]pool of Siloam, (which is by interpretation, Sent.) [b]He went his way therefore, and washed, and [c]came seeing.

8 The neighbours therefore, and they which before had seen him that he was blind, said, Is not this he that sat and begged?

9 Some said, This is he: others *said*, He is like him: *but* he said, I am *he*.

10 Therefore said they unto him, [d]How were thine eyes opened?

11 He answered and said, A man that is called Jesus made clay, and anointed mine eyes, and said unto me, Go to the pool of Siloam, and wash: and I went and washed, and I received sight.

12 Then said they unto him, Where is he? He said, I know not.

13 They brought to the Pharisees him that aforetime was blind.

14 And it was the [e]sabbath day when Jesus made the clay, and opened his eyes.

15 Then again the Pharisees also asked him how he had received his sight. He said unto them, He put clay upon mine eyes, and I washed, and do see.

16 Therefore said some of the Pharisees, This man is not of God, because he keepeth not the sabbath day. Others said, [f]How can a man that is a [g]sinner do such miracles? And there was a [h]division among them.

17 They say unto the blind man again, What sayest thou of him, that he hath opened thine eyes? He said, [i]He is a prophet.

18 But the Jews did not believe concerning him, that he had been blind, and received his sight, until they called the parents of him that had received his sight.

19 And they asked them, saying, Is this your son, who ye say was born blind? how then doth he now see?

20 His parents answered them and said, We know that this is our son, and that he was born blind:

21 But by what means he now seeth, we know not; or who hath opened his eyes, we know not: he is of age; ask him: he shall speak for himself.

22 These *words* spake his parents, because [j]they feared the Jews: for the Jews had agreed already, that if any man did confess that he was Christ, [k]he should be put out of the synagogue.

A.D. 32.

a Neh. 3:15.
b 2 Ki. 5:14.
c *Miracles* (N.T.). vs. 1-7; John 11:43, 44. (Mt. 8:2, 3; Acts 28:8, 9.)
d John 3:4.
e John 5:9.
f v. 33; John 3:2.
g *Sin.* Rom. 3:23, *note.*
h John 7:12, 43; 10:19.
i John 4:19; 6:14.
j John 7:13; 12:42; 19:38; Acts 5:13.
k v. 34; John 16:2.
l Josh. 7:19; 1 Sam. 6:5.
m v. 16.
n John 5:45-47; Acts 13:27.
o John 7:27, 28; 8:14.
p John 3:10.
q Job 27:9; 35:12; Psa. 18:41; 34:15; 66:18; Prov. 15:29; 28:9; Mic. 3:4; Zech. 7:13; Acts 19:13-16.
r i.e. *ages.*
s John 5:19; 14;10, 11.
t v. 2; Psa. 51:5; Lk. 18:11, 12.
u v. 22.
v Mt. 14:33; 16:16; Mk. 1:1; John 10:36; Acts 9:20; 1 John 5:13.
w John 4:26.
x John 14:9; 20:16, 17, 28.
y *kosmos* (Mt. 4:8) = mankind.
z Mt. 13:13; Acts 7:51-53.
aa Rom. 2:19.

23 Therefore said his parents, He is of age; ask him.

24 Then again called they the man that was blind, and said unto him, [l]Give God the praise: we [m]know that this man is a [g]sinner.

25 He answered and said, Whether he be a [g]sinner *or no*, I know not: one thing I know, that, whereas I was blind, now I see.

26 Then said they to him again, What did he to thee? how opened he thine eyes?

27 He answered them, I have told you already, and ye did not hear: wherefore would ye hear *it* again? will ye also be his disciples?

28 Then they reviled him, and said, Thou art his disciple; but we are [n]Moses' disciples.

29 We know that God spake unto Moses: *as for* this *fellow*, we know not from [o]whence he is.

30 The man answered and said unto them, [p]Why herein is a marvellous thing, that ye know not from whence he is, and *yet* he hath opened mine eyes.

31 Now we know that [q]God heareth not [g]sinners: but if any man be a worshipper of God, and doeth his will, him he heareth.

32 Since the [r]world began was it not heard that any man opened the eyes of one that was born blind.

33 If this man were not of God, he could do [s]nothing.

34 They answered and said unto him, Thou wast altogether [t]born in [g]sins, and dost thou teach us? And they [u]cast him out.

35 Jesus heard that they had cast him out; and when he had found him, he said unto him, Dost thou believe on the [v]Son of God?

36 He answered and said, Who is he, Lord, that I might believe on him?

37 And Jesus said unto him, Thou hast both seen him, and [w]it is he that talketh with thee.

38 And he said, Lord, I believe. And he [x]worshipped him.

39 And Jesus said, For judgment I am come into this [y]world, [z]that they which see not might see; and that they which see might be made blind.

40 And *some* of the Pharisees which were with him heard these words, and said unto him, [aa]Are we blind also?

41 Jesus said unto them, [a]If ye were blind, ye should have no [b]sin: but now ye say, We see; therefore your sin remaineth.

CHAPTER 10.

Discourse on the Good Shepherd.
(Cf. Psa. 23; Heb. 13:20; 1 Pet. 5:4.)

Verily, verily, I say unto you, He that entereth not by the door into the sheepfold, but climbeth up some other way, the same is a [c]thief and a robber.

2 But he that entereth in by the door is the shepherd of the sheep.

3 To him [d]the porter openeth; and the sheep [e]hear his voice: and he calleth his own sheep by [f]name, and [g]leadeth them out.

4 And when he putteth forth his own sheep, he goeth [h]before them, and the sheep follow him: for they know his voice.

5 And a [i]stranger will they not follow, but will flee from him: for they know not the voice of strangers.

6 This parable spake Jesus unto them: but they [j]understood not what things they were which he spake unto them.

7 Then said Jesus unto them again, Verily, verily, I say unto you, [1]I am the door of the sheep.

8 All that ever came before me are thieves and robbers: but the sheep did not hear them.

9 I am the door: by me if any man enter in, he shall be [k]saved, and shall go in and out, and find pasture.

10 The thief cometh not, but for to steal, and to kill, and to destroy: I am come that they might have [l]life, and that they might have *it* more [m]abundantly.

11 I am the [n]good shepherd: the good shepherd giveth his life for the sheep.

12 But he that is an hireling, and not the shepherd, whose own the sheep are not, seeth the wolf coming, and leaveth the sheep, and fleeth: and the wolf catcheth them, and scattereth the sheep.

A.D. 32.

- *a* John 15:22, 24.
- *b* *Sin.* Rom. 3:23, *note.*
- *c* v. 8.
- *d* Isa. 42:1-4; Mt. 3:13-17.
- *e* v. 27; John 6:44.
- *f* Ex. 28:9, 10, 21; Isa. 43:1; John 20:16.
- *g* John 9:34-38; Heb. 13:13.
- *h* John 17:19; Col. 2:11-15.
- *i* vs. 12, 13; Gal. 1:8; 2 Cor. 11:13-15.
- *j* John 8:43.
- *k* Rom. 1:16, *note.*
- *l* *Life (eternal).* vs. 10, 28; John 11:25. (Mt. 7:14; Rev. 22:19.)
- *m* John 6:33; 7:37-39.
- *n* Isa. 40:11; Ezk. 34:11-13, 22-25; Heb. 13:20; 1 Pet. 2:25; 5:4.
- *o* v. 27; Nah. 1:7; John 6:64; 2 Tim. 2:19.
- *p* v. 4; 2 Tim. 1:12.
- *q* vs. 17, 18; John 15:13; 1 John 3:16.
- *r* i.e. not of the Jewish fold, but Gentiles. See v. 4. *refs.;* Isa. 56:8; John 17:20; Acts 15:7-9.
- *s* *flock.* John 11:52; Eph. 2:13-16; 3:1-6; Col. 3:10, 11.
- *t* Gen. 49:24; Isa. 40:11; Ezk. 34:23.
- *u* John 5:20; Eph. 5:2; Phil. 2:9.
- *v* Mt. 26:53; John 18:6.
- *w* John 2:19; Heb. 10:5-9.
- *x* John 14:31; 17:4.
- *y* John 9:16.
- *z* *demon.* Mt. 7:22, *note.*
- *aa* *is demonized.*
- *bb* Mt. 21:23-27.
- *cc* *Faith.* John 11:25, 26. (Gen. 3:20; Heb. 11:39.)
- *dd* John 6:44; 8:47; 1 John 4:6.
- *ee* vs. 14, 15.
- *ff* John 8:12.
- *gg* John 3:16; 17:3; Rom. 6:23.
- *hh* Or, in no wise ever perish. Cf. John 6:37.

13 The hireling fleeth, because he is an hireling, and careth not for the sheep.

14 I am the good shepherd, and [o]know my *sheep*, and [p]am known of mine.

15 As the Father knoweth me, even so know I the Father: and [q]I lay down my life for the sheep.

16 And [r]other sheep I have, which are not of this fold: them also I must bring, and they shall hear my voice; and there shall be one [s]fold, *and* [t]one shepherd.

17 Therefore doth my [u]Father love me, because I lay down my life, that I might take it again.

18 No man taketh it from me, but I lay it down of [v]myself. I have [w]power to lay it down, and I have power to take it again. [x]This commandment have I received of my Father.

19 There was a [y]division therefore again among the Jews for these sayings.

20 And many of them said, He hath a [z]devil, and is mad; why hear ye him?

21 Others said, These are not the words of him that [aa]hath a devil. Can a [z]devil open the eyes of the blind?

Jesus asserts his deity.
(Cf. John 14:9; 20:28, 29.)

22 And it was at Jerusalem the feast of the dedication, and it was winter.

23 And Jesus walked in the temple in Solomon's porch.

24 Then came the Jews round about him, and said unto him, How long dost thou make us to doubt? If thou be the Christ, tell us [bb]plainly.

25 Jesus answered them, I told you, and ye believed not: the works that I do in my Father's name, they bear witness of me.

26 But ye [cc]believe not, [dd]because ye are not of my sheep, as I said unto you.

27 My sheep hear my voice, and [ee]I know them, and they [ff]follow me:

28 And I [gg]give unto them [l]eternal life; and they shall [hh]never perish,

[1] **(10:7)** The shepherd work of our Lord has three aspects: (1) As the "Good" Shepherd He gives His life for the sheep (John 10:11), and is, therefore, "the door" by which "if any man enter in he shall be saved" (John 10:9). This answers to Psa. 22. (2) He is the "Great" Shepherd, "brought again from the dead" (Heb. 13:20), to care for and make perfect the sheep. This answers to Psa. 23. He is the "Chief" Shepherd who is coming in glory to give crowns of reward to the faithful shepherds (1 Pet. 5:4). This answers to Psa. 24.

neither shall any *man* [a]pluck them out of my hand.

29 My Father, which gave *them* me, is greater than all; and no *man* is able to pluck *them* out [b]of my Father's hand.

30 I and *my* Father [c]are one.

31 Then the Jews took up stones again to [d]stone him.

32 Jesus answered them, Many good works have I shewed you from my Father; for which of those works do ye stone me?

33 The Jews answered him, saying, For a good work we stone thee not; but for [e]blasphemy; and because that thou, being a man, makest thyself God.

34 Jesus answered them, Is it not written in your law, I said, [f]Ye are gods?

35 If he called them gods, unto whom the word of God came, and the scripture [g]cannot be broken;

36 Say ye of him, whom the Father hath [h]sanctified, and sent into the [i]world, Thou blasphemest; because I said, I am the Son of God?

37 If I do not the works of my Father, believe me not.

38 But if I do, though ye believe not me, believe the works: that ye may know, and believe, that the Father *is* [j]in me, and I in him.

39 Therefore they sought again to take him: but he [k]escaped out of their hand,

Jesus goes to the place where he was baptized. (Cf. Mt. 3:1, 13, 17.)

40 And went away again beyond Jordan into the place where John at first baptized; and there he abode.

41 And many resorted unto him, and said, John did no miracle: but all things that John spake of this man were true.

42 And many believed on him there.

CHAPTER 11.

The raising of Lazarus.

Now a certain *man* was sick, *named* Lazarus, of Bethany, the town of [l]Mary and her sister Martha.

2 ([m]It was *that* Mary which anointed the Lord with ointment, and wiped his feet with her hair, whose brother Lazarus was sick.)

3 Therefore his sisters [n]sent unto him, saying, Lord, behold, he whom thou lovest is sick.

4 When Jesus heard *that*, he said, This sickness is [o]not unto death, but for the glory of God, that the Son of God might be glorified thereby.

5 Now Jesus loved Martha, and her sister, and Lazarus.

6 When he had heard therefore that he was sick, he [p]abode two days still in the same place where he was.

7 Then after that saith he to *his* disciples, Let us go into Judæa again.

8 *His* disciples say unto him, Master, the Jews of late sought to [q]stone thee; and goest thou thither again?

9 Jesus answered, Are there not twelve hours in the day? If any man walk in the day, he stumbleth not, [r]because he seeth the light of this world.

10 But [s]if a man walk in the night, he stumbleth, because there is no light in him.

11 These things said he: and after that he saith unto them, Our friend Lazarus [t]sleepeth; but I go, that I may [u]awake him out of sleep.

12 Then said his disciples, Lord, if he sleep, he shall do well.

13 Howbeit Jesus spake of his death: but they thought that he had spoken of taking of rest in sleep.

14 Then said Jesus unto them plainly, Lazarus is [v]dead.

15 And I am [w]glad for your sakes that I was not there, to the intent ye may believe; nevertheless let us go unto him.

16 Then said [x]Thomas, which is called Didymus, unto his fellowdisciples, Let us also go, that we may die with him.

17 Then when Jesus came, he found that he had *lain* in the grave four days already.

18 Now Bethany was nigh unto Jerusalem, about fifteen [y]furlongs off:

19 And many of the Jews came to Martha and Mary, to [z]comfort them concerning their brother.

20 Then Martha, as soon as she heard that Jesus was coming, went and met him: but Mary sat *still* in the house.

21 Then said Martha unto Jesus, Lord, if thou hadst been here, my brother had not died.

22 But I know, that even now, whatsoever thou [aa]wilt ask of God, God will give *it* thee.

A.D. 33.

a John 6:39; Rom. 8:35-39; 1 Pet. 1:5.
b *Assurance.* vs. 10, 14, 28, 29; John 11:26. (Isa. 32:17; Jude 1.)
c John 14:9; 15:23, 24; 17:21-24.
d vs. 31, 39; Psa. 2:2; John 8:59.
e Mt. 9:3; John 19:7.
f Psa. 82:6.
g Mt. 5:17-19; Acts 13:29.
h *Sanctify, holy (persons)* (N.T.). John 17:11, 17, 19. Mt. 4:5; Rev. 22:11.)
i *kosmos* (Mt. 4:8) = mankind.
j John 14:10; 17:22, 23.
k Or, *went forth out of their hand.* Lk. 4:30; John 8:59.
l Lk. 10:38, 39; 24:50.
m Mt. 26:7; Mk. 14:3; John 12:3.
n Lk. 7:3; John 4:46, 47.
o v. 11; Mt. 9:24; John 9:3.
p Mt. 15:23; Lk. 18:7; John 10:40.
q John 8:59; 10:31.
r John 7:30; 9:4.
s John 12:35.
t Mt. 9:24; 27:52; Acts 7:60; 1 Cor. 15:51.
u 1 Thes. 4:13-17.
v *Death (physical).* vs. 11-14; Rom. 5:12-14. (Gen. 3:19; Heb. 9:27.)
w John 9:3; 2 Cor. 12:9, 10.
x John 14:5; 20:24-29.
y One furlong = 1/8 of a mile.
z vs. 31, 33, 45.
aa John 9:31.

23 Jesus saith unto her, Thy brother shall rise again.

24 Martha saith unto him, I know that he shall rise again in the [a]resurrection at the last day.

25 Jesus said unto her, [b]I am the resurrection, and the [c]life: he that [d]believeth in me, [e]though he were [f]dead, yet shall he live:

26 And whosoever liveth and believeth in me [g]shall [h]never die. Believest thou this?

27 She saith unto him, Yea, Lord: I believe that [i]thou art the Christ, the Son of God, which should come into the [j]world.

28 And when she had so said, she went her way, and called Mary her sister secretly, saying, The Master is come, and calleth for thee.

29 As soon as she heard *that*, she arose quickly, and came unto him.

30 Now Jesus was not yet come into the town, but was in that place where Martha met him.

31 The Jews then which were with her in the house, and comforted her, when they saw Mary, that she rose up hastily and went out, followed her, saying, She goeth unto the grave to weep there.

32 Then when Mary was come where Jesus was, and saw him, she fell down at his feet, saying unto him, [k]Lord, if thou hadst been here, my brother had not died.

33 When Jesus therefore saw her [l]weeping, and the Jews also weeping which came with her, he groaned in the spirit, and was troubled,

34 And said, Where have ye laid him? They said unto him, Lord, come and see.

35 Jesus [m]wept.

36 Then said the Jews, Behold how he loved him!

37 And some of them said, Could not this man, which [n]opened the eyes of the blind, have caused that even this man should not have died?

Jesus at the grave of Lazarus.

38 Jesus therefore again groaning in himself cometh to the grave. It was a cave, and a [o]stone lay upon it.

39 Jesus said, Take ye away the stone. Martha, the sister of him that was dead, saith unto him, Lord, by this time [p]he stinketh: for he hath been *dead* four days.

40 Jesus saith unto her, Said I not unto thee, that, if thou wouldest believe, thou shouldest see the [q]glory of God?

41 Then they took away the stone *from the place* where the dead was laid. And Jesus lifted up *his* eyes, and [r]said, Father, I thank thee that thou hast heard me.

42 And I knew that [s]thou hearest me always: but because of the people which [t]stand by I said *it*, that they may believe that thou hast sent me.

43 And when he thus had spoken, he [u]cried with a loud voice, Lazarus, come forth.

44 And [v]he that was dead [w]came forth, bound hand and foot with [x]graveclothes: and his face was bound about with a napkin. Jesus saith unto them, [y]Loose him, and let him go.

The friends of Mary of Bethany are converted. (Cf. Lk. 10:38-42; John 12:1-7.)

45 Then many of the Jews which came to Mary, and had seen the things which Jesus did, [z]believed on him.

46 But some of them went their ways to the Pharisees, and [aa]told them what things Jesus had done.

The Pharisees plot to put Jesus to death.

47 Then gathered the chief priests and the Pharisees a [bb]council, and said, What do we? [cc]for this man doeth many miracles.

48 If we let him thus alone, [dd]all *men* will believe on him: and the [ee]Romans shall come and take away both our place and nation.

49 And one of them, *named* [ff]Caiaphas, being the high priest that same year, said unto them, Ye know nothing at all,

50 Nor consider that it is expedient for us, that [gg]one man should die for the people, and that the whole nation perish not.

51 And this spake he not of himself: but being high priest that year, he [hh]prophesied that Jesus should die for that nation;

52 And [ii]not for that nation only, but that also he should [jj]gather together in one the children of God that were scattered abroad.

53 Then from that day forth they took counsel together for to put him to death.

54 Jesus therefore walked [kk]no more openly among the Jews; but went thence unto a country near to the wilderness,

A.D. 33.

a Lk. 14:14; Acts 23:8.
b John 5:21; 6:39, 40; Rev. 1:18.
c *Life (eternal).* John 12:25, 50. (Mt. 7:14; Rev. 22:19.)
d *Faith.* vs. 25, 26; John 14:1. (Gen. 3:20; Heb. 11:39.)
e *even though he die, shall live again.*
f John 5:28; 1 Cor. 15:22, 23.
g *Assurance.* John 17:11. (Isa. 32:17; Jude 1.)
h i.e. the "second death." Cf. Rev. 2:11; 20:6.
i Mt. 16:16; John 6:68, 69.
j *kosmos* (Mt. 4:8) = mankind.
k v. 21.
l Acts 8:2.
m Lk. 19:41; Heb. 4:15.
n John 9:6, 7.
o Mt. 27:60, 66.
p *Contra,* Acts 13:36, 37.
q v. 4; John 17:4.
r *Bible prayers* (N.T.). John 12:27, 28. (Mt. 6:9; Rev. 22:20.)
s v. 22; John 8:29.
t John 12:29, 30.
u Mt. 8:8; John 5:25.
v *Resurrection.* vs. 11-14, 23-25, 42:44; Lk. 24:1-7. (Job 19:25; 1 Cor. 15:52.)
w *Miracles* (N.T.). vs. 38-44; John 20:19. (Mt. 8:2, 3; Acts 28:8, 9.)
x John 20:5-7; cf. Gal. 4:10.
y Rom. 8:2; Acts 18:25, 26; Gal. 5:1.
z John 8:30, 31; Acts 9:42.
aa John 5:15.
bb vs. 47-53; Psa. 2:2; Mt. 26:3.
cc John 3:19; 12:19; Acts 4:16.
dd John 6:15; 18:36, 37.
ee Acts 21:28.
ff Mt. 26:3.
gg Isa. 53:8; John 18:14.
hh Num. 27:21.
ii Isa. 49:6; 1 John 2:2.
jj Psa. 22:27; John 10:16; Rom. 1:16; 16:26; Eph. 2:14-17.
kk John 7:1.

into a city called Ephraim, and there continued with his disciples.

55 And the Jews' [a]passover was nigh at hand: and many went out of the country up to Jerusalem before the passover, to [b]purify themselves.

56 Then [c]sought they for Jesus, and spake among themselves, as they stood in the temple, What think ye, that he will not come to the feast?

57 Now both the chief priests and the Pharisees had given a commandment, that, if any man knew where he were, he should shew *it*, that [d]they might take him.

CHAPTER 12.

The supper at Bethany (Mt. 26:6-13; Mk. 14:3-9. Cf. Lk. 7:37, 38).

Then Jesus six days before the passover came to [e]Bethany, where Lazarus was which had been dead, whom he raised from the dead.

2 There they made him a supper; and [f]Martha served: but Lazarus was one of them that [g]sat at the table with him.

3 [h]Then took [i]Mary a pound of ointment of [j]spikenard, very costly, and anointed the [k]feet of Jesus, and wiped his feet with her hair: and the house was filled with the odour of the ointment.

4 Then saith one of his disciples, [l]Judas Iscariot, Simon's *son*, which should betray him,

5 Why was not this ointment sold for three hundred pence, and given to the poor?

6 This he said, not that he cared for the poor; but because he was a [m]thief, and had the bag, and bare what was put therein.

7 Then said Jesus, Let her alone: against the day of my burying hath she kept this.

8 For the poor always ye have with you; but [n]me ye have not always.

9 [o]Much people of the Jews therefore knew that he was there: and they came not for Jesus' sake only, but that they might see Lazarus also, whom he had raised from the dead.

10 But the chief priests consulted that they might put [p]Lazarus also to death;

11 Because that by reason of him [q]many of the Jews went away, and believed on Jesus.

The triumphal entry (Mt. 21:4-9; Mk. 11:7-10; Lk. 19:35-38).

12 On the next day much people that were come to the feast, [r]when they heard that Jesus was coming to Jerusalem,

13 Took branches of palm trees, and went forth to meet him, and cried, [s]Hosanna: Blessed *is* the King of Israel that cometh in the name of the [t]Lord.

14 [u]And Jesus, when he had found a young ass, sat thereon; as [v]it is written,

15 Fear not, daughter of Sion: behold, thy King cometh, sitting on an ass's colt.

16 These things [w]understood not his disciples at the first: but when Jesus was glorified, then remembered they that these things were written of him, and *that* they had done these things unto him.

17 The people therefore that was with him when he called Lazarus out of his grave, and raised him from the dead, [x]bare record.

18 For this cause the people also met him, for that they heard that he had done this miracle.

19 The Pharisees therefore said among themselves, Perceive ye how ye prevail nothing? behold, the [y]world is [z]gone after him.

Certain Greeks would see Jesus.

20 And there were certain [aa]Greeks among them that came up to worship at the feast:

21 The same came therefore to [bb]Philip, which was of Bethsaida of Galilee, and desired him, saying, Sir, we would see Jesus.

22 Philip cometh and telleth Andrew: and again Andrew and Philip tell Jesus.

Jesus' answer.

23 And Jesus [1]answered them, saying, [cc]The hour is come, that the [dd]Son of man should be glorified.

24 Verily, verily, I say unto you,

A.D. 33.

a Cf. John 2:13; 6:4; 18:28.
b Num. 9:10-13; Isa. 29:13; John 18:28.
c John 7:11.
d Mt. 26:14-16; John 18:2, 3.
e John 11:1.
f Lk. 10:40, 41; cf. Mt. 11:29, 30.
g Mk. 5:43; Lk. 15:23, 24.
h Lk. 7:37, 38; John 11:2.
i As Martha stands for service, and Lazarus for communion, so Mary shows us the worship of a grateful heart. Others before her had come to his feet to have their need met; she came to give Him His due. Though two of the evangelists record her act, John alone gives her name.
j Song 4:16.
k See *note* on Mt. 26:7.
l Mt. 26:8.
m John 6:70, 71; 13:29.
n v. 35; Mk. 14:7.
o v. 12; Mk. 12:37.
p John 9:34; 15, 20.
q John 11:45.
r See Mt. 21:4, *note*.
s Psa. 118:25, 26.
t *Jehovah* Psa. 118:26.
u Mt. 21:7.
v Zech. 9:9. Mt. 21:1-7.
w Lk. 18:34; John 2:22; 13:7; 14:26.
x v. 11; Lk. 19:37.
y *kosmos* (Mt. 4:8) = mankind.
z John 11:47, 48.
aa Psa. 72:9-11; Mk. 7:26; John 10, 16; Acts 10:34, 35.
bb John 1:43, 44; 14:8-11.
cc John 13:32; 17:1.
dd Mt. 8:20, *note*.

1 (12:23) He does not receive these Gentiles. A Christ in the flesh, King of the Jews, could be no proper object of faith to the Gentiles, though the Jews should have believed on Him as such. For Gentiles the corn of wheat must fall into the ground and die; Christ must be lifted up on the cross and believed in as a sacrifice for sin, as Seed of Abraham, not David (vs. 24, 32; Gal. 3:7-14; Eph. 2:11-13).

[1]Except a corn of wheat fall into the
ground and die, it abideth alone: but if it
[a]die, it bringeth forth [b]much fruit.
25 [c]He that loveth his life shall lose it;
and he that hateth his life in this [d]world
shall keep it unto life eternal.
26 If any man serve me, let him [e]fol-
low me; and [f]where I am, there shall also
my servant be: if any man serve me, him
will *my* Father [g]honour.
27 Now is my soul troubled; and what
shall I say? [h]Father, save me from this
hour: [i]but for this cause came I unto this
hour.
28 Father, [j]glorify thy name. [k]Then
came there a voice from heaven, *saying*, I
have both glorified *it*, and will glorify *it*
again.
29 The people therefore, that stood by,
and heard *it*, said that it thundered: others said, An [l]angel spake to him.
30 Jesus answered and said, [m]This
voice came not because of me, but for
your sakes.
31 Now is the [2]judgment of this
[d]world: now shall the [n]prince of this
world be cast out.
32 And I, if I be [o]lifted up from the
earth, will draw all *men* unto me.
33 This he said, signifying what death
he should die.
34 The people answered him, We have
heard out of the law that [p]Christ abideth
for ever: and how sayest thou, The Son
of man must be lifted up? who is this
Son of man?
35 Then Jesus said unto them, [q]Yet a
little while is the light with you. Walk
while ye have the light, lest darkness
come upon you: for [r]he that walketh in
darkness knoweth not whither he goeth.
36 While ye have light, believe in the
light, that ye may be [s]the children of light.
These things spake Jesus, and departed,
and [t]did hide himself from them.
37 But [u]though he had done so many
miracles before them, yet they believed
not on him:
38 That the saying of Esaias the
prophet might be fulfilled, which he
spake, [v]Lord, [w]who hath believed our
report? and to whom hath the arm of the
Lord been revealed?
39 Therefore they could not believe,
because that [x]Esaias said again,
40 He hath blinded their eyes, and
hardened their heart; that they should
not see with *their* eyes, nor understand
with *their* [y]heart, and [z]be converted, and
I should heal them.
41 [aa]These things said Esaias, when he
saw his glory, and spake of him.
42 Nevertheless among the chief
rulers also many believed on him; but
because of the Pharisees they did not
confess *him*, lest they should be put out
of the synagogue:
43 For they loved the praise of men
more than the praise of God.
44 Jesus cried and said, He that
believeth on me, believeth not on me,
but on [bb]him that sent me.
45 And [cc]he that seeth me seeth him
that sent me.
46 [dd]I am come a light into the [ee]world,
that whosoever believeth on me should
not abide in darkness.
47 And if any man hear my words,
and believe not, [ff]I judge him not: for [gg]I
came not to judge the world, but to save
the world.
48 He that rejecteth me, and receiveth
not my words, hath one that judgeth
him: [hh]the word that I have spoken, the
same shall judge him in the last day.

A.D. 33.

a *Sacrifice (of Christ)*. John 19:34. (Gen. 4:4; Heb. 10:18.)
b Gen. 3:3.
c Mt. 10:39; 16:25; Mk. 8:35; Lk. 9:24; 17:33.
d *kosmos* = world-system. John 14:17, 19, 22, 27, 30. (John 7:7; Rev. 13:8.)
e Mt. 16:24; John 13:36-38.
f John 14:3; 17:24.
g John 14:21, 23; 16:27; 2 Tim. 4:7, 8.
h *Bible prayers (N.T.)*. John 17. (Mt. 6:9; Rev. 22:20.)
i Lk. 22:53; John 18:37.
j Lk. 22:42; John 5:30.
k Mt. 3:17.
l Heb. 1:4, *note*.
m John 11:42.
n Mt. 12:29; Lk. 10:18; John 14:30; Heb. 2:14.
o John 3:14; 8:28; Rom. 5:8.
p Psa. 72:17; 102:23-27; Isa. 9:7.
q John 7:33.
r John 11:10; 1 John 2:11.
s Lk. 16:8.
t John 8:59; 11:54.
u John 11:47-53.
v *Jehovah*. Isa. 53:1.
w Isa. 53:1; Rom. 10:16.
x Isa. 6:10.
y Psa. 69:23.
z i.e. *should turn*.
aa Isa. 6:1.
bb Mk. 9:37; John 5:24.
cc John 14:9.
dd vs. 35, 36; John 1:4, 5; 8:12.
ee *kosmos* (Mt. 4:8) = mankind.
ff John 5:45; 8:15, 26.
gg John 3:17.
hh *Inspiration*. John 13:18. (Ex. 4:15; Rev. 22:19.)

1 (12:24) Chapters 12–17 are a progression according to the order of approach to God in the tabernacle types: Chapter 12, in which Christ speaks of His death, answers to the brazen altar of burnt-offering, type of the cross. Passing from the altar toward the holy of holies, the laver is next reached (Ex. 30:17-21), answering to Chapter 13. With His associate priests, now purified, the High Priest approaches and enters the holy place, in the high communion of Chapters 14–16. Entering alone the holy of holies (17:1), the High Priest intercedes. (Cf. Heb. 7:24-28.) That intercession is not for the salvation, but the keeping and blessing of those for whom He prays. His death (assumed as accomplished, 17:4) has saved them.

2 (12:31) The Seven Judgments. (1) Of Jesus Christ as bearing the believer's sins. The sins of believers have been judged in the person of Jesus Christ "lifted up" on the cross. The result was death for Christ, and justification for the believer, who can never again be put in jeopardy (John 5:24; Rom. 5:9; 8:1; 2 Cor. 5:21; Gal. 3:13; Heb. 9:26-28; 10:10, 14-17; 1 Pet. 2:24; 3:18). See other judgments, 1 Cor. 11:31, *note;* 2 Cor. 5:10, *note;* Mt. 25:32, *note;* Ezk. 20:37, *note;* Jude 6, *note;* Rev. 20:12, *note*.

49 For [a]I have not spoken of myself; but the Father which sent me, he gave me a commandment, what I should say, and what I should speak.

50 And I know that his commandment is [b]life everlasting: whatsoever I speak therefore, even as the Father said unto me, so I speak.

CHAPTER 13.

The last passover. (Cf. Mt. 26:7-30; Mk. 14:17-26; Lk. 22:14-39.)

Now [1]before the feast of the passover, when Jesus knew that his [c]hour was come that he should depart out of this [d]world unto the Father, having loved his own which were in the world, he [e]loved them [f]unto the end.

Jesus washes the disciples' feet.

2 And [g]supper being ended, the [h]devil having now put into the heart of Judas Iscariot, Simon's *son*, to betray him;

3 Jesus knowing that the Father had [i]given all things into his hands, and that he was [j]come from God, [k]and went to God;

4 He riseth from supper, and [l]laid aside his garments; and took a towel, and girded himself.

5 After that he poureth [m]water into a bason, and began to wash the disciples' feet, and to wipe *them* with the towel wherewith he was girded.

6 Then cometh he to Simon Peter: and Peter saith unto him, Lord, [n]dost thou wash my feet?

7 Jesus answered and said unto him, What I do thou [o]knowest not now; but thou shalt know hereafter.

8 Peter saith unto him, Thou shalt never wash my feet. Jesus answered him, If I [p]wash thee not, thou hast [q]no part with me.

9 Simon Peter saith unto him, Lord, not my feet only, but also *my* hands and *my* head.

10 Jesus saith to him, He that is [r]washed [2]needeth not save to wash *his* feet, but is clean [s]every whit: and ye are clean, but not all.

11 For [t]he knew who should betray him; therefore said he, Ye are not all clean.

12 So after he had washed their feet, and had taken his garments, and was set down again, he said unto them, Know ye what I have done to you?

13 [u]Ye call me Master and Lord: and ye say well; for *so* I am.

14 If I then, *your* Lord and Master, have washed your feet; [v]ye also ought to wash one another's feet.

15 For I [w]have given you an example, that ye should do as I have done to you.

16 Verily, verily, I say unto you, [x]The servant is not greater than his lord; neither he that is sent greater than he that sent him.

17 [y]If ye know these things, happy are ye if ye do them.

18 I speak not of you all: I know whom I have chosen: but that the [z]scripture may be fulfilled, [aa]He that eateth bread with me hath lifted up his heel against me.

19 Now I tell you [bb]before it come, that, when it is come to pass, ye may believe that I am *he*.

20 Verily, verily, I say unto you, He that receiveth whomsoever I send receiveth me; and [cc]he that receiveth me receiveth him that sent me.

Jesus foretells his betrayal (Mt. 26:2-25; Mk. 14:17-21; Lk. 22:21, 22).

21 [dd]When Jesus had thus said, he was troubled in spirit, and testified, and said, Verily, verily, I say unto you, that [ee]one of you shall betray me.

22 Then the disciples looked one on another, doubting of whom he spake.

23 Now there was leaning on Jesus'

A.D. 33.

- a John 8:38; 14:10, 31.
- b *Life (eternal).* vs. 25, 50; John 14:6. (Mt. 7:14; Rev. 22:19.)
- c John 7:8; 12:23; 17:1.
- d i.e. *earth.*
- e v. 34; John 10:11, 28-30; Rom. 8:35-39.
- f Or, *to the uttermost.*
- g Gr. *during supper.*
- h *diabolos.* Rev. 20:10, *note.*
- i John 5:20-23; 17:2.
- j John 8:42, 16:28.
- k John 17:11; 20:17.
- l Lk. 22:27; Phil. 2:7, 8.
- m Eph. 5:26.
- n See Mt. 3:14.
- o vs. 12, 36; John 12:16; Heb. 12:11.
- p Ex. 30:17-21.
- q Gen. 35:2, 3; Eph. 4:30; 1 John 2:1, 2.
- r Lit. *bathed.* The Gr. word signifies a complete ablution. "Wash" is another word.
- s 1 Cor. 1:30; 6:11; 1 John 3:9.
- t John 6:64.
- u Mt. 23:8, 10; Lk. 6:46; Eph. 6:9.
- v Rom. 12:10; Gal. 6:1, 2; 1 Pet. 5:5.
- w Mt. 11:29; Phil. 2:5; 1 Pet. 2:21; 1 John 2:6.
- x John 15:20.
- y Jas. 1:25.
- z *Inspiration.* John 14:10. (Ex. 4:15; Rev. 22:19.)
- aa Psa. 41:9.
- bb Mt. 11:3.
- cc 2 Cor. 5:20.
- dd Mt. 26:21; Mk. 14:18; Lk. 22:21.
- ee Psa. 41:9.

[1] **(13:1)** For order of events during the night of the last passover, see Mt. 26:20, *note.*

[2] **(13:10)** The underlying imagery is of an oriental returning from the public baths to his house. His feet would contract defilement and require cleansing, but not his body. So the believer is cleansed as before the law from all sin "once for all" (Heb. 10:1-12), but needs ever to bring his daily sins to the Father in confession, that he may abide in unbroken fellowship with the Father and with the Son (1 John 1:1-10). The blood of Christ answers forever to all the law could say as to the believer's *guilt,* but he needs constant cleansing from the *defilement* of sin. See Eph. 5:25-27; 1 John 5:6. Typically, the order of approach to the presence of God was, first; the brazen altar of sacrifice, and then the laver of cleansing (Ex. 40:6, 7). See, also, the order in Ex. 30:17-21. Christ cannot have communion with a defiled saint, but He can and will cleanse him.

bosom [a]one of his disciples, whom Jesus loved.

24 Simon Peter therefore beckoned to him, that he should ask who it should be of whom he spake.

25 He then lying on Jesus' breast saith unto him, Lord, who is it?

26 Jesus answered, He it is, to whom I shall give a sop, when I have dipped *it*. And when he had dipped the sop, he gave *it* to Judas Iscariot, *the son* of Simon.

27 And after the sop [b]Satan entered into him. Then said Jesus unto him, That thou doest, do quickly.

28 Now no man at the table knew for what intent he spake this unto him.

29 For some *of them* thought, because Judas had the bag, that Jesus had said unto him, Buy *those things* that we have need of against the feast; or, that he should give something to the poor.

30 He then having received the sop went immediately out: and it was night.

31 Therefore, when he was gone out, Jesus said, Now is the [c]Son of man glorified, and God is glorified in him.

32 If God be glorified in him, God shall also glorify him in himself, and shall straightway glorify him.

33 Little children, yet a little while I am with you. Ye shall seek me: and [d]as I said unto the Jews, Whither I go, ye cannot come; so now I say to you.

34 A [e]new commandment I give unto you, That ye love one another; as I have loved you, that ye also love one another.

35 By this shall all *men* know that ye are my disciples, if ye have love one to another.

Jesus foretells Peter's denial (Mt. 26:33-35; Mk. 14:29-31; Lk. 22:33, 34).

36 Simon Peter said unto him, Lord, whither goest thou? Jesus answered him, Whither I go, thou canst not follow me now; [f]but thou shalt follow me afterwards.

37 Peter said unto him, Lord, why cannot I follow thee now? I will [g]lay down my life for thy sake.

38 Jesus answered him, Wilt thou lay down thy life for my sake? Verily, verily, I say unto thee, The cock shall not crow, till thou hast denied me thrice.

CHAPTER 14.

Spoken in the passover chamber: Jesus foretells his coming for his own.
(Cf. 1 Thes. 4:14-17.)

[h]Let not your heart be troubled: ye [i]believe in God, believe also in me.

2 In my Father's house are many mansions: if *it were* not *so*, I would have told you. I go to prepare a place for you.

3 And if I go and prepare a place for you, [j]I will come again, and receive [1]you unto myself; that where I am, *there* ye may be also.

4 And whither I go ye know, and the way ye know.

5 Thomas saith unto him, Lord, we know not whither thou goest; and how can we know the way?

6 Jesus saith unto him, I am the way, the truth, and the [k]life: no man cometh unto the Father, but by me.

Jesus and the Father are one.

7 If ye had known me, ye should have known my Father also: and from henceforth ye know him, and have seen him.

8 Philip saith unto him, Lord, shew us the Father, and it sufficeth us.

9 Jesus saith unto him, Have I been so long time with you, and yet hast thou not known me, Philip? [l]he that hath seen me hath seen the Father; and how sayest thou *then*, Shew us the Father?

10 Believest thou not that [m]I am in the Father, and the Father in me? the [n]words that I speak unto you [o]I speak not of myself: but the Father that dwelleth in me, he doeth the works.

11 Believe me that I *am* in the Father, and the Father in me: or else believe me for the [p]very works' sake.

12 Verily, verily, I say unto you, He that believeth on me, the works that I do shall he do also; and greater *works* than these shall he do; because I go unto my Father.

A.D. 33.

a John 21:7, 20, 24.
b *Satan.* vs. 2, 27; Acts 5:3. (Gen. 3:1; Rev. 20:10.)
c Mt. 8:20, *note.*
d John 7:34; 8:21.
e *Law, (of Christ),* John 14:15, 21, 23. (Gal. 6:2; 2 John 5.)
f John 21:18; 2 Pet. 1:14.
g Mt. 26:33; Mk. 14:29; Lk. 22:33.
h v. 27; Isa. 43;1, 2.
i *Faith.* John 16:9. (Gen. 3:20; Heb. 11:39.)
j *Christ (Second Advent).* vs. 2, 3; Rom. 11:25, 26. (Deut. 30:3; Acts 1:9-11.)
k *Life (eternal).* John 17:2, 3. (Mt. 7:14; Rev. 22:19.)
l Col. 1:15.
m v. 20; John 10:38; 17:21, 23.
n *Inspiration.* John 15:27. (Ex. 4:15; Rev. 22:19.)
o John 5:19; 7:16; 8:28; 12:49.
p John 5:36; 10:38; Acts 2:22.

[1]**(14:3)** This promise of a second advent of Christ is to be distinguished from His return in glory to the earth; it is the first intimation in Scripture of "the day of Christ" (1 Cor. 1:8, *note*). Here He comes for His saints (1 Thes. 4:14-17), there (e.g. Mt. 24:29, 30) He comes to judge the nations, etc.

The new promise and privilege in prayer.

13 And whatsoever ye shall ask in [a]my name, that will I do, that the Father may be [b]glorified in the Son.

14 If ye shall ask any thing in my name, I will do *it*.

15 [c]If ye love me, keep my commandments.

The promise of the Spirit.

16 [d]And I will pray the Father, and he shall give you another [1e]Comforter, that he may abide with you for ever;

17 *Even* the [f]Spirit of truth; whom the [g]world [h]cannot receive, because it seeth him not, neither knoweth him: but ye know him; for he dwelleth with you, and [i]shall be in you.

18 I will not leave you [j]comfortless: I will come to you.

19 Yet a little while, and the [g]world seeth me no more; but ye see me: [k]because I live, ye shall live also.

20 At that day ye shall know that [l]I *am* in my Father, and ye in me, and I in you.

21 [m]He that hath my commandments, and keepeth them, he it is that loveth me: and he that loveth me shall be loved of my Father, and I will love him, and will [n]manifest myself to him.

22 Judas saith unto him, not Iscariot, Lord, how is it that thou wilt manifest thyself unto us, and not unto the [g]world?

23 Jesus answered and said unto him, [o]If a man [p]love me, he will keep my words: and my Father will love him, and we will come unto him, and make our abode with him.

24 He that [q]loveth me not keepeth not my sayings: and the [r]word which ye hear is not mine, but the Father's which sent me.

25 These things have I spoken unto you, being *yet* present with you.

26 But the Comforter, *which is* the [s]Holy Ghost, whom the Father will send in my name, he shall teach you all things, and [t]bring all things to your remembrance, whatsoever I have said unto you.

The bequest of peace.

27 [u]Peace I leave with you, [v]my peace I give unto you: not as the [g]world giveth, give I unto you. Let not your heart be [w]troubled, neither let it be afraid.

28 Ye have heard how I said unto you, I go away, and come *again* unto you. If ye loved me, ye would rejoice, because I said, I go unto the Father: for my Father is greater than I.

29 And now I have told you before it come to pass, that, when it is come to pass, ye might believe.

30 Hereafter I will not talk much with you: for the prince of this world cometh, and hath nothing in me.

31 But that the [x]world may know that I love the Father; and [y]as the Father gave me commandment, even so I do. Arise, let us go hence.

CHAPTER 15.

Spoken on the way to the garden: the vine and branches.

I am the [z]true vine, and my Father is the husbandman.

2 Every branch in me that beareth not fruit he taketh away: and every *branch* that [aa]beareth fruit, he [2]purgeth it, that it may bring forth more fruit.

3 Now ye are [bb]clean through the word which I have spoken unto you.

4 [3cc]Abide in me, and I in you. As the branch cannot bear fruit of itself, except it abide in the vine; no more can ye, except ye abide in me.

5 I am the vine, ye *are* the branches: He that abideth in me, and I in him, the same

A.D. 33.

a John 15:16; 16:23, 24.
b John 13:31; 15:8.
c vs. 21-23; John 15:10; 1 John 5:3.
d See Lk. 11:13, *note.*
e *Advocacy.* John 16:7. (John 14:16, 26; 1 John 2:1, 2.)
f John 15:26; 16:13; Rom. 8:15, 26; 1 John 4:6.
g *kosmos* = world-system. John 15:18, 19. (John 7:7; Rev. 13:8, *note.*)
h 1 Cor. 2:14.
i John 7:37; 1 Cor. 6:19; 2 Cor. 6:16; 1 John 3:24.
j Or, *orphans.*
k Rom. 5:10; 2 Cor. 4:10, 11; Heb. 7:25.
l v. 10; John 10:38.
m vs. 15, 23; 1 John 2:5.
n John 7:4; 2 Cor. 3:18; Heb. 2:9.
o *Law (of Christ).* vs. 15, 21, 23; John 15:12, 17. (Gal. 6:2; 2 John 5.)
p Cf. vs. 15, 21.
q Gal. 5:6; Jas. 2:14-17.
r Deut. 18:18.
s *Holy Spirit.* vs. 17, 26; John 15:26, (Mt. 1:18; Acts 2:4.)
t John 2:22.
u Cf. Mt. 10:34, *note.*
v John 16:33; Col. 3:15.
w v. 1.
x *kosmos* (Mt. 4:8) = mankind.
y John 10:18; Phil. 2:8.
z "True" in contrast with Israel. Isa. 5:1-7.
aa Mt. 13:12; John 17:17; Rom. 5:3, 4; Heb, 12:5-11.
bb Lev. 13:6; John 13:10; Eph. 5:26.
cc vs. 5-7; John 17:23; Eph. 3:17; 1 John 2:28.

[1] **(14:16)** Gr. *Parakletos,* "one called alongside to help." Translated "advocate," 1 John 2:1. Christ is the believer's Paraclete with the Father when he sins; the Holy Spirit the believer's indwelling Paraclete to help his ignorance and infirmity, and to make intercession (Rom. 8:26, 27). (See "Holy Spirit," N.T. doctrine, Mt. 1:18; Acts 2:4.)

[2] **(15:2)** Three conditions of the fruitful life: Cleansing, vs. 2, 3; John 13:10, *note;* abiding, v. 4, *note;* obedience, vs. 10, 12. (See "Law of Christ," Gal. 6:2; 2 John 5, *note.*)

[3] **(15:4)** To abide in Christ is, on the one hand, to have no known sin unjudged and unconfessed, no interest into which He is not brought, no life which He cannot share. On the other hand, the abiding

bringeth forth much [a]fruit: for [b]without
me ye can do nothing.
6 If a man abide not in me, he is cast
forth [c]as a branch, and is withered; and
men gather them, and cast *them* into the
fire, and they are burned.
7 If ye abide in me, and [d]my words
abide in you, ye shall ask what ye will,
and it shall be done unto you.
8 Herein is my Father glorified, that
ye bear [1]much fruit; so shall ye be my
disciples.
9 As the Father hath [e]loved me, so have
I loved you: continue ye in my love.
10 If [f]ye keep my commandments, ye
shall abide in my love; even as I have
kept my Father's commandments, and
abide in his love.
11 These things have I spoken unto
you, that my joy might remain in you,
and *that* your joy might be full.
12 [g]This is my commandment, That ye
love one another, as I have loved you.
13 Greater love hath no man than this,
that a man lay down his life for his
friends.
14 Ye are my friends, if ye do whatsoever I command you.

The new intimacy.

15 [2]Henceforth I call you not servants;
for the servant knoweth not what his
lord doeth: but I have called you friends;
for all things that I have heard of my
Father I have made known unto you.
16 Ye have not chosen me, but I have
[h]chosen you, and ordained you, that ye
should go and bring forth fruit, and *that*
your fruit should remain: that whatsoever ye shall ask of the Father [i]in my
name, he may give it you.
17 These things I [j]command you, that
ye love one another.

The believer and the world.

18 If the [k]world hate you, ye know
that it hated me before *it hated* you.

A.D. 33.

a The fruit. Gal. 5:22, 23; cf. Col. 3:12-17.

b Phil. 1:11; 4:13.

c v. 2; Mt. 25:30.

d John 14:13; Col. 3:16; 1 John 2:14.

e John 5:20; 10:14, 15; 17:26.

f John 14:21, 23.

g John 13:34.

h *Election (personal).* Acts 9:15. (Deut. 7:6; 1 Pet. 1:2.)

i John 14:13; 16:23, 24.

j *Law (of Christ).* vs. 12, 17; Rom. 5:5. (Gal. 6:2; 2 John 5.)

k *kosmos* = world-system. John 16:11, 33. (John 7:7; Rev. 13:8, *note.*)

l *Separation.* John 17:6, 14-16. (Gen. 12:1; 2 Cor. 6:14-17.)

m *Election (corporate).* Rom. 8:33. (Deut. 7:6; 1 Pet. 1:2.)

n *kosmos* (Mt. 4:8) = mankind.

o *Sin.* Rom. 3:23, *note.*

p Psa. 35:19; 69:4.

q *Holy Spirit.* John 16:13. (Mt. 1:18; Acts 2:4.)

r *Inspiration.* John 16:12, 13. (Ex. 4:15; Rev. 22:19.)

19 If ye [l]were of the [k]world, the
[k]world would love his own: but because
ye are not of the [k]world, but I have
[m]chosen you out of the [n]world, therefore
the [k]world hateth you.
20 Remember the word that I said unto
you, The servant is not greater than his
lord. If they have persecuted me, they
will also persecute you; if they have kept
my saying, they will keep yours also.
21 But all these things will they do
unto you for my name's sake, because
they know not him that sent me.
22 If I had not come and spoken unto
them, they had not had [o]sin: but now
they have no cloke for their sin.
23 He that hateth me hateth my Father
also.
24 If I had not done among them the
works which none other man did, they
had not had [o]sin: but now have they
both seen and hated both me and my
Father.
25 But *this cometh to pass*, that the word
might be fulfilled that is written in their
law, They hated me [p]without a cause.

The believer and the Spirit.

26 But when the Comforter is come,
whom I will send unto you from the
Father, *even* the [q]Spirit of truth, which
proceedeth from the Father, he shall testify of me:
27 And ye also shall bear witness, [r]be-
cause ye have been with me from the
beginning.

CHAPTER 16.

The disciples warned of persecutions.
(Cf. Mt. 24:9, 10; Lk. 21:16-19.)

These things have I spoken unto you,
that ye should not be offended.
2 They shall put you out of the
synagogues: yea, the time cometh, that

one takes all burdens to Him, and draws all wisdom, life and strength from Him. It is not unceasing *consciousness* of these things, and of Him, but that nothing is allowed in the life which separates from Him. See "Fellowship," 1 John 1:3; "Communion," 1 Cor. 10:16.

[1] **(15:8)** Three degrees in fruit-bearing: "Fruit," v. 2; "more fruit," v. 21 "much fruit," vs. 5, 8. As we bear "much fruit" the Father is glorified in us. The minor moralities and graces of Christianity are often imitated, but never the ninefold "fruit" of Gal. 5:22, 23. Where such fruit is the Father is glorified. The Pharisees were moral and intensely "religious," but not one of them could say with Christ, "I have glorified thee on the earth" (John 17:4).

[2] **(15:15)** Progressive intimacy in John: Servants, John 13:13; Friends, John 15:15; Brethren, John 20:17.

whosoever killeth you will think that he doeth God service.

3 And these things will they do unto you, because they have not known the Father, nor me.

4 But these things have I told you, that when the time shall come, ye may remember that I told you of them. And these things I said not unto you at the beginning, because I was with you.

5 But now I go my way to him that sent me; and none of you asketh me, Whither goest thou?

6 But because I have said these things unto you, sorrow hath filled your heart.

Threefold work of the Spirit toward the world.

7 Nevertheless I tell you the truth; It is expedient for you that I go away: for if I go not away, [a]the Comforter will not come unto you; but if I depart, I will send him unto you.

8 And when he is come, he will reprove the [b]world of [c]sin, and of righteousness, and of judgment:

9 Of sin, because they [d]believe not on me;

10 Of righteousness, because I go to my Father, and ye see me no more;

11 Of judgment, because the prince of this [e]world is judged.

New truth to be revealed by the Spirit.

12 [1]I have yet many things to say unto you, but ye cannot bear them now.

13 Howbeit when he, the [f]Spirit of truth, is come, he will guide you into all truth: for he shall not speak [g]of himself; [h]but whatsoever he shall hear, *that* shall he speak: and he will shew you things to come.

14 He shall glorify me: for he shall receive of mine, and shall shew *it* unto you.

15 All things that the Father hath are mine: therefore said I, that he shall take of mine, and shall shew *it* unto you.

A.D. 33.

a Advocacy. 1 John 2:1, 2. (John 14:16, 26; 1 John 2:1, 2.)

b *kosmos* (Mt. 4:8) = mankind.

c *Sin.* Rom. 3:23, *note.*

d *Faith.* John 20:31. (Gen. 3:20; Heb. 11:39.)

e *kosmos* = world-system. John 17:14. (John 7:7; Rev. 13:8, *note.*)

f *Holy Spirit.* John 20:22. (Mt. 1:18; Acts 2:4.)

g *from himself.* Cf. next clause.

h *Inspiration.* John 17:8, 17, 20. (Ex. 4:15; Rev. 22:19.)

i John 14:19.

j Lk. 24:17.

k *kosmos* (Mt. 4:8) = mankind.

l John 20:20; Lk. 24:41.

m 1 Pet. 1:8.

n Mt. 7:7, 8; Jas. 4:2, 3; 1 John 3:22; 5:14.

o John 14:21, 23.

Jesus speaks of his death, resurrection, and second advent.

16 A little while, and ye shall not see me: and again, a little while, and ye shall see me, because I go to the Father.

17 Then said *some* of his disciples among themselves, What is this that he saith unto us, A little while, and ye shall not see me: and again, a little while, and ye shall see me: and, Because I go to the Father?

18 They said therefore, What is this that he saith, A little while? we cannot tell what he saith.

19 Now Jesus knew that they were desirous to ask him, and said unto them, Do ye enquire among yourselves of that I said, A [i]little while, and ye shall not see me: and again, a little while, and ye shall see me?

20 Verily, verily, I say unto you, That [j]ye shall weep and lament, but the [k]world shall rejoice: and ye shall be sorrowful, but your sorrow shall be turned into joy.

21 A woman when she is in travail hath sorrow, because her hour is come: but as soon as she is delivered of the child, she remembereth no more the anguish, for joy that a man is born into the [k]world.

22 And ye now therefore have sorrow: but I will see you again, and [l]your heart shall rejoice, and your [m]joy no man taketh from you.

23 And in that day ye shall ask me nothing. Verily, verily, I say unto you, Whatsoever ye shall ask the Father in my name, he will give *it* you.

24 Hitherto have ye asked nothing in my name: [n]ask, and ye shall receive, that your joy may be full.

25 These things have I spoken unto you in proverbs: but the time cometh, when I shall no more speak unto you in proverbs, but I shall shew you plainly of the Father.

26 At that day ye shall ask in my name: and I say not unto you, that I will pray the Father for you:

27 For the [o]Father himself loveth you,

[1]**(16:12)** Christ's pre-authentication of the New Testament: (1) He expressly declared that He would leave "many things" unrevealed (v. 12). (2) He promised that this revelation should be completed ("all things") after the Spirit should come, and that such additional revelation should include new prophecies (v. 13). (3) He chose certain persons to receive such additional revelations, and to be His witnesses to them (Mt. 28:19; John 15:27; 16:13; Acts 1:8; 9:15-17). (4) He gave to their words when speaking for Him in the Spirit precisely the same authority as His own (Mt. 10:14, 15; Lk. 10:16; John 13:20; 17:20; see e.g., 1 Cor. 14:37, and "Inspiration," Ex. 4:15; Rev. 22:19).

because ye have loved me, and have
believed that I came out from God.
28 I came forth from the Father, and
am come into the [a]world: again, I leave
the world, and go to the Father.
29 His disciples said unto him, Lo,
now speakest thou plainly, and speakest
no proverb.
30 Now are we sure that thou knowest
all things, and needest not that any man
should ask thee: by this we believe that
thou camest forth from God.
31 Jesus answered them, Do ye now
believe?
32 [b]Behold, the hour cometh, yea, is
now come, that ye shall be scattered,
every man to his own, and shall leave
me alone: and yet I am not alone,
because the Father is with me.
33 These things I have spoken unto you,
that in me ye might have peace. In the
[c]world ye shall have tribulation: but be of
good cheer; I have overcome the world.

CHAPTER 17.

The prayer of intercession.

These words spake Jesus, and lifted
up his eyes to heaven, and [d]said,
Father, the hour is come; [1]glorify thy
Son, that thy Son also may glorify thee:
2 As thou hast given him power over
all flesh, that he should [2]give eternal
[e]life to as many as thou hast [3]given him.
3 And this is [e]life eternal, that they
might know [f]thee the only true God, and
Jesus Christ, whom thou hast sent.
4 I have glorified thee on the earth: [g]I
have finished the work which thou
gavest me to do.
5 And now, O Father, glorify thou me
with thine own self with the glory which
[h]I had with thee before the [i]world was.

A.D. 33.

a kosmos (Mt. 4:8 = mankind.
b Zech. 13:7; Mt. 26:31; Acts 8:1.
c kosmos = world-system, John 17:14, 16. (John 7:7; Rev. 13:8, *note.*)
d Bible prayers (N.T.). Acts 1:24, 25. (Mt. 6:9; Rev. 22:20.)
e Life (eternal). vs. 2, 3; John 20:31. (Mt. 7:14; Rev. 22:19.)
f Jer. 9:23, 24.
g John 19:30; Dan. 9:24.
h John 1:1, 2; Phil. 2:6; Heb. 1:3, 10.
i i.e. *earth.*
j Inspiration. vs. 8, 17, 20; Acts 1:8, 16. (Ex. 4:15; Rev. 22:19.)
k Deut. 18:15, 18, 19.
l Assurance. Acts 13:38, 39. (Isa. 32:17; Jude 1.)
m Psa. 119:42, 50, 161; Mk. 16:15; Acts 4:29.
n kosmos = world-system. John 18:36. (John 7:7; Rev. 13:8, *note.*)
o Separation vs. 6, 14-16, Rom. 12:2. (Gen. 12:1; 2 Cor. 6:14-17.)

6 I have manifested thy name unto the
men which thou gavest me out of the
[a]world: thine they were, and thou gavest
them me; and they have kept thy word.
7 Now they have known that all
things whatsoever thou hast given me
are of thee.
8 For I have given unto them the
[j]words which thou gavest me; and they
have received *them,* and have known
surely that I came out from thee, and they
have believed that [k]thou didst send me.
9 I pray for them: I pray not for the
[c]world, but for them which thou hast
given me; for they are thine.
10 And all mine are thine, and thine
are mine; and I am glorified in them.
11 And now I am no more in the
[a]world, but these are in the world, and I
come to thee. Holy Father, [l]keep through
thine own name those whom thou hast
given me, that they may be one, as we *are.*
12 While I was with them in the
[a]world, I kept them in thy name: those
that thou gavest me I have kept, and
none of them is lost, but the son of
perdition; that the scripture might be
fulfilled.
13 And now come I to thee; and these
things I speak in the [a]world, that they
might have my joy fulfilled in themselves.
14 I have given them [m]thy word; and
the [n]world hath hated them, because
they are not of the world, even as I am
not of the world.
15 I pray not that thou shouldest take
them out of the [a]world, but that thou
shouldest keep them from the evil.
16 They are [o]not of the [n]world, even as
I am not of the world.
17 Sanctify them through thy truth:
thy word is truth.

[1] **(17:1)** Seven petitions: (1) That Jesus may be glorified as the Son who has glorified the Father (v. 1; Phil. 2:9-11); (2) for restoration to the eternal glory (v. 5); (3) for the safety of believers from *(a)* the world (v. 11), *(b)* the evil one (v. 15); (4) for the sanctification of believers (v. 17); (5) for the spiritual unity of believers (v. 21); (6) that the world may believe (v. 21); (7) that believers may be with Him in heaven to behold and share His glory (v. 24).

[2] **(17:2)** Christ's gifts to those whom the Father gave Him: Eternal life (v. 2); the Father's name (vs. 6, 26; John 20:17); the Father's words (vs. 8, 14); His own joy (v. 13); His own glory (v. 22).

[3] **(17:2)** Seven times Jesus speaks of believers as given to Him by the Father (vs. 2, 6 [twice], 9, 11, 12, 24). Jesus Christ is God's love-gift to the world (John 3:16), and believers are the Father's love-gift to Jesus Christ. It is Christ who commits the believer to the Father for safe-keeping, so that the believer's security rests upon the Father's faithfulness to His Son Jesus Christ.

18 As thou hast sent me into the
[a]world, even so have I also sent them
into the world.
19 And for their sakes I [b]sanctify
myself, that they also might be sanctified
through the truth.
20 Neither pray I for these alone, but
for them also which shall believe on me
through their word;
21 That they all may be one; [c]as thou,
Father, *art* in me, and I in thee, that they
also may be one in us: that the [a]world
may believe that thou hast sent me.
22 And the [d]glory which thou gavest
me I have given them; that they may be
one, even as we are one:
23 I in them, and thou in me, that they
may be made [e]perfect in one; and that
the [a]world may know that thou hast sent
me, and hast loved them, as thou hast
loved me.
24 Father, I will that they also, whom
thou hast given me, [f]be with me where I
am; that they may behold my glory,
which thou hast given me: for thou
lovedst me before the foundation of the
[g]world.
25 O righteous Father, the [a]world hath
not known thee: but I have known thee,
and these have known that thou hast
sent me.
26 And I have declared unto them thy
[h]name, and will declare *it*: [i]that the love
wherewith thou hast loved me may be
in them, and I in them.

CHAPTER 18.

Jesus arrives at Gethsemane. (Cf. Mt. 26:36-46; Mk. 14:32-42; Lk. 22:39-46.)

When Jesus had spoken these words,
he went forth with his disciples
over the brook Cedron, where was a garden, into the which he entered, and his
disciples.

The betrayal and arrest (Mt. 26:47-56; Mk. 14:43-50; Lk. 22:47-53).

2 And [j]Judas also, which betrayed
him, knew the place: for Jesus ofttimes
resorted thither with his disciples.
3 Judas then, having received a band
of men and officers from the chief priests
and Pharisees, cometh thither with
lanterns and torches and weapons.
4 Jesus therefore, [k]knowing all things
that should come upon him, went forth,
and said unto them, Whom seek ye?
5 They answered him, Jesus of
Nazareth. Jesus saith unto them, I am *he*.
And Judas also, which [l]betrayed him,
stood with them.
6 As soon then as he had said unto
them, I am *he*, they went backward, and
fell to the ground.
7 Then asked he them again, Whom
seek ye? And they said, Jesus of Nazareth.
8 Jesus answered, I have told you that
I am *he*: if therefore ye [m]seek me, let
these go their way:
9 That the saying might be fulfilled,
which he [n]spake, Of them which thou
gavest me have I lost none.
10 Then Simon Peter having a sword
drew it, and smote the high priest's servant, and cut off his right ear. The servant's name was Malchus.
11 Then said Jesus unto Peter, Put up
thy sword into the sheath: the cup which
my Father hath given me, shall I not
drink it?

Jesus brought before the high priest (Mt. 26:57-68; Mk. 14:53-65; Lk. 22:66-71).

12 Then the band and the captain and
officers of the Jews took Jesus, and
bound him,
13 And led him away to [o]Annas first;
for he was father in law to Caiaphas,
which was the high priest that same year.
14 Now Caiaphas was he, which gave
[p]counsel to the Jews, that it was expedient
that one man should die for the people.

Peter's denial (also vs. 25-27) (Mt. 26:69-75; Mk. 14:66-72; Lk. 22:54-62).

15 And [q]Simon Peter followed Jesus,
and *so did* another disciple: that disciple
was known unto the high priest, and
went in with Jesus into the palace of the
high priest.
16 But Peter stood at the door without.
Then went out that other disciple, which
was known unto the high priest, and
spake unto her that kept the door, and
brought in Peter.
17 Then saith the damsel that kept the
door unto Peter, Art not thou also *one* of
this man's disciples? He saith, I am [r]not.
18 And the servants and officers stood
there, who had made a fire of coals; for it
was cold: and they warmed themselves:
and Peter stood with them, and warmed
himself.

A.D. 33.

a *kosmos* (Mt. 4:8) = mankind.
b *Sanctify, holy (persons).* vs. 11, 17, 19; Acts 3:21. Mt. 4:5; Rev. 22:11.)
c Rom. 12:5; Eph. 4:1, 6.
d 2 Cor. 3:18.
e Mt. 5:48, *note.*
f 1 Thes. 4:17.
g i.e. *earth.*
h Ex. 34:5, 7.
i Eph. 3:16, 19.
j Mt. 26:47; Mk. 14:43; Lk. 22:47.
k John 13:1, 3; Lk. 9:51; Acts 20:22; Heb. 12:2.
l Psa. 41:9.
m Isa. 53:6; Eph. 5:25.
n John 17:12; 1 Cor. 10:13.
o Lk. 3:2.
p John 11:49, 50; Lk. 24:46, 47.
q Mt. 26:58; Mk. 14:54; Lk. 22:54.
r Prov. 29:25; Mt. 10:28; 2 Tim 2:12.

(*Jesus before the high priest*, continued.)

19 [a]The high priest then asked Jesus of his disciples, and of his doctrine.

20 Jesus answered him, I spake openly to the [b]world; I ever taught in the synagogue, and in the temple, whither the Jews always resort; and in secret have I said nothing.

21 Why askest thou me? ask them which heard me, what I have said unto them: behold, they know what I said.

22 And when he had thus spoken, one of the officers which stood by struck Jesus with the palm of his hand, saying, Answerest thou the high priest so?

23 Jesus answered him, If I have spoken evil, bear witness of the evil: [c]but if well, why smitest thou me?

24 Now Annas had sent him bound unto Caiaphas the high priest.

25 And Simon Peter stood and warmed himself. They said therefore unto him, Art not thou also *one* of his disciples? He denied *it*, and said, I am not.

26 One of the servants of the high priest, being *his* kinsman whose ear Peter cut off, saith, Did not I see thee in the garden with him?

27 Peter then denied again: and [d]immediately the cock crew.

Jesus brought before Pilate (Mt. 27:1-14; Mk. 15:1-5; Lk. 23:1-7, 13, 16).

28 [e]Then led they Jesus from Caiaphas unto the hall of judgment: and it was early; and they themselves went not into the judgment hall, [f]lest they should be defiled; but that they might eat the passover.

29 Pilate then went out unto them, and said, What accusation bring ye against this man?

30 They answered and said unto him, If he were not a malefactor, we would not have delivered him up unto thee.

31 Then said Pilate unto them, Take ye him, and judge him according to your law. The Jews therefore said unto him, It is not lawful for us to put any man to death:

32 That the saying of Jesus might be fulfilled, which he [g]spake, signifying what death he should die.

33 Then Pilate entered into the judgment hall again, and called Jesus, and said unto him, Art thou the King of the Jews?

34 Jesus answered him, Sayest thou this thing of thyself, or did others tell it thee of me?

35 Pilate answered, Am I a Jew? Thine own nation and the chief priests have delivered thee unto me: what hast thou done?

36 [h]Jesus answered, [i]My kingdom is not [j]of this [k]world: if my kingdom were of this world, then would my servants fight, that I should not be delivered to the Jews: but now is my kingdom not from hence.

37 Pilate therefore said unto him, Art thou a king then? Jesus answered, Thou sayest that I am a king. To this end was I born, and for this cause came I into the [b]world, that I should bear [l]witness unto the truth. Every one that is of the truth heareth my voice.

38 Pilate saith unto him, What is truth? And when he had said this, he went out again unto the Jews, and saith unto them, I find in him [m]no fault *at all*.

Jesus condemned: Barabbas released (Mt. 27:15-26; Mk. 15:6-15; Lk. 23:18-25).

39 But ye have a custom, that I should release unto you one at the passover: will ye therefore that I release unto you the King of the Jews?

40 Then cried they all again, saying, Not this man, but Barabbas. Now Barabbas was a robber.

CHAPTER 19.

Jesus crowned with thorns (Mt. 27:27-30; Mk. 15:16-20).

Then [n]Pilate therefore took Jesus, and scourged *him*.

2 And the soldiers platted a crown of thorns, and put *it* on his head, and they put on him a [o]purple robe,

3 And said, Hail, King of the Jews! and they smote him with their hands.

Pilate brings Jesus before the multitude.

4 Pilate therefore went forth again, and saith unto them, Behold, I bring him forth to you, that ye may know [p]that I find no fault in him.

5 Then came Jesus forth, wearing the crown of thorns, and the purple robe. And *Pilate* saith unto them, [q]Behold the man!

6 When the chief priests therefore and officers saw him, they cried out, saying, Crucify *him*, crucify *him*. Pilate saith

A.D. 33.

a For order of events on the day of the crucifixion, see Mt. 26:57, *note.*

b *kosmos* (Mt. 4:8.) = mankind.

c 1 Pet. 2:19, 23.

d John 13:38; Mt. 26:34, 74; Mk. 14:68; Lk. 22:60, 61.

e Mt. 27:2; Mk. 15:1; Lk. 23:1.

f Mt. 23:23; Acts 10:28.

g John 19:7; Lev. 24:16; Mt. 20:19; Rev. 13:10.

h 1 Tim. 6:13.

i Psa. 45:3, 6; Isa. 9:6, 7; Dan. 2:44; Zech. 9:9; Rom. 14:17; Col. 1:13.

j Gk. *ek*, out of, or according to.

k *kosmos* = world-system. 1 Cor. 1:20. (John 7:7; Rev. 13:8, *note.*)

l Isa. 55:4.

m Isa. 53:9; 1 Pet. 2:22.

n Mt. 27:26; Mk. 15:15.

o Mt. 27:28.

p Isa. 53:9; John 18:38.

q John 1:29.

unto them, Take ye him, and crucify *him*: for I find no fault in him.

7 The Jews answered him, [a]We have a law, and by our law he ought to die, because he made himself the Son of God.

8 When Pilate therefore heard that saying, he was the more afraid;

9 And went again into the judgment hall, and saith unto Jesus, Whence art thou? But [b]Jesus gave him no answer.

10 Then saith Pilate unto him, Speakest thou not unto me? knowest thou not that I have power to crucify thee, and have power to release thee?

11 Jesus answered, [c]Thou couldest have no power *at all* against me, except it were given thee from above: [d]therefore he that delivered me unto thee hath the greater [e]sin.

12 And from thenceforth Pilate sought to release him: but the Jews cried out, saying, If thou let this man go, thou art not Cæsar's friend: [f]whosoever maketh himself a king speaketh against Cæsar.

13 [g]When Pilate therefore heard that saying, he brought Jesus forth, and sat down in the judgment seat in a place that is called the Pavement, but in the Hebrew, Gabbatha.

The final rejection of the King by the Jewish authorities and people.

14 And it was the preparation of the passover, and about the [h]sixth hour: and he saith unto the Jews, Behold your King!

15 But they cried out, Away with *him*, away with *him*, crucify him. Pilate saith unto them, Shall I crucify your King? The chief priests answered, [i]We have no king but Cæsar.

The crucifixion of Jesus Christ (Mt. 27:33-54; Mk. 15:22-39; Lk. 23:33-47).

16 [j]Then delivered he him therefore unto them to be crucified. And they took Jesus, and led *him* away.

17 And he bearing his cross [k]went forth into a place called *the place* of a skull, which is called in the Hebrew Golgotha:

18 Where they [l]crucified him, and two other with him, [m]on either side one, and Jesus in the midst.

19 And Pilate wrote a title, and put *it* on the cross. And the writing was, JESUS OF NAZARETH THE KING OF THE JEWS.

20 This title then read many of the Jews: for the place where Jesus was crucified was nigh to the city: and it was written in Hebrew, *and* Greek, *and* Latin.

21 Then said the chief priests of the Jews to Pilate, Write not, The King of the Jews; but that he said, I am King of the Jews.

22 Pilate answered, What I have written I have written.

23 Then the soldiers, when they had crucified Jesus, [n]took his garments, and made four parts, to every soldier a part; and also *his* coat: now the coat was without seam, woven from the top throughout.

24 They said therefore among themselves, [o]Let us not rend it, but cast lots for it, whose it shall be: that the scripture might be fulfilled, which saith, [p]They parted my raiment among them, and for my vesture they did cast lots. These things therefore the soldiers did.

25 [q]Now there stood by the cross of Jesus his mother, and his mother's sister, Mary the *wife* of Cleophas, and Mary Magdalene.

26 When Jesus therefore saw his mother, and the [r]disciple standing by, whom he loved, he saith unto his mother, Woman, [s]behold thy son!

27 Then saith he to the disciple, Behold thy mother! And from that hour that disciple took her unto his own *home*.

28 After this, Jesus knowing that all things were now accomplished, [t]that the scripture might be fulfilled, saith, I thirst.

29 Now there was set a vessel full of vinegar: and they filled a spunge with [u]vinegar, and put *it* upon hyssop, and put *it* to his mouth.

30 When Jesus therefore had received the vinegar, he said, [v]It is finished: and he bowed his head, [w]and [x]gave up the ghost.

"Not a bone of him broken."

31 The Jews therefore, because it was the [y]preparation, that the bodies should not remain upon the cross on the sabbath day, (for that sabbath day was an [z]high day,) besought Pilate that [aa]their legs might be broken, and *that* they might be taken away.

32 Then came the soldiers, and brake the legs of the first, and of

A.D. 33.

a Lev. 24:16.
b Isa. 53:7.
c John 7:30; Lk. 22:53; Acts 4:27, 28.
d John 18:3, 28; Mk. 14:44.
e *Sin.* Rom. 3:23, *note.*
f Lk. 23:2.
g Prov. 29:25; Acts 4:19.
h Cf. Mk. 15:25, *note.*
i Hos. 3:4.
j For order of events, see Mt. 27:33, *note.*
k Num. 15:36; Heb. 13:12.
l *Judgments (the seven).* vs. 16-18; Acts 17:31. (2 Sam. 7:14; Rev. 20:12.)
m Isa. 53:12.
n Psa. 22:18.
o Lk. 5:36; 2 Cor. 5:17.
p Psa. 22:18.
q Mt. 27:55; Mk. 15:40; Lk. 23:49.
r John 18:15.
s John 2:4; 21:15-17.
t vs. 24, 36, 37.
u Psa. 69:21.
v It is the Victor's cry. John 4:34; 17:4; Rom. 10:4; Gal. 3:13; Heb. 10:5-10.
w See Mt. 27:50, *note.*
x *delivered up his spirit.*
y v. 42.
z Ex. 12:16; John 16:20.
aa Deut. 21:23.

the other which was crucified with him.

33 But when they came to Jesus, and saw that he was [a]dead already, they brake not his legs:

34 But one of the soldiers with a spear [b]pierced his side, and forthwith [c]came there out [d]blood and water.

35 And he that saw *it* bare record, and his record is true: and he knoweth that he saith true, that ye might believe.

36 For these things were done, that the scripture should be fulfilled, [e]A bone of him shall not be broken.

37 And again another scripture saith, [f]They shall look on him whom they pierced.

The entombment (Mt. 27:57-60; Mk. 15:43-47; Lk. 23:50-56).

38 And after this Joseph of Arimathaea, being a disciple of Jesus, but [g]secretly for fear of the Jews, besought Pilate that he might take away the body of Jesus: and Pilate gave *him* leave. He came therefore, and took the body of Jesus.

39 And there came also [h]Nicodemus, which at the first came to Jesus by night, and brought a mixture of [i]myrrh and aloes, about an hundred [j]pound *weight*.

40 Then took they the body of Jesus, and wound it in [k]linen clothes with the spices, as the manner of the Jews is to bury.

41 Now in the place where he was crucified there was a garden; and in the garden a new sepulchre, wherein was [l]never man yet laid.

42 There laid they Jesus therefore because of the [m]Jews' preparation *day*; for the sepulchre was nigh at hand.

CHAPTER 20.

The resurrection of Jesus Christ (Mt. 28:1-10; Mk. 16:1-14; Lk. 24:1-43).

The first *day* of the week cometh [n]Mary Magdalene early, when it was yet dark, unto the sepulchre, and seeth the stone taken away from the sepulchre.

2 Then she runneth, and cometh to Simon Peter, and to the [o]other disciple, whom Jesus loved, and saith unto them, They have [p]taken away the Lord out of the sepulchre, and we know not where they have laid him.

3 Peter therefore went forth, and that other disciple, and came to the sepulchre.

4 So they ran both together: and the [q]other disciple did outrun Peter, and came first to the sepulchre.

5 And he stooping down, *and looking in*, saw the linen clothes lying; yet went he not in.

6 Then cometh Simon Peter following him, and [r]went into the sepulchre, and seeth the linen clothes lie,

7 And the [s]napkin, that was about his head, not lying with the linen clothes, but wrapped together in a place by itself.

8 Then went in also that other disciple, which came first to the sepulchre, and he saw, and believed.

9 [t]For as yet they knew not the scripture, that he must rise again from the dead.

10 Then the disciples [u]went away again unto their own home.

Jesus appears to Mary Magdalene.

11 But Mary stood without at the sepulchre [v]weeping: and as she wept, she stooped down, *and looked* into the sepulchre,

12 And seeth [w]two angels in white sitting, the one at the head, and the other at the feet, where the body of Jesus had lain.

13 And they say unto her, Woman, why weepest thou? She saith unto them, Because they have taken away my Lord, and I know not where they have laid him.

14 And when she had thus said, she turned herself back, and saw Jesus standing, and [x]knew not that it was Jesus.

15 Jesus saith unto her, Woman, why weepest thou? [y]whom seekest thou? She, supposing him to be the gardener, saith unto him, Sir, if thou have borne him hence, tell me where thou hast laid him, and I will take him away.

16 Jesus saith unto her, [z]Mary. She turned herself, and saith unto him, Rabboni; which is to say, Master.

17 Jesus saith unto her, [1aa]Touch me

A.D. 33.

a John 10:18.
b John 20:20, 25-27.
c *Sacrifice (of Christ).* Acts 20:28. (Gen. 4:4; Heb. 10:18.)
d 1 John 1:7; 5:6, 8; Tit. 3:5; Eph. 5:26.
e Ex. 12:46; Num. 9:12; Psa. 34:20.
f Zech. 12:10; Rev. 1:7.
g John 7:13; 12:42.
h John 3:2; 7:50.
i Psa. 45:8; Song 4:14.
j Ex. 16:16.
k John 11:44; 20:7; Acts 5:6.
l Isa. 53:9; Mk. 11:2.
m v. 31.
n For order of events on the resurrection day, see Mt. 28:1, *note*.
o John 13:23; 19:26; 21:7, 20, 24.
p vs. 11-13; Lk. 24:21.
q John 21:20.
r John 21:7.
s John 11:44.
t Psa. 16:10; Lk. 24:24-26; Acts 2:25, 31; 13:34, 35.
u Cf. John 21:3.
v v. 13.
w Lk. 24:4.
x Lk. 24:16; John 21:4.
y John 1:38; 18:4.
z John 10:3.
aa Or, *do not detain me*.

[1] **(20:17)** Cf. Mt. 28:9, "and they came and held him by the feet." A contradiction has been supposed. Three views are held: (1) That Jesus speaks to Mary as the High Priest fulfilling the day of atonement (Lev. 16). Having accomplished the sacrifice, He was on His way to present the sacred blood in heaven, and that, between the meeting with Mary in the garden and the meeting of Mt. 28:9, He had

not; for I am not yet [a]ascended to my Father: but go to my [b]brethren, and say unto them, I ascend unto [c]my Father, and [d]your Father; and *to* my God, and your God.

18 [e]Mary Magdalene came and told the disciples that she had seen the Lord, and *that* he had spoken these things unto her.

Jesus appears to the disciples: Thomas not present (Lk. 24:36-49).

19 Then the same day at evening, being the first *day* of the week, when the doors were shut where the disciples were assembled for [f]fear of the Jews, came Jesus and [g]stood in the midst, and saith unto them, [h]Peace *be* unto you.

20 And when he had so said, he [i]shewed unto them *his* hands and his side. [j]Then were the disciples glad, when they saw the Lord.

21 Then said Jesus to them again, Peace *be* unto you: [k]as *my* Father hath sent me, even so send I you.

22 And when he had said this, he [l]breathed on *them*, and saith unto them, Receive ye the [m]Holy Ghost:

23 Whose soever [n]sins ye remit, they are remitted unto them; *and* whose soever *sins* ye retain, they are retained.

Jesus appears to the disciples: Thomas present.

24 But Thomas, one of the twelve, called [o]Didymus, was not with them when Jesus came.

25 The other disciples therefore said unto him, We have seen the Lord. But he said unto them, [p]Except I shall see in his hands the print of the nails, and put my finger into the print of the nails, and thrust my hand into his side, I will not believe.

26 And after eight days again his disciples were within, and Thomas with them: *then* came Jesus, the doors being shut, and stood in the midst, and said, [q]Peace *be* unto you.

27 Then saith he to Thomas, Reach hither thy finger, and behold my hands; and reach hither thy hand, and thrust *it* into my side: and be not faithless, but believing.

28 And Thomas answered and said unto him, [r]My [1]Lord and my God.

29 Jesus saith unto him, Thomas, because thou hast seen me, thou hast believed: [s]blessed *are* they that have not seen, and *yet* have believed.

Conclusion: why John's Gospel was written.

30 And many other signs truly did Jesus in the presence of his disciples, which are not written in this book:

31 But these are written, that ye might [t]believe that Jesus is the Christ, the Son of God; and that believing ye might have [u]life through his name.

CHAPTER 21.

Epilogue: "If I will." The risen Christ is Master of our service.

After these things Jesus shewed himself again to the disciples at the [v]sea of Tiberias; and on this wise shewed he *himself*.

2 There were together Simon Peter, and Thomas called Didymus, and [w]Nathanael of Cana in Galilee, and the *sons* of Zebedee, and two other of his disciples.

(1) *Service in self-will, under human leadership.*

3 Simon Peter saith unto them, [x]I go a fishing. They say unto him, We also go with thee. They went forth, and entered into a ship immediately; and that night they caught [y]nothing.

A.D. 33.

a Lk. 24:51; Heb. 41:14, 15.
b Heb. 2:11.
c John 17:11; Eph. 1:3.
d Gal. 4:6.
e Mt. 28:10; Lk. 24:10.
f John 19:38; Acts 12:12-17.
g *Miracles* (N.T.). John 21:6. (Mt. 8:2, 3; Acts 28:8, 9.)
h John 14:27; Eph. 2:17.
i Lk. 24:40; Col. 1:20.
j John 16:22.
k Mt. 28:18-20; John 17:18.
l Gen. 2:7; 1 Cor. 15:45.
m *Holy Spirit.* Acts 1:2, 5, 8, 16. (Mt. 1:18; Acts 2:4.)
n Mt. 16:19; 18:18.
o John 11:16.
p Zech. 12:10; John 4:48.
q v. 19.
r John 1:1, 49; 9:35-38; Phil. 2:10, 11.
s Rom. 4:18-20; 2 Cor. 5:7.
t *Faith.* Acts 3:16. (Gen. 3:20; Heb. 11:39.)
u *Life (eternal).* Acts 2:28. (Mt. 7:14; Rev. 22:19.)
v John 6:1.
w John 1:45; 2:1.
x *Contra,* Num. 9:17-23.
y Lk. 5:3-7.

so ascended and returned: a view in harmony with types. (2) That Mary Magdalene, knowing as yet only Christ after the flesh (2 Cor. 5:15-17), and having found her Beloved, sought only to hold Him so; while He, about to assume a new relation to His disciples in ascension, gently teaches Mary that now she must not seek to hold Him to the earth, but rather become His messenger of the new joy. (3) That He merely meant: "Do not detain me now; I am not yet ascended; you will see me again; run rather to my brethren," etc.

[1] **(20:28)** The deity of Jesus Christ is declared in Scripture: (1) In the intimations and explicit predictions of the O.T. *(a)* The theophanies intimate the appearance of God in human form, and His ministry thus to man (Gen. 16:7-13; 18:2-23, especially v. 17; 32:28 with Hos. 12:3-5; Ex. 3:2-14). *(b)* The Messiah is expressly declared to be the Son of God (Psa. 2:2-9), and God (Psa. 45:6, 7 with Heb. 1:8, 9; Psa. 110:1 with Mt. 22:44; Acts 2:34 and Heb. 1:13; Psa. 110:4 with Heb. 5:6; 6:20; 7:17-21; and Zech. 6:13).

4 But when the morning was now come, Jesus stood on the shore: but the disciples [a]knew not that it was Jesus.

(2) *Service in self-will tested: the barren result.*

5 Then Jesus saith unto them, Children, have ye any meat? They answered him, No.

(3) *Christ-directed service, and the result.*

6 And he said unto them, [b]Cast the net on the right side of the ship, and ye shall find. They cast therefore, and now [c]they were not able to draw it for the multitude of fishes.

7 Therefore that disciple whom Jesus loved saith unto Peter, It is the [d]Lord. Now when Simon Peter heard that it was the Lord, he girt *his* fisher's coat *unto him*, (for he was naked,) and did [e]cast himself into the sea.

8 And the other disciples came in a little ship; (for they were not far from land, but as it were two hundred [f]cubits,) dragging the net with fishes.

9 As soon then as they were come to land, they saw a [g]fire of coals there, and fish laid thereon, and bread.

10 Jesus saith unto them, Bring of the fish which ye have now caught.

11 Simon Peter went up, and drew the net to land full of great fishes, an hundred and fifty and three: and for all there were so many, yet [h]was not the net broken.

(4)*The Master enough for the need of his servants.* (Cf. Lk. 22:35; Phil. 4:19.)

12 Jesus saith unto them, [i]Come *and* [j]dine. And none of the disciples durst ask him, Who art thou? knowing that it was the Lord.

13 Jesus then cometh, and [k]taketh bread, and giveth them, and fish likewise.

14 This is now the [l]third time that Jesus shewed himself to his disciples, after that he was risen from the dead.

(5) *The only acceptable motive in service.* (Cf. 2 Cor. 5:14; Rev. 2:4, 5.)

15 So when they had [m]dined, Jesus saith to Simon Peter, Simon, *son* of Jonas, [n]lovest thou me more than

A.D. 33.

a John 20:14.
b Lk. 5:3-7; John 9:7.
c *Miracles* (N.T.). Acts 3:1-10. (Mt. 8:2, 3; Acts 28:8, 9.)
d Lk. 24:30, 31.
e John 13:37; 20:6.
f One cubit = about 18 in.
g John 18:18.
h *Contra*, Lk. 5:6.
i John 6:10.
j Lit. *break your fast.*
k Lk. 24:30, 31.
l John 20:19, 26.
m Lit. *break-fasted.*
n Gr. *agapas, deeply love;* used of divine love (John 14:21) and of that love which the law demands (Lk. 10:27).

(c) His virgin birth was foretold as the means through which God could be "Immanuel," God with us (Isa. 7:13, 14 with Mt. 1:22, 23). *(d)* The Messiah is expressly invested with the divine names (Isa. 9:6, 7). *(e)* In a prophecy of His death He is called Jehovah's "fellow" (Zech. 13:7 with Mt. 26:31). *(f)* His eternal being is declared (Mic. 5:2 with Mt. 2:6; John 7:42).

(2) Christ Himself affirmed His deity. *(a)* He applied to Himself the Jehovistic I AM. (The pronoun "he" is not in the Greek; cf. John 8:24; John 8:56-58. The Jews correctly understood this to be our Lord's claim to full deity [v. 59]. See, also, John 10:33; 18:4-6, where, also, "he" is not in the original.) *(b)* He claimed to be the Adonai of the O.T. (Mt. 22:42-45. See Gen. 15:2, *note*). *(c)* He asserted His identity with the Father (Mt. 28:19; Mk. 14;62; John 10:30; that the Jews so understood Him is shown by vs. 31, 32; John 14:8, 9; 17:5). *(d)* He exercised the chief prerogative of God (Mk. 2:5-7; Lk. 7:48-50). *(e)* He asserted omnipresence (Mt. 18:20; John 3:13); omniscience (John 11:11-14, when Jesus was fifty miles away; Mk. 11:6-8); omnipotence (Mt. 28:18; Lk. 7:14; John 5:21-23; 6:19); mastery over nature, and creative power (Lk. 9:16, 17; John 2:9; 10:28). *(f)* He received and approved human worship (Mt. 14:33; 28:9; John 20:28, 29).

(3) The N.T. writers ascribe divine titles to Christ (John 1:1; 20:28; Acts 20:28; Rom. 1:4; 9:5; 2 Thes. 1:12; 1 Tim. 3:16; Tit. 2:13; Heb. 1:8; 1 John 5:20).

(4) The N.T. writers ascribe divine perfections and attributes to Christ (e.g. Mt. 11:28; 18:20; 28:20; John 1:2; 2:23-25; 3:13; 5:17; 21:17; Heb. 1:3, 11, 12 with Heb. 13:8; Rev. 1:8, 17, 18; 2:23; 11:17; 22:13).

(5) The N.T. writers ascribe divine works to Christ (John 1:3, 10; Col. 1:16, 17; Heb. 1:3).

(6) The N.T. writers teach that supreme worship should be paid to Christ (Acts 7:59, 60; 1 Cor. 1:2; 2 Cor. 13:14; Phil. 2:9, 10; Heb. 1: 6; Rev. 1:5, 6; 5:12, 13).

(7) The holiness and resurrection of Christ prove His deity (John 8:46; Rom. 1:4).

these? He saith unto him, Yea, Lord;
thou knowest that I [a]love thee. He saith
unto him, [b]Feed my lambs.
16 He saith to him again the second
time, Simon, *son* of Jonas, [c]lovest thou
me? He saith unto him, Yea, Lord; thou
knowest that I [a]love thee. He saith unto
him, [d]Feed my sheep.
17 He saith unto him the third time,
Simon, *son* of Jonas, [e]lovest thou me?
Peter was [f]grieved because he said unto
him the third time, Lovest thou me? And
he said unto him, Lord, thou knowest all
things; thou knowest that I [a]love thee.
Jesus saith unto him, [g]Feed my sheep.

(6) *The Master appoints the time and manner of the servant's death.*

18 Verily, verily, I say unto thee, When
thou wast young, thou girdedst thyself,
and walkedst whither [h]thou wouldest:
but when thou shalt be old, thou shalt
stretch forth thy hands, and another
shall gird thee, and carry *thee* whither
thou wouldest not.
19 This spake he, signifying [i]by what
death he should glorify God. And when
he had spoken this, he saith unto him,
[j]Follow me.

(7) *If the Lord returns the servants will not die.* (Cf. 1 Cor. 15:51, 52; 1 Thes. 4:14-18.)

20 Then Peter, turning about, seeth the
[k]disciple whom Jesus loved following;
which also leaned on his breast at supper, and said, Lord, which is he that
betrayeth thee?
21 Peter seeing him saith to Jesus,
Lord, and [l]what *shall* this man *do*?
22 Jesus saith unto him, If I will that
he tarry [m]till I come, what *is that* to thee?
follow thou me.
23 Then went this saying abroad
among the brethren, that that disciple
[n]should not die: yet Jesus said not unto
him, He shall not die; but, If I will that
he tarry till I come, what *is that* to thee?
24 This is the disciple which [o]testifieth
of these things, and wrote these things:
and we know that his testimony is true.
25 And there are also [p]many other
things which Jesus did, the which, if
they should be written every one, I suppose that even the [q]world itself [r]could
not contain the books that should be
written. Amen.

A.D. 33.

a Gr. *phileo, am fond of.* it is a lesser degree of love than *agapas.*
b 1 Pet. 5:2.
c Gr. *agapas, deeply love;* used of divine love (John 14:21) and of that love which the law demands (Lk. 10:27).
d *tend;* 1 Pet. 5:1-3.
e Our Lord here takes Peter's word, *phileis.*
f John 13:38.
g v. 15; John 10:9.
h vs. 3, 7.
i 2 Pet. 1:14.
j Mt. 4:19; 16:24.
k John 13:23; 20:2.
l Gal. 2:7-9.
m John 14:3; 1 Thes. 1:10; 5, 23.
n 1 Cor. 15:51; 1 Thes. 4:15, 17.
o John 15:27; 19:35.
p John 20:30.
q i.e. *earth.*
r Eph. 3:19; cf. 2 Cor. 3:3 with Eph. 1:22, 23.

THE ACTS OF THE APOSTLES

WRITER. In the Acts of the Apostles Luke continues the account of Christianity begun in the Gospel which bears his name. In the "former treatise" he tells what Jesus "began both to do and teach"; in the Acts, what Jesus continued to do and teach through His Holy Spirit sent down.

Date. The Acts concludes with the account of Paul's earliest ministry in Rome, A.D. 65, and appears to have been written at or near that time.

Theme. This book records the ascension and promised return of the Lord Jesus, the descent of the Holy Spirit at Pentecost, Peter's use of the keys, opening the kingdom (considered as the sphere of profession, as in Mt. 13) to the Jews at Pentecost, and to the Gentiles in the house of Cornelius; the beginning of the Christian church and the conversion and ministry of Paul.

The Holy Spirit fills the scene. As the presence of the Son, exalting and revealing the Father, is the great fact of the Gospels, so the presence of the Spirit, exalting and revealing the Son, is the great fact of the Acts.

Acts is in two chief parts: In the first section (1–9:43) Peter is the prominent personage, Jerusalem is the centre, and the ministry is to Jews. Already in covenant relations with Jehovah, they had sinned in rejecting Jesus as *the Christ*. The preaching, therefore, was directed to that point, and repentance (i.e. "a changed mind") was demanded. The apparent failure of the Old Testament promises concerning the Davidic kingdom was explained by the promise that the kingdom would be set up at the return of Christ (Acts 2:25-31; 15:14-16). This ministry to Israel fulfilled Lk. 19:12-14. In the persecutions of the apostles and finally in the martyrdom of Stephen, the Jews sent after the king the message, "We will not have this man to reign over us." In the second division (10:1–28:31) Paul is prominent, a new centre is established at Antioch, and the ministry is chiefly to Gentiles who, as "strangers from the covenants of promise" (Eph. 2:12), had but to "believe on the Lord Jesus Christ" to be saved. Chapters 11, 12, and 15 of this section are transitional, establishing finally the distinction, doctrinally, between law and grace. Galatians should be read in this connection.

The events recorded in The Acts cover a period of 32 years.

CHAPTER 1.

Introduction (vs. 1, 2)

The [a]former treatise have I made, O [b]Theophilus, of all that Jesus began both to do and teach,

2 Until the day in which he was [c]taken up, after that he through the Holy Ghost had given commandments unto the apostles whom he had chosen:

The resurrection-ministry of Christ.

3 [d]To whom also he shewed himself alive after his passion by many infallible proofs, being seen of them forty days, and speaking of the things pertaining to the kingdom of God:

4 And, [e]being assembled together with *them*, commanded them that they should not depart from Jerusalem, but wait for the promise of the Father, which, *saith he*, [f]ye have heard of me.

5 For John truly baptized [g]with water; but ye shall be baptized [g]with the Holy Ghost not many days hence.

6 When they therefore were come together, they asked of him, saying, Lord, wilt thou at this time [h]restore again the [1i]kingdom to Israel?

7 And he said unto them, [j]It is not for you to know the times or the seasons, which the Father hath put in his own power.

A.D. 33.

- a i.e. the Gospel according to Luke.
- b Lk. 1:3.
- c Lit. *received up.*
- d Lk. 24:49; John 14:16, 26, 27; Acts 2:33.
- e Or, *eating with them.*
- f Or, *heard from me.*
- g Or, *in.*
- h Mt. 3:2, *note.*
- i *Kingdom* (N.T.). vs. 6, 7; Acts 2:29-32. (Lk. 1:31-33; 1 Cor. 15:24.)
- j Mt. 24:36; Mk. 13:32; 1 Thes. 5:1.

---

[1] **(1:6)** Forty days the risen Lord had been instructing the apostles "of the things pertaining to the kingdom of God," doubtless, according to His custom (Lk. 24:27, 32, 44, 45), teaching them out of the Scriptures. One point was left untouched, viz., the *time* when He would restore the kingdom to Israel; hence the apostles' question. The answer was according to His repeated teaching; the *time* was God's secret (Mt. 24:36, 42, 44; 25:13; cf. 1 Thes. 5:1).

The apostolic commission.
(Cf. Mt. 28:18-20; Mk. 16:15-18;
Lk. 24:47, 48; John 20:21-23.)

8 But ye shall receive power, after that
the Holy Ghost is come upon you: and
ye shall be [a]witnesses unto me both in
Jerusalem, and in all Judæa, and in
Samaria, and unto the uttermost part of
the earth.
9 And when he had spoken these
things, while they beheld, [b]he was taken
up; and a cloud received him out of their
sight.

The promise of the return of
Jesus to the earth.

10 And [c]while they looked stedfastly
toward [d]heaven as he went up, behold,
two men stood by them in white apparel;
11 Which also said, Ye men of Galilee,
why stand ye gazing up into heaven?
this same Jesus, which [e]is taken up from
you into heaven, [f]shall so [1]come in like
manner as ye have seen him go into
heaven.

The ten days' waiting for the Spirit.

12 Then returned they unto Jerusalem
from the mount called Olivet, which is
from Jerusalem a sabbath day's [g]journey.
13 And when they were come in, they
went up into [h]an upper room, where
abode both Peter, and James, and John,
and Andrew, Philip, and Thomas,
Bartholomew, and Matthew, James *the
son* of Alphaeus, and Simon [i]Zelotes,
and Judas *the brother* of James.
14 These all continued with one
accord in prayer and supplication, with
the women, and Mary the mother of
Jesus, and with his brethren.

The choice of Matthias.

15 And in those days Peter stood up in
the midst of the [j]disciples, and said, (the
number of names together were about
an hundred and twenty,)
16 Men *and* brethren, this scripture
must needs have been fulfilled, [k]which
the [l]Holy Ghost by the mouth of David
spake before concerning [m]Judas, which
was guide to them that took Jesus.
17 For he was numbered with us, and
had [n]obtained part of this ministry.

A.D. 33.

a v. 22; Lk. 24:48; John 15:27; Acts 2:32.
b *Christ (First Advent).* Gen. 3:15.
c Or, *as they were looking.*
d 2 Cor. 12:2.
e Or, *was received up.*
f *Christ (Second Advent).* (Deut. 30:3.)
g About 4854 ft.
h *the;* cf. Mk. 14:15; John 20:19.
i *The Zealot.*
j Or, *brethren.*
k *Inspiration.* vs. 8, 16; Acts 9:15. (Ex. 4:15; Rev. 22:19.)
l *Holy Spirit.* vs. 2, 5, 8, 16; Acts 2:17, 18, 33, 38. (Mt. 1:18; Acts 2:4.)
m Psa. 41:9.
n Or, *received.*

[1] **(1:11)** The two Advents—Summary: (1) The O.T. foreview of the coming Messiah is in two aspects—that of rejection and suffering (as, e.g. in Isa. 53), and that of earthly glory and power (as, e.g. in Isa. 11; Jer. 23; Ezk. 37). Often these two aspects blend in one passage (e.g. Psa. 2). The prophets themselves were perplexed by this seeming contradiction (1 Pet. 1:10, 11). It was solved by partial fulfilment. In due time the Messiah, born of a virgin according to Isaiah, appeared among men and began His ministry by announcing the predicted kingdom as "at hand" (Mt. 4:17, *note*). The rejection of King and kingdom followed. (2) Thereupon the rejected King announced His approaching crucifixion, resurrection, departure, and return (Mt. 12:38-40; 16:1-4, 21, 27; Lk. 12:35-46; 17:20-36; 18:31-34; 19:12-27; Mt. 24, 25). (3) He uttered predictions concerning the course of events between His departure and return (Mt. 13:1-50; 16:18; 24:4-26). (4) This promised return of Christ becomes a prominent theme in the Acts, Epistles, and Revelation.

Taken together, the N.T. teachings concerning the return of Jesus Christ may be summarized as follows: (1) That return is an event, not a process, and is personal and corporeal (Mt. 23:39; 24:30; 25:31; Mk. 14:62; Lk. 17:24; John 14:3; Acts 1:11; Phil. 3:20, 21; 1 Thes. 4:14-17). (2) His coming has a threefold relation: to the church, to Israel, to the nations.

(a) To the church the descent of the Lord into the air to raise the sleeping and change the living saints is set forth as a constant expectation and hope (Mt. 24:36, 44, 48-51; 25:13; 1 Cor. 15:51, 52; Phil. 3:20; 1 Thes. 1:10; 4:14-17; 1 Tim. 6:14; Tit. 2:13; Rev. 22:20).

(b) To Israel, the return of the Lord is predicted to accomplish the yet unfulfilled prophecies of her national regathering, conversion, and establishment in peace and power under the Davidic Covenant (Acts 15:14-17 with Zech. 14:1-9). See "Kingdom (O.T.)," 2 Sam. 7:8-17; Zech. 13:8, *note;* Lk. 1:31-33; 1 Cor. 15:24, *note.*

(c) To the Gentile nations the return of Christ is predicted to bring the destruction of the present political world-system (Dan. 2:34, 35; Rev. 19:11, *note*); the judgment of Mt. 25:31-46, followed by world-wide Gentile conversion and participation in the blessings of the kingdom (Isa. 2:2-4; 11:10; 60:3; Zech. 8:3, 20, 23; 14:16-21).

18 Now this man purchased a field
with the [a]reward of iniquity; and falling
headlong, he burst asunder in the midst,
and all his bowels gushed out.
19 And it was known unto all the
dwellers at Jerusalem; insomuch as that
field is called in their proper tongue,
Aceldama, that is to say, The field of
blood.
20 For it is written in the book of
Psalms, [b]Let his habitation be desolate,
and let no man dwell therein: and his
[c]bishoprick let another [d]take.
21 Wherefore of these men which have
companied with us all the time that the
Lord Jesus went in and out among us,
22 Beginning from the baptism of
John, unto that same day that he was
[e]taken up from us, must one [f]be
ordained to be a witness with us of his
resurrection.
23 And they [g]appointed two, Joseph
called Barsabas, who was surnamed
Justus, and Matthias.
24 And they [h]prayed, and said, Thou,
Lord, which knowest the hearts of all
men, shew whether of these two thou
hast chosen,
25 That he may take [i]part of this ministry and apostleship, from which Judas
by [j]transgression fell, that he might go to
his own place.
26 And they gave forth their lots; and
the lot fell upon Matthias; and he was
numbered with the eleven apostles.

A.D. 33.

a Zech. 11:12, 13.
b Psa. 69:25.
c Gr. *episkopen, overseership.* See Tit. 1:5-9, *note.*
d Psa. 109:8.
e Lit. *received up.*
f Lit. *become a witness.*
g Lit. *made two stand up.*
h *Bible prayers* (N.T.). Acts 4:24-30. (Mt. 6:9; Rev. 22:20.)
i *the place in.*
j *Sin.* Rom. 3;23, *note.*
k Lev. 23:15, 16, *note;* Deut. 16:9. Acts 20:16.
l *tongues, as of fire, parting and sitting upon each of them.*
m Psa. 68:18.
n *Holy Spirit.* (Mt. 1:18.)

CHAPTER 2.

Pentecost: Peter's first use of the keys (Mt. 16:18, 19); *the Gospel given to the Jews.* (Cf. Acts 10:1-48.)

And when [k]the day of Pentecost was
fully come, they were all with one
accord in one place.
2 And suddenly there came a sound
from heaven as of a rushing mighty
wind, and it filled all the house where
they were sitting.
3 And there appeared unto them
[l]cloven tongues like as of fire, and it sat
upon each of them.
4 And they were all filled with the
[1]Holy Ghost, and began to speak with
[m]other tongues, as the [n]Spirit gave them
utterance.
5 And there were dwelling at Jerusalem Jews, devout men, out of every
nation under heaven.
6 Now when this was noised abroad,
the multitude came together, and were
confounded, because that every man
heard them speak in his own language.
7 And they were all amazed and marvelled, saying one to another, Behold,
are not all these which speak Galilæans?

[1] **(2:4)** The Holy Spirit, N.T. Summary (see Mal. 2:15, *note*):

(1) The Holy Spirit is revealed as a divine Person. This is expressly declared (e.g. John 14:16, 17, 26; 15:26; 16:7-15; Mt. 28:19), and everywhere implied.

(2) The revelation concerning Him is progressive: *(a)* In the O.T. (see Mal. 2:15, *note*) He comes upon whom He will, apparently without reference to conditions in them. *(b)* During His earth-life, Christ taught His disciples (Lk. 11:13) that they might receive the Spirit through prayer to the Father. *(c)* At the close of His ministry He promised that He would Himself pray the Father, and that in answer to His prayer the Comforter would come to abide (John 14:16, 17). *(d)* On the evening of His resurrection He came to the disciples in the upper room, and breathed on them saying, "Receive ye the Holy Ghost" (John 20:22), but instructed them to wait before beginning their ministry till the Spirit should come *upon* them (Lk. 24:49; Acts 1:8) *(e)* On the day of Pentecost the Spirit came upon the whole body of believers (Acts 2:1-4). *(f)* After Pentecost, so long as the Gospel was preached to Jews only, the Spirit was imparted to such as believed by the laying. on of hands (Acts 8:17; 9:17, etc.). *(g)* When Peter opened the door of the kingdom to the Gentiles (Acts 10), the Holy Spirit, without delay, or other condition than faith, was given to those who believed. (Acts 10:44; 11:15-18). This is the permanent fact for the entire church-age. Every believer is born of the Spirit (John 3:3, 6; 1 John 5:1), indwelt by the Spirit, whose presence makes the believer's body a temple (1 Cor. 6:19; Rom. 8:9-15; 1 John 2:27; Gal. 4:6), and baptized by the Spirit (1 Cor. 12:12, 13; 1 John 2:20, 27), thus sealing him for God (Eph. 1:13; 4:30).

(3) The N.T. distinguishes between having the Spirit, which is true of all believers, and being filled with the Spirit, which is the believer's privilege and duty (cf. Acts 2:4 with 4:29-31; Eph. 1:13, 14 with 5:18)—"One baptism, many fillings."

8 And how hear we every man in our
own [a]tongue, wherein we were born?
9 Parthians, and Medes, and Elamites,
and the dwellers in Mesopotamia, and in
Judæa, and Cappadocia, in Pontus, and
Asia,
10 Phrygia, and Pamphylia, in Egypt,
and in the parts of Libya about Cyrene,
and strangers [b]of Rome, Jews and proselytes,
11 Cretes and Arabians, we do hear
them speak in our [c]tongues the wonderful works of God.
12 And they were all amazed, and
were [d]in doubt, saying one to another,
What meaneth this?
13 Others mocking said, These men
are full of new wine.

A.D. 33.

a language.
b from.
c languages.
d perplexed.
e through.

Peter's sermon.

Theme: Jesus is Lord and Christ (v. 36).

14 But Peter, standing up with the
eleven, lifted up his voice, and [1]said
unto them, Ye men of Judæa, and all *ye*
that dwell at Jerusalem, be this known
unto you, and hearken to my words:

(1) *Introductory. Joel's prophecy fulfilled.*

15 For these are not drunken, as ye
suppose, seeing it is *but* the third hour of
the day.
16 But this is that which was spoken
[e]by the prophet Joel;
17 And it shall come to pass in the

(4) The Holy Spirit is related to Christ in His conception (Mt. 1:18-20; Lk. 1:35), baptism (Mt. 3:16; Mk. 1:10; Lk. 3:22; John 1:32, 33), walk and service (Lk. 4:1-14), resurrection (Rom. 8:11), and as His witness throughout this age (John 15:26; 16:8-11, 13, 14).

(5) The Spirit forms the church (Mt. 16:18; Heb. 12:23, *note*) by baptizing all believers into the body of Christ (1 Cor. 12:12, 13), imparts gifts for service to every member of that body (1 Cor. 12:7-11, 27, 30), guides the members in their service (Lk. 2:27; 4:1; Acts 16: 6, 7), and is Himself the power of that service (Acts 1:8; 2:4; 1 Cor. 2:4).

(6) The Spirit abides in the company of believers who constitute a local church, making of them, corporately, a temple (1 Cor. 3:16, 17).

(7) Christ indicates a threefold personal relationship of the Spirit to the believer: "With," "in," "upon" (John 14:17; Lk. 24:49; Acts 1:8). "With" indicates the approach of God to the soul, convicting of sin (John 16:9), presenting Christ as the object of faith (John 16:14), imparting faith (Eph. 2:8), and regenerating (John 3:3-16). "In" describes the abiding presence of the Spirit in the believer's body (1 Cor. 6:19) to give victory over the flesh (Rom. 8:2-4; Gal. 5:16, 17), to create the Christian character (Gal. 5:22, 23), to help infirmities (Rom. 8:26), to inspire prayer (Eph. 6:18), to give conscious access to God (Eph. 2:18), to actualize to the believer his sonship (Gal. 4:6), to apply the Scriptures in cleansing and sanctification (Eph. 5:26; 2 Thes. 2:13; 1 Pet. 1:2), to comfort and intercede (Acts 9:31; Rom. 8:26), and to reveal Christ (John 16:14).

(8) Sins against the Spirit committed by unbelievers are: To blaspheme (Mt. 12:31), resist (Acts 7:51, insult (Heb. 10:29, "despite," lit. *insult*). Believers' sins against the Spirit are: To grieve Him by allowing evil in heart or life (Eph. 4:30, 31), and to quench Him by disobedience (1 Thes. 5:19). The right attitude toward the Spirit is yieldedness to His sway in walk and service, and in constant willingness that He shall "put away" whatever grieves Him or hinders His power (Eph. 4:31).

(9) The *symbols* of the Spirit are: *(a)* oil (John 3:34; Heb. 1:9); *(b)* water (John 7:38, 39); *(c)* wind (Acts 2:1; John 3:8); *(d)* fire (Acts 2:3); *(e)* a dove (Mt. 3:16); *(f)* a seal (Eph. 1:13; 4:30); *(g)* an earnest or pledge (Eph. 1:14).

[1]**(2:14)** The theme of Peter's sermon at Pentecost is stated in verse 36. It is, that Jesus is the Messiah. No message could have been more unwelcome to the Jews who had rejected His Messianic claims, and crucified Him. Peter, therefore, does not announce his theme until he has covered every possible Jewish objection. The point of difficulty with the Jews was the apparent failure of the clear and repeated prophetic promise of a regathered Israel established in their own land under their covenanted King (e.g. Isa. 11:10-12; Jer. 23:5-8; Ezk. 37:21-28). Instead of explaining, as Rome first taught, followed by some Protestant commentators, that the covenant and promises were to be fulfilled in the church in a so-called "spiritual" sense, Peter shows (vs. 25-32) from Psa. 16 that David himself understood that the dead and risen Christ would fulfil the covenant and sit on his throne (Lk. 1:32, 33). In precisely the same way James (Acts 15:14-17) met the same difficulty. See "Kingdom (O.T.)," Zech. 12:8; (N.T.), Lk. 1:33; 1 Cor. 15:24.

[1]last days, saith God, I will [a]pour out of my [b]Spirit upon all flesh: and your sons and your daughters shall prophesy, and your young men shall see visions, and your old men shall dream dreams:

18 And on my [c]servants and on my handmaidens I will pour out in those days of my [d]Spirit; and they shall prophesy:

19 And I will shew wonders in heaven above, and signs in the earth beneath; blood, and fire, and vapour of smoke:

20 The sun shall be turned into darkness, and the moon into blood, before that [e]great and notable day of the [f]Lord come:

21 And it shall come to pass, *that* whosoever shall call on the name of the [g]Lord shall be [h]saved.

(2) *The works of Jesus prove that he is Lord and Christ.*

22 Ye men of Israel, hear these words; Jesus of Nazareth, a man approved of God among you by miracles and wonders and signs, which God did by him in the midst of you, as ye yourselves also know:

23 Him, being delivered by the determinate counsel and [i]foreknowledge of God, ye have taken, and by wicked hands have crucified and slain:

24 Whom God hath raised up, having loosed the pains of death: because it was not possible that he should be holden of it.

(3) *David foretold Messiah's kingship after resurrection.*

25 For [j]David speaketh concerning him, I foresaw the [k]Lord always before my face, for he is on my right hand, that I should not be moved:

26 Therefore did my heart rejoice, and my tongue was glad; moreover also my flesh shall rest in hope:

27 Because thou wilt not leave my soul in [l]hell, neither wilt thou suffer thine [m]Holy One to see corruption.

28 Thou hast made known to me the ways of [n]life; thou shalt make me full of joy with thy countenance.

29 Men *and* brethren, let me freely speak unto you of the patriarch [o]David, that he is both dead and buried, and his sepulchre is with us unto this day.

30 Therefore being a prophet, and knowing that God had sworn with an oath to him, that of the fruit of his loins, according to the flesh, [p]he would raise up Christ to sit on his [q]throne;

31 He seeing this before spake of the resurrection of [r]Christ, that his soul was not left in [s]hell, neither his flesh did see corruption.

(4) *His resurrection proves that he is Lord and Christ.*

32 This Jesus hath God [t]raised up, whereof we all are witnesses.

33 Therefore being by the right hand of God exalted, and having received of the Father the promise of the Holy Ghost, he hath shed forth this, which ye now see and hear.

34 For David is not ascended into the heavens: but he saith himself, The LORD said unto my [u]Lord, Sit thou on my right hand,

35 Until I make thy foes thy footstool.

36 Therefore let all the house of Israel know assuredly, that God hath made that same Jesus, whom ye have crucified, both Lord and Christ.

(5) *What Israel must do.*

37 Now when they heard *this*, they were pricked in their heart, and said unto Peter and to the rest of the apostles, Men *and* brethren, what shall we do?

38 Then Peter said unto them, [v]Repent, and be baptized every one of you in the name of Jesus Christ [w]for the [x]remission of [y]sins, and ye

A.D. 33.

a vs. 17-21; Joel 2:28-32.
b *Holy Spirit.* vs. 17, 18, 33, 38; Acts 4:8, 31. (Mt. 1:18; Acts 2:4.)
c *bondmen.*
d Joel 2:29.
e *Day (of Jehovah),* vs. 19, 20; 1 Thes. 5:1-3. (Isa. 2:10-22; Rev. 19:11-21.)
f *Jehovah.* Joel 2:31.
g *Jehovah.* Joel 2:32.
h Rom. 1:16, *note.*
i *Foreknowledge.* Acts 26:5. (Acts 2:23; 1 Pet. 1:20.)
j Psa. 16:8-11.
k *Jehovah.* Psa. 16:8.
l *Hades.* Lk. 16:23, *note.*
m *Holy One.* Psa. 16:10.
n *Life (eternal).* Acts 3:15. (Mt. 7:14 Rev. 22:19.)
o 1 Ki. 2:10; Acts 13:36.
p *Israel (prophecies).* vs. 29-32; Acts 15:14-17. (Gen. 12:2, 3; Rom. 11:26.)
q *Kingdom* (N.T.). vs. 29-32; Acts 15:14-17. (Lk. 1:31-33; 1 Cor. 15:24.)
r *the Christ.*
s *Hades.* Lk. 16:23, *note.*
t *Resurrection.* Acts 4:2, 33. (Job 19:25; 1 Cor. 15:52.)
u *Adonai.* Psa. 110:1; Mt. 22:44.
v *Repentance.* Acts 3:19. (Mt. 3:2; Acts 17:30.)
w *unto.*
x Mt. 26:28, *note.*
y *Sin.* Rom. 3:23, *note.*

1 (2:17) A distinction must be observed between "the last days" when the prediction relates to Israel, and the "last days" when the prediction relates to the church (1 Tim. 4:1-3; 2 Tim. 3:1-8; Heb. 1:1, 2; 1 Pet. 1:4, 5; 2 Pet. 3:1-9; 1 John 2:18, 19; Jude 17-19). Also distinguish the expression the "last days" (plural) from "the last day" (singular); the latter expression referring to the resurrections and last judgment (John 6:39, 40, 44, 54; 11:24; 12:48). The "last days" as related to the church began with the advent of Christ (Heb. 1:2), but have especial reference to the time of declension and apostasy at the end of this age (2 Tim. 3:1; 4:4). The "last days" as related to Israel are the days of Israel's exaltation and blessing, and are synonymous with the kingdom-age (Isa. 2:2-4; Mic. 4:1-7). They are "last" not with reference to this dispensation, but with reference to the whole of Israel's history.

shall receive the gift of the Holy Ghost.

39 For the promise is unto you, and to your children, and to all that are afar off, *even* as many as the [a]Lord our God shall call.

40 And with many other words did he testify and exhort, saying, Save yourselves from this untoward generation.

41 Then they [b]that gladly received his word were baptized: and the same day there were [c]added *unto them* about three thousand souls.

The first church. (Cf. Acts 4:32-37.)

42 And they continued stedfastly in the apostles' [d]doctrine and fellowship, and in breaking of bread, and in prayers.

43 And fear came upon every soul: and many wonders and signs were done [e]by the apostles.

44 And all that believed were together, and had all things common;

45 And sold their possessions and goods, and parted them to all *men,* as every man had need.

46 And they, continuing daily with one accord in the temple, and breaking bread from house to house, did [f]eat their meat with gladness and singleness of heart,

47 Praising God, and having favour with all the people. [g]And the Lord added to the [h]church daily such as should be [i]saved.

CHAPTER 3.

The first apostolic miracle: the lame man healed.

Now Peter and John [j]went up together into the temple at the hour of [k]prayer, *being* the ninth *hour.*

2 And a [l]certain man lame from his mother's womb was carried, whom they laid daily at the gate of the temple which is called Beautiful, [m]to ask alms of them that entered into the temple;

3 Who seeing Peter and John about to go into the temple asked an alms.

4 And Peter, fastening his eyes upon him with John, said, Look on us.

5 And he gave heed unto them, expecting to receive something of them.

6 Then Peter said, Silver and gold have I none; but such as I have give I thee: [n]In the name of Jesus Christ of Nazareth rise up and walk.

7 And he took him by the right hand, and lifted *him* up: and [o]immediately his feet and ankle bones received strength.

8 And he [p]leaping up stood, and [q]walked, and entered with them into the temple, walking, and leaping, and praising God.

9 And [r]all the people saw him walking and praising God:

10 And they knew that it was he which sat for alms at the Beautiful gate of the temple: and they were filled with wonder and amazement at that which had happened unto him.

11 And as the lame man which was healed held Peter and John, all the people ran together unto them in the [s]porch that is called Solomon's, greatly wondering.

Peter's second sermon.
Theme: the covenants will be fulfilled.

12 And when Peter saw *it,* he answered unto the people, Ye men of Israel, why marvel ye at this? or why look ye so earnestly on us, as though by our own power or [t]holiness we had made this man to walk?

13 The God of Abraham, and of Isaac, and of Jacob, the God of our fathers, hath glorified his Son Jesus; whom ye delivered up, and denied him in the presence of Pilate, when he was determined to let *him* go.

14 But ye denied the [u]Holy One and the Just, and desired a murderer to be granted unto you;

15 And killed the [v]Prince of [w]life, whom God hath raised from the dead; whereof we are witnesses.

16 And his name through [x]faith in his name hath made this man strong, whom ye see and know: yea, the faith which is [y]by him hath given him this perfect soundness in the presence of you all.

17 And now, brethren, I wot that through ignorance ye did *it,* as *did* also your rulers.

18 But those things, which God before had shewed by the mouth of all his prophets, that [z]Christ should suffer, he hath so fulfilled.

19 [aa]Repent ye therefore, and [bb]be converted, that your [cc]sins may be blotted out, [dd]when the times of [1]refreshing shall come from the presence of the Lord;

A.D. 33.

a *Jehovah.* Joel 2:32.
b *having received.*
c *Churches (local).* Acts 8:1-8. (Acts 2:41; Phil. 1:1)
d *teaching.*
e *through.*
f *partake of their food.*
g *Moreover the Lord was adding to the church day by day those being saved.* Cf. 1 Cor. 12:12, 13; Eph. 1:22, 23.
h *Church, true.* 1 Cor. 12:12-28. (Mt. 16:18; Heb. 12:23.)
i Rom. 1:16, *note.*
j *were going.*
k Psa. 55:17.
l Acts 14:8.
m John 9:8.
n Acts 4:10.
o *Miracles* (N.T.). vs. 1-10; Acts 5:12. (Mt. 8:2, 3; Acts 28:8, 9.)
p Isa. 35:6.
q *began to walk, and entered.*
r Acts 4:16, 21.
s John 10:23; Acts 5:12.
t *godliness.*
u Or, *Holy and Righteous One.*
v Or, *Author.*
w *Life (eternal).* Acts 5:20. (Mt. 7:14; Rev. 22:19.)
x *Faith.* Acts 13:39 (Gen. 3:20; Heb. 11:39.)
y *through.*
z *his Christ.*
aa *Repentance.* Acts 5:31. (Mt. 3:2; Acts 17:30.)
bb *turn again.* Lk. 22:32.
cc *Sin.* Rom. 3:23, *note.*
dd *that so may come times of refreshing from the face of the Lord, and* [that] *he may send ... Jesus Christ.*

[1](3:19) "Namely, seasons in which, through the appearance of the Messiah in His kingdom, there

20 [1]And he shall send Jesus Christ,
which before was preached unto you:
21 Whom the heaven must receive
until the times of [2]restitution of all
things, which God hath spoken by the
mouth of all his [a]holy prophets [b]since
the world began.
22 For Moses truly said unto the
fathers, [c]A prophet shall the Lord your
God raise up unto you [d]of your
brethren, like unto me; [e]him shall ye
hear in all things whatsoever he shall
say unto you.
23 And it shall come to pass, *that*
every soul, which will not hear that
prophet, shall be [f]destroyed from among
the people.
24 Yea, and all the prophets from
Samuel and those that follow after, as
many as have spoken, have likewise
foretold of these days.
25 Ye are the [g]children of the prophets,
and of the covenant which God made
with [h]our fathers, saying unto Abraham,
And in thy seed shall all the kindreds of
the earth be blessed.
26 Unto you first God, having raised
up his Son Jesus, sent him to bless you,
in turning away every one of you from
[h]his iniquities.

CHAPTER 4.

The first persecution.

And as they spake unto the people,
the priests, and the captain of the
temple, and the [i]Sadducees, came upon
them,
2 Being [j]grieved that they taught the
people, and preached through Jesus the
resurrection from the dead.

A.D. 33.

a Sanctify, holy (persons) Acts 4:27-30. (Mt. 4:5; Rev. 22:11.)
b *from old time.*
c Deut. 18:15, 18, 19.
d *from among.*
e Acts 7:37.
f *utterly destroyed.*
g Gr. *huioi, sons.*
h *your.*
i Mt. 3:7, *note.*
j *sore troubled.*
k *came to be.*
l Lk. 3:2; John 11:49; 18:13.
m Ex. 2:14; Mt. 21:23; Acts 7:27.
n Lk. 12:11, 12.
o *in.*
p Acts 3:6, 16.
q Acts 2:24.
r *Christ (as Stone).* Eph. 2:20. (Ex. 17:6; 1 Pet. 2:8.)
s Psa. 118:22.
t Rom. 1:16, *note.*
u *wherein.*
v Mt. 11:25; 1 Cor. 1:27.

3 And they laid hands on them, and
put *them* in hold unto the next day: for it
was now eventide.
4 Howbeit many of them which heard
the word believed; and the number of
the men [k]was about five thousand.

Peter's address to the Sanhedrin.

5 And it came to pass on the morrow,
that their rulers, and elders, and scribes,
6 And [l]Annas the high priest, and
Caiaphas, and John, and Alexander, and
as many as were of the kindred of the
high priest, were gathered together at
Jerusalem.
7 And when they had set them in the
midst, they asked, [m]By what power, or
by what name, have ye done this?
8 Then [n]Peter, filled with the Holy
Ghost, said unto them, Ye rulers of the
people, and elders of Israel,
9 If we this day be examined of the
good deed done to the impotent man, by
what means he is made whole;
10 Be it known unto you all, and to all
the people of Israel, that [o]by the [p]name
of Jesus Christ of Nazareth, whom ye
crucified, [q]whom God raised from the
dead, *even* [o]by him doth this man stand
here before you whole.
11 This is the [r]stone which was set [s]at
nought of you builders, which is become
the head of the corner.
12 Neither is there [t]salvation in any
other: for there is none other name
under heaven given among men,
[u]whereby we must be saved.

Preaching in the name of Jesus forbidden.

13 Now when they saw the boldness
of Peter and John, and perceived that
they were [v]unlearned and ignorant men,

shall occur blessed rest and refreshment for the people of God."—*Heinrich A. W. Meyer.*

[1] **(3:20)** The appeal here is national to the Jewish people as such, not individual as in Peter's first sermon (Acts 2:38, 39). There those who were pricked in heart were exhorted to save themselves from (among) the untoward nation; here the whole people is addressed, and the promise to *national* repentance is *national* deliverance: "and he shall send Jesus Christ" to bring in the times which the prophets had foretold (see Acts 2:14, *note*). The official answer was the imprisonment of the apostles, and the inhibition to preach, so fulfilling Lk. 19:14.

[2] **(3:21)** Gr. *apokatastaseos* = restoration, occurring here and Acts 1:6 only. The meaning is limited by the words: "Which God hath spoken by the mouth of all his holy prophets." The prophets speak of the restoration of Israel to the land (see "Israel," Gen. 12:2, 3; Rom. 11:26; also "Palestinian Covenant," Deut. 30:1-9, *note*); and of the restoration of the theocracy under David's Son. (See "Davidic Covenant," 2 Sam. 7:8-17, *note;* "Kingdom," Gen. 1:26-28; Zech. 12:8, *note.*) No prediction of the conversion and restoration of the wicked dead is found in the prophets, or elsewhere. Cf. Rev. 20:11-15.

they marvelled; and they took knowledge of them, that they had been with Jesus.

14 And beholding the man which was healed standing with them, they could say nothing against it.

15 But when they had commanded them to go aside out of the council, they conferred among themselves,

16 Saying, [a]What shall we do to these men? for that indeed a notable [b]miracle hath been done by them *is* manifest to all them that dwell in Jerusalem; and we cannot deny *it*.

17 But that it spread no further among the people, let us straitly threaten them, that they speak henceforth to no man in this name.

18 And they called them, and commanded them not to speak at all nor teach in the name of Jesus.

19 But Peter and John answered and said unto them, Whether it be right in the sight of God to [c]hearken unto you more than unto God, judge ye.

20 For we [d]cannot but speak the things which we [e]have seen and heard.

21 So when they had further threatened them, they let them go, finding nothing how they might punish them, because of the people: for all *men* glorified God for that which was done.

22 For the man was above forty years old, on whom this miracle of healing was shewed.

The Christians again filled with the Spirit.
(Cf. Acts 2:1-4.)

23 And being let go, [f]they went to their own company, and reported all that the chief priests and elders had said unto them.

24 And when they heard that, they [g]lifted up their voice to God with one accord, and said, Lord, [h]thou *art* God, which hast made heaven, and earth, and the sea, and all that in them is:

25 Who by the mouth of thy servant David hast [i]said, Why did the [j]heathen [k]rage, and the people imagine vain things?

26 The kings of the earth stood up, and the rulers were gathered together against the [l]Lord, and against his [m]Christ.

27 For of a truth against thy [n]holy child Jesus, whom thou hast anointed, both [o]Herod, and Pontius Pilate, with the Gentiles, and the people of Israel, were gathered together,

28 For to do whatsoever thy hand and thy counsel [p]determined before to be done.

29 And now, Lord, behold their threatenings: and grant unto thy servants, that with all boldness they may speak thy word,

30 By stretching forth thine hand to heal; and that signs and wonders may be done by the name of thy holy child Jesus.

31 And when they had prayed, the place was shaken where they were assembled together; and they were all filled with the [q]Holy Ghost, and they spake the word of God with boldness.

State of the church at Jerusalem.
(Cf. Acts 2:42-47.)

32 And the multitude of them that believed were of one heart and of one soul: neither said any *of them* that ought of the things which he possessed was his own; but they had all things common.

33 And with great power gave the apostles witness of the [r]resurrection of the Lord Jesus: and great grace was upon them all.

34 Neither was there any among them that lacked: for as many as were possessors of lands or houses sold them, and brought the prices of the things that were sold,

35 And laid *them* down at the apostles' feet: and distribution was made unto every man according as he had need.

36 And Joses, who by the apostles was surnamed Barnabas, (which is, being interpreted, The son of [s]consolation,) a Levite, *and* of the country of Cyprus,

37 Having land, sold *it*, and brought the money, and laid *it* at the apostles' feet.

CHAPTER 5.

The sin and death of Ananias and Sapphira.

But a certain man named Ananias, with Sapphira his wife, sold a possession,

2 And [t]kept back *part* of the price, his wife also being privy *to it*, and brought [u]a certain part, and laid *it* at the apostles' feet.

3 But Peter said, Ananias, [v]why hath [w]Satan filled thine heart to lie to the Holy Ghost, and to keep back *part* of the price of the land?

4 Whiles it remained, was it not thine own? and after it was sold, was it not in thine own power? why hast thou

A.D. 33.

a John 11:47.
b Gr. *semeion, sign.*
c Acts 5:29; Mt. 28:19; 1 Cor. 9:16; Gal. 1:10.
d Job 32:19; Jer. 20:9.
e 1 John 1:1, 3.
f Acts 2:44-46.
g *Bible Prayers.* Acts 7:59, 60. (Mt. 6:9; Rev. 22:20.)
h Isa. 51:12, 13.
i Psa. 2:2, 6, *note.*
j i.e. *Gentiles.*
k vs. 25, 26; Psa. 2:1, 2.
l *Jehovah.* Psa. 2:2.
m *Anointed.* Psa. 2:2.
n *Sanctify, holy (persons)* (N.T.). vs. 27, 30; Acts 20:32. (Mt. 4, 5; Rev. 22:11.)
o See Mt. 14:1, *ref.*
p *Predestination,* trans. *predestinated.* Rom. 8:29. (Acts 4:28; Eph. 1:5, 11)
q *Holy Spirit.* vs. 8, 31; Acts 5:3, 9, 32. (Mt. 1:18; Acts 2:4.)
r *Resurrection.* vs. 2, 33; Acts 9:36-42. (Job 19:25; 1 Cor. 15:52.)
s Or, *exhortation.*
t Josh. 7:11, 12; Mal. 3:8, 9; 1 Tim. 6:10.
u Acts 4:34-37.
v 1 Chr. 21:1; Mt. 13:19; John 13:2, 27; Eph. 6:11, 16; 1 Pet. 5:8.
w *Satan.* Acts 10:38. (Gen. 3:1; Rev. 20:10.)

conceived this thing in thine heart? thou
hast not lied unto men, [a]but unto God.
5 And Ananias [b]hearing these words
fell down, and gave up the ghost: and
great fear came on all them that heard
these things.
6 And the [c]young men arose, wound
him up, and carried *him* out, and buried
him.
7 And it was about the space of three
hours after, when his wife, not knowing
what was done, came in.
8 And Peter answered unto her, Tell
me whether ye sold the land for so
much? And she said, Yea, for so much.
9 Then Peter said unto her, How is it
that ye have agreed together to [d]tempt
the Spirit of the Lord? behold, the feet of
them which have buried thy husband *are*
at the door, and shall carry thee out.
10 Then fell she down straightway at
his feet, and yielded up the ghost: and
the young men came in, and found her
dead, and, carrying *her* forth, buried *her*
by her husband.
11 And great fear came upon all the
church, and upon as many as heard
these things.

The power of a holy church.
(See 1 Thes. 1:1-10.)

12 And by the hands of the apostles
were [e]many signs and wonders [f]wrought
among the people; (and they were all
with one accord in Solomon's porch.
13 And of the rest durst no man join
himself to them: but the people magnified them.
14 And believers were the more added
to the Lord, multitudes both of men and
women.)
15 Insomuch that they brought forth
the sick [g]into the streets, and laid *them*
on beds and couches, that at the least the
shadow of Peter passing by might overshadow some of them.
16 There came also a multitude *out* of
the cities round about unto Jerusalem,
[h]bringing sick folks, and them which
were vexed with unclean spirits: and
they were healed every one.

The second persecution.

17 Then the high priest rose up, and
all they that were with him, (which is
the [i]sect of the Sadducees,) and were
filled with [j]indignation,
18 And laid their hands on the apostles,
and put them in the common prison.
19 But [k]the [l]angel of the Lord by night
opened the prison doors, and brought
them forth, and said,
20 Go, stand and speak in the temple
to the people all the words of this [m]life.
21 And when they heard *that*, they
entered into the temple early in the
morning, and taught. But the high priest
came, and they that were with him, and
called the council together, and all the
senate of the children of Israel, and sent
to the prison to have them brought.
22 But when the officers came, and
found them not in the prison, they
returned, and told,
23 Saying, The prison truly found we
shut with all safety, and the keepers
standing without before the doors: but
when we had opened, we found no man
within.
24 Now when the high priest and the
captain of the temple and the chief
priests heard these things, they doubted
of them whereunto this would grow.
25 Then came one and told them, saying, Behold, the men whom ye put in
prison are standing in the temple, and
teaching the people.
26 Then went the captain with the officers, and brought them without violence: for they feared the people, lest
they should have been stoned.
27 And when they had brought them,
they set *them* before the council: and the
high priest asked them,
28 Saying, Did not we straitly command you that ye should not teach in this
name? and, behold, ye have filled Jerusalem with your [n]doctrine, and intend to
bring this man's blood upon us.

The answer of the apostles.

29 Then Peter and the *other* apostles
answered and said, We ought to obey
God rather than men.
30 The God of our fathers raised up
Jesus, whom ye slew and hanged on a
tree.
31 Him hath God exalted with his
right hand *to be* a Prince and a [o]Saviour,
for to give [p]repentance to Israel, and
[q]forgiveness of [r]sins.
32 And we are his witnesses of these
things; and *so is* also the [s]Holy Ghost,
whom God hath given to them that obey
him.
33 When they heard *that*, they were

A.D. 33.

a Num. 16:11; 1 Sam, 8:7; 2 Ki. 5:25,27; Lk. 10:16; 1 Thes. 4:8.
b Num. 16:26, 33; 2 Ki. 1:10, 14; 2:24; 2 Cor. 13:2, 10.
c Gr. *younger.*
d *Temptation.* Acts 15:10. (Gen. 3:1; Jas. 1:14.)
e Acts 2:43; 4:29, 30.
f *Miracles* (N.T.). vs. 12:15, 16, 19, 20; Acts 6:8. (Mt. 8:2, 3; Acts 28:8, 9.)
g Or, *in every street.*
h Mk. 16:17.
i Gr, *heresy.*
j Lit. *jealousy.* Cf. Mt. 27:18.
k *an angel.*
l Heb. 1:4, *note.*
m *Life (eternal).* Acts 11:18. (Mt. 7:14; Rev. 22:19.)
n *teaching.*
o Rom. 1:16, *note.*
p *Repentance.* Acts. 8:22. (Mt. 3:2; Acts 17:30.)
q See Mt. 26:28, *note.*
r *Sin.* Rom. 3:23, *note.*
s *Holy Spirit.* v. 3, 9, 32 ; Acts 6:3, 5, 10. (Mt. 1:18; Acts 2:4.)

A.D. 33.

[a]cut *to the heart*, and took counsel to slay them.

The warning of Gamaliel.

34 Then stood there up one in the council, a Pharisee, named Gamaliel, a doctor of the law, had in reputation among all the people, and commanded to put the apostles forth a little space;

35 And said unto them, Ye men of Israel, take heed to yourselves what ye intend to do as touching these men.

36 For before these days rose up Theudas, boasting himself to be somebody; to whom a number of men, about four hundred, joined themselves: who was slain; and all, as many as [b]obeyed him, were scattered, and brought to nought.

37 After this man rose up Judas of Galilee [c]in the days of the taxing, and drew away much people after him: [d]he also perished; and all, *even* as many as obeyed him, were dispersed.

38 And now I say unto you, Refrain from these men, and let them alone: [e]for if this counsel or this work be of men, it will come to nought:

39 But [f]if it be of God, ye cannot overthrow it; lest haply ye be found even to fight against God.

The apostles beaten.

40 And to him they agreed: and when they had called the apostles, and [g]beaten *them*, they commanded that they should not speak in the name of Jesus, and let them go.

41 And they departed from the presence of the council, rejoicing that they were counted worthy to suffer [h]shame for his name.

42 And daily in the temple, and in every house, they ceased not to teach and preach Jesus Christ.

CHAPTER 6.

The first deacons.

And in those days, when the number of the disciples was multiplied, there arose a murmuring of the [i]Grecians against the Hebrews, because their widows were neglected in the daily ministration.

2 Then the twelve called the multitude of the disciples *unto them*, and said, It is not reason that we should leave the word of God, and serve tables.

3 Wherefore, brethren, look ye out among you seven men of honest report, full of the Holy Ghost and wisdom, whom we may appoint over this business.

4 But we will give ourselves continually to prayer, and to the ministry of the word.

5 And the saying pleased the whole multitude: and they [j]chose Stephen, a man full of faith and of the Holy Ghost, and [k]Philip, and Prochorus, and Nicanor, and Timon, and Parmenas, and Nicolas a proselyte of Antioch:

6 Whom they set before the apostles: and when they had prayed, they laid *their* hands on them.

7 And the word of God increased; and the number of the disciples multiplied in Jerusalem greatly; and a great company of the priests were obedient to the faith.

The third persecution:
Stephen brought before the council.

8 And Stephen, full of faith and power, did great wonders and [l]miracles among the people.

9 Then there arose certain of the synagogue, which is called *the synagogue* of the Libertines, and Cyrenians, and Alexandrians, and of them of Cilicia and of Asia, disputing with Stephen.

10 And they were not able to resist the wisdom and the [m]spirit by which he spake.

11 [n]Then they suborned men, which said, We have heard him speak blasphemous words against Moses, and *against* God.

12 And they stirred up the people, and the elders, and the scribes, and came upon *him*, and caught him, and brought *him* to the council,

13 And set up false witnesses, which said, This man ceaseth not to speak blasphemous words against this [o]holy place, and the law:

14 [p]For we have heard him say, that this Jesus of Nazareth shall destroy this place, and shall change the customs which Moses delivered us.

15 And all that sat in the council, looking stedfastly on him, [q]saw his face as it had been the face of an [r]angel.

CHAPTER 7.

Then said the high priest, Are these things so?

Address of Stephen before the council.
Theme: The unbelief of Israel.

2 And he said, [s]Men, brethren, and

a Cf. Acts 2:37. The Gospel when preached in the power of the Spirit convicts or enrages.

b Or, *believed.*

c Lk. 2:1.

d Lk. 13:1, 2.

e Isa. 8:10; Mt. 15:13.

f Isa. 46:9, 10; 1 Cor. 1:25.

g Mt. 10:17.

h Or, *dishonour for the Name.*

i *Hellenists*, i.e. Grecian Jews.

j It is beautiful to see that these were all Hellenists, as the Grecian names show.

k Acts 8:5; 21:8.

l *Miracles* (N.T.). Acts 8:6. (Mt. 8:2, 3; Acts 28:8, 9.)

m *Holy Spirit.* vs. 3, 5,10; Acts 7:51, 55. (Mt. 1:18; Acts 2:4.)

n 1 Ki. 21:10, 13; Mt. 26:59, 60.

o *Sanctify, holy (things)* (N.T.). Acts 21:28. (Mt. 4:5; Rev. 22:11.)

p Acts 25:8.

q Ex. 34:29, 30; Acts. 4:13; 2 Cor. 3:18; 1 John 3:2.

r Heb. 1:4, *note.*

s Acts 22:1.

fathers, hearken; The [a]God of glory
appeared unto our father Abraham,
when he was in Mesopotamia, before he
dwelt in [b]Charran,
3 And said unto him, [c]Get thee out of
thy country, and from thy kindred, and
come into the land which I shall shew
thee.
4 Then came he out of the land of the
Chaldæans, and dwelt in [b]Charran: and
from thence, when [d]his father was dead,
[e]he removed him into this land, wherein
ye now dwell.
5 And he gave him [f]none inheritance
in it, no, not *so much as* to set his foot on:
yet he [g]promised that he would give it
to him for a possession, and to his seed
after him, when *as yet* he had no child.
6 And God spake on this wise, That
his [h]seed should sojourn in a strange
land; and that they should bring them
into [i]bondage, and entreat *them* evil four
hundred years.
7 And the nation to whom they shall
be in bondage will I judge, said God:
and after that shall they [j]come forth, and
serve me in this place.
8 And he gave him the [k]covenant of
circumcision: and so *Abraham* begat
Isaac, and circumcised him the eighth
day; and Isaac *begat* Jacob; and Jacob
begat the twelve patriarchs.
9 And the patriarchs, moved with
[l]envy, [m]sold Joseph into Egypt: but
[n]God was with him,
10 And delivered him out of all his
afflictions, and gave him favour and
wisdom in the sight of Pharaoh king of
Egypt; and he made him governor over
Egypt and all his house.
11 [o]Now there came a dearth over all
the land of Egypt and [p]Chanaan, and
great affliction: and our fathers found no
sustenance.
12 But when [q]Jacob heard that there
was corn in Egypt, he sent out our
fathers first.
13 And at the [r]second *time* Joseph was
made known to his brethren; and Joseph's
kindred was made known unto Pharaoh.
14 Then sent Joseph, and called his
father Jacob to *him*, and all his [1]kindred,
threescore and fifteen souls.
15 So Jacob went down into Egypt,
and died, he, and our fathers,

16 And were carried over [s]into Sychem,
and laid in the [t]sepulchre that Abraham
bought for a sum of money of the sons of
Emmor [u]the *father* of Sychem.
17 But when the [v]time of the promise
drew nigh, which God had sworn to
Abraham, the [w]people grew and multiplied in Egypt,
18 Till another king arose, which knew
not Joseph.
19 The same dealt subtilly with our
kindred, and evil entreated our fathers,
so that they cast out their young children, to the end they might not live.
20 In which time Moses was born, and
was [x]exceeding fair, and nourished up
in his father's house three months:
21 And when he was cast out,
[y]Pharaoh's daughter took him up, and
nourished him for her own son.
22 And Moses was learned in all the
wisdom of the Egyptians, and was
[z]mighty in words and in deeds.
23 And [aa]when he was full forty years
old, it came into his heart to visit his
brethren the children of Israel.
24 And seeing one *of them* suffer wrong,
he defended *him*, and avenged him that
was oppressed, and smote the Egyptian:
25 For he supposed his brethren
would have [bb]understood how that God
by his hand would deliver them: but
they understood not.
26 And the [cc]next day he shewed himself unto them as they strove, and would
have set them at one again, saying, Sirs,
ye are brethren; why do ye wrong one to
another?
27 But he that did his neighbour
wrong thrust him away, saying, [dd]Who
made thee a ruler and a judge over us?
28 Wilt thou kill me, as thou diddest
the Egyptian yesterday?
29 [ee]Then fled Moses at this saying,
and was a stranger in the land of
Madian, where he begat two sons.
30 And when forty years were
expired, there appeared to him in the
wilderness of mount Sina an [ff]angel of
the Lord in a [gg]flame of fire in a bush.
31 When Moses saw *it*, he wondered
at the sight: and as he drew near to
behold *it*, the voice of the Lord came
unto him,

A.D. 33.

a *God (of glory).* Psa. 29:3.
b Or, *Haran.* Gen. 11:31, 32.
c Gen. 12:1; Heb. 11:8-10.
d Gen. 12:5.
e Or, *God.*
f Heb. 11:9, 10.
g Gen. 12:7; 15:7; 17:8; 18:10; Heb. 11:11, 12.
h Gen. 15:13, 14; 47:11, 12.
i Ex. 1:8-14; 12:40, 41.
j Ex. 14:29, 30.
k Gen. 17:9-14.
l Or, *jealousy.*
m Gen. 37:11.
n *Jehovah.* Gen. 39:2.
o Gen. 41:54.
p *Canaan.*
q Gen. 42:1.
r Gen. 45:4, 16.
s *unto Shechem.*
t See Gen. 23:4 *note.*
u Or, *in Shechem.*
v vs. 6, 7; Ex. 2:23-25.
w Ex. 1:7-9; Psa. 105:24, 25.
x Or, *fair unto God.*
y Ex. 2:5-10.
z Lk. 24:19.
aa Ex. 2:11-15.
bb Lk. 24:49; *contra,* John 2:4.
cc Ex. 2:13.
dd Ex. 2:14; Lk. 12:14.
ee Ex. 2:15; Heb. 11:27.
ff Heb. 1:4, *note.*
gg Ex. 3:2.

[1]**(7:14)** Cf. Gen. 46:26, *note.* There is no real contradiction. The "house of Jacob" numbered seventy, but the "kindred" would include the wives of Jacob's sons.

32 *Saying,* I *am* the [a]God of thy fathers, the God of Abraham, and the God of Isaac, and the God of Jacob. Then Moses trembled, and durst not behold.

33 Then said the Lord to him, [b]Put off thy shoes from thy feet: for the place where thou standest is holy ground.

34 [c]I have seen, I have seen the affliction of my people which is in Egypt, and I have heard their groaning, and am come down to deliver them. And now come, [d]I will send thee into Egypt.

35 This Moses whom they refused, saying, Who made thee a ruler and a judge? the same did God send *to be* a ruler and a deliverer by the hand of the [e]angel which appeared to him in the bush.

36 He brought them out, after that he had shewed wonders and signs in the land of Egypt, and in the Red sea, and in the wilderness forty years.

37 This is that Moses, which said unto the children of Israel, [f]A prophet shall the [g]Lord your God raise up unto you of your brethren, like unto me; him shall ye hear.

38 This is he, that was in the [1]church in the wilderness with the [e]angel which spake to him in the mount Sina, and *with* our fathers: who received the [h]lively oracles to give unto us:

39 To whom our fathers [i]would not obey, but thrust *him* from them, and in their hearts turned back again into Egypt,

40 Saying unto Aaron, [j]Make us gods to go before us: for *as for* this Moses, which brought us out of the land of Egypt, we wot not what is become of him.

41 And they made a calf in those days, and offered sacrifice unto the idol, and [k]rejoiced in the works of their own hands.

42 Then God turned, and [l]gave them up to worship the host of heaven; as it is written in the book of the prophets, [m]O ye house of Israel, have ye offered to me slain beasts and sacrifices *by the space of* forty years in the wilderness?

43 Yea, ye took up the tabernacle of Moloch, and the star of your god [n]Remphan, figures which ye made to worship them: and [o]I will carry you away beyond Babylon.

44 Our fathers had the [p]tabernacle of witness in the wilderness, as he had appointed, speaking unto Moses, that he should make it [q]according to the fashion that he had seen.

45 Which also our fathers that came after brought in with [r]Jesus into the possession of the [s]Gentiles, whom God drave out before the face of our fathers, unto the days of David;

46 Who found favour before God, and [t]desired to find a tabernacle for the God of Jacob.

47 [u]But Solomon built him an house.

48 Howbeit the most High dwelleth not in temples made with hands; as saith the prophet,

49 [v]Heaven *is* my throne, and earth *is* my footstool: what house will ye build me? saith the [w]Lord: or what *is* the place of my rest?

50 Hath not my hand [x]made all these things?

51 Ye stiffnecked and uncircumcised in heart and ears, ye do always resist the Holy Ghost: as your fathers *did,* so *do* ye.

52 Which of the [y]prophets have not your fathers persecuted? and they have slain them which shewed before of the coming of the [z]Just One; of whom ye have been now the betrayers and murderers:

53 Who have received the law by the disposition of [e]angels, and have not kept *it.*

The first martyr: first mention of Paul.

54 [aa]When they heard these things, they were cut to the heart, and they gnashed on him with *their* teeth.

55 But he, being full of the [bb]Holy Ghost, looked up stedfastly into heaven, and saw the glory of God, and Jesus standing on the right hand of God,

56 And said, Behold, I see the [cc]heavens opened, and the Son of man standing on the right hand of God.

57 Then they cried out with a loud voice, and stopped their ears, and ran upon him with one accord,

58 And cast *him* out of the city, and stoned *him*: and the witnesses laid down

A.D. 33.

a *God.* Ex. 3:6.
b Ex. 3:4, 5; Josh. 5:15.
c Ex. 2:24, 25; 3:7.
d Psa. 105:26.
e Heb. 1:4, *note.*
f Deut. 18:15, 18, 19.
g *Jehovah.* Deut. 18:15.
h Or, *living.* Rom. 3:1, 2; 9:4, 5.
i Psa. 95:8-11.
j Ex. 32:1.
k Ex. 32:6, 18; Psa. 66:6.
l Jud. 2:11-14; Rom. 1:24, 28.
m Amos 5:25-27.
n Or, *Rephan.*
o 2 Chr. 36:11-21; Jer. 25:9-12.
p Or, *tent of testimony.*
q Ex. 25:40; 26:30; Heb. 8:5.
r i.e. *Joshua.*
s *nations, whom God drave out.*
t 1 Ki. 8:17; 1 Chr. 22:7; Psa. 132:4, 5.
u 2 Sam. 7:1-13; 1 Ki. 8:20.
v Isa. 66:1, 2; cf. 1 Ki. 8:27; Acts 17:24.
w *Jehovah.* Isa. 66:1, 2.
x Psa. 102:25-27.
y Jer. 2:30; Mt. 23:34-36; Lk. 20:9-15.
z *Righteous One.*
aa They had brought false witnesses against Stephen; he bears true witness against them, quoting the testimony of writers they owned to be inspired. He speaks of the persistent rejection of God and His servants by the nation till at last it is brought home to themselves, and arouses the maddened enmity of their hearts. It was the final trial of the nation.
bb *Holy Spirit.* vs. 51, 55; Acts 8:15. (Mt. 1:18; Acts 2:4.)
cc Mt. 3:16; Acts 9:3; Heb. 2:9.

[1]**(7:38)** Israel *in the land* is never called a church. *In the wilderness* Israel was a true church (Gr. *ecclesia* = called-out assembly), but in striking contrast with the N.T. *ecclesia* (Mt. 16:18, *note*).

their clothes at a young man's feet, whose name was Saul.

59 And they stoned Stephen, [a]calling upon [b]*God*, and saying, Lord Jesus, [c]receive my spirit.

60 And he kneeled down, and cried with a loud voice, Lord, lay not this [d]sin to their charge. And when he had said this, [e]he fell asleep.

CHAPTER 8.

The fourth persecution: Saul chief persecutor.

[f]And Saul was consenting unto his death. And at that time there was a great persecution against the church which was at Jerusalem; and they were all [g]scattered abroad throughout the regions of Judæa and Samaria, except the apostles.

2 And devout men carried Stephen *to his burial*, and made great lamentation over him.

3 As for Saul, he made havock of the [h]church, entering into every house, and haling men and women committed *them to* prison.

The first missionaries.

4 Therefore [i]they that were scattered abroad went every where preaching the word.

The ministry of Philip.
(See Acts 6:5; 21:8.)

5 Then [j]Philip went down to the [k]city of Samaria, and preached Christ unto them.

6 And the [l]people with one accord gave heed unto those things which Philip spake, hearing and seeing the [m]miracles which he did.

7 For [n]unclean spirits, crying with loud voice, came out of many that were possessed *with them*: and many taken with palsies, and that were lame, were healed.

8 And there was great joy in that city.

(The case of Simon the sorcerer.)

9 But there was a certain man, called Simon, which beforetime in the same city [o]used sorcery, and bewitched the people of Samaria, giving out that himself was some great one:

10 To whom they all gave heed, from the least to the greatest, saying, This man is the great power of God.

11 And to him they had regard, because that of long time he had bewitched them with sorceries.

12 But when they [p]believed Philip preaching the things concerning the kingdom of God, and the name of Jesus Christ, they were baptized, both men and women.

13 Then Simon himself believed also: and when he was baptized, he continued with Philip, and wondered, beholding the miracles and signs which were done.

14 Now when the [q]apostles which were at Jerusalem heard that Samaria had received the word of God, they sent unto them Peter and John:

15 Who, when they were come down, prayed for them, that they might receive the [r]Holy Ghost:

16 (For as yet [s]he was fallen upon none of them: only they were baptized in the name of the Lord Jesus.)

17 Then [t]laid they *their* hands on them, and they received the Holy Ghost.

18 And when Simon saw that through laying on of the apostles' hands the Holy Ghost was given, he offered them money,

19 Saying, Give me also this power, that on whomsoever I lay hands, he may receive the Holy Ghost.

20 But Peter said unto him, Thy money [u]perish with thee, because thou hast thought that the gift of God may be purchased with money.

21 Thou hast neither part nor lot in this [v]matter: for thy [w]heart is not right in the sight of God.

22 [x]Repent therefore of this thy wickedness, and pray [y]God, if perhaps the thought of thine heart may be forgiven thee.

23 For I perceive that thou [z]art in the gall of bitterness, and *in* the bond of iniquity.

24 Then answered Simon, and said, Pray ye to the Lord for me, [aa]that none of these things which ye have spoken come upon me.

25 And they, when they had testified and preached the word of the Lord, returned to Jerusalem, and preached the [bb]gospel in many [cc]villages of the Samaritans.

Philip and the Ethiopian.

26 And the [dd]angel of the Lord spake unto Philip, saying, Arise, and go toward the south unto the way that goeth down from Jerusalem unto Gaza, which is [ee]desert.

27 And he arose and went: and, behold, a man of [ff]Ethiopia, an eunuch of great

A.D. 34.

a *Bible prayers.* Acts 9:6, 11. (Mt. 6:9; Rev. 22:20.)
b *Omit God.* Lit. *And were stoning Stephen as he was invoking and saying, Lord Jesus, give welcome unto my spirit.*
c Lk. 23:46; 1 Pet. 4:19.
d *Sin.* Rom. 3:23, *note.*
e Lk. 8:52; 2 Tim. 1:10; 1 Thes. 4:13-18.
f Acts 7:58.
g Acts 11:19.
h *Churches (local).* vs. 1-8; Acts 9:31. (Acts 2:41; Phil. 1:1.)
i Mt. 10:23; Acts 11:19.
j Acts 6:5.
k The Jews having rejected Stephen's witness to, and of, them, the Gospel now begins to go out to "all nations." Cf. v. 1; Lk. 24:47.
l *multitude.*
m Gr. *signs. Miracles* (N.T.). Acts 9:18, 36-41. (Mt. 8:2, 3; Acts 28:8, 9.)
n Mk. 16:17.
o Acts 13:6.
p Acts 13:38, 39.
q v. 1; John 4:22.
r *Holy Spirit.* vs. 15, 17, 18, 19, 29, 39; Acts 9:17, 31. (Mt. 1:18; Acts 2:4.)
s Acts 2:38.
t Acts 19:6; Deut. 34:9.
u 2 Ki. 5:16, 26, 27; Heb. 13:5, 6.
v Gr. *word.*
w Mt. 15:8, 19.
x *Repentance.* Acts 11:18. (Mt. 3:2; Acts 17:30.)
y *the Lord.*
z *wilt become.*
aa Ex. 9:28.
bb *Gospel.* Acts 14:7, 21. (Gen. 12:1-3; Rev. 14:6.)
cc Acts. 1:8.
dd Heb. 1:4, *note.*
ee *Contra,* vs. 6-8.
ff Psa. 68:31; Jer. 38:7; Acts 28:28.

authority under Candace queen of the Ethiopians, who had the charge of all her treasure, and had come to [a]Jerusalem for to worship,

28 Was returning, and sitting in his chariot read Esaias the prophet.

29 Then the [b]Spirit said unto Philip, Go near, and join thyself to this chariot.

30 And Philip ran thither to *him*, and heard him read the prophet Esaias, and said, [c]Understandest thou what thou readest?

31 And he said, How can I, except some man should guide me? And he [d]desired Philip that he would come up and sit with him.

32 The place of the scripture which he read was this, [e]He was led as a sheep to the slaughter; and like a lamb dumb before his shearer, so opened he not his mouth:

33 In his humiliation his judgment was taken away: and who shall declare his generation? for his life is taken from the earth.

34 And the eunuch answered Philip, and said, I pray thee, [f]of whom speaketh the prophet this? of himself, or of some other man?

35 Then Philip opened his mouth, and [g]began at the same scripture, and preached unto him Jesus.

36 And as they went on *their* way, they came unto a certain water: and the eunuch said, See, *here is* water; what doth hinder me to be baptized?

37 [h]And Philip said, If thou believest with all thine heart, thou mayest. And he answered and said, I believe that Jesus Christ is the Son of God.

38 And he commanded the chariot to stand still: and they went down both into the water, both Philip and the eunuch; and he [i]baptized him.

39 And when they were come up out of the water, the [j]Spirit of the [k]Lord caught away Philip, that the eunuch saw him no more: and he went on his way [l]rejoicing.

40 But Philip was found at Azotus: and passing through he preached [m]in all the cities, till he came to Cæsarea.

A.D. 34.

a 1 Ki. 8:41, 42; John 12:20.
b Acts 10:19; 13:2; 20:23.
c Lk. 24:45; Rom. 10:14, 15; 2 Cor. 3:15.
d *besought.*
e Isa. 53:7, 8.
f Acts 2:30, 31; 1 Pet. 1:10, 11; Rev. 19:10.
g Lk. 24:27-45; Acts 10:43; 17:2, 3.
h The best authorities omit v. 37.
i Acts 16:23.
j 1 Ki. 18:12; Ezk. 8:3.
k *Jehovah.*
l v. 8.
m Or, *the gospel to all the cities.*
n Acts 8:1, 3; 26:10, 11.
o Acts 22:5.
p *that were of the Way,* i.e. Christ. John 14:6.
q 2 Cor. 4:6; 1 John 1:5.
r Zech. 2:8; John 15:20, 21; Eph. 5:29, 30.
s The Lord identifies Himself with His people.
t Acts 2:33-36; Heb. 2:9.
u *Bible prayers* (N.T.). Eph. 1:17-20. (Mt. 6:9; Rev. 22:20.)
v *the voice.*
w Or, *nothing.*
x Acts 22:12.
y Lk. 15:7; 18:13.

CHAPTER 9.

The conversion of Saul.
(Cf. Acts 22:1-16; 26:9-18.)

And Saul, [n]yet breathing out threatenings and slaughter against the disciples of the Lord, went unto the high priest,

2 And desired of him [o]letters to Damascus to the synagogues, that if he found any [p]of this way, whether they were men or women, he might bring them bound unto Jerusalem.

3 And as he journeyed, he came near Damascus: and suddenly there shined round about him a [q]light from heaven:

4 And he fell to the earth, and heard a voice saying unto him, Saul, Saul, [r]why persecutest thou [s]me?

5 And he said, Who art thou, Lord? And the Lord said, I am [t]Jesus whom thou persecutest: *it is* hard for thee to kick against the pricks.

6 And he trembling and astonished [u]said, Lord, what wilt thou have me to do? And the Lord *said* unto him, Arise, and go into the city, and it shall be told thee what thou must do.

7 And the men which journeyed with him stood speechless, hearing [v]a [1]voice, but seeing no man.

8 And Saul arose from the earth; and when his eyes were opened, he saw no man: but they led him by the hand, and brought *him* into Damascus.

9 And he was three days without sight, and neither did eat nor drink.

10 And there was a certain disciple at Damascus, named [x]Ananias; and to him said the Lord in a vision, Ananias. And he said, Behold, I *am here*, Lord.

11 And the Lord *said* unto him, Arise, and go into the street which is called Straight, and enquire in the house of Judas for *one* called Saul, of Tarsus: for, behold, he [y]prayeth,

12 And hath seen in a vision a man named Ananias coming in, and putting *his* hand on him, that he might receive his sight.

13 Then Ananias answered, Lord

[1] **(9:7)** Cf. Acts 22:9; 26:14. A contradiction has been imagined. The three statements should be taken together. The men heard the "voice" as a sound (Gr. *phone*), but did not hear the "voice" as articulating the *words*, "Saul, Saul," etc.

I have [a]heard by many of this man, how
much evil he hath done to thy saints at
Jerusalem:
14 And here he hath authority from
the chief priests to bind all that call on
thy name.
15 But the Lord said unto him, Go thy
way: [b]for he is a [c]chosen vessel unto me,
to bear my name before the [d]Gentiles,
and [e]kings, and the [f]children of Israel:
16 For [g]I will shew him how great
things he must suffer for my name's sake.

Paul filled with the Spirit.

17 And Ananias went his way, and
entered into the house; and putting his
hands on him said, Brother Saul, the
Lord, *even* Jesus, that appeared unto thee
in the way as thou camest, hath sent me,
that thou mightest receive thy sight, and
be filled with the [h]Holy Ghost.

Paul baptized.

18 And immediately there fell from his
eyes as it had been scales: and he
received [i]sight forthwith, and arose, and
was baptized.
19 And when he had received meat,
he was strengthened. Then was Saul certain days with the disciples which were
at Damascus.

Paul preaches.

20 [j]And straightway he preached
Christ in the synagogues, [1]that he is the
Son of God.
21 But all that heard *him* were amazed,
and said; Is not this he that destroyed
them which called on this name in
Jerusalem, and came hither for that
intent, that he might bring them bound
unto the chief priests?

A.D. 35.

a vs. 1, 2; Gal. 1:23.
b *Inspiration.* Acts 28:25. (Ex. 4:15; Rev. 22:19.)
c Gr. *vessel elected. Election (personal).* Acts 10:41. (Deut. 7:6; 1 Pet. 1:2.)
d Rom. 1:5; 11:13; Eph. 3:7, 8.
e Acts 26:1, 5; 2 Tim. 4:16, 17.
f Acts 21:40; Rom. 1:16; 9:1-5.
g Acts 20:23; 2 Cor. 11:23-28; Gal. 6:17; Phil. 1:29.
h *Holy Spirit* (N.T.). vs. 17, 31; Acts 10:19, 38, 44, 45, 47. (Mt. 1:18; Acts 2:4.)
i *Miracles* (N.T.). vs. 18, 36-41; Acts 13:6-12. (Mt. 8:2, 3; Acts 28:8, 9.)
j Lit. *And straightway, in the synagogues, was he proclaiming Jesus, that he is the Son of God.*
k *the very Christ.*
l Josh. 2:15; 1 Sam. 19:12; 2 Cor. 11:32, 33.
m vs. 13, 14.
n Acts 4:36; 11:22-26.
o vs. 20, 22.
p *Hellenists,* i.e. Grecian Jews.
q *Churches (local).* Acts 11:1-26. (Acts. 2:41; Phil. 1:1.)
r Eph. 4:16.
s Psa. 34:9; Heb. 12:28.
t John 14,16; Phil. 2:1, 2.
u v. 42; Acts 16:5.

22 [2]But Saul increased the more in
strength, and confounded the Jews
which dwelt at Damascus, proving that
this is [k]very Christ.
23 And after that many days were fulfilled, the Jews took counsel to kill him:
24 But their laying await was known
of Saul. And they watched the gates day
and night to kill him.
25 Then the disciples took him by
night, and [l]let *him* down by the wall in a
basket.

Paul visits Jerusalem.

26 And when Saul was [3]come to
Jerusalem, he assayed to join himself to
the disciples: but they were all [m]afraid of
him, and believed not that he was a
disciple.
27 But [n]Barnabas took him, and
brought *him* to the apostles, and
declared unto them how he had seen the
Lord in the way, and that he had spoken
to him, and how he had preached [o]bold-
ly at Damascus in the name of Jesus.
28 And he was with them coming in
and going out at Jerusalem.
29 And he spake boldly in the name of
the Lord Jesus, and disputed against the
[p]Grecians: but they went about to slay
him.

Paul returns to Tarsus.

30 *Which* when the brethren knew,
they brought him down to Cæsarea, and
sent him forth to Tarsus.
31 Then had the [q]churches rest throughout all Judæa and Galilee and Samaria,
and were [r]edified; and walking in the
[s]fear of the Lord, and in the [t]comfort of
the Holy Ghost, were [u]multiplied.

1 (9:20) Cf. Acts 2:36. Peter, while maintaining the deity of Jesus—"God hath made that same Jesus, whom ye have crucified, both Lord and Christ"—gives especial prominence to His Messiahship. Paul, fresh from the vision of the glory, puts the emphasis on His Deity. Peter's charge was that the Jews had crucified the Son of David (Acts 2:25-30); Paul's that they had crucified the Lord of glory (1 Cor. 2:8). In the A.V. the sense is largely lost. The point was, not that the Christ was God, a truth plainly taught by Isaiah (7:14; 9:6, 7), but that *Jesus,* the crucified Nazarene, was the Christ and therefore God the Son.

2 (9:22) It seems probable that verses 22-25 refer to Paul's labours in Damascus after his return from Arabia (Gal. 1:17). The "many days" of verse 23 may represent the "three years" of Gal. 1:18, which intervened between Paul's return to Damascus and his visit to Peter.

3 (9:26) The Acts records four visits of Paul to Jerusalem after his conversion: (1) Acts 9:23-30. This seems identical with the visit of Gal. 1:18, 19. The "apostles" of verse 27 were Peter, and James, the Lord's brother. (2) Acts 11:30. Paul may have been in Jerusalem during the events of Acts 12:1-24. (See v. 25.) (3) Acts 15:1-30; Gal. 2:2-10. (4) Acts 21:17–23:35.

The healing of Æneas.

32 And it came to pass, as Peter passed
throughout all *quarters*, he came down
also to the saints which dwelt at Lydda.
33 And there he found a certain man
named Æneas, which had kept his bed
eight years, and was [a]sick of the palsy.
34 And Peter said unto him, Æneas,
[b]Jesus Christ maketh thee whole: arise,
and make thy bed. And he arose immediately.
35 And all that dwelt at Lydda and
[c]Saron saw him, and [d]turned to the Lord.

Tabitha raised from the dead.

36 Now there was at Joppa a certain
disciple named Tabitha, which by interpretation is called [e]Dorcas: this woman
was [f]full of good works and almsdeeds
which she did.
37 And it came to pass in those days,
that she was sick, and died: whom when
they had washed, they laid *her* in an
upper chamber.
38 And forasmuch as Lydda was nigh
to Joppa, and the disciples had heard
that Peter was there, they sent unto him
two men, desiring *him* that he would not
delay to come to them.
39 Then Peter arose and went with
them. When he was come, they brought
him into the upper chamber: and all the
[g]widows stood by him weeping, and
shewing the coats and garments which
Dorcas made, while she was with them.
40 But Peter put them all forth, and
[h]kneeled down, and prayed; and turning
him to the body said, Tabitha, arise. And
she opened her eyes: and when she saw
Peter, she sat up.
41 And he gave her *his* hand, and lifted her up, and when he had called the
saints and widows, presented her [i]alive.
42 And it [j]was known throughout all
Joppa; [k]and many believed in the Lord.
43 And it came to pass, that he tarried
many days in Joppa with one [l]Simon a
tanner.

CHAPTER 10.

Peter's second use of the keys:
the gospel given to Gentiles.
(Cf. Mt. 16:19; Acts 2:14-41).

Cornelius' vision.

There was a certain man in Cæsarea
called Cornelius, a [m]centurion of the
[n]band called the Italian *band*,
2 *A* devout *man*, and one that [o]feared
God with all his house, which gave
much alms to the people, and prayed to
God alway.
3 He saw in a [p]vision evidently about
the ninth hour of the day an [q]angel of
God coming in to him, and saying unto
him, Cornelius.
4 And when he looked on him, he was
afraid, and said, What is it, Lord? And
he said unto him, Thy prayers and thine
alms are come up for a [r]memorial before
God.
5 And now [s]send men to Joppa, and
call for *one* Simon, whose surname is
Peter:
6 He lodgeth with one Simon a tanner,
whose house is by the sea side: he shall
tell thee what thou oughtest to do.

Cornelius sends for Peter.

7 And when the [q]angel which spake
unto Cornelius was departed, he called
two of his household servants, and a
devout soldier of them that waited on
him continually;
8 And when he had declared all *these*
things unto them, he sent them to Joppa.

Peter's vision of the great sheet.

9 On the morrow, as they [t]went on
their journey, and drew nigh unto the
city, Peter went up upon the housetop to
pray about the sixth hour:
10 And he became very hungry, and
would have eaten: but while they made
ready, he fell into a trance,
11 And saw [u]heaven opened, and a
certain vessel descending unto him, as it
had been a great sheet knit at the four
corners, and let down to the earth:
12 Wherein were all manner of four-
footed beasts of the earth, and wild
beasts, and creeping things, and fowls of
the air.
13 And there came a voice to him,
Rise, Peter; kill, and eat.
14 But Peter said, Not so, Lord; for I
have never eaten any thing that is [v]com-
mon or unclean.
15 And the voice *spake* unto him again
the second time, [w]What God hath
cleansed, *that* call not thou common.
16 This was done thrice: and the vessel
was received up again into heaven.

A.D. 38.

a Mt. 9:2-8.
b Acts 3:6, 16; 4:10.
c *Sharon.*
d Acts 11:21.
e *i.e. gazelle.*
f 1 Tim. 2:10.
g *Contra,* Acts 6:1.
h Mt. 9:25.
i *Resurrection.* vs. 36-42; Acts 17:3. (Job 19:25; 1 Cor. 15:52.)
j *came to be.*
k John 14:45; 12:11.
l Acts 10:6,28.
m Lk. 7:2-10.
n Or, *cohort.*
o v. 35; Acts 16:14.
p Cf. 10-17; Acts 9:10.
q Heb. 1:4, *note.*
r Mt. 26:13; Heb. 6:9, 10.
s Acts 11:13, 14.
t Acts 8:26-39.
u Acts 7:56; Eph. 3:5, 6.
v Lev. 11:1; Isa. 66:17; Ezk. 4:14.
w v. 28; Mt. 15:11; Rom. 14:14, 17, 20; 1 Cor. 10:25; 1 Tim. 4:4; Tit. 1:15.

Peter and the messengers of Cornelius.

17 Now while Peter [a]doubted in himself what this vision which he had seen
should mean, behold, the men which
were sent from Cornelius had made
enquiry for Simon's house, and stood
before the gate,
18 And called, and asked whether
Simon, which was surnamed Peter, were
lodged there.
19 While Peter thought on the vision,
the Spirit said unto him, Behold, three
men seek thee.
20 Arise therefore, and get thee down,
and go with them, [b]doubting nothing:
for I have sent them.
21 Then Peter went down to the men
which were sent unto him from
Cornelius; and said, Behold, I am he
whom ye seek: [c]what *is* the cause wherefore ye are come?
22 And they said, [d]Cornelius the centurion, a just man, and one that feareth
God, and of [e]good report among all the
nation of the Jews, was warned from God
by an holy angel to send for thee into his
house, and to hear words of thee.

Peter goes to Cæsarea.

23 Then called he them in, and lodged
them. And on the morrow Peter went
away with them, and [f]certain brethren
from Joppa accompanied him.
24 And the morrow after they entered
into Cæsarea. And Cornelius [g]waited for
them, and had called together his kinsmen and near friends.
25 And as Peter was coming in,
Cornelius met him, and [h]fell down at his
feet, and worshipped *him*.
26 But Peter took him up, saying,
[i]Stand up; I myself also am a man.
27 And as he talked with him, he went
in, and found many that were come
together.
28 And he said unto them, Ye know
how that it is an [j]unlawful thing for a
man that is a Jew to keep company, or
come unto one of another nation; but
[k]God hath shewed me that I should not
call any man common or unclean.
29 Therefore came I *unto you* without
gainsaying, as soon as I was sent for: I
ask therefore for [l]what intent ye have
sent for me?
30 And Cornelius said, Four days ago
I was fasting until this hour; and at the
ninth hour I prayed in my house, and,
behold, a man stood before me in
[m]bright clothing,
31 And said, Cornelius, thy [n]prayer is
heard, and [o]thine alms are had in
remembrance in the sight of God.
32 Send therefore to Joppa, and call
hither Simon, whose surname is Peter;
he is lodged in the house of *one* Simon a
tanner by the sea side: who, when he
cometh, shall speak unto thee.
33 Immediately therefore I sent to
thee; and thou hast well done that thou
art come. Now therefore are [p]we all here
[q]present before God, to hear all things
that are commanded thee of [r]God.

Peter's sermon to Gentiles in the house of Cornelius. Theme: Salvation through faith.
(Cf. Acts 2:14-41.)

34 Then Peter opened *his* mouth, and
said, Of a truth I perceive that God is no
[s]respecter of persons:
35 But in [t]every nation he that feareth
him, and worketh [u]righteousness, is
accepted with him.
36 The word which *God* sent unto the
children of Israel, preaching [v]peace by
Jesus Christ: (he is Lord of all:)
37 That word, *I say*, ye know, which
was published throughout all Judæa,
and began from Galilee, after the baptism which John preached;
38 How [w]God anointed Jesus of
Nazareth with the [x]Holy Ghost and with
power: who went about doing good, and
healing all that were oppressed of the
[y]devil; for [z]God was with him.
39 And we are [aa]witnesses of all things
which he did both in the land of the
Jews, and in Jerusalem; whom they
[bb]slew and hanged on a tree:
40 Him God [cc]raised up the third day,
and shewed him openly;
41 Not to all the people, but unto witnesses [dd]chosen before of God, *even* to
us, who did [ee]eat and drink with him
after he rose from the dead.
42 And he commanded us to preach
unto the people, and to testify that it is
he which was ordained of God *to be* the
Judge of quick and dead.
43 To him give all the prophets witness, that through his name whosoever
believeth [ff]in him shall receive remission
of [gg]sins.

A.D. 41.

a *was much perplexed.*
b Acts 16:9, 10.
c v. 29; Lk. 18:41.
d vs. 1, 2.
e Acts 22:12.
f v. 45; Acts 11:12.
g *was waiting.* Mk. 5:19; Lk. 8:40; John 4:29.
h Acts 16:29.
i Acts 14:14, 15; Rev. 19:10; 22:9.
j John 4:9; 18:28; Acts 11:3; Gal. 2:12, 14.
k v. 15; Acts 15:8, 9; Eph. 3:6.
l v. 21.
m Mt. 28:3; Mk. 16:5; Lk. 24:4.
n v. 4; Dan. 10:12.
o Heb. 6:10.
p Lk. 8:18; Gal. 4:14; 1 Thes. 2:13.
q *in the sight of.*
r *the Lord.*
s Deut. 10:17; Rom. 2:11; 3:29, 30; 10:12, 13.
t Psa. 15:1, 2; Acts 15:7-11; Rom. 2:27-29.
u Rom. 10:10, *note.*
v Lk. 2:14; Eph. 2:17; Col. 1:20.
w *Jehovah.* Isa. 61:1.
x *Holy Spirit* (N.T.). vs. 19, 38, 44, 45, 47; Acts 11:12, 15, 16, 24, 28. (Mt. 1:18; Acts 2:4.)
y *Satan.* Acts 13:10. (Gen. 3:1; Rev. 20:10.)
z Isa. 61:1-3; John 3:2; 8:29.
aa Acts 1:22.
bb Acts 2:23; 13:27, 28.
cc Acts 2:24.
dd *Election (personal).* Acts 15:7. (Deut. 7:6; 1 Pet. 1:2.)
ee Lk. 24:30, 41-43; John 21:9-13; 1 John 1:1.
ff *on him.*
gg *Sin.* Rom. 3:23, *note.*

The Holy Spirit given to Gentile believers.

44 [1]While Peter yet spake these words, the [a]Holy Ghost fell on all them which heard the word.

45 And they of the circumcision which believed were astonished, as many as came with Peter, because that on the Gentiles also was poured out the gift of the Holy Ghost.

46 For they heard them speak with [b]tongues, and magnify God. Then answered Peter,

47 Can any man forbid water, that these should not be baptized, which have received the Holy Ghost as well as we?

48 And he commanded them to be baptized in the name of [c]the Lord. Then prayed they him to tarry certain days.

CHAPTER 11.

Peter vindicates his ministry to Gentiles.

And the apostles and brethren that were in Judæa heard that the Gentiles had also received the word of God.

2 And when Peter was come up to Jerusalem, they that were of the circumcision contended with him,

3 Saying, Thou wentest in to men uncircumcised, and didst eat with them.

4 But Peter rehearsed *the matter* from the beginning, and expounded *it* [d]by order unto them, saying,

5 I was in the city of [e]Joppa praying: and in a trance I saw a vision, A certain vessel descend, as it had been a great sheet, let down from heaven by four corners; and it came even to me:

6 Upon the which when I had fastened mine eyes, I considered, and saw fourfooted beasts of the earth, and wild beasts, and creeping things, and fowls of the [f]air.

7 And I heard a voice saying unto me, Arise, Peter; slay and eat.

8 But I said, Not so, Lord: for nothing common or unclean hath at any time entered into my mouth.

9 But the voice answered me again from heaven, What God hath cleansed, *that* call not thou common.

10 And this was done three times: and all were drawn up again into heaven.

11 And, behold, immediately there were three men already come unto the house where I was, sent from Cæsarea unto me.

12 And the [g]Spirit bade me go with them, [h]nothing doubting. Moreover these six brethren accompanied me, and we entered into the man's house:

13 And he shewed us how he had seen an [i]angel in his house, which stood and said unto him, Send men to Joppa, and call for Simon, whose surname is Peter;

14 Who shall tell thee words, whereby thou and all thy house shall be [j]saved.

15 And as I began to speak, the Holy Ghost fell on them, [k]as on us at the beginning.

16 Then [l]remembered I the word of the Lord, how that he [m]said, John indeed baptized with water; but ye shall be baptized with the Holy Ghost.

17 [n]Forasmuch then as God gave them the like gift as *he did* unto us, who believed on the Lord Jesus Christ; what was I, that I could withstand God?

18 When they heard these things, they held their peace, and glorified God, saying, Then hath God also to the Gentiles granted [o]repentance unto [p]life.

The church at Antioch: the new name.

19 Now they which were scattered abroad upon the [q]persecution that arose about Stephen travelled as far as [r]Phenice, and Cyprus, and Antioch, preaching the word to none but unto the Jews only.

20 And some of them were men of Cyprus and Cyrene, which, when they were come to Antioch, spake unto the [s]Grecians, preaching the Lord Jesus.

21 And the hand of the Lord was with them: and a great number believed, and turned unto the Lord.

22 Then tidings of these things came unto the ears of the church which was in Jerusalem: and they sent forth Barnabas, that he should go as far as Antioch.

A.D. 41.

a Acts 15:8; 26:18; Rom. 10:11; Gal. 3:22.
b Psa. 68:18.
c *Jesus Christ.*
d *in.*
e Acts 10:9-48.
f *heaven.*
g John 16:13.
h *making no distinction.*
i Heb. 1:4, *note.*
j Rom. 1:16, *note.*
k *even as on us.* Cf. Acts 2:1-4; 15:7-9.
l John 14:26.
m *used to be saying.*
n Or, *if therefore the equal free gift God gave to them having believed, even as to us.*
o *Repentance.* Acts 13:24. (Mt. 3:2; Acts 17:30.)
p *Life (eternal).* Acts 13:46-48. (Mt. 7:14; Rev. 22:19.)
q Lit. *tribulation.*
r *Phoenicia.*
s *Hellenists,* i.e. Grecian Jews.

[1] **(10:44)** Verse 44 is one of the pivotal points of Scripture. Heretofore the Gospel has been offered to Jews only, and the Holy Spirit bestowed upon believing Jews through apostolic mediation. But now the normal order for this age is reached: the Holy Spirit is given without delay, mediation, or other condition than simple faith in Jesus Christ. Cf. Acts 2:4, *note;* 1 Cor. 6:19.

A.D. 42.

23 Who, when he came, and had seen the grace of God, was glad, and exhorted them all, that with purpose of heart they would cleave unto the Lord.

24 For he was a good man, and full of the [a]Holy Ghost and of faith: and much people was added unto the Lord.

25 Then departed Barnabas to Tarsus, for to seek Saul:

26 And when he had found him, he brought him unto Antioch. And it came to pass, that a whole year they assembled themselves with the [b]church, and taught much people. And the disciples were called Christians first in Antioch.

The church at Antioch sends relief to Jerusalem.

27 And in these days came prophets from Jerusalem unto Antioch.

28 And there stood up one of them named Agabus, and signified by the Spirit that there should be great dearth throughout all the [c]world: which came to pass in the days of Claudius Cæsar.

29 Then the disciples, every man according to his ability, determined to send relief unto the brethren which dwelt in Judæa:

30 Which also they did, and sent it to the [d]elders by the hands of Barnabas and Saul.

CHAPTER 12.

The fifth persecution: arrest of Peter.

NOW about that time [e]Herod the king stretched forth *his* hands to vex certain of the church.

2 And he killed James the brother of John with the sword.

3 And because he saw it pleased the Jews, he proceeded further to take [f]Peter also. (Then were the days of unleavened bread.)

4 And when he had apprehended him, he put *him* in prison, and delivered *him* to four quaternions of soldiers to keep him; intending after [g]Easter to bring him forth to the people.

Prayer for Peter's deliverance: an angel sent.

5 Peter therefore was kept in prison: but [h]prayer was made without ceasing of the church unto God for him.

6 And when Herod would have brought him forth, the same night Peter was sleeping between two soldiers, bound with two chains: and the keepers before the door kept the prison.

7 And, behold, [i]the angel of the Lord came upon *him*, and a light shined in the prison: and he smote Peter on the side, and [j]raised him up, saying, Arise up quickly. And his chains fell off from *his* hands.

8 And the [k]angel said unto him, Gird thyself, and bind on thy sandals. And so he did. And he saith unto him, Cast thy garment about thee, and follow me.

9 And he went out, and followed him; and wist not that it was true which was done by the [k]angel; but thought he saw a vision.

10 When they were past the first and the second ward, they came unto the iron gate that leadeth unto the city; which opened to them of his own accord: and they went out, and passed on through one street; and forthwith the [k]angel departed from him.

11 And when Peter was come to himself, he said, Now I know of a surety, that the Lord hath sent [l]his [k]angel, and hath delivered me out of the hand of Herod, and *from* all the expectation of the people of the Jews.

12 And when he had considered *the thing*, he came to the house of Mary the mother of John, whose surname was Mark; [m]where many were gathered together praying.

13 And as Peter knocked at the door of the gate, a damsel came to [n]hearken, named Rhoda.

14 And when she knew Peter's voice, she opened not the gate for gladness, but ran in, and told how Peter stood before the gate.

15 And they said unto her, Thou art mad. But she constantly affirmed that it was even so. Then said they, It is his [o]angel.

16 But Peter continued knocking: and when they had opened *the door*, and saw him, they were astonished.

17 But he, beckoning unto them with the hand to hold their peace, [p]declared unto them how the Lord had brought him out of the prison. And he said, Go shew these things unto James, and to the brethren. And he departed, and went into another place.

18 Now as soon as it was day, there was no small stir among the soldiers, what was become of Peter.

19 And when Herod had sought

a *Holy Spirit.* vs. 12, 15, 16, 24, 28; Acts 13:2, 4, 9, 52. (Mt. 1:18; Acts 2:4.)

b *Churches (local).* vs. 12, 15, 16, 24, 26; Acts 13:1-3. (Acts 2:41; Phil. 1:1.)

c *oikoumene* = inhabited earth (Lk. 2:1).

d *Elders.* Acts 14:23. (Acts 11:30; Tit. 1:5-9.)

e Herod Agrippa I, grandson of Herod the Great (Mt. 2:1, *note*), a strict observer of the law, and popular with the Jews (see v. 21). Herod Agrippa II, Paul's Agrippa, was his son.

f John 21:18.

g *the passover.*

h Or, *instant and earnest prayer was made.* 2 Cor. 1:11; Eph. 6:18.

i *an angel,* etc.

j *awakened him.*

k Heb. 1:4, *note.*

l 2 Chr. 16:9; Psa. 34:7; Dan. 3:28; 6:22; Heb. 1:14.

m v. 5; Isa. 65:24; Dan. 9:21.

n *answer.*

o Mt. 18:10.

p Psa. 66:16.

for him, and found him not, he examined the keepers, and commanded that *they* should be [a]put to death. And he went down from Judæa to Cæsarea, and *there* abode.

Death of Herod.

20 And Herod was highly displeased with them of Tyre and Sidon: but they came with one accord to him, and, having made Blastus the [b]king's chamberlain their friend, desired peace; because their country was nourished by the king's *country*.

21 And upon a set day Herod, arrayed in royal apparel, sat upon his throne, and made an oration unto them.

22 And the people gave a shout, *saying, It is* the voice of a god, and not of a man.

23 And [c]immediately [d]the angel of the Lord smote him, because he gave not God the glory: and he was eaten of worms, and gave up the ghost.

24 But the word of God grew and multiplied.

25 And Barnabas and Saul returned [e]from Jerusalem, when they had fulfilled *their* ministry, and took with them John, whose surname was Mark.

CHAPTER 13.

Paul and Barnabas called by the Holy Spirit.

Now there were in the [f]church that was at Antioch certain prophets and teachers; as Barnabas, and Simeon that was called Niger, and Lucius of Cyrene, and Manaen, [g]which had been brought up with [h]Herod the tetrarch, and Saul.

2 As they ministered to the Lord, and fasted, the [i]Holy Ghost said, Separate me Barnabas and Saul for the work whereunto I have called them.

Paul's first missionary journey.

3 And when they had fasted and prayed, and laid *their* hands on them, they sent *them* away.

4 So they, being sent forth by the Holy Ghost, departed unto Seleucia; and from thence they sailed to Cyprus.

5 And when they were at Salamis, they preached the word of God in the synagogues of the Jews: and they had also John [j]to *their* minister.

A.D. 44.

a *led away to death.* Cf. Acts 16:27.

b *that was over the king's bedchamber.*

c Dan. 4:37.

d *an.*

e Cf. Acts 12:1.

f *Churches (local).* vs. 1-3; Acts 14:19-23, 26-28. (Acts 2:41; Phil. 1:1.)

g *the foster-brother of.*

h See Mt. 14:1, *ref.*

i *Holy Spirit.* vs. 2, 4, 9, 52; Acts 15:8, 28. (Mt. 1:18; Acts 2:4.)

j *as their attendant.*

k Gr. *magos.* See Mt. 2:1, "wise men." The same word was used for a vulgar magician, and for a true wise man of the East.

l *proconsul* (Roman).

m *son.*

n *Satan.* Acts 26:18. (Gen. 3:1; Rev. 20:10.).

o *Miracles* (N.T.), vs. 6-12; Acts 14:8-10. (Mt. 8:2, 3; Acts 28:8, 9.)

p *teaching.*

q *Election (corporate).* Rom. 9:11. (Deut. 7:6; 1 Pet. 1:2.)

Opposition from Satan. (Cf. vs. 44, 50.)

6 And when they had gone through the isle unto Paphos, they found a certain [k]sorcerer, a false prophet, a Jew, whose name *was* Bar-jesus:

7 Which was with the [l]deputy of the country, Sergius Paulus, a prudent man; who called for Barnabas and Saul, and desired to hear the word of God.

8 But Elymas the sorcerer (for so is his name by interpretation) withstood them, seeking to turn away the deputy from the faith.

9 Then Saul, (who also *is called* Paul,) filled with the Holy Ghost, set his eyes on him,

10 And said, O full of all subtilty and all mischief, *thou* [m]child of the [n]devil, *thou* enemy of all righteousness, wilt thou not cease to pervert the right ways of the Lord?

11 And now, behold, the hand of the Lord *is* upon thee, and thou shalt be blind, not seeing the sun for a season. And immediately there [o]fell on him a mist and a darkness; and he went about seeking some to lead him by the hand.

12 Then the [l]deputy, when he saw what was done, believed, being astonished at the [p]doctrine of the Lord.

13 Now when Paul and his company loosed from Paphos, they came to Perga in Pamphylia: and John departing from them returned to Jerusalem.

Paul's sermon in the synagogue at Antioch in Pisidia.

Theme: Justification by faith, vs. 38, 39.

14 But when they departed from Perga, they came to Antioch in Pisidia, and went into the synagogue on the sabbath day, and sat down.

15 And after the reading of the law and the prophets the rulers of the synagogue sent unto them, saying, *Ye* men *and* brethren, if ye have any word of exhortation for the people, say on.

16 Then Paul stood up, and beckoning with *his* hand said, Men of Israel, and ye that fear God, give audience.

17 The God of this people of Israel [q]chose our fathers, and exalted the people when they dwelt as strangers in the land of Egypt, and with an high arm brought he them out of it.

18 And about the time of forty

years suffered he their manners in the
wilderness.
19 And when he had destroyed seven
nations in the land of [a]Chanaan, [b]he
divided their land to them by lot.
20 And after that he gave *unto them*
judges about the space of four hundred
and fifty years, until Samuel the prophet.
21 And afterward they desired a king:
and God gave unto them Saul the son of
[c]Cis, a man of the tribe of Benjamin, by
the space of forty years.
22 And when he had removed him, he
raised up unto them David to be their
king; to whom also he gave testimony,
and [d]said, I have found David the *son* of
Jesse, a man after mine own heart, which
shall fulfil all my will.
23 Of this man's seed hath God
according to *his* promise raised unto
Israel a [e]Saviour, Jesus:
24 When John had first preached
before his coming the baptism of [f]repen-
tance to all the people of Israel.
25 And as John fulfilled his course, he
said, Whom think ye that I am? I am not
he. But, behold, there cometh one after
me, whose shoes of *his* feet I am not
worthy to loose.
26 Men *and* brethren, children of the
stock of Abraham, and [g]whosoever
among you feareth God, [h]to you is the
word of this [i]salvation sent.
27 For they that dwell at Jerusalem,
and their rulers, because they knew him
not, nor yet the voices of the prophets
which are read every sabbath day, they
have fulfilled *them* in condemning *him*.
28 And though they found no cause of
death *in him*, yet desired they Pilate that
he should be slain.
29 And when they had fulfilled all that
was written of him, they took *him* down
from the tree, and laid *him* in a sepulchre.
30 But God raised him from the dead:
31 And he was [j]seen many days of
them which came up with him from
Galilee to Jerusalem, who are his witnesses unto the people.
32 And we declare unto you [k]glad tidings, how that the promise which was
made unto the fathers,
33 God hath fulfilled the same unto us
their children, in that he hath raised up
Jesus again; as it is also written in the
second psalm, [l]Thou art my Son, this
day have I begotten thee.

A.D. 45.

a *Canaan.*
b *He gave them their land.*
c *Kish.*
d 1 Sam. 13:14; Psa. 89:20. See *"Kingdom"* (Zech. 12:8; 1 Cor. 15:28); also 2 Sam. 7:8-17, *note.*
e Rom. 1:16, note.
f *Repentance.* Acts 19:4. (Mt. 3:2; Acts 17:30.)
g Isa. 55:1.
h Mt. 10:6.
i Rom. 1:16, *note.*
j Acts 1:3, 11.
k Lk. 2:10, 11.
l Psa. 2:7.
m Isa. 55:3.
n Psa. 16:10. See Lk. 1:31, 32; Acts 2:30, 31.
o Psa. 16:8-11.
p Psa. 16:10.
q *Forgiveness.* vs. 38, 39; Rom. 4:7. (Lev. 4:20; Mt. 26:28.)
r *Sin.* Rom. 3:23, *note.*
s *Faith.* Acts 13:48. (Gen. 3:20; Heb. 11:39.)
t *Assurance.* vs. 38, 39; Acts 17:31. (Isa. 32:17; Jude 1.)
u Rom. 1:16, *note.*
v *Justification.* Rom. 4:2, 5. (Lk. 18:14; Rom. 3:28.)
w *Law (of Moses).* Acts 15:5, 10, 11, 28, 29. (Ex. 19:1; Gal. 3:1-29.)
x See Hab. 1:5.
y *as they went out.*
z Acts 11:23; 14:22; Rom. 5:2; Heb. 6:11, 12; 12:15.
aa Lit. *thrust.*

34 And as concerning that he raised
him up from the dead, *now* no more to
return to corruption, he said on this
wise, [m]I will give you the sure mercies of
David.
35 Wherefore he saith also in [n]another
psalm, Thou shalt not suffer thine [o]Holy
One to see corruption.
36 For David, after he had served his
own generation by the will of God, fell
on sleep, and was laid unto his fathers,
and saw corruption:
37 But he, whom God [p]raised again,
saw no corruption.
38 Be it known unto you therefore,
men *and* brethren, that through this man
is preached unto you the [q]forgiveness of
[r]sins:
39 And by him all that [s]believe are
[t]justified from [u]all things, from which ye
could not be [v]justified by [w]the law of
Moses.
40 Beware therefore, lest that come
upon you, which is spoken of in the
prophets;
41 Behold, ye despisers, and wonder,
and perish: for I [x]work a work in your
days, a work which ye shall in no wise
believe, though a man declare it unto
you.
42 And [y]when the Jews were gone out
of the synagogue, the Gentiles besought
that these words might be preached to
them the next sabbath.
43 Now when the congregation was
broken up, many of the Jews and religious proselytes followed Paul and
Barnabas: who, speaking to them, persuaded them to [z]continue in the grace of
God.

Opposition from the Jews. (Cf. vs. 6, 50.)

44 And the next sabbath day came
almost the whole city together to hear
the word of God.
45 But when the Jews saw the multitudes, they were filled with envy, and
spake against those things which were
spoken by Paul, contradicting and blas-
pheming.

Paul and Barnabas turn to the Gentiles.
(Cf. Acts 18:6; 28:25-29.)

46 Then Paul and Barnabas waxed
bold, and said, It was necessary that the
word of God should first have been spoken to you: but seeing ye [aa]put it from
you, and judge yourselves unworthy of

everlasting life, lo, we turn to the Gentiles.

47 For so hath the Lord commanded us, *saying,* [a]I have set thee to be a light of the Gentiles, that thou shouldest be for salvation unto the ends of the earth.

48 And when the Gentiles heard this, they were glad, and glorified the word of the Lord: and as many as were ordained to [b]eternal life [c]believed.

49 And the word of the Lord was published throughout all the region.

Opposition from devout and honourable women, and chief citizens. (Cf. vs. 6, 45.)

50 But the Jews stirred up the devout and honourable women, and the chief men of the city, and raised persecution against Paul and Barnabas, and expelled them out of their coasts.

51 But they shook off the dust of their feet against them, and came unto Iconium.

52 And the disciples were filled with [d]joy, and with the Holy Ghost.

CHAPTER 14.

The work in Iconium.

And it came to pass in Iconium, that they went both together into the synagogue of the Jews, and so spake, that a great multitude both of the Jews and also of the Greeks believed.

2 But the unbelieving Jews stirred up the Gentiles, and made their minds evil affected against the brethren.

3 Long time therefore abode they speaking boldly in the Lord, which gave testimony unto the word of his grace, and granted signs and wonders to be done by their hands.

4 But the multitude of the city was divided: and part held with the Jews, and part with the apostles.

5 And when there was an assault made both of the Gentiles, and also of the Jews with their rulers, to use *them* despitefully, and to stone them,

The work in Derbe and Lystra.

6 They were ware of *it,* and fled unto [e]Lystra and Derbe, cities of Lycaonia, and unto the region that lieth round about:

7 And there they preached the gospel.

The impotent man at Lystra healed.

8 And there sat a certain man at Lystra, impotent in his feet, being a cripple from his mother's womb, who never had walked:

9 The same heard Paul speak: who stedfastly beholding him, and perceiving that he had [f]faith to be healed,

10 Said with a loud voice, Stand upright on thy feet. And he [g]leaped and walked.

11 And when the people saw what Paul had done, they lifted up their voices, saying in the speech of Lycaonia, The gods are come down to us in the likeness of men.

12 And they called Barnabas, [h]Jupiter; and Paul, [i]Mercurius, because he was the chief speaker.

13 Then the priest of Jupiter, which was before their city, brought oxen and garlands unto the gates, and would have done sacrifice with the people.

14 *Which* when the apostles, Barnabas and Paul, heard *of,* they rent their clothes, and [j]ran in among the people, crying out,

15 And saying, Sirs, why do ye these things? [k]We also are men of like passions with you, and preach unto you that ye should turn from these [l]vanities unto the living God, which made heaven, and earth, and the sea, and all things that are therein:

16 Who in times past suffered all nations to walk in their own ways.

17 Nevertheless he left not himself without witness, in that he did good, and gave us rain from heaven, and fruitful seasons, filling our hearts with food and gladness.

18 And with these sayings scarce restrained they the people, that they had not done sacrifice unto them.

Paul stoned at Lystra.

19 And there came thither *certain* Jews from Antioch and Iconium, who persuaded the people, and, having stoned Paul, [m]drew *him* out of the city, supposing he had been dead.

Further ministry of the first missionary journey.

20 Howbeit, as the disciples stood round about him, he rose up, and came into the city: and the next day he departed with Barnabas to Derbe.

A.D. 45.

a vs. 47, 48; Isa. 42:6, 7; 1 Pet. 1:6-9.

b *Life (eternal).* vs. 46-48; Rom. 2:7. (Mt. 7:14; Rev. 22:19.)

c *Faith.* Acts 14:9. (Gen. 3:20; Heb. 11:39.)

d Mt. 5:12; 1 Thes. 1:6.

e Mt. 10:23.

f *Faith.* Acts 16:31. (Gen. 3:20; Heb. 11:39.)

g *Miracles* (N.T.). vs. 8-10; Acts 16:16-18, 25, 26. (Mt. 8:2, 3; Acts 28:8, 9.)

h Latin for Gr. *Zeus,* the national god of the Greeks.

i Gr. *Hermes.*

j Lit. *sprang forth among.*

k Acts 10:26;. Jas. 5:17; Rev. 22:9.

l Isa. 44:9, 10; 1 Cor. 8:4.

m Lit. *dragged.*

A.D. 46.

21 And when they had preached the
[a]gospel to that city, and had [b]taught
many, they returned again to Lystra, and
to Iconium, and Antioch,
22 Confirming the souls of the disciples,
and exhorting them to continue in the
faith, and that we must through [c]much
tribulation enter into the kingdom of God.

Elders appointed in every church: the return to Antioch.

23 And when they had [d]ordained them
[e]elders in every [f]church, and had prayed
with fasting, they commended them to
the Lord, on whom they believed.
24 And after they had passed throughout Pisidia, they came to Pamphylia.
25 And when they had preached the
word in Perga, they went down into
Attalia:
26 And thence sailed to Antioch, from
whence they had been [g]recommended to
the grace of God for the work which
they fulfilled.
27 And when they were come, and
had gathered the [f]church together, they
rehearsed all that God had done with
them, and how he had opened the door
of faith unto the Gentiles.
28 And there they abode long time
with the disciples.

CHAPTER 15.

Council at Jerusalem: the question of circumcision.

The legalizers from Judæa.

And [h]certain men which came down
from Judæa taught the brethren, *and*
said, [i]Except ye be circumcised [j]after the
manner of Moses, ye cannot be saved.

Paul, Barnabas, and others go to Jerusalem.

2 When therefore Paul and Barnabas
had no small dissension and disputation
with them, they determined that Paul
and Barnabas, and certain other of them,
should go up to Jerusalem unto the
apostles and elders about this question.
3 And being brought on their way by
the church, they passed through
[k]Phenice and Samaria, declaring the conversion of the Gentiles: and they caused
great joy unto all the brethren.
4 And when they were come to
Jerusalem, they were received of the
church, and *of* the apostles and elders,
and they declared all things that God
had done with them.

The questions at issue.

5 But there rose up certain of the sect of
the Pharisees which believed, saying, That
it was needful to circumcise them, and to
command *them* to keep [l]the law of Moses.
6 And the apostles and elders came
together for to consider of this matter.

Peter's argument for Christian liberty: why put under law those to whom God has given the Spirit?

7 And when there had been much
[m]disputing, Peter rose up, and said unto
them, Men *and* brethren, ye know how
that a good while ago God made [n]choice
among us, that the Gentiles by [o]my
mouth should hear the word of the
[p]gospel, and believe.
8 And God, which knoweth the hearts,
bare them witness, giving them the Holy
Ghost, even as *he did* unto us;
9 And put no difference between us
and them, purifying their hearts by faith.
10 Now therefore why [q]tempt ye God,
to put a yoke upon the neck of the disciples, which neither our fathers nor we
were able to bear?
11 But we believe that through the
grace of the Lord Jesus Christ we shall
be saved, even as they.

Paul and Barnabas testify.

12 Then all the multitude kept silence,
and gave audience to Barnabas and
Paul, declaring what miracles and wonders God had wrought among the
Gentiles by them.

James declares the result: (1) the outcalling of the Gentiles agrees with the promises to Israel.

13 And after they had held their
peace, James answered, saying, [1]Men
and brethren, hearken unto me:
14 Simeon hath declared how God

a *Gospel.* vs. 7, 21; Acts 15:7. (Gen. 12:1-3; Rev. 14:6.)

b *made many disciples.*

c *many tribulations.* 2 Tim. 3:12.

d Gr. *cheirotonesantes,* to designate by stretching out (or pointing with) the hand.

e *Elders.* Acts 15:2, 4, 6, 22, 23. (Acts 11:30; Tit. 1:5-9.)

f *Churches (local).* vs. 19-23, 26-28; Acts 15:1, 32, 36-41. (Acts 2:41; Phil. 1:1.)

g *committed.*

h Gal. 2:12.

i Col. 2:11, 14.

j Lev. 12:3.

k *Phoenicia.*

l *Law (of Moses).* vs. 5, 10, 11, 28, 29; Rom. 2:12-27. (Ex. 19:1; Gal. 3:1-29.)

m *questioning.*

n *Election (personal).* Acts 22:14. (Deut. 7:6; 1 Pet. 1:2.)

o Mt. 16:19. Peter used the keys first for the Jews on the day of Pentecost; secondly, in the house of Cornelius for the Gentiles. But Paul was distinctively the apostle to the Gentiles. Gal. 2:7, 8.

p *Gospel.* Acts 16:10. (Gen. 12:1-3; Rev. 14:6.)

q *Temptation.* Acts 20:19. (Gen. 3:1; Jas. 1:14.)

[1] **(15:13)** Dispensationally, this is the most important passage in the N.T. It gives the divine purpose for this age, and for the beginning of the next. (1) The taking out from among the Gentiles of a people for His name, the distinctive work of the present, or church-age. The church is the *ecclesia*—

[a]at the first did visit the Gentiles, to take out of them a people for his name.

15 And to this agree the words of the prophets; as it is written,

16 After this I will return, and will build again the tabernacle of [b]David, which is fallen down; and I will build again the ruins thereof, and I will set it up:

17 That the residue of men might seek after the [c]Lord, and all the Gentiles, upon whom my name is called, saith the Lord, [d]who doeth all these things.

18 Known unto God are all his works from the beginning of the [e]world.

(2) *The Gentiles are not under the law.*

19 [1]Wherefore my [f]sentence is, that we trouble not them, which from among the Gentiles are turned to God:

20 But that we write unto them, that they abstain from pollutions of idols, and *from* fornication, and *from* things strangled, and *from* blood.

21 For Moses of old time hath in every city them that preach him, being read in the synagogues every sabbath day.

22 Then pleased it the apostles and elders, with the whole church, to send chosen men of their own company to Antioch with Paul and Barnabas; *namely,* Judas surnamed Barsabas, and Silas, chief men among the brethren:

23 And they wrote *letters* by them after this manner; The apostles and [g]elders and brethren *send* greeting unto the brethren which are of the Gentiles in Antioch and Syria and Cilicia:

A.D. 52.

a Lit. *for the first time,* i.e. in the house of Cornelius. vs. 8-11; Acts 10:34-48; 11:12-18.

b *Kingdom* (N.T.). vs. 14-17; Rev. 3:21. (Lk. 1:31-33; 1 Cor. 15:24.)

c *Jehovah.* vs. 16, 17; Amos 9:11, 12.

d *Israel (prophecies).* vs. 14-17; Rom. 9:1-8. (Gen. 12:2, 3; Rom. 11:26.)

e i.e. *ages.*

f *judgment.*

g *Elders.* vs. 2, 4, 6, 22, 23; Acts 16:4. (Acts 11:30; Tit. 1:5-9.)

h Gal. 5:2, 4.

i Mt. 5:17, 20; Col. 2:14; Heb. 10:1.

j Acts 13:50; 14:19; 1 Cor. 15:30; 2 Cor. 11:23, 26.

k *Holy Spirit* (N.T.). vs. 8, 28; Acts 16:6, 7. (Mt. 1:18; Acts 2:4.)

l *things sacrificed.*

m 1 Cor. 8; 10:19-22.

n Gen. 9:4; Lev. 22:8.

o 1 Cor. 5:1, 13; 7:2; 1 Thes. 4:3-8.

p *It shall be well with you.*

q Acts 11:23.

r 1 Cor. 14:3 defines the N.T. gift of prophecy.

24 Forasmuch as we have heard, that certain which went out from us have troubled you with words, [h]subverting your souls, saying, *Ye must* be circumcised, and keep the law: [i]to whom we gave no *such* commandment:

25 It seemed good unto us, being assembled with one accord, to send chosen men unto you with our beloved Barnabas and Paul,

26 [j]Men that have hazarded their lives for the name of our Lord Jesus Christ.

27 We have sent therefore Judas and Silas, who shall also tell *you* the same things by mouth.

But Gentile believers must not give offence to godly Jews.

28 For it seemed good to the [k]Holy Ghost, and to us, to lay upon you no greater burden than these necessary things;

29 That ye abstain from [l]meats offered to [m]idols, and from blood, and from [n]things strangled, and from [o]fornication: from which if ye keep yourselves, [p]ye shall do well. Fare ye well.

30 So when they were dismissed, they came to Antioch: and when they had gathered the multitude together, they delivered the epistle:

31 *Which* when they had read, [q]they rejoiced for the consolation.

32 And Judas and Silas, being [r]prophets also themselves, exhorted the brethren with many words, and confirmed *them.*

33 And after they had tarried *there* a space, they were let go in peace from the brethren unto the apostles.

the "called-out assembly." Precisely this has been in progress since Pentecost. The Gospel has never anywhere converted all, but everywhere has called out *some.* (2) "After this [viz. the outcalling] I will return." James quotes from Amos 9:11, 12. The verses which follow in Amos describe the final regathering of Israel, which the other prophets invariably connect with the fulfilment of the Davidic Covenant (e.g. Isa. 11:1, 10-12; Jer. 23:5-8). (3) "And will build again the tabernacle of David," i.e. re-establish the Davidic rule over Israel (2 Sam. 7, 8-17; Lk. 1:31-33). (4) "That the residue of men [Israelites] may seek after the Lord" (cf. Zech. 12:7, 8; 13:1, 2). (5) "And all the Gentiles," etc. (cf. Mic. 4:2; Zech. 8:21, 22). This is also the order of Rom. 11:24-27.

[1]**(15:19)** The scope of the decision goes far beyond the mere question of circumcision. The whole question of the relation of the law to Gentile believers had been put in issue (v. 5), and their exemption is declared in the decision (vs. 19, 24). The decision might be otherwise stated in the terms of Rom. 6:14: "Ye are not under the law, but under grace." Gentile believers were to show grace by abstaining from the practices offensive to godly Jews (vs. 20, 21, 28, 29; cf. Rom. 14:12-17; 1 Cor. 8:1-13).

34 Notwithstanding it pleased Silas to
abide there still.
35 [a]Paul also and Barnabas continued
in Antioch, teaching and preaching the
word of the Lord, with many others also.

Paul's second missionary journey: Silas chosen.

36 And some days after [b]Paul said
unto Barnabas, Let us go again and visit
our brethren in every city where we
have preached the word of the Lord, *and*
see how they do.
37 And Barnabas [c]determined to take
with them [d]John, whose surname was
Mark.
38 But Paul thought not good to take
him with them, who [e]departed from
them from Pamphylia, and went not
with them to the work.
39 And the contention was so sharp
between them, that they departed asunder one from the other: and so [f]Barnabas
took Mark, and sailed unto [g]Cyprus;
40 And Paul chose Silas, and departed,
[h]being recommended by the brethren
unto the grace of God.
41 And he went through Syria and
Cilicia, [i]confirming the churches.

CHAPTER 16.

Paul finds Timothy.

Then came he to [j]Derbe and Lystra:
and, behold, a certain disciple was
there, named Timotheus, the son of a
certain [k]woman, which was a Jewess,
and believed; but his father *was* a Greek:
2 Which was [l]well reported of by the
brethren that were at Lystra and Iconium.
3 Him would Paul have to go forth
with him; and took and [m]circumcised
him because of the Jews which were in
those quarters: for they knew all that his
father was a Greek.
4 And as they went through the cities,
they delivered them the decrees for to
keep, that were ordained of the apostles
and [n]elders which were at Jerusalem.
5 And so were the churches [o]estab-
lished in the faith, and increased in
number daily.

The Spirit guides: the Macedonian vision.

6 Now when they had gone throughout Phrygia and the region of Galatia,
and were forbidden of the [p]Holy Ghost
to preach the word in Asia,
7 After they were come to Mysia, they
assayed to go into Bithynia: but the
Spirit [q]suffered them not.
8 And they passing by Mysia came
down to Troas.
9 And a vision appeared to Paul in the
night; There stood a man of Macedonia,
and [r]prayed him, saying, Come over
into Macedonia, and help us.
10 And after he had seen the vision,
immediately [1]we endeavoured to go
[s]into Macedonia, assuredly gathering
that the Lord had called us for to preach
the [t]gospel unto them.
11 Therefore loosing from Troas, we
came with a straight course to Samothracia, and the next *day* to Neapolis;

Paul and Silas at Philippi.

12 And from thence to [u]Philippi,
which is the chief city of that part of
Macedonia, *and* a [v]colony: and we were
in that city abiding certain days.
13 And on the sabbath we went out of
the city by a river side, where prayer
[w]was wont to be made; and we sat
down, and spake unto the women which
resorted *thither.*

The first convert in Europe.

14 And a certain woman named Lydia,
a seller of purple, of the city of Thyatira,
which worshipped God, heard *us:*
whose [x]heart the Lord opened, that she
attended unto the things which were
spoken [y]of Paul.
15 And when she was baptized, and
her household, she besought *us,* saying,
If ye have judged me to be [z]faithful to
the Lord, come into my house, and abide
there. And [aa]she constrained us.

A demon cast out: Paul and Silas beaten.

16 And it came to pass, as we went to
prayer, a certain damsel possessed with
a [bb]spirit of divination met us, which
brought her masters [cc]much gain by
soothsaying:
17 The same followed Paul and us,

A.D. 52.

a Acts 11:26.
b Acts 13:2.
c *was minded.*
d Acts 12:12, 25; 13:5; Col. 4:10; 2 Tim. 4:11; Phm. 24.
e *withdrew.*
f And is heard of no more in the Bible story.
g Acts 4:36; 13:4.
h Cf. Acts 13:3 with 14:26.
i *Churches (local).* vs. 1-32, 36-41; Acts 18:22. (Acts 2:41; Phil. 1:1.)
j Acts 14:6.
k 1 Cor. 7:14; Eph. 6:4; 2 Tim. 1:5; 3:15.
l 1 Tim. 3:7; 3 John 12.
m 1 Cor. 9:19, 20; Gal. 2:3; 5:6; 6:15.
n *Elders.* Acts 20:17. (Acts 11:30; Tit. 1:5-9.)
o *strengthened.*
p *Holy Spirit* (N.T.). vs. 6, 7; Acts 18:25. (Mt. 1:18; Acts. 2:4.)
q R.V. adds *of Jesus,* as in the best authorities.
r *beseeching him.* Here the Gospel turns toward Europe.
s 2 Cor. 2:13.
t *Gospel.* Acts 20:24. (Gen. 12:1-3; Rev. 14:6.)
u Phil. 1:1.
v i.e. a Roman colony.
w *might legally,* i.e. a legal meeting-place for Jews where there was no synagogue.
x John 6:44; Acts 11:18; 2 Cor. 4:6.
y *by Paul.*
z 2 Sam. 20:16-22; Phil. 4:3; 2 John 4-11.
aa Gen. 19:3; 33:11; Jud. 19:21; Lk. 24:29; Heb. 13:2.
bb Gr. *a spirit, a Python.*
cc Acts 19:24.

1(16:10) The change here from "they," as in the preceding verses, to "we" indicates that at Troas Luke, the narrator, joined Paul's company.

and cried, saying, These men are the servants of the [a]most high God, which
shew unto us the way of [b]salvation.
18 And this did she many days. But
Paul, being grieved, turned and said to
the spirit, [c]I command thee in the name
of Jesus Christ to come out of her. And
he [d]came out the same hour.
19 And when her masters [e]saw that
the hope of their gains was gone, they
caught Paul and Silas, and [f]drew *them*
into the marketplace unto the rulers,
20 And brought them to the [g]magis-
trates, saying, These men, being Jews,
[h]do exceedingly trouble our city,
21 And teach customs, which are not
lawful for us to receive, neither to
observe, being Romans.
22 And the multitude rose up together
against them: and the magistrates rent
off their clothes, and [i]commanded to
beat *them*.
23 And when they had laid many
stripes upon them, they cast *them* into
[j]prison, charging the jailor to keep them
safely:
24 Who, having received such a
charge, thrust them into the inner prison,
and made their feet fast in the stocks.

Conversion of the Philippian jailor.

25 And at midnight Paul and Silas
[k]prayed, and sang praises unto God: and
the prisoners [l]heard them.
26 And suddenly there was a great
[m]earthquake, so that the foundations of
the prison were shaken: and immediately all the [n]doors were opened, and every
one's bands were loosed.
27 And the keeper of the prison awak-
ing out of his sleep, and seeing the prison
doors open, he drew out his sword, and
would have [o]killed himself, supposing
that the prisoners had been fled.
28 But Paul cried with a loud voice,
saying, Do thyself no harm: for we are
all here.
29 Then he called for a light, and
sprang in, and came trembling, and fell
down before Paul and Silas,

The only condition of salvation.

30 And brought them out, and said,
Sirs, [p]what must I do to be [b]saved?
31 And they said, [q]Believe [r]on the
Lord Jesus Christ, and thou shalt be
[b]saved, and thy [s]house.
32 And they spake unto him the word
of the Lord, and to all that were in his
house.
33 And he took them the same hour of
the night, and washed *their* stripes; and
was baptized, he and all his, straightway.
34 And when he had brought them
into his house, he set meat before them,
and [t]rejoiced, [u]believing in God with all
his house.

Paul refuses to depart privily.

35 And when it was day, the magistrates sent the [v]serjeants, saying, Let
those men go.
36 And the keeper of the prison told
this saying to Paul, The magistrates have
sent to let you go: now therefore depart,
and go in peace.
37 But Paul said unto them, They have
beaten us openly uncondemned, being
[w]Romans, and have cast *us* into prison;
and now do they thrust us out privily?
nay verily; but let them come themselves
and fetch us out.
38 And the serjeants told these words
unto the magistrates: and they feared,
when they heard that they were Romans.
39 And they came and besought them,
and brought *them* out, and [x]desired *them*
to depart out of the city.
40 And they went out of the prison,
and entered into *the house of* Lydia: and
when they had seen the brethren, they
[y]comforted them, and departed.

CHAPTER 17.

Founding of the church at Thessalonica.
(Cf. 1 and 2 Thes.)

Now when they had passed through
Amphipolis and Apollonia, they
came to Thessalonica, where was a synagogue of the Jews:
2 And Paul, [z]as his manner was, went
in unto them, and three sabbath days
reasoned with them out of the scriptures,
3 Opening and alleging, that [aa]Christ
must [bb]needs have suffered, and [cc]risen
again from the dead; and that this [dd]Jesus,
whom I preach unto you, is Christ.
4 And some of them [ee]believed, and
consorted with Paul and Silas; and of the

A.D. 53.

- a Cf. Mt. 7:22, *note*. This marks the "spirit" (v. 18) as being a demon.
- b Rom. 1:16, *note*.
- c Mk. 5:8.
- d *Miracles* (N.T.). vs. 16-18, 25, 26; Acts 19:11, 12. (Mt. 8:2, 3; Acts 28:8, 9.)
- e Mk. 5:16-17; Acts 19:25, 26.
- f Gr. *dragged* probably by the feet. Cf. Acts 14:19.
- g Gr. *praetors*, Roman magistrates.
- h 1 Ki. 18:17; Acts 17:6.
- i 2 Cor. 6:5; 11:23, 25; 1 Thes. 2:2.
- j Acts 8:3.
- k Lit. *were praying and singing hymns*.
- l *were listening*.
- m Acts 4:31; Rev. 6:12-17.
- n Acts 5:19; 12:4-7.
- o Acts 12:19.
- p Acts 2:37; 2 Cor. 7:10.
- q *Faith*. Acts 27:25. (Gen. 3:20; Heb. 11:39.)
- r John 3:16; 6:28, 29; Acts 13:38, 39; Rom. 10:6-11; 1 Pet. 1:21.
- s Isa. 54:13; Acts 2:39; 11:14.
- t Acts 2:46; Rom. 15:13.
- u *having believed God*.
- v Gr. *lictors*.
- w v. 21; Acts 22:25-29; 23:6; 25:11, 12.
- x Lk. 8:37.
- y Acts 14:22; Phil. 2:1, 2.
- z v. 10; Lk. 4:16; Acts 9:20; 13:5, 14; 14:1; 16:13; 19:8.
- aa *the Christ*, i.e. that, according to the Scriptures, the Messiah must die and rise again. That Jesus was the Messiah was the second part of his argument.
- bb Cf. Lk. 24:26, 46.
- cc *Resurrection*. vs. 3, 31; Acts 20:9, 12. (Job 19:25; 1 Cor. 15:52.)
- dd Acts 18:5, 28.
- ee *were persuaded*.

devout Greeks a great multitude, and of
the [a]chief women not a few.

Jewish opposition at Thessalonica.

5 But the Jews which believed not,
moved with envy, took unto them certain [b]lewd fellows [c]of the baser sort, and gathered a company, and set all the city on an uproar, and assaulted the house of [d]Jason, and sought to bring them out to the people.
6 And when they found them not,
they [e]drew Jason and certain brethren unto the rulers of the city, crying, These that have turned the world upside down are come hither also;
7 Whom Jason hath received: and
these all do contrary to the decrees of Cæsar, saying that there is [f]another king, *one* Jesus.
8 And they troubled the people and
the rulers of the city, when they heard these things.
9 And when they had taken security of
Jason, and of the other, they let them go.

Paul and Silas at Berea.

10 And the brethren immediately sent
away Paul and Silas by night unto Berea: who coming *thither* went into the synagogue of the Jews.
11 These were more noble than those
in Thessalonica, in that they received the word with all [g]readiness of mind, and [h]searched the scriptures daily, whether those things were so.
12 [i]Therefore many of them believed;
also of [j]honourable women which were Greeks, and of men, not a few.
13 But when the Jews of Thessalonica
had knowledge that the word of God was preached of Paul at Berea, they came thither also, and stirred up the people.
14 And then immediately the brethren
sent away Paul to go as it were to the sea: but Silas and Timotheus abode there still.

Paul at Athens.

15 And they that conducted Paul
brought him unto Athens: and [k]receiving a commandment unto Silas and Timotheus for to come to him with all speed, they departed.
16 Now while Paul waited for them at
Athens, his spirit was [l]stirred in him, when he saw the city wholly given to idolatry.
17 Therefore [m]disputed he in the synagogue with the Jews, and with the devout persons, and in the market daily with them that met with him.
18 Then certain philosophers of the
[n]Epicureans, and of the [o]Stoicks, encountered him. And some said, What will this babbler say? other some, He seemeth to be a setter forth of strange gods: because he preached unto them [p]Jesus, and the resurrection.
19 And they took him, and brought
him unto [q]Areopagus, saying, May we know what this new doctrine, whereof thou speakest, *is*?
20 For thou bringest certain strange
things to our ears: we would know therefore what these things mean.
21 (For all the Athenians and strangers
which were there spent their time in nothing else, but either to tell, or to hear some new thing.)

The sermon from Mars' hill. Theme: God will judge the world by Jesus Christ.

22 Then Paul stood in the midst of
Mars' hill, and said, *Ye* men of Athens, I perceive that in all things ye are too superstitious.
23 For as I passed by, and beheld
[r]your devotions, I found an altar with this inscription, [s]TO THE UNKNOWN GOD. Whom therefore ye ignorantly worship, him declare I unto you.
24 [t]God that made the [u]world and all
things therein, seeing that he is Lord of heaven and earth, [v]dwelleth not in temples made with hands;
25 Neither is [w]worshipped with men's
hands, as though he needed any thing, seeing he [x]giveth to all life, and breath, and all things;
26 And hath made of one [y]blood all
nations of men for to dwell on all the face of the earth, and hath determined the times before appointed, and the [z]bounds of their habitation;
27 That they should [aa]seek the Lord, if
haply they might feel after him, and find him, though he be [bb]not far from every one of us:
28 For in him we live, and move, and
have our being; as certain also of your own poets have said, [cc]For we are also his offspring.
29 Forasmuch then as we are the

A.D. 53.

a Acts 13:50; Phil. 4:3.
b *vile.*
c *of the rabble.*
d Rom. 16:21.
e *dragged.* Acts 16:19, *refs.*
f Lk. 23:2; John 19:12; 1 Pet. 2:13.
g Acts 16:14.
h Lk. 16:29; John 5:39; Acts 26:22, 23.
i Illustrates John 5:46. Believing the O.T. they believed the Gospel.
j *Greek Women of honourable estate.*
k Acts 18:5.
l *provoked within him as he beheld the city full of idols.*
m *reasoned.*
n Disciples of Epicurus, B.C. 342-271, who abandoned as hopeless the search by reason for pure truth (cf. John 18:38), seeking instead true pleasure through experience.
o Disciples of Zeno, B.C. 280, and Chrysippus, B.C. 240. This philosophy was founded on human self-sufficiency, inculcated stern self-repression, the solidarity of the race, and the unity of Deity. Epicureans and Stoics divided the apostolic world.
p 1 Cor. 2:2; 15:12.
q *Mars' hill.*
r *the objects of your worship.*
s Rom. 1:19-21; 1 Cor. 1:21; 1 Thes. 4:5.
t *The God who made,* etc.
u i.e. *earth.*
v Acts 7:48-50.
w *he served by.* Psa. 50:8.
x *Gen. 2:7; Num. 16:22; Isa. 42:5; Dan. 5:23.*
y "blood" is not in the best manuscripts. R.V. omits.
z Deut. 32:8.
aa *God, if haply,* etc.
bb Psa. 139:7-10; Jer. 23:23, 24; Acts 14:17.
cc Found in the writings of Aratus and Cleanthes.

[1a]offspring of God, we ought not to think that the Godhead is like unto [b]gold, or silver, or stone, graven by art and man's device.

30 And the times of this ignorance God [c]winked at; but now commandeth all men every where to [2d]repent:

31 Because he hath appointed a [e]day, in the which he will [f]judge the [g]world in righteousness by *that* man whom he hath ordained; *whereof* he hath given [h]assurance unto all *men*, in that he hath [i]raised him from the dead.

32 And when they heard of the resurrection of the dead, some [j]mocked: and others said, We will hear thee [k]again of this *matter*.

33 So Paul departed from among them.

34 Howbeit certain men clave unto him, and believed: among the which *was* Dionysius the Areopagite, and a woman named Damaris, and others with them.

CHAPTER 18.

Paul at Corinth.

After these things Paul departed from Athens, and came to Corinth;

2 And found a certain Jew named [l]Aquila, born in Pontus, lately come from Italy, with his wife Priscilla; (because that Claudius had commanded all Jews to depart from Rome:) and came unto them.

3 And because he was of the same craft, he abode with them, and wrought: for by their occupation they were [m]tentmakers.

Founding of the church at Corinth.
(Cf. the Corinthian Epistles.)

4 And he reasoned in the synagogue every sabbath, and [n]persuaded the Jews and the Greeks.

5 And when Silas and Timotheus were come from Macedonia, Paul was [o]pressed in the spirit, and testified to the Jews *that* Jesus *was* Christ.

6 And [p]when they opposed themselves, and blasphemed, he shook *his* raiment, and said unto them, Your blood *be* upon your own heads; I *am* clean: from [q]henceforth I will go unto the Gentiles.

7 And he departed thence, and entered into a certain *man's* house, named [r]Justus, *one* that worshipped God, whose house joined hard to the synagogue.

8 And [s]Crispus, the chief ruler of the synagogue, believed on the Lord with all his house; and many of the Corinthians hearing believed, and were baptized.

9 Then spake the Lord to Paul in the night by a vision, Be not afraid, but speak, and hold not thy peace:

10 For I am with thee, and no man shall set on thee to hurt thee: for I have [t]much people in this city.

11 And he continued *there* a year and six months, teaching the word of God among them.

The careless Gallio.

12 And when Gallio was the [u]deputy of Achaia, the Jews made insurrection with one accord against Paul, and brought him to the judgment seat,

13 Saying, This *fellow* persuadeth men to worship God contrary to the law.

14 And when Paul was now about to open *his* mouth, Gallio said unto the Jews, If it were a matter of wrong or [v]wicked lewdness, O *ye* Jews, reason would that I should bear with you:

15 But if it be a question of [w]words and names, and *of* your law, look ye

A.D. 54.

a Num. 16:22; Lk. 3:38.
b Psa. 115:4-7; Isa. 40:18, 19; Dan. 3:1.
c *overlooked.* Cf. Rom. 3:25.
d *Repentance.* (Mt. 3:2.)
e *Day of judgment.* Heb. 9:27. (Mt. 10:15; Rev. 20:11.)
f *Judgments (the seven).* Rom. 8:1, R.V. (2 Sam. 7:14; Rev. 20:12.)
g *oikoumene* = inhabited earth. (Lk. 2:1.)
h *Assurance.* Rom. 8:29-34. (Isa. 32:17; Jude 1.)
i v. 18; Rom. 1:4; Rev. 1:18.
j 1 Cor. 1:18; 15:12.
k Acts 5:38, 39; 24:25.
l Rom. 16:3; 1 Cor. 16:19; 2 Tim. 4:19.
m Acts 20:34; 1 Cor. 4:12; 1 Thes. 2:9; 2 Thes. 3:8.
n Gr. *sought to persuade.*
o Or, *constrained by the Word.* Cf. 2 Cor. 5:14.
p Cf. Acts 13:46; 28:25-29.
q Acts 13:45-47; 28:24-28; Rom. 11:11-15.
r *Titus Justus.*
s 1 Cor. 1:14.
t Acts 11:24; 13:48; *contra,* 17:34.
u *proconsul.*
v *wicked villany.*
w Acts 23:29; 25:19.

1 (17:29) Gr. *genos* = "race." The reference is to the creation-work of God in which He made man (i.e. mankind, the race in Adam) in His own likeness, Gen. 1:26, 27, thus rebuking the thought that "the Godhead is like unto gold," etc. The word "Father" is not used, nor does the passage affirm anything concerning fatherhood or sonship, which are relationships based upon faith, and the new birth. Cf. John 1:12, 13; Gal. 3:26; 4:1-7; 1 John 5:1.

2 (17:30) Repentance is the trans. of a Gr. word (*metanoia—metanoeo*) meaning, "to have another mind," "to change the mind," and is used in the N.T. to indicate a change of mind in respect of sin, of God, and of self. This change of mind may, especially in the case of Christians who have fallen into sin, be preceded by sorrow (2 Cor. 7:8-11), but sorrow for sin, though it may "work" repentance, is not repentance. The son in Mt. 21:28, 29, illustrates true repentance. Saving faith (Heb. 11:39, *note*) includes and implies that change of mind which is called repentance.

to it; for I will be no judge of such *matters*.

16 And he drave them from the judgment seat.

17 Then all the Greeks took [a]Sosthenes, the chief ruler of the synagogue, and beat *him* before the judgment seat. And Gallio [b]cared for none of those things.

The author of Rom. 6:14; 2 Cor. 3:7-14; and Gal. 3:23-28 takes a Jewish vow.

18 And Paul *after this* tarried *there* yet a good while, and then took his leave of the brethren, and sailed thence into Syria, and with him Priscilla and Aquila; having [c]shorn *his* head in Cenchrea: for he had a vow.

19 And he came to Ephesus, and left them there: but he himself entered into the synagogue, and [d]reasoned with the Jews.

20 When they desired *him* to tarry longer time with them, he consented not;

21 But bade them farewell, saying, I must by all means keep this feast that cometh in [e]Jerusalem: but I will return again unto you, if God will. And he sailed from Ephesus.

22 And when he had landed at Cæsarea, and gone up, and [f]saluted the church, he went down to Antioch.

23 And after he had spent some time *there*, he departed, and went over *all* the country of Galatia and Phrygia in order, [g]strengthening all the disciples.

Apollos at Ephesus.

24 And a certain Jew named Apollos, born at Alexandria, an eloquent man, *and* [h]mighty in the scriptures, came to Ephesus.

25 This man was [i]instructed in the way of the Lord; and being fervent in the [j]spirit, he spake and taught diligently the things of the Lord, knowing [k]only the baptism of John.

26 And he began to speak boldly in the synagogue: whom when Aquila and Priscilla had heard, they took him unto *them*, and expounded unto him the way of God more [l]perfectly.

27 And when he was disposed to pass into Achaia, the brethren [m]wrote, exhorting the disciples to receive him: who, when he was come, helped them much which had believed through grace:

28 For he [n]mightily convinced the Jews, *and that* publickly, shewing by the scriptures [o]that Jesus was [p]Christ.

CHAPTER 19.

Paul at Ephesus: the disciples of John become Christians.

And it came to pass, that, while Apollos was at Corinth, Paul having passed through the upper coasts came to Ephesus: and finding certain disciples,

2 He [q]said unto them, [1]Have ye received the [r]Holy Ghost [s]since ye believed? And they said unto him, We have not so much as heard whether there be any Holy Ghost.

3 And he said unto them, Unto what then were ye baptized? And they said, Unto John's baptism.

4 Then said Paul, John verily baptized with the baptism of [t]repentance, saying unto the people, that they should believe on him which should come after him, that is, on Christ Jesus.

5 When they heard *this*, they were baptized in the [u]name of the Lord Jesus.

6 And when Paul had laid *his* hands upon them, the [r]Holy Ghost came on them; and they spake with tongues, and prophesied.

7 And all the men were about twelve.

Paul in the synagogue at Ephesus; and in the school of Tyrannus.

8 And he went into the synagogue, and spake boldly for the space of three months, disputing and persuading the things concerning the kingdom of God.

9 But when divers were hardened, and believed not, but spake evil of that way before the multitude, he departed from them, and separated the disciples, disputing daily in the school of one Tyrannus.

A.D. 54.

- a 1 Cor. 1:1.
- b *Contra*, John 19:13-16; Acts 24:26, 27.
- c Acts 21:24; Num. 6:18.
- d Acts 17:2, 3; 19:18.
- e Rom. 1:10; 1 Cor. 4:19; Phil. 2:19, 24; Heb. 6:3; Jas. 4:15.
- f *Churches (local).* Acts 20:7, 17-32. (Acts 2:41; Phil. 1:1.)
- g 1 Thes. 3:2, 13.
- h Col. 3:16.
- i *taught by word of mouth*, or, *hearsay*, i.e. not by revelation. Cf. Gal. 1:11, 12. The N.T. Scriptures were not then written.
- j *Holy Spirit.* Acts 19:2, 6. (Mt. 1:18; Acts 2:4.)
- k Acts 19:4.
- l Or, *thoroughly.*
- m *encouraged him and wrote.*
- n *powerfully confuted.*
- o Apollos' ministry seems to have gone no further; Jesus was the long expected Messiah. Of Paul's doctrine of justification through the blood, and sanctification through the Spirit, he seems at that time to have known nothing. See Acts 19:3-6.
- p *the.*
- q *said unto them, Did ye receive the Holy Spirit when ye believed?*
- r *Holy Spirit.* vs. 2, 6; Acts 20:23, 28. (Mt. 1:18; Acts 2:4.)
- s Lit. *received ye the Holy Spirit when Ye believed?*
- t *Repentance*, Acts 20:21 (Mt. 3:2; Acts 17:30.)
- u Acts 8:16.

[1]**(19:2)** Not as in A.V., "since ye believed," but as in R.V. and *marg.*: "Did ye receive the Holy Spirit when ye believed?" Paul was evidently impressed by the absence of spirituality and power in these so-called disciples. Their answer brought out the fact that they were Jewish proselytes, disciples of John the Baptist, looking forward to a coming King, not Christians looking backward to an accomplished redemption. See Rom. 8:9; 1 Cor. 6:19; Eph. 1:13, *marg.*

A.D. 56.

10 And this continued by the space of two years; so that all they which dwelt in Asia heard the word of the Lord Jesus, both Jews and Greeks.

Miracles by Paul.

11 And God wrought special [a]miracles by the hands of Paul:

12 So that from his body were brought unto the sick handkerchiefs or aprons, and the diseases departed from them, and the evil spirits went out of them.

13 Then certain of the vagabond Jews, exorcists, took upon them to call over them which had evil spirits the name of the Lord Jesus, saying, We adjure you by Jesus whom Paul preacheth.

14 And there were seven sons of *one* Sceva, a Jew, *and* chief of the priests, which did so.

15 And the evil spirit answered and said, [b]Jesus I know, and Paul I know; but who are ye?

16 And the man in whom the evil spirit was leaped on them, and [c]overcame them, and [d]prevailed against them, so that they fled out of that house naked and wounded.

17 And this was known to all the Jews and Greeks also dwelling at Ephesus; and [e]fear fell on them all, and the name of the Lord Jesus was magnified.

18 And many that believed came, and [f]confessed, and shewed their deeds.

19 Many of them also which used [g]curious arts brought their books together, and burned them before all *men*: and they counted the price of them, and found *it* fifty thousand *pieces* of silver.

20 So [h]mightily grew the word of God and prevailed.

21 After these things were ended, Paul purposed in the [i]spirit, when he had passed through Macedonia and Achaia, to go to Jerusalem, saying, After I have been there, I must also see [j]Rome.

22 So he sent into Macedonia two of them that ministered unto him, [k]Timotheus and [l]Erastus; but he himself stayed in Asia for a season.

The uproar of the silversmiths at Ephesus.

23 And the same time there arose no small stir [m]about that way.

24 For a certain *man* named Demetrius, a silversmith, which made silver shrines for Diana, brought no small gain unto the craftsmen;

25 Whom he called together with the workmen of like occupation, and said, Sirs, ye know that by this [n]craft we have our wealth.

26 Moreover ye see and hear, that not alone at Ephesus, but almost throughout all Asia, this Paul hath persuaded and turned away much people, saying that they be [o]no gods, which are made with hands:

27 So that not only this our craft is in danger to be set at nought; but also that the temple of the great goddess Diana should be despised, and her magnificence should be destroyed, whom all Asia and the [p]world worshippeth.

28 And when they heard *these sayings*, they were full of wrath, and cried out, saying, Great *is* [q]Diana of the Ephesians.

29 And the whole city was filled with confusion: and having caught [r]Gaius and [s]Aristarchus, men of Macedonia, Paul's companions in travel, they rushed with one accord into the theatre.

30 And when Paul would have entered in unto the people, the disciples suffered him not.

31 And certain of the chief of Asia, which were his friends, sent unto him, desiring *him* that he would not adventure himself into the theatre.

32 Some therefore cried one thing, and some another: for the assembly was confused; and the more part knew not wherefore they were come together.

33 And they drew [t]Alexander out of the multitude, the Jews putting him forward. And Alexander beckoned with the hand, and would have made his defence unto the people.

34 But when they knew that he was a Jew, all with one voice about the space of two hours cried out, Great *is* Diana of the Ephesians.

35 And when the townclerk had appeased the people, he said, *Ye* men of Ephesus, what man is there that knoweth not how that the [u]city of the Ephesians is a worshipper of the great goddess Diana, and of the *image* which fell down from Jupiter?

36 Seeing then that these things cannot be spoken against, ye ought to be quiet, and to do nothing rashly.

37 For ye have brought hither these men, which are [v]neither robbers of

a *Miracles* (N.T.). Acts 28:3-6, 8, 9. (Mt. 8:2, 3; Acts 28:8, 9.)
b Mk. 1:23,24; Acts 16:16-18; Jas. 2:19.
c The sons of Sceva sought to imitate a power to which they were strangers, only to their own confusion. This striking witness from another side caused fear to fall on all.
d Lk. 11:21, 22; *contra,* 1 John 4:4.
e Lk. 1:65; 7:16; Acts 5:5, 11.
f Mt. 3:6; 1 Cor. 14:24, 25.
g *magical.* Cf. Deut. 18:10-14.
h Acts 6:7; 12:24; 1 Cor. 16:8, 9.
i i.e. *in his own mind.* Cf. Acts 20:22, *note.*
j Rom. 1:13; 15:22-29.
k 1 Tim. 1:2.
l Rom. 16:23; 2 Tim. 4:20.
m *concerning the Way,* i.e. Christ. John 14:6.
n Acts 16:16, 19.
o Acts 17:29; Rev. 13:14, 15.
p *oikoumene* = inhabited earth. (Lk. 2:1.)
q Gr. *Artemis.* Not anciently of the Greek pantheon, but an Eastern goddess. Cf. Jud. 2:13, *note.* But "Diana of the Ephesians" was rather a particular image of Artemis, reputed to have fallen from heaven; v. 35.
r Acts 20:4; 3 John 1.
s Acts 20:4; 27:2; Col. 4:10.
t 1 Tim. 1:20: 2 Tim. 4:14.
u Acts 17:21.
v Rom. 2:22; cf. 1 Thes. 1:9 with 1 Cor. 1:23, 24.

churches, nor yet blasphemers of your goddess.

38 Wherefore if Demetrius, and the craftsmen which are with him, have a matter against any man, the law is open, and there are deputies: let them implead one another.

39 But if ye enquire any thing concerning other matters, it shall be determined in a lawful assembly.

40 For we are in danger to be [a]called in question for this day's uproar, there being no cause whereby we may give an account of this concourse.

41 And when he had thus spoken, he dismissed the assembly.

CHAPTER 20.

Paul's last visit to Jerusalem: (1) *he goes into Macedonia and Greece.*

And after the uproar was ceased, Paul called unto *him* the disciples, and embraced *them*, and departed for to go into [b]Macedonia.

2 And when he had gone over those parts, and had given them much exhortation, he came into [c]Greece,

3 And *there* abode three months. And when [d]the Jews [e]laid wait for him, as he was about to sail into Syria, he purposed to return through Macedonia.

4 And there accompanied him into Asia [f]Sopater of Berea; and of the Thessalonians, [g]Aristarchus and Secundus; and [h]Gaius of Derbe, and [i]Timotheus; and of Asia, [j]Tychicus and [k]Trophimus.

5 These going before tarried for us at Troas.

(2) *Paul at Troas.*

6 And [l]we sailed away from Philippi after the [m]days of unleavened bread, and came unto them to Troas in five days; where we abode seven days.

7 And upon [n]the first *day* of the week, when the [o]disciples came together to break bread, Paul preached unto them, ready to depart on the morrow; and continued his speech until midnight.

8 And there were many lights in [p]the upper chamber, where they were gathered together.

9 And there sat in a window a certain young man named Eutychus, being fallen into a deep sleep: and as Paul was long preaching, he sunk down with sleep, and fell down from the third loft, and was taken up dead.

10 And Paul went down, and [q]fell on him, and embracing *him* said, [r]Trouble not yourselves; for his life is in him.

11 When he therefore was come up again, and had broken bread, and eaten, and talked a long while, even till break of day, so he departed.

12 And they brought the young man [s]alive, and were not a little comforted.

(3) *From Troas to Miletus.*

13 And we went before to ship, and sailed unto Assos, there intending to take in Paul: for so had he appointed, minding himself to go afoot.

14 And when he met with us at Assos, we took him in, and came to Mitylene.

15 And we sailed thence, and came the next *day* over against Chios; and the next *day* we arrived at Samos, and tarried at Trogyllium; and the next *day* we came to Miletus.

16 For Paul had determined to sail by Ephesus, [t]because he would not spend the time in Asia: for he hasted, if it were possible for him, to be at Jerusalem the day of [u]Pentecost.

(4) *Paul and the Ephesian elders.*

17 And from Miletus he sent to Ephesus, and called the [v]elders of the church.

18 And when they were come to him, he said unto them, Ye know, from the first day that I came into Asia, after what manner I have been with you at all seasons,

19 Serving the Lord with all humility of mind, and with many tears, and [w]temptations, which befell me by the lying in wait of the Jews:

20 *And* how I [x]kept back nothing that was profitable *unto you*, but have shewed you, and have taught you publickly, and from house to house,

21 Testifying both to the Jews, and also to the Greeks, [y]repentance toward God, and faith toward our Lord Jesus Christ.

22 And now, behold, I go bound

A.D. 59.

a Acts 21:31, 32.
b 1 Cor. 16:5; 1 Tim. 1:3.
c Acts 17:15; 18:1
d Or, *a plot, was formed against him by the Jews.*
e Acts 9:23; 23:12; 25:3; 2 Cor. 11:26.
f Rom. 16:21.
g Acts 19:29.
h Rom. 16:23; 3 John 1.
i Acts 19:22.
j Eph. 6:21; Col. 4:7, 8; 2 Tim. 4:12; Tit. 3:12.
k Acts 21:29; 2 Tim. 4:20.
l From the use of the pronoun, Luke here rejoins the apostle.
m Acts 12:3; 18:18.
n It was the breaking of bread for which the disciples were assembled. The passage indicates the use by the apostolic churches of the first day, not the seventh. Cf. 1 Cor. 16:2.
o Mt. 26:26-28; Acts 2:42; 1 Cor. 11:23-33.
p Acts 1:13.
q 1 Ki. 17:21, 22; 2 Ki. 4:34, 35; Acts 9:40, 41.
r *Make ye no ado.*
s *Resurrection.* vs. 9-12; Acts 24:14, 15, 21. (Job 19:25; 1 Cor. 15:52.)
t *that he might not have to.*
u Acts 2:1; 19:21; Gal. 4:10, 11.
v *Elders.* Acts 21:18. (Acts 11:30; Tit. 1:5-9.)
w *Temptation.* 1 Cor. 7:5. (Gen. 3:1; Jas. 1:14.)
x *shrank not from declaring.*
y *Repentance.* Acts 26:20. (Mt. 3:2; Acts 17:30.)

in the [1]spirit unto Jerusalem, not knowing the things that shall befall me there:

23 Save that the Holy Ghost witnesseth in every city, saying that bonds and afflictions abide me.

24 But none of these things move me, [a]neither count I my life dear unto myself, so that I might finish my course with joy, and the ministry, which I have received of the Lord Jesus, to testify the [b]gospel of the grace of God.

25 And now, behold, I know that ye all, among whom I have gone preaching the kingdom of God, shall see my face no more.

26 Wherefore I take you to record this day, that I *am* [c]pure from the blood of all *men*.

27 [d]For I have not shunned to declare unto you all the counsel of God.

28 [e]Take heed therefore unto yourselves, and to all the [f]flock, over the which the [g]Holy Ghost hath made you overseers, to feed the church of God, which he hath [h]purchased with his own blood.

29 For I know this, that after my departing shall grievous [i]wolves enter in among you, not sparing the flock.

30 Also [j]of your own selves shall men arise, speaking perverse things, to draw away disciples after them.

31 Therefore watch, and remember, that by the space of three years I ceased not to warn every one night and day with tears.

32 And now, brethren, [k]I commend you to God, and to the word of his grace, which is able to build you up, and to give you an inheritance among all them which are [l]sanctified.

33 I have coveted no man's silver, or gold, or apparel.

34 Yea, ye yourselves know, that these hands have ministered unto my necessities, and to them that were with me.

35 [m]I have shewed you all things, how that so labouring ye ought to support the weak, and to remember the words of the Lord Jesus, how he said, [n]It is more blessed to give than to receive.

36 And when he had thus spoken, he kneeled down, and prayed with them all.

37 And they all wept sore, and fell on Paul's neck, and kissed him,

38 Sorrowing most of all for the words which he spake, that they should see his face no more. And they accompanied him unto the ship.

CHAPTER 21.

(5) *From Miletus to Tyre.*

And it came to pass, that after we were gotten from them, and had launched, we came with a straight course unto [o]Coos, and the *day* following unto Rhodes, and from thence unto Patara:

2 And finding a ship sailing over unto Phenicia, we went aboard, and set forth.

3 Now when we had [p]discovered Cyprus, we left it on the left hand, and sailed into Syria, and landed at Tyre: for there the ship was to unlade her burden.

(6) *The Holy Spirit forbids Paul to go to Jerusalem.*

4 And finding disciples, we tarried there seven days: who said to Paul through the Spirit, that he should not [q]go up to Jerusalem.

5 And when we had accomplished those days, we departed and went our way; and they all brought us on our way, with wives and children, till *we were* out of the city: and we kneeled down on the shore, and prayed.

6 And when we had taken our leave one of another, we took ship; and they returned home again.

7 And when we had finished *our* course from Tyre, we came to Ptolemais, and saluted the brethren, and abode with them one day.

8 And the next *day* we that were of Paul's company departed, and came unto Cæsarea: and we entered into the house of [r]Philip the evangelist, which was *one* of the seven; and abode with him.

9 And the same man had four daughters, virgins, which did prophesy.

A.D. 60.

a *Or, I hold not my life of any account, as unto myself, in comparison with accomplishing my course.* See 1 Cor. 9:26; Phil. 3:13, 14; 2 Tim. 4:7, 8.

b *Gospel.* Rom. 1:1, 9, 15, 16. (Gen. 12:1-3; Rev. 14:6.)

c Ezk. 3:17.

d 2 Cor. 4:2; Gal. 1:10.

e 1 Cor. 9:27; Col. 4:17; 1 Tim. 4:16.

f Isa. 40:11; Lk. 12:32.

g *Holy Spirit.* vs. 23, 28; Acts 21:4-11. (Mt. 1:18; Acts 2:4.)

h *Sacrifice (of Christ).* Rom. 3:25. (Gen. 4:4;. Heb. 10:18.)

i The two sources of the apostasy: false teachers from without (2Cor. 11:13-15; 2 Pet. 2:1-3); ambitious leaders from within (3 John 9:10; Rev. 2:6, 15). Also, 1 Tim. 1:20; 1 John 2:19.

j 1 Tim. 1:19, 20; 2 Tim. 1:15; 1 John 2:19.

k *Churches (local).* vs. 7, 17-32; Rom. 16:1-5, 16, 23. (Acts 2:41; Phil. 1:1.)

l *Sanctify, holy (persons)* (N. T.) Acts 26:18. (Mt. 4:5; Rev. 22:11.)

m *In all things I have given you an example.*

n Lk. 14:12.

o *Cos.*

p *come In sight of.*

q Lit. *set foot in.* Not, as in Acts 20:23, a warning of danger, but now an imperative command. See Acts 22:17, 18.

r Acts 6:5; 8:5.

1(20:22) Cf. Acts 21:4. In Acts 20:22 Paul's own spirit (1 Thes. 5:23, *note*) is meant; in Acts 21:4 the Holy Spirit. Paul's motive in going to Jerusalem seems to have been his great affection for the Jews (Rom. 9:1-5), and his hope that the gifts of the Gentile churches, sent by him to poor saints at Jerusalem (Rom. 15:25-28), would open the hearts of the law-bound Jewish believers to the "gospel of the grace of God" (Acts 20:24).

A.D. 60.

(7) *The Holy Spirit again warns Paul.*

10 And as we tarried *there* many days, there came down from Judæa a certain prophet, named Agabus.

11 And [a]when he was come unto us, he took Paul's girdle, and bound his own hands and feet, and said, Thus saith the [b]Holy Ghost, So shall the Jews at Jerusalem bind the man that owneth this girdle, and shall deliver *him* into the hands of the Gentiles.

12 And when we heard these things, both we, and they of that place, besought him not to go up to Jerusalem.

13 Then Paul answered, What mean ye to weep and to break mine heart? for I am [c]ready not to be bound only, but also to die at Jerusalem for the name of the Lord Jesus.

(8) *Paul at Jerusalem.*

14 And when he would not be persuaded, we ceased, saying, The [d]will of the Lord be done.

15 And after those days we took up our [e]carriages, and went up to Jerusalem.

16 There went with us also *certain* of the disciples of Cæsarea, and brought with them one Mnason of Cyprus, an [f]old disciple, with whom we should lodge.

17 And when we were come to Jerusalem, the brethren received us gladly.

Paul takes a Jewish vow involving a Jewish sacrifice. (Cf. Heb. 10:2, 9-12.)

18 And the *day* following Paul went in with us unto James; and all the [g]elders were present.

19 And when he had saluted them, he [h]declared particularly what things God had wrought among the Gentiles by his ministry.

20 And when they heard *it*, they glorified the Lord, and said unto him, Thou seest, brother, how many [i]thousands of Jews there are which believe; and [j]they are all zealous of the law:

21 And they are informed of thee, that thou teachest all the Jews which are among the Gentiles to forsake Moses, saying that they ought not to circumcise *their* children, neither to walk after the customs.

22 What is it therefore? the multitude must needs come together: for they will hear that thou art come.

23 Do therefore this that we say to thee: We have four men which have a [k]vow on them;

24 Them take, and purify thyself with them, and be at [l]charges with them, that they may shave *their* heads: and all may know that those things, whereof they were informed concerning thee, are nothing; but *that* thou thyself also [m]walkest orderly, and keepest the law.

25 As touching the Gentiles which believe, we have written *and* concluded that they observe no such thing, save only that they keep themselves from *things* offered to idols, and from blood, and from strangled, and from fornication.

26 Then [n]Paul took the men, and the next day purifying himself with them entered into the temple, to signify the accomplishment of the days of purification, until that an [n]offering should be offered for every one of them.

Paul seized in the temple by the Jews.

27 And when the seven days were almost ended, the Jews which were of Asia, when they saw him in the temple, stirred up all the people, and laid hands on him,

28 Crying out, Men of Israel, help: This is the man, that teacheth all *men* every where against the people, and the law, and this place: and further brought Greeks also into the temple, and hath polluted this [o]holy place.

29 (For they had seen before with him in the city Trophimus an Ephesian, whom they supposed that Paul had brought into the temple.)

30 And all the city was moved, and the people ran together: and they took Paul, and [p]drew him out of the temple: and forthwith the doors were shut.

31 And as they went [q]about to kill him, tidings came unto the chief captain of the band, that all Jerusalem was in an uproar.

32 [r]Who immediately took soldiers and centurions, and ran down unto them: and when they saw the chief captain and the soldiers, they left beating of Paul.

a *coming to us and taking Paul's girdle he bound his own feet and hands.*

b *Holy Spirit.* vs. 4, 11; Acts 28:25. (Mt. 1:18; Acts 2:4.)

c Rom. 1:15; 2 Tim. 4:6.

d Mt. 6:10; 26:42.

e *baggage.*

f *early.*

g *Elders.* Phil. 1:1. (Acts 11:30; Tit. 1:5-9.)

h *rehearsed one by one.*

i Gr. *myriads.*

j Cf. Rom. 10:2-4; Gal. 1:14.

k Probably according to Num. 6:1-7. Cf. Col. 2:14-17.

l Lit. *spend something on them.*

m Lit. *art keeping in the ranks, guarding the law.* Cf. Rom. 10:1-12.

n *Contra,* Acts 21:4 (cf. Gal. 2:2-6). See Rom. 3:9, 10, 19, 20, 28; 4:3-5; 5:1, 2; 6:14; 7:1-4, 6; 8:3, 4; Gal. 2:15, 16, 18, 19; 3:10, 24, 25; 4:9-11, 21-31; Phil. 3:7-9; Heb. 9:14, 15, 28; 10:1-4, 17, 18; 13:11-14.

o *Sanctify, holy (things)* (N.T.). Rom. 1:2. (Mt. 4:5; Rev. 22:11.)

p *dragged.* Acts 14:19; 16:19.

q 2 Cor. 11:23.

r Acts 23:27; 24:7.

Paul bound with chains.

33 Then the chief captain came near, and took him, and commanded *him* to be bound with two chains; and demanded who he was, and what he had done.

34 And some cried one thing, some another, among the multitude: and when he could not know the certainty for the tumult, he commanded him to be carried into the castle.

35 And when he came upon the stairs, so it was, that he was borne of the soldiers for the violence of the people.

36 For the multitude of the people followed after, crying, [a]Away with him.

37 And as Paul was to be led into the castle, he said unto the [b]chief captain, May I speak unto thee? Who said, Canst thou speak Greek?

38 Art not thou [c]that Egyptian, which before these days madest an uproar, and leddest out into the wilderness four thousand men that were murderers?

39 But Paul said, I am a man *which am* a Jew of Tarsus, *a city* in Cilicia, a [d]citizen of no mean city: and, I beseech thee, suffer me to speak unto the people.

40 And when he had given him licence, Paul stood on the stairs, and beckoned with the hand unto the people. And when there was made a great silence, he spake unto *them* in the Hebrew tongue, saying,

CHAPTER 22.

Paul's defence before the multitude: recounts his conversion. (Cf. Acts 9:1-18; 26:9-18.)

Men, brethren, and fathers, hear ye my defence [e]*which I make* now unto you.

2 (And when they heard that he spake in the Hebrew tongue to them, they kept the more silence: and he saith,)

3 I am [f]verily a man *which am* a Jew, born in Tarsus, *a city* in Cilicia, yet brought up in this city at the feet of [g]Gamaliel, *and* [h]taught according to the perfect manner of the law of the fathers, and was zealous toward God, as ye all are this day.

4 And I [i]persecuted this way unto the death, binding and delivering into prisons both men and women.

5 As also the high priest doth bear me witness, and all the estate of the elders: from whom also I received letters unto the brethren, and went to Damascus, [j]to bring them which were there bound unto Jerusalem, for to be punished.

6 And it came to pass, that, as I made my journey, and was come nigh unto Damascus about noon, suddenly there shone from heaven a great light round about me.

7 And I fell unto the ground, and heard a voice saying unto me, Saul, Saul, why persecutest [k]thou me?

8 And I answered, Who art thou, Lord? And he said unto me, I am Jesus of Nazareth, whom thou persecutest.

9 And they that were with me [l]saw indeed the light, and were afraid; but they heard not the [m]voice of him that spake to me.

10 And I said, What shall I [n]do, Lord? And the Lord said unto me, Arise, and go into Damascus; and there it shall be told thee of all things which are appointed for thee to do.

11 And when I could not see for the glory of that light, being led by the hand of them that were with me, I came into Damascus.

12 And one Ananias, a devout man according to the law, having [o]a good report of all the Jews which dwelt *there*,

13 Came unto me, and stood, and said unto me, Brother Saul, receive thy sight. And the same hour I looked up upon him.

14 And he said, The God of our fathers hath [p]chosen thee, that thou shouldest know his will, and see that Just One, and shouldest hear the voice of his mouth.

15 For [q]thou shalt be his witness unto all men of what thou hast seen and heard.

16 And now why tarriest thou? arise, and be baptized, and [r]wash away thy [s]sins, calling on the name of the Lord.

The Lord had warned Paul to keep away from Jerusalem.

17 And it came to pass, that, [t]when I was come again to Jerusalem, even while I prayed in the temple, I was in a trance;

18 And saw him saying unto me, Make haste, and get thee quickly [u]out of Jerusalem: for they will not receive thy testimony concerning me.

19 And I said, Lord, [v]they know that

A.D. 60.

- a Acts 22:22; Lk. 23:18.
- b Gr. *chiliarch*, the Roman tribune. There were six such "chief captains" in each legion of 6000 men.
- c Acts 5:36.
- d Acts 22:25.
- e Lk. 12:11; 1 Pet. 3:15.
- f 2 Cor. 11:22; Phil. 3:5, 6.
- g Acts 5:34.
- h *Instructed according to the strict manner.*
- i Acts 8:3; 26:9-11; 1 Tim. 1:13.
- j Acts 9:2.
- k Isa. 63:9; Zech. 2:8; Mt. 25:45; 1 Cor. 12:26.
- l Dan. 10:7.
- m Cf. Acts 9:7, *note.*
- n Acts 2:37; 1 Tim. 3:7.
- o 1 Tim. 3:7-10.
- p *Election (personal).* Rom. 16:13. (Deut. 7:6; 1 Pet. 1:2.)
- q 2 Cor. 11:22.
- r Acts 2:38.
- s *Sin.* Rom. 3:23, *note.*
- t i.e. probably on his first visit to Jerusalem after his conversion.
- u v. 21; so also Acts 21:4.
- v Acts 8:3.

I imprisoned and beat in every synagogue them that believed on thee:

20 And when the blood of thy martyr Stephen was shed, [a]I also was standing by, and consenting unto his death, and kept the raiment of them that slew him.

21 And he said unto me, Depart: [b]for I will send thee far hence unto the Gentiles.

22 [c]And they gave him audience unto this word, and *then* lifted up their voices, and said, Away with such a *fellow* from the earth: for it is not fit that he should live.

23 And as they cried out, and cast off *their* clothes, and threw dust into the air,

24 The chief captain commanded him to be brought into the castle, and bade that he should be examined by scourging; that he might know [d]wherefore they cried so against him.

Paul a Roman citizen.

25 And [e]as they bound him with thongs, Paul said unto the centurion that stood by, Is it lawful for you to scourge a man that is a [f]Roman, and uncondemned?

26 When the centurion heard *that*, he went and told the chief captain, saying, Take heed what thou doest: for this man is a Roman.

27 Then the chief captain came, and said unto him, Tell me, art thou a Roman? He said, Yea.

28 And the chief captain answered, With a great sum obtained I this [g]freedom. And Paul said, But I [h]was *free* born.

29 Then straightway they departed from him which should have [i]examined him: and the chief captain also was afraid, after he knew that he was a Roman, and because he had bound him.

30 On the morrow, because he would have known the certainty wherefore he was accused of the Jews, he loosed him from *his* bands, and commanded the chief priests and all their council to appear, and brought Paul down, and set him before them.

CHAPTER 23.

Paul before the Sanhedrin.

And Paul, earnestly beholding the council, said, Men *and* brethren, [j]I have lived in all good conscience before God until this day.

2 And the high priest Ananias commanded them that stood by him to smite him on the mouth.

3 [k]Then said Paul unto him, God shall smite thee, *thou* whited wall: for sittest thou to judge me after the law, and commandest me to be smitten contrary to the law?

4 And they that stood by said, Revilest thou God's high priest?

5 Then said Paul, I wist not, brethren, that he was the high priest: for it is written, [l]Thou shalt not speak evil of the ruler of thy people.

Paul appeals to the Pharisees.

6 But when Paul perceived that the one part were [m]Sadducees, and the other Pharisees, he cried out in the council, Men *and* brethren, I am a Pharisee, the son of a Pharisee: of the hope and resurrection of the dead I am called in question.

7 And when he had so said, there arose a dissension between the Pharisees and the Sadducees: and the multitude was divided.

8 For the Sadducees say that there is no resurrection, neither angel, nor spirit: but the Pharisees confess both.

9 And there arose a great [n]cry: and the [o]scribes *that were* of the Pharisees' part arose, and strove, saying, We find no evil in this man: but if a spirit or an angel hath spoken to him, let us not fight against God.

10 And when there arose a great dissension, the chief captain, fearing lest Paul should have been pulled in pieces of them, commanded the soldiers to go down, and to take him by force from among them, and to bring *him* into the castle.

The Lord's grace to Paul.

11 And the night following the Lord [p]stood by him, and said, Be of good cheer, Paul: for as thou hast testified of me in Jerusalem, so must thou bear witness also at Rome.

The conspiracy to kill Paul.

12 And when it was day, [q]certain of the Jews banded together, and bound themselves under a curse, saying that they would neither eat nor drink till they had killed Paul.

a Acts 7:58; 8:1.
b Acts 13:2, 47; Rom. 11:13; Gal. 2:7, 8; Eph. 3:7, 8.
c 1 Thes. 2:16.
d *for what cause they so shouted.*
e *when they had tied him up with thongs.*
f Acts 25:16.
g *citizenship.*
h *am a Roman born*, i.e. of a father who had obtained citizenship.
i Or, *tortured him.*
j Acts 24:16; 2 Cor. 1:12; 2 Tim. 1:3; Heb. 13:18; 1 Pet. 3:15, 16; 1 John 3:21.
k Cf. John 18:23.
l Ex. 22:28.
m See Mt. 3:7, *note.*
n *clamour.*
o See Mt. 2:4, *note.*
p Acts 18:9; 27:23, 24; Psa. 46:1, 77.
q John 16:2, 3.

13 And they were more than forty which had made this conspiracy.

14 And they came to the chief priests and elders, and said, We have bound ourselves under a great curse, that we will eat nothing until we have slain Paul.

15 Now therefore ye with the council signify to the chief captain that he bring him down unto you to morrow, as though ye would enquire something more perfectly concerning him: and we, or ever he come near, are [a]ready to kill him.

16 And when Paul's sister's son heard of their lying in wait, he went and entered into the castle, and told Paul.

17 [b]Then Paul called one of the centurions unto *him*, and said, Bring this young man unto the chief captain: for he hath a certain thing to tell him.

18 So he took him, and brought *him* to the chief captain, and said, Paul the prisoner [c]called me unto *him*, and prayed me to bring this young man unto thee, who hath something to say unto thee.

19 Then the chief captain took him by the hand, and went *with him* aside privately, and asked *him*, What is that thou hast to tell me?

20 And he said, The Jews have agreed to desire thee that thou wouldest bring down Paul to morrow into the council, as though they would enquire somewhat of him more perfectly.

21 But do not thou yield unto them: for there lie in wait for him of them more than forty men, which have bound themselves with an oath, that they will neither eat nor drink till they have killed him: and now are they ready, looking for a promise from thee.

22 So the chief captain *then* let the young man depart, and charged *him*, *See thou* tell no man that thou hast shewed these things to me.

Paul sent to Felix at Cæsarea.

23 And he called unto *him* two centurions, saying, Make ready two hundred soldiers to go to Cæsarea, and horsemen threescore and ten, and spearmen two hundred, at the third hour of the night;

24 And provide *them* beasts, that they may set Paul on, and bring *him* safe unto Felix the governor.

25 And he wrote a letter after this manner:

A.D. 60.

a Psa. 37:32, 33.
b Acts 27:24, 31.
c Eph. 3:1.
d *seized by*. Acts 21:30, 33.
e *I came upon them with the soldiers.*
f Acts 22:30.
g Acts 25:25; 26:31.
h Acts 21:39.
i *palace.*
j Acts 23:2, 30, 35; 25:2.

26 Claudius Lysias unto the most excellent governor Felix *sendeth* greeting.

27 This man was [d]taken of the Jews, and should have been killed of them: then [e]came I with an army, and rescued him, having understood that he was a Roman.

28 [f]And when I would have known the cause wherefore they accused him, I brought him forth into their council:

29 Whom I perceived to be accused of questions of their law, but to have [g]nothing laid to his charge worthy of death or of bonds.

30 And when it was told me how that the Jews laid wait for the man, I sent straightway to thee, and gave commandment to his accusers also to say before thee what *they had* against him. Farewell.

31 Then the soldiers, as it was commanded them, took Paul, and brought *him* by night to Antipatris.

32 On the morrow they left the horsemen to go with him, and returned to the castle:

33 Who, when they came to Cæsarea, and delivered the epistle to the governor, presented Paul also before him.

34 And when the governor had read *the letter*, he asked of what province he was. And when he understood that *he was* of [h]Cilicia;

35 I will hear thee, said he, when thine accusers are also come. And he commanded him to be kept in Herod's [i]judgment hall.

CHAPTER 24.

Paul before Felix.

And after five days [j]Ananias the high priest descended with the elders, and *with* a certain orator *named* Tertullus, who informed the governor against Paul.

(The accusation.)

2 And when he was called forth, Tertullus began to accuse *him*, saying, Seeing that by thee we enjoy great quietness, and that very worthy deeds are done unto this nation by thy providence,

3 We accept *it* always, and in all places, most noble Felix, with all thankfulness.

4 Notwithstanding, that I be not further tedious unto thee, I pray thee that thou wouldest hear us of thy clemency a few words.

A.D. 62.

5 For we have found this man *a* pestilent [a]*fellow*, and a mover of sedition
among all the Jews throughout the
[b]world, and a ringleader of the sect of
the Nazarenes:
6 Who also hath gone about to [c]profane
the temple: whom we took, and would
have [d]judged according to our law.
7 But the chief [e]captain Lysias came
upon us, and with great violence took
him away out of our hands,
8 Commanding his accusers [f]to come
unto thee: by examining of whom thyself mayest take knowledge of all these
things, whereof we accuse him.
9 And the Jews also assented, saying
that these things were so.

(Paul's defence before Felix.)

10 Then Paul, after that [g]the governor
had beckoned unto him to speak,
answered, Forasmuch as I know that
thou hast been of many years a judge
unto this nation, I do the more cheerful-
ly answer [h]for myself:
11 Because that thou mayest understand, that there are yet but twelve days
since I went up [i]to Jerusalem for to
worship.
12 And they neither found me in the
temple disputing with any man, neither
raising up the people, neither in the synagogues, nor in the city:
13 Neither can they [j]prove the things
whereof they now accuse me.
14 But this I confess unto thee, that
after the way which they call heresy, so
worship I the God [k]of my fathers, believing all things [l]which are written in the
law and in the prophets:
15 And have [m]hope toward God,
which they themselves also allow, that
there shall be a resurrection of the dead,
both of the just and unjust.
16 And herein do I exercise myself, [n]to
have always a conscience void of offence
toward God, and *toward* men.
17 Now after many years [o]I came to
bring alms to my nation, and offerings.
18 [p]Whereupon certain Jews from Asia
found me purified in the temple, neither
with multitude, nor with tumult.
19 Who ought to have been here
before thee, and object, if they had ought
against me.
20 Or else let these same *here* say, if
they have found any evil doing in me,
while I stood before the council,
21 Except it be for this one voice, that I
cried standing among them, Touching
the [q]resurrection of the dead I am called
in question by you this day.
22 And when Felix heard these things,
having more perfect knowledge [r]of *that*
way, he deferred them, and said, When
Lysias the chief captain shall come
down, I will know the uttermost of your
matter.
23 And he commanded a centurion to
keep Paul, and to let *him* have liberty,
and that he should forbid none of his
acquaintance to minister or come unto
him.

(Paul before Felix the second time.)

24 And after certain days, when Felix
came with his wife Drusilla, which was
a Jewess, he sent for Paul, and heard him
concerning the faith in Christ.
25 And as he reasoned of [s]righteous-
ness, temperance, and judgment to
come, Felix [t]trembled, and answered, Go
thy way for this time; when I have a convenient season, I will call for thee.
26 He hoped also that money should
have been given him of Paul, that he
might loose him: wherefore he sent for
him the oftener, and communed with
him.

The silent two years at Cæsarea.

27 [u]But after two years Porcius Festus
came into Felix' room: and Felix, willing
to [v]shew the Jews a pleasure, left Paul
bound.

CHAPTER 25.

Paul before Festus.

Now when Festus was come into the
province, after three days he
ascended from Cæsarea to Jerusalem.
2 Then the high priest and the chief of
the Jews informed him against Paul, and
besought him,
3 And desired favour against him, that
he would send for him to Jerusalem,
[w]laying wait in the way to kill him.
4 But Festus answered, that Paul

a 1 Pet. 2:12,19.
b *oikoumene* = inhabited earth (Lk. 2:1).
c Acts 21:28.
d John 18:31.
e Acts 21:33.
f Acts 23:30.
g Felix made procurator over Judaea, A.D. 53.
h 1 Pet. 3:15.
i Acts 21:15.
j 1 Pet. 3:16.
k 2 Tim. 1:3.
l Acts 26:22, 23; Lk. 24:27.
m Acts 23:6; 26:6, 7; 28:20.
n Acts 23:1.
o Acts 11:29, 30.
p Acts 21:26.
q *Resurrection.* vs. 14, 15, 21; Rom. 8:10, 11. (Job 19:25; 1 Cor. 15:52.)
r *concerning the Way.* See John 14:6.
s Rom. 10:10, *note.*
t *becoming afraid;* Gr. *emphobos, afraid.*
u *But when two years were fulfilled, Felix was succeeded by Porcius Festus and desiring to gain favour with the Jews, Felix left Paul in bonds.*
v Mk. 15:15.
w Acts 23:14, 15.

A.D. 62.

should be kept at Cæsarea, and that he himself would depart shortly *thither*.

5 Let them therefore, said he, which among you are able, go down with *me*, and accuse this man, if there be any wickedness in him.

6 And when he had tarried among them [a]more than ten days, he went down unto Cæsarea; and the next day sitting on the judgment seat commanded Paul to be brought.

7 And when he was come, the Jews which came down from Jerusalem stood round about, and laid many and grievous complaints against Paul, [b]which they could not prove.

8 While he answered for himself, Neither against the law of the Jews, neither against the temple, nor [c]yet against Cæsar, have I offended any thing at all.

9 But Festus, willing to do the Jews a pleasure, answered Paul, and said, Wilt thou go up to Jerusalem, and there be judged of these things before me?

Paul appeals to Cæsar.

10 Then said Paul, I stand at Cæsar's judgment seat, where I ought to be judged: to the Jews have I done no wrong, as thou very well knowest.

11 For if I be an offender, or have committed any thing worthy of death, I refuse not to die: but if there be none of these things whereof these accuse me, no man may deliver me unto them. [d]I appeal unto Cæsar.

12 Then Festus, when he had conferred with the council, answered, Hast thou appealed unto Cæsar? unto Cæsar shalt thou go.

13 And after certain days king [e]Agrippa and Bernice came unto Cæsarea to salute Festus.

14 And when they had been there many days, Festus declared Paul's cause unto the king, saying, There is a certain man left in bonds by Felix:

15 About whom, when I was at Jerusalem, the chief priests and the elders of the Jews informed *me*, desiring *to have* judgment against him.

16 To whom I answered, It is not the manner of the Romans to deliver any man to die, before that he which is accused have the accusers face to face, and have licence to answer for himself concerning the crime laid against him.

17 Therefore, when they were come hither, without any delay on the morrow I sat on the judgment seat, and commanded the man to be brought forth.

18 Against whom when the accusers stood up, they brought none accusation of such things as I supposed:

19 But had certain questions against him of [f]their own superstition, and of one Jesus, which was dead, whom Paul affirmed to be alive.

20 And because I doubted of such manner of questions, I asked *him* whether he would go to Jerusalem, and there be judged of these matters.

21 But when Paul had appealed to be [g]reserved unto the hearing of Augustus, I commanded him to be kept till I might send him to Cæsar.

22 Then Agrippa said unto Festus, I would also hear the man myself. To morrow, said he, thou shalt hear him.

23 And on the morrow, when Agrippa was come, and Bernice, with great pomp, and was entered into the place of hearing, with the chief captains, and principal men of the city, at Festus' commandment [h]Paul was brought forth.

24 And Festus said, King Agrippa, and all men which are here present with us, ye see this man, about whom all the multitude of the Jews have dealt with me, both at Jerusalem, and *also* here, crying that he ought not to live any longer.

25 But when I found that he had committed [i]nothing worthy of death, and that he himself hath appealed to Augustus, I have determined to send him.

26 Of whom I have no certain thing to write unto my lord. Wherefore I have brought him forth before you, and specially before [j]thee, O king Agrippa, that, after examination had, I might have somewhat to write.

27 For it seemeth to me unreasonable to send a prisoner, and not withal to signify the crimes *laid* against him.

CHAPTER 26.

Paul's defence before Agrippa.

(Cf. Acts 9:1-18; 22:1-16.)

Then Agrippa said unto Paul, Thou art permitted to speak for thyself. Then

a Or, as some copies read, *no more than eight or ten days.*

b Acts 24:5, 13; Mt. 5:11, 12; 1 Pet. 4:12, 16.

c Rom. 13:1-5.

d Acts 23:11; 26:32; 27:24.

e This (v. 13) was Herod Agrippa II, son of the Herod Agrippa I of Acts 12:1, and great-grandson of Herod the Great. Mt. 2:1, *note.* Bernice, or Berenice, was the sister of Herod Agrippa II (v. 13).

f Lit. *their peculiar demon-worship.*

g *kept for the decision of the emperor.*

h Acts 9:15.

i Acts 23:9, 29; 26:31.

j See Acts 26:2, 3.

A.D. 62.

Paul stretched forth the hand, and answered for himself:

2 I think myself happy, king Agrippa, because I shall answer for myself this day before thee touching all the things whereof I am accused of the Jews:

3 Especially *because I know* thee to be expert in all customs and questions which are among the Jews: wherefore I beseech thee to hear me patiently.

4 My manner of life from my youth, which was at the first among mine own nation at Jerusalem, know all the Jews;

5 Which [a]knew me from the beginning, if they would testify, that after the most straitest sect of our religion I lived a [b]Pharisee.

6 And now [c]I stand and am judged for the hope of the [d]promise made of God unto our fathers:

7 Unto which *promise* our twelve tribes, instantly serving *God* day and night, hope to come. For which hope's sake, king Agrippa, I am accused of the Jews.

8 Why should it be [e]thought a thing incredible with you, that God should raise the dead?

9 I [f]verily thought with myself, that I ought to do many things contrary to the name of Jesus of Nazareth.

10 Which thing I also did [g]in Jerusalem: and many of the saints did I shut up in prison, having received [h]authority from the chief priests; and when they were put to death, I gave my [i]voice against *them*.

11 And I punished them oft in every synagogue, and compelled *them* to blaspheme; and being exceedingly mad against them, I persecuted *them* even unto strange cities.

12 Whereupon as I [j]went to Damascus with authority and commission from the chief priests,

13 At midday, O king, I saw in the way a light from heaven, above the brightness of the sun, shining round about me and them which journeyed with me.

14 And when we were all fallen to the earth, I [k]heard a voice speaking unto me, and saying in the Hebrew tongue, Saul, Saul, why persecutest thou me? *it is* hard for thee to kick against the [l]pricks.

15 And I said, Who art thou, Lord? And he said, I am Jesus whom thou persecutest.

16 But rise, and stand upon thy feet: for I have appeared unto thee for this purpose, to make thee a minister and a witness both of these things which thou hast seen, and of those things in the which I will appear unto thee;

17 Delivering thee from the people, and *from* the Gentiles, unto whom now I send thee,

18 To open their eyes, *and* to turn *them* from darkness to light, and *from* the power of [m]Satan unto God, that they may receive forgiveness of [n]sins, and inheritance among them which are [o]sanctified by faith that is in me.

19 Whereupon, O king Agrippa, I was not disobedient unto the heavenly vision:

20 But shewed first unto them of Damascus, and at Jerusalem, and throughout all the coasts of Judæa, and *then* to the Gentiles, that they should [p]repent and turn to God, and do works meet for repentance.

21 For these causes the Jews caught me in the temple, and went about to kill *me*.

22 Having therefore obtained help of God, I continue unto this day, witnessing both to small and great, saying none other things than those which the prophets and Moses did say should come:

23 That [q]Christ should suffer, *and* that he should be the first that should rise from the dead, and should shew light unto the people, and to the Gentiles.

24 And as he thus spake for himself, Festus said with a loud voice, Paul, thou art [r]beside thyself; much learning doth make thee mad.

25 But he said, I am not mad, most noble Festus; but speak forth the words of truth and soberness.

26 For the king knoweth of these things, before whom also I speak freely: for I am persuaded that none of these things are hidden from him; for this thing was not done in a corner.

27 King Agrippa, believest thou the prophets? I know that thou [s]believest.

28 Then Agrippa said unto Paul, [t]Almost thou persuadest me to be a Christian.

29 And Paul said, I would to God, that not only thou, but also all that hear me this day, were [u]both almost, and altogether such as I am, except these bonds.

30 And when he had thus spoken,

a *Foreknowledge*, trans. foreknow. Rom. 8:29. (Acts 2:23; 1 Pet. 1:20.)

b Acts 22:3.

c Acts 23:6.

d Acts 13:32, 33; Gen. 3:15; 22:18; 49:10.

e *judged a thing incredible with you, if God doth raise the dead?*

f John 16:2; 1 Tim. 1:12.

g Acts 8:1, 3; Gal. 1:13.

h Acts 9:14.

i *vote.*

j Acts 9:3.

k Cf. Acts 9:7, *note.*

l *goads.*

m *Satan.* Rom. 16:20. (Gen. 3:1; Rev. 20:10.)

n *Sin.* Rom. 3:23, *note.*

o *Sanctity, holy (persons)* (N.T.). Rom. 12:1. (Mt. 4:5; Rev. 22:11.)

p *Repentance.* Rom. 2:4. (Mt. 3:2; Acts 17:30.)

q *the Christ must suffer.* See Acts 3:18, *ref.*; 17:3, *ref.*

r Lit. *Thou art raving, Paul! thy great learning is turning thee round into raving madness.*

s Jas. 2:19.

t R.V. *With but little persuasion thou wouldest fain make me a Christian.* The answer might be paraphrased: "It will require more than this," etc., or, "A little more and you will make," etc.

u Lit. *both in a little and in much.*

the king rose up, and the governor, and Bernice, and they that sat with them:

31 And when they were gone aside, they talked between themselves, saying, This man doeth nothing worthy of death or of bonds.

32 Then said Agrippa unto Festus, This man might have been set at liberty, [a]if he had not appealed unto Cæsar.

CHAPTER 27.

Paul is sent to Rome.

And when it was determined that we should sail into Italy, they delivered [b]Paul and certain other prisoners unto *one* named Julius, a [c]centurion of Augustus' band.

2 And entering into a ship of Adramyttium, we launched, meaning to sail by the coasts of Asia; *one* [d]Aristarchus, a Macedonian of Thessalonica, being with us.

3 And the next *day* we touched at Sidon. And [e]Julius courteously entreated Paul, and gave *him* liberty to go unto his friends to refresh himself.

4 And when we had launched from thence, we sailed under Cyprus, because the winds were contrary.

5 And when we had sailed over the sea of Cilicia and Pamphylia, we came to Myra, *a city* of Lycia.

6 And there the centurion found a ship of Alexandria sailing into Italy; and he put us therein.

7 And when we had sailed slowly many days, and scarce were come over against Cnidus, the wind not suffering us, we sailed under [f]Crete, over against Salmone;

8 And, hardly passing it, came unto a place which is called The fair havens; nigh whereunto was the city *of* Lasea.

9 Now when much time was spent, and when sailing was now dangerous, because the [g]fast was now already past, Paul admonished *them*,

10 And said unto them, Sirs, I [h]perceive that this voyage will be with hurt and much damage, not only of the lading and ship, but also of our lives.

11 Nevertheless the centurion believed the master and the owner of the ship, more than those things which were spoken by Paul.

12 And because the haven was not commodious to winter in, the more part advised to depart thence also, if by any means they might attain to Phenice, *and there* to winter; *which is* an haven of Crete, and lieth toward the south west and north west.

13 And when the south wind blew softly, supposing that they had obtained *their* purpose, loosing *thence*, they sailed close by Crete.

The storm.

14 But not long after there [i]arose against it a [j]tempestuous wind, called Euroclydon.

15 And when the ship was caught, and could not bear up into the wind, we let *her* drive.

16 And running under a certain island which is called Clauda, we had much work to come by the boat:

17 Which when they had taken up, they used helps, undergirding the ship; and, fearing lest they should [k]fall into the quicksands, strake sail, and so were driven.

18 And we being exceedingly tossed with a tempest, the next *day* they lightened the ship;

19 And the third *day* we cast out with our own hands the tackling of the ship.

20 And when neither sun nor stars in many days appeared, and no small tempest lay on *us*, all hope that we should be saved was then taken away.

The moral ascendency of Paul.

21 But after long abstinence Paul stood forth in the midst of them, and said, Sirs, ye should have [l]hearkened unto me, and not have loosed from Crete, and to have gained this harm and loss.

22 And now [m]I exhort you to be of good cheer: for there shall be no loss of *any man's* life among you, but of the ship.

23 For there stood by me this night [n]the angel of God, whose I am, and whom I serve,

24 Saying, Fear not, Paul; thou must be brought before Cæsar: and, lo, God hath given thee all them that sail with thee.

25 Wherefore, sirs, be of good cheer: for I [o]believe God, that it shall be even as it was told me.

26 Howbeit we must be cast upon a certain island.

27 But when the fourteenth night was come, as we were driven up and down in Adria, about midnight the shipmen

A.D. 62.

a Acts 23:11; 25:11.
b Acts 25:12, 25.
c Commander of 100 soldiers.
d Acts 19:29.
e Acts 24:23; 28:16.
f Tit. 1:5, 12.
g The fast was on the tenth day of the seventh month. Lev. 23:27, 29.
h Amos 3:7.
i Or, *beat.*
j Psa. 107:25.
k *be cast upon the* Syrtis.
l vs. 9, 10.
m 1 Sam. 30:6; Psa. 112:7; 2 Cor. 1:4; 4:8, 9.
n *an angel of the God whose I am, whom also I serve.* Heb. 1:4, *note.*
o *Faith.* Rom. 1:16. (Gen. 3:20; Heb. 11:39.)

deemed that they drew near to some country;

28 And sounded, and found *it* twenty [a]fathoms: and when they had gone a little further, they sounded again, and found *it* fifteen fathoms.

29 Then fearing lest we should have fallen upon rocks, they cast four anchors out of the stern, and wished for the day.

30 And as the [b]shipmen were about to flee out of the ship, when they had let down the boat into the sea, under colour as though they would have cast anchors out of the foreship,

31 Paul said to the centurion and to the soldiers, [c]Except these abide in the ship, ye cannot be saved.

32 Then the soldiers cut off the ropes of the boat, and let her fall off.

33 And while the day was coming on, Paul besought *them* all to take meat, saying, This day is the fourteenth day that ye have tarried and continued fasting, having taken nothing.

34 Wherefore I pray you to take *some* meat: [d]for this is for your health: [e]for there shall not an hair fall from the head of any of you.

35 And when he had thus spoken, he took bread, and gave thanks to God in presence of them all: and when he had broken *it*, he began to eat.

36 Then were they all of good cheer, and they also took *some* meat.

37 And we were in all in the ship [f]two hundred threescore and sixteen souls.

38 And when they had eaten enough, they lightened the ship, and cast out the wheat into the sea.

39 And when it was day, they knew not the land: but they discovered a certain creek with a shore, into the which they were minded, if it were possible, to thrust in the ship.

40 And when they had [g]taken up the anchors, they committed *themselves* unto the sea, and loosed the rudder bands, and hoised up the mainsail to the wind, and made toward shore.

41 And falling into a place where two seas met, they ran the ship aground; and the forepart stuck fast, and remained unmoveable, but the hinder part [h]was broken with the violence of the waves.

42 And the soldiers' counsel was to kill the prisoners, lest any of them should swim out, and escape.

43 But the centurion, willing to save [i]Paul, kept them from *their* purpose; and commanded that they which could swim should cast *themselves* first *into the sea*, and get to land:

44 And the rest, some on boards, and some on *broken pieces* of the ship. And [j]so it came to pass, that they escaped all safe to land.

CHAPTER 28.

The landing on Melita: miracle of the viper's bite. (Cf. Mk. 16:18.)

And when they were escaped, then they knew that the island was called Melita.

2 And the barbarous people shewed us no little kindness: for they kindled a fire, and [k]received us every one, because of the present rain, and because of the cold.

3 And when Paul had gathered a bundle of sticks, and laid *them* on the fire, there came a viper out of the heat, and [l]fastened on his hand.

4 And when the barbarians saw the *venomous* beast hang on his hand, they said among themselves, No doubt this man is a murderer, whom, though he hath escaped the sea, yet [m]vengeance suffereth not to live.

5 And he shook off the beast into the fire, and felt no harm.

6 Howbeit they looked when he should have swollen, or fallen down dead suddenly: but after they had looked a great while, and saw no harm come to him, they changed their minds, and said that he was a god.

Miracle of the healing of Publius' father.

7 In the same quarters were possessions of the chief man of the island, whose name was Publius; who received us, and lodged us three days courteously.

8 And it came to pass, that the father of Publius lay sick of a fever and of a bloody flux: to [n]whom Paul entered in, and prayed, and [o]laid his hands on him, and [l]healed him.

9 So when this was done, others also, which had diseases in the island, came, and were healed:

10 Who also honoured us with many honours; and when we departed,

A.D. 62.

a One fathom = between 6 and 7 ft.

b *sailors were seeking to flee out of the ship and had lowered the boat.*

c v. 22; Ezk. 36:36, 37; Lk. 4:9-12.

d Mt. 15:32.

e Mt. 10:30; Lk. 21:18.

f Some ancient authorities read, *about threescore and sixteen souls.*

g Or, *cut the anchors, they left them in the sea, etc.*

h *began to break up.*

i Prov. 16:7.

j v. 22; Psa. 107:28, 30; 2 Cor. 1:8, 10.

k Heb. 13:2.

l *Miracles* (N.T.). vs. 3-6, 8, 9. (Mt. 8:2, 3.)

m *justice.*

n Jas. 5:14, 15.

o Acts 19:11; Mk. 16:18; 1 Cor. 12:9, 28.

they laded *us* with such things as were
necessary.
11 And after three months we departed in a ship of Alexandria, which had
wintered in the isle, whose sign was
Castor and Pollux.
12 And landing at Syracuse, we tarried *there* three days.
13 And from thence we fetched a compass, and came to Rhegium: and after
one day the south wind blew, and we
came the next day to Puteoli:
14 Where we found brethren, and
were desired to tarry with them seven
days: and so we went toward Rome.
15 And from thence, when [a]the
brethren heard of us, they came to meet
us as far as [b]Appii forum, and The three
taverns: whom when Paul saw, he
thanked God, and took [c]courage.

Paul arrives at Rome.

16 And when we came to Rome, the
centurion delivered the prisoners to the
captain of the guard: but Paul was suffered to dwell by himself with [d]a soldier
that kept him.

Paul in Rome: his ministry there to the Jews.

17 And it came to pass, that after three
days Paul called the chief of the Jews
together: and when they were come
together, he said unto them, Men *and*
brethren, though I have committed nothing against the people, or customs of our
fathers, yet was I [e]delivered prisoner from
Jerusalem into the hands of the Romans.
18 Who, [f]when they had examined
me, would have let *me* go, because there
was no cause of death in me.
19 But when the Jews spake against *it*,
I was constrained to [g]appeal unto
Cæsar; not that I had ought to accuse my
nation of.
20 For this cause therefore [h]have I
called for you, to see *you*, and to speak
with *you*: because that for the [i]hope of
Israel I am bound with this [j]chain.
21 And they said unto him, We neither
received letters out of Judæa concerning
thee, neither any of the brethren that
came shewed or spake any harm of thee.
22 But we desire to hear of thee what
thou thinkest: for as concerning this sect,
we know that [k]every where it is spoken
against.
23 And when they had appointed him
a day, there came many to him into *his*
lodging; to whom he [l]expounded and
testified the kingdom of God, persuading them concerning Jesus, both out of
the law of Moses, and *out of* the
prophets, from morning till evening.
24 And some believed the things which
were spoken, and some believed not.

Paul turns to the Gentiles.

25 And [m]when they agreed not among
themselves, they departed, after that
Paul had spoken one word, Well spake
the [n]Holy Ghost [o]by Esaias the prophet
unto our fathers,
26 Saying, Go unto this people, and
say, Hearing ye shall hear, and [p]shall not
understand; and seeing ye shall see, and
not perceive:
27 For the heart of this people is
waxed gross, and their ears are dull of
hearing, and their eyes have they closed;
lest they should see with *their* eyes, and
hear with *their* ears, and understand
with [q]*their* heart, and should be [r]con-
verted, and I should heal them.
28 Be it known therefore unto you,
that the [s]salvation of God is sent unto
the Gentiles, and *that* they will hear it.
29 And when he had said these words,
the Jews departed, and had great reasoning among themselves.
30 And Paul dwelt two whole years in
[1]his own hired house, and received all
that came in unto him,
31 Preaching the kingdom of God, and
teaching those things which concern the
Lord Jesus Christ, [t]with all confidence,
no man forbidding him.

A.D. 63.

a Rom. 1:8, 12.
b *the market of Appius.*
c Josh. 1:6, 7, 9; 1 Sam. 30:6; Psa. 27:14.
d *the soldier that guarded him.* Acts 24:23; 27:3.
e Acts 21:33.
f Acts 26:31-32.
g Acts 25:11.
h *did I entreat you to see and speak with me.*
i Acts 26:6, 7.
j Eph. 3:1; 6:20; 2 Tim. 1:8,12.
k Lk. 2:34; 1 Pet. 2:12; 4:14.
l Acts 17:3; Gen. 49:10; Num. 24:17; Mal. 3:1; 4:2; Lk. 24:27; John 1:45; 5:39; Rev. 19:10.
m Cf. Acts 13:46; 18:6.
n *Holy Spirit.* Rom. 1:4. (Mt. 1:18; Acts 2:4.)
o *Inspiration.* Rom. 16:25, 26. (Ex. 4:15; Rev. 22:19.)
p 2 Cor. 4:4, 6.
q vs. 26, 27; Isa. 6:9, 10.
r i.e. *turn again.*
s Rom. 1:16. *note.*
t Acts 20:25; Eph. 6:19; Phil. 1:13, 14.

[1] **(28:30)** It has been much disputed whether Paul endured two Roman imprisonments, from A.D. 62 to 68, or one. The tradition from Clement to Eusebius favours two imprisonments with a year of liberty between. Erdman (W.J.) has pointed out that the leaving of Trophimus sick at Miletus, mentioned in 2 Tim. 4:20, could not have been an occurrence of Paul's last journey to Jerusalem, for then Trophimus was not left (Acts 20:4; 21:29), nor of the journey to Rome to appear before Caesar, for then he did not touch at Miletus. To make this incident possible there must have been a release from the first imprisonment, and an interval of ministry and travel.

THE EPISTLES OF PAUL.

THE Epistles of the Apostle Paul have a very distinctive character. All Scripture, up to the Gospel accounts of the crucifixion, looks forward to the cross, and has primarily in view Israel, and the blessing of the earth through the Messianic kingdom. But "hid in God" (Eph. 3:9) was an unrevealed *fact*—the interval of time between the crucifixion and resurrection of Christ and His return in glory; and an unrevealed purpose—the outcalling of the *ecclesia,* the church which is Christ's body. In Mt. 16 our Lord announced that purpose, but wholly without explanation as to how, when, or of what materials, that church should be built, or what should be its position, relationships, privileges, or duties.

All this constitutes precisely the scope of the Epistles of Paul. They develop the doctrine of the church. In his letters to seven Gentile churches (in Rome, Corinth, Galatia, Ephesus, Philippi, Colosse, and Thessalonica), the church, the "mystery which from the beginning of the world hath been hid in God" (Eph. 3:9), is fully revealed, and fully instructed as to her unique place in the counsels and purposes of God.

Through Paul alone we know that the church is not an organization, but an organism, the body of Christ; instinct with His life, and heavenly in calling, promise, and destiny. Through him alone we know the nature, purpose, and form of organization of local churches, and the right conduct of such gatherings. Through him alone do we know that "we shall not all sleep," that "the dead in Christ shall rise first," and that living saints shall be "changed" and caught up to meet the Lord in the air at His return.

But to Paul was also committed the unfolding of the doctrines of grace which were latent in the teachings of Jesus Christ. Paul originates nothing, but unfolds everything, concerning the nature and purpose of the law; the ground and means of the believer's justification, sanctification, and glory; the meanings of the death of Christ, and the position, walk, expectation, and service of the Christian.

Paul, converted by the personal ministry of the Lord in glory, is distinctively the witness to a glorified Christ, Head over all things to the church which is His body, as the Eleven were to Christ in the flesh, the Son of Abraham and of David.

The chronological order of Paul's Epistles is believed to be as follows: 1 and 2 Thessalonians, 1 and 2 Corinthians, Galatians, Romans, Philemon, Colossians, Ephesians, Philippians, 1 Timothy, Titus, 2 Timothy. Hebrews has a distinctive place, nor can the order of that book amongst the writings of Paul be definitely fixed.

THE TWO SILENCES

TWO periods in the life of Paul after his conversion are passed over in a silence which is itself significant—the journey into Arabia, from which the Apostle returned in full possession of the Gospel explanation as set forth in Galatians and Romans; and the two silent years in prison in Caesarea, between his arrest in the temple at Jerusalem and his deportation to Rome.

It was inevitable that a trained intellect like that of Paul, a convinced believer in Mosaism and, until his conversion on the Damascus road, an eager opposer of Christianity, must seek the underlying principles of the Gospel. Immediately after his conversion he preached Jesus as the Messiah; but the relation of the Gospel to the Law, and, in a lesser degree, to the great Jewish promises, needed clear adjustment if Christianity was to be a reasonable faith, and not a mere dogma. In Arabia Paul sought and found that adjustment through revelation by the Spirit. Out of it came the doctrinal explanation of salvation by grace through faith, wholly apart from the law, embodied in Galatians and Romans.

But the Gospel brings the believer into great relationships—to the Father, to other believers, to Christ, and to the future purposes of God. It is not only a salvation from sin and the consequences of sin, but into an amazing place in the Divine counsels. Furthermore, the new thing, the church in its various aspects and functions, demanded clear revelation. And these are the chief themes of the Epistles written by Paul from Rome, and commonly called the Prison Epistles—Ephesians, Philippians, Colossians. It is contrary to the method of inspiration, as explained by Paul himself, to suppose that these crowning revelations were made apart from deep meditation, demanding quietness, and earnest seeking. It seems most congruous with the events of Paul's life to suppose that these great revelations came during the silent years at Caesarea—often spoken of as wasted.

HOW TO USE THE SUBJECT REFERENCES.

THE subject references lead the reader from the first clear mention of a great truth to the last. The first and last references (in parenthesis) are repeated each time, so that wherever a reader comes upon a subject he may recur to the first reference and follow the subject, or turn at once to the Summary at the last reference.

ILLUSTRATION

(at Mark 1:1.)

b Gospel. vs. 1, 14, 15; Mk. 8:35. (Gen. 12:1-3; Rev. 14:6.)

Here *Gospel* is the subject; vs. 1, 14, 15 show where it is at that particular place; Mk. 8:35 is the next reference in the chain, and the references in parenthesis are the first and last.

THE EPISTLE OF PAUL THE APOSTLE TO THE
ROMANS

WRITER. The Apostle Paul (1:1). *Date.* Romans, the sixth in chronological order of Paul's Epistles, was written from Corinth during the apostle's third visit to that city (2 Cor. 13:1), in A.D. 60. The Epistle has its occasion in the intention of the apostle soon to visit Rome. Naturally, he would wish to announce before his coming the distinctive truths which had been revealed to and through him. He would desire the Christians in Rome to have his own statement of the great doctrines of grace so bitterly assailed everywhere by legalistic teachers.

Theme. The theme of Romans is "the Gospel of God" (1:1), the very widest possible designation of the whole body of redemption truth, for it is He with whom is "no respect of persons"; and who is not "the God of the Jews only," but "of the Gentiles also" (2:11; 3:29). Accordingly, "all the world" is found guilty (3:19), and a redemption is revealed as wide as the need, upon the alone condition of faith. Not only does Romans embody in the fullest way the doctrines of grace in relation to salvation, but in three remarkable chapters (9–11) the great promises to Israel are reconciled with the promises concerning the Gentiles, and the fulfilment of the former shown to await the completion of the church and coming of the Deliverer out of Zion (11:25-27). The key-phrase is "the righteousness of God" (1:17; 3:21, 22).

The Epistle, exclusive of the introduction (1:1-17), is in seven parts: I. The whole world guilty before God, 1:18–3:20. II. Justification through the righteousness of God by faith, the Gospel remedy for guilt, 3:21–5:11. III. Crucifixion with Christ, the resurrection life of Christ, and the walk in the Spirit, the Gospel provision for inherent sin, 5:12–8:13. IV. The full result in blessing of the Gospel, 8:14-39. V. Parenthesis: the Gospel does not abolish the covenant promises to Israel, 9:1–11:36. VI. Christian life and service, 12:1–15:33. VII. The outflow of Christian love, 16:1-27.

CHAPTER 1.

Introduction (vs. 1-15); *theme* (vs. 16, 17).

Paul, a [a]servant of Jesus Christ, called
to be an apostle, separated unto the
gospel of God,
2 (Which he had promised afore [b]by
his prophets in the [c]holy scriptures,)
3 Concerning his Son Jesus Christ our
Lord, [d]which was made of the [e]seed of
David according to the flesh;
4 And declared *to be* the [f]Son of God
with power, according to the [g]spirit of
holiness, by the resurrection [h]from the
dead:
5 [i]By whom we have received grace
and apostleship, [j]for obedience to the
faith among all nations, for his name:
6 Among whom are ye also the called
of Jesus Christ:
7 To all that be in Rome, beloved of
God, called *to be* saints: Grace to you and
peace from God our Father, and the Lord
Jesus Christ.
8 First, I thank my God through Jesus
Christ for you all, [k]that your faith is spoken of throughout the whole [l]world.
9 For God is my witness, whom I
serve with my spirit in the gospel of his
Son, that without ceasing I make mention of you always in my prayers;
10 Making request, if by any means
now at length I might have a prosperous
journey [m]by the will of God to come
unto you.
11 For I long to see you, that I may
impart unto you some spiritual gift, to
the end ye may be established;
12 That is, that I may be comforted
together with you by the mutual faith
both of you and me.
13 Now I would not have you ignorant, brethren, that oftentimes I purposed to come unto you, (but was [n]let
hitherto,) that I might have some fruit
among you also, even as among other
Gentiles.
14 I am debtor both to the Greeks, and
to the Barbarians; both to the wise, and
to the unwise.
15 So, as much as in me is, I am

A.D. 60.

a *bondman.* Acts 7:58; 1 Tim. 1:12.
b *through.*
c *Sanctify, holy (things)* (N.T.). Rom. 7:12. (Mt. 4:5; Rev. 22:11.)
d *who was born.*
e See, on the Davidic descent of Christ, Lk. 3:23, *note.*
f Acts 9:20; Heb. 1:2.
g *Holy Spirit.* Rom. 5:5. (Mt. 1:18; Acts 2:4.)
h Or, *of such as were dead.*
i *through.*
j *unto obedience to faith,* i.e. faith as a principle, or method of divine dealing. Cf. Rom. 10:1-11.
k *because.*
l *kosmos* (Mt. 4:8) = mankind.
m *in.*
n *hindered.*

ready to preach the gospel to you that are at Rome also.

16 For I am not ashamed of the [a]gospel of Christ: for it is the power of God unto [1]salvation to every one that [b]believeth; to the Jew first, and also to the Greek.

17 For therein is [c]the righteousness of God revealed from faith to [d]faith: as it is written, [e]The just shall live by faith.

Part I. The guilty world.

(1) *The wrath of God revealed.*

18 For [f]the wrath of God is revealed from heaven against all ungodliness and unrighteousness of men, who [g]hold the [h]truth in unrighteousness;

(2) *The universe a revelation of the power and deity of God.*

19 Because that which may be known of God is manifest in them; for God hath shewed *it* unto them.

20 For the invisible things of him [i]from the creation of the [j]world are clearly seen, being understood by the things that are made, *even* his eternal power and [k]Godhead; so that they are [l]without excuse:

(3) *The seven stages of Gentile world apostasy.*

21 Because that, when they knew God, they glorified *him* not as God, neither were thankful; but became vain in their [m]imaginations, and their foolish heart was darkened.

22 Professing themselves to be [n]wise, they became fools,

23 And changed the glory of the [o]uncorruptible God into an image made like to corruptible man, and to birds, and fourfooted beasts, and creeping things.

(4) *The result of the Gentile world apostasy.*

24 Wherefore [p]God also gave them up to uncleanness through the lusts of their own hearts, to dishonour their own bodies between themselves:

25 [q]Who changed the truth of God into a lie, and worshipped and served the creature more than the Creator, who is blessed for ever. Amen.

26 For this cause God gave them up unto vile affections: for even their women did change the natural use into that which is against nature:

27 And likewise also the men, leaving the natural use of the woman, burned in their lust one toward another; men with men working that which is unseemly, and receiving in themselves that recompence of their error which was meet.

28 And even as they [r]did not like to retain God in *their* knowledge, God gave them over to a reprobate mind, to do those things [s]which are not convenient;

29 Being filled with all unrighteousness, fornication, wickedness, covetousness, maliciousness; full of envy, murder, debate, deceit, malignity; whisperers,

30 Backbiters, haters of God, [t]despiteful, proud, boasters, inventors of evil things, disobedient to parents,

31 Without understanding, covenantbreakers, without natural affection, implacable, unmerciful:

32 Who [u]knowing the judgment of God, that they which commit such things are worthy of death, not only do the same, but [v]have pleasure in them that do them.

CHAPTER 2.

(5) *The Gentile pagan moralizers no better than other pagans.*

Therefore thou art [w]inexcusable, O man, whosoever thou art that judgest: [x]for wherein thou

A.D. 60.

a Gospel. vs. 1, 9, 15, 16; Rom. 2:16. (Gen. 12:1-3 ; Rev. 14:6.)
b Faith. Rom. 1:17. (Gen. 3:20; Heb. 11:39.)
c a righteousness, etc.
d Faith. Rom. 3:22. (Gen. 3:20; Heb. 11:39.)
e Hab. 2:4; Gal. 3:11; Heb. 10:38.
f a wrath, etc.
g hold down.
h v. 25.
i since.
j i.e. *earth.*
k Deity.
l Rom. 2:14,15.
m reasonings, and their senseless heart was darkened.
n Isa. 19:11, 12; Acts 7:22.
o 1 Tim. 1:17; 6:15, 16.
p vs. 26, 28; Psa. 81:12; Acts 7:42; Eph. 4:18, 19; 2 Thes. 2:11, 12.
q For that they exchanged the truth of God for a lie, and worshipped and served the creature more than, etc.
r refused to have. Lit. *did not approve God.*
s Eph. 5:4.
t insolent, haughty, boastful.
u Rom. 2:2.
v also consent with them that practise them.
w Rom. 1:20; 3:19.
x 2 Sam. 12:5-7; Mt. 7:1-5; John 8:9.

[1] **(1:16)** The Heb. and Gr. words for salvation imply the ideas of *deliverance, safety, preservation, healing,* and *soundness.* Salvation is the great inclusive word of the Gospel, gathering into itself all the redemptive acts and processes: as *justification, redemption, grace, propitiation, imputation, forgiveness, sanctification,* and *glorification.* Salvation is in three tenses: (1) The believer *has been* saved from the guilt and penalty of sin (Lk. 7:50; 1 Cor. 1:18; 2 Cor. 2:15; Eph. 2:5, 8; 2 Tim. 1:9) and is *safe.* (2) The believer is *being* saved from the habit and dominion of sin (Rom. 6:14; Phil. 1:19; 2:12, 13; 2 Thes. 2:13; Rom. 8:2; Gal. 2:19, 20; 2 Cor. 3:18). (3) The believer is *to be* saved in the sense of entire conformity to Christ (Rom. 13:11; Heb. 10:36; 1 Pet. 1:5; 1 John 3:2). Salvation is by grace through faith, is a free gift, and wholly without works (Rom. 3:27, 28; 4:1-8; 6:23; Eph. 2:8). The divine order is: first salvation, then works (Eph. 2:9, 10; Tit. 3:5-8).

judgest another, thou condemnest thyself; for thou that judgest doest the same things.

2 But we are sure that the [a]judgment of God is according to truth against them which commit such things.

3 And thinkest thou this, O man, that judgest them which do such things, and doest the same, that thou shalt escape the judgment of God?

4 Or despisest thou the [b]riches of his goodness and [c]forbearance and [d]longsuffering; not knowing that the goodness of God leadeth thee to [e]repentance?

5 But after thy hardness and impenitent heart treasurest up unto thyself wrath [f]against the day of wrath and revelation of the righteous judgment of God;

6 Who will [g]render to every man according to his deeds:

7 To them who by patient continuance in well doing seek for glory and honour and [h]immortality, [i]eternal life:

8 But unto them that are [j]contentious, and do not obey the truth, but obey unrighteousness, indignation and wrath,

9 Tribulation and anguish, upon every soul of man that doeth evil, of the Jew first, and also of the [k]Gentile;

10 But glory, honour, and peace, to every man that worketh good, to the Jew first, and also to the [k]Gentile:

11 For [l]there is no respect of persons with God.

12 For as many as have [m]sinned without [n]law shall also perish without law: and as many as have sinned [o]in the law shall be judged by the law;

13 (For not the hearers of the law *are* just before God, but the doers of [p]the law shall be justified.

14 For when the Gentiles, which have not the law, do by nature the things contained in the law, these, having not the law, are a law unto themselves:

15 [q]Which shew the [r]work of the law written in their hearts, their [s]conscience also bearing witness, and *their* [t]thoughts the mean while accusing or else excusing one another;)

16 In the day when God shall judge the secrets of men by Jesus Christ according to my [u]gospel.

(6) *The Jew, knowing the law, is condemned by the law.*

17 Behold, thou art called a Jew, and [v]restest in the law, and makest thy boast of God,

18 And [w]knowest *his* will, and approvest the things that are more excellent, being instructed out of the law;

19 And art confident that thou thyself art a guide of the blind, a light of them which are in darkness,

20 An instructor of the foolish, a teacher of babes, which hast the form of knowledge and of the truth in the law.

21 Thou therefore which teachest another, teachest thou not thyself? thou that preachest a man should not steal, dost thou steal?

22 Thou that sayest a man should not commit adultery, dost thou commit adultery? thou that abhorrest idols, dost thou [x]commit sacrilege?

23 Thou that makest thy boast of the law, through [y]breaking the law dishonourest thou God?

24 For [z]the name of God is blasphemed among the Gentiles [aa]through you, as it is [bb]written.

25 For circumcision verily profiteth, if thou keep the law: but if thou be a [y]breaker of the law, thy circumcision is made uncircumcision.

26 Therefore if the uncircumcision keep the [cc]righteousness of the law, shall not his uncircumcision be counted for circumcision?

27 And shall not [dd]uncircumcision which is by nature, if it fulfil the [ee]law, judge thee, who by the letter and circumcision dost [y]transgress the law?

28 [ff]For he is not a Jew, which is one outwardly; neither *is that* circumcision, which is outward in the flesh:

29 But he *is* a Jew, which is one inwardly; and circumcision *is that* of the heart, [gg]in the spirit, *and* not in the letter; whose praise *is* not of men, but of God.

CHAPTER 3.

(7) *The advantage of the Jew works his greater condemnation.*

What advantage then hath the Jew? or what profit *is there* of circumcision?

2 Much every way: chiefly, because that unto them were committed the oracles of God.

A.D. 60.

- *a* Rom. 3:6, 19; 1 Cor. 6:9, 10.
- *b* Rom. 9:23; Eph. 1:7; 2:4, 7.
- *c* Rom. 3:25.
- *d* Ex. 34:6.
- *e* *Repentance.* Rom. 11:29. (Mt. 3:2; Acts 17:30.)
- *f* *in.*
- *g* Prov. 24:12; Jer. 17:10; Rev. 20:12,13.
- *h* *incorruption.* See 1 Cor. 15:42, 53-54.
- *i* *Life (eternal).* Rom. 5:10-21. (Mt. 7:14; Rev. 22:19.)
- *j* Acts 7:51;17:5, 32.
- *k* *Greek.*
- *l* Deut. 10:17; Acts 10:34.
- *m* *Sin.* Rom. 3:23, *note.*
- *n* 1 Cor. 9:21; Gal. 2:15.
- *o* *under.* See Rom. 3:19.
- *p* *a law.* The statement is general, true of "a law," any law.
- *q* *in that they.*
- *r* 1 Cor. 5:1.
- *s* Acts 24:25; 1 Cor. 5:1.
- *t* *their reasonings one with another accusing or else excusing them.*
- *u* *Gospel.* Rom. 10:8,15, 16. (Gen. 12:1-3; Rev. 14:6.)
- *v* v. 23; John 5:45; 9:28, 29.
- *w* Rom. 3:2; Lk. 12:47, 48.
- *x* Or, *rob temples.*
- *y* *Sin.* Rom. 3:23, *note.*
- *z* Isa. 52:5.
- *aa* *because of.*
- *bb* 2 Sam. 12:14; Isa. 52:5.
- *cc* Rom. 10:3, *note.*
- *dd* *the uncircumcision,* i.e. the Gentiles.
- *ee* *Law (of Moses).* vs. 12-27; Rom. 3:19, 20, 21, 27, 28, 31; 4:13-16. (Ex. 19:1; Gal. 3:1-29.)
- *ff* See Rom. 9:6, *note.*
- *gg* See Rom. 7:6, *note.*

3 For what if some did not believe? shall their unbelief make the [a]faith of God without effect?

4 God forbid: yea, let God be [b]true, but every man a liar; as it is written, [c]That thou mightest be justified in thy sayings, and mightest overcome when thou art judged.

5 But if our unrighteousness commend the [d]righteousness of God, what shall we say? *Is* God unrighteous who taketh vengeance? (I speak as a man)

6 God forbid: for then how shall God judge the [e]world?

7 For if the truth of God hath more abounded through my lie unto his glory; why yet am I also judged as a [f]sinner?

8 And not *rather*, (as we be slanderously reported, and as some affirm that we say,) Let us do evil, that good may come? whose [g]damnation is just.

(8) *The final verdict: the whole world guilty before God.*

9 What then? are we better *than they*? No, in no wise: for we have before proved both Jews and Gentiles, that they are all under [f]sin;

10 As it is written, [h]There is none [i]righteous, no, not one:

11 There is none that [j]understandeth, there is none that seeketh after [k]God.

12 They are all gone out of the [l]way, they are together become unprofitable; there is none that doeth good, no, not one.

13 Their throat *is* an open [m]sepulchre; with their tongues they have used deceit; the poison of asps *is* under their lips:

14 Whose mouth *is* full of cursing and [n]bitterness:

15 Their feet *are* swift to shed [o]blood:

16 Destruction and misery *are* in their ways:

17 And the way of peace have they not [p]known:

18 There is no fear of [q]God before their [r]eyes.

19 Now we know that what things soever the [s]law saith, it saith to them who are under the law: that every mouth may be stopped, and all the world may [t]become guilty before God.

20 Therefore by the deeds of the law [u]there shall no flesh be [v]justified in his sight: for by the law *is* the knowledge of [w]sin.

Part II. Justification by faith in Christ crucified,the alone remedy for sins
(Rom. 3:21–5:11).

(1) *Justification defined.*

21 But now [x]the [1]righteousness of God without the law is manifested, being witnessed by the law and the prophets;

22 Even the [y]righteousness of God *which is* [z]by [aa]faith of Jesus Christ unto all and upon all them that believe: for there is no difference:

23 For all have [2]sinned, and come short of the glory of God;

24 Being justified freely by his

A.D. 60.

a faithfulness.
b found true.
c Psa. 51:4.
d v. 21, *note.*
e *kosmos* (Mt. 4:8) = mankind.
f *Sin.* v. 23, *note.*
g i.e. condemnation.
h Psa. 14:1, 3.
i Rom. 10:10, *note.*
j Psa. 14:2.
k *God.* Psa. 14:2.
l Psa. 14:3.
m Psa. 5:9; 10:7; 140:3.
n Psa. 10:7.
o Isa. 59:7.
p Isa. 59:7, 8.
q *God.* Psa. 36:1.
r Psa. 36:1.
s *Law (of Moses).* vs. 20, 21, 27, 28, 31; Rom. 4:13-16. (Ex. 19:1; Gal. 3:1-29.)
t *be brought under the judgment of God.*
u Psa. 143:2. Cf. Gal. 2:16.
v *Justification.* vs. 20-28. (Lk. 18:14.)
w *Sin.* v. 23, *note.*
x *apart from the law a righteousness of God hath been manifested.*
y *Righteousness (garment).* Rev. 19:8. (Gen. 3:21; Rev. 19:8.)
z *through faith in.*
aa *Faith.* vs. 22, 25, 26, 28, 31; Rom. 3:25, 26. (Gen. 3:20; Heb. 11:39.)

[1] **(3:21)** The righteousness of God is neither an attribute of God, nor the changed character of the believer, but Christ Himself, who fully met in our stead and behalf every demand of the law, and who is, by the act of God called imputation (Lev. 25:50; Jas. 2:23), "made unto us . . . righteousness" (1 Cor. 1:30). "The believer in Christ is now, by grace, shrouded under so complete and blessed a righteousness that the law from Mt. Sinai can find neither fault nor diminution therein. This is that which is called the righteousness of God by faith."—*Bunyan.* See 2 Cor. 5:21; Rom. 4:6; 10:4; Phil. 3:9. See Rom. 3:26.

[2] **(3:23)** Sin, Summary: The literal meanings of the Heb. and Gr. words variously rendered "sin," "sinner," etc., disclose the true nature of sin in its manifold manifestations. Sin is *transgression,* an overstepping of the law, the divine boundary between good and evil (Psa. 51:1; Lk. 15:29); *iniquity,* an act inherently wrong, whether expressly forbidden or not; *error,* a departure from right (Psa. 51:9; Rom. 3:23); *missing the mark,* a failure to meet the divine standard; *trespass,* the intrusion of self-will into the sphere of divine authority (Eph. 2:1); *lawlessness,* or spiritual anarchy (1 Tim. 1:9); *unbelief,* or an insult to the divine veracity (John 16:9). Sin originated with Satan (Isa. 14:12-14); entered the world through Adam (Rom. 5:12); was, and is, universal, Christ alone excepted (Rom. 3:23; 1 Pet. 2:22); incurs the penalties of spiritual and physical death (Gen. 2:17; 3:19; Ezk. 18:4, 20; Rom. 6:23); and has no remedy but in the sacrificial death of Christ (Heb. 9:26; Acts 4:12) availed of by faith (Acts 13:38, 39). Sin may be summarized as threefold: An *act,* the violation of, or want of obedience to the revealed will of God; a *state,* absence of righteousness; a *nature,* enmity toward God.

[a]grace through the [1]redemption that is
in Christ Jesus:
25 Whom God hath set forth *to be* a
[2]propitiation through [b]faith in his
[c]blood, to declare his righteousness for
the [d]remission of sins that are past,
through the forbearance of God;
26 To declare, *I say*, at this time his
[3]righteousness: that he might be just,
and the justifier of him which believeth
in Jesus.
27 Where *is* boasting then? It is
excluded. By what law? of works? Nay:
but by the law of faith.
28 Therefore we conclude that a man
is [4]justified by [e]faith [f]without the deeds
of the law.

(2) *Justification a universal remedy.*

29 *Is he* the God of the Jews only? *is he*
not also of the Gentiles? Yes, of the
Gentiles also:
30 Seeing *it is* one God, which shall
justify the circumcision by faith, and
uncircumcision through faith.

(3) *Justification by faith honours the law.*

31 [5]Do we then make void the law
through [g]faith? God forbid: yea, we
establish the law.

A.D. 60.

a Grace (in salv.). Rom. 4:4-16. (Rom. 3:24; John 1:17, *note*.)
b Faith. Rom. 3:28. (Gen. 3:20; Heb. 11:39.)
c Sacrifice (of Christ). Rom. 5:9. (Gen. 4:4; Heb. 10:18.)
d passing over of sins done aforetime. i.e. since Adam. Cf. Heb. 9:15.
e Faith. Rom. 3:31. (Gen. 3:20; Heb. 11:39.)
f apart from.
g Faith. Rom. 4:3, 5. (Gen. 3:20; Heb. 11:39.)

[1]**(3:24)** Redemption, "to deliver by paying a price." The N.T. doctrine. The N.T. records the fulfilment of the O.T. types and prophecies of redemption through the sacrifice of Christ. The completed truth is set forth in the three words which are translated redemption: (1) *agorazo*, "to purchase in the market." The underlying thought is of a slave-market. The subjects of redemption are "sold under sin" (Rom. 7:14), but are, moreover, under sentence of death (Ezk. 18:4; John 3:18, 19; Rom. 3:19; Gal. 3:10), and the purchase price is the blood of the Redeemer who dies in their stead (Gal. 3:13; 2 Cor. 5:21; Mt. 20:28; Mk. 10:45; 1 Tim. 2:6; 1 Pet. 1:18); (2) *exagorazo*, "to buy out of the market." The redeemed are never again to be exposed to sale; (3) *lutroo*, "to loose," "to set free by paying a price" (John 8:32; Gal. 4:4, 5, 31; 5:13; Rom. 8:21). Redemption is by sacrifice and by power (Ex. 14:30, *note*); Christ paid the price, the Holy Spirit makes deliverance actual in experience (Rom. 8:2). See also Ex. 14:30, *note;* Isa. 59:20, *note;* Rom. 1:16, *note.*

[2]**(3:25)** Lit. a *propitiatory* [sacrifice], *through faith by his blood;* Gr. *hilasterion*, "place of propitiation." The word occurs, 1 John 2:2; 4:10, as the trans. of *hilasmos*, "that which propitiates," "a propitiatory sacrifice." *Hilasterion* is used by the Septuagint, and in Heb. 9:5 for "mercy-seat." The mercy-seat was sprinkled with atoning blood on the day of atonement (Lev. 16:14), in token that the righteous sentence of the law had been (typically) carried out, so that what must else have been a judgment-seat could righteously be a mercy-seat (Heb. 9:11-15; 4:14-16), a place of communion (Ex. 25:21, 22). In fulfilment of the type, Christ is Himself the *hilasmos*, "that which propitiates," and the *hilasterion*, "the place of propitiation"—the mercy-seat sprinkled with His own blood—the token that in our stead He so honoured the law by enduring its righteous sentence that God, who ever foresaw the cross, is vindicated in having "passed over" sins from Adam to Moses (Rom. 5:13) and the sins of believers under the old covenant (Ex. 29:33, *note*), and just in justifying sinners under the new covenant. There is no thought in propitiation of placating a vengeful God, but of doing right by His holy law and so making it possible for Him righteously to show mercy.

[3]**(3:26)** "His righteousness" here is God's consistency with His own law and holiness in freely justifying a sinner who believes in Christ; that is, one in whose behalf Christ has met every demand of the law (Rom. 10:4).

[4]**(3:28)** Justification, Summary: Justification and righteousness are inseparably united in Scripture by the fact that the same word (*dikaios*, "righteous"; *dikaioo*, "to justify") is used for both. The believing sinner is justified because Christ, having borne his sins on the cross, has been "made unto him righteousness" (1 Cor. 1:30). Justification originates in grace (Rom. 3:24; Tit. 3:4, 5); is through the redemptive and propitiatory work of Christ, who has vindicated the law (Rom. 3:24, 25; 5:9); is by faith, not works (Rom. 3:28-30; 4:5; 5:1; Gal. 2:16; 3:8, 24); and may be defined as the judicial act of God whereby He justly declares righteous one who believes on Jesus Christ. It is the Judge Himself (Rom. 8:31-34) who thus declares. The justified believer has been in court, only to learn that nothing is laid to his charge (Rom. 8:1, 33, 34).

[5]**(3:31)** The sinner establishes the law in its right use and honour by confessing his guilt, and acknowledging that by it he is justly condemned. Christ, on the sinner's behalf, establishes the law by enduring its penalty, death. Cf. Mt. 5:17, 18.

CHAPTER 4.

(4) *Justification by faith illustrated.*

What shall we say then that Abraham our father, as pertaining to the flesh, hath found?

2 For if Abraham were [a]justified by [1]works, he hath *whereof* to glory; but not before God.

3 For what saith the scripture? Abraham [b]believed [c]God, and it was [d]counted unto him for [e]righteousness.

4 Now to him that worketh is the reward not reckoned of [f]grace, but of debt.

(5) *Justifying faith defined.* (See also vs. 18-21.)

5 But to him that worketh not, but believeth on him that justifieth the ungodly, his [g]faith is [d]counted for righteousness.

6 Even as David also describeth the blessedness of the man, unto whom God [d]imputeth righteousness without works,

7 *Saying*, Blessed *are* they whose [h]iniquities are [i]forgiven, and whose [h]sins are covered.

8 Blessed *is* the man to whom the [j]Lord will not [d]impute sin.

(6) *Justification is apart from ordinances.*

9 *Cometh* this blessedness then upon the circumcision *only*, or upon the uncircumcision also? for we say that faith was reckoned to Abraham for righteousness.

10 How was it then reckoned? when he was in circumcision, or in uncircumcision? Not in circumcision, but in uncircumcision.

11 And he received the sign of circumcision, a seal of the righteousness of the faith which *he had yet* being uncircumcised: that he might be the father of all them that believe, though they be not circumcised; that righteousness might be [d]imputed unto them also:

12 And the father of circumcision to them who are not of the circumcision only, but who also walk in the steps of that faith of our father Abraham, which *he had* being *yet* uncircumcised.

(7) *Justification is apart from the law.*

13 For the promise, that he should be the heir of the [k]world, *was* not to Abraham, or to his seed, through the law, but through the righteousness of faith.

14 For if they which are of the law *be* heirs, faith is made void, and the promise made of none effect:

15 Because the law worketh wrath: for where no law is, *there is* no [h]transgression.

16 Therefore *it is* of faith, that *it might be* by grace; to the end the promise might be sure to all the seed; not to that only which is of the [l]law, but to that also which is of the faith of Abraham; who is the father of us all,

17 (As it is written, [m]I have made thee a father of many nations,) before him whom he believed, *even* God, who quickeneth the dead, and calleth those things which be not as though they were.

18 Who against hope believed in hope, that he might become the father of many nations; according to that which was spoken, [n]So shall thy seed be.

19 And being not weak in faith, he considered not his own body now dead, when he was about an hundred years old, neither yet the deadness of Sara's womb:

20 He staggered not at the promise of God through unbelief; but was strong in faith, giving glory to God;

21 And being fully persuaded that, what he had promised, he was able also to perform.

22 And therefore it was [d]imputed to him for righteousness.

23 Now it was not written for his sake alone, that it was [o]imputed to him;

24 But for us also, to whom it shall be [p]imputed, if we believe on him that raised up Jesus our Lord from the dead;

25 Who was delivered for our

A.D. 60.

a *Justification.* Rom. 5:1, 9. (Lk. 18:14; Rom. 3:28.)
b *Faith.* Rom. 5:1, 2. (Gen. 3:20; Heb. 11:39.)
c *Jehovah.* Gen. 15:6.
d Or, *reckoned*, or *imputed*, i.e. put to the account of. See Phm. 18, same word.
e *Righteousness.* vs. 5, 6, 9, 11, 13, 22. See Rom. 3:21, *note.*
f *Grace (in salv.).* vs. 4, 5, 16; Rom. 5:2, 15-21. (Rom. 3:24; John 1:17.)
g *Faith.* Rom. 5:1, 2. (Gen. 3:20; Heb. 11:39.)
h *Sin.* Rom. 3:23, *note.*
i *Forgiveness.* 2 Cor. 2:7-10. (Lev. 4:20; Mt. 26:28.)
j *Jehovah.* vs. 7, 8; Psa. 32:2.
k i.e. *earth.*
l *Law (of Moses).* vs. 13-16; Rom. 5:13, 20. (Ex. 19:1; Gal. 3:1-29.)
m Gen. 17:5.
n Gen. 15:5.
o i.e. *reckoned.*
p *Imputation.* vs. 6, 8, 9, 10, 11, 23, 24; Rom. 5:13. (Lev. 25:50; Jas. 2:23.)

[1] **(4:2)** Cf. Jas. 2:24. These are two aspects of one truth. Paul speaks of that which justifies man *before God*, viz. faith alone, wholly apart from works; James of the proof *before men*, that he who professes to have justifying faith really has it. Paul speaks of what God sees—faith; James of what men see—works, as the visible evidence of faith. Paul draws his illustration from Gen. 15:6; James from Gen. 22:1-19. James' key-phrase is "ye see" (Jas. 2:24), for men cannot see faith except as manifested through works.

offences, and was [1]raised again for our
justification.

CHAPTER 5.

The seven results of justification.

Therefore being justified by [a]faith, we
have peace with God through our
Lord Jesus Christ:
2 [b]By whom also we [c]have access by
faith into this grace wherein we stand,
and rejoice in hope of the glory of God.
3 And not only *so*, but we glory in
tribulations also: knowing that tribulation worketh patience;
4 And patience, experience; and experience, hope:
5 And hope maketh not ashamed;
because the [d]love of God is shed abroad
in our hearts by the [e]Holy Ghost which
is given unto us.
6 For when we were yet without
strength, in due time Christ died for the
ungodly.
7 For scarcely for a [f]righteous man
will one die: yet peradventure for a good
man some would even dare to die.
8 But God commendeth his [g]love
toward us, in that, while we were yet
sinners, Christ died for us.
9 Much more then, being now [h]justi-
fied by his blood, we [i]shall be saved
from wrath through him.
10 For if, when we were enemies, we
were [j]reconciled to God by the death of
his Son, much more, being reconciled,
we shall be saved [k]by his life.
11 And not only *so*, but we also joy in
God through our Lord Jesus Christ, by
whom we have now received the [l]atone-
ment.

Part III. Sanctification: indwelling sin, and the Gospel remedy (to 8:13).

(1) *Through Adam, sin and death.*

12 [2]Wherefore, as by one man sin
entered into the world, and death by sin;
and so death passed upon all men, for
that all [3]have sinned:
13 (For until the law sin was in the
world: but sin is not [m]imputed when
there is no law.
14 Nevertheless [n]death reigned from
[4]Adam to Moses, even over them that
had not sinned after the similitude of
Adam's transgression, who is the figure
of him that was to come.

(2) *Through Christ, righteousness and life.*

15 But not as the offence, so also *is* the
free gift. For if through the offence of
[o]one many be dead, much more the
grace of God, and the gift by grace,
which is by one man, Jesus Christ, hath
abounded unto many.
16 And not as *it was* by one that
sinned, *so is* the gift: for the judgment *was* by one to condemnation,

A.D. 60.

a *Faith.* Rom. 10:4, 6, 8, 9, 10, 17. (Gen. 3:20; Heb. 11:39.)
b *through.*
c *have had our access.*
d *Law (of Christ).* Rom. 13:8, 10. (Gal. 6:2; 2 John 5.)
e *Holy Spirit.* Rom. 8:1-27. (Mt. 1:18; Acts 2:4.)
f *Righteousness.* vs. 1, 19. See Rom. 10:10, *note.*
g *own.* John 3:16-17.
h *Justification.* vs. 1, 9; Rom. 8:30, 33. (Lk. 18:14; Rom. 3:28.)
i *Sacrifice (of Christ).* vs. 1, 9; 1 Cor. 5:7. (Gen. 4:4; Heb. 10:18.)
j *Reconciliation.* vs. 10, 11. See 2 Cor. 5:18, 19, 20; Col. 1:21.
k *in his life.* John 14:19; Col. 3:3, 4.
l *reconciliation.* See v. 10, *refs.*
m *Imputation.* Rom. 6:11. (Lev. 25:50; Jas. 2:23.)
n *Death (physical).* 1 Cor. 15:21, 22. (Gen. 3:19; Heb. 9:27.)
o *the one the many died.*

[1] **(4:25)** Christ died under our sins (1 Pet. 2:24; 2 Cor. 5:21); that He was raised and exalted to God's right hand, "now to appear in the presence of God for us" (Heb. 9:24), is the token that our sins are gone, that His work for us has the divine approbation and that we, for whom He suffered, are completely justified.

[2] **(5:12)** The "wherefore" relates back to Rom. 3:19-23, and may be regarded as a continuation of the discussion of the universality of sin, interrupted (Rom. 3:24–5:11) by the passage on justification and its results.

[3] **(5:12)** The first sin wrought the moral ruin of the race. The demonstration is simple. (1) Death is universal (vs. 12, 14), all die: sinless infants, moral people, religious people, equally with the depraved. For a universal effect there must be a universal cause; that cause is a state of universal sin (v. 12). (2) But this universal state must have had a cause. It did. The consequence of Adam's sin was that "the many were made sinners" (v. 19)—"By the offence of one judgment came upon all men unto condemnation" (v. 18). (3) Personal sins are not meant here. From Adam to Moses death reigned (v. 14), although, there being no law, personal guilt was not imputed (v. 13). Accordingly, from Gen. 4:7 to Ex. 29:14 the sin-offering is not once mentioned. Then, since physical death from Adam to Moses was not due to the sinful acts of those who die (v. 13), it follows that it was due to a universal sinful *state*, or nature, and that state is declared to be our inheritance from Adam. (4) The moral state of fallen man is described in Scripture (Gen. 6:5; 1 Ki. 8:46; Psa. 14:1-3; 39:5; Jer. 17:9; Mt. 18:11; Mk. 7:20, 23; Rom. 1:21; 2; 3:9-19; 7:24; 8:7; John 3:6; 1 Cor. 2:14; 2 Cor. 3:14; 4:4; Gal. 5:19-21; Eph. 2:1-3, 11, 12; 4:18-22; Col. 1:21; Heb. 3:13; Jas. 4:14). See 1 Cor. 15:22.

[4] **(5:14)** Broadly, the contrast is: Adam: sin, death; Christ: righteousness, life. Adam drew down into his ruin the old creation (Rom. 8:19-22) of which he was lord and head. Christ brings into moral unity

but the free gift *is* of many [a]offences unto justification.

17 For if by one man's [a]offence death reigned by one; much more they which receive abundance of grace and of the gift of [b]righteousness shall reign in life by one, Jesus Christ.)

18 Therefore as by the [a]offence of one *judgment came* upon all men to condemnation; even so by the righteousness of one *the free gift came* upon all men unto [c]justification of life.

19 For as by one man's disobedience many were made [a]sinners, so by the obedience of one shall many be made righteous.

20 Moreover the [d]law [e]entered, that the offence might abound. But where sin abounded, grace did much more abound:

21 That as [1]sin hath reigned unto death, even so might [f]grace reign through righteousness unto [g]eternal life by Jesus Christ our Lord.

CHAPTER 6.

(3) *Deliverance from the power of indwelling sin.*

(a) *By union with Christ in death and resurrection.*

What shall we say then? Shall we continue in [a]sin, that [h]grace may abound?

2 God forbid. How shall we, that are dead to [a]sin, live any longer therein?

3 Know ye not, that [i]so many of us as were baptized into Jesus Christ were baptized into his death?

4 Therefore we are buried with him by baptism into death: that like as Christ was raised up from the dead by the glory of the Father, even so we also should walk in newness of life.

A.D. 60.

a *Sin.* Rom. 3:23, *note.*
b *Righteousness.* vs. 17, 18, 21. See Rom. 3:21, *note.*
c vs. 15-18; Isa. 53:11.
d *Law (of Moses).* Rom. 6:14, 15. (Ex. 19:1; Gal. 3:1-29.
e *came in by the way.* Gal. 3:19-25.
f *Grace (in salv.).* vs. 2, 15-21; Rom. 11:5, 6. (Rom. 3:24; John 1:17, *note.*)
g *Life (eternal).* vs. 10-21. Rom. 6:4, 22, 23. (Mt. 7:14; Rev. 22:19.)
h *Grace (imparted).* vs. 1, 14, 15; Rom. 12:3, 6. (Rom. 6:1-15; 2 Pet. 3:18, *note.*)
i *all we who were baptized.*
j Or, *become united with him by,* etc.
k *was.*
l *done away.*
m *hath died.*
n Lit. *once for all.* Heb. 10:10-12, 14.
o *the life that Jesus liveth.*
p *even so.*
q *Imputation.* Rom. 8:18. (Lev. 25:50; Jas. 2:23.)
r *Righteousness.* vs. 13, 16, 18, 19, 20. See Rom. 10:10, *note.*
s *Law (of Moses).* Rom. 7:1-9, 12-14, 16, 25. (Ex. 19:1; Gal. 3:1-29.)

5 For if we have [j]been planted together in the likeness of his death, we shall be also *in the likeness* of *his* resurrection:

6 Knowing this, that our [2]old man [k]is crucified with *him*, that the body of sin might be [l]destroyed, that henceforth we should not serve sin.

7 For he that [m]is dead is freed from sin.

8 Now if we be dead with Christ, we believe that we shall also live with him:

9 Knowing that Christ being raised from the dead dieth no more; death hath no more dominion over him.

10 For in that he died, he died unto [a]sin [n]once: but [o]in that he liveth, he liveth unto God.

(b) *By counting the old life to be dead, and by yielding the new life to God.*

11 [p]Likewise [q]reckon ye also yourselves to be dead indeed unto sin, but alive unto God through Jesus Christ our Lord.

12 Let not [a]sin therefore reign in your mortal body, that ye should obey it in the lusts thereof.

13 Neither yield ye your members *as* instruments of [r]unrighteousness unto [a]sin: but yield yourselves unto God, as those that are alive from the dead, and your members *as* instruments of righteousness unto God.

(c) *By deliverance from the law through death, and by the Spirit* (i.e. *as in Rom. 8:2*).

14 For sin shall not have dominion over you: for ye are not under the [s]law, but under grace.

15 [3]What then? shall we [a]sin, because we are not under the law, but under [h]grace? God forbid.

16 Know ye not, that to whom ye

---

with God, and into eternal life, the new creation of which He is Lord. and Head (Eph. 1:22, 23). Even the animal and material creation, cursed for man's sake (Gen. 3:17), will be delivered by Christ (Isa. 11:6-9; Rom. 8:19-22).

[1]**(5:21)** "Sin" in Rom. 6, 7 is the nature in distinction from "sins," which are manifestations of that nature. Cf. 1 John 1:8 with 1 John 1:10, where this distinction also appears.

[2]**(6:6)** The expression occurs elsewhere, in Eph. 4:22 and Col. 3:9, and always means the man of old, corrupt human nature, the inborn tendency to evil in all men. In Rom. 6:6 it is the natural man himself; in Eph. 4:22; Col. 3:9 his *ways. Positionally,* in the reckoning of God, the old man is crucified, and the believer is exhorted to make this good in *experience,* reckoning it to be so by definitely "putting off" the old man and "putting on" the new (Col. 3:8-14. See Eph. 4:24, *note* 3).

[3]**(6:15)** The old relation to the law and sin, and the new relation to Christ and life are illustrated by

yield yourselves servants to obey, his
[a]servants ye are to whom ye obey;
whether of [b]sin unto death, or of obedience unto righteousness?
17 But God be thanked, that ye were
the servants of [b]sin, but ye have obeyed
from the heart that form of doctrine
which was delivered you.
18 Being then made free from [b]sin, ye
became the servants of righteousness.
19 I speak after the manner of men
because of the infirmity of your flesh: for
as ye have yielded your members servants to uncleanness and to [c]iniquity
unto iniquity; even so now yield your
members servants to righteousness unto
[d]holiness.
20 For when ye were the servants of
sin, ye were free from righteousness.
21 What fruit had ye then in those
things whereof ye are now ashamed? for
the end of those things *is* death.
22 But now being made free from [b]sin,
and become servants to God, ye have
your fruit unto [d]holiness, and the end
everlasting life.
23 For the wages of [b]sin *is* death; but
the gift of God *is* [e]eternal life [f]through
Jesus Christ our Lord.

CHAPTER 7.

Know ye not, brethren, (for I speak to
them that know the law,) how that
the law hath dominion over a man as
long as he liveth?
2 For the woman which hath an
husband is bound by the law to [g]*her*
husband so long as he liveth; but if the
husband be dead, she is loosed from the
law of [g]*her* husband.
3 So then if, while [g]*her* husband liveth,
she be married to another man, she shall
be called an adulteress: but if [g]her husband be dead, she is free from that law;
so that she is no adulteress, though she
be married to another man.
4 Wherefore, my brethren, ye also [h]are
become dead to the law [i]by the body of
Christ; that ye should be [j]married to
another, *even* to him who is raised from
the dead, that we should bring forth
fruit unto God.
5 For when we were in the flesh, the
motions of sins, which were by the law,
did work in our members to bring forth
fruit unto death.
6 But now we [k]are delivered from the
law, [l]that being dead wherein we were
held; that we should serve in [1]newness of
spirit, and not *in* the oldness of the letter.

(d) *The believer is not made holy by the law.*

7 What shall we say then? *Is* the law
[b]sin? God forbid. Nay, I had not known
sin, but by the law: for I had not known
[m]lust, except the law had said, [n]Thou
shalt not covet.
8 But [o]sin, taking occasion by the commandment, wrought in me all manner of
concupiscence. For without the law sin
was dead.
9 For I was alive without the law once:
but [2]when the commandment came, [o]sin
revived, and I died.
10 And the commandment, which *was*
ordained to life, I found *to be* unto death.

A.D. 60.

a *bond-servants.*
b *Sin.* Rom. 3:23, *note.*
c *lawlessness.*
d *Sanctification.* Rev. 22:11, *note.*
e *Life (eternal).* vs. 4:22, 23; Rom. 8:2, 6, 10. (Mt. 7:14; Rev. 22:19.)
f *in.*
g *the.*
h *were made dead.*
i *through.*
j *joined.* Eph. 5:31, same Greek word. *Bride (of Christ).* 2 Cor. 11:1-3. (John 3:29; Rev. 19:6-8.)
k *have been discharged.*
l *having died to that wherein.*
m *coveting.* Cf. Mt. 5:27-30.
n Ex. 20:17.
o *Sin.* Rom. 5:21, *note.*

the effect of death upon servitude (6:16-23), and marriage (7:1-6). (1) The old servitude was nominally to the law, but, since the law had no delivering power, the real master continued to be sin in the nature. The end was death. The law could not give life, and "sin" (here personified as the old self) is in itself deathful. But death in another form, i.e. crucifixion with Christ, has intervened (v. 6) to free the servant from his double bondage to sin (vs. 6, 7), and to the law (7:4, 6). (2) This effect of death is further illustrated by widowhood. Death dissolves the marriage relation (7:1-3). As natural death frees a wife from the law of her husband, so crucifixion with Christ sets the believer free from the law. See Gal. 3:24, *note.*

[1]**(7:6)** Cf. Rom. 2:29; 2 Cor. 3:6. "The letter" is a Paulinism for the law, as "spirit" in these passages is his word for the relationships and powers of new life in Christ Jesus. In 2 Cor. 3 a series is presented of contrasts of law with "spirit," of the old covenant and the new. The contrast is not between two methods of interpretation, literal and spiritual, but between two methods of divine dealing: one through the law, the other through the Holy Spirit.

[2]**(7:9)** The passage (vs. 7-25) is autobiographical. Paul's religious experience was in three strongly marked phases: (1) He was a godly Jew under the law. That the passage does not refer to that period is clear from his own explicit statements elsewhere. At that time he held himself to be "blameless" as concerned the law (Phil. 3:6). He had "lived in all good conscience" (Acts 23:1). (2) With his conversion

11 For [a]sin, taking occasion by the commandment, deceived me, and by it slew *me*.

12 Wherefore the law *is* [b]holy, and the commandment holy, and just, and good.

13 Was then that which is good made death unto me? God forbid. But [a]sin, [c]that it might appear [a]sin, working death in me by that which is good; that sin by the commandment might become exceeding [a]sinful.

14 For we know that the law is spiritual: but I am [1d]carnal, sold under [a]sin.

(e) *The strife of the two natures under the law.*

15 For that which [2]I do I allow not: for what I would, that do I not; but what I hate, that do I.

16 If then I do that which I would not, I consent unto the law that *it is* good.

17 Now then it is no more I that do it, but [a]sin that dwelleth in me.

18 For I know that in me (that is, in my flesh,) dwelleth no good thing: for to will is present with me; but *how* to perform that which is good I find not.

19 For the good that I would I do not: but the evil which I would not, that I do.

20 Now if I do that I would not, it is no more I that do it, but [a]sin that dwelleth in me.

21 I find then a [3]law, that, when I would do good, evil is present with me.

22 For I delight in the law of God after the inward man:

23 But I see another law in my members, warring against the law of my mind, and bringing me into captivity to the law of [a]sin which is in my members.

24 O wretched man that I am! who shall deliver me [e]from the body of this death?

25 I thank God through Jesus Christ our Lord. So then with the mind I myself serve the [f]law of God; but with the [g]flesh the law of [a]sin.

A.D. 60.

a *Sin.* Rom. 5:21, *note.*

b *Sanctify, holy (things)* (N.T.). Rom. 16:16. (Mt. 4:5; Rev. 22:11.)

c *that it might be shewn to be sin by working death, etc.*

d i.e. *fleshly.*

e Or, *out of this body of death.* Rom. 8:11; 1 Cor. 15:51, 52; 1 Thes. 4:14-17.

f *Law (of Moses).* Rom. 8:2, 3, 4, 7. (Ex. 19:1; Gal. 3:1-29.)

g *Flesh.* vs. 14, 18, 23, 25; Rom. 8:1, 3, 4-11. (John 1:13; Jude 23.)

came new light upon the law itself. He now perceived it to be "spiritual" (v. 14). He now saw that, so far from having kept it, he was condemned by it. He had supposed himself to be "alive," but now the commandment really "came" (v. 9) and he "died." Just when the apostle passed through the experience of Rom. 7:7-25 we are not told. Perhaps during the days of physical blindness at Damascus (Acts 9:9); perhaps in Arabia (Gal. 1:17). It is the experience of a renewed man, under the law, and still ignorant of the delivering power of the Holy Spirit (cf. Rom. 8:2). (3) With the great revelations afterward embodied in Galatians and Romans, the apostle's experience entered its third phase. He now knew himself to be "dead to the law by the body of Christ," and, in the power of the indwelling Spirit, "free from the law of sin and death" (8:2); while "the righteousness of the law" was wrought in him (not *by* him) while he walked after the Spirit (8:4). Romans 7 is the record of past conflicts and defeats experienced as a renewed man under law.

[1]**(7:14)** Cf. 1 Cor. 3:1, 4. "Carnal"= "fleshly" is Paul's word for the Adamic nature, and for the believer who "walks," i.e. lives, under the power of it. "Natural" is his characteristic word for the unrenewed man (1 Cor. 2:14), as "spiritual" designates the renewed man who walks in the Spirit (1 Cor. 3:1; Gal. 6:1).

[2]**(7:15)** The apostle personifies the strife of the two natures in the believer, the old or Adamic nature, and the divine nature received through the new birth (1 Pet. 1:23; 2 Pet. 1:4; Gal. 2:20; Col. 1:27) The "I" which is Saul of Tarsus, and the "I" which is Paul the apostle are at strife, and "Paul" is in defeat. In Chapter 8 this strife is effectually taken up on the believer's behalf by the Holy Spirit (8:2; Gal. 5:16, 17) and Paul is victorious. *Contra,* Eph. 6:12, where the conflict is not fleshly, but spiritual.

[3]**(7:21)** Six "laws" are to be distinguished in Romans: The law of *Moses,* which condemns (3:19); "law" as a *principle* (3:21); the law of *faith,* which excludes self-righteousness (3:27); the law of *sin* in the members, which is victorious over the law of the mind (7:21, 23, 25); the law of *the mind,* which consents to the law of Moses but cannot do it because of the law of sin in the members (7:16, 23); and the "law of *the Spirit,*" having power to deliver the believer from the law of sin which is in his members, and his conscience from condemnation by the Mosaic law. Moreover the Spirit works in the yielded believer the very righteousness which Moses' law requires (8:2, 4).

CHAPTER 8.

There is therefore now no [a]condemnation to them which are in Christ Jesus, [b]who walk not after the flesh, but after the Spirit.

(f) *The new law of the Spirit delivers* (v. 2), *makes righteous* (v. 4).

2 For the law of the [1]Spirit of life in Christ Jesus hath made me free from the law of [c]sin and death.

3 For what the law could not do, in that it was weak through the flesh, God sending his own Son in the likeness of sinful flesh, and [d]for [c]sin, condemned sin in the flesh:

4 That the righteousness of the law might be fulfilled in us, who walk not after the flesh, but after the Spirit.

(g) *Conflict of the Spirit with the flesh.* (Cf. Gal. 5:16-18.)

5 For they that are after the flesh do mind the things of the flesh; but they that are after the Spirit the things of the Spirit.

6 For to be [e]carnally minded *is* death; but to be spiritually minded *is* life and peace.

7 Because the [e]carnal mind *is* enmity against God: for it is not subject to the [f]law of God, neither indeed can be.

8 So then they that are in the flesh cannot please God.

9 But ye are not in the flesh, but in the Spirit, if so be that the Spirit of God dwell in you. Now if any man have not the Spirit of Christ, he is none of his.

10 And if Christ *be* in you, the body *is* dead because of [c]sin; but the Spirit *is* [g]life because of righteousness.

11 But if the Spirit of him that raised up Jesus from the dead dwell in you, he that [h]raised up Christ from the dead shall also quicken your mortal bodies [i]by his Spirit that dwelleth in you.

12 Therefore, brethren, we are debtors, not to the flesh, to live after the flesh.

13 For if ye live after the [j]flesh, ye shall die: but if ye through the Spirit do [k]mortify the deeds of the body, ye shall live.

A.D. 60.

a *Judgments (the seven).* Rom. 14:10. (2 Sam. 7:14; Rev. 20:12.)

b The statement ends with "Christ Jesus"; the last ten words are interpolated.

c *Sin.* Rom. 5:21, *note.*

d *as an offering.*

e i.e. *fleshly.*

f *Law (of Moses).* vs. 2, 3, 4, 7; Rom. 9:31, 32. (Ex. 19:1; Gal. 3:1-29.)

g *Life (eternal).* vs. 2, 6, 10; 2 Cor. 2:16. (Mt. 7:14; Rev. 22:19.)

h *Resurrection.* Phil. 3:20, 21. (Job 19:25; 1 Cor. 15:52.)

i Or, *because of.*

j *Flesh.* vs. 1, 3, 4-9, 12, 13; Rom. 13:14. (John 1:13; Jude 23.)

k *make to die the doings of the body.* Col. 3:5-10.

l *Adoption.* vs. 15, 23; Rom. 9:4. (Rom. 8:15, 23; Eph. 1:5.)

m *Imputation.* 2 Cor. 5:19. (Lev. 25:50; Jas. 2:23.)

n *creation.* vs. 20-23; cf. Gen. 3:17-19.

o Lit. *unveiling.* Mt. 13:40-43; 1 John 3:2.

p Lit. *placing as sons.* See *Adoption,* v. 15, *ref.*

q Eph. 1:14; 4:30 Phil. 3:20, 21.

r Or, *in that hope were we saved.*

Part IV. Full result of the Gospel.

(1) *The believer a son and heir.* (Cf. Gal. 4:4.)

14 For as many as are led by the Spirit of God, they are the sons of God.

15 For ye have not received the spirit of bondage again to fear; but ye have received the Spirit of [l]adoption, whereby we cry, Abba, Father.

16 The Spirit itself beareth witness with our spirit, that we are the [2]children of God:

17 And if children, then heirs; heirs of God, and joint-heirs with Christ; if so be that we suffer with *him,* that we may be also glorified together.

(2) *The creation, delivered from suffering and death, kept for the sons of God.* (Cf. Gen. 3:18,19.)

18 For I [m]reckon that the sufferings of this present time *are* not worthy *to be compared* with the glory which shall be revealed in us.

19 For the earnest expectation of the [n]creature waiteth for the [o]manifestation of the sons of God.

20 For the [n]creature was made subject to vanity, not willingly, but by reason of him who hath subjected *the same* in hope,

21 Because the [n]creature itself also shall be delivered from the bondage of corruption into the glorious liberty of the children of God.

22 For we know that the whole creation groaneth and travaileth in pain together until now.

23 And not only *they,* but ourselves also, which have the firstfruits of the Spirit, even we ourselves groan within ourselves, waiting for the [p]adoption, *to wit,* the [q]redemption of our body.

24 For [r]we are saved by hope: but hope that is seen is not hope: for what a man seeth, why doth he yet hope for?

25 But if we hope for that we see not, *then* do we with patience wait for *it.*

[1] **(8:2)** Hitherto in Romans the Holy Spirit has been mentioned but once (Rom. 5:5); in this chapter He is mentioned nineteen times. Redemption is by blood and by power (Ex. 14:30, *note*). Rom. 3:21–5:11 speaks of the redemptive price; Rom. 8 of redemptive power.

[2] **(8:16)** Gr. *teknon,* "one born," a child (and so in vs. 17, 21); not, as in verse 14, "sons" (Gr. *huios*). See Gal. 4:1, 7, where babyhood and sonhood are contrasted. Also "Adoption" (Rom. 8:15, 23; Eph. 1:5).

(3) *The Spirit an indwelling Intercessor.* (Cf. Heb. 7:25.)

26 Likewise the Spirit also helpeth our infirmities: for we know not [a]what we should pray for as we ought: but the Spirit [b]itself maketh intercession for us with groanings which cannot be uttered.

27 And he that searcheth the hearts knoweth what *is* the mind of the [c]Spirit, because he maketh intercession for the saints according to *the will of* God.

(4) *The unfailing purpose of God through the Gospel.*

28 And we know that all things work together for good to them that love God, to them who are the called according to *his* purpose.

29 For whom he did [d]foreknow, he also did predestinate *to be* conformed to the image of his Son, that he might be the firstborn among many brethren.

30 Moreover whom he did [e]predestinate, them he also called: and whom he called, them he also [f]justified: and whom he justified, them he also glorified.

31 What shall we then say to these things? If God *be* for us, who *can be* against us?

32 He that spared not his own Son, but delivered him up for us all, how shall he not with him also freely give us all things?

33 Who shall lay any thing to the charge of God's [g]elect? [h]*It is* God that [i]justifieth.

34 Who *is* he that condemneth? [j]*It is* Christ that died, yea rather, that is risen again, who is even at the right hand of God, who also maketh intercession for us.

(5) *The believer secure.*

35 Who shall separate us from the love of Christ? *shall* tribulation, or distress, or persecution, or famine, or nakedness, or peril, or sword?

36 As it is written, [k]For thy sake we are killed all the day long; we are accounted as sheep for the slaughter.

37 Nay, in all these things we are more than conquerors through him that loved us.

38 For I am persuaded, that neither death, nor life, nor [l]angels, nor principalities, nor powers, nor things present, nor things to come,

39 Nor height, nor depth, nor any other [m]creature, shall be able to separate us from the love of God, which is in Christ Jesus our Lord.

A.D. 60.

a how to pray.
b himself.
c Holy Spirit. vs. 1, 2, 5, 9, 10, 11, 13, 14, 15, 16, 23, 26, 27; Rom. 9:1. (Mt. 1:18; Acts 2:4.)
d Foreknowledge. Rom. 11:2. (Acts 2:23; 1 Pet. 1:20.)
e Predestination. vs. 29, 30; 1 Cor. 2:7. (Acts 4:28; Eph. 1:5, 11.)
f Assurance. 1 Cor. 12:12, 13. (Isa. 32:17; Jude 1.)
g Election (corporate). 1 Cor. 1:27, 28. (Deut. 7:6; 1 Pet. 1:2.)
h Or, *Shall God that justifieth?*
i Justification. vs. 30, 33; 1 Cor. 4:4. (Lk. 18:14; Rom. 3:28.)
j Or, *Shall Christ Jesus who died?*
k Psa. 44:22.
l Heb. 1:4, *note.*
m Or, *created thing.*
n Holy Spirit. Rom. 14:17. (Mt. 1:18; Acts 2:4.)
o Israel (prophecies). vs. 1-8; Rom. 10:1-4. (Gen. 12:2, 3; Rom. 11:26.)
p Adoption. Gal. 4:5. (Rom. 8:15, 23; Eph. 1:5.)
q Also v. 8; Gr. *teknon, child.* See Rom. 8:16, *note.*
r Gen. 21:12.

CHAPTER 9.

Part V. Parenthetic (Rom. 9-11).
The Gospel does not set aside the covenants with Israel.

(1) *The apostolic solicitude for Israel.*

I say the truth in Christ, I lie not, my conscience also bearing me witness in the [n]Holy Ghost,

2 That I have great heaviness and continual sorrow in my heart.

3 For I could wish that myself were accursed from Christ for my brethren, my kinsmen according to the flesh:

(2) *The sevenfold privilege of Israel.*

4 Who are Israelites; [o]to whom *pertaineth* the [p]adoption, and the glory, and the covenants, and the giving of the law, and the service *of God,* and the promises;

5 Whose *are* the fathers, and of whom as concerning the flesh Christ *came,* who is over all, God blessed for ever. Amen.

(3) *The distinction between Jews who are mere natural descendants from Abraham, and Jews who are also of his spiritual seed.*

6 Not as though the word of God hath taken none effect. [1]For they *are* not all Israel, which are of Israel:

7 Neither, because they are the seed of Abraham, *are they* all [q]children: but, [r]In Isaac shall thy seed be called.

(*The distinction illustrated.*)

8 That is, They which are the children

[1] **(9:6)** The distinction is between Israel after the flesh, the mere natural posterity of Abraham, and Israelites who, through faith, are also Abraham's spiritual children. Gentiles who believe are also of Abraham's spiritual seed; but here the apostle is not considering them, but only the two kinds of Israelites, the natural and the spiritual Israel (Rom, 4:1-3; Gal. 3:6, 7. Cf. John 8:37-39). See Rom. 11:1, *note.*

of the flesh, these *are* not the children of God: but the children of the promise are counted for the seed.

9 For this *is* the word of promise, [a]At this time will I come, and Sara shall have a son.

10 And not only *this;* but when Rebecca also had conceived by one, *even* by our father Isaac;

11 (For *the children* being not yet born, neither having done any good or evil, that the purpose of God according to [b]election might stand, not of works, but of him that calleth;)

12 It was said unto her, [c]The elder shall serve the younger.

13 As it is written, [d]Jacob have I loved, but Esau have I hated.

(4) *God's mercy is under his sovereign will.*

14 What shall we say then? *Is there* unrighteousness with God? God forbid.

15 For he saith to Moses, [e]I will have mercy on whom I will have mercy, and I will have compassion on whom I will have compassion.

16 So then *it is* not of him that willeth, nor of him that runneth, but of God that sheweth mercy.

17 For the scripture saith unto Pharaoh, [f]Even for this same purpose have I raised thee up, that I might shew my power in thee, and that my name might be declared throughout all the earth.

18 Therefore hath he mercy on whom he will *have mercy,* and whom he will he hardeneth.

19 Thou wilt say then unto me, Why doth he yet find fault? For who hath resisted his will?

20 Nay but, O man, who art thou that repliest against God? Shall the thing formed say to him that formed *it,* Why hast thou made me thus?

21 Hath not the potter power over the clay, of the same lump to make one vessel unto honour, and another unto dishonour?

22 *What* if God, willing to shew *his* wrath, and to make his power known, endured with much longsuffering the vessels of wrath fitted to destruction:

23 And that he might make known the

A.D. 60.

a Gen. 18:10; Heb. 11:11.

b *Election (corporate).* Rom. 11:5, 7, 28. (Deut. 7:6; 1 Pet. 1:2.)

c Gen. 25:23.

d Mal. 1:2, 3.

e Ex. 33:19.

f Ex. 9:16.

g vs. 24-30; Isa. 42:6, 7.

h *from among.* Cf. Acts 15:14.

i Hos. 2:23.

j Hos. 1:10.

k Gr. *huioi, sons.* Eph. 1:5, *note.*

l Hos. 1:10.

m vs. 27, 28; Isa. 10:22, 23.

n Rom. 1:16, *note.*

o *Adonai Jehovah.* Isa. 10:23.

p *LORD of hosts.* Isa. 1:9.

q *Remnant.* vs. 25-29; Rev. 6:9-11. (Isa. 1:9; Rom. 11:5.)

r Rom. 10:10, *note.*

s Rom. 10:3, *note.*

t *Law (of Moses).* vs. 31, 32 ; Rom. 10:4, 5. (Ex. 19:1; Gal. 3:1-29.)

u *Christ (as Stone).* vs. 32, 33; 1 Cor. 1:23. (Ex. 17:6; 1 Pet. 2:8.)

v Psa. 118:22; Isa. 8:14; 28:16; Mt. 21:42; 1 Pet. 2:6.

w *Israel (prophecies).* vs. 1-4; Rev. 7:4. (Gen. 12:2, 3; Rom. 11:26.)

x Rom. 1:16, *note.*

y Cf. Rom. 3:21, *note.*

riches of his glory on the vessels of mercy, which he had afore prepared unto glory,

24 Even us, whom he hath called, [g]not of the Jews only, but also [h]of the Gentiles?

(5) *The prophets foretold the blinding of Israel, and mercy to Gentiles.*

25 As he saith also in Osee, [i]I will call them my people, which were not my people; and her beloved, which was not beloved.

26 And it shall come to pass, *that* in the place where it was said unto them, [j]Ye *are* not my people; there shall they be called the [k]children of the living [l]God.

27 Esaias also crieth concerning Israel, [m]Though the number of the children of Israel be as the sand of the sea, a remnant shall be [n]saved:

28 For he will finish the work, and cut *it* short in righteousness: because a short work will the [o]Lord make upon the earth.

29 And as Esaias said before, Except the [p]Lord of Sabaoth had left us a [q]seed, we had been as Sodoma, and been made like unto Gomorrha.

30 What shall we say then? That the Gentiles, which followed not after [r]righteousness, have attained to righteousness, even the righteousness which is of faith.

31 But Israel, which followed after the law of righteousness, hath not attained to the law of [s]righteousness.

32 Wherefore? Because *they sought it* not by faith, but as it were by the works of the [t]law. For they stumbled at that [u]stumblingstone;

33 As it is written, [v]Behold, I lay in Sion a [u]stumblingstone and rock of offence: and whosoever believeth on him shall not be ashamed.

CHAPTER 10.

(6) *The apparent failure of the promises to Israel explained by their unbelief.*

Brethren, my heart's desire and prayer to God [w]for Israel is, that they might be [x]saved.

2 For I bear them record that they have a zeal of God, but not according to knowledge.

3 For they being ignorant of God's righteousness, and going about to establish their own [1y]righteousness,

[1](10:3) The word "righteousness" here, and in the passages having marginal references to this, means legal, or self-righteousness; the futile effort of man to work out under law a character which God can approve (Rev. 19:8, *note*).

have not submitted themselves unto the righteousness of God.

4 For Christ *is* the end of the [a]law for righteousness to every one that believeth.

5 For Moses describeth the righteousness which is of the [a]law, [b]That the man which doeth those things shall live by them.

6 But the [c]righteousness which is of faith speaketh on this wise, Say not in thine heart, [d]Who shall ascend into heaven? (that is, to bring Christ down *from above*:)

7 Or, Who shall descend into the deep? (that is, to bring up Christ again from the dead.)

8 But what saith it? [e]The word is nigh thee, *even* in thy mouth, and in thy heart: that is, the word of faith, which we preach;

9 [f]That if thou shalt confess with thy mouth the [g]Lord Jesus, and shalt believe in thine heart that God hath raised him from the dead, thou shalt be [h]saved.

10 For with the heart man [i]believeth unto [1]righteousness; and with the mouth confession is made unto salvation.

11 For the scripture saith, [j]Whosoever believeth on him shall not be ashamed.

12 For [k]there is no difference between the Jew and the Greek: for the same Lord over all is rich unto all that call upon him.

13 For whosoever shall call upon the name of the [l]Lord shall be [h]saved.

14 How then shall they call on him in whom they have not believed? and how shall they believe in him of whom they have not heard? and how shall they hear without a preacher?

15 And how shall they preach, except they be sent? as it is written, [m]How beautiful are the feet of them that preach the [n]gospel of peace, and bring glad tidings of good things!

16 But they have not all obeyed the gospel. For Esaias saith, [o]Lord, who hath believed our report?

17 So then faith *cometh* by hearing, and hearing by the word of God.

18 But I say, Have they not heard? Yes verily, [p]their sound went into all the earth, and their words unto the ends of the [q]world.

19 But I say, Did not Israel know? First Moses saith, [r]I will provoke you to jealousy by *them that are* no people, *and* by a foolish nation I will anger you.

20 But Esaias is very bold, and saith, [s]I was found of them that sought me not; I was made manifest unto [t]them that asked not after me.

21 But to Israel he saith, [u]All day long I have stretched forth my hands unto a disobedient and gainsaying people.

CHAPTER 11.

(7) *But spiritual Israel is finding salvation.*

I say then, [v]Hath [w]God [2]cast away [x]his people? God forbid. For I also am an Israelite, of the seed of Abraham, *of* the tribe of Benjamin.

2 [w]God hath not cast away his people which he [y]foreknew. Wot ye not what the scripture saith of Elias? how he maketh intercession to God against Israel, saying,

3 [z]Lord, they have killed thy prophets, and digged down thine altars; and I am left alone, and they seek my life.

4 But what saith the answer of God unto him? [aa]I have reserved to myself seven thousand men, who

A.D. 60.

a *Law (of Moses).* vs. 4, 5; Rom. 13:8, 10. (Ex. 19:1; Gal. 3:1-29.)
b Lev. 18:5.
c See v. 10.
d Deut. 30:12, 13.
e Deut. 30:14.
f Mt. 10:32; Lk. 12:8; Acts 8:37.
g *Jesus as Lord.* Cf. 1 Cor. 12:3.
h Rom. 1:16, *note.*
i *Faith.* vs. 4, 6, 8, 9, 10, 17; Rom. 14:23. (Gen. 3:20; Heb. 11:39.)
j Isa. 28:16; 49:23.
k Rom. 3:22; Gal. 3:28.
l *Jehovah.* Joel 2:32.
m Isa. 52:7; Nah. 1:15.
n *Gospel.* vs. 8, 15, 16; Rom. 11:28. (Gen. 12:1-3; Rev. 14:6.)
o Isa. 53:1.
p Psa. 19:4.
q *oikoumene* = inhabited earth. (Lk. 2:1.)
r Deut. 32:21.
s Isa. 65:1.
t vs. 19, 20; Isa. 42:6, 7.
u Isa. 65:2.
v Or, *Did God cast off.*
w *Jehovah.* Psa. 94:14.
x *Remnant.* vs. 1-5.
y *Foreknowledge.* 2 Pet. 3:17. (Acts 2:23; 1 Pet. 1:20.)
z 1 Ki. 19:10, 14.
aa 1 Ki. 19:18.

[1] **(10:10)** Righteousness here, and in the passages which refer to Rom. 10:10, means that righteousness of God which is judicially reckoned to all who believe on the Lord Jesus Christ; believers *are* the righteous. See Rom. 3:21, *note.*

[2] **(11:1)** That Israel has not been forever set aside is the theme of this chapter. (1) The salvation of Paul proves that there is still a remnant (v. 1). (2) The doctrine of the remnant proves it (vs. 2-6). (3) The present national unbelief was foreseen (vs. 7-10). (4) Israel's unbelief is the Gentile opportunity (vs. 11-25). (5) Israel is judicially broken off from the good olive tree, Christ (vs. 17-22). (6) They are to be grafted in again (vs. 23, 24). (7) The promised Deliverer will come out of Zion and the nation will be saved (vs. 25-29). That the Christian now inherits the distinctive Jewish promises is not taught in Scripture. The Christian is of the heavenly seed of Abraham (Gen. 15:5, 6; Gal. 3:29), and partakes of the spiritual blessings of the Abrahamic Covenant (Gen. 15:18, *note*); but Israel as a nation always has its own place, and is yet to have its greatest exaltation as the earthly people of God. See "Israel" (Gen. 12:2; Rom. 11:26); "Kingdom" (Gen. 1: 26-28; Zech. 12:8).

have not bowed the knee to *the image of*
Baal.
5 Even so then at this present time also
there is a [1a]remnant according to the
[b]election of grace.
6 And if [c]by grace, then *is it* no more of
works: otherwise grace is no more grace.
But if *it be* of works, then is it no more
grace: otherwise work is no more work.

(8) *National Israel is judicially blinded.*

7 What then? [d]Israel hath not obtained
that which he seeketh for; but the [e]elec-
tion hath obtained it, and the rest were
blinded
8 (According as it is written, [f]God hath
given them the spirit of slumber, eyes
that they should not see, and ears that
they should not hear;) unto this day.
9 And David saith, [g]Let their table be
made a snare, and a trap, and a stumblingblock, and a recompence unto them:
10 Let their eyes be darkened, that
they may not see, and bow down their
back alway.
11 I say then, Have they stumbled that
they should fall? God forbid: but *rather*
through their fall salvation *is come* unto
the [h]Gentiles, for to provoke them to
[i]jealousy.
12 Now if the fall of them *be* the riches
of the [j]world, and the diminishing of
them the riches of the Gentiles; [k]how
much more their fulness?

(9) *The Gentiles warned.*

13 For I speak to you Gentiles, inasmuch as I am the apostle of the Gentiles,
I magnify mine office:
14 If by any means I may provoke to
emulation *them which are* my flesh, and
might [l]save some of them.
15 For if the casting away of them *be*
the reconciling of the [j]world, what *shall*
the receiving *of them be*, [m]but life from
the dead?
16 For if the firstfruit *be* holy, the lump
is also *holy*: and if the root *be* holy, so *are*
the branches.
17 And if some of the branches be broken off, and thou, being a wild olive
tree, wert graffed in among them, and
with them partakest of the root and fatness of the olive tree;
18 Boast not against the branches. But
if thou boast, thou bearest not the root,
but the root thee.
19 Thou wilt say then, The branches
were broken off, that I might be graffed in.
20 Well; because of [n]unbelief they
were broken off, and thou [o]standest by
faith. Be not [p]highminded, but fear:
21 For if God spared not the natural
branches, *take heed* lest he also spare not
thee.
22 Behold therefore the goodness and
severity of God: on them which fell,
severity; but toward thee, goodness, if
thou continue in *his* goodness: otherwise
thou also shalt be cut off.
23 And they also, if they [q]abide not
still in unbelief, shall be graffed in: for
God is able to graff them in again.
24 For if thou wert cut out of the olive
tree which is wild by nature, and wert
graffed contrary to nature into a good
olive tree: how much more shall these,
which be the natural *branches*, be graffed
into their own olive tree?
25 For I would not, brethren, that ye
should be ignorant of this [r]mystery, lest
ye should be wise in your own conceits;
that blindness in part is happened to
Israel, until the [2s]fulness of the Gentiles
be come in.

A.D. 60.

a *Remnant.* (Isa. 1:9.) See *note.*
b *Grace (in salv.).* 2 Cor. 8:9. (Rom. 3:24; John 1:1, 17, *note.*)
c Rom. 4:4, 5; Gal. 5:4.
d Rom. 9:31; 10:3.
e *Election (corporate).* John 15:19. (Deut. 7:6; 1 Pet. 1:2.)
f *Jehovah.* Isa. 29:10; John 12:40.
g vs. 9, 10; Psa. 69:22.
h Isa. 42:6, 7; Acts 28:24, 28.
i Deut. 32:21.
j *kosmos* (Mt. 4:8) = mankind.
k Psa. 72:8-11; Isa. 49:6; 60:3.
l Rom. 1:16, *note.*
m Isa. 26:16-19; Ezk. 37:1-14; Hos. 6:1-3.
n Heb. 3:19.
o 1 Cor. 10:1-13; 2 Cor. 1:24.
p Prov. 28:14; Heb. 4:1-13.
q Jer. 3:21-25; 50:4, 5; 2 Cor. 3:16.
r Mt. 13:11, *note.*
s Lk. 21:24; 2 Pet. 3:9.

1 (11:5) Remnant, Summary: In the history of Israel a "remnant" may be discerned, a spiritual Israel within the national Israel. In Elijah's time 7,000 had not bowed the knee to Baal (1 Ki. 19:18). In Isaiah's time it was the "very small remnant" for whose sake God still forbore to destroy the nation (Isa. 1:9). During the captivities the remnant appears in Jews like Ezekiel, Daniel, Shadrach, Meshach, and Abednego, Esther and Mordecai. At the end of the 70 years of Babylonian captivity it was the remnant which returned under Ezra and Nehemiah. At the advent of our Lord, John the Baptist, Simeon, Anna, and "them that looked for redemption in Jerusalem" (Lk. 2:38), were the remnant. During the church-age the remnant is composed of believing Jews (Rom. 11:4, 5). But the chief interest in the remnant is prophetic. During the great tribulation a remnant out of all Israel will turn to Jesus as Messiah, and will become His witnesses after the removal of the church (Rev. 7:3-8). Some of these will undergo martyrdom (Rev. 6:9-11), some will be spared to enter the millennial kingdom (Zech. 12:6–13:9). Many of the Psalms express, prophetically, the joys and sorrows of the tribulation remnant.

2 (11:25) The "fulness of the Gentiles" is the completion of the purpose of God in this age,

(10) *Israel is yet to be saved nationally.*

26 And so all Israel shall be saved: as
it is written, [a]There shall come out of
Sion the [b]Deliverer, and shall turn away
ungodliness from [1]Jacob:
27 For this *is* my [c]covenant unto [d]them,
when I shall take away their [e]sins.
28 As concerning the [f]gospel, *they are*
enemies for your sakes: but as touching
the election, *they are* beloved for the
fathers' sakes.
29 For the gifts and calling of God *are*
without [g]repentance.
30 For as ye in times past have not
[h]believed God, yet have now obtained
mercy through their [i]unbelief:
31 Even so have these also now not
[h]believed, that through your mercy they
also may obtain mercy.
32 For God hath concluded them [j]all
in unbelief, that he might have mercy
upon all.
33 O the depth of the riches both of
the wisdom and knowledge of God!
how unsearchable *are* his judgments,
and his ways past finding out!
34 For who hath known the [k]mind
of the Lord? or who hath been his
counsellor?
35 Or [l]who hath first given to him,
and it shall be recompensed unto him
again?
36 For [m]of him, and through him, and
to him, *are* all things: to whom *be* glory
for ever. Amen.

CHAPTER 12.

Part VI. Christian life and service
(Rom. 12:1–15:33).

(1) *Consecration.*

I beseech you therefore, brethren, by
the [n]mercies of God, that ye [o]present
your bodies a living [p]sacrifice, [q]holy,
acceptable unto God, *which is* your reasonable [r]service.
2 [s]And be not conformed to this
[t]world: but be ye [u]transformed by the
renewing of your mind, that ye may
prove what *is* that good, and acceptable,
and perfect, will of God.

(2) *Service.*

3 For I say, through the [v]grace given
unto me, to every man that is among
you, not to think *of himself* more highly
than he ought to think; but to think
soberly, according as God hath dealt to
every man the measure of faith.
4 For as we have many members in
one body, and all members have not the
same office:
5 So we, *being* many, are one body in
Christ, and every one members one of
another.
6 Having then gifts differing according to the grace that is given to us,
whether prophecy, *let us prophesy* according to the proportion of faith;
7 Or ministry, *let us wait* on *our* ministering: or he that teacheth, on teaching;
8 Or he that exhorteth, on exhortation:
he that giveth, *let him do it* with simplicity; he that ruleth, with diligence; he that
sheweth mercy, with cheerfulness.

(3) *The Christian and those within.*

9 *Let* love be without [w]dissimulation.
Abhor that which is evil; cleave to that
which is good.
10 *Be* kindly affectioned one to another with brotherly love; in honour preferring one another;
11 Not slothful in business; fervent in
spirit; serving the Lord;
12 Rejoicing in hope; patient in tribulation; continuing instant in prayer;

A.D. 60.

a *Christ (Second Advent).* vs. 25, 26; Phil. 3:20, 21. (Deut. 30:3; Acts 1:9-11.)
b *Redeemer.* Isa. 59:20, 21.
c Isa. 27:9; Jer. 31:31-37; Heb. 8:8; 10:16.
d *Israel (prophecies).* vs. 1:27; Gen. 12:2, 3.
e *Sin.* Rom. 3:23, *note.*
f *Gospel.* Rom. 15:16, 19, 20, 29. (Gen. 12:1-3; Rev. 14:6.)
g *Repentance.* 2 Cor. 7:9, 10. (Mt. 3:2; Acts 17:30.)
h Or, *obeyed.*
i Or, *disobedience.*
j Rom. 3:9,19; Gal. 3:22.
k *Spirit of the LORD.* Isa. 40:13.
l 1 Chr. 29:11-14; Job 41:11; Psa. 50:9-12.
m 1 Cor. 11:3; 15:28; Heb. 2:10.
n i.e. The "mercies" described in Rom. 3:22; 8:39.
o Or, *yield.*
p *Sacrifice (the believer-priest's).* Phil. 4:18. (Gen. 4:4; Heb. 10:18.)
q *Sanctify, holy (persons)* (N. T.). Rom. 15:16. (Mt. 4:5; Rev. 22:11.)
r Gr. *latreian,* trans. "divine service," Heb. 9:1.)
s *Separation.* 1 Cor. 5:1, 2, 9-13. (Gen. 12:1; 2 Cor. 6:14-17.)
t *age.*
u Trans. *transfigured,* Mt. 17:2.
v *Grace (imparted).* vs. 3, 6; Rom. 15:15. (Rom. 6:1; 2 Pet. 3:18.)
w *hypocrisy.*

viz. the outcalling from among the Gentiles of a people for Christ's name, "the church which is His body" (Eph. 1:22, 23). Cf. Acts 15:14; Eph. 4:11-13; 1 Cor. 12:12, 13. It must be distinguished from "the times of the Gentiles" (Lk. 21:24).

[1] **(11:26)** Summary: Israel, so named from the grandson of Abraham, was chosen for a fourfold mission: (1) To witness to the unity of God in the midst of universal idolatry (Deut. 6:4, with Isa. 43:10, 12); (2) to illustrate to the nations the blessedness of serving the true God (Deut. 33:26-29; 1 Chr. 17:20, 21; Psa. 144:15); (3) to receive, preserve, and transmit the Scriptures (Deut. 4:5-8; Rom. 3:1, 2); (4) to produce, as to His humanity, the Messiah (Gen. 3:15; 12:3; 22:18; 28:10-14; 49:10; 2 Sam. 7:12-16; Isa. 7:14; 9:6; Mt. 1:1; Rom. 1:3). According to the prophets, Israel, regathered from all nations, restored to her own land and converted, is yet to have her greatest earthly exaltation and glory. See "Kingdom (O.T.)" (Gen. 1:26; Zech. 12:8; N.T., Lk. 1:31-33; 1 Cor. 15:24); "Davidic Covenant" (2 Sam. 7:8-17, *note*).

13 [a]Distributing to the necessity of
saints; given to hospitality.
14 [b]Bless them which persecute you:
bless, and curse not.
15 Rejoice with them that do rejoice,
and weep with them that weep.
16 *Be* of the same mind one toward
another. Mind not high things, but condescend to [c]men of low estate. Be not
wise in your own conceits.

(4) *The Christian and those without.*

17 Recompense to no man evil for evil.
[d]Provide things honest in the sight of all
men.
18 If it be possible, as much as lieth in
you, live peaceably with all men.
19 Dearly beloved, avenge not yourselves, but *rather* give place unto wrath:
for it is written, [e]Vengeance *is* mine; I
will repay, saith the Lord.
20 Therefore [f]if thine enemy hunger,
feed him; if he thirst, give him drink: for
in so doing thou shalt heap coals of fire
on his head.
21 Be not overcome of evil, but overcome evil with good.

CHAPTER 13.

Let every soul be [g]subject unto the
higher powers. For there is no
power but of God: the powers that be
are ordained of God.
2 Whosoever therefore resisteth the
power, [h]resisteth the ordinance of God:
and they that resist shall receive to themselves [i]damnation.
3 For rulers are not a terror to good
works, but to the evil. Wilt thou then not
be afraid of the power? [j]do that which is
good, and thou shalt have praise of the
same:
4 For he is the minister of God to thee
for good. But if thou do that which is
evil, be afraid; for he beareth not the
sword in vain: for he is the minister of
God, a [k]revenger to *execute* wrath upon
him that doeth evil.
5 Wherefore *ye* must needs be subject,
not only for wrath, but also for conscience sake.
6 For for this cause pay ye [l]tribute also:
for they are God's ministers, attending
continually upon this very thing.
7 Render therefore to [m]all their dues:
tribute to whom tribute *is due;* custom to
whom custom; fear to whom fear; honour to whom honour.

(5) *The law of love toward the neighbour.*
(Cf. Lk. 10:29-37.)

8 [n]Owe no man any thing, but to [o]love
one another: for he that loveth another
hath fulfilled the law.
9 For this, [p]Thou shalt not commit
adultery, Thou shalt not kill, Thou shalt
not steal, Thou shalt not bear false witness, Thou shalt not covet; and if *there be*
any other commandment, it is briefly
comprehended in this saying, namely,
Thou shalt love thy neighbour as thyself.
10 Love worketh no ill to his neighbour: therefore [q]love *is* the fulfilling of
the [r]law.
11 And that, knowing the time, that
now *it is* high time to awake out of sleep:
for now *is* our salvation [s]nearer than
when we believed.
12 The night is far spent, the day is at
hand: [t]let us therefore cast off the works
of darkness, and [u]let us put on the
armour of light.
13 Let us walk honestly, as in the day;
not in [v]rioting and drunkenness, not in
chambering and wantonness, not in
strife and [w]envying.
14 But put ye on the Lord Jesus Christ,
and make not provision for the [x]flesh, to
fulfil the lusts *thereof.*

CHAPTER 14.

(6) *The law of love concerning doubtful things.* (Cf. 1 Cor. 8:1–10:33.)

Him that is weak in the faith receive
ye, *but* not [y]to doubtful disputa-
tions.
2 For one believeth that he may eat all
things: another, who is weak, eateth
herbs.
3 Let not him that eateth despise him
that eateth not; and let not him which
eateth not judge him that eateth: for God
hath received him.
4 Who art thou that judgest [z]another
man's servant? to his own master he
standeth or falleth. Yea, he shall be holden
up: for God is able to make him stand.
5 One man esteemeth one day above
another: another esteemeth every day
alike. [aa]Let every man be fully persuaded
in his own mind.
6 He that regardeth the day, regardeth
it unto the Lord; and he that regardeth

A.D. 60.

a Heb. 13:16; 1 Pet. 4:9.
b v. 20; Mt. 5:44; Lk. 6:28.
c *them that are lowly.*
d *Take thought for things honourable,* etc.
e Deut. 32:35.
f Prov. 25:21, 22; cf. Mt. 5:44.
g Prov. 24:21; 1 Pet. 2:13.
h Acts 23:2-5; 2 Pet. 2:10, 11.
i *Condemnation,* i.e. in the sense of judgment by the magistrate.
j 1 Pet. 2:14; 3:13; 4:15.
k 2 Chr. 19:6; 1 Tim. 1:8-10.
l Mt. 17:27.
m Mk. 12:17; 1 Pet. 2:17, 18.
n Lev. 19:13; Prov. 22:7.
o Col. 1:4; 1 Pet. 1:22.
p Ex. 20:13-17; Lev. 19:18.
q *Law (of Christ).* vs. 8-10; 1 Cor. 8:9-13. (Gal. 6:2; 2 John 5.)
r *Law (of Moses).* vs. 9, 10; 1 Cor. 15:56. (Ex. 19:1; Gal. 3:1-29.)
s "Nearer" in the sense of the full result of salvation in glory. Rom. 1:16, *note;* 1 John 3:2.
t Eph. 5:11; Col. 3:8.
u Eph. 6:13; 1 Thes. 5:8.
v *revelling.*
w Or, *jealousy.*
x *Flesh.* 1 Cor. 3:4. (John 1:13; Jude 23.)
y *for decisions of doubts,* i.e. doubts about meats, etc. The church has no authority to decide questions of personal liberty in things not expressly forbidden in Scripture. vs. 2-6.
z Jas. 4:11, 12.
aa vs. 14, 23.

not the day, to the Lord he doth not
regard *it*. He that eateth, eateth to the
Lord, for he giveth God thanks; and he
that eateth not, to the Lord he eateth not,
and giveth God thanks.
7 For [a]none of us liveth to himself, and
no man dieth to himself.
8 For whether we [b]live, we live unto
the Lord; and whether we die, we [c]die
unto the Lord: whether we live therefore, or die, we are the Lord's.
9 For to this end Christ both died, and
rose, and revived, that he might be
[d]Lord both of the dead and living.
10 But why dost thou judge thy
brother? or why dost thou set at nought
thy brother? for we shall all stand before
the [e]judgment seat of Christ.
11 For it is written, [f]As I live, saith the
Lord, every knee shall bow to me, and
every tongue shall confess to God.
12 So then every one of us shall give
account of himself to God.
13 Let us not therefore judge one
another any more: but judge this rather,
that no man put a [g]stumblingblock or an
occasion to fall in *his* brother's way.
14 I know, and am persuaded by the
Lord Jesus, that *there is* [h]nothing unclean
of itself: but [i]to him that esteemeth any
thing to be unclean, to him *it is* unclean.
15 But if thy brother be [j]grieved with
thy meat, now walkest thou not charita-
bly. Destroy not him with thy meat, for
whom Christ died.
16 Let not then your [k]good be evil
spoken of:
17 For the [l]kingdom of God is not
meat and drink; but [m]righteousness, and
peace, and joy in the [n]Holy Ghost.
18 For he that in these things serveth
Christ *is* [o]acceptable to God, and [p]ap-
proved of men.
19 Let us therefore follow after the
things which make for peace, and things
wherewith one may [q]edify another.
20 [r]For meat destroy not the work of
God. All things indeed *are* pure; but *it is*
evil for that man who eateth with offence.
21 *It is* good neither to eat [s]flesh, nor
to drink wine, nor *any thing* whereby thy
brother stumbleth, or is offended, or is
made weak.
22 Hast thou faith? have *it* to thyself

A.D. 60.

a 1 Cor. 6:19, 20.
b 2 Cor. 5:13-15; Gal. 2:20.
c Acts 20:24; 21:13; Phil. 1:20, 21.
d Rev. 1:17, 18; 1 Thes. 4:13-18.
e *Judgments (the seven).* 1 Cor. 3:11-15. (2 Sam. 7:14; Rev. 20:12.)
f Isa. 45:23; Phil. 2:10, 11.
g Lk. 17:1, 2; 1 Cor. 8:7-13; 10:23; Rev. 2:14.
h vs. 2, 20; Tit. 1:15.
i v. 23; 1 Cor. 10:24-33.
j 1 Cor. 8:11.
k Rom. 3:8.
l Gal. 4:9-11; Col. 2:20-23. See Mt. 6:33, *note*.
m Rom. 10:10, *note*.
n *Holy Spirit.* Rom. 15:13, 16, 19, 30. (Mt. 1:18; Acts 2:4.)
o 2 Cor. 5:9.
p Lk. 2:52; Acts 2:47.
q Rom. 15:2; 1 Thes. 5:11.
r *Overthrow not for meat's sake a work which God is doing.*
s 1 Cor. 8:13; 10:33; 2 Cor. 6:3.
t 2 Tim. 1:3; 1 John 3:21.
u *condemned,* i.e. as in v. 22.
v John 7:17.
w *Faith.* 1 Cor. 12:9. (Gen. 3:20; Heb. 11:39)
x *Sin.* Rom. 3:23, *note*.
y Mt. 17:27; Lk. 9:51; Phil. 2:5-8
z Psa. 69:9; 1 Pet. 2:23.
aa Rom. 4:23, 24; 1 Cor. 9:9, 10; 10:11; 2 Tim. 3:16, 17; 2 Pet. 1:19.
bb 1 Cor. 1:10; Phil. 1:27.
cc 1 Cor. 10:31; 1 Pet. 4:11.
dd Rom. 14:1, 3.
ee Mt. 2:2; John 19:15, 19-22; Rom. 1:3.
ff Psa. 18:49.
gg Isa. 42:6, 7.
hh Deut. 32:43.
ii *Jehovah.* Psa. 117:1.
jj Isa. 11:1, 10.
kk *hope.*
ll v. 5 ; Heb. 13:20
mm Rom. 12:12; 14:17.

before God. Happy *is* he that [t]condem-
neth not himself in that thing which he
alloweth.
23 And he that doubteth is [u]damned if
he eat, because *he eateth* not of faith: [v]for
whatsoever *is* not of [w]faith is [x]sin.

CHAPTER 15.

(*The law of love concerning doubtful things,* continued.)

We then that are strong ought to
bear the infirmities of the weak,
and not to please ourselves.
2 Let every one of us please *his* neighbour for *his* good to edification.
3 For [y]even Christ pleased not himself;
but, as it is written, [z]The reproaches of
them that reproached thee fell on me.

(7) *Jewish and Gentile believers are one in salvation.*

4 For [aa]whatsoever things were written aforetime were written for our learning, that we through patience and comfort of the scriptures might have hope.
5 Now the God of patience and consolation grant you to be [bb]likeminded one
toward another according to Christ Jesus:
6 That ye may with one mind *and* one
mouth [cc]glorify God, even the Father of
our Lord Jesus Christ.
7 Wherefore [dd]receive ye one another,
as Christ also received us to the glory of
God.
8 Now I say that Jesus Christ was a
[ee]minister of the circumcision for the
truth of God, to confirm the promises
made unto the fathers:
9 And that the Gentiles might glorify
God for *his* mercy; as it is written, [ff]For
this cause I will confess to thee among
the [gg]Gentiles, and sing unto thy name.
10 And again he saith, [hh]Rejoice, ye
Gentiles, with his people.
11 And again, Praise the [ii]Lord, all ye
Gentiles; and laud him, all ye people.
12 And again, Esaias saith, [jj]There
shall be a root of Jesse, and he that shall
rise to reign over the Gentiles; in him
shall the Gentiles [kk]trust.
13 Now the [ll]God of hope fill you with
all [mm]joy and peace in believing, that ye
may abound in hope, through the power
of the Holy Ghost.

(8) *The apostle speaks of his ministry and coming journey.*

14 And I myself also am persuaded of you, my brethren, that ye also are full of goodness, filled with all knowledge, able also to admonish one another.

15 Nevertheless, brethren, I have written the more boldly unto you in some sort, as putting you in mind, because of [a]the grace that is given to me of God,

16 That I should be the [b]minister of Jesus Christ to the Gentiles, ministering the gospel of God, that the [c]offering up of the Gentiles might be acceptable, being [d]sanctified by the Holy Ghost.

17 I have therefore whereof I may glory through Jesus Christ in those things which pertain to God.

18 For I will not dare to speak of any of those things which Christ hath not wrought by me, to make the Gentiles obedient, by word and deed,

19 Through mighty signs and wonders, by the power of the Spirit of God; so that from Jerusalem, and round about unto Illyricum, I have fully preached the gospel of Christ.

20 Yea, [e]so have I strived to preach the [f]gospel, not where Christ was named, lest I should [g]build upon another man's foundation:

21 But as it is written, [h]To whom he was not spoken of, they shall see: and they that have not heard shall understand.

22 For which cause also I have been much hindered from coming to you.

23 But now having no more place in these parts, and having a [i]great desire these many years to come unto you;

24 Whensoever I take my journey into Spain, I will come to you: for I [j]trust to see you in my journey, and to be brought on my way thitherward by you, if first I be somewhat filled with your *company*.

25 But now I go unto Jerusalem to [k]minister unto the saints.

26 For it hath pleased them of Macedonia and Achaia to make a certain contribution for the poor saints which are at Jerusalem.

27 It hath pleased them verily; and their debtors they are. For if the Gentiles have been made partakers of their spiritual things, their duty is also to minister unto them in [l]carnal things.

28 When therefore I have performed this, and have sealed to them this fruit, I will come by you into Spain.

29 And I am sure that, when I come unto you, I shall come in the [m]fulness of the blessing of the gospel of Christ.

30 Now I beseech you, brethren, for the Lord Jesus Christ's sake, and for the love of the [n]Spirit, that ye strive together with me in *your* prayers to God for me;

31 That I may be delivered from them that do not believe in Judaea; and that my [o]service which *I have* for Jerusalem may be accepted of the saints;

32 That I may come unto you with [p]joy by the will of God, and may with you be refreshed.

33 Now the [q]God of peace *be* with you all. Amen.

CHAPTER 16.

Part VII. The outflow of Christian love.

I [r]commend unto you Phebe our sister, which is a [s]servant of the church which is at Cenchrea:

2 That ye receive her in the Lord, [t]as becometh saints, and that ye assist her in whatsoever business she hath need of you: for she hath been a [u]succourer of many, and of myself also.

3 Greet [v]Priscilla and Aquila my helpers in Christ Jesus:

4 Who have for my life laid down their own necks: unto whom not only I give thanks, but also all the churches of the Gentiles.

5 Likewise *greet* the church that is in their house. Salute my wellbeloved Epaenetus, who is the firstfruits of [w]Achaia unto Christ.

6 Greet Mary, who bestowed [x]much labour on us.

7 Salute Andronicus and Junia, my [y]kinsmen, and my fellowprisoners, who are of note among the apostles, who also were [z]in Christ before me.

8 Greet Amplias my beloved in the Lord.

9 Salute Urbane, our helper in Christ, and Stachys my beloved.

10 Salute Apelles approved in Christ. Salute them which are of Aristobulus' *household*.

11 Salute Herodion my [aa]kinsman. Greet them that be of the *household* of

A.D. 60.

a *Grace (imparted).* 1 Cor. 1:4. (Rom. 6:1; 2 Pet. 3:18.)
b Rom. 11:13; Gal. 2:7-10; Eph. 3:8.
c Num. 8:5-16; Isa. 66:20.
d *Sanctify, holy (persons)* (N.T.). 1 Cor. 1:2. (Mt. 4:5; Rev. 22:11.)
e *being ambitious to preach,* etc.
f *Gospel.* vs. 16, 19, 20, 29; Rom. 16:25. (Gen. 12:1-3; Rev. 14:6.)
g 1 Cor. 3:10; 2 Cor. 10:13-18.
h Isa. 52:15.
i Acts 19:21, 22; 23:11; Rom. 1:10, 11.
j *hope.*
k Acts 24:17.
l *things for the body.*
m Rom. 1:11; Eph. 3:8, 19.
n *Holy Spirit.* vs. 13, 16, 19, 30; 1 Cor. 2:4, 10, 11, 12, 14. (Mt. 1:18; Acts 2:4.)
o *ministration.*
p 2 John 4; 3 John 4; Phm. 20.
q Rom. 16:20; 1 Cor. 14:33; 2 Cor. 13:11; Phil. 4:9; 1 Thes. 5:23; 2 Thes. 3:16; Heb. 13:20.
r Acts 18:27; 2 Cor. 3:1-3; Phil. 2:29, 30.
s Lit. *deaconess.*
t Eph. 5:3; Phil. 1:27.
u *helper.*
v Acts 18:2, 18, 26; 1 Cor. 16:19; 2 Tim. 4:19.
w Or, *Asia.*
x v. 12; Phil. 4:3.
y vs. 11, 21.
z 1 Cor. 15:8; Gal. 1:22.
aa vs. 7, 21.

Narcissus, which are in the Lord.
12 Salute Tryphena and Tryphosa,
who labour in the Lord. Salute the
beloved Persis, which laboured much in
the Lord.
13 Salute Rufus [a]chosen in the Lord,
and his mother and mine.
14 Salute Asyncritus, Phlegon, Hermas,
Patrobas, Hermes, and the brethren
which are with them.
15 Salute Philologus, and Julia,
Nereus, and his sister, and Olympas,
and all the saints which are with them.
16 Salute one another with an [b]holy
kiss. The churches of Christ salute you.
17 Now I beseech you, brethren, mark
them which cause divisions and offences
contrary to the doctrine which ye have
learned; and avoid them.
18 For they that are such serve not our
Lord Jesus Christ, but their own belly;
and by good words and fair speeches
deceive the hearts of the simple.
19 For your obedience is come abroad
unto all *men*. I am glad therefore on your
behalf: but yet I would have you wise
unto that which is good, and simple concerning evil.
20 And the God of peace shall bruise
[c]Satan under your feet shortly. The grace
of our Lord Jesus Christ *be* with you.
Amen.
21 Timotheus my workfellow, and
Lucius, and Jason, and Sosipater, my
kinsmen, salute you.
22 I Tertius, who wrote *this* epistle,
salute you in the Lord.
23 Gaius mine host, and of the whole
[d]church, saluteth you. Erastus the chamberlain of the city saluteth you, and
Quartus a brother.
24 The grace of our Lord Jesus Christ
be with you all. Amen.
25 Now to him that is of power to stablish you according to my [e]gospel, and
the preaching of Jesus Christ, according
to the revelation of the [f]mystery, which
[g]was kept secret since the [h]world began,
26 But now is made manifest, and [i]by
the scriptures of the prophets, according
to the commandment of the everlasting
God, made known to all nations for the
[j]obedience of faith:
27 To God only wise, *be* glory through
Jesus Christ for ever. Amen.

A.D. 60.

a *Election (personal).* 1 Pet. 2:9. (Deut. 7:6; 1 Pet. 1:2.)
b *Sanctify, holy (things)* (N.T.). 1 Cor. 9:13. (Mt. 4:5; Rev. 22:11.)
c *Satan.* 1 Cor. 5:5. (Gen. 3:1; Rev. 20:10.)
d *Churches (local).* vs. 1-5, 16, 23; 1 Cor. 1:2, 10-17, 26-31. (Acts 2:41; Phil. 1:1.)
e *Gospel.* 1 Cor. 1:17. (Gen. 12:1-3; Rev. 14:6.)
f Mt. 13:11, *note.* The "mystery" here is the Church; Eph. 3:1-9.
g Lit. *hath been kept in silence through times eternal.*
h i.e. *ages.*
i *inspiration.* vs. 25, 26; 1 Cor. 2:7-16. (Ex. 4:15; Rev. 22:19.)
j Rom. 1:5, *marg.* Faith as a system in contrast with law as a system.

THE FIRST EPISTLE OF PAUL THE APOSTLE TO THE

CORINTHIANS

WRITER. The Apostle Paul. His relation to the church at Corinth is set forth in Acts 18:1-18, and in the Epistles to the Corinthians.

Date. First Corinthians was written in A.D. 59, at the close of Paul's three years' residence in Ephesus (Acts 20:31; 1 Cor. 16:5-8).

Theme. The subjects treated are various, but may all be classified under the general theme, Christian conduct. Even the tremendous revelation of the truth concerning resurrection is made to bear upon that theme (1 Cor. 15:58). The occasion of the Epistle was a letter of inquiry from Corinth concerning marriage, and the use of meats offered to idols (1 Cor. 7:1; 8:1-13), but the apostle was much more exercised by reports of the deepening divisions and increasing contentions in the church, and of a case of incest which had not been judged (1:10-12; 5:1).

The factions were not due to heresies, but to the carnality of the restless Corinthians, and to their Greek admiration of "wisdom" and eloquence. The abomination of human leadership in the things of God is here rebuked. Minor disorders were due to vanity, yielding to a childish delight in tongues and the sign gifts, rather than to sober instruction (1 Cor. 14:1-28). Paul defends his apostleship because it involved the authority of the doctrine revealed through him.

A rigid analysis of First Corinthians is not possible. The Epistle is not a treatise, but came from the Spirit through the apostle's grief, solicitude, and holy indignation. The following analysis may, however, be helpful. I. Introduction: The believer's standing in grace, 1:1-9. II. The contrast of their present factious state, 1:10–4:21. III. Immorality rebuked; discipline enjoined, 5:1–6:8. IV. The sanctity of the body, and Christian marriage, 6:9–7:40. V. Meats, and the limitations of Christian liberty, 8:1–11:1. VI. Christian order and the Lord's Supper, 11:2-34. VII. Spiritual gifts in relation to the body, the church, and Christian ministry, 12:1–14:40. VIII. The resurrection of the dead, 15:1-58. IX. Special directions and greetings, 16:1-24.

CHAPTER 1.

Part I. The believer's position in grace.
(Cf. Rom. 5:1, 2; Eph. 1:3-14.)

Paul, [a]called *to be* an apostle of Jesus
Christ through [b]the will of God, and
[c]Sosthenes *our* brother,
2 Unto the [d]church of God which is at
Corinth, to [1]them that are [e]sanctified in
Christ Jesus, [f]called *to be* saints, with all
that in every place call upon the name of
Jesus Christ our Lord, both theirs and
ours:
3 Grace *be* unto you, and peace, from
God our Father, and *from* the Lord Jesus
Christ.
4 I thank my God always on your
behalf, [g]for the grace of God which is
given you by Jesus Christ;
5 That in every thing ye are enriched
by him, [h]in all utterance, and *in* all
knowledge;
6 Even as the testimony of Christ was
confirmed in you:
7 So that ye come behind in no

A.D. 59.

a Lit. *a called apostle.*
b 2 Cor. 1:1; Eph. 1:1; Col. 1:1.
c Acts 18:17.
d *Churches (local).* vs. 2, 10-17, 26:31. 1 Cor. 6:4, 5. (Acts 2:41; Phil. 1:1.)
e *Sanctify, holy (persons)* (N.T.). 1 Cor. 3:17. (Mt. 4:5; Rev. 22:11.)
f *called saints.*
g *Grace (imparted).* 1 Cor. 3:10. (Rom. 6:1; 2 Pet. 3:18.)
h 1 Cor. 12:8; 2 Cor. 8:7.

[1] **(1:2)** Verses 2-9, in contrast with vs. 10-13, illustrate a distinction constantly made in the Epistles between the believer's position in Christ Jesus, in the family of God, and his walk, or actual state. Christian position in grace is the result of the work of Christ, and is fully entered the moment that Christ is received by faith (John 1:12, 13; Rom. 8:1, 15-17; 1 Cor. 1:2, 30; 12:12, 13; Gal. 3:26; Eph. 1:3-14; 2:4-9; 1 Pet. 2:9; Rev. 1:6; 5:9, 10). The weakest, most ignorant, and fallible believer has precisely the same relationships in grace as the most illustrious saint. All the after work of God in his behalf, the application of the word to walk and conscience (John 17:17; Eph. 5:26), the divine chastenings (1 Cor. 11:32; Heb. 12:10), the ministry of the Spirit (Eph. 4:11, 12), the difficulties and trials of the path (1 Pet. 4, 12, 13), and the final transformation at the appearing of Christ (1 John 3:2), have for their object to make the believer's character conform to his exalted position in Christ. He grows *in* grace, not *into* grace.

gift; waiting for the [1a]coming of our
Lord Jesus Christ:
8 Who shall also confirm you unto the
end, *that ye may be* [b]blameless in the
[2]day of our Lord Jesus Christ.
9 [c]God *is* faithful, by whom ye were
called unto the fellowship of his Son
Jesus Christ our Lord.

Part II. The contrast of the unspiritual state of the Corinthian saints with their exalted standing in Christ.

10 Now I beseech you, brethren, by
the name of our Lord Jesus Christ, that
ye all speak the same thing, and *that*
there be no [d]divisions among you; but
that ye be perfectly joined together in the
same mind and in the same judgment.

(1) *They were following human leaders, thus dividing the body of Christ.*

11 For it hath been declared unto me
of you, my brethren, by them *which are of*
the house of Chloe, that there are contentions among you.
12 Now this I say, that every one of
you saith, I am of Paul; and I of
[e]Apollos; and I of [f]Cephas; and I of
Christ.
13 [g]Is Christ divided? was Paul crucified for you? or were ye baptized in the
name of Paul?
14 I thank God that I baptized none of
you, but Crispus and Gaius;
15 Lest any should say that [h]I had
baptized in mine own name.
16 And I baptized also the household
of Stephanas: besides, I know not
whether I baptized any other.
17 For Christ sent me not to baptize,
but to preach the [i]gospel: not with wisdom of words, lest the cross of Christ
should be made of none effect.

(2) *They were exulting in human wisdom, which is foolishness in the things of God.*

18 For the preaching of the cross is to
them that perish foolishness; but unto us
which are [j]saved it is the power of God.
19 For it is written, [k]I will destroy the
wisdom of the wise, and will bring to
nothing the understanding of the prudent.
20 Where *is* the wise? where *is* the
scribe? where *is* the disputer of this
[l]world? hath not God made foolish the
wisdom of this [m]world?
21 For after that in the wisdom of God
the world by wisdom knew not God, it
pleased God by the foolishness of
[n]preaching to [j]save them that believe.
22 For the Jews require a sign, and the
[o]Greeks seek after wisdom:
23 But we preach [p]Christ crucified,
unto the Jews a [q]stumblingblock, and
unto the Greeks foolishness;
24 But unto them which are called,
both Jews and Greeks, Christ the power
of God, and the wisdom of God.
25 Because the foolishness of God is
wiser than men; and the weakness of
God is stronger than men.

(3) *Any way the Corinthian believers were not of the wise.*

26 For ye see your calling, brethren,
how that not many wise men after the
flesh, not many mighty, not many noble,
are called:
27 But God hath [r]chosen the foolish
things of the [s]world to confound the
wise; and God hath chosen the weak

A.D. 59.

a Gr. *apokalupsin, revelation, unveiling.*
b Col. 1:22; 1 Thes. 3:15; 5:23.
c Isa. 49:7; 1 Cor. 10:13; 1 Thes. 5:24.
d Gr. *schism, a cleft, or rent.*
e Acts 19:1.
f John 1:42.
g Or, *Christ is divided.*
h *ye were baptized into my name.*
i *Gospel.* 1 Cor. 4:15. (Gen. 12:1-3; Rev. 14:6.)
j Rom. 1:16, *note.*
k Isa. 29:14.
l *age.*
m *kosmos* = world-system. 1 Cor. 2:12. (John 7:7; Rev. 13:3-8, *note.*)
n *of the thing preached.*
o *Gentiles,* and so in vs. 23, 24.
p Or, *a Messiah crucified.*
q *Christ (as Stone).* 1 Pet. 2:8. (Ex. 17:6; 1 Pet. 2:4-8.)
r Psa. 8:2; Mt. 11:25.
s *kosmos* (Mt. 4:8) = mankind.

[1](1:7) Three words are used in connection with the return of the Lord: (1) *Parousia.* "personal presence," also used by Paul of the "coming" of Stephanas (1 Cor. 16:17), of Titus (2 Cor. 7:6, 7), and of his own "coming" to Philippi (Phil. 1:26). The word means simply personal presence, and is used of the return of the Lord as that event relates to the blessing of saints (1 Cor. 15:23; 1 Thes. 4:14, 19), and to the destruction of the man of sin (2 Thes. 2:8). (2) *Apokalupsis,* "unveiling," "revelation." The use of this word emphasizes the *visibility* of the Lord's return. It is used of the Lord (2 Thes. 1:7; 1 Pet. 1:7, 13; 4:13), of the sons of God in connection with the Lord's return (Rom. 8:19), and of the man of sin (2 Thes. 2:3, 6, 8), and always implies visibility. (3) *Epiphaneia,* "appearing," trans. "brightness" (2 Thes. 2:8, A.V.; "manifestation," R.V.), and means simply an appearing. It is used of both advents (2 Tim. 1:10; 2 Thes. 2:8; 1 Tim. 6:14; 2 Tim. 4:1, 8; Tit. 2:13).

[2](1:8) The expression, "day of Christ," occurs in the following passages: 1 Cor. 1:8; 5:5; 2 Cor. 1:14; Phil. 1:6, 10; 2:16. A.V. has "day of Christ," 2 Thes. 2:2, incorrectly, for "day of the LORD" (Isa. 2:12; Rev. 19:11-21). The "day of Christ" relates wholly to the reward and blessing of saints at His coming, as "day of the LORD" is connected with judgment.

things of the [a]world to confound the
things which are mighty;
28 And base things of the world, and
things which are despised, hath God
[b]chosen, *yea*, and things which are not,
to bring to nought things that are:
29 That no flesh should glory in his
presence.
30 But of him are ye in Christ Jesus,
who of God is made unto us [c]wisdom,
and [d]righteousness, and sanctification,
and [e]redemption:
31 That, according as it is written, He
that glorieth, let him glory in the [f]Lord.

CHAPTER 2.

(4) *They are reminded that the Christian revelation owes nothing to human wisdom.*

(a) Paul did not use it.

And I, brethren, when I came to you,
came not with excellency of speech
or of wisdom, declaring unto you the
testimony of God.
2 For I determined not to know any
thing among you, save Jesus Christ, and
him crucified.
3 And I was with you in weakness,
and in fear, and in much trembling.
4 And my speech and my preaching
was not with [g]enticing words of man's
wisdom, but in demonstration of the
Spirit and of power:
5 That your faith should not stand in
the wisdom of men, but in the power of
God.
6 Howbeit we speak wisdom among
them that are [h]perfect: yet not the wisdom of this [i]world, nor of the [j]princes of
this [i]world, that come to nought:
7 [k]But we speak the wisdom of God in
a [l]mystery, *even* the hidden *wisdom*,
which God [m]ordained before the [n]world
unto our glory:
8 Which none of the princes of this
[i]world knew: for had they known *it*,
they would not have crucified the Lord
of glory.

(b) Spiritual verities are not discoverable by human wisdom.

9 But as it is written, Eye hath not seen,
nor ear heard, neither have entered into
the heart of man, the things which God
hath prepared for them that love him.

(c) But God has revealed them to prepared men.

10 But God hath revealed *them* unto us
by his Spirit: for the Spirit searcheth all
things, yea, the deep things of God.
11 For what man knoweth the things
of a man, save the spirit of man which is
in him? even so the things of God
knoweth no man, but the [o]Spirit of God.
12 Now we have received, not the
spirit of the [p]world, but the spirit which
is of God; that we might know the things
that are freely given to us of God.

(d) The revealed things are taught in words given by the Spirit.

13 Which things also we speak, not in
the [1]words which man's wisdom teacheth, but which the Holy Ghost teacheth; comparing spiritual things with
spiritual.

(e) The revealed things are spiritually discerned.

14 But the [2]natural man receiveth not
the things of the [o]Spirit of God: for they
are foolishness unto him: neither can he
know *them*, because they are spiritually
discerned.

A.D. 59.

a *Kosmos* (Mt. 4:8.) = mankind.
b *Election (corporate).* vs. 27, 28; Eph. 1:4, (Deut. 7:6; 1 Pet. 1:2.)
c *from God*, or, *wisdom from God, even righteousness and sanctification, and redemption.*
d Rom. 3:21, *note.*
e Rom. 3;24, *note.*
f *Jehovah.* Jer. 9:24.
g *Or, persuasive.*
h *i.e. full grown.* Mt. 5:48, *note.*
i *age.*
j *rulers of this age.*
k *Inspiration.* vs. 7, 16; 1 Cor. 14:37. (Ex. 4:15; Rev. 22:19.)
l Mt. 13:11, *note.*
m *Predestination*, trans. *predestinated*, Rom. 8:29, 30; Eph. 1:5, 11. (Acts 4:28; Eph. 1:5, 11.)
n *foreordained before the ages.* Cf. Rom. 16:25, *marg.*
o *Holy Spirit.* vs. 4, 10, 11, 12, 13, 14; 1 Cor. 3:16. (Mt. 1:18; Acts 2:4.)
p *kosmos* = world-system. 1 Cor. 7:31, 33. (John 7:7; Rev. 13:3-8, *note.*)

[1]**(2:13)** (1) The writers of Scripture invariably affirm, where the subject is mentioned by them at all, that the *words* of their writings are divinely taught. This, of necessity, refers to the original documents, not to translations and versions; but the labours of competent scholars have brought our English versions to a degree of perfection so remarkable that we may confidently rest upon them as authoritative. (2) 1 Cor. 2:9-14 gives the process by which a truth passes from the mind of God to the minds of His people. *(a)* The unseen things of God are undiscoverable by the natural man (v. 9). *(b)* These unseen things God has revealed to chosen men (vs. 10-12). *(c)* The revealed things are communicated in Spirit-taught words (v. 13). This implies neither mechanical dictation nor the effacement of the writer's personality, but only that the Spirit infallibly guides in the choice of words from the writer's own vocabulary (v. 13). *(d)* These Spirit-taught words, in which the revelation has been expressed, are discerned, as to their true spiritual content, only by the spiritual among believers (1 Cor. 2:15, 16). See also Rev. 22:19, *note.*

[2]**(2:14)** Paul divides men into three classes: *psuchikos*, "of the senses" (Jas. 3:15; Jude 19), or "natural," i.e. the Adamic man, unrenewed through the new birth (John 3:3, 5); *pneumatikos*, "spiritual," i.e. the renewed man as Spirit-filled and walking in the Spirit in full communion with God (Eph. 5:18-20);

15 But he that is spiritual [a]judgeth all things, yet he himself is judged of no man.

16 For who hath known the [b]mind of the Lord, that he may instruct him? But we have the mind of Christ.

CHAPTER 3.

(5) *A carnal state prevents spiritual growth.*

And I, brethren, could not speak unto you as unto spiritual, but as unto [c]carnal, *even* as unto babes in Christ.

2 I have fed you with milk, and not with meat: for hitherto ye were not able *to bear it*, neither yet now are ye able.

3 For ye are yet [d]carnal: for whereas *there is* among you envying, and strife, and divisions, are ye not carnal, and walk [e]as men?

4 For while one saith, I am of Paul; and another, I *am* of Apollos; are ye not [f]carnal?

(6) *God only is any thing in Christian service.* (Cf. vs. 7.)

5 Who then is Paul, and who *is* Apollos, but ministers [g]by whom ye believed, even as the Lord gave to every man?

6 I have planted, Apollos watered; but [h]God gave the increase.

7 So then [i]neither is he that planteth any thing, neither he that watereth; but God that giveth the increase.

8 Now he that planteth and he that watereth are [1]one: and every man shall receive his own [j]reward according to his own labour.

(7) *Christian service and its reward.*

9 For we are [k]labourers together with God: ye are God's husbandry, *ye are* God's building.

10 According to the [l]grace of God which is given unto me, as a wise masterbuilder, I have laid the foundation, and another buildeth thereon. But let every man take heed how he buildeth thereupon.

(a) *The only foundation.*

11 For other foundation can no man lay than that is laid, which is Jesus Christ.

(b) *Two kinds of ministry and their result.*

12 Now if any man build upon this foundation gold, silver, precious stones, wood, hay, stubble;

13 Every man's work shall be made manifest: for the day shall declare it, because it shall be revealed by fire; and the fire shall try every man's work of what sort it is.

14 If any man's work abide which he hath built thereupon, he shall receive a [2j]reward.

15 If any man's work shall be burned, he shall suffer loss: but he himself shall be [m]saved; yet [n]so as [o]by fire.

16 Know ye not that ye are the temple of God, and *that* the [p]Spirit of God dwelleth in you?

17 If any man defile the temple of God, him shall God destroy; for the temple of God is [q]holy, which *temple* ye are.

18 Let no man deceive himself. If any man among you seemeth to be wise in this [r]world, let him become a fool, that he may be wise.

19 For the wisdom of this world is foolishness with God. For it is written, [s]He taketh the wise in their own craftiness.

20 And again, [t]The Lord knoweth the [u]thoughts of the wise, that they are vain.

A.D. 59.

a *discerneth all things, yet he himself is discerned of no man.*
b *Spirit of the LORD.* Isa. 40:13; Rom. 11:34.
c See Rom. 7:14, *note.*
d i.e. *fleshly.*
e *after the manner of men.*
f *Flesh.* vs. 1-3; 2 Cor. 1:12, 17. (John 1:13; Jude 23.)
g *through.*
h 1 Cor. 15:10; Acts 16:14.
i John 15:5.
j *Rewards.* 1 Cor. 9:17. (Dan. 12:3; 1 Cor. 3:14.)
k *God's fellow workers.*
l *Grace (imparted).* 1 Cor. 15:10. (Rom 6:1; 2 Pet. 3:18.)
m Rom. 1:16, *note.*
n *Judgments (the seven)* 1 Cor. 4:5. (2 Sam. 7:14; Rev. 20:12.)
o *through.*
p *Holy Spirit.* 1 Cor. 6:11, 19. (Mt. 1:18; Acts 2:4.)
q *Sanctify, holy (persons)* (N.T.). 1 Cor. 6:11. (Mt. 4:5; Rev. 22:11.)
r *age.*
s Job 5:13.
t *Jehovah.* Psa. 94:11.
u *reasonings.*

---

and *sarkikos,* "carnal," "fleshly," i.e. the renewed man who, walking "after the flesh," remains a babe in Christ (1 Cor. 3:1-4). The natural man may be learned, gentle, eloquent, fascinating, but the spiritual content of Scripture is absolutely hidden from him; and the fleshly, or carnal, Christian is able to comprehend only its simplest truths, "milk" (1 Cor. 3:1-2).

[1] **(3:8)** Paul refutes the notion that he and Cephas and Apollos are at variance, mere theologians and rival founders of sects: they are "one." See v. 22, and 1 Cor. 16:12.

[2] **(3:14)** God, in the N.T. Scriptures, offers to the *lost,* salvation, and, for the faithful service of the *saved,* rewards. The passages are easily distinguished by remembering that salvation is invariably spoken of as a free gift (e.g. John 4:10; Rom. 6:23; Eph. 2:8, 9); while rewards are earned by works (Mt. 10:42; Lk. 19:17; 1 Cor. 9:24, 25; 2 Tim. 4:7, 8; Rev. 2:10; 22:12). A further distinction is that salvation is a present possession (Lk. 7:50; John 3:36; 5:24; 6:47), while rewards are a future attainment, to be given at the coming of the Lord (Mt. 16:27; 2 Tim. 4:8; Rev. 22:12).

21 Therefore let no man glory in men.
For all things are yours;
22 Whether Paul, or Apollos, or Cephas,
or the [a]world, or life, or death, or things
present, or things to come; all are yours;
23 And ye are Christ's; and Christ *is*
God's.

CHAPTER 4.

(c) Judgment of Christ's servants is not committed to men.

Let a man so account of us, as of the
ministers of Christ, and stewards of
the mysteries of God.
2 Moreover it is required in stewards,
that a man be found faithful.
3 But with me it is a very small thing
that I should be judged of you, or of
man's judgment: yea, I judge not mine
own self.
4 For I know nothing [b]by myself; yet
am I not hereby [c]justified: but he that
judgeth me is the Lord.
5 Therefore judge nothing before the
time, until the Lord come, who both will
bring to light the hidden things of darkness, and [d]will make manifest the counsels of the hearts: and then shall every
man have praise of God.
6 And these things, brethren, I have in
a figure transferred to myself and *to*
Apollos for your sakes; that ye might
learn in us not to think *of men* above that
which is written, that no one of you be
puffed up for one against another.
7 For who maketh thee to differ *from
another*? and [e]what hast thou that thou
didst not receive? now if thou didst
receive *it*, why dost thou glory, as if thou
hadst not received *it*?
8 [f]Now ye are full, now ye are rich, ye
have reigned as kings without us: and I
would to God ye did reign, [g]that we also
might reign with you.

(8) The apostolic example of humility and patience.

9 For I think that God hath set forth us
the apostles last, as it were appointed to
death: for we are made a spectacle unto
the [h]world, and to angels, and to men.
10 We *are* [i]fools for Christ's sake, but
ye *are* wise in Christ; we *are* weak, but ye
are strong; ye *are* honourable, but we *are*
despised.
11 Even unto this present hour we
both hunger, and thirst, and are naked,
and are buffeted, and have no certain
dwellingplace;
12 And [j]labour, working with our own
hands: being [k]reviled, we bless; being
persecuted, we suffer it:
13 Being defamed, we intreat: we are
made as the filth of the [l]world, *and are* the
[m]offscouring of all things unto this day.
14 I write not these things to shame
you, but as my beloved [n]sons I warn *you*.
15 For though ye have ten thousand
instructors in Christ, yet *have ye* not
many fathers: for in Christ Jesus I have
begotten you through the [o]gospel.
16 Wherefore I beseech you, be ye followers of me.
17 For this cause have I sent unto you
Timotheus, who is my beloved [n]son, and
faithful in the Lord, who shall bring you
into remembrance of my ways which be
in Christ, as I teach every where in every
church.

(9) But there is such a thing as apostolic authority.

18 Now some are puffed up, as
though I [p]would not come to you.
19 But I will come to you shortly, if the
Lord will, and will know, not the speech
of them which are puffed up, but the
power.
20 For the kingdom of God *is* not in
word, but in power.
21 What will ye? shall I come unto you
with a rod, or in love, and *in* the spirit of
meekness?

CHAPTER 5.

Part III. Immorality rebuked, discipline enjoined (1 Cor. 5:1–6:8).

It is [q]reported commonly *that there is*
fornication among you, and such fornication as is not so much as named
among the Gentiles, that one [r]should
have his father's wife.

Indifference to evil in the church the result of divisions.

2 [1]And ye are puffed up, and have

A.D. 59.

a *kosmos* = earth. Rom. 8:19-21.
b *against.*
c *Justification.* 1 Cor. 6:11. (Lk. 18:14; Rom. 3:28.)
d *Judgments (the seven).* 1 Cor. 5:5. (2 Sam. 7:14; Rev. 20:12.)
e 1 Cor. 12:4, 11; Jas. 1:17.
f *Already are ye filled; already are ye become rich. Contra,* vs. 9-12; 1 Pet. 1:4.
g Cf. Rev. 3:21; 5:10.
h *kosmos* (Mt. 4:8) = mankind.
i Acts 26:24, 25.
j Acts 20:34.
k Mt. 5:44; Acts 7:60.
l *kosmos* (Mt. 4:8) = mankind.
m Acts 22:22.
n Gr. *teknon, child, "born one."*
o *Gospel.* 1 Cor. 9:12, 14, 16-18, 23. (Gen. 12:1-3; Rev. 14:6.)
p *were not coming.*
q *actually reported.*
r *of you hath.*

[1] **(5:2)** What contempt this pours upon the divisions among the Corinthians: "Apollonians," and "Paulinians," and "Cephasites," all alike indifferent to this instance of gross sin!

not rather mourned, that he that hath done this deed might be taken away from among you.

3 For I verily, as absent in body, but present in spirit, have judged already, as though I were present, *concerning* him that hath so done this deed,

4 In the name of our Lord Jesus Christ, when ye are gathered together, and my spirit, with the power of our Lord Jesus Christ,

5 [a]To deliver such an one unto [b]Satan for the [1]destruction of the flesh, that the spirit may be [c]saved in the day of the Lord [d]Jesus.

6 Your glorying *is* not good. Know ye not that a little leaven leaveneth the whole lump?

7 Purge out therefore the old leaven, that ye may be a new lump, as ye are unleavened. For even Christ our passover is [e]sacrificed for us:

8 Therefore let us keep the feast, not with old [f]leaven, neither with the leaven of malice and wickedness; but with the unleavened *bread* of sincerity and truth.

9 I wrote unto you in an epistle not to company with fornicators:

10 Yet not altogether with the fornicators of this [g]world, or with the covetous, or extortioners, or with idolaters; for then must ye needs go out of the [g]world.

11 But now I have written unto you not to keep company, if any man that is called a brother be a fornicator, or covetous, or an idolater, or a railer, or a drunkard, or an extortioner; with such an one no not to eat.

12 For what have I to do to judge them also that are [h]without? do not ye judge them that are within?

13 But them that are without God judgeth. Therefore put away from among [i]yourselves that wicked person.

CHAPTER 6.

Saints forbidden to go to law with each other.

Dare any of you, having a matter against another, go to law before the unjust, and not before the saints?

2 Do ye not know that the saints shall judge the [j]world? and if the world shall be judged by you, are ye unworthy to judge the smallest matters?

3 Know ye not that we shall [k]judge [l]angels? how much more things that pertain to this life?

4 If then ye have judgments of things pertaining to this life, set them to judge [m]who are least esteemed in the church.

5 I speak to your shame. Is it so, that there is not a wise man among you? no, not one that shall be able to judge between his brethren?

6 But brother goeth to law with brother, and that before the unbelievers.

7 Now therefore there is utterly a fault among you, because ye go to law one with another. Why do ye not rather take wrong? why do ye not rather *suffer yourselves to* be defrauded?

8 Nay, ye do wrong, and defraud, and that *your* brethren.

Part IV. The sanctity of the body, and marriage (1 Cor. 6:9–7:40).

(1) *The body is holy: because washed and justified.*

9 Know ye not that the unrighteous shall not inherit the kingdom of God? Be not deceived: neither fornicators, nor idolaters, nor adulterers, nor effeminate, nor abusers of themselves with mankind,

10 Nor thieves, nor covetous, nor drunkards, nor revilers, nor extortioners, shall inherit the kingdom of God.

11 And such were some of you: but ye [n]are washed, but ye are [o]sanctified, but ye are [p]justified in the name of the Lord Jesus, and by the Spirit of our God.

12 All things are lawful unto me, but all things are not expedient: all things are lawful for me, but I will not be brought under the power of any.

(2) *Because the body is the Lord's.*

13 Meats for the belly, and the belly for meats: but God shall destroy both it and them. Now the body *is* not for fornication, but for the Lord; and the Lord for the body.

14 And God hath both raised up the Lord, and will also raise up us by his own power.

15 Know ye not that your bodies are the members of Christ? [q]shall I then

A.D. 59.

a *Judgments (the seven).* 1 Cor. 6:2, 3. (2 Sam. 7:14; Rev. 20:12.)

b *Satan.* 1 Cor. 7:5. (Gen. 3:1; Rev. 20:10.)

c Rom. 1:16, *note.*

d Some ancient authorities omit *Jesus.*

e *Sacrifice (of Christ).* 1 Cor. 11:25. (Gen. 4:4; Heb. 10:18.)

f *Leaven.* vs. 6, 7, 8; Gal. 5:9. (Gen. 19:3; Mt. 13:33.)

g *kosmos* (Mt. 4:8) = mankind.

h Mk. 4:11.

i *Separation.* vs. 1, 2, 9-13; 1 Cor. 10:20, 21. (Gen. 12:1; 2 Cor. 6:14-17.)

j *kosmos* (Mt. 4:8) = mankind.

k *Judgments (the seven).* vs. 2, 3; 1 Cor. 11:31, 32. (2 Sam. 7:14; Rev. 20:12.)

l Heb. 1:4, *note.*

m *Churches (local).* 1 Cor. 7:17. (Acts 2:41; Phil. 1:1.)

n *were,* and so throughout the verse.

o *Sanctify, holy (persons)* (N.T.). 1 Cor. 7:14, 34. (Mt. 4:5; Rev. 22:11.) .

p *Justification.* Gal. 2:16. (Lk. 18:14; Rom. 3:28.)

q Paul does not invoke the authority of the seventh commandment, but appeals to the believer's sacredness as a member of Christ.

[1] **(5:5)** Gr. *olethros,* used elsewhere, 1 Thes. 5:3; 2 Thes. 1:9; 1 Tim. 6:9, never means annihilation.

take the members of Christ, and make *them* the members of an harlot? God forbid.

16 What? know ye not that he which is joined to an harlot is one body? for [a]two, saith he, shall be one flesh.

17 But he that is joined unto the Lord is one spirit.

18 Flee fornication. Every sin that a man doeth is without the body; but he that committeth fornication sinneth against his own body.

(3) *Because the body is a temple.*

19 What? know ye not that your body is [b]the temple of the [c]Holy Ghost *which is* in you, which ye have [d]of God, and ye are not your own?

20 For ye [e]are bought with a price: therefore glorify God in your body, [f]and in your spirit, which are God's.

CHAPTER 7.

(4) *Because God has established marriage.*

Now concerning the things whereof ye wrote unto me: *It is* good for a man not to touch a woman.

2 Nevertheless, *to avoid* fornication, let every man have his own wife, and let every woman have her own husband.

3 Let the husband render unto the wife due benevolence: and likewise also the wife unto the husband.

4 The wife hath not [g]power of her own body, but the husband: and likewise also the husband hath not power of his own body, but the wife.

5 Defraud ye not one the other, except *it be* with consent for a time, that ye may give yourselves to fasting and prayer; and come together again, that [h]Satan [i]tempt you not [j]for your incontinency.

6 But I speak this by [k]permission, *and* not of commandment.

7 For I would that all men were even as I myself. [l]But every man hath his proper gift of God, one after this manner, and another after that.

8 I say therefore to the unmarried and widows, It is good for them if they abide even as I.

A.D. 59.

a Gen. 2:24; Mt. 19:5.
b *a temple.*
c *Holy Spirit.* vs. 11, 19; 1 Cor. 7:40. (Mt. 1:18; Acts 2:4.)
d *from.*
e *were.*
f Some authorities end verse with "body."
g *authority over.*
h *Satan.* 2 Cor. 2:11. (Gen. 3:1; Rev. 20:10.)
i *Temptation.* 1 Cor. 10:9, 13. (Gen. 3:1; Jas. 1:14.)
j *because of your lack of self-control.*
k *concession.*
l *Howbeit, each man hath his own gift from God, etc.*
m John 2:1, 2; 1 Tim. 5:14; Heb. 13:4.
n *leave.*
o *leave her.*
p *Sanctify, holy (persons)* (N.T.). vs. 14, 34; Eph. 1:4. (Mt. 4:5; Rev. 22:11.)
q Gr. *tekna, born ones.*
r Rom. 1:16, *note.*
s *each.*
t *Churches (local).* vs. 17, 18; 1 Cor. 10:32. (Acts 2:41; Phil. 1:1.)
u *the churches.*
v Lk. 3:10, 14.

9 But if they cannot contain, [m]let them marry: for it is better to marry than to burn.

The regulation of marriage among Gentile believers.

10 And unto the married I command, *yet* not I, but the Lord, Let not the wife depart from *her* husband:

11 But and if she depart, let her remain unmarried, or be reconciled to *her* husband: and let not the husband [n]put away *his* wife.

12 But to the rest [1]speak I, not the Lord: If any brother hath a wife that believeth not, and she be pleased to dwell with him, let him not [o]put her away.

13 And the woman which hath an husband that believeth not, and if he be pleased to dwell with her, let her not leave him.

14 For the unbelieving husband is [p]sanctified by the wife, and the unbelieving wife is sanctified by the husband: else were your [q]children unclean; but now are they holy.

15 But if the unbelieving depart, let him depart. A brother or a sister is not under bondage in such *cases*: but God hath called us to peace.

16 For what knowest thou, O wife, whether thou shalt save *thy* husband? or how knowest thou, O man, whether thou shalt [r]save *thy* wife?

17 But as God hath distributed to [s]every man, as the Lord hath called [s]every one, so let him walk. And so ordain I [t]in all [u]churches.

18 Is any man called being circumcised? let him not become uncircumcised. Is any called in uncircumcision? let him not be circumcised.

19 Circumcision is nothing, and uncircumcision is nothing, but the keeping of the commandments of God.

20 Let every man [v]abide in the same calling wherein he was called.

21 Art thou called *being* a servant? care not for it: but if thou mayest be made free, use *it* rather.

22 For he that is called in the Lord,

[1] **(7:12)** So far from disclaiming inspiration, the apostle associates his teaching with the Lord's. Cases had arisen (e.g. vs. 12-16), as the Gospel overflowed Jewish limitations, not comprehended in the words of Jesus (Mt. 5:31, 32; 19:5-9) which were an instruction, primarily, to Israel. These new conditions demanded authoritative settlement, and only the inspired words of an apostle could give that. See v. 40.

being a servant, [a]is the Lord's [b]freeman: likewise also he that is called, *being* free, is Christ's servant.

23 Ye are [c]bought with a price; be not ye the servants of men.

24 Brethren, let every man, wherein he is called, therein abide with [d]God.

25 Now concerning virgins I have no commandment of the Lord: yet I give my judgment, as one that hath obtained mercy of the Lord to be faithful.

26 I suppose therefore that this is good for the present distress, *I say*, that *it is* good for a man so to be.

27 Art thou bound unto a wife? seek not to be loosed. Art thou loosed from a wife? seek not a wife.

28 But and if thou marry, thou hast not [e]sinned; and if a virgin marry, she hath not sinned. Nevertheless such shall have trouble in the flesh: [f]but I spare you.

29 But this I say, brethren, the [g]time *is* short: it remaineth, that both they that have wives be as though they had none;

30 And they that weep, as though they wept not; and they that rejoice, as though they rejoiced not; and they that buy, as though they possessed not;

31 And they that use this [h]world, as not abusing *it*: for the fashion of this world passeth away.

32 But I would have you [i]without carefulness. He that is unmarried careth for the things that belong to the Lord, how he may please the Lord:

33 But he that is married careth for the things that are of the [h]world, how he may please *his* wife.

34 There is difference *also* between a wife and a virgin. The unmarried woman careth for the things of the Lord, that she may be holy both in body and in spirit: but she that is married careth for the things of the [j]world, how she may please *her* husband.

35 And this I speak for your own profit; not that I may [k]cast a snare upon you, but for that which is comely, and that ye may attend upon the Lord without distraction.

36 But if any man think that he behaveth himself uncomely toward his virgin, if she pass the flower of *her* age, and need so require, let him do what he will, he [l]sinneth not: let them marry.

37 Nevertheless he that standeth stedfast in his heart, having no necessity, but hath power over his own will, and hath so decreed in his heart that he will keep his virgin, doeth well.

38 So then he that giveth *her* in marriage doeth well; but he that giveth *her* not in marriage doeth better.

39 The wife is bound by the law as long as her husband liveth; but if her husband be dead, she is at liberty to be married to whom she will; [m]only in the Lord.

40 But she is happier if she so abide, after my judgment: and I think [n]also that I have the [o]Spirit of God.

CHAPTER 8.

Part V. Meats, and the limitations of Christian liberty (1Cor. 8:1–11:1).

Now [p]as touching things offered unto idols, we know that we all have knowledge. Knowledge puffeth up, but [q]charity edifieth.

2 And if any man think that he knoweth any thing, he knoweth nothing yet as he ought to know.

3 But if any man love God, the same is known of him.

4 As concerning therefore the eating of those things that are offered in sacrifice unto idols, we know that an idol *is* nothing in the [r]world, and that *there is* none other God but one.

5 For though there be that are called gods, whether in heaven or in earth, (as there be gods many, and lords many,)

6 But [s]to us *there is but* one God, the Father, of whom *are* all things, and we in him; and one Lord Jesus Christ, by [t]whom *are* all things, and [u]we by him.

7 Howbeit *there is* not in every man that knowledge: for some with conscience of the idol unto this hour eat *it* as a thing offered unto an idol; and their conscience being weak is defiled.

8 But meat commendeth us not to God: for neither, if we eat, are we the better; neither, if we eat not, are we the worse.

9 But take heed lest by any means this [v]liberty of yours become a stumblingblock to them that are weak.

10 For if any man see thee which hast knowledge sit at meat in the idol's temple, [w]shall not the conscience of him

A.D. 59.

a John 8:36; Rom. 6:18, 22.
b *made free.*
c 1 Cor. 6:20; 1 Pet. 1:18, 19.
d Eph. 6:5, 8; Col. 3:22, 24.
e *Sin.* Rom. 3:23, *note.*
f *and I would spare you.*
g 1 Pet. 4:7; 2 Pet. 3:8.
h *kosmos* = world-system. 2 Cor. 7:10. (John 7:7; Rev. 13:3-8, *note.*)
i *free from cares.*
j *kosmos* (Mt. 4:8) = mankind.
k *put constraint upon you.*
l *Sin.* Rom. 3:23, *note.*
m 2 Cor. 6:14.
n *that I also have the Spirit of God.*
o *Holy Spirit.* 1 Cor. 12:3, 4, 7, 8, 9, 11, 13. (Mt. 1:18; Acts 2:4.)
p *concerning things sacrificed to.*
q *love buildeth up.*
r i.e. *earth.*
s Mal. 2:10; Eph. 4:6.
t John 1:3; Heb. 1:2.
u Rom. 5:11; Rev. 4:11; 5:9, 10.
v *Law (of Christ).* vs. 9-13; 1 Cor. 9:21. (Gal. 6:2; 2 John 5.)
w *will not his conscience if he is weak be builded up,* etc.

A.D. 59.

which is weak be emboldened to eat those things which are offered to idols;

11 And through thy knowledge shall the weak brother perish, for [a]whom Christ died?

12 But when ye [b]sin so against the brethren, and wound their weak conscience, ye sin against Christ.

13 Wherefore, if meat make my brother to [c]offend, I will eat no flesh while the [d]world standeth, [e]lest I make my brother to offend.

CHAPTER 9.

Paul vindicates his apostleship.
(Cf. Gal. 1:11–2:14.)

Am I not an apostle? am I not free? have I not seen Jesus Christ our Lord? are not ye my work in the Lord?

2 If I be not an apostle unto others, yet doubtless I am to you: for the seal of mine apostleship are ye in the Lord.

3 Mine answer to them that do examine me is this,

4 Have we [f]not power to eat and to drink?

5 Have we [f]not power to lead about a [g]sister, a wife, as well as other apostles, and *as* the brethren of the Lord, and Cephas?

6 Or I only and Barnabas, have not we [h]power to forbear working?

They who preach the Gospel are to live of the Gospel.

7 Who goeth a warfare any time at his own charges? who planteth a vineyard, and eateth not of the fruit thereof? or who feedeth a flock, and eateth not of the milk of the flock?

8 Say I these things as a man? or saith not the law the same also?

9 For [i]it is written in the law of Moses, Thou shalt not muzzle the mouth of the ox that treadeth out the corn. Doth God take care for oxen?

10 Or saith he *it* altogether for our sakes? [j]For our sakes, no doubt, *this* is written: that he that ploweth should plow in hope; and that he that thresheth [k]in hope should be partaker of his hope.

11 If we have sown unto you spiritual things, *is it* a great thing if we shall reap your [l]carnal things?

12 If others be partakers of *this* power over you, *are* not we rather? [m]Nevertheless we have not used this power; but suffer all things, lest we should hinder the gospel of Christ.

13 Do ye not know that they which minister about [n]holy things [o]live *of the things* of the temple? and they which wait at the altar are partakers with the altar?

14 Even so hath the Lord ordained that they which preach the gospel should live of the gospel.

15 But I have used none of these things: neither have I written these things, that it should be so done unto me: for *it were* better for me to die, than that any man should make my glorying void.

16 For though I preach the gospel, I have nothing to glory of: for necessity is laid upon me; yea, woe is unto me, if I preach not the gospel!

17 For if I do this thing willingly, I have a [p]reward: but if against my will, a dispensation *of the gospel* is committed unto me.

18 What is my reward then? *Verily* that, when I preach the gospel, I may make the gospel of Christ without charge, that I abuse not my power in the gospel.

The method and reward of true ministry.

19 For though I be free from all *men*, yet have I made myself servant unto all, that I might gain the more.

20 And unto the Jews I became as a Jew, that I might gain the Jews; to them that are under the law, as under the law, that I might gain them that are under the law;

21 To them that are without law, as without law, (being not [1]without law to God, but [q]under the law to Christ,) that I might gain them that are without law.

22 To the weak became I as weak, that I might gain the weak: I am made all things to all *men*, that I might by all means [r]save some.

23 And this I do for the [s]gospel's sake, that I might be partaker thereof with *you*.

24 Know ye not that they which run in a [t]race run all, but one receiveth the

a *whose sake.*
b *Sin.* Rom. 3:23, *note.*
c *stumble.*
d *the age lasteth.*
e Rom. 14:21; 1 Cor. 9:22.
f *no right.*
g *a wife who is a sister.*
h 2 Thes. 3:8, 9.
i Deut. 25:4; 1 Tim. 5:18.
j 2 Tim. 3:16.
k Or, *in hope of partaking of it.*
l i.e. *things for the body.*
m 2 Cor. 11:7, 9, 12, 14.
n *Sanctify, holy (things)* (N.T.). 1 Cor. 16:20. (Mt. 4:5; Rev. 22:11.)
o Or, *eat.*
p *Rewards.* Phil. 4:1. (Dan. 12:3; 1 Cor. 3:14.)
q *Law (of Christ).* 1 Cor. 13:1-13. (Gal. 6:2; 2 John 5.)
r Rom. 1:16, *note.*
s *Gospel.* vs. 12, 14, 16-18, 23; 1 Cor. 15:1-4. (Gen. 12:1-3; Rev. 14:6.)
t *race-course.*

[1] **(9:21)** The expression is peculiar and might be literally rendered, "not lawless toward God, but inlawed to Christ." See "Law (of Christ)," Gal. 6:2; 2 John 5. It is another way of saying, "not under the law, but under [the rule of] grace" (Rom. 6:14).

prize? [a]So run, that ye may obtain.
25 And every man that striveth for the
mastery is temperate in all things. Now
they *do it* to obtain a corruptible crown;
but we an [b]incorruptible.
26 I therefore so run, [c]not as uncertainly; so fight I, [d]not as one that beateth the
air:
27 But I [e]keep under my body, and
bring *it* into subjection: lest that by any
means, when I have preached to others, I
myself should be [f]a [1]castaway.

CHAPTER 10.

Israel in the wilderness a warning example.

Moreover, brethren, I would not that
ye should be ignorant, how that
all our fathers were under the cloud, and
all passed through the sea;
2 And were all baptized unto Moses in
the cloud and in the sea;
3 And did all eat the same spiritual
meat;
4 And did all drink the same spiritual
drink: for they drank of [g]that spiritual
[h]Rock that followed them: and that Rock
was Christ.
5 But with many of them God was not
well pleased: for they were overthrown
in the wilderness.
6 Now these things [i]were our examples, to the intent we should not lust
after evil things, as they also lusted.
7 Neither be ye idolaters, as *were* some
of them; as it is written, [j]The people sat
down to eat and drink, and rose up to
play.
8 Neither let us commit fornication, as
[k]some of them committed, and [2]fell in
one day three and twenty thousand.
9 Neither let us [l]tempt Christ, as some
of them also tempted, and were
destroyed of [m]serpents.
10 Neither murmur ye, as some of
them also [n]murmured, and were
destroyed of the destroyer.
11 Now all these things happened
unto them [o]for ensamples: and they are
written for our admonition, upon whom
the ends of the [p]world are come.
12 Wherefore let him that thinketh he
standeth take heed lest he fall.
13 There hath no [q]temptation taken you
but such as is common to man: but God *is*
faithful, who will not suffer you to be
tempted above that ye are able; but will
with the temptation [r]also make a way to
escape, that ye may be able to bear *it*.
14 Wherefore, my dearly beloved, flee
from idolatry.
15 I speak as to wise men; judge ye
what I say.

Fellowship at the Lord's table demands separation.

16 The cup of blessing which we bless,
is it not the communion of the blood of
Christ? The bread which we break, is it
not the communion of the body of Christ?
17 For we *being* many are one [s]bread,
and one body: for we are all partakers of
that one bread.
18 Behold Israel after the flesh: are not
they which eat of the sacrifices partakers
of the altar?
19 What say I then? that the [t]idol is
any thing, or that which is offered in sacrifice to idols is any thing?
20 But I *say*, that the things which the
Gentiles sacrifice, they sacrifice to [u]devils,
and not to [v]God: and I would not that ye
should have [w]fellowship with devils.
21 [x]Ye cannot drink the cup of the
Lord, and the cup of devils: ye cannot

A.D. 59.

a Phil. 3:14; 1 Tim. 6:12.
b 2 Tim. 4:8; Jas. 1:12; 1 Pet. 5:4; Rev. 2:10; 3:11.
c *as not uncertainly.*
d *as not beating the air.*
e *buffet my body, and lead it captive.*
f i.e. *disapproved.*
g *a spiritual rock.*
h *Christ (as Stone).* John 4:13, 14. (Ex. 17:6; 1 Pet. 2:8.)
i *happened as types for us.*
j Ex. 32:6.
k Num. 25:1, 9.
l Ex. 17:2, 7.
m Num. 21:6.
n Num. 14:2; 29; 26:63, 65.
o *as types.*
p i.e. *ages.*
q *Temptation.* vs. 9, 13; 2 Cor. 11:3, 4. (Gen. 3:1; Jas. 1:14.)
r *make the issue also.*
s Or, *loaf.* Cf. 1 Cor. 11:23-26; 12:12, 13.
t 1 Cor. 8:4.
u Gr. *demons;* also v. 21. See Mt. 7:22, *note.*
v Deut. 32:17.
w See v. 16, trans. *communion.*
x *Separation.* 2 Thes. 3:6, 14. (Gen. 12:1; 2 Cor. 6:14-17.)

[1]**(9:27)** Gr. *adokimos,* "disapproved." *Dokimos,* without the privative *a,* is translated "approved" in Rom. 14:18; 16:10; 1 Cor. 11:19; 2 Cor. 10:18; 2 Tim. 2:15, and in Jas. 1:12 by the word "tried." The prefix simply changes the word to a negative, i.e. not approved, or, disapproved. The apostle is writing of *service,* not of *salvation.* He is not expressing fear that he may fail of salvation but of his crown. See "Rewards" (Dan. 12:3; 1 Cor. 3:14).

[2]**(10:8)** Cf. Num. 25:9. A discrepancy has been imagined. 1 Cor. 10:8 gives the number of deaths in "one day"; Num. 25:9, the total number of deaths "in the plague." Some discrepant statements concerning numbers are, however, found in the existing manuscripts of the Hebrew Scriptures. These are most naturally ascribed to the fact that the Hebrews used letters in the place of numerals. The letters from *Koph* to *Tau* express hundreds up to four hundred. Five certain Hebrew letters, written in a different form, carry hundreds up to nine hundred, while thousands are expressed by two dots over the proper unit letter: e.g. the letter *Teth,* used alone, stands for 9; with two dots it stands for nine thousand. Error in transcription of Hebrew numbers thus becomes easy, preservation of numerical accuracy difficult.

be partakers of the Lord's table, and of the table of devils.

22 Do we provoke the Lord to jealousy? are we stronger than he?

The law of love in relation to eating and drinking. (Cf. Rom. 14:1-23.)

23 All things are lawful for me, but all things are not expedient: all things are lawful for me, but all things edify not.

24 Let no man seek his [a]own, but every man another's *wealth.*

25 Whatsoever is sold in the shambles, *that* eat, asking no question for conscience sake:

26 For the earth *is* the [b]Lord's, and the fulness thereof.

27 If any of them that believe not bid you *to a feast,* and ye be disposed to go; whatsoever is set before you, eat, asking no question for conscience sake.

28 But if any man say unto you, This is offered in sacrifice unto idols, [c]eat not for his sake that shewed it, and for conscience sake: for the earth *is* the Lord's, and the fulness thereof:

29 Conscience, I say, not thine own, but of the other: for why is my liberty judged of another *man's* conscience?

30 For if I [d]by grace be a partaker, why am I evil spoken of for that for which I give thanks?

31 Whether therefore ye eat, or drink, or whatsoever ye do, do all to the glory of God.

32 Give none offence, neither to the Jews, nor to the Gentiles, nor to [e]the [f]church of God:

33 Even as I please all *men* in all *things,* not seeking mine own profit, but the *profit* of many, that they may be [g]saved.

CHAPTER 11.

Be ye [h]followers of me, even as I also *am* of Christ.

Part VI. Christian order and the Lord's supper. (vs.2-34).

2 Now I praise you, brethren, that ye remember me in all things, and keep the [i]ordinances, as I delivered *them* to you.

3 But I would have you know, that the head of every man is Christ; and the head of the [j]woman *is* the man; and the head of Christ *is* God.

4 Every man praying or prophesying, having *his* head covered, dishonoureth his head.

5 But [k]every woman that prayeth or prophesieth with *her* head uncovered dishonoureth her head: for that is even all one as if she were shaven.

6 For if the woman be not covered, let her also be shorn: but if it be a shame for a woman to be shorn or shaven, let her be covered.

7 For a man indeed ought not to cover *his* head, forasmuch as he is the [l]image and glory of [m]God: but the woman is the glory of the man.

8 For the man is not of the woman; but the woman of the man.

9 Neither was the man created for the woman; but the woman for the man.

10 For this cause ought the woman to have [n]power on *her* head because of the [o]angels.

11 Nevertheless neither is the man without the woman, neither the woman without the man, in the Lord.

12 For as the woman *is* of the man, even so *is* the man also by the woman; but all things of God.

13 Judge in yourselves: is it [p]comely that a woman pray unto God uncovered?

14 Doth not even nature itself teach you, that, if a man have long hair, it is a shame unto him?

15 But if a woman have long hair, it is a glory to her: for *her* hair is given her for a [q]covering.

16 But if any man seem to be contentious, we have no such custom, neither the churches of God.

Disorders at the Lord's table rebuked.

17 Now in this that I declare *unto you* I praise *you* not, that ye come together not for the better, but for the worse.

18 For first of all, when ye come together in the church, [r]I hear that there be [s]divisions among you; and I partly believe it.

19 For there must be also [t]heresies among you, that they which are approved may be made manifest among you.

20 When ye come together therefore into one place, [u]*this* is not to eat the Lord's supper.

21 For in eating every one taketh before *other* his own supper: and one is [v]hungry, and another is drunken.

A.D. 59.

a *own advantage, but that of the other.*

b *Jehovah.* Psa. 24:1.

c 1 Cor. 8:10, 12.

d *partake with thanksgiving.*

e *Churches (local).* 1 Cor. 11:16-34. (Acts 2:41; Phil. 1:1.)

f *Church (visible).* 1 Cor. 12:28. (1 Cor. 10:32; 1 Tim. 3:15.)

g Rom. 1:16, *note.*

h *imitators.* 1 Cor. 4:16.

i *things delivered;* often trans. *traditions.*

j Cf. Gen. 3:16. The woman's veil, or head-covering, is a symbol of this subordination.

k Acts 21:9.

l Gen. 5:1.

m Gen. 1:27.

n *authority,* i.e. the sign of the husband's authority.

o i.e. of the presence of the angels.

p Or, *seemly.*

q Or, *veil.*

r 1 Cor. 1:11, 12.

s Or, *schisms.*

t Or, *sects.*

u Or, *ye cannot eat.*

v Jude 12.

22 What? have ye not houses to eat
and to drink in? or despise ye the church
of God, and shame them that have not?
What shall I say to you? shall I praise
you in this? I praise *you* not.

The order and meaning of the Lord's table.

23 For I have received of the Lord that
which also I delivered unto you, That
the Lord Jesus the *same* night in which
he was betrayed took bread:
24 And when he had given thanks, he
brake *it*, and said, Take, eat: this is my
body, which [a]is broken for you: this do
in remembrance of me.
25 After the same manner also *he took*
the cup, when he had supped, saying,
This cup is the new [b]testament [c]in my
blood: this do ye, as oft as ye drink *it*, in
remembrance of me.
26 For as often as ye eat this bread,
and drink this cup, ye [d]do shew the
Lord's death till he come.
27 Wherefore whosoever shall eat this
bread, and drink *this* cup of the Lord,
[e]unworthily, shall be guilty of the body
and blood of the Lord.
28 But let a man examine himself, and
so let him eat of *that* bread, and drink of
that cup.
29 For he that eateth and drinketh
unworthily, eateth and drinketh [f]damnation to himself, not discerning the Lord's
body.
30 For this cause many *are* weak and
sickly among you, and many sleep.
31 For if we would [1g]judge ourselves,
we should not be [h]judged.
32 But when we are judged, we are
chastened of the Lord, that we [i]should
not be condemned with the [j]world.
33 Wherefore, my brethren, when ye
come together to eat, tarry one for
another.
34 And if any man hunger, let him eat
at home; that ye [k]come not together
[l]unto condemnation. And the rest will I
set in order when I come.

CHAPTER 12.

Part VII. Spiritual gifts in the body of Christ for ministry and worship (1 Cor. 12:1–14:40).

NOW concerning [2]spiritual *gifts*,
brethren, I would not have you
ignorant.
2 Ye know that [m]ye were Gentiles, carried away unto these dumb idols, even
as ye were led.
3 Wherefore I give you to understand,
that no man speaking [n]by the Spirit of
God calleth Jesus accursed: and *that* no
man can say that Jesus is the Lord, but
[n]by the Holy Ghost.

True ministry is the exercise of spiritual gift (Cf. Eph. 4:7-16.)

4 Now there are diversities of [o]gifts,
but the same Spirit.
5 And there are differences of administrations, but the same Lord.
6 And there are diversities of [p]operations, but it is the same God which
worketh all in all.
7 But [q]the manifestation of the Spirit is
given to every man to profit withal.
8 For to one is given by the Spirit the

A.D. 59.

a *is for you.*
b *covenant.*
c *Sacrifice (of Christ).* 2 Cor. 5:14, 18, 19, 21. (Gen. 4:4; Heb. 10:18.)
d *declare.*
e i.e. in an unworthy manner; cf. vs. 20-22.
f *judgment,* in the sense of v. 32.
g Lit. *discern.*
h *Judgments (the seven).* vs. 31, 32; 2 Cor. 5:8-10. (2 Sam. 7:14; Rev. 20:12.)
i *may not.*
j *kosmos* (Mt. 4:8) = mankind.
k *Churches (local).* 1 Cor. 12:28-31. (Acts 2:41; Phil. 1:1.)
l *for judgment.*
m *when ye were Gentiles.*
n *in.*
o Cf. Eph. 4:8, 11, 12. The Spirit gives gifts for service to men, Christ gives the gifted men to the churches.
p *workings.*
q *to each the manifestation is given for profit.*

[1] **(11:31)** Self-judgment is not so much the believer's moral condemnation of his own ways or habits, as of *himself*, for allowing such ways. Self-judgment avoids chastisement. If neglected, the Lord judges, and the result is chastisement, but never condemnation (v. 32; 2 Sam. 7:14, 15; 12:13, 14; 1 Cor. 5:5; 1 Tim. 1:20; Heb. 12:7). See other judgments, John 12:31 *note;* 2 Cor. 5:10, *note;* Mt. 25:32, *note;* Ezk. 20:37, *note;* Jude 6, *note;* Rev. 20:12, *note.*

[2] **(12:1)** The word *pneumatika,* lit. "spirituals," i.e. matters of or from the Holy Spirit, gives the key to Chapters 12, 13, 14. Chapter 12 concerns the Spirit in relation to the body of Christ. This relation is twofold: (1) The baptism with the Spirit forms the body by uniting believers to Christ the risen and glorified Head, and to each other (vs. 12, 13). The symbol of the body thus formed is the natural, human body (v. 12), and all the analogies are freely used (vs. 14-26). (2) To each believer is given a spiritual enablement and capacity for specific service. No believer is destitute of such gift (vs. 7, 11, 27), but in their distribution the Spirit acts in free sovereignty (v. 11). There is no room for self-choosing, and Christian service is simply the ministry of such gift as the individual may have received (cf. Rom. 12:4-8). The gifts are diverse (vs. 6, 8-10, 28-30), but all are equally honourable because bestowed by the same Spirit, administered under the same Lord, and energized by the same God.

word of wisdom; to another the word of knowledge by the same Spirit;

9 To another [a]faith by the same Spirit; to another the gifts of healing by the same Spirit;

10 To another the working of miracles; to another [1]prophecy; to another [b]discerning of spirits; to another *divers* kinds of [c]tongues; to another the interpretation of tongues:

11 But all these worketh that one and the selfsame Spirit, dividing to every man severally as he will.

Every believer is a member of Christ's body and as such has a definite ministry.

12 For as the body is one, and hath many members, and all the members of that one body, being many, are one body: so also *is* Christ.

13 For by one [d]Spirit are we all baptized into one body, whether *we be* Jews or [e]Gentiles, whether *we be* bond or free; [f]and have been all [g]made to drink into one Spirit.

14 For the body is not one member, but many.

15 If the foot shall say, Because I am not the hand, I am not of the body; is it therefore not of the body?

16 And if the ear shall say, Because I am not the eye, I am not of the body; is it therefore not of the body?

17 If the whole body *were* an eye, where *were* the hearing? If the whole *were* hearing, where *were* the smelling?

18 But now hath God set the members every one of them in the body, as it hath pleased him.

19 And if they were all one member, where *were* the body?

20 But now *are they* many members, yet but one body.

21 And the eye cannot say unto the hand, I have no need of thee: nor again the head to the feet, I have no need of you.

22 Nay, much more those members of the body, which seem to be more feeble, are necessary:

23 And those *members* of the body, which we think to be less honourable, upon these we [h]bestow more abundant honour; and our uncomely *parts* have more abundant comeliness.

24 For our comely *parts* have no need: but God hath tempered the body together, having given more abundant honour to that *part* which lacked:

25 That there should be no [i]schism in the body; but *that* the members should have the same care one for another.

26 And whether one member suffer, all the members suffer with it; or one member be honoured, all the members rejoice with it.

27 Now ye are the body of Christ, and [j]members in particular.

28 [k]And God hath [l]set some in [m]the [n]church, first apostles, secondarily prophets, thirdly teachers, after that miracles, then gifts of healings, helps, governments, diversities of tongues.

29 *Are* all apostles? *are* all prophets? *are* all teachers? *are* all workers of miracles?

30 Have all the gifts of healing? do all speak with tongues? do all interpret?

31 But covet earnestly the best gifts: and yet shew I unto you a [2]more excellent way.

CHAPTER 13.

The ministry gifts must be governed by love.

Though I speak with the tongues of men and of [o]angels, and have not [p]charity, I am become *as* sounding brass, or a [q]tinkling cymbal.

2 And though I have *the gift of* prophecy, and understand all mysteries, and all knowledge; and though I have all faith, so that I could remove mountains, and have not [r]charity, I am nothing.

3 And though I bestow all my goods to feed *the poor*, and though I give my body to be burned, and have not [p]charity, it profiteth me nothing.

A.D. 59.

a *Faith.* 1 Cor. 15:14, 17. (Gen. 3:20; Heb. 11:39.)
b 1 John 4:1.
c Acts 2:4-11.
d *Holy Spirit.* vs. 3, 4, 7, 8, 9, 11, 13; 1 Cor. 14:16. (Mt. 1:18; Acts 2:4.)
e *Greeks.*
f *Assurance.* vs. 12, 13; 2 Cor. 1:10. (Isa. 32:17; Jude 1.)
g *given to drink of.*
h Or, *put on.*
i Or, *division.*
j Eph. 5:30.
k vs. 8, 11; Acts 5:4.
l *Churches (local).* vs. 28-31; 1 Cor. 14:1-5. (Acts 2:41; Phil 1:1.)
m *Church (true).* vs. 12-28, 31; 2 Cor. 11:2, 3. (Mt. 16:18; Heb. 12:23.)
n *Church (visible).* 1 Cor. 15:9. (1 Cor. 10:32; 1 Tim. 3:15.)
o Heb. 1:4, *note.*
p i.e. *love;* and so in vs. 2, 3, 4, 8, 13.
q *clanging.*
r *Law (of Christ).* vs. 1-13; 2 Cor. 5:13, 14. (Gal. 6:2; 2 John 5.)

[1] **(12:10)** The N.T. prophet is not ordinarily a foreteller, but rather a forth-teller, one whose gift enabled him to speak "to edification, and exhortation, and comfort" (1 Cor. 14:3).

[2] **(12:31)** Chapter 13 continues the *pneumatika* begun in Chapter 12. Gifts are good, but only if ministered in love (13:1, 2) Benevolence is good, but not apart from love (13:3). Love is described (13:4-7). Love is better than our present incomplete knowledge (13:8-12), and greater than even faith and hope (v. 13).

4 [a]Charity suffereth long, *and* is kind; charity envieth not; charity vaunteth not itself, is not puffed up,

5 Doth not behave itself unseemly, seeketh not her own, is not easily provoked, thinketh no evil;

6 Rejoiceth not in iniquity, but rejoiceth [b]in the truth;

7 Beareth all things, believeth all things, hopeth all things, endureth all things.

8 [a]Charity [c]never faileth: but whether *there be* prophecies, they shall fail; whether *there be* tongues, they shall cease; whether *there be* knowledge, it shall vanish away.

9 For we know [d]in part, and we prophesy in part.

10 [e]But when that which is perfect is come, then that which is in part shall be done away.

11 When I was a child, I spake as a child, I understood as a child, I [f]thought as a child: but when I became a man, I put away childish things.

12 For now we see [g]through a glass, darkly; but then face to face: now I know in part; but then shall I know even as also I am known.

13 And now abideth faith, hope, [a]charity, these three; but the greatest of these *is* charity.

CHAPTER 14.

Prophecy is the greatest of the gifts.

Follow after [h]charity, and desire spiritual *gifts*, but [1]rather that ye may prophesy.

2 For he that speaketh in [i]an *unknown* tongue speaketh not unto men, but unto God: for no man [j]understandeth *him;* howbeit in the spirit he speaketh mysteries.

3 But he that prophesieth speaketh unto men *to* edification, and exhortation, and comfort.

A.D. 59.

a i.e. *love;* and so in vs. 2, 3, 4, 8, 13.
b *with.*
c Eph. 3:17, 19.
d 1 Cor. 8:2.
e 1 John 3:2.
f *reasoned.*
g *in a mirror in an enigma.*
h *love.*
i Or, *a tongue;* and so in vs. 4, 13, 14, 19, 27.
j Gr. *heareth.*
k *Churches (local).* vs. 1-5; 1 Cor. 14:35. (Acts 2:41; Phil. 1:1.)
l i.e. *earth.*
m Rom. 14:19; Eph. 4:29.
n John 4:24.

4 He that speaketh in an *unknown* tongue edifieth himself; but he that prophesieth edifieth the church.

5 I would that ye all spake with tongues, but rather that ye prophesied: for greater *is* he that prophesieth than he that speaketh with tongues, except he interpret, that the [k]church may receive edifying.

6 Now, brethren, if I come unto you speaking with tongues, what shall I profit you, except I shall speak to you either by revelation, or by knowledge, or by prophesying, or by doctrine?

7 And even things without life giving sound, whether pipe or harp, except they give a distinction in the sounds, how shall it be known what is piped or harped?

8 For if the trumpet give an uncertain sound, who shall prepare himself to the battle?

9 So likewise ye, except ye utter by the tongue words easy to be understood, how shall it be known what is spoken? for ye shall speak into the air.

10 There are, it may be, so many kinds of voices in the [l]world, and none of them *is* without signification.

11 Therefore if I know not the meaning of the voice, I shall be unto him that speaketh a barbarian, and he that speaketh *shall be* a barbarian unto me.

12 Even so ye, forasmuch as ye are zealous of spiritual *gifts*, seek that ye may excel to the [m]edifying of the church.

13 Wherefore let him that speaketh in an *unknown* tongue pray that he may interpret.

14 For if I pray in an *unknown* tongue, my spirit prayeth, but my understanding is unfruitful.

15 What is it then? I will pray with the spirit, and I will pray [n]with the

[1] **(14:1)** The subject is still the *pneumatika.* Chapter 12 described the gifts and the Body; Chapter 13 the love which alone gives ministry of gift any value; Chapter 14 regulates the ministry of gift in the primitive, apostolic assembly of saints. (1) The important gift is that of prophecy (v. 1). The N.T. prophet was not merely a preacher, but an inspired preacher, through whom, until the N.T. was written, new revelations suited to the new dispensation were given (1 Cor. 14:29, 30). (2) Tongues and the sign gifts are to cease, and meantime must be used with restraint, and only if an interpreter be present (vs. 1-19, 27, 28). (3) In the primitive church there was liberty for the ministry of all the gifts which might be present, but for prophecy more especially (vs. 23-26, 31, 39). (4) In such meetings, when "the whole church" came together "in one place," women were required to keep silence (vs. 34, 35; cf. 1 Cor. 11:3-16; 1 Tim. 2:11-14). (5) These injunctions are declared to be "the commandments of the Lord" (vs. 36, 37).

understanding also: I will [a]sing with the
spirit, and I will sing with the understanding also.
16 Else when thou shalt bless with the
[b]spirit, how shall he that occupieth the
room of the unlearned say Amen at thy
giving of thanks, seeing he understandeth not what thou sayest?
17 For thou verily givest thanks well,
but the other is not edified.
18 I thank my God, I speak with
tongues more than ye all:
19 Yet in the church I had rather speak
five words with my understanding, that
by my voice I might teach others also,
than ten thousand words in an *unknown*
tongue.
20 Brethren, be not [c]children in understanding: howbeit in malice be ye [d]chil-
dren, but in understanding be men.
21 In the law it is written, [e]With *men of*
other tongues and other lips will I speak
unto this people; and yet for all that will
they not hear me, saith the Lord.
22 Wherefore tongues are for a [f]sign,
not to them that believe, but to them that
believe not: but prophesying *serveth* not
for them that believe not, but for them
which believe.

The order of the ministry of gift in the local church.

23 If therefore the whole church be
come together into one place, and all
speak with tongues, and there come in
those that are unlearned, or unbelievers,
will they not say that [g]ye are mad?
24 But if all prophesy, and there come in
one that believeth not, or *one* unlearned,
he is convinced of all, he is judged of all:
25 And thus are the secrets of his heart
made manifest; and so falling down on
his face he will worship [h]God, and
report that God is in you of a truth.
26 How is it then, brethren? when ye
come together, every one of you hath a
psalm, hath a doctrine, hath a tongue,
hath a revelation, hath an interpretation.
[i]Let all things be done unto edifying.
27 If any man speak in an *unknown*
tongue, *let it be* by two, or at the most *by*
three, and *that* [j]by course; and let one
interpret.
28 But if there be no interpreter, let
him keep silence in the church; and let
him speak to himself, and to God.
29 [k]Let the prophets speak two or
three, and let the other judge.
30 If *any thing* be revealed to another
that sitteth by, let the first hold his peace.
31 For ye may all prophesy one by
one, that all may learn, and all may be
comforted.
32 And the spirits of the prophets are
[l]subject to the prophets.
33 For God is not *the author* of confusion, but of peace, as in all churches of
the saints.
34 Let your women keep silence in the
churches: for it is not permitted unto them
to speak; but *they are commanded* to be
under [m]obedience, as also saith the law.
35 And if they will learn any thing, let
them ask [n]their husbands at home: for it
is a shame for women to speak in the
[o]church.
36 What? [p]came the word of God out
from you? or came it unto you only?
37 If any man [q]think himself to be a
prophet, or spiritual, let him acknowledge that the things that I write unto you
[r]are the commandments of the Lord.
38 But if any man be ignorant, let him
be ignorant.
39 Wherefore, brethren, covet to prophesy, and forbid not to speak with tongues.
40 Let all things be done decently and
in order.

CHAPTER 15.

Part VIII. The coming of the Lord and the first resurrection. (Cf. Rev. 20:5, 11-15.)

(1) *The fact of Christ's resurrection.*

MOREOVER, brethren, I declare unto
you the [s]gospel which I preached
unto you, which also ye have received,
and wherein ye stand;
2 By which also ye are [t]saved, if ye
[u]keep in memory what I preached unto
you, unless ye have believed in vain.
3 For I delivered unto you first of all
that which I also received, how that
Christ died for our [v]sins according to the
scriptures;
4 And that he was buried, and that he
rose again the third day according to the
scriptures:
5 And that he was seen of Cephas,
[w]then of the twelve:
6 After that, he was seen of above

A.D. 59.

a Eph. 5:19; Col. 3:16.
b *Holy Spirit.* vs. 2, 15, 16; 2 Cor. 1:22. (Mt. 1:18; Acts 2:4.)
c Gr. *paidon, youths.* Heb. 5:12.
d *babes.*
e Isa. 28:11, 12; Deut. 28:49.
f Mk. 16:17; Acts 2:6.
g Acts 2:13.
h Isa. 45:14.
i v. 40; also vs. 26, 33.
j Or, *in turn.*
k 1 Thes. 5:19, 20.
l Psa. 39:2, 3.
m Cf. Gen. 3:16.
n *their own husbands.*
o *Churches (local).* 1 Cor. 15:9. (Acts 2:41; Phil. 1:1.)
p Isa. 2:3; Lk. 24:47; Rom. 15:19.
q 1 John 4:6.
r *Inspiration.* Gal. 1:11, 12. (Ex. 4:15; Rev. 22:19.)
s *Gospel* vs. 1-4; 2 Cor. 2:12. (Gen. 12:1-3; Rev. 14:6.)
t Rom. 1:16, *note.*
u *hold fast the word which I announced unto you as the glad tidings.*
v *Sin.* Rom. 3:23, *note.*
w See Mk. 16:14, *note.*

five hundred brethren at once; of whom
the greater part remain unto this present, but some are fallen asleep.
7 After that, he was seen of James;
then of all the apostles.
8 And last of all he was seen of me
also, as of one [1]born out of due time.
9 For I am the least of the apostles,
that am not meet to be called an apostle,
because I persecuted the [a]church [b]of
God.
10 But by the [c]grace of God I am what
I am: and his grace which *was bestowed*
upon me was not in vain; but I laboured
more abundantly than they all: yet not I,
but the grace of God which was with
me.
11 Therefore whether *it were* I or they,
so we preach, and so ye believed.

(2) *The importance of Christ's resurrection.*

12 Now if Christ be preached that he
rose from the dead, [d]how say some
among you that there is no resurrection
of the dead?
13 But if there be no resurrection of the
dead, then is Christ not risen:
14 And if Christ be not risen, then *is*
our preaching vain, and your faith *is*
also vain.
15 Yea, and we are found false witnesses of God; because we have testified
of God that he raised up Christ: whom

A.D. 59.

a *Church (visible).* Gal. 1:13. (1 Cor. 10:32; 1 Tim. 3:15.)
b *Churches(local).* 1 Cor. 16:1, 19. (Acts 2:41; Phil. 1:1.)
c *Grace (imparted).* 2 Cor. 1:12. (Rom. 6:1; 2 Pet. 3:18.)
d Acts 26:8.
e *Faith* vs. 14, 17; 2 Cor. 5:7. (Gen. 3:20; Heb. 11:39.)
f *Sin.* Rom. 3:23, *note.*
g *pitiable.*
h *Death (physical).* vs. 21, 22; 2 Cor. 5:1-8. (Gen. 3:19; Heb. 9:27.)
i John 5:28, 29; 1 Tim. 4:10.
j *Christ (Second Advent).* vs. 23, 51, 52; 2 Thes. 1:7-10. (Deut. 30:3; Acts 1:9-11.)
k *Then, finally, when he delivers up the kingdom to God, even the Father; when he has done away with every rule, and every authority and power (for he must reign till he has put all enemies under his feet), the last enemy, death, is destroyed.*
l *Kingdom* (N.T.). vs. 24-28. (Lk. 1:31-33.)
m Psa. 110:1; Mt. 22:44.

he raised not up, if so be that the dead
rise not.
16 For if the dead rise not, then is not
Christ raised:
17 And if Christ be not raised, your
[e]faith *is* vain; ye are yet in your [f]sins.
18 Then they also which are fallen
asleep in Christ are perished.
19 If in this life only we have hope in
Christ, we are of all men most [g]miser-
able.

(3) *The order of the resurrections.*

20 But now is Christ risen from the
dead, *and* become the firstfruits of them
that slept.
21 For since by man *came* [h]death, by
man *came* also the resurrection of the
dead.
22 For as in [2]Adam all die, even so in
Christ shall all [i]be made alive.
23 But every man in his own order:
[j]Christ the firstfruits; afterward they that
are Christ's at his coming.
24 [k]Then *cometh* the end, when he
shall have delivered up the [3][l]kingdom to
God, even the Father; when he shall
have put down all rule and all authority
and power.
25 For he must reign, [m]till he hath put
all enemies under his feet.

[1] **(15:8)** Gr. *to ektromati,* "before the due time." Paul thinks of himself here as an Israelite whose time to be born again had not come, nationally (cf. Mt. 23:39), so that his conversion by the appearing of the Lord in glory (Acts 9:3-6) was an illustration, or instance before the time, of the future national conversion of Israel. See Ezek. 20:35-38; Hos. 2:14-17; Zech. 12:10–13:6; Rom. 11:25-27.

[2] **(15:22)** Adam was a contrasting type of Christ (vs. 45-47; cf. Rom. 5:14-19). (1) "The first man Adam was *made* a living soul" (Gen. 2:7), i.e. he *derived* life from another, that is, God. "The last Adam was a life-giving spirit." So far from deriving life, He was Himself the fountain of life, and He gave that life to others (John 1:4; 5:21; 10:10; 12:24; 1 John 5:12). (2) In origin the first man was of the earth, earthy; the Second Man is the Lord from heaven. (3) Each is the head of a creation, and these also are in contrast: in Adam all die; in Christ all will be made alive; the Adamic creation is "flesh"; the new creation, "spirit" (John 3:6).

[3] **(15:24)** Kingdom (N.T.), Summary: See "Kingdom (O.T.)" (Gen. 1:26-28; Zech. 12:8, *note*). Kingdom truth is developed in the N.T. in the following order: (1) The promise of the kingdom to David and his seed, and described in the prophets (2 Sam. 7:8-17, *refs.;* Zech. 12.8), enters the N.T. absolutely unchanged (Lk. 1:31-33). The King was born in Bethlehem (Mt. 2:1; Mic. 5:2), of a virgin (Mt. 1:18-25; Isa. 7:14). (2) The kingdom announced as "at hand" (Mt. 4:17, *note*) by John the Baptist, by the King, and by the Twelve, was rejected by the Jews, first morally (Mt. 11:20, *note*), and afterward officially (Mt. 21:42, 43), and the King, crowned with thorns, was crucified. (3) In anticipation of His official rejection and crucifixion, the King revealed the "mysteries" of the kingdom of heaven (Mt. 13:11, *note*) to be fulfilled in the interval between His rejection and His return in glory. (Mt. 13:1-50). (4) Afterward He announced His purpose to "build" His church (Mt. 16:18, *refs.*), another "mystery" revealed through Paul which is being fulfilled contemporaneously with the mysteries of the kingdom. The "mysteries of the kingdom of heaven" and

A.D. 59.

26 The last enemy *that* shall be destroyed *is* death.

27 For he hath put [a]all things under his feet. But when he saith all things are put under *him, it is* manifest that he is excepted, which did put all things under him.

28 And when all things shall be subdued unto him, [b]then shall the Son also himself be subject unto him that put all things under him, that God may be all in all.

29 Else what shall they do which are baptized for the [c]dead, if the dead rise not at all? why are they then baptized for the dead?

30 And why stand we in jeopardy every hour?

31 I protest by your [d]rejoicing which I have in Christ Jesus our Lord, I [e]die daily.

32 If [f]after the manner of men I have fought with beasts at Ephesus, what advantageth it me, if the dead rise not? [g]let us eat and drink; for to morrow we die.

33 Be not deceived: [h]evil communications corrupt good manners.

34 [i]Awake to righteousness, and [j]sin not; for some have not the knowledge of God: I speak *this* to your shame.

(4) *The method of resurrection.*

35 But some *man* will say, [k]How are the dead raised up? and with what body do they come?

36 *Thou* fool, that which thou sowest is not quickened, except it die:

37 And that which thou sowest, thou sowest not that body that shall be, but bare grain, it may chance of wheat, or of some other *grain*:

38 But God giveth it a body as it hath pleased him, and to every seed his own body.

39 All flesh *is* not the same flesh: but *there is* one *kind of* flesh of men, another flesh of beasts, another of fishes, *and* another of birds.

40 *There are* also celestial bodies, and bodies terrestrial: but the glory of the celestial *is* one, and the *glory* of the terrestrial *is* another.

41 *There is* one glory of the sun, and another glory of the moon, and another glory of the stars: for *one* star differeth from *another* star in glory.

42 So also *is* the resurrection of the dead. It is sown in corruption; it is raised in incorruption:

43 It is [l]sown in dishonour; it is raised in glory: it is sown in weakness; [m]it is raised in power:

44 It is sown a natural body; it is raised a spiritual body. There is a natural body, and there is a spiritual body.

45 And so it is written, [n]The first man Adam [o]was made a living soul; the last Adam [p]*was made* a [q]quickening spirit.

46 Howbeit that *was* not first which is spiritual, but that which is natural; and afterward that which is spiritual.

47 The first man *is* of the earth, earthy: the second man *is* the Lord from heaven.

48 As *is* the earthy, such *are* they also that are earthy: and as *is* the heavenly, such *are* they also that are heavenly.

49 And as we have borne the image of the earthy, we shall [r]also bear the image of the heavenly.

50 Now this I say, brethren, that flesh and blood cannot inherit the kingdom of God; neither doth corruption inherit incorruption.

(5) *All believers will not die.*
(Cf. 1 Thes. 4:14-17.)

51 Behold, I [s]shew you a [t]mystery; We shall not all sleep, but we shall all be changed,

52 In a moment, in the twinkling of

a Psa. 8:6.
b vs. 24.
c i.e. who, through the introductory rite of baptism, are taking the places in the ranks left vacant by Christians who have died.
d Phil. 3:3.
e Rom. 8:36, 37; 2 Cor. 4:10-12.
f *to speak after.*
g Isa. 22:13.
h Prov. 13:20; Eph. 4:29; 2 Tim. 2:16, 17.
i Rom. 13:11.
j *Sin.* Rom. 3:23, *note.*
k Ezk. 37:3.
l Gen. 3:19.
m Lk. 20:35, 36.
n Gen. 2:7.
o *became.*
p Omit italicized words.
q Or, *lifegiving.*
r Rom. 8:29.
s *tell.*
t Mt. 13:11, note.

the "mystery" of the church (Eph. 3:9-11) occupy, historically, the same period, i.e. this present age. (5) The mysteries of the kingdom will be brought to an end by the "harvest" (Mt. 13:39-43, 49, 50) at the return of the King in glory, the church having previously been caught up to meet Him in the air (1 Thes. 4:14-17). (6) Upon His return the King will restore the Davidic monarchy in His own person, re-gather dispersed Israel, establish His power over all the earth, and reign one thousand years (Mt. 24:27-30; Lk. 1:31-33; Acts 15:14-17; Rev. 20:1-10). (7) The kingdom of heaven (Mt. 3:2, *note*), thus established under David's divine Son, has for its object the restoration of the divine authority in the earth, which may be regarded as a revolted province of the great kingdom of God (Mt. 6:33, *note*). When this is done (vs. 24, 25) the Son will deliver up the kingdom (of heaven, Mt. 3:2) to "God, even the Father," that "God" (i.e. the triune God, Father, Son, and Holy Spirit) "may be all in all" (v. 28). The eternal throne is that "of God, and of the Lamb" (Rev. 22:1). The kingdom-age constitutes the seventh Dispensation (Eph. 1:10, *note*).

an eye, at the last trump: for the trumpet
shall sound, and the dead shall be [1a]raised
incorruptible, and we shall be changed.
53 For this corruptible must put on
[b]incorruption, and this mortal *must* put
on immortality.

(6) *The final victory over death.*

54 So when this corruptible shall have
put on [b]incorruption, and this mortal
shall have put on immortality, then shall
be brought to pass the saying that is
written, [c]Death is swallowed up in victory.
55 [d]O death, where *is* thy sting? O
[e]grave, where *is* thy victory?
56 The sting of death *is* [f]sin; and the
strength of sin *is* the [g]law.
57 But thanks *be* to God, which giveth
us the victory through our Lord Jesus
Christ.

(7) *The ultimate victory a motive to service.*

58 Therefore, my beloved brethren, be
ye stedfast, unmoveable, always abounding in the work of the Lord, forasmuch as
ye know that your labour is not in vain
in the Lord.

CHAPTER 16.

Part IX. Closing instructions and greetings.

Now concerning the collection for the
saints, as I have given order to the
churches of Galatia, even so do ye.
2 Upon the first *day* of the week let
every one of you lay by him in store, [h]as
God hath prospered him, that there be no
[i]gatherings when I come.
3 And when I come, whomsoever ye
shall approve [j]by *your* letters, them will I
send to bring your liberality unto
Jerusalem.
4 And if it be meet that I go also, they
shall go with me.
5 Now I will come unto [k]you, when I
shall pass through Macedonia: for I do
pass through Macedonia.
6 And it may be that I will abide, yea,
and winter with you, that ye may bring
me on my journey whithersoever I go.
7 For I will not see you now by the
way; but I [l]trust to tarry a while with
you, [m]if the Lord permit.
8 But I will tarry at Ephesus until
Pentecost.
9 For a great door and effectual is
opened unto me, and *there are* many [n]ad-
versaries.
10 Now if [o]Timotheus come, see that
he may be with you without fear: for he
[p]worketh the work of the Lord, as I also
do.
11 Let no man therefore [q]despise him:
but conduct him forth in peace, that he
may come unto me: for I look for him
with the brethren.
12 As touching *our* brother [r]Apollos, I
greatly desired him to come unto you
with the brethren: but his will was not at
all to come at this time; but he will come
when he shall have convenient time.

A.D. 59.

a *Resurrection.* vs. 1-52. (Job 19:25.)
b *incorruptibility.* Cf. 2 Tim. 1:10.
c Isa. 25:8.
d Hos. 13:14.
e *death.*
f *Sin.* Rom. 3:23, *note.*
g *Law (of Moses).* Gal. 2:15, 16, 19, 21. (Ex. 19:1; Gal. 1:29.)
h vs. 1, 2; 2 Cor. 8:1, *note.*
i *collections made.*
j *them will I send with letters.*
k 2 Cor. 1:15.
l *hope.*
m Jas. 4:15.
n Phil. 3:18.
o Acts 19:22; 2 Tim. 1:2.
p Phil. 2:19, 22.
q Lk. 10:16; 1 Thes. 4:8.
r Acts 19:1.

[1] **(15:52)** Resurrection, Summary: (1) The resurrection of the dead was believed by the patriarchs (Gen. 22:5 with Heb. 11:19; Job 19:25-27), and revealed through the prophets (Isa. 26:19; Dan. 12:2, 13; Hos. 13:14), and miracles of the dead restored to life are recorded in the O.T. (2 Ki. 4:32-35; 13:21). (2) Jesus Christ restored life to the dead (Mt. 9:25; Lk. 7:12-15; John 11:43, 44), and predicted His own resurrection (John 10:18; Lk. 24:1-8). (3) A resurrection of bodies followed the resurrection of Christ (Mt. 27:52, 53); and the apostles raised the dead (Acts 9:36-41; 20:9, 10). (4) Two resurrections are yet future, which are inclusive of "all that are in the graves" (John 5:28). These are distinguished as "of life" (1 Cor. 15:22, 23; 1 Thes. 4:14-17; Rev. 20:4), and "of judgment" (John 5:28, 29; Rev. 20:11-13). They are separated by a period of one thousand years (Rev. 20:5). The "first resurrection," that "unto life," will occur at the second coming of Christ (1 Cor. 15:23), the saints of the O.T. and church ages meeting Him in the air (1 Thes. 4:16, 17); while the martyrs of the tribulation, who also have part in the first resurrection (Rev. 20:4), are raised at the end of the great tribulation. (5) The mortal body will be related to the resurrection body as grain sown is related to the harvest (1 Cor. 15:37, 38); that body will be incorruptible, glorious, powerful, and spiritual (1 Cor. 15:42-44, 49). (6) The bodies of living believers will, at the same time, be instantaneously changed (1 Cor. 15:50-53; Phil. 3:20, 21). This "change" of the living, and resurrection of the dead in Christ, is called the "redemption of the body" (Rom. 8:23; Eph. 1:13, 14). (7) After the thousand years the "resurrection unto judgment" (John 5:29) occurs. The resurrection-body of the wicked dead is not described. They are judged according to their works, and cast into the lake of fire (Rev. 20:7-15).

13 [a]Watch ye, [b]stand fast in the faith,
quit you like men, be strong.
14 Let all [c]your things be done with
charity.
15 I beseech you, brethren, (ye know
the house of Stephanas, that it is the
[d]firstfruits of Achaia, and *that* they have
addicted themselves to the ministry of
the saints,)
16 That ye [e]submit yourselves unto
such, and to every one that helpeth with
us, and laboureth.
17 I am glad of the [f]coming of
Stephanas and Fortunatus and Achaicus:
for that which was [g]lacking on your part
they have supplied.
18 For they have refreshed my spirit
and yours: therefore acknowledge ye
them that are such.
19 The churches of Asia salute you.
Aquila and Priscilla salute you much in
the Lord, with the [h]church that is in their
house.
20 All the brethren greet you. Greet ye
one another with an [i]holy kiss.
21 The salutation of *me* Paul with mine
own hand.
22 If any man love not the Lord Jesus
Christ, let him be [j]Anathema Maranatha.
23 The grace of our Lord Jesus Christ
be with you.
24 My love *be* with you all in Christ
Jesus. Amen.

A.D. 59.

a 1 Pet. 5:8.
b 2 Thes. 2:15.
c *all things be done by you in love.*
d Rom. 16:5.
e Heb. 13:17.
f Gr. *parousia, personal presence.*
g Phil. 2:30.
h *Churches (local).* vs. 1, 19; 2 Cor. 1:1. (Acts 2:41; Phil. 1:1.)
i *Sanctify, holy (things)* (N.T.) Col. 2:16. (Mt. 4:5; Rev. 22:11.)
j *Accursed; our Lord cometh.* Christ is God's final test.

THE SECOND EPISTLE OF PAUL THE APOSTLE TO THE CORINTHIANS

WRITER. The Apostle Paul (1:1).

Date. A.D. 60; probably from Philippi, after the events of Acts 19:23–20:1-3.

Theme. The Epistle discloses the touching state of the great apostle at this time. It was one of physical weakness, weariness, and pain. But his spiritual burdens were greater. These were of two kinds—solicitude for the maintenance of the churches in grace as against the law-teachers, and anguish of heart over the distrust felt toward him by Jews and Jewish Christians. The chilling doctrines of the legalizers were accompanied by detraction, and by denial of his apostleship.

It is evident that the really dangerous sect in Corinth was that which said, "and I of Christ" (1 Cor. 1:12). They rejected the new revelation through Paul of the doctrines of grace; grounding themselves, probably, on the kingdom teachings of our Lord as "a minister of the circumcision" (Rom. 15:8); seemingly oblivious that a new dispensation had been introduced by Christ's death. This made necessary a defence of the origin and extent of Paul's apostolic authority.

The Epistle is in three parts: I. Paul's principles of action, 1:1–7:16. II. The collection for the poor saints at Jerusalem, 8:1–9:15. III. Paul's defence of his apostolic authority, 10:1–13:14.

CHAPTER 1.

Part I. Paul's principles of action
(2 Cor. 1:1–7:16).

(1) *The explanation.*

Paul, an apostle of Jesus Christ by the
will of God, and [a]Timothy *our*
brother, unto the church of God which is
at Corinth, with all the [b]saints which are
in all Achaia:
2 Grace *be* to you and peace from God
our Father, and *from* the Lord Jesus Christ.
3 Blessed *be* [c]God, even the Father of
our Lord Jesus Christ, the Father of
[d]mercies, and the God of all [e]comfort;
4 Who [f]comforteth us in all our tribulation, that we may be able to comfort
them which are in any trouble, by the
comfort wherewith we ourselves are
comforted of God.
5 For as the sufferings of Christ
abound in us, so our consolation also
aboundeth by Christ.
6 And whether we be afflicted, *it is* for
your consolation and [g]salvation, which
is [h]effectual in the enduring of the same
sufferings which we also suffer: or
whether we be comforted, *it is* for your
consolation and salvation.
7 And our hope of you *is* stedfast,
knowing, that [i]as ye are partakers of the
sufferings, so *shall ye be* also of the consolation.
8 For we would not, brethren, have
you ignorant of [j]our trouble which came
to us in Asia, that we were pressed out
of measure, above strength, insomuch
that we despaired even of life:
9 But we had the sentence of death in
ourselves, that we should not [k]trust in
ourselves, but in God which raiseth the
dead:
10 Who delivered us from so great a
[l]death, and doth deliver: in whom we
[m]trust that he will yet [n]deliver *us*;
11 Ye also helping together by prayer
for us, that for the gift *bestowed* upon us
by the means of many persons thanks
may be given by many on our behalf.
12 For our rejoicing is this, the [o]testi-
mony of our conscience, that in simplicity and godly sincerity, not with fleshly
wisdom, but by [p]the grace of God, we
have had our conversation in the [q]world,
and more abundantly to you-ward.
13 For we write none other things
unto you, than what ye read or acknowledge; and I [m]trust ye shall acknowledge
even to the end;
14 As also ye have acknowledged us
in part, that we are your rejoicing, even
as ye also *are* ours in the [r]day of the Lord
Jesus.
15 And in this confidence I was minded to come unto you before, that ye
might have a second benefit;

A.D. 60.

a *the brother Timothy.* 1 Cor. 16:10.
b *Churches (local).* 2 Cor. 8:1, 18, 19, 23, 24. (Acts 2:41; Phil. 1:1.)
c *the God and Father.*
d *compassions.*
e *encouragement.*
f *encourages;* and so also where "comfort," etc., occurs in following verses.
g Rom. 1:16, *note.*
h Or, *wrought.*
i Rom. 8:17.
j Acts 19:23.
k Jer. 17:5, 7.
l Psa. 34:19, 22.
m *hope.*
n *Assurance.* Eph. 1:13. (Isa. 32:17; Jude 1.)
o Acts 24:16.
p *Grace (imparted).* 2 Cor. 4:15. (Rom. 6:1; 2 Pet. 3:18.)
q *kosmos* (Mt. 4:8) = mankind.
r 1 Cor. 1:8, *note.*

16 And to pass by you into Macedonia,
and to come again out of Macedonia
unto you, and of you to be brought [a]on
my way toward Judaea.
17 When I therefore was thus minded,
did I use lightness? or the things that I
purpose, do I purpose according to the
[b]flesh, that with me there should be yea
yea, and nay nay?
18 But *as* God *is* true, our word toward
you was not yea and nay.
19 For the [c]Son of God, Jesus Christ,
who was preached among you by us,
even by me and Silvanus and Timotheus,
was not yea and nay, but in him was yea.
20 For all the promises of God [d]in him
are yea, and in him Amen, unto the glory
of God by us.
21 Now he which stablisheth us with
you in Christ, and hath [e]anointed us, *is*
God;
22 Who hath also sealed us, and given
the earnest of the [f]Spirit in our hearts.
23 Moreover I call God for a record
upon my soul, that to spare you I came
not as yet unto Corinth.
24 Not for that we have dominion
over your faith, but are helpers of your
joy: for by faith ye stand.

CHAPTER 2.

The explanation, continued.

But I determined this with myself, that
I would not come again to you in
[g]heaviness.
2 For if I make you sorry, who is he
then that maketh me glad, but the same
which is made sorry by me?
3 And I wrote this same unto you, lest,
when I came, I should have sorrow from
them of whom I ought to rejoice; having
confidence in you all, that my joy is *the*
joy of you all.
4 For out of much affliction and
anguish of heart I wrote unto you with
many tears; not that ye should be grieved,
but that ye might know the love which I
have more abundantly unto you.
5 But if any have caused grief, he hath
not grieved me, but in part: that I may
not overcharge you all.
6 Sufficient to such a man *is* this [h]pun-
ishment, which *was* [i]*inflicted* of many.
7 So that contrariwise ye *ought* rather
to [j]forgive *him*, and comfort *him*, lest
perhaps such a one should be swallowed up with overmuch sorrow.
8 Wherefore I beseech you that ye
would confirm *your* love toward him.
9 For to this end also did I write, that I
might know the proof of you, whether
ye be obedient in all things.
10 To whom ye forgive any thing, I *for-*
give also: for if I forgave any thing, to
whom [k]I forgave *it*, for your sakes *for-*
gave I it in the person of Christ;
11 Lest [l]Satan should get an advantage
of us: for we are not ignorant of his
devices.
12 Furthermore, when I came to Troas
to *preach* Christ's [m]gospel, and a door
was opened unto me of the Lord,
13 I had no rest in my spirit, because I
found not Titus my brother: but taking
my leave of them, I went from thence
into Macedonia.

(2) *The ministry* (to 6:10):
(*a*) *Triumphant.*

14 Now thanks *be* unto God, which
always [n]causeth us to triumph in Christ,
and maketh manifest the savour of his
knowledge by us in every place.
15 For we are unto God a sweet
savour of Christ, in them that are [o]saved,
and in them that [p]perish:
16 To the one *we are* the savour of
death unto death; and to the other the
savour of life unto [q]life. And who *is* sufficient for these things?
17 For we are not as many, which [r]cor-
rupt the word of God: but as of sincerity,
but as of God, in the sight of God speak
we in Christ.

CHAPTER 3.

The ministry: (b) accredited.

Do we begin again to commend our
selves? or need we, as some *others,*
epistles of commendation to you, or *let-*
ters of commendation from you?
2 Ye are our epistle written in our
hearts, known and read of all men:
3 *Forasmuch as ye are* manifestly
declared to be the epistle of Christ ministered by us, written not with ink, but
with the [s]Spirit of the living God; not [t]in
[u]tables of stone, but in [v]fleshy tables of
the heart.
4 And such trust have we through
Christ to God-ward:

A.D. 60.

a Acts 21:5.
b *Flesh.* vs. 12, 17; 2 Cor. 5:16. (John 1:13; Jude 23.)
c Acts 8:37.
d Rom. 15:8, 9.
e 1 John 2:20.
f *Holy Spirit.* 2 Cor. 3:3, 6, 8, 17, 18. (Mt. 1:18; Acts 2:4.)
g 2 Cor. 13:10.
h Or, *censure.*
i 1 Cor. 5:4, 5.
j *show grace and encourage.*
k *Forgiveness.* vs. 7-10; Eph. 4:32. (Lev. 4:20; Mt. 26:28.)
l *Satan.* 2 Cor. 11:3, 14. (Gen. 3:1; Rev. 20:10.)
m *Gospel.* 2 Cor. 4:3, 4. (Gen. 12:1-3; Rev. 14:6.)
n *leadeth us in triumph.*
o Rom. 1:16, *note.*
p *are perishing.*
q *life (eternal).* 2 Cor. 4:10-12. (Mt. 7:14; Rev. 22:19.)
r *make a trade of.*
s *Holy Spirit.* vs. 3, 6, 8, 17, 18; 2 Cor. 4:13. (Mt. 1:18; Acts 2:4.)
t Ex. 24:12.
u i.e. the ten commandments.
v Jer. 31:33; Ezk. 11:19.

5 Not that we are sufficient of ourselves to think any thing as of ourselves; but our sufficiency *is* of God;

The ministry: (c) Spiritual and glorious—not legal.

6 Who also hath made us [a]able ministers of the new testament; not of the letter, but of the spirit: [b]for the letter killeth, but the spirit giveth life.

7 But if the ministration of death, written *and* engraven in stones, [c]was glorious, so that the children of Israel could not stedfastly behold the face of Moses for the glory of his countenance; which *glory* was to be done away:

8 How shall not the ministration of the spirit be rather glorious?

9 For if the ministration of condemnation *be* glory, much more doth the ministration of [d]righteousness exceed in glory.

10 For even that which was made glorious had no glory in this respect, by reason of the [e]glory that excelleth.

11 For if that which is done away *was* glorious, much more that which remaineth *is* glorious.

12 Seeing then that we have such hope, we use great [f]plainness of speech:

13 And not as [g]Moses, *which* put a vail over his face, that the children of Israel could not stedfastly look to the end of that which is [h]abolished:

14 But their minds were blinded: for until this day remaineth the same vail untaken away in the reading of the old testament; which [i]*vail* is done away in Christ.

15 But even unto this day, when Moses is read, [j]the vail is upon their heart.

16 Nevertheless when [k]it shall turn to the [l]Lord, the vail shall be taken away.

17 Now the Lord is that Spirit: and where the Spirit of the Lord *is*, there *is* liberty.

18 But we all, [m]with open face beholding as in a glass the glory of the [n]Lord, are [o]changed into the same image from glory to glory, *even* as by the Spirit of the Lord.

CHAPTER 4.

The ministry: (d) *honest.*

Therefore seeing we have this ministry, as we have received mercy, we faint not;

(Because the truth taught is commended by the life.)

2 But have renounced the hidden things of dishonesty, not walking in craftiness, nor handling the word of God deceitfully; but by manifestation of the truth commending ourselves to every man's conscience in the sight of God.

(Because not self but Christ Jesus as Lord is preached.)

3 But if our [p]gospel be [q]hid, it is hid to them that are lost:

4 In whom [r]the god of this [s]world hath blinded the minds of them which believe not, lest the [t]light of the glorious gospel of Christ, who is the image of God, should shine unto them.

5 For we preach not ourselves, but Christ Jesus the Lord; and ourselves your [u]servants for Jesus' sake.

6 For God, who commanded the light to shine out of darkness, hath shined in our hearts, to *give* the light of the knowledge of the glory of God in the face of Jesus Christ.

(Because the power is of God alone. Cf. 1 Cor. 2:1-5.)

7 But we have this treasure in earthen vessels, that the excellency of the power may be of God, and not of us.

The ministry: (e) suffering.

8 *We are* troubled on every side, yet not distressed; *we are* perplexed, but not in despair;

9 Persecuted, but not forsaken; cast down, but not destroyed;

10 Always bearing about in the body the [v]dying of the Lord Jesus, that the [w]life also of Jesus might be made manifest in our body.

11 For we which live are alway delivered unto death for Jesus' sake, that the life also of Jesus might be made manifest in our mortal flesh.

12 So then death worketh in us, but life in you.

13 We having the same [x]spirit of faith, according as it is written, [y]I believed, and therefore have I spoken; we also believe, and therefore speak;

14 Knowing that he which raised up the Lord Jesus shall raise up us also by Jesus, and shall present *us* with you.

15 For all things *are* for your sakes, that the [z]abundant grace might through

A.D. 60.

a *sufficient as ministers of the new covenant.*
b See Rom. 7:6, *note.*
c *began with glory.*
d Rom. 3:21, *note.*
e *surpassing glory.*
f Or, *boldness.*
g Ex. 34:33.
h *annulled.*
i Omit the italicized word.
j Psa. 69:22, 23; Isa. 6:9, 10.
k i.e. *the heart.*
l *Jehovah.* Ex. 34:34.
m *unveiled.*
n *Jehovah,* Ex. 16:7.
o *transformed.* The same Greek word is rendered *transfigured* in Mt. 17:2 and Mk. 9:2.
p *Gospel.* vs. 3, 4; 2 Cor. 8:18. (Gen. 12:1-3; Rev. 14:6.)
q *veiled.*
r John 12:31.
s i.e. *age.*
t *radiance of the gospel of the glory.*
u *bondmen.*
v Lit. *putting to death,* i.e., crucifixion. v. 11; 1 Cor. 15:31
w *Life (eternal).* vs. 10:12; 2 Cor. 5:4. (Mt. 7:14; Rev. 22:19.)
x *Holy Spirit.* 2 Cor. 5:5. Mt. 1:18; Acts 2:4.)
y Psa. 116:10.
z *Grace (imparted).* 2 Cor. 6:1-3. Rom. 6:1; 2 Pet. 3:18.)

the thanksgiving of many redound to
the glory of God.
16 For which cause we faint not; but
though our outward man perish, yet the
[a]inward *man* is renewed day by day.
17 For our [b]light affliction, which is but
for a moment, worketh for us a far more
exceeding *and* eternal weight of glory;
18 While we look not at the things
which are seen, but at the things which
are [c]not seen: for the things which are
seen *are* temporal; but the things which
are not seen *are* eternal.

CHAPTER 5.

(*Why death itself has no terrors for the servant of the Lord.*)

For we know that if our earthly [d]house
of *this* tabernacle were dissolved,
we have a building of God, an house
not made with hands, eternal in the
heavens.
2 For in this we groan, earnestly desiring to be clothed upon with our house
which is from heaven:
3 If so be that being clothed we shall
not be found naked.
4 For we that are in *this* tabernacle do
groan, being burdened: not for that we
would be unclothed, but clothed upon,
that mortality might be swallowed up of
[e]life.
5 Now he that hath wrought us for the
selfsame thing *is* God, who also hath
given unto us the earnest of the [f]Spirit.
6 Therefore *we are* always confident,
knowing that, whilst we are at home in
the body, we are absent from the Lord:
7 (For we walk by [g]faith, not by sight:)
8 We are confident, *I say*, and willing
rather to be [h]absent from the body, and
to be present with the Lord.
9 Wherefore we [i]labour, that, whether
present or absent, we may be [j]accepted
of him.
10 [1]For we must all [k]appear before the
[l]judgment seat of Christ; that every one
may receive the things *done* in *his* body,
according to that he hath done, whether
it be good or bad.
11 Knowing therefore the terror of the
Lord, we persuade men; but we are made
manifest unto God; and I [m]trust also are
made manifest in your consciences.
12 For we commend not ourselves
again unto you, but give you occasion to
glory on our behalf, that ye may have
somewhat to *answer* them which glory in
appearance, and not in heart.
13 For whether we be beside ourselves, *it is* to God: or whether we be
sober, *it is* for your cause.

The ministry: (f) *motive and object.*

14 For the [n]love of Christ constraineth
us; because we thus judge, that if one
died for all, then were all dead:
15 And *that* he died for all, that they
which live should [o]not henceforth live
unto themselves, but unto him which
died for them, and rose again.
16 Wherefore henceforth know we no
man after the [p]flesh: yea, though we
have known Christ after the flesh, yet
now henceforth [q]know we *him* no more.
17 Therefore if any man *be* in Christ, *he*
is a new [r]creature: old things are passed
away; behold, all things are become new.
18 And all things *are* of God, who hath
reconciled us to himself by Jesus Christ,
and hath given to us the ministry of [s]rec-
onciliation;
19 To wit, that God was in Christ, reconciling the [t]world unto himself, not
[u]imputing their [v]trespasses unto them;
and hath committed unto us the word of
[s]reconciliation.
20 Now then we are ambassadors for
Christ, as though God did beseech *you*
by us: we pray *you* in Christ's stead, be
ye [s]reconciled to God.
21 For he hath made [w]him *to be*

A.D. 60.

a Psa. 84:7; Col. 3:10.
b Rom. 8:18.
c Heb. 11:1; cf. 2 Cor. 5:7.
d Or, *tent-house.*
e *Life (eternal).* Gal. 2:20. (Mt. 7:14; Rev. 22:19.)
f *Holy Spirit.* 2 Cor. 6:6. (Mt. 1:18; Acts 2:4.)
g *Faith.* Gal. 2:16, 20. (Gen. 3:20; Heb. 11:39.)
h *Death (physical).* vs. 1-8; Phil. 1:21-23. (Gen. 3:19; Heb. 9:27.)
i Gr. *are ambitious.*
j *well pleasing to.*
k *be manifested.*
l *Judgments (the seven).* vs. 8-10; Gal. 3:13. (2 Sam. 7:14; Rev. 20:12.)
m *hope.*
n *Law (of Christ).* vs. 13, 14; 2 Cor. 10:5. (Gal. 6:2; 2 John 5.)
o *no longer.*
p *Flesh.* 2 Cor. 7:1. (John 1:13; Jude 23.)
q *know we him so no more.*
r *creation.*
s *Reconciliation.* vs. 18, 19, 20. See Eph. 2:16.
t *kosmos* (Mt. 4:8) = mankind.
u *Imputation.* Gal. 3:6. (Lev. 25:50; Jas. 2:23.)
v *Sin.* Rom. 3:23, *note.*
w *Sacrifice (of Christ).* vs. 14, 18, 19, 21; Gal. 3:10-14. (Gen. 4:4; Heb. 10:18.)

[1] **(5:10)** The judgment of the believer's works, not sins, is in question here. These have been atoned for, and are "remembered no more forever" (Heb. 10:17); but every *work* must come into judgment (Mt. 12:36; Rom. 14:10; Gal. 6:7; Eph. 6:8; Col. 3:24, 25). The result is "reward" or "loss" (of the reward), "but he himself shall be saved" (1 Cor. 3:11-15). This judgment occurs at the return of Christ (Mt. 16:27; Lk. 14:14; 1 Cor. 4:5; 2 Tim. 4:8; Rev. 22:12). See other judgments, John 12:31, *note;* 1 Cor. 11:31, *note;* Mt. 25:32, *note;* Ezk. 20:37, *note;* Jude 6, *note;* Rev. 20:12, *note.*

[a]sin for us, who knew no sin; that we
might [b]be made the [c]righteousness of
God in him.

CHAPTER 6.

The ministry: (g) summary.

We then, *as* [d]workers together *with*
him, beseech *you* also that ye
receive not the [e]grace of God in vain.
2 (For he saith, [f]I have heard thee in a
time accepted, and in the day of salvation have I succoured thee: behold, now
is the accepted time; behold, now *is* the
day of [g]salvation.)
3 Giving no offence in any thing, that
the ministry be not blamed:
4 But in all *things* [h]approving ourselves as the [i]ministers of God, in much
patience, in afflictions, in necessities, in
distresses,
5 In stripes, in imprisonments, in
tumults, in labours, in watchings, in fastings;
6 By pureness, by knowledge, by longsuffering, by kindness, by the [j]Holy
Ghost, by love unfeigned,
7 By the word of truth, by the power
of God, by the armour of [k]righteousness
on the right hand and on the left,
8 By honour and dishonour, by evil
report and good report: [l]as deceivers,
and *yet* true;
9 As unknown, and *yet* well known; as
dying, and, behold, we live; as chastened, and not killed;
10 As sorrowful, yet alway rejoicing; as
poor, yet making many rich; as having
nothing, and *yet* [m]possessing all things.

A.D. 60.

a *Sin.* Rom. 3:23, *note.*
b *become.*
c Rom. 3:21, *note.*
d *fellow-workmen.*
e *Grace (imparted).* 2 Cor. 8:1, 6, 7, 19. (Rom. 6:1; 2 Pet. 3:18.)
f Isa. 49:8.
g Rom. 1:16, *note.*
h *commending.*
i 1 Cor. 4:1.
j *Holy Spirit.* 2 Cor. 12:18. (Mt. 1:18; Acts 2:4.)
k 1 John 3:7, *note.*
l John 7:12.
m Psa. 84:11.
n Deut. 7:2, 3; 1 Cor. 7:39; Eph. 5:6-7.
o Rom. 10:10, *note.*
p *Sin.* Rom. 3:23, *note.*
q *unbeliever.*
r Gr. *naos* the sanctuary itself.
s Lev. 26:11, 12.
t Isa. 52:11.
u *Separation.* vs. 14-17. (Gen. 12:1.)
v Jer. 31:9. Rev. 21:7.
w *Flesh.* 2 Cor. 10:2, 3, 4. (John 1:13; Jude 23.)
x Mt. 5:48, *note.*
y *Open your hearts to us.*

(3) *The appeal to separation and cleansing*
(2 Cor. 6:11–7:1).

11 O *ye* Corinthians, our mouth is
open unto you, our heart is enlarged.
12 Ye are not straitened in us, but ye
are straitened in your own bowels.
13 Now for a recompence in the same,
(I speak as unto *my* children,) be ye also
enlarged.
14 Be ye not [n]unequally yoked together with unbelievers: for what fellowship
hath [o]righteousness with [p]unrighteous-
ness? and what communion hath light
with darkness?
15 And what concord hath Christ with
Belial? or what part hath he that
believeth with an [q]infidel?
16 And what agreement hath the [r]tem-
ple of [s]God with idols? for ye are the
temple of the living God; as God hath
said, I will dwell in them, and walk in
them; and I will be their God, and they
shall be my people.
17 [t]Wherefore [1]come out from among
them, and be ye [u]separate, saith the
Lord, and touch not the unclean *thing*;
and I will receive you,
18 And will [v]be a Father unto you,
and ye shall be my sons and daughters,
saith the Lord Almighty.

CHAPTER 7.

Having therefore these promises,
dearly beloved, let us cleanse ourselves from all filthiness of the [w]flesh
and spirit, [x]perfecting holiness in the
fear of God.

(4) *The heart of Paul* (vs. 2-16.)

2 [y]Receive us; we have wronged no

[1]**(6:17)** Separation, Summary: (1) Separation in Scripture is twofold: "from" whatever is contrary to the mind of God; and "unto" God Himself. The underlying principle is that in a moral universe it is impossible for God to fully bless and use His children who are in compromise or complicity with evil. The unequal yoke is anything which unites a child of God and an unbeliever in a common purpose (Deut. 22:10). (2) Separation from evil implies *(a)* separation in desire, motive, and act, from the world, in the ethically bad sense of this present world-system (see Rev. 13:8, *note*); and *(b)* separation from believers, especially false teachers, who are "vessels unto dishonour" (2 Tim. 2:20, 21; 2 John 9-11). (3) Separation is not from *contact* with evil in the world or the church, but from complicity with and conformity to it (John 17:15; 2 Cor. 6:14-18; Gal. 6:1). (4) The reward of separation is the full manifestation of the divine fatherhood (2 Cor. 6:17, 18); unhindered communion and worship (see Heb. 13:13-15), and fruitful service (2 Tim. 2:21), as world-conformity involves the loss of these, though not of salvation. Here, as in all else, Christ is the model. He was "holy, harmless, undefiled, and separate from sinners" (Heb. 7:26), and yet in such contact with them for their salvation that the Pharisees, who illustrate the mechanical and ascetic conception of separation (Mt. 3:7, *note*), judged Him as having lost His Nazarite character (Lk. 7:39). Cf. 1 Cor. 9:19-23; 10:27.

man, we have corrupted no man, we have defrauded no man.

3 I speak not *this* to condemn *you*: for I have said before, that ye are in our hearts to die and live with *you*.

4 Great *is* my boldness of speech toward you, great *is* my glorying of you: I am filled with comfort, I am exceeding joyful in all our tribulation.

5 For, when we were come into Macedonia, our flesh had no rest, but we were troubled on every side; without *were* fightings, within *were* fears.

6 Nevertheless God, that [a]comforteth those that are cast down, comforted us by the coming of Titus;

7 And not by his coming only, but by the consolation wherewith he was comforted in you, when he told us your earnest desire, your mourning, your fervent mind toward me; so that I rejoiced the more.

8 For though I made you sorry with a letter, I do not [b]repent, though I did repent: for I perceive that the same epistle hath made you sorry, though *it were* but for a season.

9 Now I rejoice, not that ye were made sorry, but that ye sorrowed to [c]repentance: for ye were made sorry after a godly manner, that ye might receive damage by us in nothing.

10 For godly [d]sorrow worketh repentance to [e]salvation [f]not to be repented of: but the sorrow of the [g]world worketh death.

11 For behold this selfsame thing, that ye sorrowed after a godly sort, what carefulness it wrought in you, yea, *what* [h]clearing of yourselves, yea, *what* indignation, yea, *what* fear, yea, *what* vehement desire, yea, *what* zeal, yea, *what* revenge! In all *things* ye have approved yourselves to be clear in this matter.

12 Wherefore, though I wrote unto you, *I did it* not for his cause that had done the wrong, nor for his cause that suffered wrong, but that our care for you in the sight of God might appear unto you.

13 Therefore we were comforted in your comfort: yea, and exceedingly the more joyed we for the joy of Titus, because his spirit was refreshed by you all.

14 For if I have boasted any thing to him of you, I am not ashamed; but as we spake all things to you in truth, even so our boasting, which *I made* before Titus, is found a truth.

15 And his inward affection is more abundant toward you, whilst he remembereth the obedience of you all, how with fear and trembling ye received him.

16 I rejoice therefore that I have confidence in you in all *things*.

CHAPTER 8.

Part II. The collection for the poor (2 Cor. 8:1–9:15).

(1) *The example of Macedonia.*

[1]Moreover, brethren, we do you to wit of the grace of God bestowed on the churches of Macedonia;

2 How that in a great trial of affliction the [i]abundance of their joy and their deep poverty abounded unto the riches of their liberality.

3 For to *their* power, I bear record, yea, and beyond *their* power *they were* willing of themselves;

4 Praying us with much intreaty [j]that we would receive the gift, and *take upon us* the fellowship of the ministering to the saints.

5 And *this they did*, not as we hoped, [k]but first gave their own selves to the Lord, and unto us by the will of God.

6 Insomuch that we desired Titus, that as he had begun, so he would also finish in you the same [l]grace also.

(2) *The exhortation.*

7 Therefore, as ye abound in every

A.D. 60.

a *encourageth; so* in v. 7.
b *regret.*
c *Repentance.* vs. 9, 10; 2 Cor. 12:21. (Mt. 3:2; Acts 17:30.)
d Psa. 32:10.
e Rom. 1:16, *note.*
f *never to be regretted.*
g *kosmos* = world-system. Gal. 6:14. (John 7:7; Rev. 13:3-8, *note.*)
h Eph. 5:11.
i Neh. 8:10, 12.
j *[to give effect to] the grace and fellowship of the service to the saints.*
k Rom. 12:1.
l 1 Cor. 15:10.

[1](8:1) In 2 Cor. 8, 9, the apostle sums up the Christian doctrine of giving. It may be thus summarized: (1) It is a "grace," i.e. a disposition created by the Spirit (8:7). (2) In contrast with the law, which imposed giving as a divine requirement, Christian giving is voluntary, and a test of sincerity and love (8:8-12; 9:1, 2, 5, 7). (3) The privilege is universal, belonging, according to ability, to rich and poor (8:1-3, 12-15. Cf. 1 Cor. 16:1, 2). (4) Giving is to be proportioned to income (8:12-14. Cf. 1 Cor. 16:2). The O.T. proportion was the tithe, a proportion which antedates the law (Gen. 14:20). (5) The rewards of Christian giving are *(a)* joy (8:2); *(b)* increased ability to give in proportion to that which has been already given (9:7-11); *(c)* increased thankfulness to God (9:12); *(d)* God and the Gospel glorified (9:13, 14).

thing, in faith, and utterance, and knowledge, and *in* all diligence, and *in* your love to us, *see* that ye abound in this grace also.

8 I [a]speak not by commandment, but by occasion of the forwardness of others, and to prove the sincerity of your love.

9 For ye know the [b]grace of our Lord Jesus Christ, that, though he was rich, yet for your sakes he became [c]poor, that ye through his poverty might be [d]rich.

10 And herein I give *my* advice: for this is expedient for you, who have begun before, not only to do, but also to be forward a year ago.

11 Now therefore [e]perform the doing *of it;* that as *there was* a readiness to will, so *there may be* a [f]performance also out of that which ye have.

12 For if there be first a [g]willing mind, *it is* accepted according to that a man hath, *and* not according to that he hath not.

13 For *I mean* not that other men be eased, and ye burdened:

14 But by an equality, *that* now at this time your abundance *may be a supply* for their want, that their abundance also may be *a supply* for your want: that there may be equality:

15 As it is written, [h]He that *had gathered* much had nothing over; and he that *had gathered* little had no lack.

(3) *The messengers.*

16 But thanks *be* to God, which put the same earnest care into the heart of Titus for you.

17 For indeed he accepted the exhortation; but being [i]more forward, [j]of his own accord he went unto you.

18 And we have sent with him the brother, whose praise *is* in the [k]gospel throughout all the churches;

19 And not *that* only, but who was also chosen of the churches to travel with us with [l]this grace, which is administered by us to the glory of the same Lord, and [m]*declaration* of your ready mind:

20 Avoiding this, that no man should blame us in this abundance which is administered by us:

21 [n]Providing for honest things, not only in the sight of the Lord, but also in the sight of men.

22 And we have sent with them our brother, whom we have oftentimes proved diligent in many things, but now much more diligent, upon the great confidence which *I have* in you.

23 Whether *any do enquire* of Titus, *he is* my partner and fellowhelper concerning you: or our brethren *be enquired of, they are* the messengers of the churches, *and* the glory of Christ.

24 Wherefore shew ye to them, and before the [o]churches, the proof of your love, and of our boasting on your behalf.

CHAPTER 9.

For as touching the [p]ministering to the saints, it is [q]superfluous for me to write to you:

2 For I know the forwardness of your mind, for which I boast of you to them of Macedonia, that Achaia was ready a year ago; and your zeal hath provoked very many.

3 Yet have I sent the brethren, lest our boasting of you should be in vain in this behalf; that, as I said, ye may be ready:

4 Lest haply if they of Macedonia come with me, and find you unprepared, we (that we say not, ye) should be ashamed in this same confident boasting.

5 Therefore I thought it necessary to exhort the brethren, that they would go before unto you, and make up beforehand your bounty, [r]whereof ye had notice before, that the same might be ready, as *a matter of* bounty, and not as *of* covetousness.

(4) *The encouragement: God loves a cheerful giver: if we give, he will give.*

6 But this *I say,* He which soweth sparingly shall reap also sparingly; and he which soweth [s]bountifully shall reap also bountifully.

7 Every man according as he purposeth in his heart, *so let him give;* not grudgingly, or of necessity: for God loveth a [t]cheerful giver.

8 And God *is* able to make all grace abound toward you; that ye, always having all sufficiency in all *things,* may abound to every good work:

9 (As it is written, [u]He hath dispersed abroad; he hath given to the poor: his [v]righteousness remaineth for ever.

10 Now he that ministereth seed to the sower both minister bread for *your* food,

A.D. 60.

a 2 Cor. 9:7; cf. 1 Cor. 7:6.

b *Grace (in salv.).* Gal. 1:3-15. (Rom. 13:24; John 1:17, *note.*)

c Lk. 9:58; Phil. 2:6, 7.

d Rev. 3:18.

e *complete.*

f *completion.*

g vs. 10-12; 2 Cor. 8:1, *note.*

h Ex. 16:18.

i *full of zeal.*

j Phil. 2:26.

k *Gospel.* 2 Cor. 9:13. (Gen. 12:1-3; Rev. 14:6.)

l *Grace (imparted).* vs. 1, 6, 7, 19; 2 Cor. 9:8, 14. (Rom. 6:1; 2 Pet. 3:18.)

m *for a witness of our readiness.*

n Prov. 3:4; 1 Pet. 2:12.

o *Churches (local).* vs. 1, 18, 19, 23, 24; 2 Cor. 11:8, 28. (Acts 2:41; Phil. 1:1.)

p 2 Cor. 8:4.

q 1 Thes. 4:9, 10.

r Or, *which hath been so much spoken of before.*

s *with blessings.*

t Gr. *hilarious.*

u Psa. 112:9.

v vs. 9, 10. See 1 John 3:7, *note.*

A.D. 60.

and multiply your seed sown, and increase the fruits of your righteousness;)

11 Being enriched in every thing to all bountifulness, which causeth through us thanksgiving to God.

12 For the administration of this service not only supplieth the want of the saints, but is abundant also by many thanksgivings unto God;

13 Whiles by the experiment of this ministration they glorify God for your professed subjection unto the [a]gospel of Christ, and for *your* liberal distribution unto them, and unto all *men;*

14 And by their prayer for you, which long after you for the exceeding [b]grace of God in you.

15 Thanks *be* unto God for his unspeakable gift.

CHAPTER 10.

Part III. The vindication of Paul's apostleship (2 Cor. 10:1–13:14). (Cf. Gal. 1:11–2:14.)

(1) *The divine authentication.*

Now I Paul myself [c]beseech you by the meekness and gentleness of Christ, who in [d]presence *am* base among you, but being absent am bold toward you:

2 But I beseech *you,* that I may not be bold when I am present with that confidence, [e]wherewith I think to be bold against some, which think of us as if we walked according to the flesh.

3 For though we walk in the [f]flesh, we do not war after the flesh:

4 (For the weapons of our warfare *are* not [g]carnal, but mighty through God to the pulling down of strong holds;)

5 [h]Casting down imaginations, and every high thing that exalteth itself against the knowledge of God, and [i]bringing into captivity every thought [j]to the obedience of Christ;

6 And having in a readiness to revenge all disobedience, when your obedience is fulfilled.

7 Do ye look on things after the [k]outward appearance? If any man trust to himself that he is Christ's, let him of himself think this again, that, as he *is* Christ's, even so *are* we Christ's.

8 For though I should boast somewhat more of our [l]authority, which the Lord hath given us for [m]edification, and not for your [n]destruction, I should not be ashamed:

9 That I may not seem as if I would terrify you by letters.

10 For *his* letters, say they, *are* weighty and powerful; but *his* bodily presence *is* weak, and *his* speech contemptible.

11 Let such an one think this, that, such as we are in word by letters when we are absent, such *will we be* also in deed when we are present.

12 For [o]we dare not make ourselves of the number, or compare ourselves with some that commend themselves: but they measuring themselves by themselves, and comparing themselves among themselves, are not wise.

13 But we will not boast of things without *our* measure, but according to the measure of the rule which God hath distributed to us, a measure to reach even unto you.

14 For we stretch not ourselves beyond *our measure,* as though we reached not unto you: for we are come as far as to you also in *preaching* the [p]gospel of Christ:

15 Not boasting of things without *our* measure, *that is,* [q]of other men's labours; but having hope, when your faith is increased, that we shall be enlarged by you according to our rule abundantly,

16 To preach the gospel in the *regions* beyond you, *and* not to boast in another man's line of things made ready to our hand.

17 But he that glorieth, let him glory in the [r]Lord.

18 For not he that commendeth himself is approved, but whom the Lord commendeth.

CHAPTER 11.

(2) *The godly jealousy.*

Would to God ye could bear with me a little in *my* folly: and indeed bear with me.

2 For I am jealous over you with godly jealousy: for I have [s]espoused you to one husband, that I may present *you* [t]*as* a chaste virgin to Christ.

3 But I fear, lest by any means, as the serpent [u]beguiled Eve through his subtilty, so your minds should be corrupted from the simplicity that is in Christ.

4 For if he that cometh preacheth another Jesus, whom we have not preached, or *if* ye receive another spirit, which ye have not received, or [v]another gospel, which ye

a *Gospel.* 2 Cor. 10:14, 16. (Gen. 12:1-3; Rev. 14:6.)
b *Grace (imparted).* vs. 8, 14; 2 Cor. 12:9. (Rom. 6:1; 2 Pet. 3:18.)
c Rom. 12:1.
d v. 10.
e 1 Cor. 4:21.
f *Flesh.* vs. 3, 4; 2 Cor. 11:18. (John 1:13; Jude 23.)
g *fleshly.*
h *Overthrowing reasonings.*
i *leading captive every thought.*
j *Law (of Christ).* Eph. 5:2. (Gal. 6:2; 2 John 5.)
k John 7:24; 1 Cor. 2:3, 4.
l 2 Cor. 13:2, 3.
m *building up*
n *overthrow.*
o 2 Cor. 3:1.
p *Gospel.* vs. 14, 16; 2 Cor. 11:4, 7. (Gen. 12:1-3; Rev. 14:6.)
q Rom. 15:20.
r *Jehovah.* Jer. 9:24; 1 Cor. 1:31.
s *Bride (of Christ).* Eph. 5:25-32. (John 3:29; Rev. 19:6-8.)
t *Church (true).* vs. 2, 3; Eph. 1:22, 23, (Mt. 16:18; Heb. 12:23.)
u *Temptation.* vs. 3, 4; Gal. 4:14. (Gen. 3:1; Jas. 1:14.)
v *Gospel.* vs. 4, 7; Gal. 1:6-12. (Gen. 12:1-3; Rev. 14:6.)

have not accepted, ye might well bear with *him*.

5 For I suppose I was not a whit behind the very chiefest apostles.

6 But though *I be* [a]rude in speech, yet not in knowledge; but we have been throughly made manifest among you in all things.

7 Have I committed an [b]offence in abasing myself that ye might be exalted, because I have preached to you the [c]gospel of God freely?

8 I robbed other churches, taking wages *of them*, to do you service.

9 And when I was present with you, and wanted, I was chargeable to no man: for that which was lacking to me the brethren which came from Macedonia supplied: and in all *things* I have kept myself from being burdensome unto you, and *so* will I keep *myself*.

10 As the truth of Christ is in me, no man shall stop me of this boasting in the regions of Achaia.

11 Wherefore? because I love you not? God knoweth.

12 But what I do, [d]that I will do, that I may cut off occasion from them which desire occasion; that wherein they glory, they may be found even as we.

(3) *The warning against false teachers.*

13 For such *are* [e]false apostles, deceitful workers, transforming themselves into the apostles of Christ.

14 And no marvel; for [f]Satan himself [g]is transformed into an angel of light.

15 Therefore *it is* no great thing if his ministers also [h]be transformed as the ministers of [i]righteousness; whose end shall be according to their works.

(4) *The enforced boasting* (to 12:18).

16 I say again, Let no man think me a fool; if otherwise, yet as a fool receive me, that I may boast myself a little.

17 That which I speak, I speak *it* not after the Lord, but as it were foolishly, in this confidence of boasting.

18 Seeing that many glory after the [j]flesh, I will glory also.

19 For ye suffer fools gladly, seeing ye *yourselves* are wise.

20 For ye suffer, [k]if a man bring you into bondage, [l]if a man devour *you*, [m]if a man take *of you*, [n]if a man exalt himself, if a man smite you on the face.

A.D. 60.

a *a simple person in speech.*

b *Sin.* Rom. 3:23, *note.*

c *Gospel.* vs. 4, 7; Gal. 1:6-12. (Gen. 12:1-3; Rev. 14:6.)

d Gal. 6:14.

e Mt. 7:15; 24:11, 24; Gal. 2:4; 1 John 4:1.

f *Satan.* 2 Cor. 12:7. (Gen. 3:1; Rev. 20:10.)

g *transformeth himself.*

h *transform themselves.*

i 1 John 3:7, *note.*

j *Flesh.* Gal. 3:3. (John 1:13; Jude 23.)

k Gal. 2:4; 4:9.

l Mt. 23:14.

m Rom. 16:18.

n 1 Pet. 5:3.

o 2 Cor. 10:10.

p v. 5.

q Deut. 25:3.

r Acts 16:22.

s Acts 14:19.

t Acts 27.

u Acts 14:5.

v *Gentiles.*

w Acts 20:31.

x Acts 15:36.

y *Churches (local).* 2 Cor. 12:13. (Acts 2:41; Phil. 1:1.)

z 2 Cor. 12:5, 9, 10.

aa Rom. 9:5.

bb Acts 9:24, 25.

cc *know.*

dd First heaven, of clouds; second, of stars; third, God's abode.

21 I speak as concerning [o]reproach, as though we had been weak. Howbeit whereinsoever any is bold, (I speak foolishly,) I am bold also.

22 Are they [p]Hebrews? so *am* I. Are they Israelites? so *am* I. Are they the seed of Abraham? so *am* I.

23 Are they ministers of Christ? (I speak as a fool) I *am* more; in labours more abundant, in stripes above measure, in prisons more frequent, in deaths oft.

24 Of the Jews five times received I forty [q]*stripes* save one.

25 Thrice was I [r]beaten with rods, once was I [s]stoned, thrice I suffered shipwreck, a [t]night and a day I have been in the deep;

26 *In* journeyings often, *in* [u]perils of waters, *in* perils of robbers, *in* perils by *mine own* countrymen, *in* perils by the [v]heathen, *in* perils in the city, *in* perils in the wilderness, *in* perils in the sea, *in* perils among false brethren;

27 In weariness and painfulness, in [w]watchings often, in hunger and thirst, in fastings often, in cold and nakedness.

28 Beside those things that are without, that which cometh upon me daily, the [x]care of all the [y]churches.

29 Who is weak, and I am not weak? who is offended, and I burn not?

30 If I must needs glory, [z]I will glory of the things which concern mine infirmities.

31 The God and Father of our Lord Jesus Christ, [aa]which is blessed for evermore, knoweth that I lie not.

32 In [bb]Damascus the governor under Aretas the king kept the city of the Damascenes with a garrison, desirous to apprehend me:

33 And through a window in a basket was I let down by the wall, and escaped his hands.

CHAPTER 12.

It is not expedient for me doubtless to glory. I will come to visions and revelations of the Lord.

2 I [cc]knew a man in Christ above fourteen years ago, (whether in the body, I cannot tell; or whether out of the body, I cannot tell: God knoweth;) such an one caught up to the [dd]third heaven.

3 And I knew such a man, (whether in the body, or out of the body, I cannot tell: God knoweth;)

4 How that he was caught up into [a]paradise, and heard unspeakable words, which it is not [b]lawful for a man to utter.

5 Of such an one will I glory: [c]yet of myself I will not glory, but in mine infirmities.

6 For though I would desire to glory, I shall not be a fool; for I will say the truth: but *now* I forbear, lest any man should think of me above that which he seeth me *to be*, or *that* he heareth of me.

7 And lest I should be exalted above measure through the abundance of the revelations, there was given to me a [1d]thorn in the flesh, the messenger of [e]Satan to buffet me, lest I should be exalted above measure.

8 For this thing I besought the Lord thrice, that it might depart from me.

9 And he said unto me, [f]My grace is sufficient for thee: for my strength is made [g]perfect in weakness. Most gladly therefore will I rather glory in my [h]infirmities, that the power of Christ may rest upon me.

10 Therefore I take pleasure in [h]infirmities, in reproaches, in necessities, in persecutions, in [i]distresses for Christ's sake: for when I am weak, then am I strong.

11 I am become a fool in glorying; ye have compelled me: for I ought to have been commended of you: for in nothing am I behind the very chiefest apostles, [j]though I be nothing.

12 Truly the [k]signs of an apostle were wrought among you in all patience, in signs, and wonders, and mighty deeds.

13 For what is it wherein ye were inferior to other [l]churches, except *it be* that I myself was not burdensome to you? forgive me this wrong.

14 Behold, the third time I am ready to come to you; and I will not be burdensome to you: [m]for I seek not yours, but you: for the children ought not to lay up for the parents, but the parents for the children.

15 And I will very gladly spend and be spent for [n]you; though the more abundantly I love you, the less I be loved.

16 But be it so, I did not burden you: nevertheless, being crafty, I caught you with guile.

17 Did I make a gain of you by any of them whom I sent unto you?

18 I desired Titus, and with *him* I sent a brother. Did Titus make a gain of you? walked we not in the same [o]spirit? *walked we* not in the same steps?

(5) *The warning.*

19 Again, think ye that we excuse [p]ourselves unto you? we speak before God in Christ: but *we do* all things, dearly beloved, for your edifying.

20 For I fear, lest, [q]when I come, I shall not find you such as I would, and *that* I shall be found unto you such as ye would not: lest *there be* debates, envyings, wraths, strifes, backbitings, whisperings, swellings, tumults:

21 *And* lest, when I come again, my God will humble me among you, and *that* I shall bewail many which have [r]sinned already, and have not [s]repented of the uncleanness and fornication and lasciviousness which they have committed.

CHAPTER 13.

This *is* the third *time* I am coming to you. [t]In the mouth of two or three witnesses shall every word be established.

2 I told you before, and foretell you, as if I were present, the second time; and being absent now I write to them which heretofore have [r]sinned, and to all other, that, if I come again, I will not spare:

3 Since ye seek a proof of Christ speaking in me, which to you-ward is not weak, but is mighty in you.

4 For [u]though he was crucified through weakness, yet he liveth by the power of God. For we also are weak in him, but we shall live with him by the power of God toward you.

5 [v]Examine yourselves, whether ye be

A.D. 60.

a See Lk. 16:23, *note* on hades.
b *allowed to man.*
c 2 Cor. 11:30.
d Ezk. 28:24; Gal. 4:14.
e *Satan.* Eph. 4:27. (Gen. 3:1; Rev. 20:10.)
f *Grace (imparted).* Gal. 2:9. (Rom. 6:1; 2 Pet. 3:18.)
g Mt. 5:48, *note.*
h Or, *weaknesses.*
i *straits.*
j Lk. 17:10; 1 Cor. 3:7; Eph. 3:8.
k 1 Cor. 9:2.
l *Churches (local).* Gal. 1:2, 13, 22. (Acts 2:41; Phil. 1:1.)
m 1 Cor. 10:24, 33; 1 Thes. 2:8.
n *your souls.*
o *Holy Spirit.* 2 Cor. 13:14. (Mt. 1:18; Acts 2:4.)
p 2 Cor. 5:12.
q 2 Cor. 13:2, 10; 1 Cor. 4:21.
r *Sin.* Rom. 3:23, *note.*
s *Repentance.* 2 Tim. 2:25. (Mt. 3:2; Acts 17:30.)
t Deut. 19:15.
u Phil. 2:7, 8. 1 Pet. 3:18.
v 1 Cor. 11:28; 1 John 3:20.

1 (12:7) It has been conjectured that Paul's "thorn in the flesh" was chronic ophthalmia, inducing bodily weakness, and a repulsive appearance (Gal. 4:15; 1 Cor. 2:3, 4; 2 Cor. 10:10). This cannot be positively known, and the reserve of Scripture is as sure a mark of inspiration as its revelations. Paul's particular "thorn" is not described that his consolations may avail for all to whom *any* thorn is given.

in the faith; prove your own selves.
[a]Know ye not your own selves, how that
Jesus Christ is in you, except ye be
reprobates?
6 But I [b]trust that ye shall know that
we are not reprobates.
7 Now I pray to God that ye do no
evil; not that we should appear
approved, but that ye should do that
which is honest, though we be as reprobates.
8 [c]For we can do nothing against the
truth, but for the truth.
9 For we are glad, when we are weak,
and ye are strong: and this also we wish,
even your [d]perfection.
10 Therefore I write these things being
absent, lest being present I should use
sharpness, according to the power which
the Lord hath given me to edification,
and not to destruction.

(6) *Conclusion.*

11 Finally, brethren, [e]farewell. Be [f]per-
fect, be of good comfort, be of one mind,
live in peace; and the God of love and
peace shall be with you.
12 [g]Greet one another with an holy
kiss.
13 All the saints salute you.
14 The grace of the Lord Jesus Christ,
and the love of God, and the communion of the [h]Holy Ghost, *be* with you all.
Amen.

A.D. 60.

a *Do ye not recognize yourselves that.*

b i.e. *hope.*

c Prov. 21:30.

d *Perfecting.* Mt. 5:48, *note.*

e *rejoice.*

f *perfected;* cf. Mt. 5:48, *note.*

g Rom. 16:16.

h *Holy Spirit.* Gal. 3:2, 3, 5, 14. (Mt. 1:18; Acts 2:4.)

THE EPISTLE OF PAUL THE APOSTLE TO THE

GALATIANS

WRITER. The Apostle Paul (1:1).

Date. Galatians was probably written A.D. 60, during Paul's third visit to Corinth. The occasion of the Epistle is evident. It had come to Paul's knowledge that the fickle Galatians, who were not Greeks, but Gauls, "a stream from the torrent of barbarians which poured into Greece in the third century before Christ," had become the prey of the legalizers, the Judaizing missionaries from Palestine.

Theme. The theme of Galatians is the vindication of the Gospel of the grace of God from any admixture of law-conditions, which qualify or destroy its character of pure grace.

The Galatian error had two forms, both of which are refuted. The first is the teaching that obedience to the law is mingled with faith as the ground of the sinner's justification; the second, that the justified believer is made perfect by keeping the law. Paul meets the first form of the error by a demonstration that justification is through the Abrahamic Covenant (Gen. 15:18), and that the law, which was four hundred and thirty years after the confirmation of that covenant, and the true purpose of which was condemnation, not justification, cannot disannul a salvation which rests upon the earlier covenant. Paul meets the second and more subtle form by vindicating the office of the Holy Spirit as Sanctifier.

The book is in seven parts: I. Salutation, 1:1-5. II. Theme, 1:6-9. III. Paul's Gospel is a revelation, 1:10–2:14. IV. Justification is by faith without law, 2:15–3:24. V. The rule of the believer's life is gracious, not legal, 3:25–5:15. VI. Sanctification is through the Spirit, not the law, 5:16-24. VII. Exhortations and conclusion, 5:25–6:18.

CHAPTER 1.

Part I. Salutation (vs. 1-5).

Paul, an apostle, (not of men, neither
by man, but by Jesus Christ, and
God the Father, who raised him from the
dead;)
2 And all the brethren which are with
me, unto the [a]churches [b]of Galatia:
3 [c]Grace *be* to you and peace from God
the Father, and *from* our Lord Jesus
Christ,
4 Who [d]gave himself for our [e]sins, that
he might [f]deliver us from this present
evil [g]world, [h]according to the will of
God and our Father:
5 To whom *be* glory for ever and ever.
Amen.

Part II. Theme and occasion of the Epistle (vs. 6-9).

6 I marvel that ye are so soon removed
from him that called you into the [1]grace
of Christ unto another gospel:
7 Which is not [i]another; but there be
some that [j]trouble you, and would [k]pervert the gospel of Christ.
8 But though we, or an [l]angel from
heaven, preach any other gospel unto
you than that which we have preached
unto you, let him be [m]accursed.
9 As we said before, so say I now
again, If any *man* preach any other
gospel unto you than that ye have
received, let him be accursed.

Part III. Paul's gospel is a revelation, not a tradition from the other apostles (Gal. 1.10–2:14).

10 [2]For do I now persuade men, or
God? or do I seek to [n]please men? for if I
yet pleased men, I should not be the
[o]servant of Christ.

A.D. 58.

a *Churches (local).* vs. 2, 13, 22; Col. 4:15, 16. (Acts 2:41; Phil. 1:1.)
b 1 Cor. 16:1; Acts 16:6.
c *Grace (in salv.).* vs. 6, 15; Gal. 2:21. (Rom. 3:24; John 1:17, *note.*)
d Gal. 2:20; 1 Cor. 15:3; 1 Pet. 2:24.
e *Sin.* Rom. 3:23, *note.*
f Gal. 6:14; Rom. 12:2; Col. 2:20.
g i.e. *age.*
h 1 John 2:15-17.
i Acts 4:12.
j Gal. 5:10, 12; Acts 15:24.
k 2 Cor. 2:17; 11:13, 14.
l 1 Ki. 13:18.
m 1 Cor. 16:22.
n 1 Thes. 2:4.
o Phil. 1:1.

[1] **(1:6)** The test of the Gospel is grace. If the message excludes grace, or mingles law with grace as the means either of justification or sanctification (Gal. 2:21; 3:1-3), or denies the fact or guilt of sin which alone gives grace its occasion and opportunity, it is "another" gospel, and the preacher of it is under the anathema of God (vs. 8, 9).

[2] **(1:10)** The demonstration is as follows: (1) The Galatians know Paul, that he is no seeker after popularity (v. 10). (2) He puts his known character back of the assertion that his Gospel of grace was a revelation from God (vs. 11, 12). (3) As for the

11 But I certify you, brethren, that the [a]gospel which was preached of me is not after [b]man.

12 For I neither received it of man, neither was I taught *it*, but by the [c]revelation of Jesus Christ.

13 For ye have heard of my conversation in time past in the [1d]Jews' religion, how that beyond measure I persecuted [e]the church of God, and wasted it:

14 And profited in the Jews' [2]religion above many my equals in mine own nation, being more exceedingly zealous of the traditions of my fathers.

15 But when it pleased God, who [f]separated me from my mother's womb, and [g]called *me* by his grace,

16 To reveal his Son [h]in me, that I might preach him among the [i]heathen; immediately I [j]conferred not with flesh and blood:

17 Neither went I up to Jerusalem to them which were apostles before me; but I went into Arabia, and returned again unto Damascus.

18 Then after three years I [k]went up to Jerusalem to see Peter, and abode with him fifteen days.

19 But other of the apostles saw I none, save James the Lord's [l]brother.

20 Now the things which I write unto you, behold, before God, I lie not.

21 Afterwards I came into the regions of Syria and Cilicia;

22 And was unknown by face unto the churches of Judaea which were in Christ:

23 But they had [m]heard only, That he which persecuted us in times past now preacheth the faith which once he destroyed.

24 And they [n]glorified God in me.

CHAPTER 2.

Then [o]fourteen years after I went up again to Jerusalem with Barnabas, and took [p]Titus with *me* also.

2 And I went up by [q]revelation, and communicated unto them that gospel which I preach among the Gentiles, but [r]privately to them which were of reputation, lest by any means I should run, or had run, in [s]vain.

3 But neither Titus, who was with me, being a Greek, was compelled to be circumcised:

4 And that because of [t]false brethren unawares brought in, who came in privily to spy out our [u]liberty which we have in Christ Jesus, that they might bring us into bondage:

5 To whom we [v]gave place by subjection, no, not for an hour; that the [w]truth of the gospel might continue with you.

6 But of these who seemed to be somewhat, (whatsoever they were, it maketh no matter to me: God [x]accepteth no man's person:) for they who seemed *to be somewhat* in conference added nothing to me:

7 But contrariwise, when they saw that the gospel of the [y]uncircumcision was committed unto me, as *the gospel* of the [z]circumcision *was* unto Peter;

8 (For he that wrought effectually in Peter to the apostleship of the circumcision, the same was mighty in me toward the Gentiles:)

9 And when [aa]James, Cephas, and John, who seemed to be pillars, perceived the [bb]grace that was given unto me, they gave to me and Barnabas the [cc]right hands of fellowship; that we *should go* unto the [dd]heathen, and they unto the circumcision.

10 Only *they would* that we should remember the poor; the same which I also was forward to do.

11 But when Peter was come to [ee]Antioch, I withstood him to the face, because he was to be blamed.

12 For before that certain came from James, he did [ff]eat with the Gentiles: but when they were come, he withdrew and [gg]separated himself,

A.D. 58.

a *Gospel.* v. 6-12; Gal. 2:2-5, 7-14. (Gen. 12:1-3; Rev. 14:6.)
b *Inspiration.* vs. 11, 12; Eph. 3:3, 5. (Ex. 4:15; Rev. 22:19.)
c Acts 9:1-20; Gal. 1:16; Eph. 3:3-5.
d Acts 9:1-3.
e *Church (visible).* Phil. 3:6. (1 Cor. 10:32; 1 Tim. 3:15.)
f Jer. 1:5.
g Rom. 8:30.
h 2 Cor. 4:6.
i *Gentiles.*
j v. 1.
k Acts 9:26.
l Mt. 12:46; 13:55.
m Acts 9:21, 27, 28.
n Acts 11:18.
o Acts 15:1, 2.
p 2 Cor. 8:16, 23.
q Acts 16:9.
r Acts 15:4.
s Phil. 2:16.
t 2 Cor. 11:26; Jude 4.
u Gal. 5:1, 13.
v Cf. v. 11.
w v. 14; Gal. 3:1.
x Acts 10:34; Rom. 2:11.
y Acts 22:21; Rom. 11:13.
z 1 Pet. 1:1.
aa Acts 15:13.
bb *Grace (imparted).* Eph. 3:2-8. (Rom. 6:1; 2 Pet. 3:18.)
cc Acts 13:3.
dd *Gentiles.*
ee Acts 11:19-26; 15:1.
A.D. 52.]
ff Acts 11:3.
gg Gen. 12:11-13.

Judaizers, Paul himself had been a foremost Jew, and had forsaken Judaism for something better (vs. 13, 14). (4) He had preached grace years before he saw any of the other apostles (vs. 15-24). (5) When he did meet the other apostles they had nothing to add to his revelations (2:1-6). (6) The other apostles fully recognized Paul's apostleship (2:7-10). (7) If the legalizers pleaded Peter's authority, the answer was that he himself had claimed none when rebuked (2:11-14).

1 (1:13) The new dispensation of grace having come in, the Mosaic system, if still persisted in, becomes a mere "Jews' religion."

2 (1:14) In verses 13 and 14 the Greek word for "the Jews' religion" is *Ioudaismos* (Judaism). In Acts 26:5 and Jas. 1:26, 27, *threskeia*—religious service— is translated "religion," and in Col. 2:18 "worshipping." Excepting Jas. 1:27, "religion" has always a bad sense, and nowhere is it synonymous with salvation or spirituality.

fearing them which were of the circumcision.

13 And the other Jews dissembled likewise with him; insomuch that [a]Barnabas also was carried away with their dissimulation.

14 But when I saw that they walked not uprightly according to the truth of the [b]gospel, I said unto Peter before *them* all, If thou, being a Jew, livest after the manner of Gentiles, and not as do the Jews, why compellest thou the Gentiles to live as do the Jews?

Part IV. Justification is by faith without law (Gal. 2:15–3:24).

(1) *Even Jews must be so justified.*

15 [1]We *who are* [c]Jews by nature, and not [d]sinners of the Gentiles,

16 Knowing that a man is not [e]justified by the works of the law, but by the [f]faith of Jesus Christ, even we have believed in [g]Jesus Christ, that we might be [h]justified by the faith of Christ, and [i]not by the works of the law: for by the works of the law shall no flesh be justified.

17 But if, while [2]we seek to be justified [j]by Christ, we ourselves also are found [d]sinners, *is* therefore Christ the [k]minister of sin? God forbid.

18 For if I [l]build again the things which I destroyed, I make myself a [d]transgressor.

(2) *The law has already executed its sentence upon the believer.*

19 For I through the law am [m]dead to the law, that I might live unto God.

(3) *The Christian life is the outliving of the inliving Christ.* (Cf. Gal. 5:15-23.)

20 I am [n]crucified with Christ: nevertheless [o]I live; yet [p]not I, but Christ liveth in me: and the [q]life which I now live in the flesh I live by the faith of the Son of God, who loved me, and gave himself for me.

A.D. 58.

a Acts 15:37-39.
b *Gospel.* Gal. 3:8 (Gen. 12:1-3; Rev. 14:6.)
c Phil. 3:5.
d *Sin.* Rom 3:23, *note.*
e *Justification.* Gal. 3:8, 11, 24. (Lk. 18:14; Rom. 3:28.)
f *Faith.* Gal. 3:6, 7, 9, 11, 12, 22-26. (Gen. 3:20; Heb. 11:39.)
g *Christ Jesus.*
h Psa 143:2; Rom. 3:20, 28.
i *Law (of Moses).* vs. 15, 16, 19, 21; Gal. 4:21-30. (Ex. 19:1; Gal. 3:1-29.)
j Rom. 8:1; Gal. 5:6.
k Rom 6:1.
l Gal. 5:2-4.
m Rom. 7:4.
n Gal. 6:14; Col. 2:11, 12, 20.
o Rom. 6:8-11; Col. 3:1; Eph. 2:5, 6.
p Eph. 4:24, *note.*
q *Life (eternal).* Gal. 6:8. (Mt. 7:14; Rev. 22:19.)
r *Grace (in salv.).* Gal. 5:4. (Rom. 3:24; John 1:17, *note.*)
s Rom. 10:10, *note.*
t Gal. 3:4; 5:2; cf. 1 Cor. 15:17.
u Rom. 10;17.
v Mt. 5:48, *note.*
w *Flesh.* Gal. 4:23, 29. (John 1:13; Jude 23.)
x Acts 9:17; 10:44.
y *Faith.* vs. 7, 9, 11, 12, 22-26; Eph. 2:8. (Gen. 3:20; Heb. 11:39.)
z *Jehovah.* Gen. 15:6.
aa *Imputation.* Jas. 2:23. (Lev. 25:50; Jas. 2:23.)
bb *sons.*
cc *Gentiles.*
dd *Gospel.* Gal. 4:13. (Gen. 12:1-3; Rev. 14:6.)
ee Gen. 12:3.
ff *believing.*
gg Deut. 27:26.

(4) *To mingle law-works with grace in justification frustrates grace.*

21 I do not frustrate the [r]grace of God: for if [s]righteousness *come* by the law, then Christ is dead [t]in vain.

CHAPTER 3.

(5) *The gift of the Spirit is by faith, not by law-works.*

O foolish Galatians, who hath bewitched you, that ye should not obey the truth, before whose eyes Jesus Christ hath been evidently set forth, crucified among you?

2 This only would I learn of you, Received ye the Spirit by the works of the law, or by the [u]hearing of faith?

3 Are ye so foolish? having begun in the Spirit, are ye now made [v]perfect by the [w]flesh?

4 Have ye suffered so many things in vain? if *it be* yet in vain.

5 He therefore that [x]ministereth to you the Spirit, and worketh miracles among you, *doeth he it* by the works of the law, or by the hearing of faith?

(6) *The Abrahamic Covenant is a by-faith covenant.* (Cf.Rom. 4:1-22.)

6 Even as Abraham [y]believed [z]God, and it was [aa]accounted to him for righteousness.

7 Know ye therefore that they which are of faith, the same are [bb]the children of Abraham.

8 And the scripture, foreseeing that God would justify the [cc]heathen through faith, preached before the [dd]gospel unto Abraham, *saying,* [ee]In thee shall all nations be blessed.

9 So then they which be of faith are blessed with [ff]faithful Abraham.

(7) *The man under law-works is under the curse of the law.*

10 For as many as are of the works of the law are under the curse: for it is written, [gg]Cursed *is* every one that continueth

[1] **(2:15)** Paul here quotes from his words to Peter when he withstood him at Antioch to show the Galatians that, whatever the legalists may have pretended, Peter and he were in perfect accord doctrinally. Paul appealed to the common *belief* of Peter and himself as a rebuke of Peter's inconsistent *practice.*

[2] **(2:17)** That is, "we" Jews. (See Rom. 3:19-23.) The passage might be thus paraphrased: If we Jews, in seeking to be justified by faith in Christ, take our places as mere sinners, like the Gentiles, is it therefore Christ who makes us sinners? By no means. It is by putting ourselves again under law after seeking justification through Christ, that we act as if we were still unjustified sinners, seeking to become righteous through law-works. (Cf. Gal. 5:1-4.)

not in all things which are written in the
book of the law to do them.
11 But that no man is [a]justified by the
law in the sight of God, *it is* evident: for,
[b]The just shall live by faith.
12 And the law is [c]not of faith: but,
[d]The man that doeth them shall live in
them.

(8) *Christ has borne our law-curse that we might have the faith-blessing.*

13 Christ hath [e]redeemed us from the
curse of the law, being [f]made a [g]curse
for us: for it is written, [h]Cursed *is* every
one that hangeth on a tree:
14 That the [i]blessing of Abraham
might come on the [j]Gentiles through
[k]Jesus Christ; that we might receive the
promise of the [l]Spirit through faith.
15 Brethren, I speak after the manner
of men; Though *it be* but a man's
covenant, yet *if it be* confirmed, no man
disannulleth, or addeth thereto.
16 Now to [m]Abraham and his seed
were the promises made. He saith not,
And to [n]seeds, as of many; but as of
[o]one, And to thy seed, which is Christ.

(9) *The law does not add a new condition to the Abrahamic covenant of faith.*

17 And this I say, *that* the covenant,
that was confirmed before of [p]God in
Christ, the law, which was [q]four hundred and thirty years after, cannot
disannul, that it should make the
promise of none effect.
18 For [r]if the inheritance *be* of the law,
it is no more of promise: but God [s]gave
it to Abraham by promise.

(10) *The true intent of the law is condemnation, and as a preparatory discipline.*

19 [1]Wherefore then *serveth* the law? It
was added [t]because of transgressions,
till the [u]seed should come to whom the
promise was made; *and it was* ordained
by angels in the hand of a mediator.
20 Now a mediator is not *a mediator* of
one, but God is one.
21 *Is* the law then against the promises
of God? God forbid: for if there had been
a law given which could have given life,
verily [v]righteousness should have been
by the law.
22 But the scripture hath concluded all
under sin, that the promise by faith of
Jesus Christ might be given to them that
believe.
23 But before faith came, we were kept
under the law, shut up unto the faith
which should afterwards be revealed.
24 Wherefore the [2w]law was our
schoolmaster [x]*to bring us* [y]unto

A.D. 58.

- a *Justification.* vs. 8, 11, 24; Gal. 5:4. (Lk. 18:14; Rom. 3:28.
- b Hab. 2:4; Rom. 1:17.
- c Rom. 9:31, 32.
- d Lev. 18:5.
- e Gal. 4:5; Eph. 1:7.
- f *Sacrifice (of Christ).* Gal. 4:4, 5. (Gen. 4:4; Heb. 10:18.)
- g *Judgments (the seven).* 1 Tim. 1:20. (2 Sam. 7:14; Rev. 20:12.)
- h Deut. 21:23.
- i v. 8; Rom. 4:2-5.
- j Rom. 3:29, 30.
- k *Christ Jesus.*
- l *Holy Spirit.* vs. 2, 3, 5, 14; Gal. 4:6, 29. (Mt. 1:18; Acts 2:4.)
- m Gen. 13:15.
- n Gen. 25:5, 6.
- o Gen. 22:18.
- p Rom. 4:9, 10, 13, 14.
- q Ex. 12:40, 41.
- r Rom. 4:13; 11:5.
- s Gen. 22:16, 17.
- t *for the sake,* i.e. in order that sin might be made manifest as transgression. See Rom. 4:15; 5:20; 7:7, 13.
- u Gal. 4:4; Heb. 10:8, 9.
- v Rom. 10:10, *note.*
- w *Law (of Moses).* vs. 1-29. (Ex. 19:1.)
- x Omit *"to bring us."*
- y *up to,* or *until.*

[1] **(3:19)** The answer is sixfold: (1) The law was added because of transgressions, i.e. to give to sin the character of transgression. *(a)* Men had been sinning before Moses, but in the absence of law their sins were not put to their account (Rom. 5:13); the law gave to sin the character of "transgression," i.e. of personal guilt. *(b)* Also, since men not only continued to transgress after the law was given, but were provoked to transgress by the very law which forbade it (Rom. 7:8), the law conclusively proved the inveterate sinfulness of man's nature (Rom. 7:11-13). (2) The law, therefore, "concluded all under sin" (cf. Rom. 3:19, 20, 23). (3) The law was an *ad interim* dealing, "till the seed should come" (v. 19). (4) The law shut sinful man up to faith as the only avenue of escape (v. 23). (5) The law was to the Jews what the pedagogue was in a Greek household, a ruler of children in their minority, and it had this character "unto" (i.e. until) Christ (v. 24). (6) Christ having come, the believer is no longer under the pedagogue (v. 25).

[2] **(3:24)** I. The law of Moses, Summary: (1) The Mosaic Covenant was given to Israel in three parts: the commandments, expressing the righteous will of God (Ex. 20:1-26); the "judgments," governing the social life of Israel (Ex. 21:1–24:11), and the "ordinances," governing the religious life of Israel (Ex. 24:12; 31:18). (2) The commandments and ordinances were one complete and inseparable whole. When an Israelite sinned, he was held "blameless" if he brought the required offering (Lk. 1:6; Phil. 3:6). (3) Law, as a method of the divine dealing with man, characterized the dispensation extending from the giving of the law to the death of Jesus Christ (Gal. 3:13, 14, 23, 24). (4) The attempt of legalistic teachers (e.g. Acts 15:1-31; Gal. 2:1-5) to mingle law with grace as the divine method for this present dispensation of grace, brought out the true relation of the law to the Christian, viz.

II. The Christian doctrine of the law: (1) Law is in contrast with grace. Under the latter God

Christ, that we might be [a]justified by faith.

Part V. The rule of the believer's life is gracious, not legal (Gal. 3:25–5:15).

25 But after that faith is come, we are no longer under a [1]schoolmaster.

(1) *The justified believer is a son in the family of God, not a servant under the law.*

26 For ye are all [b]the children of God by faith in Christ Jesus.

27 For as many of you as have been [c]baptized [d]into Christ have put on Christ.

28 There is [e]neither Jew nor Greek, there is neither [f]bond nor free, there is neither [g]male nor female: for ye are all [h]one in Christ Jesus.

29 And if ye *be* Christ's, then are ye [i]Abraham's seed, and [j]heirs according to the promise.

CHAPTER 4.

Now I say, *That* the heir, as long as he is a child, differeth nothing from a servant, though he be lord of all;

2 But is under tutors and governors until the time appointed of the father.

3 Even so [k]we, when we were children, were in bondage under the [l]elements of the [m]world:

(2) *The believer is redeemed from under the law.*

4 But when the [n]fulness of the time was come, [o]God sent forth his Son, made of a [p]woman, made under the law,

5 To [q]redeem them that were [r]under the law, that we might receive the [s]adoption of sons.

(3) *The Spirit actualizes the believer's sonship.* (See Eph. 1:5, *note.*)

6 And because ye are sons, God hath sent forth the [t]Spirit of his Son into your hearts, crying, Abba, Father.

7 Wherefore thou art no more a servant, but a son; and if a son, then an [u]heir of God through Christ.

(4) *To lapse into legality is to go back to an elementary religion.*

8 Howbeit then, when ye knew not God, ye [v]did service unto them which by nature are no gods.

9 But now, after that ye have known God, or rather are known of God, how turn ye again to the [w]weak and beggarly elements, whereunto ye [x]desire again to be in bondage?

10 Ye [y]observe days, and months, and times, and years.

A.D. 58.

a Rom. 10:4.
b Gr. *huioi = sons.* See Eph. 1:5, *note.*
c Rom. 6:3.
d *unto.*
e Rom. 10:12; Col. 3:11.
f 1 Cor. 7:20-24.
g Acts 1:14.
h Eph. 2:15, 16; 1 Cor. 12:13.
i Rom. 4:11.
j Gal. 4:7; Heb. 9:15.
k i.e. Jews.
l v. 9; Col. 2:8, 20.
m *kosmos* (Mt. 4:8) = mankind.
n Gen. 18:10; Heb. 9:26.
o John 16:28.
p Gen. 3:15.
q *Sacrifice (of Christ).* vs. 4, 5; Eph. 1:7. (Gen. 4:4; Heb. 10:18.)
r Gal. 3:13.
s *Adoption.* Eph. 1:5. (Rom. 8:15, 23; Eph. 1:5.)
t *Holy Spirit.* vs. 6, 29; Gal. 5:5, 16, 17-25. (Mt. 1:18; Acts 2:4.)
u Eph. 1:14; 1 Pet. 1:4.
v 1 Thes. 1:9.
w Rom. 8:3; Heb. 7:18, 19.
x Gen. 3:1-3.
y Col. 2:16.

bestows the righteousness which, under law, He demanded (Ex. 19:5; John 1:17; Rom. 3:21, *note;* 10:3-10; 1 Cor. 1:30). (2) The law is, in itself, holy, just, good, and spiritual (Rom. 7:12-14). (3) Before the law the whole world is guilty, and the law is therefore of necessity a ministry of condemnation, death, and the divine curse (Rom. 3:19; 2 Cor. 3:7-9; Gal. 3:10). (4) Christ bore the curse of the law, and redeemed the believer both from the curse and from the dominion of the law (Gal. 3:13; 4:5-7). (5) Law neither justifies a sinner nor sanctifies a believer (Gal. 2:16; 3:2, 3, 11, 12). (6) The believer is both dead to the law and redeemed from it, so that he is "not under the law, but under grace" (Rom. 6:14; 7:4; Gal. 2:19; 4:4-7; 1 Tim. 1:8, 9). (7) Under the new covenant of grace the principle of obedience to the divine will is inwrought (Heb. 10:16). So far is the life of the believer from the anarchy of self-will that he is "inlawed to Christ" (1 Cor. 9:21), and the new "law of Christ" (Gal. 6:2; 2 John 5) is his delight; while, through the indwelling Spirit, the righteousness of the law is fulfilled in him (Rom. 8:2-4; Gal. 5:16-18). The commandments are used in the distinctively Christian Scriptures as an instruction in righteousness (2 Tim. 3:16; Rom. 13:8-10; Eph. 6:1-3; 1 Cor. 9:8, 9).

[1] **(3:25)** Gr. *paidagogos,* "child-conductor." "Among the Greeks and Romans, persons, for the most part slaves, who had it in charge to educate and give constant attendance upon boys till they came of age."—*H. A. W. Meyer.* The argument does not turn upon the extent or nature of the pedagogue's authority, but upon the fact that it wholly ceased when the "child" (4:1) became a *"son"* (4:1-6), when the *minor* became an *adult.* The adult *"son"* does voluntarily that which formerly he did in fear of the pedagogue. But even if he does not, it is no longer a question between the son and the pedagogue (the law), but between the son and his Father—God. (Cf. Heb. 12:5-10; 1 John 2:1, 2.)

11 I am afraid of you, lest I have bestowed upon you labour in vain.

12 Brethren, I [a]beseech you, be as I *am*; for I *am* as ye *are*: ye have not [b]injured me at all.

13 Ye know how through infirmity of the flesh I preached the [c]gospel unto you at the first.

14 And my [d]temptation which was in my flesh ye despised not, nor rejected; but received me as an angel of God, *even* as Christ Jesus.

(5) *In legality the Galatians have lost their blessing.*

15 Where is then the blessedness ye spake of? for I bear you record, that, if *it had been* possible, ye would have [e]plucked out your own eyes, and have given them to me.

16 Am I therefore become your [f]enemy, because I tell you the truth?

17 They zealously affect you, *but* not well; yea, they would [g]exclude you, that ye might affect them.

18 But *it is* good to be zealously affected always in *a* good *thing*, and [h]not only when I am present with you.

(6) *The two systems, law and grace, cannot co-exist.*

19 My [1]little children, of whom I travail in birth again until Christ be formed in you,

20 I desire to be [i]present with you now, and to change my voice; for I stand in [j]doubt of you.

21 Tell me, ye that desire to be under the [k]law, do ye not [l]hear the law?

22 For it is written, [m]that Abraham had two sons, the one by a bondmaid, the other by a freewoman.

23 But he *who was* of the bondwoman was born after the [n]flesh; but he of the freewoman *was* by [o]promise.

24 Which things are an allegory: for these are the [p]two covenants; the one from the mount [q]Sinai, which gendereth to [r]bondage, which is [s]Agar.

25 For this [s]Agar is mount Sinai in Arabia, and answereth to Jerusalem which now is, and is in [t]bondage with her children.

26 But Jerusalem which is [u]above is free, which is the [v]mother of us all.

27 For it is written, [w]Rejoice, *thou* barren that bearest not; break forth and cry, thou that travailest not: for the desolate hath many more children than she which hath an husband.

28 Now [x]we, brethren, as Isaac was, are the children of promise.

29 But as then he that was born after the flesh [y]persecuted him *that was born* after the Spirit, even so *it is* now.

30 Nevertheless what saith the scripture? [z]Cast out the bondwoman and her son: for the son of the bondwoman shall not be heir with the son of the freewoman.

31 So then, brethren, we are [aa]not children of the bondwoman, but of the [bb]free.

CHAPTER 5.

Application of the allegory.

[cc]Stand fast therefore in the liberty wherewith Christ hath made us free, and be not entangled again with the [dd]yoke of bondage.

2 Behold, I Paul say unto you, that [ee]if ye be circumcised, Christ shall profit you nothing.

3 For I testify again to every man that is circumcised, that he is a [ff]debtor to do the whole law.

4 Christ is become of [gg]no effect unto you, whosoever of you are [hh]justified by the law; ye are [ii]fallen from [jj]grace.

5 For we through the Spirit [kk]wait for the hope of [ll]righteousness by faith.

6 For in [mm]Jesus Christ neither [nn]circumcision availeth any thing, nor uncircumcision; but [oo]faith which [pp]worketh by love.

7 Ye [qq]did run well; who did hinder you that ye should not obey the truth?

8 This persuasion *cometh* not of him that calleth you.

9 A little [rr]leaven leaveneth the whole lump.

10 I have confidence in you through the Lord, that ye will be none otherwise minded: but he that troubleth you shall bear his judgment, whosoever he be.

A.D. 58.

a 2 Cor. 6:11, 13.
b 2 Cor. 2:5.
c *Gospel.* Eph. 1:13. (Gen. 12:1-3; Rev. 14:6.)
d *Temptation.* Gal. 6:1. (Gen. 3:1; Jas. 1:14.)
e Acts 20:37, 38.
f 2 Cor. 12:15.
g 2 Tim. 1:15.
h Phil. 2:12.
i 1 Cor. 4:21; 2 Cor. 13:1, 2.
j v. 11.
k *Law (of Moses).* vs. 21-30. Eph. 2:15. (Ex. 19:1; Gal. 3:1-29.)
l Rom. 3:19, 20.
m Gen. 16:15; 21:2.
n *Flesh.* vs. 23-29; Gal. 5:13, 16-21, 24. (John 1:13; Jude 23.)
o v. 28; Gen. 17:15-19.
p Heb. 8:6, 7; 9:15.
q Ex. 24:6, 8.
r Gal. 5:1.
s *Hagar.*
t John 8:32-36.
u Heb. 11:10; 12:22; Rev. 21:2.
v Phil. 3:20.
w Isa. 54:1.
x Gal. 3:29; Rom. 9:8.
y Gen. 21:9.
z Gen. 21:10.
aa Rom. 6:14.
bb *freewoman.*
cc Phil. 4:1; Gal. 2:5.
dd Acts 15:10; Col. 2:8.
ee Acts 15:1.
ff Rom. 2:25.
gg i.e. of no *experimental* effect: the sense of liberty is lost. Gal. 2:21; Col. 1:23.
hh *Justification.* Titus 3:7. (Lk. 18:14; Rom. 3:28.)
ii *fallen away.* Gal. 4:9.
jj *Grace (in salv.).* Gal. 1:6, *note;* Eph. 1:6, 7. (Rom. 3:24; John 1:17, *note.*)
kk Rom. 5:2, 5.
ll Rom. 10:10, *note.*
mm *Christ Jesus.*
nn Gal. 6:15; 3:28; Rom. 10:12.
oo Rom. 3:22; 5:1.
pp 1 Thes. 1:3; Jas. 2:20-26.
qq Gal. 3:3.
rr *Leaven.* Mt. 13:33. (Gen. 19:3; Mt. 13:33.)

1(4:19) The allegory (vs. 22-31) is addressed to justified but immature believers (cf. 1 Cor. 3:1, 2), who, under the influence of legalistic teachers, "desire to be under the law," and has, therefore, no application to a sinner seeking justification. It raises and answers, for the fifth time in this Epistle, the question, Is the believer under the law? (Gal. 2:19-21; 3:1-3; 3:25, 26; 4:4-6; 4:9-31).

11 And I, brethren, if I yet preach circumcision, why do I yet suffer [a]persecu-
tion? then is the [b]offence of the cross
ceased.
12 I would they were even cut off
which trouble you.
13 For, brethren, ye have been [c]called
unto liberty; only *use* not liberty for an
[d]occasion to the flesh, but by [e]love serve
one another.
14 For all the law is fulfilled in one
word, *even* in this; [f]Thou shalt love thy
neighbour as thyself.
15 But if ye [g]bite and devour one
another, take heed that ye be not [h]con-
sumed one of another.

Part VI. Sanctification is through the Spirit, not the law (vs.16-24).

16 *This* I say then, [i]Walk in the Spirit,
and ye shall not fulfil the lust of the flesh.

(1) *The Spirit gives victory over sin.* (Cf. Rom. 8:2. See Rom. 7:15, *note*.)

17 For the flesh [j]lusteth against the
Spirit, and the Spirit against the flesh:
and these are contrary the one to the
other: so that ye [k]cannot do the things
that ye would.
18 But if ye be [l]led of the Spirit, ye are
not [m]under the law.
19 Now the [n]works of the flesh are
manifest, which are *these*; Adultery, fornication, uncleanness, lasciviousness,
20 Idolatry, witchcraft, hatred, variance, emulations, wrath, strife, seditions,
heresies,
21 Envyings, murders, drunkenness,
revellings, and such like: of the which I
tell you before, as I have also told *you* in
time past, that they which do such things
shall [o]not inherit the kingdom of God.

(2) *Christian character is produced by the Holy Spirit, not by self-effort.* (Cf. John 15:1-5; Gal. 2:20.)

22 [1]But the fruit of the Spirit is love,
joy, peace, longsuffering, gentleness,
goodness, [p]faith,
23 Meekness, temperance: against
[q]such there is no law.
24 And they that are Christ's have crucified the [r]flesh with the affections and
lusts.

Part VII. The outworking of the new life in Christ Jesus (Gal. 5:25–6:18).

25 If we live in the [s]Spirit, let us also
walk in the Spirit.
26 Let us not be desirous of [t]vain
glory, provoking one another, envying
one another.

CHAPTER 6.

(1) *The new life as a brotherhood:*
(*a*) *the case of a sinning brother.*

Brethren, if a man be overtaken in a
[u]fault, ye which are [v]spiritual,
[w]restore such an one in the spirit of
[x]meekness; considering thyself, lest thou
also be [y]tempted.

(*b*) *The case of a burdened brother.*

2 [z]Bear ye one another's burdens, and
so fulfil the [aa]law of Christ.
3 For if a man [bb]think himself to be
something, when he is nothing, he [cc]de-
ceiveth himself.
4 But let every man [dd]prove his own
work, and then shall he have rejoicing in
[ee]himself alone, and not in another.
5 For every man shall [ff]bear his own
burden.

(*c*) *The case of a teaching brother.*

6 Let him that is taught in the word
[gg]communicate unto him that teacheth
in all good things.

(2) *The new life as a husbandry.*

7 [hh]Be not deceived; God is not
mocked: for [ii]whatsoever a man soweth,
that shall he also reap.
8 For he that soweth to his flesh shall
of the flesh reap corruption; but he that
soweth to the [jj]Spirit shall of the Spirit
reap [kk]life everlasting.
9 And let us not be [ll]weary in well
doing: for in due season we shall
[mm]reap, if we faint not.

A.D. 58.

a Gal. 6:12.
b 1 Cor. 1:23; 2 Tim. 3:11, 12.
c v. 1; Rom. 8:2.
d Rom. 6:1, 15-22; 1 Pet. 2:16.
e 1 Pet. 1:22; 1 John 3:16-18.
f Lev. 19:18.
g Jas. 3:13-16.
h Isa. 9:18-21.
i v. 25; Rom. 8:12, 13.
j Rom. 7:22, 23.
k *should not.*
l Rom. 8:14.
m i.e. not under bondage of effort to please God by law-works. 2 Cor. 3:17.
n Rom. 1:26-31; Eph. 5:11, 12; 2 Tim. 3:1-4.
o 1 Cor. 6:9, 10; Rev. 21:8.
p *faithfulness.*
q *such things.*
r *Flesh.* vs. 13, 16-21, 24; Gal. 6:8, 13. (John 1:13; Jude 23.)
s *Holy Spirit.* vs. 5, 16, 17, 18, 22, 25; Gal. 6:8. (Mt. 1:18; Acts 2:4.)
t Phil. 2:3.
u i.e. *sin.* Rom. 3:23, *note.*
v Rom. 15:1; Gal. 5:25.
w John 13:12-15.
x John 21:15-17.
y *Temptation.* 1 Thes. 3:5. (Gen. 3:1; Jas. 1:14.)
z Acts 20:35; 1 Thes. 5:14.
aa *Law (of Christ).* Lk. 6:27-38. (Gal. 6:2; 2 John 5.)
bb Rom. 12:3.
cc Jas. 1:22.
dd Rom. 12:2; 1 Cor. 11:28.
ee 2 Cor. 10, 12-18.
ff Rom. 14:12.
gg Or, *share with him.* 1 Cor. 9:7-15; 1 Tim. 5:18.
hh Jas. 1:16.
ii 1 Cor. 3:10-15.
jj *Holy Spirit.* Eph. 1:13, 17. (Mt. 1:18; Acts 2:4.)
kk *Life (eternal).* Eph. 4:18. (Mt. 7:14; Rev. 22:19.)
ll 1 Cor. 15:58; 2 Thes. 3:13.
mm Jas. 5:7, 8.

[1] **(5:22)** Christian character is not mere moral or legal correctness, but the possession and manifestation of nine graces: love, joy, peace—character as an inward state; longsuffering, gentleness, goodness—character in expression toward man; faith, meekness, temperance—character in expression toward God. Taken together they present a moral portrait of Christ, and may be taken as the apostle's explanation of Gal. 2:20, "Not I, but Christ," and as a definition of "fruit" in John 15:1-8. This character is possible because of the believer's vital union to Christ (John 15:5; 1 Cor. 12:12, 13), and is wholly the fruit of the Spirit in those believers who are yielded to Him (Gal. 5:22, 23).

(3) *The new life as a beneficence.*
(Cf. Acts 10:38)

10 As we have therefore opportunity,
let us do good unto all *men*, [a]especially
unto them who are of the household of
faith.

(4) *The new life in sacrificial love.*

11 Ye see how [1]large a letter I have
written unto you with mine own hand.
12 As many as desire to make a fair
[b]shew in the flesh, they [c]constrain you to
be circumcised; only lest they should
suffer persecution for the cross of Christ.
13 For neither they themselves who
are circumcised keep the law; but desire
to have you circumcised, that they may
glory in your [d]flesh.

(5) *The new exultation of the new life.*

14 But [e]God forbid that I should glory,
save in the [f]cross of our Lord Jesus
Christ, by whom the [g]world is crucified
unto me, and [h]I unto the [i]world.
15 For [j]in Christ Jesus neither circumcision availeth any thing, nor uncircumcision, but a new [k]creature.

(6) *The peace of the new life.*

16 And as many as walk according to
this rule, peace *be* on them, and mercy,
and upon the [l]Israel of God.

(7) *The new fellowship of suffering.*

17 From henceforth let no man trouble
me: for I bear in my body the marks of
the Lord Jesus.
18 Brethren, the grace of our Lord
Jesus Christ *be* with your spirit. Amen.

A.D. 58.

a Rom. 12:13; 1 John 3:17.
b Phil. 3:4, 6.
c "Circumcision" stands here for externality in religion—form rather than spirit. Col. 2:16-23.
d Flesh. v. 13; Eph. 2:3; John 1:13; Jude 23.)
e Phil. 3:8.
f 1 Cor. 1:18.
g Gal. 1:4; 2:20.
h Col. 2:20; John 17:9, 15.
i *kosmos* = world-system. Eph. 2:2. (John 7:7; Rev. 13:3-8, *note*.)
j Gal. 5:6.
k *creation.*
l Rom. 4:12; 9:6-8.

[1] **(6:11)** Gr. *"with how large letters . . . mine own hand."* The apostle was, it appears from many considerations, afflicted with ophthalmia, a common disease in the East, to the point almost of total blindness (e.g. Gal. 4:13-15). Ordinarily, therefore, he dictated his letters. But now, having no amanuensis at hand, but urged by the spiritual danger of his dear Galatians, he writes, we cannot know with what pain and difficulty, with his own hand, in the "large letters" his darkened vision compelled him to use.

THE EPISTLE OF PAUL THE APOSTLE TO THE

EPHESIANS

WRITER. The Apostle Paul (1:1).

Date. Ephesians was written from Rome in A.D. 64. It is the first in order of the Prison Epistles (Acts 20–27; see Acts 28:30, *note*), and was sent by Tychicus, concurrently with Colossians and Philemon. It is probable that the two greater letters had their occasion in the return of Onesimus to Philemon. Ephesians is the most impersonal of Paul's letters. Indeed the words, "to the Ephesians," are not in the best manuscripts. Colossians (4:16) mentions an epistle to the Laodiceans. It has been conjectured that the letter known to us as Ephesians is really the Laodicean letter. Probably it was sent to Ephesus and Laodicea without being addressed to any church. The letter would then be "to the saints and the faithful in Christ Jesus" anywhere.

Theme. The doctrine of the Epistle confirms this view. It contains the highest church truth, but has nothing about church order. The church here is the true church, "His body," not the local church, as in Philippians, Corinthians, etc. Essentially, three lines of truth make up this Epistle: the believer's exalted position through grace; the truth concerning the body of Christ; and a walk in accordance with that position.

There is a close spiritual affinity between Ephesians and Joshua, the "heavenlies" answering in Christian position to Canaan in Israel's experience. In both there is conflict, often failure, but also victory, rest, and possession (Josh. 21:43-45; Eph. 1:3; 3:14-19; 6:16, 23). As befits a complete revelation, the number seven is conspicuous in the structure of Ephesians.

The divisions are, broadly, four: I. The apostolic greeting, 1:1, 2. II. Positional; the believer's standing "in Christ" and "in the heavenlies" through pure grace, 1:3–3:21. III. Walk and service, 4:1–5:17. IV. The walk and warfare of the Spirit-filled believer, 5:18–6:24.

CHAPTER 1.

Part I. The apostolic salutation (vs. 1, 2).

Paul, an apostle of Jesus Christ by the
[a]will of God, to the saints which are
at [b]Ephesus, and to the [c]faithful [1]in
Christ Jesus:
2 [d]Grace *be* to you, and peace, from
God our Father, and *from* the Lord Jesus
Christ.

A.D. 64.

a Acts 9:15; Gal. 1:1, 15.
b Acts 19:1; 20:17-38.
c Rev. 2:11.
d Rom. 1:7; 1 Tim. 1:2.
e v. 17; 1 Pet. 1:3.
f Rom. 8:29-32; 1 Cor. 3:21-23; Col. 1:12, 13.
g v. 20; Eph. 2:6; 3:10; 6:12.
h Election *(corporate)*. Col. 3:12. (Deut. 7:6; 1 Pet. 1:2.)

Part II. The believer's position in grace (Eph. 1:3–3:21).

(1) *The seven elements of the believer's position.*

3 [e]Blessed *be* the God and Father of
our Lord Jesus Christ, who [f]hath blessed
us with all spiritual blessings [2]in [g]heav-
enly *places* in Christ:
4 According as he hath [h]chosen
us in him before the foundation

[1] **(1:1)** The believer's place as a member of the body of Christ, vitally united to Him by the baptism with the Holy Spirit (1 Cor. 12:12, 13).

[2] **(1:3)** Literally, *the heavenlies.* The same Greek word is used in John 3:12, where "things" is added. In both places the word signifies that which is heavenly in contradistinction to that which is earthly. In Ephesians "places" is especially misleading. "The heavenlies" may be defined as the sphere of the believer's spiritual experience as identified with Christ in nature (2 Pet. 1:4); life (Col. 3:4; 1 John 5:12); relationships (John 20:17; Heb. 2:11); service (John 17:18; Mt. 28:20); suffering (Phil. 1:29; 3:10; Col. 1:24); inheritance (Rom. 8:16, 17); and future glory in the kingdom (Rom. 8:18-21; 1 Pet. 2:9; Rev. 1:6; 5:10). The believer is a heavenly man, and a stranger and pilgrim on the earth (Heb. 3:1; 1 Pet. 2:11).

of the [a]world, that we should be [b]holy
and without blame before him in love:
5 Having [1]predestinated us unto the
[2c]adoption of children by Jesus Christ to
himself, according to the good pleasure
of his will,
6 To the praise of the glory of his
grace, wherein he hath made us accepted in the beloved.
7 In whom we have redemption
[d]through his blood, the forgiveness of
[e]sins, according to the riches of his
[f]grace;
8 Wherein he hath abounded toward
us in all wisdom and prudence;
9 Having made known unto us the
[g]mystery of his will, according to his
good pleasure which he hath purposed
in himself:
10 That in the [3]dispensation of the fulness of times he might gather together in
one all things in Christ, both which are
in heaven, and which are on earth; *even*
in him:
11 In whom also we have obtained
an inheritance, being [h]predestinated
according to the purpose of him who
worketh all things after the [i]counsel of
his own will:
12 That we should be to the [j]praise of
his glory, who first [k]trusted in Christ.
13 In whom ye also *trusted*, after that
ye heard the word of truth, the [l]gospel
of your salvation: in whom also [m]after
that ye believed, [n]ye were [4]sealed with
that [o]holy Spirit of promise,
14 Which is the earnest of our inheritance until the redemption of the purchased possession, unto the praise of his
glory.

(2) *The prayer for knowledge and power.*

15 Wherefore I also, after I heard of
your faith in the Lord Jesus, and love
unto all the saints,
16 Cease not to give thanks for you,
making mention of you in my [p]prayers;
17 That the God of our Lord Jesus
Christ, the Father of glory, may give
unto you the spirit of wisdom and revelation in the knowledge of him:
18 The eyes of your understanding
being enlightened; that ye may know
what is the hope of his calling, and what
the riches of the glory of his inheritance
in the saints,
19 And what *is* the exceeding greatness of his power to us-ward who
believe, according to the working of his
mighty power,
20 Which he wrought in Christ,
when he raised him from the dead,

A.D. 64.

a *i.e. earth.*
b *Sanctify. holy (persons)* (N.T.). Eph. 2:21. (Mt. 4:5; Rev. 22:11.)
c *Adoption.* (Rom. 8:15, 23.)
d *Sacrifice (of Christ).* Col. 1:14, 20. (Gen. 4:4; Heb. 10:18.)
e *Sin.* Rom. 3:23, *note.*
f *Grace (in salv.).* vs. 6, 7; Eph. 2:5, 7, 8. (Rom. 3:24; John 1:17, *note.*)
g Rom. 16:25, 26; Eph. 3:3; Mt. 13:11, *note.*
h *Predestination,* vs. 5, 11. (Acts 4:28.)
i Isa. 40:14; 46:10; Dan. 4:35.
j vs. 6, 14; Eph. 3:21.
k *hoped.*
l *Gospel.* Eph. 3:1-10. (Gen. 12:1-3; Rev. 14:6.)
m *having believed.*
n *Assurance.* Eph. 4:30. (Isa. 32:17; Jude 1.)
o *Holy Spirit.* vs. 13, 17; Eph. 2:18, 22. (Mt. 1:18; Acts 2:4.)
p *Bible prayers* (N.T.). Eph. 3:14-21. (Mt. 6:9; Rev. 22:20.)

[1] **(1:5)** Predestination is that effective exercise of the will of God by which things before determined by Him are brought to pass. See *Election,* 1 Pet. 1:2, *note; Foreknowledge,* 1 Pet. 1:20, *note.*

[2] **(1:5)** Adoption (*huiothesia,* "placing as a son") is not so much a word of *relationship* as of *position.* The believer's relation to God as a child results from the new birth (John 1:12, 13), whereas adoption is the act of God whereby one already a child is, through redemption from the law, placed in the position of an adult son (Gal. 4:1-5). The indwelling Spirit gives the realization of this in the believer's present experience (Gal. 4:6); but the full manifestation of the believer's sonship awaits the resurrection, change, and translation of saints, which is called "the redemption of the body" (Rom. 8:23; 1 Thes. 4:14-17; Eph. 1:14; 1 John 3:2).

[3] **(1:10)** The Dispensation of the Fulness of Times. This, the seventh and last of the ordered ages which condition human life on the earth, is identical with the kingdom covenanted to David (2 Sam. 7:8-17; Zech. 12:8, Summary; Lk. 1:31-33; 1 Cor. 15:24, Summary), and gathers into itself under Christ all past "times": (1) The time of oppression and misrule ends by Christ taking His kingdom (Isa. 11:3, 4). (2) The time of testimony and divine forbearance ends in judgment (Mt. 25:31-46; Acts 17:30, 31; Rev. 20:7-15). (3) The time of toil ends in rest and reward (2 Thes. 1:6, 7). (4) The time of suffering ends in glory (Rom. 8:17, 18). (5) The time of Israel's blindness and chastisement ends in restoration and conversion (Rom. 11:25-27; Ezk. 39:25-29). (6) The times of the Gentiles end in the smiting of the image and the setting up of the kingdom of the heavens (Dan. 2:34, 35; Rev. 19:15-21). (7) The time of creation's thraldom ends in deliverance at the manifestation of the sons of God (Gen. 3:17; Isa. 11:6-8; Rom. 8:19-21).

[4] **(1:13)** The Holy Spirit is Himself the seal. In the symbolism of Scripture a seal signifies: (1) A finished transaction (Jer. 32:9, 10; John 17:4; 19:30). (2) Ownership (Jer. 32:11, 12; 2 Tim. 2:19). (3) Security (Esth. 8:8; Dan. 6:17; Eph. 4:30).

and set *him* at his own right hand in the heavenly *places*,

21 Far above all principality, and power, and might, and dominion, and every name that is named, not only in this [a]world, but also in that which is to come:

(3) *Christ exalted to be the Head of his body, the church.*

22 And hath [b]put all *things* under his feet, and gave him *to be* the head over all *things* to the church,

23 Which is his [c]body, the [d]fulness of him that filleth all in all.

CHAPTER 2.

(4) *The method of Gentile salvation.*

And you *hath he quickened,* who were dead in trespasses and sins;

2 Wherein in time past ye walked according to the course of this [e]world, according to the [f]prince of the power of the air, the spirit that now worketh in the [g]children of disobedience:

3 Among whom also we all had our conversation in times past in the lusts of our [h]flesh, fulfilling the desires of the [i]flesh and of the [j]mind; and were by nature the children of [k]wrath, even as others.

4 But God, who is [l]rich in mercy, for his [m]great love wherewith he loved us,

5 Even when we were [1n]dead in sins, hath [o]quickened us together with Christ, (by grace ye are [p]saved;)

6 And hath raised *us* up together, and made *us* sit together in heavenly *places* in Christ Jesus:

7 That in the [q]ages to come he might shew the exceeding riches of his grace in *his* [r]kindness toward us through Christ Jesus.

8 For by [s]grace are ye [p]saved through [t]faith; and that not of yourselves: *it is* the [u]gift of God:

9 Not of [v]works, lest any man should [w]boast.

10 For we are his workmanship, [x]created in Christ Jesus unto good works, which God hath before ordained that we should walk in them.

(5) *The Gentile position by nature.*

11 Wherefore remember, that ye *being* in time past Gentiles in the flesh, who are called Uncircumcision by that which is called the Circumcision in the flesh made by hands;

12 That at that time ye were without Christ, being aliens from the commonwealth of Israel, and strangers from the covenants of promise, having no hope, and without God in the [y]world:

13 But now in Christ Jesus ye who sometimes were far off are made nigh by the blood of Christ.

(6) *Jew and Gentile one body in Christ.*

14 For he is our peace, who hath made both one, and hath broken down the middle wall of partition *between us;*

15 Having abolished in his flesh the enmity, *even* the [z]law of commandments *contained* in ordinances; for to make in himself of twain one [2]new man, *so* making peace;

16 And that he might [aa]reconcile both unto God in one body by the cross, having slain the enmity thereby:

17 And came and preached peace to you which were afar off, and to them that were nigh.

18 For through him we [bb]both have access by one Spirit unto the Father.

(7) *The church a temple for the habitation of God through the Spirit.*

19 Now therefore ye are no more strangers and foreigners, but [cc]fellowcitizens with the saints, and of the household of God;

20 And are built upon the foundation of the apostles and prophets, Jesus Christ himself being the chief corner [dd]*stone;*

21 In whom all the building fitly

A.D. 64.

a i.e. *age.*
b Psa. 8:6; 110:1; 1 Cor. 15:27; Heb. 2:8.
c *Church (true).* vs. 22, 23; Eph. 2:19-22. (Mt. 16:18; Heb. 12:23.)
d Or, *complement.* Gen. 2:18; Eph. 5:28-30, 32.
e *kosmos* = world-system. Col. 2:20. (John 7:7; Rev. 13:3-8, *note.*)
f John 12:31; 1 John 5:19.
g *sons.*
h *Flesh.* Eph. 6:12. (John 1:13; Jude 23.)
i Jas. 1:21; 2 Pet. 2:14.
j Col. 2:8.
k Rom. 1:18; Eph. 5:6.
l Eph. 1:7; 2:7; Psa. 103:8-11.
m John 3:16; 1 John 4:9, 10.
n *Death (spiritual).* vs. 1-5. (Gen. 2:17.)
o Eph. 2:1; Col. 2:13; John 5:25, 26.
p Rom. 1:16, *note.*
q Eph. 1:21; 3:21; Rev. 20:4; 21:1-4.
r Tit. 3:4.
s *Grace (in salv.).* vs. 5, 7, 8; Col. 1:6. (Rom. 3:24; John 1:17, *note.*)
t *Faith.* Eph. 3:17. (Gen. 3:20; Heb. 11:39.)
u John 1:12, 13.
v Rom. 4:4, 5; 11:6.
w Rom. 3:27; 1 Cor. 1:26-31.
x Eph. 4:24, *note.*
y *kosmos* (Mt. 4:8.) = mankind.
z *Law (of Moses).* Phil. 3:4-9. (Ex. 19:1; Gal. 3:1-29.)
aa *Reconciliation.* See Col. 1:20, 21.
bb *Holy Spirit.* vs. 18, 22: Eph. 3:5, 16. (Mt. 1:18; Acts 2:4.)
cc *Church (true).* vs. 19-22; Eph. 3:1-10. (Mt. 16:18; Heb. 12:23.)
dd *Christ (as stone).* Rom. 9:32, 33. (Ex. 17:6; 1 Pet. 2:8.)

[1] **(2:5)** Death (spiritual), Summary: Spiritual death is the state of the natural or unregenerate man as still in his sins (Eph. 2:1), alienated from the life of God (Eph. 4:18, 19), and destitute of the Spirit. Prolonged beyond the death of the body, spiritual death is a state of eternal separation from God in conscious suffering. This is called "the second death" (Rev. 2:11; 20:6, 14; 21:8).

[2] **(2:15)** Here the "new man" is not the individual believer but the church, considered as the body of Christ in the sense of Eph. 1:22, 23; 1 Cor. 12:12, 13; Col. 3:10, 11. (See Heb. 12:23, *note.*)

framed together [a]groweth unto an [b]holy temple in the Lord:

22 In whom ye also are builded together for an [c]habitation of God through the Spirit.

CHAPTER 3.

The church a mystery hidden from past ages.

For this cause I Paul, the prisoner of [d]Jesus Christ for you Gentiles,

2 If ye have heard of the dispensation of the [e]grace of God which is given me to you-ward:

3 How that by [f]revelation he made known unto me the [g]mystery; (as I [h]wrote afore in few words,

4 Whereby, when ye read, ye may understand my knowledge in the mystery of Christ)

5 Which in other [i]ages was not made known unto the sons of men, as it is [j]now revealed unto his [k]holy apostles and prophets by the Spirit;

6 [1]That the Gentiles should be fellowheirs, and of the same body, and partakers of his promise in Christ by the [l]gospel:

7 Whereof I was made a minister, according to the gift of the grace of God given unto me by the effectual working of his power.

8 Unto me, who am less than the [m]least of all saints, is this grace given, that I should preach among the [n]Gentiles the [o]unsearchable riches of Christ;

9 And to make all *men* see what *is* the fellowship of the [g]mystery, which [p]from the beginning of the world hath been [q]hid in God, who [r]created all things by Jesus Christ:

10 To the intent that now unto the [s]principalities and powers in heavenly *places* might be known by the [t]church the manifold wisdom of God,

11 [u]According to the eternal purpose which he purposed in Christ Jesus our Lord:

12 In whom we have [v]boldness and access with confidence by the faith of him.

(*Parenthetic: the prayer for inner fulness and knowledge.*)

13 Wherefore I desire that ye faint not at my tribulations for you, which is your glory.

14 For this cause I [w]bow my knees unto the [x]Father of our Lord Jesus Christ,

15 Of whom [y]the whole family in heaven and earth is named,

16 That he would grant you, according to the [z]riches of his glory, to be [aa]strengthened with might by his [bb]Spirit in the inner man;

17 That [cc]Christ may dwell in your hearts by [dd]faith; that ye, being rooted and grounded in love,

18 May be [ee]able to comprehend with all saints [ff]what *is* the breadth, and length, and depth, and height;

19 And to know the love of Christ, which passeth knowledge, that ye might be filled with all the fulness of God.

20 Now unto him that is able to do exceeding abundantly above all that we ask or think, according to the power that worketh in us,

21 Unto him *be* glory in the church by Christ Jesus throughout all ages, world without end. Amen.

CHAPTER 4.

Part III. The walk and service of the believer as in Christ, and as having the Spirit (Eph. 4:1–5:17).

(1) *The walk to be worthy the position.*

I therefore, the prisoner of the Lord, beseech you that ye walk worthy of the vocation wherewith ye are called,

2 With all lowliness and meekness, with longsuffering, forbearing one another in love;

3 Endeavouring to keep the unity of the Spirit in the bond of peace.

(2) *The seven unities to be kept.*

4 *There is* one body, and one Spirit, even as ye are called in one hope of your calling;

A.D. 64.

a 1 Cor. 3:16, 17.
b *Holy, sanctify (persons)* (N.T.). v. 21; Eph. 3:5. (Mt. 4:5; Rev. 22:11.)
c Ex. 25:8; 1 Ki. 5:3, 5; John 2:19-21; 2 Cor. 6:16.
d *Christ Jesus.*
e *Grace (imparted).* vs. 2-8; Eph. 4:7, 29. (Rom. 6:1; 2 Pet. 3:18.)
f Rom. 16:25, 26; Gal. 1:12, 15, 16.
g Mt. 13:11, *note.*
h Eph. 1:9, 10, 18-22.
i *generations.*
j *Inspiration.* vs. 3-5; Eph. 6:17. (Ex. 4:15; Rev. 22:19.)
k *Sanctify, holy (persons)* (N.T.). Eph. 5:26, 27. (Mt. 4:5; Rev. 22:11.)
l *Gospel.* vs. 1:10; Eph. 6:15-19. (Gen. 12:1-3; Rev. 14:6.)
m 1 Cor. 15:9; 1 Tim. 1:15.
n Acts 9:15; Rom. 11:13.
o vs. 18, 19; Col. 2:2, 3.
p *throughout the ages.*
q v. 5; Col. 1:26.
r John 1:3; Col. 1:16; Heb. 1:2.
s Eph. 1:21; 1 Pet. 1:12.
t *Church (true).* vs. 1-10; Eph. 5:23, 25-27, 29-32. (Mt. 16:18; Heb. 12:23.)
u Eph. 1:4, 11.
v Heb. 10:19; 1 John 4:18.
w *Bible prayers* (N.T.). Phil. 1:9-11. (Mt. 6:9; Rev. 22:20.)
x Eph. 1:3.
y *every family.*
z Eph. 1:7; 2:4; Phil. 4:19.
aa Col. 1:11.
bb *Holy Spirit.* vs. 5, 16; Eph. 4:3, 4, 30. (Mt. 1:18; Acts 2:4.)
cc John 14:23; Col. 1:27.
dd *Faith.* Phil. 3:9. (Gen. 3:20; Heb. 11:39.)
ee Eph. 1:18.
ff Rom. 10:3, 11, 12; cf. 2 Tim. 2:7.

[1] **(3:6)** That the Gentiles were to be *saved* was no mystery (Rom. 9:24-33; 10:19-21). The mystery "hid in God" was the divine purpose to make of Jew and Gentile a wholly new thing—"the church, which is his [Christ's] body," formed by the baptism with the Holy Spirit (1 Cor. 12:12, 13) and in which the earthly distinction of Jew and Gentile disappears (Eph. 2:14, 15; Col. 3:10, 11). The revelation of this mystery, which was foretold but not explained by Christ (Mt. 16:18), was committed to Paul. In his writings alone we find the doctrine, position, walk, and destiny of the church.

5 [a]One Lord, [b]one faith, [c]one baptism,
6 One [d]God and Father of all, who *is*
above all, and through all, and in you
all.

(3) *The ministry gifts of Christ to his body.*

7 But unto every one of us is given
grace according to the measure of the
gift of Christ.
8 Wherefore he saith, [e]When he
ascended up on high, he led captivity
captive, and gave gifts unto men.
9 (Now that he ascended, what is it
but that he also descended first into the
lower parts of the earth?
10 He that descended is the same also
that ascended up far above all heavens,
that he might fill all things.)
11 And he [1]gave [2]some, apostles; and
some, prophets; and some, evangelists;
and some, pastors and teachers;

(4) *The purpose of the ministry gifts.*

12 For the [f]perfecting of the saints,
[g]for the work of the ministry, for the edifying of the body of Christ:
13 Till we all come in the unity of the
faith, and of the knowledge of the Son of
God, unto a [h]perfect man, unto the measure of the stature of the fulness of
Christ:
14 That we *henceforth* be no more children, tossed to and fro, and carried
about with every [i]wind of doctrine, by
the sleight of men, *and* cunning craftiness, whereby they lie in wait to deceive;
15 But [j]speaking the truth in love, may
grow up [k]into him in all things, which is
the [l]head, *even* Christ:
16 From whom the whole body fitly
joined together and compacted by [m]that
which every joint supplieth, according to
the effectual working in the [n]measure of
every part, maketh [o]increase of the body
unto the edifying of itself in love.

(5) *The walk of the believer as a new man in Christ Jesus.*

17 This I say therefore, and testify in
the Lord, that ye henceforth [p]walk not as
other Gentiles walk, in the vanity of
their mind,
18 Having the understanding darkened, being [q]alienated from the [r]life of
God through the ignorance that is in
them, because of the blindness of their
heart:
19 [s]Who being past feeling have given
themselves over unto lasciviousness, to
work all uncleanness with greediness.
20 But ye have not so [t]learned Christ;
21 If so be that ye have heard him, and
have been taught by him, as the truth is
in Jesus:
22 That ye [u]put off concerning the former conversation the [v]old man, which is
corrupt according to the deceitful lusts;
23 [w]And be renewed in the spirit of
your mind;
24 And that ye [x]put on the [3]new man,
which after God is created in [y]righteous-
ness and true holiness.
25 Wherefore putting away lying,
[z]speak every man truth with his neighbour: for we are members one of another.
26 [aa]Be ye angry, and [bb]sin not: let not
the sun go down upon your wrath:
27 [cc]Neither give place to the [dd]devil.
28 Let him that stole steal no more: but
rather let him labour, working with *his*

A.D. 64.

a 1 Cor. 1:13; 8:5, 6.
b Gal. 1:23; 1 Cor. 15:1-8.
c 1 Cor. 12:12, 13; Eph. 5:30.
d 1 Cor. 8:6; 12:6.
e Psa. 68:18.
f Mt. 5:48, *note.*
g *unto the doing of service.*
h Eph. 1:23; 2:15.
i Mt. 11:7.
j *holding.* 2 Tim. 1:13.
k *unto.*
l Eph. 1:22.
m *every joint of supply.*
n v. 12.
o Col. 2:19.
p Eph. 2:2.
q *Death (spiritual).* vs. 18, 19; Col. 2:13. (Gen. 2:17; Eph. 2:5)
r *Life (eternal).* Phil. 2:16, (Mt. 7:14; Rev. 22:19.)
s 1 Tim. 4:2.
t Acts 2:36.
u *have put off.*
v Rom. 6:6. *note.*
w *being.*
x *have put on.*
y Rom. 10:10, *note.*
z Zech. 8:16.
aa Psa. 4:4.
bb *Sin.* Rom. 3:23, *note.*
cc 2 Cor. 2:10, 11.
dd *Satan.* Eph. 6:11. (Gen. 3:1; Rev. 20:10.)

[1] **(4:11)** In 1 Cor. 12:8-28 the Spirit is seen as enduing the members of the body of Christ with spiritual gifts, or enablements for a varied service; here certain Spirit-endued men, viz. apostles, prophets, evangelists, pastors, and teachers, are themselves the gifts whom the glorified Christ bestows upon His body the church. In Corinthians the gifts are spiritual enablements for specific service; in Ephesians the gifts are men who have such enablements.

[2] **(4:11)** The Lord, in bestowing the gifted men, determines, providentially (e.g. Acts 11:22-26), or directly through the Spirit (e.g. Acts 13:1, 2; 16:6, 7), the places of their service. "Some" (churches or places) need one gift, as, e.g. evangelist; "some" (churches or places) need rather a pastor or teacher. Absolutely nothing in Christ's service is left to mere human judgment or self-choosing. Even an apostle was not permitted to choose his place of service (Acts 16:7, 8).

[3] **(4:24)** The new man is the regenerate man as distinguished from the old man (Rom. 6:6, *note*), and is a new man as having become a partaker of the divine nature and life (2 Pet. 1:4; Col. 3:3, 4), and in no sense the old man made over, or improved (2 Cor. 5:17; Gal. 6:15; Eph. 2:10; Col. 3:10). The new man is Christ, "formed" in the believer (Gal. 2:20; 4:19; Col. 1:27; 1 John 4:12).

hands the thing which is good, that he may have to [a]give to him that needeth.

29 Let no corrupt communication proceed out of your mouth, but that which is good to the use of [b]edifying, that it may minister [c]grace unto the hearers.

(6) *The walk of the believer as indwelt by the Spirit.*

30 And grieve not the [d]holy Spirit of God, whereby ye [e]are sealed unto the day of redemption.

31 Let all bitterness, and wrath, and anger, and clamour, and evil speaking, be put away from you, with all malice:

32 And be ye kind one to another, tenderhearted, [f]forgiving one another, even as God [g]for Christ's sake hath [h]forgiven you.

CHAPTER 5.

(7) *The walk of the believer as God's dear child.*

Be ye therefore [i]followers of God, as dear children;

2 And [j]walk in love, as Christ also hath loved us, and hath given himself for us an offering and a sacrifice to God for a [k]sweetsmelling savour.

3 But fornication, and all uncleanness, or covetousness, let it not be once named among you, as becometh saints;

4 Neither filthiness, nor [l]foolish talking, nor jesting, which are not [m]convenient: but rather [n]giving of thanks.

5 For this ye know, that no whoremonger, nor unclean person, nor covetous man, who is an [o]idolater, hath any inheritance in the kingdom of Christ and of God.

6 Let no man deceive you with vain words: for because of these things cometh the wrath of God upon the [p]children of disobedience.

7 Be not ye therefore [q]partakers with them.

8 For ye were sometimes darkness, but now *are ye* [r]light in the Lord: walk as children of light:

9 (For the [s]fruit of the [t]Spirit *is* in all goodness and [u]righteousness and truth;)

10 Proving what is acceptable unto the Lord.

11 And have [v]no fellowship with the unfruitful works of darkness, but rather reprove *them*.

12 For it is a [w]shame even to speak of those things which are done of them in secret.

13 But all things that are reproved are [x]made manifest by the light: for whatsoever doth make manifest is light.

14 Wherefore he saith, [y]Awake thou that sleepest, and arise from the dead, and Christ shall give thee light.

15 See then that ye walk circumspectly, not as fools, but as wise,

16 [z]Redeeming the time, because the days are evil.

17 Wherefore be ye not unwise, [aa]but understanding what the will of the Lord *is*.

Part IV. The walk and warfare of the believer as filled with the Spirit (Eph. 5:18–6:24).

18 And be not drunk with wine, wherein is excess; but be filled with the [bb]Spirit;

(1) *The inner life of the Spirit-filled believer.*

19 Speaking to yourselves in psalms and hymns and spiritual songs, singing and making [cc]melody in your heart to the Lord;

20 [dd]Giving thanks always for all things unto God and the Father in the name of our Lord Jesus Christ;

(2) *The married life of Spirit-filled believers as illustrating Christ and the church.*

21 [ee]Submitting yourselves one to another in the fear of God.

22 Wives, [ff]submit yourselves unto your own husbands, as unto the Lord.

23 For the husband is [gg]the head of the wife, even as Christ is the head of the [hh]church: and he is the [ii]saviour of the body.

24 Therefore as the church is [jj]subject unto Christ, so *let* the wives *be* to their own husbands in every thing.

25 [kk]Husbands, love your wives, [1]even as Christ also loved the [ll]church, and gave himself for it;

A.D. 64.

a Lk. 3:11.
b Rom. 15:2.
c *Grace (imparted).* Phil. 1:7. (Rom. 6:1; 2 Pet. 3:18.)
d *Holy Spirit.* vs. 4, 23, 30; Eph. 5:9, 18. (Mt. 1:18; Acts 2:4.)
e *Assurance.* Eph. 5:29, 30. (Isa. 32:17; Jude 1.)
f Lk. 6:33-37.
g *in Christ.*
h *Forgiveness.* Col. 2:13. (Lev. 4:20; Mt. 26:28.)
i *imitators.* Cf. 1 Cor. 11:1
j *Law (of Christ).* 1 Pet. 1:8, 22. (Gal. 6:2; 2 John 5.)
k Lev. 1:9, 13, 17; 2:2.
l 2 Tim. 2:23; Tit. 3:9.
m Rom. 1:28.
n v. 20; 1 Thes. 5:18.
o 1 Cor. 5:11.
p *sons.*
q 1 Tim. 5:22.
r 1 Thes. 5:5.
s 1 John 2:9.
t *light*
u See 1 John 3:7, *note.*
v 2 Cor. 6:14.
w v. 3.
x John 3:20, 21; Heb. 4:13.
y Isa. 60:1, 2.
z Col. 4:5.
aa Rom. 12:2; Col. 1:9.
bb *Holy Spirit.* Eph. 6:17, 18. (Mt. 1:18; Acts 2:4.)
cc Psa. 101:1.
dd Psa. 34:1; Isa. 63:7; Phil. 4:6; Col. 3:17; 1 Thes. 5:18.
ee Phil. 2:3; 1 Pet. 5:5.
ff Cf. Gen. 3:16.
gg Col. 1:18.
hh *Church (true).* vs. 23, 25-27, 29-32; Col. 1:18, 24. (Mt. 16:18; Heb. 12:23.)
ii Rom. 1:16, *note.*
jj Col. 3:18; 1 Pet. 3:1, 5.
kk Col. 3:19.
ll v. 2; cf. Gal. 2:20.

[1] **(5:25)** Christ's love-work for the church is threefold: past, present, future: (1) For love He gave Himself to redeem the church (v. 25); (2) in love He is sanctifying the church (v. 26); (3) for the reward of His sacrifice and labour of love He will present the church to Himself in flawless perfection, "one pearl of great price" (v. 27; Mt. 13:46).

26 That he might [a]sanctify and cleanse it with the washing of water [b]by the word,

27 That he might present it to himself a glorious church, [c]not having spot, or wrinkle, or any such thing; but that it should be holy and without blemish.

28 So ought men to love their wives as their own bodies. He that loveth his wife loveth himself.

29 For no man ever yet hated his own flesh; but nourisheth and cherisheth it, even as [d]the Lord the church:

30 For we are [e]members of his body, of his flesh, and of his bones.

31 [f]For this cause shall a man leave his father and mother, and shall be joined unto his wife, and they two shall be one flesh.

32 This is a great [g]mystery: but I speak concerning Christ and the [1h]church.

33 Nevertheless let every one of you in particular so love his wife even as himself; and the wife *see* that she [i]reverence *her* husband.

CHAPTER 6.

(3) *The domestic life of Spirit-filled believers as children and servants.*

Children, [j]obey your parents in the Lord: for this is right.

2 [k]Honour thy father and mother; (which is the first commandment with promise;)

3 That it may be well with thee, and thou mayest live long on the earth.

4 And, ye fathers, [l]provoke not your children to wrath: but bring them up in the [m]nurture and admonition of the Lord.

5 [n]Servants, be obedient to them that are *your* masters according to the flesh, with fear and trembling, in singleness of your heart, as unto Christ;

6 Not with [o]eyeservice, as menpleasers; but as the servants of Christ, doing the will of God from the heart;

7 With good will doing service, as to the Lord, and not to men:

8 Knowing that whatsoever good thing any man doeth, the same shall he [p]receive of the Lord, whether *he be* bond or free.

9 And, ye masters, do the same things unto them, [q]forbearing threatening: knowing that [r]your Master also is in heaven; neither is there [s]respect of persons with him.

(4) *The warfare of Spirit-filled believers.*

(a) *The warrior's power.*

10 Finally, my brethren, [t]be strong in the Lord, and in the power of his might.

(b) *The warrior's armour.*

11 Put on the whole [u]armour of God, that ye may be able to stand against the wiles of the [v]devil.

(c) *The warrior's foes.*

12 For we wrestle not against [w]flesh and blood, but against principalities, against powers, against the [x]rulers of the darkness of this world, against spiritual wickedness in [y]high *places*.

13 Wherefore take unto you the [z]whole armour of God, that ye may be able to withstand in the evil day, and having done all, to stand.

14 Stand therefore, having [aa]your loins girt about with truth, and having on the [bb]breastplate of righteousness;

15 And your [cc]feet shod with the preparation of the gospel of peace;

16 Above all, taking the [dd]shield of faith, wherewith ye shall be able to quench all the fiery darts of the [ee]wicked.

17 And take the helmet of [ff]salvation, and the sword of the Spirit, which is the [gg]word of God:

(d) *The warrior's resource.*

18 [hh]Praying always with all prayer and supplication in the [ii]Spirit, and watching thereunto with all perseverance and supplication for all saints;

A.D. 64.

- a *Sanctify, holy (persons)* (N.T.). vs. 26, 27; Col. 1:22. (Mt. 4:5; Rev. 22:11.)
- b John 15:3; 17:17.
- c Song 4:7.
- d *Christ.*
- e *Assurance.* vs. 29, 30; Phil. 1:6. (Isa. 32:17; Jude 1.)
- f Gen. 2:24.
- g Mt. 13:11, *note.*
- h *Bride (of Christ).* Rev. 19:6-8. (John 3:29; Rev. 19:6-8.)
- i 1 Pet. 3:2.
- j Col. 3:20.
- k Ex. 20:12; Deut. 5:16.
- l Col. 3:21.
- m Or, *discipline.*
- n 1 Pet. 2:18.
- o Col. 3:22.
- p Col. 3:24, 25.
- q 1 Pet. 2:23.
- r Col. 4:1.
- s Col. 3:25.
- t Josh. 1:5, 6, 9.
- u Rom. 13:12; 2 Cor. 6:7.
- v *Satan.* 1 Thes. 2:18. (Gen. 3:1; Rev. 20:10.)
- w *Flesh.* Phil. 3:3, 4. (John 1:13; Jude 23.)
- x *world-rulers of this darkness.*
- y *the heavenlies*
- z v. 11; 2 Cor. 10:4.
- aa Isa. 11:5; Lk. 12:35; 1 Pet. 1:13.
- bb Isa. 59:17; 2 Cor. 6:7; 1 Thes. 5:8.
- cc Isa. 52:7; Rom. 10:15.
- dd 1 John 5:4.
- ee *wicked one.*
- ff Rom. 1:16, *note.*
- gg *Inspiration.* 1 Tim. 4:1. (Ex. 4:15; Rev. 22:19.)
- hh Col. 4:2; 1 Thes. 5:17, 18.
- ii *Holy Spirit.* vs. 17, 18; Phil. 1:19. (Mt. 1:18; Acts 2:4.)

[1] **(5:32)** Verses 30, 31 are quoted from Gen. 2:23, 24, and exclude the interpretation that the reference is to the church merely as the body of Christ. Eve, taken from Adam's body, was truly "bone of his bones, and flesh of his flesh," but she was also his wife, united to him in a relation which makes of "twain . . . one flesh" (Mt. 19:5, 6), and so a clear type of the church as bride of Christ (see 2 Cor. 11:2, 3). The bride types are Eve (Gen. 2:23, 24); *Rebecca* (Gen. 24:1-7, *note*); *Asenath* (Gen. 41:45; *note* under Gen. 37:2); *Zipporah* (Ex. 2:21). See Hos. 2:1-23, *note.*

19 And for me, [a]that utterance may be given unto me, that I may open my mouth boldly, to make known the [b]mystery of the [c]gospel,

20 For which I am an ambassador in bonds: that therein I may speak boldly, as I ought to speak.

21 But that ye also may know my affairs, *and* how I do, [d]Tychicus, a beloved brother and [e]faithful minister in the Lord, shall make known to you all things:

22 Whom I have sent unto you for the same purpose, that ye might know our affairs, and *that* he might [f]comfort your hearts.

23 Peace *be* to the brethren, and [g]love with faith, from God the Father and the Lord Jesus Christ.

24 Grace *be* with all them that love our Lord Jesus Christ in sincerity. Amen.

A.D. 64.

a Acts 4:29; Col. 4:2.
b Mt. 13:11, *note.*
c *Gospel.* Phil. 1:5-7, 17:27. (Gen. 12:1-3; Rev. 14:6.)
d Acts 20:4; 2 Tim. 4:12; Col. 1:7; Tit. 3:12.
e 1 Cor. 4:1, 2; Col. 1:7.
f 2 Cor. 1:6; 7:13.
g 1 Cor. 16:24.

THE EPISTLE OF PAUL THE APOSTLE TO THE
PHILIPPIANS

WRITER. The Apostle Paul (1:1).

Date. The date of Philippians cannot be positively fixed. It is one of the prison letters. Whether Paul was twice imprisoned, and if so, whether Philippians was written during the first or second imprisonment, affects in no way the message of the Epistle. A.D. 64 is the commonly received date. The immediate occasion of the Epistle is disclosed in Phil. 4:10-18.

Theme. The theme of Philippians is Christian experience. Soundness of doctrine is assumed. There is nothing in church order to set right. Philippi is a normal New Testament assembly—" saints in Christ Jesus, with the bishops (elders) and deacons." The circumstances of the apostle are in striking contrast with his Christian experience. As to the former, he was Nero's prisoner. As to the latter, there was the shout of victory, the paean of joy. Christian experience, he would teach us, is not something which is going on around the believer, but something which is going on within him.

The key-verse is, "For to me to live is Christ, and to die is gain" (1:21). Right Christian experience, then, is the outworking, whatever one's circumstances may be, of the life, nature, and mind of Christ living in us (1:6, 11; 2:5, 13).

The divisions are indicated by the chapters: I. Christ, the believer's life, rejoicing in suffering, 1:1-30. II. Christ, the believer's pattern, rejoicing in lowly service, 2:1-30. III. Christ, the believer's object, rejoicing despite imperfections, 3:1-21. IV. Christ, the believer's strength, rejoicing over anxiety, 4:1-23.

CHAPTER 1.

Part I. Christ, the believer's life, rejoicing in spite of suffering (Phil. 1:1-30)

(1) *Salutation*

Paul and Timotheus, the servants of
Jesus Christ, to [a]all the saints in
Christ Jesus [1]which are at Philippi, with
the [b]bishops and deacons:
2 Grace *be* unto you, [c]and peace, from
God our Father, and *from* the Lord Jesus
Christ.
3 I thank my God upon every
[d]remembrance of you,
4 Always in every [e]prayer of mine for
you all making request with joy,
5 For your fellowship in the gospel
from the first day until now;
6 Being confident of this very thing,
that he which hath [f]begun a good work
in you will perform *it* until the [g]day of
Jesus Christ:
7 Even as it is meet for me to think this
of you all, because I have you in my
heart; inasmuch as both in my bonds,
and in the defence and confirmation of
the gospel, ye all are partakers of [h]my
grace.

(2) *Joy triumphing over suffering.*

8 For God is my record, how greatly I
long after you all in the bowels of Jesus
Christ.
9 And this I [i]pray, that your love may
abound yet more and more in knowledge and *in* all judgment;
10 That ye may approve things that
are excellent; that ye may be sincere and
without offence till the [g]day of Christ;
11 Being filled with the fruits of [j]right-
eousness, which are by Jesus Christ,
unto the glory and praise of God.
12 But I would ye should understand, brethren, that the things

A.D. 64.

a *Churches (local).* (Acts 2:41.)

b Or, *overseers.* See *Elders.* 1 Tim. 3:1, 2. (Acts 11:30; Tit. 1:5-9.)

c Eph. 1:2.

d Or, *mention.*

e Eph. 1:16; 1 Thes. 1:2.

f *Assurance.* Col. 2:2. (Isa. 32:17; Jude 1.)

g 1 Cor. 1:8, *note.*

h *Grace (imparted).* Col. 3:16. (Rom. 6:1; 2 Pet. 3:18.)

i *Bible prayers (N.T.).* Col. 1:9-11. (Mt. 6:9; Rev. 22:20.)

j 1 John 3:7, *note.*

[1] **(1:1)** Churches (local), Summary: A local church is an assembly of professed believers on the Lord Jesus Christ, living for the most part in one locality, who assemble themselves together in His name for the breaking of bread, worship, praise, prayer, testimony, the ministry of the word, discipline, and the furtherance of the Gospel (Heb. 10:25; Acts 20:7; 1 Cor. 14:26; 1 Cor. 5:4, 5; Phil. 4:14-18; 1 Thes. 1:8; Acts 13:1-4). Such a church exists where two or three are thus gathered (Mt. 18:20). Every such local church has Christ in the midst, is a temple of God, and indwelt by the Holy Spirit (1 Cor. 3:16, 17). When perfected in organization a local church consists of "saints, with the bishops [elders] and deacons."

which happened unto me have fallen out
rather unto the furtherance of the gospel;
13 So that my bonds [a]in Christ are
manifest in all [b]the palace, [c]and in all
other *places;*
14 And many of the brethren in the
Lord, waxing confident by my bonds,
are much more bold to speak the word
without fear.
15 Some indeed preach Christ even of
envy and strife; and some also of good
will:
16 The one preach Christ of contention, not sincerely, supposing to add
affliction to my bonds:
17 But the other of love, knowing that
I am set for the defence of the gospel.
18 What then? notwithstanding, every
way, whether in pretence, or in truth,
Christ is preached; and I therein do
rejoice, yea, and will rejoice.
19 For I know that [d]this shall turn to
my [e]salvation through your prayer, and
the supply of the [f]Spirit of Jesus Christ,
20 According to my earnest expectation and *my* hope, that in nothing I shall
be ashamed, but *that* with all [g]boldness,
as always, *so* now also Christ shall be
magnified in my body, whether *it be* by
life, or by death.
21 For to me to live *is* Christ, and to
[h]die *is* gain.
22 But if I live in the flesh, this *is* the
fruit of my labour: yet what I shall
choose I wot not.
23 For I am in a strait betwixt two,
having a [i]desire to depart, and to be
with Christ; which is [j]far better:
24 Nevertheless to abide in the flesh *is*
more needful for you.
25 And having this confidence, I know
that I shall abide and continue with you
all for your furtherance and joy of faith;
26 That your rejoicing may be more
abundant in [k]Jesus Christ for me by my
coming to you again.
27 Only let your [l]conversation be as it
becometh the [m]gospel of Christ: that
whether I come and see you, or else be
absent, I may hear of your affairs, that ye
stand fast in one spirit, with one mind
striving together for the faith of the
gospel;
28 And in nothing terrified by your
adversaries: which is to them an evident
token of perdition, but to you of [e]salva-
tion, and that of God.
29 For unto you it is [n]given in the
behalf of Christ, not only to believe on
him, but also to suffer for his sake;
30 Having the same conflict which ye
[o]saw in me, and now hear *to be* in me.

CHAPTER 2.

Part II. Christ the believer's pattern, rejoicing in lowly service (Phil. 2:1-30).

(1) *Exhortation to unity and meekness.*

If *there be* therefore any consolation in
Christ, if any comfort of love, if any
fellowship of the [p]Spirit, if any [q]bowels
and mercies,
2 Fulfil ye my joy, that ye be likemind-
ed, having the same love, *being* of one
accord, of one mind.
3 *Let* [r]nothing *be done* through [s]strife or
[t]vainglory; but in lowliness of mind let
each esteem other better than themselves.
4 Look not every man on [u]his own
things, but every man also on the things
of others.

(2) *The sevenfold self-humbling of Christ.*

5 Let [v]this mind be in you, which was
also in Christ Jesus:
6 Who, being in the [1]form of God,
thought it not [w]robbery to be equal with
God:
7 But [x]made himself of no reputation,
and took upon him the form of a servant,
and [y]was made in the likeness of men:
8 And being found in fashion as a
man, [z]he humbled himself, and became
obedient unto death, even the death of
the cross.

(3) *The exaltation of Jesus.*

9 [aa]Wherefore God also hath highly

A.D. 64.

a Or, *for.*
b Or, *Caesar's court.* Phil. 4:22.
c Or, *to all others.*
d Job 13:16, Septuagint.
e Rom. 1:16, *note.*
f *Holy Spirit.* Phil. 2:1. (Mt. 1:18; Acts 2:4.)
g Eph. 6:19, 20.
h *Death (physical).* vs. 21-23; 2 Pet. 1:13, 14. (Gen. 3:19; Heb. 9:27.)
i 2 Cor. 5:2, 8.
j Psa. 16:11.
k *Christ Jesus.*
l *manner of life.*
m *Gospel.* vs. 5, 7, 12, 17, 27; Phil. 2:22. (Gen. 12:1-3; Rev. 14:6.)
n Acts 5:41; cf. Mt. 5:12.
o Acts 16:19; 1 Thes 2:2.
p *Holy Spirit.* Phil. 3:3. (Mt. 1:18; Acts 2:4.)
q Col. 3:12.
r Gal. 5:26; Jas. 3:14.
s *faction.*
t *ostentation.*
u 1 Cor. 13:5.
v John 13:14; 1 Pet. 2:21.
w *a thing to be grasped after.* See Gen. 3:5-6, 22.
x Or, *emptied himself.*
y Psa. 8:4-6.
z Psa. 40:6-8.
aa Heb. 2:9; Rev. 3:21.

[1] **(2:6)** "Form," etc., Gr. *en morphe,* "the form by which a person or thing strikes the vision, the external appearance."—*Thayer.* Cf. John 17:5: "The glory which I had with Thee before the world was." Nothing in this passage teaches that the Eternal Word (John 1:1) emptied Himself of either His divine nature, or His attributes, but only of the outward and visible manifestation of the Godhead. "He emptied, stripped Himself of the insignia of Majesty."—*Lightfoot.* "When occasion demanded He exercised His divine attributes.—*Moorehead.* Cf. John 1:1, *note;* 20:28, *note.*

exalted him, and given him a name
which is above every name:
10 That at the name of Jesus [a]every
knee should bow, of *things* in heaven, and
things in earth, and *things* under the earth;
11 And *that* every tongue should confess that Jesus Christ [b]*is* Lord, to the
glory of God the Father.

(4) *The outworking of the inworked salvation.*

12 Wherefore, my beloved, as ye have
always obeyed, not as in my presence
only, but now much more in my
absence, [c]work out your own [d]salvation
with fear and trembling.
13 For it is [e]God which worketh in you
both to will and to do of *his* good pleasure.
14 Do all things without [f]murmurings
and disputings:
15 That ye may be blameless and
harmless, the [g]sons of God, without
rebuke, in the midst of a crooked and
perverse [h]nation, among whom ye shine
as lights in the [i]world;
16 Holding forth the word of [j]life; that
I may rejoice in [k]the day of Christ, that I
have not run in vain, neither laboured in
vain.

(5) *The apostolic example.*

17 Yea, and if I be [l]offered upon the
sacrifice and service of your faith, I joy,
and rejoice with you all.
18 For the same cause also do ye joy,
and rejoice with me.
19 But I [m]trust in the Lord Jesus to
send [n]Timotheus shortly unto you, that I
also may be of good comfort, when I
know your state.
20 For I have no man [o]likeminded,
who will naturally care for your state.
21 For all seek their own, not the
things which are Jesus Christ's.
22 But ye know the proof of him, that,
as a son with the father, he hath served
with me in the [p]gospel.
23 Him therefore I hope to send
presently, so soon as I shall see how it
will go with me.
24 But I trust in the Lord that I also
myself shall come shortly.
25 Yet I supposed it necessary to send
to you [q]Epaphroditus, my brother, and
companion in labour, and fellowsoldier,
but your messenger, and he that ministered to my wants.
26 For he longed after you all, and was
full of heaviness, because that ye had
heard that he had been sick.
27 For indeed he was sick nigh unto

A.D. 64.

a Isa. 45:23; Rev. 5:13.
b John 13:13; Rom. 14:9.
c John 6:27, 29; Heb. 4:11; 2 Pet. 1:5, 10.
d Rom. 1:16, *note.*
e Heb. 13:21.
f 1 Cor. 10:10.
g *children.*
h *generation.* Deut. 32:5.
i *kosmos* (Mt. 4:8) = mankind.
j *Life (eternal).* Phil. 4:3. (Mt. 7:14; Rev. 22:19.)
k 1 Cor. 1:8, *note.*
l *poured out as a drink-offering.*
m *hope.*
n 1 Thes. 3:2.
o Or, *so dear unto me.*
p *Gospel.* Phil. 4:3, 15. (Gen. 12:1-3; Rev. 14:6.)
q Phil. 4:18.
r Mt. 10:40.
s 1 Thes. 5:16.
t 2 Pet. 1:12, 15.
u Isa. 56:10, 11.
v Psa. 119:115.
w Gal. 5:1, 3.
x *Holy Spirit.* Col. 1:8. (Mt. 1:18; Acts 2:4.)
y *Flesh.* vs. 3, 4; Col. 2:11, 23. (John 1:13; Jude 23.)
z Acts 23:6.
aa *Church (visible).* 1 Tim. 3:15. (1 Cor. 10:32; 1 Tim. 3:15.)
bb Rom. 10:3, *note.*
cc Isa. 53:11; Jer. 9:23, 24; John 17:3; 1 Cor. 2:2.
dd 2 Cor. 11:25, 27.
ee *Law (of Moses).* 1 Tim. 1:8, 9. (Ex. 19:1; Gal. 3:1-29.)
ff *Faith.* 1 Thes. 4:14. (Gen. 3:20; Heb. 11:39.)
gg Rom. 3:21, *note.*

death: but God had mercy on him; and
not on him only, but on me also, lest I
should have sorrow upon sorrow.
28 I sent him therefore the more carefully, that, when ye see him again, ye
may rejoice, and that I may be the less
sorrowful.
29 [r]Receive him therefore in the Lord
with all gladness; and hold such in reputation:
30 Because for the work of Christ he
was nigh unto death, not regarding his
life, to supply your lack of service
toward me.

CHAPTER 3.

Part III. Christ, object of the believer's faith, desire, and expectation (Phil. 3:1-21).

(1) *Warning against Judaizers.*

Finally, my brethren, [s]rejoice in the
Lord. To write the [t]same things to
you, to me indeed *is* not grievous, but
for you *it is* safe.
2 Beware of [u]dogs, beware of [v]evil
workers, beware of the [w]concision.
3 For we are the circumcision, which
worship God in the [x]spirit, and rejoice in
Christ Jesus, and have no confidence in
the [y]flesh.

(2) *Warning against trusting in legal righteousness.*

4 Though I might also have confidence
in the flesh. If any other man thinketh
that he hath whereof he might trust in
the flesh, I more:
5 Circumcised the eighth day, of the
stock of Israel, *of* the tribe of Benjamin,
an Hebrew of the Hebrews; as touching
the law, a [z]Pharisee;
6 Concerning zeal, persecuting [aa]the
church; touching the [bb]righteousness
which is in the law, blameless.

(3) *Christ, object of the believer's faith for righteousness.*

7 But what things were gain to me,
those I counted loss for Christ.
8 Yea doubtless, and I count all things
but loss [cc]for the excellency of the knowledge of Christ Jesus my Lord: for whom
I have [dd]suffered the loss of all things,
and do count them *but* dung, that I may
win Christ,
9 And be found in him, not having
mine own righteousness, which is of the
[ee]law, but that which is through [ff]the
faith of Christ, [gg]the righteousness
which is of God by faith:

(4) *Christ, object of the believer's desire for fellowship in resurrection power.*

10 That I may know him, and the power of his resurrection, and the [a]fellowship of his sufferings, being made conformable unto his death;

11 If by any means I might attain unto the resurrection [b]of the dead.

12 Not as though I had already attained, either were already [c]perfect: but I follow after, if that I may apprehend that for which also I am apprehended of Christ Jesus.

13 Brethren, I count not myself to have apprehended: but *this* one thing *I do*, forgetting those things which are behind, and reaching forth unto those things which are before,

14 I [d]press toward the [e]mark for the prize of the [f]high calling of God in Christ Jesus.

(5) *The appeal for unity in the walk.*

15 Let us therefore, as many as be [c]perfect, be [g]thus minded: and if in any thing ye be otherwise minded, [h]God shall reveal even this unto you.

16 Nevertheless, whereto we have already attained, let us walk by the same rule, let us mind the same thing.

(6) *But truth is not to be compromised for the sake of unity.*

17 Brethren, be followers together of me, and mark them which walk so as ye have us [i]for an ensample.

18 (For many walk, of whom I have told you often, and now tell you even weeping, *that they are* the enemies of the cross of Christ:

19 Whose [j]end *is* destruction, whose God *is their* belly, and *whose* glory *is* in their shame, who mind earthly things.)

(7) *Christ, object of the believer's expectation.*

20 For our [k]conversation is in heaven; [l]from whence also we look for the [m]Saviour, the Lord Jesus Christ:

21 Who shall [n]change our [o]vile body, that it may be fashioned like unto his [p]glorious body, according to the working whereby he is able even to subdue all things unto himself.

A.D. 64.

a 2 Cor. 1:5; 1 Pet. 4:13.
b *from among.*
c Mt. 5:48, *note.*
d 1 Cor. 9:24; Heb. 12:1.
e *goal.*
f *upward.*
g Gal. 5:10.
h Hos. 6:3; Jas. 1:5.
i 1 Pet. 5:3.
j 2 Pet. 2:1.
k *citizenship.*
l *Christ (Second Advent).* vs. 20, 21; 1 Thes. 1:9, 10. (Deut. 30:3; Acts 1:9-11.)
m Rom. 1:16, *note.*
n *Resurrection.* 1 Thes. 4:13-17. (Job 19:25, 1 Cor. 15:52.)
o *body of humiliation.*
p *body of glory.*
q *Rewards.* Col. 3:24. (Dan. 12:3; 1 Cor. 3:14.)
r *Life (eternal).* Col. 1:27. (Mt. 7:14; Rev. 22:19.)
s *gentleness.*
t Jas. 5:7, 9; Rev. 22:7, 20.
u Mt. 6:25; 1 Pet. 5:7.
v Cf. Mt. 10:34, *note.*
w Eph. 4:25.
x 2 Cor. 8:21.
y Deut. 16:20.
z Jas. 3:17.
aa 1 Cor. 13.
bb Heb. 13:20.
cc Or, *is revived.*
dd Omit *"therewith"*.
ee Heb. 13:5.

CHAPTER 4.

Part IV. Christ, the believer's strength, rejoicing over anxiety (Phil. 4:1-23).

(1) *Exhortation to unity and joy.*

Therefore, my brethren dearly beloved and longed for, my joy and [q]crown, so stand fast in the Lord, *my* dearly beloved.

2 I beseech Euodias, and beseech Syntyche, that they be of the same mind in the Lord.

3 And I intreat thee also, true yokefellow, help those women which laboured with me in the gospel, with Clement also, and *with* other my fellowlabourers, whose names *are* in the book [r]of life.

4 Rejoice in the Lord alway: *and* again I say, Rejoice.

(2) *The secret of the peace of God.*

5 Let your [s]moderation be known unto all men. [t]The Lord *is* at hand.

6 [u]Be careful for nothing; but in every thing by prayer and supplication with thanksgiving let your requests be made known unto God.

7 And the [v]peace of God, which passeth all understanding, shall keep your hearts and minds through Christ Jesus.

(3) *The presence of the God of peace.*

8 Finally, brethren, whatsoever things are [w]true, whatsoever things are [x]honest, whatsoever things *are* [y]just, whatsoever things *are* [z]pure, whatsoever things *are* [aa]lovely, whatsoever things *are* of good report; if *there be* any virtue, and if *there be* any praise, think on these things.

9 Those things, which ye have both learned, and received, and heard, and seen in me, do: and [bb]the God of peace shall be with you.

(4) *The victory over anxious care.*

10 But I rejoiced in the Lord greatly, that now at the last your care of me [cc]hath flourished again; wherein ye were also careful, but ye lacked opportunity.

11 Not that I speak in respect of want: for I have learned, in whatsoever state I am, [dd]*therewith* to be [ee]content.

12 I know both how to be abased, and I know how to abound: every where and in all things I am instructed both to be

full and to be hungry, both to abound and to suffer need.

13 I can do all things [a]through Christ which strengtheneth me.

14 Notwithstanding ye have well done, that ye did communicate with my affliction.

15 Now ye Philippians know also, that in the beginning of the [b]gospel, when I departed from Macedonia, no church communicated with me as concerning giving and receiving, but ye only.

16 For even in Thessalonica ye sent once and again unto my necessity.

17 Not because I desire a gift: but I desire fruit that may abound to your account.

18 But I [c]have all, and abound: I am full, having received of Epaphroditus the things *which were sent* from you, an odour of a sweet smell, a [d]sacrifice acceptable, wellpleasing to God.

19 But my God shall [e]supply all your need according to his riches in glory by Christ Jesus.

20 Now unto God and our Father *be* glory for ever and ever. Amen.

21 Salute every saint in Christ Jesus. The brethren which are with me greet you.

22 All the saints salute you, chiefly they that are of Caesar's household.

23 The grace of our Lord Jesus Christ *be* with you all. Amen.

A.D. 64.

a John 15:5; 2 Cor. 12:9.

b *Gospel.* vs. 3, 15; Col. 1:5; 6:23. (Gen. 12:1-3; Rev. 14:6.)

c Or, *have received.*

d *Sacrifice (the believer-priest's).* Heb. 13:15, 16. (Gen. 4:4; Heb. 10:18.)

e Psa. 23:1; 2 Cor. 9:8.

THE EPISTLE OF PAUL THE APOSTLE TO THE

COLOSSIANS

WRITER. The Apostle Paul (1:1).

Date. Colossians was sent by the same messenger who bore Ephesians and Philemon, and was probably written at the same time.

Theme. Epaphras, who laboured in the Word in the assembly at Colosse, was Paul's fellow-prisoner at Rome. Doubtless from him Paul learned the state of that church. As to fundamentals that state was excellent (1:3-8), but in a subtle way two forms of error were at work: The first was legality in its Alexandrian form of asceticism, "touch not, taste not," with a trace of the Judaic observance of "days"; the object of which was the mortification of the body (cf. Rom. 8:13). The second form of error was false mysticism, "intruding into those things which he hath not seen"—the result of philosophic speculation. Because these are ever present perils, Colossians was written, not for that day only, but for the warning of the church in all days.

The Epistle is in seven divisions: I. Introduction, 1:1-8. II. The apostolic prayer, 1:9-14. III. The exaltation of Christ, Creator, Redeemer, Indweller, 1:15-29. IV. The Godhead incarnate in Christ, in whom the believer is complete, 2:1-23. V. The believer's union with Christ in resurrection life and glory, 3:1-4. VI. Christian living, the fruit of union with Christ, 3:5–4:6. VII. Christian fellowship, 4:7-18.

CHAPTER 1.

Part I. Introduction: the apostolic greeting (vs. 1-8).

Paul, an apostle of Jesus Christ by the will of God, and Timotheus *our* brother,

2 To the saints and faithful brethren in Christ which are at Colosse: Grace *be* unto you, and peace, from God our Father and the Lord Jesus Christ.

3 We give thanks to God and the Father of our Lord Jesus Christ, praying always for you,

4 Since we heard of your faith in Christ Jesus, and of the love *which ye have* to all the saints,

5 For the hope which is laid up for you in heaven, whereof ye heard before in the word of the truth of the gospel;

6 Which is come unto you, as *it is* in all the [a]world; and [b]bringeth forth fruit, as *it doth* also in you, since the day ye heard *of it,* and knew the [c]grace of God in truth:

7 As ye also learned of [d]Epaphras our dear fellowservant, who is for you a [e]faithful minister of Christ;

8 Who also declared unto us your love in the [f]Spirit.

Part II. The apostle's sevenfold prayer (vs. 9-14).

9 For this cause we also, since the day we heard *it,* do not cease to [g]pray for you, and to desire that ye might be filled with the [h]knowledge of his will in [i]all wisdom and spiritual understanding;

10 [j]That ye might walk worthy of the Lord unto all [k]pleasing, being [l]fruitful in every good work, and increasing in the [m]knowledge of God;

11 [n]Strengthened with all might, according to his glorious power, unto all [o]patience and longsuffering [p]with joyfulness;

12 Giving thanks unto the Father, which hath made us meet to be partakers of the inheritance of the saints in light:

13 Who hath delivered us from the power of darkness, and hath translated *us* into the kingdom of [q]his dear Son:

14 In whom we have [r]redemption through his blood, *even* the [s]forgiveness of sins:

Part III. The exaltation of Christ (vs. 15-29).

(1) *The seven superiorities of Christ.*

15 Who is the [t]image of the invisible God, the [u]firstborn of every creature:

16 For [v]by him were all things created, that are in heaven, and that are in earth, visible and invisible, whether *they be* thrones, or

A.D. 64.

a i.e. *earth.*
b Mk. 4:8; John 15:16; Phil. 1:11.
c *Grace (in salv.).* 2 Thes. 2:16. (Rom. 3:24; John 1:17, *note.*)
d Col. 4:12; Phm. 23.
e 1 Cor. 4:1, 2; Eph. 6:21.
f *Holy Spirit.* 1 Thes. 1:5, 6. (Mt. 1:18; Acts 2:4.)
g *Bible prayers (N.T.).* 1 Thes. 3:10-13. (Mt. 6:9; Rev. 22:20.)
h Rom. 12:2; Eph. 5:10, 17.
i Eph. 1:8.
j Eph. 4:1; Phil. 1:27; 1 Thes. 2:12.
k Rom. 15:2; 1 Cor. 10:33; 1 Thes. 4:1.
l John 15:16; 2 Cor. 9:8; Phil. 1:11; Tit. 3:1; Heb. 13:21.
m 2 Pet. 3:18.
n Eph. 3:16; 6:10.
o 2 Cor. 6:4; 12:12; Eph. 4:2.
p 2 Cor. 8:2; Heb. 10:34.
q *the Son of his love.*
r Rom. 3:24. *note.*
s Eph. 1:7.
t 2 Cor. 4:4; Heb. 1:3.
u Rev. 3:14.
v John 1:3; Heb. 1:3.

dominions, or principalities, or powers: [a]all things were created by him, and for him:

17 And [b]he is before all things, and by him [c]all things consist.

18 And he is the [d]head of the body, the church: who is the beginning, the firstborn [e]from the dead; that in all *things* he might have the preeminence.

19 [f]For it pleased *the Father* that in him should all fulness dwell;

(2) *The reconciling work of Christ.*

20 And, having made peace [g]through the blood of his cross, by him to reconcile all things unto himself; by him, *I say*, whether *they be* things in earth, or things in heaven.

21 And you, that were sometime alienated and enemies in *your* mind by wicked works, yet now hath he [1h]reconciled

22 [i]In the body of his flesh through death, to present you [j]holy and unblameable and unreproveable [k]in his sight:

23 If ye continue in the faith grounded and settled, and *be* not moved away from the hope of the [l]gospel, which ye have heard, *and* which was [m]preached to every creature which is under heaven; whereof I Paul [n]am made a minister;

(3) *The mystery of the indwelling Christ.*

24 Who now rejoice in my sufferings for you, and fill up that which is behind of the afflictions of Christ in my flesh for his body's sake, which is the [o]church:

25 Whereof I am made a minister, according to the dispensation of God which is given to me for you, to [p]fulfil the word of God;

26 *Even* the [q]mystery which hath been hid from [r]ages and from generations, but now is made manifest to his saints:

27 To whom God would make known what *is* the riches of the glory of this [s]mystery among the Gentiles; which is [t]Christ [u]in you, the hope of glory:

A.D. 64.

a Rom. 11:36; Heb. 2:10.
b John 17:5.
c Heb. 1:3.
d Eph. 1:22.
e Rev. 1:5.
f *For in him all the fulness of the Godhead was pleased to dwell.*
g *Sacrifice (of Christ).* Heb. 7:27. (Gen. 4:4; Heb. 10:18.)
h *Reconciliation.* vs. 20, 21; see Rom. 5:10.
i Eph. 2:14-16.
j *Sanctify, holy (persons)* (N. T.). Col. 3:12. (Mt. 4:5; Rev. 22:11.)
k Eph. 5:27.
l *Gospel.* vs. 5, 6, 23; 1 Thes. 1:5. (Gen. 12:1-3; Rev. 14:6.)
m Col. 1:6.
n 1 Cor. 1:17; Gal. 2:2.
o *Church (true).* vs. 18-24; Heb. 2:12. (Mt. 16:18; Heb. 12:23.)
p *complete.*
q Mt. 13:11, *note.*
r Eph. 3:2-6.
s Mt. 13:11, *note.*
t Eph. 4:24, *note.*
u *Life (eternal).* Col. 3:3, 4. (Mt. 7:14; Rev. 22:19.)
v Acts 20:20, 27.
w Mt. 5:48, *note.*
x Phil. 1:30; Col. 1:29; 1 Thes. 2:2.
y 2 Cor. 1:6.
z Col. 3:14.
aa *Assurance.* 1 Thes. 1:5. (Isa. 32:17; Jude 1.)
bb The best authorities omit "and of the Father, and of Christ."
cc Eph. 1:9; 3:9.
dd vs. 8, 18; Rom. 16:18; 2 Cor. 11:13; Eph. 4:14; 5:6.
ee 1 Cor. 14:40.
ff 1 Pet. 5:9.
gg *kosmos* (Mt. 4:8) = mankind.

28 Whom we preach, [v]warning every man, and teaching every man in all wisdom; that we may present every man [w]perfect in Christ Jesus:

29 Whereunto I also labour, striving according to his working, which worketh in me mightily.

CHAPTER 2.

Part IV. The Godhead incarnate in Christ, in whom the believer is complete (Col. 2:1-23).

For I would that ye knew what [x]great conflict I have for you, and *for* them at Laodicea, and *for* as many as have not seen my face in the flesh;

2 [y]That their hearts might be comforted, being [z]knit together in love, and unto all riches of the [aa]full assurance of understanding, to the acknowledgement of the [2s]mystery of God, [bb]and of the Father, and of Christ;

3 [cc]In whom are hid all the treasures of wisdom and knowledge.

(1) *The danger from enticing words.* (Cf. Rom. 16:17, 18; 1 Cor. 2:4; 2 Pet. 2:3.)

4 And this I say, [dd]lest any man should beguile you with enticing words.

5 For though I be absent in the flesh, yet am I with you in the spirit, joying and [ee]beholding your order, and the [ff]stedfastness of your faith in Christ.

6 As ye have therefore received Christ Jesus the Lord, *so* walk ye in him:

7 Rooted and built up in him, and stablished in the faith, as ye have been taught, abounding therein with thanksgiving.

(2) *The twofold warning against (a) philosophy, (b) legality.*

8 Beware lest any man spoil you through philosophy and vain deceit, after the tradition of men, after the rudiments of the [gg]world, and not after Christ.

[1] **(1:21)** Reconciliation. The Greek word signifies "to change thoroughly from," and occurs, Rom. 5:10; 11:15; 1 Cor. 7:11; 2 Cor. 5:18, 19, 20. Reconciliation looks toward the effect of the death of Christ upon man, as propitiation (Rom. 3:25, *note*) is the Godward aspect, and is that effect of the death of Christ upon the believing sinner which, through divine power, works in him a "thorough change" toward God from enmity and aversion to love and trust. It is never said that God is reconciled. God is propitiated, the sinner reconciled (cf. 2 Cor. 5:18-21).

[2] **(2:2)** The "mystery of God" is Christ, as incarnating the fulness of the Godhead, and all the divine wisdom and knowledge for the redemption and reconciliation of man.

(3) *Nothing can be added to completeness.*

9 For in him [a]dwelleth all the fulness of the Godhead bodily.

10 And ye are complete in him, which is the [b]head of all principality and power:

11 In whom also ye are [c]circumcised with the circumcision made without hands, in putting off the body of [d]the sins of the flesh by the circumcision of Christ:

12 [e]Buried with him in baptism, wherein also ye are risen with *him* through the faith of the [f]operation of God, who hath raised him from the dead.

13 And you, being [g]dead in your sins and the uncircumcision of your flesh, hath he quickened together with him, having [h]forgiven you all trespasses;

(4) *Law observances were abolished in Christ.* (Cf. Mt. 5:17.)

14 [i]Blotting out the handwriting of ordinances that was against us, which was contrary to us, and took it out of the way, nailing it to his cross;

15 *And* having [j]spoiled principalities and powers, he made a shew of them openly, triumphing over them in it.

16 Let no man therefore [k]judge you in meat, or in drink, or in respect of an [l]holyday, or of the new moon, or of the sabbath *days*:

17 Which are a [m]shadow of things to come; but the body *is* of Christ.

(5) *Warning against false mysticism.*

18 Let no man beguile you of your reward in a voluntary humility and worshipping of [n]angels, [1]intruding into those things which he hath not seen, vainly puffed up by his fleshly mind,

19 And not [o]holding the [p]Head, from which all the body by joints and bands having nourishment ministered, and knit together, increaseth with the increase of God.

(6) *Warning against asceticism.*

20 Wherefore if ye be dead with Christ from the rudiments of the [q]world, why, as though living in the world, are ye subject to ordinances,

21 (Touch not; taste not; handle not;

22 Which all are to perish with the using;) after the commandments and doctrines of men?

23 Which things have indeed a shew of wisdom in will worship, and humility, and neglecting of the body; [r]not in any honour to the satisfying of the [s]flesh.

CHAPTER 3.

Part V. The believer's union with Christ, now and hereafter (vs. 1-4).

If ye then be [t]risen with Christ, seek those things which are above, where [u]Christ sitteth on the right hand of God.

2 Set your affection on things above, not on things on the earth.

3 [v]For ye are dead, and your life is hid with Christ in God.

4 When Christ, *who is* our [w]life, [x]shall appear, then shall ye also appear with him in glory.

Part VI. Christian living, the fruit of union with Christ (Col. 3:5–4:6).

5 [y]Mortify therefore your members which are upon the earth; fornication, uncleanness, inordinate affection, evil concupiscence, and covetousness, which is [z]idolatry:

6 For which things' sake the [aa]wrath of God cometh on the [bb]children of disobedience:

7 In the which [cc]ye also walked some time, when ye lived in them.

8 [dd]But now ye also put off all these; anger, wrath, malice, blasphemy, filthy communication out of your mouth.

9 Lie not one to another, seeing that ye have put off the [ee]old man with his deeds;

10 And have put on the new *man*,

A.D. 64.

a John 1:14: Col. 1:19.
b Eph. 1:21; 1 Pet. 3:22.
c Deut. 10:16; Jer. 4:4; Rom. 2:29; Phil. 3:3.
d Omit "the sins of."
e Rom. 6:4.
f Eph. 1:20.
g *Death (spiritual)* Eph. 2:1-5. (Gen. 2:17; Eph. 2:5.)
h *Forgiveness.* Col. 3:13. (Lev. 4:20; Mt. 26:28.)
i Eph. 2:15, 16.
j Eph. 6:12; Heb. 2:14.
k Rom. 14:3.
l *Sanctify, holy (things)* (N.T.) 2 Tim. 3:15. (Mt. 4:5; Rev. 22:11.)
m Heb. 8:5; 9:9; 10:1.
n Heb. 1:4, *note.*
o *holding fast.*
p Eph. 4:15, 16.
q *kosmos* = world-system. Jas. 1:27. (John 7:7; Rev. 13:3-8, *note.*)
r Or, "which do not really honour God. but only satisfy the flesh" (i.e. by creating a reputation for superior sanctity).
s *Flesh.* vs. 11, 23; 1 Pet. 3:21. (John 1:13; Jude 23.)
t Rom. 6:5; Eph. 2:6; Col. 2:12.
u Rom. 8:34; Eph: 1:20.
v Rom. 6:2; Gal. 2:20; Col. 2:20.
w *Life (eternal).* vs. 3, 4; 1 Tim. 1:16. (Mt. 7:14; Rev. 22:19.).
x Phil. 3:21; 1 John 3:2.
y Rom. 8:13; Gal. 5:24.
z Eph. 5:5.
aa Rom. 1:18; Eph. 5:6; Rev. 22:15.
bb *sons.*
cc Eph. 2:2; Tit. 3:3.
dd Eph. 4:22; Heb. 12:1; Jas. 1:21; 1 Pet. 2:1.
ee Rom. 6:6, *note.*

[1]**(2:18)** The errorists against whom Paul warns the Colossians, and against whom, *in principle,* the warning has perpetual significance, were called "Gnostics," from *gnosis,* "knowledge." These Gnostics "came most keenly into conflict with the exalted rank and redeeming work of Christ, to whom they did not leave His full divine dignity, but assigned to Him merely the highest rank in the order of spirits, while they exalted angels as concerned in bringing in "the Messianic salvation."—*H. A. W. Meyer.* Paul's characteristic word in Colossians for the divine revelation is *epignosis,* i.e. "full-knowledge" (1:9, 10; 3:10), as against the pretended "knowledge" of the errorists. The warnings apply to all extra-biblical forms, doctrines, and customs, and to all ascetic practices.

which is renewed in knowledge after the
image of him that [a]created him:
11 Where there is neither Greek nor
Jew, circumcision nor uncircumcision,
Barbarian, Scythian, bond *nor* free: [b]but
Christ *is* all, and in all.
12 Put on therefore, as the [c]elect of
God, [d]holy and beloved, [e]bowels of mercies, kindness, humbleness of mind,
meekness, longsuffering;
13 Forbearing one another, and forgiving one another, if any man have a quarrel against any: even as Christ [f]forgave
you, so also *do* ye.
14 And [g]above all these things *put on*
[h]charity, which is the bond of [i]perfectness.
15 And let the peace of [j]God [k]rule in
your hearts, to the which also ye are
called in one body; and [l]be ye thankful.
16 Let the word of Christ dwell in you
richly in all wisdom; [m]teaching and
admonishing one another in psalms and
hymns and spiritual songs, singing with
[n]grace in your hearts to the Lord.
17 And [o]whatsoever ye do in word or
deed, *do* all in the name of the Lord
Jesus, giving thanks to God and the
Father by him.
18 Wives, [p]submit yourselves unto your
own husbands, as [q]it is fit in the Lord.
19 Husbands, [r]love *your* wives, and be
not bitter against them.
20 Children, obey *your* parents in all
things: for this is [s]well pleasing unto the
Lord.
21 [t]Fathers, provoke not your children
to anger, lest they be discouraged.
22 [u]Servants, obey in all things *your*
masters according to the flesh; not with
eyeservice, as menpleasers; but in singleness of heart, fearing God:
23 And [v]whatsoever ye do, do *it* heartily, as to the Lord, and not unto men;
24 Knowing that of the Lord ye shall
receive the [w]reward of the inheritance:
for ye serve the Lord Christ.
25 But he that doeth wrong shall
receive for the wrong which he hath
done: and there is no respect of persons.

A.D. 64.

a Eph. 4:24, *note.*
b Eph. 1:23.
c *Election (corporate).* 1 Thes. 1:4. (Deut. 7:6; 1 Pet. 1:2.)
d *Sanctify, holy (persons)* (N.T.). 1 Thes. 5:23. (Mt. 4:5; Rev. 22:11.)
e Eph 4:24; Phil. 2:1, 2..
f *Forgiveness* Heb. 9:22. Lev. 4:20; Mt. 26:28.)
g John 13:34; 1 Cor. 13; Eph. 5:2; 1 Pet. 4:8.
h *love.*
i Mt. 5:48, *note.*
j *Christ.*
k John 14:27; Rom. 14:17; Phil. 4:7.
l v. 17; Phil. 4:6; Col. 2:7; 1 Thes. 5:18.
m Eph. 5:19, 20.
n *Grace (imparted).* Col. 4:6. (Rom. 6:1; 2 Pet. 3:18.)
o 1 Cor. 10:31.
p Cf. Gen. 3:16.
q Eph. 5:22; 1 Pet. 3:1.
r Eph. 5:25.
s Eph. 6:1.
t Eph. 6:4.
u Eph. 6:5; 1 Tim. 6:1; Tit. 2:9; 1 Pet. 2:18.
v Eccl. 9:10; Eph. 6:6-8.
w *Rewards.* 1 Thes. 2:19. (Deut. 12:3; 1 Cor. 3:14.)
x Eph. 6:18; 1 Thes. 5:17.
y Mt. 13:11, *note.*
z *Grace (imparted).* 2 Thes. 1:12. (Rom. 6:1; 2 Pet. 3:18.)
aa Acts 20:4; Eph. 6:21; 2 Tim. 4:12; Tit. 3:12.
bb Eph. 6:22.
cc Phm. 10.
dd Acts 19:29; 20:4; 27:2; Phm. 24.
ee Acts 15:37; 2 Tim. 4:11.
ff Col. 1:7; Phm. 23.
gg Mt. 5:48, *note.*
hh 2 Tim. 4:11.
ii 2 Tim. 4:10; Phm. 24.

CHAPTER 4.

Masters, give unto *your* servants that
which is just and equal; knowing
that ye also have a Master in heaven.
2 [x]Continue in prayer, and watch in
the same with thanksgiving;
3 Withal praying also for us, that God
would open unto us a door of utterance,
to speak the [y]mystery of Christ, for
which I am also in bonds:
4 That I may make it manifest, as I
ought to speak.
5 Walk in wisdom toward them that
are without, redeeming the time.
6 Let your speech *be* alway with [z]grace,
seasoned with salt, that ye may know
how ye ought to answer every man.

Part VII. Christian fellowship (vs. 7-18).

7 All my state shall [aa]Tychicus declare
unto you, *who is* a beloved brother, and a
faithful minister and fellowservant in
the Lord:
8 [bb]Whom I have sent unto you for the
same purpose, that he might know your
estate, and comfort your hearts;
9 With [cc]Onesimus, a faithful and
beloved brother, who is *one* of you. They
shall make known unto you all things
which *are done* here.
10 [dd]Aristarchus my fellowprisoner
saluteth you, and [ee]Marcus, sister's son
to Barnabas, (touching whom ye
received commandments: if he come
unto you, receive him;)
11 And Jesus, which is called Justus,
who are of the circumcision. These only
are my fellowworkers unto the kingdom
of God, which have been a comfort unto
me.
12 [1][ff]Epaphras, who is *one* of you, a
servant of Christ, saluteth you, always
labouring fervently for you in prayers,
that ye may stand [gg]perfect and complete in all the will of God.
13 For I bear him record, that he hath a
great zeal for you, and them *that are* in
Laodicea, and them in Hierapolis.
14 [hh]Luke, the beloved physician, and
[ii]Demas, greet you.
15 Salute the brethren which are

[1] **(4:12)** A touching illustration of priestly service (see 1 Pet. 2:9, *note*) as distinguished from ministry of gift. Shut up in prison, no longer able to preach, Epaphras was still, equally with all believers, a priest. No prison could keep him from the throne of grace, so he gave himself wholly to the priestly work of intercession.

in Laodicea, and Nymphas, and the
[a]church which is in his house.
16 And when this epistle is read
among you, cause that it be read also in
the church of the Laodiceans; and that
ye likewise read the *epistle* from
Laodicea.
17 And say to [b]Archippus, Take heed
to the ministry which thou hast received
in the Lord, that thou fulfil it.
18 The salutation by the hand of me
Paul. [c]Remember my bonds. Grace *be*
with you. Amen.

A.D. 64.

a *Churches (local).* vs. 15, 16; 1 Thes. 1:1. (Acts 2:41; Phil. 1:1.)

b Phm. 2

c Heb. 13:3.

THE FIRST EPISTLE OF PAUL THE APOSTLE TO THE
THESSALONIANS

WRITER. The Apostle Paul (1:1).

Date. The Epistle was written from Corinth, A.D. 54, shortly after Paul's departure from Thessalonica (Acts 16, 17), and is the earliest of his letters.

Theme. The theme of the Epistle is threefold: (1) To confirm young disciples in the foundational truths already taught them; (2) to exhort them to go on to holiness; (3) to comfort them concerning those who had fallen asleep. The second coming of Christ is prominent throughout. The Epistle is incidentally most interesting as showing the richness in doctrine of the primitive evangelism. During a mission of about one month the apostle had taught all the great [1]doctrines of the Christian faith.

The divisions of the Epistle are sufficiently indicated by the chapters: I. The model church, and the three tenses of the Christian life, 1:1-10, II. The model servant and his reward, 2:1-20. III. The model brother, and the believer's sanctification, 3:1-13. IV. The model walk, and the believer's hope, 4:1-18. V. The model walk, and the day of Jehovah, 5:1-28.

CHAPTER 1.

Part I. The model church, and the three tenses of the Christian life.

Paul, and Silvanus, and Timotheus, unto the [a]church of the [b]Thessalonians *which is* in God the Father and *in* the Lord Jesus Christ: Grace *be* unto you, and peace, from God our Father, and the Lord Jesus Christ.

2 We give thanks to God always for you all, making mention of you in our prayers;

3 Remembering without ceasing your [c]work of faith, and labour of love, and patience of hope in our Lord Jesus Christ, in the sight of God and our Father;

4 Knowing, brethren beloved, your [d]election of God.

5 For our [e]gospel came not unto you in word only, but also in power, and in the Holy Ghost, and in much [f]assurance; as ye know what manner of men we were among you for your sake.

6 And ye became followers of us, and of the Lord, having received the word in much affliction, with [g]joy of the [h]Holy Ghost:

7 So that ye were ensamples to all that believe in Macedonia and Achaia.

8 For from you [i]sounded out the word of the Lord not only in Macedonia and Achaia, but also [j]in every place your faith to God-ward is spread abroad; so that we need not to speak any thing.

9 For they themselves shew of us what manner of entering in we had unto you, and [2]how ye [k]turned to God from idols to serve the living and true God;

10 And [l]to wait for his Son [m]from heaven, whom he raised from the dead, *even* Jesus, which delivered us from the [n]wrath to come.

A.D. 54.

a *Churches (local).* 1 Thes. 2:14. (Acts 2:41; Phil. 1:1.)
b Acts 17:1-9.
c Lit. *operative faith, and laborious love, and hope-filled patience.*
d *Election (corporate).* 2 Thes. 2:13. (Deut. 7:6; 1 Pet. 1:2.)
e *Gospel.* 1 Thes. 2:4, 8, 9. Gen. 12:1-3; Rev. 14:6.)
f *Assurance.* 2 Tim. 1:12. (Isa. 32:17; Jude 1.)
g Acts 13:52.
h *Holy Spirit.* vs. 5, 6; 1 Thes. 4:8. (Mt. 1:18; Acts 2:4.)
i Rom. 10:18.
j 2 Thes. 1:4.
k 1 Cor. 12:2; Gal. 4:8.
l *Christ (Second Advent).* vs. 9, 10; 1 Thes. 2:19. Deut. 30:3; Acts 1:9-11.)
m *from among.*
n Mt. 3:7; Rom. 5:9.

CHAPTER 2.

Part II. The model servant, and his reward.

For yourselves, brethren, know our entrance in unto you, that it was not in vain:

[1] **(***See Introductory notes***).** That is: *election,* 1:4; *Holy Spirit,* 1:5, 6; 4:8; 5:19; *assurance,* 1:5; *Trinity,* 1:1, 5, 6; *conversion,* 1:9; *second advent of Christ,* 1:10; 2:19; 3:13; 4:14-17; 5:23; *walk,* 2:12; 4:1; *sanctification,* 4:3; 5:23; *day of Jehovah,* 5:1-3; *resurrection,* 4:14-18; *the tripartite nature of man,* 5:23.

[2] **(1:9)** The tenses of the believer's life here indicated are logical and give the true order. They occur also in v. 3. The "work of faith" is to "turn to God from idols" (cf. John 6:28, 29); the "labour of love" is to "serve the living and true God"; and the "patience of hope" is to "wait for his Son from heaven" (cf. Mt. 24:42; 25:13; Lk. 12:36-48; Acts 1:11; Phil. 3:20, 21). Paul repeats this threefold sequence in Tit. 2:11-13.

2 But even after that we had suffered before, and were shamefully entreated, as ye know, at [a]Philippi, we were [b]bold in our God to speak unto you the gospel of God with much contention.

3 For our exhortation *was* not of [c]deceit, nor of uncleanness, nor in guile:

4 But as we were allowed of God to be put in trust with the gospel, even so we speak; not as pleasing men, but God, which trieth our hearts.

5 For [d]neither at any time used we flattering words, as ye know, nor a cloke of covetousness; God *is* witness:

6 Nor of men [e]sought we glory, neither of you, nor *yet* of others, when we might have been burdensome, as the apostles of Christ.

7 But we were gentle among you, even as a nurse cherisheth [f]her children:

8 So being affectionately desirous of you, we were willing to [g]have imparted unto you, not the gospel of God only, but also our own souls, because ye were dear unto us.

9 For ye remember, brethren, our [h]labour and travail: for labouring night and day, because we would not be chargeable unto any of you, we preached unto you the [i]gospel of God.

10 Ye *are* witnesses, and God *also*, how holily and justly and unblameably we behaved ourselves among you that believe:

11 As ye know how we exhorted and comforted and charged every one of you, as a father *doth* his children,

12 That ye would walk [j]worthy of God, [k]who hath called you unto his kingdom and glory.

13 For this cause also thank we God without ceasing, because, when ye received the word of God which ye heard of us, ye received *it* not *as* the word of men, but as it is in truth, the word of God, which effectually [l]worketh also in you that believe.

14 For ye, brethren, became [m]followers of the [n]churches of God which in Judaea are in Christ Jesus: for ye also have suffered like things of your own countrymen, even as they *have* of the Jews:

15 Who both killed the Lord Jesus, and [o]their own prophets, and have persecuted us; and they please not God, and are contrary to all men:

16 [p]Forbidding us to speak to the Gentiles that they might be [q]saved, to fill up their [r]sins alway: for the wrath is come upon them to the uttermost.

17 But we, brethren, being taken from you for a short time in presence, not in heart, endeavoured the more abundantly to see your face with great desire.

18 Wherefore we would have come unto you, even I Paul, once and again; but [s]Satan hindered us.

19 For what *is* our hope, or joy, or [t]crown of rejoicing? *Are* not even ye [u]in the presence [v]of our Lord Jesus Christ [w]at his coming?

20 For ye are our glory and joy.

CHAPTER 3.

Part III. The model brother, and the believer's sanctification.

Wherefore when we could no longer forbear, we thought it good to be left at Athens alone;

2 And sent [x]Timotheus, our brother, and minister of God, and our fellowlabourer in the [y]gospel of Christ, to establish you, and to comfort you concerning your faith:

3 [z]That no man should be moved by these afflictions: for yourselves know that [aa]we are appointed thereunto.

4 For verily, when we were with you, we told you before that we should suffer tribulation; even as it came to pass, and ye know.

5 For this cause, [bb]when I could no longer forbear, I sent to know your faith, [cc]lest by some means the tempter have [dd]tempted you, and our labour [ee]be in vain.

6 But now when Timotheus came from you unto us, and brought us good tidings of your faith and [ff]charity, and that ye have good remembrance of us always, [gg]desiring greatly to see us, as we also *to see* you:

7 Therefore, brethren, we were [hh]comforted over you in all our affliction and distress by your faith:

8 For now we live, if ye stand [ii]fast in the Lord.

9 For what thanks can we render to God again for you, for all the joy wherewith we joy for your sakes before our God;

10 Night and day [jj]praying exceedingly that we might see your face, and might [kk]perfect that which is lacking in your faith?

11 Now God himself and our Father,

A.D. 54.

a Acts 16:12.
b Acts 17:2, 3.
c 2 Pet. 1:16.
d 2 Cor. 2:17.
e John. 5:41, 44; Gal. 1:10.
f *her own.*
g Rom. 1:11.
h Acts 20:34, 35; 2 Thes. 3:7, 8.
i *Gospel.* vs. 4, 8, 9; 1 Thes. 3:2. (Gen. 12:1-3; Rev. 14:6.)
j Eph. 4:1.
k 1 Cor. 1:9; 2 Thes. 2:14; 2 Tim. 1:9.
l Jas. 1:18; 1 Pet. 1:23.
m *imitators.*
n *Churches (local).* 2 Thes. 1:1, 4. (Acts 2:41; Phil. 1:1.)
o Acts 7:52.
p Acts 17:5, 13; 18:12.
q Rom. 1:16, *note.*
r *Sin.* Rom. 3:23, *note.*
s *Satan.* 2 Thes. 2:9. (Gen. 3:1; Rev. 20:10.)
t *Rewards.* 2 Tim. 4:8. (Dan. 12:3; 1 Cor. 3:14.)
u 2 Cor. 1:14; Phil. 4:1.
v Jude 24.
w *Christ (Second Advent).* 1 Thes. 3:13. (Deut. 30:3; Acts 1:9-11.)
x Acts 17:15.
y *Gospel.* 2 Thes. 1:8. (Gen. 12:1-3; Rev. 14:6.)
z Eph. 3:13.
aa John 16:2; 1 Cor. 4:9; 2 Tim. 3:12; 1 Pet. 2:21.
bb v. 1.
cc 2 Cor. 11:2, 3.
dd *Temptation.* 1 Tim. 6:9. (Gen. 3:1; Jas. 1:14.)
ee Gal. 4:11.
ff *love.*
gg Phil. 1:8.
hh 2 Cor. 7:6, 7.
ii Eph. 6:13, 14; Phil. 4:1.
jj *Bible prayers (N.T.).* 2 Thes. 1:11, 12. (Mt. 6:9; Rev. 22:20.)
kk Mt. 5:48, *note.*

and our Lord Jesus Christ, [a]direct our way
unto you.
12 And the Lord make you to increase
and abound [b]in love one toward another, and toward all *men*, even as we *do*
toward you:
13 To the end he may stablish [c]your
hearts unblameable in holiness before
God, even our Father, [d]at the coming of
our Lord Jesus Christ with all his saints.

CHAPTER 4.

Part IV. The model walk, and the believer's hope.

Furthermore then we [e]beseech you,
brethren, and [f]exhort *you* by the Lord
Jesus, that as ye have received of us how
ye ought [g]to walk and to please God, *so*
ye would [h]abound more and more.
2 For ye know what commandments
we gave you by the Lord Jesus.
3 For this is the will of God, *even* your
sanctification, [i]that ye should abstain
from fornication:
4 That every one of you should know
how to possess his vessel in sanctification and honour;
5 Not in the lust of concupiscence, even
as the [j]Gentiles which know not God:
6 That no *man* go beyond and [k]defraud
his brother [l]in *any* matter: because that
the Lord *is* the avenger of all such, as we
also have forewarned you and testified.
7 For God hath not called us unto
uncleanness, [m]but unto holiness.
8 He therefore that [n]despiseth,
despiseth not man, but God, who hath
also given unto us his [o]holy Spirit.
9 But as touching brotherly love ye
need not that I write unto you: for ye
yourselves are [p]taught of God to love
one another.
10 And indeed ye do it toward all the
brethren which are in all Macedonia: but
we beseech you, brethren, that ye
increase more and more;
11 And that ye study to be quiet, and
[q]to do your own business, and to work
with your own hands, as we commanded
you;
12 That ye may walk [r]honestly toward
them that are without, and *that* ye may
have lack of nothing.
13 But I would not have you to be
ignorant, brethren, concerning them
which are [s]asleep, that ye sorrow not,
even as others which have no hope.
14 For if we [t]believe that Jesus died and
[u]rose again, even so [v]them also which
sleep in Jesus will God bring with him.
15 For this we say unto you by the
word of the Lord, that we which are
alive *and* remain unto the coming of the
Lord shall not [w]prevent them which are
asleep.
16 [x]For the Lord himself shall descend
from heaven with a shout, with the voice
of the archangel, and with the trump of
God: and the dead in Christ [y]shall rise
first:
17 [z]Then we which are alive *and*
remain shall be [1]caught up together
[aa]with them in the clouds, to meet the
Lord in the air: and so shall we ever [bb]be
with the Lord.
18 Wherefore comfort one another
with these words.

CHAPTER 5.

Part V. The model walk, and the day of Jehovah. (Cf. Rev. 19:11-21, *note.*)

But of the times and the seasons,
brethren, ye have no need that I
write unto you.
2 For yourselves know perfectly that
the [cc]day of the Lord [dd]so cometh as a
thief in the night.
3 For when they shall say, Peace and
safety; then [ee]sudden destruction cometh
upon them, as travail upon a woman
with child; and they shall not escape.
4 But [ff]ye, brethren, are not in darkness, that that day should overtake you
as a thief.
5 Ye are all [gg]the children of light, and
the children of the day: we are not of the
night, nor of darkness.
6 [hh]Therefore let us not sleep, as *do*
others; but let us watch and be [ii]sober.
7 For they that sleep sleep in the night;
and they that be drunken are drunken in
the night.
8 But let us, who are of the day, be
sober, putting on the [jj]breastplate of
faith and love; and for an helmet, the
hope of [kk]salvation.
9 For God hath not appointed us to

A.D. 54.

a Or, *guide.*
b John 13:34-35; 1 John 4:7, 12.
c 2 Thes. 2:17; 1 John 3:20.
d *Christ (Second Advent).* 1 Thes. 4:14-17. (Deut. 30:3; Acts 1:9-11.)
e Or, *request.*
f Or, *beseech.*
g Col. 1:10.
h 1 Cor. 15:58.
i 1 Cor. 6:15, 18.
j Eph. 4:17, 18.
k Or, *oppress,* or, *overreach.*
l Or, *in the.*
m Lev. 11:44; Heb. 12:14; 1 Pet. 1:14, 16.
n Or, *rejecteth.*
o *Holy Spirit.* 1 Thes. 5:19. (Mt. 1:18; Acts 2:4.)
p John 15:12, 17.
q 1 Pet. 4:15.
r 1 Pet. 2:12
s *fallen asleep.*
t *Faith.* 2 Thes. 2:11, 12. (Gen. 3:20; Heb. 11:39.)
u *Resurrection.* vs. 13-17; 2 Tim. 2:18. (Job 9:25; 1 Cor. 15:52.)
v 1 Cor. 15:20.
w *precede.*
x *Christ (Second Advent)* vs. 14-17; 1 Cor. 15:23, 51, 52. (Deut. 30:3; Acts 1:9-11.)
y Rev. 20:5, 6.
z 1 Cor. 15:51.
aa *Church (true).* Heb. 12:23. (Mt. 16:18; Heb. 12:23.)
bb John 14:3.
cc *Day (of Jehovah).* vs. 1-3; 2 Thes. 2:1-8. (Isa. 2:10-22; Rev. 19:11-21.)
dd Lk. 12:39, 40; 2 Pet. 3:10; Rev. 16:15.
ee Gen. 7:11; Mt. 24:27; Lk. 17:26, 27; 2 Pet. 2:5; 3:6.
ff Eph. 5:8; 1 John 2:8.
gg *sons.*
hh Mt. 25:5; Rom. 13:12, 13.
ii 1 Pet. 5:8.
jj Isa. 59:17; Eph. 6:14, 17.
kk Rom. 1:16, *note.*

[1] **(4:17)** Not church saints only, but all bodies of the saved, of whatever dispensation, are included in the first resurrection (see 1 Cor. 15:52, *note*), as here described, but it is peculiarly the "blessed hope" of the Church (cf. Mt. 24:42; 25:13; Lk. 12:36-48; Acts 1:11; Phil. 3:20, 21; Tit. 2:11-13).

wrath, but to obtain [a]salvation by our
Lord Jesus Christ,
10 Who died for us, that, [b]whether we
wake or sleep, we should live together
with him.
11 Wherefore comfort yourselves
together, and edify one another, even as
also ye do.
12 And we beseech you, brethren, to
know [c]them which labour among you,
and are over you in the Lord, and
admonish you;
13 And to esteem them very highly in
love for their work's sake. *And* [d]be at
peace among yourselves.
14 Now we [e]exhort you, brethren,
warn them that are unruly, comfort the
feebleminded, support the [f]weak, be
[g]patient toward all *men*.
15 See that none [h]render evil for evil
unto any *man*; but ever follow that
which is good, both among yourselves,
and to all *men*.
16 Rejoice evermore.
17 Pray without ceasing.

18 In every thing give thanks: for this
is the will of God in Christ Jesus concerning you.
19 Quench not the [i]Spirit.
20 Despise not prophesyings.
21 Prove all things; hold fast that
which is good.
22 Abstain from [j]all appearance of
evil.
23 And the very God of peace [k]sancti-
fy you wholly; and *I pray God* your
[1]whole spirit and soul and body be preserved [l]blameless unto the coming of
our Lord Jesus Christ.
24 Faithful *is* [m]he that calleth you,
who also will do *it*.
25 Brethren, pray for us.
26 Greet all the brethren with an holy
kiss.
27 I [n]charge you by the Lord that this
epistle be read unto all the holy
brethren.
28 The grace of our Lord Jesus Christ
be with you. Amen.

A.D. 54.

a Rom. 1:16, *note.*
b Rom. 14:8, 9; 2 Cor. 5:15.
c Heb. 13:7, 17.
d Mk. 9:50.
e *beseech.*
f Rom. 15:1.
g Eph. 4:2.
h Prov. 20:22; 24:29; Mt. 5:39, 44.
i *Holy Spirit.* 2 Thes. 2:13. (Mt. 1:18; Acts 2:4.)
j *every form of.*
k *Sanctify, holy (persons)* (N.T.). 1 Tim. 4:5. (Mt. 4:5; Rev. 22:11.)
l 1 Cor. 1:8, 9.
m 1 Cor. 10:13; 2 Thes. 3:3.
n *adjure.*

[1](5:23) Man a trinity. That the human soul and spirit are not identical is proved by the facts that they are divisible (Heb. 4:12), and that soul and spirit are sharply distinguished in the burial and resurrection of the body. It is sown a natural body (*soma psuchikon* = "soul-body"), it is raised a spiritual body (*soma pneumatikon*), 1 Cor. 15:44. To assert, therefore, that there is no difference between soul and spirit is to assert that there is no difference between the mortal body and the resurrection body. In Scripture use, the distinction between spirit and soul may be traced. Briefly, that distinction is that the spirit is that part of man which "knows" (1 Cor. 2:11), his mind; the soul is the seat of the *affections, desires,* and so of the *emotions,* and of the active *will,* the self. "My soul is exceeding *sorrowful*" (Mt. 26:38; see also Mt. 11:29; and John 12:27). The word translated "soul" in the O.T. (*nephesh*) is the exact equivalent of the N.T. word for soul (Gr. *psuche*), and the use of "soul" in the O.T. is identical with the use of that word in the N.T. (see, e.g. Deut. 6:5; 14:26; 1 Sam. 18:1; 20:4, 17; Job 7:11, 15; 14:22; Psa. 42:6; 84:2). The N.T. word for spirit (*pneuma*), like the O.T. *ruach,* is trans. "air," "breath," "wind," but predominantly "spirit," whether of God (e.g. Gen. 1:2; Mt. 3:16) or of man (Gen. 41:8; 1 Cor. 5:5). Because man is "spirit" he is capable of God-consciousness, and of communication with God (Job 32:8; Psa. 18:28; Prov. 20:27); because he is "soul" he has self-consciousness (Psa. 13:2; 42:5, 6, 11); because he is "body" he has, through his senses, world-consciousness. See Gen. 1:26, *note*.

THE SECOND EPISTLE OF PAUL THE APOSTLE TO THE
THESSALONIANS

WRITER. The Apostle Paul (1:1).

Date. Second Thessalonians was evidently written very soon after Paul's first letter to that church. The occasion may well have been the return of the bearer of the former Epistle, and his report.

Theme. The theme of Second Thessalonians is, unfortunately, obscured by a mistranslation in the A.V. of 2:2, where "day of Christ is at hand" (1 Cor. 1:8, *note*) should be, "day of the LORD is now present" (Isa. 2:12, *refs.*). The Thessalonian converts were "shaken in mind" and "troubled," supposing, perhaps on the authority of a forged letter as from Paul, that the persecutions from which they were suffering were those of the "great and terrible day of the LORD," from which they had been taught to expect deliverance by "the day of Christ, and our gathering together unto him" (2:1).

The present letter, then, was written to instruct the Thessalonians concerning the day of Christ, "and our gathering together unto him" (1 Thes. 4:14-17) and the relation of the "day of Christ" to the "day of the LORD." First Thessalonians had more in view the "day of Christ"; the present Epistle the "day of the LORD."

The Epistle is in five divisions: I. Salutation, 1:1-4. II. Comfort, 1:5-12. III, Instruction concerning the day of the LORD and the man of sin, 2:1-12. IV. Exhortations and apostolic commands, 2:13–3:15. V. Benediction and authentication, 3:16-18.

CHAPTER 1.

Part I. Salutation.

Paul, and Silvanus, and Timotheus,
[a]unto the church of the Thessalonians in God our Father and the Lord
Jesus Christ:
2 Grace unto you, and peace, from
God our Father and the Lord Jesus
Christ.
3 We are bound to thank God always
for you, brethren, as it is meet, because
that your faith groweth exceedingly, and
the [b]charity of every one of you all
toward each other aboundeth;
4 So that we ourselves [c]glory in you in
the [d]churches of God for your patience
and faith in all your persecutions and
tribulations that ye [e]endure:

Part II. Comfort in persecution.

5 [f]*Which is* a manifest token of the
righteous judgment of God, that ye may
be counted worthy of the kingdom of
God, for which ye also [g]suffer:
6 [h]Seeing *it is* a righteous thing with
God to recompense tribulation to them
that trouble you;
7 And to you who are troubled rest
with us, when the Lord Jesus [i]shall be
revealed from heaven with [j]his mighty
[k]angels,
8 In flaming fire taking [l]vengeance on
them that know not God, and that obey
not the [m]gospel of our Lord Jesus Christ:
9 Who shall be punished with everlasting [n]destruction from the presence of
the Lord, and from [o]the glory of his
power;
10 When he shall come [p]to be glorified
in his saints, and to be admired in all
them that believe (because our testimony among you was believed) in that day.
11 Wherefore also we [q]pray always for
you, that our God would [r]count you
worthy of *this* calling, and fulfil all the
good pleasure of *his* goodness, and the
work of faith with power:
12 [s]That the name of our Lord Jesus
Christ may be glorified in you, and ye in
him, according to the [t]grace of our God
and the Lord Jesus Christ.

CHAPTER 2.

Part III. The day of the LORD
and the man of sin.

Now we beseech you, brethren, by
the coming of our Lord Jesus
Christ, and *by* our gathering together
unto him,
2 That ye be not soon shaken in
mind, or be troubled, neither by

A.D. 54.

a 1 Thes. 1:1.
b *love.*
c 2 Cor. 9:2.
d *Churches (local).* vs. 1, 4; 1 Tim. 3:5, 15, 16. (Acts 2:41; Phil. 1:1.)
e Jas. 5:11.
f Phil. 1:28.
g 1 Thes. 2:14; Heb. 10:32, 33.
h Rev. 6:10.
i *Christ (Second Advent).* vs. 7-10; 2 Thes. 2:8. (Deut. 30:3; Acts 1:9-11.)
j *the angels of his might.*
k Heb. 1:4, *note.*
l *Day (of destruction).* vs. 7-10; Rev. 19:19, 20. (Job 21:30; Rev. 20:11-15.)
m *Gospel.* 2 Thes. 2:14. (Gen. 12:1-3; Rev. 14:6.)
n Phil. 3:19; 2 Pet. 3:7.
o Isa. 2:19.
p Mt. 25:31.
q *Bible prayers (N.T.).* 2 Thes. 2:16, 17. (Mt. 6:9; Rev. 22:20.)
r Col. 1:12; Rev. 3:4.
s 1 Pet. 1:7.
t *Grace (imparted).* 2 Tim. 2:1. (Rom. 6:1; 2 Pet. 3:18.)

spirit, nor by word, nor by letter as from
us, as that the [a]day of Christ is [b]at hand.
3 Let no man deceive you by any
means: [1]for *that day shall not come*, except
there come [c]a falling away first, and that
[d]man of sin be revealed, the son of
perdition;
4 Who opposeth and exalteth himself
above all that is called God, or that is
worshipped; so that he as God sitteth in
the temple of God, shewing himself that
he is God.
5 Remember ye not, that, when I was
yet with you, I told you these things?
6 And now ye know [e]what withholdeth that he might be revealed in his time.
7 For the [f]mystery of [g]iniquity doth
already work: only he who now [h]letteth
will [i]*let*, until he be taken out of the way.
8 And then shall [j]that [k]Wicked be
revealed, [l]whom the Lord shall consume
with the spirit of his mouth, and shall
destroy [m]with the brightness of his coming:
9 *Even him*, whose coming is after the
working of [n]Satan with all power and
signs and lying wonders,
10 And with all deceivableness of
unrighteousness in them that perish;
because they received not [o]the love of
the truth, that they might be [p]saved.
11 And for this cause God shall send
them strong delusion, that they should
believe a lie:
12 That they all might be [q]damned
who [r]believed not the truth, but had
pleasure in [s]unrighteousness.

Part IV. Exhortation and instruction
(to 3:15).

13 But we are bound to give thanks
alway to God for you, brethren beloved
of the Lord, because God hath from the
beginning [t]chosen you to [u]salvation
through sanctification of the [v]Spirit and
belief of the truth:
14 Whereunto he called you by our

A.D. 54.

a *Day of the LORD.* See Isa. 2:12, *ref.*
b *now present.*
c *the apostasy.*
d Or, *lawless one.*
e Or, *that which restrains.*
f Mt. 13:11, *note.*
g *lawlessness.*
h *hindereth.*
i *hinder.*
j *The Beast.* vs. 3-8: Rev. 13:1-8. (Dan. 7:8; Rev. 19:20.)
k *Lawless one.*
l *Day (of Jehovah).* vs. 1-8; 2 Pet. 3:10. (Isa. 2:10-22; Rev. 19:11-21.)
m *Christ (Second Advent).* 1 Tim. 6:14, 15. (Deut. 30:3; Acts 1:9-11.)
n *Satan.* 1 Tim. 1:20. (Gen. 3:1; Rev. 20:10.)
o 1 Cor. 16:22.
p Rom. 1:16, *note.*
q *judged.*
r *Faith.* vs. 11, 12; 2 Tim. 1:12. (Gen. 3:20; Heb. 11:39.)
s *Apostasy.* 1 Tim. 4:1-3. (Lk. 18:8; 2 Tim. 3:1-8.)
t *Election (corporate).* 2 Tim. 2:10. (Deut. 7:6; 1 Pet. 1:2.)
u Rom. 1:16, *note.*
v *Holy Spirit.* 1 Tim. 3:16. (Mt. 1:18; Acts 2:4.)
w *Gospel.* 1 Tim. 1:11. (Gen. 12:1-3; Rev. 14:6.)
x Rom. 6:17; Jude 3.
y *Bible prayers* (N.T.). 2 Thes. 3:5. (Mt. 6:9; Rev. 22:20.)
z *Grace (in salv.).* 1 Tim. 1:14, 15. (Rom. 3:24; John 1:17, *note.*)
aa *Bible prayers* (N.T.). Heb. 13:20, 21. (Mt. 6:9; Rev. 22:20.)

[w]gospel, to the obtaining of the glory of
our Lord Jesus Christ.
15 Therefore, brethren, stand fast, and
hold the [x]traditions which ye have been
taught, whether by word, or our epistle.
16 [y]Now our Lord Jesus Christ himself, and God, even our Father, which
hath loved us, and hath given *us* everlasting consolation and good hope
[z]through grace,
17 Comfort your hearts, and stablish
you in every good word and work.

CHAPTER 3.

Finally, brethren, pray for us, that the
word of the Lord may have *free*
course, and be glorified, even as *it is*
with you:
2 And that we may be delivered from
unreasonable and wicked men: for all
men have not faith.
3 But the Lord is faithful, who shall
stablish you, and keep *you* from evil.
4 And we have confidence in the Lord
touching you, that ye both do and will
do the things which we command you.
5 And the [aa]Lord direct your hearts
into the love of God, and into the patient
waiting for Christ.
6 Now we command you, brethren, in
the name of our Lord Jesus Christ, that ye
withdraw yourselves from every brother
that walketh disorderly, and not after the
tradition which he received of us.
7 For yourselves know how ye ought
to follow us: for we behaved not ourselves disorderly among you;
8 Neither did we eat any man's bread
for nought; but wrought with labour
and travail night and day, that we might
not be chargeable to any of you:
9 Not because we have not power, but
to make ourselves an ensample unto you
to follow us.
10 For even when we were with you,
this we commanded you, that if any
would not work, neither should he eat.

[1] **(2:3)** The order of events is: (1) The working of the mystery of lawlessness under divine restraint which had already begun in the apostle's time (v. 7); (2) the apostasy of the professing church (v. 3; Lk. 18:8; 2 Tim. 3:1-8); (3) the removal of that which restrains the mystery of lawlessness (vs. 6, 7). The restrainer is a person—"he," and since a "mystery" always implies a supernatural element (Mt. 13:11, *note*), this Person can be no other than the Holy Spirit in the church, to be "taken out of the way" (v. 7; 1 Thes. 4:14-17); (4) the manifestation of the lawless one (vs. 8-10; Dan. 7:8; 9:27; Mt. 24:15; Rev. 13:2-10); (5) the coming of Christ in glory and the destruction of the lawless one (v. 8; Rev. 19:11-21); (6) the day of Jehovah (vs. 9-12; Isa. 2:12, *refs.*).

11 For we hear that there are some
which walk among you disorderly,
working not at all, but are [a]busybodies.
12 Now them that are such we command and exhort by our Lord Jesus
Christ, that with quietness they [b]work,
and eat their own bread.
13 But ye, brethren, [c]be not weary in
well doing.
14 And if any man obey not our word
by this epistle, note that man, and [d]have
no company with him, that he may be
ashamed.

A.D. 54.

a 1 Tim. 5:13; 1 Pet. 4:15.
b Eph. 4:28; 1 Thes. 4:11-12.
c 1 Cor. 15:58; Jas. 5:7, 11.
d *Separation.* vs. 6, 14; 1 Tim. 6:3-11. (Gen. 12:1; 2 Cor. 6:14-17.)
e Lev. 19:17.
f John 14:27.
g 1 Cor. 16:21.
h Rom. 16:24.

15 Yet count *him* not as an enemy, but
admonish *him* [e]as a brother.

Part V. Benediction and subscription.

16 Now the [f]Lord of peace himself
give you peace always by all means. The
Lord *be* with you all.
17 The [g]salutation of Paul with mine
own hand, which is the token in every
epistle: so I write.
18 The [h]grace of our Lord Jesus Christ
be with you all. Amen.

THE FIRST EPISTLE OF PAUL THE APOSTLE TO
TIMOTHY

WRITER. The Apostle Paul, (1:1).

Date. The date of this Epistle turns upon the question of the two imprisonments of Paul. If there were two (see Acts 28:30, *note*), then it is clear that First Timothy was written during the interval. If Paul endured but one Roman imprisonment, the Epistle was written shortly before Paul's last journey to Jerusalem.

Theme. As the churches of Christ increased in number, the questions of church order, of soundness in the faith, and of discipline became important. At first the apostles regulated these things directly, but the approaching end of the apostolic period made it necessary that a clear revelation should be made for the guidance of the churches. Such a revelation is in First Timothy, and in Titus. The key-phrase of this Epistle is, "That thou mayest know how thou oughtest to behave thyself in the house of God." Well had it been with the churches if they had neither added to nor taken from the divine order.

The divisions are five: I. Legality and unsound doctrine rebuked, 1:1-20. II. Prayer and the divine order of the sexes enjoined, 2:1-15. III. The qualifications of elders and deacons, 3:1-16. IV. The walk of the "good minister," 4:1-16. V. The work of the "good minister," 5:1–6:21.

CHAPTER 1.

Part I. Legalism and unsound teaching rebuked.

Paul, an apostle of Jesus Christ by the commandment of God our [a]Saviour, and [b]Lord Jesus Christ, *which is* our hope;

2 Unto Timothy, *my* [c]own son in the faith: Grace, mercy, *and* peace, from God our Father and [d]Jesus Christ our Lord.

3 As I besought thee to abide still at Ephesus, when I [e]went into Macedonia, that thou mightest charge some that they teach no other doctrine,

4 Neither give [f]heed to fables and endless genealogies, which minister questions, rather than godly edifying which is in faith: *so do.*

5 Now [g]the end of the commandment is [h]charity out of a [i]pure heart, and *of* a good conscience, and *of* faith unfeigned:

6 From which some [j]having swerved have turned aside unto vain jangling;

7 Desiring to be teachers of the law; understanding neither what they say, nor whereof they affirm.

8 But we know that the law *is* [k]good, if a man use it lawfully;

9 Knowing this, that the [l]law is not made for a righteous man, but for the lawless and disobedient, for the ungodly and for sinners, for unholy and profane, for [m]murderers of fathers and murderers of mothers, for manslayers,

10 For whoremongers, for them that defile themselves with mankind, for menstealers, for liars, for perjured persons, and if there be any other thing that is contrary to [n]sound doctrine;

11 According to the [o]glorious [p]gospel of the [q]blessed God, which was [r]committed to my trust.

12 And I thank Christ Jesus our Lord, who hath [s]enabled me, for that he counted me [t]faithful, [u]putting me into the ministry;

13 Who was [v]before a blasphemer, and a persecutor, and injurious: but I obtained mercy, because I did *it* [w]ignorantly in unbelief.

14 And the grace of our Lord was exceeding abundant with faith and love which is in Christ Jesus.

15 This *is* a [x]faithful saying, and worthy of all acceptation, that Christ Jesus came into the [y]world to [z]save [aa]sinners; of whom I am chief.

16 Howbeit for this cause I obtained mercy, that in me first Jesus Christ might shew forth all longsuffering, for a [bb]pattern to them which should hereafter believe on him to [cc]life everlasting.

17 Now unto the King eternal, [dd]immortal, [ee]invisible, the only wise

A.D. 65.

- a Rom. 1:16, *note.*
- b *Christ Jesus our hope.*
- c *true child.*
- d *Christ Jesus.*
- e Acts 20:1, 3.
- f 1 Tim. 6:3, 4, 20.
- g Rom. 13:8, 10; Gal. 5:14.
- h *love.*
- i Eph. 6:24.
- j 2 Tim. 4:10.
- k Rom. 7:12.
- l *Law (of Moses).* vs. 8, 9; Heb. 7:19. (Ex. 19:1; Gal. 3:1-29.)
- m *smiters.*
- n 2 Cor. 2:17.
- o *gospel of the glory.*
- p *Gospel.* 2 Tim. 1:8, 10. (Gen. 12:1-3; Rev. 14:6.)
- q 1 Tim. 6:15.
- r 1 Cor. 9:17.
- s 1 Cor. 15:10.
- t 1 Cor. 7:25.
- u Col. 1:25.
- v Acts 8:3; 1 Cor. 15:9.
- w Lk. 23:34.
- x John 3:16, 17.
- y *kosmos* (Mt. 4:8) = mankind.
- z Rom. 1:16, *note.*
- aa *Grace (in salv.).* vs. 14, 15; 2 Tim. 1:9. (Rom. 3:24; John 1:17, *note.*)
- bb Rom. 15:4.
- cc *Life (eternal).* 1 Tim. 4:8. (Mt. 7:14; Rev. 22:19.)
- dd *Incorruptible.*
- ee Cf. John 1:18, *note.*

God, *be* honour and glory for ever and ever. Amen.

18 This charge I commit unto thee, [a]son Timothy, according to the prophecies which went before on thee, that thou by them mightest war [b]a good warfare;

19 Holding faith, and a good conscience; which some having put away concerning faith have made shipwreck:

20 Of whom is [1c]Hymenaeus and Alexander; whom I have [d]delivered unto [e]Satan, that they may learn not to blaspheme.

CHAPTER 2.

Part II. Prayer, and the divine order of the sexes.

I exhort therefore, that, first of all, supplications, prayers, intercessions, *and* giving of thanks, be made for all men;

2 For [f]kings, and *for* all that are in authority; that we may lead a quiet and peaceable life in all godliness and [g]honesty.

3 For this *is* good and acceptable in the sight of God our [h]Saviour;

4 [i]Who will have all men to be [j]saved, and to come unto the knowledge of the truth.

5 For *there is* one God, and one mediator between God and men, the man Christ Jesus;

6 Who gave himself a [k]ransom for all, to be testified in due time.

7 Whereunto I am ordained a preacher, and an apostle, (I speak the truth in Christ, *and* lie not;) a teacher of the Gentiles in faith and verity.

8 I will therefore that [l]men pray every where, lifting up holy hands, without wrath and doubting.

9 In like manner also, that women adorn themselves in modest apparel, with shamefacedness and sobriety; not with [m]broided hair, or gold, or pearls, or costly array;

10 But (which becometh women professing godliness) with good works.

11 Let the [n]woman learn in [o]silence with all [p]subjection.

12 But I suffer not a woman to teach, nor to usurp authority over the man, but to be in [q]silence.

13 For Adam was first formed, then Eve.

14 And Adam was not deceived, but the woman being deceived was in the [r]transgression.

15 Notwithstanding she shall be [s]saved in childbearing, if they continue in faith and [t]charity and holiness with sobriety.

CHAPTER 3.

Part III. The qualifications of elders and deacons.

This *is* a true saying, If a man desire the office of a [u]bishop, he desireth a good work.

2 [v]A [w]bishop then must be blameless, the husband of one wife, [x]vigilant, sober, of good behaviour, given to hospitality, apt to teach;

3 Not given to wine, no striker, not greedy of filthy lucre; but [y]patient, not a brawler, not covetous;

4 One that ruleth [z]well his own house, having his children in subjection with all gravity;

5 (For if a man know not how to rule his own house, how shall he take care of the church of God?)

6 Not a novice, lest being [aa]lifted up with pride he fall into the condemnation of the [bb]devil.

7 Moreover he must have a good report of [cc]them which are without; lest he fall into reproach and the [dd]snare of the [ee]devil.

8 Likewise *must* the [ff]deacons *be* grave, not doubletongued, not given to much wine, not greedy of filthy lucre;

9 Holding the [gg]mystery of the faith in a pure conscience.

10 And let these also first be proved; then let them use the office of a deacon, being *found* blameless.

11 [hh]Even so *must their* wives *be* grave, not slanderers, sober, faithful in all things.

12 Let the deacons be the husbands of one wife, [ii]ruling their children and their own houses well.

13 For they that have [jj]used the office of a deacon [kk]well purchase to themselves a good degree, and great boldness in the faith which is in Christ Jesus.

14 These things write I unto thee, hoping to come unto thee shortly:

A.D. 65.

a *child.*
b *the.*
c 2 Tim. 2:17, 18.
d *Judgments (the seven).* 2 Tim. 4:1. (2 Sam. 7:14; Rev. 20:12.)
e *Satan.* 1 Tim. 3:6, 7. (Gen. 3:1; Rev. 20:10.)
f Rom. 13:1.
g *gravity.*
h Rom. 1:16, *note.*
i John 3:15, 16; 2 Pet. 3:9.
j Rom. 1:16, *note.*
k Mt. 20:28.
l *the men.*
m Or, *plaited.* 1 Pet. 3:3.
n 1 Cor. 14:34.
o *quietness.* 1 Cor. 14:34.
p Cf. Gen. 3:16.
q *quietness.*
r *Sin.* Rom. 3:23, *note.*
s *preserved.*
t *love.*
u *an overseer.*
v *an overseer.*
w *Elders.* 1 Tim. 5:1, 17, 19. (Acts 11:30; Tit. 1:5-9.)
x *discreet.*
y 2 Tim. 2:24,
z Psa. 101:2.
aa Prov. 16:18.
bb Jude 6.
cc Acts 22:12.
dd I Tim. 6:9; 2 Tim. 2:26.
ee *Satan.* 1 Tim. 5:15. (Gen. 3:1; Rev. 20:10.)
ff Acts 6:3.
gg v. 16; Mt. 13:11, *note.*
hh Or, *Women in like manner must.*
ii v. 4.
jj Or, *ministered.*
kk Mt. 25:21.

[1] **(1:20)** It is significant as bearing upon the seriousness of all false teaching, and particularly as related to resurrection, that Paul calls it blasphemy to teach that "the resurrection is past already" (2 Tim. 2:17, 18).

15 But if I tarry long, that thou mayest know how thou oughtest to behave thyself [a]in the house of God, which is the [1b]church [c]of the living God, the pillar and ground of the truth.

16 And without controversy great is the [d]mystery of godliness: God was manifest in the flesh, justified in the [e]Spirit, seen of [f]angels, preached unto the Gentiles, believed on in the [g]world, received up into glory.

CHAPTER 4.

Part IV. The walk of a "good minister of Jesus Christ."

Now the [h]Spirit [i]speaketh expressly, that in the latter times some shall [j]depart from the faith, giving heed to seducing spirits, and doctrines of [k]devils;

2 Speaking lies in hypocrisy; having their conscience seared with a hot iron;

3 Forbidding to marry, *and commanding* to abstain from meats, which God hath created to be received with thanksgiving of them which believe and know the truth.

4 For every creature of God *is* good, and nothing to be refused, if it be received with thanksgiving:

5 For it is [l]sanctified by the word of God and prayer.

6 If thou put the brethren in remembrance of these things, thou shalt be a good minister of [m]Jesus Christ, nourished up in the words of [n]faith and of good doctrine, whereunto thou hast attained.

7 But refuse profane and old wives' fables, and exercise thyself *rather* unto godliness.

8 For bodily exercise profiteth [o]little: but godliness is profitable unto all things, having promise of the life that now is, and of [p]that which is to come.

9 This *is* a faithful saying and worthy of all acceptation.

10 For therefore we both labour and suffer reproach, because we [q]trust in the living God, who is the [r]Saviour of all men, specially of those that believe.

11 These things command and teach.

12 [s]Let no man despise thy youth; but be thou an example of the believers, in word, in conversation, in [t]charity, in spirit, in faith, in purity.

13 Till I come, give attendance to reading, to exhortation, to doctrine.

14 [u]Neglect not the gift that is in thee, which was given thee by prophecy, with the [v]laying on of the hands of the presbytery.

15 Meditate upon these things; give thyself wholly to them; that thy profiting may appear to all.

16 Take heed unto thyself, and unto the doctrine; continue in them: for in doing this thou shalt both [w]save thyself, and them that hear thee.

CHAPTER 5.

Part V. The work of a "good minister of Jesus Christ."

Rebuke not an elder, but intreat *him* as a father; *and* the younger men as brethren;

2 The elder women as mothers; the younger as sisters, with all purity.

3 Honour widows that are [x]widows indeed.

4 But if any widow have children or [y]nephews, let them learn first to shew piety at home, and to requite their parents: for that is good and acceptable before God.

5 Now she that is a widow indeed, and desolate, [z]trusteth in God, and continueth in supplications and prayers night and day.

6 But she that liveth in pleasure is [aa]dead while she liveth.

7 And these things give in charge, that they may be blameless.

8 But if any provide not for his own, and [bb]specially for those of his own house, he hath denied the faith, and is worse than an [cc]infidel.

A.D. 65.

- *a* Heb. 3:6.
- *b* *Churches (local).* vs. 5, 15, 16; Phm. 2. (Acts 2:41; Phil. 1:1.)
- *c* *Church (visible).* (1 Cor. 10:32.)
- *d* Mt. 13:11, *note.*
- *e* *Holy Spirit.* 1 Tim. 4:1. (Mt. 1:18; Acts 2:4.)
- *f* Heb. 1:4, *note.*
- *g* *kosmos* (Mt. 4:8) = mankind.
- *h* *Holy Spirit.* 2 Tim. 1:7, 14. (Mt. 1:18; Acts 2:4.)
- *i* *Inspiration.* 2 Tim. 3:16. (Ex. 4:15; Rev. 22:19.)
- *j* *Apostasy.* vs. 1-3; 2 Tim. 4:3, 4. (Lk. 18:8; 2 Tim. 3:1-8.)
- *k* *demons.*
- *l* *Sanctify, holy (persons)* (N.T.). Tit. 1:8. (Mt. 4:5; Rev. 22:11.)
- *m* *Christ Jesus.*
- *n* *the faith.*
- *o* *for a little.*
- *p* *Life (eternal).* 1 Tim. 6:12, 19. (Mt. 7:14; Rev. 22:19.)
- *q* *hope.*
- *r* *Preserver.*
- *s* Tit. 2:7, 15.
- *t* *love.*
- *u* 2 Tim. 1:6.
- *v* Deut. 34:9.
- *w* Rom. 1:16, *note.*
- *x* vs. 5, 16.
- *y* *descendants.*
- *z* *hopeth.*
- *aa* Rev. 3:1.
- *bb* 2 Cor. 12:14.
- *cc* *unbeliever.*

1 **(3:15)** Church (visible), Summary: The passages under this head (1 Cor. 10:32; 1 Tim. 3:15) refer to that visible body of professed believers called, collectively, "the Church," of which history takes account as such, though it exists under many names and divisions based upon differences in doctrine or in government. Within, for the most part, this historical "Church" has existed the true Church, "which is his body, the fulness of him that filleth all in all" (Eph. 1:22, 23; Heb. 12:23, *note*), like the believing Remnant within Israel (Rom. 11:5, *note*). The predicted future of the visible Church is apostasy (Lk. 18:8; 2 Tim. 3:1-8); of the true Church, glory (Mt. 13:36-43; Rom. 8:18-23; 1 Thes. 4:14-17).

9 Let not a widow be taken into the
number under threescore years old, having been the wife of one man,
10 Well reported of for good works; if
she have brought up children, if she
have [a]lodged strangers, if she have
washed the saints' feet, if she have
relieved the afflicted, if she have diligently followed every good work.
11 But the younger widows refuse: for
when they have begun to wax wanton
against Christ, they will marry;
12 [b]Having damnation, because they
have cast off their first faith.
13 And withal they learn *to be* idle,
wandering about from house to house;
[c]and not only idle, but tattlers also and
busybodies, speaking things which they
ought not.
14 I will therefore that the younger
women marry, bear children, guide the
house, give none occasion to the adversary to speak reproachfully.
15 For some are already turned aside
after [d]Satan.
16 If any man or woman that believeth
have widows, let them relieve them, and
let not the church be charged; that it may
relieve them that are widows indeed.
17 [e]Let the elders that rule well be
counted worthy of double honour, especially they who labour in the word and
doctrine.
18 For the scripture saith, [f]Thou shalt
not muzzle the ox that treadeth out the
corn. [g]And, The labourer *is* worthy of
his reward.
19 Against an [h]elder receive not an
accusation, but [i]before two or three witnesses.
20 Them that [j]sin rebuke before all,
that others also may fear.
21 I [k]charge *thee* before God, and the
Lord Jesus Christ, and the elect [l]angels,
that thou observe these things without
[m]preferring [n]one before another, doing
nothing by partiality.
22 [o]Lay hands suddenly on no man,
neither be partaker of other men's [j]sins:
keep thyself pure.
23 Drink no longer [p]water, but use a
little wine for thy stomach's sake and
thine often infirmities.
24 Some men's [q]sins are [r]open beforehand, going before to judgment; and
some *men* they follow after.
25 Likewise also the good works *of*
some are manifest beforehand; and they
that are otherwise cannot be hid.

CHAPTER 6.

Part V. continued.

Let as many [s]servants as are under the
yoke count their own masters worthy of all honour, that the name of God
and *his* doctrine be not blasphemed.
2 And they that have believing masters, let them not despise *them*, because
they are brethren; but rather do *them* service, because they are faithful and
beloved, partakers of the benefit. These
things teach and exhort.
3 If any man teach otherwise, and consent not to [t]wholesome words, *even* the
words of our Lord Jesus Christ, and to the
doctrine which is [u]according to godliness;
4 He is proud, [v]knowing nothing, but
doting about questions and strifes of
words, whereof cometh envy, strife, rail-
ings, evil surmisings,
5 Perverse disputings of men of corrupt minds, and destitute of the truth,
supposing that gain is godliness: from
[w]such withdraw thyself.
6 But [x]godliness with [y]contentment is
great gain.
7 For we brought nothing into *this*
[z]world, *and it is* [aa]certain we can carry
nothing out.
8 And having food and raiment let us
be therewith [bb]content.
9 But they that [cc]will be rich fall into
[dd]temptation and a snare, and *into* many
foolish and hurtful lusts, which drown
men in destruction and perdition.
10 For the love of money is [ee]the root
of [ff]all evil: which while some coveted
after, they have erred from the faith, and
pierced themselves through with many
sorrows.
11 But thou, O man of God, [gg]flee
these things; and follow after [hh]right-
eousness, godliness, faith, love, patience,
meekness.
12 Fight the good fight of faith, lay
hold on [ii]eternal life, whereunto thou art
also called, and hast [jj]professed a good
profession before many witnesses.
13 I give thee [kk]charge in the sight of
God, who quickeneth all things, and
before Christ Jesus, [ll]who before Pontius
Pilate witnessed a good confession;
14 That thou keep *this* commandment
without spot, unrebukeable, until

A.D. 65.

a Acts 16:15.
b *being guilty.*
c 2 Thes. 3:11.
d *Satan.* 2 Tim. 2:6. (Gen. 3:1; Rev. 20:10.)
e Gal. 6:6; 1 Thes. 5:12, 13.
f Deut. 25:4; 1 Cor. 9:7, 11.
g Lk. 10:7.
h *Elders.* vs. 1, 17, 19; Jas. 5:14. (Acts 11:30; Tit. 1:5-9.)
i Deut. 19:15.
j *Sin.* Rom. 3:23, *note.*
k 2 Tim. 4:1.
l Heb. 1:4, *note.*
m Or, *prejudice.*
n Deut. 1:17.
o Acts 13:3.
p *water only.*
q *Sin.* Rom. 3:23, *note.*
r Gal. 5:19.
s Eph. 6:5.
t 2 Tim. 1:13.
u Tit. 1:1.
v 1 Cor. 8:2.
w 2 Tim. 3:5.
x Prov. 15:16.
y Heb. 13:5.
z *earth.*
aa Psa. 49:17.
bb Gen. 28:20; Prov. 30:8-9.
cc *will to be.* Prov. 28:20.
dd *Temptation.* Heb. 2:18. (Gen. 3:1; Jas. 1:14.)
ee *a root.*
ff *every.*
gg *Separation.* 2 Tim. 2:19-21. (Gen. 12:1; 2 Cor. 6:14-17.)
hh 1 John 3:7, *note.*
ii *Life (eternal).* vs. 12, 19; 2 Tim. 1:1, 10. (Mt. 7:14; Rev. 22:19.)
jj Heb. 10:23.
kk 1 Tim. 5:21.
ll John 18:36, 37.

[a]the appearing of our Lord Jesus Christ:

15 Which in his times he shall shew, *who is* [b]the blessed and only Potentate, the [c]King of kings, and Lord of lords;

16 Who only hath immortality, dwelling in the light which no man can approach unto; [d]whom no man hath seen, nor can see: to whom *be* honour and power everlasting. Amen.

17 Charge them that are rich in this [e]world, that they be not highminded, nor [f]trust in uncertain riches, but in the living God, who giveth us richly all things [g]to enjoy;

18 That they do good, that they be rich in good works, ready to distribute, willing to communicate;

19 Laying up in store for themselves a good foundation against the time to come, that they may [h]lay hold [i]on eternal life.

20 O Timothy, keep that which is committed to thy trust, [j]avoiding profane *and* vain babblings, and oppositions of [k]science falsely so called:

21 Which some professing have erred concerning the faith. Grace *be* with thee. Amen.

A.D. 65.

a *Christ (Second Advent).* Tit. 2:13. (Deut. 30:3; Acts 1:9-11.)
b 1 Tim. 1:17.
c Rev. 17:14.
d Cf. John 1:18, *note.*
e *age.*
f *hope.*
g Eccl. 5:18, 19.
h Phil. 3:14.
i *on what is really life.*
j Tit. 1:14.
k *the knowledge which is.*

THE SECOND EPISTLE OF PAUL THE APOSTLE TO

TIMOTHY

WRITER. The Apostle Paul (1:1).

Date. This touching letter was written by Paul to his "dearly beloved son" shortly before his martyrdom (4:6-8), and contains the last words of the great apostle which inspiration has preserved.

Theme. Second Timothy (in common with Second Peter, Jude, and Second and Third John) has to do with the personal walk and testimony of a true servant of Christ in a day of apostasy and declension. The key-phrases are, "All they which are in Asia be turned away from me" (1:15); and, "A good soldier of Jesus Christ" (2:3). The Asian churches had not disbanded, nor ceased to call themselves Christian, but they had turned away from the doctrines of grace distinctively revealed through the Apostle Paul (see Introduction, p. 1189). This was the proof that already the apostasy had set in in its first form, legalism.

The natural divisions are four: I. The Apostle's greeting, 1:1-18. II. The pathway of an approved servant in a day of apostasy, 2:1-26. III. Apostasy and the Word, 3:1-17. IV. A faithful servant and his faithful Lord, 4:1-22.

CHAPTER 1.

Part I. The apostolic greeting.

Paul, an apostle of Jesus Christ by the
will of God, according to the
[a]promise of life which is in Christ Jesus,
2 To Timothy, *my* dearly [b]beloved
[c]son: Grace, mercy, *and* peace, from God
the Father and Christ Jesus our Lord.
3 I thank God, whom I [d]serve from *my*
forefathers with pure [e]conscience, that
without ceasing I have remembrance of
thee in my prayers night and day;
4 Greatly [f]desiring to see thee, being
mindful of thy tears, that I may be filled
with joy;
5 When I call to remembrance the
unfeigned [g]faith that is in thee, which
dwelt first in thy grandmother Lois, and
thy [h]mother Eunice; and I am persuaded
that in thee also.
6 Wherefore I put thee in remembrance that thou stir up [i]the gift of God,
which is in thee by the putting on of my
hands.
7 For God hath not given us the spirit
of [j]fear; but of [k]power, and of love, and
of a sound mind.
8 Be not thou therefore ashamed of the
testimony of our Lord, nor of me his
prisoner: but be thou [l]partaker of the

A.D. 66.

a Tit. 1:2.
b 1 Tim. 1:2.
c *child.*
d Acts 23:1.
e Heb. 13:18.
f 2 Tim. 4:9, 21.
g 1 Tim. 4:6.
h Acts 16:1.
i 1 Tim. 4:14.
j Rom. 8:15; 1 John 4:18.
k Lk. 24:49; cf. Acts 1:8.
l Col. 1:24.
m Rom. 1:16, *note.*
n *Grace (in salv.).* Tit. 2:11. (Rom. 3:24; John 1:17, *note.*)
o i.e. *ages.*
p Rom. 1:16, *note.*
q *Life (eternal).* Tit. 1:2. (Mt. 7:14; Rev. 22:19.)
r *incorruptibility.*
s *Gospel.* vs. 8, 10; 2 Tim. 2:8. (Gen. 12:1-3; Rev. 14:6.)
t Rom. 1:16.
u *Assurance.* 2 Tim. 4:8, 18. (Isa. 32:17; Jude 1.)
v *Faith.* Heb. 4:2, 3; 10:22. (Gen. 3:20; Heb. 11:39.)
w *pattern,* or, *outline.*
x 1 Tim. 6:3.
y Holy Spirit. vs. 7, 14; Tit. 3:5. (Mt. 1:18; Acts 2:4.)
z Acts 19:10.
aa 2 Tim. 4:10, 16.

afflictions of the gospel according to the
power of God;
9 Who hath [m]saved us, and called *us*
with an holy calling, not according to
our works, but according to his own
purpose and [n]grace, which was given us
in Christ Jesus before the [o]world began,
10 But is now made manifest by the
appearing of our [p]Saviour Jesus Christ,
who hath abolished death, and hath
brought [q]life and [r]immortality to light
through the [s]gospel:
11 Whereunto I am appointed a
preacher, and an apostle, and a teacher
of the Gentiles.
12 For the which cause I also [1]suffer
these things: [t]nevertheless I am not
ashamed: for I [u]know whom I have [v]be-
lieved, and am persuaded that he is able
to keep that which I have committed
unto him against that day.
13 Hold fast the [w]form [x]of sound
words, which thou hast heard of me, in
faith and love which is in Christ Jesus.
14 That good thing which was committed unto thee keep by the [y]Holy
Ghost which dwelleth in us.
15 This thou knowest, that [z]all they
which are in Asia be [aa]turned away from
me; of whom are Phygellus and
Hermogenes.

[1] **(1:12)** The believer's resources in a day of general declension and apostasy are: (1) Faith (1:5); (2) the Spirit (1:6, 7); (3) the word of God (1:13; 3:1-17; 4:3, 4); (4) the grace of Christ (2:1); (5) separation from vessels unto dishonour (2:4, 20, 21); (6) the Lord's sure reward (4:7, 8); (7) the Lord's faithfulness and power (2:13, 19).

16 The Lord give mercy unto the house of Onesiphorus; [a]for he oft refreshed me, and was not ashamed of my [b]chain:

17 But, when he was in Rome, he sought me out very diligently, and found *me*.

18 The Lord grant unto him that he may find mercy of the Lord [c]in that day: and in how many things he [d]ministered unto me at Ephesus, thou knowest very well.

CHAPTER 2.

Part II. The path of a "good soldier" in the time of apostasy.

Thou therefore, my [e]son, be strong in the [f]grace that is in Christ Jesus.

2 And the things that thou hast heard of me among many witnesses, the same [g]commit thou to faithful men, who shall be able to teach others also.

3 Thou therefore [h]endure hardness, as a good soldier of Jesus Christ.

4 No man that [i]warreth entangleth himself with the affairs of *this* life; that he may please him who hath [j]chosen him to be a soldier.

5 And if a man also strive for masteries, *yet* is he not crowned, except he strive lawfully.

6 The husbandman [k]that laboureth must be first partaker of the fruits.

7 Consider what I say; and [l]the Lord give thee understanding in all things.

8 Remember that [m]Jesus Christ of the seed of David was raised from the dead according to my [n]gospel:

9 Wherein I suffer trouble, as an evil doer, *even* unto [o]bonds; but the word of God is not bound.

10 Therefore I endure all things for the [p]elect's sakes, that they may also obtain the [q]salvation which is in Christ Jesus with eternal glory.

11 *It is* a faithful saying: For if we [r]be dead with *him*, we shall also live with *him*:

12 If we suffer, we shall also reign with *him*: if we [s]deny *him*, he also will deny us:

13 If we [t]believe not, *yet* he abideth faithful: he [u]cannot deny himself.

14 Of these things [v]put *them* in remembrance, charging *them* before the Lord that they [w]strive not about words to no profit, *but* to the subverting of the hearers.

15 [x]Study to shew thyself approved unto God, a workman that needeth not to be ashamed, [y]rightly dividing the word of truth.

16 But shun profane *and* vain babblings: for they will increase unto more ungodliness.

17 And their word will eat as doth a canker: of whom is Hymenaeus and Philetus;

18 Who concerning the truth have [z]erred, [aa]saying that the [bb]resurrection is past already; and overthrow the faith of some.

19 Nevertheless the [cc]foundation of God standeth sure, having this seal, The [dd]Lord knoweth them that are his. And, Let every one that nameth the name of [ee]Christ depart from iniquity.

20 But in a great house there are not only [ff]vessels of gold and of silver, but also of wood and of earth; and some to honour, and some to dishonour.

21 If a man therefore [gg]purge himself from these, he shall be a vessel unto honour, sanctified, and meet for the master's use, *and* [hh]prepared unto every good work.

22 Flee also youthful lusts: but follow [ii]righteousness, faith, [jj]charity, peace, with them that call on the Lord out of a pure heart.

23 But foolish and unlearned [kk]questions avoid, knowing that they do gender strifes.

24 And the servant of the Lord must not strive; but be gentle unto all *men*, apt to teach, [ll]patient,

25 In [mm]meekness instructing those that oppose themselves; if God peradventure will give them [nn]repentance to the acknowledging of the truth;

26 And *that* they may recover themselves out of the snare of the [oo]devil, who are taken captive by him at his will.

CHAPTER 3.

Part III. The apostasy predicted: the believer's resource—the Scriptures.

This [1]know also, [pp]that in the last days perilous times shall come.

A.D. 66.

a 2 Tim. 4:19.
b Acts 28:20.
c Mt. 25:34.
d Heb. 6:10.
e *child.*
f *Grace (imparted).* Heb. 4:16. (Rom. 6:1; 2 Pet. 3:18.)
g 1 Tim. 1:18.
h 2 Tim. 4:5.
i *goeth as a soldier.* 1 Cor. 9:25, 26.
j *enlisted.*
k *must labour, before partaking of the fruits.*
l Prov. 2:6.
m Rom. 1:3, 4.
n *Gospel.* Phm. 13. (Gen. 12:1-3; Rev. 14:6.)
o Eph. 6:20.
p *Election (corporate).* Tit. 1:1. (Deut. 7:6; 1 Pet. 1:2.)
q Rom. 1:16, *note.*
r *have died.*
s Mt. 10:33.
t *are unfaithful.*
u Num. 23:19.
v 2 Pet. 1:13.
w Tit. 3:9, 10.
x 2 Pet. 1:10.
y Mt. 13:52.
z 1 Tim. 6:21.
aa 1 Cor. 15:12.
bb *Resurrection.* Heb. 11:19. (Job 19:25; 1 Cor. 15:52.)
cc Prov. 10:25.
dd *Jehovah.* Num. 16:5.
ee *the Lord.*
ff Rom. 9:21.
gg *Separation.* vs. 19, 21; Heb. 11:24, 25. (Gen. 12:1; 2 Cor. 6:14-17.)
hh 2 Tim. 3:17.
ii 1 John 3:7, *note.*
jj *love.*
kk v. 16.
ll Or, *forbearing.*
mm Gal. 6:1.
nn Repentance. Heb. 6:1, 6. (Mt. 3:2; Acts 17:30.)
oo *Satan.* Heb. 2:14. (Gen. 3:1; Rev. 20:10.)
pp 1 Tim. 4:1; 2 Pet. 3:3; 1 John 2:18; Jude 17, 18.

[1] **(3:1)** Apostasy, Summary: Apostasy, "falling away," is the act of professed Christians who deliberately reject revealed truth (1) as to the deity of Jesus Christ, and (2) redemption through His atoning and redeeming sacrifice (1 John 4:1-3; Phil. 3:18; 2 Pet. 2:1). Apostasy differs therefore from error

2 [a]For men shall be lovers of their own
selves, covetous, boasters, proud, blasphemers, disobedient to parents, unthankful,
unholy,
3 Without natural affection, truce-
breakers, false accusers, incontinent,
fierce, despisers of those that are good,
4 [b]Traitors, heady, highminded, lovers
of pleasures more than lovers of God;
5 [c]Having a form of godliness, but
denying the power thereof: from such
turn away.
6 For of this sort [d]are they which creep
into houses, and lead captive silly
women laden with [e]sins, led away with
divers lusts,
7 Ever learning, and never able to
come to the knowledge of the truth.
8 Now as Jannes and [f]Jambres withstood Moses, so do these also resist the
truth: [g]men of corrupt minds, [h]reprobate
concerning the faith.
9 But they shall proceed no further: for
their folly shall be manifest unto all *men*,
as theirs also was.
10 But thou hast fully known my doctrine, manner of life, purpose, faith,
longsuffering, [i]charity, patience,
11 Persecutions, afflictions, which
came unto me at [j]Antioch, at [k]Iconium,
at Lystra; what persecutions I endured:
but out of *them* all the Lord delivered me.
12 Yea, and all that will live godly in
Christ Jesus shall suffer persecution.
13 But evil men and [l]seducers shall
wax worse and worse, deceiving, and
being deceived.
14 But continue thou in the things
which thou hast learned and hast been
assured of, knowing of whom thou hast
learned *them*;
15 And that from a child thou hast
known the [m]holy scriptures, which are
able to make thee wise unto [n]salvation
through faith which is in Christ Jesus.
16 [o]All scripture *is* given by inspiration of God, and *is* profitable for doc-

A.D. 66.

a Rom. 1:24-32.
b 2 Pet. 2:10.
c Tit. 1:16.
d Tit. 1:11.
e *Sin.* Rom. 3:23, *note.*
f Ex. 7:11, 12, 22; 8:7; 9:11.
g 1 Tim. 6:5.
h *Apostasy.* vs. 1-8. (Lk. 18:8.)
i *love.*
j Acts 13:45, 50.
k Acts 14:5, 6, 19.
l *juggling impostors.*
m *Sanctify, holy (things)* (N.T.). Heb. 9:12. (Mt. 4:5; Rev. 22:11.)
n Rom. 1:16, *note.*
o *Inspiration.* 1 Pet. 1:10-12, 25. (Ex. 4:15; Rev. 22:19.)
p 1 John 3:7, *note.*
q *complete.* See Mt. 5:48, *note.*
r *Judgments (the seven).* Heb. 9:27. (2 Sam. 7:14; Rev. 20:12.)
s Tit. 2:15.
t *Apostasy.* vs. 3, 4: Heb. 6:4-8. (Lk. 18:8; 2 Tim. 3:1-8.)
u 2 Tim. 2:3.
v 1 Tim. 4:12, 15.
w Phil. 1:23; 2 Pet. 1:14.
x 1 Tim. 6:12.
y *the.*
z *Assurance.* vs. 8, 18; Heb. 6:11. (Isa. 32:17; Jude 1.)
aa *Rewards.* Heb. 11:6. (Dan. 12:3; 1 Cor. 3:14.)
bb 1 John 3:7, *note.*
cc 1 Cor. 2:9.
dd Cf. Col. 4:14; Phm. 24.
ee *age.*
ff Tit. 3:12.

trine, for reproof, for correction, for
instruction in [p]righteousness:
17 That the man of God may be [q]per-
fect, throughly furnished unto all good
works.

CHAPTER 4.

Part IV. A faithful servant and his faithful Lord.

I charge *thee* therefore before God, and
the Lord Jesus Christ, who shall
[r]judge the quick and the dead at his
appearing and his kingdom;
2 Preach the word; be instant in season,
out of season; [s]reprove, rebuke, exhort
with all longsuffering and doctrine.
3 For the time will come when they
will not endure sound doctrine; but after
their own lusts shall they heap to themselves teachers, having itching ears;
4 [t]And they shall turn away *their* ears
from the truth, and shall be turned unto
fables.
5 But watch thou in all things, [u]endure
afflictions, do the work of an evangelist,
make [v]full proof of thy ministry.
6 For I am now ready to be offered,
and the time of my [w]departure is at
hand.
7 I have [x]fought [y]a good fight, I have
finished *my* course, I have kept the faith:
8 Henceforth there is [z]laid up for me a
[aa]crown of [bb]righteousness, which the
Lord, the righteous judge, shall give me
at that day: and not to me only, but unto
all [cc]them also that love his appearing.
9 Do thy diligence to come shortly
unto me:
10 For [dd]Demas hath forsaken me,
having loved this present [ee]world, and is
departed unto Thessalonica; Crescens to
Galatia, Titus unto Dalmatia.
11 Only Luke is with me. Take Mark,
and bring him with thee: for he is profitable to me for the ministry.
12 And [ff]Tychicus have I sent to
Ephesus.

concerning truth, which may be the result of ignorance (Acts 19:1-6), or heresy, which may be due to the snare of Satan (2 Tim. 2:25, 26), both of which may consist with true faith. The apostate is perfectly described in 2 Tim. 4:3, 4. Apostates depart from the faith, but not from the outward profession of Christianity (3:5). Apostate teachers are described in 2 Tim. 4:3; 2 Pet. 2:1-19; Jude 4, 8, 11-13, 16. Apostasy in the church, as in Israel (Isa. 1:5, 6; 5:5-7), is irremediable, and awaits judgment (2 Thes. 2:10-12; 2 Pet. 2:17, 21; Jude 11-15; Rev. 3:14-16).

13 The cloke that I left at Troas with
Carpus, when thou comest, bring *with
thee*, and the books, *but* especially the
parchments.
14 Alexander the coppersmith did me
much evil: the [a]Lord reward him according
to his works:
15 Of whom be thou ware also; for he
hath greatly withstood our words.
16 At my first answer no man stood
with me, but [b]all *men* forsook me: *I pray
God* that it may not be laid to their
charge.
17 Notwithstanding [c]the Lord stood
with me, and strengthened me; that by
me the preaching might be fully known,
and *that* all the Gentiles might hear: and
I was delivered out of the [d]mouth of the
lion.
18 And the Lord shall deliver me from
every evil work, and will preserve *me*
unto his heavenly kingdom: to whom *be*
glory for ever and ever. Amen.
19 Salute Prisca and Aquila, and the
household of Onesiphorus.
20 Erastus abode at Corinth: but
Trophimus have I left at Miletum sick.
21 Do thy diligence to come before
winter. Eubulus greeteth thee, and
Pudens, and Linus, and Claudia, and all
the brethren.
22 The Lord Jesus Christ *be* with thy
spirit. Grace *be* with you. Amen.

A.D. 66.

a *Jehovah.* 2 Sam. 3:39.

b 2 Tim. 1:15,

c Deut. 31:6; Mt. 10:19; Acts 23:11.

d Psa. 22:21.

THE EPISTLE OF PAUL THE APOSTLE TO
TITUS

WRITER. The Apostle Paul (1:1).

Date. Practically the same with First Timothy.

Theme. Titus has much in common with First Timothy. Both Epistles are concerned with the due order of the churches. The distinction is that in First Timothy sound doctrine is more prominent (1 Tim. 1:3-10), in Titus the divine order for the local churches (Tit. 1:5). The permanent use of these Epistles lies in this twofold application, on the one hand to churches grown careless as to the *truth* of God, on the other, to churches careless as to the *order* of God's house. The importance of this order is made solemnly emphatic in that the tests by which true elders and deacons may be known are repeated (1 Tim. 3:1-7; Tit. 1:6-9).

There are two divisions: I. The qualifications and functions of elders, 1:1-16. II. The pastoral work of the true elder, 2:1–3:15.

CHAPTER 1.

Part I. The divine order for the local churches.

Paul, a [a]servant of God, and an apostle of Jesus Christ, according to the faith of God's [b]elect, and the acknowledging of the truth which is after godliness;

2 In hope of [c]eternal life, which God, that cannot lie, promised before the [d]world began;

3 But hath in [e]due times manifested his word through preaching, which is committed unto me according to the commandment of [f]God our [g]Saviour;

4 To Titus, *mine* own son [h]after the common faith: Grace, mercy, *and* peace, from God the Father and the Lord Jesus Christ our [g]Saviour.

5 For this cause left I thee in Crete, that thou shouldest set in order the things that are [1]wanting, and ordain [2][i]elders in every city, as I had appointed thee:

6 If any be blameless, the husband of one wife, having faithful children not accused of riot or unruly.

7 For a [i]bishop must be blameless, as the steward of God; not selfwilled, not soon angry, not given to wine, no striker, [j]not given to filthy lucre;

8 But a lover of hospitality, a lover of good men, sober, just, [k]holy, temperate;

9 [l]Holding fast the faithful word as he hath been taught, that he may be able by sound doctrine both to exhort and to convince the gainsayers.

10 For there are many unruly and vain [m]talkers and deceivers, specially they of the circumcision:

11 Whose mouths must be stopped,

A.D. 65.

a bondman.
b Election (corporate). 1 Pet. 5:13. (Deut. 7:6; 1 Pet. 1:2.)
c Life (eternal). Tit. 3:7. (Mt. 7:14; Rev. 22:19.)
d age-times.
e its own due season.
f our Saviour-God.
g Rom. 1:16, *note.*
h 1 Tim. 1:1, 2.
i Elders. vs. 5-9. (Acts 11:30.)
j no seeker of base gain.
k Sanctify, holy (persons) (N.T.). Heb. 2:11. (Mt. 4:5; Rev. 22:11.)
l 2 Thes. 2:15.
m Jas. 1:26.

[1] **(1:5)** It is not at all a question of the presence in the assembly of persons having the qualifications of elders, made overseers by the Holy Spirit (Acts 20:28); that such persons were in the churches of Crete is assumed; the question is altogether one of the *appointment* of such persons. These assemblies were not destitute of elders; but were "wanting," in that they were not duly appointed. There is a progress of doctrine in respect of the appointing of elders. Cf. v. 5, *note.*

[2] **(1:5)** Elder (*presbuteros*) and bishop (*episcopos* = "overseer") designate the same office (cf. v. 7; Acts 20:17; cf. v. 28), the former referring to the man, the latter to a function of the office. The eldership in the apostolic local churches was always plural. There is no instance of one elder in a local church. The functions of the elders are: to rule (1 Tim. 3:4, 5; 5:17), to guard the body of revealed truth from perversion and error (Tit. 1:9), to "oversee" the church as a shepherd his flock (Acts 20:28; John. 21:16; Heb. 13:17; 1 Pet. 5:2). Elders are made or "set" in the churches by the Holy Spirit (Acts 20:28), but great stress is laid upon their due *appointment* (Acts 14:23; Tit. 1:5). At first they were ordained (Gr. *cheirotoneo*, "to elect," "to designate with the hand,") by an apostle; e.g. Acts 14:23, but in Titus and 1 Timothy the qualifications of an elder become part of the Scriptures for the guidance of the churches in such appointment (1 Tim. 3:1-7).

who [a]subvert whole houses, teaching
things which they ought not, for [b]filthy
lucre's sake.
12 One of themselves, *even* a prophet
of their own, said, The Cretians *are*
alway liars, evil beasts, [c]slow bellies.
13 This witness is true. Wherefore
[d]rebuke them sharply, that they may be
sound in the faith;
14 Not giving heed to Jewish fables,
and commandments of men, that turn
from the truth.
15 [e]Unto the pure all things *are* pure:
but unto them that are defiled and unbelieving *is* nothing pure; but even their
mind and conscience is defiled.
16 They [f]profess that they [g]know God;
but in works they deny *him*, being abominable, and [h]disobedient, and unto every
good work reprobate.

CHAPTER 2.

Part II. The pastoral work of a true minister (Tit. 2:1–3:15).

But speak thou the things which
become sound doctrine:
2 That the aged men be sober, grave,
temperate, sound in faith, in [i]charity, in
patience.
3 The aged women likewise, that *they*
be in behaviour as becometh holiness,
not false accusers, not given to much
wine, teachers of good things;
4 That they may teach the young
women to be sober, to love their husbands, to love their children,
5 *To be* discreet, chaste, [j]keepers at
home, good, [k]obedient to their own husbands, that the word of God be not blasphemed.
6 Young men likewise exhort to be
sober minded.
7 In all things shewing thyself a [l]pat-
tern of good works: in doctrine *shewing*
uncorruptness, gravity, sincerity,
8 [m]Sound speech, that cannot be condemned; that he that is of the contrary
part may be ashamed, having no evil
thing to say of you.
9 *Exhort* servants to be obedient unto
their own masters, *and* to please *them*
well in all *things*; not answering again;
10 Not purloining, but shewing all
good fidelity; that they may adorn the
doctrine of [n]God our Saviour in all
things.
11 For the [o]grace of God that bringeth
salvation hath appeared to all men,

A.D. 65.

a Mt. 23:14.
b *the sake of base gain.*
c *lazy gluttons.*
d 2 Tim. 4:2.
e Rom. 14:14, 20; cf. Lk. 11:41.
f 2 Tim. 3:5, 7.
g Mt. 7:20, 21, 23; 25:12; 1 John 2:4.
h Or, *void of judgment.*
i *love.*
j Or, *diligent at home.*
k Cf. Gen. 3:16.
l 1 Tim. 4:12.
m 1 Tim. 6:3.
n *our Saviour God.*
o *Grace (in salv.).* Tit. 3:7. (Rom 3:24; John 1:17, *note.*)
p *age.*
q *Christ (Second Advent).* Jas. 5:7, 8. (Deut. 30:3; Acts 1:9-11.)
r Rom. 1:16, *note.*
s Rom. 3:24, *note.*
t *lawlessness.*
u Deut. 7:6; 14:2; 1 Pet. 2:9.
v 1 Tim. 4:12.
w Rom. 13:1.
x Eph. 4:2.
y 1 Cor. 6:11; 1 Pet. 4:3.
z *our Saviour-God.*
aa Eph. 2:4, 8, 9.
bb Rom. 10:3, *note.*
cc Rom. 1:16, *note.*
dd *Holy Spirit.* Heb. 2:4, (Mt. 1:18; Acts 2:4.)
ee Rom. 1:16, *note.*
ff *having been.*
gg *Justification.* Rom. 3:20-28. (Lk. 18:14; Rom. 3:28.)
hh *Grace (in salv.).* Heb. 2:9. (Rom. 3:24; John 1:17, *note.*)
ii *Life (eternal).* Heb. 7:3, 16. (Mt. 7:14; Rev. 22:19.)
jj vs. 1, 14.
kk 2 Tim. 2:23.
ll Mt. 18:17.
mm *Sin.* Rom. 3:23, *note.*

12 Teaching us that, denying ungodliness and worldly lusts, we should live
soberly, righteously, and godly, in this
present [p]world;
13 [q]Looking for that blessed hope, and
the glorious appearing of the great God
and our [r]Saviour Jesus Christ;
14 Who gave himself for us, that he
might [s]redeem us from all [t]iniquity, and
purify unto himself a [u]peculiar people,
zealous of good works.
15 These things speak, and exhort, and
rebuke with all authority. [v]Let no man
despise thee.

CHAPTER 3.

Part II. continued.

Put them in mind to be [w]subject to
principalities and powers, to obey
magistrates, to be ready to every good
work,
2 To speak evil of no man, to be no
brawlers, *but* gentle, shewing all [x]meek-
ness unto all men.
3 For [y]we ourselves also were sometimes foolish, disobedient, deceived,
serving divers lusts and pleasures, living
in malice and envy, hateful, *and* hating
one another.
4 But after that the kindness and love of
[z]God our Saviour toward man appeared,
5 [aa]Not by works of [bb]righteousness
which we have done, but according to
his mercy he [cc]saved us, by the washing
of regeneration, and renewing of the
[dd]Holy Ghost;
6 Which he shed on us abundantly
through Jesus Christ our [ee]Saviour;
7 That [ff]being [gg]justified [hh]by his
grace, we should be made heirs according to the hope of [ii]eternal life.
8 *This is* a faithful saying, and these
things I will that thou affirm constantly,
that they which have believed in God
might be [jj]careful to maintain good
works. These things are good and profitable unto men.
9 But [kk]avoid foolish questions, and
genealogies, and contentions, and strivings about the law; for they are unprofitable and vain.
10 A man that is an heretick after the
first and second admonition [ll]reject;
11 Knowing that he that is such is sub-
verted, and [mm]sinneth, being condemned
of himself.
12 When I shall send Artemas unto

thee, or Tychicus, be diligent to come
unto me to Nicopolis: for I have determined there to winter.
13 Bring Zenas the lawyer and Apollos
on their journey diligently, that nothing
be wanting unto them.

A.D. 65.

a Phil. 1:11.

14 And let ours also learn to maintain
[a]good works for necessary uses, that
they be not unfruitful.
15 All that are with me salute thee.
Greet them that love us in the faith.
Grace *be* with you all. Amen.

THE EPISTLE OF PAUL THE APOSTLE TO
PHILEMON

WRITER. The Apostle Paul (1:1).

Date. Probably A.D. 64. It is one of the Prison Epistles. See Introductions to Ephesians and Colossians.

Theme. Onesimus ("profitable"), a slave of Philemon, a Christian of Colosse, had robbed his master and fled to Rome. There he became a convert through Paul, who sent him back to Philemon with this letter. It is of priceless value as a teaching (1) in practical righteousness; (2) in Christian brotherhood; (3) in Christian courtesy; (4) in the law of love.

The divisions are four: I. Greeting, 1-3. II. The character of Philemon, 4-7. III. Intercession for Onesimus, 8-21. IV. Salutations and conclusion, 22-25.

A.D. 64.

Part I. The apostolic greeting.

Paul, a [a]prisoner of Jesus Christ, and Timothy *our* brother, unto Philemon our dearly beloved, and fellowlabourer,

2 And to *our* beloved Apphia, and [b]Archippus our fellowsoldier, and to the [c]church in thy house:

3 [d]Grace to you, and peace, from God our Father and the Lord Jesus Christ.

Part II. The character of Philemon.

4 [e]I thank my God, making mention of thee always in my prayers,

5 Hearing of thy love and faith, which thou hast toward the Lord Jesus, and toward all saints;

6 That the communication of thy faith may become [f]effectual by the acknowledging of [g]every good thing which is in you in Christ Jesus.

7 For we have great joy and consolation in thy love, because the bowels of the saints are refreshed by thee, brother.

Part III. Intercession for Onesimus.

8 Wherefore, though I might be much bold in Christ to enjoin thee that [h]which is [i]convenient,

9 Yet for love's sake I rather beseech *thee*, being such an one as Paul the aged, and now also a prisoner of Jesus Christ.

10 I beseech thee for my son [j]Onesimus, whom I have [k]begotten in my bonds:

11 [l]Which in time past was to thee unprofitable, but now profitable to thee and to me:

12 Whom I have sent again: thou therefore receive him, that is, mine own bowels:

13 Whom I would have retained with me, that in thy stead he might have ministered unto me in the bonds of the [m]gospel:

14 But without thy mind would I do nothing; that thy benefit should not be as it were of necessity, but willingly.

15 For perhaps he therefore departed for a season, that thou shouldest receive him for ever;

16 Not now as a [n]servant, but above a servant, a brother beloved, specially to me, but how much more unto thee, both in the flesh, and in the Lord?

17 If thou count me therefore a [o]partner, receive him as myself.

18 If he hath wronged thee, or oweth *thee* ought, put that on mine [1][p]account;

19 I Paul have written *it* with mine own hand, I will repay *it*: albeit I do not say to thee how thou owest unto me even thine own self besides.

20 Yea, brother, let me have joy of thee in the Lord: refresh my bowels [q]in the Lord.

21 Having [r]confidence in thy obedience I wrote unto thee, knowing that thou wilt also do more than I say.

a Eph. 3:1.
b Col. 4:17.
c *Churches (local).* Jas. 5:14. (Acts 2.41; Phil. 1:1.)
d Eph. 1:2.
e Eph. 1:16.
f Jas. 2:14-17.
g Phil. 4:8; 2 Pet. 1:5-8.
h v. 19.
i *fitting.*
j Col. 4:9.
k 1 Cor. 4:15.
l 1 Pet. 2:10.
m *Gospel.* Heb. 4:2. (Gen. 12:1-3; Rev. 14:6.)
n *bondman.*
o 2 Cor. 8:23.
p Lk. 14:14.
q *in Christ.*
r 2 Cor. 7:16.

[1] **(Ver. 18)** Verses 17, 18 perfectly illustrate imputation: "Receive him as myself"—reckon to him my merit; "If he hath wronged thee or oweth thee ought, put that on mine account"—reckon to me his demerit. See "Imputation," Lev. 25:50; Jas. 2:23, *note.*

Part IV. Salutations and conclusion.

22 But withal prepare me also a lodging: for I [a]trust that [b]through your
prayers I shall be given unto you.

A.D. 64.

a hope.
b Acts 12:5, 11, 12.
c Col. 1:7.
d Acts 12:12, 25.
e Acts 19:29.
f 2 Tim. 4:10.
g 2 Tim. 4:22.

23 There salute thee [c]Epaphras, my
fellowprisoner in Christ Jesus;
24 [d]Marcus, [e]Aristarchus, [f]Demas,
Lucas, my fellowlabourers.
25 The [g]grace of our Lord Jesus Christ
be with your spirit. Amen.

HOW TO USE THE SUBJECT REFERENCES.

THE subject references lead the reader from the first clear mention of a great truth to the last. The first and last references (in parenthesis) are repeated each time, so that wherever a reader comes upon a subject he may recur to the first reference and follow the subject, or turn at once to the Summary at the last reference.

ILLUSTRATION
(at Mark 1:1.)

b Gospel. vs. 1,
14, 15; Mk. 8:35.
(Gen. 12:1-3;
Rev. 14:6.)

Here *Gospel* is the subject; vs. 1, 14, 15 show where it is at that particular place; Mk. 8:35 is the next reference in the chain, and the references in parenthesis are the first and last.

THE JEWISH-CHRISTIAN EPISTLES.

In Hebrews, James, First and Second Peter, and Jude we have a group of inspired writings differing in important respects from Paul's Epistles. But this difference is in no sense one of conflict. All present the same Christ, the same salvation, the same morality. The difference is one of extension, of development. The Jewish-Christian writings deal with the elementary and foundational things of the Gospel, while to Paul were given the revelations concerning the church, her place in the counsels of God, and the calling and hope of the believer as vitally united to Christ in the one body.

The other characteristic difference is that while Paul has in view the body of true believers, who are therefore assuredly saved, the Judæo-Christian writers view the church as a professing body in which, during this age, the wheat and tares are mingled (Mt. 13:24-30). Their writings, therefore, abound in warnings calculated to arouse and alarm the mere professor. A word of caution is, however, needful at this point. The persons warned are neither mere hypocrites, nor mere formalists. So far as they have gone their experiences are perfectly genuine. It is said of the supposed persons in Heb. 6:4-9 that they had been "enlightened," and the same word is used in Heb. 10:32, translated "illuminated." They are said, too, to have "tasted" of the heavenly gift, and again a word importing reality is used, for it occurs in Heb. 2:9 of the death of Christ. The true point of the divine solicitude is expressed in verses 1 and 2. It is that they shall go on. They have made a real beginning, but it is not said of them that they have faith, and it *is* said (verse 9) that "things that accompany salvation" are "better." This fear lest beginners will "come short" is the theme of Heb. 3:7–4:3. The men in Mt. 7:21-23 are not conscious hypocrites—they are utterly surprised at their exclusion. Characteristic contrasts are, Heb. 6:4-6 with Rom. 8:29-39; 2 Pet. 1:10 with Phil. 1:6. In this respect these Epistles group with Mt. 13–23; Acts 2–9. The two Epistles of Peter, however, are less Jewish and more truly catholic than the other Jewish-Christian writings. He addresses, in his first Epistle, neither Jews as such, nor even Christian Jews of Jerusalem, or Judæa, but of the dispersion; while Second Peter is not distinctively Jewish at all.

HOW TO USE THE SUBJECT REFERENCES.

THE subject references lead the reader from the first clear mention of a great truth to the last. The first and last references (in parenthesis) are repeated each time, so that wherever a reader comes upon a subject he may recur to the first reference and follow the subject, or turn at once to the Summary at the last reference.

ILLUSTRATION
(at Mark 1:1.)

b Gospel. vs. 1, 14, 15; Mk. 8:35. (Gen. 12:1-3; Rev. 14:6.)

Here *Gospel* is the subject; vs. 1, 14, 15 show where it is at that particular place; Mk. 8:35 is the next reference in the chain, and the references in parenthesis are the first and last.

THE EPISTLE OF PAUL THE APOSTLE TO THE
HEBREWS

WRITER. The authorship of Hebrews has been in controversy from the earliest times. The book is anonymous, but the reference in 2 Pet. 3:15 seems conclusive that Paul was the writer. See also Heb. 13:23. All agree that, whether by Paul or another, the point of view is Pauline. We undoubtedly have here the method of Paul's synagogue addresses. No book of Scripture more fully authenticates itself as inspired.

Date. From internal evidence it is clear that Hebrews was written before the destruction of the Temple, A.D. 70 (cf. 10:11).

Theme. The doctrinal passages reveal the purpose of the book. It was written with a twofold intent: (1) To confirm Jewish Christians by showing that Judaism had come to an end through the fulfilment by Christ of the whole purpose of the law; and (2) the hortatory passages show that the writer had in view the danger ever present to Jewish professed believers of either lapsing back into Judaism, or of pausing short of true faith in Jesus Christ. It is clear from the Acts that even the strongest of the believers in Palestine were held to a strange mingling of Judaism and Christianity (e.g. Acts 21:18-24), and that snare would be especially apt to entangle professed Christians amongst the Jews of the dispersion.

The key-word is "better." Hebrews is a series of contrasts between the good things of Judaism and the better things of Christ. Christ is "better" than angels, than Moses, than Joshua, than Aaron; and the New Covenant than the Mosaic Covenant. Church truth does not appear, the ground of gathering only being stated (13:13). The whole sphere of Christian profession is before the writer; hence exhortations necessary to warn and alarm a mere professor.

Hebrews is in six divisions, but these include five parenthetic passages of exhortation. I. The great salvation, 1:1–2:18 (2:1-4, parenthetic). II. The rest of God, 3:1–4:16. (all parenthetic). III. Our great High Priest, 5:1–8:6 (5:11–6:12, parenthetic). IV. The new covenant and the heavenly sanctuary, 8:7–10:39 (10:26-39, parenthetic). V. The superiority of the faith-way, 11:1-40. VI. The worship and walk of the believer-priest, 12:1–13:25 (12:3-17, parenthetic).

CHAPTER 1.

Part I. The great salvation
(Heb. 1:1–2:18).

(1) *The Son better than the prophets.*

God, who [a]at sundry times and in
divers manners spake in time past
unto the fathers by the prophets,
2 Hath in these last days spoken unto
us [b]by *his* Son, whom he hath appointed
heir of all things, by whom also he made
the [c]worlds;
3 Who being the [d]brightness of *his*
glory, and the [e]express image of his person, and upholding all things by the
word of his power, when he had by himself purged our sins, [f]sat down [g]on the
right hand of the Majesty on high;

(2) *The Son better than the angels.*

4 Being made so much better than the
[1]angels, as he hath by inheritance
obtained a more excellent name than
they.
5 For unto which of the angels

A.D. 64.

a in many parts and in many ways.
b lit. *in Son.*
c ages.
d effulgence.
e expression of his substance.
f sat himself down.
g Eph. 1:20, 21.

[1] **(1:4)** Angel, Summary: Angel, "messenger," is used of God, of men, and of an order of created spiritual beings whose chief attributes are strength and wisdom (2 Sam. 14:20; Psa. 103:20; 104:4). In the O.T. the expression "the angel of the LORD" (sometimes "of God") usually implies the presence of Deity in angelic form (Gen. 16:1-13; 21:17-19; 22:11-16; 31:11-13; Ex. 3: 2-4; Jud. 2:1; 6:12-16; 13:3-22). See Mal. 3:1, *note.* The word angel is used of men in Lk. 7:24; Jas. 2:25; Rev. 1:20; 2:1, 8, 12, 18; 3:1, 7, 14. In Rev. 8:3-5 Christ is evidently meant. Sometimes angel is used of the spirit of man (Mt. 18:10; Acts 12:15). Though angels are spirits (Psa. 104:4; Heb. 1:14), power is given them to become visible in the semblance of human form (Gen. 19:1, cf. v. 5; Ex. 3:2; Num. 22:22-31; Jud. 2:1; 6:11, 22; 13:3, 6; 1 Chr. 21:16, 20; Mt. 1:20; Lk. 1:26; John 20:12; Acts 7:30; 12:7, 8, etc.). The word is always

said he at any time, Thou art my [a]Son, this day have I begotten thee? And again, [b]I will be to him a Father, and he shall be to me a Son?

6 And again, when he [c]bringeth in the firstbegotten into the [d]world, he saith, [e]And let all the angels of God worship him.

7 And of the angels he saith, [f]Who maketh his angels spirits, and his ministers a flame of fire.

8 But unto the Son *he saith*, Thy throne, O [g]God, *is* for ever and ever: a sceptre of [h]righteousness *is* the sceptre of thy kingdom.

9 Thou hast loved [i]righteousness, and hated [j]iniquity; therefore God, *even* thy God, hath anointed thee with the oil of gladness above thy fellows.

10 And, [k]Thou, Lord, in the beginning hast laid the foundation of the earth; and the heavens are the works of thine hands:

11 They shall perish; but thou remainest; and they all shall wax old as doth a garment;

12 And as a vesture shalt thou fold them up, and they shall be changed: but thou art the same, and thy years shall not fail.

13 But to which of the angels said he at any time, [l]Sit on my right hand, until I make thine enemies thy footstool?

14 Are they not all ministering spirits, sent forth to minister for them who shall be heirs of [m]salvation?

CHAPTER 2.

(Parenthesis: hearers warned.)

Therefore we ought to give the more earnest heed to the things which we have heard, lest at any time we should [n]let *them* slip.

2 For if the word spoken by angels was stedfast, and every [o]transgression and [o]disobedience received a just recompence of reward;

3 How shall we escape, if we neglect so great [m]salvation; which at the first began to be spoken by the Lord, and was confirmed unto us by them that heard *him*;

4 God also bearing *them* witness, both with signs and wonders, and with divers miracles, and gifts of the [p]Holy Ghost, according to his own will?

(3) *The earth to be put under the man Christ Jesus.*

5 For unto the angels hath he not put in subjection the [q]world to come, whereof we speak.

6 But one in a certain place testified,

A.D. 64.

a Psa. 2:7.
b 2 Sam. 7:14.
c Or, *bringeth back.*
d *oikoumene = inhabited earth.*
e Deut. 32:43, Septuagint.
f Psa. 104:4.
g vs. 8, 9; Psa. 45:6, 7.
h *uprightness.*
i 1 John 3:7, *note.*
j *lawlessness.* See Rom. 3:23, *note.*
k vs. 10-12; Psa. 102:25-27.
l Psa. 110:1; Mt. 22:44.
m Rom. 1:16, *note.*
n *slip away from them.*
o *Sin.* Rom. 3:23, *note.*
p *Holy Spirit.* Heb. 3:7. (Mt. 1:18; Acts 2:4.)
q *oikoumene = inhabited earth.*

used in the masculine gender, though sex, in the human sense, is never ascribed to angels (Mt. 22:30; Mk. 12:25). They are exceedingly numerous (Mt. 26:53; Heb. 12:22; Rev. 5:11; Psa. 68:17). Their power is inconceivable (2 Ki. 19:35). Their place is about the throne of God (Rev. 5:11; 7:11). Their relation to the believer is that of "ministering spirits, sent forth to minister for them who shall be heirs of salvation," and this ministry has reference largely to the *physical* safety and well-being of believers (1 Ki. 19:5; Psa. 34:7; 91:11; Dan. 6:22; Mt. 2:13, 19; 4:11; Lk. 22:43; Acts 5:19; 12:7-10). From Heb. 1:14, with Mt. 18:10; Psa. 91:11, it would seem that this care for the heirs of salvation begins in infancy and continues through life. The angels observe us (1 Cor. 4:9; Eph. 3:10; Eccl. 5:6), a fact which should influence conduct. They receive departing saints (Lk. 16:22). Man is made "a little lower than the angels," and in incarnation Christ took "for a little" (time) this lower place (Psa. 8:4, 5; Heb. 2:6, 9) that He might lift the believer into His own sphere above angels (Heb. 2:9, 10). The angels are to accompany Christ in His second advent (Mt. 25:31). To them will be committed the preparation of the judgment of the nations (see Mt. 13:30, 39, 41, 42; 25:32, *note*). The kingdom-age is not to be subject to angels, but to Christ and those for whom He was made a little lower than the angels (Heb. 2:5). An archangel, Michael, is mentioned as having a particular relation to Israel and to the resurrections (Dan. 10:13, 21; 12:1, 2; Jude 9; 1 Thes. 4:16). The only other angel whose name is revealed, Gabriel, was employed in the most distinguished services (Dan. 8:16; 9:21; Lk. 1:19, 26).

Fallen angels. Two classes of these are mentioned: (1)"The angels which kept not their first estate [place], but left their own habitation," are "chained under darkness," awaiting judgment (2 Pet. 2:4; Jude 6; 1 Cor. 6:3; John 5:22). See Gen. 6:4, *note.* (2) The angels who have Satan (Gen. 3:1; Rev. 20:10, *note*) as leader. The origin of these is nowhere explicitly revealed. They may be identical with the demons (Mt. 7:22, *note*). For Satan and his angels everlasting fire is prepared (Mt. 25:41; Rev. 20:10).

saying, [a]What is man, that thou art
mindful of him? or the son of man, that
thou visitest him?
7 Thou madest him a little lower than
the angels; thou crownedst him with
glory and honour, and didst set him
over the works of thy hands:
8 Thou hast put all things in subjection
under his feet. For in that he put all in
subjection under him, he left nothing
that is not put under him. But now we
see not yet all things put under him.

(4) *Jesus, made for a little time lower than the angels, dies for man that he may lift men above angels into the family of God.*

9 But we see Jesus, who was made [b]a
little lower than the angels for the suffering of death, crowned with glory and
honour; that he by the [c]grace of God
should taste death for every man.
10 For it became him, for whom *are* all
things, and by whom *are* all things, in
bringing many sons unto glory, to make
the [d]captain of their salvation perfect
through sufferings.
11 For both he that [e]sanctifieth and
they who are sanctified *are* all of one: for
which cause he is not ashamed to call
them brethren,
12 Saying, [f]I will declare thy name
unto my brethren, in the midst of the
[g]church will I sing praise unto thee.
13 And again, [h]I will put my trust in
him. And again, Behold I and the children which [i]God hath given me.
14 Forasmuch then as the children are
partakers of flesh and blood, he also himself likewise [j]took part of the same; that
through death he might [k]destroy him that
had the power of death, that is, [l]the devil;
15 And deliver them who through fear
of death were all their lifetime subject to
bondage.
16 For verily [m]he took not on *him the*
nature of angels; but he took on *him* the
seed of Abraham.
17 Wherefore in all things it behoved
him to be made like unto *his* brethren,
that he might be a merciful and faithful
high priest in things *pertaining* to God, to
make [n]reconciliation for the sins of the
people.
18 For in that he himself hath suffered
being [o]tempted, he is able to succour
them that are tempted.

CHAPTER 3.

Part II. Parenthetic: The rest of God (Heb. 3:1–4.16).

(1) *Christ the Son better than Moses the Servant.*

Wherefore, [p]holy brethren, [q]partakers
of the heavenly calling, consider
the Apostle and High Priest of our
[r]profession, Christ Jesus;
2 Who was faithful to him that
appointed him, as also [s]Moses *was faith-*
ful in all his house.
3 For this *man* was counted worthy of
more glory than Moses, inasmuch as he
who hath [t]builded the house hath more
honour than the house.
4 For every house is builded by some
man; but he that built all things *is* God.
5 And [u]Moses verily *was* faithful in all
his house, as a servant, for a [v]testimony
of those things which were to be spoken
after;
6 But Christ as a son over his own
house; whose house are we, if we hold
fast the confidence and the rejoicing of
the hope firm unto the end.

(2) *Exhortation: the generation that came out of Egypt did not enter the Canaan-rest because of unbelief.*

7 Wherefore (as the [w]Holy Ghost saith,
[x]To day if ye will hear his voice,
8 Harden not your hearts, as in the
provocation, in the day of temptation in
the wilderness:
9 When your fathers [y]tempted me,
proved me, and saw my works forty
years.
10 Wherefore I was grieved with that
generation, and said, They do alway err
in *their* heart; and they have not known
my ways.
11 So I sware in my wrath, They shall
not enter into my rest.)
12 Take heed, brethren, lest there be in
any of you an evil heart of unbelief, in
departing from the living God.
13 But exhort one another daily, while
it is called To day; lest any of you be
hardened through the deceitfulness of
[z]sin.
14 For we are made [q]partakers of
Christ, if we hold the beginning of our
confidence stedfast unto the end;
15 While it is said, [aa]To day if ye

A.D. 64.

a vs. 6-8; Psa. 8:4-6.
b Or, *for a little,* i.e. little time.
c *Grace (in salv.).* Heb. 10:29. (Rom. 3:24; John 1:17, *note.*)
d *leader,* or, *originator,* i.e. one who initiates and carries through. Trans. *author* in Heb. 12:2.
e *Sanctify, holy (persons)* (N.T.). Heb. 3:1. (Mt. 4:5; Rev. 22:11.)
f Psa. 22:22.
g *Church (true)* 1 Thes. 4:16, 17. (Mt. 16:18; Heb. 12:23.)
h Isa. 8:17. Septuagint.
i *Jehovah.* Isa. 8:18. Septuagint.
j The word trans. *took part* is not the same as that trans. *partakers,* but implies taking part in something outside one's self.
k *bring to naught.*
l *Satan.* Jas. 4:7. (Gen. 3:1; Rev. 20:10.)
m *not of angels doth he take hold, but he taketh hold of.* Cf. Isa. 41:9, Septuagint.
n Gr. *hilaskomai, propitiation.* See Rom. 3:25, *note.*
o *Temptation.* Heb. 3:8, 9. (Gen. 3:1; Jas. 1:14.)
p *Sanctify, holy (persons)* (N.T.) Heb. 10:10, 14, 29. (Mt. 4:5; Rev. 22:11.)
q *companions;* the same word trans. *fellows* in Heb. 1:9.
r *confession.*
s Num. 12:7.
t Zech. 6:12, 13.
u Num. 12:7.
v Deut. 18:15, 19.
w *Holy Spirit.* Heb. 6:4. (Mt. 1:18; Acts 2:4.)
x vs. 7-11; Psa. 95:7-11.
y *Temptation.* vs. 8:9; Heb. 4:15. (Gen 3:1; Jas. 1:14.)
z *Sin.* Rom. 3:23, *note.*
aa Psa. 95:7, 8.

will hear his voice, harden not your hearts, as in the provocation.

16 For some, when they had heard, did provoke: howbeit not all that came out of Egypt by Moses.

17 But with whom was he grieved forty years? *was it* not with them that had [a]sinned, whose carcases fell in the wilderness?

18 And to whom sware he that they should not enter into his rest, but to them that believed not?

19 So we see that they could not enter in because of unbelief.

CHAPTER 4.

(3) *But there is a better rest for the believer, of which God's creation-rest is the type.*

Let us therefore fear, lest, a promise being left *us* of entering into his rest, any of you should seem to come short of it.

2 For unto us was the [b]gospel preached, as well as unto them: but the word preached did not profit them, not being mixed with [c]faith in them that heard *it*.

3 For we which have believed do enter into rest, as he said, [d]As I have sworn in my wrath, if they shall enter into my rest: although the works were finished from the foundation of the [e]world.

4 For he spake in a certain place of the seventh *day* on this wise, And [f]God did rest the seventh day from all his works.

5 And in this *place* again, If they shall enter into my rest.

6 Seeing therefore it remaineth that some must enter therein, and they to whom [g]it was first preached entered not in because of unbelief:

7 Again, he limiteth a certain day, saying in David, To day, after so long a time; as it is [h]said, To day if ye will hear his voice, harden not your hearts.

8 For if [i]Jesus had given them rest, then would he not afterward have spoken of another day.

(4) *The believer rests in a perfect work of redemption, as God rested from a perfect work of creation.*

9 There remaineth therefore a [j]rest to the people of God.

10 For he that is entered into his rest, he also hath ceased from his own works, as God *did* from his.

11 [k]Let us labour therefore to enter into that rest, lest any man [l]fall after the same example of [m]unbelief.

12 [n]For the word of God *is* [o]quick, and powerful, and sharper than any two-edged sword, piercing even to the dividing asunder of soul and spirit, and of the joints and marrow, and *is* a discerner of the thoughts and intents of the heart.

13 Neither is there any creature that is not manifest in his sight: but all things *are* [p]naked and opened unto the eyes of him with whom we have to do.

(5) *The believer is kept in perfect rest by mercy and grace, through the Son of God.*

14 Seeing then that we have a great high priest, that is [q]passed into the heavens, Jesus the Son of God, [r]let us hold fast *our* [s]profession.

15 For we have not an high priest which cannot be [t]touched with the feeling of our infirmities; but was in all points [u]tempted like as *we are*, [v]*yet* without [w]sin.

16 Let us therefore come boldly unto the [x]throne of grace, that we may obtain mercy, and find grace [y]to help in time of need.

CHAPTER 5.

Part III. Our great High Priest (Heb. 5:1–8:6).

(1) *The office of high priest.*

For every high priest taken from among men is ordained for men in things *pertaining* to God, that he may offer both gifts and sacrifices for [w]sins:

2 Who can have compassion on the ignorant, and on them that are out of the way; for that he himself also is [z]compassed with infirmity.

3 And by reason hereof he ought, as for the people, so also for himself, to offer for [w]sins.

4 And no man taketh this honour unto himself, but he that is called of God, as *was* [aa]Aaron.

(2) *Christ a high priest after the order of Melchisedec.*

5 So also Christ glorified not himself to be made an high priest; but he that said unto him, [bb]Thou art my Son, to day have I begotten thee.

6 As he saith also in another *place*,

A.D. 64.

a *Sin.* Rom. 3:23, *note.*
b *Gospel.* 1 Pet. 1:12, 25. (Gen. 12:1-3; Rev. 14:6.)
c *Faith.* Heb. 10:22, 38. (Gen. 3:20; Heb. 11:39.)
d Psa. 95:11.
e i.e. *earth.*
f Gen. 2:2.
g Or, *the gospel.*
h Psa. 95:7, 8.
i *Joshua.*
j Or, *keeping of a sabbath.*
k 2 Pet. 1:10.
l Heb. 10:38..
m Or, *disobedience.*
n Isa. 49:2.
o *living and operative.* 1 Pet. 1:23.
p Prov. 15:11.
q Heb. 9:12, 24.
r Heb. 10:23.
s *confession.*
t Hos. 11:8.
u *Temptation.* Heb. 11:37. (Gen. 3:1; Jas. 1:14.)
v *apart from sin.*
w *Sin.* Rom. 3:23, *note.*
x *Grace (imparted).* Heb. 12:15, 28. (Rom. 6:1; 2 Pet. 3:18.)
y *for seasonable help.*
z *clothed with.*
aa Ex. 28:1; Num. 16:40.
bb Psa. 2:7.

[a]Thou *art* a priest for ever after the order of [1]Melchisedec.

7 Who in the days of his flesh, when he had offered up [b]prayers and supplications with strong crying and tears unto him that was [c]able to save him [d]from death, and was heard [e]in that he [f]feared;

8 Though he were a Son, yet learned he [g]obedience by the things which he suffered;

9 And [h]being made perfect, he became the author of eternal [i]salvation unto all them that obey him;

10 [j]Called of God an high priest after the order of Melchisedec.

(*Parenthetic: appeal and warning,* to 6:12.)

11 Of whom we have many things to say, and hard to be uttered, seeing ye are dull of hearing.

12 For when for the time ye ought to be teachers, ye have need that one teach you again which *be* the first principles of the oracles of God; and are become such as have need of [k]milk, and not of strong meat.

13 For every one that useth milk *is* [l]unskilful in the word of righteousness: for he is a babe.

14 But strong meat belongeth to them that are of full age, *even* those who by reason of use have their senses exercised to discern both good and evil.

CHAPTER 6.

Therefore leaving the [m]principles of the doctrine of Christ, let us go on unto [n]perfection; not laying again [o]the foundation of [p]repentance from [q]dead works, and of faith toward God,

2 Of the doctrine of [r]baptisms, and of laying on of hands, and of [s]resurrection of the dead, and of eternal judgment.

3 And this will we do, if God permit.

4 [t]For *it is* [2]impossible for those who were once enlightened, and have tasted of the heavenly gift, and were made [u]partakers of the [v]Holy Ghost,

5 And have tasted the good word of God, and the powers of the [w]world to come,

6 If they shall fall away, to renew them again unto [x]repentance; seeing they crucify to themselves the Son of God afresh, and put *him* to an open shame.

7 For the earth which drinketh in the rain that cometh oft upon it, and bringeth forth herbs meet for them by whom it is dressed, receiveth [y]blessing from God:

8 But that which beareth thorns and briers *is* rejected, and *is* nigh unto cursing; whose end *is* to be burned.

9 But, beloved, we are persuaded better things of you, and things that accompany [z]salvation, though we thus speak.

10 [aa]For God *is* not unrighteous to forget your work and labour of love, which ye have shewed toward his name, in that ye have ministered to the saints, and do minister.

11 And we desire that every one of you do shew the same diligence to the full [bb]assurance of hope unto the end:

12 That ye be not slothful, but [cc]followers of them who through faith and patience inherit the promises.

Part III Resumed.

(3) *Our High Priest within the veil assures our coming there too.*

13 For when God made promise to Abraham, because he could

A.D. 64.

a v. 5, 6; Psa. 110:4.
b Mt. 26:39, 44.
c Mt. 26:53.
d *out of.*
e *because of his piety.*
f Psa. 19:9, *note.*
g Phil. 2:8.
h Heb. 2:10.
i Rom. 1:16, *note.*
j *saluted.*
k 1 Cor. 3:1-3.
l *hath no experience.*
m *word of the beginning of the Christ.*
n Mt. 5:48, *note.*
o a.
p *Repentance.* vs. 1, 6; Heb. 6:6. (Mt. 3:2; Acts 17:30.)
q Heb. 9:14.
r Acts 19:4, 5.
s Acts 17:31.
t *Apostasy.* vs. 1, 6; Heb. 10:26-31. (Lk. 18:8; 2 Tim. 3:1-8.)
u Gr. *metochous, going along with.*
v *Holy Spirit.* Heb. 9:14. (Mt. 1:18; Acts 2:4.)
w i.e. *age.*
x *Repentance.* Heb. 12:17. (Mt. 3:2; Acts 17:30.)
y Psa. 65:10.
z Rom. 1:16, *note.*
aa Mt. 25:40.
bb *Assurance.* Heb. 7:25. (Isa. 32:17; Jude 1.)
cc *imitators.*

[1]**(5:6)** See Gen. 14:18, *note.* Melchisedec was a suitable type of Christ as High Priest, because: (1) he was a king-priest (Gen. 14:18 with Zech. 6:12, 13); (2) his name means, "my king is righteous" (cf. Isa. 11:5), and he was king of Salem (i.e. "peace," cf. Isa. 11:6-9); (3) he had no (recorded) "beginning of days" (cf. John 1:1), nor "end of life" (cf. Rom. 6:9; Heb. 7:23-25); nor (4) was he made a high priest by human appointment (Psa. 110:4). But the contrast between the high priesthood of Melchisedec and Aaron is only as to *person, "order"* (or appointment), and *duration.* In His *work* Christ follows the Aaronic pattern, the "shadow" of which Christ was the substance (Heb. 8:1-6; 9:1-28).

[2]**(6:4)** Heb. 6:4-8 presents the case of Jewish professed believers who halt short of faith in Christ after advancing to the very threshold of salvation, even "going along with" the Holy Spirit in His work of enlightenment and conviction (John 16:8-10). It is not said that they had faith. This supposed person is like the spies at Kadesh-barnea (Deut. 1:19-26) who saw the land and had the very fruit of it in their hands, and yet turned back.

swear by no greater, he sware by himself,

14 Saying, [a]Surely blessing I will bless thee, and multiplying I will multiply thee.

15 And so, after he had patiently endured, he obtained the promise.

16 For men verily swear by the greater: and an oath for confirmation *is* to them an end of all strife.

17 Wherein God, willing more abundantly to shew unto the [b]heirs of promise the immutability of his counsel, [c]confirmed *it* by an oath:

18 That by two immutable things, in which *it was* impossible for God to lie, we might have a strong [d]consolation, who have fled for refuge to lay hold upon the hope set before us:

19 Which *hope* we have as an anchor of the soul, both sure and stedfast, and which entereth into that [e]within the veil;

20 [f]Whither the forerunner is for us entered, *even* Jesus, made an high priest for ever after the order of [g]Melchisedec.

CHAPTER 7.

The Melchisedec high priesthood resumed.

(4) *The historic Melchisedec a type of Christ.*

For this Melchisedec, king of Salem, priest of the most high [h]God, who met Abraham returning from the slaughter of the kings, and blessed him;

2 To whom also Abraham gave a tenth part of all; first being by interpretation King of righteousness, and after that also King of Salem, which is, King of peace;

3 Without father, without mother, without [i]descent, having neither beginning of days, nor end of life; but made like unto the Son of God; abideth a priest continually.

(5) *Melchisedec high priesthood greater than the Aaronic.*

(a) Because Aaron in Abraham paid Melchisedec tithes.

4 Now consider how great this man *was*, unto whom even the patriarch Abraham gave the tenth of the spoils.

5 And verily they that are of the [j]sons of Levi, who receive the office of the priesthood, have a commandment to take tithes of the people according to the law, that is, of their brethren, though they come out of the loins of Abraham:

6 But he whose [k]descent is not counted from them [l]received tithes of Abraham, and blessed him that had the promises.

7 And without all contradiction the less is blessed of the better.

8 And here men that die receive tithes; but there he *receiveth them*, of [m]whom it is witnessed that he liveth.

9 And as I may so say, Levi also, who receiveth tithes, payed tithes in Abraham.

10 For he was yet in the loins of his father, when Melchisedec met him.

(b) Because the Aaronic priesthood made nothing perfect.

11 [n]If therefore perfection were by the Levitical priesthood, (for under it the people received the law,) what further need *was there* that another priest should rise after the order of Melchisedec, and not be called after the order of Aaron?

12 For the priesthood being changed, there is made of necessity a change also of the law.

13 For he of whom these things are spoken pertaineth to another tribe, of which no man [o]gave attendance at the altar.

14 For *it is* [p]evident that our Lord sprang out of Juda; of which tribe Moses spake nothing concerning priesthood.

15 And it is yet far more evident: for that after the similitude of Melchisedec there ariseth another priest,

16 Who is made, not after the law of a [q]carnal commandment, but after the power [r]of an [s]endless life.

17 For he testifieth, Thou *art* a priest for ever after the order of [t]Melchisedec.

18 For there is verily a [u]disannulling of the commandment going before for the weakness and unprofitableness thereof.

19 [v]For the [w]law made nothing [x]perfect, but the bringing in of a better hope *did*; by the [y]which we draw nigh unto God.

20 And inasmuch as not without an oath *he was made priest*:

21 (For those priests were made without an oath; but this with an oath by him that said unto him, [z]The Lord sware and will not repent, Thou *art* a priest for ever after the order of Melchisedec:)

A.D. 64.

a Gen. 22:16, 17.
b Heb. 11:9; Rom. 8:17.
c *intervened by, or, interposed himself.*
d *encouragement.*
e Lev. 16:15.
f Heb. 4:14.
g Gen. 14:17-19; Psa. 110:4.
h *Most high God.* Gen. 14:18.
i *genealogy.*
j Num. 18:21, 26.
k *pedigree.*
l Gen. 14:20.
m Heb. 5:6; Rev. 1:18.
n vs. 18, 19; Heb. 8:7; Gal. 2:21.
o *hath been attached to the service of.*
p Gen. 49:8, 10.
q *fleshly,* i.e. addressed to the carnal or natural man. Cf. Heb. 9:10.
r *of indissoluble life.*
s *Life (eternal),* vs. 3, 16; Jas. 1:12. (Mt. 7:14; Rev. 22:19.)
t Psa. 110:4.
u *setting aside.*
v *For the law perfected nothing, but it was the bringer in of a better hope.*
w *Law (of Moses).* Heb. 8:10. (Ex. 19:1; Gal. 3:1-29.)
x Mt. 5:48, *note.*
y Rom. 5:2.
z Psa. 110:4.

22 By so much was Jesus made a surety of a better [a]testament.

(c) Because the Aaronic priests died: Christ ever liveth.

23 And they truly were many priests, because they were not suffered to continue by reason of death:

24 But this *man*, because he continueth ever, hath an unchangeable priesthood.

25 Wherefore he is [b]able also to [c]save them [d]to the [e]uttermost that come unto God by him, seeing he ever liveth to make intercession for them.

26 For such an high priest became us, *who is* holy, harmless, undefiled, separate from [f]sinners, and made higher than the heavens;

27 Who needeth not daily, as those high priests, to offer up sacrifice, first for his own [f]sins, and then for the people's: for this he did [g]once, when he offered up himself.

28 For the law maketh men high priests which have infirmity; but the word of the oath, which was since the law, *maketh* the Son, who is [h]consecrated for evermore.

CHAPTER 8.

(d) Because the Aaronic priests served the shadows of which Christ serves the realities.

NOW of the things which we have spoken *this is* the sum: We have such an high priest, who is set on the right hand of the throne of the Majesty in the heavens;

2 A minister of the [i]sanctuary, and of the [j]true tabernacle, which the Lord pitched, and not man.

3 For every high priest is ordained to offer gifts and sacrifices: wherefore *it is* of necessity that this man have somewhat also to offer.

4 For if he were on earth, he should not be a priest, seeing that there are priests that offer gifts according to the law:

5 Who [k]serve unto the example and shadow of heavenly things, as Moses was [l]admonished of God when he was about to make the tabernacle: for, [m]See, saith he, *that* thou make all things according to the pattern shewed to thee in the mount.

(e) Because Christ mediates a better covenant.

6 But now hath he obtained a more excellent ministry, by how much also he is the mediator of a better [n]covenant, which was established upon better promises.

Part IV. The new covenant better than the old (Heb. 8:7–10:39).

7 For if [o]that first *covenant* had been faultless, then should no place have been sought for the second.

8 For finding fault with them, he saith, Behold, the days come, saith the [p]Lord, when I will [q]make a [1r]new [2s]covenant with the house of Israel and with the house of Judah:

9 Not according to the covenant that I made with their fathers in the day when I took them by the hand to lead them out of the land of Egypt; because they continued

A.D. 64.

- a *covenant.*
- b Jude 24.
- c Rom. 1:16, *note.*
- d *completely.*
- e *Assurance.* Heb. 8:10-13. (Isa. 32:17; Jude 1.)
- f *Sin.* Rom. 3:23, *note.*
- g *Sacrifice (of Christ).* Heb. 9:11-15, 22, 26. (Gen. 4:4; Heb. 10:18.)
- h *perfected.*
- i Or, *holy things.*
- j Heb. 9:11, 24; 10:21; 1 Tim. 3:15.
- k *serve the representation and.*
- l *oracularly told.*
- m Ex. 25:40.
- n Or, *testament.*
- o Ex. 3:8; 19:5.
- p *Jehovah.* vs. 8-12; Jer. 31:31-34.
- q *consummate,* or, *perfect.*
- r *Covenant (new).* (Isa. 61:8.)
- s *The Eight Covenants.* (Gen. 1:28.)

[1]**(8:8)** The New Covenant, Summary: (1) "Better" than the Mosaic Covenant, not morally, but efficaciously (Heb. 7:19; Rom. 8:3, 4). (2) Established on "better" (i.e. unconditional) promises. In the Mosaic Covenant God said, "If ye will" (Ex. 19:5); in the New Covenant He says, "I will" (Heb. 8:10, 12). (3) Under the Mosaic Covenant obedience sprang from fear (Heb. 2:2; 12:25-27); under the New from a willing heart and mind (v. 10). (4) The New Covenant secures the personal revelation of the Lord to every believer (v. 11); (5) the complete oblivion of sins (v. 12; Heb. 10:17; Cf. Heb. 10:3); (6) rests upon an accomplished redemption (Mt. 26:27, 28; 1 Cor. 11:25; Heb. 9:11, 12, 18-23); (7) and secures the perpetuity, future conversion, and blessing of Israel (Jer. 31:31-40; see also "Kingdom (O.T.)," and 2 Sam. 7:8-17). The New Covenant is the eighth, thus speaking of resurrection and of eternal completeness.

[2]**(8:8)** I. The Eight Covenants, Summary: (1) The Edenic Covenant (Gen. 1:26-28, *note*) conditioned the life of man in innocency. (2) The Adamic Covenant (Gen. 3:14-19, *note*) conditions the life of fallen man and gives promise of a Redeemer. (3) The Noahic Covenant (Gen. 9:1, *note*) establishes the principle of human government. (4) The Abrahamic Covenant (Gen. 15:18, *note*) founds the nation of Israel, and confirms, with specific additions, the Adamic promise of redemption. (5) The Mosaic Covenant (Ex. 19:25, *note*) condemns all men, "for that all have sinned." (6) The Palestinian Covenant (Deut. 28:1–30:3, *note*) secures the final restoration and conversion of Israel. (7) The Davidic Covenant (2 Sam. 7:8-17, *note*) establishes the perpetuity of the Davidic family (fulfilled in Christ, Mt. 1:1;

not in my covenant, and I regarded them not, saith the Lord.

10 For this *is* the covenant that I will make with the house of Israel after those days, saith the [a]Lord; I will put my [b]laws into their mind, and write them in their hearts: and I [c]will be to them a [d]God, and they shall be to me a people:

11 And they shall not teach every man his neighbour, and every man his brother, saying, Know the [e]Lord: for all shall know me, from the least to the greatest.

12 For I will be [f]merciful to their [g]unrighteousness, and their sins and their [h]iniquities will I remember no more.

13 In that he saith, A new *covenant*, he hath made the first old. Now that which [i]decayeth and waxeth old *is* ready to vanish away.

CHAPTER 9.

(1) *The ordinances and sanctuary of the old covenant were mere types.*

Then verily the first *covenant* had also ordinances of divine service, and a [j]worldly sanctuary.

2 For there was a tabernacle made; the first, wherein *was* the candlestick, and the table, and the [k]shewbread; which is called the [l]sanctuary.

3 And after the second veil, the tabernacle which is called the [m]Holiest of all;

4 Which had the [n]golden censer, and the [o]ark of the covenant overlaid round about with gold, wherein *was* the [p]golden pot that had manna, and [q]Aaron's rod that budded, and the [r]tables of the covenant;

5 And over it the cherubims of glory shadowing the [s]mercyseat; of which we cannot now speak [t]particularly.

6 Now when these things were thus ordained, the priests went always into the first tabernacle, accomplishing the service *of God*.

7 But into the second *went* the high priest alone once every year, not without blood, which he offered for himself, and *for* the [u]errors of the people:

8 The Holy Ghost this signifying, that the way into the holiest of all was not yet made manifest, while as the first tabernacle [v]was yet standing:

9 Which *was* a figure for the time then present, in which were offered both gifts and sacrifices, that could not make him that did the service [w]perfect, as pertaining to the conscience;

10 *Which stood* only in meats and drinks, and divers washings, and [x]carnal ordinances, imposed *on them* until the time of [y]reformation.

(2) *The sanctuary, and sacrifice of the new covenant are realities.*

11 But Christ being come an high priest [z]of good things to come, by a greater and more perfect tabernacle, not made with hands, that is to say, not of this [aa]building;

12 Neither by the blood of goats and calves, but [bb]by his own blood he entered in once into the [cc]holy place, having obtained eternal redemption *for us*.

13 For if the blood of bulls and of

A.D. 64.

a *Jehovah.* Jer. 31:33.
b *Law (of Moses).* Heb. 10:28. (Ex. 19:1; Gal. 3:1-29.)
c *Assurance.* vs. 10-13; Heb. 9:26. (Isa. 32:17; Jude 1.)
d Jer. 31:33.
e *Jehovah.* Jer. 31:34.
f Gr. *hileos propitious.* See 1 John 2:2; Rom. 3:25, *note.*
g *Sin.* Rom. 3:23, *note.*
h *lawlessnesses.*
i *grows old and aged is near to disappearing.*
j *an earthly.*
k Ex. 25:30, *note.*
l *holy.*
m *Holy of holies.*
n Lev. 16:12.
o Ex. 25:10.
p Ex. 16:33.
q Num. 17:10.
r Ex. 34:29; Deut. 10:2, 5.
s Gr. *hilasterion, place of propitiation.* See 1 John 2:2; Rom. 3:25, *note.*
t *in detail.*
u i.e. *sins of Ignorance.*
v *as yet had its standing.*
w Mt. 5:48, *note.*
x *fleshly.* Cf. Heb. 7:16.
y *setting things right.*
z Heb. 10:1; Eph. 1:3, 11.
aa *creation.*
bb 1 Pet. 1:18, 19.
cc *Sanctify, holy (things)* (N.T.). vs. 12, 24, 25; 2 Pet. 1:18. (Mt. 4:5; Rev. 22:11.)

Lk. 1:31-33; Rom. 1:3), and of the Davidic kingdom, over Israel and over the whole earth; to be fulfilled in and by Christ (2 Sam. 7:8-17; Zech. 12:8; Lk. 1:31-33; Acts 15:14-17; 1 Cor. 15:24). (8) The New Covenant rests upon the sacrifice of Christ, and secures the eternal blessedness, under the Abrahamic Covenant (Gal. 3:13-29), of all who believe. It is absolutely unconditional, and, since no responsibility is by it committed to man, it is final and irreversible.

II. The relation of Christ to the eight covenants is as follows: (1) To the Edenic Covenant, Christ, as the "second Man," the "last Adam" (1 Cor. 15:45-47), takes the place over all things which the first Adam lost (Col. 2:10; Heb. 2:7-8). (2) He is the "Seed of the woman" of the Adamic Covenant (Gen. 3:15; John 12:31; 1 John 3:8; Gal. 4:4; Rev. 20:10), and fulfilled its conditions of toil (Mk. 6:3) and obedience. (3) As the greatest son of Shem, in Him was fulfilled supremely the promise to Shem in the Noahic Covenant (Gen. 9:1, *note;* Col. 2:9). (4) He is the "Seed to whom the promises were made" in the Abrahamic Covenant; the son of Abraham obedient unto death (Gen. 22:18; Gal. 3:16; Phil. 2:8). (5) He lived sinlessly under the Mosaic Covenant and bore for us its curse (Gal. 3:10-13). (6) He lived obediently as a Jew in the land under the Palestinian Covenant, and will yet perform its gracious promises (Deut. 28-30:1-9). (7) He is the "Seed," "Heir," and "King" under the Davidic Covenant (Mt. 1:1; Lk. 1:31-33). (8) His sacrifice is the foundation of the New Covenant (Mt. 26:28; 1 Cor. 11:25).

goats, and the ashes of an heifer sprinkling the unclean, sanctifieth to the purifying of the flesh:

14 How much more shall the blood of Christ, who through the [a]eternal Spirit offered himself without spot to God, purge your conscience from dead works to [b]serve the living God?

15 And for this cause he is the mediator of the new [c]testament, that [d]by means of death, for the [e]redemption of the [f]transgressions *that were* under the first testament, they which are called might receive the promise of eternal inheritance.

(3) *The new covenant is also the last will and testament of Christ, sealed by his blood.*

16 For where a testament *is,* there must also of necessity [g]be the death of the testator.

17 For a testament *is* of force after men are dead: otherwise it is of no strength at all while the testator liveth.

18 Whereupon neither the first *testament* was [h]dedicated without blood.

19 [i]For when Moses had spoken every precept to all the people according to the law, he took the blood of calves and of goats, with water, and scarlet wool, and hyssop, and sprinkled both the book, and all the people,

20 Saying, This *is* the blood [j]of the testament which [k]God hath enjoined unto you.

21 [l]Moreover he sprinkled with blood both the tabernacle, and all the vessels of the ministry.

22 And almost all things are by the law purged with blood; and without shedding of blood is no [m]remission.

(4) *The heavenly sanctuary purged with a better sacrifice* (Lev. 16:33).

23 *It was* therefore necessary that the [n]patterns of things in the heavens should be purified with these; but the heavenly things themselves with better sacrifices than these.

24 For Christ is not entered into the holy places made with hands, *which are* the figures of the true; but into heaven itself, now to [o]appear in the presence of God for us:

(5) *The one sacrifice of the new covenant is better than the many sacrifices of the old.*

25 Nor yet that he should offer himself often, as the high priest entereth into the holy place every year with blood [p]of others;

26 For then must he often have suffered since the foundation of the world: but now once in the [q]end of the world hath he appeared [r]to put away [s]sin by the sacrifice of himself.

27 And as it is appointed unto men once to [1][t]die, but [u]after this [v]the judgment:

28 So Christ was once offered to bear the [s]sins of many; and unto them that look for him shall he appear the second time [w]without sin unto [x]salvation.

CHAPTER 10.

For the law having a shadow of good things to come, *and* not the very image of the things, can never with those sacrifices which they offered year by year continually make the comers thereunto [y]perfect.

2 For then would they not have ceased to be offered? because that the worshippers once purged should have had no more conscience of [s]sins.

3 But in those *sacrifices there is* a remembrance again *made* of [s]sins every year.

A.D. 64.

- a *Holy Spirit.* Heb. 10:1-5, 29. (Mt. 1:18; Acts 2:4.)
- b *worship.*
- c *covenant.*
- d *Sacrifice (of Christ).* vs. 11-15, 22, 26; Heb. 11:4. (Gen. 4:4; Heb. 10:18.)
- e Rom. 3:24, *note.*
- f *Sin.* Rom. 3:23, *note.*
- g Or, *be brought in.*
- h *inaugurated.*
- i v. 14:16.
- j Mt. 26:28.
- k *Jehovah.* Ex. 24:8.
- l Ex. 29:12, 36.
- m *Forgiveness.* Mt. 26:28. (Lev. 4:20; Mt. 26:28.)
- n *representations.* Heb. 8:5.
- o Rom. 8:34.
- p *not his own.*
- q *consummation of the ages.*
- r *Assurance.* Heb. 10:16-18, 22. (Isa. 32:17; Jude 1.).
- s *Sin.* Rom. 3:23, *note.*
- t *Death (physical).* (Gen. 3:19.)
- u *Judgments (the seven).* Heb. 12:5-11. (2 Sam. 7:14; Rev. 20:12.)
- v *Day of judgment.* 2 Pet. 2:9. (Mt. 10:15; Rev. 20:11.)
- w Or, *apart from.*
- x Rom. 1:16, *note.*
- y Mt. 5:48, *note.*

[1] **(9:27)** Death, physical, Summary: (1) Physical death is a consequence of sin (Gen. 3:19), and the universality of death proves the universality of sin (Rom. 5:12-14). (2) Physical death affects the body only, and is neither cessation of life nor of consciousness (Hab. 2:5, *note;* Lk. 16:23, *note;* Rev. 6:9, 10). (3) All physical death ends in the resurrection of the body. See "Resurrection" (Job 19:25; 1 Cor. 15:52, *note*). (4) Because physical death is a consequence of sin, it is not inevitable to the redeemed (Gen. 5:24; 1 Cor. 15:51, 52; 1 Thes. 4:15-17). (5) Physical death has for the believer a peculiar qualification. It is called "sleep," because his body may be "awakened" at any moment (Phil. 3:20, 21; 1 Thes. 4:14-18). (6) The soul and spirit live, independently of the death of the body, which is described as a "tabernacle" (tent), in which the "I" dwells, and which may be put off (2 Cor. 5:1-8; cf. 1 Cor. 15:42-44; 2 Pet. 1:13-15). (7) At the believer's death he is "clothed upon" with a "house from heaven" pending the resurrection of the "earthly house," and is at once "with the Lord" (2 Cor. 5:1-8; Phil. 1:23; Lk. 23:43). As to the death of Christ, see Mt. 27:50, *note.*

4 For *it is* not possible that the blood of bulls and of goats should take away [a]sins.

5 Wherefore when he cometh into the [b]world, he saith, [c]Sacrifice and offering thou wouldest not, but a [1]body hast thou prepared me:

6 In burnt offerings and *sacrifices* for [a]sin thou hast had no pleasure.

7 Then said I, Lo, I come (in the volume of the book it is written of me,) to do thy will, O [d]God.

8 Above when he said, Sacrifice and offering and burnt offerings and *offering* for [a]sin thou wouldest not, neither hadst pleasure *therein*; which are offered by the law;

9 Then said he, Lo, I come to do thy will, O God. He taketh away the first, that he may establish the second.

10 By the which will [e]we are [f]sanctified through the offering of the body of Jesus Christ once *for all*.

11 And every priest standeth daily ministering and offering oftentimes the same sacrifices, which can never take away [a]sins:

12 But this man, after he had offered one [f]sacrifice for sins [g]for ever, sat down [h]on the right hand of God;

13 From henceforth expecting till his enemies be made his footstool.

14 For by one offering he hath [i]perfected for ever [j]them that are sanctified.

15 *Whereof* the [k]Holy Ghost also is a witness to us: for after that he had said before,

16 This *is* the covenant that I will make with them after those days, saith the [l]Lord, I will put my laws into their hearts, and in their minds will I write them;

17 And their [m]sins and iniquities will I remember no more.

18 Now where remission of these *is*, *there is* no more [2]offering for [m]sin.

(6) *The believer worships in the holiest.*

19 Having therefore, brethren, boldness to enter into the [n]holiest by the blood of Jesus,

20 By a new and [o]living way, which he hath [p]consecrated for us, through the veil, that is to say, his flesh;

21 And *having* an high priest over the house of God;

22 Let us draw near with a true heart in full [q]assurance of [r]faith, having our hearts sprinkled from an evil conscience, and our bodies washed with pure water.

23 Let us hold fast the [s]profession of *our* faith without wavering; (for [t]he *is* faithful that promised;)

24 And let us consider one another to provoke unto love and to good works:

25 Not forsaking the assembling of ourselves together, [u]as the manner of some *is*; but [v]exhorting *one another*: and so much the more, [w]as ye see the day approaching.

(*Parenthetic: The wavering warned: the Jewish sacrifices had lost their efficacy; it is Christ or judgment.*)

26 For if we [m]sin [x]wilfully after that we have received the knowledge of the truth, there remaineth no more sacrifice for sins,

27 But a certain fearful looking for of judgment and fiery indignation, which shall devour the adversaries.

28 He that despised [y]Moses' law

A.D. 64.

a *Sin.* Rom. 3:23, *note.*
b *kosmos* (Mt. 4:8) = mankind.
c vs. 5, 7; Psa. 40:6-8.
d Psa. 40:8.
e v. 14.
f *Sacrifice (of Christ).* (Gen. 4:4.)
g *sat down in perpetuity.*
h vs. 12, 13; Psa. 110:1.
i Mt. 5:48, *note.*
j v. 10.
k *Holy Spirit.* vs. 15, 29; Jas. 4:5. (Mt. 1:18; Acts 2:4.)
l *Jehovah.* vs. 16, 17; Jer. 31:33, 34.
m *Sin.* Rom. 3:23, *note.*
n Heb. 9:8, 12.
o John 14:6; Heb. 7:24.
p *dedicated.*
q *Assurance.* vs. 16-18, 22; 1 Pet. 3:18. (Isa. 32:17; Jude 1.)
r *Faith.* vs. 22, 38; Heb. 12:2. (Gen. 3:20; Heb. 11:39.)
s *confession of the hope.*
t 1 Thes. 5:24.
u Mt. 10:32.
v *encouraging.*
w Mt. 24.
x 2 Pet. 2:20, 21.
y *Law (of Moses).* Jas. 2:10. (Ex. 19:1; Gal. 3:1-29.)

[1] **(10:5)** Cf. Psa. 40:6; the rule, applicable to *all* modifications of the form of quotations in the N.T. from O.T. writings, is that the divine Author of both Testaments is perfectly free, in using an earlier statement, to recast the mere literary form of it. The variant form will be found invariably to give the deeper meaning of the earlier statement.

[2] **(10:18)** Sacrifice, Summary: (1) The first intimation of sacrifice is Gen. 3:21, the "coats of skins" having obviously come from slain animals. The first clear *instance* of sacrifice is Gen. 4:4, explained in Heb. 11:4. Abel's righteousness was the result of his sacrifice, not of his character. (2) Before the giving of the law the head of the family was the family priest. By the law an order of priests was established who alone could offer sacrifices. Those sacrifices were "shadows," types, expressing variously the guilt and need of the offerer in reference to God, and all pointing to Christ and fulfilled in Him. (3) As foreshadowed by the types and explained by the N.T., the sacrifice of Christ is *penal* (Gal. 3:13; 2 Cor. 5:21); *substitutional* (Lev. 1:4; Isa. 53:5, 6; 2 Cor. 5:21; 1 Pet. 2:24); *voluntary* (Gen. 22:9; John 10:18); *redemptive* (Gal. 3;13; Eph. 1:7; 1 Cor. 6:20); *propitiatory* (Rom. 3:25); *reconciling* (2 Cor. 5:18, 19; Col. 1:21, 22); *efficacious* (John 12:32, 33; Rom. 5:9, 10; 2 Cor. 5:21; Eph. 2:13; Heb. 9:11, 12, 26; 10:10-17; 1 John 1:7; Rev. 1:5); and *revelatory* (John 3:16; 1 John 4:9, 10).

died without mercy under two or three witnesses:

29 [a]Of how much sorer punishment, suppose ye, shall he be thought worthy, [b]who hath trodden under foot the Son of God, and hath counted the blood of the covenant, wherewith he was [c]sanctified, [d]an unholy thing, and hath done despite unto the [e]Spirit of grace?

30 For we know him that hath said, Vengeance *belongeth* unto me, I will recompense, saith the [f]Lord. And again, The Lord shall judge his people.

31 *It is* a fearful thing to fall into the hands of the living God.

32 But call to remembrance the former days, in which, after ye were illuminated, ye endured a great fight of afflictions;

33 Partly, whilst ye were made a gazingstock both by reproaches and afflictions; and partly, whilst ye became companions of them that were so used.

34 For ye had compassion of me [g]in my bonds, and took joyfully the spoiling of your goods, knowing in yourselves that ye have [h]in heaven a better and an enduring substance.

35 Cast not away therefore your confidence, which hath great recompence of reward.

36 For ye have need of patience, that, [i]after ye have done the will of God, ye might receive the promise.

37 For yet a little while, and he that shall come [j]will come, and will not tarry.

38 Now the [k]just shall live by faith: but if *any man* draw back, my soul shall have no pleasure in him.

39 But we are not of them who draw back unto perdition; but of them that believe to the saving of the soul.

CHAPTER 11.

Part V. The superiority of the faith way (Heb. 11:1-40).

(1) *The sphere of faith.*

Now faith is the [l]substance of things hoped for, the [m]evidence of things not seen.

2 For by it the elders obtained a good report.

3 Through faith we understand that the [n]worlds were framed by the word of God, so that things which are seen were not made of things which do appear.

(2) *Instances of faith: Abel.*

4 By faith Abel offered unto God a more excellent [o]sacrifice than Cain, by which he obtained witness that he was [p]righteous, God testifying of his gifts: and by it he being dead yet speaketh.

Enoch.

5 By faith [q]Enoch was translated that he should not see death; and was not found, because God had translated him: for before his translation he had this testimony, that he [r]pleased God.

6 But without faith *it is* impossible to please *him*: for he that cometh to God must believe that he is, and *that* he is a [s]rewarder of them that diligently seek him.

Noah.

7 By faith [t]Noah, being warned of God of things not seen as yet, moved with fear, prepared an ark to the [u]saving of his house; by the which he condemned the [v]world, and became heir of the righteousness which is by faith.

Abraham and Sara.

8 By faith [w]Abraham, when he was called to go out into a place which he should after receive for an inheritance, obeyed; and he went out, not knowing whither he went.

9 By faith he sojourned in the land of promise, as *in* a strange country, [x]dwelling in [y]tabernacles with Isaac and Jacob, the heirs with him of the same promise:

10 For he [z]looked for a city which hath foundations, whose [aa]builder and maker *is* God.

11 Through faith also [bb]Sara herself received strength to conceive seed, and was delivered of a child when she was past age, because she judged him faithful who had promised.

12 Therefore sprang there even of one, and him as good as dead, *so many* as the [cc]stars of the sky in multitude, and as the sand which is by the sea shore innumerable.

13 These all died in faith, not having received the [dd]promises, but having seen them afar off, and were persuaded of *them*, and embraced *them*, and [ee]confessed that they were strangers and pilgrims on the earth.

14 For they that say such things declare plainly that they seek a country.

A.D. 64.

a Heb. 2:3.
b *Apostasy.* 2 Pet. 2:1-3. (Lk. 18:8; 2 Tim. 3:1-8.)
c *Sanctify, holy (persons)* (N.T.). vs. 10, 14, 29; Heb. 13:12. (Mt. 4:5; Rev. 22:11.)
d *Gr. a common thing.*
e *Grace (in salv.).* 1 Pet. 1:10, 13. (Rom. 3:24; John 1:17, *note.*
f *Jehovah.* Deut. 32:35, 36.
g *that ye have for yourselves.*
h Lk. 12:33.
i Lk. 21:19.
j *Christ (Second Advent)* 2 Pet. 3:3, 4. (Deut. 30:3; Acts 1:9-11.)
k Hab. 2:3, 4; Rom. 1:17.
l *substantiating.*
m *conviction.*
n *ages were planned.*
o Sacrifice *(of Christ).* Heb. 13:11, 12. (Gen. 4:4; Heb. 10:18.)
p vs. 4, 7. See Rom. 10:10, *note.*
q Gen. 5:22, 24.
r *had pleased.*
s *Rewards.* Jas. 1:12. (Dan. 12:3; 1 Cor. 3:14.)
t Gen. 6:14, 22.
u Rom. 1:16, *note.*
v *kosmos* (Mt. 4:8) = mankind.
w Gen. 12:1, 4.
x Gen. 13:3, 18.
y *tents.*
z *waited for.*
aa *architect and builder.*
bb Gen. 21:1, 2.
cc Gen. 22:17.
dd Gen. 3:15; 12:7.
ee i.e. acted upon them.

15 And truly, if they had been mindful of [a]that *country* from whence they came out, they might have had opportunity to have returned.

16 But now they desire a better *country*, that is, an heavenly: wherefore God is not ashamed to be called their God: for he hath prepared for them a city.

17 By faith Abraham, when he was [b]tried, offered up Isaac: and he that had received the promises offered up his only begotten *son*,

18 [c]Of whom it was said, [d]That in Isaac shall thy seed be called:

19 Accounting that God *was* able to raise *him* up, [e]even from the dead; from whence also he received him [f]in a figure.

Isaac and Jacob.

20 By faith [g]Isaac blessed Jacob and Esau concerning things to come.

21 By faith Jacob, when he was a dying, blessed both the sons of Joseph; and worshipped, [h]*leaning* upon the top of his staff.

Joseph.

22 By faith [i]Joseph, when he died, made mention of the departing of the children of Israel; and gave commandment concerning his bones.

Moses and his parents.

23 By faith Moses, when he was born, was hid three months of his parents, because they saw [j]*he was* a proper child; and they were not afraid of the king's [k]commandment.

24 By faith Moses, when he was come to years, refused to be called the son of Pharaoh's daughter;

25 Choosing rather to suffer affliction with the people of God, [l]than to enjoy the pleasures of [m]sin for a season;

26 Esteeming the reproach of Christ greater riches than the treasures in Egypt: for he had respect unto the recompence [n]of the reward.

27 By faith he forsook Egypt, not fearing the wrath of the king: for he endured, as seeing him who is invisible.

A.D. 64.

a Gen. 11:31.
b Gen. 22:1; Jas. 2:21.
c Or, *to.*
d Gen. 21:12.
e *Resurrection.* Rev. 20:4, 5. (Job 19:25; 1 Cor. 15:52.)
f Gen. 22:4; Mt. 20:19.
g Gen. 27:27.
h Gen. 47:31.
i Gen. 50:24, 25.
j *the child was beautiful.*
k Ex. 1:16; 2:2.
l *Separation.* Heb. 13:10-14. (Gen. 12:1; 2 Cor. 6:14-17.)
m *Sin.* Rom. 3:23, *note.*
n Omit *of the reward.*
o Ex. 12:21.
p Ex. 14:13; Jas. 5:15, 16; Jude 5.
q Josh. 6:12, 20.
r Josh. 6:23; Jas. 2:25.
s Jud. 6:11.
t Jud. 4:6.
u Jud. 15:16.
v Jud. 11:32.
w 1 Sam. 7:9.
x 1 John 3:7, *note.*
y 1 Ki. 17:22; 2 Ki. 4:35.
z vs. 24, 26.
aa *Temptation.* 1 Pet. 1:6. (Gen. 3:1; Jas. 1:14.)
bb *evil treated.*
cc *kosmos* (Mt. 4:8) = mankind.
dd *Faith.* (Gen. 3:20.)

28 Through faith he kept the [o]passover, and the sprinkling of blood, lest he that destroyed the firstborn should touch them.

29 [p]By faith they passed through the Red sea as by dry *land*: which the Egyptians assaying to do were drowned.

Joshua and Israel.

30 By faith the walls of [q]Jericho fell down, after they were compassed about seven days.

Rahab.

31 By faith the harlot [r]Rahab perished not with them that believed not, when she had received the spies with peace.

The many heroes of faith.

32 And what shall I more say? for the time would fail me to tell of [s]Gedeon, and *of* [t]Barak, and *of* [u]Samson, and *of* [v]Jephthae; *of* David also, and [w]Samuel, and *of* the prophets:

33 Who through faith subdued kingdoms, wrought [x]righteousness, obtained promises, stopped the mouths of lions,

34 Quenched the violence of fire, escaped the edge of the sword, out of weakness were made strong, waxed valiant in fight, turned to flight the armies of the aliens.

35 Women [y]received their dead raised to life again: and others were tortured, not [z]accepting deliverance; that they might obtain a better resurrection:

36 And others had trial of *cruel* mockings and scourgings, yea, moreover of bonds and imprisonment:

37 They were stoned, they were sawn asunder, were [aa]tempted, were slain with the sword: they wandered about in sheepskins and goatskins; being destitute, afflicted, [bb]tormented;

38 (Of whom the [cc]world was not worthy:) they wandered in deserts, and *in* mountains, and *in* dens and caves of the earth.

39 And these all, having obtained a good report through [1dd]faith, received not the promise:

[1] **(11:39)** The essence of faith consists in receiving what God has revealed, and may be defined as that trust in the God of the Scriptures and in Jesus Christ whom He hath sent, which receives Him as Saviour and Lord, and impels to loving obedience and good works (John 1:12; Jas. 2:14-26). The particular *uses* of faith give rise to its secondary definitions: (1) For salvation, faith is personal trust, apart from meritorious works, in the Lord Jesus Christ, as delivered for our offences and raised again for our justification (Rom. 4:5, 23-25). (2) As used in prayer, faith is the "confidence that we have in him, that if we ask anything according to his will, he heareth us" (1 John 5:14, 15). (3) As used in reference to

40 God having provided some better thing for us, that they without us should not be made [a]perfect.

CHAPTER 12.

Part VI. The walk and worship of the believer-priest (Heb. 12:1–13:25).

(1) *Jesus the example.*

Wherefore seeing we also are compassed about with so great a cloud of witnesses, let us [b]lay aside every weight, and [c]the sin which doth so easily beset *us*, and let us run with patience the race that is set before us,

2 Looking unto Jesus the [d]author and [e]finisher of *our* [f]faith; who for the joy that was set before him endured the cross, despising the shame, and is set down at the right hand of the throne of God.

(*Parenthetic* (to v. 17): *(a) The Father's chastening*.)

3 For [g]consider him that endured such contradiction of [h]sinners against himself, lest ye be wearied and faint in your minds.

4 Ye have not yet resisted unto blood, striving against [h]sin.

5 And ye have forgotten the exhortation which speaketh unto you as unto [i]children, My son, despise not thou the chastening of the [j]Lord, nor faint when thou art rebuked of him:

6 For whom the [k]Lord loveth he chasteneth, and scourgeth every son whom he receiveth.

7 If ye endure chastening, God dealeth with you as with sons; for what [l]son is he whom the father chasteneth not?

8 But if ye be without chastisement, whereof all are partakers, then are ye bastards, and not sons.

9 Furthermore we have had fathers of our flesh which corrected *us*, and we gave *them* reverence: shall we not much rather be in subjection unto the Father of spirits, and live?

10 For they verily for a few days chastened *us* [m]after their own pleasure; but he for *our* profit, that *we* might be partakers of his holiness.

11 Now no [n]chastening for the present seemeth to be joyous, but grievous: nevertheless afterward it yieldeth the peaceable fruit of [o]righteousness unto them which are exercised thereby.

12 Wherefore [p]lift up the hands which hang down, and the [q]feeble knees;

13 And make [r]straight paths for your feet, lest that which is lame be turned out of the way; but [s]let it rather be healed.

14 Follow [t]peace with all *men*, and holiness, without which no man shall see the Lord:

15 [u]Looking diligently lest any man fail of the grace of God; lest any root of bitterness springing up trouble *you*, and thereby many be defiled;

(b) Esau a warning to professors lest they miss the priesthood. (Cf. Gen. 25:31, *note*.)

16 Lest there *be* any [v]fornicator, or profane person, as Esau, [w]who for one morsel of meat sold his birthright.

17 For ye know how that afterward, when he would have inherited the blessing, he was rejected: for he found no place of [x]repentance, though he sought [y]it carefully with tears.

(2) *The believer-priest does not come to Mount Sinai.*

18 For ye are not come unto the [z]mount that might be touched, and that burned with fire, nor unto blackness, and darkness, and tempest,

19 And the sound of a trumpet, and the voice of words; which [aa]*voice* they that heard intreated that the word should not be spoken to them any more:

20 (For they could not endure that which was commanded, And if so much as a beast touch the mountain, it shall be stoned, or thrust through with a dart:

21 And so terrible was the sight, *that* Moses said, I exceedingly fear and quake:)

A.D. 64.

a Mt. 5:48, *note.*
b Heb. 10:39; 1 Pet. 5:7.
c Omit *the.*
d *leader,* or, *originator.* See Heb. 2:10, *ref.*
e *perfecter.*
f *Faith* Jas. 2:17, 18, 20. (Gen. 3:20; Heb. 11:39.)
g *consider well,* i.e. weigh so as to judge its value.
h *Sin.* Rom. 3:23, *note.*
i *sons.*
j *Jehovah.* Prov. 3:11, 12.
k *Jehovah,* Prov. 3:12.
l Prov. 13:24.
m Or, *as seemed good or meet to them.*
n *Judgments (the seven).* 1 Pet. 2:24. (2 Sam. 7:14; Rev. 20:12.)
o 1 John 3:7, *note.*
p Isa. 35:3.
q *failing.*
r Or, *even.*
s Gal. 6:1.
t Psa. 34:14.
u *watching lest there be any one who lacks the grace of God.*
v 1 Cor. 6:13, 18.
w Gen. 25:33.
x *Repentance.* 2 Pet. 3:9. (Mt. 3:2; Acts 17:30.)
y i.e. the blessing.
z Ex. 19:12.
aa Ex. 20:18, 19.

unseen things of which Scripture speaks, faith "gives substance" to them, so that we act upon the conviction of their reality (Heb. 11:1-3). (4) As a working principle in life, the uses of faith are illustrated in Heb. 11:1-39.

22 But ye are [a]come unto mount Sion, and unto the city of the living God, the heavenly Jerusalem, and to [b]an innumerable company of [c]angels,

23 To the general assembly [d]and [1]church of the firstborn, which are written in heaven, and to God the Judge of all, and to the spirits of just men made [e]perfect,

24 And to Jesus the [f]mediator of the new covenant, and to [g]the blood of sprinkling, that speaketh better things than *that of* Abel.

(3) *Warnings and instructions.*

25 [h]See that ye refuse not him that speaketh. For if they escaped not who refused him that spake on earth, much more *shall not* we *escape*, if we turn away from him that *speaketh* from heaven:

26 Whose voice then shook the earth: but now he hath promised, saying, [i]Yet once more I shake not the earth only, but also heaven.

27 And this *word*, Yet once more, signifieth the removing of those things that are shaken, as of things that are made, that those things which cannot be shaken may remain.

28 Wherefore we receiving a kingdom which cannot be [j]moved, let us [k]have [l]grace, whereby we may serve God acceptably with reverence and godly fear:

29 For our God *is* a consuming fire.

CHAPTER 13.

Let brotherly love continue.

2 Be not forgetful to entertain strangers: for thereby some have entertained [c]angels unawares.

3 Remember them that are in [m]bonds, as bound with them; *and* them which suffer adversity, as being yourselves also in the body.

4 [n]Marriage *is* honourable in all, and the bed undefiled: but whoremongers and adulterers God will judge.

5 *Let your* conversation *be* without [o]covetousness; *and be* content with such things as ye have: for [p]he hath said, [q]I will never leave thee, nor forsake thee.

6 So that we may boldly say, [r]The Lord *is* my helper, and I will not fear what man shall do unto me.

7 Remember [s]them which have the rule over you, who have spoken unto you the word of God: [t]whose faith follow, considering the end of *their* conversation.

8 Jesus Christ the same yesterday, and to day, and [u]for ever.

9 Be not carried about with divers and strange doctrines. For *it is* a good thing that the heart be established [v]with grace; not with meats, which have not profited them that have been occupied therein.

(4) *Christian separation and worship.*

10 We have an altar, whereof they have no right to eat which serve the tabernacle.

11 For the bodies of those beasts, whose blood is brought into the sanctuary by the high priest for sin, are burned without the camp.

12 Wherefore Jesus also, that he might [w]sanctify the people [x]with his own blood, suffered without the gate.

13 Let us go forth therefore unto him without the camp, [y]bearing his reproach.

14 For here have we no [z]continuing city, but [aa]we seek [bb]one to come.

(5) *The believer-priest's sacrifice.*

15 By him therefore let us offer the [cc]sacrifice of praise to God continually, that is, the fruit of *our* lips giving thanks to his name.

16 But to do good and to [dd]communicate forget not: for with such [ee]sacrifices God is well pleased.

(6) *The believer-priest's obedience.*

17 Obey them that [ff]have the rule over you, and submit yourselves: for they [gg]watch for your souls, as they that must give account, that they may do it with joy, and not with grief: for that *is* unprofitable for you.

A.D. 64.

a Eph. 2:19; Phil. 3:20.
b *myriads of angels, the universal gathering.*
c Heb. 1:4, *note.*
d *Church (true).* (Mt. 16:18.)
e Mt. 5:48, *note.*
f Heb. 8:6.
g Ex. 24:8.
h Acts 13:46.
i Hag. 2:6.
j *shaken.*
k *hold fast.*
l *Grace (imparted).* vs. 15, 28; Heb. 13:9. (Rom. 6:1; 1 Pet. 3:18.)
m Mt. 25:36.
n Prov. 5:18-23.
o *love of money.*
p *himself.*
q Deut. 31:6.
r Psa. 118:6.
s *your guides.*
t Lit. *considering the issue of the conversation of whom, imitate the faith.*
u *to the ages* [to come].
v *Grace (imparted).* Jas. 4:6. (Rom. 6:1; 2 Pet. 3:18.)
w *Sanctify, holy (persons)* (N.T.). 1 Pet. 1:15, 16. (Mt. 4:5; Rev. 22:11.)
x *Sacrifice (of Christ).* 1 Pet. 1:18, 19. (Gen. 4:4; Heb. 10:18.)
y Acts 5:41.
z *abiding.*
aa *Separation.* vs. 10-14; 1 John 2:15-17. (Gen. 12:1; 2 Cor. 6:14-17.)
bb *the coming one.*
cc *Sacrifice (the believer-priest's).* vs. 15, 16; 1 Pet. 2:5. (Gen. 4:4; Heb. 10:18.)
dd Or, *share what you have with others.* Cf. Rom. 12:13; Gal. 6:6.
ee Phil. 4:18.
ff *guide you.*
gg Ezk. 3:17.

[1]**(12:23)** Church (true), Summary: The true church, composed of the whole number of regenerate persons from Pentecost to the first resurrection (1 Cor. 15:52), united together and to Christ by the baptism with the Holy Spirit (1 Cor. 12:12, 13), is the body of Christ of which He is the Head (Eph. 1:22, 23). As such, it is a holy temple for the habitation of God through the Spirit (Eph. 2:21, 22); is "one flesh" with Christ (Eph. 5:30, 31); and espoused to Him as a chaste virgin to one husband (2 Cor. 11:2-4).

Conclusion: the apostolic benediction.

18 Pray for us: for we trust we have a
good [a]conscience, in all things willing to
live honestly.
19 But I beseech *you* the rather to do
this, that I may be restored to you the
sooner.
20 [b]Now the [c]God of peace, that
brought again [d]from the dead our Lord
Jesus, that great shepherd of the sheep,
through the blood of the [e]everlasting
covenant,
21 [f]Make you [g]perfect in every good
work to do his will, working in you that
which is wellpleasing in his sight,
through Jesus Christ; to whom *be* glory
for ever and ever. Amen.
22 And I beseech you, brethren, suffer
the word of exhortation: for I have written a letter unto you in few words.
23 Know ye that *our* brother Timothy
is set at liberty; with whom, if he come
shortly, I will see you.
24 Salute all them that [h]have the rule
over you, and all the saints. They of Italy
salute you.
25 Grace *be* with you all. Amen.

A.D. 64.

a Acts 24:16.
b *Bible prayers* (N.T.). Rev. 22:20. (Mt. 6:9; Rev. 22:20.)
c Rom. 5:1, 2, 10.
d *from among.*
e *eternal.*
f *perfect you.*
g Mt. 5:48, *note.*
h *guide you.*

THE GENERAL EPISTLE OF JAMES

WRITER. James. (Mt. 4:21, *note*), called "the Just," mentioned by Paul with Cephas and John as "pillars" in the church at Jerusalem (Gal. 2:9). He seems to have been, as a religious man, austere, legal, ceremonial (Acts 21:18-24).

Date. Tradition fixes the martyrdom of James in the year 62, but his Epistle shows no trace of the larger revelations concerning the church and the distinctive doctrines of grace made through the Apostle Paul, nor even of the discussions concerning the relation of Gentile converts to the law of Moses, which culminated in the first council (Acts 15), over which James presided. This presumes the very early date of James, which may confidently be set down as "the first Epistle to Christians."—*Weston.*

Theme. By "the twelve tribes scattered abroad" we are to understand, not Jews, but Christian Jews of the Dispersion. The church began with such (Acts 2:5-11), and James, who seems not to have left Jerusalem, would feel a particular pastoral responsibility for these. scattered sheep. They still resorted to the synagogues, or called their own assemblies by that name (Jas. 2:2, where "assembly" is "synagogue" in the Gr.). It appears from Jas. 2:1-8 that they still held the synagogue courts for the trial of causes arising amongst themselves. The Epistle, then, is elementary in the extreme. To suppose that Jas. 2:14-26 is a polemic against Paul's doctrine of justification is absurd. Neither Galatians nor Romans was yet written.

James' theme, then, is "religion" (Gr. *threskeia,* "outward religious service") as the expression and proof of faith. He does not exalt works as against faith, but faith as producing works. His style is that of the Wisdom-books of the O.T.

The divisions are five: I. The testing of faith, 1:1–2:26. II. The reality of faith tested by the tongue, 3:1-18. III. The rebuke of worldliness, 4:1-17. IV. The rich warned, 5:1-6. V. Hortatory, 5:7-20.

CHAPTER 1.

Part I. The testings of faith (Jas. 1:1–2:26).

(1) *The purpose of testings.*

James, a [a]servant of God and of the Lord Jesus Christ, to the twelve tribes which are [b]scattered abroad, greeting.

2 My brethren, count it all joy when ye fall into divers [c]temptations;

3 Knowing *this,* that the trying of your faith [d]worketh patience.

4 But let patience have *her* perfect work, that ye may be [e]perfect and [f]entire, wanting nothing.

5 If any of you lack wisdom, let him ask of God, [g]that giveth to all *men* liberally, and upbraideth not; and it shall be given him.

6 [h]But let him ask in faith, nothing wavering. For he that wavereth is like a wave of the sea driven with the wind and tossed.

A.D. 60.

a bondman.
b *in the dispersion.* 1 Pet. 1:1.
c i.e. *testings.*
d Rom. 5:3.
e *mature and complete.* Mt. 5:48, *note.*
f *complete.*
g Prov. 2:3-6.
h Mk. 11:24.
i Prov. 3:5.
j Jas. 2:5.
k Isa. 57:15.
l *Temptation.* vs. 2, 12, 13, 14. (Gen. 3:1.)
m *Rewards.* 1 Pet. 5:4. (Dan. 12:3; 1 Cor. 3:14.)
n *Life (eternal).* 1 Pet. 3:7. (Mt. 7:14; Rev. 22:19.)

7 For let not that man think that he shall receive any thing of the Lord.

8 A [i]double minded man *is* unstable in all his ways.

9 [j]Let the brother of low degree rejoice in that he is exalted:

10 But the rich, [k]in that he is made low: because as the flower of the grass he shall pass away.

11 For the sun is no sooner risen with a burning heat, but it withereth the grass, and the flower thereof falleth, and the grace of the fashion of it perisheth: so also shall the rich man fade away in his ways.

12 Blessed *is* the man that endureth [l]temptation: for when he is tried, he shall receive the [m]crown of [n]life, which the Lord hath promised to them that love him.

(2) *Solicitation to do evil is not of God.*

13 Let no man say when he is tempted, I am tempted of God:

for God cannot be tempted with evil,
neither tempteth he any man:
14 But every man is [1]tempted, when
he is drawn away of his own lust, and
enticed.
15 Then when lust hath conceived, it
bringeth forth [a]sin: and sin, when it is
finished, bringeth forth death.
16 Do not err, my beloved brethren.
17 Every good [b]gift and every perfect
gift is from above, and cometh down
from the Father of lights, with whom is
no [c]variableness, neither shadow of
turning.
18 [d]Of his own will begat he us with
the word of truth, that we should be a
kind of firstfruits of his creatures.
19 Wherefore, my beloved brethren,
let every man be swift to hear, slow to
speak, slow to wrath:
20 For the wrath of man worketh not
the [e]righteousness of God.
21 Wherefore lay apart all filthiness
and [f]superfluity of naughtiness, and
receive with meekness the engrafted
word, which is able to [g]save your souls.

(3) *The test of obedience.*

22 But be ye [h]doers of the word, and
not hearers only, deceiving your own
selves.
23 For if any be a hearer of the word,
and not a doer, he is like unto a man
beholding his natural face in a glass:
24 For he beholdeth himself, and
goeth his way, and straightway forgetteth what manner of man he was.
25 But whoso [i]looketh into the [j]perfect
law of liberty, and continueth *therein*, he
being not a forgetful hearer, but a doer
of the work, this man shall be blessed in
his deed.

(4) *The test of true religion.*

26 If any man among you seem to be
[k]religious, and bridleth not his [l]tongue,
but deceiveth his own heart, this man's
religion *is* vain.
27 [m]Pure religion and undefiled before
God and the Father is this, To visit the
fatherless and widows in their affliction,
and to keep [n]himself unspotted from the
[o]world.

CHAPTER 2.

(5) *The test of brotherly love.*

My brethren, have not the faith of
our Lord Jesus Christ, [p]*the Lord* of
glory, [q]with respect of persons.
2 For if there come unto your assembly a man with a gold ring, in goodly
apparel, and there come in also a poor
man in vile raiment;
3 And ye have respect to him that
weareth the gay clothing, and say unto
him, Sit thou here in a good place; and
say to the poor, Stand thou there, or sit
here under my footstool:
4 [r]Are ye not then partial in yourselves, and are become judges [s]of evil
thoughts?
5 Hearken, my beloved brethren,
[t]Hath not God chosen the poor of this
[u]world [v]rich in faith, and heirs of the
kingdom which he hath promised to
them that love him?
6 But ye have despised the poor. Do
not rich men oppress you, and draw you
before the judgment seats?
7 Do not they blaspheme that [w]worthy
name by the which ye are called?
8 If ye fulfil the royal law according to
the scripture, [x]Thou shalt love thy
neighbour as thyself, ye do well:
9 But [y]if ye have respect to persons, ye
commit [z]sin, and are convinced of the
law as transgressors.
10 For whosoever shall keep the
whole [aa]law, and yet [bb]offend in one
point, he is guilty of all.
11 For he that said, [cc]Do not commit
adultery, said also, Do not kill. Now if
thou commit no adultery, yet if thou kill,
thou art become a [z]transgressor of the
law.
12 So speak ye, and so do, as they that
shall be judged by the [dd]law of liberty.
13 For he shall have judgment
without mercy, that hath shewed

A.D. 60.

a *Sin.* Rom. 3:23, *note.*
b Two words are used in the original for "gift," the first meaning *the act of giving;* the second, *the thing given.*
c *variation.*
d John 1:13; 1 Pet. 1:23.
e Rom. 3:21, *note.*
f *overflowing of wickedness.*
g Rom. 1:16, *note.*
h Mt. 7:21.
i 2 Cor. 3:18.
j *Law (of Christ).* 1 John 2:7, 8, 15. (Gal. 6:2; 2 John 5.).
k Gr. *threskos* = *outwardly religious.*
l Psa. 34:13.
m Mt. 25:34-36.
n *oneself.*
o *kosmos* = world-system. Jas. 4:4. (John 7:7; Rev. 13:3-8, *note.*)
p *the Glory*, i.e. in the sense of Heb. 1:3, as taking the place of the shekinah.
q In the presence of Christ the Glory, earthly distinctions disappear.
r *Have ye not made a difference among yourselves*
s *with.*
t John 7:48; 1 Cor. 1:26, 28.
u *kosmos* (Mt. 4:8) = mankind.
v Lk. 12:21; 1 Tim. 6:18.
w *excellent*, or, *beautiful.*
x Lev. 19:18.
y v. 1.
z *Sin.* Rom. 3:23, *note.*
aa *Law (of Moses).* Rev. 12:17. (Ex. 19:1; Gal. 3:1-29.)
bb Mt. 5:19; Gal. 3:10.
cc Ex. 20:13, 14.
dd Jas. 1:25; 1 Pet. 2:16.

[1] **(1:14)** "Temptation" is used in two senses: (1) Solicitation to evil (e.g. Gen. 3:1-6; Mt. 4:1; 1 Cor. 10:13; 2 Cor. 11:3, 4; Jas. 1:14). (2) Testing under trial (e.g. Gen. 22:1; Lk. 22:28; cf. Lk. 4:2). Cf. Mt.6:13 (solicitation to evil) and 1 Pet. 1:6 (testing under trial).

no mercy; and [a]mercy [b]rejoiceth against
judgment.

(6) *The test of good works.*

14 What *doth it* profit, my brethren,
though a man say he hath faith, and
have not works? can [c]faith [d]save him?
15 If a brother or sister be naked, and
destitute of daily food,
16 And [e]one of you say unto them,
Depart in peace, be *ye* warmed and
filled; notwithstanding ye give them not
those things which are needful to the
body; what *doth it* profit?
17 Even so [f]faith, if it hath not works,
is [g]dead, being alone.
18 Yea, a man may say, Thou hast
faith, and I have works: [h]shew me thy
faith without thy works, and I will shew
thee my faith by my works.
19 Thou believest that [i]there is one
God; thou doest well: the [j]devils also
believe, and tremble.
20 But wilt thou know, O vain man,
that [k]faith without works is dead?

(7) *The illustration of Abraham.*
(Cf. Rom. 4:1-25.)

21 Was not Abraham our father [l]justi-
fied by works, when he had offered
Isaac his son upon the altar?
22 Seest thou how faith wrought with
his works, and by works was faith made
[m]perfect?
23 And the scripture was fulfilled which
saith, Abraham believed [n]God, and it was
[1o]imputed unto him for [p]righteousness:
and he was called the [q]Friend of God.
24 Ye see then how that by works a
man is justified, and not by faith only.
25 Likewise also was not [r]Rahab the
harlot justified by works, when she had
received the messengers, and had sent
them out another way?
26 For as the [s]body without the spirit is
dead, so faith without works is dead also.

CHAPTER 3.

Part II. A true faith will control the tongue.

My brethren, be not many [t]masters,
knowing that we shall receive
the greater condemnation.
2 For in many things [u]we offend all. If
any man offend not in word, the same *is*
a [m]perfect man, *and* able also to bridle
the whole body.
3 Behold, we put [v]bits in the horses'
mouths, that they may obey us; and we
turn about their whole body.
4 Behold also the ships, which though
they be so great, and *are* driven of fierce
winds, yet are they turned about with a
very small helm, whithersoever the governor listeth.
5 Even so [w]the tongue is a little
member, and boasteth great things.
Behold, how great a matter a little fire
kindleth!
6 [x]And the tongue *is* a fire, a world of
iniquity: so is the tongue among our
members, that it [y]defileth the whole
body, and setteth on fire the course of
nature; and it is set on fire of [z]hell.
7 For every kind of beasts, and of
birds, and of [aa]serpents, and of things in
the sea, is tamed, and hath been tamed
of mankind:
8 But the tongue can no man tame; *it is*
an unruly evil, [bb]full of deadly poison.
9 Therewith bless we [cc]God, even the
Father; and therewith curse we men,
which are made [dd]after the similitude of
God.
10 Out of the same mouth proceedeth
blessing and cursing. My brethren, these
things ought not so to be.
11 Doth a fountain send forth at the
same place sweet *water* and bitter?
12 Can the [ee]fig tree, my brethren, bear
olive berries? either a vine, figs? so *can*
no fountain both yield salt water and
fresh.
13 Who *is* a wise man and endued
with knowledge among you? let him
shew out of a good [ff]conversation his
works with meekness of wisdom.
14 But if ye have bitter envying and
strife in your hearts, glory not, and lie
not against the truth.

A.D. 60.

a Mic. 7:18.
b *glorieth over.*
c *can [that] faith save him?*
d Rom. 1:16, *note.*
e 1 John 3:18.
f *Faith.* vs. 17, 18, 20; Jas. 5:15. (Gen. 3:20; Heb. 11:39.)
g v. 26; cf. John 15:2.
h Col. 1:6; 1 Thes. 1:3; Heb. 6:10.
i *God is one.*
j *demons.* Mt. 8:29; Mk. 1:24; Acts 16:17; 19:15.
k vs. 17, 26.
l Rom. 4:2, *note.*
m Mt. 5:48, *note.*
n *Jehovah.* Gen. 15:6.
o *Imputation.* (Lev. 25:50.)
p Rom. 3:21, *note.*
q 2 Chr. 20:7; Isa. 41:8.
r Josh. 2:1-21; Heb. 11:31.
s vs. 17, 20.
t *teachers, knowing that we shall have the more severe judgment.* Cf. Mk. 12:40.
u *we all offend.*
v Psa. 32:9.
w Prov. 12:18; 15:2.
x Prov. 16:27.
y Mt. 15:18.
z Mt. 5:22, *note.*
aa *creeping things.*
bb Psa. 140:3; Rom. 3:13.
cc *God.* Gen. 1:27.
dd Gen. 1:26; 5:1; 9:6.
ee Mt. 7:16-20.
ff *behaviour.*

[1] **(2:23)** Imputation is the act of God whereby He accounts righteousness to the believer in Christ, who has borne the believer's sins in vindication of the law. See Phm. 17, 18, *note.*

15 [a]This wisdom descendeth not from above, but *is* earthly, [b]sensual, devilish.

16 For where envying and strife *is*, there *is* confusion and every evil work.

17 But the [c]wisdom that is from above is first pure, then peaceable, gentle, *and* easy to be intreated, full of mercy and good fruits, without partiality, and [d]without hypocrisy.

18 And the fruit of [e]righteousness is sown in peace [f]of them that make peace.

CHAPTER 4.

Part III. The rebuke of worldliness.

From whence *come* wars and fightings among you? *come they* not hence, *even* of your lusts [g]that war in your members?

2 Ye lust, and have not: ye kill, and desire to have, and cannot obtain: ye fight and war, yet ye have not, because ye ask not.

3 Ye ask, and receive not, [h]because ye ask [i]amiss, that ye may consume *it* upon your lusts.

4 Ye adulterers and adulteresses, know ye not that the [j]friendship of the [k]world is enmity with God? [l]whosoever therefore will be a friend of the world is the enemy of God.

5 Do ye think that the scripture [m]saith in vain, [n]The [o]spirit that dwelleth in us lusteth to envy?

6 But he giveth more [p]grace. Wherefore he saith, [q]God resisteth the proud, but giveth grace unto the humble.

7 Submit yourselves therefore to God. Resist the [r]devil, and he will flee from you.

8 [s]Draw nigh to God, and he will draw nigh to you. Cleanse *your* hands, *ye* [t]sinners; and purify *your* hearts, *ye* double minded.

9 Be afflicted, and mourn, and weep: let your laughter be turned to mourning, and *your* joy to heaviness.

10 [u]Humble yourselves in the sight of the Lord, and he shall lift you up.

11 [v]Speak not evil one of another, brethren. He that speaketh evil of *his* brother, and judgeth his brother, speaketh evil of the law, and judgeth the law: but if thou judge the law, thou art not a doer of the law, but a judge.

12 There is one lawgiver, [w]who is able to [x]save and to destroy: who art thou that judgest another?

A.D. 60.

a Phil. 3:19; Jas. 1:17.
b Or, *natural.*
c 1 Cor. 2:6, 7.
d Rom. 12:9; 1 Pet. 1:22.
e 1 John 3:7, *note.*
f *for them.*
g Rom. 7:23; Gal. 5:17; 1 Pet. 2:11.
h 1 John 5:14.
i *evilly.*
j 1 John 2:15.
k *kosmos* = world-system. 2 Pet. 1:4. (John 7:7; Rev. 13:3-8, *note.*)
l John 15:19; 17:14; Gal. 1:4.
m *speaketh in vain?*
n *Doth the Spirit . . . desire enviously?*
o *Holy Spirit.* 1 Pet. 1:2, 11, 12, 22. (Mt. 1:18; Acts 2:4.)
p *Grace (imparted).* 1 Pet. 2:19. (Rom. 6:1; 2 Pet. 3:18.)
q Prov. 3:34.
r *Satan* 1 Pet. 5:8. (Gen. 3:1; Rev. 20:10.)
s 2 Chr. 15:2; Mal. 3:7; Heb. 10:19-22.
t *Sin.* Rom. 3:23, *note.*
u Job 22:29; Lk. 14:11; 18:14; 1 Pet. 5:6.
v Eph. 4:31; 1 Pet. 2:1.
w Mt. 10:28.
x Rom. 1:16, *note.*
y Prov. 27:1; Lk. 12:18.
z Job 7:7; Psa. 102:3; 1 Pet. 1:24.
aa Acts 18:21; 1 Cor. 4:19.
bb Lk. 12:47; 2 Pet. 2:21.
cc Prov. 11:28; Lk. 6:24.
dd Jer. 17:11.
ee *in the last days.*
ff i.e. *Jehovah of hosts.*
gg *luxuriously.*
hh *indulged yourselves.*
ii Mt. 5:39.
jj Or, *be long patient,* or, *suffer with long patience.*
kk *Christ (Second Advent).* Heb. 10:37, 38. (Deut. 30:3; Acts 1:9, 11.)
ll *complain.*

13 [y]Go to now, ye that say, To day or to morrow we will go into such a city, and continue there a year, and buy and sell, and get gain:

14 Whereas ye know not what *shall be* on the morrow. For what *is* your life? [z]It is even a vapour, that appeareth for a little time, and then vanisheth away.

15 For that ye *ought* to say, [aa]If the Lord will, we shall live, and do this, or that.

16 But now ye rejoice in your boastings: all such rejoicing is evil.

17 Therefore to him that [bb]knoweth to do good, and doeth *it* not, to him it is [t]sin.

CHAPTER 5.

Part IV. The rich warned.

Go to now, *ye* [cc]rich men, weep and howl for your miseries that shall come upon *you.*

2 Your [dd]riches are corrupted, and your garments are motheaten.

3 Your gold and silver is cankered; and the rust of them shall be a witness against you, and shall eat your flesh as it were fire. Ye have heaped treasure [ee]together for the last days.

4 Behold, the hire of the labourers who have reaped down your fields, which is of you kept back by fraud, crieth: and the cries of them which have reaped are entered into the ears of [ff]the Lord of sabaoth.

5 Ye have lived [gg]in pleasure on the earth, and [hh]been wanton; ye have nourished your hearts, as in a day of slaughter.

6 Ye have condemned *and* killed the just; *and* he doth not [ii]resist you.

Part V. Exhortations in view of the coming of the Lord.

7 [jj]Be patient therefore, brethren, unto the coming of the Lord. Behold, the husbandman waiteth for the precious fruit of the earth, and hath long patience for it, until he receive the early and latter rain.

8 Be ye also patient; stablish your hearts: for [kk]the coming of the Lord draweth nigh.

9 [ll]Grudge not one against another, brethren, lest ye be condemned: behold, the judge standeth before the door.

10 Take, my brethren, the prophets,
who have spoken in the name of the
Lord, for an example of suffering [a]afflic-
tion, and of patience.
11 Behold, we count them [b]happy
which endure. Ye have heard of the [c]pa-
tience of Job, and have seen the [d]end of
the Lord; that the Lord is very pitiful,
and of tender mercy.
12 But above all things, my brethren,
[e]swear not, neither by heaven, neither
by the earth, neither by any other oath:
but let your yea be yea; and *your* nay,
nay; lest ye fall into condemnation.
13 Is any among you afflicted? let him
pray. Is any merry? let him sing [f]psalms.
14 Is any sick among you? [g]let him call
for the [h]elders of the church; and let
them pray over him, anointing him with
oil in the name of the Lord:
15 And the prayer of [i]faith shall save
the sick, and the Lord shall raise him up;
and if he have committed [j]sins, they
shall be forgiven him.
16 Confess *your* [j]faults one to another,
and pray one for another, that ye may be
healed. The [k]effectual fervent prayer of a
[l]righteous man availeth much.
17 Elias was a man subject to like passions as we are, and [m]he prayed earnestly that it might not rain: and it rained
not on the earth by the space of three
years and six months.
18 And he prayed [n]again, and the
heaven gave rain, and the earth brought
forth her fruit.
19 Brethren, if any of you do err from
the truth, and one convert him;
20 Let him know, that he which converteth the sinner from the error of his
way shall save a soul from death, and
shall [o]hide a multitude of [j]sins.

A.D. 60.

a Heb. 11:35.
b Psa. 94:12; Mt. 5:10.
c Job 1:21.
d Job 42:10.
e Mt. 5:34.
f Eph. 5:19.
g *Churches (local).* 3 John 6, 9, 10. (Acts 2:41; Phil. 1:1.)
h *Elders.* 1 Pet. 5:1. (Acts 11:30; Tit. 1:5-9.)
i *Faith.* 1 Pet. 1:5, 9. (Gen. 3:20; Heb. 11:39.)
j *Sin.* Rom. 3:23, *note.*
k Or, *fervent supplication.*
l Rom. 10:10, *note.*
m 1 Ki. 17:1.
n 1 Ki. 18:1, 42.
o Prov. 10:12.

THE FIRST EPISTLE GENERAL OF

PETER

WRITER. The Apostle Peter (1:1).

Date. Probably A.D. 60. That "Babylon" refers to the former city on the Euphrates, or to Rome, cannot be inferred from 5:13. The text is obscure.

Theme. While Peter undoubtedly has scattered Jewish believers in mind, his Epistles comprehend Gentile believers also (1 Pet. 2:10). The present Epistle, written from a church on Gentile ground (5:13), presents all the foundational truths of the Christian faith, with special emphasis on the atonement. The distinctive note of First Peter is preparation for victory over suffering. The last-named word occurs about fifteen times, and is the key-word of the Epistle.

The Epistle is in three parts: I. Christian suffering and conduct in the light of full salvation, 1:1–2:8. II. The believer's life in view of his sevenfold position, and of the vicarious suffering of Christ, 2:9–4:19. III. Christian service in the light of the coming of the Chief Shepherd, 5:1-14.

CHAPTER 1.

Part I. Christian suffering and conduct in the light of full salvation (1Pet. 1:1–2:8).

Peter, an apostle of Jesus Christ, to the [a]strangers scattered throughout Pontus, Galatia, Cappadocia, Asia, and Bithynia,

2 [1][b]Elect according to the foreknowledge of God the Father, through [c]sanctification of the Spirit, unto obedience and sprinkling of the blood of Jesus Christ: Grace unto you, and peace, be multiplied.

3 Blessed *be* the God and Father of our Lord Jesus Christ, which according to his abundant mercy hath begotten us again unto a [d]lively hope by the resurrection of Jesus Christ [e]from the dead,

4 To an inheritance incorruptible, and undefiled, and that fadeth not away, reserved in heaven for you,

5 Who are [f]kept by the power of God through [g]faith unto salvation ready to be revealed in the last time.

6 Wherein ye greatly rejoice, though now for a season, if need be, ye are in heaviness through manifold [h]temptations:

7 That the trial of your faith, being much more precious than of gold that perisheth, though it be tried with fire, [2]might be found unto praise and honour and glory at the [i]appearing of Jesus Christ:

8 Whom having not seen, ye love; in whom, though now ye see *him* not, yet believing, ye rejoice with joy unspeakable and full of glory:

9 Receiving the end of your faith, *even* the [j]salvation of *your* souls.

A.D. 60.

a *sojourners of the dispersion of.*
b *Election (personal).* (Deut. 7:6.)
c 2 Thes. 2:13.
d *living.*
e *from among.*
f *guarded.*
g *Faith.* 1 Pet. 2:6, 7. (Gen. 3:20; Heb. 11:39.)
h *Temptation.* 2 Pet. 2:9. (Gen. 3:1; Jas. 1:14.)
i Or, *revelation.*
j Rom. 1:16, *note.*

[1] **(1:2)** Election, Summary: In both Testaments the Hebrew and Greek words are rendered "elect," "election," "choose," "chosen." In all cases they mean, simply, "chosen," or "to choose"; and are used of both human and divine choices. (1) In the latter use election is: *(a) corporate,* as of the nation of Israel, or the church (Isa. 45:4; Eph. 1:4); and *(b) individual* (1 Pet. 1:2). (2) Election is according to the foreknowledge of God (1 Pet. 1:2), and wholly of grace, apart from human merit (Rom. 9:11; 11:5, 6). (3) Election proceeds from the divine volition (John 15:16).

Election is, therefore: (1) The sovereign act of God in grace whereby certain are chosen from among mankind for Himself (John 15:19). (2) The sovereign act of God whereby certain elect persons are chosen for distinctive service for Him (Lk. 6:13; Acts. 9:15; 1 Cor. 1:27, 28).

[2] **(1:7)** Suffering, in First Peter, is set in the light of: (1) assured salvation, 1:2-5; (2) the greater glory at Christ's appearing, 1:7; (3) Christ's sufferings and coming glories, 1:11; (4) the believer's association with Him in both, 2:20, 21; 3:17, 18; 4:12, 13; (5) the purifying effect of suffering, 1:7; 4:1, 2; 5:10; (6) that Christ is now glorified in the believer's patient suffering, 4:16; (7) that suffering is disciplinary, 4:17-19. (1 Cor. 11:31, 32; Heb. 12:5-13.)

10 Of which [a]salvation the prophets
have inquired and searched diligently,
[b]who prophesied of the grace *that should*
come unto you:
11 Searching what, or what manner of
time the [c]Spirit of Christ which was in
them did signify, when it testified
beforehand the sufferings of Christ, and
the glory that should follow.
12 Unto whom it was revealed, that not
unto themselves, but unto us they did
minister the things, which are now reported unto you by them that have preached
the gospel unto you with the [d]Holy Ghost
sent down from heaven; which things the
angels desire to look into.
13 Wherefore gird up the loins of your
mind, be sober, and hope to the end [e]for
the grace that is to be brought unto you
at the revelation of Jesus Christ;
14 As obedient children, not [f]fashion-
ing yourselves according to the former
lusts in your ignorance:
15 But as he which hath called you is
holy, so be ye holy in all manner of conversation;
16 Because it is written, [g]Be ye [h]holy;
for I am holy.
17 And if ye call on the Father, who
without respect of persons judgeth
according to every man's work, pass the
time of your sojourning *here* in fear:
18 Forasmuch as ye know that ye were
not [i]redeemed with corruptible things,
as silver and gold, from your vain conversation *received* by tradition from your
fathers;
19 But [j]with the precious blood of
Christ, as of a lamb without blemish and
without spot:
20 Who verily was [1k]foreordained
before the foundation of the [l]world, but
was manifest in [m]these last times for you,
21 Who by him do believe in God, that
raised him up from the dead, and gave
him glory; that your faith and hope
might be in God.
22 Seeing ye have purified your souls
in obeying the truth through the Spirit
[n]unto unfeigned love of the brethren, *see*
that ye love one another with a pure
heart fervently:
23 Being born again, not of corruptible
seed, but of incorruptible, by the word of
God, which liveth and abideth for ever.
24 For [o]all flesh *is* as grass, and all the
glory of man as the flower of grass. The
grass withereth, and the flower thereof
falleth away:
25 But the [p]word of the [q]Lord endureth
for ever. And this is the word which by
the [r]gospel is preached unto you.

CHAPTER 2.

Part I. continued.

Wherefore laying aside all malice,
and all guile, and hypocrisies,
and envies, and all evil speakings,
2 As newborn babes, desire the sincere
milk of the word, that ye may grow
thereby:
3 If so be ye have [s]tasted that the Lord
is gracious.
4 To whom coming, [t]*as unto* a living
stone, [u]disallowed indeed of men, but
chosen of God, *and* precious,
5 Ye also, as lively stones, [v]are built up
a spiritual house, an holy priesthood, to
offer up [w]spiritual sacrifices, acceptable
to God by Jesus Christ.
6 Wherefore also it is contained in the
[x]scripture, Behold, I lay in Sion a chief
corner stone, elect, precious: and he that
believeth on him shall not be confounded.
7 Unto you therefore which [y]believe
[z]*he is* precious: but unto them which be
disobedient, the stone which the
builders [u]disallowed, the same is made
the head of the corner,
8 And a [2aa]stone of stumbling, and

A.D. 60.

a Rom. 1:16, *note.*
b *Inspiration.* vs. 10-12, 25; 2 Pet. 1:21. (Ex. 4:15; Rev. 22:19.)
c 2 Pet. 1:21.
d *Holy Spirit.* vs. 2, 11, 12, 22; 1 Pet. 3:18. (Mt. 1:18; Acts 2:4.)
e *Grace (in salv.).* 1 Pet. 5:12. (Rom. 3:24; John 1:17, *note.*)
f Rom. 12:2.
g Lev. 11:44.
h *Sanctify, holy (persons) (N. T.).* vs. 15, 16; 1 Pet. 2:5, 9. (Mt. 4:5; Rev. 22:11.)
i Rom. 3:24, *note.*
j *Sacrifice (of Christ).* 1 Pet. 2:24. (Gen. 4:4;. Heb. 10:18.)
k *foreknown. Foreknowledge.* vs. 2, 20. (Acts 2:23.)
l *ages.*
m *at this end of times.*
n *Law (of Christ).* vs. 8, 22; Jas. 1:25. (Gal. 6:2; 2 John 5.)
o vs. 24, 25; Isa. 40:6-8.
p Lit. *saying.*
q *God.* Isa. 40:8.
r *Gospel.* vs. 12, 25; 1 Pet. 4:6, 17. (Gen. 12:1-3; Rev. 14:6.)
s Psa. 34:8.
t 1 Cor. 3:11.
u *rejected.* Psa. 118:22.
v *are being built up.*
w *Sacrifice (the believer-priest's).* Heb. 10:1-18. (Gen. 4:4; Heb. 10:18.)
x Isa. 28:16.
y *Faith.* vs. 6, 7; 1 John 5:1, 4, 5, 10. (Gen. 3:20; Heb. 11:39.)
z *Is the preciousness.*
aa *Christ (as Stone).* vs. 4, 8. (Ex. 17:6.)

[1] **(1:20)** The divine order is foreknowledge, election, predestination. That foreknowledge determines the election or choice is clear from 1 Pet. 1:2, and predestination is the bringing to pass of the election. "Election looks back to foreknowledge; predestination forward to the destiny." But Scripture nowhere declares what it is in the divine foreknowledge which determines the divine election and predestination. The foreknown are elected, and the elect are predestinated, and this election is certain to every believer by the mere fact that he believes (1 Thes. 1:4, 5). See "Predestination," Eph. 1:5.

[2] **(2:8)** Christ crucified is the Rock: (1) *Smitten* that the Spirit of life may flow from Him to all who will drink (Ex. 17:6; 1 Cor. 10:4; John 4:13, 14; 7:37-39). (2) To the *church* the foundation and chief corner Stone (Eph. 2:20). (3) To the *Jews* at His first coming a "stumbling stone" (Rom. 9:32, 33; 1 Cor. 1:23) (4) To *Israel*

a rock of offence, *even to them* which
stumble at the word, being disobedient:
whereunto also they were appointed.

Part II. The believer's life in view of his sevenfold position, and of the vicarious suffering of Christ.

9 But ye *are* a [a]chosen generation, a
royal [1]priesthood, an [b]holy nation, a
[c]peculiar people; that ye should shew
forth the [d]praises of him who hath called
you out of darkness into his marvellous
light:
10 Which in time past *were* not a people, but *are* now the people of [e]God:
which had not obtained mercy, but now
have obtained mercy.
11 Dearly beloved, I beseech *you* as
[f]strangers and pilgrims, abstain from
fleshly lusts, which [g]war against the
soul;
12 Having your conversation honest
among the Gentiles: that, whereas they
speak against you as evildoers, they may
by *your* [h]good works, which they shall
behold, glorify God in the day of visitation.
13 Submit [i]yourselves to every ordinance of man for the Lord's sake:
whether it be to the king, as supreme;
14 Or unto governors, as unto them
that are sent by him for the punishment
of evildoers, and for the praise of them
that do well.
15 For so is the will of God, that with
well doing ye may put to silence the
ignorance of foolish men:
16 [j]As free, and not using *your* liberty
for a cloke of maliciousness, but as the
[k]servants of God.
17 Honour all *men*. Love the brotherhood. Fear [l]God. Honour the king.
18 [m]Servants, *be* subject to *your* masters with all fear; not only to the good
and gentle, but also to the froward.
19 For [n]this *is* [o]thankworthy, if a man
for conscience toward God endure grief,
suffering wrongfully.
20 For what glory *is it*, if, when ye be
buffeted for your [p]faults, ye shall take it
patiently? but if, when ye do well, and
suffer *for it*, ye take it patiently, this *is*
acceptable with God.

(*The vicarious suffering of Christ.*)

21 For even [q]hereunto were ye called:
because Christ also suffered for us, leaving us an example, that ye should follow
his steps:
22 [r]Who did no [p]sin, neither was guile
found in his mouth:
23 Who, [s]when he was reviled, reviled
not again; when he suffered, he threatened not; but committed *himself* to him
that judgeth righteously:
24 [t]Who his own self [u]bare our [p]sins
in his own body on the tree, that we,
being dead to sins, should live unto
[v]righteousness: by whose stripes ye
were healed.
25 For ye were as sheep going astray;
but are now returned unto the
[w]Shepherd and [x]Bishop of your souls.

A.D. 60.

a *Election (personal)*. 2 John 1:13. (Deut. 7:6; 1 Pet. 1:2.)
b *Sanctify, holy (persons)* (N.T.). vs. 5, 9; 1 Pet. 3:5, 15. (Mt. 4:5; Rev. 22:11.)
c *people for a possession.*
d *virtues*, or, *excellencies.*
e *God.* Hos. 1:10.
f Psa. 119:19; cf. Heb. 11:9-10.
g Rom. 8:13.
h Mt. 5:16.
i Mt. 22:21; Rom. 13:1, 7.
j Rom. 6:14, 20, 22.
k *bondmen.* 1 Cor. 6:20.
l *Jehovah.* Prov. 24:21.
m Eph. 6:5.
n *Grace (imparted).* 1 Pet. 3:7. (Rom. 6:1; 2 Pet. 3:18.)
o *grace.*
p *Sin.* Rom. 3:23, *note.*
q Mt. 16:24; 1 Thes. 3:3, 4.
r Isa. 53:9.
s Isa. 53:7.
t *Sacrifice (of Christ).* 1 Pet. 3:18. (Gen. 4:4; Heb. 10:18.)
u *Judgments (the seven).* 1 Pet. 3:18. (2 Sam. 7:14; Rev. 20:12.)
v Rom. 10:10, *note.*
w Ezk. 34:11; Heb. 13:20.
x *overseer.*

at His second coming the "headstone of the corner" (Zech. 4:7). (5) To the *Gentile world-power* the smiting "stone cut out without hands" (Dan. 2:34). (6) In the divine purpose the Stone which, after the destruction of Gentile world-power, is to grow and fill the earth. (7) To *unbelievers* the crushing Stone of judgment (Mt. 21:44).

[1] **(2:9)** The New Testament priesthood, Summary: (1) Until the law was given the head of each family was the family priest (Gen. 8:20; 26:25; 31:54). (2) When the law was proposed, the promise to perfect obedience was that Israel should be unto God "a kingdom of priests" (Ex. 19:6); but Israel violated the law, and God shut up the priestly office to the Aaronic family, appointing the tribe of Levi to minister to them, thus constituting the typical priesthood (Ex. 28:1). (3) In the dispensation of grace, all believers are unconditionally constituted a "kingdom of priests" (1 Pet. 2:9; Rev. 1:6), the distinction which Israel failed to achieve by works. The priesthood of the believer is, therefore, a birthright; just as every descendant of Aaron was born to the priesthood (Heb. 5:1). (4) The chief privilege of a priest is access to God. Under law the high priest only could enter "the holiest of all," and that but once a year (Heb. 9:7). But when Christ died, the veil, type of Christ's human body (Heb. 10:20), was rent, so that now the believer-priests, equally with Christ the High Priest, have access to God in the holiest (Heb. 10:19-22). The High Priest is corporeally there (4:14-16; Heb. 9:24; 10:19-22). (5) In the exercise of his office the New Testament believer-priest is (1) a sacrificer who offers a threefold sacrifice: (*a*) his own living body (Rom. 12:1; Phil. 2:17; 2 Tim. 4:6; 1 John 3:16; Jas. 1:27); (*b*) praise to God, "the fruit of the

CHAPTER 3.

Part II. continued.

Likewise, ye wives, *be* in [a]subjection to your own husbands; that, if any obey not the word, they also may without the word be won by the [b]conversation of the wives;

2 While they behold your chaste [b]conversation *coupled* with fear.

3 Whose [c]adorning let it not be that outward *adorning* of plaiting the hair, and of wearing of gold, or of putting on of apparel;

4 But *let it be* the hidden man [d]of the heart, in [e]that which is not corruptible, *even the ornament* of a meek and quiet spirit, which is in the sight of God of great price.

5 For after this manner in the old time the holy women also, who [f]trusted in God, adorned themselves, being in subjection unto their own husbands:

6 Even as Sara obeyed Abraham, [g]calling him lord: whose daughters ye are, as long as ye do well, and [h]are not afraid with any amazement.

7 Likewise, ye husbands, dwell with *them* according to knowledge, giving honour unto the wife, as unto the weaker vessel, and as being heirs together of the [i]grace of [j]life; that your prayers be not hindered.

8 Finally, *be ye* all of one mind, having compassion one of another, [k]love as brethren, *be* pitiful, *be* courteous:

9 Not [l]rendering evil for evil, or railing for railing: but contrariwise blessing; [m]knowing that ye are thereunto called, that ye should inherit a blessing.

10 For [n]he that will love life, and see good days, let him refrain his tongue from evil, and his lips that they speak no guile:

11 Let him eschew evil, and do good; let him seek peace, and [o]ensue it.

12 For the eyes of the [p]Lord *are* over the [q]righteous, and his ears *are open* unto their prayers: but the face of the [r]Lord *is* [s]against them that do evil.

13 And who *is* he that will harm you, if ye be followers of that which is good?

A.D. 60.

- a vs. 1, 5, 6; cf. Gen. 3:16.
- b *behaviour.*
- c 1 Tim. 2:9, 10.
- d Rom. 2:29.
- e *the incorruptible (ornament) of a meek, etc.*
- f *hoped.*
- g Gen. 18:12.
- h Prov. 29:25.
- i *Grace (imparted).* 1 Pet. 4:10. (Rom. 6:1; 2 Pet. 3:18.)
- j *Life (eternal).* 2 Pet. 1:3. (Mt. 7:14; Rev. 22:19.)
- k 1 John 3:18.
- l Mt. 5:44.
- m *because ye have been hereunto called.*
- n Psa. 34:12.
- o *pursue.*
- p *Jehovah.* Psa. 34:12-16.
- q Rom. 10:10, *note.*
- r *Jehovah.* Psa. 34:16.
- s *upon.*
- t 1 John 3:7, *note.*
- u *Sanctify, holy (persons).* (N.T.). vs. 5, 15; 2 Pet. 1:21. (Mt. 4:5; Rev. 22:11.)
- v Psa. 119:46.
- w Tit. 3:4, 7.
- x 1 Pet. 2:21.
- y *Sacrifice (of Christ).* 1 Pet. 4:1. (Gen. 4:4; Heb. 10:18.)
- z *Judgments (the seven).* 1 Pet. 4:17. (2 Sam. 7:14; Rev. 20:12.)
- aa *Sin.* Rom. 3:23, *note.*
- bb *Assurance.* 1 John 2:2. (Isa. 32:17; Jude 1.)
- cc *Holy Spirit.* 1 Pet. 4:6, 14. (Mt. 1:18; Acts 2:4.)
- dd Heb. 11:7; 2 Pet. 1:21; 2:5.
- ee Omit "once."
- ff Rom. 8:1.
- gg Mk. 16:16; Acts 18:8; Eph. 5:26.
- hh *Flesh.* 1 Pet. 4:6. (John 1:13; Jude 23.)
- ii *demand as before God of a good conscience.*
- jj Heb. 1:4, *note.*
- kk *Sacrifice (of Christ).* 1 John 1:7. (Gen. 4:4; Heb. 10:18.)
- ll 2 Cor. 5:15.

14 But and if ye suffer for [t]righteousness' sake, happy *are ye*: and be not afraid of their terror, neither be troubled;

15 But [u]sanctify the Lord God in your hearts: and *be* [v]ready always to *give* an answer to every man that asketh you a reason of the [w]hope that is in you with meekness and fear:

16 Having a good conscience; that, whereas they speak evil of you, as of evildoers, they may be ashamed that falsely accuse your good conversation in Christ.

17 For *it is* better, if the will of God be so, that ye suffer for well doing, than for evil doing.

(*The vicarious suffering of Christ, preached by Christ through the Spirit in Noah.*)

18 [x]For Christ also [y]hath [z]once suffered for [aa]sins, the just for the unjust, [bb]that he might bring us to God, being put to death in the flesh, but quickened by the [cc]Spirit:

19 [dd]By which also he went and preached unto the spirits in prison;

20 Which sometime were disobedient, when [ee]once the longsuffering of God waited in the days of Noah, while the ark was a preparing, wherein few, that is, eight souls were saved by water.

21 [ff]The like figure whereunto *even* [gg]baptism doth also now save us (not the putting away of the filth of the [hh]flesh, but the [ii]answer of a good conscience toward God,) by the resurrection of Jesus Christ:

22 Who is gone into heaven, and is on the right hand of God; [jj]angels and authorities and powers being made subject unto him.

CHAPTER 4.

Part II. continued.

Forasmuch then as Christ hath [kk]suffered for us in the flesh, arm yourselves likewise with the same mind: for he that hath suffered in the flesh hath ceased from [aa]sin;

2 [ll]That he no longer should live the rest of *his* time in the flesh to the lusts of men, but to the will of God.

lips that make mention of His name" (R.V.), to be offered "continually" (Heb. 13:15; Ex. 25:22; "I will commune with thee from above the mercy seat"); (*c*) his substance (Heb. 13:16; Rom. 12:13; Gal. 6:6; 3 John 5-8; Heb. 13:2; Gal. 6:10; Tit. 3:14). (2) The N.T. priest is also an *intercessor* (1 Tim. 2:1; Col. 4:12).

3 For the time past of *our* life may suffice us to have wrought the will of the Gentiles, when we walked in lasciviousness, lusts, excess of wine, revellings, banquetings, and abominable idolatries:

4 Wherein they think it strange that ye run not with *them* to the same excess of riot, speaking evil of *you*:

5 Who shall give account to him that is ready to judge the quick and the dead.

6 [a]For for this cause was the gospel preached also to them [b]that are dead, that they might be [c]judged according to men in the [d]flesh, but [e]live according to God in the spirit.

7 But the [f]end of all things is [g]at hand: be ye therefore sober, and watch unto prayer.

8 And above all things have fervent [h]charity among yourselves: for charity shall cover the multitude of [i]sins.

9 Use hospitality one to another without grudging.

10 As every man hath [j]received the gift, *even so* minister the same one to another, as [k]good stewards of the manifold [l]grace of God.

11 [m]If any man speak, *let him speak* as the oracles of God; if any man minister, *let him do it* as of the ability which God giveth: that God in [n]all things may be glorified through Jesus Christ, to whom be praise and dominion for ever and ever. Amen.

12 Beloved, think it not strange concerning the fiery trial which is to try you, as though some strange thing happened unto you:

13 But rejoice, [o]inasmuch as ye are partakers of Christ's sufferings; that, [p]when his glory shall be revealed, ye may be glad also with exceeding joy.

14 [q]If ye be reproached for the name of Christ, happy *are ye;* for the [r]spirit of glory and of God resteth upon you: on their part he is evil spoken of, [s]but on your part he is glorified.

15 But let none of you suffer as a murderer, or *as* a thief, or *as* an evildoer, or as a busybody in other men's matters.

16 Yet if *any man suffer* as a Christian, let him not be ashamed; but let him glorify God on this behalf.

17 For the time *is come* that [t]judgment must [u]begin at the house of God: and if *it* first *begin* at us, what shall the end *be* of them that obey not the [v]gospel of God?

18 And if the [w]righteous [x]scarcely be [y]saved, where shall the ungodly and the [i]sinner appear?

19 Wherefore let them that suffer according to the will of God [z]commit the keeping of their souls *to him* in well doing, as unto a faithful Creator.

CHAPTER 5.

Part III. Christian service in view of the coming again of the Chief Shepherd.

The [aa]elders which are among you I exhort, who am also an elder, and a [bb]witness of the sufferings of Christ, and also a partaker of the [cc]glory that shall be revealed:

2 [dd]Feed the flock of God which is among you, taking the oversight *thereof,* not by constraint, but willingly; not for filthy lucre, but of a ready mind;

3 Neither as being [ee]lords over *God's* heritage, but being ensamples to the flock.

4 And when the chief [ff]Shepherd shall appear, ye shall receive a [gg]crown of glory that fadeth not away.

5 Likewise, ye younger, submit yourselves unto the elder. Yea, [hh]all *of you* be subject one to another, and be clothed with humility: for [ii]God resisteth the proud, and giveth grace to the humble.

6 [jj]Humble yourselves therefore under the mighty hand of God, that he may exalt you in due time:

7 [kk]Casting all your care upon him; for he careth for you.

8 Be sober, be vigilant; because your adversary the [ll]devil, as a roaring lion, walketh about, seeking whom he may devour:

9 Whom [mm]resist stedfast in the faith, knowing that the same afflictions are accomplished in your brethren that are in the [nn]world.

10 But the God of [oo]all grace, who hath called us unto his eternal glory by Christ Jesus, [pp]after that ye have suffered a while, make you [qq]perfect, stablish, strengthen, settle *you*.

11 To him *be* glory and dominion for ever and ever. Amen.

12 By Silvanus, a faithful brother unto you, as I suppose, I have written

A.D. 60.

a Acts 2:38, 41; 8:1; 9:1.
b i.e. *it was preached to them that are now dead.*
c Mt. 24:9; 1 Cor. 4:3, 5.
d *Flesh.* 2 Pet. 2:10, 11, 18. (John 1:13; Jude 23.)
e Rom. 8:9, 13; Gal. 5:25.
f Jas. 5:8, 9.
g 2 Thes. 2:2; 2 Pet. 3:8.
h *love.*
i *Sin.* Rom. 3:23, *note.*
j Rom. 12:6, 8.
k 1 Tim. 6:17, 18.
l *Grace (imparted).* 1 Pet. 5:5, 10. (Rom. 6:1; 2 Pet. 3:18.)
m 2 Cor. 4:2; Eph. 4:29.
n 1 Cor. 10:31.
o Jas. 1:2.
p 2 Tim. 2:12.
q Mt. 5:11.
r *Holy Spirit.* vs. 6, 14; 2 Pet. 1:21. (Mt. 1:18; Acts 2:4.)
s Mt. 5:16.
t *Judgments (the seven).* 2 Pet. 2:4. (2 Sam. 7:14; Rev. 20:12.)
u Lk. 12:47, 48.
v *Gospel.* vs. 6, 17; Jude 3. (Gen. 12:1-3; Rev. 14:6.)
w Rom. 10:10, *note.*
x *with difficulty.*
y Rom. 1:16, *note.*
z Psa. 37:5, 7.
aa *Elders.* 2 John 1. (Acts 11:30; Tit. 1:5-9.)
bb Mt. 26:37.
cc Rom. 8:17, 18.
dd *tend.* Cf. John 21:15-17.
ee *lording it over your possessions.*
ff Isa. 40:11.
gg *Rewards.* 2 John 8. (Dan. 12:3; 1 Cor. 3:14.)
hh Eph. 5:21.
ii Prov. 3:34; 18:12; Jas. 4:6.
jj Isa. 57:15.
kk Psa. 55:22.
ll *Satan.* 1 John 3:8, 10. (Gen. 3:1; Rev. 20:10.)
mm Jas. 4:7.
nn *kosmos* (Mt. 4:8) = mankind.
oo *Grace (imparted).* vs. 5, 10; 2 Pet. 1:2. (Rom. 6:1; 2 Pet. 3:18.)
pp *when ye have suffered a little while, himself shall perfect,* etc.
qq Mt. 5:48, *note.*

briefly, exhorting, and testifying that this
is the [a]true grace of God wherein ye
stand.
13 [b]The *church that is* at Babylon,
[c]elected together with *you,* saluteth you;
and *so doth* Marcus my son.
14 Greet ye one another with a kiss of
charity. Peace *be* with you all that are in
Christ Jesus. Amen.

A.D. 60.

a *Grace (in salv.).* John 1:16, 17. (Rom. 3:24; John 1:17, *note.*)

[b] *She that is elected with you in Babylon.* Cf. 2 John 1.

[c] *Election (personal),* Lk 6:13. (Deut. 7:6; 1 Pet. 1:2.)

THE SECOND EPISTLE GENERAL OF

PETER

WRITER. The Apostle Peter (1:1).

Date. Probably A.D. 66.

Theme. Second Peter and Second Timothy have much in common. In both, the writers are aware that martyrdom is near (2 Tim. 4:6; 2 Pet. 1:14 with John 21:18, 19); both are singularly sustained and joyful; both foresee the apostasy in which the history of the professing church will end. Paul finds that apostasy in its last stage when the so-called laity (Rev. 2:6, *note*) have become infected (2 Tim. 3:1-5; 4:3, 4); Peter traces the origin of the apostasy to false teachers (2 Pet. 2:1-3, 15-19). In Peter the false teachers deny *redemption* truth (2:1); we shall find in First John a deeper depth—denial of the truth concerning Christ's *person* (1 John 4:1-5). In Jude all phases of the apostasy are seen. But in none of these Epistles is the tone one of dejection or pessimism. God and His promises are still the resource of the believer.

The Epistle is in four divisions: I. The great Christian virtues, 1:1-14. II. The Scriptures exalted, 1:15-21. III. Warnings concerning apostate teachers, 2:1-22. IV. The second coming of Christ and the day of Jehovah, 3:1-18.

CHAPTER 1.

Part I. The great Christian virtues.

Simon Peter, a [a]servant and an apostle
of Jesus Christ, to them that have
obtained like precious faith with us
through the [b]righteousness of God and
our [c]Saviour Jesus Christ:
2 [d]Grace and peace be multiplied unto
you through the knowledge of God, and
of Jesus our Lord,
3 According as his divine power hath
given unto us all things that *pertain* unto
[e]life and godliness, through the knowledge of him that hath called us to [f]glory
and virtue:
4 [g]Whereby are given unto us exceeding great and precious promises: that by
these ye might be [h]partakers of the
divine nature, having [i]escaped the corruption that is in the [j]world through lust.
5 And beside this, giving all diligence,
[k]add to your faith virtue; [l]and to virtue
knowledge;
6 And to knowledge temperance; and
to temperance patience; and to patience
godliness;
7 And to godliness brotherly kindness;
and to brotherly kindness [m]charity.
8 For if these things be in you, and
abound, they make *you that ye shall* neither *be* [n]barren nor unfruitful in the
knowledge of our Lord Jesus Christ.

A.D. 66.

a bondman.
b Rom. 3:21, *note.*
c Rom. 1:16, *note.*
d *Grace (imparted).* 2 Pet. 3:18. (Rom. 6:1; 2 Pet. 3:18.)
e *Life (eternal).* 1 John 1:1, 2. (Mt. 7:14; Rev. 22:19.)
f *by.*
g 2 Cor. 1:20.
h Heb. 12:10.
i 2 Pet. 2:18-20.
j *kosmos* = world-system. 2 Pet. 2:20. (John 7:7, Rev. 13:3-8, *note.*)
k *in your faith provide virtue.*
l *and in.*
m *love.*
n *idle.*
o 1 John 2:9, 11.
p *Sin.* Rom. 3:23, *note.*
q 1 John 3:19.
r 2 Pet. 3:1.
s *Death (physical).* vs. 13, 14; Rev. 6:9, 10, (Gen. 3:19; Heb. 9:27.)
t John 21:18, 19.
u 2 Cor. 4:2.
v Mt. 28:18; Eph. 1:20-22.
w Jude 14.

9 But he that lacketh these things is
[o]blind, and cannot see afar off, and hath
forgotten that he was purged from his
old [p]sins.
10 Wherefore the rather, brethren, give
diligence to make your calling and election sure: [q]for if ye do these things, ye
shall never fall:
11 For so an entrance shall be ministered unto you abundantly into the everlasting kingdom of our Lord and
Saviour Jesus Christ.
12 Wherefore I will not be negligent to
put you always in remembrance of these
things, though ye know *them*, and be
established in the present truth.
13 Yea, I think it meet, as long as I am
in this tabernacle, [r]to stir you up by
putting *you* in remembrance;
14 Knowing that shortly I must [s]put
off *this* my tabernacle, even as our Lord
Jesus Christ hath [t]shewed me.

Part II. The Scriptures exalted.

15 Moreover I will endeavour that ye
may be able after my decease to have
these things always in remembrance.
16 For we have not followed cunningly devised [u]fables, when we
made known unto you the [v]power
and [w]coming of our Lord Jesus

Christ, but were [a]eyewitnesses of his majesty.

17 For he received from God the Father honour and glory, when there came such a voice to him from the excellent glory, [b]This is my beloved Son, in whom I am well pleased.

18 And this voice which came from heaven we heard, when we were with him in the [1c]holy mount.

19 We have also [d]a more sure word of prophecy; [2]whereunto ye do well that ye take heed, as unto a light that shineth in a [e]dark place, [f]until the day dawn, and the [g]day star arise in your hearts:

20 Knowing this first, that no prophecy of the scripture is of [h]any private interpretation.

21 For the prophecy came not in [i]old time by the will of man: but [j]holy men of God [k]spake *as they were* moved by the [l]Holy Ghost.

CHAPTER 2.

Part III. Warnings concerning apostate teachers.

(1) *They will deny redemption by blood: many will follow them.*

But there were false prophets also among the people, even as there shall be [m]false teachers among you, who privily shall bring in [n]damnable heresies, even [o]denying the [p]Lord that bought them, and bring upon themselves swift destruction.

2 And many shall follow their pernicious ways; by reason of whom the way of truth shall be evil spoken of.

3 And through covetousness shall they with feigned words make merchandise of you: whose judgment now of a long time lingereth not, and their [q]damnation slumbereth not.

4 For if God [r]spared not the angels that sinned, but cast *them* down to hell, and delivered *them* into chains of darkness, to be reserved unto judgment;

5 And spared not the old world, but saved Noah the eighth *person*, a preacher of righteousness, bringing in the flood upon the [s]world of the ungodly;

6 And turning the cities of Sodom and Gomorrha into ashes condemned *them* with an overthrow, making *them* an ensample unto those that after should live ungodly;

7 And delivered just Lot, vexed with the filthy conversation of the wicked:

8 (For that righteous man dwelling among them, in seeing and hearing, vexed *his* righteous soul from day to day with *their* unlawful deeds;)

9 The Lord knoweth how [t]to deliver the godly out of [u]temptations, and to reserve the unjust unto the [v]day of judgment to be punished:

10 But chiefly them that walk after the flesh in the lust of uncleanness, and despise government. Presumptuous *are they*, selfwilled, they are not afraid to speak evil of dignities.

11 Whereas angels, which are greater in power and might, bring not railing accusation against them before the Lord.

12 But these, as [w]natural brute beasts, made to be taken and destroyed, speak evil of the things that they understand not; and shall utterly perish in their own corruption;

13 And shall receive the reward of unrighteousness, *as* they that count it pleasure to riot in the day time. Spots *they are* and blemishes, sporting themselves with their own deceivings while they feast with you;

A.D. 66.

a Mt. 17:1-5.
b Mk. 1:11.
c *Sanctify, holy (things)* (N.T.). Mt. 25:31. (Mt. 4:5; Rev. 22:11.)
d Or, *the word of prophecy made more sure.*
e Or, *squalid place. Psa. 119:105; John 1:4, 9.*
f Prov. 4:18; Eph. 1:13, 14.
g Rev. 2:28.
h *its own interpretation;* i.e. not isolated from all that the Word has given elsewhere.
i Lk. 1:70.
j *Sanctify, holy (persons)* (N.T.). Jude 1, 20. (Mt. 4:5; Rev. 22:11.)
k *Inspiration.* Rev. 1:1, 19. (Ex. 4:15; Rev. 22:19.)
l *Holy Spirit.* 1 John 3:24. (Mt. 1:18; Acts 2:4.)
m Mt. 24:5, 24; Acts 20:29, 30; 1 Tim. 4:1.
n i.e. *destructive.*
o Mt. 20:28.
p *Master.*
q i.e. *destruction.*
r *Judgments (the seven).* Jude 6, 14, 15. (2 Sam. 7:14; Rev, 20:12.)
s *kosmos* (Mt. 4:8) mankind.
t Psa. 34:15, 18.
u *Temptation.* Rev. 3:10. (Gen. 3:1; Jas. 1:14.)
v *Day (of judgment).* 2 Pet. 3:7. (Mt. 10:15; Rev. 20:11.)
w Jude 10. *natural animals without reason.*

[1] **(1:18)** Where the reference is to *things,* the meaning of *"holy"* or *"sanctified"* is, simply, set apart for the use of God, or rendered sacred by the divine presence.

[2] **(1:19)** That is, made more sure by fulfilment in part. Fulfilled prophecy is a proof of inspiration because the Scripture predictions of future events were uttered so long before the events transpired that no merely human sagacity or foresight could have anticipated them, and these predictions are so detailed, minute, and specific, as to exclude the possibility that they were mere fortunate guesses. Hundreds of predictions concerning Israel, the land of Canaan, Babylon, Assyria, Egypt, and numerous personages—so ancient, so singular, so seemingly improbable, as well as so detailed and definite that no mortal could have anticipated them—have been fulfilled by the elements, and by men who were ignorant of them, or who utterly disbelieved them, or who struggled with frantic desperation to avoid their fulfilment. It is certain, therefore, that the Scriptures which contain them are inspired. "Prophecy came not in olden time by the will of man; but holy men of God spake as they were moved by the Holy Ghost" (2 Pet. 1:21).

14 Having eyes full of adultery, and that cannot cease from [a]sin; beguiling unstable souls: an heart they have exercised with covetous practices; cursed children:

(2) *The marks of the false teachers.*
(a) They are like Balaam.

15 Which have forsaken the right way, and are gone astray, following the way of [1b]Balaam *the son* of Bosor, who loved the wages of unrighteousness;
16 But was rebuked for his iniquity: the dumb ass speaking with man's voice forbad the madness of the prophet.

(b) They are destitute of the Spirit.
(Cf. John 4:14; 7:37–39; Rom. 8:9.)

17 These are wells without water, [c]clouds that are carried with a tempest; to whom the mist of darkness is reserved for ever.

(c) Their words are learned and pretentious. (Cf. 1 Cor. 2:1–5)

18 [d]For when they speak great swelling *words* of vanity, they allure through the lusts of the [e]flesh, *through much* wantonness, those that were clean escaped from them who live in error.

(d) They affect liberality.

19 While they promise them liberty, they themselves are the servants of corruption: [f]for of whom a man is overcome, of the same is he brought in bondage.
20 For if after they have escaped the pollutions of the [g]world through the knowledge of the Lord and [h]Saviour Jesus Christ, they are [i]again entangled therein, and overcome, the latter end is worse with them than the beginning.
21 For it had been [j]better for them not to have known the way of righteousness, than, [k]after they have known *it*, to turn from the holy commandment delivered unto them.

(e) Unsaved professors run after them.

22 But it is happened unto them according to the true [l]proverb, The dog *is* turned to his own vomit again; and the sow that was washed to her wallowing in the mire.

A.D. 66.

a Sin. Rom. 3:23, *note.*
b Num. 22:5.
c Jude 12.
d Apostasy. vs. 1-3, 12-18; 1 John 4:1-5. (Lk. 18:8; 2 Tim. 3:1-8.)
e Flesh. vs. 10, 11, 18. 1 John 2:16. (John 1:13; Jude 23.)
f John 8:34; Rom. 6:16.
g kosmos = world-system. 1 John 2:15-17. (John 7:7; Rev. 13:3-8, *note.*)
h Rom. 1:16. *note.*
i Lk. 11:26; Heb. 6:4-6.
j Mt. 11:23; Lk. 12:47, 48.
k knowing it, to turn back.
l Prov. 26:11.
m 2 Cor. 1:12.
n 2 Pet. 1:21.
o of the Lord and Saviour by your apostles.
p Rom. 1:16, *note.*
q Isa. 5:20; Jude 10.
r Christ (Second Advent). vs. 3, 4; 1 John 3:2. (Deut. 30:3; Acts 1:9-11.)
s is hidden from them through their own wilfulness.
t Gen. 1:6, 9.
u kosmos (Mt. 4:8) = mankind.
v Gen. 7:21-23; Mt. 24:37, 39; Lk. 17:26, 27; 2 Pet. 2:5.
w Day (of judgment). 1 John 4:17. (Mt. 10:15; Rev. 20:11.)
x destruction.
y Psa. 90:4.
z Hab. 2:3.
aa Psa. 86:15; Isa. 30:18.
*bb not wishing.*Cf. Ezk. 33:11.
cc Mt. 20:28; 1 Tim. 2:4.
dd Repentance. Rev. 2:5, 16, 21, 22. (Mt. 3:2; Acts 17:30.)
ee Day (of Jehovah). Jude 6. (Isa. 2:10-22; Rev. 19:11-21.)
ff Mt. 24:42; 1 Thes. 5:2; Rev. 16:15.
gg Gen. 1:6-8; Psa. 102:26; Isa. 51:6; Rev. 20:11.

CHAPTER 3.

Part IV. The return of the Lord and the day of the Lord (Isa. 2:12, *refs*).

This second epistle, beloved, I now write unto you; in *both* which I stir up your [m]pure minds by way of remembrance:
2 That ye may be mindful of the words [n]which were spoken before by the holy prophets, and of the commandment [o]of us the apostles of the Lord and [p]Saviour:
3 Knowing this first, that there shall come in the last days [q]scoffers, walking after their own lusts,

(1) *The return of the Lord to be generally disbelieved.*

4 And saying, [r]Where is the promise of his coming? for since the fathers fell asleep, all things continue as *they were* from the beginning of the creation.
5 For this [s]they willingly are ignorant of, that [t]by the word of God the heavens were of old, and the earth standing out of the water and in the water:
6 Whereby the [u]world that then was, being overflowed with water, [v]perished:
7 But the heavens and the earth, which are now, by the same word are kept in store, reserved unto fire against the [w]day of judgment and [x]perdition of ungodly men.
8 But, beloved, be not ignorant of this one thing, that one day *is* with the Lord as [y]a thousand years, and a thousand years as one day.
9 The Lord is not [z]slack concerning his promise, as some men count slackness; but is [aa]longsuffering to us-ward, [bb]not willing that any [cc]should perish, but that all should come to [dd]repentance.

(2) *The day of the Lord* (Isa. 2:12, *refs.*).

10 But the [ee]day of the Lord will come [ff]as a thief in the night; in the which the [gg]heavens shall pass away with a great noise, and the elements shall melt with fervent heat, the earth also and the works that are therein shall be burned up.
11 *Seeing* then *that* all these things shall be dissolved, what manner

[1] **(2:15)** Balaam (see Num. 22:5, *refs.*) was the typical hireling prophet, anxious only to make a market of his gift. This is the "way" of Balaam. See the "error" of Balaam, Jude 11, *note;* and the "doctrine" of Balaam, Rev. 2:14, *note.*

of persons ought ye to be in *all* holy conversation and godliness,

12 Looking for and [a]hasting unto the coming of the day of God, wherein the heavens being on fire shall be dissolved, and the elements shall melt with fervent heat?

13 Nevertheless we, according to his promise, [b]look for [c]new heavens and a new earth, wherein dwelleth [d]righteousness.

14 Wherefore, beloved, seeing that ye look for such things, [e]be diligent that ye may be found of him in peace, without spot, and blameless.

15 And account *that* the longsuffering of our Lord *is* [f]salvation; even as our beloved brother Paul also according to the wisdom given unto him hath written unto you;

16 As also in all *his* [g]epistles, speaking in them of these things; in which are some things hard to be understood, which they that are unlearned and unstable wrest, as *they do* [h]also the other scriptures, unto their own destruction.

17 Ye therefore, beloved, seeing ye [i]know *these things* before, beware lest ye also, being led away with the error of the wicked, fall from your own stedfastness.

18 But grow in [1j]grace, and *in* the knowledge of our Lord and Saviour Jesus Christ. To him *be* glory both now and for ever. Amen.

A.D. 66.

a hastening the coming.
b wait.
c Rev. 21:1, 27.
d 1 John 3:7, *note.*
e 2 Pet. 1:10, 11; 1 Cor. 1:8; 1 Thes. 5:23.
f Rom. 1:16, *note.*
g Rom. 8:19; 1 Cor. 15:24; 1 Thes. 4:5; 2 Thes. 1:5, 10.
h 2 Tim. 3:16.
i *Foreknowledge* [trans. *foreknow,* Rom. 8:29]; 1 Pet. 1:2, 20. (Acts 2:23; 1 Pet. 1:20.)
j *Grace (imparted).* (Rom. 6:1.)

[1]**(3:18)** Grace (imparted), Summary (see "Grace," John 1:17): Grace is not only dispensationally a method of divine dealing in salvation (John 1:17, *note*), but is also the method of God in the believer's life and service. As saved, he is "not under the law, but under grace" (Rom. 6:14). Having by grace brought the believer into the highest conceivable position (Eph. 1:6), God ceaselessly works through grace, to impart to, and perfect in him, corresponding graces (John 15:4, 5; Gal. 5:22, 23). Grace, therefore, stands connected with *service* (Rom. 12:6; 15:15, 16; 1 Cor. 1:3-7; 3:10; 15:10; 2 Cor. 12:9, 10; Gal. 2:9; Eph. 3:7, 8; 4:7; Phil. 1:7; 2 Tim. 2:1, 2; 1 Pet. 4:10); with Christian *growth* (2 Cor. 1:12; Eph. 4:29; Col. 3:16; 4:6; 2 Thes. 1:12; Heb. 4:16; 12:28, 29; 13:9; Jas. 4:6; 1 Pet. 1:2; 3:7; 5:5, 10; 2 Pet. 3:18; Jude 4); and with *giving* (2 Cor. 4:15; 8:1, 6, 7, 19; 9:14).

THE FIRST EPISTLE GENERAL OF
JOHN

WRITER. The Apostle John, as unbroken tradition affirms, and as internal evidence and comparison with the Gospel of John prove.

Date. Probably A.D. 90.

Theme. First John is a family letter from the Father to His "little children" who are in the world. With the possible exception of the Song of Solomon, it is the most intimate of the inspired writings. The world is viewed as without. The sin of a believer is treated as a child's offence against his Father, and is dealt with as a family matter (1:9; 2:1). The moral government of the universe is not in question. The child's sin as an offence against the law has been met in the Cross, and "Jesus Christ the righteous" is now his "Advocate with the Father." John's Gospel leads across the threshold of the Father's house; his first Epistle makes us at home there. A tender word is used for "children," *teknia,* "born ones," or "bairns." Paul is occupied with our public position as sons; John with our nearness as born-ones of the Father.

First John is in two principal divisions: I. The family with the Father, 1:1–3:24. II. The family and the world, 4:1–5:21. There is a secondary analysis, in each division of which occurs the phrase, "My little children," as follows: (I.) Introductory, the incarnation, 1:1, 2. (II.) The little children and fellowship, 1:3–2:14. (III.) The little children and the secular and "religious" world, 2:15-28. (IV.) How the little children may know each other, 2:29–3:10. (V.) How the little children must live together, 3:11-24. (VI.) Parenthetic: How the little children may know false teachers, 4:1-6. (VII.) The little children assured and warned, 4:7–5:21.

CHAPTER 1.

Part I. The family with the Father: fellowship.

(1) *The incarnation makes fellowship possible.*

That which was [a]from the beginning, which we have [b]heard, which we have [c]seen with our eyes, which we have [d]looked upon, and our hands have [e]handled, of the [f]Word of life;

2 (For the [g]life was manifested, and we have seen *it,* and bear witness, and shew unto you that [h]eternal life, which was [i]with the Father, and was manifested unto us;)

(2) *Fellowship is with the Father and with the Son.*

3 That which we have seen and heard declare we unto you, that ye also may have fellowship with us: and truly our fellowship *is* [j]with the Father, and with his Son Jesus Christ.

4 And these things write we unto you, that [k]your joy may be full.

(3) *The conditions of fellowship.*

(a) *The walk in the light.*

5 This then is the message which we have heard of him, and declare unto you, that [l]God is light, and in him is no darkness at all.

6 If we [m]say that we have fellowship with him, and walk in darkness, we lie, and [n]do not the truth:

7 But if we walk in the [1][o]light, as he is in the light, we have fellowship [p]one with another, and [q]the blood of Jesus Christ his Son cleanseth us from all sin.

(b) *The fact of indwelling sin admitted.* (Cf. 1 Cor. 11:31, *note.*)

8 If we say that we have no sin,

After A.D. 90.

a John 1:1; 1 John 2:13.
b John 5:24; Acts 4:20.
c John 1:14; 19:35.
d 2 Pet. 1:16, 17.
e Lk. 24:39; John 20:27.
f John 1:1, 14.
g Rom. 16:26; 1 Tim. 3:16.
h *Life (eternal)* vs. 1, 2; 1 John 2:25. (Mt. 7:14; Rev. 22:19.)
i John 1:1, 18; 16:28.
j John 17:21; 1 Cor. 1:9; 1 John 2:24.
k John 15:11; 16:24; 1 Pet. 1:8.
l John 3:20, 21; 1 Tim. 6:16.
m 1 John 2:9-11.
n *practise not.*
o Ex. 27:20, *note.*
p v. 3; 2 Tim. 2:22.
q *Sacrifice (of Christ).* Rev. 1:5. (Gen. 4:4; Heb. 10:18.)

[1] **(1:7)** What it is to "walk in the light" is explained by vs. 8-10. "All things . . . are made manifest by the light" (Eph. 5:13). The presence of God brings the consciousness of sin in the nature (v. 8), and sins in the life (vs. 9, 10). The blood of Christ is the divine provision for both. To walk in the light is to live in fellowship with the Father and the Son. Sin interrupts, but confession restores that fellowship. Immediate confession keeps the fellowship unbroken.

we deceive ourselves, and the truth is not in us.

(c) Sins confessed, forgiven, and cleansed.

9 If we confess our sins, he is [a]faithful and [b]just to forgive us *our* sins, and to cleanse us from all unrighteousness.

10 If we say that we have not sinned, [c]we make him a liar, and his word is not in us.

CHAPTER 2.

(d) Fellowship maintained by Christ's advocacy.

My little children, these things write I unto you, that ye [d]sin not. And if any man sin, [e]we have an [1f]advocate with the Father, Jesus Christ the righteous:

2 And he is the [g]propitiation for our sins: and not for ours only, [h]but also for [i]*the sins of* the whole [j]world.

(e) The tests of fellowship: obedience and love.

3 And hereby we do know that we know him, if we keep his [2]commandments.

4 He that saith, I know him, and keepeth not his commandments, is a liar, and the truth is not in him.

5 But whoso [k]keepeth his word, in him verily is the love of God [l]perfected: hereby know we that we are in him.

6 He that saith he abideth in him [m]ought himself also so to walk, even as he walked.

7 Brethren, [n]I write no new commandment unto you, but an old commandment which ye had [o]from the beginning. The [p]old commandment is the word which ye have heard from the beginning.

8 Again, a [q]new commandment I write unto you, which thing is true in him and in you: because the darkness is past, and the [r]true light now shineth.

9 He that [s]saith he is in the light, and hateth his brother, is in darkness even until now.

10 He that loveth his brother abideth in the light, and there is none occasion of stumbling in him.

11 But he that [t]hateth his brother is in darkness, and [u]walketh in darkness, and knoweth not whither he goeth, because that darkness hath blinded his eyes.

12 I write unto you, little children, because your [d]sins are [v]forgiven you for his name's sake.

13 I write unto you, fathers, because ye have [w]known him *that is* from the beginning. I write unto you, young men, because ye have [x]overcome the wicked one. I write unto you, [y]little children, because ye have [z]known the Father.

14 I have written unto you, fathers, because ye have known him *that is* from the beginning. I have written unto you, young men, because ye are strong, and the word of God abideth in you, and ye have overcome the wicked one.

The children must not love the present world (Rev. 13:8, *note*).

15 [aa]Love not the [bb]world, neither the things *that are* in the world. [cc]If any man love the world, [dd]the love of the Father is not in him.

16 For all that *is* in the world, the lust of the [ee]flesh, and the lust of the eyes, and the pride of life, is not of the Father, but is of the world.

17 And the world passeth away, and the lust thereof: [ff]but he that doeth the will of God abideth for ever.

The children warned against apostates who deny the true deity of Christ.

18 Little children, it is the last time: and as ye have heard that antichrist shall come, even now are there many antichrists; whereby we know that it is the last time.

19 They [3]went out from us, but they were not of us; for if they had been of us, they would *no doubt* have continued

After A.D. 90.

a Rom. 3:25, 26; 2 Cor. 5:21.
b *righteous.*
c 1 John 5:10; John 3:33; Rom. 3:4.
d *Sin.* Rom. 3:23, *note.*
e *Advocacy.* (John 14:16, 26.)
f *Paraclete,* trans. *Comforter* in John 14:16.
g Gr. *hilasmos, that which propitiates.* See Rom. 3:25, *note.*
h *Assurance.* 1 John 3:1, 2. (Isa. 32:17; Jude 1.)
i Omit italicized words.
j *kosmos* (Mt. 4:8) = mankind.
k John 14:23; Col. 3:16.
l Mt. 5;48, *note.*
m John 13:15; 1 Pet. 2:21.
n 2 John 5.
o 1 John 3:11.
p John 15:10.
q John 15:12.
r John 1:9; 8:12; 12:35.
s v. 4; 1 John 3:14,15.
t 1 John 3:15; 4:20.
u John 12:35.
v Acts 10:43; Col. 2:13.
w 1 John 1:1; Rev. 22:13.
x 1 John 4:4; Heb. 2:14; Eph. 6:11.
y The little ones of the family; see v. 28, *marg.*
z Rom. 8:15-17; Gal. 4:6.
aa Rom. 12:2; Gal. 1:4; Jas. 4:4.
bb *kosmos* = world-system. 1 John 3:13. (John 7:7; Rev. 13:3-8, *note.*)
cc Mt. 6:24; Gal. 1:10.
dd *Law (of Christ).* vs. 7, 8, 15; 1 John 3:23, 24. (Gal. 6:2; 2 John 5.)
ee *Flesh.* Jude 23. (John 1:13; Jude 23.)
ff *Separation.* vs. 15-17; 1 John 5:21. (Gen. 12:1; 2 Cor. 6:14-17.)

[1] **(2:1)** Advocacy is that work of Jesus Christ for sinning saints which He carries on with the Father whereby, because of the eternal efficacy of His own sacrifice, He restores them to fellowship (cf. Psa. 23:3; John 13:10, *note*).

[2] **(2:3)** John uses "commandments" (1) in the general sense of the divine will, however revealed, "his word" (v. 5); and (2) especially of the law of Christ (Gal. 6:2; 2 John 5). See, also, John 15:10-12.

[3] **(2:19)** "Went out from us," that is, *doctrinally.* Doubtless then, as now, the deniers of the Son (vs. 22, 23) still called themselves Christians. Cf. 2 Tim. 1:15.

with us: but *they went out,* [a]that they
might be made manifest that [b]they were
not all of us.
20 But ye have an [c]unction from the
Holy One, and ye know all things.
21 I have not written unto you because
ye know not the truth, but [d]because ye
know it, and that no lie is of the truth.
22 Who is [e]a liar but he that denieth
that [f]Jesus is the Christ? He is [g]anti-
christ, that [h]denieth the Father and the
Son.
23 Whosoever denieth the Son, the
same hath not the Father: *(but) he that
acknowledgeth the Son hath the Father also.*
24 Let that therefore abide in you,
which ye have heard from the beginning. If that which ye have heard from
the beginning shall remain in you, ye
also shall [i]continue in the Son, and in the
Father.
25 And this is the [j]promise that he
hath promised us, *even* [k]eternal life.
26 These *things* have I written unto
you concerning them that [l]seduce you.
27 But the [m]anointing which ye have
received of him abideth in you, and ye
need not that any man teach you: but as
the same anointing teacheth you of all
things, and is truth, and is no lie, and
even as it hath taught you, ye shall abide
in him.
28 And now, [n]little children, abide in
him; that, when [o]he shall appear, we
may have confidence, and not be
ashamed before him at his coming.

How the little children may know each other.

29 If ye know that he is [p]righteous, ye
know that every one that [q]doeth righteousness is born of him.

CHAPTER 3.

Behold, [r]what manner of love the
Father hath bestowed upon us, [s]that
we should be called the [t]sons of God:
therefore the [u]world knoweth us not,
because it knew him not.
2 Beloved, now are we the [t]sons of
God, and it doth not yet appear what we
shall be: but we know that, [v]when he
shall appear, [w]we shall be like him; for
we shall see him as he is.
3 And every man that hath this hope
in him purifieth himself, even as he is
pure.
4 Whosoever [x]committeth [y]sin transgresseth also the law: for sin is the transgression of the law.
5 And ye know that he was manifested to [z]take away our sins; and [aa]in him
is no sin.
6 Whosoever abideth in him sinneth
not: whosoever sinneth hath not seen
him, neither known him.
7 Little children, let no man deceive
you: he that doeth [1]righteousness is
righteous, even as he is righteous.
8 He that committeth sin is of the
[bb]devil; for the devil sinneth from the
beginning. For this purpose the Son of
God was manifested, [cc]that he might
[dd]destroy the works of the devil.
9 Whosoever is [ee]born of God doth not
[ff]commit sin; for his seed remaineth in
him: and he cannot sin, because he is
born of God.
10 In this the children of God are manifest, and the children of the devil:
whosoever [gg]doeth not [hh]righteousness
is not of God, neither he that loveth not
his brother.

How the little children must live together.

11 For this is the [ii]message that ye
heard from the beginning, that [jj]we
should love one another.
12 Not as Cain, *who* was of that
wicked one, and slew his brother. And
wherefore slew he him? Because his own
works were evil, and his brother's righteous.
13 Marvel not, my brethren, if the
[kk]world [ll]hate you.
14 We know that we have passed from
death unto life, because we love the
brethren. He that loveth not *his* brother
abideth in death.
15 Whosoever hateth his brother

After A.D. 90.

a 1 Cor. 11:19.
b John 10:28.
c 2 Cor. 1:21.
d 2 Pet. 3:1; Jude 5.
e *the liar.*
f 1 John 4:3.
g *Antichrist.* vs. 18, 22; 1 John 4:3. (1 John 2:18; Rev. 13:11-17.)
h John 14:9-11.
i John 15:5; Col. 1:23.
j John 3:16; 17:2, 3.
k *Life (eternal).* 1 John 3:14, 15. (Mt. 7:14; Rev. 22:19.)
l *lead you astray.*
m v. 20; John 14:26; 16:13.
n The general term for all children.
o 1 John 3:2; 4:17.
p 1 John 3:7.
q *practiseth.*
r 1 John 4:10; Eph. 2:4-7.
s *Assurance.* vs. 1, 2; Jude 1, R.V. (Isa. 32:17; Jude 1.)
t *children.*
u *kosmos* (Mt. 4:8) = mankind.
v *Christ (Second Advent).* Jude 14, 15. (Deut. 30:3; Acts 1:9-11.)
w Rom. 8:29; 1 Cor. 15:49; Phil. 3:21.
x *practiseth sin practiseth also lawlessness; and sin is lawlessness.*
y *Sin.* Rom. 3:23, *note.*
z John 1:29; Heb. 9:26.
aa 2 Cor. 5:21; Heb. 7:26; 1 Pet. 1:19.
bb *Satan.* vs. 8, 10; Jude 9. (Gen. 3:1; Rev. 20:10.)
cc Heb. 2:14.
dd *undo.*
ee *1 John 5:18; John 3:6.*
ff *practise.*
gg *does not practise.*
hh See v. 7, *note.*
ii 1 John 1:5; 2:7.
jj v. 23; John 13:34; 15:12; 1 John 4:7, 21; 2 John 5.
kk kosmos = world-system. 1 John 4:3-5. (John 7:7; Rev. 13:3-8, *note.*)
ll John 15:18-20.

[1] **(3:7)** "Righteousness" here, and in the passages having marginal references to this, means the righteous life which is the result of salvation through Christ. The righteous man under law became righteous by doing righteously; under grace he does righteously because he has been made righteous (Rom. 3:22; Rom. 10:3, *note*).

is a murderer: and ye know that no murderer hath [a]eternal life abiding in him.

16 Hereby [b]perceive we the love *of God*, [c]because he laid down his life for us: and we ought to [d]lay down *our* lives for the brethren.

17 But whoso hath this world's good, and seeth his brother have need, and shutteth up his bowels *of compassion* from him, how [e]dwelleth the love of God in him?

18 [f]My little children, let us not love in word, neither in tongue; but in deed and in truth.

19 And hereby we know that we are of the truth, and shall assure our hearts before him.

20 [g]For if our heart condemn us, God is greater than our heart, and knoweth all things.

21 Beloved, if our heart condemn us not, [h]*then* have we confidence toward God.

22 And [i]whatsoever we ask, we receive of him, because we keep his commandments, and do those things that are pleasing in his sight.

23 And [j]this is his commandment, That we should [k]believe on the name of his Son Jesus Christ, and [l]love one another, as he gave us commandment.

24 And he that keepeth his commandments [m]dwelleth in him, and he in him. And hereby we know that he abideth in us, by the [n]Spirit which he hath given us.

CHAPTER 4.

Part II. The family and the world.

Parenthetic: The children warned against false teachers.

Beloved, believe not every spirit, but [o]try the spirits whether they are of God: because many false prophets are gone out into the [p]world.

The marks of false teachers.

(a) The false doctrine of Christ's person.

2 Hereby know ye the [q]Spirit of God: Every spirit that confesseth that [r]Jesus Christ is come in the flesh is of God:

3 And every spirit that confesseth not that Jesus Christ is come in the flesh is not of God: and this is that *spirit* of [s]antichrist, whereof ye have heard that it should come; and even now already is it in the [t]world.

4 Ye are of God, little children, and have overcome them: because [u]greater is he that is in you, than [v]he that is in the world.

(b) The world-marks of false teachers.

5 [w]They are of the world: therefore speak they of the world, and [x]the world heareth them.

6 We are of God: he that knoweth God heareth us; he that is not of God heareth not us. [y]Hereby know we the spirit of truth, and the spirit of error.

The true children are born of God through faith in the propitiation of the Son of God.

7 [z]Beloved, let us love one another: for love is of God; and every one that [aa]loveth is born of God, and knoweth God.

8 He that loveth not knoweth not God; for [bb]God is love.

9 In this was [cc]manifested the love of God toward us, because that God sent his only begotten [dd]Son into the [ee]world, that we might live through him.

10 Herein is love, [ff]not that we loved God, but that he loved us, and sent his Son *to be* the [gg]propitiation for our sins.

The love-life is shown by the life of love.

11 Beloved, if God so loved us, we ought also to love one another.

12 No man hath seen God at any time. [hh]If we love one another, God dwelleth in us, and his love is [ii]perfected in us.

13 Hereby know we that we dwell in him, and he in us, because he hath given us of his Spirit.

14 And we have seen and do testify that the Father sent the Son *to be* the [jj]Saviour of the [kk]world.

15 Whosoever shall confess that Jesus is the Son of God, God dwelleth in him, and he in God.

16 And we have known and believed the love that God hath to us. God is love; and he that dwelleth in love dwelleth in God, and God in him.

17 Herein [ll]is our love made perfect, that we may have boldness in the [mm]day of judgment: because as he is, so are we in this world.

18 There is no fear in love; but perfect love casteth out fear: because fear hath

After A.D. 90.

a *Life (eternal).* vs. 14, 15; 1 John 5:11, 12, 13, 16, 20. (Mt. 7:14; Rev. 22:19.)
b *we know love.*
c John 15:13; Gal. 2:20.
d Rom. 16:4.
e 1 John 4:20.
f Rom. 12:9; Jas. 2:15, 16; 1 Pet. 1:22.
g 1 Cor. 4:4.
h 2 Cor. 1:12; Heb. 10:19.
i John 15:7.
j *Law (of Christ).* vs. 23, 24; 1 John 4:12. (Gal. 6:2; 2 John 5.)
k John 6:29.
l John 13:34.
m John 14:21.
n *Holy Spirit.* 1 John 4:2, 13. (Mt. 1:18; Acts 2:4.)
o *prove.*
p *earth.*
q *Holy Spirit.* vs. 2, 13; 1 John 5:6, 7. (Mt. 1:18; Acts 2:4.)
r Rom. 10:9, 10; 1 John 5:1.
s *Antichrist.* 2 John 7. (1 John 2:18; Rev. 13:11-17.)
t *kosmos* = world-system. 1 John 5:4, 5, 19. (John 7:7; Rev. 13:3-8, *note.*)
u Rom. 8:31.
v John 14:30; 16:11; 1 Cor. 2:12.
w *Apostasy.* vs. 1-5; Jude 3-19. (Lk. 18:8; 2 Tim. 3:1-8.)
x John 15:19; 17:14.
y 1 Cor. 2:12, 16.
z 1 John 3:10, 11, 23.
aa 1 John 3:14; 1 Thes. 4:9.
bb v. 16; 1 John 1:5.
cc Rom. 5:8.
dd Isa. 9:6; John 3:16.
ee *kosmos* (Mt. 4:8) = mankind.
ff Tit. 3:5.
gg Gr. *hilasmos.* See 1 John 2:2.
hh *Law (of Christ).* 2 John 5. (Gal. 6:2; 2 John 5.)
ii Mt. 5:48, *note.*
jj Rom. 1:16, *note.*
kk *kosmos* (Mt. 4:8) = mankind.
ll *hath love been perfected with us.*
mm *Day of judgment.* Rev. 20:11. (Mt. 10:15; Rev. 20:11.)

torment. He that feareth is not made [a]perfect in love.

19 [b]We love him, because he first loved us.

20 [c]If a man say, I love God, and hateth his brother, he is a liar: for he that loveth not his brother whom he hath seen, how can he love God whom he hath not seen?

21 And [d]this commandment have we from him, That he who loveth God love his brother also.

CHAPTER 5.

Faith is the overcoming principle in the world-conflict.

Whosoever [e]believeth that [f]Jesus is the Christ is [g]born of God: and [h]every one that loveth him that begat loveth him also that is begotten of him.

2 By this we know that we love the children of God, when we love God, and [i]keep his commandments.

3 For this is the love of God, that we keep his commandments: and his commandments [j]are not grievous.

4 For whatsoever is born of God overcometh the [k]world: and this is the victory that overcometh the world, *even* our faith.

5 Who is he that overcometh the world, but he that [l]believeth that Jesus is the Son of God?

6 This is he that came by [m]water and blood, *even* Jesus Christ; not by water only, but by water and blood. And it is the [n]Spirit that beareth witness, because the Spirit is truth.

7 [o]For there are three that bear record in heaven, the Father, the Word, and the Holy Ghost: and these three are one.

8 [p]And there are three that bear witness [q]in earth, the [r]Spirit, and the water, and the blood: and these three [s]agree in one.

9 If we receive the [t]witness of men, the witness of God is greater: for this is the witness of God which he hath testified of his Son.

10 He that believeth on the Son of God [u]hath the witness in himself: he that believeth not God [v]hath made him a liar; because he believeth not the record that God gave of his Son.

11 And this is the record, that God hath given to us eternal life, and this life is in his Son.

12 He that [w]hath the Son hath life; *and* he that hath not the Son of God hath not life.

13 These things have I written unto you that [x]believe on the name of the Son of God; that ye may know that ye have eternal life, and that ye may believe on the name of the Son of God.

14 And this is the confidence that we have in him, that, [y]if we ask any thing according to his will, he heareth us:

15 And if we know that he hear us, whatsoever we ask, we know that we have the petitions that we desired of him.

16 If any man see his brother [z]sin a sin *which is* not unto death, he shall ask, and he shall give him life for them that sin not unto death. There is a sin unto death: I do not say that he shall pray for it.

17 [aa]All unrighteousness is sin: and there is a sin not unto death.

18 We know that whosoever is [bb]born of God sinneth not; but he that is begotten of God keepeth himself, and that wicked one toucheth him not.

19 *And* we know that we are of God, and [cc]the whole world lieth [dd]in wickedness.

20 And we know that the [ee]Son of God is come, and hath given us an understanding, that we may [ff]know him that is true, and we are in him that is true, *even* in his Son Jesus Christ. This is the true God, and [gg]eternal life.

21 [hh]Little children, [ii]keep yourselves from idols. Amen.

After A.D. 90.

a Mt. 5:48, *note.*
b vs. 10; 2 Cor. 5:14, 15.
c 1 John 2:4; 3:17.
d John 13:34; 15:12; 1 John 3:23.
e John 1:12.
f 1 John 2:22, 23; 4:2, 15.
g John 1:13.
h John 15:23.
i 2 John 6; Rev. 3:19.
j Mt. 11:30.
k *kosmos* = world-system. Rev. 11:15. (John 7:7; Rev. 13:3-8, *note.*)
l *Faith.* vs. 1, 4, 5, 10; Heb. 11:1-39. (Gen. 3:20; Heb. 11:39.)
m John 19:34, 35; Eph. 5:26-27; Heb. 10:5-7.
n Heb. 2:4.
o It is generally agreed that v. 7 has no real authority, and has been inserted.
p *for.*
q Omit "in earth."
r *Holy Spirit.* vs. 6-8; Jude 19, 20. (Mt. 1:18; Acts 2:4.)
s Or, *are to one point or purpose.*
t John 8:17, 18.
u Rom. 8:16; Gal. 4:6.
v 1 John 1:10.
w John 3:36; 6:47, 48; 17:2, 3.
x *ye may know that ye have eternal life who believe the name of.*
y 1 John 3:22.
z Rom. 3:23, *note.*
aa 1 John 3:4.
bb 1 John 3:9.
cc Lk. 4:6; 2 Cor. 4:4.
dd *in the wicked one.*
ee 1 John 4:2.
ff 1 John 2:20, 27.
gg *Life (eternal).* vs. 11, 12, 13, 16, 20; Jude 21. (Mt. 7:14; Rev. 22:19.)
hh *Dear children, guard yourselves.*
ii *Separation.* 2 John 10, 11. (Gen. 12:1; 2 Cor. 6:14-17.)

THE SECOND EPISTLE OF
JOHN

WRITER. The Apostle John.

Date. Probably A.D. 90.

Theme. Second John gives the essentials of the personal walk of the believer in a day when "many deceivers are entered into the world" (v. 7). The key-phrase is "the truth," by which John means the body of revealed truth, the Scriptures. The Bible, as the only authority for doctrine and life, is the believer's resource in a time of declension and apostasy.

The Epistle is in three divisions: I. The pathway of truth and love, vs. 1-6. II. The peril of unscriptural ways, vs. 7-11. III. Superscription, vs. 12, 13.

Part I. "The truth" and love inseparable in the Christian life.

The [a]elder unto the [b]elect lady and her children, whom I love in the truth; and not I only, but also all they that have known the truth;

2 For the truth's sake, [c]which dwelleth in us, and [d]shall be with us for ever.

3 Grace be with you, mercy, *and* peace, from God the Father, and from the Lord Jesus Christ, the Son of the Father, in truth and love.

4 I [e]rejoiced greatly that I found of thy children walking in truth, as we have received a commandment from the Father.

5 And now I beseech thee, lady, not as though I wrote a new commandment unto thee, but that which we had from the beginning, [1][f]that we love one another.

6 And this is [g]love, that we walk after his commandments. This is the commandment, That, as ye have heard from the beginning, ye should walk in it.

Part II. Doctrine the final test of reality. (Cf. John 6:60–66.)

7 For many deceivers are [h]entered into the [i]world, who confess not [j]that Jesus Christ is come in the flesh. This is [k]a deceiver and [k]an [l]antichrist.

8 Look to yourselves, that we lose not those things which we have wrought, but that we receive a full [m]reward.

9 Whosoever [n]transgresseth, and abideth not in the doctrine of Christ, hath not God. He that abideth in the doctrine of Christ, he hath both the Father and the Son.

10 If there come any unto you, and bring not this doctrine, receive him [o]not into *your* house, neither [p]bid him God speed:

11 For he that [q]biddeth him God speed is partaker of his evil deeds.

Part III. Superscription.

12 Having many things to write unto you, I would not *write* with paper and ink: but I [r]trust to come unto you, and speak face to face, that our joy may be full.

13 The children of thy [b]elect sister greet thee. Amen.

After A.D. 90.

a *Elders.* 3 John 1. (Acts 11:30; Tit. 1:5-9.)
b *Election (personal).* Rev. 17:14. (Deut. 7:6; 1 Pet. 1:2.)
c Col. 3:16.
d 1 Pet. 1:23.
e 1 Thes. 2:19, 20; 3 John 3-4.
f *Law (of Christ).* (Gal. 6:2.)
g John 14:15; 1 John 5:3.
h *gone forth.*
i *kosmos* (Mt. 4:8) = mankind.
j *Jesus Christ coming in flesh.*
k *the.*
l *Antichrist.* Rev. 16:13. (1 John 2:18; Rev. 13:11-17.)
m *Rewards.* Rev. 2:10. (Dan. 12:3; 1 Cor. 3:14.)
n *Sin.* Rom. 3:23, *note.*
o *Separation.* Rev. 18:4. (Gen. 12:1; 2 Cor. 6:14-17.)
p *greet him.*
q *greeteth him is.*
r *hope.*

[1]**(v. 5)** Law (of Christ), Summary: The new "law of Christ" is the divine love, as wrought into the renewed heart by the Holy Spirit (Rom. 5:5; Heb. 10:16), and outflowing in the energy of the Spirit, unforced and spontaneous, toward the objects of the divine love (2 Cor. 5:14-20; 1 Thes. 2:7, 8). It is, therefore, "the law of liberty" (Jas. 1:25; 2:12), in contrast with the external law of Moses. Moses' law demands love (Lev. 19:18; Deut. 6:5; Lk. 10:27); Christ's law is love (Rom. 5:5; 1 John 4:7, 19, 20), and so takes the place of the external law by fulfilling it (Rom. 13:10; Gal. 5:14). It is the "law written in the heart" under the New Covenant (Heb. 8:8, *note*).

THE THIRD EPISTLE OF
JOHN

WRITER. The Apostle John.

Date. Probably about A.D. 90.

Theme. The aged Apostle had written to a church which allowed one Diotrephes to exercise an authority common enough in later ages, but wholly new in the primitive churches. Diotrephes had rejected the apostolic letters and authority. It appears also that he had refused the ministry of visiting brethren (v. 10), and cast out those who received them. Historically, this letter marks the beginning of that clerical and priestly assumption over the churches in which the primitive church order disappeared. This Epistle reveals, as well, the believer's resource in such a day. No longer writing as an apostle, but as an elder, John addresses this letter, not to the church as such, but to a faithful man in the church for the comfort and encouragement of those who were standing fast in the primitive simplicity. Second John conditions the personal walk of a Christian in a day of apostasy; Third John the personal responsibility in such a day of the believer as a member of the local church. The key-phrase is "the truth" (see 2 John, Introduction).

There are three divisions: I. Personal greetings, vs. 1-4. II. Instructions concerning ministering brethren, vs. 5-8. III. The apostate leader, and the good Demetrius, vs. 9-14.

Part I. Personal greetings.

The [a]elder unto the wellbeloved
Gaius, whom I love in the truth.
2 Beloved, I wish [b]above all things
[c]that thou mayest prosper and be in
health, even as thy soul prospereth.
3 For I rejoiced greatly, when the
brethren came and testified of the truth
that is in thee, even as thou walkest in
the truth.
4 I have no greater [d]joy than to hear
that [e]my children walk in [f]truth.

Part II. Concerning ministering brethren.

5 Beloved, thou doest faithfully whatsoever thou doest to the brethren, and to
strangers;
6 Which have borne witness of thy
[g]charity before the church: whom if thou
bring [h]forward on their journey [i]after a
godly sort, thou shalt do well:
7 Because that for his name's sake they
went forth, [j]taking nothing of the
Gentiles.
8 We therefore ought to [k]receive such,
that we might be fellowhelpers to the
truth.

Part III. The domineering Diotrephes.

9 I wrote unto the church: but
Diotrephes, who loveth to have the [l]pre-
eminence among them, receiveth us not.
10 Wherefore, if I come, I will remember his deeds which he doeth, [m]prating
against us with malicious words: and
not content therewith, neither doth he
himself receive the brethren, and forbid-
deth them that would, and casteth *them*
out of the [n]church.
11 Beloved, [o]follow not that which is
evil, but that which is good. He that
doeth good is of God: but he that doeth
evil hath not seen God.

The good Demetrius.

12 Demetrius hath good report of all
men, and of the truth itself: yea, and we
also bear [p]record; and ye know that our
[p]record is true.
13 I had many things to write, but I
will not with ink and pen write unto
thee:
14 But I [q]trust I shall shortly see thee,
and we shall speak face to face. Peace *be*
to thee. *Our* friends salute thee. Greet
the friends by name.

After A.D. 90.

a *Elders.* Rev. 4:4, 5, 9-11. (Acts 11:30; Tit. 1:5-9.)
b *that in all things.*
c Mt. 6:33.
d 1 Thes. 2:19, 20; 2 John 4.
e 1 Cor. 4:15.
f *the truth.*
g *love.*
h Acts 15:3.
i Mt. 25:40; Phil. 1:27.
j 1 Cor. 9:15, 18.
k Mt. 10:40.
l Mt. 23:8.
m Prov. 10:8, 10.
n *Churches (local).* vs. 6, 9, 10; Rev. 1:4, 11, 20. (Acts 2:41; Phil. 1:1.)
o Psa. 37:27.
p *witness.*
q *hope.*

THE GENERAL EPISTLE OF

JUDE

WRITER. Jude, the brother of James (1:1).

Date. Probably A.D. 66.

Theme. It is not so much Jude who speaks, as the constraining Spirit (v. 3), and the theme is, "Contending for the faith" (Lk. 18:8, *refs.*). In this brief letter the apostasy (2 Thes. 2:3, *note*) of the professing church is predicted, and the cause and course described. As in Second Timothy and Second Peter the apostasy is treated as having already set in.

The Epistle is in five divisions: I. Introduction, vs. 1, 2. II. Occasion of the Epistle, vs. 3, 4. III. Apostasy is possible, vs. 5-7. IV. Apostate teachers described, vs. 8-19. V. The saints assured and comforted, vs. 20-25.

Part I. Introduction.

Jude, the servant of Jesus Christ, and brother of James, to [a]them that are sanctified by God the Father, [b]and [1]preserved in Jesus Christ, *and* [c]called:

2 Mercy unto you, and peace, and love, be multiplied.

Part II. Occasion of the Epistle: the apostasy.

3 Beloved, when I gave all diligence to write unto you of the common [d]salvation, [e]it was needful for me to write unto you, and exhort *you* that ye should earnestly contend for the [f]faith which was [g]once delivered unto the saints.

4 For there are certain men crept in unawares, [h]who were before of old ordained to this condemnation, ungodly men, turning the grace of our God into lasciviousness, and denying [i]the only Lord God, and our Lord Jesus Christ.

Part III. Historical instances of apostasy.

5 I will therefore put you in remembrance, though ye once knew this, how that the Lord, having [d]saved the people out of the land of Egypt, afterward destroyed them that believed not.

6 And the [j]angels which kept not their first estate, but left their own habitation, he hath reserved in everlasting chains under darkness unto the judgment of [k]the [2]great day.

7 Even as Sodom and Gomorrha, and the cities about them in like manner, giving themselves over to fornication, and going after strange flesh, are set forth for an example, suffering the [l]vengeance of eternal fire.

Part IV. Apostate teachers described.

8 Likewise also these *filthy* dreamers [m]defile the flesh, despise dominion, and speak evil of dignities.

9 Yet Michael the archangel, when contending with the [n]devil he disputed about the body of Moses, durst not bring against him a railing [o]accusation, but said, The [p]Lord rebuke thee.

10 But these speak evil of those things which they know not: but what they know naturally, as brute beasts, in those things they corrupt themselves.

11 Woe unto them! [q]for they have gone in the way of [3]Cain, and ran

A.D. 66.

a *the called ones, beloved in God the Father, and preserved in Jesus Christ.*
b Or, *kept for Jesus Christ.*
c *Assurance.* (Isa. 32:17.)
d Rom. 1:16, *note.*
e Lit. constraint was upon me, i.e. of the Spirit.
f *Gospel.* Rev. 14:6. (Gen. 12:1-3; Rev. 14:6.)
g *once for all.*
h vs. 14, 15; Jas. 1:13, 15.
i *our only Master and Lord Jesus Christ.*
j Heb. 1:4, *note.*
k *Day (of Jehovah).* Rev. 2:26, 27. (Isa. 2:10-22; Rev. 19:11-21.)
l *judgment.*
m 2 Pet. 2:10.
n *Satan.* Rev. 2:9, 10, 13, 24. (Gen. 3:1; Rev. 20:10.)
o *judgment.*
p *Jehovah.* Zech. 3:2.
q *Apostasy.* Rev. 3:14-16. (Lk. 18:8; 2 Tim. 3:1-8.)

[1]**(v. 1)** Assurance is the believer's full conviction that, through the work of Christ alone, received by faith, he is in possession of a salvation in which he will be eternally kept. And this assurance rests only upon the Scripture promises to him who believes.

[2]**(v. 6)** The judgment of the fallen angels. The "great day" is the day of the Lord (Isa. 2:9-22, *refs.*). As the final judgment upon Satan occurs after the thousand years, and preceding the final judgment (Rev. 20:10), it is congruous to conclude, as to the time, that other fallen angels are judged with him (2 Pet. 2:4; Rev. 20:10). Christians are associated with Christ in this judgment (1 Cor. 6:3). See other judgments, Rev. 20:12, *note.*

[3]**(v. 11)** Cain (cf. Gen. 4:1), type of the religious natural man, who believes in a God,

greedily after the [1]error of Balaam for reward, and perished in the [a]gainsaying of [2]Core.

12 These are spots in your [b]feasts of charity, when they feast with you, [c]feeding themselves without fear: clouds *they are* without water, carried about of winds; [d]trees whose fruit withereth, without fruit, twice dead, plucked up by the roots;

13 Raging waves of the sea, foaming out their own shame; wandering stars, to whom is reserved the blackness of darkness for ever.

14 And Enoch also, the seventh from Adam, prophesied of these, saying, Behold, [e]the Lord [f]cometh with ten thousands of his saints,

15 To execute [g]judgment upon all, and to [h]convince all that are ungodly among them of all their ungodly deeds which they have ungodly committed, and of all their hard [i]*speeches* which ungodly [j]sinners have spoken against him.

16 These are murmurers, complainers, walking after their own lusts; and their mouth speaketh great swelling *words*, having men's persons in admiration because of advantage.

17 But, beloved, remember ye the words which were spoken before of the apostles of our Lord Jesus Christ;

18 How that they told you there should be mockers in the last time, who should walk after their own ungodly lusts.

19 These be they who separate themselves, [k]sensual, having [l]not the Spirit.

Part V. True believers assured and comforted: their sevenfold duty.

20 But ye, beloved, building up yourselves on your most [m]holy faith, praying in the [n]Holy Ghost,

21 Keep yourselves in the love of God, looking for the mercy of our Lord Jesus Christ unto [o]eternal life.

22 And of some have compassion, making a difference:

23 And others save with fear, [p]pulling *them* out of the fire; hating even the garment spotted by the [3q]flesh.

24 Now unto him that is able to keep you from [r]falling, and to present *you* faultless before the presence of his glory with exceeding joy,

25 To the only wise God our [s]Saviour, [t]*be* glory and majesty, dominion and power, both now and ever. Amen.

A.D. 66.

a *antilogia = against the Word.*
b *love feasts.*
c *shepherds that without fear feed themselves.*
d *autumn trees without fruit.*
e *Jehovah.* Deut. 33:2.
f *Christ (Second Advent).* vs. 14, 15; Rev. 1:7, 8. (Deut. 30:3; Acts 1:9-11.)
g *Judgments (the seven).* vs. 6, 14, 15; Rev. 22:12. (2 Sam. 7:14; Rev. 20:12.)
h *convict.*
i *things.*
j *Sin.* Rom. 3:23, *note.*
k *natural.*
l See Rom. 8:8, 9.
m *Sanctify, holy (persons).* (N.T.). Rev. 22:11. (Mt. 4:5; Rev. 22:11.)
n *Holy Spirit.* vs. 19, 20; Rev. 1:4, 10. (Mt. 1:18; Acts 2:4.)
o *Life (eternal).* Rev. 2:7, 10. (Mt. 7:14; Rev. 22:19.)
p *snatching.*
q *Flesh.* (John 1:13; 8:15.)
r *stumbling.*
s Rom. 1:16.
t *through Jesus Christ our Lord.*

and in "religion," but after his own will, and who rejects redemption by blood. Compelled as a teacher of religion to explain the atonement, the apostate teacher explains it away.

[1]**(v. 11)** Balaam. The "error" of Balaam must be distinguished from his "way" (2 Pet. 2:15, *note*), and his "doctrine" (Rev. 2:14, *note*). The "error" of Balaam was that, reasoning from natural morality, and seeing the evil in Israel, he supposed a righteous God *must* curse them. He was blind to the higher morality of the Cross, through which God maintains and enforces the authority and awful sanctions of His law, so that He can be just and the justifier of a believing sinner. The "reward" of v. 11 may not be money, but popularity, or applause.

[2]**(v. 11)** See Num. 16. The sin of Korah was denial of the authority of Moses as God's chosen spokesman, and intrusion into the priest's office.

[3]**(v. 23)** Flesh, Summary: "Flesh," in the ethical sense, is the whole natural or unregenerate man, spirit, soul, and body, as centered upon self, prone to sin, and opposed to God (Rom. 7:18). The regenerate man is not "in [the sphere of] the flesh, but in [the sphere of] the Spirit" (Rom. 8:9); but the flesh is still in him, and he may, according to his choice, "walk after the flesh" or "in the Spirit" (1 Cor. 3:1-4; Gal. 5:16, 17). In the first case he is a "carnal," in the second a "spiritual," Christian. Victory over the flesh will be the habitual experience of the believer who walks in the Spirit (Rom. 8:2, 4; Gal. 5:16, 17).

THE REVELATION

OF

ST. JOHN THE DIVINE

WRITER. The Apostle John (1:1).

Date. A.D. 96.

Theme. The theme of the Revelation is Jesus Christ (1:1), presented in a threefold way: (1) As to *time:* "which is, and which was, and which is to come" (1:4); (2) as to *relationships*—to the churches (1:9–3:22), to the tribulation (4:1–19:21), to the kingdom (20:1–22:21); (3) in His *offices*—High Priest (8:3-6), Bridegroom (19:7-9), King-Judge (20:1-15).

But while Christ is thus the central *theme* of the book, all of the *events* move toward one consummation, the bringing in of the covenanted kingdom. The key-phrase is the prophetic declaration of the "great voices in heaven" (11:15), lit. "The world kingdom of our Lord and of his Christ has come." The book is, therefore, a prophecy (1:3).

The three major *divisions* of Revelation must be clearly held if the interpretation is to be sane and coherent. John was commanded to "write" concerning three classes of "things" (1:19): I. Things past, "the things which thou hast seen," i.e. the Patmos vision, 1:1-20. II. Things present, "the things which are," i.e. things then existing—obviously the churches. The temple had been destroyed, the Jews dispersed: the testimony of God had been committed to the churches (1 Tim. 3:15). Accordingly we have seven messages to seven representative churches, 2:1–3:22. It is noteworthy that the church is not mentioned in chapters 5–18. III. Things future, "things which shall be hereafter," lit. "after these," i.e. after the church period ends, 4:1–22:21. The third major division, as Erdman (W. J.) has pointed out, falls into a series of six sevens, with five parenthetical passages, making, with the church division, seven sevens. The six sevens are: 1. The seven seals, 4:1–8:1. 2. The seven trumpets, 8:2–11:19. 3. The seven personages, 12:1–14:20. 4. The seven vials (bowls), 15:1–16:21. 5. The seven dooms, 17:1–20:15. 6. The seven new things, 21:1–22:21.

The parenthetical passages are: (I) The Jewish remnant and the tribulation saints, 7:1-17. (II) The angel, the little book, the two witnesses, 10:1–11:14. (III) The Lamb, the Remnant, and the everlasting Gospel, 14:1-13. (IV) The gathering of the kings at Armageddon, 16:13-16. (V) The four alleluias in heaven, 19:1-6. These passages do not advance the prophetic narrative. Looking backward and forward they sum up results accomplished, and speak of results yet to come as if they had already come. In 14:1, for example, the Lamb and Remnant are seen prophetically on Mount Sion, though they are not actually there till 20:4-6.

The end of the church period (2–3) is left indeterminate. It will end by the fulfilment of 1 Thes. 4:14-17. Chapters 4–19 are believed to synchronize with Daniel's Seventieth Week (Dan. 9:24, *note*). The great tribulation begins at the middle of the "week," and continues three and a half years (Rev. 11:3-19:21). The tribulation is brought to an end by the appearing of the Lord and the battle of Armageddon (Mt. 24:29, 30; Rev. 19:11-21). The kingdom follows (Rev. 20:4, 5); after this the "little season" (Rev. 20:7-15), and then eternity.

Interpreters of the Revelation should bear in mind two important passages: 1 Pet. 1:12; 2 Pet. 1:20, 21. Doubtless much which is designedly obscure to us will be clear to those for whom it was written as the time approaches.

CHAPTER 1.

Part I. "The things which thou hast seen" (Rev. 1:1-20).

(1) *Introduction.*

THE [a]Revelation of Jesus Christ, which
God gave unto him, to shew unto
his servants things which must shortly
come to pass; and he sent and signified
it by his [b]angel unto his servant John:
2 Who bare record of the word of God,
and of the testimony of Jesus Christ, and
of all things that he saw.
3 Blessed *is* he that readeth, and they
that hear the words of this prophecy,
and keep those things which are written
therein: for the time *is* at hand.

A.D. 96.

a *Inspiration.* vs. 1, 19; Rev. 2:1, 8, 12, 18. (Ex. 4:15; Rev. 22:19.)

b Heb. 1:4, *note.*

(2) Salutation.

4 John to the seven [a]churches which are
in Asia: Grace *be* unto you, and peace,
from him which is, and which was, and
which is to come; and from the seven
[b]Spirits which are before his throne;
5 And from Jesus Christ, *who is* the
faithful [c]witness, *and* the [d]first begotten
of the dead, and the [e]prince of the kings
of the earth. Unto him that [f]loved us,
and [g]washed us from our [h]sins in his
own blood,
6 And hath made us [i]kings and priests
unto God and his Father; to him *be* glory
and dominion for ever and ever. Amen.
7 Behold, he cometh with clouds; and
[j]every eye shall see him, and they *also*
which pierced him: and all kindreds of
the earth shall wail because of him. Even
so, Amen.
8 I am [k]Alpha and Omega, the beginning and the ending, saith the Lord,
which is, and which was, and which is
to come, the [l]Almighty.

(3) The Patmos vision.

9 I John, who also am your brother,
and companion in [m]tribulation, and in
the kingdom and patience [n]of Jesus
Christ, was in the [1]isle that is called
Patmos, for the word of God, and for the
testimony of Jesus Christ.
10 I [o]was in the [p]Spirit on the Lord's
day, and heard behind me a great [q]voice,
as of a trumpet,
11 Saying, I am Alpha and Omega, the
first and the last: and, What thou seest,
write in a book, and send *it* unto the
seven churches which are in Asia; unto
Ephesus, and unto Smyrna, and unto
Pergamos, and unto Thyatira, and unto
Sardis, and unto Philadelphia, and unto
Laodicea.
12 And I turned to see the voice that
spake with me. And being turned, I saw
seven golden [r]candlesticks;
13 And in the midst of the seven
[r]candlesticks *one* like unto the Son of
man, clothed with a garment down to
the foot, and girt about the paps with a
golden girdle.
14 His head and *his* hairs *were* [s]white
like wool, as white as snow; and his eyes
were as a flame of fire;
15 And his feet like unto fine brass, as
if they burned in a furnace; and his voice
as the sound of many waters.
16 And he had in his right hand [t]seven
stars: and out of his mouth went a sharp
twoedged sword: and his countenance
was as the sun shineth in his strength.
17 And when I saw him, I fell at his
feet as dead. And he laid his right hand
upon me, saying unto me, Fear not; I am
the first and the last:
18 *I am* he that liveth, and was dead;
and, behold, I am alive for evermore,
Amen; and have the keys of [u][v]hell and
of death.

(4) The command to write.

19 Write the things which thou hast
seen, and the things which are, and the
things which shall be [w]hereafter;
20 The [x]mystery of the seven stars
which thou sawest in my right hand,
and the seven golden [y]candlesticks. The
seven stars are the [2][z]angels of the seven
[aa]churches: and the seven candlesticks
which thou sawest are the seven
[3]churches.

A.D. 96.

a v. 20.
b Cf. 1 Cor. 12:4, 13; Isa. 11:2; Rev. 3:1.
c Isa. 55:4.
d *firstborn from among.*
e *ruler.*
f *loveth.*
g *Sacrifice (of Christ).* Rom. 12:1. (Gen. 4:4; Heb. 10:18.)
h *Sin.* Rom. 3:23, *note.*
i *a kingdom, priests.*
j *Christ (Second Advent).* Rev. 2:25-28. (Deut. 30:3; Acts 1:9-11.)
k Rev. 22:12, 13.
l Isa. 9:6.
m *the tribulation and kingdom.*
n *of Jesus.*
o *became.*
p *Holy Spirit.* vs. 4, 10; Rev. 2:7, 11, 17, 29. (Mt. 1:18; Acts 2:4.)
q *The theophanies.* vs. 9-20. (Gen. 12:7.)
r *lampstands.*
s *as white wool, as snow.*
t v. 20.
u Lk. 16:23, *note.*
v *hades.*
w *things that are to be after these,* i.e. after the church-es.
x Mt. 13:11, *note.*
y *lampstands.*
z *messengers.*
aa *Churches (local).* vs. 4, 11, 20, Rev. 2:1, 7, 8, 11, 12-29. (Acts 2:41; Phil. 1:1.)

[1] **(1:9)** From 1:1 to 1:20 the Seer is on the earth, looking at the vision of Christ. From 2:1 to 3:22 he is on the earth looking forward through the church-age. From 4:1 to 11:1 he is "in the Spirit" (4:2; cf. Ezk. 3:12-14) observing things in heaven and on earth. From 11:1 to 11:12 he is in Jerusalem with the two witnesses. From 11:13 to the end he is in heaven observing and recording things in heaven and upon the earth.

[2] **(1:20)** The natural explanation of the "messengers" is that they were men sent by the seven churches to ascertain the state of the aged apostle, now an exile in Patmos (cf. Phil. 4:18); but they figure any who bear God's messages to a church.

[3] **(1:20)** The messages to the seven churches have a fourfold application: (1) Local, to the churches actually addressed; (2) admonitory, to all churches in all time as tests by which they may discern their true spiritual state in the sight of God; (3) personal, in the exhortations to him "that hath an ear," and in the promises "to him that overcometh"; (4) prophetic, as disclosing seven phases of the *spiritual* history of the church from, say, A.D. 96 to the end. It is incredible that in a prophecy covering the church period there should be no such foreview. These messages must contain that foreview if it is in the book at all, for the church does not appear after 3:22. Again, these messages by their very terms go beyond the local assemblies mentioned. Most conclusively of all, these messages do present an exact foreview

CHAPTER 2.

Part II. "The things which are": the seven churches.

(1) *The message to Ephesus. The church at the end of the apostolic age; first love left.*

Unto the [a]angel of the church [b]of Ephesus write; These things saith he [c]that holdeth the seven stars in his right hand, who walketh in the midst of the seven golden [d]candlesticks;

2 I know thy works, and thy labour, and thy patience, and how thou canst not bear them which are evil: and thou hast [e]tried them which say they are apostles, and are not, and hast found them liars:

3 And hast borne, and hast patience, and for my name's sake hast laboured, and hast not [f]fainted.

4 Nevertheless I have *somewhat* against thee, [g]because thou hast left thy first love.

5 Remember therefore from whence thou art fallen, and [h]repent, and do the first works; or else I will come unto thee quickly, and will remove thy [i]candlestick out of his place, except thou repent.

6 But this thou hast, that thou hatest the deeds of the [1][j]Nicolaitans, which I also [k]hate.

7 He that hath an ear, let him hear what the Spirit saith unto the churches; To him that overcometh will I give to eat of the tree [l]of life, which is [m]in the midst of the paradise of God.

(2) *The message to Smyrna. Period of the great persecutions, to A.D.* 316.

8 And unto the [n]angel of the church in Smyrna write; These things saith the [o]first and the last, which was [p]dead, and is [q]alive;

9 I know thy [r]works, and tribulation, and poverty, (but thou art rich) and *I know* the blasphemy of them which [s]say they are Jews, and are not, but *are* the [t]synagogue of Satan.

10 Fear none of those things which thou shalt suffer: behold, the devil shall cast *some* of you into prison, that ye may be tried; and ye shall have tribulation ten days: be thou [u]faithful unto death, and I will give thee [v]a [w]crown of life.

11 He that hath an ear, let him hear what the Spirit saith unto the churches; He that overcometh shall not be hurt of the [x]second death.

(3) *The message to Pergamos. The church under imperial favour, settled in the world, A.D.* 316 *to the end.*

12 And to the [n]angel of the church in Pergamos write; These things saith he which hath the sharp sword with two edges;

13 I know thy works, and where thou dwellest, *even* where [y]Satan's [z]seat *is*: and thou holdest fast my name, and hast not [aa]denied my faith, even in those days wherein Antipas *was* my faithful [bb]martyr, who was slain among you, where Satan dwelleth.

14 But I have a few things against thee, because thou hast there them that hold the doctrine of [2]Balaam, who taught Balac to cast a [cc]stumblingblock before the [dd]children of Israel, to eat things sacrificed unto idols, and to commit fornication.

15 So hast thou also them that hold the doctrine of the [ee]Nicolaitans, [ff]which thing I hate.

16 Repent; or else I will come unto

A.D. 96.

a *messenger.*
b *in.*
c Rev. 1:16, 20.
d *lampstands.*
e 1 John 4:1.
f Gal. 6:9.
g *that thou.*
h *Repentance.* vs. 5, 16, 21, 22; Rev. 3:3, 19. (Mt. 3:2; Acts 17:30.)
i *lampstand.*
j v. 15; *contra,* 1 Pet. 5:2, 3; cf. Mt. 24:49.
k Cf. Mt. 18:1-11; Mt. 20:25-28.
l *Life (eternal).* vs. 7, 10; Rev. 3:5. (Mt. 7:14; Rev. 22:19.)
m *in the paradise.*
n Heb. 1:4, *note.*
o Rev. 1:17, 18.
p 1 Thes. 4:14.
q 1 Cor. 15:20.
r *tribulation and poverty.*
s Rev. 3:9; cf. Gal. 6:12, 13; John 16:33.
t Cf. 2 Cor. 11:14, 15; Mt. 16:22, 23; Gal. 1:8.
u Cf. Col. 1:23; Mk. 13:13.
v *the.*
w *Rewards.* Rev. 3:11. (Dan. 12:3; 1 Cor. 3:14.)
x *Death (the second).* Rev. 20:6-14. (John 8:21; Rev. 21:8.)
y *Satan.* vs. 9, 10, 13, 24; Rev. 3:9. (Gen. 3:1; Rev. 20:10.)
z *throne.*
aa 2 Tim. 2:12.
bb *witness.*
cc *snare.*
dd *sons.*
ee v. 6.
ff *in like manner.*

of the spiritual history of the church, and in this precise order. Ephesus gives the general state at the date of the writing; Smyrna, the period of the great persecutions; Pergamos, the church settled down in the world, "where Satan's throne is," after the conversion of Constantine, say, A.D. 316. Thyatira is the Papacy, developed out of the Pergamos state: Balaamism (worldliness) and Nicolaitanism (priestly assumption) having conquered. As Jezebel brought idolatry into Israel, so Romanism weds Christian doctrine to pagan ceremonies. Sardis is the Protestant Reformation, whose works were not "fulfilled." Philadelphia is whatever bears clear testimony to the Word and the Name in the time of self-satisfied profession represented by Laodicea.

[1] **(2:6)** From *nikao,* "to conquer," and *laos,* "the people," or "laity." There is no ancient authority for a sect of the Nicolaitanes. If the word is symbolic it refers to the earliest form of the notion of a priestly order, or "clergy," which later divided an equal brotherhood (Mt. 23:8), into "priests" and "laity." What in Ephesus was "deeds" (2:6) had become in Pergamos a "doctrine" (Rev. 2:15).

[2] **(2:14)** The "doctrine" of Balaam (cf. 2 Pet. 2:15, *note;* Jude 11, *note*) was his teaching Balak to corrupt the people who could not be cursed (Num. 31:15, 16; 22:5; 23:8), by tempting them to marry women of

thee quickly, and will fight against them
with the sword of my mouth.
17 He that hath an [a]ear, let him hear
what the Spirit saith unto the churches;
To him that overcometh will I give to eat
of the [b]hidden manna, and will give him
[c]a white stone, and in the stone [d]a new
name written, which no man knoweth
saving he that [e]receiveth *it*.

(4) *The message to Thyatira.*
A.D. 500–1500: *the triumph of Balaamism and Nicolaitanism; a believing remnant* (vs. 24-28).

18 And unto the [f]angel of the church
in Thyatira write; [g]These things saith the
Son of God, who hath his eyes like unto
a flame of fire, and his feet *are* like fine
brass;
19 I know thy works, and [h]charity, and
service, and faith, and thy patience, and
thy [i]works; and the last *to be* more than
the first.
20 Notwithstanding I have [j]a few
things against thee, because thou sufferest
that woman [k]Jezebel, which calleth herself
a prophetess, to teach and to seduce my
servants to commit fornication, and to eat
things sacrificed unto idols.
21 And I gave her space to repent of
her fornication; and she repented not.
22 Behold, I will cast her into a bed,
and them that commit adultery with her
into great tribulation, except they repent
of [l]their deeds.
23 And I will kill her children with
death; and all the churches shall know
that I am he which [m]searcheth the reins
and hearts: and I will give unto every
one of you according to your works.
24 But unto you I say, [n]and unto the
rest in Thyatira, as many as have not this
doctrine, and which have not known the
[o]depths of Satan, as they speak; I will
put upon you none other burden.
25 But that which ye have *already* hold
fast [p]till I come.
26 And he that overcometh, and keepeth my works unto the end, to him will I
give [q]power over the nations:

A.D. 96.

- *a* v. 29.
- *b* Ex. 16:33, 34; John 6:49-51; Heb. 9:4; cf. Phil. 3:10.
- *c* Signifies approval.
- *d* John 1:42; cf. Rev. 3:12.
- *e* Rev. 14:3; cf. Song 6:3.
- *f* Heb. 1:4, *note.*
- *g* *Inspiration.* vs. 1, 8, 12, 18; Rev. 3:1, 7, 14. (Ex. 4:15; Rev. 22:19.)
- *h* *love.*
- *i* *last works to be.*
- *j* *against thee that.*
- *k* 1 Ki. 16:31, 32; cf. Prov. 6:24.
- *l* *her.*
- *m* Jer. 17:10.
- *n* *the rest.*
- *o* 2 Tim. 3:1-8; cf. 2 Tim. 2:17, 18.
- *p* *Christ (Second Advent).* Rev. 16:15. (Deut. 30:3; Acts 1:9-11.)
- *q* *authority.*
- *r* *are broken to shivers.*
- *s* *Day (of Jehovah).* vs. 26, 27; Rev. 6:12-17. (Isa. 2:10-22; Rev. 19:11-21.)
- *t* Rev. 22:16; 2 Pet. 1:19; cf. 1 Thes. 4:13-18.
- *u* *Holy Spirit.* vs. 7, 11, 17, 29; Rev. 3:1, 6, 13, 22. (Mt. 1:18; Acts 2:4.)
- *v* *Churches (local).* vs. 1, 7, 8, 11, 12-29; Rev. 3:1, 6, 7, 13, 22. (Acts 2:41; Phil. 1:1.)
- *w* Heb. 1:4, *note.*
- *x* Rev. 1:4, 16; cf. Acts 2:33.
- *y* Cf. Mt. 13:24-26.
- *z* See Mt. 5:48, *note.*
- *aa* Rev. 2:5; cf. 2 Tim. 1:13.
- *bb* Rev. 16:15; cf. Mt. 24:43; 1 Thes. 5:2-5.
- *cc* Mt. 7:14; 2 Tim. 4:9-11; cf. Jas. 1:27.
- *dd* Rev. 6:11.
- *ee* *Life (eternal).* Rev. 13:8. (Mt. 7:14; Rev. 22:19.)
- *ff* Lk. 12:8.
- *gg* Cf. Lk. 1:35; John 10:36.
- *hh* Rev. 19:11; John 14:6.
- *ii* Isa. 22:22.
- *jj* Cf. Rev. 2:9.

27 And he shall rule them with a rod
of iron; as the vessels of a potter [r]shall
they be broken to shivers: even as [s]I
received of my Father.
28 And I will give him the morning
[t]star.
29 He that hath an ear, let him hear
what the [u]Spirit saith unto the [v]churches.

CHAPTER 3.

(5) *The message to Sardis. The period of the Reformations; a believing remnant* (vs. 4, 5).

And unto the [w]angel of the church in
Sardis write; These things saith he
that [x]hath the seven Spirits of God, and
the seven stars; I know thy works, that
thou hast [y]a name that thou livest, and
art dead.
2 Be watchful, and strengthen the
things which remain, that are ready to
die: for I have not found thy works [z]per-
fect before God.
3 [aa]Remember therefore how thou hast
received and heard, and hold fast, and
repent. If therefore thou shalt not watch,
I will come on thee [bb]as a thief, and thou
shalt not know what hour I will come
upon thee.
4 Thou hast [cc]a few names even in
Sardis which have not defiled their garments; and [dd]they shall walk with me in
white: for they are worthy.
5 He that overcometh, the same shall
be clothed in white raiment; and I will
not blot out his name out of the book of
[ee]life, but I will [ff]confess his name before
my Father, and before his [w]angels.
6 He that hath an ear, let him hear
what the Spirit saith unto the churches.

(6) *The message to Philadelphia. The true church in the professing church.*

7 And to the [w]angel of the church in
Philadelphia write; These things saith he
that is [gg]holy, he that is [hh]true, he that
hath [ii]the key of David, he that openeth,
and no man shutteth; and shutteth, and
no man openeth;
8 I [jj]know thy works: behold, I have set
before thee an open door, and no man

Moab, defile their separation, and abandon their pilgrim character. It is that union of the world and the church which is spiritual unchastity (Jas. 4:4). Pergamos had lost the pilgrim character and was "dwelling" (v. 13) "where Satan's throne is," in the world (John 12:31; 14:30; 16:11).

can shut it: for thou hast a little strength, and hast kept my word, and hast not denied my name.

9 Behold, I will make them of the synagogue of [a]Satan, which say they are Jews, and are not, but do lie; behold, I will make them to come and [b]worship before thy feet, and to know that I have loved thee.

10 Because thou hast kept the word of my patience, I also will keep thee from the [c]hour of [d]temptation, which shall come upon all the [e]world, to try them that dwell upon the earth.

11 Behold, I come quickly: hold that fast which thou hast, that no man take thy [f]crown.

12 Him that [g]overcometh will I make a pillar in the temple of my God, and he shall [h]go no more out: and I will [i]write upon him the name of my God, and the name of the city of my God, *which is* new Jerusalem, which cometh down out of heaven from my God: and *I will write upon him* [j]my new name.

13 He that [k]hath an ear, let him hear what the Spirit saith unto the churches.

(7) *The message to Laodicea.*
The final state of apostasy.

14 And unto the angel of the church [l]of the Laodiceans [m]write; These things saith the [n]Amen, the faithful and true witness, the beginning of the creation of God;

15 I know thy works, that thou art neither cold nor hot: I would thou wert cold or hot.

16 So then because thou art lukewarm, and neither cold nor hot, [o]I will spue thee out of my mouth.

17 Because thou sayest, I am rich, and increased with goods, and have need of nothing; and [p]knowest not that thou art wretched, and miserable, and poor, and blind, and naked:

18 I counsel thee to buy of me gold tried in the fire, that thou mayest be rich; and white raiment, that thou mayest be clothed, and *that* the shame of thy nakedness do not appear; and [q]anoint thine eyes with eyesalve, that thou mayest see.

19 As many as I love, I rebuke and chasten: be zealous therefore, and [r]repent.

Place and attitude of Christ at the end of the church-age.

20 Behold, I stand at the door, and knock: if any man hear my voice, and open the door, I will come in to him, and will sup with him, and he with me.

21 To him that overcometh will I grant to sit with me in my [s]throne, even as I also overcame, and am set down with my [1]Father in his throne.

22 He that hath an ear, let him hear what the [t]Spirit saith unto the [u]churches.

CHAPTER 4.

Part III. "Things which shall be hereafter" (Rev. 4:1–22:21).

The seven seals (Rev. 4:1–8:1).

(a) Introduction (to Rev. 5:14).

The throne in heaven.

After this I looked, and, behold, a [v]door *was* opened in heaven: and the first voice which I heard *was* as it were of a [w]trumpet talking with me; which said, [2]Come up hither, and I will shew thee things which must be [x]hereafter.

2 And immediately I [y]was in the spirit: and, behold, a [z]throne was set in heaven, and *one* sat on the throne.

3 And he that sat was to look upon [aa]like a jasper and a sardine stone: and *there was* a [bb]rainbow round about the throne, in sight like unto an emerald.

The enthroned elders.

4 And round about the throne *were* four and twenty [cc]seats: and upon the seats I saw four and twenty elders sitting, clothed in [dd]white raiment; and they had on their heads [ee]crowns of gold.

5 And out of the throne proceeded lightnings and thunderings and voices: and *there were* seven lamps of fire burning

A.D. 96.

a *Satan.* Rev. 12:9, 14, 15. (Gen. 3:1; Rev. 20:10.)
b Isa. 49:23.
c *Tribulation (the great).* Rev. 7:13, 14. (Psa. 2:5; Rev. 7:14.)
d *Temptation.* Jas. 1:2, 12, 13, 14. (Gen. 3:1; Jas. 1:14.)
e *oikoumene Inhabited earth.* (Lk. 2:1.)
f *Rewards.* Rev. 11:18. (Dan. 12:3; 1 Cor. 3:14.)
g v. 5; cf. Gal. 2:9; 1 Ki. 7:21.
h Psa. 23:6; *contra,* Heb. 13:14.
i Rev. 22:4; cf. Ex. 28:36.
j Rev. 2:17; 19:12.
k vs. 22.
l *in Laodicea.*
m *Inspiration.* vs. 1, 7, 14; Rev. 14:13. (Ex. 4:15; Rev. 22:19.)
n 2 Cor. 1:20.
o *Apostasy.* 2 Tim. 3:1-8.
p Cf. Hos. 9:7; John 9:39-41.
q *eyesalve to anoint thine eyes.*
r *Repentance.* vs. 3, 19; Rev. 9:20, 21. (Mt. 3:2; Acts 17:30.)
s *Kingdom* (N.T.). Rev. 5:1-10. (Lk. 1:31-33; 1 Cor. 15:24.)
t *Holy Spirit.* vs. 1, 6, 13, 22; Rev. 4:2, 5. (Mt. 1:18; Acts 2:4.)
u *Churches (local).* Rev. 22:16. (Acts 2:41; Phil. 1:1.)
v Lk. 23:45; cf. Heb. 10:19, 20.
w Rev. 1:10.
x *after these.*
y *became.*
z Rev. 3:21; cf. Rev. 22:3.
aa Rev. 21:11; cf. Ezk. 1:26, 27.
bb Ezk. 1:28; cf. Gen. 9:13-17.
cc *thrones.*
dd Rev. 3:4, 5; cf. Rev. 19:8,14.
ee Rev. 2:10; cf. 2 Tim. 4:8.

[1] **(3:21)** This passage, in harmony with Lk. 1:32, 33; Mt. 19:28; Acts 2:30, 34, 35; 15:14-16, is conclusive that Christ is not now seated upon His own throne. The Davidic Covenant, and the promises of God through the prophets and the Angel Gabriel concerning the Messianic kingdom await fulfilment.

[2] **(4:1)** This call seems clearly to indicate the fulfilment of 1 Thes. 4:14-17. The word "church" does not again occur in the Revelation till all is fulfilled.

before the throne, which are the seven [a]Spirits of God.

The four living creatures.

6 And before the throne *there was* [b]a sea of glass like unto crystal: and in the midst of the throne, and round about the throne, *were* four [c]beasts full of eyes before and behind.

7 And the first [c]beast *was* like a lion, and the second beast like a calf, and the third beast had a face as a man, and the fourth beast *was* like a flying eagle.

8 And the four [c]beasts had each of them six wings about *him;* and *they were* full of eyes [d]within: and they rest not day and night, saying, Holy, holy, holy, Lord God Almighty, which was, and is, and is to come.

The living creatures and elders worship because of creation. (Cf. Rev. 5:8-10.)

9 And when those [c]beasts give glory and honour and thanks to him that [f]sat on the throne, who liveth for ever and ever,

10 The four and twenty [g]elders fall down before him that sat on the throne, and worship him that liveth for ever and ever, and cast their crowns before the throne, saying,

11 Thou art worthy, [h]O Lord, to receive glory and honour and power: for thou hast [i]created all things, and for [j]thy pleasure they are and were created.

CHAPTER 5.

The seven-sealed book.

And I saw [k]in the right hand of him that sat on the throne a [l]book written within and on the backside, sealed with seven seals.

2 And I saw a strong [m]angel proclaiming with a loud voice, [n]Who is worthy to open the book, and to loose the seals thereof?

3 And [o]no man in heaven, nor in earth, neither under the earth, was able to open the book, neither to look thereon.

4 And I wept much, because no man was found worthy to open and to read the book, neither to look thereon.

Christ in his kingly character (Isa. 11:1; Jer. 23:5; Lk. 1:32, 33) *opens the book.*

5 And one of the elders saith unto me, Weep not: behold, the Lion of the tribe of Juda, the [p]Root of David, hath [q]prevailed to open the book, and to loose the seven seals thereof.

6 And I beheld, and, lo, in the midst of the throne and of the four [c]beasts, and in the midst of the elders, stood a [r]Lamb as it had been slain, having seven horns and seven [s]eyes, which are the seven Spirits of God sent forth into all the earth.

7 And he [1]came and took the book out of the right hand of him that sat upon the throne.

The living creatures and elders worship because of redemption. (Cf. Rev. 4:9-11.)

8 And when he had taken the book, the four [c]beasts and four *and* twenty elders [t]fell down before the Lamb, having every one of them harps, and golden vials full of [u]odours, which are the prayers of saints.

9 And they sung [v]a new song, saying, Thou art worthy to take the book, and to open the seals thereof: for thou wast slain, and hast [w]redeemed us to God [x]by thy blood out of every kindred, and tongue, and people, and nation;

10 And hast made us unto our [y]God kings and priests: and we shall [z]reign [aa]on the earth.

The angels exalt the Lamb.

11 And I beheld, and I heard the voice of many angels round about the throne and the [bb]beasts and the elders: and the number of them was ten thousand times ten thousand, and thousands of thousands;

12 Saying with a loud voice, [cc]Worthy is the Lamb that was slain to receive power, and riches, and wisdom, and strength, and honour, and glory, and blessing.

Universal adoration of the Lamb who is King.

13 And every creature which is in heaven, and on the earth, and under the earth, and such as are [dd]in the sea, and all that are in them, heard I saying, Blessing, and honour, and glory, and power, *be* unto him that [ee]sitteth upon the throne,

A.D. 96.

a *Holy Spirit.* vs. 2, 5; Rev. 11:11. (Mt. 1:18; Acts 2:4.)
b Rev. 15:2.
c *living creatures.* See Ezk. 1:5, *note.*
d *around and within.*
e *Jehovah of hosts.* Isa. 6:3.
f *sitteth.*
g *Elders.* vs. 4, 5, 9-11; Rev. 5:5, 6, 8, 11, 14. (Acts 11:30; Tit. 1:5-9.)
h *O, our Lord and God.*
i Gen. 1:1; cf. John 1:3.
j Cf. Col. 1:16; cf. Psa. 19:1.
k *on.*
l Ezk. 2:9, 10; cf. Dan. 12:4.
m Heb. 1:4, *note.*
n Psa. 15:1, with Rom. 3:10-12.
o Cf. Isa. 63:5.
p Isa. 11:1, 10; Rev. 22:16; Mt. 1:1.
q Rev. 3:21; Isa. 53:12; 63:1-3.
r John 1:29.
s Cf. Zech. 3:8, 9; 4:10.
t Rev. 4:8, 10; 19:4.
u *incense.* Psa. 141:2.
v Rev. 4:11; 14:3; cf. Psa. 33:3.
w Rom. 3:24, *note.*
x Heb. 9:12; 1 Pet. 1:18, 19.
y *Jehovah.* Isa. 61:6.
z *Kingdom* (N.T.) vs. 1-10; Rev. 19:11-21. (Lk. 1:31-33; 1 Cor. 15:24.)
aa *over.*
bb *living creatures.* See Ezk. 1:5, *note.*
cc v. 9; cf. Phil. 2:9-11.
dd *upon.*
ee Rev. 4:2, 3; 6:16.

1(5:7) Cf. Dan. 7:13, 14. The two visions are identical; the Revelation adding that which was hidden

and unto the [a]Lamb for ever and ever.
14 And the four [b]beasts said, Amen.
And the four *and* twenty [c]elders fell
down and worshipped him that liveth
for ever and ever.

CHAPTER 6.

(b) The seals (to Rev. 8:1).

(1) *The first seal.*

And I saw when the Lamb opened
[d]one of the seals, and I heard, as it
were the noise of thunder, one of the
four [b]beasts saying, [e]Come and see.
2 And I saw, and behold [f]a white horse:
and he that sat on him had a [g]bow; and a
crown was given unto him: and he went
forth [h]conquering, and to conquer.

(2) *The second seal: peace taken from earth.*

3 And when he had opened the second seal, I heard the second [b]beast say,
[i]Come and see.
4 And there went out another horse
that was [j]red: and *power* was given to
him that sat thereon to [k]take peace from
the earth, and that they should kill one
another: and there was given unto him a
great sword.

(3) *The third seal: famine.*

5 And when he had opened the third
seal, I heard the third [b]beast say, [l]Come
and see. And I beheld, and lo a [m]black
horse; and he that sat on him had a pair
of [n]balances in his hand.
6 And I heard a voice in the midst of
the four [b]beasts say, A [o]measure of
wheat for a [p]penny, and three measures
of barley for a penny; and *see* thou hurt
not the oil and the wine.

(4) *The fourth seal: death.*

7 And when he had opened the fourth
seal, I heard the voice of the fourth
[b]beast say, [q]Come and see.
8 And I looked, and behold a pale
horse: and his name that sat on him was
[r]Death, and [s]Hell followed with him.
And power was given unto [t]them over
the [u]fourth part of the earth, to kill with
sword, and with hunger, and with death,
and with the beasts of the earth.

(5) *The fifth seal: the martyred remnant.*

9 And when he had opened the fifth
seal, I saw under the altar the souls of
them that were [v]slain for the word of
God, and for the testimony which they
held:
10 And they cried with a loud voice,
saying, [w]How long, O Lord, holy and
true, dost thou not judge and avenge our
blood on them that dwell on the earth?
11 And white robes were given unto
[x]every one of them; and it was said unto
them, that they should rest yet for a little
season, until their fellowservants also
and their brethren, that should be killed
as they *were*, should be [y]fulfilled.

(6) *The sixth seal: anarchy.*

12 And I beheld when he had opened
the sixth seal, and, lo, there was a great
[z]earthquake; and the sun became [aa]black
as sackcloth of hair, and the moon
became as blood;
13 And the stars of heaven fell unto
the earth, even as a fig tree casteth her
untimely figs, when she is shaken of a
mighty wind.
14 And the [bb]heaven departed as a
scroll when it is rolled together; and
every [cc]mountain and island were
moved out of their places.
15 And the [dd]kings of the earth, and
the great men, and the rich men, and the
chief captains, and the mighty men, and
every bondman, and every free man,
[ee]hid themselves in the dens and in the
rocks of the mountains;
16 And said to the mountains and
rocks, Fall on us, and hide us from the
face of him that [ff]sitteth on the throne,
and from the [gg]wrath of the Lamb:
17 [hh]For the great [ii]day of his wrath is
come; and who shall be able to stand?

CHAPTER 7.

(c) (Parenthetical: the saved of the tribulation period.)

And after these things I saw four
[jj]angels standing on the four corners of the earth, holding the four
[kk]winds of the earth, that the wind
should not blow on the earth, nor on the
sea, nor on any tree.
2 And I saw another [jj]angel ascending
from the east, having the [ll]seal of the living God: and he cried with a loud voice

A.D. 96.

a Cf. John 5:23.
b *living creatures.* See Ezk. 1:5, *note.*
c *Elders.* Rev. 7:11, 13. (Acts 11:30; Tit. 1:5-9.)
d vs. 3, 5.
e *Come!* Omit "and see." So vs. 3, 5, 7.
f Zech. 6:3; cf. Christ in 19:11, whom the Beast imitates.
g Isa. 66:19.
h Dan. 7:7, 8.
i *Come.*
j Zech. 6:2; cf. Nah. 2:3; cf. 2 Ki. 3:22, 23.
k Jud. 7:22; cf. 2 Chr. 20:23.
l *Come.*
m Zech. 6:2; cf. Isa. 60:3.
n Ezk. 4:9, 10, 16, 17.
o One measure = nearly 1 qt.
p Or, *shilling;* lit. *a denarius.*
q *Come.*
r Cf. Acts 3:15; cf. Rom. 6:23.
s *hades;* Lk. 16:23, *note.*
t *him.*
u Cf. Ezk. 14:21.
v *Death (physical).* Heb. 9:27. (Gen. 3:19; Heb. 9:27.)
w Psa. 13:1.
x *Remnant.* vs. 9-11; Rev. 7:4-8. (Isa. 1:9; Rom. 11:5.)
y i.e. *their number filled up.*
z Mt. 24:7.
aa Cf. Joel 2:10, 31.
bb Isa. 34:4.
cc Jer. 3:23; Rev. 16:20.
dd Psa. 2:2; cf. Dan. 2:21.
ee Isa. 2:19.
ff Rev. 20:11.
gg Rev. 5:6, 9, 12.
hh Cf. Isa. 13:6; Mt. 24:8.
ii *Day (of Jehovah).* vs. 15-17; Rev. 16:12-17. (Isa. 2:10-22; Rev. 19:11-21.)
jj Heb. 1:4, *note.*
kk Cf. Dan. 7:2; cf. Eph. 2:2.
ll *Contra,* Eph. 1:13.

from Daniel, that the kings and priests of the church-age are to be associated with the "Son of Man," the "Lamb as it had been slain," in His reign "on the earth" (vs. 9, 10).

to the four angels, to whom it was given
to hurt the earth and the sea,
3 Saying, [a]Hurt not the earth, neither
the sea, nor the trees, till we have sealed
the servants of our God in their foreheads.

(1) *The remnant out of Israel sealed.*

4 And I heard the number of them
which were sealed: [b]*and there were* sealed
an hundred *and* forty *and* four thousand
[c]of all the tribes of the children of Israel.
5 Of the tribe of Juda *were* sealed
twelve thousand. Of the tribe of Reuben
were sealed twelve thousand. Of the tribe
of Gad *were* sealed twelve thousand.
6 Of the tribe of Aser *were* sealed
twelve thousand. Of the tribe of
Nepthalim *were* sealed twelve thousand.
Of the tribe of Manasses *were* sealed
twelve thousand.
7 Of the tribe of Simeon *were* sealed
twelve thousand. Of the tribe of Levi
were sealed twelve thousand. Of the tribe
of Issachar *were* sealed twelve thousand.
8 Of the tribe of Zabulon *were* sealed
twelve thousand. Of the tribe of Joseph
were sealed twelve thousand. Of the tribe
of Benjamin *were* sealed twelve thousand.

(2) *Vision of the Gentiles who are to be saved during the great tribulation.*

9 After this I beheld, and, lo, [d]a great
multitude, which no man could number,
of all nations, and kindreds, and people,
and tongues, stood before the throne,
and before the Lamb, clothed with white
robes, and palms in their hands;
10 And cried with a loud voice, saying, [e]Salvation to our God which sitteth
upon the throne, and unto the Lamb.
11 And all the [f]angels stood round
about the throne, and *about* the elders
and the four [g]beasts, and fell before the
throne on their faces, and worshipped
God,
12 Saying, Amen: Blessing, and glory,
and wisdom, and thanksgiving, and
honour, and power, and might, *be* unto
our God for ever and ever. Amen.
13 And one of the [h]elders answered,
saying unto me, [i]What are these which
are arrayed in white robes? and whence
came they?
14 And I said unto him, [j]Sir, thou
knowest. And he said to me, [k]These are
they which came [l]out of [m]great [1]tribula-
tion, and have washed their robes, and
made them [n]white in the blood of the
Lamb.
15 Therefore are they [o]before the
throne of God, and serve him day and
night in his temple: and he that sitteth
on the throne shall dwell among them.
16 They shall hunger no more, neither
thirst any more; neither shall the sun
[p]light on them, nor any [q]heat.
17 For the [r]Lamb which is in the midst
of the throne shall feed them, and shall
lead them unto [s]living fountains of

A.D. 96.

a Cf. 2 Thes. 2:7.
b *Israel (prophecies).* Rev. 21:12. (Gen. 12:2, 3; Rom. 11:26.)
c Gen. 49:1-27; cf. Deut. 33:6-25; cf. Ezk. 48:1-7, 23-28.
d Cf. Rom. 11:25; cf. Isa. 60:5.
e Rom. 1:16, *note.*
f Heb. 1:4, *note.*
g *living creatures.*
h *Elders.* vs. 11, 13, 14; Rev. 11:16. (Acts 11:30; Tit. 1:5-9.)
i *who.*
j *My Lord.*
k *Remnant.* vs. 4-8, 12, 17; Rev. 12:17. (Isa. 1:9; Rom. 11:5.)
l Lit. *out of the great tribulation.*
m *Tribulation (the great).* vs. 13, 14. (Psa. 2:5.)
n 1 John 1:7; cf. Zech. 3:3-5.
o v. 9.
p *strike upon.*
q *burning heat.*
r *Shepherd.* Ezk. 34:23.
s *fountains of waters of life.*

[1] **(7:14)** The great tribulation is the period of unexampled trouble predicted in the passages cited under that head from Psa. 2:5 to Rev. 7:14 and described in Rev. 11–18. Involving in a measure the whole earth (Rev. 3:10), it is yet distinctively "the time of Jacob's trouble" (Jer. 30:7), and its vortex Jerusalem and the Holy Land. It involves the people of God who will have returned to Palestine in unbelief. Its duration is three and a half years, or the last half of the seventieth week of Daniel (Dan. 9:24-27, *note;* Rev. 11:2, 3) The *elements* of the tribulation are: (1) The cruel reign of the "beast out of the sea" (Rev. 13:1), who, at the beginning of the three and a half years, will break his covenant with the Jews (by virtue of which they will have re-established the temple worship, Dan. 9:27), and show himself in the temple, demanding that he be worshipped as God (Mt. 24:15; 2 Thes. 2:4). (2) The active interposition of Satan "having great wrath" (Rev. 12:12), who gives his power to the Beast (Rev. 13:4, 5). (3) The unprecedented activity of demons (Rev. 9:2, 11); and (4) the terrible "bowl" judgments of Rev. 16.

The great tribulation will be, however, a period of salvation. An election out of Israel is seen as sealed for God (Rev. 7:4-8), and, with an innumerable multitude of Gentiles (Rev. 7:9), are said to have come "out of the great tribulation" (Rev. 7:14). They are not of the priesthood, the church, to which they seem to stand somewhat in the relation of the Levites to the priests under the Mosaic Covenant. The great tribulation is immediately followed by the return of Christ in glory, and the events associated therewith (Mt. 24:29, 30). See "Remnant" (Isa. 1:9; Rom. 11:5, *note*); "Beast" (Dan. 7:8; Rev. 19, 20, *note*); "Armageddon" (Rev. 16:14; 19:17, *note*).

waters: and [a]God shall wipe away all
tears from their eyes.

CHAPTER 8.

The seals resumed: the seventh seal, out of which the trumpets come.

And when he had opened the seventh
seal, there was silence in heaven
about the space of half an hour.

The seven trumpets (Rev. 8:2–11:19).

(a) Introduction: Christ as High Priest.

2 And I saw the seven [b]angels which
stood before God; and to them were
given seven [c]trumpets.
3 And another [b]angel came and stood
at the altar, having a golden censer; and
there was given unto him much incense,
that he should [d]offer *it* with the prayers
of all saints upon the golden altar which
was before the throne.
4 And the [e]smoke of the incense, *which*
came with the prayers of the saints,
ascended up before God out of the [b]an-
gel's hand.
5 And the [b]angel took the censer, and
[f]filled it with fire of the altar, and cast *it*
[g]into the earth: [h]and there were voices,
and thunderings, and lightnings, and an
earthquake.
6 And the seven [b]angels which had
the seven trumpets prepared themselves
to sound.

(b) The trumpet judgments.

(1) *The first trumpet.*

7 The first [b]angel sounded, and there
followed [i]hail and fire mingled with
blood, and they were cast upon the earth:
and [j]the third part of trees was burnt up,
and all green grass was burnt up.

(2) *The second trumpet.*

8 And the second [b]angel sounded, and
as it were [k]a great mountain burning
with fire was cast into the sea: and the
third part of the sea became [l]blood;
9 And the third part of the [m]creatures
which were in the sea, and had life, died;
and the third part of the ships were
destroyed.

(3) *The third trumpet.*

10 And the third [b]angel sounded, and
there fell a great [n]star from heaven,
burning [o]as it were a lamp, and it fell
upon the third part of the rivers, and
upon the [p]fountains of waters;

A.D. 96.

a *Adonai Jehovah.* Isa. 25:8.
b Heb. 1:4, *note.*
c These are trumpets of angels; contrast *"the trump of God"* (1 Thes. 4:16; 1 Cor. 15:52). Cf. Joel 2:1; Amos 3:6.
d Cf. Heb. 7:25; cf. John 14:13.
e Ex. 30:7; cf. Psa. 141:2.
f Cf. Lev. 16:12; cf. Num. 16:46.
g *upon.*
h Rev. 4:5; Psa. 97:3, 4; cf. Ex. 19:18, 19.
i Ex. 9:23, 24; Psa. 18:13; cf. Ezk. 38:22; cf. Job 38:22, 23.
j vs. 8, 10.
k Cf. Jer. 51:25; *contra,* Isa. 2:2.
l Ex. 7:19, 20; Rev. 11:6.
m Cf. 2 Chr. 20:23; Rev. 6:4.
n Cf. Rev. 9:1; cf. Isa. 14:12; *contra,* Dan. 12:3.
o *as a torch.*
p Cf. Rev. 16:4; cf. 2 Cor. 2:17.
q Cf. Deut. 29:18; cf. Jer. 23:15.
r Cf. Joel 2:31; Isa. 13:10; cf. Ex. 10:21-23; John 12:35.
s *in mid-heaven.*
t Rev. 9:12.
u *about.*
v Isa. 14:12-19; Heb. 2:14.
w *fallen.*
x *pit of the abyss.*
y *Contra,* Rev. 21:24; cf. Joel 2:10.
z Ex. 10:12-15.
aa Cf. Num. 21:6.
bb Rev. 7:2, 3; *contra.* Rev. 13:16, 17.
cc Cf. Deut. 28:67.
dd Cf. Jer. 8:3.
ee *likenesses.*
ff Cf. Nah. 3:17; cf. Rev. 16:12.
gg Cf. Rev. 13:18.

11 And the name of the star is called
Wormwood: and the third part of the
waters became [q]wormwood; and many
men died of the waters, because they
were made bitter.

(4) *The fourth trumpet.*

12 And the fourth [b]angel sounded,
and the third part [r]of the sun was smitten, and the third part of the moon, and
the third part of the stars; so as the third
part of them was darkened, and the day
shone not for a third part of it, and the
night likewise.
13 And I beheld, and heard an [b]angel
flying [s]through the midst of heaven, saying with a loud voice, [t]Woe, woe, woe,
to the inhabiters of the earth by reason
of the other voices of the trumpet of the
three angels, which are [u]yet to sound!

CHAPTER 9.

(5) *The fifth trumpet: the first woe.*

And the fifth [b]angel sounded, and I
saw a [v]star [w]fall from heaven unto
the earth: and to him was given the key
of the [x]bottomless pit.
2 And he opened the [x]bottomless pit;
and there arose a [y]smoke out of the pit,
as the smoke of a great furnace; and the
sun and the air were darkened by reason
of the smoke of the pit.
3 And there came out of the smoke
[z]locusts upon the earth: and unto them
was given power, as the [aa]scorpions of
the earth have power.
4 And it was commanded them that
they should not hurt the grass of the
earth, neither any green thing, neither any
tree; but only those men [bb]which have not
the seal of God in their foreheads.
5 And to them it was given that they
should not kill them, but that they
should be [cc]tormented five months: and
their torment *was* as the torment of a
scorpion, when he striketh a man.
6 And in those days shall men [dd]seek
death, and shall not find it; and shall
desire to die, and death shall flee from
them.
7 And the [ee]shapes of the locusts *were*
like unto horses prepared unto battle;
and on their heads *were* as it were
[ff]crowns like gold, and their [gg]faces *were*
as the faces of men.
8 And they had hair as the hair of

women, and their [a]teeth were as *the teeth* of lions.

9 And they had [b]breastplates, as it were breastplates of iron; and the sound of their wings *was* as the sound of [c]chariots of many horses running to battle.

10 And they had tails like unto scorpions, and [d]there were stings in their tails: and their power *was* to hurt men five months.

11 And they had [e]a king over them, *which is* the [f]angel of the [g]bottomless pit, whose name in the Hebrew tongue *is* [h]Abaddon, but in the Greek tongue hath *his* name [h]Apollyon.

12 One woe is past; *and*, behold, there come two woes more [i]hereafter.

(6) *The sixth trumpet.*

13 And the sixth [f]angel sounded, and I heard a voice from the four horns of the [j]golden altar which is before God,

14 Saying to the sixth [f]angel which had the trumpet, Loose the four angels which are bound in the great river Euphrates.

15 And the four [f]angels were loosed, which were [k]prepared for [l]an hour, and a day, and a month, and a year, for to slay the [m]third part of men.

16 And the number of the army of the horsemen *were* two hundred [n]thousand thousand: and I heard the number of them.

17 And thus I saw the horses in the vision, and them that sat on them, having [o]breastplates of fire, and of jacinth, and brimstone: and the heads of the horses *were* as the [p]heads of lions; and out of their mouths [q]issued fire and smoke and brimstone.

18 By these [r]three was the third part of men killed, by the fire, and by the smoke, and by the brimstone, which issued out of their mouths.

19 For [s]their power is in their mouth, and in their [t]tails: for their tails *were* like unto serpents, and had heads, and with them they do hurt.

20 And the rest of the men which were not killed by these plagues yet repented not of the works of their hands, that they should not [u]worship [v]devils, and idols of gold, and silver, and brass, and stone, and of wood: which neither can [w]see, nor hear, nor walk:

A.D. 96.

a Joel 1:6.
b v. 17; *contra*, Eph. 6:14.
c Joel 2:5.
d *stings; and their authority was in their tails to hurt.*
e Cf. Eph. 2:2; cf. John 14:30.
f Heb. 1:4, *note.*
g *abyss.*
h i.e. *Destroyer.* Cf. Job 26:6; cf. 1 Pet. 5:8.
i *after these things.*
j Cf. Rev. 8:3.
k Cf. Jon. 1:17.
l *the hour and day and month and year.*
m Cf. Rev. 8:7-9.
n Jud. 7:12.
o v. 9.
p Cf. Isa. 5:29, 30.
q Cf. Acts 9:1: cf. Psa. 27:2, 12.
r *three plagues.*
s *the power of the horses.*
t Cf. Isa. 9:15; Mic. 3:5.
u 1 Cor. 10:20: Deut. 32:17.
v *demons.*
w Psa. 115:4-7.
x Repentance. vs. 20, 21; Rev. 16:9, 11. (Mt. 3:2; Acts 17:30.)
y Cf. Rev. 21:8.
z Cf. Rev. 18:9.
aa Rev. 8:3.
bb *coming.*
cc Cf. Rev. 1:7; cf. Acts 1:9.
dd Rev. 4:3; Ezk. 1:28.
ee Cf. Rev. 1:16.
ff *Contra*, Rev. 5:1; cf. Psa. 40:7; cf. 2 Pet. 1:19-21.
gg Psa. 95:5; cf. Hag. 2:6.
hh Psa. 29:3-9.
ii Cf. Dan. 8:26; 12:4, 9.
jj Rev. 4:11; Gen. 1:1.
kk *delay.*
ll *is about to sound.*
mm Mt. 13:11, *note.*
nn *also shall be completed.*
oo *by.*
pp Cf. Rev. 4:1.
qq Cf. Ezk. 2:8, 9; 3:1-3.
rr Cf. Jer. 15:10; 20:14-18.
ss Cf. Psa. 19:10; 119:103.
tt *it was said.*

21 Neither [x]repented they of their murders, nor of their [y]sorceries, nor of their [z]fornication, nor of their thefts.

CHAPTER 10.

(c) *Parenthetical* (to Rev. 11:14).

(1) *The mighty angel and the "little book."*

AND I saw another mighty [aa]angel [bb]come down from heaven, [cc]clothed with a cloud: and a [dd]rainbow *was* upon his head, and his [ee]face *was* as it were the sun, and his feet as pillars of fire:

2 And he had in his hand [ff]a little book open: and he set his [gg]right foot upon the sea, and *his* left *foot* on the earth,

3 And cried with a loud voice, as *when* a lion roareth: and when he had cried, seven [hh]thunders uttered their voices.

4 And when the seven thunders had uttered their voices, I was about to write: and I heard a voice from heaven saying unto me, [ii]Seal up those things which the seven thunders uttered, and write them not.

5 And the [ff]angel which I saw stand upon the sea and upon the earth lifted up his hand to heaven,

6 And sware by him that liveth for ever and ever, who [jj]created heaven, and the things that therein are, and the earth, and the things that therein are, and the sea, and the things which are therein, that there should be [kk]time no longer:

7 But in the days of the voice of the seventh [ff]angel, when he [ll]shall begin to sound, the [mm]mystery of God [nn]should be finished, as he hath declared [oo]to his servants the prophets.

(2) *The "little book" eaten.*

8 And the [pp]voice which I heard from heaven spake unto me again, and said, Go *and* take the little book which is open in the hand of the [ff]angel which standeth upon the sea and upon the earth.

9 And I went unto the [ff]angel, and said unto him, Give me the little book. And he said unto me, [qq]Take *it*, and eat it up; and it shall make thy belly [rr]bitter, but it shall be in thy mouth [ss]sweet as honey.

10 And I took the little book out of the [ff]angel's hand, and ate it up; and it was in my mouth sweet as honey: and as soon as I had eaten it, my belly was bitter.

11 And [tt]he said unto me, Thou must

[a]prophesy again [b]before many peoples, and nations, and tongues, and [c]kings.

CHAPTER 11.

(3) *The "times of the the Gentiles" to end in forty-two months.*

And there was given me a [d]reed like unto a rod: and [e]the angel stood, saying, Rise, and measure the temple of God, and the altar, and them that worship therein.

2 But the [f]court which is without the temple leave out, and measure it not; for it is given unto the Gentiles: and the holy city shall they [g]tread under foot forty *and* two months.

(4) *The two witnesses to prophesy forty-two months.*

3 And I will give *power* unto my two [h]witnesses, and they shall prophesy a thousand two hundred *and* threescore days, clothed in sackcloth.

4 [i]These are the two olive trees, and the two [j]candlesticks standing before the [k]God of the earth.

5 And if any man will hurt them, [l]fire proceedeth out of their mouth, and devoureth their enemies: and if any man will hurt them, he must in this manner be killed.

6 These have power to [m]shut heaven, that it rain not in the days of their prophecy: and have power over waters [n]to turn them to blood, and to [o]smite the earth with all plagues, as often as they will.

7 And when they shall have finished their testimony, the [p]beast that ascendeth out of the [q]bottomless pit shall make [r]war against them, and shall overcome them, and kill them.

8 And their dead bodies *shall lie* in the street of the great [s]city, which spiritually is called Sodom and Egypt, where also [t]our Lord was crucified.

9 And they of the people and kindreds and tongues and nations shall [u]see their dead bodies three days and an half, and shall not suffer their dead bodies to be put in graves.

10 And they that dwell upon the earth shall [v]rejoice over them, and make merry, and shall send gifts one to another; because these two prophets tormented them that dwelt on the earth.

11 And after three days and an half the [w]Spirit of life from God entered into them, and they stood upon their feet; and great [x]fear fell upon them which saw them.

12 And they heard a great voice from heaven saying unto them, [y]Come up hither. And they ascended up to heaven in a cloud; and their enemies [z]beheld them.

The second woe.

13 And the same hour was there a great earthquake, and the tenth part of the city fell, and in the earthquake were slain of men seven thousand: and the remnant were affrighted, and gave glory to the [aa]God of heaven.

14 The second woe is past; *and,* behold, the third woe cometh quickly.

End of the second parenthetical passage.
The trumpet judgments resumed.

(7) *The seventh trumpet.*

15 And the seventh [bb]angel sounded; and there were great voices in heaven, saying, [cc]The kingdoms of this [dd]world are become *the kingdoms* of our Lord, and of his Christ; and he shall reign for ever and ever.

16 And the four and twenty [ee]elders, which sat before God on their [ff]seats, fell upon their faces, and worshipped God,

17 Saying, We give thee thanks, O Lord God Almighty, which art, and wast, and art to come; [gg]because thou hast taken to thee thy great power, and hast reigned.

18 And the nations were angry, and thy wrath is come, and the time of the [hh]dead, that they should be judged, and that thou shouldest give [ii]reward unto thy servants the prophets, and to the saints, and them that fear thy name, small and great; and shouldest destroy them which destroy the earth.

19 [jj]And the temple of God was opened in heaven, and there was seen in his temple the ark of his [kk]testament: and there were lightnings, and voices, and thunderings, and an earthquake, and great hail.

CHAPTER 12.

The seven personages.

(1) *The woman: Israel.*

The woman clothed with the sun, and the man-child.

And there appeared a great [ll]wonder in heaven; a woman clothed with the sun, and the moon under her feet,

A.D. 96.

a Cf. Jer. 25:15-26.
b *of peoples.*
c *many kings.*
d A reed = about 10 ft.
e *it was said, Rise.*
f Cf. Ezk. 8:5-9; 40:17.
g *See Times of the Gentiles.* Lk. 21:24; Rev. 16:14.
h Cf. Isa. 43:10, 12.
i Zech. 4:2, 3.
j *lampstands.*
k *Adonai.* Zech. 4:14.
l Cf. 2 Ki. 1:10, 12; Jer. 5:14; *contra,* Lk. 9:54, 55.
m Cf. 1 Ki. 17:1; cf. Jas. 5:17.
n Cf. Ex. 7:19.
o Cf. Ex. 7-10.
p Cf. Rev. 13:1; 17:8.
q *abyss.*
r Cf. Dan. 7:21.
s i.e. *Jerusalem.*
t *their.*
u *Contra,* Isa. 66:24.
v Cf. Psa. 79:2-4; cf. John 16:20; cf. 1 Ki. 21:16.
w *Holy Spirit.* Rev. 14:13. (Mt. 1:18; Acts 2:4.)
x Cf. Acts 5:11.
y Cf. Rev. 20:4-6.
z *Contra,* v. 9.
aa Dan. 2:18.
bb Heb. 1:4, *note.*
cc *The world-kingdom of our Lord and of his Christ has come.*
dd *kosmos* = world-system. Rev. 13:3-8, *note.* (John 7:7; Rev. 13:3-8, *note.*)
ee *Elders.* Rev. 14:3. (Acts 11:30; Tit. 1:5-9.)
ff *thrones.*
gg *that thou hast taken.*
hh Rev. 20:12.
ii *Rewards.* Rev. 22:12. (Dan. 12:3; 1 Cor. 3:14.)
jj v. 19 properly belongs with Chapter 12.
kk *covenant.* Heb. 9:4; Ezk. 37:1, etc.
ll *sign.*

and upon her head a [a]crown of twelve
stars:
2 And she being with child cried,
[b]travailing in birth, and pained to be
delivered.

(2) *Satan.*

3 And there appeared another [c]wonder
in heaven; and behold [d]a great red dragon, having seven heads and ten horns,
and seven [e]crowns upon his heads.
4 And his tail drew the third part of
the [f]stars of heaven, and did cast them to
the earth: and the dragon stood before
the woman which was ready to be delivered, for [g]to devour her child as soon as
it was born.

(3) *The Child: Christ.*

5 And she brought forth a man child,
[h]who was to rule all nations with a rod
of iron: and her child was [i]caught up
unto God, and *to* his throne.
6 And the woman fled into the
[j]wilderness, where she hath a place prepared of God, that they should feed her
there [k]a thousand two hundred *and*
threescore days.

(4) *The archangel.*

7 And there was [l]war in heaven:
[m]Michael and his [n]angels [o]fought
against the dragon; and the dragon
fought and his angels,
8 And prevailed not; neither was their
place found any more in heaven.
9 And the great [p]dragon was cast out,
[q]that old serpent, called the [r]Devil, and
[s]Satan, which [t]deceiveth the whole
[u]world: he was cast out into the earth,
and his [v]angels were cast out with him.
10 And I heard a loud voice saying in
heaven, Now is come [w]salvation, and
[x]strength, and the [1]kingdom of our God,
and the [y]power of his Christ: for the
accuser of our brethren is cast down,
which accused them before our God day
and night.

A.D. 96.

a Cf. Rev. 7:4-8.
b Cf. Isa. 66:7-10; Mic. 4:10.
c *sign.*
d See v. 9.
e *diadems.*
f Rev. 8:12.
g Cf. Mt. 2:16.
h *Christ.* Psa. 2:9; Rev. 2:27; 19:15.
i Lk. 24:51; Acts 1:9-11; 7:55, 56; Rev. 3:21.
j v. 14.
k Rev. 11:2, 3; 13:5; Dan. 9:27; 7:14, *note.*
l *Contra,* Lk. 19:38.
m Cf. Jude 9; cf. Dan. 10:21.
n Heb. 1:4, *note.*
o *went to war with.*
p *Satan.* vs. 3, 4, 7-17; Rev. 20:2, 7, 10. (Gen. 3:1; Rev. 20:10.)
q *the ancient serpent.* Gen. 3:1; Isa. 14:12-19.
r Cf. 1 Pet. 5:8.
s Cf. 1 Cor. 5:5.
t Cf. 2 Cor. 4:4; 11:14.
u *oikoumene = inhabited earth.* (Lk. 2:1.)
v Heb. 1:4, *note.*
w *the salvation.* Rom. 1:16, *note.*
x *the power.*
y *authority.*
z *because of.*
aa Heb. 2:14.
bb v. 17; cf. 1 Pet. 5:8.
cc *Contra,* John 9:4; cf. Lk. 9:42.
dd Cf. Mt. 24:9.
ee Cf. Ex. 19:4; cf. Isa. 40:31.
ff v. 6; cf. Hos. 2:14, 15.
gg Cf. Isa. 8:7, 8; cf. Jer. 46:8; cf. Isa. 17:12, 13.
hh Cf. 2 Chr. 20:23, 24.
ii *Remnant,* Rev. 14:1-5. (Isa. 1:9; Rom. 11:5.).
jj *Law (of Moses).* Rev. 14:12. (Ex. 19:1; Gal. 3:1-29.)
kk *Jesus.*
ll *The Beast.* vs. 1-8; Rev. 19:19, 20. (Dan. 7:8; Rev. 19:20.)
mm *diadems.*
nn *names.*

11 And they overcame him [z]by the
[aa]blood of the Lamb, and [z]by the word
of their testimony; and they loved not
their lives unto the death.
12 Therefore rejoice, *ye* heavens, and
ye that dwell in them. Woe to the inhabiters of the earth and of the sea! for the
devil is come down unto you, having
great [bb]wrath, because he knoweth that
he hath [cc]but a short time.

Satan and Israel in the tribulation.

13 And when the dragon saw that he
was cast unto the earth, he [dd]persecuted
the woman which brought forth the man
child.
14 And to the woman were given two
[ee]wings of a great eagle, that she might
fly into the wilderness, into her [ff]place,
where she is nourished for a time, and
times, and half a time, from the face of
the serpent.
15 And the serpent [gg]cast out of his
mouth water as a flood after the woman,
that he might cause her to be carried
away of the flood.
16 And the earth helped the woman,
and the earth opened her mouth, and
[hh]swallowed up the flood which the
dragon cast out of his mouth.

(5) *The Jewish remnant.*

17 And the dragon was wroth with the
woman, and went to make war with the
[ii]remnant of her seed, which keep the
[jj]commandments of God, and have the
testimony of [kk]Jesus Christ.

CHAPTER 13.

(6) *The Beast out of the sea.*

AND I stood upon the sand of the sea,
and saw a [ll]beast [2]rise up out of
the sea, having seven heads and ten
horns, and upon his horns ten
[mm]crowns, and upon his heads the
[nn]name of blasphemy.
2 And the beast which I saw was [3]like
unto a leopard, and his feet were as

[1] **(12:10)** The Dispensation of the Kingdom (2 Sam. 7:16, *refs.*) begins with the return of Christ to the earth, runs through the "thousand years" of His earth-rule, and ends when He has delivered up the kingdom to the Father (1 Cor. 15:24, *note*).

[2] **(13:1)** Daniel's fourth beast (Dan. 7:26, *note*). The "ten horns" are explained in Dan. 7:24, Rev. 17:12, to be ten kings, and the whole vision is of the last form of Gentile world-power, a confederated ten-kingdom empire covering the sphere of authority of ancient Rome. Rev. 13:1-3 refers to the ten-kingdom *empire;* vs. 4-10 to the *emperor,* who is emphatically "*the* Beast" (Rev. 19:20, *note*).

[3] **(13:2)** The three animals, leopard, bear, and lion, are found in Dan. 7:4-6 as symbols of the empires which preceded Rome, and whose characteristics all entered into the qualities of the Roman empire: Macedonian swiftness of conquest, Persian tenacity of purpose, Babylonish voracity.

the feet of a bear, and his mouth as the
mouth of a lion: and the [a]dragon gave
him his power, and his [b]seat, and great
authority.
3 And I saw [c]one of his heads as it
were [1]wounded to death; and his deadly
wound was [d]healed: and all the [e]world
[f]wondered after the beast.
4 And they worshipped the dragon
which gave [g]power unto the beast: and
they worshipped the beast, saying, Who
is like unto the beast? who is able to
make war with him?
5 And there was given unto him a
mouth speaking great things and blasphemies; and [g]power was given unto
him to continue forty *and* two months.
6 And he opened his mouth in blasphemy against God, to blaspheme his
name, and his tabernacle, and them that
[h]dwell in heaven.
7 And it was given unto him to make
[i]war with the saints, and to overcome
them: and [g]power was given him over
all kindreds, and tongues, and nations.
8 And all that dwell upon the earth
shall worship him, [j]whose names are not
written [k]in the book of life [l]of the Lamb
slain from the foundation of the [2]world.
9 If any man have an ear, let him hear.
10 He that leadeth into captivity shall
go into captivity: he that killeth with the
sword must be killed with the sword.
Here is the [m]patience and the faith of the
saints.

(7) *The Beast out of the earth.*

11 And I beheld another beast coming
up out of the earth; and he had two horns
[n]like a lamb, and he spake as a dragon.

A.D. 96.

- a Rev. 12:3.
- b *throne.*
- c Cf. Rev. 6:2 with Rev. 9:1-11.
- d Cf. Dan. 7:8.
- e *ge.* = earth. vs. 8, *note.* (John 7:7.)
- f Cf. Acts 8:10, 11.
- g *authority.*
- h Cf. Rev. 12:12.
- i Rev. 11:7, 12; cf. Dan. 7:21, 22.
- j Rev. 3:5; cf. Phil. 4:3; cf. Rev. 20:12, 15.
- k *from the foundation of the world in the book of life of the Lamb slain.*
- l *Life (eternal).* Rev. 17:8. (Mt. 7:14; Rev. 22:19.)
- m Rev. 14:12; cf. Rev. 1:9.
- n *Contra,* John 1:29.
- o v. 8.
- p *signs.*
- q Cf. 2 Ki. 1:10.
- r Cf. 1 John 4:1-3.
- s *it was given him to do.*
- t *It was given to him to give breath unto.*
- u *Contra,* Rev. 7:2, 3; cf. Rev. 14:9.
- v Cf. Dan. 12:10; cf. 1 Cor. 2:14-15.
- w Cf. Psa. 9:20; cf. Psa. 10:18.
- x Cf. Dan. 3:1; cf. 1 Sam. 17:4.
- y *the.*

12 And he exerciseth all the [g]power of
the first beast before him, and causeth
the earth and them which dwell therein
to [o]worship the first beast, whose deadly
wound was healed.
13 And he doeth great [p]wonders, so
that he maketh [q]fire come down from
heaven on the earth in the sight of men,
14 And [r]deceiveth them that dwell on
the earth by *the means of* those [p]miracles
which [s]he had power to do in the sight
of the beast; saying to them that dwell
on the earth, that they should make an
image to the beast, which had the
wound by a sword, and did live.
15 And [t]he had power to give life unto
the image of the beast, that the image of
the beast should both speak, and cause
that as many as would not worship the
image of the beast should be killed.
16 And [3]he causeth all, both small and
great, rich and poor, free and bond, to
receive [u]a mark in their right hand, or in
their foreheads:
17 And that no man might buy or sell,
save he that had the mark, or the name
of the beast, or the number of his name.
18 Here is wisdom. Let him that hath
[v]understanding count the number of the
beast: for it is the number of a [w]man;
and his number *is* [x]Six hundred threescore *and* six.

CHAPTER 14.

Parenthetical: vision of the Lamb and the one hundred and forty and four thousand.

And I looked, and, lo, [y]a Lamb stood
on the mount Sion, and with him
an hundred forty *and* four thousand,

[1] **(13:3)** Fragments of the ancient Roman empire have never ceased to exist as separate kingdoms. It was the imperial form of government which ceased; the one head wounded to death. What we have prophetically in Rev. 13:3 is the restoration of the imperial form as such, though over a federated empire of ten kingdoms; the "head" is "healed," i.e. restored; there is an emperor again—the Beast.

[2] **(13:8)** *Kosmos,* Summary: In the sense of the present world-system, the ethically bad sense of the word, refers to the "order," "arrangement," under which Satan has organized the world of unbelieving mankind upon his cosmic principles of force, greed, selfishness, ambition, and pleasure (Mt. 4:8, 9; John 12:31; 14:30; 18:36; Eph. 2:2; 6:12; 1 John 2:15-17). This world-system is imposing and powerful with armies and fleets; is often outwardly religious, scientific, cultured, and elegant; but, seething with national and commercial rivalries and ambitions, is upheld in any real crisis by armed force, and is dominated by Satanic principles.

[3] **(13:16)** Antichrist the *person* is to be distinguished from the "many antichrists" (1 John 2:18), and the "spirit of antichrist" (1 John 4:3) which characterizes all. The supreme mark of all is the denial of the Christian truth of the incarnation of the *Logos,* the eternal Son in Jesus as the Christ (John 1:1, 14; Mt. 1:16, *note*). The "many antichrists" precede and prepare the way for *the* Antichrist, who is

having [a]his Father's name [b]written in
their foreheads.
2 And I heard a voice from heaven, as
the voice of [c]many waters, and as the
voice of a great thunder: and I heard the
voice of [d]harpers harping with their
harps:
3 And they sung as it were a new song
before the throne, and before the four
[e]beasts, and the [f]elders: and no man
could learn that song but the hundred
and forty *and* four thousand, which were
[g]redeemed from the earth.
4 These are they which were not
defiled with women; for they are virgins.
These are they which follow the Lamb
whithersoever he goeth. These were [g]re-
deemed from among men, [h]*being* the
firstfruits unto God and to the Lamb.
5 And in their mouth was found no
guile: for [i]they are without fault before
the throne of God.

Vision of the angel with the everlasting Gospel.

6 And I saw another [j]angel fly in [k]the
midst of heaven, having the everlasting
[1l]gospel to preach unto them that dwell
on the earth, and to every nation, and
kindred, and tongue, and people,
7 Saying with a loud voice, Fear

A.D. 96.

a *his name and his Father's.*
b Rev. 7:3; cf. Rev. 22:4; *contra,* Rev. 13:16.
c Rev. 19:6.
d Cf. Rev. 15:2.
e *living creatures.*
f *Elders.* Rev. 19:4. (Acts 11:30; Tit. 1:5-9.)
g Rom. 3:24, *note.*
h *to be.*
i *Remnant.* vs. 1-5; Rev. 20:4. (Isa. 1:9; Rom. 11:5.)
j Heb. 1:4, *note.*
k *mid-heaven.*
l *Gospel.* (Gen. 12:1-3.)

"the Beast out of the earth" of Rev. 13:11-17, and the "false prophet" of Rev. 16:13; 19:20; 20:10. He is the last ecclesiastical head, as the Beast of Rev. 13:1-8 is the last civil head. For purposes of persecution he is permitted to exercise the autocratic power of the emperor-Beast (Rev. 19:20, *note*).

[1]**(14:6)** Gospel. This great theme may be summarized as follows:

I. In itself the word Gospel means good news.

II. Four *forms* of the Gospel are to be distinguished:

(1) The Gospel of the kingdom. This is the good news that God purposes to set up on the earth, in fulfilment of the Davidic Covenant (2 Sam. 7:16, and *refs.*), a kingdom, political, spiritual, Israelitish, universal, over which God's Son, David's heir, shall be King, and which shall be, for one thousand years, the manifestation of the righteousness of God in human affairs. See Mt. 3:2, *note.*

Two *preachings* of this Gospel are mentioned, one past, beginning with the ministry of John the Baptist, continued by our Lord and His disciples, and ending with the Jewish rejection of the King. The other is yet future (Mt. 24:14), during the great tribulation, and immediately preceding the coming of the King in glory.

(2) The Gospel of the grace of God. This is the good news that Jesus Christ, the rejected King, has died on the cross for the sins of the world, that He was raised from the dead for our justification, and that by Him all that believe are justified from all things. This form of the Gospel is described in many ways. It is the Gospel "of God" (Rom. 1:1) because it originates in His love; "of Christ" (2 Cor. 10:14) because it flows from His sacrifice, and because He is the alone Object of Gospel faith; of "the grace of God" (Acts 20:24) because it saves those whom the law curses; of "the glory" (1 Tim. 1:11; 2 Cor. 4:4) because it concerns Him who is in the glory, and who is bringing the many sons to glory (Heb. 2:10); of "our salvation" (Eph. 1:13) because it is the "power of God unto salvation to every one that believeth" (Rom. 1:16); of "the uncircumcision" (Gal. 2:7) because it saves wholly apart from forms and ordinances; of "peace" (Eph. 6:15) because through Christ it makes peace between the sinner and God, and imparts inward peace.

(3) The everlasting Gospel (Rev. 14:6). This is to be preached to the earth-dwellers at the very end of the great tribulation and immediately preceding the judgment of the nations (Mt. 25:31, *refs.*). It is neither the Gospel of the kingdom, nor of grace. Though its burden is judgment, not salvation, it is good news to Israel and to those who, during the tribulation, have been saved (Rev. 7:9-14; Lk. 21:28; Psa. 96:11-13; Isa. 35:4-10).

(4) That which Paul calls, "my Gospel" (Rom. 2:16, *refs.*). This is the Gospel of the grace of God in its fullest development, but includes the revelation of the result of that Gospel in the outcalling of the church, her relationships, position, privileges, and responsibility. It is the *distinctive* truth of Ephesians and Colossians, but interpenetrates all of Paul's writings.

III. There is "another Gospel" (Gal. 1:6; 2 Cor. 11:4) "which is not another," but a perversion of the Gospel of the grace of God, against which we are warned. It has had many seductive forms, but the test is one—it invariably denies the sufficiency of grace alone to save, keep, and perfect, and mingles with grace some kind of human merit. In Galatia it was law, in Colosse fanaticism (Col. 2:18, etc.). In any form its teachers lie under the awful anathema of God.

God, and give glory to him; for the hour
of his judgment is come: and worship
him that made heaven, and earth, and
the sea, and the fountains of waters.

The fall of Babylon announced.

8 And there followed another [a]angel,
saying, Babylon is fallen, is fallen, that
great city, [b]because she made all nations
drink of the wine of the wrath of her fornication.

The doom of the Beast-worshippers announced.

9 And the third [a]angel followed them,
saying with a loud voice, If any man worship the beast and his image, and receive
his mark in his forehead, or in his hand,
10 The same shall [c]drink of the wine
of the wrath of God, which is poured out
without mixture into the cup of his
indignation; and he shall be [d]tormented
with fire and brimstone in the [e]presence
of the holy [a]angels, and in the presence
of the Lamb:
11 And the smoke of their torment
ascendeth up [f]for ever and ever: and they
have [g]no rest day nor night, who worship
the beast and his image, and whosoever
receiveth the mark of his name.
12 Here is the patience of the saints:
[h]here *are* they that keep the [i]command-
ments of God, and the faith of Jesus.

The blessedness of the holy dead.

13 And I heard a voice from heaven
saying unto me, [j]Write, [k]Blessed *are* the
dead which die in the Lord from henceforth: Yea, saith the [l]Spirit, that they may
rest from their labours; and their works
do follow [m]them.

Vision of Armageddon.

14 And I looked, and behold a white
cloud, and upon the cloud *one* sat [n]like
unto the Son of man, having on his head
a [o]golden crown, and in his hand a
[p]sharp sickle.
15 And another [a]angel came out of the
temple, crying with a loud voice to him
that sat on the cloud, Thrust in thy sickle,
and reap: [q]for the time is come for thee to
reap; for the harvest of the earth is [r]ripe.
16 And he that sat on the cloud thrust
in his sickle on the earth; and the [s]earth
was reaped.
17 And another [a]angel came out of the
temple which is in heaven, he also having a sharp sickle.
18 And another [a]angel came out from
the altar, which had [t]power over fire;
and cried with a loud cry to him that
had the sharp sickle, saying, Thrust in
thy sharp sickle, and gather the clusters
of the vine of the earth; for her grapes
are [u]fully ripe.
19 And the [a]angel thrust in his sickle
into the earth, and gathered the vine of
the earth, and cast *it* into the great winepress of the wrath of God.
20 And the [v]winepress was trodden
without the city, and blood came out of
the winepress, even unto the horse bridles, by the space of a thousand *and* six
hundred [w]furlongs.

CHAPTER 15.

The seven vials (to Rev. 16:21).

(1) *Vision of the angels of the seven last plagues: the bowls of the wrath of God.*

And I saw another sign in heaven,
great and marvellous, seven [x]an-
gels having the seven [y]last plagues; for
in them is [z]filled up the wrath of God.
2 And I saw as it were a [aa]sea of glass
mingled with [bb]fire: and them that had
gotten the [cc]victory over the beast, and
over his image, [dd]and over his mark, *and*
over the number of his name, stand on the
sea of glass, having the [ee]harps of God.
3 And they sing the [ff]song of Moses
the servant of God, and the song of the
[gg]Lamb, saying, [hh]Great and marvellous
are thy works, Lord God Almighty; [ii]just
and true *are* thy ways, thou King of
[jj]saints.
4 Who shall not fear thee, O Lord, and
glorify thy name? for *thou* only *art*
[kk]holy: for all nations shall come and
worship before thee; for thy [ll]judgments
are made manifest.
5 And after that I looked, and, behold,
the [mm]temple of the tabernacle of the testimony in heaven was opened:
6 And the seven [x]angels came out of
the temple, having the seven plagues,
[nn]clothed in pure and white linen, and
having their breasts [oo]girded with golden
girdles.
7 And one of the four [pp]beasts gave
unto the seven [x]angels seven golden
vials full of the [qq]wrath of God, who
liveth for ever and ever.
8 And the temple was [rr]filled with
smoke from the glory of God, and from
his power; and no man was able to enter
into the temple, till the seven plagues of
the seven [x]angels were fulfilled.

A.D. 96.

a Heb. 1:4, *note.*
b *which made.*
c Rev. 16:19; cf. Jer. 25:15.
d Cf. Rev. 20:10.
e Cf. Isa. 66:23, 24; cf. 2 Thes. 1:9.
f Cf. Rev. 19:3; cf. Mk. 9:48.
g *Contra,* Rev. 4:8.
h *those that keep.*
i *Law (of Moses).* Gal. 3:1-29. (Ex. 19:1; Gal. 3:1-24.)
j *Inspiration.* Rev. 19:9. (Ex. 4:15; Rev. 22:19.)
k *Contra,* 1 Cor. 15:51; cf. Phil. 1:23.
l *Holy Spirit.* Rev. 17:3. (Mt. 1:18; Acts 2:4.)
m *with them.*
n Cf. Mt. 26:64; *Contra,* 1 Thes. 4:16, 17.
o Cf. Rev. 19:12.
p Cf. Mk. 4:29.
q Cf. Jer. 51:33.
r *dried.*
s Cf. Mt. 13:30, 36-43; cf. Lk. 3:17.
t Cf. Rev. 16:5, 8
u Cf. 2 Thes. 2:7-12.
v Cf. Rev. 19:15; cf. Isa. 63:1-6.
w One furlong = 582 ft.
x Heb. 1:4, *note.*
y *plagues, the last.*
z *completed.*
aa Cf. Rev. 4:6.
bb Cf. 1 Pet. 1:7.
cc Cf. Rev. 12:11.
dd *and over the number of his name.*
ee Cf. Rev. 5:8; cf. Psa. 150:3.
ff Cf. Ex. 15:1.
gg Cf. Psa. 22:22.
hh Deut. 32:3, 4; Psa. 92:5; Rom. 11:33.
ii Rev. 16:7.
jj *Or, ages.*
kk Rev. 4:8.
ll *righteous acts.*
mm Cf. Rev. 11:19.
nn Cf. Rev. 19:8, 14.
oo Cf. Rev. 1:13.
pp *living creatures.*
qq Cf. Rev. 14:10; cf. Jer. 25:15.
rr Ex. 40:34, 35; Isa. 6:4; 1 Ki. 8:10, 11.

CHAPTER 16.

(2) The vials of the wrath of God upon the earth.

And I heard a great voice out of the
temple saying to the seven [a]angels,
Go your ways, and pour out the [b]vials of
the wrath of God upon the earth.

The first vial.

2 And the [c]first went, and poured out
his vial upon the earth; and there fell a
noisome and grievous [d]sore upon the
men which had the mark of the beast, and
upon them which worshipped his image.

The second vial.

3 And the [e]second [a]angel poured out
his vial upon the [f]sea; and it became [g]as
the blood of a dead *man*: and every living soul died in the sea.

The third vial.

4 And the [h]third [a]angel poured out his
vial upon the [i]rivers and fountains of
waters; and they became blood.
5 And I heard the angel of the waters
say, Thou art [j]righteous, O Lord, which
art, and wast, and shalt be, because thou
hast judged thus.
6 For they have [k]shed the blood of
saints and prophets, and thou hast given
them blood to drink; for they are [l]worthy.
7 And I heard [m]another out of the
altar say, Even so, Lord God Almighty,
true and righteous *are* thy judgments.

The fourth vial.

8 And the [n]fourth [a]angel poured out
his vial upon the [o]sun; and [p]power was
given unto him to scorch men with fire.
9 And men were scorched with great
heat, and blasphemed the name of God,
[q]which hath power over these plagues:
and they repented not to give him glory.

The fifth vial.

10 And the [r]fifth [a]angel poured out his
vial upon the [s]seat of the beast; and his
kingdom [t]was full of darkness; and they
gnawed their tongues for pain,
11 And blasphemed the [u]God of heav-
en because of their pains and their sores,
and [v]repented not of their deeds.

The sixth vial.

12 And the sixth [w]angel poured out
his vial [x]upon the great river Euphrates;
and the water thereof was dried up, that
the [y]way of the kings of the east might
be prepared.

(*Parenthetical*, vs. 13-16.)

13 And I saw three unclean [z]spirits like
frogs *come* out of the mouth of the dragon, and out of the mouth of the beast, and
out of the mouth of the [aa]false prophet.
14 For they are the spirits of [bb]devils,
working [cc]miracles, *which* go forth unto
the [dd]kings of the earth and of the whole
[ee]world, to gather them to the [ff]battle of
that great day of God Almighty.
15 Behold, [gg]I come as a thief. Blessed
is he that watcheth, and keepeth his garments, lest he walk naked, and they see
his shame.
16 And he gathered them together into
a place called in the Hebrew tongue
[hh]Armageddon.

The seventh vial.

17 And the seventh [w]angel poured out
his vial [ii]into the air; and there came a
great voice out of the temple of heaven,
from the throne, saying, [jj]It is done.
18 [kk]And there were voices, and thunders, and lightnings; and there was a
great [ll]earthquake, such as was not since
men were upon the earth, so mighty an
earthquake, *and* so great.
19 And the great city was divided into
three parts, and the cities of the [mm]na-
tions fell: and great [1nn]Babylon came in
remembrance before God, to give unto
her [oo]the cup of the wine of the fierceness of his wrath.
20 And every [pp]island fled away, and
the mountains were not found.
21 And there fell upon men a great hail
out of heaven, *every stone* about the
weight of a talent: and men blasphemed
God because of the plague of the hail; for
the plague thereof was exceeding great.

A.D. 96.

a Heb. 1:4, *note.*
b Lit. *bowls.*
c Cf. Rev. 6:1; 8:7.
d Cf. Ex. 9:8-11; cf. Isa. 1:6.
e Cf. Rev. 6:3, 4; cf. Rev. 8:8, 9.
f Cf. Rev. 17:15.
g *blood as of a.*
h Cf. Rev. 6:5, 6; cf. Rev. 8:10, 11.
i Cf. Ex. 7:17-21.
j Cf. Rom. 3:3-6.
k Cf. Rev. 18:24; cf. Mt. 23:35.
l *Contra,* Rev. 5:12.
m *the altar say.*
n Cf. Rev. 6:7, 8; cf. Rev. 8:12.
o *Contra,* Mal. 4:2.
p *it was given to it.*
q *who had authority.*
r Cf. Rev. 6:9-11; 9:1-11.
s *throne.*
t *became darkened.*
u Dan. 2:18.
v *Repentance.* vs. 9:11; (Mt. 3:2: Acts 17:30.)
w Heb. 1:4, *note.*
x Rev. 9:14.
y Isa. 41:2, 25; 44:27.
z Ex. 8:1-6; 1 Tim. 4:1; 1 John 4:1-3.
aa *Antichrist.* Rev. 19:20. (1 John 2:18; Rev. 13:11-17.)
bb *demons.*
cc *signs.*
dd *Times of the Gentiles.* Rev. 16:19. (Lk. 21:24; Rev. 16:19.)
ee *oikoumene = inhabited earth.* (Lk. 2:1.)
ff *Armageddon (battle of).* Isa. 10:27-34. (Rev. 16:14; 19:11-21.)
gg *Christ. (Second Advent).* Rev. 19:11-21. (Deut. 30:3; Acts 1:9-11.)
hh i.e. *Mount of Slaughter.*
ii *upon.*
jj *Day (of Jehovah).* vs. 12-17; Rev. 19:11-21. (Isa. 2:10-22; Rev. 19:11-21.)
kk Rev. 11:19.
ll Rev. 6:12; 11:13.
mm *Times of the Gentiles.* (Lk. 21:24.)
nn See Isa. 13:1, *note.*
oo Isa. 51:21-23; Rev. 14:10; 18:5.
pp Rev. 6:14.

[1] **(16:19)** Summary: The Times of the Gentiles is that long period beginning with the Babylonian captivity of Judah, under Nebuchadnezzar, and to be brought to an end by the destruction of Gentile world-power by the "stone cut out without hands". (Dan. 2:34, 35, 44), i.e. the coming of the Lord in glory (Rev. 19:11, 21), until which time Jerusalem is politically subject to Gentile rule (Lk. 21:24).

CHAPTER 17.

The seven dooms:
(1) *The doom of "Babylon."*

The divine view of "Babylon."
(Cf. Rev. 18:1-8.)

AND there came one of the seven [a]angels which had the seven vials, and talked with me, saying unto me, Come hither; I will shew unto thee the judgment of the [b]great whore that sitteth upon many waters:

2 With whom the [c]kings of the earth have committed fornication, and the inhabitants of the earth have been made drunk with the wine of her fornication.

3 So he carried me away in the [d]spirit into the wilderness: and I saw a woman sit upon a [e]scarlet coloured beast, full of [f]names of blasphemy, having seven heads and ten horns.

4 And the woman was [g]arrayed in purple and scarlet colour, and decked with gold and precious stones and pearls, having a [h]golden cup in her hand full of abominations and filthiness of her fornication:

5 And upon her forehead *was* a name written, [i]MYSTERY, [j]BABYLON THE GREAT, THE MOTHER OF HARLOTS AND ABOMINATIONS OF THE EARTH.

6 And I saw the woman drunken [k]with the blood of the saints, and with the blood of the martyrs of Jesus: and when I saw her, I wondered with great [l]admiration.

7 And the [a]angel said unto me, Wherefore didst thou marvel? I will tell thee the [i]mystery of the woman, and of the beast that carrieth her, which hath the seven heads and ten horns.

The last form of Gentile world-power.

8 The beast that thou sawest was, and is not; and [m]shall ascend out of the [n]bottomless pit, and go into perdition: and they that dwell on the earth [o]shall wonder, whose names were not written in the book of [p]life from the foundation of the [q]world, when they behold the beast [r]that was, and is not, and [s]yet is.

9 And [t]here *is* the mind which hath wisdom. [u]The seven heads are seven mountains, on which the woman sitteth.

10 And there are seven kings: five are fallen, and one is, *and* the other is not yet come; and when he cometh, he must [v]continue a short space.

11 And the [w]beast that was, and is not, even he is the eighth, and is of the seven, and goeth into perdition.

12 And the ten horns which thou sawest are ten kings, which have received no kingdom as yet; but receive [x]power as kings one hour with the beast.

13 These have one mind, and shall give their power and [x]strength unto the beast.

14 These shall make [y]war with the Lamb, and the Lamb shall [z]overcome them: for he is [aa]Lord of lords, and King of kings: and they that are with him *are* called, and [bb]chosen, and faithful.

15 And he saith unto me, The [cc]waters which thou sawest, where the whore sitteth, are peoples, and multitudes, and nations, and tongues.

16 And the ten horns which thou sawest [dd]upon the beast, these shall [ee]hate the whore, and shall make her desolate and naked, and shall eat her flesh, and [ff]burn her with fire.

17 For God hath put in their hearts to fulfil [gg]his will, and to agree, and give their kingdom unto the beast, until the words of God shall be fulfilled.

18 And the woman which thou sawest is [hh]that great city, which reigneth over the kings of the earth.

CHAPTER 18.

The last form of apostate Christendom: the warning to God's people.

AND after these things I saw another [ii]angel come down from heaven, having great [x]power; and the earth was lightened with his glory.

2 And he cried mightily with a strong voice, saying, [1]Babylon the great is

A.D. 96.

a Heb. 1:4, *note.*
b Nah. 3:4; Rev. 19:2.
c Rev. 18:3, 9.
d *Holy Spirit.* Rev. 21:10. (Mt. 1:18; Acts 2:4.)
e Rev. 12:3.
f Rev. 13:1.
g Rev. 18:16.
h Rev. 18:6.
i Mt. 13:11, *note.*
j See Isa. 13:1, *note.*
k Rev. 16:6.
l *wonder.*
m *is about to.*
n *abyss.*
o Rev. 13:3.
p *Life (eternal).* Rev. 20:12, 15. (Mt. 7:14; Rev. 22:19.)
q *earth.*
r *that it was.*
s *shall be.*
t Rev. 13:18.
u Rev. 13:1.
v Rev. 13:5.
w Rev. 13:1, 3.
x *authority.*
y Rev. 19:19; 16:14.
z Rev. 19:20; cf. 2 Thes. 2:8, 9.
aa Rev. 19:16; cf. 1 Tim. 6:15.
bb *Election (personal).* 1 Pet. 1:2. (Deut. 7:6; 1 Pet. 1:2.)
cc Cf. Rev. 13:1; cf. Dan. 7:2 with Psa. 2:1.
dd *and*
ee Cf. Jud. 9:23, 24; cf. 2 Ki. 9:30-37.
ff Cf. Lev. 21:9 with Jas. 4:4.
gg Cf. Rev. 18:8, 20.
hh the v. 9; *contra,* Psa. 48:2.
ii Heb. 1:4, *note.*

[1] **(18:2)** Babylon, "confusion," is repeatedly used by the prophets in a symbolic sense (see Isa. 13:1, *note*). Two "Babylons" are to be distinguished in the Revelation: ecclesiastical Babylon, which is apostate Christendom, headed up under the Papacy; and political Babylon, which is the Beast's confederated empire, the last form of Gentile world-dominion. Ecclesiastical Babylon is "the great whore" (Rev. 17:1), and is destroyed by political Babylon (Rev. 17:15-18), that the beast may be the alone object of worship (2 Thes. 2:3, 4; Rev. 13:15). The power of political Babylon is destroyed by the return of the Lord in glory.

fallen, is fallen, and is become the habitation of [a]devils, and the hold of every
foul spirit, and a cage of every unclean
and hateful bird.
3 For all nations have [b]drunk of the
wine of the wrath of her fornication, and
the kings of the earth have committed
fornication with her, and the [c]merchants
of the earth are waxed rich through the
[d]abundance of her delicacies.
4 And I heard [e]another voice from
heaven, saying, [f]Come out of her, my people, that ye be not partakers of her [g]sins,
and that ye receive not of her plagues.
5 For her [g]sins have reached unto
heaven, and God hath remembered her
iniquities.
6 [h]Reward her even as she [i]rewarded
you, and double unto her double according to her works: in the cup which she
hath filled fill to her double.
7 How much she hath glorified herself, and lived [j]deliciously, so much torment and sorrow give her: for she saith
in her heart, I sit a [k]queen, and am no
widow, and shall see no sorrow.
8 Therefore shall her plagues come in
one day, death, and mourning, and
famine; and she shall be utterly burned
with fire: for [l]strong *is* the Lord God
who judgeth her.

The human view of "Babylon."
(Cf. Rev. 17:1-7.)

9 And the kings of the earth, who have
committed fornication and lived [j]deli-
ciously with her, [m]shall bewail her, and
lament for her, when they shall see the
smoke of her burning,
10 Standing afar off for the fear of her
torment, saying, [n]Alas, alas, that great
city [o]Babylon, that mighty city! for in
one hour is thy judgment come.
11 And the [p]merchants of the earth
shall weep and mourn over her; for no
man buyeth their merchandise any more:
12 The merchandise of gold, and silver, and precious stones, and of pearls,
and fine linen, and purple, and silk, and
scarlet, and all thyine wood, and [q]all
manner vessels of ivory, and all manner
vessels of most precious wood, and of
brass, and iron, and marble,
13 And cinnamon, and odours, and
ointments, and frankincense, and wine,
and oil, and fine flour, and wheat, and
[r]beasts, and sheep, and horses, and chariots, and [s]slaves, and souls of men.
14 And the fruits that thy soul lusted
after are [t]departed from thee, and all
things which were dainty and goodly
are departed from thee, and [u]thou shalt
find them no more at all.
15 The merchants of these things,
which were made rich by her, shall
[v]stand afar off for the fear of her torment, weeping and wailing,
16 And saying, [w]Alas, alas, [x]that great
city, that was clothed in fine linen, and
purple, and scarlet, and decked with
gold, and precious stones, and pearls!
17 For in [y]one hour so great riches is
come to nought. And every shipmaster,
and [z]all the company in ships, and
sailors, and as many as trade by sea,
stood afar off,
18 And cried when they saw the
smoke of her burning, saying, What *city*
is like unto this great city!
19 And they cast [aa]dust on their heads,
and cried, weeping and wailing, saying,
[bb]Alas, alas, that great city, wherein were
made rich all that had ships in the sea by
reason of her costliness! for in one hour
is she made desolate.

The angelic view of "Babylon."
(Cf. Rev. 17:1-7; 18:1-8.)

20 [cc]Rejoice over her, *thou* heaven, and
ye [dd]holy apostles and prophets; for God
hath [ee]avenged you on her.
21 And a [ff]mighty angel took up a
stone like a great [gg]millstone, and cast *it*
into the sea, saying, Thus with violence
shall that great city Babylon be thrown
down, and shall be found no more at all.
22 And the [hh]voice of harpers, and
musicians, and of pipers, and trumpeters, shall be heard no more at all in
thee; and no [ii]craftsman, of whatsoever
craft *he be*, shall be found any more in
thee; and the [jj]sound of a millstone shall
be heard no more at all in thee;
23 And the light of a [kk]candle shall
shine no more at all in thee; and the
voice of the [ll]bridegroom and of the
bride shall be heard no more at all

A.D. 96.

a *demons.*
b Rev. 17:4; cf. Jer. 51:7.
c vs. 11, 12.
d *power of her luxury.*
e Cf. Rev. 16:7.
f *Separation.* 2 Cor. 6:14-17. (Gen. 12:1; 2 Cor. 6:14-17.)
g *Sin.* Rom. 3:23, *note.*
h *Render to.*
i *hath rendered.*
j *luxuriously.*
k Cf. Isa. 47:7, 8.
l Cf. Jer. 50:34; cf. Heb. 10:31.
m Cf. Jer. 50:46.
n *Woe, woe.*
o See Isa. 13:1, *note.*
p vs. 3, 15.
q *every article.*
r *cattle.*
s *bodies.*
t Cf. Rev. 17:16.
u *they shall.*
v vs. 10, 17.
w *Woe, woe.*
x *the.* Rev. 17, 18.
y vs. 10, 19.
z *every voyager.*
aa Cf. 1 Sam. 4:12.
bb *Woe, woe.*
cc Cf. Jer. 51:48; cf. Isa. 44:23; Rev. 12:12.
dd *saints and apostles.*
ee *judged your judgment upon her.*
ff Rev. 10:1.
gg Cf. Jer. 51:63, 64.
hh Cf. Isa. 24:8; *contra,* Rev. 14:1-3.
ii Cf. Lk. 17:28.
jj Cf. Jer. 25:10.
kk *lamp.*
ll Cf. Jer. 16:9.

(See "Armageddon," Rev. 16:14; 19:17) The notion of a literal Babylon to be rebuilt on the site of ancient Babylon is in conflict with Isa. 13:19-22. But the language of Rev. 18 (e.g. vs. 10, 16, 18) seems beyond question to identify "Babylon," the "city" of luxury and traffic, with "Babylon" the ecclesiastical centre, viz. Rome. The very kings who hate ecclesiastical Babylon deplore the destruction of commercial Babylon.

in thee: for thy merchants were the great men of the earth; for by thy [a]sorceries were all nations deceived.

24 And in her was found the [b]blood of prophets, and of saints, and of all that were slain upon the earth.

CHAPTER 19.

(*Parenthetical: the four alleluias of the glorified saints.* Cf. Rev. 17:1-7; 18:1-8)

And after these things I heard a great [c]voice of much people in heaven, saying, Alleluia; [d]Salvation, and glory, and [e]honour, and power, unto the Lord our God:

2 For true and righteous *are* his judgments: for he hath judged the great [f]whore, which did corrupt the earth with her fornication, and hath [g]avenged the blood of his servants at her hand.

3 And again they said, [h]Alleluia. And her [i]smoke rose up for ever and ever.

4 And the four and twenty [j]elders and the four [k]beasts fell down and worshipped God that sat on the throne, saying, Amen; Alleluia.

5 And a [l]voice came out of the throne, saying, [m]Praise our God, all ye his servants, and ye that fear him, both small and great.

6 And I heard as it were the voice of a great multitude, and as the voice of many waters, and as the voice of mighty [n]thunderings, saying, Alleluia: for the Lord God omnipotent reigneth.

The marriage of the Lamb.

7 Let us be glad and rejoice, and give honour to him: for the marriage of the Lamb is come, and his [1o]wife hath made herself ready.

8 And to her [p]was granted that she should be arrayed in fine linen, clean and white: for the fine linen is the [2q]righteousness of saints.

9 And he saith unto me, Write, [r]Blessed *are* they which are called unto the marriage supper of the Lamb. And he saith unto me, [s]These are the true sayings of God.

10 And I fell at his feet to worship him. And he said unto me, See *thou do it* not: I am thy [t]fellowservant, and of thy brethren that have the testimony of Jesus: worship God: for the [u]testimony of Jesus is the spirit of prophecy.

The second coming of Christ in glory. (Cf. Mt. 24:16-30.)

11 And I [3]saw heaven opened, and behold a [v]white horse; and [w]he that sat upon him *was* called [x]Faithful and True, and in righteousness he doth judge and make war.

12 His [y]eyes *were* as a flame of fire, and on his head *were* many [z]crowns; and he had a name written, [aa]that no man knew, but he himself.

13 And he *was* clothed with a vesture [bb]dipped in blood: and his name is called The Word of God.

14 And the armies *which were* in heaven followed him upon white horses, clothed in fine linen, white and clean.

15 And out of his mouth goeth a [cc]sharp sword, that with it he should smite the nations: and he shall rule them with a rod of iron: and [dd]he treadeth the winepress of the fierceness and wrath of Almighty God.

16 And he hath on *his* vesture and on his thigh a name written, [ee]KING OF KINGS, AND LORD OF LORDS.

The battle of Armageddon (Rev. 16:14; 19:17, *note*).

17 And I saw an angel standing in the sun; and he cried with a loud voice, saying to all the fowls that fly in [ff]the midst of heaven, [4]Come and gather yourselves

A.D. 96.

a Cf. Nah. 3:4.
b Rev. 17:6.
c Rev. 18:20; 11:15.
d *the salvation.* See Rom. 1:16, *note.*
e *power of our God.*
f Rev. 17:1.
g Cf. Rev. 6:10; cf. Lk. 18:7, 8.
h v. 1.
i Cf. Rev. 18:9, 18; cf. Mk. 9:48.
j *Elders.* Tit. 1:5-9.
k *living creatures.*
l Cf. Rev. 18:4.
m Cf. Psa. 134:1.
n Cf. Ex. 20:18.
o *Bride (of Christ).* vs. 6-8; Rev. 21:9. (John 3:29; Rev. 19:6-8.)
p Cf. 1 Cor. 15:10.
q *righteousnesses. Righteousness (garment).* (Gen. 3:21.)
r Cf. Lk. 14:15.
s *Inspiration.* Rev. 21:5. (Ex. 4:15; Rev. 22:19.)
t Cf. Heb. 1:14.
u Cf. Eph. 1:9, 10; cf. 1 Pet. 1:10-12.
v *Contra,* Rev. 6:2; cf. Psa. 45:4; *contra,* Mt. 21:2-5.
w *Christ (Second Advent).* vs. 11-21; Rev. 20:4-6. (Deut. 30:3; Acts 1:9-11.)
x Cf. Rev. 3:7.
y Rev. 1:14.
z *diadems.*
aa Cf. vs. 13, 16; cf. Mt. 11:27; cf. 1 Tim. 6:16.
bb Cf. Isa. 63:2, 3.
cc v. 21; cf. Rev. 1:16; cf. 2 Thes. 2:8.
dd Rev. 14:20; Isa. 63:3, 6; cf. Mt. 21:44.
ee Rev. 17:14; 1:5.
ff *mid-heaven.*

[1] **(19:7)** The "Lamb's wife" here is the "bride" (Rev. 21:9), the Church, identified with the "heavenly Jerusalem" (Heb. 12:22, 23), and to be distinguished from Israel, the adulterous and repudiated "wife" of Jehovah, yet to be restored (Isa. 54:1-10; Hos. 2:1-17), who is identified with the earth (Hos. 2:23): A forgiven and restored *wife* could not be called either a *virgin* (2 Cor. 11:2, 3), or a *bride.*

[2] **(19:8)** The garment in Scripture is a symbol of righteousness. In the bad ethical sense it symbolizes self-righteousness (e.g. Isa. 64:6; see Phil. 3:6-8, the best that a moral and religious man under law could do). In the good ethical sense the garment symbolizes "the righteousness of God . . . upon all them that believe." See Rom. 3:21, *note.*

[3] **(19:11)** The vision is of the departure from heaven of Christ and the saints and angels preparatory to the catastrophe in which Gentile world-power, headed up in the Beast, is smitten by the "stone cut out without hands" (Dan. 2:34, 35).

[4] **(19:17)** Armageddon (the ancient hill and valley of Megiddo, west of Jordan in the plain of Jezreel) is the appointed place for the beginning of the great battle in which the Lord, at His coming in glory,

together unto the [a]supper of the great God;

18 That ye may [b]eat the flesh of kings, and the flesh of captains, and the flesh of mighty men, and the flesh of horses, and of them that sit on them, and the flesh of all *men, both* free and bond, both small and great.

19 And I saw the [c]beast, and the kings of the earth, and their armies, gathered together to [1d]make war against him that sat on the horse, and against his army.

(2) *Doom of the Beast,*
(3) *and of the False Prophet.*

20 And the [2]beast was taken, and with him the [e]false prophet that wrought [f]miracles before him, with which he deceived them that had received the mark of the beast, and [g]them that worshipped his image. These both [h]were cast alive into [i]a lake of fire burning with brimstone.

(4) *Doom of the kings.*

21 And the remnant were slain with the sword of [j]him that sat upon the horse, which *sword* proceeded out of his mouth: [k]and all the fowls were filled with their flesh.

CHAPTER 20.

Satan bound in the abyss during the kingdom-age.

AND I saw an angel come down from heaven, having the key of the bottomless pit and a great chain in his hand.

2 And he laid hold on the dragon, that old serpent, which is the Devil, and [l]Satan, and bound him a [3]thousand years,

3 And cast him into the bottomless pit, and shut him up, and set a seal upon him, that he should [m]deceive the nations no more, till the thousand years should be fulfilled: and after that he must be loosed a little season.

The first resurrection (1 Cor. 15:52, *note*), *and the kingdom-age.*

4 And I saw thrones, and they sat upon them, and judgment was given unto them: and *I saw* the souls of

A.D. 96.

a *great supper of God.* Cf. Ezk. 39:17-20.
b Cf. Dan. 7:5; cf. Ezk. 32:21-31.
c *The Beast.* vs. 19, 20. (Dan. 7:8.)
d *Armageddon (battle of).* Rev. 16:14; 19:17, *note.*
e *Antichrist.* Rev. 13:11-17. (1 John 2:18; Rev. 13:11-17.)
f *signs.*
g Rev. 13:12, 15.
h *Day (of destruction).* vs. 19, 20; Rev. 20:11-15. (Job 21:30; Rev. 20:11-45.)
i *the.*
j *Kingdom.* (N.T.). vs. 11-21; Rev. 20:1-15. (Lk. 1:31-33; 1 Cor. 15:24.)
k *Day (of Jehovah).* vs. 11-21. (Isa. 2:10-22.)
l *Satan.* vs. 2, 7, 10. (Gen. 3:1.)
m v. 8; 2 Cor. 4:4.

will deliver the Jewish remnant besieged by the Gentile world-powers under the Beast and False Prophet (Rev. 16:13-16; Zech. 12:1-9). Apparently the besieging hosts, whose approach to Jerusalem is described in Isa. 10:28-32, alarmed by the signs which precede the Lord's coming (Mt. 24:29, 30), have fallen back to Megiddo, after the events of Zech. 14:2, where their destruction begins; a destruction consummated in Moab and the plains of Idumea (Isa. 63:1-6). This battle is the first event in "the day of Jehovah" (Isa. 2:12, *refs.*), and is the fulfilment of the smiting-stone prophecy of Dan. 2:35.

[1] **(19:19)** The day of Jehovah (called, also, "that day," and "the great day") is that lengthened period of time beginning with the return of the Lord in glory, and ending with the purgation of the heavens and the earth by fire preparatory to the new heavens and the new earth (Isa. 65:17-19; 66:22; 2 Pet. 3:13; Rev. 21:1). The order of events appears to be: (1) The return of the Lord in glory (Mt. 24:29, 30); (2) the destruction of the Beast and his host, "the kings of the earth and their armies," and the false prophet, which is the "great and terrible" aspect of the day (Rev. 19:11-21); (3) the judgment of the nations (Zech. 14:1-9; Mt. 25:31-46); (4) the thousand years, i.e. the kingdom-age (Rev. 20:4-6); (5) the Satanic revolt and its end (Rev. 20:7-10); (6) the second resurrection and final judgment (Rev. 20:11-15); and (7) the "day of God," earth purged by fire (2 Pet. 3:10-13).

The day of the LORD is preceded by seven signs: (1) The sending of Elijah (Mal. 4:5; Rev. 11:3-6); (2) cosmical disturbances (Joel 2:1-12; Mt. 24:29; Acts 2:19, 20; Rev. 6:12-17); (3) the insensibility of the professing church (1 Thes. 5:1-3); (4) the apostasy of the professing church, then become "Laodicea" (2 Thes. 2:3); (5) the rapture of the true church (1 Thes. 4:17); (6) the manifestation of the "man of sin," the Beast (2 Thes. 2:1-8); (7) the apocalyptic judgments (Rev. 11–18).

[2] **(19:20)** The Beast, Summary: This "Beast" is the "little horn" of Dan. 7:24-26, and "desolator" of Dan. 9:27; the "abomination of desolation" of Mt. 24:15; the "man of sin" of 2 Thes. 2:4-8; earth's last and most awful tyrant, Satan's fell instrument of wrath and hatred against God and the Jewish saints. He is, perhaps, identical with the rider on the white horse of Rev. 6:2, who begins by the peaceful conquest of three of the ten kingdoms into which the former Roman empire will then be divided, but who soon establishes the ecclesiastical and governmental tyranny described in Dan. 7, 9, 11; Rev. 13. To him Satan gives the power which he offered to Christ (Mt. 4:8, 9; Rev. 13:4). See "The great tribulation," Psa. 2:5; Rev. 7:14, *note.*

[3] **(20:2)** The duration of the kingdom of heaven in its mediatorial form (1 Cor. 15:24, *note*).

[a]them that were beheaded for the witness of Jesus, and for the word of God,
and which had not [b]worshipped the
beast, neither his image, neither had
received *his* mark upon their foreheads,
or in their hands; and they lived and
[c]reigned with Christ a thousand years.
5 But the rest of the dead lived not
again until the thousand years were finished. This *is* the [1]first [d]resurrection.
6 [e]Blessed and holy *is* he that hath part
in the first resurrection: on such the second death hath no power, but they shall
be [f]priests of [g]God and of Christ, and
shall reign with him a thousand years.

Satan loosed:
(5) *the doom of Gog and Magog.*

7 And when the thousand years are
expired, Satan [h]shall be loosed out of his
prison,
8 And shall go out to deceive the
nations which are in the four quarters of
the earth, [i]Gog and Magog, to gather
them together to [j]battle: the number of
whom *is* as the sand of the sea.
9 And they went up on the breadth of
the earth, and compassed the camp of
the saints about, and the beloved city:
and fire came down from God out of
heaven, and devoured them.

(6) *The doom of Satan.*

10 And the [2k]devil that deceived them
was cast into the lake of fire and brimstone, [l]where the beast and the false
prophet *are,* and [m]shall be tormented
day and night for ever and ever.

(7) *Doom of the unbelieving dead:*
the last judgment.

11 [n]And I saw a [3o]great white throne,
and him that sat on it, from whose face
the earth and the heaven fled away; and
[4]there was found no place for them.

A.D. 96.

a *Remnant.* Rom. 11:1-5. (Isa. 1:9; Rom. 11:5.)
b Rev. 13:15-17; 14:9-13.
c *Christ (Second Advent).* vs. 4-6; Rev. 22:12. (Deut. 30:3; Acts 1:9-11.)
d *Resurrection.* vs. 4, 5; 1 Cor. 15:1-52. (Job 19:25; 1 Cor. 15:52.)
e Rev. 14:13.
f Rev. 1:6.
g *Jehovah.* Isa. 61:6.
h v. 3.
i Ezk. 38:2, *note.*
j *the war.*
k *Satan.* vs. 2, 7, 10. (Gen. 3:1.)
l Rev. 19:20.
m *they shall.*
n v. 12, *note.*
o *Day of Judgment.* (Mt. 10:15.)

[1]**(20:5)** The "resurrection of the just" is mentioned in Lk. 14:13, 14, and the resurrection of "life" distinguished from the "resurrection unto damnation" in John 5:29. We here learn for the first time what interval of time separates these two resurrections. See 1 Cor. 15:52, *note.*

[2]**(20:10)** Satan, Summary: This fearful being, apparently created one of the cherubim (Ezk. 1:5, *note;* 28:12-14, *note*) and anointed for a position of great authority, perhaps over the primitive creation (Gen. 1:2, *note.* 3; Ezk. 28:11-15), fell through pride (Isa. 14:12-14). His "I will" (Isa. 14:13) marks the introduction of sin into the universe. Cast out of heaven (Lk. 10:18), he makes earth and air the scene of his tireless activity (Eph. 2:2; 1 Pet. 5:8). After the creation of man he entered into the serpent (Gen. 3:1, *note*), and, beguiling Eve by his subtilty, secured the downfall of Adam and through him of the race, and the entrance of sin into the world of men (Rom. 5:12-14). The Adamic Covenant (Gen. 3:14-19, *note*) promised the ultimate destruction of Satan through the "Seed of the woman." Then began his long warfare against the work of God in behalf of humanity, which still continues. The present world-system (Rev. 13:8), organized upon the principles of force, greed, selfishness, ambition, and sinful pleasure, is his work and was the bribe which he offered to Christ (Mt. 4:8, 9). Of that world-system he is prince (John 14:30; 16:11), and god (2 Cor. 4:4). As "prince of the power of the air" (Eph. 2:2) he is at the head of a vast host of demons (Mt. 7:22, *note*). To him, under God, was committed upon earth the power of death (Heb. 2:14). Cast out of heaven as his proper sphere and "first estate," he still has access to God as the "accuser of the brethren" (Rev. 12:10), and is permitted a certain power of sifting or testing the self-confident and carnal among believers (Job 1:6-11; Lk. 22:31, 32; 1 Cor. 5:5; 1 Tim. 1:20), but this is a strictly permissive and limited power, and believers so sifted are kept in faith through the advocacy of Christ (Lk. 22:31, 32; 1 John 2:1, *note*). At the beginning of the great tribulation Satan's privilege of access to God as accuser will be withdrawn (Rev. 12:7-12). At the return of Christ in glory Satan will be bound for one thousand years (Rev. 20:1); after which he will be "loosed for a little season" (Rev. 20:3, 7, 8), and will become the head of a final effort to overthrow the kingdom. Defeated in this, he will be finally cast into the lake of fire, his final doom. The notion that he reigns in hell is Miltonic, not biblical. He is prince of this present world-system, but will be tormented in the lake of fire.

[3]**(20:11)** The expressions, "the judgment," or, "day of judgment," as the passages and their contexts show, refer to the final judgment of Rev. 20:11-15.

[4]**(20:11)** The "day of destruction" is that aspect of the day of Jehovah (Isa. 2:12; Rev. 19:19, Summary) which visits final and eternal judgment upon the wicked. Three such "days" are included

12 And I saw the [a]dead, small and great, stand before [b]God; [c]and the books were opened: and another [d]book was opened, which is *the book* of life: and the dead were [1]judged out of those things which were written in the books, according to their works.

13 And the sea gave up the dead which were in it; and death and [e]hell delivered up the dead which were in them: and they were judged every man according to their works.

14 And death and [f]hell were cast into the lake of fire. [g]This is the [2h]second death.

15 And [i]whosoever was not found written in the book of [j]life was [k]cast into the lake of fire.

CHAPTER 21.

The seven new things: (1) *the new heaven, and* (2) *the new earth.*

And I saw a [l]new heaven and a new earth: for the [m]first heaven and the first earth were passed away; and there was no more sea.

2 And I John saw [n]the holy city, new Jerusalem, coming down from God out of heaven, prepared [o]as a bride adorned for her husband.

(3) *The new peoples.*

3 And I heard a great voice out of heaven saying, Behold, the tabernacle of God *is* with men, and he will dwell with them, and they shall be his people, and God himself shall be with them, *and be* their God.

4 And God shall wipe away all tears from their eyes; and there shall be no more death, neither sorrow, nor crying, neither shall there be any more pain: for the former things are passed away.

5 And he that sat upon the [p]throne said, Behold, I make all things new. And he said unto me, Write: [q]for these words are true and faithful.

6 And he said unto me, It is done. I am Alpha and Omega, the beginning and the end. I will give unto him that is athirst of the fountain of the water of life freely.

7 He that overcometh shall inherit all things; and I will be his God, and he shall be my son.

8 But the fearful, and unbelieving, and the abominable, and murderers, and whoremongers, and sorcerers, and idolaters, and all liars, shall have their part in the lake which burneth with fire and brimstone: which is [r]the [2]second death.

(4) *The Lamb's wife: the new Jerusalem.*

9 And there came unto me one of the seven angels which had the seven vials full of the seven last plagues, and talked with me, saying, Come hither, I will shew thee [s]the bride, the Lamb's wife.

10 And he carried me away in the [t]spirit to a great and high mountain, and shewed me that great city, the holy Jerusalem, descending out of heaven from God,

11 Having the glory of God: and

A.D. 96.

- a *Judgments (the seven).* 2 Sam. 7:14.
- b *the throne.*
- c Dan. 7:10; Mt. 12:36.
- d Lk. 10:20; Phil. 4:3.
- e Lk. 16:23, *note.*
- f *hades.*
- g *Death (the second).* vs. 6, 14, 15; Rev. 21:8. (John 8:21, 24; Rev. 21:8.)
- h *second death, the lake of fire.*
- i *Kingdom* (N.T.). vs. 1-15; Rev. 21:1-6. (Lk. 1:31-33; 1 Cor. 15:24.)
- j *Life (eternal).* vs. 12, 15; Rev. 21:6, 27. (Mt. 7:14; Rev. 22:19.)
- k *Day (of destruction).* (Job 21:30.)
- l 2 Pet. 3:13; Isa. 65:7; 66:22.
- m Heb. 12:26, 27; 2 Pet. 3:10-12.
- n Rev. 22:19; vs. 10, 27; cf. Heb. 11:10, 16.
- o Rev. 19:7, 8; cf. Eph. 5:25-27; cf. Psa. 45:13-15.
- p *Kingdom* (N.T.). vs. 1-6; 1 Cor. 15:28. (Lk. 1:31-33; 1 Cor. 15:24.)
- q *Inspiration.* Rev. 22:17-19. (Ex. 4:15; Rev. 22:19.)
- r *Death (the second).* (John 8:21.)
- s *Bride (of Christ).* Rev. 19:6-8.
- t *Holy Spirit.* Rev. 22:17. (Mt. 1:18; Acts 2:4.)

in the "day" of Jehovah, and are described in the references beginning with Isa. 34:1-9. (See Mt. 25:32, *note;* Rev. 20:11, *refs.*)

[1] **(20:12)** The final judgment. The subjects are the "dead." As the redeemed were raised from among the dead one thousand years before (v. 5), and have been in glory with Christ during that period, the "dead" can only be the wicked dead, from the beginning to the setting up of the great white throne in space. As there are degrees in punishment (Lk. 12:47, 48), the dead are judged according to their works. The book of life is there to answer such as plead theirs works for justification, e.g. Mt. 7:22, 23; an awful blank where the name might have been.

The Judgments, Summary: Among the many judgments mentioned in Scripture, seven are invested with especial significance. These are: (1) The judgment of the believers' *sins* in the cross of Christ (John 12:31, *note*); (2) the believers' *self*-judgment (1 Cor. 11:31, *note*); (3) the judgment of the believers' *works* (2 Cor. 5:10, *note*); (4) the judgment of the nations at the return of Christ (Mt. 25:32, *note*); (5) the judgment of Israel at the return of Christ (Ezk. 20:37, *note*); (6) the judgment of angels after the one thousand years (Jude 6, *note*); and (7) the judgment of the wicked dead with which the history of the present earth ends.

[2] **(21:8)** Second death, Summary: "The second death" and the "lake of fire" are identical terms (Rev. 20:14) and are used of the eternal state of the wicked. It is "second" relatively to the preceding physical death of the wicked in unbelief and rejection of God; their eternal state is one of eternal "death" (i.e. separation from God) in sins (John 8:21, 24). That the second death is not annihilation is shown by a comparison of Rev. 19:20 with Rev. 20:10. After one thousand years in the lake of fire the Beast and False Prophet are still there, undestroyed. The words "forever and forever"

her [a]light *was* like unto a stone most precious, even like a jasper stone, clear as crystal;

12 And had a wall great and high, *and* had twelve gates, and at the gates twelve [b]angels, and names written thereon, which are [c]*the names* of the [d]twelve tribes of the [e]children of Israel:

13 On the east three gates; on the north three gates; on the south three gates; and on the west three gates.

14 And the wall of the city had twelve [f]foundations, and in them [g]the names of the twelve [h]apostles of the Lamb.

15 And he that talked with me had a golden [i]reed to measure the city, and the gates thereof, and the wall thereof.

16 And the city lieth [j]foursquare, and the length is as large as the breadth: and he measured the city with the reed, twelve thousand [k]furlongs. The length and the breadth and the height of it are equal.

17 And he measured the wall thereof, an hundred *and* forty *and* four cubits, *according to* the measure of a man, that is, of the [b]angel.

18 And the building of the wall of it was *of* jasper: and the city *was* [l]pure gold, like unto clear glass.

19 And the foundations of the wall of the city *were* garnished with all manner of precious stones. The first foundation *was* jasper; the second, sapphire; the third, a chalcedony; the fourth, an emerald;

20 The fifth, sardonyx; the sixth, sardius; the seventh, chrysolite; the eighth, beryl; the ninth, a topaz; the tenth, a chrysoprasus; the eleventh, a jacinth; the twelfth, an amethyst.

21 And the twelve gates *were* twelve [m]pearls; every several gate was of one pearl: and the [n]street of the city *was* pure gold, as it were transparent glass.

(5) *The new temple.*

22 And I saw no temple therein: for the Lord God Almighty [o]and the Lamb are the temple of it.

(6) *The new light.*

23 And the city had no need of the sun, neither of the moon, to shine in it: for the glory of [p]God did lighten it, and the Lamb *is* the [q]light thereof.

24 And the nations of them which are [r]saved [s]shall walk in the light of it: and the kings of the earth do bring their glory and honour [t]into it.

25 And the gates of it shall not be shut

A.D. 96.

- *a brightness.*
- *b* Heb. 1:4, *note.*
- *c Israel (prophecies).* Rom. 11:1-27. (Gen. 12:2, 3; Rom. 11:26.)
- *d* Cf. Ezk. 48:31-34.
- *e sons.*
- *f* Cf. Heb. 11:10.
- *g twelve names.*
- *h* Cf. Eph. 2:20, cf. Lk. 22:29, 30.
- *i* A reed = about 10 ft., also v. 16.
- *j* Cf. 1 Ki. 6:20.
- *k* One furlong = 582 ft.
- *l* Cf. 2 Chr. 3:8.
- *m* Cf. Mt. 13:45, 46 with Eph 5:25.
- *n* Rev. 22:2; cf. Rev. 3:4.
- *o is the temple of it and the Lamb.*
- *p* Isa. 60:19.
- *q lamp.*
- *r* Rom. 1:16, *note.*
- *s shall walk by the light of it.*
- *t unto.*
- *u* Cf. Rev. 22:15.
- *v he that.*
- *w they only, which.*
- *x Life (eternal)* vs. 6, 27; Rev. 22:1, 2, 14, 17, 19. (Mt. 7:14; Rev. 22:19.)
- *y a river;* cf. Rev. 20:15.
- *z* Rev. 4:2, 3.
- *aa* Rev. 21:21.
- *bb Contra,* Gen. 3:6, 7.
- *cc* Cf. Zech. 14:11; *contra,* Gen. 3:17-19.
- *dd* v. 1.
- *ee* Rev. 7:15.
- *ff no more night.*
- *gg lamp.*
- *hh Jehovah.* Isa. 60:19.
- *ii spirits of the prophets.*
- *jj* Rev. 1:1.
- *kk* Heb. 10:37.
- *ll* Heb. 1;4, *note.*
- *mm* Cf. Heb. 1:14.
- *nn Contra,* Rev. 10:4; 5:9.
- *oo* Rev. 1:3; cf. 1 Cor. 7:29.
- *pp doeth unrighteously.*
- *qq do unrighteously*

at all by day: for there shall be no night there.

26 And they shall bring the glory and honour of the nations into it.

27 And there shall in no wise [u]enter into it any thing that defileth, neither [v]*whatsoever* worketh abomination, or *maketh* a lie: but [w]they which are written in the Lamb's [x]book of life.

CHAPTER 22.

(7) *The new Paradise and its river of the water of life.*

And he shewed me [y]a pure river of water of life, clear as crystal, proceeding out of the [z]throne of God and of the Lamb.

2 In the midst of the [aa]street of it, and on either side of the river, *was there* the tree of life, which bare twelve *manner of* fruits, *and* yielded her fruit every month: and the leaves of the tree *were* for the [bb]healing of the nations.

3 And there shall be [cc]no more curse: but [dd]the throne of God and of the Lamb shall be in it; and his [ee]servants shall serve him:

4 And they shall see his face; and his name *shall be* in their foreheads.

5 And there shall be [ff]no night there; and they need no [gg]candle, neither light of the sun; for the [hh]Lord God giveth them light: and they shall reign for ever and ever.

6 And he said unto me, These sayings *are* faithful and true: and the Lord God of the [ii]holy prophets [jj]sent his angel to shew unto his servants the things which must [kk]shortly be done.

7 Behold, I come quickly: blessed *is* he that keepeth the sayings of the prophecy of this book.

The last message of the Bible.

8 And I John saw these things, and heard *them.* And when I had heard and seen, I fell down to worship before the feet of the [ll]angel which shewed me these things.

9 Then saith he unto me, See *thou do it* not: for I am thy [mm]fellowservant, and of thy brethren the prophets, and of them which keep the sayings of this book: worship God.

10 And he saith unto me, [nn]Seal not the sayings of the prophecy of this book: for [oo]the time is at hand.

11 He that [pp]is unjust, let him [qq]be

("to the ages of the ages") are used in Heb. 1:8 for the duration of the throne of God, eternal in the sense of unending.

unjust still: and he which is filthy, let
him be filthy still: and he that is [1]right-
eous, let him be righteous still: and he
that is [2a]holy, let him be holy still.
12 And, behold, I [b]come quickly; and
my [c]reward *is* with me, to give every
man [d]according as his work shall be.
13 I am Alpha and Omega, the beginning and the end, the first and the last.
14 Blessed *are* they that [e]do his commandments, that they may have right to
the tree of life, and may enter in through
the gates into the city.
15 For without *are* dogs, and sorcerers,
and whoremongers, and murderers, and
idolaters, and whosoever loveth and
maketh a lie.
16 I Jesus have sent mine angel to testify unto you these things in [f]the churches. I am the root and the offspring of
David, *and* the bright and morning star.
17 And the [g]Spirit and the bride say,
Come. And let him that heareth say,
Come. And let him that is athirst come.
And whosoever will, let him take the
water of life freely.
18 [h]For I testify unto every man that
heareth the words of the prophecy of
this book, If any man shall add unto
these things, God shall add unto him the
plagues that are written in this book:
19 And if any man shall take away
from the [3]words of the book of this
prophecy, God shall take away his part
out of the [i]book of [4]life, and out of the
holy city, and *from* the things which are
written in this book.

The last promise and the last prayer of the Bible.

20 He which testifieth these things
saith, Surely [j]I come quickly. [k]Amen.
Even so, come, Lord Jesus.
21 The grace of our Lord Jesus Christ
be with you all. Amen.

A.D. 96.

a *Sanctify, holy (persons)* (N.T.). (Mt. 4:5.)
b See v. 20.
c *Rewards.* 1 Cor. 3:14. (Dan. 12:3; 1 Cor. 3:14.)
d *Judgments (the seven).* Rev. 20:12. (2 Sam. 7:14; Rev. 20:12.)
e *wash their robes.*
f *Churches (local).* Phil. 1:1. (Acts 2:41; Phil. 1:1.)
g *Holy Spirit.* Acts 2:4. (Mt. 1:18; Acts 2:4.)
h *Inspiration.* (Ex. 4:15.)
i *Life (eternal).* vs. 1, 2, 14, 17, 19. (Mt. 7:14.)
j *Christ (Second Advent).* vs. 7, 20. (Acts 1:10, 11.)
k *Bible prayers* (N.T.). (Mt. 6:9.)

[1] **(22:11)** See *definitions* O.T. righteousness (Lk. 2:25); N.T. righteousness (Rom. 3:21, *note;* 10:10); righteous living (1 John 3:7); self-righteousness (Rom. 10:3).

[2] **(22:11)** Sanctification, holiness, Summary: (1) In both Testaments the same Hebrew and Greek words are rendered by the English words "sanctify" and "holy," in their various grammatical forms. The one uniform meaning is, "to set apart for God." (2) In both Testaments the words are used of *things* and of *persons.* (3) When used of things no moral quality is implied; they are sanctified or made holy because set apart for God.

(4) Sanctification when used of persons has a threefold meaning. *(a)* In *position,* believers are eternally set apart for God by redemption, "through the offering of the body of Jesus Christ once" (Heb. 10:9, 10). Positionally, therefore, believers are "saints" and "holy" from the moment of believing (Phil. 1:1; Heb. 3:1). *(b)* In *experience,* the believer is *being* sanctified by the work of the Holy Spirit through the Scriptures (John 17:17; 2 Cor. 3:18; Eph. 5:25, 26; 1 Thes. 5:23, 24). *(c)* In *consummation,* the believer's complete sanctification awaits the appearing of the Lord (Eph, 5:27; 1 John 3:2). See "Salvation," Rom. 1:16, *note.*

[3] **(22:19)** Inspiration: Summary. The testimony of the Bible to itself.

(1) The writers affirm, where they speak of the subject at all, that they speak by direct divine authority. (2) They invariably testify that the *words,* and not the ideas merely, are inspired. The most important passage is 1 Cor. 2:7-15, which see. (3) The whole attitude of Jesus Christ toward the Old Testament, as disclosed in His words, both before His death and after His resurrection, confirms its truth and divine origin, and He explicitly ascribes the Pentateuch to Moses. (4) In promising subsequent revelations after the predicted advent of the Spirit (John 16:12-15), our Lord prepared the way for the New Testament. (5) The writers of the New Testament invariably treat the Old Testament as authoritative and inspired. See 2 Pet. 1:19, *note;* 1 Cor. 2:13, *note.*

[4] **(22:19)** Eternal life, Summary of the teaching:

(1) The life is called "eternal" because it was from the eternity which is past unto the eternity which is to come—it is the life of God revealed in Jesus Christ, who is God (John 1:4; 5:26; 1 John 1:1, 2). (2) This life of God, which was revealed in Christ, is imparted in a new birth by the Holy Spirit, acting upon the word of God, to every believer on the Lord Jesus Christ (John 3:3-15). (3) The life thus imparted is not a new life except in the sense of human possession; it is still "that which was from the beginning." But the recipient is a "new creation" (2 Cor. 5:17; Gal. 6:15). (4) The life of God which is in the believer is an unsevered part of the life which eternally was, and eternally is, in Christ Jesus—one life, in Him and in the believer—Vine and branches; Head and members (1 Cor. 6:17; Gal. 2:20; Col. 1:27; 3:3, 4; 1 John 5:11, 12; John 15:1-5; 1 Cor. 12:12-14).

THE END

THE USE OF THE INDEX;

Its Value to the
Preacher, Sunday School Teacher, Evangelist, Christian Worker.

THE Index covers all of the editorial matter in the Scofield Study Bible except the Introductions to the Books and the running Analysis which constitutes the new system of paragraphing, and which has been one of the most acceptable features of this Bible.

In arranging the Index the Editor, who is himself a preacher, has had largely in view the helping of preachers to sermonic material. Experience had taught him the need and the best way to meet the need.

These main features are prominent:—

(1) The suggestion of a theme. The demands upon the time of the modern minister are so various as to leave the mind, often, in some measure of distraction when the time comes for preparing the two inevitable sermons for the Lord's day.

It will be found that simply to go over the Index thoughtfully will afford a wealth of suggestion for topical, expository, and thematic sermons, from which the preacher may choose.

(2) The editorial notation to which the Index gives reference will often be found to suggest at once the *logical and biblical outline* which a sermon on that theme should follow, while the passages referred to in the note or summary will give both the background and a wealth of *biblical illustration.*

(3) But perhaps the best service of the Index to the Bible preacher is in the suggestion of *series of sermons* on the great themes of Scripture.

The experience of the great constructive ministers is conclusive that no other form of teaching so permanently interests congregations. They soon come to feel that they are "getting somewhere."

Take, for example, the central theme of the Bible—Christ. The Index will be found to refer to *one hundred and thirty-four* distinct lines of truth concerning Christ. From these may be selected series of sermon subjects which will enable the preacher to give connected studies of that supreme Person once a year through many years without repetition. And this is true of the Holy Spirit, as also of all the great words of the Bible.

And not the preacher only, but the Sunday School teacher, or Evangelist—indeed any Christian worker, will find the Index the open door to the mighty riches of the Bible.

INDEX

TO THE
INTRODUCTION, ANALYSES, NOTES, DEFINITIONS, SUMMARIES, AND SUBJECT REFERENCES
IN THE
SCOFIELD STUDY BIBLE.

(Subject-references are indicated by italics.)

DICTIONARY OF
SCRIPTURE PROPER NAMES

SUBJECT–INDEX

CONCORDANCE

MAPS

DICTIONARY OF
SCRIPTURE PROPER NAMES

TOGETHER WITH COMPENDIOUS REFERENCES TO SOME OF THE PRINCIPAL INCIDENTS CONNECTED WITH THE PERSONS AND PLACES MENTIONED IN HOLY SCRIPTURE

[NOTE.— *The accent (´) shows where the stress of the voice should fall. (?) denotes meanings which are conjectural. Modern research has caused some of the older interpretations given in this list to be questioned.*]

AARON, a´-ron, light (?). Ex. 4:14.
Brother of MOSES, the FIRST HIGH PRIEST, cometh forth to meet Moses; can speak well. appointed by God to be Moses' spokesman. Ex. 4:14, 16, 27.
with Moses appeals to Pharaoh; chided by him. Ex. 5:1.
his rod becomes a serpent. Ex. 7:10.
changes the waters into blood. Ex. 7:20.
causes the plagues of frogs, lice, flies. Ex. 8:5, 17, 24.
with Moses—the plague of boils. Ex. 9:10.
with Hur holds up Moses' hands. Ex. 17:12.
set apart for priest's office. Ex. 28.
makes the golden calf. Ex. 32:4; God's anger thereat. Ex. 32:7; Deut. 9:20.
his excuse to Moses. Ex. 32:22.
consecration. Ex. 29; Lev. 8.
offers sacrifice. Lev. 9.
his sons (Nadab and Abihu) offer strange fire, and die. Lev. 10:1; Num. 3:4.
his sons (Eleazar and Ithamar) censured by Moses. Lev. 10:16.
not to drink wine when going into the tabernacle. Lev. 10:8.
speaks against Moses. Num. 12.
rebuked by God. Num. 12:9.
spoken against by Korah. Num. 16:3.
makes atonement, and the plague is stayed. Num. 16:46-48.
his rod buds, and is kept in ark for a token. Num. 17:8.
for unbelief excluded from the promised land. Num. 20:12.
dies on mount Hor. Num. 20:28.
chosen by God. Ps. 105:26; Heb. 5:4.
his line. 1 Chr. 6:49.

AARONITES, a´-ron-ites, descendants of Aaron. 1 Chr. 12:27.

ABADDON, a-bad´-don, destruction.
angel of the bottomless pit. Rev. 9:11.

ABAGTHA, a-bag´-thah, given by fortune. Esth. 1:10.

ABANA, a-ba´-nah, stony.
river of Damascus. 2 Kin. 5:12.

ABARIM, a-ba´-rim, regions beyond. Num. 27:12.
mountains of, including Nebo, Pisgah, Hor. Deut. 32:49.

ABBA, ab´-bah, father. Mark 14:36; Rom. 8:15; Gal. 4:6.

ABDA, ab´-dah, servant. 1 Kin. 4:6.

ABDEEL, ab´-de-el, same as ABDIEL. Jer. 36:26.

ABDI, ab´-di, servant of Jehovah. 1 Chr. 6:44.

ABDIEL, ab´-di-el, *s.* of God. 1 Chr. 5:15.

ABDON, ab´-don, servile. A judge. Judg. 12:13.

ABED-NEGO, a-bed´-ne-go, servant or worshipper of Nebo. Dan. 1:7.
saved in fiery furnace. Dan. 3. *See* Is. 43:2.

ABEL, a´-bel, (1) vanity. Gen. 4:2. (2) A meadow. 2 Sam. 20:14.
second son of Adam. Gen. 4:2.

ABEL—*cont.*
his offering accepted. Gen. 4:4.
slain by Cain. Gen. 4:8.
righteous. Matt. 23:35; 1 John 3:12.
blood of. Luke 11:51; Heb. 12:24.
faith of. Heb. 11:4.

ABEL-BETH-MAACHAH, a´-bel-beth-ma´-a-kah, meadow of the house of Maachah. 1 Kin. 15:20.

ABEL-MAIM, a´-bel-ma´-im, *m.* of the waters. 2 Chr. 16:4.

ABEL-MEHOLAH, a´-bel-me-ho´-lah, *m.* of dancing. Judg. 7:22; 1 Kin. 4:12; 19:16.

ABEL-MIZRAIM, a´-bel-miz-ra´-im, *m.* of Egypt.
Mourning of the Egyptians. Gen. 50:11.

ABEL-SHITTIM, a´-bel-shit´-im, *m.* of acacias. Num. 33:49.

ABEZ, a´-bez, whiteness. Josh. 19:20.

ABI, a´-bi, shortened form of ABIAH. 2 Kin. 18:2.

ABIA, a-bi´-ah, Greek form of following. Matt. 1:7.

ABIAH, a-bi´-ah, same as ABIJAH. 2 Kin. 18:2.

ABI-ALBON, a´-bi-al´-bon, father of strength. 2 Sam. 23:31.

ABIASAPH, a-bi´-a-saf, *f.* of gathering. Ex. 6:24.

ABIATHAR, ab-ia´-thar, *f.* of plenty. 1 Sam. 22:20.

ABIB, a´-bib, an ear of corn, or green ear. Ex. 13:4.
the Hebrew passover month. Ex. 23:15; 34:18.

ABIDAH, a-bi´-dah, father of knowledge. Gen. 25:4.

ABIDAN, a-bi´-dan, *f.* of a judge. Num. 1:11.

ABIEL, a-bi´-el, *f.* of strength. 1 Sam. 9:1.

ABIEZER, a´-bi-e´-zer, *f.* of help. Josh. 17:2.
ancestor of Gideon. Judg. 6.

ABIEZRITE, a´-bi-ez´-rite, a descendant of ABIEZER. Judg. 6:11.

ABIGAIL, a-bi-ga´-le, father of exultation. 1 Sam. 25:14.
wife of Nabal, and afterwards of David. 1 Sam. 25:39.
mother of Chileab, according to 2 Sam. 3:3, or Daniel, according to 1 Chr. 3:1.

ABIHAIL, a-bi-ha´-le, *f.* of strength. Num. 3:35.

ABIHU, a-bi´-hoo, He (*i.e.* God) is my *f.* Ex. 6:23.
brother of Nadab, offers strange fire, and dies. Lev. 10:2.

ABIHUD, a-bi´-hood, *f.* of Judah. 1 Chr. 8:3.

ABIJAH, a-bi´-jah, *f.* of Jehovah. 1 Kin. 14:1.
king of Judah, walked in the sins of his father. 1 Kin. 15:3.
makes war against Israel. 2 Chr. 13.
——(son of Jeroboam), his death foretold by Ahijah the prophet. 1 Kin. 14:12.

ABIJAM, a-bi´-jam, another mode of spelling ABIJAH. 1 Kin. 14:31.

ABILENE, a´-bi-le´-ne, a grassy place (?). Luke 3:1.

ABIMAEL, a-bi-ma´-el, father of Mael. Gen. 10:28.

ABIMELECH, a-bi´-me-lek, *f.* of the king. Gen. 20:2.
(king of Gerar) reproved by God about Abraham's wife. Gen. 20:3.
rebukes Abraham and restores Sarah. Gen. 20:9, 14.
healed at Abraham's prayer. Gen. 20:17.

ABIMELECH—*cont.*
——(another), Isaac rebuked by, for denying his wife. Gen. 26:10.
covenants with Isaac. Gen. 26:27.
——(king at Shechem), son of the judge Gideon. Judg. 8:31.
murders his brethren. Judg. 9:5.
his death. Judg. 9:54.
ABINADAB, a-bi´-na-dab, *f.* of nobility. 1 Sam. 7:1.
receives the ark from Philistines. 2 Sam. 6:3.
ABINER, ab´-ner, same as ABNER. 1 Sam. 14:50.
ABINOAM, a-bi-no´-am, *f.* of pleasantness. Judg. 4:6.
ABIRAM, a-bi´-ram, *f.* of loftiness. Num. 16:1.
with Korah and Dathan, rebels against Moses. Num. 16.
his punishment. Num. 16:31; 26:10.
ABISHAG, a-bi´-shag, *f.* of error (?). 1 Kin. 1:3.
the Shunammite, ministers to David, cause of breach between Solomon and Adonijah. 1 Kin. 2:22.
ABISHAI, a-bi´-shai, *f.* of a gift. 1 Sam. 26:6.
brother of Joab. 1 Chr. 2:16.
with David carries off Saul's spear. 1 Sam. 26:6-9.
slays three hundred men. 2 Sam. 23:18. *See also* 1 Chr. 11:20; 18:12.
ABISHALOM, a-bi´-sha-lom´, *f.* of peace. 1 Kin. 15:2.
ABISHUA, a-bi-sho´o-ah, *f.* of welfare. 1 Chr. 6:4.
ABISHUR, a-bi´-shoor, *f.* of the wall. 1 Chr. 2:28.
ABITAL, a-bi´-tal, *f.* of dew. 2 Sam. 3:4.
ABITUB, a-bi´-toob, *f.* of goodness. 1 Chr. 8:11.
ABIUD, a-bi´-ood, Greek form of ABIHUD. Matt. 1:13.
ABNER, ab´-ner, *f.* of light. 1 Sam. 14:50.
cousin of Saul, commander of his army. 1 Sam. 14:50.
reproved by David. 1 Sam. 26:5, 14.
makes Ish-bosheth king. 2 Sam. 2:8.
goes over to David. 2 Sam. 3:8.
slain by Joab. 2 Sam. 3:27.
mourned by David. 2 Sam. 3:31.
ABRAM, ab´-ram, a high *f.* Gen. 11:26.
ABRAHAM, a´-bra-ham, *f.* of a great multitude. Gen. 17:5.
——(Abram) begotten by Terah. Gen. 11:27.
blessed by God, and sent to Canaan. Gen. 12:5.
goes down to Egypt. Gen. 12:10.
causes his wife to pass as his sister. Gen. 12:13; 20:2.
strife between him and Lot. Gen. 13:7.
separates from Lot. Gen. 13:11.
his seed to be as the dust of the earth. Gen. 13:16.
delivers Lot from captivity, and refuses the spoil. Gen. 14:16.
blessed by Melchizedek, king of Salem. Gen. 14:19; Heb. 7:4.
his faith counted for righteousness. Gen. 15:6.
God's covenant with. Gen. 15:18; Ps. 105:9.
he and house circumcised. Gen. 17.
entertains angels. Gen. 18.
pleads for Sodom. Gen. 18:23.
sends away Hagar and Ishmael. Gen. 21:14.
his faith in offering Isaac. Gen. 22.
buys Machpelah of Ephron the Hittite for a burying place. Gen. 23.
sends for a wife for his son. Gen. 24.
gives his goods to Isaac. Gen. 25:5.
dies (in a good old age). Gen. 25:8.
his faith and works. Is. 41:8; 51:2; John 8:31; Acts 7:2; Rom. 4; Gal. 3:6; Heb. 11:8; James 2:21.
his posterity. Gen. 25:1.
ABSALOM, ab´-sa-lom, *f.* of peace. 2 Sam. 3:3.
David's son. 2 Sam. 3:3.
slays Amnon. 2 Sam. 13:28.
conspires against David. 2 Sam. 15.
David flies from. 2 Sam. 15:17.
caught by head in an oak. 2 Sam. 18:9.
slain by Joab. 2 Sam. 18:14.
wept by David. 2 Sam. 18:33; 19:1.

ACCAD, ak´-ad, fortress (?). Gen. 10:10.
ACCHO, ak´-o, sand-heated. Judg. 1:31.
ACELDAMA, a-kel´-da-mah´, field of blood. Matt. 27:8; Acts 1:19.
ACHAIA, a-ka´-yah, Greece. Acts 18:12.
Paul in. Acts 18.
contribution for poor by. Rom. 15:26; 2 Cor. 9:2. *See* 1 Cor. 16:15; 2 Cor. 11:10.
ACHAICUS, a-ka´-ik-us, belonging to Achaia. 1 Cor. 16:17.
ACHAN, or ACHAR, a´-kan, a´-kar, troubler. Josh. 7:18.
takes the accursed thing; is stoned. Josh. 7; 22:20; 1 Chr. 2:7.
ACHAZ, a´-kaz, Greek form of AHAZ. Matt. 1:9.
ACHBOR, ak´-bor, a mouse. Gen. 36:38.
ACHIM, a´-kim, short form of JACHIN (?). Matt. 1:14.
ACHISH, a´-kish, angry (?).
king of Gath, succours David. 1 Sam. 21:10; 27:2, 28:1; 29:6. *See* 1 Kin. 2:39.
ACHMETHA, ak´-me-thah, fortress (?). Ezra 6:2.
ACHOR, a´-kor, trouble. Josh. 7:24.
valley of, Achan slain there. Josh. 7:26. *See* Hos. 2:15.
ACHSA, ak´-sah, same as following. 1 Chr. 2:49.
ACHSAH, ak´-sah, anklet. Josh. 15:16.
Caleb's daughter, won in marriage by Othniel. Judg. 1:13.
asks her father's blessing. Judg. 1:15.
ACHSHAPH, ak´-shaf, enchantment. Josh. 11:1.
ACHZIB, ak´-zib, deceit. Josh. 15:44.
ADADAH, a´d-a-dah, festival (?). Josh. 15:22.
ADAH, a´-dah, ornament. Gen. 4:19.
ADAIAH, a-da´-yah, whom Jehovah adorns. 2 Kin. 22:1.
ADALIA, a-da´lyah, upright (?). Esth. 9:8.
ADAM, a´-dam, red. Gen. 2:19.
created. Gen. 1.
called the son of God. Luke 3:38.
blessed. Gen. 1:28.
placed in Eden. Gen. 2:8.
first called Adam. Gen. 2:19.
creatures named by. Gen. 2:19.
calls his wife Eve. Gen. 3:20.
his fall and punishment. Gen. 3.
hides from God. Gen. 3:8.
ground cursed for his sake. Gen. 3:17.
his death. Gen. 5:5.
his transgression. Job 31:33; Rom. 5:14.
first Adam. 1 Cor. 15:45; 1 Tim. 2:13.
in, all die. 1 Cor. 15:22.
ADAM, the last. 1 Cor. 15:45.
ADAMAH, a-dah´-mah, red earth. Josh. 19:36.
ADAMI, a-da´h-mi, human. Josh. 19:33.
ADAR, a´-dar, fire (?). Esth. 3:7.
ADBEEL, ad´-be-el, miracle of God (?). Gen. 25:13.
ADDAN, a´d-dahn, humble (?).
a city of the captivity. Ezra 2:59.
ADDAR, a´d-dar, greatness (?). 1 Chr. 8:3.
ADDI, a´d-di, ornament (?). Luke 3:28.
ADDON, a´d-don, same as ADDAN. Neh. 7:61.
ADER, a´-der, flock. 1 Chr. 8:15.
ADIEL, a´-di-el, ornament of God. 1 Chr. 4:36.
ADIN, a´-din, slender. Ezra 2:15.
ADINA, a-di´-nah, same as preceding. 1 Chr. 11:42.
ADINO, a-di´-no. 2 Sam. 23:8.
ADITHAIM, a-di-tha´-im, twofold ornament. Josh. 15:36.
ADLAI, a´d-lai, just (?). 1 Chr. 27:29.
ADMAH, ad´-mah, same as ADAMAH. Gen. 10:19.
city of the plain. *See* SODOM.
ADMATHA, ad´-math-ah. Esth. 1:14.
ADNA, ad´-nah, pleasure. Ezra 10:30.
ADNAH, same as preceding. 2 Chr. 17:14.
ADONI-BEZEK, a-do´-ni-be´-zek, lord of Bezek. Judg. 1:5.
ADONIJAH, a´-do-ni´-jah, Jehovah is my Lord. 2 Sam. 3:4.
fourth son of David, usurps the kingdom. 1 Kin. 1:5, 11, 25.

ADONIJAH—*cont.*
is pardoned by Solomon. 1 Kin. 1:53.
seeking to obtain Abishag, is slain. 1 Kin. 2:17-25.
ADONIKAM, a´-do-ni´-kam, lord of enemies. Ezra 2:13.
ADONIRAM, a´-do-ni´-ram, lord of height. 1 Kin. 4:6.
ADONI-ZEDEC, a-do´-ni-ze´-dek, lord of justice.
king of Jerusalem, resists Joshua. Josh. 10:1.
his death. Josh. 10:26.
ADORAIM, a-do-ra´-im, two chiefs (?). 2 Chr. 11:9.
ADORAM, a-do´-ram, contracted from ADONIRAM. 2 Sam. 20:24.
ADRAMMELECH, ad-ram´-me-lek, magnificence of the king (?), king of fire (?). 2 Kin. 17:31.
ADRAMYTTIUM, ad´-ra-mit´-ti-um. Acts 27:2.
ADRIA, a´-dri-ah. Acts 27:27.
ADRIEL, a´d-ri-el, flock of God. 1 Sam. 18:19.
ADULLAM, a-dul´-am, justice of the people. Josh. 12:15.
cave of. 1 Sam. 22:1; 1 Chr. 11:15.
ADULLAMITE, a-dul´-am-ite, a native of Adullam. Gen. 38:1.
ADUMMIM, a-dum´-im, the red (men ?). Josh. 15:7.
ÆNEAS, e´-ne-as, praiseworthy (?).
healing of. Acts 9:33.
ÆNON, e´-non, springs. John baptizes at. John 3:23.
AGABUS, ag´-ab-us, probably Greek form of HAGAB.
famine and Paul's sufferings foretold by. Acts 11:28; 21:10.
AGAG, a´-gag, flaming (?). Num. 24:7.
king of Amalek, spared by Saul, slain by Samuel. 1 Sam. 15.
spoken of by Balaam. Num. 24.
AGAGITE, a´-gag-ite. Esth. 3:1.
AGAR, a´-gar, same as HAGAR. Gal. 4:24.
AGEE, a´-gee, fugitive (?). 2 Sam. 23:11.
AGRIPPA, a-grip´-ah. Acts 25:13.
Paul's defence before. Acts 25:22; 26.
almost persuaded. Acts 26:28.
AGUR, a´-goor, an assembler.
prophecy. Prov. 30.
AHAB, a´-hab, uncle.
king of Israel. 1 Kin. 16:29.
marries Jezebel; his idolatry. 1 Kin. 16:31.
meets Elijah. 1 Kin. 18:17.
defeats the Syrians. 1 Kin. 20.
punished for sparing Ben-hadad. 1 Kin. 20:42.
takes Naboth's vineyard. 1 Kin. 21:17.
his repentance. 1 Kin. 21:27.
trusts false prophets, and is mortally wounded at Ramoth-gilead. 1 Kin. 22:6, 34; 2 Chr. 18.
——(son of Kolaiah), and Zedekiah, lying prophets. Jer. 29:21.
AHARAH, a´-har-ah, after the brother. 1 Chr. 8:1.
AHARHEL, a-har´-hel, behind the breastwork. 1 Chr. 4:8.
AHASAI, a´-ha-zai, probably a corruption of JAHZERAH. Neh. 11:13.
AHASBAI, a-ha´s-bai. 2 Sam. 23:34.
AHASUERUS, a-haz-u-e´-rus, king (?).
reigns from India to Ethiopia. Esth. 1:1.
Vashti's disobedience to, and divorce. Esth. 1:12; 2:4.
makes Esther queen. Esth. 2:17.
advances Haman. Esth. 3:1.
his decree to destroy the Jews. Esth. 3:12.
rewards Mordecai's loyalty. Esth. 6.
hangs Haman. Esth. 7:9; 8:7.
advances Mordecai. Esth. 9:4; 10.
AHAVA, a´-ha-vah. Ezra 8:15.
AHAZ, a´-haz, possessor. 2 Kin. 15:38.
king of Judah. 2 Kin. 16.
spoils the temple. 2 Kin. 16:17.
his idolatry. 2 Chr. 28:2.
afflicted by Syrians. 2 Chr. 28:5.
comforted by Isaiah. Is. 7.
will not ask a sign. Is. 7:12.
AHAZIAH, a´-haz-i´-ah, whom Jehovah upholds. 1 Kin. 22:40.

AHAZIAH—*cont.*
king of Judah, his wicked reign. 2 Kin. 8:25.
goes with Joram to meet Jehu. 2 Kin. 9:21.
smitten by Jehu. 2 Kin. 9:27; 2 Chr. 22:9.
——king of Israel. 1 Kin. 22:40, 49.
his sickness and idolatry. 2 Kin. 1.
his judgment by Elijah. 2 Kin. 1.
AHBAN, ah´-ban, brotherly. 1 Chr. 2:29.
AHER, a´-her, following. 1 Chr. 7:12.
AHI, a´-hi, brother. 1 Chr. 5:15.
AHIAH, a-hi´-ah, brother of Jehovah. 1 Sam. 14:3.
AHIAM, a-hi´-am, *b.* of the father (?). 2 Sam. 23:33.
AHIAN, a-hi´-an, brotherly. 1 Chr. 7:19.
AHIEZER, a´-hi-e´-zer, brother of help. Num. 1:12.
AHIHUD, a-hi´-hood, *b.* of (?). Num. 34:27.
AHIJAH, a-hi´-jah, same as AHIAH. 1 Kin. 11:29.
prophesies to Jeroboam against Solomon. 1 Kin. 11:31; against Jeroboam, and foretells his son's death. 1 Kin. 14:7.
AHIKAM, a-hi´-kam, *b.* of the enemy. 2 Kin. 22:12.
protects Jeremiah. Jer. 26:24.
AHILUD, a-hi´-lood, *b.* of one born. 2 Sam. 8:16.
AHIMAAZ, a-hi-ma´-az, *b* of anger.
son of Zadok, serves David. 2 Sam. 15:27; 17:17; 18:19.
AHIMAN, a-hi´-man, *b.* of a gift. Num. 13:22.
AHIMELECH, a-hi´-me-lek, *b.* of the king. 1 Sam. 21:1.
slain by Saul's order, for assisting David. 1 Sam. 22:18.
AHIMOTH, a-hi´-moth, *b.* of death. 1 Chr. 6:25.
AHINADAB, a-hi´na-dab, *b.* of a nobleman. 1 Kin. 4:14.
AHINOAM, a-hi-no´-am, *b.* of grace. 1 Sam. 14:50.
AHIO, a-hi´-o, brotherly. 2 Sam. 6:3.
AHIRA, a-hi´-rah, *b.* of a wicked man. Num. 1:15.
AHIRAM, a-hi´-ram, *b.* of a tall man. Num. 26:38.
AHIRAMITE, a-hi´-ram-ite, a descendant of Ahiram. Num. 26:38.
AHISAMACH, a-hi´-sa-mak, *b.* of aid. Ex. 31:6.
AHISHAHAR, a-hi´-sha-har, *b.* of the dawn. 1 Chr. 7:10.
AHISHAR, a-hi´-shar, *b.* of the singer. 1 Kin. 4:6.
AHITHOPHEL, a-hi´-tho-fel, *b.* of impiety. 2 Sam. 15:12.
his treachery. 2 Sam. 15:31; 16:20.
disgrace, and suicide. 2 Sam. 17:1, 23. *See* Ps. 41:9; 55:12; 109.
AHITUB, a-hi´-toob, *b.* of goodness. 1 Sam. 14:3.
AHLAB, ah´-lab, fertility. Judg. 1:31.
AHLAI, ah´-lai, sweet (?). 1 Chr. 2:31.
AHOAH, a-ho´-ah, same as AHIJAH (?). 1 Chr. 8:4.
AHOHLTE, a-hoh´-ite, a descendant of Ahoah. 2 Sam. 23:9.
AHOLAH, a-ho´-lah, (she has) her own tent.
——(Samaria), and Aholibah (Jerusalem), their adulteries. Ezek. 23:4.
AHOLIAB, a´-holi-a´b, father's tent. Ex. 31:6.
inspired to construct the tabernacle. Ex. 35:34; 36, &c.
AHOLIBAH, a´-holi-b´ah, my tent is in her. Ezek. 23:4.
AHOLIBAMAH, a´-holi-ba´-mah, tent of the high place. Gen. 36:2.
AHUMAI, a-hoo´-mai, brother of (*i.e.* dweller near) water. 1 Chr. 4:2.
AHUZAM, a-hooz´-am, their possession. 1 Chr. 4:6.
AHUZZATH, a-hooz´-ath, possession. Gen. 26:26.
AI, a´i, a heap of ruins. Josh. 7:2.
men of, contend with Israel. Josh. 7:5.
AIAH, ai´-ah, hawk. 2 Sam. 3:7.
AIJA, ai´-jah, same as AI. Neh. 11:31.
AJAH, a´-jah, same as AIAH. Gen. 36:24.
AIATH, ai´-ath, ruins. Is. 10:28.
AIJALON, ai´-ja-lon, place of gazelles. Josh. 21:24.
AIJELETH SHAHAR, ai-ye´-leth sha´-har, morning hind. Ps. 22 Title.
AIN, a´-in, an eye, or fountain. Num. 34:11.
AJALON, ad´-jal-on, same as AIJALON. Josh. 19:42.
AKAN, a´-kan. Gen. 36:27.
AKKUB, a´k-kub, insidious. 1 Chr. 3:24.

AKRABBIM, ak-rab-´bim, scorpions. Num. 34:4.
ALAMETH, a-la-´meth, covering. 1 Chr. 7:8.
ALAMMELECH, a-la´m-me-lek, king's oak. Josh. 19:26.
ALAMOTH, a-la-moth´, virgins (?). Ps. 46 title.
ALEMETH, a-le-´meth, same as ALAMETH. 1 Chr. 8:36.
ALEXANDER, al-´ex-an-´der, defending men. Mark 15:21.
——a member of the council. Acts 4:6.
——an Ephesian Jew. Acts 19:33.
——the coppersmith. 1 Tim. 1:20; 2 Tim. 4:14.
ALEXANDRIA, al-´ex-an-´dri-a, the city named after Alexander. Acts 18:24.
ALIAH, a´l-iah, same as ALVAH. 1 Chr. 1:51.
ALIAN, a´l-ian, same as ALVAN. 1 Chr. 1:40.
ALLELUIA, al-el-oo-´ya, praise ye the Lord. Rev. 19:1.
ALLON, al-´on, an oak. 1 Chr. 4:37.
ALLON-BACHUTH, al-on-bak-´ooth, oak of weeping. Gen. 35:8; 1 Kin. 13:14.
ALMODAD, al-mo-´dad, extension (?). Gen. 10:26.
ALMON, al-´mon, hidden. Josh. 21:18.
ALMON-DIBLATHAIM, al-´mon-dib-´ath-a-´im, hiding of the two cakes (?). Num. 33:46.
ALOTH, a-´loth, yielding milk (?). 1 Kin. 4:16.
ALPHA, al-´fah, the first letter of the Greek alphabet. Rev. 1:8; 21:6; 22:13.
ALPHÆUS, al-fee-´us, successor. Matt. 10:3.
AL-TASCHITH, al-´tash-kith´, 'do not destroy.' Ps. 57 title.
ALUSH, a-´loosh. Num. 33:13.
ALVAH, al-´vah. Gen. 36:40.
ALVAN, a´l-vahn, tall. Gen. 36:23.
AMAD, a´m-ad, eternal people (?). Josh. 19:26.
AMAL, a-´mal, labour, sorrow. 1 Chr. 7:35.
AMALEK, am-´al-ek. Gen. 36:12.
fights with Israel in Rephidim, and is defeated. Ex. 17:8, 13.
perpetual war declared against. Ex. 17:16; Deut. 25:17.
smitten by Gideon. Judg. 7:12.
by Saul. 1 Sam. 14:48; 15:8.
by David. 1 Sam. 27:9; 30:17.
AMALEKITE, am-al-´ek-ite, self-accused of killing Saul, slain by David. 2 Sam. 1:10, 15.
AMALEKITES, am-al-´ek-ites, descendants of Amalek. Gen. 14:7.
AMAM, a-´mam, metropolis (?). Josh. 15:26.
AMANA, a-ma-´nah, fixed (?). Cant. 4:8.
AMARIAH, a-´mar-i-´ah, Jehovah has said. 1 Chr. 6:7.
AMASA, a-ma-´sa, burden.
captain of the host of Absalom. 2 Sam. 17:25.
slain by Joab. 2 Sam. 20:9, 10; 1 Kin. 2:5.
AMASAI, a-ma-´sai, burdensome. 1 Chr. 6:25.
AMASHAI, a-ma´sh-ai. Neh. 11:13.
AMASIAH, a-´mas-i-´ah, burden of Jehovah. 2 Chr. 17:16.
AMAZIAH, a-´maz-i-´ah, Jehovah strengthens.
king of Judah, his good reign. 2 Kin. 14:1; 2 Chr. 25:1.
defeats Edom. 2 Chr. 25:11.
defeated by Joash king of Israel. 2 Chr. 25:21.
slain at Lachish. 2 Kin. 14:19.
——priest of Beth-el. Amos 7:10.
AMI, a-´mi, probably same as AMON. Ezra 2:57.
AMINADAB, a-mi-´na-dab, same as AMMINADAB. Matt. 1:4.
AMITTAI, a-mi´t-tai, true. 2 Kin. 14:25.
AMMAH, am-´ah. 2 Sam. 2:24.
AMMI, am-´i, my people. Hos. 2:1.
AMMIEL, am-´i-el, people of God. Num. 13:12.
AMMIHUD, am-i-´hood, *p.* of praise (?). Num. 1:10.
AMMINADAB, am-i-´na-dab, *p.* of the prince. Ex. 6:23.
AMMINADIB, am-i-´na-dib, same as preceding. Cant. 6:12.
AMMISHADDAI, a´m-sha´d-ai, *p.* of the Almighty. Num. 1:12.
AMMIZABAD, am-i-´za-bad, *p.* of the giver (*i.e.* Jehovah). 1 Chr. 27:6.

AMMON, am-´on, son of my *p.* (?).
children of. Gen. 19:38.
not to be meddled with. Deut. 2:19.
not to enter the congregation. Deut. 23:3.
make war on Israel, and are conquered by Jephthah. Judg. 11:4, 33.
slain by Saul. 1 Sam. 11:11.
outrage David's servants. 2 Sam. 10.
tortured by David. 2 Sam. 12:26.
prophecies concerning. Jer. 25:21; 49:1; Ezek. 21:28; 25:2, 3; Amos 1:13; Zeph. 2:8.
AMMONITES, am-´on-ites, a tribe descended from Ammon. Deut. 2:20.
AMMONITESS, am-´on-ite-ess, feminine of preceding. 2 Chr. 12:13.
AMNON, am-´non, faithful.
son of David. 2 Sam. 3:2.
outrages Tamar. 2 Sam. 13.
slain by Absalom. 2 Sam. 13:28.
AMOK, a-´mok, deep. Neh. 12:7.
AMON, a-´mon. 2 Kin. 21:18.
king of Judah. 2 Kin. 21:19; 2 Chr. 33:20.
his idolatry. 2 Kin. 21:21; 2 Chr. 33:23.
killed by his servants. 2 Kin. 21:23.
AMORITE, am-´or-ite, mountaineer. Gen. 10:16.
AMORITES, am-´or-ites, their iniquities, Gen. 15:16; Deut. 20:17; Josh. 3:10.
AMOS, a-´mos, burden.
declares God's judgment upon the nations. Amos 1:1, 2.
and upon Israel. Amos 3:1, &c.
his call. Amos 7:14, 15.
foretells Israel's restoration. Amos 9:11.
AMOZ, a-´moz, strong. Is. 1:1.
AMPHIPOLIS, am-phi-´pol-is, named from the river Strymon flowing *round the city*. Acts 17:1.
AMPLIAS, am-´pli-as, short form of AMPLIATUS, enlarged. Rom. 16:8.
AMRAM, am-´ram, people of the Highest (*i.e.* God). Ex. 6:18.
AMRAMITES, am-´ram-ites, the descendants of Amram. Num. 3:27.
AMRAPHAEL, am-´ra-fel. Gen. 14:1.
AMZI, am-´zi, strong. 1 Chr. 6:46.
ANAB, a-´nab, place fertile in grapes. Josh. 11:21.
ANAH, a-´nah. Gen. 36:2.
ANAHARATH, a-na-´har-ath. Josh. 19:19.
ANAIAH, an-ai-´ah, Jehovah has answered. Neh. 8:4.
ANAK, a-´nak, long-necked (?). Num. 13:22.
ANAKIM, a-´nak-im, a tribe called after Anak. Deut. 1:28.
——(giants). Num. 13:33; Deut. 9:2.
cut off by Joshua. Josh. 11:21.
ANAMIM, a-´nam-im. Gen. 10:13.
ANAMMELECH, a-nam-´me-lek, idol of the king (?), or shepherd and flock (?). 2 Kin. 17:31.
ANAN, a-´nan, a cloud. Neh. 10:26.
ANANI, an-a-´ni, shortened form of ANANIAH. 1 Chr. 3:24.
ANANIAH, an-an-i-´ah, whom Jehovah covers. Neh. 3:23.
ANANIAS, an-an-i-´as, Greek form of HANANIAH.
——(and Sapphira), their lie and death. Acts 5:1.
——(disciple), sent to Paul at Damascus. Acts 9:10; 22:12.
——(high priest), Paul brought before. Acts 22:30.
Paul smitten by order of. Acts 23:2.
rebuked by Paul. Acts 23:3.
ANATH, a-´nath, an answer to prayer. Judg. 3:31.
ANATHEMA, an-ath-´em-ah, something accursed. 1 Cor. 16:22.
ANATHOTH, a-´nath-oth, answers to prayer. Josh. 21:18.
men of, condemned for persecuting Jeremiah. Jer. 11:21. *See* 1 Kin. 2:26.
ANDREW, an-´droo. Mark 1:29.
the APOSTLE. Matt. 4:18; Mark 13:3; John 1:40; 6:8; 12:22; Acts 1:13.
ANDRONICUS, an-´dro-ni-´kus, disciple at Rome, Rom. 16:7.

ANEM, a´-nem, same as EN-GANNIM (?). 1 Chr. 6:73.
ANER, a´-ner, a young man (?). Gen. 14:13.
ANETHOTHITE, a´n-e-tho-thite, or ANETOTHITE, a´n-e-to-thite, aman of Anathoth. 2 Sam. 23:27.
ANIAM, a-ni´-am. 1 Chr. 7:19.
ANIM, a´-nim, fountains. Josh. 15:50.
ANNA, an´-ah, grace. A prophetess. Luke 2:36.
ANNAS, an´-as, Greek form of HANANIAH.
high priest. Luke 3:2.
Christ brought to. John 18:13, 24.
Peter and John before. Acts 4:6.
ANTICHRIST, an´-ti-christ, adversary to Christ. 1 John 2:18, 22; 2 John 7. *See* 2 Thess. 2:9; 1 Tim. 4:1.
ANTIOCH, an´-ti-ok, named in honour of Antiochus. Acts 6:5.
——(Syria), disciples first called Christians at. Acts 11:26.
Barnabas and Saul called to apostleship at. Acts 13:1.
Paul withstands Peter at. Gal. 2:11.
——(Pisidia), Paul's first address at. Acts 13:16.
Paul and Barnabas persecuted at. Acts 13:50.
ANTIPAS, an´-tip-as, contraction of Antipater.
Martyr. Rev. 2:13.
ANTIPATRIS, an´-tip-atr´-is, from the foregoing. Acts 23:31.
ANTOTHIJAH, an´-to-thi´-jah, prayers answered by Jehovah (?). 1 Chr. 8:24.
ANTOTHITE, an´-toth-ite, a man of Anathoth. 1 Chr. 11:28.
ANUB, a´-noob, bound together (?). 1 Chr. 4:8.
APELLES, a-pel´-es. Saluted by Paul. Rom. 16:10.
APHARSACHITES, a-far-sa-kites. Ezra 5:6.
APHARSATHCHITES, a-far-sath´-kites. Ezra 4:9.
APHARSITES, a-far´-sites. Ezra 4:9.
APHEK, a´-fek, strength. Josh. 12:18.
defeat of Saul at. 1 Sam. 29:1. *See* Josh. 13:4; 1 Sam. 4:1; 1 Kin. 20:26.
APHEKAH, a-fe´-kah, same as preceding. Josh. 15:53.
APHIAH, af-i´-ah. 1 Sam. 9:1.
APHIK, a´-fik, same as APHEK. Judg. 1:31.
APHRAH, af´-rah, dust. Mic. 1:10.
APHSES, af´-sees, dispersion. 1 Chr. 24:15.
APOLLONIA, ap´-ol-o´-ni-ah. Acts 17:1.
APOLLOS, ap-ol´-os, another form of APOLLONIUS or APOLLODORUS.
eloquent and mighty in the Scriptures. Acts 18:24; 19:1; 1 Cor. 1:12; 3:4.
APOLLYON, ap-ol´-yon, one that exterminates. Rev. 9:11.
APPAIM, ap-a´-m, the nostrils. 1 Chr. 2:30.
APPHIA, af´-yah, the Greek form of APPIA. Philem. 2.
APPII FORUM, ap´-py-i fo´-rum, forum or marketplace of Appius. Acts 28:15.
AQUILA, ak´-wil-ah, an eagle.
——(and Priscilla) go with Paul from Corinth to Ephesus. Acts 18:2, 19.
their constancy. Rom. 16:3; 1 Cor. 16:19.
Apollos instructed by. Acts 18:26.
AR, city. Num. 21:15.
ARA, a´-ra, lion (?). 1 Chr. 7:38.
ARAB, a´-rab, ambush. Josh. 15:52.
ARABAH, a-ra´h-bah, a plain. Josh. 18:18.
ARABIA, a-ra´-bi-a. Ps. 72:10, 15. Gal. 1:17.
kings of, pay tribute. 2 Chr. 9:14; 17:11; 26:7.
ARABIAN, a-ra´-bi-an, a person from Arabia. Neh. 2:19.
ARABIANS, Is. 13:20; 21:13; Jer. 25:24;—Acts 2:11.
ARAD, a´-rad, wild ass. 1 Chr. 8:15.
ARAH, a´-rah, wandering. 1 Chr. 7:39.
ARAM, a´-ram, height. Gen. 10:22.
ARAMITESS, a´-ram-ite-ess, a female inhabitant of Aram. 1 Chr. 7:14.
ARAN, a´-ran, wild goat. Gen. 36:28.
ARARAT, a´-ra-rat.
ark rested on. Gen. 8:4. *See* Jer. 51:27.
ARAUNAH, a-raw´-nah, calf (?). 2 Sam. 24:18.
——(Ornan), Jebusite, sells to David site for temple.

ARAUNAH (Ornan)—*cont.*
2 Sam. 24:16; 1 Chr. 21:15, 18; 22:1.
ARBA, or ARBAH, ar´-bah. Gen. 35:27.
ARBATHITE, ar´-bath-ite. 1 Chr. 11:32.
ARBEL, *see* BETH-ARBEL.
ARBITE, arb´-ite, an inhabitant of Arab. 2 Sam. 23:35.
ARCHELAUS, ar´-ke-la´-us, prince, king of Judæa, feared by Joseph. Matt. 2:22.
ARCHEVITES, ar´-kev-ites, the men of ERECH (?), q.v. Ezra 4:9.
ARCHI, ar´-ki, an inhabitant of Erech. Josh. 16:2.
ARCHIPPUS, at-kip´-us, master of the horse. Col. 4:17.
ARCHITE, ark´-ite, a native of Erech. 2 Sam. 15:32.
ARCTURUS, ark-tu´-rus, probably the constellations known as the Great and Little Bear. Job 9:9; 38:32.
ARD, fugitive (?). Gen. 46:21.
ARDITES, ard´-ites, descendants of Ard. Num. 26:40.
ARDON, ar´-don, fugitive. 1 Chr. 2:18.
ARELI, a-re´-li, heroic. Gen. 46:16.
ARELITES, a´-rel-ites, a family descended from Areli. Num. 26:17.
AREOPAGITE, a´-re-op´-ag-ite, belonging to the Council held on Areopagus. Acts 17:34.
AREOPAGUS, a´-re-op´-ag-us, hill of Mars, at Athens; Paul preaches on. Acts 17:19.
ARETAS, ar´-e-tas, a husbandman (?). 2 Cor. 11:32.
ARGOB, ar´-gobe, a rocky district. Deut. 3:4.
ARIDAI, a-ri´-dai. Esth. 9:9.
ARIDATHA, ar-ri´-dah-thah. Esth. 9:8.
ARIEH, ar´-ieh, lion. 2 Kin. 15:25.
ARIEL, a´-ri-el, lion of God. Ezra 8:16.
ARIMATHÆA, a´-rim-ath-ee´-ah, the same as RAMAH. Matt. 27:57.
ARIOCH, a´-ri-ok. Gen. 14:1.
ARISAI, a-ris´-ai. Esth. 9:9.
ARISTARCHUS, a-ris-tark´-us, best ruling.
fellow-prisoner of Paul, Acts 19:29; 20:4; 27:2; Col. 4:10; Philem. 24.
ARISTOBULUS, a´-ris-to-bewl´-us, best counsellor.
his household greeted by Paul. Rom. 16:10.
ARKITE, ark´-ite, fugitive (?). Gen. 10:17.
ARMAGEDDON, ar´-ma-ged´-on, height of Megiddo. Rev. 16:16.
ARMENIA, ar-me´-ni-a, land of Aram. 2 Kin. 19:37.
ARMONI, ar-mo´-ni, belonging to a palace. 2 Sam. 21:8.
ARNAN, ar´-nan, active. 1 Chr. 3:21.
ARNON, ar´-non, swift. Num. 21:13.
AROD, a´-rod, wild ass. Num. 26:17.
ARODI, a´-rod-i, same as preceding. Gen. 46:16.
ARODITES, a´-rod-ites, descendants of Arod. Num. 26:17.
AROER, a-ro´-er, ruins (?). Deut. 2:36.
built by children of Gad. Num. 32:34.
boundary of Reuben. Josh. 13:16.
AROERITE, ar-o´-er-ite, a man ofAroer. 1 Chr. 11:44.
ARPAD, ar´-pad. 2 Kin. 18:34.
ARPHAD, ar´-fad, same as preceding. Is. 36:19.
ARPHAXAD, ar-fax´-ad. Gen. 10:22.
ARTAXERXES, ar´-ta-xerk´-ses, honoured king (?). Ezra 4:8.
(king of Persia), oppresses the Jews. Ezra 4.
——(Longimanus), permits Ezra to restore the temple, Ezra 7; and Nehemiah to rebuild Jerusalem. Neh. 2.
ARTEMAS, ar´-te-mas, shortened form of ARTEMIDORUS (?). Tit. 3:12.
ARUBOTH, a-roob´-oth, windows. 1 Kin. 4:10.
ARUMAH, a-room´-ah, elevated. Judg. 9:41.
ARVAD, ar´-vad, wandering. Ezek. 27:8.
ARVADITES, ar´-vad-ites, inhabitants of Arvad. Gen. 10:18.
ARZA, ar´-zah, earth. 1 Kin. 16:9.
ASA, a´-sah, physician.
his good reign. 1 Kin. 15:8.
wars with Baasha. 1 Kin. 15:16.
his prayer against the Ethiopians. 2 Chr. 14:11.
his zeal. 2 Chr. 15.

ASA—*cont.*
seeks aid of the Syrians. 2 Chr. 16.
reproved by Hanani the seer. 2 Chr. 16:7.
reigns forty years, and dies much honoured. 2 Chr. 16:10.

ASAHEL, a´sa-hel, whom God made.
his rashness; slain by Abner in self-defence. 2 Sam. 2:18; 3:27; 23:24; 1 Chr. 11:26.

ASAHIAH, a-sah´-ah. 2 Kin. 22:12.

ASAIAH, a-sai´-ah. 1 Chr. 4:36.

ASAPH, a´-saf, collector. 2 Kin. 18:18.
a Levite, musical composer, and leader of David's choir, 1 Chr. 6:39; 2 Chr. 5:12; 29:30; 35:15; Neh. 12:46; Psalms 50 and 73 to 83 ascribed to him.

ASAREEL, a-sa´r-eel, whom God has bound. 1 Chr. 4:16.

ASARELAH, a-sar-e´l-ah, same as JESHARELAH. 1 Chr. 25:2.

ASENATH, a´-se-nath, she who is of Neith *(i.e.* a goddess of the Egyptians) (?). Gen. 41:45.
wife of Joseph. Gen. 41:45; 46:20.

ASER, a´-ser, same as ASHER. Luke 2:36.

ASHAN, a´-shan, smoke. Josh. 15:42.

ASHBEA. ash´-be-ah, I conjure. 1 Chr. 4:21.

ASHBEL, ash´-bel, blame (?). Gen. 46:21.

ASHBELITES, ash´-bel-ites, the descendants of Ashbel. Num. 26:38.

ASHCHENAZ, ash´-ken-az, same as ASHKENAZ. 1 Chr. 1:6.

ASHDOD, ash´-dod, a strong place. Josh. 15:46.
city of Philistines; the ark carried there; men of, smitten. 1 Sam. 5.
reduced by Uzziah. 2 Chr. 26:6.
predictions concerning. Jer. 25:20; Amos 1:8; Zeph. 2:4; Zech. 9:6.

ASHDODITES, ash´-dod-ites, the inhabitants of Ashdod. Neh. 4:7.

ASHDOTH-PISGAH, ash´-doth-piz´gah, springs of Pisgah. Josh. 12:3.

ASHDOTHITES, ash´-doth-ites, same as ASHDODITES. Josh. 13:3.

ASHER, ash´-er, fortunate, happy.
son of Jacob. Gen. 30:13.
his descendants. Num. 1:40; 26:44; 1 Chr. 7:30; their inheritance, Josh. 19:24; Judg. 5:17. *See* Ezek. 48:34; Rev. 7:6.
Anna, prophetess, descended from. Luke 2:36.

ASHERAH, ash-er´-ah, the goddess Ashtoreth. 2 Kin. 17:10.

ASHERITES, a´-sher-ites, descendants of Asher. Judg. 1:32.

ASHIMA, a-shi´-ma. 2 Kin. 17:30.

ASHKELON, ash´-kel-on, migration.
——(Askelon) taken. Judg. 1:18; 14:19; 1 Sam. 6:17; 2 Sam. 1:20.
prophecies concerning. Jer. 25:20; 47:5; Amos 1:8; Zeph. 2:4; Zech. 9:5.

ASHKENAZ, ash´-ken-az. Gen. 10:3.

ASHNAH, ash´-nah, strong. Josh. 15:33.

ASHPENAZ, ash´-pen-az. Dan. 1:3.

ASHRIEL, ash´-ri-el, same as ASRIEL. 1 Chr. 7:14.

ASHTAROTH, ash´-tar-oth, statutes of Ashtoreth. Josh. 9:10.
idolatrous worship of, by Israel. Judg. 2:13; 1 Sam. 12:10; by Solomon, 1 Kin. 11:5, 33.

ASHTERATHITE, ash-ter´-ath-ite, a native of Ashteroth. 1 Chr. 11:44.

ASHTEROTH KARNAIM, ash´-ter-oth kar-na´-im, Ashteroth of the two horns. Gen. 14:5.

ASHTORETH, ash-tor´-eth, she who enriches. 1 Kin. 11:5.

ASHUR, ash´-oor. 1 Chr. 2:24.

ASHURITES, ash´-oor-ites. 2 Sam. 2:9.

ASHVATH, ash´-vath. 1 Chr. 7:33.

ASIA, a´-shah. Acts 2:9.

ASIEL, a´-si-el, created by God. 1 Chr. 4:35.

ASKELON, *see* ASHKELON. Judg. 1:18.

ASNAH, as´-nah, bramble. Ezra 2:50.

ASNAPPER, as-nap´-er, same as ASSUR-BANI-PAL, Assur has formed a son. Ezra 4:10.

ASPATHA, as-pa´h-thah. Esth. 9:7.

ASRIEL, as´-ri-el, the prohibition of God. Num. 26:31.

ASRIELITES, as´-ri-el-ites, the family of Asriel. Num. 26:31.

ASSHUR, ash´-oor, the gracious One (?). Gen. 10:22.

ASSHURIM, ash-oor´-im. Gen. 25:3.

ASSIR, as´-eer, captive. Ex. 6:24.

ASSOS, as´-os. Acts 20:13.

ASSYRIA, as-ir´-ya, the land so named from ASSHUR. Gen. 2:14.
Israel carried captive to. 2 Kin. 15:29; 17.
army of, miraculously destroyed. 2 Kin. 19:35; Is. 37:36.
prophecies concerning. Is. 8; 10:5; 14:24; 30:31; 31:8; Mic. 5:6; Zeph. 2:13.
its glory. Ezek. 31:3.

ASSYRIANS, as-ir´-yans, inhabitants of Assyria. Is. 10:5.

ASTAROTH, as´-tar-oth, same as ASHTORETH. Deut. 1:4.

ASUPPIM, a-soop´-im. 1 Chr. 26:15.

ASYNCRITUS, a-sin´-krit-us, incomparable, disciple. Rom. 16:14.

ATAD, a´-tad, buckthorn. Gen. 50:10.

ATARAH, a-ta´h-rah, a crown. 1 Chr. 2:26.

ATAROTH, a-ta´h-roth, crowns. Num. 32:3.

ATER, a´-ter, bound, shut up. Ezra 2:16.

ATHACH, a´-thak, lodging-place. 1 Sam. 30:30.

ATHAIAH, a-thai´-ah, whom Jehovah made (?). Neh. 11:4.

ATHALIAH, ath´-al-i´-ah, whom Jehovah has afflicted.
daughter of Ahab, mother of Ahaziah. 2 Kin. 8:26.
slays the seed royal, Joash only saved. 2 Kin. 11:1; 2 Chr. 22:10.
slain by order of Jehoiada. 2 Kin. 11:16; 2 Chr. 23:15.

ATHLAI, a´th-lai, shortened form of ATHALIAH. Ezra 10:28.

ATHENIANS, ath-e´-ni-ans, natives of Athens. Acts 17:21.

ATHENS, ath´-ens.
Paul preaches to the philosophers at. Acts. 17:15; 1 Thess. 3:1.
men of, described. Acts 17:21.

ATROTH, at´-roth, same as ATAROTH. Num. 32:35.

ATTAI, a´-t-tai, opportune. 1 Chr. 2:35.

ATTALIA, at´-ta-li´-a, so called from Attalus, the royal founder of the city, sea-port. Acts 14:25.

AUGUSTUS, aw-gust´-us, venerable. Luke 2:1.

AVAH, a´-vah. 2 Kin. 17:24.

AVEN, a´-ven, nothingness. Ezek. 30:17.

AVIM, av´-im, ruins. Josh. 18:23.

AVITH, a´-vith. Gen. 36:35.

AZAL, a´-zal, root of a mountain. Zech. 14:5.

AZALIAH, a´-zal-i´-ah, whom Jehovah has reserved. 2 Kin. 22:3.

AZANIAH, a´-zan-i´-ah, whom Jehovah hears. Neh. 10:9.

AZARAEL, a-zar´-eel, whom God helps. Neh. 12:36.

AZAREEL, a-zar´-eel, same as preceding. 1 Chr. 12:6.

AZARIAH, a´-zar-i´-ah, whom Jehovah aids. 2 Chr. 22:6.
——(Uzziah), king of Judah, his good reign. 2 Kin. 14:21; 2 Chr. 26.
his wars. 2 Chr. 26.
invades the priest's office. 2 Chr. 26:16.
struck with leprosy. 2 Kin. 15:5; 2 Chr. 26:20.
——prophet, exhorts Asa. 2 Chr. 15.

AZAZ, a´-zaz, strong. 1 Chr. 5:8.

AZAZIAH, a´-zaz-i´-ah, whom Jehovah strengthened. 1 Chr. 15:21.

AZBUK, az´-book. Neh. 3:16.

AZEKAH, a-ze´-kah, dug over. Josh. 10:10.

AZEL, a´-zel, noble. 1 Chr. 8:37.

AZEM, a´-zem, strength, bone. Josh. 15:29.

AZGAD, az´-gad, strong in fortune. Ezra 2:12.

AZIEL, az´-i-el, whom God strengthens. 1 Chr. 15:20.

AZIZA, a-zi´-zah, strong. Ezra 10:27.

AZMAVETH, az-ma´-veth, strength (?). 2 Sam. 23:31.

AZMON, az´-mon, robust. Num. 34:4.

AZNOTH-TABOR, az´-noth-ta´-bor, ears (*i.e.* summits) of Tabor. Josh. 19:34.

AZOR, a´-zor, helper. Matt. 1:13.

AZOTUS, a-zo´-tus, the Greek form of ASHDOD. Acts 8:40.

AZRIEL, az´-ri-el, help of God. 1 Chr. 5:24.

AZRIKAM, az-ri´-kam, help against an enemy. 1 Chr. 3:23.

AZUBAH, a-zoob´-ah, forsaken. 1 Kin. 22:42.

AZUR, a´-zoor, same as AZOR. Jer. 28:1.

AZZAH, az´-ah, strong, fortified. Deut. 2:23.

AZZAN, az´-an, strong. Num. 34:26.

AZZUR, az´-oor, same as AZOR. Neh. 10:17.

BAAL, ba´-al, lord, master, possessor, owner.
worshipped. Num. 22:41; Judg. 2:13; 8:33; 1 Kin. 16:32; 18:26; 2 Kin. 17:16; 19:18; 21:3; Jer. 2:8; 7:9; 12:16; 19:5, 23:13; Hos. 2:8; 13:1, &c.
his altars and priests destroyed by Gideon. Judg. 6:25; by Elijah. 1 Kin. 18:40; by Jehu. 2 Kin. 10:18; by Jehoiada. 2 Kin. 11:18; by Josiah. 2 Kin. 23:4; 2 Chr. 34:4.

BAALAH, ba´-al-ah, mistress. Josh. 15:10.

BAALATH, ba´-al-ath, same as preceding. Josh. 19:44.

BAALATH-BEER, ba´-al-ath-be´-er, having a well. Josh. 19:8.

BAAL-BERITH, ba´-al-be-ri´th, lord of covenant. Judg. 8:33.

BAALE, ba´-al-ay, plural of Baal. 2 Sam. 6:2.

BAAL-GAD, ba´-al-gad´, lord of fortune. Josh. 11:17.

BAAL-HAMON, ba´-al-ha´-mon, place of a multitude. Cant. 8:11.

BAAL-HANAN, ba´-al-ha´-nan, lord of benignity. Gen. 36:38.

BAAL-HAZOR, ba´-al-ha´-zor, having a village. 2 Sam. 13:23.

BAAL-HERMON, ba´-al-her´-mon, place of Hermon. Judg. 3:3.

BAALI, ba´-al-i, my lord. Hos. 2:16.

BAALIM, ba´-al-im, lords. Judg. 2:11; 2 Chr. 28:2.

BAALIS, ba´-al-is. Jer. 40:14.

BAAL-MEON, ba´-al-me´-on, place of habitation. Num. 32:38.

BAAL-PEOR, ba´-al-pe´-or, lord of the opening. Num. 25:3.
the trespass of Israel concerning. Num:25; Deut. 4:3; Ps. 106:28; Hos. 9:10.

BAAL-PERAZIM, ba´-al-pe-raz´-im, place of breaches.
David's victory over Philistines at. 2 Sam. 5:20.

BAAL-SHALISHA, ba´-al-sha-lish´-ah, lord (or place) of Shalisha. 2 Kin. 4:42.

BAAL-TAMAR, ba´-al-ta´-mar, place of palm trees. Judg. 20:33.

BAAL-ZEBUB, ba´-al-ze-bo´ob, lord of flies.
false god of Ekron, Ahaziah rebuked for sending to enquire of. 2 Kin. 1:2.

BAAL-ZEPHON, ba´-al-ze-pho´n, place of Zephon, or sacred to Zephon. Ex. 14:2.

BAANA, ba´-a-nah. 1 Kin. 4:12.

BAANAH, ba´-a-nah.
and Rechab, for murdering Ish-bosheth, slain by David. 2 Sam. 4:2.

BAARA, ba´-a-rah, foolish. 1 Chr. 8:8.

BAASEIAH, ba´-as-i´-ah, work of Jehovah. 1 Chr. 6:40.

BAASHA, ba´-ash-ah, wicked (?).
king of Israel, destroys the house of Jeroboam. 1 Kin. 15:16, 27; Jehu's prophecy concerning him. 1 Kin. 16:1.

BABEL, ba´-bel, confusion.
Nimrod king of. Gen. 10:10.
confusion of tongues at the building of. Gen. 11:9.

BABYLON, bab´-il-on, Greek form of BAB-ILU, the gate of God. Gen. 10:10; 2 Kin. 17:30; 20:12.
ambassadors from, to Hezekiah. 2 Kin. 20:12; 2 Chr. 32:31; Is. 39.
Jewish captivity there. 2 Kin. 25; 2 Chr. 36; Jer. 39; 52.
return from. Ezra 1; Neh. 2.

BABYLON—*cont.*
greatness of. Dan. 4:30.
taken by the Medes. Dan. 5:30.
fall of. Is. 13:14; 21:2; 47; 48; Jer. 25:12; 50; 51.
church in. 1 Pet. 5:13.
——the Great. Rev. 14:8; 17; 18.

BABYLONISH, bab´-il-one-ish, of, or belonging to, Babylon. Josh. 7:21.

BACA, ba´-kah, weeping.
valley of misery. Ps. 84:6.

BACHRITES, bak´-rites, the family of Becher. Num. 26:35.

BAHARUMITE, ba-ha-r´um-ite, an inhabitant of Bahurim. 1 Chr. 11:33.

BAHURIM, ba-hoor´-im, (town of) young men. 2 Sam. 16:5.

BAJITH, ba´-yith (same as BETH), house. Is. 15:2.

BAKBAKKAR, bak-bak´-ar. 1 Chr. 9:15.

BAKBUK, bak´-book, a bottle. Ezra 2:51.

BAKBUKIAH, bak´-book-i´-ah, emptying (*i.e.* wasting) of Jehovah. Neh. 11:17.

BALAAM, ba´-la-am, destruction (?). Num. 22:5.
requested by Balak to curse Israel, is forbidden. Num. 22:13.
his anger. Num. 22:27.
blesses Israel. Num. 23:19; 24.
his prophecies. Num. 23:9, 24; 24:17.
his wicked counsel. Num. 31:16; Deut. 23:4. *See* Josh. 24:9; Judg. 11:25; Mic. 6:5; 2 Pet. 2:15; Jude 11; Rev. 2:14.
slain. Num. 31:8; Josh. 13:22.

BALAC, ba´-lac, same as BALAK. Rev. 2:14.

BALADAN, ba´-la-dan, He has given a son. 2 Kin. 20:12.

BALAH, ba´-lah. Josh. 19:3.

BALAK, ba´-lak, to make empty. Num. 22:2.

BAMAH, ba´-mah, high place. Ezek. 20:29.

BAMOTH, ba´-moth, high places. Num. 21:19.

BAMOTH-BAAL, ba´-moth-ba´-al, *h.p.* of Baal. Josh. 13:17.

BANI, ba´-ni, built. 2 Sam. 23:36.

BARABBAS, bar-a´b-as, son of Abba or father. Mark 15:7.
a robber, released instead of Jesus. Matt. 27:16; Mark 15:6; Luke 23:18; John 18:40.

BARACHEL, ba´-rak-el, whom God blessed. Job 32:6.

BARACHIAS, ba-rak-i´-as, whom Jehovah blesses. Matt. 23:35.

BARAK, ba´-rak, thunderbolt, lightning. Judg. 4:6.
delivers Israel from Sisera. Judg. 4:5; Heb. 11:32.

BARHUMITE, bar´-hoom-ite, same as BAHARUMITE. 2 Sam. 23:31.

BARIAH, ba-ri´-ah, a fugitive. 1 Chr. 3:22.

BAR-JESUS, bar-je´-sus, son of JESUS.
(Elymas) smitten with blindness by Paul. Acts 13:6.

BAR-JONA, bar-jo´-nah, son of Jona (Simon). Matt. 16:17.

BARKOS, bar´-kos, painter (?). Ezra 2:53.

BARNABAS, bar´-na-bas, son of exhortation.
Levite of Cyprus, sells his lands. Acts 4:36.
preaches at Antioch. Acts 11:22.
accompanies Paul. Acts 11:30; 12:25; 13; 14; 15; 1 Cor. 9:6.
his contention. Acts 15:36.
his error. Gal. 2:13.

BARSABAS, bar´-sa-bas, *s.* of Seba. Acts 1:23.

BARTHOLOMEW, bar-thol´-o-mew, *s.* of Talmai.
the apostle. Matt. 10:3; Mark 3:18; Luke 6:14; Acts 1:13.

BARTIMÆUS, bar´-ti-me´-us, *s.* of Timai.
blindness cured near Jericho. Mark 10:46.

BARUCH, ba´-rook, blessed. Jer. 32:12.
receives Jeremiah's evidence. Jer. 32:13; 36.
discredited by Azariah, and carried into Egypt. Jer. 43:6.
God's message to. Jer. 45.

BARZILLAI, bar-zi´l-ai, of iron.
loyalty to David. 2 Sam. 17:27.

BARZILLAI—*cont.*
David's recognition of. 2 Sam. 19:31; 1 Kin. 2:7.
BASHAN, ba´shan, soft rich soil.
conquered. Num. 21:33; Deut. 3:1; Ps. 68:15, 22; 135:10; 136:20.
BASHAN-HAVOTH-JAIR, ba´shan-hav´oth-ja´yir, Bashan of the villages of Jair. Deut. 3:14.
BASHEMATH, ba´shem-ath, sweet-smelling. Gen. 26:34.
BASMATH, same as BASHEMATH. 1 Kin. 4:15.
BATH-RABBIM, bath-rab´im, daughter many. Cant. 7:4.
BATH-SHEBA, bath´she-bah, *d.* of the oath. 2 Sam. 11:3.
wife of Uriah, taken by David. 2 Sam. 11; 12.
appeals to David for Solomon against Adonijah. 1 Kin. 1:15.
intercedes with Solomon for Adonijah. 1 Kin. 2:19.
BATH-SHUA, bath´shoo-ah. 1 Chr. 3:5.
BAVAI, ba´vai. Neh. 3:18.
BAZLITH, baz´lith, a making naked (?). Neh. 7:54.
BAZLUTH, baz´looth, same as BAZLITH. Ezra 2:52.
BEALIAH, be-al-i´ah, whom Jehovah rules. 1 Chr. 12:5.
BEALOTH, be-a´h-loth, citizens (?), plural of BAALAH. Josh. 15:24.
BEBAI, be´bai. Ezra 8:11.
BECHER, be´ker, a young camel. Gen. 46:21.
BECHORATH, be-kor´ath, offspring of the first birth. 1 Sam. 9:1.
BEDAD, be´dad, separation, part. Gen. 36:35.
BEDAN, be´dan, son of Dan (?). 1 Sam. 12:11.
BEDEIAH, be-di´ah. Ezra 10:35.
BEELIADA, be-el´ya-dah´, whom Baal has known. 1 Chr. 14:7.
BEELZEBUB, be-el´ze-bub´, same as BAALZEBUB. Matt. 10:25.
prince of devils. Matt. 12:24; Mark 3:22; Luke 11:15.
Christ's miracles ascribed to. Matt. 12:24, &c.
BEER, be´er, a well. Num. 21:16.
BEERA, be-er´ah, same as BEER. 1 Chr. 7:37.
BEERAH, be-er´ah, same as BEER. 1 Chr. 5:6.
BEER-ELIM, be´er-el´im, well of heroes. Is. 15:8.
BEERI, be´er-i, man of the *w.* Gen. 26:34.
BEER-LAHAI-ROI, be´er-la-hai´ro´i, *w.* of vision (of God) to the living. Gen. 16:14.
BEEROTH, be-er´oth, wells. Josh. 9:17.
BEEROTHITE, be-er´oth-ite, a native of Beeroth. 2 Sam. 23:37.
BEER-SHEBA, be´er-she´bah, well of the oath.
Abraham dwells at. Gen. 21:31; 22:19; 28:10.
Hagar relieved at. Gen. 21:14.
Jacob comforted at. Gen. 46:1.
Elijah flees to. 1 Kin. 19:3.
BEESH-TERAH, be-esh´te-rah, house or temple of Astarte (?). Josh. 21:27.
BEHEMOTH, be-he´moth, the water-ox. Job 40:15.
BEKAH, be´kah, part, half. Ex. 38:26.
BEL, bel, another form of BAAL, an idol. Is. 46:1; Jer. 50:2.
BELA, be´lah, destruction. Gen. 14:2.
BELAH, be´lah, same as BELA. Gen. 46:21.
BELAITES, be´la-ites, descendants of BELA. Num. 26:38.
BELIAL, be´li-al, worthless.
men of, wicked men so called. Deut. 13:13; Judg. 19:22.
sons of. 1 Sam. 10:27.
BELSHAZZAR, bel-shaz´ar, Bel protect the king. Dan. 5:1.
his profane feast, warning, and death. Dan. 5.
BELTESHAZZAR, bel´te-shaz´ar, preserve his life.
Daniel so named. Dan. 1:7; 4:8, &c.
BEN, ben, son. 1 Chr. 15:18.
BENAIAH, ben-ai´ah, whom Jehovah has built. 2 Sam. 8:18.
valiant acts of. 2 Sam. 23:20; 1 Chr. 11:22; 27:5.
proclaims Solomon king. 1 Kin. 1:32.

BENAIAH—*cont.*
slays Adonijah, Joab, and Shimei. 1 Kin. 2:25-46.
BEN-AMMI, ben´am-i, son of my own kindred. Gen. 19:38.
BEN-BERAK, be-ne´be-rak´, sons of Barak, or of lightning. Josh. 19:45.
BENE-JAAKAN, be-ne-ja´ak-an, *s.* of Jaakan. Num. 33:31.
BEN-HADAD, ben-ha´dad, *s.* of Hadad.
king of Syria, his league with Asa against Baasha. 1 Kin. 15:18.
——wars with Ahab. 1 Kin. 20.
baffled by Elisha. 2 Kin. 6:8.
besieges Samaria. 2 Kin. 6:24; 7.
slain by Hazael. 2 Kin. 8:7.
——son of Hazael, wars with Israel. 2 Kin. 13:3, 25. *See* Jer. 49:27; Amos 1:4.
BEN-HAIL, ben-ha´yil, son of the host. 2 Chr. 17:7.
BEN-HANAN, ben-ha´nan, *s.* of one who is gracious. 1 Chr. 4:20.
BENINU, be-ni´noo, our *s.* Neh. 10:13.
BENJAMIN, ben´ja-min, *s.* of the right hand, *i.e.* fortunate. Gen. 35:18.
(first named Ben-oni, 'son of my sorrow'), Patriarch, youngest son of Jacob, his birth at Bethlehem. Gen. 35:16.
goes into Egypt. Gen. 43:15.
Joseph's stratagem to detain. Gen. 44.
Jacob's prophecy concerning. Gen. 49:27.
HIS DESCENDANTS. Gen. 46:21; 1 Chr. 7:6.
twice numbered. Num. 1:36; 26:38.
blessed by Moses. Deut. 33:12.
their inheritance. Josh. 18:11.
their wickedness chastised. Judg. 20; 21.
the first king chosen from. 1 Sam. 9; 10.
support the house of Saul. 2 Sam. 2.
afterwards adhere to that of David. 1 Kin. 12:21; 1 Chr 11.
the tribe of Paul. Phil. 3:5. *See* Ps. 68:27; Ezek. 48:32; Rev. 7:8.
BENJAMITE, ben´jam-ite, a man of the tribe of Benjamin. Judg. 20:35.
BENO, ben-o´, his son. 1 Chr. 24:26.
BEN-ONI, be´n-o´ni, *s.* of my sorrow. Gen. 35:18.
BEN-ZOHETH, ben-zo´heth, *s.* of Zoheth. 1 Chr. 4:20.
BEON, be´on, contracted from BAAL-MEON. Num. 32:3.
BEOR, be´or. Gen. 36:32.
BERA, be´rah. Gen. 14:2.
BERACHAH, be´rak-ah, blessing. 1 Chr. 12:3.
valley of, why so named. 2 Chr. 20:26.
BERACHIAH, be´rak-i´ah, whom Jehovah hath blessed. 1 Chr. 6:39.
BERAIAH, be-rai´ah, whom Jehovah created. 1 Chr. 8:21.
BEREA, be-re´ah.
city of Macedonia, Paul preaches at. Acts 17:10.
people 'more noble'. Acts 17:11.
BERECHIAH, be´rek-i´ah, same as BERACHIAH. 1 Chr. 3:20.
BERED, be´red, hail. Gen. 16:14.
BERI, be´ri, man of the well. 1 Chr. 7:36.
BERIAH, be-ri´ah, in evil (?). Gen. 46:17.
BERIITES, be-ri´ites, descendants of Beriah. Num. 26:44.
BERITES, ber´ites. 2 Sam. 20:14.
BERITH, be´rith, a covenant. Judg. 9:46.
BERNICE, ber-ni´see, Victoria. Acts 25:13,
BERODACH-BALADAN, be´ro-dak-bal´a-dan, Bero-dach (same as MERODACH) has given a son. 2 Kin. 20:12.
BEROTHAH, be-ro´thah, wells. Ezek. 47:16.
BEROTHAI, be-to´thai, my wells. 2 Sam. 8:8.
BEROTHITE, be-ro´thite, same as BEEROTHITE. 1 Chr. 11:39.
BESAI, be´sai, sword (?), or victory (?). Ezra 2:49.
BESODEIAH, be´sod-i´ah, in the secret of Jehovah. Neh. 3:6.
BESOR, be´sor, cool. 1 Sam. 30:9.
BETAH, be´tah, confidence. 2 Sam. 8:8.

BETEN, be´-ten. Josh. 19:25.

BETHABARA, beth-ab´ar-ah, house of passage.
  place where John baptized. John 1:28.

BETH-ANATH, beth´-an-ath, echo. Josh. 19:38.

BETH-ANOTH, beth´-an-oth. Josh. 15:59.

BETHANY, beth´-an-y, house of dates.
  visited by Christ, Matt. 21:17; 26:6; Mark 11:1; Luke 19:29; John 12:1.
  raising of Lazarus at, John 11:18.
  ascension of Christ at. Luke 24:50.

BETH-ARABAH, beth-a-ra´h-bah, *h.* of the desert. Josh. 15:6.

BETH-ARAM, beth-a´-ram, *h.* of the height. Josh. 13:27.

BETH-ARBEL, beth-arb´-el, *h.* of the ambush of God. Hos. 10:14.

BETH-AVEN, beth-a´-ven, *h.* of vanity (*i.e.* of idols). Josh. 7:2.

BETH-AZMAVETH, beth´-az-ma´-veth, *h.* of strength. Neh. 7:28.

BETH-BAAL-MEON, beth´-ba´-al-me-on´, *h.* of Baalmeon. Josh. 13:17.

BETH-BARAH, beth-ba´-rah, same as BETHABARA. Judg. 7:24.

BETH-BIREI, beth-bir´-i, house of my creation. 1 Chr. 4:31.

BETH-CAR, beth´-kar, *h.* of pasture. 1 Sam. 7:11.

BETH-DAGON, beth-da´-gon, *h.* of Dagon. Josh. 15:41.

BETH-DIBLATHAIM, beth´-dib-la-tha´-im, *h.* of the two cakes. Jer. 48:22.

BETH-EL, beth´-el, *h.* of God. Gen. 12:8.
  (Luz), city of Palestine, named Beth-el by Jacob. Gen. 28:19; 31:13.
  altar built by Jacob at. Gen. 35:1.
  occupied by the house of Joseph. Judg. 1:22.
  sons of prophets resident there. 2 Kin. 2:2, 3; 17:28.
  the king's chapel. Amos 7:13.
  idolatry of Jeroboam at. 1 Kin. 12:28; 13:1.
  reformation by Josiah at. 2 Kin. 23:15.

BETHELITE, beth´-el-ite, a native of Bethel. 1 Kin. 16:34.

BETH-EMEK, beth-e´-mek, house of the valley. Josh. 19:27.

BETHER, be´-ther, separation. Cant. 2:17.

BETHESDA, beth-esd´-ah, house of mercy.
  pool of, at Jerusalem, miracles wrought at. John 5:2.

BETH-EZEL, beth-e´-zel, house of firmness (?). Mic. 1:11.

BETH-GADER, beth-ga´-der, *h.* of the wall. 1 Chr. 2:51.

BETH-GAMUL, beth-ga´-mool, *h.* of the weaned. Jer. 48:23.

BETH-HACCEREM, beth-hak-er´-em, *h.* of the vineyard. Neh. 3:14.

BETH-HARAN, beth-ha´-ran. Num. 32:36.

BETH-HOGLAH, beth-hog´-lah, *h.* of the partridge. Josh. 15:6.

BETH-HORON, beth-ho´-ron, *h.* of the hollow. Josh. 10:10.

BETH-JESIMOTH, beth-je-shim´-oth, *h.* of the deserts. Num. 33:49.

BETH-LEBAOTH, beth´-le-ba´-oth, *h.* of lionesses. Josh. 19:6.

BETH-LEHEM, beth´-le-hem, *h.* of bread. Gen. 35:19.

BETH-LEHEM EPHRATAH, beth´-le-hem ef´-ra-tah, B. the fruitful (?).
  (originally Ephratah), Naomi and Ruth return to. Ruth 1—4.
  David anointed at. 1 Sam. 16:13; 20:6.
  well of. 2 Sam. 23:15; 1 Chr. 11:17.
  Christ's birth at. Matt. 2:1; Luke 2:4; John 7:42; predicted. Mic. 5:2 (Ps. 132:5, 6).
  babes of, slain. Matt. 2:16.

BETH-LEHEMITE, beth´-le-hem-ite, a man of Beth-lehem. 1 Sam. 16:1.

BETH-LEHEM-JUDAH, beth´-le-hem-joo´-dah, B. of Judah. Judg. 17:7.

BETH-MAACHAH, beth´-ma´-ak-ah, house of Maachah. 2 Sam. 20:14.

BETH-MARCABOTH, beth´-mar´-kab-oth, *h.* of chariots. Josh. 19:5.

BETH-MEON, be´th-me-o´n, *h.* of habitation. Jer. 48:23.

BETH-NIMRAH, beth-nim´-rah, *h.* of sweet water. Num. 32:36.

BETH-PALET, beth´-pa´-let, *h.* of escape, or of Pelet. Josh. 15:27.

BETH-PAZZEZ, beth´-paz´-ez, *h.* of dispersion. Josh. 19:21.

BETH-PEOR, beth´-pe´-or, temple of Peor. Deut. 3:29.

BETHPHAGE, be´th-fa-gee, house of unripe figs. Matt. 21:1.

BETH-PHELET, beth´-fe´-let, same as BETH-PALET. Neh. 11:26.

BETH-RAPHA, beth´-ra´-fah, house of Rapha. 1 Chr. 4:12.

BETH-REHOB, beth´-re´-hob, *h.* of Rehob. Judg. 18:28.

BETHSAIDA, beth´-sai´-dah, *h.* of fishing.
  of Galilee, native place of Philip, Peter, and Andrew. Mark 6:45; John 1:44; 12:21.
  blind man cured at. Mark 8:22.
  condemned for unbelief. Matt. 11:21.
  Christ feeds the five thousand at. Luke 9:10-17.

BETH-SHAN, beth´-shan´, *h.* of rest. 1 Sam. 31:10.

BETH-SHEAN, beth´-she´-an, same as BETH-SHAN. Josh. 17:11.

BETH-SHEMESH, beth´-she´-mesh, house of the sun. Josh. 15:10.
  men of, punished for looking into the ark. 1 Sam. 6:19.
  great battle at. 2 Kin. 14:11.

BETHSHEMITE, beth´-shem´-ite, a native of Beth-shemesh. 1 Sam. 6:14.

BETH-SHITTAH, beth´-shit´-ah, house of acacias. Judg. 7:22.

BETH-TAPPUAH, beth´-tap-oo´-ah, *h.* of apples. Josh. 15:53.

BETHUEL, beth´-oo-el, house of God. Gen. 22:22.

BETHUL, beth-ool´, same as BETHEL (?). Josh. 19:4.

BETH-ZUR, beth´-zoor´, house of the rock. Josh. 15:58.

BETONIM, be-to´-nim, pistachio nuts. Josh. 13:26.

BEULAH, be-ool´-ah, married. Is. 62:4.

BEZAI, be´-zai. Ezra 2:17.

BEZALEEL, be-zal´-e-el, in the shadow of God (?).
  constructs the tabernacle. Ex. 31:2; 35:30; 36—38.

BEZEK, be´-zek, lightning (?). Judg. 1:4.

BEZER, be´-zer, ore of precious metal. Deut. 4:43.

BICHRI, bik´-ri, young. 2 Sam. 20:1.

BIDKAR, bid´-kar, cleaver (?). 2 Kin. 9:25.

BIGTHA, big´-thah. Esth. 1:10.

BIGTHAN, big´-than, given by God.
  and Teresh, their conspiracy against Ahasuerus. Esth. 2:21.

BIGTHANA, big-thah´-nah, same as BIGTHAN. Esth. 6:2.

BIGVAI, big´-vai. Ezra 2:2.

BILDAD, bil´-dad, son of contention (?). Job 2:11.
  his answers to Job. Job 8; 18; 25.

BILEAM, bil´-e-am, same as BALAAM (?), or IBLEAM (?). 1 Chr. 6:70.

BILGAH, bil´-gah, cheerfulness. 1 Chr. 24:14.

BILGAI, bil´-gai, same as BILGAH. Neh. 10:8.

BILHAH, bil´-hah, modesty. Gen. 29:29.
  Jacob's children by. Gen. 30:5.

BILHAN, bil´-han, modest. Gen. 36:27.

BILSHAN, bil´-shan, seeker (?). Ezra 2:2.

BIMHAL, bim´-hal. 1 Chr. 7:33.

BINEA, bi´-ne-ah. 1 Chr. 8:37.

BINNUI, bin´-oo-i, a building. Ezra 8:33.

BIRSHA, bir´-shah. Gen. 14:2.

BIRZAVITH, bir´-za-vith, wounds (?). 1 Chr. 7:31.

BISHLAM, bish´-lam. Ezra 4:7.

BITHIAH, bith´-yah, daughter (*i.e.* worshipper) of Jehovah. 1 Chr. 4:18.

BITHRON, bith´-ron, a broken place. 2 Sam. 2:29.

BITHYNIA, bi-thin´yah. Acts 16:7.
BIZJOTHJAH, biz-joth´jah, contempt of Jehovah. Josh. 15:28.
BIZTHA, biz´thah. Esth. 1:10.
BLASTUS, blast´us, a shoot. Acts 12:20.
BOANERGES, bo´an-er´jes, sons of thunder.
James and John surnamed by Christ. Mark 3:17.
BOAZ, bo´az, fleetness. Ruth 2:1.
his conduct towards Ruth. Ruth 2; 3; 4.
ancestor of David and Christ. Ruth 4:17, 22; Matt. 1:5; Luke 3:23, 32.
——and Jachin (strength and stability), pillars of the temple. 2 Chr. 3:17.
BOCHERU, bo´ke-roo, firstborn (?). 1 Chr. 8:38.
BOCHIM, bo´kim, weepers. Judg. 2:1.
Israel rebuked by an angel at. Judg. 2:1-3.
Israel repent at. Judg. 2:4, 5.
BOHAN, bo´han, thumb (?). Josh. 15:6.
BOOZ, bo´oz, same as BOAZ. Matt. 1:5.
BOSCATH, bos´kath, stony, elevated ground. 2 Kin. 22:1.
BOSOR, bo´sor, Greek and Aramaic form of BEOR. 2 Pet. 2:15.
BOZEZ, bo´zez, shining. 1 Sam. 14:4.
BOZKATH, boz´kath, same as BOSCATH. Josh. 15:39.
BOZRAH, boz´rah, sheepfold. Gen. 36:33.
prophecies concerning. Is. 34:6; 63:1; Jer. 48:24; 49:13; Amos 1:12.
BUKKI, book´i, wasting. Num. 34:22.
BUKKIAH, book´yah, wasting from Jehovah. 1 Chr. 25:4.
BUL, bool, rain. 1 Kin. 6:38.
BUNAH, boon´ah, prudence. 1 Chr. 2:25.
BUNNI, boon´i, built. Neh. 9:4.
BUZ, booz, contempt. Gen. 22:21.
BUZI, booz´i, descended from Buz. Ezek. 1:3.
BUZITE, booz´ite, a descendant of Buz. Job. 32:2.

CABBON, kab´on, cake. Josh. 15:40.
CABUL, cah´bool, displeasing (?). Josh. 19:27.
CÆSAR, see´zar. Matt. 22:17.
Augustus. Luke 2:1.
Tiberius. Luke 3:1.
Claudius, time of dearth. Acts 11:28.
Paul appeals to. Acts 25:11.
household of. Phil. 4:22.
CÆSAREA, see´zar-e´a, named after Augustus.
Cæsar. Acts 8:40.
CÆSAREA PHILIPPI, see´zar-e´a fil-ip´i, named after
Philip the tetrarch.
visited by Christ. Matt. 16:13; Mark 8:27.
——(Stratonis), Peter sent there. Acts 10.
Paul visits. Acts 21:8.
Paul sent to Felix there. Acts 23:23.
CAIAPHAS, kai´a-fas, depression (?).
high priest, prophesies concerning Christ. John 11:49.
his counsel. Matt. 26:3.
he condemns Him. Matt. 26:65; Mark 14:63; Luke 22:71.
CAIN, kane, possession. Gen. 4:1. Josh. 15:57.
his anger. Gen. 4:5.
murders Abel. Gen. 4:8; 1 John 3:12.
his punishment. Gen. 4:11; Jude 11.
CAINAN, kay´nan, possessor. Gen. 5:9.
CALAH, ka´lah. Gen. 10:11.
CALCOL, kal´kol. 1 Chr. 2:6.
CALEB, ka´leb, a dog.
faith of. Num. 13:30; 14:6.
permitted to enter Canaan. Num. 26:65; 32:12; Deut. 1:36.
his request. Josh. 14:6.
his possessions. Josh. 15:13.
gives his daughter to Othniel to wife. Judg. 1:13.
CALEB-EPHRATAH, ka´leb-ef´rat-ah, C. the fruitful. 1 Chr. 2:24.
CALNEH, kal´nay. Gen. 10:10.
CALNO, kal´no, same as CALNEH. Is. 10:9.
CALVARY, kal´va-ry, skull. Luke 23:33.
CAMON, ka´mon, abounding in stalks. Judg. 10:5.
CANA, ka´nah.
Christ turns water into wine at. John 2.
nobleman visits Christ at. John 4:47.
CANAAN, ka´na-an, low region. Gen. 9:18.
land of. Ex. 23:31; Josh. 1:4; Zeph. 2:5.
promised to Abraham. Gen. 12:7; 13:14; 17:8.
inhabitants of. Ex. 15:15.
their wickedness at Sodom and Gomorrah. Gen. 13:13; 19.
Israelites not to walk in the ways of. Lev. 18:3, 24, 30; 20:23.
daughters of. Gen. 28:1, 6, 8.
language of. Is. 19:18.
kingdoms of. Ps. 135:11.
king of. Judg. 4:2, 23, 24; 5:19.
wars of. Judg. 3:1.
dwelling of Abraham in. Gen. 12:6. Isaac and Jacob. Gen. 28. Esau. Gen. 36. Joseph. Gen. 37.
allotted to children of Israel. Josh. 14.
the spies visit, and their report. Num. 13.
Moses sees, from Pisgah. Num. 27:12; Deut. 3:27; 34:1.
——a son of Ham, grandson of Noah, cursed on account of his father's mockery of Noah. Gen. 9:25.
CANAANITE., ka´na-an-ite, a zealot. Mark 3:18.
CANAANITES, ka´na-an-ites, inhabitants of Canaan. Judg. 1:1.
CANAANITESS, ka´na-an-ite-ess, feminine of preceding. 1 Chr. 2:3.
CANDACE, kan´da-see, Queen of Ethiopia. Acts 8:27.
CANNEH, kan´ay, probably same as CALNEH. Ezek. 27:23.
CAPERNAUM, ka-per´na-um, city of consolation (?).
Christ dwells at. Matt. 4:13; John 2:12.
preaches at. Matt. 4:17; Mark 1:21.
miracles at. Matt. 8:5; 17:24; John 4:46; 6:17.
parables at. Matt. 13:18, 24; Mark 4.
condemned for impenitence. Matt. 11:23; Luke 10:15.
CAPHTHORIM, kaf´thor-im, same as CAPHTORIM. 1 Chr. 1:12.
CAPHTOR, kaf´tor. Deut. 2:23.
CAPHTORIM, kaf´tor-im, inhabitants of Caphtor. Gen. 10:14.
CAPPADOCIA, kap´ad-o´sha. Acts 2:9; 1 Pet. 1:1.
CARCAS, kar´kas. Esth. 1:10.
CARCHEMISH, kar´kem-ish, fortress of Chemosh. Jer. 46:2.
CAREAH, ka-re´ah, bald. 2 Kin. 25:23.
CARMEL, karm´el, park. Josh. 12:22.
Nabal's conduct to David at. 1 Sam. 25.
mount, Elijah and the prophets of Baal. 1 Kin. 18.
the Shunammite woman goes to Elisha at. 2 Kin. 4:25.
her child restored to life by Elisha. 2 Kin. 4:34.
CARMELITE, karm´el-ite, a native of Carmel. 1 Sam. 30:5.
CARMELITESS, karm´el-ite-ess, feminine of preceding. 1 Sam. 27:3.
CARMI, karm´i, a vine-dresser. Gen. 46:9.
CARMITES, karm´ites, descendants of Carmi. Num. 26:6.
CARPUS, karp´us, fruit (?). 2 Tim. 4:13.
CARSHENA, kar´shen-ah. Esth. 1:14.
CASIPHIA, ka-sif´yah, silver (?). Ezra 8:17.
CASLUHIM, kas´loo-him. Gen. 10:14.
CASTOR, kas´tor.
and Pollux, Paul's ship. Acts 28:11.
CEDRON, keed´ron, same as KIDRON. John 18:1.
CENCHREA, ken´kre-ah, millet, small pulse.
Paul shaves his head at. Acts 18:18.
seaport of Corinth, church there. Rom. 16:1.
CEPHAS, kee´fas.
(Peter), a stone. John 1:42; 1 Cor. 1:12; 3:22; 9:5; 15:5; Gal. 2:9. *See* PETER.
CHALCOL, kal´kol, same as CALCOL. 1 Kin. 4:31.
CHALDEA, kal-de´ah. Jer. 50:10.
CHALDEANS, kal-de´ans, inhabitants of Chaldea.
afflict Job. Job. 1:17.
besiege Jerusalem. 2 Kin. 24:2; 25:4; Jer. 37—39.

CHALDEANS—*cont.*
wise men of, preserved by Daniel. Dan. 2:24.
prophecies concerning. Is. 23:13; 43:14; 47:1; 48:14; Hab. 1:5.
CHALDEES, kal-dees´, same as preceding. Gen. 11:28.
CHANAAN, ka-na-an, another form of CANAAN. Acts 7:11.
CHARASHIM, kar-ash-im, craftsmen. 1 Chr. 4:14.
CHARCHEMISH, same as CARCHEMISH. 2 Chr. 35:20.
CHARRAN, kar-an, same as HARAN. Acts 7:2.
CHEBAR, ke-bar, great (?).
the river, Ezekiel's visions at. Ezek. 1; 3:15; 10:15.
CHEDORLAOMER, ke-dor-la-o-mer, glory of Laomer (?).
king of Elam, takes Lot prisoner, but subdued by Abram. Gen. 14.
CHELAL, ke-al, completion. Ezra 10:30.
CHELLUH, kel-oo. Ezra 10:35.
CHELUB, kel-oob, bird-trap. 1 Chr. 4:11.
CHELUBAI, kel-oo-bai, same as CALEB. 1 Chr. 2:9.
CHEMARIMS, kem-ah-rims, persons dressed in black attire. Zeph. 1:4.
CHEMOSH, keem-osh, subduer.
god of Moab. Num. 21:29; Judg. 11:24; Jer. 48:7, 13, 46.
worshipped by Solomon. 1 Kin. 11:7.
CHENAANAH. KE-NA-AN-AH, probably fem. of Canaan. 1 Kin. 22:11.
CHENANI, ke-nane-i, probably same as CHENANIAH. Neh. 9:4.
CHENANIAH, ke-nan-i-ah, whom Jehovah supports. 1 Chr. 15:22.
CHEPHAR-HAAMMONI, ke-far-hah-am-on-ai, village of the Ammonites. Josh. 18:24.
CHEPHIRAH, ke-fi-rah, same as CAPHAR. Josh. 9:17.
CHERAN, ke-ran. Gen. 36:26.
CHERETHIMS, ke-reth-ims, Cretans (?). Ezek. 25:16.
CHERETHITES, ke-reth-ites, probably same as preceding. 2 Sam. 8:18.
(and Pelethites), David's guard. 2 Sam. 15:18.
CHERITH, ke-rith, gorge (?). 1 Kin. 17:3.
CHERUB, cher-ub, blessing (?), strong (?). Ezra 2:59.
CHERUBIM, cher-oob-im, plural of CHERUB.
in garden of Eden. Gen. 3:24.
for the mercy seat and the temple. Ex. 25:18; 37:7; 1 Kin. 6:23; 2 Chr. 3:10; Ps. 80:1; Ezek. 41:18.
Ezekiel's visions of. Ezek. 1; 10.
CHESALON, ke-sah-lon, hope. Josh. 15:10.
CHESED, ke-sed, conqueror (?). Gen. 22:22.
CHESIL, ke-sil, a fool. Josh. 15:30.
CHESULLOTH, ke-sool-oth, confidences. Josh. 19:18.
CHEZIB, ke-zib, false. Gen. 38:5.
CHINON, ki-don, javelin. 1 Chr. 13:9.
CHILEAB, kil-e-ab, probably another form of CALEB. 2 Sam. 3:3.
CHILION, kil-yon, wasting away. Ruth 1:2.
CHILMAD, kil-mad. Ezek. 27:23.
CHIMHAM, kim-ham, longing. 2 Sam. 19:37.
CHINNERETH, kin-er-eth, a lyre. Josh. 19:35.
CHINNEROTH, kin-er-oth, plural of CHINNERETH. Josh. 11:2.
CHIOS, ki-os. Acts 20:15.
CHISLEU, kis-lew. Neh. 1:1.
CHISLON, kis-lon, confidence, hope. Num. 34:21.
CHISLOTH-TABOR, kis-loth-ta-bor, flanks (?) of Tabor. Josh. 19:12.
CHITTIM, kit-im, probably Cyprus.
prophecies of. Num. 24:24; Is. 23:1, 12; Dan. 11:30.
CHIUN, ki-oon, image. Amos 5:26.
CHLOE, klo-ee. 1 Cor. 1:11.
CHOR-ASHAN, kor-ash-an, smoking furnace. 1 Sam. 30:30.
CHORAZIN, ko-ra-zin. Matt. 11:21.
CHOZEBA, ko-ze-bah, deceiver. 1 Chr. 4:22.
CHRIST, the anointed. See *Subject-Index*, p. 1413.
CHUB, choob. Ezek. 30:5.
CHUN, choon, establishment. 1 Chr. 18:8.
CHUSHAN-RISHATHAIM, koosh-an-rish-a-tha-im.
Oppresses Israel. Judg. 3:8, 9, 10.
CHUZA, koo-zah. Luke 8:3.
CILICIA, si-lish-ya.
disciples there. Acts 15:23, 41.
the country of Paul. Acts 21:39; Gal. 1:21.
Paul born at Tarsus in. Acts 22:3.
CINNEROTH, kin-er-oth, same as CHINNEROTH. 1 Kin. 15:20.
CIS, kis. Acts 13:21, same as KISH.
CLAUDA, klawd-ah. Acts 27:16.
CLAUDIA, klawd-yah. 2 Tim. 4:21.
CLAUDIUS, klawd-yus. Acts 11:28.
CLAUDIUS LYSIAS, klawd-yus-lis-yas.
chief captain, rescues Paul. Acts 21:31; 22:24; 23:10.
sends him to Felix. Acts 23:26.
CLEMENT, klem-ent.
fellow labourer of Paul. Phil. 4:3.
CLEOPAS, kle-op-as, either a shortened form of CLEOPATROS, or a Greek form of ALPHÆUS.
a disciple. Luke 24:18. *See* EMMAUS.
CLEOPHAS, kle-of-as, probably same as preceding. John 19:25.
CNIDUS, kni-dus, nettle (?). Acts 27:7.
COL-HOZEH, kol-ho-zeh, every one that seeth. Neh. 3:15.
COLOSSE, ko-los-ee.
brethren at, encouraged and warned. Col. 1; 2.
exhorted to holiness. Col. 3; 4.
COLOSSIANS, ko-los-yans, people of Colosse.
CONANIAH. 2 Chr. 35:9, same as CONONIAH.
CONIAH, ko-ni-ah, contracted from JECONIAH. Jer. 22:24.
CONONIAH, kon-on-i-ah, whom Jehovah has set up. 2 Chr. 31:12.
COOS, ko-os.
Paul sails to. Acts 21:1.
CORE, ko-re, Greek form of KORAH. Jude 11.
CORINTH, kor-inth.
Paul and Apollos at. Acts 18; 19:1.
CORINTHIANS, kor-inth-yans, inhabitants of Corinth. Acts 18:8.
their divisions, &c., censured. 1 Cor. 1; 5; 11:18.
their faith and graces. 2 Cor. 3.
instructed concerning spiritual gifts. 1 Cor. 14; and the resurrection. 1 Cor. 15.
exhorted to charity, &c. 1 Cor. 13; 14:1; 2 Cor. 8; 9.
their false teachers exposed. 2 Cor. 11:3, 4, 13.
Paul commends himself to. 2 Cor. 11; 12.
CORNELIUS, kor-neel-yus. Acts 10:1.
devout centurion, his prayer answered. Acts 10:3; sends for Peter, 10:9; baptized, 10:48.
COSAM, ko-sam. Luke 3:28.
COZ, koz, thorn. 1 Chr. 4:8.
COZBI, kos-bi, deceitful, slain by Phineas. Num. 25:15.
CRESCENS, kres-ens, growing.
goes to Dalmatia. 2 Tim. 4:10.
CRETE, kreet.
visited by Paul. Acts 27:7.
CRETES OR CRETIANS, kreet-yans, inhabitants of Crete. Acts 2:11; Tit. 1:12.
CRISPUS, krisp-us, curled.
baptized by Paul. Acts 18:8; 1 Cor. 1:14.
CUMI, koom-i, arise. Mark 5:41.
CUSH, koosh, black. Gen. 10:6.
CUSHAN, koosh-an, same meaning as CUSH. Hab. 3:7.
CUSHI, koosh-i, same meaning as CUSH.
announces Absalom's death. 2 Sam. 18:21.
CUTH, kooth. 2 Kin. 17:30.
CUTHAH, kooth-ah, same as CUTH. 2 Kin. 17:24.
CYPRUS, si-prus. Acts 4:36.
disciples there. Acts 11:19.
Paul and Barnabas preach there. Acts 13:4.
Barnabas and Mark go there. Acts 15:39.
CYRENE, si-re-nee. Matt. 27:32.
disciples of. Acts 11:20; 13:1.

CYRENE—*cont.*
Simon of. Mark 15:21.
CYRENIAN, si-reen´-yan, a native of Cyrene. Acts 6:9.
CYRENIUS, si-reen´-yus, Greek form of the Roman name Quirinus.
governor of Syria. Luke 2:2.
CYRUS, si´-rus, the sun. 2 Chr. 36:22.
king of Persia, prophecies concerning. Is. 44:28; 45:1. *See* Dan. 6:28; 10:1.
his proclamation for rebuilding the temple. 2 Chr. 36:22; Ezra 1.

DARAREH, da´-bar-ay, pasture. Josh. 21:28.
DABBASHETH, dab-ash´-eth, hump of a camel. Josh. 19:11.
DABERATH, da´-ber-ath. Josh. 19:12, same as DABAREH.
DAGON, da´-gon, fish.
national idol-god of the Philistines, sacrificed to. Judg. 16:23.
smitten down in temple at Ashdod. 1 Sam. 5:3, 4.
Saul's head fastened in house of. 1 Chr. 10:10.
DALAIAH, da-ai´-ah, whom Jehovah hath delivered. 1 Chr. 3:24.
DALMANUTHA, dal´-ma-noo´-thah. Mark 8:10.
DALMATIA, dal´-ma´-shah. 2 Tim. 4:10.
DALPHON, dal´-fon, proud (?). Esth. 9:7.
DAMARIS, dam-ar-is, calf (?).
cleaves to Paul. Acts 17:34.
DAMASCENES, dam´-as-eens´, people of Damascus. 2 Cor. 11:32.
DAMASCUS, dam-ask´-us, activity (?). Gen. 14:15.
mentioned. Gen. 15:2.
subjugated by David. 2 Sam. 8:6; 1 Chr. 18:6.
Elisha's prophecy there. 2 Kin. 8:7.
taken by Tiglath-pileser, king of Assyria. 2 Kin. 16:9.
restored to Israel by Jeroboam. 2 Kin. 14:28.
king Ahaz copies an altar there. 2 Kin. 16:10.
Paul's journey to. Acts 9; 22:6.
Paul restored to sight, and baptized there. Acts 9:17, 18.
prophecies concerning. Is. 7:8; 8:4; 17:1; Jer. 49:23; Amos 1:3.
DAN, judge.
son of Jacob, by Rachel's handmaid. Gen. 30:6.
——TRIBEof, numbered. Num. 1:38; 26:42.
their inheritance. Josh. 19:40.
blessed by Jacob. Gen. 49:16.
blessed by Moses. Deut. 33:22.
win Laish, and call it Dan. Judg. 18:29.
set up idolatry. Judg. 18:30; 1 Kin. 12:29.
DAN-JAAN, dan´-ja´-an, woodland (?) Dan. 2 Sam. 24:6.
DANIEL, dan´-yel, God's judge. Dan. 1:6.
(Belteshazzar), with other captives, taken from Jerusalem to Babylon. Dan. 1:3.
taught the learning of the Chaldeans. Dan. 1:4.
will not take the king's meat or drink. Dan. 1:8.
has understanding in dreams. Dan. 1:17.
interprets the royal dreams. Dan. 2; 4; and handwriting on wall. Dan. 5:17.
made chief president by Darius. Dan. 6:2.
conspired against by the princes. Dan. 6:4.
idolatrous decree against, issued. Dan. 6:9; breach thereof, Dan. 6:10.
cast into the lions' den. Dan. 6:16; preservation in, Dan. 6:22.
his vision of the four beasts. Dan. 7:12; ram and he-goat. Dan. 8:3.
his prayer. Dan. 9:3.
promise of return from captivity. Dan. 9:20; 10:10; 12:13.
name mentioned. Ezek. 14:14, 20; 28:3.
DANITES, dan´-ites, descendants of Dan. Judg. 13:2.
DANNAH, dan´-ah. Josh. 15:49.
DARA, da´-rah, probably contracted from the next word. 1 Chr. 2:6.
DARDA, dar´-dah, pearl of wisdom (?). 1 Kin. 4:31.
DARIUS, da-ri´-us, governor (?). Ezra 4:5.

DARIUS—*cont.*
decree concerning the rebuilding of the temple. Ezra 6.
——(the Median) takes Babylon. Dan. 5:31; his decree to fear the God of Daniel. Dan. 6:25.
DARKON, dark´-on, scatterer (?). Ezra 2:56.
DATHAN, da´-than. Num. 16:1.
DAVID, da´-vid, beloved.
King, son of Jesse. Ruth 4:22; 1 Chr. 2; Matt. 1.
anointed by Samuel. 1 Sam. 16:8.
plays the harp before Saul. 1 Sam. 16:19.
his zeal and faith. 1 Sam. 17:26, 34.
kills Goliath of Gath. 1 Sam. 17:49.
at first honoured by Saul. 1 Sam. 18.
Saul jealous of, tries to kill. 1 Sam. 18:8, 12.
afterwards persecuted by him. 1 Sam:19; 20.
loved by Jonathan. 1 Sam. 18:1; 19:2; 20; 23:16; and by Michal. 1 Sam. 18:28; 19:11.
overcomes the Philistines. 1 Sam. 18:27; 19:8.
flees to Naioth. 1 Sam. 19:18.
eats of the shewbread. 1 Sam. 21; Ps. 52; Matt. 12:4.
flees to Gath, and feigns madness. 1 Sam. 21:10, 13; Ps. 34; 56.
dwells in the cave of Adullam. 1 Sam. 22; Ps. 63; 142.
escapes Saul's pursuit. 1 Sam. 23; Ps. 57.
twice spares Saul's life. 1 Sam. 24:4; 26:5.
his wrath against Nabal appeased by Abigail. 1 Sam. 25:23.
dwells at Ziklag. 1 Sam. 27.
dismissed from the army by Achish. 1 Sam. 29:9.
chastises the Amalekites, and rescues the captives. 1 Sam. 30:16.
kills messenger who brings news of Saul's death. 2 Sam. 1:15.
laments the death of Saul and Jonathan. 2 Sam. 1:17.
becomes king of Judah. 2 Sam. 2:4.
forms a league with Abner. 2 Sam. 3:13.
laments Abner's death. 2 Sam. 3:31.
avenges the murder of Ish-bosheth. 2 Sam. 4:9.
becomes king of all Israel. 2 Sam. 5:3; 1 Chr. 1:11.
his victories. 2 Sam. 2; 5; 8; 10; 12:29; 21:15; 1 Chr. 18—20; Ps. 60.
brings the ark to Zion. 2 Sam. 6; 1 Chr. 13; 15.
his psalms of thanksgiving. 2 Sam. 22; 1 Chr. 16:7; Ps. 18; 103; 105.
Michal despises him for dancing before the ark. 2 Sam. 6:20.
reproves her. 2 Sam. 6:21.
desires to build God a house. 2 Sam. 7:2; and is forbidden by Nathan. 1 Chr. 17:4.
God's promises to him. 2 Sam. 7:11; Chr. 17:10.
his prayer and thanksgiving. 2 Sam. 7:18; 1 Chr. 17:16.
his consideration for Mephibosheth. 2 Sam. 9.
his sin concerning Bath-sheba and Uriah. 2 Sam. 11; 12.
repents at Nathan's parable of the ewe lamb. 2 Sam. 12; Ps. 51.
Absalom conspires against. 2 Sam. 15; Ps. 3.
Ahithophel's treachery against. 1 Sam. 15:31; 16; 17.
Shimei curses. 2 Sam. 16:5; Ps. 7.
Barzillai's loyalty. 2 Sam. 17:27.
grieves over Absalom's death. 2 Sam. 18:33; 19:1.
returns to Jerusalem. 2 Sam. 19:15.
pardons Shimei. 2 Sam. 19:16.
Sheba's conspiracy against. 2 Sam. 20.
atones for the Gibeonites. 2 Sam. 21.
his mighty men. 2 Sam. 23:8; 1 Chr. 11:10.
tempted by Satan, numbers the people. 2 Sam. 24; 1 Chr. 21.
regulates the service of the tabernacle. 1 Chr. 23—26.
exhorts the congregation to fear God. 1 Chr. 28.
appoints Solomon his successor. 1 Kin. 1; Ps. 72.
his charge to Solomon. 1 Kin. 2; 1 Chr. 28:9; to

DAVID—*cont.*
build a house for the sanctuary. 1 Chr. 22:6; 28:10.
his last words. 2 Sam. 23.
his death. 1 Kin. 2; 1 Chr. 29:26.
the progenitor of Christ. Matt. 1:1; 9:27; 21:9; comp. Ps. 110, with Matt. 22:41; Luke 1:32; John 7:42; Acts 2:25; 13:22; 15:15; Rom. 1:3; 2 Tim. 2:8; Rev. 5:5; 22:16.
prophecies concerning. Ps. 89; 132; Is. 9:7; 22:22; 55:3; Jer. 30:9; Hos. 3:5; Amos 9:11.

DEBIR, de-bee´r, a recess. Josh. 10:3.

DEBORAH, deb-or-ah, bee.
the prophetess judges and delivers Israel. Judg. 4.
her song. Judg. 5.
——Rebekah's nurse, death of. Gen. 35:8.

DECAPOLIS, de-ka-pol-is, ten cities. Matt. 4:25.

DEDAN, de-dan. Gen. 10:7.

DEDANIM, de-dah-nim, inhabitants of Dedan. Is. 21:13.

DEHAVITES, de-hav-ites. Ezra 4:9.

DEKAR, de-kar, piercing. 1 Kin. 4:9.

DELAIAH, de-lai-ah, whom Jehovah has freed. 1 Chr. 24:18.

DELILAH, de-li-lah, delicate. Judg. 16:4.

DEMAS, de-mas, probably same as following. Col. 4:14.

DEMETRIUS, de-me-tri-us, belonging to Demeter.
silversmith. Acts 19:24.
disciple. 3 John 12.

DERBE, der-bee, juniper (?). Acts 14:6.

DEUEL, doo-el, the same as REUEL (?). Num. 1:14.

DEUTERONOMY, a recapitulation of the law.

DIANA, di-an-ah.
of Ephesians, tumult concerning. Acts 19:24.

DIBLAIM, dib-la-im, two cakes. Hos. 1:3.

DIBLATHAIM, dib-la-thah-im, same as DIBLAIM. Num. 33:46.

DIBLATH, dib-ath, supposed to be the same as RIBLAH. Ezek. 6:14.

DIBON, di-bon, wasting. Num. 21:30.

DIBOH-GAD, di-bon-gad´, wasting of Gad. Num. 33:45.

DIBRI, dib-ri, eloquent. Lev. 24:11.

DIDYMUS, did-im-us, twin. John 11:16.
(Thomas). John 20:24.

DIKLAH, dik-lah, a palm tree. Gen. 10:27.

DILEAN, dil-e-an, cucumber field (?). Josh. 15:38.

DIMHAH, dim-nah, dunghill. Josh. 21:35.

DIMON, di-mon, same as DIBON. Is. 15:9.

DIMONAH, di-mo-nah, probably same as preceding. Josh. 15:22.

DINAH, di-nah, vindicated.
Jacob's daughter. Gen. 30:21; outraged by Shechem, Gen. 34:2; avenged by Simeon and Levi, Gen. 34:25.

DINAITES, di-na-ites. Ezra 4:9.

DINHABAH, din-hab-ah. Gen. 36:32.

DIONYSIUS, di-o-nis-yus, belonging to Dionysus.
the Areopagite, believes. Acts 17:34.

DIOTREPHES, di-ot-ref-ees, nourished by Zeus, loveth preeminence. 3 John 9.

DISHAN, di-shan, antelope (?). Gen. 36:28.

DISHON, di-shon, same as preceding. Gen. 36:21.

DIZAHAB, di-za-hab, a place abounding in gold (?). Deut. 1:1.

DODAI, do-dai, loving. 1 Chr. 27:4.

DODANIM, do-dah-nim. Gen. 10:4.

DODAVAH, do-dah-vah, love of Jehovah. 2 Chr. 20:37.

DODO, do-do, same as DODAI. 2 Sam. 23:9.

DOEG, do-eg, anxious. 1 Sam. 21:7.
the Edomite slays the priests. 1 Sam. 22:9.

DOPHKAH, dof-kah. Num. 33:12.

DOR, dor, dwelling. Josh. 11:2.

DORCAS, dor-kas, gazelle. Acts 9:36.
(Tabitha), raised from death by Peter. Acts 9:40.

DOTHAN, do-than, two wells or cisterns. Gen. 37:17.

DRUSILLA, droo-sil-ah. Acts 24:24.

DUMAH, doom-ah, silence. Gen. 25:14.

DURA, doo-rah, town.
plain of, golden image set up. Dan. 3:1.

EBAL, e-bal, stony (?). Gen. 36:23.
mount, curses delivered from. Deut. 27:13; Josh. 8:33.

EBED, e-bed, servant. Judg. 9:26.

EBED-MELECH, e-bed-me-lek, servant of the king.
Ethiopian eunuch, intercedes with king Zedekiah for Jeremiah. Jer. 38:7; 39:16.

EBEN-EZER, e-ben-e-zer, stone of help.
Israelites smitten by Philistines at. 1 Sam. 4:1.
'hitherto hath the Lord helped us,' (stone raised by Samuel in memory of defeat of the Philistines). 1 Sam. 7:12.

EBER, e-ber, the region beyond. Gen. 10:21.

EBIASAPH, e-bi-a-saf, same as ABIASAPH. 1 Chr. 6:23.

EBRONAH, eb-ro-nah, passage (?). Num. 33:34.

ECCLESIASTES, ek-lee-zy-ast-ees, preacher.

ED, witness. Josh. 22:34.

EDAR, e-dar, flock. Gen. 35:21.

EDEN, e-den, pleasantness. Gen. 2:8.
Adam driven from. Gen. 3:24.
mentioned. Is. 51:3; Ezek. 28:13; 31:9; 36:35; Joel 2:3.

EDER, e-der, flock, same as EDAR. 1 Chr. 23:23.

EDOM, e-dom, red. Gen. 25:30.
——(Idumea), the land of Esau. Gen. 32:3; Is. 63:1.
prophecies concerning. Is. 34; Jer. 25:21; 49:7; Ezek. 25:13; 35; Amos 1:11; Obad. 1.

EDOMITES, e-dom-ites, inhabitants of Edom. Gen. 36:9.
the descendants of Esau. Gen. 36.
deny Moses passage through Edom. Num. 20:18.
their possessions. Deut. 2:5; Josh. 24:4.
not to be abhorred. Deut. 23:7.
subdued by David. 2 Sam. 8:14.
revolt. 2 Kin. 8:20; 2 Chr. 21:8.
subdued by Amaziah. 2 Kin. 14:7; 2 Chr. 11:25.

EDREI, ed-re-i, strong. Num. 21:33.

EGLAH, eg-lah, heifer. 2 Sam. 3:5.

EGLAIM, eg-la-im, two pools. Is. 15:8.

EGLON, eg-on. Judg. 3:12.
oppresses Israel. Judg. 3:14; slain by Ehud. Judg. 3:21.

EGYPT, e-jipt, black.
Abram goes down into. Gen. 12:10.
Joseph sold into. Gen. 37:36; his advancement, fall, imprisonment, and restoration there. Gen. 39; 40; 41.
Jacob's sons go to buy corn in. Gen. 42.
Jacob and all his seed go there. Gen. 46:6.
children of Israel wax mighty there. Ex. 1:7; afflicted, and build treasure cities. Ex. 1:11.
plagued on account of Israelites. Ex. 7—11.
children of Israel depart from. Ex. 13:17.
army of, pursue and perish in the Red sea. Ex. 14.
kings of, harass Judah. 1 Kin. 14:25; 2 Kin. 23:29; 2 Chr. 12:2; 35:20; 36:3; Jer. 37:5.
the 'remnant of Judah' go there. Jer. 43:7.
Jesus taken to. Matt. 2:13.
prophecies concerning. Gen. 15:13; Is. 11:11; 19; 20; 27:12; 30:1; Jer. 9:26; 25:19; 43:8; 44:28; 46; Ezek. 29—32; Dan. 11:8; Hos. 9:3; 11; Joel 3:19; Zech. 10:10; 14:18.

EGYPTIAN, e-jip-shan, a native of Egypt. 1 Sam. 30:11.

EHI, e-hi, shortened from AHIRAM. Gen. 46:21.

EHUD, e-hud, joined together (?).
judge, delivers Israel. Judg. 3:15.

EKER, e-ker, same as ACHAR. 1 Chr. 2:27.

EKRON, ek-ron, eradication. Josh. 13:3.
taken. Judg. 1:18.
men of, smitten with emerods. 1 Sam. 5:12.
their trespass offering for recovery. 1 Sam. 6:17.
prophecies concerning. Amos 1:8; Zeph. 2:4; Zech. 9:5.

EKRONITES, ek-ron-ites, inhabitants of Ekron. Josh. 13:3.

ELADAH, el´-a-dah, whom God clothes. 1 Chr. 7:20.
ELAH, e´-lah, terebinth. Gen. 36:41.
king of Israel. 1 Kin. 16:8, 10.
——valley of, Saul sets the battle in array against the Philistines. 1 Sam. 17:2.
David slays Goliath there. 1 Sam. 17:49.
ELAM, e´-am.
son of Shem. Gen. 10:22.
Chedorlaomer, king of. Gen. 14.
ELAMITES, e´-lam-ites, inhabitants of Elam. Ezra 4:9; Acts 2:9.
ELASAH, el´-a-sah, whom God made. Ezra 10:22.
ELATH, e´-lath, a grove. Deut. 2:8.
EL-BETH-EL, el-beth´-el, the house of God. Gen. 35:7.
ELDAAH, el´-da-ah, whom God called. Gen. 25:4.
ELDAD, el´-dad, whom God loves. Num. 11:26.
ELEAD, el´-e-ad, whom God praises. 1 Chr. 7:21.
ELEALEH, el´-e-a´-lay, whither God ascends. Num. 32:3.
ELEASAH, e´l-e-a´-sah, same as ELASAH. 1 Chr. 2:39.
ELEAZAR, el´-e-a´-zar, whom God aids.
son of Aaron, and chief priest. Ex. 6:23; 28; 29; Lev. 8; Num. 3:2; 4:16; 16:36; 20:26, 28; 27:22; 31:13; 34:17; Josh. 17:4; 24:33.
——son of Abinadab, keeps the ark. 1 Sam. 7:1.
——one of David's captains. 2 Sam. 23:9; 1 Chr. 11:12.
EL-ELOHE-ISRAEL, el´-el-o´-he-iz´-ra-el, God, the God of Israel.
the altar erected by Jacob at Shalem. Gen. 33:20.
ELEPH, e´-lef, ox. Josh. 18:28.
ELHANAN, el´-ha´-nan, whom God gave.
one of David's warriors. 2 Sam. 21:19; 23:24; 1 Chr. 11:26; 20:5.
ELI, e´-li, my God.
Eli, Eli, lama sabachthani? Matt. 27:46; Mark 15:34.
ELI, e´-li, height. 1 Sam. 1:3.
high priest and judge, blesses Hannah, who bears Samuel. 1 Sam. 1:17, 20.
Samuel brought to. 1 Sam. 1:25.
wickedness of his sons. 1 Sam. 2:22.
rebuked by man of God. 1 Sam. 2:27.
ruin of his house shewed to Samuel by God. 1 Sam. 3:11.
his sons slain. 1 Sam. 4:10.
his death. 1 Sam. 4:18.
ELIAB, el-i´-ab, whose father is God. Num. 1:9.
ELIADA, ELIADAH, el´-i´-ya-dah, whom God cares for. 2 Sam. 5:16.
ELIAH, el-i´-ah, same name as ELIJAH. 1 Chr. 8:27.
ELIAHBA, e´l-i-ah´-bah, whom God hides. 2 Sam. 23:32.
ELIAKIM, el-i´-a-kim, whom God establishes. 2 Kin. 18:18.
chief minister of Hezekiah; his conference with Rabshakeh's ambassadors; mission to Isaiah. 2 Kin. 18; 19.
prefigures kingdom of Christ. Is. 22:20-25.
——son of Josiah, made king by Pharaoh, and named Jehoiakim. 2 Kin. 23:34; 2 Chr. 36:4.
ELIAM, el-i´-am, same as AMMIEL. 2 Sam. 11:3.
ELIAS, el-i´-as, same as ELIJAH. Matt. 27:47, 49; Mark 15:35, 36; John 1:21. *See* ELIJAH.
ELIASAPH, el-i´-a-saf, whom God added. Num. 1:14.
ELIASHIB, el-i´-a-shib, whom God restores.
high priest, builds the wall. Neh. 3:1.
allied unto Tobiah. Neh. 13:4.
ELIATHAH, el-i´-a-thah, to whom God comes. 1 Chr. 25:4.
ELIDAD, el-i´-dad, whom God loves. Num. 34:21.
ELIEL, el-i´-el, to whom God is strength. 1 Chr. 5:24.
ELIENAI, el-i-e´-nai, unto Jehovah my eyes are raised (?). 1 Chr. 8:20.
ELIEZER, el´-i-e´-zer, my God is help.
Abraham's steward. Gen. 15:2.
——son of Moses. Ex. 18:4; 1 Chr. 23:15.
——prophet. 2 Chr. 20:37.
ELIHOENAI, el´-i-ho-e´-nai, same as ELIOENAI. Ezra 8:4.

ELIHOREPH, el´-i-ho´-ref, to whom God is the reward. 1 Kin. 4:3.
ELIHU, el-i´-hoo, whose God is He. 1 Sam. 1:1.
reproves Job's friends, Job 32; and Job's impatience, Job 33:8; and self-righteousness, Job 34:5.
declares God's justice, Job 33:12; 34:10; 35:13; 36; power, Job 33—37; and mercy, Job 33:23; 34:28.
ELIJAH, el-i´-jah, my God is Jehovah.
the Tishbite, prophet, predicts great drought. 1 Kin. 17:1; Luke 4:25; James 5:17.
hides at the brook Cherith, and is fed by ravens. 1 Kin. 17:5. (19:5).
raises the widow's son. 1 Kin. 17:21.
his sacrifice at Carmel. 1 Kin. 18:38.
slays the prophets of Baal at the brook Kishon. 1 Kin. 18:40.
flees from Jezebel into the wilderness of Beer-sheba. 1 Kin. 19; Rom. 11:2.
anoints Elisha. 1 Kin. 19:19.
by God's command denounces Ahab in Naboth's vineyard. 1 Kin. 21:17.
his prediction fulfilled. 1 Kin. 22:38; 2 Kin. 9:36; 10:10.
condemns Ahaziah for enquiring of Baal-zebub. 2 Kin. 1:3, 16.
two companies sent to take him burnt with fire from heaven. 2 Kin. 1:10; Luke 9:54.
divides Jordan. 2 Kin. 2:8.
taken up by chariot of fire. 2 Kin. 2:11.
his mantle taken by Elisha. 2 Kin. 2:13.
appears at Christ's transfiguration. Matt. 17:3; Mark 9:4; Luke 9:30.
precursor of John the Baptist. Mal. 4:5; Matt. 11:14; 16:14; Luke 1:17; 9:8, 19; John 1:21.
ELIKA, el-i´-kah, whom God purifies (?). 2 Sam. 23:25.
ELIM, eel´-im, oaks. Ex. 15:27.
ELIMELECH, el-i´-me-lek, to whom God is king. Ruth 1:2.
ELIOENAI, el´-i-o-e´-nai, unto Jehovah my eyes are turned. 1 Chr. 3:23.
ELIPHAL, el´-i-fal, whom God judges. 1 Chr. 11:35.
ELIPHALET, el-i´-fa-let, to whom God is salvation. 2 Sam. 5:16.
ELIPHAZ, el´-i-faz, to whom God is strength. Gen. 36:4.
reproves Job. Job 4; 5; 15; 22.
God's wrath against him. Job 42:7; he offers a burnt offering, and Job prays for him. Job 42:8.
ELIPHELEH, el-i´-fe-lay, whom God distinguishes. 1 Chr. 15:18.
ELIPHELET, el-l´-fe-let, same as ELIPHALET. 1 Chr. 3:8.
ELISABETH, el-iz´-a-beth, same as ELISHEBA.
cousin of Virgin Mary, and mother of John the Baptist. Luke 1:5.
angel promises her a son. Luke 1:13.
her salutation to Mary. Luke 1:42.
ELISEUS, el´-i-se´-us, Greek form of ELISHA. Luke 4:27.
ELISHA, el-i´-shah, to whom God is salvation.
——(Eliseus), succeeds Elijah. 1 Kin. 19:16.
receives his mantle, and divides Jordan. 2 Kin. 2:13.
heals the waters with salt. 2 Kin. 2:22.
bears destroy the children who mock him. 2 Kin. 2:24.
his miracles: water, 2 Kin. 3:16; oil, 4:4; Shunammite's son, 4:32; death in the pot, 4:40; feeds a hundred men with twenty loaves, 4:44; Naaman's leprosy, 5:14; iron swims, 6:5; Syrians struck blind, 6:18.
prophesies plenty in Samaria when besieged. 2 Kin. 7:1.
sends to anoint Jehu. 2 Kin. 9:1.
his death. 2 Kin. 13:20.
miracle wrought by his bones. 2 Kin. 13:21.
ELISHAH, el-i´-shah. Gen. 10:4.

ELISHAMA, el-i´sha-mah, whom God hears. Num. 1:10.
ELISHAPHAT, el-i´sha-fat, whom God judges. 2 Chr. 23:1.
ELISHEBA, el-i´she-bah, to whom God is the oath. Ex. 6:23.
ELISHUA, el-i´shoo´ah, same as ELISHA. 2 Sam. 5:15.
ELIUD, el-i´ood, God of Judah. Matt. 1:14.
ELIZAPHAN, el-i´za-fan, whom God protects. Num. 3:30.
ELIZUR, el-i´zoor, God is a Rock. Num. 1:5.
ELKANAH, el-ka´nah, whom God possessed. Ex. 6:24.
  Samuel's father. 1 Sam. 1.
ELKOSHITE, el´kosh-ite, inhabitant of Elkosh. Nah. 1:1.
ELLASAR, el-ah´sar. Gen. 14:1.
ELMODAM, el-mo´dam, same as ALMODAD. Luke 3:28.
ELNAAM, el-na´am, whose pleasure God is. 1 Chr. 11:46.
ELNATHAN, el-na´than, whom God gave. 2 Kin. 24:8.
ELOI, el-o´i, my God. Mark 15:34.
ELON, e-lon, oak. Gen. 26:34.
  judges Israel. Judg. 12:11.
ELON-BETH-HANAN, e´lon-beth´ha-nan, oak of the house of grace. 1 Kin. 4:9.
ELONITES, e´lon-ites, descendants of Elon. Num. 26:26.
ELOTH, e´loth, same as ELATH. 1 Kin. 9:26.
ELPAAL, el-pa´al, to whom God is the reward. 1 Chr. 8:11.
ELPALET, el-pa´let, same as ELIPHALET. 1 Chr. 14:5.
EL-PARAN, el-par´an, oak of Paran. Gen. 14:6.
ELTEKEH, el´te-kay, whose fear is God. Josh. 19:44.
ELTEKON, el´te-kon, whose foundation is God. Josh. 15:59.
ELTOLAD, el-to´lad, whose posterity is from God. Josh. 15:30.
ELUL, el´ool. Neh. 6:15.
ELUZAI, el-oo´zai, God is my praises. 1 Chr. 12:5.
ELYMAS, el´im-as, a wise man. Acts 13:8.
  (Bar-jesus). Acts 13:6.
ELZABAD, el-za´bad, whom God gave. 1 Chr. 12:12.
ELZAPHAN, el-za´fan, whom God protects. Ex. 6:22.
EMIMS, eem´ims, terrible men, giants. Gen. 14:5; Deut. 2:10.
EMMANUEL, em-an´u-el, same as IMMANUEL.
  God with us. Is. 7:14; 8:8; Matt. 1:23.
EMMAUS, em-a´us, hot springs (?). Luke 24:13.
  Christ talks with Cleopas and another on the way to. Luke 24:15.
EMMOR, em´or, same as HAMOR. Acts 7:16.
ENAM, e´nam, two fountains. Josh. 15:34.
ENAN, e´nan, having eyes. Num. 1:15.
EN-DOR, en´dor, fountain of Dor. Josh. 17:11.
  witch of. 1 Sam. 28:7.
ENEAS, e´ne-as. Acts 9:33, 34.
EN-EGLAIM, en´eg-la´im, *f.* of two calves. Ezek. 47:10.
EN-GANNIM, en-gan´im, *f.* of gardens. Josh. 15:34.
EN-GEDI, en´ged-i, *f.* of the kid.
  city of Judah. Josh. 15:62.
  David dwells there. 1 Sam. 23:29; 24:1.
EN-HADDAH, en-had´ah, *f.* of sharpness, *i.e.* swift *f.* Josh. 19:21.
EN-HAKKORE, en´hak-o´ree, *f.* of him that calleth. Judg. 15:19.
EN-HAZOR, en-ha´zor, *f.* of the village. Josh. 19:37.
EN-MISHPAT, en-mish´pat, *f.* of judgment. Gen. 14:7.
ENOCH, e´nok, experienced (?). Gen. 4:17.
  his faith, Heb. 11:5; prophecy, Jude 14; translation, Gen. 5:24.
ENOS, e´nos, man. Gen. 4:26.
ENOSH, enosh, same as ENOS. 1 Chr. 1:1.
EN-RIMMON, en´rim´on, fountain of the pomegranate. Neh. 11:29.
EN-ROGEL, en´ro´gel, *f.* of the fuller.
  fountain. Josh. 15:7; 18:16; 2 Sam. 17:17; 1 Kin. 1:9.
EN-SHEMESH, en-she´mesh, *f.* of the sun. Josh. 15:7.
EN-TAPPUAH, en´tap-oo´ah, *f.* of the apple tree. Josh. 17:7.
EPÆNETUS, e-pe´net-us, laudable. Rom. 16:5.
EPAPHRAS, ep´af-ras, contracted from the next word (?).
  commended. Col. 1:7; 4:12.
EPAPHRODITUS, ep-af´ro-di´tus, handsome.
  Paul's joy at his recovery, Phil. 2:25; his kindness, Phil. 4:18.
EPENETUS, same as EPÆNETUS. Rom. 16:5.
EPHAH, e´fah. Gen. 25:4.
EPHAI, e´phai, languishing. Jer. 40:8.
EPHER, e´fer, calf. Gen. 25:4.
EPHES-DAMMIM, e´fez-dam´im, boundary of blood. 1 Sam. 17:1.
EPHESIANS, e-fe´zi-ans, inhabitants of Ephesus. Acts 19:28.
  Paul's epistle to. Eph. 1.
  election. Eph. 1:4.
  adoption of grace. Eph. 1:6.
  dead in sin quickened. Eph. 2:1, 5.
  Gentiles made nigh. Eph. 2:13.
  unity and kindness enjoined. Eph. 4—6.
EPHESUS, ef´es-us.
  visited by Paul. Acts 18:19; 19:1.
  miracles there. Acts 19:11.
  tumult there. Acts 19:24.
  Paul's address at Miletus to the elders of. Acts 20:17.
  Paul fights with beasts there. 1 Cor. 15:32.
  tarries there. 1 Cor. 16:8.
EPHLAL, ef´lal, judgment. 1 Chr. 2:37.
EPHOD, e´fod. Num. 34:23.
EPHPHATHA, ef´ath-ah, be opened. Mark. 7:34.
EPHRAIM, ef´ra-im, fruitful (?).
  younger son of Joseph. Gen. 41:52.
  Jacob blesses Ephraim and Manasseh. Gen. 48:14.
  his descendants numbered. Num. 1:10, 32; 2:18; 26:35; 1 Chr. 7:20.
  their possessions. Josh. 16:5; 17:14; Judg. 1:29.
  chastise the Midianites. Judg. 7:24.
  quarrel with Gideon. Judg. 8:1; and Jephthah. Judg. 12.
  revolt from the house of David. 1 Kin. 12:25.
  chastise Ahaz and Judah. 2 Chr. 28:6, 7.
  release their prisoners. 2 Chr. 28:12.
  carried into captivity. 2 Kin. 17:5; Ps. 78:9, 67; Jer. 7:15.
  repenting, called God's son. Jer. 31:20.
  prophecies concerning. Is. 7; 9:9; 11:13; 28:1; Hos. 5—14; Zech. 9:10; 10:7.
EPHRAIMITES, ef´ra-im-ites, inhabitants of Ephraim. Judg. 12:4.
EPHRAIN, ef-ra´in, same as EPHRON. 2 Chr. 13:19.
EPHRATH, or EPHRATAH, ef´rat-ah, fruitful (?). 1 Chr. 2:50.
  ——(Beth-lehem). Gen. 35:16; Ps. 132:6; Micah 5:2.
EPHRATHITES, ef´rath-ites, inhabitants of Ephrath. Ruth. 1:2.
EPHRON, ef´ron, of or belonging to a calf. Gen. 23:8.
  the Hittite, sells Machpelah to Abraham. Gen. 23:10.
EPICUREANS, ep´ik-u-re´ans, followers of Epicurus.
  philosophers, encounter Paul at Athens. Acts 17:18.
ER, watchful. Gen. 38:3.
ERAN, e´ran. Num. 26:36.
ERANITES, e´ran-ites, posterity of Eran. Num. 26:36.
ERASTUS, e-rast´us, beloved.
  ministers to Paul. Acts 19:22; Rom. 16:23; 2 Tim. 4:20.

ERECH, e´rek. Gen. 10:10.
ERI, e´ri, same as ER. Gen. 46:16.
ERITES, er´ites, descendants of Eri. Num. 26:16.
ESAIAS, e-sai-as, same as ISAIAH. Matt. 3:3.
ESAR-HADDON, e-sar-had´on, Assur giveth a brother.
  powerful king of Assyria. 2 Kin. 19:37; Ezra 4:2; Is. 37:38.
ESAU, e´saw, hairy.
  son of Isaac. Gen. 25:25; (Mal. 1:2; Rom. 9:13).
  sells his birthright. Gen. 25:29 (Heb. 12:16).
  deprived of the blessing. Gen. 27:38.
  his anger against Jacob. Gen. 27:41; and reconciliation. Gen. 33.
  his riches and descendants. Gen. 36; 1 Chr. 1:35.
ESEK, e´sek, strife. Gen. 26:20.
ESH-BAAL, esh-ba´al, man of Baal. 1 Chr. 8:33.
ESHBAN, esh´ban. Gen. 36:26.
ESHCOL, esh´kol, cluster. Gen. 14:13.
  grapes of. Num. 13:23.
ESHEAN, esh´e-an, support (?). Josh. 15:52.
ESHEK, e´shek, oppression. 1 Chr. 8:39.
ESHKALONITES, esh´ka-lon-ites, men of Ashkalon. Josh. 13:3.
ESHTAOL, esh´ta-ol. Josh. 15:33.
ESHTAULITES, esh-ta´ool-ites, inhabitants of Eshtaol. 1 Chr. 2:53.
ESHTEMOA, esh´tem-o-´ah, obedience. Josh. 21:14.
ESHTEMOH, esh´te-mo´, same as ESHTEMOA. Josh. 15:50.
ESHTON, esh´ton, womanly. 1 Chr. 4:11.
ESLI, es´li, same as AZALIAH (?). Luke 3:25.
ESROM, es´rom, same as HEZRON. Matt. 1:3.
ESTHER, es´ter, star. Esth. 2:7.
  (Hadassah), made queen in the place of Vashti. Esth. 2:17.
  pleads for her people. Esth. 7:3, 4.
ETAM, e´tam, a place of ravenous creatures. Judg. 15:8.
ETHAM, e´tham, boundary of the sea (?). Ex. 13:20.
ETHAN, e´than, firmness. 1 Kin. 4:31.
ETHANIM, e-thah´nim, gifts (?). 1 Kin. 8:2.
ETHBAAL, eth-ba´al, living with Baal. 1 Kin. 16:31.
ETHER, e´ther, plenty. Josh. 15:42.
ETHIOPIA, e´thi-ope´yah, (region of) burnt faces. Gen. 2:13.
ETHIOPIAN, e´thi-ope´yan, a native of Ethiopia. Jer. 13:23.
ETHIOPIANS, e´thi-ope´yans, invading Judah, subdued by Asa. 2 Chr. 14:9. *See* Num. 12:1; 2 Kin. 19:19; Esth. 1:1; Job 28:19.
  prophecies concerning. Ps. 68:31; 87:4; Is. 18; 20; 43:3; 45:14; Jer. 46:9; Ezek. 30:4; 38:5; Nah. 3:9; Zeph. 3:10.
ETHNAN, eth´nan, a gift. 1 Chr. 4:7.
ETHNI, eth´ni, bountiful. 1 Chr. 6:41.
EUBULUS, eu-bew´us, good counsellor. 2 Tim. 4:21.
EUNICE, eu-ni´see.
  commended (Acts 16:1); 2 Tim. 1:5.
EUODIAS, eu-ode´yas, success. Phil. 4:2.
EUPHRATES, eu-fra´tes, the fertile river (?).
  river. Gen. 2:14; 15:18; Deut. 11:24; Josh. 1:4; 2 Sam. 8:3; Jer. 13:4; 46:2; 51:63.
  typical. Rev. 9:14; 16:12.
EUROCLYDON, eu-rok´ly-don, storm from the east.
  a wind. Acts 27:14.
EUTYCHUS, eu´tyk-us, fortunate. Acts 20:9.
  restored. Acts 20:7.
EVE, eve, life. Gen. 3:20.
  created. Gen. 1:27; 2:18.
  her fall and fate. Gen. 3. *See* ADAM.
EVI, e´vi. Num. 31:8.
EVIL-MERODACH, e´vil-me´ro-dak, man of Merodach. 2 Kin. 25:27.
  king of Babylon, restores Jehoiachin. 2 Kin. 25:27; Jer. 52:31.
EXODUS, ex´od-us, departure.
EZAR, e´zar, treasure. 1 Chr. 1:38.
EZBAI, ez´bai. 1 Chr. 11:37.
EZBON, ez´bon. Gen. 46:16.
EZEKIAS, ez´ek-i´as, same as HEZEKIAH. Matt. 1:9.
EZEKIEL, ez-e´ki-el, whom God will strengthen. Ezek. 1:3.
  sent to house of Israel. Ezek. 2; 3; 33:7.
  his visions of God's glory. Ezek. 1; 8; 10; 11:22.
    of the Jews' abominations, &c. Ezek. 8:5.
    their punishment. Ezek. 9; 11.
    of the resurrection of dry bones. Ezek. 37.
  his vision of the measuring of the temple. Ezek. 40.
  intercedes for Israel. Ezek. 9:8; 11:13.
  his dumbness. Ezek. 3:26; 24:26; 33:22.
  his parables. Ezek. 15; 16; 17; 19; 23; 24.
  exhorts Israel against idols. Ezek. 14:1; 20:1; 33:30.
  rehearses Israel's rebellions. Ezek. 20; and the sins of the rulers and people of Jerusalem, 22; 23; 24.
  predicts Israel's and the nations' doom. Ezek. 21; 25.
EZEL, e´zel, departure. 1 Sam. 20:19.
EZEM, e´zem, bone. 1 Chr. 4:29.
EZER, e´zer, help. 1 Chr. 4:4.
EZION-GABER, or EZION-GEBER, e´zi-on-ga´ber, the backbone of a giant.
  on the Red Sea. Num. 33:35; 1 Kin. 9:26.
EZNITE, ez´nite. 2 Sam. 23:8.
EZRA, ez´rah, help. Ezra 7:1.
  scribe, goes up from Babylon to Jerusalem. Ezra 7:1; 8:1.
  his commission from Artaxerxes to rebuild the temple. Ezra 7:11.
  fast ordered by. Ezra 8:21.
  reproves the people. Ezra 10:9.
  reads the book of the law. Neh. 8.
  reforms corruptions. Ezra 10; Neh. 13.
EZRAHITE, ez´rah-ite, a descendant of Zerah. 1 Kin. 4:31.
EZRI, ez´ri, the help of Jehovah (?). 1 Chr. 27:26.
FAIR HAVENS. Acts 27:8.
FELIX, fe´lix, happy. Acts 23:24.
  governor of Judæa, Paul sent to. Acts 23:23.
  Paul's defence before him. Acts 24:10.
  trembles at Paul's preaching, but leaves him bound. Acts 24:25.
FESTUS, fest´us, joyful. Acts 24:27.
  governor of Judæa. Acts 24:27.
  Paul brought before him. Acts 25.
  Paul's defence before. Acts 25:8; 26.
  acquits Paul. Acts 25:14; 26:31.
FORTUNATUS, for´tu-na´tus, prosperous.
  succours Paul. 1 Cor. 16:17.
GAAL, ga´al, loathing. Judg. 9:26.
GAASH, ga´ash, shaking. Josh. 24:30.
GABA, ga´bah, hill. Josh. 18:24.
GABBAI, gab´ai, a collector of tribute. Neh. 11:8.
GABBATHA, gab´ath-ah, height (pavement). John 19:13.
GABRIEL, ga´bri-el, man of God.
  archangel, appears to Daniel. Dan. 8:16; 9:21.
  to Zacharias. Luke 1:19.
  to Mary. Luke 1:26.
GAD, gad, a troop, good fortune.
  birth of. Gen. 30:11.
  his descendants. Gen. 46:16.
  blessed by Jacob. Gen. 49:19.
——tribe of, blessed by Moses. Deut. 33:20.
  numbered. Num. 1:24; 26:15.
  their possessions. Num. 32; 34:14.
  divers commands to. Deut. 27:13; Josh. 4:12.
  commended by Joshua. Josh. 22:1.
  charged with idolatry. Josh. 22:11.
  their defence. Josh. 22:21.
——seer, his message to David. 2 Sam. 24:11; 1 Chr. 21:9; 2 Chr. 29:25.
GADARENES, gad´ar-eens´, inhabitants of Gadara.
  or Gergesenes, Christ's miracle in the country of, Matt. 8:28; Mark 5:1; Luke 8:26.
GADDI, gad´i, fortunate. Num. 13:11.
GADDIEL, gad´i-el, fortune sent from God. Num. 13:10.

GADI, ga-´di. 2 Kin. 15:14.
GADITES, gad-´ites, persons belonging to the tribe of Gad. Deut. 3:12.
GAHAM, ga-´ham, sunburnt (?). Gen. 22:24.
GAHAR, ga-´har, hiding-place. Ezra 2:47.
GAIUS, ga-´yus. The Greek form of CAIUS. Acts 19:29.
his piety. 3 John.
GALAL, ga-´al, worthy (?). 1 Chr. 9:15.
GALATIA, ga-la-´shah, a place colonised by Gauls. Acts 16:6.
GALATIANS, ga-la-´shans, inhabitants of Galatia. Gal. 3:1.
Paul visits. Acts 16:6.
reproved. Gal. 1:6; 3.
exhorted. Gal. 5; 6.
their love to Paul. Gal. 4:13.
GALEED, gal-´e-ed, witness-heap. Gen. 31:47.
GALILEANS, gal-´il-e-´yans, slaughter of. Luke 13:1.
disciples so called. Acts 1:11; 2:7.
GALILEE, gal-´il-ee, circuit. Josh. 20:7.
Isaiah's prophecy concerning. Is. 9:1; Matt. 4:15.
work of Christ there. Matt. 2:22; 15:29; 26:32; 27:55; 28:7; Mark 1:9; Luke 4:14; 23:5; 24:6; Acts 10:37; 13:31.
GALLIM, gal-´im, heaps. 1 Sam. 25:44.
GALLIO. gal-´yo.
dismisses Paul. Acts 18:12.
GAMALIEL, ga-ma-´li-el, benefit of God. Num. 1:10.
advises the council. Acts 5:34.
Paul brought up at feet of. Acts 22:3.
GAMMADIMS, gam-ah-´dims, warriors (?). Ezek. 27:11.
GAMUL, ga-´mool, weaned. 1 Chr. 24:17.
GAREB, ga-´reb, scabby. 2 Sam. 23:38.
GARMITE, garm-´ite, bony. 1 Chr. 4:19.
GASHMU, gash-´moo, same as GESHEM. Neh. 6:6.
GATAM, ga-´tam. Gen. 36:11.
GATH, gath, wine-press. Josh. 11:22.
Goliath of. 1 Sam. 17:4.
men of, smitten with emerods. 1 Sam. 5:8.
David a refugee there. 1 Sam. 27:4.
taken by David. 1 Chr. 18:1.
by Hazael. 2 Kin. 12:17.
Uzziah breaks down the wall of. 2 Chr. 26:6.
GATH-HEPHER, gath-he-´fer, the wine-press of the well. 2 Kin. 14:25.
GATH-RIMMON, gath-rim-´on, wine-press of the pomegranate. Josh. 19:45.
GAZA, ga-´zah, same as AZZAH. Gen. 10:19.
Samson carries away the gates of. Judg. 16.
destruction of, foretold. Jer. 47; Amos 1:6; Zeph. 2:4; Zech. 9:5.
GAZATHITES, ga-´zath-ites, inhabitants of Gaza. Josh. 13:3.
GAZER, ga-´zer, place cut off. 2 Sam. 5:25.
GAZEZ, ga-´zez, shearer. 1 Chr. 2:46.
GAZITES, ga-´zites, inhabitants of Gaza. Judg. 16:2.
GAZZAM, gaz-´am, eating up. Ezra 2:48.
GEBA, ge-´bah, hill. Josh. 21:17.
GEBAL, ge-´bal, mountain. Ps. 83:7.
GEBER, ge-´ber, man. 1 Kin. 4:13.
GEBIM, ge-´bim, trenches. Is. 10:31.
GEDALIAH, ged-´al-i-´ah, whom Jehovah has made great.
governor of the remnant of Judah. 2 Kin. 25:22 (Jer. 40:5).
treacherously killed by Ishmael. 2 Kin. 25:25 (Jer. 41).
GEDEON, ged-´e-on, Greek form of GIDEON. Heb. 11:32.
GEDER, ged-´er, wall. Josh. 12:13.
GEDERAH, ged-er-´ah, enclosure, sheep-fold. Josh. 15:36.
GEDERATHITE, ged-er-´ath-ite, an inhabitant of Gederah. 1 Chr. 12:4.
GEDERITE, ged-´er-ite, native of Geder. 1 Chr. 27:28.
GEDEROTH, ged-er-´oth, sheep-folds. Josh. 15:41.
GEDEROTHAIM, ged-er-´oth-a-´m, two sheep-folds. Josh. 15:36.
GEDOR, ged-´or, wall. Josh. 15:58.
conquered by Simeonites. 1 Chr. 4.
GEHAZI, ge-ha-´zi, valley of vision.
servant of Elisha. 2 Kin. 4:12.
his covetousness. 2 Kin. 5:20.
GELILOTH, gel-il-´oth, regions. Josh. 18:17.
GEMALLI, ge-mal-´i, possessor of camels. Num. 13:12.
GEMARIAH, gem-´ar-´i-´ah, whom Jehovah has completed. Jer. 29:3.
GENESIS, jen-´es-is, generation, or beginning.
GENNESARET, gen-es-´a-ret. Matt. 14:34.
a lake of Palestine, miracles wrought there. Matt. 17:27; Luke 5:1; John 21:6.
GENTILES, jen-´tiles.
origin of. Gen. 10:5.
their state by nature. Rom. 1:21; 1 Cor. 12:2; Eph. 2; 4:17; 1 Thess. 4:5.
God's judgments on. Joel 3:9.
their conversion predicted. Is. 11:10; 42:1; 49:6 (Matt. 12:18; Luke 2:32; Acts 13:47); 62:2; Jer. 16:19; Hos. 2:23; Mal. 1:11; Matt. 8:11.
prediction fulfilled. John 10:16; Acts 8:37; 10; 14; 15; Eph. 2; 1 Thess. 1:1.
calling of. Rom. 9:24. *See* Is. 66:19.
become fellow-citizens of the saints. Eph. 2:11.
Christ made known to. Col. 1:27.
GENUBATH, ge-noob-´ath. 1 Kin. 11:20.
GERA, ge-´ra, a grain. Gen. 46:21.
GERAH, ge-´rah. Ex. 30:13.
GERAR, ge-´rar, sojourning. Gen. 10:19.
herdmen of, strive with Isaac's. Gen. 26:20.
GERGESENES, ger-´ge-seens', inhabitants of Gerasa. Matt. 8:28.
GERIZIM, ge-rize-´im, persons living in a desert.
mount of blessing. Deut. 11:29; 27:12; Josh. 8:33.
GERSHOM, ger-´shom, expulsion.
son of Moses. Ex. 2:22; 18:3.
(Gershon), son of Levi. Gen. 46:11; Num. 3:17.
GERSHONITES, ger-´shon-ites, descendants of Gershon. Num. 3:21.
their duties in the service of the tabernacle. Num. 4; 7; 10:17.
GESHAM, ge-´sham. 1 Chr. 2:47.
GESHEM, ge-´shem, stout (?). Neh. 2:19.
GESHUR, ge-´shoor, bridge. 2 Sam. 3:3.
Absalom takes refuge there after killing Amnon. 2 Sam. 13:37; 14:23 (Josh. 13:13).
GESHURI, ge-shoor-´i, inhabitants of Geshur. Deut. 3:14.
GESHURITES, ge-shoor-´ites, same as preceding. Josh. 12:5.
GETHER, ge-´ther, dregs (?). Gen. 10:23.
GETHSEMANE, geth-sem-´an-e, oil-press.
garden of, our Lord's agony there. Matt. 26:36; Mark 14:32; Luke 22:39; John 18:1.
GEUEL, goo-´el, majesty of God. Num. 13:15.
GEZER, ge-´zer, precipice. Josh. 10:33.
GEZRITES, gez-´rites, dwelling in a desert land. 1 Sam. 27:8.
GIAH, gi-´ah, gushing forth. 2 Sam. 2:24.
GIBBAR, gib-´ar, a hero. Ezra 2:20.
GIBBETHON, gib-´eth-on, a lofty place. Josh. 19:44.
GIBEA, gib-´e-ah, hill. 1 Chr. 2:49.
GIBEAH, gib-´e-ah, hill. Josh. 15:57.
a city of Benjamin. Judg. 19:14.
sin of its inhabitants. Judg. 19:22.
their punishment. Judg. 20.
the city of Saul. 1 Sam. 10:26; 11:4; 14:2; 15:34; 2 Sam. 21:6.
GIBEATH, gib-´e-ath, hill. Josh. 18:28.
GIBEON, gib-´e-on, pertaining to a hill. Josh. 9:3.
its inhabitants deceive Joshua. Josh. 9.
delivered by him from the five kings. Josh. 10.
Saul persecutes them. 2 Sam. 21:1.
David makes atonement. 2 Sam. 21:3-9.
Solomon's dream at. 1 Kin. 3:5.
tabernacle of the Lord kept at. 1 Chr. 16:39; 21:29.
GIBEONITES, gib-´e-on-ites, inhabitants of Gibeon. 2 Sam. 21:1.

GIBLITES, gib´-lites, inhabitants of Gebal. Josh. 13:5.
GIDDALTI, gid-al´-ti, I have increased. 1 Chr. 25:4.
GIDDEL, gid´-el, gigantic. Ezra 2:47.
GIDEON, gid´-e-on, one who cuts down. Judg. 6:11.
God appoints him to deliver Israel from the Midianites. Judg. 6:14.
destroys the altar and grove of Baal. Judg. 6:25, 27.
called Jerubbaal. Judg. 6:32.
God gives him two signs. Judg. 6:36-40.
his army reduced, and selected by a test of water. Judg. 7:2-7.
his stratagem. Judg. 7:16.
subdues the Midianires. Judg. 7:19; 8.
makes an ephod of the spoil. Judg. 8:24.
his death. Judg. 8:32. *See* Heb. 11:32.
GIDEONI, gid´-e-on-i, cutting down. Num. 1:11.
GIDOM, gi´-dom. Judg. 20:45.
GIHON, gi´-hon, a river. Gen. 2:13.
GILALAI, gil´-a-lai, dungy (?). Neh. 12:36.
GILBOA, gil-bo´-ah, bubbling fountain. 1 Sam. 28:4.
mount, Saul slain there. 1 Sam. 31:2; 2 Sam. 1:21.
GILEAD, gil´-e-ad, hill of witness. Gen. 31:21.
land of, granted to the Reubenites, &c. Num. 32.
invaded by the Ammonites. Judg. 10:17.
Jephthah made captain of. Judg. 11.
GILEADITE, gil´-e-ad-ite, inhabitant of Gilead. Judg. 10:3.
GILGAL, gil´-gal, a circle.
Joshua encamps there. Josh. 4:19; 9:6.
Saul made king there. 1 Sam. 10:8; 11:14.
Saul sacrifices at. 1 Sam. 13:8; 15:12.
GILOH, gi´-lo, exile. Josh. 15:51.
GILONITE, gi´-lon-ite, an inhabitant of Giloh. 2 Sam. 15:12.
GIMZO, gim´-zo, a place abounding with sycamores. 2 Chr. 28:18.
GINATH, gi´-nath, garden. 1 Kin. 16:21.
GINNETHO, gin´-eth-o, garden. Neh. 12:4.
GINNETHON, gin´-eth-on, same as preceding. Neh. 10:6.
GIRGASHITE, gir´-gash-ite, dwelling in a clayey soil. 1 Chr. 1:14.
GIRGASHITES, gir´-gash-ites, descendants of Canaan. Gen. 10:15; 15:21.
communion with, forbidden. Deut. 7:1.
driven out. Josh. 3:10; 24:11.
GIRGASITE, gir´-gas-ite, same as preceding. Gen. 10:16.
GISPA, gis´-pah, flattery. Neh. 11:21.
GITTAH-HEPHER, git´-tah-he´-fer, wine-press of the well. Josh. 19:13.
GITTAIM, git´-a-im, two wine-presses. 2 Sam. 4:3.
GITTITES, git´-ites, inhabitants of Gath. Josh. 13:3.
GITTITH, git´-ith, after the manner of Gittites. Ps:8, title.
GIZONITE, gi´-zon-ite. 1 Chr. 11:34.
GOATH, go´-ath, lowing. Jer. 31:39.
GOB, gobe, pit, cistern. 2 Sam. 21:18.
GOG. 1 Chr. 5:4.
GOG and MAGOG. Ezek. 38; 39; Rev. 20:8.
GOLAN, go´-lan, exile. Deut. 4:43.
GOLGOTHA, gol´-goth-ah, place of a skull. Matt. 27:33; Mark 15:22; Luke 23:33; John 19:17.
GOLIATH, go-li´-ath, exile (?). 1 Sam. 17:4.
of Gath. 1 Sam. 17; 21:9; 22:10.
GOMER, go´-mer, complete. Gen. 10:2.
GOMORRAH, go-mor´-ah. Gen. 10:19.
(and Sodom). Gen. 18:20; 19:24, 28; Is. 1:9; Matt. 10:15; Mark 6:11.
GOMORRHA, go-mor´-ah, same as preceding. Matt. 10:15.
GOSHEN, go´-shen, land of (Egypt), Israelites placed there. Gen. 45:10; 46:34; 47:4.
no plagues there. Ex. 8:22; 9:26.
——(Canaan). Josh. 10:41; 11:16.
GOZAN, go´-zan. 2 Kin. 17:6.
GREECE, grees, country of the Greeks. Acts 20:2.
prophecies of. Dan. 8:21; 10:20; 11:2; Zech. 9:13.

GREECE—*cont.*
Paul preaches in. Acts 16; 20.
GRECIA, greesh´-ah, same as GREECE. Dan. 8:21.
GRECIAN, greesh´-an, a Jew who speaks Greek. Acts 11:20.
GREEK, the language of Greece. Acts 21:37.
GREEKS, inhabitants of Greece. Acts 18:17.
would see Jesus. John 12, 20.
believe in Him. Acts 11:21; 17:4.
GUDGODAH, gud-go´-dah, thunder (?). Deut. 10:7.
GUNI, goon´-i, painted with colours. Gen. 46:24.
GUNITES, goon´-ites, descendants of Guni. Num. 26:48.
GUR, goor, a young lion. 2 Kin. 9:27.
GUR-BAAL, goor-ba´-al, Gur of Baal. 2 Chr. 26:7.

HAAHASHTARI, ha´-a-hash´-tar-i, the muleteer (?). 1 Chr. 4:6.
HABAIAH, hab-ai´-ah, whom Jehovah hides. Ezra 2:61.
HABAKKUK, ha-bak´-ook, embrace. Hab. 1:1.
prophet, his burden, complaint to God, his answer, and faith. Hab. 1; 2; 3.
HABAZINIAH, hab´-az-in-i´-ah, lamp of Jehovah (?). Jer. 35:3.
HABOR, ha´-bor, joining together. 2 Kin. 17:6.
HACHALIAH, hak-al-i´-ah, whom Jehovah disturbs. Neh. 1:1.
HAGHILAH, hak-i´-lah, dark. 1 Sam. 23:19.
HACHMONI, hak´-mon-i, wise. 1 Chr. 27:32.
HACHMONITE, hak´-mon-ite, a descendant of Hachmoni. 1 Chr. 11:11.
HADAD, ha´-dad. Gen. 36:35.
Edomite. 1 Kin. 11:14.
HADADEZER, had´-ad-e´-zer, whose help is Hadad. 2 Sam. 8:3.
——(Hadarezer), king of Zobah, David's wars with. 2 Sam. 8; 10:15; 1 Chr. 18.
HADADRIMMON, had´-ad-rim´-on, named from Hadad and Rimmon. Zech. 12:11.
HADAR, ha´-dar, enclosure. Gen. 25:15.
HADAREZER, had´-ar-e´-zer, same as HADADEZER. 1 Chr. 18:3.
HADASHAH, had-ash´-ah, new. Josh. 15:37.
HADASSAH, had-as´-ah, myrtle. Esth. 2:7.
HADATTAH, had-at´-ah, new. Josh. 15:25.
HADID, ha´-did, sharp. Ezra 2:33.
HADLAI, had´-lai, rest. 2 Chr. 28:12.
HADORAM, had-or´-am. Gen. 10:27.
HADRACH, had´-rak. Zech. 9:1.
HAGAB, ha´-gab, locust. Ezra 2:46.
HAGABA, hag-a´-ba, same as HAGAR. Neh. 7:48.
HAGAR, ha´-gar, flight. Gen. 16:3.
mother of Ishmael. Gen. 16.
fleeing from Sarah is comforted by an angel. Gen. 16:10, 11.
sent away with her son, Gen. 21:14; allegory of, Gal. 4:24.
HAGARENES, hag´-ar-e´-nes, inhabitants of Hagar. Ps. 83:6.
HAGARITES, hag´-ar-ites, same as preceding. 1 Chr. 5:10.
HAGERITE, hag´-er-ite, same as HAGARENE. 1 Chr. 27:31.
HAGGAI, hag´-ai, festive.
prophet. Ezra 5; 6:14. *See* Hag. 1; 2.
HAGGI, hag´-i, same as preceding. Gen. 46:16.
HAGGERI, hag´-er-i. 1 Chr. 11:38.
HAGGIAH, hag-i´-ah, festival of Jehovah. 1 Chr. 6:30.
HAGGITES, hag´-ites, the posterity of Haggi. Num. 26:15.
HAGGITH, hag´-ith, festive. 2 Sam. 3:4.
HAI, hai, same as AI. Gen. 12:8.
HAKKATAN, hak´-ah-tan, the small. Ezra 8:12.
HAKKOZ, hak´-oz, the thorn. 1 Chr. 24:10.
HAKUPHA, ha-koo´-fah. Ezra 2:51.
HALAH, ha´-lah, same as CALAH (?). 2 Kin. 17:6.
HALAK, ha´-lak, smooth. Josh. 11:17.
HALHUL, hal´-hool. Josh. 15:58.
HALI, ha´-li, necklace. Josh. 19:25.

HALLELUIAH, hal-el-oo´ya, praise the Lord. Rev. 19:1.
HALLELUJAH (Alleluia). Ps. 106; 111; 113; 146; 148; 149; 150; REV. 19:1, 3, 4, 6.
HALLOHESH, hal-o´hesh, same as following. Neh. 10:24.
HALOHESH, hal-o´hesh, the enchanter. Neh. 3:12.
HAM, ham, warm. Gen. 9:18.
son of Noah, cursed. Gen. 9:22.
his descendants. Gen. 10:6; 1 Chr. 1:8; Ps. 105:23; smitten by the Simeonites. 1 Chr. 4:40.
HAMAN, ha´man. Esth. 3:1.
HAMAN'S advancement. Esth. 3.
anger against Mordecai. Esth. 3:8.
his fall. Esth. 7.
HAMATH, ha´math, fortress.
——(Syria). Num. 34:8; Josh. 13:5; 2 Kin. 14:28; 17:24.
conquered. 2 Kin. 18:34; Is. 37:13; Jer. 49:23.
HAMATHITE, ha´math-ite, a dweller at Hamath. Gen. 10:18.
HAMATH-ZOBAH, ha´math-zo´bah, fortress of Zobah. 2 Chr. 8:3.
HAMMATH, ham´ath, warm springs. Josh. 19:35.
HAMMEDATHA, ham´ed-ah´thah, given by the moon (?). Esth. 3:1.
HAMMELECH, ham-me´lek, the king. Jer. 36:26.
HAMMOLEKETH, ham´mo-le´keth, the queen. 1 Chr. 7:18.
HAMMON, ham´on, warm. Josh. 19:28.
HAMMOTH-DOR, ham´oth-dor´, warm springs of Dor. Josh. 21:32.
HAMONAH, ha-mo´nah, multitude. Ezek. 39:16.
HAMON-GOG, ham´on-gog´, *m.* of Gog. Ezek. 39:11.
HAMOR, ha´mor, ass. Gen. 33:19.
father of Shechem. Gen. 34; Acts 7:16.
HAMUEL, ham´oo-el, heat (wrath) of God. 1 Chr. 4:26.
HAMUL, ha´mool, who has experienced mercy. Gen. 46:12.
HAMULITES, ha´mool-ites, the posterity of Hamul. Num. 26:21.
HAMUTAL, ha-moo´tal, refreshing like dew. 2 Kin. 23:31.
HANAMEEL, han´am-e´el, probably another form of HANANEEL. Jer. 32:7.
HANAN, ha´nan, merciful. 1 Chr. 8:23.
HANANEEL, han´an-e´el, whom God graciously gave. Neh. 3:1.
HANANI, ha-na´ni, probably same as HANANIAH. 1 Kin. 16:1.
prophet. 2 Chr. 16:7.
——brother of Nehemiah. Neh. 1:2; 7:2; 12:36.
HANANIAH, han´an-i´ah, whom Jehovah graciously gave. 1 Chr. 3:19.
false prophet. Jer. 28.
his death. Jer. 28:16.
HANES, ha´nees. Is. 30:4.
HANIEL, han´i-el, favour of God. 1 Chr. 7:39.
HANNAH, han´ah, gracious.
her song. 1 Sam. 2.
vow and prayer. 1 Sam. 1:11; answered. 1 Sam. 1:19.
HANNATHON, han-a´thon, gracious. Josh. 19:14.
HANNIEL, han´i-el, same as HANIEL. Num. 34:23.
HANOCH, ha´nok, same as ENOCH. Gen. 25:4.
HANOCHITES, ha´nok-ites, descendants of Hanoch. Num. 26:5.
HANUN, ha´noon, whom (God) pities. 2 Sam. 10:1.
king of the Ammonites, dishonours David's messengers. 2 Sam. 10:4.
chastised. 2 Sam. 12:30.
HAPHRAIM, haf-ra´im, two pits. Josh. 19:19.
HARA, ha´ra, mountainous. 1 Chr. 5:26.
HARADAH, har-a´dah, fear. Num. 33:24.
HARAN, ha´ran, mountaineer. Gen. 11:27.
son of Terah. Gen. 11:26.
——(city of Nahor), Abram comes to. Gen. 11:31; departs from. Gen. 12:4.
Jacob flees to Laban at. Gen. 27:43; 28:10; 29.
HARARITE, ha´rar-ite, a mountaineer. 2 Sam. 23:11.
HARBONAH, har-bo´nah. Esth. 7:9.
HAREPH, ha´ref, plucking. 1 Chr. 2:51.
HARETH, ha´reth, thicket. 1 Sam. 22:5.
HARHAIAH, har-hai´ah, dried up (?). Neh. 3:8.
HARHAS, har´has. 2 Kin. 22:14.
HARHUR, har´hoor, inflammation. Ezra 2:51.
HARIM, ha´rim, flat-nosed. 1 Chr. 24:8.
HARIPH, ha´rif, autumnal showers. Neh. 7:24.
HARNEPHER, har-ne´fer. 1 Chr. 7:36.
HAROD, ha´rod, terror. Judg. 7:1.
HARODITE, har´od-ite, inhabitant of Harod. 2 Sam. 23:25.
HAROEH, har-ro´eh, the seer. 1 Chr. 2:52.
HARORITE, har´or-ite, probably another form of HARODITE. 1 Chr. 11:27.
HAROSHETH, ha-rosh´eth, carving. Judg. 4:2.
HARSHA, har´shah, enchanter, magician. Ezra 2:52.
HARUM, ha´room, high (?). 1 Chr. 4:8.
HARUMAPH, ha-roo´maf, flat-nosed. Neh. 3:10.
HARUPHITE, ha-roof´ite. 1 Chr. 12:5.
HARUZ, ha´rooz, active. 2 Kin. 21:19.
HASADIAH, ha´sad-i´ah, whom Jehovah loves. 1 Chr. 3:20.
HASENUAH, ha´se-noo´ah, she that is hated. 1 Chr. 9:7.
HASHABIAH, ha´shab-i´ah, whom Jehovah esteems. 1 Chr. 6:45.
HASHABNAH, ha-shab´nah, same as preceding (?). Neh. 10:25.
HASHABNIAH, ha´shab-ni´ah, same as HASHABIAH. Neh. 3:10.
HASHBADANA, hash´bad-a´na. Neh. 8:4.
HASHEM, ha´shem, fat. 1 Chr. 11:34.
HASHMONAH, hash-mo´nah, fatness, fat soil. Num. 33:29.
HASHUB, hash´oob, thoughtful. Neh. 3:11.
HASHUBAH, hash-oob´ah, same as preceding. 1 Chr. 3:20.
HASHUM, hash´oom, rich. Ezra 2:19.
HASHUPHA, hash-oof´ah, another form of HASUPHA. Neh. 7:46.
HASRAH, haz´rah, probably same as HARHAS. 2 Chr. 34:22.
HASSENAAH, has-en-a´ah, the thorny. Neh. 3:3.
HASSHUB, hash´oob, same as HASHUB. 1 Chr. 9:14.
HASUPHA, has-oof´ah, one of the Nethinims. Ezra 2:43.
HATACH, ha´tak. Esth. 4:5.
HATHATH, ha´thath, terror. 1 Chr. 4:13.
HATIPHA, ha-tee´fah, seized. Ezra 2:54.
HATITA, ha-tee´tah, digging. Ezra 2:42.
HATTIL, hat´il, wavering. Ezra 2:57.
HATTUSH, hat´oosh, assembled (?). 1 Chr. 3:22.
HAURAN, how´ran, hollow land. Ezek. 47:16.
HAVILAH, ha-vil´ah. Gen. 10:7.
HAVOTH-JAIR, hav´oth-ja´ir, villages of Jair. Num. 32:41.
HAZAEL, ha´za-el, whom God watches over.
king of Syria. 1 Kin. 19:15.
Elisha's prediction. 2 Kin. 8:7.
slays Ben-hadad. 2 Kin. 8:15.
oppresses Israel. 2 Kin. 9:14; 10:32; 12:17; 13:22.
HAZAIAH, ha-zai´ah, whom Jehovah watches over. Neh. 11:5.
HAZAR-ADDAR, ha´zar-ad´ar, Addar-town. Num. 34:4.
HAZAR-ENAN, ha´zar-e´nan, fountain-town. Num. 34:9.
HAZAR-GADDAH, ha´zar-gad´ah, luck-town. Josh. 15:27.
HAZAR-HATTICON, ha´zar-hat´ik-on, middle-town. Ezek. 47:16.
HAZARMAVETH, ha´zar-ma´veth, death-town. Gen. 10:26.
HAZAR-SHUAL, ha´zar-shoo´al, jackal-town. Josh. 15:28.
HAZAR-SUSAH, ha´zar-soo´sah, mare-town. Josh. 19:5.
HAZAR-SUSIM, ha´zar-soo-sim, horses-town. 1 Chr. 4:31.

HAZELELPONI, haz´-lel-po´-ni, the shadow looking on me. 1 Chr. 4:3.
HAZERIM, haz-e´-rim, villages. Deut. 2:23.
HAZEROTH, haz-e´-roth, same as HAZERIM. Num. 11:35.
HAZEZON-TAMAR, ha´-ze-zon-ta´-mar, pruning of the palm. Gen. 14:7.
HAZIEL, ha´-zi-el, the vision of God. 1 Chr. 23:9.
HAZO, ha´-zo, vision. Gen. 22:22.
HAZOR, ha´-zor, castle. Josh. 11:1.
Canaan, burnt. Josh. 11:10; 15:25.
HEBER, he´-ber. Gen. 10:21; Luke 3:35.
——the Kenite. Judg. 4:11.
(1) same as EBER. 1 Chr. 5:13; (2) fellowship. Gen. 46:17.
HEBERITES, he´-ber-ites, descendants of Heber. Num. 26:45.
HEBREW, he´-broo, the (name of Abraham), Gen. 14:13; the language spoken by the Jews: John 19:20. Or a Jew: Jer. 34:9.
HEBREWESS, he´-broo-ess´, a Jewess. Jer. 34:9.
HEBREWS, he´-broos, descendants of Abraham. Gen. 40:15; 43:32; Ex. 2:6; 2 Cor. 11:22; Phil. 3:5.
HEBRON, heb´-ron, alliance.
——(Mamre), in Canaan, Abraham dwells there. Gen. 13:18; 23:2.
the spies come to. Num. 13:22.
taken. Josh. 10:36.
given to Caleb. Josh. 14:13; 15:13.
David reigns there. 2 Sam. 2:1; 3:2; 5:1; 1 Chr. 11; 12:38; 29:27.
HEBRONITES, he´-bron-ites, the people of Hebron. Num. 3:27.
HEGAI, or HEGE, he´-gai. Esth. 2:3, 8.
HELAH, he´-lah, rust. 1 Chr. 4:5.
HELAM, he´-lam, stronghold. 2 Sam. 10:16.
HELBAH, hel´-bah, fatness. Judg. 1:31.
HELBON, hel´-bon, fertile. Ezek. 27:18.
HELDAI, hel´-dai, terrestrial. 1 Chr. 27:15.
HELEB, he´-leb, fat, fatness. 2 Sam. 23:29.
HELED, he´-led, the world. 1 Chr. 11:30.
HELEK, he´-lek, portion. Num. 26:30.
HELEKITES, he´-lek-ites, descendants of Helek. Num. 26:30.
HELEM, he´-lem, another form of HELDAI. 1 Chr. 7:35.
HELEPH, he´-lef, exchange. Josh. 19:33.
HELEZ, he´-lez, liberation. 2 Sam. 23:26.
HELI, he´-li, the Greek form of ELI. Luke 3:23.
HELKAI, hel´-kai, another form of HILKIAH. Neh. 12:15.
HELKATH, hel´-kath, a portion. Josh. 19:25.
HELKATH-HAZZURIM, hel´-kath-haz´-oor-im, the field of swords (?). 2 Sam. 2:16.
HELON, he´-lon, strong. Num. 1:9.
HEMAM, he´-mam, same as HOMAM. Gen. 36:22.
HEMAN, he´-man, faithful. 1 Kin. 4:31.
HEMATH, he´-math; (1) fortress, 1 Chr. 2:55; (2) same as HAMATH, Amos 6:14.
HEMDAN, hem´-dan, pleasant. Gen. 36:26.
HEN, hen, favour. Zech. 6:14.
HENA, he´-nah. 2 Kin. 18:34.
HENADAD, hen´-a-dad, favour of Hadad (?). Ezra 3:9.
HENOCH, he´-nok, same as ENOCH. 1 Chr. 1:3.
HEPHER, he´-fer, pit. Josh. 12:17.
HEPHERITES, he´-fer-ites, descendants of Hepher. Num. 26:32.
HEPHZI-BAH, heph´-zi-bah, in whom is my delight.
queen of Hezekiah, and mother of Manasseh. 2 Kin. 21:1.
the restored Jerusalem. Is. 62:4.
HERES, he´-res, the sun. Judg. 1:35.
HERESH, he´-resh, artificer. 1 Chr. 9:15.
HERMAS, and HERMES, her´-mas and her´-mes, of Rome, saluted by Paul. Rom. 16:14.
HERMOGENES, her-mog´-e-nees. 2 Tim. 1:15.
HERMON, her´-mon, lofty. Deut. 3:8.
mount. Deut. 4:48; Josh. 12:5; 13:5; Ps. 89:12; 133:3.
HERMONITES, her´-mon-ites, the summits of Hermon. Ps. 42:6.
HEROD, her´-od (the Great), king of Judæa. Matt. 2:1.
troubled at Christ's birth. Matt. 2:3.
slays the babes of Bethlehem. Matt. 2:16.
——(Antipas) reproved by John the Baptist, imprisons him, Luke 3:19; beheads him. Matt. 14; Mark 6:14.
desires to see Christ. Luke 9:9.
scourges Him, and is reconciled to Pilate. Luke 23:7; Acts 4:27.
——(Agrippa) persecutes the church. Acts 12:1.
his pride and miserable death. Acts 12:23.
HERODIANS, he-ro´-di-ans, partisans of Herod, a sect, rebuked by Christ. Matt. 22:16; Mark 12:13.
plot against him. Mark 3:6; 8:15; 12:13.
HERODIAS, he-ro´-di-as. Matt. 14:3.
married to Herod Antipas. Mark 6:17.
plans the death of John the Baptist. Matt. 14; Mark 6:24.
HERODION, he-ro´-di-on. Rom. 16:11.
Paul's kinsman. Rom. 16:11.
HESED, he´-sed, mercy. 1 Kin. 4:10.
HESHBON, hesh´-bon, counting. Num. 21:25.
city of Sihon, taken. Num. 21:26; Deut. 2:24; Neh. 9:22; Is. 16:8.
HESHMON, hesh´-mon, fatness. Josh. 15:27.
HETH, sons of. Gen. 10:15.
their kindness to Abraham. Gen. 23:7; 25:10.
HETHLON, heth´-lon, hiding-place. Ezek. 47:15.
HEZEKI, hez´-ek-i, shortened from HIZKIAH. 1 Chr. 8:17.
HEZEKIAH, hez´-ek-i´-ah, the might of Jehovah. 2 Kin. 18:1.
king of Judah. 2 Kin. 16:19 (2 Chr. 28:27).
abolishes idolatry. 2 Kin. 18.
attacked by the Assyrians, his prayer and deliverance. 2 Kin. 19.
his life lengthened, shadow of dial goes backward, displays his treasure, Isaiah's prediction. 2 Kin. 20 (Is. 38); his passover. 2 Chr. 30:13.
his piety, and good reign. 2 Chr. 29.
his death. 2 Kin. 20:20.
HEZION, hez´-yon, vision. 1 Kin. 15:18.
HEZIR, he´-zir, swine. 1 Chr. 24:15.
HEZRAI, hez´-rai, enclosed wall. 2 Sam. 23:35.
HEZRO, hez-ro, same as preceding. 1 Chr. 11:37.
HEZRON, hez´-ron, same as HEZRAI. Gen. 46:12.
HEZRONITES, hez´-ron-ites, descendants of Hezron. Num. 26:6.
HIDDAI, hid´-ai, the rejoicing of Jehovah. 2 Sam. 23:30.
HIDDEKEL, hid-ek´-el. Gen. 2:14.
HIEL, hi´-el, God liveth. 1 Kin. 16:34.
——*See* JERICHO.
HIERAPOLIS, hi´-e-ra´-pol-is, a sacred or holy city. Col. 4:13.
HIGGAION, hig-a´-yon, meditation. Ps. 9:16.
HILEN, hi´-len. 1 Chr. 6:58.
HILKIAH, hilk-i´-ah, portion of Jehovah. 2 Kin. 18:18.
finds the book of the law. 2 Kin. 22:8.
HILLEL, hil´-el, praising. Judg. 12:13.
HINNOM, hin´-ome, valley of (Josh. 15:8); 2 Kin. 23:10; 2 Chr. 28:3; 33:6; Jer. 7:31; 19:11; 32:35. *See* TOPHET AND MOLOCH.
HIRAH, hi´-rah, nobility. Gen. 38:1.
HIRAM, hi´-ram, noble (?) (Huram), king of Tyre, sends aid to David and Solomon. 2 Sam. 5:11; 1 Kin. 5; 9:11; 10:11; 1 Chr. 14:1; 2Chr. 2:11.
——principal brass-worker to Solomon. 1 Kin. 7:13.
HITTITES, hit´-ites, descendants of Heth. Gen. 15:20; Judg. 1:26; 3:5.
HIVITES, hive´-ites, villagers. Gen. 10:17; Ex. 3:8, 17.
deceive Joshua. Josh. 9.
HIZKIAH, hizk-i´-ah, might of Jehovah. Zeph. 1:1.
HIZKIJAH, hizk-i´-jah, same as preceding. Neh. 10:17.
HOBAB, ho´-bab, beloved. Num. 10:29. *See* JETHRO.
HOBAH, ho´-bah, a hiding-place. Gen. 14:15.

HOD, hode, splendour. 1 Chr. 7:37.
HODAIAH, ho-dai´-ah, praise of Jehovah. 1 Chr. 3:24.
HODAVIAH, ho´-dav-i´-ah, Jehovah is his praise. 1 Chr. 5:24.
HODESH, ho´-desh, new moon. 1 Chr. 8:9.
HODEVAH, ho´-de-vah, same as HODAVIAH. Neh. 7:43.
HODIAH, ho-di´-ah, same as HODAIAH. 1 Chr. 4:19.
HODIJAH, ho-di-jah, same as preceding. Neh. 8:7.
HOGLAH, hog´-lah, partridge. Num. 26:33.
HOHAM, ho´-ham. Josh. 10:3.
HOLON, ho´-lon, sandy. Josh. 15:51.
HOMAM, ho´-mam, destruction. 1 Chr. 1:39.
HOPHNI, hof´-ni, pugilist; and PHINEHAS, sons of Eli. 1 Sam. 1:3.
their sin and death. 1 Sam. 2:12, 22; 4:11.
HOPHRA, hof´-rah, priest of the sun. Jer. 44:30.
HOR, mountain. Num. 20:23.
mount, Aaron dies on. Num. 20:25.
HORAM, ho´-ram. Josh. 10:33.
HOREB, ho´-reb, desert, mount (Sinai). Ex. 3:1; 17:6; 33:6; Deut. 1:6; 4:10.
law given. Ex. 19; 20; Deut. 4:10; 5:2; 18:16; 1 Kin. 8:9; Mal. 4:4.
Moses twice there for forty days. Ex. 24:18; 34:28; Deut. 9:9.
Elijah there for forty days. 1 Kin. 19:8.
HOREM, ho´-rem. Josh. 19:38.
HOR-HAGIDGAD, hor´-hag-gid´-gad, mountain of Gudgodah. Num. 33:32.
HORI, ho´-ri, cave-dweller. Gen. 36:22.
HORIMS, hor´-ims, descendants of Hori. Deut. 2:12.
HORITES, hor´-ites, same as preceding. Gen. 14:6.
HORMAH, hor´-mah, a devoting, a place laid waste. Num. 14:45.
destruction of. Num. 21:3; Judg. 1:17.
HORONAIM, hor´-o-na´-im, two caverns. Is. 15:5.
HORONITE, hor´-on-ite, native of Beth-horon. Neh. 2:10.
HOSAH, ho´-sah, fleeing to Jehovah for refuge (?). Josh. 19:29.
HOSANNA, ho-san´-nah, save us we pray, children sing, to Christ. Matt. 21:9, 15; Mark 11:9; John 12:13; (Ps. 118:25, 26).
HOSEA, ho-ze´-ah, salvation. Hos. 1:1.
prophet, declares God's judgment against idolatrous Israel. Hos. 1; 2; 4; and his reconciliation. Hos. 2:14; 11; 13; 14.
HOSHAIAH, ho-shai´-ah, whom Jehovah has set free. Neh. 12:32.
HOSHAMA, ho´-sha-mah. 1 Chr. 3:18.
HOSHEA, ho-she´-ah, same as HOSEA. Deut. 32:44.
last king of Israel, his wicked reign, defeat by the king of Assyria, and captivity. 2 Kin. 15:30; 17.
HOTHAM, ho´-tham, signet ring. 1 Chr. 7:32.
HOTHAN, ho´-than. 1 Chr. 11:44.
HOTHIR, ho´-thir. 1 Chr. 25:4.
HUKKOK, hook´-oke, decreed. Josh. 19:34.
HUKOK, hook´-oke, same as preceding. 1 Chr. 6:75.
HUL, hool, circle. Gen. 10:23.
HULDAH, hool´-dah, weasel. 2 Kin. 22:14.
HIMTAH, hoom´-tah, fortress (?). Josh. 15:54.
HUPHAM, hoo´-fam, inhabitant of the shore (?). Num. 26:39.
HUPHAMITES, hoo´-fam-ites, descendants of Hupham. Num. 26:39.
HUPPAH, hoop´-ah, covering. 1 Chr. 24:13.
HUPPIM, hoop´-im, same as HUPHAM (?). Gen. 46:21.
HUR, hoor, cavern. Ex. 17:10.
HURAI, hoo´-rai, another way of writing Hiddai. 1 Chr. 11:32.
HURAM, hoo´-ram, the older way of spelling Hiram. 2 Chr. 2:13.
HURI, hoo´-ri, linen-worker (?). 1 Chr. 5:14.
HUSHAH, hoo´-shah, haste. 1 Chr. 4:4.
HUSHAI, hoo´-shai, hasting, loyalty. 2 Sam. 15:32.
defeats Ahithophel's counsel. 2 Sam. 16:16; 17:5.
HUSHAM, hoo´-sham, haste. Gen. 36:34.
HUSHATHITE, hoo´-shath-ite, inhabitant of Hushah. 2 Sam. 23:27.
HUSHIM, hoosh´-im, those who make haste. Gen. 46:23.
HUZ. Gen. 22:21.
HUZZAB, hooz´-ab, it is decreed. Nah. 2:7.
HYMENÆUS, hi´-men-e´-us, belonging to Hymen. 1 Tim. 1:20; 2 Tim. 2:17.

IBHAR, ib´-har, whom God chooses. 2 Sam. 5:15.
IBLEAM, ib´-le-am, He destroys the people. Josh. 17:11.
IBNEIAH, ib-ni´-ah, whom Jehovah will build up. 1 Chr. 9:8.
IBNIJAH, ib-ni´-jah, same as preceding. 1 Chr. 9:8.
IBRI, ib´-ri, Hebrew. 1 Chr. 24:27.
IBZAN, ib´-zan, active (?). Judg. 12:8.
I-CHABOD, i´-ka-bod, inglorious. 1 Sam. 4:21; 14:3.
ICONIUM, i-kon´-yum, gospel preached at. Acts 13:51; 14:1; 16:2.
Paul persecuted at. 2 Tim. 3:11.
IDALAH, id´-al-ah, snares (?). Josh. 19:15.
IDBASH, id´-bash, honeyed. 1 Chr. 4:3.
IDDO, id´-o, (1) loving, 1 Chr. 27:21; (2) Ezra 8:17; (3) seasonable, Zech. 1:1.
IDUMEA, i´-du-me´-ah, same as EDOM. Is. 34:5.
IGAL, i´-gal, whom God will avenge. Num. 13:7.
IGDALIAH, ig´-dal-i´-ah, whom Jehovah shall make great. Jer. 35:4.
IGEAL, i´-ge-al, same as IGAL. 1 Chr. 3:22.
IIM, i´-im, ruins. Num. 33:45.
IJE-ABARIM, i-je-a-bar´-im, ruinous heaps of Abarim. Num. 21:11.
IJON, i´-jon, a ruin. 1 Kin. 15:20.
IKKESH, ik´-esh, perverseness of mouth. 2 Sam. 23:26.
ILAI, ee´-lai, most high. 1 Chr. 11:29.
ILLYRICUM, il-ir´-ik-um, gospel preached there. Rom. 15:19.
IMLA, im´-lah, same as IMLAH. 2 Chr. 18:7.
IMLAH, im´-lah, whom (God) will fill up. 1 Kin. 22:8.
IMMANUEL, im-an´-u-el (*see* EMMANUEL), God with us. Is. 7:14; Matt. 1:23.
IMMER, im´-er, talkative. 1 Chr. 9:12.
IMNA, im´-nah, whom (God) keeps back. 1 Chr. 7:35.
IMNAH, im´-nah, whom (God) assigns (?). 1 Chr. 7:30.
IMRAH, im´-rah, stubborn. 1 Chr. 7:36.
IMRI, im´-ri, eloquent. 1 Chr. 9:4.
INDIA, ind´-ya. Esth. 1:1.
IPHEDEIAH, if´-ed-i´-ah, whom Jehovah frees. 1 Chr. 8:25.
IR, eer, city. 1 Chr. 7:12.
IRA, i´-rah, watchful. 2 Sam. 20:26.
IRAD, i´-rad. Gen. 4:18.
IRAM, i´-ram, belonging to a city. Gen. 36:43.
IRI, i´-ri, same as IRAM. 1 Chr. 7:7.
IRIJAH, i-ri´-jah, whom Jehovah looks on. Jer. 37:13.
IR-NAHASH, ir-na´-hash, snake-town. 1 Chr. 4:12.
IRON, i´-ron, reverence. Josh. 19:38.
IRPEEL, ir´-pe-el, which God heals. Josh. 18:27.
IR-SHEMESH, ir-she´-mesh, sun-town. Josh. 19:41.
IRU, i´-roo, same as IRAM. 1 Chr. 4:15.
ISAAC, i´-zak, laughter. Gen. 17:19.
his birth promised. Gen. 15:4; 17:16; 18:10; born. Gen. 21:2.
offered by Abraham. Gen. 22:7.
marries Rebekah. Gen. 24:67.
blesses his sons, Gen. 27:28; dies, Gen. 35:29.
ISAIAH, i-zai´-ah, salvation of Jehovah (Esaias), prophet. Is. 1:1; 2:1.
sent to Ahaz. Is. 7; and Hezekiah. Is. 37:6; 38:4; 39:3.
prophesies concerning various nations. Is. 7; 8; 10; 13—23; 45—47.
referred to in Matt. 3:3; 4:14; 8:17; 12:17; 13:14; 15:7; Mark 1:3; Luke 3:4; 4:17; John 1:23; 12:38; Acts 8:32; 28:25; Rom. 9:27; 10:16; 15:12.
ISCAH, is´-kah. Gen. 11:29.
ISCARIOT, is-kar´-i-ot, man of Kerioth. Judas, Matt. 10:4; Mark 3:19.

ISCARIOT—*cont.*
his treachery. Matt. 26:21; Mark 14:18; Luke 22:47; John 18:3.
death, Matt. 27:5; Acts 1:18.
ISHBAH, ish´-bah, praising. 1 Chr. 4:17.
ISHBAK, ish´-bak. Gen. 25:2.
ISHBI-BENOB, ish´-bi-ben-ob´e, one who dwells at Nob. 2 Sam. 21:16.
ISH-BOSHETH, ish-bo´-sheth, man of shame. 2 Sam. 2:8; 3:7; 4:5, 8.
ISHI, eesh´-i, my husband. Hos. 2:16.
ISHI, yish´-i, salutary. 1 Chr. 2:31.
ISHIAH, ish-i´-ah, whom Jehovah lends. 1 Chr. 7:3.
ISHIJAH, ish-i´-jah, same as ISHIA. Ezra 10:31.
ISHMA, ish´-mah. 1 Chr. 4:3.
ISHMAEL, ish´-ma-el, whom God hears, son of Abram. Gen. 16:15; 17:20; 21:17; 25:17; his descendants. Gen. 25:12; 1 Chr. 1:29.
——son of Nethaniah, slays Gedaliah. 2 Kin. 25:25; Jer. 40:14; 41.
ISHMAELITES, ish´-ma-el-ites, descendants of Ishmael. Judg. 8:24.
ISHMAIAH ISH-MAI´-AH, whom Jehovah hears. 1 Chr. 27:19.
ISHMEELITES, ish´-me-el-ites, same as ISHMAELITES. Gen. 37:25.
ISHMERAI, ish´-mer-ai, whom Jehovah keeps. 1 Chr. 8:18.
ISHOD, ish´-hode, man of glory. 1 Chr. 7:18.
ISHPAN, ish´-pan, cunning (?). 1 Chr. 8:22.
ISH-TOB, ish´-tobe, men of Tob. 2 Sam. 10:6.
ISHUAH, ish´-oo-ah, level. Gen. 46:17.
ISHUAI, ish´-oo-ai, same as ISUI. 1 Chr. 7:30.
ISHUI, ish´-oo-i, same as ISHUAH. 1 Sam. 14:49.
ISMACHIAH, is-mak-i´-ah, whom Jehovah upholds. 2 Chr. 31:13.
ISMAIAH, is-mai´-ah, same as ISHMAIAH. 1 Chr. 12:4.
ISPAH, is´-pah, bald. 1 Chr. 8:16.
ISRAEL, iz´-ra-el, soldier of God. Jacob so called after wrestling with God. Gen. 32:28; 35:10; Hos. 12:3.
ISRAELITES, iz´-ra-el-ites, descendants of Israel. Ex. 9:7.
in Egypt. Ex. 1—12.
the first passover instituted. Ex. 12.
flight from Egypt. Ex. 12:31.
pass through the Red Sea. Ex. 14.
their journeys. Ex. 14:1, 19; Num. 9:15; Ps. 78:14.
fed by manna and water in the wilderness. Ex. 16:4; 17:1; Num. 11; 20.
God's covenant with at Sinai. Ex. 19; 20; Deut. 29:10.
their idolatry. Ex. 32. *See also* 2 Kin. 17; Ezra 9; Neh. 9; Ezek. 20; 22; 23; Acts 7:39; 1 Cor. 10:1.
their rebellious conduct rehearsed by Moses. Deut. 1; 2; 9.
conquer and divide Canaan under Joshua. Josh. 1; 12; 13.
governed by judges. Judg. 2; by kings. 1 Sam. 10; 2 Sam.; 1 & 2 Kin.; 1 & 2 Chr.
their captivity in Assyria, 2 Kin. 17; in Babylon, 2 Kin. 25; 2 Chr. 36; Jer. 39; 52; their return, Ezra; Neh.; Hag.; Zech.
God's wrath against. Ps. 78; 106; deliverances of. Ps. 105.
their sufferings our examples. 1 Cor. 10:6.
ISRAELITISH, iz´-ra-el-ite-ish, after the fashion of an Israelite. Lev. 24:10.
ISSACHAR, is´-ak-ar, he is hired (?). Gen. 30:18; 35:23.
descendants of. Gen. 46:13; Judg. 5:15; 1 Chr. 7:1. *See* Num. 1:28; 26:23; Gen. 49:14; Deut. 33:18; Josh. 19:17; Ezek. 48:33; Rev. 7:7.
ISSHIAH, ish-hi´-ah, same as ISHIAH. 1 Chr. 24:21.
ISUAH, is´-oo-ah, same as ISHUAH. 1 Chr. 7:30.
ISUI, is´-oo-i, same as ISHUI. Gen. 46:17.
ITALIAN, it-al´-yan, belonging to Italy. Acts 10:1.
ITALY, it´-a-ly. Acts 18:2.
ITHAI, ee´-thai, ploughman. 1 Chr. 11:31.
ITHAMAR, i´-tha-mar, island of palms. Ex. 6:23; Lev. 10:6; his charge. Num. 4.
ITHIEL, ith´-i-el, God is with me. Neh. 11:7; Prov. 30:1.
ITHMAH, ith´-mah, bereavedness. 1 Chr. 11:46.
ITHNAN, ith´-nan. Josh. 15:23.
ITHRA, ith´-rah, excellence. 2 Sam. 17:25.
ITHRAN, ith´-ran, same as ITHRA. Gen. 36:26.
ITHREAM, ith´-re-am, remainder of the people. 2 Sam. 3:5.
ITHRITE, ith´-rite, descendant of Jether (?). 2 Sam. 23:38.
ITTAH-KAZIN, it´-ah-ka´-zin, time of the chief. Josh. 19:13.
ITTAI, it´-tai, same as ITHAI (the Gittite). 2 Sam. 15:19; 18:2.
ITURÆA, i´-tu-re´-ah, a province so named from Jetur. Luke 3:1.
IVAH, i´-vah. 2 Kin. 18:34.
IZEHAR, iz´-e-har, oil. Num. 3:19.
IZEHARITES, i´-ze-har´-ites, the descendants of Izehar. Num. 3:27.
IZHAR, iz´-har, same as IZEHAR. Ex. 6:18.
IZHARITES, iz´-har-ites, the same as IZEHARITES. 1 Chr. 26:23.
IZRAHIAH, iz-rah-i´-ah, whom Jehovah brought to light. 1 Chr. 7:3.
IZRAHITE, iz´-rah-ite, probably same as ZARHITE. 1 Chr. 27:8.
IZRI, iz´-ri, a descendant of Jezer. 1 Chr. 25:11.

JAAKAN, ja´-ak-an, one who turns. Deut. 10:6.
JAAKOBAH, ja´-ak-o-bah, same as JACOB. 1 Chr. 4:36.
JAALA, ja´-a-lah, wild she-goat. Neh. 7:58.
JAALAH, ja´-a-lah, same as JAALA. Ezra 2:56.
JAALAM, ja´-a-lam, whom God hides. Gen. 36:5.
JAANAI, ja´-a-nai, whom Jehovah answers. 1 Chr. 5:12.
JAARE-OREGIM, ja´-ar-e-or´-eg-im, forests of the weavers. 2 Sam. 21:19.
JAASAU, ja´-a-saw. Ezra 10:37.
JAASIEL, ja-as´-i-el, whom God created. 1 Chr. 27:21.
JAAZANIAH, ja´-az-an-i´-ah, whom Jehovah hears. 2 Kin. 25:23.
JAAZER, ja´-a-zer, whom (God) aids. Num. 21:32.
JAAZIAH, ja´-az-i´-ah, whom Jehovah strengthens. 1 Chr. 24:26.
JAAZIEL, ja´-az´-i-el, whom God strengthens. 1 Chr. 15:18.
JABAL, ja´-bal. Gen. 4:20.
JABBOK, jab´-ok, pouring out, river. Gen. 32:22; Num. 21:24; Deut. 3:16; Josh. 12:2.
JABESH, ja´-besh, dry. 2 Kin. 15:10.
JABESH-GILEAD, ja´-besh-gil´-e-ad, Jabesh of Gilead. Judg. 21:8.
inhabitants smitten by Israel. Judg. 21.
threatened by Ammonites. 1 Sam. 11:1; delivered by Saul. 1 Sam. 11:11.
JABEZ, ja´-bez, causing pain, prayer of. 1 Chr. 4:9.
JABIN, ja´-bin, whom He (God) considered. Judg. 4:2.
king of Hazor, conquered by Joshua. Josh. 11.
——(another), destroyed by Barak. Judg. 4.
JABNEEL, jab´-ne-el, may God cause to be built. Josh. 15:11.
JABNEH, jab´-nay, which (God) causes to be built. 2 Chr. 26:6.
JACHAN, ja´-kan, troubled. 1 Chr. 5:13.
JACHIN, ja´-kin, whom (God) strengthens, one of the pillars of the porch of the temple. 1 Kin. 7:21; 2 Chr. 3:17.
JACHINITES, ja´-kin-ites, descendants of Jachin. Num. 26:12.
JACOB, ja´-kob, supplanter, his birth, Gen. 25:26; birthright, 25:33; blessing, 27:27; sent to Padan-aram, 27:43; 28:1; his vision of the ladder, and vow, 28:10; marriages, 29; sons, 29:31; 30; dealings with Laban, 31; his vision of God's host, 32:1; his prayer, 32:9; wrestles with an angel, 32:24; Hos. 12:4; reconciled

JACOB,—*cont.*
with Esau. Gen. 33; builds an altar at Beth-el, 35:1; his grief for Joseph and Benjamin, 37; 42:38; 43; goes down to Egypt, 46; brought before Pharaoh, 47:7; blesses his sons, 48; 49.
his death, and burial. Gen. 49:33; 50. *See* Ps. 105:23; Mal. 1:2; Rom. 9:10; Heb. 11:21.
JACOB'S WELL. John 4:5.
JADA, ja´dah, wise. 1 Chr. 2:28.
JADAU, ja´daw. Ezra 10:43.
JADDUA, jad´oo-ah, skilled. Neh. 10:21.
JADON, ja´don, a judge. Neh. 3:7.
JAEL, ja´el, same as JAALA, kills Sisera. Judg. 4:17; 5:24.
JAGUR, ja´goor, a lodging. Josh. 15:21.
JAH, poetic form of JEHOVAH. Ps. 68:4.
JAHATH, ja´hath. 1 Chr. 6:20.
JAHAZ, ja´haz, a place trodden down. Num. 21:23.
JAHAZA, ja´haz-ah, same as JAHAZ. Josh. 13:18.
JAHAZAH, same as JAHAZA. Josh. 21:36.
JAHAZIAH, ja´haz-i´ah, whom Jehovah watches over. Ezra 10:15.
JAHAZIEL, ja-haz´i-el, whom God watches over. 1 Chr. 16:6.
comforts Jehoshaphat. 2 Chr. 19:14.
prophecies against Moab and Ammon. 2 Chr. 20:14.
JAHDAI, jah´dai, whom Jehovah directs. 1 Chr. 2:47.
JAHDIEL, jah´di-el, whom God makes glad. 1 Chr. 5:24.
JAHDO, jah´do, union. 1 Chr. 5:14.
JAHLEEL, jah´le-el, hoping in God. Num. 26:26.
JAHLEELITES, jah´le-el-ites, descendants of Jahleel. Num. 26:26.
JAHMAI, jah´mai. 1 Chr. 7:2.
JAHZAH, ja´zah, same as JAHAZ. 1 Chr. 6:78.
JAHZEEL, jah´ze-el, whom God allots. Gen. 46:24.
JAHZEELITES, jah´ze-el-ites, descendants of Jahzeel. Num. 26:48.
JAHZERAH, jah-ze´rah, may he bring back. 1 Chr. 9:12.
JAHZIEL, jah´zi-el, same as JAHZEEL. 1 Chr. 7:13.
JAIR, ja´er, (*i.e.* God) enlightens. Num. 32:41.
Gileadite, judge. Judg. 10:3.
JAIRITE, ja´er-ite, a descendant of JAIR. 2 Sam. 20:26.
JAIRUS, ja-i´rus, Greek form of JAIR, daughter of, raised. Matt. 9:18; Mark 5:22; Luke 8:41.
JAKAN, ja´kan, same as JAAKAN. 1 Chr. 1:42.
JAKEH, ja´kay, pious (?). Prov. 30:1.
JAKIM, ja´kim, (God) sets up. 1 Chr. 8:19.
JALON, ja´lon, passing the night. 1 Chr. 4:17.
JAMBRES, jam´brees. 2 Tim. 3:8.
JAMES, the English equivalent for Jacob in the New Testament.
——(APOSTLE), son of Zebedee, called. Matt. 4:21; Mark 1:19; Luke 5:10.
ordained one of the twelve. Matt. 10:2; Mark 3:14; Luke 6:13.
witnessed Christ's transfiguration. Matt. 17:1; Mark 9:2; Luke 9:28.
present at the passion. Matt. 26:36; Mark 14:33.
slain by Herod. Acts 12:2.
——(APOSTLE), son of Alphæus. Matt. 10:3; Mark 3:18; 6:3; Luke 6:15; Acts 1:13; 12:17.
his judgment respecting ceremonial. Acts 15:13-29; *See* 1 Cor. 15:7; Gal. 1:19; 2:9.
his teaching. James 1—5.
mentioned. Acts 21:18; 1 Cor. 15:7; Gal. 1:19; 2:9.
JAMIN, ja´min, right hand. Gen. 46:10.
JAMINITES, ja´min-ites, descendants of Jamin. Num. 26:12.
JAMLECH, jam´lek, He makes to reign. 1 Chr. 4:34.
JANNA, jan´nah, probably another form of JOHN. Luke 3:24.
JANNES AND JAMBRES, magicians of Egypt. 2 Tim. 3:8 (Ex. 7:11).
JANOAH, ja-no´ah, rest. 2 Kin. 15:29.
JANOHAH, ja-no´hah, same as preceding. Josh. 16:6.
JANUM, ja´noom, sleep. Josh. 15:53.
JAPHETH, ja´feth, extension. Gen. 5:32.
son of Noah, blessed. Gen. 9:27.
his descendants. Gen. 10:1; 1 Chr. 1:4.
JAPHIA, ja-fi´ah, splendid. Josh. 19:12.
JAPHLET, jaf´let, may he deliver. 1 Chr. 7:32.
JAPHLETI, jaf-le´ti, the Japhletite, or descendant of Japhlet. Josh. 16:3.
JAPHO, ja´fo, beauty. Josh. 19:46.
JARAH, ja´rah, forest. 1 Chr. 9:42.
JAREB, ja´reb, one who is contentious. Hos. 5:13.
JARED, ja´red, descent. Gen. 5:15; Luke 3:37.
JARESIAH, ja´res-i´ah, whom Jehovah nourishes. 1 Chr. 8:27.
JARHA, jar´hah. 1 Chr. 2:34.
JARIB, ja´rib, adversary. 1 Chr. 4:24.
JARMUTH, jar´mooth, height. Josh. 10:3.
JAROAH, ja-ro´ah, moon (?). 1 Chr. 5:14.
JASHEN, ja´shen, sleeping. 2 Sam. 23:32.
JASHER, ja´sher, upright, book of. Josh. 10:13; 2 Sam. 1:18.
JASHOBEAM, ja-shob´e-am, the people returns, valour of. 1 Chr. 11:11.
JASHUB, ja´shoob, he returns. Num. 26:24.
JASHUBI-LEHEM, ja-shoob´i-le´hem, giving bread (?). 1 Chr. 4:22.
JASHUBITES, ja´shoob´ites, descendants of Jashub. Num. 26:24.
JASIEL, ja-si´el, whom God made. 1 Chr. 11:47.
JASON, ja´son, Græco-Judæan equivalent of Joshua.
persecuted at Thessalonica. Acts 17:5; Rom. 16:21.
JATHNIEL, jath´ni-el, God gives. 1 Chr. 26:2.
JATTIR, jat´yer, excelling. Josh. 15:48.
JAVAN, ja´van, wine (?), son of Japheth. Gen. 10:2.
JAZER, ja´zer, same as JAAZER. Num. 32:1.
JAZIZ, ja´ziz, wanderer (?). 1 Chr. 27:31.
JEARIM, je-ar´im, forests. Josh. 15:10.
JEATERAI, je-at´er-ai´. 1 Chr. 6:21.
JEBERECHIAH, je-ber´ek-i´ah, whom Jehovah blesses. Is. 8:2.
JEBUS, je´boos, a place trodden down (?). Judg. 19:10.
JEBUSI, je-boo´si, a Jebusite. Josh. 18:16.
JEBUSITES, je-boo´sites, the descendants of Jebus, the son of Canaan. Gen. 15:21; Num. 13:29; Josh. 15:63; Judg. 1:21; 19:11; 2 Sam. 5:6.
JECAMIAH, jek´am-i´ah. 1 Chr. 3:18.
JECHOLIAH, jek´ol-i´ah, Jehovah is strong. 2 Kin. 15:2.
JECHONIAS, jek´on-i´as, the Greek way of spelling Jeconiah. Matt. 1:11, 12; 1 Chr. 3:17.
JECOLIAH, jek´ol-i´ah, same as JECHOLIAH. 2 Chr. 26:3.
JECONIAH, jek´on-i´ah, Jehovah establishes. 1 Chr. 3:16.
JEDAIAH, jed-ai´ah, (1) Jehovah—(?). 1 Chr. 4:37.
(2) Jehovah knoweth. 1 Chr. 24:7.
JEDIAEL, je-di´a-el, known of God. 1 Chr. 7:6.
JEDIDAH, jed-i´dah, beloved. 2 Kin. 22:1.
JEDIDIAH, jed-id-i´ah (beloved of the Lord), a name of Solomon. 2 Sam. 12:25.
JEDUTHUN, jed-ooth´oon, friendship (?). 1 Chr. 16:38, 41; 25:6.
JEEZER, je-e´zer, contracted from ABIEZER. Num. 26:30.
JEEZERITES, je-ez´er-ites, descendants of Jeezer. Num. 26:30.
JEGAR-SAHADUTHA, je-gar´sa-ha-doo´thah, the heap of testimony. Gen. 31:47.
JEHALELEEL, je-hal´el-e´el, he praises God. 1 Chr. 4:16.
JEHALELEL, je-hal´e-lel, same as preceding. 2 Chr. 29:12.
JEHDEIAH, jed-i´ah, whom Jehovah makes glad. 1 Chr. 24:20.
JEHEZEKEL, je-hez´e-kel, same as EZEKIEL. 1 Chr. 24:16.
JEHIAH, je-hi´ah, Jehovah lives. 1 Chr. 15:24.
JEHIEL, je-hi´el, God liveth. 1 Chr. 15:18.

JEHIELI, je-hi´el-i, a Jehielite. 1 Chr. 26:21.
JEHIZKIAH, je´hizk-i´ah, same as HEZEKIAH. 2 Chr. 28:12.
JEHOADAH, je-ho´a-dah, whom Jehovah adorns. 1 Chr. 8:36.
JEHOADDAN, je-ho´ad-an. Jehovah is beauteous (?). 2 Kin. 14:2.
JEHOAHAZ, je-ho´a-haz, whom Jehovah holds fast.
son of Jehu, king of Israel. 2 Kin. 10:35; 13:4.
——(Shallum), king of Judah, his evil reign. 2 Kin. 23:31; 2 Chr. 36:1.
JEHOASH, je-ho´ash, Jehovah supports. 2 Kin. 11:21.
JEHOHANAN, je-ho´han-an, Jehovah is gracious. 1 Chr. 26:3.
JEHOIACHIN, je-ho´ya-kin, Jehovah has established.
king of Judah, his defeat and captivity. 2 Kin. 24:6; 2 Chr. 36:8.
JEHOIADA, je-ho´ya-dah, Jehovah knoweth. 2 Sam. 8:18.
high priest, deposes and slays Athaliah, and restores Jehoash: 2 Kin. 11:4; 2 Chr. 23; repairs the temple. 2 Kin. 12:7; 2 Chr. 24:6.
abolishes idolatry. 2 Chr. 23:16.
JEHOIAKIM, je-ho´ya-kim, Jehovah has set up.
——(Eliakim), made king of Judah by Pharaoh-nechoh, his evil reign and captivity. 2 Kin. 23:34; 24:1; 2 Chr. 36:4; Dan. 1:2. *See* Jer. 22:18.
JEHOIARIB, je-ho´ya-rib, Jehovah will contend. 1 Chr. 9:10.
JEHONADAB, je-ho´na-dab, Jehovah is bounteous. 2 Kin. 10:15.
JEHONATHAN, je-ho´na-than, same as JONATHAN. 1 Chr. 27:25.
JEHORAM, je-ho´ram, Jehovah is high.
——(son of Jehoshaphat), king of Judah. 1 Kin. 22:50; 2 Kin. 8:16; his cruelty and death, 2 Chr. 21:4, 18.
——(Joram), king of Israel, son of Ahab. 2 Kin. 1:17; 3:1; his evil reign. 2 Kin. 3:2; slain by Jehu. 2 Kin. 9:24.
JEHOSHABEATH, je-ho´shab´e-ath, Jehovah is the oath. 2 Chr. 22:11.
JEHOSHAPHAT, je-hosh´af-at, whom Jehovah judges.
king of Judah, his good reign. 1 Kin. 15:24; 2 Chr. 17; his death. 1 Kin. 22:50; 2 Chr. 21:1.
——valley of. Joel 3:2.
JEHOSHEBA, je-ho´she-bah, same as JEHOSHABEATH. 2 Kin. 11:2; 2 Chr. 22:11.
JEHOSHUA, je-hosh´oo-ah, same as JOSHUA. Num. 13:16.
JEHOSHUAH, je-hosh´oo-ah, same as JOSHUA. 1 Chr. 7:27.
JEHOVAH, je-ho´vah, the Eternal One.
JEHOVAH, (ELOHIM, I AM THAT I AM). Ex. 6:3; Ps. 83:18; Is. 12:2; 26:4.
JEHOVAH-JIREH, je-ho´vah-ji´ray, Jehovah will provide. Gen. 22:14.
JEHOVAH-NISSI, je-ho´vah-nis´i, Jehovah my banner. Ex. 17:15.
JEHOVAH-SHALOM, je-ho´vah-sha´lom, Jehovah send peace. Judg. 6:24.
——SHAMMAH, je-ho´vah-sham´mah (the LORD is there). Ezek. 48:35.
——TSIDKENU, je-ho´vah-tsid-ke´nu (the LORD is our righteousness). Jer. 23:6.
JEHOZABAD, je-ho´za-bad, Jehovah gave. 2 Kin. 12:21.
JEHOZADAK, je-ho´za-dak, Jehovah is just. 1 Chr. 6:14.
JEHU, je´hu, Jehovah is He (?), son of Hanani, prophesies against Baasha. 1 Kin. 16:1.
rebukes Jehoshaphat. 2 Chr. 19:2; 20:34.
——son of Nimshi, to be anointed king of Israel. 1 Kin. 19:16; 2 Kin. 9:1.
his reign. 2 Kin. 9:10.
JEHUBBAH, je-hoob´ah, hidden. 1 Chr. 7:34.
JEHUCAL, je-hoo-kal, Jehovah is mighty. Jer. 37:3.
JEHUD, je´hood, praise. Josh. 19:45.
JEHUDI, je-hood´i, a Jew. Jer. 36:14.
JEHUDIJAH, je-hood-i´jah, a Jewess. 1 Chr. 4:18.
JEHUSH, je´hoosh, to whom God hastens. 1 Chr. 8:39.
JEIEL, ji´el. 1 Chr. 5:7.
JEKABZEEL, je-kab´ze-el, God gathers. Neh. 11:25.
JEKAMEAM, je-kam´e-am. 1 Chr. 23:19.
JEKAMIAH, jek´am-i´ah, same as JECAMIAH. 1 Chr. 2:41.
JEKUTHIEL, je-koo´thi-el, the fear of God. 1 Chr. 4:18.
JEMIMA, je-mi´mah, dove. Job 42:14.
JEMUEL, jem-oo´el, day of God. Gen. 46:10.
JEPHTHAE, jef´thah, Greek way of writing Jephthah. Heb. 11:32.
JEPHTHAH, jef´thah, God opens. Judg. 11:1.
judge, his dealings with the Gileadites. Judg. 11:4.
defeats the Ammonites. Judg. 11:14.
his rash vow. Judg. 11:30, 34.
chastises the Ephraimites. Judg. 12.
JEPHUNNEH, je-foon´eh, for whom it is prepared. Num. 13:6.
JERAH, je´rah, the moon. Gen. 10:26.
JERAHMEEL, je-rah´me-el, whom God loves. 1 Chr. 2:9.
JERAHMEELITES, je-rah´me-el-ites, descendants of Jerahmeel. 1 Sam. 27:10.
JERED, je´red, descent. 1 Chr. 1:2.
JEREMAI, jer-e´mai, dwelling in heights. Ezra 10:33.
JEREMIAH, jer´em-i´ah, whom Jehovah has appointed.
(prophet), his call and visions. Jer. 1.
his mission. Jer. 1:17; 7.
his complaint. Jer. 20:14.
his message to Zedekiah. Jer. 21:3; 34:1.
foretells the seventy years' captivity. Jer. 25:8.
arraigned, condemned, but delivered. Jer. 26.
denounces the false prophet Hananiah. Jer. 28:5.
writes to the captives in Babylon. Jer. 29.
his promises of comfort and redemption to Israel. Jer. 31.
writes a roll of a book. Jer. 36:4; Baruch reads it. Jer. 36:8.
imprisoned by Zedekiah. Jer. 32; 37; 38.
released. Jer. 38:7.
predicts slaughter of innocents. Jer. 31:15; fulfilled. Matt. 2:17.
with all the remnant of Judah carried into Egypt. Jer. 43:4.
various predictions. Jer. 46—51; 51:59.
mentioned. Matt. 16:14; 27:9.
JEREMIAS, jer´em-i´as, Greek form of JEREMIAH. Matt. 16:14.
JEREMOTH, je-re´moth, high places. 1 Chr. 8:14.
JEREMY, jer´em-y, shortened English form of JEREMIAH. Matt. 2:17.
JERIAH, jer-i´ah, whom Jehovah regards (?). 1 Chr. 23:19.
JERIBAI, jer-ee´bai, contentious. 1 Chr. 11:46.
JERICHO, jer´ik-o, a fragrant place. Num. 22:1.
the spies at. Josh. 2:1.
capture of. Josh. 6:20 (Heb. 11:30).
rebuilt by Hiel. 1 Kin. 16:34. *See* Josh. 6:26.
JERIEL, je-ri´el, founded by God. 1 Chr. 7:2.
JERIJAH, jer-i´jah, same as JERIAH. 1 Chr. 26:31.
JERIMOTH, jer-ee´moth, same as JEREMOTH. 1 Chr. 7:7.
JERIOTH, je-ri´oth, curtains. 1 Chr. 2:18.
JEROBOAM I, jer´ob-o´am, whose people are many. 1 Kin. 11:26.
promoted by Solomon. 1 Kin. 11:28.
Ahijah's prophecy to. 1 Kin. 11:29.
made king. 1 Kin. 12:20 (2 Chr. 10).
his idolatry, withered hand, denunciation. 1 Kin. 12; 13; 14.
death. 1 Kin. 14:20.
evil example. 1 Kin. 15:34.
JEROBOAM II. 2 Kin. 13:13; 14:23-29.
JEROHAM, je-ro´ham, who is loved. 1 Sam. 1:1.
JERUBBAAL, jer-oob-ba´al, let Baal plead. Judg. 6:32.
JERUBBESHETH, jer-oob-be´sheth, let shame plead, another name for JERUBBAAL. 2 Sam. 11:21.

JERUEL, je-roo´-el, same as JERIEL. 2 Chr. 20:16.
JERUSALEM, je-roo´-sa-lem, founded in peace (?). Josh. 10:1.
——Adoni-zedec, king of, slain by Joshua. Josh. 10.
borders of. Josh. 15:8.
David reigns there. 2 Sam. 5:6.
the ark brought there. 2 Sam. 6.
saved from the pestilence. 2 Sam. 24:16.
temple built at. 1 Kin. 5—8; 2 Chr. 1—7.
sufferings from war. 1 Kin. 14:25; 2 Kin. 14:14; 25; 2 Chr. 12; 25:24; 36; Jer. 39; 52.
capture and destruction by Nebuchadrezzar. Jer. 52:12—15.
captives return: and rebuilding of the temple begun by Cyrus. Ezra 1—3; continued by Artaxerxes. Neh. 2.
wall rebuilt and dedicated by Nehemiah. Neh. 12:38.
abominations there. Ezek. 16:2.
presentation of Christ at. Luke 2:22.
the child Jesus tarries at. Luke 2:42.
Christ rides into. Matt. 21:1; Mark 11:7; Luke 19:35; John 12:14.
laments over it. Matt. 23:37; Luke 13:34; 19:41.
foretells its destruction. Matt. 24; Mark 13; Luke 13:34; 17; 23; 19:41; 21.
disciples filled with the Holy Ghost at. Acts 2:4.
which is above. Gal. 4:26.
the new. Rev. 21:2.
JERUSHA, je-roo´-shah, possession. 2 Kin. 15:33.
JERUSHAH, je-roo´-shah, same as preceding. 2 Chr. 27:1.
JESAIAH, je-sai´-ah, same as ISAIAH. 1 Chr. 3:21.
JESHAIAH, je-shai´-ah, same as preceding. 1 Chr. 25:3.
JESHANAH, je-shan´-ah, old. 2 Chr. 13:19.
JESHARELAH, jesh´-ar-el´-ah, right before God (?). 1 Chr. 25:14.
JESHEBEAB, je-sheb´-e-ab, father's seat. 1 Chr. 24:13.
JESHER, je´-sher, uprightness. 1 Chr. 2:18.
JESHIMON, je-shim´-on, the waste. Num. 21:20.
JESHISHAI, je-shee´-shai, like an old man. 1 Chr. 5:14.
JESHOHAIAH, je-sho-hai´-ah, whom Jehovah humbles. 1 Chr. 4:36.
JESHUA (Joshua), jesh´-oo-ah, Jehovah is salvation. Ezra 2:2; Neh. 8:17. *See* JOSHUA.
JESHUAH, jesh´-oo-ah, help. 1 Chr. 24:11.
JESHURUN, jesh-oor´-oon, righteous, symbolical name of Israel. Deut. 32:15; 33:5, 26; Is. 44:2.
JESIAH, je-si´-ah. 1 Chr. 12:6.
JESIMIEL, je-sim´-i-el, whom God founds (?). 1 Chr. 4:36.
JESSE, jes´-sy, gift (?). Ruth 4:17.
David's father. Ruth 4:22.
and his sons sanctified by Samuel. 1 Sam. 16:5.
his son David anointed to be king. 1 Sam. 16:13. *See* Is. 11:1.
his posterity. 1 Chr. 2:13.
JESUI, je-soo´-i, same as ISHUA. Num. 26:44.
JESUITES, je´-soo-ites, the posterity of Jesui. Num. 26:44.
JESURUN, je-soor´-oon, wrongly printed for Jeshurun. Is. 44:2.
JESUS, je´-sus, Saviour. Matt. 1:21. *See* CHRIST, *Subject-Index*, p. 1413.
JETHER, je´-ther, same as ITHRA. Judg. 8:20.
JETHETH, je´-theth. Gen. 36:40.
JETHLAH, jeth´-lah, lofty. Josh. 19:42.
JETHRO, jeth´-ro, same as ITHRA. Ex. 3:1.
Moses' father-in-law. Ex. 18:12.
JETUR, je´-toor, an enclosure. Gen. 25:15.
JEUEL, je-oo´-el, same as JEIEL. 1 Chr. 9:6.
JEUSH, je´-oosh, same as JEHUSH. Gen. 36:5.
JEUZ, je´-ooz, counsellor. 1 Chr. 8:10.
JEW, joo, an Israelite. Esth. 2:5.
JEWESS, joo´-ess, a female Jew. Acts 16:1.
JEWISH, joo´-ish, of or belonging to Jews. Tit. 1:14.
JEWRY, joo´-ry, Old English name for Judea. Dan. 5:13.
JEWS, joos, inhabitants of Judea (Israelites first so called). 2 Kin. 16:6.
Christ's mission to. Matt. 15:24; 21:37; Acts 3:26.
Christ's compassion for. Matt. 23:37 ;Luke 19:41.
Christ rejected by. Matt. 11:20; 13:15, 58; John 5:16, 38, 43; Acts 3:13; 13:46; 1 Thess. 2:15.
gospel first preached to, Matt. 10:6; Luke 24:47; Acts 1:8.
St. Paul's teaching rejected by, Acts 13:46; 28:24, 26, &c.
JEZANIAH, jez´-an-i´-ah, Jehovah adorns (?). Jer. 40:8.
JEZEBEL, jez´-e-bel, unmarried.
wife of Ahab. 1 Kin. 16:31.
kills the prophets, 1 Kin. 18:4; 19:2.
causes Naboth to be put to death. 1 Kin. 21.
her violent death. 2 Kin. 9:30.
JEZER, je´-zer, anything made. Gen. 46:24.
JEZERITES, je´-zer-ites, descendants of Jezer. Num. 26:49.
JEZIAH, jez-i´-ah, whom Jehovah assembles. Ezra 10:25.
JEZIEL, jez-i´-el, the assembly of God. 1 Chr. 12:3.
JEZLIAH, jez-li´-ah, deliverance (?). 1 Chr. 8:18.
JEZOAR, je-zo´-ar, splendid. 1 Chr. 4:7.
JEZRIHIAH, jez´-rah-i´-ah, Jehovah shines forth. Neh. 12:42.
JEZREEL, jez´-re-el, God scatters. 1 Chr. 4:3. *See* AHAB.
JEZREELITE, jez´-re-el-ite, an inhabitant of Jezreel. 1 Kin. 21:6.
JEZREELITESS, jez´-re-el-ite-ess, feminine of preceding. 1 Sam. 27:3.
JIBSAM, jib´-sam, fragrant. 1 Chr. 7:2.
JIDLAPH, jid´-laf, weeping (?). Gen. 22:22.
JIMNA, jim´-nah, same as IMNA. Num. 26:44.
JIMNAH, jim´-nah, same as IMNAH. Gen. 46:17.
JIMNITES, jim´-nites, descendants of Jimnah. Num. 26:44.
JIPHTAH, jif´-tah, same as JEPHTHAH. Josh. 15:43.
JIPHTHAH-EL, jif´-thah-el, which God opens. Josh. 19:14.
JOAB, jo´-ab, Jehovah is father. 2 Sam. 2:13.
nephew of David, and captain of the host. 2 Sam. 8:16.
kills Abner. 2 Sam. 3:23.
intercedes for Absalom, 2 Sam. 14; slays him in an oak, 2 Sam. 18:14.
reproves David's grief. 2 Sam. 19:5.
slays Amasa. 2 Sam. 20:9.
unwillingly numbers the people. 2 Sam. 24:3 (1 Chr. 21:3).
joins Adonijah's usurpation. 1 Kin. 1:7.
slain by Solomon's command. 1 Kin. 2:5, 28.
JOAH, jo´-ah, Jehovah is brother. 2 Kin. 18:18; 2 Chr. 34:8.
JOAHAZ, jo´-a-haz, whom Jehovah holds. 2 Chr. 34:8.
JOANNA, jo-an´-ah, Greek way of writing Jehonan. Luke 3:27; 8:2, 3; 24:10.
JOASH, jo´-ash, whom Jehovah supports (?). 2 Kin. 11:2.
(Jehoash), king of Israel. 2 Kin. 13:10.
visits Elisha sick. 2 Kin. 13:14.
defeats the Syrians. 2 Kin. 13:25.
chastises Amaziah. 2 Kin. 14:8; 2 Chr. 25:17.
——king of Judah. 2 Kin. 11:4; 2 Chr. 23.
repairs the temple. 2 Kin. 12; 2 Chr. 24.
kills Zechariah. 2 Chr. 24:17.
slain by his servants. 2 Kin. 12:19; 2 Chr. 24:23.
JOATHAM, jo´-ath-am, Greek form of JOTHAM. Matt. 1:9.
JOB, jobe, (1) a desert, Gen. 46:13; (2) one persecuted.
his character, Job 1:1, 8; 2:3 (Ezek. 14:14, 20).
his afflictions and patience. Job. 1:13, 20; 2:7, 10 (James 5:11).
complains of his life. Job 3.
reproves his friends. Job 6; 7; 9; 10; 12—14; 16; 17; 19; 21; 23; 24; 26—30.
solemnly protests his integrity. Job. 31.

JOB—*cont.*
humbles himself. Job 40:3; 42:1.
God accepts and doubly blesses. Job 42:10.

JOBAB, job´-bab, a desert. Gen. 10:29.

JOCHEBED, jo´-ke-bed, Jehovah is glorious (?).
mother of Moses. Ex. 6:20; Num. 26:59.

JOED, jo´-ed, for whom Jehovah is witness. Neh. 11:7.

JOEL, jo´-el, Jehovah is might.
delivers God's judgments. Joel 1—3.
proclaims a fast, and declares God's mercy. Joel 1:14; 2:12; 3.
quoted. Acts 2:16.

JOELAH, jo´-el-ah, He helps (?). 1 Chr. 12:7.

JOEZER, jo´-e-zer, Jehovah is help. 1 Chr. 12:6.

JOGBEHAH, jog´-be-hah, lofty. Num. 32:35.

JOGLI, jo´-gli, an exile. Num. 34:22.

JOHA, jo´-hah, Jehovah lives (?). 1 Chr. 8:16.

JOHANAN, jo-ha´-nan, Jehovah is gracious. 2 Kin. 25:23; Jer. 40:8, 15; 41:11; 42; 43.

JOHN, English way of spelling Johanan. Matt. 3:1.
the APOSTLE, called, Matt. 4:21; Mark 1:19; Luke 5:10.
ordained. Matt. 10:2; Mark 3:17.
enquires of Jesus. Mark 13:3.
reproved. Matt. 20:20; Mark 10:35-40; Luke 9:50.
sent to prepare the passover. Luke 22:8.
declares the divinity and humanity of Jesus Christ. John 1; 1 John 1; 4; 5.
Christ's love for. John 13:23; 19:26; 21:7, 20, 24.
his care for Mary the Lord's mother. John 19:27.
meets for prayer. Acts 1:13.
accompanies Peter before the council. Acts 3; 4.
exhorts to obedience and warns against false teachers. 1 John 1—5.
sees Christ's glory in heaven. Rev. 1:13.
writes the Revelation. Rev. 1:19.
forbidden to worship the angel. Rev. 19:10; 22:8.

——(MARK). Acts 12:12, 25. *See* MARK.

——the BAPTIST, his coming foretold. Is. 40:3; Mal. 4:5; Luke 1:17.
his birth and circumcision. Luke 1:57.
office, preaching, and baptism. Matt. 3; Mark 1; Luke 3; John 1:6; 3:26; Acts 1:5; 13:24.
baptizes Christ. Matt. 3; Mark 1; Luke 3; John 1:32; 3:26.
imprisoned by Herod, Matt. 4:12; Mark 1:14; Luke 3:20; and beheaded, Matt. 14; Mark. 6:14.
sends his disciples to Christ. Matt. 11:1; Luke 7:18.
Christ's testimony to. Matt. 11:11, 14; 17:12; Mark 9:11; Luke 7:27.
his disciples receive the Holy Ghost. Acts 18:24; 19:1.

JOIADA, jo´-ya-dah, Jehovah knows. Neh. 12:10.

JOIAKIM, jo´-ya-kim, shortened from JEHOIAKIM. Neh. 12:10.

JOIARIB, jo´-ya-rib, whom Jehovah defends. Ezra 8:16.

JOKIM, jo´-kim, shortened from JEHOIAKIM. 1 Chr. 4:22.

JOKDEAM, jok´-de-am, burning of the people. Josh. 15:56.

JOKMEAM, jok´-me-am. 1 Chr. 6:68.

JOKNEAM, jok´-ne-am, possessed by the people. Josh. 12:22.

JOKSHAN, jok´-shan, fowler. Gen. 25:2.

JOKTAN, jok´-tan, small. Gen. 10:25.

JOKTHEEL, jok´-the-el, subdued by God. Josh. 15:38.

JONA, jo´-nah, a Greek way of spelling Johanan. John 1:42.

JONADAB, jo´-na-dab, same as JEHONADAB. 2 Sam. 13:3.

——(Jehonadab), son of Rechab. 2 Kin. 10:15.

JONAH, jo´-nah, dove.
prophet. 2 Kin. 14:25.
his disobedience, punishment, prayer, and repentance. Jonah 1—4.
a type of Christ. Matt. 12:39; Luke 11:29.

JONAN, jo´-nan, contracted from JOHANAN. Luke 3:30.

JONAS, jo´-nas, (1) same as JONA. John 21:15. (2) Or JONAH. Matt. 12:39.

JONATH-ELEM-RECHOKIM, jo´-nath-e´-lem-re-ko-kim´, the silent dove afar off. Title of Ps. 56.

JONATHAN, jo´-na-than, whom Jehovah gave.
son of Saul, smites the Philistines. 1 Sam. 13:2; 14.
his love for David. 1 Sam. 18:1; 19; 20; 23:16.
slain by the Philistines. 1 Sam. 31:2.
David's lamentation for. 2 Sam. 1:17.

——son of Abiathar. 2 Sam. 15:27; 1 Kin. 1:42.

——one of David's nephews, his deeds. 2 Sam. 21:21; 1 Chr. 20:7.

——a Levite, hired by Micah. Judg. 17:7; 18.

JOPPA, jop´-ah, beauty (?).
(Jaffa). 2 Chr. 2:16; Jonah 1:3.
Tabitha raised at. Acts 9:36.
Peter dwells at. Acts 10:5; 11:5.

JORAH, jo´-rah, watering (?). Ezra 2:18.

JORAI, jo´-rai, archer (?). 1 Chr. 5:13.

JORAM, jo´-ram, same as JEHORAM. 2 Sam. 8:10.

JORDAN, jor´-dan, flowing down. Gen. 13:10.
river, waters of, divided for the Israelites. Josh. 3; 4; Ps. 114:3; by Elijah and Elisha. 2 Kin. 2:8, 13.
Naaman's leprosy cured at. 2 Kin. 5:10.
John baptizes there. Matt. 3; Mark 1:5; Luke 3:3; *See* Job 40:23; Ps. 42:6; Jer. 12:5; 49:19; Zech. 11:3.

JORIM, jo´-rim, a form of JORAM (?). Luke 3:29.

JORKOAM, jor´-ko-am, spreading of the people (?). 1 Chr. 2:44.

JOSABAD, jo´-sa-bad, same as JEHOZABAD. 1 Chr. 12:4.

JOSAPHAT, jo´-saf-at, Greek form of JEHOSHAPHAT. Matt. 1:8.

JOSEDECH, jo´-se-dek, same as JEHOZADAK. Hag. 1:1.

JOSEPH, jo´-sef, he shall add.
son of Jacob. Gen. 30:24. *See* Ps. 105:17; Acts 7:9; Heb. 11:22.
his dreams, and the jealousy of his brethren. Gen. 37:5.
sold to the Ishmeelites. Gen. 37:28.
slave to Potiphar. Gen. 39.
resists Potiphar's wife. Gen. 39:7.
interprets the dreams of Pharaoh's servants. Gen. 40; and of Pharaoh, predicting famine. Gen. 41:25.
made ruler of Egypt. Gen. 41:39.
prepares for the famine. Gen. 41:48.
receives his brethren and father. Gen. 42—46.
gives direction concerning his bones. Gen. 50:25.
his death. Gen. 50:26.

——son of Heli, husband of the Virgin. Matt. 1:19; 2:13, 19; Luke 1:27; 2:4.

——of Arimathæa. Matt. 27:57; Mark 15:42; Luke 23:50; John 19:38.

——(Barsabas), Justus. Acts 1:23.

JOSES, jo´-ses. Matt. 13:55.

JOSHAH, jo´-shah, Jehovah presents (?). 1 Chr. 4:34.

JOSHAPHAT, jo´-sha-fat, shortened from JEHOSHAPHAT. 1 Chr. 11:43.

JOSHAVIAH, jo´-shav-i´-ah, same as JOSHAH. 1 Chr. 11:46.

JOSHBEKASHAH, josh´-be-ka´-shah, seat of hardship (?). 1 Chr. 25:4.

JOSHUA, josh´-you-ah, Jehovah is salvation. Num. 14:6.
(Hoshea, Oshea, Jehoshua, Jeshua, and Jesus), son of Nun. 1 Chr. 7:27; Heb. 4:8.
discomfits Amalek. Ex. 17:9.
ministers to Moses. Ex. 24:13; 32:17; 33:11.
spies out Canaan. Num. 13:16.
ordained to succeed Moses. Num. 27:18; 34:17; Deut. 1:38; 3:28; 34:9.
reassured by God. Josh. 1.
harangues his officers. Josh. 1:10.
crosses river Jordan. Josh. 3.
erects memorial pillars. Josh. 4.
re-enacts circumcision. Josh. 5.

JOSHUA—*cont.*
assaults and destroys Jericho. Josh. 6.
condemns Achan. Josh. 7.
subdues Ai. Josh. 8.
his victories. Josh. 10—12.
apportions the land. Josh. 14—21; Heb. 4:8.
his charge to the Reubenites. Josh. 22.
exhortation to the people. Josh. 23.
reminds them of God's mercies. Josh. 24.
renews the covenant. Josh. 24:14.
his death. Josh. 24:29; Judg. 2:8.
his curse, Josh. 6:26; fulfilled, 1 Kin. 16:34.

JOSIAH, jo-si´ah, whom Jehovah heals. 2 Kin. 21:24.
prophecy concerning, 1 Kin. 13:2; fulfilled, 2 Kin. 23:15.
reigns well. 2 Kin. 22.
repairs the temple. 2 Kin. 22:3.
hears the words of the book of the law. 2 Kin. 22:8.
Huldah's message from God to him. 2 Kin. 22:15.
ordains the reading of the book. 2 Kin. 23.
keeps a signal passover to the Lord. 2 Chr. 35.
slain by Pharaoh-nechoh at Megiddo. 2 Kin. 23:29.

JOSIAS, jo-si´as, Greek form of Josiah. Matt. 1:10.

JOSIBIAH, jos´ib-i´ah, to whom God gives a dwelling. 1 Chr. 4:35.

JOSIPHIAH, jos´if-i´ah, whom Jehovah will increase. Ezra 8:10.

JOTBAH, jot´bah, pleasantness (?). 2 Kin. 21:19.

JOTBATH, jot´bath, same as JOTBAH. Deut. 10:7.

JOTBATHAH, jot-bah´thah, same as JOTBAH. Num. 33:33.

JOTHAM, jo´tham, Jehovah is upright. Judg. 9:5.
son of Gideon, his apologue. Judg. 9:7.
——king of Judah. 2 Kin. 15:32; 2 Chr. 27.

JOZABAD, jo´za-bad, same as JEHOZABAD. 1 Chr. 12:20.

JOZACHAR, jo´za-kar, whom Jehovah has remembered. 2 Kin. 12:21.

JOZADAK, jo´za-dak, same as JEHOZADAK. Ezra 3:2.

JUBAL, joo´bal, music (?).
inventor of harp and organ. Gen. 4:21.

JUCAL, joo´kal, same as JEHUCAL. Jer. 38:1.

JUDA, joo´dah, same as JUDAH. Luke 3:30.

JUDAH, joo´dah, praised.
son of Jacob. Gen. 29:35.
his descendants. Gen. 38; 46:12; Num. 1:26; 26:19; 1 Chr. 2—4.
pledges himself for Benjamin. Gen. 43:3.
his interview with Joseph. Gen. 44:18;—46:28.
blessed by Jacob. Gen. 49:8.
——tribe of, their blessing by Moses. Deut. 33:7.
their inheritance. Josh. 15.
they make David king, 2 Sam. 2:4; and adhere to his house. 1 Kin. 12; 2 Chr. 10; 11. *See* JEWS.

JUDAS, joo´das, Greek form of JUDAH. Matt. 10:4.
(JUDE, Lebbæus, Thaddæus), APOSTLE, brother of James. Matt. 10:3; Mark 3:18; Luke 6:16; Acts 1:13.
his question to our Lord. John 14:22.
enjoins perseverance. Jude 3:20.
denounces false disciples. Jude 4.
——the Lord's brother. Matt. 13:55; Mark 6:3.
——(Barsabas). Acts 15:22.

JUDAS ISCARIOT. Matt. 10:4; Mark 3:19; Luke 6:16; John 6:70.
betrays Jesus. Matt. 26:14, 47; Mark 14:10, 43; Luke 22:3, 47; John 13:26; 18:2.
hangs himself. Matt. 27:5 (Acts 1:18).

JUDE, jood, abbreviated from Judas. Jude 1.

JUDEA, joo-de´ah (land of Judah). Ezra 5:8.

JUDITH, joo´dith (probably from the same). Gen. 26:34.

JULIA, joo´li-ah, *feminine* form of JULIUS. Rom. 16:15.

JULIUS, joo´li-us, downy. Acts 27:1.

JUNIA, joo´ni-ah.
saluted by Paul. Rom. 16:7.

JUPITER, joo´pit-er.
Barnabas addressed as. Acts 14:12;—19:35.

JUSHAB-HESED, joo´shab-he´sed, whose love is returned. 1 Chr. 3:20.

JUSTUS, just´us, upright. Acts 1:23.

JUTTAH, joot´ah, extended. Josh. 15:55.

KABZEEL, kab´ze-el, God has gathered. Josh. 15:21.

KADESH, ka´desh, consecrated. Gen. 20:1.

KADESH-BARNEA, ka´desh-bar´ne-ah. Num. 34:4.
Israelites murmur against Moses and Aaron, threaten to stone Caleb and Joshua, and provoke God's anger. Num. 13; 14; Deut. 1:19; Josh. 14:6.

KADMIEL, kad´mi-el, eternity of God (?). Ezra 2:40.

KADMONITES, kad´mon-ites, Orientals. Gen. 15:19.

KALLAI, kal´ai, swift. Neh. 12:20.

KANAH, ka´nah, a place of reeds. Josh. 19:28.

KAREAH, ka-re´ah, bald. Jer. 40:8.

KARKAA, kar-ka´ah, floor. Josh. 15:3.

KARKOR, kar´kor, plain (?). Judg. 8:10.

KARNAIM, kar-na´im, two horns. Gen. 14:5.

KARTAH, kar´tah, city. Josh. 21:34.

KARTAN, kar´tan, double city. Josh. 21:32.

KATTATH, kat´ath, small (?). Josh. 19:15.

KEDAR, ke´dar, black-skinned.
son of Ishmael. Gen. 25:13; 1 Chr. 1:29; Ps. 120:5; Cant. 1:5; Jer. 2:to; Ezek. 27:21.
——tribe of, prophecies concerning. Is. 21:16; 42:11; 60:7; Jer. 49:28.

KEDEMAH, ke-de´mah, eastward. Gen. 25:15.

KEDEMOTH, ke-de´moth, eastern parts. Josh. 13:18.

KEDESH, ke´desh, sanctuary. Josh. 12:22.

KEDRON (Kidron, Cedron), ke´dron, brook and ravine, near garden of Gethsemane, frequented by our Lord. John 18:1.
crossed by David. 2 Sam. 15:23.
idols destroyed there. 1 Kin. 15:13; 2 Kin. 23:6; 2 Chr. 29:16; Jer. 31:40. *See* KIDRON.

KEHELATHAH, ke-he-lah´thah, assembly. Num. 33:22.

KEILAH, ke-ee-lah, sling (?). Josh. 15:44.
David there. 1 Sam. 23:1, 12.

KELAIAH, ke-lai´ah, contempt (?). Ezra 10:23.

KELITA, ke-li´tah, dwarf. Neh. 8:7.

KEMUEL, ke-moo´el, congregation of God. Gen. 22:21.

KENAN, ke´nan, smith (?). 1 Chr. 1:2.

KENATH, ke´nath, possession. Num. 32:42.

KENAZ, ke´naz, hunting. Gen. 36:11.

KENEZITE, ke´nez-ite, descendant of Kenaz. Num. 32:12.

KENITES, keen´ites, descendants of an unknown man named Kain. Gen. 15:19.
their fate foretold. Num. 24:22.

KENIZZITES, ke´niz-ites, same as KENEZITE. Gen. 15:19.

KEREN-HAPPUCH, ke´ren-hap´ook, horn of paint.
one of Job's daughters. Job 42:14.

KERIOTH, ke-ri´oth, cities.
city of Judah. Josh. 15:25; Jer. 48:24, 41; Amos 2:2.

KEROS, ke´ros, crook (?). Ezra 2:44.

KETURAH, ke-too´rah, incense.
Abraham's wife, Gen. 25; her children, 1 Chr. 1:32.

KEZIA, ke-zi´ah, cassia. Job 42:14.

KEZIZ, ke´ziz, cut off. Josh. 18:21.

KIBROTH-HATTAAVAH, kib´roth-hat-ta´a-vah, graves of lust. Num. 11:34.

KIBZAIM, kib-za´im, two heaps. Josh. 21:22.

KIDRON, kid´ron, turbid. 2 Sam. 15:23.

KINAH, ki´nah, song of mourning, lamentation. Josh. 15:22.

KIR, kir, town. 2 Kin. 16:9; Is. 15:1; 22:6; Amos 1:5; 9:7.

KIR-HARASETH, kir´ha-ras´eth, brick-town. 2 Kin. 3:25; Is. 16:7, 11.

KIR-HARESETH, kir´ha-res´eth, same as preceding. Is. 16:7.

KIR-HARESH, kir-har´esh, same as preceding. Is. 16:11.

KIR-HERES, kir-her´es, same as preceding. Jer. 48:31.

KIRIATHAIM, kir´yath-a´im, same as KIRJATHAIM. Ezek. 25:9.

KIRIOTH, ki-ri-´oth, cities. Amos 2:2.
KIRJATH, kir-´jath, city (?). Josh. 18:28.
KIRJATHAIM, kir-´jath-a-´im, double city. Num. 32:37.
KIRJATH-ARBA, kir-´jath-ar-´bah, city of Arba. Gen. 23:2.
KIRJATH-ARIM, kir-´jath-ar-´im, contracted from KIRJATH-JEARIM. Ezra 2:25.
KIRJATH-BAAL, kir-´jath-ba-´al, city of Baal. Josh. 15:60.
KIRJATH-HUZOTH, kir-´jath-hooz-´oth, *c.* of streets. Num. 22:39.
KIRJATH-JEARIM, kir-´jath-je-´ar-im, *c.* of woods. Josh. 9:17; 18:14; 1 Chr. 13:6.
 the ark brought to. 1 Sam. 7:1.
 ark fetched from. 1 Chr. 13:5; 2 Chr. 1:4.
KIRJATH-SANNAH, kir-jath-san-´ah, *c.* of thorns. Josh. 15:49.
KIRJATH-SEPHER, kir-jath-se-´fer, book-city. Josh. 15:15.
KISH, kish, bow.
 Saul's father. 1 Sam. 9:1.
KISHI, kish-´i, bow of Jehovah. 1 Chr. 6:44.
KISHION, kish-´i-on, hardness. Josh. 19:20.
KISHON, ki-´shon, tortuous.
 waters of Megiddo. Judg. 4:7; 5:21; 1 Kin. 18:40.
KISON, ki-´son, same as KISHON. Ps. 83:9.
KITHLISH, kith-´lish, fortified. Josh. 15:40.
KITRON, kit-´ron, burning. Judg. 1:30.
KITTIM, kit-´im, same as CHITTIM. Gen. 10:4.
KOA, ko-´ah, prince. Ezek. 23:23.
KOHATH, ko-´hath, assembly.
 son of Levi. Gen. 46:11.
 his descendants. Ex. 6:18; 1 Chr. 6:2.
 their duties. Num. 4:15; 10:21; 2 Chr. 29:12; 34:12.
KOHATHITES, ko-´hath-ites, descendants of Kohath. Num. 3:27.
KOLAIAH, kol-ai-´ah, voice of Jehovah (?). Neh. 11:7.
KORAH, ko-´rah, bald.
 Dathan, &c., their sedition and punishment. Num. 16; 26:9; 27:3.
 (Core), Jude 11.
KORAHITES, ko-´rah-ites, descendants of Korah. 1 Chr. 9:19.
KORATHITES, ko-´rath-ites, same as preceding. Num. 26:58.
KORE, ko-´re, partridge. 1 Chr. 9:19.
KORHITE, kor-´ite, same as KORATHITE. 2 Chr. 20:19.
KOZ, thorn. Ezra 2:61.
KUSHAIAH, kush-ai-´ah, longer form of KISHI. 1 Chr. 15:17.

LAADAH, la-´ad-ah, order (?). 1 Chr. 4:21.
LAADAN, la-´ad-an, put in order (?). 1 Chr. 7:26.
LABAN, la-´ban, white.
 hospitality of. Gen. 24:29.
 gives Jacob his two daughters. Gen. 29.
 envies and oppresses him. Gen. 30:27; 31:1.
 his dream. Gen. 31:24.
 his covenant with Jacob. Gen. 31:43.
LACHISH, la-´kish, impregnable. Josh. 10:3.
 conquered. Josh. 10:31; 12:11.
 Amaziah slain at. 2 Kin. 14:19.
LAEL, la-´el, (devoted) to God. Num. 3:24.
LAHAD, la-´had, oppression. 1 Chr. 4:2.
LAHAI-ROI, la-hai-ro-´i, to the living is sight. Gen. 24:62.
LAHMAM, lah-´mam. Josh. 15:40.
LAHMI, lah-´mi, warrior. 1 Chr. 20:5.
LAISH, la-´ish, lion. 1 Sam. 25:44.
 taken. Judg. 18:14.
LAKUM, la-´koom, fort (?). Josh. 19:33.
LAMA, lam-´ah, why ? Matt. 27:46.
LAMECH, la-´mek, destroyer.
 descendant of Cain. Gen. 4:18.
——father of Noah. Gen. 5:25, 29.
LAODICEA, la-´od-i-se-´ah. Col. 2:1.
LAODICEANS, la-´od-i-se-´ans, inhabitants of Laodicea. Rev. 1:11; 3:14.
LAODICEANS—*cont.*
 Paul's epistle to. Col. 4:16.
LAPIDOTH, la-´pid-oth, torches. Judg. 4:4.
LASEA, la-se-´ah. Acts 27:8.
LASHA, la-´shah, fissure. Gen. 10:19.
LASHARON, la-sha-´ron, of the plain. Josh. 12:18.
LATIN, lat-´in, the language spoken by Romans. John 19:20.
LAZARUS, laz-´ar-us, Greek form of ELEAZAR. Luke 16:20.
 and the rich man. Luke 16:19.
LAZARUS, brother of Mary and Martha, raised from the dead. John 11; 12:1.
LEAH, le-´ah, languid. Gen. 29:16, 31; 30:17; 31:4; 33:2; 49:31.
 See Ruth 4:11.
LEBANAH, le-bah-´nah, white. Ezra 2:45.
LEBANON, leb-´an-on, the white (mountain). Deut. 1:7.
 forest and mountain. Deut. 3:25; Judg. 3:3; 1 Kin. 5:14.
 its cedars. 2 Kin. 14:9; 2 Chr. 2:8; Ps. 92:12; Cant. 3:9; Is. 40:16; Hos. 14:5.
LEBAOTH, le-ba-´oth, lionesses. Josh. 15:32.
LEBBÆUS, leb-e-´us. Matt. 10:3. *See* JUDE.
LEBONAH, leb-o-´nah, frankincense. Judg. 21:19.
LECAH, le-´kah, journey (?). 1 Chr. 4:21.
LEHABIM, le-hah-´bim. Gen. 10:13.
LEHI, le-´hi, jaw-bone. Judg. 15:9.
LEMUEL, lem-´oo-el, (devoted) to God (?).
 king, his lesson. Prov. 31:1.
LESHEM, le-´shem, precious stone. Josh. 19:47.
LETUSHIM, le-toosh-´m, the hammered. Gen. 25:3.
LEUMMIM, le-oom-´im, peoples. Gen. 25:3.
LEVI, le-´vi, associate (?).
 son of Jacob. Gen. 29:34.
 avenges Dinah. Gen. 34:25; 49:5.
——*See* MATTHEW.
LEVIATHAN, le-vi-´a-than, a water monster. Ps. 104:26.
LEVITES, le-´vites, descendants of Levi, mentioned. Ex. 6:25; 32:26.
 their service. Ex. 38:21.
 appointed over the tabernacle. Num. 1:47.
 their divisions, Gershonites, Kohathites, Merarites. Num. 3.
 duties of. Num. 3:23; 4; 8:23; 18.
 their consecration. Num. 8:5.
 inheritance of. Num. 35; Deut. 18; Josh. 21.
 not to be forsaken. Deut. 12:19; 14:27.
 their genealogies. 1 Chr. 6; 9.
 charged with the temple service. 1 Chr. 23—27.
 twenty-four courses, instituted by David, 1 Chr. 23:6; re-divided by Ezra, Ezra 6:18.
 their sin censured. Mal. 1:2; Ezek. 22:26.
LEVITICUS, le-vit-´ic-us, the book which treats of the affairs of the Levitical law.
LIBERTINES, lib-´ert-ines, freedmen. Acts 6:9.
LIBNAH, lib-´nah, whiteness. Num. 33:20.
 subdued. Josh. 10:29; 21:13.
 rebels. 2 Kin. 8:22.
 attacked by Assyrians. 2 Kin. 19:8; Is. 37:8.
LIBNI, lib-´ni, white. Ex. 6:17.
LIBNITES, lib-´nites, descendants of Libni. Num. 3:21.
LIBYA, lib-´yah. Jer. 46:9; Ezek. 30:5; Dan. 11:43; Acts 2:10.
LIKHI, lik-´hi, fond of learning (?). 1 Chr. 7:19.
LINUS, li-´nus, flax. 2 Tim. 4:21.
LO-AMMI, lo-am-´i, not my people. Hos. 1:9.
LOD, lode, strife (?). 1 Chr. 8:12.
LO-DEBAR, lo-´de-bar, without pasture (?). 2 Sam. 9:4.
LOIS, lo-´is. 2 Tim. 1:5.
LO-RUHAMAH, lo-ru-hah-´mah, not having obtained mercy. Hos. 1:6.
LOT, veil. Gen. 11:27.
 (Abram's nephew), separates from Abram. Gen. 13:10.
 captured by four kings, and rescued by Abram. Gen. 14.

LOT—*cont.*
entertains angel visitors. Gen. 19:1.
saved from Sodom. Gen. 19:16; 2 Pet. 2:7.
his wife turned into a pillar of salt. Gen. 19:26; Luke 17:28, 32.

LOTAN, lo´-tan, veiling. Gen. 36:20.
LUBIMS, loob´-ims, same as LEHABIM. 2 Chr. 12:3.
LUCAS, loo´-kas, same as LUKE Phil. 24.
LUCIFER, loo´-sif-er, light-bearer. Is. 14:12.
LUCIUS, loosh´-yus, a noble (?).
of Cyrene, a teacher. Acts 13:1; Rom. 16:21.
LUD, lood, strife (?). Gen. 10:22.
LUDIM, lood´-im. Gen. 10:13.
LUHITH, loo-hith, abounding in boards. Is. 15:5.
LUKE, of or belonging to Lucania.
the beloved physician, companion of Paul. Col. 4:14; 2 Tim. 4:11; Phil. 24 (Acts 16:12; 20:5).
LUZ, looz, almond tree. Gen. 28:19.
LYCAONIA, li-ka-o´-ni-ah. Acts 14:6.
LYCLA, lish´-yah. Acts 27:5.
LYDDA, lid´-ah, Greek form of LOD (?).
miracle at. Acts 9:32.
LYDIA, lid´-yah.
of Thyatira, piety of. Acts 16:14, 40.
LYSANIAS, li-sa´-ni-as, ending sorrow. Luke 3:1.
LYSIAS, lis´-yas, a person of Lysia. Acts 23:26.
LYSTRA, lis´-trah. Acts 14:6.
miracle at. Acts 14:8.
Paul and Barnabas taken for gods at. Acts 14:11.
Paul stoned at, by Jews. Acts 14:19.

MAACAH, ma´-ak-ah (same as MAACHAH). 2 Sam. 3:3.
MAACHAH, ma´-ak-ah, royal (?). 1 Kin. 2:39.
——queen, her idolatry. 1 Kin. 15:13; 2 Chr. 15:16.
MAACHATHI, ma´-a-chah´-thi, an inhabitant of Maachah. Deut. 3:14.
MAACHATHITES, ma-ak´-ath-ites, plural of preceding. Josh. 12:5.
MAADAI, ma´-a-dai, adorned. Ezra 10:34.
MAADIAH, ma´-ad-i´-ah, ornament of Jehovah. Neh. 12:5.
MAAI, ma´-ai, compassionate (?). Neh. 12:36.
MAALEH-ACRABBIM, ma´-al-eh-ak´-rab-im, ascent of scorpions. Josh. 15:3.
MAARATH, ma´-ar-ath, a treeless place. Josh. 15:59.
MAASEIAH, ma´-as-i´-ah, work of Jehovah. Ezra 10:18.
MAASIAI, ma´-as-i-ai, same as AMASHAI (?). 1 Chr. 9:12.
MAATH, ma´-ath, small (?). Luke 3:26.
MAAZ, ma´-az, wrath. 1 Chr. 2:27.
MAAZIAH, ma´-az-i´-ah. 1 Chr. 24:18.
MACEDONIA, mas´-ed-o´-ni-ah.
Paul's mission there. Acts 16:9; 17.
liberality of. 2 Cor. 8; 9; 11:9; Phil. 4:15.
its churches. 1 & 2 Thess.
MACHBANI, mak-ban´-ai, cloak. 1 Chr. 12:13.
MACHBENAH, mak´-be-nah´, clad with a cloak (?). 1 Chr. 2:49.
MACHI, ma´-ki. Num. 13:15.
MACHIR, ma´-kir, sold. Gen. 50:23.
MACHIRITES, ma´-kir-ites, the descendants of Machir. Num. 26:29.
MACHNADEBAI, mak-nad´-eb-ai. Ezra 10:40.
MACHPELAH, mak-pe´-lah, a doubling. Gen. 23:9.
field of. Gen. 23.
patriarchs buried there. Gen. 23:19; 25:9; 35:29; 49:30; 50:12.
MADAI, ma´-dai. Gen. 10:2.
MADIAN, ma´-di-an, Greek form of MIDIAN. Acts 7:29.
MADMANNAH, mad-man´-ah, dunghill. Josh. 15:31.
MADMEN, mad´-men, dungheap. Jer. 48:2.
MADMENAH, mad-may´-nah, same as MADMEN. Is. 10:31.
MADON, ma´-don, place of contention. Josh. 11:1.
MAGBISH, mag´-bish, congregating. Ezra 2:30.
MAGDALA, mag´-dal-ah, tower. Matt. 15:39.
MAGDALENE, mag´-dal-e´-ne, inhabitant of Magdala. Matt. 27:56.
MAGDIEL, mag´-di-el, praise of God. Gen. 36:43.
MAGOG, ma´-gog. Gen. 10:2.
MAGOR-MISSABIB, ma´-gor-mis´-a-bib, fear round about. Jer. 20:3.
MAGPIASH, mag´-pi-ash. Neh. 10:20.
MAHALAH, mah´-hal-ah, disease. 1 Chr. 7:18.
MAHALALEEL, ma´-ha-lal´-e-el, praise of God. Gen. 5:12.
MAHALATH, mah´-al-ath, a musical instrument. Gen. 28:9.
MAHALATH LEANNOTH, m. le-an-oth´. Ps. 88, title.
MAHALI, ma´-ha-li, weak. Ex. 6:19.
MAHANAIM, ma´-han-a´-im, two camps. Gen. 32:2.
Jacob's vision at. Gen. 32.
Ish-bosheth made king at. 2 Sam. 2:8.
David takes refuge from Absalom at. 2 Sam. 17:24.
MAHANEH-DAN, ma´-han-e-dan´, camp of Dan. Judg. 18:12.
MAHARAI, ma´-ha-rai, impetuous. 2 Sam. 23:28.
MAHATH, ma´-hath, taking hold (?). 1 Chr. 6:35.
MAHAVITE, ma´-hav-ite. 1 Chr. 11:46.
MAHAZIOTH, ma-haz´-i-oth, visions. 1 Chr. 25:4.
MAHER-SHALAL-HASH-BAZ, ma´-her-sha´-lal-hash´-baz, the spoil hastens, the prey speeds. Is. 8:1.
MAHLAH, mah´-lah, same as MAHALAH. Num. 26:33.
MAHLI, mah´-li, same as MAHALI. 1 Chr. 6:19.
MAHLITES, mah´-lites, the descendants of Mahli. Num. 3:33.
MAHLON, mah´-lon, a sick person.
and Chilion die in Moab. Ruth 1:2.
MAHOL, ma´-hol, a dance. 1 Kin. 4:31.
MAKAZ, ma´-kaz, end (?). 1 Kin. 4:9.
MAKHELOTH, mak´-hel-oth, assemblies. Num. 33:25.
MAKKEDAH, mak´-ed-ah, place of shepherds (?). Josh. 10:10.
cave of, five kings hide in. Josh. 10:16.
MAKTESH, mak´-tesh, a mortar. Zeph. 1:11.
MALACHI, mal´-ak-i, the messenger of Jehovah.
deplores and reproves Israel's ingratitude. Mal. 1; 2.
foretells the Messiah and His messenger. Mal. 3; 4.
MALCHAM, mal´-kam, their king. 1 Chr. 8:9.
MALCHIAH, malk-i´-ah, Jehovah's king. 1 Chr. 6:40.
MALCHIEL, malk´-i-el, God's king. Gen. 46:17.
MALCHIELITES, malk´-i-el-ites, the descendants of Malchiel. Num. 26:45.
MALCHIJAH, malk-i´-jah, same as MALCHIAH. 1 Chr. 9:12.
MALCHIRAM, malk-i´-ram, king of height (?). 1 Chr. 3:18.
MALCHI-SHUA, malk´-i-shoo´-ah, king of aid. 1 Chr. 8:33.
MALCHUS, mal´-kus, Greek form of MALLUCH. John 18:10.
wounded by Peter. John 18:10; Matt. 26:51; Mark 14:47.
healed by Jesus. Luke 22:51.
MALELEEL, ma´-le-le-el´, same as MAHALELEEL. Luke 3:37.
MALLOTHI, mal-o´-thi. 1 Chr. 25:4.
MALLUCH, mal´-ook, counsellor. 1 Chr. 6:44.
MAMMON, mam´-on, fulness.
worship of. Matt. 6:24; Luke 16:9.
MAMRE, mam´-re, fatness.
Abram dwells there. Gen. 13:18; 14; 18; 23:17; 35:27.
MANAEN, ma-na´-en, Greek form of MENAHEM. Acts 13:1.
MANAHATH, ma-na´-hath, rest. Gen. 36:23.
MANAHETHITES, ma-na´-heth-ites, inhabitants of Manahath (?). 1 Chr. 2:52.
MANASSEH, ma-nas´-ay, one who causes to forget.
firstborn son of Joseph. Gen. 41:51.
his blessing. Gen. 48.
his descendants numbered, &c. Num. 1:34; 26:29; Josh. 22:1; 1 Chr. 5:23; 7:14.
their inheritance. Num. 32:33; 34:14; Josh. 13:29; 17.
incline to David's cause. 1 Chr. 9:3; 12:19; 2 Chr. 15:9; 30:11.

MANASSEH—*cont.*
——king of Judah, his reign. 2 Kin. 21; 2 Chr. 33.
MANASSES, ma-nas´es, Greek form of MANASSEH. Matt. 1:10.
MANASSITES, ma-nas´ites, members of the tribe of Manasseh. Deut. 4:43.
MANEH, ma´ne, a weight. Ezek. 45:12.
MANOAH, ma-no´ah, rest.
(father of Samson). Judg. 13; 16:31.
MAOCH, ma´ok, oppressed (?). 1 Sam. 27:2.
MAON, ma´on, habitation. Josh. 15:55.
MAONITES, ma´on-ites. Judg. 10:12.
MARA, ma´rah, sad. Ruth 1:20.
MARAH, ma´rah, bitter.
bitter waters healed there. Ex. 15:23.
MARALAH, mar´al-ah, trembling. Josh. 19:11.
MARANATHA, ma´ran-ah´thah, our lord cometh. 1 Cor. 16:22.
MARCUS, mar´kus. Col. 4:10.
MARESHAH, ma-resh´ah, capital. Josh. 15:44.
MARK, English form of MARCUS.
EVANGELIST. Acts 12:12.
goes with Paul and Barnabas. Acts 12:25; 13:5.
leaves them at Perga. Acts 13:13.
contention about him. Acts 15:37.
approved by Paul. 2 Tim. 4:11.
MAROTH, mar´oth, bitterness. Mic. 1:12.
MARS' HILL, English of Areopagus. Acts 17:22.
MARSENA, mar´se-nah. Esth. 1:14.
MARTHA, mar´thah, lady.
instructed by Christ. John 11:5, 21.
reproved by Him. Luke 10:38.
MARY, Greek form of MIRIAM. Matt. 1:16.
the VIRGIN, mother of Jesus, visited by the angel Gabriel. Luke 1:26.
believes, and magnifies the Lord. Luke 1:38, 46; John 2:5.
Christ born of. Matt. 1:18; Luke 2.
witnesses the miracle at Cana. John 2:1.
desires to speak with Christ. Matt. 12:46; Mark 3:31; Luke 8:19.
commended to John by Christ at His crucifixion. Matt. 27:56; John 19:25.
MARY MAGDALENE, Luke 8:2.
at the cross. Matt. 27:56; Mark 15:40; John 19:25.
Christ appears first to. Matt. 28:1; Mark 16:1; Luke 24:10; John 20:1.
——sister of Lazarus, commended. Luke 10:42.
Christ's love for. John 11:5, 33.
anoints Christ's feet, John 12:3; (head), Matt. 26:6; Mark 14:3.
MARYS, THE THREE, at the cross. John 19:25.
MASCHIL, mas´kil, understanding. Ps. 53, title.
MASH. Gen. 10:23.
MASHAL, ma´shal, entreaty (?). 1 Chr. 6:74.
MASREKAH, mas-rek´ah, vineyard. Gen. 36:36.
MASSA, mas´ah, burden. Gen. 25:14.
MASSAH, mas´ah, temptation.
the rebellion at. Ex. 17:7; Deut. 9:22; 33:8.
MATHUSALA, ma-thoo´sa-lah, Greek form of METHUSELAH. Luke 3:37.
MATRED, ma´tred, pushing forward. Gen. 36:39.
MATRI, ma´tri, rainy. 1 Sam. 10:21.
MATTAN, mat´an, a gift.
slain. 2 Kin. 11:18; 2 Chr. 23:17.
MATTANAH, mat´an-ah, same as preceding. Num. 21:18.
MATTANIAH, mat´an-i´ah, gift of Jehovah. 2 Kin. 24:17.
MATTATHA, mat´ath-ah, a Greek form of above. Luke 3:31.
MATTATHAH, mat´ath-ah, gift of Jehovah. Ezra 10:33.
MATTATHIAS, mat´ath-i´as, a Greek form of the preceding. Luke 3:26.
MATTENAI, mat´en-ai, liberal. Ezra 10:33.
MATTHAN, mat´than, gift. Matt. 1:15.
MATTHAT, mat´that, another form of MATTHAN. Luke 3:24.
MATTHEW, English way of spelling Mattathiah.
(Levi), APOSTLE and EVANGELIST, called. Matt. 9:9; Mark 2:14; Luke 5:27.
sent out. Matt. 10:3; Mark 3:18; Luke 6:15;—Acts 1:13.
MATTHIAS, math-i´as, another Greek form of MATTATHIAS, apostle. Acts 1:23; 26.
MATTITHIAH, mat-ith-i´ah, another form of MATTATHIAS. 1 Chr. 9:31.
MAZZAROTH, maz´ar-oth, the signs of the zodiac. Job 38:32.
MEAH, me´ah, a hundred. Neh. 3:1.
MEARAH, me-ar´ah, cave. Josh. 13:4.
MEBUNNAI, me-boon´ai, built (?). 2 Sam. 23:27.
MECHERATHITE, me-ker´ath-ite, inhabitant of Mecherah (?). 1 Chr. 11:36.
MEDAD, me´dad.
prophesies. Num. 11:26.
MEDAN, me´dan, contention. Gen. 25:2.
MEDEBA, me´deb-ah, flowing water (?). Num. 21:30.
MEDES, inhabitants of Media. 2 Kin. 17:6.
capture Babylon (Is. 21:2). Dan. 5:28, 31.
MEDIA, me´di-ah, Greek form of MADAI. Esth. 1:3.
Israel taken captive to. 2 Kin. 17:6; 18:11; Esth. 2:6.
Daniel's prophecy of. Dan. 8:20.
MEGIDDO, me-gid´o, place of troops. Josh. 12:21; 17:11; Judg. 1:27; 5:19.
Ahaziah and Josiah slain there. 2 Kin. 9:27; 23:29; Zech. 12:11.
MEGIDDON, me-gid´on, same as preceding. Zech. 12:11.
MEHETABEEL, me-het´ab-e´el, lengthened form of the following. Neh. 6:10.
MEHETABEL, me-het´ab-el, God makes happy. Gen. 36:39.
MEHIDA, me-hi´dah. Ezra 2:52.
MEHIR, me´hir, price. 1 Chr. 4:11.
MEHOLATHITE, me-ho´lath-ite, native of Meholah. 1 Sam. 18:19.
MEHUJAEL, me-hoo´ja-el, struck by God. Gen. 4:18.
MEHUMAN, me-hoo´man. Esth. 1:10.
MEHUNIM, me-hoon´im. Ezra 2:50.
MEHUNIMS, me-hoon´ims, the people of Maon (?). 2 Chr. 26:7.
ME-JARKON, me´jar´kon, waters of yellowness. Josh. 19:46.
MEKONAH, me-ko´nah, a base. Neh. 11:28.
MELATIAH, mel´at-i´ah, whom Jehovah freed. Neh. 3:7.
MELCHI, melk´i, Greek form of MELCHIAH. Luke 3:24.
MELCHIAH, melk-i´ah, Jehovah's king. Jer. 21:1.
MELCHISEDEC, melk-is´ed-ek, Greek form of MELCHIZEDEK. Heb. 5:6.
MELCHI-SHUA, melk´i-shoo´ah, same as MALCHISHUA. 1 Sam. 14:49.
MELCHIZEDEK, melk-iz´ed-ek, king of righteousness.
king of Salem, blesses Abram. Gen. 14:18.
his priesthood and Aaron's. Ps. 110:4; Heb. 5:6, 10; 6:20; 7:1.
MELEA, mel´e-ah, fulness (?). Luke 3:31.
MELECH, mel´ech, king. 1 Chr. 8:35.
MELICU, me-lee´koo, same as MALLUCH. Neh. 12:14.
MELITA, mel´it-ah.
Paul shipwrecked near, and lands at, Acts 28:1; received kindly by the people, Acts 28:2; shakes off the viper at, Acts 28:5; heals Publius' father and others at, Acts 28.
MELZAR, mel´zar, steward.
favours Daniel. Dan. 1:11.
MEMPHIS, mem´fis, in Egypt. Hos. 9:6.
MEMUCAN, me-moo´kan. Esth. 1:14.
MENAHEM, me-na´hem, comforter.
king of Israel, his evil rule. 2 Kin. 15:14, 18.

MENAN, me´nan. Luke 3:31.
MENE, me´ne, numbered.
MENE, TEKEL, UPHARSIN. Dan. 5:25—28.
MEONENIM, me-o´nen-im. Judg. 9:37.
MEONOTHAI, me-o´no-thai´, my habitations. 1 Chr. 4:14.
MEPHAATH, me-fa´ath, beauty. Josh. 13:18.
MEPHIBOSHETH, mef-ib´osh-eth, destroying shame.
son of Jonathan, his lameness. 2 Sam. 4:4.
cherished by David. 2 Sam. 9:1.
slandered by Ziba. 2 Sam. 16:1; 19:24.
spared by David. 2 Sam. 21:7.
MERAB, me´rab, increase.
Saul's daughter. 1 Sam. 14:49; 18:17.
her five sons hanged by the Gibeonites. 2 Sam. 21:8.
MERAIAH, me-rai´ah, contumacy. Neh. 12:12.
MERAIOTH, me-rai´oth, rebellions. 1 Chr. 6:6.
MERARI, me-rah´ri, bitter. Gen. 46:11.
MERARITES, descendants of Levi. Ex. 6:19; 1 Chr. 6:1; 23:21; 24:26.
their duties and dwellings. Num. 4:29; 7:8; 10:17; Josh. 21:7; 1 Chr. 6:63.
MERATHAIM, mer-ath-a´im, rebellions. Jer. 50:21.
MERCURIUS, mer-ku´ri-us.
Paul so called. Acts 14:12.
MERED, me´red, rebellion. 1 Chr. 4:17.
MEREMOTH, mer-e´moth, elevations. Ezra 8:33.
MERES, me´res, worthy (?). Esth. 1:14.
MERIBAH, me-ree´bah, water of strife.
Israel rebels there. Ex. 17:7; Num. 20:13; 27:14; Deut. 32:51; 33:8; Ps. 81:7.
MERIB-BAAL, me´rib-ba´al, contender (?) against Baal. 1 Chr. 8:34.
MERODACH, me´ro-dak. Jer. 50:2.
MERODACH-BALADAN, me´ro-dak-bal´a-dan, Merodach gives a son.
(or Berodach) BALADAN, sends messengers to Hezekiah. 2 Kin. 20:12; 2 Chr. 32:31; Is. 39;—Jer. 50:2.
MEROM, me´rom, a high place.
waters of. Josh. 11:5.
MERONOTHITE, me-ro´noth-ite, an inhabitant of Meronoth. 1 Chr. 27:30.
MEROZ, me´roz, refuge (?).
cursed. Judg. 5:23.
MESECH, me´sech, same as MESHECH. Ps. 120:5.
MESHA, me´shah, deliverance. 2 Kin. 3:4.
MESHACH, me´shak. Dan. 1:7. *See* SHADRACH.
MESHECH, me´shek, tall (?).
son of Japheth. Gen. 10:2.
traders of. Ezek. 27:13; 32:26; 38:2; 39:1.
MESHELEMIAH, me-shel´em-i´ah, Jehovah repays. 1 Chr. 9:21.
MESHEZABEEL, me-she´zab-eel, God delivers. Neh. 3:4.
MESHILLEMITH, me-shil´em-ith, recompense. 1 Chr. 9:12.
MESHILLEMOTH, me-shil´em-oth, retribution. 2 Chr. 28:12.
MESHOBAB, me-sho-bab, brought back. 1 Chr. 4:34.
MESHULLAM, me-shool´am, friend. 2 Kin. 22:3.
MESHULLEMETH, me-shool-e´meth, feminine of preceding. 2 Kin. 21:19.
MESOBAITE, me-so´ba-ite, inhabitant of Mesoba (?). 1 Chr. 11:47.
MESOPOTAMIA, mes´o-pot-a´mi-ah, amidst the rivers. (Ur), country of the two rivers.
Abram leaves. Gen. 11:31; 12:1; 24:4, 10. *See* Acts 2:9; 7:2.
king of, slain by Othniel. Judg. 3:8.
MESSIAH, mes-i´ah, anointed (anointed CHRIST).
Prince, prophecy about. Dan. 9:25.
MESSIAS, mes-i´as, Greek form of the above. John 1:41; 4:25. *See* Is. 9:6.
METHEG-AMMAH, me´theg-am´ah, bridle of Ammah. 2 Sam. 8:1.
METHUSAEL, me-thoo´sa-el, man of God. Gen. 4:18.
METHUSELAH, me-thoo´se-lah, man of the dart (?). Gen. 5:21.
his great age. Gen. 5:27.
MEUNIM, me-oon´im, same as MEHUNIM. Neh. 7:52.
MEZAHAB, me´za-hab, water of gold. Gen. 36:39.
MIAMIN, mi´ya-min, on the right hand. Ezra. 10:25.
MIBHAR, mib´har, choicest. 1 Chr. 11:38.
MIBSAM, mib´sam, sweet odour. Gen. 25:13.
MIBZAR, mib´zar, a fortress. Gen. 36:42.
MICAH, mi´kah, who (is) like unto Jehovah? Judg. 17:1.
makes and worships idols. Judg. 17; 18.
——prophet (Jer. 26:18); denounces Israel's sin. Mic. 1—3; 6; 7.
predicts the Messiah. Mic. 4; 5; 7.
MICAIAH, mi-kai´ah, fuller form of MICAH.
forewarns Ahab. 1 Kin. 22; 2 Chr. 18.
MICHAEL, mi´ka-el, who (is) like unto God? Dan. 10:13, 21; 12:1.
Archangel. Jude 9; Rev. 12:7.
MICHAH, mi´kah, same as MICAH. 1 Chr. 24:24.
MICHAIAH, mi-kai´ah, same as MICAIAH. Neh. 12:35.
MICHAL, mi´kal, brook. 1 Sam. 14:49.
David's wife. 1 Sam. 18:20.
given to another. 1 Sam. 25:44.
restored to David. 2 Sam. 3:13.
mocks his religious dancing, and is rebuked. 2 Sam. 6:16, 20; 1 Chr. 15:29.
MICHMAS, mik´mas, later form of MICHMASH. Ezra 2:27.
MICHMASH, mik´mash, treasured. 1 Sam. 13:2.
MICHMETHAH, mik´meth-ah, hiding place (?). Josh. 16:6.
MICHRI, mik´ri, precious (?). 1 Chr. 9:8.
MICHTAM, mik´tam, writing (?). Ps. 16, title.
MIDDIN, mid´in, extensions. Josh. 15:61.
MIDIAN, mid´yan, strife. Gen. 25:2.
sons of. Gen. 25:4.
——land of. Ex. 2:15. *See* 1 Kin. 11:18; Is. 60 6; Hab. 3:7.
MIDIANITES, mid´yan-ites, people of Midian. Gen. 37:28.
their cities destroyed by Moses. Num. 31:1.
subdued by Gideon. Judg. 6—8. *See* Ps. 83:9; Is. 9:4; 10:26.
MIGDAL-EL, mig´dal-el, tower of God. Josh. 19:38.
MIGDAL-GAD, mig´dal-gad, tower of Gad. Josh. 15:37.
MIGDOL, mig´dol. Ex. 14:2.
MIGRON, mig´ron, a precipice. Is. 10:28.
MIJAMIN, mi´ja-min, same as MIAMIN. 1 Chr. 24:9.
MIKLOTH, mik´loth, staves, lots. 1 Chr. 8:32.
MIKNEIAH, mik-ni´ah, possession of Jehovah. 1 Chr. 15:18.
MILALAI, mil´al-ai, eloquent (?). Neh. 12:36.
MILCAH, mil´kah, counsel (?). Gen. 11:29; 22:20.
MILCOM, mil´kom, same as MOLOCH.
false god. 1 Kin. 11:5, 33; 2 Kin. 23:13.
MILETUM, mi-le´tum, improper form of MILETUS. 2 Tim. 4:20.
MILETUS, mi-le´tus.
Paul takes leave of elders at. Acts 20:15.
Trophimus left at. 2 Tim. 4:20.
MILLO, mil´o, a mound.
house of. Judg. 9:6; 1 Sam. 5:9.
MINIAMIN, min´ya-min, full form of MIAMIN. 2 Chr. 31:15.
MINNI, min´i, Armenia. Jer. 51:27.
MINNITH, min´ith, allotment. Judg. 11:33.
MIPHKAD, mif´kad, place of meeting. Neh. 3:31.
MIRIAM, mir´yam, rebellion (?).
sister of Moses and Aaron. Ex. 15:20; Num. 26:59.
song of. Ex. 15:20, 21.
murmurs against Moses. Num. 12:1, 2.
is smitten with leprosy, and shut out of the camp. Num. 12:10, 15.
her death. Num. 20:1.
MIRMA, mir´mah, fraud. 1 Chr. 8:10.
MISGAB, mis´gab, height. Jer. 48:1.
MISHAEL, mish´a-el, who is what God is ? Ex. 6:22.
MISHAL, mi´shal, prayer. Josh. 21:30.

MISHEAL, mi´-she-al, same as MISHAL. Josh. 19:26.
MISHAM, mi´sham, cleansing. 1 Chr. 8:12.
MISHMA, mish´-mah, report. Gen. 25:14.
MISHMANNAH, mish-man´-ah, fatness. 1 Chr. 12:10.
MISHRAITES, mish´-ra-ites. 1 Chr. 2:53.
MISPERETH, mis-per´-eth, number. Neh. 7:7.
MISREPHOTH-MAIM, mis´-re-foth-ma´-im, burning of waters. Josh. 11:8.
MITHCAH, mith´-kah, place of sweetness. Num. 33:28.
MITHNITE, mith´-nite. 1 Chr. 11:43.
MITHREDATH, mith´-re-dath, given by Mithra. Ezra 1:8.
MITYLENE, mit´-il-e´-ne. Acts 20:14.
MIZAR, mi´-zar, smallness. Ps. 42:6.
MIZPAH, miz´-pah (Gilead), a look out.
Jacob and Laban meet at. Gen. 31:49.
Jephthah at. Judg. 10:17; 11:11; 20:1.
Samuel at. 1 Sam. 7:5.
——(Moab). 1 Sam. 22:3.
MIZPAR, miz´-par, number. Ezra 2:2.
MIZPEH, miz´-peh, watch-tower. Josh. 11:3.
MIZRAIM, miz-ra´-im, fortresses. Gen. 10:6.
MIZZAH, miz´-ah. Gen. 36:13.
MNASON, na´-son, an old disciple. Acts 21:16.
MOAB, mo´-ab, progeny of a father. Gen. 19:37.
his descendants, and territory. Deut. 2:9, 18; 34:5.
MOABITES, mo´-ab-ites, people of Moab. Deut. 2:9.
excluded from the congregation. Deut. 23:3.
conquered by Ehud. Judg. 3:12; by David. 2 Sam. 8:2; by Jehoshaphat and Jehoram. 2 Kin. 1:1; 3.
their overthrow. 2 Chr. 20:23.
prophecies concerning. Ex. 15:15; Num. 21:29; 24:17; Ps. 60:8; 83:6; Is. 11:14; 15; 16; 25:10; Jer. 9:26; 25:21; 48; Ezek. 25:8; Amos 2:1; Zeph. 2:8.
MOABITESS, mo´-ab-ite-ess, a lady of Moab. Ruth 4:5.
MOADIAH, mo´-ad-i´-ah, festival of Jehovah. Neh. 12:17.
MOLADAH, mo-la´-dah, birth. Josh. 15:26.
MOLECH, mo´-lek, English form for Moloch. Lev. 18:21; 20:2.
worship of. 1 Kin. 11:7; 2 Kin. 23:10; Jer. 32:35; Amos 5:26; Acts 7:43.
MOLOCH, mo´-lok, king. Amos 5:26.
MOLID, mo´-lid, begetter. 1 Chr. 2:29.
MORASTHITE, mo´-rasth-ite, native of Moresheth. Jer. 26:18.
MORDECAI, mor´-dek-ai, worshipper of Merodach (?). Esth. 2:5.
reveals conspiracy against king Ahasuerus. Esth. 2:21.
is hated by Haman. Esth. 3:5.
honoured by the king. Esth. 6.
advanced. Esth. 8—10 (Ezra 2:2; Neh. 7:7).
MOREH, mo´-reh, archer. Gen. 12:6.
MORESHETH-GATH, mo-resh´-eth-gath´, the possession of Gath. Mic. 1:14.
MORIAH, mor-i´-ah, provided by Jehovah. Gen. 22:2.
mount. Gen. 22.
David's sacrifice there. 2 Sam. 24:18; 1 Chr. 21:18; 22:1.
temple built on. 2 Chr. 3:1.
MOSERA, mo-se´-rah, bond. Deut. 10:6.
MOSEROTH, mo-se´-roth, bonds. Num. 33:30.
MOSES, mo´-zes, saved from the water.
born, and hidden. Ex. 2 (Acts 7:20; Heb. 11:23).
escapes to Midian. Ex. 2:15.
revelation from God. Ex. 3; confirmed by signs. Ex. 4.
returns to Egypt. Ex. 4:20.
intercedes with Pharaoh for Israel. Ex. 5—12.
leads Israel forth. Ex. 14.
meets God in mount Sinai. Ex. 19:3 (24:18).
brings the law to the people. Ex. 19:25; 20—23; 34:10; 35:1; Lev. 1; Num. 5; 6; 15; 27—30; 36; Deut. 12—26.
instructed to build the tabernacle. Ex. 25—31; 35:40; Num. 4; 8—10; 18; 19.

MOSES—*cont.*
his grief at Israel's idolatry. Ex. 32:19.
his intercession. Ex. 32:11 (33:12).
again meets God in the mount. Ex. 34:2.
skin of his face shines. Ex. 34:29 (2 Cor. 3:7, 13).
sets apart Aaron. Lev. 8; 9.
numbers the people. Num. 1; 26.
sends out the spies to Canaan. Num. 13.
intercedes for the murmuring people. Num. 14:13.
Korah's sedition against. Num. 16.
for his unbelief suffered not to enter Canaan. Num. 20:12; 27:12; Deut. 1:35; 3:23.
his government of Israel in the wilderness. Num. 20; 21.
makes the brazen serpent. Num. 21:9 (John 3:14).
recounts Israel's history, and exhorts to obedience. Deut. 1; 3—12; 27—31.
his charge to Joshua. Deut. 3:28; 31:7, 23.
his death. Deut. 34:5; his body, Jude 9.
seen at Christ's transfiguration. Matt. 17:3; Mark 9:4; Luke 9:30.
his meekness, Num. 12:3; dignity, Deut. 34:10; faithfulness, Num. 12:7; Heb. 3:2.
MOZA, mo´-zah, fountain. 1 Chr. 2:46.
MOZAH, mo´-zah, same as MOZA. Josh. 18:26.
MUPPIM, moop´-im, probably written for Shupham. Gen. 46:21.
MUSHI, moo´-shi, withdrawn. Ex. 6:19.
MUTH-LABBEN, mooth´-la-ben´, death to the son (?). Ps. 9, title.
MYRA, mi´-rah, balsam. Acts 27:5.
MYSIA, mish´-yah. Acts 16:7.

NAAM, na´-am, pleasantness. 1 Chr. 4:15.
NAAMAH, na´-am-ah, pleasant. Gen. 4:22.
NAAMAN, na´-am-an, pleasantness. 2 Kin. 5:1.
the Syrian, his anger. 2 Kin. 5:11.
his leprosy healed. 2 Kin. 5:14.
his request. 2 Kin. 5:17. *See* Luke 4:27.
NAAMATHITE, na-am´-ath-ite. Job. 2:11.
NAAMITES, na´-am-ites, descendants of Naaman. Num. 26:40.
NAARAH, na´-ar-ah, a girl. 1 Chr. 4:5.
NAARAI, na´-ar-ai, youthful. 1 Chr. 11:37.
NAARAN, na´-ar-an, same as NAARAH. 1 Chr. 7:28.
NAARATH, na´-ar-ath, to Naarah. Josh. 16:7.
NAASHON, na´-ash-on, enchanter. Ex. 6:23.
NAASSON, na-as´-on, Greek form of NAASHON. Matt. 1:4.
NABAL, na´-bal, foolish. 1 Sam. 25:3.
conduct to David. 1 Sam. 25:10.
Abigail, intercedes for. 1 Sam. 25:18.
his death. 1 Sam. 25:38.
NABOTH, na´-both, fruits (?).
slain by Jezebel. 1 Kin. 21.
his murder avenged. 2 Kin. 9:21.
NACHON, na´-kon, prepared. 2 Sam. 6:6.
NACHOR, na´-kor, snorting. Josh. 24:2.
NADAB, na´-dab, liberal. Ex. 6:23.
son of Aaron, offers strange fire. Lev. 10:1, 2.
——king of Israel, slain by Baasha. 1 Kin. 14:20; 15:25, 28.
NAGGE, nag´-e, Greek form of NOGAH. Luke 3:25.
NAHALAL, na´-hal-al, a pasture. Josh. 21:35.
NAHALIEL, na-hal´-i-el, valley of God. Num. 21:19.
NAHALLAL, na´-hal-al, same as NAHALAL. Josh. 19:15.
NAHALOL, na´-hal-ol, same as preceding. Judg. 1:30.
NAHAM, na´-ham, consolation. 1 Chr. 4:19.
NAHAMANI, na´-ham-a´-ni, comforter. Neh. 7:7.
NAHARAI, na´-ha-rai, one who snores. 1 Chr. 11:39.
NAHARI, na´-har-i, same as preceding. 2 Sam. 23:37.
NAHASH, na´-hash, serpent.
the Ammonite, invades Jabesh-Gilead. 1 Sam. 11.
NAHATH, na´-hath, descent. Gen. 36:13.

NAHBI, nah´-bi, hidden. Num. 13:14.
NAHOR, na´-hor, another way of spelling Nachor. Gen. 11:22.
Abram's brother. Gen. 11:26; 22:20; 24:10.
NAHSHON, nah´-shon, same as NAASHON. Num. 1:7.
NAHUM, na´-hoom, comforter.
vision of. Nah. 1:1-3.
NAIN, na´-in, pasture.
miracle at. Luke 7:11.
NAIOTH, nai´-oth, habitations. 1 Sam. 19:18.
school of prophets. 1 Sam. 19:23; 20:1.
NAOMI, na´-om-i, pleasant. Ruth 1:2.
NAPHISH, na´-fish, cheerful. Gen. 25:15.
NAPHTALI, naf´-tal-i, my wrestling.
son of Jacob. Gen. 30:8; 35:25; 46:24; 49:21; Deut. 33:23.
——tribe of, numbered. Num. 1:42; 10:27; 13:14; 26:48; Judg. 1:33.
subdue the Canaanites. Judg. 4:10; 5:18; 6:35; 7:23.
carried captive. 2 Kin. 15:29. *See* Is. 9:1; Matt. 4:13.
NAPHTUHIM, naf´-too-him. Gen. 10:13.
NARCISSUS, nar-sis´-us, benumbing.
household of. Rom. 16:11.
NATHAN, na´-than, gift.
the prophet. 2 Sam. 7.
shews David his sin. 2 Sam. 12:1.
anoints Solomon king. 1 Kin. 1:34; 1 Chr. 29:29; 2 Chr. 9:29.
——son of David. 2 Sam. 5:14; Zech. 12:12; Luke 3:31.
NATHANAEL, na-than´-a-el, gift of God.
'Israelite indeed.' John 1:45; 21:2.
NATHAN-MELECH, na´-than-me´-lek, gift of the king. 2 Kin. 23:11.
NAUM, na´-oom, same as NAHUM. Luke 3:25.
NAZARENE, naz´-ar-een´, a native of Nazareth. Acts 24:5.
NAZARETH, naz´-ar-eth, branch. Luke 1:26.
Jesus of. Matt. 2:23; 21:11; Luke 1:26; 2:39, 51; 4:16; John 1:45; 18:5; Acts 2:22; 3:6.
NAZARITE, naz´-ar-ite, one separated. Num. 6:2.
NAZARITES, law of the. Num. 6.
NEAH, ne´-ah, of a slope. Josh. 19:13.
NEAPOLIS, ne-a´-po-lis, new city. Acts 16:11.
NEARIAH, ne´-ar-i´-ah, servant of Jehovah. 1 Chr. 3:22.
NEBAI, ne´-bai, fruitful. Neh. 10:19.
NEBAIOTH, ne-bai´-oth, high places. 1 Chr. 1:29.
NEBAJOTH, ne-ba´-joth, same as NEBAIOTH. Gen. 25:13.
NEBALLAT, ne-bal´-at. Neh. 11:34.
NEBAT, ne´-bat, aspect. 1 Kin. 11:26.
NEBO, ne´-bo, a lofty place. Deut. 32:49.
NEBUCHADNEZZAR, neb´-u-kad-nez´-ar, another way of spelling the following. 2 Kin. 24:1.
king of Babylon. Jer. 20; 21; 25; 27; 28; 32; 34; Ezek. 26:7; 29:19.
captures Jerusalem. 2 Kin. 24; 25; 2 Chr. 36; Jer. 37—39; 52; Dan. 1:1.
his dreams. Dan. 2; 4.
sets up the golden image. Dan. 3.
his madness. Dan. 4:33.
his restoration and confession. Dan. 4:34.
NEBUCHADREZZAR, neb´-u-kad-rez´-ar, Nebo protect the land-mark. Jer. 21:2.
NEBUSHASBAN, neb´-u-shas´-ban, Nebo will save me. Jer. 39:13.
NEBUZAR-ADAN, neb´-u-zar´-a-dan´, Nebo gives posterity. 2 Kin. 25:8.
his care of Jeremiah. Jer. 39:11; 40:1.
NECHO, ne´-ko, conqueror (?). Jer. 46:2.
NECHOH, same as NECHO. 2 Kin. 23:29.
NEDABIAH, ned´-ab-i´-ah, Jehovah is bountiful (?). 1 Chr. 3:18.
NEGINAH, neg-een´-ah, a stringed instrument. Ps. 61, title.
NEGINOTH, neg-een´-oth, stringed instruments. Ps. 4; 54; 55; 76; 77, title.
NEGO, ne´-go, same as NEBO. Dan. 1:7.
NEHELAMITE, ne-he-lam´-ite. Jer. 29:24.
NEHEMIAH, ne´-hem-i´-ah, Jehovah comforts.
his grief for Jerusalem. Neh. 1.
his prayer for. Neh. 1:5.
his visit to. Neh. 2:5, 9, 17.
his conduct at. Neh. 4—6; 8—10; 13.
NEHILOTH, ne-hil´-oth, flutes. Ps. 5, title.
NEHUM, ne´-hoom, consolation. Neh. 7:7.
NEHUSHTA, ne-hoosh´-tah, bronze. 2 Kin. 24:8.
NEHUSHTAN, ne-hoosh´-tan, brazen.
the brazen serpent of Moses, idolatrously used by Israelites, so called by Hezekiah, and destroyed by him. 2 Kin. 18:4.
NEIEL, ni´-el, moved by God. Josh. 19:27.
NEKEB, ne´-keb, cavern. Josh. 19:33.
NEKODA, ne-ko´-dah, a herdman. Ezra 2:48.
NEMUEL, ne-moo´-el, same as JEMUEL (?). Num 26:9.
NEMUELITES, ne-moo´-el-ites, descendants of Nemuel. Num. 26:12.
NEPHEG, ne´-feg, sprout. Ex. 6:21.
NEPHISH, ne´-fish, same as NAPHISH. 1 Chr. 5:19.
NEPHISHESIM, ne-fish´-es-im, expansions. Neh. 7:52.
NEPHTHALIM, nef´-tal-im, Greek form of NAPHTALI. Matt. 4:13.
NEPHTOAH, nef-to´-ah, opened. Josh. 15:9.
NEPHUSIM, nefoos´-im, a better form for Nephishesim. Ezra 2:50.
NER, light. 1 Sam. 14:50.
NEREUS, ne´-roos, liquid (?). Rom. 16:15.
NERGAL, ner´-gal, lion. 2 Kin. 17:30.
NERGAL-SHAREZER, ner´-gal-shar-e´-zer, Nergal protect the king. Jer. 39:3.
NERI, ne´-ri, Greek form of NERIAH. Luke 3:27.
NERIAH, ner-i´-ah, lamp of Jehovah. Jer. 32:12.
NETHANEEL, neth-an´-e-el, same as NATHANAEL. Num. 1:8.
NETHANIAH, neth´-an-i´-ah, whom Jehovah gave. 2 Kin. 25:23.
NETHINIMS, neth´-in-ims, the appointed. 1 Chr. 9:2; Ezra 2:43; 7:7, 24; 8:17; Neh. 10:28.
NETOPHAH, ne-to´-phah, dropping. Ezra 2:22.
NETOPHATHI, net-of´-ath-i, an inhabitant of Netophah. Neh. 12:28.
NETOPHATHITE, net-of´-ath-ite, same as the preceding. 2 Sam. 23:28.
NEZIAH, ne-zi´-ah, illustrious. Ezra 2:54.
NEZIB, ne´-zib, garrison. Josh. 15:43.
NIBHAZ, nib´-haz. 2 Kin. 17:31.
NIBSHAN, nib´-shan, level (?). Josh. 15:62.
NICANOR, ni-ka´-nor, one of the seven deacons. Acts 6:5.
NICODEMUS, nik´-o-de´-mus, Pharisee and ruler.
goes to Jesus by night. John 3:1.
takes His part. John 7:50.
assists at Christ's burial. John 19:39.
NICOLAITANES, nik´-o-la´-it-ans, named after Nicolas. Rev. 2:6.
NICOLAS, nik´-o-las. Acts 6:5.
NICOPOLIS, nik-o´-pol-is, city of victory. Tit. 3:12.
NIGER, ni´-ger, black. Acts 13:1.
NIMRAH, nim´-rah, limpid (water). Num. 32:3.
NIMRIM, nim´-rim, clear waters. Is. 15:6.
NIMROD, nim´-rod, an inhabitant of Marad (?). Gen. 10:8.
mighty hunter. Gen. 10:9.
NIMSHI, nim´-shi, discloser (?). 1 Kin. 19:16.
NINEVEH, nin´-ev-ay, dwelling (?). Gen. 10:11.
Jonah's mission to. Jonah 1:1; 3:2.
denounced by Jonah. Jonah 3:4.
repenting, is spared by God. Jonah 3:5-10 (Matt. 12:41; Luke 11:32).
the burden of. Nah. 1:1; 2; 3.
NINEVITES, nin´-ev-ites, inhabitants of Nineveh. Luke 11:30.
NISAN, ni´-san, month. Neh. 2:1; Esth. 3:7.
NISROCH, nis´-rok, eagle (?). 2 Kin. 19:37; Is. 37:38.
NO, abode (?). Nah. 3:8.
multitude of, threatened. Jer. 46:25; Ezek. 30:14.
NO AMON, no a´-mon, abode of Amon. Jer. 46:25.

NOADIAH, no-ad-i-ah, whom Jehovah meets. Neh. 6:14.
NOAH, no-ah, (1) rest. Gen. 5:29. (2) wandering. Num. 26:33.
son of Lamech. Gen. 5:29.
finds grace with God. Gen. 6:8.
ordered to build the ark. Gen. 6:14.
with his family and living creatures enters into the ark. Gen. 7.
flood assuaging, goes forth. Gen. 8:18.
God blesses and makes a covenant with. Gen. 9:1, 8.
is drunken, and mocked of Ham. Gen. 9:22.
his death. Gen. 9:29.
NOB, nobe, high place.
city of, David comes to, and eats hallowed bread at. 1 Sam. 21:1.
smitten by Saul. 1 Sam. 22:19.
NOBAH, no-bah, a barking. Num. 32:42.
NOD, node, flight, wandering. Gen. 4:16.
NODAB, no-dab, nobility. 1 Chr. 5:19.
NOE, no-e, Greek form of NOAH. Matt. 24:37.
NOGAH, no-gah, brightness. 1 Chr. 3:7.
NOHAH, no-hah, rest. 1 Chr. 8:2.
NON, none, same as NUN. 1 Chr. 7:27.
NOPH, nofe, same as MEMPHIS.
city, warned. Is. 19:13; Jer. 2:16; 46:14; Ezek. 30:13.
NOPHAH, no-fah, windy. Num. 21:30.
NUN, noon, fish. Ex. 33:11.
NYMPHAS, nim-fas, shortened form of NYMPHODORUS. Col. 4:15.

OBADIAH, ob-ad-i-ah, worshipper of Jehovah. Obad. 1.
prophet, his prediction. Obad. 17.
——Levite, porter in the temple. Neh. 12:25.
——sent by Ahab to find water. 1 Kin. 18:3.
meets Elijah. 1 Kin. 18:7.
how he hid a hundred prophets, 1 Kin. 18:4, 13.
OBAL, o-bal, hill (?). Gen. 10:28.
OBED, o-bed, worshipping (God.). Ruth 4:17.
OBED-EDOM, o-bed-e-dom, serving Edom.
prospered while taking charge of the ark. 2 Sam. 6:10; 1 Chr. 13:14; 15:18, 24; 16:5.
his sons. 1 Chr. 26:4, 5.
OBIL, o-bil, camel keeper. 1 Chr. 27:30.
OBOTH, o-both, bottles (of skin). Num. 21:10.
OCRAN, ok-ran, troublesome. Num. 1:13.
ODED, o-ded, setting up (?).
prophet. 2 Chr. 15:1; 28:9.
OG, circle (?).
king of Bashan. Num. 21:33; Deut. 3:1; Ps. 135:11; 136:20.
OHAD, o-had, might. Gen. 46:10.
OHEL, o-hel, tent. 1 Chr. 3:20.
OLIVET, ol-iv-et, place of olives.
(Olives) mount. 2 Sam. 15:30; Matt. 21:1; 24:3; Mark 11:1; 13:3; Luke 21:37; John 8:1; Acts 1:12.
OLYMPAS, o-limp-as, bright (?). Rom. 16:15.
OMAR, o-mar, talkative. Gen. 36:11.
OMEGA, o-meg-ah, great O. Rev. 1:8, 11; 21:6; 22:13.
OMRI, om-ri, like a sheaf (?).
king of Israel. 1 Kin. 16:16, &c.; Mic. 6:16.
ON, the sun. Gen. 41:45.
ONAM, o-nam, wealthy. Gen. 36:23.
ONAN, o-nan, strong. Gen. 38:4.
ONESIMUS, o-ne-sim-us, profitable. Col. 4:9; Philem. 10.
ONESIPHORUS, o-nes-if-or-us, bringing profit. 2 Tim. 1:16.
ONO, o-no, strong. 1 Chr. 8:12.
OPHEL, o-fel, a hill. 2 Chr. 27:3.
OPHIR, o-feer.
gold of. Gen. 10:29; 1 Kin. 9:28; 10:11; 22:48; 1 Chr. 29:4; 2 Chr. 8:18; Job 22:24; Ps. 45:9; Is. 13:12.
OPHNI, of-hi, man of the hill. Josh. 18:24.
OPHRAH, of-rah, fawn. 1 Chr. 4:14.
OREB, o-reb, raven. Judg. 7:25.
OREN, o-ren, pine tree. 1 Chr. 2:25.
ORION, o-ri-on. Job 9:9.
ORNAN, or-nan (Araunah). 2 Sam. 24:16; 1 Chr. 21:15.
ORPAH, orp-ah, hind (?). Ruth. 1:4.
OSEE, o-zee, same as HOSEA. Rom. 9:25.
OSHEA, o-she-ah, same as JOSHUA. Num. 13:8.
OTHNI, oth-ni, powerful (?). 1 Chr. 26:7.
OTHNIEL, oth-ni-el, powerful man of God. Josh. 15:17; Judg. 1:13; 3:9.
OZEM, o-zem, strength. 1 Chr. 2:15.
OZIAS, o-zi-as, Greek form of UZZIAH. Matt. 1:8.
OZNI, oz-ni, hearing. Num. 26:16.
OZNITES, oz-nites, descendants of Ozni. Num. 26:16.

PAARAI, pah-a-rai, devoted to Peor (?). 2 Sam. 23:35.
PADAN-ARAM, pa-dan-a-ram, the plain of Syria. Gen. 25:20; 28:2.
PADON, pa-don, redemption. Ezra 2:44.
PAGIEL, pag-i-el, intervention of God. Num. 1:13.
PAHATH-MOAB, pa-hath-mo-ab, governor of Moab. Ezra 2:6.
PAI, pa-i, bleating. 1 Chr. 1:50.
PALAL, pa-lal, judge. Neh. 3:25.
PALESTINA, pal-es-ti-nah, land of strangers (?).
predictions about. Ex. 15:14; Is. 14:29, 31.
PALLU, pal-oo, distinguished. Ex. 6:14.
PALLUITES, pal-oo-ites, descendants of Pallu. Num. 26:5.
PALTI, pal-ti, deliverance of Jehovah. Num. 13:9.
PALTIEL, pal-ti-el, deliverance of God. Num. 34:26.
PALTITE, palt-ite, a descendant of Palti. 2 Sam. 23:26.
PAMPHYLIA, pam-fil-yah.
Paul preaches there. Acts 13:13; 14:24; 27:5.
PAPHOS, pa-fos.
Paul at. Acts 13:6.
Elymas the sorcerer at. Acts 13:8.
PARAH, pa-rah, heifer. Josh. 18:23.
PARAN, pa-ran, cavernous.
mount. Gen. 21:21; Num. 10:12; 12:16; 13:26; Deut. 33:2; Hab. 3:3.
PARBAR, par-bar, open apartment. 1 Chr. 26:18.
PARMASHTA, par-mash-tah, superior (?). Esth. 9:9.
PARMENAS, par-men-as, standing firm. Acts 6:5.
PARNACH, par-nak. Num. 34:25.
PAROSH, pa-rosh, flea. Ezra 2:3.
PARSHANDATHA, par-shan-da-thah, given to Persia (?). Esth. 9:7.
PARTHIANS, parth-yans. Acts 2:9.
PARUAH, par-oo-ah, flourishing. 1 Kin. 4:17.
PARVAIM, parv-a-im, oriental regions (?). 2 Chr. 3:6.
PASACH, pa-sak, divider. 1 Chr. 7:33.
PAS-DAMMIM, pas-dam-im, shortened from EPHESDAMMIM. 1 Chr. 11:13.
PASEAH, pa-se-ah, lame. 1 Chr. 4:12.
PASHUR, pash-oor, prosperity round about.
his cruelty to Jeremiah. Jer. 20.
PATARA, pat-ar-ah. Acts 21:1.
PATHROS, path-ros.
in Egypt. Is. 11:11; Jer. 44:1, 15; Ezek. 29:14; 30:14.
PATHRUSIM, path-roos-im, people of Pathros. Gen. 10:14.
PATMOS, pat-mos.
place of St. John's exile. Rev. 1:9.
PATROBAS, pat-ro-bas. Rom. 16:14.
PAU, pa-oo, older form of PAI. Gen. 36:39.
PAUL, or PAULUS, little. Acts 13:9.
as a persecutor. Acts 7:58; 8:1; 9:1; 22:4; 26:9; 1 Cor. 15:9; Gal. 1:13; Phil. 3:6; 1 Tim. 1:13.
as a convert to the Gospel. Acts 9:3; 22:6; 26:12.
as a preacher. Acts 9:19, 29; 13:1, 4, 14; 17:18 (2 Cor. 11:32; Gal. 1:17).
stoned at Lystra. Acts 14:8, 19.
contends with Barnabas. Acts 15:36.
is persecuted at Philippi. Acts 16.
the Holy Ghost given by his hands to John's disciples at Ephesus. Acts 19:6.

PAUL—*cont.*
restores Eutychus. Acts 20:10.
his charge to the elders of Ephesus, at Miletus. Acts 20:17.
his return to Jerusalem, and persecution there. Acts 21.
his defence before the people and the council. Acts 22; 23.
before Felix, Acts 24; Festus, Acts 25; and Agrippa, Acts 26.
appeals to Cæsar at Rome. Acts 25.
his voyage and shipwreck. Acts 27.
miracles by, at Melita. Acts 28:3, 8.
at Rome, reasons with the Jews. Acts 28:17.
his love to the churches. Rom. 1:8; 15; 1 Cor. 1:4; 4:14; 2 Cor. 1; 2; 6; 7; Phil. 1; Col. 1; 1 & 2 Thess.
his sufferings. 1 Cor. 4:9; 2 Cor. 11:23; 12:7; Phil. 1:12; 2 Tim. 3:11.
divine revelations to. 2 Cor. 12:1.
defends his apostleship. 1 Cor. 9; 2 Cor. 11; 12; 2 Tim. 3:10.
commends Timothy, &c. 1 Cor. 16:10; Phil. 2:19; 1 Thess. 3:2.
commends Titus. 2 Cor. 7:13; 8:23.
blames Peter. Gal. 2:14.
pleads for Onesimus. Philem. his epistles mentioned by St. Peter. 2 Pet. 3:15.
PEDAHEL, pe-dah´-el, God redeemed. Num. 34:28.
PEDAHZUR, pe-dah´-zoor, the Rock redeemed. Num. 1:10.
PEDAIAH, pe-dah-i´-ah, whom Jehovah redeemed. 1 Chr. 27:20.
PEKAH, pe´-kah, open-eyed.
king of Israel. 2 Kin. 15:25.
his victory over Judah. 2 Chr. 28:6.
denounced in prophecy. Is. 7:1.
PEKAHIAH, pe´-kah-i´-ah, whose eyes Jehovah opened.
king of Israel. 2 Kin. 15:22.
PEKOD, pe´-kod, visitation. Jer. 50:21.
PELAIAH, pe-la´-yah, whom Jehovah made distinguished. 1 Chr. 3:24.
PELALIAH, pe-lal-i´-ah, whom Jehovah judged. Neh. 11:12.
PELATIAH, pe-lat-i´-ah, whom Jehovah delivered. Ezek. 11:1.
PELEG, pe´-leg, division. Gen. 10:25.
PELET, pe´-let, liberation. 1 Chr. 2:47.
PELETH, pe´-leth, swiftness. Num. 16:1.
PELETHITES, pel´-eth-ites, runners. 2 Sam. 8:18.
PELONITE, pel´-on-ite. 1 Chr. 11:27.
PENIEL, pe-nee´-el, the face of God.
scene of Jacob's wrestling with an angel. Gen. 32:30.
Gideon's vengeance upon. Judg. 8:17.
PENINNAH, pe-nin´-ah, coral. 1 Sam. 1:2. *See* HANNAH.
PENTECOST, pen´-te-kost, fiftieth.
(feast of weeks), how observed. Lev. 23:15; Deut. 16:9.
Holy Spirit given at. Acts 2.
PENUEL, pe-noo´-el, old form of PENIEL. Gen. 32:31.
PEOR, pe´-or, point.
(Baal), Num. 23:28; 25:3, 18; Josh. 22:17.
PERAZIM, pe-raz´-im, breaches. Is. 28:21.
PERES, pe´-res, divided. Dan. 5:28.
PERESH, pe´-resh, distinction. 1 Chr. 7:16.
PEREZ, pe´-rez, breach. 1 Chr. 27:3.
PEREZ-UZZA, pe´-rez-uz´-ah, same as following. 1 Chr. 13:11.
PEREZ-UZZAH, pe´-rez-uz´-ah, breach of Uzzah. 2 Sam. 6:8.
PERGA, per´-gah.
visited by Paul. Acts 13:13; 14:25.
PERGAMOS, per´-ga-mos, citadel (?).
epistle to. Rev. 1:11; 2:12.
PERIDA, pe-ree´-dah, a recluse. Neh. 7:57.
PERIZZITES, per´-iz-ites, belonging to a village. Gen. 13:7; 15:20; 34:30; Judg. 1:4; 2 Chr. 8:7.
PERSIA, per´-shah.

PERSIA—*cont.*
kingdom of. 2 Chr. 36:20; Esth. 1:3; Ezek. 27:10; 38:5; Dan. 6.
prophecies concerning. Is. 21:2; Dan. 5:28; 8:20; 10:13; 11:2.
PERSIAN, per´-shan, belonging to Persia. Dan. 6:28.
PERSIS, per´-sis, a Persian woman.
the beloved. Rom. 16:12.
PERUDA, pe-roo´-dah, same as PERIDA. Ezra 2:55.
PETER, pe´-ter, a stone. Matt. 16:18.
APOSTLE, called. Matt. 4:18; Mark 1:16; Luke 5; John 1:35.
sent forth. Matt. 10:2; Mark 3:16; Luke 6:14.
tries to walk to Jesus on the sea. Matt. 14:29.
confesses Jesus to be the Christ. Matt. 16:16; Mark 8:29; Luke 9:20.
witnesses the transfiguration. Matt. 17; Mark 9; Luke 9:28; 2 Pet. 1:16.
his self-confidence reproved. Luke 22:31; John 13:36.
thrice denies Christ. Matt. 26:69; Mark 14:66; Luke 22:57; John 18:17.
his repentance. Matt. 26:75; Mark 14:72; Luke 22:62.
the assembled disciples addressed by. Acts 1:15.
the Jews preached to by. Acts 2:14; 3:12.
brought before the council. Acts 4.
condemns Ananias and Sapphira. Acts 5.
denounces Simon the sorcerer. Acts 8:18.
restores Æneas and Tabitha. Acts 9:32, 40.
sent for by Cornelius. Acts 10.
instructed by a vision not to despise the Gentiles. Acts 10:9.
imprisoned, and liberated by an angel. Acts 12.
his decision about circumcision. Acts 15:7.
rebuked by Paul. Gal. 2:14.
bears witness to Paul's teaching. 2 Pet. 3:15.
comforts the church, and exhorts to holy living by his epistles. 1 & 2 Pet.
his martyrdom foretold by Christ. John 21:18; 2 Pet. 1:14.
PETHAHIAH, pe´-thah-i´-ah, whom Jehovah looses. 1 Chr. 24:16.
PETHOR, pe´-thor. Num. 22:5.
PETHUEL, pe-thoo´-el, God's opening (?). Joel. 1:1.
PEULTHAI, pe-ool´-thai, deed of Jehovah. 1 Chr. 26:5.
PHALEC, fa´-lek, Greek form of PELEG. Luke 3:35.
PHALLU, fal´-oo, an English way of spelling Pallu. Gen. 46:9.
PHALTI, fal´-ti, deliveranceof Jehovah. 1 Sam. 25:44.
PHALTIEL, fal´-ti-el, deliverance of God. 2 Sam. 3:15.
PHANUEL, fan-oo´-el, Greek form of PENUEL. Luke 2:36.
PHARAOH, fa´-roh, the sun (title of rulers of Egypt). Gen. 12:14; Ezek. 29:3.
Abram's wife taken into house of. Gen. 12:15.
Pharaoh plagued because of her. Gen. 12:17.
——(patron of Joseph), his dreams, &c. Gen. 40.
his hospitality to Joseph's father and brethren. Gen. 47.
——(oppressor of the Israelites). Ex. 1:8.
daughter preserves Moses. Ex. 2:5, 10; Acts 7:21.
miracles performed before, and plagues sent. Ex. 7—10.
grants Moses' request. Ex. 12:31.
repenting, pursues Israel, and perishes in the Red sea. Ex. 14 (Neh. 9:10; Ps. 135:9; 136:15; Rom. 9:17).
——(father-in-law of Solomon). 1 Kin. 3:1.
shelters Hadad, Solomon's adversary. 1 Kin. 11:19.
PHARAOH-HOPHRA, fa´-roh-hof´-rah, Pharaoh the priest of the sun.
his fate predicted. Jer. 44:30. *See* Ezek. 30—32.
compared to a dragon. Ezek. 29:3.
PHARAOH-NECHO, fa´-roh-ne´-ko, Pharaoh the lame. slays Josiah. 2 Kin. 23:29; 2 Chr. 35:20.
his wars with Israel. 2 Kin. 23:33; 2 Chr. 36:3.
PHARES, fa´-res, Greek form of PHAREZ. Luke 3:33.

PHAREZ, fa´-rez, breach. Gen. 38:29; Ruth 4:18.
PHARISEES, far´-is-ees, the separated.
celebrated ones: Nicodemus, John 3:1; Simon, Luke 7; Gamaliel, Acts 5:34; Saul of Tarsus, Acts 23:6; 26:5; Phil. 3:5.
Christ entertained by. Luke 7:36; 11:37; 14:1.
Christ utters woes against. Matt. 23:13; Luke 11:42.
Christ questioned by, about divorce, Matt. 19:3; eating, Matt. 9:11; 15:1; Mark 2:16; Luke 5:30; forgiveness of sin, Luke 5:21; sabbath, Matt. 12:2, 10; fasting, Mark 2:18; tribute, Matt. 22:17.
deride Christ. Luke 16:14.
murmur against Christ. Matt. 9:34; Luke 15:2.
denounced by Christ. Matt. 5:20; 16:6; 21:43; 23:2; Luke 11:39.
people cautioned against. Mark 8:15; Luke 12:1.
seek a sign from Christ. Matt. 12:38; 16:1.
take counsel against Christ. Matt. 12:14; Mark 3:6.
Nicodemus remonstrates with. John 7:51.
cast out the man cured of blindness. John 9:13.
dissensions about. John 9:16.
send officers to take Christ. John 7:32.
contend about circumcision. Acts 15:5.
their belief in the resurrection, &c. Acts 23:8.
and publican. Luke 18.
PHAROSH, fa´-rosh, same as PAROSH. Ezra 8:3.
PHARPAR, far´-par, swift. 2 Kin. 5:12.
PHARZITES, farz´-ites, descendants of Pharez. Num. 26:20.
PHASEAH, fa-se´-ah, same as PASEAH. Neh. 7:51.
PHEBE, fe´-be, moon. Rom. 16:1.
PHENICE, fe-ni´-see, palm tree. Acts 11:19; 15:3; 27:12.
PHENICIA, fe-nish´-yah, land of palms. Acts 21:2.
PHICHOL, fi´-kol, attentive (?). Gen. 21:22.
PHILADELPHIA, fil´-a-delf´-yah, brotherly love.
church of, commended. Rev. 1:11; 3:7.
PHILEMON, fil-e´-mon, affectionate.
Paul's letter to, concerning Onesimus. Philem.
PHILETUS, fil-e´-tus, beloved. 2 Tim. 2:17.
PHILIP, fil´-ip, lover of horses.
APOSTLE, called. John 1:43.
sent forth. Matt. 10:3; Mark 3:18; Luke 6:14; John 12:22; Acts 1:13.
remonstrated with by Christ. John 14:8.
——deacon, elected. Acts 6:5.
preaches in Samaria. Acts 8:5.
baptizes the eunuch. Acts 8:27.
his four virgin daughters prophesy. Acts 21:8.
——(brother of Herod). Matt. 14:3; Mark 6:17; Luke 3:1, 19.
PHILIPPI, fil-ip´-i, a town so called after Philip of Macedon.
Paul persecuted at. Acts 16:12.
church at, commended and exhorted. Phil. 1—4.
PHILIPPIANS, fil-ip´-yans, the people of Philippi. Phil. 4:15.
PHILISTIA, fil-ist´-yah, the land of the Philistines. Gen. 21:34; Ex. 13:17; Josh. 13:2; 2 Kin. 8:2; Ps. 60:8.
PHILISTIM, fil´-ist-im, wanderers. Gen. 10:14.
PHILISTINES, fil´-ist-ines, same as PHILISTIM. Gen. 21:34.
origin of. Gen. 10:14; 1 Chr. 1:12.
fill up Isaac's wells. Gen. 26:15.
contend with Joshua. Josh. 13; Shamgar, Judg. 3:31; Samson, Judg. 14—16; Samuel, 1 Sam. 4; 7; Jonathan, 1 Sam. 14; Saul, 1 Sam. 17; David, 1 Sam. 18.
their wars with Israel. 1 Sam. 4:1; 28; 29; 31; 2 Chr. 21:16.
mentioned. Ps. 60:8; 83:7; 87:4; 108:9; Is. 2:6; 9:12; 11:14; Jer. 25:20.
their destruction predicted. Jer. 47; Ezek. 25:15; Amos 1:8; Obad. 19; Zeph. 2:5; Zech. 9:6.
PHILOLOGUS, fil-o´-log-us, talkative.
Julia, and all saints with them. Rom. 16:15.
PHINEHAS, fin´-e-as, serpent's mouth. Ex. 6:25.

PHINEHAS—*cont.*
slays Zimri and Cozbi. Num. 25:7, 11; Ps. 106:30.
sent against the Midianites, Reubenites, and Benjamites. Num. 31:6; Josh. 22:13; Judg. 20:28.
——son of Eli, his sin and death. 1 Sam. 1:3; 2:22; 4:11.
PHLEGON, fleg´-on, zealous, burning. Rom. 16:14.
PHRYGIA, frij´-yah. Acts 2:10; 16:6; 18:23.
PHURAH, foor´-ah, branch (?). Judg. 7:10.
PHUT, foot. Gen. 10:6.
PHUVAH, foo´-vah, mouth. Gen. 46:13.
PHYGELLUS, fi-gel´-us, little fugitive.
and Hermogenes turned away from Paul. 2 Tim. 1:15.
PI-BESETH, pi-be´-seth, the city of Bast. Ezek. 30:17.
PI-HAHIROTH, pi´-ha-hi´-roth, where sedge grows. Ex. 14:2.
PILATE, pi´-lat, armed with a javelin (?). Matt. 27:2.
Pontius, governor of Judæa during our Lord's ministry, sufferings, and death. Luke 3:1.
Christ delivered to, admonished by his wife, examines Jesus, washes his hands, but delivers Him to be crucified. Matt. 27; Mark 15; Luke 23; John 18; 19.
grants request of Joseph of Arimathæa. Matt. 27:57; Mark 15:42; Luke 23:50; John 19:38. *See* Acts 3:13; 4:27; 13:28; 1 Tim. 6:13.
PILDASH, pil´-dash, steel (?). Gen. 22:22.
PILEHA, pi´-le-hah, ploughman (?). Neh. 10:24.
PILTAI, pil´-tai, whom Jehovah delivers. Neh. 12:17.
PINON, pi´-non, darkness. Gen. 36:41.
PIRAM, pi´-ram, like a wild ass. Josh. 10:3.
PIRATHON, pir-ah´-thon, leader. Judg. 12:15.
PIRATHONITE, pir-ah´-thon-ite, an inhabitant of Pirathon. Judg. 12:13.
PISGAH, piz´-gah, a part, boundary.
mount. Num. 21:20; 23:14; Deut. 3:27; 34:1.
PISIDIA, pi-sid´-yah. Acts 13:14; 14:24.
PISON, pi´-son, flowing stream (?), a river in Eden. Gen. 2:11.
PISPAH, pis´-pah, expansion. 1 Chr. 7:38.
PITHOM, pi´-thom.
(and Raamses), cities built by Israelites in Egypt. Ex. 1:11.
PITHON, pi´-thon, simple (?). 1 Chr. 8:35.
PLEIADES, pli´-ad-ees, (coming at) the sailing season (?). Job 9:9; 38:31; Amos 5:8.
POCHERETH OF ZEBAIM, po-ke´-reth of Ze-ba´-im, offspring of gazelles (?). Ezra 2:57.
POLLUX, pol´-ux. Acts 28:11.
PONTIUS, pon´-shus, belonging to the sea. Matt. 27:2. *See* PILATE.
PONTUS, pont´-us, sea. Acts 2:9.
PORATHA, po-rah´-thah, having many chariots (?). Esth. 9:8.
PORCIUS FESTUS, por´-shus fest´-us. Acts 24:27.
POTIPHAR, pot´-i-far, belonging to the sun. Gen. 37:36.
Joseph's master. Gen. 39.
POTI-PHERAH, pot´-i-fer´-ah, same as POTIPHAR. Gen. 41:45.
PRISCA, pris´-kah, ancient. 2 Tim. 4:19.
PRISCILLA, pris-il´-ah, diminutive of PRISCA. Acts 18:2.
(and AQUILA). Acts 18; Rom. 16:3; 1 Cor. 16:19.
PROCHORUS, prok´-or-us, he that presides over the choir. Acts 6:5.
PTOLEMAIS, tol´-em-a´-is, city of Ptolemy.
Paul at. Acts 21:7.
PUA, poo´-ah, same as PHUVAH. Num. 26:23.
PUAH, poo´-ah, splendour. Ex. 1:15.
PUBLIUS, pub´-li-us.
entertains Paul. Acts 28:7.
PUDENS, pu´-dens, shamefaced. 2 Tim. 4:21.
PUHITES, poo´-hites. 1 Chr. 2:53.
PUL, pool, (1) a short name for Tiglath-Pileser (?). 2 Kin. 15:19. (2) son (?). Is. 66:19.
king of Assyria. 1 Chr 5:26.
PUNITES, poon´-ites, descendants of Pua. Num. 26:23.
PUNON, poon´-on, same as PINON. Num. 33:42.

PUR, poor, a lot. Esth. 3:7.
PURIM, poor´-im, lots. Esth. 9:26.
feast of. Esth. 9:20.
PUT, poot, same as PHUT. 1 Chr. 1:8.
PUTEOLI, poo-te-´o-li, wells.
(Pozzuoli), seaport of Italy. Acts 28:13.
PUTIEL, poot´-i-el. Ex. 6:25.

QUARTUS, kwart´-us, the fourth. Rom. 16:23.

RAAMAH, ra´-am-ah, trembling. Gen. 10:7.
RAAMIAH, ra´-am-i´-ah, trembling of Jehovah. Neh. 7:7.
RAAMSES, ra-am´-ses, son of the sun. Ex. 1:11.
RABBAH, rab´-ah, capital city. Josh. 13:25.
city. 2 Sam. 11; 12:26; Jer. 49:2; Ezek. 21:20; 25:5; Amos 1:14.
RABBATH, rab´-ath, same as RABBAH. Deut. 3:11.
RABBI, rab´-i, master. Matt. 23:7, 8; John 1:38; 3:2.
RABBITH, rab´-ith, populous. Josh. 19:20.
RABBONI, rab-o´-ni, my master.
title addressed to Christ by Mary. John 20:16.
RAB-MAG, rab´-mag, most exalted. Jer. 39:3.
RAB-SARIS, rab´-sar-is, chief eunuch. 2 Kin. 18:17.
RAB-SHAKEH, rab´-sha-kay, chief of the cupbearers. 2 Kin. 18:17.
reviles Hezekiah. 2 Kin. 18:19; 19:1; Is. 36:4.
RACHAB, ra´-kab, Greek form of RAHAB. Matt. 1:5.
RACHAL, ra´-kal, traffic. 1 Sam. 30:29.
RACHEL, ra´-chel, ewe. Gen. 29:6.
(Rahel) and Jacob. Gen. 29:10, 28; 30; 31:4, 19, 34; 35:16.
RADDAI, rad´-ai, subduing. 1 Chr. 2:14.
RAGAU, ra´-gaw, Greek form of REU. Luke 3:35.
RAGUEL, ra-goo´-el, friend of God. Num. 10:29.
RAHAB, ra´-hab, (1) broad. Josh. 2:1. (2) violence. Ps. 87:4.
the harlot. Josh. 2; 6:22. *See* Matt. 1:5; Heb. 11:31; James 2:25.
——(EGYPT). Ps. 87:4; 89:10; Is. 51:9.
RAHAM, ra´-ham. 1 Chr. 2:44.
RAHEL, ra´-hel, same as RACHEL. Jer. 31:15.
RAKEM, ra´-kem, variegated. 1 Chr. 7:16.
RAKKATH, rak´-ath, shore. Josh. 19:35.
RAKKON, rak´-on, same as RAKKATH. Josh. 19:46.
RAM, high. Ruth 4:19.
RAMA, ra´-mah, Greek form of RAMAH. Matt. 2:18.
RAMAH, ra´-mah, high place. Josh. 18:25; Judg. 4:5; 1 Sam. 1:19; 7:17; 8:4; 19:18; 25:1; Jer. 31:15.
RAMATH, ra´-math, same as preceding. Josh. 19:8.
RAMATHAIM, ra´-math-a´-im, double high place. 1 Sam. 1:1.
RAMATHITE, ra´-math-ite, a native of Ramah. 1 Chr. 27:27.
RAMATH-LEHI, ra´-math-le´-hi, height of Lehi. Judg. 15:17.
RAMATH-MIZPEH, ra´-math-miz´-peh, height of Mizpeh. Josh. 13:26.
RAMESES, ra´-me-sees, same as RAAMSES. Gen. 47:11.
RAMIAH, ram-i´-ah, Jehovah is high. Ezra 10:25.
RAMOTH, ra´-moth, plural of Ramah. 1 Chr. 6:73.
RAMOTH-GILEAD, ra´-moth gil´-yad, heights of Gilead. Deut. 4:43; 1 Kin. 4:13, 22; 2 Kin. 8:28; 9:1; 2 Chr. 18; 22:5.
RAPHA, ra´-fah, giant (?). 1 Chr. 8:37.
RAPHU, ra´-foo, healed. Num. 13:9.
REAIA, re-ai´-ah, Jehovah has seen. 1 Chr. 5:5.
REAIAH, correct form of REAIA. 1 Chr. 4:2.
REBA, re´-bah, a fourth part. Num. 31:8.
REBECCA, Greek form of REBEKAH. Rom. 9:10.
REBEKAH, re-bek´-ah, a noose.
history of. Gen. 22:23; 24:15, 67; 27:6, 42; 49:31; Rom. 9:10.
RECHAB, re´-kab, horseman. 2 Kin. 10:15.
RECHABITES, re´-kab-ites, descendants of Rechab. Jer. 35:2.
RECHAH, re´-kah, side (?). 1 Chr. 4:12.
REELAIAH, re´-el-ai´-ah, trembling caused by Jehovah. Ezra 2:2.
REGEM, re´-gem, friend. 1 Chr. 2:47.
REGEM-MELECH, re´-gem-me´-lek, friend of the king. Zech. 7:2.
REHABIAH, re´-hab-i´-ah, Jehovah enlarges. 1 Chr. 23:17.
REHOB, re´-hob, street. 2 Sam. 8:3.
REHOBOAM, re´-hob-o´-am, who enlarges the people. 1 Kin. 11:43.
king of Judah. 1 Kin. 11; 12; 14; 2 Chr. 9—12.
REHOBOTH, re-ho´-both, roominess. Gen. 10:11; 26:22.
REHUM, re´-hoom, merciful. Ezra 4:8.
REI, re´-i, friendly. 1 Kin. 1:8.
REKEM, re´-kem, same as RAKEM. Num. 31:8.
REMALIAH, rem´-al-i´-ah, whom Jehovah adorned. 2 Kin. 15:25.
REMETH, re´-meth, a high place. Josh. 19:21.
REMMON, rem´-on, more correctly spelt RIMMON. Josh. 19:7.
REMMON-METHOAR, rem´-on-me-tho´-ar, R. stretching (to Neah). Josh. 19:13.
REMPHAN, rem´-fan. Acts 7:43.
REPHAEL, re´-fa-el, whom God healed. 1 Chr. 26:7.
REPHAH, re´-fah, riches. 1 Chr. 7:25.
REPHAIAH, ref-ai´-ah, whom Jehovah healed. 1 Chr. 3:21.
REPHAIM, re-fa´-m, giants. 2 Sam. 5:18.
REPHAIMS, re-fa´-ims, same as REPHAIM. Gen. 14:5.
REPHIDIM, re-fee´-dim, supports.
Amalek subdued there by Joshua. Ex. 17.
RESEN, re´-sen, bridle. Gen. 10:12.
RESHEPH, re´-shef, flame. 1 Chr. 7:25.
REU, re-oo´, same as RAGUEL. Gen. 11:18.
REUBEN, roo´-ben, behold a son (?).
son of Jacob. Gen. 29; 30; 35; 37; 42; 49; 1 Chr. 5:1.
REUBENITES, roo´-ben-ites, descendants of Reuben.
their number and possessions. Num. 1; 2; 26; 32; Deut. 3:12; Josh. 13:15; 1 Chr. 5:18.
dealings of Moses and Joshua with. Num. 32; Deut. 33; Josh. 1; 22.
go into captivity. 1 Chr. 5:26 (Rev. 7:5).
REUEL, roo´-el, friend of God. 1 Chr. 9:8.
REUMAH, room´-ah, exalted. Gen. 22:24.
REZEPH, re´-zef, a stone. 2 Kin. 19:12.
REZIA, rez´-yah, delight. 1 Chr. 7:39.
REZIN, re´-zin, firm.
king of Syria. 2 Kin. 15:37; 16:5, 9; Is. 7:1.
REZON, re´-zon, lean.
of Damascus. 1 Kin. 11:23.
RHEGIUM, re´-ji-um. Acts 28:13.
RHESA, re´-sah, chieftain (?). Luke 3:27.
RHODA, ro´-dah, a rose. Acts 12:13.
RHODES, rodes.
island of. Acts 21:1.
RIBAI, rib´-ai, contentious. 2 Sam. 23:29.
RIBLAH, rib´-lah, fertility. Num. 34:11.
in Syria. 2 Kin. 23:33; 25:6; Jer. 39:5; 52:9.
RIMMON, rim´-on, (1) pomegranate, 2 Sam. 4:2; (2) idol, 2 Kin. 5:18.
RIMMON-PAREZ, rim´-on-pa´-rez, pomegranate of the breach. Num. 33:19.
RINNAH, rin´-ah, shout. 1 Chr. 4:20.
RIPHATH, ri´-fath. Gen. 10:3.
RISSAH, ris´-ah, ruin. Num. 33:21.
RITHMAH, rith´-mah, broom. Num. 33:18.
RIZPAH, riz´-pah, hot coal. 2 Sam. 3:7.
ROBOAM, rob-o´-am, Greek form of REHOBOAM. Matt. 1:7.
ROGELIM, ro´-gel-im, fullers. 2 Sam. 17:27.
ROHGAH, ro´-gah, outcry. 1 Chr. 7:34.
ROMAMTI-EZER, ro-mam´-ti-e´-zer, I have exalted help. 1 Chr. 25:4.
ROMANS, ro´-mans, men of Rome. John 11:48.
St. Paul's teaching to. *See* Epistle to Romans, *also* FAITH, WORK, RIGHTEOUSNESS.
ROME, strength (?).
strangers of, at Pentecost. Acts 2:10.
Jews ordered to depart from. Acts 18:2.
Paul preaches there. Acts 28.
ROSH, head. Gen. 46:21.
RUFUS, roo´-fus, red. Mark 15:21.

RUFUS—*cont.*
(chosen in the Lord). Rom. 16:13.
RUHAMAH, roo-hah´-mah, compassionated. Hos. 2:1.
RUMAH, roo´-mah, height. 2 Kin. 23:36.
RUTH, tooth, friendship (?). Ruth 1:4.
story of. Ruth 1—4.
Christ descended from, Matt. 1:5.

SABACHTHANI, sa-bac-thah´-ni, thou hast forsaken me. Mark 15:34.
SABAOTH, sab-a´-oth (Hosts), the Lord of. Rom. 9:29; James 5:4.
SABEANS, sab-e´-ans, people of Seba. Job 1:15; Is. 45:14.
SABTAH, sab´-tah, rest (?). Gen. 10:7.
SABTECHA, sab´-te-kah. 1 Chr. 1:9.
SABTECHAH, sab´-te-kah. Gen. 10:7.
SACAR, sa´-kar, hire, reward. 1 Chr. 11:35.
SADDUCEES, sad´-u-sees (named from ZADOK, founder of the sect).
their controversies with Christ, Matt. 16:1; 22:23; Mark 12:18; Luke 20:27; with the apostles, Acts 4:1; with Paul, Acts 23:6.
their doctrines. Matt. 22:23; Mark 12:18; Acts 23:8.
SADOC, sa´-dok, Greek form of ZADOK. Matt. 1:14.
SALA, sa´-ah, Greek form of SALAH. Luke 3:35.
SALAH, sa´-lah, sprout (?). Gen. 10:24.
SALAMIS, sal´-am-is. Acts 13:5.
SALATHIEL, sa-la´-thi-el, Greek form of SHEALTIEL. 1 Chr. 3:17.
SALCAH, or SALCHAH, sal´-kah, road. Deut. 3:10.
SALEM, sa´-lem, perfect. Gen. 14:18; Heb. 7:1.
SALIM, sa´-lim, Greek form of SALEM. John 3:23.
SALLAI, sal´-ai, exaltation. Neh. 11:8.
SALLU, sal´-oo, same as SALLAI. 1 Chr. 9:7.
SALMA, sal´-mah, garment. 1 Chr. 2:11.
SALMON, sal´-mon, shady. Ps. 68:14.
SALMONE, sal-mo´-ne. Acts 27:7.
SALOME, sal-o´-me, perfect. Mark 15:40; 16:1.
SALU, sa´-loo, same as SALLU. Num. 25:14.
SAMARIA, sa-ma´-ri-ah, Greek equivalent of Shomron which means guard.
(city of). 1 Kin. 16:24; 20:1; 2 Kin. 6:24.
——(region of), visited by Christ. Luke 17:11; John 4.
gospel preached there. Acts 8.
SAMARITAN, sa-mar´-it-an.
parable of the good. Luke 10:33.
miracle performed on. Luke 17:16.
SAMARITANS, sa-mar´-it-ans, inhabitants of Samaria. 2 Kin. 17:29.
SAMGAR-NEBO, sam-gar´-ne-bo, Be gracious, Nebo. Jer. 39:3.
SAMLAH, sam´-lah, garment. Gen. 36:36.
SAMOS, sa´-mos, a height (?). Acts 20:15.
SAMOTHRACIA, sa´mo-thra´-shah. Acts 16:11.
SAMSON, sam´-son, like the sun. Judg. 13—16.
delivered up to Philistines. Judg. 16:21.
his death. Judg. 16:30.
SAMUEL, sam´-u-el, name of God, or, heard of God. 1 Sam. 1:20.
born, and presented to the Lord. 1 Sam. 1:19, 26.
ministers to the Lord. 1 Sam. 3.
the Lord speaks to. 1 Sam. 3:11.
judges Israel. 1 Sam. 7; 8:1; Acts 13:20.
anoints Saul king. 1 Sam. 10:1.
rebukes Saul for sin. 1 Sam. 13:13; 15:16.
anoints David 1 Sam. 16; 19:18.
his death. 1 Sam. 25:1; 28:3.
his spirit consulted by Saul. 1 Sam. 28:12.
as a prophet. Ps. 99:6; Acts 3:24; Heb. 11:32.
SANBALLAT, san-bal´-at, Sin (the moon) giveth life (?). Neh. 2:10; 4; 6:2; 13:28.
SANSANNAH, san-san´-ah, palm branch. Josh. 15:31.
SAPH, threshold. 2 Sam. 21:18.
SAPHIR, saf´-ir, beautiful. Mic. 1:11.
SAPPHIRA, saf-i´-rah, Greek form of the above (feminine). Acts 5:1.

SARA, sa´-rah, Greek form of SARAH. Heb. 11:11.
SARAH, sa´-rah, princess. Gen. 17:15.
(Sarai). Gen. 11; 12; 20:2. *See* ABRAHAM.
her death and burial. Gen. 23 (Heb. 11:11; 1 Pet. 3:6).
SARAI, sa´-rai, contentious (?). Gen. 11:29.
SARAPH, sa´-raf, burning. 1 Chr. 4:22.
SARDIS, sard´-is.
church of. Rev. 1:11; 3:1.
SARDITES, sard´-ites, descendants of Sered. Num. 26:26.
SAREPTA, sa-rep´-tah, Greek form of ZAREPHATH. Luke 4:26.
SARGON, sar´-gon, [God] appoints the king. Is. 20:1.
SARID, sa´-rid, survivor. Josh. 19:10.
SARON, sa´-ron, Greek form of SHARON. Acts 9:35.
SARSECHIM, sar´-se-kim. Jer. 39:3.
SARUCH, sa´-rook, Greek form of SERUG. Luke 3:35.
SATAN, sa´-tan, adversary. 1 Chr. 21:1. *See* DEVIL, *Subject-Index,* p. 1419.
SAUL, asked for. 1 Sam. 9:2.
king of Israel, his parentage, anointing by Samuel, prophesying, and acknowledgment as king. 1 Sam. 9; 10.
his disobedience, and rejection by God. 1 Sam. 14:31; 15.
possessed by an evil spirit, quieted by David. 1 Sam. 16:14, 15, 23.
favours David, 1 Sam. 18:5; seeks to kill him, 1 Sam. 18:10; pursues him, 1 Sam. 20; 23; 24; 26.
slays priests for succouring David. 1 Sam. 22:9.
enquires of the witch of En-dor. 1 Sam. 28:7.
his ruin and suicide. 1 Sam. 28:15; 31; 1 Chr. 10.
his posterity. 1 Chr. 8:33.
——of Tarsus. *See* PAUL.
SCEVA, se´-vah, left-handed. Acts 19:14.
SCYTHIAN, sith´-yan. Col. 3:11.
SEBA, se´-bah, man (?). Gen. 10:7.
SEBAT, se´-bat, rest (?). Zech. 1:7.
SECACAH, se-kah´-kah, enclosure. Josh. 15:61.
SECHU, se´-koo, watch-tower. 1 Sam. 19:22.
SECUNDUS, se-cun´-dus, second. Acts 20:4.
SEGUB, se´-goob, elevated. 1 Kin. 16:34.
SEIR, se´-ir, hairy.
mount, Edom, land of Esau. Gen. 14:6; 32:3; 36:8, 20; Deut. 33:2; Josh. 24:4; Is. 21:11; Ezek. 25:8.
predictions about. Num. 24:18; Ezek. 35:2.
SEIRATH, se-ir´-ath, well wooded. Judg. 3:26.
SELA, se´-ah, rock. Is. 16:1.
SELA-HAMMAHLEKOTH, se´-lah-ham-ah´-lek-oth, rock of escapes. 1 Sam. 23:28.
SELAH, se´-lah, forte (?), a musical direction, pause. Ps. 3:2; 4:2; 24:6; 39:5, 11; 46:3; 48:8; 50:6; Hab. 3:3, 9, 12, &c.
SELED, se´-led, exultation, or burning. 1 Chr. 2:30.
SELEUCIA, se-loo´-shah, called after Seleucus.
apostles at. Acts 13:4.
SEM, Greek form of SHEM. Luke 3:36.
SEMACHIAH, sem´-ak-i´-ah, whom Jehovah sustains. 1 Chr. 26:7.
SEMEI, sem´-e-i, Greek form of SHIMEI. Luke 3:26.
SENAAH, sen-a´-ah, perhaps thorny. Ezra 2:35.
SENEH, se´-nay, crag, thorn. 1 Sam. 14:4.
SENIR, se´-nir, coat of mail. 1 Chr. 5:23.
SENNACHERIB, sen-ak´-er-ib, Sin (the moon) multiplies brethren. 2 Kin. 18:13; 2 Chr. 32; Is. 36:37.
SENUAH, se-noo´-ah, bristling (?). Neh. 11:9.
SEORIM, se-or´-im, barley. 1 Chr. 24:8.
SEPHAR, se´-far, a numbering. Gen. 10:30.
SEPHARAD, se-far´-ad. Obad. 20.
SEPHARVAIM, se´-far-va´-im. 2 Kin. 17:24; 18:34; 19:13.
SERAH, se´-rah, abundance. Gen. 46:17.
SEPAIAH, ser-ai´-ah, soldier of Jehovah (?). 2 Sam. 8:17.
SERAPHIMS, ser´-af-ims, burning ones. Is. 6:2.
SERED, se´-red, fear. Gen. 46:14.
SERGIUS, ser´-ji-us. Acts 13:7.
SERUG, se´-roog, shoot. Gen. 11:20.
SETH, substitute.

SETH—*cont.*
son of Adam. Gen. 4:25; 5:3.
SETHUR, se´-thoor, hidden. Num. 13:13.
SHAALABBIN, sha´-al-ab´-in, earths of foxes. Josh. 19:42.
SHAALBIM, sha-alb´-im, same as preceding. Judg. 1:35.
SHAALBONITE, sha-alb´-on-ite, inhabitant of Shaalbim. 2 Sam. 23:32.
SHAAPH, sha´-af, anger (?). 1 Chr. 2:47.
SHAARAIM, sha-ar-a´-im, two gates. 1 Sam. 17:52.
SHAASHGAZ, sha-ash´-gaz, beauty's servant (?). Esth. 2:14.
SHABBETHAI, shab´-e-thai, born on the sabbath. Ezra 10:15.
SHACHIA, sha´-ki-ah, lustful. 1 Chr. 8:10.
SHADDAI, shad´-ai, Almighty. Num. 1:6.
SHADRACH, shad´-rak. Dan. 1:7.
Meshach, and Abed-nego, their faith and sufferings, and deliverance. Dan. 1; 3.
SHAGE, sha´-ge, wanderer. 1 Chr. 11:34.
SHAHARAIM, sha´-har-a´-im, two dawns. 1 Chr. 8:8.
SHAHAZIMAH, sha-ha-zee´-mah, lofty places. Josh. 19:22.
SHALEM, sha´-lem, safe, perfect. Gen. 33:18.
SHALIM, sha´-lim, foxes. 1 Sam. 9:4.
SHALISHA, sha-lish´-ah, a third part. 1 Sam. 9:4.
SHALLECHETH, shal-e´-keth, felling. 1 Chr. 26:16.
SHALLUM, shal´-oom, retribution. 2 Kin. 15:10; 22:14; 2 Chr. 34:22; Jer. 22:11.
SHALLUN, shal´-oon, spoliation. Neh. 3:15.
SHALMAI, shal´-mai, peaceful (?). Ezra 2:46.
SHALMAN, shal´-man, shortened form of following. Hos. 10:14.
SHALMANESER, shal´-man-e´-zer, Shalman be propitious. 2 Kin. 17:3.
carries ten tribes captive. 2 Kin. 17; 18:9.
SHAMA, sha´-mah, obedient. 1 Chr. 11:44.
SHAMARIAH, sha´-mar-i´-ah, whom Jehovah guards. 2 Chr. 11:19.
SHAMED, sha´-med, destroyer. 1 Chr. 8:12.
SHAMER, sha´-mer, keeper. 1 Chr. 6:46.
SHAMGAR SHAM´-GAR, destroyer (?).
judges Israel. Judg. 3:31; 5:6.
SHAMHUTH, sham´-hooth, notoriety (?). 1 Chr. 27:8.
SHAMIR, sha´-mir, a thorn. 1 Chr. 24:24.
SHAMMA, sham´-ah, desert. 1 Chr. 7:37.
SHAMMAH, sham´-ah, same as SHAMMA. Gen. 36:13.
his valour. 2 Sam. 23:11.
SHAMMAI, sham´-ai, wasted. 1 Chr. 2:28.
SHAMMOTH, sham´-oth, deserts. 1 Chr. 11:27.
SHAMMUA, sham´-oo-ah, famous. Num. 13:4.
SHAMMUAH, same as preceding. 2 Sam. 5:14.
SHAMSHERAI, sham´-sher-ai. 1 Chr. 8:26.
SHAPHAM, sha´-fam, bald. 1 Chr. 5:12.
SHAPHAN, sha´-fan, coney.
repairs the temple. 2 Kin. 22:3; 2 Chr. 34:8.
SHAPHAT, sha´-fat, judge. Num. 13:5.
SHAPHER, sha´-fer, pleasantness. Num. 33:23.
SHARAI, shar´-ai, free. Ezra 10:40.
SHARAIM, shar-a´-im, same as SHAARAIM. Josh. 15:36.
SHARAR, shar´-ar, firm. 2 Sam. 23:33.
SHAREZER, shar-e´-zer, [God] protect the king. 2 Kin. 19:37.
SHARON, sha´-ron, plain. 1 Chr. 27:29.
rose of. Cant. 2:1.
SHARONITE, sha´-ron-ite, one who lives in Sharon. 1 Chr. 27:29.
SHARUHEN, sha-roo´-hen. Josh. 19:6.
SHASHAI, shash´-ai, pale. Ezra 10:40.
SHASHAK, sha´-shak, activity (?). 1 Chr. 8:14.
SHAUL, sha´-ool, same as SAUL. Gen. 46:10.
SHAULITES, sha´-ool-ites, the family of Shaul. Num. 26:13.
SHAVEH, sha´-vay, plain. Gen. 14:17.
SHAVEH KIRIATHAIM, sha´-vay kir-iath-a´-im, plain of Kiriathaim. Gen. 14:5.
SHAVSHA, shav´-shah, another name of Seraiah. 1 Chr. 18:16.

SHEAL, she´-al, prayer. Ezra 10:29.
SHEALTIEL, she-al´-ti-el, I asked from God. Ezra 3:2.
SHEARIAH, she´-ar-i´-ah, gate of Jehovah. 1 Chr. 8:38.
SHEAR-JASHUB, she´-ar-ja´-shoob, the remnant shall return. Is. 7:3.
SHEBA, she´-bah, an oath. Gen. 25:3; 2 Sam. 20:1; Job 6:19; Ps. 72:10; Jer. 6:20; Ezek. 27:22; 38:13.
queen of. 1 Kin. 10; 2 Chr. 9; Matt. 12:42.
——(Benjamite) revolts. 2 Sam. 20.
SHEBAH, seven. Gen. 26:33.
SHEBAM, she´-bam, fragrance. Num. 32:3.
SHEBANIAH, she´-ban-i´-ah, whom Jehovah hides. 1 Chr. 15:24.
SHEBARIM, she-bar´-im, breaches. Josh. 7:5.
SHEBER, she´-ber, breaking. 1 Chr. 2:48.
SHEBNA, sheb´-nah, youth (?).
the scribe. 2 Kin. 18:18; 19:2; Is. 22:15; 36:3; 37:2.
SHEBUEL, she-boo´-el, captive of God. 1 Chr. 23:16.
SHECANIAH, she´-kan-i´-ah, same as following. 1 Chr. 24:11.
SHECHANIAH, she´-kan-i´-ah, Jehovah dwells. 1 Chr. 3:21.
SHECHEM, she´-kem, back, shoulder. Gen. 34:2.
the Hivite. Gen. 34.
——city of. Josh. 17:7; Ps. 60:6.
charge of Joshua at. Josh. 24.
its treachery and penalty. Judg. 9:1, 41
SHECHEMITES, she´-kem-ites, people of Shechem. Num. 26:31.
SHEDEUR, she´-de-oor, giving forth of light. Num. 1:5.
SHEHARIAH, she´-har-i´-ah, Jehovah seeks. 1 Chr. 8:26.
SHELAH, she´-lah, petition.
son of Judah. Gen. 38:5.
SHELANITES, she´-lan-ites, descendants of Shelah. Num. 26:20.
SHELEMIAH, she´-lem-i´-ah, whom Jehovah repays. 1 Chr. 26:14.
SHELEPH, she´-lef, drawing out. Gen. 10:26.
SHELESH, she´-lesh, triad. 1 Chr. 7:35.
SHELOMI, she-lo´-mi, peaceful. Num. 34:27.
SHELOMITH, she-lo´-mith, peacefulness. Lev. 24:11.
SHELOMOTH, she-lo´-moth, same as SHELOMITH. 1 Chr. 24:22.
SHELUMIEL, she-loom´-i-el, friend of God. Num. 1:6.
SHEM, name. Gen. 5:32; 9:26; 10:21; 11:10; 1 Chr. 1:17.
SHEMA, she´-mah, (1) echo (?), Josh. 15:26; (2) fame, 1 Chr. 2:43.
SHEMAAH, she-ma´-ah, fame. 1 Chr. 12:3.
SHEMAIAH, she-mai´-ah, Jehovah has heard.
prophet. 1 Kin. 12:22; 2 Chr. 11:2; 12:5 (Jer. 29:24).
SHEMARIAH, she´-mar-i-ah, Jehovah guards. 1 Chr. 12:5.
SHEMEBER, shem-e´-ber, soaring on high (?). Gen. 14:2.
SHEMER, she´-mer, guardian. 1 Kin. 16:24.
SHEMIDA, shem-i´-dah, fame of wisdom. Num. 26:32.
SHEMIDAH, shem-i´-dah, same as preceding. 1 Chr. 7:19.
SHEMIDAITES, shem-id´-a-ites, descendants of Shemida. Num. 26:32.
SHEMINITH, she-mi´-nith, eighth. 1 Chr. 15:21.
SHEMIRAMOTH, she-mi´-ram-oth, most high name. 1 Chr. 15:18.
SHEMUEL, she´-moo-el, same as SAMUEL. Num. 34:20.
SHEN, tooth. 1 Sam. 7:12.
SHENAZAR, she-na´-zar. 1 Chr. 3:18.
SHENIR, she´-nir, same as SENIR. Deut. 3:9.
SHEPHAM, she´-fam, nakedness. Num. 34:10.
SHEPHATHIAH, she´-fat-i´-ah, an incorrect way of spelling the next word. 1 Chr. 9:8.
SHEPHATIAH, she´-fat-i´-ah, whom Jehovah defends. 2 Sam. 3:4.

SHEPHI, she´-fi, baldness. 1 Chr. 1:40.
SHEPHO, she´-fo, same as SHEPHI. Gen. 36:23.
SHEPHUPHAN, she´-foof-an, serpent (?). 1 Chr. 8:5.
SHERAH, she´-rah, consanguinity. 1 Chr. 7:24.
SHEREBIAH, she´-reb-i´-ah, heat of Jehovah. Ezra 8:18.
SHERESH, she´-resh, root. 1 Chr. 7:16.
SHEREZER, sher-e´-zer, same as SHAREZER (?). Zech. 7:2.
SHESHACH, she´-shak, a name for Babel. Jer. 25:26; 51:41.
SHESHAI, shesh´-ai, clothed in white (?). Num. 13:22.
SHESHAN, she´-shan, lily (?). 1 Chr. 2:31.
SHESHBAZZAR, shesh-baz´-ar. Ezra 1:8; 5:14.
SHETH, shayth, tumult. Num. 24:17.
SHETHAR, she´-thar, star. Esth. 1:14.
SHETHAR-BOZNAI, she´-thar-boz´-nai, bright star. Ezra 5:3.
 and Tatnai oppose rebuilding of temple. Ezra 5:6.
SHEVA, she´-vah, vanity. 2 Sam. 20:25.
SHIBBOLETH, shib´-ol-eth, an ear of corn, or a flood. Judg. 12:6.
SHIBMAH, shib´-mah, fragrant. Num. 32:38.
SHICRON, shik´-ron, drunkenness. Josh. 15:11.
SHIGGAION, shig-ai´-on, irregular. Ps. 7, title.
SHIGIONOTH, shig´-i-o´-noth. Hab. 3:1.
SHIHON, shi´-hon, ruin. Josh. 19:19.
SHIHOR, shi´-hor, black. 1 Chr. 13:5.
SHIHOR-LIBNATH, shi´-hor-lib´-nath. Josh. 19:26.
SHILHI, shil´-hi, darter. 1 Kin. 22:42.
SHILHIM, shil´-him, aqueducts. Josh. 15:32.
SHILLEM, shil´-em, requital. Gen. 46:24.
SHILOAH, shi-lo´-ah, outlet of water. Is. 8:6.
SHILOH, shi´-lo, rest, Messiah. Gen. 49:10.
——site of tabernacle. Josh. 18:1; Judg. 21:19; 1 Sam. 1:3; 2:14; 3:21; Ps. 78:60; Jer. 7:12; 26:6.
SHILONI, shi´-lo-ni, native of Shiloh. Neh. 11:5.
SHILONITE, shi´-lo-nite, same as preceding. 1 Kin. 11:29.
SHILSHAH, shil´-shah, triad. 1 Chr. 7:37.
SHIMEA, shim´-e-ah, famous. 1 Chr. 3:5.
SHIMEAH, shim´-e-ah, same as SHEMAAH. 2 Sam. 21:21.
SHIMEAM, shim´-e-am, same as preceding. 1 Chr. 9:38.
SHIMEATH, shim´-e-ath, fame. 2 Kin. 12:21.
SHIMEATHITE, shi´-me-ath-ite. 1 Chr. 2:55.
SHIMEI, shim´-e-i, my fame. Num. 3:18.
 curses David. 2 Sam. 16:5.
 slain by Solomon. 1 Kin. 2:36.
SHIMEON, shim´-e-on, a hearkening. Ezra 10:31.
SHIMHI, shim´-hi, same as SHIMEI. 1 Chr. 8:21.
SHIMI, shim´-i, same as preceding. Ex. 6:17.
SHIMITES, shim´-ites, descendants of Shimei. Num. 3:21.
SHIMMA, shim´-ah, rumour. 1 Chr. 2:13.
SHIMON, shi´-mon. 1 Chr. 4:20.
SHIMRATH, shim´-rath, watchfulness. 1 Chr. 8:21.
SHIMRI, shim´-ri, watchful. 1 Chr. 4:37.
SHIMRITH, shim´-rith, vigilant. 2 Chr. 24:26.
SHIMROM, shim´-rome, watch-post. 1 Chr. 7:1.
SHIMRON, shim´-rone, watchful. Josh. 11:1.
SHIMRONITES, shim´-ron-ites, descendants of Shimron. Num. 26:24.
SHIMRON-MERON, shim´-ron-me´-ron. Josh. 12:20.
SHIMSHAI, shim´-shai, sunny. Ezra. 4:8.
SHINAB, shi´-nab, hostile (?). Gen. 14:2.
SHINAR, shi´-nar. Gen. 10:10.
SHIPHI, shi´-fi, abundant. 1 Chr. 4:37.
SHIPHMITE, shif´-mite, a native of Shephan. 1 Chr. 27:27.
SHIPHRAH, shif´-rah, beauty. Ex. 1:15.
SHIPTAN, shif´-tan, judicial. Num. 34:24.
SHISHA, shi´-shah, brightness. 1 Kin. 4:3.
SHISHAK, shi´-shak, illustrious. 1 Kin. 11:40.
 invades and spoils Jerusalem. 1 Kin. 14:25; 2 Chr. 12.
SHITRAI, shit´-rai, official. 1 Chr. 27:29.
SHITTIM, shit´-im, acacias. Num. 25:1.
SHIZA, shi´-zah, cheerful (?). 1 Chr. 11:42.
SHOA, sho´-ah, opulent. Ezek. 23:23.
SHOBAB, sho´-bab, apostate. 2 Sam. 5:14.
SHOBACH, sho´-bak, pouring. 2 Sam. 10:16.
SHOBAI, sho´-bai, bright (?). Ezra 2:42.
SHOBAL, sho´-bal, stream. Gen. 36:20.
SHOBEK, sho´-bek, forsaker. Neh. 10:24.
SHOBI, sho´-bi, taking captive. 2 Sam. 17:27.
SHOCHO, sho´-ko, same as the next word. 2 Chr. 28:18.
SHOCHOH, sho´-ko, a hedge. 1 Sam. 17:1.
SHOCO, sho´-ko, same as the preceding. 2 Chr. 11:7.
SHOHAM, sho´-ham, onyx. 1 Chr. 24:27.
SHOMER, sho´-mer, watchman. 2 Kin. 12:21.
SHOPHACH, sho´-fak, same as SHOBAK. 1 Chr. 19:16.
SHOPHAN, sho´-fan, baldness. Num. 32:35.
SHOSHANNIM, sho-shan´-im, lilies. Ps. 45, title.
SHOSHANNIM-EDUTH, sh.-e´-dooth, lilies a testimony. Ps. 80, title.
SHUA, shoo´-ah, wealth. 1 Chr. 2:3.
SHUAH, shoo´-ah, depression. Gen. 25:2.
SHUAL, shoo´-al, jackal. 1 Chr. 7:36.
SHUBAEL, shoo´-ha-el, same as SHEBUEL (?). 1 Chr. 24:20.
SHUHAM, shoo´-ham, pitman (?). Num. 26:42.
SHUHAMITES, shoo´-ham-ites, the descendants of Shuham. Num. 26:42.
SHUHITE, shoo´-hite, a descendant of Shua. Job 8:1.
SHULAMITE, shoo´-lam-ite, same as SHELOMITH. Cant. 6:13.
SHUMATHITES, shoo´-math-ites, people of Shumah. 1 Chr. 2:53.
SHUNAMMITE, shoon´-am-ite, an inhabitant of Shunem. 1 Kin. 1:3.
SHUNEM, shoon´-em, two resting-places. Josh. 19:18; 1 Sam. 28:4; 2 Kin. 4:8.
SHUNI, shoon´-i, quiet. Gen. 46:16.
SHUNITES, shoon´-ites, descendants of Shuni. Num. 26:15.
SHUPHAM, shoo´-fam, serpent. Num. 26:39.
SHUPHAMITES, shoo´-fam-ites, the descendants of Shupham. Num. 26:39.
SHUIPPIM, shoop´-im. 1 Chr. 7:12.
SHUR, shoor, a fort. Gen. 16:7.
SHUSHAN, shoo´-shan.
 city, Artaxerxes at. Neh. 1:1; Esth. 2:8; 3:15.
SHUSHAN-EDUTH, sh.-e´-dooth, lily of the testimony. Ps. 60, title.
SHUTHALHITES, shoo´-thal-ites, the descendants of Shuthelah. Num. 26:35.
SHUTHELAH, shoo-theel´-ah, plantation (?). Num. 26:35.
SIA, si´-ah, assembly. Neh. 7:47.
SIAHA, si´-a-hah, council. Ezra 2:44.
SIBBECAI, sib´-e-kai, entangling. 1 Chr. 11:29.
SIBBECHAI, same as preceding. 2 Sam. 21:18.
SIBBOLETH, sib´-o-leth, same as SHIBBOLETH. Judg. 12:6.
SIBMAH, sib´-mah, same as SHIBMAH. Josh. 13:19.
SIBRAIM, sib-ra´-im, two hills (?). Ezek. 47:16.
SICHEM, si´-kem, the shoulder-blade. Gen. 12:6.
SIDDIM, sid´-im, the plains. Gen. 14:3.
SIDON, si´-don, fishing.
 son of Canaan. Gen. 10:15.
——(Zidon), city of. Josh. 19:28; 1 Kin. 5:6; Acts 27:3.
SIDONIANS, si-do´-ni-ans, persons living in Sidon. Deut. 3:9.
SIHON, si´-hon, brush.
 king of the Amorites. Num. 21:21; Deut. 1:4; 2:26; Ps. 135:11; 136:19.
SIHOR, si´-hor, same as SHICHOR. Josh. 13:3.
SILAS, si´-las, shortened form of SILVANUS. Acts 15:22; 16:19; 17:4. *See* 2 Cor. 1:19; 1 Thess. 1:1; 1 Pet. 5:12.
SILLA, sil´-ah, way, highway (?). 2 Kin. 12:20.
SILOAM, si-lo´-am, same as SHILOAH. 1 John 9:7.
SILVANUS, sil-vane´-us, of the forest. 2 Cor. 1:19.

SIMEON, sim´-e-on, same as SHIMEON.
son of Jacob. Gen. 29:33; 34:7, 25; 42:24.
his descendants. Gen. 46:10; Ex. 6:15; Num. 1:22; 26:12; 1 Chr. 4:24; 12:25.
prophecy concerning. Gen. 49:5.
——blesses Christ. Luke 2:25.
SIMON, si´-mon, same as preceding.
brother of Christ. Matt. 13:55; Mark 6:3.
——(Zelotes), APOSTLE. Matt. 10:4; Mark 3:18; Luke 6:15.
——(Pharisee), reproved. Luke 7:36.
——(leper). Matt. 26:6; Mark 14:3.
——(of Cyrene), bears the cross of Jesus. Matt. 27:32; Mark 15:21; Luke 23:26.
——(a tanner), Peter's vision in his house. Acts 9:43; 10:6.
——(a sorcerer), baptized. Acts 8:9; rebuked by Peter. Acts 8:18.
——PETER. *See* PETER.
SIMRI, sim´-ri, same as SHIMRI. 1 Chr. 26:10.
SIN, clay. Ex. 16:1.
(Zin), wilderness of. Ex. 16; Num. 13:21; 20; 27:14.
SINA, si´-nah, Greek form of SINAI. Acts 7:30.
SINAI, si´-nai, pointed. Ex. 19:1.
mount. Deut. 33:2; Judg. 5:5; Ps. 68:8, 17; Gal. 4:24.
SINIM, sin´-im. Chinese (?). Is. 49:12.
SINITE, sin´-ite. Gen. 10:17.
SION, si´-on, (1) lifted up, Deut. 4:48; (2) Greek name for Mount Zion, Matt. 21:5.
SIPHMOTH, sif´-moth, bare places (?). 1 Sam. 30:28.
SIPPAI, sip´-ai, belonging to the doorstep (?). 1 Chr. 20:4.
SIRAH, si´-rah, withdrawing. 2 Sam. 3:26.
SIRION, sir´-i-on, a coat of mail.
mount. Deut. 8:9; Ps. 29:6.
SISAMAI, sis´-a-mai, fragrant (?). 1 Chr. 2:40.
SISERA, si´-ser-ah, binding in chains (?). Judg. 4:2, 21; 5:24; 1 Sam. 12:9; Ps. 83:9.
SITNAH, sit´-nah, contention. Gen. 26:21.
SIVAN, si´-van, bright. Esth. 8:9.
SMYRNA, smir´-nah, myrrh. Rev. 1:11.
SO, Hebrew form of EGYPTIAN word Sevech. 2 Kin. 17:4.
SOCHO, so´-ko, same as SHOCHO. 1 Chr. 4:18.
SOCHOH, same as SHOCHOH. 1 Kin. 4:10.
SOCOH, same as SHOCO. Josh. 15:35.
SODI, so´-di, an acquaintance. Num. 13:10.
SODOM, sod´-om, burning. Gen. 10:19.
its iniquity and destruction. Gen. 13:13; 18:20; 19:4-24; Deut. 23:17; 1 Kin. 14:24.
Lot's deliverance from. Gen. 19.
a warning. Deut. 29:23; 32:32; Is. 1:9; 13:19; Lam. 4:6; Matt. 10:15; Luke 17:29; Jude 7; Rev. 11:8.
SODOMA, sod´-om-ah, Greek form of the preceding. Rom. 9:29.
SODOMITES, sod´-om-ites, persons who were as wicked as the men of Sodom. 1 Kin. 15:12.
SOLOMON, sol´-om-on, peaceable. 2 Sam. 5:14.
king of Israel. 2 Sam. 12:24; 1 Kin. 1; 2:24; 1 Chr. 28:9; 29.
asks of God wisdom. 1 Kin. 3:5 (4:29); 2 Chr. 1:7.
the wise judgment of. 1 Kin. 3:16.
his league with Hiram for building the temple. 1 Kin. 5; 2 Chr. 2.
builds the temple (2 Sam. 7:12; 1 Chr. 17:11); 1 Kin. 6; 7; 2 Chr. 3—5; the dedication, 1 Kin. 8; 2 Chr. 6.
God's covenant with. 1 Kin. 9; 2 Chr. 7:12.
the queen of Sheba visits. 1 Kin. 10; 2 Chr. 9; Matt. 6:29; 12:42.
David's prayer for. Ps. 72.
his idolatry, rebuke, and death. 1 Kin. 11:1, 9, 14, 31, 41; 2 Chr. 9:29; Neh. 13:26.
his Proverbs and Canticles. Prov. 1:1; Eccles. 1:1; Cant. 1:1.
SON of GOD. *See* CHRIST.
——of MAN. *See* CHRIST.
SOPATER, so´-pa-ter. Acts 20:4.
SOPHERETH, so-fer´-eth, scribe. Ezra 2:55.
SOREK, so´-rek, choice vine. Judg. 16:4.
SOSIPATER, so-si´-pat-er. Rom. 16:21.
SOSTHENES, sos´-then-ees. Acts 18:17.
SOTAI, so´-tai, deviator. Ezra 2:55.
SPAIN. Rom. 15:24.
STACHYS, sta´-kis, an ear of corn. Rom. 16:9.
STEPHANAS, ste´-fan-as, crowned. 1 Cor. 1:16.
STEPHEN, ste´-ven, English form of STEPHANAS.
deacon and protomartyr. Acts 6:5, 8; 7:58.
STOICKS, sto´-ics, philosophers whose founder taught in a famous porch or Stoa. Acts 17:18.
SUAH, soo´-ah, sweepings. 1 Chr. 7:36.
SUCCOTH, sook´-oth, booths.
(Canaan). Gen. 33:17; Josh. 13:27; 1 Kin. 7:46; Ps. 60:6.
punished by Gideon. Judg. 8:5, 16.
——(in Egypt). Ex. 12:37; 13:20.
SUCCOTH-BENOTH, suc-coth´-be-noth. 2 Kin. 17:30.
SUCHATHITES, sook´-ath-ites. 1 Chr. 2:55.
SUKKIIMS, sook´-i-ims, nomads. 2 Chr. 12:3.
SUR, soor. 2 Kin. 11:6.
SUSANCHITES, soo´-sank-ites, inhabitants of Susa or Susinak. Ezra. 4:9.
SUSANNA, su-san´-ah, lily. Luke 8:3.
SUSI, soo´-si, horseman. Num. 13:11.
SYCHAR, si´-kar, drunken (?). John 4:5.
SYCHEM, si´-kem, Greek form of SHECHEM. Acts 7:16.
SYENE, si-e´-ne, opening. Ezek. 29:10.
SYNTYCHE, sin´-ty-kee, fortunate. Phil. 4:2.
SYRACUSE, si´-ra-kuse. Acts 28:12.
SYRIA, sir´-yah. Judg. 10:6.
SYRIAN, sir´-yan, inhabitant of Syria. Gen. 25:20.
SYRIANS, sir´-yans. Gen. 25:20; Deut. 26:5.
subdued by David. 2 Sam. 8; 10.
contend with Israel. 1 Kin. 10:29; 11:25; 20; 22; 2 Kin. 6:24; 7; 8:13; 13:7; 16:6; 2 Chr. 18.
employed to punish Joash. 2 Chr. 24:23 *See* 2 Chr. 28:23; Is. 7:2; Ezek. 27:16; Hos. 12:12; Amos 1:5.
gospel preached to. Matt. 4:24; Acts 15:23; 18:18; Gal. 1:21.
SYROPHENICIAN, si´-ro-fee-nish´-yan, Phenician living in Syria. Mark 7:26.
TAANACH, ta´-a-nak, castle (?). Josh. 12:21.
TAANATH-SHILOH, ta´-a-nath-shi-lo, fig-tree of Shiloh (?). Josh. 16:6.
TABBAOTH, tab´-a-oth, rings. Ezra 2:43.
TABBATH, tab´-ath, pleasantness. Judg. 7:22.
TABEAL, tab´-e-al, God is good. Is. 7:6.
TABEEL, tab´-e-el, another way of writing Tabeal. Ezra 4:7.
TABERAH, tab-er´-ah, burning. Num. 11:3.
TABITHA, tab´-ith-ah, gazelle. Acts 9:36.
TABOR, ta´-bor, height. Josh. 19:22.
(mount). Judg. 4:14. *See* Judg. 8:18; 1 Sam. 10:3; Ps. 89:12; Jer. 46:18; Hos. 5:1.
TABRIMON, tab´-rim-on, Rimmon is good. 1 Kin. 15:18.
TACHMONITE, tak´-mon-ite, same as HACHMONITE (?). 2 Sam. 23:8.
TADMOR, tad´-mor, city of palms (?).
(Palmyra), built by Solomon. 1 Kin. 9:18.
TAHAN, ta´-han, camp. Num. 26:35.
TAHANITES, ta´-han-ites, descendants of Tahan. Num. 26:35.
TAHAPANHES, ta´-ha-pan´-es, head of the land. Jer. 2:16.
TAHPANHES, same as preceding. Jer. 43:7.
TAHPENHES, tah´-pen-es. 1 Kin. 11:19.
TAHATH, ta´-hath, substitute. 1 Chr. 6:24.
TAHREA, tah-re´-ah, cunning (?). 1 Chr. 9:41.
TAHTIM-HODSHI, tah´-tim-hod´-shi, nether land newly inhabited (?). 2 Sam. 24:6.
TALITHA, ta-li´-tha, girl. Mark. 5:41.
TALMAI, tal´-mai, abounding in furrows. Num. 13:22.
TALMON, tal´-mon, oppressed. 1 Chr. 9:17.

TAMAH, ta´mah, joy. Neh. 7:55.
TAMAR, ta´mar, a palm tree. Gen. 38:6.
TAMMUZ, tam´ooz, son of life (?).
women weeping for. Ezek. 8:14.
TANACH, ta´nak, same as TAANACH. Josh. 21:25.
TANHUMETH, tan-hoom´eth, consolation. 2 Kin. 25:23.
TAPHATH, ta´fath, a drop (?). 1 Kin. 4:11.
TAPPUAH, tap-oo´ah, apple. 1 Chr. 2:43.
TARAH, ta´rah, station. Num. 33:27.
TARALAH, ta´ra-lah, reeling (?). Josh. 18:27.
TAREA, ta-re´ah, same as TAHREA. 1 Chr. 8:35.
TARPELITES, tar´pel-ites, people of Tarpel. Ezra 4:9.
TARSHISH, tar´shish. Gen. 10:4; 1 Kin. 10:22; 2 Chr. 9:21; 20:36; Jer. 10:9; Ezek. 27:12; 38:13.
Jonah going there. Jonah 1:3.
prophecies concerning. Ps. 48:7; 72:10; Is. 2:16; 23; 60:9; 66:19.
TARSUS, tar´sus, city of the apostle Paul. Acts 9:11; 11:25; 21:39.
TARTAK, tar´tak. 2 Kin. 17:31.
TARTAN, tar´tan, military chief. 2 Kin. 18:17.
TATNAI, tat´nai, gift (?).
and Shethar-boznai hinder the rebuilding of the temple. Ezra 5:3; 6:13.
TEBAH, te´bah, slaughter. Gen. 22:24.
TEBALIAH, te-bal-i´ah, whom Jehovah has immersed. 1 Chr. 26:11.
TEBETH, te´beth. Esth. 2:16.
TEHAPHNEHES, te-haph´ne-hes, same as TAHAPANES. Ezek. 30:18.
TEHINNAH, te-hin´ah, cry for mercy. 1 Chr. 4:12.
TEKEL, te´kel, weighed. Dan. 5:25.
TEKOA, te-ko´ah, sound of trumpet (1 Chr. 2:24; 4:5).
widow of. 2 Sam. 14 (Jer. 6:1).
TEKOAH, te-ko´ah, same as TEKOA. 2 Sam. 14:2.
TEKOITE, te-ko´ite, inhabitant of Tekoah. 2 Sam. 23:26.
TEL-ABIB, tel-a´bib, hill of ears of corn. Ezek. 3:15.
TELAH, te´lah. 1 Chr. 7:25.
TELAIM, te-la´im, lambs. 1 Sam. 15:4.
TELASSAR, tel-as´ar, Assyrian hill. Is. 37:12.
TELEM, te´lem, oppression. Ezra 10:24.
TEL-HARESHA, tel-har´e-shah, forest-hill. Neh. 7:61.
TEL-HARSA, tel-har´sah, same as preceding. Ezra 2:59.
TEL-MELAH, tel-me´lah, salt-hill. Ezra 2:59.
TEMA, te´mah, a desert. Gen. 25:15; Job 6:19; Is. 21:14; Jer. 25:23.
TEMAN, te´man, on the right hand. Gen. 36:11; Jer. 49:7, 20; Ezek. 25:13; Amos 1:12; Obad. 9; Hab. 3:3.
TEMANI, te´man-i, descendants of Teman. Gen. 36:34.
TEMANITE, te´man-ite, same as preceding. Job 2:11.
TEMENI, te´men-i, same as TEMANI. 1 Chr. 4:6.
TERAH, te´rah, a station (?). Gen. 11:24.
TERAPHIM, ter´af-im, nourishers.
of Laban. Gen. 31:34.
of Micah. Judg. 17:5; 18:14.
of Michal. 1 Sam. 19:13.
TERESH, te´resh, severe (?). Esth. 2:21.
TERTIUS, ter´shus, the third. Rom. 16:22.
TERTULLUS, ter-tul´us (*dim.* of TERTIUS). Acts 24:1.
TETRARCH, tet´rark, ruler of a fourth part of a country. Matt. 14:1.
THADDÆUS, thad-e´us, Greek form of THEUDAS. Matt. 10:3.
THAHASH, tha´hash, seal (?). Gen. 22:24.
THAMAH, tha´mah, laughter. Ezra 2:53.
THAMAR, tha´mar, Greek equivalent of Tamar. Matt. 1:3.
THARA, tha´rah, Greek form of TERAH. Luke 3:34.
THARSHISH, thar´shish, same as TARSHISH. 1 Kin. 10:22.
THEBEZ, the´bez, brightness.
Abimelech wounded at. Judg. 9:50.
THELASAR, thel´as´ar, same as TELASSAR. 2 Kin. 19:12.
THEOPHILUS, the-ó´fil-us, loved of God. Luke 1:3.
THESSALONICA, thes´al-on-i´kah.
Paul at. Acts 17.
church there instructed. 1 & 2 Thess.
THEUDAS, thoo´das, praise (?). Acts 5:36.
THIMNATHAH, thim-nah´thah, portion. Josh. 19:43.
THOMAS, tom´as, a twin.
APOSTLE. Matt. 10:3; Mark 3:18; Luke 6:15; Acts 1:13.
his zeal. John 11:16.
his unbelief and confession. John 20:24.
THUMMIM, thoom´im, truth (?).
on high priest's breastplate. Ex. 28:30; Lev. 8:8; Deut. 33:8; Ezra 2:63; Neh. 7:65.
THYATIRA, thi´at-i´rah (Acts 16:14).
angel of. Rev. 1:11; 2:18.
TIBERIAS, ti-be´ri-as, a place named after Tiberius. John 6:1.
TIBERIUS, ti-be´ri-us. Luke 3:1.
TIBHATH, tib´hath, butchery. 1 Chr. 18:8.
TIBNI, tib´ni, made of straw (?). 1 Kin. 16:21.
TIDAL, ti´dal, dread. Gen. 14:1.
TIGLATH-PILESER, tig´lath-pil-e´zer, the son of the temple of Sarra is a ground of confidence (?).
(Tilgath-pilneser, 1 Chr. 5:6, 26), 2 Kin. 15:29; 16:7; 2 Chr. 28:20.
TIKVAH, tik´vah, expectation. 2 Kin. 22:14.
TIKVATH, tik´vath, same as TIKVAH. 2 Chr. 34:22.
TILGATH-PILNESER, til´gath-pil-ne´ser, same as TIGLATH-PILESER. 1 Chr. 5:6.
TILON, ti´lon, gift (?). 1 Chr. 4:20.
TIMÆUS, ti-me´us, polluted (?). Mark 10:46.
TIMNA, tim´nah, unapproachable. Gen. 36:12.
TIMNAH, tim´nah, a portion. Josh. 15:10.
TIMNATH, tim´nath, same as TIMNAH. Gen. 38:12.
TIMNATH-HERES, tim´nath-he´res, portion of the sun. Judg. 2:9.
TIMNATH-SERAH, tim´nath-se´rah, portion of the remainder. Josh. 19:50.
Joshua buried there. Josh. 24:30.
TIMNITE, tim´nite, a man of Timna. Judg. 15:6.
TIMON, ti´mon. Acts 6:5.
TIMOTHEUS, ti-mo´the-us, honouring God. Acts 16:1.
TIMOTHY, tim´oth-y, English form of the above.
accompanies Paul. Acts 16:3; 17:14, 15; Rom. 16:21; 2 Cor. 1:1, 19.
commended. 1 Cor. 16:10; Phil. 2:19.
instructed in letters by Paul. 1 & 2 Tim.
TIPHSAH, tif´sah, passage. 1 Kin. 4:24.
TIRAS, ti´ras, crushing (?). Gen. 10:2.
TIRATHITES, ti´rath-ites. 1 Chr. 2:55.
TIRHAKAH, tir-hah´kah, distance (?).
Sennacherib's war with. 2 Kin. 19:9.
TIRHANAH, tir´han-ah, murmuring (?). 1 Chr. 2:48.
TIRIA, tir´i-ah, fear. 1 Chr. 4:16.
TIRSHATHA, tir-sha´thah, the feared (?). Ezra 2:63; Neh. 7:70.
TIRZAH, tir´zah, pleasantness. Num. 26:33; 1 Kin. 14:17; 15:21; 16:8, 15; 2 Kin. 15:16; Cant. 6:4 (Josh. 12:24).
TISHBITE, tish´bite, inhabitant of Tishbe. 1 Kin. 17:1.
TITUS, ti´tus, protected. Gal. 2:3.
Paul's love for. 2 Cor. 2:13; 7:6, 13.
instructed by Paul. Tit. 1—3.
TIZITE, ti´zite. 1 Chr. 11:45.
TOAH, to´ah, low. 1 Chr. 6:34.
TOB, tobe, good. Judg. 11:3.
TOB-ADONIJAH, tob´a-do-ni´jah, good is my lord Jehovah. 2 Chr. 17:8.
TOBIAH, tob-i´ah, Jehovah is good. Ezra 2:60.
the Ammonite, vexes the Jews. Neh. 4:3; 6:1, 12, 14; 13:4.
TOBIJAH, tob-i´jah, same as TOBIAH. 2 Chr. 17:8.
TOCHEN, to´ken, a measure. 1 Chr. 4:32.
TOGARMAH, to-gar´mah, rugged. Gen. 10:3.
TOHU, to´hoo, same as TOAH. 1 Sam. 1:1.
TOI, to´i, wanderer. 2 Sam. 8:9.

TOLA, to´-lah, worm. Gen. 46:13.
TOLAD, to´-lad, birth. 1 Chr. 4:20.
TOLAITES, to´-la-ites, descendants of Tola. Num. 26:23.
TOPHEL, to´-fel, lime. Deut. 1:1.
TOPHET, to´-fet, burning. Is. 30:33.
TOPHETH, to´-feth, same as TOPHET. 2 Kin. 23:10. *See* MOLOCH.
TORMAH, torm´-ah, privily. Judg. 9:31.
TOU, to´-oo, older form of TOI. 1 Chr. 18:9.
TRACHONITIS, tra-ko-ni´-tis, rugged. Luke 3:1.
TROAS, tro´-as, so called from Tros.
visited by Paul. Acts 16:8; 20:5; 2 Cor. 2:12; 2 Tim. 4:13.
TROGYLLIUM, tro-gil´-yum. Acts 20:15.
TROPHIMUS, trof´-im-us, master of the house (?).
companion of Paul. Acts 20:4; 21:29; 2 Tim. 4:20.
TRYPHENA, tri-fe´-nah, delicate. Rom. 16:12.
TRYPHOSA, tri-fo´-sah, delicate. Rom. 16:12.
TUBAL, too´-bal, production (?). Gen. 10:2; Is. 66:19; Ezek. 27:13; 32:26; 38; 39.
TUBAL-CAIN, too´-bal-kane´, producer of weapons (?). Gen. 4:22.
TYCHICUS, tik´-ik-us, fortuitous.
companion of Paul. Acts 20:4; 2 Tim. 4:12; Tit. 3:12.
commended. Eph. 6:21; Col. 4:7.
TYRANNUS, ti-ran´-us, tyrant. Acts 19:9.
TYRE, tire, rock. Josh. 19:29.
its wealth. Ezek. 27.
fall. Ezek. 26:7.
Christ visits coasts of. Matt. 15:21.
Paul lands at. Acts 21:3.
TYRUS, ti´-rus, Latin name of Tyre. Jer. 25:22.

UCAL, oo´-kal, I shall prevail. Prov. 30:1.
UEL, oo´-el, will of God (?). Ezra 10:34.
ULAI, oo´-lai. Dan. 8:2.
ULAM, oo´-lam, foremost. 1 Chr. 7:16.
ULLA, ool´-ah, yoke. 1 Chr. 7:39.
UMMAH, oom´-ah, community. Josh. 19:30.
UNNI, oon´-i, depressed. 1 Chr. 15:18.
UPHARSIN, oo-far´-sin, and dividers. Dan. 5:25.
UPHAZ, oo´-faz, gold of. Jer. 10:9; Dan. 10:5.
UR, oor, light.
land of. Gen. 11:28; 15:7.
URBANE, ur´-ban, pleasant. Rom. 16:9.
URI, oo´-ri, fiery. Ex. 31:2.
URIAH, oo-ri´-ah, light of Jehovah.
the HITTITE. 2 Sam. 11; 1 Kin. 15:5; Matt. 1:6.
URIAS, oo-ri´-as, Greek form of URIAH. Matt. 1:6.
URIEL, oo´-ri-el, light of God. 1 Chr. 6:24.
URIJAH, oo´-ri-jah, same as URIAH.
(priest). 2 Kin. 16:10, 16.
——(prophet). Jer. 26:20.
URIM, oo´-rim, light. Ex. 28:30. *See* THUMMIM.
UTHAI, oo´-thai, helpful. 1 Chr. 9:4.
UZ, fertile. Gen. 10:23.
UZAI, oo´-zai, hoped for (?). Neh. 3:25.
UZAL, ooz´-al, wanderer. Gen. 10:27.
UZZA, ooz´-ah, strength. 2 Kin. 21:18.
UZZAH, another form of UZZA.
his trespass. 2 Sam. 6:3.
his death. 1 Chr. 13:7.
UZZEN-SHERAH, ooz´-en-she´-rah. 1 Chr. 7:24.
UZZI, ooz´-i, shortened form of UZZIAH. 1 Chr. 6:5.
UZZIA, ooz-i´-ah, another form of UZZIAH. 1 Chr. 11:44.
UZZIAH, ooz-i´-ah, might of Jehovah. 2 Kin. 15:13. *See* AZARIAH.
UZZIEL, ooz´-i-el, power of God. Ex. 6:18.
UZZIELITES, ooz´-i-el-ites, descendants of Uzziel. Num. 3:27.

VAJEZATHA, va-je-za´-thah, strong as the wind (?). Esth. 9:9.
VANAIH, va-ni´-ah, distress (?). Ezra 10:36.
VASHNI, vash´-ni, strong (?); but perhaps not a proper name. 1 Chr. 6:28.
VASHTI, vash´-ti, beautiful. Esth. 1:9.
VOPHSI, vof´-si, expansion (?). Num. 13:14.

ZAANAIM, za´-an-a´-im, wanderings (?). Judg. 4:11.
ZAANAN, za´-a-nan, place of flocks. Mic. 1:11.
ZAANANNIM, za´-a-nan´-im, same as ZAANAIM. Josh. 19:33.
ZAAVAN, za´-av-an, disturbed. Gen. 36:27.
ZABAD, za´-bad, gift. 1 Chr. 2:36.
ZABBAI, zab´-ai. Ezra 10:28.
ZABBUD, zab´-ood, given. Ezra 8:14.
ZABDI, zab´-di, the gift of Jehovah. Josh. 7:1.
ZABDIEL, zab´-di-el, the gift of God. 1 Chr. 27:2.
ZABUD, za´-bood, same as ZABBUD. 1 Kin. 4:5.
ZABULON, Greek form of ZEBULUN. Matt. 4:13.
ZACCAI, zak´-ai, pure. Ezra 2:9.
ZACCHÆUS, zak-e´-us, Greek form of ZACCAI. Luke 19:2.
ZACCHUR, zak´-oor, mindful. 1 Chr. 4:26.
ZACCUR, zak´-oor, same as preceding. Num. 13:4.
ZACHARIAH, zak´-ar-i´-ah, whom Jehovah remembers.
last king of Israel of Jehu's race, as foretold by the word of the Lord, begins to reign. 2 Kin. 14:29.
smitten by Shallum, who succeeds him. 2 Kin. 15:10.
ZACHARIAS, zak´-ar-i´-as, Greek form of preceding.
father of John the Baptist, with Elisabeth his wife, accounted righteous before God. Luke 1:6.
is promised a son. Luke 1:13.
doubting, is stricken with dumbness. Luke 1:18, 22.
his recovery and song. Luke 1:64, 68.
——'son of Barachias', slain 'between the temple and the altar'. Matt. 23:35; Luke 11:51. *See* ZECHARIAH.
ZACHER, za´-ker, memorial. 1 Chr. 8:31.
ZADOK, za´-dok, just.
priest. 2 Sam. 8:17; 15:24; 20:25.
anoints Solomon king. 1 Kin. 1:39.
ZAHAM, za´-ham, loathing. 2 Chr. 11:19.
ZAIR, za´-ir, small. 2 Kin. 8:21.
ZALAPH, za´-laf, wound (?). Neh. 3:30.
ZALMON, zal´-mon, shady. 2 Sam. 23:28.
ZALMONAH, zal-mo´-nah, same as preceding. Num. 33:41.
ZALMUNNA, zal-moon´-ah, shelter denied. Judg. 8:5.
ZAMZUMMIMS, zam-zoom´-ims, giant race, destroyed by the Ammonites. Deut. 2:20, 21.
ZANOAH, za-no´-ah, marsh. Josh. 15:34.
ZAPHNATH-PAANEAH, zaf´-nath-pa´-a-ne´-ah, prince of the life of the age. Gen. 41:45.
ZAPHON, za´-fon, north. Josh. 13:27.
ZARA, za´-rah, Greek form of ZARAH. Matt. 1:3.
ZARAH, za´-rah, sunrise (?). Gen. 38:30.
ZAREAH, za´-re-ah, hornet. Neh. 11:29.
ZAREATHITES, za´-re-ath-ites, inhabitants of Zareah. 1 Chr. 2:53.
ZARED, za´-red, exuberant growth. Num. 21:12.
ZAREPHATH, zar´-ef-ath, workshop for refining metals.
(Sarepta), Elijah there. 1 Kin. 17:10. *See* ELIJAH.
ZARETAN, za´-ret-an, same as ZARTHAN. Josh. 3:16.
ZARETH-SHAHAR, za´-reth-sha´-har, the splendour of the morning. Josh. 13:19.
ZARHITES, zar´-hites, persons descended from ZERAH. Num. 26:13.
ZARTANAH, zar-tah´-nah. 1 Kin. 4:12.
ZARTHAN, zar´-than, same as ZARETAN. 1 Kin. 7:46.
ZATTHU, zat´-thoo, same as ZATTU. Neh. 10:14.
ZATTU, zat´-oo, irascible (?). Ezra 2:8.
ZAVAN, za´-van, same as ZAAVAN. 1 Chr. 1:42.
ZAZA, za´-zah. 1 Chr. 2:33.
ZEBADIAH, zeb´-ad-i´-ah, full form of ZABDI. 1 Chr. 8:15.
ZEBAH, ze´-bah, sacrifice.
and Zalmunna. Judg. 8:5, 21; Ps. 83:11.
ZEBAIM, ze-ba´-im, same as ZEBOIM. Ezra 2:57.
ZEBEDEE, zeb´-ed-ee, Greek form of ZEBADIAH. Matt. 4:21; Mark 1:20.

ZEBINA, ze-bi´-nah, bought. Ezra 10:43.
ZEBOIM, ze-bo´-im, gazelles. Gen. 10:19; 14:2; 19:25; Deut. 29:23; Hos. 11:8.
ZEBUDAH, ze-boo´-dah, given. 2 Kin. 23:36.
ZEBUL, ze´-bool, habitation. Judg. 9:28.
ZEBULONITE, ze-bool´-on-ite, a member of the tribe of Zebulun. Judg. 12:11.
ZEBULUN, ze-bool´-un. Gen. 30:20; 35:23; 49:13; Num. 1:30; 26:26; Deut. 33:13; Josh. 19:10; Judg. 4:6; 5:14, 18; 6:35; 2 Chr. 30:11, 18; Ps. 68:27; Ezek. 48:26; Rev. 7:8.
Christ preaches in the land of (Is. 9:1); Matt. 4:13.
ZEBULUNITES, ze-bool´-un-ites, a less correct way of spelling Zebulonites. Num. 26:27.
ZECHARIAH, zek´-ar-i´-ah, a better way of spelling Zachariah.
son of Jehoiada, stoned in the court of the Lord's house. 2 Chr. 24:20, 21.
——son of Jeberechiah. Is. 8:2.
——the prophet, his exhortations to repentance, his visions and predictions. Zech. 1—14.
ZEDAD, ze´-dad, hunting (?). Num. 34:8.
ZEDEKIAH, zed´-ek-i´-ah, justice of Jehovah.
false prophet. 1 Kin. 22:11; 2 Chr. 18:10, 23.
——another. Jer. 29:22.
——(Mattaniah), king of Judah. 2 Kin. 24:17; 25; 2 Chr. 36:10, 11; Jer. 37; 38; 39; 52.
ZEEB, ze´-eb, wolf. Judg. 7:25.
ZELAH, ze´-ah, side. Josh. 18:28.
ZELEK, ze´-lek, fissure. 2 Sam. 23:37.
ZELOPHEHAD, ze-lo´-fe-had, fracture. Num. 26:33.
ZELOTES, ze-lo´-tees, Greek equivalent of Canaanite, an emulator. Luke 6:15.
ZELZAH, zel´-zah, shade in the heat. 1 Sam. 10:2.
ZEMARAIM, zem´-ar-a´-im, two fleeces. Josh. 18:22.
ZEMARITE, zem´-ar-ite. Gen. 10:18.
ZEMIRA, ze-mi´-rah. 1 Chr. 7:8.
ZENAN, ze´-nan, same as ZAANAN. Josh. 15:37.
ZENAS, ze´-nas, contraction of Zenodorus. Tit. 3:13.
ZEPHANIAH, zef´-an-i´-ah, whom Jehovah hid. 2 Kin. 25:18.
priest. Jer. 29:25; 37:3.
——prophet. Zeph. 1; 2; 3.
ZEPHATH, ze´-fath, watch-tower (?). Judg. 1:17.
ZEPHATHAH, ze´-fath-ah. 2 Chr. 14:10.
ZEPHI, ze´-fi, same as ZEPHATH. 1 Chr. 1:36.
ZEPHO, ze´-fo, older form of ZEPHI. Gen. 36:11.
ZEPHON, ze´-fon, a looking out. Num. 26:15.
ZEPHONITES, ze´-fon-ites, descendants of Zephon. Num. 26:15.
ZER, flint (?). Josh. 19:35.
ZERAH, ze´-rah, dawn. 2 Chr. 14:9; 16:8.
ZERAHIAH, zer´-ah-i´-ah, whom Jehovah caused to rise. 1 Chr. 6:6.
ZERED, ze´-red, same as ZARED. Deut. 2:13.
ZEREDA, ze-re´-dah, cool. 1 Kin. 11:26.
ZEREDATHAH, ze-re-dah´-thah, same as preceding. 2 Chr. 4:17.
ZERERATH, ze-re´-rath. Judg. 7:22.
ZERESH, ze´-resh, gold. Esth. 5:10.
ZERETH, ze´-reth, gold (?). 1 Chr. 4:7.
ZERI, ze´-ri, same as IZRI. 1 Chr. 25:3.
ZEROR, ze´-ror, bundle. 1 Sam. 9:1.
ZERUAH, ze-roo´-ah, leprous. 1 Kin. 11:26.
ZERUBBABEL, ze-roob´-ab-el, scattered in Babylon.
(Zorobabel), prince of Judah. Ezra 2:2.
restores the worship of God. Ezra 3:1; Neh. 12:47; Hag. 1:1, 14; 2:1; Zech. 4:6.
ZERUIAH, ze-roo´-yah. 1 Sam. 26:6.
ZETHAM, ze´-tham, olive. 1 Chr. 23:8.
ZETHAN, ze´-than, same as ZETHAM 1 Chr. 7:10.
ZETHAR, ze´-thar. Esth. 1:10.
ZIA, zi´-ah, motion. 1 Chr. 5:13.
ZIBA, zi´-bah, planter. 2 Sam. 9:2.
ZIBEON, zib´-e-on, dyed. Gen. 36:2.
ZIBIA, zib´-i-ah, gazelle (?). 1 Chr. 8:9.
ZIBIAH, zib´-i-ah, same as ZIBIA. 2 Kin. 12:1.
ZICHRI, zik´-ri, famous. 2 Chr. 23:1; 28.
ZIDDIM, zid´-im, sides. Josh. 19:35.
ZIDKIJAH, zid-ki´-jah, justice of Jehovah. Neh. 10:1.
ZIDON, zi´-don, fishing. Gen. 49:13; Josh. 11:8; Judg. 10:6; 18:7; 1 Kin. 11:1; Ezra 3:7; Luke 4:26; Acts 12:20.
prophecies concerning. Is. 23; Jer. 25:22; 27:3; 47:4; Ezek. 27:8; 28:21; 32:30; Joel 3:4; Zech. 9:2.
ZIDONIANS, zi-done´-yans, inhabitants of Zidon. Judg. 10:12; 18:7; 1 Kin. 11:1.
ZIF, blossom. 1 Kin. 6:1.
ZIHA, zi´-hah, drought. Ezra 2:43.
ZIKLAG, zik´-lag. Josh. 15:31; 1 Sam. 27:6; 30:1; 2 Sam. 1:1; 1 Chr. 12:1.
ZILLAH, zil´-ah, shade. Gen. 4:19.
ZILPAH, zil´-pah, dropping. Gen. 29:24.
ZILTHAI, zil´-thai, shady. 1 Chr. 8:20.
ZIMMAH, zim´-ah, planning. 1 Chr. 6:20.
ZIMRAN, zim´-ran, celebrated. Gen. 25:2.
ZIMRI, zim´-ri, same as ZIMRAN. 1 Kin. 16:9.
ZIN, thorn.
wilderness of. Num. 13:21; Josh. 15:1.
ZINA, zi´-nah, abundance (?). 1 Chr. 23:10.
ZION, zi´-on, sunny.
(mount). 2 Sam. 5:7; 1 Kin. 8:1; Rom. 11:26; Heb. 12:22; Rev. 14:1.
ZIOR, zi´-or, smallness. Josh. 15:54.
ZIPH, zif, flowing. 1 Chr. 4:16.
ZIPHUAH, zi´-fah, feminine of ZIPH. 1 Chr. 4:16.
ZIPHIMS, zif´-ims, inhabitants of Ziph. Ps. 54, title.
ZIPHITES, zif´-ites, same as ZIPHIMS. 1 Sam. 23:19.
ZIPHION, zif´-yon, same as ZEPHON. Gen. 46:16.
ZIPHRON, zif´-ron, sweet smell. Num. 34:9.
ZIPPOR, zip´-or, bird. Num. 22:2.
ZIPPORAH, zip-or´-ah, *fem.* of ZIPPOR. Ex. 2:21; 4:20.
ZITHRI, zith´-ri, protection of Jehovah (?). Ex. 6:22.
ZIZ, a flower. 2 Chr. 20:16.
ZIZA, zi´-zah, abundance. 1 Chr. 4:37.
ZIZAH, fulness. 1 Chr. 23:11.
ZOAN, zo´-an, low region. Num. 13:22; Ps. 78:12.
ZOAR, zo´-ar, smallness. Gen. 13:10; 14:2; 19:22 (Is. 15:5); Deut. 34:3; Jer. 48:34.
ZOBA, zo´-bah, a plantation. 2 Sam. 10:6.
ZOBAH, same as preceding.
kings of, subdued. 1 Sam. 14:47; 2 Sam. 8:3; 1 Kin. 11:23.
ZOBEBAH, zo-be´-bah, walking slowly. 1 Chr. 4:8.
ZOHAR, zo´-har, light. Gen. 23:8.
ZOHELETH, zo-he´-eth, serpent stone. 1 Kin. 1:9.
ZOHETH, zo´-heth, strong (?). 1 Chr. 4:20.
ZOPHAH, zo´-fah, a cruse (?). 1 Chr. 7:35.
ZOPHAI, zo´-phai, honeycomb. 1 Chr. 6:26.
ZOPHAR, zo´-far, chatterer. Job. 2:11; 11; 20; 42:9.
ZOPHIM, zo´-fim, watchers. Num. 23:14.
ZORAH, zo´-rah, a place of hornets.
city of Samson. Josh. 19:41; Judg. 13:2, 25; 16:31.
ZORATHITES, zo´-rath-ites, people of Zorah. 1 Chr. 4:2.
ZOREAH, zo´-re-ah, same as ZORAH. Josh. 15:33.
ZORITES, zor´-ites, same as ZORATHITES. 1 Chr. 2:54.
ZOROBABEL, zo-rob´-ab-el, Greek form of ZERUBBABEL. Matt. 1:12.
ZUAR, zoo´-ar, same as ZOAR. Num. 1:8.
ZUPH, zoof, flag, sedge. 1 Sam. 1:1.
ZUR, zoor, rock. Num. 25:15.
ZURIEL, zoor´-i-el, God is the Rock. Num. 3:35.
ZURISHADDAI, zoor´-i-shad´-ai, whose Almighty is the Rock. Num. 1:6.
ZUZIMS, zooz´-ims, giants. Gen. 14:5.

OMEGA, the end. Rev. 1:8, 11; 21:6; 22:13.

SUBJECT–INDEX

TO THE HOLY SCRIPTURES

[1]It is the opinion of some eminent commentators that the sermons on the mount and on the plain were one and the same.

CONCORDANCE

TO THE HOLY SCRIPTURES

ABASE. Ezek. 21:26, and *a.* him that is high.
Dan. 4:37, walk in pride, he is able to *a.*
Mat. 23:12; Lu. 14:11; 18:14, whosoever exalteth himself shall be *a.*
Phil. 4:12, I know how to be *a.*
See Job 40:11; Isa. 31:4; 2 Cor. 11:7.
ABATED. Gen. 8:3; Lev. 27:18; Deut. 34:7; Judg. 8:3.
ABHOR. Ex. 5:21, made our savour to be *a.*
Job 19:19, my inward friends *a.*
Ps. 78:59, Lord wroth, and *a.* Israel.
89:38, thou hast cast off and *a.*
107:18, soul *a.* all manner of meat.
119:163, I hate and *a.* lying.
Prov. 22:14, *a.* of the Lord shall fall there.
Isa. 7:16, land thou *a.* shall be forsaken.
66:24, they shall be an *a.* unto all flesh.
Ezek. 16:25, made thy beauty to be *a.*
Amos 6:8, I *a.* the excellency of Jacob.
See Lev. 26:11; Job 42:6; Rom. 12:9.
ABIDE. Gen. 44:33, let servant *a.* instead of lad.
Ex. 16:29, *a.* every man in his place.
Num. 24:2, he saw Israel *a.* in tents.
31:19, *a.* without camp seven days.
1 Sam. 5:7, ark of God not *a.* with us.
Job 24:13, nor *a.* in the paths thereof.
Ps. 15:1, Lord, who shall *a.* in thy tabernacle.
91:1, shall *a.* under the shadow.
Prov. 15:31, reproof *a.* among wise.
Eccl. 1:4, the earth *a.* for ever.
Jer. 42:10, if ye will still *a.* in this land.
49:18, 33; 50:40, there shall no man *a.*
Hos. 3:3, thou shalt *a.* many days.
Joel 2:11, day very terrible, who can *a.* it.
Mat. 10:11; Mk. 6:10; Lu. 9:4, there *a.* till ye go.
Lu. 2:8, shepherds *a.* in field.
19:5, to-day I must *a.* at thy house.
24:29, *a.* with us, it is toward evening.
John 3:36, wrath of God *a.* on him.
5:38, not his word *a.* in you.
14:16, another Comforter that he may *a.*
15:4, *a.* in me.
5, he that *a.* in me bringeth.
10, *a.* in my love.
Acts 16:15, come to my house and *a.*
1 Cor. 3:14, if any man's work *a.*
13:13, now *a.* faith, hope, charity.
2 Tim. 2:13, if we believe not he *a.*
See Gen. 29:19; Num. 35:25; Eccl. 8:15.
ABILITY. Ezra 2:69, they gave after their *a.*
Dan. 1:4, had *a.* to stand in the palace.
Mat. 25:15, to teach according to *a.*
1 Pet. 4:11, as of the *a.* God giveth.
See Lev. 27:8; Neh. 5:8; Acts 11:29.
ABJECTS. Ps. 35:15, the *a.* gathered themselves together.
ABLE. Deut. 16:17, every man give as he is *a.*
Josh. 23:9, no man *a.* to stand before you.
1 Sam. 6:20, who is *a.* to stand before God.
1 Kings 3:9, who is *a.* to judge.
2 Chron. 2:6, who is *a.* to build.
Prov. 27:4, who is *a.* to stand before envy.
Amos 7:10, land not *a.* to bear his words.
Mat. 3:9, God is *a.* of these stones.
9:28, believe ye that I am *a.*
20:22, are ye *a.* to drink of cup.
Lu. 12:26, not *a.* to do least.
Acts 6:10, not *a.* to resist wisdom.
Rom. 4:21, what he had promised he was *a.*
8:39, *a.* to separate us from love of God.
1 Cor. 10:13, tempted above that ye are *a.*
2 Cor. 3:6, *a.* ministers of new testament.
Eph. 3:18, *a.* to comprehend with all saints.
Phil. 3:21, *a.* to subdue all things.
Heb. 2:18, *a.* to succour tempted.
Jas. 4:12, *a.* to save and destroy.
Jude 24, *a.* to keep you from falling.
Rev. 5:3, no man *a.* to open book.
6:17, who shall be *a.* to stand.
See Ex. 18:21.
ABOARD. Acts 21:2.
ABODE (*n.*). John 14:23, we will come and make our *a.*
See 2 Kings 19:27; Isa. 37:28.
ABODE (*v.*). Gen. 49:24, his bow *a.* in strength.
Ex. 24:16, glory of the Lord *a.* on Sinai.
Judg. 21:2, the people *a.* there before God.
Lu. 1:56, Mary *a.* with her three months.
John 1:32, the Spirit, and it *a.* on him.
39, they came and *a.* with him.
8:44, a murderer, and *a.* not in truth.
Acts 14:3, long time *a.*, speaking boldly.
18:3, Paul *a.* with them and wrought.
See 1 Sam. 7:2; Ezra 8:15.
ABOLISH. 2 Cor. 3:13, the end of that which is *a.*
Eph. 2:15, *a.* in his flesh the enmity.
2 Tim. 1:10, Christ, who hath *a.* death.
See Isa. 2:18; 51:6; Ezek. 6:6.
ABOMINABLE. 1 Kings 21:26, Ahab *a.* in following idols.
Job 15:16, how much more *a.* is man.
Ps. 14:1; 53:1, they have done *a.* works.
Isa. 14:19, cast out like *a.* branch.
65:4; Jer. 16:18, broth of *a.* things.
Jer. 44:4, this *a.* thing that I hate.
Tit. 1:16, in works they deny him, being *a.*
1 Pet. 4:3, walked in *a.* idolatries.
See Lev. 11:43; Deut. 14:3; Rev. 21:8.
ABOMINATION. Gen. 43:32; 46:34, *a.* to Egyptians.
Lev. 18:26, shall not commit any *a.*
Deut. 7:26, nor bring *a.* into house.
18:9, after the *a.* of nations.
12, because of *a.* the Lord doth drive.
25:16, do unrighteously are *a.* to God.
1 Sam. 13:4, Israel had in *a.* with Philistines.
Prov. 3:32; 11:20, froward *a.* to the Lord.
8:7, wickedness an *a.* to my lips.
15, 8, 9, 26; 21:27, sacrifice, etc. of wicked are *a.*
28:9, even his prayer shall be *a.*
Isa. 44:19, residue thereof an *a.*
Jer. 4:1, put away thine *a.* out of sight.
6:15; 8:12, ashamed when committed *a.*
Ezek. 5:9, the like, because of all thine *a.*
33:29, land desolate because of *a.*
Dan. 11:31; Mat. 24:15; Mk. 13:14, *a.* of desolation.
Lu. 16:15, esteemed among men *a.* with God.
Rev. 21:27, in no wise enter that worketh *a.*
See Lev. 7:18; 11:41; Mal. 2:11; Rev. 17:4.
ABOUND. Prov. 28:20, faithful shall *a.* with blessings.
Rom. 15:13, that ye may *a.* in hope.
1 Cor. 15:58, always *a.* in work.
2 Cor. 1:5, as sufferings *a.* so consolation *a.*
See Rom. 3:7; 5:15; Phil. 4:12.
ABOVE. Deut. 28:13, *a.* only and not beneath.
Job 31:2, portion of God from *a.*
Prov. 15:24, way of life *a.* to wise.

Mat. 10:24; Lu. 6:40, disciple not *a.* master.
John 3:31, cometh from *a.* is *a.* all.
8:23, I am from *a.*
Rom. 14:5, one day *a.* another.
1 Cor. 4:6, *a.* that which is written.
Gal. 4:26, Jerusalem *a.* is free.
See Gen. 48:22; Ps. 138:2; Jas. 1:17.
ABSENT. 1 Cor. 5:3; Col. 2:5, *a.* in body.
2 Cor. 5:6, *a.* from Lord.
See Gen. 31:49; 2 Cor. 10:1.
ABSTAIN. Acts 15:20, 29, *a.* from pollutions of idols.
1 Thess. 5:22, *a.* from all appearance of evil.
1 Pet. 2:11, *a.* from fleshly lusts.
See 1 Thess. 4:3; 1 Tim. 4:3.
ABSTINENCE. Acts 27:21, after long *a.* Paul stood forth.
ABUNDANCE. 1 Sam. 1:16, out of *a.* of my complaint.
1 Kings 18:41, sound of *a.* of rain.
1 Chron. 29:21, offered sacrifices in *a.*
Ps. 52:7, trusted in *a.* of riches.
72:7; Jer. 33:6, *a.* of peace.
Eccl. 5:10, loveth *a.* with increase.
12, *a.* of rich not suffer to sleep.
Mat. 12:34; Lu. 6:45, out of *a.* of heart.
13:12; 25:29, he shall have more *a.*
Lu. 12:15, life consisteth not in *a.*
2 Cor. 8:2, of affliction the *a.* of their joy.
12:7, through *a.* of revelations.
See Job 36:31; Rom. 5:17; Rev. 18:3.
ABUNDANT. Job 36:28, clouds drop and distil *a.*
Ps. 145:7, *a.* utter the memory.
Isa. 56:12, as this day and more *a.*
1 Cor. 15:10; 2 Cor. 11:23, laboured more *a.* than all.
1 Tim. 1:14, grace was exceeding *a.*
Tit. 3:6, shed *a.* through Jesus Christ.
2 Pet. 1:11, entrance administered *a.*
See Ex. 31:6; Isa. 55:7; 1 Pet. 1:3.
ABUSE. 1 Cor. 7:31, use world as not *a.*
9:18, that I *a.* not my power.
See 1 Sam. 31:4; 1 Chron. 10:4.
ACCEPT. Gen. 4:7, shalt thou not be *a.*
Ex. 28:38; Lev. 10:19, *a.* before the Lord.
Deut. 33:11, *a.* the work of his hands.
1 Sam. 18:5, *a.* in sight of all people.
2 Sam. 24:23, the Lord thy God *a.* thee.
Esth. 10:3, *a.* of his brethren.
Job 13:8; 32:21, will ye *a.* his person.
42:8, 9, him will I *a.*
Prov. 18:5, not good to *a.* wicked.
Jer. 14:12; Amos 5:22, I will not *a.* them.
37:20; 42:2, supplication be *a.*
Ezek. 20:40; 43:27, I will *a.*
Mal. 1:13, should I *a.* this.
Lu. 4:24, no prophet is *a.*
Acts 10:35, he that worketh righteousness is *a.*
Rom. 15:31, service *a.* of saints.
2 Cor. 5:9, present or absent we may be *a.*
See Ps. 119:108; Eccl. 12:10; Mal. 1:8.
ACCESS. Rom. 5:2; Eph. 2:18; 3:12.
ACCOMPLISH. Job 14:6, *a.* as an hireling.
Ps. 64:6, they *a.* diligent search.
Prov. 13:19, desire *a.* is sweet.
Isa. 40:2, her warfare is *a.*
Lu. 12:50, straitened till it be *a.*
1 Pet. 5:9, afflictions are *a.* in brethren.
See Isa. 55:11; Lu. 18:31; 22:37.
ACCORD. Acts 1:14; 4:24; 8:6; Phil. 2:2.
ACCORDING. Ex. 12:25, *a.* as he hath promised.
Deut. 16:10, *a.* as God hath blessed thee.
Job 34:11; Jer. 17:10; 25:14; 32:19, *a.* to ways.
Mat. 16:27; Rom. 2:6; 2 Tim. 4:14, *a.* to works.
John 7:24, *a.* to the appearance.
Rom. 8:28, called *a.* to his purpose.
12:6, gifts differing *a.* to grace.
2 Cor. 8:12, *a.* to that a man hath.
See Mat. 9:29; Tit. 3:5.
ACCOUNT. Mat. 12:36, give *a.* in day of judgment.
Lu. 16:2, give *a.* of stewardship.
Lu. 20:35, *a.* worthy to obtain.
Rom. 14:12, every one give *a.* to God.
Gal. 3:6, *a.* to him for righteousness.
Heb. 13:17, watch as they that give *a.*
See Job 33:13; Ps. 144:3; 1 Pet. 4:5.
ACCURSED. Josh. 6:18; 7:1; 22:20; 1 Chron. 2:7, *a.* thing.
Rom. 9:3, wish myself *a.* from Christ.
1 Cor. 12:3, no man calleth Jesus *a.*
Gal. 1:8, 9, preach other gospel, let him be *a.*
See Deut. 21:23; Josh. 6:17; Isa. 65:20.
ACCUSATION. Lu. 19:8, anything by false *a.*
1 Tim. 5:19, against elder receive not *a.*
2 Pet. 2:11; Jude 9, railing *a.*
See Mat. 27:37; Mk. 15:26; Lu. 6:7.
ACCUSE. Prov. 30:10, *a.* not servant to his master.
Mat. 27:12, when *a.* he answered nothing.
Lu. 16:1, was *a.* that he had wasted.
John 5:45, I will *a.* you to the Father.
Tit. 1:6, not *a.* of riot or unruly.
See Mat. 12:10; Mk. 3:2; Lu. 11:54; Rev. 12:10.
ACKNOWLEDGE. Ps. 32:5; 51:3, I *a.* my sin.
Prov. 3:6, in all thy ways *a.* him.
Isa. 63:16, though Israel *a.* us not.
1 John 2:23, he that *a.* the Son.
See Dan. 11:39; Hos. 5:15.
ACQUAINT. Job 22:21; Ps. 139:3; Eccl. 2:3; Isa. 53:3.
ACQUAINTANCE. Job. 19:13; Ps. 31:11; 55:13.
ACQUIT. Job 10:14; Nah. 1:3.
ACTIONS. 1 Sam. 2:3.
ACTIVITY. Gen. 47:6.
ADDER. Gen. 49:17; Ps. 58:4; 91:13; 140:3; Prov. 23:32.
ADDICTED. 1 Cor. 16:15.
ADDITION. 1 Kings 7:29, 30, 36.
ADJURE. Josh. 6:26; 1 Sam. 14:24; 1 Kings 22:16; 2 Chron. 18:15; Mat. 26:63; Mk. 5:7; Acts 19:13.
ADMINISTER. 1 Cor. 12:5; 2 Cor. 8:19, 20; 9:12.
ADMIRE. 2 Thess. 1:10; Jude 16; Rev. 17:6.
ADMONISH. Acts 27:9, Paul *a.* them.
Rom. 15:14; Col. 3:16, *a.* one another.
1 Thess. 5:12, over you in Lord, and *a.* you.
2 Thess. 3:15, *a.* him as a brother.
Heb. 8:5, Moses was *a.* of God.
See Eccl. 4:13; 12:12; Jer. 42:19.
ADMONITION. 1 Cor. 10:11; Eph. 6:4; Tit. 3:10.
ADO. Mk. 5:39.
ADOPTION. Rom. 8:15, 23; 9:4; Gal. 4:5; Eph. 1:5.
ADORN. Isa. 61:10; Rev. 21:2, bride *a.* herself.
1 Tim. 2:9; 1 Pet. 3:3, 5, women *a.*
Tit. 2:10. *a.* doctrine of God.
See Jer. 31:4; Lu. 21:5.
ADVANCED. 1 Sam. 12:6; Esth. 3:1; 5:11; 10:2.
ADVANTAGE. Lu. 9:25, what is a man *a.*
Rom. 3:1; 1 Cor. 15:32, what *a.*?
2 Cor. 2:11, lest Satan get *a.*
See Job 35:3; Jude 16.
ADVENTURE. Deut. 28:56; Judg. 9:17; Acts 19:31.
ADVERSARY. Deut. 32:43; Ps. 89:42; Isa. 59:18; Jer. 46:10; Nah. 1:2; Lu. 13:17, his *a.*
Ex. 23:22, I will be *a.* to thy *a.*
Num. 22:22, angel stood for *a.*
1 Kings 5:4, neither *a.* nor evil.
11:14, 23, Lord stirred up *a.*
Job 31:35, that mine *a.* had written.
Ps. 38:20; 69:19; 109:4, 20, 29; Isa. 1:24, my *a.*
74:10, how long shall *a.* reproach.
Isa. 50:8, who is mine *a.*
64:2; Jer. 30:16; Mic. 5:9, thy *a.*
Amos 3:11, *a.* shall be round the land.
Mat. 5:25, agree with thine *a.*
Lu. 12:58, when thou goest with thine *a.*
1 Cor. 16:9, there are many *a.*
Phil. 1:28, terrified by your *a.*
1 Tim. 5:14, give no occasion to *a.*
Heb. 10:27, indignation shall devour *a.*
1 Pet. 5:8, 9, because your *a.* the devil.
See 1 Sam. 2:10; Isa. 9:11; 11:13.
ADVERSITY. 1 Sam. 10:19; 2 Sam. 4:9; 2 Chron. 15:6, all *a.*

Ps. 10:6, I shall never be in *a.*
94:13; Prov. 24:10; Eccl. 7:14, day of *a.*
Prov. 17:17, brother is born for *a.*
Isa. 30:20, bread of *a.*
Heb. 13:3, remember them which suffer *a.*
See Ps. 31:7; 35:15.
ADVERTISE. Num. 24:14; Ruth 4:4.
ADVICE. 1 Sam. 25:33, blessed be thy *a.*
2 Sam. 19:43, that our *a.* should not be first.
2 Chron. 10:9, 14, what *a.* give ye.
Prov. 20:18, with good *a.* make war.
2 Cor. 8:10, herein I give my *a.*
See Judg. 19:30; 20:7; 2 Chron. 25:17.
ADVISE. Prov. 13:10, with the well *a.* is wisdom.
Acts 27:12, the more part *a.* to depart.
See 2 Sam. 24:13; 1 Kings 12:6; 1 Chron. 21:12.
ADVISEMENT. 1 Chron. 12:19.
ADVOCATE. 1 John 2:1, an *a.* with the Father.
AFAR-OFF. Jer. 23:23, a God *a.*
30:10; 46:27, I will save them from *a.*
Mat. 26:58; Mk. 14:54; Lu. 22:54, followed *a.*
Acts 2:39, promise to all *a.*
Eph. 2:17, preached to you *a.*
Heb. 11:13, seen the promises *a.*
See Gen. 22:4; Ezra 3:13.
AFFAIRS. 1 Chron. 26:32, pertaining to God and *a.* of king.
2 Tim. 2:4, entangleth himself with *a.*
See Dan. 2:49; 3:12; Eph. 6:21, 22.
AFFECTED. Acts 14:2, minds evil *a.* against brethren.
Gal. 4:17, 18 zealously *a.*
See Lam. 3:51.
AFFECTION. 1 Chron. 29:3, have set *a.* to house of God.
Rom. 1:26, vile *a.*
31; 2 Tim. 3:3, without natural *a.*
12:10, be kindly *a.* one to another.
Gal. 5:24, crucified with *a.*
Col. 3:2, set your *a.* on things above.
5, inordinate *a.*
See 2 Cor. 7:15.
AFFINITY. 1 Kings 3:1; 2 Chron. 18:1; Ezra 9:14.
AFFIRM. Acts 25:19, Jesus, whom Paul *a.* to be alive.
See Rom. 3:8; 1 Tim. 1:7; Tit. 3:8.
AFFLICT. Lev. 16:29, 31; Num. 29:7; Isa. 58:3, 5, *a.* your souls.
Num. 11:11, wherefore hast thou *a.*
Ruth 1:21, Almighty hath *a.* me.
1 Kings 11:39, I will *a.* seed of David.
2 Chron. 6:26; 1 Kings 8:35, turn when thou dost *a.*
Job 6:14, to *a.* pity should be showed.
Ps. 44:2, how thou didst *a.* people.
55:19, God shall hear and *a.*
82:3, do justice to the *a.*
90:15, the days wherein thou hast *a.*
119:67, before I was *a.*
140:12, maintain cause of *a.*
Prov. 15:15, days of the *a.* evil.
22:22, neither oppress the *a.*
31:5, pervert judgment of *a.*
Isa. 51:21, hear thou *a.* and drunken.
53:4, 7, smitten of God and *a.*
54:11, thou *a.* tossed with tempest.
63:9, in all their *a.* he was *a.*
Lam. 1:5, 12, the Lord hath *a.*
Nah. 1:12, I will *a.* no more.
Zeph. 3:12, I will leave an *a.* people.
2 Cor. 1:6, *a.* it is for consolation.
1 Tim. 5:10, if she have relieved the *a.*
Heb. 11:37, destitute, *a.*, tormented.
Jas. 4:9, be *a.* and mourn and weep.
5:13, is any *a.*, let him pray.
See Ex. 1:11, 12; 22:22, 23.
AFFLICTION. Gen. 29:32; Deut. 26:7; Ps. 25:18, looked on *a.*
Ex. 3:7; Acts 7:10, 11, 34, have seen *a.* of people.
Deut. 16:3; 1 Kings 22:27; 2 Chron. 18:26, bread of *a.*
2 Chron. 20:9, cry to thee in *a.*
33:12, in *a.* besought the Lord.
Job 5:6, *a.* cometh not forth of the dust.
30:16, 27, days of *a.*
Job 36:8, cords of *a.*
Ps. 34:19, many are *a.* of righteous.
119:50, this my comfort in *a.*
132:1 remember David and all his *a.*
Isa. 30:20, water of *a.*
48:10, furnace of *a.*
Jer. 16:19, refuge in day of *a.*
Lam. 3:1 man that hath seen *a.*
Hos. 5:15, in their *a.* they will seek.
Mk. 4:17, *a.* ariseth for the word's sake.
Acts 20:23, bonds and a abide me.
2 Cor. 2:4, out of much *a.* I wrote.
4:17, light *a.* for moment.
8:2, great trial of *a.*
Phil. 1:16, add *a.* to bonds.
Heb. 10:32, great fight of *a.*
11:25, suffer *a.* with people.
Jas. 1:27, visit fatherless in *a.*
See 2 Kings 14:26; Col. 1:24.
AFFRIGHT. Isa. 21:4, fearfulness *a.* me.
Mk. 16:5; Lu. 24:37, they were *a.*
Mk. 16:6, be not *a.* ye seek Jesus.
See Deut. 7:21; 2 Chron. 32:18; Jer. 51:32.
AFOOT. Mk. 6:33; Acts 20:13.
AFORETIME. Dan. 6:10, prayed as *a.*
Rom. 15:4, things were written *a.*
See Isa. 52:4; Jer. 30:20.
AFRAID. Mat. 14:27; Mk. 5:36; 6:50; John 6:20, be not *a.*
Gen. 20:8; Ex. 14:10; Mk. 9:6; Lu. 2:9, sore *a.*
Lev. 26:6; Job 11:19; Isa. 17:2; Ezek. 34:28; Mic. 4:4; Zeph. 3:13, none make *a.*
Judg. 7:3, whosoever is fearful and *a.*
1 Sam. 18:29, Saul yet the more *a.*
Neh. 6:9, they all made us *a.*
Job 3:25, that I was *a.* of is come.
9:28, I am *a.* of sorrows.
Ps. 27:1, of whom shah I be *a.*
56:3, 11, what time I am *a.*
65:8, *a.* at thy tokens.
91:5, *a.* for terror by night.
112:7, *a.* of evil tidings.
Isa. 51:12, be *a.* of a man that shall die.
Mk. 9:32; 10:32, *a.* to ask him.
John 19:8, Pilate was more *a.*
Gal. 4:11, I am *a.* of you.
Heb. 11:23, not *a.* of commandment.
See Deut. 1:17; Ps. 3:6.
AFRESH. Heb. 6:6.
AFTERNOON. Judg. 19:8.
AFTERWARDS. 1 Sam 24:5, *a.* David's heart smote him.
Ps. 73:24, *a.* receive me to glory.
Prov. 20:17, deceit sweet, but *a.*
24:27, prepare work and *a.* build.
29:11, wise man keepeth till *a.*
John 13:36, thou shalt follow me *a.*
1 Cor. 15:23, *a.* they that are Christ's.
See Ex. 11:1; Mat. 21:32; Gal. 3:23.
AGAINST. Lu. 2:34; Acts 19:36; 28:22, spoken *a.*
See Gen. 16:12; Mat. 12:30; Lu. 11:23.
AGATE. Ex. 28:19; 39:12, an *a.*
Isa. 54:12, make thy windows of *a.*
Ezek. 27:16, and *a.*
AGED. 2 Sam. 19:32; Job 15:10; Tit. 2:2, *a.* men.
Philem. 9, Paul the *a.*
See Job 12:20; 29:8; 32:9.
AGES. Eph. 2:7; 3:5, 21; Col. 1:26.
AGONE. 1 Sam. 30:13.
AGONY. Lu. 22:44.
AGREE. Amos 3:3, except they be *a.*
Mat. 5:25, *a.* with adversary.
18:19, two of you shall *a.*
Mk. 14:56, 59, witness *a.* not.
Acts 15:15, to this *a.* words of the prophets.
1 John 5:8, these three *a.* in one.
See Mat. 20:2; Lu. 5:36; Acts 5:9; Rev. 17:17.
AGREEMENT. Isa. 28:15; 2 Cor. 6:16.
AGROUND. Acts 27:41.

AHA. Ps. 35:21; 40:15; 70:3; Isa. 44:16; Ezek. 25:3; 26:2; 36:2.
AILETH. Gen. 21:17; Judg. 18:23; 1 Sam. 11:5; 2 Sam. 14:5; Ps. 114:5; Isa. 22:1.
AIR. Job 41:16, no *a.* can come between.
1 Cor. 9:26, as one that beateth the *a.*
14:9, ye shall speak into *a.*
1 Thess. 4:17, meet Lord in *a.*
See 2 Sam. 21:10; Eccl. 10:20; Acts 22:23; Rev. 9:2.
ALARM (how sounded). Num. 10:5, when ye blow an *a.*
Jer. 4:19; 49:2, *a.* of war.
Joel 2:1, sound *a.* in holy mountain.
See 2 Chron. 13:12; Zeph. 1:16.
ALAS. 2 Kings 6:5, 15, *a.* my master.
Ezek. 6:11, stamp and say *a.*
See Num. 24:23; Jer. 30:7; Rev. 18:10.
ALBEIT. Ezek. 13:7; Philem. 19.
ALIEN. Deut. 14:21, sell it to an *a.*
Ps. 69:8, an *a.* unto my mother's children.
Eph. 2:12, *a.* from commonwealth.
Heb. 11:34, armies of the *a.*
See Ex. 18:3; Job 19:15; Isa. 61:5; Lam. 5:2.
ALIENATED. Ezek. 23:17; Eph. 4:18; Col. 1:21.
ALIKE. Job 21:26, lie down *a.* in dust.
Ps. 33:15, fashioneth hearts *a.*
Eccl. 9:2, things cometh *a.* to all.
See Ps. 139:12; Eccl. 11:6; Rom. 14:5.
ALIVE. Lev. 16:10, scapegoat presented *a.*
Num. 16:33, went down *a.* into pit.
Deut. 4:4, are *a.* every one of you.
32:39; 1 Sam. 2:6, I kill and I make *a.*
Ezek. 13:18; 18:27, save soul *a.*
Mk. 16:11, heard that he was *a.*
Lu. 15:24, 32, son was dead and is *a.*
24:23, angels who. said he was *a.*
Acts 1:3, showed himself *a.*
Rom. 6:11, 13 *a.* to God.
1 Cor. 15:22, all be made *a.*
1 Thess. 4:15, we who are *a.* and remain.
Rev. 1:18, I am *a.* for evermore.
See 2 Kings 5:7; Dan. 5:19; Rev. 2:8; 19:20.
ALLEGING. Acts 17:3.
ALLEGORY. Gal. 4:24, which things are an *a.*
ALLOW. Lu. 11:48; Acts 24:25; Rom. 7:15; 14:22.
ALLOWANCE. 2 Kings 25:30.
ALL THINGS. 1 Cor. 6:12, *a.* are lawful, but not expedient.
ALLURE. Hos. 2:14; 2 Pet. 2:18.
ALMIGHTY. Ex. 6:3, by the name of God *A.*
Job 11:7, canst thou find out the *A.*
29:5, when *A.*was yet with me.
Ezek. 1:24; 10:5, I heard as voice of *A.*
Rev. 1:8; 4:8; 11:17, *A.* who was, and is.
See Gen. 17:1; Job 21:15; Ps. 91:1.
ALMS. Mat. 6:1; Lu. 11:41; 12:33; Acts 10:2.
ALMOND. Num. 17:8, and yielded *a.*
Jer. 1:11, a rod of an *a.* tree.
Eccl. 12:5, *a.* tree shall flower.
ALOES. Ps. 45:8, smell of .... and *a.*
Cant. 4:14, *a.*, with all the chief spices.
John 19:39, a mixture of myrrh and *a.*
ALONE. Num. 11:14; Deut. 1:9, bear all these people *a.*
1 Kings 11:29, they two *a.* in field.
Job 1:15, escaped *a.* to tell.
Ps. 136:4, *a.* doeth great wonders.
Mat. 4:4; Lu. 4:4, not live by bread *a.*
Lu. 9:18, 36; John 6:15, Jesus was *a.*
13:8, let *a.* this year also.
See Gen. 2:18; Mat. 18:15; Jas. 2:17.
ALREADY. Eccl. 1:10; Mal. 2:2; John 3:18; Phil. 3:16.
ALTAR. Mat. 5:23, bring gift to *a.*
23:18, swear by *a.*
1 Cor. 9:13; 10:18, wait at *a.*
Heb. 13:10, we have an *a.*
See 1 Kings 13:2; Isa. 19:19; Acts 17:23.
ALTER. Ps. 89:34, nor *a.* thing gone out of my lips.
Lu. 9:29, fashion of countenance *a.*
See Lev. 27:10; Dan. 6:8.
ALTOGETHER. Ps. 14:3; 53:3, *a.* become filthy.
Ps. 50:21, *a.* such an one as thyself.
Cant. 5:16, he is *a.* lovely.
See Ps. 19:9; 39:5; 139:4.
ALWAYS. Job 7:16, I would not live *a.*
Ps. 103:9, not *a.* chide.
Mat. 28:20, I am with you *a.*
Mk. 14:7; John 12:8, me ye have not *a.*
Phil. 4:4, rejoice in Lord *a.*
See Ps. 16:8; Isa. 57:16; John 11:42.
AMAZED. Mat. 19:25, disciples exceedingly *a.*
Mk. 2:12; Lu. 5:26, *a.*, and glorified God.
14:33, he began to be sore *a.*
Lu. 9:43, *a.* at mighty power of God.
See Ezek. 32:10; Acts 3:10; 1 Pet. 3:6.
AMBASSADORS. 2 Chron. 32:31, the business of the *a.*
2 Cor. 5:20, we are *a.* for Christ.
See Prov. 13:17; Isa. 18:2; 33:7; Jer. 49:14; Obad. 1; Eph. 6:20.
AMBER. Ezek. 1:4, 27; 8:2, as the colour of *a.*
AMEN (tantamount to an oath). Num. 5:22, the woman shall say, *A.*
Deut. 27:15-26, the people shall say, *A.*
Ps. 41:13; 72:19; 89:52, *A.* and *A.*
106:48, let all the people say, *A.*
Mat. 6:13, and the glory for ever, *A.*
1 Cor. 14:16, of the unlearned say, *A.*
2 Cor. 1:20, and in him, *A.*
Rev. 3:14, These things saith the *A.*
See Rev. 22:20.
AMEND. Jer. 7:3; 26:13; 35:15; John 4:52.
AMIABLE. Ps. 84:1.
AMISS. 2 Chron. 6:37; Dan. 3:29; Lu. 23:41; Jas. 4:3.
ANCHOR. Heb. 6:19, have as an *a.* of the soul.
ANCIENT OF DAYS. Dan. 7:22, until the *a.* came.
ANGEL. Gen. 48:16, the *A.* who redeemed me.
Ps. 34:7, *a.* of Lord encampeth.
78:25, man did eat *a.* food.
Eccl. 5:6, nor say before *a.* it was error.
Isa. 63:9, *a.* of his presence saved them.
Hos. 12:4, he had power over *a.*
Mat. 13:39, reapers are the *a.*
Mk. 12:25; Lu. 20:36, are as *a.* in heaven.
Lu. 22:43, an *a.* strengthening him.
John 5:4, *a.* went down at a certain season.
Acts 12:15, it is his *a.*
1 Cor. 6:3, we shall judge *a.*
2 Cor. 11:14, transformed into *a.* of light.
Heb. 2:2, word spoken by *a.*
16, not nature of *a.*
13:2, entertained *a.* unawares.
1 Pet. 1:12, *a.* desire to look into.
See Gen. 19:1; Ps. 8:5; Mat. 25:41; Heb. 2:7.
ANGER. Gen. 49:7, cursed be their *a.*
Neh. 9:17, slow to *a.*
Ps. 6:1; Jer. 10:24, rebuke me not in *a.*
30:5, *a.* endureth but a moment.
Prov. 15:1, grievous words stir up *a.*
19:11, discretion deferreth *a.*
Eccl. 7:9, *a.* resteth in bosom of fools.
Mk. 3:5, he looked on them with *a.*
Col. 3:8, put off *a.*, wrath, malice.
See Ps. 37:8; 85:3; 90:7; Prov. 16:32.
ANGRY. Ps. 7:11, God is *a.* with the wicked.
Prov. 14:17, he that is soon *a.*
22:24, make no friendship with *a.* man.
25:23, so doth an *a.* countenance.
Jon. 4:4, doest thou well to be *a.*
Mat 5:22, whosoever is *a.* with brother.
John 7:23, are ye *a.* at me.
Eph. 4:26, be *a.* and sin not.
Tit. 1:7, bishop not soon *a.*
See Gen. 18:30; Prov. 21:19; Eccl. 5:6; 7:9.
ANGUISH. Ex. 6:9, hearkened not for *a.*
Job 7:11, I will speak in *a.* of spirit.
Rom. 2:9, tribulation and *a.* on every soul.
2 Cor. 2:4, out of much *a.* of heart.
See Gen. 42:21; Isa. 8:22; John 16:21.
ANOINT. Deut. 28:40; 2 Sam. 14:2, *a.* not thyself.

Lu. 16:3, to beg. I am *a.*
Rom. 1:16, not *a.* of Gospel.
5:5, hope maketh not *a.*
9:33; 10:11, believeth shall not be *a.*
2 Tim. 1:8, not *a.* of testimony.
2:15, workman that needeth not to be *a.*
Heb. 2:11, not *a.* to call them brethren.
11:16, not *a.* to be called their God.
1 Pet. 4:16, suffer as Christian, not be *a.*
See Gen. 2:25; 2 Tim. 1:12.
ASHES. Gen. 18:27, which am but dust and *a.*
Job 2:8, and he sat down among the *a.*
13:12, remembrances are like unto *a.*
30:19, and become like dust and *a.*
42:6, and repent in dust and *a.*
Ps. 102:9, I have eaten *a.* like bread.
Isa. 44:20, he feedeth on *a.*
Jon. 3:6, king sat in *a.*
Heb. 9:13, if the *a.* of an heifer.
See 2 Sam. 13:19; Esth. 4:1; Isa. 58:5; Mat. 11:21.
ASIDE. 2 Kings 4:4; Mk. 7:33; Heb. 12:1.
ASK. Ps. 2:8; Isa. 45:11, *a.* of me.
Isa. 65:1, sought of them that *a.* not.
Mat. 7:7; Lu. 11:9, *a.* and it shall be given.
21:22, whatsoever ye *a.*
Mk. 6:22, *a.* what thou wilt.
John 14:13; 15:16, *a.* in my name.
Jas. 1:5, let him *a.* of God.
1 Pet. 3:15, *a.* reason of hope.
1 John 3:22; 5:14, whatsoever we *a.*
See Deut. 32:7; John 4:9, 10; 1 Cor. 14:35.
ASLEEP. Mat. 8:24; Mk. 4:38, but he was *a.*
26:40; Mk. 14:40, disciples *a.*
1 Cor. 15:6, some are fallen *a.*
1 Thess. 4:13, 15, them that are *a.*
2 Pet. 3:4, since fathers fell *a.*
See Cant. 7:9.
ASP. Deut. 32:33, the cruel venom of *a.*
Job 20:14, 16, it is the gall of *a.*
Isa. 11:8, play on the hole of the *a.*
Rom. 3:13, the poison of *a.*
ASS. Num. 22:30, am not I thine *a.*
Prov. 26:3, bridle for *a.*
Isa. 1:3, *a.* his master's crib.
Jer. 22:19, burial of an *a.*
Zech. 9:9; Mat. 21:5, riding on *a.*
Lu. 14:5, *a.* fallen into pit.
2 Pet. 2:16, dumb *a.* speaking.
See Gen. 49:14; Ex. 23:4; Deut. 22:10.
ASSAULT. Esth. 8:11; Acts 14:5; 17:5.
ASSAY. Acts 9:26, Saul *a.* to join disciples.
16:7, their *a.* to go to Bithynia.
Heb. 11:29, Egyptians *a.* to do.
See Deut. 4:34; 1 Sam. 17:39; Job 4:2.
ASSENT. 2 Chron. 18:12; Acts 24:9.
ASSIGNED. Gen. 47:22; Josh. 20:8; 2 Sam. 11:16.
ASSIST. Rom. 16:2.
ASSOCIATE. Isa. 8:9.
ASSURANCE. Isa. 32:17, effect of righteousness *a.*
Col. 2:2, full *a.* of understanding.
1 Thess. 1:5, gospel came in much *a.*
Heb. 6:11; 10:22, full *a.* of hope.
See Deut. 28:66; Acts 17:31.
ASSURE. 2 Tim. 3:14; 1 John 3:19.
ASSWAGE. Gen. 8:1; Job 16:5.
ASTONIED. Ezra 9:3; Job 17:8; Dan. 3:24; 4:19.
ASTONISHED. Mat. 7:28; 22:33; Mk. 1:22; 6:2; 11:18; Lu. 4:32, *a.* at his doctrine.
Lu. 2:47, *a.* at his understanding.
5:9, *a.* at draught of fishes.
24:22, women made us *a.*
Acts 9:6, Saul trembling and *a.*
12:16, saw Peter, they were *a.*
13:12, deputy believed, being *a.*
See Job 26:11; Jer. 2:12.
ASTONISHMENT. 2 Chron. 29:8; Jer. 25:9, *a.* and hissing.
Ps. 60:3, made us drink wine of *a.*
Jer. 8:21, *a.* hath taken hold.
See Deut. 28:28, 37; Ezek. 5:15.
ASTROLOGERS. Isa. 47:13, let now the *a.*
Dan. 2:2; 4:7; 5:7, the *a.*
ATHIRST. Mat. 25:44; Rev. 21:6; 22:17.
ATONEMENT. Lev. 23:28; 25:9, a day of *a.*
2 Sam. 21:3, wherewith shall I make *a.*
Rom. 5:11, by whom we received *a.*
See Lev. 4:20; 16:17; Num. 8:21.
ATTAIN. Ps. 139:6, I cannot *a.* to it.
2 Sam. 23:19; 1 Chron. 11:26, he *a.* not to first three.
Rom. 9:30, Gentiles *a.* to righteousness.
Phil. 3:11, 12, 16, that I might *a.*
See Gen. 47:9; Prov. 1:5; Ezek. 46:7; 1 Tim. 4:6.
ATTEND. Ps. 17:1; 61:1; 142:6, *a.* to my cry.
Prov. 4:20, my son *a.* to my words.
See Ps. 55:2; 86:6.
ATTENDANCE. 1 Tim. 4:13; Heb. 7:13.
ATTENT. 2 Chron. 6:40; 7:15.
ATTENTIVE. Neh. 1:6; Job 37:2; Ps. 130:2; Lu. 19:48.
ATTIRE. Jer. 2:32; Ezek. 23:15.
AUDIENCE. 1 Chron. 28:8, in *a.* of our God.
Lu. 7:1; 20:45, in *a.* of people.
Acts 13:16, ye that fear God give *a.*
See Ex. 24:7; Acts 15:12.
AUGMENT. Num. 32:14.
AUSTERE. Lu. 19:21.
AUTHOR. 1 Cor. 14:33; Heb. 5:9; 12:2.
AUTHORITY. Mat. 7:29; Mk. 1:22, as one having *a.*
8:9; Lu. 7:8, I am a man under *a.*
21:23; Lu. 4:36, by what *a.*
Lu. 9:1, power and *a.* over devils.
19:17, have *a.* over ten cities.
John 5:27, *a.* to execute judgment.
1 Cor. 15:24, put down all *a.*
1 Tim. 2:2, kings and all in *a.*
12, suffer not a woman to usurp *a.*
Tit. 2:15, rebuke with all *a.*
1 Pet. 3:22, angels and *a.* subject.
See Prov. 29:2; 2 Cor. 10:8; Rev. 13:2.
AVAILETH. Esth. 5:13; Gal. 5:6; Jas. 5:16.
AVENGE. Deut. 32:43, he will *a.* blood.
Josh. 10:13, sun stayed till people *a.*
1 Sam. 24:12, the Lord judge and *a.*
2 Sam. 22:48; Ps. 18:47, it is God that *a.* me.
Esth. 8:13, Jews *a.* themselves.
Isa. 1:24, I will *a.* me of mine enemies.
Lu. 18:3, *a.* me of my adversary.
See Gen. 4:24; Lev. 19:18; Jer. 5:9; 9:9.
AVENGER. Ps. 8:2; 44:16, enemy and *a.*
1 Thess. 4:6, the Lord is. the *a.*
See Num. 35:12; Deut. 19:6; Josh. 20:5.
AVERSE. Mic. 2:8.
AVOID. Prov. 4:15, *a.* it, pass not by it.
1 Tim. 6:20; 2 Tim. 2:23; Tit. 3:9, *a.* babblings.
See Rom. 16:17; 2 Cor. 8:20.
AVOUCHED. Deut. 26:17, 18.
AWAKE. Ps. 17:15, when I *a.*, with thy likeness.
73:20, as a dream when one *a.*
Prov. 23:35, *a.* I will seek it again.
Isa. 51:9, *a.*, *a.*, put on strength.
Joel 1:5, *a.* ye drunkards.
Zech. 13:7, *a.* O sword.
Lu. 9:32, when *a.* they saw his glory.
Rom. 13:11, high time to *a.*
1 Cor. 15:34, *a.* to righteousness.
Eph. 5:14, *a.* thou that sleepest.
See Jer. 51:57; John 11:11.
AWARE. Cant. 6:12; Jer. 50:24; Lu. 11:44.
AWE. Ps. 4:4; 33:8; 119:161.
AWL. Ex. 21:6; Deut. 15:17.
AXE. Ps. 74:5, famous as he had lifted up *a.*
Isa. 10:15, shall the *a.* boast.
Mat. 3:10; Lu. 3:9, the *a.* is laid to root.
See 1 Sam. 13:20; 1 Kings 6:7; 2 Kings 6:5.

B

BABBLER. Eccl. 10:11; Acts 17:18.
BABBLING. Prov. 23:29; 1 Tim. 6:20; 2 Tim. 2:16.
BABE. Ps. 8:2; Mat. 21:16, out of mouth of *b*.
17:14, leave their substance to *b*.
Isa. 3:4, *b*. shall rule over them.
Mat. 11:25; Lu. 10:21, revealed to *b*.
Rom. 2:20, teacher of *b*.
1 Cor. 3:1, *b*. in Christ.
1 Pet. 2:2, newborn *b*.
See Ex. 2:6; Lu. 2:12, 16; Heb. 5:13.
BACK. Josh. 8:26, drew not his hand *b*.
1 Sam. 10:9, he turned his *b*.
Neh. 9:26, cast law behind *b*.
Ps. 129:3, plowers plowed upon my *b*.
Prov. 10:13; 19:29; 26:3, rod for *b*.
Isa. 38:17, cast sins behind *b*.
50:6, gave *b*. to smiters.
See Num. 24:11; 2 Sam. 19:10; Job 26:9.
BACKBITERS. Rom. 1:30.
BACKBITING. Ps. 15:3; Prov. 25:23; 2 Cor. 12:20.
BACKSLIDER. Prov. 14:14, *b*. in heart filled with his own ways.
Jer. 3:6, 8, 11, 12, *b*. Israel.
8:5, perpetual *b*.
14:7, our *b*. are many.
Hos. 4:16, as a *b*. heifer.
11:7, bent to *b*. from me.
14:4, will heal their *b*.
See Jer. 2:19; 5:6; 31:22; 49:4.
BACKWARD. 2 Kings 20:10; Isa. 38:8, let shadow return *b*.
Job 23:8, *b*., but I cannot perceive.
Ps. 40:14; 70:2, driven *b*.
Isa. 59:14, judgment is turned *b*.
Jer. 7:24, they went *b*. and not forward.
See Gen. 9:23; 49:17; John 18:6.
BAD. Gen. 24:50; 31:24, 29; Lev. 27:12, 14, 33; Num. 13:19; 24:13; 2 Sam. 13:22; 14:17; 1 Kings 3:9; Mat. 22:10; 2 Cor. 5:10, good or *b*.
See Lev. 27:10; Ezra 4:12; Jer. 24:2; Mat. 31:48.
BADGERS' SKINS. Ex. 25:5, and *b*.
26:14, a covering above of *b*.
BADNESS. Gen. 41:19.
BAG. Deut. 25:13; Prov. 16:11; Mic. 6:11, *b*. of weights.
Job 14:17, transgression sealed in *b*.
Isa. 46:6, lavish gold out of *b*.
Hag. 1:6, *b*. with holes.
Lu. 12:33, *b*. that wax not old.
John 12:6; 13:29, a thief, and had the *b*.
See 1 Sam. 17:40; 2 Kings 5:23; Prov. 7:20.
BAKE. Gen. 19:3; Lev. 26:26; 1 Sam. 28:24; Isa. 44:15, *b*. bread.
Ex. 12:39; Lev. 24:5, *b*. cakes.
See Gen. 40:17; Ex. 16:23; Lev. 2:4; Num. 11:8.
BAKER. Gen. 40:1; 41:10; 1 Sam. 8:13; Jer. 37:21; Hos. 7:4.
BALANCE. Lev. 19:36; Prov. 16:11; Ezek. 45:10, just *b*.
Job 37:16, the *b*. of clouds.
Ps. 62:9, laid in *b*., lighter than vanity.
Prov. 11:1; 20:23; Hos. 12:7; Amos 8:5; Mic. 6:11, false *b*.
Isa. 40:12, 15, weighed hills in *b*.
46:6, weigh silver in the *b*.
Rev. 6:5, a pair of *b*.
See Job 6:2; 31:6; Jer. 32:10.
BALD. 2 Kings 2:23, go up, thou *b*. head.
Jer. 48:37; Ezek. 29:18, every head *b*.
See Lev. 13:40; Jer. 16:6; Ezek. 27:31.
BALDNESS. Isa. 3:24, instead of well set hair *b*.
22:12, call to weeping and *b*.
Mic. 1:16, enlarge thy *b*. as eagle.
See Lev. 21:5; Deut. 14:1; Ezek. 7:18; Amos 8:10.
BALL. Isa. 22:18.
BALM. Jer. 8:22; 46:11, *b*. in Gilead.
See Gen. 37:25; 43:11; Jer. 51:8; Ezek. 27:17.
BANDS. Ps. 2:3; 107:14, break their *b*. asunder.
73:4, there are no *b*. in their death.
Hos. 11:4, drew them with *b*. of love.
Zech. 11:7, two staves, Beauty and *B*.
Mat. 27:27; Mk. 15:16, gathered to him whole *b*.
See Job 38:31; Eccl. 7:26; Lu. 8:29; Col. 2:19.
BANISHED. 2 Sam. 14:13; Ezra 7:26; Lam. 2:14.
BANK. Lu. 19:23, gavest not money into *b*.
See Gen. 41:17; 2 Sam. 20:15; Ezek. 47:7.
BANNER. Ps. 20:5, in name of God set up *b*.
See Ps. 60:4; Cant. 2:4; 6:4; Isa. 13:2.
BANQUET. Esth. 5:4; Job 41:6; Cant. 2:4; Dan. 5; Amos 6:7.
BAPTISM. Mat. 20:22; Mk. 10:38; Lu. 12:50, to be baptized with *b*.
21:25; Mk. 11:30; Lu. 7:29; 20:4; Acts 1:22; 18:25; 19:3, *b*. of John.
Mk. 1:4; Lu. 3:3; Acts 13:24; 19:4, *b*. of repentance.
Rom. 6:4; Col. 2:12, buried with him by *b*.
Eph. 4:5, one Lord, one faith, one *b*.
Heb. 6:2, doctrine of *b*.
See Mat. 3:7; 1 Pet. 3:21.
BAPTIZE. Mat. 3:11; Mk. 1:8; Lu. 3:16; John 1:26, *b*. with Holy Ghost.
14, I have need to be *b*.
16, Jesus when *b*. went up.
Mk. 16:16, he that believeth and is *b*.
Lu. 3:7, multitude came to be *b*.
12; 7:29, publicans to be *b*.
21, Jesus being *b*., and praying.
7:30, Pharisees and lawyers being not *b*.
John 1:33, he that sent me to *b*.
3:22, 23, tarried with them and *b*.
4:1, 2, Jesus made and *b*. more.
Acts 2:38, repent and be *b*.
41, gladly received word were *b*.
8:12, *b*. both men and women.
16, *b*. in name of Jesus.
36, what doth hinder to be *b*.
9:18, Saul arose and was *b*.
10:47, can any forbid *b*.
16:15, 33, *b*. and household.
18:8, many believed and were *b*.
22:16, be *b*. and wash away thy sins.
Rom. 6:3; Gal. 3:27, were *b*. into Jesus.
1 Cor. 1:13, were ye *b*. in name of Paul.
10:2, were all *b*. in cloud.
12:13, all *b*. into one body.
15:29, *b*. for the dead.
See Mat. 28:19; John 1:25, 28, 31.
BARBARIANS. Acts 28:4; Rom. 1:14; 1 Cor. 14:11.
BARBAROUS. Acts 28:2.
BARBED. Job 41:7.
BARBER. Ezek. 5:1.
BARE (*v*.). Ex. 19:4; Deut. 1:31; Isa. 53:12; 63:9; Mat. 8:17; 1 Pet. 2:24.
BARE (*ad*.). Isa. 52:10; 1 Cor. 15:37.
BARLEY. Ex. 9:31, *b*. was in the ear.
Deut. 8:8, a land of wheat and *b*.
Ruth 1:22, beginning of *b*. harvest.
John 6:9, five *b*. loaves.
Rev. 6:6, three measures of *b*.
BARKED. Joel 1:7.
BARN. Job 39:12, gather thy seed into *b*.
Mat. 6:26; Lu. 12:24, nor gather into *b*.
13:30, gather wheat into *b*.
Lu. 12:18, pull down my *b*.
See 2 Kings 6:27; Joel 1:17; Hag. 2:19.
BARREL. 1 Kings 17:12, 14; 18:33.
BARREN. 2 Kings 2:19, water naught and ground *b*.
Ps. 107:34, turneth fruitful land into *b*.
Isa. 54:1, sing, O *b*., thou that didst not bear.
2 Pet. 1:8, neither *b*. nor unfruitful.
See Ex. 23:26; Job 24:21; Lu. 23:29.
BARS. Job 17:16, down to the *b*. of the pit.
Ezek. 38:11, having neither *b*. nor gates.
See 1 Sam. 23:7; Job 38:10; Ps. 107:16; Isa. 45:2.
BASE. Job 30:8, children of *b*. men.
Mal. 2:9, I have made you *b*.
Acts 17:5, fellows of *b*. sort.
1 Cor. 1:28, *b*. things of the world.
2 Cor. 10:1, in presence am *b*.
See 2 Sam. 6:22; Isa. 3:5; Ezek. 17:14; Dan. 4:17.

BASKET. Deut. 28:5, 17, blessed be thy *b.*
Amos 8:1, *b.* of summer fruit.
Mat. 14:20; Mk. 6:43; Lu. 9:17; John 6:13, twelve *b.*
15:37; Mk. 8:8, seven *b.*
16:9; Mk. 8:19, how many *b.*
See Gen. 40:16; Ex. 29:23; Judg. 6:19; Jer. 24:2.
BASON. John 13:5, poureth water into a *b.*
See Ex. 12:22; 24:6; 1 Chron. 28:17; Jer. 52:19.
BASTARD. Deut. 23:2, a *b.* shall not enter.
Zech. 9:6, *b.* shall dwell in Ashdod.
Heb. 12:8, *b.* and not sons.
BATH (a measure). 1 Kings 7:26, it contained two thousand *b.*
2 Chron. 2:10, twenty thousand *b.* of. wine.
Ezra 7:22, an hundred *b.* of wine.
Isa. 5:10, shall yield one *b.*
BATHE. Lev. 15:5; 17:16; Num. 19:7; Isa. 34:5.
BATS. Lev. 11:19; Deut. 14:18; Isa. 2:20.
BATTLE, 1 Sam. 17:20, host shouted for *b.*
47; 2 Chron. 20:15, the *b.* is the Lord's.
1 Chron. 5:20, they cried to God in *b.*
Ps. 18:39, strength to *b.*
55:18, delivered my soul from *b.*
Eccl. 9:11, nor *b.* to strong.
Jer. 50:22, sound of *b.* in land.
See Job 39:25; 41:8; Ps. 76:3; 140:7.
BATTLEMENTS. Deut. 22:8; Jer. 5:10.
BAY TREE. Ps. 37:35.
BEACON. Isa. 30:17.
BEAM. Ps. 104:3, who layeth *b.* in waters.
Mat. 7:5; Lu. 6:42, cast out *b.*
See Judg. 16:14; 2 Kings 6:2; Hab. 2:11.
BEAR (*v.*). Gen. 4:13, greater than I can *b.*
13:6; 36:7, land not able to *b.*
43:9; 44:32, let me b blame.
Ex. 20:16; 1 Kings 21:10; Lu. 11:48; John 1:7; 5:31; 8:19; 15:27; Acts 23:11; Rom. 8:16; 1 John 1:2; 5:8, *b.* witness.
28:12, Aaron *b.* names before Lord.
Lev. 24:15; Ezek. 23:49; Heb. 9:28, *b.* sin.
Num. 11:14; Deut. 1:9, not able to *b.* people.
Esth. 1:22; Jer. 5:31; Dan. 2:39, *b.* rule.
Ps. 91:12; Mat. 4:6; Lu. 4:11, they shall *b.* thee up.
Prov. 18:14, wounded spirit who can *b.*
Isa. 52:11, clean that *b.* vessels.
Jer. 31:19, *b.* reproach of youth.
Lam. 3:27, good to *b.* yoke in youth.
Mat. 3:11, not worthy to *b.*
27:32; Mk. 15:21; Lu. 23:26, *b.* cross.
John 16:12, cannot *b.* them now.
Rom. 13:4, *b.* not sword in vain.
15:1, *b.* infirmities of the weak.
1 Cor. 13:7, charity *b.* all things.
15:49, *b.* image of the heavenly.
Gal. 6:2, 5, *b.* burdens.
17, *b.* in my body.
See Ex. 28:38; Deut. 1:31; Prov. 12:24.
BEAR (*n.*). Isa. 11:7, cow and *b.* shall feed.
59:11, roar like *b.*
Hos. 13:8, as a *b.* bereaved.
Amos 5:19, as if a man did flee from *b.*
See 1 Sam. 17:34; 2 Sam. 17:8; Prov. 17:12.
BEARD. 2 Sam. 10:5; 1 Chron. 19:5, till *b.* be grown.
Ps. 133:2, even Aaron's *b.*
Ezek. 5:1, cause razor to pass on *b.*
See Lev. 13:29; 1 Sam. 21:13; 2 Sam. 20:9.
BEARING. Ps. 126:6, *b.* precious seed.
John 19:17, *b.* cross.
Rom. 2:15; 9:1, conscience *b.* witness.
2 Cor. 4:10, *b.* about in body dying of Jesus.
Heb. 13:13, *b.* his reproach.
See Gen. 1:29; Num. 10:17; Mk. 14:13.
BEAST. Job 12:7, ask *b.*, they shall teach.
Job 18:3, counted as *b.*
Ps. 49:12, like *b.* that perish.
73:22, as *b.* before thee.
Prov. 12:10, regardeth life of *b.*
Eccl. 3:19, no pre-eminence above *b.*
1 Cor. 15:32, fought with *b.*
Jas. 3:7, every kind of *b.* is tamed.
2 Pet. 2:12, as natural brute *b.*
See Lev. 11:47; Ps. 50:10; 147:9; Rom. 1:23.
BEAT. Isa. 2:4; Joel 3:10; Mic. 4:3, *b.* swords.
Lu. 12:47, *b.* with many stripes.
1 Cor. 9:26, as one that *b.* the air.
See Prov. 23:14; Mic. 4:13; Mk. 12:5; 13:9.
BEAUTIFUL. Ps. 48:2, *b.* for situation is Zion.
Eccl. 3:11, everything *b.* in his time.
Cant. 6:4, thou art *b.*, O my love.
Isa. 4:2, the branch of the Lord be *b.*
52:1, O Zion, put on thy *b.* garments.
7; Rom. 10:15, how *b.* are the feet.
64:11, *b.* house is burnt up.
Jer. 13:20, where is thy *b.* flock?
Mat. 23:27, sepulchres which appear *b.*
Acts 3:2, 10, at the gate called *B.*
BEAUTY. 1 Chron. 16:29; 2 Chron. 20:21; Ps. 29:2; 96:9; 110:3, *b.* of holiness.
Ezra 7:27, to *b.* the Lord's house.
Ps. 27:4, behold *b.* of the Lord.
39:11, *b.* to consume away.
50:2, perfection of *b.*
Prov. 31:30, *b.* is vain.
See 2 Sam. 1:19; Ps. 90:17; Zech. 9:17.
BEAUTY AND BANDS. Zech. 11:7, two staves, *B.*
BECKON. Lu. 1:22; John 13:24; Acts 12:17; 21:40.
BECOMETH. Ps. 93:5, holiness *b.* thy house.
Rom. 16:2; Eph. 5:3, as *b.* saints.
Phil. 1:27; 1 Tim. 2:10; Tit. 2:3, as *b.* gospel.
See Prov. 17:7; Mat. 3:15.
BED. Job 7:13, when I say my *b.* shall comfort.
33:15, in slumberings upon *b.*
Ps. 63:6, when I remember thee upon my *b.*
Mat. 9:6; Mk. 2:9; John 5:11, take up *b.*
See 2 Kings 4:10; Isa. 28:20; Mk. 4:21; Lu. 8:16.
BEDSTEAD. Deut. 3:11, was a *b.* of iron.
BEES. Deut. 1:44; Judg. 14:8; Ps. 118:12; Isa. 7:18.
BEEVES. Lev. 22:19; Num. 31:28, 38.
BEFALL. Gen. 42:4; 44:29, mischief *b.* him.
49:1; Deut. 31:29; Dan. 10:14, *b.* in last days.
Judg. 6:13, why is all this *b.* us?
Ps. 91:10, no evil *b.* thee.
Eccl. 3:19, *b.* men, *b.* beasts, one thing *b.*
See Lev. 10:19; Deut. 31:17; Acts 20:19.
BEG. Ps. 37:25; 109:10; Prov. 20:4; Lu. 16:3.
BEGGARLY. Gal. 4:9.
BEGIN. Ezek. 9:6, *b.* at my sanctuary.
1 Pet. 4:17, judgment *b.* at house of God.
See 1 Sam. 3:12; 2 Cor. 3:1.
BEGINNING. Gen. 1:1, in the *b.* God created heaven.
Job 8:7, though thy *b.* was small.
Ps. 111:10; Prov. 1:7; 9:10, *b.* of wisdom.
119:160, word true from *b.*
Eccl. 7:8, better end than *b.*
Mat. 19:8, from *b.* not so.
Lu. 24:47, *b.* at Jerusalem.
John 1:1, in the *b.* was the Word.
2:11, this *b.* of miracles.
Heb. 3:14, hold *b.* of confidence.
Rev. 1:8; 21:6; 22:13, I am the *b.*
See 1 Chron. 17:9; Prov. 8:22, 23; Col. 1:18.
BEGOTTEN. Ps. 2:7; Acts 13:33; Heb. 1:5; 5:5, this day have I *b.* thee.
1 Pet. 1:3, *b.* to a lively hope.
See Job 38:28; 1 Cor. 4:15; Philem. 10.
BEGUILE. Gen. 29:25; Josh. 9:22, wherefore hast thou *b.* me.
2 Pet. 2:14, *b.* unstable souls.
See Num. 25:18; 2 Cor. 11:3.
BEGUN. Gal. 3:3, having *b.* in Spirit.
Phil. 1:6, hath *b.* good work.
See Deut. 3:24; 2 Cor. 8:16; 1 Tim. 5:11.
BEHALF. Job 36:2, speak on God's *b.*
Phil. 1:29, in *b.* of Christ.
See 2 Chron. 16:9; 2 Cor. 1:11; 5:12.
BEHAVE. 1 Sam. 18:5, 14, 15, 30, David *b.* wisely.

1 Chron. 19:13, *b.* ourselves valiantly.
Ps. 101:2, I will *b.* wisely.
Isa. 3:5, child shall *b.* proudly.
1 Thess. 2:10, how unblameably we *b.*
1 Tim. 3:2, bishop of good *b.*
See Ps. 131:2; 1 Cor. 13:5; Tit. 2:3.
BEHEADED. Mat. 14:10; Mk. 6:16; Lu. 9:9; Rev. 20:4.
BEHIND. Ex. 10:26, not hoof be left *b.*
Phil. 3:13, things which are *b.*
Col. 1:24, fill up what is *b.*
See 1 Kings 14:9; Neh. 9:26; 2 Cor. 11:5.
BEHOLD. Ps. 37:37, *b.* the upright.
Mat. 18:10, their angels always *b.*
John 17:24, that they may *b.* glory.
2 Cor. 3:18, *b.* as in a glass.
See Num. 24:17; Ps. 91:8; 119:37.
BEHOVED. Lu. 24:46; Heb. 2:17.
BELIEF. 2 Thess. 2:13.
BELIEVE. Num. 14:11, how long ere they *b.* me.
2 Chron. 20:20, *b.* Lord, *b.* prophets.
Ps. 78:22, they *b.* not in God.
Prov. 14:15, simple *b.* every word.
Mat. 8:13, as thou hast *b.* so be it.
9:28, *b.* ye that I am able.
21:25; Mk. 11:31, why then did ye not *b.*
27:42, come down and we will *b.*
Mk. 5:36; Lu. 8:50, only *b.*
9:23, canst *b.* all things possible.
11:24, *b.* that ye receive.
16:13, neither *b.* they them.
Lu. 1:1, things most surely *b.*
8:13, which for a while *b.*
24:25, slow of heart to *b.*
41, *b.* not for joy.
John 1:7, all through him might *b.*
2:22, they *b.* the scripture.
3:12 *b.* heavenly things.
5:44, how can ye *b.* which receive honour.
47, how shall ye *b.* my words.
6:36, seen me and *b.* not.
7:5, neither did his brethren *b.*
48, have any of the rulers *b.*?
10:38, *b.* the works.
11:15, to intent ye may *b.*
26, never die, *b.* thou this?
48, all men will. *b.*
12:36, *b.* in the light.
17:21, the world may *b.*
20:25, I will not *b.*
29, have not seen yet have *b.*
Acts 4:32, multitude of them that *b.*
13:39, all that *b.* are justified.
48, ordained to eternal life *b.*
16:34, *b.* with all his house.
Rom. 4:11, father of all that *b.*
18, against hope *b.* in hope.
9:33, *b.* not ashamed.
10:14, how shall they *b.*
1 Cor. 7:12, wife that. *b.* not.
2 Cor. 4:13, we *b.* and therefore speak.
Gal. 3:22, promise to them that *b.*
2 Thess. 1:10, admired in all that *b.*
Heb. 10:39, b, to saving of soul.
11:6, must *b.* that he is.
Jas. 2:19, devils *b.* and tremble.
1 Pet. 2:6, he that *b.* shall not be confounded.
See Ex. 4:5; 19:9; Isa. 43:10; Mat. 21:22; John 8:24; 10:37; Acts 9:26.
BELLY. Gen. 3:14; Job 15:2; Mat. 15:17; Mk. 7:19; John 7:38; Rom. 16:18; Phil. 3:19; Tit. 1:12.
BELONGETH. Deut. 32:35; Ps. 94:1; Heb. 10:30.
BELOVED. Deut. 33:12, *b.* dwell in safety.
Ps. 127:2, giveth his *b.* sleep.
Dan. 9:23; 10:11, 19, greatly *b.*
Mat. 3:17; 17:5; Mk. 1:11; 9:7; Lu. 3:22; 9:35; 2 Pet. 1:17, *b.* son.
Rom. 11:28, *b.* for fathers' sakes.
Eph. 1:6, accepted in the *b.*
Col. 4:9; Philem. 16, *b.* brother.
See Neh. 13:26; Cant. 2:16; Rom. 16:9.
BEMOAN. Job 42:11; Jer. 15:5; Nah. 3:7.
BEND. Ps. 11:2; Isa. 60:14; Ezek. 17:7.
BENEATH. Prov. 15:24, depart from hell *b.*
Isa. 14:9, hell from *b.* is moved.
John 8:23, ye are from *b.*
See Deut. 4:39; Jer. 31:37.
BENEFACTORS. Lu. 22:25.
BENEFIT. Ps. 68:19, loadeth us with *b.*
1 Tim. 6:2, partakers of the *b.*
See 2 Chron. 32:25; Ps. 103:2; 2 Cor. 1:15; Philem. 14.
BENEVOLENCE. 1 Cor. 7:3.
BEREAVE. Gen. 42:36; 43:14, *b.* of children.
Eccl. 4:8, *b.* my soul of God.
Jer. 15:7; 18:21, I will *b.* thee.
See Ezek. 5:17; 36:12; Hos. 13:8.
BESEECH. Job 42:4, hear I *b.* thee.
Mat. 8:5; Lu. 7:3, centurion *b.* him.
Lu. 9:38, I *b.* thee, look on my son.
2 Cor. 5:20, as though God did *b.* you.
Eph. 4:1, *b.* you to walk.
Philem. 9, for love's sake *b.* thee.
See Ex. 33:18; Jon. 1:14; Rom. 12:1.
BESET. Ps. 22:12; 139:5; Hos. 7:2; Heb. 12:1.
BESIDE. Mk. 3:21; Acts 26:24; 2 Cor. 5:13.
BESIEGE. Deut. 28:52; Eccl. 9:14; Isa. 1:8.
BESOUGHT. Ex. 32:11; Deut. 3:23; 1 Kings 13:6; 2 Chron. 33:12; Jer. 26:19, *b.* the Lord.
Mat. 8:31; Mk. 5:10; Lu. 8:31, devils *b.* him.
34; Lu. 8:37, *b.* him to depart.
John 4:40, *b.* that he would tarry.
2 Cor. 12:8, I *b.* the Lord thrice.
See Gen. 42:21; Esth. 8:3.
BEST. 1 Sam. 15:9, 15, spared *b.* of sheep.
Ps. 39:5, at *b.* state vanity.
Lu. 15:22, *b.* robe.
1 Cor. 12:31, *b.* gifts.
See Gen. 43:11; Deut. 23:16; 2 Sam. 18:4.
BESTEAD. Isa. 8:21.
BESTIR. 2 Sam. 5:24.
BESTOW. Lu. 12:17, no room to *b.* my fruits.
1 Cor. 15:10, grace *b.* on us not in vain.
Gal. 4:11, lest I have *b.* labour in vain.
1 John 3:1, manner of love Father *b.*
See 1 Chron. 29:25; Isa. 63:7; John 4:38.
BETHINK. 1 Kings 8:47; 2 Chron. 6:37.
BETIMES. Gen. 26:31; 2 Chron. 36:15; Job 8:5; Prov. 13:24.
BETRAY. Mat. 26:16; Mk. 14:11; Lu. 22:21, 22, opportunity to *b.*
27:4, I *b.* innocent blood.
1 Cor. 11:23, same night he was *b.*
See Mat. 24:10; Mk. 14:18; John 6:64; 21:20.
BETROTH. Hos. 2:19, 20.
BETTER. 1 Sam. 15:22, to obey *b.* than sacrifice.
1 Kings 19:4, I am not *b.* than my fathers.
Ps. 63:3, lovingkindness *b.* than life.
Eccl. 4:9, two are *b.* than one.
7:10, former days *b.* than these.
Mat. 12:12, man b, than a sheep.
Lu. 5:39, he saith, the old is *b.*
Phil. 2:3, each esteem other *b.* than himself.
Heb. 1:4, much *b.* than angels.
11:16, a *b.* country.
2 Pet. 2:21, *b.* not have known the way.
See Eccl. 2:24; Cant. 1:2; Jon. 4:3.
BEWAIL. Lu. 8:52, all wept and *b.* her.
Lu. 23:27, of women which also *b.*
2 Cor. 12:21, *b.* many who have sinned.
See Deut. 21:13; Judg. 11:37; Rev. 18:9.
BEWARE. Judg. 13:4, *b.* and drink not wine.
Job 36:18, *b.* lest he take thee away.
Mat. 16:6; Mk. 8:15; Lu. 12:1, *b.* of leaven.
Mk. 12:38; Lu. 20:46, *b.* of scribes.
Lu. 12:15, *b.* of covetousness.
Phil. 3:2, *b.* of dogs, *b.* of evil workers.
See Deut. 6:12; 8:11; 15:9.
BEWITCHED. Acts 8:9; Gal. 3:1.

BEWRAY. Isa. 16:3; Prov. 27:16; 29:24; Mat. 26:73.
BEYOND. Num. 22:18; 2 Cor. 8:3; Gal. 1:13; 1 Thess. 4:6.
BIER, 2 Sam. 3:31; Lu. 7:14.
BILLOWS. Ps. 42:7; Jon. 2:3.
BIND. Prov. 6:21, *b.* them continually upon heart.
  Isa. 61:1, *b.* up brokenhearted.
  Mat. 12:29; Mk. 3:27, *b.* strong man.
    16:19; 18:18, *b.* on earth.
  See Num. 30:2; Job 26:8; 38:31.
BIRD. 2 Sam. 21:10, suffered not *b.* to rest.
  Cant. 2:12, time of the singing of *b.*
  Jer. 12:9, heritage like a speckled *b.*
  Mat. 8:20; Lu. 9:58, *b.* of the air have nests.
  See Ps. 11:1; 124:7; Prov. 1:17; Eccl. 10:20.
BIRTH. John 9:1, blind from *b.*
  Gal. 4:19, of whom I travail in *b.*
  See Eccl. 7:1; Isa. 66:9; Lu. 1:14.
BIRTHDAY. Gen. 40:20, which was Pharaoh's *b.*
  Mat. 14:6; Mk. 6:21, when Herod's *b.* was kept.
BIRTHRIGHT. Gen. 25:31; 27:36; Heb. 12:16.
BISHOP (qualifications of). 1 Tim. 3:1, if a man desire office of *b.*
  Tit. 1:7, *b.* must be blameless.
  1 Pet. 2:25, Shepherd and *B.* of your souls.
  See Acts 1:20; Phil. 1:1.
BIT. Ps. 32:9; Jas. 3:3.
BITE, Prov. 23:32, at last it *b.* like serpent.
  Mic. 3:5, prophets that *b.* with teeth.
  Gal. 5:15, if ye *b.* and devour one another.
  See Eccl. 10:8; Amos 5:19; 9:3.
BITTER. Ex. 12:8; Num. 9:11, with *b.* herbs.
  Deut. 32:24, devoured with *b.* destruction.
  Job. 13:26, writest *b.* things.
  Isa. 5:20, that put *b.* for sweet.
    24:9, drink *b.* to them that drink it.
  Jer. 2:19, an evil thing and *b.*
  Mat. 26:75; Lu. 22:62, Peter wept *b.*
  Col. 3:19, be not *b.* against them.
  See Ex. 1:14; 15:23, 2 Kings 14:26.
BITTERNESS. Job 10:1; 21:25; Isa. 38:15, in *b.* of soul.
  Prov. 14:10, heart knoweth own *b.*
  Acts 8:23, in the gall. of *b.*
  Eph. 4:31, let all *b.* be put away.
  Heb. 12:15, lest any root of *b.*
  See 1 Sam. 15:32; Prov. 17:25; Rom. 3:14.
BLACK. Mat. 5:36; Jude 13; Rev. 6:5.
BLADE. Judg. 3:22; Mat. 13:26; Mk. 4:28.
BLAME. 2 Cor. 6:3; 8:20; Gal. 2:11; Eph. 1:4.
BLAMELESS. 1 Cor. 1:8, be *b.* in day of the Lord.
  Phil. 2:15, that ye may be *b.*
  See Mat. 12:5; Phil. 3:6; Tit. 1:6, 7.
BLASPHEME. 2 Sam. 12:14, occasion to enemies to *b.*
  Isa. 52:5, my name continually is *b.*
  Mat. 9:3, scribes said, this man *b.*
  Mk. 3:29, *b.* against Holy Ghost.
  Acts 26:11, I compelled them to *b.*
  Rom. 2:24, name of God is *b.* through you.
  Jas. 2:7, *b.* that worthy name.
  See 1 Kings 21:10; Ps. 74:10, 18; 1 Tim. 1:20.
BLASPHEMY. Mat. 12:31, all manner of *b.*
    26:65; Mk. 14:64, he hath spoken *b.*
  Lu. 5:21, who is this which speaketh *b.*?
  See 2 Kings 19:3; Ezek. 35:12; Mat. 15:19.
BLAST. Gen. 41:6; Deut. 28:22; 1 Kings 8:37.
BLAZE. Mk. 1:45.
BLEATING. Judg. 5:16; 1 Sam. 15:14.
BLEMISH. Dan. 1:4, children in whom was no *b.*
  Eph. 5:27, holy and without *b.*
  1 Pet. 1:19, a lamb without *b.* and spot.
  See Lev. 21:17; Deut. 15:21; 2 Sam. 14:25.
BLESS. Deut. 28:3, *b.* in city, *b.* in field.
  1 Chron. 4:10, Oh that thou wouldest *b.* me.
  Prov. 10:7, memory of just is *b.*
  Isa. 32:20, *b.* are ye that sow.
    65:16, *b.* himself in God of truth.
  Mat. 5:44; Lu. 6:28; Rom. 12:14, *b.* them that curse.
  Acts 20:35, more *b.* to give than receive.
  2 Cor. 11:32, *b.* for evermore.
  Tit. 2:13, looking for that *b.* hope.
  Rev. 14:12, *b.* are dead that die in Lord.
  See Gen. 22:17; Hag. 2:19; Jas. 3:9, 10.
BLESSING. Deut. 23:5; Neh. 13:2, turned curse into *b.*
  Job 19:13, *b.* of him that was ready to perish.
  Prov. 10:22, *b.* of Lord maketh rich.
    28:20, faithful man shall abound with *b.*
  Isa. 65:8, destroy it not, a *b.* is in it.
  Mal. 2:2, I will curse your *b.*
    3:10, pour you out a *b.*
  Rom. 15:29, fulness of *b.* of Gospel.
  1 Cor. 10:16, cup of *b.* which we bless.
  Jas. 3:10, proceed *b.* and cursing.
  Rev. 5:12, worthy to receive honour and *b.*
  See Gen. 27:35; 39:5; Deut. 11:26, 29.
BLIND (*v.*). Ex. 23:8, the gift *b.* the wise.
  2 Cor. 3:14; 4:4, their minds were *b.*
  1 John 2:11, darkness hath *b.*
  See Deut. 16:19; 1 Sam. 12:3.
BLINDNESS. Eph. 4:18, because of *b.* of their heart.
  See Deut. 28:28; 2 Kings 6:18; Zech. 12:4.
BLOOD. Gen. 9:6, whoso sheddeth man's *b.*
  Josh. 2:19; 1 Kings 2:32, *b.* on head.
  Ps. 51:14, deliver me from *b.* guiltiness.
    72:14, precious shall *b.* be in his sight.
  Prov. 29:10, the *b.* thirsty hate upright.
  Isa. 9:5, garments rolled in *b.*
  Jer. 2:34, the *b.* of poor innocents.
  Ezek. 9:9, land is full of *b.*
    18:13; 33:5, his *b.* be upon him.
  Hab. 2:12, buildeth a town with *b.*
  Mat. 9:20; Mk. 5:25; Lu. 8:43, issue of *b.*
    16:17, flesh and *b.* hath not revealed.
    27:4, I have betrayed innocent *b.*
    25, his *b.* be on us and our children.
  Mk. 14:24; Lu. 22:20, my *b.* shed.
  Lu. 22:20; 1 Cor. 11:25, new testament in my *b.*
    44, sweat as drops of *b.* falling.
  John 1:13, born not of *b.*
    6:54, 55, 56, drinketh my *b.*
  Acts 15:20; 21:25, abstain from *b.*
    17:26, made of one *b.*
    20:28, church purchased with his *b.*
  Rom. 3:25, through faith in his *b.*
    5:9, justified by his *b.*
  1 Cor. 10:16, communion of *b.* of Christ.
    11:27, guilty of body and *b.* of the Lord.
    15:50, flesh and *b.* cannot inherit.
  Eph. 1:7; Col. 1:14, redemption through his *b.*
  Heb. 9:22, without shedding of *b.*
    10:29; 13:20, *b.* of the covenant.
  1 Pet. 1:19, with precious *b.* of Christ.
  Rev. 7:14; 12:11, in the *b.* of the Lamb.
  See Gen. 9:4; Ex. 4:9; 12:13; Lev. 3:17; Ps. 55:23; Rev. 16:6; 17:6.
BLOSSOM. Isa. 35:1, desert shall *b.* as the rose.
  Hab. 3:17, fig tree shall not *b.*
  See Gen. 40:10; Num. 17:5; Isa. 27:6.
BLOT. Ex. 32:32; Ps. 69:28; Rev. 3:5, *b.* out of book.
  Isa. 44:22, *b.* out as thick cloud.
  Acts 3:19, repent that sins may be *b.* out.
  Col. 2:14, *b.* out handwriting.
  See Deut. 9:14; 2 Kings 14:27; Jer. 18:23.
BLUSH. Ezra 9:6; Jer. 6:15; 8:12.
BOAST (*n.*). Ps. 34:2; Rom. 2:17, 23; 3:27.
BOAST (*v.*). 1 Kings 20:11, not *b.* as he that putteth it off.
  Ps. 49:6; 94:4, *b.* themselves.
  Prov. 27:1, *b.* not of to-morrow.
  2 Cor. 11:16, that I may *b.* myself a little.
  Eph. 2:9, lest any man should *b.*
  Jas. 3:5, tongue *b.* great things.
  See 2 Chron. 25:19; Prov. 20:14; Jas. 4:16.
BOATS. John 6:22; Acts 27:16, 30.
BODY. Job 19:26, worms destroy this *b.*
  Prov. 5:11, when thy flesh and *b.* are consumed.
  Mat. 5:29, *b.* cast into hell.

Mat. 6:22; Lu. 11:34, *b.* full of light.
25; Lu. 12:22, take no thought for *b.*
Mk. 5:29, felt in *b.* that she was healed.
Lu. 17:37, wheresoever the *b.* is.
John 2:21, the temple. of his *b.*
Acts 19:12, from his *b.* were brought.
Rom. 6:6, *b.* of sin destroyed.
7:24, *b.* of this death.
12:1, present your *b.* a living sacrifice.
4; 1 Cor. 12:14, many members, one *b.*
1 Cor. 9:27, I keep under my *b.*
13:3, though I give my *b.* to. be burned.
2 Cor. 5:8, absent from the *b.*
12:2, whether in *b.* or out of the *b.*
Gal. 6:17, I bear in *b.* marks.
Phil. 3:21, like to his glorious *b.*
1 Pet. 2:24, in his own *b.* on tree.
See Gen. 47:18; Deut. 28:4; Rom. 12:5.
BODILY. Lu. 3:22; 2 Cor. 10:10; Col. 2:9; 1 Tim. 4:8.
BOLD. Eccl. 8:1, the *b.* of face changed.
John 7:26, he speaketh *b.*
2 Cor. 10:2, I may not be *b.*
Eph. 3:12, we have *b.* and access.
Heb. 4:16, let us come *b.* to throne.
1 John 4:17, have *b.* in day of judgment.
See Prov. 28:1; Acts 13:46; Rom. 10:20.
BOND. Acts 8:23, in *b.* of iniquity.
Eph. 4:3, *b.* of peace.
Col. 3:14, *b.* of perfectness.
See Num. 30:2; Ezek. 20:37; Lu. 13:16.
BONDAGE. John 8:33, never in *b.* to any man.
See Rom. 8:15; Gal. 5:1; Heb. 2:15.
BONDMAID. Lev. 19:20, a woman that is a *b.*
25:44, and thy *b.*
BONDMAN. Deut. 15:15; 16:12; 24:18.
BONDMEN. Lev. 25:39, both thy *b.*
BONDWOMAN. Gen. 21:10; Gal. 4:30.
BONE. Ex. 12:46; Num. 9:12, neither shall ye break a *b.* thereof.
Job 20:11, *b.* full of sin.
40:18, *b.* as pieces of brass.
Ps. 51:8, the *b.* broken may rejoice.
Prov. 12:4, as rottenness in his *b.*
Mat. 23:27, full of dead men's *b.*
Lu. 24:39, spirit hath not flesh and *b.*
See Gen. 2:23; Ezek. 37:7; John 19:36.
BOOK. Job 19:23, printed in a *b.*
31:35, adversary had written a *b.*
Isa. 34:16, seek out of the *b.* of the Lord.
Mal. 3:16, *b.* of remembrance.
Lu. 4:17, when he had opened *b.*
John 21:25, world could not contain *b.*
Phil. 4:3; Rev. 3:5; 13:8; 17:8; 20:12; 21:27; 22:19, *b.* of life.
Rev. 22:19, take away from words of *b.*
See Ex. 17:14; Ezra 4:15; Acts 19:19; 2 Tim. 4:13.
BOOTH. Job 27:18; Jon. 4:5.
BOOTHS. Lev. 23:42, ye shall dwell in *b.*
Neh. 8:14, Israel shall dwell in *b.*
BOOTY. Num. 31:32; Jer. 49:32; Hab. 2:7; Zeph. 1:13.
BORN. Job 5:7, man *b.* to trouble.
14:1; 15:14; 25:4; Mat. 11:11, *b.* of a woman.
Ps. 87:4, this man was *b.* there.
Isa. 9:6, unto us a child is *b.*
66:8, shall a nation be *b.* at once.
John 1:13; 1 John 4:7; 5:1, 4, 18, *b.* of God.
3:3; 1 Pet. 1:23, *b.* again.
6:8, *b.* of Spirit.
1 Cor. 15:8, as one *b.* out of due time.
1 Pet. 2:2, as new-*b.* babes.
See Job 3:3; Prov. 17:17; Eccl. 3:2.
BORNE. Ps. 55:12, an enemy, then I could have *b.* it.
Isa. 53:4, *b.* our griefs, carried our sorrows.
Mat. 23:4; Lu. 11:46, grievous to be *b.*
See Job 34:31; Lam. 5:7; Mat. 20:12.
BORROW. Deut. 15:6; 28:12, lend but not *b.*
Ps. 37:21, wicked *b.* and payeth not.
Prov. 22:7, the *b.* is servant.
Mat. 5:42, him that would *b.* of thee.
See Ex. 3:22; 11:2; 22:14; 2 Kings 4:3.
BOSOM. Ps. 35:13, prayer returned into own *b.*
Prov. 6:27, take fire in his *b.*
Isa. 40:11, carry lambs in *b.*
Lu. 16:22, carried into Abraham's *b.*
John 1:18, in the *b.* of the Father.
13:23, leaning on Jesus' *b.*
See Ex. 4:6; Deut. 13:6; Job 31:33.
BOSSES. Job 15:26.
BOTCH. Deut. 28:27, 35.
BOTTLE. Judg. 4:19, a *b.* of milk.
1 Sam. 1:24; 10:3; 16:20; 2 Sam. 16:1, a *b.* of wine.
Ps. 56:8, put thou my tears into thy *b.*
119:83, like a *b.* in the smoke.
See Gen. 21:14, 15; Hab. 2:15.
BOTTLES. Josh. 9:13, these *b.* of wine.
1 Sam. 25:18, and two *b.* of wine.
Job 32:19, ready to burst like new *b.*
Hos. 7:5, sick with *b.* of wine.
Mat. 9:17; Mk. 2:22; Lu. 5:37, new wine in old *b.*
BOTTOMLESS. Rev. 9:1; 11:7; 17:8; 20:1, 2, the *b.* pit.
BOUGH. Gen. 49:22; Judg. 9:48; Deut. 24:20; Job 14:9; Ps. 80:10; Ezek. 31:30.
BOUGHT. Lu. 14:18; 1 Cor. 6:20; 7:23; 2 Pet. 2:1.
BOUND Ps. 107:10, being *b.* in affliction.
Prov. 22:15, foolishness *b.* in heart of child.
Acts 20:22, *b.* in spirit to Jerusalem.
1 Cor. 7:27, art thou *b.* to a wife.
2 Tim. 2:9, word of God is not *b.*
Heb. 13:3, in bonds as *b.* with them.
See Gen. 44:30; Mat. 16:19; Mk. 5:4.
BOUNTY. 1 Kings 10:13; 2 Cor. 9:5.
BOUNTIFUL. Prov. 22:9, a *b.* eye shall be blessed.
Isa. 32:5, nor churl said to be *b.*
See Ps. 13:6; 116:7; 119:17; 2 Cor. 9:6.
BOWELS. Gen. 43:30, his *b.* did yearn.
Isa. 63:15, where is sounding of thy *b.*
2 Cor. 6:12, straitened in *b.*
Col. 3:12, *b.* of mercies.
Phil. 1:8, after you in *b.* of Christ.
2:1, if there be any *b.*
1 John 3:17, *b.* of compassion.
See Acts 1:18; Philem. 12.
BOWLS. Num. 7:25, one silver *b.*
Eccl. 12:6, golden *b.* be broken.
Amos 6:6, that drink wine in *b.*
Zech. 4:2, with a *b.* upon the top of it.
BRACELET. Gen. 24:30; Ex. 35:22; Isa. 3:19.
BRAKE. 2 Kings 23:14; 2 Chron. 34:4, Josiah *b.* images.
Mat. 14:19; 15:36; 26:26; Mk. 6:41; 8:6; 14:22; Lu. 9:16; 22:19; 24:30; 1 Cor. 11:24, blessed and *b.*
See Ex. 32:19; 1 Sam. 4:18; Lu. 5:6; John 19:32.
BRAMBLE. Judg. 9:14; Isa. 34:13; Lu. 6:44.
BRANCH. Job 14:7, tender *b.* not cease.
Prov. 11:28, righteous flourish as *b.*
Jer. 23:5, will raise a righteous *b.*
Mat. 13:32; Lu. 13:19, birds lodge in *b.*
21:8; Mk. 11:8; John 12:13, cut down *b.*
See Zech. 3:8; 6:12; John 15:2, 4, 5, 6; Rom. 11:16.
BRAND. Judg. 15:5, set the *b.* on fire.
Zech. 3:2, as a fire *b.* plucked out.
BRASS. Deut. 8:9; 28:23; 1 Cor. 13:1.
BRAVERY. Isa. 3:18.
BRAWLER. Prov. 25:24; 1 Tim. 3:3; Tit. 3:2.
BRAY. Job 6:5; 30:7; Prov. 27:22.
BREACH. Isa. 58:12, the repairer of the *b.*
Lam. 2:13, thy *b.* is great like the sea.
See Lev. 24:20; Ps. 106:23; Amos 4:3; 6:11.
BREAD. Deut. 8:3; Mat. 4:4; Lu. 4:4, not live by *b.* alone.
Ruth 1:6, visited people in giving them *b.*
1 Kings 17:6, ravens brought *b.* and flesh.
Job 22:7, withholden *b.* from hungry.
33:20, soul abhorreth *b.*
Ps. 132:15, satisfy poor with *b.*
Prov. 9:17, *b.* eaten in secret.
12:11; 20:13; 28:19, satisfied with *b.*

Prov. 31:27, eateth not *b.* of idleness.
Eccl. 11:1, cast *b.* on waters.
Isa. 33:16, *b.* given and waters sure.
55:2, money for that which is not *b.*
10, seed to sower, *b.* to eater.
Mat. 4:3; Lu. 4:3, stones made *b.*
6:11; Lu. 11:11, give us daily *b.*
15:26; Mk. 7:27, take children's *b.*
Lu. 24:35, known in breaking *b.*
Acts 2:42; 20:7; 27:35, breaking *b.*
2 Thess. 3:8, eat any man's *b.* for nought.
See Ex. 16:4; 23:25; Josh. 9:5; Judg. 7:13.
BREAK. Cant. 2:17; 4:6, day *b.* and shadows flee.
Isa. 42:3; Mat. 12:20, bruised reed shall he not *b.*
Jer. 4:3; Hos. 10:12, *b.* up fallow ground.
Acts 21:13, to weep and *b.* my heart.
See Ps. 2:3; Mat. 5:19; 9:17; 1 Cor. 10:16.
BREATH. Gen. 2:7; 6:17; 7:15, *b.* of life.
Isa. 2:22, cease from man whose *b.*
Ezek. 37:5, 10, I will cause *b.* to enter.
Acts 17:25, he giveth to all life and *b.*
See Job 12:10; 33:4; Ps. 146:4; 150:6.
BREATHE. Ps. 27:12; Ezek. 37:9; John 20:22.
BREECHES. Ex. 28:42; Lev. 6:10; 16:4; Ezek. 44:18.
BRETHREN. Mat. 23:8, all ye are *b.*
Mk. 10:29; Lu. 18:29, no man left house or *b.*
Col. 1:2, faithful *b.* in Christ.
1 John 3:14, because we love the *b.*
See Gen. 42:8; Prov. 19:7; John 7:5.
BRIBE. 1 Sam. 12:3, have I received any *b.*
Ps. 26:10, right hand is full of *b.*
See 1 Sam. 8:3; Isa. 33:15; Job 15:34.
BRICK. Gen. 11:3; Ex. 1:14; 5:7; Isa. 9:10; 65:3.
BRIDE. Isa. 61:10; Jer. 2:32; Rev. 21:2; 22:17.
BRIDEGROOM. Mat. 25:1, to meet the *b.*
John 3:29, because of *b.* voice.
See Ps. 19:5; Isa. 62:5; Mat. 9:15.
BRIDLE. Prov. 26:3, a *b.* for the ass.
Jas. 1:26, *b.* not his tongue.
3:2, able to *b.* whole body.
See 2 Kings 19:28; Ps. 39:1; Isa. 37:29.
BRIGANDINE. Jer. 46:4; 51:3.
BRIGHT. Job 37:21, *b.* light in the clouds.
Isa. 60:3, to *b.* of thy rising.
62:1, righteousness go forth as *b.*
Mat. 17:5, *b.* cloud overshadowed.
2 Thess. 2:8, *b.* of his coming.
Heb. 1:3, the *b.* of his glory.
Rev. 22:16, the *b.* and morning star.
See Lev. 13:2; Jer. 51:11; Zech. 10:1.
BRIMSTONE. Gen. 19:24, rained upon Sodom and Gomorrah *b.*
Isa. 30:33, like a stream of *b.*
Rev. 9:17, issued fire and *b.*
14:10, tormented with fire and *b.*
19:20, a lake of fire and *b.*
BRINK. Gen. 41:3; Ex. 2:3; 7:15; Josh. 3:8.
BROAD. Ps. 119:96; Mat. 7:13; 23:5.
BROIDERED. Ezek. 16:10, 13; 27:7, 16, 24, *b.* work.
See Ex. 28:4; 1 Tim. 2:9.
BROILED. Lu. 24:42.
BROKEN. Ps. 34:18; 51:17; 69:20, *b.* heart.
John 10:35, scripture cannot be *b.*
19:36, bone shall not be *b.*
Eph. 2:14, *b.* down middle wall.
See Job 17:11; Prov. 25:19; Jer. 2:13.
BROOD. Lu. 13:34.
BROOK. 1 Sam. 17:40; Ps. 42:1; 110:7.
BROTH. Judg. 6:19; Isa. 65:4.
BROTHER. Prov. 17:17, *b.* born for adversity.
18:9, slothful *b.* to waster.
19, *b.* offended harder to be won.
24. friend closer than *b.*
Eccl. 4:8, neither child nor *b.*
Mat. 10:21, *b.* shall deliver up *b.*
1 Cor. 6:6, *b.* goeth to law with *b.*
2 Thess. 3:15, admonish as *b.*
See Gen. 4:9; Mat. 5:23; 12:50; Mk. 3:35.
BROTHERLY. Rom. 12:10; 1 Thess. 4:9; Heb. 13:1, *b.* love.
See Amos 1:9; 2 Pet. 1:7.
BROW. Isa. 48:4; Lu. 4:29.
BRUISE (*n.*). Isa. 1:6; Jer. 30:12; Nah. 3:19.
BRUISE (*v.*). 2 Kings 18:21, staff of this *b.* reed.
Isa. 42:3; Mat. 12:20, *b.* reed shall he not break.
53:5, *b.* for our iniquities.
See Gen. 3:15; Isa. 53:10; Rom. 16:20.
BRUIT. Jer. 10:22; Nah. 3:19.
BRUTISH. Ps. 92:6, a *b.* man knoweth not.
Prov. 30:2, I am more *b.* than any.
Jer. 10:21, pastors are become *b.*
See Ps. 49:10; Jer. 10:8; Ezek. 21:31.
BUCKET. Num. 24:7; Isa. 40:15.
BUCKLER. 2 Sam. 22:31; Ps. 18:2; 91:4; Prov. 2:7.
BUD. Num. 17:8. Isa. 18:5; 61:11; Hos. 8:7.
BUFFET. Mat. 26:67; 1 Cor. 4:11; 2 Cor. 12:7; 1 Pet. 2:20.
BUILD. Ps. 127:1, labour in vain that *b.*
Eccl. 3:3, a time to *b.* up.
Isa. 58:12, *b.* old waste places.
Mat. 7:24; Lu. 6:48, wise man *b.* on rock.
Lu. 14:30, began to *b.*, not able to finish.
Acts 20:32, able to *b.* you up.
Rom. 15:20, lest I *b.* on another.
1 Cor. 3:12, if any *b.* on this foundation.
Eph. 2:22, in whom ye are *b.* together.
See 1 Chron. 17:12; 2 Chron. 6:9; Eccl. 2:4.
BUILDER. Ps. 118:22; Mat. 21:42; Mk. 12:10; Lu. 20:17; Acts 4:11; 1 Pet. 2:7, *b.* refused.
1 Cor. 3:10, as a wise master-*b.*
Heb. 11:10, whose *b.* and maker is God.
See 1 Kings 5:18; Ezra 3:10.
BUILDING. 1 Cor. 3:9; 2 Cor. 5:1; Eph. 2:21; Col. 2:7.
BULRUSH. Ex. 2:3; Isa. 18:2; 58:5.
BULWARK, Isa. 26:1, salvation for walls and *b.*
See Deut. 20:20; Ps. 48:13; Eccl. 9:14.
BUNDLE. Gen. 42:35; 1 Sam. 25:29; Mat. 13:30; Acts 28:3.
BURDEN. Ps. 55:22, cast thy *b.* on the Lord.
Eccl. 12:5, grasshopper shall be a *b.*
Mat. 11:30, my *b.* is light.
20:12, borne *b.* and heat of day.
23:4; Lu. 11:46, bind heavy *b.*
Gal. 6:2, 5, bear his own *b.*
See Num. 11:11; Acts 15:28; 2 Cor. 12:16.
BURDENSOME. Zech. 12:3; 2 Cor. 11:9; 1 Thess. 2:6.
BURIAL. Eccl. 6:3; Jer. 22:19; Mat. 26:12; Acts 8:2.
BURN. Ps. 39:3, musing the fire *b.*
Prov. 26:23, *b.* lips and wicked heart.
Isa. 9:18, wickedness *b.* as fire.
33:14, dwell with everlasting *b.*
Mal. 4:1, day that shall *b.* as oven.
Mat. 13:30, bind tares to *b.* them.
Lu. 3:17, chaff *b.* with fire unquenchable.
12:35, loins girded and lights *b.*
24:32, did not our heart *b.*
John 5:35, he was a *b.* and shining light.
1 Cor. 13:3, give my body to be *b.*
Heb. 6:8, whose end is to be *b.*
Rev. 4:5, lamps b, before throne.
19:20, into a lake *b.*
See Gen. 44:18; Ex. 3:2; 21:25.
BURNT-OFFERING. Ps. 40:6, *b.* thou hast not required.
Isa. 61:8, I hate robbery for *b.*
Jer. 6:20, your *b.* not acceptable.
Hos. 6:6, knowledge more than *b.*
Mk. 12:33, love neighbour more than *b.*
See Gen. 22:7; Lev. 1:4; 6:9.
BURST. Job 32:19; Prov. 3:10; Mk. 2:22; Lu. 5:37.
BURY. Mat. 8:21; Lu. 9:59, suffer me to *b.* my father.
22; Lu. 9:60, let dead *b.* dead.
John 19:40, manner of the Jews is to *b.*
Rom. 6:4; Col. 2:12, *b.* with him by baptism.
1 Cor. 15:4, he was *b.* and rose again.
See Gen. 23:4; 47:29; Mat. 14:12.
BUSHEL. Mat. 5:15; Mk. 4:21; Lu. 11:38.
BUSINESS. 1 Sam. 21:8, king's *b.* requireth haste.

CATCH. Ps. 10:9, to *c.* the poor.
Mat. 13:19, devil *c.* away what was sown.
Lu. 5:10, from henceforth thou shalt *c.* men.
John 10:12, wolf *c.* and scattereth sheep.
See 2 Kings 7:12; Ezek. 19:3; Mk. 12:13.
CATTLE. Gen. 46:32, their trade to feed *c.*
Ex. 10:26, our *c.* shall go with us.
Deut. 2:35; 3:7; Josh. 8:2, the *c.* ye shall take for prey.
Ps. 50:10, *c.* upon a thousand hills.
See Gen. 1:25; 30:43; Jon. 4:11.
CAUGHT. Gen. 22:13, ram *c.* by horns.
John 21:3, that night they *c.* nothing.
2 Cor. 12:2, *c.* up to third heaven.
16, I *c.* you with guile.
1 Thess. 4:17, be *c.* up together with them.
See 2 Sam. 18:9; Prov. 7:13; Rev. 12:5.
CAUSE (*n.*). Mat. 19:5; Mk. 10:7; Eph. 5:31, for this *c.* shall a man leave.
1 Cor. 11:30, for this *c.* many are sickly.
1 Tim. 1:16, for this *c.* I obtained mercy.
See Prov. 18:17; 2 Cor. 4:16; 5:13.
CAUSE (*v.*). Ezra 6:12, God *c.* his name to dwell.
Ps. 67:1; 80:3, *c.* his face to shine.
Rom. 16:17, them. who *c.* divisions.
See Deut. 1:38; 12:11; Job 6:24.
CAUSELESS. 1 Sam. 25:31; Prov. 26:2.
CAVES. 1 Kings 18:4, Obadiah hid them by fifty in *c.*
19:9, and he came thither into a *c.*
Isa. 2:19, go into a *c.* for fear of the Lord.
See Gen. 19:30; 23:19; 49:29; Josh. 10:16; 1 Sam. 13:6; 22:1; 24:10.
CEASE. Deut. 15:11, poor never *c.* out of land.
Job 3:17, the wicked *c.* from troubling.
Ps. 46:9, he maketh wars to *c.*
Prov. 26:20, strife *c.*
Eccl. 12:3, grinders *c.* because few.
Acts 20:31, I *c.* not to warn.
1 Cor. 13:8, tongues they shall. *c.*
1 Thess. 5:17, pray without *c.*
1 Pet. 4:1, hath *c.* from sin.
See Gen. 8:22; Isa. 1:16; 2:22.
CEDAR. 1 Kings 5:6, they hew me *c.* trees out of Lebanon.
6:15, with boards of *c.*
Job 40:17, he moveth his tail like a *c.*
Ps. 92:12, grow like a *c.* in Lebanon.
CEDARS (of Lebanon). Judg. 9:15, devour the *c.* of Lebanon.
Isa. 2:13, upon all the *c.* of Lebanon.
See Ps. 104:16; 148:9; Cant. 5:15; Ezek. 17:3.
CELEBRATE. Lev. 23:32; Isa. 38:18.
CELESTIAL. 1 Cor. 15:40.
CENSER. Ezek. 8:11, every man his *c.*
Heb. 9:4, holiest had the golden *c.*
Rev. 8:3, angel having a golden *c.*
5, angel took the *c.* and filled.
See Lev. 10:1; 16:12; Num. 16:36; 1 Kings 7:30.
CEREMONIES. Num. 9:3.
CERTAIN. Ex. 3:12, *c.* I will be with thee.
1 Cor. 4:11, no *c.* dwelling-place.
Heb. 10:27, a *c.* looking for of judgment.
See Deut. 13:14; 1 Kings 2:37; Dan. 2:45.
CERTIFY. 2 Sam. 15:28; Gal. 1:11.
CHAFF. Mat. 3:12; Lu. 3:17, burn up *c.* with fire.
See Jer. 23:28; Hos. 13:3; Zeph. 2:2.
CHAIN. Mk. 5:3, no, not with *c.*
Acts 12:7, Peter's *c.* fell off.
2 Tim. 1:16, not ashamed of my *c.*
2 Pet. 2:4, into *c.* of darkness.
Jude 6, everlasting *c.* under darkness.
See Ps. 73:6; Lam. 3:7; Isa. 40:19.
CHALCEDONY. Rev. 21:19, the third, a *c.*
CHALLENGETH. Ex. 22:9.
CHAMBER. 2 Kings 4:10, little *c.* on wall.
Ps. 19:5, as bridegroom coming out of *c.*
Isa. 26:20, enter into thy *c.*
Ezek. 8:12, *c.* of imagery.
Mat. 24:26, in secret *c.*
Acts 9:37; 20:8 in upper *c.*
See Dan. 6:10; Joel 2:16; Prov. 7:27.
CHAMPION. 1 Sam. 17:4, 51.
CHANCE. 1 Sam. 6:9; 2 Sam. 1:6; Eccl. 9:11; Lu. 10:31.
CHANGE (*n.*). Job 14:14, till my *c.* come.
Prov. 24:21, meddle not with them given to *c.*
See Judg. 14:12; Zech. 3:4; Heb. 7:12.
CHANGE (*v.*). Ps. 15:4, sweareth and *c.* not.
102:26, as vesture shalt thou *c.* them.
Lam. 4:1, fine gold. *c.*
Mal. 3:6, I the Lord *c.* not.
Rom. 1:23, *c.* glory of uncorruptible God.
1 Cor. 15:51, we shall all be *c.*
2 Cor. 3:18, *c.* from glory to glory.
See Job 17:12; Jer. 2:36; 13:23.
CHANT. Amos 6:5.
CHAPEL. Amos 7:13, for it is the king's *c.*
CHAPMEN. 2 Chron. 9:14.
CHAPT. Jer. 14:4.
CHARGE. Job 1:22, nor *c.* God foolishly.
4:18, angels he *c.* with folly.
Mat. 9:30; Mk. 5:43; Lu. 9:21, Jesus *c.* them.
Acts 7:60; 2 Tim. 4:16, lay not sin to their *c.*
Rom. 8:33, who shall lay any thing to *c.*
1 Cor. 9:18, gospel without *c.*
1 Tim. 1:3, *c.* that they teach no other.
5:21; 2 Tim. 4:1, I *c.* thee before God.
6:17, *c.* them that are rich.
See Ex. 6:13; Ps. 35:11; 91:11; Mk. 9:25.
CHARGEABLE. 2 Sam. 13:25; 2 Cor. 11:9; 1 Thess. 2:9.
CHARIOT. 2 Kings 2:11, there appeared a *c.* of fire.
CHARIOTS. Ex. 14:6, he made ready his *c.*
1 Sam. 13:5, Philistines gathered thirty thousand *c.*
2 Sam. 10:18, David slew the men of seven hundred *c.*
Ps. 20:7, some trust in *c.*
Nah. 3:2, and of the jumping *c.*
See 2 Kings 6:14, 17; Ps. 68:17.
CHARITY. Rom. 14:15, now walkest not *c.*
Col. 3:14, put on *c.*
2 Thess. 1:3, *c.* aboundeth.
1 Tim. 1:5, end of commandment is *c.*
2 Tim. 2:22, follow faith, *c.*, peace.
Tit. 2:2, sound in faith, in *c.*
1 Pet. 4:8, *c.* cover sins.
2 Pet. 1:7, to brotherly kindness *c.*
Jude 12, spots in feasts of *c.*
See 1 Cor. 8:1; 13:1; 14:1; 16:14; Rev. 2:19.
CHARMER. Deut. 18:11; Ps. 58:5; Jer. 8:17.
CHASE. Lev. 26:8, five *c.* hundred.
Deut. 32:30; Josh. 23:10, one *c.* thousand.
See Job 18:18; Ps. 35:5; Lam. 3:52.
CHASTE. 2 Cor. 11:2; Tit. 2:5; 1 Pet. 3:2.
CHASTEN. Deut. 8:5, as a man *c.* son.
Ps. 6:1; 38:1, nor *c.* me in displeasure.
94:12, blessed is the man whom thou *c.*
Prov. 19:18, *c.* thy son while there is hope.
2 Cor. 6:9, as *c.* and not killed.
Heb. 12:6; Rev. 3:19, whom the Lord loveth he *c.*
11, no *c.* seemeth to be joyous.
See Ps. 69:10; 73:14; 118:18.
CHASTISEMENT. Deut. 11:2; Job 34:31; Isa. 53:5.
CHATTER. Isa. 38:14.
CHEEK. Mat. 5:39; Lu. 6:29, smiteth on right *c.*
See Job 16:10; Isa. 50:6; Lam. 3:30.
CHEER. Prov. 15:13, maketh a *c.* countenance.
Zech. 9:17, corn make young men *c.*
John 16:33, be of good *c.*, I have overcome.
Acts 23:11; 27:22, 25, be of good *c.*
Rom. 12:8, he that showeth mercy with *c.*
2 Cor. 9:7, God loveth a *c.* giver.
See Judg. 9:13; Mat. 9:2; 14:27; Mk. 6:50.
CHERISHETH. Eph. 5:29; 1 Thess. 2:7.
CHICKENS. Mat. 23:37.
CHIDE. Ex. 17:2; Judg. 8:1; Ps. 103:9.
CHIEFEST. Cant. 5:10; Mk. 10:44; 2 Cor. 11:5.
CHILD. Gen. 42:22, do not sin against the *c.*
Ps. 131:2, quieted myself as a weaned *c.*
Prov. 20:11, a *c.* is known by his doings.

Prov. 22:6, train up a *c.* in way.
15, foolishness in heart of *c.*
Isa. 9:6, to us a *c.* is born.
65:20, *c.* shall die an hundred years old.
Lu. 1:66, what manner of *c.*
John 4:49, come ere my *c.* die.
1 Cor. 13:11, when I was a *c.*
2 Tim. 3:15, from a *c.* hast known.
See Ex. 2:2; Eccl. 4:13; 10:16; Heb. 11:23.
CHILDREN. 1 Sam. 16:11, are here all thy *c.*
Ps. 34:11, come ye *c.* hearken to me.
45:16, instead of fathers shall be *c.*
128:3, thy *c.* like olive plants.
Isa. 8:18; Heb. 2:13, I and *c.* given me.
30:9, lying *c.*, *c.* that will not hear.
63:8, *c.* that will not lie.
Jer. 31:15; Mat. 2:18, Rachel weeping for her *c.*
Ezek. 18:2, *c.* teeth on edge.
Mat. 15:26; Mk. 7:27; not take *c.* bread.
17:26, then are the *c.* free.
19:14; Mk. 10:14; Lu. 18:16, suffer little *c.*
Lu. 16:8, *c.* of this world wiser than *c.* of light.
20:36, *c.* of God and the resurrection.
John 12:36; Eph. 5:8; 1 Thess. 5:5, *c.* of light.
Rom. 8:16; Gal. 3:26; 1 John 3:10, witness that we are the *c.* of God.
Eph. 4:14, be henceforth no more *c.*
5:6; Col. 3:6, *c.* of disobedience.
6:1; Col. 3:20, *c.* obey your parents.
1 Tim. 3:4, having his *c.* in subjection.
See Num. 16:27; Esth. 3:13; Mat. 14:21.
CHODE. Gen. 31:36; Num. 20:3.
CHOICE. 1 Sam. 9:2, Saul a *c.* young man.
Acts 15:7, God made *c.* among us.
See Gen. 23:6; 2 Sam. 10:9; Prov. 8:10.
CHOKE. Mat. 13:22; Mk. 4:19; Lu. 8:14.
CHOLER. Dan. 8:7; 11:11.
CHOSE. Ps. 33:12, people *c.* for his inheritance.
89:19, exalted one *c.* out of people.
Prov. 16:16; 22:1, rather to be *c.*
Jer. 8:3, death *c.* rather than life.
Mat. 20:16; 22:14, many called, few *c.*
Lu. 10:42, hath *c.* that good part.
14:7, they *c.* the chief rooms.
John 15:16, ye have not *c.* me.
Acts 9:15, he is a *c.* vessel.
Rom. 16:13, *c.* in the Lord.
1 Cor. 1:27, 28, God hath *c.* foolish things.
Eph. 1:4, according as he hath *c.* us.
1 Pet. 2:4, *c.* of God and precious.
9, a *c.* generation.
See Ex. 18:25; 2 Sam. 6:21; 1 Chron. 16:13.
CHRIST. Mat. 16:16, thou art the C.
24:5, many shall come, saying, I am C.
John 4:25, the Messias which is called C.
29, is not this the C.?
6:69, we are sure that thou art that C.
Phil. 1:15, 16, some preach C. of contention.
1 Pet. 1:11, the Spirit of C. did signify.
1 John 2:22, denieth that Jesus is the C.?
5:1, whoso believeth Jesus is the C.
Rev. 20:4, they reigned with C. a thousand years.
6, priests of God and C.
See Mat. 1:16; 2:4; Lu. 2:26.
CHRISTIAN. Acts 11:26; 26:28; 1 Pet. 4:16.
CHRYSOLITE. Rev. 21:20, the seventh *c.*
CHRYSOPRASUS. Rev. 21:20, the tenth, a *c.*
CHURCH. Mat. 18:17, tell it to the *c.*
Acts 2:47, added to *c.* daily.
7:38, the *c.* in the wilderness.
19:37, neither robbers of *c.*
20:28, feed the *c.* of God.
Rom. 16:5; 1 Cor. 16:19; Philem. 2, *c.* in house.
1 Cor. 14:28, 34, keep silence in the *c.*
Eph. 5:24, the *c.* is subject to Christ.
25, as Christ loved the *c.*
Col. 1:18, 24, head of the body the *c.*
Heb. 12:23, the *c.* of the firstborn.
See Mat. 16:18; Rev. 1:4; 2:1; 22:16.
CHURLISH. 1 Sam. 25:3, but the man was *c.*
CIELED. 2 Chron. 3:5; Jer. 22:14; Hag. 1:4.
CIRCLE. Isa. 40:22.
CIRCUIT. 1 Sam. 7:16; Job 22:14; Ps. 19:6; Eccl. 1:6.
CIRCUMCISE. Rom. 4:11, though not *c.*
Gal. 5:2, if ye be *c.* Christ shall profit nothing.
Phil. 3:5, *c.* the eighth day.
See Deut. 30:6; John 7:22; Acts 15:1.
CIRCUMCISION. Rom. 3:1, what profit is there of *c.*
15:8, Jesus Christ minister of *c.*
Gal. 5:6; 6:15, in Christ neither *c.* availeth.
Phil. 3:3, the *c.* which worship God.
Col. 2:11, *c.* without hands.
3:11, neither *c.* nor uncircumcision.
See Ex. 4:26; John 7:22; Acts 7:8.
CIRCUMSPECT. Ex. 23:13; Eph. 5:15.
CISTERN. Eccl. 12:6, the wheel broken at the *c.*
Jer. 2:13, hewed out *c.*, broken *c.*
See 2 Kings 18:31; Prov. 5:15; Isa. 36:16.
CITIZEN. Lu. 15:15; 19:14; Acts 21:39; Eph. 2:19.
CITY. Num. 35:6; Josh. 15:59, *c.* of refuge.
2 Sam. 19:37, I may die in mine own *c.*
Ps. 46:4, make glad the *c.* of God.
107:4, found no *c.* to dwell in.
127:1, except Lord build *c.*
Prov. 8:3, wisdom crieth in *c.*
16:32, than he that taketh a *c.*
Eccl. 9:14, a little *c.* and few men.
Isa. 33:20, *c.* of solemnities.
Zech. 8:3, a *c.* of truth.
Mat. 5:14, *c.* set on a hill.
21:10, all the *c.* was moved.
Lu. 24:49, tarry in the *c.*
Acts 8:8, great joy in that *c.*
Heb. 11:10, a *c.* that hath foundations.
12:22, the *c.* of living God.
13:14, no continuing *c.*
Rev. 16:19, the *c.* of the nations fell.
20:9, compassed the beloved *c.*
See Gen. 4:17; 11:4; Jon. 1:2; Rev. 14:8; 21:10.
CLAD. 1 Kings 11:29; Isa 59:17.
CLAMOUR Prov. 9:13; Eph. 4:31.
CLAP. Ps. 47:1, *c.* your hands all ye people.
98:8, let the floods *c.* their hands.
Isa. 55:12, the trees shall *c.* their hands.
Lam. 2:15, all that pass by *c.* their hands.
See 2 Kings 11:12; Job 27:23; 34:37.
CLAVE. Ruth 1:14, Ruth *c.* to her mother-in-law.
2 Sam. 23:10, his hand *c.* to the sword.
Neh. 10:29, they *c.* to their brethren.
Acts 17:34, certain men *c.* to Paul.
See Gen. 22:3; Num. 16:31; 1 Sam. 6:14.
CLAWS. Deut. 14:6; Dan. 4:33; Zech. 11:16.
CLAY. Job 10:9, thou hast made me as *c.*
13:12, bodies like to bodies of *c.*
33:6, I also am formed out of *c.*
Ps. 40:2, out of the miry *c.*
Dan. 2:33, part of iron, part of *c.*
John 9:6, made *c.* and anointed.
Rom. 9:21, power over the *c.*
See Isa. 29:16; 41:25; 45:9; 64:8; Jer. 18:4.
CLEAN. 2 Kings 5:12, may I not wash and be *c.*
Job 14:4, who can bring *c.* out of unclean.
15:15, heavens not *c.* in his sight.
Ps. 24:4, he that hath *c.* hands.
51:10, create in me a *c.* heart.
77:8, is his mercy *c.* gone for ever?
Prov. 16:2, *c.* in his own eyes.
Isa. 1:16, wash you, make you *c.*
52:11, be *c.* that bear vessels of the Lord.
Ezek. 36:25, then will I sprinkle *c.* water.
Mat. 8:2; Mk. 1:40; Lu. 5:12, thou canst make me *c.*
23:25; Lu. 11:39, make *c.* the outside.
Lu. 11:41, all things *c.* unto you.
John 13:11, ye are not all *c.*

John 15:3, *c.* through word I have spoken.
Acts 18:6, I am *c.*
Rev. 19:8, arrayed in fine linen *c.* and white.
See Lev. 23:22; Josh. 3:17; Prov. 14:4.
CLEANNESS. 2 Sam. 22:21; Ps. 18:20; Amos 4:6.
CLEANSE. Ps. 19:12, *c.* me from secret faults.
73:13, I have *c.* my heart in vain.
Prov. 20:30, blueness of wound *c.* evil.
Mat. 8:3, immediately his leprosy was *c.*
10:8; 11:5; Lu. 7:22, *c.* lepers.
23:26, *c.* first that which is within.
Lu. 4:27, none was *c.* saving Naaman.
17:17, were not ten *c.*
Acts 10:15; 11:9, what God hath *c.*
2 Cor. 7:1, let us *c.* ourselves.
Jas. 4:8, *c.* your hands, ye sinners.
1 John 1:7, 9, *c.* us from all sin.
See Ezek. 36:25; Mk. 1:44.
CLEAR. Gen. 44:16, how shall we *c.* ourselves?
Ex. 34:7, by no means *c.* the guilty.
2 Sam. 23:4, *c.* shining after rain.
Job 11:17, age shall be *c.* than noonday.
Ps. 51:4, be *c.* when thou judgest.
Mat. 7:5; Lu. 6:42, see *c.* to pull out mote.
Mk. 8:25, saw every man *c.*
Rom. 1:20, things from creation *c.* seen.
Rev. 21:11; 22:1, light *c.* as crystal.
See Gen. 24:8; Cant. 6:10; Zech. 14:6.
CLEAVE. Josh. 23:8, *c.* to the Lord your God.
2 Kings 5:27, leprosy shall *c.* to thee.
Job 29:10; Ps. 137:6; Ezek. 3:26, *c.* to roof of mouth.
Ps. 119:25, my soul *c.* to dust.
Eccl. 10:9, he that *c.* wood shall be endangered.
Acts 11:23, with purpose of heart *c.*
Rom. 12:9, *c.* to that which is good.
See Gen. 2:24; Mat. 19:5; Mk. 10:7.
CLEFTS. Cant. 2:14; Isa. 2:21; Jer. 49:16; Amos 6:11; Obad. 3.
CLEMENCY. Acts 24:4.
CLERK. Acts 19:35.
CLIMB. John 10:1, but *c.* up some other way.
See 1 Sam. 14:13; Amos 9:2; Lu. 19:4.
CLODS. Job 21:33, the *c.* of the valley shall be sweet.
See Job 7:5; Isa. 28:24; Hos. 10:11; Joel 1:17.
CLOKE. Mat. 5:40; Lu. 6:29, let him have thy *c.* also.
1 Thess. 2:5, a *c.* of covetousness.
1 Pet. 2:16, a *c.* of maliciousness.
CLOSE (*v.*). Gen. 2:21; Isa. 29:10; Mat. 13:15.
CLOSE. Prov. 18:24, sticketh *c.* than a brother.
Lu. 9:36, they kept it *c.*
See Num. 5:13; 1 Chron. 12:1; Job 28:21.
CLOSET. Mat. 6:6; Lu. 12:3.
CLOTH. 1 Sam. 19:13; 21:9; Mat. 9:16; Mk. 2:21.
CLOTHE. Ps. 65:13, pastures *c.* with flocks.
109:18, *c.* himself with cursing.
132:9, *c.* with righteousness.
16, *c.* with salvation.
Prov. 23:21, drowsiness shall *c.* a man.
31:21, household *c.* with scarlet.
Isa. 50:3, *c.* heavens with blackness.
61:10, *c.* with garments of salvation.
Mat. 6:30; Lu. 12:28, *c.* grass of field.
31, wherewithal shall we be *c.*
11:8; Lu. 7:25, man *c.* in soft raiment.
25:36, 43, naked and ye *c.* me.
Mk. 1:6, *c.* with camel's hair.
5:15; Lu. 8:35, *c.* and in right mind.
15:17, *c.* Jesus with purple.
Lu. 16:19, *c.* in purple and fine linen.
2 Cor. 5:2, desiring to be *c.* upon.
1 Pet. 5:5, be *c.* with humility.
Rev. 3:18, that thou mayest be *c.*
12:1, woman *c.* with the sun.
19:13, *c.* with a vesture dipped in blood.
See Gen. 3:21; Ex. 40:14; Esth. 4:4.
CLOTHES. Deut. 29:5; Neh. 9:21, *c.* not waxen old.
Mk. 5:28, if I touch but his *c.*
Lu. 2:7, in swaddling *c.*
Lu. 8:27, a man that ware no *c.*
19:36, spread *c.* in the way.
24:12; John 20:5, linen *c.* laid.
John 11:44, bound with grave-*c.*
Acts 7:58, laid down *c.* at Saul's feet.
22:23, cried out and cast off *c.*
See Gen. 49:11; 1 Sam. 19:24; Neh. 4:23.
CLOTHING. Ps. 45:13, her *c.* of wrought gold.
Prov. 27:26, lambs are for thy *c.*
31:22, her *c.* is silk and purple.
25, strength and honour are her *c.*
Isa. 3:7, in my house is neither bread nor *c.*
23:18, merchandise for durable *c.*
59:17, garments of vengeance for *c.*
Mat. 7:15, in sheep's *c.*
Mk. 12:38, love to go in long *c.*
Acts 10:30, a man in bright *c.*
Jas. 2:3, to him that weareth gay *c.*
See Job 22:6; 24:7; 31:19; Ps. 35:13.
CLOUD. Ex. 13:21; 14:24; Neh. 9:19, a pillar of *c.*
1 Kings 18:44, 45, a little *c.*
Ps. 36:5, faithfulness reacheth to *c.*
97:2, *c.* and darkness round about him.
99:7, spake in *c.* pillar.
Prov. 3:20, *c.* dropped down dew.
Eccl. 11:4, regardeth the *c.* not reap.
12:2, nor *c.* return after rain.
Isa. 5:6, command *c.* rain not.
44:22, blotted out as thick *c.*
60:8, fly as a *c.*
Dan. 7:13; Lu. 21:27, Son of man with *c.*
Hos. 6:4; 13:3, goodness as morning *c.*
Mat. 17:5; Mk. 9:7; Lu. 9:34, *c.* overshadowed.
24:30; 26:64; Mk. 13:26; 14:62, in *c.* with power.
1 Cor. 10:1, fathers under *c.*
1 Thess. 4:17, caught up in *c.*
2 Pet. 2:17, *c.* carried with tempest.
Jude 12, *c.* without water.
Rev. 1:7, he cometh with *c.*
14:14-16, white *c.*
See Gen. 9:13; Ex. 24:15; 40:34.
CLOUT. Josh. 9:5; Jer. 38:11.
CLOVEN. Lev. 11:3; Deut. 14:7; Acts 2:3.
CLUSTER. Isa. 65:8, new wine in *c.*
See Num. 13:23; Cant. 1:14; Rev. 14:18.
COAL. Prov. 6:28, hot *c.* and not be burned.
25:22; Rom. 12:20, heap *c.* of fire.
John 18:18; 21:9, fire of *c.*
See Job 41:21; Ps. 18:8; Isa. 6:6.
COAST. 1 Chron. 4:10; Mat. 8:34; Mk. 5:17.
COAT. Mat. 5:40, take away thy *c.*
10:10; Mk. 6:9, neither provide two *c.*
Lu. 6:29, thy *c.* also.
John 19:23, *c.* without seam.
21:7, fisher's *c.*
Acts 9:39, the *c.* which Dorcas made.
See Gen. 3:21; 37:3; 1 Sam. 2:19.
COCK. Mat. 26:34; Mk. 13:35; 14:30; Lu. 22:34.
COCKATRICE. Isa. 11:8; 14:29; 59:5.
COCKLE. Job 31:40.
COFFER. 1 Sam. 6:8, 11, 15.
COFFIN. Gen. 50:26.
COGITATIONS. Dan. 7:28.
COLD. Prov. 20:4, by reason of *c.*
25:13, *c.* of snow in harvest.
20, garment in *c.* weather.
25, *c.* waters to thirsty soul.
Mat. 10:42, cup of *c.* water.
24:12, love of many wax *c.*
2 Cor. 11:27, in *c.* and nakedness.
Rev. 3:15, neither *c.* nor hot.
See Gen. 8:22; Job 24:7; 37:9; Ps. 147:17.
COLLECTION. 2 Chron. 24:6; Acts 11:29; Rom. 15:26; 1 Cor. 16:1.
COLLEGE. 2 Kings 22:14; 2 Chron. 34:22.
COLOUR. Prov. 23:31, *c.* in the cup.
Acts 27:30, under *c.* as though.

See Gen. 37:3; Ezek. 1:4; Dan. 10:6.
COMELY. Ps. 33:1, praise is *c.*
1 Cor. 11:13, is it *c.* that a woman.
See 1 Sam. 16:18; Prov. 30:29; Isa. 53:2.
COMFORT (*n.*). Mat. 9:22; Mk. 10:49; Lu. 8:48.
2 Cor. 13:11, be of good *c.*
Acts 9:31, *c.* of Holy Ghost.
Rom. 15:4, patience and *c.* of scriptures.
2 Cor. 1:3, God of all *c.*
7:13, were comforted in your *c.*
Phil. 2:1, if any *c.* of love.
See Job 10:20; Ps. 94:19; 119:50; Isa. 57:6.
COMFORT (*v.*). Gen. 37:35; Ps. 77:2; Jer. 31:15, refused to be *c.*
Ps. 23:4, rod and staff *c.*
Isa. 40:1, *c.* ye, *c.* ye my people.
49:13; 52:9, God hath *c.* his people.
61:2, *c.* all that mourn.
66:13, as one whom his mother *c.*
Mat. 5:4, they shall be *c.*
Lu. 16:25, he is *c.*, and thou art tormented.
John 11:19, to *c.* concerning their brother.
2 Cor. 1:4, able to *c.* them.
1 Thess. 4:18, *c.* one another with these words.
5:11, wherefore *c.* yourselves together.
14, *c.* the feeble-minded.
See Gen. 5:29; 18:5; 37:35.
COMFORTABLE. Isa. 40:2; Hos. 2:14; Zech. 1:13.
COMFORTER. Job 16:2, miserable *c.* are ye all.
Ps. 69:20, looked for *c.* but I found none.
John 14:16, give you another *C.*
15:26, when the *C.* is come.
16:7, *C.* will not come.
See 2 Sam. 10:3; 1 Chron. 19:3.
COMFORTLESS. John 14:18.
COMMAND. Ps. 33:9, he *c.* and it stood fast.
Lu. 8:25, he *c.* even the winds.
9:54, *c.* fire from heaven.
John 15:14, if ye do what I *c.* you.
Acts 17:30, *c.* all men everywhere.
See Gen. 18:19; Deut. 28:8.
COMMANDER. Isa. 55:4.
COMMANDMENT. Ps. 119:86, *c.* are faithful.
96, *c.* exceeding broad.
127, I love thy *c.*
143, thy *c.* are my delight.
Mat. 15:9; Mk. 7:7; Col. 2:22, the *c.* of men.
Lu. 23:56, rested according to *c.*
John 13:34; 1 John 2:7; 2 John 5, a new *c.*
Rom. 7:12, *c.* is holy, just, and good.
1 Cor. 7:6; 2 Cor. 8:8, by permission, not by *c.*
Eph. 6:2, first *c.* with promise.
1 Tim. 1:5, end of the *c.* is charity.
See Esth. 3:3.
COMMEND. Lu. 16:8, *c.* unjust steward.
23:46, into thy hands I *c.*
Rom. 3:5, unrighteousness *c.* righteousness of God.
5:8, God *c.* his love toward us.
1 Cor. 8:8, meat *c.* us not.
2 Cor. 3:1; 5:12, *c.* ourselves.
4:2, *c.* to every man's conscience.
10:18, not he that *c.* himself is approved.
See Prov. 12:8; Eccl. 8:15; Acts 20:32.
COMMISSION. Ezra 8:36; Acts 26:12.
COMMIT. Ps. 37:5, *c.* thy way to the Lord.
Jer. 2:13, have *c.* two evils.
John 2:24, Jesus did not *c.* himself to them.
5:22, hath *c.* judgment to Son.
Rom. 3:2, were *c.* oracles of God.
2 Cor. 5:19, had *c.* to us word of reconciliation.
1 Tim. 6:20, keep what is *c.* to thee.
2 Tim. 2:2, *c.* thou to faithful men.
1 Pet. 2:23, *c.* himself to him that judgeth.
See Job 5:8; Ps. 31:5; 1 Cor. 9:17.
COMMODIOUS. Acts 27:12.
COMMON. Eccl. 6:1, evil, and it is *c.* among men.
Mk. 12:37, the *c.* people heard him gladly.
Acts 2:44; 4:32, all things *c.*
10:14; 11:8, never eaten any thing *c.*
15; 11:9, call not thou *c.*
1 Cor. 10:13, temptation *c.* to men.
Eph. 2:12, aliens from *c.*-wealth.
See Lev. 4:27; Num. 16:29; 1 Sam. 21:4.
COMMOTION. Jer. 10:22; Lu. 21:9.
COMMUNE. Job 4:2, if we *c.* with thee.
Ps. 4:4; 77:6; Eccl. 1:16, *c.* with own heart.
Zech. 1:14, angel that *c.* with me.
See Ex. 25:22; 1 Sam. 19:3; Lu. 22:4.
COMMUNICATE. Gal. 6:6, let him that is taught *c.*
1 Tim. 6:18, be willing to *c.*
Heb. 13:16, do good and *c.*
See Gal. 2:2; Phil. 4:14, 15.
COMMUNICATION. Mat. 5:37, let your *c.* be yea.
Lu. 24:17, what manner of *c.*
1 Cor. 15:33, evil *c.* corrupt good manners.
Eph. 4:29, let no corrupt *c.* proceed.
See 2 Kings 9:11; Philem. 6.
COMMUNION. 1 Cor. 10:16; 2 Cor. 6:14; 13:14.
COMPACT. Ps. 122:3; Eph. 4:16.
COMPANY. 1 Sam. 10:5; 19:20, a *c.* of prophets.
Ps. 55:14, walked to house of God in *c.*
68:11, great was the *c.* of those.
Mk. 6:39; Lu. 9:14, sit down by *c.*
2 Thess. 3:14, have no *c.* with him.
Heb. 12:22, innumerable *c.* of angels.
See Num. 16:6; Judg. 9:37; 18:23.
COMPANION. Job 30:29, a *c.* to owls.
Ps. 119:63, a *c.* to them that fear thee.
Prov. 13:20, *c.* of fools shall be destroyed.
28:7, *c.* of riotous men.
24, the *c.* of a destroyer.
Acts 19:29, Paul's *c.* in travel.
Phil. 2:25; Rev. 1:9, brother and *c.* in labour.
See Ex. 32:27; Judg. 11:38; 14:20.
COMPARE. Prov. 3:15; 8:11, not to be *c.* to wisdom.
Isa. 40:18, what likeness will ye *c.* to him?
46:5, to whom will ye *c.* me.
Lam. 4:2, *c.* to fine gold.
Rom. 8:18, not worthy to be *c.* with glory.
1 Cor. 2:13, *c.* spiritual things with spiritual.
See Ps. 89:6; 2 Cor. 10:12.
COMPARISON. Judg. 8:2; Hag. 2:3; Mk. 4:30.
COMPASS (*n.*). 2 Sam. 5:23; 2 Kings 3:9; Isa. 44:13; Acts 28:13.
COMPASS (*v.*). 2 Sam. 22:5; Ps. 18:4; 116:3, waves of death *c.* me.
6; Ps. 18:5, sorrows of hell *c.* me.
Ps. 5:12, with favour *c.* as with a shield.
32:7, *c.* with songs of deliverance.
10, mercy shall *c.* him about.
Isa. 50:11, *c.* yourselves with sparks.
Mat. 23:15, *c.* sea and land.
Lu. 21:20, Jerusalem *c.* with armies.
Heb. 5:2, he also is *c.* with infirmity.
12:1, *c.* about with cloud of witnesses.
See Josh. 6:3; Job 16:13; Jer. 31:22.
COMPASSION. Isa. 49:15, that she should not have *c.*
Lam. 3:22, his *c.* fail not.
32; Mic. 7:19, yet will he have *c.*
Mat. 9:36; 14:14; Mk. 1:41; 6:34, Jesus moved with *c.*
18:33, *c.* on thy fellowservant.
20:34, had *c.* on them and touched.
Mk. 5:19, the Lord hath had *c.*
9:22, have *c.*, and help us.
Lu. 10:33, the Samaritan had *c.*
15:20, father had *c.*, and ran.
Rom. 9:15, I will have *c.* on whom I will.
Heb. 5:2, have *c.* on ignorant.
1 Pet. 3:8, of one mind, having *c.*
1 John 3:17, shutteth up bowels of *c.*
Jude 22, of some have *c.*, making a difference.
See Ps. 78:38; 86:15; 111:4; 112:4.
COMPEL. Mat. 5:41, *c.* thee to go a mile.
27:32; Mk. 15:21, *c.* to bear cross.

Lu. 14:23, *c.* to come in.
Acts 26:11, I *c.* them to blaspheme.
See Lev. 25:39; 2 Cor. 12:11; Gal. 2:3.
COMPLAIN. Ps. 144:14, no *c.* in our streets.
Lam. 3:39, wherefore doth a living man *c.*
Jude 16, these murmurers, *c.*
See Num. 11:1; Judg. 21:22; Job 7:11.
COMPLAINT. Job 23:2, to-day is my *c.* bitter.
Ps. 142:2, I poured out my *c.* before him.
See 1 Sam. 1:16; Job 7:13; 9:27; 10:1.
COMPLETE. Lev. 23:15; Col. 2:10; 4:12.
COMPREHEND. Job 37:5; Isa. 40:12; John 1:5; Eph. 3:18.
CONCEAL. Prov. 12:23, prudent man *c.* knowledge.
25:2, glory of God to *c.* a thing.
Jer. 50:2, publish and *c.* not.
See Gen. 37:26; Deut. 13:8.
CONCEIT. Rom. 11:25; 12:16, wise in your own *c.*
CONCEIT (reproved). Prov. 3:7; 12:15; 18:11; 20:5; 28:11; Isa. 5:21.
CONCEIVE. Ps. 7:14, *c.* mischief, brought forth falsehood.
Ps. 51:5, in sin did my mother *c.* me.
Acts 5:4, why hast thou *c.* this thing.
Jas. 1:15, when lust *c.* it bringeth forth.
See Job 15:35; Isa. 7:14; 59:4.
CONCERN. Lu. 24:27, things *c.* himself.
Rom. 9:5, as *c.* the flesh Christ came.
16:19, simple *c.* evil.
Phil. 4:15, *c.* giving and receiving.
1 Tim. 6:21, have erred *c.* the faith.
1 Pet. 4:12, *c.* fiery trial.
See Lev. 6:3; Num. 10:29; Ps. 90:13; 135:14.
CONCISION. Phil. 3:2.
CONCLUDE. Rom. 3:28; 11:32; Gal. 3:22.
CONCLUSION. Eccl. 12:13.
CONCORD. 2 Cor. 6:15.
CONCUPISCENCE. Col. 3:5; 1 Thess. 4:5, mortify evil *c.*
CONDEMN. Job 10:2, I will say to God, do not *c.* me.
Amos 2:8, drink wine of the *c.*
Mat. 12:7, ye would not have *c.* the guiltless.
37, by thy words shalt be *c.*
42; Lu. 11:31, rise in judgment and *c.*
20:18, shall *c.* him to death.
27:3, Judas when he saw he was *c.*
Mk. 14:64, all *c.* him to be guilty.
Lu. 6:37, *c.* not and ye shall not be *c.*
John 3:17, God sent not his Son to *c.*
18, believe not is *c.*
8:10, hath no man *c.* thee?
11, neither do I *c.* thee.
Rom. 2:1, thou *c.* thyself.
8:3, *c.* sin in the flesh.
34, who is he that *c.*?
14:22, that *c.* not himself.
Tit. 2:8, sound speech that cannot be *c.*
Jas. 5:6, ye *c.* and killed the just.
9, grudge not lest ye be *c.*
1 John 3:21, if our heart *c.* us not.
See Job 9:20; 15:6; Mat. 12:41.
CONDEMNATION. John 3:19, this is the *c.*, that light.
2 Cor. 3:9, the ministration of *c.*
1 Tim. 3:6, the *c.* of the devil.
Jas. 5:12, lest ye fall into *c.*
Jude 4, of old ordained to this *c.*
See Lu. 23:40; Rom. 5:16; 8:1.
CONDESCEND. Rom. 12:16.
CONDITION. 1 Sam. 11:2; Lu. 14:32.
CONDUIT. 2 Kings 18:17; 20:20; Isa. 7:3; 36:2.
CONEY. Lev. 11:5; Ps. 104:18; Prov. 30:26.
CONFECTION. Ex. 30:35; 1 Sam. 8:13.
CONFEDERATE. Gen. 14:13; Isa. 7:2; 8:12; Obad. 7.
CONFERENCE. Gal. 2:6.
CONFERRED. Gal. 1:16.
CONFESS. Prov. 28:13, whoso *c.* and forsaketh.
Mat. 10:32; Lu. 12:8, *c.* me before men.
John 9:22, if any man did *c.*
12:42, rulers did not *c.* him.
Acts 23:8, Pharisees *c.* both.
Rom. 10:9, shall *c.* with thy mouth.
14:11; Phil. 2:11, every tongue *c.*
Heb. 11:13, *c.* they were strangers.
Jas. 5:16, *c.* your faults one to another.
1 John 1:9, if we *c.* our sins.
4:2, every spirit that *c.* Christ.
15, whoso shall *c.* that Jesus is the Christ.
Rev. 3:5, I will *c.* his name before my Father.
See Lev. 16:21; 1 Kings 8:33; 2 Chron. 6:24.
CONFESSION. Rom. 10:10; 1 Tim. 6:13.
CONFIDENCE. Ps. 65:5, the *c.* of all the ends of the earth.
118:8, 9, than to put *c.* in man.
Prov. 3:26, the Lord shall be thy *c.*
14:26, in fear of the Lord is strong *c.*
Isa. 30:15, in *c.* shall be your strength.
Jer. 2:37, hath rejected thy *c.*
Eph. 3:12, access with *c.* by the faith of him.
Phil. 3:3, 4, no *c.* in flesh.
Heb. 3:6, 14, hold fast *c.*
10:35, cast not away *c.*
1 John 2:28, we may have *c.*
3:21, we have *c.* toward God.
5:14, this is the *c.* we have in him.
See Job 4:6; 18:14; 31:24; Prov. 25:19.
CONFIDENT. Ps. 27:3; Prov. 14:16; 2 Cor. 5:6; Phil. 1:6.
CONFIRM. Isa. 35:3, *c.* the feeble knees.
Mk. 16:20, *c.* the word with signs.
Acts 14:22, *c.* the souls of the disciples.
15:32, 41, exhorted brethren, and *c.* them.
Rom. 15:8, *c.* the promises made to fathers.
See 2 Kings 15:19.
CONFIRMATION. Phil. 1:7; Heb. 6:16.
CONFISCATION. Ezra 7:26.
CONFLICT. Phil. 1:30; Col. 2:1.
CONFORM. Rom. 8:29; 12:2; Phil. 3:10.
CONFOUND. Ps. 22:5, fathers trusted and were not *c.*
40:14; 70:2, ashamed and *c.*
Acts 2:6, multitude were *c.*
9:22, Saul *c.* the Jews.
See Gen. 11:7; Ps. 71:13; 129:5.
CONFUSED. Isa. 9:5; Acts 19:32.
CONFUSION. Dan. 9:7, to us belongeth *c.* of faces.
Acts 19:29, city was filled with *c.*
1 Cor. 14:33, God not author of *c.*
See Ps. 70:2; 71:1; 109:29; Isa. 24:10.
CONGEALED. Ex. 15:8.
CONGRATULATE. 1 Chron. 18:10.
CONGREGATION. Num. 14:10, all the *c.* bade stone them.
Neh. 5:13, all the *c.* said Amen.
Ps. 1:5, nor sinners in the *c.* of the righteous.
26:12, in the *c.* will I bless the Lord.
Prov. 21:16, in the *c.* of the dead.
Joel 2:16, sanctify the *c.*
Acts 13:43, when the *c.* was broken up.
See Ex. 12:6; 16:2; 39:32; Lev. 4:13.
CONIES. Ps. 104:18, the rocks for the *c.*
Prov. 30:26, the *c.* are but a feeble folk.
See Lev. 11:5; Deut. 14:7.
CONQUERORS. Rom. 8:37; Rev. 6:2.
CONSCIENCE. Acts 24:16, *c.* void of offence.
Rom. 2:15; 9:1; 2 Cor. 1:12, *c.* bearing witness.
13:5; 1 Cor. 10:25, 27, 28, for *c.* sake.
1 Cor. 8:10, 12, weak *c.*
1 Tim. 1:5, 19; Heb. 13:18; 1 Pet. 3:16, a good *c.*
3:9, mystery of faith in pure *c.*
4:2, *c.* seared with hot iron.
Heb. 9:14, purge *c.* from dead works.
10:22, hearts sprinkled from evil *c.*
See John 8:9; Acts 23:1; 2 Cor. 4:2.
CONSECRATE. 1 Chron. 29:5, to *c.* his service to the Lord.
Mic. 4:13, I will *c.*
Heb. 7:28, who is *c.* for evermore.
10:20, living way which he hath *c.*
See Ex. 28:3; 29:35; 32:29; Lev. 7:37.
CONSENT. Ps. 50:18, a thief thou *c.* with him.
Prov. 1:10, if sinners entice thee *c.* not.
Zeph. 3:9, to serve with one *c.*

Lu. 14:18, with one *c.* began to make excuse.
See Deut. 13:8; Acts 8:1; Rom. 7:16.
CONSIDER. Ps. 8:3, when I *c.* the heavens.
41:1, blessed is he that *c.* the poor.
48:13, *c.* her palaces.
50:22, *c.* this, ye that forget God.
Prov. 6:6, *c.* her ways and be wise.
23:1, *c.* diligently what is before thee.
24:12, doth not he *c.* it.?
28:22, and *c.* not that poverty.
Eccl. 5:1, they *c.* not that they do evil.
7:14, in day of adversity *c.*
Isa. 1:3, my people doth not *c.*
Jer. 23:20; 30:24, in latter days ye shall *c.*
Ezek. 12:3, it may be they will *c.*
Hag. 1:5, 7, *c.* your ways.
Mat. 6:28; Lu. 12:27, *c.* lilies of the field.
7:3, *c.* not the beam.
Lu. 12:24, *c.* the ravens.
Gal. 6:1, *c.* thyself lest thou also be tempted.
Heb. 3:1, *c.* the Apostle and High Priest.
7:4, now *c.* how great this man was.
10:21, *c.* one another to provoke.
12:3, *c.* him that endured.
13:7, *c.* the end of their conversation.
See Deut. 32:29; Judg. 18:14; 1 Sam. 12:24.
CONSIST. Lu. 12:15; Col. 1:17.
CONSOLATION. Job 15:11, are the *c.* of God small.
Lu. 6:24, ye have received your *c.*
Rom. 15:5, the God of *c.*
Phil. 2:1, if there be any *c.* in Christ.
2 Thess. 2:16, everlasting *c.*
Heb. 6:18, strong *c.*
See Jer. 16:7; Lu. 2:25; Acts 4:36.
CONSPIRACY. 2 Sam. 15:2; Jer. 11:9; Acts 23:13.
CONSTANTLY. 1 Chron. 28:7; Prov. 21:28; Tit. 3:8.
CONSTRAIN. Job 32:18; Lu. 24:29; 2 Cor. 5:14; 1 Pet. 5:2.
CONSULT. Ps. 83:3; Mk. 15:1; Lu. 14:31; John 12:10.
CONSUME. Ex. 3:2, bush was not *c.*
Deut. 4:24; 9:3; Heb. 12:29, a *c.* fire.
1 Kings 18:38; 2 Chron. 7:1, fire fell and *c.* the sacrifice.
Job 20:26, fire not blown shall *c.* him.
Ps. 39:11, *c.* away like a moth.
Mal. 3:6, therefore ye are not *c.*
Lu. 9:54, *c.* them as Elias did.
Gal. 5:15, take heed ye be not *c.*
Jas. 4:3, that ye may *c.* it on your lusts.
See Ex. 32:10; 33:3; Deut. 5:25; Josh. 24:20.
CONSUMMATION. Dan. 9:27.
CONSUMPTION. Lev. 26:16; Deut. 28:22; Isa. 10:22.
CONTAIN. 1 Kings 8:27; 2 Chron. 2:6; 6:18; 1 Cor. 7:9.
CONTEMN. Ps. 10:13; 15:4; 107:11; Ezek. 21:10.
CONTEMPT. Prov. 18:3, wicked cometh, then cometh *c.*
Dan. 12:2, awake to everlasting *c.*
See Esth. 1:18; Job 31:34; Ps. 119:22.
CONTEMPTIBLE. Mal. 1:7, 12; 2:9; 2 Cor. 10:10.
CONTEND. Isa. 49:25, I will *c.* with him that *c.*
50:8, who will *c.* with me.
Jer. 12:5, how canst thou *c.* with horses.
See Job 10:2; 13:8; Eccl. 6:10; Jude 3, 9.
CONTENT. Mk. 15:15, willing to *c.* the people.
Lu. 3:14, be *c.* with your wages.
Phil. 4:11, I have learned to be *c.*
1 Tim. 6:6, godliness with *c.* is great gain.
8, having food let us be *c.*
Heb. 13:5, be *c.* with such things as ye have.
See Gen. 37:27; Josh. 7:7; Job 6:28; Prov. 6:35.
CONTENTION. Prov. 18:18, the lot causeth *c.* to cease.
19:13; 27:15, *c.* of a wife.
23:29, who hath *c.*
Acts 15:39, the *c.* was sharp.
1 Cor. 1:11, there are *c.* among you.
Phil. 1:16, preach Christ of *c.*
1 Thess. 2:2, to speak with much *c.*
Tit. 3:9, avoid *c.* and strivings.
See Prov. 13:10; 17:14; 18:6; 22:10.
CONTENTIOUS. Prov. 21:19; 26:21; 27:15; Rom. 2:8; 1 Cor. 11:16.
CONTINUAL. Ps. 34:1; 71:6, praise *c.* in my mouth.
40:11, let thy truth *c.* preserve me.
73:23, I am *c.* with thee.
Prov. 6:21, bind them *c.* on thine heart.
15:15, merry heart hath a *c.* feast.
Isa. 14:6, smote with a *c.* stroke.
52:5, my name is *c.* blasphemed.
Lu. 18:5, lest by her *c.* coming.
24:53, were *c.* in the temple.
Acts 6:4, give ourselves *c.* to prayer.
Rom. 9:2, I have *c.* sorrow in my heart.
Heb. 7:3, abideth a priest *c.*
See Ex. 29:42; Num. 4:7; Job 1:5.
CONTINUANCE. Deut. 28:59; Ps. 139:16; Isa. 64:5; Rom. 2:7.
CONTINUE. Job 14:2, as a shadow and *c.* not.
Ps. 72:17, name shall *c.* as long as the sun.
Isa. 5:11, *c.* till wine inflame them.
Jer. 32:14, evidences may *c.* many days.
Lu. 6:12, he *c.* all night in prayer.
22:28, that *c.* with me in my temptation.
John 8:31, if ye *c.* in my word.
15:9, *c.* ye in my love.
Acts 1:14; 2:46, *c.* with one accord.
12:16, Peter *c.* knocking.
13:43, to *c.* in grace of God.
14:22, exhorting them to *c.* in faith.
26:22, I *c.* unto this day.
Rom. 6:1, shall we *c.* in sin?
12:12; Col. 4:2, *c.* in prayer.
Gal. 3:10, that *c.* not in all things.
Col. 1:23; 1 Tim. 2:15, if ye *c.* in the faith.
1 Tim. 4:16; 2 Tim. 3:14, *c.* in them.
Heb. 7:23, not suffered to *c.* by reason.
24, this man *c.* ever.
13:1, let brotherly love *c.*
14, here have we no *c.* city.
Jas. 4:13, and *c.* there a year.
2 Pet. 3:4, all things *c.* as they were.
1 John 2:19, no doubt have *c.* with us.
See 1 Sam. 12:14; 13:14; 2 Sam. 7:29.
CONTRADICTION. Heb. 7:7; 12:3.
CONTRARIWISE. 2 Cor. 2:7; Gal. 2:7; 1 Pet. 3:9.
CONTRARY. Acts 18:13, *c.* to the law.
26:9, many things *c.* to name of Jesus.
Gal. 5:17, *c.* the one to the other.
1 Thess. 2:15, *c.* to all men.
1 Tim. 1:10, *c.* to sound doctrine.
Tit. 2:8, he of the *c.* part may be ashamed.
See Lev. 26:21; Esth. 9:1; Mat. 14:24; Acts 17:7.
CONTRIBUTION. Rom. 15:26.
CONTRITE. Ps. 34:18; 51:17; Isa. 57:15; 66:2.
CONTROVERSY. Jer. 25:31, a *c.* with the nations.
Mic. 6:2, hath a *c.* with his people.
1 Tim. 3:16, without *c.* great is the mystery.
See Deut. 17:8; 19:17; 21:5; 25:1.
CONVENIENT. Prov. 30:8, feed me with food *c.*
Acts 24:25, when I have a *c.* season.
Rom. 1:28, things which are not *c.*
Eph. 5:4, talking, jesting, are not *c.*
See Jer. 40:4; Mk. 6:21; 1 Cor. 16:12.
CONVERSANT. Josh. 8:35; 1 Sam. 25:15.
CONVERSATION. Ps. 37:14, such as be of upright *c.*
50:23, that ordereth his *c.* aright.
Phil. 1:27, *c.* as becometh the gospel.
3:20, our *c.* is in heaven.
1 Tim. 4:12, an example in *c.*
Heb. 13:5, *c.* without covetousness.
7, considering end of their *c.*
1 Pet. 1:15; 2 Pet. 3:11, holy *c.*
18, redeemed from vain *c.*
2:12, your *c.* honest among Gentiles.
3:1, won by *c.* of wives.
2 Pet. 2:7, vexed with filthy *c.*
See Gal. 1:13; Eph. 2:3; 4:22; Jas. 3:13.
CONVERSION. Acts 15:3.

CONVERT. Ps. 19:7, perfect, *c.* the soul.
Isa. 6:10; Mat. 13:15; Mk. 4:12; John 12:40; Acts 28:27, lest they *c.*
Mat. 18:3, except ye be *c.*
Lu. 22:32, when *c.* strengthen thy brethren.
Acts 3:19, repent and be *c.*
Jas. 5:19, 20, and one *c.* him.
See Ps. 51:13; Isa. 1:27; 60:5.
CONVICTED. John 8:9.
CONVINCE. John 8:46, which of you *c.* me of sin.
Tit. 1:9, able to *c.* gainsayers.
See Job 32:12; Acts 18:28; 1 Cor. 14:24.
CONVOCATION. Ex. 12:16; Lev. 23:2; Num. 28:26.
COOK. 1 Sam. 8:13; 9:23, 24.
COOL. Gen. 3:8; Lu. 16:24.
COPPER. Ezra 8:27; 2 Tim. 4:14.
COPY. Deut. 17:18; Josh. 8:32; Prov. 25:1.
CORBAN. Mk. 7:11, it is *c.*
CORD. Prov. 5:22, holden with the *c.* of sins.
Eccl. 4:12, a threefold *c.*
12:6, silver *c.* loosed.
Isa. 5:18, draw iniquity with *c.*
54:2, lengthen *c.*
Hos. 11:4, the *c.* of a man.
John 2:15, scourge of small *c.*
See Judg. 15:13; Ps. 2:3; 118:27; Jer. 38:6.
CORN. Gen. 42:2; Acts 7:12, *c.* in Egypt.
Deut. 25:4; 1 Cor. 9:9; 1 Tim. 5:18, ox treadeth *c.*
Judg. 15:5, foxes into standing *c.*
Job 5:26, like as a shock of *c.*
Ps. 4:9, in time their *c.* increased.
65:7, prepared them *c.*
13, valleys covered over with *c.*
72:16, handful of *c.* in the earth.
Prov. 11:26, he that withholdeth *c.*
Zech. 9:17, *c.* shall make men cheerful.
Mat. 12:1; Mk. 2:23; Lu. 6:1, pluck *c.*
Mk. 4:28, full *c.* in the ear.
John 12:24, a *c.* of wheat fall into ground.
See Gen. 27:28; 41:57; Deut. 33:28; Isa. 36:17.
CORNER. Ps. 118:22; Eph. 2:20, head stone of *c.*
144:12, daughters as *c.* stones.
Isa. 28:16; 1 Pet. 2:6, a precious *c.* stone.
Mat. 6:5, pray in *c.* of the streets.
Rev. 7:1, on four *c.* of the earth.
See Job 1:19; Prov. 7:8; 21:9.
CORNET. 2 Sam. 6:5; 1 Chron. 15:28; Dan. 3:5.
CORPSE. 2 Kings 19:35; Isa. 37:36; Nah. 3:3; Mk. 6:29.
CORRECT. Prov. 3:12, whom the Lord loveth he *c.*
29:17, *c.* thy son.
19, servant will not be *c.* by words.
Jer. 10:24, *c.* me, but with judgment.
30:11; 46:28, I will *c.* thee in measure.
Heb. 12:9, we have had fathers which *c.* us.
See Job 5:17; Ps. 39:11; 94:10.
CORRECTION. Prov. 22:15, rod of *c.* shall drive it.
Jer. 2:30; 5:3; 7:28; Zeph. 3:2, receive *c.*
2 Tim. 3:16, scripture profitable for *c.*
See Job 37:13; Prov. 3:11; 7:22; 15:10.
CORRUPT. Deut. 4:16, take heed lest ye *c.*
31:29, after my death ye will *c.*
Mat. 6:19; Lu. 12:33, moth *c.*
7:17; 12:33; Lu. 6:43, a *c.* tree.
1 Cor. 15:33, evil communications *c.*
2 Cor. 2:17, not as many, which *c.* the word.
7:2, we have *c.* no man.
11:2, lest your minds be *c.*
Eph. 4:22, put off old man which is *c.*
29, let no *c.* communication.
1 Tim. 6:5; 2 Tim. 3:8, men of *c.* minds.
Jas. 5:1, your riches are *c.*
See Gen. 6:11; Job 17:1; Prov. 25:26.
CORRUPTERS. Isa. 1:4; Jer. 6:28.
CORRUPTIBLE. Rom. 1:23; 1 Cor. 9:25; 15:53; 1 Pet. 1:18; 3:4.
CORRUPTION. Ps. 16:10; 49:9; Acts 2:27; 13:35, not see *c.*
Jon. 2:6, brought up life from *c.*
Rom. 8:21, from bondage of *c.*
1 Cor. 15:42, 50, sown in *c.*
Gal. 6:8, of flesh reap *c.*
2 Pet. 1:4, the *c.* that is in world.
2:12, perish in their own *c.*
See Lev. 22:25; Job 17:14; Isa. 38:17.
CORRUPTLY. 2 Chron. 27:2; Neh. 1:7.
COST. 2 Sam. 24:24; 1 Chron. 21:24, offer of that which *c.* nothing.
Lu. 14:28, sitteth down and counteth *c.*
See 2 Sam. 19:42; 1 Kings 5:17; John 12:3; 1 Tim. 2:9.
COTTAGE. Isa. 1:8; 24:20; Zeph. 2:6.
COUCH. Lu. 5:19, let him down with *c.*
24, take up thy *c.*
Acts 5:15, laid sick on *c.*
See Gen. 49:11; Job 7:13; 38:40; Ps. 6:6; Amos 6:4.
COULD. Isa. 5:4; Mk. 6:19; 9:18; 14:8.
COULTER. 1 Sam. 13:20, 21.
COUNCIL. Mat. 5:22; 10:17; Acts 5:27; 6:12.
COUNSEL. Neh. 4:15, brought their *c.* to nought.
Job 38:2; 42:3, darkeneth *c.* by words.
Ps. 1:1, *c.* of the ungodly.
33:11; Prov. 19:21, *c.* of Lord standeth.
55:14, took sweet *c.* together.
73:24, guide me with thy *c.*
Prov. 1:25, 30, set at nought all my *c.*
11:14, where no *c.* is, people fall.
15:22, without *c.* purposes are disappointed.
21:30, there is no *c.* against the Lord.
Eccl. 8:2, I *c.* thee keep king's commandment.
Isa. 28:29, wonderful in *c.*
30:1, that take *c.*, but not of me.
40:14, with whom took he *c.*
46:10, my *c.* shall stand.
Jer. 32:19 great in *c.*, mighty in working.
Hos. 10:6, ashamed of his own *c.*
Mk. 3:6; John 11:53, took *c.* against Jesus.
Acts 2:23, determinate *c.* of God.
4:28, what thy *c.* determined before.
5:38, if this *c.* be of men.
20:27, declare all *c.* of God.
1 Cor. 4:5, make manifest *c.* of the heart.
Eph. 1:11, after the *c.* of his own will.
Heb. 6:17, the immutability of his *c.*
Rev. 3:18, I *c.* thee to buy gold tried in fire.
See Ex. 18:19; Josh. 9:14; 2 Sam. 15:31.
COUNSELLOR. Prov. 11:14; 15:22; 24:6, in multitude of *c.*
12:20, to *c.* of peace is joy.
Mic. 4:9, is thy *c.* perished?
Mk. 15:43; Lu. 23:50, an honourable *c.*
Rom. 11:34, who hath been his *c.*
See 2 Chron. 22:3; Job 3:14; 12:17.
COUNT. Gen. 15:6; Ps. 106:31; Rom. 4:3; Gal. 3:6, *c.* for righteousness.
Ps. 44:22, *c.* as sheep for the slaughter.
Prov. 17:28, even a fool is *c.* wise.
Isa. 32:15, field be *c.* for a forest.
Mat. 14:5; Mk. 11:32, they *c.* him as a prophet.
Lu. 21:36; Acts 5:41; 2 Thess. 1:5, 11; 1 Tim. 5:17, *c.* worthy.
Acts 20:24, neither *c.* I my life dear.
Phil. 3:7, 8, I *c.* loss for Christ.
13, I *c.* not myself to have apprehended.
Heb. 10:29, *c.* blood an unholy thing.
Jas. 1:2, *c.* it all joy.
2 Pet. 3:9, as some men *c.* slackness.
See Num. 23:10; Job 31:4; Ps. 139:18, 22.
COUNTENANCE. 1 Sam. 16:7, look not on his *c.* or stature.
12; 17:42, David of beautiful *c.*
Neh. 2:2, why is thy *c.* sad?
Job 14:20, thou changest his *c.*
Ps. 4:6; 44:3; 89:15; 90:8, light of thy *c.*
Prov. 15:13, merry heart maketh cheerful *c.*
27:17, sharpeneth *c.* of his friend.
Eccl. 7:3, by sadness of *c.* heart made better.
Isa. 3:9, their *c.* doth witness against them.
Mat. 6:16, hypocrites of a sad *c.*
28:3; Lu. 9:29, *c.* like lightning.
Rev. 1:16, his *c.* as the sun shineth.

Col. 2:14, nailing it to his *c.*
Heb. 12:2, for joy endured the *c.*
See Obad. 14; Mat. 10:38; John 19:17, 19.
CROUCH. 1 Sam. 2:36; Ps. 10:10.
CROWN. Job 19:9, taken the *c.* from my head.
Ps. 8:5; Heb. 2:7, 9, *c.* with glory and honour.
65:11, thou *c.* the year.
103:4, *c.* thee with lovingkindness.
Prov. 4:9, a *c.* of glory shall she deliver.
12:4, virtuous woman is a *c.*
14:18, prudent *c.* with knowledge.
16:31, hoary head a *c.* of glory.
17:6, children's children are the *c.* of old men.
Isa. 28:1, woe to the *c.* of pride.
Mat. 27:29; Mk. 15:17; John 19:2, a *c.* of thorns.
1 Cor. 9:25, to obtain a corruptible *c.*
Phil. 4:1, my joy and *c.*
1 Thess. 2:19, a *c.* of rejoicing.
2 Tim. 2:5, not *c.* except he strive.
4:8, a *c.* of righteousness.
Jas. 1:12; Rev. 2:10, *c.* of life.
1 Pet. 5:4, a *c.* of glory.
Rev. 3:11, hold fast, that no man take try *c.*
4:10, cast *c.* before throne.
19:12, on head were many *c.*
See Ex. 25:25; 29:6; Job 31:36.
CRUCIFY. Mat. 27:22, all said, let him be *c.*
Mk. 15:13; Lu. 23:21; John 19:6, 15, *c.* him.
Acts 2:23, by wicked hands ye have *c.*
Rom. 6:6, old man is *c.* with him.
1 Cor. 1:13, was Paul *c.* for you.
23, we preach Christ *c.*
2:2, save Jesus Christ and him *c.*
2 Cor. 13:4, though he was *c.* through weakness.
Gal. 2:20, I am *c.* with Christ.
3:1, Christ set forth *c.*
5:24, have *c.* the flesh.
6:14, the world is *c.* unto me.
Heb. 6:6, *c.* to themselves afresh.
See Mat. 20:19; 23:34; 27:31; Mk. 15:20.
CRUEL. Ps. 25:19, with *c.* hatred.
27:12, breathe out *c.*
74:20, full of the habitations of *c.*
Prov. 5:9, give thy years to the *c.*
11:17, *c.* troubleth his own flesh.
12:10, tender mercies of the wicked are *c.*
27:4, wrath is *c.*
Cant. 8:6, jealousy is *c.*
Heb. 11:36, trials of *c.* mockings.
See Gen. 49:7; Ex. 6:9; Deut. 32:33.
CRUMBS. Mat. 15:27; Mk. 7:28; Lu. 16:21.
CRUSE. 1 Sam. 26:11; 1 Kings 14:3; 17:12; 19:6.
CRUSH. Job 5:4, children are *c.* in the gate.
39:15, forgetteth that the foot may *c.* them.
See Lev. 22:24; Num. 22:25; Deut. 28:33.
CRY (*n.*). 1 Sam. 5:12, *c.* of the city went up to heaven.
Job 34:28, he heareth the *c.* of the afflicted.
Ps. 9:12, forgetteth not *c.* of the humble.
34:15, ears are open to their *c.*
Prov. 21:13, stoppeth his ears at the *c.* of the poor.
Mat. 25:6, at midnight there was a *c.* made.
See Gen. 18:20; Ex. 2:23; Num. 16:34.
CRY (*v.*). Ex. 14:15, wherefore *c.* thou unto me?
Lev. 13:45, cover his lip, and *c.* unclean.
Job 29:12, I delivered poor that *c.*
Ps. 147:9, food to young ravens which *c.*
Prov. 8:1, doth not wisdom *c.*
Isa. 58:1, *c.* aloud, spare not.
Mat. 12:19, he shall not strive nor *c.*
20:31; Mk. 10:48; Lu. 18:39, they *c.* the more.
Lu. 18:7, elect who *c.* day and night.
John 7:37, Jesus *c.*, if any man thirst.
Acts 19:32; 21:34, some *c.* one thing and some another.
See Ex. 5:8; 32:18; 2 Kings 8:3.
CRYING. Prov. 19:18; Isa. 65:19; Heb. 5:7; Rev. 21:4.
CRYSTAL. Job 28:17; Ezek. 1:22; Rev. 4:6; 21:11; 22:1.
CUBIT. Mat. 6:27; Lu. 12:25.
CUCUMBERS. Num. 11:5; Isa. 1:8.
CUMBER. Deut. 1:12; Lu. 10:40; 13:7.
CUNNING. Ps. 137:5, let my hand forget her *c.*
Jer. 9:17, send for *c.* women.
Eph. 4:14, carried about by *c.* craftiness.
2 Pet. 1:16, not follow *c.* devised fables.
See Gen. 25:27; Ex. 38:23; 1 Sam. 16:16; Dan. 1:4.
CUP. Ps. 116:13, take *c.* of salvation.
Mat. 10:42; Mk. 9:41, *c.* of cold water.
20:22; Mk. 10:39, drink of my *c.*
23:25, make clean outside of *c.*
26:27; Mk. 14:23; Lu. 22:17; 1 Cor 11:25, took *c.*
39; Mk. 14:36; Lu. 22:42, let this *c.* pass.
Luke 22:20; 1 Cor. 11:25 this *c.* is new testament.
John 18:11, *c.* which my father hath given.
1 Cor. 10:16, *c.* of blessing we bless.
11:26, as often as ye drink this *c.*
27, drink this *c.* unworthily.
See Gen. 40:11; 44:2; Prov. 23:31.
CURDLED. Job 10:10.
CURE. Lu. 7:21, in that hour he *c.* many.
9:1, power to *c.* diseases.
13:32, I do *c.* to-day.
See Jer. 33:6; 46:11; Hos. 5:13; Mat. 17:16.
CURIOUS. Ex. 28:8; Ps. 139:15; Acts 19:19.
CURRENT. Gen. 23:16.
CURSE (*n.*). Deut. 11:26, I set before you blessing and *c.*
23:5, turned *c.* into blessing.
Mal. 3:9, ye are cursed with a *c.*
Gal. 3:10, are under the *c.*
Rev. 22:3, no more *c.*
See Gen. 27:12; Num. 5:18.
CURSE (*v.*). Lev. 19:14, not *c.* the deaf.
Num. 23:8, how shall I *c.* whom God hath not.
Judg. 5:23, *c.* ye Meroz, *c.* ye bitterly.
Job 2:9, *c.* God, and die.
Ps. 62:4, they bless, but *c.* inwardly.
Mal. 2:2, I will *c.* your blessing.
Mat. 5:44; Lu. 6:28; Rom. 12:14, bless them that *c.* you.
26:74; Mk. 14:71, he began to *c.*
Mk. 11:21, fig tree thou *c.*
John 7:49, knoweth not the law are *c.*
Gal. 3:10, *c.* is every one that continueth not.
Jas. 3:9, therewith *c.* we men.
See Gen. 8:21; 12:3; Num. 22:6.
CURTAIN. Ex. 26:36, the length of one *c.*
CUSTOM. Mat. 9:9; Mk. 2:14; Lu. 5:27, receipt of *c.*
Mat. 17:25, of whom do kings take *c.*
Lu. 4:16, as his *c.* was, went into synagogue.
John 18:39, ye have a *c.*
Acts 16:21, teach *c.* which are not lawful.
Rom 13:7, *c.* to whom *c.*
1 Cor. 11:16, we have no such *c.*
See Gen. 31:35; Judg. 11:39; Jer. 10:3.
CUTTING. Ex. 31:5; 35:33; Isa. 38:10; Mk. 5:5.
CYMBAL. 1 Cor 13:1.
CYMBALS. 2 Sam 6:5, on cornets and on *c.*
1 Chron. 15:16, harps and *c.*
16:5, Asaph made a noise with *c.*
Ps. 150:5, praise him upon the loud *c.*

D

DAGGER. Judg. 3:16, 21:22.
DAILY. Ps. 13:2, sorrow in my heart *d.*
68:19, *d.* loadeth us.
Prov. 8:30, I was *d.* his delight.
Dan. 8:11; 11:31; 12:11, *d.* sacrifice taken away.
Mat. 6:11; Lu. 11:3, our *d.* bread.
Lu. 9:23, take up cross *d.*
Acts 2:47, added to church *d.*
6:1, the *d.* ministration.
16:5, churches increased *d.*
17:11, searched the scriptures *d.*
1 Cor. 15:31, I die *d.*
Jas. 2:15, destitute of *d.* food.
See Num. 4:16; 28:24; Neh. 5:18; Dan. 1:5.
DAINTY. Ps. 141:4, let me not eat of their *d.*

Isa. 65:20, an infant of *d.*
Joel 2:11, 31; Zeph. 1:14; Mal. 4:5; Acts 2:20, great *d.* of the Lord.
Zech. 4:10, despised *d.* of small things.
Mal. 3:2, who may abide *d.* of his coming.
Mat. 7:22, many will say in that *d.*
24:36; Mk. 13:32, that *d.* knoweth no man.
50; Lu. 12:46, in a *d.* looked not for.
25:13, ye know not the *d.* nor the hour.
Lu. 21:34, that *d.* come unawares.
23:43, to-*d.* shalt thou be with me.
John 6:39, raise it again at last *d.*
8:56, Abraham rejoiced to see my *d.*
9:4, I must work while it is *d.*
Acts 17:31, he hath appointed a *d.*
Rom. 2:5, wrath against *d.* of wrath.
14:5, esteemeth every *d.* alike.
2 Cor. 6:2, the *d.* of salvation.
Phil. 1:6, perform it until *d.* of Christ.
1 Thess. 5:2; 2 Pet. 3:10, *d.* cometh as a thief.
5, children of the *d.*
Heb. 13:8, Jesus Christ same to-*d.* and for ever.
2 Pet. 3:8, one *d.* as a thousand years.
See Gen. 1:5, 27:2; Job 1:4; Ps. 77:5; 118:24; John 11:24; 12:48; 1 Cor. 3:13; Rev. 6:17; 16:14; 20:10.
DAYS (last). Isa. 2:2, it shall come to pass in the last *d.*
See Mic. 4:1; Acts 2:17; 2 Tim. 3:1; Heb. 1:2; Jas. 5:3; 2 Pet. 3:3.
DAYSMAN. Job 9:33.
DAYSPRING. Job 38:12, *d.* to know his place.
Lu. 1:78, *d.* from on high hath visited us.
DAYSTAR. 2 Peter 1:19, *d.* arise in your hearts.
DEAD. Lev. 19:28, cuttings for the *d.*
Ruth 1:8, as ye have dealt with *d.*
1 Sam. 24:14; 2 Sam 9:8; 16:9, *d.* dog.
Ps. 31:12, forgotten as a *d.* man.
115:17, *d.* praise not the Lord.
Prov. 9:18, knoweth not that the *d.* are there.
Eccl. 4:2, the *d.* which are already *d.*
9:4, living dog better than *d.* lion.
5, *d.* know not any thing.
10:1, *d.* flies cause ointment.
Isa. 26:19, thy *d.* men shall live.
Jer. 22:10, weep not for the *d.*
Mat. 8:22, let the *d.* bury their *d.*
9:24, Mk. 5:39; Lu. 8:52, not *d.* but sleepeth.
11:5; Lu. 7:22, deaf hear *d.* raised.
22:32, not God of the *d.*
23:27, full of *d.* men's bones.
Mk. 9:10, rising from *d.* should mean.
Lu. 15:24, 32; Rev. 1:18, *d.* and is alive again.
16:31, though one rose from the *d.*
John 5:25, *d.* shall hear.
6:49, did eat manna, and are *d.*
11:25, though *d.* yet shall he live.
44, he that was *d.* came forth.
Acts 10:42; 2 Tim. 4:1, judge of quick and *d.*
26:23, first that should rise from *d.*
Rom. 6:2, 11; 1 Pet. 2:24, *d.* to sin.
7:4; Gal. 2:19, *d.* to the law.
14:9, Lord both of *d.* and living.
1 Cor. 15:15, if the *d.* rise not.
35, how are the *d.* raised.
2 Cor. 1:9, trust in God who raiseth *d.*
5:14, then were all *d.*
Eph. 2:1; Col. 2:13, *d.* in trespasses and sins.
5:14, arise from the *d.*
Col. 1:18, firstborn from the *d.*
2:20; 2 Tim. 2:11, *d.* with Christ.
1 Thess. 4:16, *d.* in Christ shall rise first.
1 Tim. 5:6, *d.* while she liveth.
Heb. 6:1; 9:14, from *d.* works.
11:4, being *d.*, yet speaketh.
13:20, brought again from the *d.*
Jas. 2:17, 20, 26, faith *d.*
1 Pet. 4:6, preached to them that are *d.*
Jude 12, twice *d.*
Rev. 1:5, first-begotten of the *d.*
Rev. 3:1, a name that thou livest, and art *d.*
14:13, blessed are the *d.*
20:5, rest of *d.* lived not again.
12, the *d.* small and great.
13, sea gave up *d.*
See Gen. 23:3; Ex. 12:30; Mk. 9:26; Rev 1:18.
DEADLY. Mk. 16:18, drink any *d.* thing.
Jas. 3:8, tongue full of *d.* poison.
See 1 Sam. 5:11; Ps. 17:9 Ezek. 30:24.
DEAF. Ps. 58:4, like *d.* adder that stoppeth.
Isa. 29:18, shall the *d.* hear the words.
Mat. 11:5; Lu. 7:22, the *d.* hear.
Mk. 7:37, he maketh the *d.* to hear.
9:25, thou *d.* spirit, come out.
See Ex. 4:11; Lev. 19:14; Isa. 42:18; 43:8.
DEAL (a measure). Ex. 29:40, with the one lamb, a tenth *d.* of flour.
Lev. 14:10, three tenth *d.* of fine flour for a meat offering.
DEAL. Lev. 19:11, nor *d.* falsely.
Job 42:8, *d.* with you after folly.
Ps. 75:4, *d.* not foolishly.
Prov. 12:22, they that *d.* truly his delight.
Isa. 21:2; 24:16, treacherous dealer *d.* treacherously.
26:10, in land of uprightness *d.* unjustly.
Jer. 6:13; 8:10, every one *d.* falsely.
Hos. 5:7, have *d.* treacherously against the Lord.
Zech. 1:6, as Lord thought, so hath he *d.*
Mk. 7:36; 10:48, the more a great *d.*
Lu. 2:48, why hast thou thus *d.* with us?
Rom. 12:3, according as God hath *d.*
See Gen. 32:9; Ex. 1:10; Deut. 7:5; 2 Chron. 2:3.
DEALING. 1 Sam. 2:23; Ps. 7:16; John 4:9.
DEAR. Jer. 31:20, is Ephraim my *d.* son.
Acts 20:24, neither count I my life *d.*
Rom. 12:19; 1 Cor 10:14; 2 Cor. 7:1; 12:19; Phil. 4:1; 2 Tim. 1:2; 1 Pet. 2:11, *d.* beloved.
Eph. 5:1, followers of God as *d.* children.
Col. 1:13, into kingdom of his *d.* Son.
1 Thess. 2:8, because ye were *d.* unto us.
See Jer. 12:7; Lu. 7:2; Philem. 1.
DEARTH. 2 Chron. 6:28, if there be a *d.* in the land.
Neh. 5:3, buy corn because of *d.*
Acts 11:28, Agabus signified a great *d.*
See Gen. 41:54; 2 Kings 4:38; Jer. 14:1; Acts 7:11.
DEATH. Num. 16:29, if these men die common *d.*
23:10, let me die *d.* of righteous.
Judg. 5:18, jeoparded lives to the *d.*
16:16, soul was vexed to *d.*
30, which he slew at his *d.* were more.
Ruth 1:17, if ought but *d.* part thee and me.
1 Sam. 15:32, the bitterness of *d.* past.
20:3, but a step between me and *d.*
2 Sam. 1:23, in *d.* not divided.
22:5; Ps. 18:4; 116:8, waves of *d.* compassed.
Job 3:21, long for *d.* but it cometh not.
7:15, my soul chooseth *d.*
30:23, thou wilt bring me to *d.*
Ps. 6:5, in *d.* no remembrance.
13:3, lest I sleep the sleep of *d.*
23:4, valley of shadow of *d.*
48:14, our guide even unto *d.*
68:20, the issues from *d.*
89:48, what man shall not see *d.*
102:20, loose those appointed to *d.*
107:10, in darkness and shadow of *d.*
116:15, precious is *d.* of his saints.
Prov. 7:27, to chambers of *d.*
8:36, that hate me love *d.*
14:32, righteous hath hope in his *d.*
24:11, deliver them drawn to *d.*
Cant. 8:6, love is strong as *d.*
Isa. 9:2; Jer. 2:6, land of the shadow of *d.*
25:8; 1 Cor. 15:56, swallow up *d.* in victory.
38:18, for *d.* cannot celebrate thee.
Jer. 8:3, *d.* chosen rather than life.
9:21, *d.* come up to our windows.
Ezek. 18:32; 33:11, no pleasure in *d.*

Hos. 13:14, O *d.* I will be thy plagues.
Mat. 15:4; Mk. 7:10, let him die the *d.*
16:28; Mk. 9:1; Lu. 9:27, not taste of *d.*
26:38; Mk. 14:34, my soul is sorrowful to *d.*
Mk. 5:23; John 4:47, lieth at point of *d.*
Lu. 2:26, should not see *d.* before.
22:33, will go to prison and *d.*
John 5:24; 1 John 3:14, passed from *d.* to life.
8:51, 52, keep my saying, shall never see *d.*
11:4, sickness not unto *d.*
12:33; 18:32; 21:19, signifying what *d.*
Acts 2:24, having loosed pains of *d.*
Rom. 1:32, such things are worthy of *d.*
5:10; Col. 1:22, reconciled by the *d.*
12, *d.* by sin and so *d.* passed on all.
14:17, *d.* reigned from Adam to Moses.
6:5, planted in likeness of his *d.*
21, end of those things is *d.*
23, wages of sin is *d.*
8:2, law of sin and *d.*
1 Cor. 3:22, life or *d.* all are yours.
11:26, show the Lord's *d.* till he come.
15:21, by man came *d.*
55:56, O *d.* where is thy sting?
2 Cor. 1:9, sentence of *d.* in ourselves.
2:16, savour of *d.* unto *d.*
4:12, *d.* worketh in us.
11:23, in *d.* oft.
Phil. 2:8, *d.*, even *d.* of the cross.
Heb. 2:9, taste *d.* for every man.
15, through fear of *d.* were.
Jas. 1:15, sin bringeth forth *d.*
1 John 5:16, a sin unto *d.*
Rev. 1:18, keys of hell and of *d.*
2:10, be faithful unto *d.*
11; 6:14, second *d.*
6:8, his name that sat on him was *d.*
9:6, seek *d.* and *d.* shall flee.
20:16, *d.* and hell delivered up.
21:4, no more *d.*
See Prov. 14:12; 16:25; John 18:31; Jas. 5:20.
DEBASE. Isa. 57:9.
DEBATE. Prov. 25:9; Isa. 58:4; Rom. 1:29; 2 Cor. 12:20.
DEBT. 2 Kings 4:7, go, pay thy *d.* and live.
Neh. 10:31, leave the exaction of every *d.*
Prov. 22:26, be not sureties for *d.*
Mat. 18:27, forgave him the *d.*
See 1 Sam 22:2; Mat. 6:12; Rom. 4:4.
DEBTOR. Mat. 6:12, as we forgive our *d.*
Lu. 7:41, creditor which had two *d.*
Rom. 1:14, I am *d.* to the Greeks.
8:12, we are *d.*, not to the flesh.
15:27, their *d.* they are.
Gal. 5:3, *d.* to do the whole law.
See Ezek. 18:7; Mat. 18:21; 23:16; Lu. 16:5.
DECAY. Lev. 25:35; Neh. 4:10; Heb. 8:13.
DECEASE. Isa. 26:14; Mat. 22:25; Lu. 9:31; 2 Pet. 1:15
DECEIT. Ps. 10:7, mouth full of *d.* and fraud.
36:3, words are iniquity and *d.*
55:23, *d.* men shall not live half their days.
Prov. 12:5, counsels of wicked are *d.*
20:17, bread of *d.* is sweet.
27:6, kisses of an enemy are *d.*
31:30, favour is *d.* and beauty vain.
Jer. 14:14; 23:26, prophesy the *d.* of their heart.
17:9, heart is *d.* above all things.
48:10, that doeth work of the Lord *d.*
Hos. 11:12, compasseth me with *d.*
Amos. 8:5, falsifying balances by *d.*
Zeph. 1:9, fill their masters' houses with *d.*
Mat. 13:22; Mk. 4:19, the *d.* of riches.
Mk. 7:22, out of heart proceed *d.*
Rom. 3:13, they have used *d.*
2 Cor. 4:2, handling word of God *d.*
11:13, false apostles, *d.* workers.
Eph. 4:22, according to *d.* lusts.
Col. 2:8, vain *d.*, after tradition.
See Ps. 50:19; Prov. 12:20; Jer. 5:27; Mic. 6:11.
DECEIVE. Deut. 11:16, take heed that your heart be not *d.*
2 Kings 19:10; Isa. 37:10, let not thy God *d.* thee.
Job 12:16, the *d.* and the *d.* are his.
Jer. 20:7, thou hast *d.* me and I was *d.*
37:9, *d.* not yourselves.
Obad. 3, pride of heart hath *d.* thee.
Mat. 24:24, if possible *d.* the very elect.
27:63, remember that that *d.* said.
John 7:12, nay, but he *d.* the people.
47, are ye also *d.*?
1 Cor. 6:9; 15:33; Gal. 6:7, be not *d.*
2 Cor. 6:8, as *d.*, and yet true.
Eph. 4:14, whereby they lie in wait to *d.*
5:6, 2 Thess. 2:3; 1 John 3:7, let no man *d.* you.
1 Tim. 2:14, Adam was not *d.*
2 Tim. 3:13, worse and worse, *d.* and being *d.*
1 John 1:8, no sin, we *d.* ourselves.
2 John 7, many *d.* entered into world.
See Gen. 31:7; Isa. 44:20; Ezek. 14:9; Rev. 12:9; 19:20.
DECENTLY. 1 Cor. 14:40.
DECISION. Joel 3:14.
DECK. Job 40:10, *d.* thyself with majesty.
Isa. 61:10, as a bridegroom *d.* himself.
Jer. 4:30, though thou *d.* thee with ornaments.
10:4, they *d.* it with silver.
See Prov. 7:16; Ezek. 16:11; Rev. 17:4; 18:16.
DECLARATION. Esth. 10:2; Job 13:17; Lu. 1:1; 2 Cor. 8:19.
DECLARE. 1 Chron. 16:24; Ps. 96:3, *d.* glory among heathen.
Job 21:31, who shall *d.* his way to his face.
31:37, I would *d.* number of my steps.
Ps. 2:7, I will *d.* decree.
9:11, *d.* among the people his doings.
19:1, heavens *d.* glory of God.
30:9, shall dust *d.* thy truth.
40:10, I have *d.* what he hath done.
66:16, I will *d.* for ever.
75:9, I will *d.* for ever.
118:17, live and *d.* the works of the Lord.
145:4, one generation shall *d.* thy mighty acts.
Isa. 3:9, they *d.* their sin as Sodom.
41:26; 45:21, who hath *d.* from beginning.
45:19, I *d.* things that are right.
46:10, *d.* end from the beginning.
53:8; Acts 8:33, who shall *d.* his generation.
66:19, *d.* my glory among Gentiles.
John 17:26 have *d.* thy name and will *d.* it.
Acts 13:32, we *d.* to you glad tidings.
17:23, him *d.* I unto you.
20:27, *d.* the counsel of God.
Rom. 1:4, *d.* to be Son of God with power.
1 Cor. 3:13, day shall *d.* it.
See Josh. 20:4; John 1:18; Heb. 11:14; 1 John 1:3.
DECLINE. Deut. 17:11, thou shalt not *d.* from sentence.
2 Chron. 34:2, *d.* neither to right nor left.
Ps. 102:11; 109:23, days like a shadow that *d.*
119:51, 157, not *d.* from thy law.
See Ex. 23:2; Job 23:11; Prov. 4:5; 7:25.
DECREASE. Gen. 8:5, Ps. 107:38; John 3:30.
DECREE. Job 22:28, thou shalt *d.* a thing and it shall be.
28:26, made a *d.* for the rain.
Ps. 148:6, a *d.* which shall not pass.
Prov. 8:15, by me princes *d.* justice.
29, he gave to the sea his *d.*
Isa. 10:1, that *d.* unrighteous *d.*
Acts 16:4, delivered the *d.* to keep.
See Dan. 2:9; 6:8; Acts 17:7; 1 Cor 7:37.
DEDICATE. Deut. 20:5, lest he die and another *d.* it.
Judg. 17:3, wholly *d.* silver to the Lord.
1 Chron. 26:27, of spoil they did *d.*
Ezek. 44:29, every *d.* thing shall be theirs.
See 1 Kings 7:51, 8:63; 15:15; 1 Chron. 18:11; Heb 9:18.
DEED. Ex. 9:16; 1 Sam 25:34; 26:4, in very *d.*
2 Sam 12:14, by this *d.* hast given occasion.
Ezra 9:13, come upon us for our evil *d.*
Neh. 13:14, wipe not out my good *d.*
Ps. 28:4; Isa. 59:18; Jer. 25:14; Rom. 2:6, according to their *d.*

Lu. 11:48, ye allow the *d.* of your fathers.
23:41, due reward of our *d.*
24:19, a prophet might in *d.*
John 3:19, because their *d.* were evil.
8:41, ye do the *d.* of your father.
Acts 7:22, Moses, mighty in word and *d.*
Rom. 3:20, by *d.* of law, no flesh justified.
28, justified without *d.* of the law.
Col. 3:9, put off old man with his *d.*
17, whatsoever ye do in word or *d.*
Jas. 1:25, shall be blessed in his *d.*
1 John 3:18, not love in word, but in *d.*
See Gen. 44:15; Lu. 23:51; Acts 19:18.
DEEMED. Acts 27:27.
DEEP. Gen. 7:11; 8:2, fountains of *d.*
Deut. 33:13, the *d.* that coucheth beneath.
Job 38:30, face of *d.* is frozen.
41:31, maketh the *d.* boil like a pot.
Ps. 36:6, thy judgments are a great *d.*
42:7, *d.* calleth to *d.*
Ps. 95:4, in his hand are the *d.* places.
107:24, see his wonders in the *d.*
Prov. 22:14; 23:27, strange women *d.* pit.
Isa. 63:13, led them through *d.*
Mat. 13:5, no *d.* of earth.
Lu. 5:4, launch into *d.*
6:48, digged *d.* and laid foundations.
8:31, command to go into the *d.*
John 4:11, the well is *d.*
1 Cor. 2:10, searcheth *d.* things of God.
See Job 4:13; 33:15; Prov. 19:15; Rom. 10:7.
DEER. Deut. 14:5; 1 Kings 4:23.
DEFAME. Jer. 20:10; 1 Cor. 4:13.
DEFEAT. 2 Sam. 15:34; 17:14.
DEFENCE. Job 22:25, the Almighty shall be thy *d.*
Ps. 7:10, my *d.* is of God
59:9, 17; 62:2, for God is my *d.*
89:18; 94:22, Lord is *d.*
Eccl. 7:12, wisdom a *d.* money a *d.*
Isa. 33:16, place of *d.* munitions of rocks.
Phil. 1:7, 17, in *d.* of the Gospel.
See Num. 14:9; Acts 19:33; 22:1.
DEFEND. Ps. 5:11, shout for joy, because thou *d.* them.
82:3, *d.* the poor and fatherless.
Zech. 9:15, Lord of hosts shall *d.* them.
Acts 7:24, *d.* him and avenged the oppressed.
See Ps. 20:1; 59:1; Is. 31:5.
DEFILE. Ex. 31:14, that *d.* sabbath be put to death.
Num. 35:33, blood *d.* the land.
2 Kings 23:13, high places did king *d.*
Neh. 13:29, they have *d.* the priesthood.
Ps. 74:7; 79:1, *d.* dwelling-place of thy name.
106:39, *d.* with their won works.
Isa. 59:3, your hands are *d.* with blood.
Jer. 2:7; 16:18, ye *d.* my land.
Ezek. 4:13, eat their *d.* bread.
23:38, they have *d.* my sanctuary.
36:17, they *d.* it by their own ways.
Dan. 1:8, would not *d.* himself with meat.
Mat. 15:11, 18:20; Mk. 7:15, 20, 23, *d.* a man.
John 18:28, lest they should be *d.*
1 Cor. 3:17, if any man *d.* temple of God.
8:7, conscience being weak is *d.*
1 Tim. 1:10, law for them that *d.* themselves.
Tit. 1:15, to *d.* nothing pure, even conscience *d.*
Heb. 12:15, thereby many be *d.*
Jude 8, filthy dreamers *d.* flesh.
Rev. 3:4, few not *d.* their garments.
See Ex. 31:41; Lev. 21:4; Jas. 3:6; Rev. 21:27.
DEFRAUD. 1 Sam. 12:3,4, whom have I *d.*?
Mk. 10:19; 1 Cor. 7:5, *d.* not.
1 Cor. 6:7, rather suffer to be *d.*
8, do wrong and *d.* your brethren.
2 Cor. 7:2, we have *d.* no man.
See Lev. 19:13; 1 Thess. 4:6.
DEGENERATE. Jer. 2:21.
DEGREE. Ps. 62:9, men of low *d.*, high *d.*
1 Tim. 3:13, purchase to themselves good *d.*
Jas. 1:9, brother of low *d.* rejoice.
See 2 Kings 20:9; 1 Chron. 17:17; Isa. 38:8; Lu. 1:52.
DELAY. Mat. 24:48; Lu. 12:45, my lord *d.* his coming.
Acts 9:38, that he would not *d.* to come.
See Ex. 22:29; 32:1; Acts 25:17.
DELECTABLE. Isa. 44:9.
DELICACY. Rev. 18:3.
DELICATE. 1 Sam 15:32, Agag came to him *d.*
Prov. 29:21, he that *d.* bringeth up servant.
Isa. 47:1, no more called tender and *d.*
Lam. 4:5, that did feed *d.* are desolate.
Lu. 7:25, that live *d.* are kings' courts.
See Deut. 28:54, 56; Jer. 6:2; Mic. 1:16.
DELICIOUSLY. Rev. 18:7.
DELIGHT (*n.*). Deut. 10:15, Lord had a *d.* in thy fathers.
1 Sam. 15:22, hath Lord as great *d.* in offerings.
2 Sam 15:26, I have no *d.* in thee.
Job 22:26, shalt thou have *d.* in the Almighty.
Ps. 1:2, his *d.* is in law of Lord.
16:3, to excellent in whom is my *d.*
119:24, testimonies my *d.* and counsel.
77, 92, 174, thy law is my *d.*
143, thy commandments are my *d.*
Prov. 8:30, I was daily his *d.*
31, my *d.* were with sons of men.
Prov. 18:2, fool hath no *d.* in understanding.
19:10, *d.* not seemly for a fool.
Cant. 2:3, under his shadow with great *d.*
Isa. 58:13, call sabbath a *d.*
See Prov. 11:1; 12:22; 15:8; 16:13.
DELIGHT (*v.*). Job 27:10, will he *d.* himself in the Almighty?
Ps. 37:4, *d.* also in the Lord.
11, meek shall *d.* in abundance of peace.
51:16, thou *d.* not in burnt offering.
94:19, thy comforts *d.* my soul.
Isa. 42:1, elect in whom my soul *d.*
55:2, soul *d.* itself in fatness.
62:4, the Lord *d.* in thee.
Mic. 7:18, he *d.* in mercy.
Rom. 7:22, I *d.* after the inward man.
See Num. 14:8; Prov. 1:22; 2:14; Mal. 3:1
DELIGHTSOME. Mal. 3:12.
DELIVER. Ex. 3:8; Acts 7:34, I am come down to *d.* them.
Numb. 35:25, congregation shall *d.* slayer.
Deut. 32:39; Isa. 43:13, any *d.* out of my hand.
2 Chron. 32:13, were gods able to *d.* their lands.
Job 5:19, shall *d.* thee in six troubles.
36:18, great ransom cannot *d.*
Ps. 33:17, nor *d.* any by great strength.
56:13, *d.* my feet from falling.
144:10, *d.* David from hurtful sword.
Prov. 24:11, forbear to *d.* them.
Eccl. 9:15, by wisdom *d.* city.
Isa. 50:2, have I no power to *d.*?
Jer. 1:8, I am with thee to *d.* thee.
39:17, I will *d.* in that day.
Dan. 3:17, for God is able to *d.* and will *d.*
6:14, king set heart on Daniel to *d.*
Amos. 2:14, neither shall mighty *d.*
9:1, he that escapeth shall not be *d.*
Mal. 3:15, they that tempt God are *d.*
Mat. 6:13; Lu. 11:4, *d.* us from evil.
11:27; Lu. 10:22, all things *d.* to me of my Father.
26:15, I will *d.* him to you.
Acts 2:23, being *d.* by the counsel of God.
Rom. 4:25, was *d.* for our offences.
7:6, we are *d.* from the law.
8:21, creature shall be *d.*
2 Cor. 4:11, *d.* to death for Jesus' sake.
2 Tim. 4:18, *d.* me from every evil work.
Jude 3, faith once *d.* to saints.
See Rom. 8:32; 2 Cor. 1:10; Gal. 1:4; 2 Pet. 2:7.
DELIVERANCE. 2 Kings 5:1, by him had given *d.* to Syria.
1 Chron. 11:14, saved by great *d.*
Ps. 32:7, compass me with songs of *d.*
Lu. 4:18, preach *d.* to the captives.

1 John 5:15, we have petitions we *d.*
See Gen. 3:6; Job 7:2; Ps. 51:6; Lu. 5:39.
DESIROUS. Prov. 23:3; Lu. 23:8; John 16:19; Gal. 5:26.
DESOLATE. Ps. 25:16, have mercy, for I am *d.*
40:15, let them be *d.* for reward.
143:4, my heart within me is *d.*
Isa. 54:1; Gal. 4:27, more are children of *d.*
62:4, nor shall thy land any more be termed *d.*
Jer. 2:12, be ye very *d.*, saith the Lord.
32:43; 33:12, *d.* without man or beast.
Ezek. 6:6, your altars may be made *d.*
Dan. 11:31; 12:11, abomination that maketh *d.*
Mal. 1:4, return and build the *d.* places.
Mat. 23:38; Lu. 13:35, house left to you *d.*
Acts 1:20, let his habitation be *d.*
1 Tim. 5:5, widow indeed, and *d.*
Rev. 18:19, in one hour is she made *d.*
See Ps. 34:22; Jer. 12:10; Joel 2:3; Zech. 7:14.
DESOLATION. 2 Kings 22:19, they should become a *d.* and a curse.
Ps. 46:8, what *d.* he hath made in the earth.
74:3; Jer. 25:9; Ezek. 35:9, perpetual *d.*
Prov. 1:27, when your fear cometh as *d.*
3:25, the *d.* of the wicked.
Isa. 61:4, raise up former *d.*, the *d.* of many generations.
Dan. 9:26, to end of war *d.* are determined.
Zeph 1:15, a day of wrath, wasting, and *d.*
Mat. 12:25; Lu. 11:17, house divided brought to *d.*
Lu. 21:20, then know *d.* is nigh.
See Lev. 26:31; Josh. 8:28; Job 30:14.
DESPAIR. 1 Sam. 27:1; Eccl. 2:20; 2 Cor. 4:8.
DESPERATE. Job 6:26; Isa. 17:11; Jer. 17:9.
DESPISE. Num. 11:20, ye have *d.* the Lord.
15:31; Prov. 13:13; Isa. 5:24; 30:12, *d.* the word.
1 Sam. 2:30, that *d.* me shall be lightly esteemed.
Neh. 4:4, hear, O God, for we are *d.*
Esth. 1:17, so that they *d.* their husbands.
Job 5:17; Prov. 3:11; Heb. 12:5, *d.* not chastening.
19:18, young children *d.* me.
36:5, God is mighty and *d.* not any.
Ps. 51:17, contrite heart thou wilt not *d.*
53:5, put to shame, because God *d.* them.
73:20, thou shalt *d.* their image.
102:17, he will not *d.* their prayer.
Prov. 1:7, fools *d.* wisdom.
30:5, 12, *d.* reproof.
6:30, men do not *d.* a thief.
15:5, fool *d.* father's instruction.
20, foolish man *d.* his mother.
32, refuseth instruction *d.* own soul.
19:16, he that *d.* his ways shall die.
30:17, *d.* to obey his mother, ravens shall.
Eccl. 9:16, poor man's wisdom is *d.*
Isa. 33:15, he that *d.* gain of oppressions.
49:7, saith Lord to him whom man *d.*
Jer. 49:15, I will make thee small and *d.*
Ezek. 20:13, 16, they *d.* my judgments.
22:8, thou hast *d.* holy things.
Amos 2:4, they *d.* they law of the Lord.
Zech. 4:10, who hath *d.* day of small things.
Mal. 1:6, wherein have we *d.* thy name?
Mat. 6:24, Lu. 16:13, hold to one, *d.* the other.
18:10, *d.* not one of these little ones.
Lu. 10:16, *d.* you, *d.* me; *d.* him that sent me.
18:9, righteous, and *d.* others.
Rom. 2:4, *d.* thou the riches of his goodness.
1 Cor. 1:28, things *d.* God hath chosen.
4:10, ye are honourable, but we are *d.*
11:22, *d.* ye the church of God.
16:11, let no man therefore *d.* him.
1 Thess. 4:8, *d.* not man, but God.
5:20, *d.* not prophesyings.
1 Tim. 4:12, let no man *d.* thy youth.
6:2, not *d.* because brethren.
Tit. 2:15, let no man *d.* thee.
Heb. 12:2, endured cross, *d.* the shame.
Jas. 2:6, ye have *d.* the poor.
See Gen. 16:4; 25:34; 2 Sam. 6:16; Rom. 14:3.
DESPISERS. Acts 13:41; 2 Tim. 3:3.
DESPITE. Ezek. 25:6, 15; 36:5; Rom. 1:30; Heb. 10:29.
DESPITEFULLY. Mat. 5:44; Lu. 6:28; Acts 14:5.
DESTITUTE. Ps. 102:17, will regard prayer of *d.*
Prov. 15:21, folly is joy to him that is *d.* of wisdom.
1 Tim. 6:5, *d.* of the truth.
Heb. 11:37, being *d.*, afflicted, tormented.
See Gen. 24:27; Ezek. 32:15; Jas. 2:15.
DESTROY. Gen. 18:23, *d.* righteous with the wicked.
Ex. 22:20, he shall be utterly *d.*
Deut. 9:14, let me alone that I may *d.* them.
1 Sam. 15:6, depart, lest I *d.* you with them.
2 Sam. 1:14, *d.* Lord's anointed.
Job 2:3, movedst me to *d.* without cause.
10:8, made me, yet thou dost *d.* me.
19:10, he hath *d.* me on every side.
26, though worms *d.* his body.
Ps. 40:14; 63:9, seek my soul to *d.* it.
145:20, all the wicked will be *d.*
Prov. 1:32, prosperity of fools shall *d.* them.
13:23, is *d.* for want of judgment.
31:3, that which *d.* kings.
Eccl. 9:18, one sinner *d.* much good.
Isa. 10:7, it is in his heart to *d.*
11:9; 65:25, *d.* in holy mountain.
19:3, I will *d.* the counsel thereof.
28:2, as a *d.* storm.
Jer. 13:14, I will not spare but *d.* them.
17:18, *d.* them with double destruction.
23:1, woe to pastors that *d.* the sheep.
Ezek. 9:1, with *d.* weapon in his hand.
22:27, *d.* souls to get dishonest gain.
Dan. 8:24, he shall *d.* wonderfully.
Hos. 13:9, thou hast *d.* thyself.
Mat. 5:17, not to *d.* but to fulfil.
10:28, fear him that is able to *d.*
12:14; Mk. 3:6; 11:18, they might *d.* him.
21:41, he will miserably *d.* those.
22:7, and *d.* those murderers.
27:20, ask Barabbas and *d.* Jesus.
Mk. 1:24; Lu. 4:34, art thou come to *d.*
12:9, Lu. 20:16, *d.* the husbandmen.
14:58, say, I will *d.* this temple.
15:29, thou that *d.* the temple.
Lu. 6:9, is it lawful to save life or *d.*
9:56, is not come to *d.* men's lives.
17:27, flood came and *d.* them all.
John 2:19, Jesus said, *d.* this temple.
Rom. 14:15, *d.* not him with thy meat.
1 Cor. 6:13, God shall *d.* both it and them.
Gal. 1:23, preacheth the faith he once *d.*
2:18, if I build the things which I *d.*
2 Thess. 2:8, *d.* with brightness of his coming.
Heb. 2:14, *d.* him that had the power.
Jas. 4:12, able to save and to *d.*
1 John 3:8, *d.* the works of the devil.
See Gen. 6:17; Isa. 65:8; Rom. 6:6; 2 Pet. 2:12; Jude 5.
DESTROYER. Ex. 12:23, not suffer *d.* to some.
Judg. 16:24, delivered the *d.* of our country.
Job 15:21, in prosperity the *d.* shall come.
Ps. 17:4, kept from paths of the *d.*
Prov. 28:24, the companion of a *d.*
See Job 33:22; Isa. 49:17; Jer. 22:7; 50:11.
DESTRUCTION. 2 Chron. 22:4, his counsellors to his *d.*
26:16, heart lifted up to *d.*
Esth. 8:6, endure to see *d.* of my kindred.
Job 5:21, neither be afraid of *d.*
21:17, how oft cometh *d.*
26:6, *d.* hath no covering.
31:3, is not *d.* to the wicked.
Ps. 9:6, *d.* are come to a perpetual end.
35:8, into that very *d.* let him fall.
73:18, thou castedst them down to *d.*
90:3, turnest man to *d.*
91:6, the *d.* that wasteth at noon day.
103:4, redeemeth thy life from *d.*

Prov. 1:27, your *d.* cometh as a whirlwind.
10:14, mouth of foolish near *d.*
15, *d.* of poor is their poverty.
14:28, want of people *d.* of the prince.
16:18, pride goeth before *d.*
17:19, exalteth gate seeketh *d.*
18:7, fool's mouth is his *d.*
27:20, hell and *d.* never full.
31:8, such as are appointed to *d.*
Isa. 14:23, the besom of *d.*
19:18, the city of *d.*
59:7, wasting and *d.* in their paths.
60:18, *d.* be no more heard.
Jer. 17:18, destroy with double *d.*
46:20, *d.* cometh out of north.
50:22, sound of great *d.* in the land.
Lam. 2:11; 3:48; 4:10, *d.* of the daughter of my people.
Hos. 13:14, O grave, I will be thy *d.*
Mat. 7:13, broad way leadeth to *d.*
Rom. 3:16, *d.* and misery in their ways.
9:22, vessels fitted to *d.*
Phil. 3:18, 19, many walk whose end is *d.*
1 Thess. 5:3, then sudden *d.* cometh.
2 Thess. 1:9, punished with everlasting *d.*
1 Tim. 6:9, lusts drown men in *d.*
2 Pet. 2:1, bring on themselves swift *d.*
3:16, wrest to their own *d.*
See Job 21:20; 31:23; Prov. 10:29; 21:15.
DETAIN. Judg. 13:15, 16; 1 Sam 21:7.
DETERMINATE. Acts. 2:23.
DETERMINATION. Zeph. 3:8.
DETERMINE. Ex. 21:22, pay as the judges *d.*
1 Sam. 20:7, be sure evil is *d.* by him.
Job 14:5, seeing his days are *d.*
Dan. 11:36, that that is *d.* shall be done.
Lu. 22:22, Son of man goeth as it was *d.*
Acts 3:13, Pilate was *d.* to let him go.
17:26, hath *d.* the times appointed.
1 Cor. 2:2, I *d.* not to know anything.
See 2 Chron. 2:1; 25:16; Isa. 19:17; Dan. 9:24.
DETEST. Deut. 7:26.
DETESTABLE. Jer. 16:18; Ezek. 5:11; 7:20; 11:18; 37:23.
DEVICE. Esth. 9:25, *d.* return on his own head.
Ps. 10:2, let them be taken in the *d.*
33:10, maketh *d.* of the people of none effect.
37:7, bringeth wicked *d.* to pass.
Prov. 1:31, be filled with their own *d.*
12:2, man of wicked *d.* will he condemn.
19:21, many *d.* in a man's heart.
Eccl. 9:10, no work nor *d.* in grave.
Jer. 18:12, will walk after our own *d.*
Dan. 11:24, 25, he shall forecast *d.*
Acts 17:29, like stone graven by man's *d.*
2 Cor. 2:11, not ignorant of his *d.*
See 2 Chron. 2:14; Esth. 8:3; Job 5:12.
DEVILISH. Jas. 3:15.
DEVILS (Sacrifices offered to). Lev. 17:7, offer their sacrifices unto *d.*
See Deut. 32:17; 2 Chron. 11:15; Ps. 106:37; 1 Cor. 10:20; Rev. 9:20.
DEVILS (confess Jesus to be Christ). Mat. 8:29; Mk 1:24; 3:11; 5:7; Lu. 4:34, 41; Acts 19:15.
Jas. 2:19, the *d.* also believe and tremble.
DEVISE. Ex. 31:4; 35:32, 35, *d.* works in gold.
Ps. 35:4, to confusion that *d.* my hurt.
36:4, he *d.* mischief on his bed.
41:7, against me do they *d.* my hurt.
Prov. 3:29, *d.* not evil against thy neighbour.
6:14, he *d.* mischief continually.
18, a heart that *d.* wicked imaginations.
14:22, err that *d.* evil, *d.* good.
16:9, man's heart *d.* his way.
Isa. 32:7, *d.* wicked devices to destroy poor.
8, the liberal *d.* liberal things.
2 Pet. 1:16, cunningly *d.* fables.
See 2 Sam. 14:14; Jer. 51:12; Lam. 2:17; Mic. 2:1.
DEVOTE. Lev. 27:21, 28; Num. 18:14; Ps. 119:38.
DEVOTIONS. Acts 17:23.
DEVOUR. Gen. 37:20, some evil beast hath *d.* him.
41:7, 24, seven thin *d.* the seven rank.
Ex. 24:17; Isa. 29:6; 30:27, 30; 33:14, *d.* fire.
Lev. 10:2, fire from Lord *d.* them.
Deut. 32:24, *d.* with burning heat.
2 Sam. 11:25, sword *d.* one as well as another.
18:8, wood *d.* more than sword *d.*
22:9; Ps. 18:8, fire out of his mouth *d.*
Job 18:13, death shall *d.* his strength.
Ps. 80:13, beasts of field *d.* it.
Prov. 20:25, man who *d.* that which is holy.
30:14, jaw teeth as knives to *d.*
Isa. 1:7, strangers *d.* it in your presence.
20, if ye rebel, be *d.* with sword.
Jer. 2:30, your sword hath *d.* prophets.
3:24, shame *d.* labour of our fathers.
30:16, that *d.* thee shall be *d.*
Ezek. 15:7, fire shall *d.* them.
23:37, pass through fire to *d.* them.
Hos. 8:14; Amos 1:14; 2:2, it shall *d.* palaces.
Joel 2:3, a fire *d.* before them.
Amos 4:9, fig trees, palmer-worm *d.* them.
Hab. 1:13, wicked *d.* man that is more righteous.
Zeph. 1:18; 3:8, *d.* by fire of jealousy.
Mal. 3:11, will rebuke the *d.* for your sakes.
Mat. 13:4; Mk. 4:4; Lu. 8:5, fowls *d.* them.
23:14; Mk. 12:40; Lu. 20:47, *d.* widows' houses.
Lu. 15:30, thy son hath *d.* thy living.
2 Cor. 11:20, if a man *d.* you.
Gal. 5:15, ye bite and *d.* one another.
Heb. 10:27, which shall *d.* adversaries.
1 Pet. 5:8, seeking whom he may *d.*
See Gen. 31:15; 2 Sam 2:26; Ps. 50:3; 52:4.
DEVOUT. Lu. 2:25, Simeon was just and *d.*
Acts 2:5; 8:2, *d.* men.
See Acts 10:2; 13:50; 17:4, 17; 22:12.
DEW. Gen. 27:28, God give thee the *d.* of heaven.
Deut. 32:2, my speech shall distil as the *d.*
33:13, for the *d.*, and for the deep.
Judg. 6:37, if the *d.* be on the fleece only.
2 Sam. 1:21, let there be no *d.*
17:12, we will light on him as *d.* falleth.
1 Kings 17:1, there shall not be *d.* nor rain.
Job 38:28, who hath begotten drops of *d.*
Prov. 3:20, clouds drop down *d.*
Isa. 18:4, like *d.* in heat of harvest.
Dan. 4:15, 23, 25, 33, wet with *d.* of heaven.
Hos. 6:4; 13:3, goodness as early *d.*
Hag. 1:10, heaven is stayed from *d.*
See Ex. 16:13; Num. 11:9; Job 29:19; Ps. 110:3; 133:3; Prov. 19:12; Isa. 26:19; Hos. 14:5.
DIADEM. Job 29:14; Isa. 28:5; 62:3; Ezek. 21:26.
DIAL. 2 Kings 20:11, it had gone down in the *d.* of Ahaz.
Isa. 38:8, gone down in the sun *d.* of Ahaz.
DIAMOND (in high priest's breastplate). Ex. 28:18; 39:11.
See Jer. 17:1; Ezek. 28:13.
DID. Mat. 13:58, he *d.* not many mighty works.
John 4:29, all things that ever I *d.*
9:26, what *d.* he to thee?
15:24, works which none other man *d.*
See Gen. 6:22; 1 Sam. 1:7; Job 1:5; 1 Pet. 2:22.
DIE. Gen. 2:17; 20:7; 1 Sam. 14:44; 22:16; 1 Kings 2:37, 42; Jer. 26:8; Ezek. 3:18; 33:8, 14, surely *d.*
3:3; Lev. 10:6; Num. 18:32, lest ye *d.*
27:4; 45:28; Prov. 30:7, before I *d.*
Ex. 21:12, smiteth a man that he *d.*
Lev. 7:24; 22:8; Deut. 14:21; Ezek. 4:14, that *d.* of itself.
Num. 16:29, if these *d.* common death.
23:10, let me *d.* death of righteous.
Deut. 31:14, days approach that thou must *d.*
Ruth 1:17, where thou *d.* will I *d.*
2 Sam. 3:33, *d.* Abner as a fool *d.*?
2 Kings 20:1; Isa. 38:1, shalt *d.* and not live.
2 Chron. 25:4; Jer. 31:30, every man *d.* for own sin.
Job 2:9, his wife said, curse God and *d.*
3:11, why *d.* I not from the womb.

Mat. 10:42, give cup of water in the name of a *d.*
12:2, thy *d.* do that which is not lawful.
15:2, why do *d.* transgress tradition.
17:16, brought to thy *d.*, and they could not cure.
19:13; Mk. 10:13, the *d.* rebuked them.
20:17, Jesus took *d.* apart.
22:16, Pharisees sent their *d.*
26:18; Mk. 14:14; Lu. 22:11, keep passover with *d.*
35, likewise also said the *d.*
56, all the *d.* forsook him and fled.
28:7, tell his *d.* he is risen.
13, say ye, his *d.* came by night.
Mk. 2:18; Lu. 5:33, why do *d.* of John fast?
4:34, he expounded all things to *d.*
7:2, *d.* eat with unwashen hands.
5, why walk not *d.* according to tradition?
Lu. 5:30, Pharisees murmured against *d.*
6:20, lifted up eyes on *d.*
11:1, as John taught his *d.*
14:26, 27, 33, cannot be my *d.*
19:37, *d.* began to rejoice and praise God.
39, Master, rebuke thy *d.*
John 2:11, his *d.* believed on him.
4:2, Jesus baptized not, but his *d.*
6:22, his *d.* were gone away alone.
66, many of his *d.* went back.
7:3, that thy *d.* may see works.
8:31; 13:35, then are ye my *d.* indeed.
9:27, will ye also be his *d.*?
28, thou art his *d.*, we are Moses' *d.*
13:5, began to wash *d.* feet.
15:8, so shall ye be my *d.*
18:15, 16, that *d.* was known.
17, 25, art not thou one of his *d.*?
19:26; 20:2; 21:7, 20, *d.* whom Jesus loved.
38, a *d.* of Jesus, but secretly for fear.
20:18, told *d.* she had seen the Lord.
21:23, that that *d.* should not die.
24, this is the *d.* which testifieth.
Acts 9:1, slaughter against *d.*
26, essayed to join himself to *d.*
11:26, *d.* called Christians first.
20:7, *d.* came together to break bread.
30, to draw away *d.* after them.
21:16, an old *d.* with whom we should lodge.
See Mat. 11:1; John 3:25; 18:1, 2; 20:26.
DISCIPLINE. Job 36:10.
DISCLOSE. Isa. 26:21.
DISCOMFITED. Judg. 4:15, Lord *d.* Sisera.
8:12, Gideon *d.* all the host.
2 Sam. 22:15; Ps. 18:14, lightnings, and *d.* them.
Isa. 31:8, his young men shall be *d.*
See Ex. 17:13; Num. 14:45; Josh. 10:10
DISCOMFITURE. 1 Sam. 14:20.
DISCONTENTED. 1 Sam. 22:2.
DISCONTINUE. Jer. 17:4.
DISCORD. Prov. 6:14, 19.
DISCOURAGE. Num. 32:7, wherefore *d.* the heart of the children of Israel.
Deut. 1:21, fear not, nor be *d.*
28, our brethren have *d.* our heart.
Col. 3:21, your children, lest they be *d.*
See Num. 21:4; 32:9; Isa. 42:4.
DISCOVER. 1 Sam. 14:8, 11, we will *d.* ourselves to them.
2 Sam. 22:16; Ps. 18:15, foundations of the world *d.*
Job 12:22, he *d.* deep things.
41:13, who can *d.* face of his garment?
Prov. 25:9, *d.* not a secret to another.
Ezek. 21:24, your transgressions are *d.*
See Ps. 29:9; Hos. 7:1; Hab. 3:13; Acts 21:3.
DISCREET. Gen. 41:33, 39; Mk. 12:34; Tit. 2:5.
DISCRETION. Ps. 112:5; Prov. 11:22; Isa. 28:26; Jer. 10:12.
DISDAINED. 1 Sam. 17:42; Job 30:1.
DISEASE. Ex. 15:26; Deut. 7:15, none of these *d.* on you.
Deut. 28:60, bring on thee all *d.* of Egypt.
2 Kings 1:2; 8:8, 9, recover of *d.*
2 Chron. 16:12, in *d.* sought not the Lord.
Job 30:18, by force of my *d.*
Ps. 103:3, who healeth all thy *d.*
Eccl. 6:2, vanity, and it is an evil *d.*
Ezek. 34:4, *d.* have ye not strengthened.
21, have pushed *d.* with your horns.
See Mat. 4:23; 14:35; Lu. 9:1; Acts 28:9.
DISFIGURE. Mat. 6:16.
DISGRACE. Jer. 14:21.
DISGUISE. 1 Sam. 28:8; 1 Kings 14:2; 20:38; 22:30; 2 Chron. 18:29; 35:22; Job 24:15.
DISH. Judg. 5:25; 2 Kings 21:13; Mat. 26:23; Mk. 14:20.
DISHONESTY. 2 Cor. 4:2.
DISHONOUR. Ps. 35:26; 71:13, clothed with shame and *d.*
Prov. 6:33, a wound and *d.* shall he get.
Mic. 7:6, son *d.* father.
John 8:49, I honour my father, ye *d.* me.
Rom. 9:21, one vessel to honour, another to *d.*
1 Cor. 15:43, sown in *d.*
2 Cor. 6:8, by honour and *d.*
2 Tim. 2:20, some to honour, some to *d.*
See Ezra 4:14; Rom. 1:24; 2:23; 1 Cor. 11:4, 5.
DISINHERIT. Num. 14:12.
DISMAYED. Deut. 31:8; Josh. 1:9; 8:1; 10:25; 1 Chron. 22:13; 28:20; 2 Chron. 20:15, 17; 32:7; Isa. 41:10; Jer. 1:17; 10:2; 23:4; 30:10; 46:27; Ezek. 2:6; 3:9, fear not nor be *d.*
Jer. 17:18, let them be *d.*, let not me be *d.*
See 1 Sam. 17:11; Jer. 8:9; 46:5; Obad. 9.
DISMISSED. 2 Chron. 23:8; Acts 15:30; 19:41.
DISOBEDIENCE. Rom. 5:19; Eph. 2:2; 5:6; Heb. 2:2.
DISOBEDIENT. Lu. 1:17, turn *d.* to wisdom of just.
Acts 26:19, not *d.* to heavenly vision.
Rom. 1:30; 2 Tim. 3:2, *d.* to parents.
1 Tim. 1:9, law for lawless and *d.*
Tit. 3:3, we ourselves were sometimes *d.*
1 Pet. 2:7, to them which be *d.*
3:20, spirits, which sometime were *d.*
See 1 Kings 13:26; Neh. 9:26; Rom. 10:21.
DISORDERLY. 1 Thess. 5:14; 2 Thess. 3:6, 7, 11.
DISPENSATION. 1 Cor. 9:17, a *d.* of the gospel is committed me.
Eph. 1:10, in the *d.* of the fulness of times.
3:2, the *d.* of the grace of God.
Col. 1:25, according to the *d.* of God.
DISPERSE. Prov. 15:7, lips of wise *d.* knowledge.
See Ps. 112:9; Jer. 25:34; Ezek. 12:15; 20:23.
DISPERSED. Esth. 3:8, and *d.* among the people.
Isa. 11:12, the *d.* of Judah.
John 7:35, go unto the *d.* among the Gentiles.
DISPERSED (prophecies concerning). Jer. 25:24; Ezek. 36:19; Zeph. 3:10.
DISPLAYED. Ps. 60:4.
DISPLEASE. Num. 11:1, it *d.* the Lord.
22:34, if it *d.* thee, I will get me back.
2 Sam. 11:27, thing David had done *d.* the Lord.
1 Kings 1:6, father had not *d.* him at any time.
Ps. 60:1, thou hast been *d.*
Prov. 24:18, lest the Lord see it, and it *d.* him.
Isa. 59:15, it *d.* him there was no judgment.
Jon. 4:1, it *d.* Jonah exceedingly.
Mat. 21:15, scribes saw it, they were *d.*
Mk. 10:14, Jesus was much *d.*
41, much *d.* with James and John.
See Gen. 48:17; 1 Sam. 8:6; 18:8; Zech. 1:2.
DISPLEASURE. Deut. 9:19; Judg. 15:3; Ps. 2:5; 6:1; 38:1.
DISPOSE. Job 34:13; 37:15; Prov. 16:33; 1 Cor. 10:27.
DISPOSITION. Acts 7:53.
DISPOSSESS. Num. 33:53; Deut. 7:17; Judg. 11:23.
DISPUTATION. Acts 15:2; Rom. 14:1
DISPUTE. Job 23:7, the righteous might *d.* with him.
Mk. 9:33, what was it ye *d.* of by the way?
1 Cor. 1:20, where is the *d.* of this world?
Phil. 2:14, do all things without *d.*
1 Tim. 6:5, perverse *d.*
See Acts 9:29; 15:7; 17:17; Jude 9.
DISQUIET. 1 Sam. 28:15, why *d.* to bring me up?
Ps. 42:5, 11; 43:5, why art thou *d.* within me?
See Ps. 38:8; 39:6; Jer. 50:34.

DISSEMBLE. Josh. 7:11; Ps. 26:4; Prov. 26:24; Jer. 42:20; Gal. 2:13.
DISSENSION. Acts 15:2; 23:7, 10.
DISSIMULATION. Rom. 12:9; Gal. 2:13.
DISSOLVE. Isa. 34:4, host of heaven shall be *d.*
Dan. 5:16, thou canst *d.* doubts.
2 Cor. 5:1, house of tabernacle *d.*
2 Pet. 3:11, all these things shall be *d.*
12, heavens being on fire shall be *d.*
See Job 30:22; Ps. 75:3; Isa. 14:31; 24:19; Dan. 5:12; Nah. 2:6.
DISTAFF. Prov. 31:19.
DISTIL. Deut. 32:2; Job 36:28.
DISTINCTION. 1 Cor. 14:7.
DISTINCTLY. Neh. 8:8.
DISTRACT. Ps. 88:15; 1 Cor. 7:35.
DISTRESS. Gen. 42:21, therefore is this *d.* come upon us.
Judg. 11:7, why are ye come when ye are in *d.*?
1 Sam. 22:2, every one in *d.* came to David.
2 Sam. 22:7; Ps. 18:6; 118:5; 120:1, in *d.* I called.
1 Kings 1:29, redeemed my soul out of all *d.*
2 Chron. 28:22, in *d.* Ahaz trespassed more.
Neh. 2:17, ye see the *d.* we are in.
Ps. 25:17; 107:6, 13, 19, 28, out of *d.*
Prov. 1:27, mock when *d.* cometh.
Isa. 25:4, a strength to needy in *d.*
Obad. 12:14; Zeph. 1:15, day of *d.*
Lu. 21:23, shall be great *d.* in the land.
25, on earth *d.* of nations.
Rom. 8:35, shall *d.* separate us?
1 Cor. 7:26, good for present *d.*
2 Cor. 6:4, approving ourselves in *d.*
12:10, take pleasure in *d.*
See Gen. 35:3; Neh. 9:37; 2 Cor. 4:8; 1 Thess. 3:7.
DISTRIBUTE. Neh. 13:13, office was to *d.* to brethren.
Job. 21:17, God *d.* sorrows in his anger.
Lu. 18:22, sell and *d.* to poor.
John 6:11, given thanks, he *d.*
Rom. 12:13, *d.* to necessity of saints.
1 Cor. 7:17, as God hath *d.* to every man.
2 Cor. 9:13, your liberal *d.*
See Josh. 13:32; Acts 4:35; 2 Cor. 10:13; 1 Tim. 6:18.
DITCH. Ps. 7:15, fallen into *d.* he made.
Mat. 15:14; Lu. 6:39, both fall into *d.*
See 2 Kings 3:16; Job 9:31; Prov. 23:27; Isa. 22:11.
DIVERS. Deut. 22:9, sow vineyard with *d.* kinds.
11, garment of *d.* sorts.
25:13, not have in bag *d.* weights.
14, *d.* measures, great and small.
Prov. 20:10, 23, *d.* weights and measures abomination.
Mat. 4:24; Mk. 1:34; Lu. 4:40, *d.* diseases.
24:7; Mk. 13:8; Lu. 21:11, in *d.* places.
Mk. 8:3, for *d.* of them came from far.
1 Cor. 12:10, to another *d.* kinds of tongues.
2 Tim. 3:6; Tit. 3:3, led away with *d.* lusts.
Jas. 1:2, joy in *d.* temptations.
See Eccl. 5:7; Heb. 1:1; 2:4; 9:10; 13:9.
DIVERSE. Esth. 3:8, laws *d.* from all people.
1 Cor. 12:6, *d.* of operations, but same God.
See Esth. 1:7; 1 Cor. 12:4, 28;
DIVIDE. Lev. 11:4, 5, 6, 7, 26; Deut. 14:7, not eat these of them that *d.* the hoof.
Josh. 19:49, and end of *d.* the land.
1 Kings 3:25, *d.* living child in two.
Job 27:17, innocent shall *d.* silver.
Ps. 68:12; Prov. 16:19; Isa. 9:3; 53:12, *d.* spoil.
Amos 7:17, thy land shall be *d.* by line.
Mat. 12:25; Mk. 3:24; Lu. 11:17, kingdom or house *d.*
26; Mk. 3:26; Lu. 11:18, *d.* against himself.
Lu. 12:13, that he *d.* inheritance with me.
14, who made me a *d.*?
52, five in one house *d.*
53, father *d.* against son.
15:12, he *d.* unto them his living.
Acts 14:4; 23:7, multitude *d.*
1 Cor. 1:13, is Christ *d.*?
12:11, *d.* to every man severally as he will.
2 Tim. 2:15, rightly *d.* word of truth.
Heb. 4:12, piercing to *d.* asunder.
See Dan. 7:25; Hos. 10:2; Mat. 25:32; Lu. 22:17.
DIVINATION. Num. 23:23, neither is any *d.* against Israel.
Acts. 16:16, damsel with a spirit of *d.*
See Deut. 18:10; 2 Kings 17:17; Ezek. 13:23.
DIVINE (*v.*). Gen. 44:15, wot ye not that I can *d.*?
1 Sam. 28:8, *d.* unto me by the familiar spirit.
Ezek. 13:9, prophets that *d.* lies.
21:29, they *d.* lies unto thee.
Mic. 3:11, prophets *d.* for money.
See Gen. 44:5; Ezek. 22:28; Mic. 3;6.
DIVINE (*ad.*). Prov. 16:10; Heb. 9:1; 2 Pet. 1:3, 4.
DIVINER. 1 Sam. 6:2; Isa. 44:25; Jer. 27:9; 29:8.
DIVISION. Ex. 8:23, will put a *d.* between my people.
Judg. 5:15, for *d.* of Reuben great thoughts of heart.
Lu. 12:51, I tell you nay, but rather *d.*
John 7:43; 9:16; 10:19, *d.* because of him.
Rom. 16:17, mark them which cause *d.*
See 1 Cor. 1:10; 3:3; 11:18.
DO. Ruth 3:5, all thou sayest I will *d.*
Eccl. 3:12, for a man to *d.* good.
Isa. 46:11, I will also *d.* it.
Hos. 6:4, what shall I *d.* unto thee?
Mat. 7:12, men should *d.* to you, *d.* ye even so.
23:3, they say, and *d.* not.
Lu. 10:28, this *d.* and thou shalt live.
22:19; 1 Cor. 11:24, this *d.* in remembrance.
John 15:5, without me ye can *d.* nothing.
Rom. 7:15, what I would, that *d.* I not.
2 Cor. 11:12, what I *d.* that I will *d.*
Gal. 5:17, ye cannot *d.* the things ye would.
Phil. 4:13, I can *d.* all things through Christ.
Heb. 4:13, with whom we have to *d.*
Jas. 1:23, a hearer, not a *d.* of the word.
See John 6:38; 10:37; Rev. 19:10; 22:9.
DOCTOR. Acts 5:34, Gamaliel, a *d.* of the law.
Lu. 2:46, sitting in the midst of the *d.*
5:17, *d.* of the law sitting by.
DOCTRINE. Prov. 4:2, I give you good *d.*
Isa. 28:9, made to understand *d.*
Jer. 10:8, the stock is a *d.* of vanities.
Mat. 15:9; Mk. 7:7, teaching for *d.* commandments of men.
16:12, the *d.* of the Pharisees.
Mk. 1:27; Acts 17:19, what new *d.* is this?
John 7:17, do his will shall know of the *d.*
Acts 2:42, continued in apostles' *d.*
5:28, filled Jerusalem with your *d.*
Rom. 6:17, obeyed that form of *d.*
16:17, contrary to the *d.*
1 Cor. 14:26, every one hath a *d.*
Eph. 4:14, every wind of *d.*
1 Tim. 1:10, contrary to sound *d.*
4:6, nourished in words of good *d.*
13, give attendance to *d.*
16, take heed to thyself and *d.*
2 Tim. 3:10, hast fully known my *d.*
16, scripture profitable for *d.*
4:2, exhort with all longsuffering and *d.*
Tit. 1:9, by sound *d.* to exhort and convince.
2:1, things which become sound *d.*
7, in *d.* showing uncorruptness.
10, adorn the *d.* of God our Saviour.
Heb. 6:1, principles of the *d.*
2, the *d.* of baptisms.
13:9, not carried about with strange *d.*
2 John 9, abideth in *d.* of Christ.
See Deut. 32:2; Job 11:4; John 7:16; 1 Tim. 5:17.
DOG. Ex. 11:7, against Israel not a *d.* move.
Deut. 23:18, not bring price of *d.* into house.
Judg. 7:5, that lappeth as *d.* lappeth.
1 Sam. 17:43; 24:14; 2 Sam. 3:8, am I a *d.*?
2 Sam. 9:8, upon such a dead *d.* as I am.
2 Kings 8:13, what, is thy servant a *d.*?
Job 30:1, disdained to set with *d.*
Ps. 22:20, darling from power of the *d.*
59:6, they make noise like a *d.*
Prov. 26:11; 2 Pet. 2:22, as a *d.* returneth.

Prov. 26:17, like one that taketh a *d.* by ears.
Eccl. 9:4, living *d.* better than dead lion.
Isa. 56:10, they are all dumb *d.*
66:3, as if he cut off a *d.* neck.
Mat. 7:6, give not that which is holy to *d.*
15:27; Mk. 7:28, the *d.* eat of crumbs.
Phil. 3:2, beware of *d.*
Rev. 22:15, without are *d.*
See Ex. 22:31; 1 Kings 14:11; 21:23; 22:28.
DOING. Ex. 15:11, fearful in praises, *d.* wonders.
Judg. 2:19, ceased not from their own *d.*
1 Sam. 25:3, churlish and evil in his *d.*
1 Chron. 22:16, arise, and be *d.*
Neh. 6:3, I am *d.* a great work.
Ps. 9:11; Isa. 12:4, declare his *d.*
66:5, terrible in *d.* toward children of men.
77:12, I will talk of thy *d.*
118:23; Mat. 21:42; Mk. 12:11, the Lord's *d.*
Mic. 2:7, are these his *d.*?
Mat. 24:46; Lu. 12:43, shall find so *d.*
Acts 10:38, went about *d.* good.
Rom. 2:7, patient continuance in well *d.*
2 Cor. 8:11, perform the *d.* of it.
Gal. 6:9; 2 Thess. 3:13, weary in well *d.*
Eph. 6:6, *d.* will of God from heart.
1 Pet. 2:15, with well *d.* put to silence.
3:17, suffer for well *d.*
4:19, commit souls in well *d.*
See Lev. 18:3; Prov. 20:11; Isa. 1:16; Jer. 4:4.
DOLEFUL. Isa. 13:21; Mic. 2:4.
DOMINION. Gen. 27:40, when thou shalt have *d.*
37:8, shalt thou have *d.* over us?
Num. 24:19, come he that shall have *d.*
Job. 25:2, *d.* and fear are with him.
38:33, canst thou set the *d.* thereof?
Ps. 8:6, *d.* over works of thy hands.
19:13; 119:133, let them not have *d.* over me.
72:8; Zech. 9:10, *d.* from sea to sea.
Isa. 26:13, other lords have had *d.* over us.
Dan. 4:34; 7:14, *d.* is an everlasting *d.*
Mat. 20:25, princes of Gentiles exercise *d.*
Rom 6:9, death hath no more *d.*
14, sin shall not have *d.*
7:1, law hath *d.* over a man.
2 Cor. 1:24, not *d.* over your faith.
Eph. 1:21, above all *d.*
Col. 1:16, whether they be thrones or *d.*
See Dan. 6:26; 1 Pet. 4:11; Jude 25; Rev. 1:6.
DOOR. Gen. 4:7, sin lieth at the *d.*
Ex. 12:7, strike blood on *d.* posts.
33:8; Num. 11:10, every man at tent *d.*
Judg. 16:3, Samson took *d.* of the gate.
Job 31:9, laid wait at neighbour's *d.*
32, I opened my *d.* to the travellers.
38:17, the *d.* of the shadow of death.
41:14, who can open *d.* of his face?
Ps. 24:7, ye everlasting *d.*
78:23, opened the *d.* of heaven.
84:10, rather be *d.*-keeper.
141:3, keep the *d.* of my lips.
Prov. 5:8, come not nigh *d.* of her house.
8:3, wisdom crieth at *d.*
26:14, as *d.* turneth on hinges.
Eccl. 12:4, *d.* shall be shut in the streets.
Isa. 6:4, posts of the *d.* moved.
26:20, enter, and shut thy *d.* about thee.
Hos. 2:15, for a *d.* of hope.
Mal. 1:10, who would shut the *d.* for nought?
Mat. 6:6, when thou hast shut thy *d.*
24:33; Mk. 13:29, near, even at the *d.*
25:10, and the *d.* was shut.
27:60; 28:2; Mk. 15:46, *d.* of sepulchre.
Mk. 1:33, city gathered at the *d.*
2:2, not so much as about the *d.*
Lu. 13:25, master hath shut to the *d.*
John 10:1, 2, entereth not by *d.*
7:9, I am the *d.*
John 18:16, Peter stood at the *d.* without.
17, damsel that kept the *d.*
20:19, 26, when *d.* were shut, Jesus came.
Acts 5:9, feet at the *d.* to carry thee out.
14:27, opened the *d.* of faith.
1 Cor. 16:9, great *d.* and effectual.
2 Cor. 2:12, *d.* opened to me of the Lord.
Col. 4:3, open a *d.* of utterance.
Jas. 5:9, judge standeth before the *d.*
Rev. 3:8, set before thee an open *d.*
20, I stand at *d.* and knock.
4:1, behold a *d.* opened in heaven.
See Ex. 21:6; Deut. 11:20; Isa. 57:8; Acts 5:19; 16:26.
DOTE. Jer. 50:36; Ezek. 23:5; 1 Tim. 6:4.
DOUBLE. Gen. 43:12, 15, take *d.* money in hand.
Ex. 22:4, 7, 9, he shall restore *d.*
Deut. 15:18, worth a *d.* hired servant.
2 Kings 2:9, a *d.* portion of thy spirit.
1 Chron. 12:33; Ps. 12:2, a *d.* heart.
Isa. 40:2, received *d.* for all her sins.
Jer. 16:18, recompense their sin *d.*
1 Tim. 3:8, deacons not *d.* tongued.
5:17, worthy of *d.* honour.
Jas. 1:8, a *d.* minded man unstable.
4:8, purify your hearts, ye *d.* minded.
See Gen. 41:32; Isa. 61:7; Ezek. 21:14; Rev. 18:6.
DOUBT. Deut. 28:66, thy life shall hang in *d.*
Job. 12:2, no *d.* ye are the people.
Ps. 126:6, shall *d.* come again, rejoicing.
Dan. 5:12, 16, dissolving of *d.*
Mat. 14:31, wherefore didst thou *d.*?
21:21, if ye have faith, and *d.* not.
Mk. 11:23, shall not *d.* in his heart.
Lu. 11:20, no *d.* kingdom of God is come.
John 10:24, how long dost thou make us to *d.*?
Acts 5:24, they *d.* whereunto this would grow.
28:4, no *d.* this man is a murderer.
Rom. 14:23, he that *d.* is damned if he eat.
Gal. 4:20, I stand in *d.* of you.
1 Tim. 2:8, pray without wrath and *d.*
1 John 2:19, would no *d.* have continued.
See Lu. 12:29; Acts 2:12; Phil. 3:8.
DOUGH. Num. 15:20, a cake of the first of your *d.*
Neh. 10:37, the firstfruits of our *d.*
Ezek. 44:30, give unto the priest the first of your *d.*
DOVE. Ps. 55:6, that I had wings like a *d.*
Isa. 59:11, mourn sore like *d.*
60:8, flee as *d.* to their windows.
Mat. 10:16, be harmless as *d.*
21:12; Mk. 11:15; John 2:14, them that sold *d.*
See Jer. 48:28; Hos. 7:11; Mat. 3:16; Mk. 1:10.
DOWN. 2 Sam. 3:35, if I taste ought till sun be *d.*
2 Kings 19:30; Isa. 37:31, again take root *d.*
Ps. 59:15, let them wander up and *d.*
109:23, I am tossed up and *d.*
Eccl. 3:21, spirit of the beast that goeth *d.*
Zech. 10:12, walk up and *d.* in his name.
See Josh. 8:29; Ps. 139:2; Ezek. 38:14.
DOWRY. Gen. 30:20; 34:12; Ex. 22:17; 1 Sam. 18:25.
DRAG. Hab. 1:15, 16; John 21:8.
DRAGON. Deut. 32:33, their wine is the poison of *d.*
Neh. 2:13, before the *d.* well.
Job 30:29, I am a brother to *d.*
Ps. 91:13, the *d.* shalt thou trample.
148:7, praise the Lord, ye *d.*
Isa. 43:20, the *d.* and owls shall honour me.
Jer. 9:11, will make Jerusalem a den of *d.*
Rev. 20:2, the *d.*, that old serpent.
See Rev. 12:3; 13:2, 11; 16:13.
DRANK. 1 Sam. 30:12, nor *d.* water three days and nights.
2 Sam. 12:3, and *d.* of his own cup.
1 Kings 17:6, and he *d.* of the brook.
Dan. 1:5, appointed of the wine he *d.*
5:4, they *d.* wine, and praised the gods.
Mk. 14:23, and they all *d.* of it.
Lu. 17:27, 28, they *d.*, they married.
John 4:12, than our father, who *d.* thereof.

1 Cor. 10:4, for they *d.* of that spiritual Rock.
See Gen. 9:21; 24:46; 27:25; Num. 20:11.
DRAUGHT. Mat. 15:17; Mk. 7:19; Lu. 5:4, 9; 21:6, 11.
DRAVE. Ex. 14:25; Josh. 24:12; Judg. 6:9.
DRAW. Job 40:23, trusteth he can *d.* up Jordan.
41:1, canst thou *d.* out leviathan?
Ps. 28:3, *d.* me not away with wicked.
37:14, wicked have *d.* out sword.
55:21, yet were they *d.* swords.
88:3, my life *d.* nigh unto the grave.
Eccl. 12:1, nor years *d.* nigh.
Cant. 1:4, *d.* me. will run after thee.
Isa. 5:18, *d.* iniquity with cords.
12:3, *d.* water from wells of salvation.
Jer. 31:3, with lovingkindness have I *d.* thee.
Mat. 15:8, people *d.* nigh me with their mouth.
Lu. 21:8, the time *d.* near.
28, your redemption *d.* nigh.
John 4:11, thou hast nothing to *d.* with.
15, thirst not, neither come hither to *d.*
John 6:44, except the Father *d.* him.
12:32, if lifted up, will *d.* all men.
Heb. 10:22, *d.* near with true heart.
38, 39, if any *d.* back.
Jas. 4:8, *d.* nigh to God, he will *d.*
See Acts 11:10; 20:30; Heb 7:19; Jas. 2:6.
DRAWER. Deut. 29:11; Josh 9:21
DREAD. Gen. 28:17, how *d.* is this place!
Deut. 2:25; 11:25, begin to put *d.* of thee.
Isa. 8:13, let him be your *d.*
Mal. 4:5, the great and *d.* day.
See Gen. 9:2; Ex. 15:16, Dan. 9:4.
DREAM. Job 20:8, shall fly away as a *d.*
33:15, 16, in a *d.* he openeth the ears.
Ps. 73:20, as a *d.* when one awaketh.
126:1, we were like them that *d.*
Eccl. 5:3, a *d.* cometh through much business.
Jer. 23:28, prophet that hath a *d.*
Joel 2:28; Acts 2:17, old men *d. d.*
Jude 8, filthy *d.* defile the flesh.
See Job 7:14; Isa. 29:8; Jer. 27:9.
DREGS. Ps. 75:8; Isa. 51:17.
DRESS. Gen. 2:15, put man in garden to *d.* it.
Deut. 28:39, plant vineyards and *d.* them.
2 Sam. 12:4, poor man's lamb and *d.* it.
See Ex. 30:7; Lu. 13:7; Heb. 6:7.
DREW. Gen. 47:29, time *d.* nigh that Israel must die.
Ex. 2:10, because I *d.* him out of the water.
Josh. 8:26, Joshua *d.* not his hand back.
1 Kings 22:34; 2 Chron. 18:33, man *d.* a bow.
2 Kings 9:24, Jehu *d.* bow with full strength.
Hos. 11:4, *d.* them with cords of a man.
Zeph. 3:2, she *d.* not near to her God.
Mat. 21:34, when time of fruit *d.* near.
Lu. 24:15, Jesus himself *d.* near.
Acts 5:37, and *d.* away much people.
See Esth. 5:2; Lam. 3:57; Acts 7:17.
DRINK (*n.*). Lev. 10:9, do not drink strong *d.* when ye go.
Num. 6:3, separate himself from strong *d.*
Deut. 14:26, bestow money for strong *d.*
29:6, strong *d.* these forty years.
Prov. 20:1, strong *d.* is raging.
31:4, not for princes to drink strong *d.*
6, give strong *d.* to him that is ready to perish.
Isa. 24:9, strong *d.* shall be bitter.
28:7, erred through strong *d.*
Mic. 2:11, prophesy of wine and strong *d.*
Hab. 2:15, that giveth his neighbour *d.*
Hag. 1:6, ye are not filled with *d.*
Mat. 25:35, 37, 42, thirsty, and ye gave me *d.*
John 4:9, a Jew, askest *d.* of me.
6:55, my blood is *d.* indeed.
Rom 12:20, if thine enemy thirst, give him *d.*
14:17, the kingdom of god is not meat and *d.*
1 Cor. 10:4, same spiritual *d.*
Col. 2:16, judge you in meat or in *d.*
See Gen. 21:19; Isa. 5:11, 22; 32:6; 43:20. Lu. 1:15; 1 Tim. 5:23.
DRINK (*v.*). Ex. 15:24, what shall we *d.*?
17:1, no water for people to *d.*
2 Sam. 23:16; 1 Chron. 11:18; David would not *d.*
Ps. 36:8, *d.* of the river of thy pleasures.
60:3, *d.* the wine of astonishment.
80:5, gavest them tears to *d.*
110:7, he shall *d.* of the brook in the way.
Prov. 5:15, *d.* waters of thine own cistern.
31:5, lest they *d.* and forget the law.
7, let him *d.*, and forget his poverty.
Eccl. 9:7, *d.* wine with merry heart.
Cant. 5:1, *d.*, yea, *d.* abundantly.
Isa. 5:22, mighty to *d.* wine.
65:13, my servants shall *d.*, but ye.
Jer. 35:2, give Rechabites wine to *d.*
6, we will *d.* no wine.
14, to this day they *d.* none.
Ezek. 4:11, thou shalt *d.* water by measure.
Amos. 2:8, *d.* the wine of the condemned.
Zech. 9:15, they shall *d.*, and make a noise
Mat. 10:42, whoso shall give to *d.*
20:22; Mk. 10:38, are ye able to *d.*?
26:27, saying, *d.* ye all of it.
29; Mk. 14:25; Lu. 22:18, when I *d.* it new.
42, may not pass except I *d.*
Mk. 9:41, shall give you cup of water to *d.*
16:18, if they *d.* any deadly thing.
John 4:10, give me to *d.*
7:37, let him come to me, and *d.*
18:11, cup given me, shall I not *d.* it?
Rom 14:21, not good to *d.* wine.
1 Cor. 10:4, did all *d.* same spiritual drink.
11:25, as oft as ye *d.* it.
12:13, made to *d.* into one Spirit.
See Mk. 2:16; Lu. 7:33; 10:7.
DRIVE. Gen. 4:14, thou hast *d.* me out.
Ex. 23:28, hornets shall *d.* out Hivite.
Deut. 4:19, lest thou be *d.* to worship them.
Job 24:3, they *d.* away ass of the fatherless.
30:5, they were *d.* forth from among men.
Prov. 14:32, wicked *d.* away in his wickedness.
22:15, rod shall *d.* it away.
25:23, north wind *d.* away rain.
Jer. 46:15, stood not, because Lord did *d.* them.
Dan. 4:25; 5:21, they shall *d.* thee from men.
Hos. 13:3, as chaff *d.* with whirlwind.
Lu. 8:29, he was *d.* of the devil.
Jas. 1:6, wave *d.* with the wind.
See 2 Kings 9:20; Jer. 8:3; Ezek. 31:11.
DROMEDARIES. 1 Kings 4:28, straw for the horses and *d.*
Esth. 8:10, and young *d.*
Isa. 60:6, the *d.* of Midian and Ephah.
Jer. 2:23, thou art a swift *d.* traversing her ways.
DROP (*n.*). Job 36:27, maketh small the *d.* of water.
Isa. 40:15, as the *d.* of a bucket.
See Job 38:28; Cant. 5:2; Lu. 22:44.
DROP (*v.*). Deut. 32:2, doctrine shall *d.* as the rain.
Job 29:22, my speech *d.* upon them.
Ps. 65:11, paths *d.* fatness.
68:8 heavens *d.* at presence of God.
Eccl. 10:18, through idleness house *d.* through.
Isa. 45:8, *d.* down, ye heavens.
Ezek. 20:46, *d.* thy word toward the south.
See 2 Sam. 21:10; Joel 3:18; Amos 9:13.
DROPSY. Lu. 14:2, a man which had the *d.*
DROSS. Ps. 119:119; Prov. 25:4; 26:23; Isa. 1:22, 25; Ezek. 22:18.
DROUGHT. Deut. 28:24; 1 Kings 17; Isa. 58:11; Jer. 17:8; Hos. 13:5; Hag. 1:11.
DROVE. Gen. 3:24; 15:11; 32:16; 33:8; John 2:15.
DROWN. Cant. 8:7, neither can floods *d.* it.
1 Tim 6:9, that *d.* men in perdition.
See Ex. 15:4; Mat. 18:6; Heb. 11:29.
DROWSINESS. Prov. 23:21.
DRUNK. 2 Sam. 11:13, David made Uriah *d.*

1 Kings 20:16, was drinking himself *d.*
Job 12:25; Ps. 107:27, stagger like a *d.* man.
Jer. 23:9, I am like a *d.* man.
Lam. 5:4, we have *d.* water for money.
Hab. 2:15, makest him *d.* also.
Mat. 24:49; Lu. 12:45, drink with the *d.*
Acts 2:15, these are not *d.*
1 Cor. 11:21, one is hungry, and another *d.*
1 Thess. 5:7, they that be *d.* are *d.* in the night.
See Lu. 5:39; John 2:10; Eph. 5:18; Rev. 17:6
DRUNKARD. Deut. 21:20, our son is a glutton and a *d.*
Prov. 23:21, *d.* and glutton come to poverty.
26:9, as a thorn goeth into hand of *d.*
1 Cor. 6:10, nor *d.* shall inherit.
See Ps. 69:12; Isa. 24:20; Joel 1:5; Nah. 1:10.
DRUNKENNESS. Deut. 29:19, to add *d.* to thirst.
Eccl. 10:17, eat for strength, not for *d.*
Ezek. 23:33, shalt be filled with *d.*
See Lu. 21:34; Rom. 13:13; Ga. 5:21.
DRY. Prov. 17:22, a broken spirit *d.* the bones.
Isa. 44:3, pour floods on *d.* ground.
Mat. 12:43; Lu. 11:24, through *d.* places.
Mk. 5:29, fountain of blood *d.* up.
See Ps. 107:33, 35; Isa. 53:2; Mk. 11:20.
DUE. Lev. 10:13, 14, it is thy *d.*, and thy sons' *d.*
26:4; Deut. 11:14, rain in *d.* season.
Ps. 104:27; 145:15; Mat. 24:45; Lu. 14:42, meat in *d.* season.
Prov. 15:23, word spoken in *d.* season.
Mat. 18:34, pay all that was *d.*
Lu. 23:41, the *d.* reward of our deeds.
Rom. 5:6, in *d.* time Christ died.
Gal. 6:9, in *d.* season we shall reap.
See Prov. 3:27; 1 Cor. 15:8; Tit. 1:3; 1 Pet. 5:6.
DULL. Mat. 13:15; Acts 28:27; Heb. 5:11.
DUMB. Ex. 4:11, who maketh the *d.*?
Prov. 31:8, open thy mouth for the *d.*
Isa. 35:6, the tongue of the *d.* shall sing.
53:7; Acts 8:32, as sheep before shearers is *d.*
56:10, they are all *d.* dogs.
Ezek. 3:26, be *d.*, and shalt not be a reprover.
Hab. 2:19, woe to him that saith to *d.* stone.
Mat. 9:32; 12:22; 15:30; Mk. 7:37; 9:17; *d.* man.
See Ps. 39:2; Dan. 10:15; Lu. 1:20; 11:14; 2 Pet. 2:16.
DUNG. 1 Sam 2:8; Ps. 113:7, lifteth beggar from *d.*-hill.
Lu. 13:8, till I dig about it, and *d.* it.
14:35, neither fit for land nor *d.*-hill.
Phil. 3:8, count all things but *d.*
See Neh. 2:13; Lam. 4:5; Mal. 2:3.
DUNGEON. Gen. 40:15; 41:14; Ex. 12:29; Jer. 38:6; Lam. 3:53.
DURABLE. Prov. 8:18; Isa. 23:18.
DURETH. Mat. 13:21.
DURST. Mat. 22:46; Mk. 12:34; Lu. 20:40, nor *d.* ask questions.
John 21:12, none of disciples *d.* ask.
See Esth. 7:5; Job 32:6; Acts 5:13; Jude 9.
DUST. Gen. 2:7, Lord God formed man of *d.*
3:14, *d.* shalt thou eat.
19, *d.* thou art.
18:27, who am but *d.* and ashes.
Job 10:9, wilt thou bring me into *d.* again?
22:24; 27:16, lay up gold as *d.*
34:15, man shall turn again to *d.*
42:6, I repent in *d.* and ashes.
Ps. 30:9, shall the *d.* praise thee?
102:14, servants favour *d.* thereof.
103:14, remembereth that we are *d.*
104:29, they die and return to their *d.*
Eccl. 3:20, all are of the *d.* and turn to *d.* again.
12:7, then shall the *d.* return to the earth.
Isa. 40:12, comprehended *d.* of the earth.
65:25, *d.* shall be serpent's meat.
Lam. 3:29, he putteth his mouth in the *d.*
Dan. 12:2, many that sleep in *d.* shall awake.
Mic. 7:17, lick the *d.* like a serpent.
Mat. 10:14; Mk. 6:11; Lu. 9:5, shake off *d.* from feet.
Lu. 10:11, even *d.* of your city.
Acts 22:23, as they threw *d.* into the air.
See Ex. 8:16; Num. 23:10; Deut. 9:21; Josh. 7:6; Job 2:12; 39:14; Lam. 2:10.
DUTY. Eccl. 12:13, the whole *d.* of man.
Lu. 17:10, that which was our *d.* to do.
Rom. 15:27, their *d.* is to minister.
See Ex. 21:10; Deut. 25:5; 2 Chron. 8:14; Ezra 3:4.
DWELL. Deut. 12:11, cause his name to *d.* there.
1 Sam. 4:4; 2 Sam. 6:2; 1 Chron. 13:6, *d.* between the cherubims.
1 Kings 8:30; 2 Chron. 6:21, heaven thy *d.* place
Ps. 23:6, will *d.* in house of the Lord.
37:3, so shalt thou *d.* in the land.
84:10, than to *d.* in tents of wickedness.
132:14, here will I *d.*
133:1, good for brethren to *d.* together.
Isa. 33:14, who shall *d.* with devouring fire?
16, he shall *d.* on high.
57:15, I *d.* in the high and holy place.
John 6:56, *d.* in me, and I in him.
14:10, the Father that *d.* in me.
17, for he *d.* with you, and shall be in you.
Rom. 7:17, sin that *d.* in me.
Col. 2:9, in him *d.* fulness of Godhead.
3:16, word of Christ *d.* in you richly.
1 Tim. 6:16, *d.* in the light.
2 Pet. 3:13, wherein *d.* righteousness.
1 John 3:17, how *d.* the love of God in him?
4:12, God *d.* in us.
See Rom. 8:9; 2 Cor. 6:16; Jas. 4:5
DYED. Ex. 25:5; Isa. 63:1; Ezek. 23:15
DYING. 2 Cor. 4:10, the *d.* of Lord Jesus.
2 Cor. 6:9, as *d.* and behold we live.
See Num. 17:13; Lu. 8:42; Heb. 11:21.

E

EACH. Isa. 57:2, *e.* one walking in his uprightness.
Ezek. 4:6, *e.* day for a year.
Acts 2:3, cloven tongues sat on *e.*
Phil. 2:3, let *e.* esteem other.
See Ex. 18:7; Ps. 85:10; 2 Thess. 1:3
EAGLE. Ex. 19:4, how I bare you on *e.* wings.
2 Sam. 1:23, were swifter than *e.*
Job 9:26, *e.* that hasteth to prey.
39:27, doth the *e.* mount up?
Ps. 103:5, youth renewed like *e.*
Isa. 40:31, mount up with wings as *e.*
Ezek. 1:10, they four also had the face of an *e.*
17:3, a great *e.* with great wings.
Obad. 4, thou shalt exalt thyself as the *e.*
Mat. 24:28; Lu. 17:37, *e.* be gathered.
Rev. 4:7, the fourth beast was like a flying *e.*
See Dan. 4:33; Rev. 12:14.
EAR (*n.*). Neh. 1:6, let thine *e.* be attentive.
Job 12:11; 34:3, doth not *e.* try words?
29:11, when the *e.* heard me, it blessed me.
42:5, heard of thee by the hearing of the *e.*
Ps. 45:10, and incline thine *e.*
58:4, like the deaf adder that stoppeth her *e.*
78:1, give *e.*, O my people.
94:9, he that planted the *e.*, shall he not hear?
Prov. 15:31, the *e.* that heareth the reproof.
17:4, liar giveth *e.* to naughty tongue.
18:15, *e.* of wise seeketh knowledge.
20:12, hearing *e.* seeing eye, Lord made.
20:17, bow down thine *e.*
25:12, wise reprover on obedient *e.*
Eccl. 1:8, nor the *e.* filled with hearing.
Isa. 48:8, from that time thine *e.* not opened.
50:4, he wakeneth my *e.* to hear.
55:3, incline your *e.* and come unto me.
59:1, nor his *e.* heavy, that it cannot.
Jer. 9:20, let your *e.* receive word of the Lord.
Amos 3:12, out of mouth of lion piece of an *e.*
1 Cor. 2:9, nor *e.* heard.
12:16, if *e.* say, because I am not the eye.
See Rev. 2:7.
EAR (*v.*). Ex. 34:21; Deut. 21:4; 1 Sam 8:12.

EARLY. Ps. 46:5, and that right *e.*
63:1, *e.* will I seek thee.
90:14, satisfy us *e.* with thy mercy.
Prov. 1:28; 8:17, seek me *e.* shall find me.
Cant. 7:12, get up *e.* to vineyards.
Hos. 6:4; 13:3, as *e.* dew.
Jas. 5:7, the *e.* and latter rain.
See Judg. 7:3; Lu. 24:22; John 20:1.
EARNEST. Job 7:2, as servant *e.* desireth shadow.
Jer. 31:20, I do *e.* remember him still.
Mic. 7:3, do evil with both hands *e.*
Lu. 22:44, in agony he prayed more *e.*
Rom. 8:19, the *e.* expectation of the creature.
1 Cor. 12:31, covet *e.* best gifts.
2 Cor. 1:22; 5:5, the *e.* of the Spirit.
5:2, *e.* desiring to be clothed.
Eph. 1:14, the *e.* of our inheritance.
Phil. 1:20, to my *e.* expectation and hope.
Jude 3, *e.* contend for the faith.
See Acts 3:12; Heb. 2:1; Jas. 5:17.
EARNETH. Hag. 1:6.
EARS. Ex. 10:2, tell it in *e.* of thy son.
1 Sam. 3:11; 2 Kings 21:12; Jer. 19:3, at which *e.* shall tingle.
2 Sam. 7:22, we have heard with our *e.*
Job 15:21, dreadful sound is in his *e.*
28:22, heard fame with our *e.*
Ps. 18:6, my cry came even into his *e.*
34:15, his *e.* are open unto their cry.
115:6; 135:17, they have *e.*, but hear not.
Prov. 21:13, stoppeth *e.* at cry of the poor.
23:9, speak not in *e.* of a fool.
26:17, one that taketh dog by the *e.*
Isa. 6:10; Mat. 13:15; Acts 28:27, make *e.* heavy.
Mat. 10:27, what ye hear in *e.*, preach.
13:16, blessed are your *e.*
26:51; Mk. 14:47, smote off *e.*
Mk. 7:33, put his fingers into *e.*
8:18, having *e.*, hear ye not?
Acts 7:51, uncircumcised in heart and *e.*
17:20, strange things to our *e.*
2 Tim. 4:3, having itching *e.*
Jas. 5:4, entered into *e.* of the Lord.
1 Pet. 3:12, his *e.* are open to prayer.
See Mat. 11:15; Mk. 4:9.
EARS (*of corn*). Deut. 23:25; Mat. 12:1.
EARTH. Gen. 8:22, while *e.* remaineth.
10:25, in his days was *e.* divided.
18:25, shall not Judge of all the *e.* do right?
Num. 14:21, all *e.* filled with glory.
16:30, if the *e.* open her mouth.
Deut. 32:1, O *e.* hear the words of my mouth.
Josh. 3:11; Zech. 6:5, Lord of all the *e.*
23:14, going way of all the *e.*
1 Kings 8:27; 2 Chron. 6:18, will God dwell on the *e.*?
2 Kings 5:17, two mules' burden of *d.*
Job 7:1, appointed time to man upon *e.*
9:24, *e.* given into hand of wicked.
19:25, stand at latter day upon *e.*
26:7, hangeth *e.* upon nothing.
38:4, when I laid foundations of the *e.*
41:33, on *e.* there is not his like.
Ps. 2:8, uttermost parts of *e.*
8:1, excellent is thy name in *e.*
16:3, to saints that are in the *e.*
25:13, his seed shall inherit the *e.*
33:5, the *e.* is full of the goodness.
34:16, cut off remembrance from the *e.*
37:9, 11, 22, wait on Lord shall inherit *e.*
41:2, shall be blessed upon the *e.*
46:2, not fear, though *e.* be removed.
6, uttered voice, the *e.* melted.
8, desolations made in the *e.*
10, will be exalted in the *e.*
47:9, shields of the *e.* belong to God.
48:2, joy of the whole *e.*
50:4, call to *e.*, that he may judge.
57:5; 108:5, glory above all the *e.*
Ps. 58:11, a God that judgeth in the *e.*
60:2, made the *e.* to tremble.
63:9, lower parts of the *e.*
65:8, dwell in uttermost parts of *e.*
9, visitest *e.*, and waterest it.
67:6; Ezek. 34:27, *e.* yield increase.
68:8, *e.* shook, heavens dropped.
71:20, bring me up from depths of the *e.*
72:6, showers that water the *e.*
16, handful of corn in the *e.*
73:9, tongue walketh through *e.*
25, none on *e.* I desire beside thee.
75:3; Isa. 24:19, *e.* dissolved.
83:18; 97:9, most high over all *e.*
90:2, or ever thou hadst formed the *e.*
97:1, Lord reigneth, let *e.* rejoice.
99:1, Lord reigneth, let *e.* be moved.
102:25; 104:5; Prov. 8:29; Isa. 48:13, laid foundation of *e.*
104:13, the *e.* is satisfied.
24, the *e.* is full of thy riches.
112:2, seed mighty upon *e.*
115:16, *e.* given to children of men.
119:19, stranger in the *e.*
64, the *e.* full of thy mercy.
90, established the *e.*, it abideth.
146:4, he returneth to the *e.*
147:8, prepareth rain for the *e.*
148:13, glory above *e.* and heaven.
Prov. 3:19; Isa. 24:1, Lord founded the *e.*
8:23, set up from everlasting, or ever *e.* was.
26, he had not yet made *e.*, nor fields.
11:31, righteous recompensed in *e.*
25:3, the *e.* for depth.
30:14, teeth as knives to devour poor from *e.*
16, the *e.* not filled with water.
21, for three things *e.* is disquieted.
24, four things little upon *e.*
Eccl. 1:4, the *e.* abideth for ever.
3:21, spirit of beast goeth to *e.*
5:9, profit of the *e.* for all.
12:7, dust return to *e.*
Isa. 4:2, fruit of *e.* excellent.
11:9, *e.* full of knowledge of the Lord.
13:13, *e.* shall remove out of her place.
14:16, is this the man that made *e.* tremble?
26:9, when thy judgments are in the *e.*
21, *e.* shall disclose her blood.
34:1, let the *e.* hear.
40:22, sitteth on circle of the *e.*
28, Creator of ends of *e.* fainteth not.
44:24, spreadeth abroad *e.* by myself.
45:22, be saved, all ends of the *e.*
49:13, be joyful, O *e.*
51:6, the *e.* shall wax old.
66:1, the *e.* is my footstool.
8, shall *e.* bring forth in one day?
Jer. 15:10, man of contention to whole *e.*
22:29; Mic. 1:2, O *e.*, *e.*, *e.*, hear word of Lord.
31:22, hath created new thing in *e.*
51:15, made the *e.* by his power.
Ezek. 9:9, the Lord hath forsaken the *e.*
43:2, the *e.* shined with his glory.
Hos. 2:22, the *e.* shall hear the corn.
Amos 3:5, bird fall in snare on *e.*
8:9, darken *e.* in the clear day.
9:9, least grain fall upon the *e.*
Jon. 2:6, *e.* with bars about me.
Mic. 6:2, ye strong foundations of the *e.*
7:2, good man perished out of the *e.*
17, move like worms of the *e.*
Nah. 1:5, *e.* burnt up at his presence
Hab. 2:14, *e.* filled with knowledge.
3:3, the *e.* full of his praise.
Hag. 1:10, *e.* stayed from her fruit.
Zech. 4:10, eyes of Lord run through *e.*
Mal. 4:6, lest I smite *e.* with a curse.
Mat. 5:5, meek shall inherit *e.*

Mat. 5:35, swear not by the *e.*
6:19, treasures upon *e.*
9:6; Mk. 2:10; Lu. 5:24, power on *e.* to forgive.
10:34, to send peace on *e.*
13:5, Mk. 4:5, not much *e.*
16:19, 18:18, shalt bind on *e.*
18:19, shall agree on *e.*
23:9, call no man father on *e.*
25:18, 25, digged in the *e.*
Mk. 4:28, *e.* bringeth forth fruit of herself.
31, less than all seeds in the *e.*
9:3, no fuller on *e.* can white them.
Lu. 2:14, on *e.* peace.
23:44, darkness over all *e.*
John 3:12, I have told you *e.* things.
31, of *e.* is *e.*, and speaketh of the *e.*
12:32, lifted up from the *e.*
17:4, I have glorified thee on the *e.*
Acts 8:33, life taken from the *e.*
9:4, 8; 26:14, Saul fell to the *e.*
22:22, away with such a fellow from *e.*
Rom. 10:18, sound went into all *e.*
1 Cor. 15:47, first man is of the *e.*, *e.*
48, as is the *e.*, such are they that are *e.*
49, the image of the *e.*
2 Cor. 4:7, treasure in *e.* vessels.
Col. 3:2, affection not on things on *e.*
Phil. 3:19, who mind *e.* things.
Heb. 6:7, *e.* drinketh in the rain.
8:4, if he were on *e.*
11:13, strangers on the *e.*
12:25, refused him that spake on *e.*
26, voice then shook the *e.*
Jas. 3:15, this wisdom is *e.*
5:5, lives in pleasure on *e.*
7, the precious fruit of the *e.*
18, and the *e.* brought forth her fruit.
2 Pet. 3:10, the *e.* shall be burnt up.
Rev. 5:10, we shall reign on the *e.*
7:3, hurt not the *e.*
18:1, *e.* lightened with his glory.
20:11, from whose face the *e.* fled.
21:1, a new *e.*
See Gen. 1:1, 11; 3:17; 7:10; Ex. 9:29; Job 12:8; Ps. 24:1; Isa. 65:16; Mic. 1:4; Zeph. 3:8; 2 Pet. 3:7, 13; Rev. 20:9.
EARTHQUAKE. 1 Kings 19:11; Isa. 29:6; Amos 1:1; Zech. 14:5; Mat. 24:7; 27:54; Acts 16:26; Rev. 6:12; 8:5; 11:13; 16:18.
EASE. Ex. 18:22, so shall it be *e.* for thyself.
Deut. 28:65, among nations find no *e.*
Job 12:5, thought of him that is at *e.*
16:6, though I forbear, what am I *e.*?
21:23, dieth, being wholly at *e.*
Ps. 25:13, his soul shall dwell at *e.*
Isa. 32:9, 11, women that are at *e.*
Amos. 6:1, woe to them that are at *e.*
Mat. 9:5; Mk. 2:9; Lu. 5:23, is *e.* to say.
19:24; Mk. 10:25; Lu. 18:25, *e.* for camel.
1 Cor. 13:5, not *e.* provoked.
Heb. 12:1, sin which doth so *e.* beset.
See Jer. 46:27; Zech. 1:15; Lu. 12:19.
EAST. Gen. 41:6; 23:27, blasted with *e.* wind.
Ex. 10:13, Lord brought an *e.* wind.
Job 1:3, greatest of all men of the *e.*
15:2, fill his belly with *e.* wind.
27:21, *e.* wind carrieth him away.
38:24, scattereth *e.* wind on the earth.
Ps. 48:7, breakest ships with *e.* wind.
75:6, promotion cometh not from *e.*
103:12, as far as *e.* from west.
Isa. 27:8, stayeth rough wind in day of *e.* wind.
Ezek. 19:12, the *e.* wind drieth up her fruit.
43:2, glory of God of Israel came from way of *e.*
47:1, house stood toward the *e.*
Hos. 12:1, Ephraim followeth *e.* wind.
13:15, though fruitful, an *e.* wind shall come.
See Jon. 4:5, 8; Mat. 2:1; 8:11; 24:27.

EASTER. Acts 12:4, intending after *E.* to bring him forth.
EASY. Prov. 14:6; Mat. 11:30; 1 Cor. 14:9; Jas. 3:17.
EAT. Gen. 2:17, in day thou *e.* thou shalt die.
9:4; Lev. 19:26; Deut. 12:16, blood not *e.*
24:33, not *e.* till I have told.
43:32, Egyptians might not *e.* with Hebrews.
Ex. 12:16, no work, save that which man must *e.*
23:11, that the poor may *e.*
29:34, shall not be *e.*, because holy.
Lev. 25:20, what shall we *e.* seventh year?
Num. 13:32, a land that *e.* up inhabitants.
Josh. 5:11, 12, *e.* of old corn of the land.
1 Sam. 14:30, if haply people had *e.* freely.
28:20, had *e.* no bread all day.
22, *e.*, that thou mayest have strength.
2 Sam. 19:42, have we *e.* at all of the king's cost?
1 Kings 19:5; Acts 10:13; 11:7, angel said, Arise and *e.*
2 Kings 4:43, 44, they shall *e.*, and leave thereof.
6:28, give thy son, that we may *e.* him.
Neh. 5:2, corn, that we may *e.*, and live.
Job 3:24, my sighing cometh before I *e.*
5:5, whose harvest the hungry *e.* up.
6:6, *e.* without salt.
21:25, another never *e.* with pleasure.
31:17, have *e.* my morsel alone.
Ps. 22:26, meek shall *e.* and be satisfied.
69:9; John 2:17, zeal hath *e.* me up.
102:9, have *e.* ashes like bread.
Prov. 1:31; Isa. 3:10, *e.* fruit of their own way.
13:25, *e.* to satisfying of soul.
18:21, they that love it shall *e.* the fruit.
23:1, sittest to *e.* with ruler.
24:13, *e.* honey, because it is good.
25:27, not good to *e.* much honey.
Eccl. 2:25, who can *e.* more than I?
4:5, fool *e.* his own flesh.
5:11, goods increase, they increased that *e.*
12, sleep be sweet, whether he *e.* little or much
17, all his days also he *e.* in darkness.
19; 6:2, not power to *e.* thereof.
10:16, thy princes *e.* in the morning.
17, blessed when princes *e.* in due season.
Isa. 4:1, we will *e.* our own bread.
7:15, 22, butter and honey shall he *e.*
11:7; 65:25, lion *e.* straw like ox.
29:8, he *e.*, awaketh, and is hungry.
51:8, worm shall *e.* them like wool.
55:1, come ye, buy and *e.*
2, *e.* ye that which is good.
10, give bread to the *e.*
65:13, my servants shall *e.*, but ye shall be.
Jer. 5:17, they shall *e.* up thine harvest.
15:16, words were found, and I did *e.* them.
24:2; 29:17, figs could not be *e.*
31:29; Ezek. 18:2, the fathers have *e.* sour grapes.
Ezek. 3:1, 2, 3, *e.* this roll.
4:10, *e.* by weight.
Dan. 4:33, *e.* grass as oxen.
Hos. 4:10; Mic. 6:14; Hag. 1:6, *e.*, and not have enough.
10:13, have *e.* the fruit of lies.
Mic. 7:1, there is not cluster to *e.*
Mat. 6:25; Lu. 12:22, what ye shall *e.*
9:11; Mk. 2:16; Lu. 15:2, why *e.* with publicans?
12:1, ears of corn, and *e.*
4, *e.* shewbread, which was not lawful to *e.*
14:16; Mk. 6:37; Lu. 9:13, give ye them to *e.*
15:20, to *e.* with unwashen hands
15:27; Mk. 7:28, dogs *e.* of crumbs.
32; Mk. 8:1, multitude have nothing to *e.*
24:49, to *e.* and drink with the drunken.
Mk. 2:16, when they saw him *e.* with.
6:31, no leisure so much as to *e.*
11:14, no man *e.* fruit of thee.
Lu. 5:33, but thy disciples *e.* and drink.
10:8, *e.* such things as are set before you.
12:19, take thine ease, *e.*, drink.
13:26, we have *e.* and drunk in thy presence.

Lu. 15:23, let us *e.* and be merry.
22:30, that ye may *e.* at my table.
24:43, he took it, and did *e.* before them.
John 4:31, Master, *e.*
32, meat to *e.* ye know not of.
6:26, because ye did *e.* of loaves.
52, can this man give us his flesh to *e.*?
53, except ye *e.* the flesh.
Acts 2:46, did *e.* their meat with gladness.
9:9, Saul did neither *e.* nor drink.
11:3, thou didst *e.* with them.
23:14, will *e.* nothing until we have slain Paul.
Rom. 14:2, one believeth he may *e.* all things; weak *e.* herbs.
6, *e.* to the Lord.
20, who *e.* with offence.
21, neither to *e.* flesh nor drink wine.
1 Cor. 5:11, with such an one no not to *e.*
8:7, *e.* it as a thing offered to idol.
8, neither if we *e.* are we better.
13, I will *e.* no flesh while world.
9:4, have we not power to *e.*?
10:3, all *e.* same spiritual meat.
27, *e.*, asking no question.
31, whether ye *e.* or drink.
11:29, he that *e.* unworthily.
2 Thess. 3:10, work not, neither should he *e.*
Heb. 13:10, whereof they have no right to *e.*
Rev. 2:7, *e.* of the tree of life.
17, will give to *e.* of hidden manna.
19:18, *e.* flesh of kings.
See Judg. 14:14; Prov. 31:27; Isa. 1:19; 65:4.
EDGE. Prov. 5:4; Heb. 4:12; Eccl. 10:10.
EDIFY. Rom. 14:19, wherewith one may *e.*
15:2, please his neighbour to *e.*
1 Cor. 8:1, charity *e.*
14:3, he that prophesieth speaketh to *e.*
4, *e.* himself, *e.* the church.
10:23, all things lawful, but *e.* not.
Eph. 4:12, for *e.* of the body of Christ.
See 2 Cor. 10:8; 13:10; 1 Tim. 1:4.
EFFECT. Num. 30:8, make vow of none *e.*
2 Chron. 7:11, Solomon prosperously *e.* all.
Ps. 33:10, devices of the people of none *e.*
Isa. 32:17, the *e.* of righteousness quietness.
Mat. 15:6; Mk. 7:13, commandment of God of none *e.*
1 Cor. 1:17, lest cross be of none *e.*
Gal. 5:4, Christ is become of none *e.*
See Rom. 3:3; 4:14; 9:6; Gal. 3:17.
EFFECTUAL. 1 Cor. 16:9, a great door and *e.* is opened.
Eph. 3:7; 4:16, the *e.* working.
Jas. 5:16, *e.* prayer of righteous man.
See 2 Cor. 1:6; Gal. 2:8; 1 Thess. 2:13.
EFFEMINATE. 1 Cor. 6:9.
EGG. Job 6:6, taste in the white of an *e.*
39:14, ostrich leaveth *e.* in earth.
Lu. 11:12, if he ask an *e.*
See Deut. 22:6; Isa. 10:14; 59:5; Jer. 17:11.
EITHER. Gen. 31:24, speak not *e.* good or bad.
Eccl. 11:6, prosper, *e.* this or that.
Mat. 6:24; Lu. 16:13, *e.* hate the one.
John 19:18, on *e.* side one.
Rev. 22:2, on *e.* side the river.
See Deut. 17:3; 28:51; Isa. 7:11; Mat. 12:33.
ELDER. 1 Sam. 15:30, honour me before *e.* of people.
Job 15:10, aged men, much *e.* than thy father.
32:4, waited, because they were *e.* than he.
Prov. 31:23, husband known among *e.*
Mat. 15:2; Mk. 7:3, tradition of the *e.*
1 Tim. 5:17, let *e.* that rule be worthy.
Tit. 1:5, ordain *e.* in every city.
Heb. 11:2, the *e.* obtained good report.
Jas. 5:14, call for *e.* of the church.
1 Pet. 5:1, the *e.* I exhort, who am an *e.*
5, younger submit to the *e.*
See John 8:9 1 Tim. 5:2; 2 John 1; 3 John 1.
ELECT. Isa. 42:1, mine *e.*, in whom my soul delighteth.
Isa. 45:4, mine *e.* I have called by name.
65:9, 22, mine *e.* shall inherit.
Mat. 24:22; Mk. 13:20, for *e.* sake days shortened.
24; Mk. 13:22, deceive very *e.*
31; Mk. 13:27, gather together his *e.*
Lu. 18:7, avenge his own *e.*
Rom. 8:33, to charge of God's *e.*
Col. 3:12, put on as the *e.* of God.
1 Tim. 5:21, charge thee before *e.* angels.
1 Pet. 1:2, *e.* according to foreknowledge.
2:6, corner stone, *e.*, precious.
See 2 Tim. 2:10; Tit. 1:1; 1 Pet. 5:13; 2 John 1:13.
ELECTION. Rom. 9:11; 11:5; 1 Thess. 1:4; 2 Pet. 1:10.
ELEMENTS. Gal. 4:3, 9; 2 Pet. 3:10.
ELEVEN. Gen. 32:22, Jacob took his *e.* sons.
37:9, and *e.* stars made obeisance.
Acts 1:26, he was numbered with the *e.*
See Mat. 28:16; Mk. 16:14; Lu. 24:9.
ELOQUENT. Ex. 4:10; Isa. 3:3; Acts 18:24.
EMBALMED. Gen. 50:2, the days of those which are *e.*
26, and they *e.* him.
See John 19:39.
EMBOLDEN. Job 16:3; 1 Cor. 8:10.
EMBRACE. Job 24:8, *e.* rock for want of shelter.
Eccl. 3:5, a time to *e.*
Heb. 11:13, seen and *e.* promises.
See Prov. 4:8; 5:20; Lam. 4:5; Acts 20:1.
EMBROIDER. Ex. 28:39; 35:35; 38:23.
EMERALDS. Ex. 28:18; 39:11; Rev. 4:3; 21:19.
EMERODS. Deut. 28:27, and with *e.*
1 Sam. 5:6, and smote them with *e.*
EMINENT. Ezek. 16:24, 31, 39; 17:22.
EMPIRE. Esth. 1:20.
EMPLOY. Deut. 20:19; 1 Chron. 9:3; Ezra. 10:15; Ezek. 39:14.
EMPTY. Gen. 31:42; Mk. 12:3; Lu. 1:53; 20:10, sent *e.* away.
Ex. 3:21, ye shall not go *e.*
23:15; 34:20; Deut. 16:16, appear before me *e.*
Deut. 15:13, not let him go away *e.*
Job 22:9, thou hast sent widows away *e.*
Eccl. 11:3, clouds *e.* themselves on the earth.
Isa. 29:8, awaketh, and his soul is *e.*
Jer. 48:11, Moab *e.* from vessel to vessel.
Nah. 2:2, the emptiers have *e.* them out.
Mat. 12:44, come, he findeth it *e.*
See 2 Sam. 1:22; 2 Kings 4:3; Hos. 10:1.
EMULATION. Rom. 11:14; Gal. 5:20.
ENABLED. 1 Tim. 1:12.
ENCAMP. Ps. 27:3, though host *e.* against me.
34:7, angel of Lord *e.* round.
See Num. 10:31; Job 19:12; Ps. 53:5.
ENCOUNTERED. Acts 17:18.
ENCOURAGE. Deut. 1:38; 3:28; 2 Sam. 11:25, *e.* him.
Ps. 64:5, they *e.* themselves in an evil matter.
See 1 Sam. 30:6; 2 Chron. 31:4; 35:2; Isa. 41:7
END. Gen. 6:13, the *e.* of all flesh before me.
Ex. 23:16; Deut. 11:12, in the *e.* of the year.
Num. 23:10, let my last *e.* be like his.
Deut. 8:16, do thee good at thy latter *e.*
32:29, consider their latter *e.*
Job 6:11, what is mine *e.*, that I should prolong?
8:7; 42:12, thy latter *e.* shall increase.
16:3, shall vain words have an *e.*?
26:10, till day and night come to an *e.*
Ps. 7:9, wickedness of wicked come to an *e.*
9:6, destructions come to perpetual *e.*
37:37, the *e.* of that man is peace.
39:4, make me to know my *e.*
73:17, then understood I their *e.*
102:27, the same, thy years have no *e.*
107:27, are at their wit's *e.*
119:96, an *e.* on all perfection.
Prov. 14:12, the *e.* thereof are ways of death.
17:24, eyes of fool in *e.* of earth.
19:20, be wise in thy latter *e.*
25:8, lest thou know not what to do in *e.*
Eccl. 3:11, find out from beginning to the *e.*
4:8, no *e.* of all his labour.

Eccl. 4:16, no *e.* of all the people.
7:2, that is the *e.* of all men.
8, better the *e.* of a thing.
10:13, the *e.* of his talk is madness.
12:12, of making books there is no *e.*
Isa. 9:7, of his government shall be no *e.*
46:10, declaring *e.* from beginning.
Jer. 5:31, what will ye do in *e.* thereof?
8:20, harvest past, summer *e.*
17:11, at his *e.* shall be a fool.
29:11, to give you an expected *e.*
31:17, there is hope in thine *e.*
Lam. 1:9, remembereth not her last *e.*
4:18; Ezek. 7:2, our *e.* is near, *e.* is come.
Ezek. 21:25; 35:5, iniquity shall have an *e.*
Dan. 8:17, 19; 11:27, at the time of *e.*
11:45, he shall come to his *e.*, and none shall help him.
12:8, what shall be the *e.*?
13, go thy way till the *e.* be.
Hab. 2:3, at the *e.* it shall speak.
Mat. 10:22; 24:13; Mk. 13:13, endureth to *e.*
13:39, harvest is *e.* of the world.
24:3, what sign of the *e.* of the world?
6; Mk. 13:7; Lu. 21:9, the *e.* is not yet.
14, then shall the *e.* come.
31, gather from one *e.* of heaven.
26:58, Peter sat to see the *e.*
28:20, I am with you, even unto the *e.*
Mk. 3:26, cannot stand, but hath an *e.*
Lu. 1:33, of his kingdom there shall be no *e.*
22:37, things concerning me have an *e.*
John 13:1, he loved them unto the *e.*
18:37, to this *e.* was I born.
Rom. 6:21, the *e.* of those things is death.
22, the *e.* everlasting life.
10:4, the *e.* of the law for righteousness.
1 Cor. 10:11, on whom *e.* of world are come.
Phil. 3:19, whose *e.* is destruction.
1 Tim. 1:5, the *e.* of the commandment.
Heb. 6:8, whose *e.* is to be burned.
16, an oath an *e.* of strife.
7:3, neither beginning nor *e.* of life.
9:26, once in the *e.* hath he appeared.
13:7, considering *e.* of their conversation.
Jas. 5:11, ye have seen *e.* of the Lord.
1 Pet. 1:9, receiving the *e.* of your faith.
13, be sober, and hope to the *e.*
4:7, the *e.* of all things is at hand.
17, what shall the *e.* be of them that obey not?
Rev. 2:26, keepeth my works unto *e.*
21:6; 22:13, the beginning and the *e.*
See Ps. 19:6; 65:5; Isa. 45:22; 52:10; Jer. 4:27
ENDAMAGE. Ezra. 4:13.
ENDANGER. Eccl. 10:9; Dan 1:10.
ENDEAVOUR. Ps. 28:4; Eph. 4:3; 2 Pet. 1:15.
ENDLESS. 1 Tim. 1:4; Heb. 7:16.
ENDUE. Gen. 30:20; 2 Chron. 2:12; Lu. 24:49; Jas. 3:13.
ENDURE. Gen. 33:14, as the children be able to *e.*
Esth. 8:6, how can I *e.* to see evil?
Job 8:15, hold it fast, but it shall not *e.*
31:23, I could not *e.*
Ps. 9:7; 102:12; 104:31, Lord shall *e.* for ever.
30:5, anger *e.* a moment, weeping *e.* for a night.
52:1, goodness of God *e.* continually.
72:5, as long as sun and moon *e.*
17, his name shall *e.* for ever.
100:5, his truth *e.* to all generations.
106:1; 107:1; 118:1; 136:1; 138:8; Jer. 33:11, his mercy *e.* for ever.
111:3; 112:3, 9, his righteousness *e.* for ever.
119:160, every one of thy judgments *e.*
135:13, thy name, O Lord, *e.* for ever.
145:13, thy dominion *e.*
Prov. 27:24, doth *e.* to every generation.
Ezek. 22:14, can thy heart *e.*?
Mat. 10:22; 24:13; Mk. 13:13, *e.* to the end.
Mk. 4:17, so *e.* but for a time.
John 6:27, meat that *e.* unto life.
Rom. 9:22, God *e.* with much longsuffering.
1 Cor. 13:7, charity *e.* all things.
2 Tim. 2:3, *e.* hardness as good soldier.
4:3, they will not *e.* sound doctrine.
5, watch, *e.* afflictions.
Heb. 10:34, in heaven a better and *e.* substance.
12:7, if ye *e.* chastening.
Jas. 1:12, blessed is man that *e.* temptation.
5:11, we count them happy which *e.*
1 Pet. 1:25, the word of the Lord *e.* for ever.
2:19, if a man for conscience *e.* grief.
See Heb. 10:32; 11:27; 12:2, 3.
ENEMY. Ex. 23:22, I will be *e.* to thine *e.*
Deut. 32:31, our *e.* themselves being judges.
Josh. 7:12, Israel turned backs before *e.*
Judg. 5:31, so let all thy *e.* perish.
1 Sam. 24:19, if man find *e.*, will he let him go?
1 Kings 21:20, hast thou found me, O mine *e.*?
Job 13:24, wherefore holdest thou me for *e.*?
Ps. 8:2, still the *e.* and avenger.
23:5, in presence of mine *e.*
38:19, mine *e.* are lively.
61:3, a strong tower from the *e.*
72:9, his *e.* shall lick the dust.
119:98, wise than mine *e.*
127:5, speak with *e.* in the gate.
139:22, I count them mine *e.*
Prov. 16:7, maketh his *e.* at peace.
24:17, rejoice not when *e.* falleth.
25:21; Rom. 12:20, if *e.* hunger, give bread.
27:6, kisses of *e.* deceitful.
Isa. 9:11, Lord shall join *e.* together.
59:19, when *e.* shall come in like a flood.
63:10, he was turned to be their *e.*
Jer. 15:11, will cause *e.* to entreat thee well.
30:14, wounded thee with wound of *e.*
Mic. 7:6, man's *e.* men of his own house.
Mat. 5:43, said, thou shalt hate thine *e.*
44; Lu. 6:27, 35, I say, love your *e.*
13:25, 28, 39, his *e.* sowed tares.
Lu. 19:43, thine *e.* shall cast a trench.
Acts 13:10, thou *e.* of all righteousness.
Rom. 5:10, if when *e.* we were reconciled.
11:28, concerning the gospel they are *e.*
Gal. 4:16, am I become your *e.*?
Phil. 3:18, the *e.* of the cross.
Col. 1:21, were *e.* in your mind.
2 Thess. 3:15, count him not as an *e.*
Jas. 4:4, friend of the world is the *e.* of God.
See Ps. 110:1; Isa. 62:8; Jer. 15:14; Heb. 10:13.
ENGAGED. Jer. 30:21.
ENGINES. 2 Chron. 26:15, and he made in Jerusalem *e.*
Ezek. 26:9, and he shall set *e.* of war.
ENGRAFTED. Jas. 1:21.
ENGRAVE. Ex. 28:11; 35:35; 38:23; Zech. 3:9; 2 Cor. 3:7.
ENJOIN. Job 36:23; Philem. 8; Heb. 9:20.
ENJOY. Lev. 26:34; 2 Chron. 36:21, land shall *e.* her sabbaths.
Eccl. 2:1, *e.* pleasure, this also is vanity.
24; 3:13; 5:18, soul *e.* good.
1 Tim. 6:17, giveth us all things to *e.*
See Num. 36:8; Isa. 65:22; Heb. 11:25.
ENLARGE. Deut. 12:20, when the Lord shall *e.* thy border.
Ps. 4:1, thou hast *e.* me in distress.
25:17, troubles of heart *e.*
119:32, when thou shalt *e.* my heart.
Isa. 5:14, hell hath *e.* herself.
2 Cor. 6:11, 13; 10:15, our heart is *e.*
See Isa. 54:2; Hab. 2:5; Mat. 23:5.
ENLIGHTEN. Ps. 19:8; Eph. 1:18; Heb. 6:4.
ENMITY. Rom. 8:7, carnal mind is *e.*
Eph. 2:15, 16, having abolished the *e.*
Jas. 4:4, friendship of world *e.* with God.
See Gen. 3:15; Num. 35:21; Lu. 23:12.
ENOUGH. Gen. 33:9, 11, I have *e.*, my brother.
45:28, it is *e.*, Joseph is alive.
Ex. 36:5, people bring more than *e.*

2 Sam. 24:16; 1 Kings 19:4; 1 Chron. 21:15; Mk. 14:41; Lu. 22:38, it is *e.*, stay thine hand.
Prov. 28:19, shall have poverty *e.*
30:15, four things say not, it is *e.*
16, fire saith not, it is *e.*
Isa. 56:11, dogs which can never have *e.*
Jer. 49:9, will destroy till they have *e.*
Hos. 4:10, eat, and not have *e.*
Obad. 5, stolen till they had *e.*
Mal. 3:10, room *e.* to receive it.
Mat. 10:25, *e.* for disciple.
25:9, lest there be not *e.*
See Deut. 1:6; 2 Chron. 31:10; Hag. 1:6; Lu. 15:17.
ENQUIRE. Ex. 18:15, people come to me to *e.* of God.
2 Sam. 16:23, as if a man had *e.* of oracle.
2 Kings 3:11, is there not a prophet to *e.*?
Ps. 78:34, returned and *e.* early after God.
Ezek. 14:3, should I be *e.* of at all by them?
20:3, 31, I will not be *e.*
36:37, I will yet for this be *e.* of.
Zeph. 1:6, those that have not *e.* for.
Mat. 10:11, *e.* who in it is worthy.
1 Pet. 1:10, of which salvation the prophets *e.*
See Deut. 12:30; Isa. 21:12; John 4:52.
ENRICH. 1 Sam. 17:25; Ps. 65:9; Ezek. 27:33; 1 Cor. 1:5; 2 Cor. 9:11.
ENSAMPLE. 1 Cor. 10:11, happened to them for *e.*
Phil. 3:17, as ye have us for an *e.*
2 Thess. 3:9, to make ourselves an *e.*
See 1 Thess. 1:7; 1 Pet. 5:3; 2 Pet. 2:6.
ENSIGN. Ps. 74:4; Isa. 5:26; 11:10; 18:3; 30:17.
ENSNARED. Job 34:30.
ENSUE. 1 Pet. 3:11
ENTANGLE. Ex. 14:3; Mat. 22:15; Ga. 5:1
ENTER. Ps. 100:4, *e.* his gates with thanksgiving.
119:130, the *e.* of thy word giveth light.
Isa. 26:2, righteous nation may *e.* in.
20, *e.* thou into thy chambers.
Ezek. 44:5, mark well *e.* in of the house.
Mat. 6:6, prayest, *e.* into thy closet.
7:13; Lu. 13:24, *e.* in at strait gate.
10:11; Lu. 10:8, 10, what city ye *e.*
18:8; Mk. 9:43, better to *e.* into life.
19:17, if thou wilt *e.* into life, keep.
25:21, well done, *e.* into joy.
Mk. 5:12; Lu. 8:32, we may *e.* into swine.
14:38; Lu. 22:46, lest ye *e.* into temptation.
Lu. 9:34, feared as they *e.* cloud.
13:24, many will seek to *e.*
John 3:4, can he *e.*?
4:38, ye are *e.* into their labours.
10:1, 2, *e.* not by the door.
Rom. 5:12, sin *e.* into world.
1 Cor. 2:9, neither have *e.* into heart of man.
Heb. 3:11, 18, shall not *e.* into rest.
4:10, he that is *e.* into rest.
6:20, forerunner is for us *e.*
2 Pet. 1:11, so an *e.* shall be ministered.
See Ps. 143:2; Prov. 17:10; Mat. 15:17.
ENTICE. Judg. 14:15; 16:5, *e.* husband that he may declare.
2 Chron. 18:19, Lord said, who shall *e.* Ahab?
Prov. 1:10, if sinners *e.* thee.
1 Cor. 2:4; Col. 2:4, with *e.* words.
See Job 31:27; Prov. 16:29; Jas. 1:14.
ENTIRE. Jas. 1:4.
ENTREAT. Mat. 22:6; Lu. 18:32, *e.* them spitefully.
ENTRY. 1 Chron. 9:19; Prov. 8:3; Ezek. 8:5; 40:38.
ENVIRON. Josh. 7:9.
ENVY. Job 5:2, *e.* slayeth the silly one.
Ps. 73:3, I was *e.* at the foolish.
Prov. 3:31, *e.* not the oppressor.
14:30, *e.* is rottenness of the bones.
23:17, let not heart *e.* sinners.
24:1, 19, be not *e.* against evil men.
27:4, who is able to stand before *e.*?
Eccl. 4:4, for this a man is *e.*
9:6, their love, hatred, and *e.* is perished.
Mat. 27:18; Mk. 15:10, for *e.* they delivered.
Acts 7:9, patriarchs moved with *e.*
13:45; 17:5, Jews filled with *e.*
Rom. 1:29, full of *e.*, murder.
13:13, walk honestly, not in *e.*
1 Cor. 3:3, among you *e.* and strife.
13:4, charity *e.* not.
2 Cor. 12:20, I fear lest there be *e.*
Gal. 5:21, works of flesh are *e.*, murders.
26, *e.* one another.
Phil. 1:15, preach Christ even of *e.*
1 Tim. 6:4, whereof cometh *e.*
Tit. 3:3, living in malice and *e.*
Jas. 4:5, spirit in us lusteth to *e.*
See Gen. 37:11; Ps. 106:16; Ezek. 31:9; 35:11.
EPHAH. Ex. 16:36, now an omer is the tenth part of an *e.*
Lev. 19:36, a just *e.* shall ye have.
Ezek. 45:10, ye shall have just balances, and a just *e.*
Zech. 5:6, this is an *e.* that goeth forth.
EPHOD. Ex. 28:6, they shall make the *e.* of gold.
Ex. 39:2, and he made the *e.* of gold.
Judg. 8:27, and Gideon made an *e.* thereof.
17:5, and made an *e.*
EPISTLE. 2 Cor. 3:1, nor need *e.* of commendation.
2, ye are our *e.*
3, to be the *e.* of Christ.
2 Thess. 2:15; 3:14, by word or *e.*
2 Pet. 3:16, as also in all his *e.*
See Acts 15:30; 23:33; 2 Cor. 7:8; 2 Thess. 3:17.
EQUAL. Ps. 17:2, eyes behold things that are *e.*
55:13, a man mine *e.*, my guide.
Prov. 26:7, legs of lame not *e.*
Isa. 40:25; 46:5, to whom shall I be *e.*?
Ezek. 18:25, 29; 33:17, 20, is not my way *e.*?
Mat. 20:12, hast made him *e.* to us.
Lu. 20:36, are *e.* to angels.
John 5:18; Phil. 2:6, *e.* with God.
Col. 4:1, give servants what is *e.*
See Ex. 36:22; 2 Cor. 8:14; Gal. 1:14.
EQUITY. Ps. 98:9, judge the people with *e.*
Prov. 1:3, receive instruction of *e.*
2:9, understand judgment and *e.*
17:26, not good to strike princes for *e.*
Eccl. 2:21, a man whose labour is in *e.*
See Isa. 11:4; 59:14; Mic. 3:9; Mal. 2:6.
ERECTED. Gen. 33:20.
ERR. Ps. 95:10, people that do *e.* in their heart.
119:21, do *e.* from thy commandments.
Isa. 3:12; 9:16, lead the cause to *e.*
28:7, they *e.* in vision.
35:8, wayfaring men shall not *e.*
Mat. 22:29; Mk. 12:24, *e.*, not knowing scriptures.
1 Tim. 6:10, have *e.* from the faith.
21, have *e.* concerning the faith.
Jas. 1:16, do not *e.* beloved brethren.
5:19, if any do *e.* from truth.
See Isa. 28:7; 29:24; Ezek. 45:20.
ERRAND. Gen. 24:33; Judg. 3:19; 2 Kings 9:5.
ERROR. Ps. 19:12, who can understand his *e.*?
Eccl. 5:6, neither say thou, it was an *e.*
10:5, evil which I have seen as an *e.*
Mat. 27:64, last *e.* worse than first.
Jas. 5:20, converteth sinner from *e.*
2 Pet. 3:17, led away with *e.* of wicked.
1 John 4:6, the spirit of *e.*
See Job 19:4; Rom. 1:27; Heb. 9:7; Jude 11.
ESCAPE. Gen. 19:17, *e.* for thy life, *e.* to mountain.
1 Kings 18:40; 2 Kings 9:15, let none of them. *e.*
Esth. 4:13, think not thou shalt *e.* in king's house.
Job 11:20, wicked shall not *e.*
19:20, *e.* with skin of my teeth.
Ps. 55:8, I would hasten my *e.*
Prov. 19:5, speaketh lies shall not *e.*
Eccl. 7:26, whoso pleaseth God shall *e.*
Isa. 20:6; Heb. 2:3, how shall we *e.*?
Ezek. 33:21, one that had *e.* came to me.
Amos. 9:1, he that *e.* shall not be delivered.

Mat. 23:33, how can ye *e.* damnation?
Lu. 21:36, worthy to *e.*
John 10:39, he *e.* out of their hands.
Acts 27:44, they *e.* all safe to land.
28:4, he *e.* sea, yet vengeance.
Heb. 11:34, through faith *e.* edge of sword.
12:25, if they *e.* not who refused.
2 Pet. 1:4, *e.* corruption in the world.
20, after they *e.* pollutions.
See Deut. 23:15; Ps. 124:7; 1 Cor. 10:13.
ESCHEW. Job 1:1; 2:3; 1 Pet. 3:11.
ESPECIALLY. Gal. 6:10; 1 Tim. 4:10; 5:8; Philem. 16.
ESPOUSE. Cant. 3:11; Jer. 2:2; 2 Cor. 11:2.
ESPY. Gen. 42:27; Josh. 14:7; Jer. 48:19;
Ezek. 20:6.
ESTABLISH. Ps. 40:2, and *e.* my goings.
90:17, *e.* work of our hands.
Prov. 4:26, let thy ways be *e.*
12:19, lip of truth *e.* for ever.
16:12, throne *e.* by righteousness.
20:18, every purpose *e.* by counsel.
24:3, by understanding is house *e.*
29:4, king by judgment *e.* the land.
Isa. 7:9, if ye will not believe, ye shall not be *e.*
16:5, in mercy shall the throne be *e.*
Jer. 10:12; 51:15, he *e.* world by wisdom.
Mat. 18:16, two witnesses every word *e.*
Rom. 3:31, yea, we *e.* the law.
10:3, to *e.* their own righteousness.
Heb. 13:9, the heart be *e.* with grace.
2 Pet. 1:12, be *e.* in the present truth.
See Amos 5:15; Hab. 2:12; Acts 16:5.
ESTATE. Ps. 136:23, remembered us in low *e.*
Eccl. 1:16, lo, I am come to great *e.*
Mk. 6:21, Herod made supper to chief *e.*
Rom. 12:16, condescend to me of low *e.*
Jude 6, angels kept not first *e.*
See Ezek. 36:11; Dan. 11:7; Lu. 1:48.
ESTEEM. Deut. 32:15, lightly *e.* rock of salvation.
1 Sam. 2:30, despise me shall be lightly *e.*
18:23, I am a poor man, and lightly *e.*
Job 23:12, I have *e.* the words of his mouth.
36:19, will he *e.* thy riches?
41:27, he *e.* iron as straw.
Ps. 119:128, I *e.* all thy precepts.
Isa. 53:4, did *e.* him smitten.
Lam. 4:2, *e.* as earthen pitchers.
Lu. 16:15, highly *e.* among men.
Rom. 14:5, one man *e.* one day above another.
14, that *e.* any thing unclean.
Phil. 2:3, let each *e.* other better.
1 Thess. 5:13, *e.* highly for work's sake.
Heb. 11:26, *e.* reproach greater riches.
See Prov. 17:28; Isa. 29:17; 1 Cor. 6:4.
ESTIMATION. Lev. 27:2-8, 13; Num. 18:16.
ESTRANGED. Job 19:13; Ps. 78:30; Jer. 19:4; Ezek. 14:5.
ETERNAL. Deut. 33:27, the *e.* God is thy refuge.
Isa. 60:15, will make thee an *e.* excellency.
Mat. 19:16; Mk. 10:17; Lu. 10:25; 18:18, what shall I do that I may have *e.* life?
25:46, righteous into life *e.*
Mk. 3:29, is in danger of *e.* damnation.
10:30, receive in world to come *e.* life.
John 3:15, believeth in him have *e.* life.
4:36, gathereth fruit unto life *e.*
5:39, scriptures, in them *e.* life.
6:54, drinketh my blood hath *e.* life.
68, thou hast words of *e.* life.
10:28, give sheep *e.* life.
12:25, hateth life, shall keep it to life *e.*
17:2, give *e.* life to as many.
3, this is life *e.*, that they might know thee.
Acts 13:48, many as were ordained to *e.* life.
Rom. 2:7, who seek for glory, *e.* life.
5:21, grace reign to *e.* life.
6:23, gift of God is *e.* life.
2 Cor. 4:17, an *e.* weight of glory.
2 Cor. 4:18, things not seen are *e.*
5:1, house *e.* in the heavens.
Eph. 3:11, according to *e.* purpose.
1 Tim. 6:12, 19, lay hold on *e.* life.
Tit. 1:2; 3:7, in hope of *e.* life.
Heb. 5:9, author of *e.* salvation.
6:2, doctrine of *e.* judgment.
9:15, promise of *e.* inheritance.
1 Pet. 5:10, called to *e.* glory by Christ.
1 John 1:2, *e.* life, which was with the Father.
2:25, this is the promise, even *e.* life.
3:15, no murderer hath *e.* life.
5:11, record, that God hath given to us *e.* life.
13, know that ye have *e.* life.
20, this is true God, and *e.* life.
Jude 7, vengeance of *e.* fire.
See Rom. 1:20; 1 Tim. 1:17; 2 Tim. 2:10; Jude 21.
ETERNITY. Isa. 57:15.
EUNUCHS. Isa. 56:4, for thus saith the Lord to the *e.*
Mat. 19:12, for there are some *e.*
Acts 8:27, an *e.* of great authority.
See Isa. 56:3.
EVANGELIST. Acts 21:8; Eph. 4:11; 2 Tim. 4:5.
EVENING. 1 Sam. 14:24, cursed that eateth till *e.*
1 Kings 17:6, brought bread morning and *e.*
Ps. 90:6, in *e.* cut down and withereth.
104:23, goeth to his labour until the *e.*
141:2, prayer as the *e.* sacrifice.
Eccl. 11:6, in *e.* withhold not thine hand.
Jer. 6:4, shadows of *e.* stretched out.
Hab. 1:8; Zeph. 3:3, *e.* wolves.
Zech. 14:7, at *e.* time shall be light.
Mat. 14:23, when *e.* was come, he was there alone.
Lu. 24:29, abide, for it is toward *e.*
See Gen. 30:16; Ps. 65:8; Mat. 16:2; Mk. 14:17.
EVENT. Eccl. 2:14; 9:2, 3.
EVER. Gen. 3:22, lest he eat, and live for *e.*
43:9; 44:32, let me bear blame for *e.*
Ex. 14:13, ye shall see them no more for *e.*
Lev. 6:13, fire *e.* burning on altar.
Deut. 5:29; 12:28, be well with them for *e.*
13:16, a heap for *e.*
32:40, lift up hand and say, I live for *e.*
Job 4:7, who *e.* perished?
Ps. 9:7, Lord shall endure for *e.*
12:7, thou wilt preserve them for *e.*
22:26, your heart shall live for *e.*
23:6, dwell in house of the Lord for *e.*
29:10, Lord sitteth king for *e.*
33:11, counsel of Lord standeth for *e.*
37:26, he is *e.* merciful, and lendeth.
48:14, our God for *e.* and *e.*
49:9, that he should still live for *e.*
51:3, my sin is *e.* before me.
52:8, trust in mercy of God for *e.* and *e.*
61:4, will abide in tabernacle for *e.*
73:26, my strength and portion for *e.*
74:19, forget not congregation of poor for *e.*
81:15, their time should have endured for *e.*
92:7, they shall be destroyed for *e.*
93:5, holiness becometh thine house for *e.*
102:12, thou shalt endure for *e.*
103:9, not keep his anger for *e.*
105:8, remember his covenant for *e.*
119:89, for *e.* thy word is settled.
132:14, this is my rest for *e.*
146:6, Lord keepeth truth for *e.*
10, Lord shall reign for *e.*
Prov. 27:24, riches not for *e.*
Eccl. 3:14, whatsoever God doeth shall be for *e.*
Isa. 26:4, trust in Lord for *e.*
32:17, assurance for *e.*
34:10; Rev. 14:11; 19:3, smoke shall go up for *e.*
40:8, word of God shall stand for *e.*
57:16, will not contend for *e.*
Lam. 3:31, Lord will not cast off for *e.*
Mat. 6:13, thine is the glory for *e.*

Mat. 21:19; Mk. 11:14, no fruit grow on thee for *e.*
John 8:35, servant abideth not for *e.*
12:34, heard that Christ abideth for *e.*
14:16, Comforter abide for *e.*
Rom. 9:5, God blessed for *e.*
1 Thess. 4:17, so shall we *e.* be with the Lord.
5:15, *e.* follow good.
2 Tim. 3:7, *e.* learning.
Heb. 7:25, he *e.* liveth to make.
13:8, same yesterday, to day, and for *e.*
See Mat. 24:21; Lu. 15:31; John 10:8.
EVERLASTING. Ex. 40:15; Num. 25:13, an *e.* priesthood.
Ps. 90:2, from *e.* to *e.* thou art God.
139:24, lead me in way *e.*
Prov. 8:23, I was set up from *e.*
10:25, righteous in an *e.* foundation.
Isa. 9:6, called the *e.* Father.
26:4, in the Lord is *e.* strength.
33:14, with *e.* burnings.
35:10; 51:11; 61:7, *e.* joy.
45:17, with *e.* salvation.
54:8, with *e.* kindness.
55:13, for an *e.* sign.
56:5; 63:12, an *e.* name.
60:19, 20, an *e.* light.
Jer. 31:3, with an *e.* love.
Hab. 3:6, the *e.* mountains.
Mat. 18:8; 25:41, into *e.* fire.
19:29, inherit *e.* life.
25:46, into *e.* punishment.
Lu. 16:9, into *e.* habitations.
18:30, in world to come *e.* life.
John 3:16, 36, believeth shall have *e.* life.
4:14, water springing up into *e.* life.
5:24, heareth my word hath *e.* life.
6:27, meat which endureth to *e.* life.
40, seeth Son may have *e.* life.
12:50, his commandment is life *e.*
Acts 13:46, unworthy of *e.* life.
Rom. 6:22, free from sin, the end *e.* life.
Gal. 6:8, of Spirit reap life *e.*
2 Thess. 1:9, punished with *e.* destruction.
2:16, given us *e.* consolation.
Jude 6, reserved in *e.* chains.
Rev. 14:6, having the *e.* gospel.
See Dan. 4:3; 7:27; 2 Pet. 1:11.
EVERMORE. Ps. 16:11, pleasures for *e.*
37:27, do good and dwell for *e.*
121:8, preserve thy going out for *e.*
133:3, the blessing, life for *e.*
John 6:34, *e.* give us this bread.
1 Thess. 5:16, rejoice *e.*
Heb. 7:28, consecrated for *e.*
Rev. 1:18, I am alive for *e.*
See 2 Kings 17:37; Ps. 77:8; 106:31.
EVERY. Gen. 4:14, *e.* one that findeth me shall slay me.
6:5, *e.* imagination of heart evil.
Lev. 19:10, neither shalt gather *e.* grape.
Deut. 4:4, alive *e.* one of you this day.
2 Kings 18:31, eat *e.* one of his fig tree.
2 Chron. 30:18, pardon *e.* one.
Ps. 29:9, *e.* one doth speak of glory.
32:6, for this shall *e.* one that is godly.
68:30, till *e.* one submit himself.
119:101, refrained from *e.* evil way.
Prov. 2:9, *e.* good path.
7:12, in *e.* corner.
14:15, simple believeth *e.* word.
20:3, *e.* fool will be meddling.
30:5, *e.* word of God is pure.
Eccl. 10:3, saith to *e.* one he is a fool.
Jer. 51:29, *e.* purpose of the Lord.
Mat. 4:4, by *e.* word that proceedeth.
7:8; Lu. 11:10, *e.* one that asketh.
Mk. 1:45, came from *e.* quarter.
Lu. 19:26, to *e.* one which hath shall be given.
Rom. 14:11, *e.* knee bow, *e.* tongue confess.

2 Cor. 10:5, *e.* thought.
Eph. 1:21; Phil. 2:9, far above *e.* name.
1 Tim. 4:4, *e.* creature of God.
2 Tim. 2:19, *e.* one that nameth.
21, *e.* good work.
Heb. 12:1, *e.* weight.
Jas. 1:17, *e.* good and perfect gift.
1 Pet. 2:13, *e.* ordinance of man.
1 John 4:1, believe not *e.* spirit.
7, *e.* one that loveth.
Rev. 6:11, robes given to *e.* one.
See Gen. 27:29; Acts 2:38; 17:27; 20:31.
EVIDENCE. Jer. 32:10; Heb. 11:1.
EVIDENT. Gal. 3:1, Christ hath been *e.* set forth.
11, that no man is justified is *e.*
Phil. 1:28, an *e.* token of perdition.
See Job 6:28; Heb. 7:14, 15.
EVIL. Gen. 6:5; 8:21, thoughts of heart only *e.*
47:9, few and *e.* have the days.
Ex. 32:14; 2 Sam. 24:16; 1 Chron. 21:15, repented of the *e.*
Deut. 28:54, eye *e.* towards his brother.
56, her eye *e.* towards husband.
Job 2:10, receive good, and not *e.*
30:26, looked for good, then *e.* came.
Ps. 34:14; 37:27; Prov. 3:7, depart from *e.*
35:12; 109:5, they rewarded me *e.*
40:12, innumerable *e.* have compassed.
Prov. 14:19, *e.* bow before the good.
15:3, beholding the *e.* and good.
17:13, whoso rewardeth *e.* for good.
Isa. 1:4, a seed of *e.*-doers.
5:20, that call *e.* good, and good *e.*
7:15, 16, refuse the *e.* and choose the good.
Jer. 2:13, have committed two *e.*
19, know it is an *e.* thing and bitter.
24:3; 29:17, *e.* figs, very *e.*
42:6, whether good or *e.*, we will obey.
Mat. 5:45, rise on *e.* and good.
6:34, sufficient unto the day is the *e.* thereof.
7:11; Lu. 11:13, if ye, being *e.*
18, good tree cannot bring forth *e.*
9:4, wherefore think *e.* in your hearts?
Mk. 9:39, lightly speak *e.* of me.
Lu. 6:22, cast out your name as *e.*
35, he is kind to the *e.*
Lu. 6:45, *e.* man bringeth forth *e.*
John 3:20, doeth *e.* hateth light.
18:23, if I have spoken *e.*
Acts 23:5, not speak *e.* of ruler.
Rom. 7:19, the *e.* I would not.
12:9, abhor that which is *e.*
17, recompense to no man *e.* for *e.*
21, overcome *e.* with good.
1 Thess. 5:22, appearance of *e.*
1 Tim. 6:10, the root of all *e.*
2 Tim. 4:18; Jas. 3:16, every *e.* work.
Tit. 3:2, speak *e.* of no man.
Jas. 3:8, tongue an unruly *e.*
1 Pet. 3:9, not rendering *e.* for *e.*
See Prov. 13:21; Isa. 45:7; Eccl. 12:1; Eph 5:16; 6:13.
EXACT. Deut. 15:2, shall not *e.* it of neighbour.
Neh. 5:7, 10, 11, you *e.* usury.
10:31, leave the *e.* of every debt.
Job 11:6, God *e.* of thee less.
Lu. 3:13, *e.* not more than what is.
See Ps. 89:22; Isa. 58:3; 60:17.
EXALT. 1 Chron. 29:11, *e.* as head above all.
Ps. 12:8, when vilest men are *e.*
34:3, let us *e.* his name together.
92:10, my horn shalt thou *e.*
97:9, *e.* far above all gods.
Prov. 4:8, *e.* her, and she shall promote thee.
11:11, by blessing of upright the city is *e.*
14:29, he that is hasty of spirit *e.* folly.
34, righteousness *e.* a nation.
17:19, he that *e.* his gate.
Isa. 2:2; Mic. 4:1, mountain of Lord's house *e.*

EXPRESSLY. 1 Sam. 20:21; Ezek. 1:3; 1 Tim. 4:1.
EXTEND. Ps. 16:2; 109:12; Isa. 66:12.
EXTINCT. Job 17:1; Isa. 43:17.
EXTOL. Ps. 30:1; 145:1, I will *e.* thee
68:4, *e.* him that rideth.
See Ps. 66:17; Isa. 52:13; Dan. 4:37.
EXTORTION. Ezek. 22:12; Mat. 23:25.
EXTORTIONER. Ps. 109:11, let *e.* catch all he hath.
Isa. 16:4, the *e.* is at an end.
1 Cor. 5:11, if any man be an *e.*
See Lu. 18:11; 1 Cor. 5:10; 6:10.
EXTREME. Deut. 28:22; Job 35:15.
EYE. Gen. 3:6, pleasant to the *e.*
7, *e.* of both were opened.
27:1, his *e.* were dim.
49:12, his *e.* shall be red with wine.
Num. 10:31, be to us instead of *e.*
16:14, wilt thou put out *e.*?
24:3, 15, man whose *e.* are open said.
Deut. 3:27, lift up *e.*, behold with thine *e.*
12:8; Judg. 17:6; 21:25, right in own *e.*
16:19, gift blind *e.* of wise.
28:32, *e.* look, and fail with longing.
32:10, kept him as apple of *e.*
34:7, his *e.* was not dim.
1 Kings 1:20, *e.* of all Israel upon thee.
8:29, 52; 2 Chron. 6:20, 40, *e.* open towards this house.
20:6, whatsoever is pleasant in thine *e.*
2 Kings 6:17, Lord opened *e.* of young man.
20, open the *e.* of these men.
2 Chron. 16:9; Zech. 4:10, *e.* of Lord run to and fro.
34:28, nor thine *e.* see all the evil.
Job 7:8; 20:9, *e.* that hath seen me.
11:20, the *e.* of wicked shall fail.
15:12, what do thine *e.* wink at?
19:27, mine *e.* shall behold, and not another.
28:7, path vulture's *e.* hath not seen.
10, his *e.* seeth every precious thing.
29:11, when the *e.* saw me.
15, I was *e.* to the blind.
31:16, caused *e.* of widow to fail.
Ps. 11:4, his *e.* try children of men.
15:4, in whose *e.* a vile person.
19:8, enlightening the *e.*
33:18, *e.* of Lord on them that fear him.
34:15; 1 Pet. 3:12, *e.* of Lord on the righteous.
36:1, no fear of God before his *e.*
69:3; 119:82, 123; Lam. 2:11, mine *e.* fail.
77:4, holdest mine *e.* waking.
116:8, delivered mine *e.* from tears.
119:18, open mine *e.*
132:4, not give sleep to mine *e.*
Prov. 10:26, as smoke to the *e.*
20:12, the seeing *e.*
22:9, a bountiful *e.*
23:29, redness of *e.*
27:20, the *e.* of man never satisfied.
30:17, the *e.* that mocketh.
Eccl. 1:8, *e.* is not satisfied with seeing.
2:14, wise man's *e.* are in his head.
6:9, better sight of *e.* than wandering of desire.
11:7, for the *e.* to behold the sun.
Isa. 1:16, I will hide mine *e.* from you.
29:10, the Lord hat closed *e.*
33:17, thine *e.* shall see the king in his beauty.
40:26; Jer. 13:20, lift up your *e.* on high.
Jer. 5:21; Ezek. 12:2, have *e.* and see not.
9:1, mine *e.* a fountain of tears.
13:17, mine *e.* shall weep sore.
14:17, let mine *e.* run down with tears.
24:6, set mine *e.* upon them for good.
Lam. 2:18, let not apple of *e.* cease.
Ezek. 24:16, 25, the desire of thine *e.*
Hab. 1:13, of purer *e.* than to behold evil.
Mat. 5:29, if right *e.* offend thee.
13:16, blessed are your *e.*
18:9; Mk. 9:47, to enter with one *e.*
Mk. 8:18, having *e.*, see ye not?
Lu. 1:2, from beginning were *e.*-witnesses.
24:16, their *e.* were holden.
John 11:37, could not this man, which opened *e.*
Gal. 4:15, have plucked out your *e.*
Eph. 1:18, the *e.* of your understanding.
2 Pet. 2:14, having *e.* full of adultery.
1 John 2:16, the lust of the *e.*
See Deut. 11:12; Ezra 5:5; Ps. 32:8; Prov. 3:7; 12:15; 15:3; 16:2; 21:2; Mat. 20:33; John 10:21; 1 Pet. 3:12.
EYESERVICE. Eph. 6:6; Col. 3:22, not with *e.* as menpleasers.

F

FABLES. 1 Tim. 1:4; 4:7; 2 Tim. 4:4; Tit. 1:14; 2 Pet. 1:16.
FACE. Gen. 4:14, from thy *f.* shall I be hid.
32:30, I have seen God *f.* to *f.*
Ex. 33:11, Lord spake to Moses *f.* to *f.*
34:29, skin of *f.* shone.
33; 2 Cor. 3:13, put vail on *f.*
Lev. 19:32, shall honour the *f.* of the old man.
Deut. 25:9, spit in *f.*, saying.
1 Sam. 5:3, Dagon was fallen on his *f.*
2 Kings 4:29, 31, lay staff on *f.* of child.
14:8, let us look one another in *f.*
Ezra 9:7; Dan. 9:7, confusion of *f.*
Neh. 8:6, worshipped with *f.* to ground.
Job 1:11; 2:5, curse thee to thy *f.*
4:15, spirit passed before my *f.*
13:24; Ps. 44:24; 88:14, wherefore hidest thou thy *f.*?
Ps. 13:1, how long wilt thou hide thy *f.*?
27:9; 69:17; 102:2; 143:7, hide not thy *f.*
34:5, *f.* not ashamed.
59:2, sins have hid his *f.* from you.
84:9, look upon *f.* of anointed.
Prov. 27:19, in water *f.* answereth to *f.*
Eccl. 8:1, wisdom maketh *f.* to shine.
Isa. 3:15, ye grind *f.* of the poor.
25:8, wipe tears from off all *f.*
50:7, set my *f.* like flint.
Jer. 2:27, turned their back, and not *f.*
5:3, their *f.* harder than a rock.
30:6, all *f.* turned into paleness.
Dan. 10:6, *f.* as appearance of lightning.
Hos. 5:5, testifieth to his *f.*
Mat. 6:17, wash thy *f.*
11:10; Mk. 1:2; Lu. 7:27, messenger before *f.*
16:3; Lu. 12:56, discern *f.* of sky.
17:2, his *f.* did shine as sun.
18:10, angels behold *f.* of my father.
Lu. 2:31, before *f.* of all people.
9:51, 53, set his *f.* to Jerusalem.
22:64, struck him on *f.*
1 Cor. 13:12, then *f.* to *f.*
2 Cor. 3:18, all, with open *f.*
Gal. 1:22, I was unknown by *f.*
2:11, withstood him to the *f.*
Jas. 1:23, beholding *f.* in glass.
Rev. 20:11, from whose *f.* earth fled away.
See 1 Kings 19:13; Dan. 1:10; Acts 6:15; 20:25.
FADE. Isa. 1:30, whose leaf *f.*
24:4, earth mourneth and *f.*, the world *f.*
40:7, the flower *f.*
64:6, all *f.* as a leaf.
Jer. 8:13, and the leaf shall *f.*
Ezek. 47:12, whose leaf shall not *f.*
1 Pet. 1:4; 5:4, inheritance that *f.* not away.
Jas. 1:11, rich man shall *f.* away.
See 2 Sam. 22:46; Ps. 18:45; Isa. 28:1.
FAIL. Gen. 47:16, if money *f.*
Deut. 28:32, thine eyes shall *f.* with longing.
Josh. 21:45; 23:14; 1 Kings 8:56, there *f.* not any good thing.
1 Sam. 17:32, let no man's heart *f.* him.
1 Kings 2:4; 8:25, shall not *f.* a man on throne.
17:14, neither shall cruse of oil *f.*
Ezra 4:22, take heed that ye *f.* not.
Job. 14:11, as waters *f.* from sea.
19:14, my kinsfolk have *f.*

Ps. 12:1, the faithful *f.* among men.
31:10; 38:10, my strength *f.* me.
77:8, doth his promise *f.*
89:33, nor suffer my faithfulness to *f.*
142:4, refuge *f.* me.
Eccl. 10:3, his wisdom *f.* him.
12:5, desire shall *f.*
Isa. 15:6, the grass *f.*
19:5, waters shall *f.*
31:3, they shall all *f.* together.
32:6, cause drink of thirsty to *f.*
10, the vintage shall *f.*
34:16, no one of these shall *f.*
38:14, eyes *f.* with looking upward.
41:17, tongue *f.* for thirst.
59:15, truth *f.*
Jer. 14:6, their eyes did *f.*
15:18, as waters that *f.*
48:33, I caused wine to *f.*
Lam. 3:22, his compassions *f.* not.
4:17, our eyes as yet *f.*
Ezek. 12:22, every vision *f.*
Amos 8:4, make poor of land to *f.*
Hab. 3:17, labour of olive shall *f.*
Lu. 12:33, treasure that *f.* not.
16:9, when ye *f.* they may receive you.
17, one tittle of law *f.*
21:26, hearts *f.* them for fear.
22:32, that thy faith *f.* not.
1 Cor. 13:8, charity never *f.*
Heb. 1:12, thy years shall not *f.*
11:32, time would *f.* me to tell.
12:15, lest any man *f.* of grace of God.
See Deut. 31:6; Ps. 40:12; 143:7; Isa. 44:12.
FAIN. Job 27:22; Lu. 15:16.
FAINT. Gen. 25:29, 30, came from field, and he was *f.*
45:26, Jacob's heart *f.*
Judg. 8:4, *f.* yet pursuing.
Job 4:5, now it is come, and thou *f.*
Ps. 27:13, I had *f.* unless I had believed.
107:5, their soul *f.* in them.
Prov. 24:10, if thou *f.* in day of adversity.
Isa. 1:5, whole heart *f.*
10:18, as when a standardbearer *f.*
40:28, Creator of earth *f.* not.
29, giveth power to the *f.*
30; Amos 8:13, even youths shall *f.*
31, walk, and not *f.*
44:12, he drinketh no water, and is *f.*
Jer. 8:18; Lam. 1:22; 5:17, my heart is *f.*
Mat. 15:32; Mk. 8:3, lest they *f.* by the way.
Lu. 18:1, pray, and not to *f.*
2 Cor. 4:1, 16, as we have received mercy, we *f.* not.
Gal. 6:9, reap, if we *f.* not.
Heb. 12:3, wearied and *f.* in your minds.
5, nor *f.* when thou art rebuked.
See Deut. 20:8; Ps. 84:2; 119:81; Mat. 9:36.
FAIR. Job 37:22, *f.* weather out of the north.
Ps. 45:2, *f.* than children of men.
Prov. 11:22, a *f.* woman without discretion.
26:25, when he speaketh *f.*, believe not.
Cant. 1:8; 5:9; 6:1, thou *f.* among women
6:10, *f.* as the moon.
Isa. 5:9, houses great and *f.*
Jer. 4:30, in vain shalt thou make thyself *f.*
12:6, though they speak *f.* words.
Dan. 1:15, their countenances appeared *f.*
Mat. 16:2, it will be *f.* weather.
Acts 7:20, Moses was exceeding *f.*
Rom. 16:18, by *f.* speeches deceive.
See Gen. 6:2; Isa. 54:11; Ezek. 27:12.
FAITH. Deut. 32:20, children in whom is no *f.*
Mat. 6:30; 8:26; 14:31; 16:8; Lu. 12:28, ye of little *f.*
8:10; Lu. 7:9, so great *f.*
9:2; Mk. 2:5; Lu. 5:20, seeing their *f.*
22; Mk. 5:34; 10:52; Lu. 8:48; 17:19, thy *f.* hath made thee whole.
Mat. 9:29, according to your *f.*
15:28, great is thy *f.*
17:20, *f.* as a grain of mustard seed.
21:21, if ye have *f.*, ye shall not only do this.
23:23, omitted judgment, mercy, and *f.*
Mk. 4:40, how is it ye have no *f.*?
11:22, have *f.* in God.
Lu. 7:50, thy *f.* hath saved thee.
8:25, where is your *f.*?
17:5, increase our *f.*
18:8, shall he find *f.* on the earth?
22:32, that thy *f.* fail not.
Acts 3:16, the *f.* which is by him.
6:5; 11:24, a man full of *f.*
14:9, perceiving he had *f.* to be healed.
27, opened the door of *f.*
15:9, purifying their hearts by *f.*
16:5, established in the *f.*
26:18, sanctified by *f.*
Rom. 1:5, grace for obedience to *f.*
17, revealed from *f.* to *f.*
3:27, boasting excluded by *f.*
28; 5:1; Gal. 2:16; 3:24, justified by *f.*
4:5, *f.* counted for righteousness.
16, it is of *f.*, which is of the *f.* of Abraham.
19, 20, being not weak in *f.*
5:2, we have access by *f.*
10:8, the word of *f.*, which we preach.
17, *f.* cometh by hearing.
12:3, the measure of *f.*
6, prophesy according to proportion of *f.*
14:1, weak in *f.* receive ye.
22, hast thou *f.*?
23, what is not of *f.* is sin.
1 Cor. 2:5, your *f.* should not stand is wisdom.
13:2, though I have all *f.*
13, now abideth *f.*
15:14, and your *f.* is also vain.
16:13, stand fast in the *f.*
2 Cor. 1:24, not have dominion over *f.*
4:13, same spirit of *f.*
5:7, we walk by *f.*
13:5, examine whether ye be in the *f.*
Gal. 2:20, I live by the *f.* of Son of God.
3:2, by the hearing of *f.*
12, law is not of *f.*
23, before *f.* came.
5:6, *f.* which worketh by love.
6:10, the household of *f.*
Eph. 3:12, access by *f.* of him.
17, dwell in your hearts by *f.*
4:5, one Lord, one *f.*
13, in the unity of the *f.*
6:16, the shield of *f.*
Phil. 1:27, striving together for the *f.* of the gospel.
Col. 1:23, if ye continue in the *f.*
2:5, the stedfastness of your *f.*
1 Thess. 1:3; 2 Thess. 1:11, your work of *f.*
5:8, the breastplate of *f.*
2 Thess. 3:2, all men have not *f.*
1 Tim. 1:2; Tit. 1:4, my own son in the *f.*
5; 2 Tim. 1:5, *f.* unfeigned.
2:15, if they continue in *f.*
3:13, great boldness in the *f.*
4:1, shall depart from the *f.*
5:8, he hath denied the *f.*
6:10, 21, erred from the *f.*
12, fight the good fight of *f.*
2 Tim. 3:8, reprobate concerning the *f.*
4:7, I have kept the *f.*
Tit. 1:1, the *f.* of God's elect.
Heb. 4:2, not being mixed with *f.*
6:1, not laying again the foundation of *f.*
12, through *f.* inherit the promises.
10:22, in full assurance of *f.*
11:1, *f.* is substance of things hoped for.
4, 5, 7, 8, 9, etc., by *f.* Abel, etc.

Heb. 11:6, without *f.* it is impossible.
13, these all died in *f.*
33, through *f.* subdued kingdoms.
39, a good report through *f.*
12:2, author and finisher of our *f.*
13:7, whose *f.* follow.
Jas. 1:3; 1 Pet. 1:7, the trying of your *f.*
6, let them ask in *f.*
2:1, I have not *f.* with respect of persons.
5, rich in *f.*
14, man say he hath *f.*, can *f.* save him?
17, *f.* without works is dead.
18, thou hast *f.*, and I have works.
22, *f.* wrought with his works.
5:15, the prayer of *f.* shall save.
1 Pet. 1:9, the end of your *f.*
5:9, resist stedfast in the *f.*
2 Pet. 1:1, like precious *f.*
5, add to your *f.* virtue.
1 John 5:4, overcometh the world, even our *f.*
Jude 3, earnestly contend for the *f.*
20, your most holy *f.*
Rev. 2:13, hast not denied my *f.*
19, I know thy works and *f.*
13:10, patience and *f.* of the saints.
14:12, they that keep the *f.* of Jesus.
See Hab. 2:4; Rom. 1:12; 1 Tim. 4:6.

FAITHFUL. 2 Sam. 20:19, one of them that are *f.* in Israel.
Neh. 7:2, a *f.* man, and feared God.
9:8, his heart *f.* before thee.
13:13, counted *f.* to distribute.
Ps. 12:1, the *f.* fail among men.
89:37, a *f.* witness in heaven.
101:6, the *f.* of the land.
119:86, commandments *f.*
138, testimonies *f.*
Prov. 11:13, *f.* spirit concealeth.
13:17, *f.* ambassador is health.
14:5; Isa. 8:2; Jer. 42:5, a *f.* witness.
20:6, a *f.* man who can find?
25:13, as snow in harvest, so is a *f.* messenger.
27:6, *f.* are wounds of a friend.
28:20, *f.* man shall abound.
Isa. 1:21, 26, *f.* city.
Mat. 24:45; Lu. 12:42, who is a *f.* and wise servant?
25:21, good and *f.* servant.
23; Lu. 19:17, *f.* in a few things.
Lu. 16:10, *f.* in least *f.* in much.
Acts 16:15, if ye have judged me *f.*
1 Cor. 4:2, required in stewards that a man be *f.*
17, Timothy *f.* in the Lord.
Gal. 3:9, blessed with *f.* Abraham.
Eph. 6:21; Col. 1:7; 4:7, a *f.* minister.
1 Thess. 5:24, *f.* is he that calleth you.
2 Thess. 3:3, Lord is *f.*, who shall stablish you.
1 Tim. 1:15; 4:9; 2 Tim. 2:11; tit. 3:8, a *f.* saying.
3:11, wives *f.* in all things.
2 Tim. 2:2, commit to *f.* men.
13, yet he abideth *f.*
Heb. 2:17, a *f.* high priest.
3:2, *f.* to him that appointed him.
10:23; 11:11, he is *f.* that promised.
1 Pet. 4:19, as unto a *f.* Creator.
1 John 1:9, he is *f.* and just to forgive.
Rev. 2:10, be thou *f.* unto death.
13, my *f.* martyr.
17:14, called and chosen, and *f.*
21:5; 22:6, these words are true and *f.*
See Deut. 7:9; Dan. 6:4; Rev. 1:5; 3:14; 19:11.

FAITHFULLY. 2 Chron. 19:9; 34:12; Jer. 23:28; 3 John 5.

FAITHFULNESS. Ps. 5:9, no *f.* in their mouths.
36:5, thy *f.* reacheth unto the clouds
40:10; 88:11, declared thy *f.*
89:33, nor suffer my *f.* to fail.
92:2, show forth thy *f.* every night.
Isa. 11:5, *f.* the girdle of his reins.
Lam. 3:23, great is thy *f.*
See 1 Sam. 26:23; Ps. 119:75; 143:1.

FAITHLESS. Mat. 17:17; Mk. 9:19; Lu. 9:41; John 20:27.

FALL (*n.*). Prov. 16:18, haughty spirit before a *f.*
Mat. 7:27, great was the *f.* of it.
Lu. 2:34, set for the rise and *f.* of many.
Rom. 11:12, if the *f.* of them be the riches.
See Jer. 49:21; Ezek. 26:15; 31:16; 32:10.

FALL (*v.*). Gen. 45:24, see ye *f.* not out by the way.
Lev. 25:35, thy brother be *f.* in decay.
1 Sam. 3:19, let none of his words *f.*
2 Sam. 1:19, 25, 27, how are the mighty *f.*!
3:38, great man *f.* this day.
24:14; 1 Chron. 21:13, *f.* into hands of God.
2 Kings 14:10, why meddle that thou shouldest *f.*?
Job 4:13; 33:15, deep sleep *f.* on men.
Ps. 5:10, let them *f.* by their own counsels.
7:15, is *f.* into ditch.
16:6, lines *f.* in pleasant places.
37:24, though he *f.*, not utterly cast down.
56:13; 116:8, deliver my feet from *f.*
72:11, kings shall *f.* down before him.
91:7, a thousand shall *f.* at thy side.
Prov. 10:8, 10, a prating fool shall *f.*
11:14, where no counsel is, the people *f.*
28, he that trusteth in riches shall *f.*
13:17; 17:20; 24:16, *f.* into mischief.
24:16, just man *f.* seven times.
17, rejoice not when thine enemy *f.*
26:27; Eccl. 10:8, diggeth a pit shall *f.* therein.
Eccl. 4:10, woe to him that is alone when he *f.*
11:3, where the tree *f.*, there it shall be.
Isa. 14:12, how art thou *f.*!
34:4, as the leaf *f.* from the vine.
40:30, the young men shall utterly *f.*
Jer. 49:26; 50:30, young men *f.* in her streets.
Ezek. 24:6, let no lot *f.* on it.
Dan. 3:5; 11:26; Mat. 4:9, *f.* down and worship.
Hos. 10:8; Lu. 23:30; Rev. 6:16, say to hills, *f.* on us.
Mic. 7:8, when I *f.*
Zech. 11:2, the cedar is *f.*
Mat. 10:29, sparrow *f.* on ground.
12:11, *f.* into pit on sabbath day.
15:14; Lu. 6:39, both *f.* into the ditch.
21:44; Lu. 20:18, *f.* on this stone.
24:29; Mk. 13:25, stars *f.* from heaven.
Lu. 8:13, in time of temptation *f.* away.
10:18, Satan as lightning, *f.* from heaven.
Rom. 14:4, to his master he standeth or *f.*
13, occasion to *f.*
1 Cor. 10:12, take heed lest he *f.*
15:6, 18, some are *f.* asleep.
Gal. 5:4, ye are *f.* from grace.
1 Tim. 3:6, *f.* into the condemnation.
7, lest he *f.* into reproach.
6:9, rich *f.* into temptation.
Heb. 4:11, lest any *f.* after same example.
6:6, if they *f.* away.
10:31, to *f.* into hands of living God.
Jas. 1:2, joy when ye *f.* into temptation.
11; 1 Pet. 1:24, flower thereof *f.*
5:12, lest ye *f.* into condemnation.
2 Pet. 1:10, ye shall never *f.*
3:17, lest ye *f.* from stedfastness.
See Isa. 21:9; Lam 5:16; Rev. 14:8; 18:2.

FALLING. Job 4:4; 2 Thess. 2:3; Jude 24.

FALLOW. Jer. 4:3; Hos. 10:12.

FALSE. Ex. 20:16; Deut. 5:20; Mat. 19:18, shalt not bear *f.* witness.
23:1, shalt not raise a *f.* report.
2 Kings 9:12, it is *f.*, tell us now.
Ps. 119:104, 128, I hate every *f.* way.
120:3, thou *f.* tongue.
Prov. 6:19; 12:17; 14:5; 19:5; 21:28; 25:18, a *f.* witness.
11:1; 20:23, a *f.* balance.
Mat. 15:19, out of heart proceed *f.* witness.
24:24; Mk. 13:22, *f.* Christs and *f.* prophets.
26:59, 60; Mk. 14:56, 57, *f.* witness against Christ.

Mk. 13:22, *f.* prophets shall rise.
Lu. 19:8, any thing by *f.* accusation.
1 Cor. 15:15, found *f.* witnesses of God.
2 Cor. 11:13, such are *f.* apostles.
11:26, perils among *f.* brethren.
2 Tim. 3:3; Tit. 2:3, *f.* accusers.
See Gal. 2:4; 2 Pet. 2:1; 1 John 4:1.
FALSEHOOD. Job 21:34, in answers remaineth *f.*
Ps. 7:14, hath brought forth *f.*
144:8, 11, right hand of *f.*
Isa. 28:15, under *f.* have we hid ourselves.
57:4, a seed of *f.*
59:13, words of *f.*
Mic. 2:11, walking in the spirit and *f.*
See 2 Sam. 18:13; Jer. 13:25; Hos. 7:1.
FALSELY. Lev. 6:3, 5; 19:12; Jer. 5:2; 7:9; Zech. 5:4, swear *f.*
Jer. 5:31; 29:9, prophets prophesy *f.*
Mat. 5:11, evil *f.*, for my sake.
1 Tim. 6:20, science *f.* so called.
See Jer. 43:2; Lu. 3:14; 1 Pet. 3:16.
FAME. Josh. 9:9, we heard the *f.* of God.
1 Kings 10:1; 2 Chron. 9:1, *f.* of Solomon.
Zeph. 3:19, get them *f.* in every land.
Mat. 4:24; Mk. 1:28; Lu. 4:14, 37; 5:15, *f.* of Jesus.
9:31, spread abroad his *f.*
14:1, Herod heard of the *f.*
See Gen. 45:16; Num. 14:15; Job 28:22; Isa. 66:19.
FAMILIAR. Job 19:14; Ps. 41:9; Jer. 20:10.
FAMILY. Gen. 12:3; 28:14, in thee all *f.* be blessed.
25:10, return every man to his *f.*
Deut. 29:18, lest a *f.* turn away from God.
1 Sam. 9:21, my *f.* the least.
18:18, what is my father's *f.*?
1 Chron. 4:38, princes in their *f.*
Ps. 68:6, setteth the solitary in *f.*
Jer. 3:14, one of a city, and two of a *f.*
10:25, on *f.* that call not.
31:1, God of all the *f.* of Israel.
Zech. 12:12, every *f.* apart.
Eph. 3:15, whole *f.* in heaven and earth.
See Num. 27:4; Judg. 1:25; Amos 3:2.
FAMINE. 2 Sam. 21:1, a *f.* in days of David.
1 Kings 8:37; 2 Chron. 20:9, if there be *f.*
18:2; 2 Kings 6:25, sore *f.* in Samaria.
2 Kings 8:1, the Lord hath called for a *f.*
Job 5:20, in *f.* he shall redeem thee.
22, at *f.* thou shalt laugh.
Ps. 33:19, to keep them alive in *f.*
37:19, in the days of *f.* shall be satisfied.
Jer. 24:10; 29:17, will send *f.* among them.
42:16, *f.* shall follow close.
Lam. 5:10, black because of *f.*
Ezek. 5:16, evil arrows of *f.*
36:29, I will lay no *f.* upon you.
Amos 8:11, a *f.*, not of bread.
Mat. 24:7; Mk. 13:8; Lu. 21:11, *f.* in divers places.
See Gen. 12:10; 41:27; 47:13; Lu. 15:14; Rom. 8:35.
FAMISH. Gen. 41:55; Prov. 10:3; Isa. 5:13; Zeph. 2:11.
FAMOUS. Ruth 4:11, 14; 1 Chron. 5:24; Ps. 74:5; Ezek. 23:10.
FAN. Isa. 30:24; Jer. 15:7; 51:2; Mat. 3:12.
FAR. Gen. 18:25; 1 Sam. 20:9, that be *f.* from thee.
Deut. 12:21; 14:24, if place too *f.* from thee.
Judg. 19:11; Mk. 6:35; Lu. 24:29, day *f.* spent.
1 Sam. 2:30; 22:15; 2 Sam. 20:20; 23:17, be it *f.* from me.
Job 5:4, children *f.* from safety.
11:14; 22:23, put iniquity *f.* away.
19:13, put my brethren *f.* from me.
34:10, *f.* be it from God to do wickedness.
Ps. 10:5, thy judgments are *f.* out of sight.
22:11; 35:22; 38:21; 71:12, be not *f.* from me.
97:9, *f.* above all gods.
103:12, *f.* as east from west.
Prov. 31:10, *f.* above rubies.
Isa. 43:6; 60:4, 9, sons from *f.*
46:12, *f.* from righteousness.
57:19, peace to him that is *f.* off.
Amos 6:3, put *f.* away evil day.
Mat. 16:22, be it *f.* from thee, Lord.
Mk. 12:34, not *f.* from the kingdom.
13:34, as a man taking a *f.* journey.
John 21:8, they were not *f.* from land.
Acts 17:27, not *f.* from every one of us.
Rom. 13:12, the night is *f.* spent.
2 Cor. 4:17, a *f.* more exceeding.
Eph. 1:21, *f.* above all principality.
2:13, *f.* off made nigh.
4:10, *f.* above all heavens.
Phil. 1:23, which is *f.* better.
Heb. 7:15, it is yet *f.* more evident.
See Isa. 33:17; Mat. 15:8; Mk. 8:3.
FARE. 1 Sam. 17:18; Jon. 1:3; Lu. 16:19.
FAREWELL. Lu. 9:61; Acts 18:21; 2 Cor. 13:11.
FARM. Mat. 22:5.
FARTHING. Mat. 5:26; 10:29; Mk. 12:42; Lu. 12:6.
FASHION. Job 10:8; Ps. 119:73, thine hands have *f.* me.
31:15, did not one *f.* us?
Ps. 33:15, he *f.* hearts alike.
139:16, in continuance were *f.*
Isa. 45:9, say to him that *f.* it.
Mk. 2:12, never saw it on this *f.*
Lu. 9:29, the *f.* of his countenance.
1 Cor. 7:31, the *f.* of this world passeth.
Phil. 2:8, found in *f.* as a man.
See Gen. 6:15; Ex. 32:4; Ezek. 42:11; Jas. 1:11.
FAST. 2 Sam. 12:23, he is dead, wherefore should I *f.*?
Ps. 33:9, he commanded, and it stood *f.*
65:6, setteth *f.* the mountains.
Isa. 58:3, why have we *f.*, and thou seest not?
4, ye *f.* for strife.
5, wilt thou call this a *f.*?
6, is not this the *f.* that I have chosen?
Joel 1:14, sanctify a *f.*?
Zech. 7:5, did ye at all *f.* unto me?
Mat. 6:16, when ye *f.*, be not.
18, appear not to *f.*
Mk. 2:19, can children of bridechamber *f.*
Lu. 18:12, I *f.* twice in the week.
See Jer. 14:12; Mat. 4:2; Acts 13:2.
FASTEN. Eccl. 12:11, as nails *f.* by the masters.
Isa. 22:23, 25, I will *f.* him as a nail.
Lu. 4:20, eyes of all were *f.* on him.
Acts 11:6, when I had *f.* mine eyes.
See 1 Sam. 31:10; Job 38:6; Acts 3:4; 28:3.
FASTING. Ps. 35:13, I humbled myself with *f.*
109:24, knees weak through *f.*
Jer. 36:6, upon the *f.* day.
Mk. 8:3, send them away *f.*
1 Cor. 7:5, give yourselves to *f.* and prayer.
2 Cor. 6:5, in stripes, in *f.*
11:27, in *f.* oft.
See Dan. 6:18; 9:3; Mat. 17:21; Mk. 9:29.
FAT. Gen. 45:18, shall eat the *f.* of the land.
49:20, his bread shall be *f.*
Deut. 32:15, Jeshurun waxed *f.*, and kicked.
Neh. 8:10, eat the *f.*, and drink the sweet.
9:25, 35, took a *f.* land, and became *f.*
Ps. 17:10, inclosed in their own *f.*
92:14, shall be *f.* and flourishing.
119:70, heart *f.* as grease.
Prov. 11:25, liberal soul made *f.*
13:4, soul of diligent made *f.*
15:30, good report maketh the bones *f.*
Isa. 10:16, among his *f.* ones leanness.
25:6, feast of *f.* things.
Hab. 1:16, by them their portion if *f.*
See Gen. 41:2; Ex. 29:13; Lev. 3:3, 17; 7:22; Num. 13:20; Judg. 3:17.
FATHER. Gen. 15:15, go to thy *f.* in peace.
17:4; Rom. 4:17, a *f.* of nations.
Ex. 15:2, he is my *f.* God, I will exalt him.
20:5; Num. 14:18, iniquity of *f.* upon children.
21:15, he that smiteth his *f.*
17; Lev. 20:9, he that curseth his *f.*
Judg. 17:10; 18:19, be to me a *f.* and a priest.

1 Sam. 10:12, who is their *f.*?
2 Sam. 10:2; 1 Chron. 19:2, as his *f.* showed kindness.
1 Kings 19:4, no better than my *f.*
2 Kings 2:12; 13:14, Elisha cried, my *f.*, my *f.*
6:21, my *f.*, shall I smite them?
1 Chron. 28:9, know thou the God of thy *f.*
2 Chron. 32:13, what I and my *f.* have done.
Ezra 7:27, blessed be the Lord God of our *f.*
Job 29:16, I was a *f.* to the poor.
31:18, brought up with me as with a *f.*
38:28, hath the rain a *f.*?
Ps. 27:10, when my *f.* and mother forsake me.
39:12, as all my *f.* were.
68:5, *f.* of fatherless.
95:9; Heb. 3:9, your *f.* tempted me.
103:13, as a *f.* pitieth his children.
Prov. 4:1, the instruction of a *f.*
3, I was my *f.* son.
10:1; 15:20, wise son maketh a glad *f.*
17:21, the *f.* of a fool hath no joy.
25; 19:13, foolish son grief to his *f.*
Isa. 9:6, the everlasting *F.*
49:23, kings shall be thy nursing *f.*
63:16; 64:8, doubtless thou art our *f.*
Jer. 3:4, wilt thou not cry, my *f.*?
31:9, I am a *f.* to Israel.
29; Ezek. 18:2, *f.* have eaten sour grapes.
Ezek. 18:4, as the soul of the *f.*
22:7, set light by *f.* and mother.
Mal. 1:6, if I be a *f.*, where is mine honour?
2:10, have we not all one *f.*?
Mat. 5:16, 45, 48, your *F.* in heaven.
6:8, 32; Lu. 12:30, your *F.* knoweth.
9; Lu. 11:2, our *F.* which art in heaven.
7:21; 12:50, the will of my *F.*
8:21; Lu. 9:59, to go and bury my *f.*
10:21, *f.* deliver up the child.
37, he that loveth *f.* or mother.
18:10, behold the face of my *F.*
14, not the will of your *F.*
23:9, call no man *f.* on earth.
25:34, ye blessed of my *F.*
Mk. 14:36; Rom. 8:15; Gal. 4:6, Abba, *F.*
Lu. 2:49, about my *F.* business.
6:36, as your *F.* is merciful.
11:11, of any that is a *f.*
12:32, it is your *F.* good pleasure.
15:21, *f.*, I have sinned.
16:27, send him to my *f.* house.
22:42, *F.* if thou be willing.
23:34, *F.*, forgive them.
46, *F.*, into thy hand.
John 1:14, as of the only begotten of the *F.*
5:21, as the *F.* raiseth up the dead.
22, the *F.* judgeth no man.
23, even as they honour the *F.*
37:8, 16; 12:49; 14:24, the *F.* which hath sent me.
6:37, all the *F.* giveth me.
46; 14:8, 9, hath seen the *F.*
8:41, we have one *F.*, even God.
44, devil is a liar, and the *f.* of it.
49, I honour my *F.*
10:15, as the *F.* knoweth me.
29, my *F.* is greater than all.
12:27, *F.* save me from this hour.
28, *F.*, glorify thy name.
13:1, should depart unto the *F.*
14:6, no man cometh to the *F.*, but by me.
16; 16:26, I will pray the *F.*
28, I am come from the *F.*
15:1, my *F.* is the husbandman.
16, whatsoever ye ask of the *F.*
16:16, because I go to the *F.*
32, the *F.* is with me.
17:1, *F.*, the hour is come.
20:17, I ascend to my *F.* and your *F.*
Acts 24:14, so worship I the God of my *f.*
Rom. 4:11, the *f.* of all that believe.
1 Cor. 4:15, yet have we not many *f.*
2 Cor. 1:3, *F.* of mercies, God of all comfort.
Gal. 1:14, zealous of the traditions of my *f.*
4:2, the time appointed of the *f.*
Eph. 4:6, one God and *F.* of all.
6:4, *f.*, provoke not your children.
Phil. 2:11, to the glory of the *F.*
22, as a son with the *f.*
Col. 1:19, it pleased the *F.* that in him.
1 Tim. 5:1, entreat him as a *f.*
Heb. 1:5, I will be to him a *F.*
7:3, without *f.*, without mother.
12:9, the *F.* of spirits.
Jas. 1:17, the *F.* of lights.
2 Pet. 3:4, since the *f.* fell asleep.
1 John 1:3, fellowship with the *F.*
2:1, an advocate with the *F.*
13, I write unto you, *f.*
15, the love of the *F.* is not in him.
23, hath not the *F.*
3:1, what manner of love the *F.* hath.
5:7, the *F.*, the Word, and Holy Ghost.
See 1 Chron. 29:10; Lu. 11:2; John 5:26; 20:7; Acts 1:4; 15:10; Rom. 4:16.

FATHERLESS. Ps. 10:14, the helper of the *f.*
Prov. 23:10, the fields of the *f.*
Isa. 1:23, they judge not the *f.*
10:2, that they may rob the *f.*
Jer. 49:11, leave thy *f.* children.
Hos. 14:3, in thee the *f.* findeth mercy.
Mal. 3:5, against those that oppress *f.*
Jas. 1:27, to visit the *f.* and widows.
See Ex. 22:22; Deut. 10:18; 14:29; 24:17; Job 31:17.

FATNESS. Ps. 36:8, the *f.* of thine house.
63:5, as with marrow and *f.*
65:11, thy paths drop *f.*
73:7, eyes stand out with *f.*
Isa. 55:2, soul delight itself in *f.*
See Gen. 27:28; Judg. 9:9; Rom. 11:17.

FAULT. Gen. 41:9, I remember my *f.* this day.
Ps. 19:12, cleanse me from secret *f.*
Dan. 6:4, find none occasion nor *f.* in him.
Mat. 18:15, tell him his *f.*
Lu. 23:4; John 18:38; 19:4, 6, I find no *f.*
Rom. 9:19, why doth he yet find *f.*?
Gal. 6:1, overtaken in a *f.*
Jas. 5:16, confess your *f.*
Rev. 14:5, are without *f.* before throne.
See Deut. 25:2; 1 Sam. 29:3; 2 Sam. 3:8.

FAULTLESS. Heb. 8:7; Jude 24.

FAULTY. 2 Sam. 14:13; Hos. 10:2.

FAVOUR. Gen. 39:21, *f.* in the sight of the keeper.
Ex. 3:21; 11:3; 12:36, *f.* in sight of Egyptians.
Deut. 33:23, satisfied with *f.*
Ps. 5:12, with *f.* wilt thou compass him.
30:5, his *f.* is life.
102:13, the set time to *f.* her.
14, *f.* the dust thereof.
112:5, a good man showeth *f.*
Prov. 13:15, good understanding giveth *f.*
14:35; 19:12, the king's *f.*
18:22, obtaineth *f.* of the Lord.
31:30 *f.* is deceitful.
Lu. 2:52, increased in *f.* with God and man.
Acts 2:47, having *f.* with all people.
See Prov. 8:35; 12:2; Eccl. 9:11; Dan. 1:9.

FAVOURABLE. Judg. 21:22; Job 33:26; Ps. 77:7; 85:1.

FEAR (*n.*). Gen. 9:2, the *f.* of you on every beast.
20:11, *f.* of God not in this place.
Deut. 2:25; 11:25; 1 Chron. 14:17, *f.* of thee on nations.
Job 4:6, is not this thy *f.*?
15:4, thou castest off *f.*
39:22, he mocketh at *f.*
Ps. 5:7, in thy *f.* will I worship.
14:5, there were they in great *f.*
19:9, *f.* of the Lord is clean.

Ps. 34:11, I will teach you the *f.* of the Lord.
36:1; Rom. 3:18, no *f.* of God before his eyes.
53:5, in *f.*, where no *f.* was.
111:10; Prov. 1:7; 9:10, *f.* beginning of wisdom.
Prov. 1:26, 27, mock when your *f.* cometh.
3:25, not afraid of sudden *f.*
10:21, *f.* of Lord prolongeth days.
14:26, in *f.* of Lord is strong confidence.
27, *f.* of Lord a fountain of life.
15:16, better little with *f.* of Lord.
19:23, *f.* of Lord tendeth to life.
29:25, *f.* of man bringeth a snare.
Eccl. 12:5, when *f.* shall be in the way.
Isa. 8:12, neither fear ye their *f.*
14:3, Lord give thee rest from *f.*
29:13, *f.* toward me taught by men.
Jer. 30:5, a voice of *f.*, not of peace.
32:40, I will put my *f.* in their hearts.
Mal. 1:6, where is my *f.*?
Mat. 14:26, disciples cried for *f.*
Lu. 21:26, hearts failing them for *f.*
John 7:13; 19:38; 20:19, for *f.* of the Jews.
1 Cor. 2:3, with you in weakness and *f.*
2 Cor. 7:11, what *f.*, what desire.
Eph. 6:5; Phil. 2:12, with *f.* and trembling.
Heb. 2:15, *f.* of death.
11:7, Noah moved with *f.*
12:28, with reverence and godly *f.*
Jude 12, feeding themselves without *f.*
23, others save with *f.*
See Ps. 2:11; 2 Cor. 7:5, 15; 1 Pet. 2:18; 3:2.
FEAR (*v.*). Gen. 22:12, I know that thou *f.* God.
42:18, this do, and live, for I *f.* God.
Ex. 1:21, because they *f.* God.
14:13, *f.* not, stand still, and see.
18:21, able men, such as *f.* God.
20:20, *f.* God is come to prove.
Deut. 4:10, that they may learn to *f.*
5:29, O that they would *f.* me.
28:58, *f.* this glorious name.
66, thou shalt *f.* day and night.
1 Chron. 16:30; Ps. 96:9, *f.* before him all earth.
Neh. 7:2, he *f.* God above many.
Job 1:9, doth Job *f.* God for nought?
11:15, put iniquity away, thou shalt not *f.*
Ps. 27:1, whom shall I *f.*?
3, my heart shall not *f.*
31:19, laid up for them that *f.* thee.
34:9, *f.* the Lord, ye his saints.
56:4; 118:6, will not *f.* what flesh can do.
66:16, come all ye that *f.* God.
76:7, thou art to be *f.*
86:11, unite my heart to *f.* thy name.
115:11, ye that *f.* the Lord, trust.
119:74, they that *f.* thee will be glad.
Prov. 3:7; 24:21, *f.* the Lord, and depart.
28:14, happy is the man that *f.* always.
31:30, woman that *f.* the Lord.
Eccl. 3:14, that men should *f.* before him.
5:7, but *f.* thou God.
9:2, as he that *f.* an oath.
12:13, *f.* God, and keep his commandments.
Isa. 8:12, neither *f.* ye their fear.
35:4, to them of fearful heart *f.* not.
41:10; 43:5, *f.* thou not, I am with thee.
14, *f.* not, thou worm Jacob.
Jer. 5:24, neither say they, let us *f.* the Lord.
10:7, who would not *f.* thee, King of nations?
33:9, they shall *f.* and tremble.
Dan. 6:26, that men *f.* before the God of Daniel.
Zeph. 3:7, I said, surely thou wilt *f.* me.
Mal. 3:16, they that *f.* the Lord spake.
4:2, to you that *f.* my name.
Mat. 1:20, *f.* not to take to thee.
10:28; Lu. 12:5, *f.* him who is able.
14:5; 21:46, Herod *f.* the multitude.
21:26; Mk. 11:32; Lu. 20:19, we *f.* the people.
Mk. 4:41, they *f.* exceedingly.
5:33, woman *f.* and trembling came.
11:18, scribes *f.* Jesus.
Lu. 9:31, *f.* as they entered cloud.
12:32, *f.* not, little flock.
18:2, judge which *f.* not God.
19:21, I *f.* thee, because thou art.
23:40, dost not thou *f.* God?
John 9:22, because they *f.* the Jews.
Acts 10:22, just, and one that *f.* God.
35, he that *f.* is accepted.
13:26, whosoever among you *f.* God.
Rom. 8:15, bondage again to *f.*
11:20, not highminded, but *f.*
2 Cor. 11:3; 12:20, I *f.* lest.
1 Tim. 5:20, rebuke, that others may *f.*
Heb. 5:7, heard in that he *f.*
13:6, I will not *f.* what man.
1 John 4:18, that *f.* not perfect in love.
See 1 Kings 18:12; Col. 3:22; Heb. 4:1.
FEARFUL. Ex. 15:11, *f.* in praises.
Ps. 139:14, *f.* and wonderfully made.
Isa. 35:4, to them of a *f.* heart.
Mat. 8:26; Mk. 4:40, why are ye *f.*?
Heb. 10:27, *f.* looking for of judgment.
31, *f.* thing to fall into the hands.
See Deut. 20:8; Judg. 7:3; Lu. 21:11; Rev. 21:8.
FEARFULNESS. Ps. 55:5; Isa. 21:4; 33:14.
FEAST. Job 1:4, his sons went and *f.* in their houses.
Ps. 35:16, hypocritical mockers in *f.*
Prov. 15:15, merry heart continual *f.*
Eccl. 7:2; Jer. 16:8, the house of *f.*
10:19, *f.* is made for laughter.
Isa. 1:14, you appointed *f.* my soul hateth.
Amos 5:21, I despise your *f.* days.
8:10, turn your *f.* into mourning.
Mat. 23:6; Mk. 12:39; Lu. 20:46, uppermost rooms at *f.*
26:5; Mk. 14:2, not on the *f.* day.
Lu. 2:42, after the custom of the *f.*
14:13, when thou makest a *f.*
John 7:8, go ye up to this *f.*
14, about the midst of the *f.*
37, that great day of the *f.*
13:29, buy what we need against the *f.*
Acts 18:21, I must by all means keep this *f.*
1 Cor. 5:8, let us keep the *f.*
10:27, if any bid you to a *f.*
See Judg. 14:10; Esth. 9:17; Mal. 2:3; Jude 12.
FEATHERS. Job 39:13; Ps. 91:4; Dan. 4:33.
FED. Gen. 48:15, who *f.* me all my life long.
Ps. 37:3, verily thou shalt be *f.*
Ezek. 34:8, shepherds *f.* themselves, not flock.
Mat. 25:37, hungred, and *f.* thee.
1 Cor. 3:2, I have *f.* you with milk.
See Deut. 8:3; Ps. 78:72; 81:16; Lu. 16:21.
FEEBLE. Neh. 4:2, what do these *f.* Jews?
Job 4:4; Isa. 35:3; Heb. 12:12, strengthened the *f.* knees.
Ps. 105:37, not one *f.* person.
Prov. 30:26, comes a *f.* folk.
Ezek. 7:17; 21:7, all hands shall be *f.*
1 Thess. 5:14, comfort the *f.* minded.
See Gen. 30:42; Jer. 47:3; 1 Cor. 12:22.
FEED. Gen. 46:32, trade hath been to *f.* cattle.
1 Kings 17:4, commanded ravens to *f.* thee.
22:27, *f.* him with bread of affliction.
Ps. 28:9, *f.* them, and lift them up for ever.
Prov. 15:14, mouth *f.* on foolishness.
30:8, *f.* me with food convenient.
Isa. 5:17, lambs shall *f.* after their manner.
11:7; 27:10, cow and bear shall *f.*
44:20, he *f.* on ashes.
61:5, strangers shall *f.* your flocks.
65:25, the wolf and lamb shall *f.*
Jer. 3:15, pastors *f.* you with knowledge.
6:3, *f.* every one in his place.
Hos. 12:1, Ephraim *f.* on wind.
Zech. 11:4, *f.* the flock of the slaughter.

Mat. 6:26, your heavenly Father *f.* them.
Lu. 12:24, sow not, yet God *f.* them.
John 21:15, 16, 17, *f.* my lambs.
Rom. 12:20, if enemy hunger, *f.* him.
1 Pet. 5:2, *f.* the flock of God.
See Cant. 1:7; Acts 20:28; Rev. 7:17.
FEEL. Gen. 27:12, 21, my father will *f.* me.
Acts 17:27, if haply they might *f.* after.
See Judg. 16:26; Job 20:20; Eccl. 8:5.
FEELING. Eph. 4:19, being past *f.*
Heb. 4:15, touched with *f.* of infirmities.
FEET. Gen. 49:10, lawgiver from between his *f.*
Deut. 2:28, I will pass through on my *f.*
Josh. 3:15, *f.* of priests dipped in Jordan.
14:9, land whereon *f.* have trodden.
Ruth 3:14, she lay at his *f.*
1 Sam. 2:9, keep *f.* of his saints.
2 Sam. 22:37; Ps. 18:36, my *f.* did not slip.
2 Kings 6:32, sound of his master's *f.*
13:21, dead man stood on his *f.*
Neh. 9:21, their *f.* swelled not.
Job 29:15, *f.* was I to the lame.
Ps. 8:6; 1 Cor. 15:27; Eph. 1:22, all things under his *f.*
22:16, pierced my hands and my *f.*
31:8, set my *f.* in a large room.
40:2, my *f.* on a rock.
56:13; 116:8, deliver my *f.* from falling.
66:9, suffered not our *f.* to be moved.
73:2, my *f.* were almost gone.
115:7, *f.* have they, but walk not.
119:105, a lamp to my *f.*
122:2, our *f.* shall stand within thy gates.
Prov. 1:16; 6:18; Isa. 59:7, *f.* run to evil.
4:26, ponder path of thy *f.*
5:5, her *f.* go down to death.
6:13, speaketh with his *f.*
28, and his *f.* not be burnt.
7:11, her *f.* abide not in house.
19:2, he that hasteth with his *f.*
Cant. 5:3, washed my *f.*, how shall I defile?
7:1; Isa. 52:7, how beautiful are *f.*
Isa. 3:16, tinkling with *f.*
6:2, with twain he covered is *f.*
23:7, her own *f.* shall carry her.
26:6, the *f.* of the poor.
49:23; Mat. 10:14; Mk. 6:11; Lu. 9:5; Acts 13:51, dust of *f.*
52:7; Nah. 1:15, the *f.* of him that bringeth.
60:13, place of my *f.* glorious.
Lam. 3:34, crush under *f.* prisoners.
Ezek. 2:1, 2; 3:24, stand upon thy *f.*
24:17, 23, shoes upon thy *f.*
25:6, stamped with thy *f.*
32:2, troublest waters with thy *f.*
34:18, 19, foul residue with *f.*
Dan. 2:33, 42, *f.* part iron and part clay.
Dan. 10:6; Rev. 1:15; 2:18, *f.* like polished brass.
Nah. 1:3, clouds are the dust of his *f.*
Zech. 14:4, *f.* shall stand on Zion.
Mat. 7:6, trample them under *f.*
18:8, rather than having two *f.*
28:9, they held him by the *f.*
Lu. 1:79, guide our *f.* into way of peace.
7:38, she kissed his *f.*, and anointed them.
8:35, sitting at the *f.* of Jesus.
10:39, Mary sat at Jesus' *f.*
24:39, 40, behold my hands and my *f.*
John 11:2; 12:3, wiped *f.* with her hair.
12:3, anointed the *f.* of Jesus.
13:5, began to wash disciples' *f.*
6, dost thou wash my *f.*?
8, thou shalt never wash my *f.*
10, needeth not save to wash his *f.*
20:12, one angel at head, other at *f.*
Acts 3:7, his *f.* received strength.
4:35, 37; 5:2, laid at apostles' *f.*
5:9, *f.* of them that buried thy husband.
Acts 14:8, a man impotent in his *f.*
21:11, Agabus bound his own hands and *f.*
222:3, at *f.* of Gamaliel.
Rom. 3:15, *f.* swift to shed blood.
10:15, the *f.* of them that preach.
16:20, bruise Satan under your *f.*
1 Cor. 12:21, nor head to the *f.*, I have no need.
Eph. 6:15, your *f.* shod with preparation.
Rev. 1:17, I fell at his *f.* as dead.
13:2, *f.* as *f.* of a bear.
19:10; 22:8, at his *f.* to worship.
See 2 Sam. 4:4; 2 Kings 9:35; 1 Tim. 5:10.
FEIGN. 1 Sam. 21:13, David *f.* himself mad.
Ps. 17:1, prayer not out of *f.* lips.
Jer. 3:10, turned to me *f.*
Lu. 20:20, *f.* themselves just men.
See 2 Sam. 14:2; 1 Kings 14:5, 6; Neh. 6:8.
FELL. Gen. 4:5, his countenance *f.*
Josh. 6:20, the wall *f.* flat.
1 Kings 18:38, fire of Lord *f.*, and consumed.
2 Kings 6:5, as one was *f.* a beam.
Dan. 4:31, then *f.* a voice from heaven.
Jon. 1:7, lot on Jonah.
Mat. 7:25; Lu. 6:49, house *f.* not.
Lu. 8:23, Jesus *f.* asleep.
10:30, 36, *f.* among thieves.
13:4, upon whom tower *f.*
Acts 1:25, from which Judas *f.*
26, lot *f.* on Matthias.
13:36, *f.* on sleep.
2 Pet. 3:4, since fathers *f.* asleep.
Rev. 16:19, cities of the nations *f.*
See Mat. 13:4; Acts 10:44; 19:35; 20:9.
FELLOW. Ex 2:13, wherefore smitest thou thy *f.*?
1 Sam. 21:15, this *f.* to play the madman.
2 Sam. 6:20, as one of the vain *f.*
2 Kings 9:11, wherefore came this mad *f.*?
Ps. 45:7; Heb. 1:9, oil of gladness above thy *f.*
Eccl. 4:10, one shall lift up his *f.*
Zech. 13:7, the man that is my *f.*
Mat. 11:16, like children calling to their *f.*
24:49, begin to smite his *f.*-servants.
26:61, this *f.* said, I am able to destroy.
71; Lu. 22:59, this *f.* was also with Jesus.
Lu. 23:2, found this *f.* perverting.
John 9:29, as for this *f.*
Acts 17:5, lewd *f.* of the baser sort.
22:22, away with such a *f.*
24:5, this man a pestilent *f.*
Eph. 2:19, *f.*-citizens with the saints.
3:6, Gentiles *f.*-heirs.
Phil. 4:3; 1 Thess. 3:2; Philem 24, *f.*-labourers.
3 John 8, *f.*-helpers to the truth.
See Col. 4:11; Philem. 2; Rev. 19:10; 22:9.
FELLOWSHIP. Acts 2:42, in doctrine and *f.*
1 Cor. 1:9, called to the *f.* of his Son.
10:20, not have *f.* with devils.
2 Cor. 6:14, what *f.* hath righteousness?
Eph. 3:9, the *f.* of mystery.
5:11, have no *f.* with.
Phil. 1:5, your *f.* in the gospel.
2:1, if any *f.* of the Spirit.
3:10, the *f.* of his sufferings.
1 John 1:3, our *f.* is with the Father.
7, we have *f.* one with another.
See Lev. 6:2; Ps. 94:20; 2 Cor. 8:4, 13, 14; Gal. 2:9.
FELT. Ex. 10:21; Prov. 23:35; Mk. 5:29; Acts 28:5.
FEMALE. Mat. 19:4; Mk. 10:6, made them male and *f.*
Gal. 3:28, in Christ neither male nor *f.*
See Gen. 7:16; Lev. 3:1; 27:4; Deut. 4:16.
FENCE. Job 10:11; 19:8; Ps. 62:3; Isa. 5:2.
FERVENT. Acts 18:25; Rom. 12:11, *f.* in spirit.
Jas. 5:16, *f.* prayer availeth much.
1 Pet. 1:22, with a pure heart *f.*
2 Pet. 3, 10, 12, melt with *f.* heat.
See 2 Cor. 7:7; Col. 4:12; 1 Pet. 4:8.
FETCH. Num. 20:10, must we *f.* water?

Job 36:3, I will *f.* my knowledge from afar.
Isa. 56:12, I will *f.* wine.
Acts 16:37, come themselves and *f.* us out.
See Deut. 19:5; 2 Sam. 14:3; Acts 28:13.
FETTERS. Judg. 16:21; Ps. 105:18; 149:8; Mk. 5:4; Lu. 8:29.
FEVER. Deut. 28:22, the Lord shall smite thee with a *f.*
Mat. 8:14; Mk. 1:30, Simon's wife's mother lay sick of a *f.*
John 4:52, at the seventh hour the *f.* left him.
FEW. Gen. 29:20, they seemed but a *f.* days.
47:9, *f.* and evil have the days of my life.
1 Sam. 14:6, to save by many or *f.*
17:28, with whom left those *f.* sheep?
2 Kings 4:3, borrow not a *f.*
Neh. 7:4, city large, people *f.*
Job 14:1, man is of *f.* days.
16:22, when a *f.* years are come.
Eccl. 5:2, let thy words be *f.*
Mat. 7:14, *f.* there be that find it.
9:37; Lu. 10:2, the labourers are *f.*
15:34; Mk. 8:7, a *f.* little fishes.
20:16; 22:14, many called, *f.* chosen.
25:21, faithful in a *f.* things.
Mk. 6:5, laid hands on a *f.* sick folk.
Lu. 12:48, beaten with *f.* stripes.
13:23, are there *f.* that be saved?
Rev. 3:4, a *f.* names even in Sardis.
See Deut. 7:7; Ps. 109:8; Heb. 12:10.
FIDELITY. Tit. 2:10, showing good *f.*
FIELD. Deut. 21:1, if one be found slain in *f.*
1 Sam. 22:7, will he give every one of you *f.*?
Prov. 24:30, the *f.* of the slothful.
Isa. 5:8, that lay *f.* to *f.*
Mat. 13:38, the *f.* is the world.
44, treasure hid in a *f.*
John 4:35, look on the *f.*
Jas. 5:4, labourers which reaped your *f.*
See Mat. 6:28; 27:7; Acts 1:19.
FIERCE. Gen. 49:7, anger, for it was *f.*
Deut. 28:50, a nation of a *f.* countenance.
Mat. 8:28, exceeding *f.*
Lu. 23:5, and they were more *f.*
2 Tim. 3:3, men shall be incontinent, *f.*
Jas. 3:4, driven of *f.* winds.
See 2 Sam. 19:43; Isa. 33:19; Dan. 8:23.
FIERY. Deut. 33:2, a *f.* law for them.
Dan. 3:6, a *f.* furnace.
Eph. 6:16, the *f.* darts of the wicked.
Heb. 10:27, judgment and *f.* indignation.
1 Pet. 4:12, concerning the *f.* trial.
See Num. 21:6; Deut. 8:15; Isa. 14:29.
FIG. 1 Kings 4:25; Mic. 4:4, dwelt under his *f.* tree.
2 Kings 18:31; Isa. 36:16, eat every one of his *f.* tree.
20:7, Isaiah said, Take a lump of *f.*
Isa. 38:21, let them take a lump of *f.*
Jer. 24:1, two baskets of *f.* were set before the temple.
Hab. 3:17, although *f.* tree shall not blossom.
Mat. 7:16; Lu. 6:44, do men gather *f.* of thistles?
Lu. 21:29, behold the *f.* tree.
Jas. 3:12, can the *f.* tree bear olive berries?
Rev. 6:13, casteth untimely *f.*
See Judg. 9:10; Jer. 8:13; Lu. 13:6; John 1:48.
FIGHT. Ex. 14:14; Deut. 1:30; 3:22; 20:4, Lord *f.* for you.
Josh. 23:10, he it is that *f.* for you.
1 Sam. 25:28, *f.* the battles of the Lord.
2 Kings 10:3, *f.* for your master's house.
Neh. 4:14, *f.* for your brethren, sons, and wives.
Ps. 144:1, teacheth my fingers to *f.*
John 18:36, then would my servants *f.*
Acts 5:39; 23:9, *f.* against God.
1 Cor. 9:26, so *f.* I.
2 Cor. 7:5, without were *f.*
1 Tim. 6:12; 2 Tim. 4:7, the good *f.*
Heb. 10:32, great *f.* of afflictions.
11:34, valiant in *f.*
Jas. 4:1, wars and *f.* among you.
2, ye *f.* and war.
See Zech. 10:5; 14:14; Rev. 2:16.
FIG-TREE. Mat. 21:19, presently the *f.* withered away.
Mk. 11:13, seeing a *f.* afar off.
FIG-TREE (parable of). Mat. 24:32; Lu. 21:29.
FIGURE. Deut. 4:16; Rom. 5:14; 1 Cor. 4:6; Heb. 9:9; 1 Pet. 3:21.
FILL. Num. 14:21; Ps. 72:19; Hab. 2:14, earth *f.* with glory.
Job 23:4, *f.* my mouth with arguments.
Ps. 81:10, open mouth, I will *f.* it.
104:28, they are *f.* with good.
Prov. 3:10, barns *f.* with plenty.
14:14, *f.* with his own ways.
30:22, a fool when *f.* with meat.
Isa. 65:20, who hath not *f.* his days.
Mat. 5:6; Lu. 6:21, they shall be *f.*
Mk. 7:27, let the children first be *f.*
Lu. 1:15; Acts 4:8; 9:17; 13:9, *f.* with Holy Ghost.
14:23, that my house may be *f.*
John 16:6, sorrow hath *f.* your heart.
Acts 5:28, ye have *f.* Jerusalem with your doctrine.
14:17, *f.* our hearts with food and gladness.
Rom. 1:29, *f.* with all unrighteousness.
15:14, *f.* with all knowledge.
Eph. 1:23, him that *f.* all in all.
3:19, *f.* with fulness of God.
5:18, be *f.* with the Spirit.
Phil. 1:11, *f.* with fruits of righteousness.
Col. 1:24, *f.* up what is behind.
Jas. 2:16, be ye warned and *f.*
Rev. 15:1, in them is *f.* up wrath of God.
See Dan 2:35; Lu. 2:40; 15:16; John 2:7.
FILTH. Isa. 4:4, washed away the *f.* of Zion.
1 Cor. 4:13, as the *f.* of the world.
FILTHINESS. 2 Cor. 7:1, cleanse from all *f.* of flesh.
Eph. 5:4, nor let *f.* be named.
Jas. 1:21, lay apart all *f.*
See Ezek. 33:15; 36:25.
FILTHY. Job 15:16, how much more *f.* is man?
Ps. 14:3; 53:3, altogether become *f.*
Isa. 64:6, as *f.* rags.
Zech. 3:3, clothed with *f.* garments.
Col. 3:8, put off *f.* communication.
1 Tim. 3:3; Tit. 1:7; 1 Pet. 5:2, *f.* lucre.
2 Pet. 2:7, vexed with *f.* conversation.
Jude 8, *f.* dreamers.
Rev. 22:11, he that is *f.*, let him be *f.*
FINALLY. 2 Cor. 13:11; Eph. 6:10; Phil. 3:1;4:8; 2 Thess. 3:1; 1 Pet. 3:8.
FIND. Num. 32:23, be sure your sin will *f.* you out.
Job 9:10; Rom. 11:33, things past *f.* out.
23:3, where I might *f.* him.
Prov. 4:22, life to those that *f.* them.
8:17; Jer. 29:13, seek me early shall *f.* me.
35, whoso *f.* me, *f.* life.
18:22, *f.* a wife, *f.* a good thing.
Eccl. 9:10, thy hand *f.* to do, do it.
11:1, *f.* it after many days.
Isa. 58:13, *f.* thine own pleasure.
Jer. 6:16; Mat. 11:20, *f.* rest to your souls.
Mat. 7:7; Lu. 11:9, seek, and ye shall *f.*
7:14, few there be that *f.* it.
10:39, loseth his life shall *f.* it.
22:9, as many as ye shall *f.*
Mk. 11:13, he might *f.* any thing thereon.
13:36, he *f.* you sleeping.
Lu. 15:4, 8, till he *f.* it.
18:8, shall he *f.* faith on earth?
John 1:41, first *f.* his brother.
Rom. 7:21, I *f.* a law that when I would.
Heb. 4:16, *f.* grace to help.
See John 7:34; 2 Tim. 1:18; Rev. 9:6.
FINE. Ps. 19:10, more to be desire than *f.* gold.
81:16; 147:14, the *f.* of the wheat.
Prov. 25:12, as an ornament of *f.* gold.
Lam. 4:1, how is the *f.* gold changed!
Mk. 15:46, Joseph brought *f.* linen.
See Job 28:1, 17; Lu. 16:19; Rev. 18:12; 19:8
FINGER. Ex. 8:19, this is the *f.* of God.

Ex. 31:18; Deut. 9:10, written with the *f.* of God.
1 Kings 12:10; 2 Chron. 10:10, little *f.* thicker.
Prov. 7:3, bind them on thy *f.*
Isa. 58:9, the putting forth of the *f.*
Dan. 5:5, the *f.* of a man's hand.
Mat. 23:4; Lu. 11:46, not move with *f.*
Lu. 16:24, the tip of his *f.*
John 8:6, with his *f.* wrote on ground.
20:25, put my *f.* into print of nails.
27, reach hither thy *f.*
See Ps. 8:3; Prov. 6:13; Isa. 2:8; 59:3; Lu. 11:20.
FINISH. 1 Chron. 28:20, till thou hast *f.*
Neh. 6:15, so the wall was *f.*
Lu. 14:28, 29, 30, whether sufficient to *f.*
John 4:34, to do his will, and *f.* his work.
5:36, which the Father hath given me to *f.*
17:4, have *f.* the work.
19:30, it is *f.*
Acts 20:24; 2 Tim. 4:7, that I might *f.* my course.
2 Cor. 8:6, *f.* in you the same grace.
Heb. 12:2, Jesus, author and *f.* of our faith.
Jas. 1:15, sin, when it is *f.*
See Dan. 9:24; Rev. 19:7; 11:7; 20:5.
FIRE. Gen. 22:7, behold the *f.* and the wood.
Ex. 3:2, bush burned with *f.*
22:6, he that kindled *f.* shall make restitution.
Lev. 10:2, *f.* from the Lord.
18:21; Deut. 19:10; 2 Kings 17:17; 23:10, pass through *f.*
Judg. 15:5, brands on *f.*, and burnt corn.
1 Kings 18:24, that answereth by *f.*
19:12, the Lord was not in the *f.*
1 Chron. 21:26, Lord answered him by *f.*
Ps. 39:3, musing, the *f.* burned.
74:7, they have cast *f.* into thy sanctuary.
Prov. 6:27, can a man take *f.*?
26:18, mad man who casteth *f.*-brands.
20, no wood, the *f.* goeth out.
21, as wood is to *f.*, so is a contentious man.
Isa. 9:19, as the fuel of the *f.*
24:15, glorify the Lord in the *f.*
43:2, walkest through *f.* not be burned.
44:16, I have seen the *f.*
64:2, the melting *f.* burneth.
66:15, the Lord will come with *f.*
16, by *f.* will the Lord plead.
24; Mk. 9:44, neither their *f.* quenched.
Jer. 20:9, word as a *f.* in my bones.
Ezek. 36:5, in the *f.* of my jealousy.
Dan. 3:27, the *f.* had no power.
Amos 4:11, as a *f.*-brand plucked out.
Nah. 1:6, fury poured out like *f.*
Zech. 2:5, a wall of *f.* round about.
3:2, a brand plucked out of the *f.*
Mal. 3:2, like a refiner's *f.*
Mat. 3:10; 7:19; Lu. 3:9; John 15:6, tree cast into *f.*
11; Lu. 3:16, baptize with *f.*
13:42, cast them into furnace of *f.*
18:8; 25:41; Mk. 9:43, 46, everlasting *f.*
Lu. 9:54, wilt thou that we command *f.*?
12:49, come to send *f.* on earth.
17:29, same day it rained *f.* and brimstone.
Acts 2:3, cloven tongues like as of *f.*
1 Cor. 3:13, revealed by *f.* and the *f.* shall try.
15, saved, yet so as by *f.*
2 Thess. 1:8, in flaming *f.* taking vengeance.
Heb. 1:7, his ministers a flame of *f.*
11:34, quenched violence of *f.*
Jas. 3:5, a little *f.* kindleth.
6, the tongue is a *f.*
1 Pet. 1:7, gold tried with *f.*
2 Pet. 3:7, reserved unto *f.*
12, heavens being on *f.*
Jude 7, vengeance of eternal *f.*
23, pulling them out of the *f.*
Rev. 3:18, buy gold tried in the *f.*
20:9, *f.* came down from God.
10, devil cast into lake of *f.*
Rev. 20:14, death and hell cast into *f.*
21:8, the lake that burneth with *f.*
See Isa. 33:14; Jer. 23:29; Heb. 12:29.
FIRM. Josh. 3:17; Job 41:24; Ps. 73:4; Heb. 3:6.
FIRMAMENT. Gen. 1:6, let there be a *f.*
Ps. 19:1, the *f.* sheweth his handywork.
Ezek. 1:22, the likeness of the *f.*
Dan. 12:3, shine as the brightness of the *f.*
FIRST. 1 Kings 17:13, make a little cake *f.*
Ezra 3:12; Hag. 2:3, the glory of the *f.* house.
Job 15:7, art thou the *f.* man born?
Prov. 3:9, honour the Lord with *f.*-fruits.
18:17, *f.* in his own cause.
Isa. 43:27, try *f.* father hath sinned.
Mat. 5:24, *f.* be reconciled.
6:33, seek ye *f.* the kingdom.
7:5, *f.* cast out the beam.
12:29; Mk. 3:27, except he *f.* bind strong man.
45, last state of that man worse than *f.*
17:10, 11; Mk. 9:12, Elias must *f.* come.
20:10, when the *f.* came, they supposed.
22:38; Mk. 12:28, 29, 30, the *f.* commandment.
Mk. 4:28, *f.* the blade.
9:35, if any desire to be *f.*, same shall be last.
13:10, gospel must *f.* be published.
Lu. 14:28, sitteth not down *f.*
17:25, but *f.* must he suffer many things.
John 1:41, *f.* findeth his brother Simon.
5:4, whosoever *f.* stepped in.
8:7, let him *f.* cast a stone.
Acts 11:26, called Christians *f.* at Antioch.
Rom. 2:9, 10, of the Jew *f.*
8:23, the *f.*-fruits of the Spirit.
29, *f.*-born among many brethren.
11:16, if the *f.*-fruit be holy.
1 Cor. 12:28, *f.* apostles, secondarily prophets.
14:30, let the *f.* hold peace.
15:20, 23, Christ the *f.*-fruits,
45, the *f.* man was made a living soul.
46, not *f.* which is spiritual.
47, *f.* man is of the earth.
2 Cor. 8:5, *f.* gave their own selves.
12, if there be *f.* a willing mind.
Eph. 6:2, the *f.* commandment with promise.
Col. 1:15, 18, the *f.*-born of every creature.
1 Thess. 4:16, dead in Christ shall rise *f.*
2 Thess. 2:3, a falling away *f.*
1 Tim. 1:16, that in me *f.*
2:13, Adam was *f.* formed.
3:10, let these *f.* be proved.
5:4, learn *f.* to show piety at home.
12, cast off their *f.* faith.
2 Tim. 4:16, at my *f.* answer no man.
Tit. 3:10, after *f.* and second admonition.
Heb. 5:12, which be the *f.* principles.
7:27, *f.* for his own sins.
10:9, taketh away the *f.*
Jas. 3:17, *f.* pure, then peaceable.
1 Pet. 4:17, if judgment *f.* begin at us.
1 John 4:19, because he *f.* loved us.
Jude 6, kept not their *f.* estate.
Rev. 2:4, left thy *f.* love.
5, do thy *f.* works.
20:5, this is the *f.* resurrection.
21:1, *f.* heaven and *f.* earth passed away.
See Ex. 4:8; Num. 18:13; John 12:16.
FIR TREE. Isa. 41:19, I will set in the desert the *f.*
55:13, instead of the thorn shall come up the *f.*
60:13, the *f.*
Hos. 14:8, I am like a green *f.*
FISH. Eccl. 9:12, *f.* taken in an evil net.
Hab. 1:14, men as the *f.* of the sea.
Mat. 7:10, if he ask a *f.*
14:17; Mk. 6:38; Lu. 9:13, five loaves and two *f.*
John 21:3, Peter saith, I go a *f.*
1 Cor. 15:39, one flesh of beasts, another of *f.*
See Jer. 16:16; Mat. 4:19; Mk. 1:17; Lu. 24:42.

FISHERS. Mat. 4:18; Mk. 1:16, for they were *f.*
John 21:7, he girt his *f.* coat unto him.
See Lu. 5:2.
FIT. Job 34:18, is it *f.* to say to a king?
Lu. 9:62, is *f.* for the kingdom.
14:35, it is not *f.* for the dunghill.
Col. 3:18, submit, as it is *f.* in the Lord.
See Lev. 16:21; Prov. 24:27; Ezek. 15:5; Rom. 9:22.
FITLY. Prov. 25:11; Eph. 2:21; 4:16.
FIXED. Ps. 57:7; 108:1; 112:7; Lu. 16:26.
FLAME. Gen. 3:24, at garden of Eden a *f.* sword.
Judg. 13:20, angel ascended in *f.*
Isa. 5:24, as the *f.* consumeth chaff.
29:6, a *f.* of devouring fire.
43:2, neither shall *f.* kindle.
66:15, rebuke with *f.* of fire.
Ezek. 20:47, the *f. f.* shall not be quenched.
Lu. 16:24, tormented in this *f.*
See Ps. 29:7; Heb. 1:7; Rev. 1:14; 2:18.
FLATTER. Job 17:5, he speaketh *f.* to his friends.
32:21, 22, give *f.* titles to man.
Ps. 5:9, they *f.* with their tongue.
12:2, *f.* lips and double heart.
Prov. 20:19, meddle not with him that *f.*
26:28, a *f.* mouth worketh ruin.
1 Thess. 2:5, neither used we *f.* words.
See Prov. 28:23; 29:5; Dan. 11:21, 32, 34.
FLATTERY. Ps. 78:36; Prov. 2:16; 24:24.
FLEE. Lev. 26:17, 36, ye shall *f.* when none pursueth.
Num. 10:35, them that hate thee *f.* before thee.
Neh. 6:11, should such a man as I *f.*?
Job 14:2, he *f.* as a shadow.
Ps. 139:7, whither shall I *f.*?
Prov. 28:1, the wicked *f.* when no man pursueth.
17, he shall *f.* to the pit.
Cant. 2:17; 4:6, till shadows *f.* away.
Isa. 35:10; 51:11, sighing shall *f.* away.
Mat. 3:7; Lu. 3:7, to *f.* from wrath to come.
10:23, in one city, *f.* to another.
24:16; Mk. 13:14; Lu. 21:21, *f.* to mountains.
26:56; Mk. 14:50, forsook him and *f.*
John 10:5, not follow, but will *f.* from him.
13, the hireling *f.*
1 Tim. 6:11, *f.* these things.
2 Tim. 2:22, *f.* youthful lusts.
Jas. 4:7, he will *f.* from you.
See 1 Cor. 6:18; 10:14; Rev. 12:6, 14.
FLEECE. Judg. 6:37, I will put a *f.* of wool in the floor.
FLESH. Gen. 2:24; Mat. 19:5; Mk. 10:8; 1 Cor. 6:16; Eph. 5:31, one *f.*
6:12, all *f.* had corrupted his way.
13, end of all *f.* is come.
7:21, all *f.* died.
Ex. 16:3, when we sat by the *f.* pots.
Lev. 17:14, the life of all *f.* is the blood.
19:28, cuttings in your *f.*
Num. 11:33, while *f.* was between their teeth.
16:22; 27:16, God of spirits of all *f.*
1 Kings 17:6, bread and *f.* in morning and evening.
2 Chron. 32:8, with him is an arm of *f.*
Neh. 5:5, our *f.* is as the *f.* of our brethren.
Job 19:26, in my *f.* shall I see God.
33:21, his *f.* is consumed away.
Ps. 16:9; Acts 2:26, my *f.* shall rest in hope.
65:2, to thee shall all *f.* come.
78:20, can he provide *f.*?
Prov. 5:11, mourn, when *f.* consumed.
11:17, the cruel troubleth his own *f.*
23:20, among riotous eaters of *f.*
Eccl. 4:5, the fool eateth his own *f.*
12:12, weariness of the *f.*
Isa. 40:5, all *f.* shall see it.
6; 1 Pet. 1:24, all *f.* is grass.
Ezek. 11:19; 36:26, a heart of *f.*
Joel 2:28; Acts 2:17, pour Spirit on all *f.*
Mat. 16:17, *f.* and blood hath not revealed it.
24:22; Mk. 13:20, there should no *f.* be saved.
Mat. 26:41; Mk. 14:38, spirit willing, *f.* weak.
Lu. 24:39, spirit hath not *f.* and bones.
John 1:14, Word made *f.*, and dwelt.
6:51, 54, 55, bread I give is my *f.*
52, can this man give us his *f.*?
63, the *f.* profiteth nothing.
8:15, ye judge after the *f.*
17:2, power over all *f.*
Rom. 6:19, because of the infirmity of your *f.*
8:3, condemned sin in the *f.*
8, they that are in *f.* cannot please God.
9, not in the *f.*, but the Spirit.
12:13, to live after the *f.*
9:3, kinsmen according to the *f.*
5, of whom as concerning the *f.*
13:14, make not provision for the *f.*
1 Cor. 1:29, that no *f.* should glory.
15:39, all *f.* not the same *f.*
50, *f.* and blood cannot inherit.
2 Cor. 12:7, a thorn in the *f.*
Gal. 1:16, I conferred not with *f.* and blood.
2:20, life I now live in the *f.*
5:17, *f.* lusteth against the Spirit.
Eph. 2:3, lusts of *f.*, desires of *f.*
Phil. 3:3, 4, no confidence in the *f.*
1 Tim. 3:16, manifest in the *f.*
1 Pet. 3:18, Christ put to death in *f.*
1 John 4:2; 2 John 7, denieth that Christ is come in *f.*
Jude 8, dreamers defile the *f.*
23, hating garment spotted by *f.*
See John 1:13; 3:6; Gal. 5:19; Heb. 2:14.
FLESHLY. 2 Cor. 1:12; 3:3; Col. 2:18; 1 Pet. 2:11.
FLIES. Ex. 8:21, I will send swarms of *f.* upon thee.
Ps. 78:45, he sent divers sorts of *f.* among thee.
105:31, he spake, and there came divers sorts of *f.*
FLIGHT. Isa. 52:12; Amos 2:14; Mat. 24:20; Heb. 11:34.
FLINT. Num. 20:11; Deut. 8:15; 32:13; Ps. 114:8; Isa. 5:28; 50:7; Ezek. 3:9; 1 Cor. 10:4.
FLOCK. Jer. 13:20, where is the *f.*, thy beautiful *f.*?
Ezek. 34:31, the *f.* of my pasture are men.
Zech. 11:7, the poor of the *f.*
Lu. 12:32, fear not, little *f.*
Acts 20:28, take heed to the *f.*
29, not sparing the *f.*
1 Pet. 5:2, feed the *f.* of God.
3, being ensamples to the *f.*
See Ezek. 36:37; Mal. 1:14; Mat. 26:31.
FLOOD. Josh. 24:2, on other side of the *f.*
Job 28:11, he bindeth *f.* from overflowing.
Ps. 32:6, in *f.* of great waters.
Cant. 8:7, neither can *f.* drown love.
Isa. 44:3, *f.* upon the dry ground.
59:19, enemy come in like a *f.*
Mat. 7:25, *f.* came, and the winds blew.
24:38, in days before the *f.*
39; Lu. 17:27, knew not till *f.* came.
See Gen. 6:17; 7:11; 8; 9:11; Ps. 90:5; 2 Pet. 2:5; Rev. 12:15.
FLOOR. 1 Sam. 23:1, they rob the threshing-*f.*
2 Sam. 24:21, to buy the threshing-*f.* of thee.
Hos. 9:1, loved a reward on every corn-*f.*
Mic. 4:12, gather as sheaves into the *f.*
Mat. 3:12; Lu. 3:17, purge his *f.*
See Deut. 15:14; Dan. 2:35; Joel 2:24.
FLOUR. Ex. 29:2, of wheaten *f.* shalt thou make them.
Lev. 2:2, take thereout his handful of the *f.*
FLOURISH. Ps. 72:7, in his days shall the righteous *f.*
90:6, in the morning it *f.*
92:12, righteous shall *f.* like a palm tree.
103:15, as flower so he *f.*
Prov. 11:28, righteous shall *f.* as branch.
14:11, tabernacle of upright *f.*
Eccl. 12:5, when the almond tree shall *f.*
Cant. 6:11; 7:12, whether the vine *f.*
Ezek. 17:24, have made dry tree to *f.*
Phil. 4:10, your care of me hath *f.*
See Ps. 92:14; Dan. 4:4.
FLOW. Ps. 147:18, wind to blow, and waters *f.*

Cant. 4:16, that the spices may *f.* out.
Isa. 2:2, all nations shall *f.* unto it.
64:1, 3, mountains *f.* at thy presence.
Jer. 31:12, shall *f.* to the goodness of the Lord.
John 7:38, shall *f.* living water.
See Job 20:28; Isa. 60:5; Joel 3:18; Mic. 4:1.
FLOWER. 1 Sam. 2:33, shall die in *f.* of age.
Job 14:2, cometh forth as a *f.*
Cant. 2:12, the *f.* appear on earth.
Isa. 28:1, 4, glorious beauty is a fading *f.*
40:6, as the *f.* of the field.
7; Nah. 1:4; Jas. 1:10; 1 Pet. 1:24, *f.* fadeth.
See Job 15:33; Isa. 18:5; 1 Cor. 7:36.
FLY. Job 5:7, as sparks *f.* upward.
Ps. 55:6, then would I *f.* away.
90:10, and we *f.* away.
Prov. 23:5, riches *f.* away.
Isa. 60:8, that *f.* as a cloud.
See Dan. 9:21; Rev. 14:6; 19:17.
FOAM. Hos. 10:7; Mk. 9:18; Lu. 9:39; Jude 13.
FOES. Ps. 27:2; 30:1; 89:23; Mat. 10:36; Acts 2:35.
FOLD. Prov. 6:10; 24:33, *f.* of the hands to sleep.
Eccl. 4:5, fool *f.* his hands and eateth.
Hab. 3:17, flock cut off from the *f.*
John 10:16, one *f.*, and one shepherd.
See Isa. 13:20; 65:10; Nah. 1:10.
FOLK. Prov. 30:26; Jer. 51:58; Mk. 6:5; John 5:3.
FOLLOW. Num. 14:24, Caleb hath *f.* me fully.
1 Kings 18:21, God, *f.* him.
Ps. 23:6, goodness and mercy shall *f.* me.
63:8, my soul *f.* hard after thee.
68:25, the players *f.* after.
Prov. 12:11; 28:19, that *f.* vain persons.
Isa. 5:11, that they may *f.* strong drink.
Hos. 6:3, if we *f.* on to know the Lord.
Amos. 7:15, took me as I *f.* the flock.
Mat. 4:19; 8:22; 9:9; 16:24; 19:21; Mk. 2:14; 8:34; 10:21; Lu. 5:27; 9:23, 59; John 1:43; 21:22, Jesus said, *f.* me.
8:19; Lu. 9:57, 61, Master, I will *f.* thee.
Mk. 10:28; Lu. 18:28, we left all, and *f.* thee.
32, as they *f.*, they were afraid.
Lu. 22:54, Peter *f.* afar off.
John 10:27, my sheep hear my voice, and *f.* me.
13:36, thou canst not *f.* me now.
Rom. 14:19, *f.* things that make for peace.
1 Cor. 10:4, the rock that *f.* them.
14:1, *f.* after charity.
Phil. 3:12, I *f.* after.
1 Thess. 5:15, ever *f.* that which is good.
1 Tim. 5:24, some men they *f.* after.
6:11; 2 Tim. 2:22, *f.* righteousness.
Heb. 12:14, *f.* peace with all men.
13:7, whose faith *f.*
1 Pet. 1:11, the glory that should *f.*
2:21, that ye should *f.* his steps.
2 Pet. 2:15, *f.* the way of Balaam.
Rev. 14:4, they that *f.* the Lamb.
13, their works do *f.* them.
See Mk. 9:38; 1 Pet. 3:13; 2 Pet. 1:16; Rev. 6:8.
FOLLOWER. Eph. 5:1, *f.* of God, as dear children.
Heb. 6:12, *f.* of them who through faith.
FOLLY. 1 Sam. 25:25, and *f.* is with him.
Job 4:18, his angels he charged with *f.*
24:12, yet God layeth not *f.* to them.
42:8, lest I deal with you after your *f.*
Ps. 49:13, this their way is their *f.*
85:8, let them not turn again to *f.*
Prov. 13:16, a fool layeth open his *f.*
14:8, the *f.* of fools is deceit.
18, the simple inherit *f.*
16:22, instruction of fools is *f.*
17:12, rather than a fool in his *f.*
26:4, answer not a fool according to his *f.*
5, answer fool according to his *f.*
Eccl. 1:17, to know wisdom and *f.*
2:13, wisdom excelleth *f.*
7:25, the wickedness of *f.*
Eccl. 10:6, *f.* is set in great dignity.
2 Cor. 11:1, bear with me a little in my *f.*
2 Tim. 3:9, their *f.* shall be manifest.
See Josh. 7:15; Prov. 14:24; Isa. 9:17.
FOOD. Gen. 3:6, tree good for *f.*
Ex. 21:10, her *f.* shall not be diminished.
Deut. 10:18, in giving him *f.* and raiment.
Job 23:12, more than my necessary *f.*
24:5, wilderness yieldeth *f.*
Ps. 78:25, did eat angels' *f.*
104:14, bring forth *f.* out of the earth.
136:25, giveth *f.* to all flesh.
Prov. 6:8, gathereth her *f.* in harvest.
13:23, much *f.* in tillage of poor.
30:8, with *f.* convenient for me.
31:14, she bringeth her *f.* from far.
2 Cor. 9:10, minister bread for your *f.*
1 Tim. 6:8, having *f.* and raiment.
Jas. 2:15, destitute of daily *f.*
See Gen. 1:29; 2:9; 6:21; 9:3; 41:35; Lev. 22:7; Ps. 145:16; 147:9.
FOOL. 2 Sam. 3:33, died Abner as a *f.* dieth?
Ps. 14:1; 53:1, *f.* said in his heart.
75:4, to *f.*, deal not foolishly.
Prov. 1:7, *f.* despise wisdom.
3:35, shame the promotion of *f.*
10:8, 10, a prating *f.* shall fall.
21, *f.* die for want of wisdom.
23, sport to a *f.* to do mischief.
11:29, the *f.* shall be servant to the wise.
12:15, way of *f.* right in own eyes.
16, *f.* wrath presently known.
13:16, *f.* layeth open his folly.
20, companion of *f.* shall be destroyed.
14:8, folly of *f.* is deceit.
9, *f.* make a mock at sin.
16, the *f.* rageth, and is confident.
15:2, mouth of *f.* poureth out foolishness.
5, a *f.* despiseth his father's instruction.
16:22, the instruction of *f.* is folly.
17:28, a *f.*, when he holdeth his peace, counted wise.
20:3, every *f.* will be meddling.
29:11, a *f.* uttereth all his mind.
Eccl. 2:14, *f.* walketh in darkness.
16, how dieth wise man? as the *f.*
19, who knoweth whether wise or a *f.*?
5:3, a *f.* voice is known by multitude of words.
10:14, a *f.* is full of words.
Isa. 35:8, wayfaring men, though *f.*
Jer. 17:11, at his end he shall be a *f.*
Hos. 9:7, the prophet is a *f.*
Mat. 5:22, shall say, thou *f.*
23:17, ye *f.* and blind.
Lu. 12:20, thou *f.*, this night.
24:25, O *f.*, and slow of heart.
1 Cor. 3:18, let him become a *f.*
2 Cor. 11:16, let no man think me a *f.*
12:11, I am a *f.* in glorying.
Eph. 5:15, walk not as *f.*, but as wise.
See Prov. 10:18; 19:1; 28:26; Eccl. 10:3
FOOLISH. Deut. 32:6, O *f.* people.
2 Sam. 24:10; 1 Chron. 21:8, I have done very *f.*
Job 2:10, as one of the *f.* women.
Ps. 73:3, I was envious at the *f.*
Prov. 9:6, forsake the *f.*, and live.
13, a *f.* woman is clamorous.
14:1, the *f.* plucketh it down.
17:25; 19:13, a *f.* son is grief.
Eccl. 7:17, neither be thou *f.*
Jer. 4:22, my people are *f.*
Mat. 7:26, unto a *f.* man.
Rom. 1:21, their *f.* heart was darkened.
1 Cor. 1:20, hath not God made *f.*
Gal. 3:1, O *f.* Galatians.
3:3, are ye so *f.*?
Eph. 5:4, nor *f.* talking.
1 Tim. 6:9, rich fall into *f.* lusts.

2 Tim. 2:23; Tit. 3:9, *f.* questions avoid.
Tit. 3:3, we were sometimes *f.*
1 Pet. 2:15, ignorance of *f.* men.
See Job 5:3; Lam. 2:14; Ezek. 13:3.
FOOLISHNESS. Ps. 69:5, thou knowest my *f.*
Prov. 22:15, *f.* is bound in heart of child.
24:9, thought of *f.* is sin.
1 Cor. 1:18, to them that perish *f.*
21, by the *f.* of preaching.
23, Christ crucified, to Greeks *f.*
25, the *f.* of God is wiser than men.
2:14, things of Spirit are *f.* to him.
3:19, wisdom of world *f.* with God.
See 2 Sam. 15:31; Prov. 27:22.
FOOT. Gen. 41:44, without thee no man lift *f.*
Deut. 2:5, not so much as *f.* breadth.
11:10, wateredst it with thy *f.*
Ps. 38:16, when my *f.* slippeth.
91:12; Mat. 4:6; Lu. 4:11, dash *f.* against stone.
94:18, my *f.* slippeth, thy mercy.
121:3, not suffer *f.* to be moved.
Prov. 3:23, thy *f.* shall not stumble.
25:17, withdraw *f.* from neighbour's house.
Eccl. 5:1, keep thy *f.* when thou goest.
Isa. 1:6, from sole of *f.* to head no soundness.
Mat. 14:13, people followed on *f.*
18:8; Mk. 9:45, if thy *f.* offend thee.
1 Cor. 12:15, if the *f.* say, because I am not.
Heb. 10:29, trodden under *f.* the Son of God.
See Jer. 12:5; Mat. 5:35; Jas. 2:3.
FORBADE. Mat. 3:14; Mk. 9:38; Lu. 9:49.
FORBEAR. Ex. 23:5, wouldest *f.* to help.
2 Chron. 35:21, *f.* from meddling with God.
Neh. 9:30, many years didst thou *f.* them.
Ezek. 2:5; 3:11, whether hear or *f.*
1 Cor. 9:6, power to *f.* working.
Eph. 4:2; Col. 3:13, *f.* one another in love.
6:9, *f.* threatening.
See Prov. 24:11; Ezek. 3:27; Zech. 11:12.
FORBID. Num. 11:28, Joshua said, *f.* them.
Mk. 9:39; Lu. 9:50, *f.* him not.
10:14; Lu. 18:16, children, *f.* them not.
Lu. 6:29, *f.* not to take coat.
23:2, *f.* to give tribute.
Acts 10:47, can any *f.* water?
1 Cor. 14:39, *f.* not to speak with tongues.
1 Tim. 4:3, *f.* to marry.
See Acts 16:6; 28:31; 1 Thess. 2:16.
FORCE. Deut. 34:7, nor natural *f.* abated.
Ezra 4:23, made them cease by *f.*
Mat. 11:12, violent take it by *f.*
John 6:15, perceived they would take him by *f.*
Heb. 9:17, a testament is of *f.* after.
See Deut. 20:19; Prov. 30:33; Amos 2:14.
FORCIBLE. Job 6:25.
FOREFATHERS. Jer. 11:10; 2 Tim. 1:3.
FOREHEAD. Ex. 28:38, it shall always be on his *f.*
1 Sam. 17:49, smote Philistine in his *f.*
Ezek. 3:8, made thy *f.* strong.
9:4, set a mark on *f.* of them that sigh.
Rev. 7:3; 9:4, sealed in their *f.*
22:4, his name shall be in their *f.*
See Rev. 13:16; 14:1; 17:5; 20:4.
FOREIGNER. Ex. 12:45; Deut. 15:3; Eph. 2:19.
FOREKNOW. Rom. 8:29; 11:2; 1 Pet. 1:2.
FOREKNOWLEDGE. Acts 2:23, delivered by *f.* of God.
FOREMOST. Gen. 32:17; 33:2; 2 Sam. 18:27.
FOREORDAINED. 1 Pet. 1:20.
FORERUNNER. Heb. 6:20.
FORESEE. Prov. 22:3; 27:12; Gal. 3:8.
FOREST. Ps. 50:10, every beast of *f.* is mine.
Isa. 29:17; 32:15, field esteemed as *f.*
Jer. 5:6, lion out of *f.* shall slay them.
26:18; Mic. 3:12, high places of the *f.*
46:23, they shall cut down her *f.*
Amos 3:4, will lion roar in the *f.*?
See Ezek. 15:6; 20:46; Hos. 2:12.

FORETELL. Mk. 13:23; Acts 3:24; 2 Cor. 13:2.
FOREWARN. Lu. 12:5; 1 Thess. 4:6.
FORGAT. Judg. 3:7, they *f.* the Lord.
Ps. 78:11, they *f.* his works.
106:13, soon *f.* his works.
Lam. 3:17, I *f.* prosperity.
See Gen. 40:23; Hos. 2:13.
FORGAVE. Mat. 18:27, 32, and *f.* him the debt.
Lu. 7:42, he frankly *f.* them both.
43, he to whom he *f.* most.
2 Cor. 2:10, if I *f.* any thing.
Col. 3:13, even as Christ *f.* you.
See Ps. 32:5; 78:38; 99:8.
FORGE. Job 13:4; Ps. 119:69.
FORGET. Deut. 4:9, lest thou *f.* things thine eyes have seen.
23, lest ye *f.* the covenant.
6:12; 8:11, beware lest thou *f.* the Lord.
Job 8:13, so are the paths of all that *f.* God.
Ps. 9:17, all nations that *f.* God.
10:12, *f.* not the humble.
45:10, *f.* thine own people.
50:22, consider, ye that *f.* God.
78:7, that they might not *f.* works of God.
88:12, in the land of *f.*
102:4, I *f.* to eat my bread.
103:2, *f.* not all his benefits.
119:16, I will not *f.* thy word.
137:5, if I *f.* thee, O Jerusalem.
Prov. 2:17, *f.* the covenant of her God.
3:1, *f.* not my law.
31:5, lest they drink and *f.*
7, let him drink, and *f.* his poverty.
Isa. 49:15, can a woman *f.*?
51:13, and *f.* the Lord thy Maker.
65:11, *f.* my holy mountain.
Jer. 2:32, maid *f.* her ornaments.
23:27, cause my people to *f.* my name.
Amos 8:7, I will never *f.* their works.
Phil. 3:13, *f.* those things which are behind.
Heb. 6:10, not unrighteous to *f.*
13:2, not *f.* to entertain.
16, to communicate *f.* not.
Jas. 1:24, *f.* what manner of man.
See Gen. 41:51; Lam. 5:20; Hos. 4:6.
FORGIVE. Ex. 32:32, if thou wilt *f.* their sin.
34:7; Num. 14:18, *f.* iniquity, transgression.
1 Kings 8:30, 39; 2 Chron. 6:21, 30, hearest *f.*
2 Chron. 7:14, then will I hear and *f.*
Ps. 32:1; Rom. 4:7, whose transgression is *f.*
86:5, good, and ready to *f.*
103:3, who *f.* all thine iniquities.
Mat. 6:12; Lu. 11:4, *f.* us, as we *f.*
14, if ye *f.*
15, if ye *f.* not.
9:6; Mk. 2:10; Lu. 5:24, power to *f.* sin.
18:21, how oft, and I *f.* him?
35, if ye from your hearts *f.*
Mk. 2:7, who can *f.* sins?
11:25, *f.* that your Father may *f.*
26, not *f.*, Father will not *f.*
Lu. 6:37, *f.*, and ye shall be *f.*
7:47, her sins, which are many, are *f.*
49, who is this *f.* sins also?
17:3, 4, if brother repent, *f.* him.
23:34, Father *f.* them, they know not.
Acts 8:22, thought of thine heart may be *f.*
2 Cor. 2:7, ye ought rather to *f.*
10, to whom ye *f.*, I *f.* also.
12:13, *f.* me this wrong.
Eph. 4:32, as God for Christ's sake hath *f.*
Col. 2:13, quickened, having *f.*
1 John 1:9, faithful and just to *f.*
See Mat. 9:2; 12:31; Mk. 3:28; Lu. 12:10.
FORGIVENESS. Ps. 130:4, *f.* with thee, that thou mayest be feared.
Mk. 3:29, hath never *f.*
Acts 5:31, exalted to give *f.*

Eph. 1:7; Col. 1:14, in whom we have *f.*
See Dan. 9:9; Acts 13:38; 26:18.
FORGOTTEN. Deut. 24:19, and hast *f.* a sheaf.
32:18, *f.* God that formed thee.
Ps. 9:18, needy not always *f.*
10:11, said, God hath *f.*
31:12, *f.* as a dead man.
42:9, why hast thou *f.* me?
44:20, if we have *f.* name of our God.
77:9, hath God *f.* to be gracious?
Eccl. 2:16, in days to come all *f.*
8:10, wicked were *f.* in city.
9:5, the memory of them is *f.*
Isa. 17:10, *f.* the God of thy salvation.
44:21, thou shalt not be *f.* of me.
49:14, my Lord hath *f.* me.
65:16, former troubles are *f.*
Jer. 2:32; 13:25; 18:15, my people have *f.*
3:21, *f.* the Lord their God.
44:9, *f.* the wickedness of your fathers.
50:6, *f.* their restingplace.
Ezek. 22:12; 23:35, thou hast *f.* me.
Mat. 16:5; Mk. 8:14, *f.* to take bread.
Lu. 12:6, not one *f.* before God.
2 Pet. 1:9, *f.* that he was purged.
See Lam. 2:6; Hos. 4:6; 8:14; 13:6.
FORM (*n.*). Gen. 1:2; Jer. 4:23, without *f.*, and void.
Job 4:16, could not discern the *f.*
Isa. 52:14, *f.* more than sons of men.
Ezek. 10:8, the *f.* of a man's hand.
Dan. 3:19, *f.* of visage changed.
25, *f.* of fourth like Son of God.
Mk. 16:12, appeared in another *f.*
Rom. 2:20, hast *f.* of knowledge and truth.
Phil. 2:6, being in the *f.* of God.
7, the *f.* of a servant.
2 Tim. 1:13, *f.* of sound words.
3:5, having *f.* of godliness.
See 1 Sam. 28:14; Ezek. 43:11; Rom. 6:17.
FORM (*v.*). Deut. 32:18, forgotten God that *f.* thee.
2 Kings 19:25; Isa. 37:26, that I have *f.* it.
Job 26:5, dead things are *f.*
13, hath *f.* crooked serpent.
33:6, I also am *f.* of clay.
Ps. 90:2, or ever thou hadst *f.*
94:9, he that *f.* the eye.
Prov. 26:10, great God that *f.* all things.
Isa. 43:1, he that *f.* thee, O Israel.
7; 44:21, I have *f.* him.
10, before me was no God *f.*
21, people have I *f.* for myself.
44:10, who hath *f.* a god?
54:17, no weapon *f.* against thee.
Amos 7:1, he *f.* grasshoppers.
Rom. 9:20, shall thing *f.* say.
Gal. 4:19, till Christ be *f.* in you.
See Gen. 2:7, 19; Ps. 95:5; Jer. 1:5.
FORMER. Ruth 4:7, manner in *f.* time.
Job 8:8, enquire of the *f.* age.
Ps. 89:49, where are they *f.* lovingkindnesses?
Eccl. 1:11, no remembrance of *f.* things.
7:10, *f.* days better than these.
Isa. 43:18, remember not the *f.* things.
46:9, remember the *f.* things of old
48:3, declared *f.* things from beginning.
65:7, measure their *f.* work.
16, *f.* troubles are forgotten.
Jer. 5:24; Hos. 6:3; Joel 2:23, *f.* and latter rain.
10:16; 51:19, the *f.* of all things.
Hag. 2:9, glory of *f.* house.
Zech. 1:4; 7:7, 12, *f.* prophets have cried.
8:11, I will not be as in *f.* days.
14:8, half of them toward *f.* sea.
Mal. 3:4, pleasant as in *f.* years.
Eph. 4:22, concerning the *f.* conversation.
Rev. 21:4, for the *f.* things are passed away.
See Gen. 40:13; Dan. 11:13; Acts 1:1

FORSAKE. Deut. 4:31; 31:6; 1 Chron. 28:20, he will not *f.*
12:19, *f.* not the Levite.
32:15, he *f.* God which made him.
Josh. 1:5; Heb. 13:5, I will not fail nor *f.*
Judg. 9:11, *f.* my sweetness and fruit.
1 Chron. 28:9, if thou *f.* him, he will cast thee off.
2 Chron. 15:2, if ye *f.* him, he will *f.* you.
Neh. 10:39, we will not *f.* house of our God.
13:11, why is house of God *f.*?
Job 6:14, he *f.* the fear of the Almighty.
20:19, oppressed and *f.* the poor.
Ps. 22:1; Mat. 27:46; Mk. 15:34, why hast thou *f.* me?
37:25, yet have I not seen the righteous *f.*
28, the Lord *f.* not his saints.
119:8, *f.* me not utterly.
138:8, *f.* not work of thine own hands.
Prov. 1:8; 6:20, *f.* not law of thy mother.
2:17, *f.* the guide of her youth.
4:6, *f.* her not, and she shall preserve thee.
27:10, thy friend, and father's friend, *f.* not.
Isa. 6:12, a great *f.* in the land.
17:9, as a *f.* bough.
32:14; Jer. 4:29; Ezek. 36:4, a *f.* city.
54:6, as a woman *f.*
7, for a small moment *f.*
62:4, no more be termed *f.*
12, a city not *f.*
Jer. 2:13; 17:13, *f.* fountain of living waters.
Mat. 19:27; Lu. 5:11, we have *f.* all
29, that hath *f.* houses.
26:56; Mk. 14:50, disciples *f.* him, and fled.
Mk. 1:18, they *f.* their nets.
Lu. 14:33, whosoever *f.* not all.
2 Cor. 4:9, persecuted, but not *f.*
2 Tim. 4:10, Demas hath *f.* me.
16, all men *f.* me.
Heb. 10:25, not *f.* assembling of ourselves.
11:27, but faith Moses *f.* Egypt.
See Ps. 71:11; Isa. 49:14; Jer. 5:7; 22:9; Ezek. 8:12.
FORSWEAR. Mat. 5:33.
FORTRESS. 2 Sam. 22:2; Ps. 18:2; Jer. 16:19, Lord is my *f.*
FORTY STRIPES. Deut. 25:3, *f. s.* he may give him.
2 Cor. 11:24, of the Jews five times received I *f. s.* save one.
FORTY YEARS. Ex. 16:35, Israel did not eat manna *f. y.*
Num. 14:33, your children shall wander in the wilderness *f. y.*
Ps. 95:10, *f. y.* long was I grieved.
See Judg. 3:11; 5:31; 8:28.
FORWARD. Jer. 7:24, backward, and not *f.*
Zech. 1:15, helped *f.* the affliction.
See 2 Cor. 8:8; 9:2; 3 John 6.
FOUL. Job 16:16; Mat. 16:3; Mk. 9:25; Rev. 18:2.
FOUND. Gen. 27:20, *f.* it so quickly.
37:2, this have we *f.*
44:16, hat *f.* out iniquity.
1 Kings 20:36, a lion *f.* him.
21:20, hast thou *f.* me?
2 Kings 22:8, I *f.* book of the law.
2 Chron. 19:3, good things *f.* in thee.
Job 28:12, 13, where shall wisdom be *f.*?
33:24, I have *f.* a ransom.
Ps. 32:6, where thou mayest be *f.*
36:2, iniquity *f.* to be hateful.
84:3, sparrow hath *f.* an house.
Prov. 25:16, hast thou *f.* honey?
Eccl. 7:28, one among a thousand have I *f.*
29, this only have I *f.*
Cant. 3:4, but I *f.* him whom my soul loveth.
Isa. 65:1; Rom. 10:20, *f.* of them that sought me not.
Jer. 2:26, thief ashamed when he is *f.*
34, in thy skirts is *f.*
41:8, ten men were *f.*
Ezek. 22:30, I sought for a man, but *f.* none.
Dan. 5:27, weighed, and *f.* wanting.
Mal. 2:6, iniquity not *f.* in his lips.
Mat. 7:25; Lu. 6:48, it was *f.* on a rock.
8:10; Lu. 7:9, have not *f.* so great faith.

Mat. 13:46, *f.* one pearl of great price.
20:6, *f.* others standing idle.
21:19; Mk. 14:40; Lu. 22:45, *f.* nothing thereon.
Mk. 7:2, they *f.* fault.
30, she *f.* the devil gone out.
Lu. 2:46, they *f.* him in the temple.
8:35, they *f.* the man clothed.
15:5, 6, *f.* the sheep.
9, *f.* the piece of money.
24, 32, was lost, and is *f.*
23:14, I have *f.* no fault.
24:2, *f.* the stone rolled away.
3:23, *f.* not the body.
John 1:41, 45, we have *f.* the Messias.
Acts 7:11, our fathers *f.* no sustenance.
9:2, if he *f.* any of this way.
17:23, I *f.* an altar.
Rom. 7:10, I *f.* to be unto death.
Gal. 2:17, we ourselves also are *f.* sinners.
Phil. 2:8, *f.* in fashion as a man.
Heb. 11:5, Enoch was not *f.*
12:17, he *f.* no place of repentance.
Rev. 3:2, not *f.* thy works perfect.
12:8, nor was their place *f.* any more.
16:20, mountains were not *f.*
See Gen. 6:8; 2 Chron. 15:4; 2 Cor. 5:3; Phil. 3:9.
FOUNDATION. Josh. 6:26; 1 Kings 16:34, lay the *f.* in his firstborn.
Job 4:19, them whose *f.* is in dust.
Ps. 11:3, if *f.* be destroyed.
82:5, all the *f.* of earth out of course.
102:25, of old laid *f.* of earth.
137:7, raise it even to the *f.*
Prov. 10:25, righteous an everlasting *f.*
Isa. 28:16, I lay in Zion a *f.*
Isa. 58:12, the *f.* of many generations.
Lu. 6:48, laid the *f.* on a rock.
49, without a *f.*
Rom. 15:20, on another man's *f.*
1 Cor. 3:10, I laid the *f.*
11, other *f.* can no man lay.
12, if any man build on this *f.*
Eph. 2:20, on the *f.* of the apostles and prophets.
1 Tim. 6:19, laying up for themselves a good *f.*
2 Tim. 2:19, the *f.* of God standeth sure.
Heb. 6:1, not laying the *f.* of repentance.
11:10, a city that hath *f.*
Rev. 21:14, the wall had twelve *f.*
See Mat. 13:35; John 17:24; Acts 16:26.
FOUNTAIN. Gen. 7:11; 8:2, *f.* of great deep.
Deut. 8:7, a land of *f.*
2 Chron. 32:3, took counsel to stop *f.* of water.
Ps. 36:9, the *f.* of life.
Prov. 5:16, let thy *f.* be dispersed.
8:24, no *f.* abounding with water.
13:14, law of the wise a *f.* of life
14:27, fear of the Lord a *f.* of life.
25:26, a troubled *f.* and corrupt spring.
Eccl. 12:6, pitcher broken at the *f.*
Cant. 4:12, a *f.* sealed.
15, a *f.* of gardens.
Jer. 2:13; 17:13, forsaken *f.* of living waters.
9:1, eyes a *f.* of tears.
Hos. 13:15, his *f.* shall be dried up.
Zech. 13:1, in that day shall be a f. opened.
Jas. 3:11, 12, doth a *f.* send forth.
Rev. 7:17, lead them to living *f.*
14:7, worship him that made *f.* of waters.
21:6, of the *f.* of life freely.
See Isa. 12:3; 44:3; 55:1; Jer. 6:7; Joel 3:18; Mk. 5:29; John 5:10.
FOWLS. Gen. 1:20, and *f.* that may fly above the earth.
7:3, of *f.* also of the air by sevens.
Ps. 104:12, the *f.* of heaven have their habitation.
148:10, creeping things, and flying *f.*
FOXES. Cant. 2:15, take us the *f.*, the little *f.*
Lam. 5:18, the *f.* walk upon it.
Mat. 8:20, the *f.* have holes.
Lu. 13:32, go ye, and tell that *f.*
See Judg. 15:4.
FRAGMENTS. John 6:12, 13, gather up *f.* that remain.
See Mat. 14:20; Mk. 6:43; 8:19; Lu. 9:17.
FRAIL. Ps. 39:4.
FRAME. Judg. 12:6, he could not *f.* to pronounce.
Ps. 94:20, *f.* mischief by a law.
103:14, he knoweth our *f.*
Isa. 29:16, shall thing *f.* say of him that *f.* it?
Eph. 2:21, building fitly *f.* together.
See Ezek. 40:2; Hos. 5:4; Heb. 11:3.
FRANKLY. Lu. 7:42.
FRAUD. Ps. 10:7; Jas. 5:4.
FRAY. Deut. 18:26; Jer. 7:33; Zech. 1:21.
FREE. Gen. 2:16, of every tree thou mayest *f.* eat.
Deut. 24:5, shall be *f.* at home one year.
Josh. 9:23, there shall none of you be *f.*
1 Sam. 14:30, if people had eaten *f.*
2 Chron. 29:31, of *f.* heart offered.
Ezra 2:68, chief fathers offered *f.*
7:15, king and counsellors offered *f.* to God.
Ps. 51:12, with thy *f.* spirit.
88:5, *f.* among the dead.
Isa. 58:6, let the oppressed go *f.*
Hos. 14:4, I will love them *f.*
Mat. 10:8, *f.* ye have received, *f.* give.
17:26, then are the children *f.*
Mk. 7:11, if a man say Corban, he shall be *f.*
John 8:32, the truth shall make you *f.*
33, how sayest thou, ye shall be *f.*?
36, Son make you *f.*, ye shall be *f.* indeed.
Acts 22:28, I was *f.* born.
Rom. 3:24, justified *f.* by his grace.
5:15, the *f.* gift.
6:18, 22, being made *f.* from sin.
20, servants of sin, *f.* from righteousness.
8:2, *f.* from the law of sin and death.
32, with him *f.* give us all things.
1 Cor. 9:1, am I not *f.*?
19, though *f.* from all men.
12:13; Eph. 6:8, whether bond or *f.*
Gal. 3:28; col. 3:11, there is neither bond nor *f.*
5:1, wherewith Christ hath made us *f.*
2 Thess. 3:1, word have *f.* course.
1 Pet. 2:16, as *f.*, and not using liberty.
Rev. 21:6, give of fountain of life *f.*
22:17, let him take water of life *f.*
See Ex. 21:2; Deut. 15:13; Jer. 34:9; Gal. 4:22.
FREEWILL. Lev. 22:18, and for all his *f.* offerings.
Num. 15:3, or in a *f.* offering.
Deut. 16:10, a tribute of a *f.* offering.
See Ezra 3:5.
FREEWOMAN. Gal. 4:22.
FRESH. Num. 11:8; Job 29:20; 33:25; Jas. 3:12.
FRET. Ps. 37:1, 7, 8; Prov. 24:19, *f.* not thyself.
Prov. 19:3, his heart *f.* against the Lord.
See 1 Sam. 1:6; Isa. 8:21; Ezek. 16:43.
FRIEND. Ex. 33:11, as a man to his *f.*
2 Sam. 19:6, lovest thine enemies, and hatest *f.*
2 Chron. 20:7, Abraham thy *f.* for ever.
Job 6:27, ye dig a pit for your *f.*
42:10, when he prayed for his *f.*
Ps. 35:14, as though he had been my *f.*
41:9, my familiar *f.* hath lifted.
88:18, lover and *f.* hast thou put far from me.
Prov. 6:1, if thou be surety for thy *f.*
3, make sure thy *f.*
14:20, the rich hath many *f.*
16:28; 17:9, whisperer separateth chief *f.*
17:17, *f.* loveth at all times.
18:24, a *f.* that sticketh closer than a brother.
19:4, wealth maketh many *f.*
27:6, faithful are wounds of a *f.*
10, thine own *f.* and father's *f.* forsake not.
17, man sharpeneth countenance of his *f.*
Cant. 5:16, this is my *f.*

Isa. 41:8, seed of Abraham my *f*
Jer. 20:4, a terror to thy *f*
Mic. 7:5, trust not in a *f*.
Zech. 13:6, wounded in house of my *f*.
Mat. 11:19; Lu. 7:34, a *f*. of publicans.
20:13, *f*. I do thee no wrong.
22:12, *f*., how camest thou hither?
26:50, *f*., wherefore art thou come?
Mk. 5:19, go home to thy *f*.,
Lu. 11:5, which of you shall have a *f*.,
8, though he give not because he is his *f*.
14:12, call not thy *f*.
15:6, 9, calleth his *f*. and neighbours.
16:9, *f*. of the mammon.
John 11:11, our *f*. Lazarus sleepeth.
15:13, lay down his life for his *f*.
14, ye are my *f*., if ye do whatsoever I command.
15, not servants, but *f*.
19:12, thou art not Caesar's *f*.
Jas. 2:23, Abraham was called the *f*. of God.
4:4, a *f*. of the world.
See Prov. 22:24; Lu. 14:10; 3 John 14.
FRINGES. Num. 15:37, that they make them *f*.
Deut. 22:12, thou shalt make thee *f*.
See Mat. 23:5.
FROGS. Ex. 8:6; Ps. 78:45; 105:30; Rev. 16:13.
FRONTLETS. Ex. 13:16; Deut. 6:8, for *f*. between thine eyes.
FROWARD. Deut. 32:20, a very *f*. generation.
Prov. 2:12, man that speaketh *f*. things.
3:32, the *f*. is abomination.
4:24, put away *f*. mouth.
11:20; 17:20, of a *f*. heart.
16:28, a *f*. man soweth strife.
21:8, the way of man is *f*.
22:5, snares are in the way of the *f*.
See Prov. 10:32; Isa. 57:17; 1 Pet. 2:18.
FRUIT. Num. 13:26, showed them the *f*. of the land.
Deut. 26:2, take the first of all *f*.
33:14, precious *f*. brought forth.
Ps. 107:37, yield *f*. of increase.
127:3, the *f* of the womb is his reward.
Prov. 8:19, my *f*. is better than gold.
11:30, *f*. of the righteous a tree of life.
12:14; 18:20, satisfied by the *f*. of his mouth.
Cant. 2:3, his *f*. was sweet to my taste.
4:13, 16, orchard with pleasant *f*.
Isa. 3:10; Mic. 7:13, the *f*. of their doings.
27:6, fill face of the world with *f*.
28:4, the hasty *f*. before summer.
57:19, I create the *f*. of the lips.
Jer. 17:10; 21:14; 32:19, according to *f*. of doings.
Hos. 10:13, eaten the *f*. of lies.
Amos 8:1, basket of summer *f*.
Mic. 6:7, *f*. of body for sin of soul.
Hab. 3:17, neither shall *f*. be in vines.
Hag. 1:10, earth is stayed from her *f*.
Mat. 3:8; Lu. 3:8, *f*. meet for repentance.
7:16, 20, by their *f*. ye shall know them.
12:33, make tree good, and his *f*. good.
13:23, is he who beareth *f*.
21:19, let no *f*. grow on thee.
34, when time of *f*. drew near.
26:29; Mk. 14:25, drink of *f*. of vine.
Mk. 4:28, 3 earth bringeth forth *f*. of herself.
12:2, receive the *f*. of the vineyard.
Lu. 13:6, he sought *f*. thereon.
7, I come seeking *f*. on this fig tree.
9, if it bear *f*., well.
John 4:36, *f*. to life eternal.
15:2, branch that beareth *f*.
4, branch cannot bear *f*. of itself.
8, that ye bear much *f*.
16, ordained that ye should bring forth *f*.
Rom. 1:13, have some *f*. among you.
6:21, what *f*. had ye then.
7:4, bring forth *f*. unto God.
2 Cor. 9:10; Phil. 1:11, the *f*. of righteousness.
Gal. 5:22; Eph. 5:9, the *f*. of the Spirit.
Phil. 1:22, this is the *f*. of my labour.
4:17, I desire *f*. that may abound.
Col. 1:6, the gospel bringeth forth *f*. in you.
2 Tim. 2:6, first partaker of the *f*.
Heb. 12:11, peaceable *f*. of righteousness.
13:15, the *f*. of our lips.
Jas. 3:17, wisdom full of good *f*.
5:7, waiteth for the precious *f*.
Jude 12, trees whose *f*. withereth, without *f*.
Rev. 22:2, yielded her *f*. every month.
See Gen. 30:2; Ps. 92:14; Jer. 12:2; Col. 1:10.
FRUSTRATE. Ezra 4:5; Isa. 44:25; Gal. 2:21.
FUEL. Isa. 9:5; Ezek. 15:4; 21:32.
FULFIL. Ps. 20:4, the Lord *f*. all thy counsel.
5, *f*. all thy petitions
145:19, he will *f*. the desire of men.
Mat. 3:15, to *f*. all righteousness.
5:17, not to destroy, but to *f*.
18; 24:34, till all be *f*.
Mk. 13:4, what the sign when these shall be *f*.?
Lu. 1:20, my words shall be *f*. in season.
21:24, times of the Gentiles be *f*.
22:16, till it be *f*. in kingdom of God.
John 3:29; 17:13, this my joy is *f*.
Acts 13:25, and as John *f*. his course.
33, God hath *f*. the same unto us.
Rom. 13:10, love is the *f*. of the law.
Gal. 5:14, all the law is *f*. in one word.
6:2, so *f*. the law of Christ.
Eph. 2:3, *f*. the desires of the flesh.
Phil. 2:2, *f*. ye my joy.
Col. 4:17, take heed thou *f*. the ministry.
2 Thess. 1:11, *f*. good pleasure of his will.
Jas. 2:8, if ye *f*. the royal law.
See Ex. 5:13; 23:26; Gal. 5:16; Rev. 17:17.
FULL. Lev. 19:29, land became *f*. of wickedness.
Deut. 6:11, houses *f*. of good things.
34:9, Joshua was *f* of spirit of wisdom.
Ruth 1:21, I went out *f*.
2 Kings 6:17, mountain was *f*. of horses.
1 Chron. 21:22, 24, for the *f*. price.
Job 5:26, come to grave in *f*. age.
11:2, a man *f*. of talk.
14:1, *f*. of trouble.
20:11, *f*. of the sins of youth.
21:23, dieth in his *f* strength.
32:18, I am *f*. of matter.
Ps. 10:7; Rom. 3:14, mouth *f*. of cursing.
65:9, which is *f*. of water.
74:20, *f*. of habitations of cruelty.
88:3, soul *f*. of troubles.
119:64, earth is *f*. of thy mercy.
127:5, happy the man that hath his quiver *f*.
Prov. 27:7, the *f*. soul loatheth an honeycomb.
20, hell and destruction are never *f*.
Prov. 30:9, lest I be *f*., and deny thee.
Eccl. 1:7, yet the sea is not *f*.
Hab. 3:3, earth *f*. of his praise.
Zech. 8:5, streets *f*. of boys and girls.
Mat. 6:22; Lu. 11:36, *f*. of light.
Lu. 6:25, woe unto you that are *f*.!
11:39, *f*. of ravening.
John 1:14, *f*. of grace and truth.
15:11; 16:24, that your joy may be *f*.
Acts 6:3; 7:55; 11:24, men *f* of the Holy Ghost.
9:36, *f*. of good works.
Rom. 15:14, ye also are *f*. of goodness.
1 Cor. 4:8, now ye are *f*.
Phil. 4:12, I am instructed to be *f*.
18, I am *f*.
2 Tim. 4:5, make *f*. proof of thy ministry.
Heb. 5:14, meat to them of *f*. age.
1 Pet. 1:8, with joy unspeakable and *f*. of glory.
Rev. 15:7, *f*. of the wrath of God.
See Lev. 2:14; 2 Kings 4:6; 10:21; Amos 2:13.
FULLY. Num. 14:24, Caleb hath followed me *f*.

Eccl. 8:11, heart is *f.* set to do evil.
Rom. 14:5, let every man be *f.* persuaded.
15:19, I have *f.* preached the gospel.
Rev. 14:18, her grapes are *f.* ripe.
See 1 Kings 11:6; Acts 2:1; Rom. 4:21.
FULNESS. Ps. 16:11, *f.* of joy.
John 1:16, of his *f.* have we received.
Rom. 11:25, the *f.* of the Gentiles.
Eph. 1:23, the *f.* of him that filleth all in all.
3:19, filled with the *f.* of God.
4:13, the stature of the *f.* of Christ.
Col. 1:19, in him should all *f.* dwell.
2:9, the *f.* of the Godhead bodily.
See Num. 18:27; Ps. 96:11; Rom. 11:12.
FURIOUS. Prov. 22:24, with a *f.* man thou shalt not go.
29:22, a *f.* man aboundeth in transgression.
Nah. 1:2, the Lord is *f.*
See 2 Kings 9:20; Ezek. 5:15; 23:25.
FURNACE. Deut. 4:20, Lord hath taken you out of *f.*
Ps. 12:6, as silver tried in a *f.*
Isa. 48:10, in the *f.* of affliction.
Mat. 13:42, into a *f.* of fire.
See Gen. 15:17; 19:28; 1 Kings 8:51; Dan. 3:6, 11, 15, etc.; Ezek. 22:18.
FURNISH. Ps. 78:19; Mat. 22:10; 2 Tim. 3:17.
FURROWS. Ps. 65:10; 129:3; Hos. 10:4; 12:11.
FURTHER. Ezra 8:36, they *f.* the people.
Job 38:11, hitherto shalt thou come, but no *f.*
Lu. 24:28, as though he would have gone *f.*
Acts 4:17, that it spread no *f.*
2 Tim. 3:9, they shall proceed no *f.*
See Mk. 5:35; Phil. 1:12, 25.
FURY. Gen. 27:44, till thy brother's *f.* turn.
Isa. 27:4, *f.* is not in me.
63:5, my *f.* uphold me.
Jer. 21:5, I will fight against thee in *f.*
25:15, the wine cup of this *f.*
Ezek. 21:17, I will cause my *f.* to rest.
See Dan. 3:13, 19; 8:6; 9:16; 11:44.

G

GAIN. Job 22:3, is it *g.* to him that thou makest thy ways perfect?
Prov. 1:19; 15:27; Ezek. 22:12, greedy of *g.*
3:14, the *g* thereof better than gold.
28:8, by usury and unjust *g.*
Ezek. 22:13, 27, at thy dishonest *g.*
Dan. 11:39, he shall divide the land for *g.*
Mic. 4:13, consecrate their *g.* to the Lord.
Mat. 16:26; Mk. 8:36; Lu. 9:25, if he *g.* the world.
18:15, thou hast *g.* thy brother.
25:17, 22, had also *g.* other two.
Lu. 19:15, 16, 18, had *g.* by trading.
Acts 16:19, hope of their *g.* was gone.
19:24, no small *g.* to the craftsmen.
1 Cor. 9:19, that I might *g.* the more.
20, that I might *g.* the Jews.
2 Cor. 12:17, 18, did I make a *g.* of you?
Phil. 1:21, to die is *g.*
3:7, *g.* to me, I counted loss.
1 Tim. 6:5, supposing that *g.* is godliness.
6, godliness with contentment is great *g.*
See Judg. 5:19; Job 27:8; Jas. 4:13.
GAINSAY. Lu. 21:15; Tit. 1:9; Jude 11.
GALL. Ps. 69:21; Lam. 3:19; Mat. 27:34; Acts 8:23.
GALLOWS. Esth. 7:10, they hanged Haman on the *g.*
GAP. Ezek. 13:5; 22:30.
GARDEN. Gen. 2:8, God planted a *g.* eastward in Eden.
13:10, as the *g.* of the Lord.
Deut. 11:10; 1 Kings 21:2, as a *g.* of herbs.
Cant. 4:12, a *g.* enclosed.
16, blow upon my *g.*
5:1, I am come into my *g.*
6:2, 11, gone down into his *g.*
Isa. 1:8, as a lodge in a *g.*
30, as a *g.* that hath no water.
51:3, her desert like the *g.* of the Lord.
Isa. 58:11; Jer. 31:12, like a watered *g.*
61:11, as the *g.* causeth things sown to spring forth.
Jer. 29:5, plant *g.*, and eat the fruit.
Ezek. 28:13, in Eden the *g.* of God.
31:8, 9, cedars in the *g.* of God.
36:35, is become like the *g.* of Eden.
Joel 2:3, land as the *g.* of Eden before them.
John 18:1, where was a *g.*
26, did not I see thee in the *g.*
19:41, there was a *g.*, and in the *g.*
See Gen. 2:15; Amos 4:9; 9:14; John 20:15.
GARMENT. Gen. 39:12, he left his *g.*, and fled.
49:11, washed his *g.* in wine.
Josh. 7:21, a goodly Babylonish *g.*
9:5, Gibeonites took old *g.*
2 Kings 5:26, is it a time to receive *g.*?
7:15, all the way was full of *g.*
Job 37:17, how thy *g.* are warm.
Ps. 22:18, they part my *g.* among them.
102:26; Isa. 50:9; 51:6; Heb. 1:11, wax old as a *g.*
104:2, with light as with a *g.*
6, coveredst it with the deep as with a *g.*
109:18, clothed himself with cursing as with his *g.*
Prov. 20:16, take his *g.* that is surety.
25:20, a *g.* in old weather.
30:4, who hath bound the waters in a *g.*?
Eccl. 9:8, let thy *g.* be always white.
Isa. 52:1, put on thy beautiful *g.*
61:3, *g.* of praise for spirit of heaviness.
10, the *g.* of salvation.
Joel 2:13, rend your heart and not your *g.*
Zech. 13:4, a rough *g.* to deceive.
Mat. 9:16; Mk. 2:21; Lu. 5:36, new cloth, old *g.*
20:14, 36; Mk. 5:27; Lu. 8:44, hem of *g.*
21:8; Mk. 11:8, spread *g.* in way.
22:11, 12, wedding *g.*
23:5, enlarge borders of *g.*
27:35; Mk. 15:24, parted *g.*, casting lots.
Mk. 11:7; Lu. 19:35, cast *g.* on colt.
13:16, not turn back again to take *g.*
Lu. 22:36, let him sell his *g.*
24:4, in shining *g.*
Acts 9:39, showing the coats and *g.*
Jas. 5:2, your *g.* are motheaten.
Jude 23, the *g.* spotted by the flesh.
Rev. 3:4, not defiled their *g.*
16:15, that watcheth, and keepeth his *g.*
GARNER. Ps. 144:13; Joel 1:17; Mat. 3:12.
GARNISH. Job 26:13; Mat. 12:44; 23:29.
GATE. Gen. 28:17, the *g.* of heaven.
Deut. 6:9; 11:20, write them on the *g.*
Ps. 9:13, the *g.* of death.
118:19, the *g.* of righteousness.
Prov. 17:19, exalteth *g.* seeketh destruction.
31:23, her husband known in the *g.*
Isa. 26:2, open the *g.*, that righteous may enter.
38:10, the *g.* of the grave.
45:1, open the two leaved *g.*
60:11, thy *g.* shall be open continually.
18, walls Salvation, and *g.* Praise.
Mat. 7:13; Lu. 13:24, strait *g.*, wide *g.*
16:18, *g.* of hell shall not prevail.
Heb. 13:12, also suffered without the *g.*
Rev. 21:25, *g.* not shut at all by day.
See Ps. 24:7; Isa. 28:6; Nah. 2:6.
GATHER. Gen. 41:35, let them *g.* all the food.
49:10, to him shall *g.* of the people be.
Ex. 16:17, *g.*, some more, some less.
Deut. 28:38, carry much out, and *g.* little in.
30:3; Ezek. 36:24, will *g.* thee from all nations.
2 Sam. 14:14, spilt which cannot be *g.* up.
Job 11:10, if he *g.* together, who can hinder?
Ps. 26:9, *g.* not my soul with sinners.
39:6, knoweth not who shall *g.* them.
Prov. 6:8, the ant *g.* her food.
10:5, he that *g.* in summer.
13:11, he that *g.* by labour shall increase.

Isa. 27:12, ye shall be *g.* one by one.
40:11, he shall *g.* the lambs.
56:8, yet will I *g.* others.
62:10, *g.* out the stones.
Mat. 3:12; Lu. 3:17, *g.* wheat into garner.
6:26, nor *g.* into barns.
7:16; Lu. 6:44, do men *g.* grapes of thorns?
12:30; Lu. 11:23, he that *g.* not scattereth.
13:28, wilt thou that we *g.* them up?
29, lest while ye *g.* up the tares.
41, shall *g.* out of his kingdom.
25:32, before him shall be *g.* all nations.
John 6:12, *g.* up fragments.
15:6, men *g.* them, and cast.
1 Cor. 16:2, that there be no *g.* when I come.
2 Thess. 2:1, by our *g.* together unto him.
See Mat. 23:37; John 4:36; 11:52.
GAVE. Gen. 3:12, the woman *g.* me.
Josh. 21:44; 2 Chron. 15:15; 20:30, Lord *g.* them rest.
1 Sam. 10:9, *g.* to Saul another heart.
Neh. 8:8., they read, and *g.* the sense.
Job 1:21, the Lord *g.*
Ps. 21:4, he asked life, and thou *g.* it.
68:11, the Lord *g.* the word.
Eccl. 12:7, to God who *g.* it.
Amos 2:12, ye *g.* the Nazarites wine.
Mat. 21:23; Mk. 11:28; Lu. 20:2, who *g.* thee this authority?
25:35, 42, ye *g.* me meat.
Lu. 15:16, no man *g.* unto him.
John 10:29, my Father, who *g.* them.
Acts 2:4, as the Spirit *g.* them utterance.
26:10, I *g.* my voice against them.
Rom. 1:28, God *g.* them over.
1 Cor. 3:6, God *g.* the increase.
Eph. 4:8, *g.* gifts unto men.
11, he *g.* some apostles.
See 2 Cor. 8:5; Gal. 1:4; Tit. 2:14.
GAY. Jas. 2:3.
GAZE. Ex. 19:21; Nah. 3:6; Acts 1:11; Heb. 10:33.
GENERATION. Deut. 1:35, not one of this evil *g.*
32:5, 20, a perverse and crooked *g.*
Ps. 14:5, God is in the *g.* of the righteous.
22:30, it shall be accounted for a *g.*
102:18, written for the *g.* to come.
145:4, one *g.* shall praise thy works.
Prov. 27:24, crown endure to every *g.*
30:11, there is a *g.* that curseth.
Eccl. 1:4, one *g.* passeth away.
Isa. 34:10, from *g.* to *g.* it shall lie waste.
Joel 1:3, children tell another *g.*
Mat. 3:7; 12:34; 23:33; Lu. 3:7, *g.* of vipers.
12:41, in judgment with this *g.*
17:17; Mk. 9:19; Lu. 9:41, perverse *g.*
23:36, shall come on this *g.*
24:34; Mk. 13:30; Lu. 21:32, this *g.* shall not pass.
Lu. 16:8, are in their *g.* wiser.
17:25, rejected of this *g.*
1 Pet. 2:9, a chosen *g.*
See Isa. 53:8; Dan. 4:3; Mat. 1:1; Lu. 11:30.
GENTILES. Mat. 10:5, go not in way of the *G.*
John 7:35, to the dispersed among *G.*
Acts 9:15, bear my name before the *G.*
13:42, *G.* besought that these words.
46, we turn to the *G.*
15:3, declaring conversion of the *G.*
18:6, from henceforth I will go to the *G.*
Rom. 3:29, is he not also of the *G.*
11:11, salvation is come to the *G.*
11:13, as the apostle of the *G.*
1 Cor. 5:1, not so much as named among *G.*
Eph. 4:17, walk not as other *G.*
2 Tim. 1:11, I am ordained a teacher of *G.*
3 John 7, taking nothing of the *G.*
See Rom. 2:9; 1 Pet. 2:12; Rev. 11:2.
GENTLE. 1 Thess. 2:7, we were *g.* among you.
2 Tim. 2:24, servant of Lord be *g.*
Tit. 3:2, *g.*, showing all meekness.
Jas. 3:17, wisdom is pure and *g.*
1 Pet. 2:18, not only to the good and *g.*
See 2 Sam. 18:5; 22:36; Gal. 5:22.
GETTETH. Prov. 3:13; 4:7; 19:8; Jer. 17:11.
GIFT. Ex. 23:8; Deut. 16:19, a *g.* blindeth.
2 Sam. 19:42, hath he given us any *g.*?
2 Chron. 19:7, with the Lord no taking of *g.*
Ps. 68:18; Eph. 4:8, *g.* unto men.
72:10, kings of Sheba and Seba offer *g.*
Prov. 6:35, not content, though many *g.*
15:27, he that hateth *g.* shall live.
17:8, a *g.* is as a precious stone.
18:16, man's *g.* maketh room for him.
21:14, a *g.* in secret pacifieth anger.
Eccl. 3:13; 5:19, enjoy good, it is God's *g.*
7:7, a *g.* destroyeth the heart.
Isa. 1:23, every one loveth *g.*
Mat. 5:23, bring thy *g.* to the altar.
24, leave thy *g.* before the altar.
7:11; Lu. 11:13, know how to give good *g.*
Lu. 21:1, casting *g.* into treasury.
John 4:10, if thou knewest the *g.* of God.
Acts 8:20, though the *g.* of God may be purchased.
Rom. 1:11, some spiritual *g.*
5:15, free *g.*, *g* by grace.
6:23, the *g.* of God is eternal life.
11:29, *g.* of God without repentance.
12:6, *g.* differing according to grace.
1 Cor. 7:7, his proper *g.* of God.
12:4, diversities of *g.*
31, covet best *g.*
14:1, 12, desire spiritual *g.*
2 Cor. 9:15, unspeakable *g.*
Eph. 2:8, faith the *g.* of God.
Phil. 4:17, not because I desire a *g.*
1 Tim. 4:14, neglect not the *g.*
2 Tim. 1:6, stir up the *g.*
Jas. 1:17, good and perfect *g.*
See Num. 18:29; Mat. 15:5; Acts 2:38; 10:45; 1 Cor. 13:2.
GIRD. 2 Sam. 22:40; Ps. 18:39, hast *g.* me with strength.
Isa. 45:5, I *g.* thee, though thou has not.
Joel 1:13, *g.* yourselves, and lament.
Eph. 6:14, having your loins *g.*
See Prov. 31:17; John 13:4; 21:18; Rev. 15:6.
GIRDLE. Ex. 28:4, and a *g*
Jer. 13:1, go and get thee a linen *g.*
See Isa. 11:5; Mat. 3:4; Mk. 1:6.
GIRL. Joel 3:3; Zech. 8:5.
GIVE. Gen. 28:22, I will *g.* the truth.
Ex. 30:15, rich shall not *g.* more, poor not *g.* less.
Deut. 15:10, thou shalt *g.* him thine heart.
16:17; Ezek. 46:5, *g.* as he is able.
1 Chron. 29:14, of thine own have we *g.* thee.
Ezra 9:9, to *g.* us a reviving.
Ps. 2:8, I shall *g.* thee the heathen.
6:5, in the grave who shall *g.* thanks?
29:11, Lord will *g* strength.
37:4, *g.* thee the desires of thy heart.
21, the righteous showeth mercy, and *g.*
84:11, Lord will *g.* grace and glory.
109:4, I *g.* myself unto prayer.
Prov. 23:26, *g.* me thine heart.
Isa. 55:10, *g.* seed to the sower.
Mat. 5:42, *g.* to him that asketh.
6:11; Lu. 11:3, *g.* daily bread.
7:9, will he *g.* him a stone?
10:8, freely *g.*
13:11; Mk. 4:11, it is *g.* to you to know.
16:26; Mk. 8:37, *g.* in exchange.
19:21; Mk. 10:21, go sell, and *g.* to the poor.
20:23; Mk. 10:40, not mine to *g.*
26:9; Mk. 14:5, sold and *g.* to the poor.
Lu. 6:38, *g.* and it shall be *g.*
John 4:7, 10, *g.* me to drink.
6:37, all that the Father *g.* me.
65, no man can come, except it were *g.* him.
10:28, I *g.* to them eternal life.

John 13:29, that he should *g.* something to poor.
14:27, not as the world *g.*, *g.* I.
Acts 3:6, such as I have *g.* I thee.
6:4, we will *g.* ourselves to prayer.
20:35, more blessed to *g.*
Rom. 12:8, he that *g.*, let him do it.
19, rather *g.* place until wrath.
1 Cor. 3:7, God *g.* the increase.
2 Cor. 9:7, *g.* not grudgingly, a cheerful *g.*
Phil. 4:15, concerning *g.* and receiving.
1 Tim. 4:13, *g.* attendance to reading.
15, *g.* thyself wholly to them.
6:17, who *g.* us richly.
Jas. 1:5, that *g.* to all men liberally.
4:6, *g.* more grace, *g.* grace to humble.
2 Pet. 1:5, *g.* all diligence.
See Mk. 12:15; Lu. 12:48; John 3:34.
GLAD. Ex. 4:14, he will be *g.* in heart.
Job 3:22, *g.* when they can find the grave.
Ps. 16:9, therefore my heart is *g.*
34:2; 69:32, humble shall hear, and be *g.*
46:4, make *g.* the city of God.
101:15, maketh *g.* the heart of man.
122:1, I was *g.* when they said.
126:3, whereof we are *g.*
Prov. 10:1; 15:20, wise son maketh a *g.* father.
24:17, let not thine heart be *g.*
Lam. 1:21, they are *g.* that thou hast done it.
Lu. 15:32, make merry, and be *g.*
John 8:56, saw my day, and was *g.*
11:15, I am *g.* for your sakes.
Acts 11:23, when he had seen grace of God, was *g.*
See Mk. 6:20; 12:37; Lu. 1:19; 8:1.
GLADNESS. Num. 10:10, in day of your *g.*
Deut. 18:47, servedst not with *g.* of heart.
Neh. 8:17, there was very great *g.*
Ps. 4:7, thou hast put *g.* in my heart.
45:7; Heb. 1:9, the oil of *g.*
97:11, *g.* is sown for the upright.
Isa. 35:10; 51:11, they shall obtain joy, and *g.*
Acts 2:46, did eat with *g.* of heart.
12:14, opened not for *g.*
14:17, filling our hearts with food and *g.*
See Ps. 100:2; Prov. 10:28; Isa. 51:3.
GLASS. 1 Cor. 13:12, we see through a *g.* darkly.
2 Cor. 3:18, beholding as in a *g.* the glory of the Lord.
Rev. 4:6; 15:2, a sea of *g.*, like unto crystal.
GLEAN. Lev. 19:10; Jer. 6:9; 49:9.
GLISTERING. 1 Chron. 29:2; Lu. 9:29.
GLITTERING. Deut. 32:41; Job 20:25; 39:23; Nah. 3:3.
GLOOMINESS. Joel 2:2; Zeph. 1:15.
GLORIFY. Lev. 10:3, before all people I will be *g.*
Ps. 50:23, whoso offereth praise *g.* me.
86:9, all nations shall *g.* thy name.
12, I will *g.* thy name for evermore.
Isa. 24:15, *g.* the Lord in the fires.
60:7, I will *g.* house of my glory.
Ezek. 28:22, I will be *g.* in midst of thee.
Dan. 5:23, God hast thou not *g.*
Mat. 5:16, *g.* your Father in heaven.
15:31, they *g.* God of Israel.
Lu. 4:15, being *g.* of all.
John 7:39, because Jesus was not yet *g.*
11:4, that the Son of God might be *g.*
12:16, but when Jesus was *g.*, they remembered.
28, Father, *g.* thy name: I have both *g.*
13:32, God shall also *g.* him.
15:8, herein is my Father *g.*
17:1, *g.* thy Son.
4, I have *g.* thee on earth.
21:19, by what death he should *g.* God.
Rom. 1:21, they *g.* him not as God.
8:17, suffer with him, that we may be *g.*
30, them he also *g.*
1 Cor. 6:20, *g.* God in body and spirit.
Gal. 1:24, they *g.* God in me.
2 Thess. 1:10, to be *g.* in his saints.
Heb. 5:5, so Christ *g.* not himself.
See Isa. 25:5; Mat. 9:8; 15:31; Lu. 7:16.
GLORIOUS. Ex. 15:11, *g.* in holiness.
Deut. 28:58; 1 Chron. 29:13, this *g.* name.
Ps. 45:13, all *g.* within.
66:2, make his praise *g.*
72:19, blessed be his *g.* name.
87:3, *g.* things are spoken.
Isa. 11:10, his rest shall be *g.*
28:1, whose *g.* beauty is a fading flower.
60:13, place of my feet *g.*
63:1, *g.* in his apparel.
14, to make thyself a *g.* name.
Jer. 17:12, a *g.* high throne.
Dan. 11:16, 41, stand in the *g.* land.
45, in the *g.* holy mountain.
Lu. 13:17, rejoiced for *g.* things done.
Rom. 8:21, *g.* liberty of children of God.
2 Cor. 3:7, 8, ministration *g.*
4:4, light of *g.* gospel.
Eph. 5:27, a *g.* church.
Phil. 3:21, like to his *g.* body.
1 Tim. 1:11, the *g.* gospel of the blessed God.
Tit. 2:13, the *g.* appearing of the great God.
See Ex. 15:1; 2 Sam. 6:20; Isa. 24:23.
GLORY. Ex. 33:18, show me thy *g.*
Num. 14:21; Ps. 72:19; Isa. 6:3, earth filled with *g.*
Ps. 8:1, thy *g.* above the heavens.
16:9, my *g.* rejoiceth.
24:7, 10, the King of *g.*
73:24, afterward receive me to *g.*
84:11, will give grace and *g.*
108:1, will give praise with my *g.*
145:11, the *g.* of thy kingdom.
Prov. 3:35, the wise shall inherit *g.*
17:6, the *g.* of children are their fathers.
20:29, the *g.* of young men is their strength.
25:2, *g.* of God to conceal.
27, for men to search their own *g.* is not *g.*
Isa. 10:2, where will ye leave your *g.*?
24:16, even *g.* to the righteous.
42:8, my *g.* will I not give to another.
43:7, have created him for my *g.*
60:7, will glorify house of my *g.*
Jer. 2:11, my people have changed their *g.*
Ezek. 20:6, 15, the *g.* of all lands.
31:18, to whom art thou thus like in *g.*?
Dan. 2:37; 7:14, God hat given power and *g.*
Hos. 4:7, change *g.* into shame.
Hag. 2:7, I will fill this house with *g.*
Mat. 6:2, that ye may have *g.* of men.
29; Lu. 12:27, Solomon in all his *g.*
16:27; Mk. 8:38, in *g.* of his Father.
19:28; Lu. 9:26, Son of man sit in his *g.*
24:30; Mk. 13:26; Lu. 21:27, power and great *g.*
Lu. 2:14; 19:38, *g.* to God in the highest.
9:31, appeared in *g.*, and spake of his decease.
9:32, they saw his *g.*
24:26, to enter into his *g.*
John 1:14, we beheld his *g.*
2:11, thus did Jesus, and manifested his *g.*
8:50, I seek not mine own *g.*
17:5, the *g.* I had with thee.
24, that they may behold my *g.*
Acts 12:23, he gave not God the *g.*
Rom. 3:23, come short of the *g.* of God.
8:18, not worthy to be compared with *g.*
11:36; Gal. 1:5; 2 Tim. 4:18; Heb. 13:21; 1 Pet. 5:11, to whom be *g.*
1 Cor. 2:8, crucified the Lord of *g.*
10:31, do all to *g.* of God.
11:7, woman is the *g.* of the man.
15, long hair, it is a *g.* to her.
15:40, *g.* of celestial, *g.* of terrestrial.
43, raised in *g.*
2 Cor. 3:18, beholding as in a glass the *g.*
4:17, eternal weight of *g.*

Eph. 1:17, the Father of *g.*
3:21, to him be *g.* in the church.
Phil. 3:19, whose *g.* is in their shame.
4:19, according to his riches, in *g.*
Col. 1:27, Christ in you, the hope of *g.*
3:4, appear with him in *g.*
2 Thess. 1:9, the *g.* of his power.
1 Tim. 3:16, received up into *g.*
Heb. 1:3, the brightness of his *g.*
2:10, in bringing many sons to *g.*
3:3, this man was counted worthy of more *g.*
1 Pet. 1:8, joy unspeakable and full of *g.*
11, the *g.* that should follow.
24, the *g.* of man as flower of grass.
4:14, the spirit of *g.* and of God.
5:10, called to eternal *g.*
2 Pet. 1:17, voice from the excellent *g.*
Rev. 4:11; 5:12, worthy to receive *g.*
7:12, blessing, and *g.*, and wisdom.
18:1, earth lightened with his *g.*
21:23, *g.* of God did lighten it.
See Lu. 17:18; 2 Cor. 3:18; Jas. 2:1; Jude 25.
GLORYING. 1 Cor. 5:6; 9:15; 2 Cor. 7:4; 12:11.
GNASH. Mat. 8:12; 13:42; 22:13; 24:51; 25:30; Lu. 13:28, *g.* of teeth.
Mk. 9:18, he foameth, and *g.* with his teeth.
See Job 16:9; Ps. 35:16; Acts 7:54.
GNAT. Mat. 23:234.
GO. Gen. 32:26, let me *g.*, for the day breaketh.
Ex. 14:15; Job 23:8, *g.* forward.
23:23; 32:34, angel shall *g.* before thee.
33:15, presence *g.* not with me.
Ruth 1:16, whither thou *g.*, I will *g.*
Ps. 139:7, whither shall I *g.*?
Prov. 22:6, the way he should *g.*
30:29, three things which *g.* well.
Mat. 5:41, to *g.* a mile, *g.* twain.
21:30, I *g.* sir, and went not.
Lu. 10:37, *g.* and do likewise.
John 14:12, I *g.* to the Father.
See Mt. 8:9; Lu. 7:8; 1 Cor. 9:7; Rev. 14:4.
GOATS. Job 39:1, the wild *g.* of the rock.
GOD. Gen. 5:22; 6:9, walked with *G.*
16:13, thou *G.* seest me.
32:28, hath power with *G.*
48:21, I die, but *G.* shall be with you.
Num. 23:19, *G.* is not a man, that he should lie.
23, what hath *G.* wrought?
Deut. 3:24, what *G.* is there that can do.
33:27, the eternal *G.* is thy refuge.
1 Sam. 17:46, may know there is a *G.* in Israel.
1 Kings 18:21, if the Lord be *G.*, follow him.
39, he is the *G.*, he is the *G.*
Job 22:13; Ps. 73:11, how doth *G.* know?
Ps. 14:1; 53:1, hath said, there is no *G.*
22:1; Mat. 27:46, my *G.*, my *G.*, why hast.
56:9, this I know, for *G.* is for me.
86:10; Isa. 37:16, thou art *G.* alone.
Eccl. 5:2, *G.* is in heaven.
Isa. 44:8, is there a *G*, beside me?
45:22; 46:9, I am *G.*, there is none else.
Hos. 11:9, I am *G*, and not man.
Amos 5:27, whose name is the *G*, of hosts.
Jon. 1:6, arise, call upon thy *G.*
Mic. 6:8, walk humbly with thy *G.*
Mat. 1:23, *G*, with us.
22:32, *G*, is not *G.* of dead.
Mk. 12:32, one *G.*, and none other.
John 3:33, that *G.* is true.
4:24, *G.* is a spirit.
13:3, come from *G.*, and went to *G.*
20:17, ascend to my *G.* and your *G.*
Rom. 3:4, let *G.* be true.
8:31, if *G.* be for us.
1 Cor. 1:9; 19:13, *G.* is faithful.
14:25, that *G.* is in you.
33, *G.* is not author of confusion.
Gal. 3:20, but *G.* is none.
6:7, *G.* is not mocked.
2 Thess. 2:4, above all that is called *G.*
1 Tim. 3:16, *G.* manifest in the flesh.
Heb. 8:10, I will be to them a *G.*
11:16, not ashamed to be called their *G.*
11:23, but ye are come to *G.*
1 John 1:5, *G.* is light.
4:8, 16, *G.* is love.
12, no man hath seen *G.*
5:19, we know that we are of *G.*
Rev. 21:3, *G.* himself shall be with them.
4, *G.* shall wipe away all tears.
7, I will be his *G.*
See Job 33:12; 36:5; Ps. 10:4; 33:12.
GOD *(an idol)*. Gen. 31:30, stolen my *g.*
Ex. 32:1, make us *g.*, which shall go before us.
4, these be thy *g.*
Judg. 5:8, they chose new *g.*
6:31, if he be a *g.*, let him plead.
10:14, go and cry to the *g.* ye have chosen.
17:5, Micah had a house of *g.*
18:24, ye have taken away my *g.*
2 Kings 17:29, every nation made *g.*
33, they feared the Lord, and served own *g.*
Isa. 44:15, maketh a *g.* and worshippeth it.
45:20, pray to a *g.* that cannot save.
Jon. 1:5, cried every man to his *g.*
Acts 12:22, the voice of a *g.*, not a man.
14:11, the *g.* are come down.
1 Cor. 8:5, there be *g.* many.
See Ex. 12:12; 20:23; Jer. 2:11; Dan. 3:28.
GODDESS. 1 Kings 11:5; Acts 19:27, 35, 37.
GODHEAD. Acts 17:29; Rom. 1:20; Col. 2:9.
GODLINESS. 1 Tim. 3:16, the mystery of *g.*
4:7, exercise thyself to *g.*
8, *g.* is profitable.
6:3, doctrine according to *g.*
5, supposing that gain is *g.*
2 Tim. 3:5, a form of *g.*
Tit. 1:1, the truth which is after *g.*
2 Pet. 1:3, pertain to life and *g.*
6, and to patience *g.*
3:11, in all holy conversation, and *g.*
See 1 Tim. 2:2, 10; 6:6, 11.
GODLY, Ps. 12:1, the *g.* man ceaseth.
Mal. 2:15, seek a *g.* seed.
2 Cor. 1:12, in *g.* sincerity.
7:9, 10, *g.* sorrow worketh repentance.
2 Tim. 3:12, all that will live *g.* in Christ.
Tit. 2:12, live *g.* in this world.
Heb. 12:28, reverence and *g.* fear.
2 Pet. 2:9, how to deliver the *g.*
3 John 6, bring forward after a *g.* sort.
See Ps. 4:3; 32:6; 2 Cor. 7:9; 11:2.
GOD SAVE THE KING. 2 Sam. 16:16, Hushai said unto Absalom, *G.*
GOING. Josh. 23:14, I am *g.* the way of all the earth.
2 Sam. 5:24; 1 Chron. 14:15, sound of *g.* in trees.
Job 33:24, 28, from *g.* down to pit.
Ps. 17:5, hold up my *g.*
40:2, establish my *g.*
Prov. 5:21, pondereth all his *g.*
20:24, man's *g.* are of the Lord.
Dan. 6:14, laboured till *g.* down of the sun.
Mic. 5:2, whose *g.* forth have been from of old.
Mat. 26:46, rise, let us be *g.*
Rom. 10:3, *g.* about to establish.
1 Tim. 5:24, *g.* before to judgment.
See Prov. 7:27; 14:15; Isa. 59:8; Hos. 6:3.
GOLD. Num. 31:22, only *g.*, etc., that may abide fire.
Deut. 8:13, when thy *g.* is multiplied.
17:17, nor shall he greatly multiply *g.*
1 Kings 20:3, silver and *g.* is mine.
Job 22:24, then shalt thou lay up *g* as dust.
28:1, a vein for silver, a place for *g.*
19, wisdom not valued with *g.*

Job 31:24, if I made *g.* my hope.
Ps. 19:10, more to be desired than *g.*
21:3, thou settest a crown of pure *g.* upon his head.
Prov. 25:11, like applies of *g.*
Isa. 46:6, they lavish *g.* out of the bag.
60:17, for brass I will bring *g.*
Hag. 2:8, the silver is mine, and the *g.* is mine.
Zech. 4:2, behold, a candlestick all of *g.*
13:9, try them as *g.* is tried.
Mal. 10:9, provide neither *g.* nor silver.
Acts 3:6, silver and *g.* have I none.
17:29, not think Godhead like to *g.*
20:33, coveted no man's *g.*
2 Tim. 2:20, in great house not only vessels of *g*
Jas. 2:2, man with a *g.* ring.
5:3, your *g.* is cankered.
1 Pet. 1:7, trial more precious than of *g.*
18, not redeemed with *g.*
Rev. 3:18, buy of me *g.* tried in the fire.
21:18, city was pure *g.*
See Gen. 2:11; Eccl. 12:6; Isa. 13:12.
GONE. Deut. 23:23, that which is *g.* out of thy lips.
1 Kings 20:40, busy here and there, he was *g.*
Ps. 42:4, I had *g.* with the multitude.
73:2, my feet were almost *g.*
77:8, mercy clean *g.* for ever.
103:16, wind passeth, and it is *g.*
109:23, I am *g.* like the shadow.
119:176; Isa. 53:6, *g.* astray like sheep.
Eccl. 8:10, come and *g.* from place of the holy.
Jer. 15:9, sun *g.* down while yet day.
Mat. 12:43; Lu. 11:24, spirit *g.* out.
25:8, lamps are *g.* out.
Mk. 5:30; Lu. 8:46, virtue had *g.* out of him.
John 12:19, the world is *g.* after him.
Acts 16:19, hope of their gains *g.*
Rom. 3:12, they are all *g.* out of the way.
Jude 11, *g.* in the way of Cain.
See Ps. 89:34; Cant. 2:11; Isa. 45:23.
GOOD (*n.*). Gen. 14:21, take the *g.* to thyself.
24:10, the *g.* of his master in his hand.
50:29, God meant it unto *g.*
Neh. 5:19; 13:31, think upon me for *g.*
Job 2:10, shall we receive *g.*
22:21, thereby *g.* shall come.
Ps. 4:6, who will show us any *g.*?
14:1; 53:1; Rom. 3:12, none doeth *g.*
34:12, loveth days that he may see *g.*
39:2, held my peace even from *g.*
86:17, a token for *g*
Prov. 3:27, withhold not *g*
Eccl. 3:12, I know there is no *g.* in them.
5:11, when *g.* increase.
9:18, destroyeth much *g.*
Mat. 12:29; Mk. 3:27, spoil his *g.*
24:27, ruler over all his *g.*
26:24, has been *g.* for that man.
Lu. 6:30, of him that taketh away thy *g*
12:19, much *g.* laid up.
15:12, the portion of *g.*
16:1, accused that he had wasted his *g.*
19:8, half of my *g.* I give.
Acts 10:38, went about doing *g.*
Rom. 8:28, work together for *g.*
13:4, minister of God for *g.*
1 Cor. 13:3, bestow all my *g.* to feed.
Heb. 10:34, joyfully the spoiling of your *g.*
1 John 3:17, this world's *g.*
Rev. 3:17, rich and increased with *g.*
See Job 5:27; 7:7; Prov. 11:17; 13:21.
GOOD (*adj.*). Gen. 1:4, 10, 12, 18, 21, 25, 31, God saw it was *g.*
2:18, not *g.* that man should be alone.
27:46, what *g.* shall my life do me?
Deut. 2:4; Josh. 23:11, take *g.* heed.
1 Sam. 2:24, no *g.* report I hear.
12:23, I will teach you the *g.* way.
25:15, men were very *g.* to us.
Ezra 7:9; Neh. 2:8, the *g.* hand of God on him.
Neh. 9:20, thy *g.* spirit to instruct.
Ps. 34:8, taste and see that the Lord is *g.*
45:1, my heart is inditing a *g.* matter.
112:5, a *g.* man showeth favour.
119:68, thou are *g.*, and doest *g.*
145:9, the Lord is *g.* to all.
Prov. 12:25, a *g.* word maketh the heart glad.
15:23, in season, how *g.* is it
20:18, with *g.* advice make war.
22:1, a *g.* name rather to be chosen.
25:25, *g.* news from a far country.
Eccl. 6:12, who knoweth what is *g.*?
Isa. 55:2, eat ye that which is *g.*
Lam. 3:26, it is *g.* that a man hope.
27, *g.* that a man bear yoke.
Zech. 1:13, answered with *g.* words.
Mat. 5:13, it is *g.* for nothing.
7:11; Lu. 11:13, how to give *g.* gifts.
9:22; Lu. 8:48, be of *g.* comfort.
19:16, what *g.* thing shall I do?
17; Lu. 18:19, none *g.*, save one.
20:15, is thine eye evil because I am *g.*?
25:21, *g.* and faithful servant.
Mk. 9:50; Lu. 14:34, salt is *g.*, but.
Lu. 1:53, filled the hungry with *g.* things.
6:38, *g.* measure, pressed down.
10:42, chosen that *g.* part.
12:32, your Father's *g.* pleasure.
16:25, thou in thy lifetime receivedst *g.* things.
23:50, Joseph was a *g.* man, and a just.
John 1:46, can any *g.* thing come out of Nazareth?
2:10, kept *g.* wine until now.
7:12, some said, he is a *g.* man.
10:11, I am the *g.* shepherd.
33, for a *g.* work we stone thee not.
Rom. 7:12, the commandment holy, just, and *g.*
18, in my flesh dwelleth no *g.* thing.
12:2, that *g.* and perfect will of God.
14:21, it is *g.* neither to eat.
1 Cor. 7:26, this is *g.* for the present.
15:33, corrupt *g.* manners.
2 Cor. 9:8, abound in every *g.* work.
Gal. 6:6, communicate in all *g.* things.
Phil. 1:6, hath begun a *g.* work.
Col. 1:10, fruitful in every *g.* work.
1 Thess. 5:15; 3 John 11, follow that which is *g.*
21, hold fast that which is *g.*
1 Tim. 1:8, the law is *g.*
3:1, desireth a *g.* work.
4:4, every creature of God is *g.*
2 Tim. 3:3, despisers of *g.*
Tit. 2:7, a pattern in *g.* works.
14, zealous of *g.* works.
Heb. 6:5, tasted the *g.* work of God.
13:9, *g.* thing that the heart be established.
Jas. 1:17, every *g.* gift.
See 2 Thess. 2:17; Tit. 1:16; 3:8.
GOODLINESS. Isa. 40:6.
GOODLY. Gen. 49:21, giveth *g.* words.
Ex. 2:2, a *g.* child.
Deut. 8:12, when thou hast built *g.* houses.
1 Sam. 9:2, a choice young man, and a *g.*
16:12, ruddy, and *g.* to look to.
Ps. 16:6; Jer. 3:19, a *g.* heritage.
Zech. 11:13, a *g.* price I was prized at.
Mat. 13:45, *g.* pearls.
Jas. 2:2, a man in *g.* apparel.
See 1 Sam. 8:16; 1 Kings 20:3; Lu. 21:5.
GOODNESS. Ex. 33:19, make all my *g.* pass.
34:6, abundant in *g.* and truth.
Ps. 16:2, my *g.* extendeth not to thee.
23:6, *g.* and mercy shall follow.
27:13, believed to see the *g.* of the Lord.
31:19; Zech. 9:17, how great is thy *g.*
33:5, earth full of thy *g.*
65:11, crownest the year with thy *g.*

Ps. 145:7, the memory of thy *g*.
Prov. 20:6, proclaim every one his own *g*.
Hos. 6:4, your *g*. is as a morning cloud.
Rom. 2:4, the riches of his *g*.
11:22, the *g*. and severity of God.
See Neh. 9:25; Isa. 63:7; Gal. 5:22; Eph. 5:9.
GOSPEL. Rom. 2:16, according to my *g*.
2 Cor. 4:3, if our *g*. be hid.
Gal. 1:8, 9, any other *g*.
2:7, the *g*. of uncircumcision, *g*. of circumcision.
Col. 1:23, the hope of the *g*.
1 Tim. 1:11, *g*. of the blessed God.
Rev. 14:6, everlasting *g*.
See Mat. 4:23; Mk. 16:15; Acts 20:24.
GOURD. Jon. 4:6, and the Lord God prepared a *g*.
See Jon. 4:7, 9, 10.
GOVERNMENT. Isa. 9:6; 1 Cor. 12:28; 2 Pet. 2:10.
GRACE. Ps. 45:2, *g*. is poured into thy lips
Prov. 1:9, an ornament of *g*.
3:22, life to thy soul, and *g*. to thy neck.
34; Jas. 4:6, giveth *g*. to the lowly.
Zech. 4:7, crying, *g*., *g*. unto it.
12:10, spirit of *g*. and supplications.
John 1:14, full of *g*. and truth.
16, all received, and *g*. for *g*.
17, *g*. and truth came by Jesus Christ.
Acts 4:33, great *g*. was upon them all.
11:23, when he had seen the *g*.
14:3, the word of his *g*.
Rom. 1:7; 1 Cor. 1:3; 2 Cor. 1:2; Gal. 1:3; Eph. 1:2; Phil. 1:2; Col. 1:2; 1 Thess. 1:1; 2 Thess. 1:2; Philem. 3; 1 Peter 1:2; 2 Pet. 1:2; Rev. 1:4, *g*. and peace.
3:24, justified freely by his *g*.
4:4, not reckoned of *g*., but of debt.
5:2, access into this *g*.
17, abundance of *g*.
20, where sin abounded, *g*. did much more abound.
6:14, 15, under *g*.
11:5, the election of *g*.
2 Cor. 8:9, know the *g*. of our Lord.
9:8, able to make all *g*. abound.
12:9, my *g*. is sufficient.
Gal. 1:6, 15, who called you by his *g*.
5:4, ye are fallen from *g*.
Eph. 2:5, 8, by *g*. ye are saved.
3:8, to me is this *g*. given.
4:29, minister *g*. to hearers.
6:24, *g*. be with all that love our Lord.
Col. 4:6, let your speech be alway with *g*.
2 Thess. 2:16, good hope through *g*.
1 Tim. 1:2; 2 Tim. 1:2; Tit. 1:4; 2 John 3, *g*., mercy and peace.
Heb. 4:16, the throne of *g*.
10:29, despite to the Spirit of *g*.
12:28, *g*. to serve God acceptably.
13:9, heart established with *g*.
Jas. 1:11, the *g*. of the fashion of it.
4:6, he giveth more *g*.
1 Pet. 3:7, heirs of *g*.
5:5, giveth *g*. to the humble.
2 Pet. 3:18, grow in *g*.
Jude 4, turning *g*. of God into lasciviousness.
See Acts 20:24; 2 Cor. 6:1; Gal. 2:21.
GRACIOUS. Gen. 43:29, God be *g*. to thee.
Ex. 22:27, I will hear, for I am *g*.
33:19, I will be *g*. to whom I will be *g*.
Neh. 9:17, 31, ready to pardon, *g*., merciful.
Ps. 77:9, hath God forgotten to be *g*.?
Prov. 11:16, a *g*. woman retaineth honour.
Isa. 30:18, wait, that he may be *g*.
Amos 5:15, may be the Lord will be *g*.
Jon. 4:2, I know thou art a *g*. God.
Lu. 4:22, wondered at the *g*. words.
1 Pet. 2:3, tasted that the Lord is *g*.
See Ex. 34:6; 2 Chron. 30:9; Hos. 14:2.
GRAFT. Rom. 11:17, 19, 23, 24.
GRAIN. Mat. 13:31; 17:20; Mk. 4:31; Lu. 13:19; 17:6, *g*. of mustard seed.
See Amos 9:9; 1 Cor. 15:37.
GRANT. Ruth 1:9, *g*. that you may find rest.
1 Chron. 4:10, God *g*. him that which he requested.
Job 6:8, *g*. the thing I long for.
Mat. 20:21; Mk. 10:37, *g*. that my two sons.
Rev. 3:21, will I *g*. to sit with me.
See Ps. 20:4; 85:7; Acts 4:29.
GRAPE. Gen. 49:11, washed clothes in the blood of *g*.
Num. 6:3, nor eat moist *g*., or dried.
Deut. 23:24, then thou mayest eat *g* thy fill.
24:21, when thou gatherest the *g*. of thy vineyard.
32:14, drink the blood of the *g*.
Cant. 2:13, 15, vines with tender *g*.
Isa. 5:2, looked it should bring forth *g*.
17:6; 24:13, yet gleaning *g*.
Jer. 8:13, there shall be no *g*.
31:29, 20; Ezek. 18:2, have eaten a sour *g*.
Amos 9:13, treader of *g*. shall overtake.
See Lev. 19:10; 25:5; Lu. 6:4; Rev. 14:18.
GRASS. Deut. 32:2, as showers upon the *g*.
2 Kings 19:26; Ps. 129:6, as *g*. on housetops.
Ps. 72:6, like rain upon mown *g*.
90:5, like *g*. which groweth up.
102:4, 11, withered like *g*.
103:15, days are as *g*.
Isa. 40:6; 1 Pet. 1:24, all flesh is *g*.
Mat. 6:30; Lu. 12:28, if God so clothe the *g*.
See Prov. 27:25; John 6:10; Rev. 8:7; 9:4.
GRASSHOPPERS. Amos 7:1, and, behold, he formed *g*.
GRAVE (*n*.). Gen. 42:38; 44:31, with sorrow to the *g*.
Ex. 14:11, no *g*. in Egypt.
Num. 19:16, or a *g*.
Job 5:26, come to *g*. in full age.
7:9, he that goeth to the *g*.
14:13, hide me in the *g*.
17:1, the *g*. are ready for me.
13, if I wait, the *g*. is mine house.
33:22, his soul draweth near to the *g*.
Ps. 6:5, in the *g*. who shall give thee thanks?
31:17, let wicked be silent in the *g*.
49:14, like sheep laid in the *g*.
15; Hos. 13:14, the power of the *g*.
Eccl. 9:10, no wisdom in the *g*.
Isa. 38:18, the *g*. cannot praise thee.
53:9, made his *g*. with the wicked.
Hos. 13:14, O *g*., I will be thy destruction.
John 5:28, all in the *g*. shall hear.
11:31, she goeth to the *g*.
1 Cor. 15:55, O *g*., where is thy victory?
See Mat. 27:52; Lu. 11:44; Rev. 11:9; 20:13.
GRAVE (*v*.). Isa. 49:16, I have *g*. thee upon the palms.
Hab. 2:18, that the maker hat *g*. it.
See Ex. 28:9; 2 Chron. 2:7; 3:7.
GRAVE (*adj*.). 1 Tim. 3:8; Tit. 2:2.
GRAVEL. Prov. 20:17; Isa. 48:19; Lam. 3:16.
GRAVITY. 1 Tim. 3:4; Tit. 2:7.
GRAY. Ps. 71:18; Prov. 20:29; Hos. 7:9.
GREAT. Gen. 12:2; 18:18; 46:3, make a *g*. nation.
48:19, he also shall be *g*.
Deut. 29:24, the heat of his *g*. anger.
1 Sam. 12:24, consider how *g* things.
2 Kings 5:13, bid thee do some *g*. thing.
2 Chron. 2:5, the house is *g*., for *g*. is our God.
Neh. 6:3, I am doing a *g*. work.
Job 32:9, *g*. men not always wise.
36:18, a *g*. ransom.
Ps. 14:5; 53:5, there were they in *g*. fear.
19:11, there is *g*. reward.
31:19, how *g*. is thy goodness
92:5, how *g*. are thy works!
139:17, how *g*. is the sum of them!
Prov. 18:16, gift bringeth before *g*. men.
25:6, stand not in place of *g*. men.
Mat. 5:12, *g*. is your reward.
19, called *g*. in kingdom of heaven.

Mat. 13:46, pearl of *g.* price.
15:28, *g.* is thy faith.
20:26, whosoever will be *g.* among you.
22:36, 38, the *g.* commandment.
Lu. 10:2, the harvest is *g.*
16:26, a *g.* gulf fixed.
Acts 8:9, giving out he was some *g.* one.
19:28, 34, *g.* is Diana.
1 Tim. 3:16, *g.* is the mystery.
Heb. 2:3, so *g.* salvation.
12:1, so *g.* a cloud of witnesses.
Jas. 3:5, how *g.* a matter a little fire kindleth!
See Deut. 9:2; Eccl. 2:9; Rev. 7:9.
GREATER. Gen. 4:13, punishment *g.* than I can bear.
1 Chron. 11:9; Esth. 9:4, waxed *g.* and *g.*
Hag. 2:9, glory of latter house *g.*
Mat. 11:11; Lu. 7:28, *g.* than he.
12:6, one *g.* than the temple.
Mk. 12:31, no commandment *g.* than these.
John 1:50; 5:20; 14:12, shalt see *g.* things.
4:12; 8:53, art thou *g.* than our father?
10:29; 14:28, my Father is *g.* than all.
13:16; 15:20, servant not *g.* than his lord.
15:13, *g.* love hat no man.
1 Cor. 15:6, the *g.* part remain.
Heb. 6:13, he could swear by no *g.*
1 John 3:20, God is *g.* than our hearts.
4:4, *g.* is he in you than he in world.
3 John 4, no *g.* joy.
See Gen. 41:40; 48:19; Heb. 9:11.
GREATEST. Mat. 13:32, it is *g.* among herbs.
18:1, 4, who is *g.* in kingdom?
Mk. 9:34; Lu. 9:46, disputed who should be *g.*
1 Cor. 13:13, the *g.* of these is charity.
See Job 1:3; Jer. 31:34; Lu. 22:24.
GREATLY. 2 Sam. 24:10; 1 Chron. 21:8, I have sinned *g.*
1 Kings 18:3, Obadiah feared the Lord *g.*
Ps. 28:7, my heart *g.* rejoiceth.
47:9, God is *g.* exalted.
89:7, *g.* to be feared in the assembly.
116:10, I was *g.* afflicted.
Dan. 9:23; 1:11, thou art *g.* beloved.
Obad. 2, thou art *g.* despised.
Mk. 12:27, ye do *g.* err.
See Ps. 62:2; Mk. 9:15; Acts 3:11; 6:7.
GREATNESS. 1 Chron. 29:11, thine is the *g.*, power, and glory.
Ps. 145:3, his *g.* is unsearchable.
Prov. 5:23, in the *g.* of his folly.
Isa. 63:1, travelling in the *g.* of his power.
Eph. 1:19, the exceeding *g.* of his power.
See 2 Chron. 9:6; Ps. 66:3; 79:11; 150:2.
GREEDILY. Prov. 21:26; Ezek. 22:12.
GREEDINESS. Eph. 4:19.
GREEDY. Prov. 1:19; 15:27, *g.* of gain.
Isa. 56:11, they are *g.* dogs.
See Ps. 17:12; 1 Tim. 3:3.
GREEN. Lev. 23:14; Judg. 16:7; Lu. 23:31.
GRIEF. 2 Chron. 6:29, every one shall know his own *g.*
Job 6:2, Oh that my *g.* were weighed!
Ps. 31:10, life spent with *g.*
Eccl. 1:18, in much wisdom is much *g.*
Isa. 53:3, acquainted with *g.*
Jer. 10:19, this is a *g.*, and I must bear it.
See Jon. 4:6; Heb. 13:17; 1 Pet. 2:19.
GRIEVE. Gen. 6:6, it *g.* him at his heart.
45:5, be not *g.* that ye sold me.
1 Sam. 2:33, the man shall be to *g.* thine heart.
Ps. 78:40, they *g.* him in the desert.
95:10, forty years was I *g.*
Lam. 3:33, doth not willingly *g.*
Mk. 3:5, being *g.* for the hardness.
10:22, he went away *g.*
John 21:17, Peter was *g.*
Rom. 14:15, brother *g.* with meat.
Eph. 4:30, *g.* not the holy Spirit of God.
See Neh. 2:10; 13:8; Ps. 119:158; 139:21.
GRIEVOUS. Gen. 21:11, thing was *g.* in Abraham's sight.
Gen. 50:11, a *g.* mourning.
Ps. 10:5, his ways are always *g.*
Prov. 15:1, *g.* words stir up anger.
Isa. 15:4, his life shall be *g.*
Jer. 30:12; Nah. 3:19, thy wound is *g.*
Mat. 23:4; Lu. 11:46, burdens *g.* to be borne.
Phil. 3:1, to me is not *g.*
Heb. 12:11, chastening *g.*
1 John 5:3, commandments not *g.*
See Eccl. 2:17; Jer. 16:4; Acts 20:29.
GRIND. Isa. 3:15, *g.* faces of the poor.
Lam. 5:13, took young men to *g.*
Mat. 21:44; Lu. 20:18, it will *g.* him to powder.
See Eccl. 12:3; Mat. 24:41; Lu. 17:35.
GROAN. Ex. 2:24, God heard their *g.*
Job 24:12, men *g.* from out the city.
Joel 1:18, how do the beasts *g.*!
Rom. 8:23, we ourselves *g.*
2 Cor. 5:2, 4, in this we *g.*
See Job 23:2; Ps. 6:6; John 11:33, 38.
GROPE. Deut. 28:29; Job 5:14; 12:25; Isa. 59:10.
GROSS. Isa. 60:2; Jer. 13:16; Mat. 13:15; Acts 28:27.
GROUND. Ex. 3:5; Acts 7:33, holy *g.*
Job 5:6, nor trouble spring out of the *g.*
Isa. 35:7, parched *g.* become a pool.
Jer. 4:3; Hos. 10:12, break up fallow *g.*
Mat. 13:8; Lu. 8:8, good *g.*
Mk. 4:16, stony *g.*
Lu. 13:7, why cumbereth it the *g.*?
14:18, bought a piece of *g.*
19:44, lay thee even with the *g.*
John 8:6, he wrote on the *g.*
See Zech. 8:12; Mal. 3:11; John 12:24.
GROUNDED. Eph. 3:17; Col. 1:23.
GROW. Gen. 48:16, let them *g.* into a multitude.
2 Sam. 23:5, though he make it not to *g.*
Ps. 92:12, *g.* like a cedar.
Isa. 53:2, he shall *g.* up before him.
Hos. 14:5, he shall *g.* as the lily.
Mal. 4:2, *g.* up as calves of the stall.
Mat. 13:30, let both *g.* together.
Mk. 4:27, seed should *g.* up, he knoweth not.
Acts 5:24, whereunto this would *g*
Eph. 2:21, *g.* unto an holy temple.
4:15 may *g.* up into him.
2 Thess. 1:3, your faith *g.* exceedingly.
1 Pet. 2:2, that ye may *g.* thereby.
2 Pet. 3:18, *g.* in grace.
See 2 Kings 19:26; Jer. 12:2; Zech. 6:12.
GRUDGE. Lev. 19:18; 2 Cor. 9:7; Jas. 5:9; 1 Pet. 4:9.
GUESTS. Zeph. 1:7; Mat. 22:10; Lu. 19:7.
GUIDE. Ps. 25:9, meek will he *g.* in judgment.
32:8, I will *g.* thee with mine eye.
48:14, our *g.* even unto death.
73:24, *g.* me with thy counsel.
Prov. 6:7, having no *g.*, overseer, or ruler.
Isa. 58:11, the Lord shall *g.* thee.
Jer. 3:4, the *g.* of my youth.
Mat. 23:16, 24, ye blind *g.*
Lu. 1:79, *g.* our feet into the way of peace.
John 16:13, *g.* you into all truth.
See Gen. 48:14; Prov. 11:3; 23:19.
GUILE. Ps. 32:2, in whose spirit is no *g.*
34:13; 1 Pet. 3:10, keep lips from speaking *g.*
John 1:47, in whom is no *g.*
2 Cor. 12:16, I caught you with *g.*
1 Pet. 2:1, laying aside *g.*
22, nor was *g.* found in his mouth.
3:10, and his lips that they speak no *g.*
See Ex. 21:14; 1 Thess. 2:3; Rev. 14:5.
GUILTLESS. Ex. 20:7; Deut. 5:11, will not hold him *g.*
Josh. 2:19, we will be *g.*
2 Sam. 3:28, are *g.* of blood
Mat. 12:7, ye would not have condemned the *g.*
See Num. 5:31; 1 Sam. 26:9; 1 Kings 2:9.
GUILTY. Gen. 42:21, verily *g.* concerning our brother.
Ex. 34:7; Num. 14:18, by no means clear the *g.*

Lev. 5:3, when he knoweth of it, he shall be *g*.
Rom. 3:19, all the world *g*. before God.
1 Cor. 11:27, *g*. of the body and blood.
Jas. 2:10, he is *g*. of all.
See Num. 35:27; Prov. 30:10; Mat. 26:66.
GULF. Lu. 16:26.
GUSH. 1 Kings 18:28; Ps. 78:20; 105:41; Jer. 9:18.

H

HABITATION. Ex. 15:13, guided them to thy holy *h*.
2 Chron. 6:2, have built an house of *h*.
Ps. 26:8, have loved the *h*.
33:14, from the place of his *h*.
69:25, let their *h*. be desolate.
74:20, full of *h*. of cruelty.
89:14, justice and judgment the *h*. of thy throne.
107:7, 36, a city of *h*.
132:13, the Lord desired it for his *h*.
Prov. 3:33, he blesseth the *h*. of the just.
Isa. 32:18, dwell in a peaceable *h*.
Jer. 21:13, who shall enter into our *h*.
25:37, the peaceable *h*. are cut down.
Lu. 16:9, into everlasting *h*.
Eph. 2:22, an *h*. of God through the Spirit.
Jude 6, angels which left their own *h*.
See Prov. 8:31; Acts 1:20; 17:26; Rev. 18:2.
HAIL. Job 38:22, the treasures of the *h*.
Isa. 28:17, *h*. sweep away refuge of lies.
See Ex. 9:18; Josh. 10:11; Rev. 8:7; 11:19; 16:21.
HAIR. Gen. 42:38; 44:29, bring down gray *h*. with sorrow.
Judg. 20:16, sling stones at *h*. breadth.
Job 4:15, the *h*. of my flesh stood up.
Ps. 40:12, more than the *h*. of my head.
Mat. 3:4; Mk. 1:6, raiment of camel's *h*
5:36, make one *h*. white or black.
10:30, *h*. of head numbered.
1 Cor. 11:14, 15, long *h*., it is a shame.
1 Tim. 2:9, broided *h*.
1 Pet. 3:3, plaiting the *h*.
See 2 Sam. 14:26; Hos. 7:9; John 11:2; Rev. 1:14.
HALE. Lu. 12:58; Acts 8:3.
HALL. John 18:28, then led they Jesus from Caiaphas unto the *h*. of judgment.
33; 19:9, then Pilate entered into the judgment *h*.
See Acts 25:23.
HALLOW. Lev. 22:32, I am the Lord which *h*. you.
25:10, shall *h*. the fiftieth year.
Num. 5:10, every man's *h*. things.
1 Kings 9:3, I have *h*. this house.
Jer. 17:22; 24:27, but *h*. ye the sabbath day.
Ezek. 20:20; 44:24, and *h*. my sabbaths.
Mat. 6:9; Lu. 11:2, *h*. be thy name.
HALT. 1 Kings 18:21, how long *h*. ye?
Ps. 38:17, I am ready to *h*.
Jer. 20:10, my familiars watched for my *h*.
See Gen. 32:31; Mic. 4:6; Zeph. 3:19.
HAND. Gen. 16:12, *h*. against every man.
24:2; 47:29, put thy *h*. under my thigh.
27:22, the *h*. are the *h*. of Esau.
31:29, in the power of my *h*. to do you hurt.
Ex. 21:24; Deut. 19:21, *h*. for *h*., foot for foot.
33:22, cover with my *h*. while I pass.
Num. 11:23; Isa. 59:1, Lord's *h*, waxed short.
22:29, would there were sword in mine *h*.
Deut. 8:27, my *h*. hath gotten this wealth.
33:2, from right *h*. went fiery law.
Judg. 7:2, saying, my own *h*. hath saved me.
1 Sam. 5:11, *h*. of God was heavy.
6:9, not his *h*. that smote us, but a chance
12:3, of whose *h*. have I received any bribe?
19:5; 28:21, put his life in his *h*.
23:16, Jonathan strengthened his *h*. in God.
26:18, what evil is in mine *h*.?
2 Sam. 14:19, is not *h*. of Joab in this?
24:14; 1 Chron. 21:13, let us fall into *h*. of Lord.
1 Kings 18:44, cloud like a man's *h*.
2 Kings 5:11, strike his *h*. over the place.
1 Chron. 12:2, could use right *h*. and left.
Ezra 7:9; 8:18; Neh. 2:8, good *h*. of God.
10:19, they gave their *h* that they would
Neh. 2:18, strengthened their *h*. for work.
6:5, with open letter in his *h*.
Job 12:10, in whose *h*. is the soul.
19:21, the *h*. of God hath touched me.
40:14, that thine own *h*. can save.
Ps. 16:11, at right *h*. pleasures for evermore.
24:4, clean *h*. and pure heart.
68:31, stretch out her *h* unto God.
90:17, establish thou the work of our *h*.
137:5, let my right *h*. forget her cunning.
Prov. 3:16, in left *h*. riches and honour.
6:10; 24:33, folding of *h*. to sleep.
10:4, that dealeth with slack *h*.
11:21; 16:5, though *h*. join *h*.
12:24, *h*. of diligent shall bear rule.
19:24; 26:15, slothful man hideth his *h*.
22:26, be not of them that strike *h*.
Eccl. 2:24, this I saw was from *h* of God.
9:10, whatsoever thy *h*. findeth.
11:6, in evening withhold not thine *h*.
Isa. 1:12, who hath required this at your *h*.?
5:25; 9:12; 10:4; 14:27, his *h*. stretched out still.
14:26, this is the *h*. that is stretched out.
40:12, measured waters in hollow of *h*.
44:5, subscribe with his *h*. to the Lord.
53:10, pleasure of Lord shall prosper in his *h*.
56:2, keepeth his *h*. from evil.
Jer. 23:14, strengthen *h*. of evil doers.
33:13, shall pass under *h*. of him that telleth.
Lam. 2:4, with his right *h*. as adversary.
4:10, *h*. of pitiful women have sodden.
Ezek. 7:17; 21:7, all *h*. shall be feeble.
10:2, fill *h*. with coals of fire.
17:18, lo, he had given his *h*.
Dan. 4:35, none can stay his *h*.
Hos. 7:5, stretched out *h*. with scorners.
Mic. 7:3, do evil with both *h*. earnestly.
Zeph. 3:16, let not thine *h*. be slack.
Zech. 13:6, what are these wounds in thine *h*.?
Mat. 3:2; 4:17; 10:7, kingdom of heaven at *h*.
12; Lu. 3:17, whose fan is in his *h*.
6:3, let not left *h*. know.
18:8; Mk. 9:43, if thy *h*. or foot offend.
26:18, my time is at *h*.
46; Mk. 14:42, he is at *h*. that doth betray.
Mk. 14:62, sitting on right *h*. of power.
16:19, sat on right *h*. of God.
Lu. 9:44, delivered into *h*. of men.
John 10:28, nor pluck out of my *h*.
29, my Father's *h*.
20:27, reach hither thy *h*.
Acts 20:34, these *h*. have ministered.
2 Cor. 5:1, house not made with *h*.
Phil. 4:5, moderation be known, the Lord is at *h*.
1 Thess. 4:11, work with your own *h*.
2 Thess. 2:2, the day of Christ is at *h*.
1 Tim. 2:8, lifting up holy *h*.
Heb. 10:31, the *h*. of living God.
Jas. 4:8, cleanse your *h*.
1 Pet. 4:7, end of all things is at *h*.
1 John 1:1, our *h*. have handled of the Word.
See Isa. 49:16; Lu. 9:62; John 18:22; Col. 2:14.
HANDLE. Judg. 5:14, that *h*. pen of the writer.
Ps. 115:7, hands, but the *h*. not.
Prov. 16:20, that *h*. a matter wisely.
Jer. 2:8, they that *h*. the law.
Mk. 12:4, sent away shamefully *h*.
Lu. 24:39, *h*. me, and see.
2 Cor. 4:2, not *h*. word deceitfully.
Col. 2:21, taste not, *h*. not.
1 John 1:1, have *h*. of Word of life.
See Gen. 4:21; 1 Chron. 12:8; Ezek. 27:29.
HANDMAID. Ps. 86:16; 116:16; Prov. 30:23; Lu. 1:38.
HANG. Deut. 21:23; Gal. 3:13, he that is *h*. is accursed.

Job 26:7, *h.* the earth on nothing.
Ps. 137:2, we *h.* our harps upon the willows.
Mat. 18:6; Mk. 9:42; Lu. 17:2, millstone *h.* about neck.
22:40, on these *h.* the law and the prophets.
27:5, went and *h.* himself.
Heb. 12:12, lift up the hands which *h.* down.
See Gen. 40:22; Esth. 7:10; Lu. 23:39.
HAPLY. 1 Sam. 14:30; Mk. 11:13; Acts 5:39; 17:27.
HAPPEN. 1 Sam. 6:9, it was a chance that *h.*
Prov. 12:21, there shall not evil *h.* to the just.
Isa. 41:22, let them show us what shall *h.*
Jer. 44:23, therefore this evil is *h.*
Mk. 10:32, to tell what should *h.*
Lu. 24:14, talked of things that had *h.*
Rom. 11:25, blindness is *h.* to Israel.
1 Cor. 10:11, things *h.* for ensamples.
Phil. 1:12, things which *h.* to me.
1 Pet. 4:12, as though some strange thing *h.*
2 Pet. 2:22, it is *h.* according to proverb.
See Eccl. 2:14; 8:14; 9:11; Acts 3:10.
HAPPY. Gen. 30:13, *h.* am I.
Deut. 33:29, *h.* art thou.
Job 5:17, *h.* is the man whom God correcteth.
Ps. 127:5, *h.* is the man that hath quiver full.
128:2, *h.* shalt thou be.
144:15, *h.* is that people.
Prov. 3:13, 18, *h.* that findeth wisdom.
14:21, he that hath mercy, *h.* is he.
28:14, *h.* is the man that feareth alway.
Jer. 12:1, why are they *h.* that deal treacherously?
Mal. 3:15, now we call proud *h.*
John 13:17, if ye know, *h.* if ye do them.
Rom. 14:22, *h.* is he that condemneth not.
Jas. 5:11, we count them *h.* that endure.
1 Pet. 3:14; 4:14, *h.* are ye.
See Ps. 146:5; Prov. 29:18; 1 Cor. 7:40.
HARD. Gen. 18:14, is any thing too *h.* for the Lord?
Deut. 1:17; 17:8, cause that is too *h.*
15:18, it shall not seem *h.* to thee.
1 Kings 10:1; 2 Chron. 9:1, prove with *h.* questions
Job 41:24, *h.* as piece of nether millstone.
Prov. 13:15, the way of transgressors is *h.*
18:19, brother offended *h.* to be won.
Jer. 32:17, 27, there is nothing too *h.* for thee.
Ezek. 3:5, 6, to a people of *h.* language.
Mat. 25:24, thou art an *h.* man.
John 6:60, this is an *h.* saying.
Acts 9:5; 26:14, *h.* to kick against the pricks.
Heb. 5:11, many things *h.* to be uttered.
2 Pet. 3:16, things *h.* to be understood.
See Deut. 15:18; 2 Kings 2:10; Mk. 10:24.
HARDEN. Ex. 4:21; 7:3; 14:4, I will *h.* Pharoah's heart.
14:17, *h.* hearts of Egyptians.
Job 6:10, I would *h.* myself in sorrow.
9:4, who hath *h.* himself against him?
Prov. 21:29, a wicked man *h.* his face.
28:14, he that *h.* his heart.
29:1, he that being often reproved *h.* his neck.
Isa. 63:17, why hast thou *h.* our heart?
Mk. 6:52; 8:17, their heart was *h.*
John 12:40, he hath *h.* their heart.
Acts 19:9, when divers were *h.*
Rom. 9:18, whom he will he *h.*
Heb. 3:13, lest any of you be *h.*
See Deut. 15:7; 2 Kings 17:14; Job 39:16.
HARDLY. Gen. 16:6; Mat. 19:23; Mk. 10:23; Lu. 18:24.
HARDNESS. Mk. 3:5, grieved for *h.* of their hearts.
16:14, upbraided them for *h.* of heart.
2 Tim. 2:3, endure *h.*, as good soldier.
See Job 38:38; Mat. 19:8; Mk. 10:5; Rom. 2:5.
HARM. Lev. 5:16, make amends for *h.*
Num. 35:23, nor sought his *h.*
1 Sam. 26:21, I will no more do thee *h.*
2 Kings 4:41, no *h.* in the pot.
1 Chron. 16:22; Ps. 105:15, do prophets no *h.*
Prov. 3:30, if he have done thee no *h.*
Acts 16:28, do thyself no *h.*
Acts 28:5, he felt no *h.*
1 Pet. 3:13, who will *h.* you?
See Gen. 31:52; Jer. 39:12; Acts 27:21.
HARMLESS. Mat. 10:16; Phil. 2:15; Heb. 7:26.
HARP. 1 Sam. 16:16, cunning player on an *h.*
Ps. 49:4, dark sayings on the *h.*
137:2, hanged *h.* on the willows.
Isa. 5:12, *h.* and viol are in their feasts.
24:8, joy of the *h.* ceaseth.
1 Cor. 14:7, what is piped or *h.*, except they give.
Rev. 14:2, harping with their *h.*
See Gen. 4:21; Ezek. 26:13; Dan. 3:5.
HARROW. 2 Sam. 12:31; 1 Chron. 20:3; Job 39:10.
HART. Deut. 12:15, and as of the *h.*
1 Kings 4:23, besides *h.* and roebucks.
See Ps. 42:1; Isa. 35:6.
HARVEST. Gen. 8:22, *h.* shall not cease.
Ex. 23:16; 34:22, the feast of *h.*
Lev. 19:19; 23:10; Deut. 24:19, when ye reap *h.*
1 Sam. 12:17, is it not wheat *h.* to-day?
Job 5:5, whose *h.* the hungry eateth up.
Prov. 6:8, the ant gathereth food in *h.*
10:5, he that sleepeth in *h.*
25:13, cold of snow in time of *h.*
26:1, as rain in *h.*
Isa. 9:3, according to joy in *h.*
16:9, they *h.* is fallen.
18:4, dew in heat of *h.*
Jer. 5:17, they shall eat up thine *h.*
24, appointed weeks of *h.*
8:20, the *h.* is past, the summer ended.
51:33, the time of her *h.* shall come.
Joel 3:13; Rev. 14:15, the *h.* is ripe.
Mat. 9:37, the *h.* is plenteous.
38; Lu. 10:2, the Lord of the *h.*
13:30, in the time of *h.* I will say.
Mk. 4:29, putteth in sickle, because *h.* is come.
Lu. 10:2, the *h.* truly is great.
John 4:35, the fields are white to *h.*
See Josh. 3:15; Isa. 23:3; Mat. 13:39.
HASTE. Ex. 12:11, shall eat it in *h.*
1 Sam. 21:8, king's business required *h.*
Ps. 31:22; 116:11, I said in my *h.*
Prov. 19:2, he that *h.* with feet sinneth.
28:22, he that *h.* to be rich.
Isa. 51:14, captive exile *h.*
60:22, will *h.* it in his time.
Jer. 1:12, I will *h.* my word.
Zeph. 1:14, day of the Lord *h.* greatly.
See 2 Kings 7:15; Ps. 16:4; 55:8; Eccl. 1:5.
HASTILY. Prov. 20:21; 25:8.
HASTY. Prov. 14:29; 21:5; 29:20; Eccl. 5:2; 7:9.
HATE. Gen. 37:4, 5, 8, *h.* Joseph yet the more.
Lev. 19:17, shall not *h.* thy brother.
1 Kings 22:8; 2 Chron. 18:7, one man, but I *h.* him.
2 Chron. 19:2, and love them that *h.* the Lord.
Ps. 34:21, they that *h.* righteous shall be desolate.
97:10, ye that love the Lord, *h.* evil.
139:21, do not I *h.* them that *h.* thee?
Prov. 1:22, how long will ye *h.* knowledge?
13:24, he that spareth his rod *h.* his son.
14:20, the poor is *h.* of his neighbour.
15:10, he that *h.* reproof shall die.
27, he that *h.* gifts shall live.
Eccl. 2:17, I *h.* life.
3:8, a time to *h.*
Isa. 1:14, your feasts my soul *h.*
61:8, I *h.* robbery for burnt offering.
Amos 5:15, *h.* the evil, and love the good.
Mic. 3:2, who *h.* the good, and love the evil.
Zech. 8:17, these are things that I *h.*
Mal. 1:3; Rom. 9:13, I loved Jacob, and *h.* Esau.
Mat. 5:44; Lu. 6:27, do good to them that *h.* you.
6:24, either he will *h.* the one.
10:22; Mk. 13:13; Lu. 21:17, ye shall be *h.*
24:10, and shall *h.* one another.
Lu. 6:22, blessed are ye when men shall *h.* you.

Lu. 14:26, and *h.* not his father.
John 3:20, *h.* the light.
7:7, the world cannot *h.* you.
12:25, he that *h.* his life.
15:18; 1 John 3:13, marvel not if world *h.* you.
24, they have both seen and *h.*
Eph. 5:29, no man ever yet *h.* his own flesh.
1 John 2:9, 11; 3:15; 4:20, *h.* his brother.
See Gen. 27:41; Deut. 1:27; Prov. 6:16; Rev. 2:6.
HATEFUL. Ps. 36:2; Ezek. 23:29; Tit. 3:3.
HATERS. Ps. 81:15; Rom. 1:30.
HAUGHTY. 2 Sam. 22:28, thine eyes are upon the *h.*
Ps. 131:1, my heart is not *h.*
Prov. 16:18, a *h.* spirit before a fall.
21:24, proud and *h.* scorner.
Isa. 10:33, the *h.* shall be humbled.
Zeph. 3:11, no more be *h.* because.
See Isa. 2:11; 13:11; 24:4; Ezek. 16:50.
HAWK. Lev. 11:16, and the *h.* after his kind.
Job 39:26, doth the *h.* fly by wisdom?
HEAD. Gen. 3:15, it shall bruise thy *h.*
Josh. 2:19, blood be on his *h.*
Judg. 11:9, shall I be your *h.*?
2 Kings 2:3, take thy master from thy *h.* to-day.
4:19, he said, My *h.*, my *h.*
Ps. 24:7, 9, lift up your *h.*
66:12, caused men to ride over our *h.*
110:7, therefore shall he lift up the *h.*
141:5, oil, which shall not break my *h.*
Prov. 10:6, blessings on *h.* of the just.
11:26, on *h.* of him that selleth corn.
25:22; Rom. 12:20, coals of fire on his *h.*
Eccl. 2:14, a wise man's eyes are in his *h.*
Isa. 1:5, the whole *h.* is sick.
35:10; 51:11, everlasting joy upon their *h.*
58:5, to bow down *h.* as bulrush.
59:17; Eph. 6:17, helmet of salvation on *h.*
Jer. 9:1, Oh that my *h.* were waters.
14:3, 4, ashamed, and covered their *h.*
Dan. 3:38, thou art this *h.* of gold.
Amos 2:7, that pant after dust on *h.*
9:1, cut them in the *h.*
Zech. 1:21, no man did lift up his *h.*
4:7, the *h.*-stone with shoutings.
Mat. 5:36, neither swear by *h.*
27:39; Mk. 15:29, reviled, wagging their *h.*
Lu. 7:46, my *h.* thou didst not anoint.
21:18, not hair of *h.* perish.
28, then look up, and lift up your *h.*
John 13:9, also my hands and my *h.*
1 Cor. 11:3, the *h.* of every man is Christ.
4, dishonoureth his *h.*
10, woman to have power on her *h.*
Eph. 1:22; 4:15; Col. 1:18, the *h.* of the church.
5:23, husband is *h.* of wife.
Col. 2:19, not holding the *h.*
See Num. 6:5; Josh. 7:6; Acts 18:6; Rev. 13:1.
HEAL. Ex. 15:26, I am the Lord that *h.* thee.
Deut. 32:39, I wound, I *h.*
2 Kings 2:22, waters were *h.*
2 Kings 20:5, 8, I will *h.* the.
Ps. 6:2, O Lord, *h.* me.
41:4, *h.* my soul, for I have sinned.
103:3, who *h.* all thy diseases.
107:20, sent his word, and *h.* them.
Isa. 6:10, lest they convert and be *h.*
53:5, with his stripes we are *h.*
Jer. 6:14; 8:11, they have *h.* the hurt slightly.
15:18, wound refuseth to be *h.*
17:14, *h.* me, and I shall be *h.*
Lam. 2:13, who can *h.* thee?
Hos. 5:13, yet could he not *h.* thee.
6:1, he hath torn, and he will *h.* us.
14:4, I will *h.* their backslidings.
Mat. 8:7, I will come and *h.* him.
8:8, speak, and my servant shall be *h.*
10:1, to *h.* all manner of sickness.
Mat. 10:8; Lu. 9:2; 10:9, *h.* the sick.
12:10; Lu. 14:3, is it lawful to *h.* on sabbath?
Mk. 3:2; Lu. 6:7, whether he would *h.* on the sabbath day.
Lu. 4:18, to *h.* broken-hearted.
23, physician, *h.* thyself.
5:17, power of the Lord present to *h.*
John 5:47, that he would come and *h.*
5:13, he that was *h.* wist not.
Acts. 4:14, beholding the man which was *h.*
5:16, they were *h.* every one.
14:9, he had faith to be *h.*
Heb. 12:13, let it rather be *h.*
Jas. 5:16, pray that ye may be *h.*
1 Pet. 2:24, by whose stripes ye were *h.*
Rev. 13:3, his deadly wound was *h.*
See Eccl. 3:3; Isa. 3:7; Mat. 4:21; 14:14.
HEALING. Jer. 14:19, there is no *h.* for us.
Nah. 3:19, no *h.* of thy bruise.
Mal. 4:2, with *h.* in his wings.
Mat. 4:23, went about *h.* all.
Lu. 9:11, that had need of *h.*
1 Cor. 12:9, 28, 30, the gift of *h.*
Rev. 22:2, for the *h.* of the nations.
See Jer. 30:13; Lu. 9:6; Acts 4:22; 10:38.
HEALTH. 2 Sam. 20:9, art thou in *h.*, my brother?
Ps. 42:11; 43:5, the *h.* of my countenance.
67:2, thy saving *h.*
Prov. 3:8, *h.* to thy navel.
4:22, they are *h.* to all their flesh.
16:24, *h.* to the bones.
Isa. 58:8, thy *h.* shall spring forth.
Jer. 8:15, looked for a time of *h.*
22, why is not *h.* recovered?
3 John 2, mayest be in *h.*
See Gen. 43:28; Jer. 30:17; Acts 27:34.
HEAP. Deut. 32:23, *h.* mischiefs upon them.
Job 16:4, I could *h.* up words.
27:16, though he *h.* up silver.
Ps. 39:6, he *h.* up riches.
Prov. 25:22; Rom. 12:20, *h.* coals of fire.
Ezek. 24:10, *h.* on wood.
Hab. 1:10, they shall *h.* dust.
Mic. 3:12, Jerusalem shall become *h.*
2 Tim. 4:3, *h.* to themselves teachers.
Jas. 5:3, ye have *h.* treasure for last days.
See Judg. 15:16; Neh. 4:2; Eccl. 2:26.
HEAR. Ex. 6:12, how shall Pharaoh *h.* me?
1 Sam. 15:14, lowing of oxen which I *h.*
1 Kings 8:42, they shall *h.* of thy great name.
18:26, O Baal, *h.* us.
2 Kings 18:28; Isa. 36:13, *h.* words of the great king.
1 Chron. 14:15, when thou *h.* a sound of going.
Neh. 8:2, all that could *h.* with understanding.
Job. 31:35, Oh that one would *h.* me!
Ps. 4:1; 39:12; 54:2; 84:8; 102:1; 143;1; Dan. 9:17, *h.* my prayer.
3; 17:6; Zech. 10:6, the Lord will *h.*
10:17, cause thine ear to *h.*
49:1, *h.* this, all ye people.
59:7, who, say they, doth *h.*?
66:18, if I regard iniquity, the Lord will not *h.* me.
85:8, I will *h.* what God the Lord will speak.
102:20, *h.* groaning of the prisoner.
Prov. 13:8, the poor *h.* not rebuke.
18:13, answereth a matter before he *h.*
22:17, *h.* the words of the wise.
Eccl. 5:1, more ready to *h.* than give.
7:5, better to *h.* rebuke of wise.
12:13, *h.* conclusion of the whole matter.
Isa. 1:2, *h*, O heavens, and give ear.
15; Jer. 7:16; 11:14; 14:12; Ezek. 8:18, make many prayers, I will not *h.*
6:9; Mk. 4:12, *h.* but understand not.
29:18, shall deaf *h.* words of the book.
33:13, *h.*, ye that are afar off.
34:1, let the earth *h.*
42:20, opening ears, but he *h.* not.
55:3; John 5:25, *h.*, and your soul shall live.

Jer. 17:9, the *h.* is deceitful above all things.
20:9, in mine *h.* as a burning fire.
24:7, I will give them a *h.* to know me.
30:21, that engaged his *h.* to approach.
49:16; Obad. 3, pride of *h.* deceived thee.
Ezek. 11:19, take stony *h.*
18:31, make you a new *h.*
36:26, will give you a *h.* of flesh.
44:7; Acts 7:51, uncircumcised in *h.*
Dan. 1:8, Daniel purposed in his *h.*
Joel 2:13, rend your *h.*
Zech. 7:12, made *h.* as adamant.
Mal. 2:2, if ye will not lay it to *h.*
4:6, turn *h.* of fathers to children.
Mat. 5:8, blessed are the pure in *h.*
6:21; Lu. 12:34, there will your *h.* be also.
11:29, meek and lowly in *h.*
12:34; Lu. 6:45, out of abundance of the *h.*
15:19, out of the *h.* proceed evil thoughts.
18:35, if ye from your *h.* forgive not.
Mk. 2:8, why reason ye in your *h.*?
8:17, have ye your *h.* yet hardened?
10:5; 16:14, hardness of *h.*
Lu. 2:19, 51, kept them in her *n.*
21:14, settle it in your *h.*
24:25, slow of *h.* to believe.
32, did not our *h.* burn within us?
John 14:1, 27, let not your *h.* be troubled.
Acts 5:23; 7:54, were cut to the *h.*
11:23, with purpose of *h.*
Rom. 10:10, with the *h.* man believeth.
1 Cor. 2:9, neither have entered into *h.*
2 Cor. 3:3, in fleshy tables of the *h.*
5:12, glory in appearance, not in *h.*
Eph. 3:17, that Christ dwell in your *h.* by faith.
5:19, singing and making melody in your *h.*
6:6, doing will of God from the *h.*
Phil. 4:7, keep your *h.* and minds.
Col. 3:22, in singleness of *h.*
2 Thess. 3:5, direct your *h.* into love of God.
Heb. 4:12, discerner of intents of the *h.*
10:22, draw near with true *h.*
13:9, good that the *h.* be established.
Jas. 3:14, if ye have strife in your *h.*
4:8, purify your *h.*
1 Pet. 3:4, the hidden man of the *h.*
15, sanctify the Lord in your *h.*
See Ps. 57:7; 108:1; Col. 3:15; 2 Pet. 1:19.
HEARTH. Gen. 18:6; Ps. 102:3; Isa. 30:14; Jer. 36:22.
HEARTILY. Col. 3:23.
HEAT. Deut. 29:24, the *h.* of this great anger.
Ps. 19:6, nothing hid from *h.* thereof.
Eccl. 4:11, two together, then they have *h.*
Isa. 4:6; 25:4, a shadow from the *h.*
18:4, *h.* upon herbs, dew in *h.* of harvest.
49:10, neither shall *h.* smite them.
Hos. 7:4, as oven *h.* by the baker.
Mat. 20:12, burden and *h.* of the day.
Jas. 1:11, sun no sooner risen with burning *h.*
2 Pet. 3:10, melt with fervent *h.*
See Dan. 3:19; Lu. 12:55; Acts 28:3.
HEATH. Jer. 17:6; 48:6.
HEATHEN. Ps. 2:1; Acts 4:25, why do the *h.* rage?
8, give *h.* for inheritance.
102:15, the *h.* shall fear name of the Lord.
Ezek. 36:24, I will take you from among *h.*
Zech. 8:13, ye were a curse among the *h.*
Mat. 6:7, repetitions, as the *h.*
18:17, let him be as *h.* man.
See Lev. 25:44; Deut. 4:27; Neh. 5:8.
HEAVEN. Gen. 28:17, the gate of *h.*
Ex. 20:22, have talked with you from *h.*
Lev. 26:19, make your *h.* as iron.
Deut. 10:14; 1 Kings 8:27; Ps. 115:16, the *h.* and *h.* of heavens.
33:13, the precious things of *h.*
2 Kings 7:2, if the Lord make windows in *h.*
Job 15:15, the *h.* are not clean in his sight.
22:12, is not God in the height of *h.*?
Ps. 8:3, when I consider thy *h.*
14:2; 53:2, had looked down from *h.*
73:25, whom have I in *h.*?
89:6, who in *h.* can be compared to the Lord?
119:89, thy word is settled in *h.*
Prov. 8:27, when he prepared the *h.* I was there.
25:3, the *h.* for height.
Eccl. 5:2, for God is in *h.*
Isa. 13:13; Hag. 2:6, will shake the *h.*
40:12, meted out *h.* with the span.
65:17; Rev. 21:1, new *h.* and new earth.
Jer. 7:18, make cakes to queen of *h.*
23:24, do not I fill *h.* and earth?
31:37, if *h.* can be measured.
Ezek. 1:1; Mat. 3:16; Mk. 1:10, the *h.* were opened.
32:7, I will cover the *h.*
Dan. 7:13, with clouds of *h.*
Hag. 1:10, *h.* over you is stayed from dew.
Mal. 3:10, if I will not open windows of *h.*
Mat. 5:18, till *h.* and earth pass.
11:23, exalted to *h.*
24:29; Mk. 13:25, the powers of *h.*
Mk. 13:32, no, not the angels in *h.*
Lu. 15:18, I have sinned against *h.*
John 1:51, ye shall see *h.* open.
6:31, 32, bread from *h.*
Acts 4:12, none other name under *h.*
Rom. 1:18, wrath of God revealed from *h.*
2 Cor. 5:1, eternal in the *h.*
2, our house that is from *h.*
Gal. 1:8, though an angel from *h.* preach.
Eph. 1:10, gather in one, things in *h.*
3:15, whole family in *h.*
6:9; Col. 4:1, your master is in *h.*
Phil. 3:20, our conversation is in *h.*
Heb. 12:23, written in *h.*
1 John 5:7, three that bear record in *h.*
Rev. 4:1, door opened in *h.*
2, throne set in *h.*
8:1, silence in *h.*
12:1, 3, a great wonder in *h.*
See 2 Cor. 12:2; 1 Thess. 4:16; 2 Thess. 1:7.
HEAVENLY. Lu. 2:13, multitude of the *h.* host.
John 3:12, I tell you of *h.* things.
Acts 26:19, the *h.* vision.
1 Cor. 15:48, as is the *h.*, such are they.
Eph. 1:3; 2:6; 3:10, in *h.* places.
Heb. 3:1, partakers of the *h.* calling.
8:5; 9:23, shadow of *h.* things.
11:16, an *h.* country.
See 2 Tim. 4:18; Heb. 6:4; 12:22.
HEAVENLY FATHER. Mat. 6:14, your *h. f.* also will forgive you.
Lu. 11:13, how much more shall your *h. f.* give the Holy Spirit to them that ask him?
HEAVINESS. Ps. 69:20, I am full of *h.*
Prov. 12:25, *h.* in the heart maketh it stoop.
14:13, the end of that mirth is *h.*
Isa. 61:3, garment of praise for spirit of *h.*
Jas. 4:9, let your joy be turned to *h.*
See Ezra 9:5; Prov. 10:1; Rom. 9:2.
HEAVY. Ex. 17:12, Moses' hands were *h.*
1 Kings 14:6, sent with *h.* tidings.
Neh. 5:18, the bondage was *h.*
Job 33:7; Ps. 32:4, hand *h.*
Prov. 25:20, songs to a *h.* heart.
31:6, wine to those of *h.* heart.
Isa. 58:6, to undo the *h.* burdens.
Mat. 11:28, all ye that are *h.* laden.
23:4, they bind *h.* burdens.
26:37, he began to be very *h.*
43; Mk. 14:33, their eyes were *h.*
See Prov. 27:3; Isa. 59:1; Lu. 9:32.
HEDGE. Job 3:23, whom God hat *h.* in.
Prov. 15:19, way of slothful an *h.* of thorns.

Eccl. 10:8, whoso breaketh an *h.*
Lam. 3:7, he hath *h.* me about.
Hos. 2:6, I will *h.* up thy way.
Mk. 12:1, he set a *h.* about it.
Lu. 14:23, the highways and *h.*
See Isa. 5:5; Ezek. 13:5; 22:30; Nah. 3:17.
HEED. 2 Sam. 20:10, took no *h.* to the sword.
Ps. 119:9, by taking *h.* thereto.
Eccl. 12:9, preacher gave good *h.*
Isa. 21:7, hearkened diligently with much *h.*
Jer. 18:18, let us not give *h.*
1 Tim. 1:4; Tit. 1:14, neither give *h.* to fables.
4:1, giving *h.* to seducing spirits.
Heb. 2:1, give more earnest *h.*
See Prov. 17:4; Acts 3:5; 8:6.
HEEL. Gen. 3:15, thou shalt bruise his *h.*
Ps. 49:5, when the iniquity of my *h.* shall compass me about.
HEIGHT. Ps. 102:19, from *h.* of his sanctuary.
Prov. 25:3, the heaven for *h.*
Isa. 7:11, ask it either in the depth, or in the *h.* above.
Eph. 3:18, 19, the *h.* of the love of Christ.
See Job 22:12; Ps. 148:1; Amos 2:9.
HEIR 2 Sam. 14:7, we will destroy the *h.*
Prov. 30:23, handmaid that is *h.* to her mistress.
Mat. 21:38; Mk. 12:7; Lu. 20:14, this is the *h.*
Rom. 8:17, *h.* of God, joint-*h.* with Christ.
Gal. 3:29, *h.* according to the promise.
4:7, an *h.* of God through Christ.
Eph. 3:6, Gentiles fellow-*h.*
Tit. 3:7, *h.* according to hope of eternal life.
Heb. 1:14, who shall be *h.* of salvation.
6:17, the *h.* of promise.
11:7, *h.* of the righteousness.
Jas. 2:5, *h.* of the kingdom.
1 Pet. 3:7, as *h.* together of the grace.
See Jer. 49:1; Mic. 1:15; Rom. 4:13.
HELL. Deut. 32:22, fire shall burn to lowest *h.*
2 Sam. 22:6; Ps. 18:5, sorrows of *h.* compassed me.
Job. 11:8, deeper than *h.*
26:6, *h.* is naked before him.
Ps. 9:17, wicked turned into *h.*
16:19; Acts 2:27, not leave soul in *h.*
55:15, let them go down quick into *h.*
139:8, if I make my bed in *h.*
Prov. 5:5, her steps take hold on *h.*
7:27, house is the way to *h.*
9:18, her guests are in the depths of *h.*
15:11, *h.* and destruction before the Lord.
24, that he may depart from *h.* beneath.
23:14, deliver his soul from *h.*
27:20, *h.* and destruction are never full.
Isa. 14:9, *h.* from beneath is moved.
28:15, 18, with *h.* are we at agreement.
Ezek. 31:16, when I cast him down to *h.*
32:21, shall speak out of the midst of *h.*
Amos 9:2, though they dig into *h.*
Jon. 2:2, out of the belly of *h.*
Hab. 2:5, enlargeth his desire as *h.*
Mat. 5:22, in danger of *h.* fire.
29, 30, whole body cast into *h.*
10:28; Lu. 12:5, destroy soul and body in *h.*
11:23; Lu. 10:15, brought down to *h.*
16:18, gates of *h.* shall not prevail.
18:9; Mk. 9:47, having two eyes to be cast into *h.*
23:15, more the child of *h.*
33, now can ye escape the damnation of *h.*?
Lu. 16:23, in *h.* he lift up.
Acts 2:31, soul not left in *h.*
Jas. 3:6, tongue set on fire of *h.*
2 Pet. 2:4, cast angels down to *h.*
See Isa. 5:14; Rev. 1:18; 6:8; 20:13.
HELP. Gen. 2:18, 20, an *h.* meet for him.
Deut. 33:29, the shield of thy *h.*
2 Chron. 26:15, he was marvellously *h.*
Job 6:13, is not my *h.* in me?
Ps. 22:11, for there is none to *h.*
Ps. 33:20, he is our *h.* and our shield.
42:5, the *h.* of his countenance.
46:1, a very present *h.* in trouble.
60:11; 108:12, vain is the *h.* of man.
89:19, laid *h.* on one that is mighty.
121:1, the hills from whence cometh my *h.*
124:8, our *h.* is in the name of the Lord.
Isa. 10:3, to whom will ye flee for *h.*?
41:6, they *h.* every one his neighbour.
Hos. 13:9, in me is thine *h.*
Mat. 15:25, Lord, *h.* me.
Mk. 9:24, *h.* thou mine unbelief.
Acts 21:28, men of Israel, *h.*
26:22, having obtained *h.* of God.
Heb. 4:16, grace to *h.* in time of need.
See Isa. 31:3; Rom. 8:26; 2 Cor. 1:24.
HELPER. Heb. 13:6.
HEM Mat. 9:20, touched the *h.* of his garment.
14:36, might only touch the *h.* of his garment.
See Num. 15:38, 39; Mat. 23:5.
HEMLOCK. Hos. 10:4, judgment springeth up as *h.*
Amos 6:12, the fruit of righteousness into *h.*
HEN. Mat. 23:37; Lu. 13:34.
HENCEFORTH. 2 Cor. 5:15; Gal. 6:17; 2 Tim. 4:8.
HERITAGE. Job 20:29, *h.* appointed by God.
Ps. 16:6; Jer. 3:19, a goodly *h.*
61:5, the *h.* of those that fear.
127:3, children are an *h.* of the Lord.
Isa. 54:17, this is the *h.* of the servants.
Mic. 7:14, feed flock of thine *h.*
1 Pet. 5:3, lords over God's *h.*
See Joel 2:17; 3:2; Mal. 1:3.
HID. 2 Kings 4:27, the Lord hath *h.* it from me.
Job 3:21, more than for *h.* treasures.
Ps. 32:5, mine iniquity have I not *h.*
69:5, my sins are not *h.*
119:11, thy word have I *h.* in mine heart.
Zeph. 2:3, it may be ye shall be *h.*
Mat. 10:26; Mk. 4:22, there is nothing *h.*
Lu. 19:42, now they are *h.* from thine eyes.
1 Cor. 2:7, even the *h.* wisdom.
2 Cor. 4:3, if our gospel be *h.*
Col. 3:3, your life is *h.* with Christ.
1 Pet. 3:4, the *h.* man of the heart.
Rev. 2:17, to eat of the *h.* manna.
See Gen. 3:8; Mat. 5:14; Mk. 7:24.
HIDE. Gen. 18:17, shall I *h.* from Abraham.
Job 14:13, *h.* me in the grave.
34:29, when he *h.* his face.
Ps. 10:11, he *h* his face.
17:8, *h.* me under the shadow of thy wings.
27:5, *h.* me in pavilion.
31:20, *h.* them in secret of thy presence.
89:46, how long wilt thou *h.* thyself?
139:12, darkness *h.* not from thee.
Isa. 1:15, I will *h.* mine eyes from you.
3:9, they *h.* not their sin.
26:20, *h.* thyself for a little moment.
32:2, a man shall be as an *h.* place.
45:15, thou art a God that *h.* thyself.
Ezek. 28:3, no secret they can *h.* from thee.
Jas. 5:20, *h.* a multitude of sins.
Rev. 6:16, *h.* us from the face of him.
See Job 13:24; Prov. 28:28; Amos 9:3.
HIGH. Job 11:8, it is as *h.* as heaven.
22:12, behold stars, how *h.* they are!
41:34, he beholdeth all *h.* things.
Ps. 62:9, men of *h.* degree are a lie.
68:18, thou hast ascended on *h.*
103:11, as the heaven is *h.* above the earth.
131:1, in things too *h.* for me.
138:6, though the Lord be *h.*
139:6, it is *h.*, I cannot attain unto it.
Eccl. 12:5, afraid of that which is *h.*
Isa. 32:15, spirit poured on us from on *h.*
33:16, he shall dwell on *h.*
35:8, an *h.*-way shall be there.

Mk. 13:11, not ye that speak, but *H.* Ghost.
Lu. 1:15, shall be filled with the *H.* Ghost.
35, that *h.* thing which shall be born of thee.
3:22, *H.* Ghost descended in bodily shape.
4:1, Jesus being full of the *H.* Ghost.
12:12, *H.* Ghost shall teach you.
John 7:39, the *H.* Ghost was not yet given.
14:26, the Comforter, which is the *H.* Ghost.
17:11, *h.* Father keep those.
20:22, receive ye the *H.* Ghost.
Acts 1:8, after the *H.* Ghost is come.
2:4; 4:31, all filled with *H.* Ghost.
4:27, 30, against thy *h* child Jesus.
5:3, to lie to the *H.* Ghost.
6:3, look out men full of the *H.* Ghost.
7:51, ye do always resist the *H.* Ghost.
8:15, prayed that they might receive *H.* Ghost.
9:31, in comfort of the *H.* Ghost.
10:44, *H.* Ghost fell on all which heard.
47, received *H.* Ghost as well as we.
15:8, giving them *H.* Ghost, as he did unto us.
28, seemed good to the *H.* Ghost.
16:6, forbidden of the *H.* Ghost.
19:2, have ye received the *H.* Ghost?
20:28, *H.* Ghost hath made you overseers.
Rom. 1:2, promised in the *h.* scriptures.
7:12, commandment is *h.*, just, and good.
9:1, bearing witness in *H.* Ghost.
11:16, if the firstfruit be *h.*, if the root be *h.*
12:1, a living sacrifice, *h.* acceptable to God.
14:17, joy in the *H.* Ghost.
16:16; 1 Cor. 16:20; 2 Cor. 13:12; 1 Thess. 5:26; 1 Pet. 5:14, with a *h.* kiss.
1 Cor. 2:13, words which the *H.* Ghost teacheth.
3:17, the temple of God is *h.*
7:14, now are they *h.*
2 Cor. 13:14, communion of the *H.* Ghost.
Eph. 1:4; 5:27, be *h.* and without blame.
2:21, groweth to an *h.* temple in the Lord.
Col. 1:22, present you *h.* and unblameable.
3:12, elect of God, *h.* and beloved.
1 Thess. 5:27, all the *h.* brethren.
1 Tim. 2:8, lifting up *h.* hands.
2 Tim. 1:9, called us with an *h.* calling.
Tit. 1:8, bishop must be *h.*
3:5, the renewing of the *H.* Ghost.
Heb. 3:1, *h.* brethren, partakers.
1 Pet. 1:12, *H.* Ghost sent down from heaven.
15; 2 Pet. 3:11, *h.* in all conversation.
2:5, an *h.* priesthood.
3:5, the *h.* women, who trusted.
2 Pet. 1:18, with him in the *h.* mount.
21, *h.* men moved by *H.* Ghost.
Rev. 3:7, saith he that is *h.*
67:10, O lord, *h.* and true.
20:6, *h.* is he that hath part.
21:10, the *h.* Jerusalem.
22:11, he that is *h.*, let him be *h.*
See 2 Tim. 3:15; Heb. 2:4; 1 Pet. 1:16; 2 Pet. 3:2; Jude 20.
HOME. Ex. 9:19, and shall not be brought *h.*
Lev. 18:9, whether born at *h.* or abroad.
Deut. 24:5, free at *h.* one year.
Ruth 1:21, the Lord hath brought me *h.* empty.
2 Sam. 14:13, fetch *h.* his banished.
1 Kings 13:7, come *h.* with me.
2 Kings 14:10; 2 Chron. 25:19, tarry at *h.*
1 Chron. 13:12, bring ark of God *h.*
Job 39:12, he will bring *h.* thy seed.
Ps. 68:12, she that tarried at *h*
Eccl. 12:5, man goeth to this long *h.*
Lam. 1:20, at *h.* there is as death.
Hag. 1:9, when ye brought it *h.*
Mk. 5:19, go *h.* to thy friends.
John 19:27, took her to his own *h.*
20:10, went away to their own *h.*
1 Cor. 11:34, let him eat at *h.*
14:35, ask their husbands at *h.*
2 Cor. 5:6, at *h.* in the body.
1 Tim. 5:4, show piety at *h.*
Tit. 2:5, keepers at *h.*
See Jer. 2:14; LU. 9:61; 15:6.
HONEST. Lu. 8:15, an *h.* and good heart.
Acts 6:3, men of *h.* report.
Rom. 12:17; 2 Cor. 8:21, provide things *h.*
Rom. 13:13, let us walk *h.*, as in the day.
Phil. 4:8, whatsoever things are *h.*
1 Pet. 2:12, conversation *h.* among Gentiles.
See 1 Thess. 4:12; 1 Tim. 2:2; Heb. 13:18.
HONOUR (*n.*). Num. 22:17, I will promote thee to *h.*
24:11, hath kept thee back from *h.*
2 Sam. 6:22, of them shall I be had in *h.*
1 Kings 3:13, also given thee riches and *h.*
1 Chron. 29:18, died full of riches and *h.*
2 Chron. 1:11, 12, thou hast not asked *h.*
26:18, neither shall it be for thy *h.*
Esth. 1:20, the wives shall give their husbands *h.*
Job 14:21, his sons come to *h.*
Ps. 7:5, lay mine *h.* in the dust.
8:5; Heb. 2:7, crowned him with *h.*
26:8, place where thine *h.* dwelleth.
49:12, man being in *h.* abideth not.
96:6, *h.* and majesty are before him.
149:9, this *h.* have all his saints.
Prov. 3:16, in left hand riches and *h.*
4:8, she shall bring thee to *h.*
5:9, lest thou give their *h.* to others.
14:28, in multitude of people is king's *h.*
20:3, an *h.* to cease from strife.
25:2, the *h.* of kings to search out.
26:1, 8, *h.* is not seemly for a fool.
31:25, strength and *h.* are her clothing.
Eccl. 6:2, to whom God hath given *h.*
Mal. 1:6, where is mine *h.*?
Mat. 13:57; Mk. 6:4; John 4:44, not without *h.*
John 5:41, I receive not *h.* from men.
44, who receive *h.* one of another.
Rom. 2:7, in well doing seek for *h.*
10, *h.* to every man that worketh good.
12:10, in *h.* preferring one another.
13:7, *h.* to whom *h.*
2 Cor. 6:8, by *h.* and dishonour.
Col. 2:23, not in any *h.* to satisfying.
1 Thess. 4:4, possess his vessel in *h.*
1 Tim. 5:17, elders worthy of double *h.*
6:1, count masters worthy of *h.*
16, to whom be *h.* and power everlasting.
2 Tim. 2:20, 21, some to *h.*, some to dishonour.
Heb. 3:3, more *h.* than the house.
5:4, no man taketh this *h.* unto himself.
1 Pet. 3:7, giving *h.* to the wife.
Rev. 4:11; 5:12, thou art worthy to receive *h.*
See Rev. 5:13; 7:12; 19:1; 21:24.
HONOUR (*v.*). Ex. 14:4, I will be *h.* upon Pharaoh.
Ex. 20:12; Deut. 5:16; Mat. 15:4; 19:19; Mk. 7:10; 10:19; Lu. 18:20; Eph. 6:2, *h.* thy father and mother.
Lev. 19:32, thou shalt *h.* the face of the old man.
1 Sam. 2:30, them that *h.* me I will *h.*
15:30, *h.* me now before elders.
Esth. 6:6, the king delighteth to *h.*
Ps. 15:4, he *h.* them that fear the Lord.
Prov. 3:9, *h.* the Lord with thy substance.
12:9, better than he that *h.* himself.
Mal. 1:6, a son *h.* his father.
Mat. 15:8; Mk. 7:6, *h.* me with their lips.
John 5:23, *h.* the Son as they *h.* the Father.
1 Tim. 5:3, *h.* widows that are widows indeed.
1 Pet. 2:17, *h.* all men, *h* the king.
See Isa. 29:13; 58:13; Acts 28:10.
HONOURABLE. Ps. 45:9, among thy *h.* women.
Isa. 3:3, take away the *h.* man.
9:15, ancient and *h.*, he is the head.
42:21, magnify the law, and make it *h.*
See Lu. 14:8; 1 Cor. 4:10; 12:23; Heb. 13:4.
HOPE (*n.*). Job 7:6, my days are spent without *h.*

Job 8:13, the hypocrite's *h.* shall perish.
17:15, where is now my *h.*?
19:10, my *h.* hath he removed.
Ps. 16:9; Acts 2:26, my flesh also shall rest in *h.*
39:7, my *h.* is in thee.
119:116, let me not be ashamed of my *h.*
Prov. 13:12, *h.* deferred maketh the heart sick.
14:32, hath *h.* in his death.
26:12; 29:20, more *h.* of a fool.
Eccl. 9:4, to all the living there is *h.*
Jer. 17:7, the man whose *h.* the Lord is.
31:17, there is *h.* in thine end.
Hos. 2:15, for a door of *h.*
Zech. 9:12, ye prisoners of *h.*
Acts 28:20, for the *h.* of Israel I am bound.
Rom. 4:18, who against *h.* believed in *h.*
8:24, we are saved by *h.*
12:12, rejoicing in *h.*
1 Cor. 13:13, faith, *h.*, charity.
15:19, if in this life only we have *h.*
Eph. 1:18, the *h.* of his calling.
2:12, having no *h.*, and without God.
Col. 1:27, Christ in you, the *h.* of glory.
1 Thess. 4:13, even as others who have no *h.*
5:8, for an helmet, the *h.* of salvation.
2 Thess. 2:16, good *h.* through grace.
Tit. 3:7, the *h.* of eternal life.
Heb. 6:18, lay hold on *h.* set before us.
19, *h.* as an anchor of the soul.
1 Pet. 1:3, begotten to a lively *h.*
3:15, a reason of the *h.* that is in you.
See Lam. 3:18; Col. 1:5; 1 John 3:3.
HOPE (*v.*). Ps. 22:9, thou didst make me *h.*
31:24, all ye that *h.* in the Lord.
42:5, 11; 43:5, *h.* thou in God.
71:14, I will *h.* continually.
Lam. 3:26, good that a man both *h.* and wait.
Rom. 8:25, if we *h.* for that we see not.
1 Pet. 1:13, *h.* to the end.
See Jer. 3:23; Acts 24:26; Heb. 11:1.
HORRIBLE. Ps. 11:6; 40:2; Jer. 2:12; Ezek. 32:10.
HOSPITALITY. Rom. 12:13; 1 Tim. 3:2; Tit. 1:8; 1 Pet. 4:9.
HOT. Ps. 39:3; Prov. 6:28; 1 Tim. 4:2; Rev. 3:15.
HOUR. Mat. 10:19; Lu. 12:12, shall be given you in that same *h.*
20:12, have wrought but one *h.*
24:36; Mk. 13:32, that *h.* knoweth no man.
26:40; Mk. 14:37, could ye not watch one *h.*?
Lu. 12:39, what *h.* the thief would come.
22:53, but this is your *h.*
John 5:25; 16:32, the *h.* is coming, and now is.
11:9, are there not twelve *h.* in the day?
12:27, save me from this *h.*
Acts 3:1, at the *h.* of prayer.
Gal. 2:5, give place, no, not for an *h.*
Rev. 3:10, the *h.* of temptation.
See Acts 2:15; 1 Cor. 4:11; 15:30; Rev. 3:3.
HOUSE. Gen. 28:17, none other but the *h.* of God.
Deut. 8:12, when thou hast built goodly *h.*
2 Kings 20:1; Isa. 38:1, set thine *h.* in order.
20:15, what have they seen in thine *h.*?
Neh. 13:11, why is the *h.* of God forsaken?
Job 30:23, *h.* appointed for all living.
Ps. 26:8, have loved the habitation of thy *h.*
65:4, satisfied with goodness of thy *h.*
69:9; John 2:17, the zeal of thine *h.*
84:3, the sparrow hath found an *h.*
92:13, planted in the *h.* of the Lord.
118:26, blessed you out of the *h.* of the Lord.
Prov. 2:18, her *h.* inclineth to death.
9:1, wisdom hath builded her *h.*
12:7, *h.* of the righteous shall stand.
19:14, *h.* and riches are inheritance.
Eccl. 7:2, *h.* of mourning, *h.* of feasting.
12:3, when keepers of the *h.* shall tremble.
Isa. 3:14, spoil of poor in your *h.*
5:8, woe unto them that join *h.* to *h.*
64:11, our holy and beautiful *h.* is burned.
Hos. 9:15, I will drive them out of mine *h.*
Hag. 1:4, and this *h.* lie waste.
9, because of mine *h.* that is waste.
Mal. 3:10, that there may be meat in mine *h.*
Mat. 7:25; Lu. 6:48, beat upon that *h.*
10:12, when ye come into an *h.*
12:25; Mk. 3:25, *h.* divided cannot stand.
23:38, your *h.* is left desolate.
24:17; Mk. 13:15, to take anything out of *h.*
Lu. 10:7, go not from *h.* to *h.*
14:23, that my *h.* may be filled.
18:14, went down to his *h.* justified.
John 12:3, *h.* filled with odour.
14:2, in my Father's *h.* are many mansions.
Acts 2:46, breaking bread from *h.* to *h.*
5:42, in every *h.* ceased not to preach.
10:2; 16:34; 18:8, with all his *h.*
20:20, I taught you from *h.* to *h.*
1 Cor. 11:22, have ye not *h.* to eat in?
2 Cor. 5:1, *h.* not made with hands.
Col. 4:15, church in his *h.*
1 Tim. 3:4, 5, 12, ruleth well his own *h.*
5:8, especially for hose of his own *h.*
2 Tim. 3:6, which creep into *h.*
Tit. 1:11, subvert whole *h.*
See Mat. 9:6; Lu. 7:44; 19:5, Acts 4:34.
HOUSEHOLD. Gen. 18:19, command his *h.* after him.
1 Sam. 17:3; 2 Sam. 2:3, every man with his *h.*
2 Sam. 6:20, returned to bless his *h.*
Prov. 31:27, looketh well to her *h.*
Mat. 10:36, a man's foes shall be of his own *h.*
Gal. 6:10, the *h.* of faith.
Eph. 2:19, of the *h.* of God.
See Gen. 31:37; 47:12; 2 Sam. 17:23.
HUMBLE. Deut. 8:2, to *h.* thee and prove thee.
2 Chron. 33:12, *h.* himself greatly.
Ps. 9:12; 10:12, forgetteth not cry of the *h.*
34:2, the *h.* shall hear thereof.
35:13, I *h.* my soul with fasting.
113:6, *h.* himself to behold things in heaven.
Prov. 16:19, better be of *h.* spirit.
Isa. 57:15, of contrite and *h.* spirit.
Mat. 18:4; 23:12; Lu. 14:11; 18:14, *h.* himself.
Phil. 2:8, he *h.* himself.
Jas. 4:6; 1 Pet. 5:5, God giveth grace to the *h.*
1 Pet. 5:6, *h.* yourselves under mighty hand of God.
See Isa. 2:11; 5:15; Lam. 3:20.
HUMBLY. 2 Sam. 16:4; Mic. 6:8.
HUMILITY. Prov. 15:33; 18:12, before honour is *h.*
22:4, by *h.* are riches.
See Acts 20:19; Col. 2:18, 23; 1 Pet. 5:5.
HUNGER. Deut. 8:3, he suffered thee to *h.*
Job 18:12, his strength shall be *h.*-bitten.
Ps. 34:10, young lions do lack, and suffer *h.*
Prov. 19:15, an idle soul shall suffer *h.*
Isa. 49:10, shall not *h.* nor thirst.
Jer. 38:9, he is like to die for *h.*
Mat. 5:6; Lu. 6:21, blessed are ye that *h.*
Lu. 6:25, woe unto ye that are full! for ye shall *h.*
John 6:35, he that cometh to me shall never *h.*
Rom. 12:20, if thine enemy *h.*
1 Cor. 4:11, we both *h.* and thirst.
11:34, if any man *h.*, let him eat at home.
Rev. 7:16, they shall *h.* no more.
See Mat. 4:2; 12:1; 25:35; Lu. 15:17.
HUNGRY. Job 22:7, withholden bread from *h.*
24:10, they take away the sheaf from the *h.*
Ps. 50:12, if I were *h.*, I would not tell thee.
107:5, *h.* and thirsty, their soul fainted in them.
9, he filled the *h.* soul with goodness.
146:7, which giveth food to the *h.*
Prov. 25:21, if thine enemy be *h.*, give him bread to eat.
27:7, to the *h.* every bitter thing is sweet.
Isa. 29:8, when a *h.* man dreameth.
58:7, is it not to deal thy bread to the *h.*?
65:13, my servants eat, but ye shall be *h.*
Ezek. 18:7, given his bread to the *h.*

Lu. 1:53, he hath filled the *h.* with good things.
Acts. 10:10, and he became very *h.*
1 Cor. 11:21, one is *h.*, and another drunken.
Phil. 4:12, instructed both to be full and to be *h.*
See Prov. 6:30; Isa. 8:21; 9:20; Mk. 11:12.
HUNT. 1 Sam. 26:20, as when one doth *h.* a partridge.
Jer. 16:16, *h.* them from every mountain.
Ezek. 13:18, *h.* souls of my people.
Mic. 7:2, they *h.* every man his brother.
See Gen. 10:9; 27:5; 1 Sam. 24:11.
HUNTING. Prov. 12:27.
HURL. Num. 35:20; 1 Chron. 12:2; Job 27:21.
HURT. Ps. 15:4, that sweareth to his own *h.*
Eccl. 8:9, ruleth over another to his own *h.*
Isa. 11:9, shall not *h.* nor destroy.
Jer. 6:14; 8:11, have healed *h.* slightly.
8:21, for the *h.* of my people.
25:6, provoke not, I will do no *h.*
Dan. 3:25, they have no *h.*
6:23, no manner of *h.* found upon him.
Mk. 16:18, deadly thing, it shall not *h.*
Lu. 10:19, nothing shall by any means *h.* you.
Acts 18:10, no man set on thee to *h.* thee.
Rev. 6:6, *h.* not the oil and the wine.
See Rev. 7:2; 9:4; 11:5.
HURTFUL. Ezra 4:15; Ps. 144:10; 1 Tim. 6:9.
HUSBAND. Ex. 4:25, a bloody *h.* art thou.
Prov. 12:4, virtuous wife a crown to her *h.*
31:11, 23, 28, her *h.* doth safely trust.
Isa. 54:5, thy Maker is thy *h.*
John 4:16, go, call thy *h.*
1 Cor. 7:16, whether thou shalt save thy *h.*
14:35, let them ask their *h.* at home.
Eph. 5:22, submit yourselves to you *h.*
25; Col. 3:19, *h.*, love your wives.
1 Tim. 3:12, the *h.* of one wife.
Tit. 2:4, teach young women to love their *h.*
5, obedient to their own *h.*
1 Pet. 3:1, be in subjection to your *h.*
7, ye *h.*, dwell with them.
See Gen. 3:6; Ruth 1:11; Esth. 1:17, 20.
HYMN. Mat. 26:30; Mk. 14:26; Eph. 5:19; Col. 3:16.
HYPOCRISY. Mat. 23:28, within ye are full of *h.*
Mk. 12:15, he, knowing their *h.*
Lu. 12:1, leaven of Pharisees, which is *h.*
Jas. 3:17, wisdom is pure, and without *h.*
See Isa. 32:6; 1 Tim. 4:2
HYPOCRITE. Job 8:13, the *h.* hope shall perish.
20:5, the joy of the *h.* but for a moment.
36:13, the *h.* in heart.
Isa. 9:17, every one is an *h.*
Mat. 6:2, 5, 16, as the *h.* do.
7:5; Lu. 6:42; 13:15, thou *h.*
15:7; 16:3; 22:8; Mk. 7:6; Lu. 12:56, ye *h.*
23:13; Lu. 11:44, woe unto you, *h.*
24:51, appoint his portion with the *h.*
See Job 13:16; 27:8; Prov. 11:9.
HYPOCRITICAL. Ps. 35:16; Isa. 10:6.

I

IDLE. Ex. 5:8, 17, they be *i.*
Prov. 19:15, an *i.* soul shall hunger.
31:27, she eateth not bread of *i.*
Mat. 12:36, every *i.* word men speak.
20:3, 6, others standing *i.*
See Eccl. 10:18; Ezek. 16:49; 1 Tim. 5:13.
IDOL. 1 Chron. 16:26; Ps. 96:5, all gods of the people are *i.*
Isa. 66:3, as if he blessed an *i.*
Jer. 50:38, they are mad upon their *i.*
Hos. 4:17, Ephraim is joined to *i.*
Acts 15:20, abstain from pollutions of *i.*
1 Cor. 8:4, we know an *i.* is nothing.
7, with conscience of the *i.*
1 Thess. 1:9, ye turned to God from *i.*
1 John 5:21, keep yourselves from *i.*
See Acts 17:16; Gal. 5:20; Col. 3:5.
IGNORANCE. Acts 3:17, through *i.* ye did it.
Acts 17:30, the times of *i.* God winked at.
Eph. 4:18, alienated through *i.*
1 Pet. 2:15, put to silence *i.* of foolish men.
See Lev. 4:2, 13, 22, 27; 5:15; Num. 15:24.
IGNORANT. Ps. 73:22, so foolish was I and *i.*
Isa. 63:16, though Abraham be *i.* of us.
Acts 4:13, perceived they were *i.* men.
Rom. 10:3, being *i.* of God's righteousness.
1 Cor. 14:38, if any man be *i.*, let him be *i.*
2 Cor. 2:11, not *i.* of his devices.
Heb. 5:2, can have compassion on the *i.*
2 Pet. 3:5, they willingly are *i.*
See Num. 15:28; Acts 17:23; 1 Tim. 1:13.
IMAGINATION. Gen. 6:5; 8:21, *i.* of heart evil.
Deut. 29:19; Jer. 23:17, walk in *i.* of heart.
1 Chron. 28:9, understandeth all the *i.* of thoughts.
Rom. 1:21, vain in their *i.*
2 Cor. 10:5, casting down *i.*
See Deut. 31:21; Prov. 6:18; Lam. 3:60.
IMAGINE. Ps. 62:3, how long will ye *i.* mischief?
Nah. 1:9, what do you *i.* against the Lord?
11, there is one that *i.* evil.
See Job 21:27; Ps. 10:2; 21:11; Acts 4:25.
IMMORTAL. 1 Tim. 1:17.
IMMORTALITY. Rom. 2:7; 1 Cor. 15:53; 1 Tim. 6:16; 2 Tim. 1:10.
IMPART. Job 39:17; Lu. 3:11; Rom. 1:11; 1 Thess. 2:8.
IMPEDIMENT. Mk. 7:32.
IMPENITENT. Rom. 2:5.
IMPLACABLE. Rom. 1:31.
IMPOSE. Ezra 7:24; Heb. 9:10.
IMPOSSIBLE. Mat. 19:26; Mk. 10:27; Lu. 18:27, with men it is *i.*
Lu. 1:37; 18:27, with God nothing *i.*
See Mat. 17:20; Lu. 17:1; Heb. 6:4, 18; 11:6.
IMPOTENT. John 5:3; Acts 4:9; 14:8.
IMPOVERISH. Judg. 6:6; Isa. 40:20; Jer. 5:17.
IMPRISONMENT. Ezra 7:26; 2 Cor. 6:5; Heb. 11:36.
IMPUDENT. Prov. 7:13; Ezek. 2:4; 3:7.
IMPUTE. Lev. 17:4, blood shall be *i.* to that man.
Ps. 32:2; Rom. 4:8, to whom the Lord *i.* not iniquity.
Hab. 1:11, *i.* his power to his god.
Rom. 5:13, sin is not *i.* when there is no law.
See 1 Sam. 22:15; 2 Sam. 19:19; 2 Cor. 5:19.
INCLINE. Josh. 24:23, *i.* your hearts to the Lord.
1 Kings 8:58, that he may *i.* hearts to keep law.
Ps. 40:1; 116:2, he *i.* unto me, and heard my cry.
119:36, *i.* my heart to thy testimonies.
Jer. 7:24; 11:8; 17:23; 34:14, nor *i.* ear.
See Prov. 2:18; Jer. 25:4; 44:5.
INCLOSED. Ps. 17:10; 22:16; Lu. 5:6.
INCONTINENT. 1 Cor. 7:5; 2 Tim. 3:3.
INCORRUPTIBLE. 1 Cor. 9:25, an *i.* crown.
1 Pet. 1:4, inheritance *i.*
23, born of *i.* seed.
See Rom. 1:23; 1 Cor. 15:42, 50, 52, 53, 54.
INCREASE (*n.*). Lev. 25:36, take no usury or *i.*
26:4, the land shall yield her *i.*
Deut. 14:22, 28, tithe all *i.*
Ps. 67:6; Ezek. 34:27, earth shall yield her *i.*
Prov. 18:20, with the *i.* of his lips.
Eccl. 510, not satisfied with *i.*
Isa. 9:7, *i.* of his government.
1 Cor. 3:6, 7, God gave the *i.*
See Jer. 2:3; Eph. 4:16; Col. 2:19.
INCREASE (*v.*). Job 8:7, thy latter end shall greatly *i.*
Ps. 4:7, that their corn and wine *i.*
62:10, if riches *i.*, set not your heart upon them.
115:14, Lord shall *i.* you more and more.
Prov. 1:5; 9:9, a wise man will *i.* learning.
11:24, there is that scattereth, and yet *i.*
Eccl. 1:18, he that *i.* knowledge *i.* sorrow.
Isa. 9:3, multiplied the nation, and not *i.* the joy.
40:29, he *i.* strength.
Ezek. 36:37, *i.* them with men like a flock.
Dan. 12:4, knowledge shall be *i.*
Hos. 12:1, he daily *i.* lies.
Hab. 2:6, that *i.* that which is not his.
Lu. 2:52, Jesus *i.* in wisdom.

Judg. 17:6, no *k.* in Israel.
1 Sam. 8:5, now make us a *k.*
19, we will have a *k.*
10:24; 2 Sam. 16:16, God save the *k.*
Job 18:14, bring him to the *k.* of terrors.
34:18, is it fit to say to a *k.*?
Ps. 5:2; 84:3, my *K.* and my God.
10:16, the Lord is *K.* for ever.
20:9, let the *k.* hear us when we call.
74:12, God is my *K.* of old.
102:15, the *k.* of the earth shall fear.
Prov. 8:15, by me *k.* reign.
22:29, the diligent shall stand before *k.*
31:3, that which destroyeth *k.*
4, it is not for *k.* to drink wine.
Eccl. 2:12, what can the man do that cometh after the *k.*?
10:16, woe to thee when thy *k.* is a child!
20, curse not the *k.*
Isa. 32:1, a *k.* shall reign in righteousness.
33:17, thine eyes shall see the *k.* in his beauty.
49:23, *k.* shall be thy nursing fathers.
Jer. 10:10, the Lord is an everlasting *k.*
Mat. 22:11, when the *k.* came in to see the guests.
Lu. 19:38, blessed be the *K.* that cometh.
23:2, saying that he himself is Christ a *k.*
John 6:15, by force, to make him a *k.*
19:14, behold your *K*!
15, we have no *k.* but Caesar.
1 Tim. 1:17, now unto the *K.* eternal.
6:15, the *K.* of *k.* and Lord of lords.
Rev. 1:6; 5:10, made us *k.* and priests unto God.
15:3, thou *K.* of saints.
See Lu. 10:24; 1 Tim. 2:2; 1 Pet. 2:17.
KINGDOM. Ex. 19:6, a *k.* of priests.
1 Chron. 29:11; Mat. 6:13, thine is the k.
Ps. 22:28, the *k.* is the Lord's.
103:19, his *k.* ruleth over all.
145:12, the glorious majesty of his *k.*
Isa. 14:16, is this the man that did shake *k.*?
Dan. 4:3, his *k.* is an everlasting *k.*
Mat. 4:23; 9:35; 24:14, gospel of the *k.*
8:12, children of the *k.* cast out.
12:25; Mk. 3:24; Lu. 11:17, *k.* divided against itself.
13:38, good seed are children of the *k.*
25:34, inherit the *k.*
Lu. 12:32, Father's good pleasure to give you the *k.*
22:29, I appoint unto you a *k.*
John 18:36, my *k.* is not of this world.
Acts 1:6, wilt thou restore the *k.* to Israel?
1 Cor. 15:24, when he shall have delivered *up* the *k.*
Col. 1:13, into the *k.* of his dear Son.
2 Tim. 4:18, to his heavenly *k.*
Jas. 2:5, heirs of the *k.* he hath promised.
2 Pet. 1:11, entrance into everlasting *k.*
See Rev. 1:9; 11:15; 16:10; 17:17.
KISS. Ps. 85:10; Prov. 27:6; Lu. 7:38; Rom. 16:16.
KNEW. Gen. 28:16, the Lord is in this place, and I *k.* it not.
Jer. 1:5, before I formed thee I *k.* thee.
Mat. 7:23, I never *k* you, depart.
John 4:10, if thou *k.* the gift of God.
2 Cor. 5:21, who *k.* no sin.
See Gen. 3:7; Deut. 34:10; John 1:10; Rom. 1:21.
KNOW. 1 Sam. 3:7, Samuel did not yet *k.* the Lord.
1 Chron. 28:9, *k.* thou the God of thy father.
Job 5:27, *k.* thou it for thy good.
8:9, we are but of yesterday, and *k.* nothing.
13:23, make me to *k.* my transgression.
19:25, I *k.* that my redeemer liveth.
22:13; Ps. 73:11, how doth God *k.*?
Ps. 39:4, make me to *k.* mine end.
46:10, be still, and *k.* that I am God.
56:9, this I *k.*, for God is for me.
103:14, he *k.* our frame.
139:23, *k.* my heart.
Eccl. 9:5, the living *k.* they shall die.
11:9, *k.* that for all these things.
Isa. 1:3, the ox *k.* his owner.
Jer. 17:9, the heart is deceitful, who can *k.* it?
31:34; Heb. 8:11, *k.* the Lord, for all shall *k.* me.
Ezek. 2:5; 33:33, *k.* there hat h been a prophet.
Hos. 2:20, thou shalt *k.* the Lord.
7:9, yet he *k.* it not.
Mat. 6:3, let not thy left hand *k.*
13:11; Mk. 4:11; Lu. 8:10, given to you to *k.*
25:12, I *k.* you not.
Mk. 1:24; Lu. 4:34, I *k.* thee, who thou art.
Lu. 19:42, if thou hadst *k.*
22:57, 60, I *k.* him not.
John 7:17, he shall *k.* of the doctrine.
10:14, I *k.* my sheep, and am *k.* of mine.
13:7, *k.* not now, but shalt *k.* hereafter.
17, if ye *k.* these things.
35, by this shall all men *k.* ye are my disciples.
Acts 1:7, it is not for you to *k.*
Rom. 8:28, we *k.* that all things work.
1 Cor. 2:14, neither can he *k.* them.
13:9, 12, we *k.* in part.
Eph. 3:19, and to *k.* the love of Christ.
2 Tim. 1:12, I *k.* the love of Christ.
1:12, I *k.* whom I have believed.
3:15, thou hast *k.* the scriptures.
1 John 2:4, he that saith, I *k.* him.
3:2, we *k.* that when he shall appear.
Rev. 2:2, 9, 13, 19; 3:1, 8, I *k.* thy works.
See Mat. 6:8; 2 Tim. 2:19; 2 Pet. 2:9; Rev. 2:17.
KNOWLEDGE. 2 Chron. 1:10, 11, 12, give me *k.*
Job 21:14, 23 desire not *k.* of thy ways.
Ps. 94:10, he that teacheth man *k.*
139:6, such *k.* is too wonderful.
144:3, that thou takest *k.* of him.
Prov. 10:14, wise men lay up *k.*
14:6, *k.* is easy to him that understandeth.
17:27, he that hath *k.* spareth words.
24:5, a man of *k.* increaseth strength.
30:3, nor have the *k.* of the holy.
Eccl. 1:18, increaseth *k.* increaseth sorrow.
9:10, nor *k.* in the grave.
Isa. 11:2, the spirit of *k.*
40:14, who taught him *k.*?
53:11, by his *k.* justify many.
Dan. 1:17, God gave them *k.*
12:4, *k.* shall be increased.
Hos. 4:6, destroyed for lack of *k.*
Hab. 2:14, earth shall be filled with the *k.*
Lu. 11:52, taken away key of *k.*
Acts 4:13, took *k.* of them.
24:22, more perfect *k.* of that way.
Rom. 10:2, zeal of God, but not according to *k.*
1 Cor. 8:1, *k.* puffeth up.
13:8, *k.* shall vanish away.
15:34, some have not the *k.* of God.
Eph. 3:19, love of Christ, which passeth *k.*
Phil. 3:8, but loss for the *k.* of Christ.
Col. 2:3, treasures of wisdom and *k.*
1 Tim. 2:4; 2 Tim. 3:7, the *k.* of the truth.
Heb. 10:26, sin after we have received *k.*
2 Pet. 1:5, 6, to virtue *k.* and to *k.* temperance.
3:18, grow in grace and *k.*
See Gen. 2:9; 1 Sam. 2:3; Prov. 19:2; Hos. 4:1.

L

LABOUR (*n.*). Ps. 90:10, yet is their strength *l.* and sorrow.
104:23, goeth to his *l.* till evening.
Prov. 13:11, he that gathereth by *l.* shall increase.
14:23, in all *l.* there is profit.
Eccl. 1:8, all things are full of *l.*
2:22, what hath man of all his *l.*
6:7, all the *l.* of man is for his mouth.
John 4:38, are entered into their *l.*
1 Cor. 15:58, your *l.* is not in vain.
1 Thess. 1:3; Heb. 6:10, your *l.* of love.
Rev. 2:2, I know thy *l.* and patience.
14:13, rest from their *l.*
See Gen. 31:42; Isa. 58:3; 2 Cor. 6:5; 11:23.

LABOUR (*v.*). Ex. 20:9; Deut. 5:13, six days shalt thou *l.*
Neh. 4:21, so we *l.* in the work.
Ps. 127:1, they *l.* in vain.
144:14, our oxen may be strong to *l.*
Prov. 16:26, he that *l. l.* for himself.
23:4, *l.* not to be rich.
Eccl. 4:8, for whom do I *l.*?
5:12, the sleep of a *l.* man is sweet.
Mat. 11:28, all ye that *l.*
John 6:27, *l.* not for the meat which perisheth.
1 Cor. 3:9, we are *l.* together with God.
Eph. 4:28, but rather *l.*, working with his hands.
1 Thess. 5:12, which *l.*, among you.
1 Tim. 5:17, they who *l.* in word and doctrine.
See Mat. 9:37; 20:1; Lu. 10:2.
LACK. Mat. 19:20; Lu. 22:35; Acts 4:34.
LADEN, Isa. 1:4; Mat. 11:28; 2 Tim. 3:6.
LAMB. Isa. 5:17, the *l.* feed after their manner.
11:6, the wolf shall dwell with the *l.*
53:7; Jer. 11:19, as *l.* to the slaughter.
John 1:29, 36, behold the *L.* of God.
1 Pet. 1:19, as of a *l.* without blemish.
Rev. 5:6; 13:8, stood a *L.* slain.
12:11, by the blood of the *L.*
22:1, the throne of God and of the *L.*
See Isa. 40:11; Lu. 10:3; John 21:15.
LAME. Job 29:15; Prov. 26:7; Isa. 35:6; Heb. 12:13.
LAMENT. Mat. 11:17; John 16:20; Acts 8:2.
LAMP. Ps. 119:105; Prov. 13:9; Isa. 62:1; Mat. 25:1.
LAP. Judg. 7:6; Prov. 16:33.
LAST. Num. 23:10, let my *l.* end be like his.
Prov. 23:32, at the *l.* it biteth like a serpent.
Mat. 12:45; Lu. 11:26, *l.* state of that man.
19:30; 20:16; Mk. 10:31; Lu. 13:30, first shall be *l.*
John 6:39; 11:24; 12:48, the *l.* day.
See Lam. 1:9; 2 Tim. 3:1; 1 Pet. 1:5; 1 John 2:18.
LATTER. Job 19:25; Prov. 19:20; Hag. 2:9.
LAUGH. Prov. 1:26; Eccl. 3:4; Lu. 6:21; Jas. 4:9.
LAW. Josh. 8:34, all the words of the *l.*
Ps. 37:31, the *l.* of his God is in his heart.
40:8, thy *l.* is within my heart.
119:70, 77, 92, 174, I delight in thy *l.*
97:113, 163, 165, how I love thy *l.*
Prov. 13:14, the *l.* of the wise is a fountain of life.
Isa. 8:20, to the *l.* and to the testimony.
Mal. 2:6, the *l.* of truth was in his mouth.
Mat. 5:17, not come to destroy the *l.*
23:23, the weightier matters of the *l.*
John 7:51, doth our *l.* judge any man.
19:7 we have a *l.*, and by our *l.*
Rom. 2:14, are a *l.* unto themselves.
3:20, by the deeds of the *l.*
7:12, the *l.* is holy.
14, the *l.* is spiritual.
16; 1 Tim. 1:8, the *l.* is good.
8:3, what the *l.* could not do.
Gal. 3:24, the *l.* was our schoolmaster.
5:14, all the *l.* is fulfilled in one word.
23, against such there is no *l.*
6:2, so fulfil the *l.* of Christ.
1 Tim. 1:9, the *l.* is not made for a righteous man.
Heb. 7:16, the *l.* of a carnal commandment.
Jas. 1:25; 2:12, perfect *l.* of liberty.
2:8, the royal *l.*
See Ps. 1:2; 19:7; Mat. 7:12; Rom. 10:4.
LAWFUL. Mat. 12:2; John 5:10; 1 Cor. 6:12.
LAWLESS. 1 Tim. 1:9.
LEAD. Deut. 4:27; 28:37, whither the Lord shall *l.* you.
Ps. 23:2, he *l.* me beside still waters.
27:11, *l.* me in a plain path.
31:3, *l.* me, and guide me.
61:2, *l.* me to the rock that is higher than I.
139:10, there shall thy hand *l.* me.
24, *l.* me in the way everlasting.
Prov. 6:22, when thou goest, it shall *l.* thee.
Isa. 11:6, a little child shall *l.* them.
42:16, I will *l.* them in paths not known.
48:17, I am the Lord which *l.* thee.
Mat. 6:13; Lu. 11:4, *l.* us not into temptation.
15:14; Lu. 6:39, if the blind *l.* the blind.
Acts 13:11, seeking some to *l.* him.
1 Tim. 2:2, we may *l.* a quiet life.
See John 10:3; 1 Cor. 9:5; 2 Tim. 3:6; Rev. 7:17.
LEAF. Lev. 26:36; Ps. 1:3; Isa. 64:6; Mat. 21:19.
LEAN. Prov. 3:5; Amos 5:19; Mic. 3:11; John 13:23; 21:20.
LEARN. Deut. 31:13, *l.* to fear the Lord.
Prov. 1:5; 9:9; 16:21, will increase *l.*
22:25, lest thou *l.* his ways.
Isa. 1:17, *l.* to do well.
2:4; Mic. 4:3, neither shall they *l.* war.
29:11, 12, deliver to one that is *l.*
John 6:45, every one that hath *l.* of the Father.
7:15, having never *l.*
Acts 7:22, *l.* in all the wisdom of the Egyptians.
26:24, much *l.* doth make thee mad.
Rom. 15:4, written for our *l.*
Eph. 4:20, ye have not so *l.* Christ.
2 Tim. 3:14, in the things thou has *l.*
Heb. 5:8, though a Son, yet *l.* he obedience.
See Mat. 9:13; 11:29; Phil. 4:11; Rev. 14:3.
LEAST. Mat. 5:19, one of these *l.* commandments.
11:11; Lu. 7:28, he that is *l.* in kingdom of heaven.
25:40, 45, done it to the *l.* of these.
Lu. 12:26, not able to do that which is *l.*
16:10, faithful in that which is *l.*
Eph. 3:8, less than the *l.* of all saints.
See Gen. 32:10; Jer. 31:34; 1 Cor. 6:4.
LEAVE. Gen. 2:24; Mat. 19:5; Mk. 10:7; Eph. 5:31, *l.* father and mother, and shall cleave.
Ps. 16:10; Acts 2:27, not *l.* my soul in hell.
27:9; 119:121, *l.* me not.
Mat. 23:23, and not to *l.* the other undone.
John 14:27, peace I *l.* with you.
Heb. 13:5, I will never *l.* thee.
See Ruth 1:16; Mat. 5:24; John 16:28.
LEES. Isa. 25:6; Jer. 48:11; Zeph. 1:12.
LEND. Deut. 15:6, thou shalt *l.* to many nations.
Ps. 37:26; 112:5, ever merciful, and *l.*
Prov. 19:17, he that hath pity on poor *l.* to the Lord.
22:7, the borrower is servant to the *l.*,
Lu. 6:34, if ye *l.* to them of whom.
See 1 Sam. 1:28; Isa. 24:2; Lu. 11:5.
LESS. Ex. 30:15; Job 11:6; Isa. 40:17.
LIARS. Ps. 116:11; John 8:44; Tit. 1:12; Rev. 2:2; 21:8.
LIBERAL. Prov. 11:25; Isa. 32:5, 8; Jas. 1:5.
LIBERTY. Ps. 119:45, I will walk at *l.*
Isa. 61:1; Jer. 34:8; Lu. 4:18, to proclaim *l.*
Rom. 8:21, the glorious *l.* of the children of God.
1 Cor. 8:9, take heed lest this *l.* of yours.
2 Cor. 3:17, where the Spirit is, there is *l.*
Gal. 5:1, stand fast in the *l.*
Jas. 1:25; 2:12, the law of *l.*
See Lev. 25:10; Gal. 5:13; 1 Pet. 2:16.
LIFE. Gen. 2:7; 6:17; 7:22, the breath of *l.*
9; 3:24; Rev. 2:7, the tree of *l.*
Deut. 30:15; Jer. 21:8, I have set before thee *l.*
Josh. 2:14, our *l.* for yours.
1 Sam. 25:29, bound in the bundle of *l.*
Ps. 16:11, show me the path of *l.*
17:14; Eccl. 9:9, their portion in this *l.*
26:9, gather not my *l.* with bloody men.
27:1, the strength of my *l.*
30:5, in his favour is *l.*
34:12, what man is he that desireth *l.*?
36:9, the fountain of *l.*
91:16, with long *l.* will I satisfy him.
133:3, even *l.* for evermore.
Prov. 3:22, so shall they be *l.* to thy soul.
8:35, whoso findeth me findeth *l.*
15:24, the way of *l.* is above to the wise.
Mat. 6:25; Lu. 12:22, take no thought for your *l.*
18:8; 19:17; Mk. 9:43, to enter into *l.*
Lu. 12:15, a man's *l.* consisteth not.
23, the *l.* is more than meat.

John 1:4, in him was *l.*
5:24; 1 John 3:14, passed from death to *l.*
26, as the Father hath *l.* in himself.
40; 10:10, will not come that ye might have *l.*
6:33, 47, 48, 54, the bread of *l.*
10:15, 17; 13:37, I lay down my *l.*
11:25; 14:6, the resurrection and the *l.*
Rom. 6:4, in newness of *l.*
11:15, *l.* from the dead.
2 Cor. 2:16, the savour of *l.* unto *l.*
Gal. 2:20, the *l.* that I now live.
Eph. 4:18, alienated from the *l.* of God.
Col. 3:3, your *l.* is hid.
1 Tim. 4:8; 2 Tim. 1:1, the promise of the *l.*
2 Tim. 1:10, brought *l.* to light by gospel.
Jas. 4:14, what is your *l.*?
1 John 1:2, the *l.* was manifested.
2:16, the pride of *l.*
5:11, this *l.* is in his Son.
Rev. 22:1, 17, river of water of *l.*
See Mat. 10:39; 20:28; Acts 5:20.
LIGHT. Ex. 10:23, Israel had *l.* in their dwellings.
Job 18:5, the *l.* of the wicked.
37:21, men see not bright *l.* in clouds.
Ps. 4:6; 90:8, the *l.* of thy countenance.
27:1, the Lord is my *l.*
36:9, in thy *l.* shall we see *l.*
97:11, *l.* is sown for the righteous.
119:105, a *l.* to my path.
Eccl. 11:7, the *l.* is sweet.
Isa. 5:20, darkness for *l.*, and *l.* for darkness.
30:26, the *l.* of the moon as *l.* of sun.
59:9, we wait for *l.*
60:1, arise, shine, for thy *l.* is come.
Zech. 14:6, the *l.* shall not be clear.
Mat. 5:15; John 8:12; 9:5, the *l.* of the world.
16, let your *l.* so shine.
6:22, the *l.* of the body is the eye.
Lu. 12:35, your loins girded, and *l.* burning.
16:8, wiser than children of *l.*
John 1:9, that was the true *L.*
3:19, *l.* is come into the world.
20, hateth the *l.*
5:35, burning and shining *l.*
12:35, yet a little while is the *l.* with you.
36, while ye have *l.*, believe in the *l.*
Acts 26:18, turn from darkness to *l.*
1 Cor. 4:5, bring to *l.* hidden things.
2 Cor. 4:4, *l.* of the gospel.
6, commanded *l.* to shine out of darkness.
11:14, an angel of *l.*
Eph. 5:8, now are ye *l.*, walk as children of *l.*
14, Christ shall give thee *l.*
1 Tim. 6:16, in *l.* which no man can approach.
2 Pet. 1:19, a *l.* shining in a dark place.
1 John 1:5, God is *l.*
7, walk in the *l.*, as he is in the *l.*
Rev. 22:5, they need no candle, neither *l.* of the sun.
See 2 Tim. 1:10; Rev. 7:16; 18:23; 21:23.
LIGHTNING. Ex. 19:16; Mat. 24:27; Lu. 10:18.
LIKENESS. Ps. 17:15, when I awake, with thy *l.*
Isa. 40:18, what *l.* will ye compare?
Acts 14:11, gods are come down in *l.* of men.
Rom. 6:5, *l.* of his death, *l.* of his resurrection.
8:3, in the *l.* of sinful flesh.
Phil. 2:7, was made in the *l.* of men.
See Gen. 1:26; 5:1; Ex. 20:4; Deut. 4:16.
LIMIT. Ps. 78:41; Ezek. 43:12; Heb. 4:7.
LINE. Ps. 16:6; Isa. 28:10, 17; 34:11; 2 Cor. 10:16.
LINGER. Gen. 19:16; 43:10; 2 Pet. 2:3.
LIP. 1 Sam. 1:13, only her *l.* moved.
Job 27:4, my *l.* shall not speak wickedness.
33:3, my *l.* shall utter knowledge.
Ps. 12:2, 3, flattering *l.*
4, our *l.* are our own.
17:1, goeth not out of feigned *l.*
31:18; 120:2; Prov. 10:18; 12:22; 17:7, lying *l.*
Prov. 15:7, the *l.* of the wise disperse knowledge.
Eccl. 10:12, the *l.* of a fool will swallow himself.
Cant. 7:9, causing *l.* of those asleep to speak.
Isa. 6:5, a man of unclean *l.*
Mat. 15:8, honoureth me with their *l.*
See Ps. 51:15; 141:3; Dan. 10:16; Hab. 3:16.
LITTLE. Ezra 9:8, for a *l.* space, a *l.* reviving.
Job 26:14, how *l.* a portion is heard?
Ps. 8:5; Heb. 2:7, a *l.* lower than angels.
37:16, a *l.* that a righteous man hath.
Prov. 6:10; 24:33, a *l.* sleep.
15:16; 16:8, better is a *l.* with fear of Lord.
30:24, four things *l.* on earth.
Isa. 28:10, here a *l.* and there a *l.*
40:15; Ezek. 16:47, as a very *l.* thing.
Hag. 1:6, bring in *l.*
Mat. 6:30; 8:26; 14:31; 16:8; Lu. 12:28, *l.* faith.
10:42; 18:6; Mk. 9:42; Lu. 17:2, *l.* ones.
Lu. 7:47, to whom *l.* is forgiven.
19:3, *l.* of stature.
1 Cor. 5:6; Gal. 5:9, a *l.* leaven.
1 Tim. 4:8, bodily exercise profiteth *l.*
5:23, use a *l.* wine.
See John 7:33; 14:19; 16:16; Rev. 3:8; 6:11.
LIVE. Gen. 17:18, O that Ishmael might *l.* before thee!
45:3, doth my father yet *l.*?
Lev. 18:5; Neh. 9:29; Ezek. 20:11, if a man do, he shall *l.*
Deut. 8:3; Mat. 4:4; Lu. 4:4, not *l.* by bread alone.
Job. 7:16, I would not *l.* alway.
14:14, shall he *l.* again?
Ps. 118:17, I shall not die, but *l.*
Isa. 38:16, make me to *l.*
55:3, hear, and your soul shall *l.*
Ezek. 3:21; 18:9; 33:13, he shall surely *l.*
16:6, when thou wast in thy blood, *l.*
Hos. 6:2, we shall *l.* in his sight.
Hab. 2:4, the just shall *l.* by faith.
Lu. 10:28, this do, and thou shalt *l.*
John 11:25, though he were dead, yet shall he *l.*
14:19, because I *l.*, ye shall *l.* also.
Acts 17:28, in him we *l.* and move.
Rom. 8:12, *l.* after the flesh.
14:8, whether we *l.*, we *l.* unto the Lord.
1 Cor. 9:14, should *l.* of the gospel.
2 Cor. 6:9, as dying, and behold we *l.*
Gal. 2:19, that I might *l.* unto God.
5:25, if we *l.* in the Spirit.
Phil. 1:21, for me to *l.* is Christ.
2 Tim. 3:12, all that will *l.* godly.
Jas. 4:15, if the Lord will, we shall *l.*
Rev. 1:18, I am he that *l.*, and was dead.
3:1, a name that thou *l.*
See Rom. 6:10; 1 Tim. 5:6; Rev. 20:4.
LIVELY. Ex. 1:19; Acts 7:38; 1 Pet. 1:3; 2:5.
LIVING. Gen. 2:7, a *l.* soul.
Job 28:13; Ps. 27:13; 52:5; 116:9, the land of the *l.*
33:30; Ps. 27:13, light of *l.*
Ps. 69:28, the book of the *l.*
Eccl. 7:2, the *l.* will lay it to heart.
9:5, the *l.* know they shall die.
Cant. 4:15; Jer. 2:13; 17:13; Zech. 14:8; John 4:10, *l.* water.
Isa. 38:19, the *l.* shall praise thee.
Lam. 3:39, wherefore doth a *l.* man complain?
Mk. 12:44, even all her *l.*
Lu. 8:43, spent all her *l.*
John 6:51, I am the *l.* bread.
Heb. 10:30, a new and *l.* way.
See Mat. 22:32; Mk. 12:27; 1 Cor. 15:43.
LOADETH. Ps. 68:19.
LOAN. 1 Sam. 2:20.
LOATHE. Num. 21:5; Job 7:16; Ezek. 6:9; 20:43; 36:31.
LODGE. Ruth 1:16; Isa. 1:21; 1 Tim. 5:10.
LOFTY. Ps. 131:1; Isa. 2:11; 57:15.
LONG. Job 3:21, which *l.* for death.
6:8, that God would grant the thing I *l.* for!
Ps. 63:1, my flesh *l.* for thee in a dry land.
84:2, my soul *l.* for courts of the Lord.

Ps. 119:174, I have *l.* for thy salvation.
See Deut. 12:20; 28:32; 2 Sam. 23:15; Phil. 1:8.
LOOK. Gen. 19:17, *l.* not behind thee.
Num. 21:8, when he *l.* on the serpent.
Job. 33:27, he *l.* on men.
Ps. 5:3, and will *l.* up.
34:5, they *l.* to him, and were lightened.
84:9, *l.* upon the face of thine anointed.
Isa. 5:7; 59:11, he *l.* for judgment.
17:7, at that day shall a man *l.* to his Maker.
45:22, *l.* unto me, and be saved.
63:5, I *l.*, and there was none to help.
66:2, to this man will I *l.*
Jer. 8:15; 14:19, we *l.* for peace.
39:12, *l.* well to him.
40:4, come with me, and I will *l.* well to thee.
Hag. 1:9, ye *l.* for much.
Mat. 11:3; Lu. 7:19, do we *l.* for another?
24:50, in a day he *l.* not for.
Lu. 9:62, no man *l.* back is fit for the kingdom.
10:32, a Levite came and *l.* on him.
22:61, the Lord turned, and *l.* on Peter.
John 13:22, disciples *l.* one on another.
Acts 3:4, 12, said, *l.* on us.
6:3, *l.* ye out seven men.
2 Cor. 4:18, we *l.* not at things seen.
10:7, *l.* upon things after outward appearance.
Phil. 2:4, *l.* not every man on his own things.
Tit. 2:13, *l.* for that blessed hope.
Heb. 11:10, he *l.* for a city.
12:2, *l.* unto Jesus.
1 Pet. 1:12, angels desire to *l.* into.
2 John 8, *l.* to yourselves.
See Prov. 14:15; Mat. 5:28; 2 Pet. 3:12.
LOOSE. Job 38:31, canst thou *l.* the bands of Orion?
Ps. 102:20, *l.* those appointed to death.
116:16, thou hast *l.* my bonds.
Eccl. 12:6, or ever the silver cord be *l.*
Mat. 16:19; 18:18, *l.* on earth be *l.* in heaven.
John 11:44, *l.* him, and let him go.
Acts 2:24, having *l.* the pains of death.
1 Cor. 7:27, art thou *l.* from a wife?
See Deut. 25:9; Isa. 45:1; 51:14; Lu. 13:12.
LORD. Ex. 34:6, the *L.*, the *L.* God, merciful.
Deut. 4:35; 1 Kings 18:39, the *L.* is God.
6:4, the *L.* our God is one *L.*
Ruth 2:4; 2 Chron. 20:17; 2 Thess. 3:16, the *L.* be with you.
1 Sam. 3:18; John 21:7, it is the *L.*
Neh. 9:6; Isa. 37:20, thou art *L.* alone.
Ps. 33:12, whose God is the *L.*
100:3, know that the *L.* he is God.
118:23, this is the *L.* doing.
Zech. 14:9, one *L.*, and his name one.
Mat. 7:21, not every one that saith *L.*, *L.*
26:22, *L.*, is it I?
Mk. 2:28; Lu. 6:5, the *L.* of the sabbath.
Lu. 6:46, why call ye me *L.*, *L.*?
John 9:36, who is he, *L*?
20:25, we have seen the *L.*
Acts 2:36, both *L.* and Christ.
9:5; 26:15, who art thou, *L.*?
Eph. 4:5, one *L.*
See Rom. 10:12; 1 Cor. 2:8; 15:47; Rev. 11:15.
LORDSHIP. Mk. 10:42; Lu. 22:25.
LOSE. Mat. 10:39; 16:25; Mk. 8:35; Lu. 9:24, shall *l.* it.
16:26; Mk. 8:36; Lu. 9:25, *l.* his own soul.
John 6:39, Father's will I should *l.* nothing.
See Judg. 18:25; Eccl. 3:6; Lu.15:4, 8.
LOSS. 1 Cor. 3:15; Phil. 3:7, 8.
LOST. Ps. 119:176; Jer. 50:6, like *l.* sheep.
Ezek. 37:11, our hope is *l.*
Mat. 10:6; 15:24, go to *l.* sheep of Israel.
18:18; Lu. 19:10, to save that which was *l.*
John 6:12, that nothing be *l.*
17:12, none of them is *l.*
18:9, have I *l.* none.
See Lev. 6:3; Deut. 22:3; 2 Cor. 4:3.

LOT. Ps. 16:5, thou maintainest my *l.*
125:3, not rest on the *l.* of the righteous.
Prov. 1:14, cast in thy *l.* among us.
16:3, *l.* is cast into the lap.
18:18, *l.* causeth contention to cease.
Dan. 12:13, stand in thy *l.*
Acts 8:21, neither part nor *l.* in this matter.
See Num. 26:55; Mat. 27:35; Acts 1:26.
LOUD. Ezra 3:13; Prov. 7:11; 27:14; Lu. 23:23.
LOVE (*n.*). 2 Sam. 1:26, wonderful, passing the *l.* of women.
Prov. 10:12, *l.* covereth all sins.
15:17, better a dinner of herbs where *l.* is.
Cant. 2:4, his banner over me was *l.*
8:6, *l.* is strong as death.
Jer. 31:3, loved thee with everlasting *l.*
Hos. 11:4, the bands of *l.*
Mat. 24:12, *l.* of many shall wax cold.
John 5:42, ye have not the *l.* of God in you.
13:35, if ye have *l.* one to another.
15:13, greater *l.* hath no man than this.
Rom. 13:10, *l.* worketh no ill.
2 Cor. 5:14, the *l.* of Christ constraineth us.
13:11, the God of *l.* shall be with you.
Eph. 3:19, the *l.* of Christ, which passeth.
1 Tim. 6:10, *l.* of money is the root of all evil.
Heb. 13:1, let brotherly *l.* continue.
1 John 4:7, *l.* is of God.
8:16, God is *l.*
10, herein is *l.*, not that we loved God.
18, no fear in *l.*
Rev. 2:4, thou hast left thy first *l.*
See Gen. 29:29; Gal. 5:22; 1 Thess. 1:3.
LOVE (*v.*). Lev. 19:18; Mat. 19:19; 22:39; Mk. 12:31, thou shalt *l.* thy neighbour.
Deut. 6:5; 10:12; 11:1; 19:9; 30:5; Mat. 22:37; Mk. 12:30; Lu. 10:27, *l.* the Lord thy God.
Ps. 18:1, I will *l.* thee, O Lord, my strength.
26:8, I have *l.* the habitation of thy house.
34:12, what man is he that *l.* many days?
69:36, they that *l.* his name.
97:10, ye that *l.* the Lord.
109:17, as he *l.* cursing.
122:6, they shall prosper that *l.* thee.
Prov. 8:17, I *l.* them that *l.* me.
17:17, a friend *l.* at all times.
Eccl. 3:8, a time to *l.*
Jer. 5:31, my people *l.* to have it so.
31:3, I have *l.* thee with an everlasting *l.*
Hos. 14:4, I will *l.* them freely.
Amos 5:15, hate the evil, and *l.* the good.
Mic. 6:8, but to *l.* mercy, and walk humbly.
Mat. 5:44; Lu. 6:27, I say, *l.* your enemies.
46, if ye *l.* them which *l.* you.
Lu. 7:42, which will *l.* him most?
John 11:3, he whom thou *l.* is sick.
15:12, 17, that ye *l.* one another.
21:15, 16, 17, *l.* thou me?
Rom. 13:8, owe no man any thing, but to *l.*
Eph. 6:24, grace be with all them that *l.* our Lord.
1 Pet. 1:8, whom having not seen, ye *l.*
2:17, *l.* the brotherhood.
1 John 4:19, we *l.* him, because he first *l.* us.
Rev. 3:19, as many as I *l.* I rebuke.
See Gen. 22:2; John 14:31; 1 John 4:20, 21.
LOVELY. 2 Sam. 1:23; Cant. 5:16; Ezek. 33:32; Phil. 4:8.
LOVER. 1 Kings 5:1; Ps. 88:18; 2 Tim. 3:4; Tit. 1:8.
LOW. Ps. 136:23; Rom. 12:16; Jas. 1:9, 10.
LOWER. Ps. 8:5; 63:9; Eph. 4:9; Heb. 2:7.
LOWEST. Deut. 32:22; Ps. 86:13; Lu. 14:9.
LOWLINESS. Eph. 4:2; Phil. 2:3.
LOWLY. Prov. 11:2, with the *l.* is wisdom.
Mat. 11:29, I am meek and *l.*
See Ps. 138:6; Prov. 3:34; 16:19; Zech. 9:9.
LUST. Deut. 12:15, 20, 21; 14:26, whatsoever thy soul *l.* after.
Ps. 81:12, gave them up to their own *l.*
Rom. 7:7, I had not known *l.*
Gal. 5:24, Christ's have crucified flesh with *l.*

1 Tim. 6:9, rich fall into hurtful *l*.
Tit. 2:12, denying worldly *l*.
Jas. 1:14, when he is drawn of his own *l*.
1 Pet. 2:11, abstain from fleshly *l*.
1 John 2:16, the *l*. of the flesh.
17, the world passeth away, and the *l*. thereof.
Jude 16, 18, walking after *l*.
See Mat. 5:28; 1 Cor. 10:6; Rev. 18:14.
LYING. Ps. 31:18, let the *l*. lips be put to silence.
119:163, I abhor *l*., but thy law I love.
Prov. 6:17, the Lord hateth a *l*. tongue.
12:9, a *l*. tongue is but for a moment.
Jer. 7:4, trust not in *l*. words.
Eph. 4:25, putting away *l*.
See 1 Kings 22:22; 2 Chron. 18:21; Dan. 2:9.

M

MAD. John 10:20; Acts 26:11, 24; 1 Cor. 14:23.
MADE. Ex. 2:14, who *m*. thee a prince over us?
Ps. 118:24, this is the day the Lord hath *m*.
Prov. 16:4, the Lord *m*. all things for himself.
Eccl. 3:11, he hath *m*. every thing beautiful.
7:29, God hath *m*. man upright.
Isa. 66:2, all these things hath mine hand *m*.
John 1:3, all things were *m*. by him.
5:6, wilt thou be *m*. whole?
2 Cor. 5:21, he hath *m*. him to be sin for us.
Eph. 2:13, *m*. nigh by the blood of Christ.
3:7; Col. 1:23, I was *m*. a minister.
Col. 1:20, having *m*. peace.
Heb. 2:17, to be *m*. like his brethren.
See Ps. 95:5; 149:2; John 19:7; Acts 17:24.
MAGNIFY. Josh. 3:7, this day will I begin to *m*. thee.
Job 7:17, what is man, that thou shouldest *m*. him?
Ps. 34:3; 40:16; Lu. 1:46, *m*. the Lord.
35:26; 38:16, that *m*. themselves.
138:2, thou hast *m*. thy word above all.
Isa. 42:21, *m*. the law.
Acts 19:17, the name of Jesus was *m*.
Rom. 11:13, I *m*. mine office.
See Dan. 8:25; 11:36; Acts 5:13; Phil. 1:20.
MAIDSERVANTS. Ex. 20:10, nor thy *m*.
21:7, if a man sell his daughter to be a *m*.
Deut. 15:17, unto thy *m*. thou shalt do likewise.
MAIL. 1 Sam. 17:5.
MAINTAIN. 1 Kings 8:45; 49:59; 2 Chron. 35:39, *m*. their cause.
Ps. 16:5, thou *m*. my lot.
Tit. 3:8, 14, careful to *m*. good works.
See Job 13:15; Ps. 9:4; 140:12.
MAINTENANCE. Ezra 4:14; Prov. 27:27.
MAKER. Job 4:17, shall a man be more pure than this *m*.?
32:22, my *m*. would soon take me away.
35:10, none saith, where is God my *m*.?
36:3, ascribe righteousness to my *m*.
Ps. 95:6, kneel before the Lord our *m*.
Prov. 14:31; 17:5, reproacheth his *m*.
22:2, the Lord is *m*. of them all.
Isa. 45:9, that striveth with his *m*.
51:13, forgettest the Lord thy *m*.
54:5, thy *m*. is thine husband.
Heb. 11:10, whose builder and *m*. is God.
See Isa. 1:31; 17:7; 22:11; Hab. 2:18.
MALICIOUSNESS. Rom. 1:29; 1 Pet. 2:16.
MAN. Gen. 3:22, the *m*. is become as one of us.
8:21, for *m*. sake.
Num. 23:19, God is not a *m*.
Neh. 6:11, should such a *m*. as I flee?
Job. 5:7, *m*. is born to trouble.
10:4, seest thou as *m*. seeth?
11:12, vain *m*. would be wise.
14:1, *m*. that is born of a woman.
15:7, art thou the first *m*. that was born?
25:6, *m*. that is a worm.
33:12, God is greater than *m*.
Ps. 10:18, the *m*. of earth.
49:12, *m*. being in honour abideth not.
89:48, what *m*. is he that liveth?
Ps. 90:3, thou turnest *m*. to destruction.
104:23, *m*. goeth forth to his labour.
118:6, I will not fear, what can *m*. do?
Prov. 12:2, a good *m*. obtaineth favour.
Eccl. 6:12, who knoweth what is good for *m*.?
Isa. 2:22, cease ye from *m*.
Jer. 10:23, it is not in *m*. to direct his steps.
Lam. 3:1, I am the *m*. that hath seen affliction.
Hos. 11:9, I am God, and not *m*.
Mat. 6:24; Lu. 16:13, no *m*. can serve.
8:4; Mk. 8:26, 30; Lu. 5:14; 9:21, tell no *m*.
17:8, they saw no *m*.
John 1:18; 1 John 4:12, no *m*. hath seen God.
19:5, behold the *m*.!
1 Cor. 2:11, what *m*. knoweth things of a *m*.?
11:8, *m*. is not of the woman.
2 Cor. 4:16, though our outward *m*. perish.
Phil. 2:8, in fashion as a *m*.
1 Tim. 2:5, the *m*. Christ Jesus.
See John 7:46; 1 Cor. 15:47; Eph. 4:24.
MANDRAKES. Gen. 30:14, found *m*. in the field.
Cant. 7:13, the *m*. give a smell.
MANEH. Ezek. 45:12.
MANGER. Lu. 2:7.
MANIFEST. Mk. 4:22, nothing hid that shall not be *m*.
John 2:11, and *m*. forth his glory.
14:22, how is it thou wilt *m*. thyself?
1 Cor. 4:5, who will make *m*. the counsels of the hearts.
2 Cor. 2:14, maketh *m*. savour of knowledge.
Gal. 5:19, the works of the flesh are *m*.
2 Thess. 1:5, a *m*. token of righteous judgment.
1 Tim. 3:16, God was *m*. in the flesh.
5:25, good works of some are *m*. beforehand.
Heb. 4:13, no creature that is not *m*.
1 John 1:2, the life was *m*.
3:5, he was *m*. to take away our sins.
4:9, in this was *m*. the love of God.
See Rom. 8:19; John 17:6; 1 John 3:10.
MANIFOLD. Ps. 104:24, how *m*. are thy works!
Eph. 3:10, the *m*. wisdom of God.
1 Pet. 1:6, through *m*. temptations.
4:10, stewards of the *m*. grace of God.
See Neh. 9:19, 27; Amos 5:12; Lu. 18:30.
MANNER. 2 Sam. 7:19, is this the *m*. of man?
Ps. 144:13, all *m*. of store.
Isa. 5:17, lambs shall feed after their *m*
Mat. 8:27; Mk. 4:41; Lu. 8:25, what *m*. of man is this!
12:31, all *m*. of sin shall be forgiven.
Acts 26:4, my *m*. of life from my youth.
1 Cor. 15:33, evil communications corrupt good *m*.
Heb. 10:25, as the *m*. of some is.
Jas. 1:24, forgetteth what *m*. of man.
1 Pet. 1:15, holy in all *m*. of conversation.
2 Pet. 3:11, what *m*. of persons ought ye to be?
See Mat. 4:23; 5:11; Lu. 9:55; Rev. 22:2.
MANTLE. 2 Kings 2:8; Job 1:20; Ps. 109:29.
MAR. Lev. 19:27, nor *m*. the corners of thy beard.
1 Sam. 6:5, images of your mice that *m*. the land.
Job 30:13, they *m*. my path.
Isa. 52:14, visage *m*. more than any man.
Mk. 2:22, wine spilled, and bottles *m*.
See Ruth 4:6; 2 Kings 3:19; Jer. 13:7; 18:4.
MARBLE. 1 Chron. 29:2, and *m*. stones in abundance.
Cant. 5:15, his legs are as pillars of *m*.
MARK. Gen. 4:15, the Lord set a *m*. on Cain.
Job 22:15, hast thou *m*. the old way?
Ps. 37:37, *m*. the perfect man.
48:13, *m*. well her bulwarks.
130:3, if thou shouldest *m*. iniquities.
Jer. 2:22, thine iniquity is *m*. before me.
23:18, who hath *m*. his word?
Phil. 3:14, I press toward the *m*. for the prize.
17, *m*. them which walk so.
See Lu. 14:7; Rom. 16:17; Rev. 13:16; 20:4.
MARROW. Job 21:24; Ps. 63:5; Prov. 3:8; Heb. 4:12.
MARVEL. Mat. 8:10; Mk. 6:6; Lu. 7:9, Jesus *m*.
Mk. 5:20, all men did *m*.

John 3:7; 5:28; 1 John 3:13, *m.* not.
See Eccl. 5:8; John 7:21; Gal. 1:6.
MARVELLOUS. Job 5:9, *m.* things without number.
Ps. 17:7, *m.* lovingkindness.
118:23; Mat. 21:42; Mk. 12:11, *m.* in our eyes.
John 9:30, herein is a *m.* thing.
1 Pet. 2:9, into his *m.* light.
See Ps. 105:5; 139:14; Dan. 11:36; Mic. 7:15.
MASTER. 2 Kings 6:32, sound of his *m.* feet behind him.
Mal. 1:6, if I be a *m.*, where is my fear?
2:12, the Lord will cut off the *m.* and the scholar.
Mat. 6:24; Lu. 16:13, no man can serve two *m.*
10:24; Lu. 6:40, disciple not above his *m.*
25, enough for the disciple that he be as his *m.*
17:24, doth not your *m.* pay tribute?
23:8, 10, one is your *M.*, even Christ.
26:25, *M.*, is it I?
Mk. 5:35; Lu. 8:49, why troublest thou the *M.*?
9:5; Lu. 9:33, *M.*, it is good for us to be here.
10:17; Lu. 10:25, good *M.*, what shall I do?
Lu. 13:25, when once the *m.* of the house is risen.
John 3:10, art thou a *m.* of Israel?
11:28, the *m.* is come, and calleth.
13:13, ye call me *M.*, and ye say well.
Rom. 14:4, to his own *m.* he standeth or falleth.
1 Cor. 3:10, as a wise *m.*-builder.
Eph. 6:5; Col. 3:22; Tit. 2:9; 1 Pet. 2:18, be obedient to *m.*
9; Col. 4:1, *m.*, do the same things to them.
1 Tim. 6:1, count their *m.* worthy of honour.
2, that have believing *m.*
Jas. 3:1, be not many *m.*
See Gen. 24:12; 39:8; Prov. 25:13; Eccl. 12:11.
MASTERY. Ex. 32:18; 1 Cor. 9:25; 2 Tim. 2:5.
MATTER. Ezra 10:4, arise, for this *m.* belongeth to thee.
Job 19:28, the root of the *m.* is found in me.
32:18, I am full of *m.*
Ps. 45:1, my heart is inditing a good *m.*
Prov. 16:20, handleth a *m.* wisely.
18:13, answereth a *m.* before he heareth it.
Eccl. 10:20, that which hath wings shall tell the *m.*
12:13, conclusion of the whole *m.*
Mat. 23:23, the weightier *m.*
Acts 18:14, if it were a *m.* of wrong.
1 Cor. 6:2, to judge the smallest *m.*
2 Cor. 9:5, as a *m.* of bounty.
Jas. 3:5, how great a *m.* a little fire kindleth!
See Gen. 30:15; Dan. 3:16; Acts 8:21; 71:32.
MAY. Mat. 9:21; 26:42; Acts 8:37.
MEAN. Ex. 12:26; Josh. 4:6, what *m.* ye by this service?
Deut. 6:20, what *m.* the testimonies?
Prov. 22:29, not stand before *m.* men.
Isa. 2:9; 5:15; 31:8, the *m.* man.
Ezek. 17:12, know ye not what these things *m.*?
Mk. 9:10, what the rising from the dead should *m.*
Acts 21:39, citizen of no *m.* city.
See Acts 10:17; 17:20; 21:13.
MEANS. Ex. 34:7; Num. 14:18, by no *m.* clear guilty.
Ps. 49:7, none can by any *m.* redeem.
Mal. 1:9, this hath been by your *m.*
Mat. 5:26, shalt by no *m.* come out.
Lu. 10:19, nothing shall by any *m.* hurt you.
John 9:21, by what *m.* he now seeth.
1 Cor. 8:9, lest by any *m.* this liberty.
9:22, that I might by all *m.* save some.
Phil. 3:11, by an *m.* attain.
2 Thess. 3:16, give you peace always by all *m.*
See Jer. 5:31; 1 Cor. 9:27; Gal. 2:2.
MEASURE (*n.*). Deut. 25:14; Prov. 20:10, thou shalt not have divers *m.*
Job 11:9, the *m.* is longer than the earth.
28:25, he weigheth the waters by *m.*
Ps. 39:4, the *m.* of my days.
Isa. 40:12, the dust of the earth in a *m.*
Jer. 30:11; 46:28, I will correct thee in *m.*
Ezek. 4:11, thou shalt drink water by *m.*
Mat. 7:2; Mk. 4:24; Lu. 6:38, with what *m.* ye mete.
13:33; Lu. 13:21, three *m.* of meal.
Mat. 23:32, fill up *m.* of your fathers.
Lu. 6:38, good *m.*, pressed down.
John 3:34, giveth not the Spirit by *m.*
Rom. 12:3, to every man the *m.* of faith.
2 Cor. 12:7, exalted above *m.*
Eph. 4:7, the *m.* of the gift of Christ.
13, to the *m.* of the stature.
16, in the *m.* of every part.
Rev. 6:6, a *m.* of wheat for a penny.
21:17, according to the *m.* of a man.
See Ps. 80:5; Isa. 5:14; Mic. 6:10.
MEASURE (*v.*). Isa. 40:12, who hath *m.* the waters?
65:7, I will *m.* former work into bosom.
Jer. 31:37, if heaven can be *m.*
33:22; Hos. 1:10, as the sand cannot be *m.*
2 Cor. 10:12, *m.* themselves by themselves.
See Ezek. 40:3; 42:15; Zech. 2:1.
MEAT. Gen. 27:4, make me savoury *m.*
1 Kings 19:8, went in strength of that *m.*
Ps. 59:15, wander up and down for *m.*
69:21, they gave me also gall for my *m.*
78:25, he sent them *m.* to the full.
145:15, *m.* in due season.
Prov. 23:3, dainties for they are deceitful *m.*
30:22, a fool when filled with *m.*
31:15, she giveth *m.* to her household.
Isa. 65:25, dust shall be the serpent's *m.*
Ezek. 4:10, thy *m.* shall be by weight.
47:12, fruit for *m.*
Dan. 1:8, not defile himself with king's *m.*
Hab. 1:16, because their *m.* is plenteous.
3:17, fields yield no *m.*
Mal. 3:10, bring tithes, that there may be *m.*
Mat. 6:25; Lu. 12:23, life more than *m.*?
10:10, workman worthy of his *m.*
15:37; Mk. 8:8, of broken *m.*
25:35, ye gave me *m.*
Lu. 3:11, he that hath *m.* let him do likewise.
24:41; John 21:5, have ye any *m.*?
John 4:32, I have *m.* to eat.
34, my *m.* is to do the will of him that sent me.
6:27, labour not for the *m.* that perisheth.
Acts 2:46, did eat *m.* with gladness.
15:29, abstain from *m.* offered to idols.
Rom. 14:15, destroy not him with thy *m.*
17, kingdom of God is not *m.* and drink.
20, for *m.* destroy not the work of God.
1 Cor. 6:13, *m.* for the belly.
8:13, if *m.* make my brother to offend.
10:3, the same spiritual *m.*
1 Tim. 4:3, to abstain from *m.*
Heb. 5:12, 14, not of strong *m.*
12:16, who for one morsel of *m.*
See Gen. 1:29; 9:3; Mat. 3:4; Col. 2:16.
MEDDLE. 2 Kings 14:10; 2 Chron. 25:19, why *m.* to thy hurt?
Prov. 20:3, every fool will be *m.*
19, *m.* not with him that flattereth.
26:17, that *m.* with strife.
See 2 Chron. 35:21; Prov. 17:14; 24:21.
MEDITATE. Gen. 24:63, Isaac went out to *m.*
Josh. 1:8, thou shalt *m.* therein.
Ps. 1:2, in his law doth he *m.*
63:6; 119:148, *m.* in the night watches.
77:12; 143:5, I will *m.* of thy works.
Isa. 33:18, thine heart shall *m.* terror.
Lu. 21:14, not to *m.* before.
1 Tim. 4:15, *m.* upon these things.
See Ps. 19:14; 104:34; 119:97, 99.
MEEK. Num. 12:3, Moses was very *m.*
Ps. 22:26, the *m.* shall eat and be satisfied.
25:9, the *m.* will he guide.
37:11; Mat. 5:5, the *m.* shall inherit the earth.
149:4, will beautify the *m.*
Isa. 29:19, the *m.* shall increase their joy.
61:1, good tidings to the *m.*
Mat. 11:29, for I am *m.*
1 Pet. 3:4, a *m.* and quiet spirit.

See Ps. 76:9; 147:6; Isa. 11:4; Mat. 21:5.
MEEKNESS. 2 Cor. 10:1, by the *m.* of Christ.
Gal. 6:1, restore in the spirit of *m.*
1 Tim. 6:11, follow after *m.*
2 Tim. 2:25, in *m.* instructing.
Tit. 3:2, showing *m.* to all men.
1 Pet. 3:15, give reason of hope in you with *m.*
See Zeph. 2:3; Gal. 5:23; Eph. 4:2.
MEET. Prov. 11:24, withholdeth more than is *m.*
Mat. 15:26, not *m.* to take children's bread.
25:1, 6, to *m.* the bridegroom.
1 Cor. 15:9, not *m.* to be called an apostle.
1 Thess. 4:17, to *m.* the Lord in the air.
See Prov. 22:2; Amos 4:12; Mat. 8:34.
MELODY. Isa. 23:16; 51:3; Amos 5:23; Eph. 5:19.
MELT. Ps. 46:6, the earth *m.*
97:5, the hills *m.*
107:26, their soul *m.*
147:18, he sendeth his word, and *m.* them.
Isa. 13:7, every man's heart shall *m.*
64:2, as when the *m.* fire burneth.
See Ex. 15:15; Josh. 14:8; Jer. 9:7.
MEMBER. Ps. 139:16, all my *m.* were written.
Rom. 6:13, 19, neither yield your *m.*
12:4, as we have many *m.*
1 Cor. 6:15, bodies *m.* of Christ.
Jas. 3:5, the tongue is a little *m.*
4:1, lusts which war in your *m.*
See Job 17:7; Mat. 5:29; Eph. 4:24; 5:30.
MEMORY. Ps. 109:15; 145:7; Prov. 10:7; Eccl. 9:5.
MEN. 2 Chron. 6:18, will God dwell with *m.*?
1 Sam. 4:9; 1 Cor. 16:13, quit yourselves like *m.*
Ps. 9:20, know themselves to be but *m.*
82:7, but ye shall die like *m.*
Eccl. 12:3, strong *m.* shall bow themselves.
Isa. 31:3, the Egyptians are *m.* and not God.
46:8, show yourselves *m.*
Gal. 1:10, do I now persuade *m.*?
1 Thess. 2:4, not as pleasing *m.*, but God.
See Ps. 116:11; 1 Tim. 2:4; 1 Pet. 2:17.
MEND. 2 Chron. 24:12; 34:10; Mat. 4:21; Mk. 1:19.
MENTION. Gen. 40:14, make *m.* of me to Pharaoh.
Ps. 71:16, I will make *m.* of thy righteousness.
Isa. 12:4, make *m.* that his name is exalted.
63:7, I will *m.* the lovingkindnesses of the Lord.
Rom. 1:9; Eph. 1:16; 1 Thess. 1:2, *m.* of you in my prayers.
See Isa. 62:6; Ezek. 18:22; 33:16.
MERCHANDISE. Prov. 3:14, *m.* of it better than *m.* of silver.
Isa. 23:18, *m.* shall be holiness to the Lord.
Mat. 22:5, one to his farm, another to his *m.*
John 2:16, my father's house an house of *m.*
2 Pet. 2:3, make *m.* of you.
See Deut. 21:14; 24:7; Ezek. 26:12; Rev. 18:11.
MERCHANT. Gen. 23:16, current money with the *m.*
Isa. 23:8, whose *m.* are princes.
47:15, even thy *m.* shall wander.
Rev. 18:3, 11, the *m.* of the earth.
23, thy *m.* were great men of the earth.
See Prov. 31:24; Isa. 23:11; Mat. 13:45.
MERCIFUL. Ps. 37:26, ever *m.*, and lendeth.
67:1, God be *m.* to us, and bless us.
Prov. 11:17, the *m.* doeth good to his own soul.
Isa. 57:1, *m.* men are taken away.
Jer. 3:12, return, for I am *m.*
Mat. 5:7, blessed are the *m.*
Lu. 6:36, be ye *m.*, as your Father is *m.*
18:13, God be *m.* to me a sinner.
Heb. 2:17, a *m.* High Priest.
See Ex. 34:6; 2 Sam. 22:26; 1 Kings 20:31.
MERCY. Gen. 32:10, not worthy the least of the *m.*
Ex. 33:19, will show *m.* on whom I will show *m.*
34:7; Dan. 9:4, keeping *m.* for thousands.
Num. 14:18; Ps. 103:11; 145:8, longsuffering and of great *m.*
1 Chron. 16:34, 41; 2 Chron. 5:13; 7:3, 6; Ezra 3:11; Ps. 106:1; 107:1; 118:1; 136:1; Jer. 33:11, his *m.* endureth for ever.
Ps. 23:6, surely goodness and *m.* shall follow.
25:7, according to thy *m.* remember me.
33:22, let thy *m.* be upon us.
52:8, I trust in the *m.* of God.
59:10, the God of my *m.*
66:20, not turned his *m.* from me.
77:8, is his *m.* clean gone for ever?
85:10, *m.* and truth are met together.
89:2, *m.* shall be built up for ever.
90:14, satisfy us early with thy *m.*
101:1, I will sing of *m.*
108:4, thy *m.* is great above the heavens.
115:1, for thy *m.*, and for thy truth's sake.
119:64, the earth is full of thy *m.*
130:7, with the Lord there is *m.*
Prov. 3:3, let not *m.* and truth forsake thee.
14:21, 31, he that hath *m.* on the poor.
16:6; 20:28, *m.* and truth.
Isa. 54:7, with great *m.* will I gather thee.
Jer. 6:23, they are cruel, and have no *m.*
Lam. 3:22, it is of the Lord's *m.*
Hos. 4:1, because there is no *m.* in the land.
6:6; Mat. 9:13, I desired *m.*, and not sacrifice.
10:12, sow in righteousness, reap in *m.*
14:3, in thee the fatherless and find *m.*
Mic. 6:8, but to do justly, and love *m.*
7:18, he delighteth in *m.*
Hab. 3:2, in wrath remember *m.*
Mat. 5:7, the merciful shall obtain *m.*
9:27; 15:22; 20:30; Mk. 10:47, 48; 18:38, 39, thou son of David have *m.* on me.
Lu. 10:37, he that showed *m.*
Rom. 9:15, 18, *m.* on whom I will have *m.*
16, of God that showeth *m.*
12:1, beseech you by the *m.* of God.
8, he that showeth *m.*, with cheerfulness.
2 Cor. 1:3, the Father of *m.*
Eph. 2:4, God, who is rich in *m.*
1 Tim. 1:13, 16, I obtained *m.*, because.
2 Tim. 1:18, that he may find *m.* in that day.
Heb. 4:16, obtain *m.*, and find grace.
Jas. 2:13, without *m.*, that showed no *m.*
1 Pet. 1:3, according to his abundant *m.*
See Prov. 12:10; Dan. 4:27; 1 Tim. 1:2.
MERRY. Gen. 43:34, were *m.* with him.
Judg. 16:25, their hearts were *m.*
Prov. 15:13, *m.* heart maketh cheerful countenance.
15, *m.* heart hath a continual feast.
17:22, *m.* heart doeth good like a medicine.
Eccl. 8:15, nothing better than to eat and be *m.*
9:7, drink thy wine with a *m.* heart.
10:19, wine maketh *m.*
Jas. 5:13, is any *m.*?
See Lu. 12:19; 15:23; Rev. 11:10.
MESSENGER. Job 33:23; Prov. 25:13; Isa. 42:19.
METE. Isa. 40:12; Mat. 7:2; Mk. 4:24; Lu. 6:38.
MIDDLE. Ezek. 1:16; Eph. 2:14.
MIDST. Ps. 102:24, in the *m.* of my days.
Prov. 23:34, lieth down in *m.* of the sea.
Dan. 9:27, in the *m.* of the week.
Mat. 18:2; Mk. 9:36, a little child in the *m.*
20, there am I in the *m.*
Lu. 24:36; John 20:19, Jesus himself in the *m.*
Phil. 2:15, in the *m.* of a crooked nation.
Rev. 2:7, in the *m.* of the Paradise of God.
4:6; 5:6; 7:17, in the *m.* of the throne.
See Gen. 2:9; Isa. 12:6; Hos. 11:9.
MIGHT. Deut. 6:5, love God with all thy *m.*
8:17, the *m.* of mine hand hath gotten.
2 Sam. 6:14, David danced with all his *m.*
Eccl. 9:10, do it with thy *m.*
Isa. 40:29, to them that have no *m.*
Jer. 9:23, mighty man glory in his *m.*
51:30, their *m.* hath failed.
Zech. 4:6, not by *m.*, nor by power.
Eph. 3:16; Col. 1:11, strengthened with *m.*
See Eph. 6:10; 2 Pet. 2:11; Rev. 7:12.
MIGHTILY. Jon 3:8; Acts 18:28; 19:20; Col. 1:29.
MIGHTY. Gen. 10:9, he was a *m.* hunter.

Judg. 5:23, to the help of the Lord against the *m*.
2 Sam. 1:19, 25, how are the *m*. fallen!
23:8, these be the names of the *m*. men whom David had.
1 Chron. 11:10, the chief of the *m*. men.
Job 9:4, wise in heart and *m*. in strength.
Ps. 24:8, strong and *m*., *m*. in battle.
89:13, thou hast a *m*. arm.
19, help upon one that is *m*.
93:4, the *m*. waves of the sea.
Isa. 1:24; 30:29; 49:26; 60:16, the *m*. One of Israel.
5:15, *m*. to drink wine.
63:1, *m*. to save.
Jer. 32:19, *m*. in work.
Amos 2:14, neither shall *m*. deliver himself.
Mat. 11:20; 13:54; 14:2; Mk. 6:2, *m*. works.
Lu. 9:43, the *m*. power of God.
24:19, prophet *m*. in deed and word.
Acts 18:24, *m*. in the scriptures.
1 Cor. 1:26, not many *m*.
2 Cor. 10:4, weapons *m*. through God.
Eph. 1:19, the working of his *m*. power.
See Num. 14:12; Eccl. 6:10; Mat. 3:11.
MILK. Gen. 49:12, teeth white with *m*.
Prov. 30:33, churning of *m*.
Isa. 55:1, buy wine and *m*.
Lam. 4:7, Nazarites were whiter than *m*.
Ezek. 25:4, shall eat thy fruit and drink thy *m*.
Heb. 5:12, 13, such as have need of *m*.
1 Pet. 2:2, the sincere *m*. of the word.
See Judg. 4:19; 5:25; Job 21:24; Joel 3:18.
MIND (*n*.). Neh. 4:6, the people had a *m*. to work.
Job 23:13, he is in one *m*., who can turn him?
34:33, should it be according to thy *m*.?
Ps. 31:12, as a dead man out of *m*.
Prov. 29:11, a fool uttereth all his *m*.
Isa. 26:3, whose *m*. is stayed on thee.
Mk. 5:15; Lu. 8:35, sitting, in his right *m*.
Lu. 12:29, neither be of doubtful *m*.
Rom. 8:7, the carnal *m*. is enmity against God.
12:16, be of the same *m*.
14:5, fully persuaded in his own *m*.
2 Cor. 8:12, if there be first a willing *m*.
13:11; Phil. 1:27; 2:2, be of one *m*.
Phil. 2:3, in lowliness of *m*.
5, let this *m*. be in you.
4:7, peace of God keep your *m*.
1 Tim. 6:5; 2 Tim. 3:8, men of corrupt *m*.
2 Tim. 1:7, spirit of sound *m*.
Tit. 3:1, put them in *m*. to be subject.
1 Pet. 1:13, the loins of your *m*.
2 Pet. 3:1, stir up your pure *m*.
See Rom. 8:6; 11:20; 1 Thess. 5:14; Jas. 1:8.
MIND (*v*.). Rom. 8:5; 12:16; Phil. 3:16, 19.
MINDFUL. Ps. 8:4; 111:5; Isa. 17:10; 2 Pet. 3:2.
MINGLE. Lev. 19:19; Isa. 5:22; Mat. 27:34; Lu. 13:1.
MINISTER (*n*.). Ps. 103:21, ye *m*. of his.
104:4; Heb. 1:7, his *m*. a flame of fire.
Isa. 61:6, men shall call you the *m*. of God.
Joel 1:9, the Lord's *m*. mourn.
Mat. 20:26; Mk. 10:43, let him be your *m*.
Rom. 13:4, he is the *m*. of God to thee.
2 Cor. 3:6, able *m*. of new testament.
Gal. 2:17, is Christ the *m*. of sin?
Eph. 3:7; Col. 1:23, whereof I was made a *m*.
6:21; Col. 1:7; 4:7, a faithful *m*.
1 Tim. 4:6, a good *m*.
See 2 Cor. 6:4; 11:23; 1 Thess. 3:2.
MINISTER (*v*.). 1 Sam. 2:11, the child did *m*. unto the Lord.
1 Chron. 15:2, chosen to *m*. for ever.
Dan. 7:10, thousand thousands *m*. to him.
Mat. 4:11; Mk. 1:13, angels *m*. to him.
20:28; Mk. 10:45, not to be *m*. unto, but to *m*.
Lu. 8:3, which *m*. of their substance.
Acts 20:34, these hands have *m*.
See 2 Cor. 9:10; Heb. 1:14; 2 Pet. 1:11.
MINISTRATION. Lu. 1:23; Acts 6:1; 2 Cor. 3:7; 9:13.
MINISTRY. Acts 6:4, give ourselves to the *m*.
2 Cor. 4:1, seeing we have this *m*.
5:18, the *m*. of reconciliation.
6:3, that the *m*. be not blamed.
Eph. 4:12, for the work of the *m*.
Col. 4:17, take heed to the *m*.
2 Tim. 4:5, make full proof of thy *m*.
See Acts 1:17; 12:25; Rom. 12:7; Heb. 8:6.
MINSTREL. 2 Kings 3:15; Mat. 9:23.
MIRACLE. Judg. 6:13, where be all his *m*.?
Mk. 9:39, no man which shall do a *m*. in my name.
Lu. 23:8, hoped to have seen some *m*.
John 2:11, beginning of *m*.
4:54, this is the second *m*.
10:41, said, John did no *m*.
Acts 2:22, approved of God by *m*. and signs.
1 Cor. 12:10, to another, the working of *m*.
See Gal. 3:5; Heb. 2:4; Rev. 13:14; 16:14; 19:20.
MIRTH. Ps. 137:3; Prov. 14:13; Eccl. 2:1; 7:4; 8:15.
MIRY. Ps. 40:2; Ezek. 47:11; Dan. 2:41.
MISCHIEF. Job 15:35; Ps. 7:14; Isa. 59:4, they conceive *m*.
Ps. 28:3, *m*. is in their hearts.
94:20, frameth *m*. by a law.
Prov. 10:23, it is as sport to a fool to do *m*.
11:27, he that seeketh *m*.
24:2, lips talk of *m*.
Ezek. 7:26, *m*. shall come upon *m*.
Acts 13:10, O full of all subtilty and all *m*.
See Prov. 24:8; Eccl. 10:13; Mic. 7:3.
MISERABLE. Job 16:2; Mat. 21:41; 1 Cor. 15:19; Rev. 3:17.
MISERY. Prov. 31:7, drink, and remember his *m*. no more.
Eccl. 8:6, the *m*. of man is great upon him.
Lam. 1:7, remembered in days of her *m*.
Jas. 5:1, howl for your *m*. that shall come.
See Judg. 10:16; Job 3:20; 11:16; Rom. 3:16.
MIXED. Prov. 23:30, they seek *m*. wine.
Isa. 1:22, thy wine *m*. with water.
Heb. 4:2, not being *m*. with faith.
See Ex. 12:38; Num. 11:4; Neh. 13:3.
MOCK. Gen. 19:14, he seemed as one that *m*.
Num. 22:29; Judg. 16:10, 13, 15, thou hast *m*. me.
1 Kings 18:27, at noon Elijah *m*. them.
2 Chron. 36:16, they *m*. the messengers of God.
Prov. 1:26, I will *m*. when your fear cometh.
17:5, whoso *m*. the poor.
30:17, the eye that *m*. at his father.
Gal. 6:7, God is not *m*.
See 2 Kings 2:23; Mat. 2:16; 27:29; Mk. 15:20.
MOCKER. Ps. 35:16; Prov. 20:1; Isa. 28:22; Jude 18.
MODERATION. Phil. 4:5.
MOISTURE. Ps. 32:4; Lu. 8:6.
MOLLIFIED. Isa. 1:16.
MOMENT. Num. 16:21, 45, consume them in a *m*.
Job 7:18, try him every *m*.
21:13, and in a *m*. they go down.
Ps. 30:5, his anger endureth but a *m*.
Isa. 26:20, hide thyself as it were a *m*.
27:3, I will water it every *m*.
54:7, for a small *m*. have I forsaken thee.
1 Cor. 15:51, 52, we shall all be changed in a *m*.
2 Cor. 4:17, affliction, which is but for a *m*.
See Ex. 33:5; Ezek. 26:16; 32:10; Lu. 4:5.
MONEY. 2 Kings 5:26, is it a time to receive *m*.?
Eccl. 7:12, *m*. is a defence.
10:19, *m*. answereth all things.
Isa. 52:3, redeemed without *m*.
55:1, he that hath no *m*.
2, wherefore do ye spend *m*.
Mat. 17:24; 22:19, the tribute *m*.
25:18, hid his lord's *m*.
Acts 8:20, thy *m*. perish with thee.
1 Tim. 6:10, the love of *m*.
See Gen. 23:9; Mk. 6:8; Lu. 9:3; Acts 4:37.
MORROW. Prov. 27:1, boast not thyself of to-*m*.
Isa. 22:13; 1 Cor. 15:32, for to-*m*. we die.
56:12, to-*m*. shall be as this day.
Mat. 6:34, take no though for the *m*.
Jas. 4:14, ye know not what shall be on the *m*.

See Josh. 5:12; 2 Kings 7:1; Prov. 3:28.
MORSEL. Job 31:17; Ps. 147:17; Prov. 17:1; Heb. 12:16.
MORTAL. Job 4:17, shall *m.* man be more just?
Rom. 6:12; 8:11, in your *m.* body.
1 Cor. 15:53, 54, this *m.* must put on immortality.
See Deut. 19:11; 2 Cor. 4:11; 5:4.
MORTAR. Prov. 27:22; Ezek. 13:11, 22, 28.
MORTIFY. Rom. 8:13; Col. 3:5.
MOTE. Mat. 7:3; Lu. 6:41.
MOTH. Job 27:18, he buildeth his house as a *m.*
Ps. 39:11, consume away like a *m.*
Isa. 50:9, the *m.* shall eat them up.
Hos. 5:12, unto Ephraim as a *m.*
Mat. 6:10, where *m.* and rust doth corrupt.
MOTHER. Judg. 5:7; 2 Sam. 20:19, a *m.* in Israel.
1 Kings 22:52, Ahaziah walked in the way of his *m.*
2 Chron. 22:3, his *m.* was his counsellor.
Job 17:14, to the worm, thou art my *m.*
Ps. 113:9, a joyful *m.* of children.
Isa. 66:13, as one whom his *m.* comforteth.
Ezek. 16:44, as is the *m.*, so is her daughter.
Mat. 12:48; Mk. 3:33, who is my *m.*?
John 2:1; Acts 1:14, the *m.* of Jesus.
See Gen. 3:20; 17:16; Gal. 4:26; 1 Tim. 1:9; 5:2.
MOULDY. Josh. 9:5, 12.
MOUNT. Ex. 18:5, the *m.* of God.
Ps. 107:26, they *m.* up to heaven.
Isa. 40:31, *m.* with wings, as eagles.
See Job 20:6; 39:27; Isa. 27:13.
MOURN. Gen. 37:35, down to the grave *m.*
Prov. 5:11, and thou *m.* at the last.
Isa. 61:2, to comfort all that *m.*
Jer. 31:13, I will turn their *m.* into joy.
Mat. 5:4, blessed are they that *m.*
24:30, then shall all the tribes of the earth *m.*
Lu. 6:25, woe to you that laugh, for ye shall *m.*
See Neh. 8:9; Zech. 7:5; Jas. 4:9.
MOURNER. 2 Sam. 14:2; Eccl. 12:5; Hos. 9:4.
MOURNFULLY. Mal. 3:14.
MOUTH. Job 9:20, mine own *m.* shall condemn me.
40:4, I will lay my hand on my *m.*
Ps. 8:2; Mat. 21:16, out of the *m.* of babes.
39:1, I will keep my *m.* with a bridle.
49:3, my *m.* shall speak of wisdom.
55:21, words of his *m.* smoother than butter.
81:10, open thy *m.* wide.
Prov. 10:14; 14:3; 15:2, the *m.* of the foolish.
13:2, good by the fruit of his *m.*
3; 21:23, he that keepeth his *m.*
Eccl. 6:7, all the labour of a man is for his *m.*
Isa. 29:13; Mat. 15:8, this people draw near with *m.*
Ezek. 33:31, with their *m.* they show much love.
Mal. 2:6, the law of truth was in his *m.*
Mat. 12:34; Lu. 6:45, the *m.* speaketh.
13:35, I will open my *m.* in parables.
Lu. 21:15, I will give you a *m.* and wisdom.
Rom. 10:10, with the *m.* confession is made.
Tit. 1:11, whose *m.* must be stopped.
Jas. 3:10, out of the same *m.* proceedeth.
See Lam. 3:29; John 19:29; 1 Pet. 2:22.
MOVE. Ps. 10:6; 16:8; 30:6; 62:2, I shall not be *m.*
Mat. 21:10; Acts 21:30, all the city was *m.*
John 5:3, waiting fro the *m.* of the water.
Acts 17:28, in him we live, and *m.*
20:24, none of these things *m.* me.
See Prov. 23:31; Isa. 7:2; 2 Pet. 1:21.
MUCH. Ex. 16:18; 2 Cor. 8:15, he that gathered *m.*
Num. 16:3, ye take too *m.* upon you.
Lu. 7:47, for she loved *m.*
12:48, to whom *m.* is given.
16:10, faithful in *m.*
See Prov. 25:16; Eccl. 5:12; Jer. 2:22.
MULTIPLY. Isa. 9:3, thou hast *m.* the nation, and not increased the joy.
Jer. 3:16, when ye be *m.* they shall say.
Dan. 4:1; 6:25; 1 Pet. 1:2; 2 Pet. 1:2; Jude 2, peace be *m.*
Nah. 3:16, thou hast *m.* thy merchants.
See Acts 6:1; 7:17; 9:31; 12:24.
MULTITUDE. Ex. 23:2, a *m.* to do evil.
Job 32:7, *m.* of years should teach wisdom.
Ps. 5:7; 51:1; 69:13; 106:7, in the *m.* of thy mercy.
33:16, no king saved by the *m.* of an host.
94:19, in the *m.* of my thoughts.
Prov. 10:19, in *m.* of words there wanteth not sin.
11:14; 15:22; 24:6, in the *m.* of counsellors.
Eccl. 5:3, through the *m.* of business.
Jas. 5:20; 1 Pet. 4:8, hide a *m.* of sins.
See Deut. 1:10; Josh. 11:4; Lu. 2:13.
MURMURINGS. Ex. 16:7; Num. 14:27; Phil. 2:14.
MUSE. Ps. 39:3; 143:5; Lu. 3:15.
MUTTER. Isa. 8:19; 59:3.
MUTUAL. Rom. 1:12.
MYSTERY. Mat. 13:11; 1 Cor. 2:7; 15:51; Eph. 5:32.

N

NAIL. Ezra 9:8, give us a *n.* in his holy place.
Isa. 22:23, fasten as a *n.* in sure place.
John 20:25, put finger into print of *n.*
Col. 2:14, *n.* it to his cross.
See Judg. 4:21; Eccl. 12:11; Dan. 4:33.
NAKED. Ex. 32:25, made *n.* to their shame.
Job 1:21, *n.* came I out, and *n.* shall I return.
Mat. 25:36, *n.*, and ye clothed me.
1 Cor. 4:11, to this present hour we are *n.*
2 Cor. 5:3, we shall not be found *n.*
Heb. 4:13, all things are *n.* to eyes of him.
See John 21:7; Jas. 2:15; Rev. 3:17; 16:15.
NAKEDNESS. Rom. 8:35; 2 Cor. 11:27; Rev. 3:18.
NAME (*n.*). Gen. 32:29; Judg. 13:18, wherefore dost thou ask after my *n.*?
Ex. 3:15, this is my *n.* for ever.
23:21, my *n.* is in him.
Josh. 7:9, what wilt thou do to thy great *n.*?
2 Chron. 14:11, in thy *n.* we go.
Neh. 9:10, so didst thou get thee a *n.*
Job 18:17, he shall have no *n.* in the street.
Ps. 20:1, the *n.* of God defend thee.
5, in the *n.* of God set up banners.
22:22; Heb. 2:12, I will declare thy *n.*
48:10, according to thy *n.* so is thy praise.
69:36, they that love his *n.*
111:9, holy and reverend is his *n.*
115:1, unto thy *n.* give glory.
138:2, thy word above all thy *n.*
Prov. 10:7, the *n.* of the wicked shall rot.
18:10, the *n.* of the Lord a strong tower.
22:1; Eccl. 7:1, good *n.* rather to be chosen.
Cant. 1:3, thy *n.* is as ointment poured forth.
Isa. 42:8, I am the Lord, that is my *n.*
55:13, it shall be to the Lord for a *n.*
56:5; 63:12, an everlasting *n.*
57:15, whose *n.* is Holy.
62:2, called by a new *n.*
64:7, there is none that calleth on thy *n.*
Jer. 10:6, thou art great, and thy *n.* is great.
14:14; 23:25; 27:15, prophesy lies in my *n.*
44:26, sworn by my great *n.*
Zech. 10:12, walk up and down in his *n.*
14:9, one Lord, and his *n.* one.
Mal. 1:6, wherein have we despised thy *n.*?
4:2, to you that fear my *n.*
Mat. 6:9; Lu. 11:2, hallowed be thy *n.*
10:22; 19:29; Mk. 13:13; Lu. 21:12; John 15:21; Acts 9:16, for my *n.* sake.
12:21, in his *n.* shall the Gentiles trust.
18:5; Mk. 9:37; Lu. 9:48, receive in my *n.*
20, gathered together in my *n.*
24:5; Mk. 13:6; Lu. 21:8, many shall come in my *n.*
Mk. 5:9; Lu. 8:30, what is thy *n.*?
9:39, do a miracle in my *n.*
Lu. 10:20, *n.* written in heaven.
John 5:43, if another shall come in his own *n.*
14:13; 15:16; 16:23, 24, 26, whatsoever ye ask in my *n.*
Acts 3:16, his *n.* through faith in his *n.*
4:12, none other *n.* under heaven.

Acts 5:28, that ye should not teach in this *n.*
41, worthy to suffer for his *n.*
Eph. 1:21, far above every *n.*
Phil. 2:9, 10, a *n.* above every *n.*
4:3, whose *n.* are in the book of life.
Col. 3:17, do all in the *n.* of the Lord Jesus.
Heb. 1:4, obtained a more excellent *n.*
Jas. 2:7, that worthy *n.*
Rev. 2:13, holdest fast my *n.*
17, a *n.* written, which no man knoweth.
3:1, thou hast a *n.* that thou livest.
4, a few *n.* in Sardis.
13:1, the *n.* of blasphemy.
14:1; 22:4, Father's *n.* in their foreheads.
See Gen. 2:20; Ex. 28:9; Isa. 45:3; John 10:3.
NAME (*v.*). Eccl. 6:10, that which hath been is *n.* already.
Isa. 61:6, ye shall be *n.* Priests of the Lord.
Rom. 15:20, not where Christ was *n.*
2 Tim. 2:19, every one that *n.* the name of Christ.
See 1 Sam. 16:3; Isa. 62:2; Lu. 2:21; 6:13.
NARROW. Isa. 28:20; 49:19; Mat. 7:14.
NATION. Gen. 10:32, by these were the *n.* divided.
20:4, wilt thou slay a righteous *n.*?
Num. 14:12; Deut. 9:14, I will make thee a greater *n.*
2 Sam. 7:23; 1 Chron. 17:21, what *n.* like thy people?
Ps. 33:12, blessed is the *n.* whose God is the Lord.
147:20, he hath not dealt so with any *n.*
Prov. 14:34, righteousness exalteth a *n.*
Isa. 2:4; Mic. 4:3, *n.* shall not lift sword against *n.*
18:2, a *n.* scattered and peeled.
26:2, that the righteous *n.* may enter in.
34:1, come near, ye *n.*, to hear.
52:15, so shall he sprinkle many *n.*
Jer. 10:7, O King of *n.*
Zech. 2:11, many *n.* shall be joined to the Lord.
8:22, strong *n.* shall seek the Lord.
Mat. 24:7; Mk. 13:8; Lu. 21:10, *n.* against *n.*
Lu. 7:5, he loveth our *n.*
21:25, distress of *n.*
John 11:50, that the whole *n.* perish not.
Acts 2:5, devout men of every *n.*
10:35, in every *n.* he that feareth.
Phil. 2:15, crooked and perverse *n.*
Rev. 5:9, redeemed out of every *n.*
See Deut. 4:27; 15:6; Jer. 2:11; 4:2; 31:10.
NATIVITY. Gen. 11:28; Jer. 46:16; Ezek. 21:30; 23:15.
NATURAL. Deut. 34:7, nor his *n.* force abated.
Rom. 1:31; 2 Tim. 3:3, without *n.* affection.
1 Cor. 2:14, the *n.* man receiveth not.
See 1 Cor. 15:44; Phil. 2:20; Jas. 1:23.
NATURE. 1 Cor. 11:14, doth not even *n.* itself teach?
Eph. 2:3, by *n.* children of wrath.
Heb. 2:16, the *n.* of angels.
2 Pet. 1:4, partakers of the divine *n.*
See Rom. 1:26; 2:14, 27; Gal. 2:15; 4:8.
NAUGHT. Prov. 20:14, it is *n.*, saith the buyer.
Isa. 49:4, spent strength for *n.*
52:3, ye have sold yourselves for *n.*
Mal. 1:10, shut the doors for *n.*
Acts 5:38, if of men, it will come to *n.*
See Deut. 15:9; Job 1:9; Rom. 14:10; 1 Cor. 1:28.
NAUGHTINESS. 1 Sam. 17:28; Prov. 11:6; Jas. 1:21.
NAUGHTY. Prov. 6:12; 17:4; Jer. 24:2.
NAY. Mat. 5:37; 2 Cor. 1:17, 18, 19; Jas. 5:12.
NEAR. Judg. 20:34, knew not evil was *n.*
Ps. 22:11, trouble is *n*
148:14, a people *n.* to him.
Prov. 27:10, better a neighbour that is *n.*
Isa. 50:8, he is *n.* that justifieth.
55:6, call upon the Lord while he is *n.*
Obad. 15; Zeph. 1:14, the day of the Lord is *n.*
Mat. 24:33, it is *n.*, even at the doors.
Mk. 13:28, ye know that summer is *n.*
See Ezek. 11:3; 22:5; Rom. 13:11.
NECESSARY. Job 23:12; Acts 15:28; 28:10; Tit. 3:14.
NECESSITIES. 2 Cor. 6:4, as the ministers of God, in *n.*
NECESSITY. Rom. 12:13, distributing to the *n.* of saints.
1 Cor. 9:16, *n.* is laid upon me.
2 Cor. 9:7; Philem. 14, give, not grudgingly, or of *n.*
See Acts 20:34; 2 Cor. 12:10; Phil. 4:16.
NECK. Prov. 3:3; 6:21, bind them about thy *n.*
Mat. 18:6; Mk. 9:42; Lu. 17:2, millstone about his *n.*
Lu. 15:20; Acts 20:37, fell on his *n.*
Acts 15:10, yoke on the *n.* of disciples.
See Neh. 9:29; Isa. 3:16; Lam. 5:5; Rom. 16:4.
NEED. 2 Chron. 20:17, ye shall not *n.* to fight.
Prov. 31:11, he shall have no *n.* of spoil.
Mat. 6:8; Lu. 12:30, what things ye have *n.* of.
9:12; Mk. 2:17; Lu. 5:31, *n.* not a physician.
14:16, they *n.* not depart.
21:3; Mk. 11:3; Lu. 19:31, 34, the Lord hath *n.* of them.
Lu. 11:8, as many as he *n.*
Acts 2:45; 4:35, as every man had *n.*
1 Cor. 12:21, cannot say, I have no *n.* of thee.
Phil. 4:12, to abound and to suffer *n.*
19, God shall supply all your *n.*
2 Tim. 2:15, that *n.* not to be ashamed.
Heb. 4:16, grace to help in time of *n.*
5:1, ye have *n.* that one teach you.
1 John 3:17, seeth his brother have *n.*
Rev. 3:17, rich, and have *n.* of nothing.
21:23; 22:5, city had no *n.* of the sun.
See Deut. 15:8; Lu. 9:11; John 2:25; Acts 17:25.
NEEDFUL. Lu. 10:42; Phil. 1:24; Jas. 2:16.
NEEDY. Deut. 15:11, thou shalt open thine hand to thy *n.*
Job 24:4, they turn the *n.* out of the way.
Ps. 9:18, the *n.* shall not alway be forgotten.
40:17; 70:5; 86:1; 109:22, I am poor and *n.*
74:21, let the poor and *n.* praise thy name.
Prov. 31:9, plead the cause of the poor and *n.*
Isa. 41:17, when the *n.* seek water.
See Ezek. 16:49; 18:12; 22:29; Amos 8:4, 6.
NEGLECT. Mat. 18:17; Acts 6:1; 1 Tim. 4:14; Heb. 2:3.
NEGLIGENT. 2 Chron. 29:11; 2 Pet. 1:12.
NEIGHBOUR. Prov. 3:28, say not to thy *n.*, go and come again.
14:20, the poor is hated even of his *n.*
21:10, his *n.* findeth no favour.
Eccl. 4:4, envied of his *n.*
Jer. 22:13, that useth his *n.* service without wages.
Hab. 2:15, that giveth his *n.* drink.
Zech. 8:16; Eph. 4:25, speak every man truth to his *n.*
Lu. 10:29, who is my *n.*?
14:12, call not thy rich *n.*
See Ex. 20:16; Lev. 19:13; Mat. 5:43; Rom. 13:10.
NEST. Num. 24:21, thou puttest thy *n.* in a rock.
Deut. 32:11, as an eagle stirreth up her *n.*
Job 29:18, I shall die in my *n.*
Ps. 84:3, the swallow hath found a *n.*
Mat. 8:20; Lu. 9:58, birds of the air have *n.*
See Prov. 27:8; Isa. 16:2; Jer. 49:16; Obad. 4; Hab. 2:9.
NET. Ps. 141:10, let the wicked fall into their own *n.*
Prov. 1:17, in vain the *n.* is spread.
Eccl. 9:12, as fishes taken in an evil *n.*
Hab. 1:16, they sacrifice unto their *n.*
Mat. 13:47, kingdom of heaven like a *n.*
Mk. 1:18, they forsook their *n.*
Lu. 5:5, at thy word I will let down the *n.*
See Mat. 4:21; Mk. 1:16; John 21:6.
NETHER. Deut. 24:6; Job 41:24.
NEVER. Lev. 6:13, the fire shall *n.* go out.
Job 3:16, as infants which *n.* saw light.
Ps. 10:11, he will *n.* see it.
15:5; 30:6, shall *n.* be moved.
Prov. 27:20; 30:15, *n.* satisfied.
Isa. 56:11, which can *n.* have enough.
Mat. 7:23, I *n.* knew you.
9:33, it was *n.* so seen in Israel.
26:33, yet will I *n.* be offended.
Mk. 2:12, we *n.* saw it on this fashion.
3:29, hath *n.* forgiveness.
14:21, if he had *n.* been born.
John 4:14; 6:35, shall *n.* thirst.
7:46, *n.* man spake like this man.
8:51; 10:28; 11:26, shall *n.* see death.

1 Cor. 13:8, charity *n.* faileth.
Heb. 13:5, I will *n.* leave thee.
2 Pet. 1:10, ye shall *n.* fall.
See Judg. 2:1; Ps. 58:5; Jer. 33:17; Dan. 2:44.
NEW. Num. 16:30, if the Lord make a *n.* thing.
Ps. 33:3; 40:3; 96:1; 98:1; 144:9; 149:1; Isa. 42:10; Rev. 5:9;
14:3, a *n.* song.
Eccl. 1:9, no *n.* thing under the sun.
Isa. 65:17; 66:22; Rev. 21:1, *n.* heavens and *n.* earth.
Lam. 3:23, *n.* every morning.
Mat. 9:16; Mk. 2:21; Lu. 5:36, *n.* cloth to old garment.
13:52, things *n.* and old.
Mk. 1:27; Acts 17:19, what *n.* doctrine is this?
John 13:34; 1 John 2:7, 8, a *n.* commandment.
Acts 17:21, to tell or hear some *n.* thing.
2 Cor. 5:17; Gal. 6:15, a *n.* creature.
Eph. 2:15; 4:24; Col. 3:10, *n.* man.
Heb. 10:20, *n.* and living way.
Rev. 2:17; 3:12, a *n.* name.
21:5, I make all things *n.*
See Isa. 24:7; 43:19; 65:8; Acts 2:13.
NEWLY. Deut. 32:17; Judg. 7:19.
NEWNESS. Rom. 6:4; 7:6.
NEWS. Prov. 25:25.
NIGH. Num. 24:17, but not *n.*
Deut. 30:14; Rom. 10:8, the word is *n.* unto thee.
Ps. 34:18, *n.* to them of broken heart.
145:18, *n.* to all that call upon him.
Eph. 2:13, made *n.* by the blood of Christ.
See Joel 2:1; Lu. 21:20; Heb. 6:8.
NIGHT. Ex. 12:42, a *n.* to be much observed.
Job 7:4, when shall I arise, and the *n.* be gone?
35:10; Ps. 77:6, songs in the *n.*
Ps. 30:5, weeping may endure for a *n.*
91:5, the terror by *n.*
136:9; Jer. 31:35, moon and stars to rule by *n.*
139:11, then *n.* shall be light about me.
Isa. 21:4, the *n.* of my pleasure.
11, watchman, what of the *n.*?
Lu. 6:12, he continued all *n.* in prayer.
John 9:4, the *n.* cometh, when no man can work.
John 11:10, walk in the *n.*, he stumbleth.
Rom. 13:12, the *n.* is far spent.
1 Thess. 5:2; 2 Pet. 3:10, cometh as a thief in the *n.*
Rev. 21:25; 22:5, no *n.* there.
See Job 7:3; Ps. 121:6; Mat. 27:64; John 3:2.
NOBLE. Neh. 3:5, the *n.* put not their neck.
Job 29:10, the *n.* held their peace.
Jer. 2:21, planted thee a *n.* vine.
14:3, their *n.* sent their little ones to the waters.
Acts 17:11, Bereans were more *n.*
1 Cor. 1:26, not many *n.*
See Num. 21:18; Ps. 149:8; Eccl. 10:17.
NOISE. Ezra 3:13, not discern *n.* of joy.
Ps. 66:1; 81:1; 95:1; 98:4; 100:1, joyful *n.*
Ezek. 1:24; 43:2, *n.* of great waters.
2 Pet. 3:10, pass away with great *n.*
See Josh. 6:27; Mat. 9:23; Mk. 2:1; Acts 2:6.
NOISOME. Ps. 91:3; Ezek. 14:21; Rev. 16:2.
NOTHING. Deut. 2:7; Neh. 9:21, thou hast lacked *n.*
2 Sam. 24:24, neither offer of that which doth cost *n.*
2 Chron. 14:11, it is *n.* with thee to help.
Neh. 8:10, portions to them for whom *n.* is prepared.
Job 8:9, but of yesterday, and know *n.*
Ps. 49:17, he shall carry *n.* away.
119:165, *n.* shall offend them.
Prov. 13:4, the sluggard desireth, and hath *n.*
7, there is that maketh himself rich, yet hath *n.*
Lam. 1:12, is it *n.* to you?
Mat. 17:20; Lu. 1:37, *n.* shall be impossible.
21:19; Mk. 11:13, *n.* but leaves.
Lu. 6:35, hoping for *n.* again.
7:42, they had *n.* to pay.
John 15:5, without me ye can do *n.*
1 Cor. 4:4, I know *n.* by myself.
2 Cor. 6:10, as having *n.*
13:8, we can do *n.* against the truth.
1 Tim. 4:4, *n.* to be refused.
6:7, brought *n.* into this world, can carry *n.* out.
See Phil. 4:6; Jas. 1:4; 3 John 7.
NOURISH. Isa. 1:2, I have *n.* and brought up children.
1 Tim. 4:6, *n.* in words of faith.
Jas. 5:5, have *n.* your hearts.
See Gen. 45:11; 50:21; Acts 12:20; Col. 2:19.
NOW. Job 4:5, *n.* it is come upon thee.
Ps. 119:67, but *n.* have I kept thy word.
Hos. 2:7, then was it better than *n.*
Lu. 14:17, all things are *n.* ready.
John 13:7, thou knowest not *n.*
16:12, ye cannot bear them *n.*
1 Cor. 13:12, *n.* I know in part.
Gal. 2:20, the life I *n.* live.
1 Tim. 4:8, the life that *n.* is.
1 Pet. 1:8, though *n.* ye see him not.
1 John 3:2, *n.* are we sons of God.
See Rom. 6:22; Gal. 3:3; Heb. 2:8.
NUMBER (*n.*). Job 5:9; 9:10, marvellous things without *n.*
25:3, is there any *n.* of his armies?
Ps. 139:18, more in *n.* than the sand.
147:4, he telleth the *n.* of the stars.
Acts 11:21, a great *n.* believed.
16:5, the churches increased in *n.* daily.
Rev. 13:17, 18, the *n.* of his name.
See Deut. 7:7; Hos. 1:10; Rom. 9:27.
NUMBER (*v.*). Gen. 41:49, gathered corn till he left *n.*
2 Sam. 24:2; 1 Chron. 21:2, *n.* the people.
Ps. 90:12, so teach us to *n.* our days.
Eccl. 1:15, that which is wanting cannot be *n.*
Isa. 53:12; Mk. 15:28, he was *n.* with transgressors.
Mat. 10:30; Lu. 12:7, hairs are all *n.*
Rev. 7:9, multitude which no man could *n.*
See Ex. 30:12; Job 14:16; Ps. 40:5; Acts 1:17.
NURSE. Gen. 35:8, Deborah Rebekah's *n.* died.
2 Sam. 4:4, and his *n.* took him up and fled.
1 Thess. 2:7, even as a *n.* cherisheth her children.
See Ex. 2:7, 9; Isa. 60:4.
NURSING. Isa. 49:23, kings shall be thy *n.* fathers, and their queens thy *n.* mothers.
NURTURE. Eph. 6:4.

O

OBEDIENCE. Rom. 5:19, by the *o.* of one.
16:26, the *o.* of faith.
Heb. 5:8, yet learned he *o.*
See Rom. 16:19; 2 Cor. 10:5; 1 Pet. 1:2.
OBEDIENT. Ex. 24:7, all will we do, and be *o.*
Prov. 25:12, wise reprover upon an *o.* ear.
Isa. 1:19, if *o.* ye shall eat.
2 Cor. 2:9, *o.* in all things.
Eph. 6:5; Tit. 2:9, be *o.* to your masters.
Phil. 2:8, *o.* unto death.
1 Pet. 1:14, as *o.* children.
See Num. 27:20; 2 Sam. 22:45; Tit. 2:5.
OBEISANCE. Gen. 37:7; 43:28; 2 Sam. 15:5.
OBEY. Deut. 11:27, a blessing if ye *o.*
Josh. 24:24, his voice will we *o.*
1 Sam. 15:22, to *o.* is better than sacrifice.
Jer. 7:23, *o.* my voice, and I will be your God.
Acts. 5:29, his servants ye are to whom ye *o.*
Rom. 6:16, his servants ye are to thom ye *o.*
Eph. 6:1; Col. 3:20, *o.* your parents in the Lord.
2 Thess. 1:8; 1 Pet. 4:17, that *o.* not the gospel.
Heb. 13:17, *o.* them that have rule over you.
1 Pet. 1:22, purified your souls in *o.* the truth.
See Ex. 5:2; 23:21; Dan. 9:10; Mat. 8:27.
OBJECT. Acts 24:19.
OBSCURE. Prov. 20:20.
OBSCURITY. Isa. 29:18; 58:10; 59:9.
OBSERVATION. Lu. 17:20.
OBSERVE. Gen. 37:11, his father *o.* the saying.
Ps. 107:43, whoso is wise, and will *o.* these things.
Prov. 23:26, let thine eyes *o.* my ways.
Eccl. 11:4, he that *o.* the wind.
Jon. 2:8, that *o.* lying vanities.

Mat. 28:20, teaching them to *o.* all things.
Mk. 6:20, Herod feared John, and *o.* him.
10:20, all these have I *o.*
See Ex. 12:42; 31:16; Ezek. 20:18; Gal. 4:10.
OBSERVER. Deut. 18:10.
OBSTINATE. Deut. 2:30; Isa. 48:4.
OBTAIN. Prov. 8:35, shall *o.* favour of the Lord.
Isa. 35:10; 51:11, shall *o.* joy and gladness.
Lu. 20:35, worthy to *o.* that world.
Acts 26:22, having *o.* help of God.
1 Cor. 9:24, so run that ye may *o.*
1 Thess. 5:9; 2 Tim. 2:10, to *o.* salvation.
1 Tim. 1:13, I *o.* mercy.
Heb. 4:16, *o.* mercy, and find grace to help.
9:12, having *o.* eternal redemption.
1 Pet. 2:10, which had not *o.* mercy, but now have *o.*
2 Pet. 1:1, *o.* like precious faith.
See Dan. 11:21; Hos. 2:23; Acts 1:17; 22:28.
OCCASION. 2 Sam. 12:14, great *o.* to enemies to blaspheme.
Dan. 6:4, sought to find *o.*
Rom. 7:8, sin, taking *o.* by the commandment.
14:13, an *o.* to fall in his brother's way.
1 Tim. 5:14, give none *o.* to the adversary.
See Gen. 43:18; Ezra 7:20; Ezek. 18:3.
OCCUPATION. Gen. 46:33; Jon. 1:8; Acts 18:3; 29:25.
OCCUPY. Ezek. 27:9; Lu. 19:13.
ODOUR. John 12:3; Phil. 4:18; Rev. 5:8.
OFFENCE. Eccl. 10:4, yielding pacifieth great *o.*
Isa. 8:14; Rom. 9:33; 1 Pet. 2:8, a rock of *o.*
Mat. 16:23, thou art an *o.* to me.
18:7; Lu. 17:1, woe to the world because of *o.*!
Acts 24:16, conscience void of *o.*
Rom. 14:20, that man who eateth with *o.*
1 Cor. 10:32; 2 Cor. 6:3, give none *o.*
Phil. 1:10, without *o.* till the day of Christ.
See 1 Sam. 25:31; Rom. 5:15; 16:17; Gal. 5:11.
OFFEND. Job 34:31, I will not *o.* any more.
Ps. 119:165, nothing shall *o.* them.
Prov. 18:19, brother *o.* is harder to be won.
Mat. 5:29; 18:9; Mk. 9:47, if thine eye *o.* thee.
13:41, gather all things that *o.*
57; Mk. 6:3, they were *o.* in him.
26:33, though all shall be *o.*, yet will I never be.
Rom. 14:21, whereby thy brother is *o.*
Jas. 2:10, yet *o.* in one point.
See Gen. 20:9; Jer. 37:18; 2 Cor. 11:29.
OFFENDER. 1 Kings 1:21; Isa. 29:21; Acts 25:11.
OFFER. Judg. 5:2, people willingly *o.* themselves.
Ps. 50:23, whoso *o.* praise.
Mat. 5:24, then come and *o.* thy gift.
Lu. 6:29, one cheek, *o.* also the other.
1 Cor. 8:1, 4, 7; 10:19, things *o.* to idols.
Phil. 2:17, *o.* in the service of your faith.
2 Tim. 4:6, now ready to be *o.*
Heb. 9:28, Christ once *o.* to bear the sins of many.
See 2 Chron. 17:16; Ezra 1:6; 2:68; Mal. 1:8.
OFFICE. 1 Sam. 2:36, put me into one of the priests' *o.*
Rom. 11:13, I magnify mine *o.*
1 Tim. 3:1, the *o.* of a bishop.
Heb. 7:5, the *o.* of the priesthood.
See Gen. 41:13; Ps. 109:8; Rom. 12:4.
OFFSCOURING. Lam. 3:45; 1 Cor. 4:13.
OFFSPRING. Job 27:14; Acts 17:28; Rev. 22:16.
OFTEN. Prov. 29:1, being *o.* reproved.
Mal. 3:16, spake *o.* one to another.
Mat. 23:37; Lu. 13:34, how *o.* would I have gathered.
1 Cor. 11:26, as *o.* as ye eat.
1 Tim. 5:23, thine *o.* infirmities.
See 2 Cor. 11:26; Heb. 9:25; 10:11.
OIL. Ps. 45:7; Heb. 1:9, with *o.* of gladness.
92:10, be anointed with fresh *o.*
104:15, *o.* to make his face to shine.
Isa. 61:3, *o.* of joy for mourning.
Mat. 25:3, took no *o.* with them.
Lu. 10:34, pouring in *o.* and wine.
See Ex. 27:20; Mic. 6:7; Lu. 7:46.
OLD. Deut. 8:4; 29:5; Neh. 9:21, waxed not *o.*
Josh. 5:11, did eat of the *o.* corn.
Ps. 37:25, I have been young, and now am *o.*
71:18, when I am *o.* forsake me not.
Prov. 22:6, when he is *o.* he will not.
Isa. 58:12, build the *o.* waste places.
Jer. 6:16, ask for the *o.* paths.
Lu. 5:39, he saith, the *o.* is better.
2 Cor. 5:17, *o.* things are passed away.
2 Pet. 2:5, God spared not the *o.* world.
1 John 2:7, the *o.* commandment is the word.
Rev. 12:9; 20:2, that *o.* serpent.
See Job 22:15; Ps. 77:5; Mat. 5:21; Rom. 7:6.
OMITTED. Mat. 23:23.
ONCE. Gen. 18:32, yet but this *o.*
Num. 13:30, let us go up at *o.*
Job 33:14; Ps. 62:11, speaketh *o.*, yea twice.
Isa. 66:8, shall a nation be born at *o.*?
Heb. 6:4, *o.* enlightened.
9:27, *o.* to die.
See Rom. 6:10; Heb. 10:10; 1 Pet. 3:18.
ONE. Job 9:3, *o.* of a thousand.
Eccl. 7:27; Isa. 27:12, *o.* by *o.*
Mk. 10:21; LU. 18:22, *o.* thing thou lackest.
Lu. 10:42, *o.* thing is needful.
John 9:25, *o.* thing I know.
17:11, 21, 22, that they may be *o.*
Gal. 3:28, all *o.* in Christ.
Eph. 4:5, *o.* Lord, *o.* faith, *o.* baptism.
See Deut. 6:4; Mk. 12:32; 1 Tim. 2:5.
ONYX. Ex. 28:20; 39:13, and an *o.*
OPEN. Num. 16:30, if the earth *o.* her mouth.
Ps. 49:4, I will *o.* my dark saying.
51:15, *o.* thou my lips.
81:10, *o.* thy mouth wide.
104:28; 145:16, thou *o.* thine hand.
119:18, *o.* thou mine eyes.
Prov. 31:8, *o.* thy mouth for the dumb.
Isa. 22:22, he shall *o.*, and none shall shut.
42:7, to *o.* the blind eyes.
60:11, thy gates shall be *o.* continually.
Ezek. 16:63, never *o.* thy mouth.
Mal. 3:10, *o.* windows of heaven.
Mat. 25:11; Lu. 13:25, Lord *o.* to us.
27:52, graves were *o.*
Mk. 7:34, that is, be *o.*
Lu. 24:32, while he *o.* to us the scriptures.
45, then *o.* he their understanding.
Acts 26:18, to *o.* their eyes, and turn them.
1 Cor. 16:9, great door and effectual is *o.*
Col. 4:3, *o.* to us a door of utterance.
See Acts 16:14; 2 Cor. 2:12; Heb. 4:13; Re. 5:2.
OPERATION. Ps. 28:5; Isa. 5:12; 1 Cor. 12:6; Col. 2:12.
OPINION. 1 Kings 18:21; Job 32:6.
OPPORTUNITY. Gal. 6:10; Phil. 4:10; Heb. 11:15.
OPPOSE. Job 30:21; 2 Thess. 2:4; 2 Tim. 2:25.
OPPOSITIONS. 1 Tim. 6:20.
OPPRESS. Ex. 22:21; 23:9, *o.* a stranger.
Lev. 25:14, 17, ye shall not *o.* one another.
1 Sam. 12:3, whom have I *o.*?
Ps. 10:18, that the man of earth may no more *o.*
Prov. 14:31; 22:16, he that *o.* the poor.
28:3, a poor man that *o.* the poor.
Jer. 7:6, if ye *o.* not the stranger.
Hos. 12:7, he loveth to *o.*
Zech. 7:10, *o.* not the widow.
See Mal. 3:5; Acts 7:24; 10:38; Jas. 2:6.
OPPRESSION. Deut. 26:7, the Lord looked on our *o.*
Ps. 62:10, trust not in *o.*
119:134, deliver me from the *o.* of man.
Eccl. 4:1, I considered the *o.*
7:7, *o.* maketh a wise man mad.
Isa. 30:12, ye trust in *o.*
See Isa. 33:15; Zech. 9:8; 10:4.
ORATOR. Isa. 3:3; Acts 24:1.
ORDAIN. 1 Chron. 17:9, I will *o.* a place for my people.
Ps. 8:2, hast thou *o.* strength.
81:5, this he *o.* in Joseph.

Ps. 132:17, I have *o*. a lamp for mine anointed.
Isa. 26:12, thou wilt *o*. peace for us.
30:33, Tophet is *o*. of old.
Jer. 1:5, I *o*. thee a prophet.
Mk. 3:14, Jesus *o*. twelve.
John 15:16, have *o*. you, that ye should bring forth.
Acts 1:22, one be *o*. to be a witness.
10:42, *o*. of God to be the Judge.
13:48, *o*. to eternal life.
14:23; Tit. 1:5, *o*. elders.
16:4, decrees that were *o*.
17:31, by that man whom he hath *o*.
Rom. 13:1, the powers that be are *o*. of God.
Gal. 3:19, the law was *o*. by angels.
Eph. 2:10, good works which God hath before *o*.
Jude 4, of old *o*. to this condemnation.
See 1 Cor. 2:7; 9:14; 1 Tim. 2:7; Heb. 5:1.
ORDER. Judg. 13:12, how shall we *o*. the child?
2 Kings 20:1; Isa. 38:1, set thine house in *o*.
Job 10:22, land without any *o*.
23:4, I would *o*. my cause.
37:19, we cannot *o*. our speech.
Ps. 40:5, they cannot be reckoned in *o*.
50:21, I will set them in *o*.
23, to him that *o*. his conversation aright.
110:4; Heb. 5:6; 6:20; 7:11, the *o*. of Melchisedec.
1 Cor. 14:40, decently and in *o*.
Tit. 1:5, that thou shouldest set in *o*.
See Ps. 37:23; Acts 21:24; 1 Cor. 15:23.
ORDINANCE. Isa. 58:2; Rom. 13:2, the *o*. of their God.
Mal. 3:14, what profit that we have kept *o*.?
Eph. 2:15, commandments contained in *o*.
Col. 2:14, handwriting of *o*.
Heb. 9:10, in carnal *o*.
See Jer. 31:36; Luke 1:6; 1 Pet. 2:13.
ORPHANS. Lam. 5:3.
OSTRICH. Job 39:13, or wings and feathers unto the *o*.
Lam. 4:3, like the *o*. in the wilderness.
OUGHT. 1 Chron. 12:32, to know what Israel *o*. to do.
Mat. 23:23; Lu. 11:42, these *o*. ye to have done.
Lu. 24:26, *o*. not Christ to have suffered?
John 4:20, the place where men *o*. to worship.
Acts 5:29, we *o*. to obey God.
Rom. 8:26, what we should pray for as we *o*.
Heb. 5:12, when ye *o*. to be teachers.
Jas. 3:10, these things *o*. not so to be.
Pet. 3:11, what manner of persons *o*. ye to be?
See Rom. 12:3; 15:1; 1 Tim. 3:15.
OURS. Mk. 12:7; Lu. 20:14; 1 Cor. 1:2; 2 Cor. 1:14.
OUT. Num. 32:23, be sure your sin will find you *o*.
Ps. 82:5, are *o*. of course.
Prov. 4:23, *o*. of it are the issues of life.
Mat. 12:34; 15:19, *o*. of abundance of heart the mouth speaketh.
2 Tim. 3:11, *o*. of them all the Lord delivered me.
4:2, instant in season, *o*. of season.
See Gen. 2:9, 23; 3:19; John 15:19; Acts 2:5.
OUTCAST. Ps. 147:2; Isa. 11:12; 27:13; Jer. 30:17.
OUTGOINGS. Josh. 17:18; Ps. 65:8.
OUTRAGEOUS. Prov. 27:4.
OUTRUN. John 20:4.
OUTSIDE. Judg. 7:11; Mat. 23:25; Lu. 11:39.
OUTSTRETCHED. Deut. 26:8; Jer. 21:5; 27:5.
OUTWARD. 1 Sam. 16:7, looketh on *o*. appearance.
Mat. 23:27, appear beautiful *o*.
Rom. 2:28, not a Jew, which is one *o*.
2 Cor. 4:16, though our *o*. man perish.
See Mat. 23:28; Rom. 2:28; 1 Pet. 3:3.
OVERCHARGE. Lu. 21:34; 2 Cor. 2:5.
OVERCOME. Gen. 49:19, he shall *o*. at last.
Jer. 23:9, like a man whom wine hath *o*.
John 16:33, I have *o*. the world.
Rom. 12:21, be not *o*. of evil, but *o*. evil.
1 John 5:4, 5, victory that *o*. the world.
Rev. 2:7, 17, 26; 3:12, 21, to him that *o*.
See Cant. 6:5; 2 Pet. 2:19; Rev. 12:11.
OVERMUCH. Eccl. 7:16; 2 Cor. 2:7.
OVERPAST. Ps. 57:1; Isa. 26:20.
OVERPLUS. Lev. 25:27.
OVERSEER. Gen. 41:34; Prov. 6:7; Acts 20:28.
OVERSHADOW. Mat. 17:5; Mk. 9:7; Lu. 1:35; Acts 5:15.
OVERSIGHT. Gen. 43:12; Neh. 11:16; 1 Pet. 5:2.
OVERSPREAD. Gen. 9:19; Dan. 9:27.
OVERTAKE. Amos 9:13, plowman shall *o*. the reaper.
Gal. 6:1, if a man be *o*. in a fault.
1 Thess. 5:4, day should *o*. you as a thief.
See Deut. 19:6; Isa. 59:9; Jer. 42:16.
OVERTHROW. Ex. 23:24, utterly *o*. them.
Job. 19:6, God hath *o*. me.
Ps. 14:4, purposed to *o*. my goings.
Prov. 13:6, wickedness *o*. the sinner.
Jon. 3:4, yet forty days, and Nineveh shall be *o*.
Acts 5:39, if it be of God, ye cannot *o*. it.
See Gen. 19:21; Prov. 29:4; 2 Tim. 2:18.
OVERTURN. Job 9:5; 12:15; 28:9; Ezek. 21:27.
OVERWHELM. Job 6:27, ye *o*. the fatherless.
Ps. 61:2, when my heart is *o*.
77:3; 142:3; 143:4, my spirit was *o*.
See Ps. 55:5; 78:53; 124:4.
OVERWISE. Eccl. 7:16.
OWE. Lu. 16:5, 7, how much *o*. thou?
Rom. 13:8, *o*. no man any thing.
See Mat. 18:24, 28; Lu. 7:41; Philem. 18.
OWN. Num. 32:42, called it after his *o*. name.
1 Chron. 29:14, of thine *o*. have we given thee.
Ps. 12:4, our lips are our *o*.
Ps. 67:6, even our *o*. God shall bless us.
Mat. 20:15, do what I will with mine *o*.
John 1:11, to his *o*., and his *o*. received him not.
13:1, having loved his *o*.
1 Cor. 6:19, ye are not your *o*.
See Acts 5:4; Phil. 3:9; 1 Tim. 5:8; Rev. 1:5.
OWNER. Ex. 21:28; 22:11; Eccl. 5:13; Isa. 1:3.

P

PACIFY. Prov. 16:14; 21:14; Eccl. 10:4; Ezek. 16:63.
PAIN. Ps. 55:4, my heart is sore *p*.
116:3, the *p*. of hell gat hold upon me.
Acts 2:24, having loosed the *p*. of death.
Rom. 8:22, creation travaileth in *p*.
Rev. 21:4, neither shall there be any more *p*.
See Ps. 73:16; Jer. 4:19; 2 Cor. 11:27.
PAINTED. 2 Kings 9:30; Jer. 4:30; 22:14; Ezek. 23:40.
PALACE. Ps. 48:13, consider her *p*.
122:7, prosperity within thy *p*.
144:12, the similitude of a *p*.
Jer. 9:21, death is entered into our *p*.
Lu. 11:21, a strong man keepeth his *p*.
Phil. 1:13, manifest in all the *p*.
See 1 Chron. 29:1; Neh. 1:1; 2:8; Isa. 25:2.
PALE. Isa. 29:22; Jer. 30:6; Rev. 6:8.
PALM. Isa. 49:16; Mat. 26:67; Mk. 14:65; Rev. 7:9.
PANT. Ps. 38:10; 42:1; 119:131; Amos 2:7.
PARCHMENTS. 2 Tim. 4:13, but especially the *p*.
PARDON. Ex. 23:21, he will not *p*.
2 Kings 5:18, the Lord *p*. thy servant.
2 Chron. 30:18, the good Lord *p*. every one.
Neh. 9:17, a God ready to *p*.
Isa. 55:7, he will abundantly *p*.
See Jer. 33:8; 50:20; Lam. 3:42; Mic. 7:18.
PARENTS. Mat. 10:21; Mk. 13:12, children rise up against *p*.
Lu. 18:29, no man that hath left *p*.
21:16, ye shall be betrayed by *p*.
John 9:2, who did sin, this man, or his *p*.?
Rom. 1:30; 2 Tim. 3:2, disobedient to *p*.
2 Cor. 12:14, not to lay up for *p*., but *p*. for children.
Eph. 6:1; Col. 3:20, children, obey your *p*.
See Lu. 2:27; 8:56; 1 Tim. 5:4; Heb. 11:23.
PART (*n*.). Josh. 22:25, 27, ye have no *p*. in the Lord.
Ps. 5:9, their inward *p*. is very wickedness.
51:6, in hidden *p*. make me to know.
118:7, the Lord taketh my *p*.
139:9, dwell in the uttermost *p*.
Mk. 9:40, he that is not against us is on our *p*.

Lu. 10:42, that good *p.*
John 13:8, thou hast no *p.* with me.
Acts 8:21, neither *p.* nor lot.
2 Cor. 6:15, what *p.* hath he that believeth?
See Tit. 2:8; Rev. 20:6; 21:8; 22:19.
PART (*v.*). Ruth 1:17, if ought but death *p.* thee and me.
2 Sam. 14:6, there was none to *p.* them.
Ps. 22:18, they *p.* my garments.
Lu. 24:51, while he blessed them he was *p.*
Acts 2:45, *p.* them to all men.
See Mat. 27:35; Mk. 15:24; Lu. 23:34; John 19:24.
PARTAKE. Ps. 50:18, hast been *p.* with adulterers.
Rom. 15:27, *p.* of their spiritual things.
1 Cor. 9:10, *p.* of his hope.
13; 10:18, *p.* with the altar.
10:17, *p.* of that one bread.
21, *p.* of the Lord's table.
1 Tim. 5:22, neither be *p.* of other men's sins.
Heb. 3:1, *p.* of the heavenly calling.
1 Pet. 4:13, *p.* of Christ's sufferings.
5:1, a *p.* of the glory.
2 Pet. 1:4, *p.* of the divine nature.
See Eph. 3:6; Phil. 1:7; Col. 1:12; Rev. 18:4.
PARTIAL. Mal. 2:9; 1 Tim. 5:21; Jas. 2:4; 3:17.
PARTICULAR. 1 Cor. 12:27; Eph. 5:33.
PARTITION. 1 Kings 6:21; Eph. 2:14.
PARTNER. Prov. 29:24; Lu. 5:7; 2 Cor. 8:23.
PASS. Ex. 12:13, when I see the blood I will *p.* over.
Isa. 43:2, when thou *p.* through waters.
Mat. 26:39; Mk. 14:36, let this cup *p.*
Lu. 16:26, neither can they *p.* to us.
1 Cor. 7:31; 1 John 2:17, fashion of this world *p.*
Eph. 3:19, love of Christ, which *p.* knowledge.
Phil. 4:7, which *p.* all understanding.
See Jer. 2:6; LU. 18:37; Rom. 5:12; Rev. 21:1.
PASSION. Acts 1:3; 14:15; Jas. 5:17.
PAST. Job 29:2, as in months *p.*
Eccl. 3:15, God requireth that which is *p.*
Cant. 2:11, the winter is *p.*
Jer. 8:20, the harvest is *p.*
Rom. 3:25, of sins that are *p.*
11:33, ways *p.* finding out.
2 Cor. 5:17, old things *p.* away.
Eph. 4:19, being *p.* feeling.
See Eph. 2:2; 2 Tim. 2:18; 1 Pet. 2:10.
PASTOR. Jer. 3:15; 17:16; 23:1; Eph. 4:11.
PASTURE. Ps. 95:7; 100:3; Ezek. 34:14; John 10:9.
PATE. Ps. 7:16.
PATH. Job 28:7, there is a *p.* which no fowl knoweth.
Ps. 16:11, show me the *p.* of life.
27:11, lead me in a plain *p.*
65:11, thy *p.* drop fatness.
77:19, thy *p.* is in the great waters.
119:105, a light to my *p.*
Prov. 4:18, the *p.* of the just.
Isa. 2:3; Mic. 4:2, we will walk in his *p.*
42:16, in *p.* they have not known.
58:12, restorer of *p.* to dwell in.
Jer. 6:16, ask for the old *p.*
Mat. 3:3; Mk. 1:3; Lu. 3:4, make his *p.* straight.
See Ps. 139:3; Prov. 3:17; Lam. 3:9; Heb. 12:13.
PATIENCE. Mat. 18:26, 29, have *p.* with me.
Lu. 8:15, bring forth fruit with *p.*
21:19, in your *p.* possess ye your souls.
Rom. 5:3, tribulation worketh *p.*
8:25, with *p.* wait for it.
15:4, through *p.* and comfort.
5, the God of *p.*
2 Cor. 6:4, as ministers of God in much *p.*
Col. 1:11, strengthened with all might to all *p.*
1 Thess. 1:3, your *p.* of hope.
2 Thess. 1:4, glory in you for your *p.*
1 Tim. 6:11, follow after *p.*
Tit. 2:2, sound in faith, charity, *p.*
Heb. 10:36, ye have need of *p.*
12:1, run with *p.*
Jas. 1:3, trying of your faith worketh *p.*
Jas. 1:4, let *p.* have her perfect work.
5:7, the husbandman hath long *p.*
10, for an example of *p.*
11, ye have heard of the *p.* of Job.
2 Pet. 1:6, add to temperance *p.*
Rev. 2:2, 19, I know thy *p.*
3:10, thou hast kept word of *p.*
13:10; 14:12, here is the *p.* of saints.
See Eccl. 7:8; Rom. 12:12; 1 Thess. 5:14.
PATIENTLY. Ps. 37:7; 40:1; Heb. 6:15; 1 Pet. 2:20.
PATTERN. 1 Tim. 1:16; Tit. 2:7; Heb. 8:5; 9:23.
PAVILION. 2 Sam. 22:12, and he made darkness *p.*
See Ps. 18:11; 27:5; 31:20; Jer. 43:10.
PAY. Ex. 22:7, let him *p.* double.
Num. 20:19, water, I will *p.* for it.
2 Kings 4:7, sell the oil, and *p.* thy debt.
Ps. 22:25; 66:13; 116:14, will *p.* my vows.
Prov. 22:27, if thou hast nothing to *p.*
Eccl. 5:4, defer not to *p.* it.
Mat. 18:26, I will *p.* thee all.
18:28, *p.* that thou owest.
23:23, ye *p.* tithe of mint.
See Ex. 21:19; Mat. 17:24; Rom. 13:6; Heb. 7:9.
PEACE. Gen. 41:16, an answer of *p.*
Num. 6:26, the Lord give thee *p.*
25:12, my covenant of *p.*
Deut. 20:10, proclaim *p.* to it.
23:6, thou shalt not seek their *p.*
1 Sam. 25:6; Lu. 10:5, *p.* be to this house.
2 Kings 9:19, what hast thou to do with *p.*?
31, had Zimri *p.*, who slew his master?
Job 5:23, beasts shall be at *p.* with thee.
22:21, acquaint thyself with him, and be at *p.*
Ps. 4:8, I will lay me down in *p.*
29:11, the Lord will bless his people with *p.*
34:14; 1 Pet. 3:11, seek *p.*, and pursue it.
37:37, the end of that man is *p.*
85:8, will speak *p.* to his people.
122:6, pray for *p.* of Jerusalem.
Eccl. 3:8, a time of *p.*
Isa. 26:3, keep him in perfect *p.*
32:17, work of righteousness shall be *p.*
45:7, I make *p.*, and create evil.
48:18, thy *p.* as a river.
22; 57:21, no *p.* to the wicked.
52:7; Nah. 1:15, that publisheth *p.*
59:8; Rom. 3:17, the way of *p.* they know not.
Jer. 6:14; 8:11, saying *p.*, *p.*, when there is no *p.*
8:15; 14:19, we looked for *p.*
34:5, thou shalt die in *p.*
Ezek. 7:25, they shall seek *p.*
Dan. 4:1; 6:25; 1 Pet. 1:2; 2 Pet. 1:2; Jude 2, *p.* be multiplied.
Hag. 2:9, in this place will I give *p.*
Mat. 10:13, let your *p.* come upon it.
34; Lu. 12:51, to send *p.* on earth.
Mk. 9:50, have *p.* one with another.
Lu. 1:79, to guide our feet into way of *p.*
2:14, on earth *p.*
19:42, things which belong to thy *p.*
John 14:27, *p.* I leave, my *p.* I give you.
16:33, that in me ye might have *p.*
Rom. 1:7; 1 Cor. 1:3; 2 Cor. 1:2; Gal. 1:3; Eph. 1:2; Phil. 1:2, *p.* from God our Father.
5:1, we have *p.* with God.
10:15; Eph. 6:15, the gospel of *p.*
14:19, follow after the things which make for *p.*
15:33; 16:20; 2 Cor. 13:11; Phil. 4:9; 1 Thess. 5:23; Heb. 13:20, the God of *p.*
1 Cor. 14:33, author of *p.*
2 Cor. 13:11, live in *p.*
Eph. 2:14, he is our *p.*
17, *p.* to you which were afar off.
4:3, in the bond of *p.*
Phil. 4:7, *p.* of God which passeth all understanding.
Col. 1:2; 1 Thess. 1:1; 2 Thess. 1:2; 1 Tim. 1:2; 2 Tim. 1:2; Tit. 1:4; Philem. 3; 2 John 3, grace and *p.* from God.
3:15, let the *p.* of God rule in your hearts.

1 Thess. 5:13, be at *p.* among yourselves.
2 Thess. 3:16, Lord of *p.* give you *p.* always.
2 Tim. 2:22; Heb. 12:14, follow *p.* with all men.
Heb. 7:2, king of *p.*
Jas. 2:16, depart in *p.*
3:18, fruit of righteousness is sown in *p.*
3:18, fruit of righteousness is sown in *p.*
2 Pet. 3:14, found of him in *p.*
See Mat. 5:9; Lu. 24:36; John 20:19; Gal. 6:16.
PEACEABLE. Isa. 32:18; 1 Tim. 2:2; Heb. 12:11; Jas. 3:17.
PEACEABLY. Gen. 37:4; 1 Sam. 16:4; Jer. 9:8; Rom. 12:18.
PEACOCKS. 2 Chron. 9:21, the ships of Tarshish bringing *p.*
Job. 39:13, gavest thou the goodly wings until the *p.*
PEELED. Isa. 18:2; Ezek. 29:18.
PEEP. Isa. 8:19; 10:14.
PELICAN. Lev. 11:18, and the swan, and the *p.*
Deut. 14:17, the *p.*, and the gier eagle.
Ps. 102:6, I am like a *p.* of the wilderness.
PEN. Judg. 5:14, they that handle the *p.*
Job 19:24, graven with an iron *p.*
Ps. 45:1, my tongue is the *p.* of a ready writer.
Isa. 8:1, write in it with a man's *p.*
Jer. 8:8, the *p.* of the scribes is in vain.
17:1, is written with a *p.* of iron.
3 John 13, I will not with ink and *p.* write.
PENCE. Mat. 18:28; Mk. 14:5; Lu. 7:41; 10:35.
PENNY. Mat. 20:13, didst not thou agree with me for a *p.*?
22:19, they brought him a *p.*
Mk. 12:15, bring me a *p.*
Rev. 6:6, a measure of wheat for a *p.*
PENURY. Prov. 14:23; Lu. 21:4.
PEOPLE. Ex. 6:7; Deut. 4:20; 2 Sam. 7:24; Jer. 13:11, I will take you to me for a *p.*
Lev. 20:24, 26, separated from other *p.*
Deut. 4:3, did ever *p.* hear voice of God and live?
33:29, O *p.* saved by the Lord.
2 Sam. 22:44; Ps. 18:43, a *p.* I knew not.
Ps. 81:11, my *p.* would not hearken.
144:15, happy is that *p.*
Prov. 30:25, the ants are a *p.* not strong.
Isa. 1:4, a *p.* laden with iniquity.
27:11, a *p.* of no understanding.
43:4, I will give *p.* for thy life.
8, blind *p.* that have eyes.
Jer. 6:22; 50:41, a *p.* cometh from the north.
Jon. 1:8, of what *p.* art thou?
Lu. 1:17, a *p.* prepared for the Lord.
Tit. 2:14, purify unto himself a peculiar *p.*
See Mat. 1:21; Rom. 11:2; Heb. 11:25.
PERCEIVE. Deut. 29:4, a heart to *p.*
Josh. 22:31, we *p.* the Lord is among us.
Job 9:11, I *p.* him not.
23:8, I cannot *p.* him.
Isa. 6:9, see indeed, but *p.* not.
33:19, deeper speech than thou canst *p.*
64:4, nor *p.* by the ear what God hath.
Mat. 22:18, Jesus *p.* their wickedness.
Mk. 8:17, *p.* ye not yet?
Lu. 8:46, I *p* that virtue is gone out.
John 4:19, I *p.* thou art a prophet.
Acts 10:34, I *p.* God is no respecter of persons.
1 John 3:16, hereby *p.* we the love of God.
See 1 Sam. 3:8; Neh. 6:12; Job 33:14; Mk. 12:28.
PERFECT. Gen. 6:9, Noah was *p.*
17:1, walk before me, and be thou *p.*
Deut. 18:13, thou shalt be *p.* with the Lord.
32:4, his work is *p.*
2 Sam. 22:31; Ps. 18:30, his way is *p.*
Ps. 19:7, law of the Lord is *p.*
37:37, mark the *p.* man.
Prov. 4:18, more and more to *p.* day.
Ezek. 28:15, thou wast *p.* in thy ways.
Mat. 5:48; 2 Cor. 13:11, be ye *p.*
19:21, if thou wilt be *p.*
John 17:23, be made *p.* in one.
Rom. 12:2, that *p.* will of God.
1 Cor. 2:6, wisdom among them that are *p.*
2 Cor. 12:9, strength made *p.* in weakness.
Eph. 4:13, unto a *p.* man.
Phil. 3:12, not as though I were already *p.*
15, let us, as many as be *p.*
Col. 1:28, present every man *p.*
4:12, may stand *p.* and complete.
2 Tim. 3:17, that the man of God may be *p.*
Heb. 2:10, make *p.* through suffering.
11:40, without us should not be made *p.*
12:23, spirits of just men made *p.*
13:21, make you *p.* in every good work.
Jas. 1:4, patience have her *p.* work.
17, every good and *p.* gift.
25, *p.* law of liberty.
3:2, the same is a *p.* man.
1 John 4:18, *p.* love casteth out fear.
See 2 Chron. 8:16; Lu. 6:40; 2 Cor. 7:1; Eph. 4:12.
PERFECTION. Job 11:7; Ps. 119:96; 2 Cor. 13:9; Heb. 6:1.
PERFECTLY. Jer. 23:20; Acts 18:26; 1 Cor. 1:10.
PERFECTNESS. Col. 3:14.
PERFORM. Ex. 18:18, not able to *p.* it thyself alone.
Esth. 5:6; 7:2, to half of kingdom it shall be *p.*
Job 5:12, cannot *p.* their enterprise.
Ps. 65:1, unto thee shall the vow be *p.*
119:106, I have sworn, and I will *p.* it.
Isa. 9:7, zeal of the Lord will *p.* this.
44:28, shall *p.* all my pleasure.
Jer. 29:10; 33:14, I will *p.* my good word.
Rom. 4:21, able also to *p.*
7:18, how to *p.* that which is good I find not.
Phil. 1:6, *p.* it until day of Christ.
See. Job 23:14; Ps. 57:2; Jer. 35:14; Mat. 5:33.
PERFORMANCE. Lu. 1:45; 2 Cor. 8:11.
PERIL. Lam. 5:9; Rom. 8:35; 2 Cor. 11:26.
PERILOUS. 2 Tim. 3:1.
PERISH. Num. 17:12, we die, we *p.*, we all *p.*
Deut. 26:5, a Syrian ready to *p.*
Job 4:7, who ever *p.*, being innocent?
29:13, blessing of him that was ready to *p.*
34:15, all flesh shall *p.* together.
Ps. 1:6, way of ungodly shall *p.*
37:20, the wicked shall *p.*
49:12, like the beasts that *p.*
80:16, they *p.* at rebuke of thy countenance.
102:26, they shall *p.*, but thou shalt endure.
Prov. 11:10; 28:28, when the wicked *p.*
29:18, no vision, the people *p.*
31:6, strong drink to him that is ready to *p.*
Isa. 27:13, they shall come that were ready to *p.*
Jer. 7:28, truth is *p.*
Jon. 1:6; 3:9, God will think on us, that we *p.* not.
14, let us not *p.* for this man's life.
Mat. 8:25; Lu. 8:24, save us, we *p.*
18:14, that one of these little ones should *p.*
26:52, shall *p.* with the sword.
Mk. 4:38, carest thou not that we *p.*?
Lu. 13:3, 5, ye shall all likewise *p.*
15:17, I *p.* with hunger.
21:18, there shall not an hair of your head *p.*
John 6:27, labour not for the meat which *p.*
Acts 8:20, thy money *p.* with thee.
Col. 2:22, which are to *p.* with the using.
2 Pet. 3:9, not willing that any should *p.*
See Ps. 2:12; Jer. 6:21; John 10:28; Rom. 2:12.
PERMISSION. 1 Cor. 7:6.
PERMIT. 1 Cor. 14:34; 16:7; Heb. 6:3.
PERNICIOUS. 2 Pet. 2:2.
PERPETUAL. Ex. 31:16, sabbath for a *p.* covenant.
Lev. 25:34, their *p.* possession.
Ps. 9:6, destructions are come to a *p.* end.
74:3; Jer. 25:9' Ezek. 35:9, the *p.* desolations.
Jer. 8:5, a *p.* backsliding.
15:18, why is my pain *p.*?
Hab. 3:6, the *p.* hills.
See Gen. 9:12; Jer. 5:22; 50:5; 51:39; Ezek. 46:14.
PERPETUALLY. 1 Kings 9:3; 2 Chron. 7:16; Amos 1:11.
PERPLEXED. Lu. 9:7; 24:4; 2 Cor. 4:8.

PERPLEXITY. Isa. 22:5; Mic. 7:4; Lu. 21:25.
PERSECUTE. Job 19:22, why do ye *p.* me?
Ps. 7:1, save me from them that *p.* me.
10:2, the wicked doth *p.* the poor.
71:11, *p.* and take him, there is none to deliver.
143:3, the enemy hath *p.* my soul.
Mat. 5:11, 12, blessed are ye when men *p.* you.
44, pray for them that *p.* you.
John 15:20, if they have *p.* me.
Acts 9:4; 22:7; 26:14, why *p.* thou me?
22:4, I *p.* this way unto death.
26:11, I *p.* them even to strange cities.
1 Cor. 4:12, being *p.*, we suffer it.
15:9; Gal. 1:13, I *p.* the church of God.
2 Cor. 4:9, *p.* but not forsaken.
Phil. 3:6, concerning zeal, *p.* the church.
See John 5:16; Acts 7:52; Rom. 12:14; Gal. 1:23; 4:29.
PERSECUTION. Mat. 13:21; Mk. 4:17, when *p.* ariseth.
2 Cor. 12:10, take pleasure in *p.*
2 Tim. 3:12, all that will live godly shall suffer *p.*
See Lam. 5:5; Acts 8;1; Gal. 6:12; 1 Tim. 1:13.
PERSEVERANCE. Eph. 6:18.
PERSON. Deut. 10:17; 2 Sam. 14:14, God, which regardeth not *p.*
2 Sam. 17:11, go to battle in thine own *p.*
Ps. 15:4; Isa. 32:5, 6, vile *p.*
26:4; Prov. 12:11; 28:19, with vain *p.*
105:37, not one feeble *p.*
Mat. 22:16; Mk. 12:14, regardest not *p.* of men.
2 Cor. 2:10, forgave I it in the *p.* of Christ.
Heb. 1:3, the express image of his *p.*
2 Pet. 3:11, what manner of *p.* ought ye to be?
See Mal. 1:8; Lu. 15:7; Heb. 12:16; Jude 16.
PERSUADE. 1 Kings 22:20, who shall *p.* Ahab?
Prov. 25:15, by long forbearing is a prince *p.*
Mat. 28:14, we will *p.* him, and secure you.
Acts 26:28, almost thou *p.* me.
Rom. 14:5, let every man be fully *p.*
2 Cor. 5:11, we *p.* men.
Gal. 1:10, do I now *p.* men or God?
Heb. 6:9, we are *p.* better things of you.
See 2 Kings 18:32; 2 Chron. 18:2; 2 Tim. 1:12.
PERTAIN. Rom. 15:17; 1 Cor. 6:3; 2 Pet. 1:3.
PERVERSE. Deut. 32:5, a *p.* and crooked generation.
Job 6:30, cannot my taste discern *p.* things?
Prov. 4:24, *p.* lips put far from thee.
12:8, *p.* heart shall be despised.
17:20, *p.* tongue falleth into mischief.
23:33, thine heart shall utter *p.* things.
Phil. 2:15, in the midst of a *p.* nation.
See Num. 23:21; Isa. 30:12; 1 Tim. 6:5.
PERVERT. Deut. 16:19, a gift doth *p.* words.
Job 8:3, doth God *p.* judgment?
Prov. 10:9, he that *p.* his ways shall be known.
19:3, the foolishness of man *p.* his way.
Jer. 3:21, they have *p.* their way.
23:36, ye have *p.* the words of God.
Acts 13:10, wilt thou not cease to *p.* right ways?
Gal. 1:7, would *p.* the gospel.
See Eccl. 5:8; Mic. 3:9; Lu. 23:2.
PESTILENCE. Ex. 5:3; 9:15; Jer. 42:17; 44:13.
PESTILENT. Acts 24:5.
PETITION. 1 Sam. 1:17, God of Israel grant thee thy *p.*
1 Kings 2:20, one small *p.*
Esth. 5:6; 7:2; 9:12, what is thy *p.*?
Dan. 6:7, whosoever shall ask a *p.*
13, maketh his *p.* three times a day.
See Esth. 7:3; Ps. 20:5; 1 John 5:15.
PHILOSOPHERS. Acts 17:18, then certain *p.* of the Epicureans.
PHILOSOPHY. Col. 2:8.
PHYLACTERIES. Mat. 23:5, they make broad their *p.*
See Ex. 13:9, 16; Num. 15:38.
PHYSICIAN. Mat. 9:12; Mk. 2:17; Lu. 5:31, they that be whole need not a *p.*
Lu. 4:23, *p.*, heal thyself.
See Jer. 8:22.
PICK. Prov. 30:17.
PICTURES. Num. 33:52; Prov. 25:11; Isa. 2:16.
PIECE. 1 Sam. 2:36; Prov. 6:26; 28:21, a *p.* of bread.
15:33, Samuel hewed Agag in *p.*
Ps. 7:2, rending in *p.* while none to deliver.
50:22, consider, lest I tear you in *p.*
Jer. 23:29, hammer that breaketh rock in *p.*
Amos 4:7, one *p.* was rained upon.
Zech. 11:12, weighed for my price thirty *p.*
13; Mat. 27:6, 9, took thirty *p.* of silver.
See Lu. 14:18; Acts 19:19; 23:10; 27:44.
PIERCE. 2 Kings 18:21; Isa. 36:6, into his hand and *p.* it.
Zech. 12:10; John 19:37, they shall look on me whom they have *p.*
1 Tim. 6:10, *p.* themselves with many sorrows.
See Isa. 27:1; Lu. 2:35; Heb. 4:12; Rev. 1:7.
PIETY. 1 Tim. 5:4, let them learn first to show *p.* at home.
PILE. Isa. 30:33; Ezek. 24:9.
PILLAR. Gen. 19:26, a *p.* of salt.
Job 9:6; 26:11, the *p.* thereof tremble.
Prov. 9:1, she hath hewn out her seven *p.*
Gal. 2:9, Cephas and John, who seemed to be *p.*
1 Tim. 3:15, the *p.* and ground of the truth.
Rev. 3:12, him that overcometh will I make a *p.*
See Isa. 19:19; Jer. 1:18; Joel 2:30; Lu. 17:32; Rev. 10:1.
PILLOW. Gen. 28:11; 1 Sam. 19:13; Ezek. 13:18; Mk. 4:38.
PILOTS. Ezek. 27:8.
PIN. Judg. 16:14; Ezek. 15:3.
PINE. Lev. 26:39; Lam. 4:9; Isa. 38:12; Ezek. 24:23.
PINE TREE. Isa. 41:19; 60:13, and the *p. t.*
PIPE. Isa. 5:12, the harp and *p.* are in their feasts.
Mat. 11:17; Lu. 7:32, we have *p.* unto you.
1 Cor. 14:7, how shall it be known what is *p.*?
Rev. 18:22, voice of *p.* shall be heard no more.
See 1 Sam. 10:5; 1 Kings 1:40; Isa. 30:29.
PIT. Gen. 37:20, cast him into some *p.*
Ex. 21:33, 34, if a man dig a *p.*
Num. 16:30, 33, go down quick into the *p.*
Job. 33:24, deliver him from going down to the *p.*
Ps. 28:1; 143:7, like them that go down into the *p.*
40:2, out of an horrible *p.*
Prov. 22:14; 23:27, a deep *p.*
28:10, shall fall into his own *p.*
Isa. 38:17, the *p.* of corruption.
Mat. 12:11; Lu. 14:5, fall into a *p.* on sabbath.
PITCHER. Gen. 24:14, let down thy *p.*
Judg. 7:16, lamps within the *p.*
Eccl. 12:6, or the *p.* be broken.
Lam. 4:2, esteemed as earthen *p.*
Mk. 14:13; Lu. 22:10, a man bearing a *p.* of water.
PITIFUL. Lam. 4:10; Jas. 5:11; 1 Pet. 3:8.
PITY. Deut. 7:16; 13:8; 19:13, thine eye shall have no *p.*
2 Sam. 12:6, because he had no *p.*
Job 19:21, have *p.* on me, my friends.
Ps. 69:20, I looked for some to take *p.*
Prov. 19:17, that hath *p.* on the poor lendeth.
28:8, gather for him that will *p.* the poor.
Isa. 13:18, they shall have no *p.* on fruit.
63:9, in his *p.* he redeemed them.
Jer. 13:14, I will not *p.* nor spare.
Ezek. 16:5, none eye *p.* thee.
24:21, I will profane what your soul *p.*
Joel 2:18, the Lord will *p.* his people.
Zech. 11:5, their own shepherds *p.* them not.
Mat. 18:33, as I had *p.* on thee.
See Ps. 103:13; Jer. 15:5; Lam. 2:2; Jon. 4:10.
PLACE. Ex. 3:5; Josh. 5:15, *p.* whereon thou standest is holy.
Judg. 18:10, a *p.* where there is no want.
2 Kings 5:11, strike his hand over the *p.*
6:1; Isa. 49:20, the *p.* is too strait for us.
Ps. 26:8, the *p.* where thine honour dwelleth.
32:7; 119:114, thou art my hiding *p.*
37:10, thou shalt diligently consider his *p.*
74:20, the dark *p.* of the earth.
90:1, our dwelling *p.*
Prov. 14:26, his children have a *p.* of refuge.
15:3, the eyes of the Lord in every *p.*
Eccl. 3:20, all go to one *p.*

Isa. 5:8, lay field to field, till there be on *p.*
60:13, the *p.* of my feet.
66:1, where is the *p.* of my rest?
Jer. 6:3, they shall feed every one in his *p.*
Mic. 1:3, the Lord cometh out of his *p.*
Zech. 10:10, *p.* shall not be found for them.
Mal. 1:11, in every *p.* incense shall be offered.
Mat. 28:6; Mk. 16:6, see the *p.* where the Lord lay.
Lu. 10:1, two and two into every *p.*
14:9, give this man *p.*
John 8:37, my word hath no *p.* in you.
18:2, Judas knew the *p.*
Acts 2:1, with one accord in one *p.*
4:31, the *p.* was shaken.
Rom. 12:19, rather give *p.* to wrath.
Eph. 4:27, neither give *p.* to the devil.
Heb. 12:17, found no *p.* of repentance.
Rev. 20:11, there was found no *p.* for them.
See Ps. 16:6; Isa. 40:4; Eph. 1:3; 2:6; 3:10.
PLAGUE. Lev. 26:21, I will bring seven times more *p.*
Deut. 28:59, will make thy *p.* wonderful.
29:22, when they see the *p.* of that land.
1 Kings 8:38, every man the *p.* of his own heart.
Ps. 73:5, nor are they *p.* like other men.
91:10, nor any *p.* come nigh thy dwelling.
Hos. 13:14, O death, I will be thy *p.*
Rev. 18:4, that ye receive not of her *p.*
22:18, shall add to him the *p.* written.
See Lev. 14:35; Num. 8:19; 16:46; Mk. 3:10.
PLAIN. Gen. 25:27, Jacob was a *p.* man.
Ps. 27:11, lead me in a *p.* path.
Prov. 8:9, they are *p.* to him t hat understandeth.
15:19, the way of the righteous is made *p.*
Isa. 40:4, rough places *p.*
Hab. 2:2, write the vision, make it *p.*
See Gen. 13:10; 19:17; Isa. 28:25; Mk. 7:35.
PLAINLY. Deut. 27:8, write the words very *p.*
Isa. 32:4, stammers shall speak *p.*
John 10:24, tell us *p.*
16:25, I shall show you *p.* of the Father.
29, now speakest thou *p.*
See Ex. 21:5; Ezra 4:18; John 11:14; 2 Cor. 3:12.
PLAITING. 1 Pet. 3:3.
PLANES. Isa. 44:13.
PLANT (*n.*). Job 14:9, bring forth boughs like a *p.*
Ps. 128:3, children like olive *p.*
144:12, sons as *p.* grown up.
Isa. 5:7; 17:10, his pleasant *p.*
16:8, broken down principal *p.*
53:2, as a tender *p.*
Ezek. 34:29, a *p.* of renown.
Mat. 15:13, every *p.* my Father hath not planted.
See Gen. 2:5; 1 Chron. 4:23; Jer. 48:32.
PLANT (*v.*). Num. 24:6, as trees which the Lord hath *p.*
2 Sam. 7:10; 1 Chron. 17:9, I will *p.* them.
Ps. 1:3; Jer. 17:8, like a tree *p.*
80:15, the vineyard thy right hand hath *p.*
92:13, *p.* in the house of the Lord.
94:9, he that *p.* the ear.
Jer. 2:21, I had *p.* thee a noble vine.
Ezek. 17:10, being *p.* shall it prosper?
Lu. 17:6, be thou *p.* in the sea.
Rom. 6:5, if we have been *p.* together.
1 Cor. 3:6, I have *p.*
See Mat. 21:33; Mk. 12:1; Lu. 20:9.
PLATE. Ex. 28:36; 39:30; Jer. 10:9.
PLATTED. Mat. 27:29; Mk. 15:17; John 19:2.
PLATTER. Mat. 23:25; Lu. 11:39.
PLAY. Ex. 32:6; 1 Cor. 10:7, people rose up to *p.*
1 Sam. 16:17, a man that can *p.* well.
2 Sam. 6:21, I will *p.* before the Lord.
10:12, let us *p.* the men.
Job 41:5, wilt thou *p.* with him?
Ps. 33:3, *p.* skilfully with a loud noise.
Isa. 11:8, the sucking child shall *p.*
Ezek. 33:32, can *p.* well on an instrument.
See 2 Sam. 2:14; 1 Chron. 15:29; Ps. 68:25; Zech. 8:5.

PLEA. Deut. 17:8.
PLEAD. Judg. 6:31, 32, will ye *p.* for Baal?
Job 9:19, who shall set me a time to *p.*?
13:19, who will *p.* with me?
16:21, that one might *p.* for a man.
23:6, will he *p.* against me with his great power?
Isa. 1:17, *p.* for the widow.
3:13, the Lord standeth up to *p.*
43:26, let us *p.* together.
59:4, none *p.* for truth.
Jer. 2:9, I will yet *p.* with you.
Lam. 3:58, thou hast *p.* the causes of my soul.
Joel 3:2, I will *p.* with them for my people.
See 1 Sam. 25:39; Job 13:6; Isa. 66:16; Hos. 2:2.
PLEASANT. Gen. 3:6, *p.* to the eyes.
2 Sam. 1:23, were *p.* in their lives.
26, very *p.* hast thou been to me.
Ps. 16:6, lines fallen in *p.* places.
106:24, they despised the *p.* land.
133:1, how *p.* for brethren to dwell together.
Prov. 2:10, knowledge is *p.* to thy soul.
15:26, the words of the pure are *p.* words.
16:24, *p.* words are as honeycomb.
Eccl. 11:7, it is *p.* to behold the sun.
Cant. 4:13, 16; 7:13, with *p.* fruits.
Isa. 64:11, our *p.* things are laid waste.
Jer. 31:20, is Ephraim a *p.* child?
Ezek. 33:32, of one that hath a *p.* voice.
Dan. 10:3, I ate no *p.* bread.
See Amos 5:11; Mic. 2:9; Nah. 2:9; Zech. 7:14.
PLEASANTNESS. Prov. 3:17.
PLEASE. 1 Kings 3:10, the speech *p.* the Lord.
Ps. 51:19, then shalt thou be *p.* with sacrifices.
115:3; 135:6; Jon. 1:14, he hath done whatsoever he *p.*
Prov. 16:7, when a man's ways *p.* the Lord.
Isa. 2:6, they *p.* themselves in children of strangers.
53:10, it *p.* the Lord to bruise him.
55:11, accomplish that which I *p.*
Mic. 6:7, will the Lord be *p.* with rams?
Mal. 1:8, offer it, will he be *p.* with thee?
John 8:29, I do always those thongs that *p.* him.
Rom. 8:8, in the flesh cannot *p.* God.
15:1, to bear, and not to *p.* ourselves.
3, even Christ *p.* not himself.
1 Cor. 1:21, it *p.* God by the foolishness of preaching.
10:33, as I *p.* men in all things.
Gal. 1:10, do I seek to *p.* men?
Eph. 6:6; Col. 3:22, as men-*p.*
Heb. 11:6, without faith it is impossible to *p.* God.
See 1 Cor. 7:32; Col. 1:19; 1 Thess. 2:4; 1 John 3:22.
PLEASURE. 1 Chron. 29:17, hast *p.* in uprightness.
Esth. 1:8, do according to every man's *p.*
Job 21:21, what *p.* hath he in his house?
25, another never eateth with *p.*
22:3, is it any *p.* to the Almighty?
Ps. 16:11, *p.* for evermore.
35:27, hath *p.* in the prosperity of his servants.
51:18, do good in thy good *p.*
102:14, thy servants take *p.* in her stones.
103:21, ye ministers of his that do his *p.*
111:2, of all them that hath *p.* therein.
147:11, taketh *p.* in them that fear him.
149:4, the Lord taketh *p.* in his people.
Prov. 21:17, he that loveth *p.* shall be poor.
Eccl. 5:4, he hath no *p.* in fools
12:1, I have no *p.* in them.
Isa. 44:28, Cyrus shall perform all my *p.*
53:10, the *p.* of the Lord shall prosper.
58:3, in the day of your fast ye find *p.*
13, doing thy *p.* on my holy day.
Jer. 22:28; 48:38; Hos. 8:8, a vessel wherein is no *p.*
Ezek. 18:23; 33:11, have I any *p.*?
Mal. 1:10, I have no *p.* in you, saith the Lord.
Lu. 8:14, choked with *p.* of this life.
12:32, Father's good *p.*
Eph. 1:5, the good *p.* of his will.
Phil. 2:13, to will and to do of his good *p.*

1 Tim. 5:6, she that liveth in *p.*
2 Tim. 3:4, lovers of *p.*
Heb. 10:38, my soul shall have no *p.* in him.
11:25, the *p.* of sin for a season.
12:10, chastened us after their own *p.*
Jas. 5:5, ye have lived in *p.* on earth.
Rev. 4:11, for thy *p.* they were created.
See Gen. 18:12; Ps. 5:4; Eccl. 2:1; Tit. 3:3; 2 Pet. 2:13.
PLENTEOUS. Ps. 86:5; 103:8, *p.* in mercy.
130:7, *p.* redemption.
Hab. 1:16, portion fat and meat *p.*
Mat. 9:37, the harvest truly is *p.*
See Gen. 41:34; Deut. 28:11; 30:9; Prov. 21:5; Isa. 30:23.
PLENTIFUL. Ps. 31:23; 68:9; Jer. 2:7; 48:33; Lu. 12:16.
PLENTY. Gen. 27:28, *p.* of corn and wine.
Job 22:26, *p.* of silver.
37:23, *p.* of justice.
Prov. 3:10, barns filled with *p.*
See 2 Chron. 31:10; Prov. 28:19; Jer. 44:17; Joel 2:26.
PLOW. Job 4:8 that *p.* iniquity shall reap.
Prov. 20:4, not *p.* by reason of cold.
21:4, the *p.* of the wicked is sin.
Isa. 2:4; Mic. 4:3, beat swords into *p.*-shares.
28:24, doth plowman *p.* all day to sow?
Joel 3:10, beat your *p.*-shares into swords.
Amos 9:13, the *p.*-man overtake the reaper.
See Deut. 22:10; 1 Sam. 14:14; Job 1:14; 1 Cor. 9:10.
PLUCK. Deut. 23:25, mayest *p.* the ears with thy hand.
2 Chron. 7:20, then will I *p.* them up.
Job 24:9, they *p.* the fatherless from the breast.
Ps. 25:15, he shall *p.* my feet out of the net.
74:11, *p.* it out of thy bosom.
Prov. 14:1, foolish *p.* it down with her hands.
Eccl. 3:2, a time to *p.* up.
Isa. 50:6, my cheeks to them that *p.*
Jer. 22:24, yet I would *p.* thee thence.
Amos 4:11; Zech. 3:2, a firebrand *p.* out.
Mat. 5:29; 18:9; Mk. 9:47, offend thee, *p.* it out.
12:1; Mk. 2:23; Lu. 6:1, began to *p.* ears.
John 10:28, nor shall any *p.* out of my hand.
See Gen. 8:11; Lu. 17:6; Gal. 4:15; Jude 12.
POINT. Jer. 17:1, written with the *p.* of a diamond.
Heb. 4:15, in all *p.* tempted.
Jas. 2:10, yet offend in one *p.*
See Gen. 25:32; Eccl. 5:16; Mk. 5:23; John 4:47.
POLE. Num. 21:8.
POLICY. Dan. 8:25.
POLISHED. Ps. 144:12; Isa. 49:2; Lam. 4:7; Dan. 10:6.
POLL. 2 Sam. 14:26; Ezek. 44:20; Mic. 1:16.
POMP. Isa. 5:14; 14:11; Ezek. 7:24; 30:18; Acts 25:23.
PONDER. Prov. 4:26, *p.* the path of thy feet.
5:6, lest thou shouldest *p.*
21, the Lord *p.* all his goings.
See Prov. 21:2; 24:12; Lu. 2:19.
POOL. Ps. 84:6; Isa. 35:7; 41:18; John 5:2; 9:7.
POOR. Ex. 30:14, the *p.* shall not give less.
Deut. 15:11, the *p.* shall never cease.
2 Kings 24:14, none remained, save *p.* sort.
Job 24:4, the *p.* of the earth hide.
29:16, I was a father to the *p.*
Ps. 10:14, the *p.* committeth himself to thee.
34:6, this *p.* man cried.
40:17; 69:29; 70:5; 86:1; 109:22, I am *p.*
49:2, rich and *p.* together.
Prov. 10:4, becometh *p.* that dealeth with slack hand.
13:23, food in the tillage of the *p.*
18:23, the *p.* useth entreaties.
22:2, rich and *p.* meet together.
30:9, lest I be *p.* and steal.
Isa. 41:17, when *p.* and needy seek water.
Amos 2:6, they sold the *p.*
Zech. 11:7, 11, I will feed even you, O *p.* of the flock.
Mat. 5:3, blessed are the *p.* in spirit.
2 Cor. 6:10, as *p.*, yet making many rich.
8:9, for your sakes he became *p.*
See Lev. 27:8; Jas. 2:2; Rev. 3:17; 13:16.
POPULOUS. Deut. 26:5; Nah. 3:8.

PORTION. Gen. 31:14, is there yet any *p.* for us?
48:22, one *p.* above thy brethren.
Deut. 32:9, the Lord's *p.* is his people.
2 Kings 2:9, a double *p.* of thy spirit.
Neh. 8:10; Esth. 9:19, send *p.* to them.
Job 20:29, this is the *p.* of a wicked man.
24:18, their *p.* is cursed.
26:14; 27:13, how little a *p.* is heard of him?
31:2, what *p.* of God is there from above?
Ps. 11:6, this shall be the *p.* of their cup.
16:5, Lord is the *p.* of mine inheritance.
17:14, have their *p.* in this life.
73:26, God is my *p.*
119:57; 142:5, thou art my *p.*, O Lord.
Prov. 31:15, giveth a *p.* to her maidens.
Eccl. 2:10, this was my *p.* of all my labour.
3:22; 5:18; 9:9, rejoice, for that is his *p.*
5:19, God hath given power to take *p.*
9:6, nor have they any more *p.* for ever.
11:2, give a *p.* to seven.
Isa. 53:12, divide a *p.* with the great.
61:7, they shall rejoice in their *p.*
Jer. 10:16; 51:19, *p.* of Jacob not like them.
12:10, my pleasant *p.* a wilderness.
52:34, every day a *p.*
Dan. 1:8, with *p.* of king's meat.
Mic. 2:4, he hath changed the *p.* of my people.
Mat. 24:51, appoint him *p.* with hypocrites.
Lu. 12:42, their *p.* in due season.
46, his *p.* with unbelievers.
15:12, he *p.* of goods that falleth.
See Gen. 47:22; Josh. 17:14; Dan. 4:15; 11:26.
POSSESS. Gen. 22:17; 24:60, thy seed shall *p.* the gate.
Job 7:3, made to *p.* months of vanity.
13:26, *p.* iniquities of my youth.
Prov. 8:22, the Lord *p.* me in beginning.
Lu. 18:12, I give tithes of all I *p.*
21:19, in patience *p.* your souls.
See Lu. 12:15; Acts 4:32; 1 Cor. 7:30; 2 Cor. 6:10.
POSSESSION. Gen. 17:8; 48:4, an everlasting *p.*
Prov. 28:10, good things in *p.*
Eccl. 2:7; Mat. 19:22; Mk. 10:22, great *p.*
Acts 2:45, and sold their *p.*
Eph. 1:14, redemption of purchased *p.*
See Lev. 25:10; 27:16; 1 Kings 21:15.
POSSIBLE. Mat. 19:26; Mk. 10:27, with God all things are *p.*
24:24; Mk. 13:22, if *p.* deceive elect.
26:39; Mk. 14:35, 36, if *p.* let this cup.
Mk. 9:23, all things are *p.* to him that believeth.
14:36; Lu. 18:27, all things are *p.* to thee.
Rom. 12:18, if *p.* live peaceably.
See Acts 2:24; 20:16; Gal. 4:15; Heb. 10:4.
POST. Deut. 6:9; Job 9:25; Jer. 51:31; Amos 9:1.
POSTERITY. Gen. 45:7; Ps. 49:13; 109:13; Dan. 11:4.
POT. 2 Kings 4:2, not anything save a *p.* of oil.
40, there is death in the *p.*
Job 41:31, maketh the deep boil like a *p.*
Zech. 14:21, every *p.* shall be holiness.
Mk. 7:4, the washing of cups and *p.*
John 2:6, six water-*p.*
See Ex. 16:33; Jer. 1:13; John 4:28; Heb. 9:4.
POTENTATE. 1 Tim. 6:15.
POUND. Lu. 19:13; John 12:13.
POUR. Job 10:10, hast thou not *p.* me out as milk.
29:6, rock *p.* out rivers of oil.
30:16, my soul is *p.* out upon me.
Ps. 45:2, grace is *p.* into thy lips.
62:8, *p.* out your heart before him.
Prov. 1:23; Isa. 44:3; Joel 2:28, 29; Acts 2:17, 18, I will *p.* out my Spirit.
Cant. 1:3, as ointment *p.* forth.
Isa. 26:16, *p.* out prayer when chastening.
32:15, till the spirit be *p.* on us.
44:3, I will *p.* water on thirsty.
53:12, *p.* out his soul unto death.
Jer. 7:20; 42:18, my fury shall be *p.* out.
Lam. 2:19, *p.* out thine heart like water.

Nah. 1:6, fury is *p.* out like fire.
Mal. 3:10, if I will not *p.* out a blessing.
Mat. 26:7; Mk. 14:3, *p.* ointment on his head.
John 2:15, he *p.* out the changers' money.
See 2 Sam. 23:16; 2 Kings 3:11; Rev. 14:10; 16:1.
POURTRAY. Ezek. 4:1; 8:10; 23:14.
POVERTY. Gen. 45:11; Prov. 20:13, lest thou come to *p.*
Prov. 6:11; 24:34, thy *p.* come as one that travelleth.
10:15, destruction of poor is *p.*
11:24, it tendeth to *p.*
13:18, *p.* to him that refuseth instruction.
28:19, shall have *p.* enough.
30:8, give me neither *p.* nor riches.
31:7, drink and forget his *p.*
See Prov. 23:21; 2 Cor. 8:2; Rev. 2:9.
POWDER. Ex. 32:20; 2 Kings 23:6; Mat. 21:44.
POWER. Gen. 32:28; Hos. 12:3, hast thou *p.* with God.
Ex. 15:6, glorious in *p.*
Lev. 26:19, the pride of your *p.*
Deut. 8:18, he giveth thee *p.* to get wealth.
2 Sam. 22:33, God is my strength and *p.*
1 Chron. 29:11; Mat. 6:13, thine is the *p.* and glory.
2 Chron. 25:8, God hath *p.* to help.
Job 26:2, him that is without *p.*
Ps. 49:15, from the *p.* of the grave.
65:6, being girded with *p.*
90:11, who knoweth *p.* of thine anger.
Prov. 3:27, when it is in *p.* to do it.
18:21, in the *p.* of the tongue.
Eccl. 5:19; 6:2, *p.* to eat thereof.
8:4, where word of king is, there is *p.*
Isa. 40:29, he giveth *p.* to the faint.
Mic. 3:8, full of *p.* by the spirit.
Hab. 3:4, the hiding of his *p.*
Zech. 4:6, not by might, nor by *p.*
Mat. 9:6; Mk. 2:10; Lu. 5:24, *p.* on earth to forgive.
8, who had given such *p.* to men.
24:30; Lu. 21:27, coming in clouds with *p.*
28:18, all *p.* is given to me.
Lu. 1:35, the *p.* of the Highest.
4:6, all this *p.* will I give thee.
14, Jesus returned in the *p.* of the Spirit.
32, his word was with *p.*
5:17, the *p.* of the Lord was present.
9:43, amazed at the mighty *p.* of God.
12:5, that hath *p.* to cast into hell.
11, bring you unto magistrates and *p.*
22:53, your hour and the *p.* of darkness.
24:49, with *p.* from on high.
John 1:12, *p.* to become sons of God.
10:18, I have *p.* to lay it down.
17:2, *p.* over all flesh.
19:10, I have *p.* to crucify thee.
Acts 1:8, *p.* after the Holy Ghost is come.
3:12, as though by our own *p.*
5:4, was it not in thine own *p.*
8:10, this man is the great *p.* of God.
19, give me also this *p.*
26:18, from the *p.* of Satan unto God.
Rom. 1:20, his eternal *p.* and Godhead.
9:17, that I might show my *p.* in thee.
13:2, whosoever resisteth the *p.*
1 Cor. 15:43, it is raised in *p.*
Eph. 2:2, prince of the *p.* of the air.
3:7, the effectual working of his *p.*
Phil. 3:10, the *p.* of his resurrection.
2 Thess. 1:9, from the glory of his *p.*
2 Tim. 1:7, spirit of *p.* and love.
3:5, form of godliness, but denying the *p.*
Heb. 2:14, him that had *p.* of death.
6:5, the *p.* of the world to come.
7:16, the *p.* of an endless life.
Rev. 2:26, to him will I give *p.*
4:11, worthy to receive *p.*
See Mat. 22:29; Lu. 22:69; Rom. 1:16.
POWERFUL. Ps. 29:4; 2 Cor. 10:10; Heb. 4:12.
PRAISE (*n.*). Ex. 15:11, fearful in *p.*
Deut. 10:21, he is thy *p.* and thy God.
Judg. 5:3; Ps. 7:17; 9:2; 57:7; 61:8; 104:33, I will sing *p.*
Neh. 9:5, above all blessing and *p.*
Ps. 22:3, that inhabitest the *p.* of Israel.
25, my *p.* shall be of thee.
33:1; 147:1, *p.* is comely for the upright.
34:1, his *p.* continually be in my mouth.
50:23, whoso offereth *p.* glorifieth me.
65:1, *p.* waiteth for thee.
66:2, make his *p.* glorious.
109:1, O God of my *p.*
148:14, the *p.* of all his saints.
Prov. 27:21, so is a man to his *p.*
Isa. 60:18, call thy gates *P.*
61:3, garment of *p.*
62:7, a *p.* in the earth.
Jer. 13:11, that they might be to me for a *p.*
49:25, how is the city of *p.*
Hab. 3:3, earth was full of his *p.*
Zeph. 3:30, a *p.* among all people.
John 9:24, give God the *p.*
12:43, the *p.* of men.
Rom. 2:29, whose *p.* is not of men.
13:3, thou shalt have *p.*
1 Cor. 4:5, every man have *p.* of God.
2 Cor. 8:18, whose *p.* is in the gospel.
Eph. 1:6, 12, *p.* of glory of his grace.
Phil. 4:8, if there be any *p.*
Heb. 13:15, offer sacrifice of *p.*
1 Pet. 2:14, *p.* of them that do well.
4:11, to whom be *p.* and dominion.
See 2 Chron. 29:30; Acts 16:25; 1 Pet. 2:9.
PRAISE (*v.*). Gen. 49:8, whom thy brethren shall *p.*
2 Sam. 14:25, none to be so much *p.*
Ps. 30:9, shall the dust *p.* thee?
42:5, 11; 43:5, I shall yet *p.* him.
45:17, therefore shall the people *p.* thee.
49:18, men will *p.* thee when thou doest well.
63:3, my lips shall *p.* thee.
67:3, 5, let the people *p.* thee.
71:14, I will yet *p.* thee more and more.
72:15, daily shall he be *p.*
76:10, the wrath of man shall *p.* thee.
88:10, shall the dead arise and *p.* thee?
107:32, *p.* him in the assembly.
115:17, the dead *p.* not.
119:164, seven times a day do I *p.* thee.
145:4, one generation shall *p.* thy works.
10, all thy works shall *p.* thee.
Prov. 27:2, let another *p.* thee.
31:31, her own works *p.* her in the gates.
Isa. 38:19, the living shall *p.* thee.
See Lu. 2:13; 24:53; Acts 2:47; 3:8.
PRANCING. Judg. 5:22; Nah. 3:2.
PRATING. Prov. 10:8; 3 John 10.
PRAY. Gen. 20:7, a prophet and shall *p.* for thee.
1 Sam. 7:5, I will *p.* for you to the Lord.
12:23, sin in ceasing to *p.* for you.
2 Chron. 7:14, if my people shall *p.*
Ezra 6:10, *p.* for the life of the king.
Job 21:15, what profit if we *p.* to him.
Ps. 5:2, to thee will I *p.*
55:17, evening, morning, and at noon will I *p.*
122:6, *p.* for the peace of Jerusalem.
Isa. 45:20, *p.* to a god that cannot save.
Jer. 7:16; 11:14; 14:11, *p.* not for this people.
37:3; 42:2, 20, *p.* now to the Lord for us.
Zech. 7:2, they sent men to *p.*
Mat. 5:44, and *p.* for them which despitefully use you.
6:5, they love to *p.* standing.
14:23; Mk. 6:46; Lu. 6:12; 9:28, apart to *p.*
26:36; Mk. 14:32, while I *p.* yonder.
Mk. 11:25, and when ye stand *p.*, forgive.
Lu. 11:1, Lord, teach us to *p.*
18:1, men ought always to *p.*
John 14:16; 16:26, I will *p.* the Father.
17:9, I *p.* for them, I *p.* not for the world.

John 17:20, neither *p.* I for these alone.
Acts. 9:11, behold he *p.*
Rom. 8:26, know not what we should *p.* for.
1 Cor. 14:15, I will *p.* with the spirit, and *p.* with understanding also.
Eph. 6:18, *p.* always with all prayer.
1 Thess. 5:17, *p.* without ceasing.
1 Tim. 2:8, that men *p.* everywhere.
Jas. 5:13, is any afflicted? let him *p.*
16, *p.* one for another.
1 John 5:16, I do not say he shall *p.* for it.
See Lu. 9:29; 1 Cor. 11:4; 14:14; 1 Thess. 5:25.
PRAYER. 2 Chron. 7:15, ears shall be attent to the *p.*
Job 15:4, thou restrainest *p.*
16:17; Ps. 4:1; 5:3; 6:9; 17:1; 35:13; 39:12; 66:19; Lam. 3:8, my *p.*
Ps. 65:2, thou that hearest *p.*
72:15, *p.* shall be made continually.
109:4, I give myself to *p.*
Prov. 15:8, the *p.* of the upright.
Isa. 1:15, when ye make many *p.*
56:7; Mat. 21:13; Mk. 11:17; Lu. 19:46, house of *p.*
Mat. 21:22, whatever ye ask in *p.*, believing.
23:14; Mk. 12:40; Lu. 20:47, long *p.*
Lu. 6:12, all night in *p.* to God.
Acts 3:1, the hour of *p.*
6:4, give ourselves continually to *p.*
12:5, *p.* was made without ceasing.
16:13, where *p.* was wont to be made.
Phil. 4:6, in everything by *p.*
Jas. 5:15, *p.* of faith shall save the sick.
16, effectual fervent *p.* of a righteous man.
1 Pet. 4:7, watch unto *p.*
Rev. 5:8; 8:3, the *p.* of the saints.
See Ps. 72:20; Dan. 9:21; Rom. 12:12; Col. 4:2.
PREACH. Neh. 6:7, appointed prophets to *p.* of thee.
Isa. 61:1, to *p.* good tidings.
Jon. 3:2, *p.* the preaching I bid thee.
Mat. 4:17; 10:7, Jesus began to *p.*
11:1, to *p.* in their cities.
5, the poor have the gospel *p.*
Mk. 2:2, he *p.* the word to them.
16:20, and *p.* everywhere.
Lu. 9:60, go thou and *p.* kingdom of God.
Acts 8:5, and *p.* Christ unto them.
10:36, *p.* peace by Jesus Christ.
13:38, through his man is *p.* forgiveness.
17:18, he *p.* Jesus and the resurrection.
Rom. 2:21, thou that *p.* a man should not steal.
10:15, how shall they *p.* except.
1 Cor. 1:18, the *p.* of the cross is foolishness.
21, by the foolishness of *p.*
23, but we *p.* Christ crucified.
9:27, lest when I have *p.* to others.
15:11, so we *p.* and so ye believed.
14, then is our *p.* vain.
2 Cor. 4:5, we *p.* not ourselves.
Phil. 1:15, some *p.* Christ of envy and strife.
2 Tim. 4:2, *p.* the word; be instant.
Heb. 4:2, word *p.* did not profit.
1 Pet. 3:19, *p.* to spirits in prison.
See Ps. 40:9; 2 Cor. 11:4; Gal. 1:8; Eph. 2:17.
PREACHER. Rom. 10:14, how shall they hear without a *p.*?
1 Tim. 2:7, whereunto I am ordained a *p.*
2 Pet. 2:5, Noah, a *p.* of righteousness.
See Eccl. 1:1; 7:27; 12:8; 2 Tim. 1:11.
PRECEPT. Neh. 9:14, commandedst them *p.*
Isa. 28:10, 13, *p.* must be upon *p.*
29:13, taught by *p.* of men.
Jer. 35:18, ye have kept Jonadab's *p.*
See Ps. 119:4, etc.; Dan. 9:5; Mk. 10:5; Heb. 9:19.
PRECIOUS. Deut. 33:13, 14, 15, 16, *p.* things.
1 Sam. 3:1, the word was *p.* in those days.
26:21, my soul was *p.* in thine eyes.
2 Kings 1:13, let my life be *p.*
Ezra 8:27, fine copper, *p.* as gold.
Ps. 49:8, the redemption of their soul is *p.*
Ps. 72:14, *p.* shall their blood be in his sight.
116:15, *p.* in sight of the Lord is death of saints.
126:6, bearing *p.* seed.
133:2, like *p.* ointment upon the head.
139:17, how *p.* are thy thoughts.
Prov. 3:15, wisdom more *p.* than rubies.
Eccl. 7:1, good name better than *p.* ointment.
Isa. 13:12, I will make a man more *p.*
28:16; 1 Pet. 2:6, a *p.* corner stone.
43:4, since thou wast *p.* in my sight.
Jer. 15:19, take the *p.* from the vile.
Lam. 4:2, the *p.* sons of Zion.
1 Pet. 1:7, trial of faith more *p.* than gold.
19, the *p.* blood of Christ.
2:7, to you which believe he is *p.*
2 Pet. 1:1, like *p.* faith.
4, great and *p.* promises.
See Mat. 26:7; Mk. 14:3; Jas. 5:7; Rev. 21:11.
PREEMINENCE. Eccl. 3:19; Col. 1:18; 3 John 9.
PREFER. Ps. 137:6; John 1:15; Rom. 12:10; 1 Tim. 5:21.
PREMEDITATE. Mk. 13:11.
PREPARATION. Prov. 16:1, *p.* of the heart.
Eph. 6:15, feet shod with *p.* of gospel.
See Mat. 27:62; Mk. 15:42; Lu. 23:54; John 19:14.
PREPARE. 1 Sam. 7:3, *p.* your hearts unto the Lord.
2 Chron. 20:33, as yet the people had not *p.*
Ps. 68:10, thou hast *p.* of thy goodness.
107:36, that they may *p.* a city.
Prov. 8:27, when he *p.* the heavens I was there.
Isa. 40:3; Mal. 3:1; Mat. 3:3; Mk. 1:2; Lu. 1:76, *p.* way of the Lord.
62:10, *p.* the way of the people.
Amos 4:12, *p.* to meet thy God.
Jon. 1:17, Lord had *p.* a great fish.
Mat. 20:23; Mk. 10:40, to them for whom *p.*
John 14:2, I go to *p.* a place for you.
Rom. 9:23, afore *p.* to glory.
1 Cor. 2:9, things God hath *p.*
Heb. 10:5, a body hast thou *p.* me.
See 1 Chron. 22:5; Ps. 23:5; Rev. 21:2.
PRESCRIBE. Ezra 7:22; Isa. 10:1.
PRESENCE. Gen. 4:16, Cain went out from the *p.* of the Lord.
47:15, why should we die in thy *p.*
Ex. 33:15, if thy *p.* go not with me.
Job 23:15, I am troubled at his *p.*
Ps. 16:11, in thy *p.* is fulness of joy.
17:2, my sentence come forth from thy *p.*
31:20, in the secret of thy *p.*
51:11, cast me not away from thy *p.*
139:7, whither shall I flee from thy *p.*?
Prov. 14:7, go from *p.* of a foolish man.
Isa. 63:9, angel of his *p.* saved them.
Jer. 23:39; 52:3, I will cast you out of my *p.*
Jon. 1:3, to flee from *p.* of the Lord.
Zeph. 1:7, hold thy peace at *p.* of the Lord.
Lu. 13:26, we have eaten and drunk in thy *p.*
Acts 3:19, times of refreshing from the *p.*
2 Cor. 10:1, 10, who in *p.* am base.
2 Thess. 1:9, destruction from the *p.* of the Lord.
See Gen. 16:12; Ps. 23:5; Prov. 25:6; Lu. 15:10.
PRESENT. 1 Sam. 10:27, they brought him no *p.*
Ps. 46:1, a very *p.* help in trouble.
John 14:25, being yet *p.* with you.
Acts 10:33, all here *p.* before God.
Rom. 7:18, to will is *p.* with me.
21, evil is *p.* with me.
8:18, sufferings of this *p.* time.
12:1, *p.* your bodies a living sacrifice.
1 Cor. 7:26, good for the *p.* distress.
2 Cor. 5:8, to be *p.* with the Lord.
9, whether *p.* or absent.
Gal. 1:4, deliver us from this *p.* world.
Col. 1:28, *p.* every man perfect.
2 Tim. 4:10, having loved this *p.* world.
Tit. 2:12, live godly in this *p.* world.
Heb. 12:11, no chastening for *p.* seemeth joyous.
2 Pet. 1:12, established in the *p.* truth.

Jude 24, able to *p.* you faultless.
See Ps. 72:10; Mat. 2:11; Lu. 2:22.
PRESENTLY. Prov. 12:16; Mat. 21:19; 26:53.
PRESERVE. Gen. 32:30, I have seen God, and my life is *p.*
45:5, did send me before you to *p.* life.
Job 29:2, as in days when God *p.* me.
Ps. 36:6, thou *p.* man and beast.
121:7, the Lord *p.* thee from evil.
8, *p.* thy going out and coming in.
Prov. 2:8, he *p.* the way of his saints.
11, discretion shall *p.* thee.
20:28, mercy and truth *p.* the king.
Jer. 49:11, I will *p.* them alive.
Lu. 17:33, lose his life shall *p.* it.
See Neh. 9:6; Isa. 49:6; Hos. 12:13; Jude 1.
PRESS. Prov. 3:10, *p.* burst with new wine.
Amos 2:13, I am *p.* under you as a cart is *p.*
Mk. 3:10, they *p.* on him to touch him.
Lu. 6:38, good measure, *p.* down.
16:16, every man *p.* into it.
Phil. 3:14, I *p.* toward the mark.
See Mk. 2:4; 5:27; Lu. 8:19; 19:3.
PRESUME. Deut. 18:20; Esth. 7:5.
PRESUMPTUOUS. Num. 15:30; Ps. 19:13; 2 Pet. 2:10.
PRETENCE. Mat. 23:14; Mk. 12:40; Phil. 1:18.
PREVAIL. Gen. 32:28; Hos. 12:4, power with God, and hast *p.*
Ex. 17:11, Moses held up hand, Israel *p.*
1 Sam. 2:9, by strength shall no man *p.*
Ps. 9:19, let not man *p.*
65:3, iniquities *p.* against me.
Eccl. 4:12, if one *p.* against him.
Mat. 16:18, gates of hell shall not *p.*
Acts. 19:20, grew word of God and *p.*
See Job 14:20; Jer. 20:7; Lam. 1:16; John 12:19.
PREVENT. 2 Sam. 22:6; Ps. 18:5, snares of death *p.* me.
Ps. 88:13, in the morning shall my prayer *p.* thee.
119:147, I *p.* the dawning of the morning.
See Ps. 21:3; 79:8; Isa. 21:14; 1 Thess. 4:15.
PREY. Isa. 49:24, shall the *p.* be taken from the mighty?
Jer. 21:9; 38:2; 39:18; 45:5, his life shall be for a *p.*
Ezek. 34:22, my flock shall no more be a *p.*
See Gen. 49:9; Num. 14:3; Neh. 4:4; Amos 3:4.
PRICE. Lev. 25:52, the *p.* of his redemption.
2 Sam. 24:24; 1 Chron. 21:22, I will buy it at a *p.*
Acts 5:2, kept back part of the *p.*
1 Cor. 6:20; 7:23, bought with a *p.*
1 Pet. 3:4, meek spirit of great *p.*
See Deut. 23:18; Prov. 31:10; Zech. 11:12.
PRICKS. Num. 33:55; Acts 9:5; 26:14.
PRIDE. Ps. 31:20, hide them from *p.* of man.
Prov. 8:13, *p.* do I hate.
14:3, in mouth of foolish is rod of *p.*
Isa. 28:1, woe to the crown of *p.*
Jer. 49:16, *p.* of thine heart hath deceived thee.
See Mk. 7:22; 1 Tim. 3:6; 1 John 2:16.
PRIEST. Gen. 14:18; Heb. 7:1, *p.* of most high God.
Ex. 19:6, a kingdom of *p.*
1 Sam. 2:35, I will raise up a faithful *p.*
2 Chron. 6:41; Ps. 132:16, *p.* clothed with salvation.
13:9, *p.* of them that are no gods.
15:3, without a teaching *p.*
Isa. 24:2, as with the people, so with the *p.*
28:7, *p.* and prophet have erred.
61:6, shall be named the *p.* of the Lord.
Jer. 13:13, will fill *p.* with drunkenness.
Mic. 3:11, the *p.* teach for hire.
Mal. 2:7, the *p.* lips should keep knowledge.
Lu. 17:14, show yourselves to the *p.*
Acts 6:7, *p.* were obedient to the faith.
Rev. 1:6; 5:10; 20:6, kings and *p.* to God.
See Heb. 2:17; 3:1; 4:15; 7:26.
PRIESTHOOD. Ex. 40:15; Num. 25:13, an everlasting *p.*
Num. 16:10, seek ye the *p.* also.
Heb. 7:24, an unchangeable *p.*
1 Pet. 2:5, an holy *p.*
9, ye are a royal *p.*
See Num. 18:1; Josh. 18:7; Neh. 13:29.

PRINCE. Gen. 32:28, as a *p.* hast thou power.
Ex. 2:14; Num. 16:13, who made thee a *p.* over us?
1 Sam. 2:8; Ps. 113:8, to set them among *p.*
2 Sam. 3:38, a *p.* fallen in Israel.
Job 12:21; Ps. 107:40, poureth contempt on *p.*
21:28, where is the house of the *p.*?
31:37, as a *p.* would I go near him.
Ps. 45:16, make *p.* in all the earth.
118:9, than to put confidence in *p.*
146:3, put not your trust in *p.*
Prov. 8:15, by me *p.* decree justice.
31:4, nor for *p.* strong drink.
Eccl. 10:7, *p.* walking as servants.
16, when thy *p.* eat in the morning.
17, blessed when *p.* eat in due season.
Isa. 34:12; 40:23, all her *p.* shall be nothing.
Hos. 3:4, abide many days without a *p.*
Mat. 9:34; 12:24; Mk. 3:22, by *p.* of devils.
John 12:31; 14:30; 16:11, the *p.* of this world.
Acts 3:15, and killed the *P.* of life.
5:31, exalted to be a *P.* and Saviour.
1 Cor. 2:6, wisdom of the *p.* of this world.
8, which none of *p.* of this world knew.
Eph. 2:2, the *p.* of the power of the air.
See Isa. 3:4; Hos. 7:5; Mat. 20:25.
PRINCIPAL. Prov. 4:7; Isa. 28:25; Acts 25:23.
PRINCIPALITY. Eph. 6:12, we wrestle against *p.* and powers.
Tit. 3:1, to be subject to *p.*
See Rom. 8:38; Eph. 1:21; 3:10; Col. 1:16.
PRINCIPLES. Heb. 5:12; 6:1.
PRINT. Lev. 19:28; Job 13:27; 19:23; John 20:25.
PRISON. Ps. 142:7, bring my soul out of *p.*
Eccl. 4:14, out of *p.* he cometh to reign.
Isa. 53:8, taken from *p.* and from judgment.
61:1, opening of the *p.*
Mat. 5:25; Lu. 12:58, thou be cast into *p.*
11:2, John heard in the *p.*
25:36, 39, in *p.* that ye came unto me.
Lu. 22:33, to go with thee to *p.* and to death.
2 Cor. 11:23, in *p.* more frequent.
1 Pet. 3:19, spirits in *p.*
See Jer. 32:2; 39:14; Lu. 3:20; Acts 5:18.
PRISONER. Ps. 79:11; Zech. 9:12; Mat. 27:16; Eph. 3:1.
PRIVATE. 2 Pet. 1:20.
PRIVATELY. Mat. 24:3; Mk. 9:28; Lu. 10:23; Gal. 2:2.
PRIVILY. Mat. 1:19; 2:7; Acts 16:37; Gal. 2:4; 2 Pet. 2:1.
PRIZE. 1 Cor. 9:24; Phil. 3:14.
PROCEED. Gen. 24:50, the thing *p.* from the Lord.
Deut. 8:3; Mat. 4:4, that *p.* out of mouth of God.
Job 40:5, I will *p.* no further.
Isa. 29:14, I will *p.* to do a marvellous work.
51:4, a law shall *p.* from me.
Jer. 9:3, they *p.* from evil to evil.
Mat. 15:18; Mk. 7:21, *p.* out of the mouth.
John 8:42, I *p.* forth from God.
Jas. 3:10, *p.* blessing and cursing.
See Lu. 4:22; John 15:26; Eph. 4:29; Rev. 22:1.
PROCLAIM. Ex. 33:19; 34:5, I will *p.* the name of the Lord.
Isa. 61:1, to *p.* liberty to captives.
2, to *p.* acceptable year.
62:11, Lord hath *p.*, thy salvation cometh.
Jer. 34:15, in *p.* liberty every man to his neighbour.
Lu. 12:3, *p.* upon the housetops.
See Deut. 20:10; Prov. 20:6; Jer. 3:12; Joel 3:9.
PROCURE. Prov. 11:27; Jer. 2:17; 4:18; 26:19; 33:9.
PRODUCE. Isa. 41:21.
PROFANE. Lev. 18:21; 19:12; 20:3; 21:6; 22:2, *p.* name of God.
Jer. 23:11, prophet and priest are *p.*
Ezek. 22:26, no difference between holy and *p.*
Mat. 12:5, priests in temple *p.* sabbath.
Acts 24:6, hath gone about to *p.* temple.
1 Tim. 1:9, law for unholy and *p.*
4:7, refuse *p.* and old wives' fables.
6:20; 2 Tim. 2:16, avoiding *p.* babblings.
Heb. 12:16, any *p.* person.
See Ps. 89:39; Jer. 23:15; Mal. 1:12; 2:10.
PROFESS. Rom. 1:22; 2 Cor. 9:13; 1 Tim. 2:10; 6:12.

PROFIT (*n*.). Gen. 25:32, what *p*. shall birthright do me?
37:26, what *p*. if we slay?
Job 21:15, what *p*. if we pray?
Prov. 14:23, in all labour there is *p*.
Eccl. 1:3; 3:9; 5:16, what *p*. of labour?
2:11, there was no *p*. under the sun.
5:9, *p*. of the earth for all.
7:11, by wisdom there is *p*.
Jer. 16:19, things wherein is no *p*.
Mal. 3:14, what *p*. that we have kept.
1 Cor. 10:33, not seeking own *p*., but *p*. of many.
2 Tim. 2:14, about words to no *p*.
Heb. 12:10, he chasteneth us for our *p*.
See Esth. 3:8; Ps. 30:9; Isa. 30:5; 1 Tim. 4:15.
PROFIT (*v*.). 1 Sam. 12:21, vain things which cannot *p*.
Job 33:27, I have sinned, and it *p*. not.
34:9, *p*. nothing to delight in God.
Prov. 10:2, treasures of wickedness *p*. nothing.
11:4, riches *p*. not in the day of wrath.
Isa. 30:5, 6, people that could not *p*.
48:17, the Lord which teacheth thee to *p*.
Jer. 2:11, changed for that which doth not *p*.
23:32, they shall not *p*. this people.
Mat. 16:26; Mk. 8:36, what is a man *p*.?
1 Cor. 12:7, to every man to *p*. withal.
Gal. 5:2, Christ shall *p*. you nothing.
1 Tim. 4:8, bodily exercise *p*. little.
Heb. 4:2, the word preached did not *p*.
See Mat. 15:5; Rom. 2:25; 1 Cor. 13:3; Jas. 2:14.
PROFITABLE. Job 22:2, can a man be *p*. to God?
Eccl. 10:10, wisdom is *p*. to direct.
Acts 20:20, I kept back nothing *p*.
1 Tim. 4:8, godliness is *p*. to all things.
2 Tim. 3:16, scripture is *p*. for doctrine.
See Mat. 5:29; 2 Tim. 4:11; Tit. 3:8; Philem. 11.
PROLONG. Deut. 4:26; 30:18, ye shall not *p*. your days.
Job 6:11, what is mine end that I should *p*. my life?
Prov. 10:27, fear of the Lord *p*. days.
Eccl. 8:12, though a sinner's days be *p*.
See Ps. 61:6; Prov. 28:2; Isa. 13:22; 53:10.
PROMISE (*n*.). Num. 14:34, ye shall know my breach of *p*.
1 Kings 8:56, hath not failed one word of *p*.
Ps. 77:8, doth his *p*. fail?
Lu. 24:49; Acts 1:4, *p*. of Father.
Acts 2:39, the *p*. is to you and your children.
26:6, for hope of the *p*.
Rom. 4:14, the *p*. made of none effect.
20, staggered not at the *p*.
9:4, to whom pertain the *p*.
8; Gal. 4:28, the children of the *p*.
2 Cor. 1:20, *p*. are yea and Amen.
Gal. 3:21, is the law against the *p*. of God?
1 Tim. 4:8; 2 Tim. 1:1, *p*. of the life that now is.
Heb. 6:12, through faith and patience inherit the *p*.
9:15; 10:36, the *p*. of eternal inheritance.
11:13, died, not having received *p*.
2 Pet. 1:4, great and precious *p*.
3:4, where is the *p*. of his coming?
9, not slack concerning his *p*.
See Eph. 1:13; 2:12; 6:2; Heb. 4:1; 11:9.
PROMISE (*v*.). Ex. 12:25, will give you as he hath *p*.
Num. 14:40, will go to place the Lord *p*.
Deut. 1:11; 15:6, the Lord bless you as he hath *p*.
9:28, not able to bring into land *p*.
19:8; 27:3, give the land he *p*. to give.
Josh. 23:15, all good things which the Lord *p*.
2 Kings 8:19; 2 Chron. 21:7, he *p*. to give him a light.
Mk. 14:11, they *p*. to give him money.
Rom. 4:21, what he *p*. he was able to perform.
Heb. 10:23; 11:11, he is faithful that *p*.
1 John 2:25, he hath *p*. eternal life.
See 1 Kings 8:24; Neh. 9:15; Ezek. 13:22.
PROMOTE. Num. 22:17; 24:11; Prov. 4:8.
PROMOTION. Ps. 75:6; Prov. 3:35.
PRONOUNCE. Judg. 12:6; Jer. 34:5.
PROOF. 2 Cor. 2:9; 8:24; 13:3; Phil. 2:22; 2 Tim. 4:5.
PROPER. 1 Chron. 29:3; 1 Cor. 7:7; Heb. 11:23.
PROPHECY. 1 Cor. 13:8, whether *p*., shall fail.
2 Pet. 1:19, sure word of *p*.
21, *p*. came not in old time.
Rev. 1:3; 22:7, the words of this *p*.
See Neh. 6:12; Prov. 31:1; 1 Tim. 4:14.
PROPHESY. Num. 11:25, they *p*. and did not cease.
2 Chron. 18:7, he never *p*. good to me.
Isa. 30:10, *p*. not to us right things.
Jer. 5:31, prophets *p*. falsely.
14:14; 23:25, prophets *p*. lies.
28:9, the prophet which *p*. of peace.
Ezek. 37:9, *p*. to the wind.
Joel 2:28; Acts 2:17, your sons shall *p*.
Amos 3:8, who can but *p*.
7:13, *p*. not again any more.
Mic. 2:11, I will *p*. of wine.
Mat. 26:68; Mk. 14:65; Lu. 22:64, *p*., thou Christ.
Rom. 12:6, let us *p*. according to the proportion.
1 Cor. 13:9, we *p*. in part.
14:39, covet to *p*.
1 Thess. 5:20, despise not *p*.
See Amos 2:12; 1 Cor. 11:5; Rev. 10:11; 11:3.
PROPHET. Ex. 7:1, Aaron shall be thy *p*.
Num. 11:29, would all Lord's people were *p*.
12:6, if there be a *p*. among you.
Deut. 13:1, if there arise a *p*. or dreamer.
18:15; Acts 3:22; 7:37, the Lord will raise up a *P*.
34:10, there arose not a *p*. like Moses.
1 Sam. 10:12; 19:24, is Saul among *p*.?
1 Kings 13:11, there dwelt an old *p*. in Beth-el.
18:22, I only remain a *p*.
22:7; 2 Kings 3:11, is there not a *p*. besides?
2 Kings 5:8, he shall know there is a *p*.
1 Chron. 16:22; Ps. 105:15, do my *p*. no harm.
2 Chron. 20:20, believe his *p*., so shall ye prosper.
Ps. 74:9, there is no more any *p*.
Isa. 3:2, the Lord taketh away the *p*.
Jer. 29:26, mad, and maketh himself a *p*.
37:19, where are now your *p*.?
Ezek. 2:5; 33:33, there hath been a *p*. among them.
Hos. 9:7, the *p*. is a fool.
Amos 7:14, I was no *p*., nor *p*. son.
Zech. 1:5, the *p*., do they live for ever?
Mat. 7:15, beware of false *p*.
10:41, that receiveth a *p*. in name of a *p*.
13:57; Mk. 6:4; Lu. 4:24; John 4:44, a *p*. not without honour.
23:29; Lu. 11:47, ye build the tombs of the *p*.
Lu. 1:76, be called the *p*. of the Highest.
7:16, a great *p*. is risen.
28, not a great *p*. than John.
39, if he were a *p*. would have known.
Lu. 13:33, it cannot be that a *p*. perish out of.
24:19, Jesus, who was a *p*. mighty.
John 4:19, I perceive thou art a *p*.
7:40, of a truth this is the *P*.
52, out of Galilee ariseth no *p*.
Acts 26:27, believest thou the *p*.?
1 Cor. 12:29, are all *p*.?
14:37, if any man think himself a *p*.
Eph. 2:20, built on foundation of *p*.
4:11, he gave some *p*.
1 Pet. 1:10, of which salvation the *p*. enquired.
Rev. 22:9, I am of thy brethren the *p*.
See 1 Kings 20:35; Neh. 6:14; 1 Cor. 14:32.
PROPORTION. 1 Kings 7:36; Job 41:12; Rom. 12:6.
PROSPER. Gen. 24:56, the Lord hath *p*. my way.
39:3, the Lord made all Joseph did to *p*.
Num. 14:41, transgress, but it shall not *p*.
Deut. 28:29, thou shalt not *p*. in thy ways.
1 Chron. 22:11, *p*. thou, and build.
2 Chron. 20:20, believe, so shall ye *p*.
26:5, God made him to *p*.
Ezra 5:8, this work *p*. in their hands.
Neh. 2:20, the God of heaven will *p*. us.
Job 9:4, who hardened himself and *p*.
Ps. 1:3, whatsoever he doeth shall *p*.

Ps. 37:7, fret not because of him who *p.*
73:12, the ungodly who *p.* in the world.
122:6, they shall *p.* that love thee.
Prov. 28:13, he that covereth sins shall not *p.*
Eccl. 11:6, knowest not whether shall *p.*
Isa. 53:10, pleasure of the Lord shall *p.*
54:17, no weapon against thee shall *p.*
55:11, it shall *p.* in the thing.
Jer. 2:37, thou shalt not *p.* in them.
12:1, wherefore doth way of wicked *p.*?
22:30, no man of his seed shall *p.*
Ezek. 17:9, 10, shall it *p.*?
15, shall he *p.*, shall he escape?
1 Cor. 16:2, lay by as God hath *p.* him.
3 John 2, in health, even as thy soul *p.*
See Prov. 17:8; Dan. 6:28; 8:12.
PROSPERITY. Deut. 23:6, thou shalt not seek their *p.*
1 Sam. 25:6, say to him that liveth in *p.*
Job 15:21, in *p.* the destroyer shall come.
Ps. 30:6, in my *p.* I said, I shall never.
73:3, when I saw the *p.* of the wicked.
Prov. 1:32, *p.* of fools shall destroy them.
Eccl. 7:14, in day of *p.* be joyful.
Jer. 22:21, I spake to thee in thy *pi.*
See 1 Kings 10:7; Job 36:11; Ps. 35:17; 122:7.
PROSPEROUS. Gen. 39:2, he was a *p.* man.
Josh. 1:8, then thou shalt make thy way *p.*
Job 8:6, make habitation of thy righteousness *p.*
Zech. 8:12, the seed shall be *p.*
See Gen. 24:21; Judg. 18:5; 2 Chron. 7:11; Rom. 1:10.
PROTECTION. Deut. 32:38.
PROTEST. Gen. 43:3; Jer. 11:7; Zech. 3:6; 1 Cor. 15:31.
PROUD. Job 38:11, here shall thy *p.* waves be stayed.
40:11, every one that is *p.*, and abase him.
Ps. 31:23, rewardeth the *p.* doer.
40:4, man that respecteth not the *p.*
94:2, render a reward to the *p.*
101:5, him that hath a *p.* heart will not I suffer.
123:4, soul filled with contempt of the *p.*
138:6, the *p.* he knoweth afar off.
Prov. 6:17, the Lord hateth a *p.* look.
15:25, the Lord will destroy house of the *p.*
16:5, *p.* in heart is abomination.
21:4, a *p.* heart is sin.
Eccl. 7:8, patient better than *p.* in spirit.
Hab. 2:5, he is a *p.* man.
Mal. 3:15, we call the *p.* happy.
Lu. 1:51, scattered the *p.*
1 Tim. 6:4, he is *p.*, knowing nothing.
Jas. 4:6; 1 Pet. 5:5, God resisteth the *p.*
See Job 9:13; 26:12; Rom. 1:30; 2 Tim. 3:2.
PROUDLY. Ex. 18:11; 1 Sam. 2:3; Neh. 9:10; Isa. 3:5; Obad. 12.
PROVE. Ex. 15:25, there he *p.* them.
Judg. 6:39, let me *p.* thee but this once.
1 Sam. 17:39, I have not *p.* them.
1 Kings 10:1; 2 Chron. 9:1, she came to *p.* Solomon.
Ps. 17:3, thou hast *p.* mine heart.
81:7, I *p.* thee at the waters.
95:9; Heb. 3:9, when your fathers *p.* me.
Mal. 3:10, *p.* me now herewith.
Lu. 14:19, I go to *p.* them.
2 Cor. 8:22, whom we have often *p.* diligent.
13:5, *p.* your own selves.
1 Thess. 5:21, *p.* all things.
See Eccl. 2:1; 7:23; Dan. 1:14; John 6:6.
PROVERB. Deut. 28:37, a *p.* and a byword.
Ps. 69:11, I became a *p.* to them.
Eccl. 12:9, set in order many *p.*
Ezek. 16:44, every one that useth *p.*
Lu. 4:23, will surely say this *p.*
John 16:29, speakest plainly, and no *p.*
See Num. 21:27; 1 Sam. 10:12; Prov. 1:6.
PROVIDE. Gen. 22:8, God will *p.* himself a lamb.
30:30, when shall I *p.* for mine own house?
Ps. 78:20, can he *p.* flesh?
Mat. 10:9, *p.* neither gold nor silver.
Lu. 12:20, whose shall those things be thou hast *p*?
Lu. 12:33, *p.* bags that wax not old.
Rom. 12:17; 2 Cor. 8:21, *p.* things honest.
1 Tim. 5:8, if any *p.* not for his own.
Heb. 11:40, having *p.* better thing for us.
See Job 38:41; Prov. 6:8; Acts 23:24.
PROVIDENCE. Acts 24:2.
PROVISION. Gen. 42:25; 45:21, *p.* for the way.
Ps. 132:15, I will abundantly bless her *p.*
Rom. 13:14, make not *p.* for the flesh.
See Josh. 9:5; 1 Kings 4:7; 2 Kings 6:23.
PROVOCATION. Job 17:2; Ps. 95:8; Ezek. 20:28.
PROVOKE. Ex. 23:21, obey his voice and *p.* him not.
Num. 14:11, how long will this people *p.* me?
Deut. 31:20, *p.* me and break my covenant.
Job 12:6, they that *p.* God are secure.
Ps. 106:7, they *p.* him at the sea.
29, they *p.* him with their inventions.
Lu. 11:53, began to urge and *p.* him to speak.
Rom. 10:19; 11:11, I will *p.* to jealousy.
1 Cor. 13:5, is not easily *p.*
Gal. 5:26, *p.* one another.
Eph. 6:4, *p.* not your children to wrath.
Heb. 10:24, to *p.* to love and good works.
See Prov. 20:2; Isa. 65:3; Jer. 7:19; 44:8.
PRUDENCE. 2 Chron. 2:12; Prov. 8:12; Eph. 1:8.
PRUDENT. Prov. 12:16, a *p.* man covereth shame.
23, a *p.* man concealeth knowledge.
14:15, the *p.* looketh well to his going.
16:21, wise in heart called *p.*
19:14, *p.* wife is from the Lord.
22:3; 27:12, *p.* man forseeth evil.
Isa. 5:21, woe unto them that are *p.* in their own sight.
Jer. 49:7, counsel perished from *p.*
Hos. 14:9, who is *p.*?
Mat. 11:25; Lu. 10:21, hast hid things from *p.*
See Isa. 52:13; Amos 5:13; Acts 13.
PRUNE. Lev. 25:3; Isa. 2:4; Joel 3:10; Mic. 4:3.
PSALTERY. Dan. 3:5, the sound of the cornet, flute, *p.*, etc.
See 2 Sam. 6:5; 2 Chron. 9:11.
PUBLIC. Mat. 1:19; Acts 18:28; 20:20.
PUBLISH. Deut. 32:3, I will *p.* the name of the Lord.
2 Sam. 1:20, *p.* it not in Askelon.
Ps. 68:11, great was the company that *p.* it.
Isa. 52:7; Nah. 1:15, that *p.* peace.
Mk. 1:45; 5:20, he began to *p.* it much.
Lu. 8:39, *p.* throughout the whole city.
See Esth. 1:20; 3:14; Jon. 3:7; Mk. 13:10.
PUFFED. 1 Cor. 4:6; 5:2; 13:4; Col. 2:18.
PUFFETH. Ps. 10:5; 12:5; 1 Cor. 8:1.
PULL. Lam. 3:11, *p* me in pieces.
Amos 9:15, shall no more be *p.* up.
Zech. 7:11, they *p.* away the shoulder.
Mat. 7:4; Lu. 6:42, *p.* mote out of thine eye.
Lu. 12:18, will *p.* down barns.
14:5, will not *p.* him out on sabbath.
2 Cor. 10:4, to the *p.* down of strong holds.
Jude 23, *p.* them out of the fire.
See Gen. 8:9; Ezra 6:11; Ps. 31:4; Isa. 22:19.
PULPIT. Neh. 8:4.
PULSE. 2 Sam. 17:28; Dan. 1:12.
PUNISH. Ezra 9:13, *p.* less than iniquities deserve.
Prov. 17:26, to *p.* the just is not good.
Isa. 13:11, I will *p.* the world for their evil.
26:21, Lord cometh to *p.* inhabitants.
Jer. 13:21, what wilt thou say when he *p.*
Acts 26:11, I *p.* them in every synagogue.
2 Thess. 1:9, *p.* with everlasting destruction.
2 Pet. 2:9, to day of judgment to be *p.*
See Lev. 26:18; Prov. 21:11; 22:3; 27:12.
PUNISHMENT. Gen. 4:13, my *p.* is greater than I can bear.
Lev. 26:41, accept the *p.* of their iniquity.
1 Sam. 28:10, no *p.* shall happen to thee.
Lam. 3:39, a man for the *p.* of his sins.
4:6, *p.* greater than *p.* of Sodom.
22, the *p.* is accomplished.
Ezek. 14:10, shall bear *p.* of their iniquity.
Mat. 25:46, everlasting *p.*

Heb. 10:29, of how much sorer *p.*
1 Pet. 2:14, the *p.* of evildoers.
See Prov. 19:19; Amos 1:3; 2:1; 2 Cor. 2:6.
PURCHASE. Ruth 4:10, have I *p.* to be my wife.
Ps. 74:2, congregation thou hast *p.*
Acts 1:18, *p.* a field with reward of iniquity.
8:20, gift of God *p.* by money.
20:28, he hath *p.* with his own blood.
Eph. 1:14, redemption of *p.* possession.
1 Tim. 3:13, *p.* to themselves a good degree.
See Gen. 49:32; Ex. 15:16; Lev. 25:33; Jer. 32:11.
PURE. Deut. 32:14, the *p.* blood of the grape.
2 Sam. 22:27; Ps. 18:26, with *p.* show thyself *p.*
Job 4:17, shall man be more *p.*?
8:6, if thou wert *p.* and upright.
11:4, my doctrine is *p.*
16:17, my prayer is *p.*
25:5, stars are not *p.* in his sight.
Ps. 12:6, the words of the Lord are *p.*
19:8, commandment of the Lord is *p.*
119:140, thy word is very *p.*
Prov. 15:26, words of the *p.* are pleasant.
20:9, who can say, I am *p.*?
Mic. 6:11, shall I count them *p.*?
Zeph. 3:9, turn to the people a *p.* language.
Acts 20:26, *p.* from blood of all men.
Rom. 14:20, all things indeed are *p.*
Phil. 4:8, whatsoever things are *p.*
1 Tim. 3:9; 2 Tim. 1:3, in a *p.* conscience.
5:22, keep thy self *p.*
Tit. 1:15, to the *p.* all things are *p.*
Jas. 1:27, *p.* religion.
3:17, first *p.*, then peaceable.
2 Pet. 3:1, stir up your *p.* minds.
1 John 3:3, even as he is *p.*
Rev. 22:1, a *p.* river of water of life.
See Ex. 27:20; Ezra 6:20; Mal. 1:11.
PURELY. Isa. 1:25.
PURENESS. Job 22:30; Prov. 22:11; 2 Cor. 6:6.
PURER. Lam. 4:7; Hab. 1:13.
PURGE. 2 Chron. 34:8, when he had *p.* the land.
Ps. 51:7, *p.* me with hyssop.
65:3, transgressions, thou shalt *p.* them.
Isa. 1:25, and purely *p.* away thy dross.
6:7, thy sin is *p.*
22:14, this iniquity shall not be *p.*
Ezek. 24:13, I have *p.* thee and thou wast not *p.*
Mal. 3:3, *p.* them as gold.
Mat. 3:12; Lu. 3:17, *p.* his floor.
John 15:2, he *p.* it, that it may bring forth.
1 Cor. 5:7, *p.* out the old leaven.
2 Tim. 2:21, if a man *p.* himself from these.
Heb. 9:14, *p.* your conscience.
22, all things are *p.* with blood.
See Prov. 16:6; Heb. 1:3; 10:2; 2 Pet. 1:9.
PURIFY. Tit. 2:14; Jas. 4:8; 1 Pet. 1:22.
PURITY. 1 Tim. 4:12; 5:2.
PURLOINING. Tit. 2:10.
PURPOSE. Job 17:11, my *p.* are broken off.
Prov. 20:18, every *p.* established by counsel.
Isa. 14:27, the Lord hath *p.*, who shall disannul?
46:11, I have *p.*, I will also do it.
Mat. 26:8, to what *p.* is this waste?
Acts 11:23, with *p.* of heart.
Rom. 8:28, called according to his *p.*
9:11, that the *p.* of God might stand.
Eph. 1:11, according to the *p.*
3:11, eternal *p.* in Christ.
See 2 Cor. 1:17; 2 Tim. 1:9; 1 John 3:8.
PURSE. Prov. 1:14; Mat. 10:9; Mk. 6:8; Lu. 10:4.
PURSUE. Lev. 26:17; Prov. 28:1, shall flee when none *p.*
Deut. 19:6; Josh. 20:5, lest avenger *p.*
Job 13:25, wilt thou *p.* the stubble?
30:15, terrors *p.* my soul.
Ps. 34:14, seek peace and *p.* it.
Prov. 11:19, he that *p.* evil *p.* it to death.
13:21, evil *p.* sinners.
Jer. 48:2, the sword shall *p.* thee.
See Ex. 15:9; 2 Sam. 24:13; 1 Kings 18:27.
PUSH. Ex. 21:29; 1 Kings 22:11; Job 30:12.
PUT. Ex. 23:1, *p.* not thine hand with the wicked.
Lev. 26:8; Deut. 32:30, *p.* ten thousand to flight.
Judg. 12:3; 1 Sam. 28:21, I *p.* my life in my hands.
1 Sam. 2:36, *p.* me into one of priests' offices.
1 Kings 9:3; 14:21, to *p.* my name there.
Eccl. 10:10, must he *p.* to more strength.
Isa. 43:26, *p.* me in remembrance.
Mat. 19:6; Mk. 10:9, let not man *p.* asunder.
Mk. 10:16, *p.* his hands on them and blessed.
Philem. 18, *p.* that on mine account.
2 Pet. 1:14, I must *p.* off this tabernacle.
See Lu. 9:62; John 13:2; 1 Thess. 5:8.
PUTRIFYING. Isa. 1:6.

Q

QUAKE. Joel 2:10; Nah. 1:5; Mat. 27:51; Heb. 12:21.
QUANTITY. Isa. 22:24.
QUARREL. Lev. 26:25; 2 Kings 5:7; Mk. 6:19; Col. 3:13.
QUARTER. Ex. 13:7; Mk. 1:45; Rev. 20:8.
QUATERNIONS. Acts 12:4, delivered him to four *q.*
QUEEN. Jer. 44:17, 25, burn incense unto the *q.*
QUENCH. Num. 11:2, the fire was *q.*
2 Sam. 21:17, *q.* not light of Israel.
Cant. 8:7, many waters cannot *q.* love.
Isa. 34:10, shall not be a *q.* night nor day.
42:3; Mat. 12:20, smoking flax not *q.*
66:24, neither shall their fire be *q.*
Mk. 9:43, 48, fire that never shall be *q.*
Eph. 6:16, able to *q.* fiery darts.
1 Thess. 5:19, *q.* not the Spirit.
Heb. 11:34, *q.* violence of fire.
See. Ps. 104:11; 118:12; Ezek. 20:27; Amos 5:6.
QUESTION. 1 Kings 10:1; 2 Chron. 9:1, to prove him with *q.*
Mat. 22:46, neither durst ask him *q.*
Mk. 9:16, what *q.* ye with them?
11:29, I will ask you one *q.*
1 Cor. 10:25, asking no *q.* for conscience.
1 Tim. 1:4, which minister *q.* rather.
6:4, doting about *q.*
2 Tim. 2:23; Tit. 3:9, unlearned *q.* avoid.
See Mk. 1:27; 9:10; Acts 18:15; 19:40.
QUICK. Num. 16:30; Ps. 55:15, go down *q.*
Isa. 11:3, of *q.* understanding.
Acts 10:42; 2 Tim. 4:1; 1 Pet. 4:5, Judge of *q.* and dead.
Heb. 4:12, the word is *q.* and powerful.
See Lev. 13:10, 24; Ps. 124:3.
QUICKEN. Ps. 71:20, thou shalt *q.* me again.
80:18, *q.* us and we will call.
119:25, *q.* me according to thy word.
37, *q.* me in thy way.
50, thy word hath *q.* me.
Rom. 8:11, shall also *q.* your bodies.
1 Cor. 15:36, that thou sowest is not *q.*
Eph. 2:1, you hath he *q.*
5; Col. 2:13, *q.* us together with Christ.
1 Pet. 3:18, to death in flesh, *q.* by Spirit.
See John 5:21; 6:63; Rom. 4:17; 1 Tim. 6:13.
QUICKLY. Ex. 32:8; Deut. 9:12, have turned aside *q.*
Num. 16:46, go *q.* to congregation.
Josh. 10:6, come *q.* and save us.
Eccl. 4:12, threefold cord not *q.* broken.
Mat. 5:25, agree with adversary *q.*
Lu. 14:21, go *q.* into streets and lanes.
John 13:27, that thou doest, do *q.*
Rev. 2:5, 16, repent, else I will come *q.*
3:11; 22:7, 12, I come *q.*
22:20, surely I come *q.*
See Gen. 18:6; 27:20; Lu. 16:6; Acts 22:18.
QUICKSANDS. Acts 27:17, fearing lest they should fall into the *q.*
QUIET. Ps. 107:30, then are they glad because *q.*
131:2, I have *q.* myself as a child.
Eccl. 9:17, words of wise are heard in *q.*
Isa. 7:4, be *q.*, fear not.

Isa. 14:7, earth is at rest and *q*.
32:18, in *q*. resting places.
33:20, a *q*. habitation.
Jer. 49:23, sorrow on the sea, it cannot be *q*.
Ezek. 16:42, I will be *q*.
Acts 19:36, ye ought to be *q*.
1 Thess. 4:11, study to be *q*.
1 Tim. 2:2, a *q*. and peaceable life.
1 Pet. 3:4, ornament of a meek and *q*. spirit.
See 2 Kings 11:20; 2 Chron. 14:1; Job 3:13; 21:23.
QUIETLY. 2 Sam. 3:27; Lam. 3:26.
QUIETNESS. Job 34:29, when he giveth *q*.
Prov. 17:1, better a dry morsel and *q*.
Eccl. 4:6, better handful with *q*. than both.
Isa. 30:15, in *q*. and confidence strength.
32:17, effect of righteousness *q*.
See Judg. 8:28; 1 Chron. 22:9; 2 Thess. 3:12.
QUIT. Ex. 21:19; Josh. 2:20; 1 Sam. 4:9; 1 Cor. 16:13.
QUITE. Gen. 31:15; Job 6:13; Hab. 3:9.
QUIVER. Ps. 127:5; Jer. 5:16; Lam. 3:13.

R

RACE. Ps. 19:5; Eccl. 9:11; 1 Cor. 9:24; Heb. 12:1.
RAGE. 2 Kings 5:12, turned away in a *r*.
Ps. 2:1; Acts 4:25, why do the heathen *r*.
Prov. 14:16, the fool *r*. and is confident.
See Prov. 6:34; 29:9; Dan. 3:13; Hos. 7:16.
RAGGED. Isa. 2:21.
RAGING. Ps. 89:9; Prov. 20:1; Lu. 8:24; Jude 13.
RAGS. Prov. 23:21; Isa. 64:6; Jer. 38:11.
RAIMENT. Gen. 28:20, if the Lord will give me *r*.
Deut. 8:4, thy *r*. waxed not old.
24:13, that he may sleep in his *r*.
17, nor take a widow's *r*. to pledge.
Job 27:16, though he prepare *r*. as the clay.
Isa. 63:3, I will stain all my *r*.
Zech. 3:4, I will clothe thee with *r*.
Mat. 6:25; Lu. 12:23, the body more than *r*.
28, why take though for *r*.
11:8; Lu. 7:25, man clothed in soft *r*.
17:2; Mk. 9:3; Lu. 9:29, his *r*. was white as light.
1 Tim. 6:8, having food and *r*., be content.
Jas. 2:2, poor man in vile *r*.
Rev. 3:18, buy white *r*.
See Mt. 3:4; Lu. 10:30; 23:34; Acts 22:20.
RAIN (*n*.). Lev. 26:4; Deut. 11:14; 28:12, *r*. in due season.
Deut. 11:11, drinketh water of the *r*. of heaven.
32:2, my doctrine shall drop as the *r*.
2 Sam. 23:4, clear shining after *r*.
1 Kings 18:41, sound of abundance of *r*.
Ezra 10:13, a time of much *r*.
Job 5:10, who giveth *r*. on earth.
37:6, to small *r*. and to great *r*.
38:28, hath the *r*. a father.
Ps. 72:6, like *r*. on mown grass.
Prov. 25:14, like clouds and wind without *r*.
23, north wind driveth away *r*.
26:1, as *r*. in harvest.
28:3, that oppresseth poor is like sweeping *r*.
Eccl. 11:3, if clouds be full of *r*.
12:2, nor clouds return after *r*.
Cant. 2:11, the *r*. is over and gone.
Isa. 4:6, covert from storm and *r*.
55:10, as the *r*. cometh down.
Ezek. 38:22, I will *r*. an overflowing *r*.
Hos. 6:3, he shall come unto us as the *r*.
Mat. 5:45, *r*. on just and unjust.
7:25, the *r*. descended and floods came.
See Jer. 5:24; Acts 14:17; 28:2; Heb. 6:7.
RAIN (*v*.). Ex. 16:4, I will *r*. bread from heaven.
Job 20:23, God shall *r*. his fury on him.
Ps. 11:6, on wicked he shall *r*. snares.
78:24, 27, and *r*. down manna.
Ezek. 22:24, thou art the land not *r*. upon.
Hos. 10:12, till he come and *r*. righteousness.
See Gen. 2:5; 7:4; Amos 4:7; Rev. 11:6.
RAINY. Prov. 27:15.
RAISE. Deut. 18:15; Acts 3:22, will *r*. up a Prophet.
Judg. 2:16, 18, the Lord *r*. up judges.
1 Sam. 2:8; Ps. 113:7, he *r*. poor out of dust.
Job 41:25, when he *r*. himself, mighty are.
Ps. 145:14; 146:8, he *r*. those that be bowed down.
Isa. 45:13, I have *r*. him in righteousness.
Hos. 6:2, in third day he will *r*. us up.
Mat. 10:8; 11:5; Lu. 7:22, *r*. the dead.
16:21; 17:23; Lu. 9:22, be *r*. the third day.
John 2:19, in three days I will *r*. it up.
6:39, 40, 44, 54, I will *r*. him up at the last day.
Acts 2:24, 32; 3:15; 4:10; 5:30; 10:40; 13:30, 33, 34; 17:31; Rom. 10:9; 1 Cor. 6:14; 2 Cor. 4:14; Gal. 1:1; Eph. 1:20, whom God hath *r*. up.
26:8, why incredible that God should *r*. the dead?
Rom. 4:25, *r*. again for our justification.
6:4, like as Christ was *r*. from the dead.
8:11, Spirit of him that *r*. up Jesus.
1 Cor. 6:14, and will also *r*. up us by his power.
15:15, *r*. up Christ, whom he *r*. not up.
16, then is not Christ *r*.
17, if Christ be not *r*.
35, how are the dead *r*.
43, it is *r*. in glory, it is *r*. in power.
2 Cor. 1:9, trust in God which *r*. the dead.
4:14, he shall *r*. up us also.
Eph. 2:6, and hath *r*. us up together.
Heb. 11:19, accounting God was able to *r*. him.
35, women received dead *r*. to life.
Jas. 5:15, and the Lord shall *r*. him up.
See Lu. 20:37; John 5:21; 2 Tim. 2:8.
RAN. Ex. 9:23; Num. 16:47; Jer. 23:21.
RANG. 1 Sam. 4:5; 1 Kings 1:45.
RANKS. 1 Kings 7:4; Joel 2:7; Mk. 6:40.
RANSOM. Ex. 21:30, give for the *r*. of his life.
30:12, every man a *r*. for his soul.
Job 33:24, I have found a *r*.
36:18, a great *r*. cannot deliver.
Ps. 49:7, nor give a *r*. for him.
Prov. 13:8, the *r*. of a man's life are his riches.
Isa. 35:10, the *r*. of the Lord shall return.
43:3, I gave Egypt for thy *r*.
Hos. 13:14, I will *r*. them from the grave.
Mat. 20:18; Mk. 10:45, to give his life a *r*.
1 Tim. 2:6, gave himself a *r*. for all.
See Prov. 6:35; Isa. 51:10; Jer. 31:11.
RARE. Dan. 2:11.
RASE. Ps. 137:7.
RASH. Eccl. 5:2; Acts 19:36.
RATHER. Job 7:15; Jer. 8:3, death *r*. than life.
Ps. 84:10, *r*. be a doorkeeper.
Mat. 10:6, go *r*. to lost sheep
28, *r*. fear him that is able.
25:9, go *r*. to them that sell.
Mk. 5:26, but *r*. grew worse.
Lu. 18:14, justified *r*. than the other.
John 3:19, loved darkness *r*. than light.
Acts 5:29, obey God *r*. than men.
Rom. 8:34, that died, yea *r*., that is risen.
12:19, *r*. give place to wrath.
1 Cor. 6:7, why do ye not *r*. take wrong.
Heb. 11:25, choosing *r*. to suffer.
12:13, let it *r*. be healed.
See Josh. 22:24; 2 Kings 5:13; Phil. 1:12.
RAVENING. Ps. 22:13; Ezek. 22:25; Mat. 7:15.
RAVENOUS. Isa. 35:9; 46:11; Ezek. 39:4.
REACH. Gen. 11:4; John 20:27; 2 Cor. 10:13.
READ. Deut. 17:19, king shall *r*. his life.
Isa. 34:16, seek out of book of Lord and *r*.
Mat. 12:3; 19:4; 21:16; 22:31; Mk. 2:25; 12:10; Lu. 6:3, have ye not *r*.
Lu. 4:16, Jesus stood up to *r*.
2 Cor. 3:2, epistle known and *r*. of all men.
1 Tim. 4:13, give attendance to *r*.
See Hab. 2:2; 2 Cor. 3:14; Rev. 1:3; 5:4.
READINESS. Acts 17:11; 2 Cor. 8:11; 10:6.
READY. Num. 32:17, we will go *r*. armed.

Deut. 26:5, a Syrian *r.* to perish.
2 Sam. 18:22, wherefore run, no tidings *r.*
Neh. 9:17, thou art a God *r.* to pardon.
Job 12:5, *r.* to slip with is feet.
17:1, the graves are *r.* for me.
29:13, blessing of him *r.* to perish.
Ps. 38:17, I am *r.* to halt.
45:1, pen of a *r.* writer.
86:5, good and *r.* to forgive.
88:15, *r.* to die from my youth.
Prov. 24:11, deliver those *r.* to be slain.
31:6, give strong drink to *r.* to perish.
Eccl. 5:1, be more *r.* to hear.
Isa. 27:13, shall come that were *r.* to perish.
32:4, stammerers *r.* to speak plainly.
38:20, the Lord was *r.* to save me.
Dan. 3:15, if ye be *r.* to fall down.
Mat. 22:4; Lu. 14:17, all things are *r.*
8, the wedding is *r.*
24:44; Lu. 12:40, be ye also *r.*
25:10, they that were *r.* went in.
Mk. 14:38, the spirit is *r.*
Lu. 22:33, I am *r.* to go with thee.
John 7:6, your time is alway *r.*
Acts 21:13, *r.* not to be bound only, but.
Rom. 1:15, I am *r.* to preach at Rome.
2 Cor. 8:19, declaration of your *r.* mind.
9:2, Achaia was *r.* a year ago.
1 Tim. 6:18, *r.* to distribute.
2 Tim. 4:6, *r.* to be offered.
Tit. 3:1, *r.* to every good work.
1 Pet. 1:5, *r.* to be revealed.
3:15, *r.* always to give an answer.
5:2, but of a *r.* mind.
Rev. 3:2, things that are *r.* to die.
See Ex. 17:4; 19:11; Ezra 7:6; Job 15:23.

REAP. Lev. 25:11, in jubilee neither sow nor *r.*
Eccl. 11:4, regardeth clouds shall not *r.*
Jer. 12:13, sown wheat, but shall *r.* thorns.
Hos. 8:7, shall *r.* the whirlwind.
10:12, sow in righteousness, *r.* in mercy.
Mic. 6:15, shalt sow, but not *r.*
Mat. 6:26; Lu. 12:24, sow not, neither *r.*
25:26; Lu. 19:21, *r.* where I sowed not.
John 4:38, *r.* whereon ye bestowed no labour.
1 Cor. 9:11, if we shall *r.* your carnal things.
2 Cor. 9:6, shall *r.* sparingly.
Gal. 6:7, that shall he also *r.*
Jas. 5:4, cried of them which *r.*
See Isa. 17:5; John 4:36, 37; Rev. 14:15.

REASON (*n.*). Job 32:11, I gave ear to your *r.*
Prov. 26:16, seven men that can render a *r.*
Eccl. 7:25, to search out the *r.* of things.
Isa. 41:21, bring forth your strong *r.*
1 Pet. 3:15, a *r.* of the hope in you.
See 1 Kings 9:15; Dan. 4:36; Acts 6:2.

REASON (*v.*). Job 9:14, choose words to *r.* with you.
13:3, I desire to *r.* with God.
15:3, should he *r.* with unprofitable talk.
Isa. 1:18, let us *r.* together.
Mat. 16:7; 21:25; Mk. 8:16; 11:31; Lu. 20:5, they *r* among themselves.
Lu. 5:22, what *r.* ye in your hearts.
24:15, while they *r.* Jesus drew near.
Acts 24:25, as he *r.* of righteousness.
See 1 Sam. 12:7; Mk. 2:6; 12:28; Acts 28:29.

REASONABLE. Rom. 12:1.

REBEL. Num. 14:9, only *r* not against the Lord.
Josh. 1:18, whosoever doth *r.* he shall die.
Neh. 2:19, will ye *r.* against the king.
Job 24:13, that *r.* against the light.
Ps. 105:28, they *r* not against his word.
Isa. 1:2, have nourished children and they *r.*
63:10, they *r.* and vexed his holy Spirit.
Lam. 3:42, we have *r.*, thou hast not pardoned.
Dan. 9:9, though we have *r.* against him.
See 1 Sam. 12:14; Ezek. 2:3; Hos. 7:14; 13:16.

REBELLION. 1 Sam. 15:23, *r.* is as the sin of witchcraft.
Job 34:37, he addeth *r.* to his sin.
Prov. 17:11, an evil man seeketh *r.*
Jer. 28:16, thou hast taught *r.*
See Deut. 31:27; Ezra 4:19; Neh. 9:17.

REBELLIOUS. Deut. 21:18, 20, a stubborn and *r.* son.
1 Sam. 20:30, son of perverse *r.* woman.
Ps. 66:7, let not the *r.* exalt themselves.
68:6, the *r.* dwell in a dry land.
Isa. 1:23, *r.*, companions of thieves.
Jer. 5:23, this people hath a *r.* heart.
See Ezek. 2:3; 3:9; 12:2; 17:12; 24:3.

REBELS. Num. 17:10; 20:10; Ezek. 20:38.

REBUKE (*n.*). 2 Kings 19:3; Isa. 37:3, this is a day of *r.*
Ps. 39:11, when thou with *r.* dost correct.
80:16, perish at *r.* of thy countenance.
104:7, at thy *r.* they fled.
Prov. 13:8, the poor heareth not *r.*
27:5, open *r.* is better than secret love.
Eccl. 7:5, better to hear *r.* of wise.
Isa. 30:17, thousand flee at *r.* of one.
Jer. 15:15, for thy sake I suffered *r.*
Phil. 2:15, without *r.*
See Deut. 28:20; Isa. 25:8; 50:2.

REBUKE (*v.*). Ps. 6:1; 38:1, *r.* me not in anger.
Prov. 9:7, he that *r.* a wicked man getteth a blot.
8, *r.* a wise man, and he will love thee.
28:23, he that *r.* a man shall find favour
Isa. 2:4; Mic. 4:3, he shall *r.* many nations.
Zech. 3:2; Jude 9, the Lord *r.* thee.
Mal. 3:11, I will *r.* the devourer for your sakes.
Mat. 8:26; Mk. 4:39; Lu. 8:24, he *r.* wind.
16:22; Mk. 8:32, Peter began to *r.* him.
Lu. 4:39, he *r.* the fever.
17:3, if thy brother trespass, *r.* him.
19:39, Master, *r.* thy disciples.
1 Tim. 5:1, *r.* not an elder.
20, them that sin, *r.* before all.
2 Tim. 4:2, *r.*, exhort, with longsuffering.
Tit. 1:13; 2:15, *r.* them sharply.
Heb. 12:5, nor faint when thou art *r.*
See Ruth 2:16; Neh. 5:7; Amos 5:10.

RECALL. Lam. 3:21.

RECEIPT. Mat. 9:9; Mk. 2:14; Lu. 5:27.

RECEIVE. 2 Kings 5:26, is it a time to *r.* money.
Job 4:12, mine ear *r.* a little.
22:22, *r.* law from his mouth.
Ps. 6:9, the Lord will *r.* my prayer.
49:15, he shall *r.* me.
68:18, hast *r.* gifts for men.
73:24, afterwards *r.* me to glory.
Prov. 2:1, if thou wilt *r.* my words.
Isa. 40:2, she hath *r.* double.
Jer. 2:30, your children *r.* no correction.
Hos. 10:6, Ephraim shall *r.* shame.
14:2, *r.* us graciously.
Mat. 11:5, the blind *r.* their sight.
14, if ye will *r.* it, this is Elias.
18:5, whoso shall *r.* one such little child.
19:12, he that is able let him *r.* it.
21:22, ask, believing ye shall *r.*
Mk. 15:23, but he *r.* it not.
16:19; Acts 1:9, he was *r.* up into heaven.
Lu. 16:9, *r.* you into everlasting habitations.
18:42; Acts 22:13, *r.* thy sight.
John 1:11, his own *r.* him not.
12, to as many as *r.* him.
3:27, can *r.* nothing, except.
5:43, in his own name, he ye will *r.*
44, which *r.* honour one of another.
16:24, ask, and ye shall *r.*
20:22, *r.* ye the Holy Ghost.
Acts 7:59, *r.* my spirit.
8:17, they *r.* the Holy Ghost.
10:43, shall *r.* remission of sins.
19:2, have ye *r.* the Holy Ghost.
20:24, which I have *r.* of the Lord.

Rom. 5:11, by whom we *r.* atonement.
14:3, for God hath *r.* him.
15:7, *r.* ye one another.
1 Cor. 3:8, every man shall *r.* his own reward.
11:23, I *r.* of the Lord that which also I delivered.
2 Cor. 4:1, as we have *r.* mercy we faint not.
5:10, every one may *r.* things done.
7:2, *r.* us; we have wronged no man.
Phil. 2:29, *r.* him in the Lord.
4:15, as concerning giving and *r.*
Col. 2:6, as ye have *r.* Christ.
1 Tim. 3:16, *r.* up into glory.
4:4, if it be *r.* with thanksgiving.
1 John 3:22, whatsoever we ask we *r.*
See Ezek. 3:10 Acts 20:35; Jas. 4:3.
RECKON. Lev. 25:50, he shall *r.* with him that bought him.
Ps. 40:5, thy thoughts cannot be *r.* up.
Mat. 18:24, when he had begun to *r.*
25:19, lord of servants *r.* with them.
Rom. 4:4, reward is not *r.* of grace.
6;11, *r.* yourselves dead to sin.
8:18, I *r.* the sufferings of this present time.
See 2 Kings 22:7; Isa. 38:13; Lu. 22:37.
RECOMMENDED. Acts 14:26; 15:40.
RECOMPENCE. Deut. 32:35, to me belongeth *r.*
Job 15:31, vanity shall be his *r.*
Isa. 35:4, God will come with a *r.*
Hos. 9:7, days of *r.* are come.
Joel 3:4, will ye render me a *r.*?
Lu. 14:12, and a *r.* be made thee.
2 Cor. 6:13, for a *r.*, be ye also enlarged.
Heb. 2:2; 10:35; 11:26, just *r.* of reward.
See Prov. 12:14; Isa. 34:8; Jer. 51:56.
RECOMPENSE. Num. 5:7, he shall *r.* his trespass.
Ruth 2:12, the Lord *r.* thy work.
2 Sam. 19:36, why should the king *r.* me?
Job 34:33, he will *r.* it, whether.
Prov. 20:22, say not, I will *r.* evil.
Isa. 65:6, but will *r.*, even *r.* into their bosom.
Jer. 25:14; Hos. 12:2, will *r.* according to deeds.
Lu. 14:14, for they cannot *r.* thee.
Rom. 11:35, it shall be *r.* to him again.
12:17, *r.* to no man evil for evil.
See 2 Chron. 6:23; Jer. 32:18; Heb. 10:30.
RECONCILE. 1 Sam. 29:4, wherewith should he *r.* himself.
Ezek. 45:20, so shall ye *r.* the house.
Mat. 5:24, first be *r.* to thy brother.
Rom. 5:10, if when enemies we were *r.*
Eph. 2:16, that he might *r.* both.
See Lev. 16:20; Rom. 11:15; 2 Cor. 5:19.
RECORD. Ex. 20:24, in places where I *r.* my name.
Deut. 30:19; 31:28, I call heaven to *r.*
Job 16:19, my *r.* on high.
John 8:13, thou bearest *r.* of thyself.
Rom. 10:2, I bare them *r.*
Phil. 1:8, God is my *r.* how greatly I long.
1 John 5:7, three that bare *r.*
10, he believeth not the *r.*
11, this is the *r.*, that God hath given.
3 John 12, we bare *r.*, and our *r.* is true.
See Acts 20:26; John 1:19; Rev. 1:2.
RECOUNT. Nah. 2:5, *r.* his worthies.
RECOVER. 2 Kings 5:3, the prophet would *r.* him.
Ps. 39:13, that I may *r.* strength.
Isa. 11:11, to *r.* remnant of his people.
Hos. 2:9, and I will *r.* my wool and flax.
Mk. 16:18, lay hands on sick, and they shall *r.*
Lu. 4:18, preach *r.* of sight to blind.
See Isa. 38:16; Jer. 8:22; 41:16; 2 Tim. 2:16.
RED. Gen. 25:30, *r.* pottage.
49:12, eyes *r.* with wine.
2 Kings 3:22, water *r.* as blood.
Ps. 75:8, wine is *r.*, full of mixture.
Prov. 23:31, look not on wine when *r.*
Isa. 1:18, though your sins be *r.* like crimson.
27:2, a vineyard of *r.* wine.
63:2, *r.* in thine apparel.
Mat. 16:2, fair weather, for the sky is *r.*
See Lev. 13:19; Num. 19:2; Nah. 2:3; Rev. 6:4.
REDEEM. Gen. 48:16, angel which *r.* me.
Ex. 6:6, I will *r.* you.
15:13, people whom thou hast *r.*
Lev. 27:28, no devoted thing, shall be *r.*
2 Sam. 4:9, the Lord hath *r.* my soul.
Neh. 5:5, nor is it in our power to *r.* them.
8, after our ability have *r.* Jews.
Job 5:20, in famine he shall *r.* thee.
6:23, to *r.* me from hand of mighty.
Ps. 25:22, *r.* Israel out of all his troubles.
34:22, the Lord *r.* the soul of his servants.
44:26, *r.* us for thy mercies' sake.
49:7, none can *r.* his brother.
15, God will *r.* my soul from the grave.
72:14, he shall *r.* their soul from deceit.
107:2, let the *r.* of the Lord say so.
130:8, he shall *r.* Israel.
Isa. 1:27, Zion shall be *r.* with judgment.
35:9, the *r.* shall walk there.
44:22, return, for I have *r.* thee.
50:2, is my hand shortened, t hat it cannot *r.*
51:11, the *r.* of the Lord shall return.
52:3, *r.* without money.
63:4, the year of my *r.* is come.
Hos. 7:13, though I *r.* them, they have spoken lies.
13:14, I will *r.* them from death.
Lu. 1:68, hath visited, and *r.* his people.
24:21, he who should have *r.* Israel.
Gal. 3:13, *r.* us from curse of the law.
4:5, *r.* them that were under the law.
Tit. 2:14, that he might *r.* us from iniquity.
1 Pet. 1:18, not *r.* with corruptible things.
Rev. 5:9, thou hast *r.* us by thy blood.
See Num. 18:15; 2 Sam. 7:23; Eph. 5:16; Col. 4:5.
REDEEMER. Job 19:25, I know that my *r.* liveth.
Ps. 19:14, O Lord, my strength and my *r.*
78:35, God was their *r.*
Prov. 23:11, their *r.* is mighty.
Isa. 47:4, as for our *r.*, the Lord of hosts is his name.
49:26; 60:16, know that I am thy *R.*
59:20, the *R.* shall come to Zion.
63:16, thou art our *r.*
See Isa. 41:14; 44:6; 48:17; 54:5; Jer. 50:34.
REDEMPTION. Lev. 25:24, grant a *r.* for the land.
Ps. 49:8, the *r.* of their soul is precious.
111:9, he sent *r.* to his people.
130:7, plenteous *r.*
Jer. 32:7, the right of *r.* is thine.
Lu. 2:38, that looked for *r.* in Jerusalem.
21:28, your *r.* draweth nigh.
Rom. 8:23, the *r.* of our body.
Eph. 4:30, sealed unto the day of *r.*
See Num. 3:49; Rom. 3:24; 1 Cor. 1:30; Heb. 9:12.
REDOUND. 2 Cor. 4:15, grace might *r.*
REFORMATION. Heb. 9:10, time of *r.*
REFORMED. Lev. 26:23, if ye will not be *r.*
REFRAIN. Gen. 45:1, Joseph could not *r.* himself.
Job 7:11, I will not *r.* my mouth.
29:9, princes *r.* talking.
Ps. 40:9, I have not *r.* my lips.
119:101, *r.* my feet from every evil way.
Prov. 1:15, *r.* thy foot from their path.
10:19, he that *r.* his lips is wise.
Acts 5:38, *r.* from these men.
See Gen. 43:31; Isa. 64:12; Jer. 31:16; 1 Pet. 3:10.
REFRESH. Ex. 31:17, he rested and was *r.*
Job 32:20, I will speak that I may be *r.*
Prov. 25:13, he *r.* the soul of his masters.
Acts 3:19, times of *r.* shall come.
1 Cor. 16:18, they *r.* my spirit.
See 1 Kings 13:7; Isa. 28:12; Rom. 15:32; 2 Cor. 7:13.
REFUSE (*n.*). 1 Sam. 15:9; Lam. 3:45; Amos 8:6.
REFUSE (*v.*). Gen. 37:35, Jacob *r.* to be comforted.
Num. 22:13, the Lord *r.* to give me leave.
1 Sam. 16:7, look not on him. for I have *r.* him.

Job 6:7, things my soul *r.* to touch.
Ps. 77:2, my soul *r.* to be comforted.
78:10, they *r.* to walk in his law.
118:22, stone the builders *r.*
Prov. 1:24, I have called and ye *r.*
8:33, be wise and *r.* it not.
10:17, he that *r.* reproof.
13:18, shame to him that *r.* instruction.
15:32, he that *r.* instruction despiseth his soul.
21:25, his hands *r.* to labour.
Isa. 7:15, 16, may know to *r.* the evil.
Jer. 8:5, they *r.* to return.
9:6, they *r.* to know me.
15:18, my wound *r.* to be healed.
25:28, if they *r.* to take the cup.
38:21, if thou *r.* to go forth.
Zech. 7:11, they *r.* to hearken.
Acts 7:35, this Moses whom they *r.*
1 Tim. 4:4, nothing to be *r.*
7, *r.* profane and old wives' fables.
5:11, the younger widows *r.*
Heb. 11:24, Moses *r.* to be called.
12:25, *r.* not him that speaketh.
See Ex. 4:23; 10:3; 1 Kings 20:35; 2 Kings 5:16.

REGARD. Gen. 45:20, *r.* not your stuff.
Ex. 5:9, let them not *r.* vain words.
Deut. 10:17, that *r.* not persons.
1 Kings 18:29, neither voice, nor any that *r.*
Job 4:20, they perish without any *r.* it.
34:19, nor *r.* rich more than poor.
39:7, neither *r.* crying of the driver.
Ps. 28:5; Isa. 5:12, they *r.* not works of the Lord.
66:18, if I *r.* iniquity in my heart.
102:17, he will *r.* prayer of the destitute.
106:44, he *r.* their affliction.
Prov. 1:24, and no man *r.*
5:2, that thou mayest *r.* discretion.
6:35, he will not *r.* any ransom.
12:10, *r.* the life of his beast.
13:18; 15:5, he that *r.* reproof.
Eccl. 11:4, he that *r.* the clouds.
Lam. 4:16, the Lord will no more *r.* them.
Dan. 11:37, *r.* God of his fathers, nor *r.* any god.
Mal. 1:9, will he *r.* your persons.
Mat. 22:16; Mk. 12:14, *r.* not the person of men.
Lu. 18:2, neither *r.* man.
Rom. 14:6, he that *r.* the day, *r.* it to the Lord.
See Deut. 28:50; 2 Kings 3:14; Amos 5:22; Phil. 2:30.

REGENERATION. Mat. 19:28, in the *r.*
Tit. 3:5, by the washing of *r.*
See John 1:13; 3:3.

REGISTER. Ezra 2:62; Neh. 7:5, 64.

REHEARSE. Judg. 5:11, *r.* the righteous acts.
Acts 14:27, they *r.* all God has done.
See Ex. 17:14; 1 Sam. 8:21; 17:31; Acts 11:4.

REIGN. Gen. 37:8, shalt thou *r.* over us?
Ex. 15:18; Ps. 146:10, Lord shall *r.* for ever.
Lev. 26:17, that hate you shall *r.* over you.
Deut. 15:6, thou shalt *r.* over many nations.
Judg. 9:8, the trees said, *r.* thou over us.
1 Sam. 11:12, shall Saul *r.* over us?
12:12, nay, but a king shall *r.* over us.
2 Sam. 16:8, in whose stead thou hast *r.*
Job. 34:30, that the hypocrite *r.* not.
Ps. 47:8, God *r* over the heathen.
93:1; 96:10; 97:1; 99:1, the Lord *r.*
Prov. 8:15, by me kings *r.*
30:22, for a servant when he *r.*
Eccl. 4:14, out of prison he cometh to *r.*
Isa. 32:1, a king shall *r.* in righteousness.
52:7, that saith unto Zion, thy God *r.*
Jer. 22:15, shalt thou *r.* because thou closest?
23:5, a king shall *r.* and prosper.
Mic. 4:7, the Lord shall *r.* over them.
Lu. 19:14, not have this man to *r.* over us.
27, that would not I should *r.*
Rom. 5:14, death *r.* from Adam to Moses.
Rom. 5:17, death *r.* by one.
21, as sin hath *r.*, so might grace *r.*
6:12, let not sin *r.* in your bodies.
1 Cor. 4:8, ye have *r.* as kings without us.
15:25, for he must *r.*
2 Tim. 2:12, if we suffer we shall also *r.* with him.
Rev. 5:10, we also shall *r.* on the earth.
11:15, he shall *r.* for ever and ever.
19:6, the Lord God omnipotent *r.*
See Isa. 24:23; Luke 1:33; Rev. 20:4; 22:5.

REINS. Job 16:13, he cleaveth my *r.* asunder.
19:27, though my *r.* be consumed.
Ps. 7:9, God trieth the *r.*
16:7, my *r.* instruct me.
26:2, examine me, try my *r.*
73:21, thus I was pricked in my *r.*
139:13, thou hast possessed my *r.*
Prov. 23:16, my *r.* shall rejoice.
Isa. 11:5, faithfulness the girdle of his *r.*
Rev. 2:23, I am he who searcheth the *r.*
See Jer. 11:20; 12:2; 17:10; 20:12; Lam. 3:13.

REJECT. 1 Sam. 8:7, they have not *r.* thee, but they have *r.* me.
10:19, ye have *r.* God who saved you.
15:23, because thou hast *r.* the word of the Lord.
16:1, I have *r.* him from being king.
Isa. 53:3, despised and *r.* of men.
Jer. 2:37, the Lord hath *r.* thy confidence.
7:29, the Lord hath *r.* the generation.
8:9, they have *r.* the word of the Lord.
14:19, thou hast utterly *r.* Judah.
Lam. 5:22, thou has utterly *r.* us.
Hos. 4:6, because thou hast *r.* knowledge, I will *r.* thee
Mat. 21:42; Mk. 12:10; Lu. 20:17, the stone which builders *r.*
Mk. 7:9, full well ye *r.* the commandment.
Lu. 7:30, lawyers *r.* the counsel of God.
17:25, must first be *r.* of this generation.
Tit. 3:10, after admonition *r.*
Heb. 12:17, when he would have inherited was *r.*
See Jer. 6:19; Mk. 6:26; 8:31; Lu. 9:22; John 12:48.

REJOICE. Deut. 12:7, shall *r.* in all ye put your hand to.
16:14, thou shalt *r.* in thy feast.
26;11, thou shalt *r.* in every good thing.
28:63; 30:9, the Lord will *r.* over you.
30:9, *r.* for good as he *r.* over thy fathers.
1 Sam. 2:1, because I *r.* in thy salvation.
1 Chron. 16:10, let the heart of them *r.* that seek the Lord.
2 Chron. 6:41, let thy saints *r.* in goodness.
Job 21:12, they *r.* at sound of the organ.
31:25, if I *r.* because my wealth was great.
29, if I *r.* at destruction of him that.
39:21, the horse *r.* in his strength.
Ps. 2:11, *r.* with trembling.
5:11, let all that trust in thee *r.*
9:14, I will *r.* in thy salvation.
19:5, *r.* as a strong man to run a race.
33:21, our heart shall *r.* in him.
35:15, in mine adversity they *r.*
26, let them be ashamed that *r.* at my hurt.
38:16, hear me, lest they should *r.* over me.
51:8, bones thou hast broken may *r.*
58:10, righteous shall *r.* when he seeth.
63:7, in shadow of thy wings will I *r.*
68:3, let righteous *r.*, yea exceedingly *r.*
85:6, that thy people may *r.* in thee.
89:16, in thy name shall they *r.* all the day.
96:11, let the heavens *r.*
97:11, the Lord reigneth, let the earth *r.*
104:31, the Lord shall *r.* in his works.
107:42, the righteous shall see it and *r.*
109:28, let thy servant *r.*
149:2, let Israel *r.* in him that made him.
Prov. 2:14, who *r.* to do evil.
5:18, *r.* with the wife of thy youth.
23:15, if thine heart be wise, mine shall *r.*
24, father of the righteous shall greatly *r.*
25, she that bare thee shall *r.*
24:17, *r.* not when thine enemy falleth.

Prov. 29:2, when righteous are in authority people *r.*
31:25, she shall *r.* in time to come.
Eccl. 2:10, my heart *r.* in all my labour.
3:12, for a man to *r.* and do good.
22; 5:19, that a man should *r.* in his works.
11:9, *r.* O young man in thy youth.
Isa. 9:3, as men *r.* when they divide the spoil.
24:8, noise of them that *r.* endeth.
29:19, poor among men shall *r.*
35:1, the desert shall *r.*
62:5, as the bridegroom *r.* over the bride.
64:5, him that *r.* and worketh righteousness.
65:13, my servants shall *r.*, but ye.
66:14, when ye see this, your heart shall *r.*
Jer. 11:15, when thou doest evil, then thou *r.*
32:41, I will *r.* over them to do them good.
51:39, that they may *r.* and sleep.
Ezek. 7:12, let not buyer *r.*
Amos 6:13, which *r.* in a thing of nought.
Mic. 7:8, *r.* not against me.
Hab. 3:18, yet I will *r.* in the Lord.
Mat. 18:13, he *r.* more of that sheep.
Lu. 1:14, many shall *r.* at his birth.
6:23, *r.* ye in that day, and leap for joy.
10:20, in this *r.* not, but rather *r.* because.
21, in that hour Jesus *r.* in spirit.
15:6, 9, *r.* with me.
John 5:35, willing for a season to *r.* in his light.
8:56, Abraham *r.* to see my day.
14:28, if ye loved me, ye would *r.*
16:20, ye shall weep, but the world shall *r.*
22, I will see you again, and your heart shall *r.*
Rom. 5:2, and *r.* in hope.
12:15, *r.* with them that do *r.*
1 Cor. 7:30, they that *r.* as though they *r.* not.
13:6, *r.* not in iniquity, but *r.* in the truth.
Phil. 1:18, I therein do *r.* and will *r.*
2:16, that I may *r.* in the day of Christ.
3:1, finally, *r.* in the Lord.
4:4, *r.* in the Lord alway, and again I say *r.*
1 Thess. 5:16, *r.* evermore.
Jas. 1:9, let the brother of low degree *r.*
2:13, mercy *r.* against judgment.
1 Pet. 1:8, *r.* with joy unspeakable.
See 1 Kings 1:40; 5:7; 2 Kings 11:14; 1 Chron. 29:9.
REJOICING. Job 8:21, till he fill thy lips with *r.*
Ps. 107:22, declare his works with *r.*
118:15, voice of *r.* is in tabernacles of the righteous.
119:111, they are the *r.* of my heart.
126:6, shall doubtless come again *r.*
Prov. 8:31, *r.* in the habitable part of his earth.
Isa. 65:18, I create Jerusalem a *r.*
Jer. 15:16, thy word was to me the *r.* of my heart.
Zeph. 2:15, this is the *r.* city.
Acts 5:41, *r.* that they were counted worthy.
Rom. 12:12, *r.* in hope.
2 Cor. 6:10, as sorrowful, yet alway *r.*
1 Thess. 2:19, what is our crown of *r.*
See Hab. 3:14; Acts 8:39; Gal. 6:4; Jas. 4:16.
RELEASE. Esth. 2:18; Mat. 27:17; Mk. 15:11; John 19:10.
RELIEVE. Lev. 25:35, then thou shalt *r.* him.
Ps. 146:9, he *r.* the fatherless and widow.
Isa. 1:17, *r.* the oppressed.
Lam. 1:16, comforter that should *r.* my soul is far from me.
See Acts 11:29; 1 Tim. 5:10, 16.
RELIGION. Acts 26:5; Gal. 1:13; Jas. 1:26, 27.
RELIGIOUS. Acts 13:43; Jas. 1:26.
RELY. 2 Chron. 13:18; 16:7, 8.
REMAIN. Gen. 8:22, while earth *r.*
14:10, they that *r.* fled to the mountain.
Ex. 12:10, let nothing of it *r.* until morning.
Josh. 13:1, there *r.* yet much land to be possessed.
1 Kings 18:22, I only *r.* a prophet.
Job 21:32, yet shall he *r.* in the tomb.
Prov. 2:21, the perfect shall *r.* in the land.
Eccl. 2:9, my wisdom *r.* with me.
Jer. 17:25, this city shall *r.* for ever.
Jer. 37:10, there *r.* but wounded men.
Lam. 2:22, in day of anger none *r.*
Mat. 11:23, would have *r.* until this day.
John 6:12, gather up the fragments that *r.*
9:41, ye say, we see, therefore your sin *r.*
Acts 5:4, whiles it *r.*, was it not thine own?
1 Cor. 15:6, the greater part *r.* to this present.
1 Thess. 4:15, we which are alive and *r.* unto coming of the Lord.
Heb. 4:9, there *r.* a rest to the people of God.
10:26, there *r.* no more sacrifice for sins.
Rev. 3:2, things which *r.* ready to die.
See Ps. 76:10; Lam. 5:19; John 1:33; 1 John 3:9.
REMEDY. 2 Chron. 36:16; Prov. 6:15; 29:1.
REMEMBER. Gen. 40:23, yet did not the butler *r.*
41:9, I do *r.* my faults this day.
Ex. 13:3, *r.* this day ye came out of Egypt.
20:8, *r.* the sabbath day.
Num. 15:39, *r.* all the commandments.
Deut. 5:15; 15:15; 16:12; 24:18, 22, *r.* thou wast a servant.
8:2, *r.* all the way the Lord led thee.
32:7, *r.* the days of old.
1 Chron. 16:12, *r.* his marvellous works.
Neh. 13:14, *r.* me, O God, concerning this.
Job 7:7, O *r.* my life is wind.
11:16, *r.* it as waters that pass away.
14:13, appoint me a set time and *r.* me.
24:20, the sinner shall be no more *r.*
Ps. 9:12, when he maketh inquisition he *r.*
20:7, he will *r.* the name of the Lord.
25:6, *r.* thy mercies, they have been ever of old.
7, *r.* not sins of my youth, by mercy *r.* me.
63:6, when I *r.* thee upon my bed.
77:3, I *r.* God and was troubled.
78:39, he *r.* that they were but flesh.
79:8, *r.* not against us former iniquities.
89:47, *r.* how short my time is.
105:8, he hath *r.* his covenant for ever.
119:55, I have *r.* thy name in the night.
136:23, who *r.* us in our low estate.
137:1, we wept when we *r.* Zion.
Prov. 31:7, drink and *r.* his misery no more.
Eccl. 5:20, not much *r.* the days of his life.
11:8, let him *r.* the days of darkness.
12:1, *r.* now thy Creator.
Cant. 1:4, we will *r.* thy love.
Isa. 23:16, sing songs that thou mayest be *r.*
43:18; 46:9, *r.* ye not the former things.
57:11, thou hast not *r.* me.
65:17, the former heavens shall not be *r.*
Jer. 31:20, I do earnestly *r.* him still.
51:50, ye that have escaped *r.* the Lord.
Lam. 1:9, she *r.* not her last end.
Ezek. 16:61; 20:43; 36:31, then shalt thou *r.* thy ways.
Amos 1:9, and *r.* not the brotherly covenant.
Hab. 3:2, in wrath *r.* mercy.
Zech. 10:9, they shall *r.* me in far countries.
Mat. 26:75, Peter *r.* the word of Jesus.
Lu. 16:25, son, *r.* that thou in thy lifetime.
17:32, *r.* Lot's wife.
23:42, Lord *r.* me when thou comest.
24:8, and they *r.* his words.
John 2:22, when he was risen, they *r.*
15:20, *r.* the word I said unto you.
Acts 11:16, then *r.* I the word of the Lord.
20:35, *r.* the words of the Lord Jesus.
Gal. 2:10, that we should *r.* the poor.
Col. 4:18, *r.* my bonds.
1 Thess. 1:3, *r.* your work of faith.
Heb. 13:3, *r.* them that are in bonds.
7, *r.* them that have the rule over you.
Rev. 2:5, *r.* from whence thou art fallen.
3:3, *r.* how thou hast received.
See Ps. 88:5; 103:14; Mat. 5:23; John 16:21.
REMEMBRANCE. Num. 5:15, bringing iniquity to *r.*
2 Sam. 18:18, no son to keep my name in *r.*
1 Kings 17:18, art thou come to call my sin to *r.*

Job 18:17, his *r.* shall perish.
Ps. 6:5, in death there is no *r.* of thee.
30:4; 97:12, give thanks at *r.* of his holiness.
77:6, I call to *r.* my song in the night.
112:6, righteous shall be in everlasting *r.*
Eccl. 1:11, there is no *r.* of former things.
2:16, no *r.* of wise more than the fool.
Isa. 43:26, put me in *r.*
57:8, behind doors hast thou set up thy *r.*
Lam. 3:20, my soul hath them still in *r.*
Ezek. 23:19, calling to *r.* days of youth.
Mal. 3:16, a book of *r.*
Lu. 22:19; 1 Cor. 11:24, this do in *r.* of me.
John 14:26, bring all things to your *r.*
Acts 10:31, thine alms are had in *r.*
2 Tim. 1:3, I have *r.* of thee in my prayers.
2:14, of these things put them in *r.*
See Heb. 10:3; 2 Pet. 1:12; 3:1; Jude 5; Rev. 16:19.
REMIT. John 20:23, whose soever sins ye *r.*, are *r.*
REMNANT. Lev. 5:13, the *r.* shall be the priest's.
2 Kings 19:4; Isa. 37:4, lift up prayer for the *r.*
Ezra 9:8, grace shewed to leave us a *r.*
Isa. 1:9, unless the Lord had left a *r.*
11:11, to recover the *r.* of his people.
16:14, the *r.* shall be very small and feeble.
Jer. 44:28, *r.* shall know whose words shall stand.
Ezek. 6:8, yet will I leave a *r.*
Joel 2:32, the *r.* whom the Lord shall call.
See Mic. 2:12; Hag. 1:12; Rom. 11:5; Rev. 11:13.
REMOVE. Deut. 19:14, shall not *r.* landmark.
Job 9:5, *r.* the mountains and they know not.
14:18, the rock is *r.* out of his place.
Ps. 36:11, let not hand of wicked *r.* me.
39:10, *r.* thy stroke away from me.
46:2, not fear though the earth be *r.*
81:6, I *r.* his shoulder from burden.
103:12, so far hath he *r.* our transgressions.
119:22, *r.* from me reproach.
125:1, as mount Zion, which cannot be *r.*
Prov. 4:27, *r.* thy foot from evil.
10:30, the righteous shall never be *r.*
Eccl. 11:10, *r.* sorrow from thy heart.
Isa. 13:13, earth shall *r.* out of her place.
24:20, earth shall be *r.* out of her place.
29:13, have *r.* their heart far from me.
54:10, the hills shall be *r.*
Jer. 4:1, return unto me, then shalt thou not *r.*
Lam. 3:17, thou hast *r.* my soul from peace.
Mat. 17:20, ye shall say, *r.* hence, and it shall *r.*
Lu. 22:42, *r.* this cup from me.
Gal. 1:6, I marvel ye are so soon *r.*
Rev. 2:5, or else I will *r.* thy candlestick.
See Job 19:10; Eccl. 10:9; Ezek. 12:3; Heb. 12:27.
REND. 1 Kings 11:11, I will *r.* the kingdom.
Isa. 64:1, that thou wouldest *r.* the heavens.
Hos. 13:8, I will *r.* the caul of their heart.
Joel 2:13, *r.* your heart.
Mat. 7:6, lest they turn again and *r.* you.
See Ps. 7:2; Eccl. 3:7; Jer. 4:30; John 19:24.
RENDER. Deut. 32:41, *r.* vengeance.
1 Sam. 26:23, *r.* to every man his faithfulness.
Job 33:26, he will *r.* to man his righteousness.
34:11, the work of a man shall be *r.* to him.
Ps. 28:4, *r.* to them their desert.
38:20, they that *r.* evil for good.
79:12, and *r.* to our neighbour sevenfold.
94:2, *r.* a reward to the proud.
116:12, what shall I *r.* to the Lord.
Prov. 24:12; Rom. 2:6, *r.* to every man according.
26:16, wiser than seven men who can *r.* a reason.
Hos. 14:2, so will we *r.* the calves of our lips.
Joel. 3:4, will ye *r.* me a recompence.
Zech. 9:12, I will *r.* double.
Mat. 21:41, *r.* fruits in their seasons.
22:21; Mk. 12:17; Lu. 20:25, *r.* unto Caesar.
Rom. 13:7, *r.* to all their dues.
1 Thess. 3:9, what thanks can we *r.*
1 Thess. 5:15, see that none *r.* evil for evil.
1 Pet. 3:9, not *r.* evil for evil, or railing.
See Num. 18:9; Judg. 9:56; Ps. 62:12; Isa. 66:6.
RENEW. Job 10:17, thou *r.* thy witnesses.
29:20, my bow was *r.* in my hand.
Ps. 51:10, and *r.* a right spirit within me.
103:5, thy youth is *r.* like the eagle's
104:30, thou *r.* the face of the earth.
Isa. 40:31, wait on Lord shall *r.* strength.
41:1, let the people *r.* their strength.
Lam. 5:21, *r.* our days as of old.
2 Cor. 4:16, the inward man is *r.* day by day.
Eph. 4:23, be *r.* in spirit of your mind.
Col. 3:10, new man which is *r.* in knowledge.
Heb. 6:6, if they fall away, to *r.* them again.
See 2 Chron. 15:8; Rom. 12:2; Tit. 3:5.
RENOUNCED. 2 Cor. 4:2, have *r.* hidden things.
RENOWN. Gen. 6:4; Num. 16:2, men of *r.*
Num. 1:16, the *r.* of the congregation.
Isa. 14:20, evil doers shall never be *r.*
Ezek. 16:14, thy *r.* went forth among the heathen.
34:29, a plant of *r.*
See Ezek. 23:23; 26:17; 39:13; Dan. 9:15.
RENT. Gen. 37:33, Joseph is *r.* in pieces.
Josh. 9:4, bottles old and *r.*
Judg. 14:5, 6, *r.* lion as he would have *r.* a kid.
1 Kings 13:3, the altar shall be *r.*
Job 26:8, the cloud is not *r.* under them.
Mat. 9:16; Mk. 2:21, the *r.* is made worse.
27:51; Mk. 15:38; Lu. 23:45, veil was *r.* in twain.
See 1 Sam. 15:27; Job 1:20; 2:12; Jer. 36:24.
REPAID. Prov. 13:21, to righteous good shall be *r.*
REPAIR. 2 Chron. 24:5, gather money to *r.* the house.
Isa. 61:4, they shall *r.* the waste cities.
See 2 Kings 12:5; Ezra 9:9; Neh. 3:4; Isa. 58:12.
REPAY. Deut. 7:10, he will *r.* to his face.
Lu. 10:35, when I come I will *r.* thee.
Rom. 12:19, vengeance is mine, I will *r.*
Philem. 19, I have written it, I will *r.* it.
See Job 21:31; 41:11; Isa. 59:18.
REPEATETH. Prov. 17:9, he that *r.* a matter.
REPENT. Gen. 6:6, it *r.* the Lord.
Ex. 13:17, lest the people *r.*
32:14; 2 Sam. 24:16; 1 Chron. 21:15; Jer. 26:19, Lord *r.* of evil he thought to do.
Num. 23:19, neither son of man that he should *r.*
Deut. 32:36, Lord shall *r.* for his servants.
1 Sam. 15:29, will not *r.*, for he is not a man that he should *r.*
Job 42:6, I *r.* in dust and ashes.
Ps. 90:13, let it *r.* thee concerning thy servants.
106:45, Lord *r.* according to his mercies.
110:4; Heb. 7:21, Lord hath sworn and will not *r.*
Jer. 8:6, no man *r.* of his wickedness.
18:8; 26:13, if that nation turn I will *r.*
31:19, after that I was turned I *r.*
Joel 2:13, he is slow to anger and *r.* him.
Mat. 12:41; Lu. 11:32, they *r.* at the preaching.
21:29, afterward he *r.* and went.
27:3, Judas *r.* himself.
Lu. 13:3, except ye *r.*
15:7, joy over one sinner that *r.*
17:3, if thy brother *r.*, forgive him.
Acts 8:22, *r.* of this thy wickedness.
Rev. 2:21, space to *r.*, and she *r.*, not.
See Acts 2:38; 17:30; Rev. 2:5; 3:3; 16:9.
REPENTANCE. Hos. 13:14, *r.* shall be hid.
Mat. 3:8; Lu. 3:8; Acts 26:2, fruits meet for *r.*
Rom. 2:4, goodness of God leadeth thee to *r.*
11:29, gifts of God are without *r.*
2 Cor. 7:10, *r.* not to be repented of.
Heb. 6:1, not laying again the foundation of *r.*
6, to renew them again to *r.*
12:17, no place of *r.*, though he sought it.
See Lu. 15:7; Acts 20:21; 2 Tim. 2:25; 2 Pet. 3:9.
REPLENISH. Gen. 1:28; 9:1; Jer. 31:25; Ezek. 26:2.
REPLIEST. Rom. 9:20, that *r.* against God.

REPORT (*n*.). Gen. 37:2, their evil. *r*.
Ex. 23:1, thou shalt not *r*. a false *r*.
Num. 13:32, an evil *r*. of the land.
1 Sam. 2:24, it is no good *r*. I hear.
1 Kings 10:6; 2 Chron. 9:5, it was a true *r*. I heard.
Prov. 15:30, a good *r*. maketh the bones fat.
Isa. 28:19, a vexation only to understand *r*.
53:1, who hath believed our *r*.
Acts 6:3, men of honest *r*.
10:22, of good *r*. among the Jews.
2 Cor. 6:8, by evil *r*. and good *r*.
Phil. 4:8, whatsoever things are of good *r*.
1 Tim. 3:7, a bishop must have a good *r*.
See Deut. 2:25; Heb. 11:2, 39; 3 John 12.
REPORT (*v*.). Neh. 6:6, it is *r*. among heathen.
Jer. 20:10, *r*., say they, and we will *r*. it.
Mat. 28:15, saying is commonly *r*.
Acts 16:2, well *r*. of by the brethren.
1 Cor. 14:25, he will *r*. that God is in you.
See Ezek. 9:11; Rom. 3:8; 1 Tim. 5:10; 1 Pet. 1:12.
REPROACH (*n*.). Gen. 30:23, hath taken away my *r*.
34:14, that were a *r*. to us.
1 Sam. 11:2, lay it for a *r*. upon all Israel.
Neh. 2:17, build that we be no more a *r*.
Ps. 15:3, that taketh not up a *r*.
22:6, a *r*. of men.
31:11, I was a *r*. among mine enemies.
44:13; 79:4; 89:41, a *r*. to our neighbours.
69:9; Rom. 15:3, the *r*. of them that reproached thee.
78:66, put them to a perpetual *r*.
Prov. 6:33, his *r*. shall not be wiped away.
14:34, sin is a *r*. to any people.
18:3, with ignominy cometh *r*.
Isa. 43:28, I have given Israel to *r*.
51:7, fear not the *r*. of men.
Jer. 23:40, I will bring an everlasting *r*.
31:19, I did bear the *r*. of my youth.
Lam. 3:30, he is filled full with *r*.
Ezek. 5:14, I will make thee a *r*. among nations.
15, Jerusalem shall be a *r*. and a taunt.
Mic. 6:16, ye shall bear the *r*. of my people.
2 Cor. 11:21, I speak as concerning *r*.
12:10, pleasure in *r*. for Christ's sake.
1 Tim. 3:7, good report lest he fall into *r*.
4:10, we labour and suffer *r*.
Heb. 11:26, the *r*. of Christ greater riches.
13:13, without the camp bearing his *r*.
See Ps. 69:10; 119:39; Jer. 6:10; 20:8; 24:9.
REPROACH (*v*.). Num. 15:30, *r*. the Lord.
Ruth 2:15, *r*. her not.
2 Kings 19:22; Isa. 37:23, whom hast thou *r*.
Job 19:3, these ten times have ye *r*. me.
27:6, my heart shall not *r*. me.
Ps. 42:10, as with a sword mine enemies *r*. me.
44:16, the voice of him that *r*.
74:22, how the foolish man *r*. thee.
119:42; Prov. 27:11, to answer him that *r*. me.
Prov. 14:31; 17:5, oppresseth poor *r*. his Maker.
Lu. 6:22, men shall *r*. you for my sake.
1 Pet. 4:14, if ye be *r*. for Christ's sake.
See Ps. 55:12; 74:18; 79:12; 89:51; Zeph. 2:8.
REPROACHFULLY. Job 16:10; 1 Tim. 5:14.
REPROVE. 1 Chron. 16:21, *r*. kings for their sakes.
Job 6:25, what doth your arguing *r*.
13:10, he will *r*. you if ye accept.
22:4, will he *r*. thee for fear.
40:2, he that *r*. God let him answer it.
Ps. 50:8, I will not *r*. thee for burnt offerings.
141:5, let him *r*. me, it shall be excellent oil.
Prov. 9:8, *r*. not a scorner lest he hate thee.
15:12, a scorner loveth not one that *r*.
19:25, *r*. one that hath understanding.
29:1, he that being often *r*.
30:6, lest he *r*. thee and thou be found.
Isa. 11:4, *r*. with equity for the meek.
Jer. 2:19, thy backslidings shall *r*. thee.
John 3:20, lest his deeds should be *r*.
John 16:8, he will *r*. the world of sin.
See Lu. 3:19; Eph. 5:11, 13; 2 Tim. 4:2.
REPROVER. Prov. 25:12; Ezek. 3:26.
REPUTATION. Eccl. 10:1, him that is in *r*. for wisdom.
Acts 5:34, had in *r*. among the people.
Phil. 2:7, made himself of no *r*.
29, hold such in *r*.
See Job 18:3; Dan. 4:35; Gal. 2:2.
REQUEST, Judg. 8:24, I would desire a *r*. of thee.
Ezra 7:6, the king granted all his *r*.
Job 6:8, Oh that I might have my *r*.
Ps. 21:2, hast not withholden *r*. of his lips.
106:15, he gave them their *r*.
Phil. 1:4, in every prayer making *r*. with joy.
4:6, let your *r*. be made known.
See 2 Sam. 14:15; Neh. 2:4; Esth. 4:8; 5:3.
REQUESTED. 1 Kings 19:4, Elijah *r*. that he might die.
REQUIRE. Gen. 9:5, blood of your lives will I *r*.
31:39, of my hand didst thou *r*. it.
Deut. 10:12; Mic. 6:8, what doth the Lord *r*.
Josh. 22:23; 1 Sam. 20:16, let the Lord himself *r*. it.
Ruth 3:11, I will do all thou *r*.
1 Sam. 21:8, the king's business *r*. haste.
2 Sam. 3:13, one thing I *r*. of thee.
19:38, whatsoever thou shalt *r*. I will do.
2 Chron. 24:22, the Lord look on it and *r*. it.
Neh. 5:12, we will restore and *r*. nothing of them.
Ps. 10:13, he hath said thou wilt not *r*. it.
40:6, sin offering hast thou not *r*.
137:3, they that wasted us *r*. of us mirth.
Prov. 30:7, two things have I *r*. of thee.
Eccl. 3:15, God *r*. that which is past.
Isa. 1:12, who hath *r*. this at your hand?
Ezek. 3:18; 33:6, his blood will I *r*. at thine hand.
34:10, I will *r*. my flock at their hand.
Lu. 11:50, may be *r*. of this generation.
12:20, this night thy soul shall be *r*.
48:, of him shall much be *r*.
19:23, I might have *r*. mine own with usury.
1 Cor. 1:22, the Jews *r*. a sign.
4:2, it is *r*. in stewards.
See 2 Chron. 8:14; Ezra 3:4; Neh. 5:18; Esth. 2:15.
REQUITE. Gen. 50:15, Joseph will certainly *r*. us.
Deut. 32:6, do you thus *r*. the Lord.
Judg. 1:7, as I have done so God hath *r*. me.
2 Sam. 2:6, I also will *r*. you this kindness.
16:12, it may be the Lord will *r*. good for his.
1 Tim. 5:4, learn to *r*. their parents.
See Ps. 10:14; 41:10; Jer. 51:56.
REREWARD. Josh. 6:9; Isa. 52:12; 58:8.
RESCUE. Ps. 35:17, *r*. my soul.
Hos. 5:14, none shall *r*. him.
See Deut. 28:31; 1 Sam. 14:45; Dan. 6:27; Acts 23:27.
RESEMBLANCE. Zech. 5:6, this is their *r*.
RESEMBLE. Judg. 8:18; Lu. 13:18.
RESERVE. Gen. 27:36, hast thou not *r*. a blessing.
Ruth 2:18, gave her mother in law that she had *r*.
Job 21:30, the wicked is *r*. to day of destruction.
38:23, which I have *r*. against time of trouble.
Jer. 3:5, will he *r*. anger for ever.
5:24, he *r*. the weeks of harvest.
50:20, I will pardon them whom I *r*.
Nah. 1:2, the Lord *r*. wrath for his enemies.
1 Pet. 1:4, an inheritance *r*. in heaven.
2 Pet. 2:4, to be *r*. to judgment.
3:7, the heavens and earth are *r*. unto fire.
See Num. 18:9; Rom. 11:4; 2 Pet. 2:9; Jude 6:13.
RESIDUE. Ex. 10:5, locusts shall eat the *r*.
Isa. 38:10, I am deprived of the *r*. of my years.
Jer. 15:9, *r*. of them will I deliver to the sword.
Ezek. 9:8, wilt thou destroy all the *r*.
Zech. 8:11, I will not be to the *r*. as in former days.
Mal. 2:15, yet had he the *r*. of the Spirit.
Acts 15:17, that the *r*. might seek the Lord.
See Neh. 11:20; Jer. 8:3; 29:1; 39:3.
RESIST. Zech. 3:1, at his right hand to *r*.
Mat. 5:39, *r*. not evil.

Lu. 21:15, adversaries shall not be able to *r.*
Rom. 9:19, who hath *r.* his will.
13:2, whoso *r.* power, *r.* ordinance of God.
Jas. 4:6; 1 Pet. 5:5, God *r.* the proud.
7, *r.* the devil, and he will flee.
1 Pet. 5:9, whom *r.* stedfast in the faith.
See Acts 6:10; 7:51; 2 Tim. 3:8; Heb. 12:4.
RESORT. Neh. 4:20, *r.* hither to us.
Ps. 71:3, whereunto I may continually *r.*
John 18:2, Jesus ofttimes *r.* thither.
See Mk. 2:13; 10:1; John 18:20; Acts 16:13.
RESPECT (*n.*). Gen. 4:4, Lord had *r.* to Abel.
Ex. 2:25, God had *r.* unto them.
1 Kings 8:28; 2 Chron. 6:19, have *r.* unto their prayer.
2 Chron. 19:7; Rom. 2:11; Eph. 6:9; Col. 3:25, there is no *r.* of persons with God.
Ps. 74:20, have *r.* unto thy covenant.
119:15, I will have *r.* unto thy ways.
138:6, yet hath he *r.* to the lowly.
Prov. 24:23; 28:31, not good to have *r.* of persons.
Isa. 17:7, his eyes shall have *r.* to Holy One.
22:11, nor had *r.* to him that fashioned it.
Phil. 4:11, not that I speak in *r.* of want.
See Heb. 11:26; Jas. 2:1, 3, 9; 1 Pet. 1:17.
RESPECT (*v.*). Lev. 19:15, shalt not *r.* person of poor.
Deut. 1:17, ye shall not *r.* persons in judgment.
Job 37:24, he *r.* not any that are wise of heart.
See Num. 16:15; 2 Sam. 14:14; Ps. 40:4; Lam. 4:16.
RESPITE. Ex. 8:15; 1 Sam. 11:3.
REST (*n.*). Gen. 49:15, Issachar saw that *r.* was good.
Ex. 31:15; 35:2; Lev. 16:31; 23:3, 32; 25:4, the sabbath of *r.*
33:14, my presence shall go with thee, and I will give thee *r.*
Lev. 25:5, a year of *r.* to the land.
Deut. 12:10, when he giveth you *r.* from your enemies.
Judg. 3:30, the land had *r.* fourscore years.
Ruth 3:1, shall not I seek *r.* for thee.
1 Chron. 22:9, a man of *r.*, and I will give him *r.*
18, hath he not given you *r.* on every side.
28:2, to build a house of *r.*
Neh. 9:28, after they had *r.* they did evil.
Esth. 9:16, the Jews had *r.* from their enemies.
Job 3:17, there the weary be at *r.*
11:18, thou shalt take thy *r.* in safety.
17:16, when our *r.* together is in the dust.
Ps. 55:6, then would I fly away and be at *r.*
95:11; Heb. 3:11, not enter into my *r.*
116:7, return to thy *r.*, O my soul.
132:8, arise into thy *r.*
14, this is my *r.* for ever.
Eccl. 2:23, his heart taketh not *r.* in the night.
Isa. 11:10, his *r.* shall be glorious.
14:7; Zech. 1:11, earth is at *r.* and quiet.
18:4, I will take my *r.*
30:15, in returning and *r.* shall ye be saved.
66:1, where is the place of my *r.*?
Jer. 6:16, ye shall find *r.* for your souls.
Ezek. 38:11, I will go to them that are at *r.*
Mic. 2:10, depart, this is not your *r.*
Mat. 11:28, I will give you *r.*
29, ye shall find *r.* to your souls.
12:43; Lu. 11:24, seeking *r.* and finding none.
26:45; Mk. 14:41, sleep on and take your *r.*
John 11:13, of taking *r.* in sleep.
Acts 9:31, then had the churches *r.*
See Prov. 29:17; Eccl. 6:5; Dan. 4:4; 2 Thess. 1:7.
REST (*v.*). Gen. 2:2, he *r.* on seventh day.
Num. 11:25, when the Spirit *r.* upon them.
2 Chron. 32:8, people *r.* on the words.
Job 3:18, there the prisoners *r.* together.
Ps. 16:9; Acts 2:26, my flesh shall *r.* in hope.
37:7, *r.* in the Lord.
Eccl. 7:9, anger *r.* in bosom of fools.
Isa. 11:2, the spirit of the Lord shall *r.* upon him.
28:12, ye may cause the weary to *r.*
57:20, like the sea when it cannot *r.*
62:1, for Jerusalem's sake I will not *r.*
Isa. 63:14, Spirit of the Lord caused him to *r.*
Jer. 47:6, *r.* and be still.
Dan. 12:13, thou shalt *r.* and stand in thy lot.
Mk. 6:31, come and *r.* awhile.
2 Cor. 12:9, power of Christ may *r.* on me.
Rev. 4:8, they *r.* not day and night.
6:11, *r.* yet for a little season.
14:13, that they may *r.* from their labours.
See Prov. 14:33; Cant. 1:7; Isa. 32:18; Lu. 10:6.
RESTORE. Ex. 22:4, he shall *r.* double.
Lev. 6:4, he shall *r.* that he took away.
Deut. 22:2, things strayed thou shalt *r.* again.
Ps. 23:3, he *r.* my soul.
51:12, *r.* to me the joy of thy salvation.
69:4, I *r.* that which I took not away.
Isa. 1:26, I will *r.* thy judges as at the first.
Jer. 27:22, I will *r.* them to this place.
30:17, I will *r.* health to thee.
Ezek. 33:15, if wicked *r.* pledge.
Mat. 17:11; Mk. 9:12, Elias shall *r.* all things.
Lu. 19:8, I *r.* him fourfold.
Acts 1:6, wilt thou at this time *r.* the kingdom.
Gal. 6:1, *r.* such an one in meekness.
See Ruth 4:15; Isa. 58:12; Joel 2:25; Mk. 8:25.
RESTRAIN. Gen. 11:6, nothing will be *r.*
Ex. 36:6, people were *r.* from bringing.
1 Sam. 3:13, his sons made themselves vile, and he *r.* them not.
Job 15:4, thou *r.* prayer before God.
8, dost thou *r.* wisdom to thyself.
Ps. 76:10, remainder of wrath shalt thou *r.*
See Gen. 8:2; Isa. 63:15; Ezek. 31:15; Acts 14:18.
RESTRAIN. Job 2:9, dost thou still *r.* integrity.
Prov. 3:18, happy is every one that *r.* her.
4:4, let thine heart *r.* my words.
11:16, a gracious woman *r.* honour.
Eccl. 8:8, no man hath power to *r.* the spirit.
John 20:23, whose soever sins ye *r.* they are *r.*
See Mic. 7:18; Rom. 1:28; Philem. 13.
RETIRE. Judg. 20:39; 2 Sam. 11:15; Jer. 4:6.
RETURN. Gen. 3:19, to dust shalt thou *r.*
Ex. 14:27, the sea *r.* to his strength.
Judg. 7:3, whosoever is fearful, let him *r.*
Ruth 1:16, entreat me not to leave thee or *r.*
2 Sam. 12:23, he shall not *r.* to me.
2 Kings 20:10, let the shadow *r.* backward.
Job 1:21, naked shall I *r.* thither.
7:10, he shall *r.* no more.
10:21; 16:22, I go whence I shall not *r.*
15:22, he believeth not he shall *r.* out of darkness.
33:25, he shall *r.* to the days of his youth.
Ps. 35:13, my prayer *r.* into mine own bosom.
73:10, his people *r.* hither.
90:3, thou sayest, *r.*, ye children of men.
104:29, they die and *r.* to their dust.
116:7, *r.* to thy rest, O my soul.
Prov. 2:19, none that go to her *r.* again.
26:11, as a dog *r.* to his vomit.
27, he that rolleth a stone, it will *r.*
Eccl. 1:7, whence rivers come, thither they *r.* again.
5:15, naked shall he *r.* to go as he came.
12:2, nor the clouds *r.* after the rain.
7, dust *r.* to earth and spirit *r.* to God.
Isa. 21:12, if ye will enquire, enquire ye; *r.*, come.
35:10; 51:11, the ransomed of the Lord shall *r.*
44:22, *r.* unto me, for I have redeemed thee.
45:23, word is gone out and shall not *r.*
55:11, it shall not *r.* to me void.
Jer. 4:1, if thou wilt *r.*, saith the Lord, *r.* unto me.
15:19, let them *r.* unto thee, but *r.* not thou.
24:7, they shall *r.* with whole heart.
31:8, a great company shall *r.* thither.
36:3, *r.* every man from his evil way.
Ezek. 46:9, he shall not *r.* by the way he came.
Hos. 2:7, I will *r.* to my first husband.
5:15, I will *r.* to my place.
7:16, they *r.*, but not to the most High.

Hos. 14:7, they that dwell under his shadow shall *r.*
Amos 4:6, yet have ye not *r.* to me.
Joel 2:14, who knoweth if he will *r.* and repent.
Zech. 1:16, I am *r.* to Jerusalem with mercies.
8:3, I am *r.* to Zion and will dwell.
Mal. 3:7, *r.* to me and I will *r.* to you.
18, then shall ye *r.* and discern.
Mat. 12:44; Lu. 11:24, I will *r.* into my house.
24:18, neither let him in the field *r.* back.
Lu. 9:10, apostles *r.* and told him all.
10:17, the seventy *r.* with joy.
12:36, when he will *r.* from wedding.
17:18, not found that *r.* to give glory.
Acts 13:34, now no more to *r.* to corruption.
Heb. 11:15, might have had opportunity to *r.*
1 Pet. 2:25, now *r.* to the Shepherd of your souls.
See Gen. 31:3; Ex. 4:18; Lev. 25:10; Isa. 55:7.
REVEAL. Deut. 29:29, things *r.* belong unto us and to our children.
1 Sam. 3:7, nor was word of Lord *r.* to him.
Job 20:27, the heaven shall *r.* his iniquity.
Prov. 11:13; 20:19, a talebearer *r.* secrets.
Isa. 22:14, it was *r.* in mine ears.
40:5, glory of the Lord shall be *r.*
53:1; John 12:38, to whom is arm of Lord *r.*
56:1, my righteousness is near to be *r.*
Jer. 11:20, unto thee have I *r.* my cause.
33:6, I will *r.* abundance of peace.
Dan. 2:22, he *r.* deep and secret things.
28, there is a God that *r.* secrets.
Amos 3:7, he *r.* his secrets to the prophets.
Mat. 10:26; Lu. 12:2, nothing covered that shall not be *r.*
11:25, hast *r.* them unto babes.
16:17, flesh and blood hath not *r.* it.
Lu. 2:35, that thoughts of many hearts may be *r.*
17:30, in day when Son of man is *r.*
Rom. 1:17, righteousness of God *r.*
18, wrath of God is *r.* from heaven.
8:18, glory which shall be *r.* in us.
1 Cor. 2:10, God hath *r.* them by his Spirit.
3:13, it shall be *r.* by fire.
14:30, if anything be *r.* to another.
Gal. 1:16, to *r.* his Son in me.
2 Thess. 1:7, when Lord Jesus shall be *r.*
2:3, man of sin be *r.*
8, that wicked one be *r.*
1 Pet. 1:5, ready to be *r.* in last time.
4:13, when his glory shall be *r.*
5:1, partaker of glory that shall be *r.*
See Eph. 3:5; Phil. 3:15; 2 Thess. 2:6.
REVELATION. Rom. 2:5, *r.* of righteous judgment.
16:25, *r.* of the mystery.
1 Cor. 14:26, every one hath a *r.*
2 Cor. 12:1, to visions and *r.*
See Gal. 2:2; Eph. 1:17; 3:3; 1 Pet. 1:13; Rev. 1:1.
REVELLINGS. Gal. 5:21; 1 Pet. 4:3.
REVENGE. Jer. 15:15, O Lord, *r.* me.
20:10, we shall take our *r.* on him.
Nah. 1:2, the Lord *r.* and is furious.
2 Cor. 7:11, what *r.* it wrought in you.
10:6, in readiness to *r.*
See Ps. 79:10; Ezek. 25:12; Rom. 13:4.
REVENUE. Prov. 8:19, my *r.* better than silver.
16:8, better than great *r.* without right.
Jer. 12:13, ashamed of your *r.*
See Ezra 4:13; Prov. 15:6; Isa. 23:3; Jer. 12:13.
REVERENCE. Ps. 89:7; Mat. 21:37; Mk. 12:6; Heb. 12:9.
REVEREND. Ps. 111:9, holy and *r.* is his name.
REVERSE. Num. 23:20; Esth. 8:5, 8.
REVILE. Isa. 51:7, neither be afraid of *r.*
Mat. 27:39, they that passed by *r.* him.
Mk. 15:32, they that were crucified *r.* him.
1 Cor. 4:12, being *r.* we bless.
1 Pet. 2:23, when he was *r.*, *r.* not again.
See Ex. 22:28; Mat. 5:11; John 9:28; Acts 23:4.
REVIVE. Neh. 4:2, will they *r.* the stones.
Ps. 85:6, wilt thou not *r.* us.
Ps. 138:7, thou wilt *r.* me.
Isa. 57:15, to *r.* spirit of the humble.
Hos. 6:2, after two days will he *r.* us.
14:7, they shall *r.* as corn.
Hab. 3:2, *r.* thy work in midst of years.
Rom. 7:9, when commandment came sin *r.*
14:9, Christ both died, rose, and *r.*
See Gen. 45:27; 2 Kings 13:21; Ezra 9:8.
REVOLT. Isa. 1:5; 31:6; 59:13; Jer. 5:23.
REWARD (*n.*). Gen. 15:1, thy exceeding great *r.*
Num. 22:7, *r.* of divination in their hand.
Deut. 10:17, God who taketh not *r.*
Ruth 2:12, full *r.* be given thee of the Lord.
2 Sam. 4:10, thought I would have given *r.*
Job 6:22, did I say, give a *r.*
7:2, as an hireling looketh for *r.*
Ps. 19:11, in keeping them there is great *r.*
58:11, there is a *r.* for the righteous.
91:8, thou shalt see the *r.* of the wicked.
127:3, fruit of womb is his *r.*
Prov. 11:18, soweth righteousness a sure *r.*
21:14, a *r.* in the bosom.
24:20, no *r.* to the evil. man.
Eccl. 4:9, they have a good *r.* for labour.
9:5, neither have they any more a *r.*
Isa. 1:23, every one followeth after *r.*
5:23, justify wicked for *r.*
40:10; 62:11, his *r.* is with him.
Ezek. 16:34, thou givest *r.*, and no *r.* is given thee.
Dan. 5:17, give thy *r.* to another.
Hos. 9:1, thou hast loved a *r.*
Mic. 3:11, the heads thereof judge for *r.*
7:3, judge asketh for a *r.*
Mat. 5:12; Lu. 6:23, great is your *r.* in heaven.
46, what *r.* have ye.
6:1, ye have no *r.* of your father.
2, 5, 16, they have their *r.*
10:41, a prophet's *r.*, a righteous man's *r.*
42; Mk. 9:41, in no wise lose *r.*
Lu. 6:35, do good and your *r.* shall be great.
23:41, we receive due *r.* of our deeds.
Acts 1:18, purchased with *r.* of iniquity.
Rom. 4:4, the *r.* is not reckoned.
1 Cor. 3:8, every man shall receive his own *r.*
9:18, what is my *r.* then.
Col. 2:18, let no man beguile you of your *r.*
3:24, the *r.* of the inheritance.
1 Tim. 5:18, labourer worthy of his *r.*
Heb. 2:2; 10:35; 11:26, recompence of *r.*
2 Pet. 2:13, the *r.* of unrighteousness.
See 2 John 8; Jude 11; Rev. 11:18; 22:12.
REWARD (*v.*). Gen. 44:4, wherefore have ye *r.*
Deut. 32:41, I will *r.* them that hate me.
1 Sam. 24:17, thou hast *r.* me good.
2 Chron. 15:7, be strong, and your work shall be *r.*
20:11, behold how they *r.* us.
Job 21:19, he *r.* him and he shall know it.
Ps. 31:23, plentifully *r.* the proud doer.
35:12; 109:5, they *r.* me evil for good.
103:10, nor *r.* us according to our iniquities.
137:8, happy is he that *r.* thee.
Prov. 17:13, whoso *r.* evil, evil shall not depart.
25:22, heap coals, and the Lord shall *r.* thee.
26:10, both *r.* the fool and *r.* transgressors.
Jer. 31:16, thy work shall be *r.*
See 2 Sam. 22:21; Mat. 6:4; 16:27; 2 Tim. 4:14.
RICH. Gen. 13:2, Abram was very *r.*
14:23, lest thou shouldest say, I have made Abram *r.*
Ex. 30:15, the *r.* shall not give more.
Josh. 22:8, return with much *r.* to your tents.
Ruth 3:10, followedst not poor or *r.*
1 Sam. 2:7, the Lord maketh poor and *r.*
1 Kings 3:11; 2 Chron. 1:11, neither hast asked *r.*
13, I have given thee both *r.* and honour.
10:23; 2 Chron. 9:22, Solomon exceeded all for *r.*
1 Chron. 29:12, both *r.* and honour come of thee.
Job 15:29, he shall not be *r.*

Job 20:15, he swallowed down *r.*
27:19, *r.* man shall lie down, but shall not be gathered.
36:19, will he esteem thy *r.*
Ps. 37:16, better than *r.* of many wicked.
39:6, he heapeth up *r.*
45:12, the *r.* shall entreat thy favour.
49:16, be not afraid when one is made *r.*
52:7, trusted in abundance of *r.*
62:10, if *r.* increase set not your heart.
73:12, the ungodly increase in *r.*
104:24, the earth is full of thy *r.*
112:3, wealth and *r.* shall be in his house.
Prov. 3:16, in left hand *r.* and honour.
8:18, *r.* and honour are with me.
10:4, hand of diligent maketh *r.*
22, blessing of the Lord maketh *r.*
11:4, *r.* profit not in day of wrath.
13:7, poor yet hath great *r.*
18:23, the *r.* answereth roughly.
21:17, he that loveth wine shall not be *r.*
23:5, *r.* make themselves wings.
28:11, *r.* man is wise in his own conceit.
30:8, give me neither poverty nor *r.*
Eccl. 5:13, *r.* kept for owners to their hurt.
10:20, curse not *r.* in thy bedchamber.
Isa. 45:3, I will give thee hidden *r.*
53:9, with the *r.* in his death.
Jer. 9:23, let not *r.* man glory in his *r.*
17:11, getteth *r.* and not by right.
Ezek. 28:5, heart lifted up because of *r.*
Hos. 12:8, Ephraim said, I am become *r.*
Zech. 11:5, blessed be the Lord, for I am *r.*
Mat. 13:22; Mk. 4:19; Lu. 8:14, deceitfulness of *r.*
Mk. 10:23, hardly shall they that have *r.*
12:41, *r.* cast in much.
Lu. 1:53, *r.* he hath sent empty away.
6:24, woe to you *r.* for ye have received.
12:21, not *r.* toward God.
14:12, call not thy *r.* neighbours.
18:23, sorrowful, for he was very *r.*
Rom. 2:4, the *r.* of his goodness.
9:23, make known the *r.* of his glory.
10:12, the Lord is *r.* to all that call.
11:12, fall of them the *r.* of the world.
33, the depth of the *r.* of the wisdom.
1 Cor. 4:8, now ye are full, now ye are *r.*
2 Cor. 6:10, poor, yet making many *r.*
8:9, *r.*, yet for your sakes.
Eph. 1:7, redemption according to the *r.* of grace.
2:4, God, who is *r.* in mercy.
7, that he might show the exceeding *r.* of grace.
3:8, unsearchable *r.* of Christ.
Phil. 4:19, according to his *r.* in glory by Christ.
Col. 1:27, *r.* of the glory of this mystery.
2:2, the *r.* of the full assurance.
1 Tim. 6:9, they that will be *r.* fall into temptation.
17, nor trust in uncertain *r.*
18, do good and be *r.* in good works.
Heb. 11:26, reproach of Christ greater *r.*
Jas. 1:10, let *r.* rejoice that he is made low.
2:5, hath not God chosen the poor, *r.* in faith.
5:2, your *r.* are corrupted.
Rev. 2:9, but thou art *r.*
3:17, because thou sayest, I am *r.*
18, buy of me gold that thou mayest be *r.*
5:12, worthy is the Lamb to receive *r.*
See Lev. 25:47; Jas. 1:11; 2:6; 5:1; Rev. 6:15.
RICHLY. Col. 3:16; 1 Tim. 6:17.
RIDDANCE. Lev. 23:22; Zeph. 1:18.
RIDDLE. Judg. 14:12; Ezek. 17:2.
RIDE. Deut. 32:13, *r.* on high places of the earth.
33:26, who *r.* upon the heaven.
Judg. 5:10, ye that *r.* on white asses.
2 Kings 4:24, slack not thy *r.* for me.
Job 30:22, causest me to *r.* upon the wind.
Ps. 45:4, in thy majesty *r.* prosperously.
66:12, hast caused men to *r.* over our heads.
Ps. 68:4, 33, extol him that *r.* on the heavens.
Isa. 19:1, the Lord *r.* on a swift could.
See Hos. 14:3; Amos 2:15; Hab. 3:8; Hag. 2:22.
RIDER. Gen. 49:17; Ex. 15:1; Job 39:18; Zech. 10:5.
RIDGES. Ps. 65:10, waterest the *r.* thereof.
RIGHT (*n.*). Gen. 18:25, shall not Judge of all do *r.*?
Deut. 6:18; 12:25; 21:9, shalt do that is *r.*
21:17, the *r.* of the firstborn is his.
2 Sam. 19:28, what *r.* have I to cry to the king.
Neh. 2:20, ye have no *r.* in Jerusalem.
Job 34:6, should I lie against my *r.*
36:6, he giveth *r.* to the poor.
Ps. 9:4, thou maintainest my *r.*
17:1, hear the *r.*, O Lord.
140:12, Lord will maintain *r.* of the poor.
Prov. 16:8, great revenues without *r.*
Jer. 17:11, that getteth riches and not by *r.*
Ezek. 21:27, till he come whose *r.* it is.
See Amos 5:12; Mal. 3:5; Heb. 13:10.
RIGHT (*adj.*). Gen. 24:48, the Lord led me in *r.* way.
Deut. 32:4, God of truth, just and *r.* is he.
1 Sam. 12:23, I will teach you the good and *r.* way.
2 Sam. 15:3, thy matters are good and *r.*
Neh. 9:13, thou gavest them *r.* judgments.
Job 6:25, how forcible are *r.* words.
34:23, he will not lay on man more than *r.*
Ps. 19:8, the statutes of the Lord are *r.*
45:6, sceptre is a *r.* sceptre.
51:10, renew a *r.* spirit within me.
107:7, he led them forth by the *r.* way.
119:75, thy judgments are *r.*
Prov. 4:11, I have led thee in *r.* paths.
8:6, opening of my lips shall be *r.* things.
12:5, thoughts of the righteous are *r.*
15:, way of a fool is *r.* in his own eyes.
14:12; 16:25, there is a way that seemeth *r.*
21:2, every way of man is *r.* in his own eyes.
24:26, kiss his lips that giveth a *r.* answer.
Isa. 30:10, prophesy not *r.* things.
Jer. 2:21, planted wholly a *r.* seed.
Ezek. 18:5, if a man do that which is *r.*
19; 21:27; 33:14, that which is lawful and *r.*
Hos. 14:9, the ways of the Lord are *r.*
Amos 3:10, they know not how to do *r.*
Mat. 20:4, whatsoever is *r.* I will give you.
Mk. 5:15; Lu. 8:35, in his *r.* mind.
Lu. 10:28, thou hast answered *r.*
Eph. 6:1, obey your parents, this is *r.*
See Judg. 17:6; Lu. 12:57; Acts 8:21; 2 Pet. 2:15.
RIGHTEOUS. Gen. 7:1, thee have I seen *r.* before me.
18:23, wilt thou destroy *r.* with wicked.
20:4, wilt thou slay also a *r.* nation?
38:26, she hath been more *r.* than I.
Ex. 23:8, gift perverteth words of the *r.*
Num. 23:10, let me die the death of the *r.*
Deut. 25:1; 2 Chron. 6:23, they shall justify the *r.*
1 Sam. 24:17, thou art more *r.* than I.
1 Kings 2:32, two men more *r.* than he.
Job 4:7, where were the *r.* cut off.
9:15, though I were *r.* yet would I not answer.
15:14, what is man that he should be *r.*
17:9, *r.* shall hold on his way.
22:3, is it any pleasure that thou art *r.*
23:7, there the *r.* might dispute with him.
34:5, Job hath said, I am *r.*
Ps. 1:5, the congregation of the *r.*
6, the Lord knoweth the way of the *r.*
7:9, the *r.* God trieth the hearts.
11:3, what can the *r.* do.
34:17, the *r.* cry, and the Lord heareth them.
19, many are the afflictions of the *r.*
37:16, a little that a *r.* man hath.
21, the *r.* showeth mercy and giveth.
25, have not seen the *r.* forsaken.
29, the *r.* shall inherit the land.
30, mouth of *r.* speaketh wisdom.
39, salvation of *r.* is of the Lord.

Acts 13:10, thou enemy of all *r.*
24:25, as he reasoned of *r.*
Rom. 1:17; 3:5; 10:3, the *r.* of God.
4:6, to whom God imputeth *r.*
11, seal of the *r.* of faith.
5:17, which receive the gift of *r.*
18, by the *r.* of one.
21, so might grace reign through *r.*
6:13, yield your members as instruments of *r.*
20, ye were free from *r.*
8:10, the Spirit is life, because of *r.*
9:30, the *r.* which is of faith.
10:3, going about to establish their own *r.*
4, Christ is the end of the law for *r.*
10, with the heart man believeth unto *r.*
14:17, kingdom of God not meat and drink, but *r.*
1 Cor. 1:30, Christ is made unto us *r.*
15:34, awake to *r.*
2 Cor. 5:21, that we might be made the *r.*
6:7, the armour of *r.*
14, what fellowship hath *r.*
Gal. 2:21, if *r.* come by the law.
5:5, we wait for the hope of *r.*
Eph. 6:14, the breastplate of *r.*
Phil. 1:11, filled with the fruits of *r.*
3:6, touching the *r.* in the law, blameless.
9, not having mine own *r.*, but the *r.* of God.
1 Tim. 6:11, follow after *r.*
2 Tim. 3:16, for instruction in *r.*
4:8, laid up for me a crown of *r.*
Tit. 3:5, not by works of *r.*
Heb. 1:8, a sceptre of *r.*
5:13, unskilful in the word of *r.*
7:2, by interpretation, King of *r.*
11:7, heir of the *r.* which is by faith.
33, through faith wrought *r.*
12:11, the peaceable fruit of *r.*
Jas. 1:20, wrath of man worketh not *r.* of God.
3:18, the fruit of *r.* is sown in peace.
1 Pet. 2:24, dead to sins should live unto *r.*
2 Pet. 2:5, a preacher of *r.*
21, better not to have known way of *r.*
3:13, new earth, wherein dwelleth *r.*
1 John 2:29, every one that doeth *r.*
See Isa. 54:14; 63:1; Zech. 8:8; Rev. 19:8.
RIGHTLY. Gen. 27:36; Lu. 7:43; 20:21; 2 Tim. 2:15.
RIGOUR. Ex. 1:13, 14; Lev. 25:43, 46, 53.
RINGLEADER. Acts 24:5, a *r.* of the sect of the Nazarenes.
RIOT. Rom. 13:13; Tit. 1:6; 1 Pet. 4:4; 2 Pet. 2:13.
RIPE. Gen. 40:10, brought forth *r.* grapes.
Ex. 22:29, offer the first of thy *r.* fruits.
Num. 18:13, whatsoever is first *r.* be thine.
Joel 3:13, put in sickle, for the harvest is *r.*
Mic. 7:1, my soul desired the first-*r* fruit.
Rev. 14:5, time to reap, for harvest of earth is *r.*
See Num. 13:20; Jer. 24:2; Hos. 9:10; Nah. 3:12.
RISE. Gen. 19:2, ye shall *r.* up early.
23, the sun was *r.* when Lot entered Zoar.
Num. 24:17, a sceptre shall *r.* out of Israel.
32:14, ye are *r.* up in your fathers' stead.
Job 9:7, commandeth the sun and it *r.* not.
14:12, man lieth down and *r.* not.
24:22, he *r.* up, and no man is sure of life.
31:14, what shall I do when God *r.* up.
Ps. 27:3, though war should *r.* up against me.
119:62, at midnight I will *r.* to give thanks.
127:2, it is vain to *r.* up early.
Prov. 31:15, she *r* up while it is yet night.
28, her children *r.* up and call her blessed.
Eccl. 12:4, he shall *r.* at the voice of the bird.
Isa. 33:10, now will I *r.*, saith the Lord.
58:10, then shall thy light *r.* in obscurity.
60:1, the glory of the Lord is *r.* upon thee.
Jer. 7:13; 25:3; 35:14, I spake unto you, *r.* up early.
25; 25:4; 26:5; 29:19; 35:15; 44:4, I sent my servants, *r.* early.
11:7, *r.* early and protesting.
25:27, fall and *r.* no more.
Lam. 3:63, sitting down and *r.* up, I am their music.
Mat. 5:45, maketh sun to *r.* on evil and good.
17:9; Mk. 9:9, until Son of man be *r.*
20:19; Mk. 9:31; 10:34; Lu. 18:33; 24:7, the third day he shall *r.* again.
26:32; Mk. 14:28, after I am *r.* I will go before you.
46, *r.*, let us be going.
Mk. 4:27, should sleep, and *r.* night and day.
9:10, what the *r.* from dead should mean.
10:49, *r.*, he calleth thee.
Lu. 2:34, this child is set for the fall and *r.*
11:7, I cannot *r.* and give thee.
22:46, why sleep ye, *r.* and pray.
24:34, the Lord is *r.* indeed.
John 11:23, thy brother shall *r.* again.
Acts 10:13, *r.*, Peter, kill and eat.
26:16, *r.*, and stand upon thy feet.
23, the first that should *r.* from the dead.
Rom. 8:34, that died, yea rather that is *r.*
1 Cor. 15:15, if so be the dead *r.* not.
20, but now is Christ *r.*
Col. 3:1, if ye than be *r.* with Christ.
1 Thess. 4:16, the dead in Christ shall *r.* first.
See Prov. 30:31; Isa. 60:3; Mk. 16:2; Col. 2:12.
RITES. Num. 9:3, according to all the *r.* of it.
RIVER. Ex. 7:19; 8:5, stretch out hand on *r.*
2 Sam. 17:13, that city, and we will draw it into the *r.*
2 Kings 5:12, are the *r.* of Damascus better.
Job 20:17, ye shall not see the *r.* of honey.
28:10, he cutteth out *r.* among the rocks.
29:6, the rock poured out *r.* of oil.
40:23, he drinketh up a *r.*, and hasteth not.
Ps. 1:3, tree planted by the *r.*
36:8, the *r.* of thy pleasures.
46:4, *r.*, the streams whereof make glad.
65:9, enrichest it with *r.* of God.
107:33, turneth *r.* into a wilderness.
119:136, *r.* of waters run down mine eyes.
137:1, by the *r.* of Babylon we sat.
Eccl. 1:7, all the *r.* run into the sea.
Isa. 32:2, shall be as *r.* of water in a dry place.
43:2, through the *r.*, they shall not overflow.
19, I will make *r.* in the desert.
48:18, then had thy peace been as a *r.*
66:12, I will extend peace like a *r.*
Lam. 2:18, let tears run down like *r.*
Mic. 6:7, be pleased with *r.* of oil.
John 7:38, shall flow *r.* of living water.
Rev. 22:1, a pure *r.* of water of life.
See Gen. 41:1; Ex. 1:22; Ezek. 47:9; Mk. 1:5.
ROAD. 1 Sam. 27:10, whither have ye made a *r.*
ROAR. 1 Chron. 16:32; Ps. 96:11; 98:7, let the sea *r.*
Job 3:24, my *r.* are poured out.
Ps. 46:3, will not fear, though waters *r.*
104:21, young lions *r.* after their prey.
Prov. 19:12; 20:2, king's wrath as the *r.* of a lion.
Isa. 59:11, we *r.* like bears.
Jer. 6:23, their *r.* like the sea.
25:30, the Lord shall *r.* from on high.
Hos. 11:10, he shall *r.* like a lion.
Joel 3:16; Amos 1:2, the Lord shall *r.* out of Zion.
Amos 3:4, will a lion *r.* when he hath no prey?
See Ps. 22:1; 32:3; Zech. 11:3; Rev. 10:3.
ROARING. Prov. 28:15, as a *r.* lion, is a wicked ruler.
Lu. 21:25, distress, the sea and waves *r.*
1 Pet. 5:8, the devil as a *r.* lion.
See Ps. 22:13; Isa. 31:4; Ezek. 22:25; Zeph. 3:3.
ROAST. Ex. 12:9, not raw, but *r.* with fire.
Prov. 12:27, slothful man *r.* not that he took.
Isa. 44:16, he *r.* *r.*, and is satisfied.
See Deut. 16:7; 1 Sam. 2:15; 2 Chron. 35:13.
ROB. Prov. 22:22, *r.* not the poor.
Isa. 10:2, that they may *r.* the fatherless.
13, I have *r.* their treasures.
42:22, this is a people *r.* and spoiled.
Ezek. 33:15, if he give again that he had *r.*
Mal. 3:8, ye have *r.* me.

ROUGH. Isa. 27:8, stayeth his *r.* wind.
40:4; Lu. 3:5, *r.* places made plain.
Zech. 13:4, wear a *r.* garment to deceive.
See Deut. 21:4; Jer. 51:27; Dan. 8:21.
ROUGHLY. Gen. 42:7, Joseph spake *r.*
Prov. 18:23, the rich answereth *r.*
See 1 Sam. 20:10; 1 Kings 12:13; 2 Chron. 10:13.
ROUND. Ex. 16:14; Isa. 3:18; Lu. 19:43.
ROWED. Jonah 1:13; Mk. 6:48; John 6:19.
ROYAL. Gen. 49:20, yield *r.* dainties.
Esth. 1:7, *r.* wine in abundance.
5:1; 6:8; 8:15; Acts 12:21, *r.* apparel.
Jas. 2:8, fulfil the *r.* law.
1 Pet. 2:9, a *r.* priesthood.
See 1 Chron. 29:25; Isa. 62:3; Jer. 43:10.
RUBIES. Job 28:18; Prov. 8:11; 31:10.
RUDDY. 1 Sam. 16:12; Cant. 5:10; Lam. 4:7.
RUDE. 2 Cor. 11:6, *r.* in speech.
RUDIMENTS. Col. 2:8, 20, *r.* of the world.
RUIN. 2 Chron. 28:23, they were the *r.* of him.
Ps. 89:40, hast brought his strong holds to *r.*
Prov. 24:22, who knoweth the *r.* of both.
26:28, a flattering mouth worketh *r.*
Ezek. 18:30, so iniquity shall not be your *r.*
21:15, that their *r.* may be multiplied.
Lu. 6:49, the *r.* of that house was great.
See Isa. 3:8; Ezek. 36:35; Amos 9:11; Acts 15:16.
RULE (*n.*). Esth. 9:1, Jews had *r.* over them.
Prov. 17:2, a wise servant shall have *r.*
19:10, servant to have *r.* over princes.
25:28, no *r.* over his own spirit.
Isa. 63:19, thou never barest *r.* over them.
1 Cor. 15:24, when he shall put down all *r.*
Gal. 6:16, as many as walk according to this *r.*
Heb. 13:7, 17, them that have the *r.* over you.
See Eccl. 2:19; Isa. 44:13; 2 Cor. 10:13.
RULE (*v.*). Gen. 1:16, to *r.* the day.
3:16, thy husband shall *r.* over thee.
Judg. 8:23, I will not *r.* over you.
2 Sam. 23:3, that *r.* over men must be just.
Ps. 66:7, he *r.* by his power for ever.
89:9, thou *r.* the raging of the sea.
103:19, his kingdom *r.* over all.
Prov. 16:32, that *r.* his spirit.
22:7, rich *r.* over the poor.
Eccl. 9:17, him that *r.* among fools.
Isa. 3:4, babes *r.* over them.
32:1, princes shall *r.* in judgment.
40:10, his arm shall *r.* for him.
Ezek. 29:15, shall no more *r.* over nations.
Rom. 12:8, he that *r.* with diligence.
Col. 3:15, peace of God *r.* in your hearts.
1 Tim. 3:4, one that *r.* well his own house.
5:17, elders that *r.* well.
See Dan. 5:21; Zech. 6:13; Rev. 2:27; 12:5.
RULER. Num. 13:2, every one a *r.* among them.
Prov. 6:7, ant, having no guide, overseer, or *r.*
23:1, when thou sittest to eat with a *r.*
28:16, a wicked *r.* over the poor.
Isa. 3:6, be thou our *r.*
Mic. 5:2, out of thee shall come *r.*
Mat. 25:21, I will make thee *r.*
John 7:26, do the *r.* know that this is Christ?
48, have any of the *r.* believed.
Rom. 13:3, *r.* not a terror to good works.
See Gen. 41:43; Neh. 5:7; Ps. 2:2; Isa. 1:10.
RUMOUR. Jer. 49:14, I have heard a *r.*
Ezek. 7:26, *r.* shall be upon *r.*
Mat. 24:6; Mk. 13:7, wars and *r.* of wars.
See 2 Kings 19:7; Obad. 1; Lu. 7:17.
RUN. 2 Sam. 18:27, the *r.* of the foremost is like.
2 Chron. 16:9, eyes of Lord *r.* to and fro.
Ps. 19:5, as a strong man to *r.* a race.
23:5, my cup *r.* over.
147:15, his word *r.* very swiftly.
Cant. 1:4, draw me, we will *r.* after thee.
Isa. 40:31, they shall *r.* and not be weary.
Isa. 55:5, nations shall *r.* to thee.
Jer. 12:5, if thou hast *r.* with the footmen.
51:31, one post shall *r.* to meet another.
Dan. 12:4, many shall *r.* to and fro.
Hab. 2:2, that he may *r.* that readeth.
Zech. 2:4, *r.*, speak to this young man.
Lu. 6:38, good measure *r.* over.
Rom. 9:16, nor of him that *r.*
1 Cor. 9:24, they which *r.* in a race *r.* all.
26, I therefore so *r.*
Gal. 2:2, lest I should *r.* or had *r.* in vain.
5:7, ye did *r.* well.
Heb. 12:1, let us *r.* with patience.
1 Pet. 4:4, that ye *r.* not to same excess.
See Prov. 4:12; Jer. 5:1; Lam. 2:18; Amos 8:12.
RUSH (*n.*). Job 8:11; Isa. 9:14; 19:15; 35:7.
RUSH (*v.*). Isa. 17:13; Jer. 8:6; Ezek. 3:12; Acts 2:2.
RUST. Mat. 6:19, 20; Jas. 5:3.

S

SABBATH. Lev. 25:8, number seven *s.* of years.
2 Kings 4:23, it is neither new moon nor *s.*
2 Chron. 36:21, as long as desolate she kept *s.*
Ezek. 46:1, on the *s.* it shall be opened.
Amos 8:5, when will the *s.* be gone.
Mk. 2:27, the *s.* was made for man.
28; Lu. 6:5, the Son of man is Lord of the *s.*
Lu. 13:15, doth not each on *s.* loose.
See Isa. 1:13; Lam. 1:7; 2:6; Mat. 28:1; John 5:18.
SACK. Gen. 42:25; 43:21; 44:1, 11, 12; Josh. 9:4.
SACKCLOTH. 2 Sam. 3:31, gird you with *s.*
1 Kings 20:32, they girded *s.* on their loins.
Neh. 9:1, assembled with fasting and *s.*
Esth. 4:1, put on *s.* with ashes.
Ps. 30:11, thou hast put off my *s.*
35:13, my clothing was *s.*
Jonah 3:5, and put on *s.*
SACRIFICE (*n.*). Gen. 31:54, Jacob offered *s.*
Ex. 5:17, let us go and do *s.* to the Lord.
Num. 25:2, called people to the *s.* of their gods.
1 Sam. 2:29, wherefore kick ye at my *s.*
9:13, he doth bless the *s.*
15:22, to obey is better than *s.*
Ps. 4:5, offer the *s.* of righteousness.
27:6, will I offer *s.* of joy.
40:6; 51:16, *s.* thou didst not desire.
51:17, the *s.* of God are a broken spirit.
118:27, bind the *s.* with cords.
Prov. 15:8, *s.* of wicked an abomination.
17:1, than a house full of *s.* with strife.
21:3, to do justice is more acceptable than *s.*
Eccl. 5:1, the *s.* of fools.
Isa. 1:11, to what purpose is multitude of *s.*
Jer. 6:20, nor are your *s.* sweet unto me.
33:18, nor want a man to do *s.*
Dan. 8:11; 9:27; 11:31; daily *s.* taken away.
Hos. 3:4, many days without a *s.*
6:6; Mat. 9:13; 12:7, I desired mercy and not *s.*
Amos 4:4, bring your *s.* every morning.
Zeph. 1:7, the Lord hath prepared a *s.*
Mal. 1:8, ye offer the blind for *s.*
Mk. 9:49, every *s.* shall be salted.
12:33, to love the Lord is more than *s.*
Lu. 13:1, blood Pilate mingled with *s.*
Acts 7:42, have ye offered *s.* forty years.
14:13, and would have done *s.*
Rom. 12:1, present your bodies a living *s.*
1 Cor. 8:4; 10:19, 28, offered in *s.* to idols.
Eph. 5:2, a *s.* to God for sweet-smelling savour.
Phil. 2:17, upon the *s.* of your faith.
4:18, a *s.* acceptable, well pleasing.
Heb. 9:26, put away sin by *s.* of himself.
10:12, offered one *s.* for sins.
10:26, there remaineth no more *s.* for sin.
11:4, a more excellent *s.*
13:15, let us offer the *s.* of praise.
16, with such *s.* God is well pleased.

1 Pet. 2:5, to offer up spiritual *s*.
See 2 Chron. 7:1; Ezra 6:10; Neh. 12:43; Jonah 1:16.
SACRIFICE (*v*.). Ex. 22:20, he that *s*. to any god.
Ezra 4:2, we seek your God, and do *s*. to him.
Neh. 4:2, will they *s*.
Ps. 54:6, I will freely *s*. to thee.
106:37, they *s*. their sons to devils.
107:22, let them *s*. sacrifices of thanksgiving.
Eccl. 9:2, to him that *s*. and that *s*. not.
Isa. 65:3, people that *s*. in gardens.
Hos. 8:13, they *s*., but the Lord accepteth not.
Heb. 1:16, they *s*. unto their net.
1 Cor. 5:7, Christ our passover is *s*. for us.
10:20, things Gentiles *s*., they *s*. to devils.
See Ex. 8:26; Deut. 15:21; 1 Sam. 1:3; 15:15.
SACRILEGE.
Rom. 2:22, dost thou commit *s*.
SAD. 1 Kings 21:5, why is thy spirit so *s*.
Eccl. 7:3, by *s*. of countenance the heart is made better.
Mat. 6:16, be not of a *s*. countenance.
Mk. 10:22, he was *s*. at that saying.
Lu. 24:17, as ye walk and are *s*.
See Gen. 40:6; 1 Sam. 1:18; Neh. 2:1; Ezek. 13:22.
SADDLE. 1 Sam. 19:26; 1 Kings 13:13.
SAFE. 2 Sam. 18:29, is the young man *s*.
Job 21:9, their houses are *s*. from fear.
Ps. 119:117, hold me up and I shall be *s*.
Prov. 18:10, righteous run and are *s*.
29:25, whoso trusteth in the Lord shall be *s*.
Ezek. 34:27, they shall be *s*. in their land.
Acts 27:44, so they escaped all *s*.
See 1 Sam. 12:11; Isa. 5:29; Lu. 15:27; Phil. 3:1.
SAFEGUARD. 1 Sam. 22:23, with me thou shalt be in *s*.
SAFELY. Ps. 78:53, he led them on *s*.
Prov. 1:33, shall dwell *s*.
3:23, shalt thou walk *s*.
31:11, doth *s*. trust in her.
Hos. 2:18, I will make them to lie down *s*.
See Isa. 41:3; Zech. 14:11; Mk. 14:44; Acts 16:23.
SAFETY. Job 3:26, I was not in *s*.
5:4, his children are far from *s*.
11:18, thou shalt take thy rest in *s*.
Prov. 11:14; 24:6, in the multitude of counsellors is *s*.
21:31, *s*. is of the Lord.
1 Thess. 5:3, when they say peace and *s*.
See Job 24:23; Ps. 12:5; 33:17; Isa. 14:30.
SAIL. Isa. 33:23; Ezek. 27:7; Lu. 8:23; Acts 27:9.
SAINTS. 1 Sam. 2:9, he will keep feet of *s*.
Job 5:1, to which of the *s*. wilt thou turn.
15:15, he putteth no trust in his *s*.
Ps. 16:3, but to the *s*. that are in the earth.
30:4, sing to the Lord, O ye *s*. of his.
37:28, the Lord forsaketh not his *s*.
50:5, gather my *s*. together.
89:5, the congregation of the *s*.
7, to be feared in assembly of *s*.
97:10, preserveth the souls of his *s*.
116:15, precious is the death of his *s*.
132:9, let thy *s*. shout for joy.
149:9, this honour have all his *s*.
Dan. 7:18, but the *s*. shall take the kingdom.
8:13, then I heard one *s*. speaking.
Mat. 27:52, many bodies of *s*. arose.
Acts 9:13, evil he hath done to thy *s*.
Rom. 1:7; 1 Cor. 1:2, called to be *s*.
8:27, he maketh intercession for the *s*.
12:13, distributing to the necessity of *s*.
16:2, receive her as becometh *s*.
1 Cor. 6:1, dare any go to law, and not before *s*.
2, the *s*. shall judge the world.
16:1, concerning collection for *s*.
16:15, the ministry of *s*.
Eph. 1:18, his inheritance in the *s*.
2:19, fellowcitizens with the *s*.
3:8, less than least of all *s*.
4:12, perfecting of the *s*.
5:3, not named among you, as becometh *s*.

Col. 1:12, the *s*. in light.
1 Thess. 3:13, at coming of our Lord with *s*.
2 Thess. 1:10, to be glorified in his *s*.
1 Tim. 5:10, if she have washed the *s*. feet.
Jude 3, faith once delivered to *s*.
Rev. 5:8; 8:3, 4, the prayers of *s*.
See Phil. 4:21; Rev. 11:18; 13:7; 14:12; 15:3.
SAKE. Gen. 3:17, cursed for thy *s*.
8:21, not curse ground for man's *s*.
12:13, be well with me for thy *s*.
18:26, I will spare for their *s*.
30:27, the Lord hath blessed me for thy *s*.
Num. 11:29, enviest thou for my *s*.
Deut. 1:37; 3:26; 4:21, angry with me for your *s*.
2 Sam. 9:1, shew kindness for Jonathan's *s*.
18:5, deal gently for my *s*.
Neh. 9:31, for thy great mercies' *s*.
Ps. 6:4; 31:16, save me for thy mercies' *s*.
23:3, he leadeth me for his name's *s*.
Ps. 44:22, for thy *s*. are we killed.
106:8, he saved them for his name's *s*.
Mat. 5:10, persecuted for righteousness' *s*.
10:18; Mk. 13:9; Lu. 21:12, for my *s*.
24:22; Mk. 13:20, for the elect's *s*.
John 11:15, I am glad for your *s*.
13:38, wilt thou lay down thy life for my *s*.
Rom. 13:5; 1 Cor. 10:25, for conscience *s*.
Col. 1:24, for his body's *s*. which is the church.
1 Thess. 5:13, for their work's *s*.
1 Tim. 5:23, for thy stomach's *s*.
Tit. 1:11, for lucre's *s*.
2 John 2, for the truth's *s*.
See Rom. 11:28; 2 Cor. 8:9; 1 Thess. 3:9.
SALUTATION. Mk. 12:38; Lu. 1:29; Col. 4. 18; 2 Thess. 3:17.
SALUTE. 1 Sam. 10:4; 2 Kings 4:29; Mk. 15:18.
SALVATION. Gen. 49:18, I have waited for thy *s*.
Ex. 14:13; 2 Chron. 20:17, see the *s*. of the Lord.
15:2, he is become my *s*.
Deut. 32:15, lightly esteemed the rock of his *s*.
1 Sam. 11:13; 19:5, the Lord wrought *s*. in Israel.
14:45, Jonathan, who hath wrought this *s*.
2 Sam. 22:51, he is the tower of *s*. for his king.
1 Chron. 16:23, show forth from day to day his *s*.
2 Chron. 6:41, let thy priests be clothed with *s*.
Ps. 3:8, *s*. belongeth to the Lord.
9:14, I will rejoice in thy *s*.
14:7, O that the *s*. of Israel were come.
25:5, thou art the God of my *s*.
27:1; 62:6; Isa. 12:2, my light and my *s*.
35:3, say unto my soul, I am thy *s*.
37:39, the *s*. of the righteous is of the Lord.
40:10, I have declared thy faithfulness and *s*.
50:23, to him will I show the *s*. of God.
51:12; 70:4, restore the joy of thy *s*.
68:20, he that is our God, is the God of *s*.
69:13, hear me in the truth of thy *s*.
29, let thy *s*. set me up on high.
71:15, my mouth shall show forth thy *s*.
74:12, working *s*. in the midst of the earth.
78:22, they trusted not in his *s*.
85:9, his *s*. is nigh them that fear him.
91:16, will satisfy him and show him my *s*.
96:2, show forth his *s*. from day to day.
98:3, ends of the earth have seen the *s*.
116:13, the cup of *s*.
118:14; Isa. 12:2, the Lord is become my *s*.
119:41, let thy *s*. come.
81, my soul fainteth for thy *s*.
123, mine eyes fail for thy *s*.
155, *s*. is far from the wicked.
174, I have longed for thy *s*.
132:16, I will clothe her priests with *s*.
144:10, that giveth *s*. unto kings.
149:4, beautify the meek with *s*.
Isa. 12:3, the wells of *s*.
26:1, *s*. will God appoint for walls.

Isa. 33:2, be thou our *s.* in time of trouble.
45:8, earth open and let them bring forth *s.*
17, saved with an everlasting *s.*
49:8, in a day of *s.* have I helped thee.
51:5, my *s.* is gone forth.
52:7, feet of him that publisheth *s.*
10, ends of the earth shall see *s.*
56:1, my *s.* is near to come.
59:11, we look for *s.*, but it is far off.
16, his arm brought *s.*
17, an helmet of *s.* on his head.
60:18, call thy walls *S.*
61:10, the garments of *s.*
62:1, the *s.* thereof as a lamp.
63:5, mine own arm brought *s.*
Jer. 3:23, in vain is *s.* hoped for.
Lam. 3:26, wait for the *s.* of the Lord.
Jonah 2:9, *s.* is of the Lord.
Hab. 3:8, ride on thy chariots of *s.*
18, I will joy in the God of my *s.*
Zech. 9:9, thy King, just, and having *s.*
Lu. 1:69, an horn of *s.* for us.
77, give knowledge of *s.* to his people.
2:30, mine eyes have seen thy *s.*
3:6, all flesh shall see the *s.* of God.
19:9, this day is *s.* come to this house.
John 4:22, *s.* is of the Jews.
Acts 4:12, neither is there *s.* in any other.
13:26, to you is the word of *s.* sent.
16:17, these men show to us the way of *s.*
Rom. 1:16, the power of God to *s.*
10:10, confession is made to *s.*
13:11, now is our *s.* nearer.
2 Cor. 1:6, comforted, it is for your *s.*
6:2, the day of *s.*
7:10, sorrow worketh repentance to *s.*
Eph. 1:13, the Gospel of your *s.*
6:17; 1 Thess. 5:8, the helmet of *s.* and sword.
Phil. 1:19, this shall turn to my *s.*
28, an evident token of *s.*
2:12, work out your own *s.*
1 Thess. 5:9, hath appointed us to obtain *s.*
2 Thess. 2:13, God hath chosen you to *s.*
2 Tim. 3:15, wise unto *s.*
Tit. 2:11, grace of God that bringeth *s.*
Heb. 1:14, for them who shall be heirs of *s.*
2:3, if we neglect so great *s.*
10, the captain of their *s.*
5:9, author of eternal *s.*
6:9, things that accompany *s.*
9:28, without sin unto *s.*
1 Pet. 1:5, kept through faith unto *s.*
9, end of faith, *s.* of your souls.
10, of which *s.* the prophets enquired.
2 Pet. 3:15, longsuffering of the Lord is *s.*
Jude 3, of the common *s.*
Rev. 7:10, saying, *s.* to our God.
See Job 13:16; 1 Sam. 2:1; 2 Sam. 22:36.

SAME. Job 4:8, sow wickedness, reap the *s.*
Ps. 102:27; Heb. 1:12, thou art the *s.*
Mat. 5:46, do not the publicans the *s.*
Acts 1:11, this *s.* Jesus shall come.
Rom. 10:12, the *s.* Lord over all.
12:16; 1 Cor. 1:10; Phil. 4:2, be of *s.* mind.
Heb. 13:8, *s.* yesterday, to-day, and for ever.
See 1 Cor. 10:3; 12:4; 15:39; Eph. 4:10.

SANCTIFY. Lev. 11:44; 20:7; Num. 11:18; Josh. 3:5; 7:13; 1 Sam. 16:5, *s.* yourselves.
Isa. 5:16, God shall be *s.* in righteousness.
13:3, I have commanded my *s.* ones.
29:23, they shall *s.* the Holy One.
66:17, *s.* themselves in gardens.
Jer. 1:5, I *s.* and ordained thee a prophet.
Ezek. 20:41; 36:23, I will be *s.* in you.
28:25; 39:27, *s.* in them in sight of heathen.
Joel 1:14; 2:15, *s.* yea fast.
John 10:36, him whom the Father *s.*
John 17:17, *s.* them through thy truth.
19, for their sakes I *s.* myself.
Acts 20:32; 26:18, inheritance among them that are *s.*
Rom. 15:16, being *s.* by the Holy Ghost.
1 Cor. 1:2, to them that are *s.*
6:11, but now ye are *s.*
7:14, husband is *s.* by the wife, and the wife is *s.*
Eph. 5:26, *s.* and cleanse the church.
1 Thess. 5:23, the very God of peace *s.* you.
1 Tim. 4:5, it is *s.* by the word of God.
2 Tim. 2:21, a vessel *s.* for the Master's use.
Heb. 2:11, he that *s.* and they who are *s.*
10:10, by the which will we are *s.*
14, perfected for ever them that are *s.*
13:12, that he might *s.* the people.
1 Pet. 3:15, *s.* the Lord God in your hearts.
Jude 1, to them that are *s.* by God the Father.
See Gen. 2:3; Ex. 13:2; Job 1:5; Mat. 23:17.

SANCTUARY. Ex. 15:17, plant them in the *s.*
25:8, let them make me a *s.*
36:1; 3:4, work for the *s.*
Num. 7:9, service of *s.* belongeth to them.
Neh. 10:39, where are the vessels of the *s.*
Ps. 74:7, they have cast fire into thy *s.*
Isa. 60:13, beautify the place of my *s.*
Lam. 2:7, the Lord hath abhorred his *s.*
See Dan. 8:11; 9:17; Heb. 8:2; 9:1.

SAND. Gen. 22:17, as the *s.* which is upon the sea shore.
Hos. 1:10; Rev. 20:8, as the *s.* of the sea.
Heb. 11:12, the *s.* which is by the sea.
See Job 6:3; Prov. 27:3; Mat. 7:26.

SANDALS. Mk. 6:9, be shod with *s.*
Acts 12:8, bind on thy *s.*

SANG. Ex. 15:1; Neh. 12:42; Job 38:7.

SANK. Ex. 15:5, they *s.* into the bottom.

SAP. Ps. 104:16, trees full of *s.*

SAPPHIRE. Ex. 24:10, a paved work of a *s.* stone.
28:18; Ezek. 28:13; Rev. 21:19, and a *s.*
Ezek. 1:26, as the appearance of a *s.* stone.
10:1, as it were a *s.* stone.

SARDINE. Rev. 4:3, like a jasper and *s.* stone.

SARDIUS. Ex. 28:17, the first row shall be a *s.*
Ezek. 28:13; Rev. 21:20, *s.* etc.

SARDONYX. Rev. 21:20, the fifth *s.*

SAT. Judg. 20:26, they *s.* before the Lord.
Job 29:25, I *s.* chief.
Ps. 26:4, have not *s.* with vain persons.
Jer. 15:17, I *s.* alone because of thy hand.
Ezek. 3:15, I *s.* where they *s.*
Mat. 4:16, the people who *s.* in darkness.
Mk. 16:19, he *s.* on the right hand of God.
Lu. 7:15, he that was dead *s.* up.
10:39, Mary *s.* at Jesus' feet.
John 4:6, *s.* thus on the well.
Acts 2:3, cloven tongues *s.* upon each.
See Ezra 10:16; Neh. 1:4; Ps. 137:1; Rev. 4:3.

SATAN. 1 Chron. 21:1, *S.* provoked David.
Ps. 109:6, let *S.* stand at his right hand.
Mat. 11:26; Mk. 3:23; Lu. 11:18, if *S.* cast out *S.*
16:23; Mk. 8:33; Lu. 4:8, get behind me, *S.*
Lu. 10:18, I beheld *S.* as lightning fall.
Acts 5:3, why hath *S.* filled thine heart.
26:18, turn them from power of *S.*
2 Cor. 12:7, messenger of *S.* to buffet me.
2 Thess. 2:9, after the working of *S.*
1 Tim. 1:20, whom I have delivered unto *S.*
5:15, already turned aside after *S.*
See Rom. 16:20; 1 Cor. 5:5; 2 Cor. 2:11; 11:14.

SATIATE. Jer. 31:14, 25; 46:10.

SATISFY. Job 38:27, to *s.* the desolate.
Ps. 17:15, I shall be *s.* when I awake.
22:26, the meek shall eat and be *s.*
36:8, they shall be *s.* with fatness.
37:19, in days of famine be *s.*
59:15, and grudge if they be not *s.*
63:5, my soul shall be *s.*
81:16, with honey should I have *s.* thee.

Ps. 90:14, *s.* us early with thy mercy.
91:16, with long life will I *s.* him.
103:5, who *s.* thy mouth with good.
104:13, the earth is *s.*
105:40, he *s.* them with bread from heaven.
107:9, he *s.* the longing soul.
132:15, I will *s.* her poor with bread.
Prov. 6:30, if he steal to *s.* his soul.
12:11, he that tilleth his land shall be *s.*
14:14, a good man shall be *s.* from himself.
19:23, he that hath it shall abide *s.*
20:13, open thine eyes and thou shalt be *s.*
30:15, three things never *s.*
Eccl. 1:8, the eye is not *s.* with seeing.
4:8, neither is his eye *s.* with riches.
5:10, shall not be *s.* with silver.
Isa. 9:20; Mic. 6:14, shall eat and not be *s.*
53:11, travail of his soul and be *s.*
58:10, if thou *s.* the afflicted soul.
11, the Lord shall *s.* thy soul in drought.
Jer. 31:14, shall be *s.* with my goodness.
Ezek. 16:28, yet thou couldest not be *s.*
Amos 4:8, wandered to drink, but were not *s.*
Hab. 2:5, as death and cannot be *s.*
See Ex. 15:9; Deut. 14:29; Job 19:22; 27:14.
SAVE. Gen. 45:7, to *s.* your lives.
47:25, thou hast *s.* our lives.
Deut. 28:29, spoiled and no man shall *s.* thee.
33:29, O people, *s.* by the Lord.
Josh. 10:6, come up quickly and *s.* us.
Judg. 6:15, wherewith shall I *s.* Israel?
1 Sam. 4:3, the ark may *s.* us.
10:27, how shall this man *s.* us?
11:3, if there be no man to *s.* us we will come.
14:6, no restraint to *s.* by many or by few.
2 Sam. 19:9, the king *s.* us, and now he is fled.
2 Kings 6:10, *s.* himself there, not once nor twice.
Job 2:6, in thine hand, but *s.* his life.
22:29, he shall *s.* the humble.
26:2, how *s.* thou.
Ps. 7:10, God who *s.* the upright.
20:6, the Lord *s.* his anointed.
34:18, he *s.* such as be of a contrite spirit.
44:3, neither did their own arm *s.* them.
60:5, *s.* with thy right hand.
72:4, he shall *s.* the children of the needy.
80:3; Prov. 28:18; Jer. 17:14; Mat. 10:22; 24:13; Mk. 13:13; 16:16; John 10:9; Acts 2:21; 16:31; Rom. 5:9; 9:27; 10:9; 11:26, shall be *s.*
86:2, *s.* thy servant that trusteth.
109:31, *s.* him from those that condemn.
118:25, *s.*, I beseech thee, send prosperity.
119:94, *s.* me, for I have sought.
146, *s.* me, and I shall keep thy testimonies.
138:7, thy right hand shall *s.*
Prov. 20:22, wait on Lord and he shall *s.* thee.
Isa. 35:4, your God will come and *s.* you.
43:12, I have declared and have *s.*
45:20, pray to a god that cannot *s.*
22, look unto me and be ye *s.*
47:15, they shall wander, none shall *s.*
49:25, I will *s.* thy children.
59:1, Lord's hand not shortened, that it cannot *s.*
63:1, mighty to *s.*
Jer. 2:28, let them arise if they can *s.*
8:20, summer is ended, and we are not *s.*
11:12, but they shall not *s.*
14:9, as a mighty man that cannot *s.*
15:20; 30:11; 42:11; 46:27, I am with thee to *s.* thee.
17:14, *s.* me and I shall be *s.*
30:10, I will *s.* thee from afar.
48:6, flee, *s.* your lives.
Lam. 4:17, a nation that could not *s.* us.
Ezek. 3:18, to warn wicked, to *s.* his life.
34:22, therefore will I *s.* my flock.
Hos. 1:7, I will *s.* them by the Lord.
13:10, is there any other that may *s.* thee.
Hab. 1:2, cry to thee and thou wilt not *s.*
Zeph. 3:17, he will *s.*
Mat. 1:21, *s.* his people from their sins.
16:25; Mk. 8:35; Lu. 9:24, will *s.* his life.
18:11; Lu. 19:10, to seek and to *s.* that which was lost.
19:25; Mk. 10:26; Lu. 18:26, who then can be *s.*?
27:40; Mk. 15:30, *s.* thyself.
42; Mk. 15:31, he *s.* others, himself he cannot *s.*
Mk. 3:4; Lu. 6:9, is it lawful to *s.*
Lu. 7:50; 18:42, thy faith hath *s.* thee.
8:12, lest they should believe and be *s.*
9:56, not to destroy but to *s.*
13:23, are there few that be *s.*?
23:35, let him *s.* himself.
39, if thou be Christ, *s.* thyself and us.
John 3:17, that the world might be *s.*
5:34, these things I say that ye might be *s.*
12:47, not to judge but to *s.*
Acts 2:47, such as should be *s.*
4:12, no other name whereby we must be *s.*
15:1, except ye be circumcised ye cannot be *s.*
16:30, what must I do to be *s.*?
27:43, the centurion willing to *s.* Paul.
Rom. 8:24, we are *s.* by hope.
10:1, my prayer is that they might be *s.*
Rom. 11:14; 1 Cor. 9:22, if I might *s.* some.
1 Cor. 1:18, to us who are *s.*
21, by foolishness of preaching to *s.* some.
3:15, *s.* yet so as by fire.
5:5, that the spirit may be *s.*
7:16, shalt *s.* thy husband.
2 Cor. 2:15, savour in them that are *s.*
Eph. 2:5, 8, by grace ye are *s.*
1 Tim. 1:15, came to *s.* sinners.
2:4, who will have all men to be *s.*
4:16, thou shalt *s.* thyself and them.
Heb. 5:7, able to *s.* him from death.
7:25, able to *s.* to the uttermost.
10:39, believe to *s.* of soul.
11:7, an ark to the *s.* of his house.
Jas. 1:21, word which is able to *s.* your souls.
2:14, can faith *s.* him?
4:12, able to *s.* and destroy.
5:15, prayer of faith shall *s.* sick.
20, shall *s.* a soul from death.
1 Pet. 3:20, souls were *s.* by water.
4:18, righteous scarcely be *s.*
Jude 23, others *s.* with fear.
See Mat. 14:30; John 12:27; 1 Pet. 3:21.
SAVE (*except*). 2 Sam. 22:32, who is God, *s.* the Lord?
Mat. 11:27, nor knoweth any *s.* the Son.
13:57, *s.* in his own country.
17:8; Mk. 9:8, *s.* Jesus only.
Lu. 17:18, *s.* this stranger.
18:19, none good *s.* one.
2 Cor. 11:24, forty stripes *s.* one.
Gal. 6:14, glory *s.* in the cross.
See Mk. 5:37; Lu. 4:26; Rev. 2:17; 13:17.
SAVIOUR. 2 Sam. 22:3, my refuge, my *s.*
2 Kings 13:5, the Lord gave Israel a *s.*
Ps. 106:21, they forgat God their *s.*
Isa. 19:20, he shall send them a *s.*
45:21, a just God and a *S.*
49:26, all shall know I am thy *S.*
63:8, so he was their *S.*
Eph. 5:23, Christ is the *s.* of the body.
1 Tim. 4:10, who is the *S.* of all men.
Tit. 2:10, adorn doctrine of God our *S.*
13, glorious appearing of our *S.*
Jude 25, the only wise God our *S.*
See Neh. 9:27; Obad. 21; John 4:42; Acts 5:31.
SAVOUR. Gen. 8:21, Lord smelled a sweet *s.*
Ex. 5:21, have made our *s.* to be abhorred.
Cant. 1:3, *s.* of thy good ointment.
Joel 2:20, his ill *s.* shall come up.
Mat. 5:13; Lu. 14:34, if salt have lost his *s.*
See Eccl. 10:1; Ezek. 6:13; 20:41; Eph. 5:2.

SAVOUREST. Mat. 16:23; Mk. 8:33.
SAVOURY. Gen. 27:4, 7, 14, 31.
SAW. Gen. 22:4, Abraham *s.* the place.
26:28, we *s.* the Lord was with thee.
Ex. 10:23, they *s.* not one another.
24:10, they *s.* the God of Israel.
2 Chron. 25:21, they *s.* one another in the face.
Job 29:11, when the eye *s.* me.
Ps. 77:16, the waters *s.* thee.
Eccl. 2:24, this I *s.*, it was from hand of God.
Cant. 3:3, *s.* ye him whom my soul loveth.
Mat. 12:22, both spake and *s.*
17:8, they *s.* no man.
Mk. 8:23, if he *s.* ought.
John 1:48, under the fig-tree I *s.* thee.
8:56, Abraham *s.* my day.
20:20, glad when they *s.* the Lord.
See 1 Sam. 19:5; Ps. 50:18; Isa. 59:16.
SAY. Ex. 3:13, what shall I *s.* unto them?
4:12, teach thee what thou shalt *s.*
Num. 22:19, know what the Lord will *s.*
Judg. 18:24, what is this ye *s.* to me?
Ezra 9:10, what shall we *s.* after this?
Mat. 3:9, think not to *s.* within yourselves.
7:22, many will *s.* in that day.
16:13; Mk. 8:27, whom do men *s.* that I am?
23:3, they *s.* and do not.
Lu. 7:40, I have somewhat to *s.* to thee.
1 Cor. 12:3, no man can *s.* that Jesus.
See Lu. 7:7; John 4:20; 8:26; 16:12.
SAYING. Deut. 1:23, the *s.* pleased me well.
1 Kings 2:38, the *s.* is good.
Ps. 49:4, my dark *s.* upon the harp.
78:2, utter dark *s.* of old.
Prov. 1:6, the dark *s.* of the wise.
Mat. 28:15, this *s.* is commonly reported.
Lu. 2:51, kept all these *s.* in her heart.
John 4:37, herein is that *s.* true.
6:60, an hard *s.*, who can hear it?
See John 21:23; Rom. 13:9; 1 Tim. 1:15.
SCAB. Lev. 13:2, a *s.* or bright spot.
Deut. 28:27, and with the *s.*
Isa. 3:17, the Lord will smite with a *s.*
SCANT. Mic. 6:10, *s.* measure.
SCARCE. Gen. 27:30; Acts 14:18.
SCARCELY. Rom. 5:7; 1 Pet. 4:18.
SCARCENESS. Deut. 8:9, bread without *s.*
SCAREST. Job 7:14, thou *s.* me with dreams.
SCATTER. Gen. 11:4, lest we be *s.* abroad.
Lev. 26:33, I will *s.* you among the heathen.
Num. 10:35; Ps. 68:1, let thine enemies be *s.*
Job 18:15, brimstone shall be *s.* on his habitation.
37:11, he *s.* his bright cloud.
38:24, which *s.* the east wind.
Ps. 68:30, *s.* thou the people that delight in war.
92:9, the workers of iniquity shall be *s.*
147:16, he *s.* the hoar frost.
Prov. 11:24, there is that *s.* and yet increaseth.
20:8, a king *s.* evil with his eyes.
26, a wise king *s.* the wicked.
Jer. 10:21, all their flocks shall be *s.*
23:1, woe to pastors that *s.* the sheep.
50:17, Israel is a *s.* sheep.
Zech. 13:7; Mat. 26:31; Mk. 14:27, sheep shall be *s.*
Mat. 9:36, *s.* as sheep having no shepherd.
12:30; Lu. 11:23, he that gathereth not with me *s.*
See John 11:52; 16:32; Acts 8:1; Jas. 1:1.
SCENT. Job 14:9; Jer. 48:11; Hos. 14:7.
SCHOLAR. 1 Chron. 25:8; Mal. 2:12.
SCHOOLMASTER. Gal. 3:24, the law was our *s.*
SCIENCE. Dan. 1:4; 1 Tim. 6:20.
SCOFF. Hab. 1:10; 2 Pet. 3:3.
SCORCH. Mat. 13:6; Mk. 4:6; Rev. 16:8.
SCORN. Esth. 3:6; Job 16:20; Ps. 44:13; 79:4.
SCORNER. Prov. 9:8, reprove not a *s.*
13:1, a *s.* heareth not rebuke.
19:25, smite a *s.*
Prov. 28, an ungodly witness *s.* judgment.
29, judgments are prepared for *s.*
21:11, when *s.* is punished simple is made wise.
24:9, the *s.* is an abomination.
Isa. 29:20, the *s.* is consumed.
Hos. 7:5, stretched out hands with *s.*
See Ps. 1:1; Prov. 1:22; 3:34; 9:12.
SCORPIONS. Deut. 8:15, fiery serpents and *s.*
Lu. 10:19, power to tread on *s.*
Rev. 9:3, as the *s.* of the earth.
SCOURGE. Job 5:21, the *s.* of the tongue.
9:23, if the *s.* slay suddenly.
Isa. 28:15, the overflowing *s.*
Mat. 10:17; 23:34, they will *s.* you.
John 2:15, a *s.* of small cords.
Acts 22:25, is it lawful to *s.* a Roman.
Heb. 12:6, the Lord *s.* every son.
See Josh. 23:13; Isa. 10:26; Mat. 27:26; John 19:1.
SCRAPE. Lev. 14:41; Job 2:8; Ezek. 26:4.
SCRIBE. 1 Chron. 27:32, a wise man and a *s.*
Isa. 33:18, where is the *s.*?
Jer. 8:8, the pen of the *s.* is in vain.
Mat. 5:20, exceed righteousness of the *s.*
7:29, authority, and not as the *s.*
13:52, every *s.* instructed unto kingdom.
Mk. 12:38; Lu. 20:46, beware of the *s.*
See Ezra 4:8; 7:6; Neh. 8:4; Mat. 8:19.
SCRIP. 1 Sam. 17:40; Mat. 10:10; Lu. 10:4; 22:35.
SEARCH (*n.*). Ps. 64:6; 77:6; Jer. 2:34.
SEARCH (*v.*). Num. 13:2, that they may *s.* the land.
1 Chron. 28:9, the Lord *s.* all hearts.
Job 11:7, canst thou by *s.* find out God?
13:9, is it good that he should *s.* you out?
28:27, he prepared it and *s.* it out.
29:16, the cause I knew not I *s.* out.
32:11, I waited whilst ye *s.* out what to say.
36:26, can number of his years be *s.* out.
Ps. 44:21, shall not God *s.* this out?
139:1, thou hast *s.* me and known me.
23, *s.* me and know my heart.
Prov. 25:2, honour of kings to *s.* out a matter.
27, for men to *s.* out their own glory.
Eccl. 1:13; 7:25, I gave my heart to *s.* wisdom.
Isa. 40:28, no *s.* of his understanding.
Jer. 17:10, I the Lord *s.* the heart.
29:13, when ye shall *s.* for me with all.
31:37, foundations of the earth *s.* out.
Lam. 3:40, let us *s.* our ways, and turn.
Ezek. 34:6, none did *s.* or seek after them.
8, neither did my shepherds *s.* for my flock.
11, I will *s.* my sheep.
Amos 9:3, I will *s.* and take them out thence.
Zeph. 1:12, I will *s.* Jerusalem with candles.
John 5:39; Acts 17:11, *s.* the scriptures.
Rom. 8:27, that *s.* hearts knoweth mind.
1 Cor. 2:10, the Spirit *s.* all things.
1 Pet. 1:10, which salvation prophets *s.* diligently.
See Job 10:6; 28:3; Prov. 2:4; 1 Pet. 1:11.
SEARED. 1 Tim. 4:2, conscience *s.*
SEASON. Gen. 1:14, for signs, and *s.*, and days.
Deut. 28:12, give rain in his *s.*
2 Chron. 15:3, for long *s.* without true God.
Job 5:26, as a shock of corn in his *s.*
Ps. 1:3, that bringeth forth fruit in his *s.*
22:2, I cry in the night *s.*
104:19, appointed the moon for *s.*
Prov. 15:23, word spoken in due *s.*
Eccl. 3:1, to everything there is a *s.* and a time.
Isa. 50:4, know how to speak a word in *s.*
Jer. 5:24, former and latter rain in his *s.*
33:20, day and night in their *s.*
Ezek. 34:26, cause shower to come down in *s.*
Dan. 2:21, changeth the times and *s.*
7:12, lives prolonged for a *s.*
Hos. 2:9, take away my wine in *s.*
Mat. 21:41, render the fruits in their *s.*
Lu. 1:20, my words shall be fulfilled in *s.*

Prov. 23:30, they that go to *s.* mixed wine.
35, I will *s.* it yet again.
Eccl. 1:13; 7:25, gave my heart to *s.* wisdom.
Cant. 3:2, I will *s.* him whom my soul loveth.
Isa. 1:17, learn to do well, *s.* judgment.
8:19, should not a people *s.* unto their God.
19:3, they shall *s.* to charmers.
34:16, *s.* ye out of the book of the Lord.
41:17, when the needy *s.* water.
45:19, I said not, *s.* ye my face in vain.
Jer. 5:1, any that *s.* the truth.
29:13, ye shall *s.* me and find when ye search.
30:17, Zion whom no man *s.* after.
38:4, this man *s.* not welfare of people.
Lam. 3:25, the Lord is good to the soul that *s.* him.
Ezek. 7:25, they shall *s.* peace.
34:16, I will *s.* that which was lost.
Dan. 9:3, I set my face to *s.* by prayer.
Amos 5:4, *s.* me and ye shall live.
Zeph. 2:3, *s.* ye the Lord, all ye meek.
Mal. 2:7, they should *s.* the law at his mouth.
Mat. 6:32, after these things do Gentiles *s.*
33; Lu. 12:21, *s.* first the kingdom of God.
7:7; Lu. 11:9, *s.* and ye shall find.
12:39; 16:4, adulterous generation *s.* a sign.
28:5; Mk. 16:6, I know that ye *s.* Jesus.
Mk. 1:37, all men *s.* for thee.
8:11, *s.* of him a sign from heaven.
Lu. 13:7, I come *s.* fruit.
24, many will *s.* to enter in.
15:8, doth she not *s.* diligently.
19:10, is come to *s.* and to save.
24:5, why *s.* ye the living among the dead?
John 1:38, what *s.* ye?
4:23, the Father *s.* such to worship him.
7:25, is not this he whom they *s.* to kill?
34, ye shall *s.* me and shall not find me.
18:8, if ye *s.* me, let these go their way.
20:15, woman, whom *s.* thou?
Rom. 3:11, there is none that *s.* after God.
1 Cor. 1:22, the Greeks *s.* after wisdom.
10:24, let no man *s.* his own.
13:5, charity *s.* not her own.
2 Cor. 12:14, I *s.* not yours, but you.
Phil. 2:21, all *s.* their own things.
Col. 3:1, *s.* those things which are above.
Heb. 11:6, a rewarder of them that *s.* him.
14, declare plainly that they *s.* a country.
13:14, but we *s.* one to come.
1 Pet. 5:8, *s.* whom he may devour.
Rev. 9:6, in those days shall men *s.* death.
See Jer. 45:5; Mat. 13:45; John 6:24; 1 Cor. 10:33.
SEEM. Gen. 19:14, he *s.* as one that mocked.
29:20, they *s.* to him but a few days.
Num. 16:9, *s.* it but a small thing.
Prov. 14:12, there is a way that *s.* right.
Lu. 8:18, taken away that he *s.* to have.
24:11, words *s.* as idle tales.
1 Cor. 3:18, if any *s.* to be wise.
11:16, if any man *s.* to be contentious.
Heb. 4:1, lest any *s.* to come short.
12:11, now no chastening *s.* to be joyous.
See Gen. 27:12; Eccl. 9:13; Acts 17:18; Gal. 2:6.
SEEMLY. Prov. 19:10; 26:1.
SEEN. Gen. 32:30, I have *s.* God face to face.
Ex. 14:13, Egyptians whom ye have *s.* to-day.
Judg. 6:22, because I have *s.* an angel.
2 Kings 20:15, what have they *s.*
Job 13:1, mine eye hath *s.* all this.
28:7, a path the vulture's eye hath not *s.*
Ps. 37:25, have I not *s.* righteous forsaken.
90:15, years wherein we have *s.* evil.
Eccl. 6:5, he hath not *s.* the sun.
Isa. 9:2, have *s.* a great light.
64:4; 1 Cor. 2:9, neither hath eye *s.*
66:8, who hath *s.* such things.
Mat. 6:1; 23:5, to be *s.* of men.
Mat. 9:33, never so *s.* in Israel.
Mk. 9:1, till they have *s.* the kingdom of God.
Lu. 5:26, we have *s.* strange things to-day.
John 1:18, no man hath *s.* God.
8:57, hast thou *s.* Abraham?
14:9, he that hath *s.* me hath *s.* the Father.
Acts 11:23, when he had *s.* the grace of God.
1 Cor. 9:1, have I not *s.* Jesus Christ.
1 Tim. 6:16, whom no man hath *s.*, nor can see.
Heb. 11:1, evidence of things not *s.*
1 Pet. 1:8, whom having not *s.*, ye love.
See John 5:37; 9:37; 15:24; 20:29; Rom. 1:20.
SEER. 1 Sam. 9:9, a prophet was beforetime called a *s.*
2 Sam. 24:11, the prophet Gad, David's *s.*
SEETHE. Ex. 23:19; 2 Kings 4:38; Ezek. 24:5.
SEIZE. Job 3:6; Ps. 55:15; Jer. 49:24; Mat. 21:38.
SELF. Tit. 1:7; 2 Pet. 2:10.
SELL. Gen. 25:31, *s.* me thy birthright.
37:27, come, let us *s.* him.
1 Kings 21:25, Ahab did *s.* himself to work.
Neh. 5:8, will ye even *s.* your brethren.
Prov. 23:23, buy the truth, and *s.* it not.
Joel 3:8, I will *s.* your sons and daughters.
Amos 8:5, that we may *s.* corn.
6, and *s.* the refuse of the wheat.
Mat. 19:21; Mk. 10:21; Lu. 12:33; 18:22, *s.* that thou hast.
Lu. 22:36, let him *s.* his garment.
Jas. 4:13, we will buy and *s.*, and get gain.
See Ps. 44:12; Prov. 11:26; 31:24; Mat. 13:44.
SELLER. Isa. 24:2; Ezek. 7:12, 13; Acts 16:14.
SEND. Gen. 24:7, God shall *s.* his angel.
12, *s.* me good speed this day.
Ex. 4:13, *s.* by hand of him whom thou wilt *s.*
2 Chron. 7:13; Ezek. 14:9, if I *s.* pestilence.
Ps. 20:2, *s.* thee help from the sanctuary.
43:3, *s.* out thy light and truth.
118:25, *s.* now prosperity.
Isa. 6:8, whom shall I *s.*? *s.* me.
Mat. 9:38; Lu. 10:2, *s.* labourers.
12:20, till he *s.* forth judgment.
15:23, *s.* her away, for she crieth after us.
Mk. 3:14, that he might *s.* them to preach.
John 14:26, whom the Father will *s.* in my name
17:8, believed that thou didst *s.* me.
Rom. 8:3, God *s.* his Son in likeness.
See Lu. 10:3; 24:49; John 20:21; 2 Thess. 2:11.
SENSUAL. Jas. 3:15; Jude 19.
SENT. Gen. 45:5, God *s.* me.
Judg. 6:14, have not I *s.* thee.
Ps. 77:17, the skies *s.* out a sound.
106:15, he *s.* leanness into their soul.
107:20, he *s.* his word and healed them.
Jer. 23:21, I have not *s.* these prophets.
Mat. 15:24, I am not *s.* but to lost sheep.
John 4:34, the will of him that *s.* me.
9:4, work the works of him that *s.* me.
17:3, life eternal to know him whom thou hast *s.*
Acts 10:29, as soon as I was *s.* for.
Rom. 10:15, preach, except they be *s.*
See Isa. 61:1; John 1:6; 3:28; 1 Pet. 1:12.
SENTENCE. Ps. 17:2, let my *s.* come forth.
Prov. 16:10, a divine *s.* in the lips of the king.
Eccl. 8:11, because *s.* is not executed speedily.
2 Cor. 1:9, *s.* of death in ourselves.
See Deut. 17:9; Jer. 4:12; Dan. 5:12; 8:23.
SEPARATE. Gen. 13:9, *s.* thyself from me.
Deut. 19:2, thou shalt *s.* three cities.
Prov. 16:28; 17:9, whisperer *s.* chief friends.
19:4, the poor is *s.* from his neighbour.
Mat. 25:32, he shall *s.* them.
Rom. 8:35, who shall *s.* us from love of God?
2 Cor. 6:17, be ye *s.*
Heb. 7:26, *s.* from sinners.
See Num. 6:2; Ezra 10:11; Isa. 56:3; 59:2.
SEPARATION. Num. 6:8; 19:9; 31:23; Ezek. 42:20.
SERPENT. Gen. 3:1, the *s.* was more subtil.
49:17, Dan shall be a *s.* by the way.

Job 26:13, his hand formed the crooked *s.*
Ps. 58:4, like the poison of a *s.*
104:3, sharpened their tongues like a *s.*
Prov. 23:32, at last it biteth like a *s.*
Eccl. 10:8, breaketh a hedge, a *s.* shall bite him.
11, *s.* will bite without enchantment.
Isa. 27:1, the Lord shall punish the *s.*
65:25, dust shall be the *s.* meat.
Jer. 8:17, I will send *s.* among you.
Amos 9:3, I will command the *s.*
Mic. 7:17, they shall lick dust like a *s.*
Mat. 7:10; Lu. 11:11, will he give him a *s.*?
10:16, be ye wise as *s.*
23:33, ye *s.*, how can ye escape.
Mk. 16:18, they shall take up *s.*
John 3:14, as Moses lifted up the *s.*
Rev. 12:9; 20:2, that old *s.* called the Devil.
See Ex. 4:3; Num. 21:8; 2 Kings 18:4; Jas. 3:7.

SERVANT. Gen. 9:25, a *s.* of *s.* shall he be.
Job 3:19, the *s.* is free.
7:2, as a *s.* desireth the shadow.
Ps. 116:16; 119:125; 143:12, I am thy *s.*
Prov. 22:7, the borrower is *s.* to the lender.
29:19, a *s.* will not be corrected with words.
Isa. 24:2, as with *s.* so with master.
Mat. 10:25, enough for *s.* to be as his lord.
25:21, good and faithful *s.*
Lu. 12:47, that *s.* which knew his lord's will.
17:10, unprofitable *s.*
John 8:35, *s.* abideth not in house for ever.
15:15, *s.* knoweth not what his lord doeth.
1 Cor. 7:21, art thou called, being a *s.*
23, be not ye the *s.* of men.
Eph. 6:5; Col. 3:22; Tit. 2:9; 1 Pet. 2:18, *s.* be obedient.
See Rom. 6:16; Col. 4:1; 1 Tim. 6:1; Rev. 22:3.

SERVE. Gen. 25:23, elder shall *s.* the younger.
Deut. 6:13; 10:12, 20; 11:13; 13:4; Josh. 22:5; 24:14; 1 Sam. 7:3; 12:14, thou shalt fear the Lord and *s.* him.
Josh. 24:15, choose ye whom ye will *s.*
1 Chron. 28:9, *s.* him with a perfect heart.
Job 21:15, what is the Almighty, that we should *s.* him?
Ps. 22:30, a seed shall *s.* him.
72:11, all nations shall *s.* him.
Isa. 43:23, I have not caused thee to *s.*
24, thou hast made me to *s.* with thy sins.
Jer. 5:19, so shall ye *s.* strangers.
Dan. 6:16, thy God whom thou *s.* will deliver.
Zeph. 3:9, to *s.* him with one consent.
Mal. 3:17, spareth his son that *s.* him.
18, between him that *s.* God and him that.
Mat. 6:24; Lu. 16:13, no man can *s.* two masters.
Lu. 10:40, hath left me to *s.* alone.
15:29, these many years do I *s.* thee.
John 12:26, if any man *s.* me, let him.
Acts 6:2, leave word of God and *s.* tables.
Rom. 6:6, henceforth we should not *s.* sin.
Gal. 5:13, by love *s.* one another.
Col. 3:24, for ye *s.* the Lord Christ.
1 Thess. 1:9, from idols to *s.* living God.
Rev. 7:15, they *s.* him day and night.
See Lu. 22:27; Acts 13:36; Heb. 9:14; 12:28.

SERVICE. Ex. 12:26, what mean ye by this *s.*?
1 Chron. 29:5, who is willing to consecrate his *s.*
John 16:2, will think he doeth God *s.*
Rom. 12:1, your reasonable *s.*
Eph. 6:7, doing *s.* as to the Lord.
Phil. 2:30, to supply your lack of *s.*
See Ezra 6:18; Ps. 104:14; Jer. 22:13.

SET. Gen. 4:15, the Lord *s.* a mark on Cain.
9:13, I do *s.* my bow in the cloud.
Deut. 1:8, I have *s.* the land before thee.
Job 33:5, *s.* thy words in order.
Ps. 16:8, I have *s.* the Lord before me.
20:5, we will *s.* up our banners.
91:14, he hath *s.* his love upon me.
Eccl. 7:14, hath *s.* the one against the other.
Cant. 8:6, *s.* me as a seal upon thine heart.
Mat. 5:14, a city *s.* on a hill.
Acts 18:10, no man shall *s.* on thee.
Heb. 6:18, the hope *s.* before us.
See Ps. 75:7; 107:41; Eph. 1:20; Col. 3:2.

SETTLE. Zeph. 1:12; Lu. 21:14; Col. 1:23.

SEVER. Lev. 20:26; Ezek. 39:14; Mat. 13:49.

SEW. Gen. 3:7; Job 14:17; Eccl. 3:7; Mk. 2:21.

SHADE. Ps. 121:5, the Lord is thy *s.*

SHADOW. Gen. 19:8, the *s.* of my roof.
Job 7:2, as servant earnestly desireth the *s.*
14:2, he fleeth as a *s.* and continueth not.
17:7, all my members are as a *s.*
Ps. 91:1, under the *s.* of the Almighty.
102:11, my days are like a *s.*
144:4; Eccl. 8:13, his days are as a *s.*
Eccl. 6:12, life which he spendeth as a *s.*
Cant. 2:3, under his *s.* with great delight.
17; 4:6, till the *s.* flee away.
Isa. 4:6, for a *s.* in the daytime.
25:4, a *s.* from the heat.
32:2, as the *s.* of a great rock.
49:2; 51:16, in the *s.* of his hand.
Jer. 6:4, the *s.* of evening are stretched out.
Lam. 4:20, under his *s.* we shall live.
Hos. 14:7, they that dwell under his *s.* shall return.
Acts 5:15, the *s.* of Peter might overshadow.
Jas. 1:17, with whom is no *s.* of turning.
See Judg. 9:15, 36; Isa. 38:8; Jonah 4:5.

SHAFT. Ex. 25:31; 37:17; Isa. 49:2.

SHAKE. Judg. 16:20, I will *s.* myself.
Ps. 29:8, voice of Lord *s.* wilderness.
72:16, fruit thereof shall *s.* like Lebanon.
Isa. 2:19, when he ariseth to *s.* the earth.
13:13; Joel 3:16; Hag. 2:6, 21, I will *s.* the heavens.
52:2, *s.* thyself from the dust.
Hag. 2:7, I will *s.* all nations.
Mat. 11:7; Lu. 7:24, a reed *s.* with the wind.
Lu. 6:38, good measure, *s.* together.
2 Thess. 2:2, be not soon *s.* in mind.
Heb. 12:26, I *s.* not earth only.
27, things which cannot be *s.*
See Job 9:6; Ezek. 37:7; Mat. 24:29.

SHAME. Ps. 4:2, turn my glory into *s.*
40:14; 83:17, let them be put to *s.*
Prov. 10:5; 17:2, a son that causeth *s.*
Isa. 61:7, for your *s.* ye shall have double.
Jer. 51:51, *s.* hath covered our faces.
Ezek. 16:52, bear thine own *s.*
Dan. 12:2, awake, some to *s.*
Zeph. 3:5, the unjust knoweth no *s.*
Lu. 14:9, with *s.* to take lowest room.
Acts 5:41, worthy to suffer *s.*
1 Cor. 6:5; 15:34, I speak this to your *s.*
Eph. 5:12, a *s.* to speak of those things.
Phil. 3:19, whose glory is in their *s.*
Heb. 6:6, put him to an open *s.*
12:2, despising the *s.*
See 1 Cor. 11:6; 14:35; 1 Thess. 2:2; 1 Tim. 2:9.

SHAPE. Lu. 3:22; John 5:37; Rev. 9:7.

SHARP. 1 Sam. 13:20, to *s.* every man his share.
21, a file to *s.* the goads.
Ps. 52:2, tongue like a *s.* razor.
140:3, they *s.* their tongues like a serpent.
Prov. 25:18, false witness is *s.* arrow.
27:17, iron *s.* iron, so a man *s.* his friend.
Isa. 41:15, a *s.* threshing instrument.
Acts 15:39, the contention was so *s.*
Heb. 4:12, *s.* than any two-edged sword.
See Mic. 7:4; 2 Cor. 13:10; Rev. 1:16; 14:14.

SHEAF. Deut. 24:19; Ruth 2:7; Ps. 126:6; 129:7.

SHEARERS. Gen. 38:12; 1 Sam. 25:7; Isa. 53:7.

SHEATH. 1 Sam. 17:51; 1 Chron. 21:27; Ezek. 21:3.

SHED. Gen. 9:6, shall his blood be *s.*
Mat. 26:28, *s.* for many for remission of sins.
Rom. 5:5, love of God *s.* in our hearts.
Tit. 3:6, which he *s.* on us abundantly.
Heb. 9:22, without *s.* of blood is no remission.

See Ezek. 18:10; 22:3; Acts 2:33.
SHEEP. Gen. 4:2, Abel was a keeper of *s.*
Num. 27:17; 1 Kings 22:17; 2 Chron. 18:16; Mat. 9:36; Mk. 6:34, as *s.* which have no shepherd.
1 Sam. 15:14, what meaneth this bleating of *s.*
Ps. 49:14, like *s.* are laid in the grave.
95:7; 100:3, we are the *s.* of his hand.
Isa. 53:6, all we like *s.* have gone astray.
Jer. 12:3, pull them out like *s.* for slaughter.
Ezek. 34:6, my *s.* wandered.
Mat. 7:15, false prophets in *s.* clothing.
10:6, go rather to lost *s.*
12:12, how much is a man better than a *s.*
John 10:2, that entereth by door is shepherd of *s.*
11, good shepherd giveth his life for the *s.*
21:16, feed my *s.*
See Mat. 10:16; 12:11; 18:12; 25:32; Heb. 13:20.
SHEET. Judg. 14:12; Acts 10:11; 11:5.
SHELTER. Job 24:8; Ps. 61:3.
SHEPHERD. Gen. 46:34, *s.* abomination to Egyptians.
Ps. 23:1, the Lord is my *s.*
Isa. 13:20, nor shall *s.* make their fold there.
40:11, he shall feed his flock like a *s.*
56:11, they are *s.* that cannot understand.
Jer. 23:4, I will set *s.* over them who shall feed.
50:6, their *s.* have caused them to go astray.
Amos 3:12, as the *s.* taketh out of the mouth.
Zech. 11:17, woe to the idol *s.*
John 10:14, I am the good *s.*
See Zech. 11:3; Lu. 2:8; 1 Pet. 2:25; 5:4.
SHIELD. Judg. 5:8, was there a *s.* seen.
Ps. 5:12, compass him as with a *s.*
33:20; 59:11; 84:9, the Lord is our *s.*
84:11, a sun and *s.*
91:4, truth shall be thy *s.*
Isa. 21:5, anoint the *s.*
Eph. 6:16, taking the *s.* of faith.
See Prov. 30:5; Jer. 51:11; Ezek. 23:24; 39:9.
SHINE. Job 22:28, the light shall *s.* upon thy ways.
29:3, when his candle *s.* upon my head.
Ps. 104:15, oil to make his face *s.*
139:12, the night *s.* as the day.
Prov. 4:18, light that *s.* more and more.
Isa. 9:2, upon them hath the light *s.*
60:1, arise, *s.*, for thy light is come.
Dan. 12:3, wise shall *s.* as the brightness.
Mat. 5:16, let your light so *s.*
13:43, the righteous *s.* as the sun.
2 Cor. 4:6, God who commanded the light to *s.*
See John 1:5; 2 Pet. 1:19; 1 John 2:8; Rev. 1:16.
SHOCK. Judg. 15:5; Job 5:26.
SHOD. Mk. 6:9; Eph. 6:15.
SHOOT. Ps. 22:7, they *s.* out the lip.
64:3, to *s.* their arrows, even bitter words.
144:6, *s.* out thine arrows and destroy them.
See 1 Chron. 12:2; Mk. 4:32; Lu. 21:30.
SHORT. Job 17:12, the light is *s.*
20:5, triumphing of wicked is *s.*
Ps. 89:47, remember how *s.* my time is.
Rom. 3:23, come *s.* of the glory of God.
1 Cor. 7:29, the time is *s.*
See Num. 11:23; Isa. 50:2; 59:1; Mat. 24:22.
SHORTER. Isa. 28:20, the bed is *s.*
SHORTLY. Gen. 41:32; Ezek. 7:8; Rom. 16:20.
SHOUT. Ps. 47:5, God is gone up with a *s.*
Lam. 3:8, when I *s.* he shutteth out my prayer.
1 Thess. 4:16, shall descend with a *s.*
See Num. 23:21; 1 Sam. 4:5; Isa. 12:6.
SHOWER. Ps. 65:10, makest it soft with *s.*
72:6, like *s.* that water the earth.
Ezek. 34:26, will cause *s.* to come in season.
See Deut. 32:2; Job 24:8; Jer. 3:3; 14:22.
SHUN. Acts 20:27; 2 Tim. 2:16.
SHUT. Gen. 7:16, the Lord *s.* him in.
Isa. 22:22, he shall open and none shall *s.*
60:11, gates shall not be *s.* day nor night.
Jer. 36:5, I am *s.* up, I cannot go to the house of the Lord.
Lam. 3:8, he *s.* out my prayer.
See Gal. 3:23; 1 John 3:17; Rev. 3:7; 20:3.
SICK. Prov. 13:12, maketh the heart *s.*
23:35, stricken me and I was not *s.*
Cant. 2:5, I am *s.* of love.
Isa. 1:5, the whole head is *s.*
Hos. 7:5, made him *s.* with bottles of wine.
Mat. 8:14, wife's mother *s.*
Jas. 5:14, is any *s.*? call elders of the church.
15, prayer of faith shall save the *s.*
SICKNESS. Ps. 41:3; Eccl. 5:17; Mat. 8:17.
SIFT. Isa. 30:28; Amos 9:9; Lu. 22:31.
SIGHT. Ex. 3:3, this great *s.*
Deut. 28:34, for *s.* of thine eyes.
Eccl. 6:9, better is *s.* of eyes.
Mat. 11:5; 20:34; Lu. 7:21, blind receive *s.*
26; Lu. 10:21, it seemed good in thy *s.*
Lu. 18:42; Acts 22:13, receive thy *s.*
21:11, fearful *s.* and signs from heaven.
Rom. 12:17, things honest in *s.* of all men.
2 Cor. 5:7, walk by faith, not by *s.*
See Eccl. 11:9; Isa. 43:4; Dan. 4:11; Heb. 4:13.
SIGN. Isa. 7:11, ask thee a *s.* of the Lord.
55:13, for an everlasting *s.*
Ezek. 12:6, I have set thee for a *s.*
Dan. 4:3, how great are his *s.*
Mat. 16:3, *s.* of the times.
Mk. 16:20, with *s.* following.
Lu. 2:34, for a *s.* which shall be spoken against.
John 4:48, except ye see *s.*
Acts 2:22, man approved of God by *s.*
4:30, that *s.* may be done by the name.
See Rom. 4:11; 15:19; 1 Cor. 1:22; Rev. 15:1.
SIGNIFY. John 12:33; Heb. 9:8; 1 Pet. 1:11.
SILENCE. Mat. 22:34; 1 Tim. 2:11; 1 Pet. 2:15.
SILENT. 1 Sam. 2:9, *s.* in darkness.
Ps. 28:1, be not *s.* to me.
31:17, let the wicked be *s.* in the grave.
Zech. 2:13, be *s.*, all flesh, before the Lord.
See Ps. 22:2; 30:12; Isa. 47:5; Jer. 8:14.
SILK. Prov. 31:22, her clothing is *s.* and purple.
Ezek. 16:10, I covered thee with *s.*
SILLY. Job 5:2; Hos. 7:11; 2 Tim. 3:6.
SILVER. 1 Kings 10:27, king made *s.* as stones.
Job 22:25, thou shalt have plenty of *s.*
Ps. 12:6; 66:10, as *s.* is tried.
Prov. 8:10, receive instruction and not *s.*
Eccl. 5:10, he that loveth *s.* shall not be satisfied.
Isa. 1:22, thy *s.* is become dross.
Jer. 6:30, reprobate *s.* shall men call them.
Mal. 3:3, sit as a refiner and purifier of *s.*
See Gen. 44:2; Eccl. 12:6; Mat. 27:6; Acts 19:24.
SIMILITUDE. Num. 12:8, the *s.* of the Lord.
Deut. 4:12, saw no *s.*
Ps. 144:12, after the *s.* of a palace.
Rom. 5:14, after the *s.* of Adam's transgression.
Jas. 3:9, made after the *s.* of God.
See Hos. 12:10; Dan. 10:16; Heb. 7:15.
SIMPLE (foolish). Ps. 19:7, making wise the *s.*
116:6, the Lord preserveth the *s.*
119:130, it giveth understanding to the *s.*
Prov. 1:22, how long, ye *s.* ones?
32, the turning away of the *s.*
7:7, and behold among the *s.*
8:5, O ye *s.* understand wisdom.
9:4, whoso is *s.*
14:15, the *s.* believeth every word.
19:25, and the *s.* will beware.
22:3; 27:12, the *s.* pass on, and are punished.
Rom. 16:18, deceive the hearts of the *s.*
SIMPLICITY. 2 Cor. 1:12, that in *s.* and godly sincerity.
11:3, from the *s.* that is in Christ.
SIN (*n.*). Gen. 4:7, *s.* lieth at the door.
Num. 27:3, died in his own *s.*
Deut. 24:16; 2 Kings 14:6; 2 Chron. 25:4, put to death for his own *s.*
Job 10:6, thou searchest after my *s.*

Ps. 19:13, from presumptuous *s.*
25:7, remember not *s.* of my youth.
32:1, blessed is he whose *s.* is covered.
38:18, I will be sorry for my *s.*
51:3, my *s.* is ever before me.
90:8, our secret *s.*
103:10, hath not dealt with us according to our *s.*
Prov. 5:22, holden with cords of *s.*
10:19, in multitude of words wanteth not *s.*
14:9, fools make a mock at *s.*
34, *s.* is a reproach to any people.
Isa. 30:1, to add *s.* to *s.*
43:25; 44:22, not remember *s.*
53:10, offering for *s.*
12, bare the *s.* of many.
Jer. 51:5, land filled with *s.*
Ezek. 33:16, none of his *s.* shall be mentioned.
Hos. 4:8, they eat up *s.* of my people.
Mic. 6:7, fruit of my body for *s.* of my soul.
Mat. 12:31, all manner of *s.* shall be forgiven.
John 1:29, the *s.* of the world.
8:7, he that is without *s.*
16:8, will reprove the world of *s.*
19:11, hath the greater *s.*
Acts 7:60, lay not this *s.* to their charge.
22:16, wash away thy *s.*
Rom. 5:20, where *s.* abounded.
6:1, shall we continue in *s.*
7:7, I had not known *s.*
14:23, whatsoever is not of faith is *s.*
2 Cor. 5:21, made him to be *s.* for us.
2 Thess. 2:3, that man of *s.*
1 Pet. 2:24, his own self bare our *s.*
See 1 John 1:8; 3:4; 4:10; 5:16; Rev. 1:5.
SIN (*v.*). Gen. 42:22, do not *s.* against the child.
Ex. 9:27; 10:16; Num. 22:34; Josh. 7:20; 1 Sam. 15:24; 26:21; 2 Sam. 12:13; Job 7:20; Ps. 41:4; Mat. 27:4; Lu. 15:18, I have *s.*
Job 10:14, if I *s.*, thou markest me.
Ps. 4:4, stand in awe and *s.* not.
39:1, that I *s.* not with my tongue.
Prov. 8:36, he that *s.* against me.
Isa. 43:27, thy first father hath *s.*
Ezek. 18:4, the soul that *s.* it shall die.
Hos. 13:2, now they *s.* more and more.
Mat. 18:21, how oft shall my brother *s.*
John 5:14; 8:11, *s.* no more.
Rom. 6:15, shall we *s.* because.
1 Cor. 15:34, awake to righteousness and *s.* not.
Eph. 4:26, be ye angry, and *s.* not.
1 John 3:9, he cannot *s.* because born of God.
See Num. 15:28; Job 1:5, 22; Rom. 3:23.
SINCERE. Phil. 1:10; 1 Pet. 2:2.
SINCERITY. Josh. 24:14; 1 Cor. 5:8; Eph. 6:24.
SINFUL. Lu. 5:8; 24:7; Rom. 7:13; 8:3.
SINGING. Ps. 100:2; 126:2; Cant. 2:12; Eph. 5:19.
SINGLE. Mat. 6:22; Lu. 11:34.
SINGLENESS. Acts 2:46; Eph. 6:5; Col. 3:22.
SINNER. Gen. 13:13, men of Sodom *s.* exceedingly.
Ps. 1:1, standeth not in way of *s.*
25:8, teach *s.* in the way.
26:9, gather not my soul with *s.*
51:13, *s.* shall be converted.
Prov. 1:10, if *s.* entice thee.
13:21, evil pursueth *s.*
Eccl. 9:18, one *s.* destroyeth much good.
Isa. 33:14, the *s.* in Zion are afraid.
Mat. 9:11; Mk. 2:16; Lu. 5:30; 15:2, eat with *s.*
13; Mk. 2:17; Lu. 5:32, call *s.* to repentance.
11:19; Lu. 7:34, a friend of *s.*
Lu. 7:37, woman who was a *s.*
13:2, suppose ye these were *s.* above all?
15:7, 10, joy over one *s.*
18:13, be merciful to me a *s.*
John 9:16, how can a man that is a *s.* do such miracles?
25, whether he be a *s.* I know not.
Rom. 5:8, while we were yet *s.*
Rom. 5:19, many were made *s.*
Heb. 7:26, separate from *s.*
See Jas. 4:8; 5:20; 1 Pet. 4:18; Jude 15.
SISTER. Job 17:14; Prov. 7:4; Mat. 12:50; 1 Tim. 5:2.
SIT. 2 Kings 7:3, why *s.* we here until we die?
Ps. 69:12, they that *s.* in the gate.
107:10, such as *s.* in darkness.
Isa. 30:7, their strength is to *s.* still.
Jer. 8:14, why do we *s.* still?
Ezek. 33:31, they *s.* before thee as thy people.
Mic. 4:4, they *s.* every man under his vine.
Mal. 3:3, he shall *s.* as a refiner.
Mat. 20:23; Mk. 10:37, to *s.* on my right hand.
See Prov. 23:1; Lam. 3:63; Acts 2:2.
SITUATION. 2 Kings 2:19; Ps. 48:2.
SKILFUL. 1 Chron. 28:21; Ps. 33:3; Ezek. 21:31; Dan. 1:4.
SKILL. 2 Chron. 2:7; Eccl. 9:11; Dan. 1:17; 9:22.
SKIN. Ex. 34:29, wist not that *s.* of his face shone.
Job 2:4, *s.* for *s.*
10:11, thou hast clothed me with *s.* and flesh.
19:26, though after my *s.* worms destroy.
Jer. 13:23, can the Ethiopian change his *s.*
Ezek. 37:6, I will cover you with *s.*
Heb. 11:37, wandered in sheep-*s.*
See Gen. 3:21; 27:16; Ps. 102:5; Mic. 3:2; Mk. 1:6.
SKIP. Ps. 29:6; 114:4; Jer. 48:27.
SKIRT. Ps. 133:2; Jer. 2:34; Zech. 8:23.
SLACK. Deut. 7:10; Prov. 10:4; Zeph. 3:16; 2 Pet. 3:9.
SLAIN. Gen. 4:23, I have *s.* a man.
Prov. 7:26, strong men have been *s.* by her.
22:13, the slothful man saith, I shall be *s.*
24:11, deliver those ready to be *s.*
Isa. 22:2, thy *s.* men are not *s.* with the sword.
26:21, earth shall no more cover her *s.*
66:16, the *s.* of the Lord shall be many.
Jer. 9:1, weep for the *s.* of my people.
Lam. 4:9, *s.* with sword better than *s.* with hunger.
Ezek. 37:9, breathe upon these *s.*
Eph. 2:16, having *s.* the enmity.
Rev. 5:6, a Lamb as it had been *s.*
See 1 Sam. 18:7; 22:21; Lu. 9:22; Heb. 11:37.
SLANDEROUSLY. Rom. 3:8, as we be *s.* reported.
SLAUGHTER. Ps. 44:22, as sheep for the *s.*
Isa. 53:7; Jer. 11:19, brought as a lamb to the *s.*
Jer. 7:32; 19:6, valley of *s.*
Ezek. 9:2, every man a *s.* weapon.
See Hos. 5:2; Zech. 11:4; Acts 9:1; Jas. 5:5.
SLAVE. Jer. 2:14; Rev. 18:13.
SLAY. Gen. 18:25, far from thee to *s.* the righteous.
Job 9:23, if scourge *s.* suddenly.
13:15, though he *s.* me.
See Gen. 4:15; Ex. 21:14; Neh. 4:11; Lu. 11:49; 19:27.
SLEEP (*n.*). 1 Sam. 26:12, deep *s.* from God.
Job 4:13; 33:15, when deep *s.* falleth.
Ps. 13:3, lest I sleep the *s.* of death.
127:2, giveth his beloved *s.*
Prov. 3:24, thy *s.* shall be sweet.
6:10; 24:33, yet a little *s.*
20:13, love not *s.*, lest.
Eccl. 5:12, the *s.* of a labouring man.
Jer. 51:39, sleep a perpetual *s.*
Lu. 9:32, heavy with *s.*
John 11:13, of taking rest in *s.*
Rom. 13:11, high time to awake out of *s.*
See Dan. 2:1; 6:18; 8:18; Acts 16:27; 20:9.
SLEEP (*v.*). Ex. 22:27, raiment, wherein shall he *s.*
Job 7:21, now shall I *s.* in the dust.
Ps. 4:8, I will lay me down and *s.*
121:4, shall neither slumber nor *s.*
Prov. 4:16, they *s.* not, except they have done.
6:22, when thou *s.* it shall keep thee.
10:5, he that *s.* in harvest is a son that causeth shame.
Cant. 5:2, I *s.*, but my heart waketh.
Dan. 12:2, many that *s.* in the dust.
Mat. 9:24; Mk. 5:39; Lu. 8:52, not dead but *s.*
13:25, while men *s.* the enemy sowed.
26:45; Mk. 14:41, *s.* on now.

Mk. 13:36, coming suddenly he find you *s.*
Lu. 22:46, why *s.* ye? rise and pray.
John 11:11, our friend Lazarus *s.*
1 Cor. 11:30, for this cause many *s.*
15:51, we shall not all *s.*
Eph. 5:14, awake thou that *s.*
1 Thess. 4:14, them which *s.* in Jesus.
5:6, let us not *s.* as do others.
7, they that *s. s.* in the night.
10, that whether we wake or *s.*
See Gen. 28:11; 1 Kings 18:27; Acts 12:6; 1 Cor. 15:20.
SLEIGHT. Eph. 4:14, the *s.* of men.
SLEW. Judg. 9:54, a woman *s.* him.
1 Sam. 17:36, *s.* both the lion and the bear.
29:5, Saul *s.* his thousands.
2 Kings 10:9, who *s.* all these?
Ps. 78:34, when he *s.* them, then they sought him.
Isa. 66:3, killeth an ox is as if he *s.* a man.
Dan. 5:19, whom he would he *s.*
Mat. 23:35, whom ye *s.* between temple and altar.
Acts 5:30; 10:39, whom ye *s.* and hanged on a tree.
22:20, kept raiment of them that *s.* him.
Rom. 7:11, sin by the commandment *s.* me.
See Gen. 4:8; Ex. 2:12; 13:15; Neh. 9:26; Lam. 2:4.
SLIDE. Deut. 32:35; Ps. 26:1; 37:31; Hos. 4:16.
SLIGHTLY. Jer. 6:14; 8:11, healed hurt *s.*
SLIME. Gen. 11:3; 14:10; Ex. 2:3.
SLIP. 2 Sam. 22:37; Ps. 18:36, feet did not *s.*
Job 12:5, he that is ready to *s.*
Ps. 17:5, that my footsteps *s.* not.
38:16, when my foot *s.* they magnify.
73:2, my steps had well nigh *s.*
Heb. 2:1, lest we should let them *s.*
See Deut. 19:5; 1 Sam. 19:10; Ps. 94:18.
SLIPPERY. Ps. 35:6; 73:18; Jer. 23:12.
SLOTHFUL. Judg. 18:9, be not *s.* to possess.
Mat. 25:26, thou *s.* servant.
Rom. 12:11, not *s.* in business.
Heb. 6:12, that ye be not *s.*
See Prov. 18:9; 19:24; 24:30; Eccl. 10:18.
SLOW. Ex. 4:10, I am *s.* of speech.
Neh. 9:17, a God *s.* to anger.
Prov. 14:29, *s.* to wrath is of great understanding.
Lu. 24:25, *s.* of heart.
See Acts 27:7; Tit. 1:12; Jas. 1:19.
SLUGGARD. Prov. 6:6, go to the ant, thou *s.*
10:26, so is the *s.* to them that send him.
13:4, the soul of the *s.* desireth.
20:4, the *s.* will not plow.
26:16, the *s.* is wiser in his own conceit.
SLUMBER. Ps. 121:3, that keepeth thee will not *s.*
Prov. 6:4, give not *s.* to thine eyelids.
10; 24:33, a little more *s.*
Isa. 5:27, none shall *s.* among them.
56:10, loving to *s.*
Nah. 3:18, thy shepherds *s.*
Rom. 11:8, hath given them the spirit of *s.*
See Job 33:15; Mat. 25:5; 2 Pet. 2:3.
SMALL. Ex. 16:14, *s.* round thing, *s.* as hoar frost.
18:22, every *s.* matter they shall judge.
Num. 16:9, a *s.* thing that God hath separated.
13, a *s.* thing that thou hast brought us.
Deut. 9:21, I ground the calf *s.*, even as *s.* as dust.
32:2, doctrine distil as *s.* rain.
2 Sam. 7:19; 1 Chron. 17:17, yet a *s.* thing in thy sight.
1 Kings 2:20, one *s.* petition of thee.
2 Kings 19:26, inhabitants of *s.* power.
Job 8:7, thy beginning was *s.*
15:11, are consolations of God *s.*?
36:27, he maketh *s.* the drops of water.
Ps. 119:141, I am *s.*
Prov. 24:10, thy strength is *s.*
Isa. 7:13, is it a *s.* thing to weary men?
16:14, remnant very *s.* and feeble.
40:15, nations as the *s.* dust.
54:7, for a *s.* moment.
60:22, a *s.* one shall become a strong nation.
Jer. 49:15, I will make thee *s.* among heathen.
Dan. 11:23, strong with a *s.* people.
Amos 7:2, by whom shall Jacob arise? for he is *s.*
Zech. 4:10, the day of *s.* things.
Mk. 8:7; John 6:9, a few *s.* fishes.
Acts 12:18; 19:23, no *s.* stir.
15:2, had no *s.* dissension.
Jas. 3:4, turned with very *s.* helm.
See Jer. 44:28; Ezek. 34:18; 1 Cor. 6:2.
SMART. Prov. 11:15, shall *s.* for it.
SMELL. Gen. 27:27, as *s.* of field which the Lord hath blessed.
Deut 4:28, gods that neither see nor *s.*
Job 39:25, he *s.* the battle.
Ps. 45:8, thy garments *s.* of myrrh.
115:6, noses have they, but they *s.* not.
Isa. 3:24, instead of sweet *s.*
Dan. 3:27, nor the *s.* of fire.
1 Cor. 12:17, hearing, where were the *s.*?
Eph. 5:2, sacrifice for sweet-*s.* savour.
Phil. 4:18, an odour of a sweet *s.*
See Cant. 1:12; 2:13; 4:10; 7:8; Amos 5:21.
SMITE. Ex. 2:13, wherefore *s.* thou?
21:12, he that *s.* a man.
1 Sam. 26:8, I will not *s.* him the second time.
2 Kings 6:18, *s.* this people with blindness.
21, shall I *s.* them?
Ps. 121:6, the sun shall not *s.* thee by day.
141:5, let the righteous *s.* me.
Prov. 19:25, *s.* a scorner.
Isa. 10:24, he shall *s.* thee with a rod.
49:10, neither shall heat *s.* thee.
50:6, gave my back to the *s.*
58:4, to *s.* with the fist of wickedness.
Jer. 18:18, let us *s.* him with the tongue.
Lam. 3:30, giveth his cheek to him that *s.*
Ezek. 7:9, know that I am the Lord that *s.*
21:14, prophesy, and *s.* thine hands together.
Nah. 2:10, the knees *s.* together.
Zech. 13:7, awake, O sword, and *s.* the shepherd.
Mal. 4:6, lest I *s.* the earth with a curse.
Mat. 5:39, *s.* thee on the right cheek.
24:49, shall begin to *s.* his fellow servants.
Lu. 22:49, shall we *s.* with sword?
John 18:23, why *s.* thou me?
See Lu. 6:29; Acts 23:2; 2 Cor. 11:20; Rev. 11:6.
SMITH. 1 Sam. 13:19; Isa. 44:12; Jer. 24:1.
SMITTEN. Num. 22:28, that thou hast *s.*
Deut. 28:25, cause thee to be *s.*
1 Sam. 4:3, wherefore hath the Lord *s.* us?
2 Kings 13:19, thou shouldest have *s.* five or six times.
Ps. 3:7, thou hast *s.* all mine enemies.
102:4, my heart is *s.*
Isa. 24:12, the gate is *s.* with destruction.
53:4, *s.* of God.
Jer. 2:30, in vain have I *s.* your children.
Hos. 6:1, he hath *s.* and he will bind.
Amos 4:9, I have *s.* you.
See Job 16:10; Ezek. 22:13; Acts 23:3.
SMOKE. Gen. 19:28, as the *s.* of a furnace.
Deut. 29:20, the anger of the Lord shall *s.*
Ps. 37:20, wicked consume into *s.*
68:2, as *s.* is driven away.
74:1, why doth thy anger *s.*?
102:3, my days are consumed like *s.*
104:32; 144:5, he toucheth the hills, and they *s.*
119:83, like a bottle in the *s.*
Prov. 10:26, as *s.* to the eyes.
Isa. 6:4, the house was filled with *s.*
34:10, the *s.* thereof shall go up for ever.
51:6, the heavens shall vanish like *s.*
65:5, these are a *s.* in my nose.
Hos. 13:3, as the *s.* out of a chimney.
See Rev. 9:2; 14:11; 15:8; 18:9; 19:3.
SMOKING. Gen. 15:17; Ex. 20:18; Isa. 42:3; Mat. 12:20.
SMOOTH. Gen. 27:11, I am a *s.* man.
1 Sam. 17:40; Isa. 57:6, five *s.* stones.

Isa. 30:10, speak unto us *s.* things.
Lu. 3:5, rough ways shall be made *s.*
See Ps. 55:21; Prov. 5:3; Isa. 41:7.
SMOTE. Num. 20:11, Moses *s.* the rock twice.
Judg. 15:8, Samson *s.* them hip and thigh.
1 Sam. 24:5, David's heart *s.* him.
Isa. 60:10, in my wrath I *s.* thee.
Jer. 31:19, I *s.* upon my thigh.
Hag. 2:17, I *s.* you with blasting and mildew.
Mat. 26:68; Lu. 22:64, who is he that *s.* thee?
Lu. 18:13, *s.* upon his breast.
Acts 12:23, immediately angel *s.* him.
See 2 Sam. 14:7; Dan. 2:34; Mat. 27:30.
SNARE. Ex. 10:7, this man be a *s.* unto us.
Deut. 7:25, nor take silver of idols, lest thou be *s.*
12:30, take heed that thou be not *s.* by them.
Josh. 23:13, they shall be *s.* unto you.
Judg. 8:27, which thing became a *s.* to Gideon.
1 Sam. 18:21, that she may be a *s.*
28:9, wherefore layest thou a *s.* for my life?
2 Sam. 22:6; Ps. 18:5, *s.* of death prevented me.
Job 18:8, he walketh on a *s.*
22:10, *s.* are round about thee.
Ps. 11:6, upon the wicked he shall rain *s.*
38:12, they lay *s.* for me.
64:5, commune of laying *s.* privily.
69:22, let their table become a *s.*
91:3, deliver thee from *s.* of fowler.
124:7, the *s.* is broken.
Prov. 6:2; 12:13, *s.* with words of thy mouth.
7:23, as a bird hasteth to the *s.*
13:14; 14:27, the *s.* of death.
18:7, a fool's lips are the *s.* of his soul.
22:25, learn his ways, and get a *s.* to thy soul.
29:8, bring city into *s.*
25, fear of man bringeth a *s.*
Eccl. 9:12, *s.* in an evil time.
Isa. 24:17; Jer. 48:43, the *s.* are upon thee.
Lam. 3:47, fear and a *s.* is come upon us.
Ezek. 12:13, he shall be taken in my *s.*
Hos. 9:8, the prophet is a *s.*
Amos 3:5, can a bird fall in a *s.*?
Lu. 21:35, as a *s.* shall it come.
1 Tim. 3:7, lest he fall into the *s.*
6:9, they that will be rich fall into a *s.*
2 Tim. 2:26, recover out of the *s.* of the devil.
See Ex. 23:33; Deut. 7:16; Judg. 2:3; Eccl. 7:26.
SNATCH. Isa. 9:20, shall *s.* and be hungry.
SNOW. Ex. 4:6; Num. 12:10; 2 Kings 5:27, leprous as *s.*
2 Sam. 23:20, slew lion in time of *s.*
Job 6:16, wherein the *s.* is hid.
9:30, wash myself in *s.* water.
24:19, drought and heat consume *s.* waters.
37:6, saith to *s.*, be thou on the earth.
38:22, the treasures of the *s.*
Ps. 51:7, I shall be whiter than *s.*
147:16, he giveth *s.* like wool.
Prov. 25:13, cold of *s.* in harvest.
26:1, as *s.* in summer.
31:21, she is not afraid of the *s.*
Isa. 1:18, your sins shall be white as *s.*
55:10, as the *s.* from heaven returneth not.
Jer. 18:14, will a man leave the *s.* of Lebanon?
Lam. 4:7, Nazarites purer than *s.*
Dan. 7:9; Mat. 28:3; Mk. 9:3, garment white as *s.*
See Ps. 68:14; 148:8; Rev. 1:14.
SNUFFED. Jer. 14:6; Mal. 1:13.
SOAKED. Isa. 34:7, land *s.* with blood.
SOAP. Jer. 2:22; Mal. 3:2.
SOBER. 2 Cor. 5:13, *s.* for your cause.
1 Thess. 5:6, let us watch and be *s.*
1 Tim. 3:2; Tit. 1:8, a bishop must be *s.*
Tit. 2:2, aged men be *s.*
4, teach young women to be *s.*
1 Pet. 4:7, be ye therefore *s.*, and watch.
See Acts 26:25; Rom. 12:3; Tit. 2:6.
SODDEN. Ex. 12:9; 1 Sam. 2:15; Lam. 4:10.
SOFT. Job 23:16, God maketh my heart *s.*
41:3, will he speak *s.* words?
Ps. 65:10, thou makest it *s.* with showers.
Prov. 15:1, a *s.* answer turneth away wrath.
25:15, a *s.* tongue breaketh the bone.
See Ps. 55:21; Mat. 11:8; Lu. 7:25.
SOFTLY. Gen. 33:14; Judg. 4:21; 1 Kings 21:27; Isa. 38:15.
SOIL. Ezek. 17:8, planted in a good *s.*
SOJOURN. Gen. 19:9, this fellow came in to *s.*
26:3, *s.* in this land, and I will be with thee.
47:4, to *s.* in the land are we come.
Deut. 26:5, *s.* with a few, and became a nation.
Judg. 17:9, I go to *s.* where I may find place.
2 Kings 8:1, *s.* wheresoever thou canst *s.*
Ps. 120:5, woe is me, that I *s.*
Isa. 23:7, feet carry her afar off to *s.*
Jer. 42:22, die in place whither ye desire to *s.*
Lam. 4:15, they shall no more *s.* there.
Heb. 11:9, by faith he *s.* in land of promise.
1 Pet. 1:17, pass time of your *s.* here in fear.
SOJOURNER. Gen. 23:4; Ps. 39:12.
SOLD. Gen. 31:15, our father hath *s.* us.
45:4, whom ye *s.* into Egypt.
Lev. 25:23, the land shall not be *s.* for ever.
42, shall not be *s.* as bondmen.
27:28, no devoted thing shall be *s.*
Deut. 15:12, if thy brother be *s.* unto thee.
32:30, except their Rock had *s.* them.
1 Kings 21:20, thou hast *s.* thyself to work evil.
Neh. 5:8, or shall they be *s.* unto us?
Esth. 7:4, for we are *s.* to be slain.
Isa. 50:1, have ye *s.* yourselves?
52:3, ye have *s.* yourselves for nought.
Lam. 5:4, our wood is *s.* unto us.
Joel 3:3, they have *s.* a girl for wine.
Amos 2:6, they *s.* the righteous for silver.
Mat. 10:29, are not two sparrows *s.* for a farthing?
13:46, went and *s.* all that he had.
18:25, his lord commanded him to be *s.*
21:12; Mk. 11:15, cast out them that *s.*
26:9; Mk. 14:5, might have been *s.* for much.
Lu. 17:28, they bought, they *s.*, they planted.
Acts 2:45, and *s.* their possessions.
Rom. 7:14, *s.* under sin.
1 Cor. 10:25, whatsoever is *s.* in the shambles.
See Lu. 19:45; John 12:5; Acts 5:1; Heb. 12:16.
SOLDIER. Ezra 8:22, ashamed to require *s.*
Mat. 8:9; Lu. 7:8, having *s.* under me.
Lu. 3:14, *s.* demanded, what shall we do?
Acts 10:7, a devout *s.*
2 Tim. 2:3, as a good *s.* of Jesus Christ.
See 2 Chron. 25:13; Isa. 15:4; Acts 27:31.
SOLE. Gen. 8:9, dove found no rest for *s.* of her foot.
2 Sam. 14:25; Isa. 1:6, from *s.* of foot to crown.
See Deut. 28:35, 56, 65; Josh. 1:3; Job 2:7.
SOLEMN. Ps. 92:3, sing praise with a *s.* sound.
See Num. 10:10; Isa. 1:13; Lam. 2:22; Hos. 9:5.
SOLEMNITY. Isa. 30:29, when a holy *s.* is kept.
See Deut. 31:10; Isa. 33:20; Ezek. 45:17; 46:11.
SOLEMNLY. Gen. 43:3; 1 Sam. 8:9.
SOLITARY. Ps. 68:6, God setteth the *s.* in families.
107:4, wandered in a *s.* way.
Isa. 35:1, the wilderness and *s.* place shall be glad.
See Job 3:7; 30:3; Lam. 1:1; Mic. 7:14; Mk. 1:35.
SOME. Gen. 37:20, *s.* evil beast.
Ex. 16:17, gathered, *s.* more, *s.* less.
1 Kings 14:13, found *s.* good thing.
Ps. 20:7, *s.* trust in chariots.
69:20, I looked for *s.* to take pity.
Dan. 12:2, *s.* to life, and *s.* to shame.
Mat. 16:14; Mk. 8:28; Lu. 9:19, *s.* say thou art John the Baptist.
28:17, *s.* doubted.
John 6:64, *s.* of you that believe not.
Acts 19:32; 21:34, *s.* cried one thing, *s.* another.
Rom. 3:3, what if *s.* did not believe?
5:7, *s.* would even dare to die.

1 Cor. 6:11, such were *s.* of you.
15:34, *s.* have not knowledge.
Eph. 4:11, *s.* prophets, *s.* evangelists.
1 Tim. 5:24, *s.* men's sins are open.
Heb. 10:25, as the manner of *s.* is.
2 Pet. 3:9, as *s.* men count slackness.
See 1 Tim. 1:19; 2 Tim. 2:18; Jude 22.
SOMEBODY. Lu. 8:46; Acts 5:36.
SOMETIMES. Eph. 2:13, *s.* far off.
5:8, ye were *s.* darkness.
Col. 1:21, *s.* alienated.
See Col. 3:7; Tit. 3:3; 1 Pet. 3:20.
SOMEWHAT. 1 Kings 2:14; Gal. 2:6; Rev. 2:4.
SON. Gen. 6:2; Job 1:6; 2:1; 38:7; John 1:12; Phil. 2:15; 1 John 3:1, *s.* of God.
Job 14:21, his *s.* come to honour.
Ps. 2:12, kiss the *S.*, lest he be angry.
86:16, save *s.* of thine handmaid.
116:16, I am the *s.* of thine handmaid.
Prov. 10:1; 13:1; 15:20; 17:2; 19:26, a wise *s.*
17:25; 19:13, a foolish *s.*
31:2, *s.* of my womb, *s.* of my vows.
Isa. 9:6, unto us a *s.* is given.
14:12, *s.* of the morning.
Jer. 35:5, *s.* of the Rechabites.
Ezek. 20:31; 23:37, *s.* pass through fire.
Hos. 1:10, the *s.* of the living God.
Mal. 3:17, as a man spareth his *s.*
Mat. 11:27, no man knoweth the *S.*
13:55; Mk. 6:3; Lu. 4:22, the carpenter's *s.*
17:5, this is my beloved *S.*
22:42, Christ, whose *s.* is he?
Lu. 7:12, only *s.* of his mother.
10:6, if the *s.* of peace.
19:9, he also is a *s.* of Abraham.
John 1:18; 3:18, only begotten *S.*
5:21, the *S.* quickeneth whom he will.
8:35, the *S.* abideth ever.
36, if the *S.* make you free.
17:12; 2 Thess. 2:3, the *s.* of perdition.
Acts 4:36, *s.* of consolation.
Rom. 1:9, serve in the gospel of his *S.*
8:3, God sending his own *S.*
29, conformed to the image of his *S.*
32, spared not his own *S.*
1 Cor. 4:14, as my beloved *s.* I warn you.
Gal. 4:5, the adoption of *s.*
7, if a *s.*, then an heir.
Col. 1:13, the kingdom of his dear *S.*
Heb. 2:10, bringing many *s.* to glory.
5:8, though a *S.*, yet learned he obedience.
11:24, refused to be called *s.*
12:6, scourgeth every *s.*
1 John 2:22, antichrist denieth the *s.*
5:12, he that hath the *S.* hath life.
See 1 John 1:7; 4:9; 5:10, 11; Rev. 21:7.
SONGS. Job 30:9, now am I their *s.*
35:10; Ps. 77:6, who giveth *s.* in the night.
Ps. 32:7, with *s.* of deliverance.
33:3; Isa. 42:10, sing unto him a new *s.*
40:3, he hath put a new *s.* in my mouth.
69:12, I was the *s.* of drunkards.
119:54, my *s.* in house of my pilgrimage.
137:4, the Lord's *s.* in a strange land.
Prov. 25:20, that singeth *s.* to an heavy heart.
Isa. 23:16, sing many *s.*
35:10, the ransomed shall come with *s.*
Ezek. 33:32, as a very lovely *s.*
Amos 8:3, *s.* of the temple.
Eph. 5:19; Col. 3:16, in psalms and spiritual *s.*
See Cant. 1:1; Rev. 5:9; 14:3; 15:3.
SOON. Ex. 2:18, how is it ye are come so *s.*?
Job 32:22, my Maker would *s.* take me away.
Ps. 37:2, shall *s.* be cut down.
58:3, go astray as *s.* as born.
68:31, Ethiopia shall *s.* stretch out her hands.
90:10, it is *s.* cut off.
Ps. 106:13, they *s.* forgat his works.
Prov. 14:17, he that is *s.* angry.
See Mat. 21:20; Gal. 1:6; 2 Thess. 2:2; Tit. 1:7.
SORE. 2 Chron. 6:29; Isa. 1:6; Lu. 16:20.
SORROW. Gen. 3:16, multiply thy *s.*
42:28, with *s.* to the grave.
Job 6:10, I would harden myself in *s.*
21:17, God distributeth *s.* in his anger.
41:22, *s.* is turned into joy.
Ps. 13:2, having *s.* in my heart daily.
90:10, yet is their strength labour and *s.*
116:3, I found trouble and *s.*
127:2, to eat the bread of *s.*
Prov. 10:22, maketh rich, addeth no *s.*
23:29, who hath *s.*?
Eccl. 2:23, all his days are *s.*
7:3, *s.* is better than laughter.
11:10, remove *s.* from thy heart.
Isa. 17:11, day of desperate *s.*
35:10; 51:11, *s.* and sighing shall flee away.
53:3, a man of *s.*
Jer. 30:15, thy *s.* is incurable.
49:23, there is *s.* on the sea.
Lam. 1:12, any *s.* like unto my *s.*
Mat. 24:8; Mk. 13:8, beginning of *s.*
Lu. 22:45, sleeping for *s.*
John 16:6, *s.* hath filled your heart.
2 Cor. 2:7, with overmuch *s.*
7:10, godly *s.* worketh repentance.
1 Thess. 4:13, *s.* not as others.
1 Tim. 6:10, pierced with many *s.*
See Prov. 15:13; Hos. 8:10; Rev. 21:4.
SORROWFUL. 1 Sam. 1:15, woman of a *s.* spirit.
Ps. 69:29, I am poor and *s.*
Prov. 14:13, even in laughter the heart is *s.*
Jer. 31, 25, replenished every *s.* soul.
Zeph. 3:18, I will gather them that are *s.*
Mat. 19:22; Lu. 18:23, went away *s.*
26:37, he began to be *s.*
38; Mk. 14:34, my soul is exceeding *s.*
John 16:20, ye shall be *s.*
See Job 6:7; 2 Cor. 6:10; Phil. 2:28.
SORRY. Ps. 38:18, I will be *s.* for my sin.
Isa. 51:19, who shall be *s.* for thee?
See 1 Sam. 22:8; Neh. 8:10; Mat. 14:9.
SORT. Gen. 6:19, two of every *s.*
1 Chron. 29:14, to offer after this *s.*
Dan. 3:29, deliver after this *s.*
Acts 17:5, fellows of the baser *s.*
2 Cor. 7:11; 3 John 6, after a godly *s.*
2 Tim. 3:6, of this *s.* are they.
See Deut. 22:11; Eccl. 2:8; Ezek. 27:24; 38:4.
SOTTISH. Jer. 4:22, they are *s.* children.
SOUGHT. Gen. 43:30, he *s.* where to weep.
Ex. 4:24, the Lord *s.* to kill him.
1 Sam. 13:14, the Lord hath *s.* him a man.
1 Chron. 15:13, we *s.* him not after due order.
2 Chron. 15:4, when they *s.* him he was found.
15, they *s.* him with their whole desire.
16:12, in his disease he *s.* not the Lord.
26:5, as long as he *s.* the Lord.
Ps. 34:4; 77:2, I *s.* the Lord, and he heard me.
111:2, *s.* out of all that have pleasure.
Eccl. 7:29, *s.* out many inventions.
12:10, the preacher *s.* to find acceptable words.
Isa. 62:12, shalt be called, *S.* out.
65:1, *s.* of them that asked not.
Jer. 10:21, pastors have not *s.* the Lord.
Lam. 1:19, they *s.* meat to relieve their souls.
Ezek. 22:30, I *s.* for a man among them.
34:4, neither have ye *s.* that which was lost.
Lu. 11:16, *s.* of him a sign.
13:6, he *s.* fruit thereon.
19:3, *s.* to see Jesus.
Rom. 9:32, *s.* it not by faith.
Heb. 12:17, though he *s.* it carefully with tears.
See Cant. 3:1; Lu. 2:44; 1 Thess. 2:6.

SOUL. Gen. 2:7, a living *s.*
Ex. 30:12, a ransom for his *s.*
Deut. 11:13, serve him with all your *s.*
13:6, thy friend, which is as thine own *s.*
30:2; Mat. 22:37, obey with all thy *s.*
Judg. 10:16, his *s.* was grieved.
1 Sam. 18:1; 20:17, loved him as his own *s.*
1 Kings 8:48, return with all their *s.*
1 Chron. 22:19, set your *s.* to seek the Lord.
Job 3:20, life unto the bitter in *s.*
12:10, in whose hand is the *s.*
16:4, if your *s.* were in my *s.* stead.
23:13, what his *s.* desireth, even that he doeth.
31:30, wishing a curse to his *s.*
33:22, his *s.* draweth near to the grave.
Ps. 33:19, to deliver their *s.* from death.
34:22, redeemeth the *s.* of his servants.
49:8, the redemption of their *s.* is precious.
62:1, my *s.* waiteth upon God.
63:1, my *s.* thirsteth for thee.
74:19, the *s.* of thy turtledove.
103:1; 104:1, bless the Lord, O my *s.*
116:7, return to thy rest, O my *s.*
8, thou hast delivered my *s.* from death.
119:175, let my *s.* live.
142:4, no man cared for my *s.*
Prov. 11:25, the liberal *s.* shall be made fat.
19:2, *s.* without knowledge.
25:25, cold waters to thirsty *s.*
Isa. 55:3, hear, and your *s.* shall live.
58:10, if thou wilt satisfy the afflicted *s.*
Jer. 20:13, hath delivered the *s.* of the poor.
31:12, their *s.* shall be as a watered garden.
Ezek. 18:4, all *s.* are mine.
22:25, they have devoured *s.*
Hab. 2:10, thou hast sinned against thy *s.*
Mat. 10:28, to destroy both *s.* and body.
16:26; Mk. 8:36, lose his own *s.*
26:38; Mk. 14:34, my *s.* is exceeding sorrowful.
Lu. 21:19, in your patience possess ye your *s.*
Acts 4:32, of one heart and *s.*
Rom. 13:1, let every *s.* be subject.
1 Thess. 5:23, that your *s.* and body be preserved.
Heb. 6:19, an anchor of the *s.*
13:17, they watch for your *s.*
Jas. 5:20, shall save a *s.* from death.
1 Pet. 2:11, which war against the *s.*
4:19, commit keeping of *s.* to him.
2 Pet. 2:14, beguiling unstable *s.*
3 John 2, even as thy *s.* prospereth.
See Prov. 3:22; Ezek. 3:19; Acts 15:24.
SOUND (*n.*). Lev. 26:36, the *s.* of a shaken leaf.
1 Kings 18:41, *s.* of abundance of rain.
Job 15:21, a dreadful *s.* is in his ears.
Ps. 89:15, that know the joyful *s.*
92:3, harp with a solemn *s.*
Eccl. 12:4, *s.* of grinding is low.
Jer. 50:22, *s.* of battle in the land.
51:54, *s.* of a cry cometh.
Ezek. 33:5, he heard *s.*, and took not warning.
John 3:8, thou hearest the *s.*, but canst not tell.
Acts 2:2, suddenly a *s.* from heaven.
Rom. 10:18, *s.* went into all the earth.
1 Cor. 14:8, an uncertain *s.*
See 2 Kings 6:32; Rev. 1:15; 9:9; 18:22.
SOUND (*adj.*). Prov. 2:7; 3:21; 8:14, *s.* wisdom.
Prov. 14:30, a *s.* heart is life of the flesh.
1 Tim. 1:10; 2 Tim. 4:3; Tit. 1:9; 2:1, *s.* doctrine.
2 Tim. 1:7, spirit of a *s.* mind.
13, form of *s.* words.
See Ps. 119:80; Lu. 15:27; Tit. 2:2, 8.
SOUND (*v.*). Ex. 19:19, the trumpet *s.* long.
Joel 2:1, *s.* an alarm in holy mountain.
Mat. 6:2, do not *s.* a trumpet before thee.
1 Thess. 1:8, from you *s.* out word of the Lord.
See Neh. 4:18; 1 Cor. 13:1; 15:52; Rev. 8:7.
SOUR. Isa. 18:5; Jer. 31:29; Ezek. 18:2; Hos. 4:18.
SOW. Job 4:8, they that *s.* wickedness.
Ps. 97:11, light is *s.* for the righteous.
126:5, *s.* in tears.
Prov. 6:16, he that *s.* discord.
Eccl. 11:4, he that observeth the wind shall not *s.*
6, in morning *s.* thy seed.
Isa. 32:20, that *s.* beside all waters.
Jer. 4:3, *s.* not among thorns.
12:13, they have *s.* wheat, but shall reap thorns.
Hos. 10:12, *s.* in righteousness, reap in mercy.
Nah. 1:14, that no more of thy name be *s.*
Hag. 1:6, ye have *s.* much, and bring in little.
Mat. 6:26, they *s.* not.
37, he that *s.* good seed.
John 4:36, both he that *s.* and he that reapeth.
1 Cor. 15:36, that which thou *s.* is not quickened.
2 Cor. 9:6, he which *s.* sparingly.
Gal. 6:7, whatsoever a man *s.*, that shall he reap.
See Lev. 26:5; Deut. 11:10; Jer. 2:2; Jas. 3:18.
SOWER. Isa. 55:10; Jer. 50:16; Mat. 13:3; Mk. 4:3; Lu. 8:5; 2 Cor. 9:10.
SPAKE. Ps. 39:3, then *s.* I with my tongue.
106:33, he *s.* unadvisedly with his lips.
Mal. 3:16, *s.* often one to another.
John 7:46, never man *s.* like this man.
1 Cor. 13:11, I *s.* as a child.
Heb. 12:25, refused him that *s.* on earth.
2 Pet. 1:21, holy men *s.* as they were moved.
See Gen. 35:15; John 9:29; Heb. 1:1.
SPAN. Ex. 28:16; Isa. 40:12; 48:13; Lam. 2:20.
SPARE. Gen. 18:26, I will *s.* for their sakes.
Neh. 13:22, *s.* me according to thy mercy.
Ps. 39:13, *s.* me, that I may recover strength.
Prov. 13:24, he that *s.* the rod.
19:18, let not thy soul *s.* for his crying.
Joel 2:17, *s.* thy people.
Mal. 3:17, I will *s.* them as a man *s.*
Lu. 15:17, bread enough and to *s.*
Rom. 8:32, *s.* not his own Son.
11:21, if God *s.* not the natural branches.
2 Pet. 2:4, if God *s.* not the angels.
See Prov. 17:27; 21:26; Isa. 54, 2; 58:1.
SPARK. Job 5:7; 18:5; Isa. 1:31; 50:11.
SPEAK. Gen. 18:37, to *s.* to God.
Ex. 4:14, I know he can *s.* well.
33:11, spake to Moses as a man *s.* to his friend.
Num. 20:8, *s.* to the rock.
1 Sam. 25:17, a man cannot *s.* to him.
Job 11:5, oh that God would *s.* against thee.
13:7, will ye *s.* wickedly for God?
32:7, days should *s.*
33:14, God *s.* once, yea, twice.
37:20, if a man *s.* he shall be swallowed up.
Ps. 85:8, I will hear what the Lord will *s.*
Prov. 23:9, *s.* not in the ears of a fool.
Cant. 7:9, causing lips of those asleep to *s.*
Isa. 19:18, shall *s.* language of Canaan.
63:1, I that *s.* in righteousness.
65:24, while they are yet *s.*, I will hear.
Jer. 20:9, I will not *s.* any more in his name.
Hab. 2:3, at the end it shall *s.*
Zech. 8:16; Eph. 4:25, *s.* every man the truth.
Mat. 8:8, *s.* the word only, and my servant.
10:19; Mk. 13:11, how or what ye shall *s.*
12:34; Lu. 6:45, of abundance of heart mouth *s.*
36, every idle word that men shall *s.*
Mk. 9:39, can lightly *s.* evil of me.
Lu. 6:26, when all men *s.* well of you.
John 3:11, we *s.* that we do know.
Acts 4:17, that they *s.* to no man in this name.
20, we cannot but *s.*
26:25, I *s.* words of truth and soberness.
1 Cor. 1:10, that ye all *s.* the same thing.
14:28, let him *s.* to himself and to God.
2 Cor. 4:13, we believe and therefore *s.*
Eph. 4:15, *s.* the truth in love.
Heb. 11:4, he being dead yet *s.*

Heb. 12:24, that *s.* better things than that of Abel.
Jas. 1:19, slow to *s.*
See 1 Cor. 14:2; 1 Pet. 2:1; 2 Pet. 2:12.
SPEAR. Josh. 8:18, stretch out the *s.*
Judg. 5:8, was there a shield or *s.* seen?
1 Sam. 13:22, nor *s.* with any but Saul.
17:7, the staff of his *s.*
45, thou comest to me with a *s.*
Ps. 46:9, he cutteth the *s.* in sunder.
Isa. 2:4; Mic. 4:3, beat *s.* into pruninghooks.
See Job 41:29; Jer. 6:23; Hab. 3:11; John 19:34.
SPECIAL. Deut. 7:6; Acts 19:11.
SPECTACLE. 1 Cor. 4:9, made a *s.* to the world.
SPEECH. Gen. 11:1, earth was of one *s.*
Ex. 4:10, I am slow of *s.*
Num. 12:8, not in dark *s.*
Deut. 32:2, my *s.* shall distil as dew.
1 Kings 3:10, Solomon's *s.* pleased the Lord.
Job 6:26, the *s.* of one that is desperate.
15:3, or with *s.* wherewith he can do no good.
Ps. 19:2, day unto day uttereth *s.*
3, there is no *s.* where their voice is not heard.
Prov. 17:7, excellent *s.* becometh not a fool.
Cant. 4:3, thy *s.* is comely.
Isa. 33:19, of deeper *s.* than thou canst perceive.
Mat. 26:73, thy *s.* bewrayeth thee.
1 Cor. 2:1, not with excellency of *s.*
4:19, not the *s.*, but the power.
2 Cor. 3:12, we use great plainness of *s.*
10:10, his *s.* is contemptible.
Col. 4, 6, let your *s.* be alway with grace.
Tit. 2:8, sound *s.*, that cannot be condemned.
See Ezek. 3:5; Rom. 16:18; 2 Cor. 11:6.
SPEECHLESS. Mat. 22:12; Lu. 1:22; Acts 9:7.
SPEED. Gen. 24:12, send me good *s.*
2 John 10, receive him not, neither bid him God *s.*
See Ezra 6:12; Isa. 5:26; Acts 17:15.
SPEEDILY. Ps. 31:2, deliver me *s.*
63:17; 143:7, hear me *s.*
Ps. 79:8, let thy mercies *s.* prevent us.
102:2, when I call, answer me *s.*
Eccl. 8:11, because sentence is not executed *s.*
Isa. 58:8, thy health shall spring forth *s.*
Zech. 8:21, let us go *s.* to pray.
Lu. 18:8, he will avenge them *s.*
See 1 Sam. 27:1; Ezra 6:13; 7:17; Joel 3:4.
SPEND. Job 21:13, they *s.* their days in wealth.
36:11, they *s.* their days in prosperity.
Ps. 90:9, we *s.* our years as a tale that is told.
Isa. 55:2, why *s.* money for that which is not bread?
2 Cor. 12:15, very gladly *s.* and be spent for you.
See Prov. 21:20; Eccl. 6:12; Lu. 10:35.
SPENT. Gen. 21:15, water was *s.* in the bottle.
Job 7:6, days *s.* without hope.
Ps. 31:10, my life is *s.* with grief.
Isa. 49:4, I have *s.* my strength for nought.
Acts 17:21, *s.* their time to tell some new thing.
See Mk. 6:35; Lu. 15:14; 24:29; Rom. 13:12.
SPILT. 2 Sam. 14:14, as water *s.*
SPIN. Ex. 35:25; Mat. 6:28; Lu. 12:27.
SPIRIT. Gen. 6:3, my *s.* shall not always strive.
Ex. 35:21, every one whom his *s.* made willing.
Num. 11:17, take of the *s.* that is on thee.
14:24, he had another *s.* with him.
16:22; 27:16, the God of the *s.* of all flesh.
27:18, a man in whom is the *s.*
Josh. 5:1, nor was there any more *s.* in them.
1 Kings 22:21; 2 Chron. 18:20, there came forth a *s.*
2 Kings 2:9, let a double portion of thy *s.*
Neh. 9:20, thou gavest thy good *s.* to instruct.
Job 4:15, a *s.* passed before my face.
15:13, thou turnest thy *s.* against God.
26:4, whose *s.* came from thee?
32:8, there is a *s.* in man.
Ps. 31:5; Lu. 23:46, into thine hand I commit my *s.*
32:2, in whose *s.* there is no guile.
51:10, renew a right *s.* within me.
Ps. 78:8, whose *s.* was not stedfast.
104:4; Heb. 1:7, who maketh his angels *s.*
106:33, they provoked his *s.*
139:7, whither shall I go from thy *s.*?
Prov. 16:2, the Lord weigheth the *s.*
18, an haughty *s.* goeth before a fall.
19; 29:23; Isa. 57:15, an humble *s.*
32, he that ruleth his *s.* better than he.
Eccl. 3:21, who knoweth *s.* of man, and *s.* of beast?
7:8, the patient in *s.* better than the proud.
8:8, no man hath power over *s.* to retain *s.*
11:5, the way of the *s.*
12:7, the *s.* shall return to God.
Isa. 4:4; 28:6, *s.* of judgment.
11:2; Eph. 1:17, the *s.* of wisdom.
34:16, his *s.* it hath gathered them.
42:1, I have put my *s.* upon him.
57:16, the *s.* should fail before me.
61:1; Lu. 4:18, the *S.* of the Lord is upon me.
Ezek. 3:14; 8:3; 11:1, I went in the heat of my *s.*
11:19; 18:31; 36:26, a new *s.*
Mic. 2:11, a man walking in the *s.* and falsehood.
Mat. 14:26; Mk. 6:49, it is a *s.*
26:41; Mk. 14:38, the *s.* is willing.
Mk. 1:10; John 1:32, the *S.* descending on him.
8:12, sighed deeply in his *s.*
Lu. 1:17, go before him in *s.* and power of Elias.
2:27, came by the *S.* into the temple.
8:55, her *s.* came again.
9:55, ye know not what manner of *s.*
10:21, Jesus rejoiced in *s.*
24:39, a *s.* hath not flesh and bones.
John 3:34, God giveth not the *S.* by measure.
4:24, God is a *S.*, worship him in *s.* and in truth.
6:63, it is the *s.* that quickeneth.
14:17; 15:26; 16:13; 1 John 4:6, *S.* of truth.
Acts 2:4, begin to speak as the *S.* gave utterance.
6:10, not able to resist the wisdom and *s.*
17:16, his *s.* was stirred within him.
23:8, say that there is neither angel nor *s.*
Rom. 8:1, walk not after the flesh, but after the *S.*
2, the law of the *S.* of life.
11, the *S.* of him that raised up Jesus.
16, the *S.* itself beareth witness.
26, the *S.* maketh intercession.
12:11, fervent in *s.*
1 Cor. 2:4, in demonstration of the *S.*
10, the *S.* searcheth all things.
4:21; Gal. 6:1, in the *s.* of meekness.
6:17, he that is joined to the Lord is one *s.*
20, glorify God in body and *s.*
12:4, diversities of gifts, but the same *S.*
10, to another discerning of *s.*
14:2, in the *s.* he speaketh mysteries.
15:45, the last Adam made a quickening *s.*
2 Cor. 3:6, the letter killeth, but the *s.* giveth life.
17, where the *S.* of the Lord is, there is liberty.
Gal. 3:3, having begun in the *S.*
5:16, walk in the *S.*
22; Eph. 5:9, the fruit of the *S.*
25, if we live in the *S.*, let us walk in the *S.*
6:8, he that soweth to the *S.* shall of the *S.* reap.
Eph. 2:2, the *s.* that worketh in children of disobedience.
18, access by one *S.*
22, habitation of God through the *S.*
3:16, strengthened by his *S.* in inner man.
4:3, the unity of the *S.*
4, one body and one *S.*
23, renewed in *s.* of your mind.
30, grieve not the holy *S.* of God.
5:18, be filled with the *S.*
6:17, take sword of the *S.*
Phil. 1:27, stand fast in one *s.*
2:1, if any fellowship of the *S.*
Col. 1:8, your love in the *s.*
2:5, absent in flesh, yet with you in the *s.*
1 Thess. 5:19, quench not the *S.*

2 Thess. 2:13, chosen through sanctification of the *S.*
1 Tim. 3:16, justified in the *S.*
4:1, giving heed to seducing *s.*
12, be thou an example in *s.*
2 Tim. 4:22, the Lord Jesus be with thy *s.*
Heb. 1:14, ministering *s.*
4:12, dividing asunder of soul and *s.*
9:14, who through the eternal *S.*
12:9, in subjection to the Father of *s.*
23, to *s.* of just men made perfect.
Jas. 2:26, the body without the *s.* is dead.
4:5, the *s.* lusteth to envy.
1 Pet. 1:2, through sanctification of the *S.*
3:4, ornament of a meek and quiet *s.*
18, but quickened by the *S.*
19, preached to *s.* in prison.
4:6, live according to God in the *s.*
1 John 3:24, by the *S.* he hath given us.
4:1, believe not every *s.*, but try the *s.*
2, hereby know ye the *S.* of God.
3, every *s.* that confesseth not.
5:6, it is the *S.* that beareth witness.
8, the *s.*, the water, and the blood.
Jude 19, sensual, having not the *S.*
Rev. 1:10, I was in the *S.* on the Lord's day.
2:7, 11, 17, 29; 3:6, 13, 22, hear what the *S.* saith.
4:2, I was in the *s.*, and, behold.
11:11, the *S.* of life from God entered.
14:13, blessed are the dead: Yea, saith the *S.*
22:17, the *S.* and the bride say, Come.
See Mat. 8:16; John 3:5; Acts 7:59; Rom. 7:6.
SPIRITUAL. Hos. 9:7, the *s.* man is mad.
Rom. 1:11, impart some *s.* gift.
7:14, the law is *s.*
15:27, partakers of their *s.* things.
1 Cor. 2:13, comparing *s.* things with *s.*
15, he that is *s.* judgeth all things.
3:1, not speak unto you as unto *s.*
10:3, all eat the same *s.* meat.
12:1; 14:1, concerning *s.* gifts.
15:44, it is raised a *s.* body.
46, that was not first which is *s.*
Gal. 6:1, ye. which are *s.*, restore such an one.
Eph. 5:19, in psalms and hymns and *s.* songs.
6:12, *s.* wickedness in high places.
1 Pet. 2:5, a *s.* house, to offer up *s.* sacrifices.
See 1 Cor. 9:11; Col. 1:9; 3:16.
SPIRITUALLY. Rom. 8:6; 1 Cor. 2:14; Rev. 11:8.
SPITE. Ps. 10:14, thou beholdest mischief and *s.*
SPOIL (*n.*). Judg. 5:30, necks of them that take *s.*
1 Sam. 14:32, people flew upon the *s.*
2 Chron. 15:11, offered to the Lord of the *s.*
20:25, three days gathering the *s.*
28:15, with the *s.* they clothed the naked.
Esth. 3:13; 8:11, take the *s.* of them for a prey.
9:10, on the *s.* laid they not their hand.
Job 29:17, I plucked the *s.* out of his teeth.
Ps. 119:162, rejoice as one that findeth great *s.*
Prov. 16:19, than to divide *s.* with the proud.
31:11, he shall have no need of *s.*
Isa. 3:14, the *s.* of the poor is in your houses.
42:24, who gave Jacob for a *s.*?
53:12, divide the *s.* with the strong.
See Isa. 9:3; Ezek. 7:21; 38:13; Nah. 2:9; Zech. 14:1.
SPOIL (*v.*). Ex. 3:22, ye shall *s.* the Egyptians.
Ps. 78:5, the stouthearted are *s.*
Cant. 2:15, the little foxes that *s.* the vines.
Isa. 33:1, woe to thee that *s.*, and thou wast not *s.*!
42:22, this is a people robbed and *s.*
Jer. 4:30, when *s.*, what wilt thou do?
Hab. 2:8, thou hast *s.* many nations.
Zech. 11:2, howl because the mighty are *s.*
Col. 2:15, having *s.* principalities.
See Ps. 35:10; Isa. 22:4; Col. 2:8; Heb. 10:34.
SPOKEN. Num. 23:19, hath he *s.*, and shall he not make it good?
1 Sam. 1:16, out of my grief have I *s.*
1 Kings 18:24, the people said, it is well *s.*
2 Kings 4:13, wouldest thou be *s.* for to the king?
Ps. 62:11, God hath *s.* once.
66:14, my mouth hath *s.* when in trouble.
87:3, glorious things are *s.* of thee.
Prov. 15:23, a word *s.* in due season.
25:11, a word fitly *s.* is like.
Eccl. 7:21, take no heed to all words *s.*
Isa. 48:15, I, even I, have *s.*
Mal. 3:13, what have we *s.* so much against?
Mk. 14:9, shall be *s.* of for a memorial.
Lu. 2:34, for a sign which shall be *s.* against.
Acts 19:36, these things cannot be *s.* against.
Rom. 1:8, your faith is *s.* of.
14:16, let not your good be evil *s.* of.
Heb. 2:2, the word *s.* by angels.
See Heb. 13:7; 1 Pet. 4:14; 2 Pet. 3:2.
SPOKESMAN. Ex. 4:16, he shall be thy *s.*
SPORT. Gen. 26:8; Isa. 57:4; 2 Pet. 2:13.
SPOT. Num. 28:3; 9:11; 29:17, lambs without *s.*
Deut. 32:5, their *s.* is not the *s.* of his children.
Job 11:15, lift up thy face without *s.*
Jer. 13:23, or the leopard his *s.*
Eph. 5:27, glorious church, not having *s.*
1 Tim. 6:14, commandment without *s.*
Heb. 9:14, offered himself without *s.*
1 Pet. 1:19, lamb without blemish or *s.*
2 Pet. 3:14, that ye may be found without *s.*
Jude 12, these are *s.* in your feasts.
See Cant. 4:7; 2 Pet. 2:13; Jude 23.
SPOUSE. Cant. 4:8; 5:1; Hos. 4:13.
SPRANG. Mk. 4:8; Acts 16:29; Heb. 7:14; 11:12.
SPREAD. Deut. 32:11, eagle *s.* abroad her wings.
2 Kings 19:14; Isa. 37:14, *s.* letter before the Lord.
Job 9:8, God who alone *s.* out the heavens.
26:9, he *s.* his cloud upon it.
29:19, my root was *s.* out by waters.
36:30, he *s.* his light upon it.
37:18, hast thou with him *s.* out the sky?
Ps. 105:39, he *s.* a cloud for a covering.
104:5, they have *s.* a net by the wayside.
Isa. 1:15, when ye *s.* forth your hands I will hide.
33:23, they could not *s.* the sail.
65:2, *s.* out hands to a rebellious people.
Jer. 8:2, they shall *s.* them before the sun.
Ezek. 26:14, a place to *s.* nets upon.
Mat. 21:8; Mk. 11:8; Lu. 19:36, *s.* garments.
Acts 4:17, but that it *s.* no further.
See Judg. 8:25; 1 Kings 8:54; Ezra 9:5.
SPRIGS. Isa. 18:5; Ezek. 17:6.
SPRING. Num. 21:17, *s.* up, O well.
1 Sam. 9:26, about the *s.* of the day.
Job 5:6, neither doth trouble *s.* out of the ground.
38:16, hast thou entered into the *s.* of the sea?
Ps. 87:7, all my *s.* are in thee.
104:10, he sendeth the *s.* into valleys.
107:33, he turneth water-*s.* into dry ground.
35, turneth dry ground into water-*s.*
Prov. 25:26, a troubled fountain, and a corrupt *s.*
Isa. 42:9, before they *s.* forth I tell you.
43:19, a new thing, now it shall *s.* forth.
45:8, let righteousness *s.* up together.
58:8, thine health shall *s.* forth.
11, shall be like a *s.* of water.
Mk. 4:27, seed should *s.* he knoweth not how.
See Joel 2:22; John 4:14; Heb. 12:15.
SPRINKLE. Job 2:12; Isa. 52:15; Ezek. 36:25.
SPROUT. Job 14:7, a tree will *s.* again.
SPUNGE. Mat. 27:48; Mk. 15:36; John 19:29.
SPY. Num. 13:16; Josh. 2:1; Gal. 2:4.
STABILITY. Isa. 33:6, the *s.* of thy times.
STABLE. 1 Chron. 16:30; Ezek. 25:5.
STAFF. Gen. 32:10, with my *s.* I passed over.
Ex. 12:11, eat it with *s.* in hand.
Num. 13:23, bare grapes between two on a *s.*
Judg. 6:21, the angel put forth end of his *s.*
2 Sam. 3:29, not fail one that leaneth on a *s.*

2 Kings 4:29, lay my *s.* on face of the child.
18:21; Isa. 36:6, thou trustest on *s.*
Ps. 23:4, thy rod and *s.* comfort me.
Isa. 3:1, the stay and *s.*, the whole stay of bread.
9:4, thou hast broken the *s.* of his shoulder.
10:5, the *s.* in their hand is mine indignation.
15, as if the *s.* should lift up itself.
14:5, the Lord hath broken the *s.* of the wicked.
Jer. 48:17, how is the strong *s.* broken?
Zech. 11:10, took my *s.*, even Beauty.
Mk. 6:8, take nothing, save *s.* only.
Heb. 11:21, leaning on the top of his *s.*
See Ex. 21:19; Num. 22:27; Isa. 28:27.
STAGGER. Job 12:25; Ps. 107:27, *s.* like a drunken man.
Isa. 29:9, they *s.*, but not with strong drink.
See Isa. 19:14; Rom. 4:20.
STAIN. Job 3:5; Isa. 23:9; 63:3.
STAIRS. 1 Kings 6:8; Neh. 9:4; Cant. 2:14.
STAKES. Isa. 33:20; 54:2.
STALK. Gen. 41:5; Josh. 2:6; Hos. 8:7.
STALL. Prov. 15:17; Hab. 3:17; Mal. 4:2.
STAMMERING. Isa. 28:11; 32:4; 33:19.
STAMP. Deut. 9:21; 2 Sam. 22:43; Jer. 47:3.
STAND. Ex. 14:13; 2 Chron. 20:17, *s.* still, and see.
Deut. 29:10, ye *s.* this day all of you before the Lord.
1 Sam. 9:27, *s.* thou still a while.
1 Kings 8:11; 2 Chron. 5:14, priests could not *s.* to minister.
17:1; 18:15; 2 Kings 3:14; 5:16, the Lord before whom I *s.*
2 Kings 10:4, two kings stood not, how shall we *s.*?
2 Chron. 34:32, caused all present to *s.* to it.
Esth. 8:11, to *s.* for their life.
Job 8:15, shall lean on his house, but it shall not *s.*
19:25, he shall *s.* at the latter day.
Ps. 1:1, nor *s.* in the way of sinners.
5, the ungodly shall not *s.* in judgment.
4:4, *s.* m awe, and sin not.
10:1, why *s.* thou afar off?
24:3, who shall *s.* in his holy place?
33:11, the counsel of the Lord *s.* for ever.
35:2, *s.* up for my help.
76:7, who may *s.* in thy sight?
94:16, who will *s.* up for me?
109:31, shall *s.* at right hand of the poor.
122:2, our feet shall *s.* within thy gates.
103:3, if thou, Lord, mark iniquities, who shall *s.*?
147:17, who can *s.* before his cold?
Prov. 22:29, shall *s.* before kings.
27:4, who is able to *s.* before envy?
Eccl. 8:3, *s.* not in an evil thing.
Isa. 7:7; 8:10, thus saith the Lord, it shall not *s.*
21:8, I *s.* continually on watchtower.
28:18, your agreement with hell shall not *s.*
40:8, the word of God shall *s.* for ever.
65:5, *s.* by thyself, I am holier than thou.
Jer. 6:16, *s.* ye in the ways, ask for the old paths.
35:19, shall not want a man to *s.* before me.
Dan. 11:16, he shall *s.* in the glorious land.
12:13, and shall *s.* in thy lot.
Mic. 5:4, he shall *s.* and feed in strength.
Nah. 2:8, *s.*, *s.*, shall they cry.
Zech. 3:1, Satan *s.* at his right hand.
Mal. 3:2, who shall *s.* when he appeareth?
Mat. 12:25; Mk. 3:24, 25; Lu. 11:18, house divided shall not *s.*
16:28; Lu. 9:27, there be some *s.* here.
20:3, others *s.* idle in the marketplace.
Rom. 5:2, this grace wherein we *s.*
14:4, God is able to make him *s.*
1 Cor. 2:5, faith should not *s.* in wisdom.
16:13, *s.* fast in the faith.
Gal. 4:20, I *s.* in doubt of you.
5:1, *s.* fast in the liberty.
Eph. 6:13, having done all, to *s.*
Phil. 1:27, *s.* fast in one spirit.
4:1; 1 Thess. 3:8, *s.* fast in the Lord.
1 Thess. 3:8, we live, if ye *s.* fast.
2 Tim. 2:19, the foundation of God *s.* sure.
Jas. 5:9, the judge *s.* before the door.
Rev. 3:20, I *s.* at the door, and knock.
6:17, is come, and who shall be able to *s.*?
20:12, the dead, small and great, *s.* before God.
See Rom. 14:4; 1 Cor. 10:12; Rev. 15:2.
STANDARD. Isa. 10:18, as when *s.*-bearer fainteth.
49:22, I will set up my *s.* to the people.
59:19, Spirit of the Lord shall lift up *s.* against.
62:10, go through, lift up a *s.*
Jer. 4:6; 50:2; 51:12, set up a *s.*
See Num. 1:52; 2:3; 10:14.
STATE. Ps. 39:5; Mat. 12:45; Lu. 11:26.
STATURE. Num. 13:32, men of great *s.*
1 Sam. 16:7, look not on height of his *s.*
Isa. 10:33, high ones of *s.* hewn down.
45:14, men of *s.* shall come.
Mat. 6:27; Lu. 12:25, not add to *s.*
Lu. 2:52, Jesus increased in *s.*
19:3, little of *s.*
Eph. 4:13, *s.* of the fulness of Christ.
See 2 Sam. 21:20; Cant. 7:7; Ezek. 17:6; 31:3.
STATUTE. Ex. 18:16, the *s.* of God.
Lev. 3:17; 16:34; 24:9, a perpetual *s.*
2 Kings 17:8, *s.* of the heathen.
Neh. 9:14, *s.* and laws.
Ps. 19:8, the *s.* of the Lord are right.
50:16, to declare my *s.*
Ezek. 5:6, hath changed my *s.*
20:25, *s.* that were not good.
33:15, walk in the *s.* of life.
Zech. 1:6, my *s.*, did they not take hold?
See Ps. 18:22; 105:45; 119:12, etc.; Ezek. 18:19.
STAVES. Num. 21:18, nobles digged with *s.*
1 Sam. 17:43, am I a dog, that thou comest with *s.*?
Hab. 3:14, strike through with his *s.*
Zech. 11:7, took unto me two *s.*
Mat. 10:10; Lu. 9:3, neither two coats, nor *s.*
See Mat. 26:47; Mk. 14:43; Lu. 22:52.
STAY (*n.*). 2 Sam. 22:19; Ps. 18:18, the Lord was my *s.*
Isa. 3:1, take away the *s.* and staff.
See Lev. 13:5; 1 Kings 10:19; Isa. 19:13.
STAY (*v.*). Gen. 19:17, neither *s.* in plain.
Ex. 9:28, ye shall *s.* no longer.
Num. 16:48; 25:8; 2 Sam. 24:25; 1 Chron. 21:22; Ps. 106:30, the plague was *s.*
2 Sam. 24:16; 1 Chron. 21:15, *s.* now thine hand.
Job 37:4, he will not *s.* them.
38:11, here shall thy proud waves be *s.*
37, who can *s.* the bottles of heaven?
Prov. 28:17, let no man *s.* him.
Isa. 26:3, whose mind is *s.* on thee.
27:8, he *s.* his rough wind.
29:9, *s.* yourselves, and wonder.
30:12, ye trust m oppression, and *s.* thereon.
50:10, trust in name of the Lord, and *s.* on his God.
Dan. 4:35, none can *s.* his hand.
Hag. 1:10, heaven is *s.*, earth is *s.*
See Josh. 10:13; 1 Sam. 24:7; Jer. 4:6; 20:9.
STEAD. Ex. 4:16, be to him in *s.* of God.
Num. 10:31, be to us in *s.* of eyes.
32:14, risen in your fathers' *s.*
Job 16:4, if your soul were in my soul's *s.*
31:40, thistles grow in *s.* of wheat.
34:24, he shall set others in their *s.*
Ps. 45:16, in *s.* of fathers shall be children.
Prov. 11:8., the wicked cometh in his *s.*
Isa. 3:24, In *s.* of girdle a rent.
55:13, in *s.* of the thorn shall come up the fir tree.
2 Cor. 5:20, we pray you in Christ's *s.*
See Gen. 30:2; 2 Kings 17:24; 1 Chron. 5:22.
STEADY. Ex. 17:12, Moses' hands were *s.*
STEAL. Gen. 31:27, wherefore didst thou *s.* away?
44:8, how then should we *s.* silver or gold?
Prov. 6:30, if he *s.* to satisfy his soul.
30:9, lest I be poor, and *s.*
Jer. 23:30, prophets that *s.* my words.
Mat. 6:19, thieves break through and *s.*

John 10:10, thief cometh not, but to *s.*
See Hos. 4:2; Mat. 27:64; Rom. 2:21.
STEALTH. 2 Sam. 19:3, by *s.* into city.
STEDFAST. Ps. 78:8, not *s.* with God.
Dan. 6:26, living God, and *s.* for ever.
Heb. 2:2, word spoken by angels was *s.*
3:14, hold our confidence *s.* to end.
6:19, hope as anchor, sure and *s.*
1 Pet. 5:9, resist *s.* in the faith.
See Acts 2:42; Col. 2:5; 2 Pet. 3:17.
STEEL. 2 Sam. 22:35; Job 20:24; Jer. 15:12.
STEEP. Ezek. 38:20; Mic. 1:4; Mat. 8:32.
STEP. 1 Sam. 20:3, but a *s.* between me and death.
Job 14:16, thou numberest my *s.*
23:11, my foot hath held his *s.*
29:6, I washed my *s.* with butter.
31:4, doth not he count my *s.*?
7, if my *s.* hath turned out of the way.
Ps. 37:23, the *s.* of a good man are ordered.
31, none of his *s.* shall slide.
44:18, nor have our *s.* declined.
56:6, they mark my *s.*
73:2, my *s.* had well nigh slipped.
85:13, set us in the way of his *s.*
119:133, order my *s.* in thy word.
Prov. 4:12, thy *s.* shall not be straitened.
5:5, her *s.* take hold on hell.
16:9, the Lord directeth his *s.*
Isa. 26:6, the *s.* of the needy shall tread it down.
Jer. 10:23, not in man to direct his *s.*
Rom. 4:12, walk in *s.* of that faith.
2 Cor. 12:18, walked we not in same *s.*?
1 Pet. 2:21, that ye should follow his *s.*
See Ex. 20:26; 2 Sam. 22:37; Lam. 4:18; Ezek. 40:22.
STEWARD. 1 Kings 16:9, drunk in house of his *s.*
Lu. 12:42, that faithful and wise *s.*
See Gen. 15:2; Lu. 8:3; 1 Cor. 4:1; 1 Pet. 4:10.
STICK. Num. 15:32, gathered *s.* on sabbath.
1 Kings 17:12, I am gathering two *s.*
Job 33:21, his bones *s.* out.
Ps. 38:2, thine arrows *s.* fast in me.
Prov. 18:24, a friend that *s.* closer than a brother.
Ezek. 37:16, take *s.*, and write on it.
See 2 Kings 6:6; Lam. 4:8; Ezek. 29:4.
STIFF. Ex. 32:9; 33:3; 34:9; Deut. 9:6, 13; 10:16, *s.*-necked people.
Ps. 75:5, speak not with *s.* neck.
Jer. 17:23, obeyed not, but made their neck *s.*
Ezek. 2:4, impudent and *s.*-hearted.
Acts 7:51, ye *s.*-necked, ye do always resist.
See Deut. 31:27; 2 Chron. 30:8; 36:13.
STILL. Ex. 15:16, as *s.* as a stone.
Num. 14:38, Joshua and Caleb lived *s.*
Josh. 24:10, Balaam blessed you *s.*
Judg. 18:9, the land is good, and are ye *s.*?
2 Sam. 14:32, good to have been there *s.*
2 Kings 7:4, if we sit *s.* here, we die also.
2 Chron. 22:9, no power to keep *s.* the kingdom.
Job 2:9, dost thou *s.* retain thine integrity?
Ps. 4:4, commune with thine heart, and be *s.*
8:2, *s.* the enemy and avenger.
23:2, beside the *s.* waters.
46:10, be *s.*, and know that I am God.
76:8, earth feared, and was *s.*
83:1, hold not thy peace, and be not *s.*, O God.
84:4, they will be *s.* praising thee.
107:29, so that the waves thereof are *s.*
139:18, when I awake, I am *s.* with thee.
Eccl. 12:9, he *s.* taught knowledge.
Isa. 5:25; 9:12; 10:4, his hand is stretched out *s.*
30:7, their strength is to sit *s.*
42:14, I have been *s.*, and refrained.
Jer. 8:14, why do we sit *s.*?
31:20, I do earnestly remember him *s.*
Zech. 11:16, nor feed that that standeth *s.*
Mk. 4:39, arose, and said, peace, be *s.*
Rev. 22:11, unjust *s.*, filthy *s.*, holy *s.*
See Num. 13:30; Ps. 65:7; 89:9; 92:14.
STING. Prov. 23:32; 1 Cor. 15:55; Rev. 9:10.
STIR. Num. 24:9, who shall *s.* him up?
Deut. 32:11, as an eagle *s.* up her nest.
1 Sam. 22:8, my son hath *s.* up my servant.
26:19, if the Lord have *s.* thee up.
1 Kings 11:14, the Lord *s.* up an adversary.
1 Chron. 5:26; 2 Chron. 36:22; Hag. 1:14, God *s.* up the spirit.
Job 17:8, the innocent shall *s.* up himself.
41:10, none dare *s.* him up.
Ps. 35:23, *s.* up thyself.
39:2, my sorrow was *s.*
Prov. 10:12, hatred *s.* up strifes.
15:18; 29:22, a wrathful man *s.* up strife.
Isa. 10:26, the Lord shall *s.* up a scourge.
14:9, hell from beneath *s.* up the dead.
64:7, none *s.* up himself to take hold.
Lu. 23:5, he *s.* up the people.
Acts 17:16, his spirit was *s.* in him.
19:23, no small *s.* about that way.
2 Tim. 1:6, *s.* up gift of God in thee.
2 Pet. 1:13, I think it meet to *s.* you up.
See Cant. 2:7; 3:5; 8:4; Isa. 22:2; Acts 12:18.
STOCK. Job 14:8, though the *s.* thereof die.
Isa. 40:24, their *s.* shall not take root.
44:19, shall I fall down to the *s.* of a tree?
Hos. 4:12, my people ask counsel at their *s.*
Nah. 3:6; Heb. 10:33, a gazing-*s.*
Acts 13:26, children of the *s.* of Abraham.
See Jer. 2:27; 10:8; 20:2; Phil. 3:5.
STOLE. 2 Sam. 15:6, Absalom *s.* the hearts.
Eph. 4:28, let him that *s.* steal no more.
See Gen. 31:20; 2 Kings 11:2; 2 Chron. 22:11; Mat. 28:13.
STOLEN. Josh. 7:11, they have *s.*, and dissembled.
2 Sam. 21:12, men had *s.* the bones of Saul.
Prov. 9:17, *s.* waters are sweet.
Obad. 5, *s.* till they had enough.
See Gen. 30:33; 31:19; Ex. 22:7; 2 Sam. 19:41.
STOMACH. 1 Tim. 5:23, for thy *s.* sake.
STONE. Gen. 11:3, they had brick for *s.*
28:18, 22; 31:45; 35:14, set up a *s.* for a pillar.
Deut. 8:9, a land whose *s.* are iron.
Josh. 24:27, this *s.* shall be a witness.
2 Sam. 17:13, till there be not one small *s.* found there.
2 Kings 3:25, cast every man his *s.*
Job 5:23, in league with *s.* of the field.
6:12, is my strength the strength of *s.*?
14:19, the waters wear the *s.*
28:3, he searcheth out the *s.* of darkness.
41:24, his heart is as firm as a *s.*
Ps. 91:12; Mat. 4:6; Lu. 4:11, lest thou dash thy foot against a *s.*
118:22; Mat. 21:42; Mk. 12:10, the *s.* which the builders refused is become the head *s.*
Prov. 27:3, a *s.* is heavy, a fool's wrath heavier.
Isa. 54:11, I will lay thy *s.* with fair colours.
60:17, bring for *s.* iron.
62:10, gather out the *s.*
Jer. 2:27, and to a *s.*, thou hast brought me forth.
Dan. 2:34, a *s.* was cut out of the mountain.
Hab. 2:11, the *s.* shall cry out of the wall.
19, that saith to the dumb *s.*, arise.
Hag. 2:15, before *s.* was laid upon *s.*
Zech. 3:9, upon one *s.* shall be seven eyes.
4:7, bring forth the head-*s.* thereof.
7:12, they made their hearts as *s.*
Mat. 7:9; Lu. 11:11, will he give him a *s.*?
21:44; Lu. 20:18, whosoever shall fall on this *s.*
24:2; Mk. 13:2; Lu. 19:44; 21:6, not one *s.* upon another.
Mk. 13:1, see what manner of *s.* are here!
16:4; Lu. 24:2, found *s.* rolled away.
Lu. 4:3, command this *s.* that it be made bread.
John 1:42, Cephas, by interpretation a *s.*
8:7, first cast a *s.*
11:39, take ye away the *s.*
Acts 17:29, that the Godhead is like to *s.*

1 Pet. 2:5, as lively *s.*, are built up.
See 1 Sam. 30:6; 1 Cor. 3:12; 2 Cor. 3:3; Rev. 2:17.
STONY. Ps. 141:6; Ezek. 11:19; 36:26; Mat. 13:5.
STOOD. Gen. 18:22, *s.* yet before the Lord.
Num. 14:19, *s.* behind them.
Josh. 3:16, waters *s.* up on an heap.
2 Kings 23:3, all the people *s.* to the covenant.
Esth. 9:16, Jews *s.* for their lives.
Ps. 33:9, he commanded, and it *s.* fast.
Lu. 24:36, Jesus himself *s.* in the midst.
2 Tim. 4:16, no man *s.* with me.
See Gen. 23:3; Job 29:8; Ezek. 37:10; Rev. 7:11.
STOOP. Gen. 49:9, Judah *s.* down.
Prov. 12:25, heaviness maketh the heart *s.*
John 8:6, *s.* down, and wrote on the ground.
See 2 Chron. 36:17; Job 9:13; Mk. 1:7; John 20:11.
STOP. Gen. 8:2, windows of heaven were *s.*
1 Kings 18:44, that the rain *s.* thee not.
Ps. 107:42, iniquity shall *s.* her mouth.
Zech. 7:11, refused, and *s.* their ears.
Acts 7:57, *s.* their ears, and ran upon him.
Rom. 3:19, that every mouth may be *s.*
Tit. 1:11, whose mouths must be *s.*
Heb. 11:33, through faith *s.* mouths of lions.
See Gen. 26:15; Job 5:16; Ps. 58:4; Prov. 21:13.
STORE. Lev. 25:22; 26:10, eat of the old *s.*
Deut. 28:5, blessed be thy basket and *s.*
2 Kings 20:17, thy fathers have laid up in *s.*
Ps. 144:13, affording all manner of *s.*
Nah. 2:9, none end of the *s.* and glory.
Mal. 3:10, bring tithes into *s.*-house.
Lu. 12:24, neither have *s.*-house nor barn.
1 Cor. 16:2, every one lay by him in *s.*
1 Tim. 6:19, laying up in *s.* a good foundation.
2 Pet. 3:7, by same word are kept in *s.*
See 1 Kings 10:10; 1 Chron. 29:16; Ps. 33:7.
STORK. Ps. 104:17, as for the *s.*, the fir trees are her house.
Jer. 8:7, yea, the *s.* in the heaven.
Zech. 5:9, like the wings of a *s.*
STORM. Ps. 55:8, escape from windy *s.*
83:15, make them afraid with thy *s.*
107:29, he maketh the *s.* a calm.
Isa. 4:6; 25:4, a covert from *s.*
28:2, as a destroying *s.*
Ezek. 38:9, shalt ascend and come like a *s.*
Nah. 1:3, the Lord hath his way in the *s.*
See Job 21:18; 27:21; Mk. 4:37; Lu. 8:23.
STORMY. Ps. 107:25; 148:8; Ezek. 13:11.
STORY. 2 Chron. 13:22; 24:27.
STOUT. Dan. 7:20, whose look was more *s.*
Mal. 3:13, words have been *s.* against me.
See Ps. 76:5; Isa. 9:9; 10:12; 46:12.
STRAIGHT. Ps. 5:8, make thy way *s.*
Prov. 4:25, let eyelids look *s.* before thee.
Eccl. 1:15; 7:13, crooked cannot be made *s.*
Isa. 40:3, make *s.* a highway.
4; 42:16; 45:2; Lu. 3:5, crooked shall be made *s.*
Jer. 31:9, cause them to walk in a *s.* way.
Mat. 3:3; Mk. 1:3; Lu. 3:4; John 1:23, make his paths *s.*
Lu. 13:13, she was made *s.*
Acts 9:11, street which is called *S.*
Heb. 12:13, make *s.* paths for your feet.
See Josh. 6:5; 1 Sam. 6:12; Ezek. 1:7; 10:22.
STRAIGHTWAY. Prov. 7:22, he goeth after her *s.*
Mat. 4:20; Mk. 1:18, they *s.* left their nets.
Jas. 1:24, *s.* forgetteth what manner of man.
See Lu. 14:5; John 13:32; Acts 9:20; 16:33.
STRAIN. Mat. 23:24, *s.* at a gnat.
STRAIT. 2 Sam. 24:14, I am in a great *s.*
Job 20:22, he shall be in *s.*
Isa. 49:20, the place is too *s.* for me, give place.
Mic. 2:7, is spirit of the Lord *s.*?
Mat. 7:13; Lu. 13:24, enter in at the *s.* gate.
Lu. 12:50, how am I *s.* till it be accomplished!
2 Cor. 6:12, ye are not *s.* in us.
Phil. 1:23, I am in a *s.* betwixt two.
See 2 Kings 6:1; Job 18:7; 37:10; Jer. 19:9.
STRAITLY. Gen. 43:7; Josh. 6:1; Acts 4:17.
STRAITNESS. Deut. 28:53; Job 36:16.
STRANGE. Gen. 42:7, Joseph made himself *s.*
Ex. 2:22; 18:3; Ps. 137:4, in a *s.* land.
Lev. 10:1; Num. 3:4; 26:61, offered *s.* fire.
1 Kings 11:1, Solomon loved many *s.* women.
Job 19:17, my breath is *s.* to my wife.
31:3, a *s.* punishment to workers.
Prov. 2:16, to deliver thee from the *s.* woman.
5:3, 20, for the lips of a *s.* woman.
21:8, the way of man is froward and *s.*
23:27, a *s.* woman is a narrow pit.
Isa. 28:21, his *s.* work, his *s.* act.
Ezek. 3:5, not sent to people of a *s.* speech.
Zeph. 1:8, clothed with *s.* apparel.
Lu. 5:26, we have seen *s.* things to-day.
Acts 17:20, thou bringest *s.* things to our ears.
26:11, persecuted them even to *s.* cities.
Heb. 13:9, carried about with *s.* doctrines.
1 Pet. 4:4, they think it *s.* ye run not.
12, not *s.* concerning the fiery trial.
See Judg. 11:2; Ezra 10:2; Prov. 2:16; Jer. 8:19.
STRANGER. Gen. 23:4; Ps. 39:12, I am a *s.* with you.
Ex. 23:9, ye know the heart of a *s.*
1 Chron. 29:15, we are *s.*, as were all our fathers.
Job 15:19, no *s.* passed among them.
31:32, the *s.* did not lodge in the street.
Ps. 54:3, for *s.* are risen up against me.
109:11, let the *s.* spoil his labour.
146:9, the Lord preserveth the *s.*
Prov. 2:16, to deliver thee even from the *s.*
5:10, lest *s.* be filled with thy wealth.
17, let them be thine own, not *s.* with thee.
6:1, stricken thy hand with a *s.*
7:5, from the *s.* which flattereth.
11:15, he that is surety for a *s.* shall smart.
14:10, a *s.* doth not intermeddle.
20:16; 27:13, garment that is surety for a *s.*
27:2, let a *s.* praise thee.
Isa. 1:7, your land, *s.* devour it.
2:6, please themselves in children of *s.*
14:1, the *s.* shall be joined with them.
56:3, neither let the son of the *s.* speak.
Jer. 14:8, why be as a *s.* in the land?
Ezek. 28:10, thou shalt die by the hand of *s.*
Hos. 7:9, *s.* have devoured his strength.
Mat. 25:35, I was a *s.*, and ye took me in.
Lu. 17:18, that returned, save this *s.*
Eph. 2:12, *s.* from the covenant.
19, no more *s.*, but fellowcitizens.
Heb. 11:13, confessed they were *s.*
13:2, be not forgetful to entertain *s.*
See Mat. 17:25; John 10:5; 1 Pet. 2:11.
STRANGLED. Nah. 2:12; Acts 15:20; 21:25.
STREAM. Ps. 124:4; Isa. 35:6; 66:12; Amos 5:24.
STREET. Prov. 1:20; Lu. 14:21; Rev. 21:21; 22:2.
STRENGTH. Ex. 15:2; 2 Sam. 22:33; Ps. 18:2; 28:7; 118:14; Isa. 12:2, the Lord is my *s.*
Judg. 5:21, thou hast trodden down *s.*
1 Sam. 2:9, by *s.* shall no man prevail.
5:29, the *S.* of Israel will not lie.
Job 9:19, if I speak of *s.*, lo, he is strong.
12:13, with him is wisdom and *s.*
Ps. 18:32, girded me with *s.*
27:1, the Lord is the *s.* of my life.
29:11, the Lord will give *s.* to his people.
33:16, mighty not delivered by much *s.*
39:13, spare me, that I may recover *s.*
46:1; 81:1, God is our refuge and *s.*
68:34, ascribe *s.* to God, his *s.* is in the clouds.
35, God giveth *s.* and power.
73:26, God is the *s.* of my heart.
84:5, the man whose *s.* is in thee.
7, they go from *s.* to *s.*
96:6, *s.* and beauty are in his sanctuary.
138:3, strengthenedst me with *s.* in my soul.
Prov. 10:29, the way of the Lord is *s.*

Eccl. 9:16, wisdom is better than *s.*
10:17, princes eat for *s.*
Isa. 25:4, a *s.* to the poor, a *s.* to the needy.
40:29, he increaseth *s.*
51:9, awake, put on *s.*
Hag. 2:22, I will destroy the *s.* of the kingdoms.
Lu. 1:51, he hath showed *s.* with his arm.
Rom. 5:6, when ye were without *s.*
1 Cor. 15:56, the *s.* of sin is the law.
Rev. 3:8, thou hast a little *s.*
See Job 21:23; Prov. 20:29; 2 Cor. 12:9.
STRENGTHEN. Job 15:25, he *s.* himself against.
Ps. 20:2, *s.* thee out of Zion.
104:15, bread which *s.* man's heart.
Eccl. 7:19, wisdom *s.* the wise.
Isa. 35:3, *s.* ye the weak hands.
Lu. 22:32, when converted, *s.* thy brethren.
Eph. 3:16; Col. 1:11, to be *s.* with might.
Phil. 4:13, all things through Christ who *s.* me.
See Lu. 22:43; 1 Pet. 5:10; Rev. 3:2.
STRETCH. Ps. 68:31, *s.* out her hands to God.
Isa. 28:20, shorter than a man can *s.* himself.
Jer. 10:12; 51:15, he *s.* out the heavens.
Ezek. 16:27, I have *s.* out my hand over thee.
Mat. 12:13, *s.* forth thine hand.
See Ps. 104:2; Prov. 1:24; Rom. 10:21; 2 Cor. 10:14.
STRIKE. Job 17:3; Prov. 22:26, *s.* hands.
Ps. 110:5, shall *s.* through kings.
Prov. 7:23, till a dart *s.* through his liver.
See Prov. 23:35; Isa. 1:5; 1 Tim. 3:3; Tit. 1:7.
STRIPES. Deut. 25:3, forty *s.* he may give.
2 Cor. 11:24, five times received I forty *s.*
STRIVE. Gen. 6:3, shall not always *s.*
Prov. 3:30, *s.* not without cause.
Lu. 13:24, *s.* to enter in at strait gate.
2 Tim. 2:5, if a man *s.* for mastery.
24, the servant of the Lord must not *s.*
See Isa. 45:9; Jer. 50:24; Mat. 12:19; Heb. 12:4.
STRONG. 1 Sam. 4:9; 1 Kings 2:2; 2 Chron.
15:7; Isa. 35:4; Dan. 10:19, be *s.*
Job 9:19, if I speak of strength, lo, he is *s.*
Ps. 19:5, as a *s.* man to run a race.
24:8, the Lord is *s.*
31:2, be thou my *s.* rock.
71:7, thou art my *s.* refuge.
Prov. 10:15, the rich man's wealth is his *s.* city.
18:10, the name of the Lord is a *s.* tower.
Eccl. 9:11, the battle is not to the *s.*
Isa. 40:26, for that he is *s.* in power.
Mat. 12:29, first bind the *s.* man.
Rom. 4:20, *s.* in faith.
1 Cor. 4:10, we are weak, ye are *s.*
2 Thess. 2:11, *s.* delusion.
Heb. 5:12, of milk, and not of *s.* meat.
6:18, we have a *s.* consolation.
See Prov. 14:26; Joel 3:10; Rom. 15:1; Rev. 5:2.
STUBBLE. Ps. 83:13, make them as *s.*
Isa. 33:11, conceive chaff, bring forth *s.*
41:2, as driven *s.*
Jer. 13:24, I will scatter them as *s.*
See Joel 2:5; Nah. 1:10; Mal. 4:1; 1 Cor. 3:12.
STUDY. Eccl. 12:12, much *s.* is a weariness of the flesh.
See 1 Thess. 4:11; 2 Tim. 2:15.
STUMBLE. Prov. 4:19, know not at what they *s.*
Isa. 28:7, they *s.* in judgment.
59:10, we *s.* at noonday.
Jer. 46:6; Dan. 11:19, *s.* and fall.
Mal. 2:8, have caused many to *s.*
1 Pet. 2:8, that *s.* at the word.
See John 11:9; Rom. 9:32; 11:11; 14:21.
SUBDUE. Ps. 47:3, he shall *s.* the people.
Mic. 7:19, he will *s.* our iniquities.
Phil. 3:21, able to *s.* all things.
Heb. 11:33, through faith *s.* kingdoms.
See Dan. 2:40; Zech. 9:15; 1 Cor. 15:28.
SUBJECT. Lu. 10:17, devils are *s.* unto us.
Rom. 8:7, not *s.* to law of God.
Rom. 8:20, creature *s.* to vanity.
13:1, *s.* to the higher powers.
1 Cor. 14:32, spirits of prophets *s.* to prophets.
15:28, then shall the Son also be *s.* to him.
Eph. 5:24, as the church is *s.* to Christ.
Heb. 2:15, all their lifetime *s.* to bondage.
Jas. 5:17, a man *s.* to like passions.
1 Pet. 2:18, servants, be *s.* to your masters.
3:22, angels and powers *s.* to him.
5:5, all of you be *s.* one to another.
See Lu. 2:51; Col. 2:20; Tit. 3:1.
SUBMIT. 2 Sam. 22:45, *s.* themselves.
Ps. 68:30, till every one *s.* himself.
Eph. 5:22, wives *s.* yourselves.
Jas. 4:7, *s.* yourselves to God.
1 Pet. 2:13, *s.* yourselves to every ordinance of man.
See Rom. 10:3; Eph. 5:21; Heb. 13:17.
SUBSCRIBE. Isa. 44:5; Jer. 32:44.
SUBSTANCE. Gen. 13:6, their *s.* was great.
Deut. 33:11, bless his *s.*
Job 30:22, thou dissolvest my *s.*
Ps. 17:14, they leave their *s.* to babes.
139:15, my *s.* was not hid from thee.
Prov. 3:9, honour the Lord with thy *s.*
28:8, he that by usury increaseth his *s.*
Cant. 8:7, give all his *s.* for love.
Jer. 15:13; 17:3, thy *s.* will I give to spoil.
Hos. 12:8, I have found me out *s.*
Mic. 4:13, I will consecrate their *s.*
Lu. 8:3, ministered to him of their *s.*
15:13, wasted his *s.*
Heb. 10:34, a better *s.*
11:1, the *s.* of things hoped for.
See Prov. 1:13; 6:31; 8:21; 12:27; 29:3.
SUBTIL. Gen. 3:1; 2 Sam. 13:3; Prov. 7:10.
SUBTILTY. Gen. 27:35; Mat. 26:4; Acts 13:10.
SUBVERT. Lam. 3:36; 2 Tim. 2:14; Tit. 1:11; 3:11.
SUCCESS. Josh. 1:8, have good *s.*
SUCK. Deut. 32:13, *s.* honey out of rock.
33:19, *s.* abundance of the seas.
Job 20:16, *s.* poison of asps.
Isa. 60:16, *s.* the milk of the Gentiles.
See Mat. 24:19; Mk. 13:17; Lu. 21:23; 23:29.
SUDDEN. Job 22:10; Prov. 3:25; 1 Thess. 5:3.
SUDDENLY. Prov. 29:1, be *s.* destroyed.
Eccl. 9:12, when it falleth *s.*
Mal. 3:1, shall *s.* come to his temple.
Mk. 13:36, lest coming *s.* he find you sleeping.
1 Tim. 5:22, lay hands *s.* on no man.
SUFFER. Job 21:3, *s.* me that I may speak.
Ps. 55:22, never *s.* righteous to be moved.
89:33, nor *s.* my faithfulness to fail.
Prov. 19:15, the idle soul shall *s.* hunger.
Eccl. 5:12, not *s.* him to sleep.
Mat. 3:15, *s.* it to be so now.
8:21; Lu. 9:59, *s.* me first to bury my father.
16:21; 17:12; Mk. 8:31; Lu. 9:22, *s.* many things.
19:14; Mk. 10:14; Lu. 18:16, *s.* little children.
23:13, neither *s.* ye them that are entering to go in.
Lu. 24:46; Acts 3:18, behoved Christ to *s.*
Rom. 8:17, if we *s.* with him.
1 Cor. 3:15, he shall *s.* loss.
10:13, will not *s.* you to be tempted.
12:26, whether one member *s.*, all *s.* with it.
Gal. 6:12, lest they should *s.* persecution.
2 Tim. 2:12, if we *s.*, we shall also reign.
3:12, shall *s.* persecution.
Heb. 13:3, remember them who *s.*
1 Pet. 2:21, *s.* for us, leaving an example.
4:1, he that hath *s.* in the flesh.
See Gal. 3:4; Phil. 3:8; Heb. 2:18; 5:8.
SUFFICIENCY. Job 20:22; 2 Cor. 3:5; 9:8.
SUFFICIENT. Isa. 40:16, not *s.* to burn.
Mat. 6:34, *s.* for the day is the evil.
2 Cor. 2:16, who is *s.* for these things?
See Deut. 15:8; John 6:7; 2 Cor. 3:5; 12:9.
SUM. Ps. 139:17; Acts 22:28; Heb. 8:1.

SUMMER. Gen. 8:22; Ps. 74:17, *s.* and winter.
Prov. 6:8; 30:25, provideth meat in *s.*
10:5, he that gathereth in *s.* is a wise son.
26:1, as snow in *s.*
Jer. 8:20, the *s.* is ended.
Mat. 24:32; Mk. 13:28, ye know *s.* is nigh.
See Dan. 2:35; Zech. 14:8; Lu. 21:30.
SUMPTUOUSLY. Lu. 16:19, fared *s.* every day.
SUN. Josh. 10:12, *s.*, stand thou still.
Judg. 5:31, as the *s.* in his might.
Job 8:16, hypocrite is green before the *s.*
Ps. 58:8, that they may not see the *s.*
84:11, a *s.* and shield.
121:6, the *s.* shall not smite thee.
Eccl. 1:9, no new thing under the *s.*
11:7, a pleasant thing it is to behold the *s.*
12:2, while the *s.* or stars be not darkened.
Cant. 1:6, because the *s.* hath looked upon me.
6:10, clear as the *s.*
Jer. 15:9, her *s.* is gone down while yet day.
Joel 2:10; 3:15, the *s.* be darkened.
Mal. 4:2, the *S.* of righteousness.
Mat. 5:45, maketh his *s.* to rise on evil.
13:43, then shall righteous shine as *s.*
Eph. 4:26, let not *s.* go down on your wrath.
See 1 Cor. 15:41; Jas. 1:11; Rev. 7:16; 21:23.
SUPERFLUITY. Jas. 1:21, *s.* of naughtiness.
SUPPLICATION. 1 Kings 9:3, I have heard thy *s.*
Job 9:15, I would make *s.* to my judge.
Ps. 6:9, the Lord hath heard my *s.*
Dan. 9:3, to seek by prayer and *s.*
Zech. 12:10, spirit of grace and *s.*
Eph. 6:18, with all prayer and *s.*
1 Tim. 2:1, that *s.* be made for all men.
See Ps. 28:6; 31:22; Phil. 4:6; Heb. 5:7.
SUPPLY. Phil. 1:19; 2:30; 4:19.
SUPPORT. Acts 20:35; 1 Thess. 5:14.
SUPREME. 1 Pet. 2:13, to the king as *s.*
SURE. Num. 32:23, be *s.* your sin will find you out.
Job 24:22, no man is *s.* of life.
Prov. 6:3, make *s.* thy friend.
Isa. 55:3; Acts 13:34, the *s.* mercies of David.
2 Tim. 2:19, the foundation of God standeth *s.*
See Isa. 33:16; Heb. 6:19; 2 Pet. 1:10, 19.
SURFEITING. Lu. 21:34, overcharged with *s.*
SURPRISED. Isa. 33:14; Jer. 48:41; 51:41.
SUSTAIN. Ps. 3:5; 55:22; Prov. 18:14; Isa. 59:16.
SWALLOW. Ps. 84:3, the *s.* a nest for her young.
Prov. 26:2, as the *s.* by flying.
Isa. 38:14, like a crane or a *s.*
Jer. 8:7, the *s.* observe the time.
SWAN. Lev. 11:8; Deut. 14:16, and the *s.*
SWEAR. Ps. 15:4, that *s.* to his hurt.
Eccl. 9:2, he that *s.*, as he that feareth an oath.
Isa. 45:23, to me every tongue shall *s.*
65:16, shall *s.* by the God of truth.
Jer. 4:2, *s.*, the Lord liveth, in truth.
23:10, because of *s.* the land mourneth.
Hos. 4:2, by *s.*, and lying, they break out.
10:4, *s.* falsely in making a covenant.
Zech. 5:3, every one that *s.* shall be cut off.
Mal. 3:5, a witness against false *s.*
See Zeph. 1:5; Mat. 26:74; Heb. 6:13.
SWEAT. Gen. 3:19; Ezek. 44:18; Lu. 22:44.
SWEET. Job 20:12, though wickedness be *s.*
Ps. 55:14, we took *s.* counsel together.
104:34, my meditation shall be *s.*
Prov. 3:24, thy sleep shall be *s.*
9:17, stolen waters are *s.*
13:19, desire accomplished is *s.*
16:24, pleasant words are *s.*
27:7, to the hungry every bitter thing is *s.*
Eccl. 5:12, sleep of labouring man is *s.*
11:7, truly the light is *s.*
Cant. 2:3, his fruit was *s.* to my taste.
Isa. 5:20, put bitter for *s.*, and *s.* for bitter.
23:16, make *s.* melody.
Jas. 3:11, at same place *s.* water and bitter.
See Judg. 14:18; Mic. 6:15; Mk. 16:1.
SWELLING. Jer. 12:5; 2 Pet. 2:18; Jude 16.
SWIFT. Eccl. 9:11, the race is not to the *s.*
Amos 2:15, the *s.* of foot shall not deliver.
Rom. 3:15, feet *s.* to shed blood.
See Job 7:6; 9:25; Jer. 46:6; Mal. 3:5.
SWIM. 2 Kings 6:6, iron did *s.*
Ezek. 47:5, waters to *s.* in.
See Ps. 6:6; Isa. 25:11; Ezek. 32:6; Acts 27:42.
SWOLLEN. Acts 28:6, when he should have *s.*
SWOON. Lam. 2:11, children *s.* in the streets.
SWORD. Ps. 57:4, their tongue a sharp *s.*
Isa. 2:4, nation shall not lift up *s.*
Ezek. 7:15, the *s.* is without, pestilence within.
Mat. 10:34, not to send peace, but a *s.*
Lu. 2:35, a *s.* shall pierce thy own soul.
Rom. 13:4, he beareth not the *s.* in vain.
Eph. 6:17, the *s.* of the Spirit.
Heb. 4:12, sharper than twoedged *s.*
Rev. 1:16; 19:15, out of his mouth a sharp *s.*
13:10, that killeth with *s.* must be killed with *s.*
See Isa. 2:4; Joel 3:10; Mic. 4:3; Lu. 22:38.

T

TABERNACLE. Ps. 15:1, abide in thy *t.*
27:5, in secret of his *t.* shall he hide me.
84:1, how amiable are thy *t.*!
Isa. 33:20, a *t.* that shall not be taken down.
See Job 5:24; Prov. 14:11; 2 Cor. 5:1.
TABLE. Ps. 23:5, thou preparest a *t.*
69:22, let their *t.* become a snare.
78:19, can God furnish a *t.* in the wilderness?
128:3, like olive plants about thy *t.*
Prov. 9:2, wisdom hath furnished her *t.*
Mat. 15:27; Mk. 7:28, from their masters' *t.*
Acts 6:2, leave word of God, and serve *t.*
2 Cor. 3:3, fleshy *t.* of the heart.
See Prov. 3:3; Jer. 17:1; Mal. 1:7; 1 Cor. 10:21.
TABRET. Gen. 31:27; 1 Sam. 18:6; Isa. 5:12, the *t.*
TAKE. Ex. 6:7, I will *t.* you to me for a people.
34:9, *t.* us for thine inheritance.
Judg. 19:30, *t.* advice, and speak your minds.
2 Kings 19:30; Isa. 37:31, shall yet *t.* root.
Job 23:10, he knoweth the way that I *t.*
Ps. 51:11, *t.* not thy holy spirit from me.
116:13, I will *t.* the cup of salvation.
Cant. 2:15, *t.* us the foxes, the little foxes.
Isa. 33:23, the lame *t.* the prey.
Hos. 14:2, *t.* with you words.
Amos 9:2, thence shall mine hand *t.* them.
Mat. 6:25, 28, 31, 34; 10:19; Mk. 13:11; Lu.
12:11, 22, 26, *t.* no thought.
11:29, *t.* my yoke.
16:5; Mk. 8:14, forgotten to *t.* bread.
18:16, then *t.* with thee one or two more.
20:14, *t.* that thine is, and go thy way.
26:26; Mk. 14:22; 1 Cor. 11:24, *t.*, eat; this is my body.
Lu. 6:29, forbid him not to *t.* thy coat also.
12:19, soul, *t.* thine ease.
John 16:15, he shall *t.* of mine.
1 Cor. 6:7, why do ye not rather *t.* wrong?
1 Tim. 3:5, how shall he *t.* care of the church?
1 Pet. 2:20, if yet. it patiently.
Rev. 3:11, that no man *t.* thy crown.
See John 1:29; 10:18; 1 Cor. 10:13; Rev. 22:19.
TALE. Ps. 90:9; Lu. 24:11.
TALK. Deut. 5:24, God doth *t.* with man.
6:7, *t.* of them when thou sittest.
Job 11:2, a man full of *t.*
13:7, will ye *t.* deceitfully for him?
15:3, reason with unprofitable *t.*
Ps. 71:24, *t.* of thy righteousness.
145:11, *t.* of thy power.
Prov. 6:22, it shall *t.* with thee.
Jer. 12:1, let me *t.* with thee of thy judgments.
Ezek. 3:22, arise, and I will *t.* with thee there.

Mat. 22:15, they might entangle him in his *t.*
Lu. 24:32, while he *t.* with us by the way.
John 9:37, it is he that *t.* with thee.
See Prov. 14:23; John 14:30; Eph. 5:4.
TALL. Deut. 1:28; 2:10; 2 Kings 19:23.
TAME. Mk. 5:4; Jas. 3:7, 8.
TARE. 2 Sam. 13:31; 2 Kings 2:24; Mk. 9:20.
TARRY. Gen. 27:44, and *t.* a few days.
Ex. 12:39, were thrust out, and could not *t.*
2 Kings 7:9, if we *t.* till morning light.
9:3, flee, and *t.* not.
Ps. 68:12, she that *t.* at home divided the spoil.
101:7, he that telleth lies shall not *t.* in my sight.
Prov. 23:30, they that *t.* long at the wine.
Isa. 46:13, my salvation shall not *t.*
Jer. 14:8, that turneth aside to *t.* for a night.
Hab. 2:3, though it *t.*, wait for it.
Mat. 25:5, while the bridegroom *t.*
26:38; Mk. 14:34, *t.* here and watch.
Lu. 24:29, he went in to *t.* with them.
49, *t.* ye in city of Jerusalem until endued.
John 21:22, if I will that he *t.*
Acts 22:16, why *t.* thou, arise, and be baptized.
1 Cor. 11:33, *t.* one for another.
Heb. 10:37, will come, and will not *t.*
See 1 Sam. 30:24; Mic. 5:7; John 3:22.
TASKMASTERS. Ex. 1:11, they did set over them *t.*
5:6, the *t.* of the people.
TASTE. Num. 11:8, the *t.* of it as *t.* of fresh oil.
Job 6:6, is any *t.* in white of egg?
12:11, doth not the mouth *t.* his meat?
34:3, trieth words as mouth *t.* meat.
Ps. 34:8, *t.* and see that the Lord is good.
119:103, how sweet are thy words to my *t.*!
Jer. 48:11, his *t.* remained in him.
Mat. 16:28; Mk. 9:1; Lu. 9:27, some, which shall not *t.* death.
Lu. 14:24, none bidden shall *t.* of my supper.
John 8:52, keep my saying, shall never *t.* of death.
Col. 2:21, touch not, *t.* not.
Heb. 2:9, *t.* death for every man.
6:4, and have *t.* of the heavenly gift.
1 Pet. 2:3, have *t.* that the Lord is gracious.
See 1 Sam. 14:43; 2 Sam. 19:35; Mat. 27:34.
TATTLERS. 1 Tim. 5:13, *t.* and busybodies.
TAUGHT. Judg. 8:16, he *t.* the men of Succoth.
2 Chron. 6:27, thou hast *t.* them the good way.
23:13, such as *t.* to sing praise.
Ps. 71:17; 119:102, thou hast *t.* me.
Prov. 4:4, he *t.* me also, and said.
11, I have *t.* thee in way of wisdom.
Eccl. 12:9, he still *t.* the people knowledge.
Isa. 29:13, their fear is *t.* by precept of men.
54:13, all thy children shall be *t.* of God.
Jer. 12:16, as they *t.* my people to swear by Baal.
32:33, *t.* them, rising up early.
Zech. 13:5, *t.* me to keep cattle.
Mat. 7:29; Mk. 1:22, *t.* as one having authority.
28:15, and did as they were *t.*
Lu. 13:26, thou hast *t.* in our streets.
John 6:45, they shall be all *t.* of God.
8:28, as my Father hath *t.* me.
Gal. 1:12, nor was I *t.* it, except by revelation.
6:6, let him that is *t.* in the word.
Eph. 4:21, if so be ye have been *t.* by him.
2 Thess. 2:15, the traditions ye have been *t.*
See Col. 2:7; 1 Thess. 4:9; Tit. 1:9; 1 John 2:27.
TAUNT. Jer. 24:9; Ezek. 5:15; Hab. 2:6.
TEACH. Ex. 4:15, I will *t.* you.
Deut. 4:10, that they may *t.* their children.
6:7; 11:19, *t.* them diligently.
Judg. 13:8, *t.* us what we shall do to the child.
1 Sam. 12:23, I will *t.* you the good way.
2 Sam. 1:18, bade them *t.* the use of the bow.
2 Chron. 15:3, without a *t.* priest.
Job 6:24, *t.* me, and I will hold my tongue.
8:10, thy fathers, shall not they *t.* thee?
Job 12:7, ask the beasts, and they shall *t.* thee.
34:32, that which I see not *t.* thou me.
36:22, God exalteth, who *t.* like him?
Ps. 25:4, *t.* me thy paths.
8, he will *t.* sinners in the way.
27:11; 86:11, *t.* me thy way, and lead me.
34:11, I will *t.* you the fear of the Lord.
51:13, then will I *t.* transgressors.
90:12, so *t.* us to number our days.
94:12, blessed is the man whom thou *t.*
Prov. 6:13, the wicked man *t.* with his finger.
Isa. 2:3; Mic. 4:2, he will *t.* us of his ways.
28:9, whom shall he *t.* knowledge?
26, God doth *t.* him discretion.
48:17, I am thy God which *t.* thee to profit.
Jer. 9:20, and *t.* your daughters wailing.
Ezek. 44:23, *t.* my people the difference.
Mic. 3:11, priests *t.* for hire.
Mat. 28:19, *t.* all nations.
Lu. 11:1, *t.* us to pray.
12:12, the Holy Ghost shall *t.* you.
John 9:34, dost thou *t.* us?
14:26, shall *t.* you all things.
Acts 5:42, they ceased not to *t.* and preach.
Rom. 12:7, he that *t.*, on *t.*
1 Cor. 4:17, as I *t.* every where.
11:14, doth not even nature *t.* you?
14:19, that by my voice I might *t.* others.
Col. 1:28, *t.* every man in all wisdom.
3:16, *t.* and admonishing one another.
1 Tim. 1:3, charge some that they *t.* no other.
2:12, I suffer not a woman to *t.*
3:2; 2 Tim. 2:24, apt to *t.*
4:11, these things command and *t.*
6:2, these things *t.* and exhort.
2 Tim. 2:2, faithful men, able to *t.*
Tit. 1:11, *t.* things they ought not.
2:4, *t.* young women to be sober.
12, *t.* us, that denying ungodliness.
Heb. 5:12, ye have need that one *t.* you again.
See Mat. 22:16; Mk. 6:34; 12:14; Rev. 2:20.
TEACHER. 1 Chron. 25:8, as well *t.* as scholar.
Ps. 119:99, more understanding than all my *t.*
Prov. 5:13, have not obeyed the voice of my *t.*
Isa. 30:20, thine eyes shall see thy *t.*
Hab. 2:18, a *t.* of lies.
John 3:2, a *t.* come from God.
Rom. 2:20, thou art a *t.* of babes.
1 Cor. 12:29, are all *t.*?
Eph. 4:11, evangelists, pastors, and *t.*
1 Tim. 1:7, desiring to be *t.* of the law.
Tit. 2:3, aged women, *t.* of good things.
See 1 Tim. 2:7; 2 Tim. 1:11; Heb. 5:12; 2 Pet. 2:1.
TEAR. Job 16:9, he *t.* me in his wrath.
18:4, he *t.* himself in his anger.
Ps. 7:2, lest he *t.* my soul.
35:15, they did *t.* me, and ceased not.
50:22, lest I *t.* you in pieces.
Hos. 5:14, I will *t.* and go away.
See Mic. 5:8; Zech. 11:16; Mk. 9:18; Lu. 9:39.
TEARS. 2 Kings 20:5; Isa. 38:5, I have seen thy *t.*
Job 16:20, mine eye poureth out *t.*
Ps. 6:6, I water my couch with *t.*
39:12, hold not thy peace at my *t.*
42:3, *t.* have been my meat.
56:8, put thou my *t.* into thy bottle.
80:5, the bread of *t.*, and *t.* to drink.
116:8, thou hast delivered mine eyes from *t.*
126:5, they that sow in *t.*
Isa. 16:9, I will water thee with my *t.*
25:8, will wipe away *t.*
Jer. 9:1, oh that mine eyes were a fountain of *t.*!
13:17; 14:17, mine eyes run down with *t.*
31:16, refrain thine eyes from *t.*
Lam. 1:2, her *t.* are on her cheeks.
2:11, mine eyes do fail with *t.*
Ezek. 24:16, neither shall thy *t.* run down.

Mal. 2:13, covering the altar with *t.*
Lu. 7:38, to wash his feet with her *t.*
Acts 20:19, serving the Lord with many *t.*
31, ceased not to warn with *t.*
2 Tim. 1:4, being mindful of thy *t.*
See 2 Cor. 2:4; Heb. 5:7; 12:17; Rev. 7:17.
TEDIOUS. Acts 24:4, that I be not further *t.*
TEETH. Gen. 49:12, *t.* white with milk.
Num. 11:33, flesh yet between their *t.*
Job 19:20, escaped with the skin of my *t.*
Prov. 10:26, as vinegar to the *t.*
Isa. 41:15, an instrument having *t.*
Jer. 31:29; Ezek. 18:2, *t.* set on edge.
Amos 4:6, cleanness of *t.*
See Mic. 3:5; Zech. 9:7; Mat. 27:44; Rev. 9:8.
TELL. Gen. 15:5, *t.* the stars.
32:29, *t.* me thy name.
2 Sam. 1:20, *t.* it not in Gath.
Ps. 48:12, *t.* the towers thereof.
50:12, if I were hungry, I would not *t.* thee.
Eccl. 6:12; 10:14, who can *t.* what shall be after?
10:20, that which hath wings shall *t.*
Jonah 3:9, who can *t.* if God will turn?
Mat. 18:15, *t.* him his fault.
17, *t.* it unto the church.
21:27; Mk. 11:33; Lu. 20:8, neither *t.* I you.
Mk. 5:19, *t.* how great things.
11:33; Lu. 20:7, we cannot *t.*
Lu. 13:32, *t.* that fox.
John 3:8, canst not *t.* whence.
12, if I *t.* you of heavenly things.
4:25, he will *t.* us all things.
18:34, did others *t.* it thee of me?
Acts 17:21, either to *t.* or hear some new thing.
See Ps. 56:8; Isa. 19:12; Mat. 28:7; 2 Cor. 12:2.
TEMPER. Ex. 29:2; 30:35; Ezek. 46:14; 1 Cor. 12:24.
TEMPEST. Job 9:17, breaketh me with a *t.*
Ps. 11:6, on wicked he shall rain a *t.*
55:8, hasten from windy storm and *t.*
Isa. 32:2, a covert from the *t.*
Heb. 12:18, not come to darkness and *t.*
2 Pet. 2:17, clouds carried with a *t.*
TEMPESTUOUS. Ps. 50:3; Jonah 1:11; Acts 27:14.
TEMPLE. 2 Sam. 22:7, hear. my voice out of his *t.*
Neh. 6:10, meet together in the *t.*
Ps. 27:4, to enquire in his *t.*
29:9, in his *t.* doth every one speak of his glory.
Isa. 6:1, his train filled the *t.*
Amos 8:3, songs of the *t.* shall be howlings.
Mal. 3:1, the Lord shall suddenly come to his *t.*
Mat. 12:6, one greater than the *t.*
John 2:19, destroy this *t.*
1 Cor. 3:16; 6:19; 2 Cor. 6:16, ye are the *t.* of God.
See Hos. 8:14; Rev. 7:15; 11:19; 21:22.
TEMPORAL. 2 Cor. 4:18, things seen are *t.*
TEMPT. Gen. 22:1, God did *t.* Abraham.
Ex. 17:2, wherefore do ye *t.* the Lord?
Num. 14:22, have *t.* me these ten times.
Deut. 6:16; Mat. 4:7; Lu. 4:12, ye shall not *t.* the Lord your God.
Ps. 78:18, they *t.* God in their heart.
Isa. 7:12, I will not ask, neither *t.* the Lord.
Mal. 3:15, they that *t.* God are delivered.
Mat. 22:18; Mk. 12:15; Lu. 20:23, why *t.* ye me?
Lu. 10:25, a lawyer, *t.* him.
Acts 5:9, agreed together to *t.* the Spirit.
15:10, why *t.* ye God to put a yoke?
1 Cor. 10:13, will not suffer you to be *t.*
Gal. 6:1, considering thyself, lest thou be *t.*
Heb. 2:18, hath suffered, being *t.*
4:15, in all points *t.* like as we are.
Jas. 1:13, cannot be *t.*, neither *t.* he any man.
See Mat. 4:1; Mk. 1:13; Lu. 4:2; John 8:6.
TEMPTATION. Mat. 6:13, lead us not into *t.*
26:41; Mk. 14:38; Lu. 22:46, lest ye enter into *t.*
Lu. 8:13, in time of *t.* fall away.
1 Cor. 10:13, there hath no *t.* taken you.
Gal. 4:14, my *t.* in flesh ye despised not.
1 Tim. 6:9, they that will be rich fall into *t.*
Jas. 1:2, when ye fall into divers *t.*
2 Pet. 2:9, how to deliver out of *t.*
See Lu. 11:4; Acts 20:19; 1 Pet. 1:6; Rev. 3:10.
TEMPTER. Mat. 4:3, and when the *t.* came to him.
1 Thess. 3:5, the *t.* have tempted you.
TEND. Prov. 11:19; 14:23; 19:23; 21:5.
TENDER. Deut. 28:54, man that is *t.*
32:2, distil as small rain on *t.* herb.
2 Kings 22:19; 2 Chron. 34:27, thy heart was *t.*
Job 14:7, the *t.* branch will not cease.
Prov. 4:3, *t.* in sight of my mother.
Cant. 2:13, 15; 7:12, vines with *t.* grapes.
Isa. 47:1, no more be called *t.*
53:2, grow up before him as a *t.* plant.
Dan. 1:9, God brought Daniel into *t.* love.
Lu. 1:78, through the *t.* mercy of our God.
Eph. 4:32, be kind and *t.*-hearted.
Jas. 5:11, the Lord is pitiful, and of *t.* mercy.
See 1 Chron. 22:5; Ezek. 17:22; Mk. 13:28.
TENOR. Gen. 43:7; Ex. 34:27.
TENT. Gen. 9:21, was uncovered within his *t.*
27, he shall dwell in the *t.* of Shem.
12:8, and pitched his *t.*
25:27, a plain man, dwelling in *t.*
Num. 24:5, how goodly are thy *t.*!
1 Sam. 4:10; 2 Sam. 18:17, fled every man to his *t.*
1 Kings 12:16, to your *t.*, O Israel.
Ps. 84:10, than to dwell in *t.* of wickedness.
Isa. 38:12, removed as a shepherd's *t.*
54:2, enlarge the place of thy *t.*
Jer. 10:20, there is none to stretch forth my *t.*
Acts 18:3, by occupation they were *t.*-makers.
See Isa. 40:22; Jer. 4:20; 35:7; Zech. 12:7; Heb. 11:9.
TENTH. Gen. 28:22; Lev. 27:32; Isa. 6:13.
TERRIBLE. Ex. 34:10, a *t.* thing I will do.
Deut. 1:19; 8:15, that *t.* wilderness.
7:21; 10:17; Neh. 1:5; 4:14; 9:32, a mighty God and *t.*
10:21, hath done for thee *t.* things.
Judg. 13:6, like an angel of God, very *t.*
Job 37:22, with God is *t.* majesty.
39:20, the glory of his nostrils is *t.*
Ps. 45:4, thy right hand shall teach thee *t.* things.
65:5, by *t.* things in righteousness.
66:3, say unto God, how *t.* art thou!
5, *t.* in his doing.
68:35, *t.* out of thy holy places.
76:12, he is *t.* to the kings of the earth.
99:3, thy great and *t.* name.
145:6, the might of thy *t.* acts.
Cant. 6:4, *t.* as an army with banners.
Isa. 25:4, blast of the *t.* ones.
64:3, when thou didst *t.* things.
Jer. 15:21, redeem thee out of hand of the *t.*
Joel 2:11, the day of the Lord is very *t.*
Heb. 12:21, so *t.* was the sight.
See Lam. 5:10; Ezek. 1:22; 28:7; Dan. 7:7.
TERRIBLENESS. Deut. 26:8; 1 Chron. 17:21; Jer. 49:16.
TERRIBLY. Isa. 2:19, 21; Nah. 2:3.
TERRIFY. Job 9:34, let not his fear *t.*
Lu. 21:9, when ye hear of wars, be not *t.*
24:37, they were *t.* and affrighted.
Phil. 1:28, in nothing *t.* by adversaries.
See Job 7:14; 2 Cor. 10:9.
TERROR. Gen. 35:5; Job 6:4, the *t.* of God.
Deut. 32:25, the sword without and *t.* within.
Josh. 2:9, your *t.* is fallen upon us.
Job 18:11, *t.* shall make him afraid.
24:17, in the *t.* of the shadow of death.
31:23, destruction was a *t.* to me.
33:7, my *t.* shall not make thee afraid.
Ps. 55:4, the *t.* of death are fallen upon me.
73:19, utterly consumed with *t.*
91:5, afraid for the *t.* by night.
Jer. 17:17, be not a *t.* to me.
20:4, a *t.* to thyself.

Ezek. 26:21; 27:36; 28:19, I will make thee a *t.*
Rom. 13:3, rulers are not *t.* to good works.
2 Cor. 5:11, knowing the *t.* of the Lord.
See Jer. 15:8; Lam. 2:22; Ezek. 21:12; 1 Pet. 3:14.
TESTIFY. Num. 35:30, one witness shall not *t.*
Deut. 31:21, this song shall *t.* against them.
Ruth 1:21, seeing the Lord hath *t.* against me.
2 Sam. 1:16, thy mouth hath *t.* against thee.
Neh. 9:30, *t.* against them by thy spirit.
Job 15:6, thine own lips *t.* against thee.
Isa. 59:12, our sins *t.* against us.
Hos. 5:5; 7:10, the pride of Israel doth *t.*
Mic. 6:3, what have I done? *t.* against me.
Lu. 16:28, send Lazarus, that he may *t.*
John 2:25, needed not that any should *t.*
3:32, seen and heard, that he *t.*
5:39, they *t.* of me.
7:7, because I *t.* of it.
15:26, he shall *t.* of me.
21:24, the disciple which *t.* of these things.
Acts 23:11, as thou hast *t.* in Jerusalem.
1 Tim. 2:6, gave himself to be *t.* in due time.
1 Pet. 1:11, it *t.* beforehand the sufferings.
1 John 4:14, we have seen and do *t.*
See 1 Cor. 15:15; 1 Thess. 4:6; Rev. 22:16.
TESTIMONY. 2 Kings 17:15, rejected his *t.*
Ps. 93:5, thy *t.* are sure.
119:22, I have kept thy *t.*
24, thy *t.* are my delight.
46, I will speak of thy *t.*
59, I turned my feet to thy *t.*
119, I love thy *t.*
129, thy *t.* are wonderful.
Isa. 8:16, bind up the *t.*
20, to the law and to the *t.*
Mat. 10:18; Mk. 13:9, for a *t.* against them.
Lu. 21:13, it shall turn to you for a *t.*
John 3:32, no man receiveth his *t.*
21:24, we know that his *t.* is true.
Acts 14:3, *t.* to the word of his grace.
1 Cor. 2:1, declaring the *t.* of God.
2 Cor. 1:12, the *t.* of our conscience.
2 Tim. 1:8, be not ashamed of the *t.*
Heb. 11:5, Enoch had this *t.*
See Rev. 1:2; 6:9; 11:7; 12:11; 19:10.
THANK. Mat. 11:25; Lu. 10:21; 18:11; John 11:41, I *t.* thee.
Acts 28:15, *t.* God, and took courage.
1 Cor. 1:4, I *t.* God on your behalf.
2 Thess. 1:3, we are bound to *t.* God.
1 Tim. 1:12, I *t.* Jesus Christ.
See 1 Chron. 23:30; Dan. 2:23; Rom. 6:17.
THANKS. Neh. 12:31, companies that gave *t.*
Mat. 26:27; Lu. 22:17, took the cup, and gave *t.*
Lu. 2:38, Anna gave *t.* to the Lord.
Rom. 14:6, eateth to the Lord, for he giveth *t.*
1 Cor. 15:57, *t.* be to God, who giveth us the victory.
Eph. 5:20, giving *t.* always for all things.
1 Thess. 3:9, what *t.* can we render?
Rev. 4:9, give *t.* to him that sat on the throne.
See 2 Cor. 1:11; 2:14; 8:16; 9:15; Heb. 13:15.
THANKSGIVING. Ps. 26:7, the voice of *t.*
95:2, come before his face with *t.*
Isa. 51:3, *t.* and melody shall be found therein.
Amos 4:5, offer a sacrifice of *t.*
Phil. 4:6, with *t.* let your requests be made.
Col. 4:2, watch in the same with *t.*
1 Tim. 4:3, to be received with *t.*
See Neh. 11:17; 12:8; 2 Cor. 4:15; 9:11.
THAT. Gen. 18:25, *t.* be far from thee.
Num. 24:13; 1 Kings 22:14, *t.* will I speak.
Job 23:13, even *t.* he doeth.
Ps. 27:4, *t.* will I seek after.
Zech. 11:9, *t. t.* dieth, let it die.
Mat. 10:15; Mk. 6:11, than for *t.* city.
13:12; 25:29; Mk. 4:25, *t.* he hath.
John 1:8, he was not *t.* light.
5:12, what man is *t.* which said?
John 13:27, *t.* thou doest, do quickly.
21:22, what is *t.* to thee?
Rom. 7:19, the evil which I would not, *t.* I do.
Jas. 4:15, we shall live, and do this or *t.*
See Mk. 13:11; 1 Cor. 11:23; 2 Cor. 8:12; Philem. 18.
THEN. Gen. 4:26, *t.* began men to call.
Josh. 14:12, if the Lord be with me, *t.* I shall be able.
Ps. 27:10, *t.* the Lord will take me up.
55:12, *t.* I could have borne it.
Isa. 58:8, *t.* shall thy light break forth.
Ezek. 39:28, *t.* shall they know.
Mat. 5:24, *t.* come and offer thy gift.
19:25; Mk. 10:26, who *t.* can be saved?
24:14, *t.* shall the end come.
2 Cor. 12:10, *t.* am I strong.
See 1 Cor. 4:5; 13:12; 1 Thess. 5:3; 2 Thess. 2:8.
THESE. Ex. 32:4, *t.* be thy gods, O Israel.
Eccl. 7:10, former days better than *t.*
Isa. 60:8, who are *t.* that fly?
Mat. 5:37, whatsoever is more than *t.*
23:23, *t.* ought ye to have done.
25:40, one of the least of *t.*
John 17:20, neither pray I for *t.* alone.
21:15, lovest thou me more than *t.*?
See Job 26:14; Ps. 73:12; Jer. 7:4.
THICK. Deut. 32:15, thou art grown *t.*
2 Sam. 18:9, the mule went under the *t.* boughs.
Ps. 74:5, lifted up axes on the *t.* trees.
Ezek. 31:3, top was among *t.* boughs.
Hab. 2:6, ladeth himself with *t.* clay.
See 1 Kings 12:10; 2 Chron. 10:10; Neh. 8:15; Job 15:26.
THICKET. Gen. 22:13; Isa. 9:18; Jer. 4:7, 29.
THIEF. Ps. 50:18, when thou sawest a *t.*
Jer. 2:26, as the *t.* is ashamed.
Joel 2:9, enter at windows like a *t.*
Lu. 12:33, where no *t.* approacheth.
John 10:1, the same is a *t.* and a robber.
1 Pet. 4:15, let none suffer as a *t.*
See Prov. 6:30; 29:24; Mat. 24:43.
THIEVES. Isa. 1:23; Lu. 10:30; John 10:8; 1 Cor. 6:10.
THIGH. Gen. 24:2; 47:29, put hand under *t.*
32:25, touched hollow of Jacob's *t.*
Judg. 15:8, smote them hip and *t.*
Cant. 3:8, every man hath sword on his *t.*
See Ps. 45:3; Jer. 31:19; Ezek. 21:12; Rev. 19:16.
THINE. Gen. 31:32, discern what is *t.*
1 Sam. 15:28, to a neighbour of *t.*
1 Kings 20:4, I am *t.*, and all I have.
1 Chron. 29:11, *t.* is the greatness.
Ps. 74:16, the day is *t.*, the night also is *t.*
119:94, I am *t.*, save me.
Isa. 63:19, we are *t.*
Mat. 20:14, take that is *t.*
Lu. 4:7, worship me, all shall be *t.*
22:42, not my will, but *t.* be done.
John 17:6, *t.* they were, and thou gavest them me.
10, all mine are *t.* and *t.* are mine.
See Gen. 14:23; Josh. 17:18; 1 Chron. 12:18; Lu. 15:31.
THING. Gen. 21:11, the *t.* was very grievous.
Ex. 18:17, the *t.* thou doest is not good.
2 Sam. 13:33, let not my lord take the *t.* to heart.
2 Kings 20:10, thou hast asked a hard *t.*
Eccl. 1:9, the *t.* that hath been.
Isa. 7:13, is it a small *t.* to weary?
41:12, as a *t.* of nought.
43:19; Jer. 31:22, a new *t.*
Mk. 1:27, what *t.* is this?
John 5:14, lest a worse *t.* come unto thee.
Phil. 3:16, let us mind the same *t.*
See Heb. 10:29; 1 Pet. 4:12; 1 John 2:8.
THINK. Gen. 40:14, but *t.* on me when it shall be well.
Neh. 5:19, *t.* on me, O my God, for good.
Ps. 40:17, I am poor, yet the Lord *t.* on me.
Prov. 23:7, as he *t.* in his heart, so is he.
Isa. 10:7, nor doth his heart *t.* so.
Jonah 1:6, if God will *t.* upon us.
Mat. 3:9, *t.* not to say within yourselves.

Mat. 6:7, *t.* they shall be heard.
9:4, why *t.* ye evil in your hearts?
17:25; 22:17, what *t.* thou?
22:42; 26:66; Mk. 14:64, what *t.* ye of Christ?
Rom. 12:3, more highly than he ought to *t.*
1 Cor. 10:12, that *t.* he standeth.
2 Cor. 3:5, to *t.* any thing as of ourselves.
Gal. 6:3, if a man *t.* himself to be something.
Eph. 3:20, able to do above all we ask or *t.*
Phil. 4:8, *t.* on these things.
Jas. 1:7, let not that man *t.* he shall receive.
1 Pet. 4:12, *t.* it not strange.
See Job 35:2; Jer. 29:11; Ezek. 38:10; Lu. 10:36.
THIRST (*n.*). Ex. 17:3, to kill us with *t.*
Deut. 29:19, to add drunkenness to *t.*
Judg. 15:18, now I shall die for *t.*
2 Chron. 32:11, doth persuade you to die by *t.*
Ps. 69:21, in my *t.* they gave me vinegar.
Isa. 41:17, when their tongue faileth for *t.*
Amos 8:11, not a *t.* for water, but of hearing.
2 Cor. 11:27, in hunger and *t.* often.
See Deut. 28:48; Job 24:11; Ps. 104:11.
THIRST (*v.*). Ps. 42:2; 63:1; 143:6, my soul *t.* for God.
Isa. 49:10; Rev. 7:16, shall not hunger nor *t.*
55:1, every one that *t.*
Mat. 5:6, *t.* after righteousness.
John 4:14; 6:35, shall never *t.*
7:37, if any man *t.*, let him come unto me.
19:28, I *t.*
See Ex. 17:3; Isa. 48:21; Rom. 12:20; 1 Cor. 4:11.
THIRSTY. Ps 63:1; 143:6, in a *t.* land.
Ps. 107:5, hungry and *t.*, their soul fainted.
Prov 25:25, as cold waters to a *t.* soul.
Isa. 21:14, brought water to him that was *t.*
29:8, as when a *t.* man dreameth.
44:3, pour water on him that is *t.*
65:13, but ye shall be *t.*
See Judg. 4:19; Isa. 32:6; Ezek. 19:13; Mat. 25:35.
THISTLE. Gen. 3:18, thorns and *t.* shall it bring forth.
Job 31:40, let *t.* grow instead of wheat.
Mat. 7:16, do men gather figs of *t.*?
See 2 Kings 14:9; 2 Chron. 25:18; Hos. 10:8.
THORN. Num. 33:55; Judg. 2:3, *t.* in your sides.
Ps. 118:12, quenched as the fire of *t.*
Prov. 15:19, way of slothful man is as an hedge of *t.*
24:31, it was all grown over with *t.*
26:9, as a *t.* goeth into hand of drunkard.
Eccl. 7:6, crackling of *t.* under a pot.
Cant. 2:2, as the lily among *t.*
Isa. 33:12, as *t.* cut up shall they be burned.
34:13, and *t.* shall come up in her palaces.
55:13, instead of the *t.* shall come up the fir tree.
Jer. 4:3, sow not among *t.*
12:13, but shall reap *t.*
Hos. 2:6, I will hedge up thy way with *t.*
9:6, *t.* shall be in their tabernacles.
10:8, the *t.* shall come up on their altars.
Mic. 7:4, most upright is sharper than *t.* hedge.
2 Cor. 12:7, a *t.* in the flesh.
See Mat. 13:7; 27:29; Mk. 15:17; John 19:2.
THOUGHT (*n.*). 1 Chron. 28:9, the Lord understandeth the *t.*
Job 4:13, in *t.* from the visions of the night.
12:5, despised in *t.* of him that is at ease.
42:2, no *t.* can be withholden from thee.
Ps. 10:4, God is not in all his *t.*
40:5, thy *t.* cannot be reckoned.
92:5, thy *t.* are very deep.
94:11, the Lord knoweth the *t.* of man.
19, in the multitude of my *t.*
139:2, thou understandest my *t.* afar off.
17, how precious are thy *t.* to me!
23, try me, and know my *t.*
Prov. 12:5, the *t.* of the righteous are right.
16:3, thy *t.* shall be established.
24:9, the *t.* of foolishness is sin.
Isa. 55:7, and the unrighteous man his *t.*
8, my *t.* are not your *t.*
Isa. 55:9, so are my *t.* higher than your *t.*
Mic. 4:12, they know not the *t.* of the Lord.
Mat. 6:25, 31, 34; 10:19; Mk. 13:11; Lu. 12:11, 22, take no *t.*
9:4; 12:25; Lu. 5:22; 6:8; 9:47; 11:17, Jesus knowing their *t.*
15:19; Mk. 7:21, out of the heart proceed evil *t.*
Lu. 2:35, the *t.* of many hearts may be revealed.
24:38, why do *t.* arise in your hearts?
Acts 8:22, if the *t.* of thine heart may be forgiven.
1 Cor. 3:20, the Lord knoweth the *t.* of the wise.
2 Cor. 10:5, bringing into captivity every *t.*
Heb. 4:12, the word of God is a discerner of the *t.*
Jas. 2:4, ye are become judges of evil *t.*
See Gen. 6:5; Jer. 4:14; 23:20; Amos 4:13.
THOUGHT (*v.*). Gen. 48:11, I had not *t.* to see thy face.
Num. 24:11, I *t.* to promote thee.
Deut. 19:19, do to him as he *t.* to have done.
2 Kings 5:11, I *t.*, he will surely come out.
Neh. 6:2, they *t.* do me mischief.
Ps. 48:9. we have *t.* of thy lovingkindness.
50:21, thou *t.* I was such an one as thyself.
73:16, when I *t.* to know this.
119:59, I *t.* on my ways.
Prov. 30:32, if thou hast *t.* evil.
Isa. 14:24, as I have *t.*, so shall it come.
Jer. 18:8, I will repent of the evil I *t.* to do.
Zech. 8:14, as *t.* to punish you.
15, I *t.* to do well.
Mal. 3:16, for them that *t.* on his name.
Mat. 1:20, but while he *t.* on these things.
Mk. 14:72, when he *t.* thereon, he wept.
Lu. 12:17, he *t.* within himself, what shall I do?
19:11, *t.* kingdom of God should appear.
John 11:13, they *t.* he had spoken of taking of rest.
Acts 10:19, while Peter *t.* on the vision.
26:8, why should it be *t.* a thing incredible?
1 Cor. 13:11, I *t.* as a child.
Phil. 2:6, *t.* it not robbery to be equal with God.
See Gen. 20:11; 50:20; 1 Sam. 1:13; Heb. 10:29.
THREAD. Gen. 14:23; Josh. 2:18; Judg. 16:9.
THREATEN. Acts 4:17; 9:1; Eph. 6:9; 1 Pet. 2:23.
THREEFOLD. Eccl. 4:12, a *t.* cord.
THRESH. Isa. 41:15, thou shalt *t.* the mountains.
Jer. 51:33, it is time to *t.* her.
Mic. 4:13, arise and *t.*
Hab. 3:12, thou didst *t.* the heathen.
1 Cor. 9:10, *t.* in hope.
See Lev. 26:5; 1 Chron. 21:20; Isa. 21:10; 28:28
THREW. 2 Kings 9:33; Mk. 12:42; Lu. 9:42; Acts 22:23.
THROAT. Ps. 5:9; 115:7; Prov. 23:2; Mat 18:28.
THRONE. Ps. 11:4, the Lord's *t.* is in heaven.
94:20, shall *t.* of iniquity have fellowship with thee?
122:5, there are set *t.* of judgment.
Prov. 20:28, his *t.* upholden by mercy.
Isa. 66:1; Acts 7:49, heaven is my *t.*
Jer. 17:12, a glorious high *t.* from the beginning.
Dan. 7:9, his *t.* was like the fiery flame.
Mat. 19:28; 25:31, the Son of man shall sit in the *t.*
Col. 1:16, whether they be *t.*
Heb. 4:16, the *t.* of grace.
Rev. 3:21, to him will I grant to sit on my *t.*
4:2, a *t.* was set in heaven.
See Rev. 6:16; 7:9; 14:3; 19:4; 20:11; 22:1.
THRONG. Mk. 3:9; 5:31; Lu. 8:42, 45.
THROW. Mic. 5:11; Mal. 1:4; Mat. 24:2.
THRUST. Job 32:13, God *t.* him down, not man.
Joel 2:8, neither shall one *t.* another.
Lu. 10:15, shall be *t.* down to hell.
13:28, and you yourselves *t.* out.
John 20:25, and *t.* my hand into his side.
Rev. 14:15, *t.* in thy sickle.
See Ex. 11:1; 1 Sam. 31:4; Ezek. 34:21.
TIDINGS. Ps. 112:7, afraid of evil *t.*
Jer. 20:15, cursed be the man who brought *t.*
Dan. 11:44, *t.* out of the east.
Lu. 1:19; 2:10; 8:1; Acts 13:32; Rom. 10:15, glad *t.*
See Ex. 33:4; 1 Kings 14:6; Jer. 49:23.
TILL. Gen. 2:5; Prov. 12:11; 28:19; Ezek. 36:9.

TILLAGE. 1 Chron. 27:26; Neh. 10:37; Prov. 13:23.
TIME. Gen. 47:29, the *t.* drew nigh.
Job 22:16, cut down out of *t.*
38:23, reserved against the *t.* of trouble.
Ps. 32:6, in a *t.* when thou mayest be found.
37:19, not ashamed in the evil *t.*
41:1, deliver him in *t.* of trouble.
56:3, what *t.* I am afraid.
69:13; Isa. 49:8; 2 Cor. 6:2, acceptable *t.*
89:47, remember how short my *t.* is.
Eccl. 3:1, there is a *t.* to very purpose.
9:11, *t.* and chance happeneth to all.
Isa. 60:22, I will hasten it in his *t.*
Jer. 46:21, the *t.* of their visitation.
Ezek. 16:8, thy *t.* was the *t.* of love.
Dan. 7:25, a *t.* and *t.* and the dividing of *t.*
Hos. 10:12, it is *t.* to seek the Lord.
Mal. 3:11, neither shall vine cast fruit before the *t.*
Mat. 16:3, the signs of the *t.*
Lu. 19:44, the *t.* of thy visitation.
Acts 3:19, the *t.* refreshing.
21, the *t.* of restitution.
Rom. 13:11, it is high *t.* to awake.
1 Cor. 7:29, the *t.* is short.
Eph. 5:16; Col. 4:5, redeeming the *t.*
Heb. 4:16, help in *t.* of need.
1 Pet. 1:11, what manner of *t.*
Rev. 1:3, the *t.* is at hand.
10:6, *t.* no longer.
See Prov. 17:17; Eph. 1:10; 1 Tim. 4:1.
TINGLE. 1 Sam. 3:11; 2 Kings 21:12; Jer. 19:3.
TINKLING. Isa. 3:16, 18; 1 Cor. 13:1.
TOGETHER. Prov. 22:2, meet *t.*
Amos 3:3, can two walk *t.*?
Mat. 18:20, where two or three are gathered *t.*
Rom. 8:28, work *t.* for good.
1 Thess. 4:17, caught up *t.*
See Mat. 19:6, Eph. 2:21; 2 Thess. 2:1.
TOIL. Gen. 5:29; 41:51; Mat. 6:28; Lu. 12:27.
TOLERABLE. Mat. 10:15; 11:24; Mk. 6:11; Lu. 10:12.
TONGUE. Job 5:21, hid from scourge of the *t.*
20:12, hide wickedness under his *t.*
Ps. 34:13; 1 Pet. 3:10, keep thy *t.* from evil.
Prov. 10:20, *t.* of the just as choice silver.
12:18; 31:26, *t.* of the wise is health.
19, the lying *t.* is but for a moment.
15:4, a wholesome *t.* is a tree of life.
18:21, death and life are in the power of the *t.*
21:23, whoso keepeth his *t.* keepeth his soul.
25:15, a soft *t.* breaketh the bone.
Isa. 30:27, his *t.* as a devouring fire.
50:4, hath given me the *t.* of the learned.
Jer. 9:5, taught their *t.* to speak lies.
18:18, let us smite him with the *t.*
Mk. 7:35, his *t.* was loosed.
Jas. 1:26, and bridleth not his *t.*
3:5, the *t.* is a little member.
6, the *t.* is a fire.
8, the *t.* can no man tame.
1 John 3:18, not love in word, neither in *t.*
See Ps. 45:1; Lu. 16:24; Rom. 14:11; Phil. 2:11.
TOOL. Ex. 20:25; 32:4; Deut. 27:5; 1 Kings 6:7.
TOOTH. Ex. 21:24; Prov. 25:19; Mat. 5:38.
TOPAZ. Ex. 28:17; Rev. 21:20.
TORCHES. Nah. 2:3; Zech. 12:6; John 18:3.
TORMENT. Mat. 8:29, to *t.* before the time.
Lu. 16:23, being in *t.*
Heb. 11:37, destitute, afflicted, *t.*
1 John 4:18, fear hath *t.*
Rev. 9:5, *t.* as *t.* of a scorpion.
14:11, the smoke of their *t.*
See Mat. 4:24; Mk. 5:7; Lu. 8:28.
TORN. Gen. 44:28, surely he is *t.* in pieces.
Ezek. 4:14, have not eaten of that which is *t.*
Hos. 6:1, he hath *t.*, and he will heal us.
See Isa. 5:25; Mal. 1:13; Mk. 1:26.
TORTOISE. Lev. 11:29, and the *t.* after his kind.

TOSS. Ps. 109:23, I am *t.* up and down.
Isa. 22:18, he will *t.* thee like a ball.
54:11, afflicted, *t.* with tempest.
Eph. 4:14, no more children, *t.* to and fro.
See Mat. 14:24; Acts 27:18; Jas. 1:6.
TOUCH. Gen. 3:3, nor *t.* it, lest ye die.
1 Sam. 10:26, a band whose hearts God had *t.*
1 Chron. 16:22; Ps. 105:15, *t.* not mine anointed.
Job 5:19, there shall no evil *t.* thee.
6:7, things my soul refused to *t.*
Isa. 6:7, lo, this hath *t.* thy lips.
Jer. 1:9, the Lord *t.* my mouth.
Zech. 2:8, he that *t.* you, *t.* the apple of his eye.
Mat. 9:21; Mk. 5:28, if I may but *t.* his garment.
Mk. 10:13; Lu. 18:15, children, that he should *t.* them.
John 20:17, *t.* me not.
2 Cor. 6:17, *t.* not the unclean thing.
Col. 2:21, *t.* not, taste not.
See Job 19:21; Lu. 7:14; 11:46; 1 Cor. 7:1.
TOWER. 2 Sam. 22:3; Ps. 18:2; 144:2, my high *t.*
Ps. 61:3, a strong *t.* from the enemy.
Prov. 18:10, the name of the Lord is a strong *t.*
Isa. 33:18, where is he that counted the *t.*?
See Isa. 2:15; 5:2; Mic. 4:8; Mat. 21:33.
TRADITION. Mat. 15:2; Mk. 7:3, they disciples transgress the *t.*
Gal. 1:14, zealous of the *t.* of my fathers.
Col. 2:8, after the *t.* of men.
1 Pet. 1:18, received by *t.* from your fathers.
TRAFFICK. Gen. 42:34; 1 Kings 10:15; Ezek. 17:4.
TRAIN. 1 Kings 10:2; Prov. 22:6; Isa. 6:1.
TRAITOR. Lu. 6:16; 2 Tim. 3:4.
TRAMPLE. Ps. 91:13; Isa. 63:3; Mat. 7:6.
TRANQUILLITY. Dan. 4:27, lengthening of thy *t.*
TRANSFORM. Rom. 12:2; 2 Cor. 11:13, 14, 15.
TRANSGRESS. Num. 14:41, wherefore do ye *t.*?
1 Sam. 2:24, make the Lord's people to *t.*
Neh. 1:8, if ye *t.*, I will scatter you abroad.
Ps. 17:3, my mouth shall not *t.*
Prov. 28:21, for a piece of bread that man will *t.*
Jer. 2:8, the pastors *t.*
3:13, only acknowledge that thou hast *t.*
Hab. 2:5, he *t.* by wine.
See Mat. 15:2; Rom. 2:27; 1 John 3:4; 2 John 9.
TRANSGRESSION. Ex. 34:7; Num. 14:18, forgiving *t.*
1 Chron. 10:13, Saul died for his *t.*
Ezra 10:6, he mourned because of their *t.*
Job 7:21, why dost thou not pardon my *t.*?
13:23, make me to know my *t.*
14:17, my *t.* is sealed up.
31:33, if I covered my *t.*
Ps. 19:13, innocent from the great *t.*
25:7, remember not my *t.*
32:1, blessed is he whose *t.* is forgiven.
51:1, blot out all my *t.*
65:3, as for our *t.*, thou shalt purge them.
107:17, fools because of their *t.* are afflicted.
Prov. 17:9, he that covereth a *t.*
Isa. 43:25; 44:22, blotteth out thy *t.*
53:5, he was wounded for our *t.*
8, for the *t.* of my people was he smitten.
58:1, show my people their *t.*
Ezek. 18:22, his *t.* shall not be mentioned.
Mic. 1:5, what is the *t.* of Jacob?
See Rom. 4:15; 5:14; 1 Tim. 2:14; Heb. 2:2.
TRANSGRESSOR. Ps. 51:13, teach *t.* thy ways.
59:5, be not merciful to any wicked *t.*
Prov. 13:15, the way of *t.* is hard.
21:18, the *t.* shall be ransom for the upright.
Isa. 48:8, thou wast called a *t.* from the womb.
53:12; Mk. 15:28; Lu. 22:37, numbered with the *t.*
See Dan. 8:23; Hos. 14:9, Gal. 2:18.
TRANSLATE. 2 Sam. 3:10; Col. 1:13; Heb. 11:5.
TRAP. Job 18:10; Ps. 69:22; Jer. 5:26; Rom. 11:9.
TRAVAIL. Ps. 7:14, he *t.* with iniquity.
Isa. 23:4, I *t.* not.
53:11, the *t.* of his soul.

Rom. 8:22, the whole creation *t.* in pain.
Gal. 4:19, my children of whom I *t.*
See Job 15:20; Isa. 13:8; Mic. 5:3; Rev. 12:2.
TRAVEL. Eccl. 1:13; 2:23; 1 Thess. 2:9; 2 Thess. 3:8.
TRAVELLER. Judg. 5:6; 2 Sam. 12:4; Job 31:32.
TREACHEROUS. Isa. 21:2; Jer. 9:2; Zeph. 3:4.
TREACHEROUSLY. Isa. 33:1, thou dealest *t.*
Jer. 12:1, why are they happy that deal *t.*?
Lam. 1:2, her friends have dealt *t.* with her.
See Hos. 5:7; 6:7; Mal. 2:10, 15.
TREAD. Deut. 11:24, whereon soles of feet *t.*
Deut. 25:4; 1 Cor. 9:9; 1 Tim. 5:18, not muzzle the ox when he *t.*
Ps. 7:5, let him *t.* down my life.
44:5, through thy name will we *t.* them under.
60:12; 108:13, shall *t.* down our enemies.
91:13, thou shalt *t.* upon lion and adder.
Isa. 10:6, to *t.* them down like mire.
16:10, shall *t.* out no wine.
63:3, I will *t.* them in mine anger.
Jer. 48:33, none shall *t.* with shouting.
Ezek. 34:18, but ye must *t.* the residue.
Hos. 10:11, loveth to *t.* out corn.
Mal. 4:3, ye shall *t.* down the wicked.
See Job 9:8; Isa. 41:25; 62:2; Rev. 19:15.
TREASURE. Gen. 43:23, God hath given you *t.*
Ex. 19:5; Ps. 135:4, a peculiar *t.* to me.
Deut. 28:12, open to thee his good *t.*
Job 3:21; Ps. 17:14; Prov. 2:4, for hid *t.*
38:22, the *t.* of the snow.
Prov. 8:21, I will fill *t.* of those that love me.
10:2, *t.* of wickedness profiteth nothing.
15:16, than great *t.* and trouble therewith.
21:20, there is a *t.* to be desired.
Eccl. 2:8, I gathered the peculiar *t.* of kings.
Isa. 2:7, neither is there any end of their *t.*
45:3, I will give thee the *t.* of darkness.
Jer. 41:8, slay us not, for we have *t.*
51:13, waters abundant in *t.*
Dan. 11:43, power over the *t.* of gold.
Mic. 6:10, the *t.* of wickedness.
Mat. 6:21; Lu. 12:34, where your *t.* is.
12:35, out of the good *t.* of the heart.
13:44, like unto *t.* hid in a field.
52, out of his *t.* things new and old.
19:21; Mk. 10:21; Lu. 18:22, thou shalt have *t.* in heaven.
Lu. 12:21, that layeth up *t.* for himself.
Col. 2:3, in whom are hid *t.* of wisdom.
2 Cor. 4:7, we have this *t.* in earthen vessels.
Heb. 11:26, greater riches than the *t.* in Egypt.
Jas. 5:3, ye have heaped *t.*
See Deut. 32:34; 33:19; Isa. 33:6; Mat. 2:11.
TREASURER. Neh. 13:13; Isa. 22:15; Dan. 3:2.
TREASURY. Mk. 12:41, the people cast money into the *t.*
Lu. 21:1, rich men casting their gifts into the *t.*
See Josh. 6:19; Jer. 38:11; Mat. 27:6.
TREE. Deut. 20:19, the *t.* is man's life.
Job 14:7, there is hope of a *t.*
24:20, wickedness shall be broken as a *t.*
Ps. 1:3; Jer. 17:8, like a *t.* planted.
104:16, the *t.* of the Lord are full of sap.
Eccl. 11:3, where the *t.* falleth.
Isa. 56:3, I am a dry *t.*
61:3, called *t.* of righteousness.
Ezek. 15:2, what is the vine *t.* more than any *t.*?
31:9, all the *t.* of Eden envied him.
See Mk. 8:24; Lu. 21:29; Jude 12; Rev. 7:3.
TREMBLE. Deut. 2:25, the nations shall *t.*
Judg. 5:4; 2 Sam. 22:8; Ps. 18:7; 77:18; 97:4, the earth *t.*
Ezra 9:4, then assembled to me every one that *t.*
Job 9:6, the pillars thereof *t.*
26:11, the pillars of heaven *t.*
Ps. 2:11, rejoice with *t.*
60:2, thou hast made earth to *t.*
99:1, the Lord reigneth, let the people *t.*
104:32, he looketh on the earth, and it *t.*
Eccl. 12:3, the keepers of the house shall *t.*
Isa. 14:16, is this the man that made earth *t.*?
64:2, that the nations may *t.* at thy presence.
66:5, ye that *t.* at his word.
Jer. 5:22, will ye not *t.* at my presence?
33:9, they shall *t.* for all the goodness.
Amos 8:8, shall not the land *t.* for this?
Acts 24:25, Felix *t.*
Jas. 2:19, devils also believe, and *t.*
See Acts 9:6; 16:29; 1 Cor. 2:3; Eph. 6:5; Phil. 2:12.
TRENCH. 1 Sam. 17:20; 26:5; 1 Kings 18:32; Lu. 19:43.
TREPASS. Gen. 31:36, what is my *t.*?
50:17, we pray thee forgive the *t.*
Ezra 9:2, rulers have been chief in this *t.*
Ps. 68:21, goeth on still in his *t.*
Mat. 6:14, if ye forgive men their *t.*
18:15, if thy brother *t.*, tell him his fault.
Lu. 17:3, if thy brother *t.* against thee.
2 Cor. 5:19, not imputing their *t.*
Eph. 2:1, dead in *t.* and sins.
Col. 2:13, having forgiven you all *t.*
See Num. 5:6; 1 Kings 8:31; Ezek. 17:20; 18:24.
TRIAL. Job 9:23, the *t.* of the innocent.
2 Cor. 8:2, a great *t.* of affliction.
See Ezek. 21:13; Heb. 11:36; 1 Pet. 1:7; 4:12.
TRIBES. Ps. 105:37, not one feeble person among their *t.*
122:4, whither the *t.* go up.
Isa. 19:13, they that are the stay of the *t.*
49:6, my servant to raise up the *t.*
Hab. 3:9, according to oaths of the *t.*
Mat. 24:30, than shall all *t.* of the earth mourn.
See Num. 24:2; Deut. 1:13; 12:5; 18:5.
TRIBULATION. Deut. 4:30, when thou art in *t.*
Judg. 10:14, let them deliver you in *t.*
Mat. 13:21, when *t.* ariseth.
24:21, then shall be great *t.*
John 16:33, in the world ye shall have *t.*
Acts 14:22, through much *t.*
Rom. 5:3, we glory in *t.* also.
12:12, patient in *t.*
See 2 Cor. 1:4; 7:4; Eph. 3:13; Rev. 7:14.
TRIBUTARY. Deut. 20:11; Judg. 1:30; Lam. 1:1.
TRIBUTE. Gen. 49:15, a servant to *t.*
Num. 31:37, the Lord's *t.*
Deut. 16:10, *t.* of freewill offering.
Ezra 7:24, not lawful to impose *t.*
Neh. 5:4, borrowed money for king's *t.*
Prov. 12:24, the slothful shall be under *t.*
See Mat 17:24; 22:17; Lu. 23:2.
TRIM. 2 Sam. 19:24; Jer. 2:33; Mat. 25:7.
TRIUMPH. Ex. 15:1, he hath *t.* gloriously.
Ps. 25:2, let not mine enemies *t.*
92:4, I will *t.* in the works of thy hands.
2 Cor. 2:14, which always causeth us to *t.*
Col. 2:15, a show of them openly, *t.* over them.
See 2 Sam. 20; Job 20:5; Ps. 47:1.
TRODDEN. Job 22:15, the old way which wicked men have *t.*
Ps. 119:118, thou hast *t.* down all that err.
Isa. 5:5, the vineyard shall be *t.* down.
63:3, I have *t.* the winepress alone.
Mic. 7:10, now shall she be *t.* as mire.
Mat. 5:13, salt to be *t.* under foot.
Lu. 21:24, Jerusalem shall be *t.* down.
Heb. 10:29, hath *t.* under foot the Son of God.
See Deut 1:36; Judg. 5:21; Isa. 18:2.
TRODE. 2 Kings 14:9, 2 Chron. 25:18; Lu. 12:1.
TROOP. 2 Sam. 22:30; Ps. 18:29; Hos. 7:1.
TROUBLE (*n.*). Deut. 31:17, many *t.* shall befall.
1 Chron. 22:14, in my *t.* I prepared for the house.
Neh. 9:32, let not the *t.* seem little.
Job 3:26, yet *t.* came.
5:6, neither doth *t.* spring out of the ground.
7, man is born to *t.*
19, shall deliver thee in six *t.*
14:1, of few days, and full of *t.*
30:25, weep for him that was in *t.*
34:29, he giveth quietness, who can make *t.*?

Job 38:23, I have reserved against the time of *t.*
Ps. 9:9, a refuge in time of *t.*
22:11, for *t.* is near.
25:17, the *t.* of mine heart are enlarged.
22, redeem Israel out of all his *t.*
27:5, in time of *t.* he shall hide me.
46:1, a very present help in *t.*
73:5, they are not in *t.* as other men.
88:3, my soul is full of *t.*
119:143, *t.* and anguish have taken hold on me.
138:7, thou I walk in the midst of *t.*
Isa. 17:14, at eveningtide *t.*
30:6, into the land of *t.* they will carry riches.
65:16, because former *t.* are forgotten.
23, they shall not bring forth for *t.*
Jer. 2:27, in time of *t.* they will say, save us.
8:15, we looked for health, and behold *t.*
1 Cor. 7:28, such shall have *t.* in the flesh.
2 Cor. 1:4, able to comfort them in *t.*
See Prov. 15:6; 25:19; Jer. 11:12; 30:7; Lam. 1:21.
TROUBLE (*v.*). Josh. 7:25, why hast thou *t.* us?
1 Kings 18:17, art thou he that *t.* Israel?
18, I have not *t.* Israel, but thou.
Job 4:5, now it toucheth thee, and thou art *t.*
Ps. 3:1, how are they increased that *t.* me!
77:4, I am so *t.* that I cannot speak.
Prov. 25:26, is as a *t.* fountain.
Isa. 57:20, the wicked are like the *t.* sea.
Dan. 5:10, let not thy thoughts *t.* thee.
11:44, tidings out of the north shall *t.* him.
Mat. 24:6, see that ye be not *t.*
26:10; Mk. 14:6, why *t.* ye the woman?
John 5:4, an angel *t.* the water.
11:33; 12:27; 13:21, Jesus groaned, and was *t.*
2 Cor. 4:8; 7:5, we are *t.* on every side.
Gal. 1:7, there be some that *t.* you.
6:17, let no man *t.* me.
See 2 Thess. 1:7; 2:2; Heb. 12:15;1 Pet. 3:14.
TROUBLING. Job 3:17; John 5:4.
TRUCE. 2 Tim. 3:3, men shall be *t.*-breakers.
TRUE. Gen. 42:11, we are *t.* men.
1 Kings 22:16, tell me nothing but that which is *t.*
2 Chron. 15:3, Israel hath been without the *t.* God.
Neh. 9:13, thou gavest them *t.* laws.
Ps. 119:160, thy word is *t.* from the beginning.
Prov. 14:25, a *t.* witness delivereth souls.
Jer. 10:10, the Lord is the *t.* God.
Mat. 22:16; Mk. 12:14, we know that thou art *t.*
Lu. 16:11, the *t.* riches.
John 1:9, that was the *t.* light.
4:23, when the *t.* worshippers.
5:31, if I bear witness of myself, my witness is not *t.*
6:32, the *t.* bread.
10:41, all things that John spake were *t.*
15:1, I am the *t.* vine.
17:3; 1 John 5:20, to know thee the only *t.* God.
2 Cor. 6:8, as deceivers, and yet *t.*
Eph. 4:24, created in *t.* holiness.
Phil. 4:8, whatsoever things are *t.*
Heb. 10:22, draw near with a *t.* heart.
See Rev. 3:7; 6:10; 15:3; 16:7; 19:9, 11; 21:5.
TRUST. Job 13:15, though he slay me, yet will I *t.*
39:11, wilt thou *t.* him, because his strength is great?
Ps. 25:2; 31:6; 55:23; 56:3; 143:8, I *t.* in thee.
37:3; 40:3; 62:8; 115:9; Prov. 3:5; Isa. 26.
4, *t.* in the Lord.
118:8, better to *t.* in the Lord.
144:2, he in whom I *t.*
Prov. 28:26, he that *t.* in his own heart is a fool.
Isa. 50:10, let him *t.* in the name of the Lord.
Jer. 49:11, let thy widows *t.* in me.
Mic. 7:5, *t.* ye not in a friend.
Nah. 1:7, the Lord knoweth them that *t.* in him.
Mat. 27:43, he *t.* in God, let him deliver him.
Lu. 18:9, certain which *t.* in themselves.
See Jer. 17:5; 2 Cor. 1:9; 1 Tim. 4:10.
TRUTH. Deut. 32:4, a God of *t.*
Ps. 15:2, speaketh the *t.* in his heart.
51:6, desirest *t.* in inward parts.
91:4, his *t.* shall be thy shield.
117:2, his *t.* endureth for ever.
119:30, I have chosen the way of *t.*
Prov. 23:23, buy the *t.*
Isa. 59:14, *t.* is fallen in the streets.
Jer. 9:3, they are not valiant for the *t.*
Zech. 8:16, speak every man *t.* to his neighbour.
Mal. 2:6, the law of *t.* was in his mouth.
John 1:14, full of grace and *t.*
8:32, know the *t.*, and the *t.* shall make you free.
14:6, I am the way, the *t.*, and the life.
16:13, Spirit of *t.* will guide you into all *t.*
18:38, what is *t.*?
Rom. 1:18, who hold the *t.* in unrighteousness.
1 Cor. 5:8, unleavened bread of sincerity and *t.*
2 Cor. 13:8, can do nothing against *t.*, but for the *t.*
Eph. 4:15, speaking the *t.* in love.
1 Tim. 3:15, the pillar and ground of *t.*
2 Tim. 2:15, rightly dividing the word of *t.*
Jas. 5:19, if any err from the *t.*
See 1 Cor. 13:6; 2 Tim. 3:7; 1 John 3:19; 5:6.
TRY. 2 Chron. 32:31, God left him to *t.* him.
Job 23:10, when he hath *t.* me.
Ps. 26:2, *t.* my reins and my heart.
Jer. 9:7; Zech. 13:9, I will melt them and *t.* them.
1 Cor. 3:13, shall *t.* every man's work.
Jas. 1:12, when *t.* he shall receive the crown.
1 John 4:1, *t.* the spirits.
See Prov. 17:3; Isa. 28:16; 1 Pet. 4:12; Rev. 3:18.
TURN. Job 23:13, who can *t.* him.
Ps. 7:12, if he *t.* not, he will whet his sword.
Prov. 1:23, *t.* at my reproof.
Jer. 31:18; Lam. 5:21, *t.* thou me, and I shall be *t.*
Ezek. 14:6; 18:30; 33:9; Hos. 12:6; Joel 2:12, repent, and *t.*
Zech. 9:12, *t.* you to the strong hold, ye prisoners.
Mat. 5:39, *t.* the other also.
Acts 26:18, to *t.* them from darkness to light.
2 Tim. 3:5, from such *t.* away.
See Prov. 21:1; 26:14; Hos. 7:8; Lu. 22:61; Jas. 1:17.
TWAIN. Isa. 6:2; Mat. 5:41; 19:5; Eph. 2:15.
TWICE. Job 33:14; Mk. 14:30; Lu. 18:12; Jude 12.
TWINKLING. 1 Cor. 15:52, in the *t.* of an eye.

U

UNADVISEDLY. Ps. 106:33, he spake *u.*
UNAWARES. Lu. 21:34; Gal. 2:4; Heb. 13:2; Jude 4.
UNBELIEF. Mk. 9:24, help thou mine *u.*
Rom. 3:3, shall *u.* make faith without effect?
11:32, concluded all in *u.*
Heb. 3:12, evil heart of *u.*
See Mat. 13:58; Mk. 6:6; 1 Tim. 1:13; Heb. 4:11.
UMBLAMEABLE. Col. 1:22; 1 Thess. 3:13.
UNCERTAIN. 1 Cor. 9:26; 14:8; 1 Tim. 6:7.
UNCLEAN. Acts 10:28; Rom. 14:14; 2 Cor. 6:17.
UNCLOTHED. 2 Cor. 5:4, not that we would be *u.*
UNCORRUPTNESS. Tit. 2:7, in doctrine showing *u.*
UNCTION. 1 John 2:20, an *u.* from the Holy One.
UNDEFILED. Ps. 119:1, blessed are the *u.*
Jas. 1:27, pure religion and *u.*
1 Pet. 1:4, an inheritance *u.*
See Cant. 5:2; 6:9; Heb. 7:26; 13:4.
UNDER. Rom. 3:9; 1 Cor. 9:27; Gal. 3:10.
UNDERSTAND. Ps. 19:12, who can *u.* his errors?
73:17, then *u.* I their end.
119:100, I *u.* more than the ancients.
139:2, thou *u.* my thought afar off.
Prov. 8:9, all plain to him that *u.*
20:24, how can a man *u.* his own way?
29:19, though he *u.* he will not answer.
Isa. 6:9, hear ye indeed, but *u.* not.
28:19, a vexation only to *u.* the report.
Jer. 9:24, let him glory in this, that he *u.* me.
Dan. 10:12, thou didst set thine heart to *u.*
12:10, wicked shall not *u.* the wise shall *u.*
Hos. 14:9, who is wise, and he shall *u.* these things?

Mat. 13:51, have ye *u.* all these things?
24:15, whoso readeth, let him *u.*
Lu. 24:45, that they might *u.* the scriptures.
John 8:43, why do ye not *u.* my speech?
Rom. 3:11, there is none that *u.*
15:21, they that have not heard shall *u.*
1 Cor. 13:2, though I *u.* all mysteries.
11, I *u.* as a child.
See 1 Cor. 14:2; Heb. 11:3; 2 Pet. 2:12; 3:16.
UNDERSTANDING. Ex. 31:3; Deut. 4:6, wisdom and *u.*
1 Kings 3:11, hast asked for thyself *u.*
4:29, gave Solomon wisdom and *u.*
7:14, filled with wisdom and *u.*
1 Chron. 12:32, men that had *u.* of the times.
2 Chron. 26:5, had *u.* in visions.
Job 12:13, he hath counsel and *u.*
20, he taketh away the *u.* of the aged.
17:4, thou hast hid their heart from *u.*
28:12, where is the place of *u.*?
32:8, the Almighty giveth them *u.*
38:36, who hath given *u.* to the heart?
39:17, neither imparted to her *u.*
Ps. 47:7, sing ye praises with *u.*
49:3, the meditation of my heart shall be of *u.*
119:34, 73, 125, 144, 169, give me *u.*
99, I have more *u.* than my teachers.
104, through thy precepts I get *u.*
147:5, his *u.* is infinite.
Prov. 2:2, apply thine heart to *u.*
11, *u.* shall keep thee.
3:5, lean not to thine own *u.*
19, by *u.* hath he established the heavens.
4:5, 7, get wisdom, get *u.*
8:1, doth not *u.* put forth her voice?
9:6, go in the way of *u.*
10, the knowledge of the holy is *u.*
14:29, he that is slow to wrath is of great *u.*
16:22, *u.* is a wellspring of life.
17:24, wisdom is before him that hath *u.*
19:8, he that keepeth *u.* shall find good.
21:30, there is no *u.* against the Lord.
24:3, by *u.* an house is established.
30:2, have not the *u.* of a man.
Eccl. 9:11, nor yet riches to men of *u.*
Isa. 11:2, the spirit of *u.* shall rest on him.
27:11, it is a people of no *u.*
29:14, the *u.* of prudent men shall be hid.
40:14, who showed him the way of *u.*?
28, there is no searching of his *u.*
Jer. 3:15, pastors shall feed you with *u.*
Ezek. 28:4, with thy *u.* thou hast gotten riches.
Dan. 4:34, mine *u.* returned.
Mat. 15:16; Mk. 7:18, are ye also without *u.*?
Mk. 12:33, to love him with all the *u.*
Lu. 2:47, astonished at his *u.*
24:45, then opened he their *u.*
1 Cor. 1:19, bring to nothing *u.* of prudent.
14:15, I will pray with the *u.* also.
20, be not children in *u.*
Eph. 4:18, having the *u.* darkened.
Phil. 4:7, peace of God, which passeth all *u.*
See Col. 1:9; 2:2; 2 Tim. 2:7; 1 John 5:20.
UNDERTAKE. Isa. 38:14, *u.* for me.
UNDONE. Josh. 11:15; Isa. 6:5; Mat. 23:23; Lu. 11:42.
UNEQUAL. Ezek. 18:25, 29; 2 Cor. 6:14.
UNFAITHFUL. Ps. 78:57; Prov. 25:19.
UNFEIGNED. 2 Cor. 6:6; 1 Tim. 1:5; 2 Tim. 1:5; 1 Pet. 1:22.
UNFRUITFUL. Mat. 13:22; Eph. 5:11; Tit. 3:14; 2 Pet. 1:8.
UNGODLINESS. Rom. 1:18; 11:26; 2 Tim. 2:16; Tit. 2:12.
UNGODLY. 2 Chron. 19:2, shouldest thou help the *u.*?
Job 16:11, God hath delivered me to the *u.*
Ps. 1:1, counsel of *u.*
6, the way of the *u.* shall perish.
43:1, plead my cause against an *u.* nation.
Prov. 16:27, an *u.* man diggeth up evil.
Rom. 5:6, Christ died for the *u.*
1 Pet. 4:18, where shall the *u.* appear?
2 Pet. 3:7, perdition of *u.* men.
See Rom. 4:5; 1 Tim. 1:9; 2 Pet. 2:5; Jude 15.
UNHOLY. Lev. 10:10; 1 Tim. 1:9; 2 Tim. 3:2; Heb. 10:29.
UNICORN. Num. 23:22, he hath as it were the strength of an *u.*
Deut. 33:17, his horns are like the horns of an *u.*
Job 39:9, will the *u.* be willing to serve thee?
Isa. 34:7, the *u.* shall come down with them.
UNITE. Gen. 49:6; Ps. 86:11.
UNITY. Ps. 133:1; Eph. 4:3, 13.
UNJUST. Ps. 43:1; Prov. 11:7; 29:27, *u.* man.
Prov. 28:8, he that by *u.* gain.
Zeph. 3:5, the *u.* knoweth no shame.
Mat. 5:44, he sendeth rain on the just and *u.*
Lu. 18:6, hear what the *u.* judge saith.
11, not as other men, *u.*
Acts 24:15, a resurrection both of the just and *u.*
1 Cor. 6:1, go to law before the *u.*
1 Pet. 3:18, suffered, the just for the *u.*
Rev. 22:11, he that is *u.*, let him be *u.* still.
See Ps. 82:2; Isa. 26:10; Lu. 16:8; 2 Pet. 2:9.
UNKNOWN. Acts 17:23; 1 Cor. 14:2; 2 Cor. 6:9; Gal. 1:22.
UNLAWFUL. Acts 10:28; 2 Pet. 2:8.
UNLEARNED. Acts 4:13; 1 Cor. 14:16; 2 Tim. 2:23; 2 Pet. 3:16.
UNMINDFUL. Deut. 32:18, thou art *u.*
UNMOVEABLE. Acts 27:41; 1 Cor. 15:58.
UNPERFECT. Ps. 139:16, yet being *u.*
UNPREPARED. 2 Cor. 9:4, find you *u.*
UNPROFITABLE. Job 15:3, *u.* talk.
Mat. 25:30; Lu. 17:10, *u.* servant.
See Rom. 3:12; Tit. 3:9; Philem. 11; Heb. 7:18; 13:17.
UNPUNISHED. Prov. 11:21; 16:5; 17:5; 19:5; Jer. 25:29; 49:12, shall not be *u.*
See Jer. 30:11; 46:28.
UNQUENCHABLE. Mat. 3:12; Lu. 3:17.
UNREASONABLE. Acts 25:27; 2 Thess. 3:2.
UNREPROVEABLE. Col. 1:22, *u.* in his sight.
UNRIGHTEOUS. Ex. 23:1, an *u.* witness.
Isa. 10:1, decree *u.* decrees.
55:7, let the *u.* man forsake his thoughts.
Rom. 3:5, is God *u.*?
Heb. 6:10, God is not *u.* to forget your work.
See Deut. 25:16; Ps. 71:4; Lu. 16:11; 1 Cor. 6:9.
UNRIGHTEOUSNESS. Lu. 16:9, mammon of *u.*
Rom. 1:18, hold the truth in *u.*
2:8, to them that obey *u.*
3:5, if our *u.* commend righteousness.
6:13, instruments of *u.*
9:14, is there *u.* with God?
2 Cor. 6:14, what fellowship with *u.*?
2 Thess. 2:12, had pleasure in *u.*
2 Pet. 2:13, receive the reward of *u.*
1 John 1:9, cleanse us from all *u.*
5:17, all *u.* is sin.
See Lev. 19:15; Ps. 92:15; Jer. 22:13; John 7:18.
UNRULY. 1 Thess. 5:14; Tit. 1:6; Jas. 3:8.
UNSAVOURY. Job 6:6, can that which is *u.* be. eaten?
UNSEARCHABLE. Job 5:9; Ps. 145:3; Rom. 11:33; Eph. 3:8.
UNSEEMLY. Rom. 1:27; 1 Cor. 13:5.
UNSKILFUL. Heb. 5:13, is *u.* in the word.
UNSPEAKABLE. 2 Cor. 9:15; 12:4; 1 Pet. 1:8.
UNSPOTTED. Jas. 1:27, *u.* from the world.
UNSTABLE. Gen. 49:4; Jas. 1:8; 2 Pet. 2:14.
UNTHANKFUL. Lu. 6:35; 2 Tim. 3:2.
UNWASHEN. Mat. 15:20; Mk. 7:2, 5.
UNWISE. Deut. 32:6; Hos. 13:13; Rom. 1:14; Eph. 5:17.
UNWORTHY. Acts 13:46; 1 Cor. 6:2; 11:27.
UPBRAID. Mat. 11:20; Mk. 16:14; Jas. 1:5.
UPHOLD. Ps. 51:12, *u.* me with thy free spirit.
54:4, with them that *u.* my soul.
119:116, *u.* me according to thy word.
145:14, the Lord *u.* all that fall.
Isa. 41:10, I will *u.* thee with right hand.
42:1, my servant, whom I *u.*
63:5, wondered there was none to *u.*
Heb. 1:3, *u.* all things by the word of his power.
See Ps. 37:17; 41:12; 63:8; Prov. 20:28.
UPPERMOST. Mat. 23:6; Mk. 12:39; Lu. 11:43.

V

VESSEL. 2 Kings 4:6, there is not a *v.* more.
Ps. 2:9, them in pieces like a potter's *v.*
31:12, I am like a broken *v.*
Isa. 66:20, bring an offering in a clean *v.*
Jer. 22:28, a *v.* wherein is no pleasure.
25:34, fall like a pleasant *v.*
Mat. 13:48, gathered the good into *v.*
25:4, the wise took oil in their *v.*
Acts 9:15, he is a chosen *v.* unto me.
Rom. 9:22, the *v.* of wrath.
23, the *v.* of mercy.
1 Thess. 4:4, to possess his *v.* in sanctification.
2 Tim. 2:21, he shall be a *v.* to honour.
1 Pet. 3:7, giving honour to the wife as to weaker *v.*
See Isa. 52:11; 65:4; Jer. 14:3; Mk. 11:16.
VESTRY. 2 Kings 10:22, him that was over the *v.*
VESTURE. Gen. 41:42; Ps. 22:18; 102:26; Mat. 27:35; Heb. 1:12; Rev. 19:13.
VEX. Ex. 22:21; Lev. 19:33, not *v.* a stranger.
Num. 33:55, those ye let remain shall *v.* you.
2 Sam. 12:18, how will he *v.* himself?
Job 19:2, how long will ye *v.* my soul?
Isa. 11:13, Judah shall not *v.* Ephraim.
Ezek. 32:9, I will *v.* the hearts of many.
Mat. 15:22, my daughter is grievously *v.*
2 Pet. 2:8, *v.* his righteous soul.
See Lev. 18:18; Judg. 16:16; Isa. 63:10; Hab. 2:7.
VEXATION. Eccl. 1:14; 2:22; Isa. 9:1; 28:19; 65:14.
VICTORY. 2 Sam. 19:2, *v.* was turned to mourning.
1 Chron. 29:11, thine is the *v.*
Ps. 98:1, hath gotten him the *v.*
Mat. 12:20, send forth judgment unto *v.*
1 John 5:4, this is the *v.*, even our faith.
See Isa. 25:8; 1 Cor. 15:54, 55, 57.
VICTUALS. Ex. 12:39, neither had they prepared *v.*
Josh. 9:14, the men took of their v.
Neh. 10:31, bring *v.* on the sabbath.
13:15, in the day wherein they sold *v.*
Mat. 14:15; Lu. 9:12, into villages to buy *v.*
See Gen. 14:11; Judg. 17:10; 1 Sam. 22:10.
VIEW. Josh. 2:7; 7:2; 2 Kings 2:7; Neh. 2:13.
VIGILANT. 1 Tim. 3:2; 1 Pet. 5:8.
VILE. 1 Sam. 3:13, made themselves *v.*
Job 18:3, wherefore are we reputed *v.*?
40:4, I am *v.*, what shall I answer thee?
Ps. 15:4; Isa. 32:5; Dan. 11:21, a *v.* person.
Jer. 15:19, take the precious from the *v.*
Lam. 1:11, see, O Lord, for I am become *v.*
Nah. 3:6, I will make thee *v.*
Rom. 1:26, gave them up to *v.* affections.
Phil. 3:21, shall change our *v.* body.
Jas. 2:2, a poor man in *v.* raiment.
See 2 Sam. 1:21; Job 30:8; Ps. 12:8; Nah. 1:14.
VILLANY. Isa. 32:6; Jer. 29:23.
VINE. Deut. 32:32, their *v.* is of the *v.* of Sodom.
Judg. 13:14, may not eat any thing that cometh of the *v.*
1 Kings 4:25, dwelt every man under his *v.*
2 Kings 18:31; Isa. 36:16, eat every man of his own *v.*
Ps. 80:8, a *v.* out of Egypt.
128:3, thy wife as a fruitful *v.*
Isa. 24:7, the new wine mourneth, the *v.* languisheth.
Hos. 10:1, Israel is an empty *v.*
Mic. 4:4, they shall sit every man under his *v.*
Mat. 26:29; Mk. 14:25; Lu. 22:18, this fruit of the *v.*
John 15:1, I am the true *v.*
See Deut. 8:8; Cant. 2:15; Joel 1:7; Hab. 3:17.
VINTAGE. Job 24:6; Isa. 16:10; 32:10; Mic. 7:1.
VIOL. Isa. 5:12; 14:11; Amos 5:23; 6:5.
VIOLENCE. Gen. 6:11, earth was filled with *v.*
Ps. 11:5, him that loveth *v.*
55:9, I have seen *v.* in the city.
58:2, weigh the *v.* of your hands.
72:14, redeem their soul from *v.*
73:6, *v.* covereth them as a garment.
Prov. 4:17, they drink the wine of *v.*
10:6, *v.* covereth the mouth of the wicked.
Isa. 53:9, because he had done no *v.*
Isa. 60:18, *v.* shall no more be heard.
Ezek. 8:17; 28:16, they have filled the land with *v.*
Amos 3:10, store up *v.* in their palaces.
Hab. 1:3, *v.* is before me.
Mal. 2:16, one covereth *v.* with his garment.
Mat. 11:12, kingdom of heaven suffereth *v.*
Lu. 3:14, do *v.* to no man.
See Mic. 2:2; 6:12; Zeph. 1:9; Heb. 11:34.
VIOLENT. Ps. 7:16, his *v.* dealing.
18:48; 140:1; Prov. 16:29, the *v.* man.
See 2 Sam. 22:49; Eccl. 5:8; Mat. 11:12.
VIOLENTLY. Isa. 22:18; Mat. 8:32; Mk. 5:13.
VIRGIN. Isa. 23:12; 47:1; 62:5; Jer. 14:17.
VIRTUE. Mk. 5:30; Lu. 6:19; 8:46; Phil. 4:8; 2 Pet. 1:5.
VIRTUOUS. Ruth 3:11; Prov. 12:4; 31:10, 29.
VISAGE. Isa. 52:14; Lam. 4:8; Dan. 3:19.
VISION. Job 20:8, as a *v.* of the night.
Prov. 29:18, where there is no *v.*, people perish.
Isa. 22:1, the valley of *v.*
28:7, they err in *v.*
Lam. 2:9, prophets find no *v.* from the Lord.
Hos. 12:10, I have multiplied *v.*
Joel 2:28; Acts 2:17, young men shall see *v.*
Zech. 13:4, ashamed every one of his *v.*
Mat. 17:9, tell the *v.* to no man.
Lu. 24:23, had seen a *v.* of angels.
Acts 26:19, not disobedient to heavenly *v.*
See Job 4:13; Ezek. 1:1; 8:3; Mic. 3:6.
VISIT. Gen. 50:24; Ex. 13:19, God will *v.* you.
Ex. 20:5; 34:7; Num. 14:18; Deut. 5:9, *v.* the iniquity of the fathers.
32:34, when I *v.*, I will *v.* their sin upon them.
Ruth 1:6, how the Lord had *v.* his people.
Job 5:24, thou shalt *v.* thy habitation.
7:18, shouldest *v.* him every morning.
Ps. 8:4; Heb. 2:6, the son of man, that thou *v.* him.
106:4, *v.* me with thy salvation.
Jer. 5:9; 9:9, shall I not *v.* for these things?
29:10, I will *v.*, and perform my good word.
Ezek. 38:8, after many days thou shalt be *v.*
Mat. 25:36, I was sick and ye *v.* me.
Acts 15:14, how God did *v.* the Gentiles.
Jas. 1:27, to *v.* the fatherless and widows.
See Job 31:14; Lu. 1:68, 78; 7:16.
VISITATION. Job 10:12, thy *v.* hath preserved.
Isa. 10:3; 1 Pet. 2:12, in the day of *v.*
Jer. 8:12; 10:15; 46:21; 50:27; Lu. 19:44, in the time of *v.*
See Num. 16:29; Jer. 11:23; Hos. 9:7.
VOCATION. Eph. 4:1, worthy of the *v.*
VOICE. Gen. 4:10, *v.* of thy brother's blood.
27:22, the *v.* is Jacob's *v.*
Ex. 23:21, obey his *v.*, provoke him not.
24:3, all the people answered with one *v.*
32:18, it is not the *v.* of them that shout.
Deut. 4:33, did ever people hear *v.* of God and live?
Josh. 6:10, nor make any noise with thy *v.*
1 Sam. 24:16; 26:17, is this thy *v.*?
1 Kings 19:12, after the fire, a still small *v.*
2 Kings 4:31, there was neither *v.* nor hearing.
Job 3:7, let no joyful *v.* come therein.
30:31, my organ into the *v.* of them that weep.
37:4, a *v.* roareth.
40:9, canst thou thunder with a *v.* like him?
Ps. 5:3, my *v.* shalt thou hear in the morning.
31:22; 86:6, the *v.* of my supplications.
42:4, with the *v.* of joy.
95:7, to day, if ye will hear his *v.*
103:20, the *v.* of his word.
Prov. 1:20, wisdom uttereth her *v.* in the streets.
5:13, not obeyed the *v.* of my teachers.
8:1, doth not understanding put forth her *v.*?
4, my *v.* is to the sons of man.
Eccl. 5:3, a fool's *v.* is known.
12:4, rise up at the *v.* of the bird.
Cant. 2:8; 5:2, the *v.* of my beloved.
12, the *v.* of the turtle is heard.
14, sweet is thy *v.*

Isa. 13:2, exalt the *v.* unto them.
40:3; Mat. 3:3; Mk. 1:3; Lu. 3:4, *v.* of him that crieth.
6, the *v.* said, cry.
48:20, with a *v.* of singing.
52:8, with the *v.* together shall they sing.
65:19, the *v.* of weeping shall be no more heard.
66:6, a *v.* of noise, a *v.* from the temple.
Jer. 7:34, the *v.* of mirth, and the *v.* of gladness.
30:19, the *v.* of them that make merry.
48:3, a *v.* of crying shall be.
Ezek. 23:42, a *v.* of a multitude at ease.
33:32, one that hath a pleasant *v.*
43:2, *v.* like a noise of many waters.
Nah. 2:7, lead her as with the *v.* of doves.
Mat. 12:19, neither shall any man hear his *v.*
Lu. 23:23, the *v.* of them and of the chief priests prevailed.
John 5:25, the dead shall hear the *v.* of Son of God.
10:4, the sheep follow, for they know his *v.*
5, they know not the *v.* of strangers.
12:30, this *v.* came not because of me.
18:37, every one that is of the truth heareth my *v.*
Acts 12:14, and when she knew Peter's *v.*
26:10, I gave my *v.* against them.
1 Cor. 14:10, there are so many *v.* in the world.
19, that by my *v.* I might teach others.
Gal. 4:20, I desire now to change my *v.*
1 Thess. 4:16, descend with *v.* of archangel.
2 Pet. 2:16, the dumb ass speaking with man's *v.*
Rev. 3:20, if any man hear my *v.*
4:5, out of the throne proceeded *v.*
See Gen. 3:17; Ps. 58:5; John 3:29; Acts 12:22.

VOID. Gen. 1:2; Jer. 4:23, without form, and *v.*
Deut. 32:28, a people *v.* of counsel.
Ps. 89:39, made *v.* the covenant.
119:126, they have made *v.* thy law.
Prov. 11:12, *v.* of wisdom.
Isa. 55:11, my word shall not return to me *v.*
Jer. 19:7, make *v.* the counsel of Judah.
Nah. 2:10, empty, *v.* and waste.
Acts 24:16, a conscience *v.* of offense.
See Num. 30:12; Rom. 3:31; 4:14.

VOLUME. Ps. 40:7; Heb. 10:7.

VOLUNTARY. Lev. 1:3; 7:16; Ezek. 46:12; Col. 2:18.

VOMIT. Job 20:15; Prov. 26:11; 2 Pet. 2:22.

VOW (*n.*). Gen. 28:20; 31:13, Jacob vowed a *v.*
Num. 29:39, these ye shall do beside your *v.*
Deut. 12:6, thither bring your *v.*
Judg. 11:30, Jephthah vowed a *v.*, and said.
39, her father did with he according to his *v.*
1 Sam. 1:21, Elkanah went up to offer his *v.*
Job 22:27, thou shalt pay thy *v.*
Ps. 22:25; 66:13; 116:14, I will pay my *v.*
50:14, pay thy *v.* unto the most High.
Ps. 56:12, thy *v.* are upon me, O God.
61:5, for thou hast heard my *v.*
8, that I may daily perform my *v.*
65:1, to thee shall the *v.* be performed.
Prov. 7:14, this day have I paid my *v.*
20:25, after *v.* to make enquiry.
31:2, the son of my *v.*
Eccl. 5:4, when thou vowest a *v.*, defer not to pay.
Isa. 19:21, they shall vow a *v.* unto the Lord.
Jonah 1:16, feared the Lord, and made *v.*
Acts 18;18, shorn his head, for he had a *v.*
21:23, four men which have a *v.* on them.
See 2 Sam. 15:7; Jer. 44:25; Nah. 1:15.

VOW (*v.*). Deut. 23:22, if forbear to *v.*, no sin.
Ps. 76:11, *v.* and pay to the Lord your God.
132:3, and *v.* to the mighty God.
See Num. 21:2; Eccl. 5:5; Jonah 2:9.

VULTURE. Lev. 11:14; Deut. 14:13, and the *v.* after his kind.
Job 28:7, which the *v.* eye hath not seen.
Isa. 34:15, there shall the *v.* be.

W

WAG. Jer. 18:16; Lam. 2:15; Zeph. 2:15.

WAGES. Gen. 29:15, what shall thy *w.* be?
Gen. 30:28, appoint me thy *w.*
31:7, changed my *w.* ten times.
Ex. 2:9, nurse this child, I will give *w.*
Jer. 33:13, useth neighbour's service without *w.*
Hag. 1:6, earneth *w.* to put in bag with holes.
Lu. 3:14, be content with your *w.*
John 4:36, he that reapeth receiveth *w.*
Rom. 6:23, the *w.* of sin is death.
2 Pet. 2:15, the *w.* of unrighteousness.
See Ezek. 29:18; Mal. 3:5; 2 Cor. 11:8.

WAGONS. Gen. 45:19; Num. 7:7; Ezek. 23:24.

WAIL. Ezek. 32:18, *w.* for the multitude.
Amos 5:16, *w.* shall be in all streets.
Mic. 1:8, therefore I will *w.* and howl.
Mat. 13:42, there shall be *w.* and gnashing.
Mk. 5:38, he seeth them that *w.* greatly.
Rev. 1:7, all kindreds of the earth shall *w.*
18:15, the merchants shall stand afar off *w.*
See Esth. 4:3; Jer. 9:10, 19, 20; Ezek. 7:11.

WAIT. Gen. 49:18, I have *w.* for thy salvation.
Num. 35:20; Jer. 9:8, by laying of *w.*
2 Kings 6:33, should I *w.* for the Lord any longer?
Job 14:14, I will *w.* till my change come.
15:22, he is *w.* for of the sword.
17:13, if I *w.*, the grave is my house.
29:21, to me men *w.*, and kept silence.
23, they *w.* for me as for rain.
30:26, when I *w.* for light, darkness came.
Ps. 25:3; 69:6, let none that *w.* be ashamed.
27:14; 37:34; Prov. 20:22, *w.* on the Lord.
33:20, our soul *w.* for the Lord.
37:7, *w.* patiently.
52:9, I will *w.* on thy name.
62:1; 130:6, my soul *w.* upon God.
5, *w.* only on God.
65:1, praise *w.* for thee in Zion.
69:3, mine eyes fail while I *w.* for God.
104:27, these all *w.* upon thee.
106:13, they *w.* not for counsel.
123:2, so our eyes *w.* on the Lord.
Prov. 27:18, he that *w.* on his master.
Isa. 30:18, the Lord *w.* to be gracious.
40:31, they that *w.* on the Lord shall renew.
42:4, the isles shall *w.* for his law.
59:9, we *w.* for light.
64:4, prepared for him that *w.* for him.
Lam. 3:26, good that a man hope and quietly *w.*
Dan. 12:12, blessed is he that *w.*, and cometh to the days.
Hab. 2:3, though the vision tarry, *w.* for it.
Zech. 11:11, poor of the flock that *w.* upon me.
Mk. 15:43, who also *w.* for the kingdom of God.
Lu. 2:25, *w.* for the consolation of Israel.
12:36, like unto men that *w.* for their lord.
Acts 1:4, but *w.* for promise of the Father.
Rom. 8:23, groan, *w.* for the adoption.
25, then do we with patience *w.* for it.
12:7, let us *w.* on our ministering.
1 Cor. 9:13, they which *w.* at the altar are partakers.
Gal. 5:5, we *w.* for the hope.
1 Thess. 1:10, to *w.* for his Son from heaven.
See Num. 3:10; Neh. 12:44; Isa. 8:17.

WAKE. Ps. 139:18, when I *w.* I am still with thee.
Jer. 51:39, sleep a perpetual sleep, and not *w.*
Joel 3:9, prepare war, *w.* up the mighty men.
Zech. 4:1, the angel came again, and *w.* me.
1 Thess. 5:10, whether we *w.* or sleep.
See Ps. 77:4; 127:1; Cant. 5:2; Isa. 50:4.

WALK. Gen. 17:1, *w.* before me, and be perfect.
24:40, the Lord before whom I *w.*
48:15, before whom my fathers did *w.*
Ex. 16:4, whether they will *w.* in my law.
18:20, the way wherein they must *w.*
Lev. 26:12, I will *w.* among you.
Deut. 23:14, God *w.* in midst of the camp.
Judg. 5:10, speak, ye that *w.* by the way.
2 Sam. 2:29, Abner and his men *w.* all that night.
Job 18:8, he *w.* on a snare.

Job 22:14, he *w.* in the circuit of heaven.
29:3, when by his light I *w.* through darkness.
Ps. 23:4, though I *w.* through the valley of the shadow of death.
26:11, as for me, I will *w.* in mine integrity.
48:12, *w.* about Zion, and go round about her.
55:14, we *w.* to house of God in company.
56:13, that I may *w.* before God in the light of the living.
84:11, from them that *w.* uprightly.
91:6, the pestilence that *w.* in darkness.
104:3, who *w.* upon wings of the wind.
116:9, I will *w.* before the Lord.
119:45, I will *w.* at liberty.
138:7, though I *w.* in the midst of trouble.
Prov. 10:9; 28:18, he that *w.* uprightly *w.* surely.
13:20, he that *w.* with wise men shall be wise.
19:1; 28:6, better is the poor that *w.* in integrity.
28:26, whoso *w.* wisely shall be delivered.
Eccl. 2:14, the fool *w.* in darkness.
Isa. 2:5, let us *w.* in the light of the Lord.
9:2, the people that *w.* in darkness.
20:3, as my servant hath *w.* naked and barefoot.
30:21, a voice saying, this is the way, *w.* in it.
35:9, the redeemed shall *w.* there.
50:10, that *w.* in darkness, and hath no light.
11, *w.* in the light of your fire.
Jer. 6:16, ask where is the good way, and *w.* therein.
10:23, it is not in man that *w.* to direct his steps.
Ezek. 28:14, hast *w.* in midst of stones of fire.
Dan. 4:37, those that *w.* in pride.
Hos. 14:9, the just shall *w.* in them.
Amos 3:3, can two *w.* together?
Mic. 6:8, to *w.* humbly with thy God.
Nah. 2:11, where the lion *w.*
Zech. 1:11, we have *w.* to and fro through the earth.
Mal. 3:14, what profit that we have *w.* mournfully?
Mat. 9:5; Mk. 2:9; Lu. 5:23; John 5:8, 11, 12; Acts 3:6, arise, and *w.*
12:43; Lu. 11:24, *w.* through dry places.
14:29, he *w.* on the water.
Mk. 16:12, he appeared to two of them, as they *w.*
Lu. 13:33, I must *w.* to day and to morrow.
John 8:12, shall not *w.* in darkness.
11:9, if any man *w.* in the day.
Rom. 4:12, who *w.* in steps of that faith.
6:4, *w.* in newness of life.
8:1, who *w.* not after the flesh, but after the Spirit.
2 Cor. 5:7, we *w.* by faith.
Gal. 6:16, as many as *w.* according to this rule.
Eph. 2:2; Col. 3:7, in time past ye *w.*
10, ordained that we should *w.* in them.
4:1, *w.* worthy of the vocation.
17, that ye *w.* not as other Gentiles.
5:15, *w.* circumspectly.
Phil. 3:17, mark them which *w.*
18, many *w.*, of whom I told you.
Col. 1:10; 1 Thess. 2:12, that ye might *w.* worthy of the Lord.
1 Thess. 4:1, how ye ought to *w.*
12, ye may *w.* honestly.
2 Thess. 3:6, from every brother that *w.* disorderly.
1 Pet. 4:3, when we *w.* in lasciviousness.
5:8, *w.* about, seeking whom he may devour.
1 John 1:7, if we *w.* in the light.
2:6, to *w.*, even as he *w.*
See Gal. 5:16; Eph. 5:2; Phil. 3:16.

WALKING. Deut. 2:7, the Lord knoweth thy *w.*
Job 31:26, the moon *w.* in brightness.
Dan. 3:25, four men loose, *w.* in the fire.
Mat. 14:25, Jesus went to them, *w.* on the sea.
Mk. 8:24, I see men as trees, *w.*
Acts 9:31, *w.* in the fear of the Lord.
See Isa. 3:16; 2 Cor. 4:2; 2 Pet. 3:3; Jude 16.

WALL. Gen. 49:22, branches run over the *w.*
Ex. 14:22, the waters were a *w.* to them.
Num. 22:24, a *w.* being on this side, a *w.* on that.
2 Sam. 22:30; Ps. 18:29, have I leaped over a *w.*
2 Kings 20:2; Isa. 36:11, turned his face to the *w.*
Ezra 5:3, who commanded you to make this *w.*?
Neh. 4:6, so built we the *w.*
Ps. 62:3, a bowing *w.* shall ye be.
122:7, peace be within thy *w.*
Prov. 24:31, the *w.* thereof was broken down.
25:28, like a city without *w.*
Isa. 26:1, salvation will God appoint for *w.*
59:10, we grope for the *w.*
60:18, thou shalt call thy *w.* Salvation.
Ezek. 8:7, a hole in the *w.*
Dan. 5:5, fingers wrote on the *w.*
Amos 5:19, leaned hand on *w.*, and serpent bit him.
Hab. 2:11, the stone shall cry out of the *w.*
Acts 23:3, thou whited *w.*
Eph. 2:14, the middle *w.* of partition.
See Ezek. 38:11; Zech. 2:4; Acts 9:25; Rev. 21:14.

WALLOW. Jer. 6:26; 25:34, *w.* in ashes.
2 Pet. 2:22, washed, to her *w.* in the mire.
See 2 Sam. 20:12; Ezek. 27:30.

WANDER. Num. 14:33, your children shall *w.*
Deut. 27:18, cursed by he that maketh blind to *w.*
Job 12:24, he causeth them to *w.*
15:23, he w. abroad for bread.
38:41, young ravens *w.* for lack of meat.
Ps. 55:7, then would I *w.* far off.
59:15, let them *w.* up and down.
119:10, let me not *w.* from thy commandments.
Prov. 27:8, as a bird that *w.* from nest.
Isa. 16:3, bewray not him that *w.*
47:15, *w.* every one to his quarter.
Jer. 14:10, thus have they loved to *w.*
Lam. 4:14, they have *w.* as blind men.
Ezek. 34:6, my sheep *w.* through mountains.
Amos 4:8, two cities *w.* to one city to drink.
See Hos. 9:17; 1 Tim. 5:13; Heb. 11:37; Jude 13.

WANT (*n.*). Deut. 28:48, thou shalt serve in *w.*
Judg. 18:10, a place where there is no *w.*
19:20, let all thy *w.* lie on me.
Job 24:8, they embrace the rock for *w.*
31:19, if I have seen any perish for *w.*
Ps. 34:9, there is no *w.* to them that fear him.
Amos 4:6, I have given you *w.* of bread.
Mk. 12:44, she of her *w.* cast in all.
Lu. 15:14, he began to be in *w.*
Phil. 2:25, that ministered to my *w.*
See Prov. 6:11; Lam. 4:9; 2 Cor. 8:14; Phil. 4:11.

WANT (*v.*). Ps. 23:1, I shall not *w.*
34:10, shall not *w.* any good thing.
Prov. 9:4, for him that *w.* understanding.
10:19, in multitude of words there *w.* not sin.
13:25, the belly of the wicked shall *w.*
Eccl. 6:2, he *w.* nothing for his soul.
Isa. 34:16, none shall *w.* her mate.
Jer. 44:18, we have *w.* all things.
Ezek. 4:17, that they may *w.* bread and water.
John 2:3, when they *w.* vine.
2 Cor. 11:9, when I *w.* I was chargeble to no man.
See Eccl. 1:15; Dan. 5:27; Tit. 1:5; Jas. 1:4.

WANTON. Isa. 3:16; Rom. 13:13; 1 Tim. 5:11; Jas. 5:5.

WAR (*n.*). Ex. 32:17, there is a noise of *w.*
Num. 32:6, shall your brethren go to *w.*, and shall ye sit here?
Deut. 24:5, taken a wife, he shall not go out to *w.*
Judg. 5:8, then was *w.* in the gates.
1 Chron. 5:22, many slain, because the *w.* was of God.
Job 10:17, changes and *w.* are against me.
38:23, reserved against the day of *w.*
Ps. 27:3, though *w.* should rise against me.
46:9, he maketh *w.* to cease.
55:21, *w.* was in his heart.
68:30, scatter the people that delight in *w.*
Prov. 20:18, with good advice make *w.*
Eccl. 3:8, a time of *w.*
8:8, no discharge in that *w.*
Isa. 2:4; Mic. 4:3, nor learn *w.* any more.
Jer. 42:14, to Egypt, where we shall see no *w.*
Mic. 2:8, as men averse from *w.*

Mat. 24:6; Mk. 13:7; Lu. 21:9, *w.* and rumours of *w.*
Lu. 14:31, what king, going to make *w.*?
Jas. 4:1, from whence come *w.*?
Rev. 12:7, there was *w.* in heaven.
See Eccl. 9:18; Ezek. 32:27; Dan. 7:21; 9:26.
WAR (*v.*). 2 Sam. 22:35; Ps. 18:34; 144:1, teacheth my hands to *w.*
2 Chron. 6:34, if thy people go to *w.*
Isa. 41:12, they that *w.* against thee.
2 Cor. 10:3, we do not *w.* after the flesh.
1 Tim. 1:18, *w.* a good warfare.
2 Tim. 2:4, no man that *w.* entangleth himself.
Jas. 4:1, lusts that *w.* in your members.
2, ye fight and *w.*, yet ye have not.
1 Pet. 2:11, from lusts which *w.* against the soul.
See 1 Kings 14:19; Isa. 37:8 Rom. 7:23.
WARDROBE. 2 Kings 22:14; 2 Chron. 34:22.
WARE. Mat. 24:50; Lu. 8:27; 2 Tim. 4:15.
WARFARE. Isa. 40:2, that her *w.* is accomplished.
2 Cor. 10:4, weapons of our *w.* are not carnal.
See 1 Sam. 28:1; 1 Cor. 9:7; 1 Tim. 1:18.
WARM. Eccl. 4:11, how can one be *w.* alone?
Isa. 47:14, there shall not be a coal to *w.* at.
Hag. 1:6, ye clothe you, but there is none *w.*
Mk. 14:54; John 18:18, Peter *w.* himself.
Jas. 2:16, be ye *w.* and filled.
See 2 Kings 4:34; Job 37:17; 39:14; Isa. 44:15.
WARN. Ezek. 3:18; Acts 20:31; 1 Thess. 5:14.
WASH. 2 Kings 5:10, go, *w.* in Jordan.
12, may I not *w.* in them, and be clean?
Job 9:30, if I *w.* myself with snow water.
14:19, thou *w.* away things which grow.
29:6, when I *w.* my steps with butter.
Ps. 26:6; 73:13, I will *w.* my hands in innocency.
51:2, *w.* me throughly from mine iniquity.
7, *w.* me, and I shall be whiter than snow.
Prov. 30:12, a generation not *w.*
Cant. 5:12, his eyes are *w.* with milk.
Isa. 1:16, *w.* you, make you clean.
Jer. 2:22, though thou *w.* thee with nitre.
4:14, *w.* thy heart.
Ezek. 16:4, nor wast *w.* in water to supple thee.
Mat. 6:17, when thou fastest, *w.* thy face.
27:24, took water, and *w.* his hands.
Mk. 7:3, except they *w.* oft, eat not.
Lu. 7:38, began to *w.* his feet with tears.
44, she hath *w.* my feet with her tears.
John 9:7, go, *w.* in the pool of Siloam.
Acts 16:33, he *w.* their stripes.
22:16, *w.* away thy sins.
1 Cor. 6:11, but ye are *w.*
Heb. 10:22, having our bodies *w.* with pure water.
2 Pet. 2:22, the sow that was *w.*
Rev. 1:5, that *w.* us from our sins.
7:14, have *w.* their robes.
See Neh. 4:23; Eph. 5:26; Tit. 3:5; Heb. 9:10.
WASTE. Deut. 32:10; Job 30:3, in *w.* wilderness.
1 Kings 17:14, the barrel of meal shall not *w.*
Ps. 80:13, the boar out of the wood doth *w.* it.
91:6, nor for the destruction that *w.* at noonday.
Isa. 24:1, the Lord maketh the earth *w.*
61:4, they shall build the old *w.*
Joel 1:10, the field is *w.*, the corn is *w.*
See Prov. 18:9; Is. 59:7; Mat. 26:8; Mk. 14:4.
WATCH (*n.*). Ps. 90:4, as a *w.* in the night.
119:148, mine eyes prevent the night *w.*
Jer. 51:12, make the *w.* strong.
Hab. 2:1, I will stand upon my *w.*
See Mat. 14:25; 24:43; 27:65; Lu. 2:8.
WATCH (*v.*). Gen. 31:49, the Lord *w.* between me and thee.
Job 14:16, dost thou not *w.* over my sin?
Ps. 37:32, the wicked *w.* the righteous.
102:7, I *w.* and am as a sparrow.
130:6, more than they that *w.* for morning.
Isa. 29:20, all that *w.* for iniquity are cut off.
Jer. 20:10, my familiars *w.* for my halting.
31:28, so will I *w.* over them, to build.
Jer. 44:27, I will *w.* over them for evil.
Ezek. 7:6, the end is come, it *w.* for thee.
Hab. 2:1, I will *w.* to see what he will say.
Mat. 24:42; 25:13; Mk. 13:35; Lu. 21:36; Acts 20:31, *w.* therefore.
26:41; Mk. 13:33; 14:38, *w.* and pray.
1 Thess. 5:6; 1 Pet. 4:7, let us *w.* and be sober.
Heb. 13:17, for they *w.* for your souls.
See 1 Cor. 16:13; 2 Tim. 4:5; Rev. 3:2; 16:15.
WATCH TOWER. 2 Chron. 20:24; Judah came toward the *w.*
Isa. 21:5, watch in the *w.*
WATER (*n.*). Gen. 26:20, the *w.* is ours.
49:4, unstable as *w.*
Deut. 8:7, a land of brooks of *w.*
11:11, the land drinketh *w.* of rain of heaven.
Josh. 7:5, their hearts melted, and became as *w.*
2 Sam. 14:14, as *w.* spilt on the ground.
1 Kings 13:22, eat no bread, and drink no *w.*
22:27; 2 Chron. 18:26, *w.* of affliction.
2 Kings 3:11, who poured *w.* on Elijah's hands.
20:20, brought *w.* into the city.
Neh. 9:11, threwest as a stone into mighty *w.*
Job 8:11, can the flag grow without *w.*?
14:9, through the scent of *w.* it will bud.
19, the *w.* wear the stones.
15:16, who drinketh iniquity like *w.*
22:7, thou hast not given *w.* to weary to drink.
26:8, he bindeth up the *w.* in his thick clouds.
38:30, the *w.* are hid as with a stone.
Ps. 22:14, I am poured out like *w.*
23:2, beside the still *w.*
33:7, he gathereth the *w.* of the sea.
46:3, though the *w.* roar and be troubled.
63:1, a dry and thirsty land, where no *w.* is.
73:10, *w.* of a full cup are wrung out to them.
77:16, the *w.* saw thee.
79:3, their blood have they shed like *w.*
124:4, then the *w.* had overwhelmed us.
148:4, praise him, ye *w.* above the heavens.
Prov. 5:15, drink *w.* out of thine own cistern.
9:17, stolen *w.* are sweet.
20:5, counsel is like deep *w.*
25:25, as cold *w.* to a thirsty soul.
27:19, as in *w.* face answereth to face.
30:4, who hath bound the *w.* in a garment?
Eccl. 11:1, cast thy bread upon the *w.*
Cant. 4:15; John 7:38, well of living *w.*
8:7, many *w.* cannot quench love.
Isa. 1:22, thy wine is mixed with *w.*
3:1, take away the whole stay of *w.*
11:9; Hab. 2:14, as the *w.* cover the seas.
19:5, the *w.* shall fail from the sea.
28:17, *w.* shall overflow the hiding place.
32:20, blessed are ye that sow beside all *w.*
33:16, his *w.* shall be sure.
35:6, in the wilderness shall *w.* break out.
41:17, when the poor seek *w.*
43:2, when thou passest through the *w.*
16, a path in the mighty *w.*
20, I give *w.* in the wilderness.
44:3, I will pour *w.* on him that is thirsty.
55:1, come ye to the *w.*
57:20, whose *w.* cast up mire and dirt.
Jer. 2:13; 17:13, the fountain of living *w.*
9:1, Oh that my head were *w.*!
14:3, their nobles sent little ones to the *w.*
47:2, behold, *w.* rise up out of the north.
Ezek. 4:17, that they may want bread and *w.*
7:17; 21:7, be weak as *w.*
31:4, the *w.* made him great.
36:25, then will I sprinkle clean *w.* upon you.
Amos 8:11, not famine of bread nor thirst for *w.*
Mat. 3:11; Mk. 1:8; Lu. 3:16; John 1:26; Acts 1:5; 11:16, baptize you with *w.*
10:42; Mk. 9:41, whoso giveth a cup of cold *w.*
14:28, bid me come to thee on the *w.*
27:24, Pilate took *w.*, and washed.

Lu. 8:23, ship filled with *w.*
24, and rebuked the raging of the *w.*
16:24, dip the tip of his finger in *w.*
John 3:5, except a man be born of *w.*
23, there was much *w.* there.
4:15, give me this *w.*
5:3, waiting for moving of the *w.*
19:34, forthwith came out blood and *w.*
Acts 10:47, can any forbid *w.*?
2 Cor. 11:26, in perils of *w.*
Eph. 5:26, cleanse it with washing of *w.*
1 Pet. 3:20, eight souls were saved by *w.*
2 Pet. 2:17, wells without *w.*
1 John 5:6, this is he that came by *w.*
Rev. 22:17, let him take the *w.* of life freely.
See Ps. 29:3; Jer. 51:13; Ezek. 32:2; 47:1.
WATER (*v.*). Gen. 2:6, mist that *w.* face of ground.
13:10, plain was well *w.*
Deut. 11:10, *w.* it with thy foot, as a garden.
Ps. 6:6, I *w.* my couch with tears.
72:6, as showers that *w.* the earth.
104:13, he *w.* the hills from his chambers.
Prov. 11:25, he that *w.*, shall be *w.*
Isa. 16:9, I will *w.* thee with my tears.
27:3, I will *w.* it every moment.
55:10, returneth not, but *w.* the earth.
58:11; Jer. 31:12, thou shalt be like a *w.* garden.
Ezek. 32:6, I will also *w.* with thy blood.
1 Cor. 3:6, Apollos *w.*, but God gave the increase.
See Ps. 65:9; Ezek. 17:7; Joel 3:18.
WAVERING. Heb. 10:23, the profession of our faith without *w.*
Jas. 1:5, ask in faith, nothing *w.*
WAVES. Ps. 42:7, all thy *w.* are gone over me.
65:7; 89:9; 107:29, stilleth noise of *w.*
93:4, the Lord is mightier than mighty *w.*
Isa. 48:18, thy righteousness as the *w.* of the sea.
Jer. 5:22, though the *w.* toss.
Zech. 10:11, shall smite the *w.* in the sea.
Jude 13, raging *w.* of the sea.
See Mat. 8:24; 14:24; Mk. 4:37; Acts 27:41.
WAX (*n.*). Ps. 22:14; 68:2; 97:5; Mic. 1:4.
WAX (*v.*). Ex. 22:24; 32:10, my wrath shall *w.* hot.
Num. 11:23, is the Lord's hand *w.* short?
Deut. 8:4; 29:5; Neh. 9:21, raiment *w.* not old.
32:15, Jeshurun *w.* fat, and kicked.
Ps. 102:26; Isa. 50:9; 51:6; Heb. 1:11, shall *w.* old as doth a garment.
Mat. 24:12, the love of many shall *w.* cold.
Lu. 12:33, bags which *w.* not old.
See Mat. 13:15; 1 Tim. 5:11; 2 Tim. 3:13.
WAY. Gen. 6:12, all flesh had corrupted his *w.*
28:20, if God will keep me in this *w.*
56, seeing the Lord hath prospered my *w.*
Num. 22:32, thy *w.* is perverse.
Deut. 8:6; 26:17; 28:9; 30:16; 1 Kings 2:3; Ps. 119:3; 128:1; Isa. 42:24, walk in his *w.*
Josh 23:14; 1 Kings 2:2, the *w.* of all the earth.
1 Sam. 12:23, teach you the good and right *w.*
2 Sam. 22:31; Ps. 18:30, as for God, his *w.* is perfect.
2 Kings 7:15, all the *w.* was full of garments.
2 Chron. 6:27, when thou hast taught them the good *w.*
Ezra 8:21, to seek of him a right *w.*
Job 3:23, to a man whose *w.* is hid.
12:24; Ps. 107:40, to wander where there is no *w.*
16:22, I go the *w.* whence I shall not return.
19:8, fenced up my *w.*
22:15, hast thou marked the old *w.*?
23:10, he knoweth the *w.* that I take.
24:13, they know not the *w.* of the light.
31:4, doth not he see my *w.*?
38:19, where is the *w.* where light dwelleth?
Ps. 1:6, the Lord knoweth the *w.* of righteous.
2:12, lest ye perish from the *w.*
25:9, the meek will he teach his *w.*
27:11; 86:11, teach me thy *w.*
36:4, in a *w.* that is not good.
Ps. 37:5, commit thy *w.* unto the Lord.
39:1, I will take heed to my *w.*
49:13, this their *w.* is their folly.
67:2, that thy *w.* may be known.
78:50, he made a *w.* to his anger.
95:10; Heb. 3:10, they have not known my *w.*
101:2, behave wisely in a perfect *w.*
119:5, O that my *w.* were directed.
30, I have chosen the *w.* of truth.
59, I thought on my *w.*
168, all my *w.* are before thee.
139:24, lead me in the *w.* everlasting.
Prov. 2:8, he preserveth the *w.* of his saints.
3:6, in all thy *w.* acknowledge him.
17, her *w.* are *w.* of pleasantness.
5:21, the *w.* of man are before the Lord.
6:6, consider her *w.*, and be wise.
23; 15:24; Jer. 21:8, the *w.* of life.
12:15, the *w.* of a fool is right in his own eyes.
15:19, the *w.* of the slothful man.
16:7, when a man's *w.* please the Lord.
22:6, train up a child in the *w.*
23:19, guide thy heart in the *w.*
26, let thine eyes observe my *w.*
26:13, there is a lion in the *w.*
Eccl. 11:5, the *w.* of the spirit.
12:5, fears shall be in the *w.*
Isa. 2:3; Mic. 4:2, he will teach us of his *w.*
30:21, this is the *w.*, walk ye in it.
35:8, and a *w.*, called the *w.* of holiness.
40:27, my *w.* is hid from the Lord.
42:16, the blind by a *w.* they knew not.
24, they would not walk in his *w.*
45:13, I will direct all his *w.*
55:8, neither are your *w.* my *w.*
58:2, they delight to know my *w.*
Jer. 6:16, where is the good *w.*?
17:10; 32:19, every man according to his *w.*
18:11, make your *w.* and doings good.
32:39, I will give them one heart and one *w.*
50:5, they shall ask the *w.* to Zion.
Ezek. 3:18, to warn the wicked from his *w.*
18:29, are not my *w.* equal? are not your *w.* unequal?
Joel 2:7, march every one on his *w.*
Nah. 1:3, the Lord hath his *w.* in the whirlwind.
Hag. 1:5, consider your *w.*
Mal. 3:1, he shall prepare the *w.* before me.
Mat. 7:13, broad is the *w.* that leadeth.
10:5, go not into *w.* of Gentiles.
22:16; Mk. 12:14; Lu. 20:21, teachest the *w.* of God.
Mk. 8:3, they will faint by the *w.*
11:8; Mat. 21:8; Lu. 19:36, spread garments in the *w.*
Lu. 15:20, when he was yet a great *w.* off.
19:4, he was to pass that *w.*
John 10:1, but climbeth up some other *w.*
14:4, and the *w.* ye know.
6, I am the *w.*, the truth, and the life.
Acts 9:2, if he found any of this *w.*
27, how he had seen the Lord in the *w.*
16:17, which show unto us the *w.* of salvation.
18:26, expounded the *w.* of God more perfectly.
19:23, no small stir about that *w.*
24:14, after the *w.* which they call heresy.
Rom. 3:12, they are all gone out of the *w.*
11:33, his *w.* are past finding out.
1 Cor. 10:13, will make a *w.* to escape.
12:31, a more excellent *w.*
Col. 2:14, took handwriting of ordinances out of the *w.*
Heb. 5:2, compassion of them out of the *w.*
9:8, the *w.* into the holiest.
10:20, by a new and living *w.*
Jas. 1:8, unstable in all his *w.*
5:20, the sinner from error of his *w.*
2 Pet. 2:2, many shall follow their pernicious *w.*
15, which have forsaken the right *w.*
21, better not to have known *w.* of righteousness.
Jude 11, they have gone in the *w.* of Cain.

See Hos. 2:6; Lu. 10:31; Rev. 15:3.
WEAK. Judg. 16:7, *w.* as other men.
2 Sam. 3:1, Saul's house waxed *w.* and *w.*
2 Chron. 15:7, let not your hands be *w.*
Job 4:3, thou hast strengthened the *w.* hands.
Ps. 6:2, I am *w.*
Isa. 14:10, art thou also become *w.* as we?
35:3, strengthen ye the *w.* hands.
Ezek. 7:17; 21:7, shall be *w.* as water.
16:30, how *w.* is thy heart!
Joel 3:10, let the *w.* say, I am strong.
Mat. 26:41; Mk. 14:38, but the flesh is *w.*
Acts 20:35, ye ought to support the *w.*
Rom. 4:19, being not *w.* in faith.
8:3, for the law was *w.*
1 Cor. 1:27, *w.* things to confound the mighty.
11:30, for this cause many are *w.*
2 Cor. 10:10, his bodily presence is *w.*
11:29, who is *w.*, and I am not *w.*?
12:10, when I am *w.*, then am I strong.
Gal. 4:9, turn again to *w.* elements.
1 Pet. 3:7, giving honour to the wife, as *w.* vessel.
See Job 12:21; Jer. 38:4; Rom. 15:1; 1 Thess. 5:14.
WEAKNESS. 1 Cor. 1:25, the *w.* of God.
2:3, I was with you in *w.*
15:43, it is sown in *w.*, raised in power.
See 2 Cor. 12:9; 13:4; Heb. 7:18; 11:34.
WEALTH. Deut. 8:18, Lord giveth power to get *w.*
1 Sam. 2:32, thou shalt see an enemy in all the *w.*
2 Chron. 1:11, thou hast not asked *w.*
Esth. 10:3, seeking the *w.* of his people.
Job 21:13, they spend their days in *w.*
31:25, if I rejoiced because my *w.* was great.
Ps. 44:12, dost not increase *w.* by price.
49:6, they that trust in *w.*
49:10, wise men die, and leave *w.* to others.
112:3, *w.* and riches shall be in his house.
Prov. 5:10, lest strangers be filled with thy *w.*
10:15; 18:11, the rich man's *w.* is his strong city.
13:11, *w.* gotten by vanity.
19:4, *w.* maketh many friends.
Acts 19:25, by this craft we have our *w.*
1 Cor. 10:24, seek every man another's *w.*
See Deut. 8:17; Ruth 2:1; Ezra 9:12; Zech. 14:14.
WEALTHY. Ps. 66:12; Jer. 49:31.
WEANED. 1 Sam. 1:22; Ps. 131:2; Isa. 11:8; 28:9.
WEAPON. Neh. 4:17, with the other hand held a *w.*
Isa. 13:5; Jer. 50:25, the *w.* of his indignation.
54:17, no *w.* formed against thee shall prosper.
Jer. 22:7, every one with his *w.*
Ezek. 9:1, with destroying *w.* in his hand.
2 Cor. 10:4, the *w.* of our warfare.
See Job 20:24; Ezek. 39:9; John 18:3.
WEAR. Job 14:19, the waters *w.* the stones.
Isa. 4:1, we will *w.* our own apparel.
Zech. 13:4, nor shall they *w.* a rough garment.
Mat. 11:8, that *w.* soft clothing.
See Deut. 22:5; Esth. 6:8; Lu. 9:12; 1 Pet. 3:3.
WEARINESS. Eccl. 12:12; Mal. 1:13; 2 Cor. 11:27.
WEARY. Gen. 27:46, I am *w.* of my life.
2 Sam. 23:10, he smote till his hand was *w.*
Job 3:17, and the *w.* be at rest.
10:1, my soul is *w.*
16:7, now he hath made me *w.*
22:7, thou hast not given water to the *w.*
Ps. 6:6, I am *w.* with groaning.
Prov. 3:11, be not *w.* of the Lord's correction.
25:17, lest he be *w.* of thee.
Isa. 5:27, none shall be *w.* among them.
7:13, will ye *w.* my God also?
28:12, cause the *w.* to rest.
32:2, as the shadow of a great rock in *w.* land.
40:28, God fainteth not, neither is *w.*
31, they shall run, and not be *w.*
43:22, thou hast been *w.* of me.
46:1, a burden to the *w.* beast.
50:4, a word in season to him that is *w.*
Jer. 6:11, I am *w.* with holding in.
15:6, I am *w.* with repenting.
20:9, I was *w.* with forbearing.
31:25, I have satiated the *w.* soul.
Lu. 18:5, lest she *w.* me.
Gal. 6:9; 2 Thess. 3:13, be not *w.* in well doing.
See Judg. 4:21; Ps. 68:9; 69:3; Hab. 2:13.
WEARY (*v.*). Isa. 43:24, thou hast *w.* me.
47:13, *w.* in the multitude of counsels.
57:10, *w.* in the greatness of thy way.
Jer. 12:5, with footmen, and they *w.* thee.
Ezek. 24:12, she hat *w.* herself with lies.
Mic. 6:3, wherein have I *w.* thee?
John 4:6, being *w.*, sat thus on the well.
Heb. 12:3, lest ye be *w.* and faint.
See Eccl. 10:10; Jer. 4:31; Mal. 2:17.
WEASEL. Lev. 11:29.
WEATHER. Job 37:22; Prov. 25:20; Mat. 16:2.
WEB. Judg. 16:13; Job 8:14; Isa. 59:5.
WEDGE. Josh. 7:21; Isa. 13:12.
WEEK. Gen. 29:27, fulfil her *w.*
Jer. 5:24, the appointed *w.* of harvest.
Dan. 9:27, in the midst of the *w.*
Mat. 28:1; Mk. 16:2, 9; Lu. 24:1; John 20:1, 19; Acts 20:7; 1 Cor. 16:2, the first day of the *w.*
See Num. 28:26; Dan. 10:2; Lu. 18:12.
WEEP. Gen. 43:30, he sought where to *w.*
1 Sam. 1:8; John 20:13, why *w.* thou?
11:5, what aileth the people that they *w.*?
30:4, no more power to *w.*
Neh. 8:9, mourn not, nor *w.*
Job 27:15, his widows shall not *w.*
30:25, did not I *w.* for him that was in trouble?
Eccl. 3:4, a time to *w.*
Isa. 15:2, he is gone up to *w.*
22:4, I will *w.* bitterly.
30:19, thou shalt *w.* no more.
Jer. 9:1, that I might *w.* day and night.
22:10, *w.* ye not for the dead.
Joel 1:5, awake, ye drunkards, and *w.*
Mk. 5:39, why make ye this ado, and *w.*?
Lu. 6:21, blessed are ye that *w.* now.
7:13; 8:52; Rev. 5:5, *w.* not.
23:28, *w.* not for me, but *w.* for yourselves.
John 11:31, she goeth to the grave to *w.* there.
Acts 21:13, what mean ye to *w.*?
Rom. 12:15, and *w.* with them that *w.*
See John 16:20; 1 Cor. 7:30; Jas. 4:9; 5:1.
WEEPING. 2 Sam. 15:30, *w.* as they went.
Ezra 3:13, could not discern noise of joy from *w.*
Job 16:16, my face is foul with *w.*
Ps. 6:8, the Lord hath heard the voice of my *w.*
30:5, *w.* may endure for a night.
102:9, I have mingled my drink with *w.*
Isa. 65:19, the voice of *w.* be no more heard.
Jer. 31:16, refrain thy voice from *w.*
48:5, continual *w.* shall go up.
Joel 2:12, turn to me with fasting and *w.*
Mat. 8:12; 22:13; 24:51; 25:30; Lu. 13:28, *w.* and gnashing of teeth.
Lu. 7:38, stood at his feet behind him *w.*
John 11:33, when Jesus saw her *w.*
20:11, Mary stood without at sepulchre *w.*
Phil. 3:18, now tell you even *w.*
See Num 25:6; Jer. 31:15; Mal. 2:13; Mat. 2:18; Acts 9:39.
WEIGH. 2 Sam. 14:26, *w.* the hair of his head.
Job 6:2, oh that my grief were *w.*!
31:6, let me be *w.* in an even balance.
Isa. 26:7, thou dost *w.* the path of the just.
40:12, who hath *w.* the mountains?
Dan. 5:27, thou art *w.* in the balances.
See Job 28:25; Prov. 16:2; Zech. 11:12.
WEIGHT. Lev. 26:26, deliver your bread by *w.*
Job 28:25, to make the *w.* for the winds.
Ezek. 4:10, thy meat shall be by *w.*
16, they shall eat bread by *w.*
2 Cor. 4:17, a more exceeding *w.* of glory.

Heb. 12:1, lay aside every *w*.
See Deut. 25:13; Prov. 16:11; Mic. 6:11.
WEIGHTY. Prov. 27:3; Mat. 23:23; 2 Cor. 10:10.
WELFARE. Neh. 2:10, to seek *w*. of Israel.
Job 30:15, my *w*. passeth away.
Ps. 69:22, which should have been for their *w*.
Jer. 38:4, seeketh not the *w*. of this people.
See Gen. 43:27; Ex. 18:7; 1 Chron. 18:10.
WELL (*n*.). Num. 21:17, spring up, O *w*.
Deut. 6:11, and *w*. which thou diggedst not.
2 Sam. 23:15; 1 Chron. 11:17, water of the *w*. of Bethlehem.
Ps. 84:6, through valley of Baca make it a *w*.
Prov. 5:15, waters out of thine own *w*.
10:11, a *w*. of life.
Cant. 4:15; John 4:14, *w*. of living waters.
Isa. 12:3, the *w*. of salvation.
John 4:6, sat thus on the *w*.
2 Pet. 2:17, *w*. without water.
See Gen. 21:19; 49:22; 2 Sam. 17:18.
WELL (*adv*.). Gen. 4:7, if thou doest *w*.
12:13, *w*. with me for thy sake.
29:6, is he *w*.? and they said, he is *w*.
40:14, think on me when it shall be *w*. with thee.
Ex. 4:14, I know he can speak *w*.
Num. 11:18, it was *w*. with us in Egypt.
Deut. 4:40; 5:16; 6:3; 12:25; 19:13; 22:7; Ruth 3:1; Eph. 6:3, that it may go *w*. with thee.
1 Sam. 20:7, if he say thus, it is *w*.
2 Kings 4:26, is it *w*. with thee, is it *w*.?
2 Chron. 12:12, in Judah things went *w*.
Ps. 49:18, when thou doest *w*. to thyself.
Prov. 11:10, when it goeth *w*. with the righteous.
14:15, looketh *w*. with the righteous.
30:29, three things which go *w*.
Eccl. 8:12, it shall be *w*. with them that fear God.
Isa. 3:10, say to the righteous, it shall be *w*.
Ezek. 33:32, one that can play *w*.
Jonah 4:4, doest thou *w*. to be angry?
Mat. 25:21; Lu. 19:17, *w*. done.
Mk. 7:37, he hath done all things *w*.
Lu. 6:26, when all men speak *w*. of you.
Gal. 5:7, ye did run *w*.
See Phil 4:14; 1 Tim. 3:5; 5:17; Tit. 2:9.
WENT. Gen. 4:16, Cain *w*. out from the presence.
Deut. 1:31, in all the way ye *w*.
2 Kings 5:26, *w*. not my heart with thee?
Ps. 42:4, I *w*. with them to the house of God.
106:32, it *w*. ill with Moses.
Mat. 21:30, I go, sir, and *w*. not.
Lu. 17:14, as they *w*. they were cleansed.
18:10, two men *w*. up into the temple to pray.
See Mat. 11:7;20:1; Lu. 6:19; John 8:9.
WEPT. 2 Kings 8:11, the man of God *w*.
Ezra 10:1; Neh. 8:9, the people *w*. very sore.
Neh. 1:4, I *w*. before God.
Lu. 7:32, we mourned, and ye have not *w*.
19:41, beheld the city, and *w*. over it.
John 11:35, Jesus *w*.
1 Cor. 7:30, that weep as though they *w*. not.
See 2 Sam. 12:22 Ps. 69:10; 137:1; Rev. 5:4.
WET. Job 24:8, Dan. 4:15; 5:21.
WHAT. Ex. 16:15, they wist not *w*. it was.
2 Sam. 16:10, *w*. have I to do with you?
Ezra 9:10, *w*. shall we say after this?
Job 7:17; 15:14; Ps. 8:4; 144:3, *w*. is man?
Isa. 38:15; John 12:27, *w*. shall I say?
Hos. 6:4, *w*. shall I do unto thee?
Mat. 5:47, *w*. do ye more than others?
Mk. 14:36, not *w*. I will, but *w*. thou wilt.
John 21:22, *w*. is that to thee?
See Acts 9:6; 10:4; 16:30; 1 Pet. 1:11.
WHATSOEVER. Ps. 1:3, *w*. he doeth shall prosper.
Eccl. 3:14, *w*. God doeth shall be for ever.
Mat. 5:37, *w*. is more than these cometh of evil.
7:12, *w*. ye would that men should do to you.
20:4, *w*. is right I will give you.
Phil. 4:8, *w*. things are true.
See John 15:16; Rom. 14:23; 1 Cor. 10:31.
WHEAT. 1 Sam. 12:17, is it not *w*. harvest to-day?
Job 31:40, let thistles grow instead of *w*.
Ps. 81:16; 147:14, the finest of the *w*.
Jer. 12:13, they have sown *w*., but reap thorns.
23:28, what is the chaff to the *w*.?
Mat. 3:12, gather his *w*. into the garner.
Lu. 22:31, that he may sift you as *w*.
See John 12:24; Acts 27:38; 1 Cor. 15:37.
WHEEL. Ex. 14:25, took off their chariot *w*.
Judg. 5:28, why tarry the *w*.?
Ps. 83:13, make them like a *w*.
Prov. 20:26, a wise king bringeth the *w*. over them.
Eccl. 12:6, or the *w*. broken at the cistern.
Isa. 28:28, nor break it with the *w*. of his cart.
Nah. 3:2, the noise of the rattling of the *w*.
See Isa. 5:28; Jer. 18:3; 47:3; Ezek. 1:16.
WHELP. 2 Sam. 17:8; Prov. 17:12; Hos. 13:8.
WHEN. 1 Sam. 3:12, *w*. I begin, I will also.
1 Kings 8:30, *w*. thou hearest, forgive.
Ps. 94:8, *w*. will ye be wise?
Eccl. 8:7, who can tell him *w*. it shall be?
Mat. 24:3; Mk. 13:4; Lu. 21:7, *w*. shall these things be?
See Deut. 6:7; John 4:25; 16:8; 1 John 2:28.
WHENCE. Gen. 42:7; Josh. 9:8, *w*. come ye?
Job 10:21, *w*. I shall not return.
Isa. 51:1, the rock *w*. ye are hewn.
Jas. 4:1, from *w*. come wars?
Rev. 7:13, *w*. came they?
See Mat. 13:54; John 1:48; 7:28; 9:29.
WHERE. Gen. 3:9, *w*. art thou?
Ex. 2:20; 2 Sam. 9:4; Job 14:10, *w*. is he?
Job 9:24, if not, *w*. and who is he?
Ps. 42:3, *w*. is thy God?
Jer. 2:6, *w*. is the Lord?
Zech. 1:5, your fathers, *w*. are they?
See Isa. 49:21; Hos. 1:10; Lu. 17:37.
WHEREBY. Lu. 1:18, *w*. shall I know this?
Acts 4:12, none other name *w*. we must be saved.
Rom. 8:15, the spirit of adoption, *w*. we cry.
See Jer. 33:8; Ezek. 18:31; 39:26; Eph. 4:30.
WHEREFORE. 2 Sam. 12:23, *w*. should I fast?
Mat. 14:31, *w*. didst thou doubt?
26:50, *w*. art thou come?
See 2 Sam. 16:10; Mal. 2:15; Acts 10:21.
WHERETO. Isa. 55:11; Phil. 3:16.
WHEREWITH. Judg. 6:5, *w*. shall I save Israel?
Ps. 119:42, so shall I have *w*. to answer.
Mic. 6:6, *w*. shall I come before the Lord?
See Mat. 5:13; Mk. 9:5; John 17:26; Eph. 2:4.
WHET. Deut. 32:41; Ps. 7:12; 64:3; Eccl. 10:10.
WHETHER. Mat. 21:31, *w*. of them did the will.
Mat. 23:17, *w*. is greater, the gold or the temple?
Rom. 14:8, *w*. we live or die.
2 Cor. 12:2, *w*. in the body, or out of the body.
See 1 Kings 20:18; Ezek. 2:5; 3:11; 1 John 4:1.
WHILE. 2 Chron. 15:2, with you, *w*. ye be with him.
Ps. 49:18, *w*. he lived he blessed his soul.
Isa. 55:6, *w*. he may be found.
Jer. 15:9, her sun is gone down *w*. it was yet day.
Lu. 18:4, he would not for a *w*.
24:44, *w*. I was yet with you.
John 9:4, work *w*. it is day.
1 Tim. 5:6, she is dead *w*. she liveth.
See 1 Sam. 9:27; 2 Sam. 7:19; Acts 20:11.
WHIP. 1 Kings 12:11; Prov. 26:3; Nah. 3:2.
WHIT. 1 Sam. 3:18; John 7:23; 13:10; 2 Cor. 11:5.
WHITE. Gen. 49:12, his teeth shall be *w*. with milk.
Num. 12:10, leprous, *w*. as snow.
Job 6:6, is any taste in the *w*. of an egg?
Eccl. 9:8, let thy garments be always *w*.
Cant. 5:10, my beloved is *w*. and ruddy.
Isa. 1:18, they shall be *w*. as snow.
Mat. 5:36, thou canst not make one hair *w*. or black.
John 4:35, *w*. already to harvest.
Rev. 2:17, a *w*. stone.
3:4, walk with me in *w*.

See Dan. 11:35; 12:10; Mat. 17:2; 28:3.
WHITED. Mat. 23:27; Acts 23:3.
WHITER. Ps. 51:7; Lam. 4:7.
WHITHER. 2 Kings 5:25; Cant. 6:1; Heb. 11:8.
WHOLE. 2 Sam. 1:9, my life is yet *w.* in me.
Eccl. 12:13, this is the *w.* duty of man.
Jer. 19:11, a vessel that cannot be made *w.*
Ezek. 15:5, when *w.* it was meet for no work.
Mat. 5:29, not that thy *w.* body be cast into hell.
9:12; Mk. 2:17, the *w.* need not a physician.
13:33; Lu. 13:21, till the *w.* was leavened.
16:26; Mk. 8:36; Lu. 9:25, gain the *w.* world.
John 11:50, expedient that the *w.* nation perish not.
1 Cor. 12:17, if the *w.* body were an eye.
1 Thess. 5:23, I pray God your *w.* spirit.
Jas. 2:10, keep the *w.* law.
1 John 2:2, for the sins of the *w.* world.
5:19, the *w.* world lieth in wickedness.
See Mat. 15:31; John 5:6; 7:23; Acts 9:34.
WHOLESOME. Prov. 15:4; 1 Tim. 6:3.
WHOLLY. Job 21:23, dieth, being *w.* at ease.
Jer. 2:21, planted thee *w.* a right seed.
46:28, not *w.* unpunished.
Acts 17:16, the city *w.* given to idolatry.
1 Thess. 5:23, sanctify you *w.*
1 Tim. 4:15, give thyself *w.* to them.
See Lev. 19:9; Deut. 1:36; Josh. 14:8.
WHOMSOEVER. Dan. 4:17, 25, 32, to *w.* he will.
Mat. 11:27, to *w.* the Son will reveal him.
21:44; Lu. 20:18, on *w.* it shall fall.
Lu. 4:6, to *w.* I will, I give it.
12:48, to *w.* much is given.
See Gen. 31:32; Judg. 11:24; Acts 8:19.
WHOSE. Gen. 32:17, *w.* art thou, *w.* are these?
Jer. 44:28, shall know *w.* words shall stand.
Mat. 22:20; Mk. 12:16; Lu. 20:24, *w.* is this image?
Lu. 12:20, then *w.* shall these things be?
Acts 27:23, *w.* I am, and whom I serve.
See 1 Sam. 12:3; Dan. 5:23; John 20:23.
WHOSOEVER. 1 Cor. 11:27, *w.* shall eat this bread.
Gal. 5:10, bear his judgment, *w.* he be.
Rev. 22:17, *w.* will, let him take.
See Mat. 11:6; 13:12; Lu. 8:18; Rom. 2:1.
WHY. 1 Sam. 2:23, *w.* do ye such things?
Jer. 8:14, *w.* do we sit still?
27:13; Ezek. 18:31; 33:11, *w.* will ye die?
Mat. 21:25; Mk. 11:31; Lu. 20:5, *w.* did ye not believe?
Mk. 5:39, *w.* make ye this ado?
Acts 9:4; 22:7; 26:14, *w.* persecutest thou me?
Rom. 9:19, *w.* doth he yet find fault?
20, *w.* hast thou made me thus?
See 2 Chron. 25:16; Lu. 2:48; John 7:45; 10:20.
WICKED. Gen. 18:23, destroy righteous with *w.*
Deut. 15:9, a thought in thy *w.* heart.
1 Sam. 2:9, the *w.* shall be silent.
Job 3:17, there the *w.* cease from troubling.
8:22, dwelling place of the *w.* shall come to nought.
9:29; 10:15, if I be *w.*, why labour I in vain?
21:7, wherefore do the *w.* live?
30, the *w.* is reserved to destruction.
Ps. 7:9, let the wickedness of the *w.* come to an end.
11, God is angry with the *w.*
9:17, the *w.* shall be turned into hell.
10:4, the *w*, will not seek God.
11:2, the *w*, bend their bow.
6, upon the *w.* he shall rain snares.
12:8, the *w.* walk on every side.
26:5, I will not sit with the *w.*
34:21, evil shall slay the *w.*
37:21, the *w.* borroweth, and payeth not.
32, the *w.* watcheth the righteous.
35, I have seen the *w.* in great power.
58:3, the *w.* are estranged from the womb.
68:2, so let the *w.* perish.
94:3, how long shall the *w.* triumph?
139:24, see if there by any *w.* way in me.
145:20, all the *w.* will he destroy.
Prov. 11:5, the *w.* shall fall by his own wickedness.
14:32, the *w.* is driven away.
28:1, the *w.* flee when no man pursueth.
Eccl. 7:17, be not overmuch *w.*
8:10, I saw the *w.* buried.
Isa. 13:11, I will punish the *w.*
53:9, he made his grave with the *w.*
55:7, let the *w.* forsake his way.
57:20, the *w.* are like the troubled sea.
Jer. 17:9, the heart is desperately *w.*
Ezek. 3:18; 33:8, to warn the *w.*
11:2, these men give *w.* counsel.
18:23, have I any pleasure that the *w.* should die?
33:15, if the *w.* restore the pledge.
Dan. 12:10, the *w.* shall do wickedly.
Mic. 6:11, with *w.* balances.
Nah. 1:3, the Lord will not at all acquit the *w.*
Mat. 12:45; Lu. 11:26, more *w.* than himself.
13:49, sever the *w.* from the just.
18:32; 25:26; Lu. 19:22, thou *w.* servant.
Acts 2:23, and by *w.* hands have crucified and slain.
1 Cor. 5:13, put away that *w.* person.
Eph. 6:16, the fiery darts of the *w.*
Col. 1:21, enemies in your mind by *w.* works.
2 Thess. 2:8, then shall that *W.* be revealed.
See Eccl. 9:2; Isa. 48:22; 2 Pet. 2:7; 3:17.
WICKEDLY. Job 13:7, will you speak *w.* for God?
34:12, God will not do *w.*
Ps. 73:8; 139:20, they speak *w.*
Dan. 12:10, the wicked shall do *w.*
Mal. 4:1, all that do *w.*
See 2 Chron. 6:37; 22:3; Neh. 9:33; Ps. 106:6.
WICKEDNESS. Gen. 39:9, this great *w.*
Judg. 20:3, how was this *w.*?
1 Sam. 24:13, *w.* proceedeth from the wicked.
1 Kings 21:25, sold himself to work *w.*
Job 4:8, they that sow *w.*, reap the same.
22:5, is not thy *w.* great?
35:8, thy *w.* may hurt a man.
Ps. 7:9, let the *w.* of the wicked come to an end.
55:11, *w.* is in the midst thereof.
15, *w.* is in their dwellings.
58:2, in heart ye work *w.*
84:10, the tents of *w.*
Prov. 4:17, they eat the bread of *w.*
8:7, *w.* is an abomination to my lips.
11:5, the wicked shall fall by his own *w.*
13:6, *w.* overthroweth the sinner.
26:26, his *w.* shall be shewed.
Eccl. 7:25, the *w.* of folly.
Isa. 9:18, *w.* burneth as the fire.
47:10, thou hast trusted in thy *w.*
Jer. 2:19, thine own *w.* shall correct thee.
6:7, she casteth out her *w.*
8:6, no man repented of his *w.*
44:9, have you forgot the *w.* of your kings?
Ezek. 3:19, if he turn not from his *w.*
7:11, violence is risen up into a rod of *w.*
31:11, I have driven him out for his *w.*
33:12, in the day he turneth from his *w.*
Hos. 9:15, for the *w.* of their doings.
10:13, ye have ploughed *w.*
Mic. 6:10, are treasures of *w.* in house.
Zech. 5:8, he said, this is *w.*
Mal. 1:4, the border of *w.*
3:15, they that work *w.* are set up.
Mk. 7:21, out of the heart proceed *w.*
Lu. 11:39, your inward part is full of *w.*
Rom. 1:29, being filled with all *w.*
1 Cor. 5:8, nor with the leaven of *w.*
Eph. 6:12, spiritual *w.* in high places.
1 John 5:19, the whole world lieth in *w.*
See Gen. 6:5; Ps. 94:23; Prov. 21:12; Jer. 23:11.
WIDE. Ps. 35:21, they opened their mouth *w.*
104:25, this great and *w.* sea.
Prov. 21:9; 25:24; Jer. 22:14, a *w.* house.
Mat. 7:13, *w.* is the gate that leadeth to destruction.

See Deut. 15:8; Ps. 81:10; Nah. 3:13.
WIFE. Prov. 5:18; Eccl. 9:9, the *w.* of thy youth.
18:22, whoso findeth a *w.* findeth a good thing.
19:14, a prudent *w.* is from the Lord.
Lu. 14:20, I have married a *w.*
17:32, remember Lot's *w.*
1 Cor. 7:14, the unbelieving *w.* is sanctified.
Eph. 5:23, the husband is the head of the *w.*
Rev. 21:9, the bride, the Lamb's *w.*
See 1 Tim. 3:2; 5:9; Tit. 1:6; 1 Pet. 3:7.
WILES. Num. 25:18; Eph. 6:11.
WILFULLY. Heb. 10:26, if we sin *w.*
WILL. Mat. 8:3; Mk. 1:41; Lu. 5:13, I *w.*, be thou clean.
18:14, not the *w.* of your Father.
26:39, not as I *w.*, but as thou wilt.
Mk. 3:35, whosoever shall do the *w.* of God.
John 1:13, born not of the *w.* of the flesh.
4:34, to do the *w.* of him that sent me.
Acts 21:14, the *w.* of the Lord be done.
Rom. 7:18, to *w.* is present with me.
Phil. 2:13, both to *w.* and to do.
1 Tim. 2:8, I *w.* that men pray every where.
Rev. 22:17, whosoever *w.*, let him take.
See Rom. 9:16; Eph. 1:11; Heb. 2:4; Jas. 1:18.
WILLING. Ex. 35:5, a *w.* heart.
1 Chron. 28:9, serve God with a *w.* mind.
29:5, who is *w.* to consecrate his service?
Ps. 110:3, *w.* in the day of thy power.
Mat. 26:41, the spirit is *w.*
2 Cor. 5:8, *w.* rather to be absent.
8:12, if there be first a *w.* mind.
1 Tim. 6:18, *w.* to communicate.
2 Pet. 3:9, not *w.* that any should perish.
See Lu. 22:42; John 5:35; Philem. 14; 1 Pet. 5:2.
WIN. 2 Chron. 32:1; Prov. 11:30; Phil. 3:8.
WIND. Job 6:26, reprove speeches which are as *w.*
7:7, remember that my life is *w.*
Prov. 11:29, he shall inherit *w.*
25:23, the north *w.* driveth away rain.
30:4, gathereth the *w.* in his fists.
Eccl. 11:4, he that observeth the *w.*
Isa. 26:18, we have brought forth *w.*
27:8, he stayeth his rough *w.*
Ezek. 37:9, prophesy to the *w.*
Hos. 8:7, they have sown *w.*
Amos 4:13, he that createth the *w.*
Mat. 11:7, a reed shaken with the *w.*
John 3:8, the *w.* bloweth where it listeth.
Eph. 4:14, carried about with every *w.* of doctrine.
See Acts 2:2; Jas. 1:6; Jude 12.
WINDOWS. Gen. 7:11; Eccl. 12:3; Jer. 9:21; Mal. 3:10.
WINGS. Ps. 17:8; 36:7; 57:1; 61:4; 68:13; 91:4, the shadow of thy *w.*
18:10; 104:3, on the *w.* of the wind.
55:6, Oh that I had *w.* like a dove!
139:9, the *w.* of the morning.
Prov. 23:5, riches make themselves *w.*
Mal. 4:2, with healing in his *w.*
See Ezek. 1:6; Zech. 5:9; Mat. 23:37; Lu. 13:34.
WINK. Job 15:12; Ps. 35:19; Prov. 6:13; 10:10; Acts 17:30.
WINTER. Gen. 8:22; Cant. 2:11; Mat. 24:20; Mk. 13:18.
WIPE. 2 Kings 21:13; Isa. 25:8; Lu. 7:38; John 13:5.
WISDOM. Job 4:21, they die without *w.*
12:2, *w.* shall die with you.
Prov. 4:7, *w.* is the principal thing.
16:16, better to get *w.* than gold.
19:8, he that getteth *w.* loveth his own soul.
23:4, cease from thine own *w.*
Eccl. 1:18, in much *w.* is much grief.
Isa. 10:13, by my *w.* I have done it.
29:14, the *w.* of their wise men shall perish.
Jer. 8:9, they have rejected the word of the Lord; and what *w.* is in them?
Mic. 6:9, the man of *w.* shall see thy name.
Mat. 11:19, *w.* is justified of her children.
1 Cor. 1:17, not with *w.* of words.
24, Christ the *w.* of God.
1 Cor. 1:30, who of God is made unto us *w.*
2:6, we speak w. among them that are perfect.
3:19, the *w.* of this world is foolishness with God.
2 Cor. 1:12, not with fleshly *w.*
Col. 1:9, that ye might be filled with all *w.*
4:5, walk in *w.* toward them.
Jas. 1:5, if any lack *w.*
3:17, the *w.* from above is pure.
Rev. 5:12, worthy is the Lamb to receive *w.*
13:18, here is *w.*
See Eccl. 1:16; Rom. 11:33; Col. 2:3; 3:16.
WISE. Gen. 3:6, to make one *w.*
Ex. 23:8, the gift blindeth the *w.*
Deut. 4:6, this nation is a *w.* people.
32:29, O that they were *w.*!
1 Kings 3:12, I have given thee a *w.* heart.
Job 9:4, he is *w.* in heart.
11:12, vain man would be *w.*
22:2, he that is *w.* may be profitable.
32:9, great men are not always *w.*
Ps. 2:10, be *w.* now, O ye kings.
19:7, making *w.* the simple.
36:3, he hath left off to be *w.*
94:8, when will ye be *w.*?
107:43, whoso is *w.*, and will observe.
Prov. 1:5, a *w.* man shall attain *w.* counsels.
3:7, be not *w.* in thine own eyes.
6:6; 8:33; 23:19; 27:11, be *w.*
9:12, thou shalt be *w.* for thyself.
11:30, he that winneth souls is *w.*
16:21, the *w.* in heart shall be called prudent.
20:26, a *w.* king scattereth the wicked.
Eccl. 7:23, I said, I will be *w.*
91, the *w.* are in the hands of God.
12:11, the words of the *w.* are as goads.
Isa. 19:11, I am the son of the *w.*
Dan. 12:3, they that be *w.* shall shine.
Mat. 10:16, be *w.* as serpents.
11:25, hid these things from the *w.*
Rom. 1:14, I am debtor to the *w.*
12:16, be not *w.* in your own conceits.
1 Cor. 1:20, where is the *w.*?
4:10, ye are *w.* in Christ.
2 Tim. 3:15, *w.* unto salvation.
See Isa. 5:21; Jer. 4:22; Mat. 25:2.
WISELY. Ps. 58:5, charmers, charming never so *w.*
101:2, I will behave myself *w.*
Prov. 16:20, that handleth a matter *w.*
See Prov. 21:12; 28:26; Eccl. 7:10; Lu. 16:8.
WISER. 1 Kings 4:31; Lu. 16:8; 1 Cor. 1:25.
WISH. Ps. 73:7, more than heart could *w.*
Rom. 9:3, I could *w.* myself accursed.
3 John 2, I *w.* above all things.
See Job 33:6; Jonah 4:8; 2 Cor. 13:9.
WITCH. Ex. 22:18, thou shalt not suffer a *w.* to live.
Deut. 18:10, or a *w.*
WITHDRAW. Job 9:13; Prov. 25:17; 2 Thess. 3:6.
WITHER. Ps. 1:3, his leaf shall not *w.*
37:2, they shall *w.* as the green herb.
129:6; Isa. 40:7; 1 Pet. 1:24, the grass *w.*
Mat. 21:19; Mk. 11:21, the fig tree *w.* away.
Jude 12, threes whose fruit *w.*
See Joel 1:12; John 15:6; Jas. 1:11
WITHHOLD. Ps. 40:11, *w.* not thy mercies.
84:11, no good thing will he *w.*
Prov. 3:27, *w.* not good from them to whom it is due.
23:13, *w.* not correction.
Eccl. 11:6, *w.* not thy hand.
Jer. 5:25, your sins have *w.* good things.
See Job 22:7; 42:2; Ezek. 18:16; Joel 1:13.
WITHIN. Mat. 23:26, cleanse first what is *w.*
Mk. 7:21, from *w.* proceed evil thoughts.
2 Cor. 7:5, *w.* were fears.
See Ps. 45:13; Mat. 3:9; Lu. 12:17; 16:3.
WITHOUT. Gen. 24:31, wherefore standest thou *w.*?
2 Chron. 15:3, for a long season *w.* the true God.
Prov. 1:20, wisdom crieth *w.*

Isa. 52:3; 55:1, *w.* money.
Jer. 33:10, *w.* man, *w.* beast *w.* inhabitant.
Hos. 3:4, Israel *w.* king, *w.* prince, *w.* sacrifice.
Eph. 2:12, *w.* God in the world.
Col. 4:5; 1 Thess. 4:12; 1 Tim. 3:7, them that are *w.*
Heb. 13:12, Jesus suffered *w.* the gate.
Rev. 22:15, for *w.* are dogs.
See Prov. 22:12; Mat. 10:29; Lu. 11:40.

WITHSTAND. Eccl. 4:12, two shall *w.* him.
Acts 11:17, what was I that I could *w.* God?
Eph 6:13, able to *w.* in evil day.
See Num. 22:32; 2 Chron. 20:6; Esth. 9:2.

WITNESS (*n.*). Gen. 31:50, God is *w.* betwixt.
Josh. 24:27, this stone shall be a *w.*
Job 16:19, my *w.* is in heaven.
Ps. 89:37, as a faithful *w.* in heaven.
Prov. 14:5, a faithful *w.* will not lie.
Isa. 55:4, I have given him for a *w.* to the people.
Jer. 42:5, the Lord be a true and faithful *w.*
Mat. 24:14, for a *w.* unto all nations.
John 1:7, the same came for a *w.*
3:11, ye receive not our *w.*
5:36, I have greater *w.* than that of John.
Acts 14:17, he left not himself without *w.*
Rom. 2:15, conscience also bearing them *w.*
1 John 5:9, the *w.* of God is greater.
10, hath the *w.* in himself.
See Isa. 43:10; Lu. 24:48; Acts 1:8; 13:31.

WITNESS (*v.*). Deut. 4:26, heaven and earth to *w.*
Isa. 3:9, countenance doth *w.* against them.
Acts 20:23, the Holy Ghost *w.* in every city.
Rom. 3:21, being *w.* by the law and prophets.
1 Tim. 6:13, before Pilate *w.* a good confession.
See 1 Sam. 12:3; Mat. 26:62; 27:13; Mk. 14:60.

WITS. Ps. 107:27, are at their *w.* end.

WITTY. Prov. 8:12, knowledge of *w.* inventions.

WIZARD. Lev. 20:27, or that is a *w.*

WOEFUL. Jer. 17:16, the *w.* day.

WOMAN. Judg. 9:54, a *w.* slew him.
Ps. 48:6; Isa. 13:8; 21:3; 26:17; Jer. 4:31; 6:24; 13:21, 22, 23; 30:6; 31:8; 48:41; 49:22, 24; 50:43, pain as of a *w.* in travail.
Prov. 6:24, to keep thee from the evil *w.*
9:13, a foolish *w.* is clamorous.
12:4; 31:10, a virtuous *w.*
14:1, every wise *w.* buildeth her house.
21:9, with a brawling *w.* in wide house.
Eccl. 7:28, a *w.* among all those have I not found.
Isa. 54:6, as a *w.* forsaken.
Jer. 31:22, a *w.* shall compass a man.
Mat. 5:28, whoso looketh on a *w.*
15:28, O w. great is thy faith.
22:27; Mk. 12:22; Lu. 20:32, the *w.* died also.
26:10, why trouble ye the *w.*?
13, shall this, that this *w.* hath done, be told.
John 2:4, *w.*, what have I to do with thee?
8:3, a *w.* taken in adultery.
19:26, *w.*, behold thy son.
Acts 9:36, this *w.* was full of good works.
Rom. 1:27, the natural use of the *w.*
1 Cor. 7:1, it is good for a man not to touch a *w.*
11:7, the *w.* is the glory of the man.
Gal. 4:4, God sent forth his Son, made of a *w.*
1 Tim. 2:12, I suffer not a *w.* to teach.
14, the *w.* being deceived.
See Isa. 49:15; Lu. 7:39; 13:16; Rev. 12:1.

WOMB. Gen. 49:25, blessings of the *w.*
1 Sam. 1:5, the Lord had shut up her *w.*
Ps. 22:9, took me out of the *w.*
10, cast upon thee from the *w.*
127:3, the fruit of the *w.* is his reward.
139:13, thou hast covered me in my mother's *w.*
Eccl. 11:5, how bones grow in the *w.*
Isa. 44:2; 49:5, the Lord formed thee from the *w.*
48:8, a transgressor from the *w.*
49:15, compassion on son of her *w.*
Hos. 9:14, give them miscarrying *w.*
Lu. 1:42, blessed is the fruit of thy *w.*
Lu. 11:27, blessed is the *w.* that bare thee.
23:29, blessed are the *w.* that never bare.
See Job 3:11; 24:20; 31:15; Prov. 30:16.

WOMEN. Judg. 5:24, blessed above *w.*
1 Sam. 18:7, the *w.* answered one another.
2 Sam. 1:26, passing the love of *w.*
Ps. 45:9, among thy honourable *w.*
Prov. 31:3, give not thy strength to *w.*
Lam. 4:10, the pitiful *w.* have sodden their children.
Mat. 11:11; Lu. 7:28, among them that are born of *w.*
24:41; Lu. 17:35, two *w.* grinding at the mill.
Lu. 1:28, blessed art thou among *w.*
1 Cor. 14:34, let your *w.* keep silence.
1 Tim. 2:9, *w.* adorn themselves.
11, let the *w.* learn in silence.
5:14, that the younger *w.* marry.
2 Tim. 3:6, lead captive silly *w.*
Tit. 2 3, the aged *w.* in behaviour as becometh holiness.
Heb. 11:35, *w.* received their dead.
See Acts 16:13; 17:4; Phil. 4:3; 1 Pet. 3:5.

WONDER (*n.*). Ps. 71:7, as *w.* unto many.
77:14, thou art the God that doest *w.*
88:12, shall thy *w.* be known in the dark?
96:3, declare his *w.* among all people.
107:24, his *w.* in the deep.
Isa. 20:3, walked barefoot for a sign and a *w.*
29:14, I will do a marvellous work and a *w.*
Joel 2:30; Acts 2:19, I will show *w.* in heaven.
John 4 48, except ye see signs and *w.*
Acts 4:30, that *w.* may be done by the name.
See Rom 15:19; 2 Cor. 12:12; 2 Thess. 2:9.

WONDER (*v.*). Isa. 29:9, stay yourselves, and *w.*
59:16, he *w.* there was no intercessor.
63:5, I *w.* there was none to uphold.
Hab. 1:5, regard, and *w.* marvellously.
Zech. 3:8, they are men *w.* at.
Lu. 4:22, all *w.* at the gracious words.
See Acts 3:11; 8:13; 13:41; Rev. 13:3; 17:6.

WONDERFUL. 2 Sam. 1:26, thy love was *w.*
Job 42:3, things too *w.* for me.
Ps. 139:6, such knowledge is too *w.* for me.
Isa. 9:6, his name shall be called *W.*
28:29, who is *w.* in counsel.
See Deut. 28:59; Jer. 5:30; Mat. 21:15.

WONDERFULLY. Ps. 139:14; Lam. 1:9; Dan. 8:24.

WONDROUS. 1 Chron. 16:9; Job 37:14; Ps. 26:7; 75:1; 78:32; 105:2; 106:22; 119:27; 145:5; Jer. 21:2, *w.* works.
Ps. 72:18; 86:10; 119:18, *w.* things.

WONT. Ex. 21:29, if the ox were *w.* to push.
Mat. 27:15, the governor was *w.* to release.
Mk. 10:1, as he was *w.*, he taught them.
Lu. 22:39, he went, as he was *w.*
Acts 16:13, where prayer was *w.* to be made.
See Num. 22:30; 2 Sam. 20:18; Dan. 3:19.

WOOD. Gen. 22:7, behold the fire and the *w.*
Deut. 29:11; Josh. 9:21; Jer. 46:22, hewer of *w.*
2 Sam. 18 8, the *w.* devoured more people.
Ps. 141:7, as one cleaveth *w.*
Prov. 26:20, where no *w.* is, the fire goeth out.
See Jer. 7:18; Hag. 1:8; 1 Cor. 3:12.

WOOL. Ps. 147:16, he giveth snow like *w.*
Isa. 1:18, your sins shall be as *w.*
Dan. 7:9; Rev. 1:14, hair like *w.*
See Prov. 31:13; Ezek. 34:3; 44:17; Hos. 9:1.

WORD. Deut. 8:3; Mat. 4:4, every *w.* of God.
30:14; Rom. 10:8, the *w.* is very nigh.
Job 12:11, doth not the ear try *w.*?
35:16, he multiplieth *w.*
38:2, by *w.* without knowledge.
Ps. 19:14, let the *w.* of my mouth be acceptable.
68:11, the Lord gave the *w.*
119:43; 2 Cor. 6:7; Eph. 1:13, Col. 1:5; 2 Tim. 2:15; Jas. 1:18, the *w.* of truth.
Prov. 15:23, a *w.* spoken in due season.
25:11, a *w.* fitly spoken.
Isa. 29:21, an offender for a *w.*
30:21, thine ears shall hear a *w.* behind thee.

Isa. 50:4, how to speak a *w.* in season.
Jer. 5:13, the *w.* is not in them.
 18:18, nor shall the *w.* perish.
 4:28, know whose *w.* shall stand.
Hos. 14:2, take with you *w.*
Mat. 8:8, speak the *w.* only.
 12:36, every idle *w.* that men shall speak.
 18:16, that every *w.* may be established.
 24:35, may *w.* shall not pass away.
Mk. 4:14, the sower soweth the *w.*
 8:38; Lu. 9:26, ashamed of my *w.*
Lu. 4:22, gracious *w.* which proceeded.
 36, amazed, saying, what a *w.* is this!
 24:19, a prophet mighty in deed and *w.*
John 6:63, the *w.* I speak are life.
 68, thou hast the *w.* of eternal life.
 12:48, the *w.* I have spoken shall judge him.
 14:24, the *w.* ye hear is not mine.
 17:8, I have given them the *w.* thou gavest me.
Acts 13:15, any *w.* of exhortation.
 20:35, remember the *w.* of the Lord Jesus.
 26:25, the *w.* of truth and soberness.
1 Cor. 1:17, not with wisdom of *w.*
 4:20, not in *w.*, but in power.
 14:9, except ye utter *w.* easy to be understood.
2 Cor. 1:18, our *w.* was not yea and nay.
 5:19, the *w.* of reconciliation.
Gal. 5:14, all the law is fulfilled in one *w.*
 6:6, him that is taught in the *w.*
Eph. 5:6, deceive you with vain *w.*
Phil. 2:16, holding forth the *w.* of life.
Col. 3:16, let the *w.* of Christ dwell in you.
1 Thess. 1:5, the gospel came not in *w.* only.
 4:18, comfort one another with these *w.*
1 Tim. 4:6, nourished in *w.* of faith.
 5:17, labour in the *w.* and doctrine.
2 Tim. 2:14, strive not about *w.*
 4:2, preach the *w.*
Tit. 1:3, in due times manifested his *w.*
 9, holding fast the faithful *w.*
Heb. 1:3, by the *w.* of his power.
 2:2, if the *w.* spoken by angels was stedfast.
 4:2, the *w.* preached did not profit.
 12, the *w.* of God is quick and powerful.
 5:13, is unskilful in the *w.*
 6:5, and have tasted the good *w.* of God.
 7:28, the *w.* of the oath.
 11:3, the worlds were framed by the *w.* of God.
 13:7, who have spoken to you the *w.*
Jas. 1:21, the engrafted *w.*
 22, be ye doers of the *w.*
 23, if any be a hearer of the *w.*
 3:2, if any man offend not in *w.*
1 Pet. 1:23, being born again by the *w.*
 25, this is the *w.* which is preached.
 2:2, the sincere milk of the *w.*
 8, them that stumble at the *w.*
 3:1, if any obey not the *w.*, they also may without the *w.*
2 Pet. 1:19, a more sure *w.* of prophecy.
 3:2, the *w.* spoken by the prophets.
 5, by the *w.* of God the heavens were of old.
 7, the heavens by the same *w.* are kept in store.
1 John 1:1, hands have handled, of W. of life.
 2:5, whoso keepeth his *w.*, in him is the love.
 3:18, let us not love in *w.*
Rev. 3:8, thou hast kept my *w.*
 10, the *w.* of my patience.
 6:9, that were slain for the *w.*
 22:19, take away from the *w.* of this prophecy.
See Isa. 8:20; Jer. 20:9; Mic. 2:7; Rev. 21:5.
WORK (*n.*). Gen. 2:2, God ended his *w.*
 5:29, shall comfort us concerning our *w.*
Ex. 20:9; 23:12; Deut. 5:13, six days thou shalt do all thy *w.*
 35:2, six days shall *w.* be done.
Deut. 3:24, what God can do according to thy *w.*?
 4:28; 27:15; 2 Kings 19:18; 2 Chron. 32:19; Ps. 115:4; 135:15, the *w.* of men's hands.
1 Chron. 16:37, as every day's *w.* required.
2 Chron. 31:21, in every *w.* he began he did it.
 34:12, the men did the *w.* faithfully.
Ezra 5:8, this *w.* goeth fast on.
 6:7, let the *w.* alone.
Neh. 3:5, their nobles put not their necks to the *w.*
 6:3, why should the *w.* cease?
 16, they perceived this *w.* was of God.
Job 1:10, thou hast blessed the *w.* of his hands.
 10:3; 14:15; Ps. 143:5, the *w.* of thine hands.
 34:11, the *w.* of a man shall he render unto him.
Ps. 8:3, the *w.* of thy fingers.
 19:1, his handy-*w.*
 33:4, all his *w.* are done in truth.
 40:5; 78:4; 107:8; 111:4; Mat. 7:22; Acts 2:11, wonderful *w.*
 90:17, establish thou the *w.* of our hands.
 101:3, I hate the *w.* of them that turn aside.
 104:23, man goeth forth to his *w.*
 111:2, the *w.* of the Lord are great.
 141:4, to practise wicked *w.*
Prov. 16:3, commit thy *w.* unto the Lord.
 20:11, whether his *w.* be pure.
 24:12; Mat. 16:27; 2 Tim. 4:14, to every man according to his *w.*
 31:31, let her own *w.* praise her.
Eccl. 1:14, I have seen all the *w.* that are done.
 3:17, there is a time for every *w.*
 5:6, wherefore should God destroy the *w.*?
 8:9, I applied my heart to every *w.*
 9:1, their *w.* are in the hand of God.
 7, God now accepteth thy *w.*
 10, there is no *w.* in the grave.
 12:14, God shall bring every *w.* into judgment.
Isa. 2:8; 37:19; Jer. 1:16; 10:3, 9, 15; 51:18, they worship the *w.* of their own hands.
 5:19, let him hasten his *w.*
 10:12, when the Lord hath performed his whole *w.*
 26:12, thou hast wrought all our *w.* in us.
 28:21, do his *w.*, his strange *w.*
 29:15, their *w.* are in the dark.
 49:4, my *w.* is with my God.
 66:18, I know their *w.* and their thoughts.
Jer. 32:19, great in counsel, and mighty in *w.*
 48:7, thou hast trusted in thy *w.*
Amos 8:7, I will never for get any of their *w.*
Hab. 1:5, I will work a *w.* in your days.
Mat. 23:3, do not ye after their *w.*
 5, all their *w.* they do to be seen of men.
Mk. 6:5, he could there do no mighty *w.*
John 5:20, greater *w.* than these.
 6:28, that we might work the *w.* of God.
 29, this is the *w.* of God. that ye believe.
 7:21, I have done one *w.*, and ye all marvel.
 9:3, that the *w.* of God should be made manifest.
 10:25, the *w.* I do in my Father's name.
 32, for which of those *w.* do ye stone me?
 14:12, the *w.* I do shall he do, and greater *w.*
 17:4, I have finished the *w.*
Acts 5:38, if this *w.* be of men, it will come to nought.
 15:38, who went not with them to the *w.*
Rom. 3:27, by what law? of *w.*?
 4:6, imputeth righteousness without *w.*
 9:11, not of *w.*, but of him that calleth.
 11:6, grace, otherwise *w.* is no more *w.*
 13:12, let us therefore cast off the *w.* of darkness.
 14:20, for meat destroy not the *w.* of God.
1 Cor. 3:13, every man's *w.* shall be made manifest.
 9:1, are not ye may *w.* in the Lord?
Gal. 2:16, by *w.* of law shall no flesh be justified.
 6:4, let every man prove his own *w.*
Eph. 2:9, not of *w.* lest any man should boast.
 4:12, the *w.* of the ministry.
 5:11, the unfruitful *w.* of darkness.
Col. 1:21, enemies in your mind by wicked *w.*
1 Thess. 5:13, esteem them in love for their *w.* sake.
2 Thess. 2:17, in every good word and *w.*
2 Tim. 1:9; Tit. 3:5, saved us, not according to our *w.*

2 Tim. 4:5, do the *w.* of an evangelist.
Tit. 1:16, in *w.* they deny him.
Heb. 6:1; 9:14, from dead *w.*
Jas. 1:4, let patience have her perfect *w.*
2:14, if he have not *w.*, can faith save him?
17, faith, if it hath not *w.*, is dead, being alone.
18, shew me thy faith without thy *w.*
21, was not Abraham justified by *w.*?
22, by *w.* was faith made perfect.
2 Pet. 3:10, earth and *w.* therein shall be burnt up.
1 John 3:8, destroy the *w.* of the devil.
Rev. 2:2, 9, 13, 19; 3:1, 8, 15, I know thy *w.*
26, he that keepeth my *w.* to the end.
3:2, I have not found thy *w.* perfect.
14:13, and their *w.* do follow them.
See Gal. 5:19; 2 Thess. 1:11; Rev. 18:6; 20:12.
WORK (*v.*). 1 Sam. 14:6, the Lord will *w.* for us.
1 Kings 21:20, sold thyself to *w.* evil.
Neh. 4:6, the people had a mind to the *w.*
Job 23:9, on the left hand, where he doth *w.*
33:29, all these things *w.* God with man.
Ps. 58:2, in heart ye *w.* wickedness.
101:7, he that *w.* deceit.
119:126, it is time for thee to *w.*
Isa. 43:13, I will *w.*, and who shall let it?
Mic. 2:1, woe to them that *w.* evil.
Hag. 2:4, *w.*, for I am with you.
Mal. 3:15, they that *w.* wickedness are set up.
Mat. 21:28, son, go *w.* to day in my vineyard.
Mk. 16:20, the Lord *w.* with them.
John 5:17, my Father *w.* hitherto, and I *w.*
6:28, that we might *w.* the works of God.
30, what dost thou *w.*?
9:4, the night cometh, when no man can *w.*
Acts 10:35, he that *w.* righteousness is accepted.
Rom. 4:15, the law *w.* wrath.
5:3, tribulation *w.* patience.
8:28, all things *w.* together for good.
1 Cor. 4:12, and labour, *w.* with our own hands.
12:6, it is the same God which *w.* all in all.
2 Cor. 4:12, death *w.* in us.
17, *w.* for us a far more exceeding weight of glory.
Gal. 5:6, faith which *w.* by love.
Eph. 1:11, who *w.* all things after the counsel.
2:2, the spirit that now *w.*
3:20, the power that *w.* in us.
4:28, *w.* with his hands the thing that is good.
Phil. 2:12, *w.* out your own salvation.
1 Thess. 4:11, *w.* with your own hands.
2 Thess. 2:7, the mystery of iniquity doth *w.*
3:10, if any would not *w.*, neither should he eat.
Jas. 1:3, the trying of your faith *w.* patience.
See Ezek. 46:1; Prov. 11:18; 31:13; Eccl. 3:9.
WORKMAN, Hos. 8:6; Eph. 2:10; 2 Tim. 2:15.
WORLD. Job 18:18, chased out of the *w.*
34:13, who hath disposed the whole *w.*?
37:12, on the face of the *w.*
Ps. 17:14, from men of the *w.*
50:12, the *w.* in mine.
73:12, the ungodly, who prosper in the *w.*
77:18; 97:4, lightnings lightened the *w.*
93:1, the *w.* also is stablished.
Eccl. 3:11, he hath set the *w.* in their heart.
Isa. 14:21, nor fill the face of the *w.* with cities.
24:4, the *w.* languisheth.
34:1, let the *w.* hear.
Mat. 4:8; Lu. 4:5, all the kingdoms of the *w.*
5:14, the light of the *w.*
13:22; Mk. 4:19, the cares of this *w.* choke.
38, the field is the *w.*
40, in the end of the *w.*
16:26; Mk. 8:36; Lu. 9:25, gain the whole *w.*
18:7, woe to the *w.* because of offences.
Mk. 10:30; Lu. 18:30; Heb. 2:5; 6:5, in the *w.* to come.
Lu. 1:70; Acts 3:21, since the *w.* began.
2:1, all the *w.* should be taxed.
16:8, 20:34, children of this *w.*
Lu. 20:35, worthy to obtain that *w.*
John 1:10, he was in the *w.*
29, which taketh away the sin of the *w.*
3:16, God so loved the *w.*
4:42, 1 John 4:14, the Saviour of the *w.*
6:33, he that giveth life unto the *w.*
7:4, shew thyself to the *w.*
7, the *w.* cannot hate you.
8:12; 9:5, I am the light of the *w.*
12:19, the whole *w.* is gone after him.
31, now is the judgment of this *w.*
47, not to judge the *w.*, but to save the *w.*
13:1, depart out of this *w.*
14:17, whom the *w.* cannot receive.
22, manifest thyself unto us, and not unto the *w.*
27, not as the *w.* giveth, give I unto you.
30, the prince of this *w.* cometh.
15:18; 1 John 3:13, if the *w.* hate you.
19, the *w.* would love his own.
16:33, in the *w.* ye shall have tribulation.
17:9, I pray not for the *w.*
16, they are not of the *w.*
21, that the *w.* may believe.
21:25, the *w.* could not contain the books.
Acts 17:6, turned the *w.* upside down.
Rom. 3:19, that all the *w.* may become guilty.
12:2, be not conformed to this *w.*
1 Cor. 1:20, where is the disputer of this *w.*?
2:6, the wisdom of this *w.*
7:31, they that use this *w.* as not abusing it.
2 Cor. 4:4, the god of this *w.* hath blinded.
Gal. 1:4, this present evil *w.*
6:14, the *w.* is crucified unto me.
Eph. 2:2, according to the course of this *w.*
12, without God in the *w.*
1 Tim. 6:7, we brought nothing into this *w.*
17, them that are rich in this *w.*
2 Tim. 4:10, having loved this present *w.*
Heb. 11:38, of whom the *w.* was not worthy.
Jas. 1:27, unspotted from the *w.*
3:6, the tongue is a *w.* of iniquity.
4:4, the friendship of the *w.*
2 Pet. 2:5, God spared not the old *w.*
3:6, the *w.* that then was.
1 John 2:15, love not the *w.*
3:1, the *w.* knoweth us not.
5:19, the whole *w.* lieth in wickedness.
See 2 Sam. 22:16; 1 Chron. 16:30; Prov. 8:26.
WORLDLY. Tit. 2:12; Heb. 9:1.
WORM. Job 7:5, my flesh is clothed with *w.*
17:14, I said to the *w.*, thou art my mother.
19:26, though *w.* destroy this body.
21:26, shall lie down, and *w.* shall cover them.
24:20, the *w.* shall feed sweetly on him.
25:6, man, that is a *w.*, etc.
Ps. 22:6, I am a *w.*, and no man.
Isa. 14:11, the *w.* is spread under thee.
41:14, fear not, thou *w.* Jacob.
66:24; Mk. 9:44, 46, 48, their *w.* shall not die.
Mic. 7:17, like *w.* of the earth.
See Jonah 4:7; Acts 12:23.
WORMWOOD. Jer. 9:15; 23:15; Amos 5:7.
WORSE. Mat. 9:16; Mk. 2:21, the rent is made *w.*
12:45:27:64; Lu. 11:26, last state *w.* than the first.
Mk. 5:26, nothing bettered, but grew *w.*
John 5:14, lest a *w.*, thing come unto thee.
1 Cor. 11:17, not for the better, but for the *w.*
1 Tim. 5:8, he is *w.* than an infidel.
2 Tim. 3:13, shall wax *w.* and *w.*
2 Pet. 2:20, the latter end is *w.* with them.
See Jer. 7:26; 16:12; Dan. 1:10; John 2:10.
WORSHIP. Ps. 95:6, let us *w.* and bow down.
97:7, *w.* him, all ye gods.
99:5, *w.* at his footstool.
Isa. 27:13, shall *w.* the Lord in the holy mount.
Jer. 44:19, did we *w.* her without our men?
Zeph. 1:5, them that *w.* the host of heaven.

Mat. 4:9; Lu. 4:7, fall down and *w.* me.
15:9, in vain they do *w.* me.
John 4:20, our fathers *w.* in this mountain.
22, ye *w.* ye know not what.
12:20, Greeks came to *w.*
Acts 17:23, whom ye ignorantly *w.*
24:14, so *w.* I the God of my fathers.
Rom. 1:25, *w.* the creature more than the Creator.
1 Cor. 14:25, so falling down he will *w.* God.
See Col. 2:18; Heb 1:6; Rev. 4:10; 9:20.
WORTH. Job 24:25; Prov. 10:20; Ezek. 30:2.
WORTHY. Gen. 32:10, I am not *w.* of the least.
1 Sam. 26:16, ye are *w.* to die.
1 Kings 1:52, if he shew himself a *w.* man.
Mat. 3:11, whose shoes I am not *w.* to bear.
8:8; Lu. 7:6, I am not *w.* that thou shouldest come.
10:10, the workman is *w.* of his meat.
37, loveth father or mother more than me is not *w.* of me.
22:8, they which were bidden were not *w.*
Mk. 1:7; Lu. 3:16; John 1:27, not *w.* to unloose.
Lu. 3:8, fruits *w.* of repentance.
7:4, that he was *w.* for whom he should do this.
10:7; 1 Tim. 5:18, the labourer is *w.* of his hire.
12:48, things *w.* of stripes.
15:19, no more *w.*, to be called thy son.
20:35, *w.* to obtain that world.
Acts 24:2, very *w.* deeds are done.
Rom. 8:18, not *w.* to be compared with the glory.
Eph. 4:1; Col. 1:10; 1 Thess. 2:12, walk *w.*
Heb. 11:38, of whom the world was not *w.*
Jas. 2:7, that *w.* name.
Rev. 3:4, for they are *w.*
See Nah. 2:5; Rev. 4:11; 5:2; 16:6.
WOULD. Num. 22:29, I *w.* there were a sword.
Ps. 81:11, Israel *w.* none of me.
Prov. 1:25, ye *w.* none of my reproof.
30, they *w.* none of my counsel.
Dan. 5:19, whom he *w.* he slew.
Mat. 7:12; Lu. 6:31, whatsoever ye *w.* that men.
Mk. 3:13, and calleth unto him whom he *w.*
Rom. 7:15, what I *w.* that do I not.
1 Cor. 7:7, I *w.* that all men were even as I.
Rev. 3:15, I *w.* thou wert cold or hot.
See Num. 11:29; Acts 26:29; Ga. 5:17.
WOUND (*n.*). Ex. 21:25, give *w.* for *w.*
Job 34:6, my *w.* is incurable.
Ps. 147:3, he bindeth up their *w.*
Prov. 23:29, who hath *w.* without cause?
27:6, faithful are the *w.* of a friend.
Isa. 1:6, but *w.* and bruises.
Jer. 15:18, why is my *w.* incurable?
30:17, I will heal thee of thy *w.*
Zech. 13:6, what are these *w.* in thy hands?
Lu. 10:34, bound up his *w.*
See Prov. 6:33; 20:30; Hos. 5:13; Rev. 13:3.
WOUND (*v.*). Deut. 32:39, I *w.*, and I heal.
1 Kings 22:34; 2 Chron. 18:33, carry me out, for I am *w.*
Job 5:18, he *w.*, and his hands make whole.
Ps. 64:7, suddenly shall they be *w.*
109:22, my heart is *w.* within me.
Prov. 7:26, she hath cast down many *w.*
18:14, a *w.* spirit who can bear?
Isa. 53:5, he was *w.* for our transgressions.
Jer. 37:10, there remained but *w.* men.
See Gen. 4:23; Mk. 12:4; Lu. 10:30; Acts 19:16.
WRAP. Isa. 28:10; Mic. 7:3; John 20:7.
WRATH. Gen. 49:7, cursed by their *w.*
Deut. 32:27, were it not I feared the *w.* of the enemy.
Job 21:30; Prov. 11:4; Zeph. 1:15; Rom. 2:5; Rev. 6:17, the day of *w.*
36:18, because there is *w.*, beware.
Ps. 76:10, the *w.* of man shall praise thee.
90:7, by thy *w.* are we troubled.
Prov. 16:14, *w.* of a king is as messengers of death.
19:19, a man of great *w.* shall suffer.
27:3, a fool's *w.* is heavier.
4, *w.* is cruel, and anger outrageous.
Eccl. 5:17, much *w.* with his sickness.
Isa. 13:9, the day of the Lord cometh with *w.*
54:8, in a little *w.* I hid my face.
Nah. 1:2, he reserveth *w.* for his enemies.
Hab. 3:2, in *w.* remember mercy.
Mat. 3:7; Lu. 3:7, from the *w.* to come.
Rom. 2:5, *w.* against the day of *w.*
Eph. 6:4, provoke not your children to *w.*
1 Thess. 5:9, God hath not appointed us to *w.*
1 Tim. 2:8, lifting up holy hands, without *w.*
See Jas. 1:19; Rev. 6:16; 12:12; 14:8.
WRATHFUL. Ps. 69:24; Prov. 15:18.
WREST. Ex. 23:2; Deut. 16:19; Ps. 56:5; 2 Pet. 3:16.
WRESTLE. Gen. 32:24; Eph. 6:12.
WRETCHED. Num. 11:15; Rom. 7:24; Rev. 3:17.
WRING. Judg. 6:38; Ps. 75:8; Prov. 30:33.
WRINKLE. Job 16:8; Eph. 5:27.
WRITE. Prov. 3:3; 7:3, *w.* on table of thy heart.
Isa. 10:1, *w.* grievousness which they have prescribed.
19, few, that a child may *w.* them.
Jer. 22:30, *w.* ye this man childless.
31:33; Heb. 8:10, I will *w.* it in their hearts.
Hab. 2:2, *w.* the vision, make it plain.
See Job 13:26; Ps. 87:6; Rev. 3:12.
WRITING. Ex. 32:16; John 5:47; Col. 2:14.
WRITTEN. Job 19:23, Oh that my words were *w.*
Ps. 69:28, let them not be *w.* with the righteous.
Ezek. 2:10, roll was *w.* within and without.
Lu. 10:20, because your names are *w.* in heaven.
John 19:22, what I have *w.* I have *w.*
1 Cor. 10:11, *w.* for our admonition.
2 Cor. 3:2, ye are our epistle *w.* in our hearts.
See Isa. 4:3; Jer. 17:1; Rev. 2:17; 13:8.
WRONG. Ex. 2:13, to him that did the *w.*
1 Chron. 12:17, there is no *w.* in mine hands.
Job 19:7, I cry out of *w.* but am not heard.
Jer. 22:3, do no *w.*
Mat. 20:13, friend, I do thee no *w.*
1 Cor. 6:7, why do ye not rather take *w.*?
2 Cor. 12:13, forgive me this *w.*
Col. 3:25, he that doeth *w.* shall receive.
Philem. 18, if he hath *w.* thee.
See Prov. 8:36; Acts 25:10; 2 Cor. 7:2.
WRONGFULLY. Job 21:27; Ezek. 22:29; 1 Pet. 2:19.
WROTE. Dan. 5:5; John 8:6; 19:19; 2 John 5.
WROTH. Gen. 4:6, why art thou *w.*?
Deut. 1:34; 3:26; 9:19; 2 Sam. 22:8; 2 Chron. 28. 9; Ps. 18:7; 78:21, heard your words, and was *w.*
2 Kings 5:11, but Naaman was *w.*, and went away.
Ps. 80:38, thou hast been *w.* with thine anointed.
Isa. 47:6, I was *w.* with my people.
54:9, I have sworn I would not be *w.*
57:16, neither will I be always *w.*
64:9, be not *w.* very sore.
Mat. 18:34, his lord was *w.*, and delivered.
See Num. 16:22; Isa. 28:21; Mat. 2:16.
WROUGHT. Num. 23:23, what hath God *w.*!
1 Sam. 6:6, when God had *w.* wonderfully.
14:45, Jonathan hath *w.* with God this day.
Neh. 4:17, with one of his hands *w.* in the work.
6:16, this work was *w.* of our God.
Job 12:9, the hand of the Lord hath *w.* this.
36:23, who can say, thou hast *w.* iniquity?
Ps. 31:19, hast *w.* for them that trust in thee.
68:28, strengthen that which thou hast *w.* for us.
139:15, curiously *w.* in lowest parts of the earth.
Eccl. 2:11, I looked on all my hands had *w.*
Isa. 26:12, thou also hast *w.* all our works in us.
41:4, who hath *w.* and done it?
Jer. 18:3, he *w.* a work on the wheels.
Ezek. 20:9, I *w.* for my name's sake.
Dan. 4:2, the wonders God hath *w.* toward me.
Mat. 20:12, these last have *w.* but one hour.
26:10; Mk. 14:6, she hath *w.* a good work on me.
John 3:21, manifest that they are *w.* in God.
Acts 15:12, what wonders God had *w.*

Acts 18:3, he abode with them, and *w.*
19:11, *w.* special miracles by hands of Paul.
Rom. 7:8, *w.* in me all manner of concupiscence.
15:18, things which Christ hath not *w.*
2 Cor. 5:5, he that hath *w.* us for the selfsame thing.
7:11, what carefulness it *w.* in you.
12:12, the signs of an apostle were *w.*
Gal. 2:8, he that *w.* effectually in Peter.
Eph. 1:20, which he *w.* in Christ.
2 Thess. 3:8, but we *w.* with labour.
Heb. 11:33, through faith *w.* righteousness.
Jas. 2:22, faith *w.* with his works.
1 Pet. 4:3, to have *w.* the will of the Gentiles.
2 John 8, lose not those things we have *w.*
Rev. 19:20, the false prophet that *w.* miracles.
See Ex. 36:4; 2 Sam. 18:13; 1 Kings 16:25.
WRUNG. Lev. 1:15; Ps. 73:10; Isa. 51:17.

Y

YARN. 1 Kings 10:28; 2 Chron. 1:16.
YE. 1 Cor. 6:11; 2 Cor. 3:2; Gal. 6:1.
YEA. Mat. 5:37; Jas. 5:12, let your communication be *y.*, *y.*
2 Cor. 1:17, there should be *y.*, *y.*, and nay, nay.
See 2 Cor. 1:18; Phil. 3:8; 2 Tim. 3:12.
YEAR. Gen. 1:14, for seasons, days and *y.*
47:9, few and evil have they *y.* of my life been.
Ex. 13:10, keep this ordinance from *y.* to *y.*
23:29, I will not drive them out in one *y.*
Lev. 16:34, make atonement once a *y.*
25:5, it is a *y.* of rest.
Num. 14:34, each day for a *y.* shall ye bear.
Deut. 14:22, thou shalt tithe the increase *y.* by *y.*
15:9, the *y.* of release is a hand.
26:12, the third *y.*, which is the *y.* of tithing.
32:7, consider the *y.* of many generations.
Judg. 11:40, to lament four days in a *y.*
1 Sam. 2:19, brought a coat from *y.* to *y.*
7:16, went from *y.* to *y.* in circuit.
2 Sam. 14:26, every *y.* he polled it.
1 Kings 17:1, there shall not be dew nor rain these *y.*
2 Chron. 14:6, the land had rest, no war in those *y.*
Job 10:5, are thy *y.* as man's days?
15:20, the number of *y.* is hidden.
16:22, when a few *y.* are come.
32:7, multitude of *y.* should teach wisdom.
36:11, they shall spend their *y.* in pleasures.
26, nor can the number of his *y.* be searched out.
Ps. 31:10, my *y.* are spent with sighing.
61:6, prolong his *y.* as many generations.
65:11, thou crownest the *y.* with thy goodness.
77:5, the *y.* of ancient times.
10, I will remember the *y.* of the right hand.
78:33, their *y.* did he consume in trouble.
90:4, a thousand *y.* in thy sight.
9, we spend our *y.* as a tale that is told.
10, the days of our *y.* are threescore and ten.
102:24, they *y.* are throughout all generations.
27, thy *y.* shall have no end.
Prov. 4:10, the *y.* of thy life shall be many.
5:9, lest thou give thy *y.* to the cruel.
10:27, the *y.* of the wicked shall be shortened.
Eccl. 12:1, nor the *y.* draw nigh.
Isa. 21:16, according to the *y.* of an hireling.
29:1, add ye *y.* to *y.*
38:15, go softly all my *y.*
61:2; Lu. 4:10, the acceptable *y.* of the Lord.
63:4, the *y.* of my redeemed is come.
Jer. 11:23; 23:12; 48:44, the *y.* of their visitation.
17:8, shall not be careful in *y.* of drought.
28:16, this *y.* thou shalt die.
51:46, a rumour shall come in one *y.*
Ezek. 4:5, I have laid on thee the *y.* of their iniquity.
22:4, thou art come even unto thy *y.*
38:8, in latter *y.* thou shalt come.
46:17, it shall be his to the *y.* of liberty.
Dan. 11:6, in the end of *y.* they shall join.
Joel 2:2, to the *y.* of many generations.
Mic. 6:6, shall I come with calves of a *y.* old?
Hab. 3:2, revive thy work in the midst of the *y.*
Mal. 3:4, the offering be pleasant, as in former *y.*
Lu. 13:8, let it alone this *y.* also.
Gal. 4:10, ye observe days and *y.*
Rev. 20:2, Satan bound for a thousand *y.*
See Zech. 14:16; Jas. 4:13; Rev. 9:15.
YEARLY. 1 Sam. 1:3; 20:6; Esth. 9:21.
YEARN. Gen. 43:30; 1 Kings 3:26.
YELL. Jer. 2:15; 51:38.
YESTERDAY. Job 8:9; Ps. 90:4; Heb. 13:8.
YET. Gen. 40:23, *y.* did not the butler remember.
Ex. 10:7, knowest thou not *y.*?
Deut. 9:29, *y.* they are thy people.
12:9, ye are not as *y.* come.
Judg. 7:4, the people are *y.* too many.
1 Kings 19:18, *y.* I have left me.
2 Kings 13:23, nor cast them from his presence as *y.*
Ezra 3:6, the foundation was not *y.* laid.
Job 1:16, while he was *y.* speaking.
13 15, though he slay me, *y.* will I trust in him.
29:5, when the Almighty was *y.* with me.
Ps. 2:6, *y.* have I set my king.
Eccl. 4:3, he which hath not *y.* been.
Isa. 28:4, while it is *y.* in his hand.
49:15, *y.* will I not forget.
Jer. 2:9, I will *y.* plead with you.
23:21, *y.* they ran.
Ezek. 11:16, *y.* will I be to them.
36:37, I will *y.* for this be enquired of.
Dan. 11:35, it is *y.* for a time appointed.
Hos. 7:9, *y.* he knoweth not.
Amos 6:10, is there *y.* any with thee?
Jonah 3:4, *y.* forty days.
Hab. 3:18, *y.* I will rejoice.
Mat. 15:17, do not ye *y.* understand?
19:20, what lack I *y.*?
24:6; Mk. 13:7, the end is not *y.*
Mk. 11:13, the time of figs was not *y.*
Lu. 24:44, while I was *y.* with you.
John 2:4; 7:6; 8:20, hour is not *y.* come.
11:25, though dead, *y.* shall he live.
Rom. 5:6, *y.* without strength.
8:24, why doth he *y.* hope for?
1 Cor. 3:15, *y.* so as by fire.
15:17, ye are *y.* in your sins.
Gal. 2:20, *y.* not I, but Christ.
Heb. 4:15, *y.* without sin.
1 John 3:2, it doth not *y.* appear.
See Acts 8:16; Rom. 9:19; 1 Cor. 3:3.
YIELD. Gen. 4:12, not henceforth *y.* strength.
Lev. 19:25, that it may *y.* the increase.
26:4, the land shall *y.* her increase.
Num. 17:8, the rod *y.* almonds.
2 Chron. 30:8, *y.* yourselves to the Lord.
Neh. 9:37, it *y.* much increase to the kings.
Ps. 67:6, the earth *y.* her increase.
107:37, plant vineyards, which may *y.* fruits.
Prov. 7:21, she caused him to *y.*
Eccl. 10:4, *y.* pacifieth great offences.
Hos. 8:7, if it *y.*, the strangers shall swallow it up.
Joel 2:22, the fig tree and vine do *y.* their strength.
Hab. 3:17, though fields shall *y.* no meat.
Mat. 27:50, cried again, and *y.* up the ghost.
Acts 23:21, do not thou *y.* to them.
Rom. 6:13, neither *y.* ye your members, but *y.* yourselves to God.
16, to whom ye *y.* yourselves servants.
Heb. 12:11, *y.* the peaceable fruits of righteousness.
See Gen. 1:29; Isa. 5:10; Dan. 3:28.
YOKE. Gen. 27:40, thou shalt break his *y.*
Lev. 26:13, I have broken the bands of your *y.*
Num. 19:2; 1 Sam. 6:7, on which never came *y.*
Deut. 28:48, he shall put a *y.* on thy neck.
1 Kings 12:4, thy father made our *y.* grievous.
Isa. 9:4; 10:27; 14:25, thou hast broken the *y.* of his burden.
58:6, that ye break every *y.*

Jer. 2:20, of old time I have broken thy *y*.
27:2; 28:13, make thee bonds and *y*.
31:18, as a bullock unaccustomed to the *y*.
Lam. 3:27, it is good to bear the *y*. in youth.
Mat. 11:29, take my *y*. upon you.
30, for my *y*. is easy.
Acts 15:10, to put a *y*. upon the neck of the disciples.
2 Cor. 6:14, not unequally *y*. with unbelievers.
Gal. 5:1, entangled with the *y*. of bondage.
Phil. 4:3, I entreat thee also, true *y*-fellow.
1 Tim. 6:1, as many servants as are under the *y*.
See Job 1:3; 42:12; Lam. 1:14; Lu. 14:19.
YONDER. Gen. 22:5; Num. 23:15; Mat. 17:20.
YOU. Gen. 48:21, God shall be with *y*.
Ruth 2:4, the Lord be with *y*.
1 Chron. 22:18, is not the Lord with *y*.?
2 Chron. 15:2, the Lord is with *y*., while ye be with him.
Jer. 19:6, cannot I do with *y*.
42:11; Hag. 1:13; 2:4, for I am with *y*.
Zech. 8:23, we will go with *y*., God is with *y*.
Mat. 7:12; Lu. 6:21, that men should do to *y*.
28:20, I am with *y*. alway.
Lu. 10:16, he that heareth *y*. heareth me.
13:28, and *y*. yourselves thrust out.
Acts 13:46, seeing ye put it from *y*.
Rom. 16:20; 1 Cor. 16:23; Phil. 4:23; Col. 4:18; 1 Thess. 5:28; 2 Thess. 3:18; 2 Tim. 4:15; Tit. 3:15; Heb. 13:25; 2 John 3; Rev. 22:21, grace be with *y*.
1 Cor. 6:11, such were some of *y*.
2 Cor. 12:14, I seek not yours, but *y*.
Eph. 2:1; Col. 2:13, *y*. hath he quickened.
Col. 1:27, Christ in *y*.
4:9, a brother, who is one of *y*.
1 Thess. 5:12, know them that are over *y*.
1 John 4:4, greater is he that is in *y*.
See Hag. 1:4; Mal. 2:1; 2 Cor. 8:13; Phil. 3:1; 1 Pet. 2:7.
YOUNG. Ex. 23:26, there shall nothing cast their *y*.
Lev. 22:28, ye shall not kill it and her *y*. in one day.
Deut. 22:6, thou shalt not take the dam with the *y*.
28:50, which will not show favour to the *y*.
57, her eyes shall be evil toward her *y*. one.
32:11, as an eagle fluttereth over her *y*.
1 Chron. 22:5; 29:1, Solomon my son is *y*.
2 Chron. 13:7, when Rehoboam was *y*. and tender.
34:3, while he was yet *y*., he began to seek God.
Job 38:41, when his *y*. ones cry to God, they wander.
39:16, the ostrich is hardened against her *y*.
Ps. 37:25, I have been *y*., and now am old.
78:71, from following ewes great with *y*.
84:3, a nest where she may lay her *y*.
147:9, he giveth food to the *y*. ravens which cry.
Prov. 30:17, the *y*. eagles shall eat it.
Cant. 2:9; 8:14, my beloved is like a *y*. hart.
Isa. 11:7, their *y*. shall lie down together.
40:11, and gently lead those that are with *y*.
Jer. 31:12, flow together for *y*. of the flock.
Ezek. 17:4, cropped off his *y*. twigs.
John 21:18, when *y*. thou girdedst thyself.
Tit. 2:4, teach the *y*. women to be sober.
See Gen. 33:13; Isa. 30:6; Mk. 7:25; John 12:14.
YOUNGER. Gen. 25:23, the elder shall serve the *y*.
Job 30:1, they that are *y*. have me in derision.
Lu. 22:26, he that is greatest, let him be as the *y*.
1 Tim. 5:1, intreat the *y*. man as brethren.
1 Pet. 5:5, ye *y*., submit yourselves to the elder
See Gen. 29:18; Lu. 15:12; 1 Tim. 5:2, 11.
YOUNGEST. Gen. 42:13; Josh. 6:26; 1 Kings 16:34.
YOURS. 2 Chron. 20:15; Lu. 6:20; 1 Cor. 3:21.
YOUTH. Gen. 8:21, imagination is evil from *y*.
46:34, about cattle from our *y*. till now.
1 Sam. 17:33, he a man of war from his *y*.
55, whose son is this *y*.?
2 Sam. 19:7, evil that befell thee from thy *y*.
1 Kings 18:12, I fear the Lord from my *y*.
Job 13:26, to possess the iniquities of my *y*.
20:11, his bones are full of the sin of his *y*.
29:4, as in days of my *y*.
30:12, on my right hand rise the *y*.
33:25, he shall return to the days of his *y*.
36:14, hypocrites die in *y*.
Ps. 25:7, remember not the sins of my *y*.
71:5, thou art my trust from my *y*.
17, thou hast taught me from my *y*.
88:15, ready to die from my *y*. up.
89:45, the days of his *y*. hast thou shortened.
103:5, thy *y*. is renewed like the eagle's.
110:3, the dew of thy *y*.
127:4, the children of thy *y*.
129:1, they have afflicted me from my *y*.
144:12, as plants grown up in *y*.
Prov. 2:17, forsaketh the guide of her *y*.
5:18, rejoice with the wife of thy *y*.
Eccl. 11:9, rejoice, young man, in thy *y*.
10, childhood and *y*. are vanity.
12:1, remember now thy Creator in days of *y*.
Isa. 47:12, wherein thou hast laboured from thy *y*.
54:4, forget the shame of thy *y*.
Jer. 2:2, the kindness of thy *y*.
3:4, thou art the guide of my *y*.
22:21, this hath been thy manner from thy *y*.
31:19, bear the reproach of my *y*.
32:30, have done evil before me from their *y*.
48:11, hath been at ease from his *y*.
Lam. 3:27, it is good that he bear the yoke in his *y*.
Ezek. 4:14, soul not polluted from *y*.
16:22, thou hast not remembered the days of thy *y*.
Hos. 2:15, she shall sing as in the days of her *y*.
Joel 1:8, lament for husband of her *y*.
Zech. 13:5, man taught me to keep cattle from my *y*.
Mat. 19:20; Mk. 10:20; Lu. 18:21, have kept from my *y*.
Acts 26:4, my manner of life from my *y*.
1 Tim. 4:12, let no man despise thy *y*.
See Prov. 7:7; Isa. 40:30; Jer. 3:24, 25.
YOUTHFUL. 2 Tim. 2:22, flee *y*. lusts.

Z

ZEAL. 2 Sam. 21:2, sought to slay them in his *z*.
2 Kings 10:16, come and see my *z*. for the Lord.
Ps. 69:9; John 2:17, the *z*. of thine house.
119:139, my *z*. hath consumed me.
Isa. 9:7, the *z*. of the Lord will perform this.
59:17, clad with *z*. as a cloak.
63:15, where is thy *z*.?
Ezek. 5:13, I have spoken it in my *z*.
Rom. 10:2, they have a *z*. of God.
2 Cor. 9:2, your *z*. hath provoked many.
Phil. 3:6, concerning *z*. persecuting the church.
Col. 4:13, he hath a great *z*. for you.
See 2 Kings 19:31; Isa. 37:32; 2 Cor. 7:11.
ZEALOUS. Num. 25:11, he was *z*. for my sake.
Acts 21:20, they are all *z*. of the law.
1 Cor. 14:12, as ye are *z*. of spiritual gifts.
Tit. 2:14, *z*. of good works.
Rev. 3:19, be *z*. therefore, and repent.
See Num. 25:13; Acts 22:3; Gal. 1:14.
ZEALOUSLY. Gal. 4:18, *z*. affected.

THE NEW OXFORD BIBLE MAPS

1 Jerusalem in Old Testament times
2 Background of the Exodus
3 Israel in Canaan: Joshua to Samuel and Saul
4 The United Monarchy
5 The Near East in the time of the Assyrian Empire
6 Central Palestine in Old Testament times
7 Palestine under the Herods
8 The Background of the New Testament: Rome and the East (including Paul's Journeys)
9 Jerusalem in New Testament times

INDEX TO MAPS

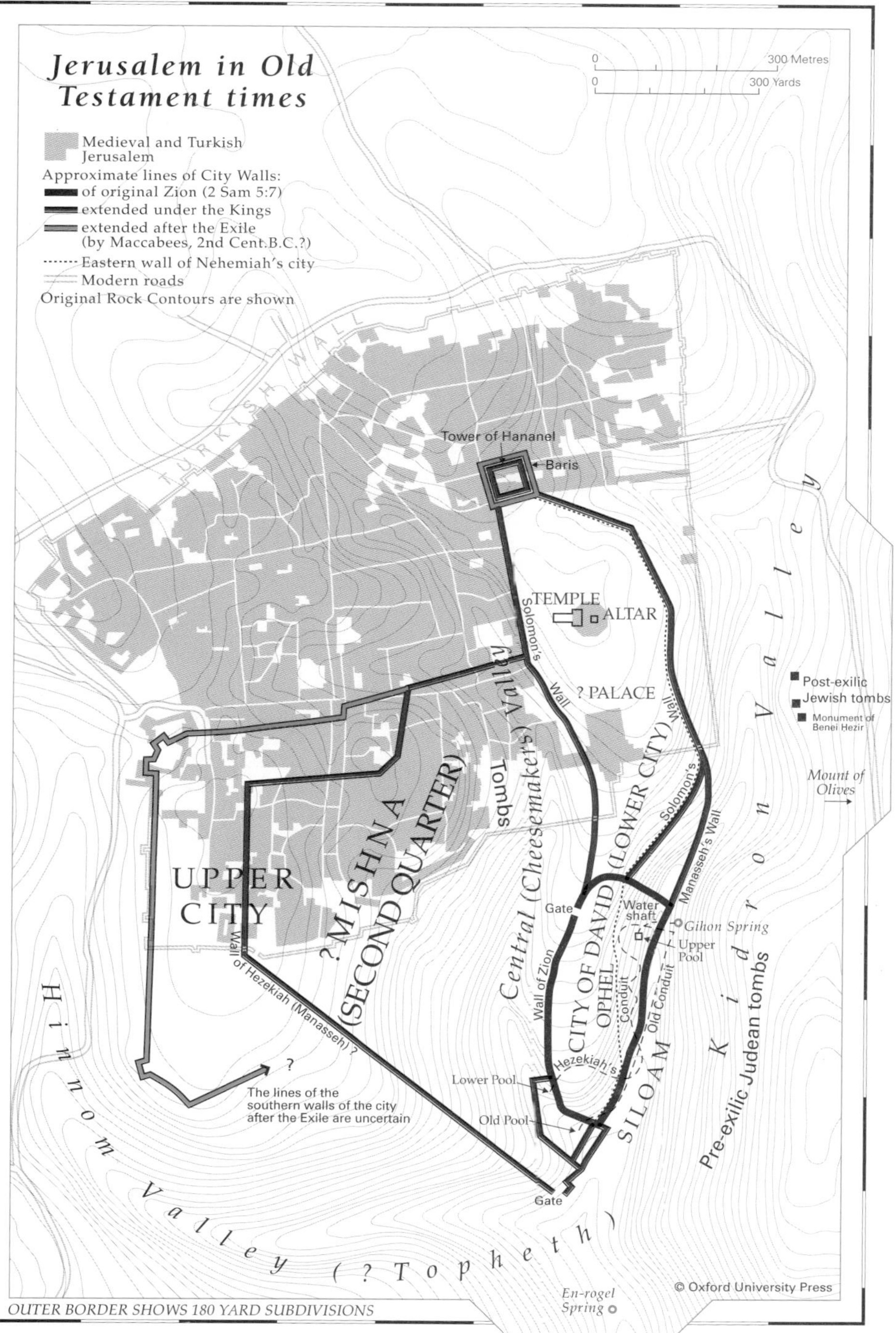
Jerusalem in Old Testament times
Medieval and Turkish Jerusalem
Approximate lines of City Walls:
of original Zion (2 Sam 5:7)
extended under the Kings
extended after the Exile (by Maccabees, 2nd Cent. B.C.?)
Eastern wall of Nehemiah's city
Modern roads
Original Rock Contours are shown
0 300 Metres
0 300 Yards
TURKISH WALL
Tower of Hananel
Baris
TEMPLE
ALTAR
Solomon's Wall
? PALACE
Post-exilic Jewish tombs
Monument of Benei Hezir
Mount of Olives
Central (Cheesemaker's) Valley
Tombs
? MISHNA (SECOND QUARTER)
UPPER CITY
Wall of Hezekiah (Manasseh) ?
CITY OF DAVID (LOWER CITY)
OPHEL
Wall
Solomon's
Manasseh's Wall
Gate
Water shaft
Gihon Spring
Upper Pool
Wall of Zion
Conduit
Old Conduit
Hezekiah's
Lower Pool
Old Pool
SILOAM
Kidron Valley
Pre-exilic Judean tombs
?
The lines of the southern walls of the city after the Exile are uncertain
Hinnom Valley (? Topheth)
Gate
En-rogel Spring
© Oxford University Press
OUTER BORDER SHOWS 180 YARD SUBDIVISIONS

NOBM 11N SW Press

MAP 2

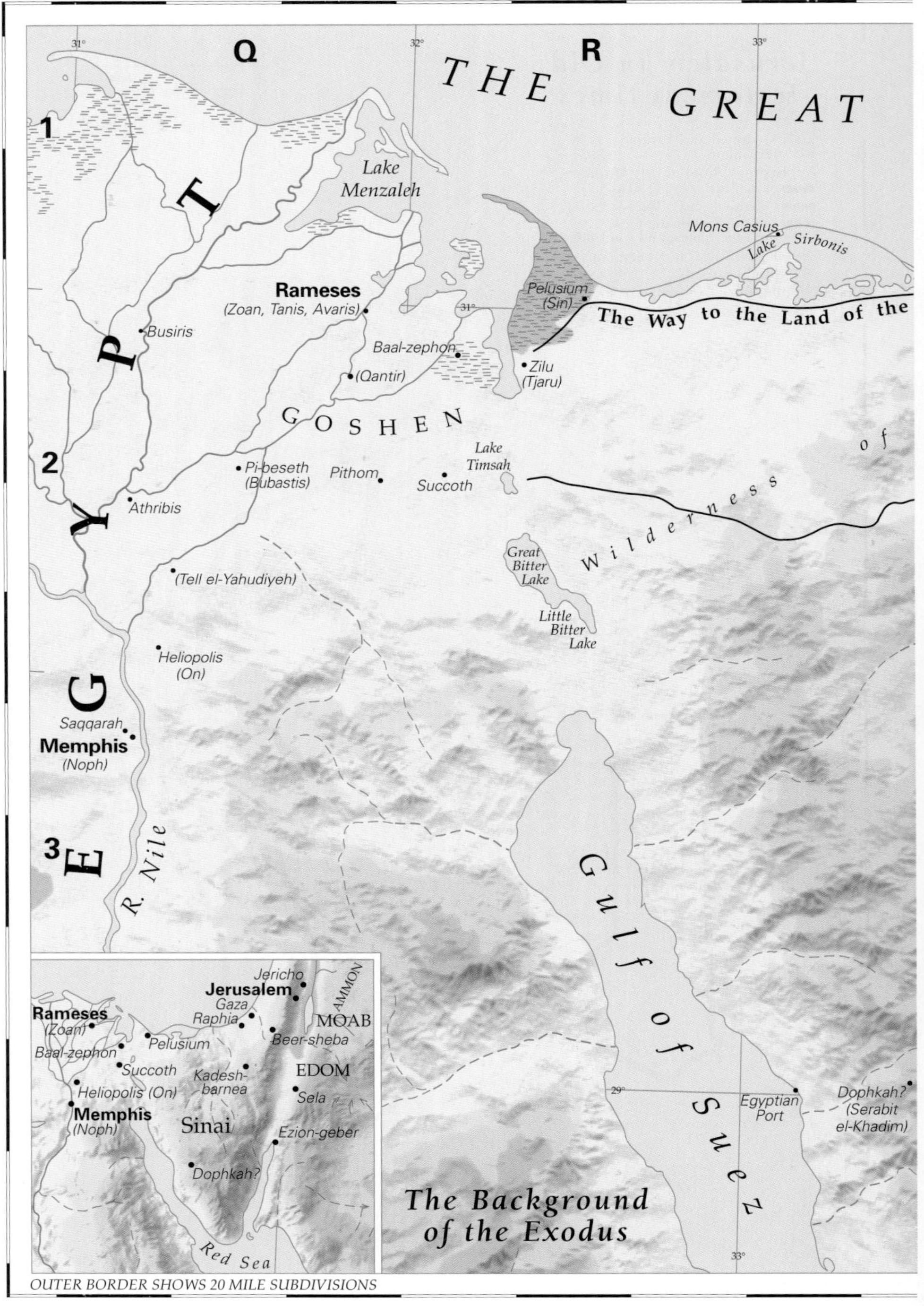

31°
Q
32°
R
33°
THE GREAT
1
2
3
EGYPT
Lake Menzaleh
Mons Casius
Lake Sirbonis
Rameses
(Zoan, Tanis, Avaris)
Pelusium
(Sin)
31°
The Way to the Land of the
Busiris
Baal-zephon
Zilu
(Tjaru)
(Qantir)
GOSHEN
Lake Timsah
Pi-beseth
(Bubastis)
Pithom
Succoth
Wilderness of
Athribis
Great Bitter Lake
(Tell el-Yahudiyeh)
Little Bitter Lake
Heliopolis
(On)
Saqqarah
Memphis
(Noph)
R. Nile
Gulf of Suez
Jericho
Jerusalem
AMMON
Gaza
Raphia
MOAB
Rameses
(Zoan)
Pelusium
Beer-sheba
Baal-zephon
Succoth
Kadesh-barnea
EDOM
Heliopolis (On)
Sela
Memphis
(Noph)
Sinai
Ezion-geber
Dophkah?
Red Sea
29°
Egyptian Port
Dophkah?
(Serabit el-Khadim)
33°
The Background of the Exodus

OUTER BORDER SHOWS 20 MILE SUBDIVISIONS

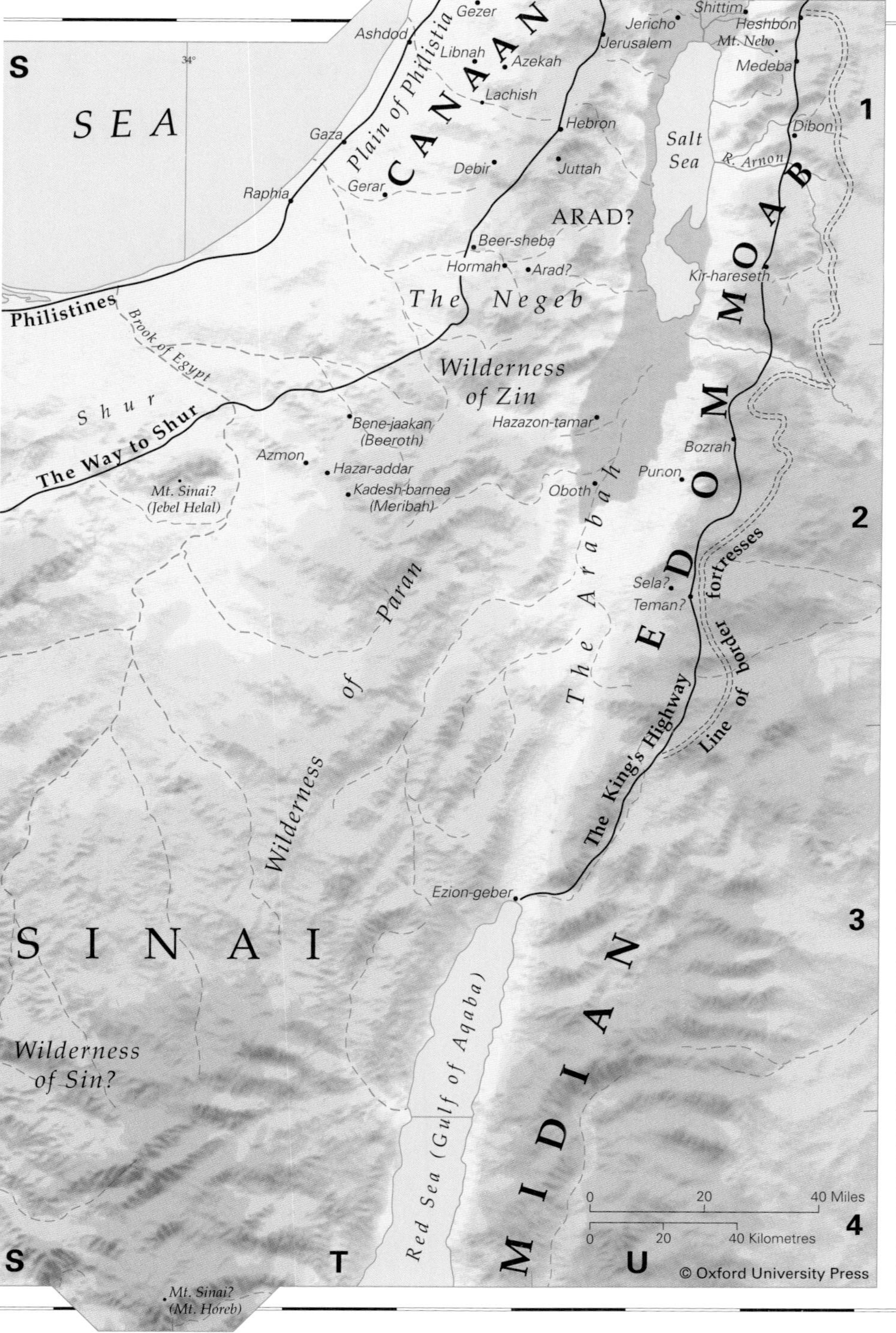

S
SEA
34°
Gezer
Ashdod
Plain of Philistia
CANAAN
Libnah
Azekah
Lachish
Jerusalem
Jericho
Shittim
Heshbon
Mt. Nebo
Medeba
Hebron
Gaza
Salt Sea
Dibon
R. Arnon
Debir
Juttah
Gerar
Raphia
ARAD?
Beer-sheba
Hormah
Arad?
Kir-hareseth
MOAB
Philistines
Brook of Egypt
The Negeb
Wilderness of Zin
Shur
The Way to Shur
Bene-jaakan (Beeroth)
Hazazon-tamar
Azmon
Hazar-addar
Kadesh-barnea (Meribah)
Bozrah
Punon
Oboth
Mt. Sinai? (Jebel Helal)
The Arabah
EDOM
Line of border fortresses
Sela?
Teman?
Wilderness of Paran
The King's Highway
Ezion-geber
SINAI
MIDIAN
Red Sea (Gulf of Aqaba)
Wilderness of Sin?
1
2
3
4
0 20 40 Miles
0 20 40 Kilometres
S
T
U
Mt. Sinai? (Mt. Horeb)

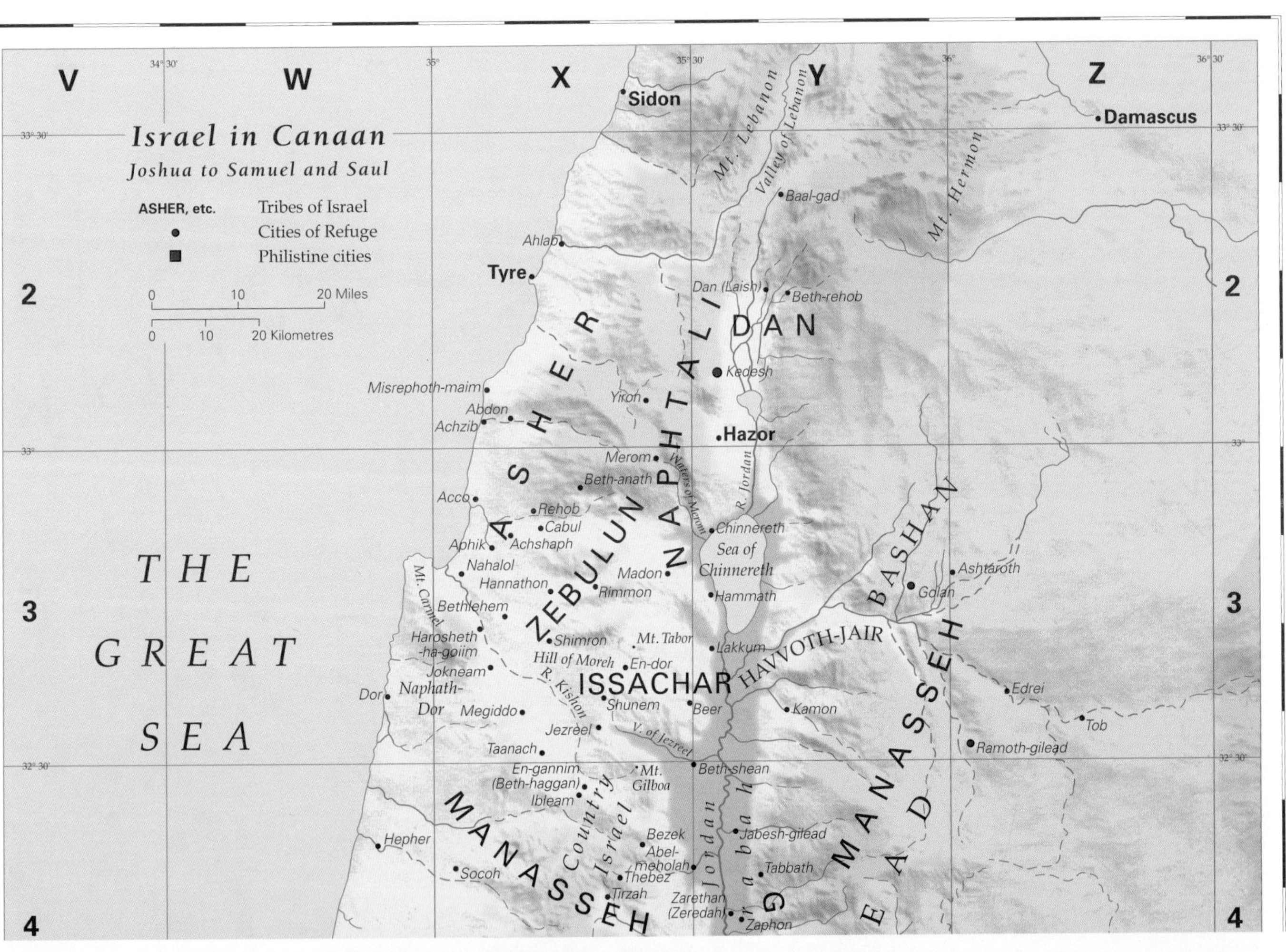
Israel in Canaan
Joshua to Samuel and Saul
ASHER, etc. Tribes of Israel
Cities of Refuge
Philistine cities
0 10 20 Miles
0 10 20 Kilometres
V
W
X
Y
Z
2
3
4
THE GREAT SEA
Sidon
Damascus
Mt. Lebanon
Valley of Lebanon
Mt. Hermon
Baal-gad
Ahlab
Tyre
Dan (Laish)
Beth-rehob
DAN
Kedesh
Misrephoth-maim
Yiron
Abdon
Achzib
Hazor
ASHER
NAPHTALI
ZEBULUN
ISSACHAR
BASHAN
HAVVOTH-JAIR
MANASSEH
GAD
Merom
Waters of Merom
R. Jordan
Beth-anath
Acco
Rehob
Cabul
Chinnereth
Sea of Chinnereth
Aphik
Achshaph
Nahalol
Hannathon
Madon
Rimmon
Hammath
Ashtaroth
Golan
Mt. Carmel
Bethlehem
Harosheth-ha-goiim
Shimron
Mt. Tabor
Lakkum
Hill of Moreh
En-dor
Jokneam
R. Kishon
Dor
Naphath-Dor
Shunem
Beer
Kamon
Edrei
Tob
Megiddo
Jezreel
V. of Jezreel
Taanach
Ramoth-gilead
En-gannim (Beth-haggan)
Mt. Gilboa
Beth-shean
Ibleam
Country Israel
Arabah
Jordan
Hepher
Bezek
Jabesh-gilead
Abel-meholah
Thebez
Tabbath
Socoh
Tirzah
Zarethan (Zeredah)
Zaphon
34° 30'
35°
35° 30'
36°
36° 30'
33° 30'
33°
32° 30'

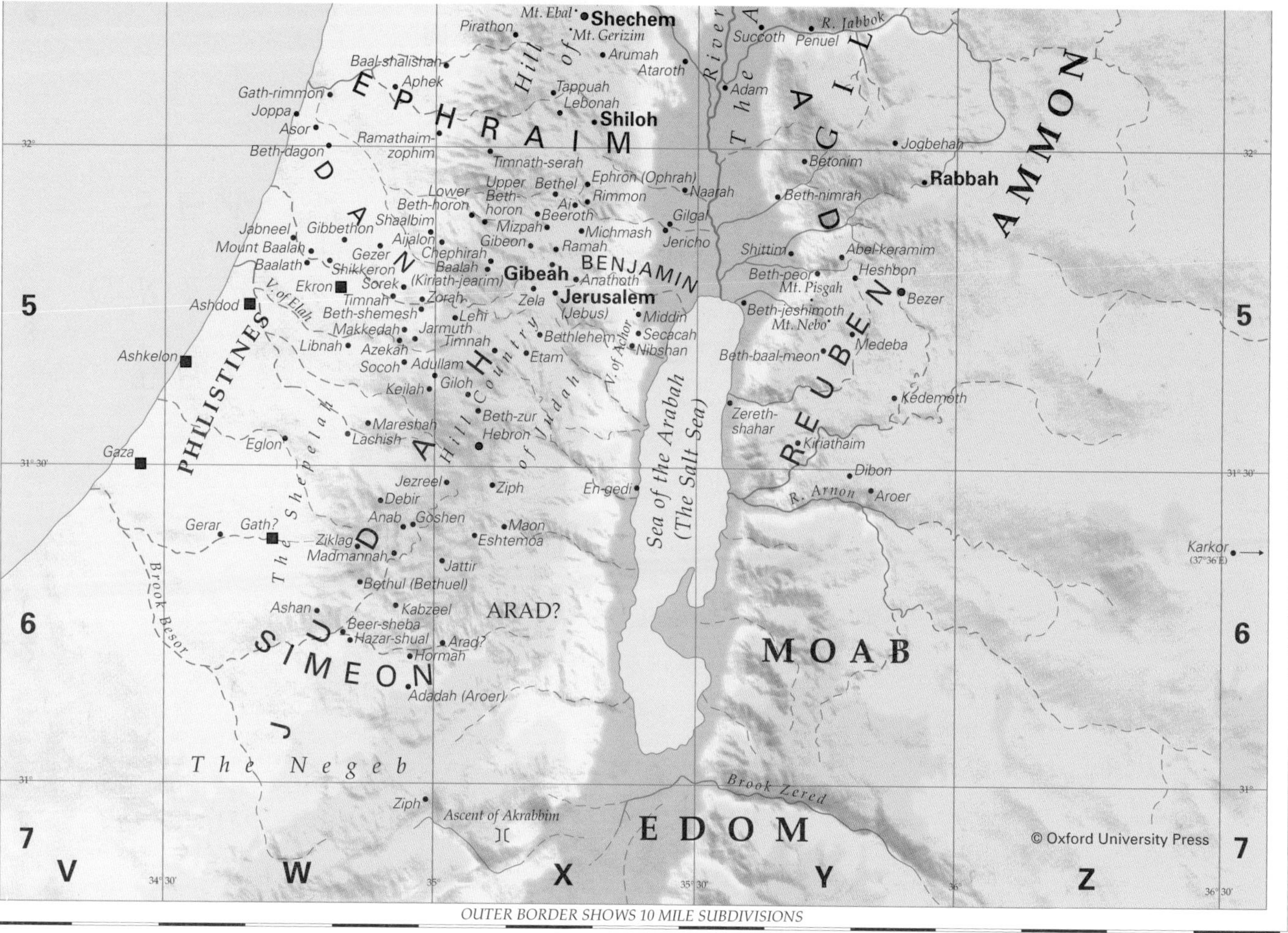
AMMON
GILEAD
EPHRAIM
DAN
BENJAMIN
JUDAH
REUBEN
SIMEON
MOAB
EDOM
PHILISTINES
ARAD?
The River Jordan
Hill of Ephraim
Hill Country of Judah
The Shephelah
The Negeb
Sea of the Arabah (The Salt Sea)
R. Jabbok
R. Arnon
Brook Zered
Brook Besor
V. of Elah
V. of Achor
Ascent of Akrabbim
Mt. Ebal
Shechem
Mt. Gerizim
Pirathon
Arumah
Ataroth
Succoth
Penuel
Adam
Baal-shalishah
Aphek
Gath-rimmon
Joppa
Asor
Beth-dagon
Ramathaim-zophim
Tappuah
Lebonah
Shiloh
Timnath-serah
Jogbehah
Betonim
Rabbah
Upper Beth-horon
Lower Beth-horon
Bethel
Ai
Ephron (Ophrah)
Rimmon
Naarah
Beth-nimrah
Beeroth
Mizpah
Michmash
Gilgal
Jericho
Gibeon
Ramah
Shittim
Abel-keramim
Jabneel
Gibbethon
Shaalbim
Aijalon
Mount Baalah
Gezer
Chephirah
Baalath
Shikkeron
Baalah (Kiriath-jearim)
Gibeah
Anathoth
Beth-peor
Mt. Pisgah
Heshbon
Ekron
Sorek
Zorah
Zela
Jerusalem (Jebus)
Bezer
Ashdod
Timnah
Beth-shemesh
Lehi
Middin
Beth-jeshimoth
Mt. Nebo
Makkedah
Jarmuth
Secacah
Nibshan
Libnah
Azekah
Bethlehem
Etam
Medeba
Beth-baal-meon
Ashkelon
Socoh
Adullam
Keilah
Giloh
Kedemoth
Beth-zur
Zereth-shahar
Mareshah
Lachish
Hebron
Eglon
Kiriathaim
Gaza
Dibon
Jezreel
Ziph
En-gedi
Aroer
Debir
Anab
Goshen
Maon
Gerar
Gath?
Ziklag
Eshtemoa
Madmannah
Karkor (37°36'E)
Jattir
Bethul (Bethuel)
Ashan
Kabzeel
Beer-sheba
Hazar-shual
Arad?
Hormah
Adadah (Aroer)
Ziph
32°
31°30'
31°
34°30'
35°
35°30'
36°
36°30'
5
6
7
V
W
X
Y
Z
© Oxford University Press
OUTER BORDER SHOWS 10 MILE SUBDIVISIONS

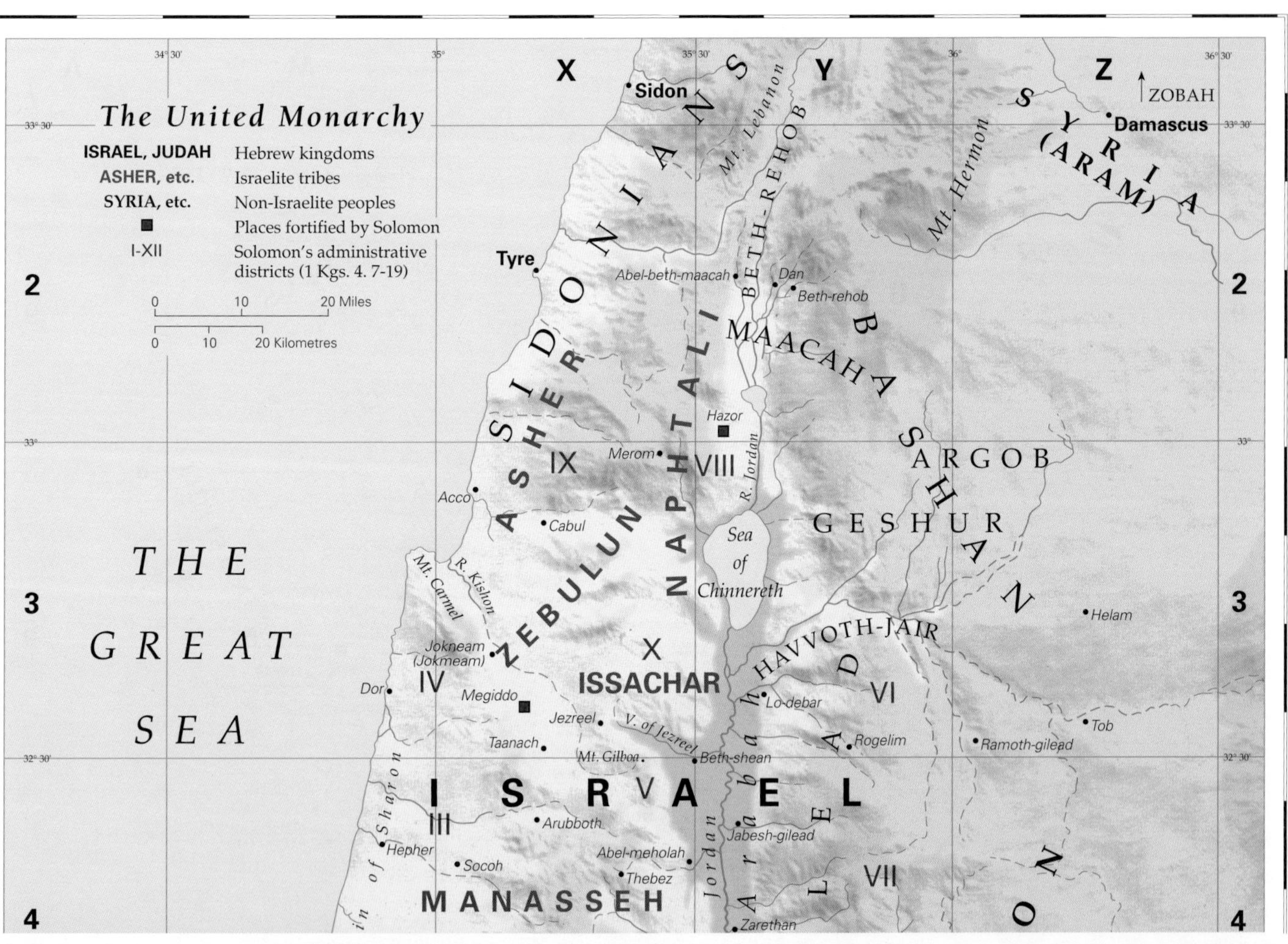
The United Monarchy
ISRAEL, JUDAH Hebrew kingdoms
ASHER, etc. Israelite tribes
SYRIA, etc. Non-Israelite peoples
Places fortified by Solomon
I-XII Solomon's administrative districts (1 Kgs. 4. 7-19)
0 10 20 Miles
0 10 20 Kilometres
THE GREAT SEA
SIDONIANS
SYRIA (ARAM)
ZOBAH
Damascus
Sidon
Tyre
Mt. Lebanon
Mt. Hermon
BETH-REHOB
Abel-beth-maacah
Dan
Beth-rehob
MAACAH
BASHAN
ASHER
NAPHTALI
ZEBULUN
ISSACHAR
Hazor
Merom
R. Jordan
Sea of Chinnereth
ARGOB
GESHUR
HAVVOTH-JAIR
GILEAD
Helam
Tob
Ramoth-gilead
Acco
Cabul
Mt. Carmel
R. Kishon
Jokneam (Jokmeam)
Dor
Megiddo
Jezreel
V. of Jezreel
Taanach
Mt. Gilboa
Beth-shean
Lo-debar
Rogelim
ISRAEL
Arubboth
Plain of Sharon
Hepher
Socoh
Abel-meholah
Thebez
Jabesh-gilead
Zarethan
Arabah
Jordan
MANASSEH
AMMON
I
III
IV
V
VI
VII
VIII
IX
X
X
Y
Z
2
3
4

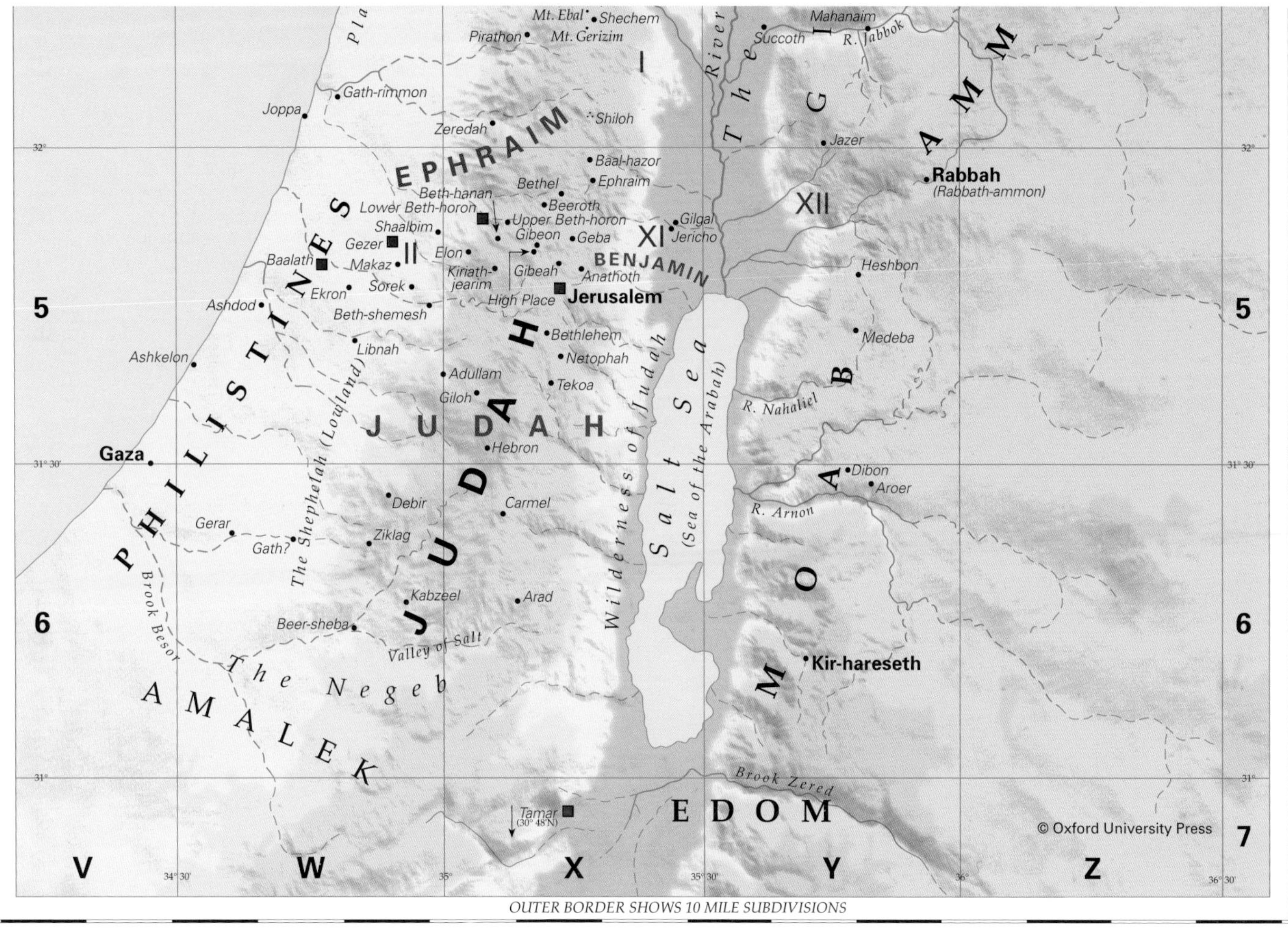
EPHRAIM
BENJAMIN
JUDAH
PHILISTINES
AMALEK
AMMON
GILEAD
MOAB
EDOM
I
II
XI
XII
Mt. Ebal
Shechem
Pirathon
Mt. Gerizim
Gath-rimmon
Joppa
Shiloh
Zeredah
Baal-hazor
Bethel
Ephraim
Beth-hanan
Lower Beth-horon
Beeroth
Upper Beth-horon
Shaalbim
Gibeon
Geba
Gezer
Elon
Baalath
Makaz
Kiriath-jearim
Gibeah
Anathoth
Ekron
Sorek
High Place
Jerusalem
Ashdod
Beth-shemesh
Gilgal
Jericho
Bethlehem
Libnah
Netophah
Ashkelon
Adullam
Tekoa
Giloh
Hebron
Gaza
Debir
Carmel
Gerar
Gath?
Ziklag
Kabzeel
Arad
Beer-sheba
Valley of Salt
The Negeb
The Shephelah (Lowland)
Brook Besor
Wilderness of Judah
Salt Sea
(Sea of the Arabah)
Tamar
(30° 48'N)
Brook Zered
The River
Pla
Succoth
Mahanaim
R. Jabbok
Jazer
Rabbah
(Rabbath-ammon)
Heshbon
Medeba
R. Nahaliel
Dibon
Aroer
R. Arnon
Kir-hareseth
© Oxford University Press
5
6
7
V
W
X
Y
Z
32°
31° 30'
31°
34° 30'
35°
35° 30'
36°
36° 30'
OUTER BORDER SHOWS 10 MILE SUBDIVISIONS

MAP 5

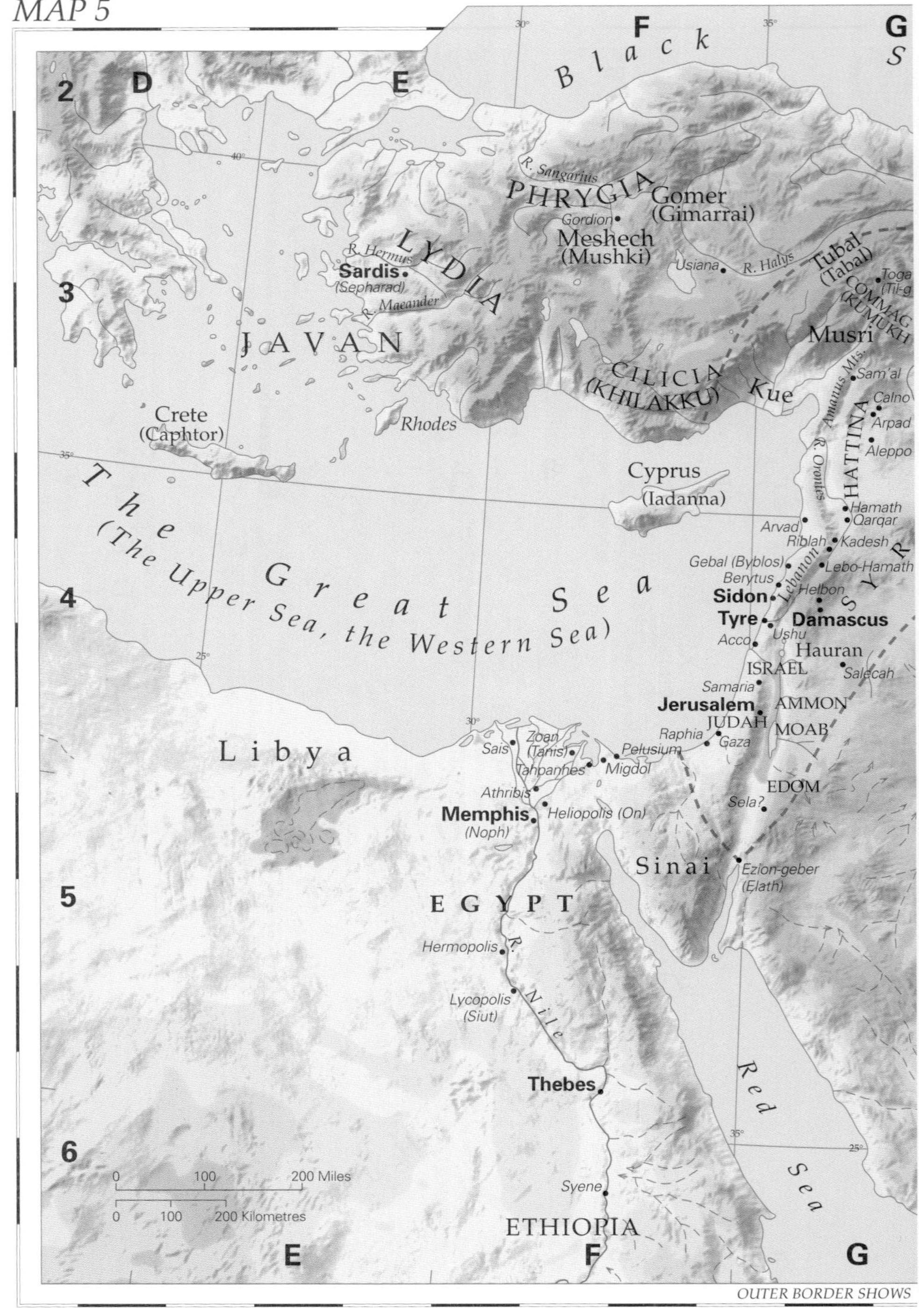

Black Sea
PHRYGIA
R. Sangarius
Gomer (Gimarrai)
Gordion
Meshech (Mushki)
LYDIA
R. Hermus
Sardis
(Sepharad)
R. Maeander
Usiana
R. Halys
Tubal (Tabal)
COMMAGENE (KUMUKH)
Musri
JAVAN
CILICIA (KHILAKKU)
Kue
Sam'al
Calno
Arpad
Aleppo
Amanus Mts.
HATTINA
R. Orontes
Crete (Caphtor)
Rhodes
Cyprus (Iadanna)
Hamath
Qarqar
Arvad
Riblah
Kadesh
Gebal (Byblos)
Lebo-Hamath
Berytus
Lebanon
Helbon
Sidon
Tyre
Damascus
Ushu
Acco
Hauran
ISRAEL
Salecah
Samaria
Jerusalem
AMMON
JUDAH
MOAB
Raphia
Gaza
The Great Sea
(The Upper Sea, the Western Sea)
Libya
Sais
Zoan (Tanis)
Pelusium
Tahpanhes
Migdol
Athribis
Memphis (Noph)
Heliopolis (On)
EDOM
Sela?
Sinai
Ezion-geber (Elath)
EGYPT
Hermopolis
R. Nile
Lycopolis (Siut)
Thebes
Red Sea
Syene
ETHIOPIA
0 100 200 Miles
0 100 200 Kilometres

OUTER BORDER SHOWS

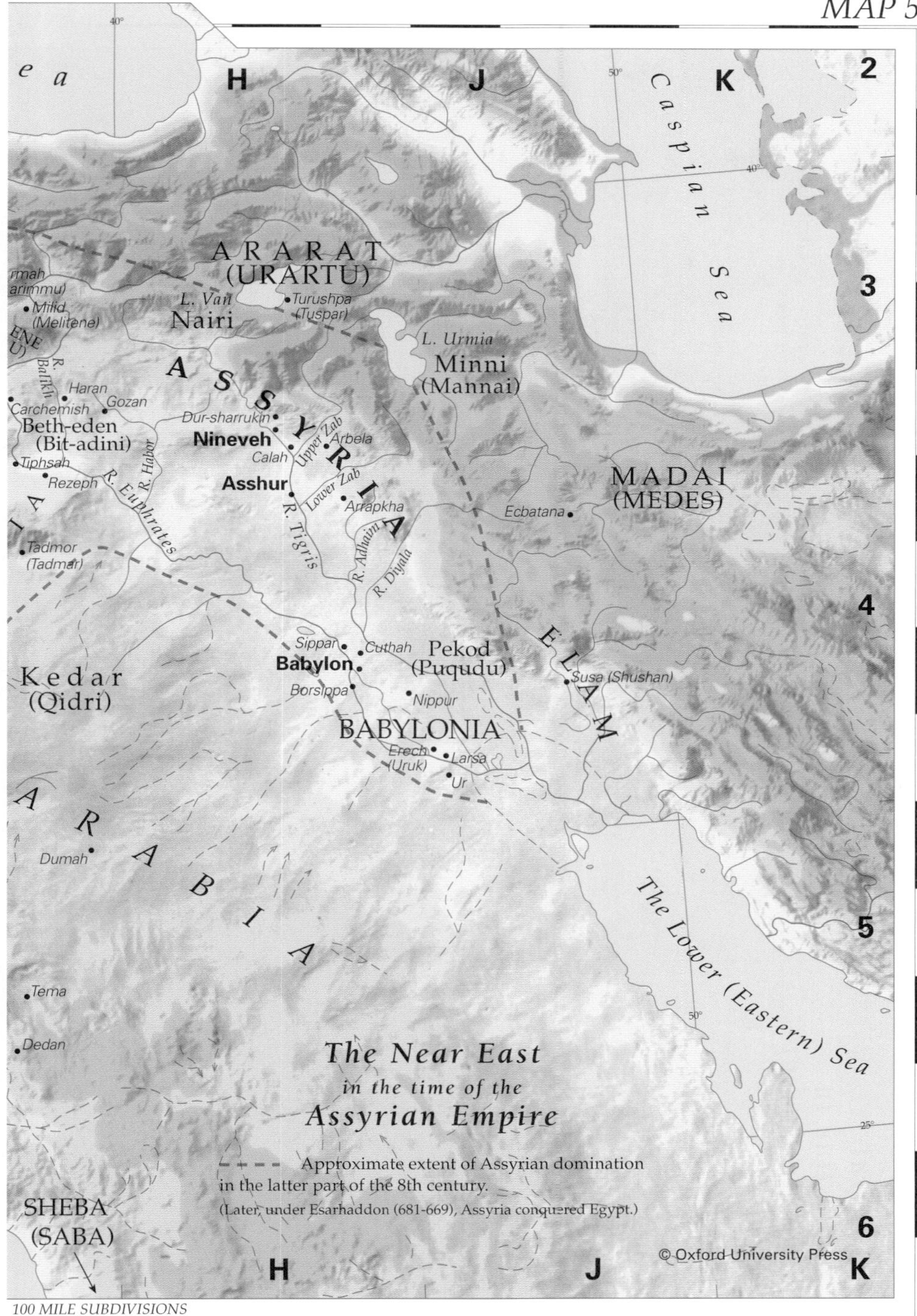
H
J
K
2
3
4
5
6
Caspian Sea
ARARAT (URARTU)
L. Van
Turushpa (Tuspar)
Nairi
Milid (Melitene)
L. Urmia
Minni (Mannai)
ASSYRIA
R. Balikh
Haran
Gozan
Carchemish
Beth-eden (Bit-adini)
Dur-sharrukin
Nineveh
Upper Zab
Arbela
Calah
Tiphsah
R. Habor
Rezeph
R. Euphrates
Asshur
Lower Zab
Arrapkha
R. Tigris
R. Adhaim
R. Diyala
MADAI (MEDES)
Ecbatana
Tadmor (Tadmar)
ELAM
Sippar
Cuthah
Pekod (Puqudu)
Babylon
Borsippa
Nippur
Susa (Shushan)
Kedar (Qidri)
BABYLONIA
Erech (Uruk)
Larsa
Ur
ARABIA
Dumah
The Lower (Eastern) Sea
Tema
Dedan
The Near East in the time of the Assyrian Empire
Approximate extent of Assyrian domination in the latter part of the 8th century.
(Later, under Esarhaddon (681-669), Assyria conquered Egypt.)
SHEBA (SABA)
100 MILE SUBDIVISIONS

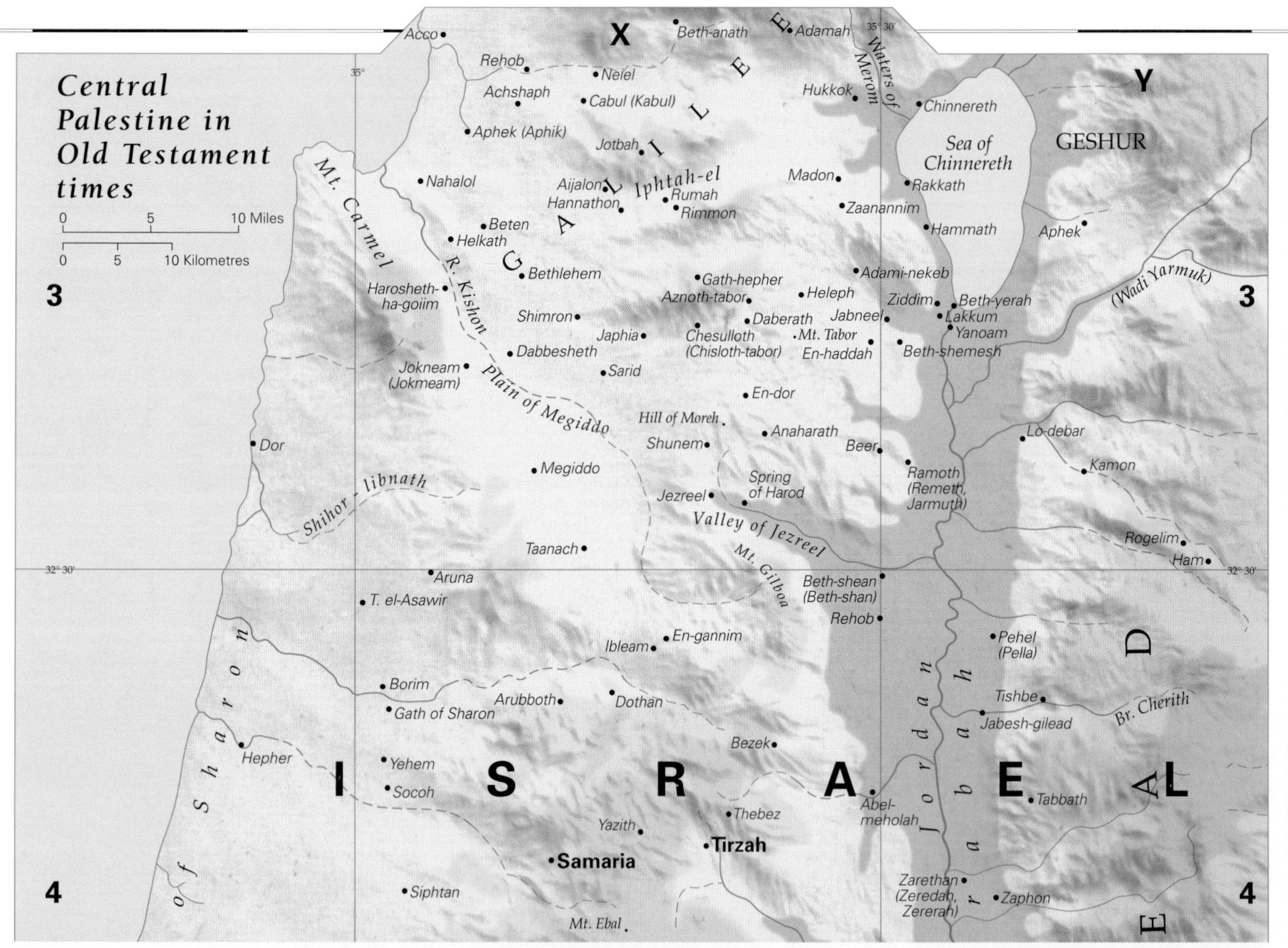
Central Palestine in Old Testament times
0 5 10 Miles
0 5 10 Kilometres
3
4
35°
35° 30'
32° 30'
GESHUR
Sea of Chinnereth
Waters of Merom
(Wadi Yarmuk)
Br. Cherith
R. Kishon
Plain of Megiddo
Valley of Jezreel
Mt. Carmel
Mt. Gilboa
Mt. Tabor
Mt. Ebal
Hill of Moreh
Shihor - libnath
Iphtah-el
Jordan
Acco
Rehob
Achshaph
Aphek (Aphik)
Neiel
Cabul (Kabul)
Beth-anath
Adamah
Hukkok
Chinnereth
Rakkath
Hammath
Madon
Zaanannim
Adami-nekeb
Ziddim
Lakkum
Beth-yerah
Yanoam
Beth-shemesh
Jabneel
En-haddah
Heleph
Daberath
Chesulloth (Chisloth-tabor)
Aznoth-tabor
Gath-hepher
Rimmon
Rumah
Jotbah
Hannathon
Aijalon
Bethlehem
Beten
Helkath
Nahalol
Shimron
Japhia
Dabbesheth
Sarid
Harosheth-ha-goiim
Jokneam (Jokmeam)
Megiddo
Taanach
Shunem
En-dor
Anaharath
Spring of Harod
Jezreel
Beer
Ramoth (Remeth, Jarmuth)
Beth-shean (Beth-shan)
Rehob
En-gannim
Ibleam
Dothan
Arubboth
Gath of Sharon
Aruna
T. el-Asawir
Borim
Yehem
Socoh
Siphtan
Dor
Hepher
of Sharon
Samaria
Yazith
Tirzah
Thebez
Bezek
Abel-meholah
Arabah
Zarethan (Zeredah, Zererah)
Zaphon
Tabbath
Jabesh-gilead
Tishbe
Pehel (Pella)
Lo-debar
Kamon
Rogelim
Ham
Aphek
X
Y
GALILEE
ISRAEL